MW01505060

The Retinal Atlas

For Elsevier
Commissioning Editor: *Russell Gabbedy*
Development Editor: *Nani Clansey*
Editorial Assistant: *Joshua Mearns*
Project Manager: *Joanna Souch*
Designer: *Christian Bilbow*
Marketing Manager: *Melissa Fogarty*

THE RETINAL ATLAS

Second Edition

K. BAILEY FREUND, MD

Vitreous Retina Macula Consultants of New York
Clinical Professor of Ophthalmology
New York University School of Medicine
New York, NY, USA

DAVID SARRAF, MD

Clinical Professor of Ophthalmology
Retinal Disorders and Ophthalmic Genetics Division
Stein Eye Institute, UCLA
Los Angeles, CA, USA

WILLIAM F. MIELER, MD

Cless Family Professor and Vice-Chairman
Director, Residency and Vitreoretinal Fellowship Training
Department of Ophthalmology & Visual Sciences
University of Illinois at Chicago
Chicago, IL, USA

LAWRENCE A. YANNUZZI, MD

Vitreous Retina Macula Consultants of New York
Professor of Clinical Ophthalmology
College of Physicians and Surgeons
Columbia University Medical School
New York, NY, USA

Special Contributor to the Second Edition

CAROL L. SHIELDS, MD

Co-Director, Ocular Oncology Service
Wills Eye Hospital
Professor of Ophthalmology
Thomas Jefferson University Hospital
Philadelphia, PA, USA

ELSEVIER

ELSEVIER

First edition 2010

Notices

Knowledge and best practice in this field are constantly changing. As new research and experience broaden our understanding, changes in research methods, professional practices, or medical treatment may become necessary.

Practitioners and researchers must always rely on their own experience and knowledge in evaluating and using any information, methods, compounds, or experiments described herein. In using such information or methods they should be mindful of their own safety and the safety of others, including parties for whom they have a professional responsibility.

With respect to any drug or pharmaceutical products identified, readers are advised to check the most current information provided (i) on procedures featured or (ii) by the manufacturer of each product to be administered, to verify the recommended dose or formula, the method and duration of administration, and contraindications. It is the responsibility of practitioners, relying on their own experience and knowledge of their patients, to make diagnoses, to determine dosages and the best treatment for each individual patient, and to take all appropriate safety precautions.

To the fullest extent of the law, neither the Publisher nor the authors, contributors, or editors, assume any liability for any injury and/or damage to persons or property as a matter of products liability, negligence or otherwise, or from any use or operation of any methods, products, instructions, or ideas contained in the material herein.

ISBN: 978-0-323-28792-0
E-Book ISBN: 978-0-323-28793-7

Printed in China

Last digit is the print number: 9 8 7 6 5 4 3 2 1

COLOR CODING—*HOW TO USE THIS BOOK*

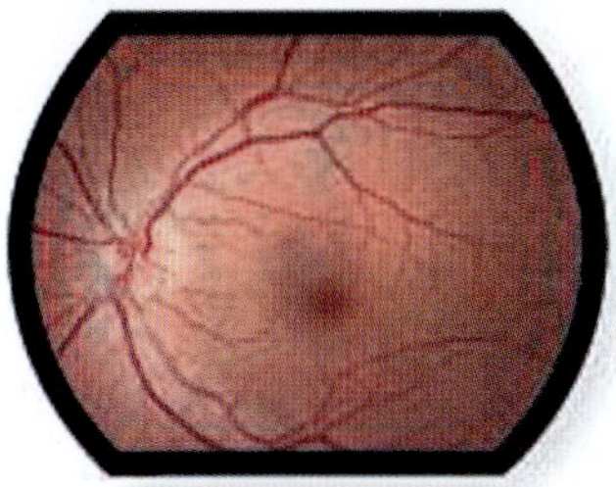

General

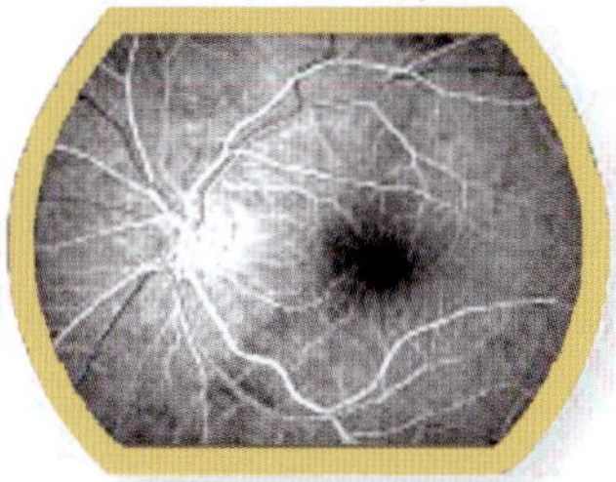

Fluorescein Angiogram (FA)

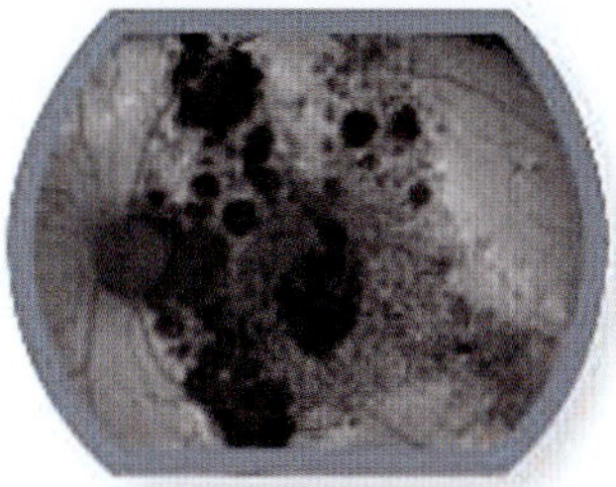

Fundus Autofluorescence (FAF)

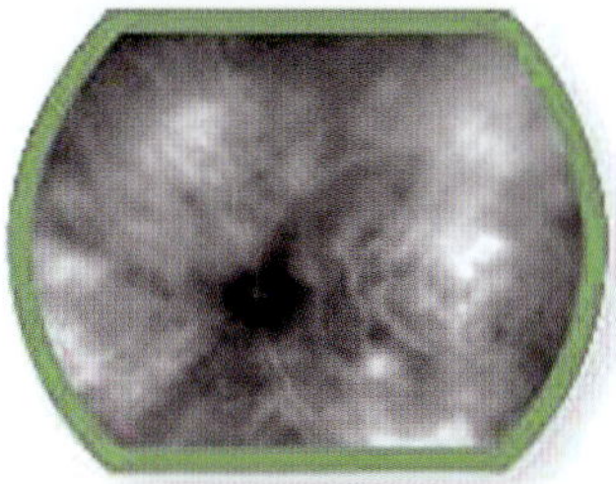

Indocyanine Green (ICG) Angiogram

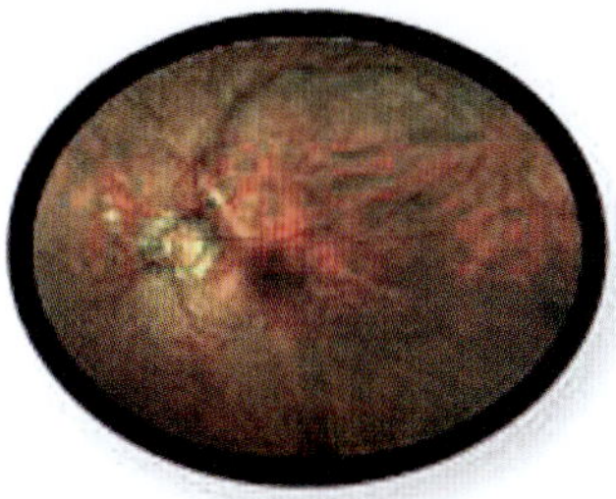

Ultra-widefield Color Photograph

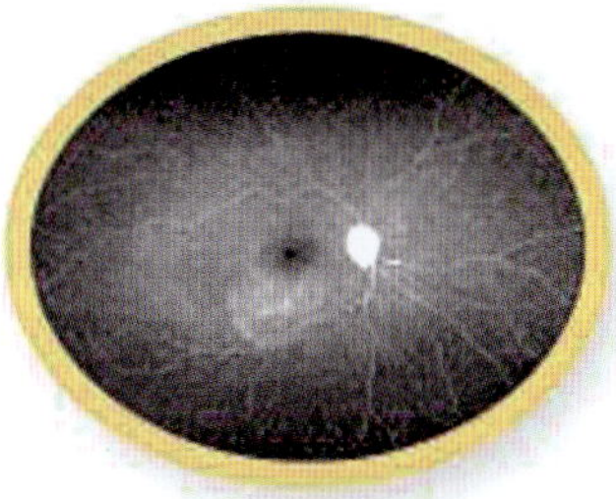

Ultra-widefield (FA)

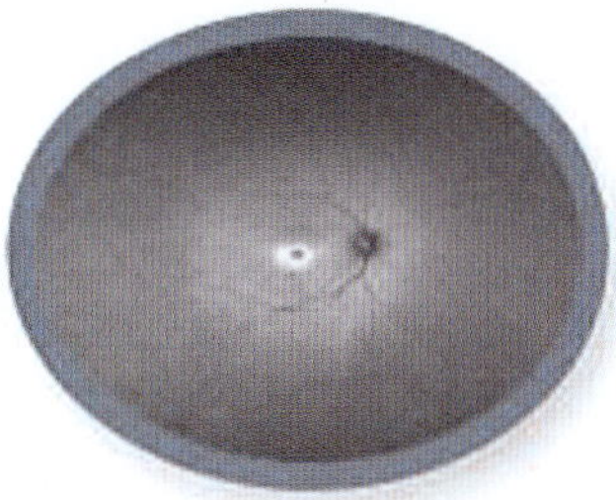

Ultra-widefield (FAF)

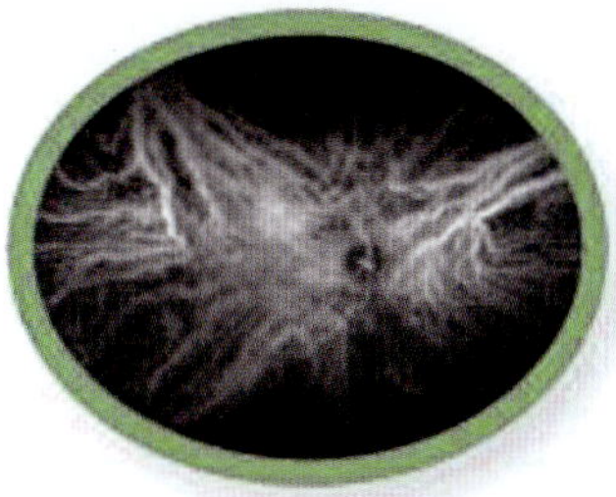

Ultra-widefield (ICG)

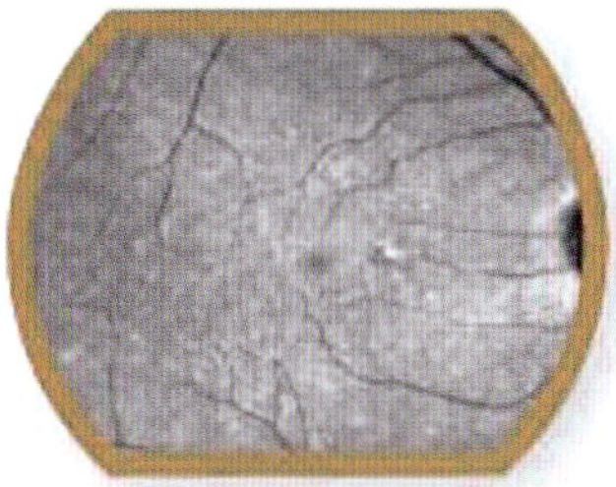

Near-infrared Reflectance (NIR)

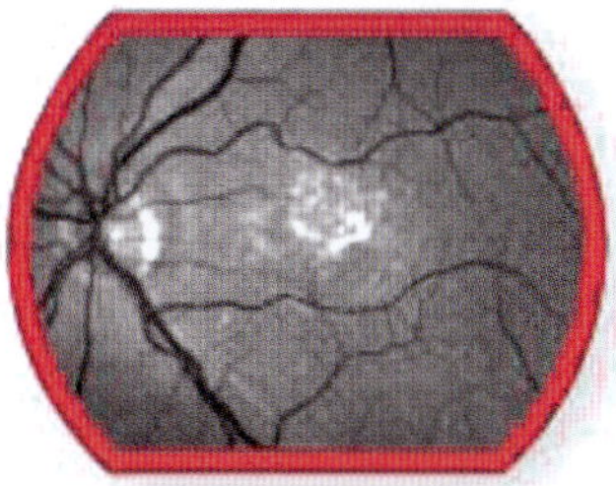

Red Free (RF) Photograph

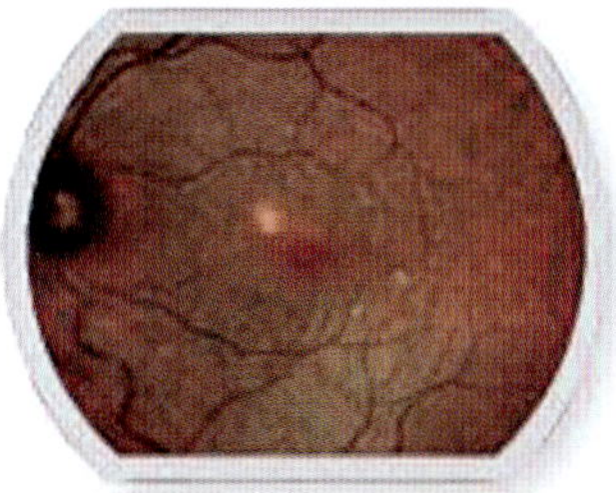

Multicolored Imaging

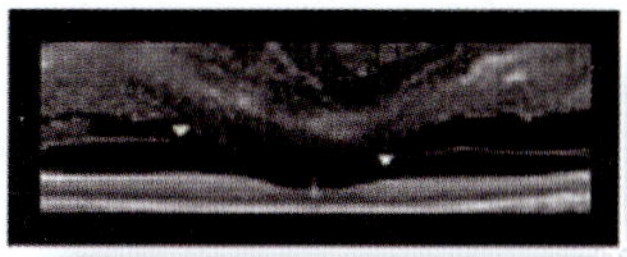

Optical Coherence Tomography (OCT)

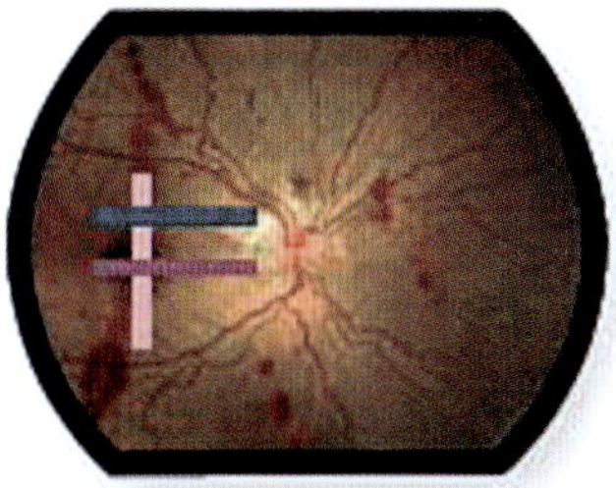

OCT scans through the corresponding colored lines in photograph

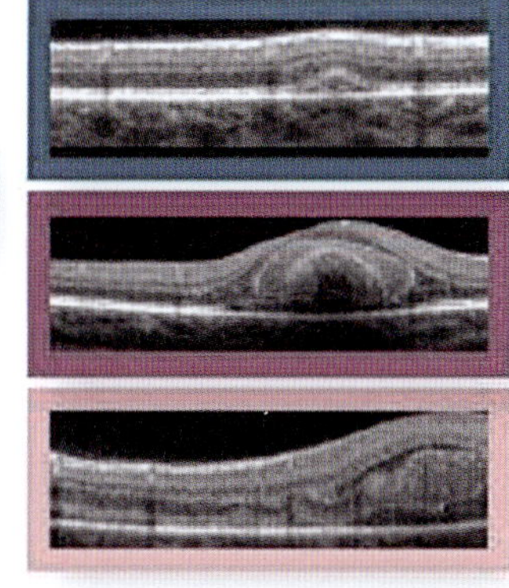

The figures in *The Retinal Atlas* have been organized using categories of imaging with color-coded borders for easy reference and identification.

DEDICATION

We would like to express our deepest gratitude and most heartfelt appreciation to our respective families whose eternal unwavering support has allowed us to complete the challenging project of editing the Atlas. Nina, Allegra and Avery Freund, Natalie, Danielle and Desiree Sarraf and Jennifer Kang-Mieler and Sabrina Derwent have been incredible pillars of strength and encouragement throughout this entire process and we are forever grateful for their love and commitment.

CONTENTS

Contributors to the First Edition

William E. Benson, MD
Attending Surgeon Wills Eye Institute
Professor of Ophthalmology
Thomas Jefferson Medical College
Philadelphia, PA, USA

K. Bailey Freund, MD
Vitreous Retina Macula Consultants of New York
Clinical Professor of Ophthalmology
New York University School of Medicine
New York, NY, USA

W. Richard Green, MD
Professor of Ophthalmology and Pathology
International Order of Odd Fellows Professor of Ophthalmology
The Wilmer Eye Institute
Johns Hopkins Hospital
Baltimore, MD, USA

Richard Hackel, MA CRA, FOPS
Clinical Instructor and Director of Ophthalmic Photography,
Kellogg Eye Center
Assistant Professor of Art, School of Art and Design
University of Michigan
Ann Arbor, MI, USA

H. Richard McDonald, MD
West Coast Retina Medical Group
San Francisco, CA, USA
Clinical Professor of Ophthalmology
California Pacific Medical Center
San Francisco, CA, USA

William F. Mieler, MD
Cless Family Professor and Vice-Chairman
Director, Residency and Vitreoretinal Fellowship Training
Department of Ophthalmology & Visual Sciences
University of Illinois at Chicago
Chicago, IL, USA

David Sarraf, MD
Clinical Professor of Ophthalmology
Retinal Disorders and Ophthalmic Genetics Division
Stein Eye Institute, UCLA
Los Angeles, CA, USA

Carol L. Shields, MD
Co-Director, Oncology Service
Wills Eye Institute
Professor of Ophthalmology
Thomas Jefferson University Hospital
Philadelphia, PA, USA

Jerry A. Shields, MD
Co-Director, Ocular Oncology Service
Wills Eye Hospital
Professor of Ophthalmology
Thomas Jefferson University Hospital
Philadelphia, PA, USA

Michael T. Trese, MD
Chief of Pediatric and Adult Vitreoretinal Surgery
Beaumont Eye Institute, Wm. Beaumont Hospital
Royal Oak, MI, USA
Clinical Professor of Biomedical Sciences
Eye Research Institute
Oakland University
Rochester, MI, USA

PREFACE TO THE SECOND EDITION

The first edition of *The Retinal Atlas* published six years ago in 2010 was at its time, and still remains, the most comprehensive retinal atlas ever published. It was the opus of our mentor, Dr. Lawrence Yannuzzi. While the first edition was the product of a team effort, it was ultimately a very personal statement, a vibrant and everlasting representation of Larry's encyclopedic mind and passionate interest in retinal disease. It has been our honor and privilege to have been entrusted with the daunting responsibility of revising this award-winning work, which is considered one of the truly classic contributions to the world's ophthalmic literature.

We co-authors each owe Larry a debt of gratitude for his many decades of mentorship, guidance, and generosity. His enthusiasm, energy, and incredible insight in the recognition of novel diseases and presentation of illustrative cases have inspired each of us and the entire retina community. Poring over the pages and pages of spectacular images in *The Retinal Atlas* reminds us of his infallible memory at work in the clinic, the conference room, and the lecture hall where he never fails to recall (always accurately) similar or related cases from the near and distant past. His discerning eye and keen analytical skills have helped us to identify that which was once invisible, to explain disease pathogenesis, and to enhance the diagnosis and treatment of retinal disease in our patients.

The first edition of *The Retinal Atlas* is a true tour de force with a vast array of spectacular images covering an enormous breadth of retinal disease. However, the fields of medical and surgical retina are amongst the fastest growing specialties in medicine. Novel therapeutics have exploded into the clinical arena providing unprecedented capacity to treat retinal disease and even improve vision. The advances in retinal imaging have been no less remarkable. The development of wide-field imaging, fundus autofluorescence, and, especially, optical coherence tomography has provided awe-inspiring insights into the structure and function of the retina. We are very proud to update the first *Atlas* with a prodigious supplement of cases with advanced imaging that will allow the *Atlas* to continue to be a worldwide comprehensive resource for the diagnosis of retinal disease.

The importance of educating, mentoring, and collaborating with younger professionals in our field has, from the beginning, been a passionate interest of Larry, which he has instilled in each of us. The first and second editions of *The Retinal Atlas* would not have been possible without the efforts of a team of amazing residents and fellows. We are grateful for the support they have provided and for the outstanding contributions they have made to the second edition. We hope and expect that each of our talented trainees will become future leaders in the worldwide retinal community. We would like to introduce each of them below to express our gratitude.

K. Bailey Freund, MD
David Sarraf, MD
William F. Mieler, MD

Contributors to the Second Edition

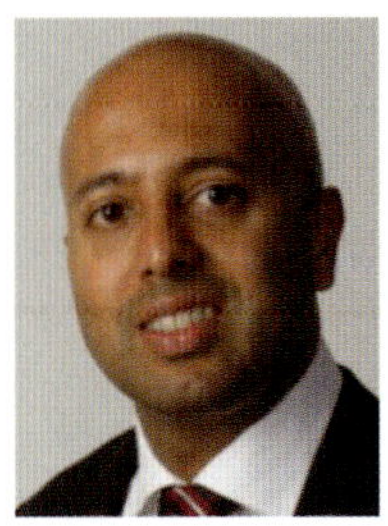

Chandrakumar Balaratnasingam, MBBS (Hons.), PhD (Dist.), FRANZCO
Associate Professor of Ophthalmology,
University of Western Australia,
Vitreoretinal Surgeon
Royal Perth Hospital, Sir Charles Gairdner Hospital and Lions Eye Institute, Perth, Australia

Chandrakumar (Chandra) Balaratnasingam received his MBBS and PhD from the University of Western Australia and then completed ophthalmology residency in Perth, Australia. Chandra finished vitreoretinal surgical training at the University of British Columbia, Vancouver, Canada and medical retina training at the Vitreous Retina Macula Consultants of New York. He was subsequently appointed as a clinical instructor in vitreoretinal surgery at Bellevue Hospital Center, New York University School of Medicine. While training in New York he made major contributions to the writing and preparation of Chapters 7, 8, 9, and 10. Chandra now lives in Australia with his wife and children. He holds clinical and academic positions at the University of Western Australia and is actively involved in laboratory-based and clinical research in retinal vascular diseases.

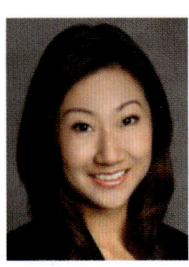

Claudine E. Pang, MBBS, MRCSEd, FRCSEd (Edinburgh), FAMS (Ophth)
Vitreoretinal Surgeon and Medical Retina Specialist,
Jerry Tan Eye Surgery, Camden Medical Centre, Singapore

Claudine Pang was born in Singapore and graduated with Distinction from the National University of Singapore (MBBS). She completed ophthalmology training in Singapore and received the Fellowship of the Royal College of Surgeons in Edinburgh (FRCSEd) and Fellowship of the Academy of Medicine, Singapore (FAMS) in Ophthalmology. She completed a Medical Retina and Research Fellowship at the Vitreous Retina Macula Consultants of New York, during which she put her heart and soul into writing and editing Chapters 7, 8, 9, and 10. Following that, she was awarded the William H. Ross Surgical Vitreoretinal Fellowship at the University of British Columbia in Vancouver, Canada and went on to receive electrophysiology training at Moorfields Eye Hospital in London, United Kingdom. She has now joined the Jerry Tan Eye Surgery in Singapore to head the Vitreoretinal Service where she hopes to provide novel retinal therapies for incurable macular diseases. She is grateful to her husband, Aaron, who has supported her in her pursuit of multi-national vitreoretinal training, and is a proud mother of their two lovely children, Nathanael and Sophie.

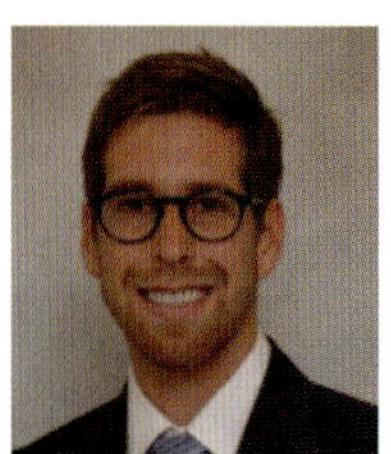

Christian J. Sanfilippo, MD
Vitreoretinal Fellow at the Stein Eye Institute, UCLA, Los Angeles, CA, USA

Christian Sanfilippo grew up in Orange County, California. He received his undergraduate degree in Human Biology from the University of California, San Diego and graduated from medical school at UCLA. After an internship in Internal Medicine at Cedars-Sinai Medical Center, Christian completed ophthalmology residency training at the Stein Eye Institute at UCLA. In addition to his important contributions to Chapters 1, 2, 3, 4, and 6, Christian has published several papers describing novel imaging findings in retinal diseases and investigating advanced retinal imaging systems such as OCT angiography. Outside of medicine, he is fortunate to have the support of his beautiful fiancé Kathryn and their rambunctious dog Joey.

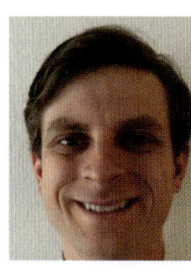

Joseph G. Christenbury, MD
PGY-4 Resident in Ophthalmology, Stein Eye Institute, UCLA, Los Angeles, CA, USA

Joseph Christenbury was born in Durham, North Carolina and completed his undergraduate and medical degrees at Duke University. As an outstanding resident at the Stein Eye Institute at UCLA, Joe completed various research and academic projects including important publications in the field of retinal imaging and remarkable contributions to Chapter 5 of the new Atlas. Joe hopes to pursue an academic career in ophthalmology and is looking forward to returning to North Carolina with his wife Kathryn and his young son Clay.

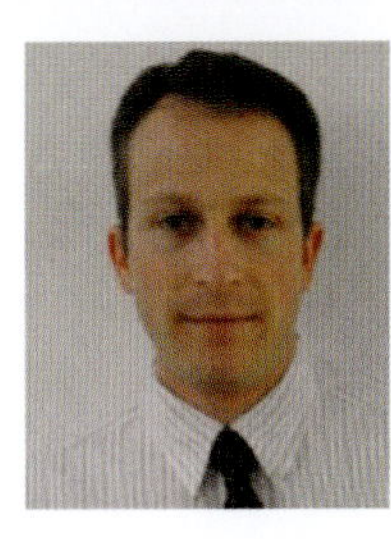

Aaron Nagiel, MD, PhD
Vitreoretinal Fellow at the Stein Eye Institute, UCLA, Los Angeles, CA, USA

Aaron Nagiel grew up in San Diego, California. He received his undergraduate degree in Biochemical Sciences from Harvard College and then completed a combined MD-PhD program at Cornell University in New York City. During his PhD training at the Rockefeller University, Aaron studied synaptogenesis in larval zebrafish. After an internship at Memorial Sloan-Kettering Cancer Center, Aaron completed ophthalmology residency training at the Stein Eye Institute. In addition to his important contribution to Chapter 6 of the new Atlas, Aaron has written many significant papers on retinal imaging and is a recipient of the Heed Ophthalmic Foundation Fellowship and the Ronald G Michels Fellowship Foundation awards. He is blessed with a beautiful wife Svetlana and two lovely daughters, Elina and Rita.

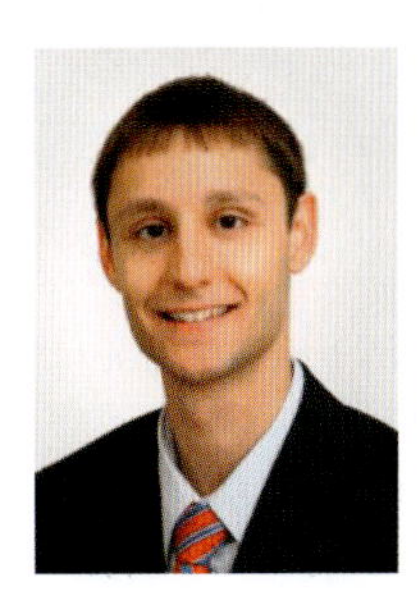

Michael T. Andreoli, MD
Vitreoretinal Fellow at the University of Illinois at Chicago, Chicago, IL, USA

Michael Andreoli was born and raised in Wheaton, Illinois. He pursued the field of ophthalmology and vitreoretinal diseases due to the complexity of pathology and intricacy of management. Michael completed his residency in ophthalmology at the University of Illinois at Chicago (UIC), and then stayed at UIC for his surgical vitreoretinal fellowship training. He contributed to The Retinal Atlas *while a surgical vitreoretinal fellow. In the future, Michael plans to stay in the Chicago area where he will practice vitreoretinal surgery and ocular oncology. Michael made significant contributions to Chapters 13 and 14.*

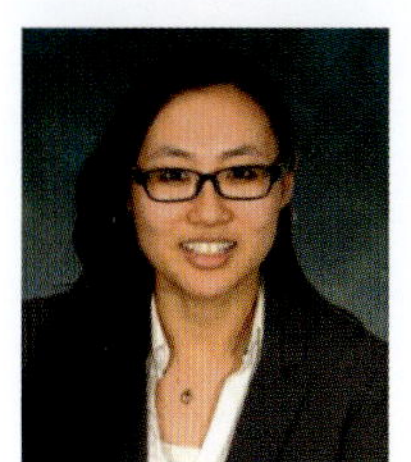

Judy J. Chen, MD
Vitreoretinal Fellow at West Coast Retina, San Francisco, CA, USA

Judy Chen was born in Taipei, Taiwan and chose to pursue a career in ophthalmology, and ultimately vitreoretinal surgery, because of the field's innovative advancements in technology and the profound impact that improving vision can have on patients' lives. While contributing to The Retinal Atlas, *Judy was a senior resident at the University of Illinois at Chicago (UIC). She is now a surgical vitreoretinal fellow with the West Coast Retina Medical group in the San Francisco bay area. In the future, she hopes to combine her interests in clinical medicine, research, and teaching into a fulfilling career. Judy made significant contributions to Chapters 11 and 12.*

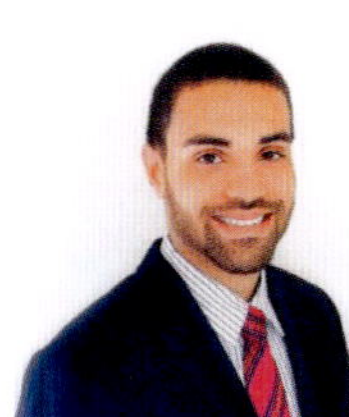

Andrew Francis, MD
Vitreoretinal Fellow at the University of California-San Francisco, San Francisco, CA, USA

Andrew Francis was born in Los Angeles, CA. He chose to pursue a career in ophthalmology as he was fascinated by the diverse range of pathology that affects both the vitreous and retina and the innovative medical and surgical interventions available to treat patients. Andrew contributed to The Retinal Atlas *while a senior resident in ophthalmology at the University of Illinois at Chicago (UIC). He is currently a surgical vitreoretinal fellow at the University of San Francisco, CA. In the future, Andrew hopes to pursue a career in academic ophthalmology and acquire an advanced level of training in the management of complex medical and surgical disorders of the retina and vitreous. He also plans to continue publishing novel research, provide excellent teaching and mentorship, and practice compassionate medicine with respect for all of his patients. Andrew made significant contributions to Chapter 15.*

Preface to the First Edition

The authors have included the original unedited Preface by Dr. Lawrence Yannuzzi in its entirety. Dr. Yannuzzi provides the important historical context for the original landmark first edition with his trademark eloquence.

The eye, specifically the retina and its contiguous interrelated tissue, provides the field of medicine with the unique opportunity to study the anatomical structure and pathophysiological nature of a critical organ in a noninvasive manner. Only the transparency of the ocular media and the accessibility of its internal vascular layers have made it possible for basic scientists, guided by clinical research retinal specialists, to develop novel and meaningful imaging devices that have led to a better understanding of known chorioretinal diseases, as well as newly discovered, clinically distinct entities, and their treatment. Historically, imaging of the fundus began with the invention of the direct ophthalmoscope by Charles Babbage in 1847[1] *(Figure 1)*. It was reinvented independently by Hermann von Helmholtz in 1851[2] *(Figure 2)*, who used a simple device: a curved mirror with a naked candle for illumination, to explain the pupillary light reflex to a physiology class. Since then, burgeoning knowledge of the ocular fundus has been provided by a series of diagnostic adjuncts through generations of creative technological advances for innovative imaging concepts, beginning with basic fundus photography, a simple snapshot of the central retina to document the macular area and the optic nerve. Following the Helmholtz discovery, several ophthalmologists experimented with photographing anesthetized animals; it wasn't until 1886 that WT Jackson and JD Webster published the first fundus photographs of the living human eye.[3] Their primitive system represented a major advance in documenting fundus details. It employed a curved ophthalmoscopic mirror with a central hole in conjunction with a 2-inch microscope objective. Illumination was provided by a carbon light source with a 2½-minute exposure *(Figure 3)*.

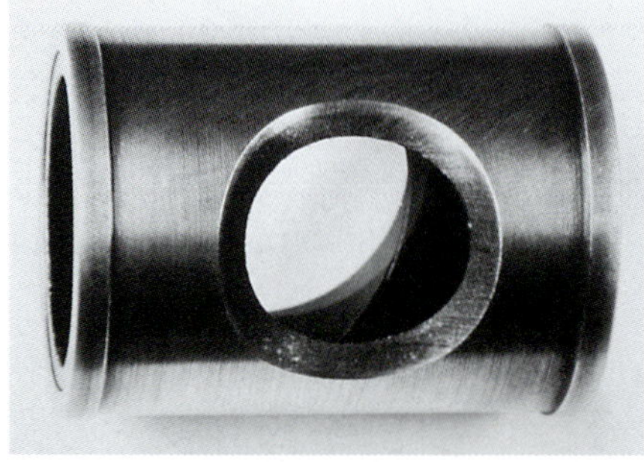

Figure 1. Charles Babbage used a plane mirror with three small spots scraped in the middle and fixed in a tube to reflect rays of light into the eye. *Courtesy of The College of Optometrists, 2003*

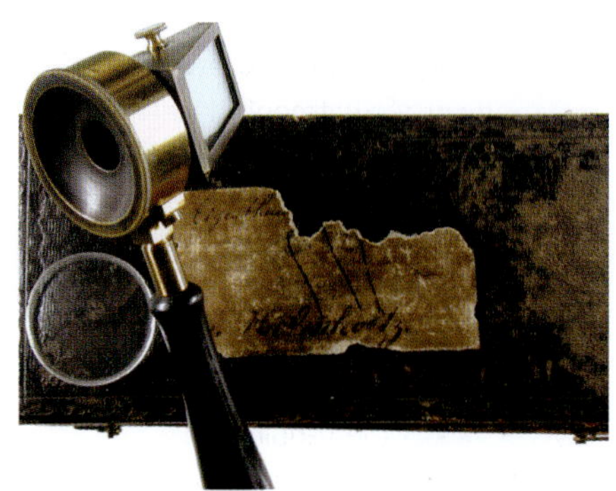

Figure 2. Helmholtz used a naked candle for a source of illumination and a curved mirror as an ophthalmoscope. *Courtesy of C. Richard Keeler*

Progress in the improvement of better quality images was made by several investigators, most notably by O Gerhoff, who used flash powder in 1891[5], and F Dimmer, who switched to a carbon arc in 1899[6] *(Figure 4)*. Dimmer's superb photographs were the basis of the first black and white fundus photography atlas in 1907.[7]

The introduction of the first modern fundus camera to the ophthalmic community was by the Carl Zeiss Company in 1926. The camera, developed by JW Nordenson,[8] was created based on Gullstrand's principles with a 10° field of view and an exposure time of 0.5 a second[9] *(Figure 5)*. AJ Bedell used this camera for the first stereo and color fundus atlas in 1929.[10] This system prevailed until AB Rizzutti adapted the electronic flash tube for use in ophthalmology in 1950.[11] P Hansell and EJG Beeson championed the use of a compact xenon arc lamp modification for the Zeiss fundus camera with Kodachrome color film with a flash 1/25 of a second,[12] which soon became the standard for high-quality color retinal photos for the modern retinal camera in 1953. Simple, singular retinal photographs with limited resolution and field have given way to full fundus photography with enhanced resolution and color balance, wide-field capability, and high-speed-stereoscopic analysis. This fundus camera generated enormous intellectual curiosity and provided numerous clinical observations, which had an impact on visual function information regarding the normal as well as the abnormal eye.

In the 1960s, the introduction of fundus fluorescein angiography provided the next greatest impact on our understanding of the retina and the development of the subspecialty, medical-retinal diseases. It was P Chao and M Flocks[13] who first investigated a method for studying the retinal circulation time in cats. This was the basis for the legendary

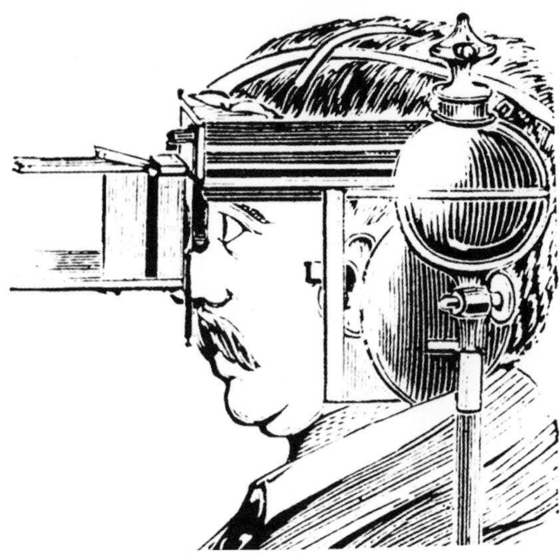

Figure 3. The first fundus photograph by WT Jackson and JD Webster was made through a stationary direct ophthalmoscope with a 2½-minute exposure time and an albo carbon burner for illumination. *Courtesy of Patrick J. Saine, CRA*[4]

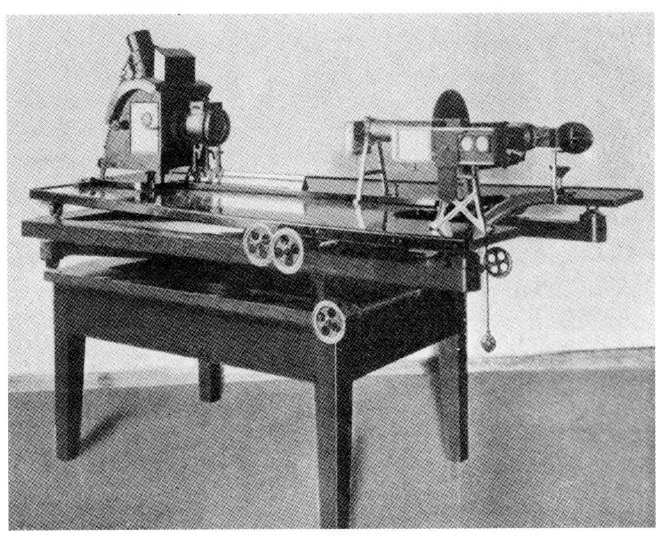

Figure 4. Dimmer's fundus camera (reproduced from Dimmer and Pillal, 1927). *Courtesy of Patrick J. Saine, CRA*[4]

discovery by HR Novotny and DL Alvis[14] *(Figure 6)*, which described retinal angiography with intravenous fluorescein dye, utilizing an excitatory filter, a matched barrier filter in the film plane, and an electronic flash to sequentially document retinal blood flow. For the first time, vascular permeability, perfusion, and vasogenic manifestations could be imaged dynamically to display physiological, as well as anatomical, abnormalities in diabetic retinopathy, retinal venous-occlusive disease, neovascular age-related macular degeneration, and other leading causes of irreversible severe vision loss. This was an important development in the medical-retina subspecialty. Expanded clinical knowledge based on that imaging system was provided by Dr. J. Donald Gass,[15] who spirited the recognition of new manifestations of known diseases, the discovery of distinct clinical entities and the development of treatment strategies such as ophthalmic laser devices; and, more recently, pharmacological therapy via intravitreal administration of drugs. No other diagnostic aid in its prime proved to be more valuable than fluorescein angiography to study permeability, perfusion, and proliferative abnormalities of the retina and choroidal circulations.

When fluorescein angiography was first introduced, the Zeiss retinal camera was the only commercially available fundus camera. It was equipped with a Zeiss camera, which required manual film advancement. The flash unit provided by the system recycled every few seconds at the required intensity. These two limitations were quickly addressed with the addition of a booster flash electronic device manufactured by a mechanic in his garage in Miami, Florida. Johnny Justice, Jr., the creative fluorescein pioneer photographer and Gass' original photographer, assisted me in obtaining one of these units for $200. I was thrilled at the ability to recycle the electronic system every second at sufficient intensity, but there was still the problem of rapid film advancement. This was mediated with an adaptor ring and a substitution Nikon SP range finder camera, which had a thumb trigger mechanism for advancing the film, soon to be supplanted by an electronic motor device. Advances continued with the introduction of camera systems by new manufacturers such as Topcon, Canon, Nidek, and Olympus, with multifocal lens systems, zoom lenses, automated stereo devices and more. At the Manhattan Eye, Ear & Throat Hospital, we introduced a systematic method to interpret fluorescein angiographs,[16] which became the basis of a text authored by H Schatz et al. to be used by a generation of retinal specialists who were to convert from surgical retinal specialists ("scleral bucklers") to medical retina angiographists.[17]

In recent years, more precise histological and physiological techniques have emerged to appreciate changes within the various layers of the vitreoretinal interface, the inner retina, the retinal pigment epithelium (RPE), and the choroid. Clearer histopathological imaging of the potential anatomic cavities in the macula, such as intraretinal cysts and

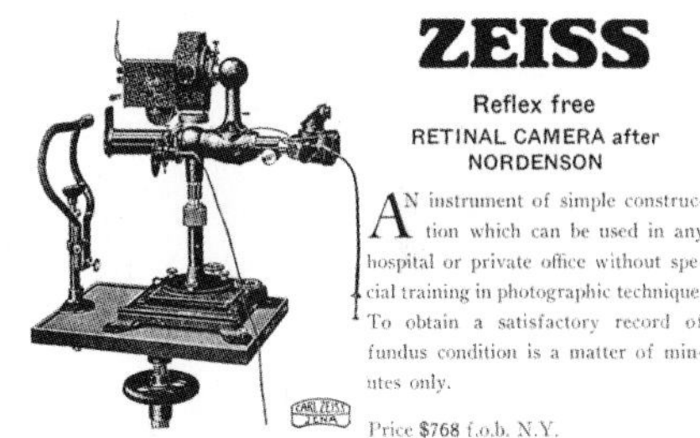

Figure 5. An advertisement for the Zeiss fundus camera from 1932. (reproduced from American Journal of Ophthalmology, 1932). *Saine PJ and Tyler ME. Ophthalmic photography: retinal photography, angiography, and electronic imaging. Second Journal of Ophthalmic Photography*

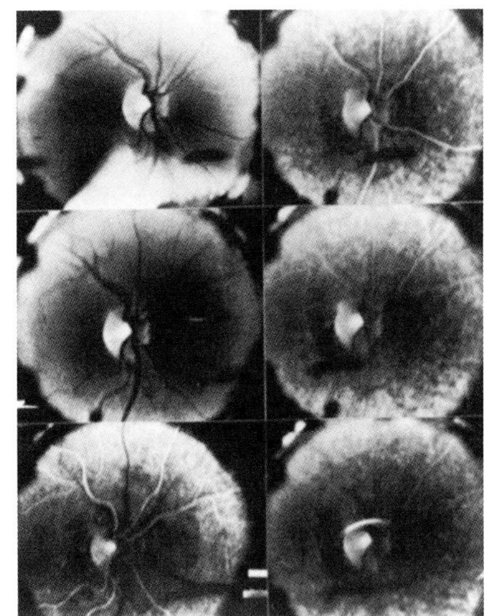

Figure 6. The first modern fluorescein angiogram was taken by Dr. Alvis in 1959. *From Novotny HR, Alvis DL. A method of photographing fluorescence in circulating blood in the human retina. Circulation 1961, 24 (1): 82-86*

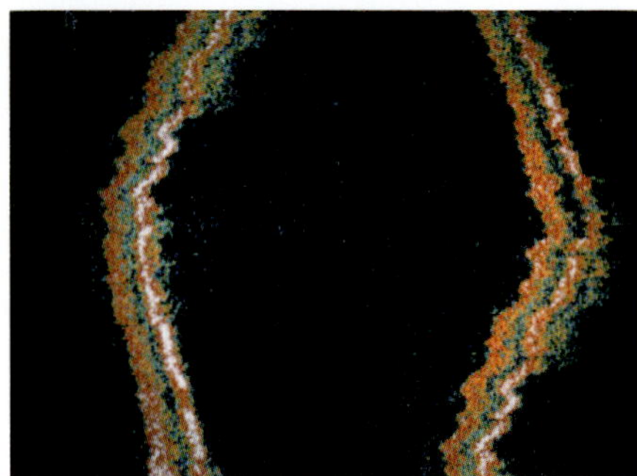

Figure 7. This is the original OCT image at 45 A-Scan/sec. *From Yannuzzi LA. Legendary Landmarks in Ophthalmic Imaging. J Ophthalmic Photogr 2009; 31:s53*

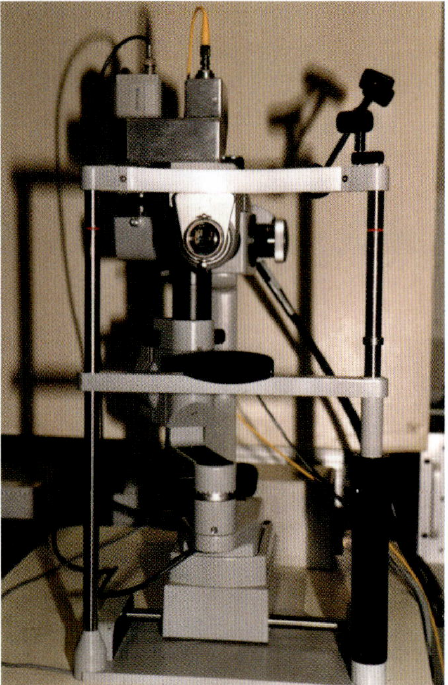

Figure 8. This is the prototype OCT on the slit lamp showing the scanner head. *From Yannuzzi LA. Legendary Landmarks in Ophthalmic Imaging. J Ophthalmic Photogr 2009; 31:s53*

detachments of the neurosensory retina and pigment epithelium, can now be studied. These new imaging systems are led by advances in optical coherence tomography (OCT),[18] now available with high-three resolution, 3-dimensional reconstruction with stored automated comparisons for point-to-point correlations. The roots for OCT imaging date back to the 1960s with the invention of autocorrelation for determination of laser pulse width, a range-finding technology *(Figure 7)*. According to John Moore, who has served ophthalmology throughout his career by developing solutions for eye disease and diagnosis, James Fujimoto (MIT) and Adolf Fercher (University of Vienna) invented the technology for retinal imaging with the MIT scanning system and the earlier Vienna A-scan length measurement in 1991. John convinced the Zeiss Company to develop the OCT-1, the first commercially available system. The technology was applied to ophthalmology by James Fujimoto, David Huang, J Izett, Eric Swanson, and CP Linn[18] *(Figure 8)*. They combined a super luminous diode, a Michelson interferometer, and a beam-scanning system. Dr. Carmen Puliafito immediately recognized the potential for retinal imaging and he recruited collaborators Dr. David Huang, Dr. Michael Hee, and Dr. Jay Duker, while Dr. Joel Schulman worked on glaucoma applications *(Figure 8)*. John Moore was kind enough to invite me to consult on the development of the slit-lamp prototype. My only meaningful suggestions were, "faster scan, longer wavelength, and, yes, get it on a fundus camera for clinical correlation and coding." The slit-lamp base was perceived to be an insurmountable challenge at the time.

Indocyanine green angiography, fundus autofluorescence, automated perimetry, and multifocal electroretinograms have also provided new dimensions for functional, as well as pathophysiological, clinical information, not previously available to retinal specialists. For sure, the intellect, intuition, and innovative minds of each new generation of retinal specialists will discover even better imaging systems than those available today with discrimination of not only tissue layers, but cellular components, normal and abnormal, and perhaps in time pathophysiological elements such as immune complex antibodies, antigens, and even pathogens.

Given the advent of these diagnostic adjuncts for imaging retinal diseases, it is rational to introduce a new retinal atlas to assemble and to incorporate the products of these technological advances. So, for this atlas, I scoured drawers of files in search of the best examples of instructive cases and used examples of current imaging systems to full advantage.

The next phase in the development of this atlas was to conceive a useful design to display these images illustrating the early and late stages of a given disease as well as phenotypic variants for full appreciation of each disorder. I must admit that I could not resist including some images from *The Retina Atlas*, cases which I considered as precious, priceless, and phenomenal. I also tried to accommodate the needs and interests of all potential readers, ranging from physicians in training, comprehensive ophthalmologists, and ophthalmic residents, to medical-retinal specialists and ancillary personnel in the eye care industry. Next, it was my purpose to obtain the assistance and cooperation of the publisher to broaden the boundaries of standard productions to minimize unutilized space or so-called "white paper." Accordingly, the margins on each page have been reduced to illustrate as much information about a given disease entity as possible, and above all, to accommodate a variety of geometric sizes which range from a magnified photograph of limited field to a panoramic image of the fundus. In some cases, normal areas of a fundus were deleted from a wide-angle photograph, to emphasize the pathology; in other cases, a wide-angle image was used as the primary photograph and a portion of it was magnified separately to show details of the pathological changes more explicitly. These publishing techniques are not unique, but they are new to an atlas involving the fundus, and they will hopefully add to the teaching value and comfort of the reader.

The design also enframes diagnostic imaging systems with a specific color: red borders are used for monochromatic red-free photos, yellow for fluorescein angiograms, green for ICG images, blue for fundus autofluorescence, and black for color photographs. This approach is meant to assist readers in identifying the exact nature of the images. Finally, in this atlas there is not much text beyond a brief description of the entity and legends to describe the illustrations. Some pertinent references were included, but more extensive discussion of the rapidly evolving nature of the disease entities will require additional reading in referenced articles and companion texts. The clinical material presented in each disorder was solely intended to provide a brief description of typical findings at various stages, initial and long-standing manifestations, and selected therapeutic outcomes. I must admit that the penalty for trying to be comprehensive and instructive within the confines of publishing deadlines led to compromise on the quality of some images where resolution was lost due to enhancement of contrast. This is particularly true when I could not locate the perfect example of each disease or manifestation. I compromised by using the best cases available. I hope that readers will only be rarely disappointed by their annoying color imbalance and limited clarity. The author, not the publisher, is to blame. If acceptance of this atlas warrants consideration for a new edition, I pledge to strive for excellence to remedy such deficiencies. Otherwise, I hope that this atlas will find a meaningful and valued place in the libraries of its readers, today and in the future.

Lawrence A. Yannuzzi, MD

References

1. Keeler, C., 1997. Evolution of the British ophthalmoscope. Doc. Ophthalmol. 94, 139–150.
2. Helmholtz, H., 1851. Bescreibung eines Augenspiegels zur Untersuchung der Netzhaut in lebenden Auge. Forstner, Berlin, p. 1.
3. Jackson, W.T., Webster, J.D., 1886. On Photographing the Retina of the Living Human Eye. Photographer, Philadelphia, 23, pp. 275–276.
4. Saine, P.J., 1993. Landmarks in the historical development of fluorescein angiography. J. Ophthalmic. Photogr. 15, 1.
5. Gerhoff, O., 1891. Ueber die Photographie des Augenhinter-grundes. Klin. Monat. Augenheilkd. 29, 397–403.
6. Dimmer, F., 1907. Ueber die Photographie des Augenhinter-grundes. Bergmann, Wiesbaden, p. 1.
7. Dimmer, F., Pillal, A., 1927. Atlas photographischer Bilder des Menschichen Augenhintergrundes. F. Deuticke, Leipzig.
8. Nordenson, J.W., 1925. Augenkamera zum stationaren Ophthalmoskop von Gullstrand. Berl. Dtsch. Ophthalm. Ges. 45, 278.
9. Gullstrand, A., 1910. Neue Methoden der reflexlosen Ophthalmoskopie. Berl. Dtsch. Ophthalm. Ges. 36, 75.
10. Bedell, A.J., 1929. Atlas of Stereoscopic Photographs of the Fundus Oculi. Davis, Philadelphia, p. 1.
11. Rizzutti, A.B., 1950. High speed photography of the anterior ocular segment. Arch. Ophthalmol. 43, 365–369.
12. Hansell, P., Beeson, E.J.G., 1953. Retinal photography in colour. Br. J. Ophthalmol. 37, 65–69.
13. Chao, P., Flocks, M., 1958. The retinal circulation time. Am. J. Ophthalmol. 46, 8–10.
14. Novotny, H.R., Alvis, D.L., 1961. A method of photographing fluorescence in circulating blood in the human retina. Circulation 24, 82–86.
15. Gass, J.D., 1967. Pathogenesis of disciform detachment of the neuroepithelium. Am. J. Ophthalmol. 63 (Suppl.), 617–645.
16. Yannuzzi, L.A., Fisher, Y., Levy, J., 1971. A classification for abnormal fundus fluorescence. Ann. Ophthalmol. 3, 711–718.
17. Schatz, H., Burton, T.C., Yannuzzi, L.A., et al., 1978. Interpretation of Fundus Fluorescein Angiography. CV Mosby, St. Louis, pp. 3–9.
18. Swanson, E.A., Izatt, J.A., Hee, M.R., et al., 1993. In vivo retinal imaging using optical coherence tomography. Opt. Lett. 18, 1864–1866.

Image References

Figures which have been previously published in other sources are listed below. Each of these figures has been given a unique copyright number (placed adjacent to the image) and readers should refer to the list below for the full copyright information.

1: Hogan MJ, Alvardo JE, Weddelm JE: Histology of the Human Eye. © Elsevier 1971.

2, 3, 4, 5, 6, 7, 8, 9, 10, 11: Graemiger RA, Niemeyer G, Schneeberger SA, et al: Wagner vitreoretinal degeneration. Follow-up of the original pedigree. Ophthalmology 1995;102(12):1830–1839. © Elsevier 1995.

12: Ho JES: Fundus Photography First Place. ASCRS 2004 Ophthalmic Photography Competition. J Ophthalmic Photogr 2004; 26(2):76.

13, 14, 15: Ober MD, Del Priore LV, Tsai J, et al: Diagnostic and therapeutic challenges. Retina 2006 Apr;26(4):462–467.

16: Renner AB, Kellner U, Fiebig B, et al: ERG variability in X-linked congenital retinoschisis patients with mutations in the RS1 gene and the diagnostic importance of fundus autofluorescence and OCT. Doc Ophthalmol 2008 Mar;116(2):97–109.

17: Lai TY, Wong VW, Lam DS: Asymmetrical ocular involvement and persistent fetal vasculature in an adult with osteoporosis pseudoglioma syndrome. Arch Ophthalmol 2006 Mar;124(3):422–423. © American Medical Association. All rights reserved.

18: Kellner U, Fuchs S, Bornfeld N, et al: Ocular phenotypes associated with two mutations (R121W, C126X) in the Norrie disease gene. Ophthalmic Genet 1996 Jun;17(2):67–74.

19, 20, 21: Soltau JB, Lueder GT: Bilateral macular lesions in incontentia pigmenti. Retina 1996;16:38–41.

22: Kellner U, Fuchs S, Bornfeld N, et al: Ocular henotypes associated with two mutations (R121W, C126X) in the Norrie disease gene. Ophthalmic Genet 1996 Jun;17(2):67–74.

23: Finley TA, Siatkowski RM: Progressive Visual Loss in a Child with Parry-Rhomberg Syndrome. Semin Ophthalmol 2004 Sep–Dec;19(3–4):91–94.

24, 25, 26, 27, 28, 29, 30: Ober MD, Del Priore LV, Tsai J, et al: Diagnostic and therapeutic challenges. Retina 2006 Apr;26(4):462–467.

31, 32, 33, 34: Kirwan M, Dokal I: Dyskeratosis congenita: a genetic disorder of many faces. Clin Genet 2008 Feb;73(2):103–112.

35: Lopez PF, Maumenee IH, de la Cruz Z, et al: Autosomal-dominant fundus flavimaculatus: clinicopathologic correlation. Ophthalmology 1990; 97:798–809. © Elsevier 1990.

36, 37, 38, 39, 40: Fishman GA, Baca W, Alexander KR, et al: Visual acuity in patients with Best vitelliform macular dystrophy. Ophthalmology 1993;100:1668. © Elsevier 1993.

41, 42: Frangieh GT, Green WR, Fine SL: A Histopathological study of Best's macular dystrophy. Arch Ophthalmol 1982;100:1115–1121. © American Medical Association. All rights reserved.

43, 44: Deutman AF, van Blommestein JD, Henkes HE, et al: Butterly-shaped pigment dystrophy of the fovea. Arch Ophthalmol 1970;83:558–569. © American Medical Association. All rights reserved.

45, 46: McGimpsey SJ, Rankin SJ: Case of Sjögren reticular dystrophy. Arch Ophthalmol 2007 Jun;125(6):850. © American Medical Association. All rights reserved.

47, 48: Guyer DR, Yannuzzi LA, Chang S, et al: Retina-Vitreous Macula. © Elsevier 1999.

49: Ulbig MR, Riordan-Eva P, Holz FG, et al: Membranoproliferative glomerulonephritis type II associated with central serous retinopathy. Am J Ophthalmol 1993;116:410–413. © Elsevier 1993.

50, 51: Navarro R, Casaroli-Marano R, Mateo C, et al: Optical Coherence Tomography Findings in Alport Syndrome. Retin Cases Brief Rep 2008;2(1):17–49.

52, 53, 54, 55: O'Donnell FE, Welch RB: Fenestrated sheen macular dystrophy. Arch Ophthalmol 1979;97:1292–1296. © American Medical Association. All rights reserved.

56, 57, 58, 59: Jean-Charles A, Cohen SY, Merle H, et al: Martinique (West Indies) crinkled retinal pigment epitheliopathy: clinical description. Retina 2013 May;33(5):1041–1048.

60: Jalili, IK: Cone-rod dystrophy and amelogenesis imperfecta (Jalili syndrome): phenotypes and environs. Eye (Lond) 2010 Nov;24(11): 1659–1668.

61, 62, 63: Reprinted by permission from Macmillan Publishers Ltd: Fleckenstein M, Charbel Issa P, Fuchs HA, et al: Discrete arcs of increased fundus autofluorescence in retinal dystrophies and functional correlate on microperimetry. Eye (Lond) 2009 Mar; 23:567–575.

64: Small KW, Letson R, Scheinman J: Ocular findings in primary hyperoxaluria. Arch Ophthalmol 1990 Jan;108(1):89–93. © American Medical Association. All rights reserved.

65: Image reprinted with permission from eMedicine.com, 2010. Available at: http://emedicine.medscape.com/article/1227488-overview

66, 67, 68: Makino S, Tampo H: Ocular findings in two siblings with Joubert syndrome. Clin Ophthalmol 2014 Jan;8:229–233.

69, 70: Abu el-Asrar AM, Kahtani ES, Tabbara KF: Retinal arteriovenous communication in retinitis pigmentosa with Refsum's disease-like findings. Doc Ophthalmol 1995;89(4):313–320. With kind permission from Springer Science + Business Media.

71: Ryan SJ: Retina, ed 2. © Elsevier 1994.

72, 73: Luckenbach MW, Green WR, Miller NR, et al: Ocular clinicopathologic correlation of Hallervorden-Spatz syndrome with acanthocytosis and pigmentary retinopathy. Am J Ophthalmol 1983 Mar;95(3):369–382. © Elsevier 1983.

74, 75, 76, 77, 78, 79: Holz FG, Spaide RF, Bird AC, et al: Fundus Autofluorescence Imaging with the Confocal Scanning Laser Ophthalmoscope. Springer Berlin Heidelberg 2007. With kind permission from Springer Science + Business Media.

80, 81, 82: Mura M, Sereda C, Jablonski MM, et al: Clinical and functional findings in choroideremia due to complete deletion of the CHM gene. Arch Ophthalmol 2007 Aug;125(8):1107–1113. © American Medical Association. All rights reserved.

83, 84, 85, 86, 87, 88: Yuan A, Kaines A, Jain A: Ultra-wide-field and autofluorescence imaging of choroidal dystrophies. Ophthalmic Surg Lasers Imaging 2010 Oct;41 Online:e1–5.

89, 90, 91: Wilson DJ, Weleber RG, Green WR: Ocular clinicopathologic study of gyrate atrophy. Am J Ophthalmol 1991;111:24–33. © Elsevier 1991.

92, 93, 94, 95: Oliveira TL, Andrade RE, Muccioli C, et al: Cystoid macular edema in gyrate atrophy of the choroid and retina: a fluorescein angiography and optical coherence tomography evaluation. Am J Ophthalmol 2005 Jul;140(1):147–149. © Elsevier 2005.

96, 97, 98, 99: Yuan A, Kaines A, Jain A, et al: Ultra-wide-field and autofluorescence imaging of choroidal dystrophies. Ophthalmic Surg Lasers Imaging 2010 Oct;41 Online:e1–5.

100, 101, 102, 103, 104: Reproduced from Noble KG, Carr RE, Siegel IM: Fluorescein angiography of the hereditary choroidal dystrophies. Br J Ophthalmol 1977;61:43–53, with permission from BMJ Publishing Group Ltd.

105, 106: Bass S, Noble K: Autosomal Dominant Pericentral Retinochoroidal Atrophy. Retina 2006; 26(1):71–81.

107: Sakamoto T, Maeda K, Sueishi K, et al: Ocular histopathologic findings in a 46-year-old man with primary hyperoxaluria. Arch Ophthalmol 1991;109:384. © American Medical Association. All rights reserved.

108, 109: Small KW, Letson R, Scheinman J: Ocular findings in primary hyperoxaluria. Arch Ophthalmol 1990 Jan;108(1):89–93. © American Medical Association. All rights reserved.

110, 111, 112, 113, 114: Jean-François E, Low JY, Gonzales CR, et al: Sjögren-Larsson syndrome and crystalline maculopathy associated with a novel mutation. Arch Ophthalmol 2007 Nov;125(11):1582–1583. © American Medical Association. All rights reserved.

115, 116, 117: Reproduced from Issacs TW, McAllister IL, Wade MS: Benign fleck retina. Br J Ophthalmol 1996 Mar;80(3):267–268, with permission from BMJ Publishing Group Ltd.

118, 119, 120, 121: Ryan SJ: Retina, ed 2. © Elsevier 1994.

122, 123: Chui HC, Green WR: Acute Retrolental Fibroplasia: A Clinical Pathological Correlation, MD Med J 1977;26:71–74, with permission.

124: Goldberg MF: Persistent fetal vasculature (PFV): an integrated interpretation of signs and symptoms associated with persistent hyperplastic primary vitreous (PHPV). LIV Edward Jackson Memorial Lecture. Am J Ophthalmol 1997 Nov;124(5):587–626. © Elsevier 1997.

125: Guyer DR, Yannuzzi LA, Chang S, et al: Retina-Vitreous Macula. © Elsevier 1999.

126, 127, 128: McHugh KL: Case Report: Cavernous Hemangioma of the Retina. J Ophthalmic Photogr 2008;30(2):64.

129, 130, 131: Sarraf D, Payne AM, Kitchen ND, et al: Familial cavernous hemangioma: An expanding ocular spectrum. Arch Ophthalmol 2000 Jul;118(7):969–973. With Permission.

132, 133, 134, 135: Tsui I, Song B, Tsang SH: A practical approach to retinal dystrophies. Retinal Physician 2007;4:18–26.

136, 137, 138: Ryan SJ: Retina, ed 2. © Elsevier 1994.

139: Spencer W: Ophthalmic pathology: an atlas and textbook, vol 2, ed 3, Philadelphia, 1993, WB Saunders.

140, 141, 142, 143: Heroman JW, Rychwalski P, Barr CC: Cherry red spot in sialidosis (mucolipidosis type I). Arch Ophthalmol 2008 Feb;126(2):270–271. © American Medical Association. All rights reserved.

144, 146, 147: Matthews JD, Weiter JJ, Kolodny EH: Macular halos associated with Niemann-Pick type B disease. Ophthalmology 1994;93:933–937. © Elsevier 1994.

145, 148: Ryan SJ: Retina, ed 2. Copyright Elsevier 1994.

149, 150: Ueno SS, Kamitani, T et al: Clinical and histopathologic studies of a case with juvenile form of Gaucher's disease. Jpn J Ophthalmol 1977;121:98–108. With kind permission from Springer Science + Business Media.

151, 152, 153, 154, 155: Shrier EM, Grabowski GA, Barr CC: Vitreous Opacities and retinal vascular abnormalities in Gaucher disease. Arch Ophthalmol 2004;122:1395–1398. © American Medical Association. All rights reserved.

156, 157, 158, 159, 160, 161, 162, 163: Coussa RG, Roos JC, Aroichane M, et al: Progression ED12 of retinal changes in Gaucher disease: a case report. Eye (Lond) 2013 Nov;27(11):1331–1333. Figure 2.

164: Albert DM, Jakobiec FA: Principles and Practice of Ophthalmology, 1st edition. © Elsevier 1994.

165, 166, 167: Slakter JS, Yannuzzi LA, Flower RW: Indocyanine Green Angiography. © Elsevier 1997.

168, 169, 170, 171, 172, 173, 174: Klufas MA, O Hearn T, Sarraf D: Optical coherence tomography angiography and widefield fundus autofluorescence in punctate inner choroidopathy. Retin Cases Brief Rep 2015l;9(4):323–326.

175, 176, 177: Slakter JS, Yannuzzi LA, Flower RW: Indocyanine Green Angiography. © Elsevier 1997.

178: Guyer DR, Yannuzzi LA, Chang S, et al: Retina-Vitreous Macula. © Elsevier 1999.

179, 180, 181: Slakter JS, Yannuzzi LA, Flower RW: Indocyanine Green Angiography. © Elsevier 1997.

182, 183, 184, 185, 186, 187, 187a–h: Mrejen S, Sarraf D, Chexal S, et al: Choroidal Involvement in Acute Posterior Multifocal Placoid Pigment Epitheliopathy. Ophthalmic Surg Lasers Imaging Retina 2016 Jan;47(1):20–26.

188, 189: Karagiannis D, Venkatadri S, Dowler J: Serpiginous Chorioidopathy with Bilateral Foveal Sparing and Good Visual Acuity after 18 years of disease. Retina 2007;27(7):989–990.

190, 191, 192, 193: Slakter JS, Yannuzzi LA, Flower RW: Indocyanine Green Angiography. © Elsevier 1997.

194, 195, 196: Reproduced from Gaudio PA, Kaye DB, Crawford JB: Histopathology of birdshot retinochoroidopathy. Br J Ophthalmol 2002;86: 1439–1441, with permission from BMJ Publishing Group Ltd.

197, 198: Koizumi H, Pozzoni MC, Spaide RF: Fundus Autofluorescence in Birdshot Chorioretinopathy. Ophthalmology 2008 May;115(5):e15–20. © Elsevier 2008.

199: Guyer DR, Yannuzzi LA, Chang S, et al: Retina-Vitreous Macula. © Elsevier 1999.

200, 201: Okwuosa TM, Lee EW, Starosta M, et al: Purtscher-like retinopathy in a patient with adult-onset Still's disease and concurrent thrombotic thrombocytopenic purpura. Arthritis Rheum 2007 Feb;57(1):182–185.

202: Agarwal M, Biswas J: Unilateral Frosted Branch Angiitis in a Patient with Abdominal Tuberculosis. Retin Cases Brief Rep 2008;2(1):39–40.

203, 206: Ryan SJ: Retina, ed 2. © Elsevier 1994.

204, 205, 205a: Spencer WH, ed: Ophthalmic pathology. An atlas and textbook, vol 2, Philadelphia, 1985, WB Saunders.

207, 208, 209, 210, 211: Guyer DR, Yannuzzi LA, Chang S, et al: Retina-Vitreous Macula. © Elsevier 1999.

212: Dreyer WB Jr, Zegarra H, Zakov ZN: Sympathetic ophthalmia. Am J Ophthalmol 1981;92:816–823. © Elsevier 1981.

213, 214, 215, 216, 217, 218: Guyer DR, Yannuzzi LA, Chang S, et al: Retina-Vitreous Macula. © Elsevier 1999.

219: Spirn MC, Regillo C: Proliferative Vitreoretinopathy. Retinal Physician Jan 2008.

220, 221, 222: Fisher JP, Lewis ML, Blumenkranz M, et al: The acute retinal necrosis syndrome. Part 1: Clinical manifest. Ophthalmology 1982;89:1309–1316. © Elsevier 1982.

223: Aizman A, Johnson MW, Elner SG: Treatment of acute retinal necrosis syndrome with oral antiviral medications. Ophthalmology 2007 Feb;114(2):307–312. © Elsevier 2007.

224, 225: Culbertson WW, Blumenkranz MS, Haines H, et al: The acute retinal necrosis syndrome. Part 2: Histopathology and etiology. Ophthalmology 1982;89:1317–1325. © Elsevier 1982.

226: Pepose JS, Flowers B, Stewart JA, et al: Herpes virus antibody levels in the etiologic diagnosis of the acute retinal necrosis syndrome. Am J Ophthalmol 1992;113:248–256. © Elsevier 1992.

227, 228, 229, 230, 231, 232, 233, 234, 235, 236, 237, 238: Cunningham ET Jr, Short GA, Irvine AR, et al: Acquired immunodeficiency syndrome—associated herpes simplex virus retinitis. Clinical description and use of a polymerase chain reaction—based assay as a diagnostic tool. Arch Ophthalmol 1996 Jul;114(7):834–840. Erratum in: Arch Ophthalmol 1997 Apr;115(4):559.

239, 240, 241: Engstrom RE, Holland GN, Margolis TP, et al: The progressive outer retinal necrosis syndrome: A variant of necrotizing herpetic retinopathy in patients with AIDS. Ophthalmology 1994;101:1488–1502. © Elsevier 1994.

242, 243: Kim SJ, Baranano DE, Grossniklaus HE, et al: Epstein-Barr Infection of the Retina: Case Report and Review of the Literature. Retin Cases Brief Rep 2011;5(1):1–5.

244, 245: Bains HS, Jampol LM, Caughron MC, et al: Vitritis and chorioretinitis in a patient with West Nile virus infection. Arch Ophthalmol 2003;121:205–207. © American Medical Association. All rights reserved.

246, 247, 248: Yannuzzi LA, Jampol LM, Rabb MF, et al: Unilateral acute idiopathic maculopathy. Arch Ophthalmol 1991;109:1411–1416. © American Medical Association. All rights reserved.

249, 250: Myers JP, Leveque TK, Johnson MW: Extensive Chorioretinitis and Severe Vision Loss Associated with West Nile Virus Meningoencephalitis. Arch Ophthalmology 2005;123:1754–1756. © American Medical Association. All rights reserved.

251: Folk JC, Weingeist TA, Corbett JJ, et al: Syphilitic neuroretinitis. Am J Ophthalmol 1983;95:480–485. © Elsevier 1983.

252, 253: Spencer WH, ed: Ophthalmic pathology. An atlas and textbook, vol 2, Philadelphia, 1985, WB Saunders.

254: Folk JC, Weingeist TA, Corbett JJ, et al: Syphilitic neuroretinitis. Am J Ophthalmol 1983;95:480–485. © Elsevier 1983.

255: Ryan SJ: Retina, ed 2. © Elsevier 1994.

256, 257: Knox DL, King J: Retinal arteritis, iridocyclitis, and giardiasis. Ophthalmology 1982;89:1303–1308. © Elsevier 1982.

258: Ryan SJ: Retina, ed 2. © Elsevier 1994.

259: Holz FG, Spaide RF, Bird AC, et al: Fundus Autofluorescence Imaging with the Confocal Scanning Laser Ophthalmoscope. Springer Berlin Heidelberg 2007. With kind permission of Springer Science + Business Media.

260: Guyer DR, Yannuzzi LA, Chang S, et al: Retina-Vitreous Macula. WB Saunders. © Elsevier 1999.

261, 262: Levecq LJ, De Potter P: Solitary choroidal tuberculoma in an immunocompetent patient. Arch Ophthalmol 2005 Jun;123(6):864–866. © American Medical Association. All rights reserved.

263, 264: Cangemi FE, Friedman AH, Josephberg R: Tuberculoma of the choroid. Ophthalmology 1980;87:252–258. © Elsevier 1980.

265: Jampol LM, Strauch BS, Albert DM: Intraocular nocardiosis. Am J Ophthalmol 1973;76:568. © Elsevier 1973.

266, 267: Gregor RJ, Chong CA, Augsburger JJ, et al: Endogenous Nocardia asteroides subretinal abscess diagnosed by transvitreal fine-needle aspiration biopsy. Retina 1989;9:118–121.

268, 269: Reproduced from Schulman JA, Leveque C, Coats M, et al: Fatal disseminated cryptococcoses following intraocular involvement. Br J Ophthalmol 1988;72:171–175, with permission from BMJ Publishing Group Ltd.

270: Folk JC, Weingeist TA, Corbett JJ, et al: Syphilitic neuroretinitis. Am J Ophthalmol 1983;95:480–485. © Elsevier 1983.

271: Wender JD, Elliot D, Jumper M, et al: How to Recognize Syphilis. Review of Ophthalmology. November 2008.

272: de Souza EC, Jalkh AE, Trempe CL, et al: Unusual central chorioretinitis as the first manifestation of early secondary syphilis. Am J Ophthalmol 1988;105:271–276. © Elsevier 1988.

273: Guyer DR, Yannuzzi LA, Chang S, et al: Retina-Vitreous Macula. © Elsevier 1999.

274: Ryan SJ: Retina, ed 2. © Elsevier 1994.

275, 277, 278, 279: Griffin JR, Pettit TH, Fishman LS, et al: Blood-borne Candida endophthalmitis: a clinical and pathologic study of 21 cases. Arch Ophthalmol 1973;89:450. © American Medical Association. All rights reserved.

276, 280, 281, 282: Snip RC, Michels RG: Pars plana vitrectomy in the management of endogenous Candida endophthalmitis. Am J Ophthalmol 1976;82:699–704. © Elsevier 1976.

283, 284: Coskuncan NM, Jabs DA, Dunn JP, et al: The eye in bone marrow transplantation: VI. Retinal complications. Arch Ophthalmol 1994;112:372–379. © American Medical Association. All rights reserved.

285, 286: Reproduced from Schulman JA, Leveque C, Coats M, et al: Fatal disseminated cryptococcoses following intraocular involvement. Br J Ophthalmol 1988;72:171–175, with permission from BMJ Publishing Group Ltd.

287, 288: Khodadoust AA, Payne JW: Cryptococcal "torular" retinitis: a clinicopathologic case report. Am J Ophthalmol 1969;67:745–750. © Elsevier 1969.

289, 290, 291, 292, 293: Lewis H, Aaberg TM, Fary DRB, et al: Latent disseminated blastomycosis with choroidal involvement. Arch Ophthalmol 1988;106:527–530. © American Medical Association. All rights reserved.

294: Zakka KA, Foos RY, Brown WJ: Intraocular coccidioidomycosis. Surv Ophthalmol 1978;22:313–321. © Elsevier 1978.

295: Rainin EA, Little HL: Ocular coccidioidomycosis: a clinical pathologic case report, Trans Am Acad Ophthalmol 1972;76:645–651.

296, 297, 298, 299: Arevalo JF, Fuenmayor-Rivera D, Giral AE, et al: Indocyanine green videoangiography of multifocal *Cryptococcus neoformans* choroiditis in a patient with acquired immunodeficiency syndrome. Retina 2001;21(5):537–541.

300: Friedman AH, Pokorny KS, Suhan J, et al: Electron microscopic observations of intravitreal *Cysticercus cellulosae (Taenia solium)*, Ophthalmologica 1980;180:267–273.

301, 304: Ryan SJ: Retina, ed 2. © Elsevier 1994.

302, 303, 307: Aghamohammadi S, Yoken J, Lauer AK, et al: Intraocular Cysticercosis By *Taenia crassiceps*. Retin Cases Brief Rep 2008;2(1):61–64.

305, 306a: Spencer W: Ophthalmic pathology: an atlas and textbook, vol 2, ed 3, Philadelphia, 1993, WB Saunders.

308: Cover, Volume 115, Issue 1, Pages A1–A40, 1–224, Opthalmology, © Elsevier January 2008.

309: Maguire AM, Green WR, Michels RG, et al: Recovery of intraocular *Toxocara canis* by pars plana vitrectomy. Ophthalmology 1990;97:675–680. © Elsevier 1990.

310, 311, 312, 313: McDonald HR, Kazacos KR, Schatz H, et al: Two cases of intraocular infection with *Alaria mesocercariae* trematodes. Am J Ophthalmol 1994;117:447. © Elsevier 1994.

314, 315: Vedantham V, Vats MM, Kakade SJ, et al: Diffuse unilateral subacute neuroretinitis with unusual findings. Am J Ophthalmol 2006 Nov;142(5):880–883. © Elsevier 2006.

316, 317: Sharifipour F, Feghhi M: Anterior ophthalmomyiasis interna: an ophthalmic emergency. Arch Ophthalmol 2008 Oct;126(10):1466–1467. © American Medical Association. All rights reserved.

318, 319, 320, 321, 322: Funata M, Custis P, de la Cruz Z, et al: Intraocular gnathostomiasis. Retina 1993;13:240–244.

323, 324, 325: Reprinted by permission from Macmillan Publishers Ltd: Sinawat S, Sanguansak T, Angkawinijwong T, et al: Ocular angiostrongyliasis: clinical study of three cases. Eye (Lond) 2008 Nov;22(11):1446–1448.

326: Image taken from de Crecchio G, Alfieri MC, Cennamo G: Congenital macular macrovessels. Graefes Arch Clin Exp Ophthalmol 2006 Sep;244(9):1183–1187.

327, 328: Images from Rahimy E, Rayess N, Talamini CL, et al: Traumatic Prepapillary loop torsion and associated branch retinal artery occlusion. JAMA Ophthalmol 2014 Nov;132(11):1376–1377.

329: Laird PW, Mohney BG, Renaud DL: Bull's-eye maculopathy in an infant with Leigh disease. Am J Ophthalmol 2006 Jul;142(1):186–187. © Elsevier 2006.

330, 331, 332, 333, 334, 335, 336, 337, 338, 339, 340, 341, 342: Images taken from Yu S, Pang CE, Gong Y: The spectrum of superficial and deep capillary ischemia in retinal artery occlusion. Am J Ophthalmol 2015 Jan;159(1):53–63.e1–2.

343, 344: Images from Rahimy E, Rayess N, Talamini CL, et al: Traumatic Prepapillary loop torsion and associated branch retinal artery occlusion. JAMA Ophthalmol 2014 Nov;132(11):1376–1377.

345, 346, 347, 348: Jarrett WH, North AW: Dynamic platelet embolization of the retinal arteriole. Arch Ophthalmol 1995 Apr;113(4):531–532. © American Medical Association. All rights reserved.

349, 350: Tsui I, Kaines A, Havunjian MA: Ischemic index and neovascularization in central retinal vein occlusion. Retina 2011 Jan;31(1):105–110.

351, 352: Green WR, Chan CC, Hutchins GM, et al: Central retinal vein occlusion: a prospective histopathologic study of 29 eyes in 28 cases. Retina 1981;1:27–55.

353, 354, 355: Images taken from Rahimy E, Sarraf D, Dollin ML: Paracentral acute middle maculopathy in nonischemic central retinal vein occlusion. Am J Ophthalmol 2014 Aug;158(2):372–380.e1.

356, 357, 358, 359: Images taken from Emmett T, Cunningham H, McDonald R, et al: Paracentral acute middle maculopathy spectral-domain optical coherence tomography feature of deep capillary ischemia. Curr Opin Ophthalmol 2014;25(3):207–212.

360, 361, 362, 363, 364, 365, 366, 367: Images taken from Eadie JA, Ip MS, Kulkarni AD: Response to aflibercept as secondary therapy in patients with persistent retinal edema due to central retinal vein occlusion initially treated with bevacizumab or ranibizumab. Retina 2014 Dec;34(12):2439–2443.

368, 369: Images taken from Maggio E, Polito A, Guerriero M, et al: Intravitreal dexamethasone implant for macular edema secondary to retinal vein occlusion: 12-month follow-up and prognostic factors. Ophthalmologica 2014;232(4):207–215.

370, 371, 372: Vaghefi HA, Green WR, Kelly JS, et al: Correlation of clinicopathologic findings in a patient: congenital night blindness, branch retinal vein occlusion, cilioretinal artery drusen of the optic nerve head, and intraretinal pigmented lesion. Arch Ophthalmol 1978;96:2097–2104. © American Medical Association. All rights reserved.

373: Images taken from Pichi F, Morara M, Torrazza C, et al: Intravitreal bevacizumab for macular complications from retinal arterial macroaneurysms. Am J Ophthalmol 2013 Feb;155(2):287–294.e1.

374, 375: Images taken from Sigler EJ, Randolph JC, Calzada JI, et al: Current management of Coats disease. Surv Ophthalmol 2014 Jan-Feb;59(1):30–46.

376, 377: Henry CR, Berrocal AM, Hess DJ, et al: Intraoperative spectral-domain optical coherence tomography in Coats' disease. Ophthalmic Surg Lasers Imaging 2012 Jul 26;43 Online:e80–4.

378: Reese AB: Telangiectasis of the retina and Coats disease. Am J Ophthalmol 1956;42:1–8. © Elsevier 1956.

379: Images taken from Sigler EJ, Randolph JC, Calzada JI, et al: Current management of Coats disease. Surv Ophthalmol 2014 Jan-Feb;59(1):30–46.

380, 381, 382: Margolis R, Folgar FA, Moussa M, et al: Diffuse retinal capillary leakage in Coats disease. Retin Cases Brief Rep 2012;6(3):285–289.

383, 384, 385, 386: Sigler EJ, Randolph JC, Calzada JI, et al: Current Management of Coats disease. Surv Ophthalmol 2014 Jan-Feb;59(1):30–46.

387, 388, 389, 390, 391, 392, 395, 396, 397, 398, 399, 400, 401, 402, 403, 404, 405, 406: Sallo FB1, Leung I, Clemons TE, et al: Multimodal imaging in type 2 idiopathic macular telangiectasia. Retina 2015 Apr;35(4):742–749.

393, 394: Balaskas K, Leung I, Sallo FB, et al: Associations between autofluorescence abnormalities and visual acuity in idiopathic macular telangiectasia type 2: MacTel project report number 5. Retina 2014 Aug;34(8):1630–1636.

407, 408, 409, 410, 411, 412: Spaide RF, Klancnik JM Jr, Cooney MJ: Retinal vascular layers in macular telangiectasia type 2 imaged by optical coherence tomographic angiography. JAMA Ophthalmol 2015 Jan;133(1):66–73.

413, 414, 415, 416, 417: Wu L, Evans T, Arevalo JF: Idiopathic macular telangiectasia type 2 (idiopathic juxtafoveolar retinal telangiectasis type 2A, MacTel 2). Surv Ophthalmol 2013 Nov-Dec;58(6):536–559.

418: Powner MB, Gillies MC, Zhu M, et al: Loss of Muller's cells and photoreceptors in macular telangiectasia type 2. Ophthalmology 2013 Nov;120(11):2344–2352.

419, 420: Powner MB, Gillies MC, Tretiach M, et al: Perifoveal Muller cell depletion in a case of macular telangiectasia type 2. Ophthalmology 2010 Dec;117(12):2407–2416.

421, 422, 423: Meleth AD, Toy BC, Nigam D, et al: Prevalence and progression of pigment clumping associated with idiopathic macular telangiectasia type 2. Retina 2013 Apr;33(4):762–770.

424: Baumüller S, Charbel Issa P, Scholl HP, et al: Outer retinal hyperreflective spots on spectral-domain optical coherence tomography in macular telangiectasia type 2. Ophthalmology 2010 Nov;117(11):2162–2168.

425, 426, 427, 428: Sallo FB, Leung I, Chung M, et al: Retinal crystals in type 2 idiopathic macular telangiectasia. Ophthalmology 2011 Dec;118(12):2461–2467.

429, 430, 431, 432, 433: Narayanan R, Chhablani J, Sinha M, et al: Efficacy of anti-vascular endothelial growth factor therapy in subretinal neovascularization secondary to macular telangiectasia type 2. Retina 2012 Nov-Dec;32(10):2001–2005.

434: Charbel Issa P, Finger RP, Kruse K, et al: Monthly ranibizumab for nonproliferative macular telangiectasia type 2: a 12-month prospective study. Am J Ophthalmol 2011 May;151(5):876-886.e1.

435, 436, 437, 438, 439: Roller AB, Folk JC, Patel NM, et al: Intravitreal bevacizumab for treatment of proliferative and nonproliferative type 2 idiopathic macular telangiectasia. Retina 2011 Oct;31(9):1848–1855.

440: Gragoudas E, et al: Radiation maculopathy after proton beam irradiation for choroidal melanoma. Ophthalmology 1992;99:1278–1285. © Elsevier 1992.

441, 442, 443: Groenewald C, Konstantinidis L, Damato B: Effects of radiotherapy on uveal melanomas and adjacent tissues. Eye (Lond) 2013 Feb;27(2):163–171.

444, 445, 446: Shah NV, Houston SK, Markoe A, et al: Combination therapy with triamcinolone acetonide and bevacizumab for the treatment of severe radiation maculopathy in patients with posterior uveal melanoma. Clin Ophthalmol 2013;7:1877–1882.

447, 448, 449, 450, 451, 452: Das T, Pathengay A, Hussain N, et al: Eales disease: diagnosis and management. Eye (Lond) 2010 Mar;24(3):472–482.

453, 454, 457, 461: Franklin RM, ed.: Proceedings of the symposium on retina and vitreous, New Orleans, La, 1993, New York, Kugler Publications.

455, 456: Wang H, Chhablani J, Freeman WR, et al: Characterization of diabetic microaneurysms by simultaneous fluorescein angiography and spectral-domain optical coherence tomography. Am J Ophthalmol 2012 May;153(5):861–867.

458, 460, 465, 466, 467: Ryan SJ: Retina, ed 2. © Elsevier 1994. Courtesy of the ETDRS Research Group.

459: Ryan SJ: Retina, ed 2. © Elsevier 1994.

462, 463: Martinez KR, Cibis GW, Tauber JT: Lipemia retinalis, Arch Ophthalmol 1992;110:1171. © American Medical Association. All rights reserved.

464: Shin JY, Byeon SH, Kwon OW: Optical coherence tomography-guided selective focal laser photocoagulation: a novel laser protocol for diabetic macular edema. Graefes Arch Clin Exp Ophthalmol 2015 Apr;253(4):527–535.

468: Pacella E, Vestri AR, Muscella R, et al: Preliminary results of an intravitreal dexamethasone implant (Ozurdex) in patients with persistent diabetic macular edema. Clin Ophthalmol 2013;7:1423–1428.

469: Romayananda N, Goldberg MF, Green WR: Histopathology of sickle cell retinopathy, Trans Am Ophthalmol Soc 1973;77:652–676. Republished with permission of the American Ophthalmological Society.

470: Cho M, Kiss S: Detection and monitoring of sickle cell retinopathy using ultra widefield color photography and fluorescein angiography. Retina 2011 Apr;31(4):738–747.

471: Sanfilippo CJ, Klufas MA, Sarraf D, et al: Optical coherence tomography angiography of sickle cell maculopathy. Retin Cases Brief Rep 2015l;9(4):360–362.

472, 473, 474, 475, 476: Buettner H, Bollins JP: Retinal arteriovenous communications in carotid occlusive disease. In: Excerpta Medica: current aspects of ophthalmology, Amsterdam, 1992.

477, 478, 479, 480: Tanaka T, Shimizu K: Retinal arteriovenous shunts in Takayasu disease. Ophthalmology 1987 Nov;94(11):1380–1388. © Elsevier 1987.

481, 482: Sugiyama K, Ijiri S, Tagawa S, Shimizu K: Takayasu disease on the centenary of its discovery. Jpn J Ophthalmol 2009 Mar;53(2):81–91. With kind permission of Springer Science + Business Media.

483: Baker PS, Garg SJ, Fineman MS, et al: Serous macular detachment in Waldenstrom macroglobulinemia: a report of four cases. Am J Ophthalmol 2013 Mar;155(3):448–455.

484, 485, 486, 487: Image courtesy of Rusu IM, Mrejen S, Engelbert M, et al: Immunogammopathies and acquired vitelliform detachments: a report of four cases. Am J Ophthalmol 2014 Mar;157(3):648–657.e1.

488, 489: Schwartz SG, Hickey M, Puliafito CA: Bilateral CRAO and CRVO from thrombotic thrombocytopenic purpura: OCT findings and treatment with triamcinolone acetonide and bevacizumab. Ophthalmic Surg Lasers Imaging 2006 Sep–Oct;37(5):420–422.

490: Guyer DR, Green WR, de Bustros S, et al: Histopathologic features of idiopathic macular holes and cysts, Ophthalmology 1990;87:1045–1051. © Elsevier 1990.

491, 491a–h: From Nemiroff et al, The spectrum of Amalric triangular choroidal infarction. Retinal Cases and Brief Reports

492: Matlach J, Freiberg FJ, Gadeholt Om et al: Vasculitis-like hemorrhagic retinal angiopathy in Wegener's granulomatosis. BMC Res Notes 2013 Sep 10;6:364.

493, 494, 495, 496, 497: Boets EP, Chaar CG, Ronday K, et al: Chorioretinopathy in primary antiphospholipid syndrome: a case report. Retina 1998;18(4):382–384.

498: Hong-Kee N, Mei-Fong C, Azhany Y, et al: Antiphospholipid syndrome in lupus retinopathy. Clin Ophthalmol 2014 Nov 24;8:2359–2363.

499, 500, 501, 502, 503, 504: Li HK, Dejean BJ, Tang RA: Reversal of visual loss with hyperbaric oxygen treatment in a patient with Susac syndrome. Ophthalmology 1996 Dec;103(12):2091–2098. © Elsevier 1996.

505, 506, 507, 508: Bui SK, O'Brien JM, Cunningham ET Jr: Purtscher retinopathy following drug-induced pancreatitis in an HIV-positive patient. Retina 2001;21(5):542–545.

509: Coady PA, Cunningham ET Jr, Vora RA: Spectral domain optical coherence tomography findings in eyes with acute ischemic retinal whitening. Br J Ophthalmol 2015 May;99(5):586–592.

510, 511: Ryan SJ: Retina, ed 2. © Elsevier 1994

512, 513, 514: Lida T, Kishi S: Choroidal vascular abnormalities in preeclampsia. Arch Ophthalmol 2002;120:1406–1407. © American Medical Association. All rights reserved.

515, 516: Park KH, Kim YK, Woo SJ, et al: Iatrogenic occlusion of the ophthalmic artery after cosmetic facial filler injections: a national survey by the Korean Retina Society. JAMA Ophthalmol 2014 Jun;132(6):714–723.

517, 518, 519, 520, 521, 522, 523, 524: From Ophthalmology 2014;121:1020–1028.

525, 526, 527: JAMA Ophthalmol 2014;132(9): 1148–1150.

528, 529: Middle East Afr J Ophthalmol 2012 Jul–Sep;19(3):346–348.

530, 531: Arch Ophthalmol 2010:128(2):206–210.

532, 533, 534: Ophthalmic Surg Lasers Imaging Retina 2014 May;45 Online:e23–25.

535, 536, 537: Korean J Ophthalmol 2013 Dec; 27(6):463–465.

538, 539, 540: Arch Ophthalmol 2011; 129(9): 1222.

541, 542, 543, 544, 545: Front Genet 2013 Apr 4;4:14.

546, 547, 548, 549: Retina 2011;31:482–491.

550: Pathologic Myopia by Yannuzzi, Spaide, Ohno-Matsui: Springer publisher.

551: Am J Ophthalmol 2013;156:958–967.

552: Caillaux V, Gaucher D, Gualino V, et al: Morphologic characterization of dome-shaped macula in myopic eyes with serous macular detachment. Am J Ophthalmol 2013 Nov;156(5):958–967.

553, 554, 555, 556: Retina 2014;34(9): 1841–1847.

557, 558, 559: Arch Ophthalmol 2006;124(12):1783–1784.

560: Retina 2010;30:1441–1454.

561, 562, 563, 564, 565, 566, 567, 568, 569, 570: Retina 2015 Jul;35(7):1339–1350.

571, 572, 573: Am J Ophthalmol 2009;147:801–810.

574, 575, 576, 577, 578, 579, 580: JAMA Ophthalmology 2014;132(7):806–813.

581, 582, 583: Eye (Lond) 2015 May;29(5):703–706.

584: Retina 2014;34(7):1289–1295.

585, 586, 587, 588, 589, 590, 591, 592: Ophthalmology 2015;122:2316–2326.

593, 594, 595, 596, 597, 598, 599, 600, 601, 602: Retina 2010;30:1039–1045.

603, 604, 605: Retina 2012;32:1057–1068.

606, 607, 608, 609: Retina 2013;32:1057–1068.

610, 611, 612: Retina 2014;32:1057–1068.

613, 614, 615, 616, 617, 618: Retina 2013;33(1):48–55.

619, 620, 621, 622, 623, 624, 625: Retina 2015;35(4):603–613.

626, 627: Nicholson DH, Green WR, Kenyon KR: Light and electron microscopic study of early lesions in angiomatous retinae, Am J Ophthalmol 1976;82:193–204. © Elsevier 1976.

628, 629: Chan CC, Collins AB, Chew EY: Molecular pathology of eyes with von Hippel-Lindau (VHL) Disease: a review. Retina 2007;27(1):1–7.

630, 630a: Spencer W: Ophthalmic pathology: an atlas and textbook, ed 3, Philadelphia, 1985, WB Saunders.

631, 632: Goldberg RE, Pheasant TR, Shields JA: Cavernous hemangiomas of the retina. Arch Ophthalmol 1979;97:2321. © American Medical Association. All rights reserved.

633: Guyer DR, Yannuzzi LA, Krupsky S, et al: Indocyanine-green angiography of intraocular tumors. Semin Ophthalmol (Dec) 1993.

634, 635, 636, 637, 638: JAMA Ophthalmol 2014;132(6):756–760.

639, 639a: Lebwohl M: Atlas of the skin and systemic disease. New York, Churchill-Livingstone, Inc. © Elsevier 1995.

640: Oliver SCN, Ciardella AP, Sands RE, et al: Retin Cases Brief Rep 2007;1(2):82–84.

641, 642, 643, 644, 645, 646: Am J Ophthalmol 2014 Dec;158(6):1253–1261.

647: Barr CC, Green WR, Payne JW, et al: Intraocular reticulum cell sarcoma: clinicopathologic study of four cases and review of literature. Surv Ophthalmol 1975;19:224–239. © Elsevier 1975.

648: Brodsky MC, Safar AN: Optic disc tuber. Arch Ophthalmol 2007 May;125(5):710–712. © American Medical Association. All rights reserved.

649, 650, 651, 652: Guyer DR, Green WR, Schachat AP, et al: Bilateral ischemic optic neuropathy and retinal vascular occlusions associated with lymphoma and sepsis, Ophthalmology 1990;97:882–888. © Elsevier 1990.

653, 654: Patikulsila D, Visaetsilpanonta S, Sinclair SH, et al: Cavernous hemangioma of the optic disk. Retina 2007 Mar;27(3):391–392.

655: Green WR, McLean IW: Retina. In Spencer WH, ed: Ophthalmic pathology, ed 4, Philadelphia, 1996, WB Saunders.

656: Rich RR (ed) et al: Clinical Immunology. © Elsevier 2008.

657, 658: Minella A, Yannuzzi LA, Slakter J, et al: Bilateral perifoveal ischemia associated with chronic granulocytic leukemia. Arch Ophthalmol 1988;106:1170. © American Medical Association. All rights reserved.

659: Ryan SJ: Retina, ed 2. © Elsevier 1994.

660, 661: Mandava N, Costakos D, Bartlett H: Chronic Myleogenous Leukemia Manifested as Bilateral Proliferative Retinopathy. Arch Ophthalmol 2005 Apr;123(4):576–577. © American Medical Association. All rights reserved.

662, 663: Retina 2014;34:1513–1523.

664, 665, 666: International Journal of retina and Vitreous, published online 2015 by Bora Chae et al.

667, 668: Retina 2011;31:13–25.

669, 670: Guyer DR, Gragoudas ES: Idiopathic macular holes. In Albert D, and Jakobiec F, eds: Principles and practices of ophthalmology. © Elsevier 1993.

671: Retina 2012;32:1719–1726.

672, 673, 674, 675, 676, 677, 678: Am J Ophthalmol 2015;159:227–231.

679, 680, 681, 682, 683: Retina 2014;34:1513–1523.

684: Guyer DR, Yannuzzi LA, Slakter JS, et al: Digital indocyanine-green videoangiography of central serous chorioretinopathy, Arch Ophthalmol 1994;112:1057–1062. © American Medical Association. All rights reserved.

685, 686, 687, 688, 689, 690, 691: Am J Ophthalmol 2014 Aug;158(2):362–371.

692, 693, 694, 695: Ophthalmic Surg Lasers Imaging Retina 2015 Sep;46(8):832–836.

696, 697, 698, 699, 700, 701, 702, 703, 704: Ophthalmology 2016 Apr 12. pii: S0161-6420(16)00354-7. doi: 10.1016/j.ophtha.2016.03.017. [Epub ahead of print]

705, 706, 707, 708, 709, 710, 711, 712, 713, 714, 715, 716, 717, 718: Retina 2015 Jan;35(1):1–9.

719, 720, 721, 722, 723, 724, 725, 726: Retina 2016 Mar;36(3):499–516.

727: Margo CE, Hamed LF, Mames RN (eds): Diagnostic Problems in Clinical Ophthalmology. Philadelphia. © Elsevier 1994.

728: Guyer DR, Yannuzzi LA, Chang S, et al: Retina-Vitreous Macula. © Elsevier 1999.

729, 730, 731: Margo CE, Hamed LF, Mames RN (eds): Diagnostic Problems in Clinical Ophthalmology. Philadelphia. © Elsevier 1994.

732, 733, 734, 735, 736, 737, 738, 739: Clin Ophthalmol 2014 Dec 30;9:43–49.

740, 741, 742, 743, 744, 745, 746, 747: Byer NE: The peripheral retina in profile: a stereoscopic atlas, Criterion Press.

748, 749: Mansour AM, Green WR, Hogge C: Histopathology of commotio retinae. Retina 1992;12:24–28.

750, 751, 752, 753, 754: Clin Exp Ophthalmol 2006;34:893–894.

755: Cover, Ophthalmology Volume 115, Issue 2. © Elsevier 2008.

756: Copyright Doheny Eye Institute 2010.

757: Lois N, Sehmi KS, Hykin PG: Giant retinal pigment epithelial tear after trabeculectomy. Arch Ophthalmol 1999 Apr;117(4):546–547. © American Medical Association. All rights reserved.

758: Sakamoto T, Maeda K, Sueishi K, et al: Ocular histopathologic findings in a 46-year-old man with primary hyperoxaluria. Arch Ophthalmol 1991;109:384. © American Medical Association. All rights reserved.

759, 760: Miller FS 3rd, Bunt-Milam AH, Kalina RE: Clinical-ultra-structural study of thioridazine retinopathy. Ophthalmology 1982;89:1478–1488. © Elsevier 1982.

761: Guyer DR, Yannuzzi LA, Chang S, et al: Retina-Vitreous-Macula. WB Saunders. Philadelphia 1999, p 862. © Elsevier 1999.

762, 763, 764, 765, 766, 767, 768, 807: Guyer DR, Tiedeman J, Yannuzzi LA, et al: Interferon-associated retinopathy. Arch Ophthalmol 1993;111:350–356. © American Medical Association. All rights reserved.

769, 770: Millay RH, Klein ML, Illingworth DR: Niacin maculopathy. Ophthalmology 1988 Jul;95(7):930–936. © Elsevier 1988.

771: Esmaeli B, Prieto VG, Butler CE, et al: Severe periorbital edema secondary to STI571 (Gleevec). Cancer 2002 Aug;95(4):881–887.

772, 773, 774, 775: Smith SV, Benz MS, Brown DM: Cystoid macular edema secondary to albumin-bound paclitaxel therapy. Arch Ophthalmol 2008 Nov;126(11):1605–1606. © American Medical Association. All rights reserved.

778: Kaiser-Kupfer MI, Kupfer C, Rodriguez MM: Tamoxifen retinopathy a clinicopathologic report. Ophthalmology 1981 Jan;88(1):89–93. © Elsevier 1981.

776, 777, 779, 780, 781, 782, 783, 784, 785, 786, 787, 788, 789, 790, 791, 792: Bourla DH, Sarraf D, Schwartz SD: Peripheral retinopathy and maculopathy in high-dose tamoxifen therapy. Am J Ophthalmol 2007 Jul;144:126–128. © Elsevier 2007.

793, 794, 795, 796, 797, 798: Novak MA, Roth AS, Levine MR: Calcium oxalate retinopathy associated with methoxyfl urane abuse, Retina 1988;8:230–236.

799, 800, 801, 802: Drenser K, Sarraf D, Jain A, et al: Crystalline retinopathies. Surv Ophthalmol 2006 Nov–Dec;51(6):535–549. © Elsevier 2006.

803, 804, 805, 806: Sarraf D, Ceron O, Rasheed K, et al: West African crystalline maculopathy. Arch Ophthalmol 2003 Mar;121(3):338–342. © American Medical Association. All rights reserved.

808, 809: Witherspoon SR, Callanan D: Celiac disease presenting as a xerophthalmic fundus. Retina 2008 Mar;28(3):525–526.

810, 811: Moore M, Salles D, Jampol LM: Progressive Optic Nerve Cupping and Neural Rim Decrease in a Patient With Bilateral Autosomal Dominant Optic Nerve Colobomas. Am J Ophth 2000 Apr;129(4):517–520. © Elsevier 2000.

812, 813: Lincoff, H, Lopez, R, Kreissig, I, et al: Retinoschisis associated with optic nerve pits. Arch Ophthalmol 1988;106:61–67. © American Medical Association. All rights reserved.

814, 815: Cohen SY, Quentel G: Uneven Distribution of Drusen in Tilted Disc Syndrome. Retina 2008;28(9):1361–1362.

816, 817, 818, 819: Oliver SCN, Mandava N: Ultrasonographic Signs in Complete Optic Nerve Avulsion. Arch Ophthalmol 2007 May;125(5):716–717. © American Medical Association. All rights reserved.

820: Albert DL, Jakobiec FA (eds): Principles and practice of ophthalmology, vol 2. © Elsevier 1994.

821: Abe S, Yamamoto T, Haneda S, et al: Three-Dimensional Features of Polypoidal Choroidal Vasculopathy Observed by Spectral-Domain OCT. Ophthalmic Surg Lasers Imaging 2010 Mar;41:1–6.

822, 823, 824, 825: Vendantham V, Vats MM, Kakade SJ, et al: Diffuse unilateral subacute neuroretinitis with unusual findings. Am J Ophthalmol 2006;142: 880–883.

CHAPTER 1

Normal

Retinal Histology

The sensory retina extends to the ora serrata, where it is continuous with the nonpigmented ciliary epithelium of the pars plana. The ora serrata is 2.1 mm wide temporally and 0.7–0.8 mm wide nasally and is located more anteriorly on the nasal versus the temporal side. The nasal ora has a irregular, or serrated border and is about 6 mm posterior to the limbus while the temporal ora has an regular or smooth border and is about 6.5 mm posterior to the limbus. The average distance from the ora serrata to the optic nerve is 32.5 mm temporally and 27 mm nasally, and 31 mm superiorly and inferiorly. The retina itself is a thin transparent tissue that is thickest near the optic nerve where it measures 0.56 mm and becomes progressively thinner at the equator (0.18 mm) and the ora serrata (0.1 mm). At the fovea, the retina is thin and measures 0.2 mm in thickness. The nerve fiber layer increases toward the edge of the disc and is the only retinal structure that continues into the disc to become the optic nerve. The sensory retina is composed of nine contiguous microscopic layers, linked by synaptic connections between axons and dendrites in the inner and outer plexiform layers. The neuronal cells are supported by Müller cells and the astrocytes from the inner portion of the retina. The retinal pigment epithelial layer is a monocellular tissue of irregular density. It has a cuboidal and hexagonal shape with villous processes that envelop the photoreceptor outer segments. It also contains melanin granules and is taller, more densely pigmented, and columnar in shape in the central macula.

Bruch membrane refers to a sheet-like condensation of the innermost portion of the choroidal stroma that consists of two layers of collagen on either side of a central layer of elastic tissue. The basement membrane of the retinal pigment epithelium (RPE) and the choriocapillaris endothelium are the boundaries of Bruch membrane, although this interpretation is controversial. Some consider Bruch membrane as a part of the choroidal stroma. The choroidal circulation is supplied by the short ciliary or choroidal arteries that are concentrated in the macula and peripapillary region. A dense anastomotic network of vessels comprises the choriocapillaris bordered by the outer part of Bruch membrane. In the macula, the choriocapillaris is composed of a lobular pattern of highly concentrated and interconnecting capillary segments supplied by a central arteriole and drained by circumferential venules.

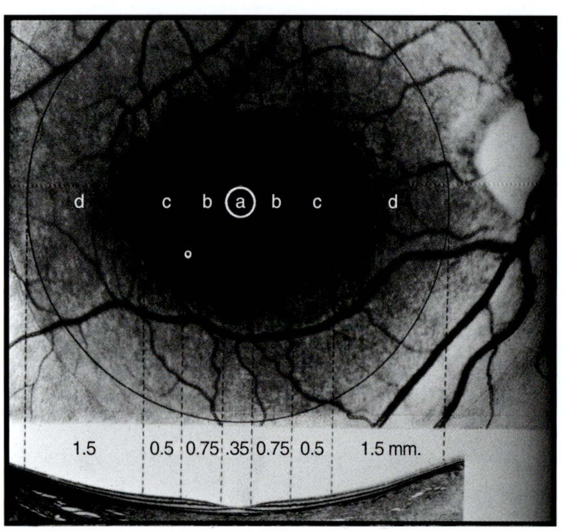

© I

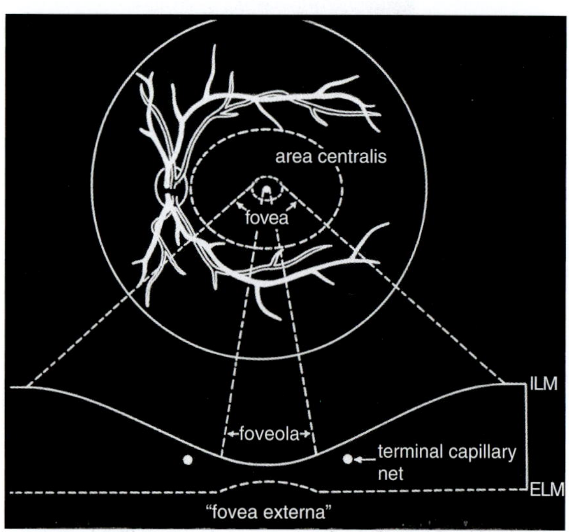

Left: fundus photograph matched with a horizontal section of the macula, delineating the (a) foveola, (b) fovea, (c) parafovea, and (d) perifovea. Right: schematic diagram showing the relative dimensions of the fovea, foveola, macula (area centralis), and peripheral fundus. ILM, internal limiting membrane; ELM, external limiting membrane.

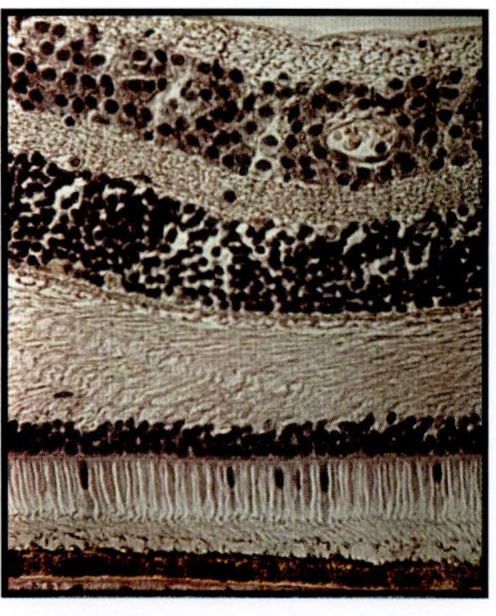

The histology of the macula is represented in this image and is defined by the multilayered ganglion cell layer. The retina is bordered anteriorly by the internal limiting membrane (ILM) comprised of Müller cell footplates. Note the nerve fiber layer (NFL) and its ganglion cells (GC), the inner plexiform layer (IPL), the inner nuclear layer (INL), middle limiting membrane (MLM), the outer plexiform layer (OPL), the outer nuclear layer (ONL), the external limiting membrane (ELM), the inner segments of the photoreceptors (IS), the outer segments of the photoreceptors (OS), and the retinal pigment epithelium (RPE). The ELM is comprised of Müller cell attachments to the inner segments.

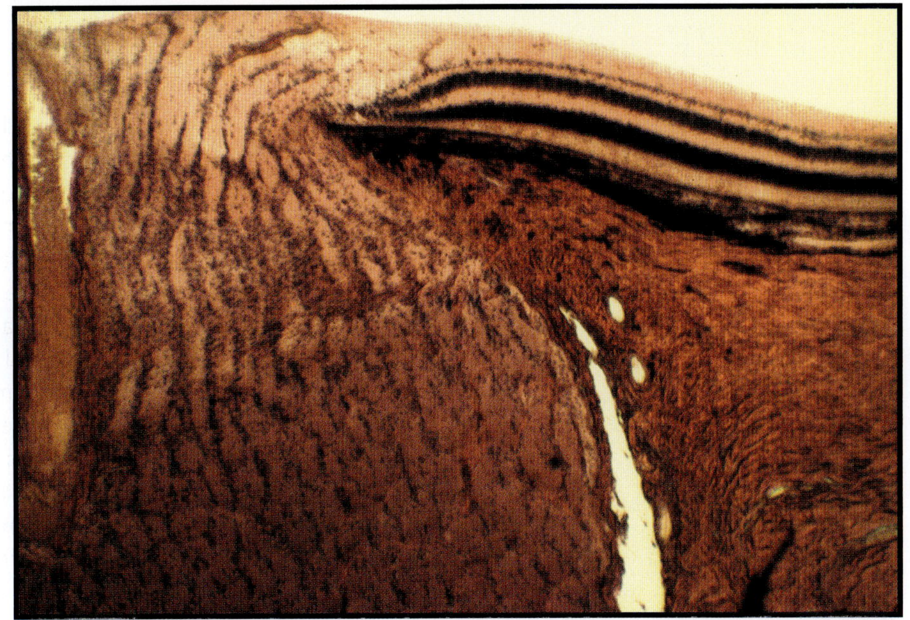

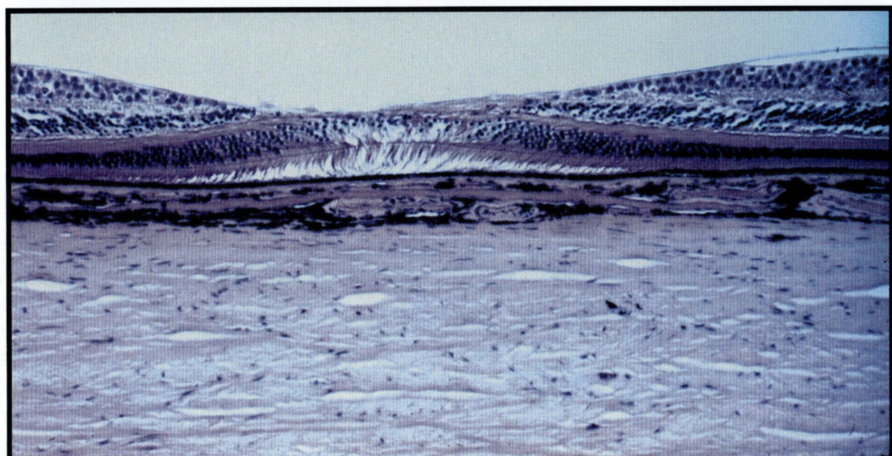

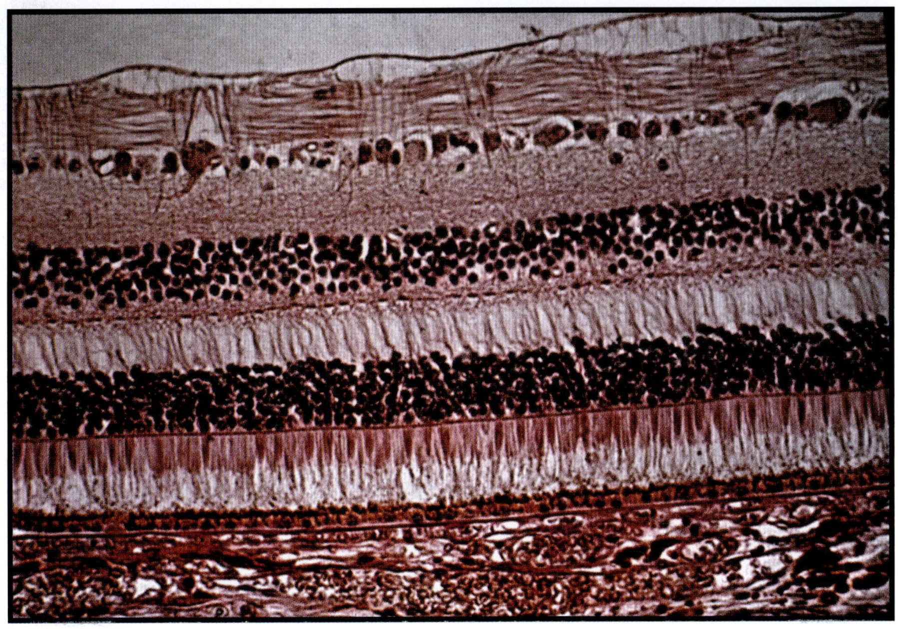

These are histological specimens of the optic nerve *(top)*, the foveal area including the sclera *(middle)*, and the peripheral retina *(bottom)* defined by the single layer of ganglion cells.

The Fundus

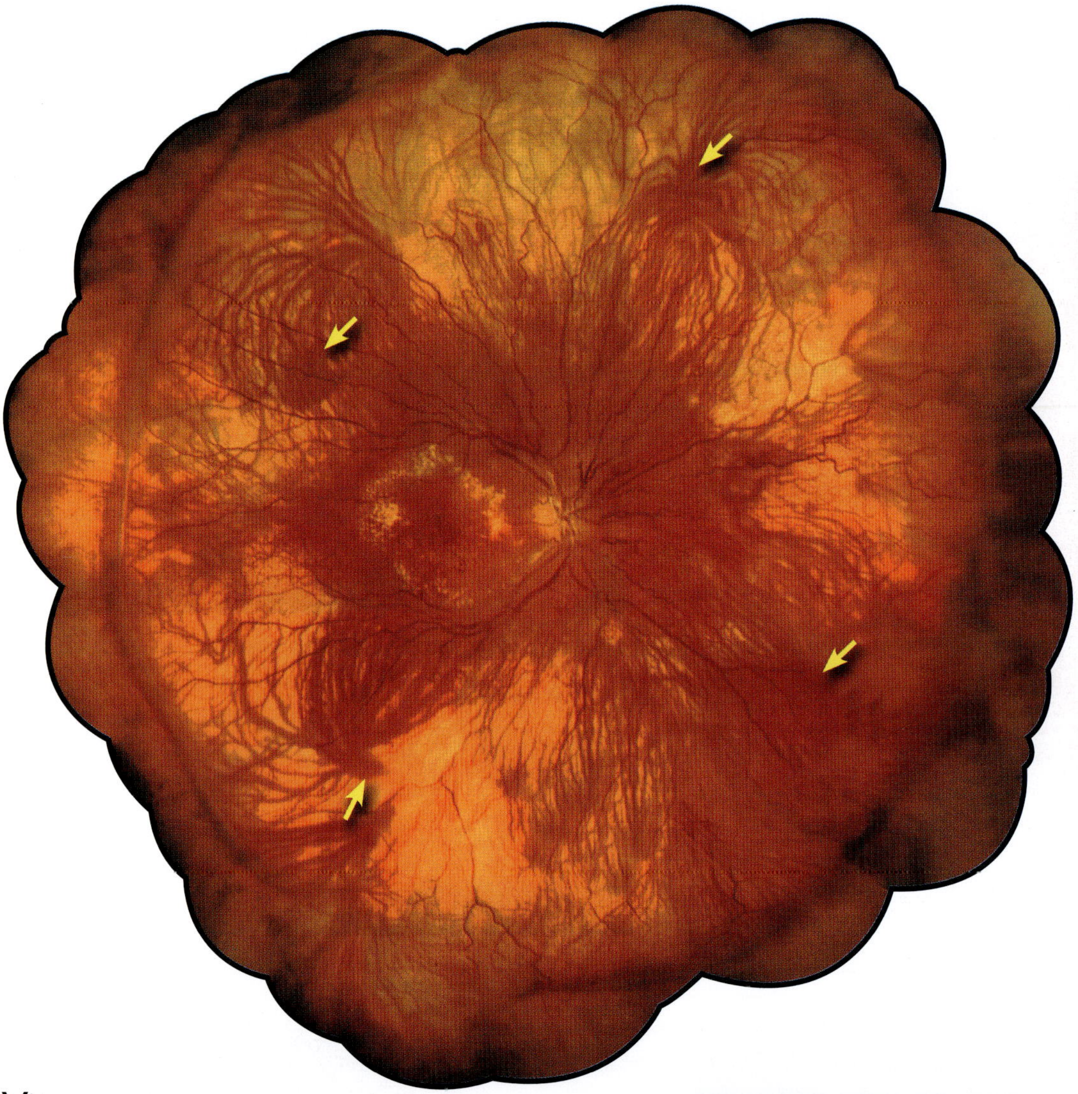

This is a color montage of a blond fundus. The choroidal circulation is visible through a mildly pigmented retinal pigment epithelium. Note the 4 vortex veins *(arrows)* in the outer choroidal circulation, which accommodate the very high flow supplied posteriorly by 10–20 short posterior ciliary branches of the ophthalmic artery. Nasal and temporal long posterior ciliary arteries supply the anterior choroid and uvea.

Vitreous

The vitreous body extends from the posterior lens to the surface of the retina. It is slightly less than 3.9 mL in volume, comprising approximately 2/3 to 3/4 of the adult globe. It is spherical posteriorly and saucer-shaped anteriorly due to a depression caused by the convexity of the posterior lens surface. The vitreous cortex is made of 3 visible components: (1) collagen-like fibers, (2) cells, and (3) mucopolysaccharides and other proteins. The vitreous cortex is covered by the hyaloid membrane, a thin enveloping structure. In the posterior pole, there is a precortical vitreous pocket, referred to as the premacular bursa, which may extend to the retinal vascular arcades.

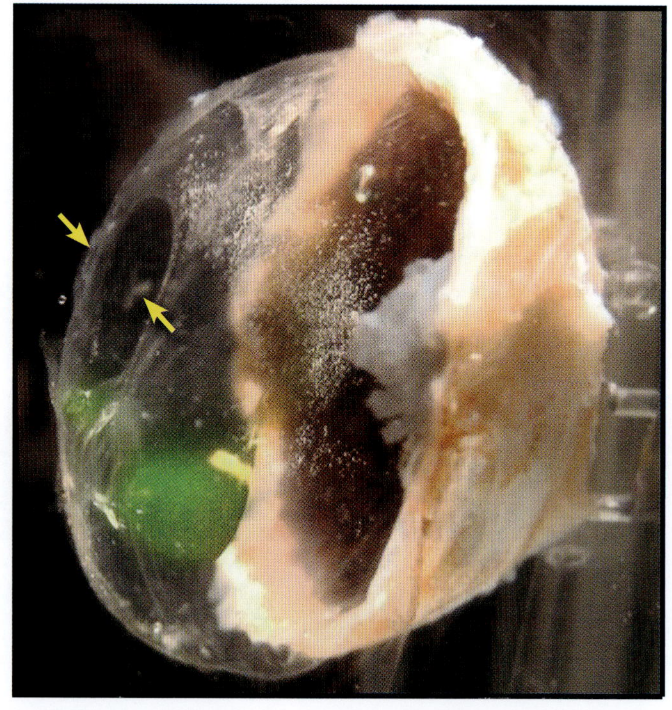

Note the posterior precortical vitreous pocket (PPVP) that forms the premacular bursa and that is located immediately anterior to the posterior fundus surrounded by the temporal vascular arcades *(arrows)*. The posterior wall of the PPVP is composed of a thin layer of vitreous cortex. The rest of its border is contoured by formed vitreous. Occasionally, the PPVP expands to become confluent with adjacent lacunae in the vitreous. This structure is inconsistently detectable clinically when there is posterior vitreous detachment. Otherwise it is consistently present in normal eyes. *Courtesy of Dr. Lennart Berglin, Dr. Louise Bergman, and Dr. Henry F. Edelhauser*

Retina

The retina lines the inner surface of the eye with neuronal connections extending to the optic nerve and the central nervous system. It is a layered diaphanous structure comprised of neurons and interconnected synapses with principal light-sensitive cells at its outer aspect in the photoreceptor layer, which contains rods and cones. There are approximately 6 million cones, most densely packed within the fovea, and 125 million rods positioned predominantly in the eccentric macula and peripheral retina.

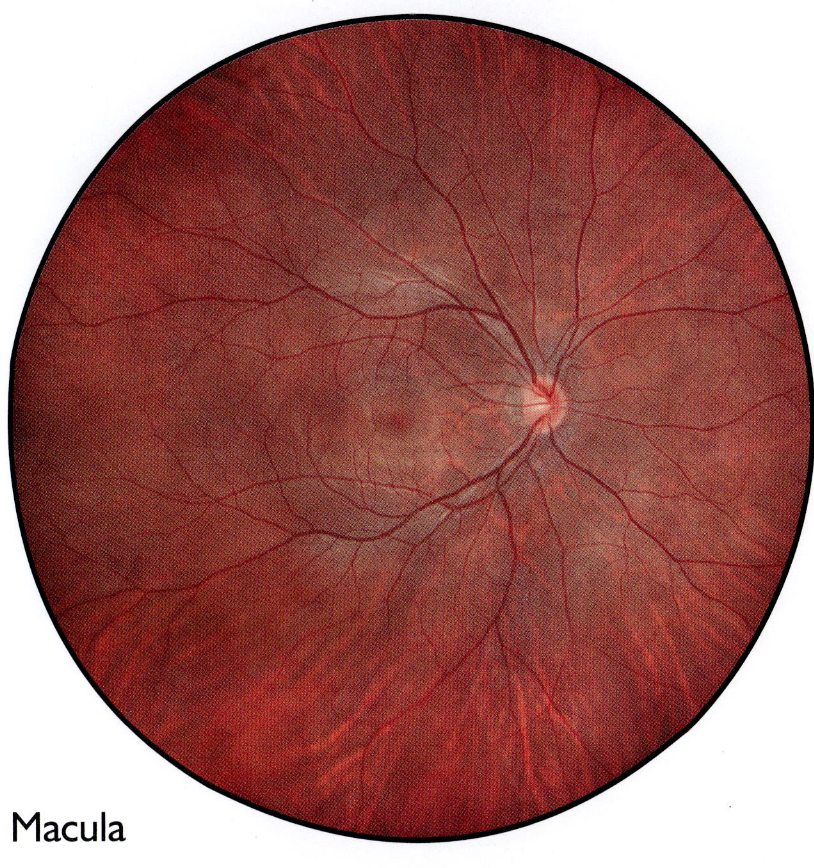

This image illustrates the distribution of the retinal vessels throughout the retina. The retinal venules are darker and more dilated (in a 3:2 ratio) than the brighter arterioles. Note the 4 major vascular arcades, 2 temporal and 2 nasal.

Macula

The macula refers to an area that includes the parafoveolar area (about 2.85 mm in diameter), but some equate the macula to the foveal area (about 1.8 mm in diameter). The fovea is a 1.5 mm depression in the center of the macula. It is located about 4 mm temporal and 0.8 mm inferior to the horizontal raphe. The average thickness of the fovea is about 0.25 mm, roughly half that of the adjacent parafoveal area. The central 0.35 mm of the fovea is the foveola, which is located in a capillary-free zone (i.e. the foveal avascular zone) that measures about 0.5 mm in diameter. A small protuberance in the center of the foveola is called the umbo, where there is a dense concentration of cell bodies of elongated cones referred to as the cone bouquet of Rochon–Duvigneaud. A 0.5 mm wide annular zone surrounding the fovea is the area where the ganglion cell layer, nuclear layers, and outer plexiform layer of Henle are the thickest. This is referred to as the parafoveal area. This area is surrounded by a 1.5 mm ring zone called the perifoveal area where the ganglion cell layer is reduced from 5–7 layers to a single layer of nuclei, as noted elsewhere in the peripheral retina.

There are several modifications in the retinal architecture in the macular area, beginning with the absence of retinal vessels in the central foveal region (i.e. foveal avascular zone). There are no rods in the foveola, and the cones are so modified that they resemble rods in form. The outer segments of the cones are long and approach the apical side of the RPE cells. At the edge of the fovea, the ganglion cell layer and the inner nuclear layer thicken, but both layers disappear within the fovea. In the foveolar area, only photoreceptor cells and Müller cell processes are present. Each cell is united with a single bipolar cell and possibly a single ganglion cell, yielding maximal transmission of the visual stimulus.

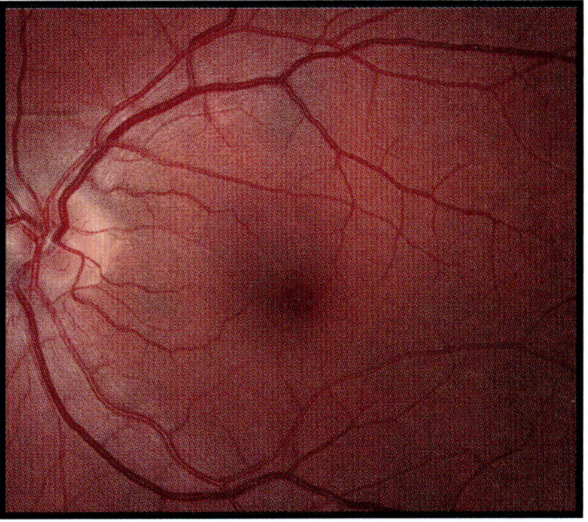

The morphological landmarks of the macula are not very distinct clinically. However, a dark zone surrounding the fovea is clearly evident due to the intrinsic pigmentation of the retina (xanthophyll) and, above all, the retinal pigment epithelium (melanin). The foveal pit and the umbo are noted by the characteristic central foveolar light reflex.

Fluorescein Angiography (FA)

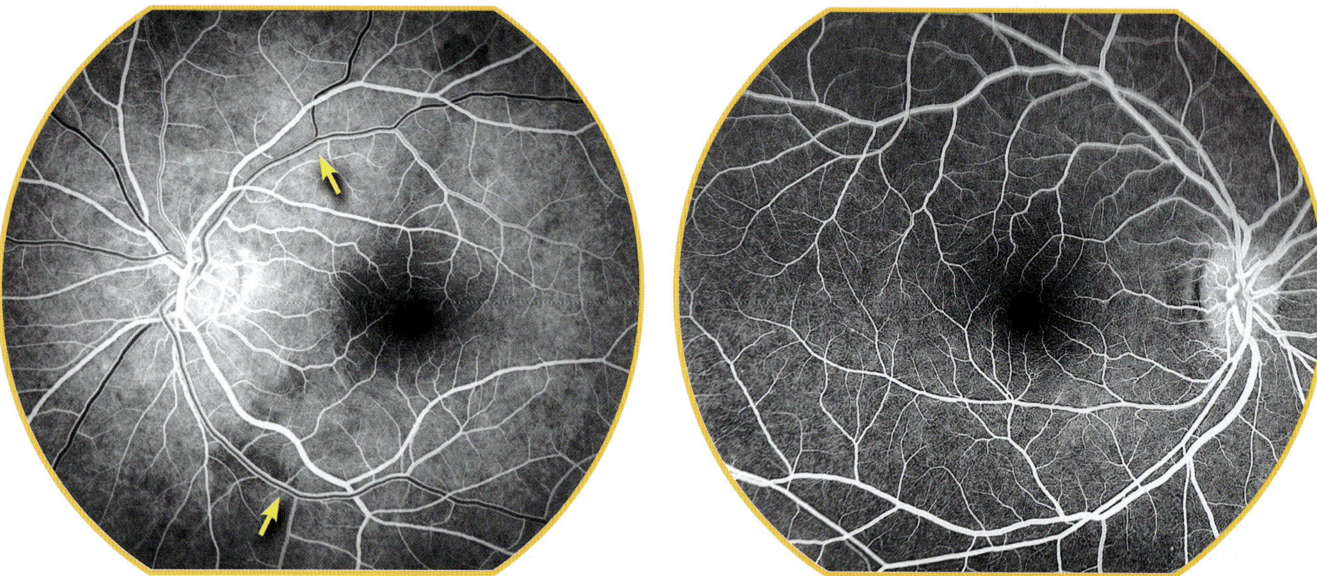

Fluorescein angiogram (FA) of the left eye *(left)* (arteriovenous phase) demonstrating lamellar flow *(yellow arrows)* in the retinal veins and FA of the right eye *(right)* during the later venous phase showing complete flow within the retinal arteries and veins. Note the presence of the hypofluorescent fovea because of the foveal avascular zone and the dense pigmentation of the retinal pigment epithelium.

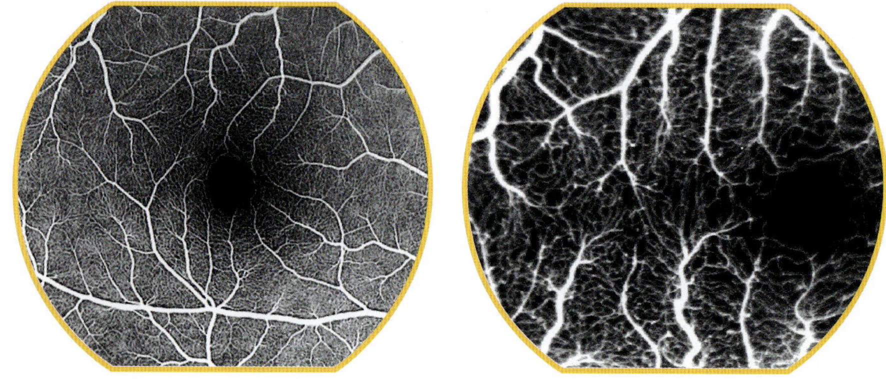

One way to study the retinal circulation is with high-speed stereo fluorescein angiography (FA). The foveal avascular zone and its marked variability are well illustrated with this form of imaging *(left and right)*. The dense foveal capillary plexus is clearly identified but is comprised predominantly by the superficial retinal capillary plexus due to obstruction of the underlying deep retinal capillary plexus with conventional dye-based angiography. *Right image courtesy of Ethan Friel*

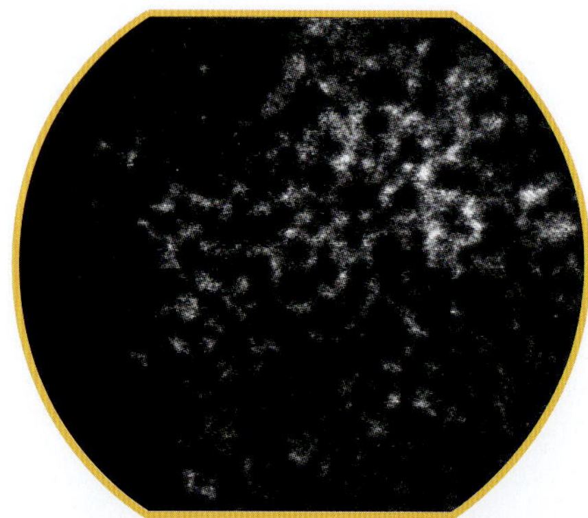

This image illustrates the fluorescein angiographic filling of the choriocapillaris with high-speed angiography and serial subtraction technique. There is a lobular filling pattern of the choriocapillaris, which is seldom appreciated, except in eyes that have ischemic choroidopathies.

Indocyanine Green (ICG)

Indocyanine green (ICG) angiography is an effective modality to image the choroidal circulation. The longer wavelength penetrates the pigment epithelium to enhance the choroidal vasculature in the normal and abnormal eye. It is not possible to image the choriocapillaris of the choroidal circulation without high-speed serial subtraction techniques. Because of the enhanced protein binding capacity of ICG, diffuse choriocapillaris leakage is not seen (as with FA), which further improves identification of the larger choroidal vessels. The pigment epithelium–Bruch membrane–choriocapillaris complex has been collectively referred to as the *tunica ruyschiana*, given commonalities in development, anatomy, and physiology.

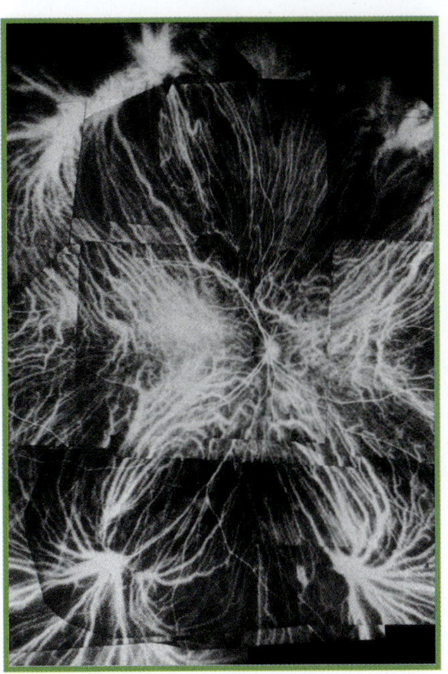

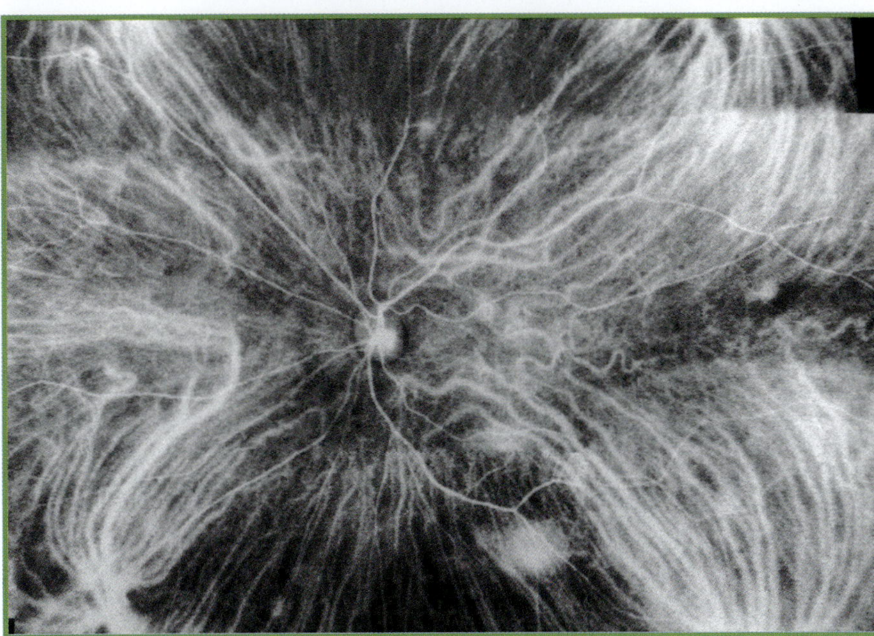

Fundus Autofluorescence (FAF)

Fundus autofluorescence (FAF) is a noninvasive imaging technique that can provide a density map of the predominant retinal fluorophore, lipofuscin, in the RPE. Autofluorescence is captured by excitation and emission filters in the camera that match the autofluorescent spectra of lipofuscin or related fluorophores. Different retinal diseases that alter the distribution of lipofuscin, mask its presence, or cause increases in levels of other fluorescent material can be associated with various signature autofluorescent patterns.

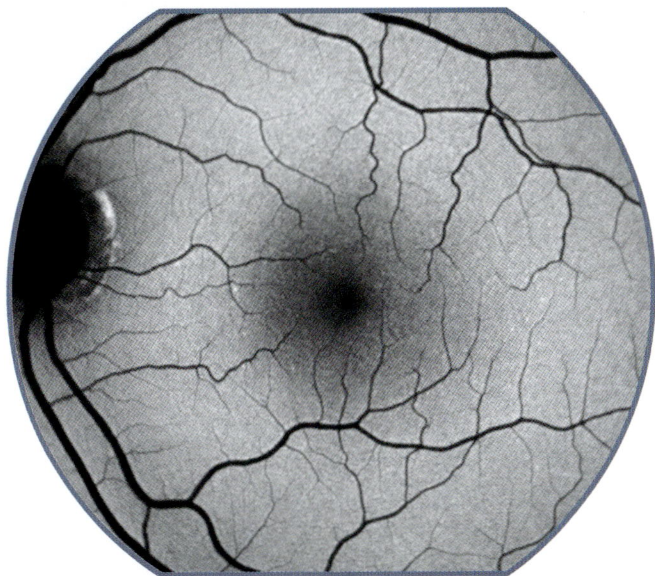

This is a normal fundus autofluorescence image. Note the decreased autofluorescence of the central macula due to blockage by the macular xanthophyll pigments (i.e. lutein, zeaxanthin).

Ultra Widefield Imaging

Ultra widefield imaging combines confocal scanning laser imaging with an elliptical mirror to achieve up to a 200 degree view of the retina with a single image capture. This technique can be combined with FAF, FA, and ICG angiography.

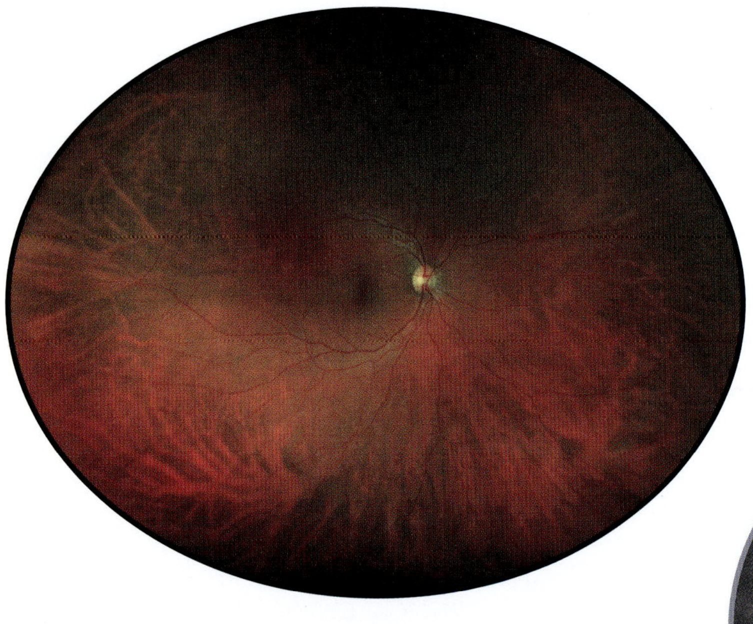

This is a normal ultra widefield pseudocolor fundus image.

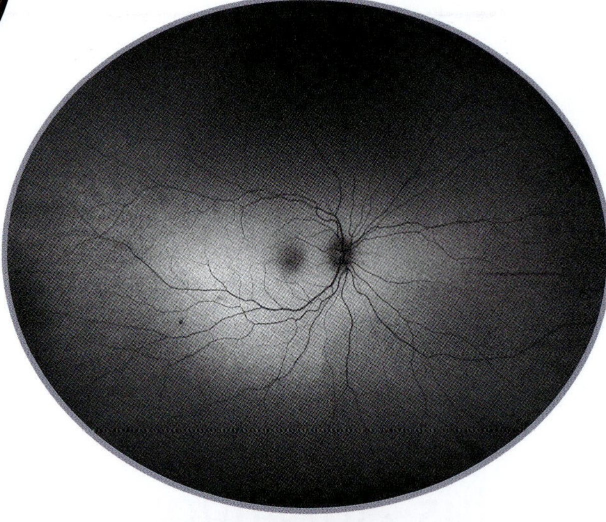

Ultra widefield imaging can be combined with autofluorescence *(top)*, fluorescein angiography *(middle)*, and ICG angiography *(bottom)*.

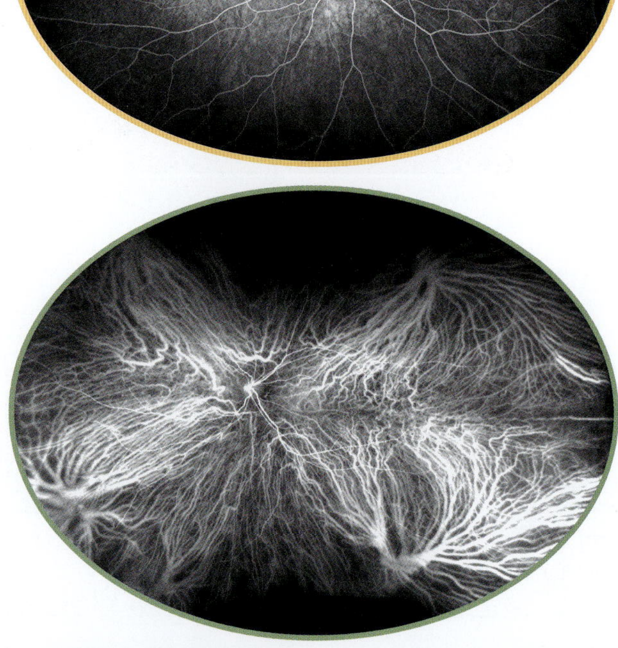

Optical Coherence Tomography (OCT)

For the past several years, optical coherence tomography (OCT) has become the most important diagnostic adjunct in imaging the macula and paramacular region. Using the basic property of interferometry, OCT can yield high-resolution cross sectional images of the macula with histological grade quality and rapid acquisition.

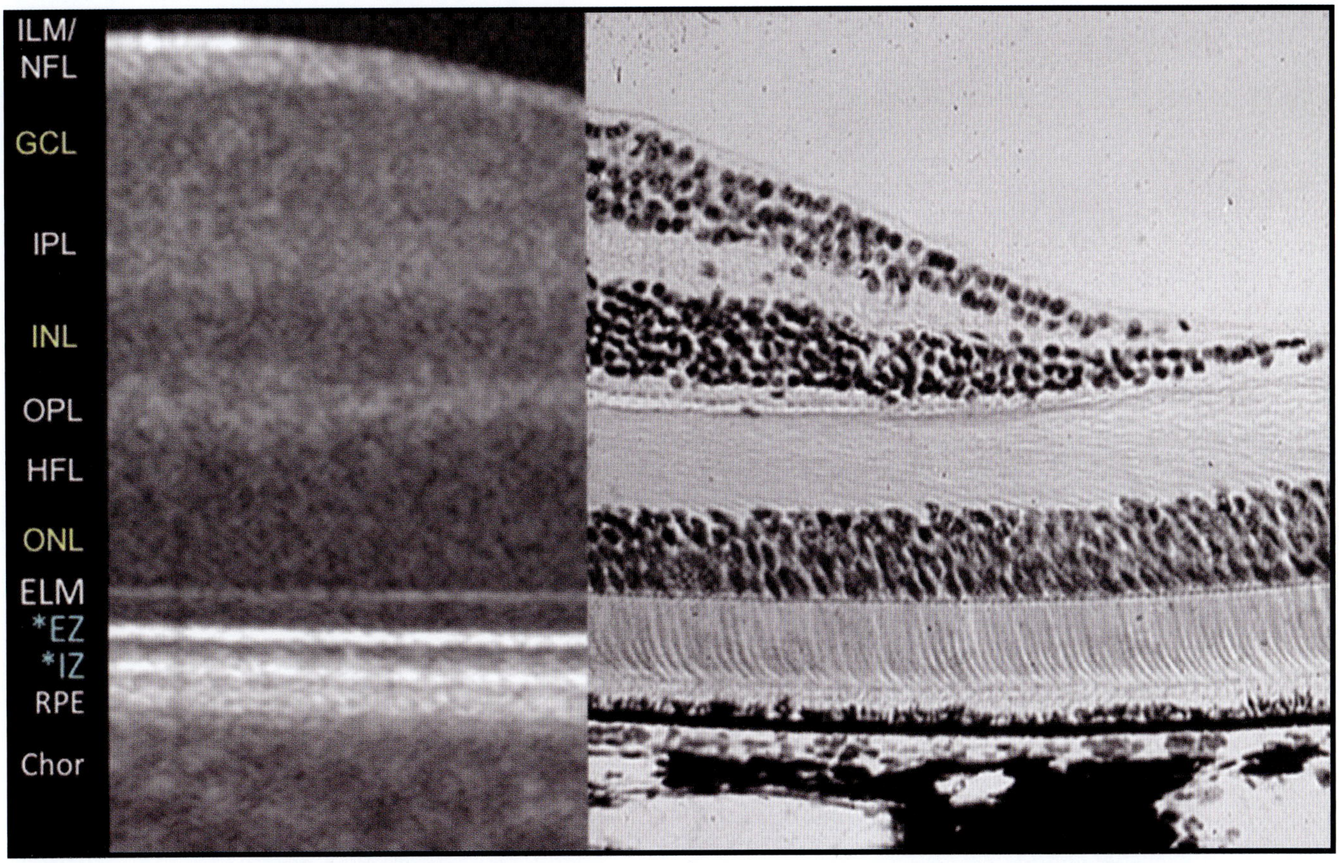

This photograph illustrates a normal spectral domain-OCT (SD-OCT) image on the left merged with a normal histology section of the retina on the right and demonstrates how the different cell layers can be distinguished with SD-OCT imaging. (ILM = internal limiting membrane; NFL = nerve fiber layer; GCL = ganglion cell layer; IPL = inner plexiform layer; INL = inner nuclear layer; OPL = outer plexiform layer; HFL = Henle fiber layer; ONL = outer nuclear layer; ELM = external limiting membrane; EZ = ellipsoid zone; IZ = interdigitation zone; RPE = retinal pigment epithelium; Chor = choroid). *Images courtesy of Brandon Lujan, MD and University of Delaware Library institutional repository*

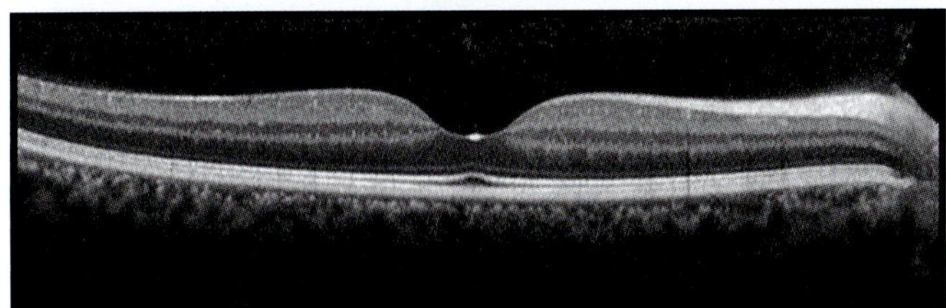

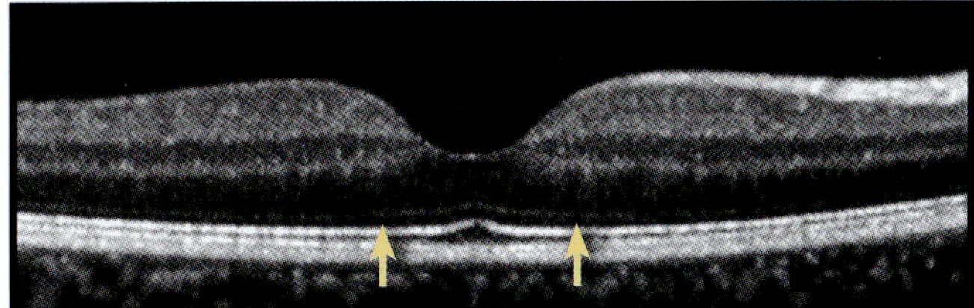

The laminated appearance of the central macula and depression of the fovea is illustrated in these SD-OCTs from normal right eyes. Also note the prominence of the nerve fiber layer in the papillomacular bundle and the integrity of the 4 outer retinal hyper-reflective bands: external limiting membrane (ELM), inner segment ellipsoid zone (EZ, *yellow arrows*), the interdigitation zone (IZ), and the retinal pigment epithelium. Note that the central fovea is identified by the central depression, the widening of the outer nuclear layer, and the vitreal bowing of the ELM and EZ due to elongation of the outer segments. *Courtesy of Dr. Gabriel Coscas*

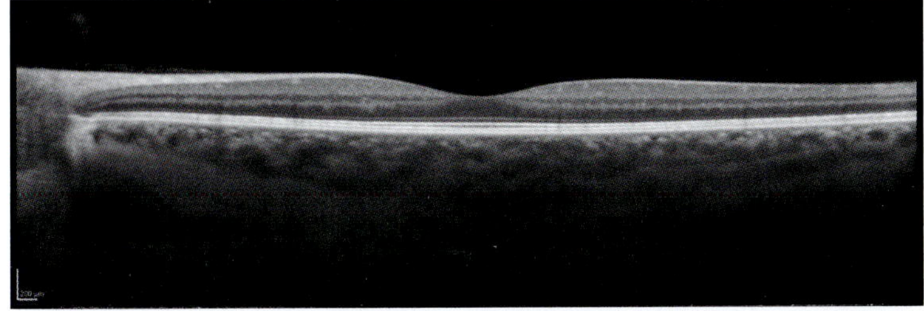

Enhanced depth imaging OCT with deeper signal penetration providing enhanced identification of the choroidal vascular layers, which include the choriocapillaris and Sattler and Haller layers. Also note the hyper-reflective dots at the inner and outer border of the inner nuclear layer indicating the intermediate and deep retinal capillary plexus, respectively.

Optical Coherence Tomography Angiography (OCTA)

Optical coherence tomography angiography (OCTA) is a new imaging modality increasingly used in both research and clinical settings. This advanced imaging technology employs amplitude- versus phase-based decorrelation algorithms and motion contrast detection through the analysis of high volume structural OCT B scans acquired in rapid succession to create images of the retinal and choroidal microvasculature without the need for contrast dye. Depth-resolved identification of the vasculature allows independent evaluation of the different retinal capillary plexuses and choroidal vessels.

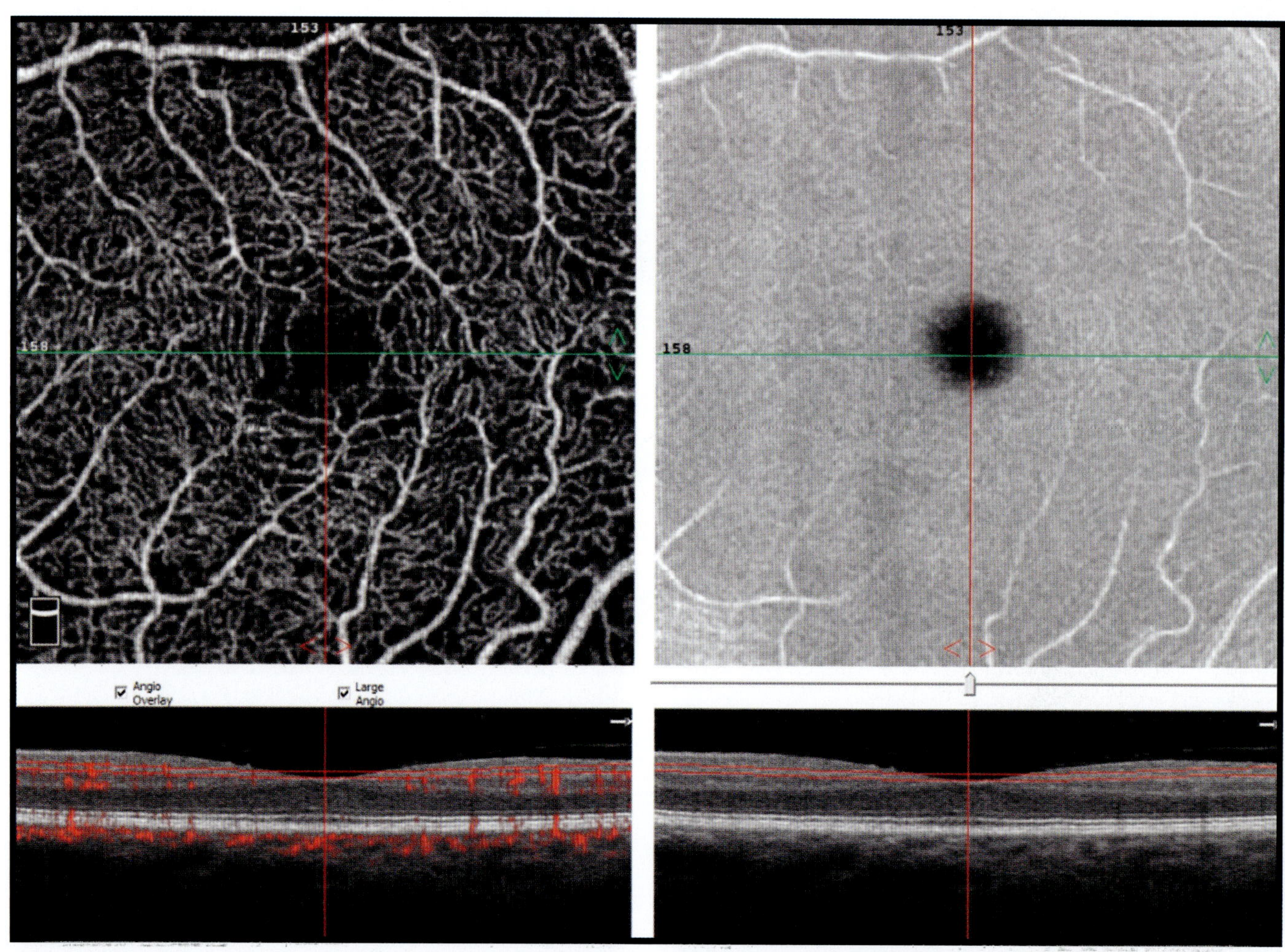

OCT angiography of the superficial retinal capillary plexus (SCP) demonstrating the large inner retinal blood vessels and the ladder-like pattern of the SCP and the associated foveal avascular zone. The corresponding B scan OCT identifies the level of segmentation (at the SCP) and also includes the cross-sectional flow overlay illustrating flow at the level of the superficial, intermediate, and deep retinal capillary plexus and the choroid.The structural *en face* OCT image is demonstrated on the right with the corresponding OCT B scan with the level of segmentation.

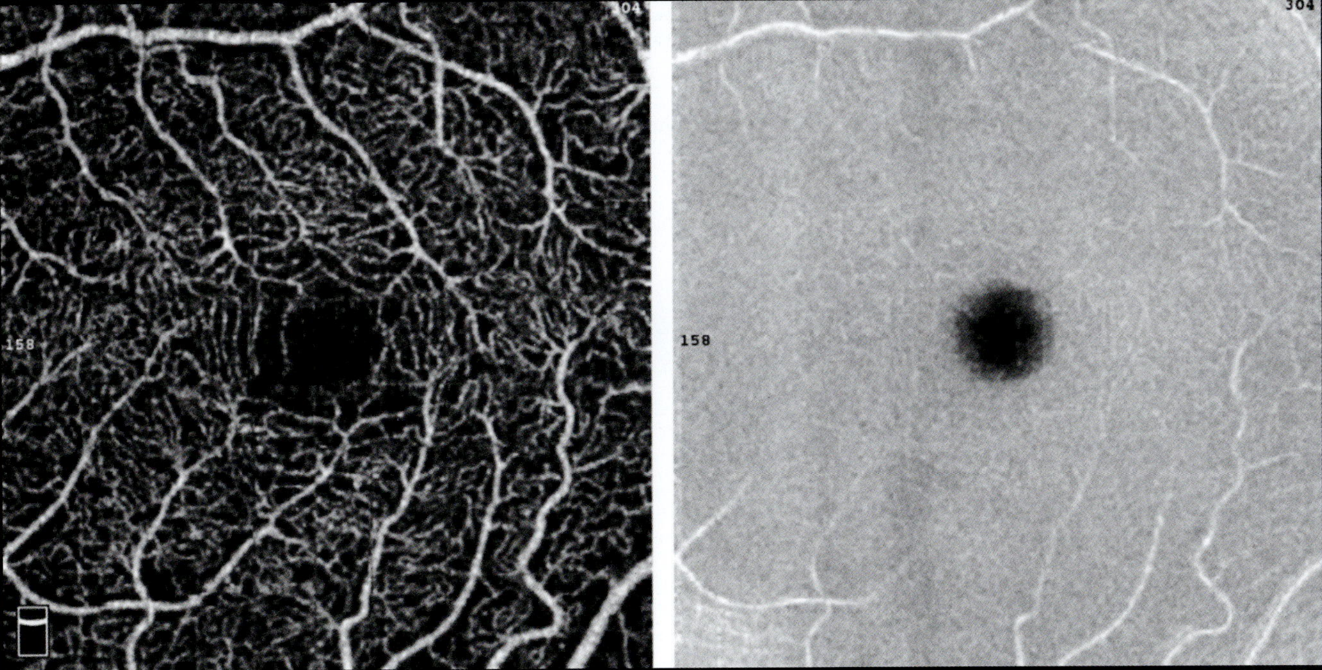

Higher magnification of the OCT angiogram of the SCP (from above), which illustrates the normal SCP. Vessels of the SCP can also be identified in the corresponding *en face* structural OCT.

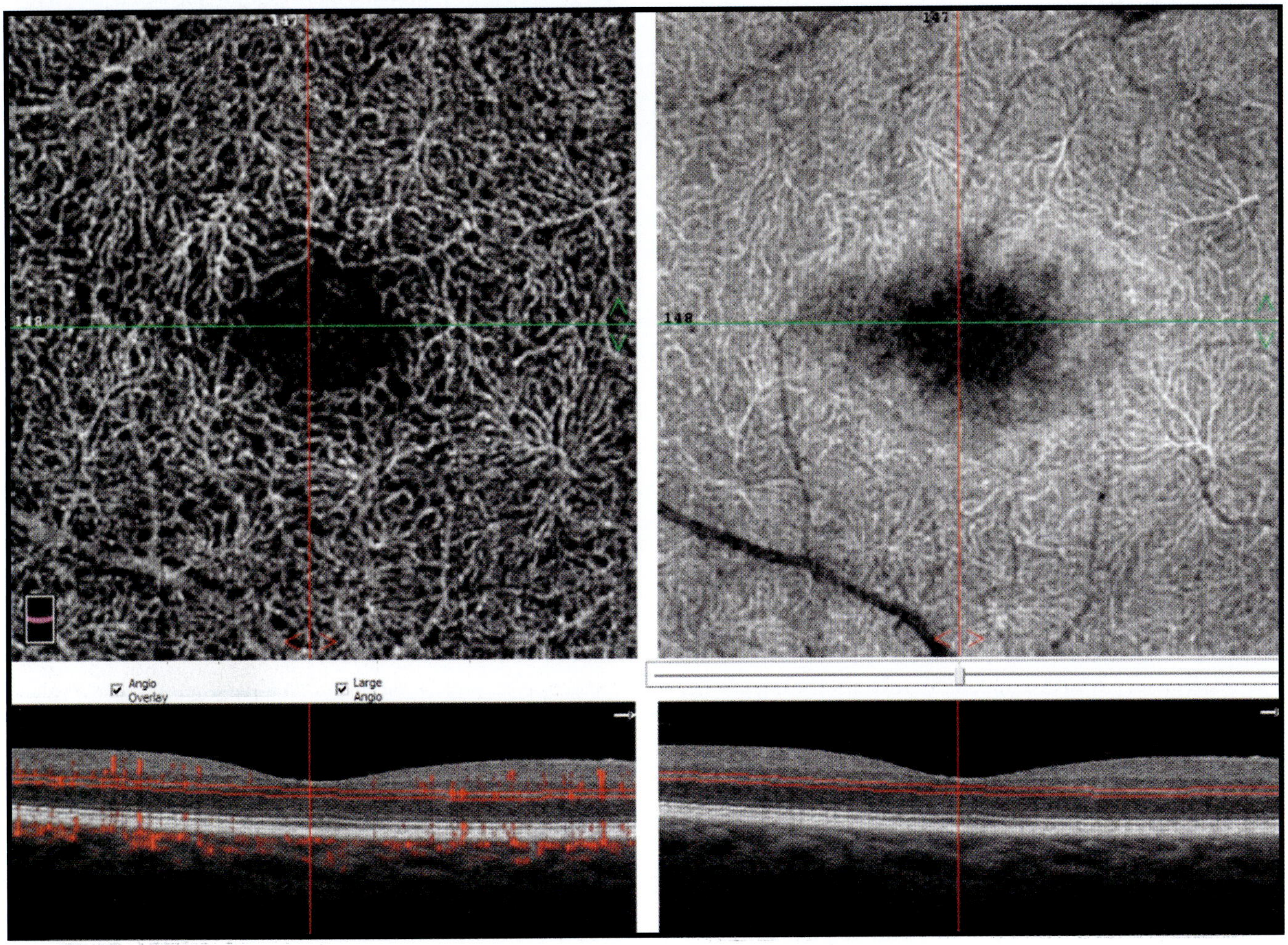

OCT angiography of the deep retinal capillary plexus (DCP) demonstrating the characteristic vortex pattern of the DCP and the associated foveal avascular zone. The corresponding B scan OCT identifies the level of segmentation (at the DCP) and also includes the cross sectional flow overlay illustrating flow at the level of the superficial, intermediate, and deep retinal capillary plexus and the choroid. The structural *en face* OCT image is demonstrated on the right with the corresponding OCT B scan with the level of segmentation. Note the capillaries of the DCP are also well illustrated in the structural *en face* OCT.

Optic Nerve

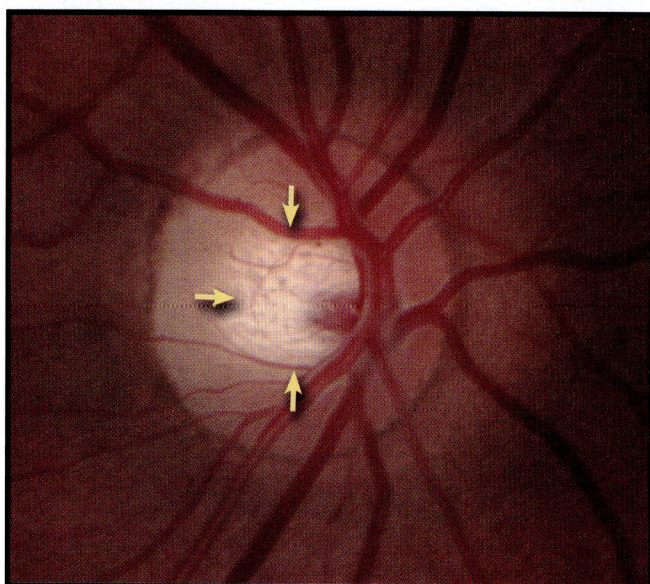

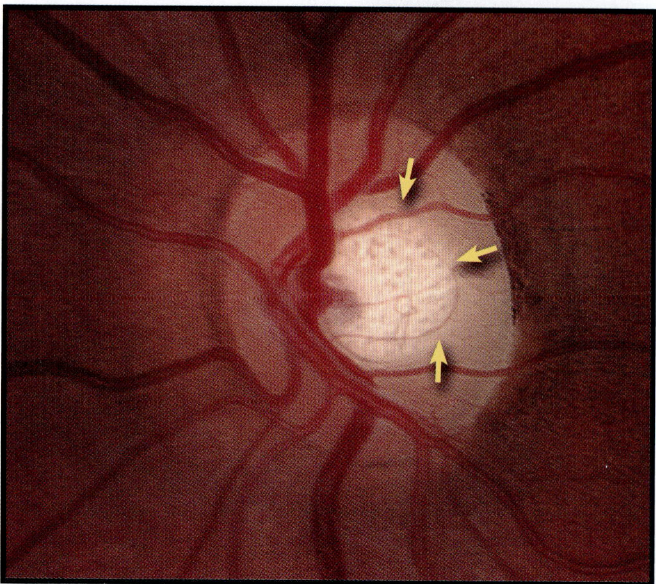

The optic nerve head is illustrated with retinal vessels emerging from the physiological cup *(yellow arrows)* in each eye. The central retinal artery gives rise to the blood supply of the nerve fiber layer. The blood supply of the optic nerve head can be divided into three plexuses: retro-laminar, laminar, and pre-laminar. The retro-laminar plexus originates mainly from the pial vessels and short posterior ciliary arteries. The laminar plexus is supplied by the arterial circle of Zinn-Haller, which itself arises from short posterior ciliary arteries. The pre-laminar optic nerve head is supplied by the short posterior ciliary arteries and recurrent choroidal arteries. This plexus can be visualized by OCT angiography. There is a rich, axonally oriented, anastomotic bed within the nerve between these circulations. The autoregulation of the optic nerve head capillary bed is comparable to that of the retinal circulation. *Courtesy of Ophthalmic Imaging Systems, Inc*

CHAPTER 2

Hereditary Chorioretinal Dystrophies

Several hereditary disorders may cause degeneration of the vitreous and the retina. Many of these disorders are limited to the eye while others have more widespread systemic manifestations.

Stickler Syndrome

Stickler syndrome is the most common cause of hereditary rhegmatogenous retinal detachment. The syndrome can be classified into at least four different subgroups, all caused by different mutations in the genes encoding components of one of the three collagen types expressed in the vitreous (types 2, 9, and 11). The different mutations in the subunits that make up these collagen types are responsible for the varied systemic and ocular manifestations. The ocular signs in Stickler syndrome consist of both anterior and posterior segment abnormalities, including myopia, megalophthalmos, early-onset wedge-shaped cataract, severe degeneration of the vitreous, radial perivascular retinal degeneration, and lattice degeneration with a high risk of rhegmatogenous retinal detachment. Systemic manifestations include a characteristic facial appearance, with midface hypoplasia, cleft palate, and bifid uvula, hearing loss, and skeletal abnormalities, including epiphyseal dysplasia, lax joints, marfanoid body habitus, arachnodactyly, kyphosis, scoliosis, and early-onset arthritis. The Pierre Robin sequence, consisting of cleft palate, micrognathia, and small tongue, can also be associated with this syndrome, and approximately 12% of patients with the Pierre Robin sequence also suffer from Stickler syndrome.

Type I Stickler syndrome is the most common and is caused by an autosomal dominant mutation in COL2A1 (encoding a structural component of type 2 collagen). Type II Stickler syndrome is caused by a mutation in COL11A1 (encoding a structural component of type eleven collagen). Type I and type II can be distinguished clinically by vitreous abnormalities; type I is characterized by a congenital membranous vestigial vitreous remnant in the retrolenticular area extending a variable distance over the pars plana and peripheral retina while type II presents with a fibrillar or beaded vitreous abnormality. Type III Stickler syndrome is caused by mutation in COL11A2 (encoding a structural component of type eleven collagen). Type III Stickler syndrome is unique in that it has no ocular findings, only systemic manifestations of the disease. Type IV Stickler syndrome is caused by a mutation in COL9A1 or COL9A2 (encoding structural components of type nine collagen). It is the only form that is inherited in an autosomal recessive pattern. There is considerable inter- and intrafamilial variability in the expression of Stickler syndrome. Furthermore, some patients with mutations in COL2A1 may only have ocular manifestations of the disease, and therefore the absence of systemic symptoms does not rule out this disorder.

Rhegmatogenous retinal detachment occurs in approximately 50% of Stickler patients during their lifetime. Retinal tears are generally caused by progressive vitreous traction and are frequently multiple and posterior in location at varying distances from the ora serrata. Surgical prognosis for repair of detachments may be complicated by difficult drainage of subretinal fluid due to nearly complete liquefaction of the vitreous, poor funduscopic view due to cataract, and increased risk of hemorrhage secondary to changes in the underlying choroid. Aggressive prophylactic laser or cryo treatment of all new tears, and treatment of all areas of lattice degeneration, are recommended due to the high rate of retinal detachment and poor surgical prognosis in these patients.

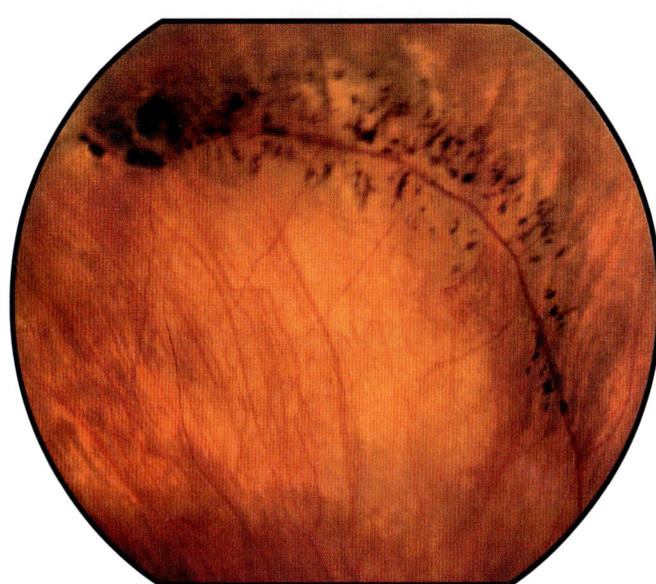

Note the radial perivascular pigmentary lattice degeneration typical of Stickler syndrome. *Courtesy of Dr. Irene Maumenee*

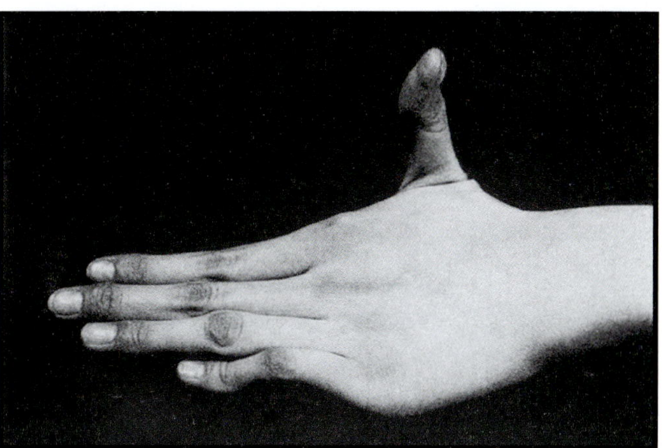

This patient with Stickler syndrome has long fingers with hyperflexibility. Loose joints, long fingers, and grooved nails are characteristic.

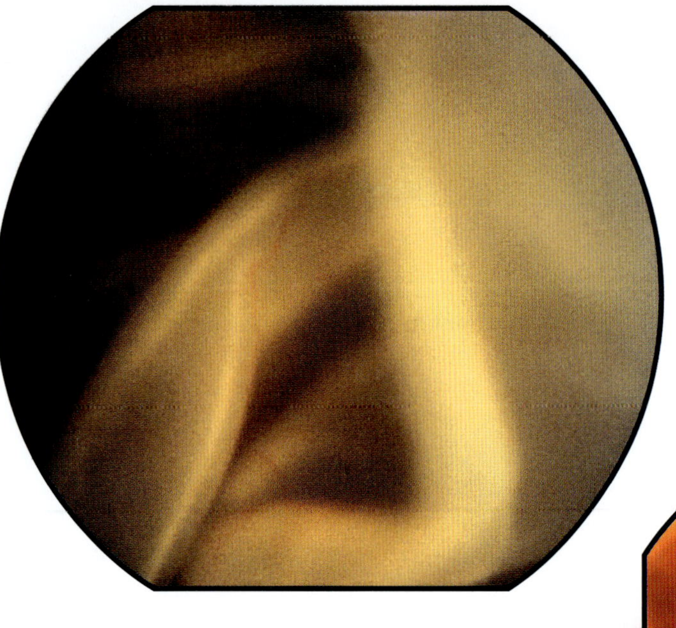

This is an image of a chronic detachment in Stickler syndrome. Stickler syndrome has a retinal detachment incidence of 50%.

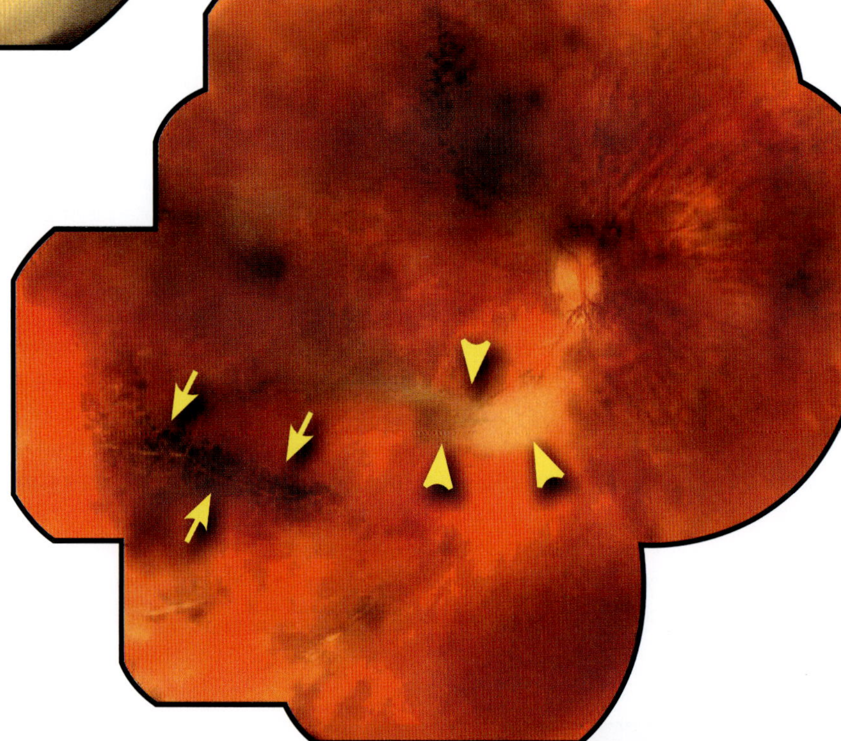

In this patient with Stickler syndrome, there is radial pigmentary perivascular lattice degeneration *(arrows)*. The montage image shows the fibrous change in the vitreous, characteristic of this disorder *(arrowheads)*.

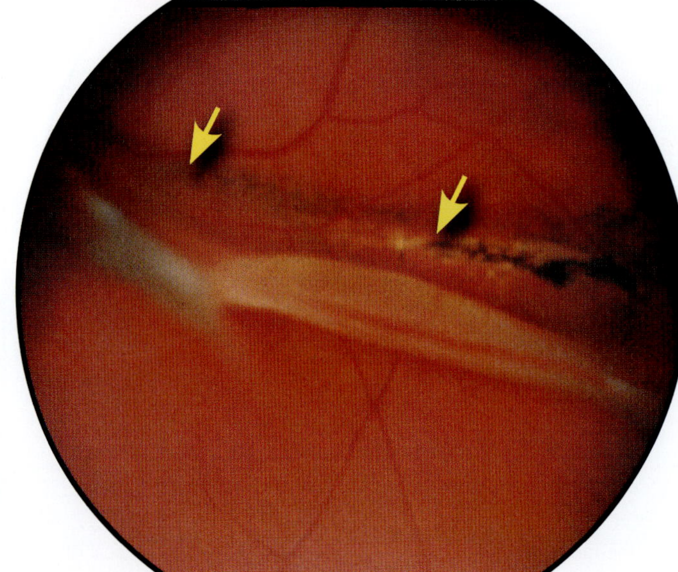

This patient has developed a retinal detachment. There is pigmentation and atrophy along the vessel, early hyperpigmented demarcation line *(arrows)*, fibrous traction, and retinal detachment.

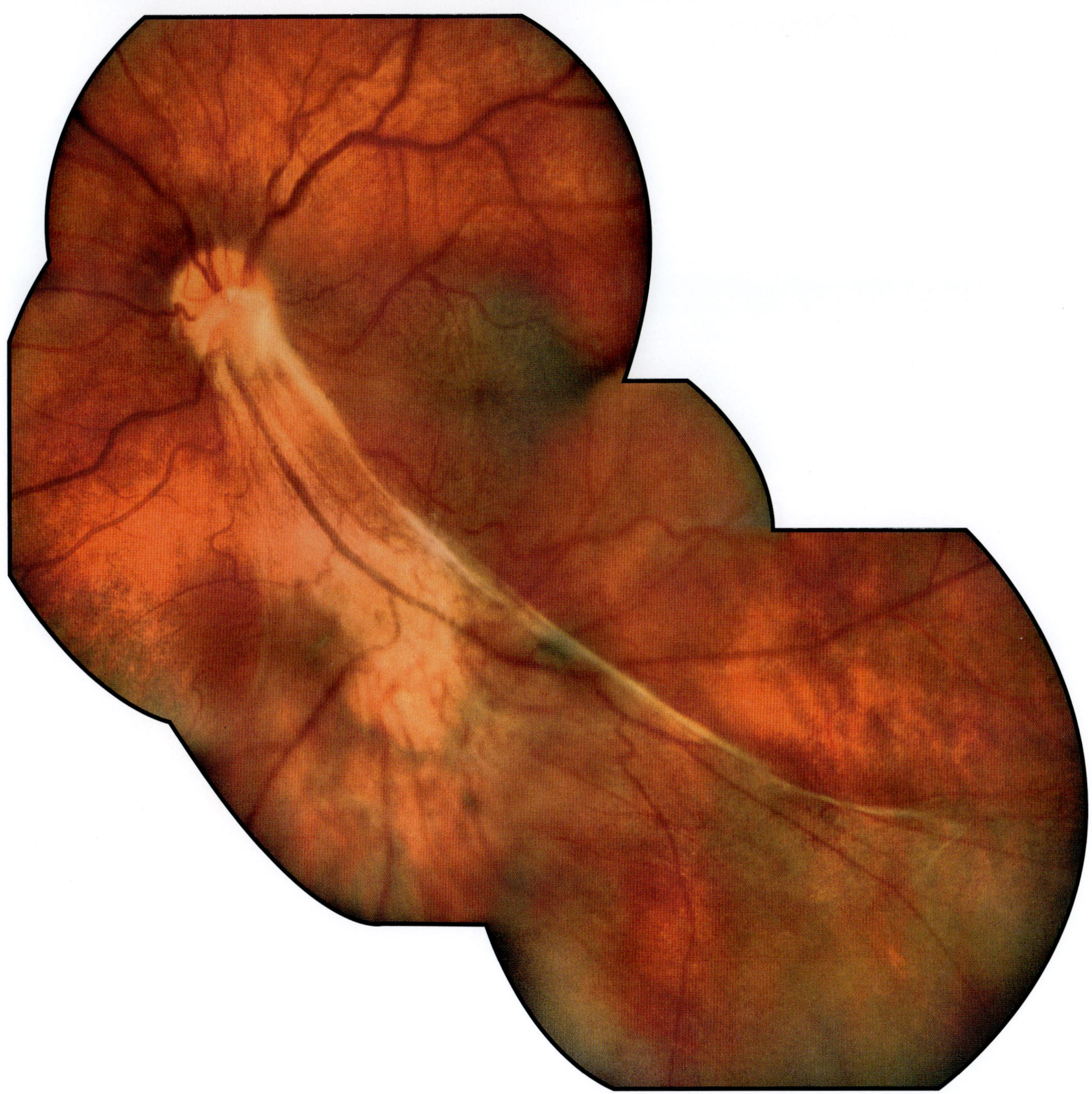

In this patient with Stickler syndrome there is fibrous proliferation and a curvilinear band that extends from the optic nerve to the inferotemporal periphery. There are tractional folds that border this huge band on the nasal side and an epiretinal membrane in the macula.

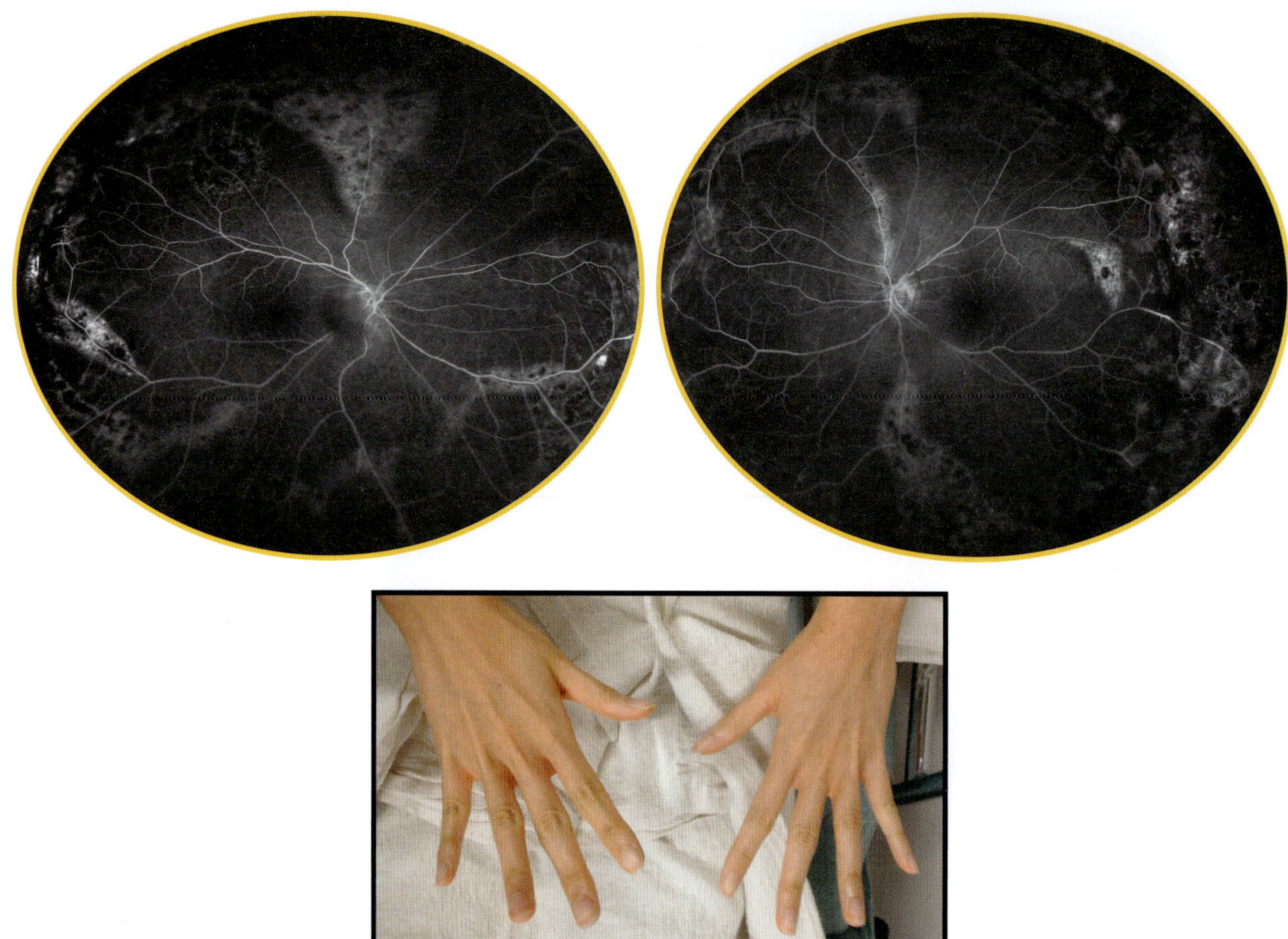

Widefield fluorescein angiography of a patient with Stickler syndrome *(top row)* shows perivascular pigmentary changes which are highlighted by window defects and late staining. The patient's hands were remarkable for long fingers with hyperflexible joints. *Images courtesy of Steven D. Schwartz, MD*

Wagner Syndrome (Wagner Vitreoretinal Degeneration)

Wagner syndrome is an autosomal dominant vitreoretinal degeneration which is caused by mutation in the gene VCAN, which encodes versican, (also known as chondroitin sulfate proteoglycan-2) a proteoglycan present in the vitreous. Controversy still exists regarding whether Wagner and Stickler syndromes are truly distinct entities. Unlike Stickler syndrome, Wagner syndrome traditionally has consisted of solely ocular findings. Nyctalopia may occur at an early age, but vision remains stable until middle age, when formation of dot-like opacities in the lens cortex can reduce visual acuity. The fundus findings in Wagner syndrome include preretinal avascular membranes, pigmentation in a perivascular distribution, peripheral vascular sheathing, myopic degeneration, temporally displaced fovea causing pseudoexotropia, and an optically empty vitreous cavity similar to that seen in Stickler syndrome. While nyctalopia, progressive chorioretinal atrophy, peripheral tractional retinal detachment, and anterior-segment dysgenesis are observed in Wagner syndrome, they are not features of Stickler syndrome. Retinal detachment is believed to be less frequent in Wagner syndrome than in Stickler syndrome.

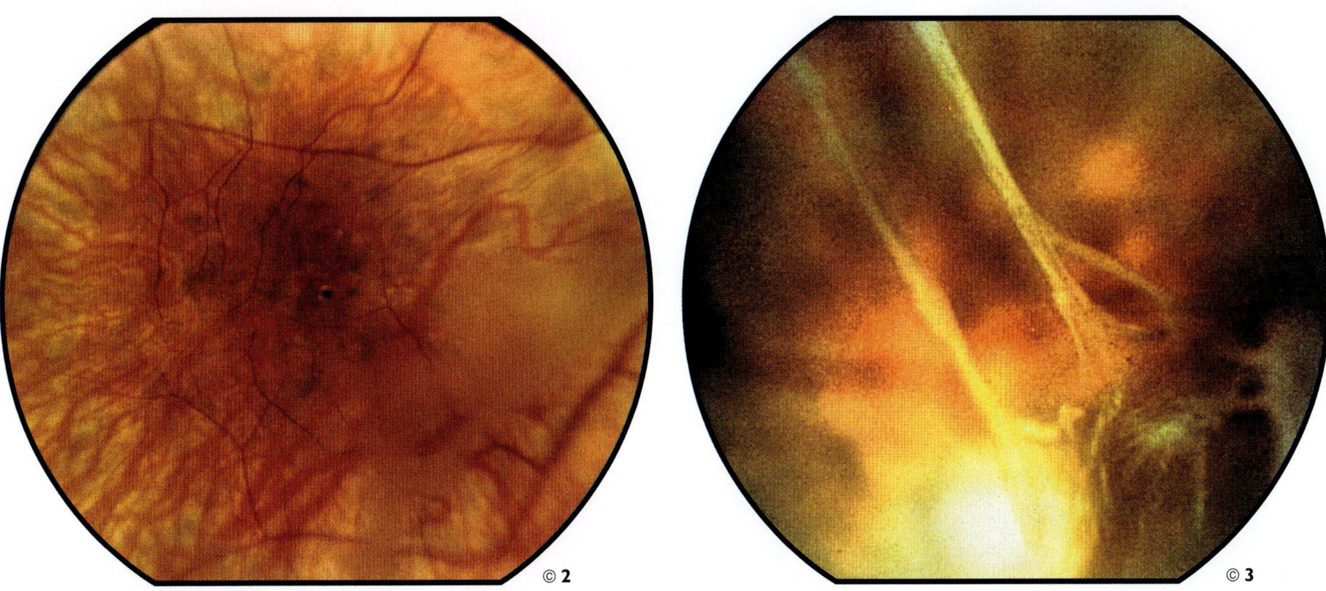

This patient with Wagner syndrome has granular pigmentation in the macula surrounded by an irregular zone of atrophy, reminiscent of choroideremia. The peripheral retina has vitreoretinal bands with retinal traction.

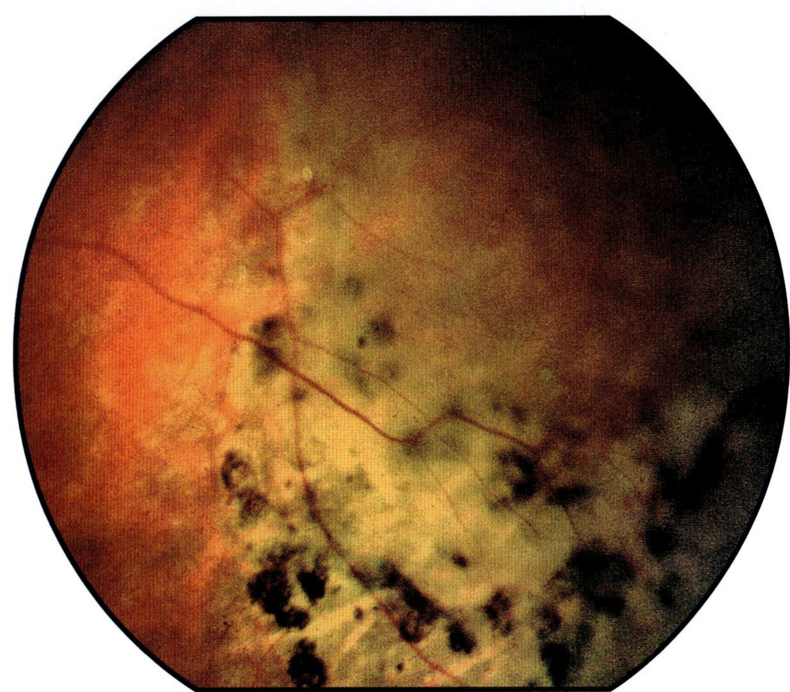

Note the presence of perivascular pigmentation and chorioretinal atrophy in this patient with Wagner syndrome.

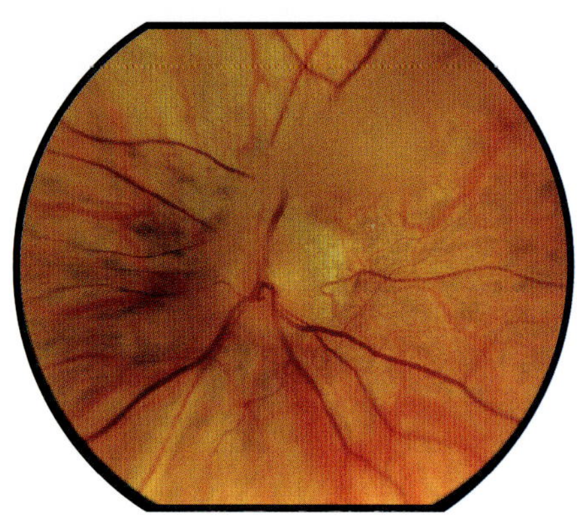

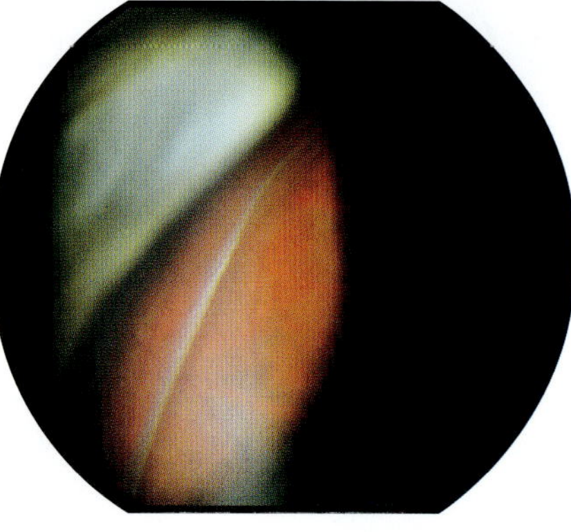

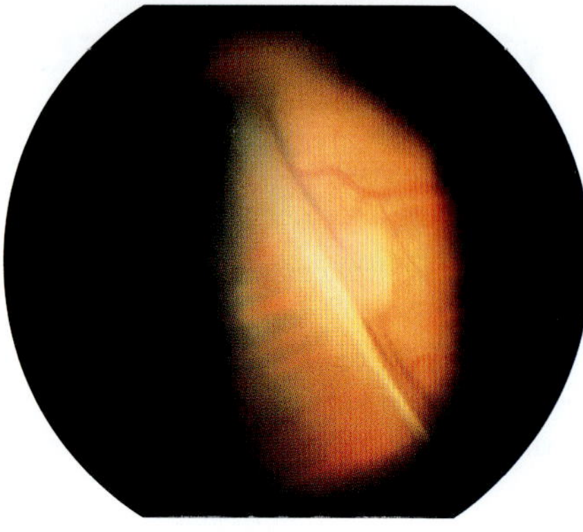

Note the presence of vitreous opacification, retinal folds, and tractional detachment in this patient with Wagner syndrome. *Middle and right images courtesy of Dr. Irene Maumenee*

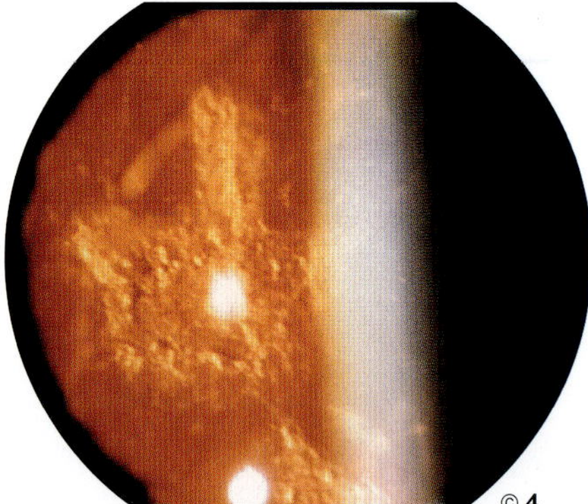

© 4

In this 41-year-old woman with Wagner syndrome, there is a visually significant posterior subcapsular cataract. Visual acuity was 20/40.

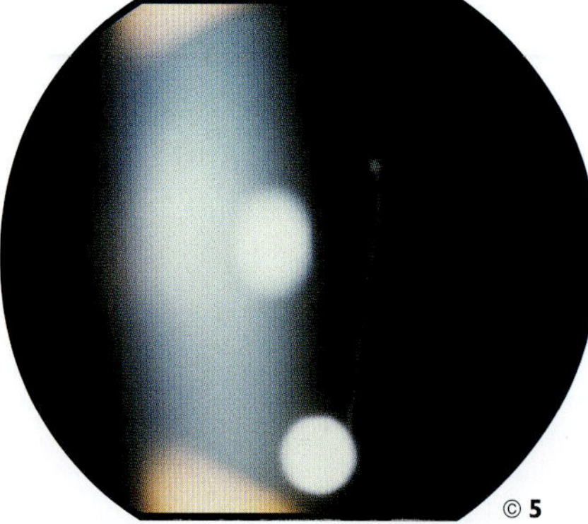

© 5

This is a slit-lamp photograph of an 11-year-old boy with Wagner syndrome showing early fibular condensation in an otherwise "empty vitreous."

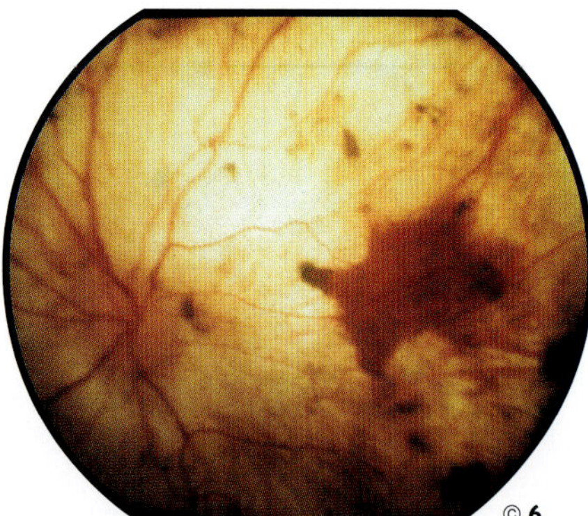

© 6

This 65-year-old man with Wagner syndrome has advanced chorioretinal atrophy, mimicking choroideremia.

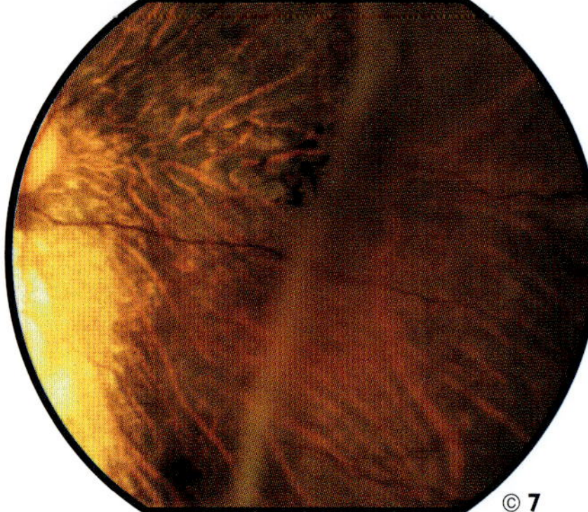

© 7

This is a 44-year-old man with Wagner syndrome with vitreoretinal adhesion to the midperipheral retina nasally.

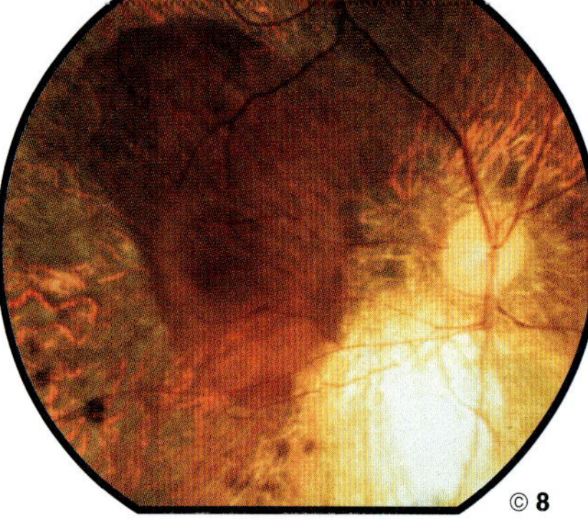

© 8

The same eye shows marked chorioretinal atrophy with pigment migration into the retina and sparing of the macular area. Visual acuity was 20/25.

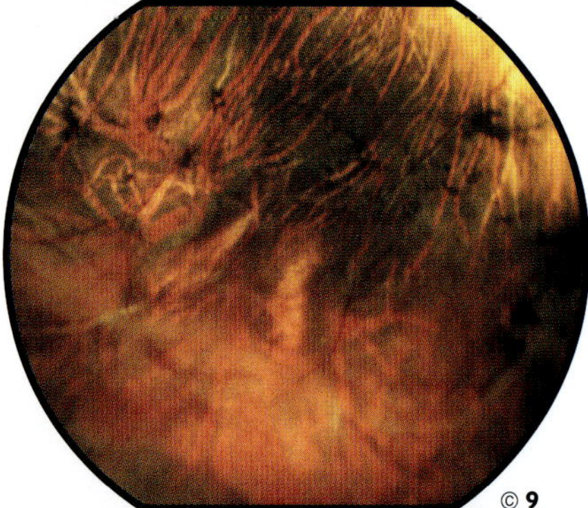

© 9

The same patient shows sheathing of vessels, atrophy, and vitreous condensation.

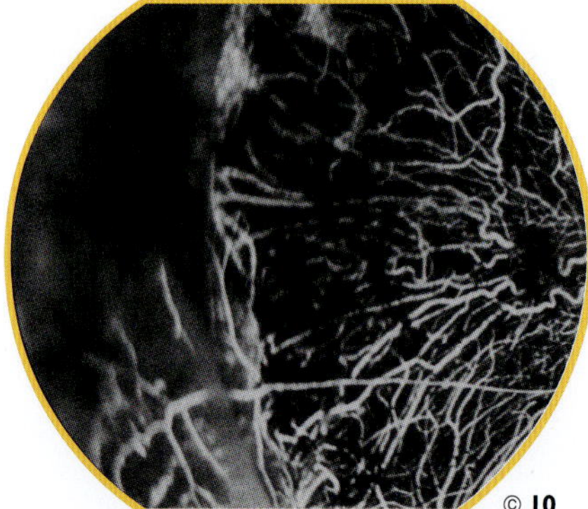

© 10

Mid-phase angiogram of the same eye shows an avascular retina in the temporal periphery.

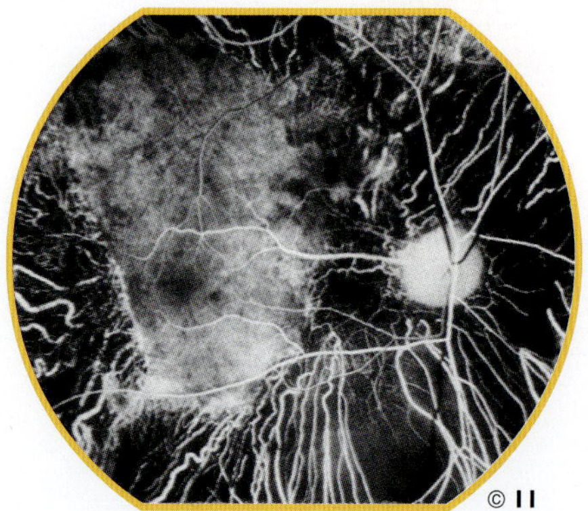

© 11

Fluorescein angiogram of the same eye in early venous phase shows extensive atrophy of the choriocapillaris, sparing only the macular area.

Marfan Syndrome

Marfan syndrome is an autosomal dominant connective tissue disorder caused by a mutation in the fibrillin-1 gene on chromosome 15. The clinical features primarily involve the skeletal, cardiovascular, and ocular systems and include increased height, long limbs, long digits (arachnodactyly), anterior chest deformity, joint laxity, vertebral column deformity, a narrow highly arched palate with crowded teeth, mitral valve prolapse, mitral regurgitation, dilatation of the aortic root, and aortic regurgitation. Ocular findings include ectopia lentis (usually superior and temporal), flat cornea, premature cataract and increased axial length of the globe, and myopic degeneration. Retinal detachment occurs in 5–20% of patients and is more common (8–38%) in eyes with ectopia lentis. In cases with retinal detachment, 69% will have bilateral involvement. A pigmentary retinopathy may also occur.

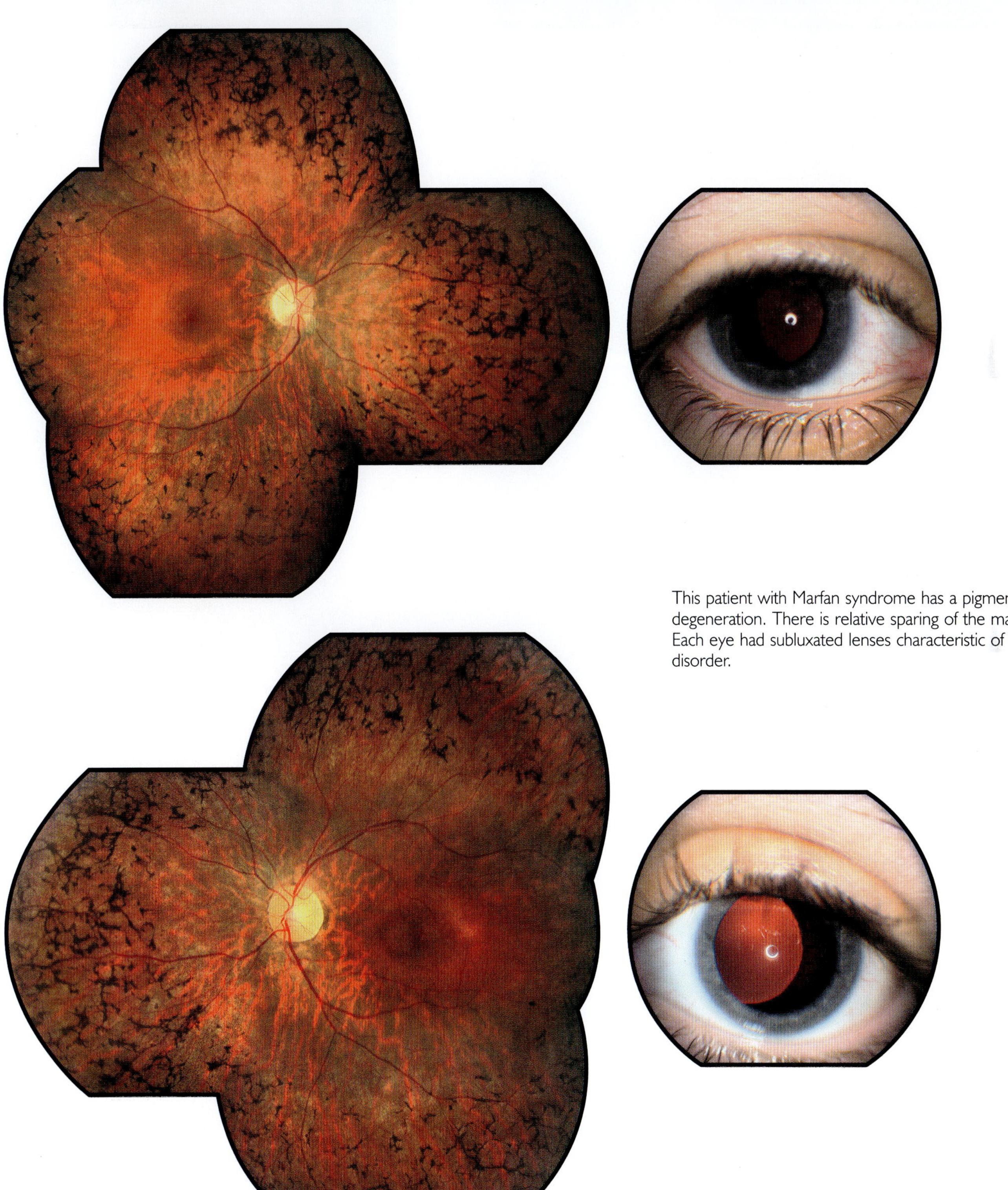

This patient with Marfan syndrome has a pigmentary degeneration. There is relative sparing of the macula. Each eye had subluxated lenses characteristic of this disorder.

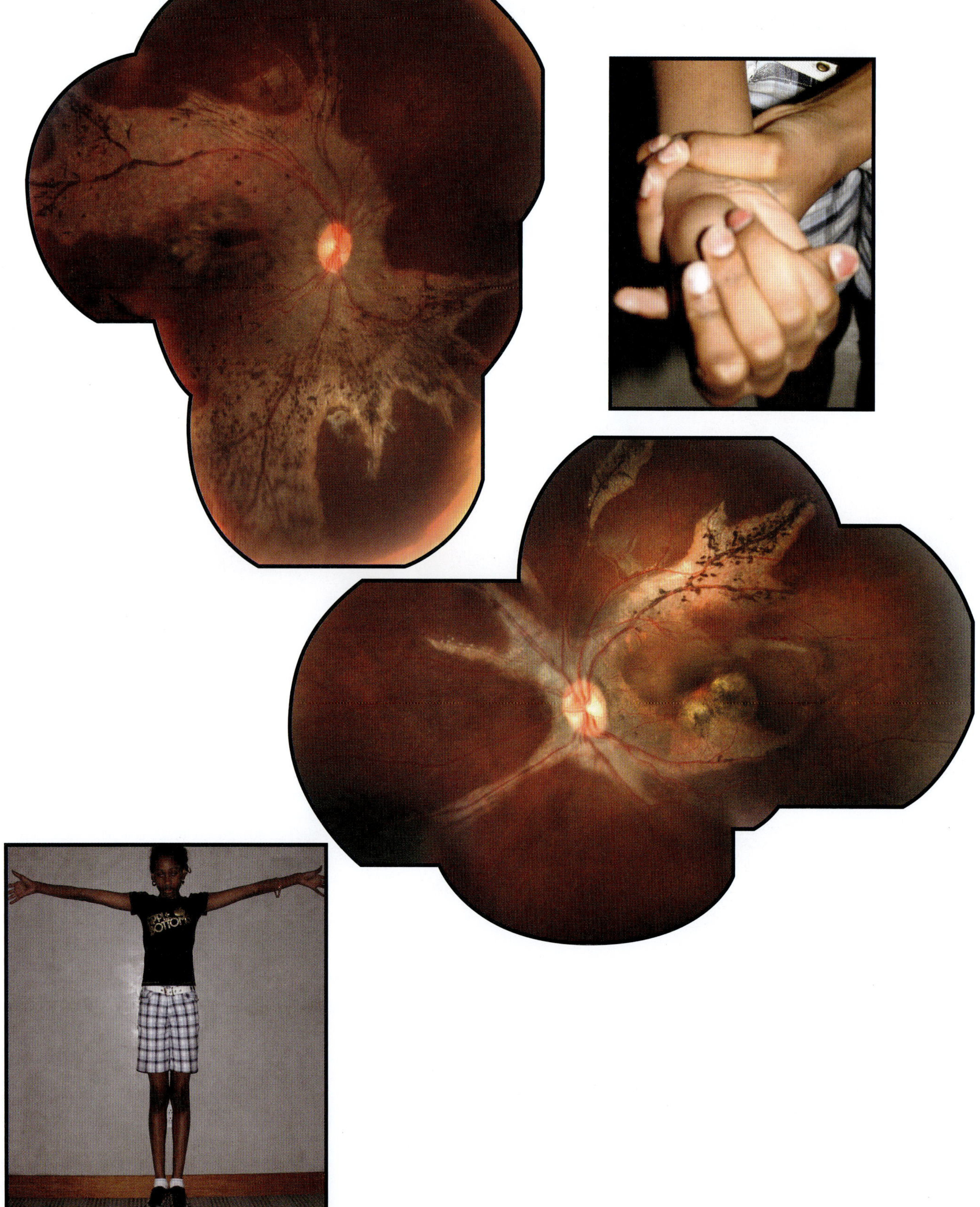

This 11-year-old girl with Marfan syndrome has all the characteristic skeletal changes. The fundus is remarkable for pigmented paravenous retinal choroidal atrophy, not the typical pigmentary retinopathy. She has a fibrillin-1 genetic mutation.

Autosomal Dominant Vitreoretinochoroidopathy

Autosomal dominant vitreoretinochoroidopathy (ADVIRC) is a rare retinal dystrophy characterized by a peripheral circumferential band of hyperpigmentation and chorioretinal atrophy extending anterior from the ora serratta to a well-defined boundary near the equator. It is one of five known bestrophinopathies, and is caused by mutation in Bestrophin 1 (BEST1). Mutations in BEST1 are also implicated in Best vitelliform macular dystrophy, adult-onset foveomacular vitelliform dystrophy, autosomal recessive bestrophinopathy, and MRCS (microcornea, rod–cone dystrophy, cataract, posterior staphyloma) syndrome. It is believed that ADVIRC-causing mutations result in alternative splicing products not present in other bestrophinopathies. Additional vitreoretinal findings include vitreous degeneration with fibrillar condensation, cystoid macular edema, epiretinal membrane, white retinal opacities, and other vascular abnormalities including arteriole narrowing and pre-retinal neovascularization. Other ocular abnormalities include hyperopia, cataract, and glaucoma. Electrooculogram (EOG) may show reduced Arden ratio. Full field electroretinogram (ERG) varies from normal to severe depression of both rods and cones. Unlike retinitis pigmentosa, nyctalopia and peripheral field loss are not prominent features.

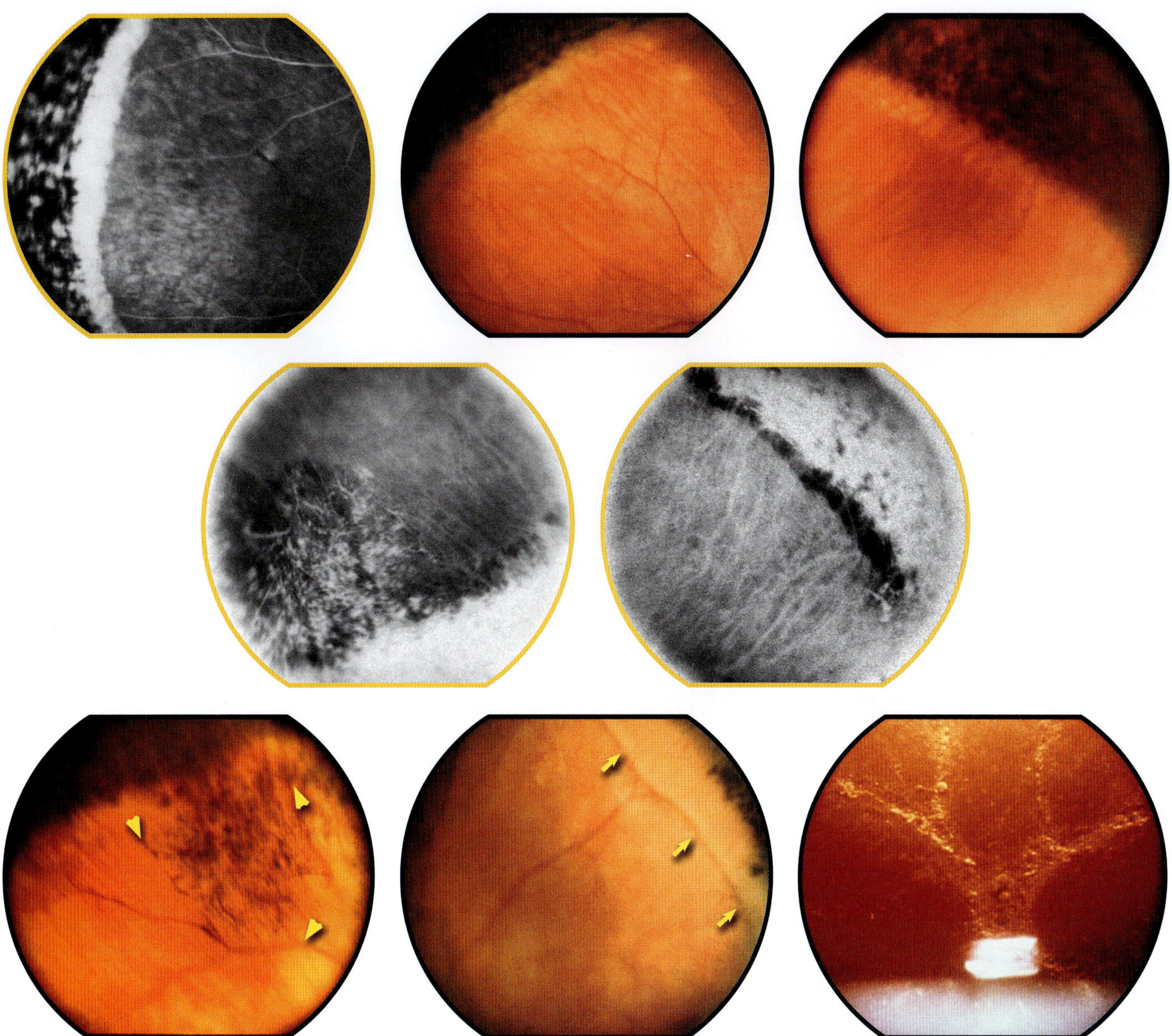

These are images from a family with autosomal dominant vitreoretinochoroidopathy. Note the sharply demarcated, peripheral zone of concentric atrophy bordered by hyperpigmentation that is very characteristic of this disease. There is also a fibrous proliferative band in one eye *(arrows)*. Early posterior subcapsular cataract is also characteristic of this disorder *(lower right photo)* and scattered pigmentation may be seen throughout the more posterior fundus *(arrowheads)*. *Courtesy of Dr. Gerald Fishman*

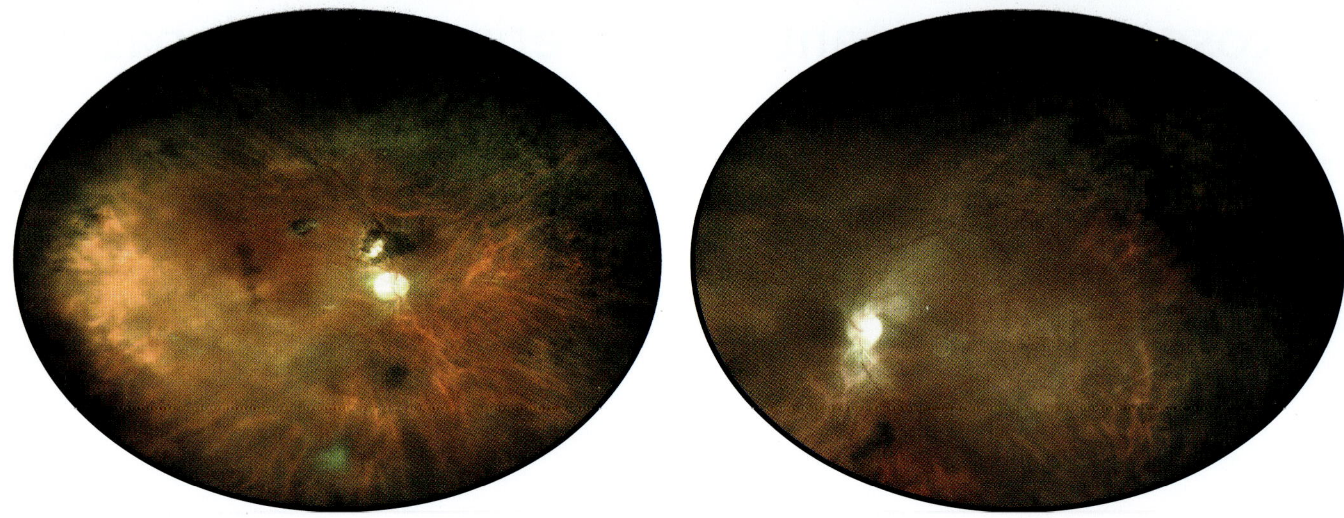

Widefield color photos of a patient with ADVIRC. Note the 360 degree pigmentary alterations extending from the ora toward the midperiphery. *Courtesy of Dr. Clement Chow and Dr. Norman Blair (UIC)*

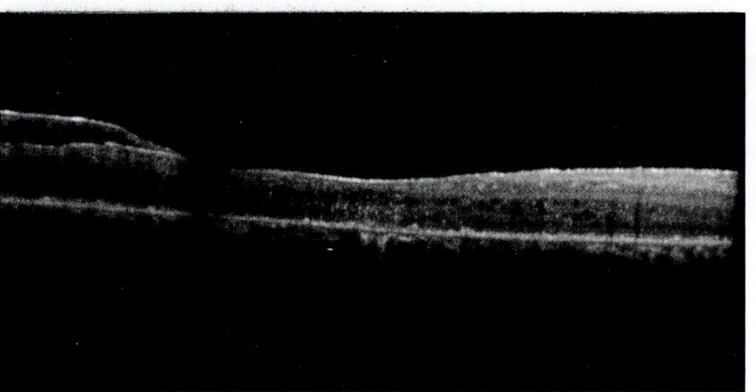

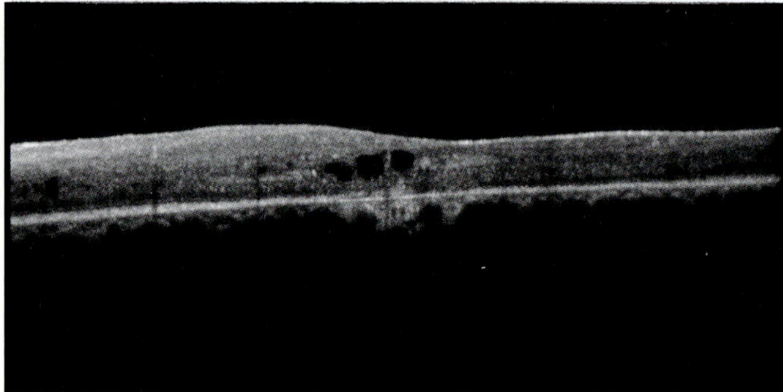

SD-OCT done in the same patient demonstrates cystoid macular edema, epiretinal membrane, drusenoid deposits, and diffuse outer retinal atrophy. *Courtesy of Dr. Clement Chow and Dr. Norman Blair (UIC)*

Snowflake Vitreoretinodegeneration

Snowflake vitreoretinodegeneration (SVD) is an autosomal dominant, distinct vitreoretinopathy caused by mutation in the KCNJ13 gene which encodes a potassium channel expressed predominantly in the retina. The disorder is characterized by corneal guttae, an abnormal-appearing optic nerve head, and retinal vascular sheathing and attenuation. Of note, an optically empty vitreous with fibrillar degeneration is associated with peripheral retinal pigmentary changes and tiny crystalline deposits visible only with high magnification in the peripheral retina (snowflakes). Rhegmatogenous retinal detachment occurs in approximately 20% of affected individuals. Unlike Stickler syndrome, there are no known systemic abnormalities.

Idiopathic Vitreoretinal Degeneration

Idiopathic vitreoretinal degeneration occurs in patients with a pigmentary retinopathy involving the posterior pole and peripheral fundus. It also may be associated with vitreoretinal bands and traction with susceptibility to breaks and detachment. The pigmentary changes resemble those seen in Goldmann–Favre syndrome, and the vitreoretinal abnormalities are very similar to Stickler syndrome. Some cases of retinitis pigmentosa may also be associated with vitreoretinal abnormalities and so it is unclear if idiopathic vitreoretinal degeneration is an independent entity.

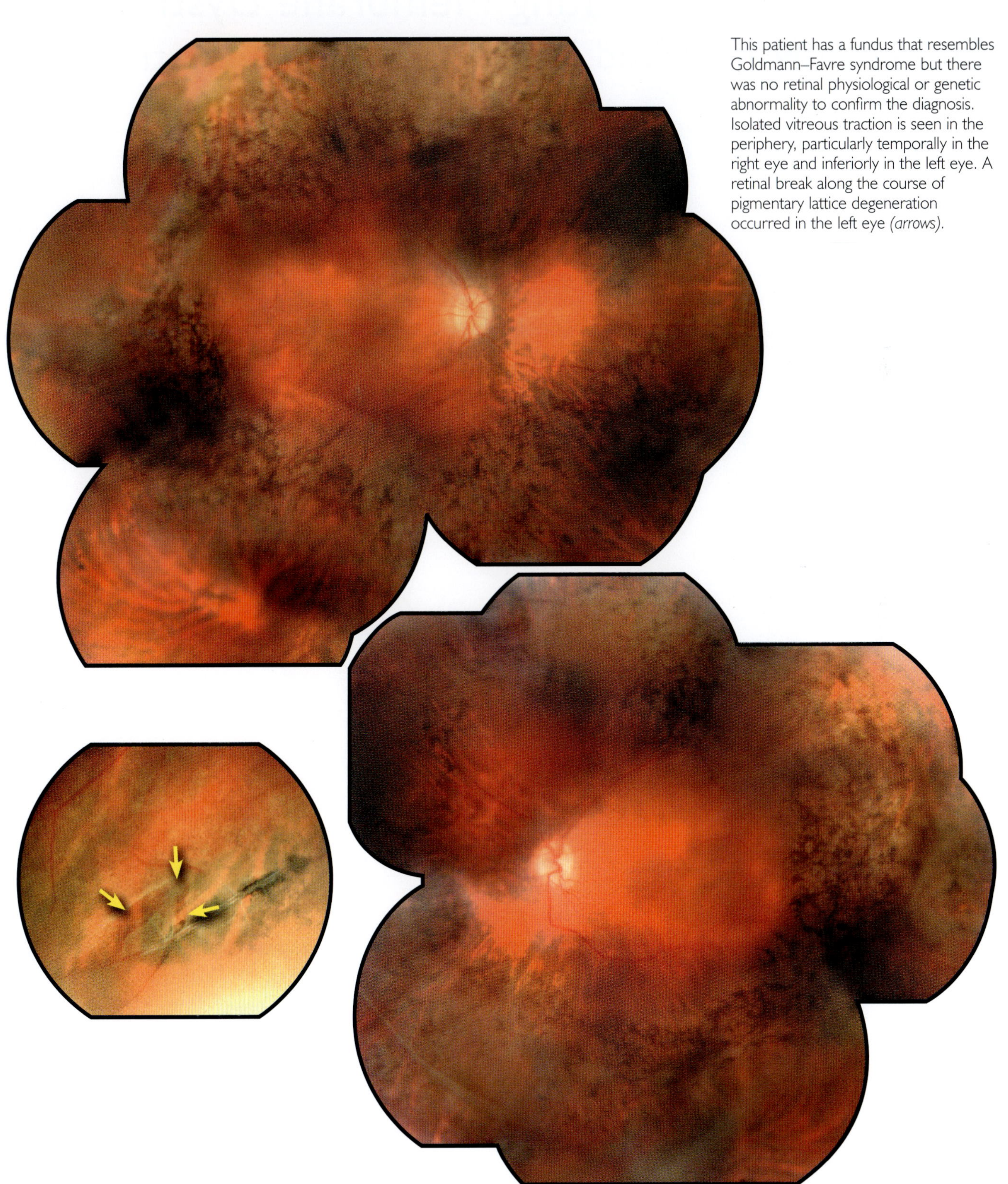

This patient has a fundus that resembles Goldmann–Favre syndrome but there was no retinal physiological or genetic abnormality to confirm the diagnosis. Isolated vitreous traction is seen in the periphery, particularly temporally in the right eye and inferiorly in the left eye. A retinal break along the course of pigmentary lattice degeneration occurred in the left eye *(arrows)*.

This section will include any of the genetic and hereditary dystrophies affecting the inner portion of the retina and involving Müller cells or bipolar cells and associated therefore with an electronegative ERG due to loss of the B wave and preservation of the A wave. We have included enhanced S-cone syndrome in this section because of its close similarity to X-linked juvenile retinoschisis, although the former disorder resides at the photoreceptor level.

Familial Internal Limiting Membrane Dystrophy (Dominantly Inherited Müller Cell Sheen Dystrophy)

Familial internal limiting membrane dystrophy is a dominantly inherited disorder that is believed to be associated with vascular permeability defects on the surface of the retina. It has also been referred to as dominantly inherited Müller cell sheen dystrophy and is presumed to be a primary defect in Müller cells. Visual loss typically does not occur until midlife. Widespread intraretinal edema, typically cystoid macular edema, and superficial microcystic changes most commonly in, but not limited to, the posterior fundus are seen. Histopathologic examination reveals thickening and undulation of the internal limiting membrane of the retina with schisis cavities in the inner retina and numerous areas of separation of the internal limiting lamina from the retina. A filamentous material is present in some of these areas. Endothelial cell swelling, pericyte degeneration, and basement membrane thickening of retinal capillaries may also be seen along with chronic edema, swelling, degeneration of Müller cells, ganglion cell atrophy, and cystic spaces in the inner nuclear layer. An ERG shows diminished B-wave amplitudes consistent with abnormal Müller cells.

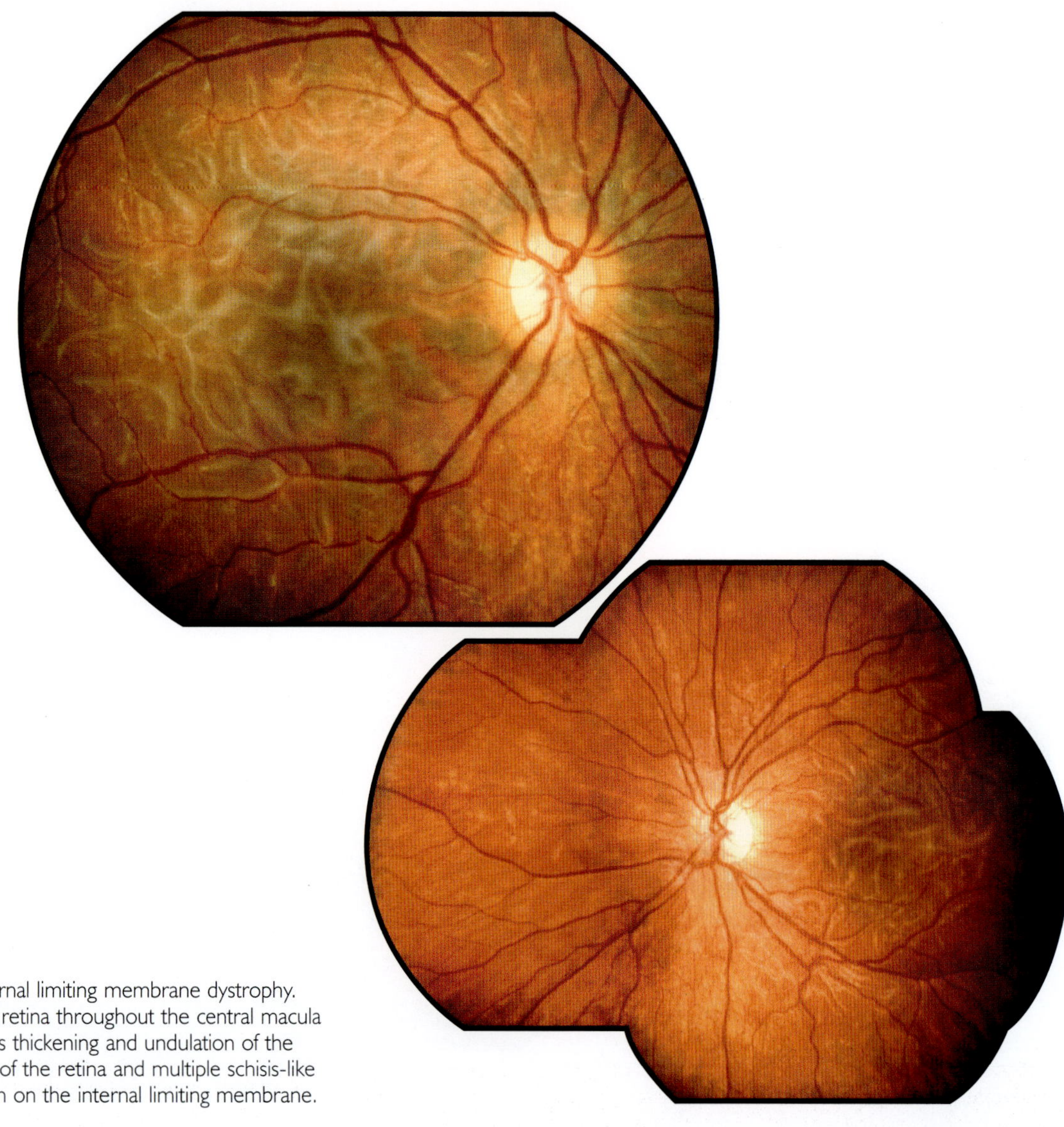

This patient has familial internal limiting membrane dystrophy. Note the folds in the inner retina throughout the central macula and posterior pole. There is thickening and undulation of the internal limiting membrane of the retina and multiple schisis-like cavities from fibrous traction on the internal limiting membrane.

X-Linked Juvenile Retinoschisis

X-linked juvenile retinoschisis is an X-linked recessive disorder in which males develop bilateral splitting of the superficial retinal layers. It is caused by mutation in the retinoschisin gene (RS1) at Xp22. While the disease was originally thought to be due to a Müller cell abnormality, the putative protein, retinoschisin, has been identified and is expressed mainly by photoreceptors and bipolar cells and is thought to be important in cell adhesion, perhaps at the photoreceptor-bipolar synaptic level. Fundus changes include a characteristic stellate or spoke-like cystic appearance of the macula referred to as "foveal schisis" which is associated with a mild to moderate decline in vision. Early anatomical reports described schisis predominantly involving the NFL. However, more recently, SD-OCT imaging has demonstrated that cystic cavities in the macula most commonly involve layers deep to the NFL, most frequently the INL. The ONL and OPL may also be involved, and parafoveal schisis may involve the NFL and GCL. Despite a cystic appearance, the macular lesions do not leak on fluorescein angiography. Peripheral retinoschisis, typically inferotemporal, occurs in about half of the affected patients who may also experience large, inner layer holes associated with "vitreous veils." Sheathed, occluded, and unsupported retinal vessels with vitreous hemorrhage may also occur. Retinal detachment may complicate 16–22% of cases. The use of topical carbonic anhydrase inhibitors has been shown to decrease the size of foveal cysts in up to two-thirds of patients; however, this does not always correlate with improved visual acuity.

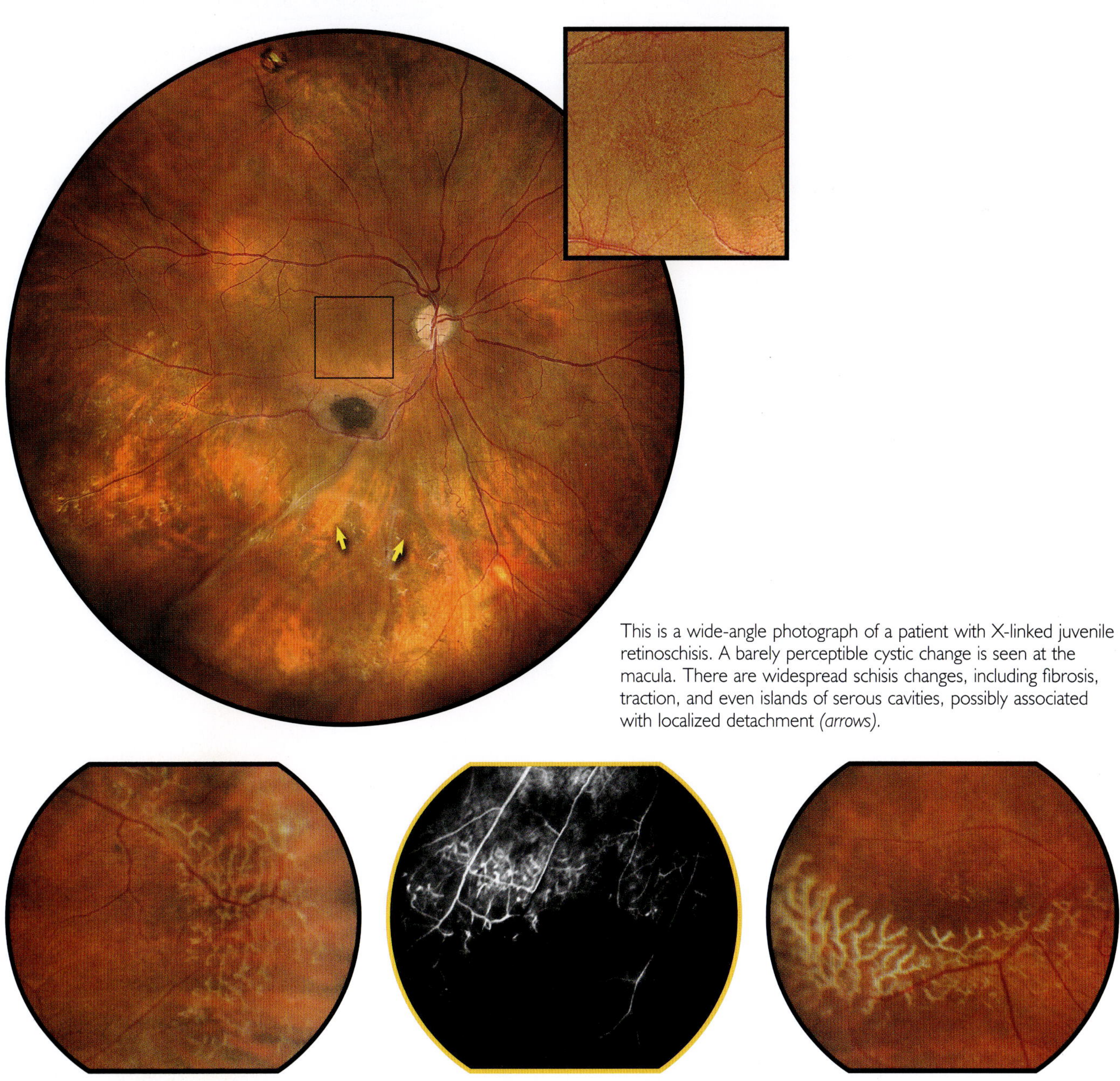

This is a wide-angle photograph of a patient with X-linked juvenile retinoschisis. A barely perceptible cystic change is seen at the macula. There are widespread schisis changes, including fibrosis, traction, and even islands of serous cavities, possibly associated with localized detachment *(arrows)*.

A delicate lacy pattern is sometimes seen in the periphery of a patient with X-linked juvenile retinoschisis. The fluorescein angiogram accentuates the delicate vascular pattern within the retina seen in these areas.

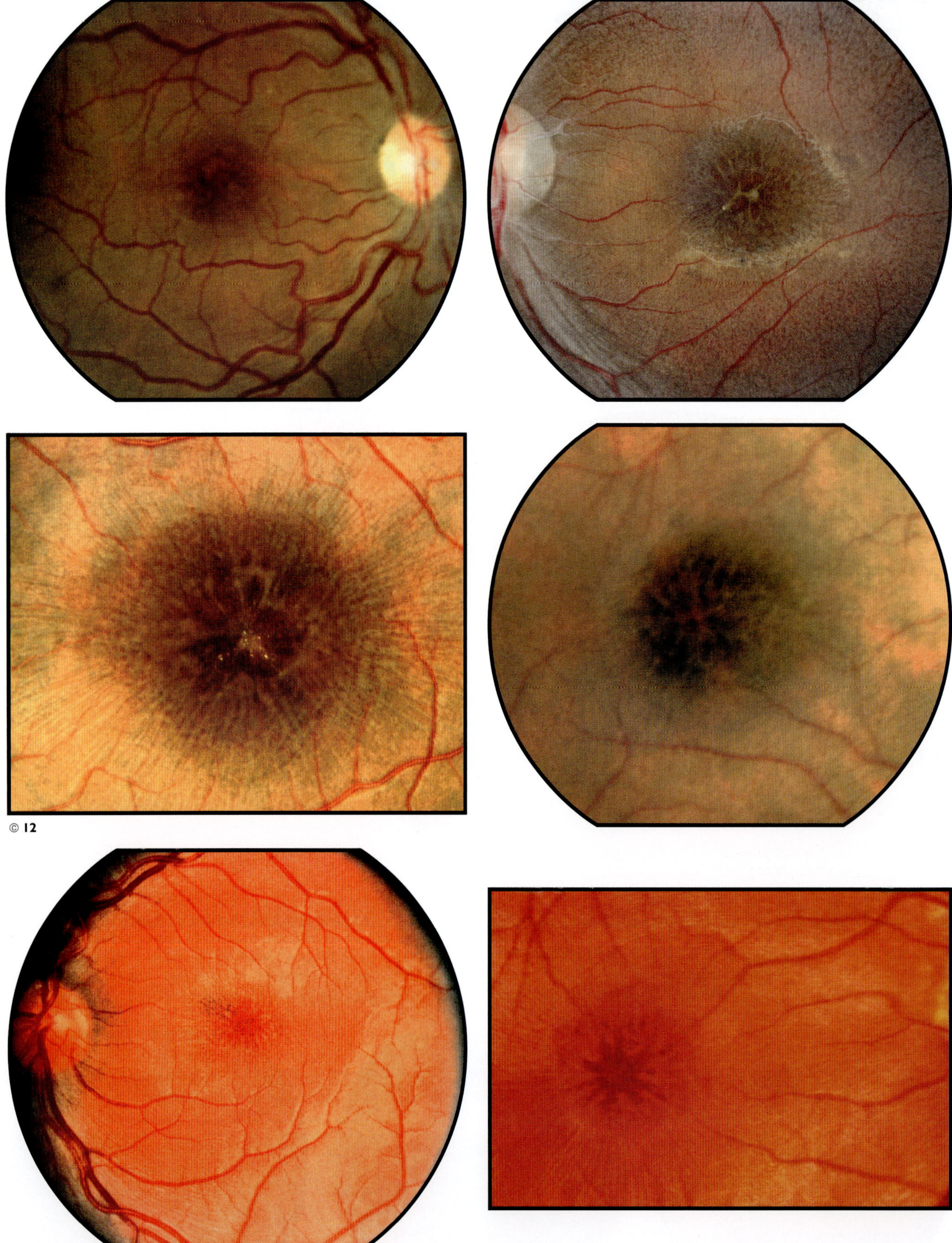

X-linked juvenile retinoschisis is associated with macular schisis in all cases. The schisis can vary from barely detectable to a very prominent cystic change at the fovea with spoke-like radial extension into the paramacular region. *Top row right image courtesy of Drs Ron Carr and Ken Noble, lower left image courtesy of Dr. Harry Flynn, lower right image courtesy of Wills Eye Hospital*

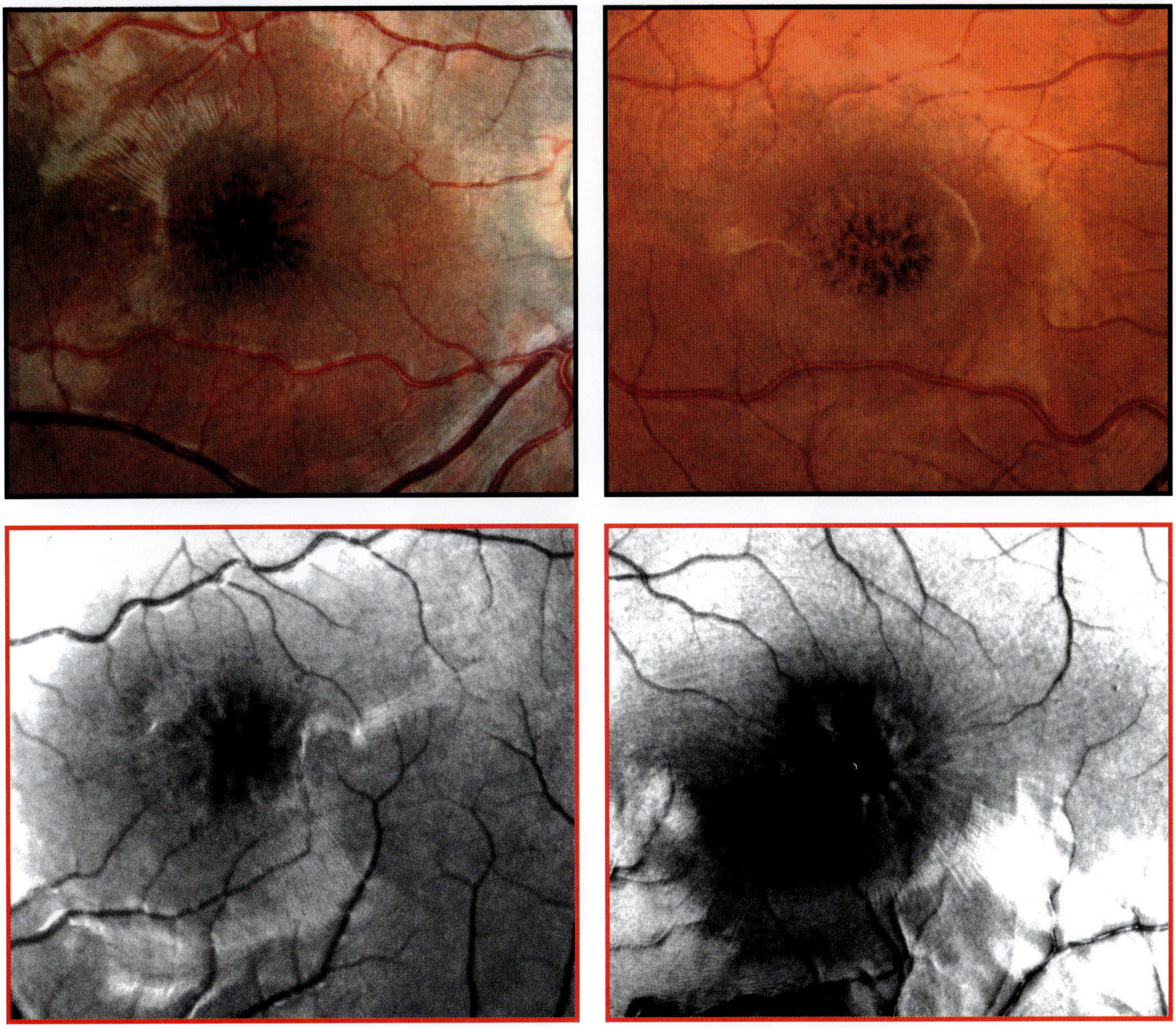

In this patient with X-linked juvenile retinoschisis, there is a schisis pattern in the fovea, but no peripheral schisis. The schisis changes are best evident on the red-free photographs *(bottom row photos)*.

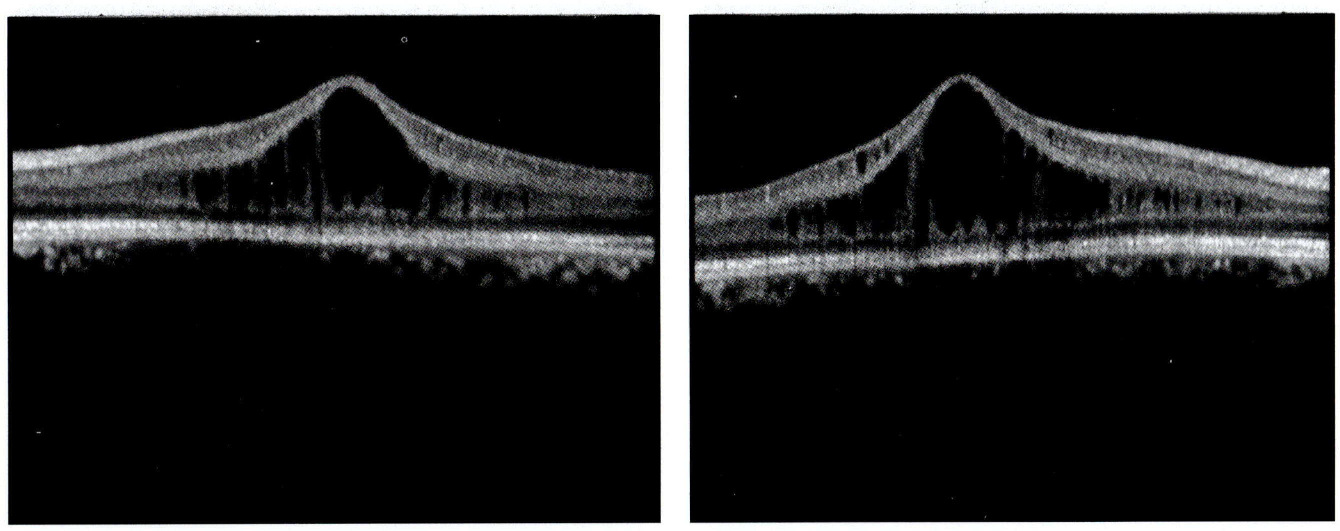

X-linked juvenile retinoschisis in a patient with large schitic cavities visible on SD-OCT. *Images courtesy of Dr. Pradeep Prasad*

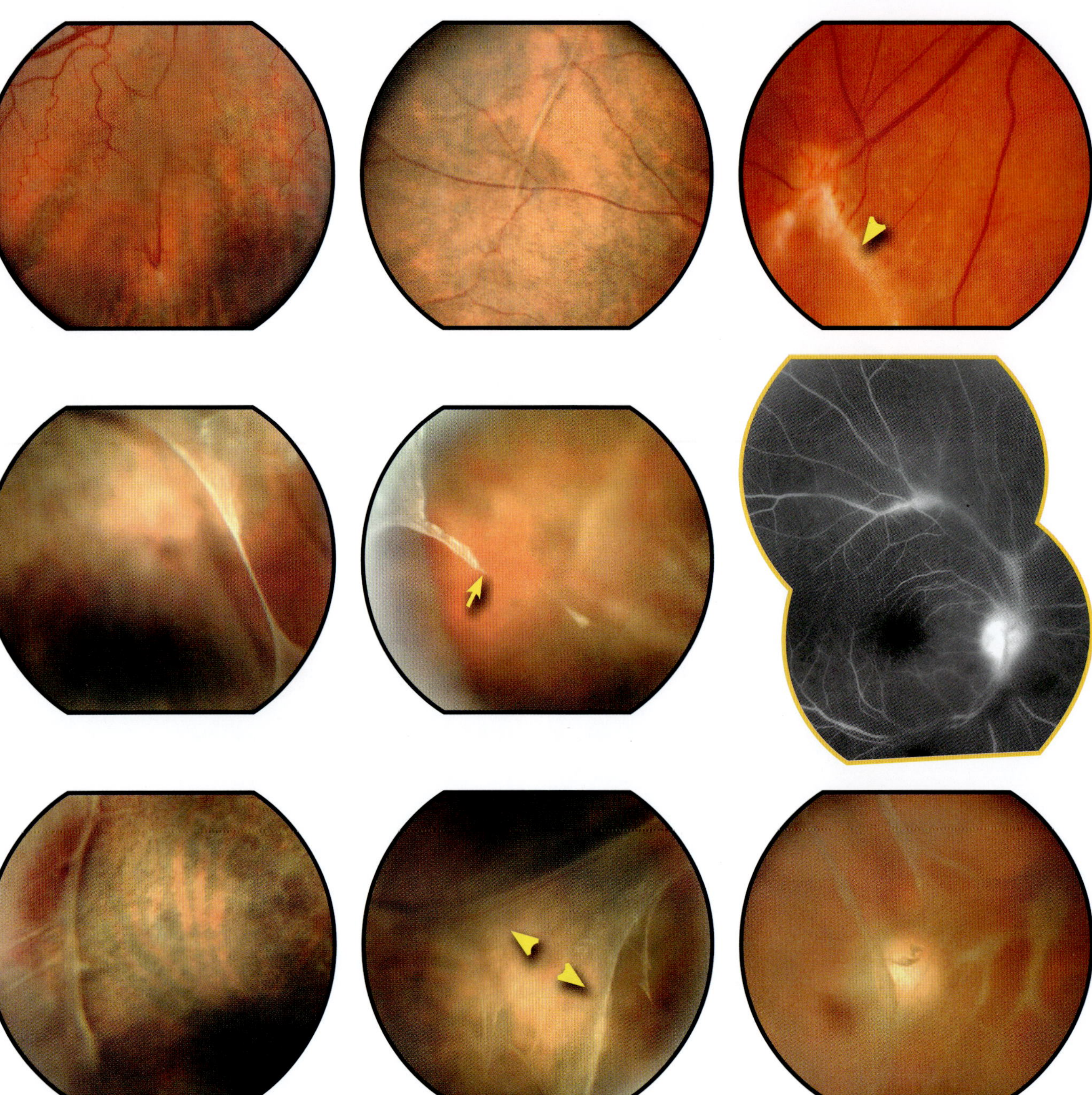

Peripheral retinoschisis is seen in X-linked juvenile retinoschisis in about 50% of cases. Note the various vitreoretinal bands, some of which released spontaneously *(arrow)*. The schisis can be extremely opaque, obliterating retinal details *(arrowheads)*. The fluorescein angiogram here shows some permeability and segmental staining from the vitreoretinal traction. *Top left image courtesy of Dr. Harold Weissman, top right image courtesy of Drs Ron Carr and Ken Noble*

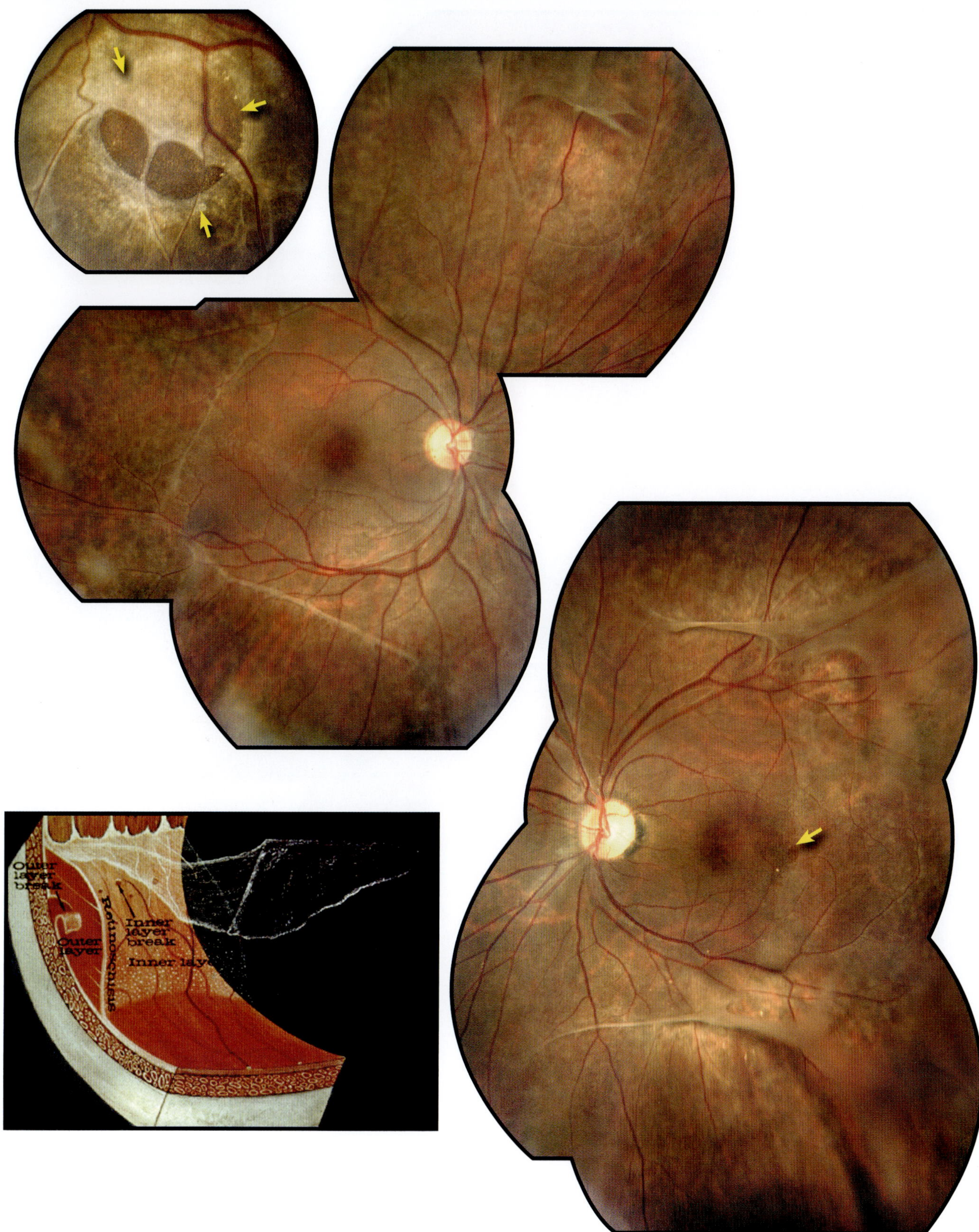

The two composite photographs illustrate extensive vitreous cavities with traction bands throughout the fundus in both eyes. Inner retinal holes are also evident. The upper left image shows two full-thickness retinal holes associated with the schisis cavity *(arrows)*. The schematic image demonstrates how vitreous traction, inner cystic cavities, and outer retinal breaks, may lead to retinal detachment.

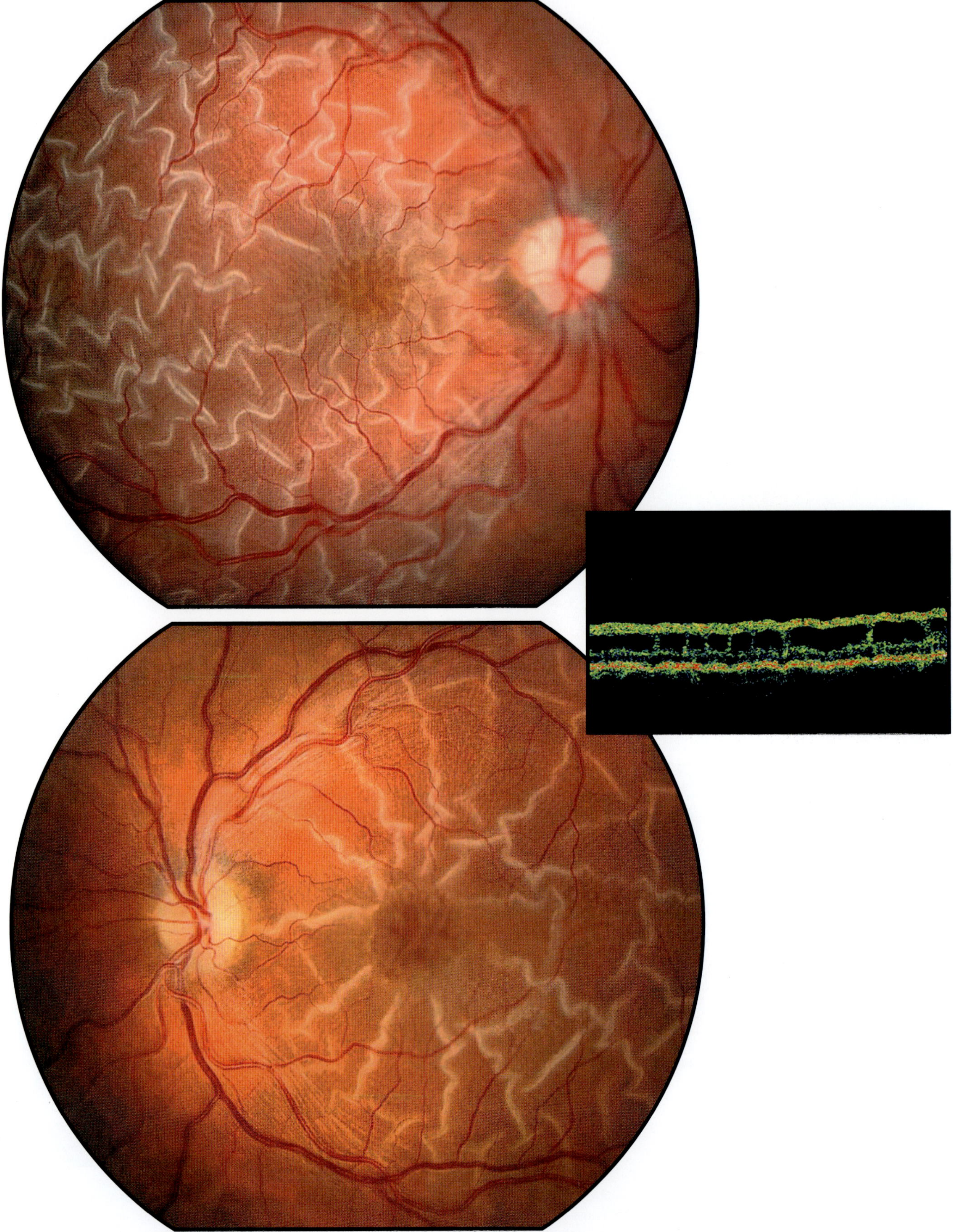

In this patient with X-linked juvenile retinoschisis, a rhegmatogenous detachment has occurred in each eye. There is a delicate pattern of outer retinal folds in the macula, extending from the macular schisis toward the periphery. Macular schisis is evident on the OCT. *Courtesy of Dr. Henry Lee*

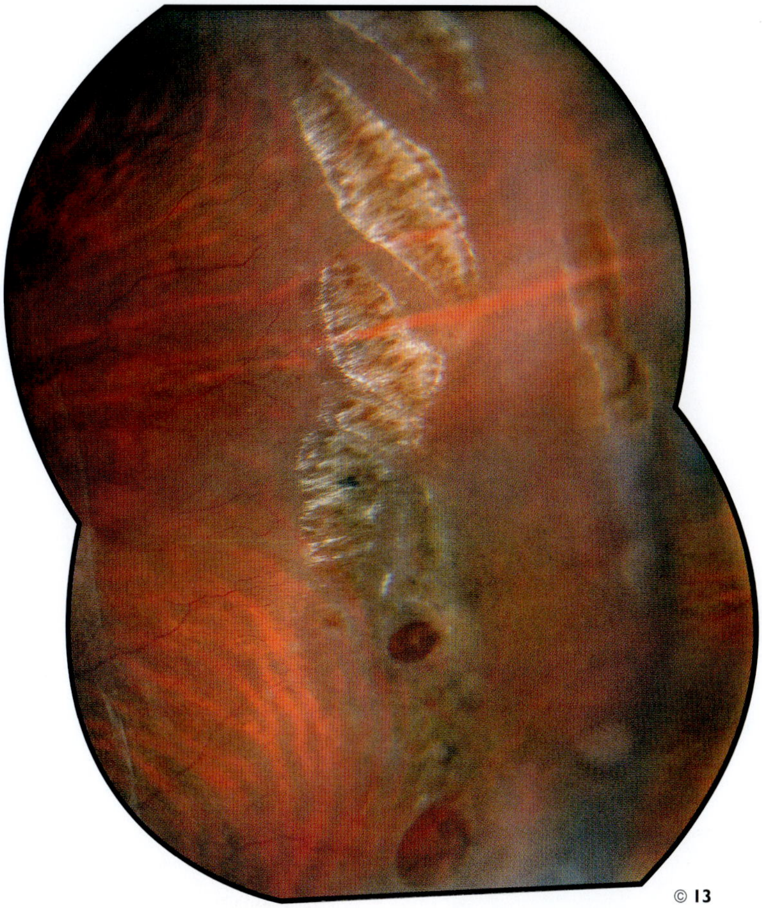

© 13

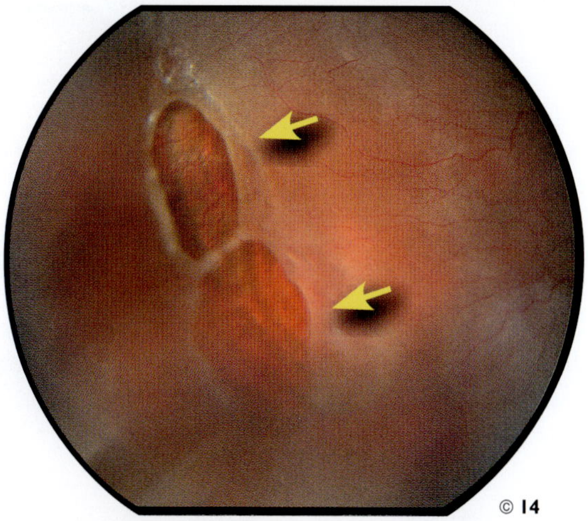

© 14

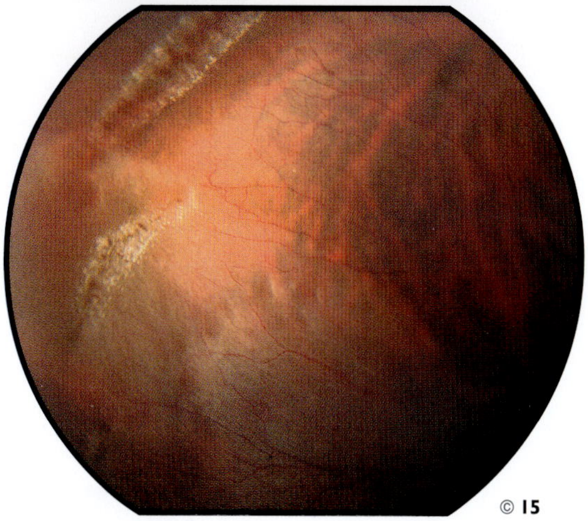

© 15

This patient has X-linked juvenile retinoschisis with peripheral lattice degeneration, inner lamellar holes, vitreous traction, and two large outer lamellar retinal holes *(arrows)*.

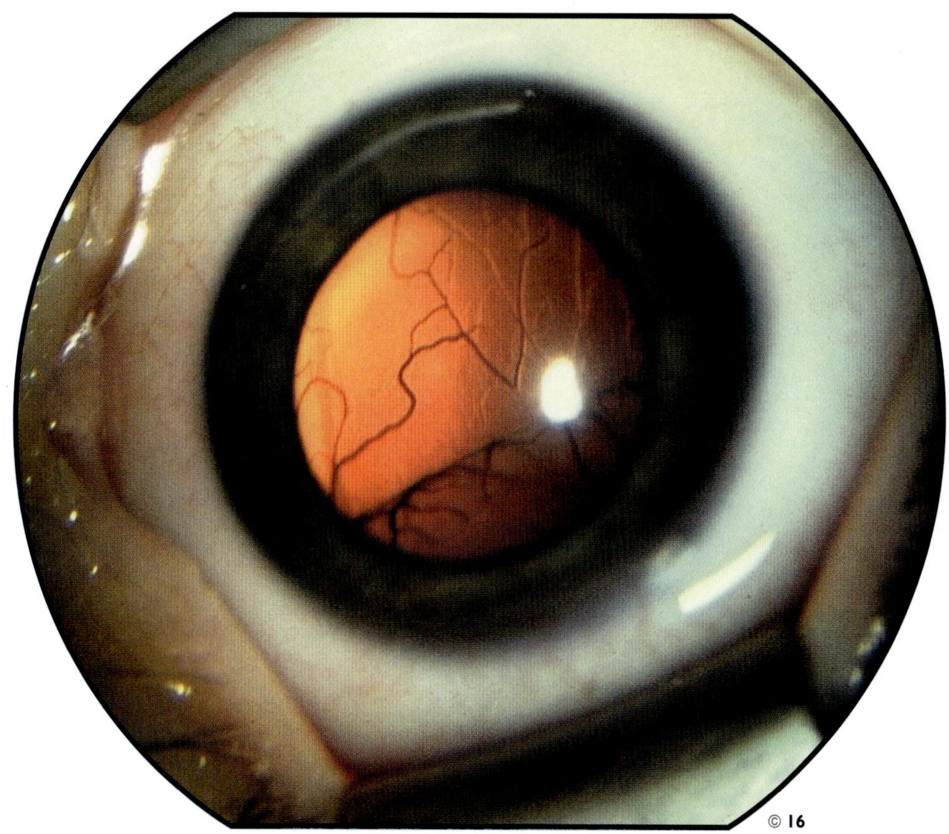

© 16

This patient with X-linked juvenile retinoschisis had a bullous retinal detachment which extended up to the lens. It is seen through the pupil, as the retinal vessels shadow the detached area.

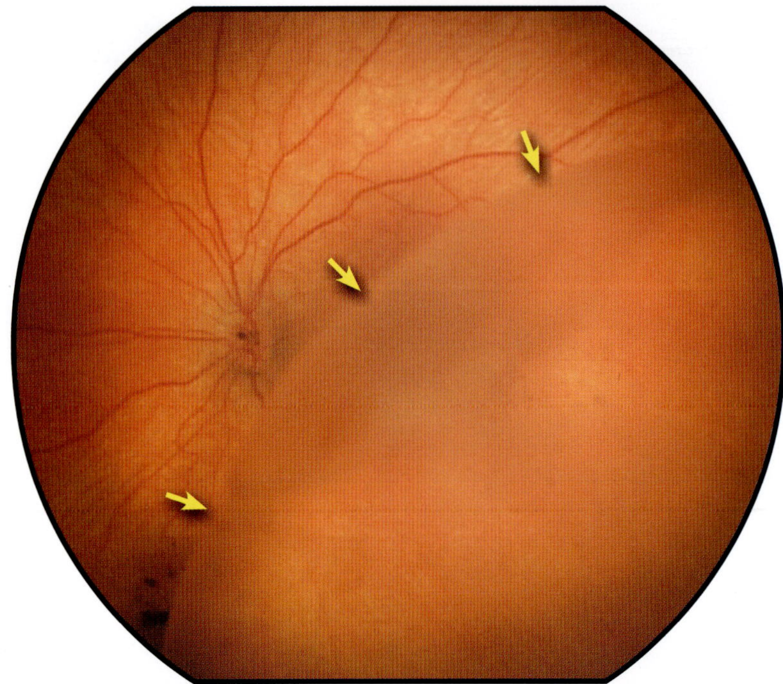

A large peripheral schisis has obstructed the visual axis of this 9-month-old boy with congenital X-linked retinal schisis *(arrows)*.

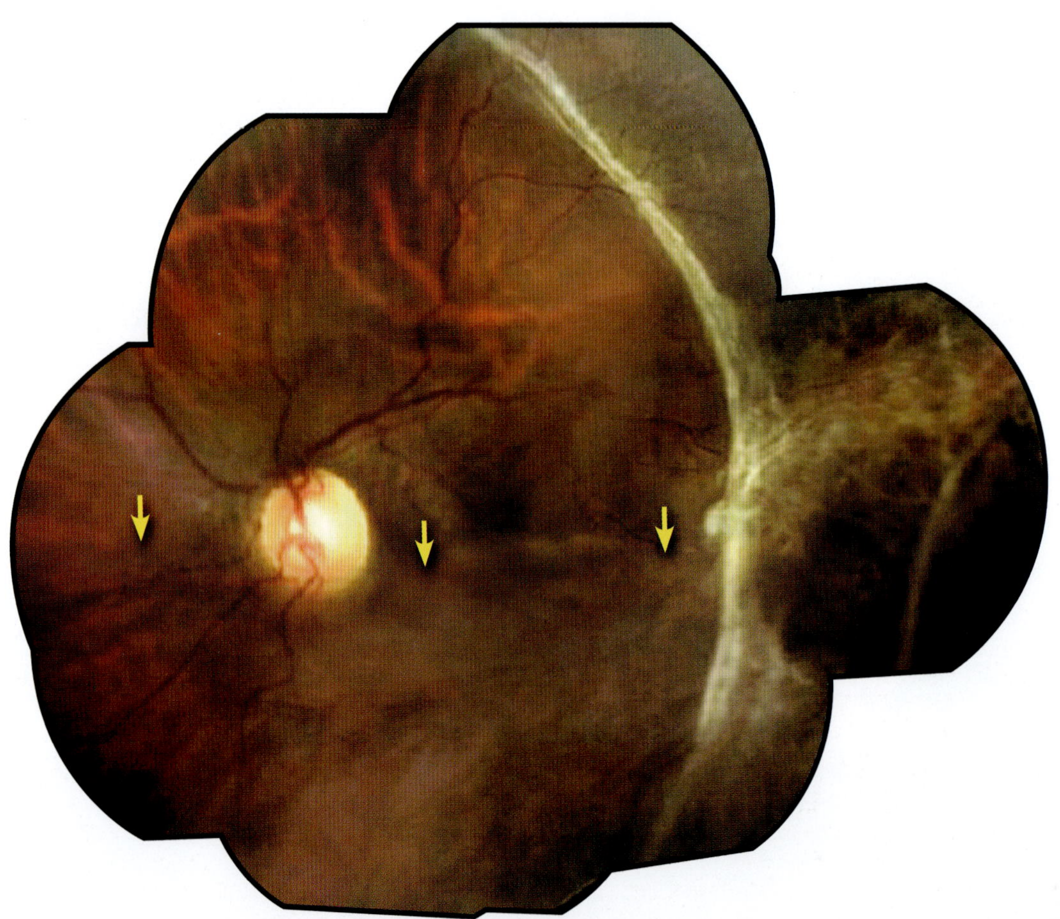

This patient has multiple retinal schisis cavities in the peripheral fundus, which are delineated by fibrous bands. A dependent retinal detachment *(arrows)* is also present inferiorly, extending toward the fovea. *Courtesy of Dr. Antonio Capone, Jr*

Stellate Nonhereditary Idiopathic Foveomacular Retinoschisis

Stellate nonhereditary idiopathic foveomacular retinoschisis (SNIFR) is a recently described disorder characterized by macular schisis in the absence of any identifiable cause or genetic etiology. Schisis may be unilateral or bilateral, and both male and female patients have been reported. Patients are most often asymptomatic with minimal or no visual deficit. Fundoscopy reveals foveal-involving macular schisis and occasionally concurrent peripheral schisis. SD-OCT localizes the macular schisis cavity most frequently to the outer plexiform layer.

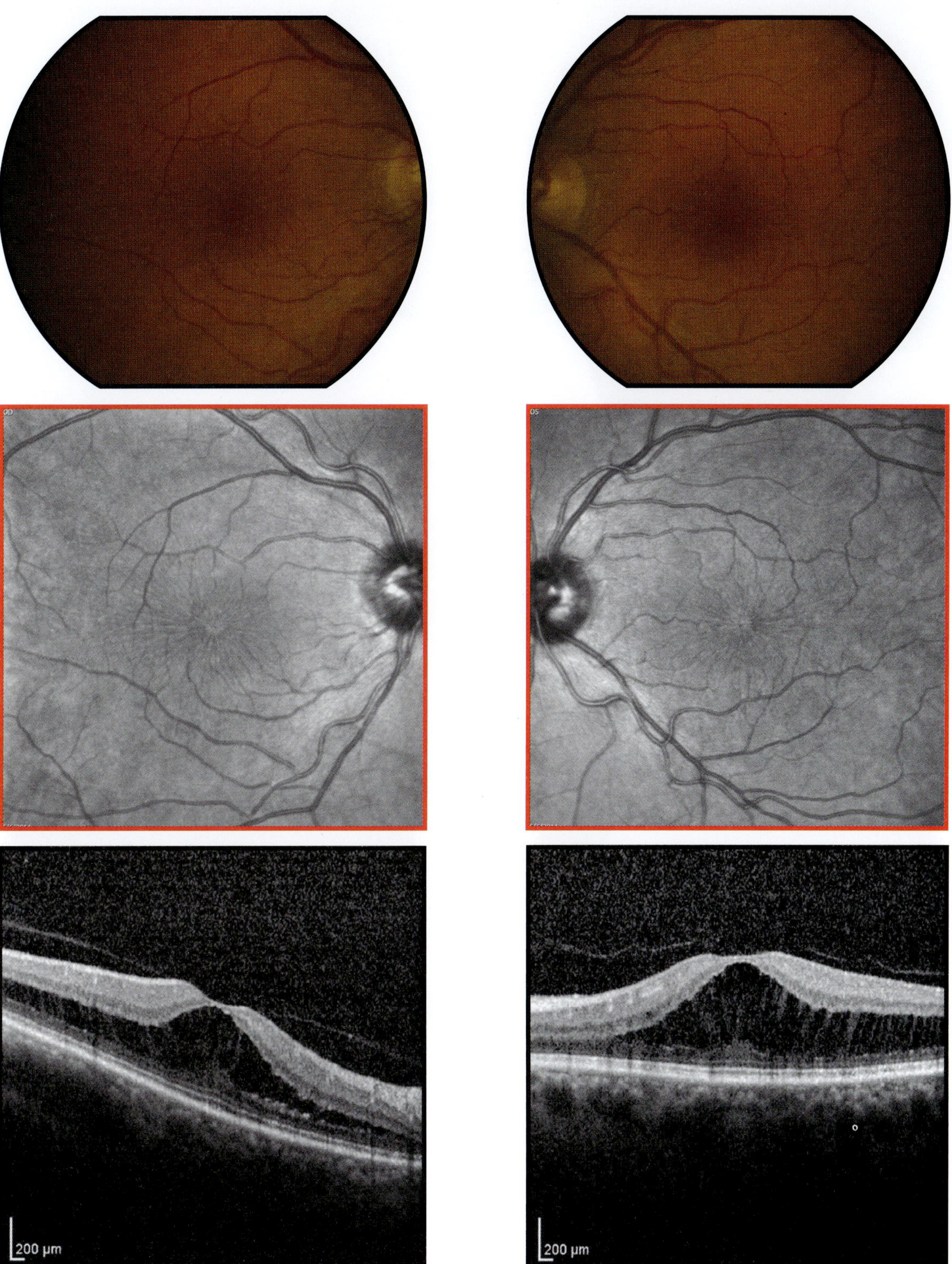

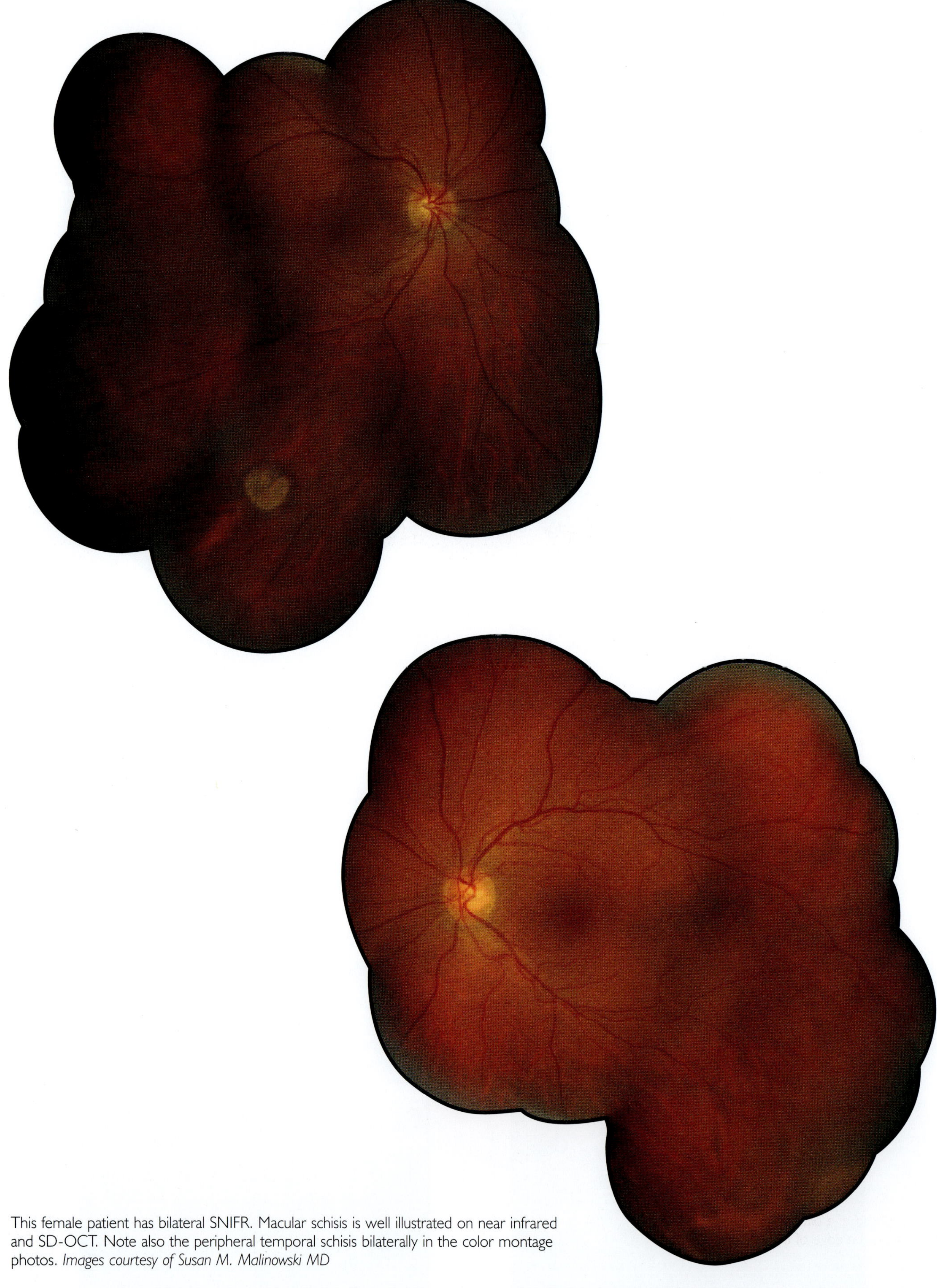

This female patient has bilateral SNIFR. Macular schisis is well illustrated on near infrared and SD-OCT. Note also the peripheral temporal schisis bilaterally in the color montage photos. *Images courtesy of Susan M. Malinowski MD*

Degenerative Retinal Schisis

X-linked juvenile schisis should be differentiated from peripheral degenerative schisis, which is typically identified in older asymptomatic individuals and is not associated with macular schisis or a genetic etiology. These thin, bullous and concave schitic cavities arise from peripheral cystoid degeneration and are typically located in the temporal quadrants, especially inferotemporal. Widefield angiography often shows associated leaking capillaries at the edge of the schitic cavities. Peripheral degenerative schisis can be complicated by inner and/or outer retinal holes and even schisis-detachment but rarely progresses into the posterior pole. Prophylactic laser therapy or surgery is rarely indicated.

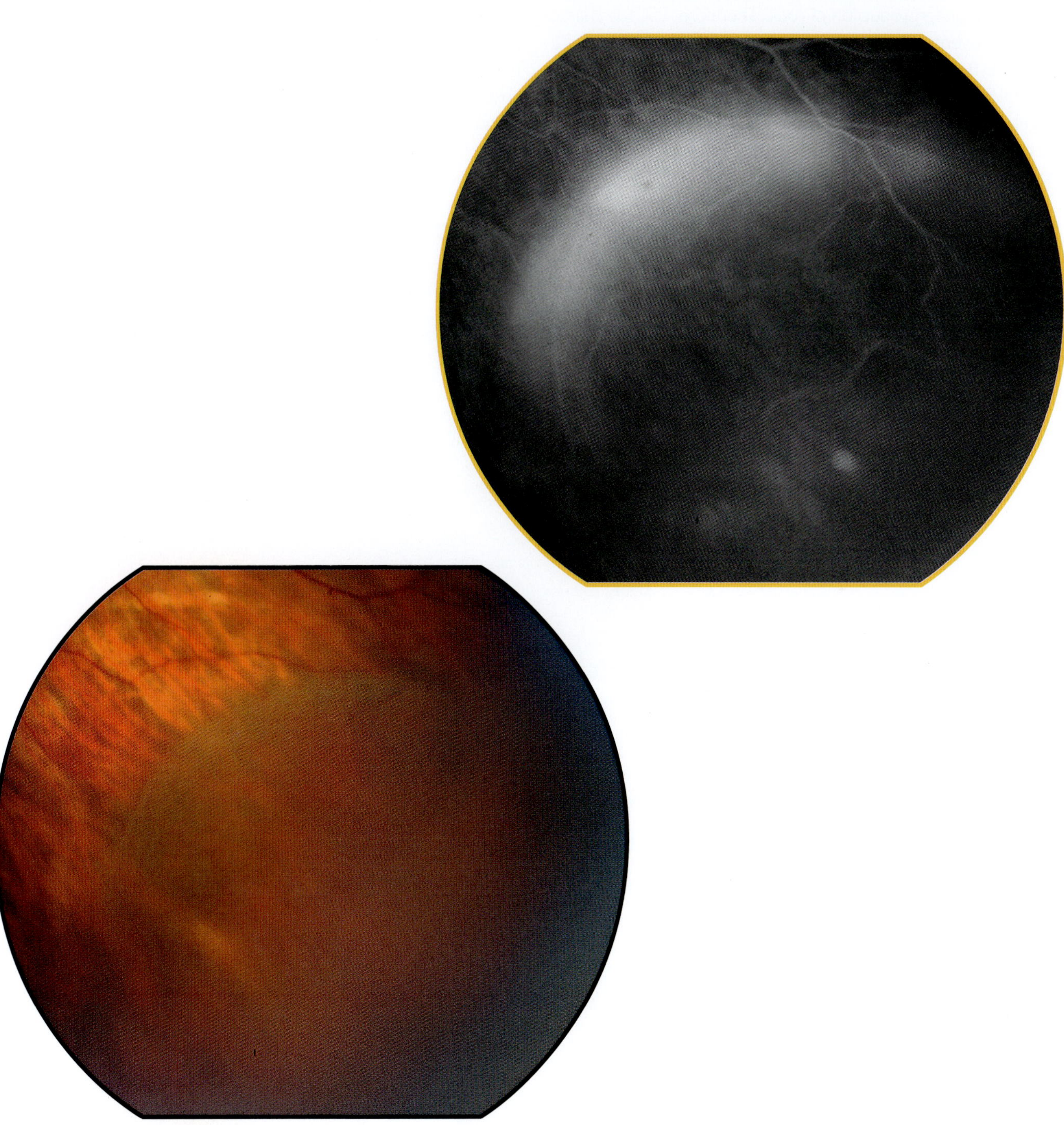

Color photo of a patient with peripheral degenerative schisis *(bottom left)* showing a thin, bullous schisis cavity. Fluorescein angiography reveals leakage at the edge of the schisis cavity *(top right)*.

Enhanced S-Cone Syndrome (Goldmann–Favre Syndrome)

The enhanced S-cone syndrome (ESCS) is an autosomal recessive disorder with some similar findings to X-linked juvenile schisis and caused by mutations in the nuclear receptor gene (NR2E3) on 15q23. Mutations in this gene alter retinal cell fate determination leading to increased differentiation of photoreceptor precursors to S-cones and underproduction of rods. Therefore, ESCS is characterized by overexpression of S (short-wavelength, blue) cones in the retina. Because S-cones may be the default pathway of cone differentiation, NR2E3 mutations may alter a signaling pathway in the genetic program that controls development of the normal ratio of S to L (long-wavelength, red) and M (middle-wavelength, green) photoreceptor subtypes.

Clinically, ESCS is a slowly progressive retinal degeneration characterized by early-onset nyctalopia, usually within the first decade of life, development of a ring of peripheral pigmentary changes along the vascular arcades with or without foveal schisis-like abnormalities. Peripheral retinal schisis may also be present. Other findings that may be noted include an optically empty vitreous with pre-retinal bands, lattice degeneration, and even retinal detachment. Patients have characteristic ERG findings that reflect the near absence of rods and a predominance of S cones. The scotopic response is therefore extinguished and the maximal rod–cone response resembles the photopic flash waveform.

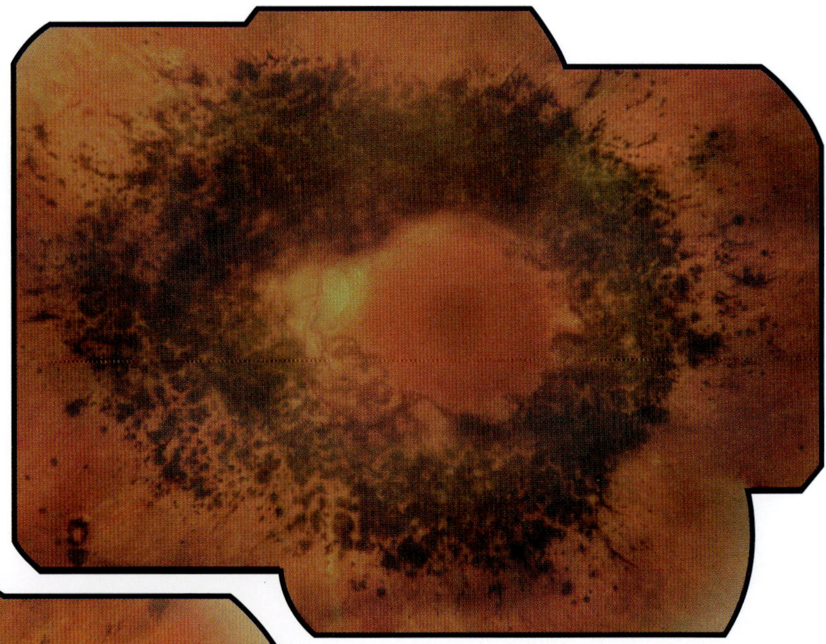

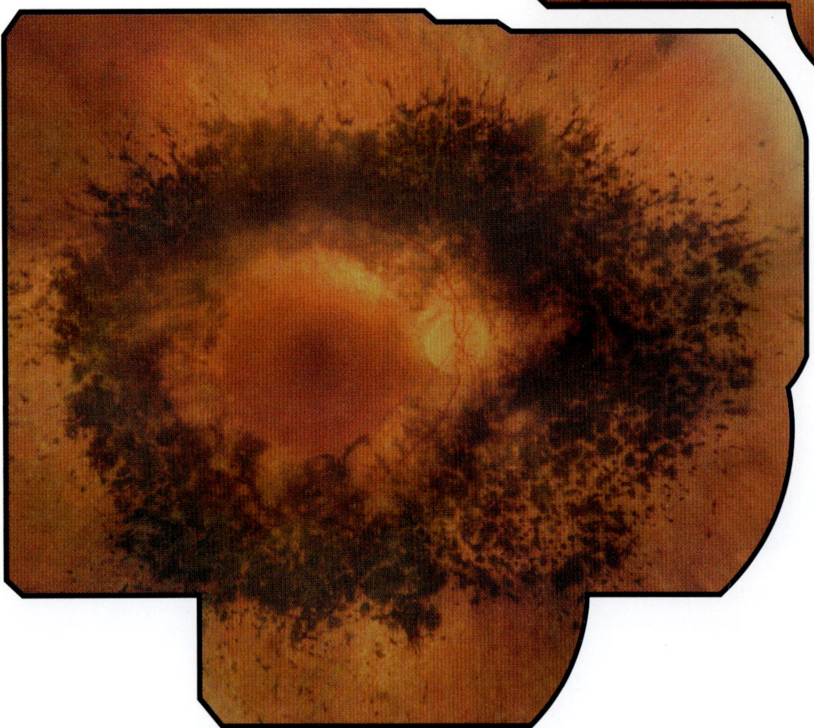

This patient with Goldman–Favre or enhanced S-cone syndrome has a wreath of very heavy pigment epithelial hyperplastic change surrounding the fundus in each eye. The manifestations are quite symmetric bilaterally. There is also schisis in the macula. Spontaneous detachment of the posterior hyaloid may relieve the macular traction and result in disappearance of the schisis and improvement in visual acuity.

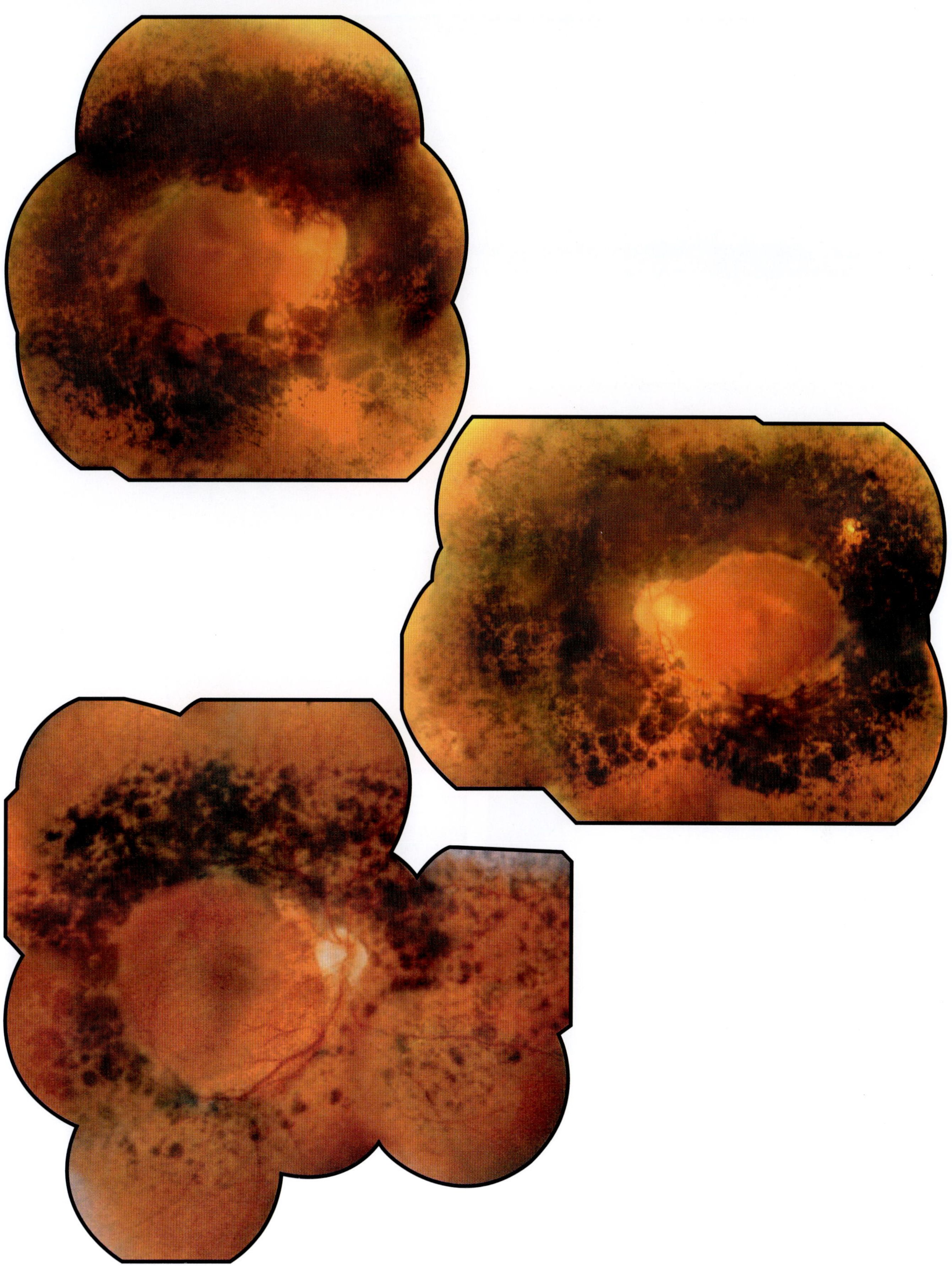

This patient with Goldmann–Favre syndrome has been followed for 25 years. Note the heavy wreath of pigmentation surrounding the posterior pole in each eye. There is minimal cystoid change in the macula. A montage image of that eye was made 25 years earlier *(lower left)*. The right eye has a dense cataract, obscuring fundus views. The patient's visual acuity is still 20/50 in spite of the cataract and some atrophic change in the macula.

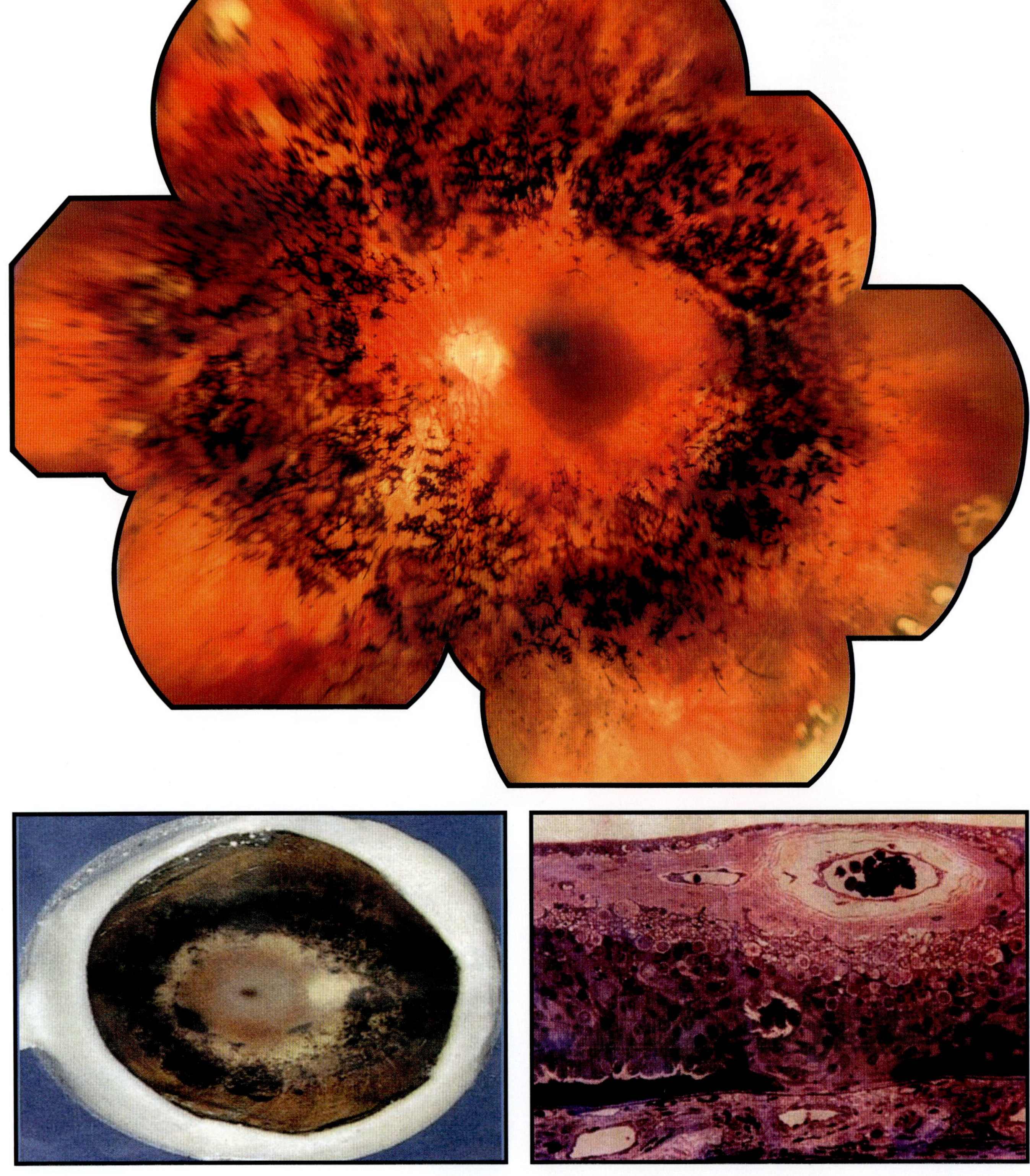

This is a montage photograph of a patient with Goldmann–Favre or enhanced S-cone syndrome. The gross pathology on another patient shows the heavy pigment epithelial hyperplastic change. The histopathology shows pigment migration into the retina and perivascular area and some atrophy of the RPE and photoreceptors. Cataract formation is characteristic of these patients. *Images courtesy of Dr. Samuel Jacobson*

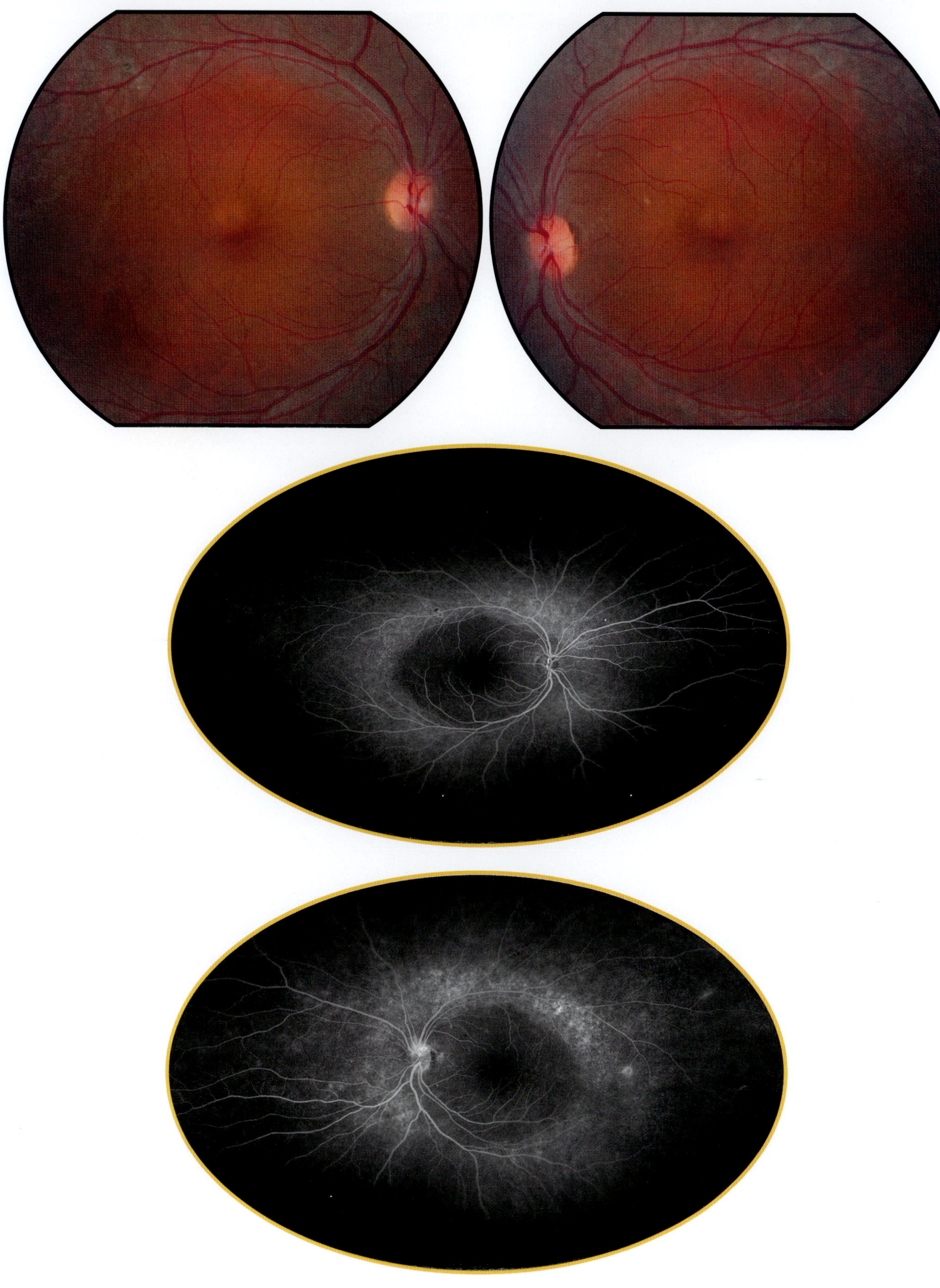

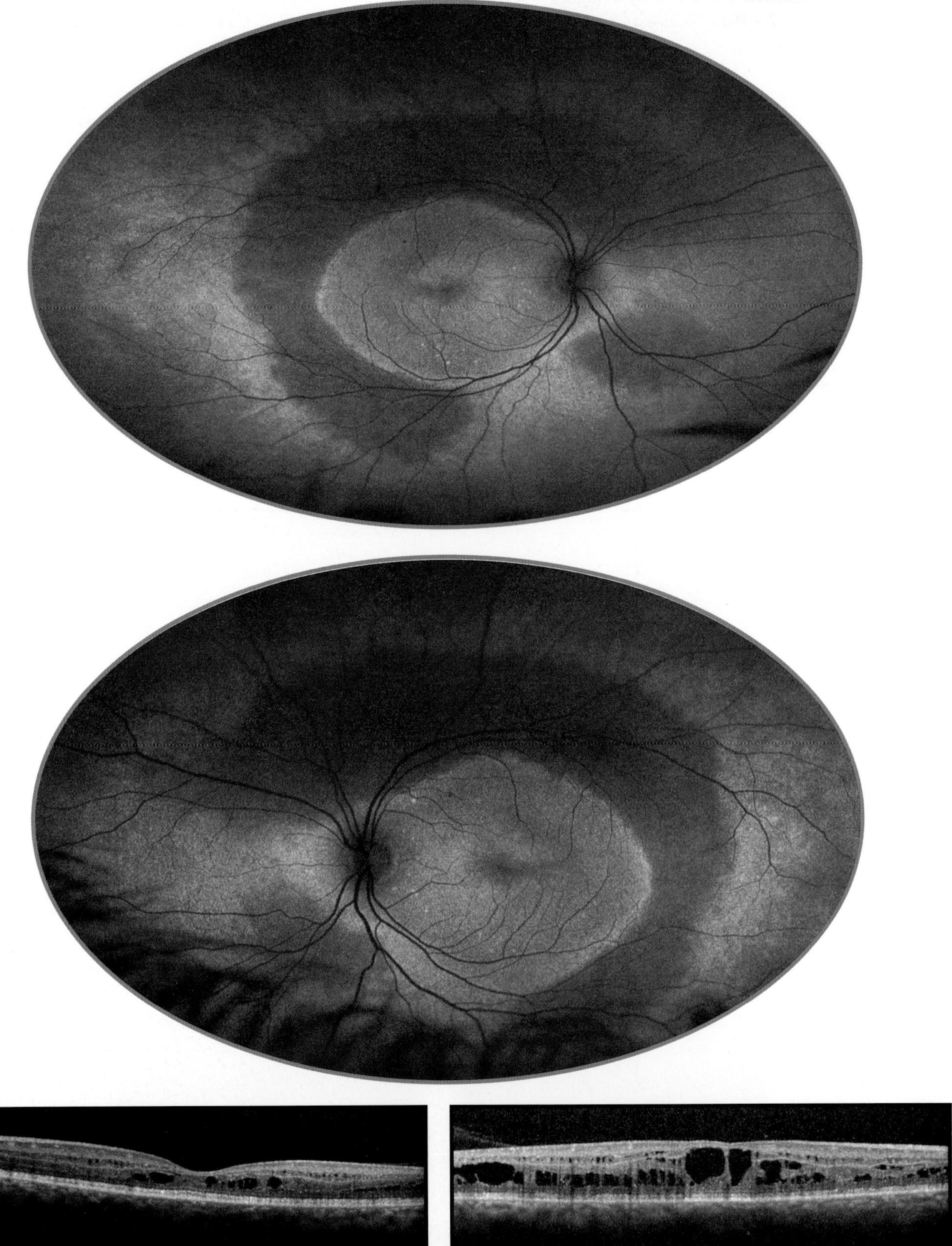

Fundus photos of this patient show midperipheral pigmentary changes that correspond to hyperfluorescent window defects and hypoautofluorescence with widefield fluorescein angiography and autofluorescence respectively. SD-OCT shows diffuse macular schisis involving inner and outer retinal layers. *Courtesy of Steven D. Schwartz, MD*

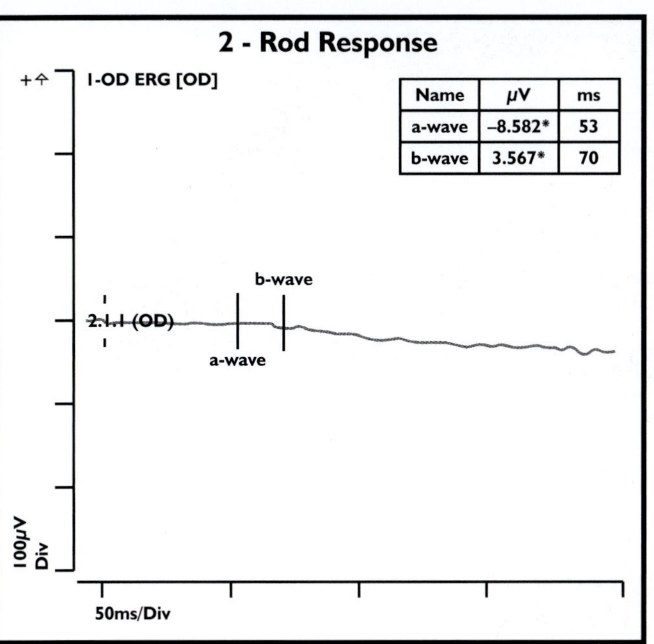

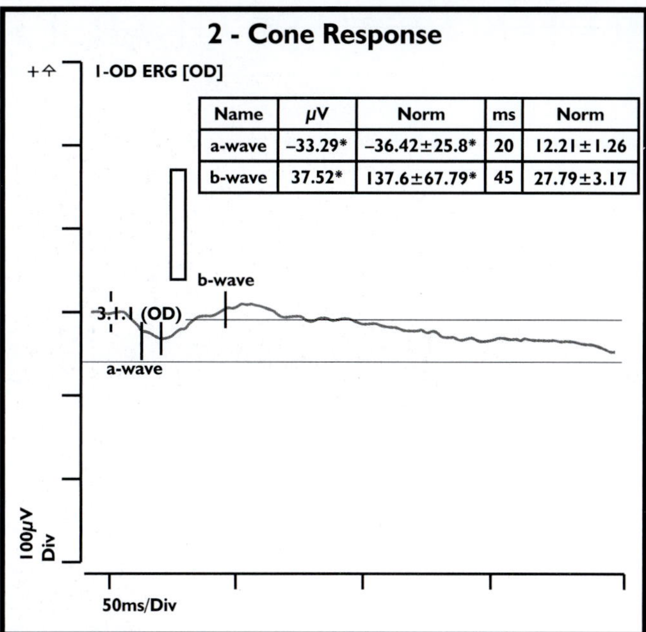

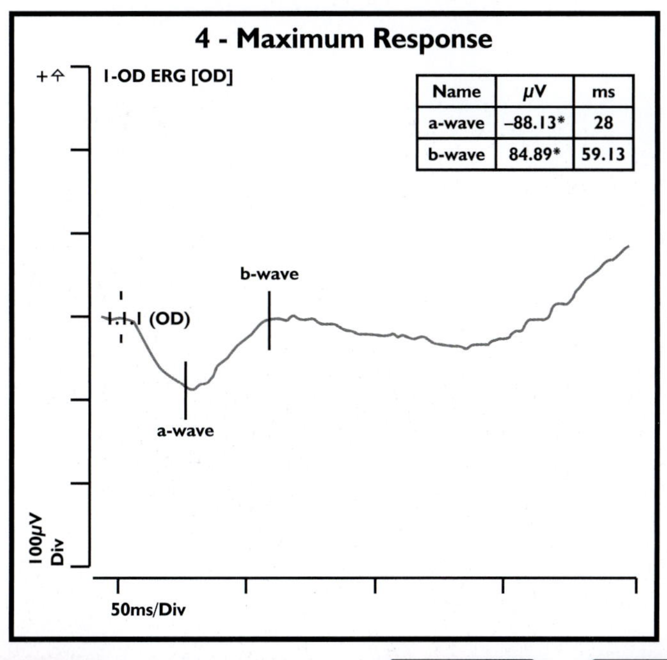

Electroretinogram of the same patient shows an absent rod response and little difference between the cone and maximum response waves. *Images courtesy of Pouya Dayani, MD*

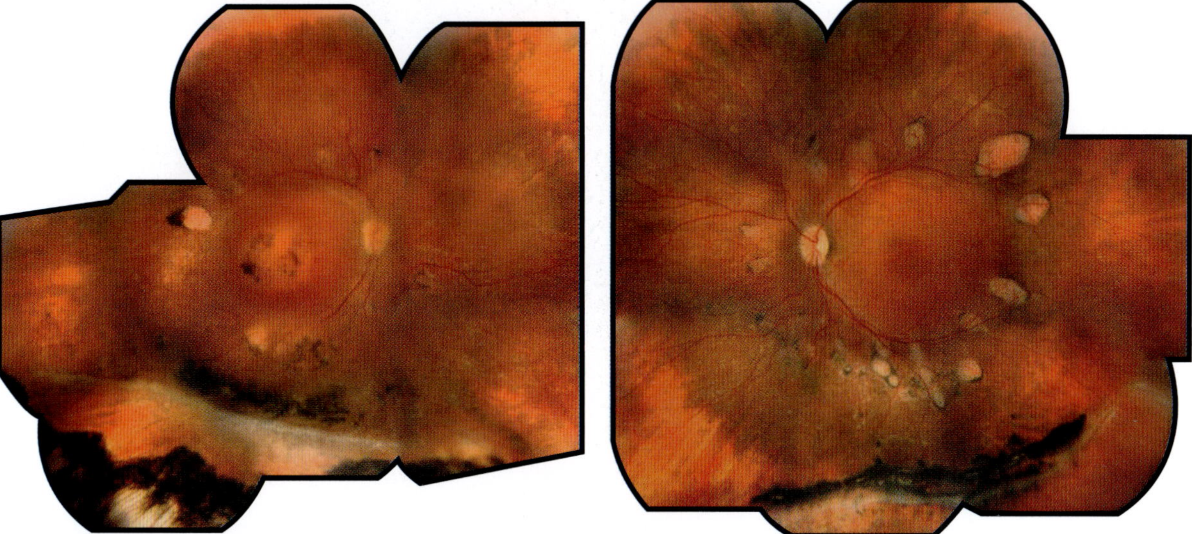

This compound heterozygous patient with Goldmann–Favre Disease experienced bilateral detachment. The vitreoretinal surgical procedure with membrane peeling relaxed the macular traction in the right eye.

Retinal Vascular Dystrophies

Numerous dystrophies of the fundus may involve predominantly the retinal circulation. They range from minor irregularities in vessel caliber to more visually significant abnormalities that are associated with hemorrhage, traction, retinal detachment, and macular abnormalities. Typically there is an underlying genetic abnormality and hereditary transmission and often associated systemic involvement.

Hereditary or Familial Retinal Artery Tortuosity

Hereditary or familial retinal artery tortuosity (FRAT) is characterized by marked tortuosity of second- and third-order retinal arteries with normal first-order artery and venous systems. It is inherited in an autosomal dominant pattern. The tortuosity primarily affects the retinal arterioles in the macular region with tortuosity increasing with age. Recurrent macular hemorrhages may occur spontaneously or after minor trauma, but typically resolve with normalization of vision. Rarely retinal vascular occlusion may complicate this syndrome. In some families, there may be systemic involvement, such as renal vascular abnormalities. Spontaneous retinal hemorrhages may occur in family members in the absence of retinal artery tortuosity or related systemic disease.

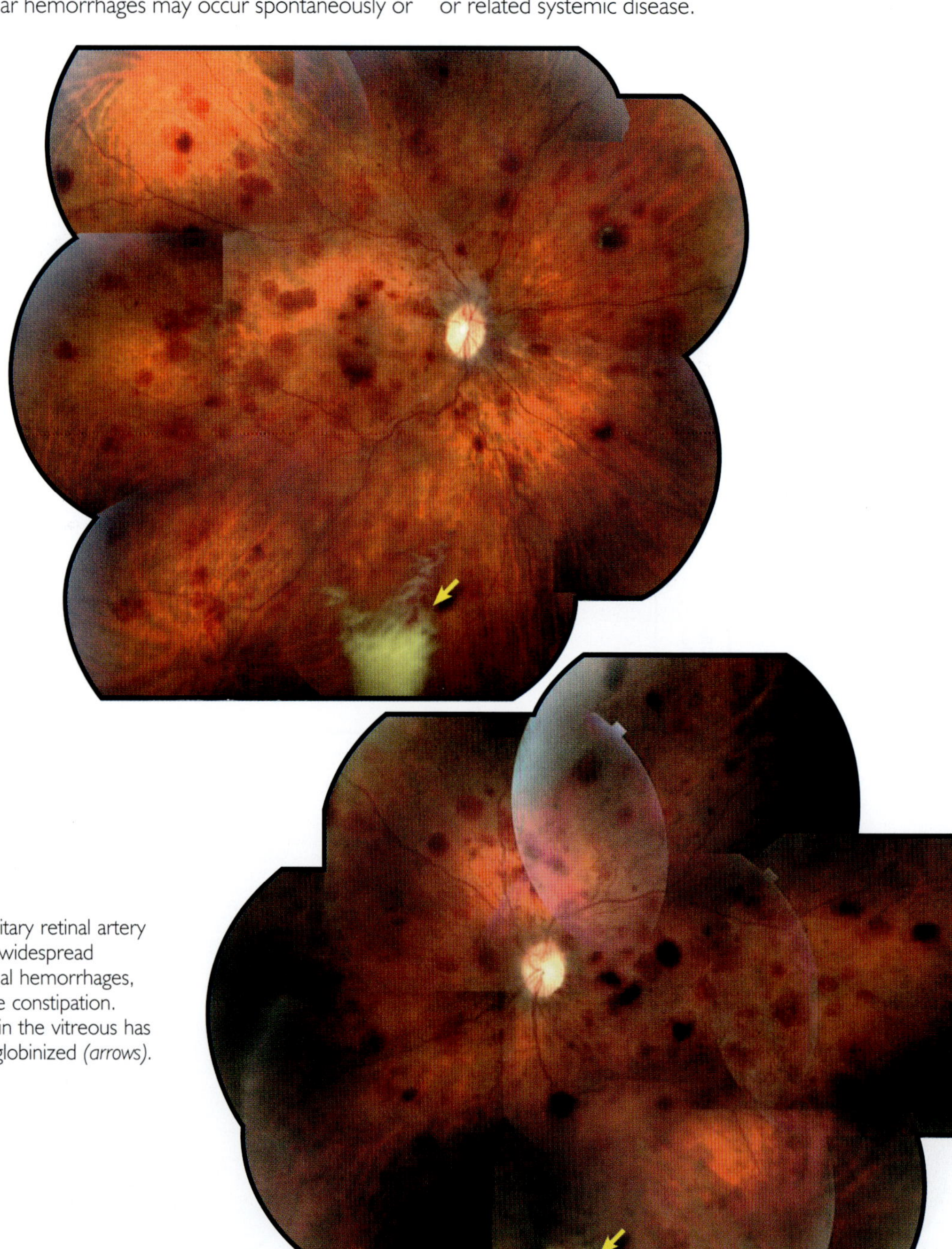

This patient with hereditary retinal artery tortuosity experienced widespread intraretinal and preretinal hemorrhages, coincidental with severe constipation. Resolving hemorrhage in the vitreous has now become dehemoglobinized *(arrows)*.

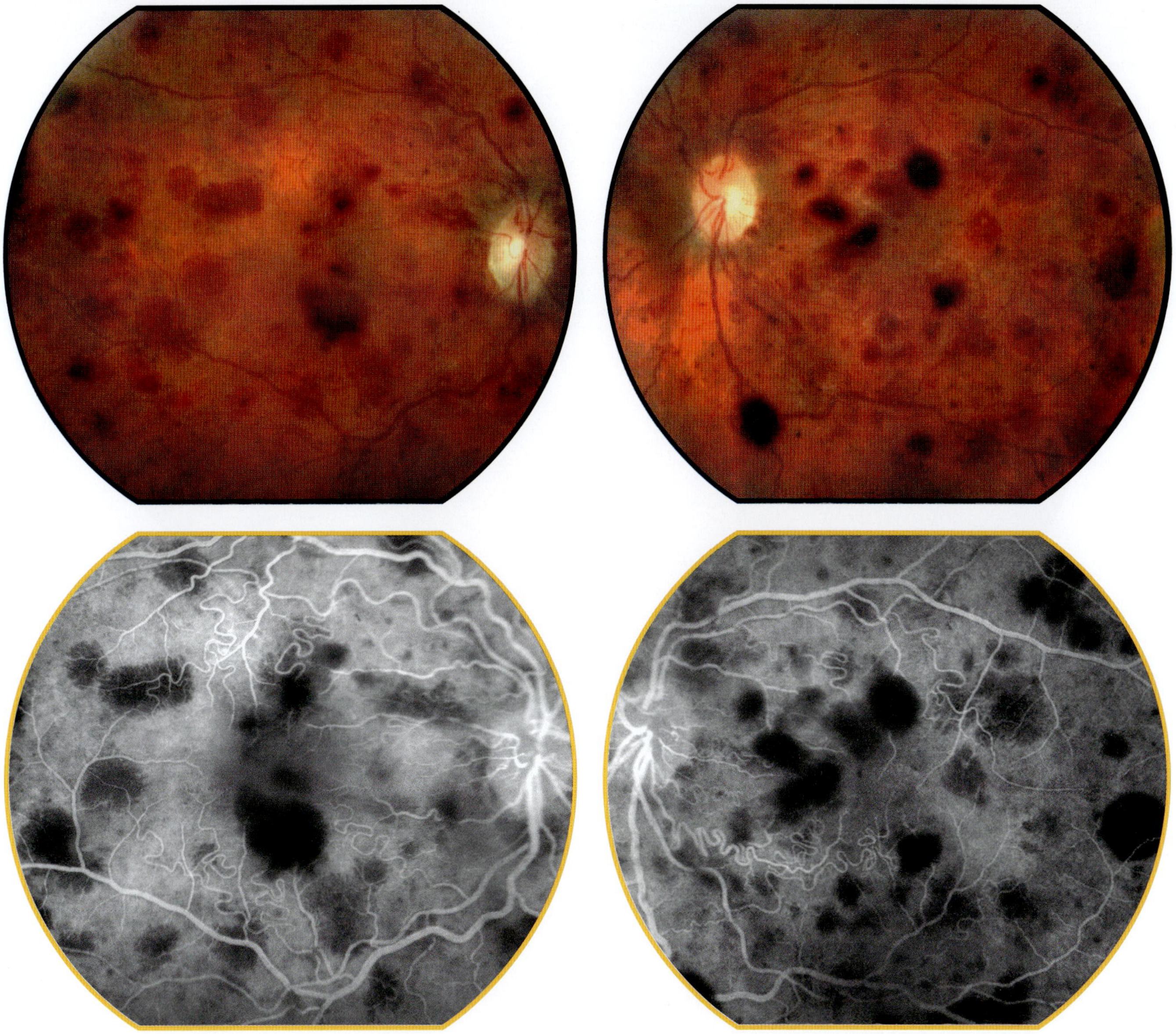

The central macula in the same patient showed multiple levels of hemorrhage: preretinal, intraretinal, and subretinal. The fluorescein angiogram showed no leakage in either eye with blockage from the heme. Note the vascular tortuosity principally involving the second-order arterioles.

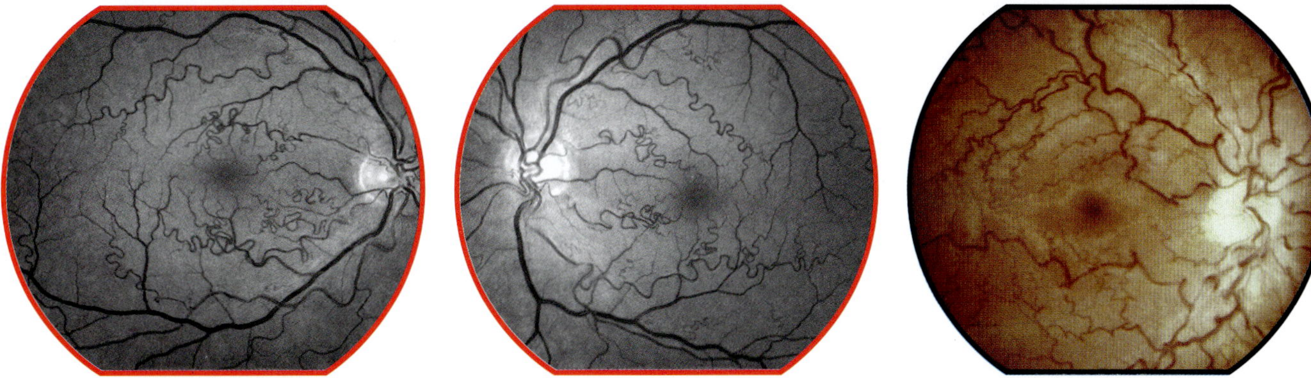

The fundus of the patient's father showed a familial nature of the abnormality with widespread tortuosity, principally on the arteriolar side of the circulation.

This case of hereditary retinal artery tortuosity shows tortuous vessels on both sides of the circulation, arteriolar and venular.

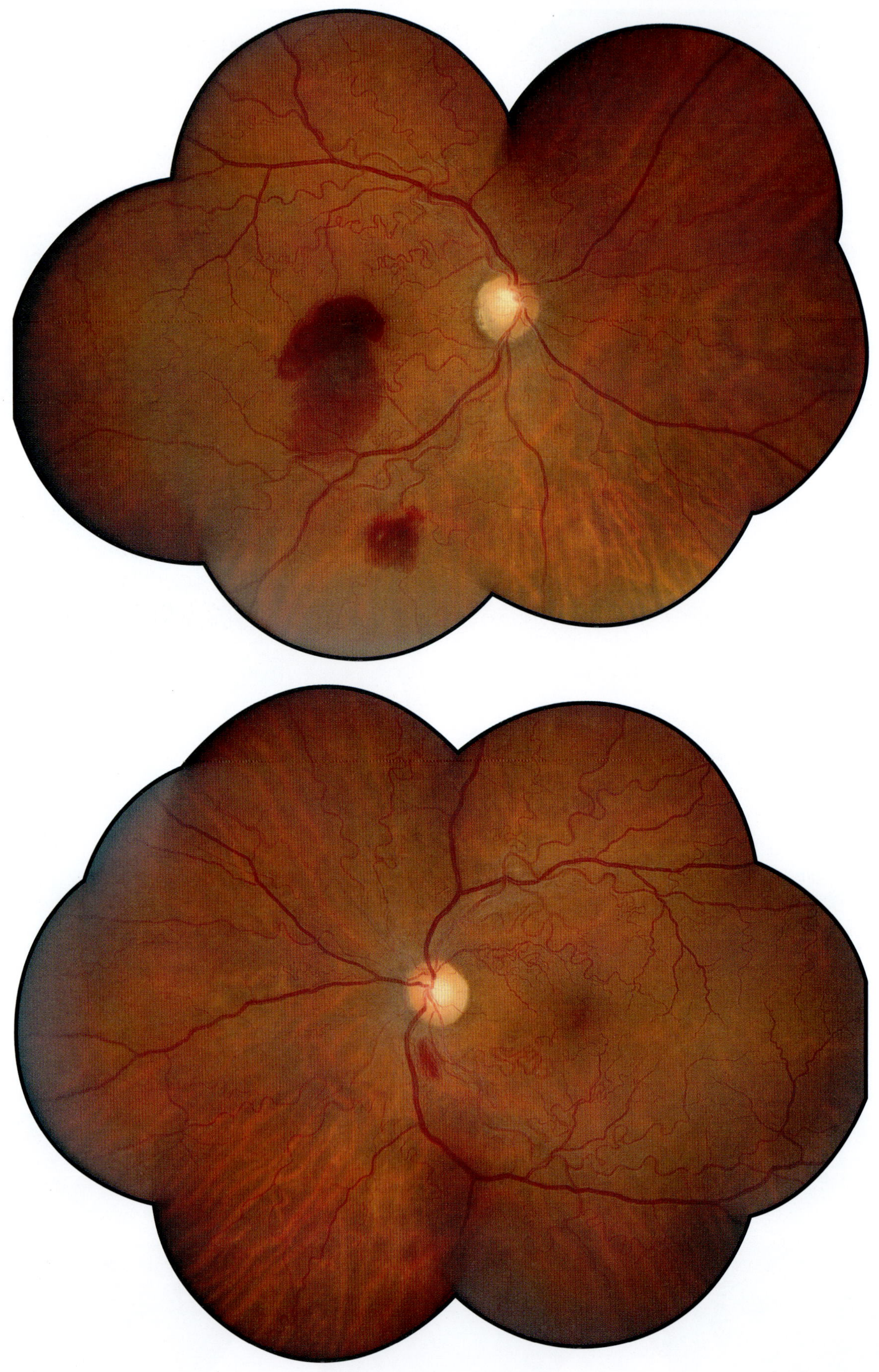

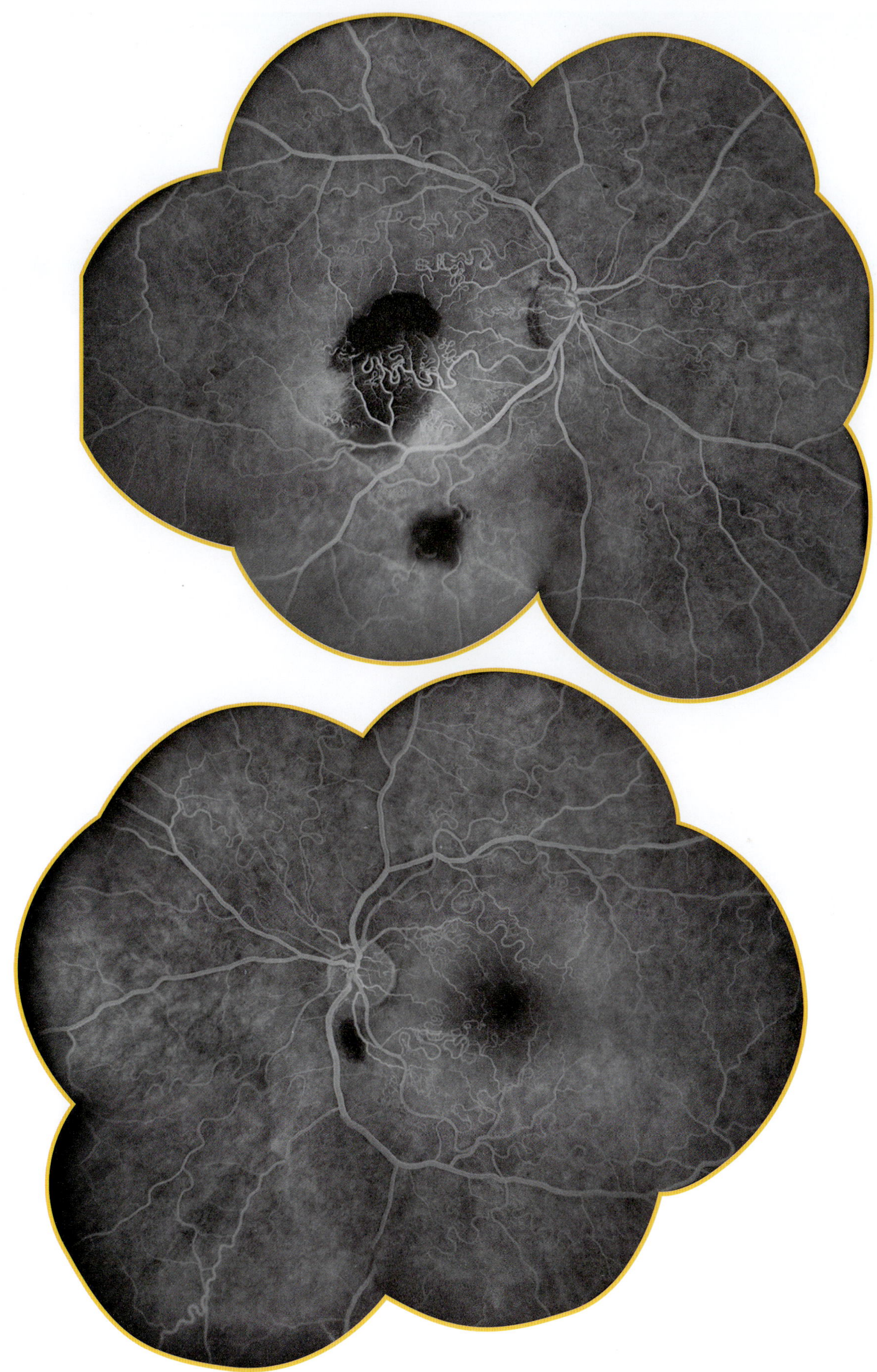

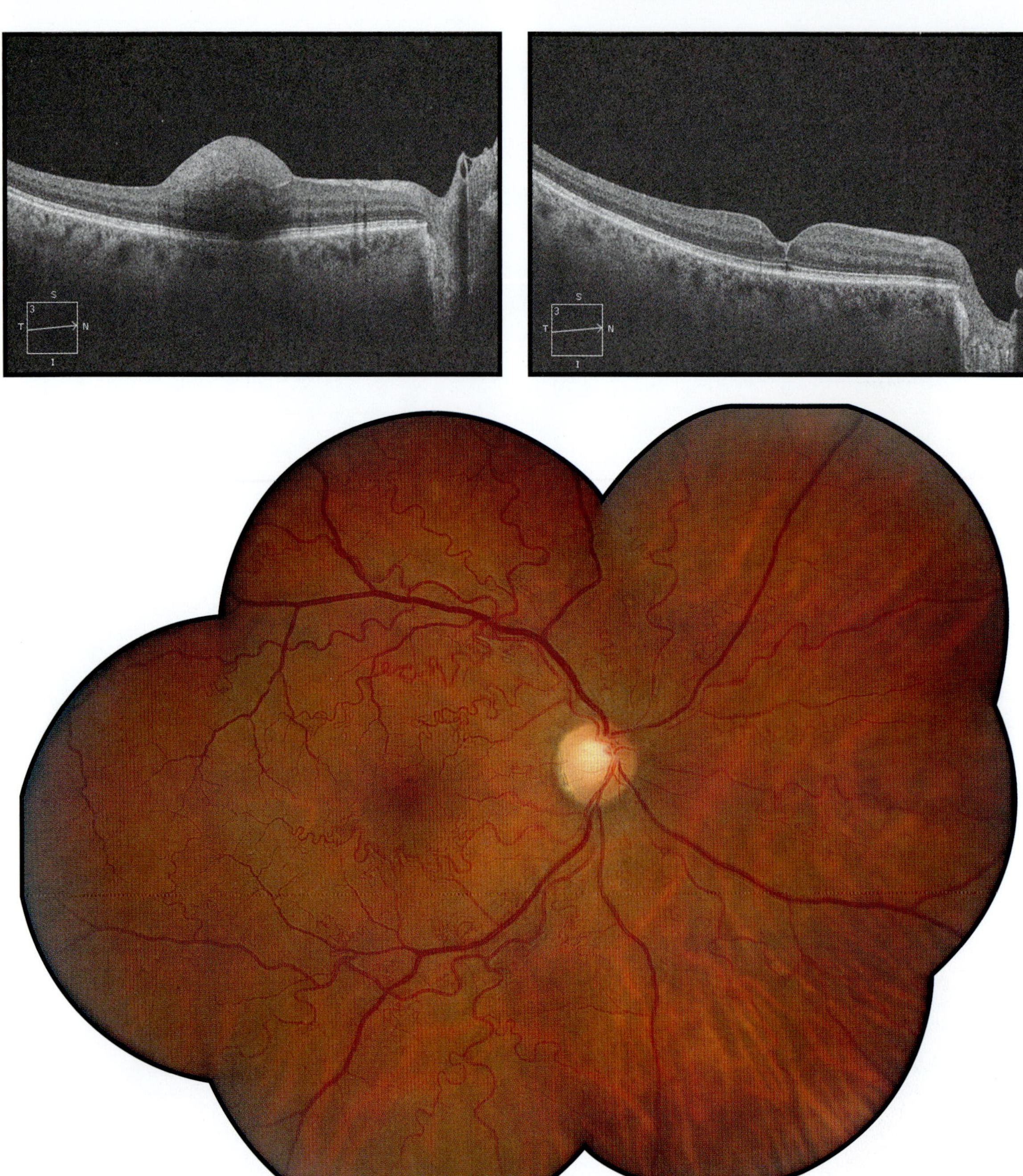

This patient with FRAT presented with a large subhyaloid hemorrhage over the macula of the right eye seen on color fundus montage, fluorescein angiography montage, and SD-OCT. Note that the subhyaloid hemorrhage resolved in the follow-up SD-OCT and color montage. *Images courtesy of Susan M. Malinowski, MD*

Fabry Disease

Fabry disease is an X-linked lysosomal storage disorder caused by a mutation in the GLA gene, which leads to insufficient levels of the enzyme α-galactosidase A. As a result, glycosphingolipids accumulate in virtually all tissues, leading to progressive dysfunction of multiple organ systems. Both males and females are affected, though female carriers typically manifest a less severe form of the disease. Marked retinal vascular tortuosity can be observed in approximately 77% of males and 19% of females. Other ocular manifestations of the disease include bulbar conjunctival vascular tortuosity, corneal verticillata, and spoke-like posterior lenticular opacity. The systemic manifestations are more concerning and include left ventricular dysfunction, cardiac arrhythmia, early stroke, and end-stage renal disease. Early diagnosis is essential as enzyme replacement therapy is now available.

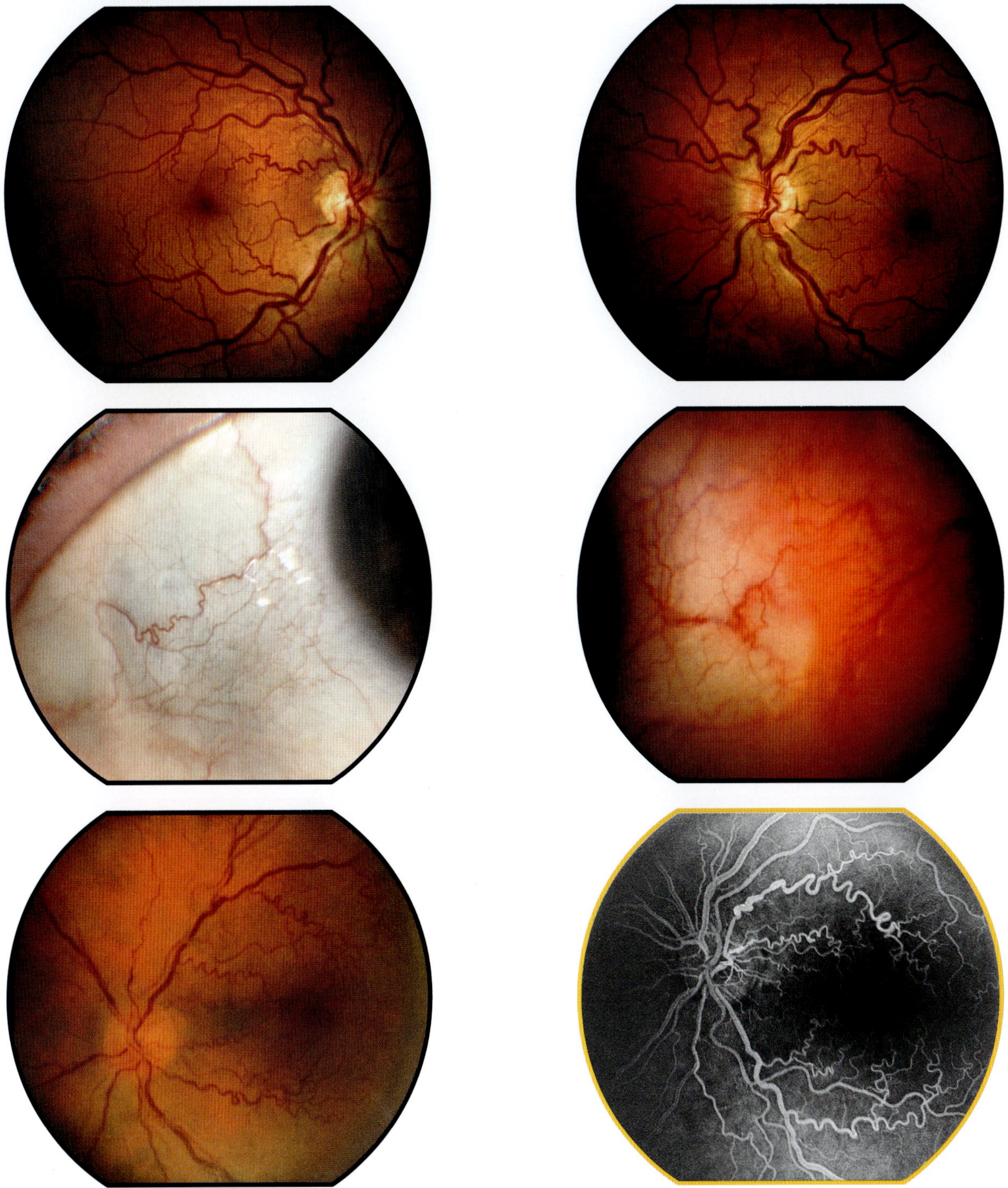

These images correspond to three patients with Fabry disease. Note the marked tortuosity of the retinal circulation. There is also conjunctival vascular tortuosity in each eye. The fluorescein angiogram shows tortuosity, but no leakage. *Top row left image, bottom row right image courtesy of Dr. Tom Weingiest*

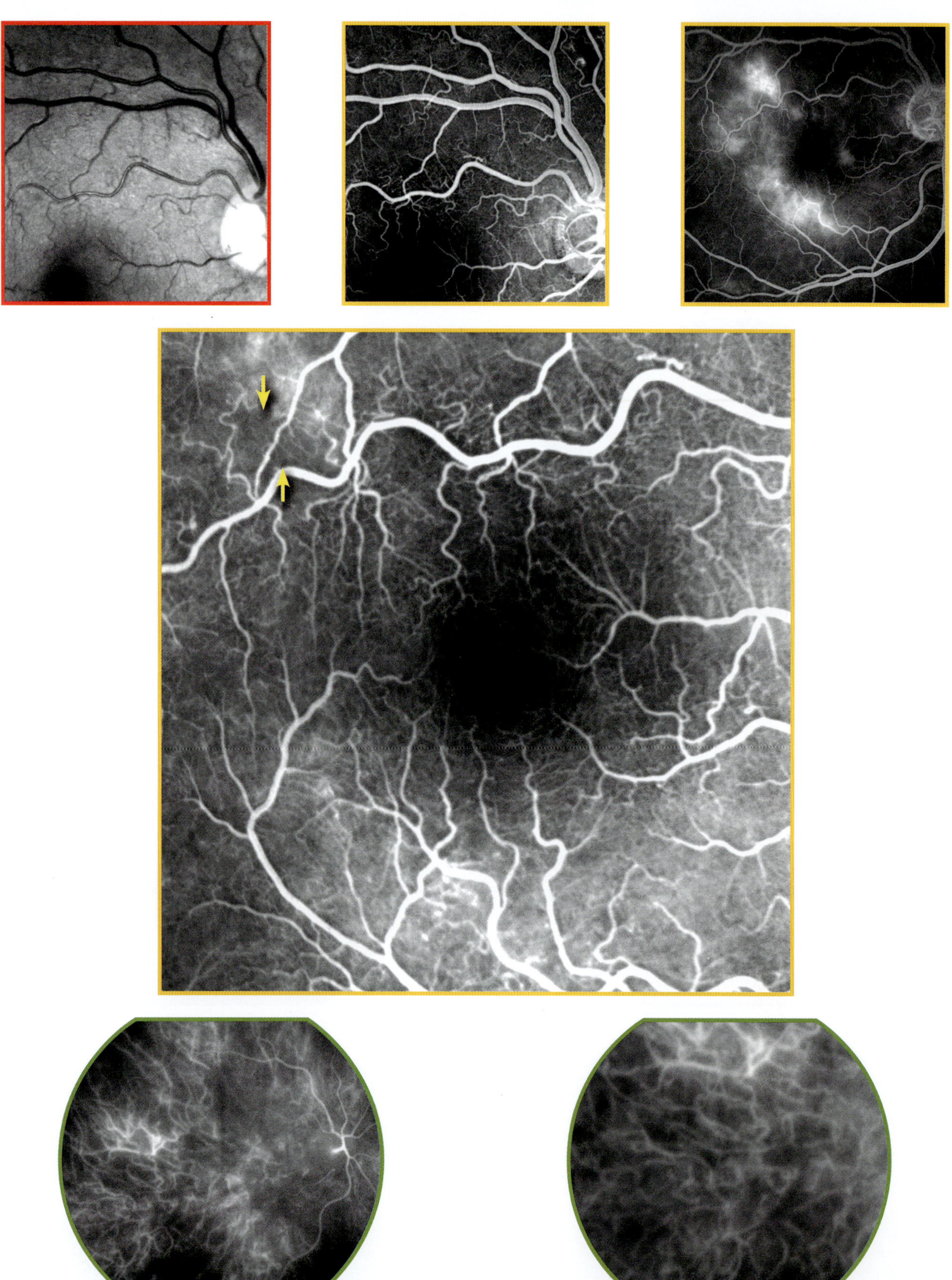

In this patient with Fabry disease, there are prominent capillaries noted on the red-free photograph *(top left)* and leakage of tortuous retinal vessels on the arteriolar and venular side of the circulation with fluorescein angiography. In the magnified image of the central macula, small islands of capillary non-perfusion can be seen *(arrows)*. The indocyanine green angiogram shows tortuosity in the inner choroidal circulation as well.

Familial Exudative Vitreoretinopathy

Exudative vitreoretinopathy 1, more commonly known as familial exudative vitreoretinopathy (FEVR), is a hereditary retinal disorder with features similar to retinopathy of prematurity (ROP); however, patients lack a history of prematurity or oxygen supplementation. Peripheral retinal vascular abnormalities include telangiectasia, aneurysms, arteriovenous shunts, and non-perfusion and ischemia. Dragging and straightening of the posterior retinal vasculature into the periphery often occurs. A variable degree of peripheral subretinal and intraretinal exudation with lipid deposition and a greater risk for tractional retinal detachment due to fibrovascular proliferation are noted.

FEVR is a genetically heterogeneous disorder that is most commonly autosomal dominant, and less commonly autosomal recessive or X-linked recessive. Approximately 50% of cases are linked to mutations in one of four genes: FZD4, LRP5, TSPAN12, and NDP. FZD4 (AD), LRP5 (AR and AD), and TSPAN12 (AD) are located on chromosome 11 while NDP, the same gene responsible for Norrie Disease, is located on the X chromosome. LRP5 and NDP mutations have systemic implications; LRP5 mutations are linked to decreased bone mineral density and NDP mutations may be linked to deafness. FEVR exhibits marked variability in penetrance, and therefore family history of known FEVR or unexplained visual loss is commonly absent. However, screening of family members with widefield angiography frequently identifies other affected individuals who may require close ophthalmologic follow-up or systemic intervention.

Patients with peripheral retinal ischemia and neovascularization may benefit from prophylactic panretinal laser photocoagulation and surgical intervention may be necessary to treat exuberant epiretinal membrane or tractional retinal detachment. Systemic intervention may be indicated, as with the LRP5 subtype, to correct low bone density.

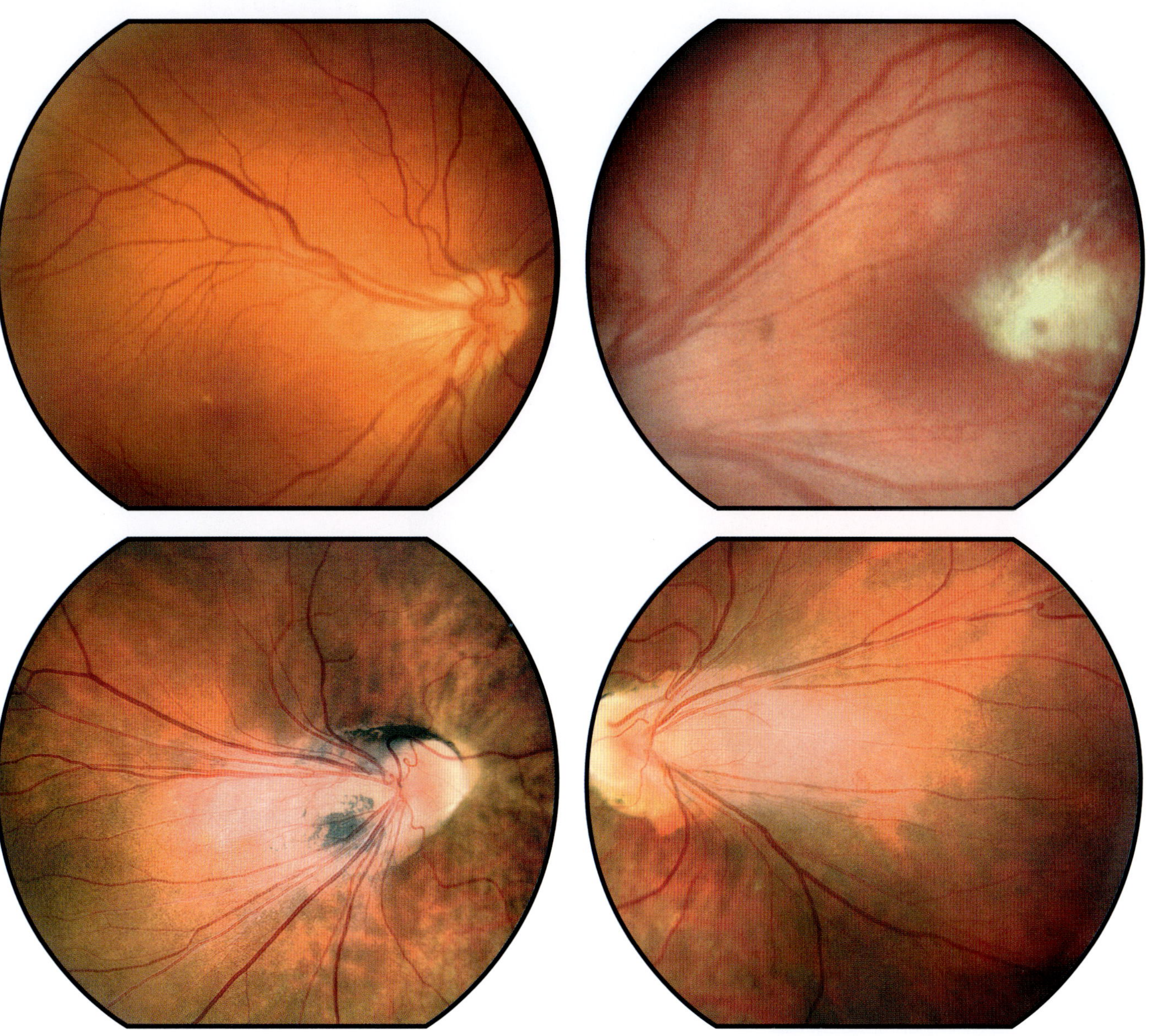

These are patients with FEVR. Note the changes in the posterior segment of the eye. There is dragging of the retinal vasculature from the disc; fibrosis and exudation with deposits of lipid into the macula; as well as localized detachment of the retina *(right bottom)*.

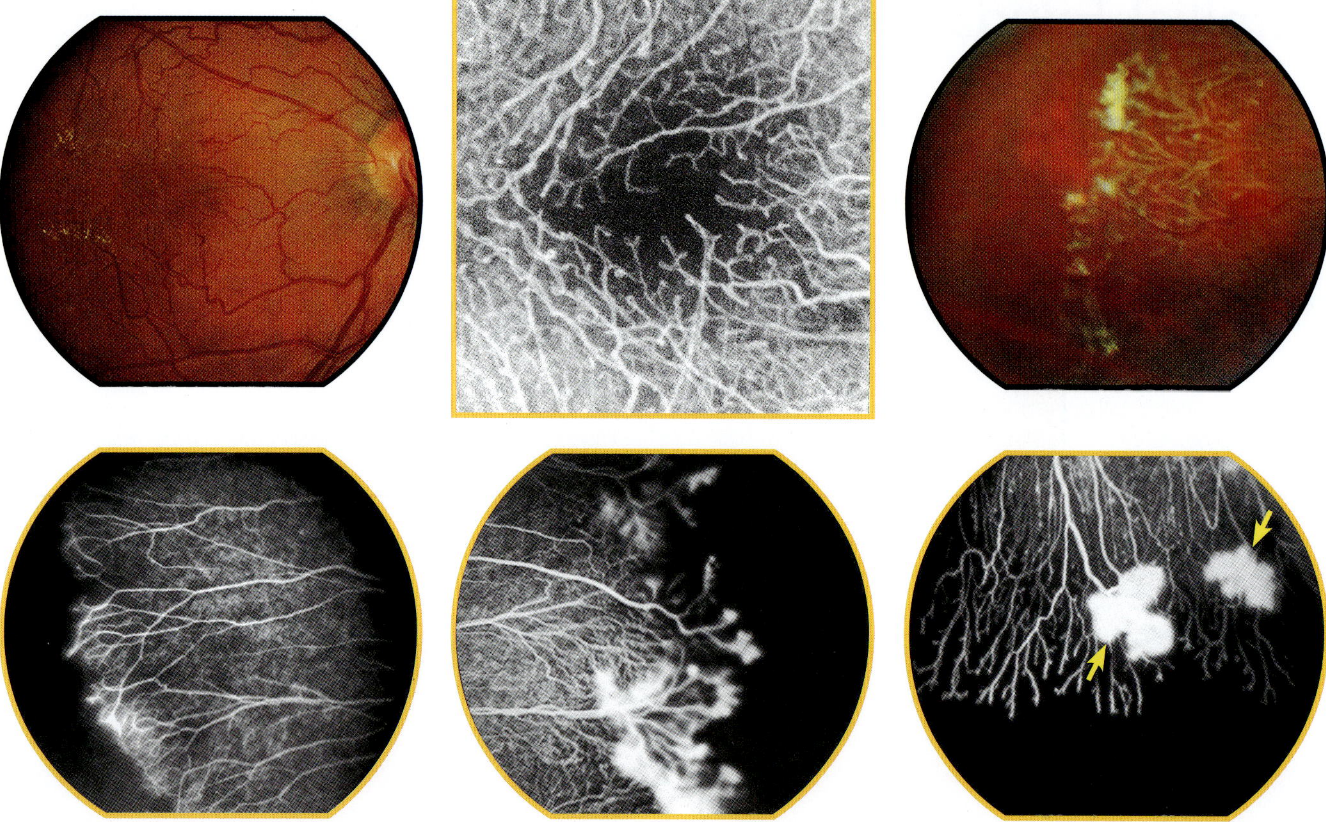

Fluorescein angiography is helpful in making a diagnosis of FEVR. Note the peculiar perifoveal capillaries which appear to have blunted endings rather than a network of communicating capillaries *(top row, middle)*. Peripheral ischemia leads to neovascularization and exudative detachment. Retinal capillaries appear to be dragged to the periphery where there is an abrupt, ischemic zone. Neovascularization may appear at the junction between perfused and non-perfused retina and well into the perfused zone *(arrows). Top row left and middle images courtesy of Dr. Alessandro Schirru, second row left and middle images courtesy of Dr. James Augsberger*

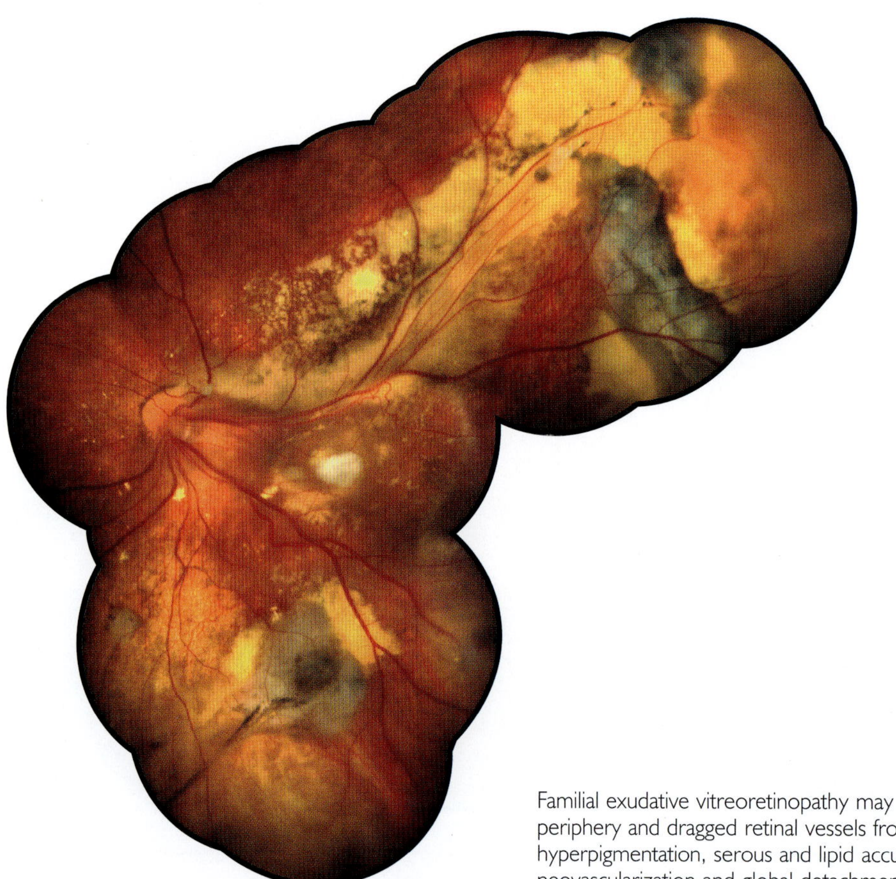

Familial exudative vitreoretinopathy may first show evidence of lipid accumulation in the periphery and dragged retinal vessels from the optic nerve, as seen in this patient; hyperpigmentation, serous and lipid accumulation under the retina and even preretinal neovascularization and global detachment may also develop.

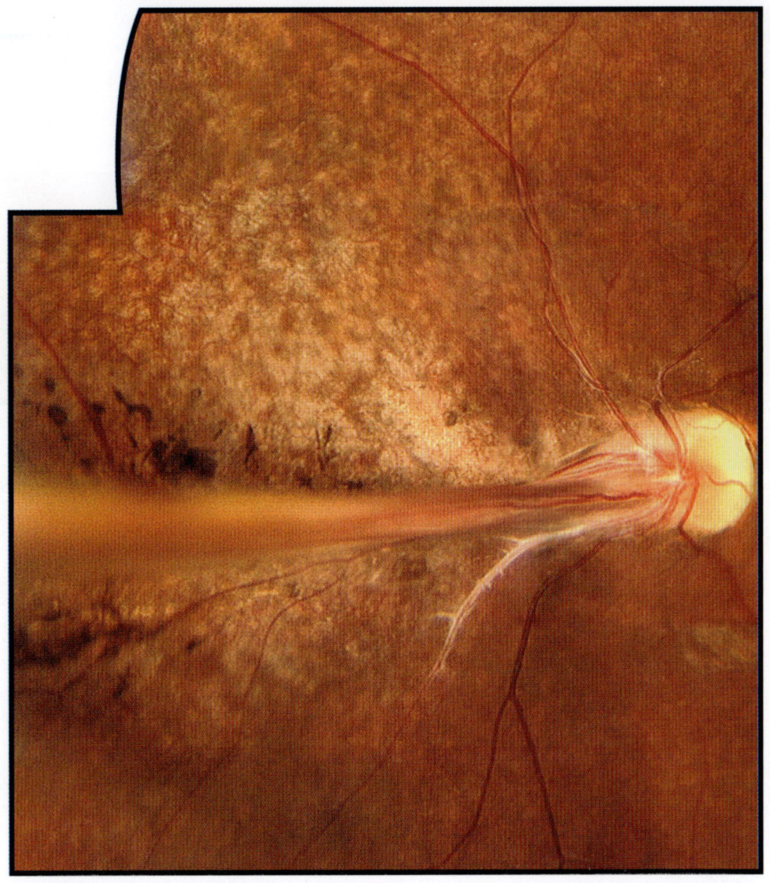
© 17

Note the retinal fold extending from the disc margin to the far periphery, where there are pigment epithelial and retinal vascular abnormalities.

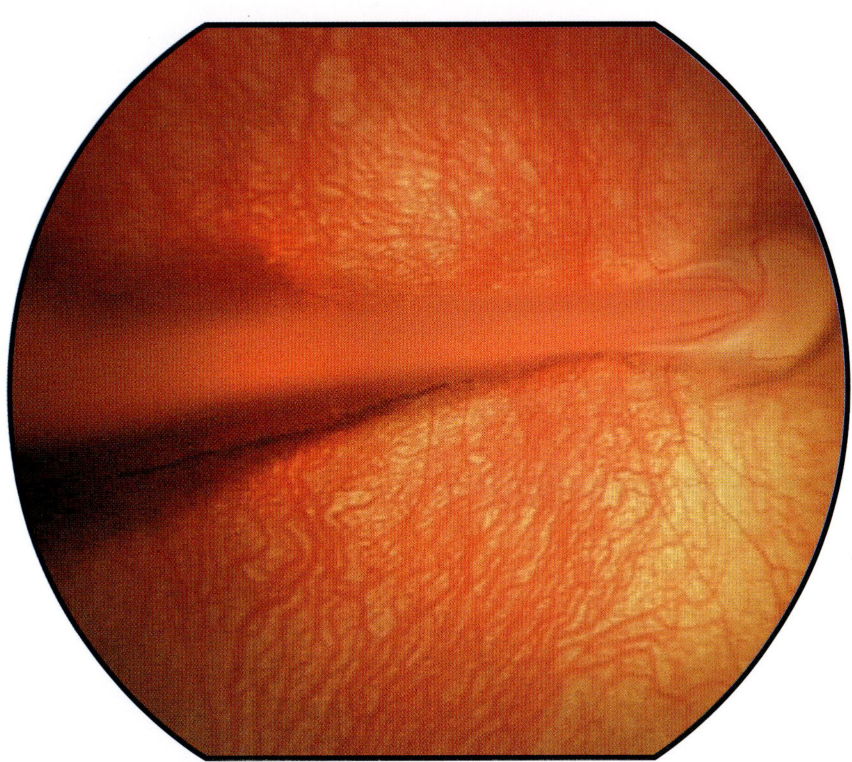

A large temporal retinal fold coursing through the macula is seen in the right eye of this 5-month-old boy with FEVR.

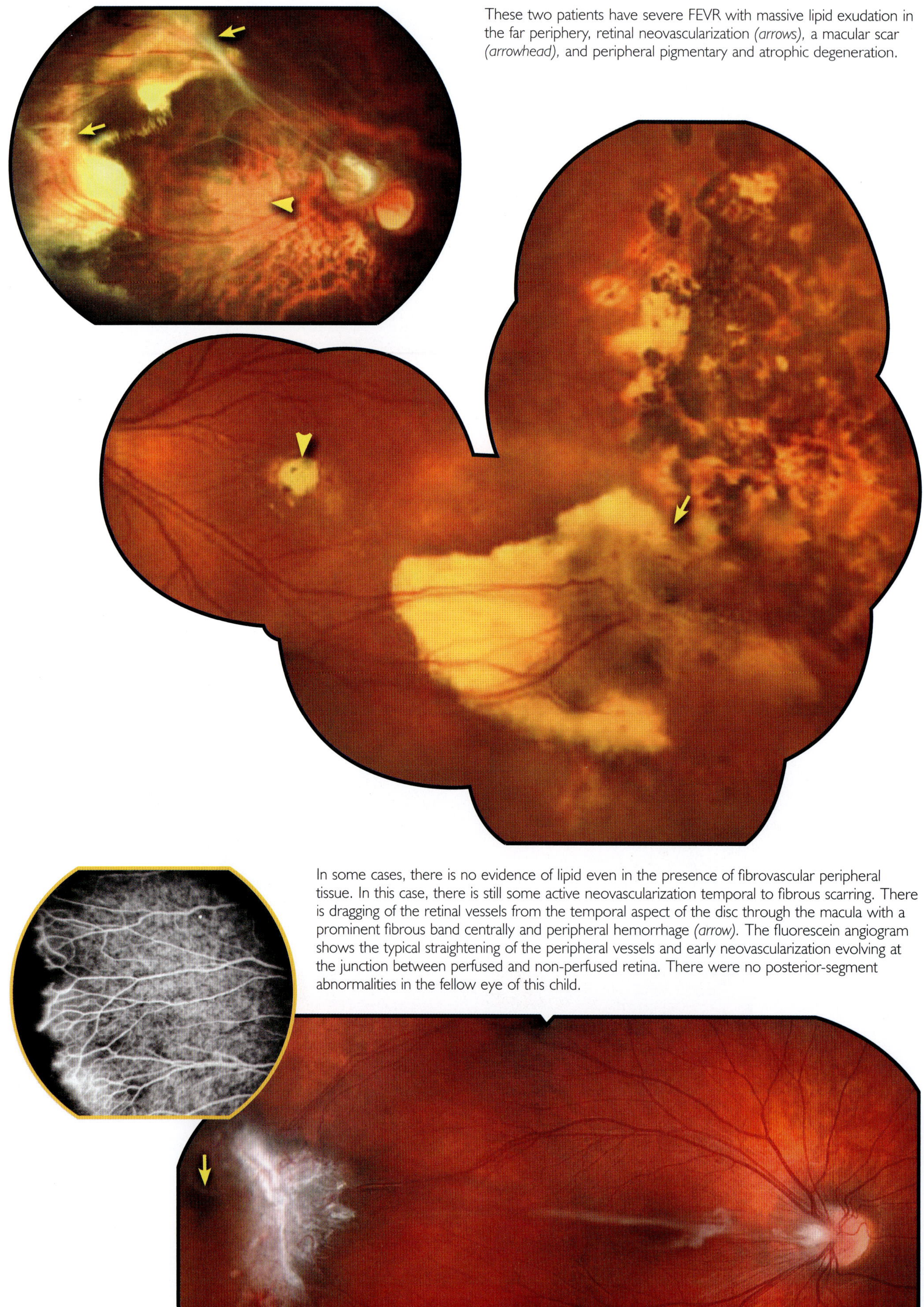

These two patients have severe FEVR with massive lipid exudation in the far periphery, retinal neovascularization *(arrows)*, a macular scar *(arrowhead)*, and peripheral pigmentary and atrophic degeneration.

In some cases, there is no evidence of lipid even in the presence of fibrovascular peripheral tissue. In this case, there is still some active neovascularization temporal to fibrous scarring. There is dragging of the retinal vessels from the temporal aspect of the disc through the macula with a prominent fibrous band centrally and peripheral hemorrhage *(arrow)*. The fluorescein angiogram shows the typical straightening of the peripheral vessels and early neovascularization evolving at the junction between perfused and non-perfused retina. There were no posterior-segment abnormalities in the fellow eye of this child.

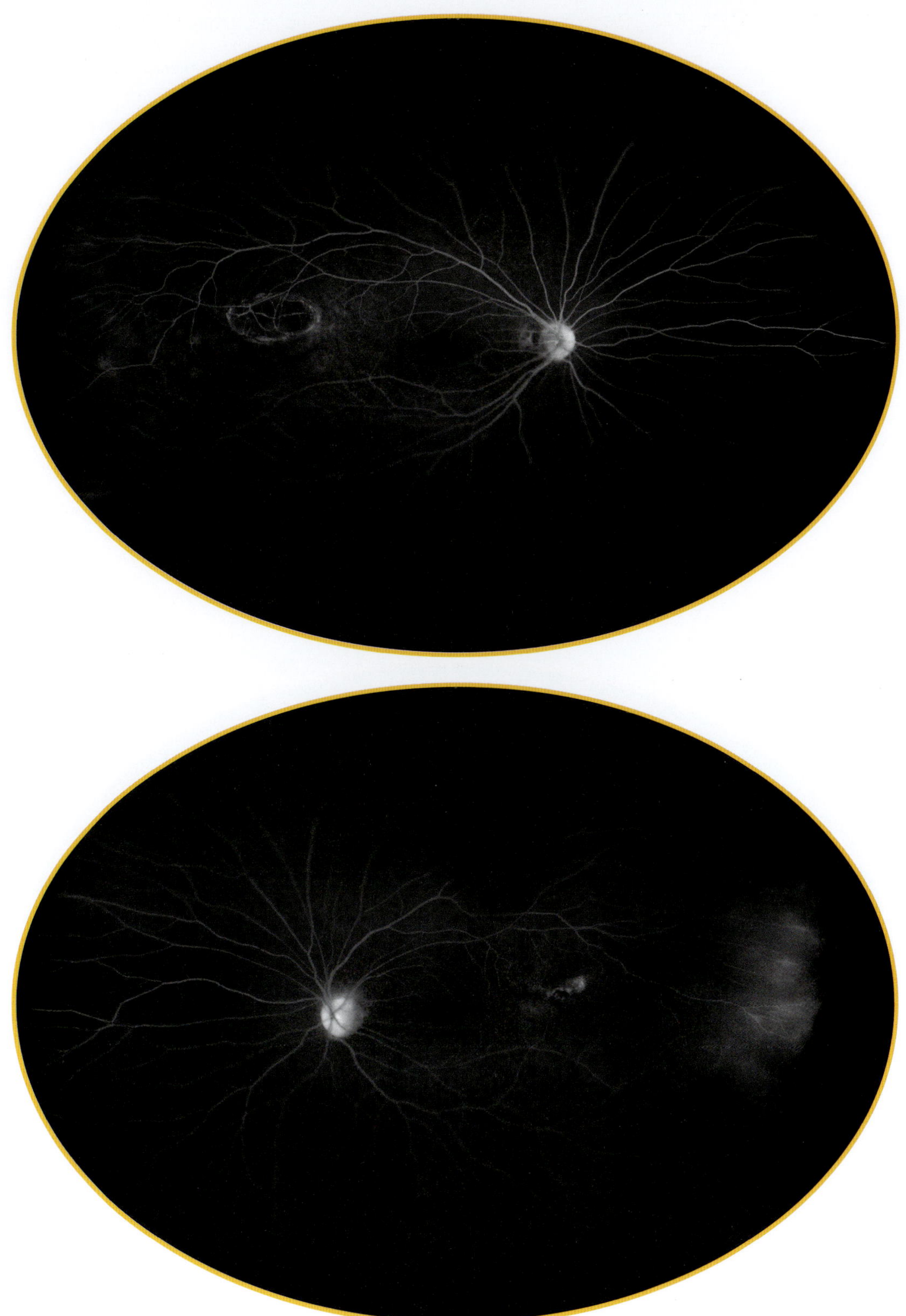

Widefield fluorescein angiography of a 14-year-old female diagnosed with FEVR showing peripheral retinal ischemia and leakage.

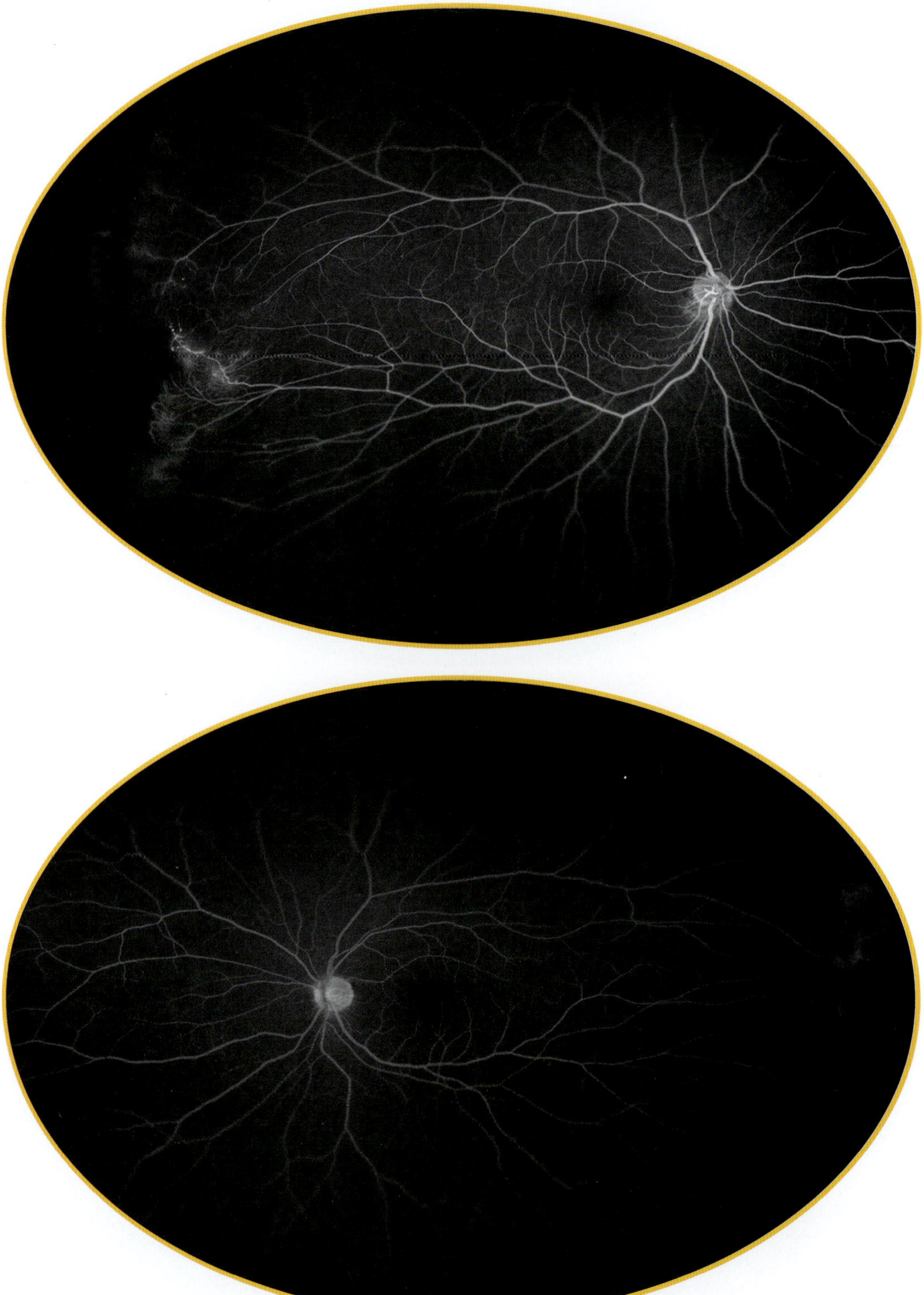

Widefield FA of asymptomatic sibling (of patient above) with similar abnormalities of FEVR.

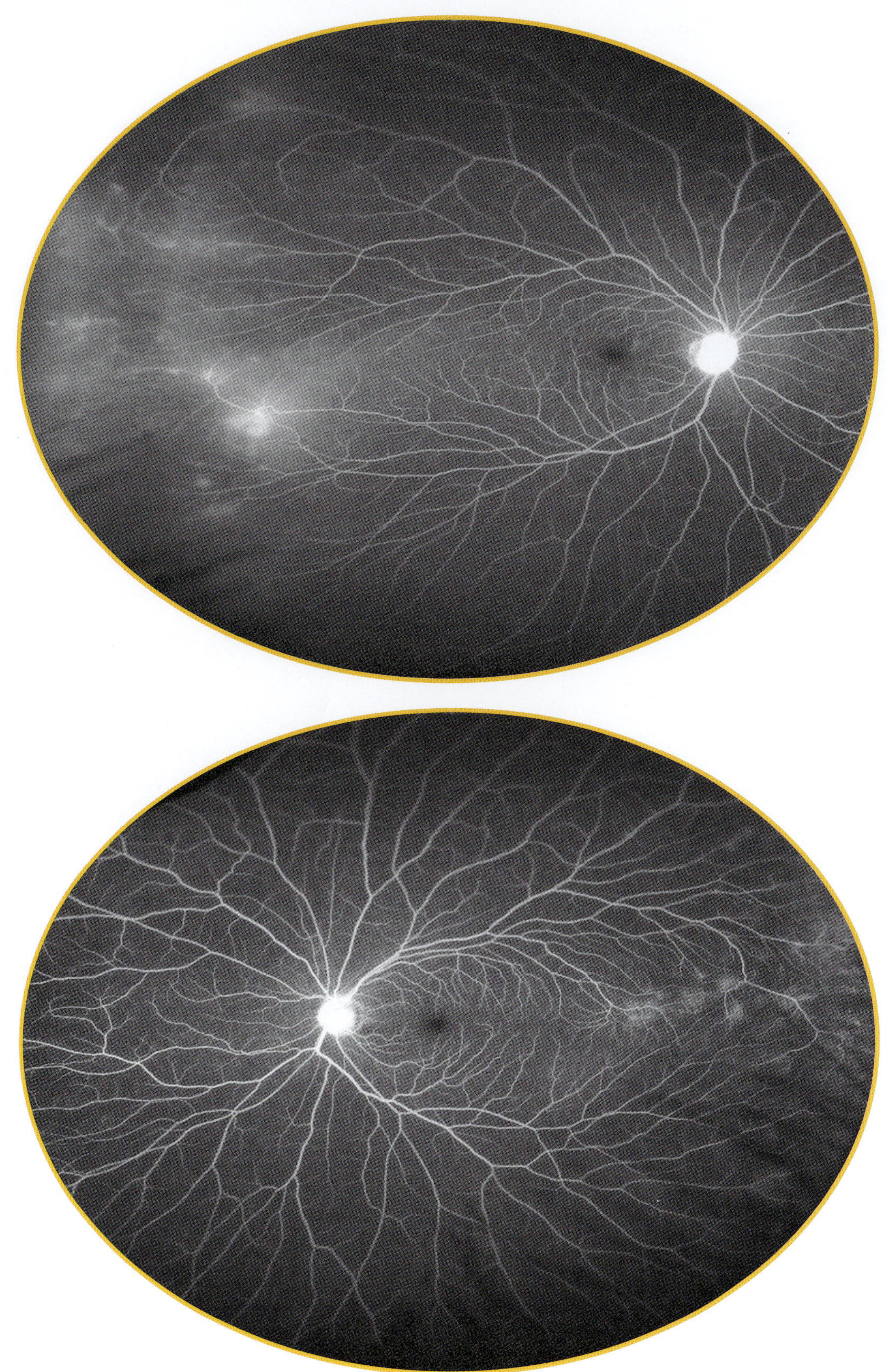

Widefield FA of asymptomatic mother of patients above with findings consistent with FEVR.

FEVR with Norrie's Gene

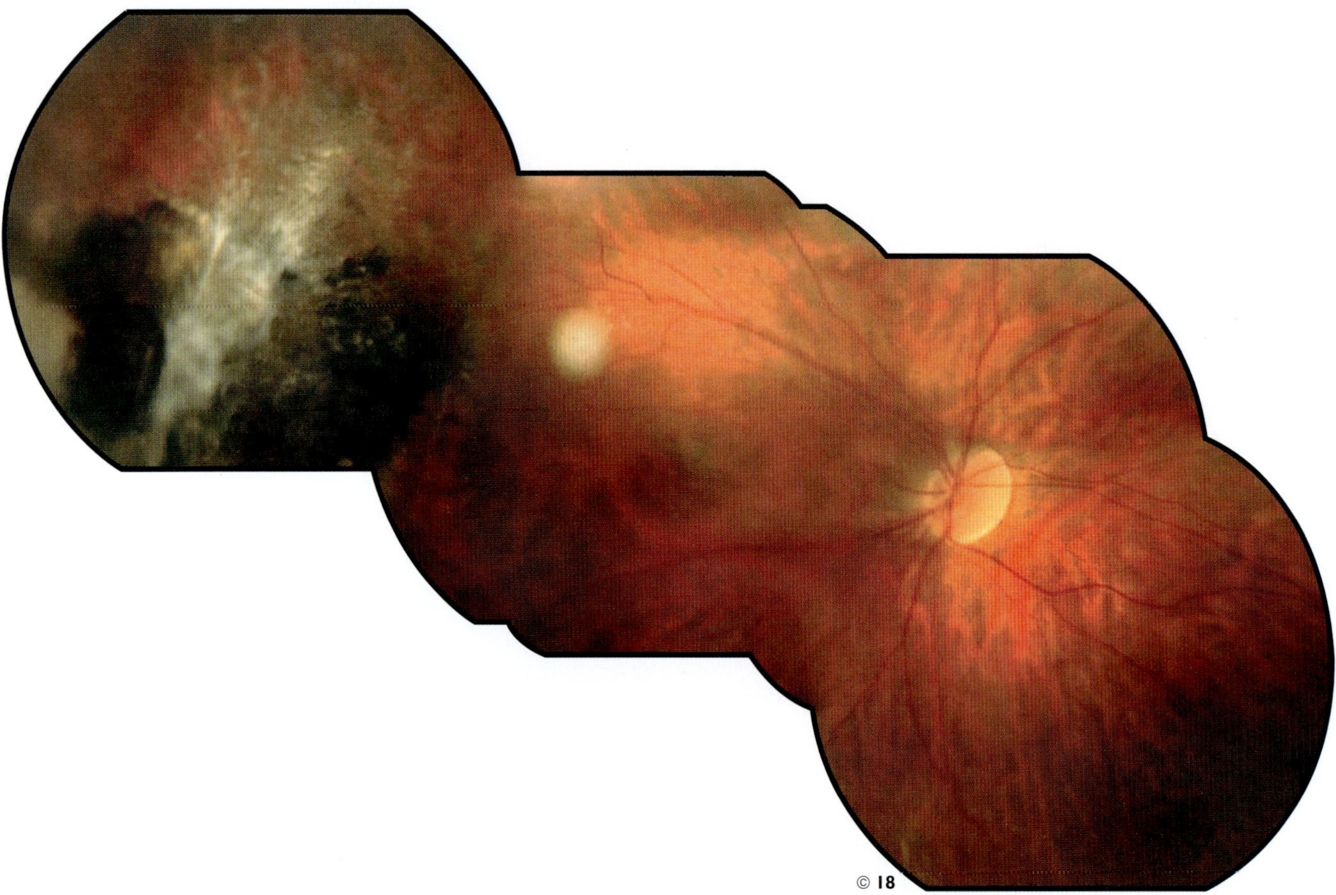

Some patients with FEVR carry the Norrie's gene. This patient originally presented with an extensive exudative peripheral detachment, which was treated with ablative therapy. The retina is now attached with pigment epithelial hyperplasia surrounding fibrotic changes. A signature phenotype for Norrie's gene does not exist.

Incontinentia Pigmenti

Incontinentia pigmenti (IP) is a rare X-linked dominant generalized ectodermal dysplasia affecting the skin, CNS, eyes and teeth. It results from a mutation in the NEMO gene, which is needed for proper functioning of nuclear factor kappa beta. This mutation is nearly uniformly fatal in males. The disease has characteristic skin findings beginning at birth. In at least 30% of cases, there is ocular involvement. The most serious ocular manifestations occur as a result of retinal ischemia, which may progress to neovascularization, fibrosis, and tractional retinal detachment in up to 20% of patients. Peripheral retinal findings may appear similar to that in ROP with large areas of avascular retina. Other ocular abnormalities include nystagmus, strabismus, myopia, cataract, diffuse mottling of the retina and retinal pigment epithelium (RPE), and optic atrophy. Alopecia, dental hypoplasia, spastic paralysis, and mental retardation may complicate 30% of cases.

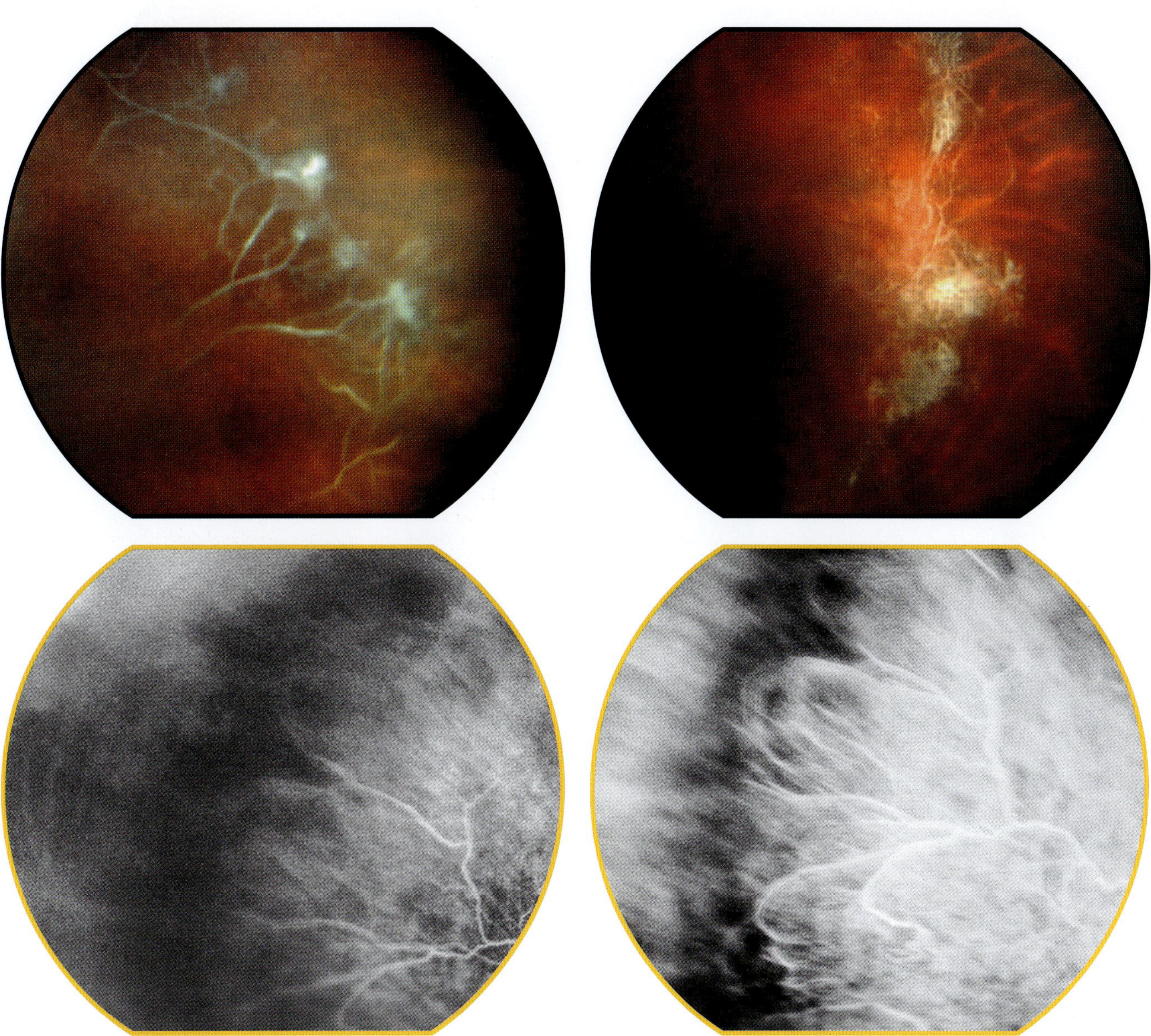

The principal ocular problem in incontinentia pigmenti involves the retina. There may be peripheral ischemia, as seen here in this patient, and neovascularization. The fluorescein angiogram shows the obliterated capillaries in the far periphery. The color images demonstrate tortuous and fibrotic preretinal neovascularization.

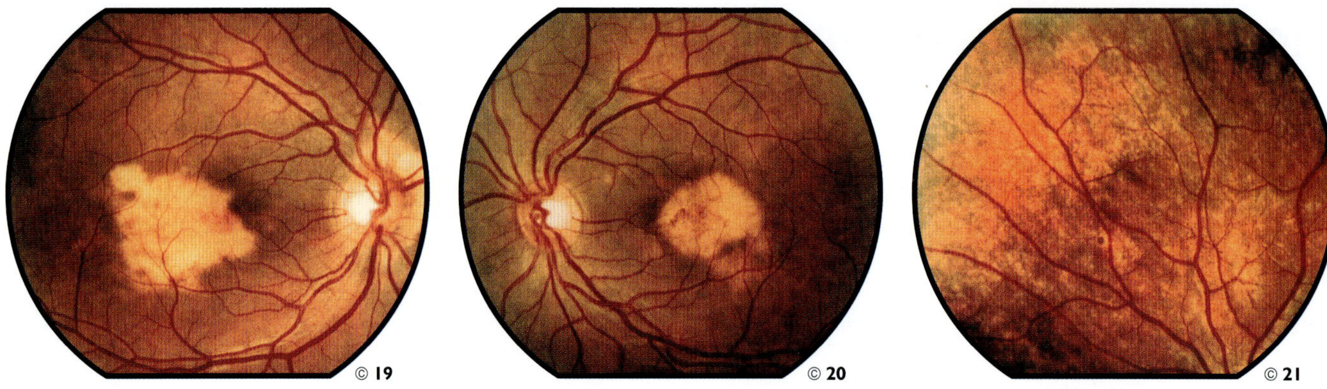

Retinal pigment epithelial granular pigmentation has been described in patients with incontinentia pigmenti, and placoid pigment epithelial atrophy has also been reported in one case of incontinentia pigmenti, as seen above.

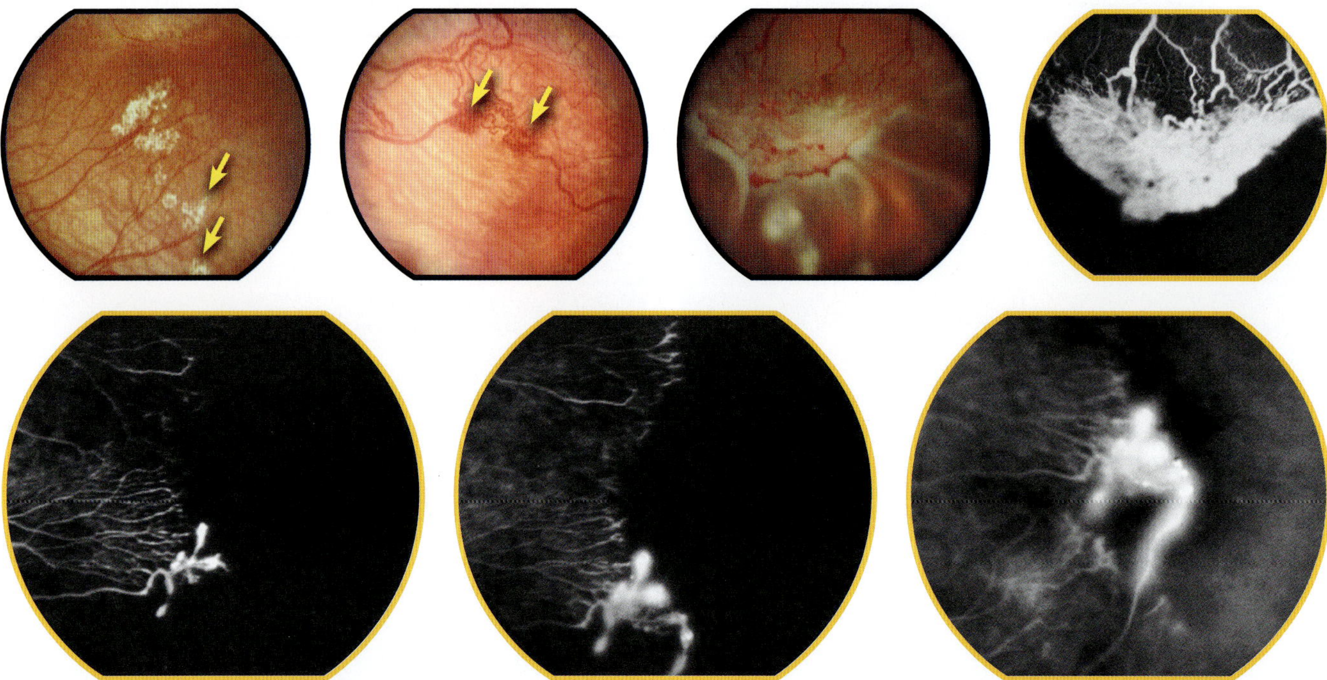

These patients with IP have peripheral retinal ischemia and neovascularization *(arrows)*. Extensive neovascularization is evident in this patient with IP, at the junction between perfused and non-perfused retina in the peripheral fundus (see fluorescein angiogram). Late staining can also be seen. Note the straightening of the peripheral vasculature and the prominence of the capillary bed. Familial exudative vitreoretinopathy may be indistinguishable from these angiographic changes.

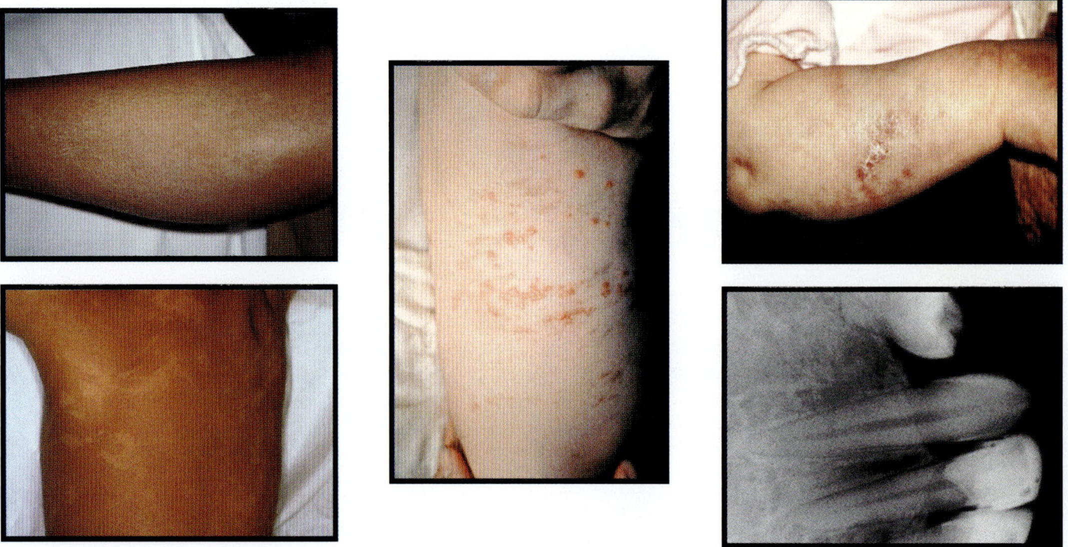

These patients with IP have patchy hypopigmentation, blistering erythematous cutaneous lesions, and dental hypoplasia.

Norrie Disease

Norrie disease is an X-linked recessive disorder caused by mutation in the NDP gene on Xp11.4, which leads to poor development and vascularization of the retina. Affected males typically present in infancy with leukocoria and severe bilateral vision loss. Funduscopic examination may reveal a total or subtotal retinal detachment often with associated disorganized, avascular retina sometimes referred to as "pseudoglioma." Persistent fetal vasculature and vitreous hemorrhage may also be present. Anterior segment manifestations include iris atrophy, elevated intraocular pressures, and corneal opacities. Systemic manifestations include progressive sensorineural hearing loss in nearly all affected individuals, and developmental delay in 30–50% of affected individuals. The carrier female may also demonstrate retinal abnormalities or mild hearing loss. A less severe mutation in NDP leading to decreased but not absent levels of the gene product is implicated in X-linked recessive FEVR. Some authors have reported success in treating patients who present without total retinal detachment with prophylactic retinal photocoagulation in order to prevent further vision loss due to retinal detachment.

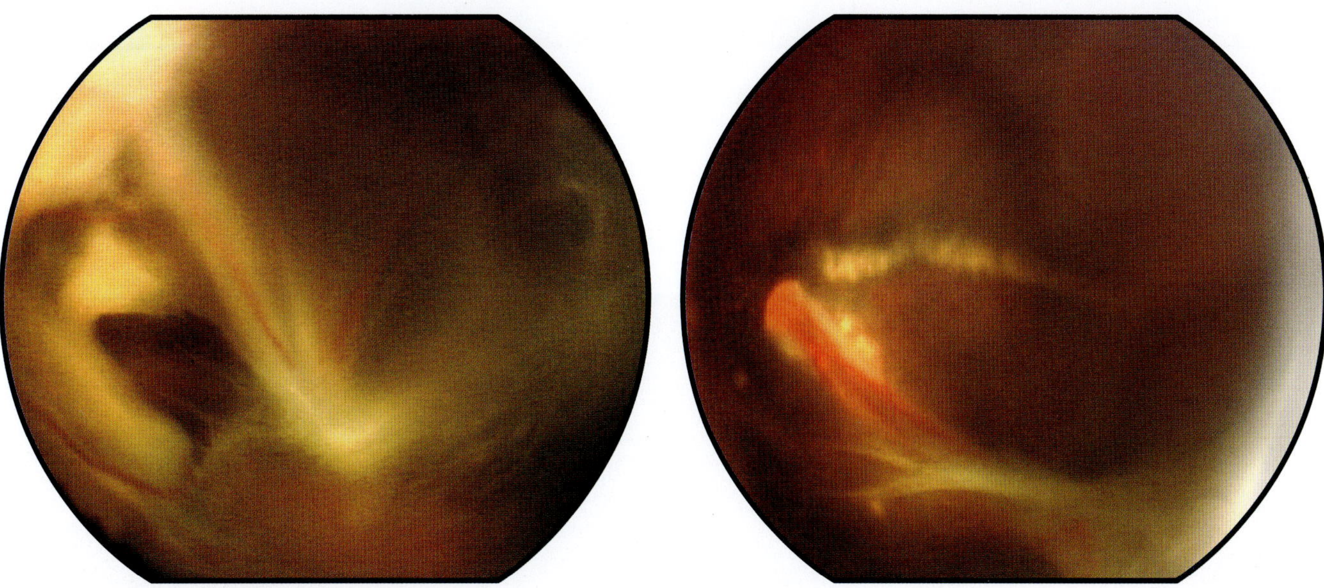

In these patients with Norrie disease, there is extensive dysplasia of the retina. Retinal detachment, fibrous traction, and overall disorganization of the posterior fundus are seen in each patient.

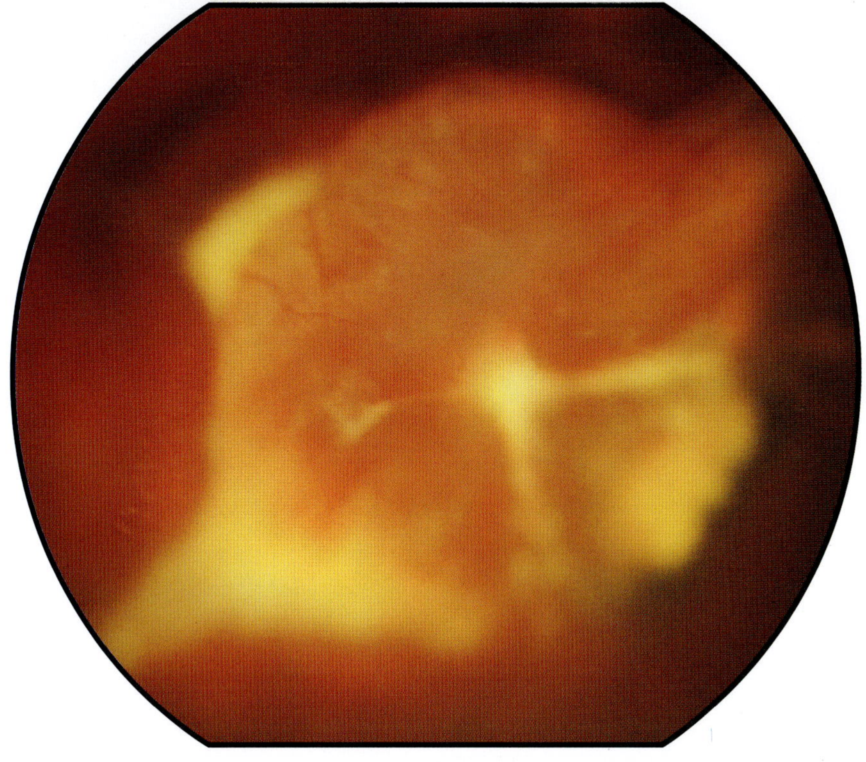

This montage of a patient with Norrie disease shows massive disorganization of the retina with an irregular-shaped detachment, lipid exudation, and fibrovascular proliferation. *Courtesy of Dr. Mark Walsh*

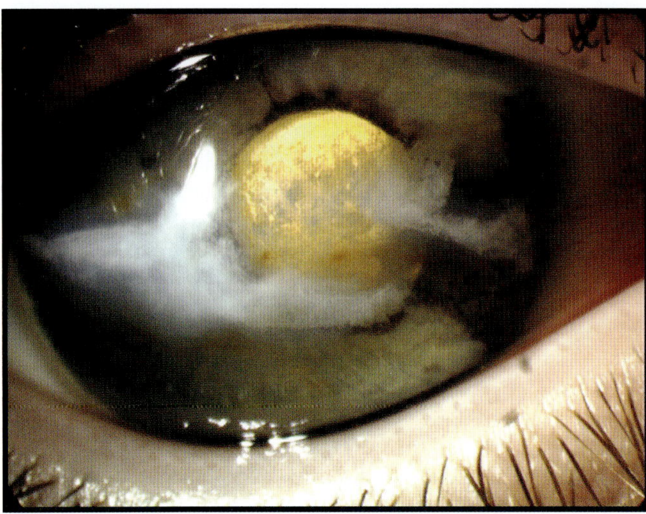

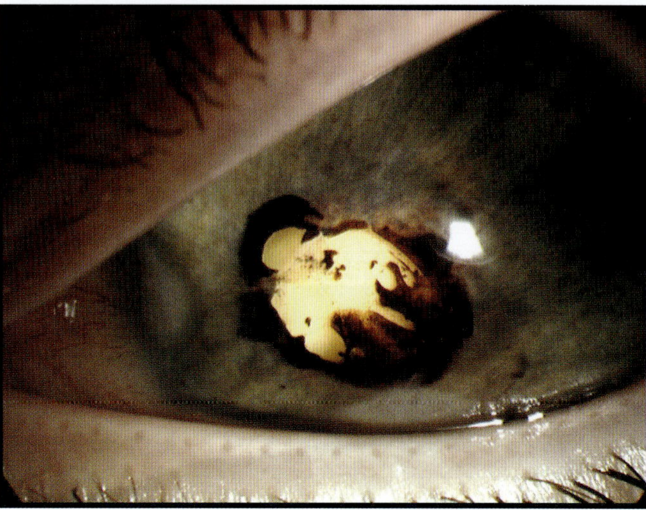

Patients with Norrie disease may present with leukocoria. Note the cornea leukoma, the mature lens cataract, and the pigment epithelial proliferation at the margins of the pupil. *Courtesy of Dr. Anthony Moore*

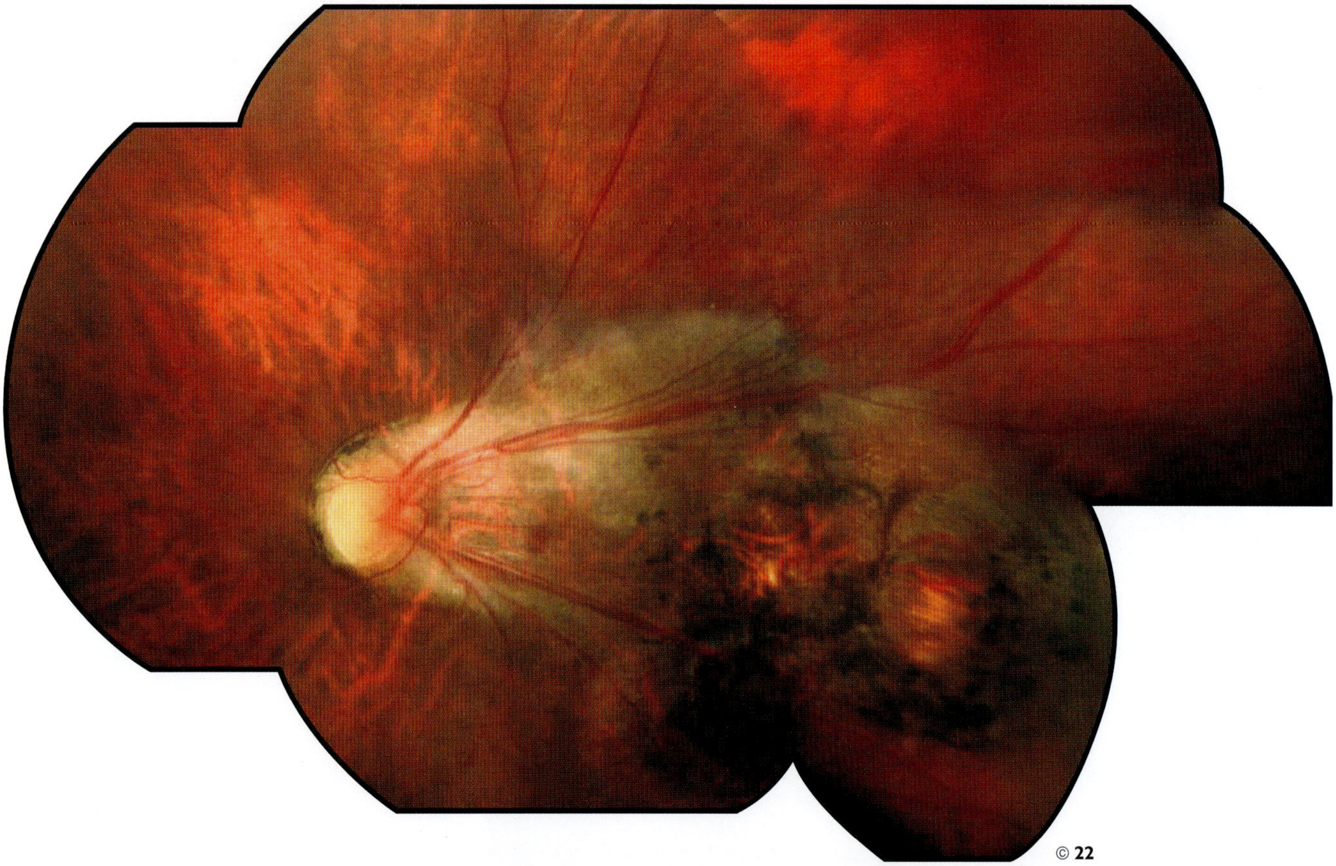

This patient is a female carrier of Norrie disease. She has a disorganized fundus that appears limited to the posterior pole. Note the dragging of the blood vessels, the fibrous proliferation, the atrophy, and pigment epithelial hyperplasia.

Facioscapulohumeral Muscular Dystrophy

Facioscapulohumeral muscular dystrophy (FSHD) is the third most common type of muscular dystrophy after Duchenne and myotonic muscular dystrophy and is characterized by a mutation localized to chromosome 4q35. It is an autosomal dominant disease in 70–90% of patients and is sporadic in the remainder. The clinical features of this condition range from minimally detectable myopathy to severe disability. There is a characteristic pattern of weakness that affects predominantly the face and shoulder muscles and later descends to involve the abdomen and the legs. Symptoms become manifest in the teen years to early adulthood and progress slowly. A variant of Coats disease with retinal telangiectasia and exudation is a common ocular finding, affecting 49–75% of patients. These findings are typically bilateral and not associated with significant visual changes; however, FSHD can rarely present with decreased visual acuity, peripheral retinal vascular ischemia, proliferative retinopathy, and even neovascular glaucoma.

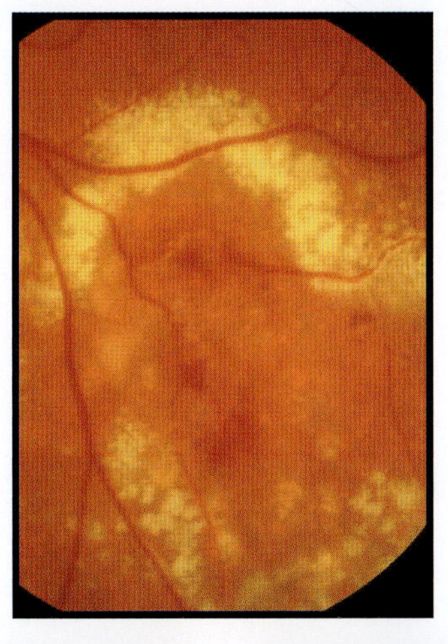

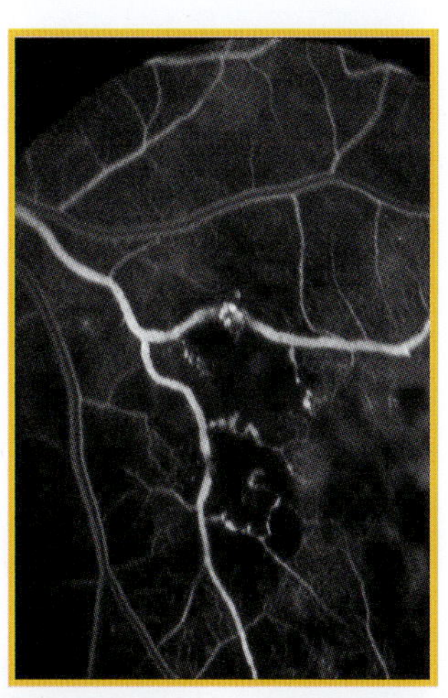

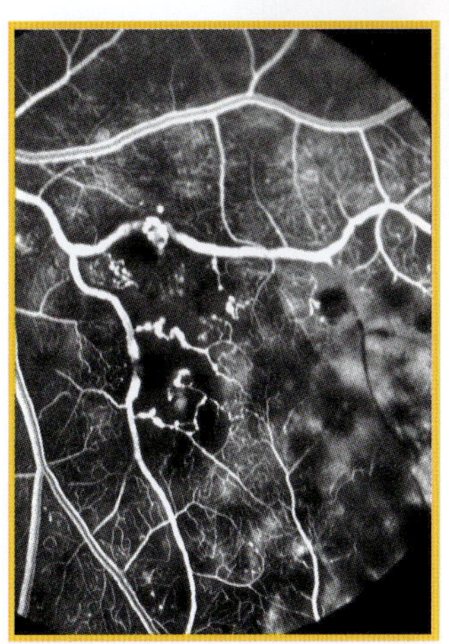

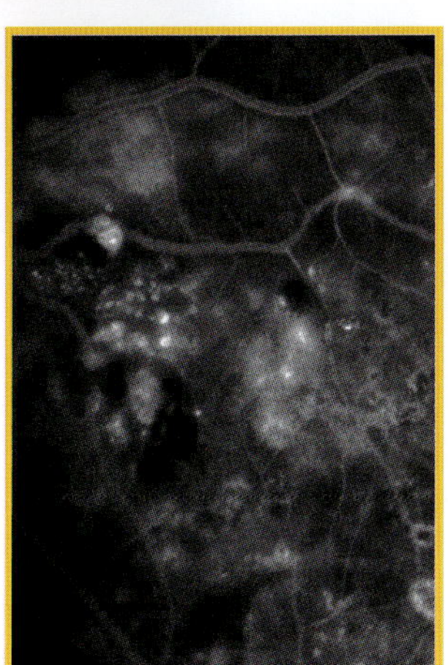

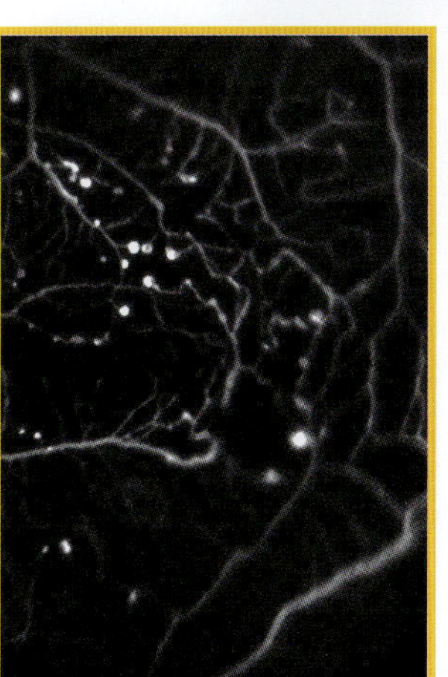

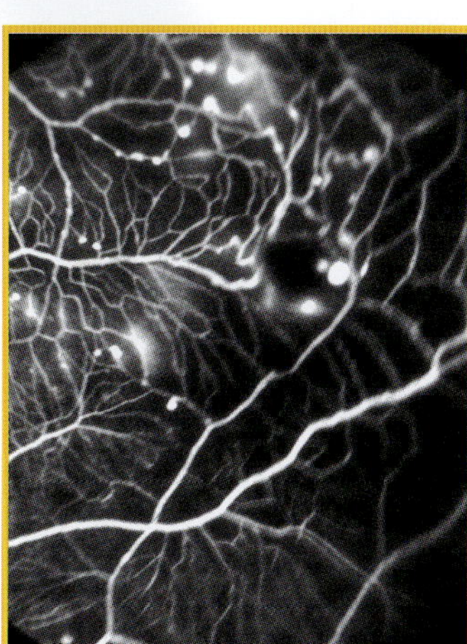

This patient has facioscapulohumeral muscular dystrophy with a Coats-like response in the retina. Note the lipid deposition surrounding the retinal abnormalities, which include telangiectasia, multiple aneurysmal changes, ischemia, and leakage.

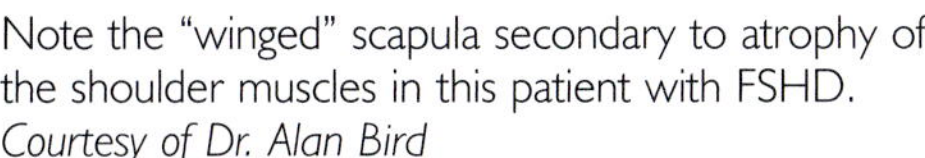

Note the "winged" scapula secondary to atrophy of the shoulder muscles in this patient with FSHD.
Courtesy of Dr. Alan Bird

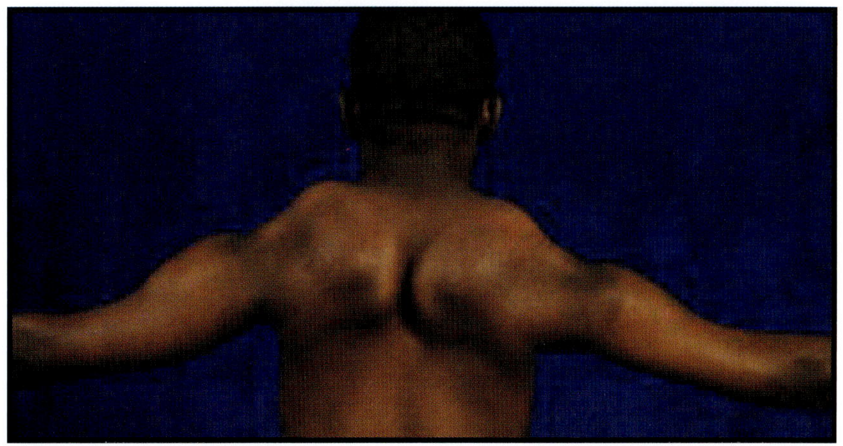

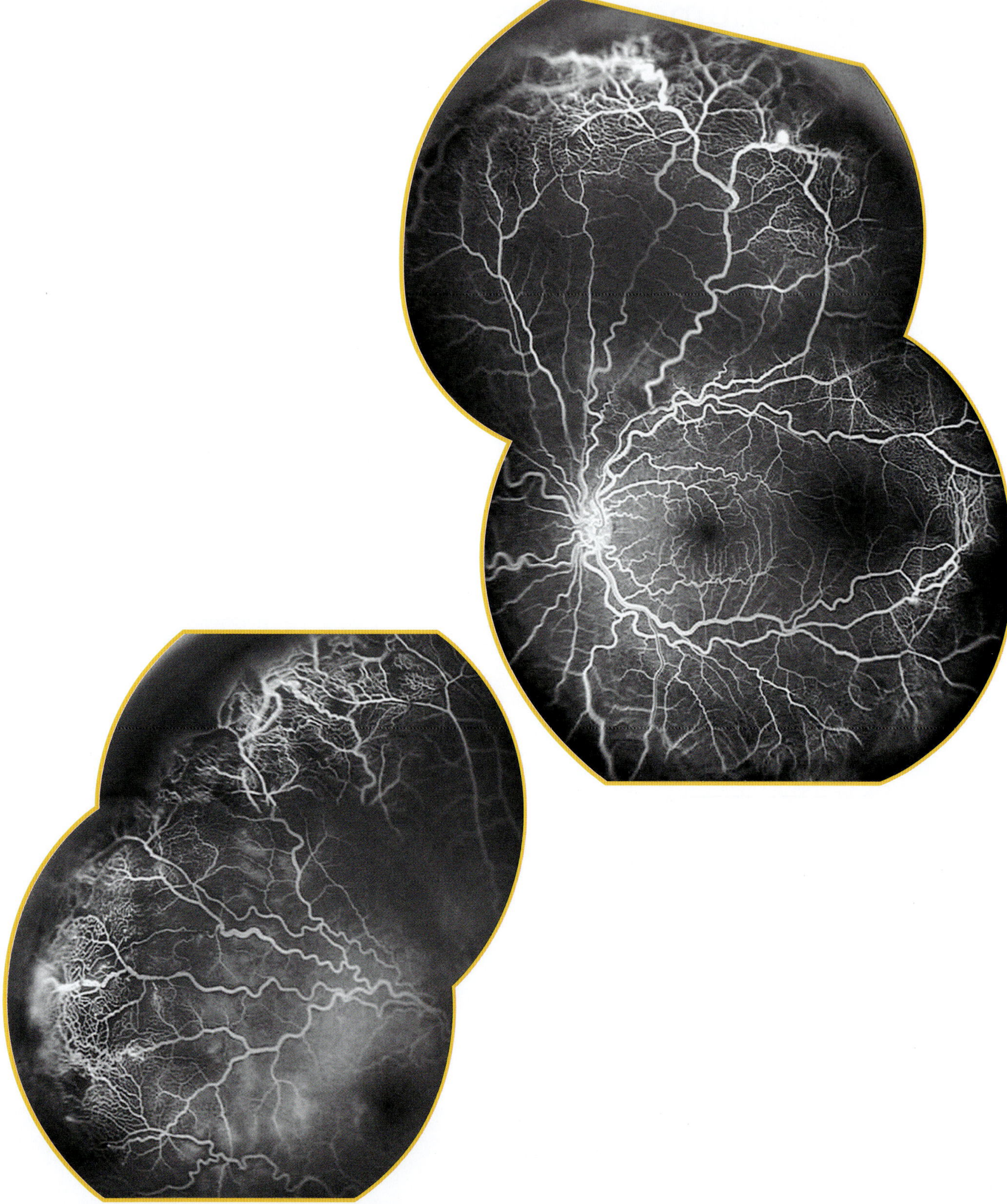

The fluorescein angiogram in this patient shows peripheral ischemia and neovascularization. At the interface between perfused and non-perfused retina, there are dilated vessels and crowding of the peripheral vasculature. Although the posterior pole in the left eye was non-revealing, the periphery indicated the presence of associated retinal vascular abnormalities. This case is referred to as infantile facioscapulohumeral muscular dystrophy with a 4q35 genetic mutation.

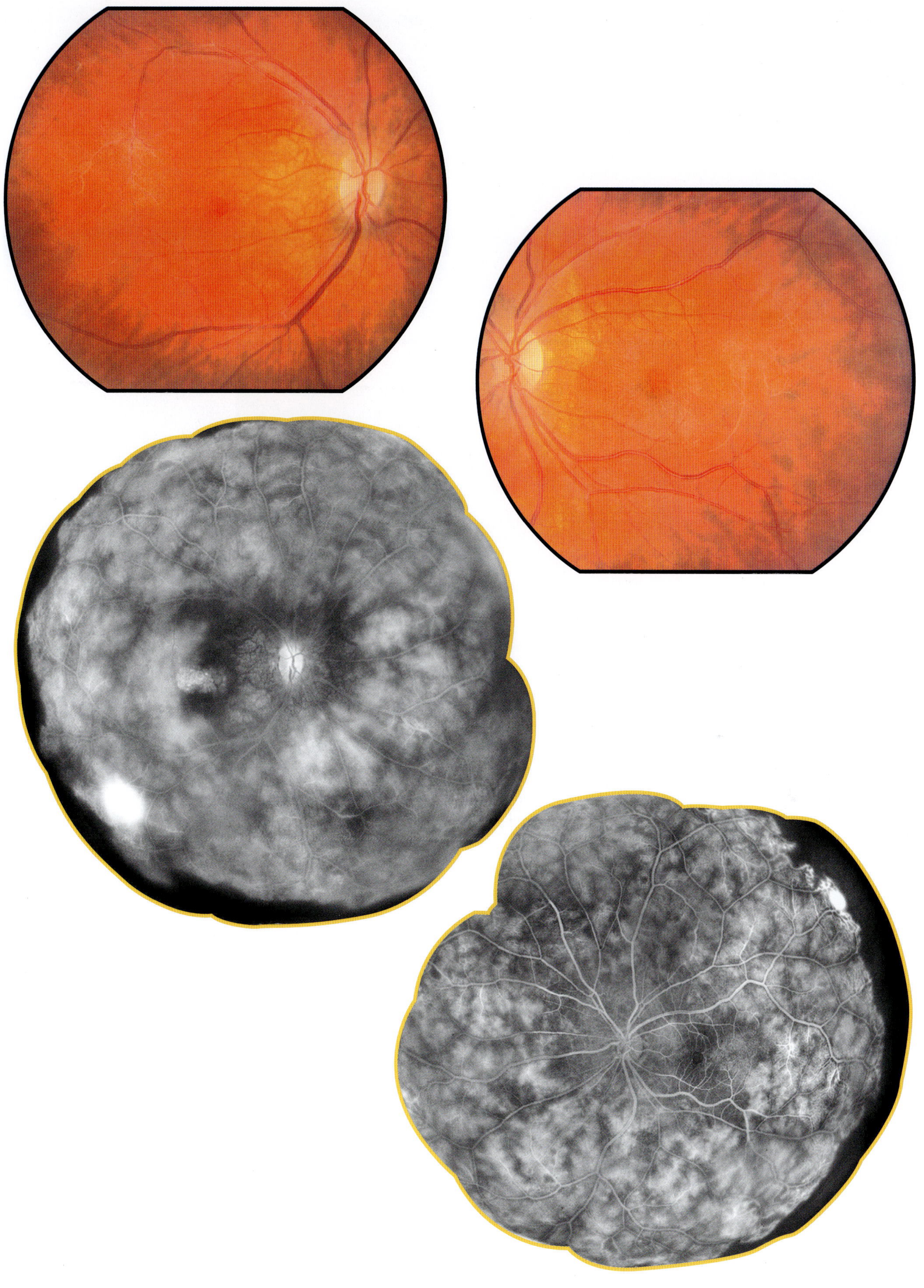

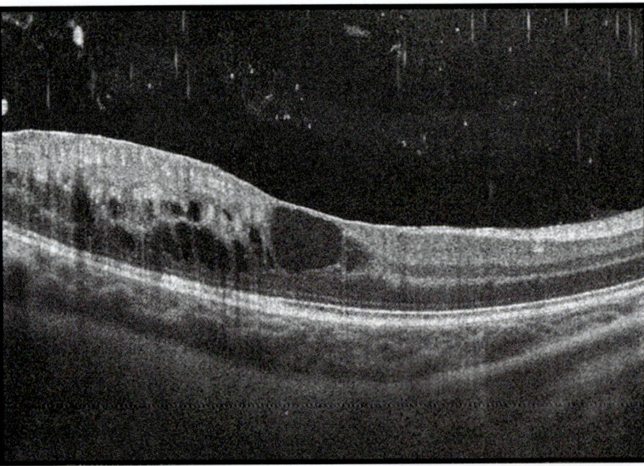

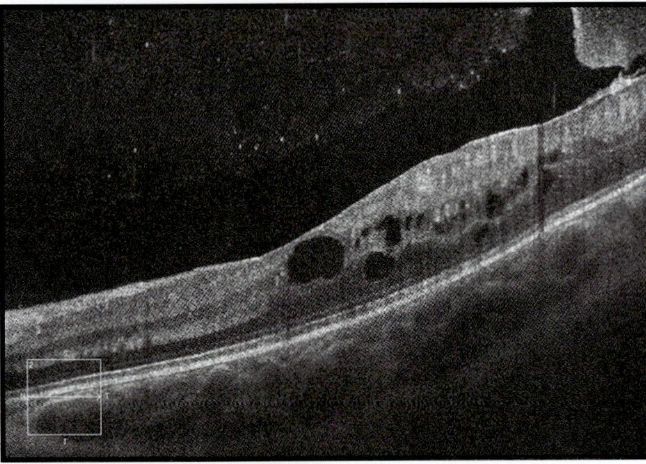

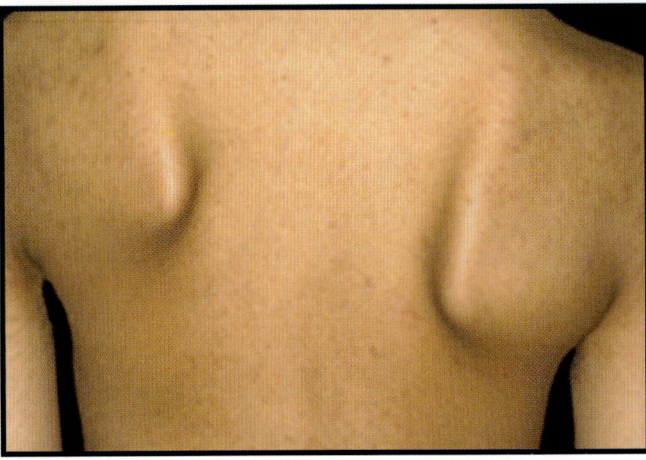

This 13-year-old boy has FSHD. Anterior segment examination was significant for neovascularization of the iris. Color fundus photos show vascular sheathing and a blunted foveal reflex. Fluorescein angiogram montage shows diffuse vascular leakage, peripheral retinal ischemia, and neovascularization in each eye. There is bilateral macular edema on SD-OCT. Physical examination revealed winged scapula. *Images courtesy of Sara J. Haug MD, PhD and H. Richard McDonald, MD*

Parry–Rhomberg Syndrome

Parry–Rhomberg syndrome is a rare craniofacial disorder characterized by slowly progressive unilateral atrophy involving the soft tissues of half of the face. Onset of the disease is usually in preadolescent years with progression for 2–10 years often followed by stabilization. The facial changes will often begin with the tissues above the upper maxilla or between the nose and lip and progress to involve the angle of the mouth, areas around the eye and brow, and the ear and neck. Dermatologic findings include vitiligo, poliosis, alopecia, and areas of hyperpigmentation. There is also an association with a localized, linear form of scleroderma affecting the forehead known as *en coup de sabre*. Patients often experience neurological abnormalities, including prolonged headaches, trigeminal neuralgia, contralateral epilepsy, and hemiatrophy of the brain. Ocular findings include motility disturbances, lid abnormalities, lacrimal drainage obstructions, iris heterochromia, Horner syndrome, and fundus pigment changes, but most patients do not experience vision loss. When vision loss does occur, it may be related to fundus abnormalities that include ipsilateral neuroretinopathy with macular and peripapillary exudation or retinal vascular changes with telangiectasia, ischemia, neovascularization, and exudative detachment.

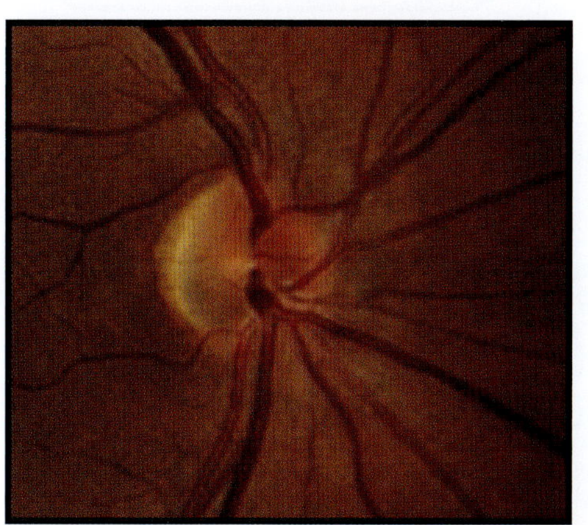

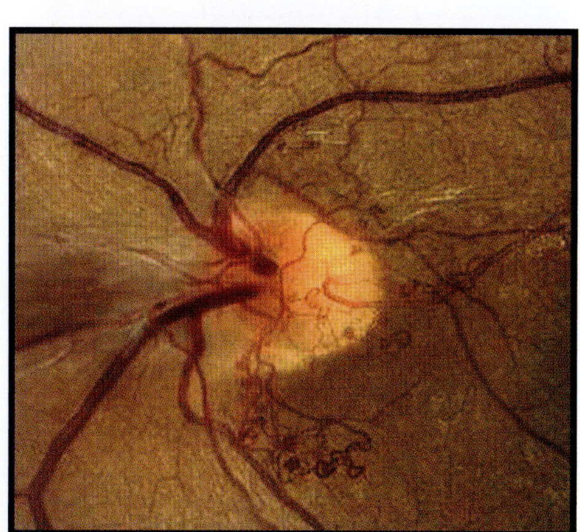

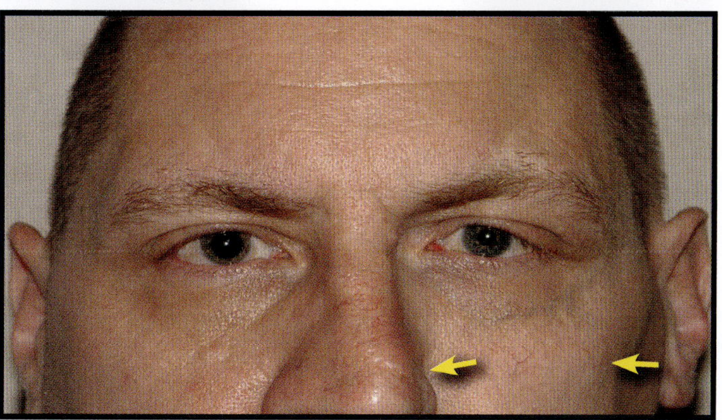

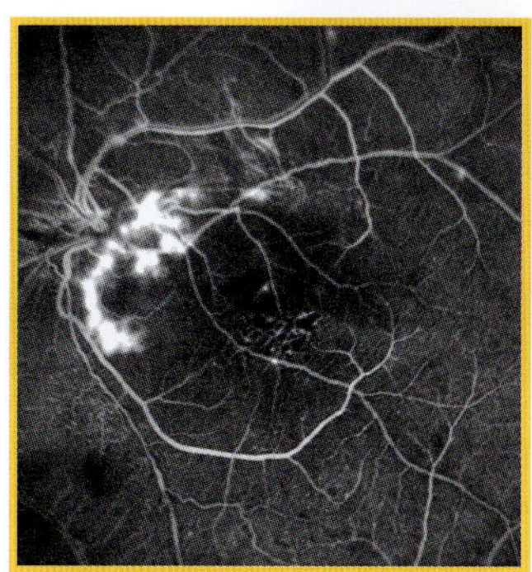

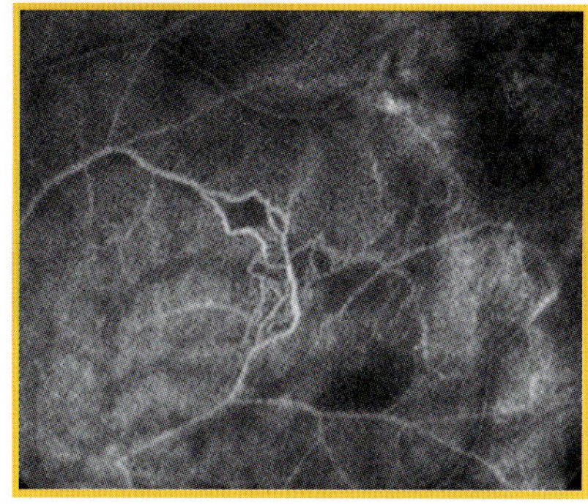

This patient with Parry–Rhomberg syndrome has hemiatrophy of the face *(arrows)*. The left eye reveals proliferating blood vessels at the disc. The right eye dilated normally, whereas the ipsilateral eye is relatively miotic from atrophy of the dilator muscle. The pupil may be pharmacologically non-reactive due to atrophy of the sphincter or dilator muscle in this disorder. Also, the iris is hazel in the right and blue in the left. The fluorescein study of the left eye demonstrates neovascularization at the disc, as seen in the photo on the lower left and ischemia in the periphery, as noted in the image on the lower right. The retinal vasculature in the right eye was normal. *Courtesy of Dr. Jose Pulido*

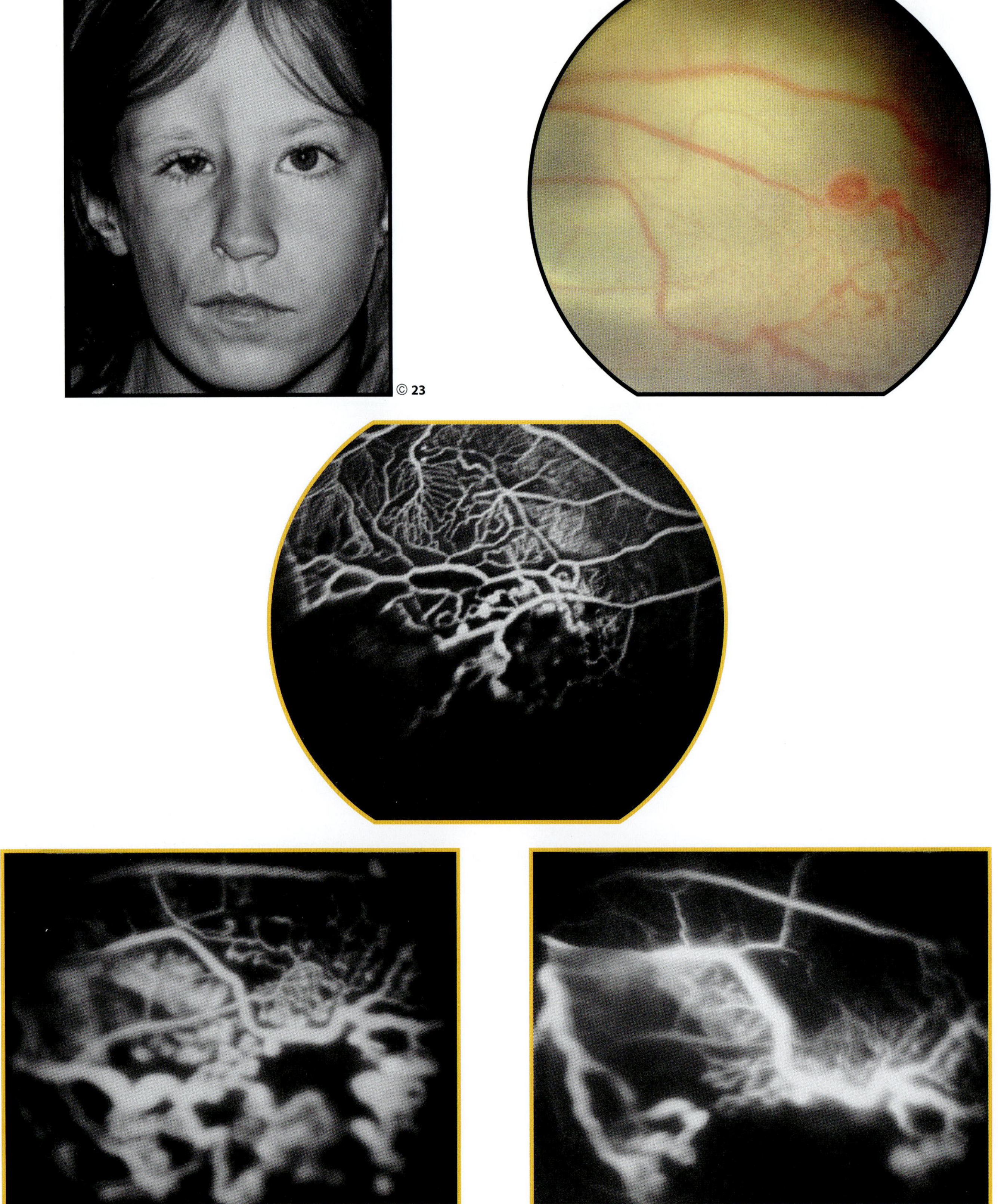

This patient with Parry–Rhomberg syndrome has hemifacial atrophy and retinal manifestations that include telangiectasia, aneurysmal formation, massive lipid exudation, ischemia, and leakage. This is indistinguishable from the congenital unilateral telangiectasia seen in Coats disease.

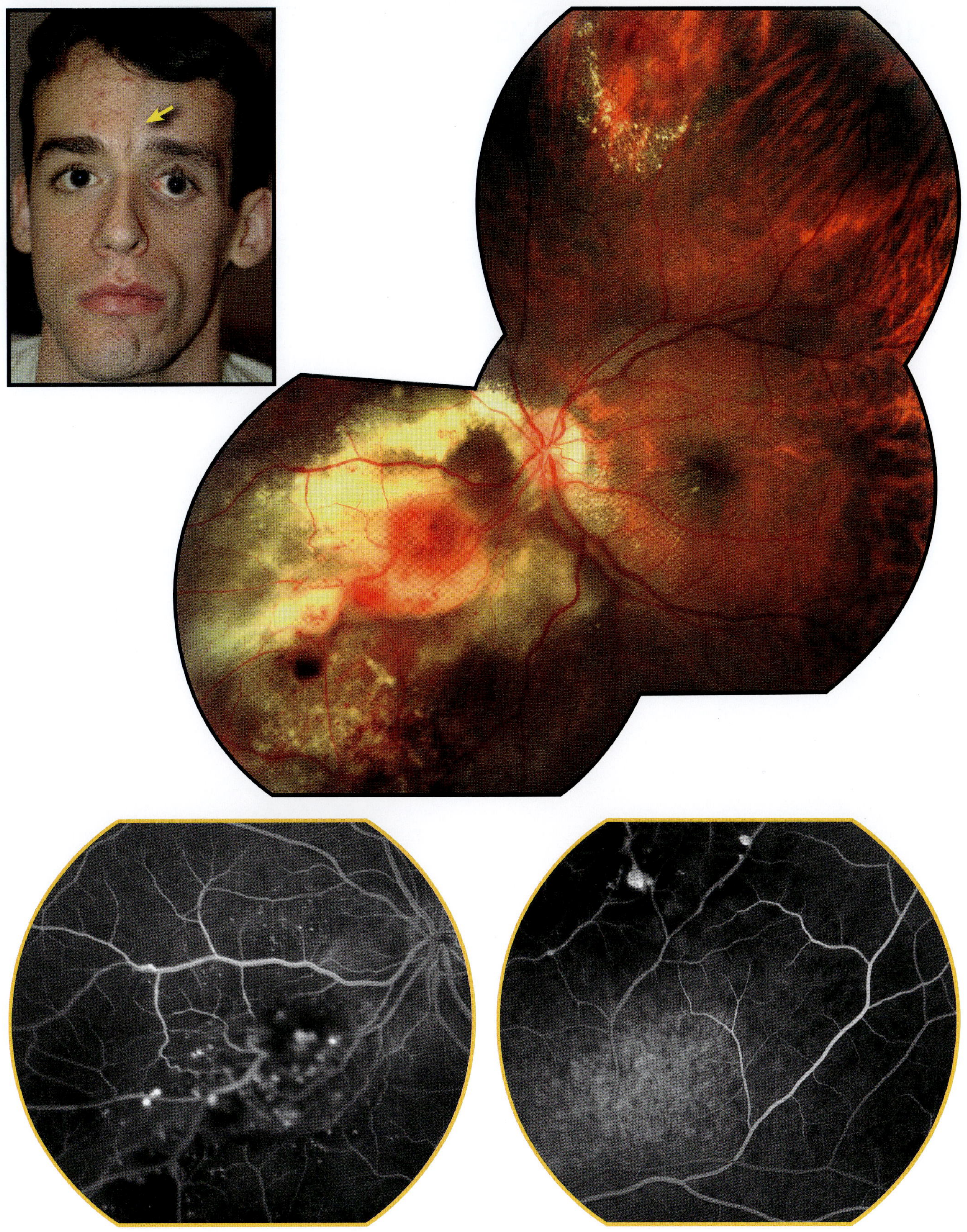

This patient with Parry–Rhomberg syndrome also has linear scleroderma confirmed by a biopsy of the hemifacial atrophy. Notice the cleft on the forehead *(arrow)*. This is commonly referred to as *en coup de sabre*. The manifestations in the fundus of the left eye are Coats-like with aneurysms, telangiectasia, heavy lipid leakage, and ischemia. *Courtesy of Dr. John J. Huang*

Duchenne Muscular Dystrophy

Duchenne muscular dystrophy is an X-linked recessive disorder caused by a mutation in the dystrophin gene localized to chromosome Xp21.2. It is characterized by progressive proximal muscular dystrophy with pseudohypertrophy of the calves and myocardium involvement. However, bulbar muscles are spared. High plasma levels of creatine kinase are seen, as well as myopathic changes on electromyography and myofiber degeneration with fibrosis and fatty infiltration on muscle biopsy. Patients begin to show symptoms before the age of 3 years old and are often wheelchair-bound by the age of 12 with death occurring by the age of 20. Dystrophin gene products are also known to localize to the retina, specifically to the presynaptic photoreceptor terminal. Its function is not completely clear, but many Duchenne patients have subtle red-green color deficits and an ERG may show an electro-negative pattern with loss of the b-wave and increased implicit times. Patients tend to have normal visual acuity, and a relatively normal fundoscopic exam with some increase in macular pigmentation. Rarely, in Duchenne patients who also have severe cardiomyopathy, there is massive proliferative retinopathy which leads to rapid and severe loss of vision, presumably due to a vasoendothelial growth factor response. Panretinal photocoagulation may be beneficial.

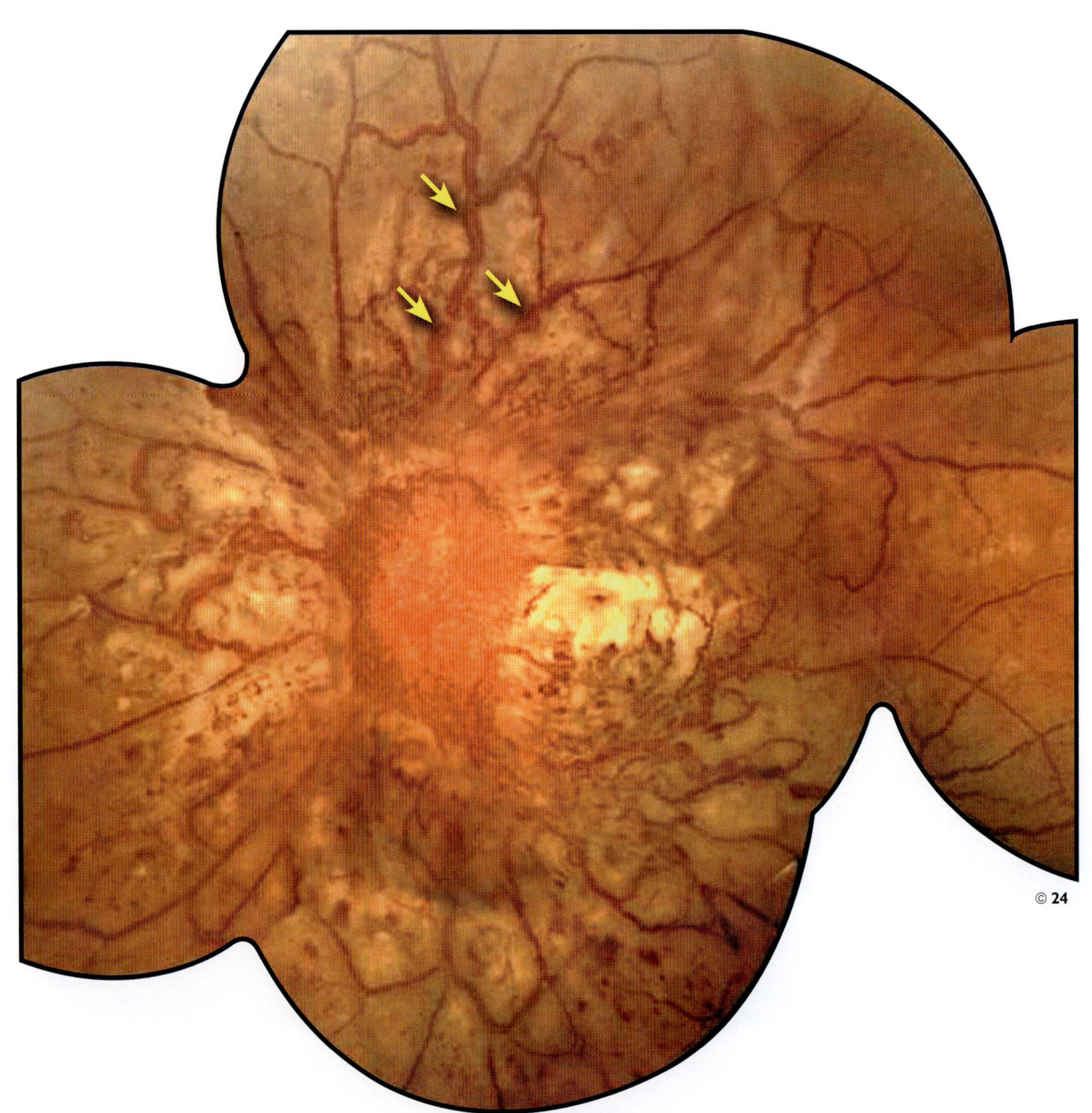

This patient has Duchenne muscular dystrophy with a rare, but known, retinal vascular proliferative abnormality. There is massive neovascularization at the disc; macular infarction and ciliary retinal vessel occlusion; and widespread retinal vascular abnormalities, including venous beading and tortuosity. Some large venules appear to have aneurysmal dilations, beading or a sausage-like configuration *(arrows)*.

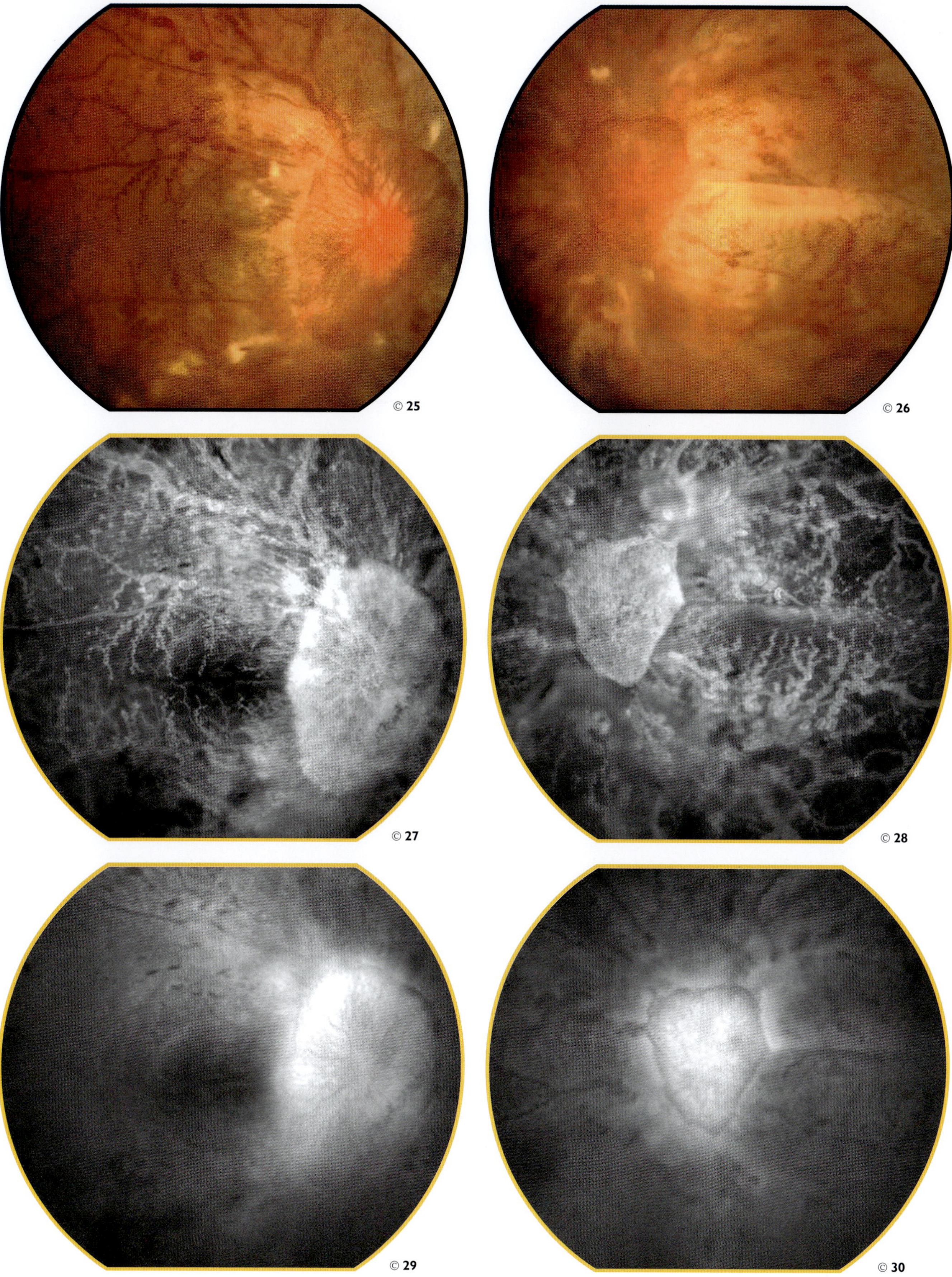

There is florid neovascularization at the disc bilaterally. The mid and late fluorescein angiograms show severe disc neovascularization bilaterally with late leakage. There are also prominent retinal vascular effects, including telangiectasia, severe venous beading, and ischemia. This vasoendothelial growth factor effect is due to cardiac hypoperfusion, the absence of an antivasogenic effect of dystrophin, and anemia.

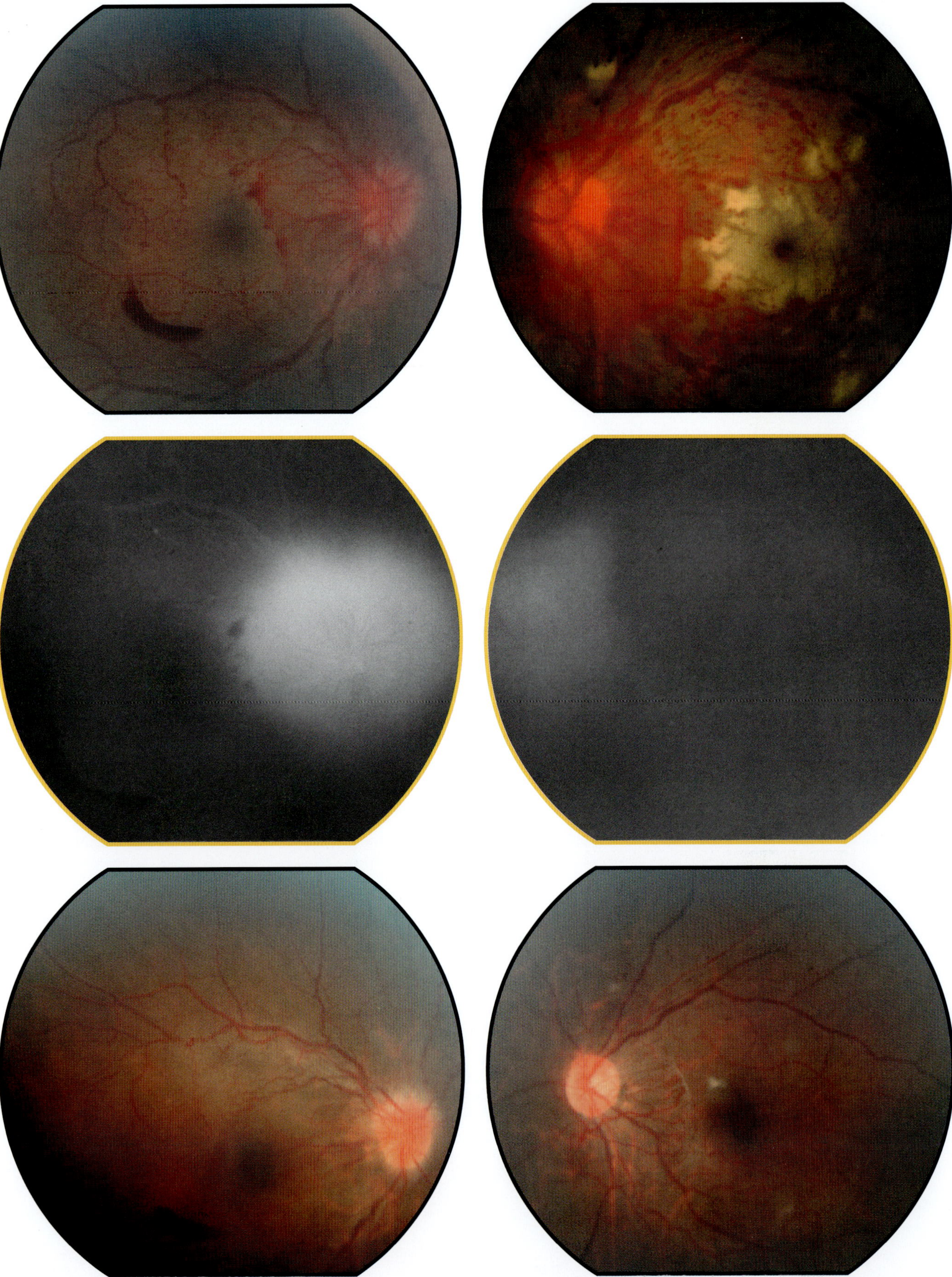

These color photos show florid neovascularization of the disk in both eyes and cilioretinal artery occlusion and macular infarction in the left eye of this patient with DMD. Late phase fluorescein angiography shows severe late leakage of neovascularization. Two weeks after treatment with panretinal photocoagulation OU and anti-VEGF injection OS, the patient showed marked improvement *(bottom row). Photos courtesy of Yannek I. Leiderman, MD, PhD and Ivana Kim, MD*

Dyskeratosis Congenita

Dyskeratosis congenita (DKC) is generally an X-linked recessive disorder caused by a mutation in dyskerin, a protein important in telomere maintenance. Tissues with high turnover rates are most affected. Patients have several cutaneous abnormalities including a mottled or reticulated skin pattern and abnormalities of the nails, such as ridges and fissures and leukoplakia of the tongue. Patients may also have a retinal vasculopathy associated with telangiectasia, aneurysms, leakage, peripheral ischemia, and neovascularization.

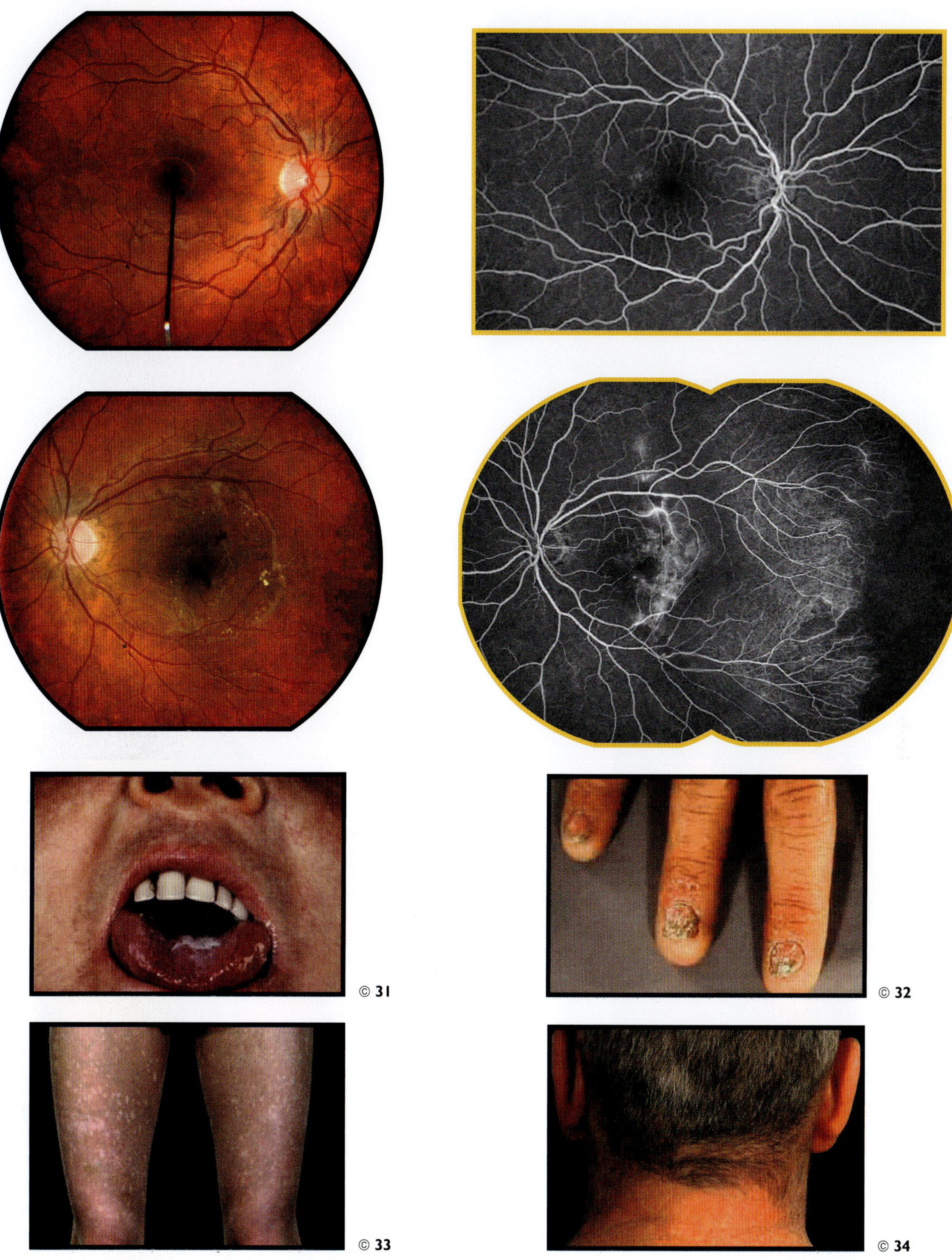

This patient with dyskeratosis congenita has macular telangiectasia and peripheral retinal ischemia. Note the fluorescein angiogram of the left eye in the macular region, showing dilated aneurysms, capillaries, ischemia, and leakage *(second row)*. The periphery of this left eye shows ischemia and non-perfusion. Similar changes are present in the right eye *(top row)* but much milder. The patient has pancytopenia, multiple malignancies. Multiple skin, hair, and nail findings were also present including leukoplakia, abnormal skin pigmentation, fissuring of the nails, premature graying of the hair, and early hair loss. The blood abnormalities may account for some of the retinal vascular changes. *Second row right image courtesy of Dr. R. Mark Hatfield*

Cohen Syndrome

Cohen syndrome is a rare autosomal recessive disorder with variable expression caused by a mutation in COH1 gene at 8q22. It is characterized by mental retardation, microcephaly, craniofacial dysmorphism, benign neutropenia, and muscle hypotonia. Truncal obesity and skeletal abnormalities are also characteristic including slender arms and legs and narrow hands and feet with slender fingers. Visual symptoms include nyctalopia and/or hemeralopia and progressively decreased visual acuity. Most patients will manifest a progressive pigmentary retinopathy often beginning before the age of 5 years old with a "bull's-eye" maculopathy which progresses to involve the entire fundus. Other ocular findings may also include myopia, nystagmus, strabismus, microphthalmia, optic atrophy, and iris/retinal coloboma, as well as retinal vascular abnormalities.

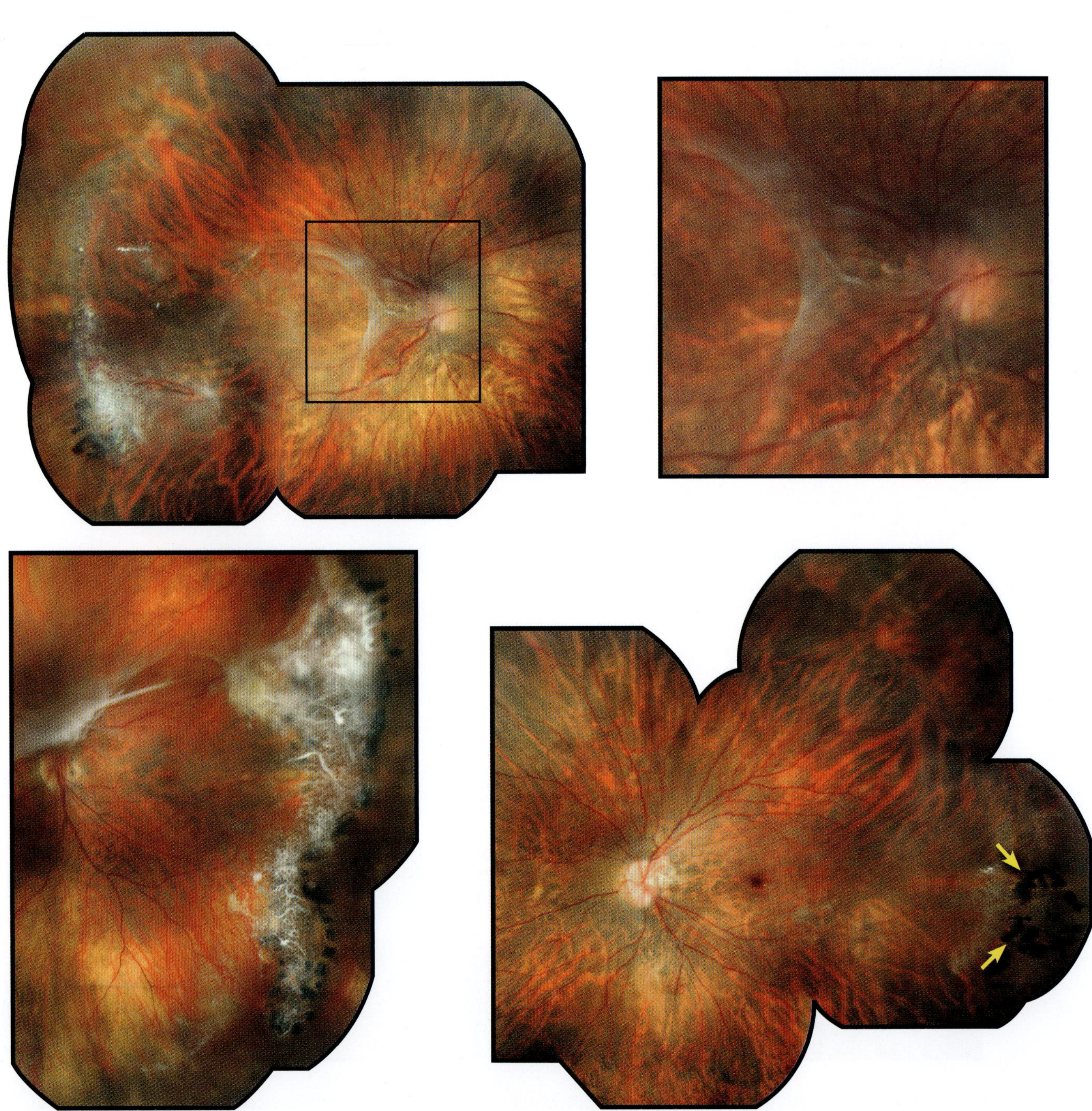

This patient with Cohen syndrome has ischemia, fibrovascular proliferation, and pigmentary degeneration of the retinal periphery. Preretinal macular fibrosis with vitreoretinal traction and shallow detachment of the posterior pole of the right eye is also noted. The left eye has lattice degeneration and retinal breaks. There is laser photocoagulation of one of the high-risk holes temporally in the left eye *(arrows)*.

Hereditary dystrophies in the fundus may involve only the macula or may involve both the posterior pole and periphery with more significant macular involvement. Macular dystrophies are bilateral and symmetrical with an underlying genetic etiology and typically with hereditary transmission.

Stargardt Disease (Stargardt Macular Dystrophy, Fundus Flavimaculatus)

Stargardt disease is the most common hereditary macular dystrophy. It is characterized by bilateral macular atrophy in a "bull's-eye" or geographic pattern, often with a "beaten-bronze" or metallic sheen. Associated yellowish pisciform or triradiate flecks may be present in the posterior pole with relative sparing of the peripapillary area. The presence of peripheral flecks is known as fundus flavimaculatus, a clinical variant of Stargardt disease with an identical genetic profile. Stargardt disease is most commonly inherited as an autosomal recessive trait, caused by mutation in the ABCA4 gene on chromosome 1p21-p13 (STGD1). Three additional autosomal dominant loci have been mapped to chromosomes 13q (STGD2) and 6q14 (STGD3) where the causative gene is ELOVL4, and 4p (STGD4). The genetics of Stargardt disease is extremely heterogeneic and hundreds of disease-causing sequences within ABCA4 alone have been described. This likely accounts for the wide variability in clinical disease severity and presentation. Point mutations affecting one allele have been associated with age related macular degeneration while large frame shift mutations affecting both alleles have been associated with cone-rod dystrophy, a much more severe variant of the disease. Patients often present with central visual loss in their teenage years, but may present much later in life with a better visual prognosis. Fundus autofluorescence is informative with hyperfluorescence of flecks. A peripapillary ring-shaped region of normal-appearing autofluorescence has been described in all stages of Stargardt disease and may aid in the recognition of this entity. A "dark" or "silent" choroid may be seen with fluorescein angiography in 70% of cases, a phenomenon caused by the diffuse accumulation of lipofuscin.

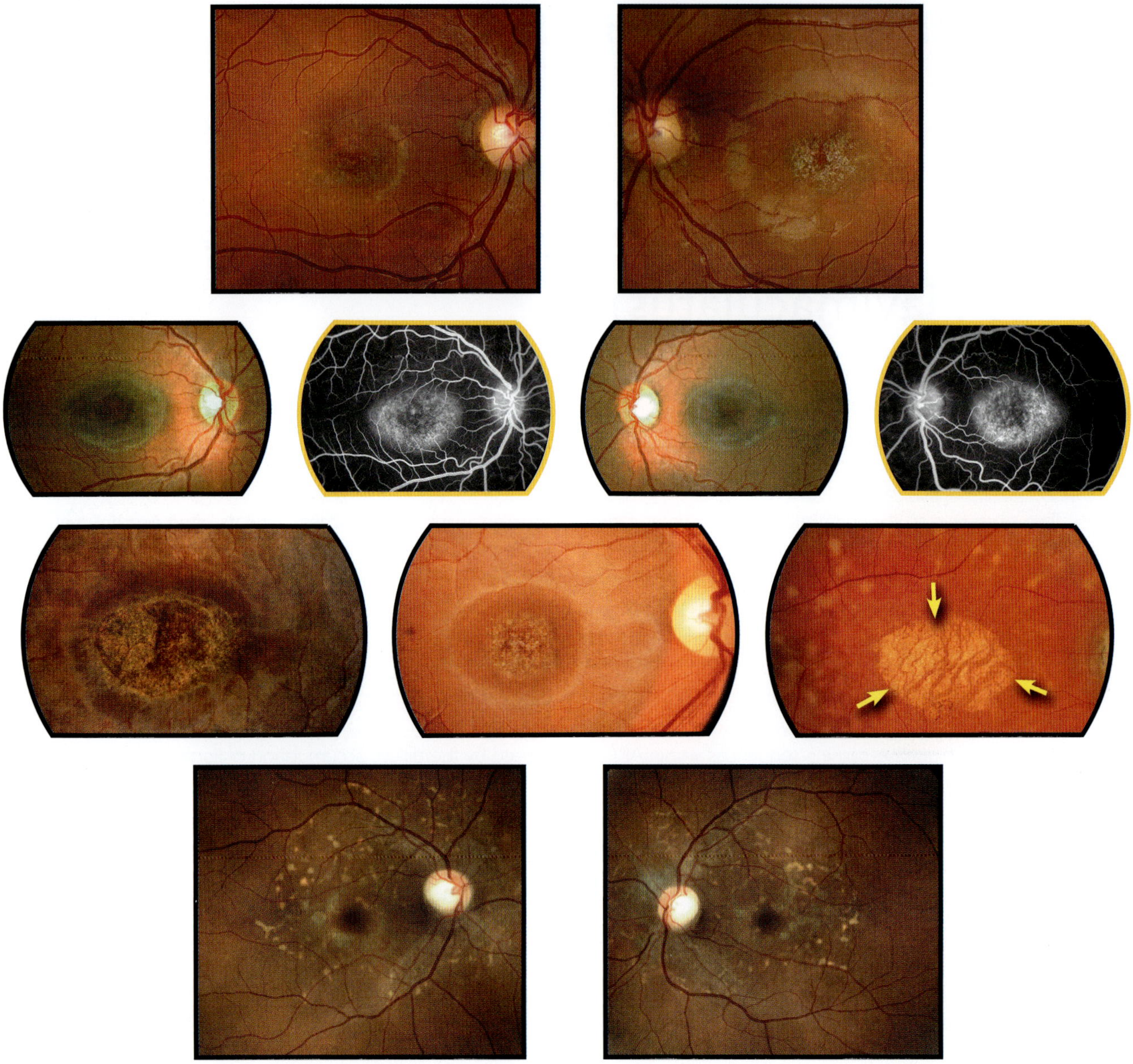

These are patients with Stargardt disease. Note the polymorphic metallic sheen in the macula that is generally ovoid in appearance surrounding the fovea and indicative of atrophy. A fluorescein angiogram in the early stages of the disease will show a "dark choroid" where there is accumulation of lipofuscin in the pigment epithelium which blocks choroidal fluorescence. Eventually more severe atrophy will develop in the central macula, as seen in the third row *(arrows)*. Some patients with Stargardt disease demonstrate flecks in the paramacular region, along the arcades and in the near peripheral fundus, seen most clearly in the bottom two photographs. *Third row first and last images courtesy of Drs Ron Carr and Ken Noble*

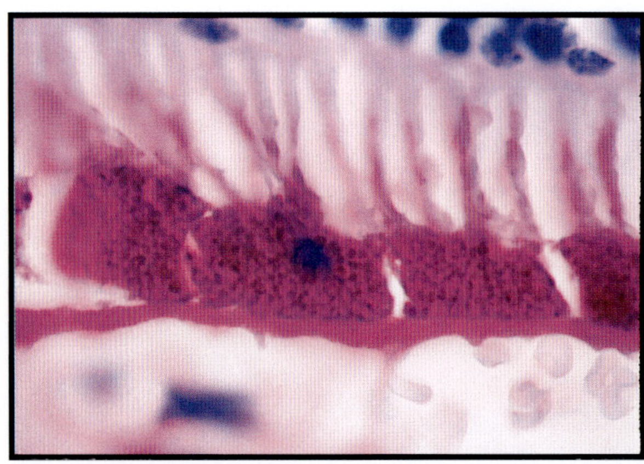

The histopathology of a patient with Stargardt disease reveals accumulation of lipofuscin in the pigment epithelium.

The Spectrum of Stargardt Disease

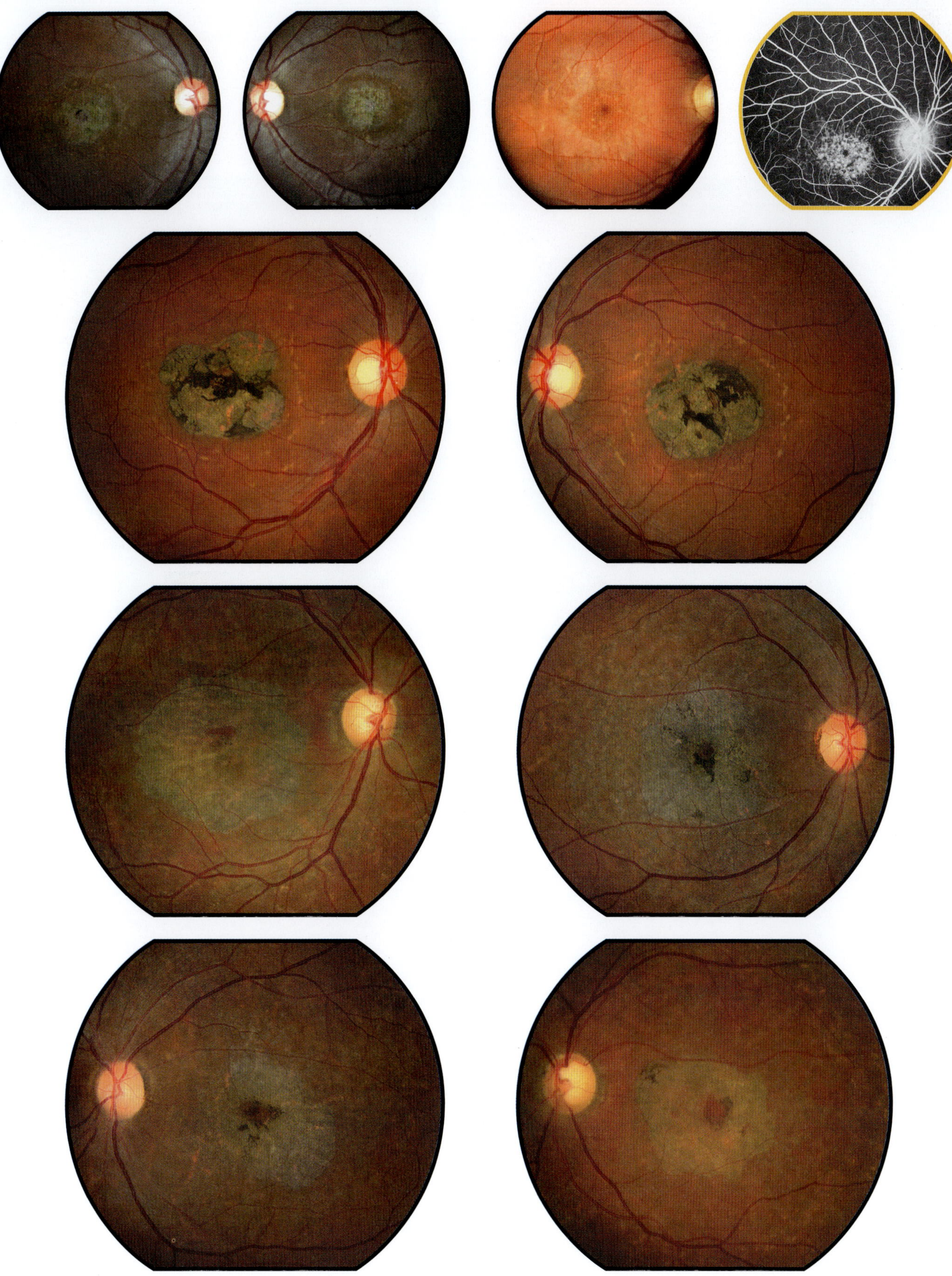

Patients with Stargardt disease have a variable refractile sheen to the macula, some pigment epithelial hyperplasia, focal and multifocal areas of atrophy, and flecks in the fundus. *Top left figure courtesy of Daniela C. Ferrara, MD, PhD*

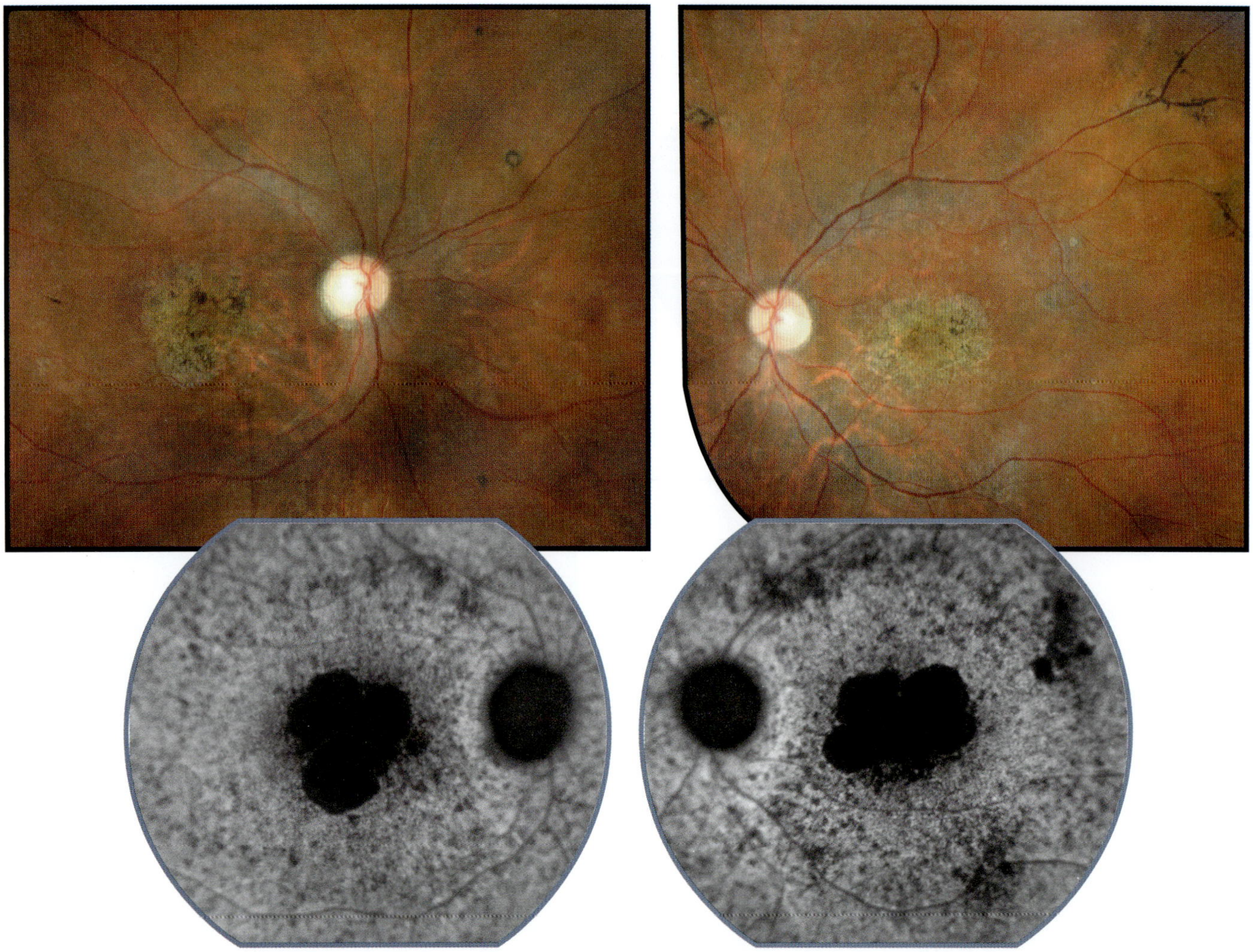

This patient has Stargardt disease, but also has pigment epithelial hyperplastic change in the near peripheral fundus. The fundus autofluorescence shows atrophy in the macula (hypoautofluorescence) and a granular area in the posterior pole which corresponds to additional, multifocal areas of less severe atrophy.

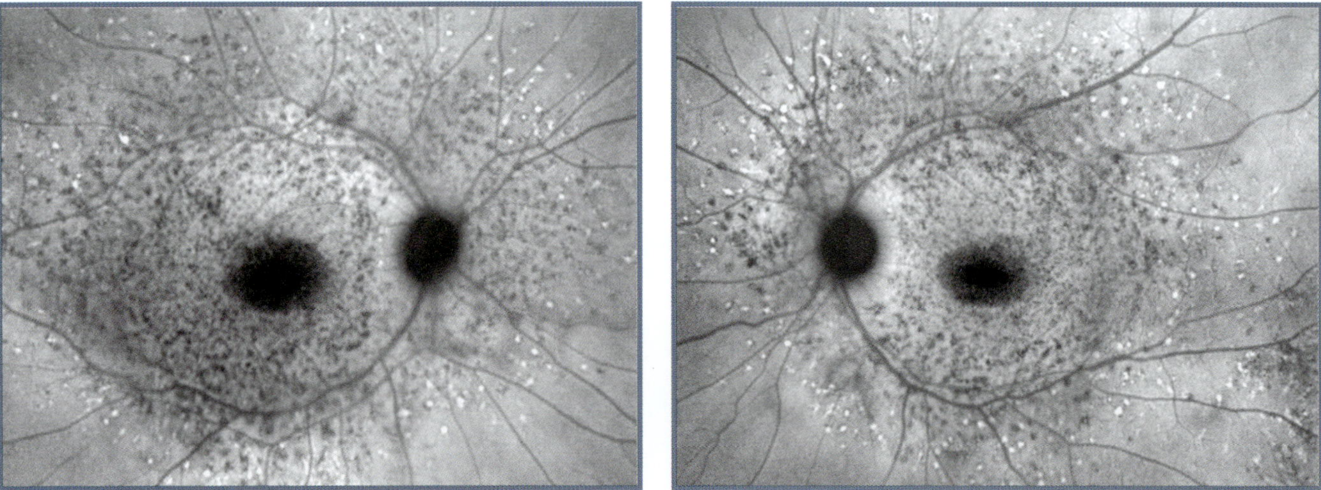

This patient has Stargardt disease with fundus flavimaculatus. Numerous flecks are present in the paramacular region and near peripheral fundus. The atrophic flecks are hypoautofluorescent. The more recently developed flecks are hyperautofluorescent, as are cells at risk of becoming atrophic. There is always atrophy in the macula and relative sparing of the peripapillary area in the typical presentation of Stargardt disease. *Courtesy of Daniela C. Ferrara, MD, PhD*

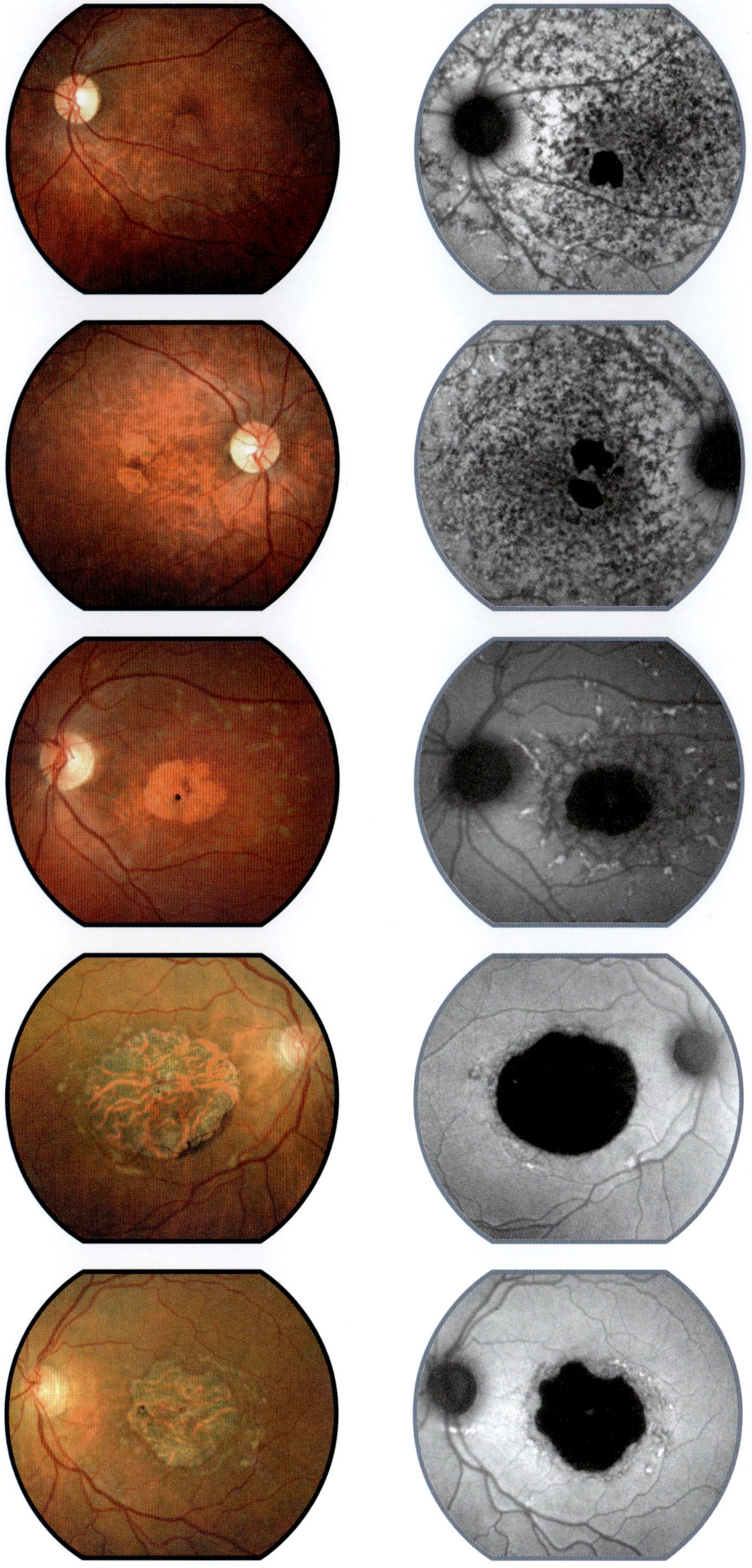

These patients with Stargardt disease have a variable degree of atrophy and fleck deposition. There is also bilaterality and some degree of symmetry but not exactly identical with respect to the macular atrophy.

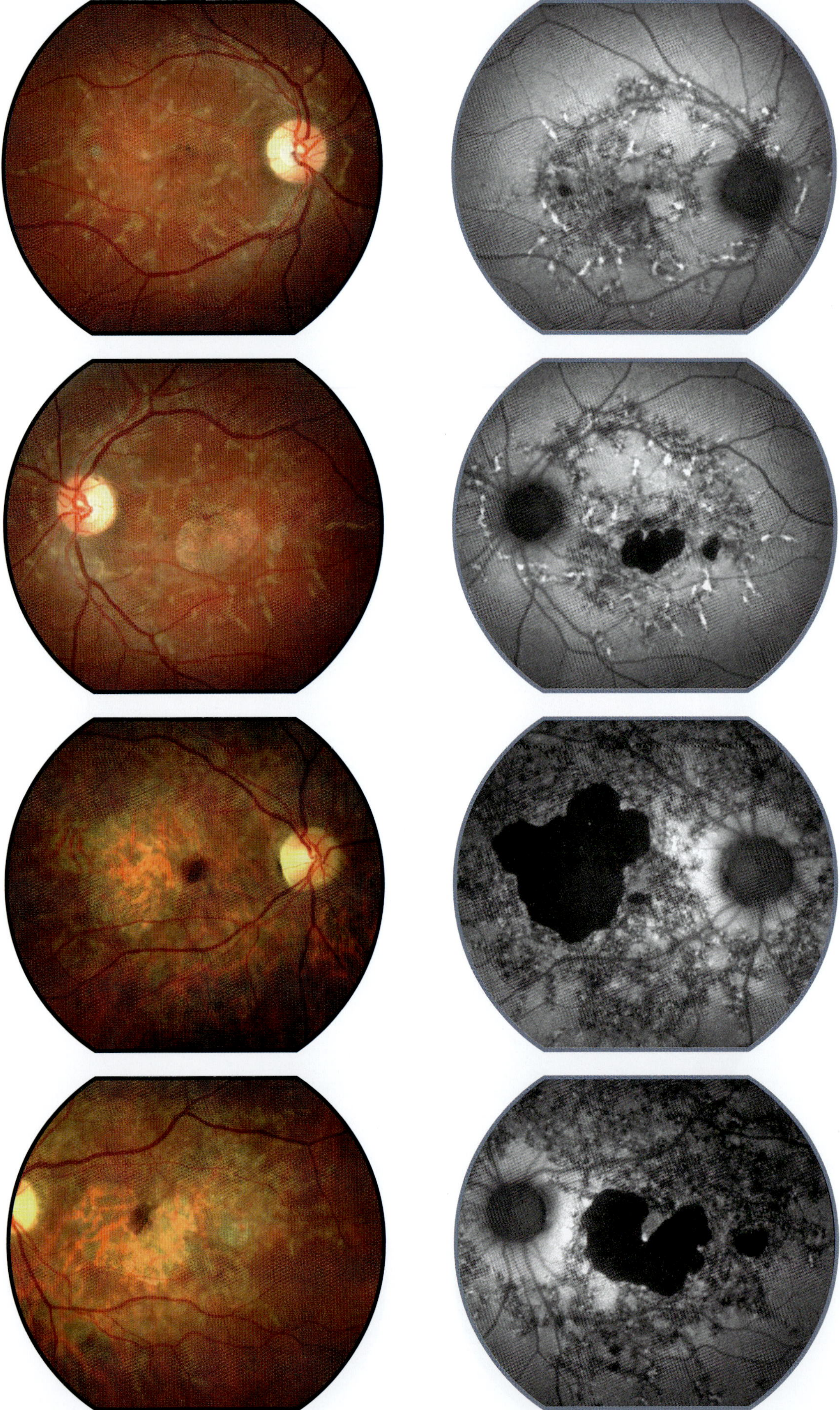

These patients with Stargardt disease also demonstrate the spectrum of macular lesions and flecks. There is also variability in the shape of macular atrophy in each eye of a given patient. Note the preservation of the pigment epithelium around the disc and the involvement of the fovea.

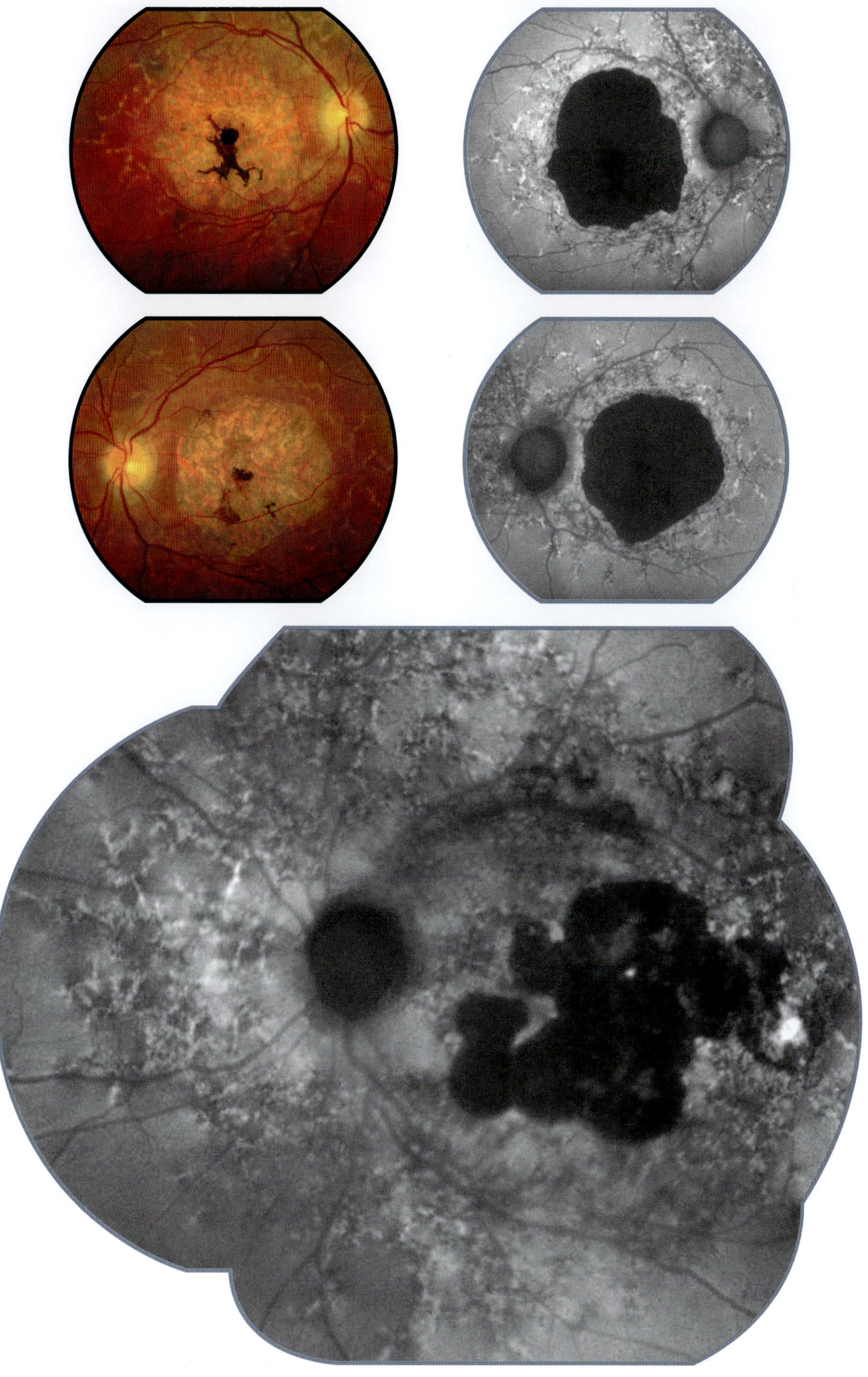

In these patients with Stargardt disease, there is severe atrophy centrally. In addition, the flecks extend beyond into the near peripheral fundus. *Top two rows courtesy of Daniela C. Ferrara, MD, PhD*

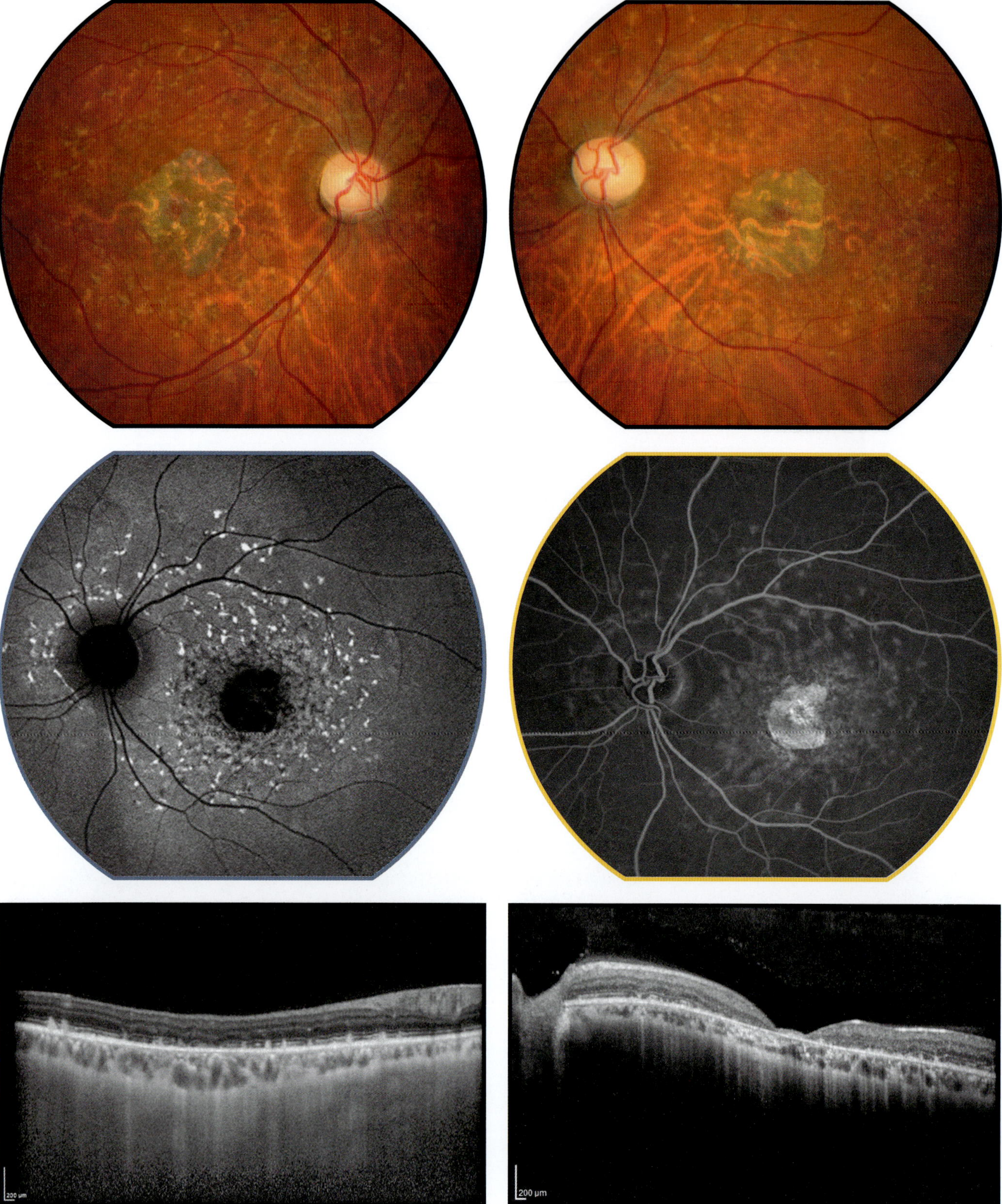

Color fundus photos of a patient with Stargardt disease confirmed by genetic testing for mutation in ABCA4 show multiple pisciform flecks with peripapillary sparing and geographic atrophy in the central macula of both eyes. Fundus autofluorescence and fluorescein angiogram highlight these changes and also show a dark choroid. Outer retinal atrophy and hyper-reflective flecks are highlighted by SD-OCT.

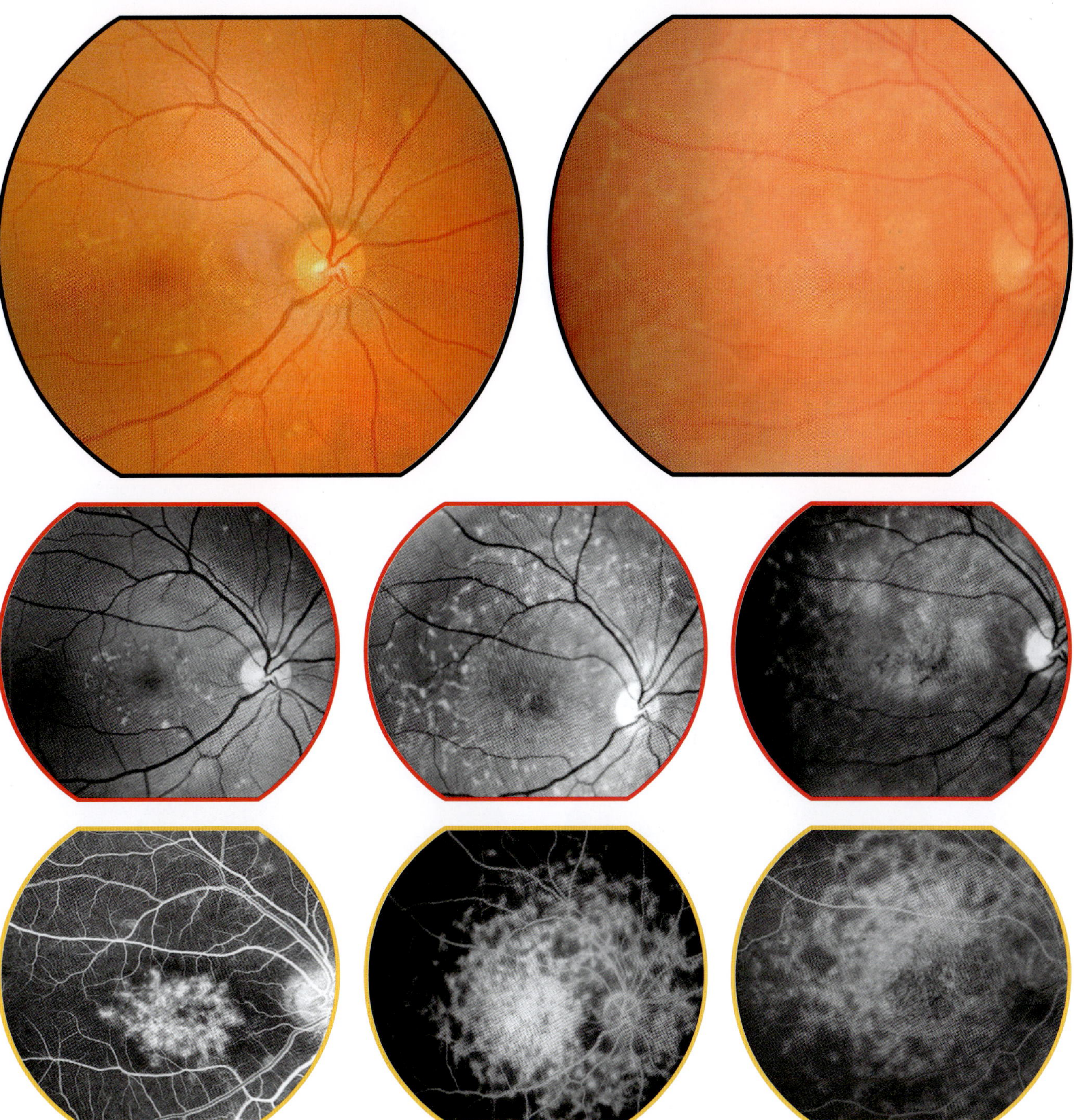

This patient with Stargardt disease was followed over several decades. Color fundus photos show an increase of yellow deposits and central atrophy from 1980 *(top left)* to 2003 *(top right)*. Red-free photos taken in 1980 *(second row left)*, 1993 *(second row middle)*, and 2003 *(second row right)* highlight these changes. Fluorescein angiogram shows progression of macular atrophy from 1980 *(bottom left)*, through 1993 *(bottom middle)*, and 2003 *(bottom right)*. *Images courtesy of Eric Souied, MD*

Best Vitelliform Macular Dystrophy

Best vitelliform macular dystrophy (VMD), or Best disease, is an heritable disorder characterized by variable deposition of yellowish material attributed to lipofuscin in the RPE and/or subretinal space of the macula. The majority of cases are inherited in an autosomal dominant pattern; however, atypical autosomal recessive cases have been reported. The basic defect in Best disease is related to a mutation in the BEST1 gene (formerly called VMD2) coding for bestrophin, a Ca^{2+}-sensitive Cl-channel protein located on the basolateral membrane of RPE cells. While virtually all patients harbor an abnormal copy of BEST1, approximately 100 different disease-causing mutations have been described with variable penetrance and expressivity. The phenotypic appearance of Best disease therefore varies with each individual, sometimes making the diagnosis difficult. Patients often present with decreased visual acuity; however, the visual acuity is generally better than would be expected given the fundus appearance.

Best disease progresses through five characteristic stages: previtelliform, vitelliform, pseudohypopyon, vitelliruptive, and atrophic. In the previtelliform stage, the macula appears normal. The vitelliform stage is characterized by a dome-shaped accumulation of yellowish material in the central macula simulating the appearance of an egg yolk. This lesion is hyperautofluorescent and shows dome-shaped hyper-reflective thickening at the level of the RPE and the subneurosensory space with spectral domain OCT, although a frank pigment epithelial detachment with subretinal fluid may be noted. In some patients, the material may be multifocal in distribution. The yellowish material may gravitate inferiorly or layer, leading to the pseudohypopyon stage. Over years, the vitelliform lesion breaks apart giving the appearance of a "scrambled-egg," known as the vitelliruptive stage. Eventually, the material dissipates and RPE mottling may ensue with isolated vitelliform deposits at the edges of the macular lesion and ultimately an oval area of RPE atrophy develops. This is the final, atrophic stage of the disease. Choroidal neovascularization can complicate 2–9% of cases and may occur at any stage of the disease and may ultimately lead to the development of a fibrovascular disciform scar. A severely abnormal electrooculogram with an Arden ratio approximating 1.0 is universally present regardless of the clinical presentation, and is therefore helpful in making the diagnosis. Very rarely the Arden ratio may be normal despite genetic confirmation of the disease. The vitelliform stage of VMD can appear similar to other conditions typically associated with yellowish macular lesions such as adult-onset vitelliform macular dystrophy (AVMD), basal laminar drusen with vitelliform macular detachment, or the rare acute exudative polymorphous vitelliform maculopathy.

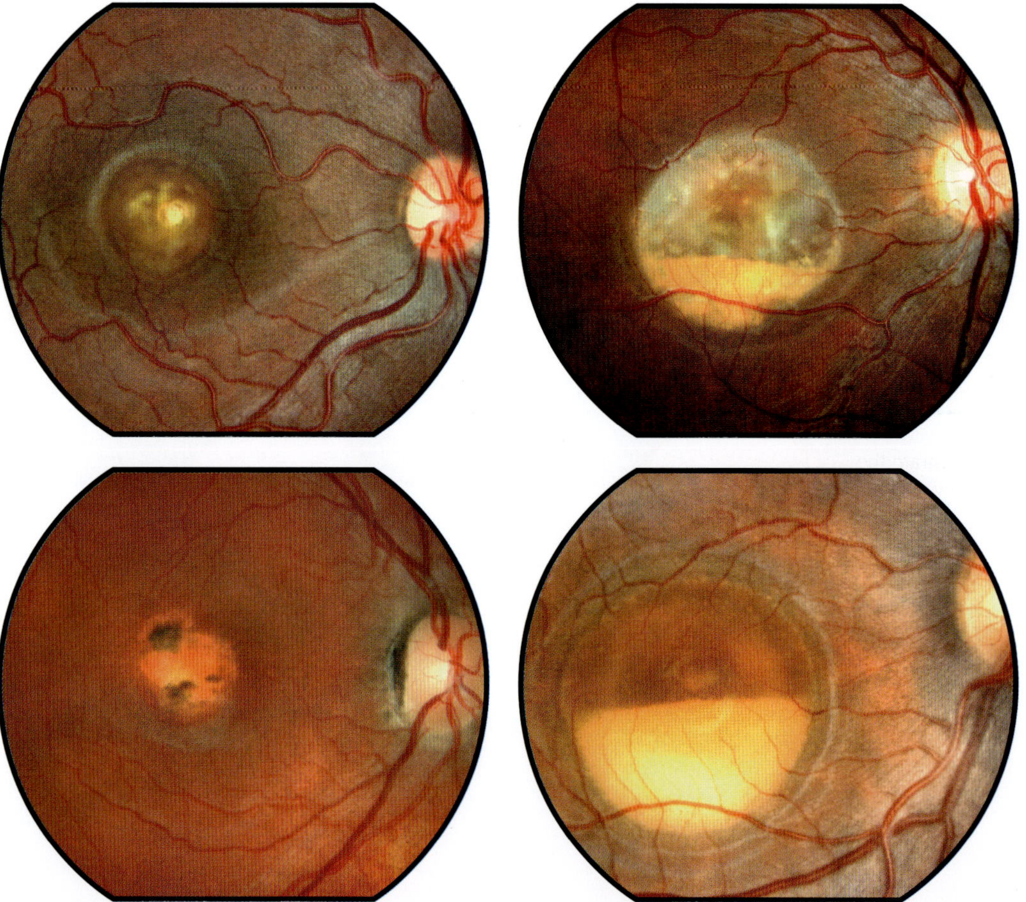

These patients with Best vitelliform macular dystrophy show a unifocal lesion in the central macula. The vitelliform abnormality may vary in size. With the accumulation of lipofuscin in the subsensory retinal space, a pseudohypopyon appearance may develop (*right photographs*) due to layering of the lipofuscin material. The lower left photograph shows the development of an early disciform scar from fibrovascular proliferation. There is also a zone of atrophy of the pigment epithelium.

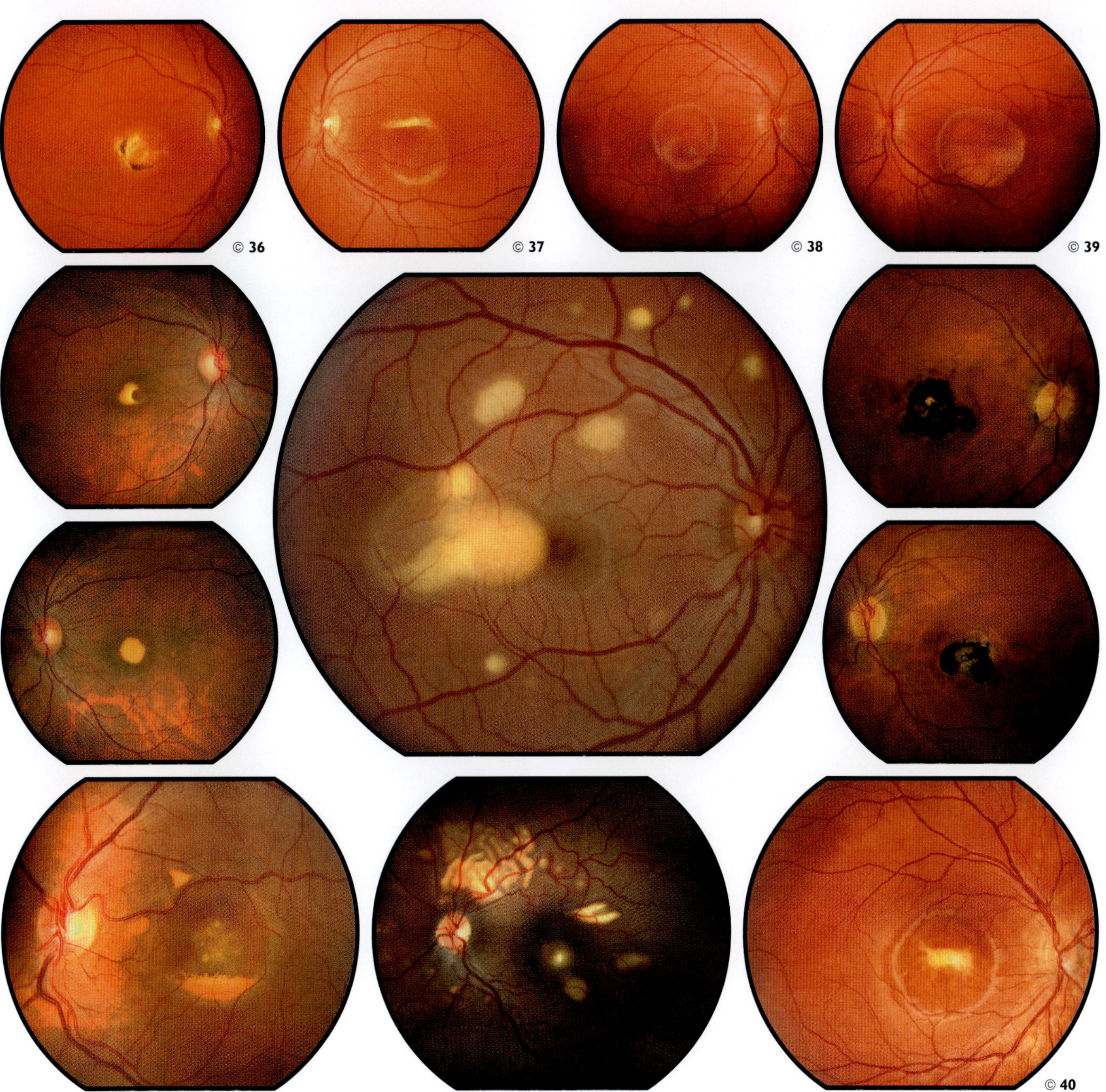

These illustrations demonstrate the variable morphology for patients with Best vitelliform macular dystrophy. There may be a clear cystic detachment of the retina with an incomplete accumulation of yellowish material, multifocal lesions, pigment epithelial hyperplasia, and scarring.

Fluorescein Angiography

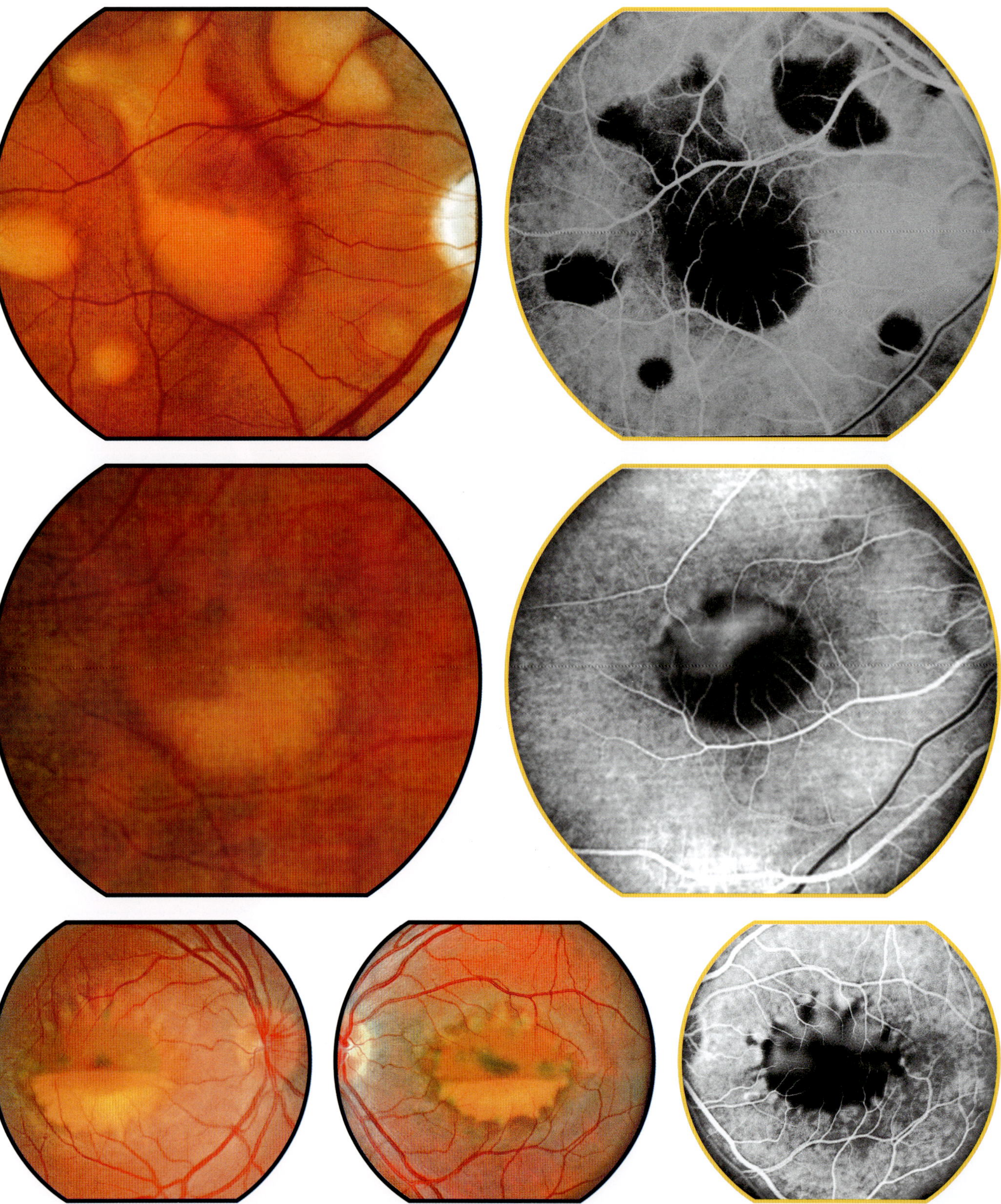

Fluorescein angiography is not very helpful in patients with Best disease. The yellowish vitelliform subretinal material will be hypofluorescent due to blockage of the underlying choriocapillaris, as seen in these patients. *Top row courtesy of Dr. Tom Weingiest*

Fundus Autofluoresence

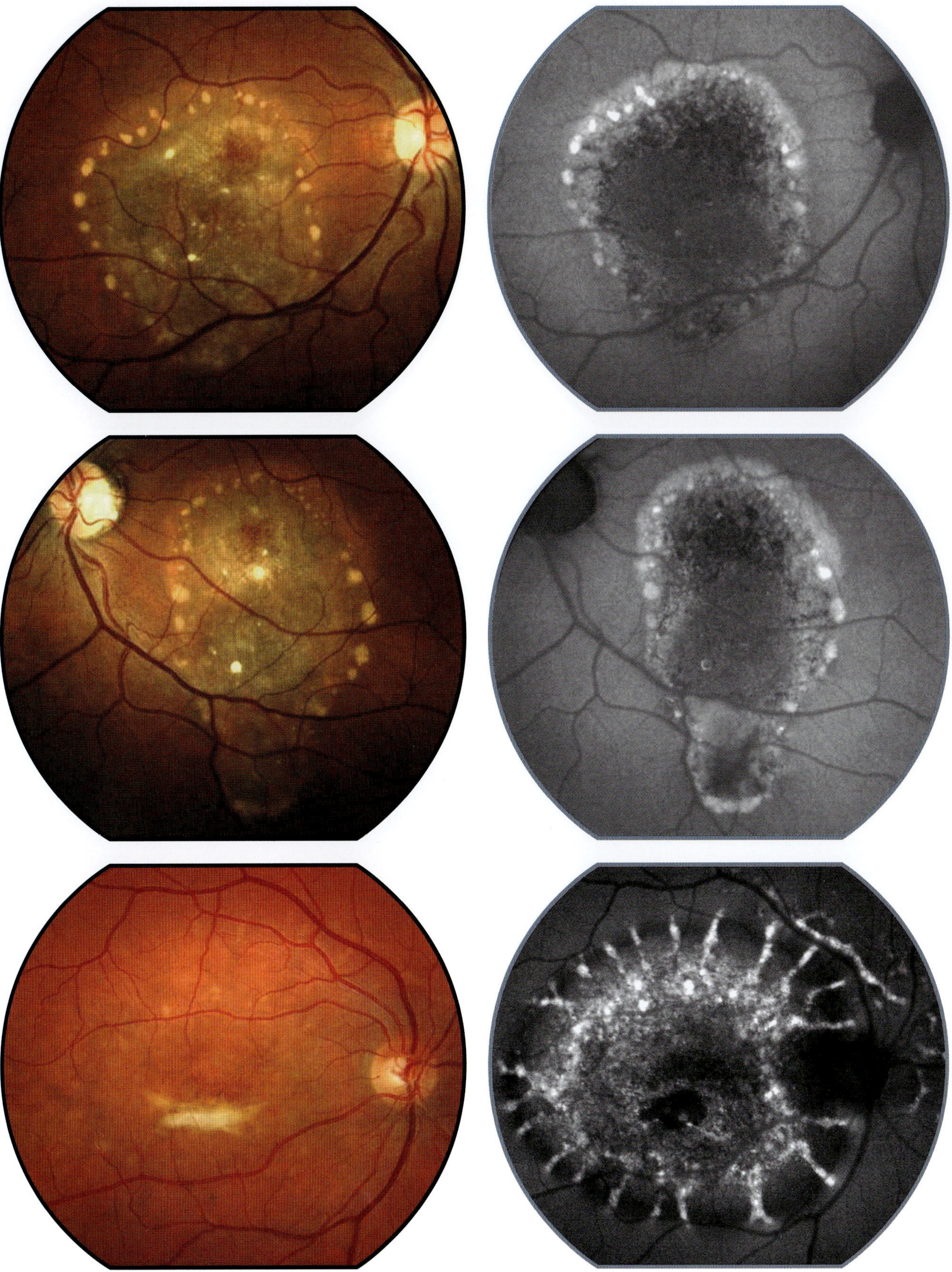

Fundus autofluorescence is a more practical and useful modality in detecting the lipofuscin accumulation in patients with Best disease. The hyperautofluorescence will correspond to the lipofuscin. Hypofluorescence will be evident where there is pigment epithelial atrophy. *Bottom row courtesy of Dr. Richard Spaide*

Optical Coherence Tomography (OCT)

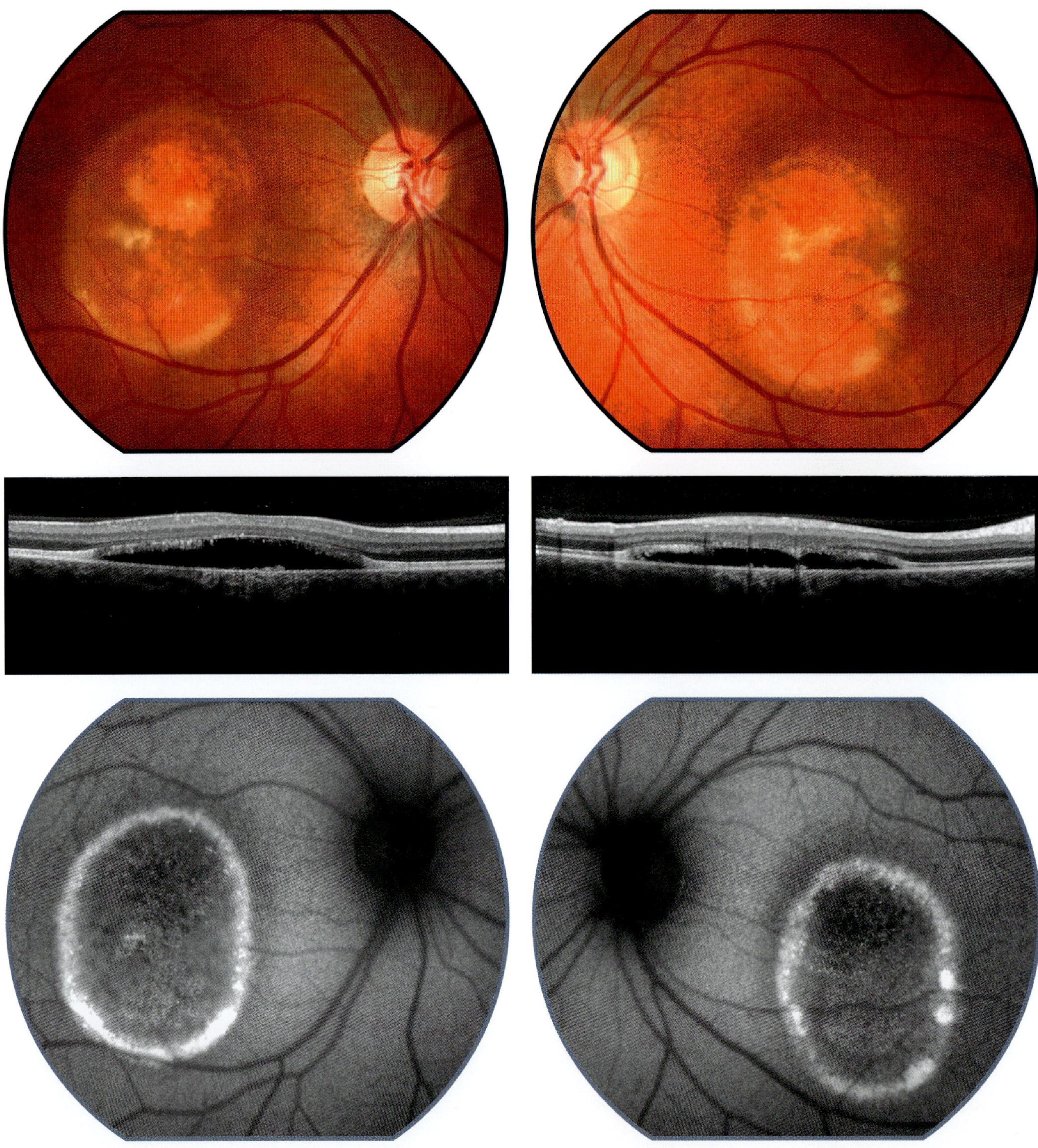

This patient with presumed Best disease was suspected of having chronic central serous chorioretinopathy. The exudative detachments in the macula were associated with lipofuscin. The OCT images revealed some photoreceptor degeneration at the site of chronic macular detachment, but no discrete pigment epithelial detachment. Fundus autofluorescence clearly delineated the hyperfluorescent margins of the detachment where lipofuscin had accumulated (ring of yellow exudate seen clinically in each eye). Hypoautofluorescence is evident where there is pigment epithelial atrophy or scarring.

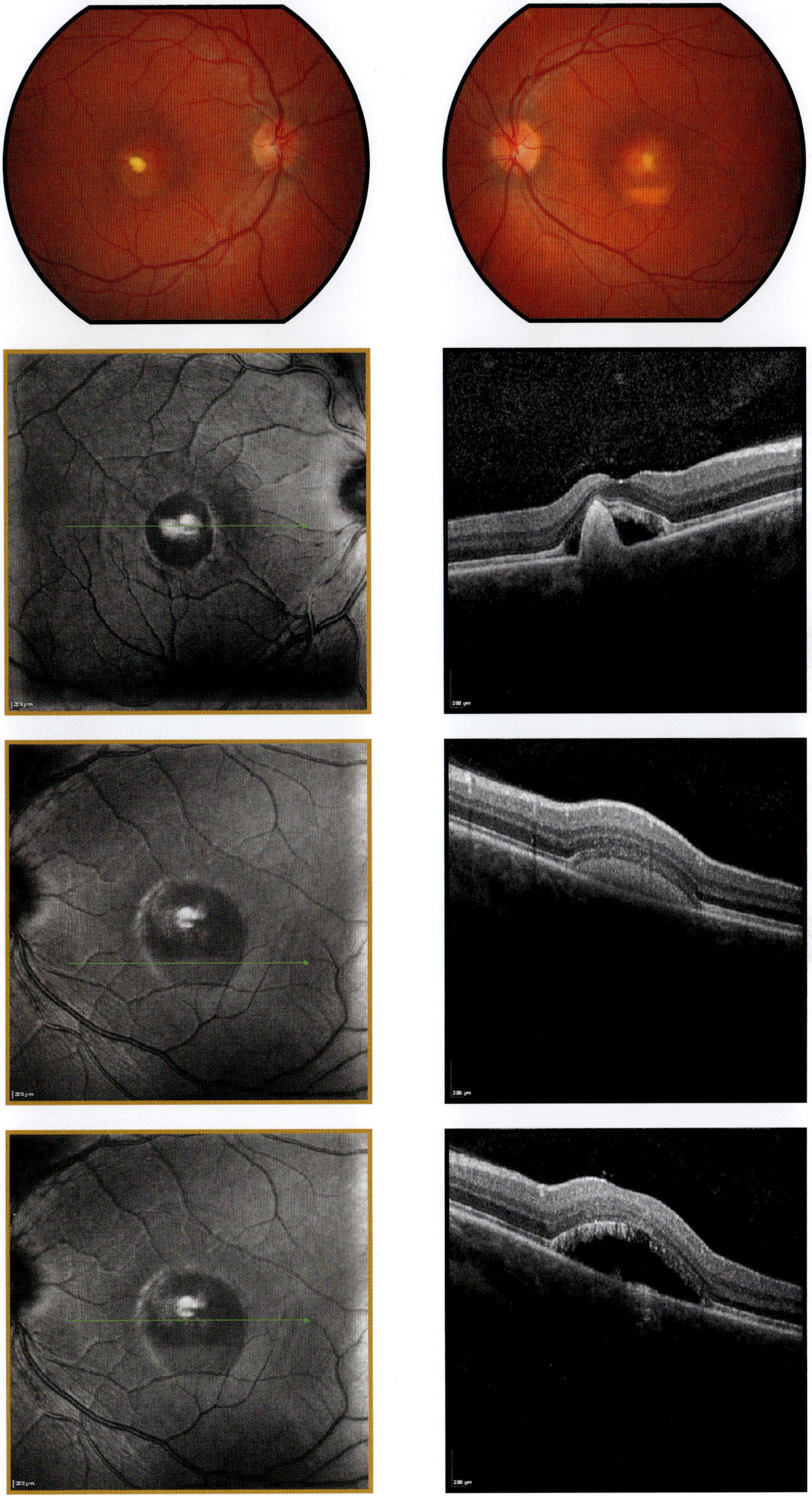

Color fundus photographs of patient with Best disease showing vitelliform stage of the right eye and pseudohypopyon of the left eye. SD-OCT images show a PED with subretinal fluid on the right and vitelliform macular detachment on the left.

Choroidal Neovascularization

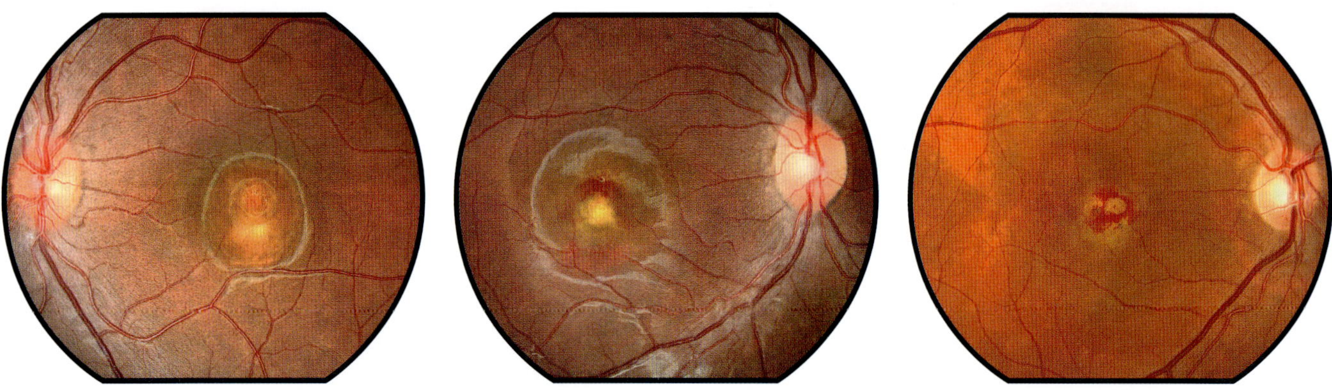

Patients with Best disease are at risk of developing choroidal neovascularization indicated by the presence of subretinal hemorrhage OD. Vitelliform maculopathy is present OS.

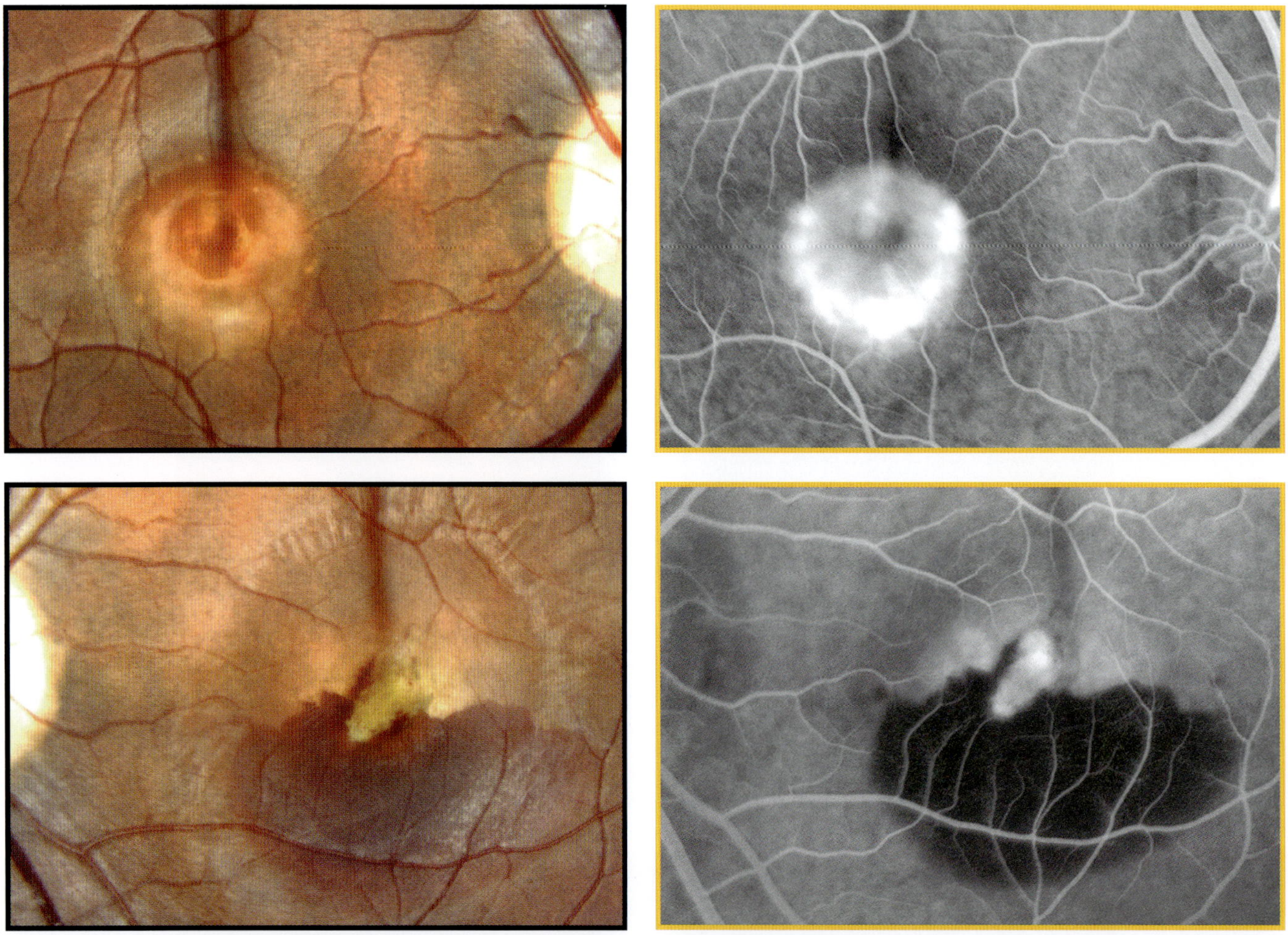

This patient has Best disease with vitelliform maculopathy and late staining on the fluorescein angiogram *(top row)*. In the left eye, there is a large macular hemorrhage secondary to a choroidal neovascularization, which is leaking on the fluorescein study.

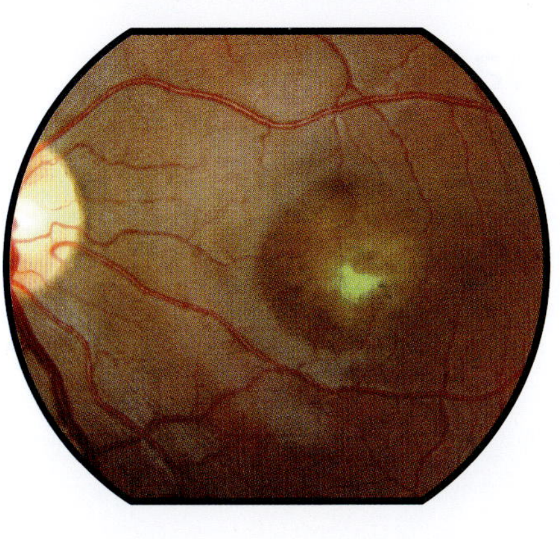
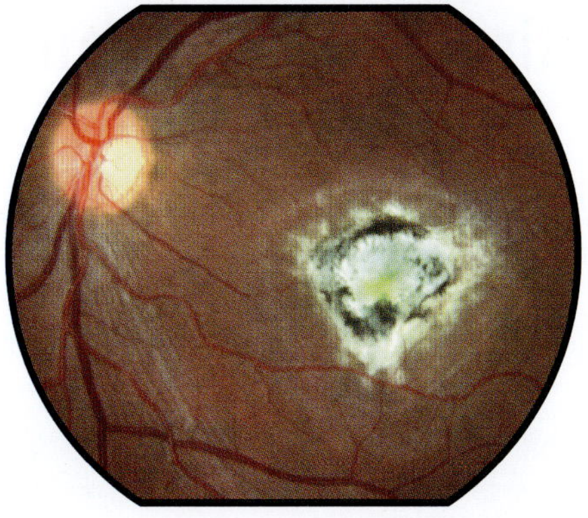
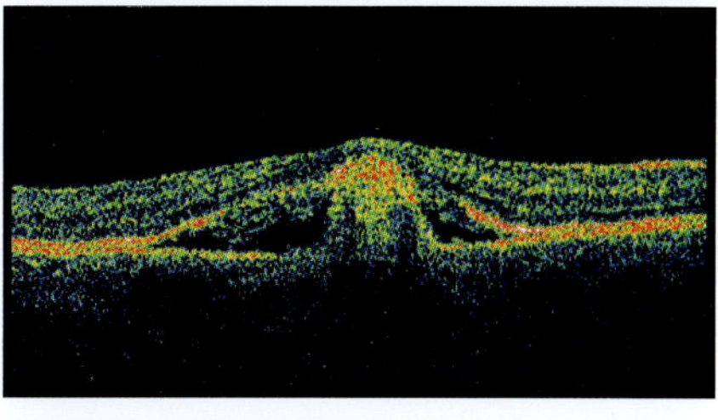

These Best patients demonstrate a disciform fibrovascular scar due to an old choroidal neovascular membrane. The OCT shows an exudative detachment of the neurosensory retina with prominent reflectance beneath the fovea, which correponds to the fibrotic scar.

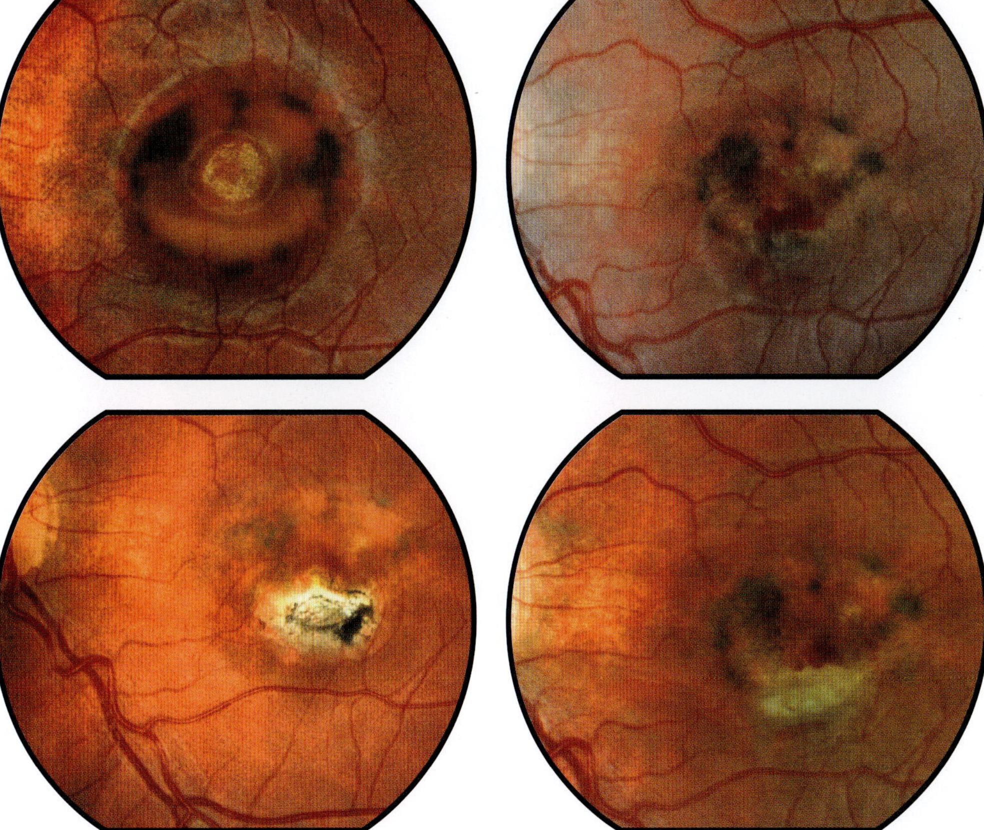

This Best patient originally presented with vitelliform maculopathy OS *(upper left)*. Years later he developed a hemorrhagic detachment of the macula *(upper right)*. Laser photocoagulation treatment was applied to the neovascularization, which was straddled between the two hemorrhages. Three years later *(lower left)*, he developed a fibrotic scar. Twenty-six years later, the scar had not progressed significantly and his visual acuity was still in the 20/40 range.

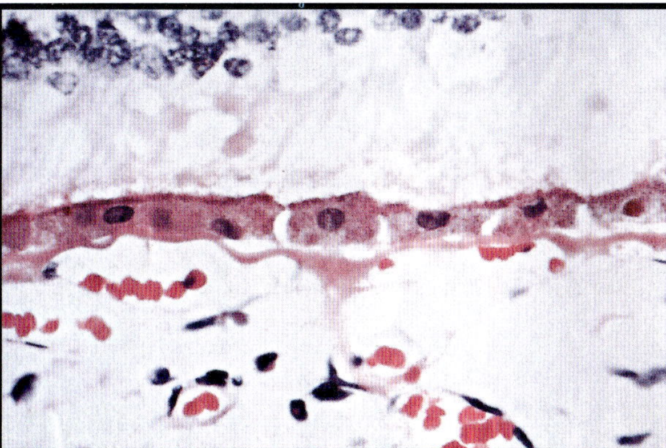

© **41**

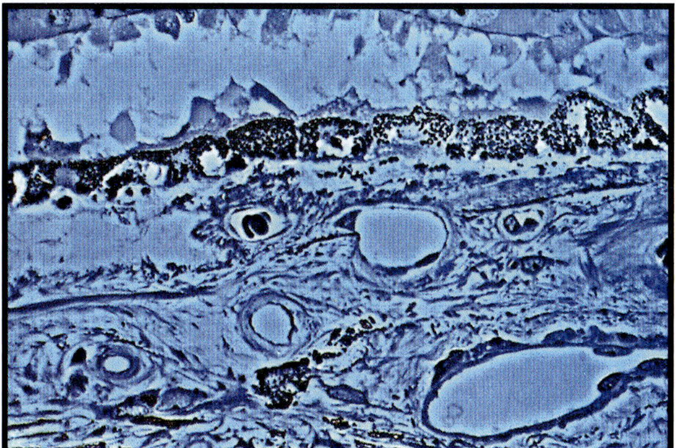

© **42**

The histopathology of Best vitelliform macular dystrophy will show prominent pigment epithelial cells and fibrous proliferation beneath the RPE when associated with neovascularization *(right)*.

Autosomal Recessive Bestrophinopathy

Autosomal recessive bestrophinopathy is a rare disorder which results from a biallelic mutation in the Best1 gene, effectively leading to the complete absence of normal functioning bestrophin. Clinically, the disorder is characterized by multifocal subretinal yellow vitelliform lesions throughout the posterior pole and mid-periphery. Fundus autoflourescence may be informative showing multiple hyperfluorescent lesions scattered throughout or concentric to the posterior pole. Since Best1 is important to the normal structural development of the eye, other ocular abnormalities are frequently observed including hyperopia with shallow anterior chamber angles predisposing patients to angle closure glaucoma. Like BVMD, EOG is severely abnormal, often with complete absence of the light rise. However, unlike BVMD, a full field ERG may demonstrate progressive photoreceptor dysfunction. Visual acuity ranges from 20/25 to 20/200 and tends to remain stable. However, cystoid macular edema and choroidal neovascularization have been reported in association with this disorder.

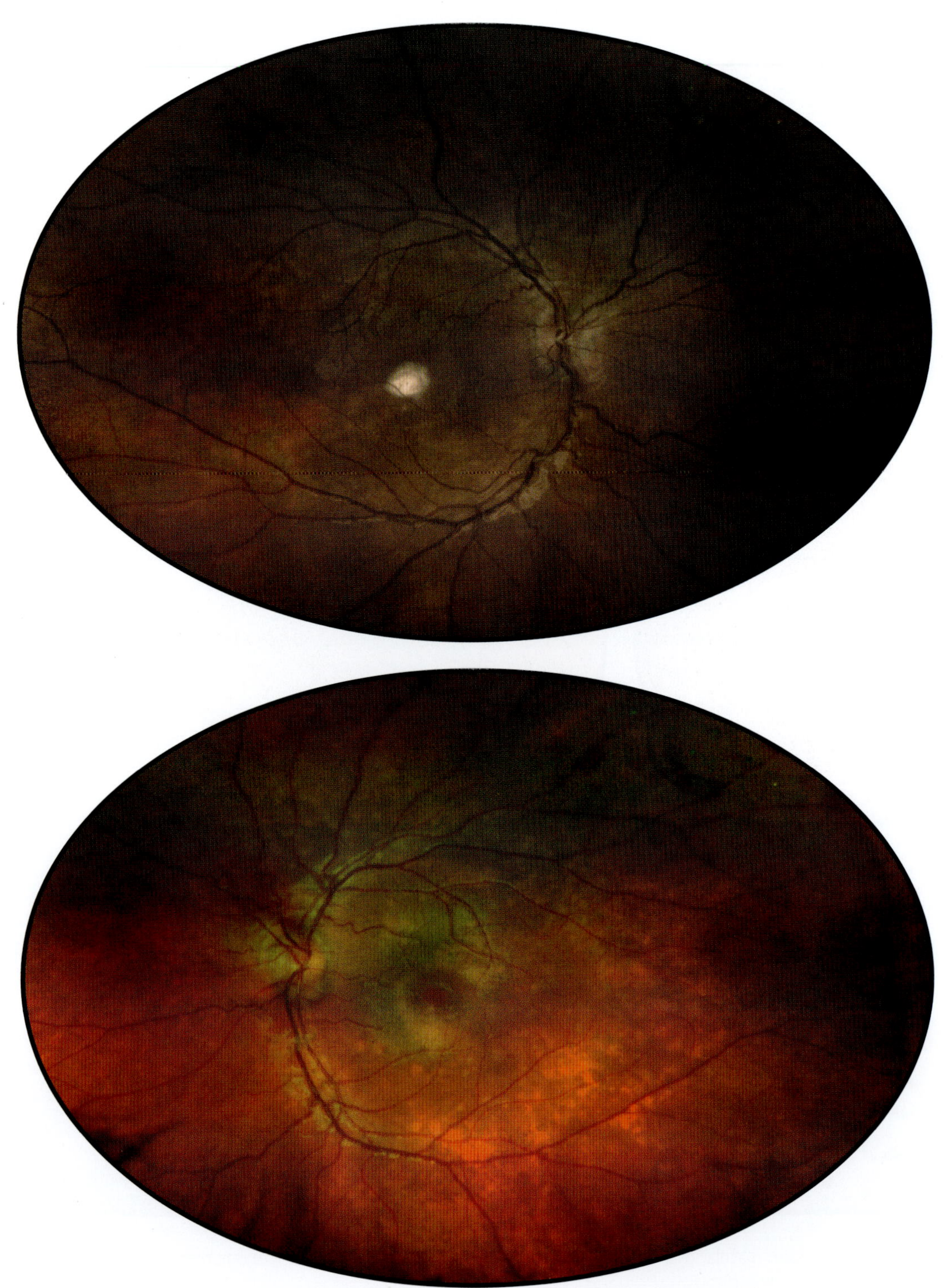

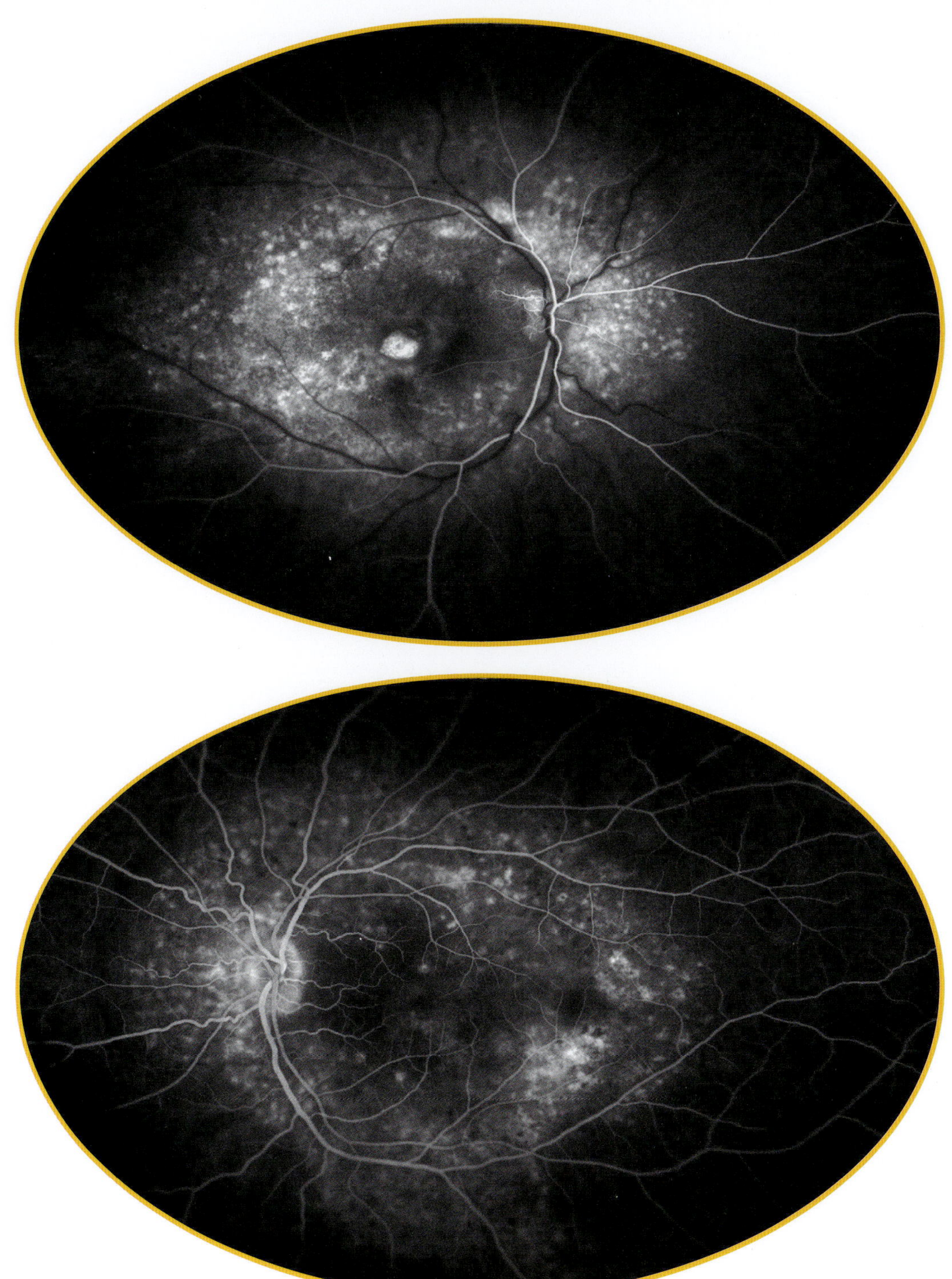

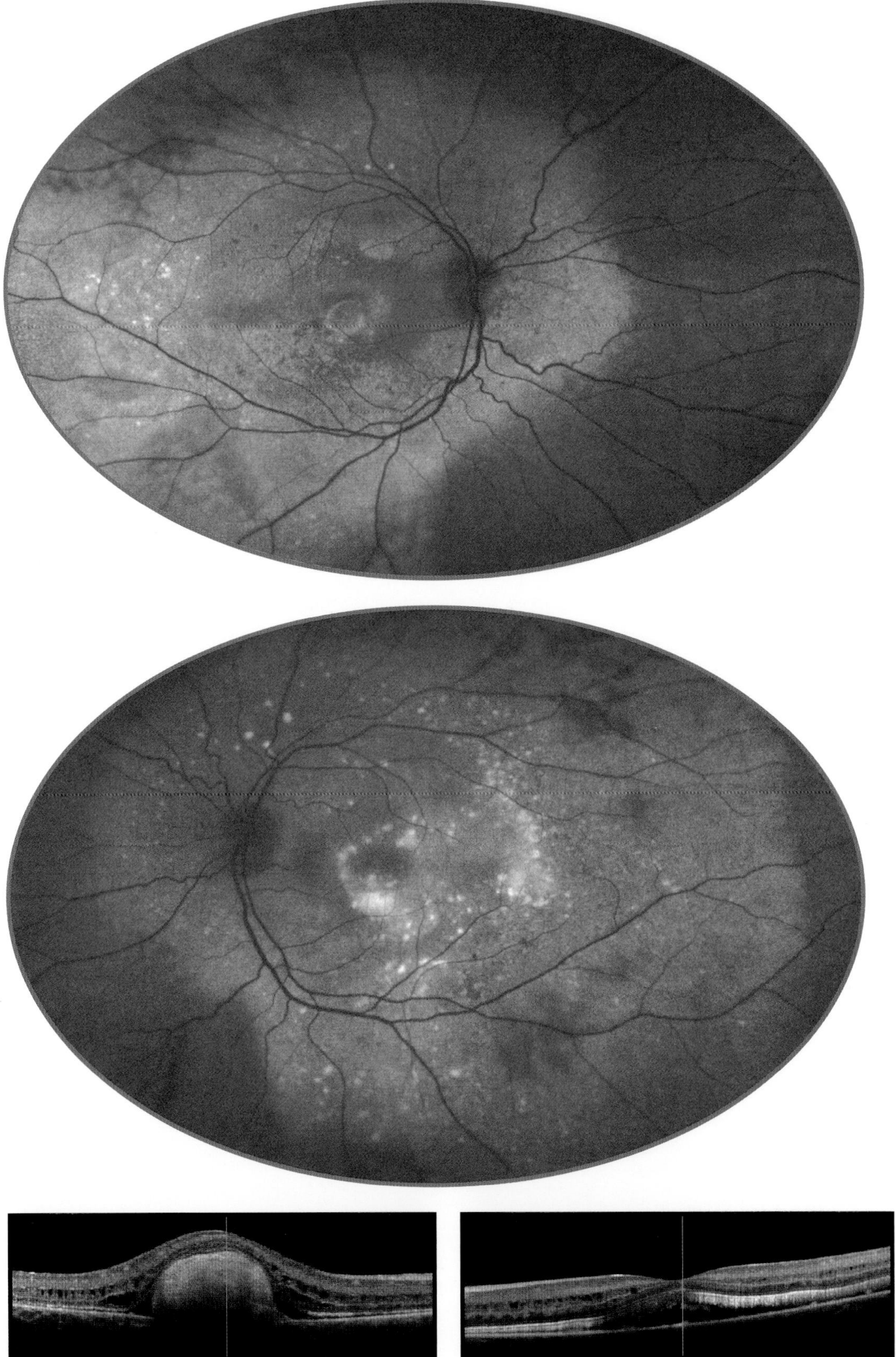

These photos are taken from a patient with autosomal recessive bestrophinopathy. Color photos show central vitelliform lesions and multifocal subretinal deposits OU. These deposits stain prominently on fluorescein angiography *(second row)* and are hyperautofluorescent *(third row)*. SD-OCT through the macula nicely demonstrates hyper-reflective subretinal material OS similar to that seen in Best disease and a dense submacular scar OD. Macular schitic changes are also noted OU. *Images courtesy of Steven D. Schwartz, MD*

Pattern Dystrophy of the RPE

Pattern dystrophy of the RPE refers to a group of disorders which may be inherited in an autosomal dominant fashion with incomplete penetrance and highly variable expression. Mutation in the RDS gene (peripherin 2, PRPH2) has been linked to some of these conditions. Symptoms and findings typically begin in the third to fifth decade with mild decrease in central vision. Yellowish subretinal deposits exhibiting fundus hyperautofluorescence may occur in a unifocal or mutlifocal pattern in one or both eyes. Categorization of these dystrophies is based upon the pattern of these lesions. Classically there are five pattern dystrophies: adult-onset vitelliform macular dystrophy (although as mentioned above, many cases of AVMD are better categorized as bestrophinopathies), butterfly-shaped pattern dystrophy, Sjögren reticular dystrophy, fundus pulverulentus, and multifocal pattern dystrophy simulating fundus flavimaculatus. In some patients, a vitelliform lesion (e.g. age-related macular degeneration) may appear very similar to that observed in Best vitelliform macular dystrophy and may be referred to as pseudovitelliform detachment. With fluorescein angiography the central lesions typically block fluorescence early but exhibit late staining as the dye slowly leaks into the subretinal space. These changes can be misinterpreted as choroidal neovascularization. Although these diseases are considered somewhat benign, macular atrophy and CNVM may complicate pattern dystrophy in 50% of patients.

Adult-Onset Vitelliform Macular Dystrophy (Adult-Onset Foveomacular Dystrophy, Pseudovitelliform Macular Degeneration)

Adult-onset vitelliform macular dystrophy (AVMD), or adult-onset foveomacular dystrophy, is characterized by a central yellow vitelliform lesion similar to that observed in Best disease, but typically smaller in size with an associated central pigment clump, a later age of onset, slower progression, and only slightly low to normal Arden ratios on electrooculography. The majority of cases are sporadic, but there are reports of familial cases inherited in an autosomal dominant pattern. Several mutations have been described including rare mutations in BEST1 and more commonly RDS (PRPH2) mutations. Patients often present in the fourth or fifth decade of life with minor decrease in visual acuity which may slowly progress due to evolving macular atrophy. Fluorescein angiography shows early blockage with late staining of the central vitelliform lesion and hyperautofluorescence is noted with fundus autofluorescence. OCT imaging shows a central hyper-reflective dome-shaped thickening at the level of the RPE and subneurosensory space. CNVM formation is rare, affecting up to 15% of patients.

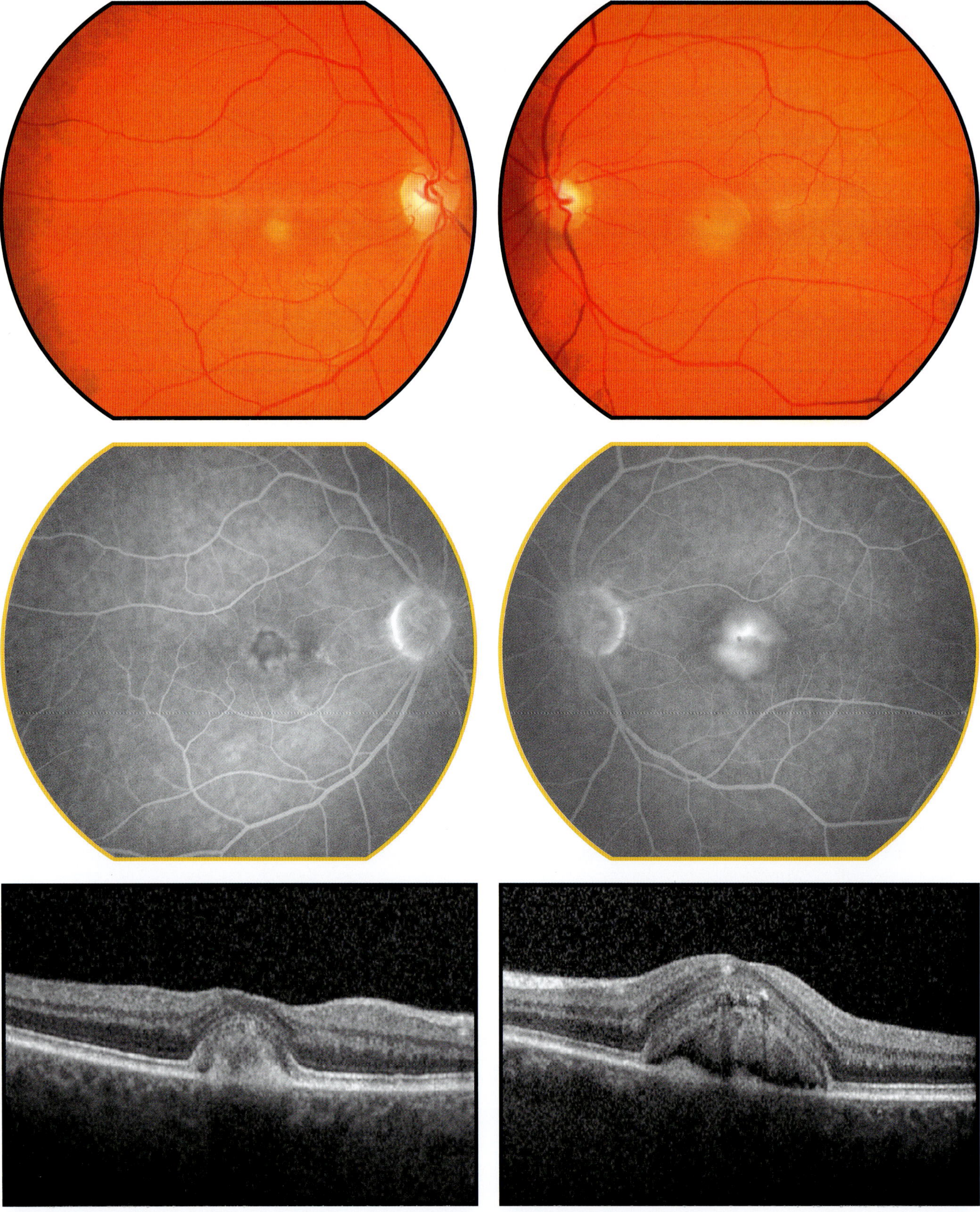

This patient has adult-onset vitelliform macular dystrophy. There is early blockage and late pooling into the vitelliform lesion on fluorescein angiogram. SD-OCT shows the hyper-reflective dome-shaped vitelliform lesion.

Butterfly-Shaped Pattern Dystrophy

Butterfly-shaped pattern dystrophy (BPD) is characterized by a butterfly-shaped pigment pattern surrounded by a zone of depigmentation in the central macula. It is a genetically heterogeneous disorder most often linked to an autosomal dominant mutation in RDS/peripherin (PRPH2), but mutations on the long arm of chromosome 5 have also been described. Fundus autofluorescence shows areas of hyper and hypofluorescence corresponding to the lesion and related to the distribution of lipofuscin. Patients most often exhibit only mild decreases in visual acuity; however, retinal atrophy may ensue leading to reduced central vision with age.

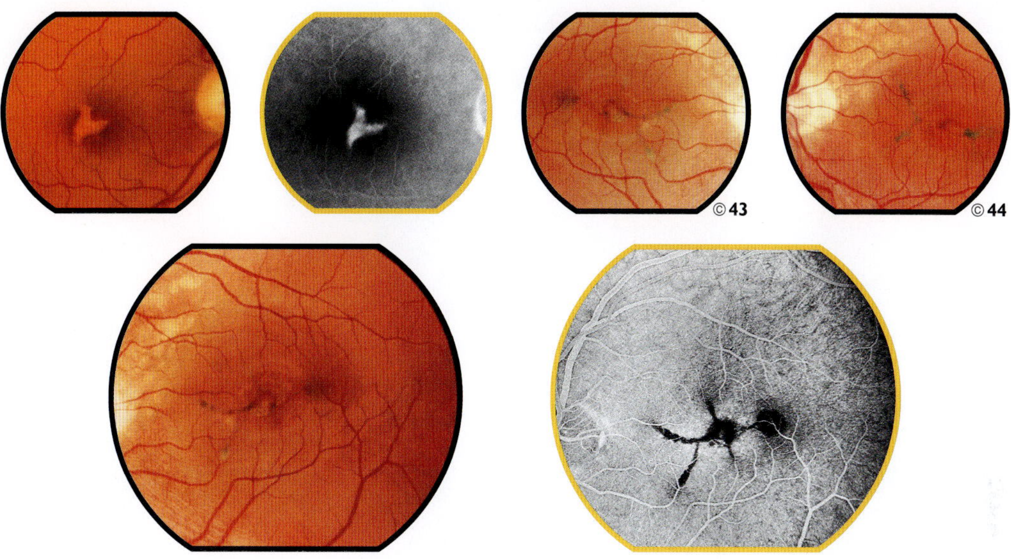

These images are all examples of adult-onset pigment epithelial dystrophy or so-called pattern dystrophy. Note the butterfly configurations of the atrophic and pigmented figures. The fluorescein angiogram shows staining of the atrophic lesion and blockage from the pigmented lesion.

Myotonic Dystrophy 1 (Dystrophia Myotonica, Steinert Disease, DM1)

Myotonic dystrophy is an autosomal dominant disorder caused by mutation in the dystrophia myotonica protein kinase gene (DMPK), located on chromosome 19q13.3. The disease results from an unstable trinucleotide repeat which exhibits the genetic phenomenon of anticipation: increasing number of tandem repeats with each generation resulting in progressive disease severity. The classic clinical findings include myotonia and progressive muscular abnormalities affecting the head and neck and distal before proximal muscle involvement. Other systemic features include frontal balding and bossing (due to temporal muscle atrophy), cognitive impairment, cardiac conduction defects, and hypogonadism. Ocular findings include ptosis, orbicularis weakness, and limitation of extraocular muscle movements, strabismus, hypotony, and iridescent multicolored cataract. Retinal findings include a slowly progressive butterfly-shaped macular pattern dystrophy; 26% of patients with myotonia show these characteristic macular changes. Reticular pigmentary changes may be extensive and present in the posterior pole and/or periphery. Peripheral atrophic polygonal changes and retinal vascular microangiopathy due to narrowing of arterioles and microthrombosis of peripheral retinal vessels may also be observed in some of these patients.

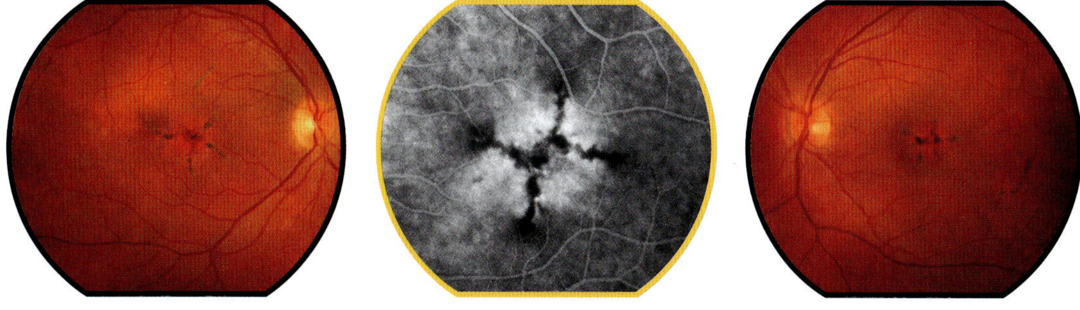

Patients with myotonic dystrophy may also have an associated butterfly-shaped pattern dystrophy. These lesions show blocking on fluorescein angiogram *(middle)* and hyperautofluorescence on autofluorescence imaging (not shown).

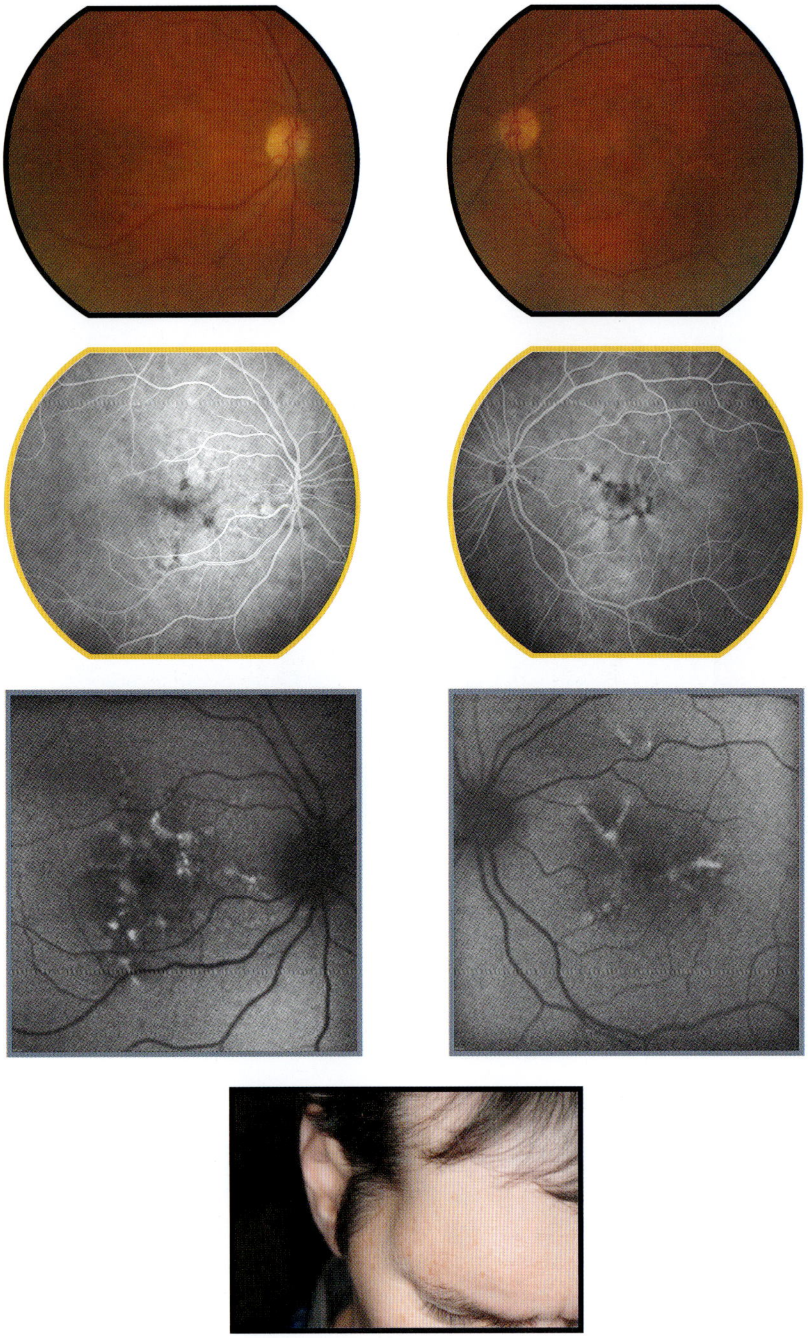

This patient with myotonic dystrophy also has a butterfly-shaped pattern dystrophy highlighted here on fundus autofluorescence and fluorescein angiography. A picture of his forehead shows classic temporal muscle wasting.

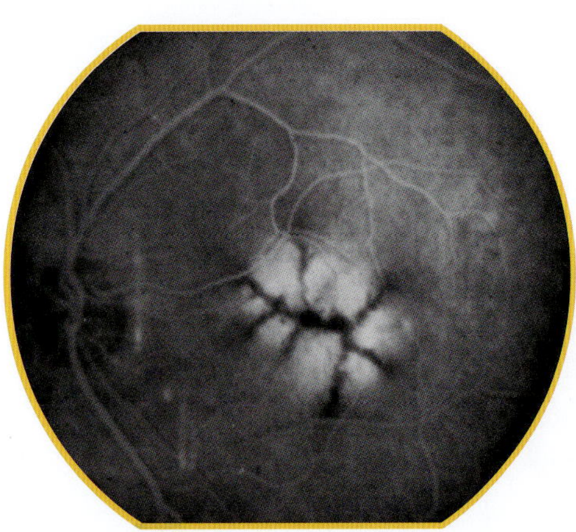
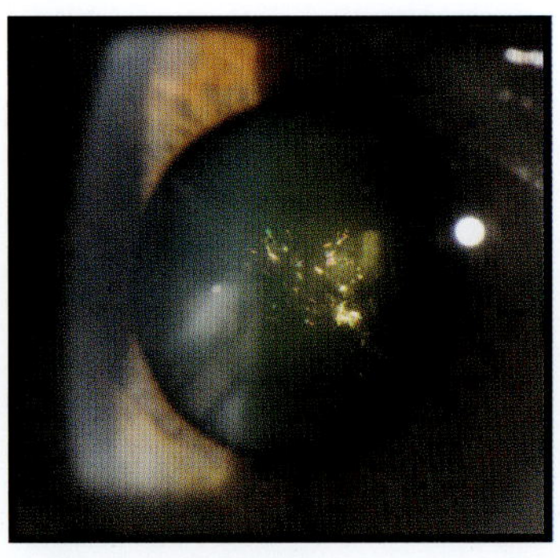
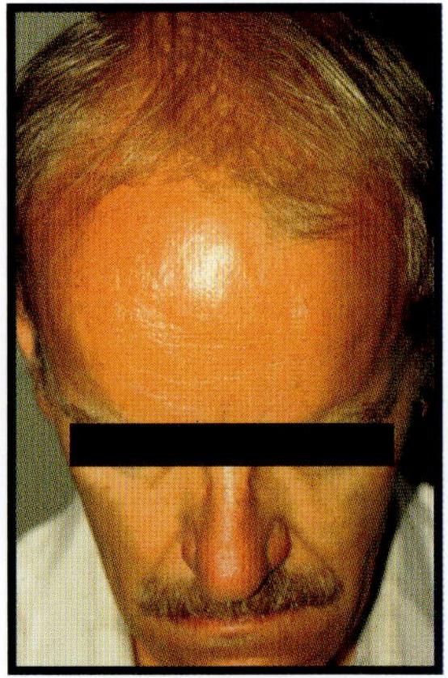

This patient with myotonic dystrophy has a pattern dystrophy of the RPE and multicolored cataract that is characteristic of this disorder. A photograph of his head shows the classic frontal bossing and frontal balding.

Sjögren Reticular Dystrophy (Reticular Pigmentary Retinal Dystrophy of the Posterior Pole)

Sjögren reticular dystrophy is an exceedingly rare condition first described by Sjögren in 1950 with both autosomal recessive and dominant modes of inheritance. A bilateral and symmetric reticular pattern of RPE clumping, hyperplasia, and associated atrophic degenerative changes is noted that may or may not be associated with a slight decrease in central vision. In the initial stages, pigment granules accumulate at the site of the fovea with a network that resembles a "fishnet with knots." The midperiphery and periphery may be spared, but in some cases this may be the principal area of involvement. In more advanced cases the shape of the network becomes irregular and bleached as the pigment gradually disappears. Fundus autofluorescence nicely highlights the hyperfluorescent reticular pattern of RPE changes that conversely block with fluorescein angiography. There are no known ERG abnormalities although the EOG Arden ratio may be reduced. The reticular changes probably appear in infancy and are often fully developed by 15 years of age. Choroidal neovascularization may explain vision loss during the adult stages of this disease.

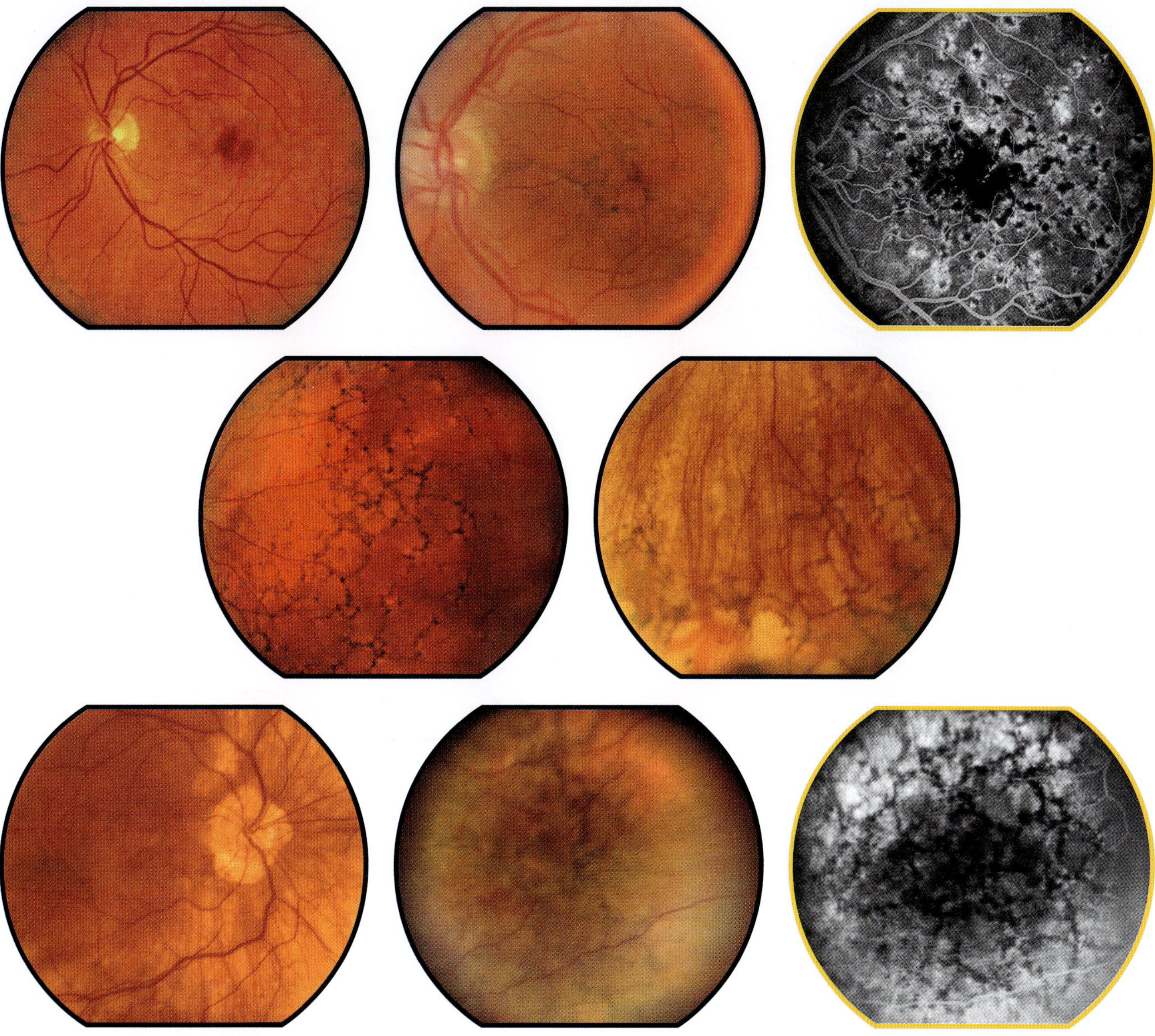

Sjögren reticular dystrophy is associated with pigment epithelial hyperplastic and atrophic degenerative changes that often form a reticular or fishnet pattern in the macula, posterior pole, and peripheral fundus. The fluorescein angiogram accentuates these changes, given the contrast induced by the pigment and the atrophy. *Courtesy of Drs Ron Carr and Ken Noble*

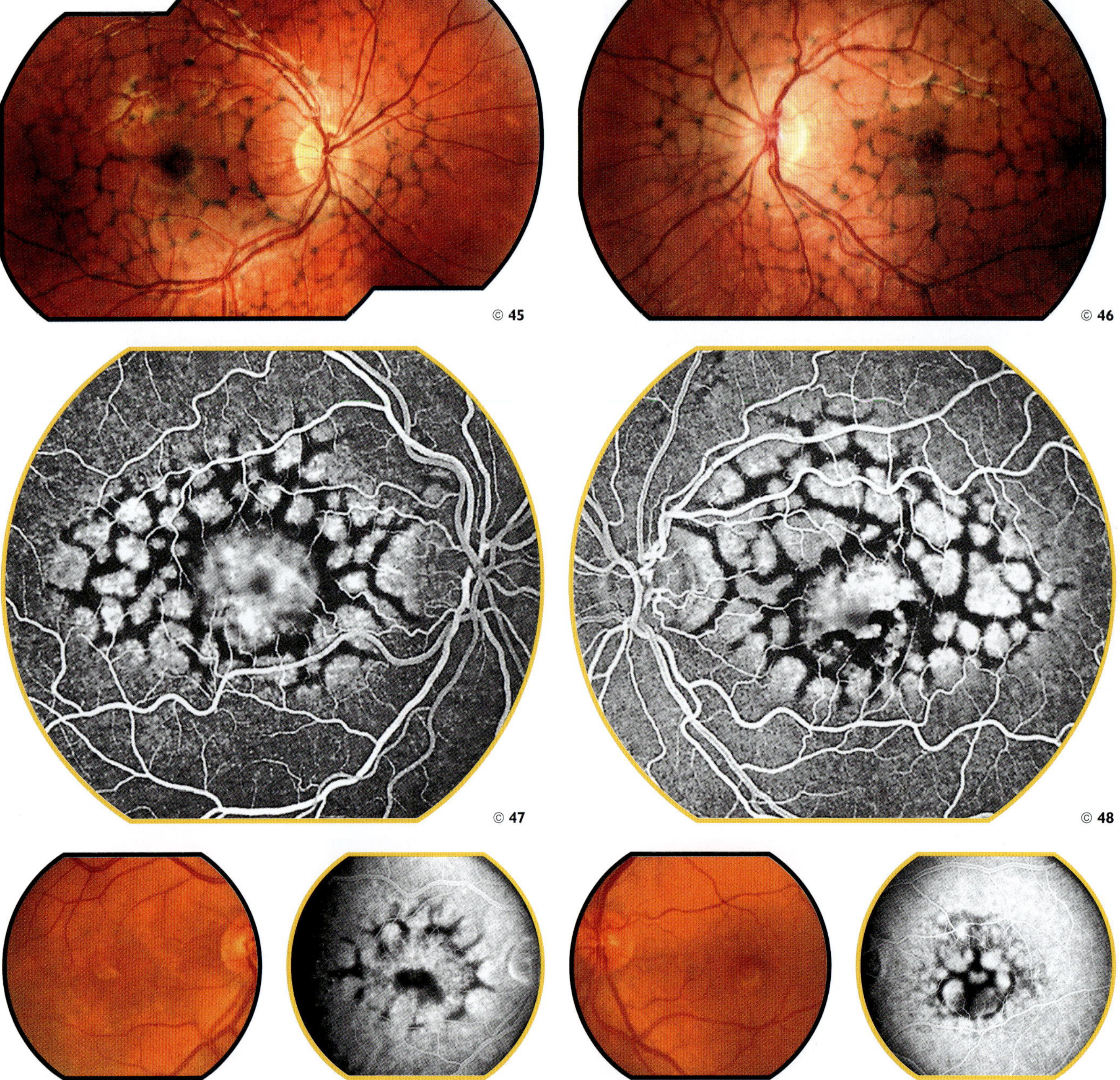

These patients demonstrate a variation in the reticular pattern that is seen in Sjögren reticular dystrophy. Note the extension of the reticular changes surrounding the disc in the top two photos. The fluorescein angiogram in the middle photos highlights the reticular pattern due to blockage by the pigmentary changes. The last patient *(bottom row)* shows that blockage on fluorescein angiogram may be present, even when there is no melanin pigmentation in the fundus. This blockage indicates the presence of lipofuscin within the reticular pattern.

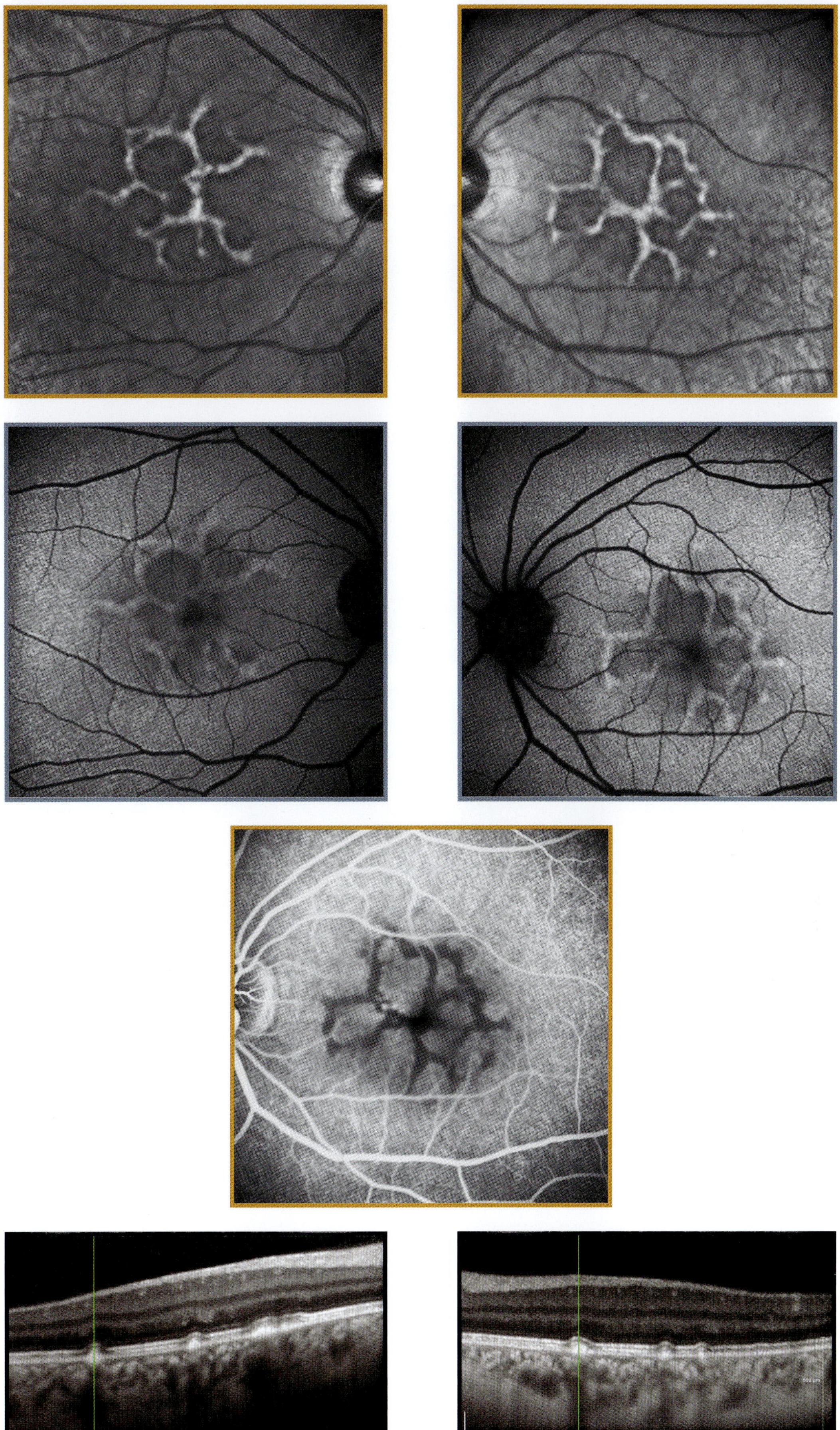

Near-infrared photos, fundus autofluorence *(second row)*, late phase fluorescein angiogram of the left eye and accompanying SD-OCT of a patient with Sjögren reticular dystrophy showing multifocal hypertrophy of the RPE. *Images courtesy of Eric Souied, MD*

Fundus Pulverulentus

Fundus pulverulentus is a rare, autosomal dominant pattern dystrophy characterized by coarse mottling and punctate pigment clumping of the RPE in the macula. Its genetic basis has not yet been identified.

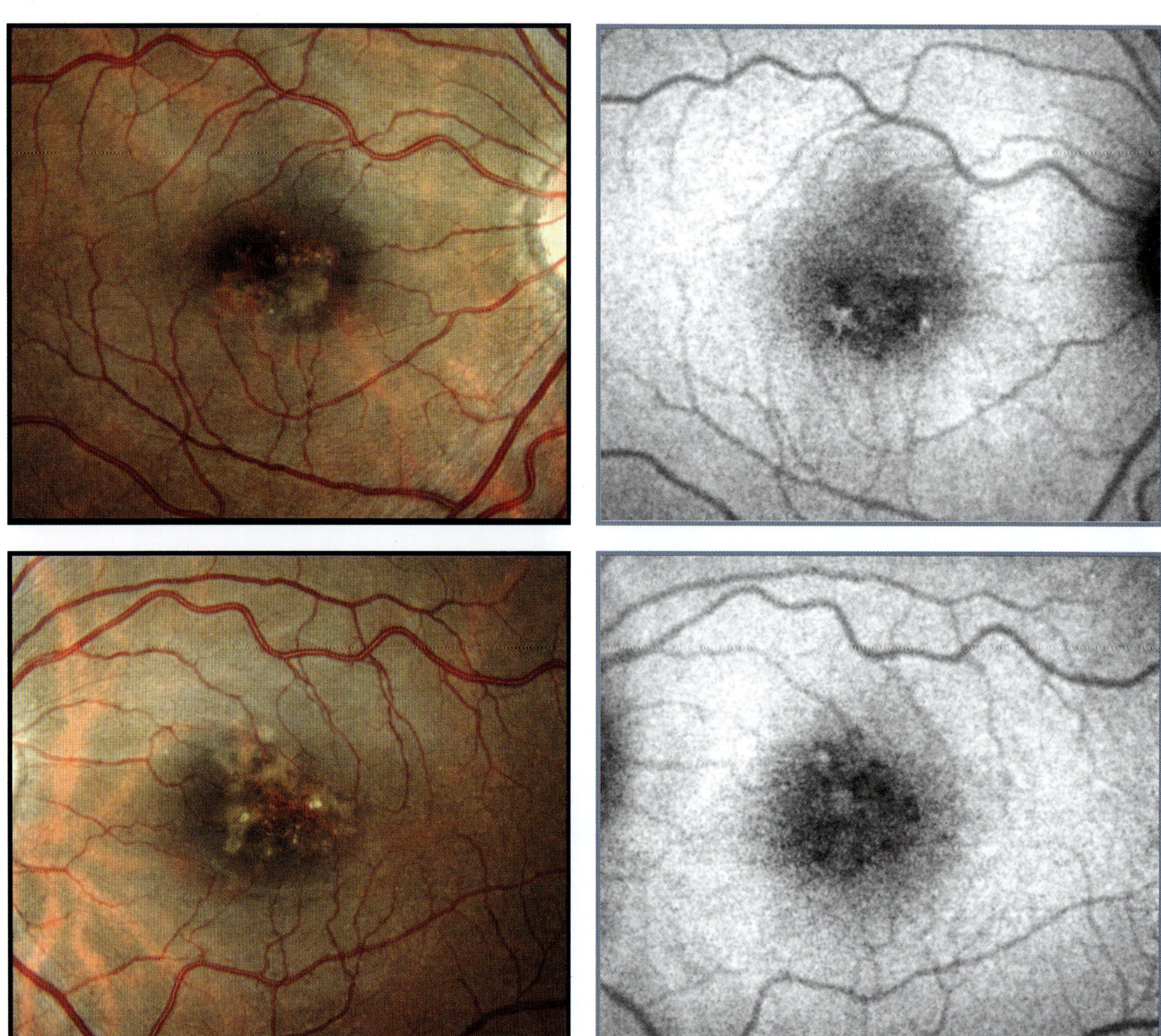

A patient with pattern dystrophy, most likely representing the pulverulentus subtype, with stippling of the RPE in the central macula. These changes are often accentuated on the fundus autofluorescent images.

Multifocal Pattern Dystrophy Simulating Fundus Flavimaculatus

Autosomal dominant mutations of the peripherin/RDS (PRPH2) gene have been demonstrated in some family members of patients with multifocal pattern dystrophy. Funduscopically, multiple irregular or triradiate yellow lesions are seen centrally or eccentrically, sometimes widely scattered and partly interconnected, simulating Stargardt disease, but in the absence of any evidence of macular atrophy or angiographic dark choroid. FA shows multifocal stellate hypofluorescent lesions surrounded by hyperfluorescence and the lesions hyperfluoresce with autofluorescent imaging. Histopathologic and electron microscopic studies have revealed minor variations in pigmentation of the RPE with distended cells containing tubulovesicular membranous material in the cytoplasm but no evidence of excess lipofuscin accumulation. Visual prognosis is excellent unless choroidal neovascularization complicates the underlying disorder.

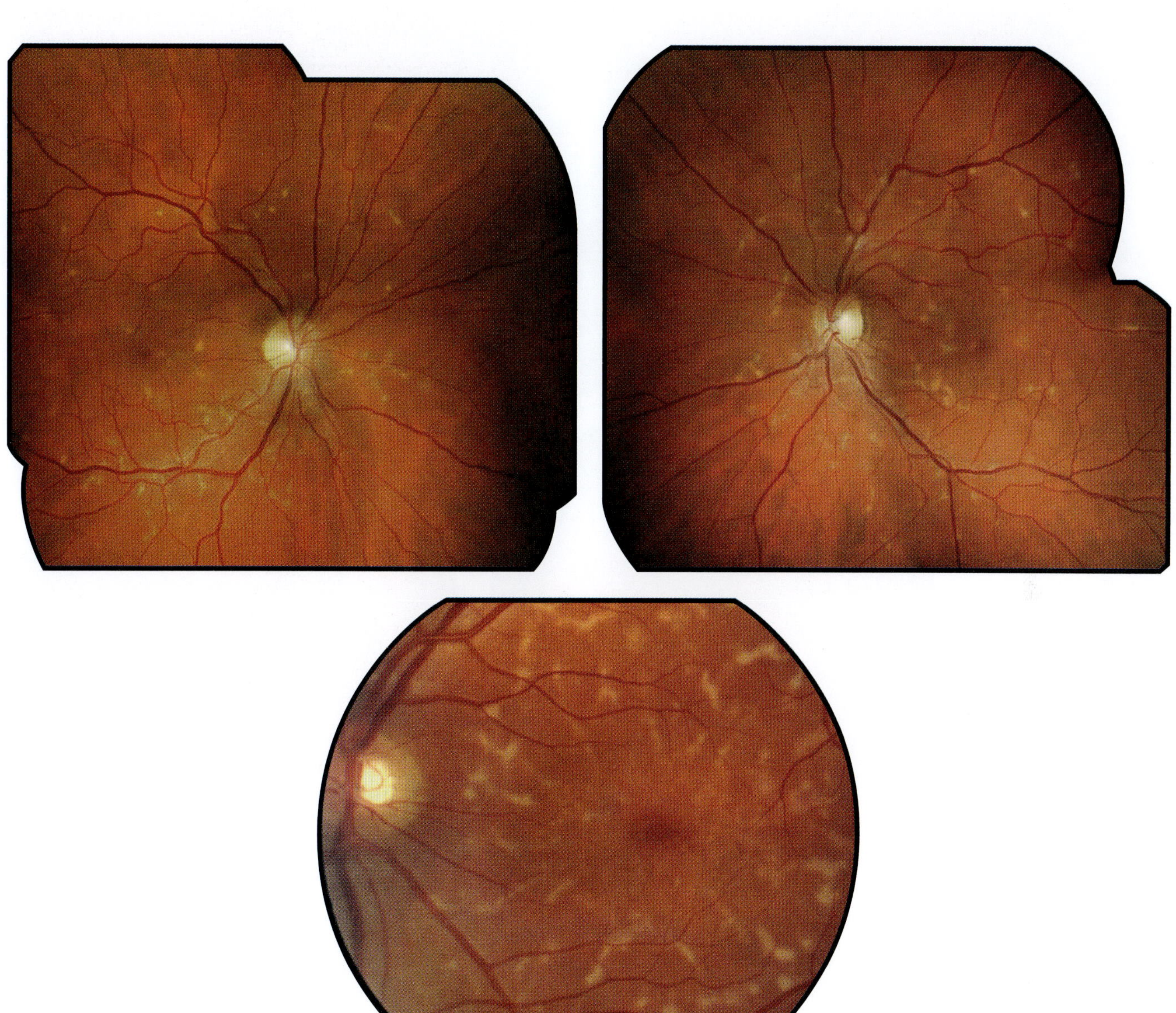

Color fundus photographs of two cases of multifocal pattern dystrophy with triradiate fleck-like lesions scattered throughout the posterior pole and beyond the arcades. Good vision is commonly associated with this disturbance in the absence of macular atrophy, in contrast to Stargardt disease.
Top row courtesy of Dr. Mark Balles

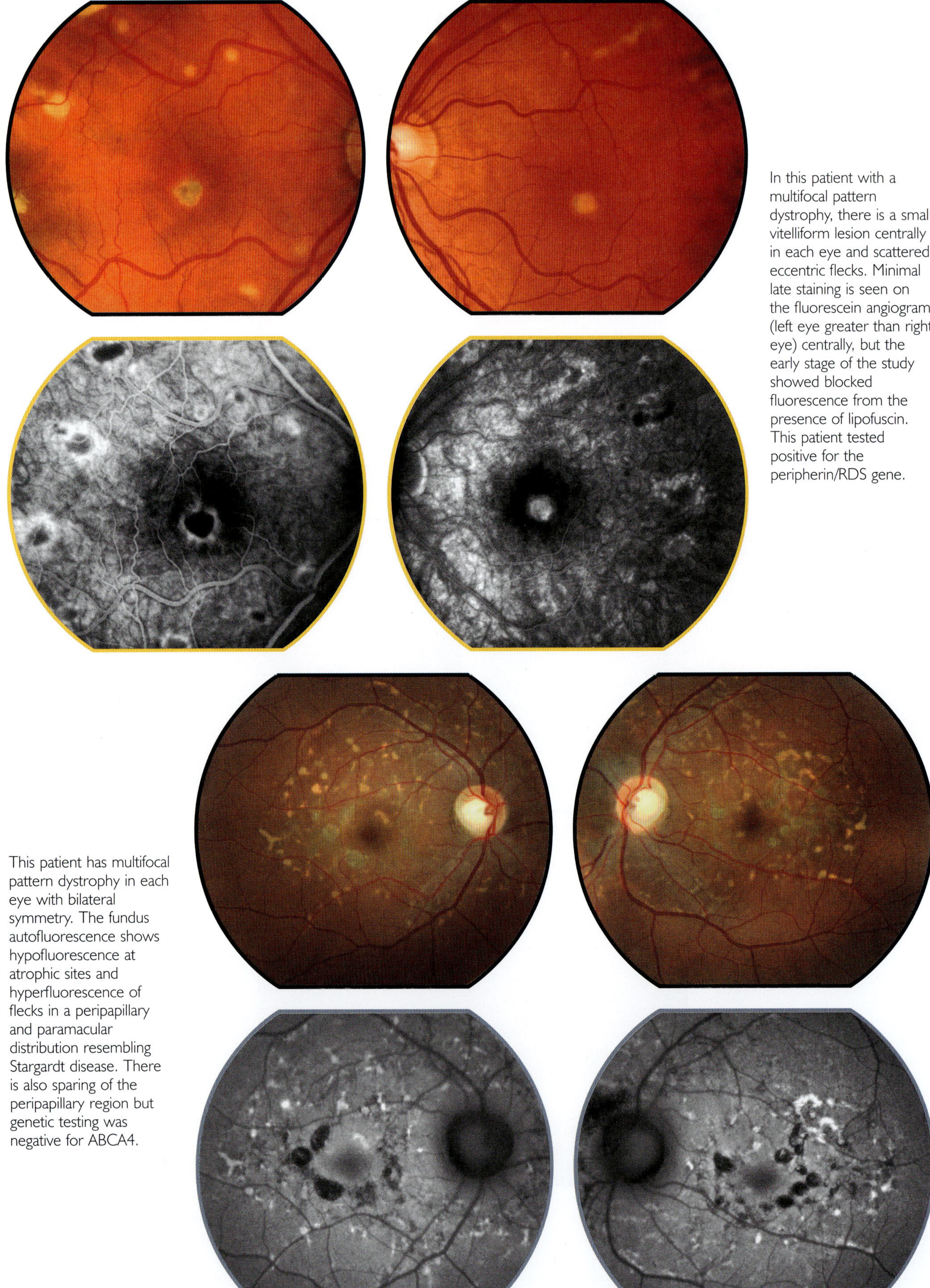

In this patient with a multifocal pattern dystrophy, there is a small vitelliform lesion centrally in each eye and scattered eccentric flecks. Minimal late staining is seen on the fluorescein angiogram (left eye greater than right eye) centrally, but the early stage of the study showed blocked fluorescence from the presence of lipofuscin. This patient tested positive for the peripherin/RDS gene.

This patient has multifocal pattern dystrophy in each eye with bilateral symmetry. The fundus autofluorescence shows hypofluorescence at atrophic sites and hyperfluorescence of flecks in a peripapillary and paramacular distribution resembling Stargardt disease. There is also sparing of the peripapillary region but genetic testing was negative for ABCA4.

Pattern Dystrophy and Choroidal Neovascularization

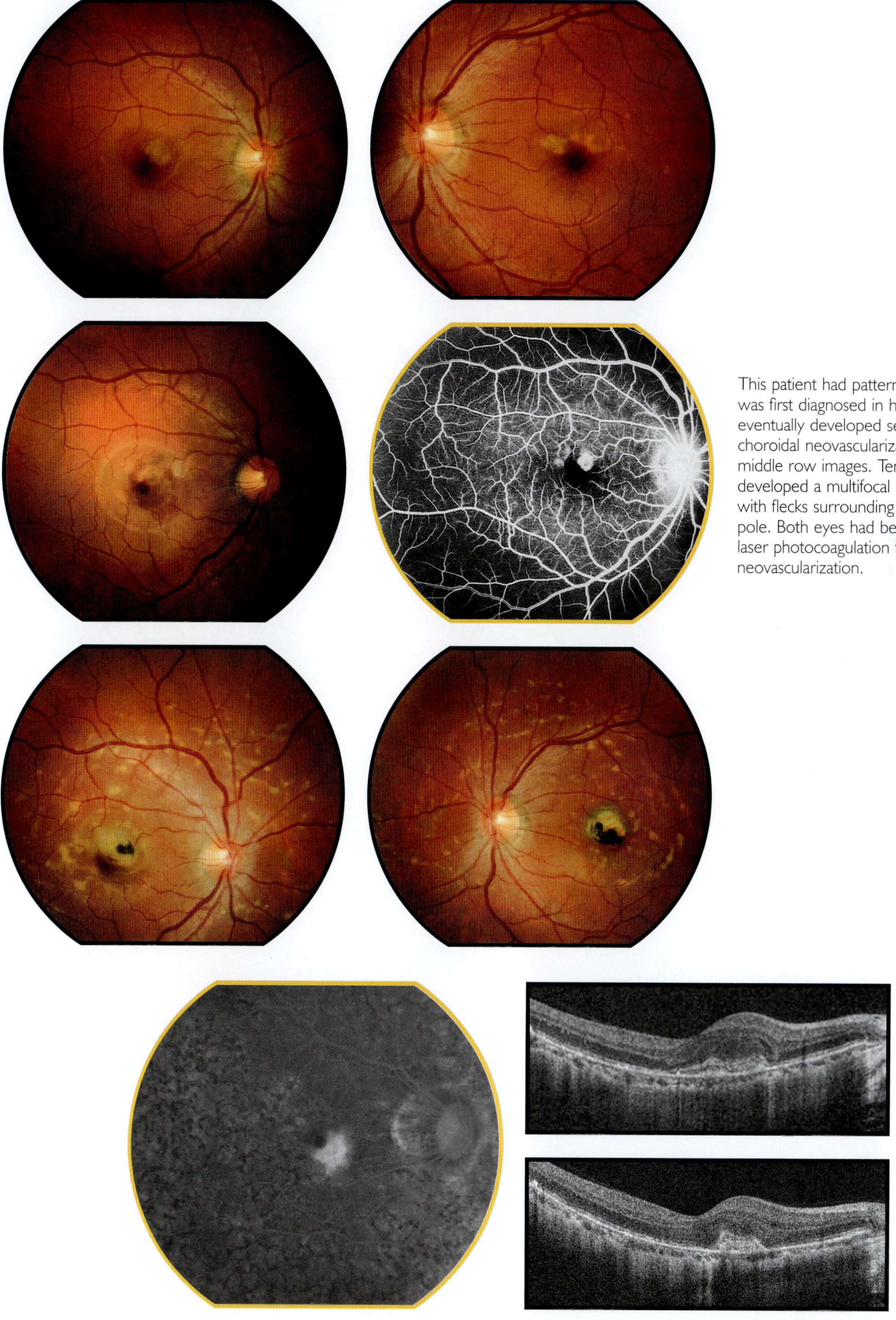

This patient had pattern dystrophy, which was first diagnosed in his 30s. He eventually developed secondary choroidal neovascularization, seen in the middle row images. Ten years later, he developed a multifocal dystrophic fundus with flecks surrounding the posterior pole. Both eyes had been treated with laser photocoagulation for choroidal neovascularization.

Fluorescein angiography of this patient with Sjögren reticular dystrophy shows late leakage of a classic choroidal neovascular membrane in the central macula. SD-OCT confirms the presence of a type II neovascular membrane, which may develop in eyes with pattern dystrophy *(top right)*. Visual acuity improved after injection of anti-VEGF agents and the type II neovascular membrane decreased in size as seen on follow-up SD-OCT *(bottom right)*. *Images courtesy of David Boyer, MD*

Malattia Leventinese (Doyne Honeycomb Retinal Dystrophy, Autosomal Dominant Radial Drusen)

Malattia leventinese is inherited in an autosomal dominant pattern due, in most cases, to mutation in the EFEMP1 (EGF-containing fibrillin-like extracellular matrix protein 1) gene, also known as the fibulin 3 gene on chromosome 2p16. The classic finding is the bilateral presence of drusen in a radiating pattern throughout the macula, most prominently on the temporal side. Drusen may also be found outside the arcades and nasal to the optic nerve, but the periphery is typically spared. Central coalescence of soft drusen may simulate a vitelliform macular dystrophy. These drusen are histologically composed of deposits between the RPE and Bruch membrane similar in composition to those found in AMD. Variable amounts of RPE hyperplasia and irregular subretinal fibrous metaplasia may be present. Drusen onset varies from childhood to old age with most patients presenting by the third or fourth decade of life often complaining of decreased vision, metamorphopsia or central scotoma. As the disorder progresses, confluence of the drusen with pigment hyperplasia, geographic atrophy, and choroidal neovascularization can lead to severe visual loss.

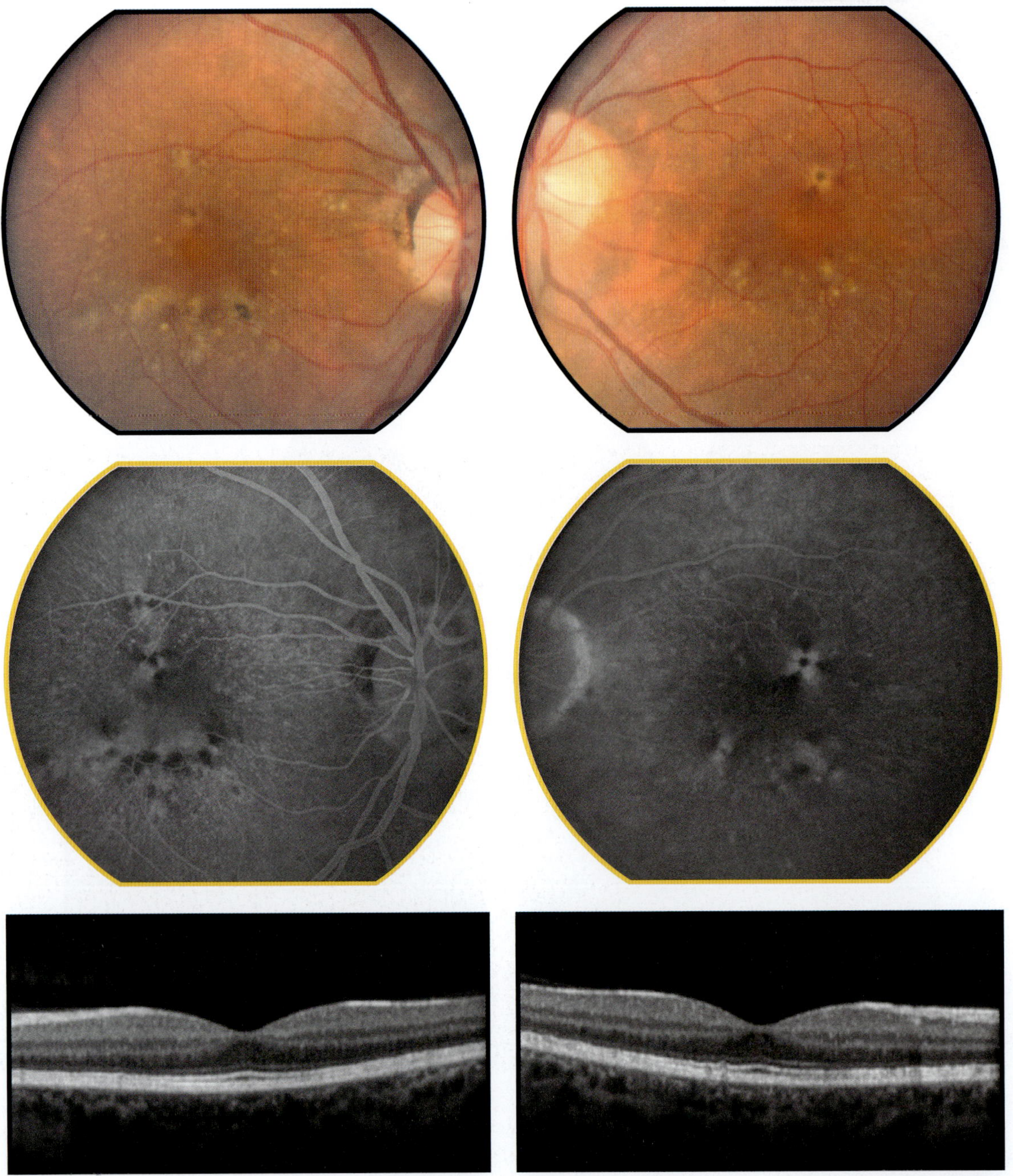

Color fundus photos showing diffuse macular drusen distributed in a radial pattern that stain with fluorescein angiography. Subtle hyper-reflective thickening of the RPE/Bruch complex may be seen on SD-OCT temporal OS.

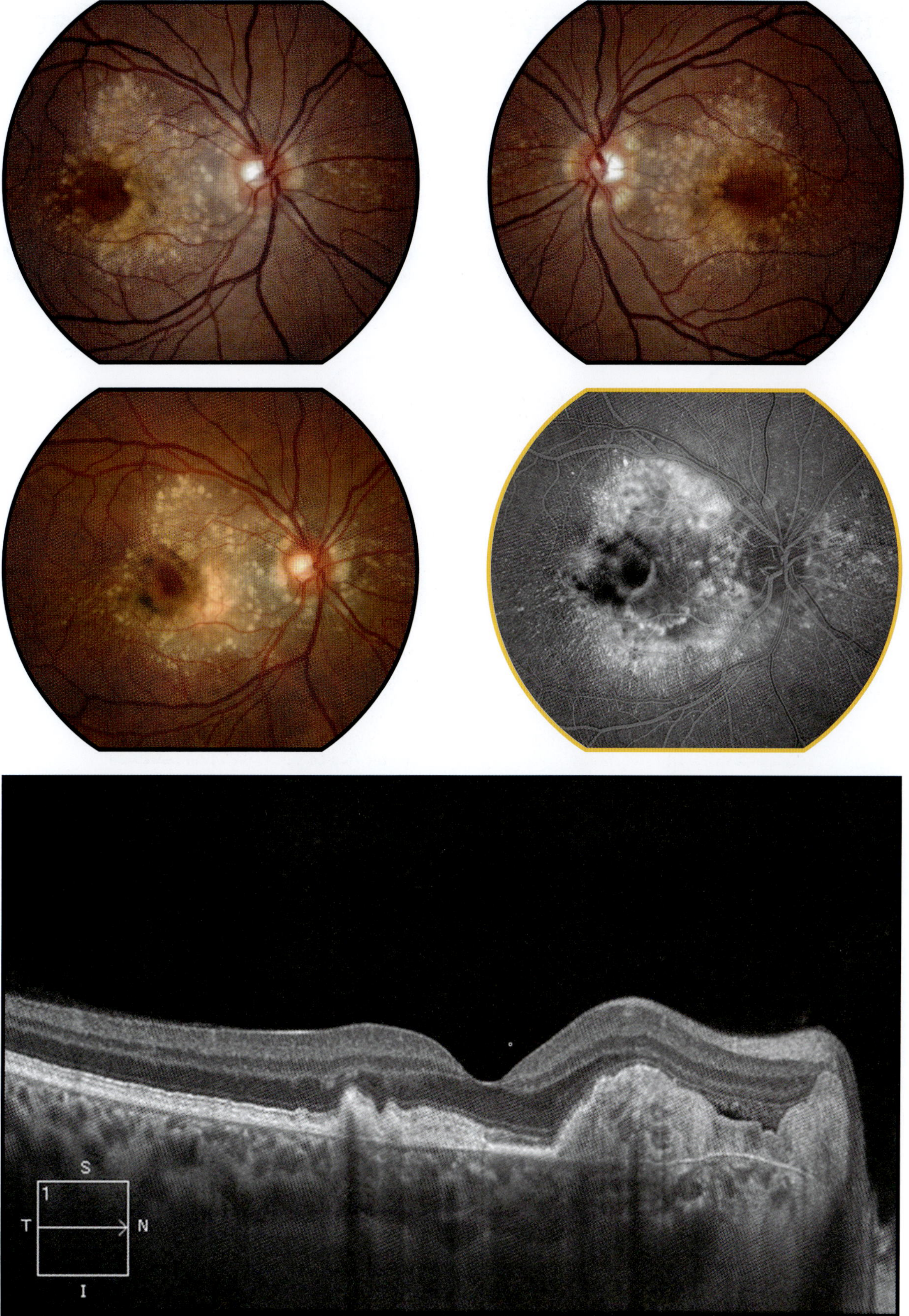

This patient shows confluent and radially oriented drusen with color fundus photography *(top row)*. Genetic testing confirmed mutation in EFEMP1. Five years after initial presentation, she developed choroidal neovascularization in the left eye and was treated with anti-VEGF therapy (not shown). Eight years after initial presentation, she developed choroidal neovascularization of the right eye. Color fundus photos at this presentation show confluent and radial drusen and hemorrhage *(middle row)*. Fluorescein angiogram shows classic choroidal neovascularization *(middle row, right)*. SD-OCT confirms the presence of a type II neovascular membrane and fibrovascular scar formation. The patient was treated with anti-VEGF therapy. *Images courtesy of Francisco Rodriguez, MD*

Membranoproliferative Glomerulonephritis (Mesangiocapillary Glomerulonephritis)

There are three types of membranoproliferative glomerulonephritis (MPGN) classified based on location and composition of the protein deposits within the kidney. Type II is the most severe and progressive type with onset in childhood or early adulthood; it often affects the fundus and recurs even after renal transplantation. Complement component C3 deficiency, partial lipodystrophy, and complement factor H deficiency are associated with this disorder. Type II MPGN is associated with basal laminar drusen as well as larger, more variably sized drusen in the macula and paramacular region; these increase in number and size with age but are not typically associated with visual sequelae. Rarely choroidal neovascularization and vision loss can develop at an early age. Histopathology and electron microscopy reveal diffuse, electron dense, focal deposits within Bruch membrane and the choriocapillaris, similar to those found in the glomerulus.

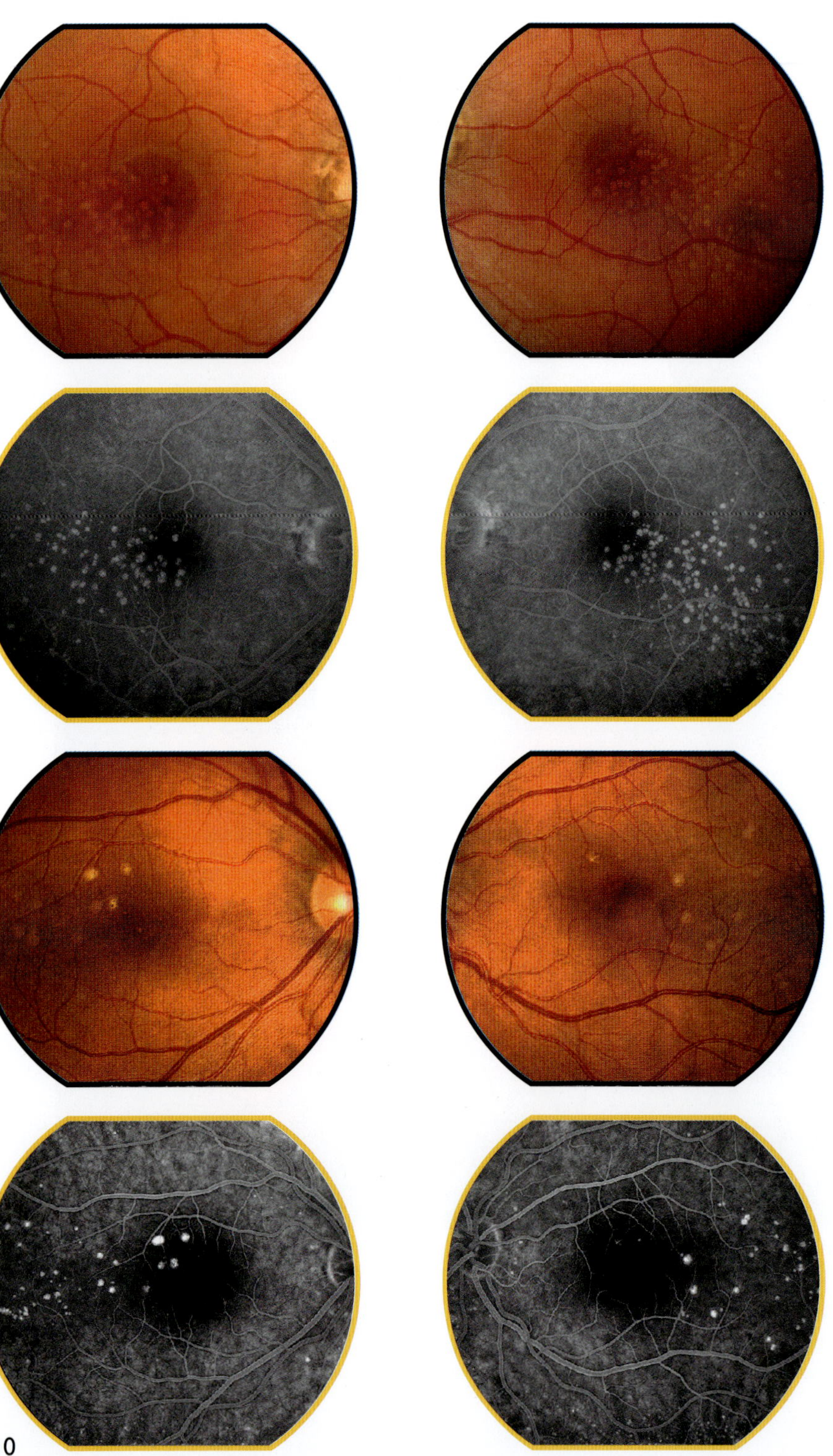

Membranoproliferative glomerulonephritis (MPGN type II) is an oculorenal syndrome which may be associated with macular abnormalities. Initially, variably sized drusenoid changes are evident in the macula and paramacular region. They may lead to neovascularization from the choroid. *Bottom two rows courtesy of Ophthalmic Imaging Systems, Inc*

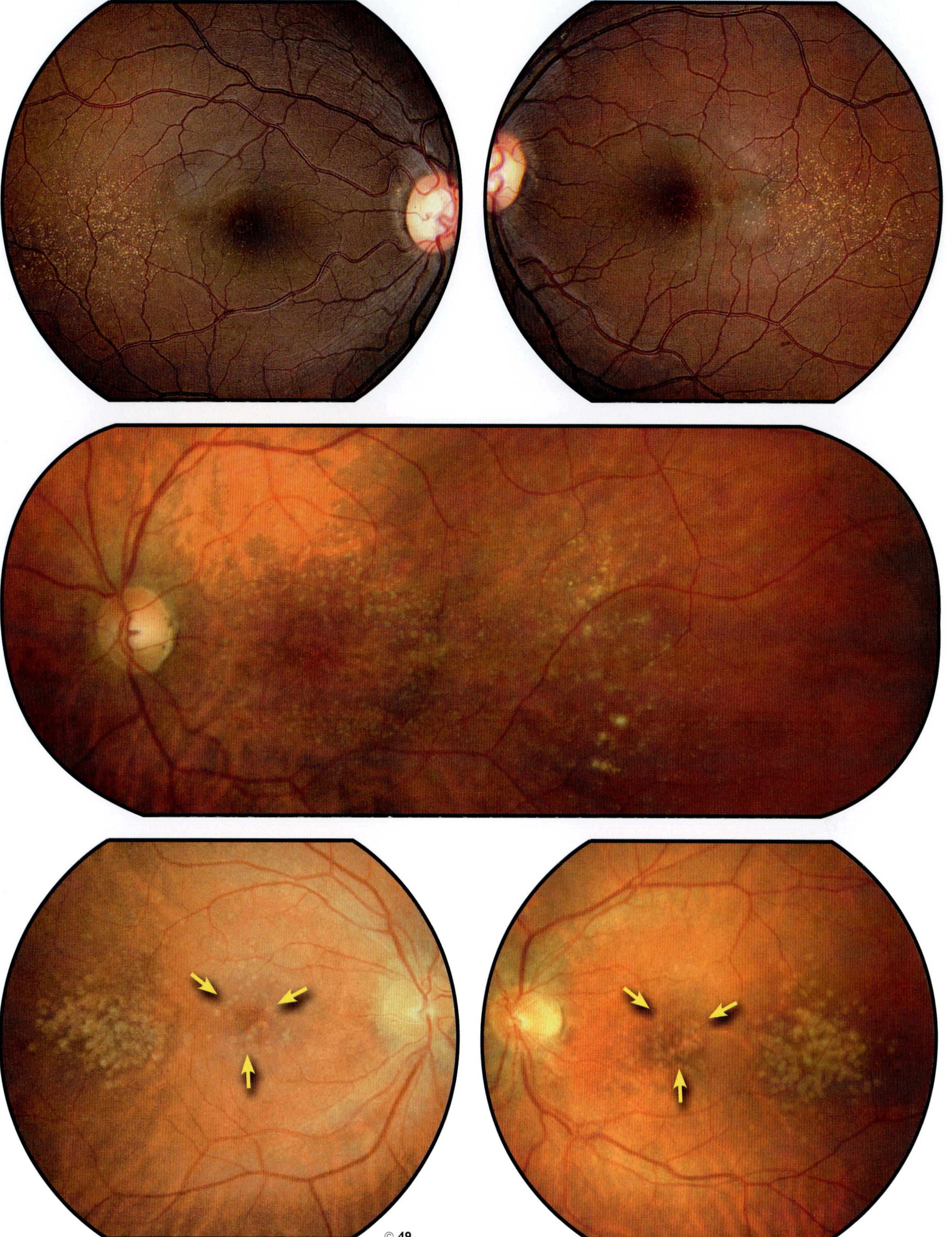

© 49

These patients have MPGN type II with variable sized drusenoid deposition symmetrically present in the central macula *(arrows)* and beyond.

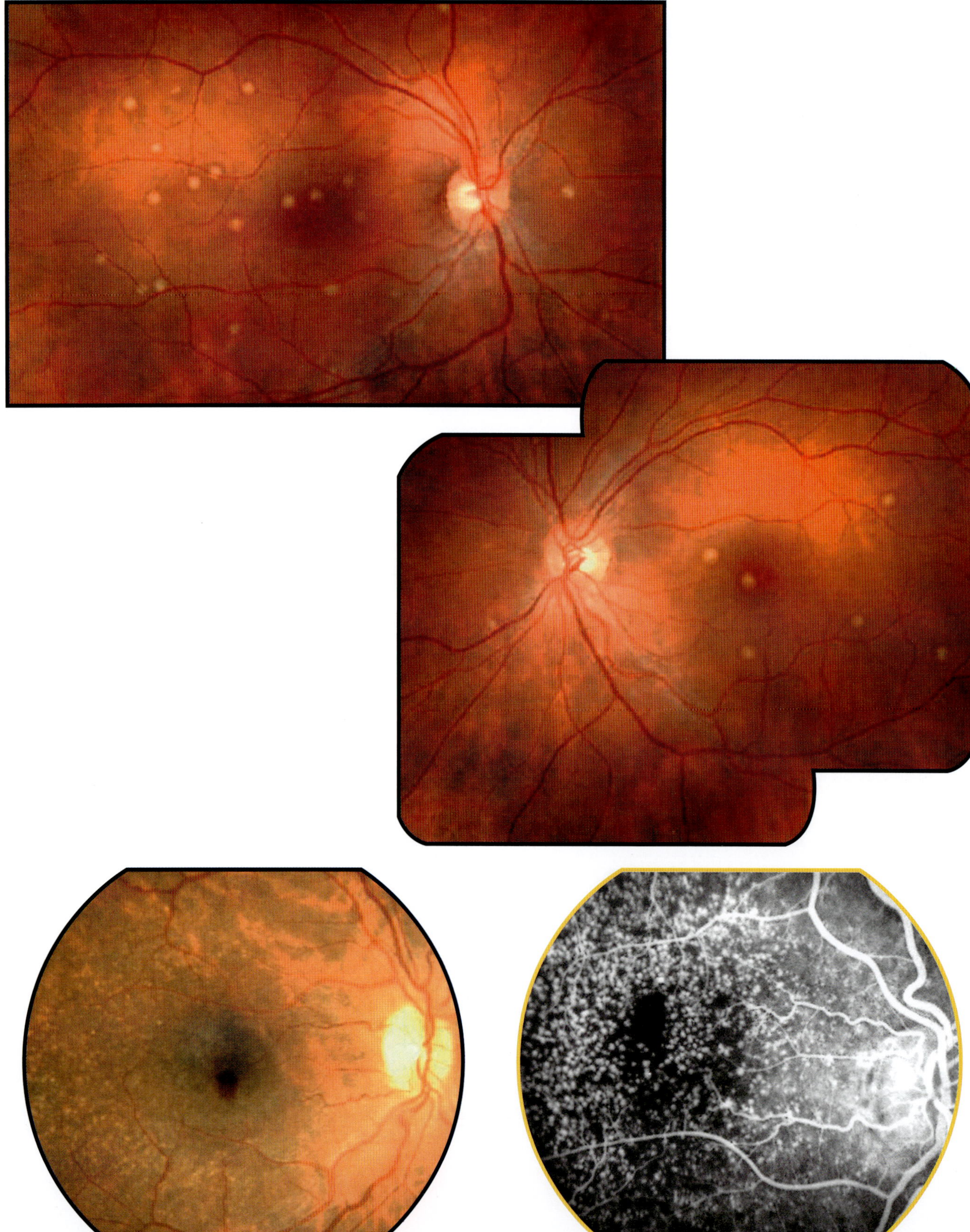

These two cases showed a marked variation in the drusenoid changes in patients with membranoproliferative glomerulonephritis type II. The patient shown in the top two images has discrete nummular drusen resembling small pigment epithelial detachments, scattered randomly throughout the macula and near temporal periphery. The patient shown in the bottom row has a multitude of small drusenoid changes of a size and dimension that are similar to basal laminar cuticular drusen or simply small drusen. *Bottom two images courtesy of Dr. Craig Mason*

Alport Syndrome

Alport syndrome is caused by mutations in collagen biosynthesis genes. Most patients with Alport syndrome have an X-linked pattern due to a mutation in the COL4A5 gene located on chromosome Xq22.3; autosomal dominant and recessive patterns of inheritance have also been reported. Systemically, Alport syndrome is characterized by childhood-onset nephritis, renal failure by the fifth decade, high-frequency, progressive sensorineural deafness, and multiple ocular manifestations. Anterior segment findings include posterior polymorphous corneal dystrophy, anterior and posterior subcapsular cataracts, anterior lenticonus, and microspherophakia. Approximately 85% of patients develop a "dot and fleck" retinopathy which is characterized by multiple, small, punctate yellow-white, sometimes refractile, deposits often in a ring-like configuration around the fovea with temporal extension. These deposits may extend to the arcades and midperiphery. Patients may present early in childhood and lesions may become more apparent with age. Spotty window defects in the RPE that are associated with the peripheral lesions may represent nodular thickening of the basement membrane of the RPE and can be seen on fluorescein angiography. Optical coherence tomography may reveal temporal macular thinning in up to 80% of patients. Macular hole formation may complicate the course of retinal disease.

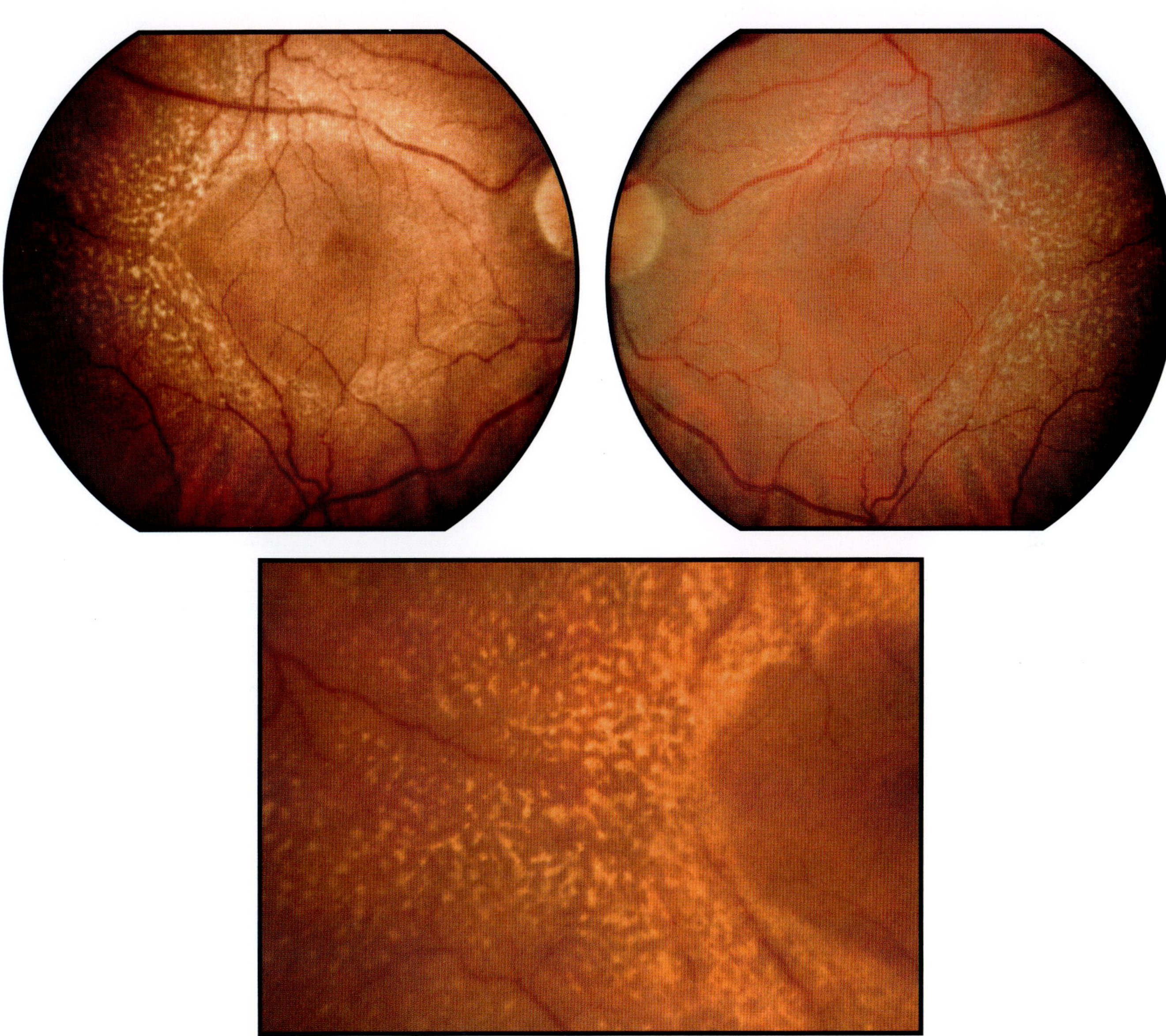

This patient with Alport syndrome has multiple crystalline-like deposits in the temporal macula, extending toward the vascular arcades and paramacular region. *Images courtesy of Dr. Scott Sneed*

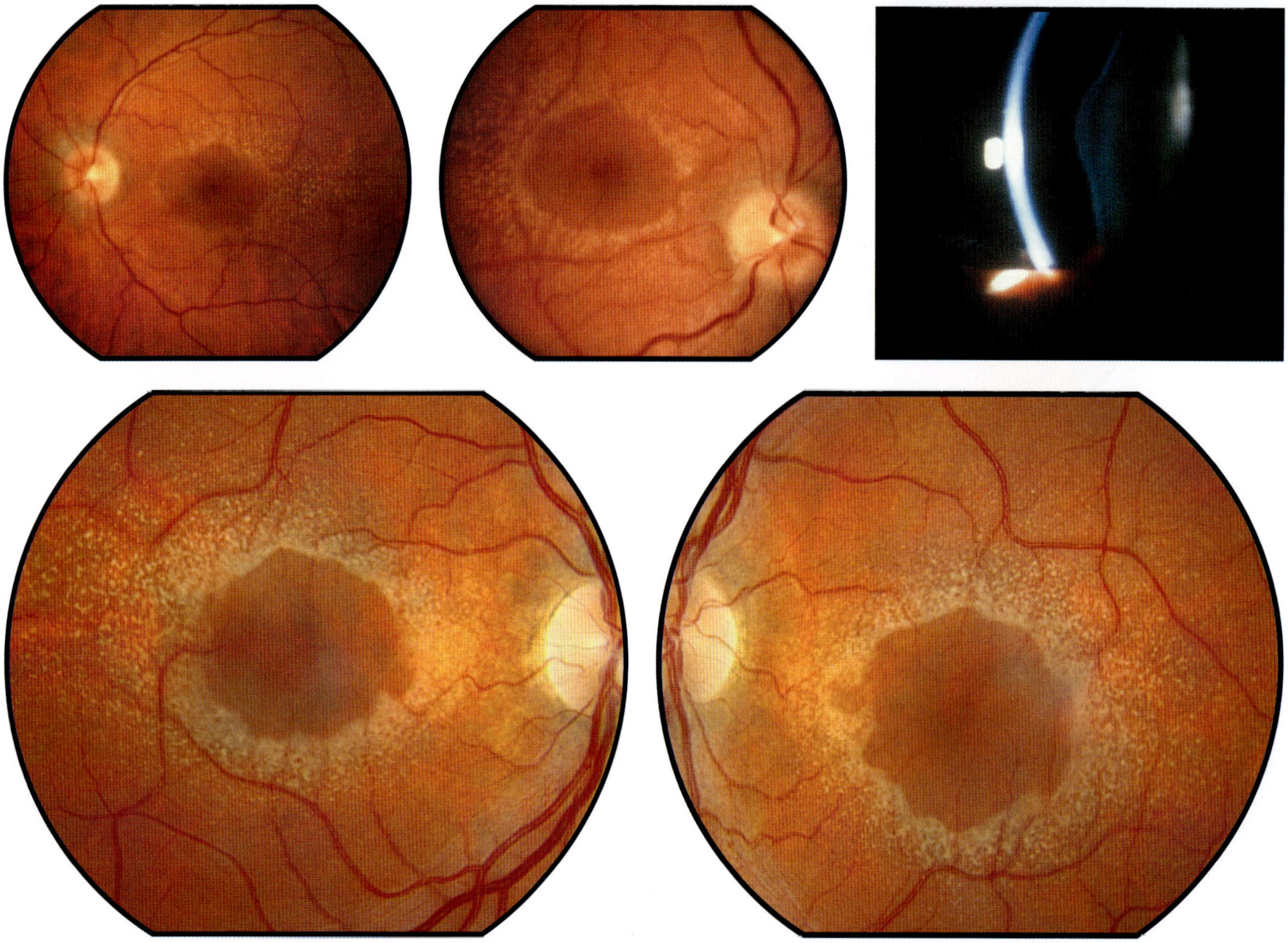

These patients demonstrate prominent crystalline-like deposits in Alport syndrome. The lesions are distributed circumferentially around the macula with temporal predilection. Note the presence of anterior lenticonus. *Courtesy of Dr. Herbert Cantrill*

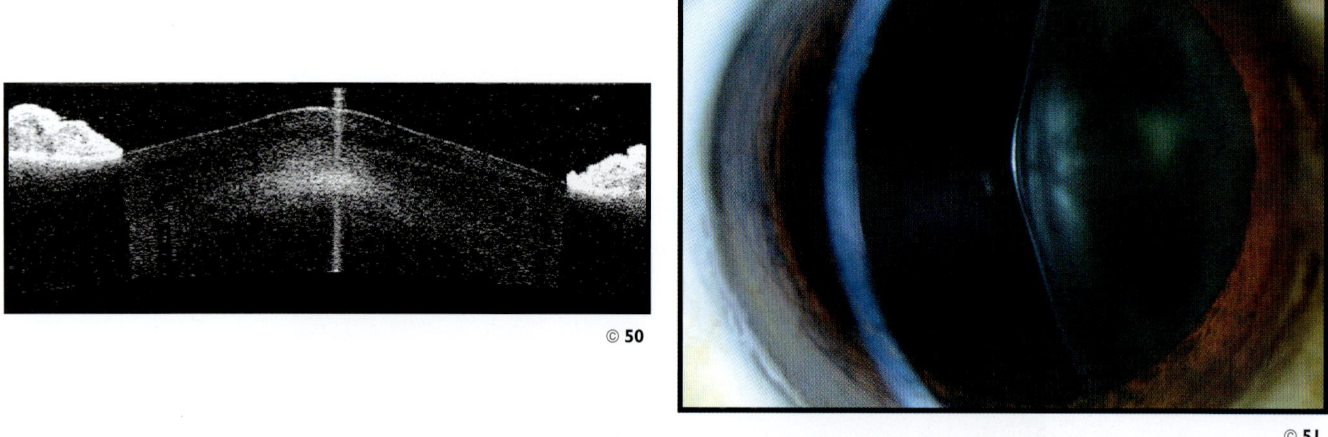

© **50**

© **51**

An OCT of the lens and a color image of the anterior segment demonstrate the anterior lenticonus in a patient with Alport syndrome.

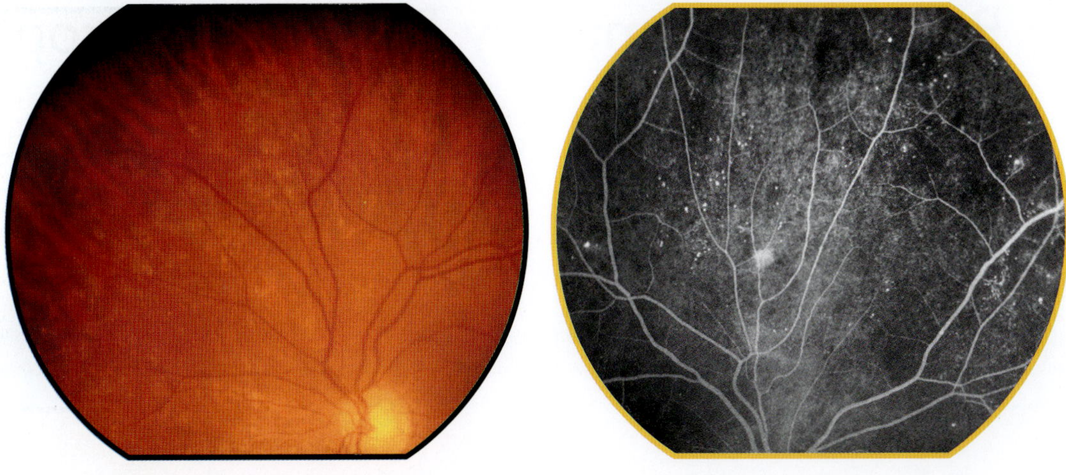

Extramacular drusenoid deposits with late staining and even some crystals may be seen in the peripheral fundus of patients with Alport syndrome.

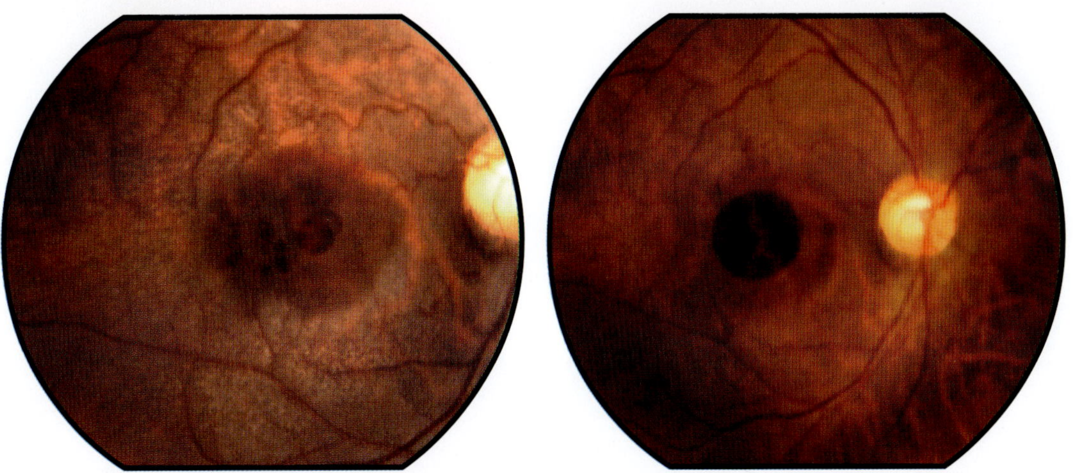

Patients with Alport syndrome may develop macular holes. This patient demonstrated a large full thickness macular hole without evidence of trauma. *Courtesy of Dr. David Weinberg*

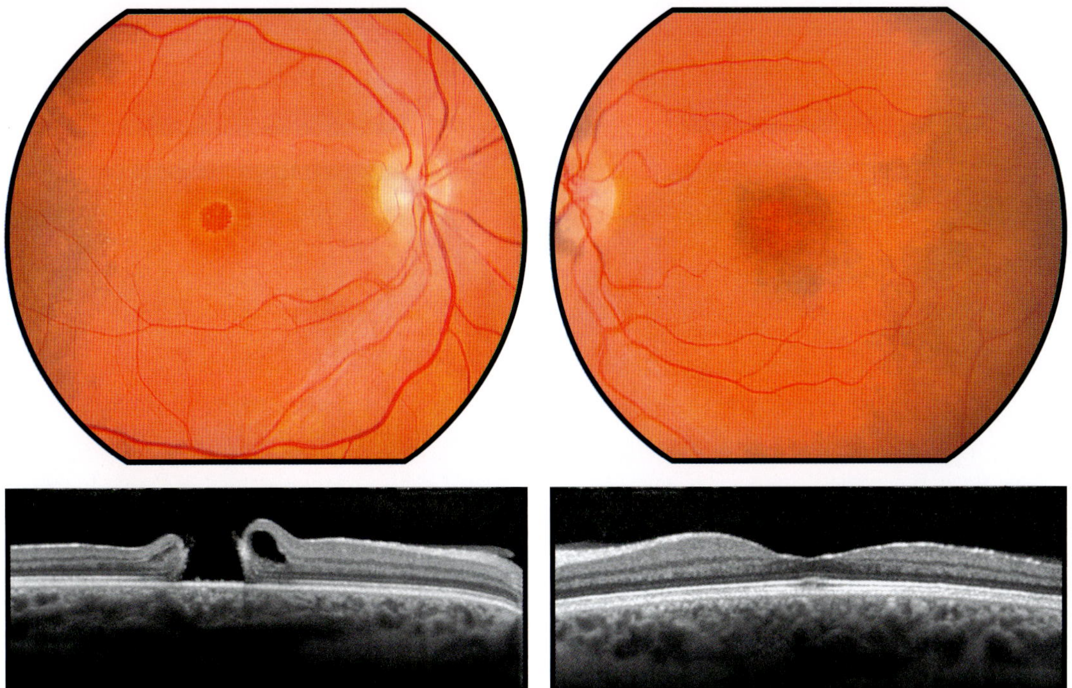

This patient with Alport syndrome developed a large macular hole in the right eye. Note the subtle deposits located in the temporal macula OU. *Photos courtesy of Arthur D. Fu, MD*

Sorsby Pseudoinflammatory Fundus Dystrophy

Sorsby pseudoinflammatory fundus dystrophy is an autosomal dominant maculopathy caused by mutation in the gene encoding for tissue inhibitor of metalloproteinase-3 (TIMP3) at 22q12.1-q13.2. The retinal changes usually become apparent in the third to fifth decade of life with the deposition of confluent yellow drusen-like material throughout the posterior pole and progression to choroidal neovascularization, hemorrhagic maculopathy, and eventual disciform fibrosis and atrophy which can extend well beyond the macula, producing profound vision loss.

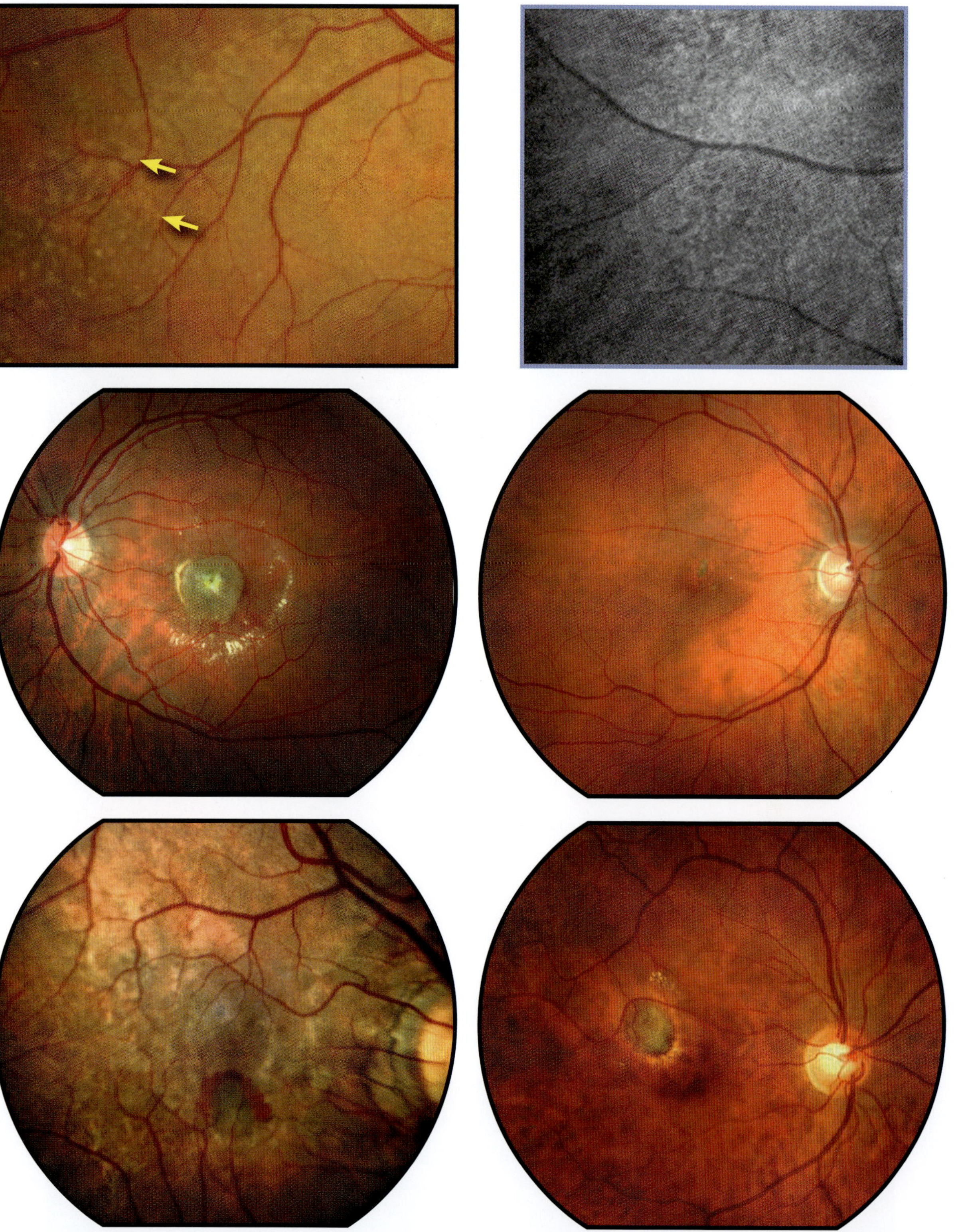

Sorsby pseudoinflammatory fundus dystrophy may initially present with multiple drusen-like spots in the paramacular region *(top two photographs, arrows)*. Choroidal neovascularization may develop, as seen in the four cases illustrated on this page. The neovascularization may be type 2 (or "classic" by fluorescein angiography), as evidenced by the gray-green membrane in each case.

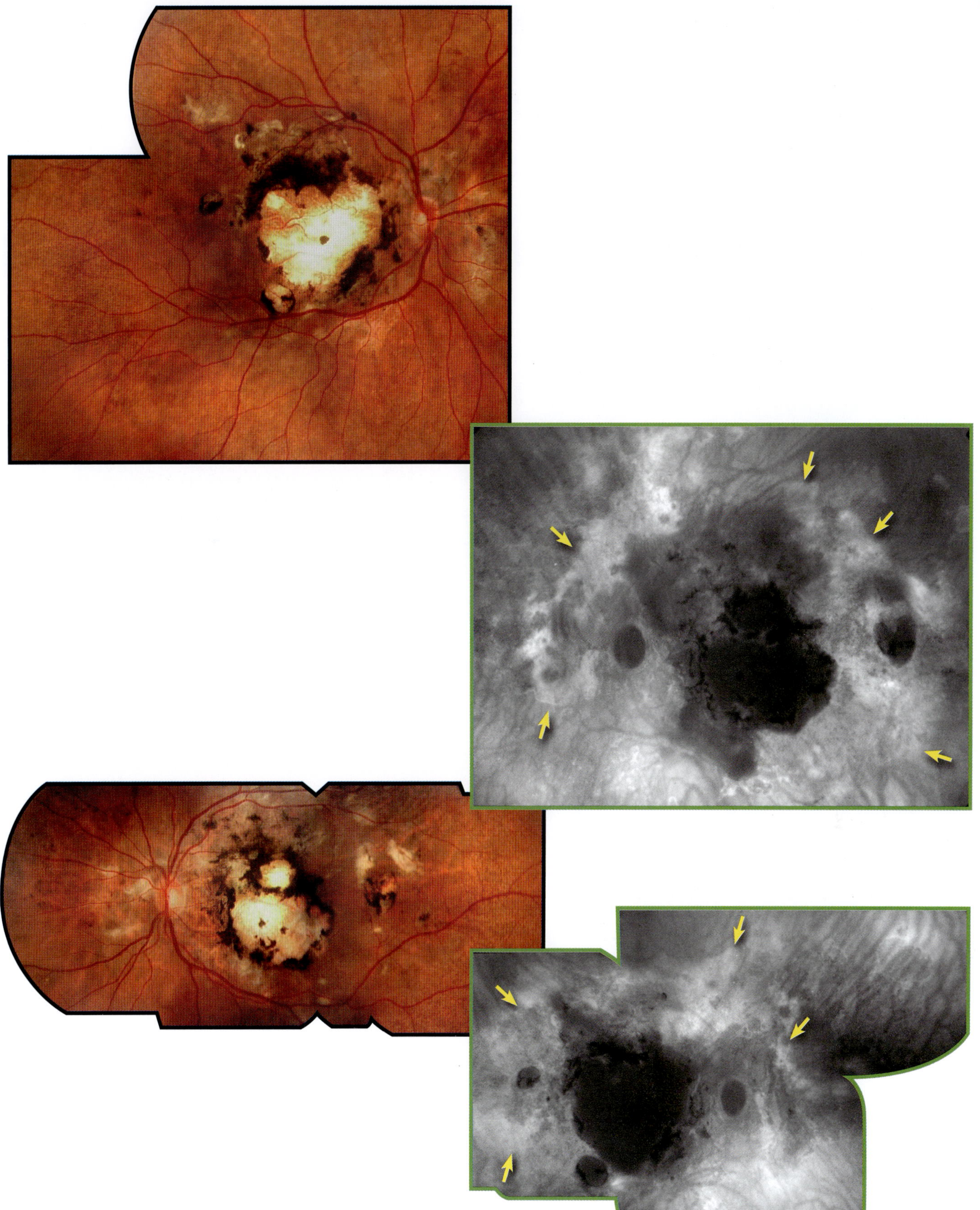

This patient with Sorsby pseudoinflammatory fundus dystrophy had photocoagulation centrally for multiple areas of choroidal neovascularization. There are large zonal areas of atrophy due to photocoagulation therapy of the proliferating new vessels. Indocyanine green angiography shows a more extensive network of neovascularization *(arrows)*. This case illustrates the aggressive angiogenic nature of this disorder.

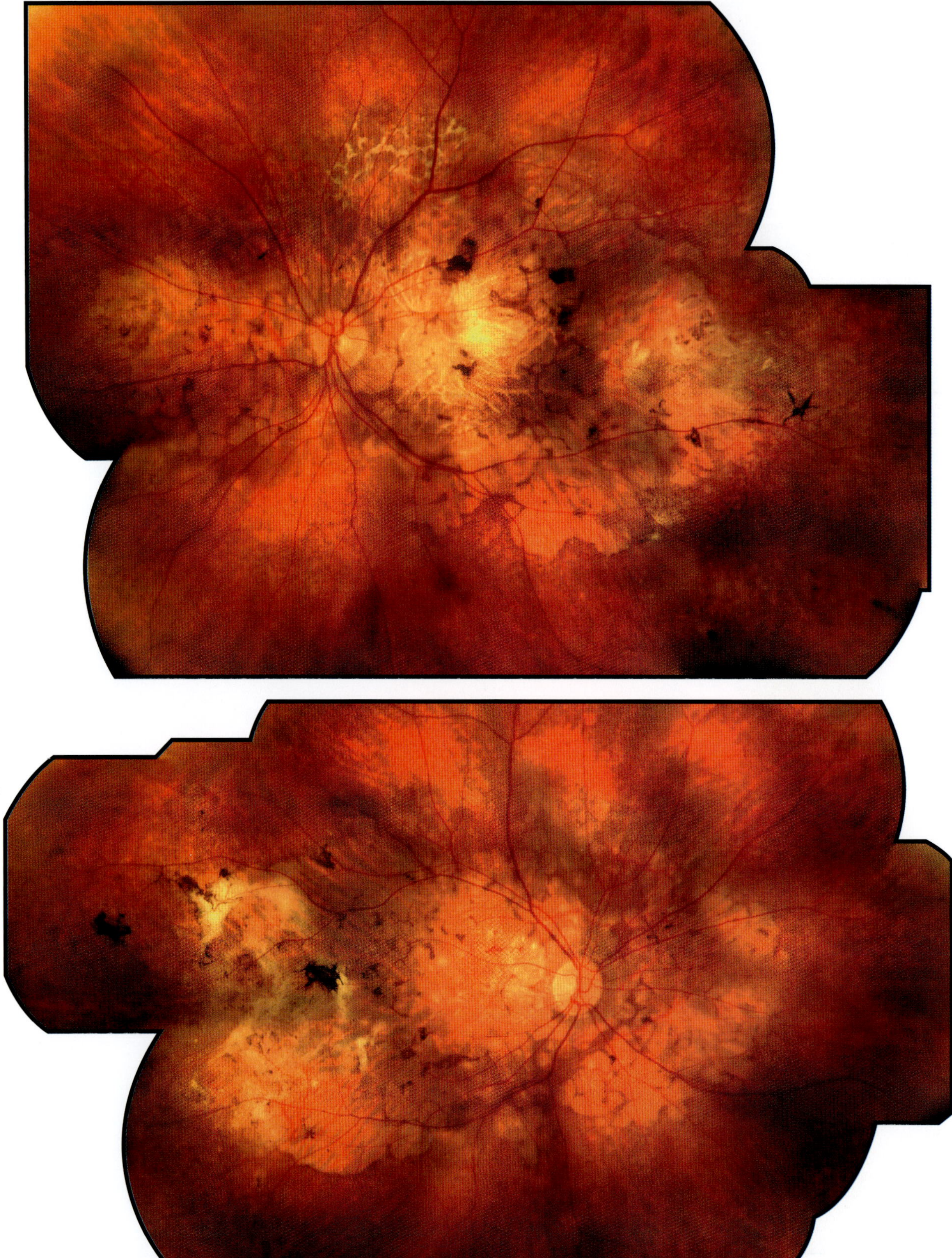

This case of Sorsby pseudoinflammatory fundus dystrophy demonstrates widespread atrophy and fibrous scarring with pigment epithelial hyperplasia. The appearance of the fundus is clinically indistinguishable from end-stage disciform neovascular age-related macular degeneration.

North Carolina Macular Dystrophy (Macular Dystrophy of the Retina Locus 1)

North Carolina macular dystrophy, (registered in Online Mendelian Inheritance in Man as macular dystrophy of the retina, locus 1) is an autosomal dominant disorder caused by a mutation within a 1.2 megabase pair region on chromosome 6p16 called the MCDR1 locus. The putative gene has recently been identified and evidence indicates that dysregulation of the retinal transcription factor PRDM13 may be the cause of this retinal dystrophy. The dystrophy was initially identified in a group of Irish settlers in the mountainous region of North Carolina, but has since been found in multiple regions of the world. Classically, it is characterized by three grades: grade 1 consists of drusen-like deposits and RPE mottling in the parafoveal area; grade 2 consists of confluent drusen, RPE atrophy and disciform scarring of the macula; grade 3 consists of severe chorioretinal atrophy centrally within the macula, which may appear similar to a chorioretinal coloboma or staphyloma or may mimic a toxoplasmosis scar. Disease onset is in infancy, reaching its maximum severity by the mid-teens. NCMD has complete penetrance but variable expressivity, therefore in some patients, disease progression halts at grade 1 with vision remaining in the 20/50 range, while others progress to almost total atrophy of the choroid, RPE, and retina with staphylomatous outpouching. Choroidal neovascularization and disciform scarring have also been described corresponding with further decline in visual acuity. Visual acuity may be much better than expected based on fundus appearance. Histopathologically, a discrete macular lesion characterized by central absence of photoreceptors and RPE and attenuation and focal atrophy of Bruch membrane and choriocapillaris have been described.

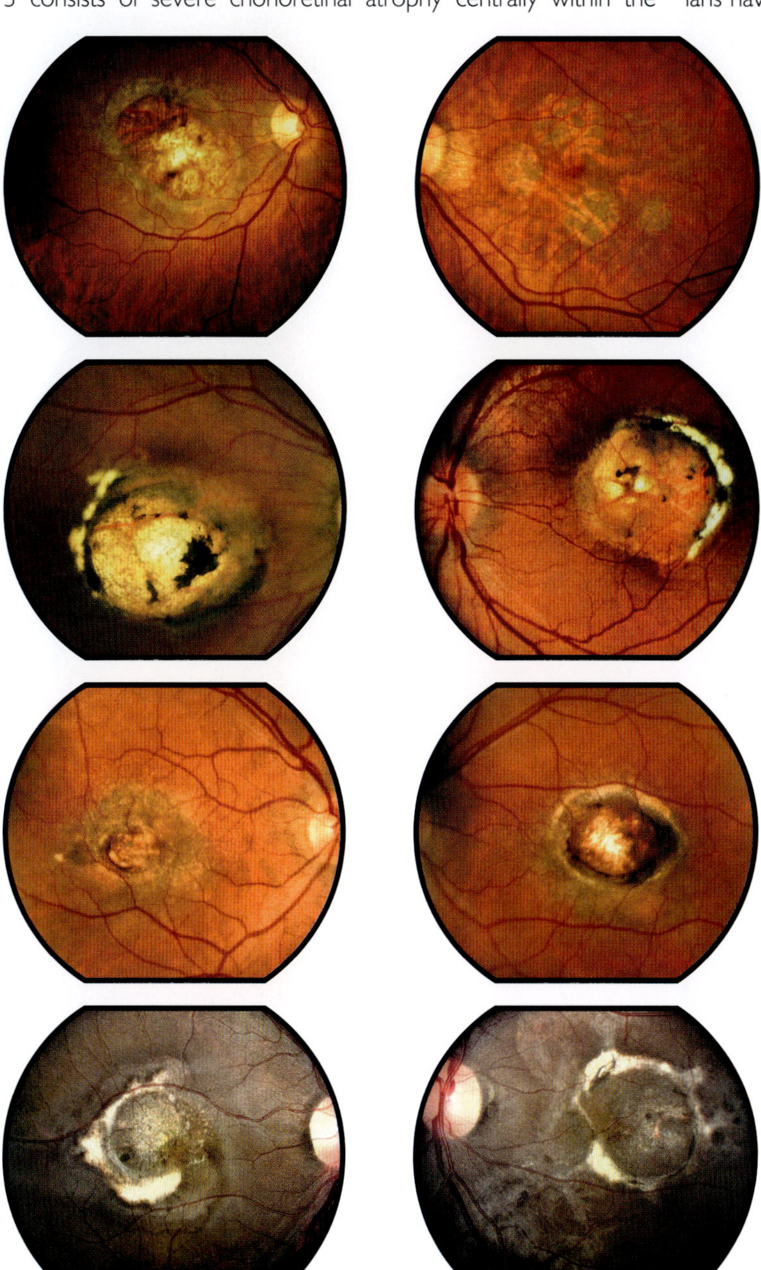

In these patients with North Carolina macular dystrophy, there is an oval to spherical zone of variable atrophy, pigment epithelial hyperplasia, and fibrous scarring. The visual acuity is surprisingly good in each eye. *Top and third rows courtesy of Dr. Mark Hughes, second row courtesy of Dr. Kent Small*

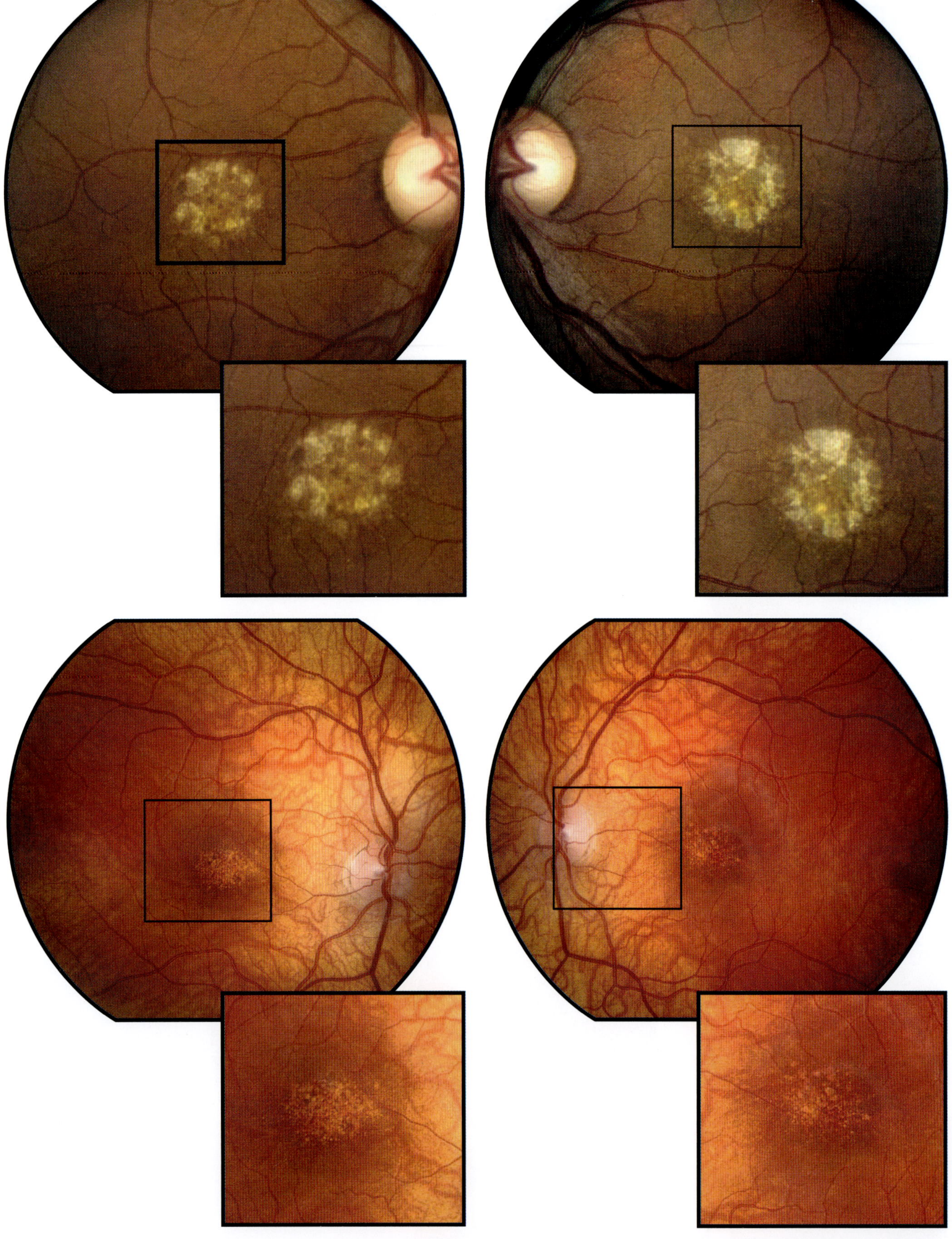

These are patients with North Carolina macular dystrophy who have unusual or atypical phenotypic macular findings. One patient has a yellowish nummular discoloration that resembles Best disease *(top row)*. Another patient has pigment epithelial granularity and mottling, which could be misdiagnosed as Stargardt disease *(bottom row)*. *Courtesy of Dr. Anita Agarwal*

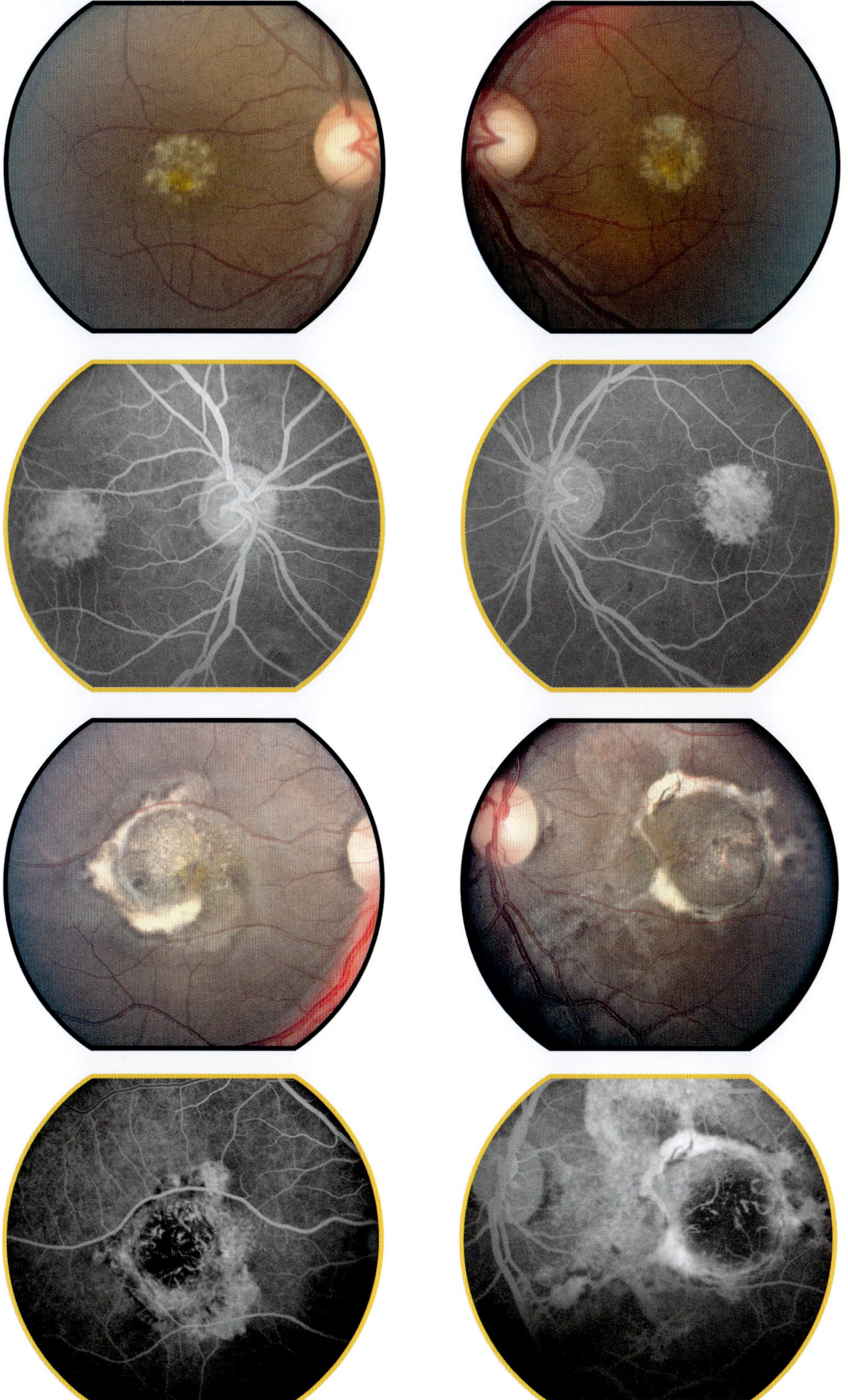

This family with North Carolina Macular Dystrophy illustrates a variable spectrum of disease. Color photograph and fluorescein angiogram images from father *(top two rows)* demonstrate smaller grade 2 lesions. Father's visual acuity was 20/40 and 20/50 in the right and left eyes respectively. Color photograph and fluorescein angiogram images from daughter *(bottom two rows)* illustrate larger coloboma-like grade 3 lesions, although her visual acuity was better at 20/25 in each eye.

Benign Concentric Annular Macular Dystrophy (BCAMD)

This is a peculiar disorder with a likely autosomal dominant inheritance pattern caused by a gene mutation localized to chromosome 6p12.3-q16. BCAMD is characterized by a "bulls-eye" pattern of macular depigmentation or atrophy similar to chloroquine retinopathy. Small drusen have been observed surrounding the depigmented ring. In most cases, vision is relatively well preserved. However, long term follow-up of at least 10 patients has revealed progressive peripheral retinopathy with bone spicules and ERG findings showing generalized cone and rod dysfunction. Waxy disc pallor, peripapillary atrophy, and attenuated arterioles can also be seen in late stages of disease suggestive of a diagnosis of retinitis pigmentosa and associated with progressive visual loss, nyctalopia, and decreased color vision.

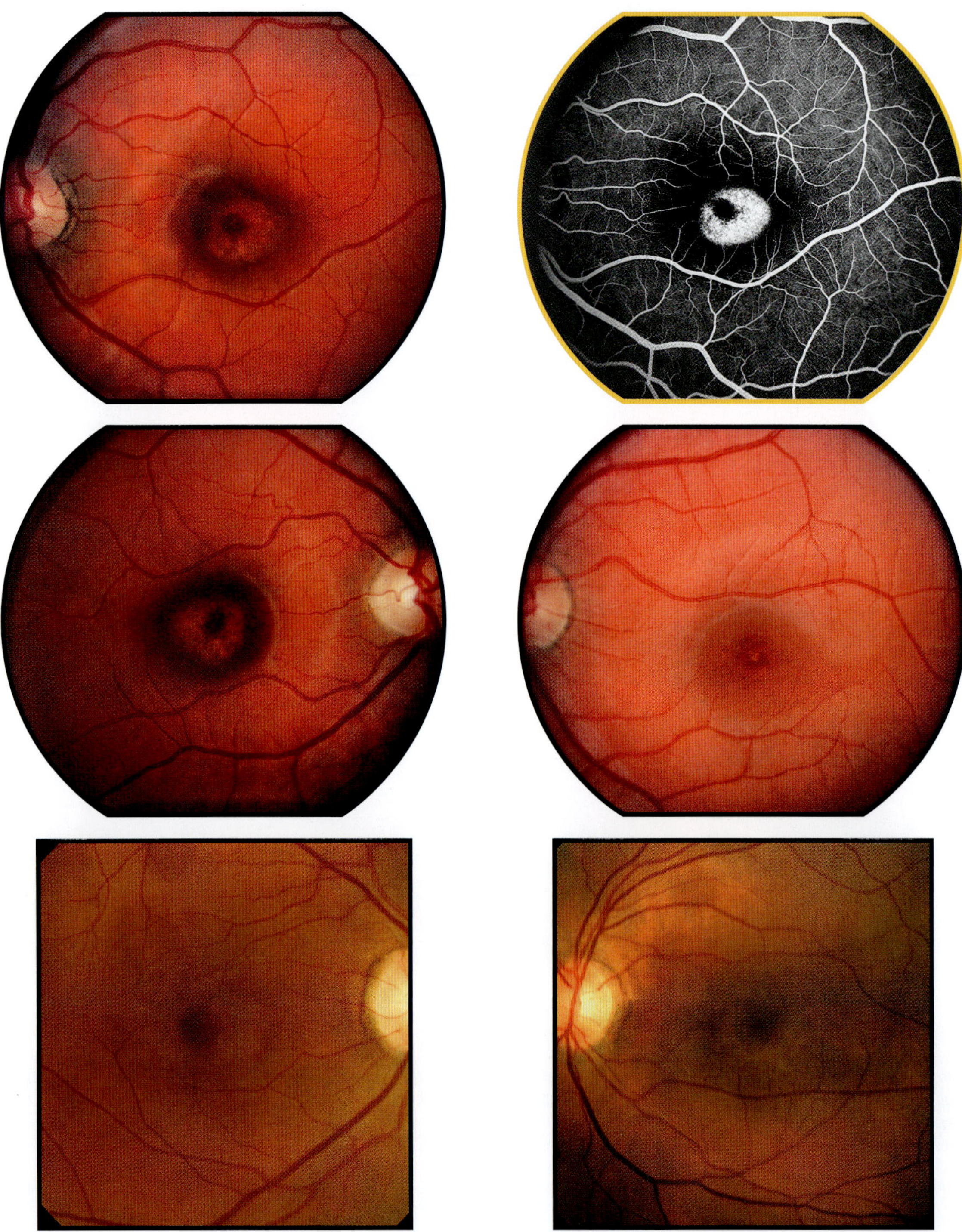

These patients have BCAMD. Early manifestations in the macula are misleading, but generally there is a peculiar "bull's-eye" appearance as the disease progresses with relative preservation otherwise of the fovea. The fluorescein angiogram shows hyperfluorescence corresponding to the atrophic changes in the macula. *Top two rows courtesy of Dr. Stuart Fine*

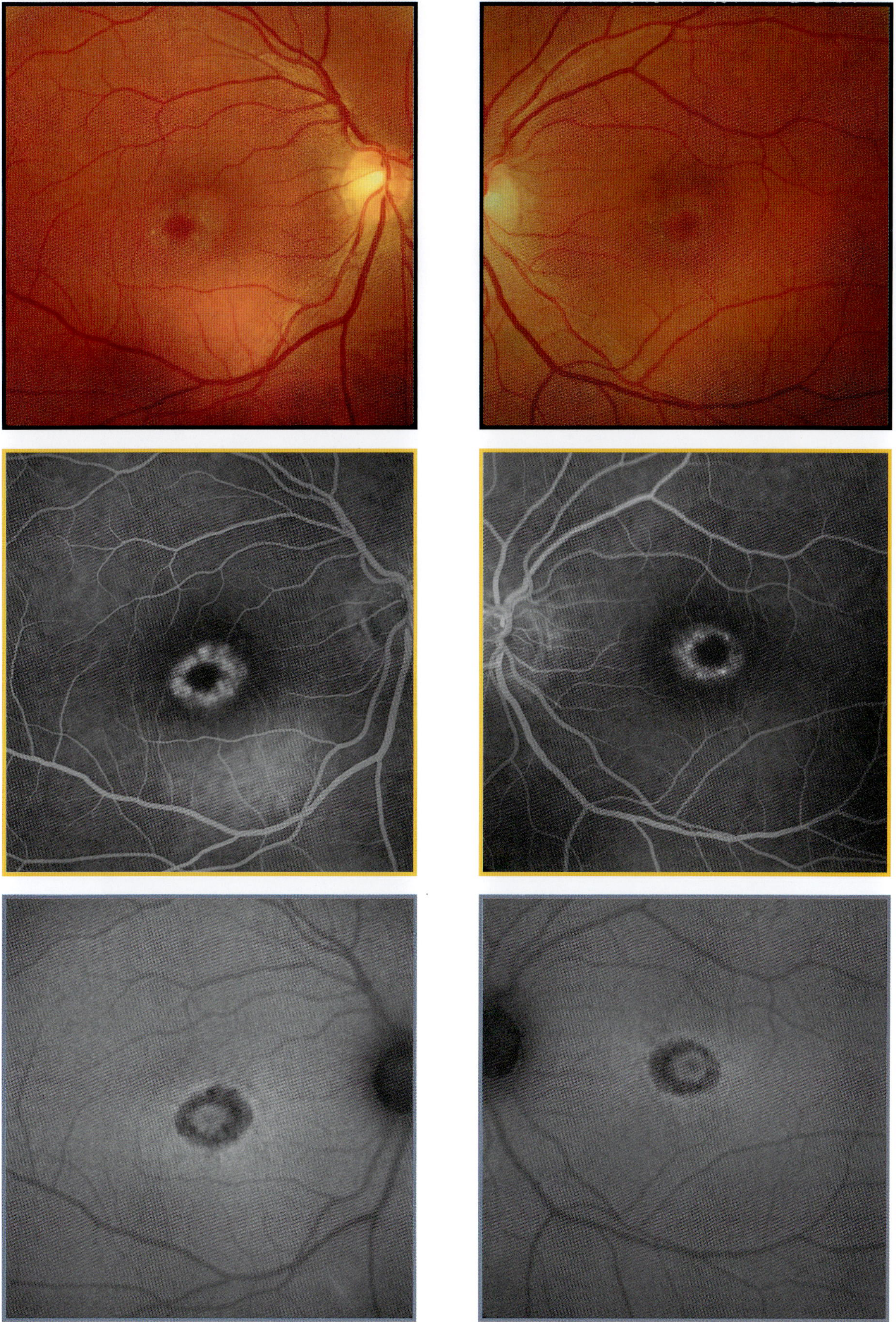

These two patients also have BCAMD. The color photographs show a ring of atrophy in a "bull's-eye" appearance surrounding the macula. The fluorescein angiogram shows a window defect with late staining resembling a "bull's-eye" pattern. Fundus autofluorescence images are a reversal of the fluorescein angiograms and show hypoautofluorescence of the atrophic RPE.

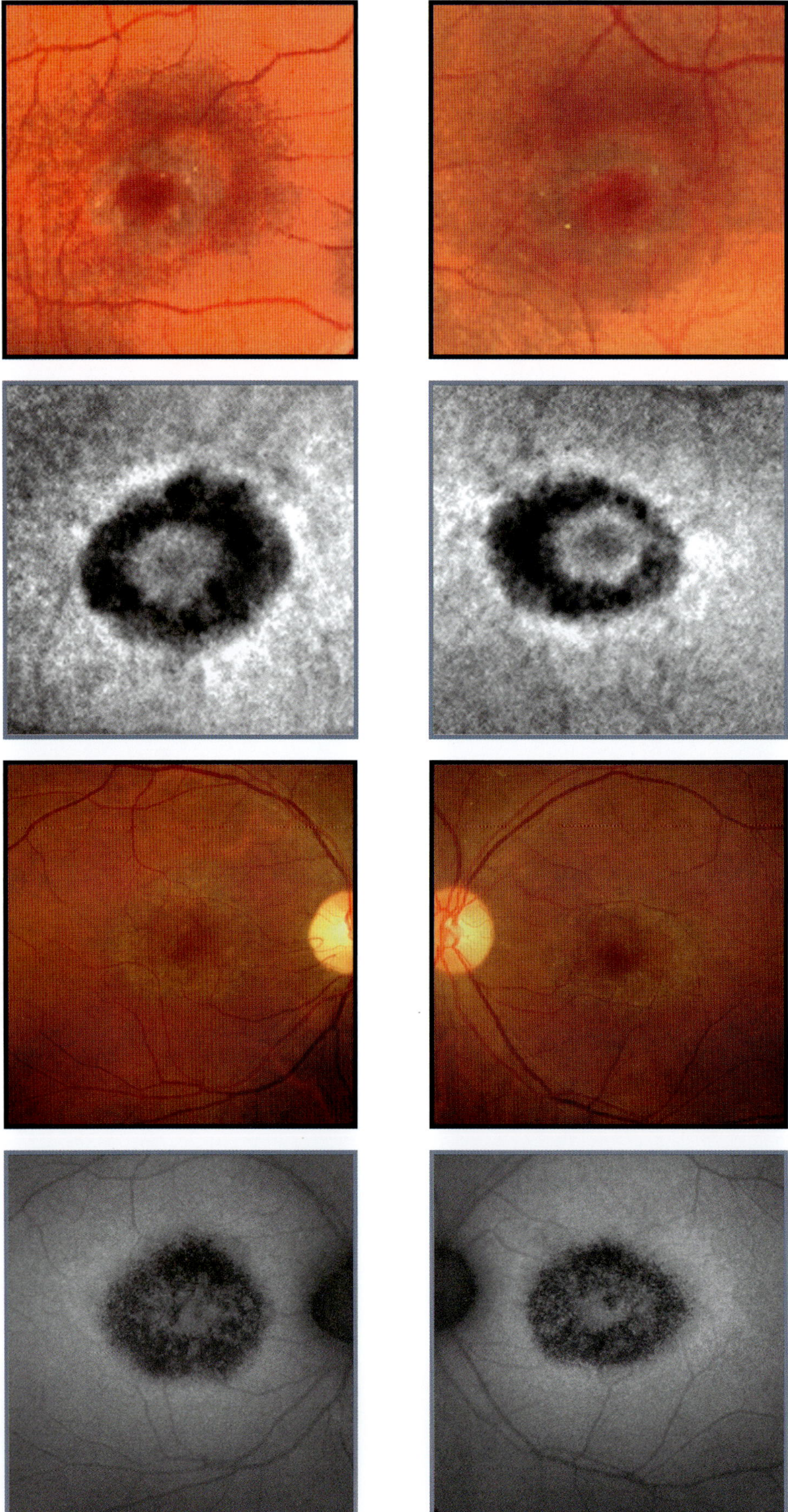

As BCAMD progresses in time to involve the central fovea, the initial good vision may decline. The color photographs shows an irregular atrophic pattern surrounding the fovea. Fluorescein angiography and fundus autofluorescence are very useful in delineating the exact state of the pigment epithelium and photoreceptors.

Fenestrated Sheen Macular Dystrophy

This is an autosomal dominant maculopathy that is associated with only a mild loss of vision, usually beginning in late adulthood. A paracentral scotoma may be the first presenting symptom. A yellowish refractile sheen is clinically evident in the macula with red fenestrations within the sensory retina. In time, an annular zone of hypopigmentation of the RPE appears, giving the lesion a "bull's-eye" appearance. The yellowish sheen persists, but the fenestrations disappear as more RPE changes occur with time. A defect in macular xanthophyll may be related to this disorder.

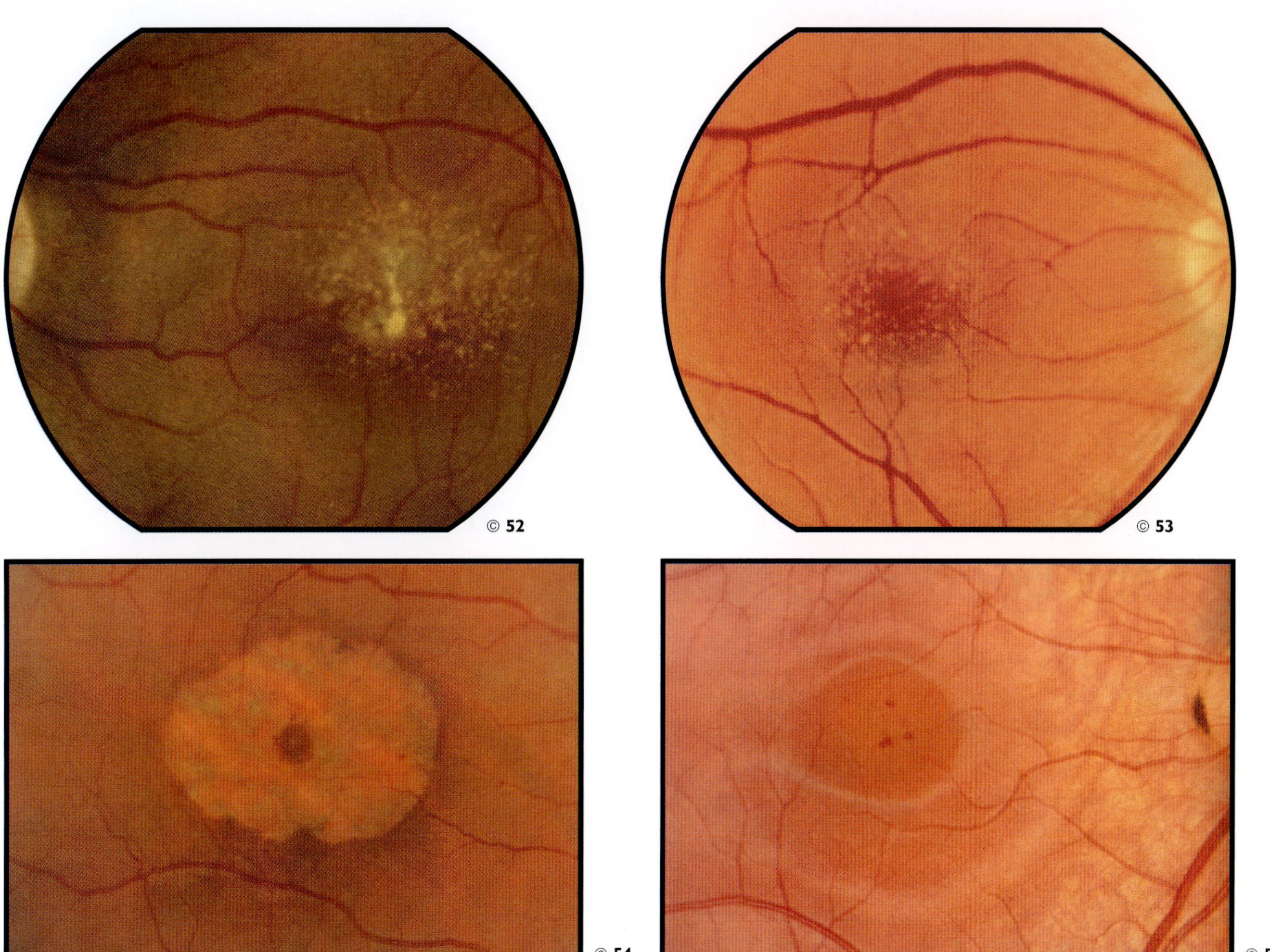

These patients with fenestrated sheen macular dystrophy show a yellowish sheen to the central macula. There is atrophy of the pigment epithelium *(lower left)* and a "bull's-eye" appearance *(upper right)* as well. The atrophy is well demarcated, and there is preservation of the fovea.

White Dot Fovea

White-dot fovea is a bilateral abnormality characterized by very fine dot-like lesions on the foveal surface, either diffusely or along its margin, forming a faint, grayish ring. Often there are no subjective symptoms or visual disturbance. It warrants recognition to differentiate these changes from more significant foveal pathology.

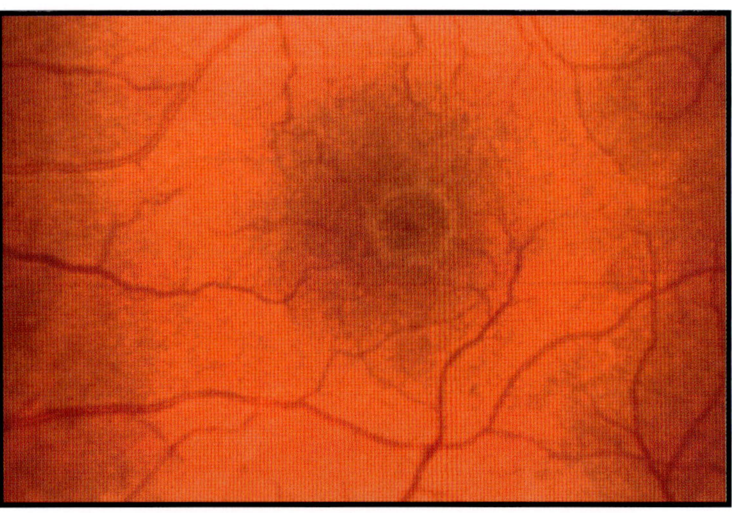

This patient has white-dot fovea, with fine punctate lesions around the foveal margin and within the fovea itself. There were no significant visual changes.

Martinique Crinkled Retinal Pigment Epitheliopathy (West Indies Crinkled Retinal Pigment Epitheliopathy)

Martinique crinkled retinal pigment epitheliopathy is a peculiar disorder identified in patients from the island of Martinique that is characterized by diffuse deep white lines in the macula visible on funduscopic examination, which give the macula a "crinkled" appearance. These lines are hyperautofluorescent and SD-OCT localizes the abnormality to the level of the RPE. The disorder appears to be autosomal dominant and may be associated with polypoidal choroidal vasculopathy and CNVM formation.

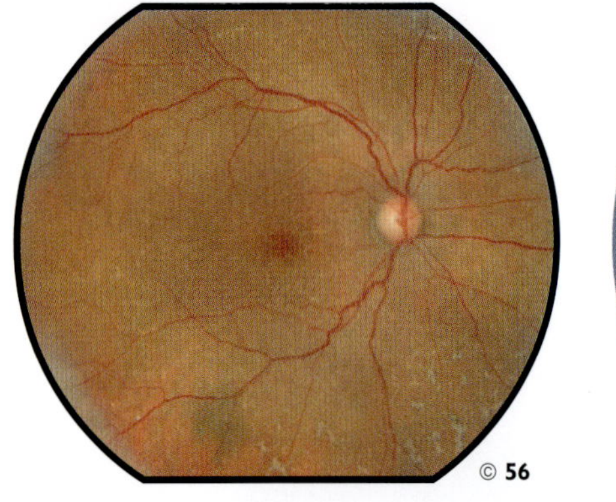

© 56

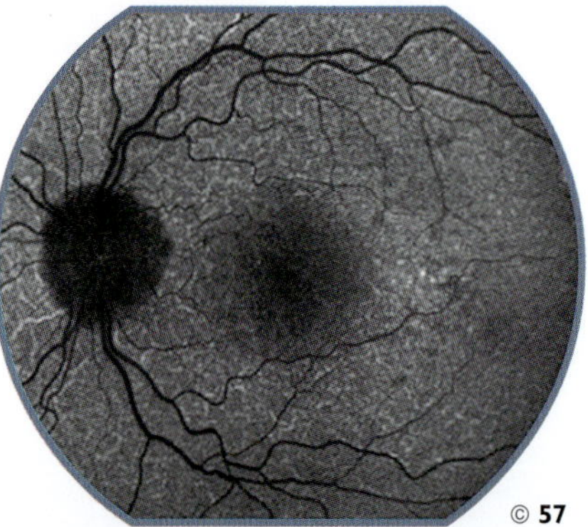

© 57

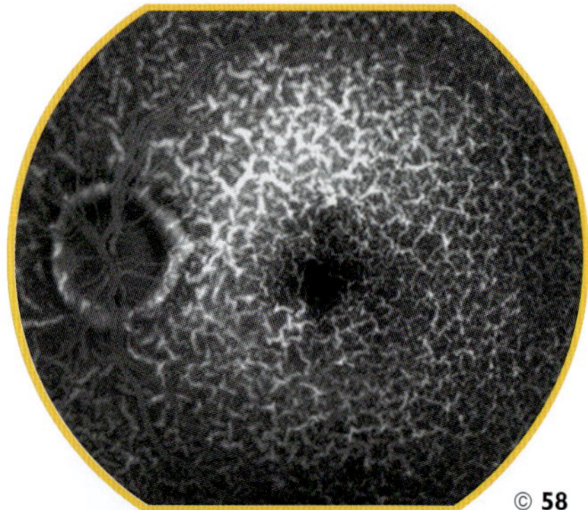

© 58

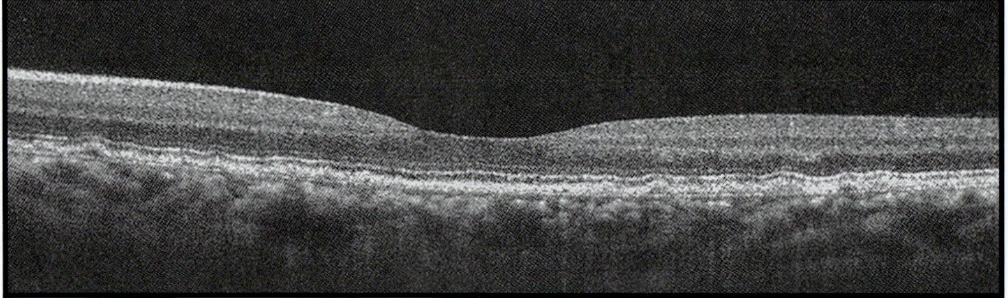

© 59

Color fundus photograph of a patient with MCRPE shows deep, reticular lines that involve the RPE and are highlighted with fundus autofluorescence and fluorescein angiogram. SD-OCT shows irregular, scalloped elevation of the PRE.

Cone Dystrophies

The cone dystrophies represent a diverse group of disorders characterized primarily by cone loss and dysfunction and associated with photophobia; central scotoma and vision loss; and color vision deficits. This group of disorders include the congenital loss of cone receptors, such as achromatopsia and cone monochromatism, as well as non-congenital progressive cone dystrophies. These conditions demonstrate signature phenotypic findings and specific electroretinographic deficits remarkable for predominant cone dysfunction.

Cone Dystrophy

Cone dystrophy is a genetically heterogeneous group of disorders characterized by progressive deterioration of cone function with normal rod function. Autosomal dominant, autosomal recessive, and X-linked modes of inheritance have all been reported, with the autosomal recessive form of the disease representing the most common form. Several genes have been implicated including ABCA4 (AR), CNGB3 (AR), KCNV2 (AR), PDE6C (AR), RPGR (XL), GUCA1A (AD), and PITPNM3 (AD). Patients typically present with decreased visual acuity and color vision deficits in the mid-teenage years with progression to legal blindness by middle age. Retinal findings are quite variable and may be normal; however, a "bull's-eye" maculopathy is common which may be associated with temporal optic nerve pallor. Fundus autofluorescence may nicely highlight a "bull's-eye" ring of hyperautofluorescence or a geographic zone of hypoautofluorescence and SD-OCT may show diffuse central ellipsoid loss. Formal visual field testing will show a central scotoma. Full-field ERG is essential for diagnosis and will demonstrate marked depression of cone responses with normal rod function. The X-linked form of cone dystrophy (RPGR mutation, COD 1) is associated with a golden tapetal fundus reflex that is very characteristic.

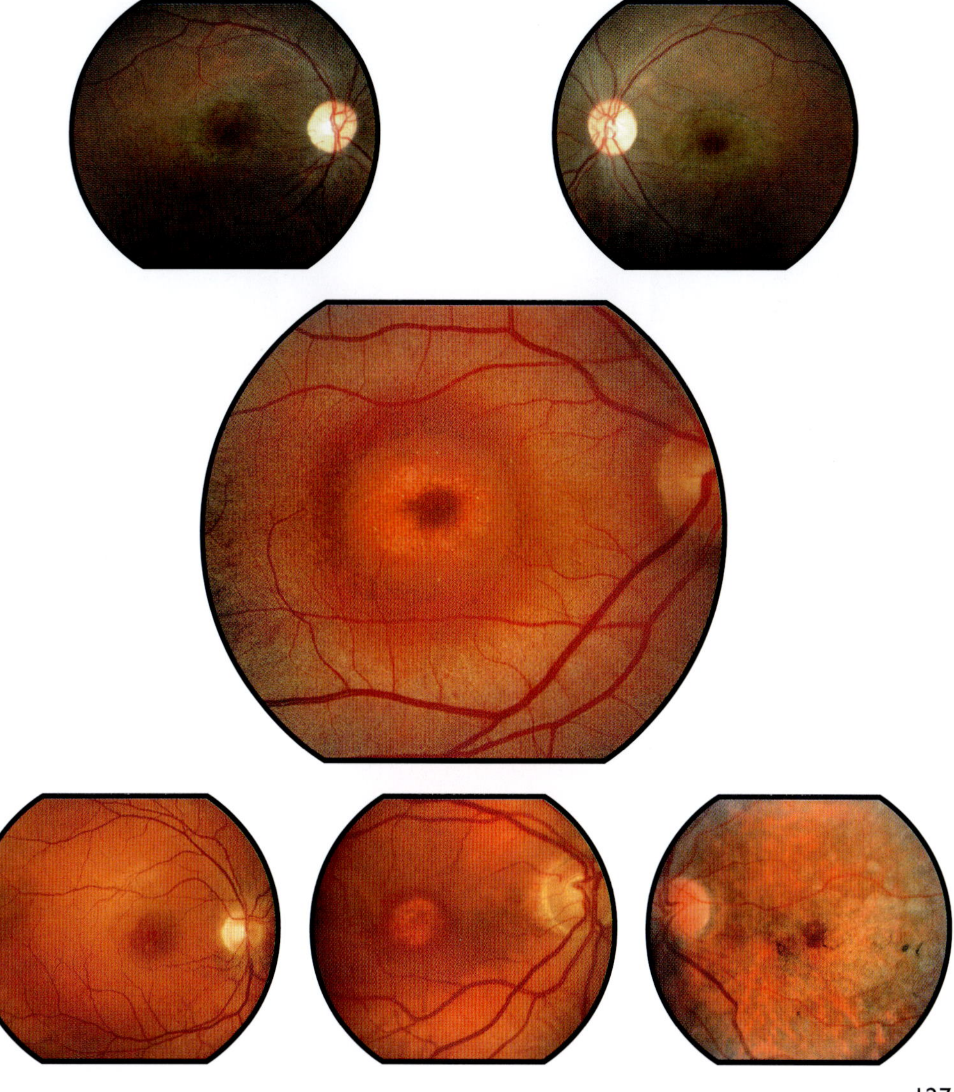

The clinical manifestations of a cone dystrophy in its early stages will vary tremendously. A ring of atrophy surrounding the foveal area producing a form of "ring maculopathy" may be seen, as in the two images in the top row. A more typical "bull's-eye" pattern in a cone dystrophy is seen in the center image, with concentric and alternating areas of normal to hyperpigmentation and hypopigmentation. In some cases, the early stage of the disease shows essentially no changes in the macula as in the lower left image. Progressive atrophy may occur around the fovea *(lower middle image)*, leading to more generalized atrophic changes, extending from the posterior pole to the mid and far periphery *(lower right image)*. *Middle and bottom rows courtesy of Drs Ron Carr and Ken Noble*

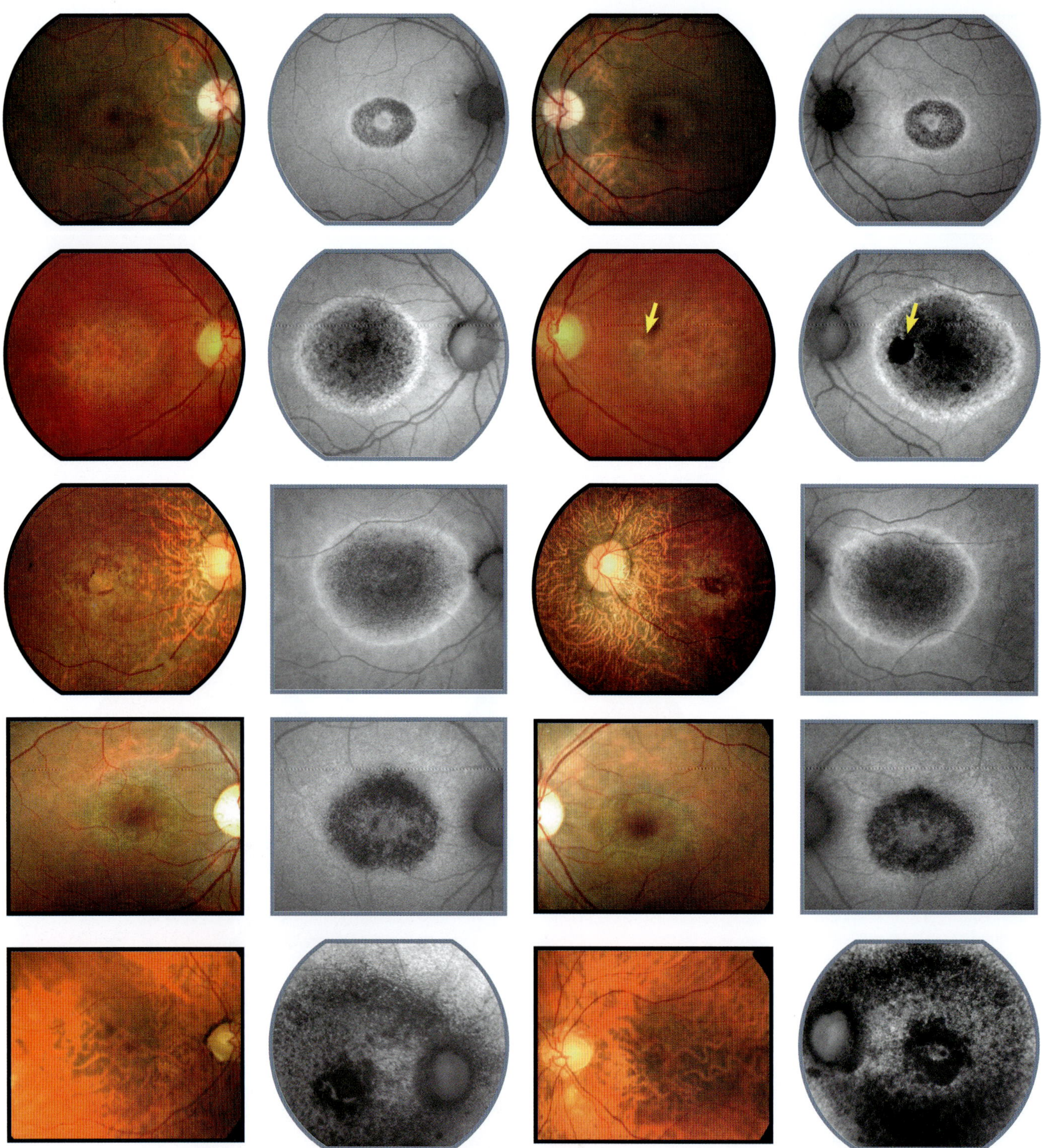

Fundus autofluorescence is sometimes helpful in establishing the clinical diagnosis of cone dystrophy. The ring maculopathy appearance is accentuated with alternating areas of hypoautofluorescence and hyperautofluorescence, as seen above. In the second row, more severe atrophy is beginning to occur in the left eye of this case *(arrows)*, whereas a more generalized milder degree of pigment epithelial loss is evident within a ring of hyperautofluorescence in each eye. As the cone dystrophy progresses, there is a more prominent hypoautofluorescence surrounding the fovea. In the later stages of the disease, the pigment epithelial atrophic change becomes granular and diffuse throughout the central and paramacular region and beyond *(bottom row)*.

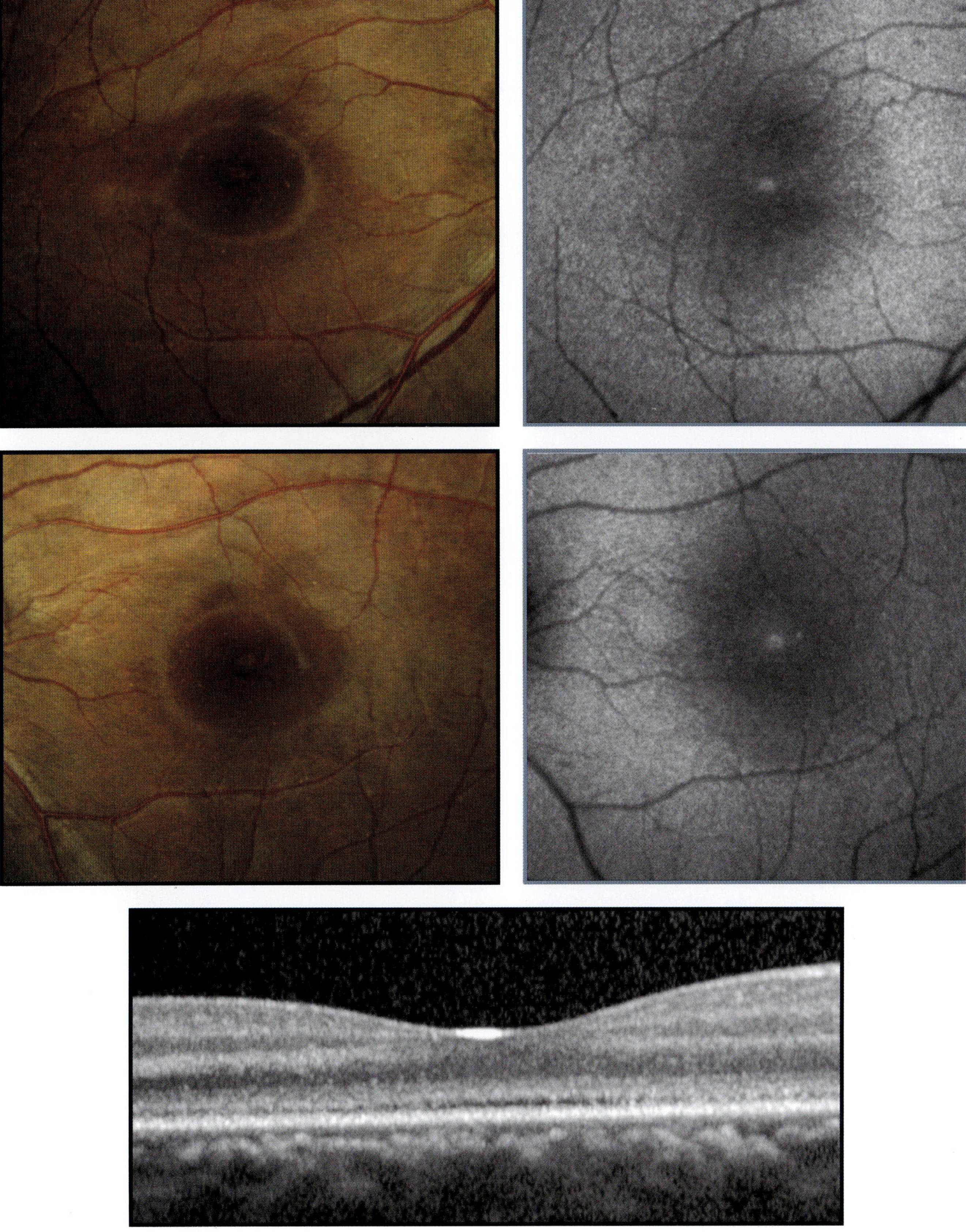

In this 31-year-old female with central vision loss the clinical examination was normal. Autofluorescence studies show slight hyperautofluorescence (central and parafoveal) of a non-specific nature, and OCT scanning illustrates foveal thinning with inner segment ellipsoid attenuation. ERG testing confirmed the diagnosis of a cone dystrophy.

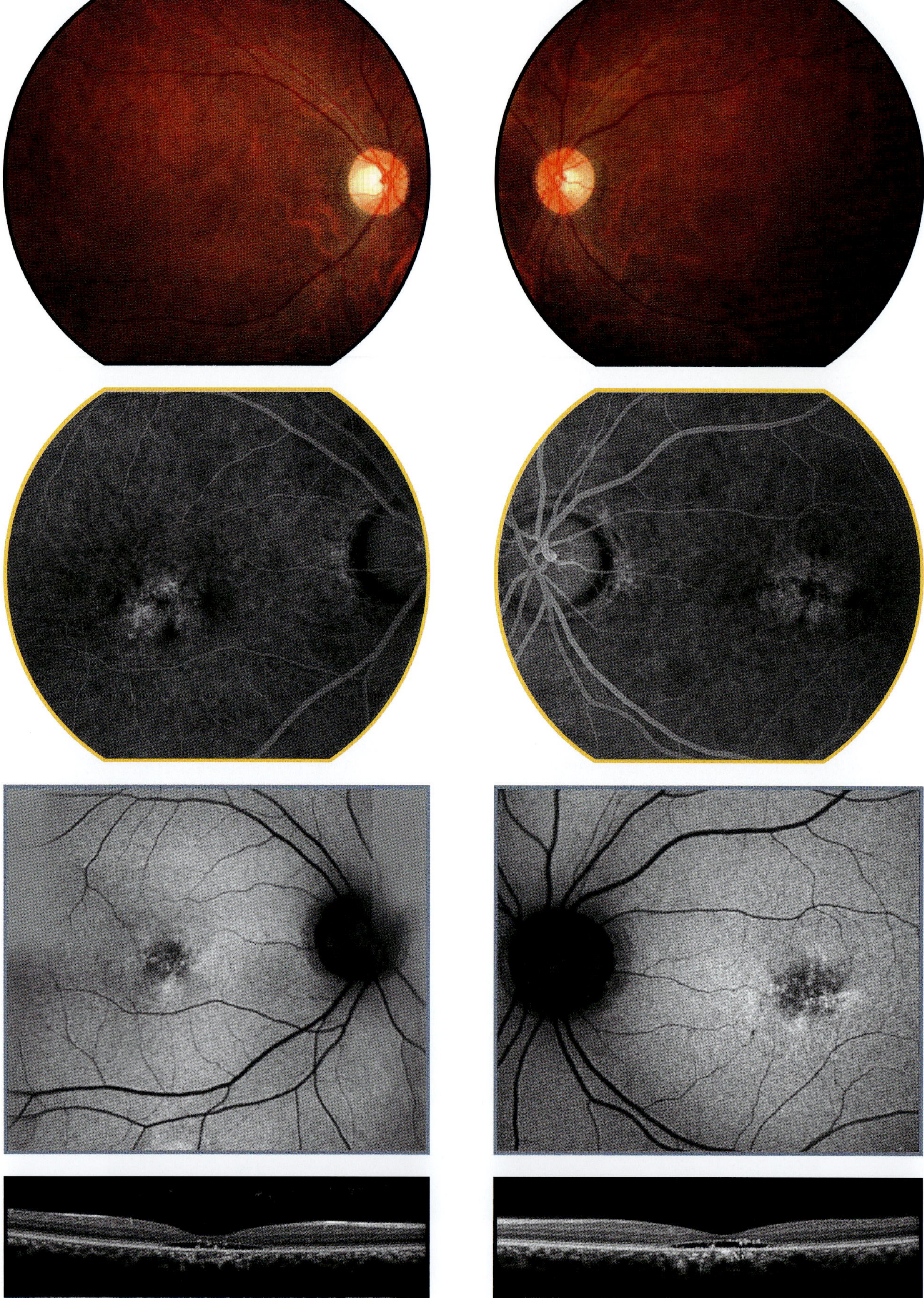

Color photos of this patient with cone dystrophy show mild pigmentary changes in the macula. Note the mottled fluorescence with angiography and predominant atrophy and hypoautofluorescence with fundus autofluorescence. SD-OCT through the macula reveals subfoveal loss of the ellipsoid layer. *Images courtesy of SriniVas Sadda, MD*

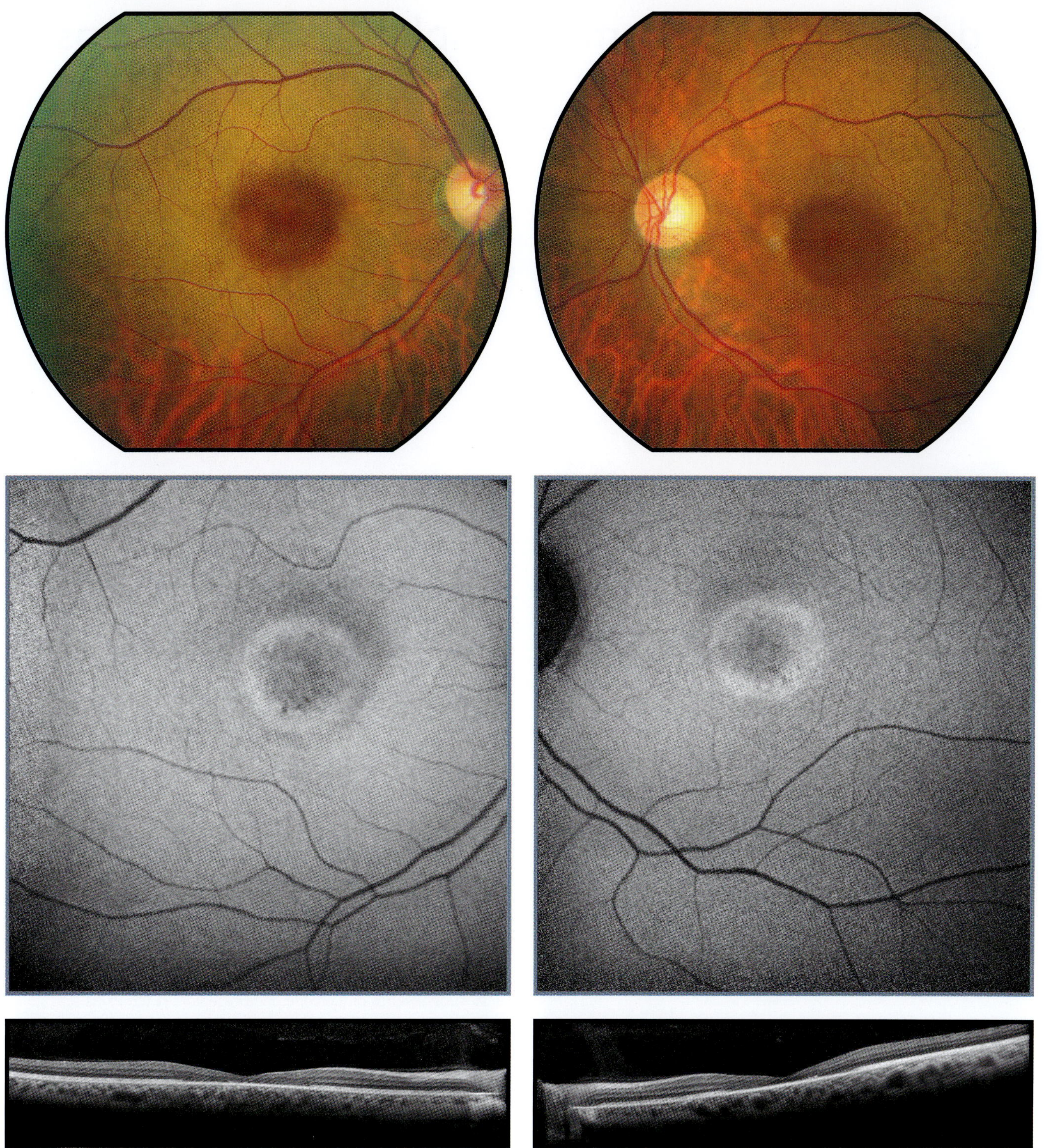

This patient with cone dystrophy has a presumed COD1 (RPGR) mutation. Note the golden tapetal fundus reflex. SD-OCT shows photoreceptor and ellipsoid atrophy beneath the fovea.

Rod Monochromatism (Complete Achromatopsia)

Rod monochromatism is an autosomal recessive disorder characterized by a complete congenital absence of cone function. Three genes, each of which encode proteins involved in the cone phototransduction cascade, have been associated with this disorder: CNGA3, CNGB3, and GNAT2. Normal rods and a marked reduction in the number of extrafoveal cones (5–10% of normal) are typically seen. The foveal cones usually are normal in number, but abnormal morphologically. Vision is poor at birth in the 20/200 range, with varying degrees of photophobia, color vision loss, and nystagmus, which is often present in infancy but may become less severe over time. Vision in ordinary lighting is severely restricted and relatively better in dim light (hemeralopia). The photophobia is often more debilitating than the reduced visual acuity. Red contact lenses have been used with excellent success in alleviating the photophobia. Fundus findings may be normal with only mild nonspecific central retinal pigment epithelial changes or a very subtle "bull's-eye" pattern of atrophy. ERG studies reveal an extinguished photopic cone response and a normal scotopic rod response.

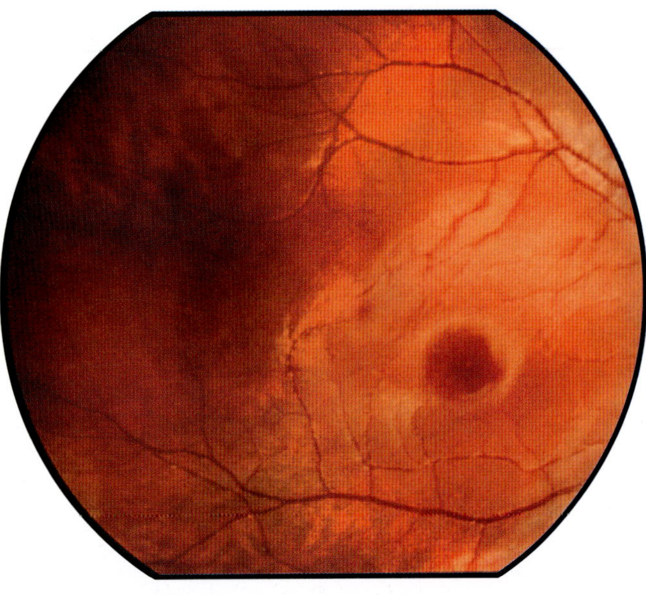

In this patient with rod monochromatism, the macula is virtually normal except for a mild degree of pigment epithelial atrophy.

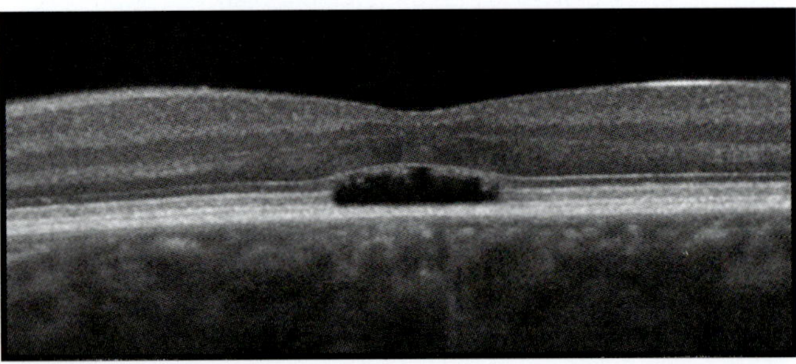

The OCT in a patient with complete achromatopsia shows a rectangular absence of the cone photoreceptors in the fovea.

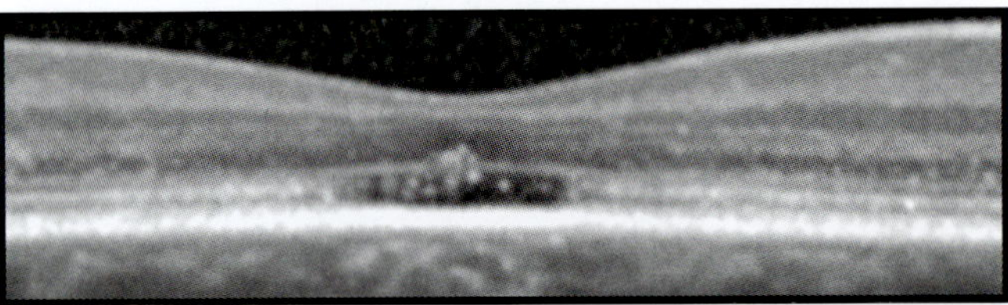

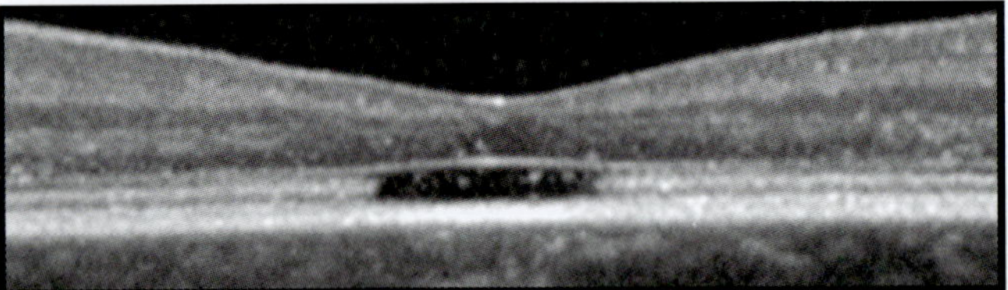

High-resolution OCT shows a degeneration of the photoreceptors in the fovea in this patient with achromatopsia.

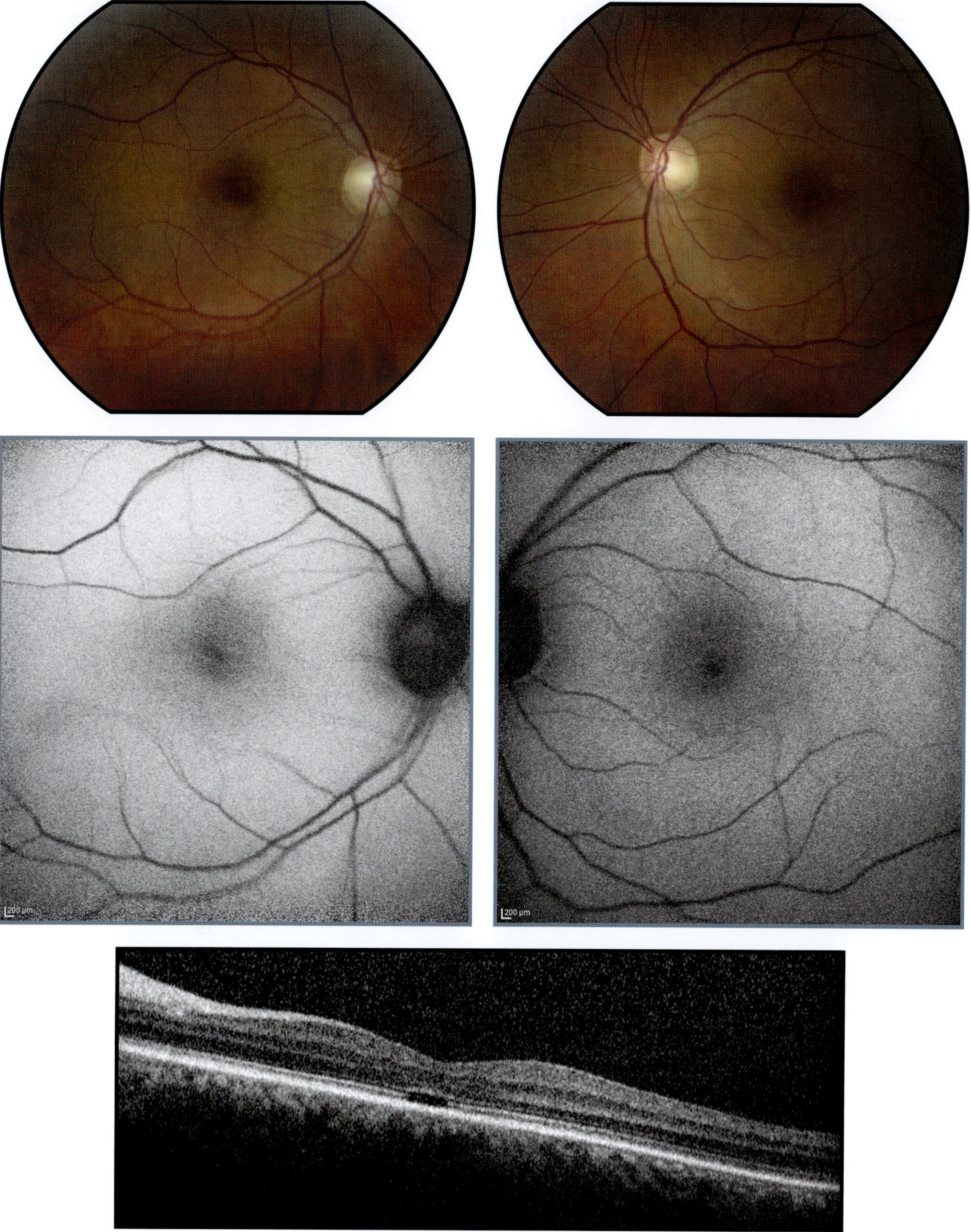

This patient with achromatopsia has subtle pigmentary changes in the macula highlighted on autofluorescence *(middle row)*. There is loss of the subfoveal ellipsoid layer leaving an optically empty rectangular space on SD-OCT. Genetic testing was positive for CNGA3 mutation. *Images courtesy of Jaclyn Kovach, MD*

Occult Macular Dystrophy

RP1L1 mutation can cause a diverse spectrum of retinal disease including autosomal recessive retinitis pigmentosa versus autosomal dominant occult macular dystrophy (OMD), a maculopathy associated with bilateral symmetric central inner segment ellipsoid loss with SD-OCT in the absence of visible funduscopic or fluorescein angiographic abnormalities. Patients with OMD are typically middle aged with central vision loss. The full-field ERG is normal but may also reveal photopic cone loss consistent with a cone dystrophy. The macular or multifocal ERG reveals diminished amplitudes typical of a cone dystrophy.

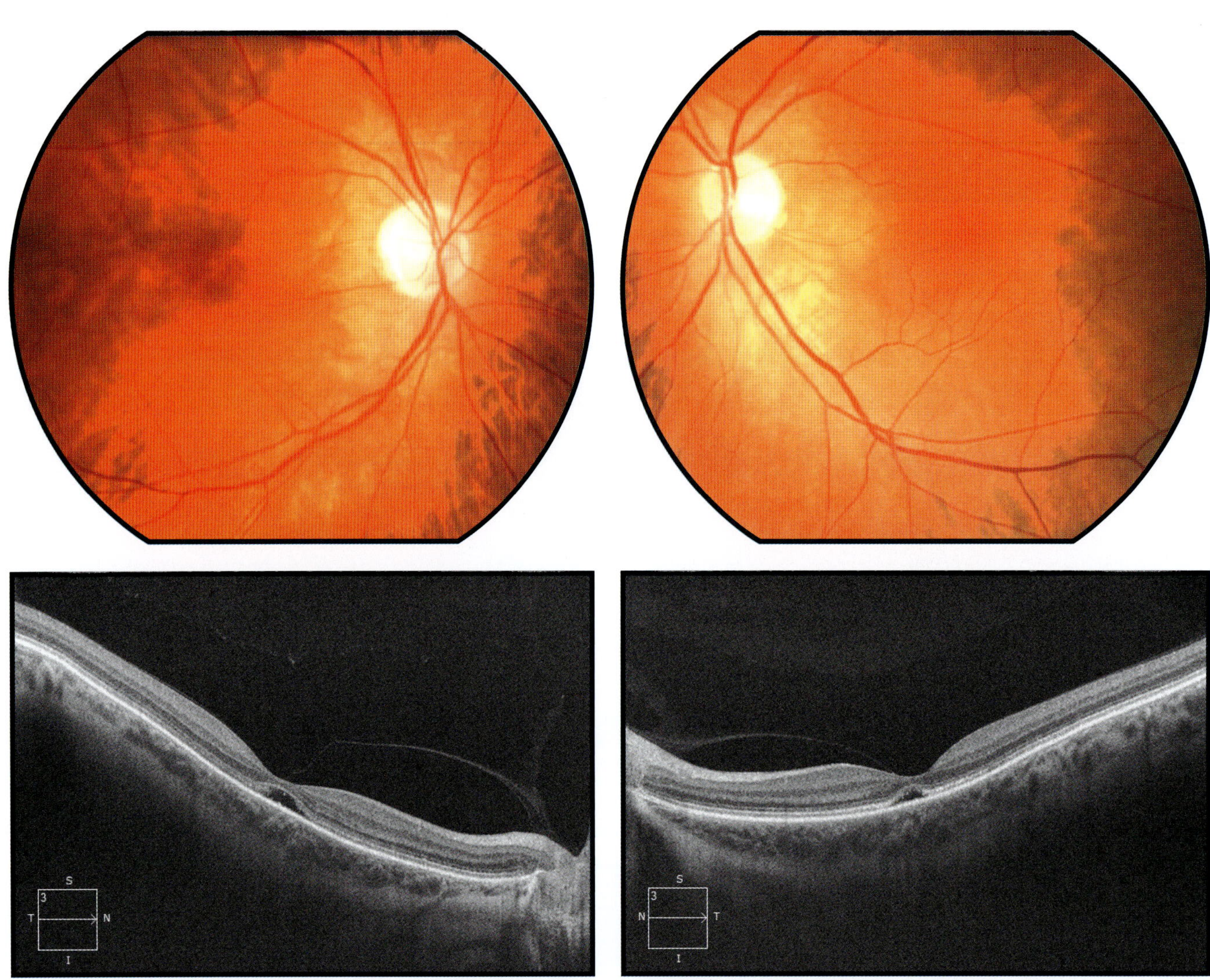

This patient with occult macular dystrophy had no apparent clinical abnormalities on funduscopic examination or fluorescein angiogram (not shown). However, visual field testing revealed central scotoma. SD-OCT shows subfoveal loss of the ellipsoid band. *Images courtesy of Rishi Doshi, MD*

Cone–Rod Dystrophies

Cone–rod dystrophies (CORD) are very similar to the cone dystrophies previously described except that there is additional rod involvement with scotopic rod loss with formal full field ERG testing. The following genetic mutations have been associated with CORD syndromes: GUCYRD (AD), AIPL1 (AD), RIM1 (AD), PERPHERIN/RDS (AD), GUCA1A (AD), CRX (AD), PITPNM3 (AD), HRG4 (AD), ABCA4 (AR), RPGRIP1 (AR), CRB1 (AR), RPGR (XL), and CACNA1F (XL).

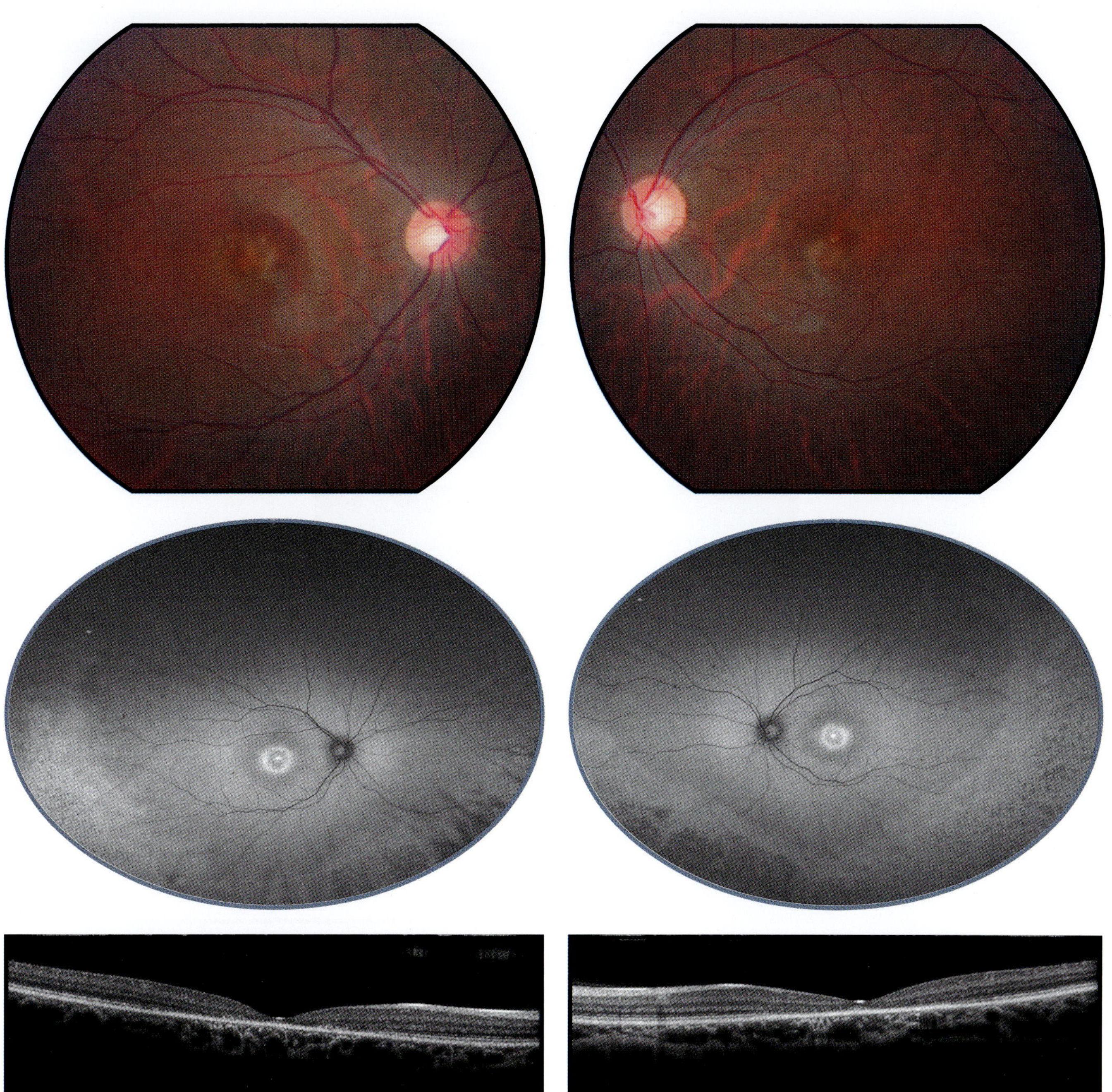

This patient with cone–rod dystrophy has a "bull's-eye" maculopathy as well as peripheral pigmentary changes which are highlighted on autofluorescence. SD-OCT through the macula shows ellipsoid loss most pronounced in the central macula.

Jalili Syndrome

Jalili syndrome is a rare disorder characterized by the combination of cone-rod dystrophy and a disorder of dental enamel causing hypoplastic and hypomineralized teeth called amelogenesis imperfecta. The disorder is linked to mutation in the CNNM4 gene on chromosome 2q11, one of the loci implicated in achromatopsia. Patients present with decreased visual acuity, dental anomalies, and photophobia in the first decade of life. Funduscopic examination may reveal a "bull's-eye" maculopathy with variable amounts of peripheral pigmentary changes. As the disease progresses, the "bull's-eye" lesion may become excavated or staphylomatous. An ERG will show cone dysfunction, which may be severe, and a variable severity of rod dysfunction.

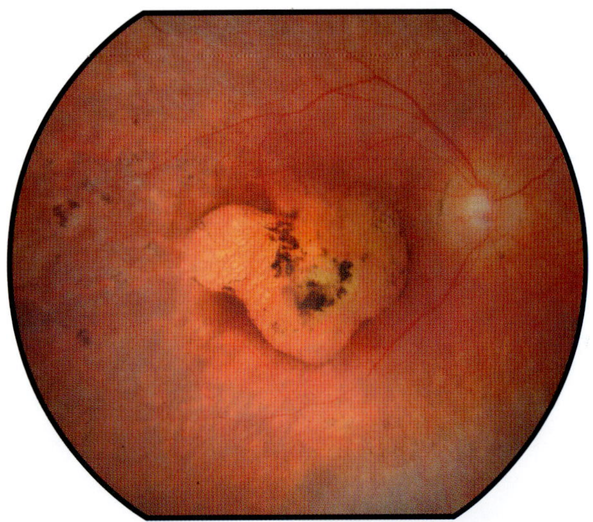

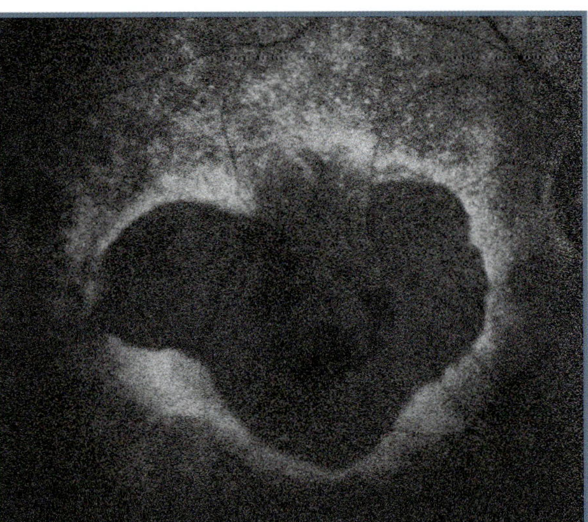

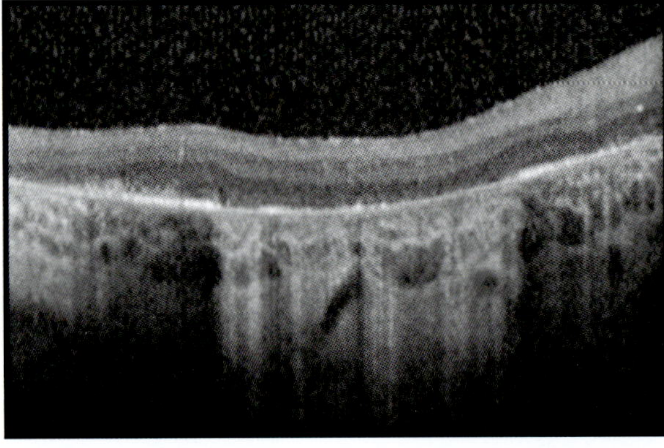

Central macular atrophy is shown on color fundus photography. Corresponding areas of central hypoautofluorescence and a ring of hyperautofluorescence characteristic of cone-rod dystrophy, are illustrated in this patient with Jalili syndrome. The SD OCT B scan shows outer retinal atrophy. *Images courtesy of Ala Moshiri, MD, PhD*

The characteristic dental anomalies of patients with Jalili syndrome are shown here.

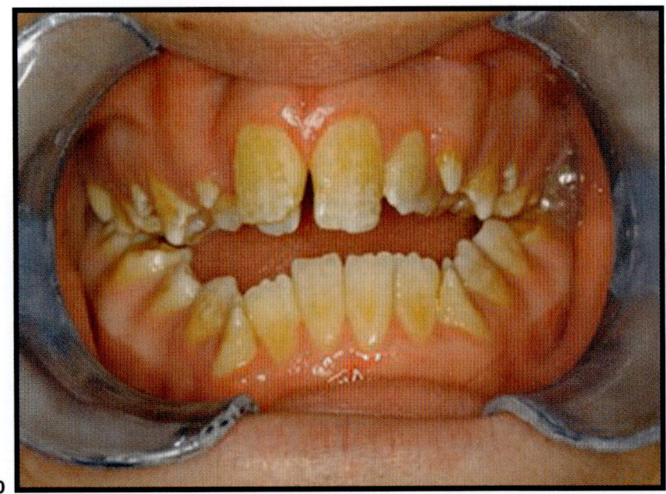

© 60

Retinitis Pigmentosa (Generalized Rod-Cone Dystrophies

Retinitis pigmentosa is the name given to a large group of hereditary retinal degenerations that share the common feature of progressive damage to the photoreceptor–pigment epithelial complex. These disorders occur in approximately 1 in 4000 people worldwide. Typical RP is heralded by night blindness or nyctalopia and problems with dark adaptation. The visual disturbance is compounded by loss of visual field, usually beginning in the midperiphery and then extending into the far periphery. An annular scotoma may progress to "tunnel vision" late in the course of the disorder. While the central retina is affected, vision loss is not as significant as that in the midperiphery. With ERG analysis the scotopic rod response is severely depressed or extinguished and the photopic cone response is less severely reduced.

Retinitis pigmentosa has various inheritance patterns which include an autosomal dominant pattern (30–40%), an autosomal recessive pattern (50–60%), and an X-linked pattern (10–15%). Retinitis pigmentosa shows considerable genetic heterogeneity with mutations identified in over 100 different genes thus far. Furthermore, many of these mutations confer different phenotypes even within the same family. Although there are many exceptions, the age of onset and degree of central vision loss may be related to the mode of familial transmission, with the autosomal dominant forms often conferring a less severe phenotype than the X-linked and recessive forms.

The typical clinical features of RP include retinal arteriolar attenuation and a generalized and diffuse pattern of mottled and moth-eaten RPE. A bone spicule pattern of intraretinal pigment located in the midperiphery is not always present (i.e., RP sine pigmento) but is typical. Waxy pallor of the disc and macular atrophy are usually signs of more advanced disease. Associated vitreous and retinal complications include vitreous veils and pigmentary cells, cystoid macular edema, epiretinal membrane formation, and a Coats-like retinal vascular response. Coats-like reactions may include retinal neovascularization and preretinal hemorrhage and even vasoproliferative tumors. Other ocular complications may include posterior subcapsular cataract and optic disc drusen. Broadly speaking, RP may be grouped into non-syndromic and syndromic forms with additional systemic manifestations that may include hearing loss, metabolic disorders, neurological syndromes, and renal or hepatic abnormalities among other systemic abnormalities.

Non-Syndromic Retinitis Pigmentosa

Retinitis pigmentosa may exist as an isolated ophthalmologic disorder. This group is genetically and phenotypically heterogeneous, and most easily broken down by inheritance patterns. While exact frequencies vary by ethnicity and geography, the most frequently identified genes involved in the autosomal recessive form are EYS, RPE65, PDE6A, PDE6B, and ABCA4. The most frequently identified genes involved in the autosomal dominant form are RHO (rhodopsin), PRPF31, and PRPH2/RDS and RP1. The most frequently identified genes in X-linked RP are RPGR and RP2.

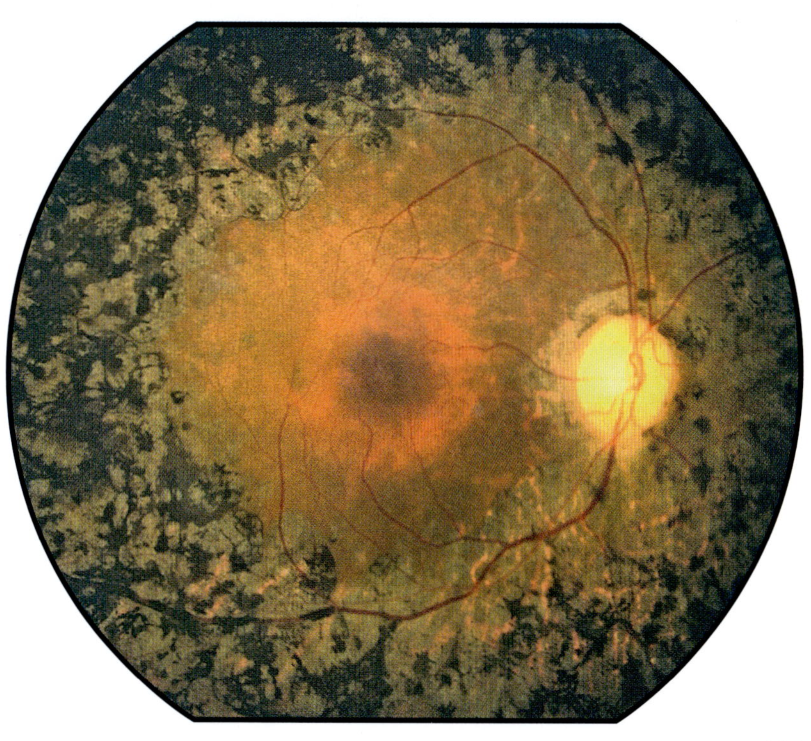

This is a posterior fundus of a typical patient with retinitis pigmentosa. Note the circumferential variable pigment epithelial hyperplastic change. Pigment has migrated into the retina, and in some areas into the perivenular space, all within a zonal area of patchy pigment epithelial atrophy. There is generalized arteriolar narrowing and some waxy pallor to the optic nerve. The fovea demonstrates a pigment epithelial granularity. This is one of many changes that can occur centrally in this disease. *Courtesy of Mark Croswell*

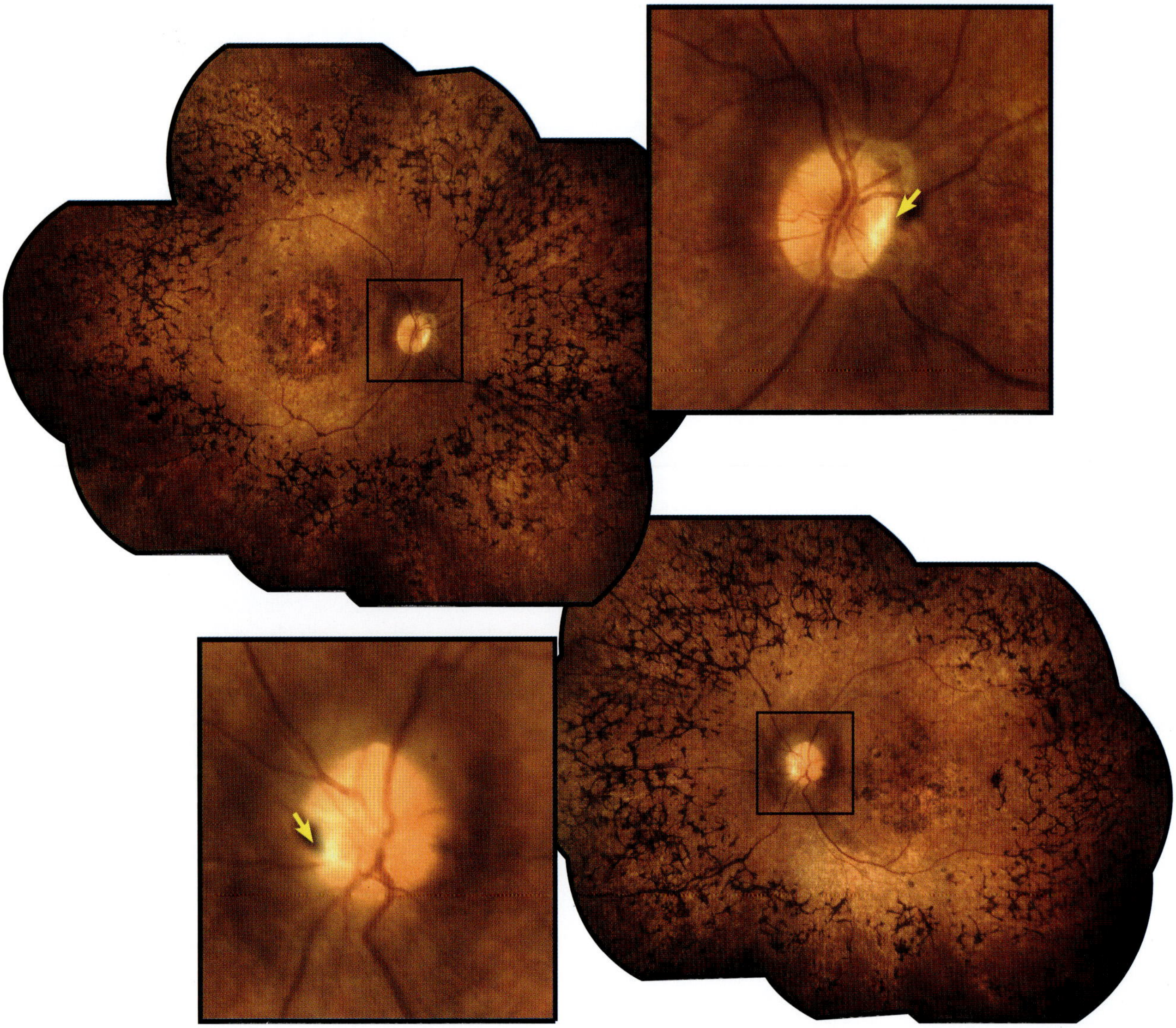

These are montage images of both eyes of a patient with retinitis pigmentosa (RP). Note the lacy-like spicules of pigment epithelial hyperplasia surrounding the posterior pole and extending into the mid and far peripheral fundus. There is a striking bilateral symmetry that is typical of RP. Note the presence of optic nerve head drusen in each eye *(arrows)*. Macular atrophy is noted, which is more typical in the later stages of disease.

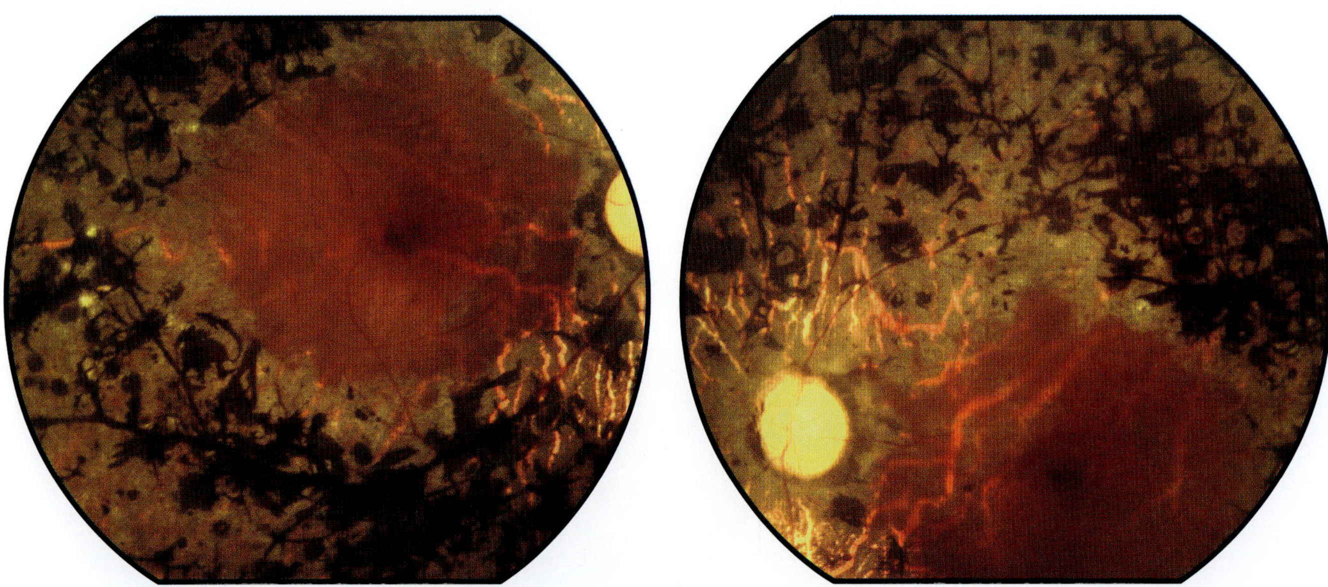

Dense pigment spiculation is present in this patient with retinitis pigmentosa. There is also dense chorioretinal atrophy extending from the disc. Waxy pallor of the disc is evident bilaterally, another late stage finding.

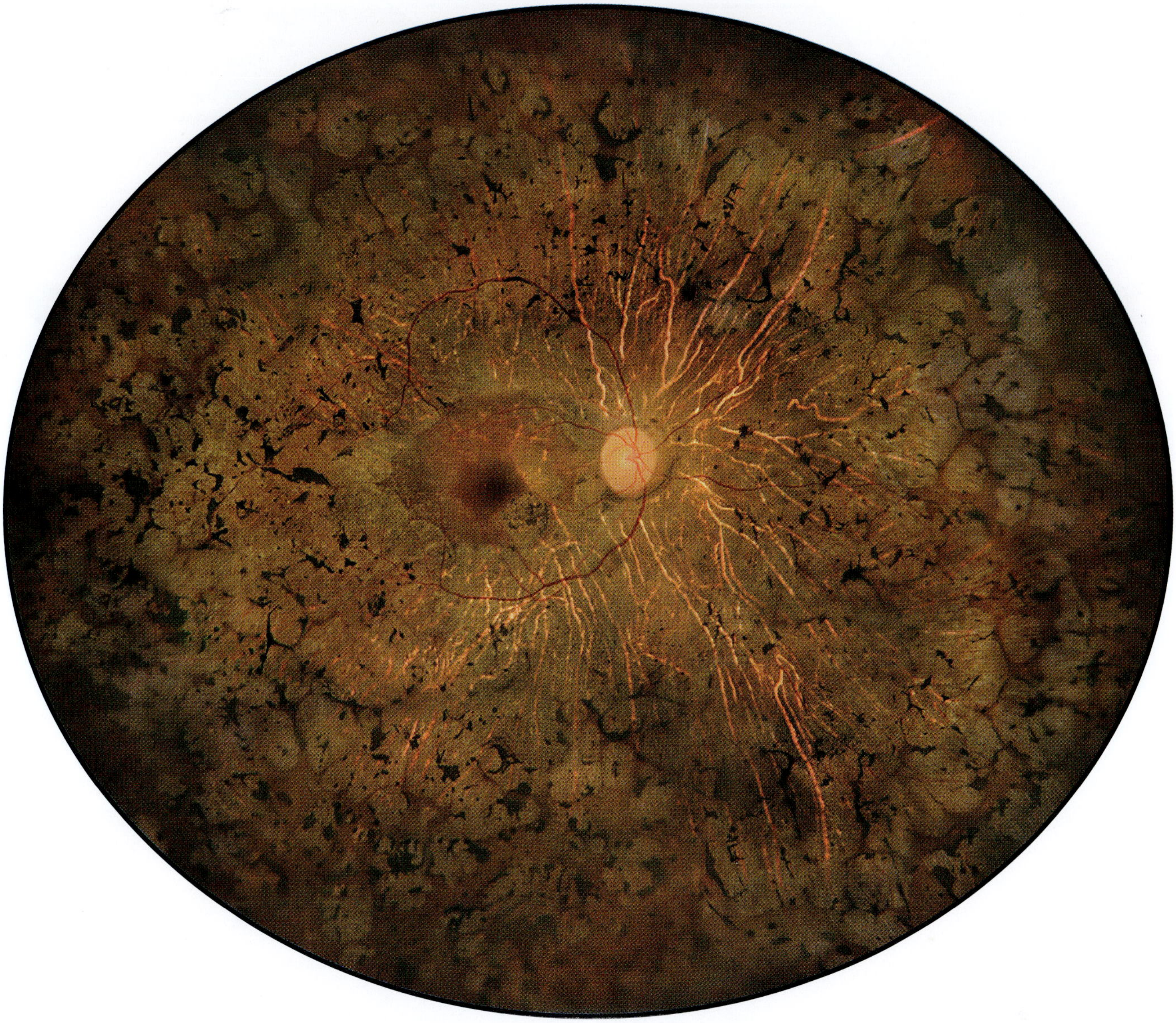

This wide-angle montage of this patient with retinitis pigmentosa shows a variation in the morphology of the pigment epithelial hyperplasia and migration. There is almost a reticular pattern, delineated by the pigment and demarcating zones of RPE atrophy. In other areas of the midperipheral fundus, the pigment epithelium is more homogeneously atrophic and there is a prominence of the choroidal architecture which appears to be sclerotic.

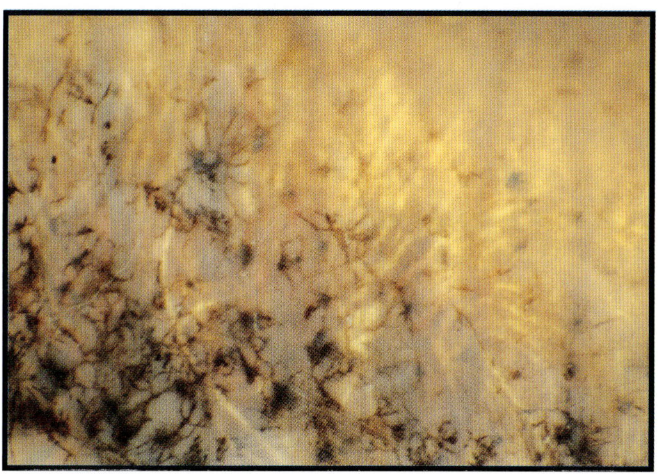

In this histopathological specimen, there is prominent pigment epithelial hyperplasia with spider-like extensions and generalized retinal pigment epithelial atrophy. Choroidal vessels can be seen.

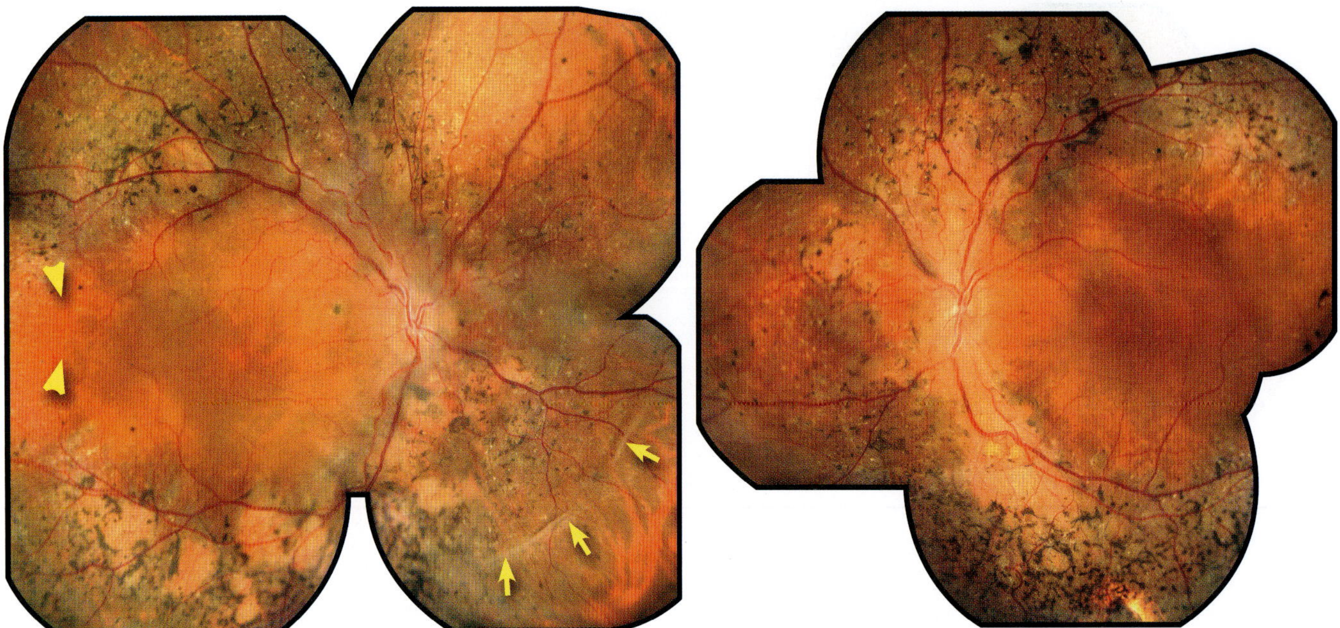

In this patient with retinitis pigmentosa, there is a midperipheral to peripheral area of pigment epithelial hyperplasia, atrophy, and multiple drusenoid spots. In the right eye, there are faintly evident radially oriented spots in the temporal macula *(arrowheads)* and also a curvilinear area of preretinal fibrosis exhibiting traction on the retina *(arrows)*. The macula has only a minor degree of atrophy but there is a translucent epiretinal membrane formation.

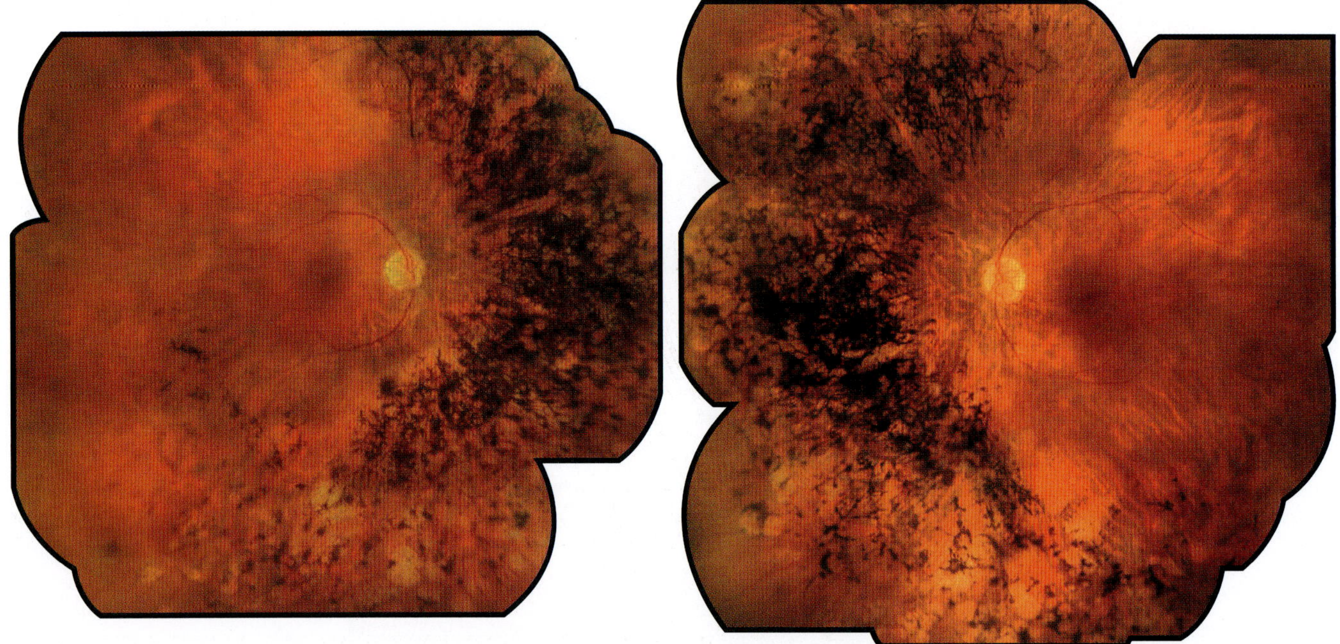

This patient with retinitis pigmentosa also illustrates the propensity for symmetric findings with dense pigmentation nasally in an arcuate pattern with relative sparing temporally in each eye.

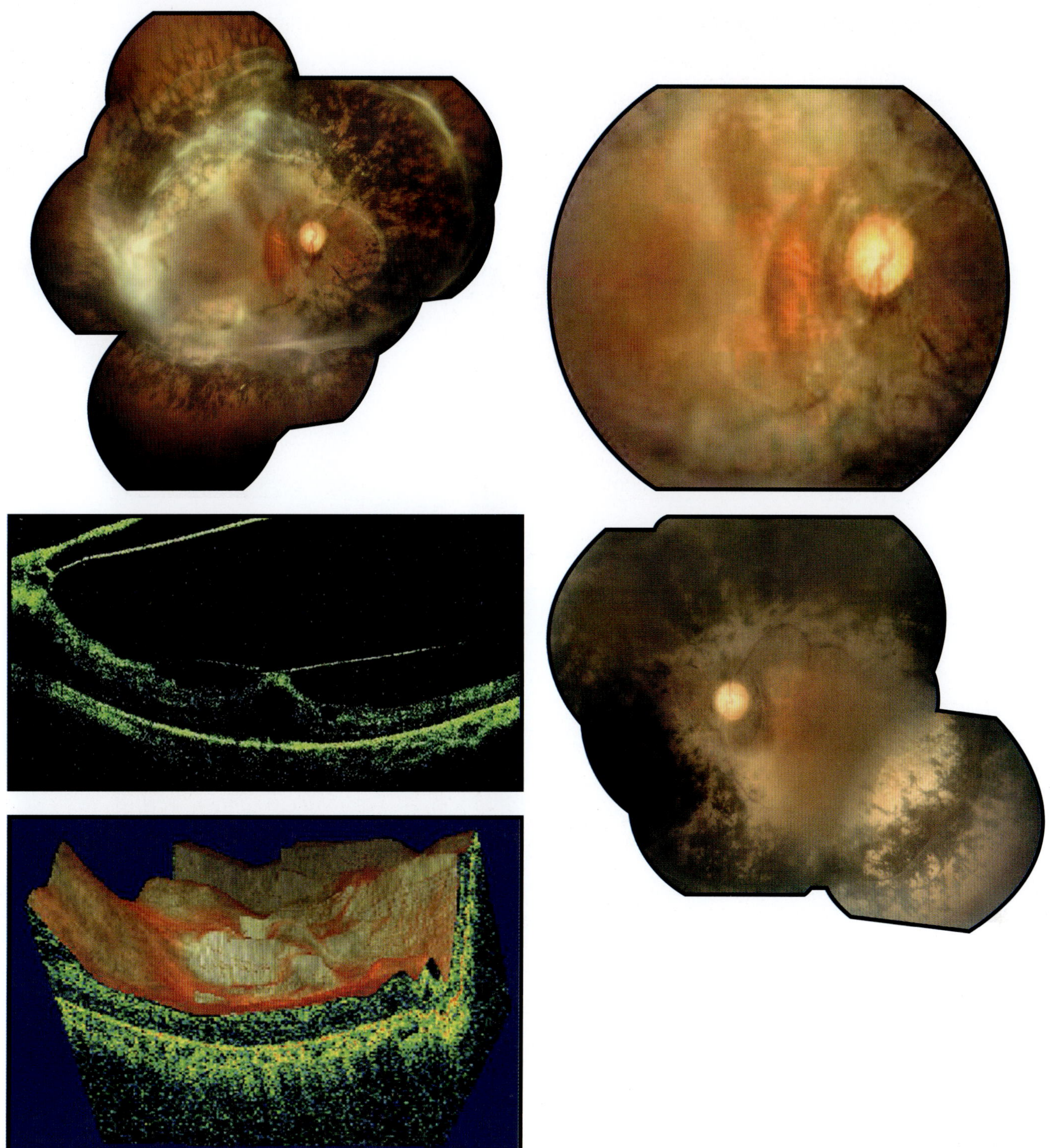

In this patient with dominantly inherited and advanced retinitis pigmentosa, as shown in the color montage of each eye, there is an extensive and prominent vitreoretinal fibrotic sheet in the right eye. The OCT image demonstrates the vitreoretinal traction and cystic change. With three-dimensional OCT, the planar contour of the retina is clearly demonstrated, as induced by the vitreous condensation and traction. *Courtesy of Dr. Iñigo Corcóstegui*

Female Carriers of X-Linked Retinitis Pigmentosa

Female carriers of X-linked retinitis pigmentosa may exhibit mosaicism with variable manifestations in the fundus that are often peripheral and zonal without clinical or electroretinographic (ERG) abnormalities. In some patients, the changes are sufficient to induce macular and electrophysiological changes and more severe forms of RP with an extinguished ERG may even be seen. A golden tapetal reflex in the macula can be very suggestive.

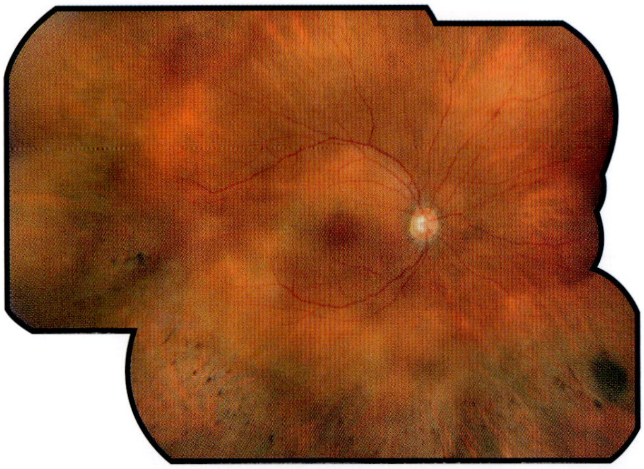

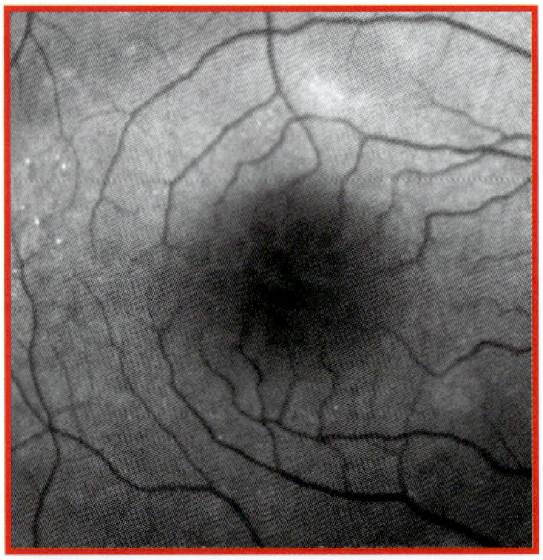

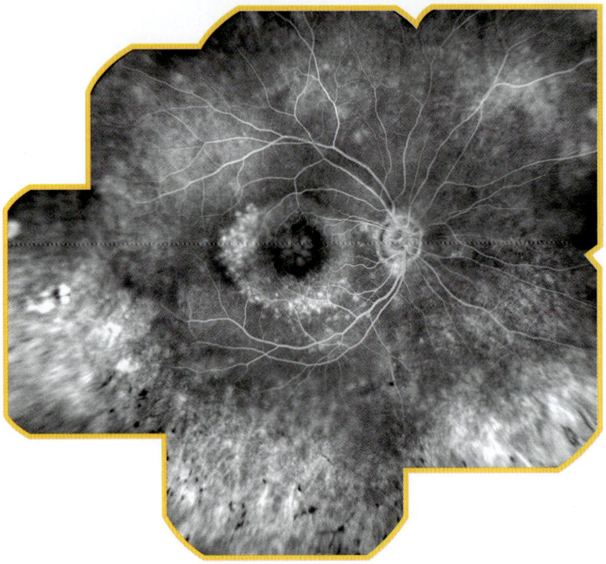

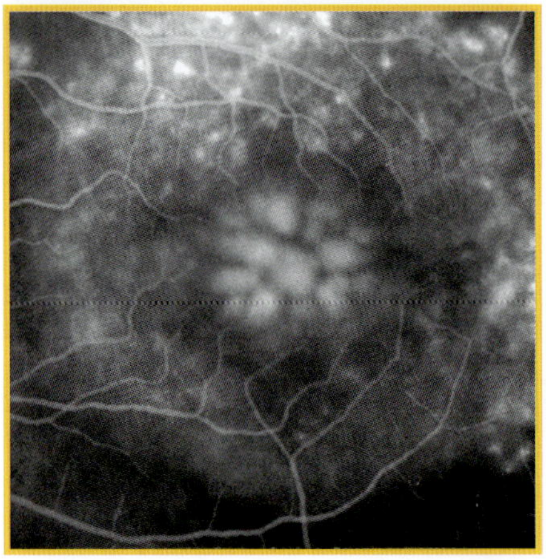

This is a female carrier of X-linked retinitis pigmentosa. The color montage photograph shows patchy peripheral pigment epithelial hyperplasia and atrophy more notable inferiorly. The red-free photograph demonstrates a cystoid pattern in the macula. Fluorescein angiography shows petaloid leakage or cystoid macular edema. There is retinal edema surrounding the central foveal leakage.

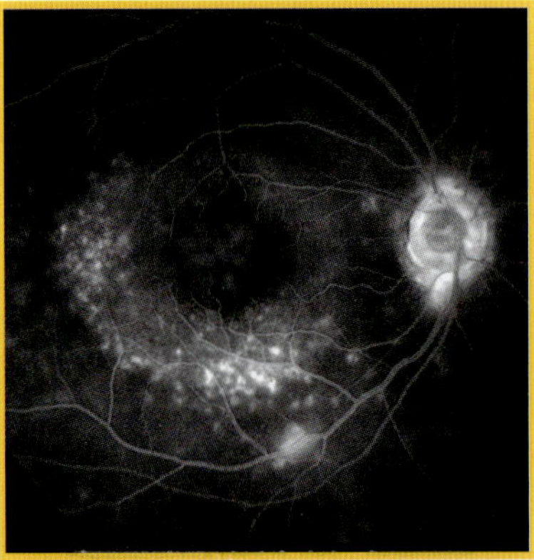
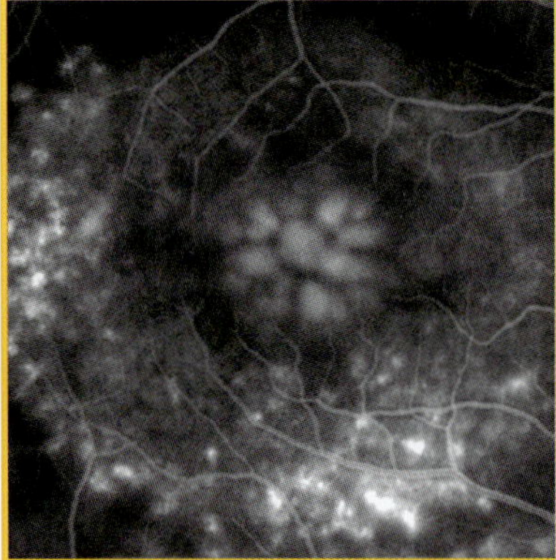
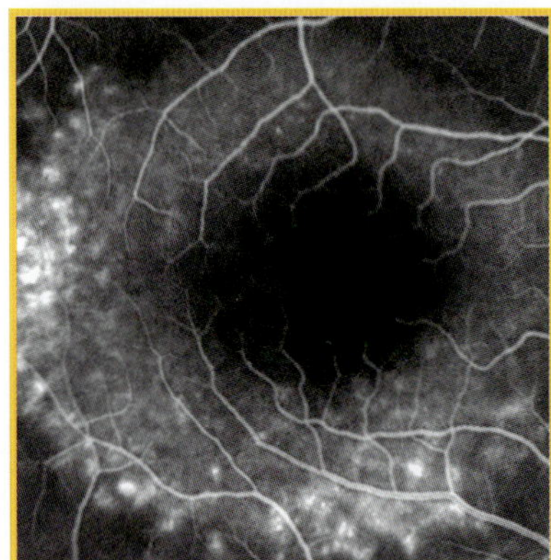

Note the resolution of CME following treatment with a topical carbonic anhydrase inhibitor. A component of leakage may be due to incontinence of the outer blood–retinal barrier or RPE.

Macular Abnormalities in Retinitis Pigmentosa

Numerous macular complications occur in retinitis pigmentosa, such as atrophy, pigmentary degeneration, epiretinal membrane formation, macular edema, and macular hole formation.

Hole

These two patients with RP demonstrate a full thickness macular hole. "Bull's-eye" atrophy is noted in the color montage due to chronicity of the hole and the concentric margin or cuff of subretinal fluid. The macular hole from the case on the left is unusually large. Note the pigmentation and atrophy of the fundus temporal to the hole indicative of RP.

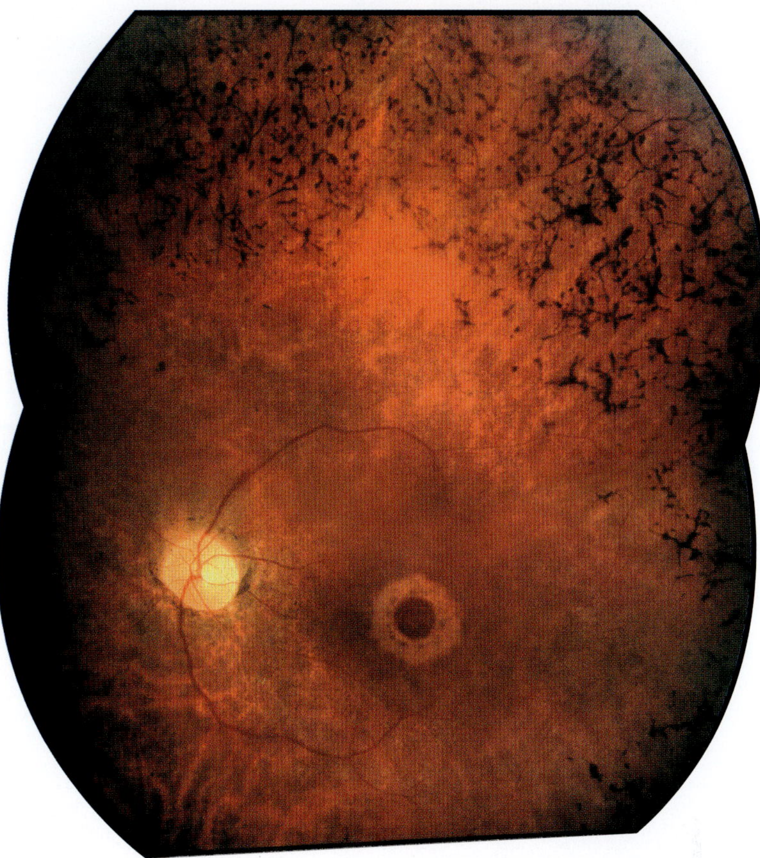

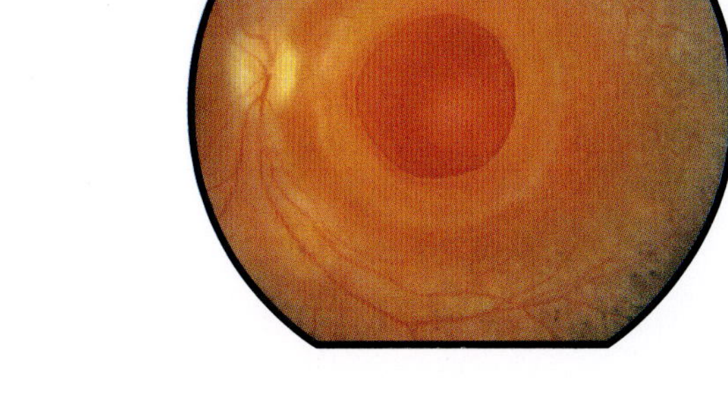

Atrophy

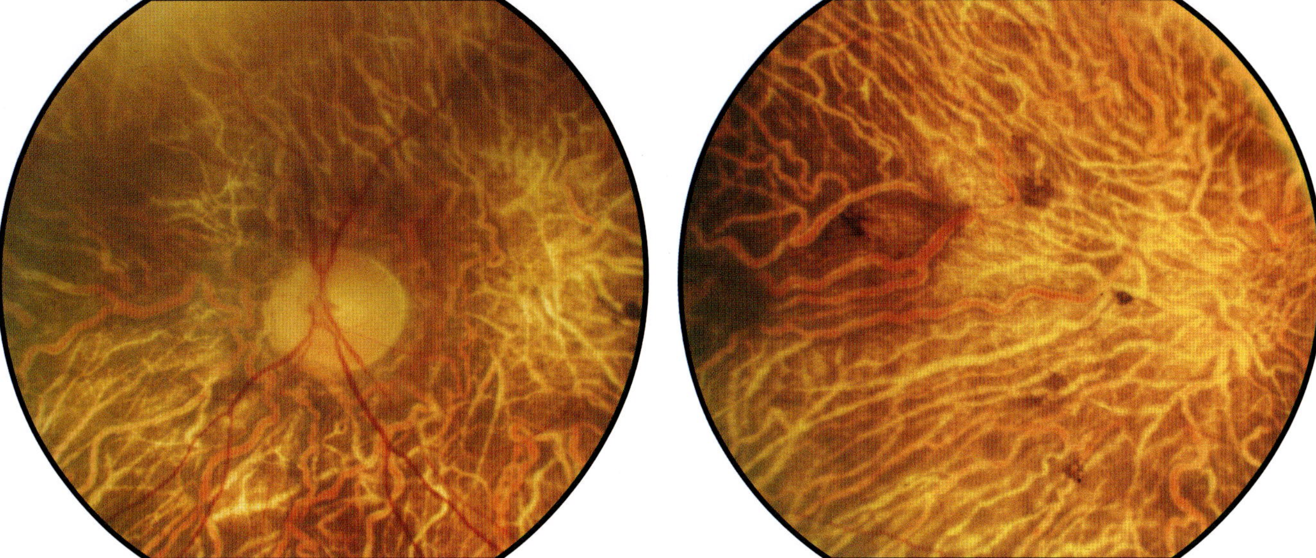

This patient has widespread chorioretinal atrophy that includes the central macula.

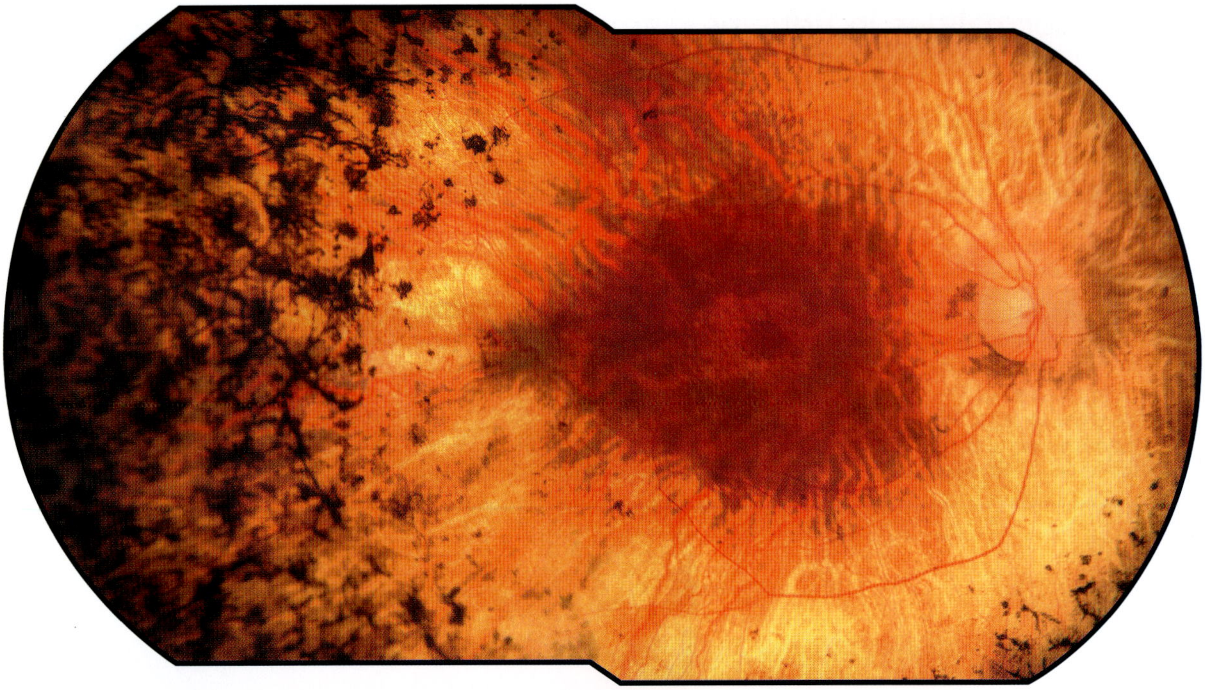

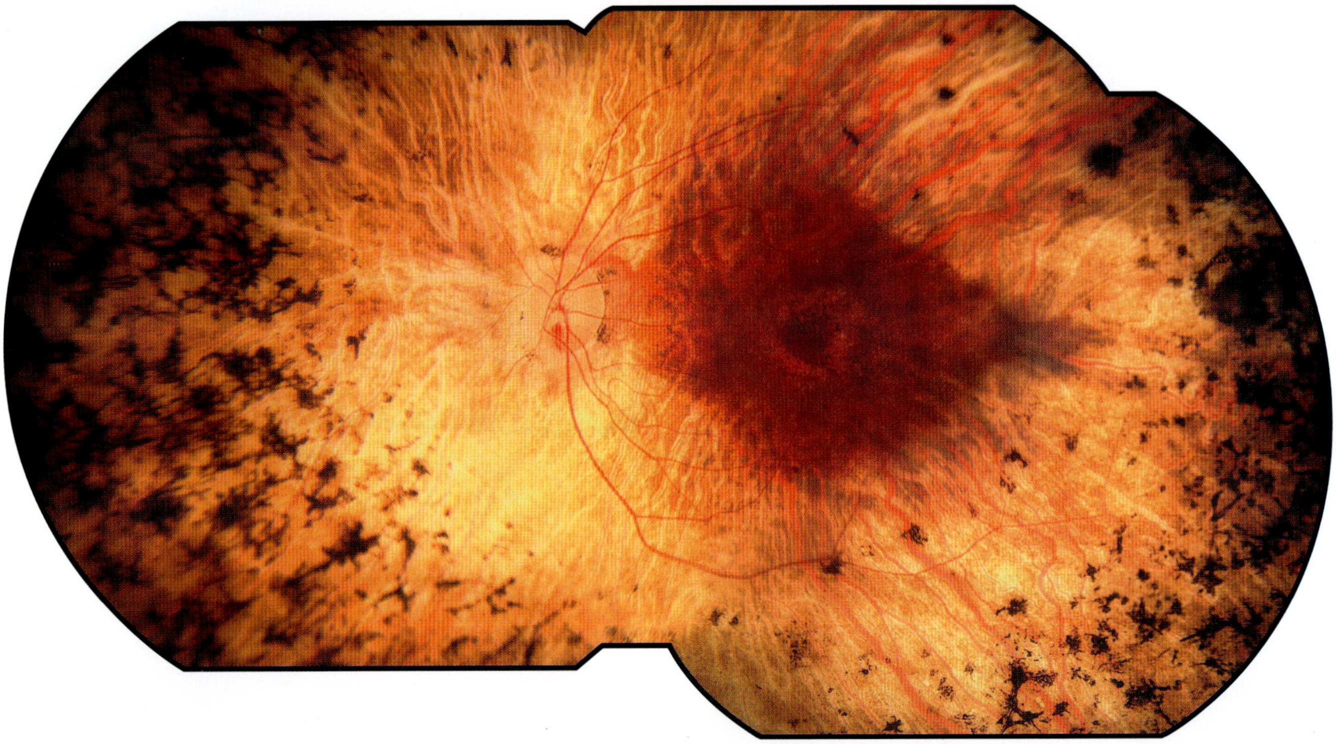

These patients with retinitis pigmentosa demonstrate a "ring maculopathy" from atrophy surrounding a relatively intact fovea. Bordering the ring of atrophy is pigment epithelium which is not yet implicated in the pathology. *Images courtesy of Drs. J.B. Bateman, G.E. Lang and Irene Maumenee*

Edema

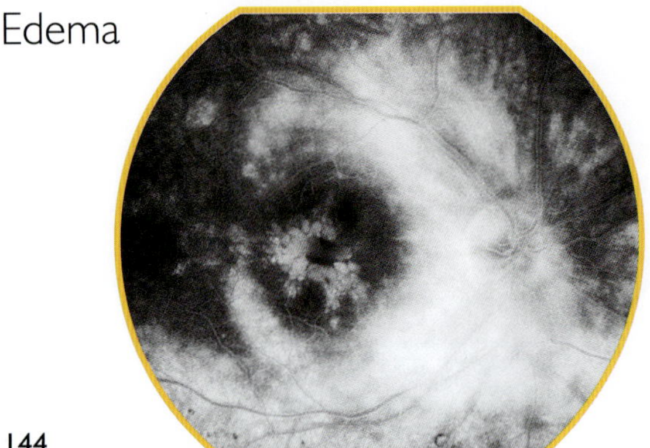

CME and diffuse retinal edema may complicate RP. A cystoid pattern of leakage is present central and diffuse peripapillary and retinal vascular leakage are also noted.

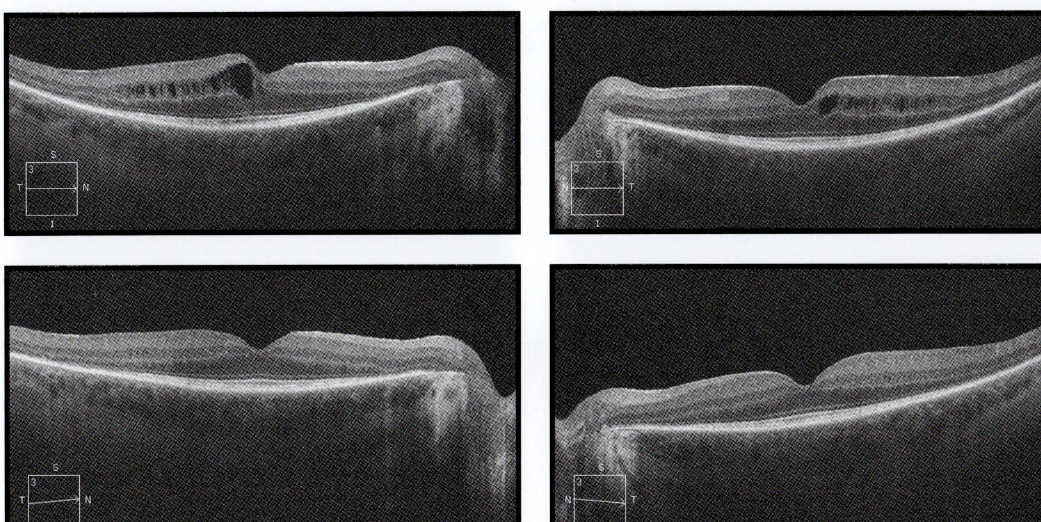

This patient with reintitis pigmentosa has cystoid macular edema. Note the paramacular loss of photoreceptors and inner segments in each eye characteristic of RP. The edema significantly improved after treatment with topical dorzolamide. *Images courtesy of Susan M. Malinowski, MD*

Ring Autofluorescence

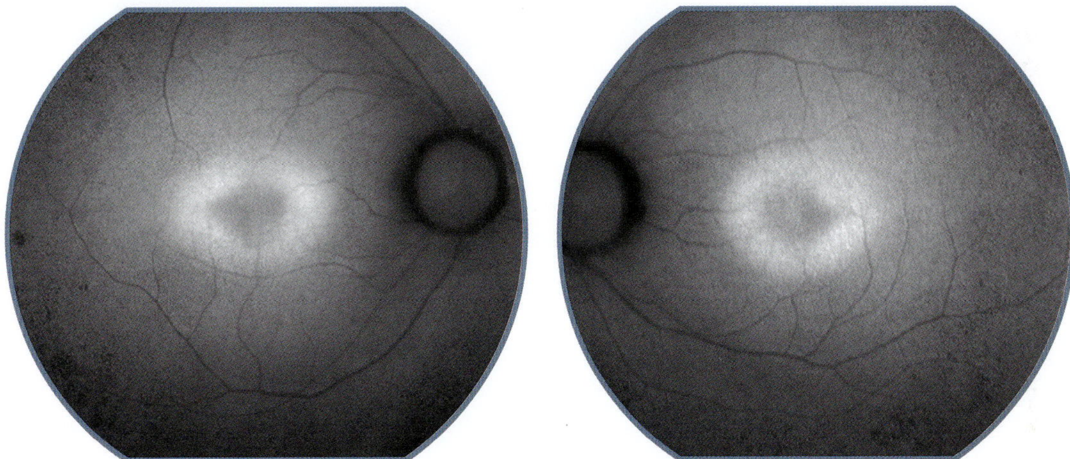

A ring of hyperautofluorescence, referred to as the Robson-Holder ring, may be seen in the macula of patients with retinitis pigmentosa.

Epiretinal Membrane

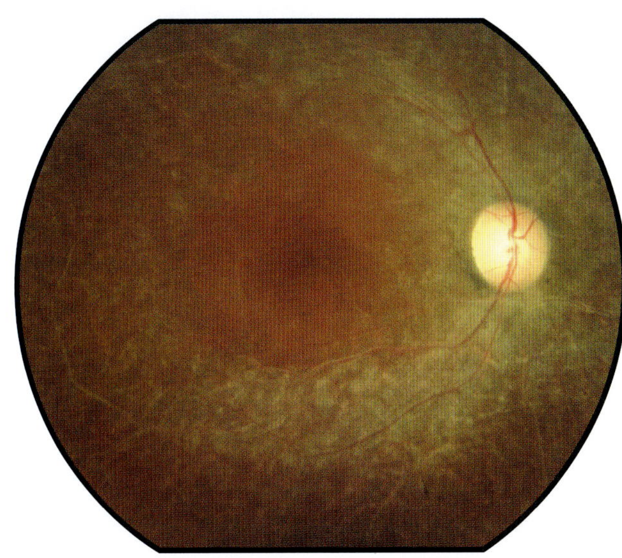

Epiretinal membrane (ERM) formation is common in RP and may manifest as a macular sheen or frank macular pucker with traction and distortion. This patient with retinitis pigmentosa has an ERM. SD-OCT is most sensitive in detecting ERMs and associated complications such as vitreomacular traction and CME.

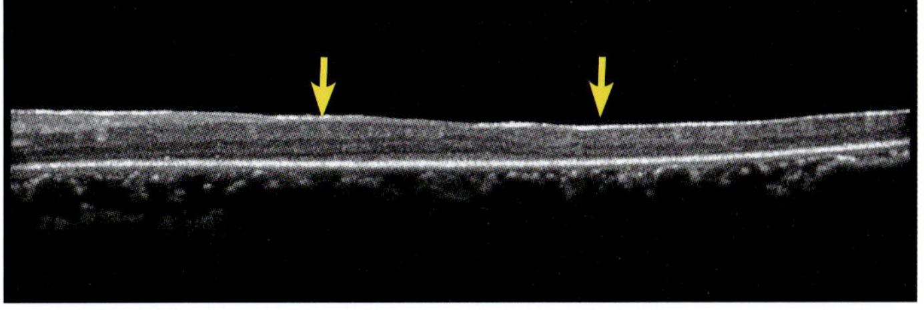

Angiomatous Proliferation in Retinitis Pigmentosa

Patients with retinitis pigmentosa may exhibit a spectrum of retinal vascular abnormalities including Coats-like retinal telangiectasia with lipid exudation. Peripheral retinal ischemia with preretinal neovascularization, severe leakage, and preretinal hemorrhage, and even vasoproliferative tumors, may also complicate RP.

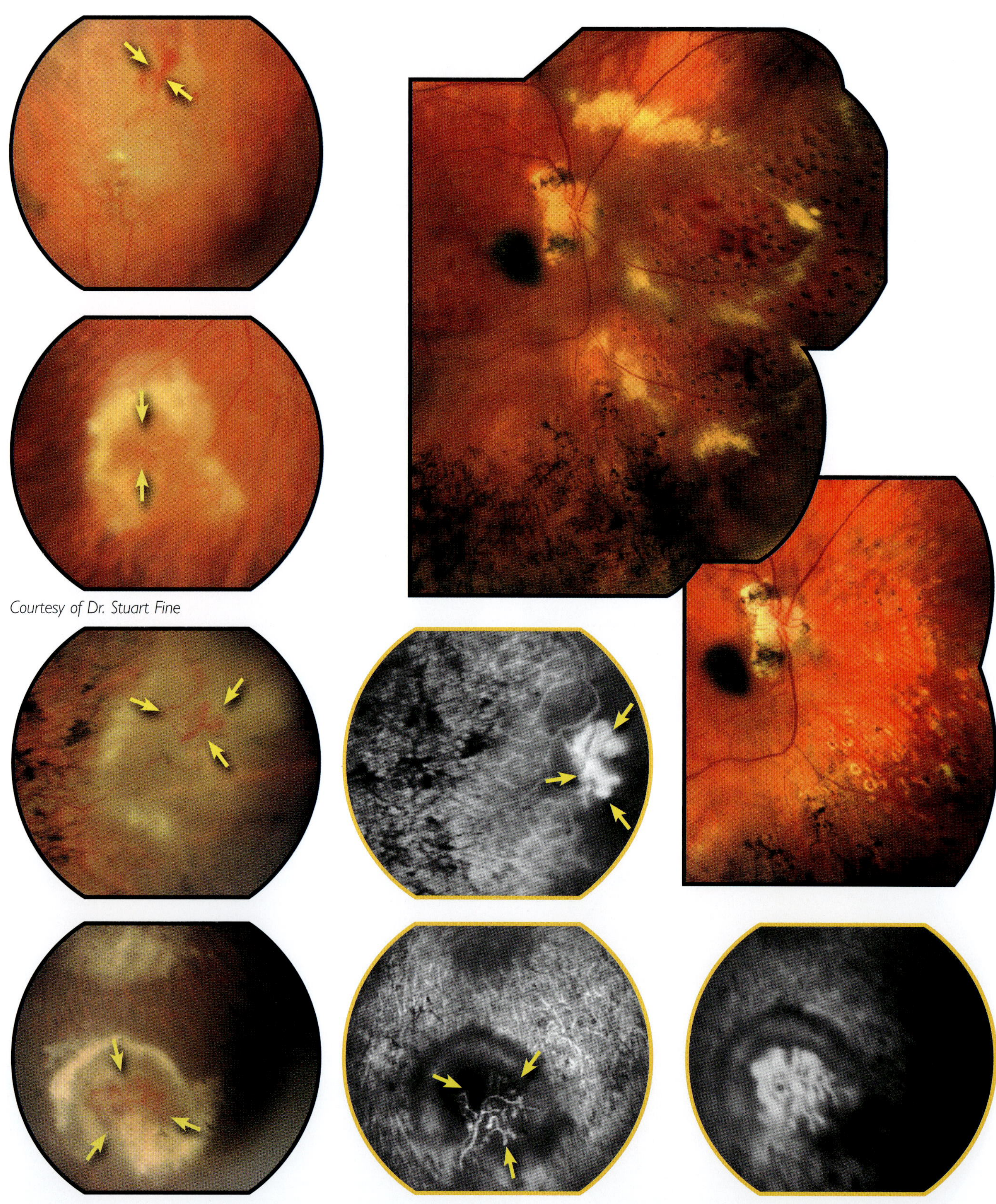

Courtesy of Dr. Stuart Fine

Patients with retinitis pigmentosa are prone to develop angiomatous proliferation with lipid exudation. Note the presence of vascular proliferation *(arrows)* evident early and late on fluorescein angiography.

Sector Retinitis Pigmentosa

Retinitis pigmentosa (RP) may rarely be localized to isolated quadrants of the retina. The most frequently involved quadrants are inferior, and patients often have bilaterally symmetric disease. Despite the fundus appearance, full-field ERG may reveal global dysfunction, although prognosis is generally better with regional or localized forms of retinitis pigmentosa such as sector RP. The most common genetic etiology of sectoral RP is a rhodopsin mutation.

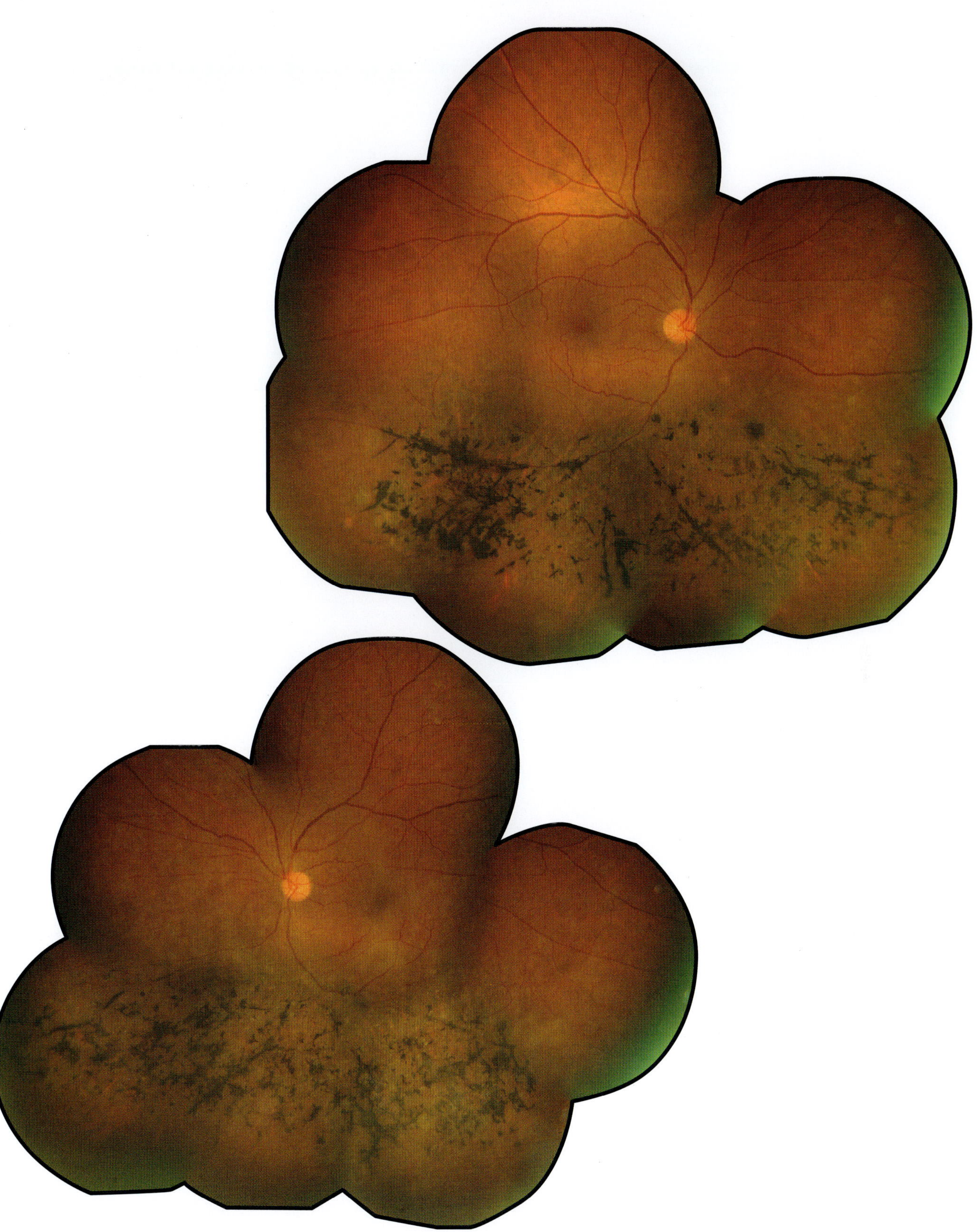

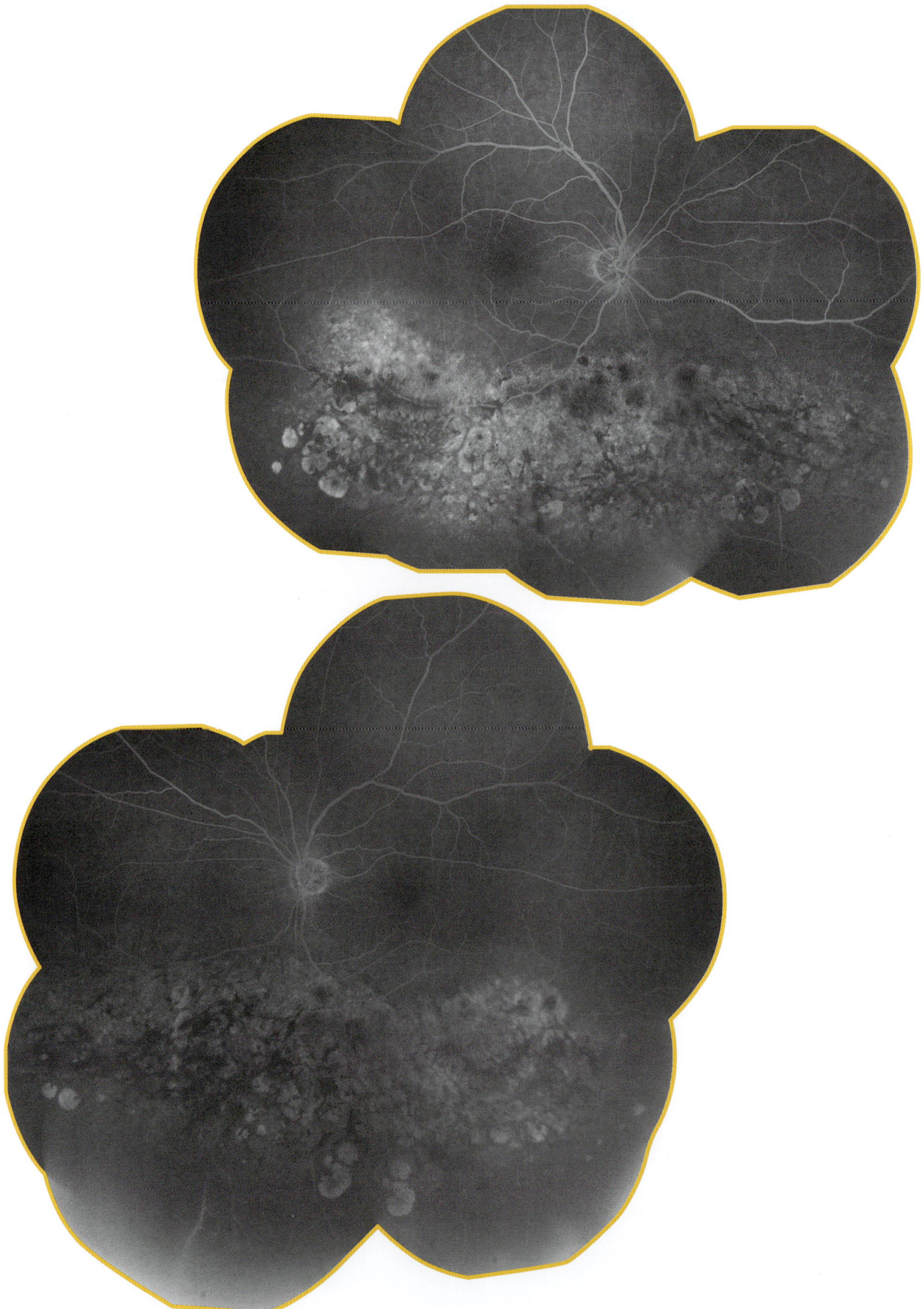

Color fundus montage and fluorescein angiogram montage of this patient with sector retinitis pigmentosa shows bone-spicule pigmentary changes and RPE atrophy in the inferior quadrants of both eyes.

Pigmented Paravenous Retinochoroidal Atrophy (PPRCA)

Pigmented paravenous retinochoroidal atrophy (PPRCA) is a bilaterally symmetric, typically stationary, disease of the retina characterized by pigment clumping and spicules in a predominantly paravenous distribution with variable amounts of retinochoroidal atrophy along the same distribution. The etiology of the condition is unclear. A male predilection has been noted and familial cases have been reported in the literature, but most cases are sporadic. It has been postulated that the disease may be a response to an inflammatory or infectious etiology with cases reported following such disorders. Patients are usually asymptomatic and relatively stable over time, although progression has been reported in one case. The optic disc, macula, and retinal vessels are typically normal, although some cases have demonstrated vascular attenuation, optic disc pallor, and CME and RPE changes in the macula. Electroretinogram and electrooculogram findings are variable: normal, borderline normal and abnormal reports of both tests are reported in the literature and tend to remain stable even with long term follow-up. On fluorescein angiography, hyperfluorescent areas of RPE atrophy may extend away from the retinal vessels and in some cases may demonstrate associated choriocapillaris atrophy. Mutation in the CRB1 gene, more commonly associated with preserved para-arteriolar RPE syndrome, has been noted to cause PPRCA in one report.

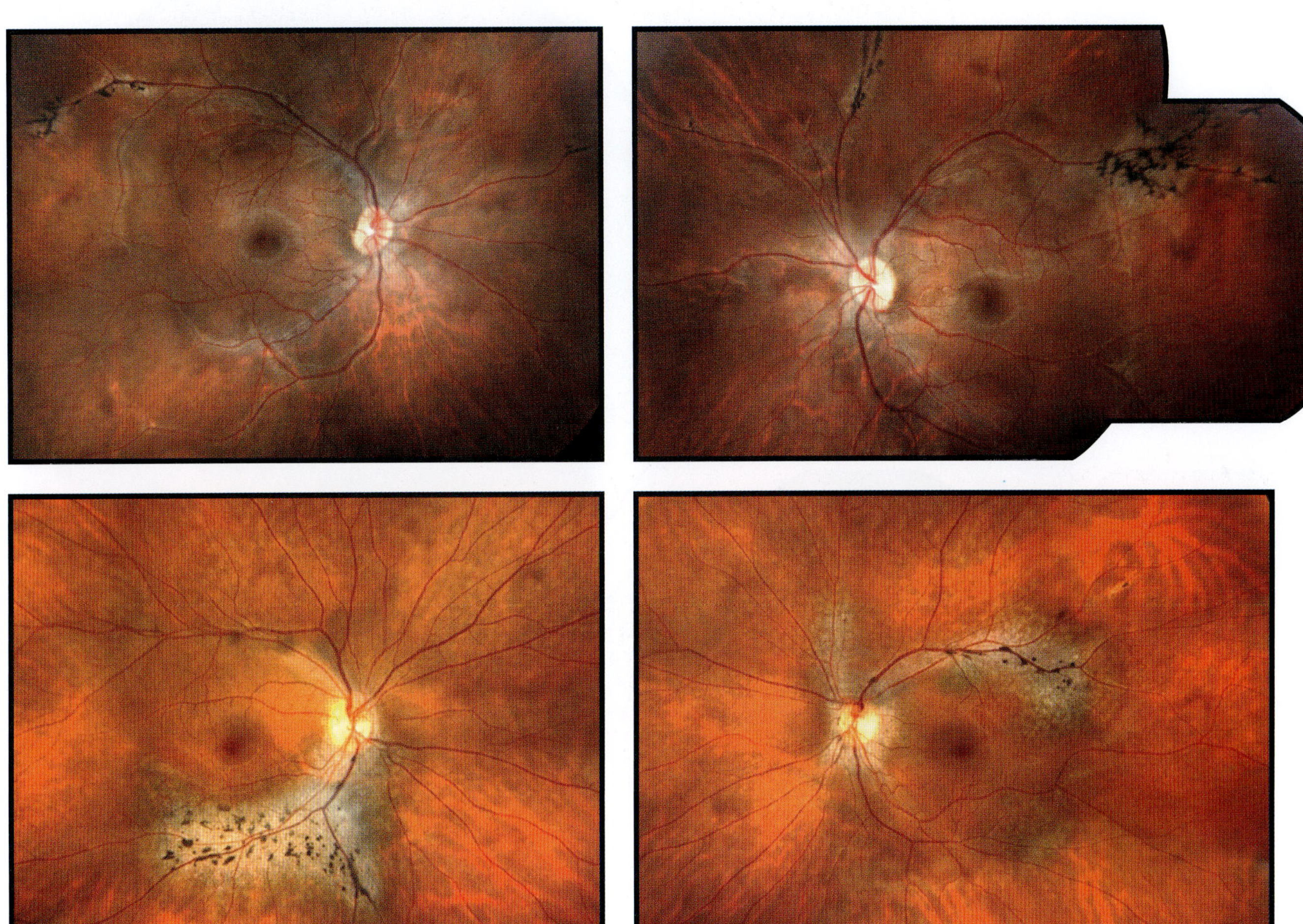

PPRCA is seen here in two patients. These two cases demonstrate the variability in the atrophy surrounding the venous arcades in both distribution and severity. This condition is often congenital and stationary, although families have been reported in which the process begins peripherally and extends posteriorly.

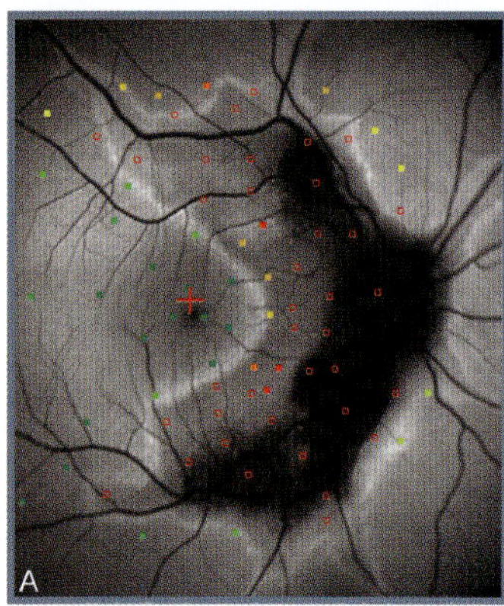

© 61

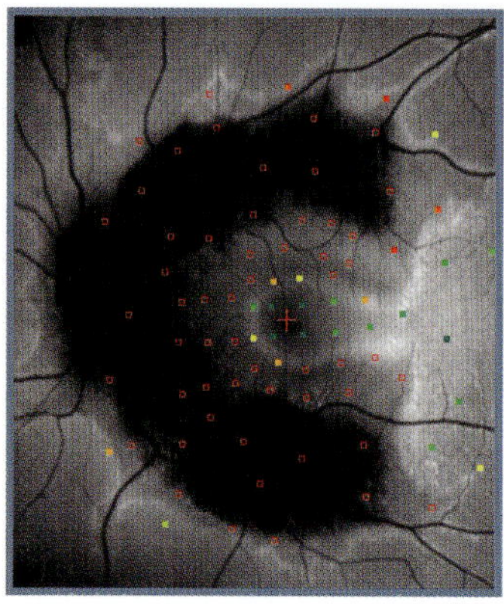

© 62

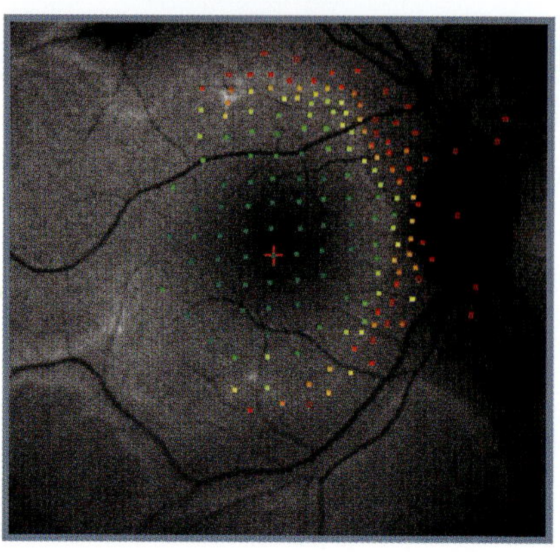

© 63

The patient on the left shows microperimetry analysis superimposed on fundus autofluorescence in each eye *(left and middle images)* and in one eye of another patient *(right image)*. Note that increased sensitivity is present in the paramacular regions while sensitivity is reduced where there is relative fundus hypofluorescence and more significantly reduced where there is more severe fundus hypofluorescence.

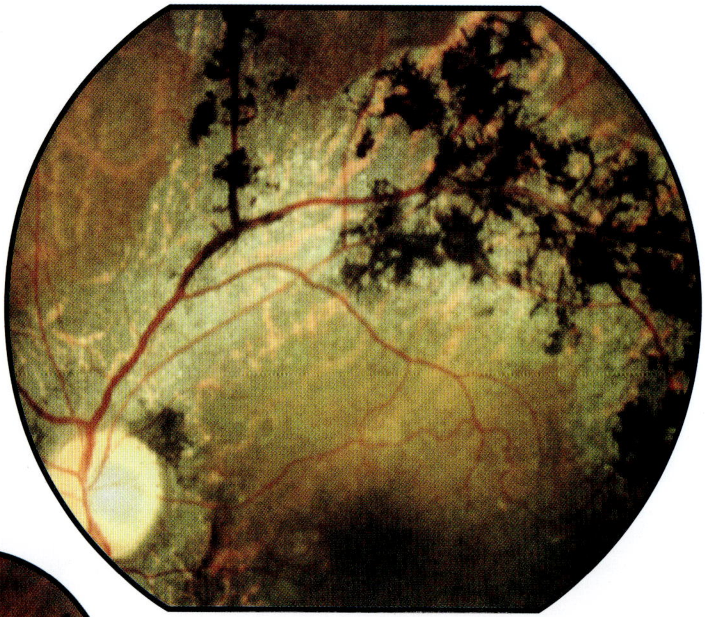

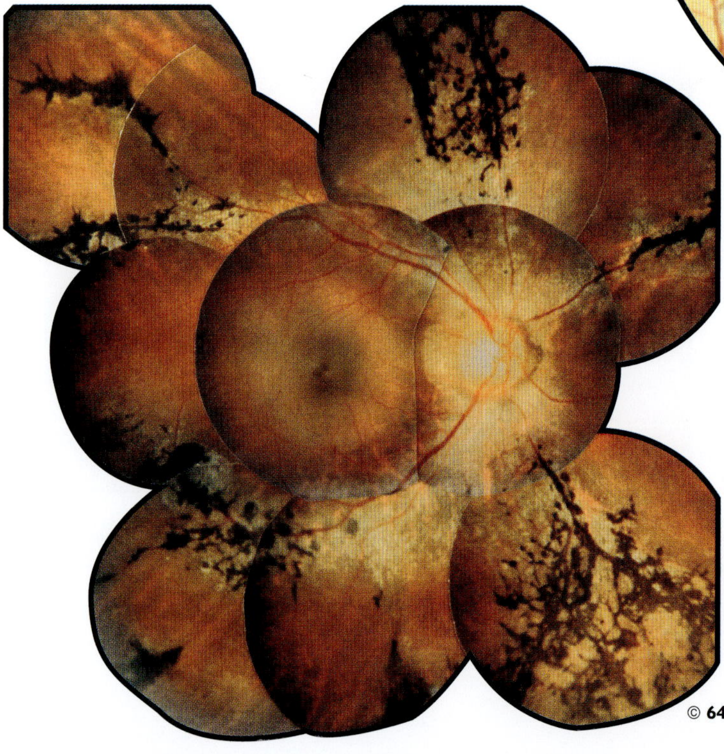

© 64

These two patients with pigmented paravenous retinochoroidal atrophy have a more prominent pattern of pigmentary epithelial hyperplasia and spiculation, extending beyond the venous system and also involving the arteriolar vasculature.

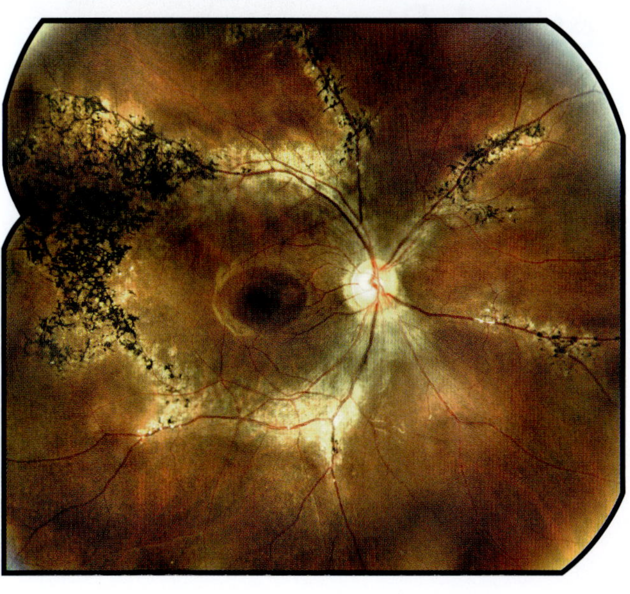

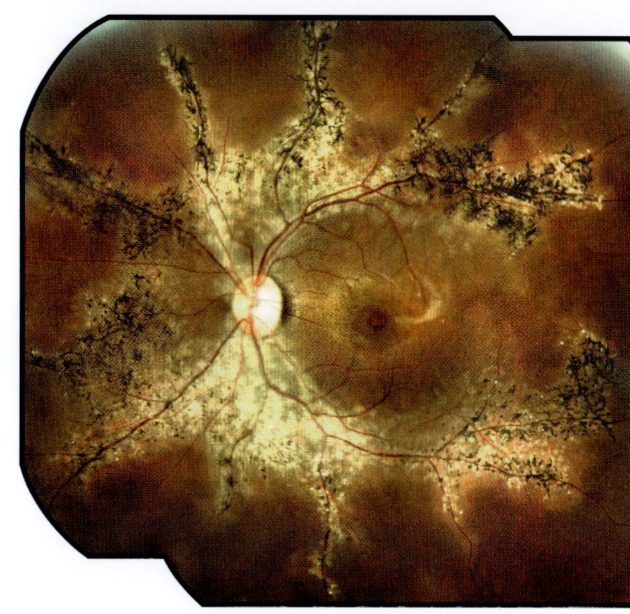

This patient with PPRCA has a striking bilateral similarity with typical sparing of the posterior pole and good vision.

In this patient with PPRCA, the process is predominantly atrophic in nature, perhaps related to the underlying "blonde fundus."

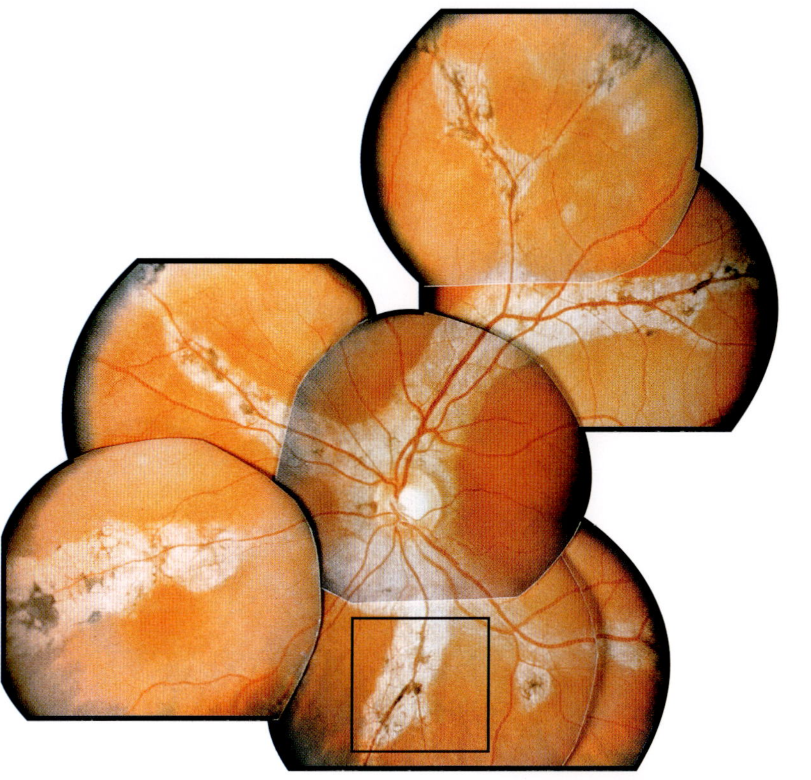

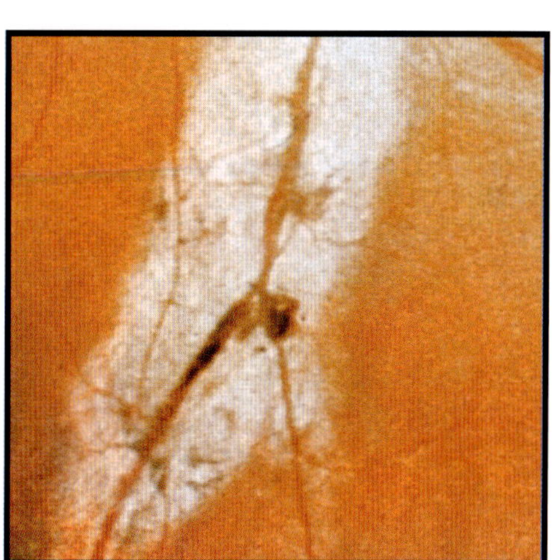

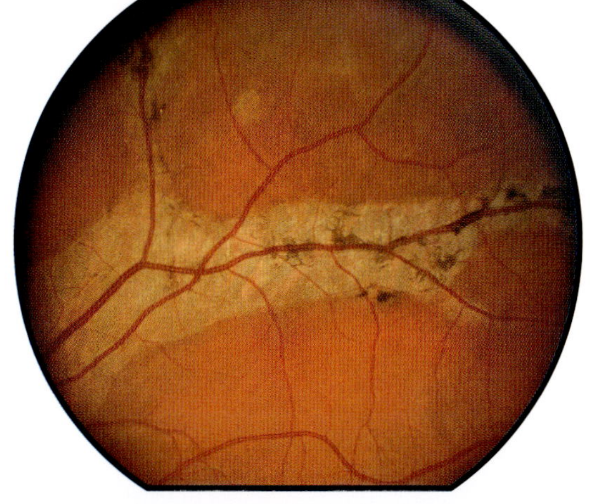

Preserved Para-arteriolar Retinal Pigment Epithelium in Retinitis Pigmentosa

In some cases of retinitis pigmentosa, there is sparing of the RPE adjacent to and along the distribution of retinal arterioles. This is typically most evident in the equatorial and peripheral areas of the retina. An association with the CRB1 mutation has been reported and associated findings of this syndrome include optic disc drusen, dense subretinal pigment clumping, Coats-like response with retinal telangiectasia and lipid exudation and vasoproliferative tumor. The CRB1 mutation is one of many genetic associations of Lebers Congenital Amaurosis.

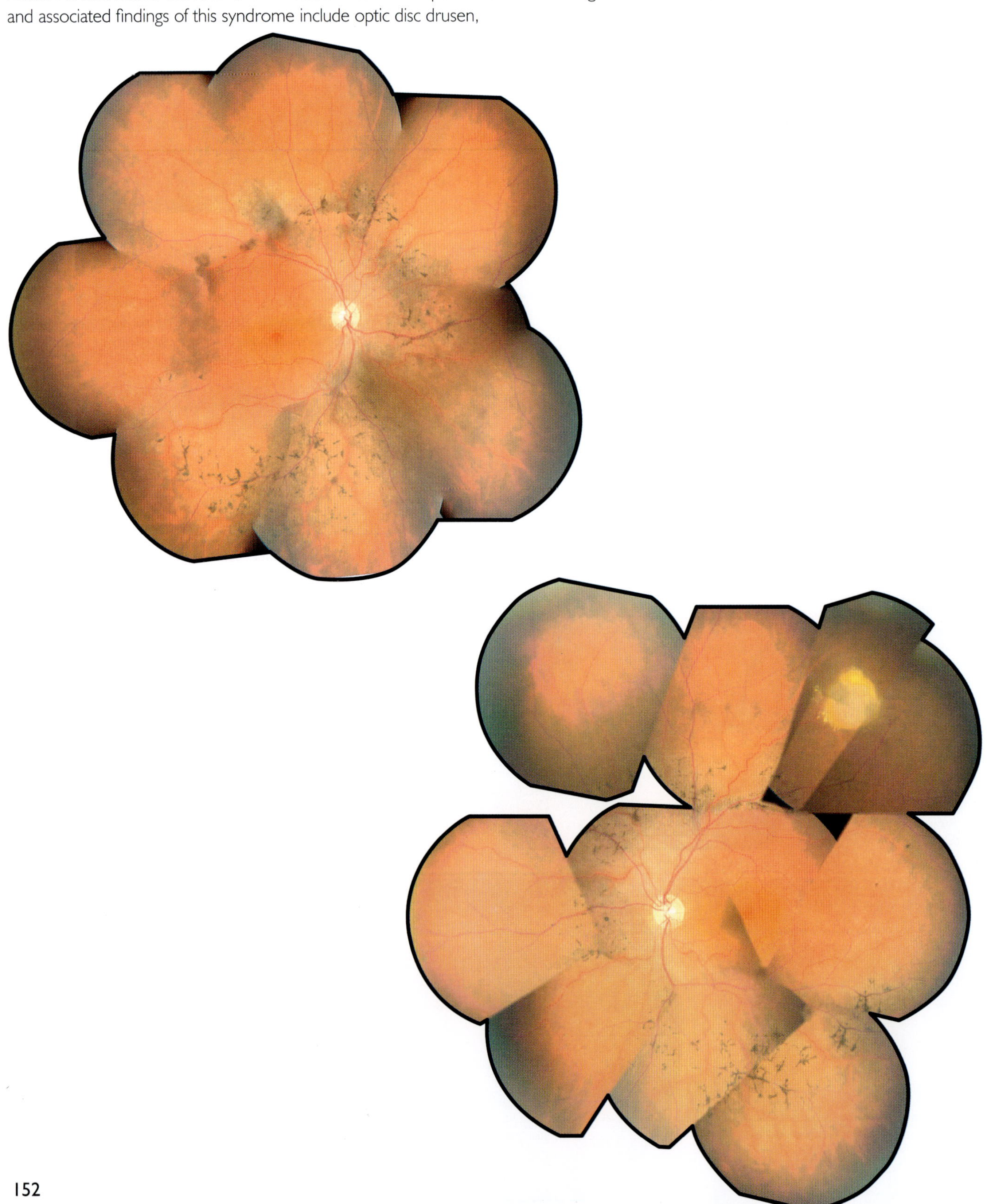

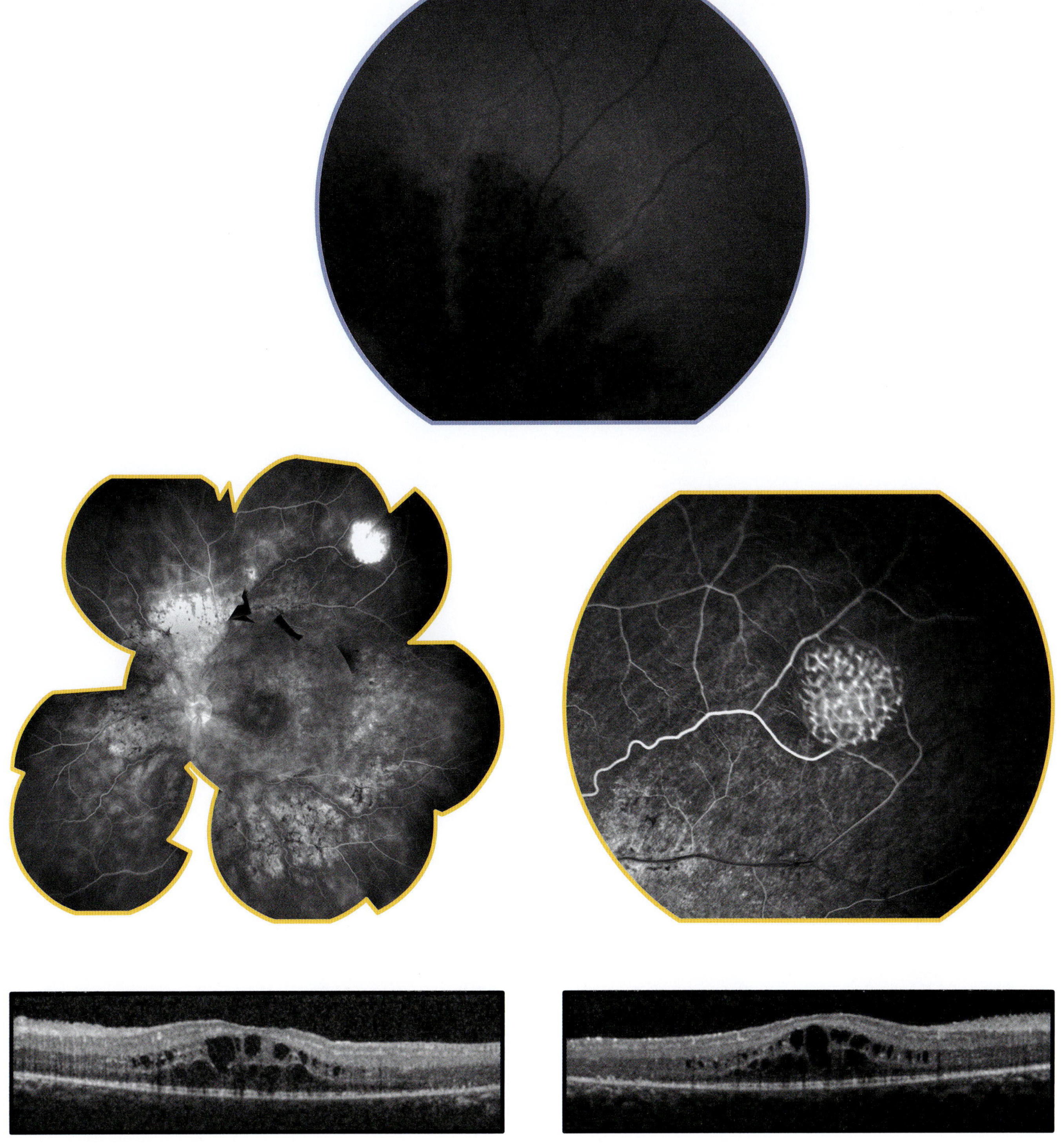

Fundus photo montage of this patient with RP shows para-arteriolar preservation of the RPE in both eyes, confirmed with fundus autofluorescence. In the superotemporal quadrant of the left eye there is also a yellow elevated mass that shows capillary filling on the early phase of fluorescein angiography, consistent with a vasoproliferative tumor. SD-OCT illustrates CME in both eyes and paramacular photoreceptor and ellipsoid loss. Genetic testing confirmed CRB1 mutation. *Images courtesy of Amani A. Fawzi, MD*

Syndromic Retinitis Pigmentosa

Retinitis pigmentosa may be part of a multisystem disorder and therefore a comprehensive systems review is an essential component of any patient presenting with RP. Associated systemic diseases include mitochondrial disorders, conditions with inborn errors of metabolism (see Chapter 3), and various other systemic syndromes.

Mitochondrial Disorders

Mitochondrial DNA encodes 37 genes essential to oxidative phosphorylation and energy production; however, it lacks the DNA repair mechanisms that protect nuclear DNA, and is therefore at least ten times more prone to mutation. These mutations are inherited in a maternal pattern and are responsible for a myriad of multisystem abnormalities. Many of these diseases affect the eye, where they most commonly cause optic neuropathy and pigmentary retinopathy. Because each cell in the body contains an assortment of wild-type mitochondria and mutated mitochondria, a phenomenon called heteroplasmy, disease phenotypes vary widely depending on the ratio of normal to mutated mitochondria. Clinical symptoms only manifest once the wild-type mitochondria can no longer keep pace with the tissue's energy demands. Numerous mutations have been associated with these diseases, and while specific mutations are nearly always present in certain disorders, such as the A3243G mutation in MIDD or MELAS, others are characterized by multiple different mutations.

Kearns–Sayre Syndrome

Kearns–Sayre syndrome is a mitochondrial disorder classically characterized by the triad of chronic progressive external ophthalmoplegia (CPEO), pigmentary retinopathy and onset before the age of 20 years old. Additionally, cardiac conduction block, increased cerebrospinal fluid protein or cerebellar ataxia must be present. CPEO is most often the presenting clinical abnormality. Retinal findings may include a salt-and-pepper pigmentary retinopathy and nummular RPE atrophy limited to the macular region or even a retinitis pigmentosa-like peripheral retinopathy. Diagnosis may be confirmed through muscle biopsy that shows "ragged red fibers" on trichrome stain.

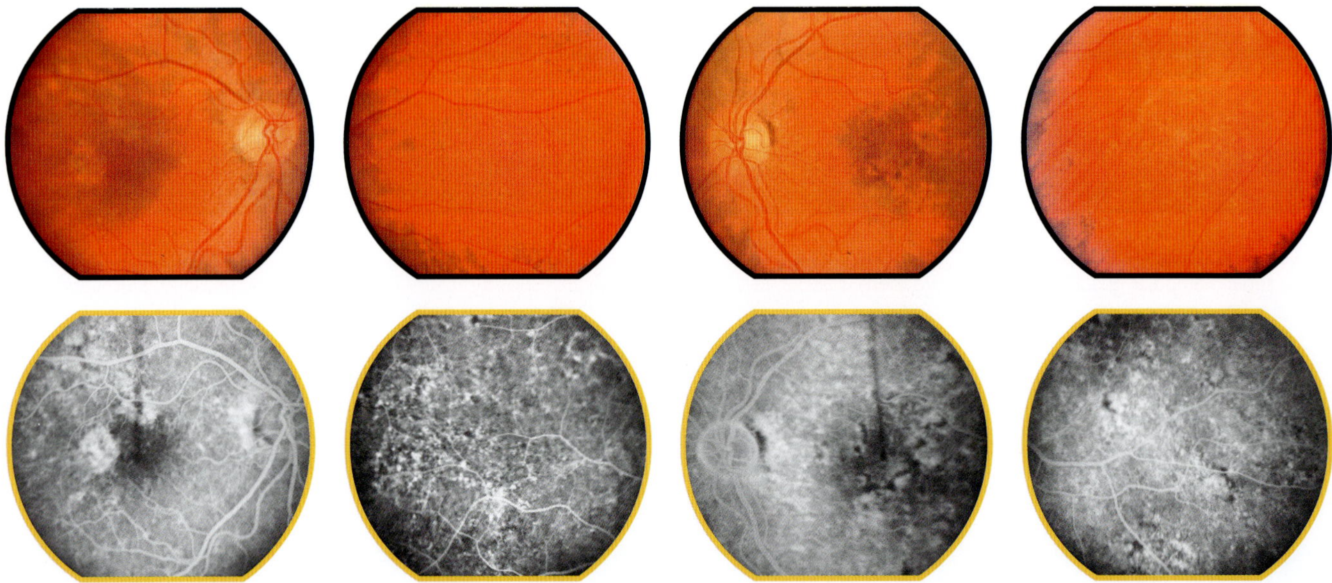

Fundus photos and fluorescein angiography of a patient with a large mitochondrial deletion and chronic progressive external ophthalmoplegia with macular atrophy OD and RPE mottling OS and diffuse pigmentary retinopathy OU.

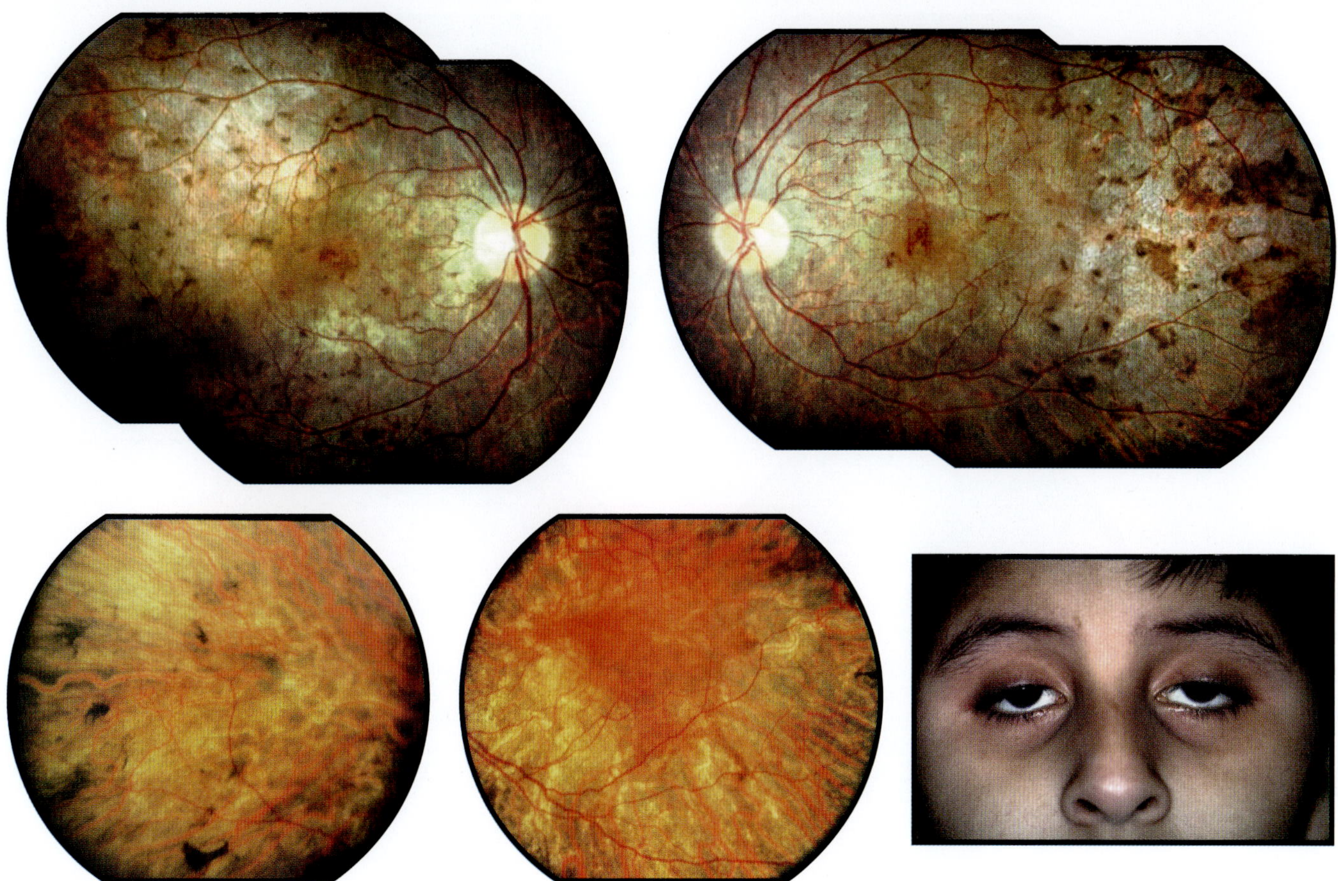

These two patients have Kearns–Sayre syndrome. There is diffuse RPE atrophy with small islands of preserved pigment epithelium and patchy pigment epithelial hyperplasia *(color montages, bottom left and middle images)*. Note the presence of ptosis in the second patient *(bottom right)*. *Montages and external photo courtesy of Dr. Richard Gieser*

MELAS and MIDD Syndromes (Retinopathy due to A3243G Mutation)

The mitochondrial mutation A3243G causes several syndromes including MELAS (mitochondrial encephalopathy, lactic acidosis, and stroke-like episodes) and MIDD (maternally inherited diabetes and deafness), both of which are associated with characteristic retinal findings. Signs and symptoms of these disorders usually appear in the second decade of life following a period of normal development. Clinically, MELAS is characterized by migraine headache, vomiting, and stroke-like episodes primarily affecting the occipital and temporal lobes causing hemianopia and hemiplegia and due principally to mitochondrial failure rather than vascular events. Other symptoms may include deafness, short stature, and diabetes mellitus. As its name implies, MIDD is clinically characterized by deafness and diabetes resulting from poor insulin secretion. As with all mitochondrial disorders, there is wide phenotypic variation in both of these disorders owing to heteroplasmy and mitotic segregation, with variable mutation load in different tissues and family members, some of whom might be asymptomatic with only retinal findings. The A3243G mutation is associated with a distinct macular dystrophy characterized by discrete circumferentially oriented patches of parafoveal atrophy that coalesce over time, but spare the fovea until late in the disease process. Mottling of the RPE with pale pigment epithelial deposits and pigment clumping may also be noted. Unlike Stargardt disease, which it resembles, the peripapillary region is not spared in this disorder. Another distinguishing feature from other macular dystrophies is that autofluorescence imaging reveals much more widespread pigment epithelial abnormality than would be expected from the fundoscopic appearance.

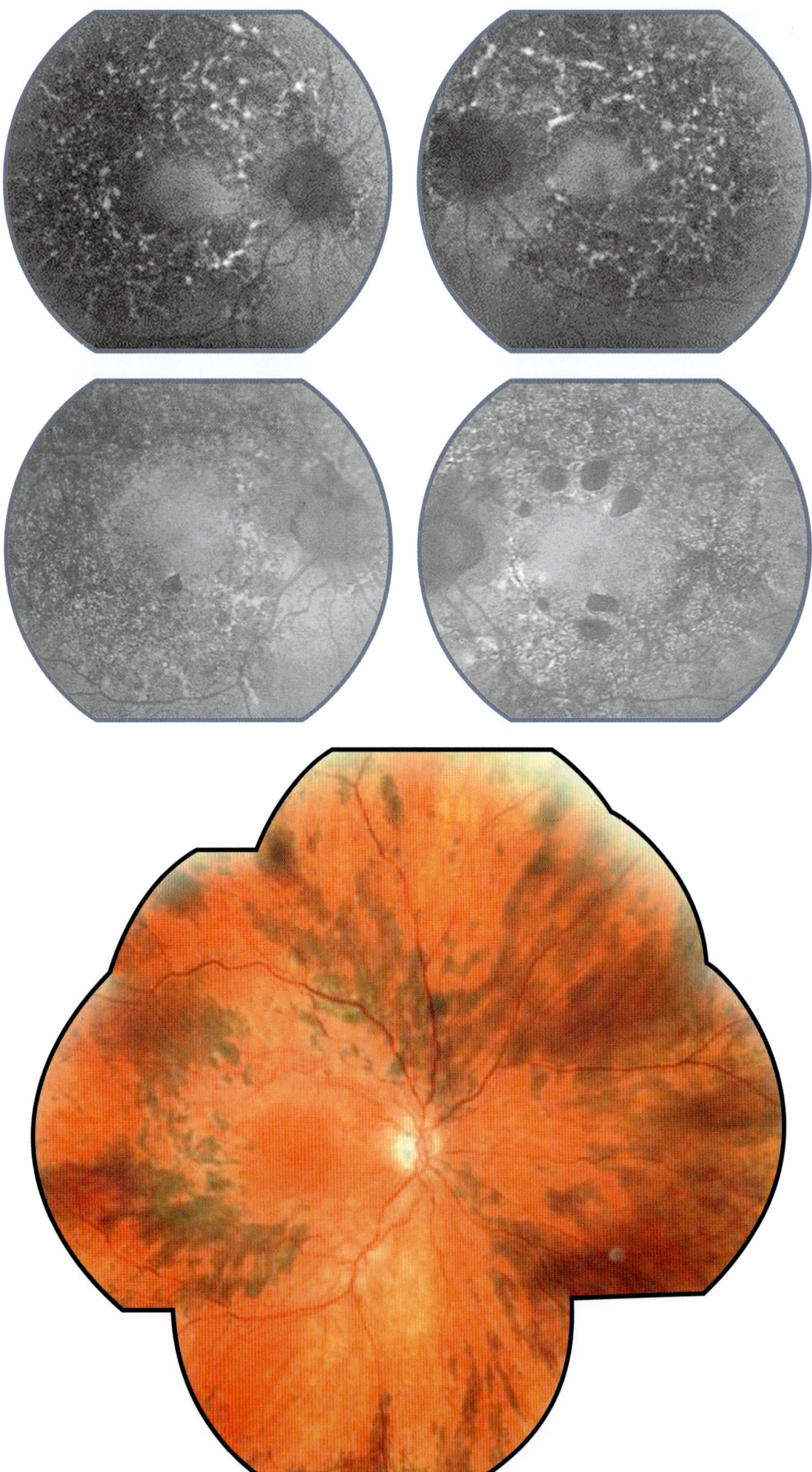

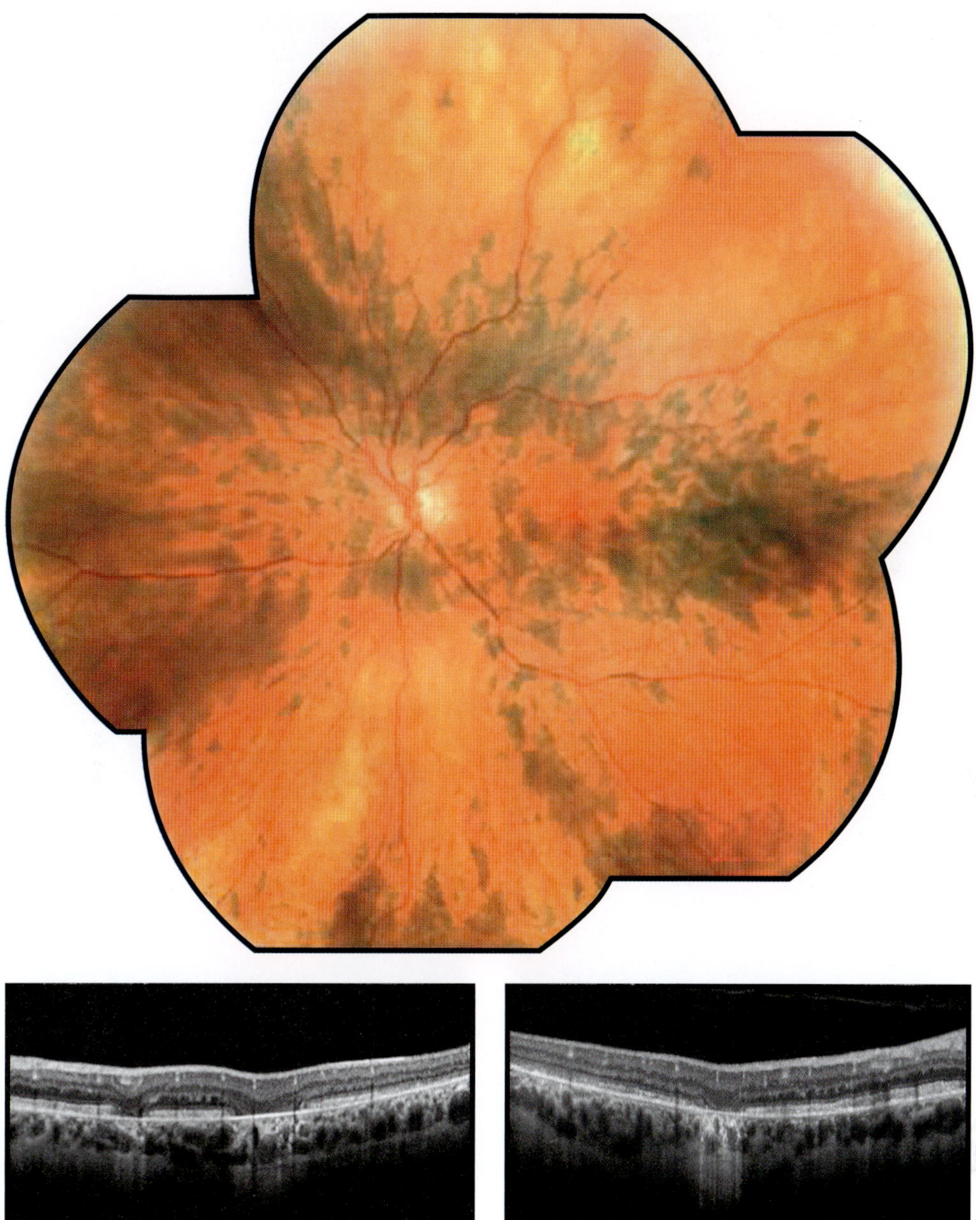

This patient with MELAS syndrome had progressive dementia, hearing loss, a cardiac abnormality, spastic paraplegia, and a pigmentary retinopathy with macular predilection. The patient initially presented with a peculiar pattern of reticular change surrounding the posterior pole extending to the peripapillary area, unlike Stargardt disease, illustrated well with fundus autofluorescence *(top row)*. Fundus autofluorescence *(second row)* and color photo montage *(third row)* four years later demonstrates progressive, multifocal, paramacular RPE, and outer retinal atrophy. SD-OCT shows outer nuclear layer thinning, ellipsoid attenuation, and areas of severe outer retinal and RPE atrophy *(bottom row)*. *Images courtesy of Daniela C. Ferrara, MD, PhD*

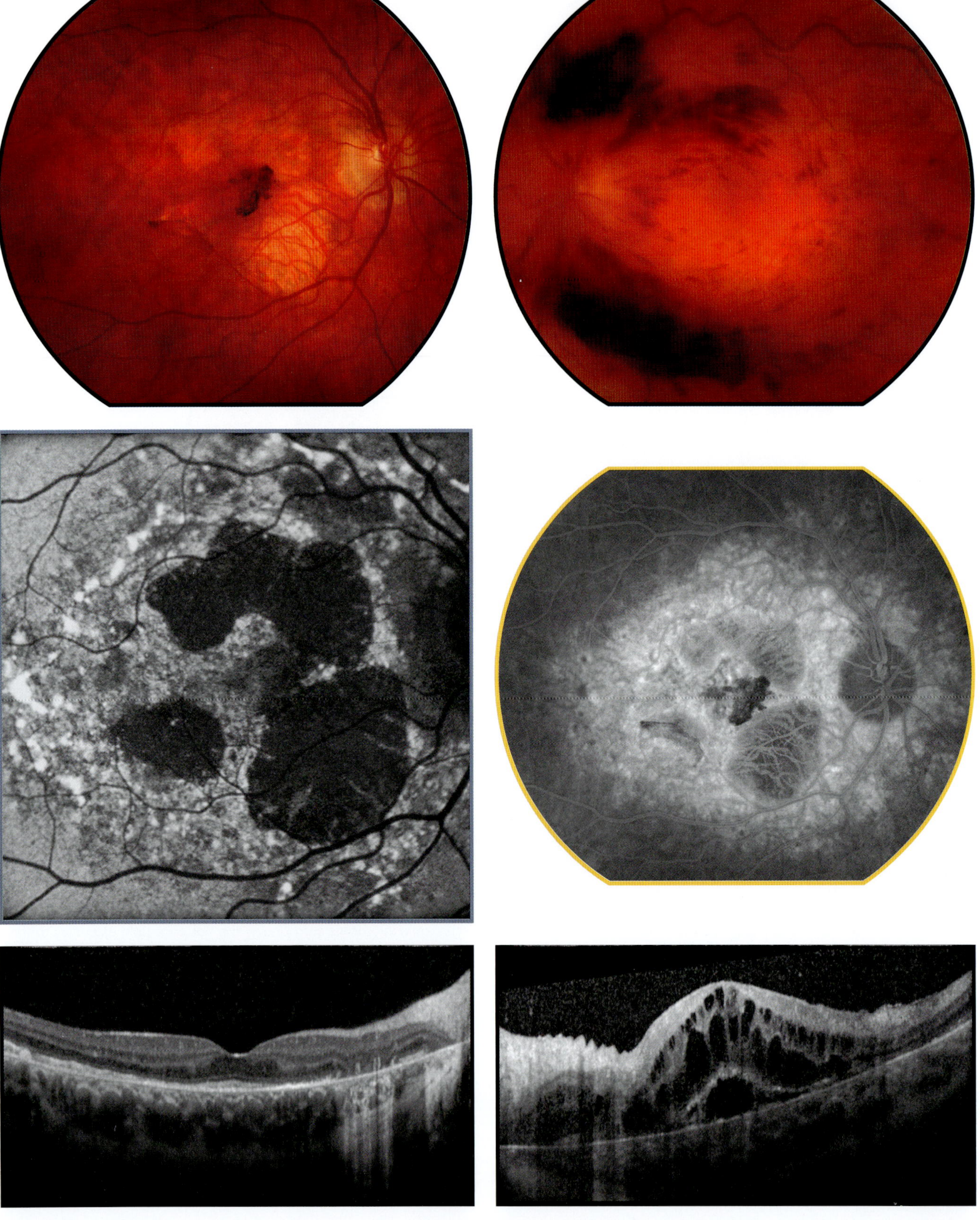

This patient with MELAS presented after developing CRVO in the left eye. Fundus photos illustrate patchy perimacular atrophy of the right eye and hemorrhagic CRVO of the left eye *(top row)*. Fundus autofluorescence and fluorescein angiogram confirm the presence of patchy outer macular atrophy in the right eye *(middle row)*. SD-OCT of the right eye shows marked outer retinal atrophy in a perifoveal distribution. There is severe CME in the left eye due to the CRVO. *Images courtesy Amani A. Fawzi, MD*

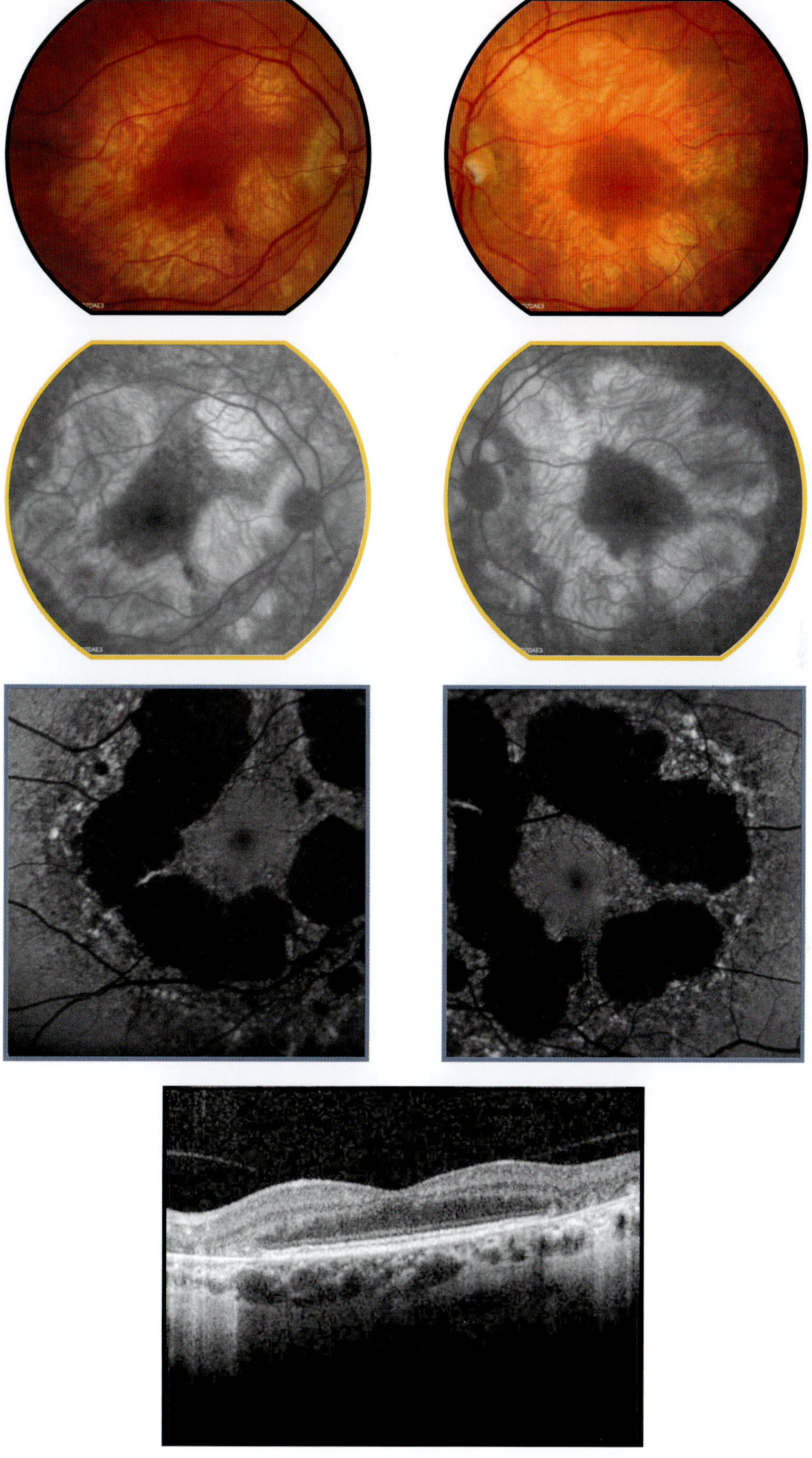

This patient with diabetes and sensorineural hearing loss illustrates the characteristic ring-like pattern of patchy perimacular RPE and outer retinal atrophy. Genetic testing showed 3243 mutation in the mitochondrial DNA confirming the diagnosis of MIDD. *Images courtesy of Herbert L. Cantrill, MD*

Neurogenic Weakness Ataxia and Retinitis Pigmentosa (NARP) Syndrome

Neurogenic weakness, ataxia and retinitis pigmentosa (NARP) syndrome is a rare mitochondrial disorder caused by mutation in the 8993 nucleotide of the mtDNA ATPase 6 gene. As the name implies, the disease is characterized primarily by ataxia, progressive motor weakness, and retinal degeneration. However, as with many mitochondrial diseases, clinical presentations are variable and symptoms may also include cognitive impairment, epileptic seizures, sensorineural hearing loss, diabetes, and cardiomyopathy. Depending on the severity of disease, patients may present in early childhood with systemic symptoms, or remain asymptomatic into early adulthood when they may present with complaints of nyctalopia or decreased vision. Like other aspects of the disease, the retinopathy is variable. Cases of typical retinitis pigmentosa as well as cone-rod dystrophy and cone dystrophy have been reported, often with large variability within affected families. Funduscopic examination may reveal typical peripheral bone-spicule findings of RP with vascular attenuation and waxy pallor of the optic nerve. However, "bull's-eye" maculopathy with temporal optic nerve pallor and with or without peripheral pigmentary changes has also been described. Likewise, electroretinography may reveal deficits that are predominantly rod versus rod–cone versus cone mediated.

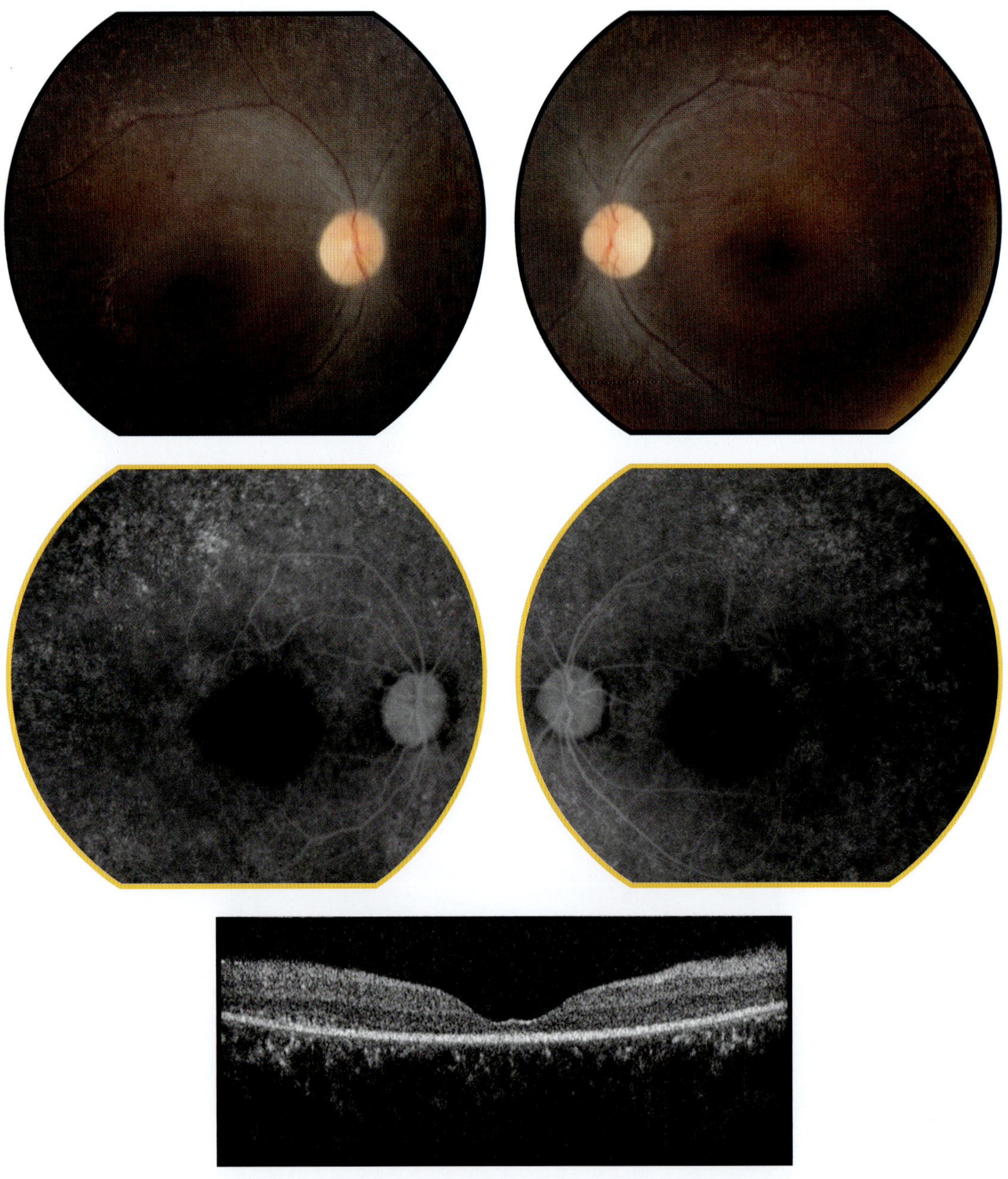

This patient had a history of sensorineural deafness, developmental delay, and ataxia. Funduscopic examination, fluorescein angiogram, and ERG (not pictured) were consistent with a rod–cone dystrophy. SD-OCT illustrates outer retinal atrophy. Mitochondrial DNA analysis showed mutation in the ATPase 6 gene, which confirmed the diagnosis of NARP syndrome. *Images courtesy of Adam S. Berger, MD*

Myoclonic Epilepsy and Ragged Red Fiber (MERRF) Syndrome

Myoclonic epilepsy and ragged red fiber (MERRF) is a rare mitochondrial disorder most commonly caused by a mutation in the 8344 nucleotide of the MT-TK mitochondrial gene. MERRF is a multisystem disorder that is characterized by myoclonus, ataxia, epilepsy and ragged red fibers on muscle biopsy. Additional features may include sensorineural hearing loss, short stature, and cardiomyopathy with Wolf–Parkinson–White syndrome. Ocular manifestations include optic atrophy and occasionally a pigmentary retinopathy occurring in approximately 20% of patients, which is similar in appearance to that seen in Kearns–Sayer syndrome.

CILIOPATHY DISORDERS

Retinal ciliopathies are a diverse group of disorders characterized by a primary defect in the function or structure of cilia, an organelle present on the cell membrane of nearly all mammalian cells. Cilia are essential for the proper function of photoreceptors in the retina and are located at the junction of the inner and outer segments. In addition to the retina, defects in these organelles cause functional deficits in multiple systemic tissues including the inner ear, kidney, pancreas, liver, spleen, bone, and central nervous system. They are also important in olfaction and during embryonic development of limbs. As a result, these diseases have a wide range of phenotypes with manifestations in multiple organ systems.

Alström Syndrome

Alström syndrome is an autosomal recessive disorder caused by a mutation in the ALMS1 gene located at the gene locus 2p13. It is characterized by a tapetoretinal degeneration in association with childhood obesity, hyperinsulinemia, type II diabetes mellitus, acanthosis nigricans, sensorineural hearing loss, renal failure, hypertriglyceridemia, dilated cardiomyopathy, dysfunction of the pulmonary, hepatic, and urologic systems, and systemic fibrosis that develops with age. Renal failure, cardiomyopathy, and liver dysfunction are the most frequent causes of death. The pigmentary retinopathy is a progressive cone–rod dystrophy with resultant early loss of central vision and profound vision loss in the first decade. ERG analysis initially shows severe cone dysfunction with progression to an extinguished panretinal response by age 10. Nystagmus results from the severe early vision loss. This disorder is similar to and often confused with Bardet–Biedl syndrome, but there is no polydactyly, hypogonadism, or mental deficit in patients with Alström syndrome.

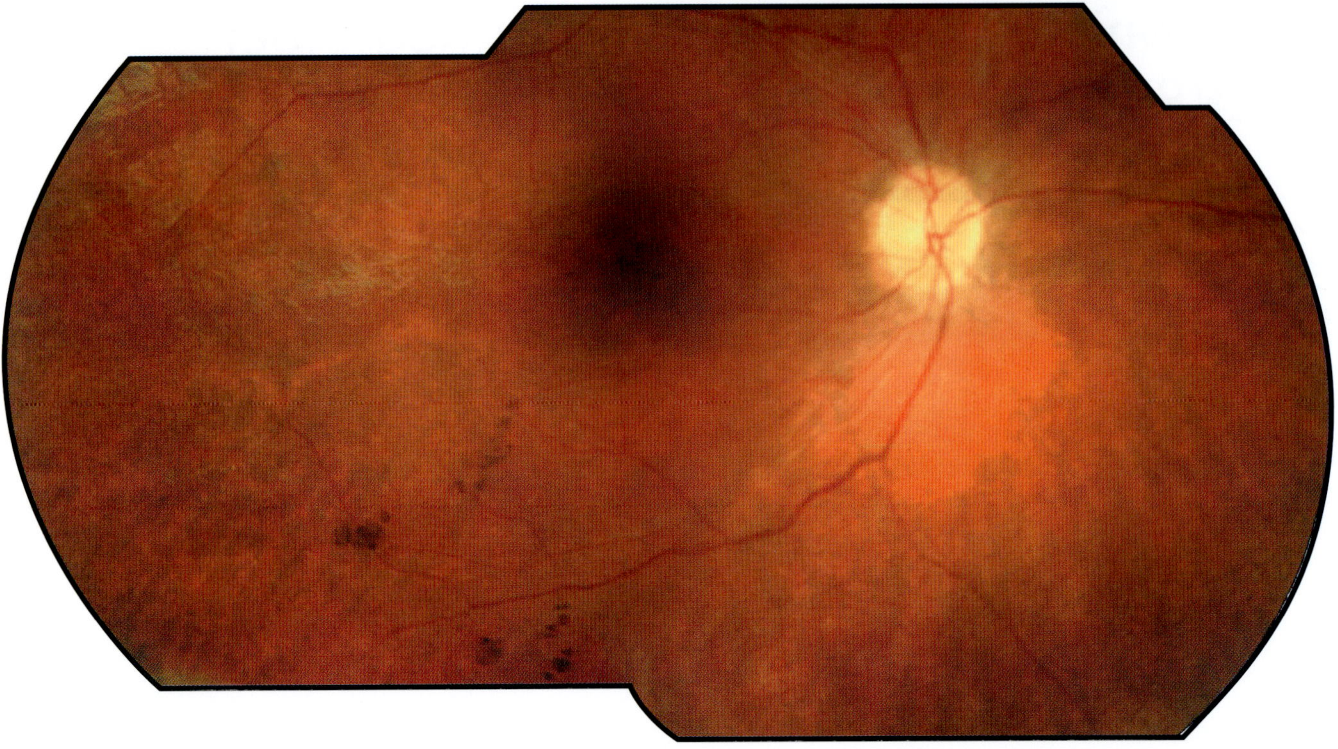

This patient with Alström syndrome has a retinitis pigmentosa-like fundus with optic nerve pallor, retinal arteriolar attenuation and multifocal areas of scattered hyperpigmentation. *Courtesy of Dr. Alessandro Iannaccone*

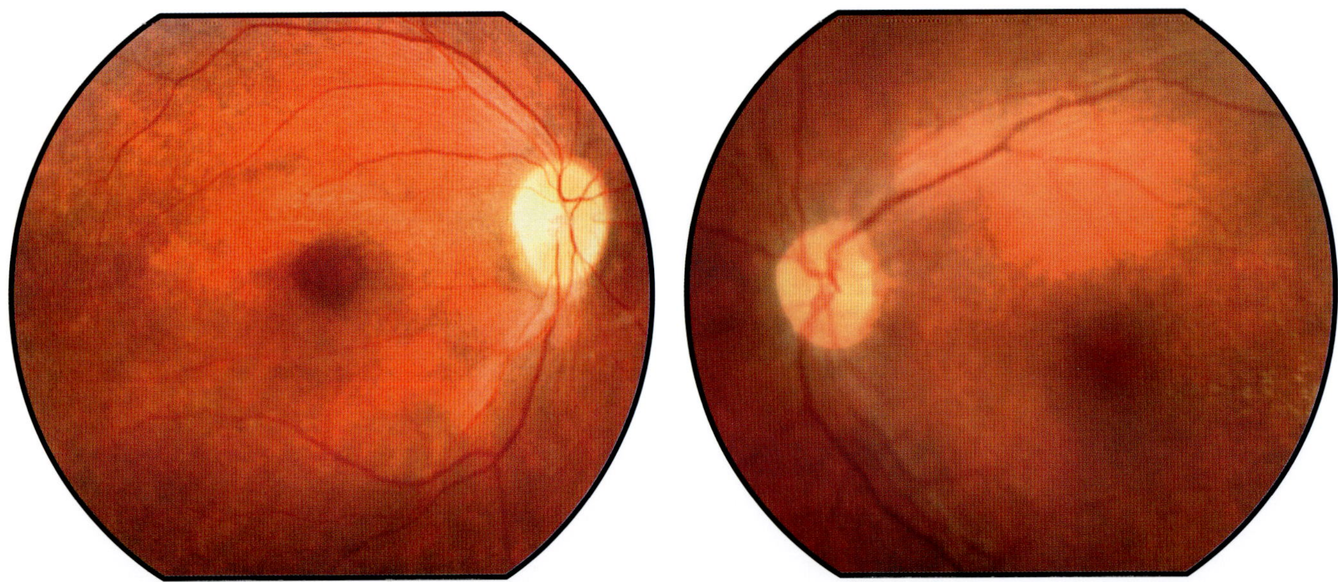

This patient with Alström syndrome has optic disc pallor and ring or "bull's-eye" macular atrophy especially affecting the right eye. There was also associated nephrotic syndrome. *Courtesy of Dr. Stephen Tsang*

Bardet–Biedl Syndrome (Laurence–Moon–Biedl–Bardet Syndrome)

Bardet–Biedl and Laurence–Moon syndromes were originally considered separate disorders, with the latter having paraplegia as a feature, but lacking polydactyly and obesity. Recent research suggests that they may not be distinct entities. To date fourteen different gene mutations have been identified that cause Bardet–Biedel syndrome, the most common of which is in the BBS1 gene on chromosome 11q13. All implicated genes are expressed in the cilia of photoreceptors as well as in other ciliated cells in the body. This autosomal recessive disorder consists of a progressive pigmentary retinopathy similar to retinitis pigmentosa (although RP sine pigmento is not unusual) and multiple systemic findings including truncal obesity, polydactyly or syndactyly, hypogonadism (seen more frequently in males), renal failure, and mental and growth retardation. Retinal dystrophy is often severe, leading to legal blindness by the second decade of life. The fundus appearance is variable and may not show the typical pigmentary retinopathy until later in life. However, ERG findings are consistent with a cone-rod or rod–cone dystrophy as early as three years of age. Macular changes with an atrophic, "bull's-eye" appearance are associated with early loss of central vision in many cases. An epiretinal membrane may also be present.

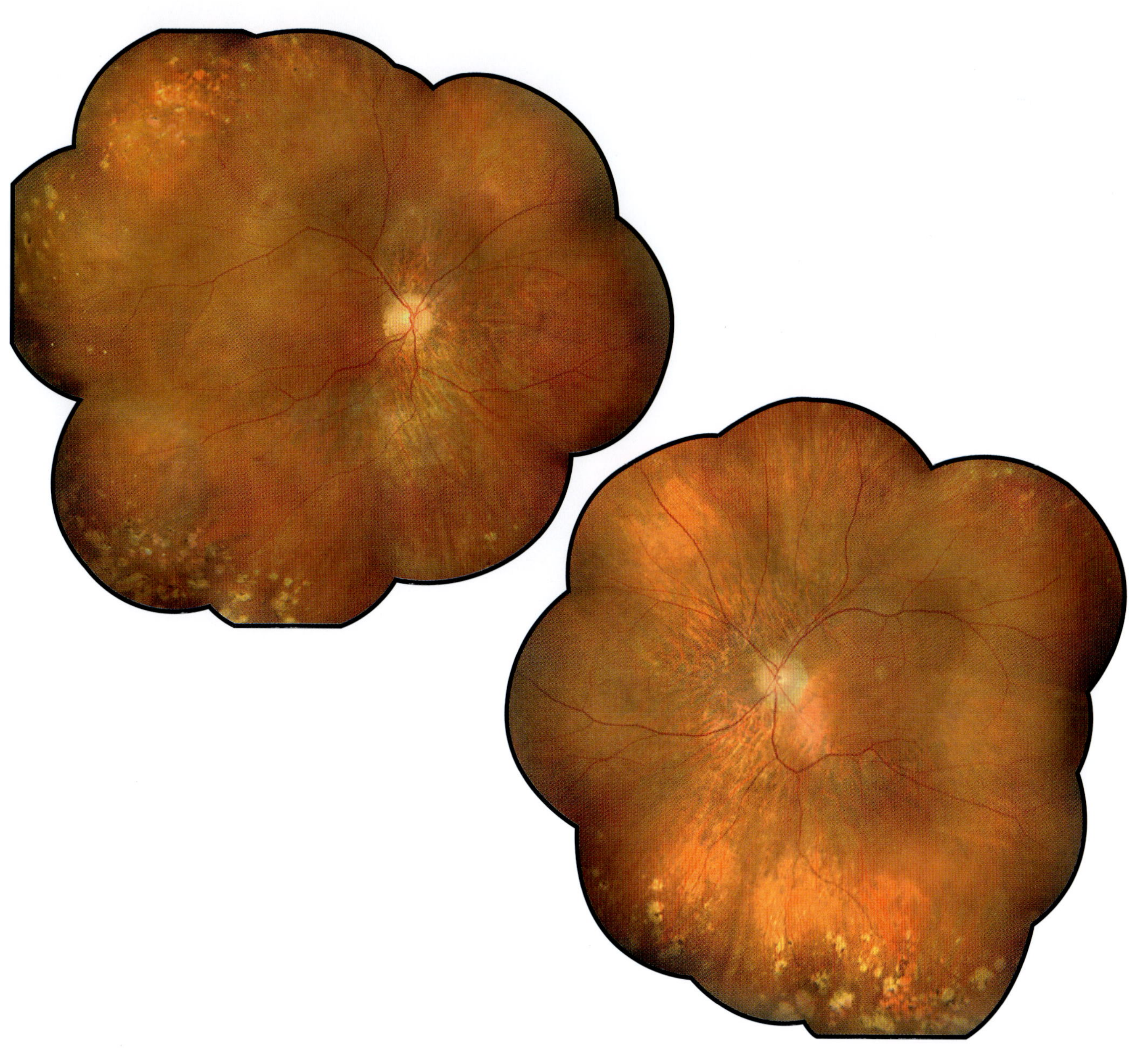

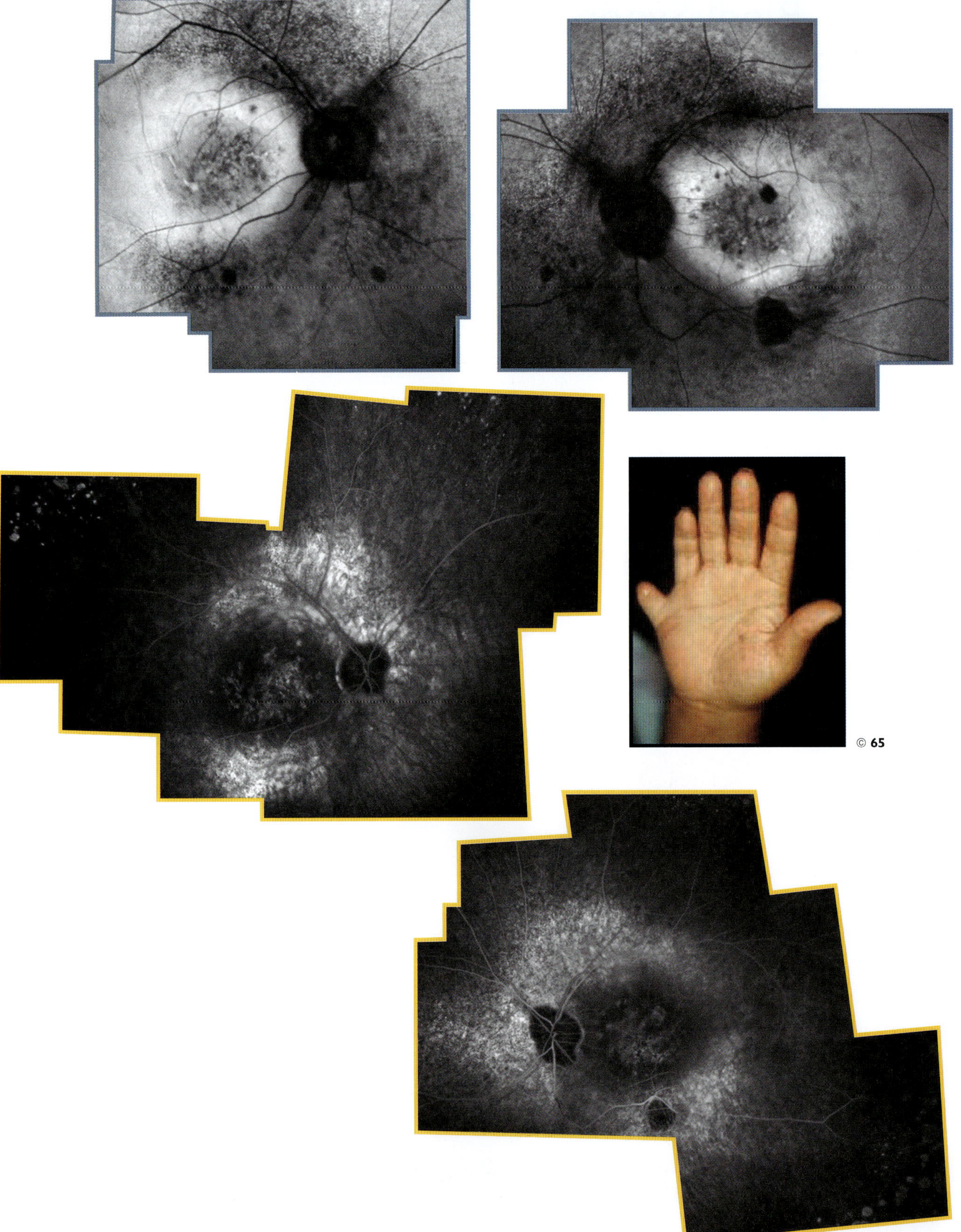

© 65

This patient with Bardet–Biedl syndrome has a peripheral pigmentary and atrophic chorioretinal degeneration. However, the fundus autofluorescence *(middle two photographs)* shows macular involvement with multifocal areas of atrophy and a wreath of pigment epithelial cells at risk, as indicated by the ring of macular hyperautofluorescence. The two lower photographs are fluorescein studies of the same patient, showing window defects in the central macula due to atrophy. The patient also had polydactyly. A sixth rudimentary digit had been incompletely surgically excised. *Courtesy of Dr. Howard Fine*

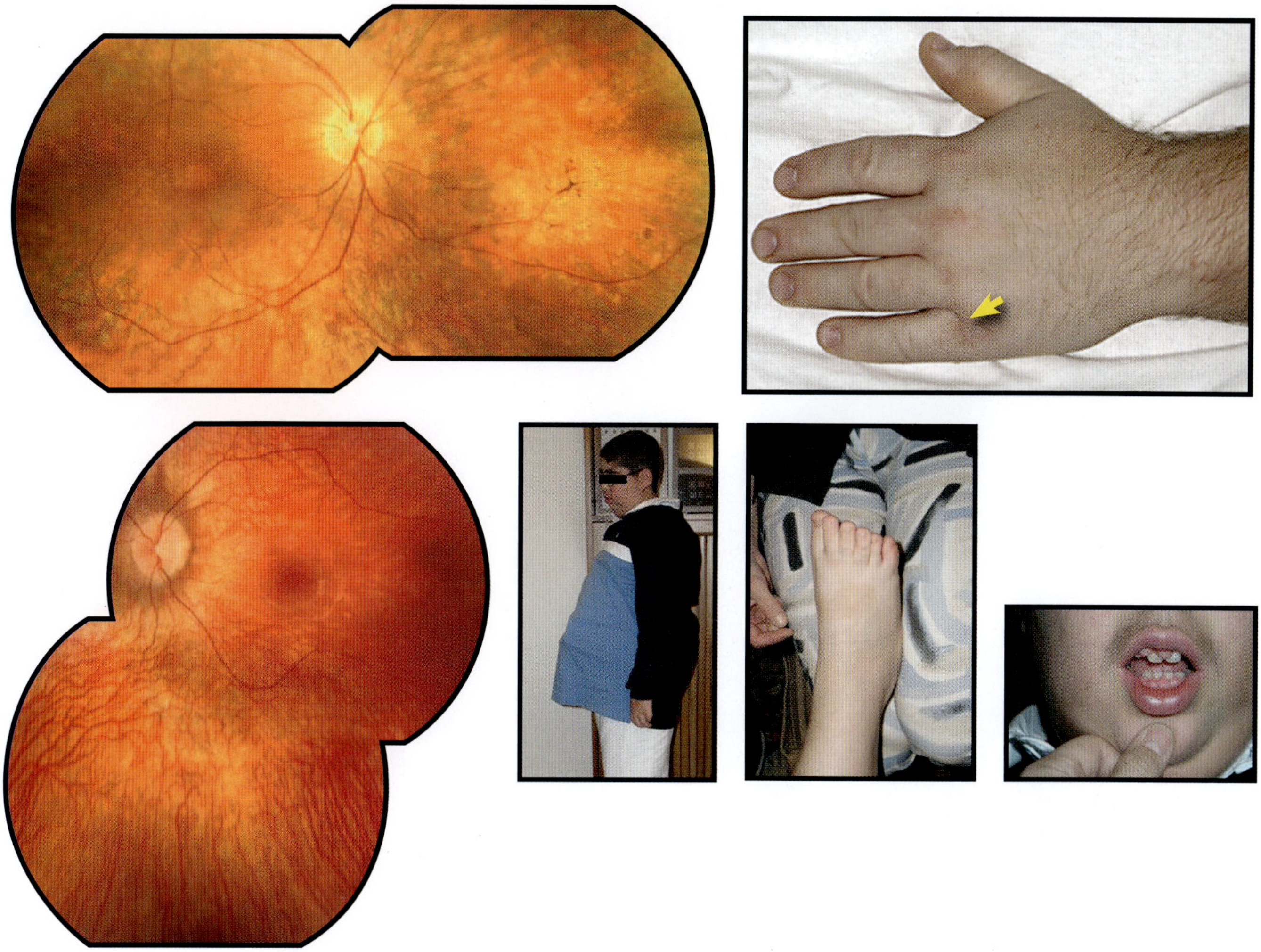

This patient with Bardet–Biedl syndrome has peripheral retinal degeneration with macular abnormalities. A small nubbin on the side of his hand corresponded to an excised sixth digit *(arrow)*. Obesity and polydactyly involving the feet were evident along with dental abnormalities. *Courtesy of Dr. Alessandro Iannaccone*

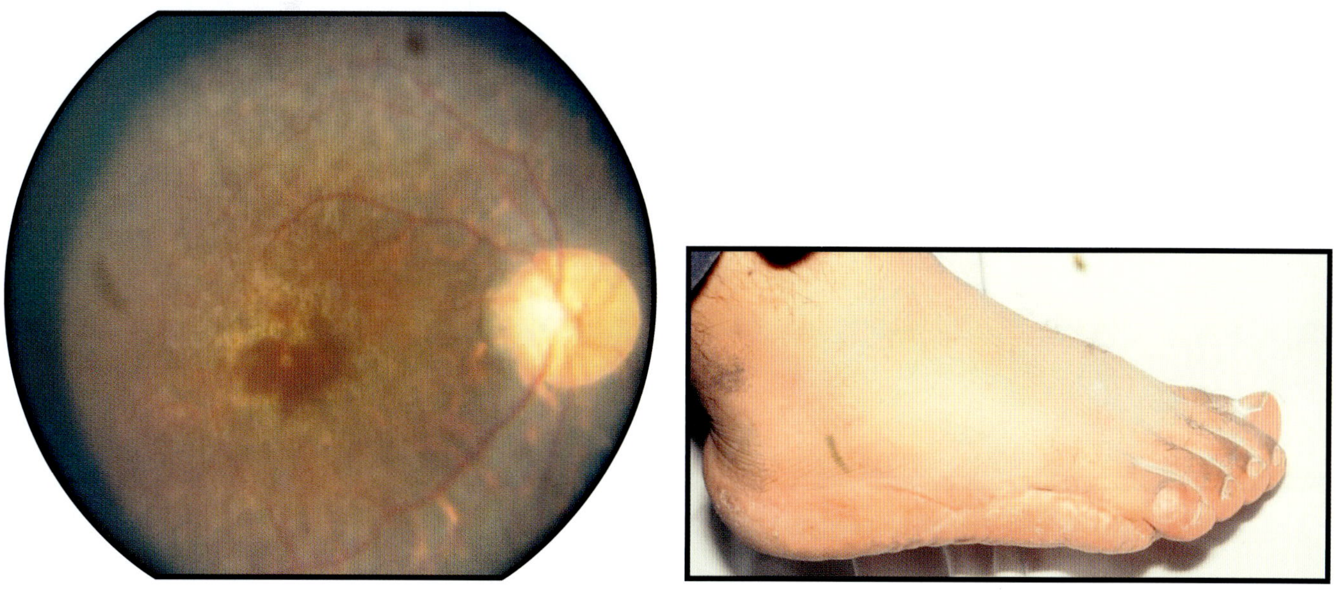

Fundus photography of a patient with Bardet–Biedl shows retinal degeneration with "bull's-eye" maculopathy. The patient had polydactyly of the right foot.

Senior–Loken Syndrome

Senior–Loken syndrome is an autosomal recessive ciliopathy that is associated with tapetoretinal degeneration and medullary cystic kidney disease called nephronophthisis which leads to renal failure by the early teenage years. Mutations in five genes, NPHP1, NPHP3, NPHP4, IQCB1, and CEP290 have all been shown to cause Senior–Loken syndrome. This is a heterogeneous disorder with a variable age of onset of the retinal abnormality. The combination of kidney dysfunction and progressive pigmentary retinopathy is the key to establishing the diagnosis. Other clinical findings that may be seen include liver fibrosis, nystagmus, amblyopia, bone dysplasia, sensorineural deafness, cerebellar vermis aplasia (Joubert syndrome), and mental retardation.

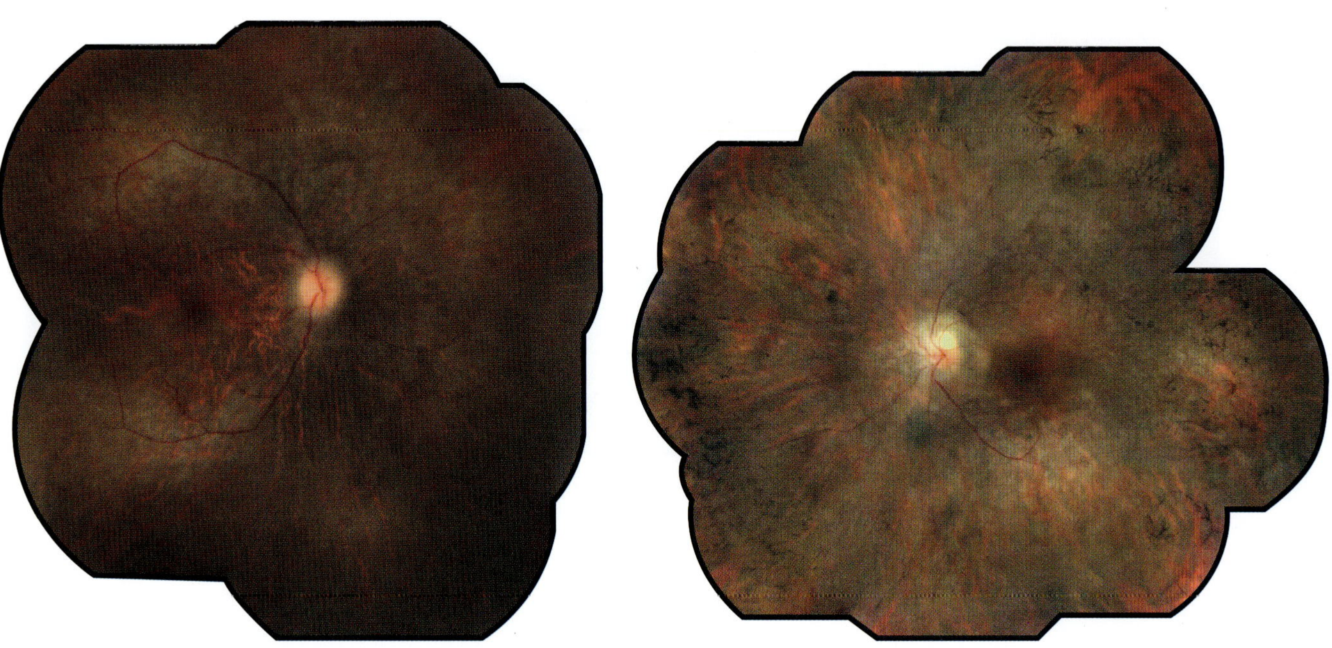

These are color montages of a patient with Senior–Loken syndrome showing a pigmentary retinopathy consistent with RP.

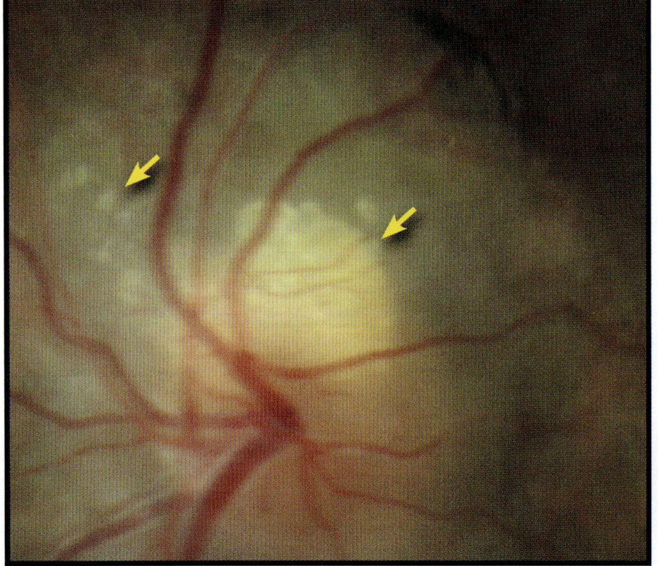

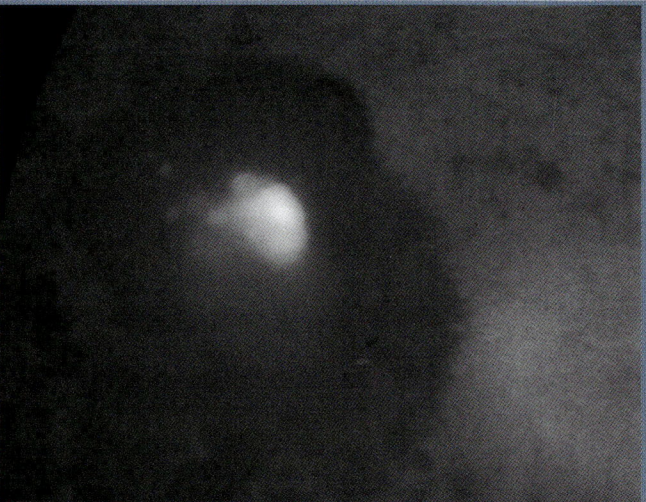

The same patient has optic nerve head drusen *(arrows)* confirmed with fundus autofluorescence.

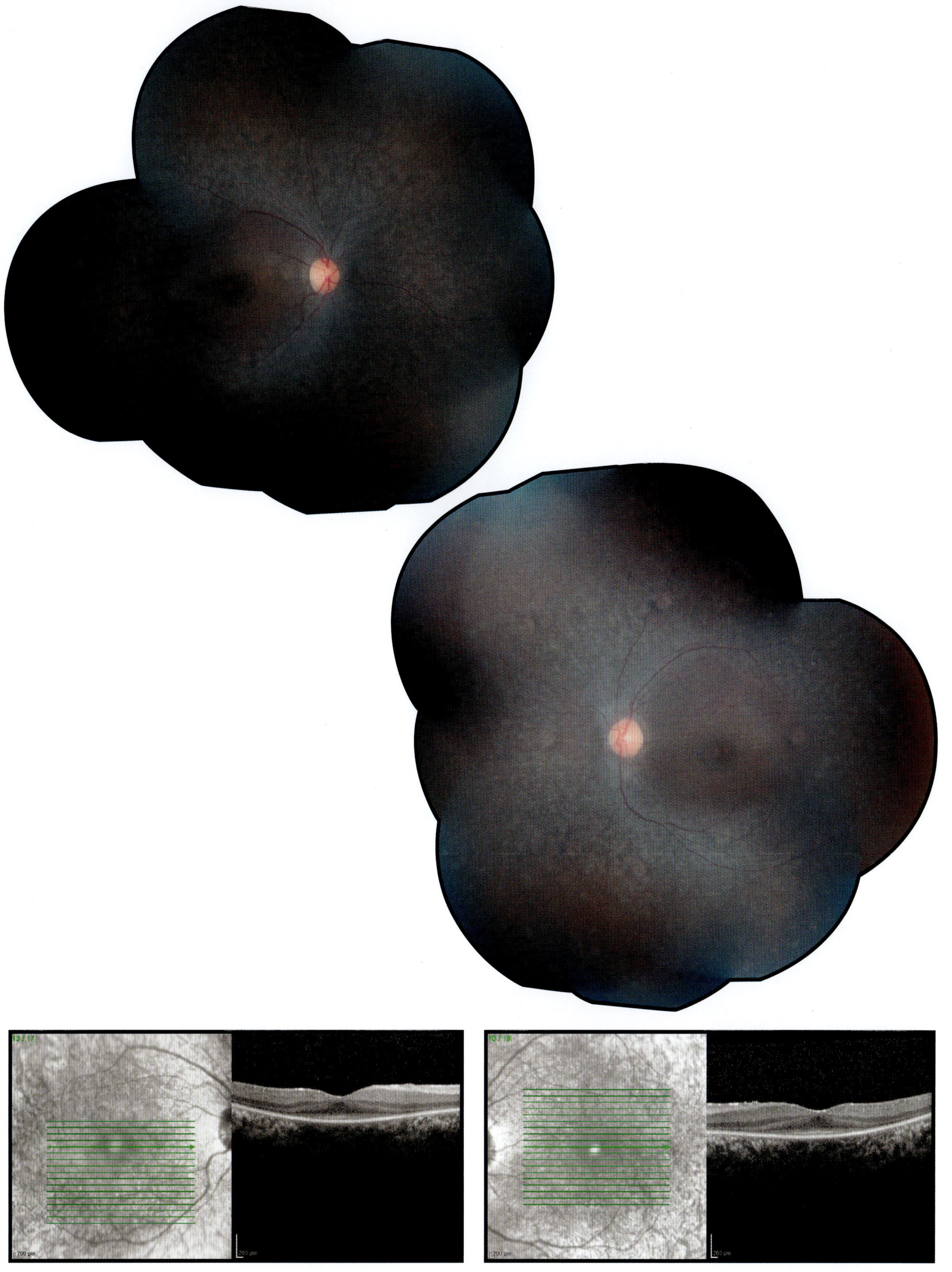

This patient has renal dysfunction and a pigmentary retinopathy illustrated with color fundus photos. The SD-OCT shows diffuse ellipsoid loss with relative sparing of the central macula. *Images courtesy of Michael Gorin, MD, PhD*

Joubert Syndrome

Joubert Syndrome (JS) is a rare, genetically heterogeneous ciliopathy characterized by developmental delay, ataxia, hypotonia, episodic hyperpnea, multiple ocular abnormalities, and structural defects of the cerebellar vermis confirmed by a pathognomonic finding on neuroimaging called the "molar tooth sign." Ocular or oculomotor abnormalities have been described in 70–100% of patients and include strabismus, nystagmus, oculomotor apraxia, vertical gaze palsy, and various fundus abnormalities that include optic nerve head drusen, coloboma, and pigmentary retinal degeneration that may be associated with profound visual loss early in life. Like the other ciliopathies, other organs are frequently affected including the kidneys, liver, and limbs, and the disease can been subclassified depending upon which organ systems are affected. These classifications may be useful clinically and prognostically. For example, pigmentary retinopathy is associated with a higher rate of multi-cystic kidney disease and decreased survival rate, whereas coloboma is more frequently seen in disease involving the liver.

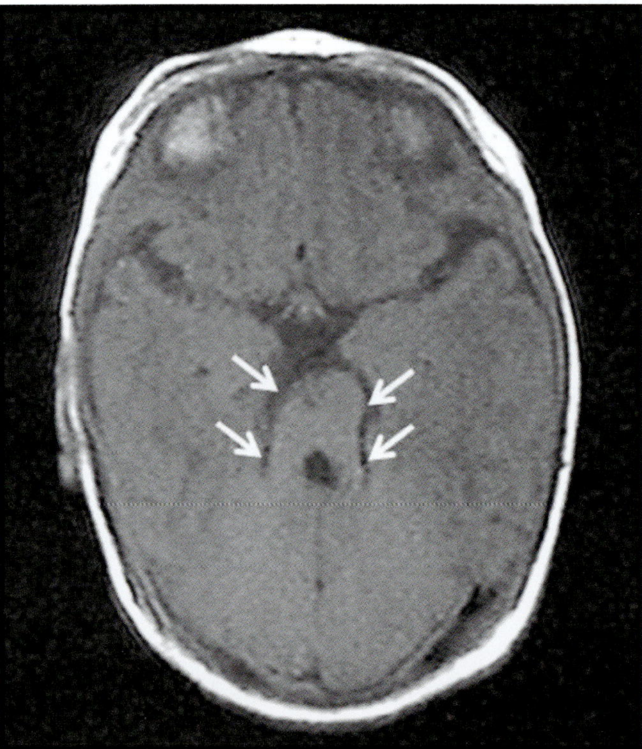

© 66

MRI of the brain showing structural abnormality of the cerebellar vermis causing the "molar tooth sign," which is pathognomonic for JS.

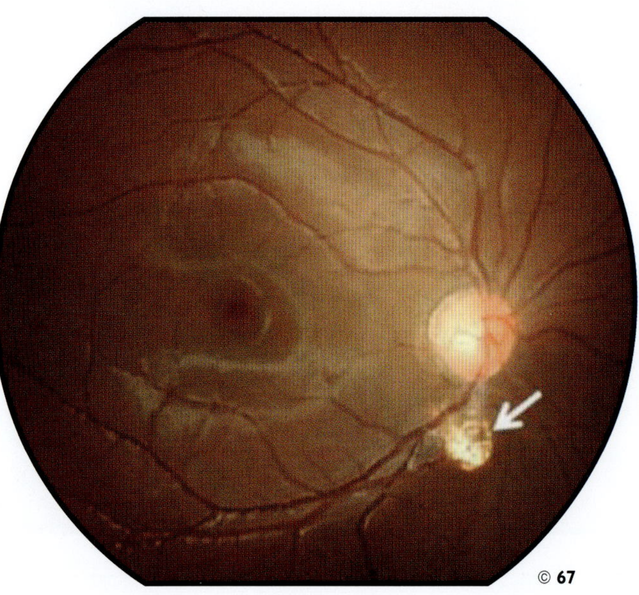

© 67

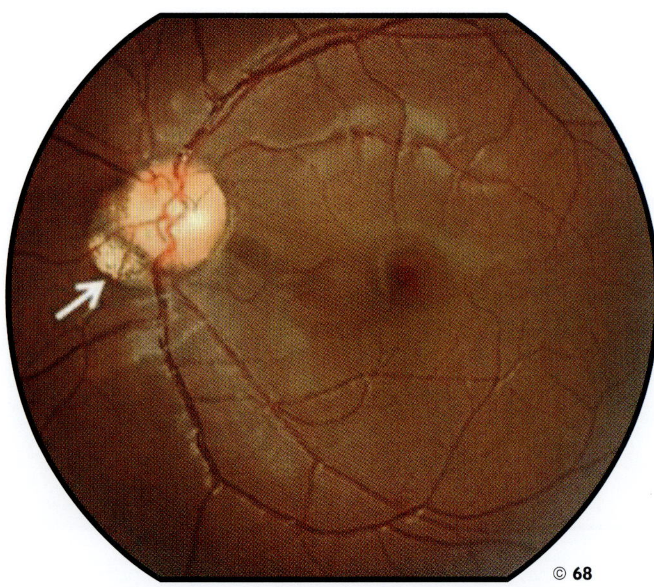

© 68

This patient with Joubert syndrome was found to have a retinal coloboma in the right eye and optic disc coloboma in the left eye.

Jeune Asphyxiating Thoracic Dystrophy

Jeune syndrome is a rare autosomal recessive inherited ciliopathy characterized by shortened ribs, shortened limbs, brachydactyly, polydactyly, renal failure, hepatic dysfunction, and retinal dystrophy. Shortened ribs cause constriction of the thoracic outlet predisposing neonates to recurrent respiratory infections and lethal respiratory distress in up to 60% of patients. The disease is most commonly associated with mutation in DYNC2H1, but five others have been described, all of which encode proteins needed in ciliary intraflagellar transport. Ophthalmologic symptoms may include progressive nyctalopia and central scotoma. Fundoscopic examination shows patchy chorioretinal atrophy, RPE mottling in the macula, peripheral pigmentary abnormalities and retinal vascular attenuation. ERG may demonstrate progressive rod and cone dysfunction.

Usher Syndrome

Usher syndrome is a clinical entity that is defined as the combination of congenital hearing loss and retinitis pigmentosa. It is the most common systemic association to occur in conjunction with retinitis pigmentosa, accounting for up to 10–20% of all retinitis pigmentosa cases. Usher syndrome is a genetically heterogeneous group of autosomal recessive conditions consisting of three major forms: type I, with childhood-onset retinopathy, and congenital profound sensorineural deafness and unintelligible speech, and constant vestibular symptoms; type II, the most common form, with milder, later-onset retinopathy and partial, non-progressive deafness and absence of vestibular symptoms; and type III, the rarest, with adult-onset retinopathy, and progressive deafness starting late in the second to fourth decades. Some forms may also be associated with anosmia. To date fifteen different genetic loci have been implicated, and while their gene products identified thus far are not primary structural components of cilia, there is growing evidence that they form scaffold networks essential to the maintenance and function of the cilia in the inner ear (hair cells) and in the photoreceptors and RPE cells. The most common genes identified so far include the myosin VIIa gene (subtype USH1B), the usherin gene (subtype USH2A) and clarin 1 (subtype USH3A).

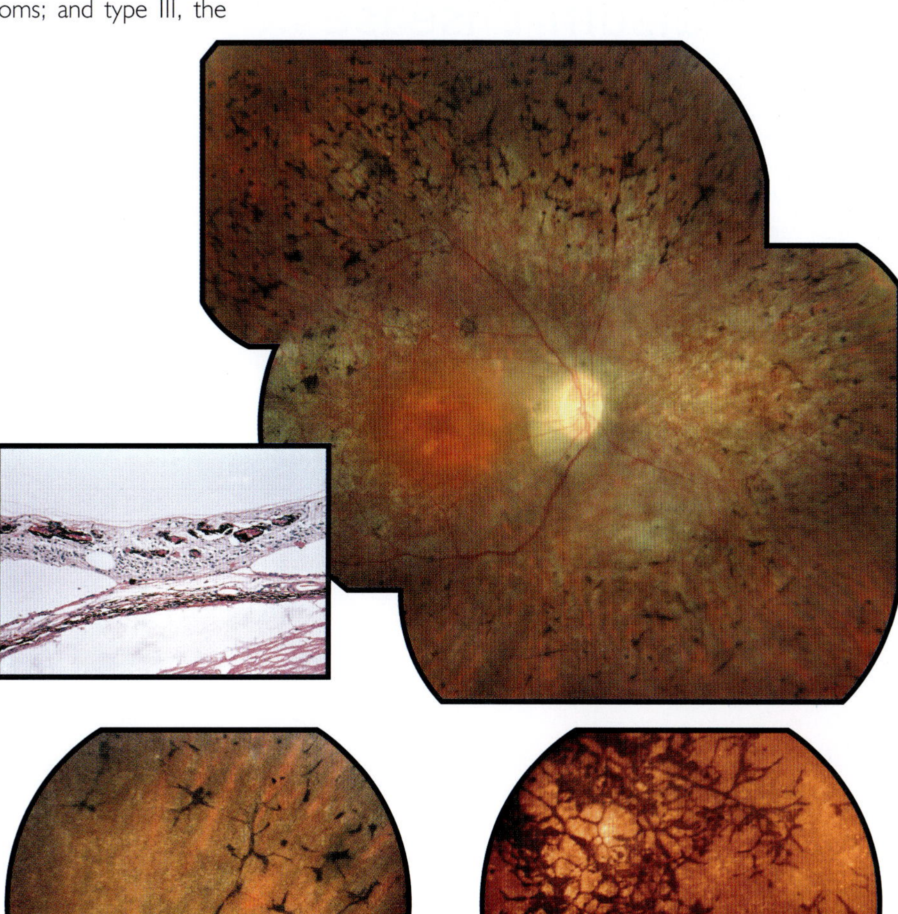

Bony spicule changes with diffuse heavy pigmentation into the retina and around retinal vessels is seen in these patients with Usher syndrome. *Courtesy of Dr. Irene Maumenee*

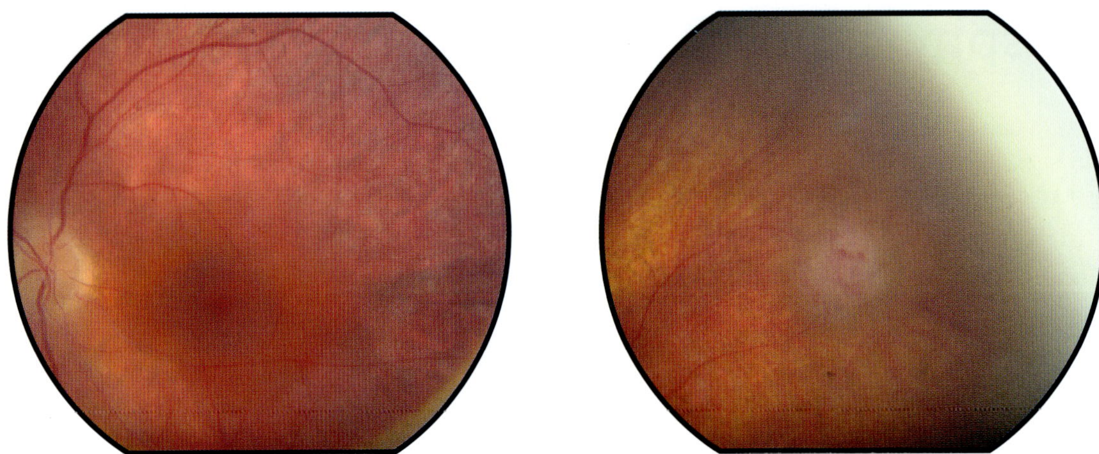

This patient has Usher syndrome with a relatively large angioma in the peripheral superotemporal quadrant of the left eye. Angiomatous malformations may be associated with retinitis pigmentosa. *Images courtesy of Eric R. Holz, MD*

Neurological Disorders

Some hereditary chorioretinal dystrophies are associated with neurological as well as other systemic abnormalities.

Adult Refsum Disease

Adult Refsum disease is an inherited disorder caused by a primary deficiency in peroxisomes leading to decreased catabolism of phytanic acid and its subsequent accumulation in fat-containing cells, most notably nervous tissue. Elevated serum phytanic acid levels is the hallmark of this disease, although it is present in many other peroxisomal disorders. Clinically, it is characterized by a progressive panretinal degeneration. If left untreated, deafness, anosmia, peripheral neuropathy, cardiac arrhythmia, and early death can ensue. Funduscopic examination often reveals diffuse retinal pigment epithelial degeneration, attenuated vasculature and waxy pallor of the optic nerve consistent with an advanced phenotype of retinitis pigmentosa; however, bone spicules may be absent. Nyctalopia is present in nearly all patients and is by far the most common ocular symptom, occurring at the onset of the disease. Visual acuity gradually decreases along with progressive constriction of the visual field. Restriction of dietary phytanic acid is the mainstay of treatment and may reduce the rate of neurological deterioration but does not influence the progression of retinal degeneration.

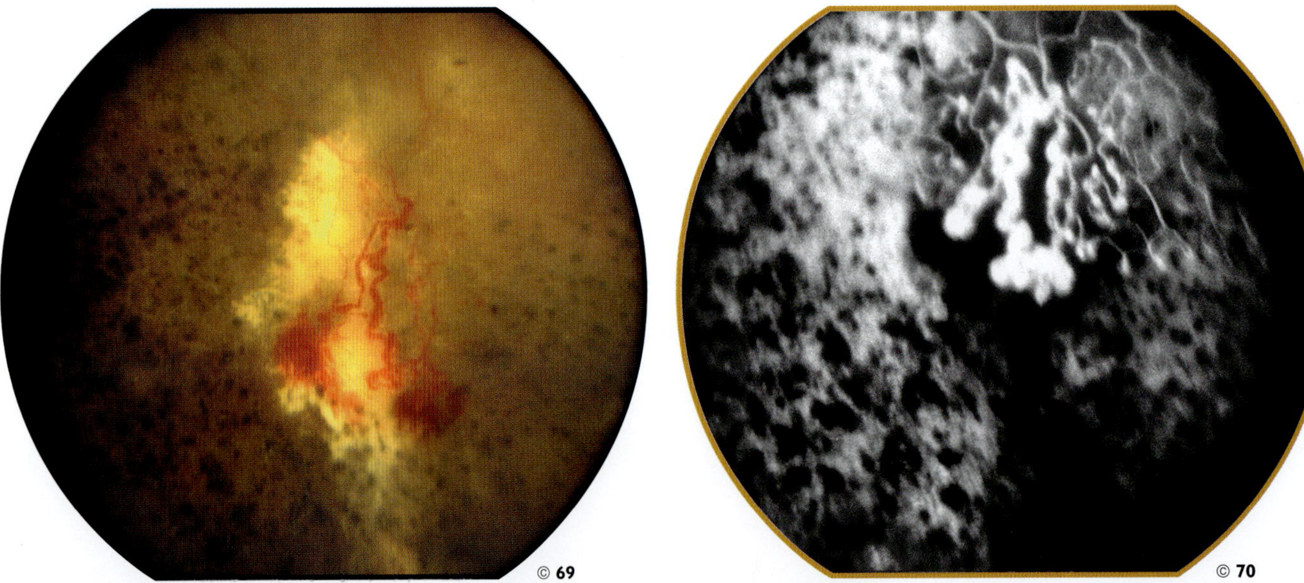

This patient with Refsum disease shows a pigmentary retinopathy and had a history of peripheral polyneuropathy and cerebellar ataxia. Note the acquired angiomatous vasoproliferative lesion in the periphery associated with exudation and hemorrhage. The fluorescein angiogram delineates the vascular nature of the abnormality.

Alagille Syndrome (Arteriohepatic Dysplasia)

Alagille syndrome is an autosomal dominant disorder caused by mutation of the JAG1 gene on chromosome 20p12-p11.23. Intrahepatic hypoplasia, neonatal jaundice, pulmonary valve stenosis, peripheral arterial stenosis, abnormal vertebrae, growth and mental retardation, hypogonadism, and characteristic triangular facies with prominent forehead are all features of this disorder. Anterior segment findings include posterior embryotoxon, Axenfeld anomaly, and corectopia. Esotropia may also be noted. Funduscopic manifestations may include diffuse peripheral hypopigmentation or atrophy or regional peri-papillary and macular hypopigmentation or atrophy in a "sleep mask" pattern. Panretinal degeneration and an RP-like phenotype may be seen along with an atrophic or "bull's-eye" maculopathy. Additional findings include chorioretinal folds and elevated or anomalous discs with or without optic disc drusen. Histopathologically, there is photoreceptor degeneration, atrophy of the outer nuclear layer, and melanin deposits within the inner nuclear layer. Ultrastructurally in the inner collagenous portion of Bruch membrane, numerous lipofuscin granules, vesicular bodies, and crystalline material are seen.

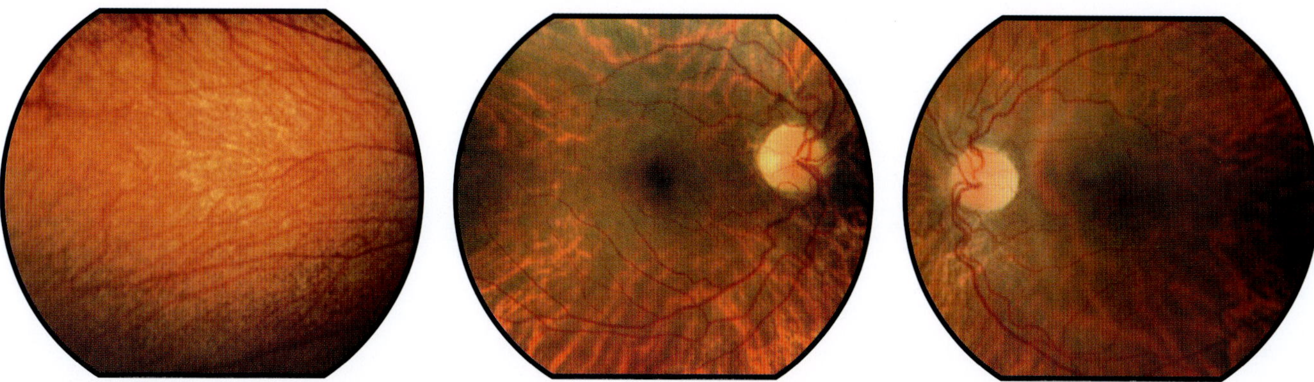

This patient with Alagille syndrome has reduced pigmentation versus chorioretinal atrophy zonally in a multifocal distribution in the fundus, characteristic of the disease. *Courtesy of Dr. Irene Maumenee*

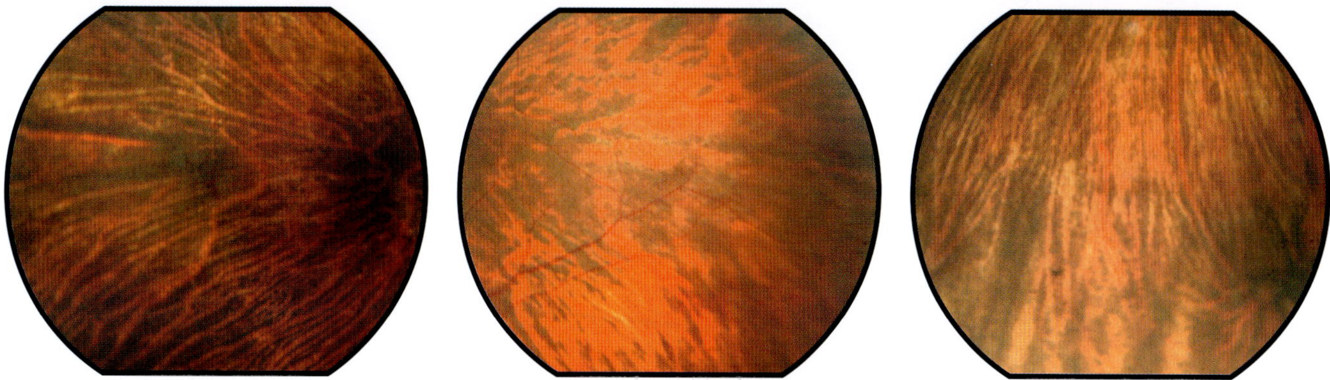

Widespread atrophic change with choroidal vessel visibility is evident in this patient with Alagille syndrome. *Courtesy of Dr. Anthony Moore*

Bassen–Kornzweig Syndrome (Abetalipoproteinemia)

Bassen–Kornzweig syndrome is a rare autosomal recessive disorder caused by a mutation in the microsomal triglyceride transfer protein gene on chromosome 4q22-q24. It is characterized by intestinal lipid malabsorption with low serum cholesterol, vitamin A and E deficiency, and absent plasma betalipoproteins. Systemic findings include acanthocytosis (crenation of red blood cells), neuropathy, and cerebellar dysfunction (Friedreich-type spinal cerebellar ataxia). The ocular findings include a pigmentary retinopathy that may resemble retinitis punctata albescens or the more typical retinitis pigmentosa. Angioid streaks may also be present. Strabismus, nystagmus, and progressive ophthalmoplegia can occur. The retinal changes are presumed to be due to a deficiency of vitamin A, and the clinical course of the retinal degeneration resembles that seen in vitamin A deficiency with rod function deteriorating earlier than cone function. Treatment with a low-fat diet and large doses of supplements of the fat-soluble vitamins A, E, and K may slow progression.

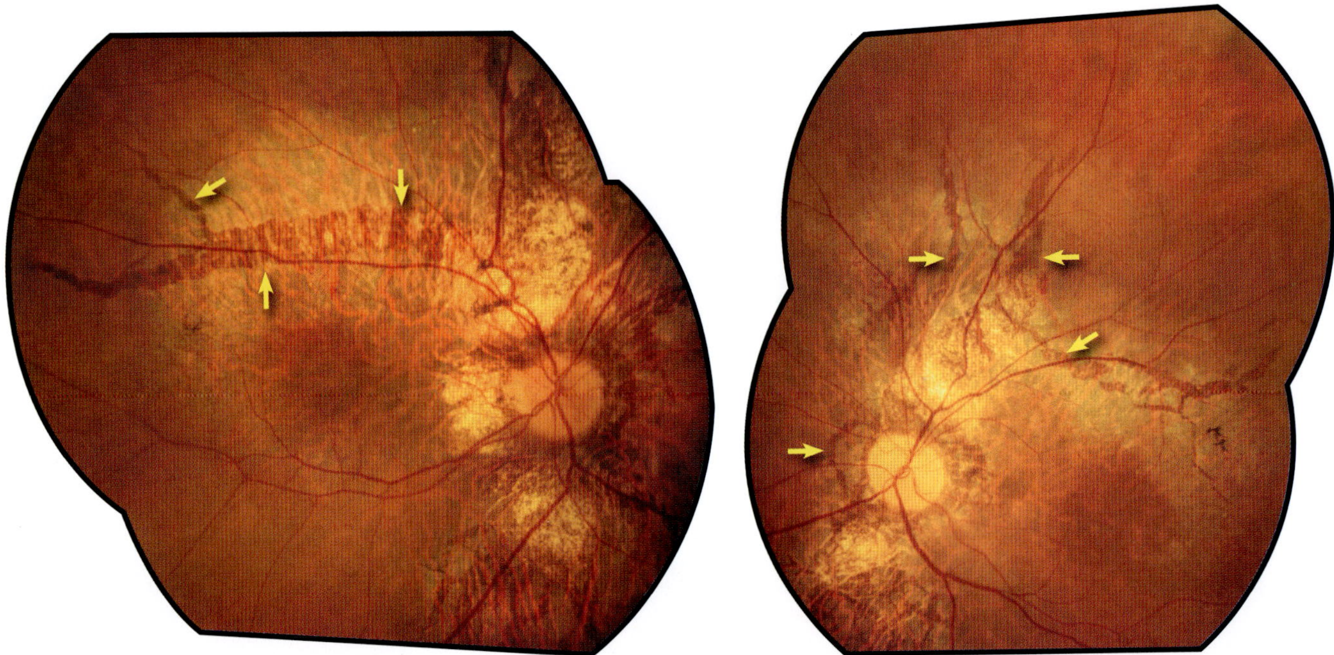

This patient with Bassen–Kornzweig syndrome has chorioretinal atrophy around the posterior pole and disc. A broad angioid streak is present superotemporally in the right eye and finer branching streaks are seen in the same area of the left eye *(arrows)*. *Courtesy of Dr. Scott Sneed*

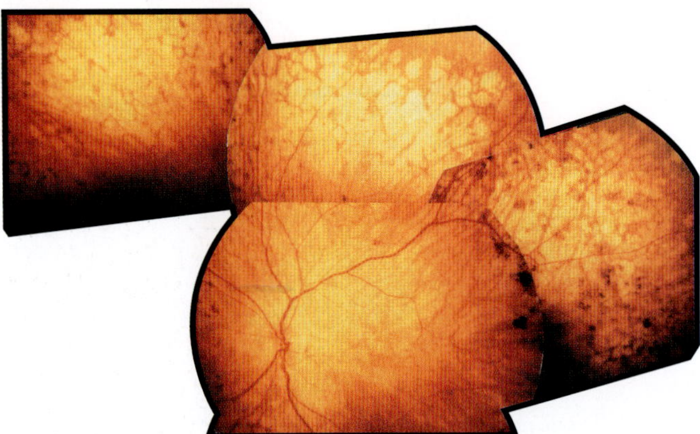

In this patient with Bassen–Kornzweig syndrome, diffuse peripheral chorioretinal atrophy and pigment epithelial hyperplasia is noted. *Courtesy of Dr. A. Rodriguez*

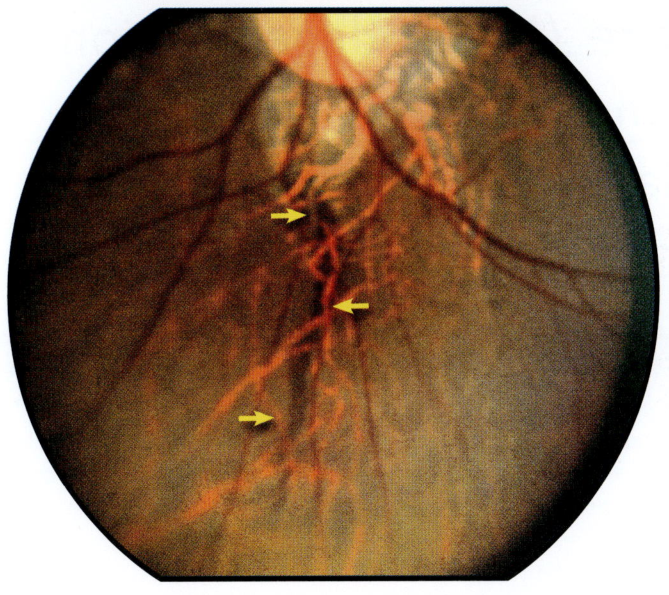

This patient with Bassen–Kornzweig syndrome has a prominent angioid streak *(arrows)* with chorioretinal atrophy around the disc and otherwise a relatively normal fundus. *Courtesy of Dr. A. Rodriguez*

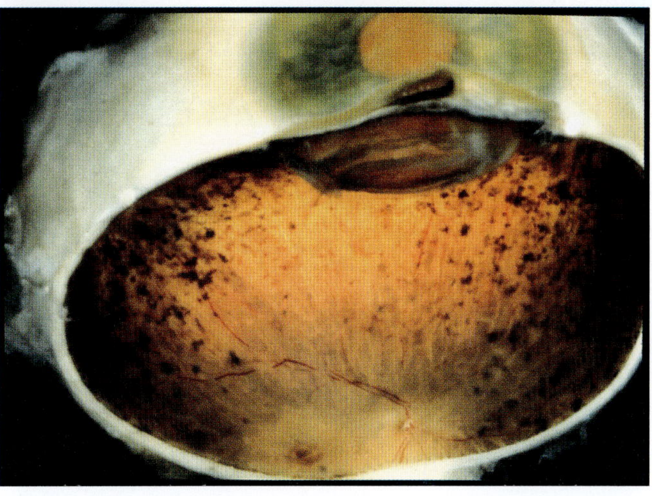

This histopathological specimen shows atrophy and pigmentation in the fundus characteristic of the pigmentary retinopathy seen in Bassen–Kornzweig syndrome. *Courtesy of Dr. Irene Maumenee*

Cockayne Syndrome

Cockayne syndrome is a rare autosomal recessive disorder caused by a primary defect in DNA repair. Clinically it is characterized by neonatal growth retardation, impaired development of the nervous system, hearing loss, premature aging, cachexia, and characteristic facies and multiple ocular problems. Anterior segment manifestations include severe tear film deficiency leading to exposure keratopathy and early cataract. A "salt and pepper" type pigmentary retinal degeneration can be documented in over 60% of patients and is considered one of the hallmarks of the disease. In some cases a retinitis pigmentosa-type picture has been described with peripheral bone spicules, vascular attenuation, and optic atrophy.

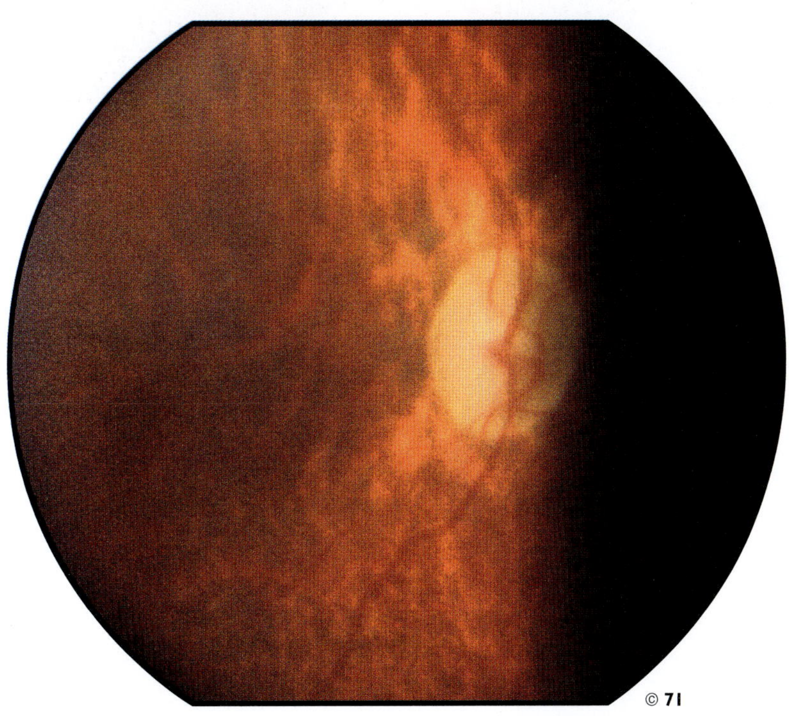

This patient with Cockayne syndrome had keratopathy, cataracts, miosis, and a pigmentary retinal degeneration. Optic atrophy is prominent in association with retinal vascular attenuation in this 9-year-old female.

Hallervorden–Spatz Disease (Neurodegeneration with Brain Iron Accumulation 1 (NBIA1), Pantothenate Kinase-Associated Neurodegeneration, Juvenile-Onset PKAN Neuroaxonal Dystrophy)

Hallervorden–Spatz disease is an autosomal recessive neurodegenerative disorder caused by a mutation in the pantothenate kinase gene (PANK2). It is characterized by early onset of extrapyramidal motor signs, dysarthria, rigidity, choreoathetosis, epilepsy, and dementia with a rapidly progressive course leading to death in early adulthood. It has been classified clinically into three forms each with a different age of onset and rate of progression. All patients with this disorder have characteristic changes on MRI in the globus pallidus. Approximately 25% of these patients develop retinal degeneration initially remarkable for mottling of the RPE, and retinal fleck formation and later remarkable for bone spicule migration and an atrophic annular "bull's-eye" maculopathy. Patients with retinal findings tend to have an earlier onset of disease that is more rapidly progressive, leading to death in late childhood. Histopathologically, there is absence of photoreceptors and atrophy of the plexiform and outer nuclear layers but the inner retinal layers are normal. Degenerative changes and accumulation of melanofuscin in the RPE are also noted. RPE clumping and extracellular pigment around equatorial blood vessels are also present.

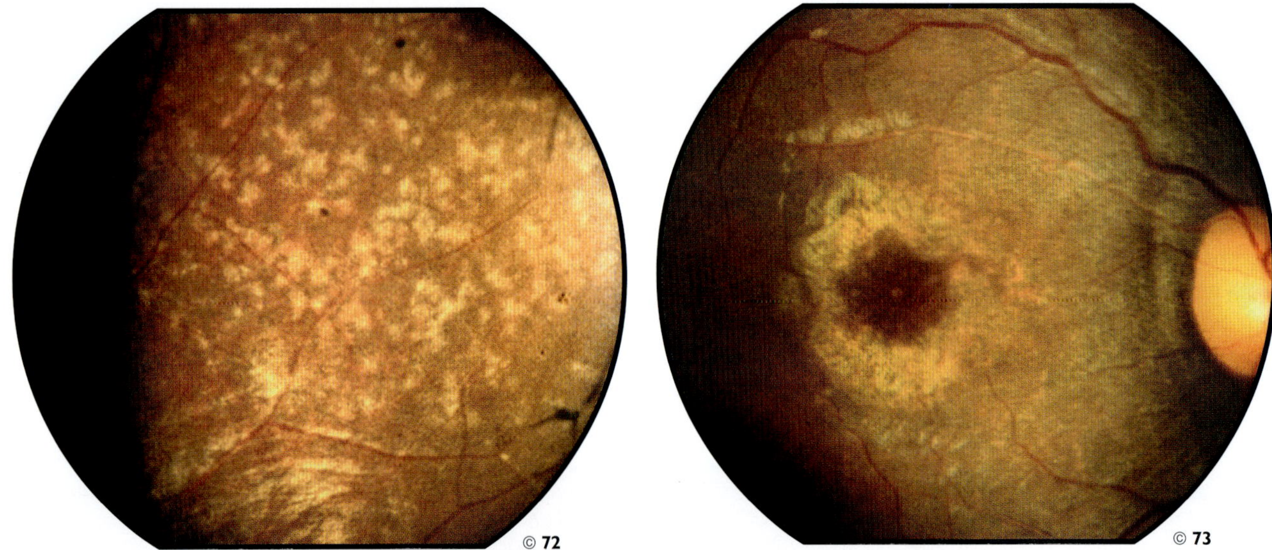

This patient had dementia, dysarthria, and rigidity consistent with Hallervorden–Spatz disease. Acanthocytosis and a pigmentary retinal degeneration were also noted and the latter occurs in about one-quarter of these patients. Retinal flecks are often seen in the peripheral fundus, as is evident in the photo on the left. Atrophic "bull's-eye" maculopathy is also present.

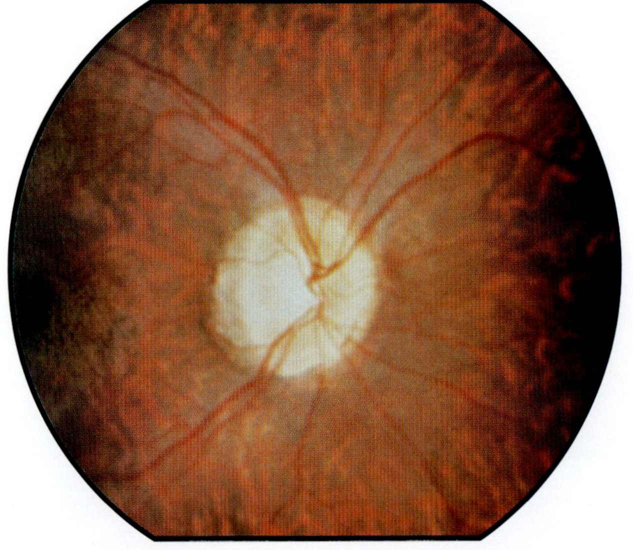

This patient with Hallervorden–Spatz disease shows severe optic atrophy and attenuated retinal vessels with a pigmentary retinopathy.

Kjellin Syndrome (Spastic Paraplegia 15, Spastic Paraplegia 11, Spastic Paraplegia and Retinal Degeneration)

Kjellin syndrome is an autosomal recessive syndrome caused by mutation in the gene encoding spastizin (ZFYVE26) on chromosome 14q24.1 or the gene encoding spatacsin (KIAA1840) on chromosome 15. It is characterized by distal amyotrophia, atrophy of the corpus callosum, progressive spasticity affecting primarily the lower limbs, cognitive impairment, and maculopathy. Fundus findings are phenotypically similar to Stargardt disease or pattern dystrophy, but with distinct differences. Multiple round yellowish flecks at the level of the RPE are noted in the posterior pole. These may be seen dramatically with fundus autofluorescence where they exhibit central hyperautofluorescence surrounded by a hypoautofluorescent halo. With fluorescein angiography, the lesions block fluorescence centrally with a hyperfluorescent halo in late phase. A "dark choroid" is not present. The central portion of the lesions exhibits late staining with indocyanine green angiography.

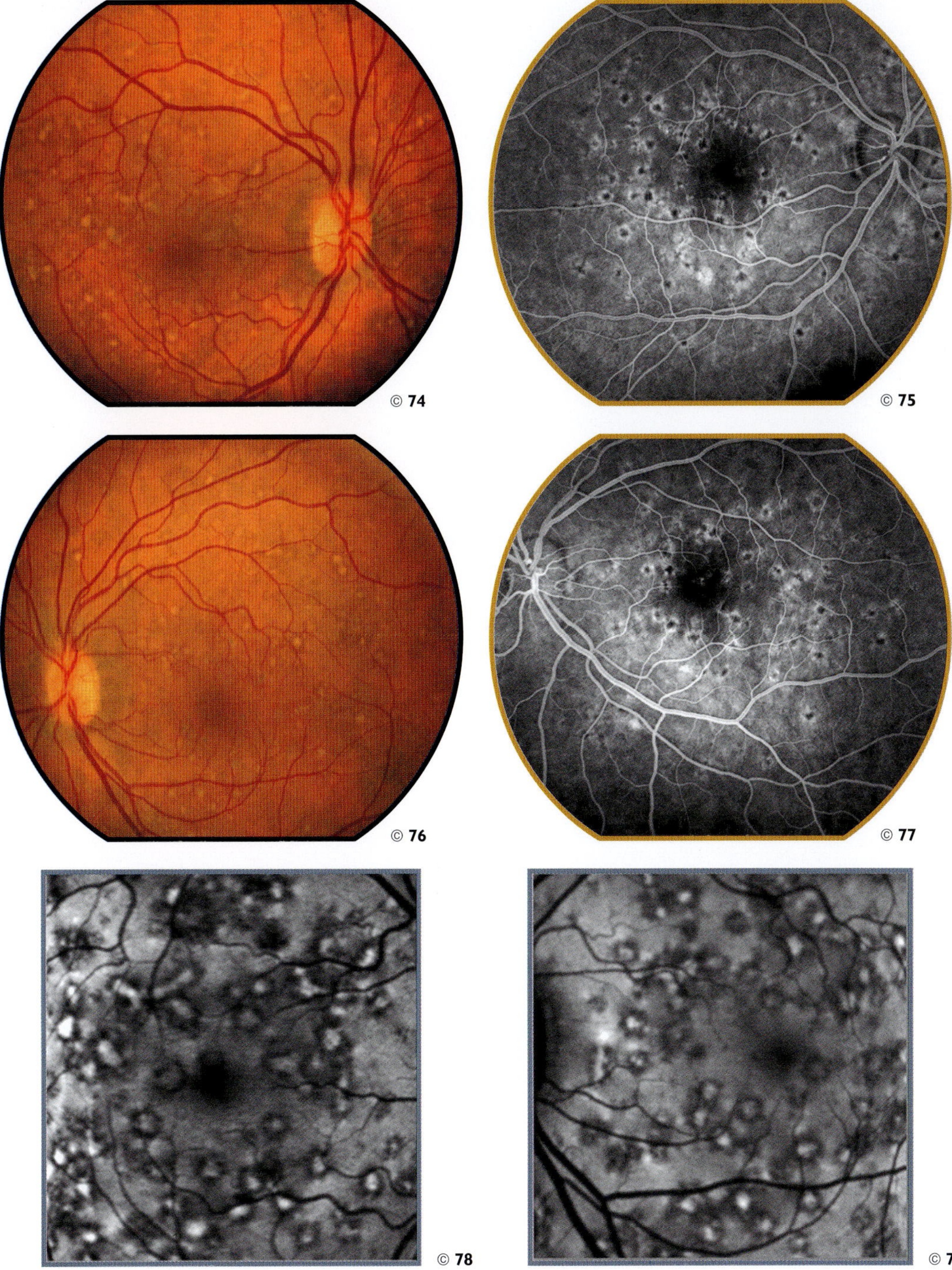

Fundus autofluorescence in this Kjellin patient demonstrates hyperautofluorescence centrally bordered by a ring of hypofluorescence of the fleck deposits, a reversal of the findings seen with fluorescein angiography. These are characteristic of the disorder, implicating the presence of lipofuscin in the central portion of the lesion.

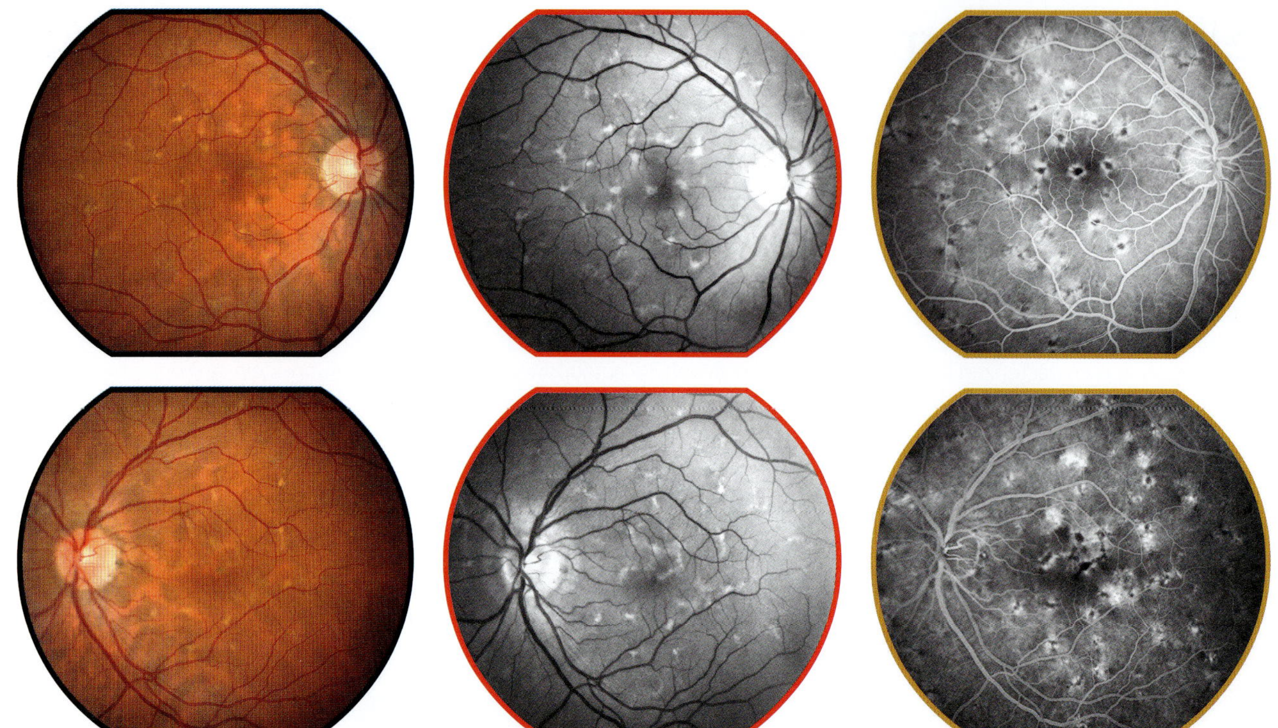

This patient had Kjellin syndrome with typical manifestations in the macula. The lesions on fluorescein angiography are dark with borders of hyperfluorescence. *Courtesy of Dr. Jose Pulido*

Spinocerebellar Ataxia (Autosomal Dominant Cerebellar Ataxia)

Spinocerebellar ataxia is a large, heterogeneous group of diseases characterized by progressive cerebellar atrophy leading to poor coordination, balance and tremor typically manifesting in the fourth decade of life. The disorder is genetically heterogeneous and typically inherited in an autosomal dominant manner with variable penetrance and many of the subtypes are a result of trinucleotide expansions. While at least 30 distinct subtypes have been described, types 1, 2, 3, 6, and 7 represent approximately 80% of diagnoses. A severe cone-rod dystrophy has been well documented in SCA7. Patients may present with progressive color and sometimes severe visual acuity deficits. Examination early in the course may reveal granular changes in the pigment epithelium, or a "bull's-eye" maculopathy, which may progress to a well circumscribed, atrophic macular lesion. Multifocal and full-field ERG may show severe cone dysfunction with less severe rod dysfunction. Funduscopy in SCA1 may reveal hypopigmentation within the macula and photoreceptor loss on optical coherence tomography.

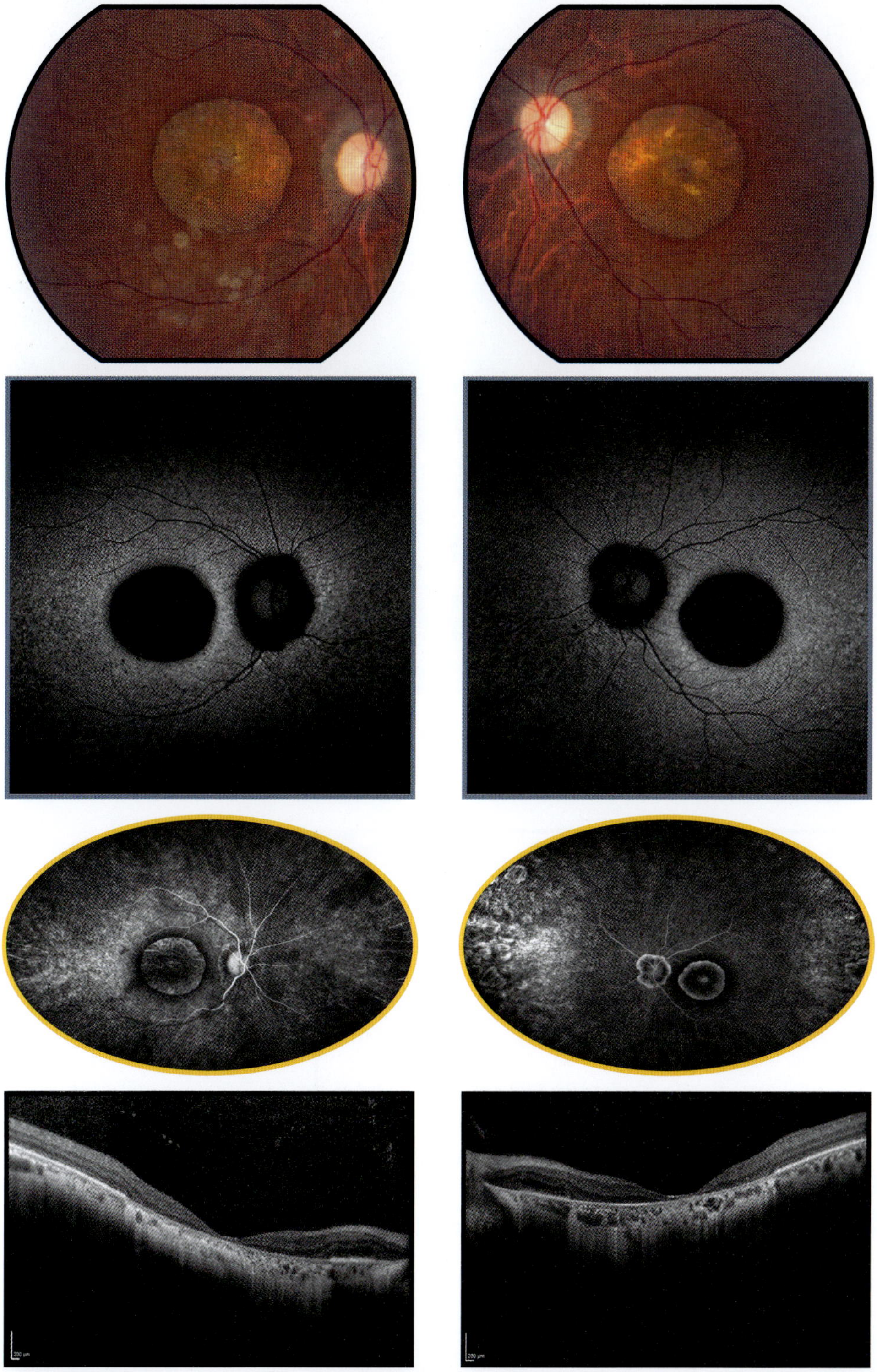

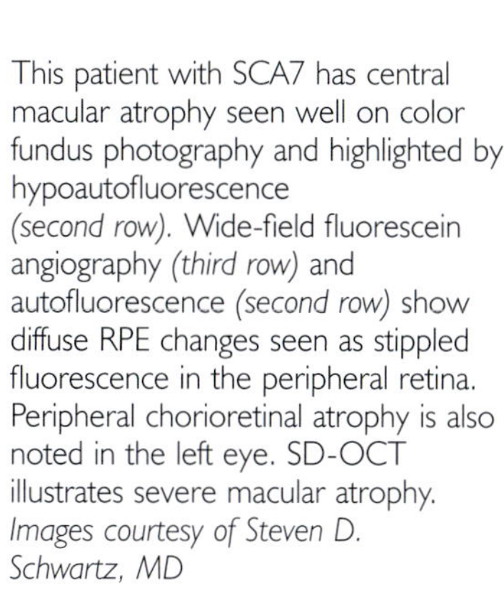

This patient with SCA7 has central macular atrophy seen well on color fundus photography and highlighted by hypoautofluorescence *(second row)*. Wide-field fluorescein angiography *(third row)* and autofluorescence *(second row)* show diffuse RPE changes seen as stippled fluorescence in the peripheral retina. Peripheral chorioretinal atrophy is also noted in the left eye. SD-OCT illustrates severe macular atrophy. *Images courtesy of Steven D. Schwartz, MD*

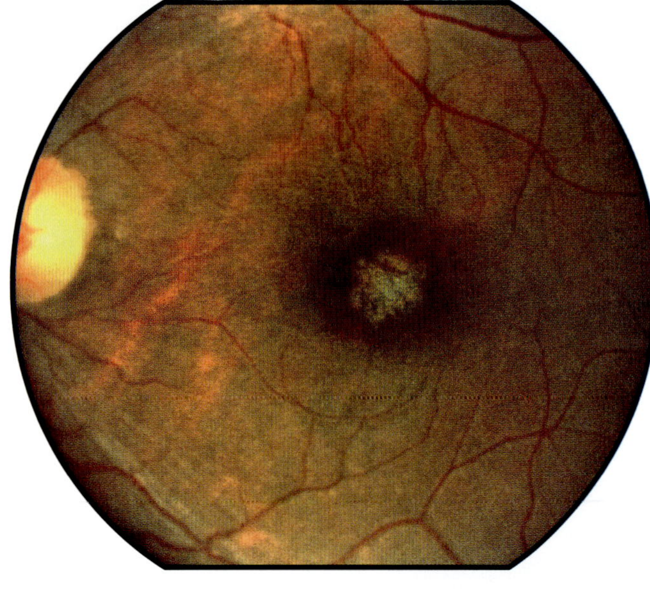

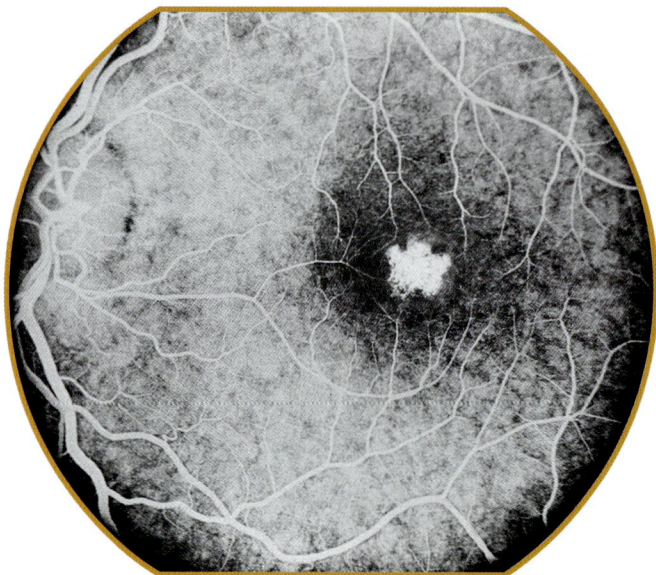

This patient with SCA type III shows an atrophic maculopathy.

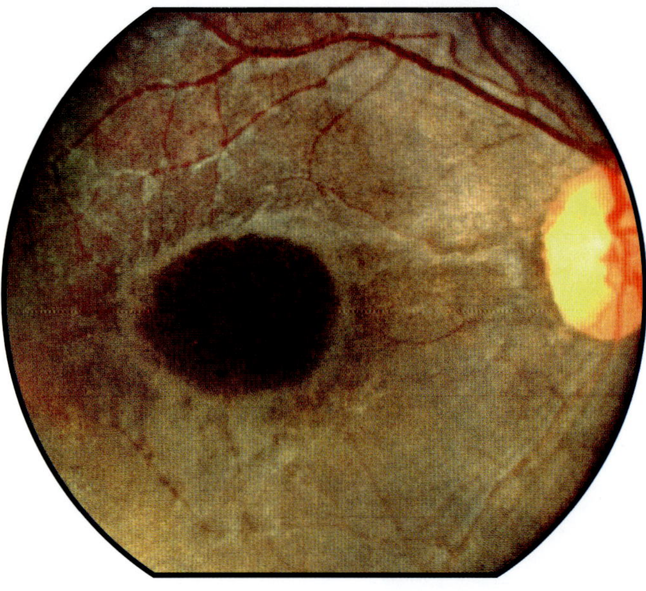

A polymorphic macular sheen is noted. This abnormality often precedes the "bull's-eye" appearance as atrophy evolves in the central macula. The optic nerve is atrophic. *Top two rows courtesy of Dr. Irene Maumenee*

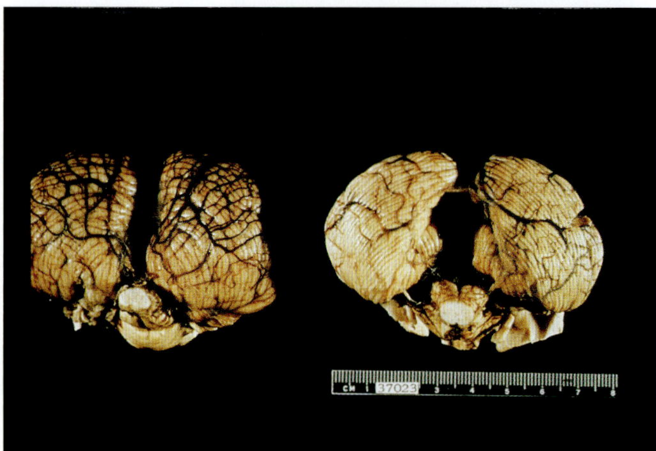

The histopathology of the brain shows cerebellar degeneration.

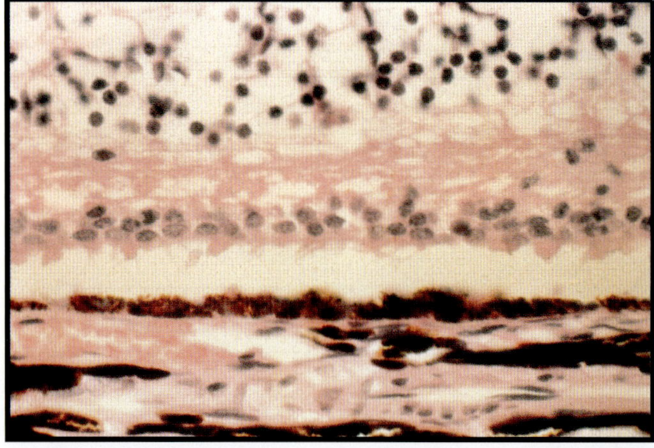

Histopathological specimen in which the RPE is relatively intact. There is a total loss of outer segments and total loss of inner segments with a reduction in the outer nuclear layer. These changes suggest that the primary defect is in the photoreceptor cells.

Pseudo Retinitis Pigmentosa

Several entities may present with a pigmentary retinopathy similar in appearance to retinitis pigmentosa. These include syphilis, congenital rubella, and phenothiazine toxicity. Congenital syphilis can cause an asymmetric pigmentary retinopathy with or without pigment spicules and associated peripheral vision loss in patients with other stigmata of this syndrome including saddle-shaped nose, peg shaped teeth, and interstitial keratitis. Congenital rubella syndrome causes a salt and pepper pigmentary retinopathy with preserved visual field and ERG. Thioridazine toxicity causes nummular loss of the RPE and choriocapillaris that may extend from the posterior pole to the periphery.

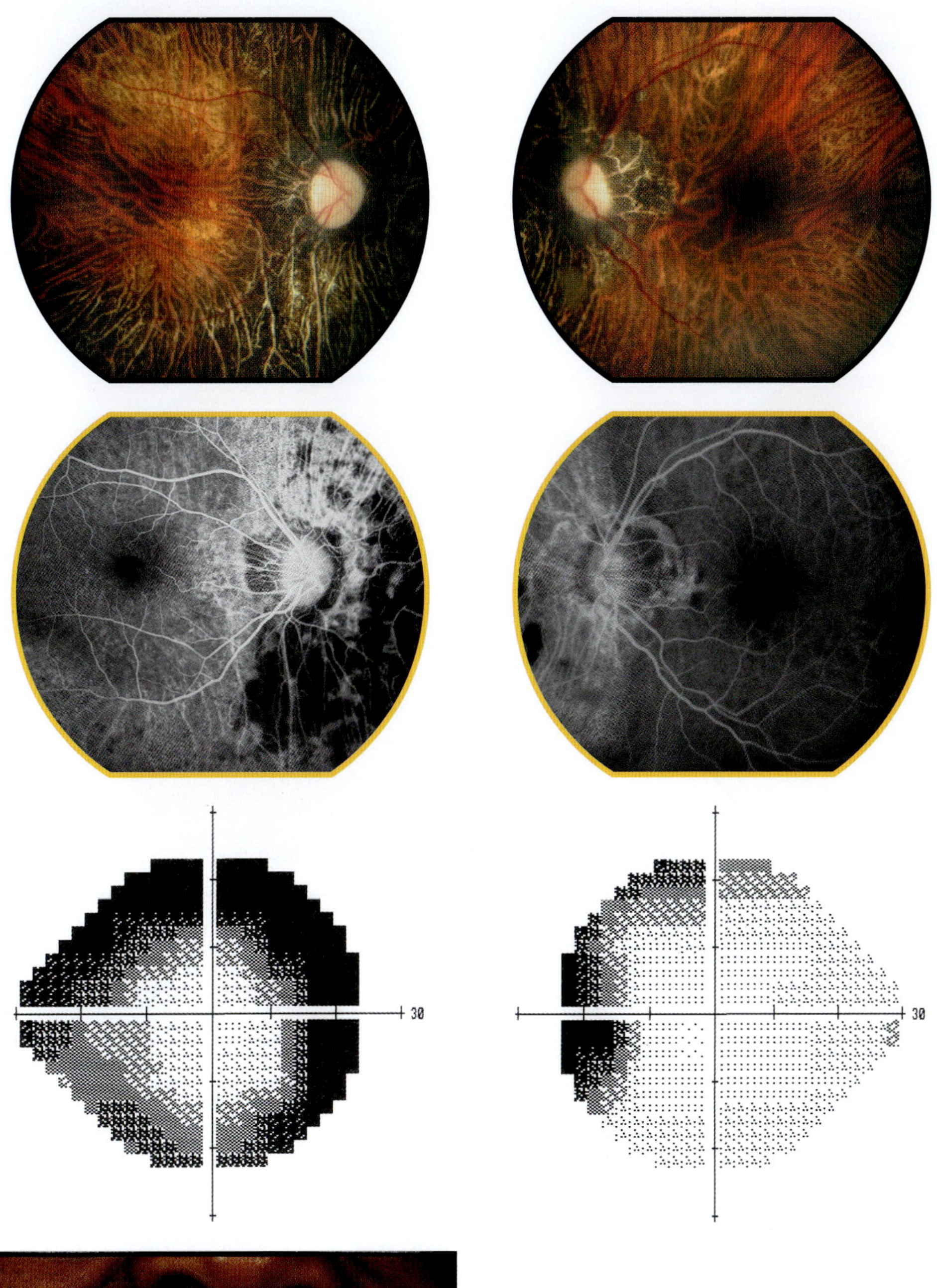

Syphilis may occasionally mimic retinitis pigmentosa with widespread and asymmetric RPE and retinal atrophy seen here on color fundus photos and fluorescein angiogram. Note the presence of retinal vascular attenuation more marked in the right eye. Peripheral visual field constriction or an annular scotoma, like that seen in retinitis pigmentosa, may also be seen as is noted in the right eye of this syphilitic patient *(third row)*. The facial photograph illustrates peg-shaped teeth with blunting of the incisors characteristic of congenital syphillis.

Oculocutaneous Albinism

Oculocutaneous albinism (OCA) is a genetically heterogeneous disorder characterized by decreased or absent pigmentation in the hair, skin, and eyes. Patients manifest various degrees of hypopigmentation in the iris and fundus with associated reduced vision, large refractive errors, nystagmus, strabismus, and foveal hypoplasia. Misrouting of the optic nerves and increased decussating axonal fibers occur at the chiasm. Ocular findings include iris transillumination defects and a hypopigmented fundus with enhanced visualization of the underlying choroid. Some pigmentation in the RPE is due to accumulation of lipofuscin. SD-OCT confirms blunting or complete absence of the foveal pit and absence of the central elongated inner segment band (foveal hypoplasia). Histopathologic sectioning through the center of the macula shows a lack of foveal differentiation.

Most forms of OCA are inherited in an autosomal recessive fashion and include OCA1 and OCA2. OCA1 (tyrosinase-negative) is caused by mutation in the tyrosinase gene with either complete absence (IA) or reduced (IB) tyrosinase activity. OCA2 (tyrosinase-positive) is also an autosomal recessive form caused by mutation in the OCA2 gene, which leads to reduced melanin production. OCA2 is the most common form of OCA in which patients typically have milder findings than OCA1.

Unique systemic syndromes that include various degrees of albinism as a feature are Hermansky–Pudlak and Chédiak–Higashi. Hermansky–Pudlak syndrome is a rare autosomal recessive disorder with oculocutaneous albinism, bleeding related to poor platelet aggregation, lysosomal ceroid accumulation in a variety of tissues, pulmonary fibrosis, granulomatous enteropathic disease, and renal failure. Chédiak–Higashi syndrome is characterized by partial oculocutaneous albinism, impaired bacteriolysis due to failure of phagolysosome formation, neutropenia, abnormal susceptibility to infection, and lymphomatous disease. Patients rarely live beyond 7 years.

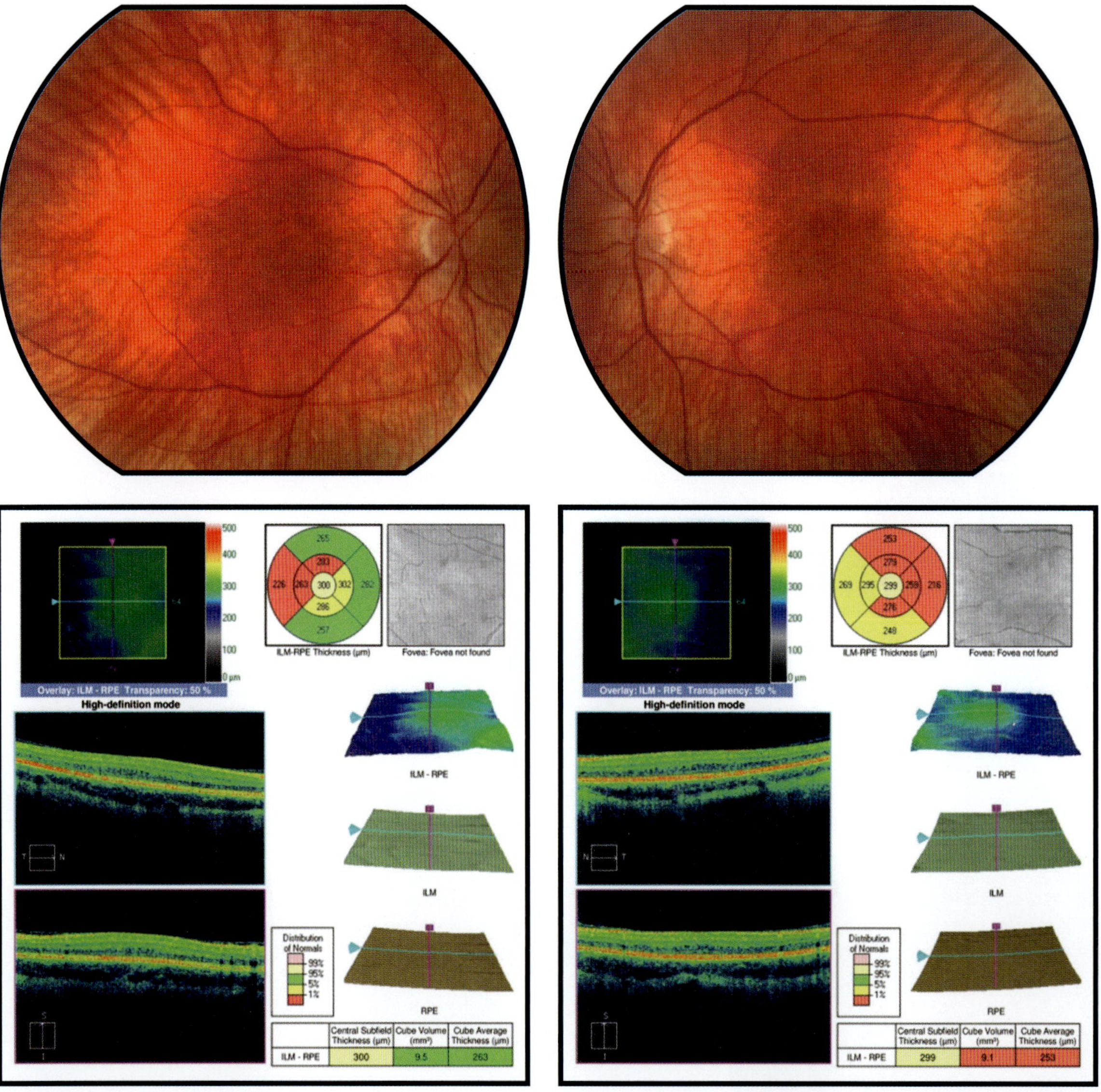

This patient with oculocutaneous albinism has a hypopigmented fundus with loss of the normal foveal reflex. SD-OCT with map analysis demonstrates near complete loss of the foveal contour. Systemic work up revealed severe thrombocytopenia and Hermansky–Pudlak syndrome. *Images courtesy of SriniVas Sadda, MD*

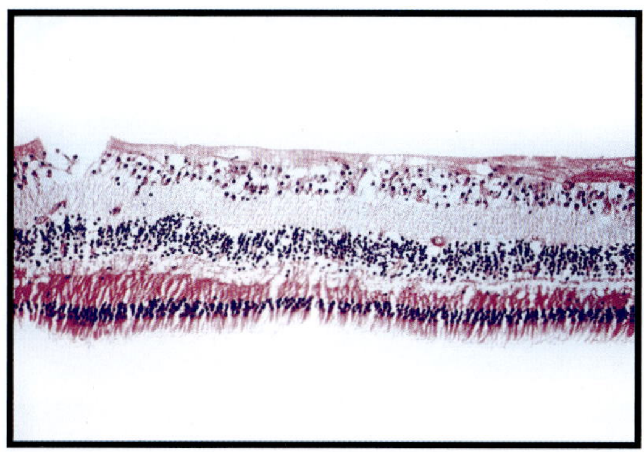

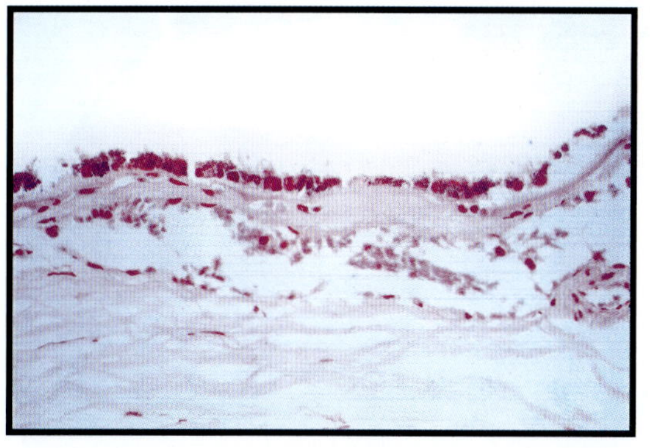

Clinical pathological correlation of a patient with oculocutaneous albinism reveals total absence of melanin pigment. The histopathological serial sectioning through the center of the macula in a patient with ocular albinism shows a lack of foveal differentiation. Some pigmentation in the RPE is due to accumulation of lipofuscin. *All images courtesy of Dr. Jeffrey Shakin*

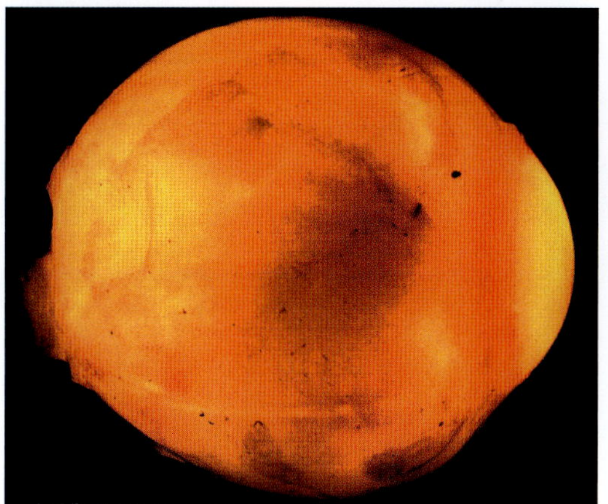

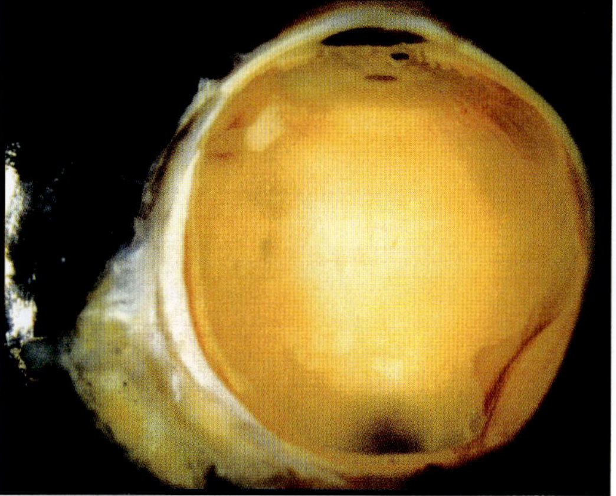

Transillumination of the globe and gross examination also show absence of substantial pigment.

Ocular Albinism Type I (Nettleship–Falls-Type Albinism)

Ocular albinism type I is an X-linked disorder caused by mutation in the OA1 gene, where affected males typically manifest abnormal melanin production limited to the eye. Findings include vision loss, nystagmus, iris transillumination defects, hypopigmented fundus with easily visible choroidal vessels, and foveal hypoplasia. Female carriers show a mosaic pigmentation pattern. In these carriers, hyperpigmented "bear-track"-like lesions may be seen. With fluorescein angiography, areas of normal pigmentation will block fluorescence adjacent to areas of increased transmission from the choroid through less pigmented areas.

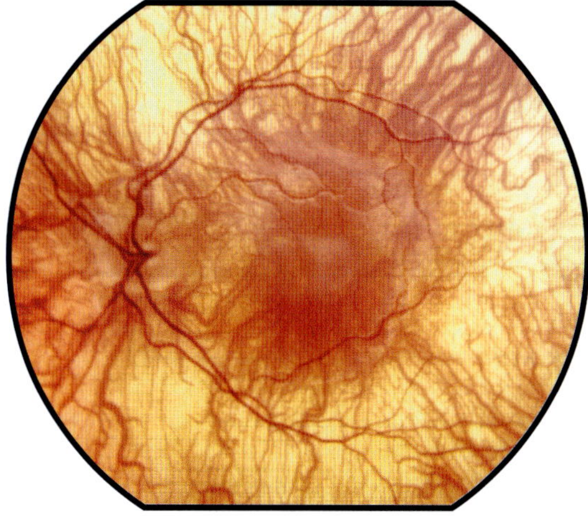

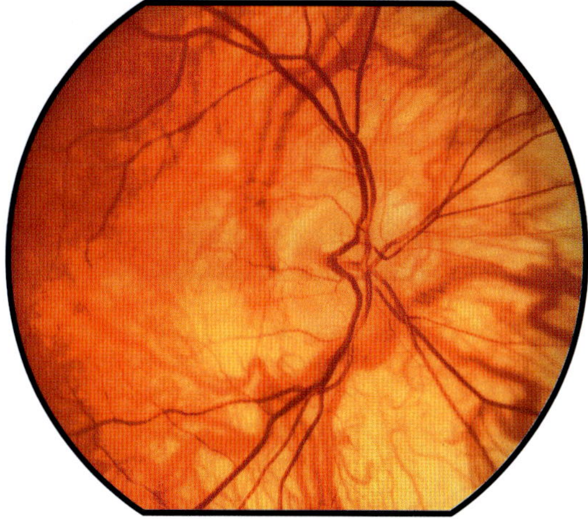

This patient with ocular albinism demonstrates the characteristic hypopigmented fundus. There is enhanced visualization of the choroidal circulation through the depigmented pigment epithelial layer.

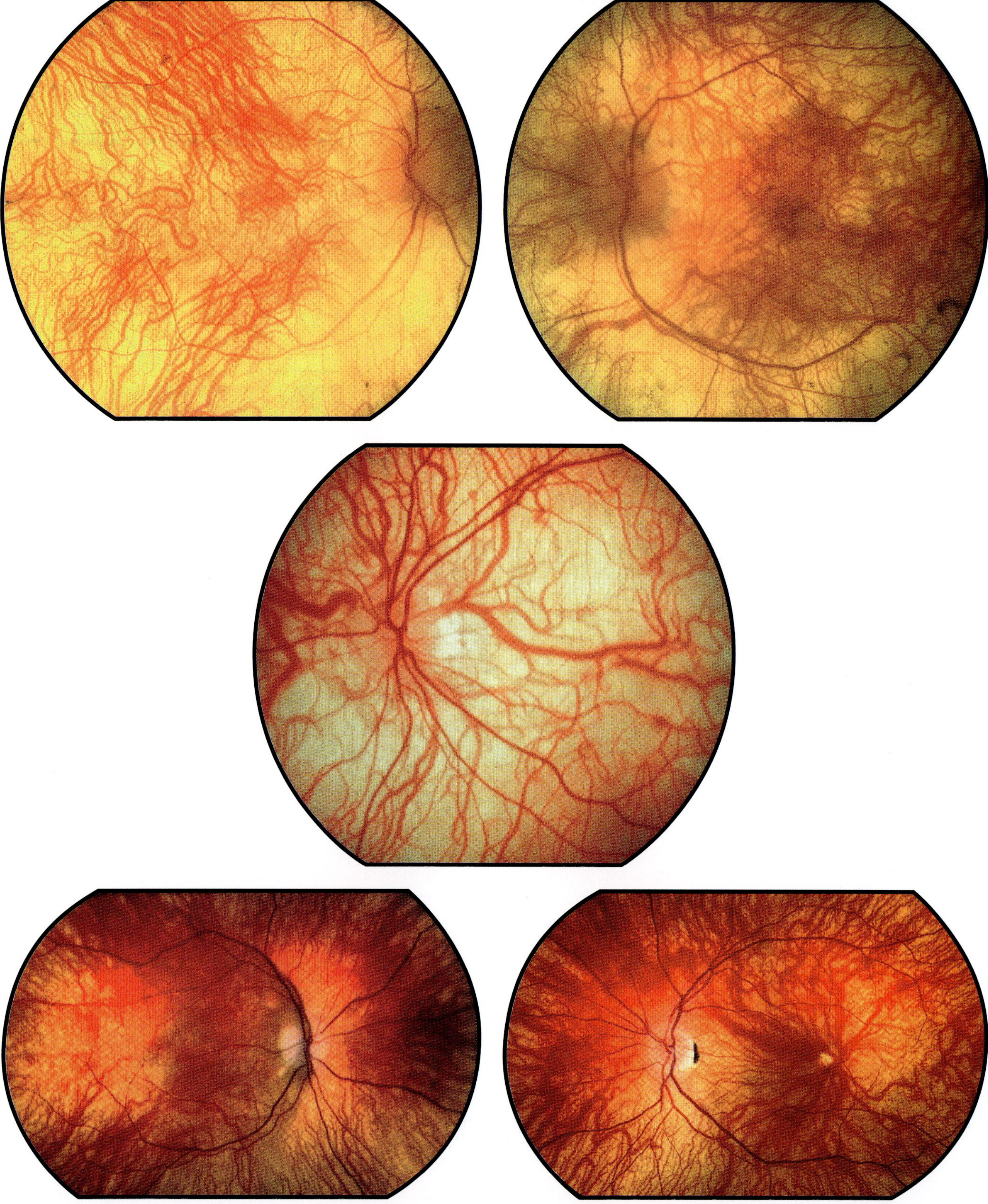

These patients show the typical features of albinism in the fundus. There is no evidence of pigmentation, prominent choroidal vessels are easily visible clinically, and there is poor differentiation of the fovea. *Bottom row courtesy of Dr. Edwin Ryan*

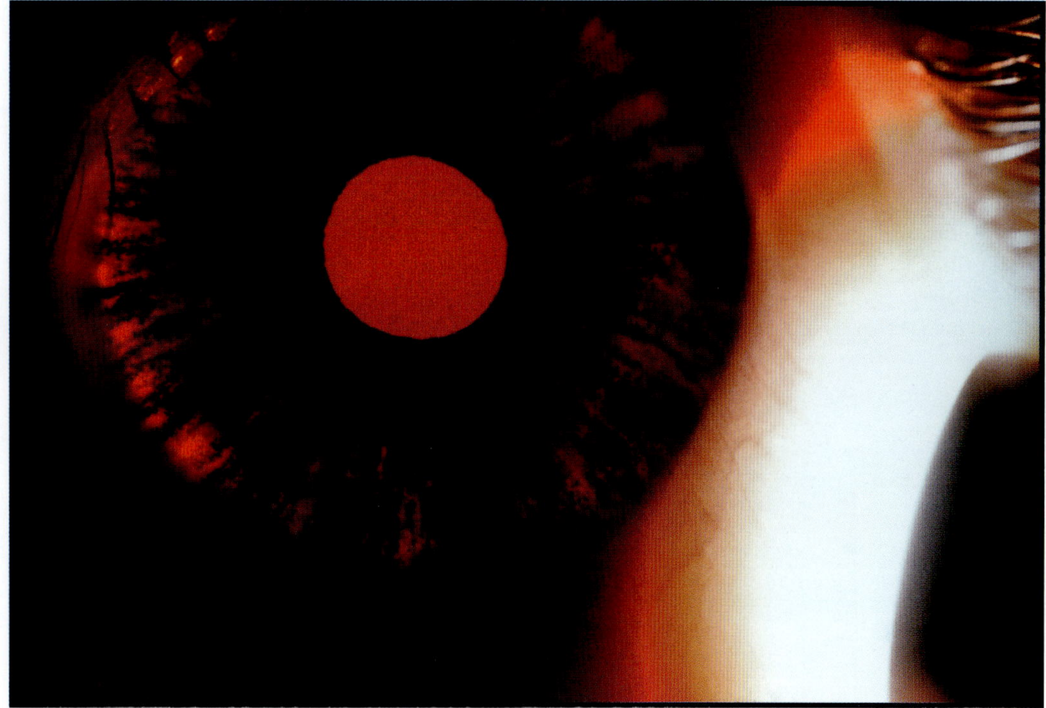

Transillumination of the iris can be noted.

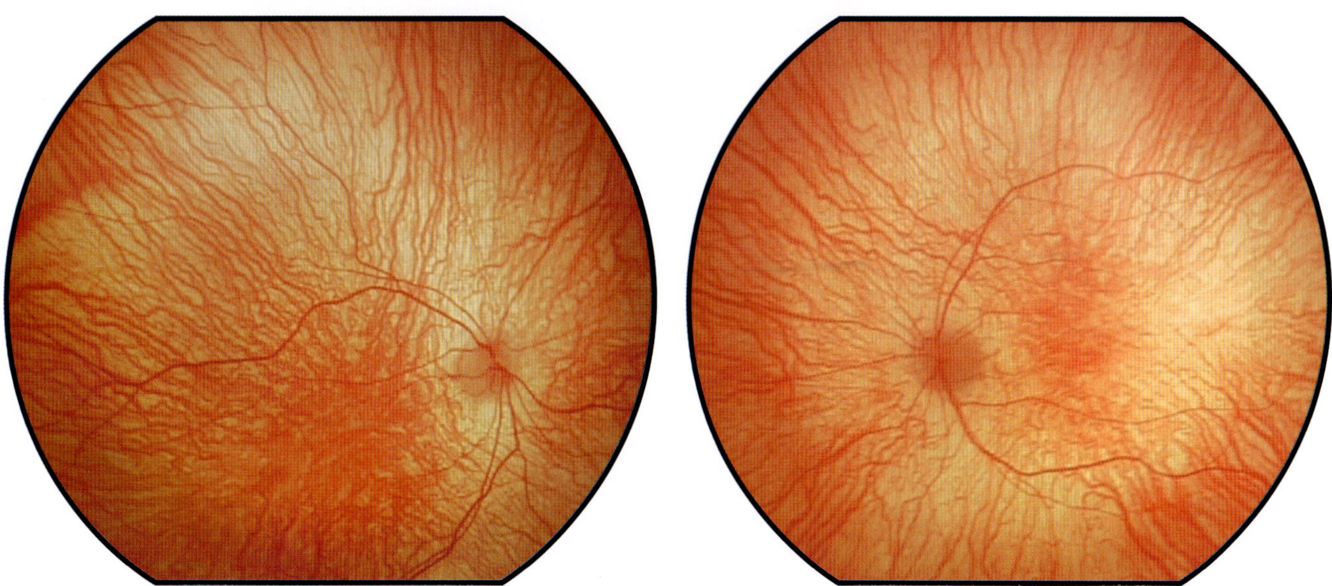

This is a 2-year-old patient with ocular albinism, showing widespread hypopigmentation and an indistinct foveal depression. A pale fundus like this may sometimes be confused with other pediatric fundus anomalies and abnormalities.

Albinism — Female Carrier

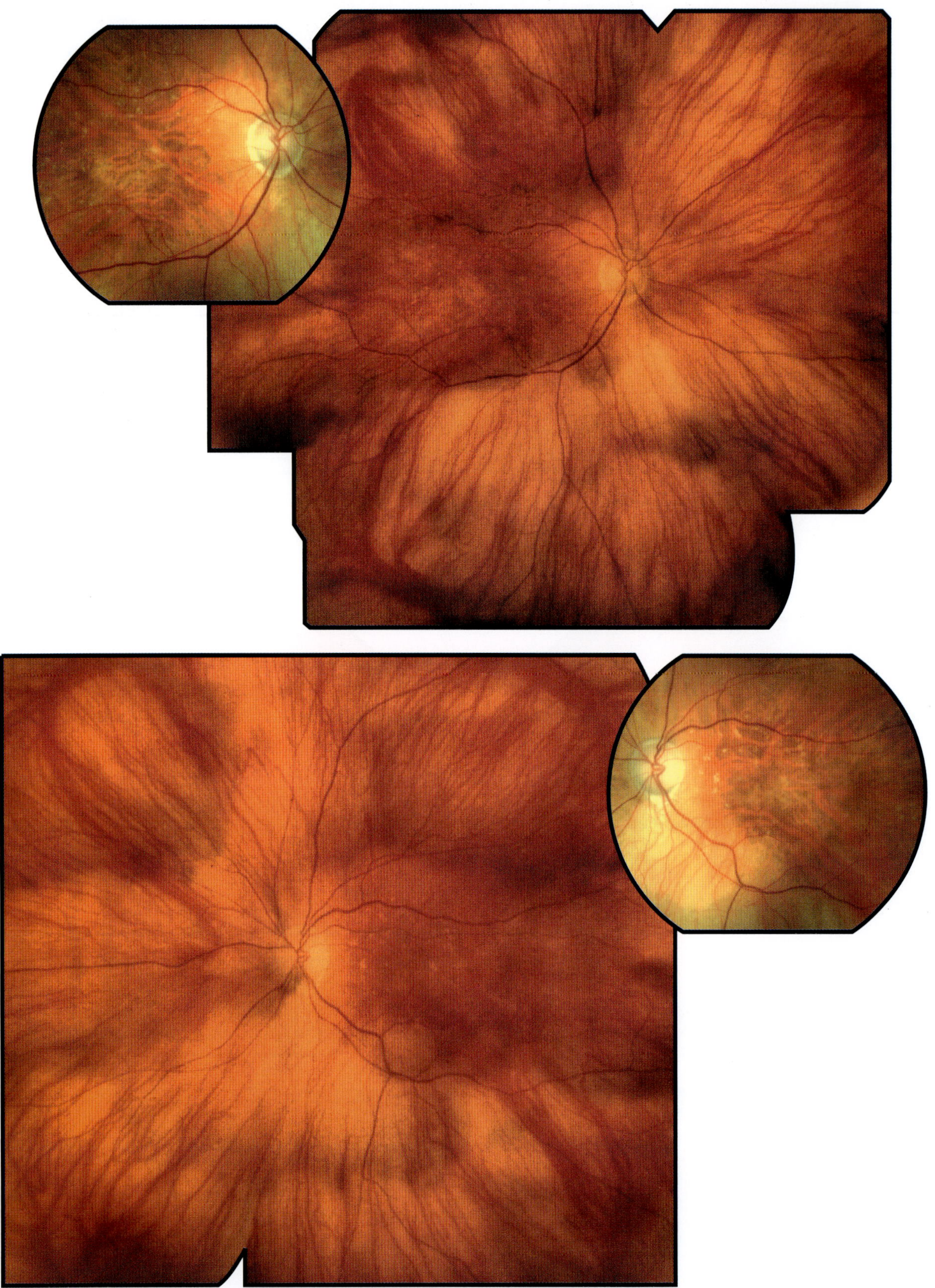

This female carrier of ocular albinism shows a pale fundus. In the macular region of each eye there are drusen, a rare but known occurrence.

Female Carrier of X-Linked Ocular Albinism

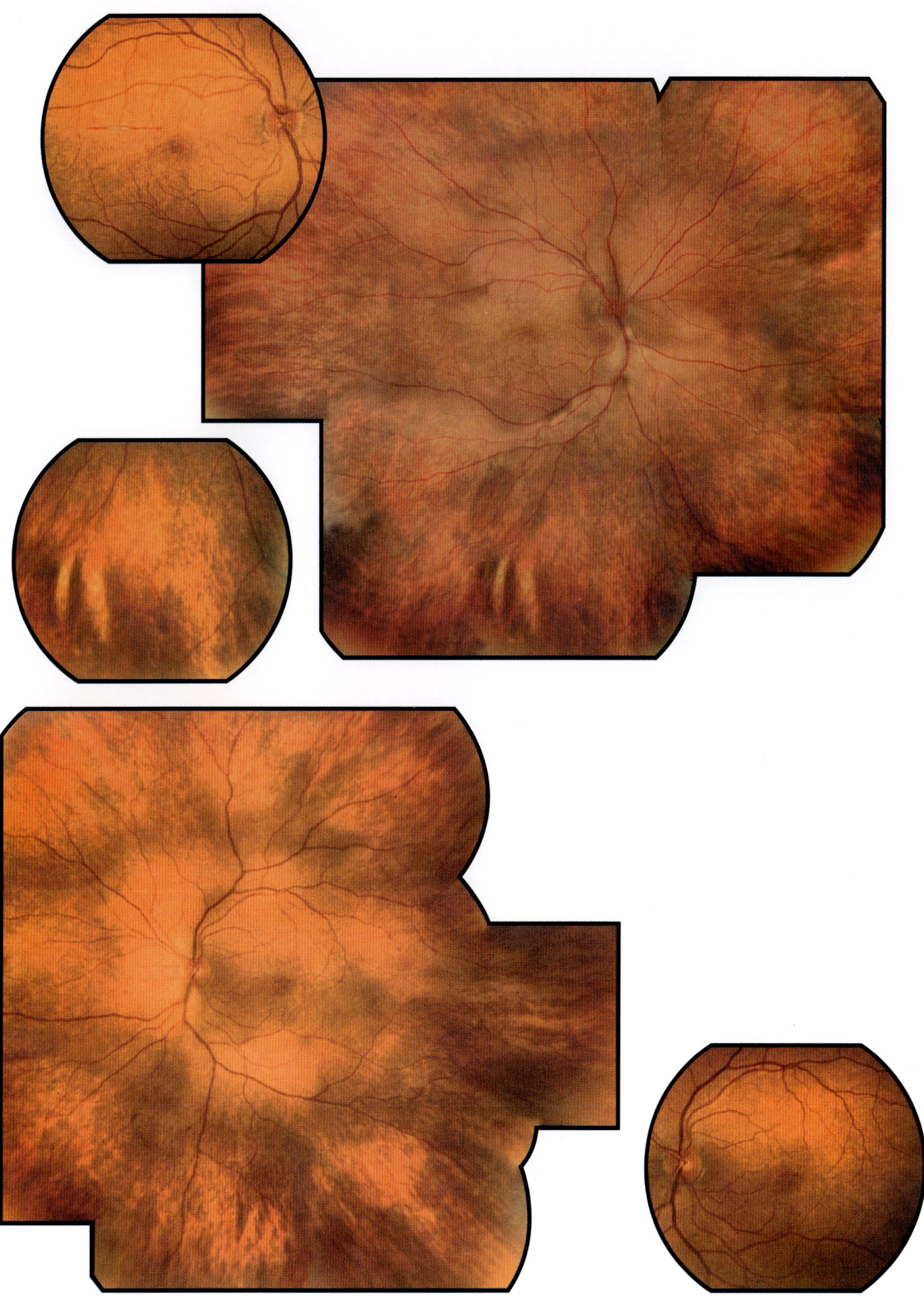

This patient is also a female carrier of X-linked ocular albinism. This is the so-called "mud-slung" fundus with alternating areas of hypo- and hyperpigmentation throughout the fundus from the central foveal area to the far periphery.

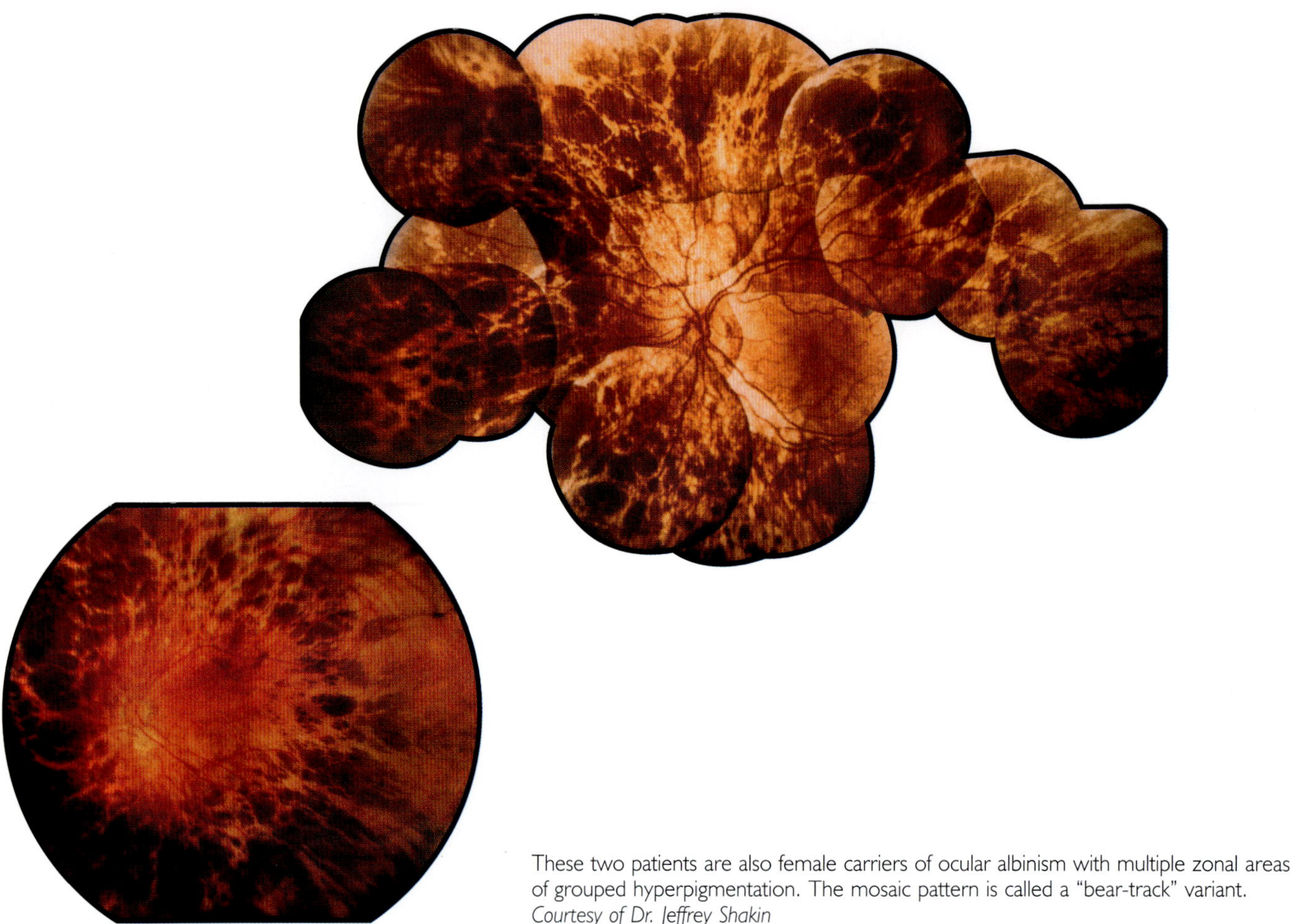

These two patients are also female carriers of ocular albinism with multiple zonal areas of grouped hyperpigmentation. The mosaic pattern is called a "bear-track" variant.
Courtesy of Dr. Jeffrey Shakin

Choroidal Dystrophies

This group of disorders can be associated with progressive peripheral and central vision loss and nyctalopia similar to RP but is primarily characterized by diffuse atrophy of the RPE and choriocapillaris. Migrating pigment spicules and vascular attenuation are not prominent features of this class of disease.

Choroideremia

Choroideremia is an X-linked recessive progressive degeneration of the RPE, retina, and choroid. It is caused by a mutation of CHM gene localized to Xq21.2, which encodes Rab escort protein-1 (REP1). It is the most common hereditary choroidal dystrophy seen in the western world. The disease follows a well-characterized course of progression with onset in the first to second decade of life. Affected male patients often present with complaints of nyctalopia. Fundus examination early in the disease course reveals "salt and pepper" pigmentary retinopathy involving the midperiphery and posterior pole, with patchy areas of pigment loss giving the underlying fundus a metallic sheen. Diffuse choroidal atrophy ensues, beginning in the midperiphery and extending toward the macula, which leaves scattered small areas of intact choriocapillaris in the central macula and periphery. This leads to progressive night blindness and constriction of visual fields. Central vision is typically spared until late in the disease course. ERG abnormalities may be detected early, showing a reduced scotopic response. Later in the disease scotopic and photopic responses become extinguished. Heterozygous females may show a diffuse pigmentary retinopathy, for example, reticular pigment degeneration, but typically demonstrate preserved visual and ERG function. Rarely carrier females may demonstrate diffuse chorioretinal atrophy similar to affected male patients. This is thought to be a result of random inactivation of the wild type X chromosome in the female carrier, a genetic phenomenon known as lyonization. Carrier females generally maintain normal vision throughout life; however, subtle progressive ERG changes may eventually develop. Histopathologically, extensive choroidal atrophy is seen in male patients with choroideremia. Tissue from female carriers may show scattered areas of photoreceptor and RPE atrophy, pigment clumping and patchy areas of choriocapillaris loss.

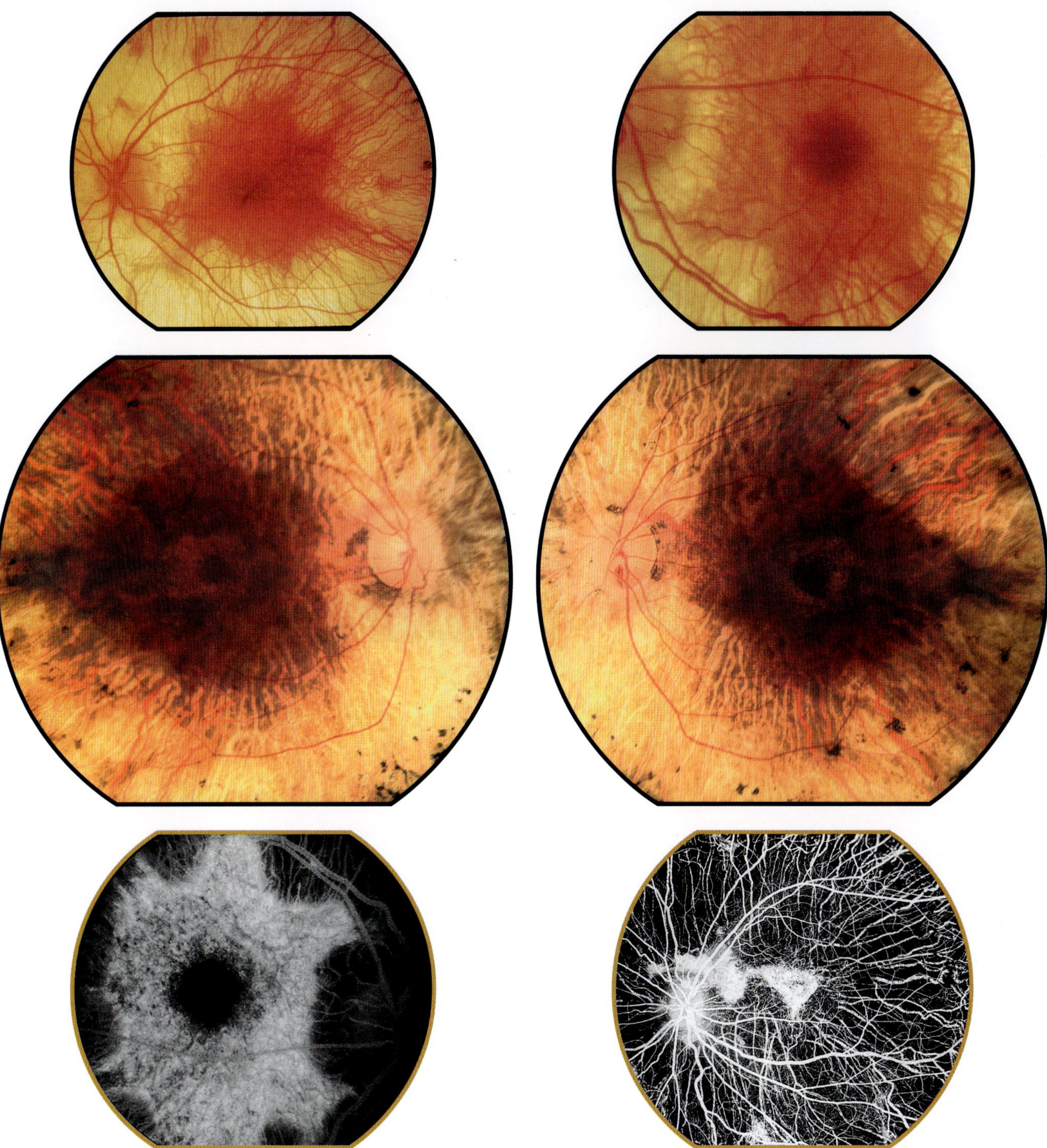

These patients have severe choroideremia. Note the pallor to the fundus, which is diffusely atrophic surrounding the posterior pole. The fluorescein angiogram shows diffuse loss of the choriocapillaris, except for a preserved central hyperfluorescent island. A ring of perifoveal pigment epithelial and choriocapillaris atrophy is noted in the middle row of color photos. *Top row right and bottom row left courtesy of Dr. Jim Tiedeman*

This patient with choroideremia had relative preservation of the macula, but widespread areas of choriocapillaris and pigment epithelial loss outside the posterior pole clearly evident on the fluorescein angiogram.

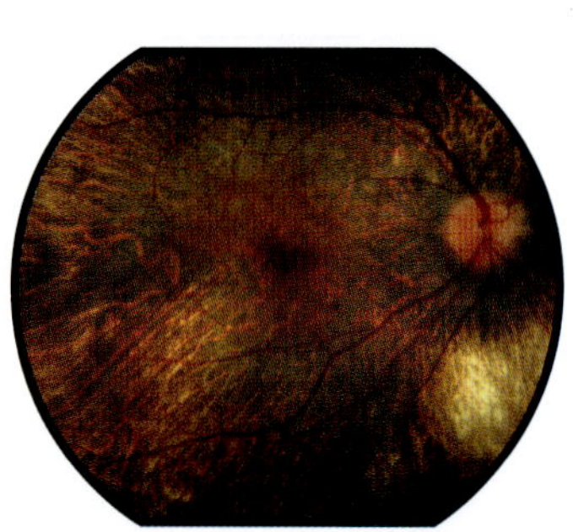

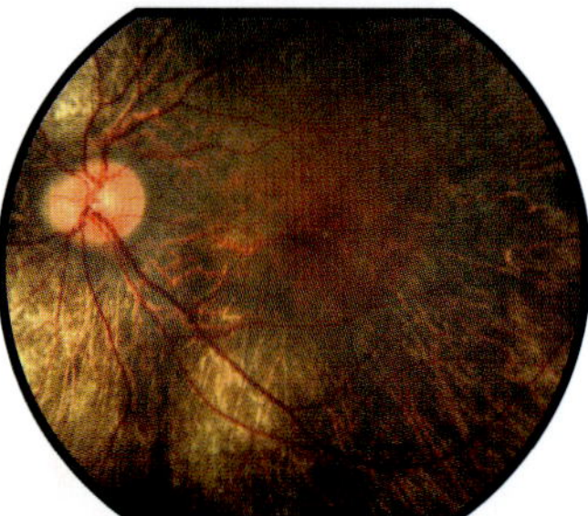

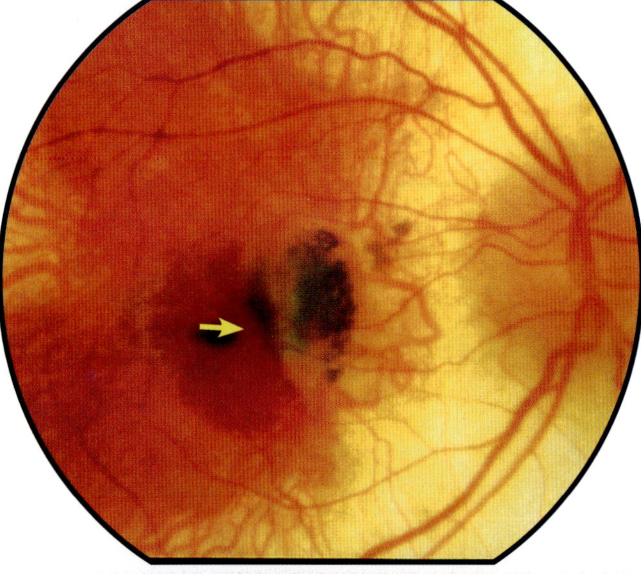

This patient had choroideremia with central preservation of the choriocapillaris but choroidal neovascularization developed – a very rare occurrence in the area of intact choriocapillaris *(arrow). Courtesy of Dr. Jim Tiedeman*

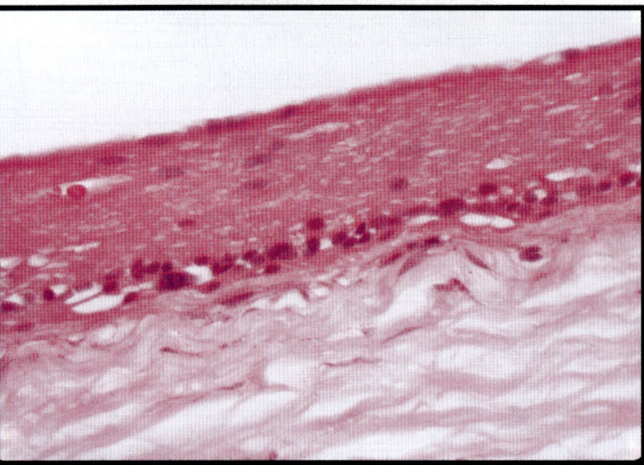

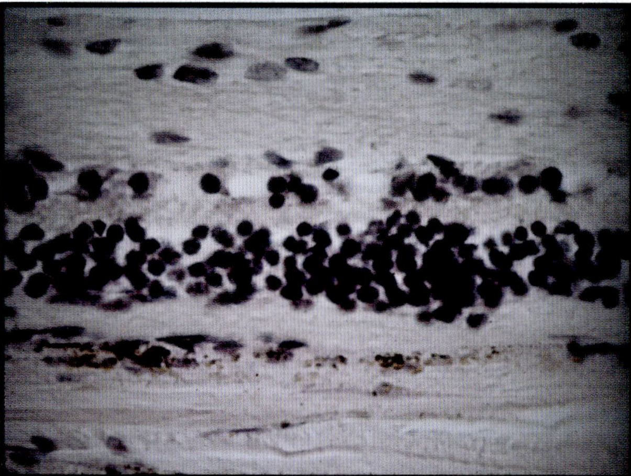

The histopathology images from a patient with choroideremia reveal loss of the choroid, retinal pigment epithelium, and outer retinal areas.

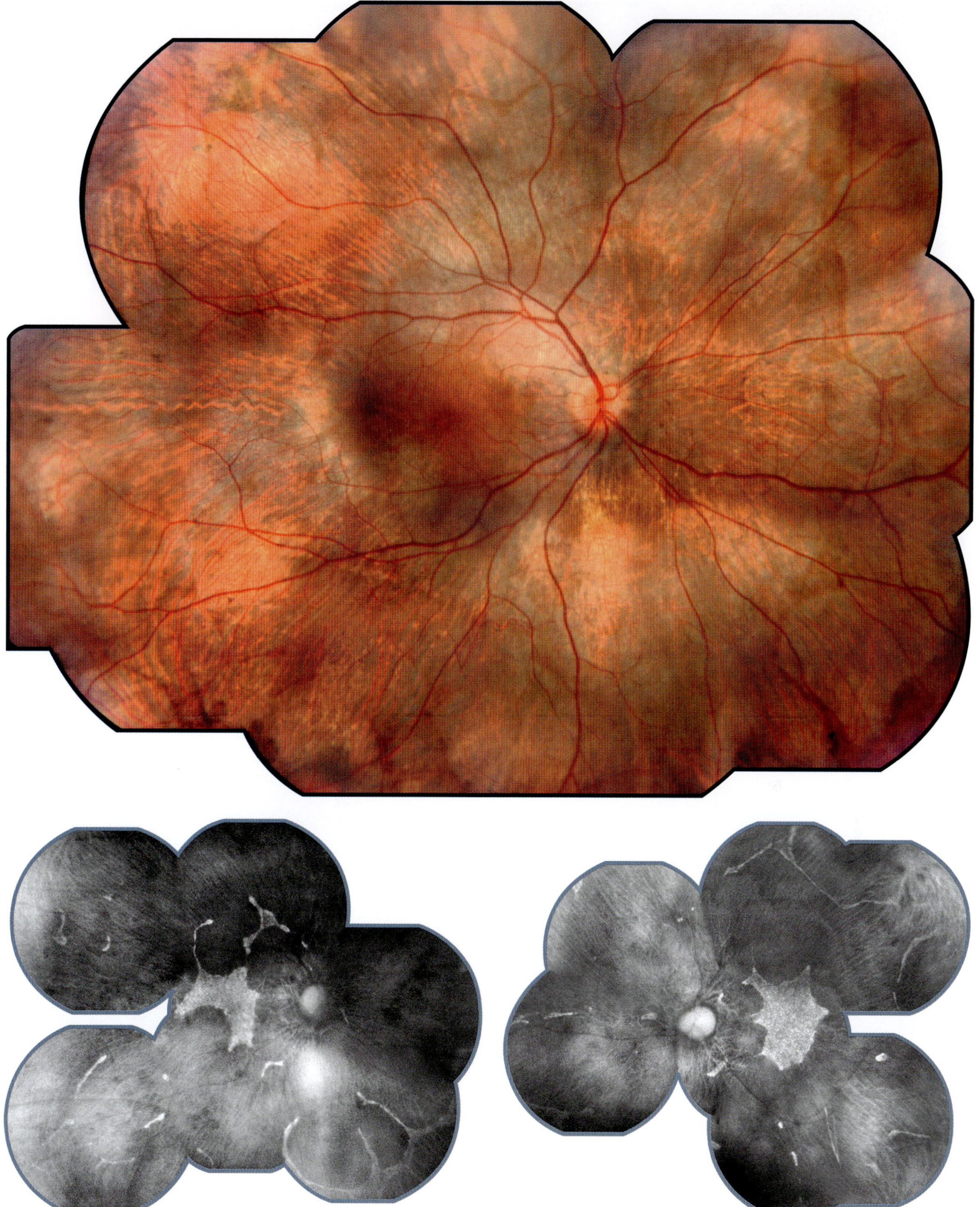

In this patient with choroideremia, zonal areas of widespread atrophy can be seen throughout the entire fundus. Note the thin islands of preserved hyperautofluorescent RPE in the periphery and in the central macular region.

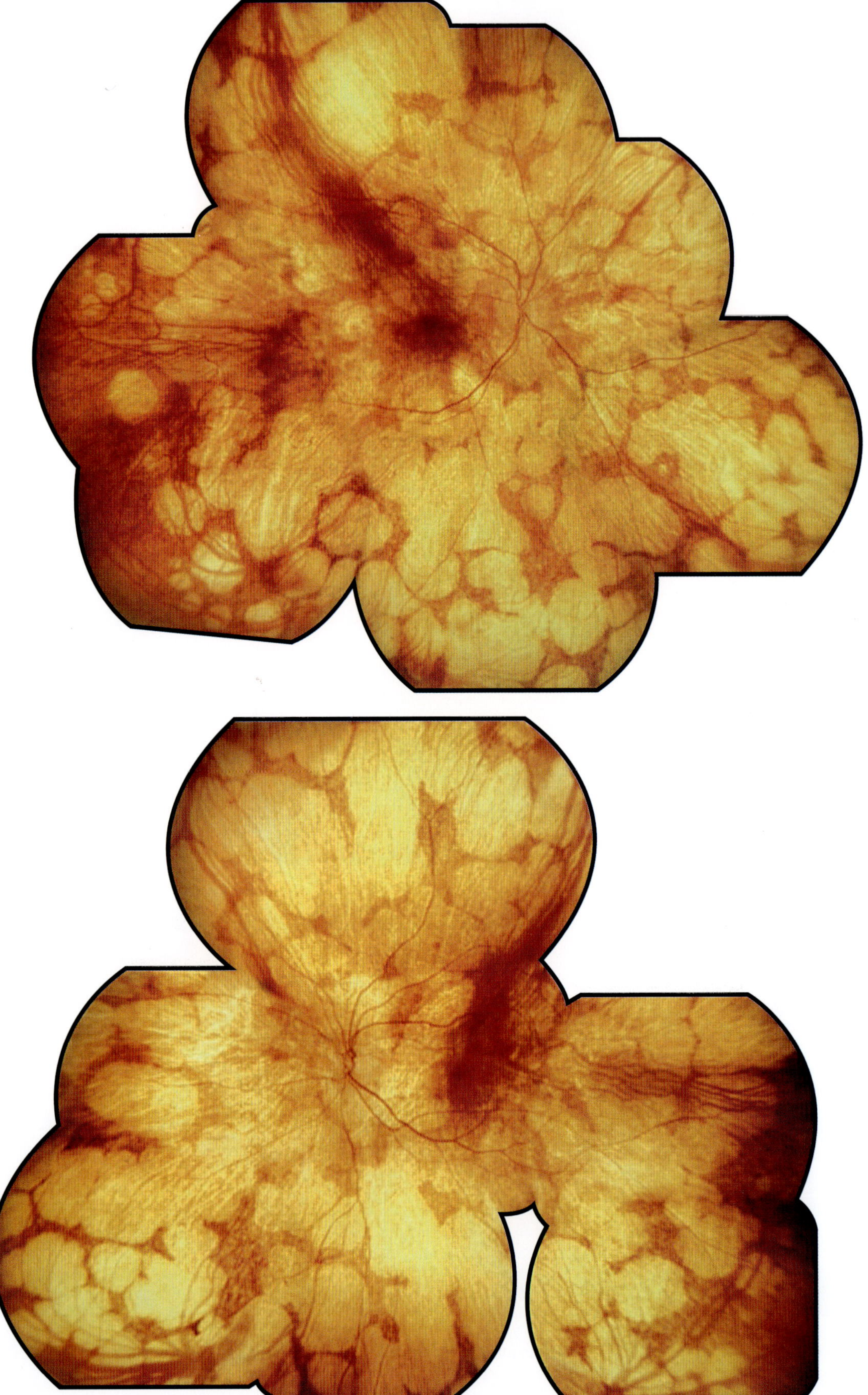

This patient with choroideremia also shows widespread chorioretinal atrophy with islands of choriocapillaris/RPE preservation scattered throughout the peripheral fundus and in the central macula of each eye.

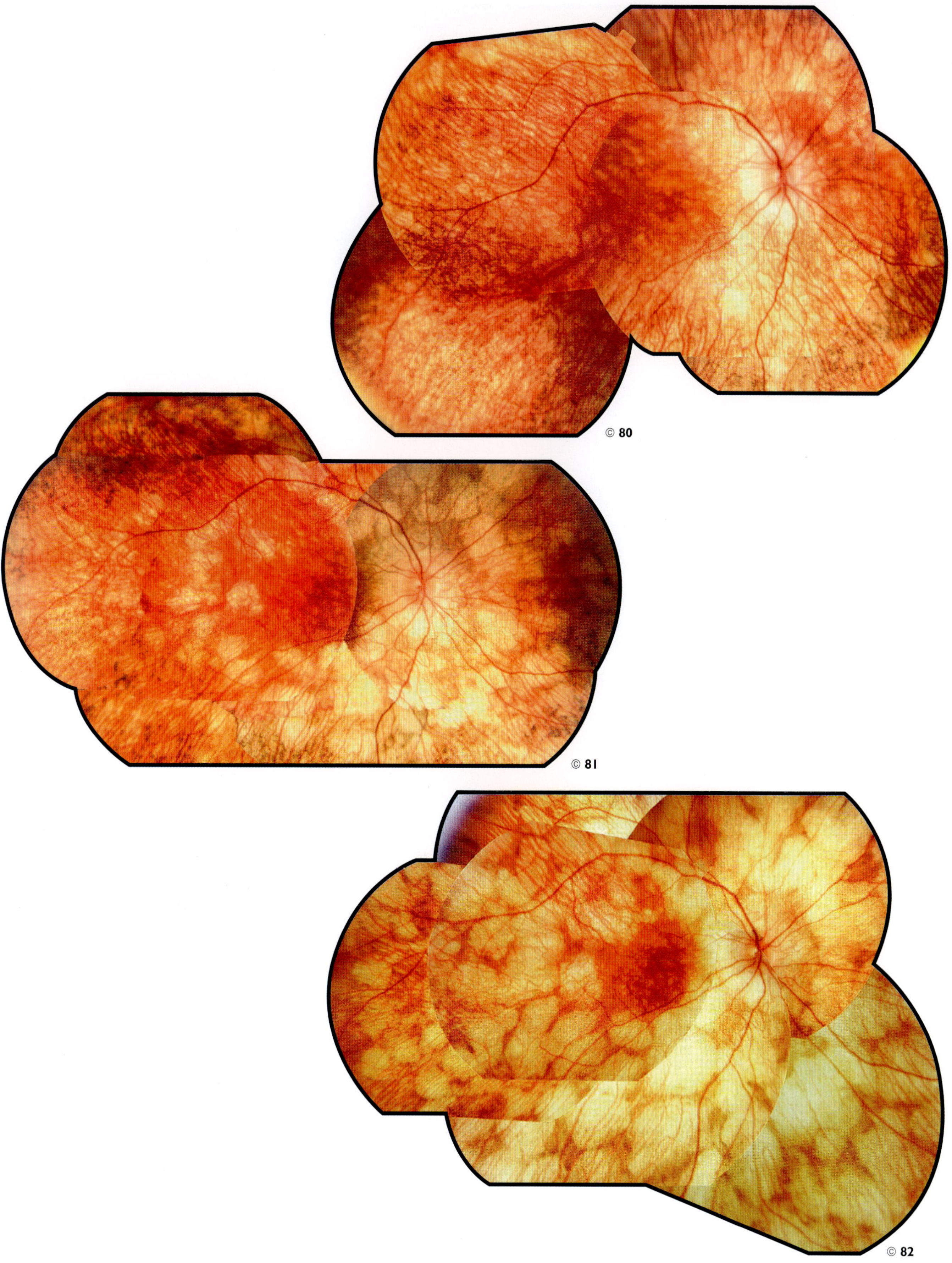

This patient with choroideremia demonstrates the progressive nature of the disease over a period of 25 years.

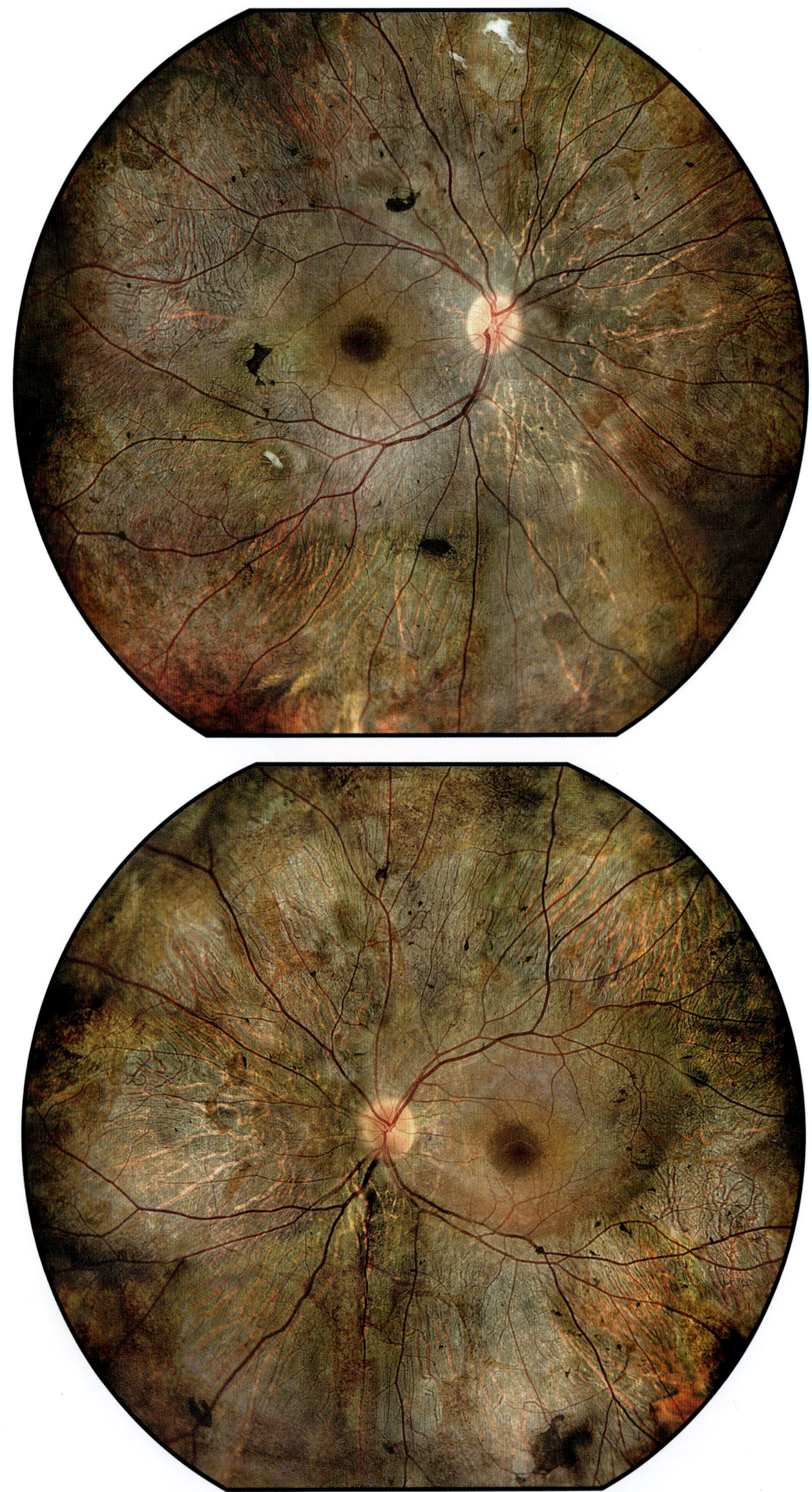

This patient with choroideremia had zonal areas of atrophy in a widespread, but patchy distribution throughout the fundus but sparing the central macular region.

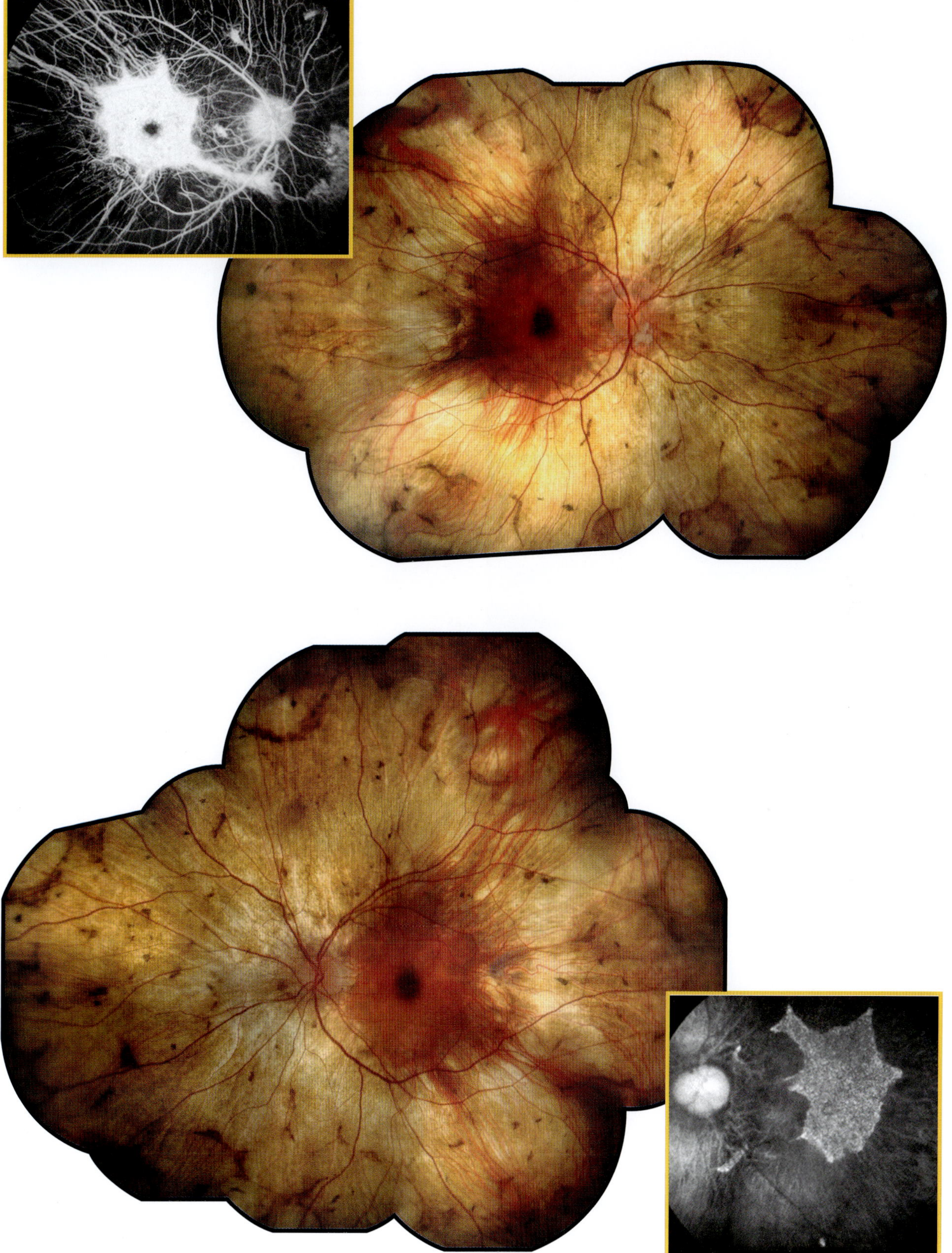

This patient with choroideremia had a peculiar type of stellate preservation of the posterior pole (color montage OD and OS) that is very characteristic of the disease. The fluorescein angiograms from a different patient show a similar stellate preservation in the macula. Presumably, this pattern may relate to conformity to the lobular architectural structure of the choriocapillaris. *Bottom images courtesy of Dr. Anita Agarwal*

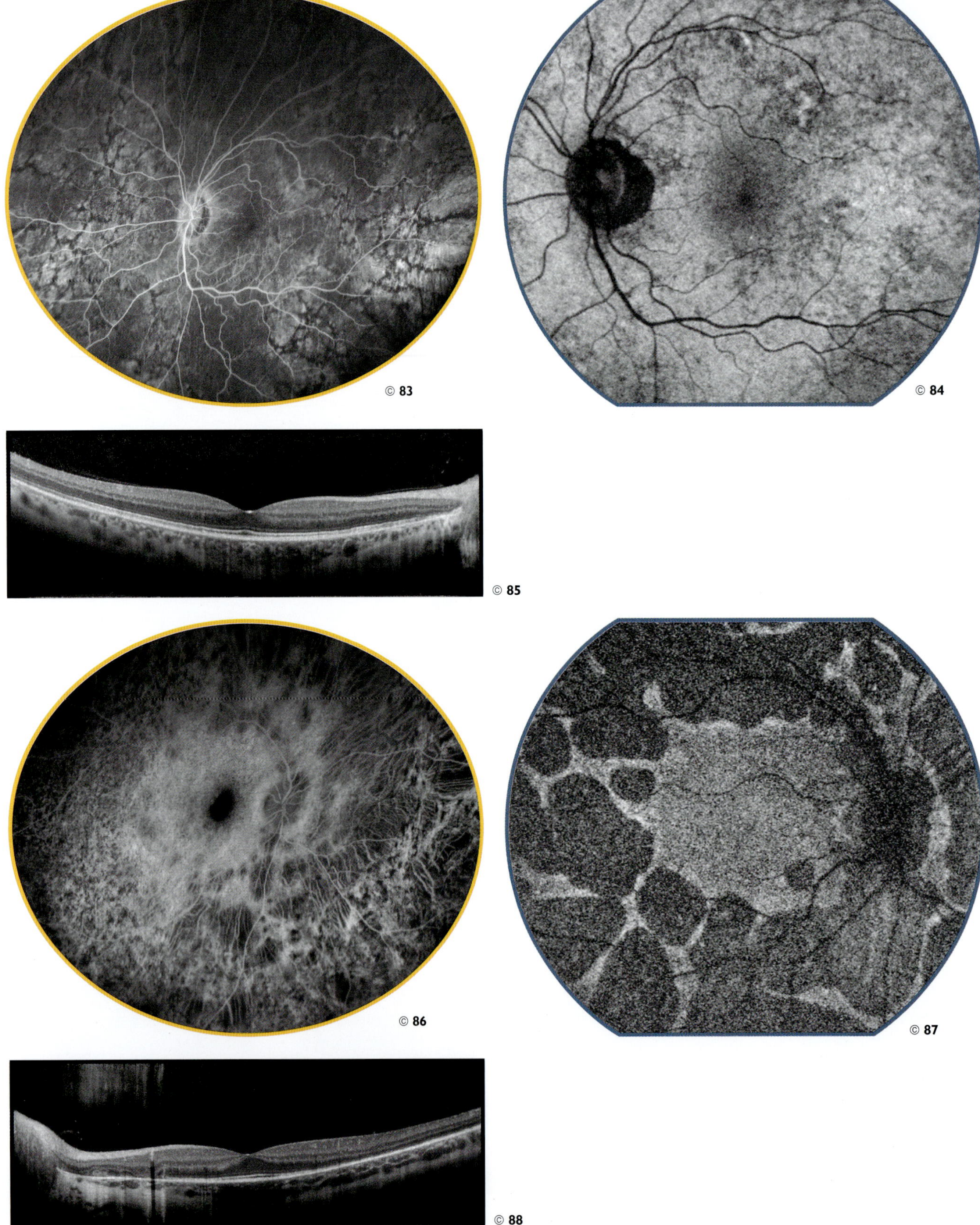

Fluorescein angiogram, corresponding fundus autofluorescence and SD-OCT of a female carrier of choroideremia *(first and second rows)*. Fluorescein angiogram and autofluorescence *(third row)* of her son shows diffuse chorioretinal atrophy. SD-OCT of this patient shows outer retinal atrophy in a paramacular distribution.

Choroideremia—Female Carrier

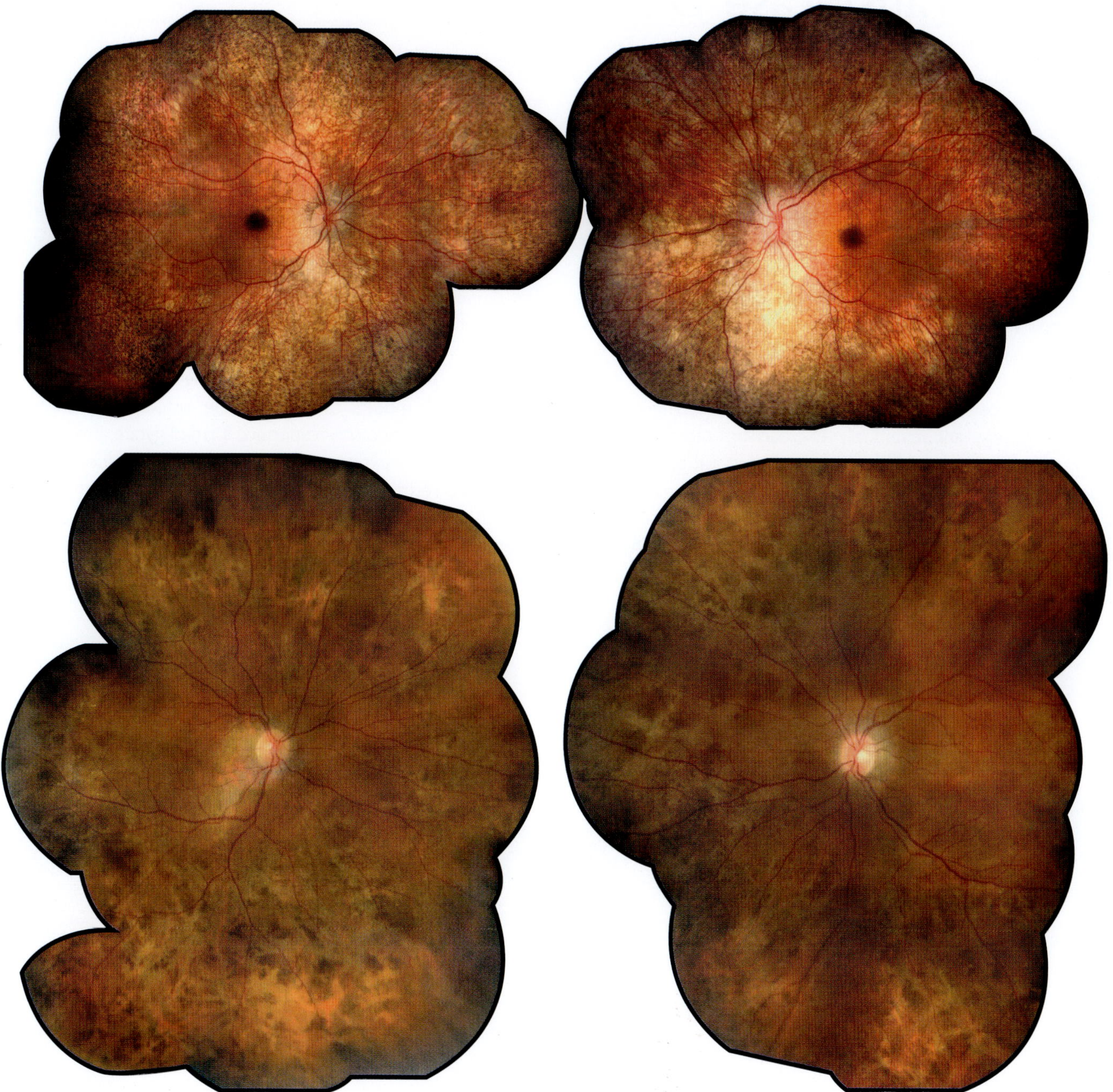

The two patients illustrated here are female carriers of choroideremia. They demonstrate similar manifestations with widespread patchy RPE atrophy and granularity, but relative preservation of the central macula in each eye. *Courtesy of Dr. Anita Agarwal*

Gyrate Atrophy (Ornithine Aminotransferase Deficiency)

Gyrate atrophy is an autosomal recessive chorioretinal dystrophy which leads to progressive retinal and choroidal degeneration. Deficiency in ornithine-delta-aminotransferase (OAT) linked to chromosome 10q26 leads to hyperornithinemia with plasma ornithine levels 10–20 times higher than those of controls. Patients generally present with nyctalopia, high myopia, and astigmatism within the first decade of life with subsequent development of posterior subcapsular cataracts by the second decade. Slowly progressive constriction of visual fields and eventual loss of central visual acuity continue into the fourth to fifth decades. Initially, circular, sharply demarcated regions of chorioretinal atrophy with hyperpigmented margins in the midperiphery are seen that slowly enlarge and coalesce in a "scalloped" pattern, spreading anteriorly and posteriorly, and eventually encroaching into the macula. Leakage at the margins of healthy and affected tissue, with hyperfluorescence within the gyrate lesions, may be seen on fluorescein angiography. Early impaired scotopic and photopic responses are seen on electrophysiologic testing, and these become extinguished as the disease progresses. Histopathologically, the earliest changes are seen in the RPE cells, with subsequent loss of photoreceptors and choriocapillaris, suggesting that this damage may be secondary to the loss of RPE integrity. Other associated findings include tubular aggregates in type II skeletal muscle fibers, subclinical skeletal muscle changes on CT and MRI, abnormalities on EEG, and premature atrophy and white-matter lesions on brain MRI. These patients usually have no muscular symptoms, but may show impaired performance when speed or acute strength is required. The disease progresses to almost complete loss of type 2 fibers, but the progression of muscular abnormalities is slower than the chorioretinal degeneration. Treatment for gyrate atrophy has been aimed toward reducing plasma ornithine levels. Ornithine reduction in mouse models can prevent the histological changes. In patients with a pyridoxine-responsive form of gyrate atrophy, supplementation with pyridoxine has been shown to reduce ornithine levels. Diets restricted in arginine (the precursor of ornithine) have been shown to delay the progression of visual deficits, although patients may demonstrate continued chorioretinal deterioration.

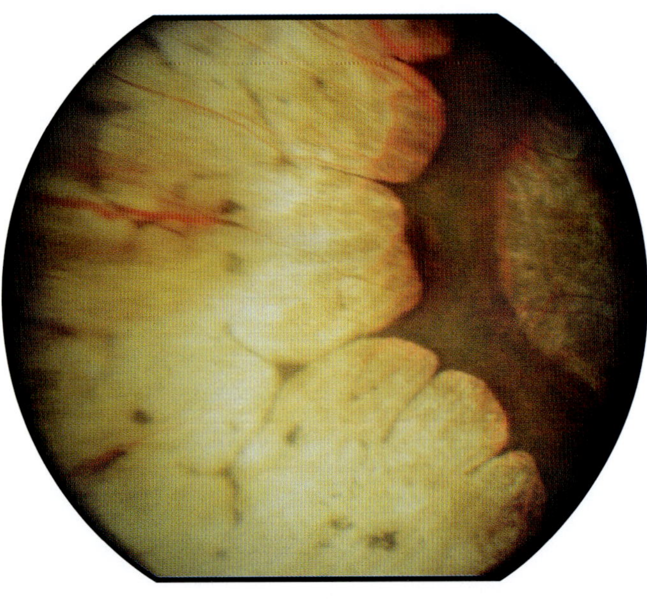
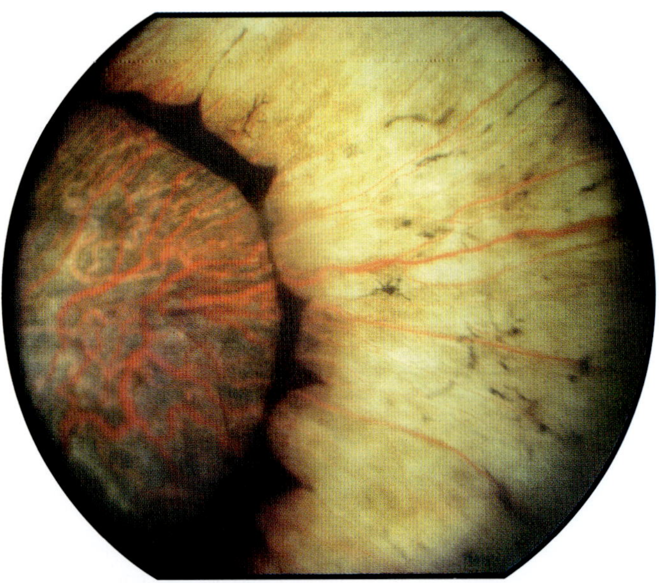

In this patient with gyrate atrophy, there is high myopia and peripheral chorioretinal atrophy with well-delineated scallop-like borders. Like choroideremia, the atrophic lesions start in the midperiphery and then extend in both directions, anteriorly and posteriorly. *Courtesy of Dr. Irene Maumenee*

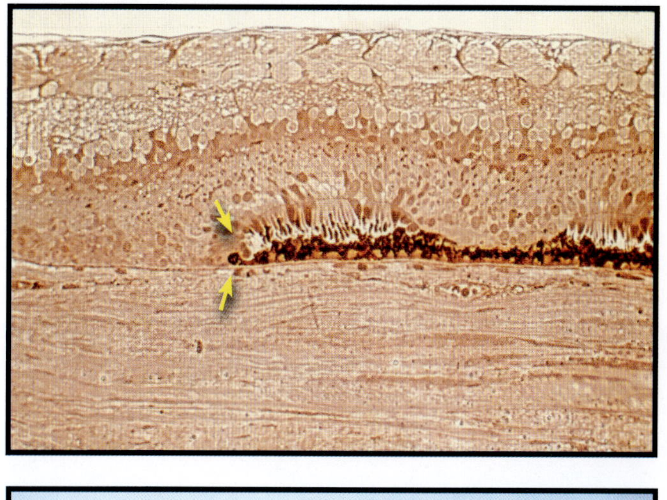

© 89

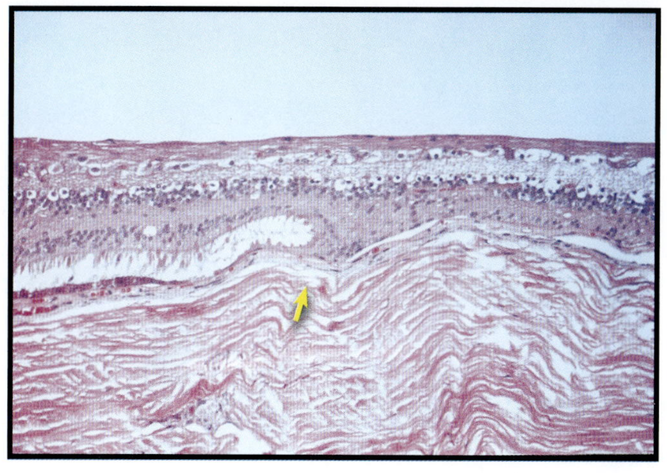

© 90

The gyrate atrophy seen in this patient has sharply circumscribed areas of atrophy with scalloped margins. On light microscopy, there is a clearly distinguishable junction between unaffected and affected areas on these phase contrast and light microscopy photographs *(arrows)*. There is also an absence of the choroid and outer retinal layers in the affected area.

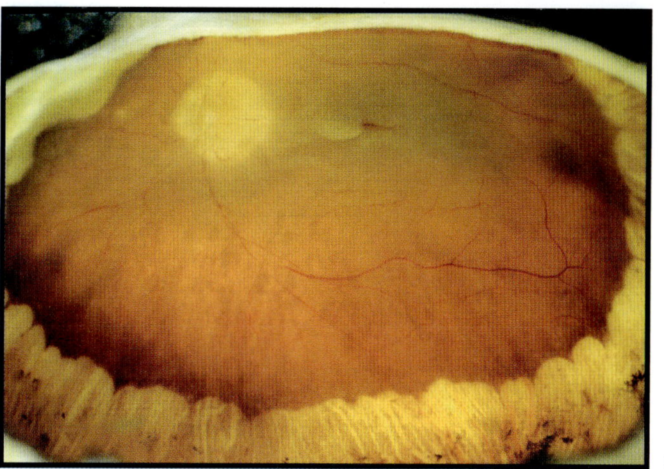

© 91

The sharply demarcated, confluent, concentric and scalloped band of peripheral atrophy in these patients is very characteristic of the disorder. Note the preservation of a few islands of RPE within atrophic areas. Optic disc drusen can also be seen.

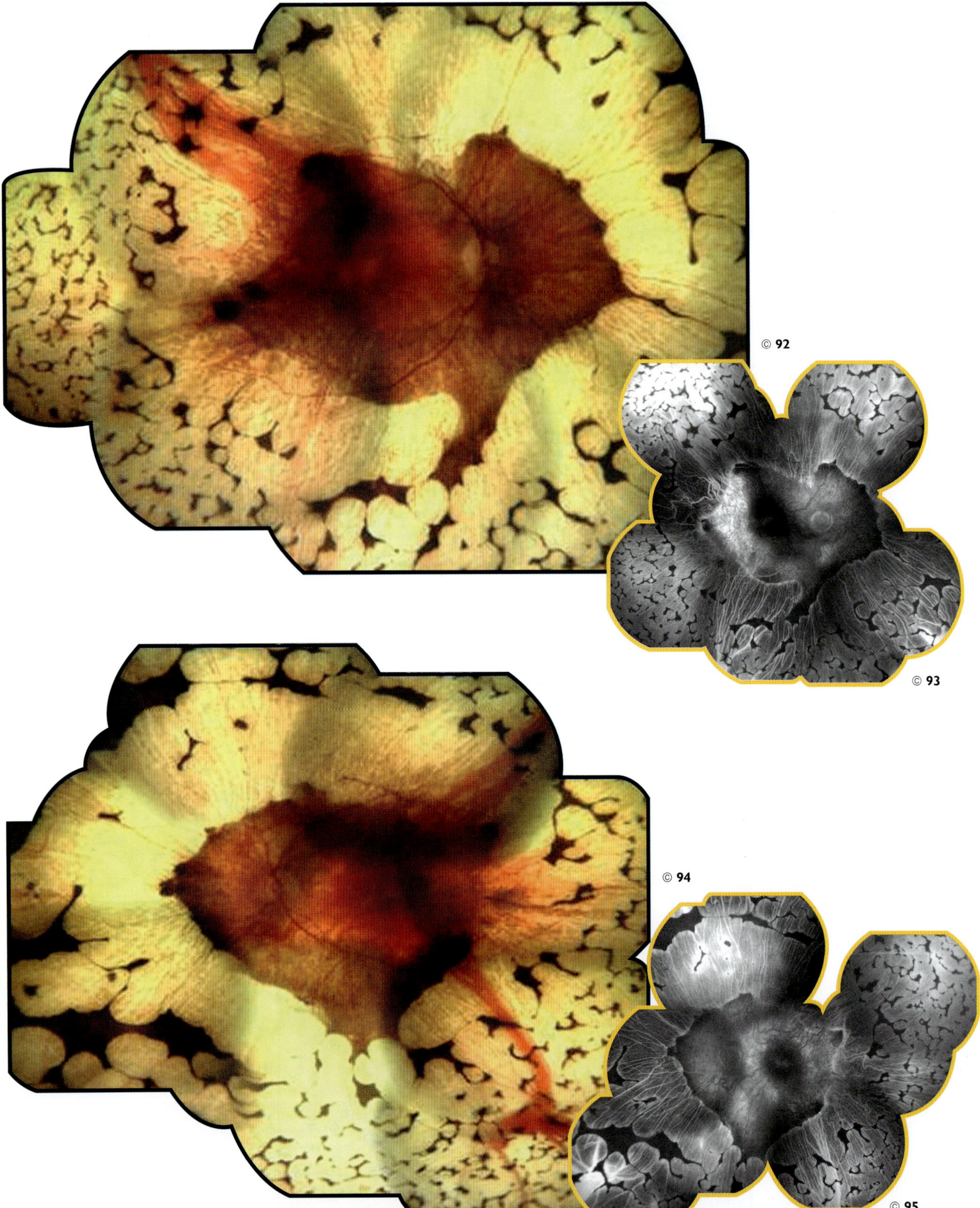

This patient with gyrate atrophy has islands of preserved RPE within the well-demarcated atrophic zones peripherally. There is also some pigment epithelial hyperplasia. This patient also has angiographic cystoid macular edema in both eyes.

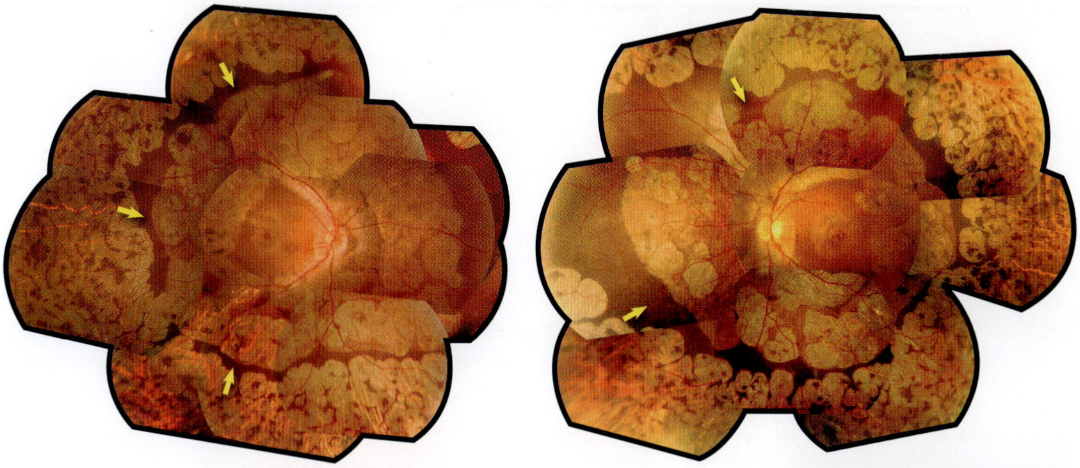

In this patient with gyrate atrophy, note the relative preservation *(arrows)* of RPE in the midperipheral fundus as the atrophic process expands posteriorly and anteriorly. *Courtesy of Dr. Ketan Laud*

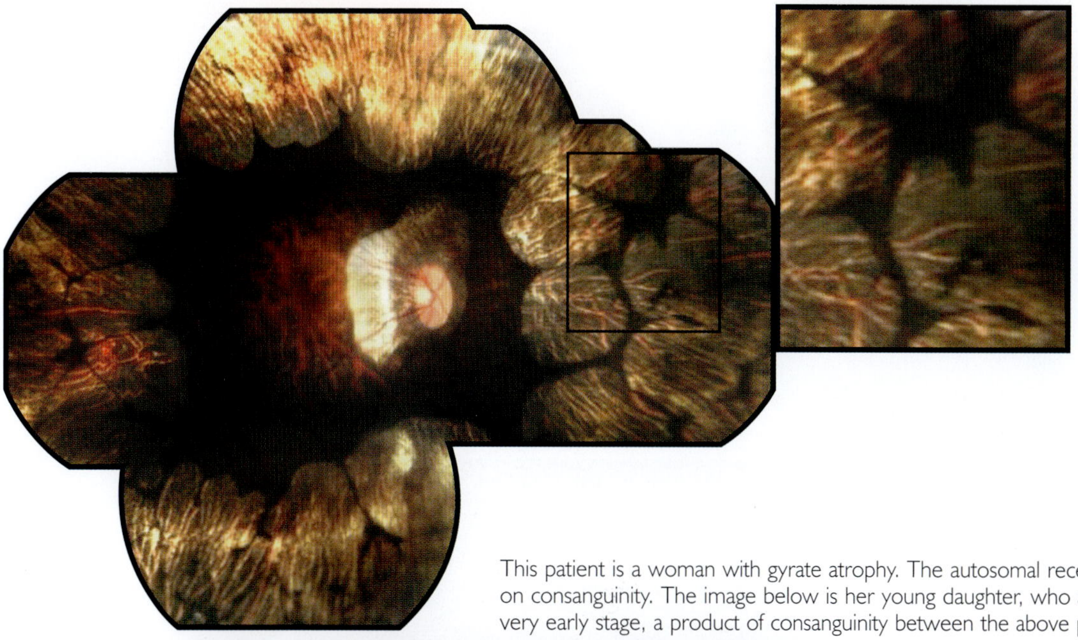

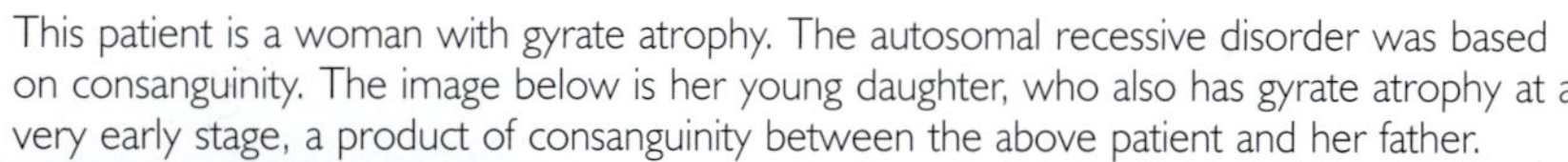
This patient is a woman with gyrate atrophy. The autosomal recessive disorder was based on consanguinity. The image below is her young daughter, who also has gyrate atrophy at a very early stage, a product of consanguinity between the above patient and her father.

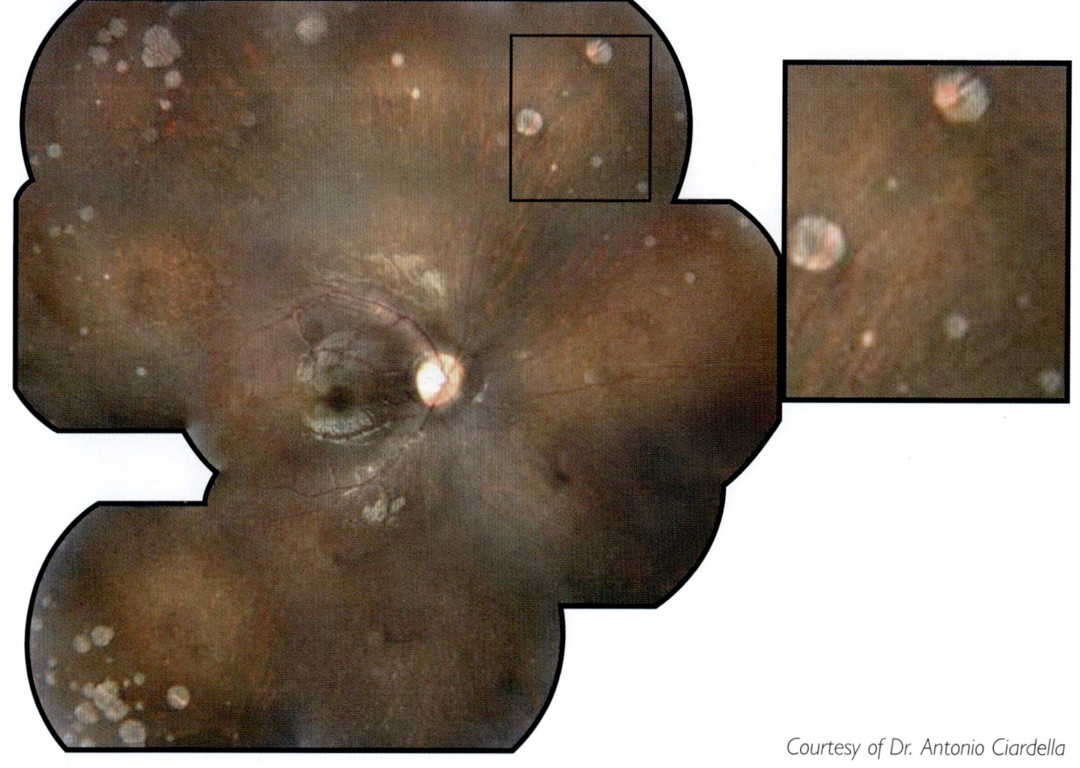

Courtesy of Dr. Antonio Ciardella

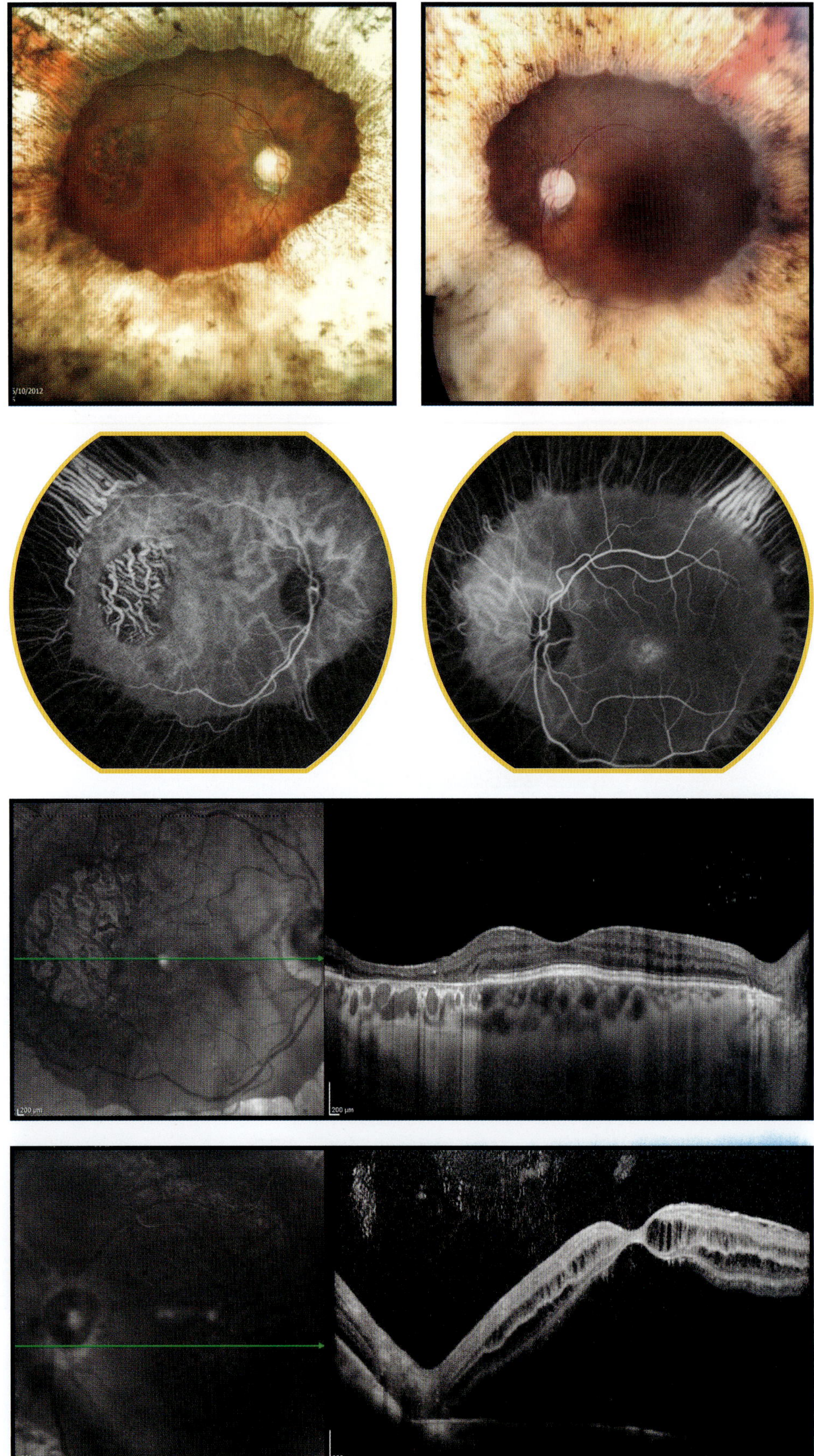

Color photo, fluorescein angiogram, and SD-OCT of a patient with gyrate atrophy who developed nasal retinal schisis and posterior retinal detachment of the left eye. *Images courtesy of Mark W. Johnson, MD*

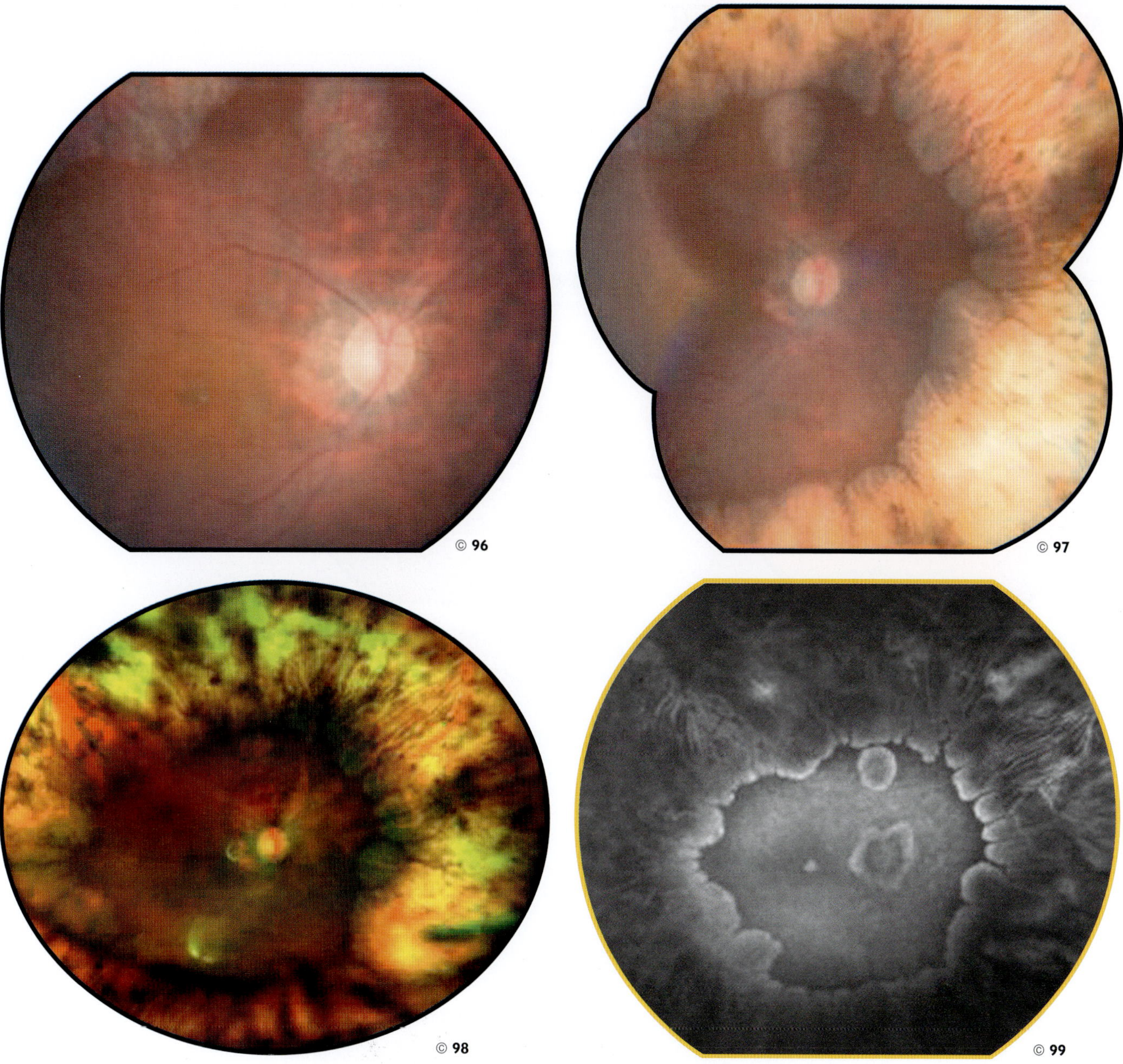

Color fundus photo, color montage, widefield color photo, and fluorescein angiogram of a patient with advanced gyrate atrophy.

Late-Onset Retinal Dystrophy (LORD)

While late-onset retinal dystrophy may begin with RPE mottling and drusenoid deposition in the posterior pole and periphery, in the advanced stages widespread chorioretinal atrophy most marked in the periphery is noted. Some patients experience a late onset of the disease. Associated ocular findings include elongated spindles extending from the ciliary body to the central position on the lens capsule, best appreciated with transillumination. The inheritance pattern is usually autosomal dominant and linked to mutation in the C1QTNF5 gene on chromosome 11.

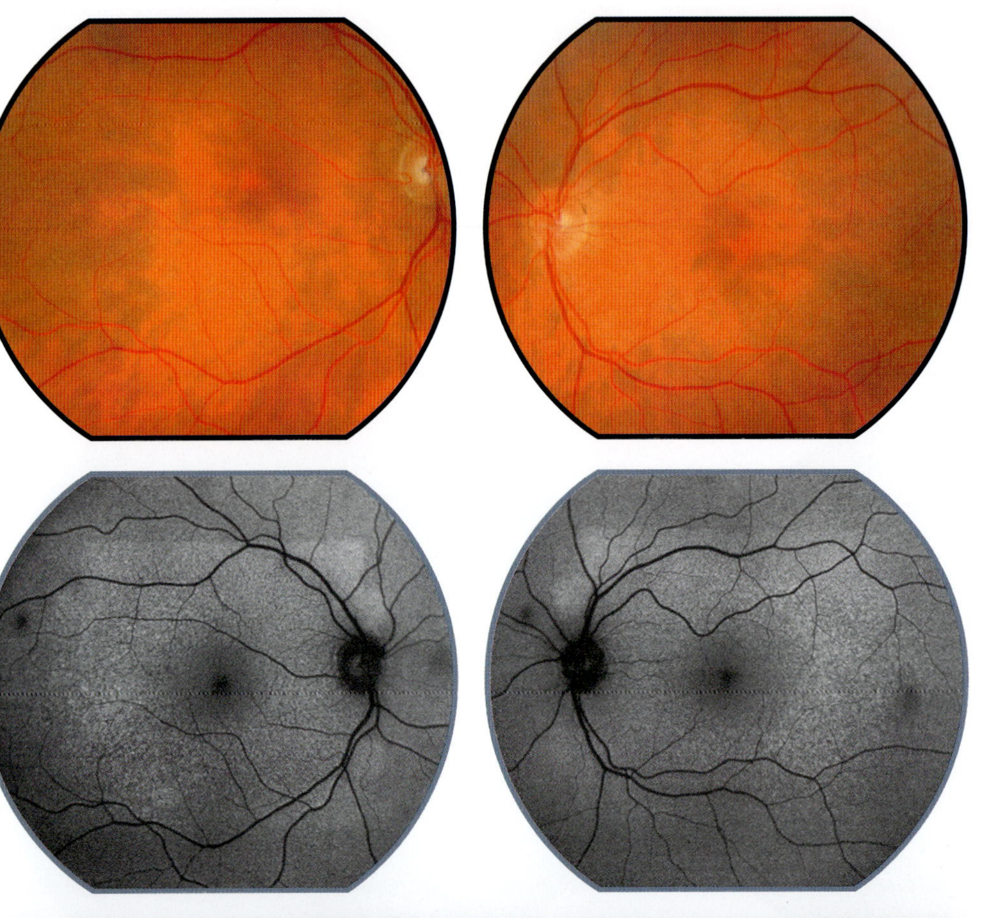

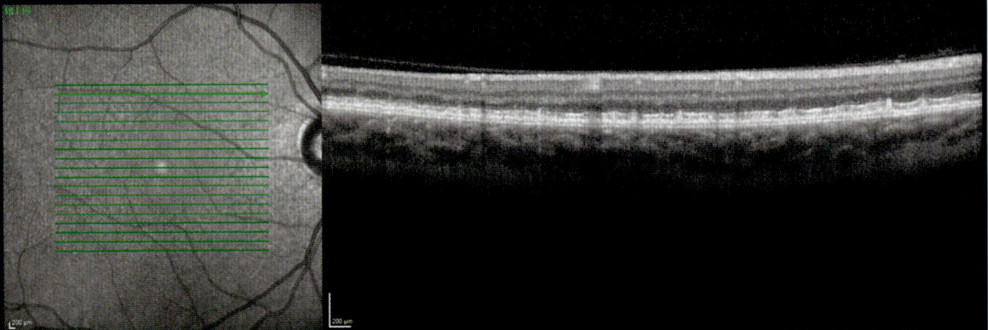

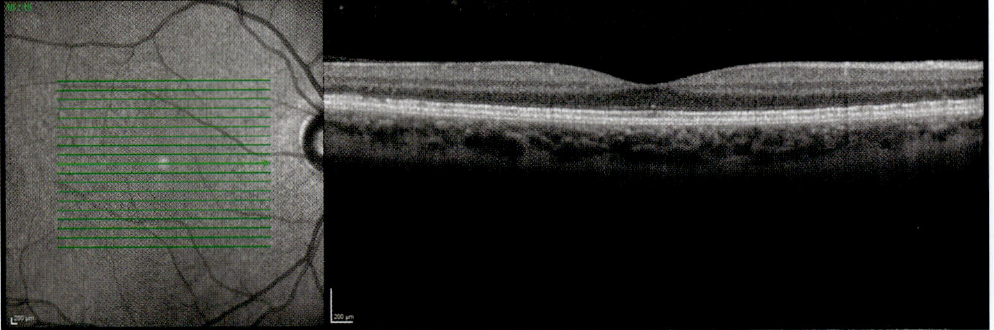

Some patients with LORD may develop reticular drusen-like deposits in the macula in early stages of the disease. These are highlighted by autofluorescence and SD-OCT. *Images courtesy of Alan Bird, MD*

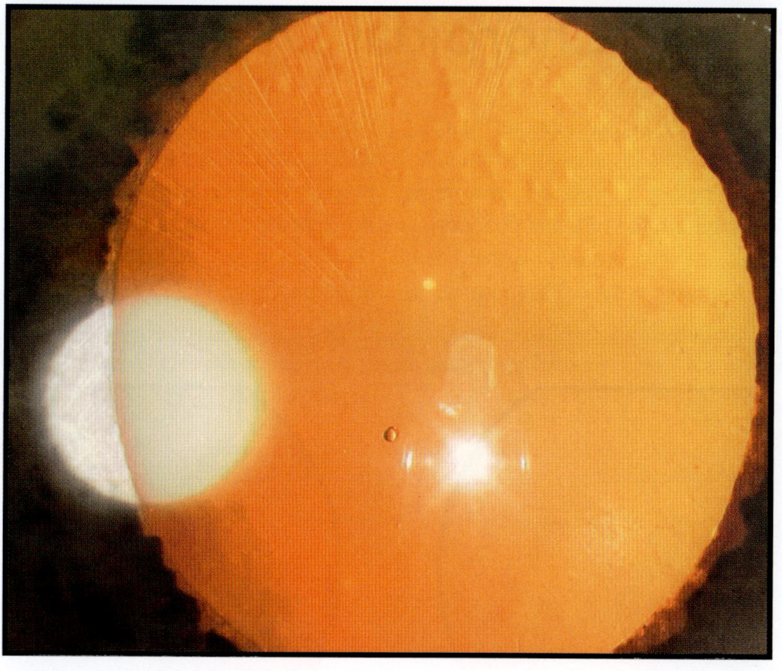

Retroillumination from the same patient with LORD reveals elongated zonules with central lens insertion and iris atrophy. *Photos courtesy of Alan Bird, MD*

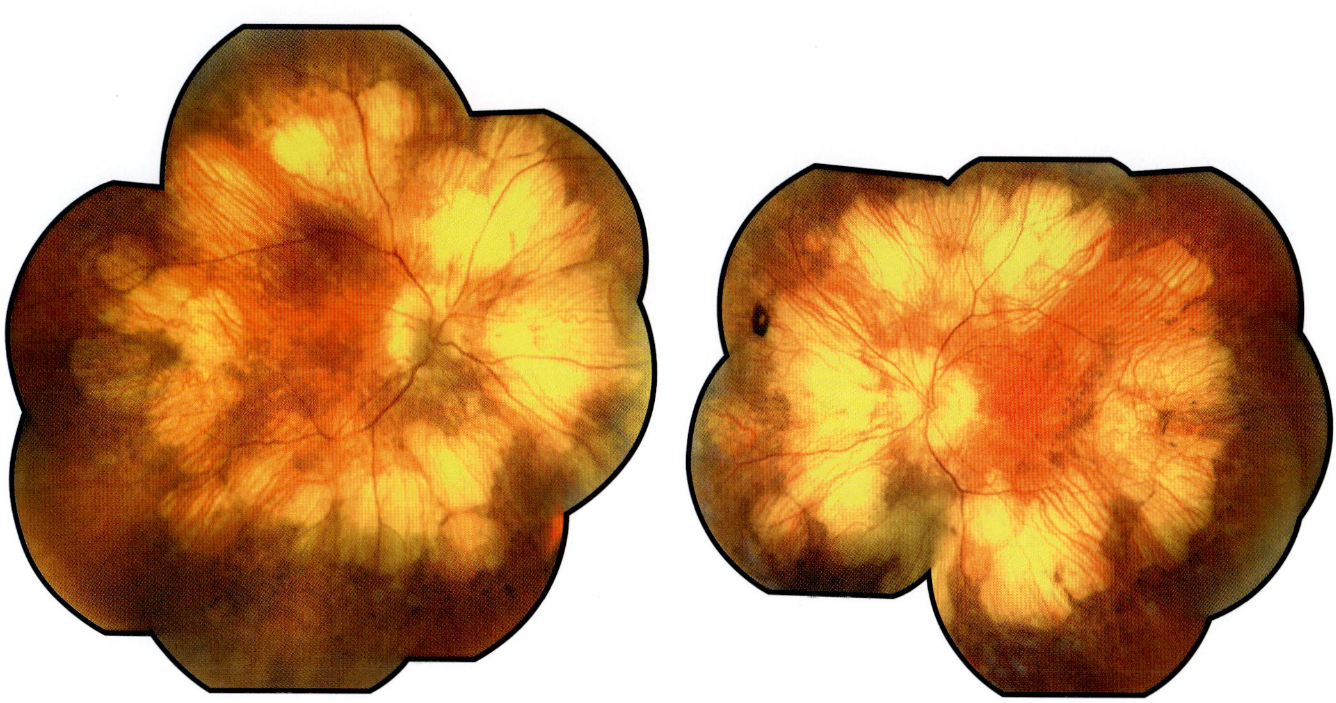

In later stages, as in this second patient with LORD, a characteristic scalloped peripheral chorioretinal degeneration develops. *Photos courtesy of Edwin Ryan, MD*

Central Areolar Choroidal Dystrophy (CACD)

Central areolar choroidal dystrophy (CACD) is an inherited macular dystrophy which begins with non-specific foveal pigment granularity that progresses into well-defined and bilaterally symmetric central regions of atrophy involving both the RPE and choriocapillaris. The large choroidal vessels are well visualized within these areas due to atrophy of the overlying tissues. The absence of drusen and flecks distinguishes CACD from other maculopathies which produce central geographic atrophy such as age related macular degeneration and Stargardt disease. It is often autosomal dominant and most frequently linked to mutation in the peripherin-2 (PRPH2) gene, although mutations at other loci have been described (e.g., GUCY2D).

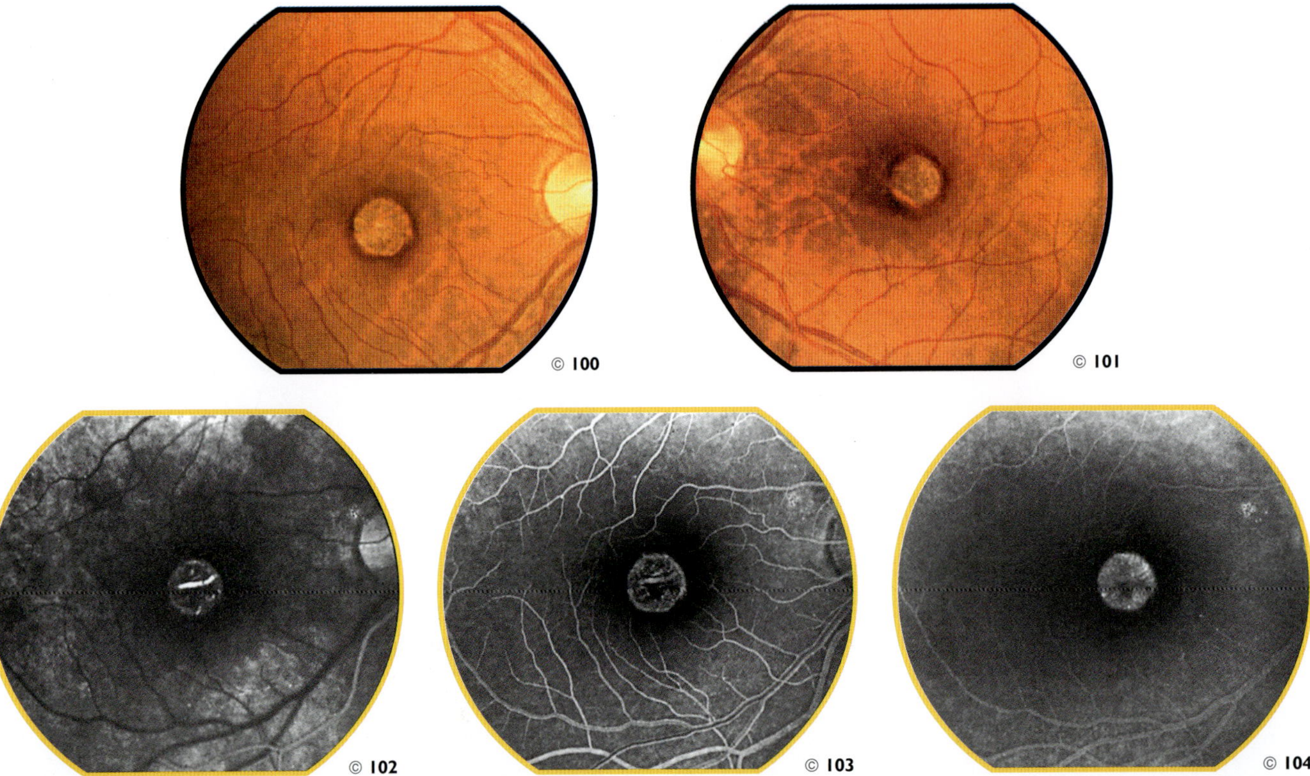

This patient with central areolar choroidal dystrophy has a bilateral symmetric loss of the RPE and choriocapillaris in the foveal region. Note the fluorescein angiogram that shows a well circumscribed geographic window defect early with late staining due to central atrophy. The very late angiogram shows staining of visible sclera and the silhouette of larger choroidal vessels. There is no leakage into the extrachoroidal tissue because of the absence of the choriocapillaris.

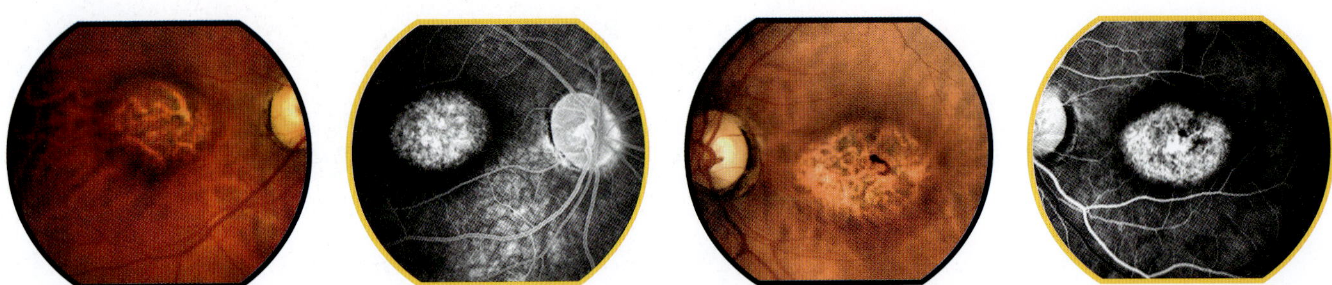

This patient with central areolar choroidal dystrophy has a larger, ovoid, symmetrical atrophic maculopathy.

Posterior Polar Central Choroidal Dystrophy

Posterior polar central choroidal dystrophy is a more extensive atrophic abnormality of the choroid that involves the posterior pole within the vascular arcades. Atrophy may even extend outside of the arcades and surround the optic nerve.

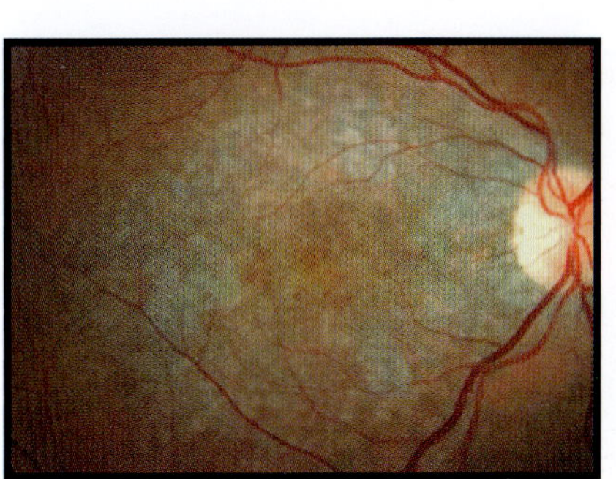

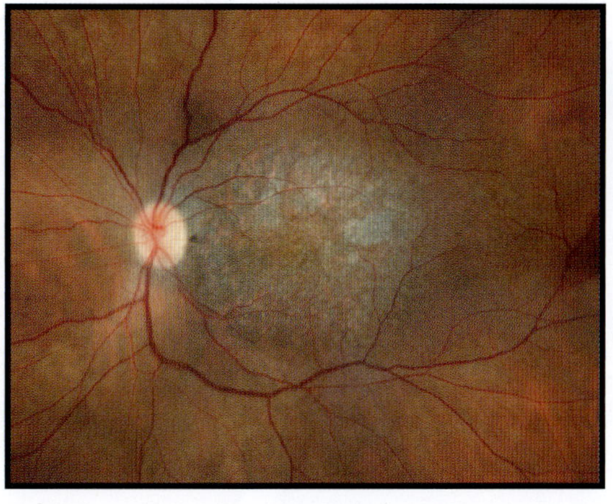

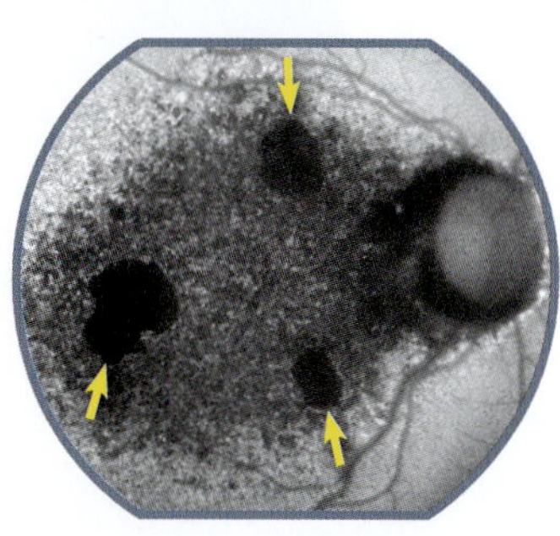

This patient with posterior polar central choroidal dystrophy has a large atrophic, ovoid zone of pigment epithelial atrophy. There are multiple areas of more pronounced atrophy, which include the choriocapillaris within the ovoid zone. These atrophic areas are more clearly evident on the fundus autofluorescence image where patchy areas of hypoautofluorescence are present *(arrows)*.

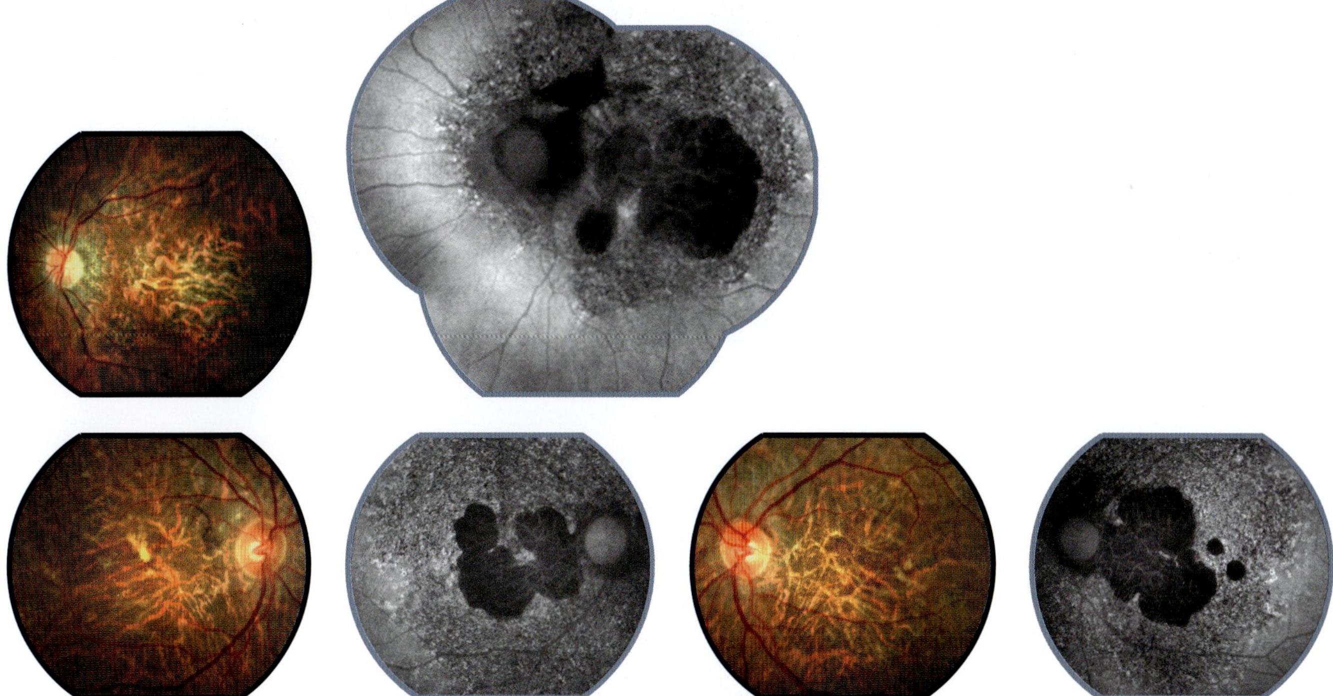

Posterior polar central choroidal dystrophy may start as a focal degenerative process in the central macula, but the area of atrophy may expand. At first, there may be patchy or zonal atrophy, followed by confluency as the entire process expands to the temporal vascular arcades and the disc and beyond.

Posterior Polar Annular Choroidal Dystrophy

Posterior polar annular choroidal dystrophy is a peculiar atrophy of the posterior segment that surrounds the vascular arcades and optic nerve.

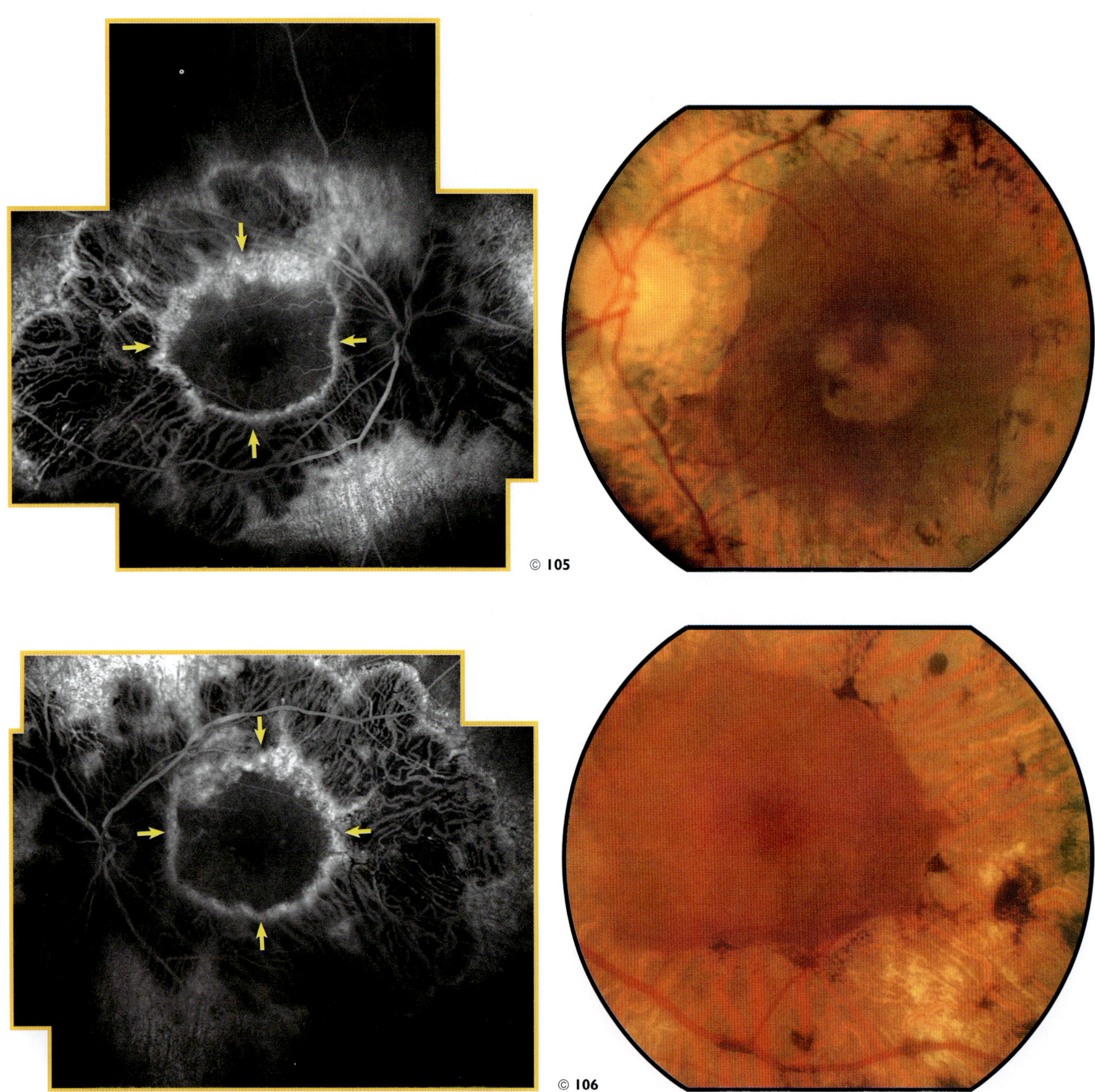

Posterior polar annular choroidal dystrophy may be associated with progressive chorioretinal atrophy surrounding the optic disc and vascular arcades, as in this patient. A fringe or ring of preserved hyperfluorescent choriocapillaris beneath atrophic RPE may be seen in the central macula *(arrows)*. The annular zone of atrophy has scalloped and indistinct margins, again with some preservation of the choriocapillaris at the junction with the normal choroid. *Courtesy of Drs Ron Carr and Ken Noble*

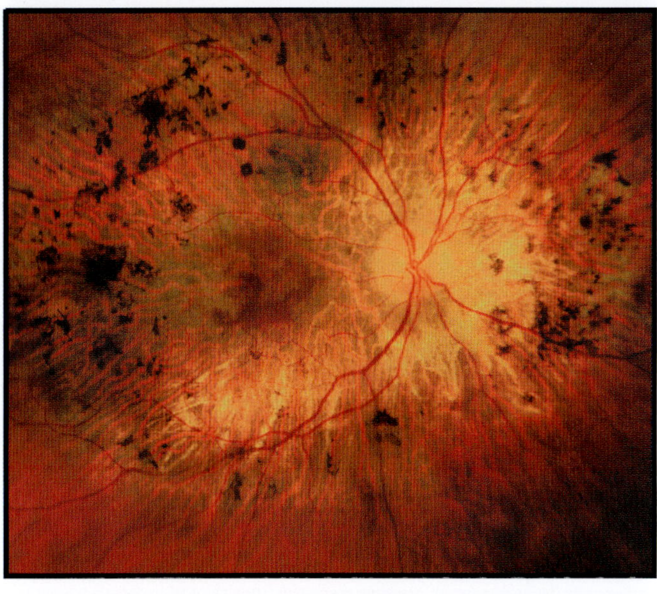
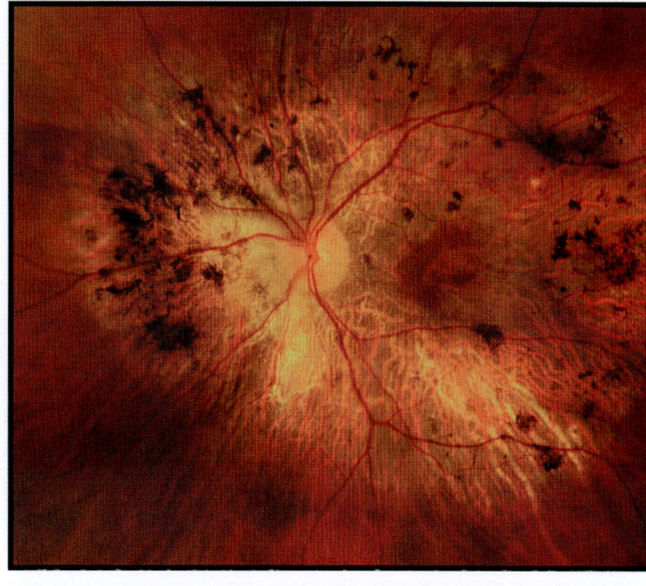

This patient with posterior polar annular choroidal dystrophy has a huge zonal area of atrophy with dense multifocal pigmentation. There is relative preservation of the immediate perifoveal area.

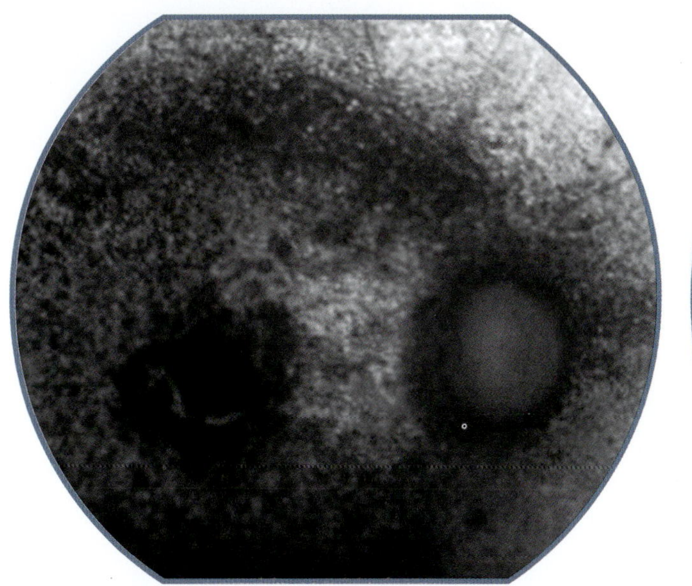
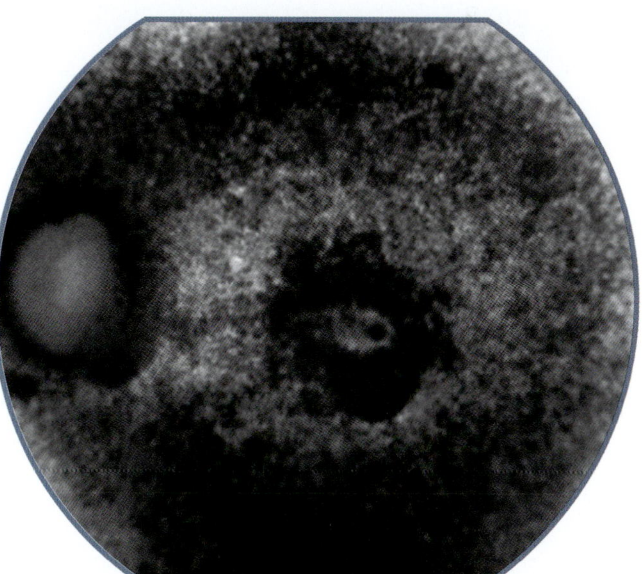

Posterior polar annular choroidal dystrophy may progress in some patients. The fundus autofluorescence images show extensive loss of the RPE and choriocapillaris which now extends to the near periphery and beyond.

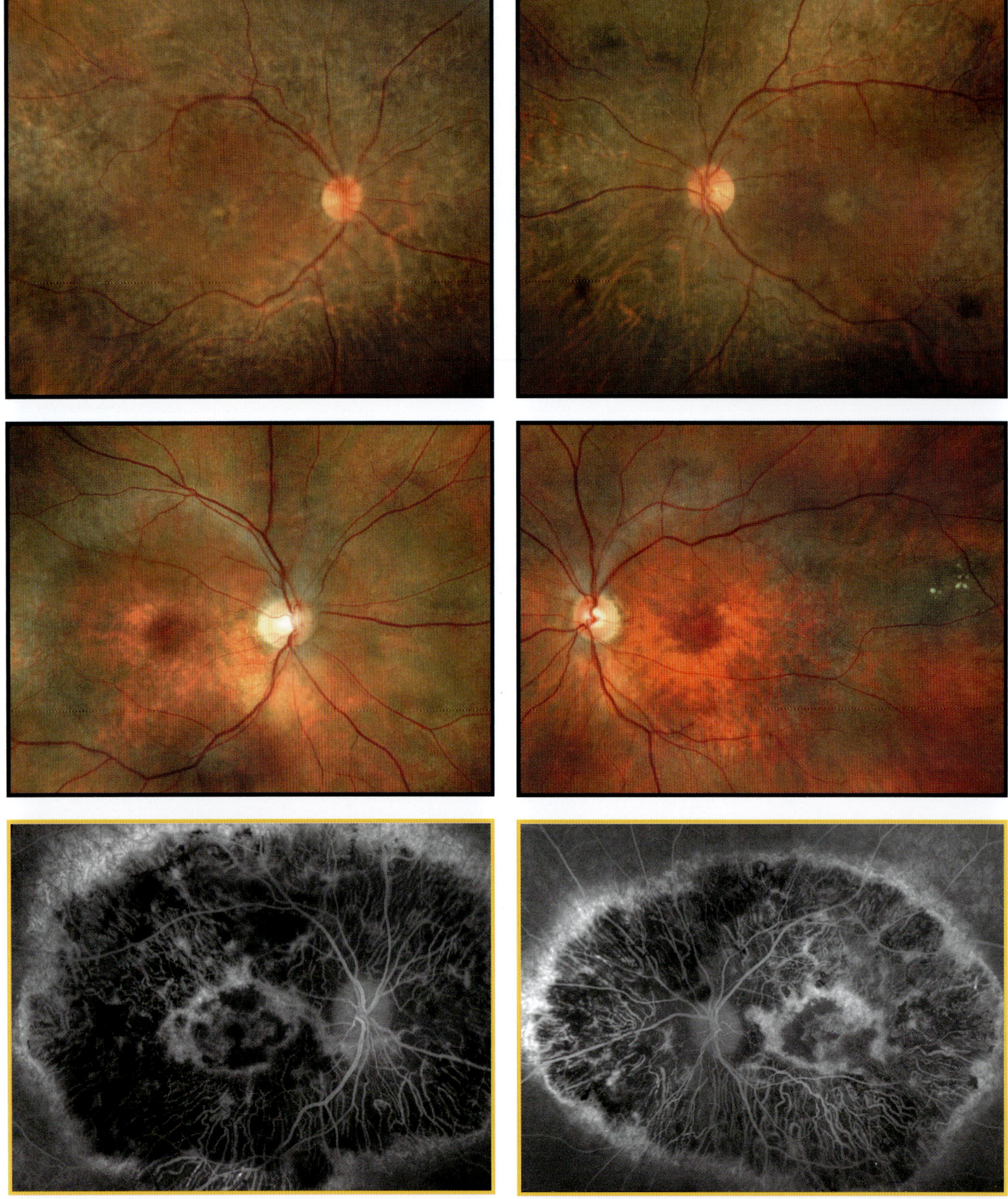

These two patients have posterior polar annular choroidal dystrophy. Note the ring of atrophy surrounding the posterior pole and the disc. Evidence of central macular atrophy is also present. The fluorescein angiogram again shows a fringe of choriocapillaris hyperfluorescence concentric to the posterior pole and central macular region.

Posterior Polar Hemispheric Choroidal Dystrophy

In posterior polar hemispheric choroidal dystrophy, the atrophic changes in the choroid involve half of the posterior segment, from the juxtafoveal area beyond the vascular arcade.

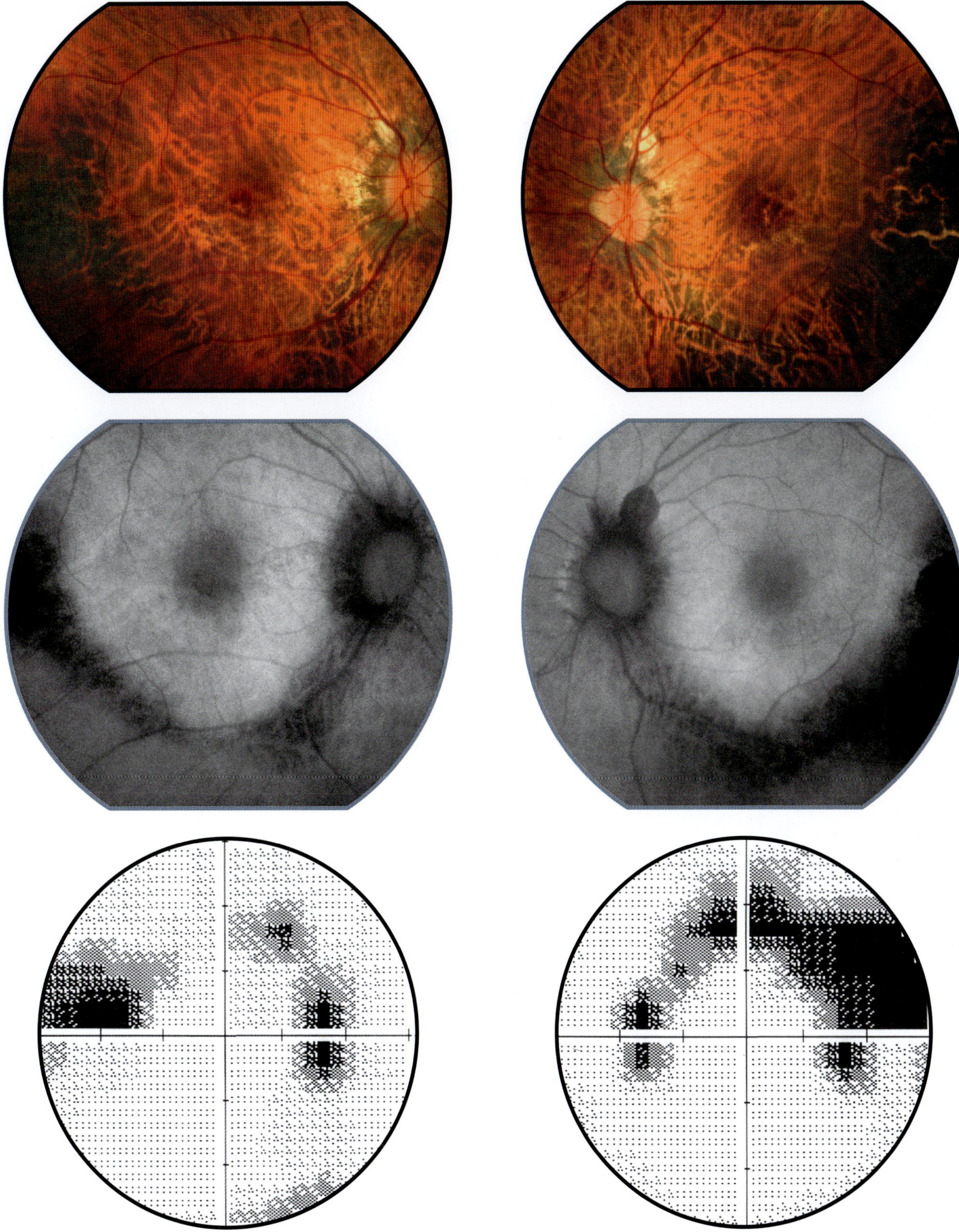

In this choroidal dystrophy, there is annular, hemispheric loss of pigment epithelium and choriocapillaris inferiorly, which is highlighted with the fundus autofluorescence images. There is field loss superiorly, which corresponds to the choroidal atrophy. *Courtesy of Dr. Richard Spaide*

Central and Peripheral Annular Choroidal Dystrophy

This very rare choroidal dystrophy is notable for central macular atrophy associated with a broad well-circumscribed ring of pigmentary and atrophic changes in the peripheral fundus.

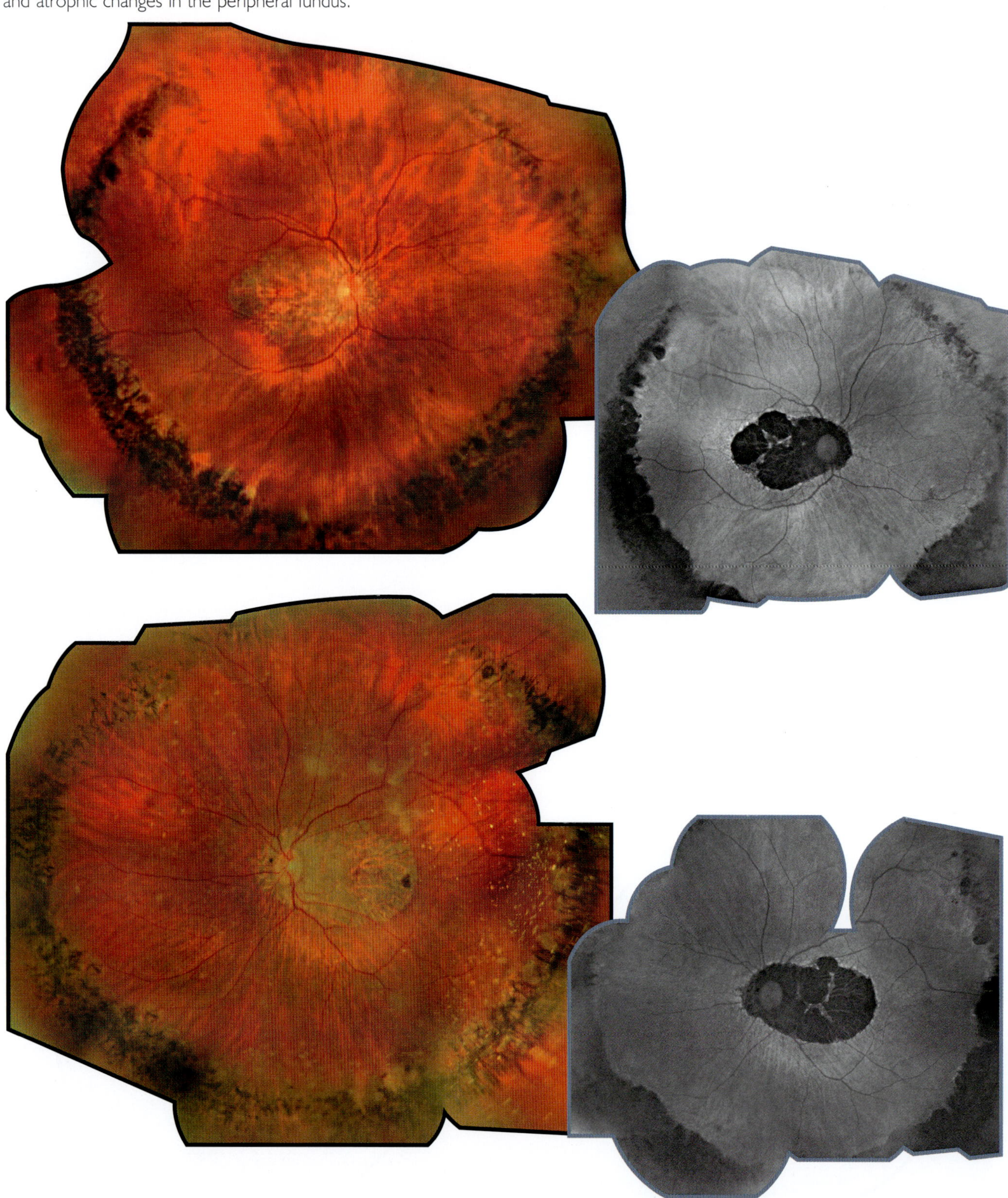

This patient has a bilateral and symmetrical central choroidal dystrophy in association with a far-peripheral annular choroidal dystrophy, which is bilateral and symmetrical. The fundus autofluorescence reveals hypoautofluorescence in areas of chorioretinal atrophy with islands of sparing in the central macula where there is preserved pigment epithelium.

This group of disorders is characterized by genetically driven inborn errors in metabolism leading to crystalline refractile deposits within the retina and in certain cases within other ocular tissues. They are all associated with systemic manifestations, most frequently renal disorders.

Bietti Crystalline Corneoretinal Dystrophy (BCD, Bietti Crystalline Retinopathy, Bietti Crystalline Tapetoretinal Dystrophy)

Bietti crystalline corneoretinal dystrophy is a rare, autosomal recessive disorder caused by mutation in the CYP4V2 gene on chromosome 4q35.1. It is characterized by numerous glistening, yellow, crystalline deposits distributed throughout the fundus and, in some cases, the superficial cornea near the limbus and the lens capsule. Patients may develop progressive nyctalopia, constriction of visual fields and decreased visual acuity progressing to legal blindness in the sixth decade. Fundus examination reveals crystalline deposits and geographic areas of RPE and choriocapillaris atrophy beginning and predominating in the posterior pole. The crystals are more prominent in the areas of preserved RPE, but they can be found anywhere in the fundus. SD-OCT reveals hyper-reflective deposits at the level of Bruch membrane corresponding to the retinal crystals in addition to areas of outer retinal atrophy and outer retinal tubulation. The disorder is more common in East Asia, in particular China and Japan.

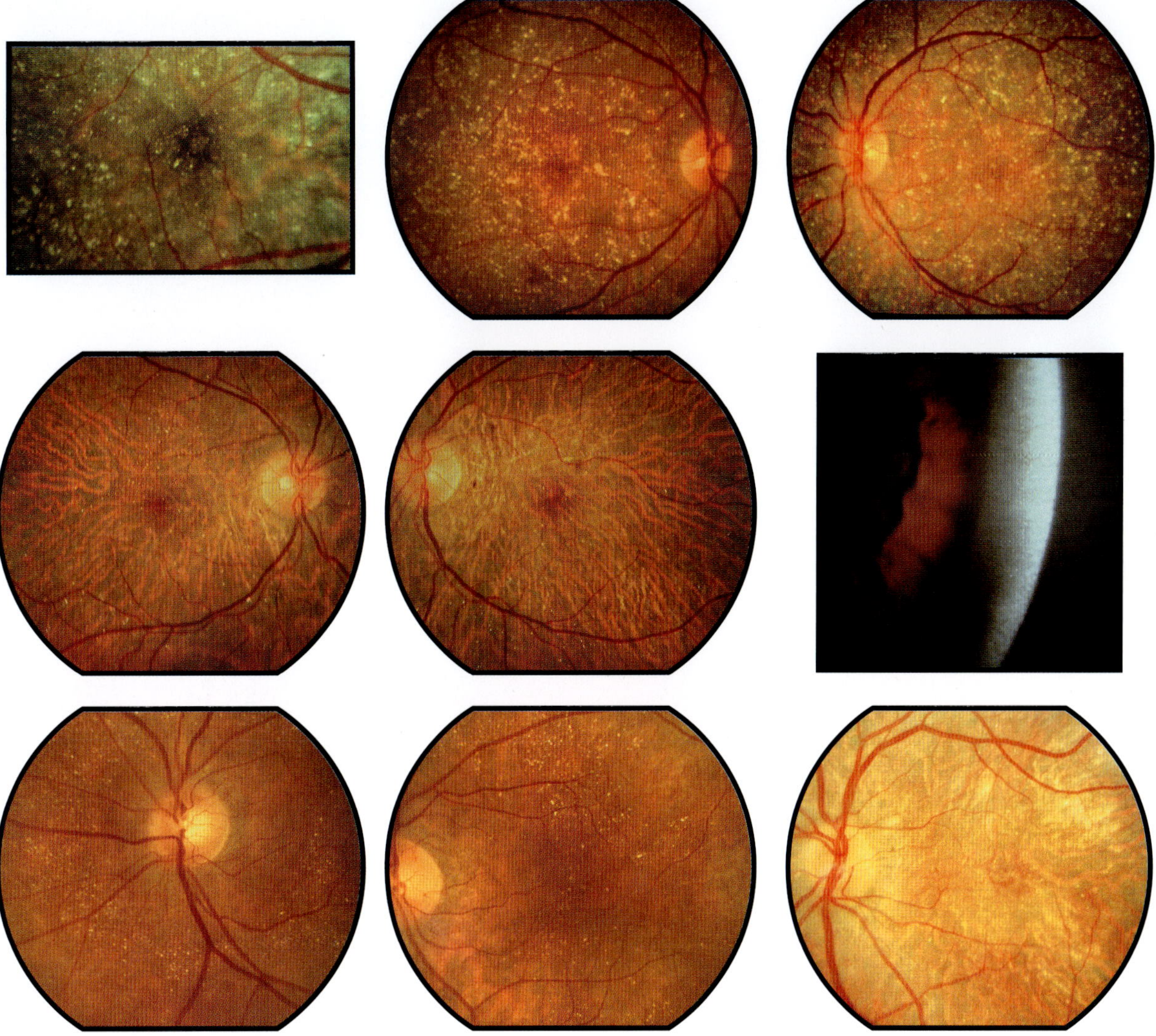

Clinical manifestations of Bietti crystalline corneoretinal dystrophy are seen in these images. There are crystalline deposits in the posterior segment and in the periphery. As RPE/choriocapillaris atrophy evolves in later stages of the disease, the crystalline deposits are not as evident *(lower right image Courtesy of Dr. Irene Maumenee)*. Crystalline deposition in the cornea is usually in the middle stroma near the limbus. *Courtesy of Dr. Jose Pulido*

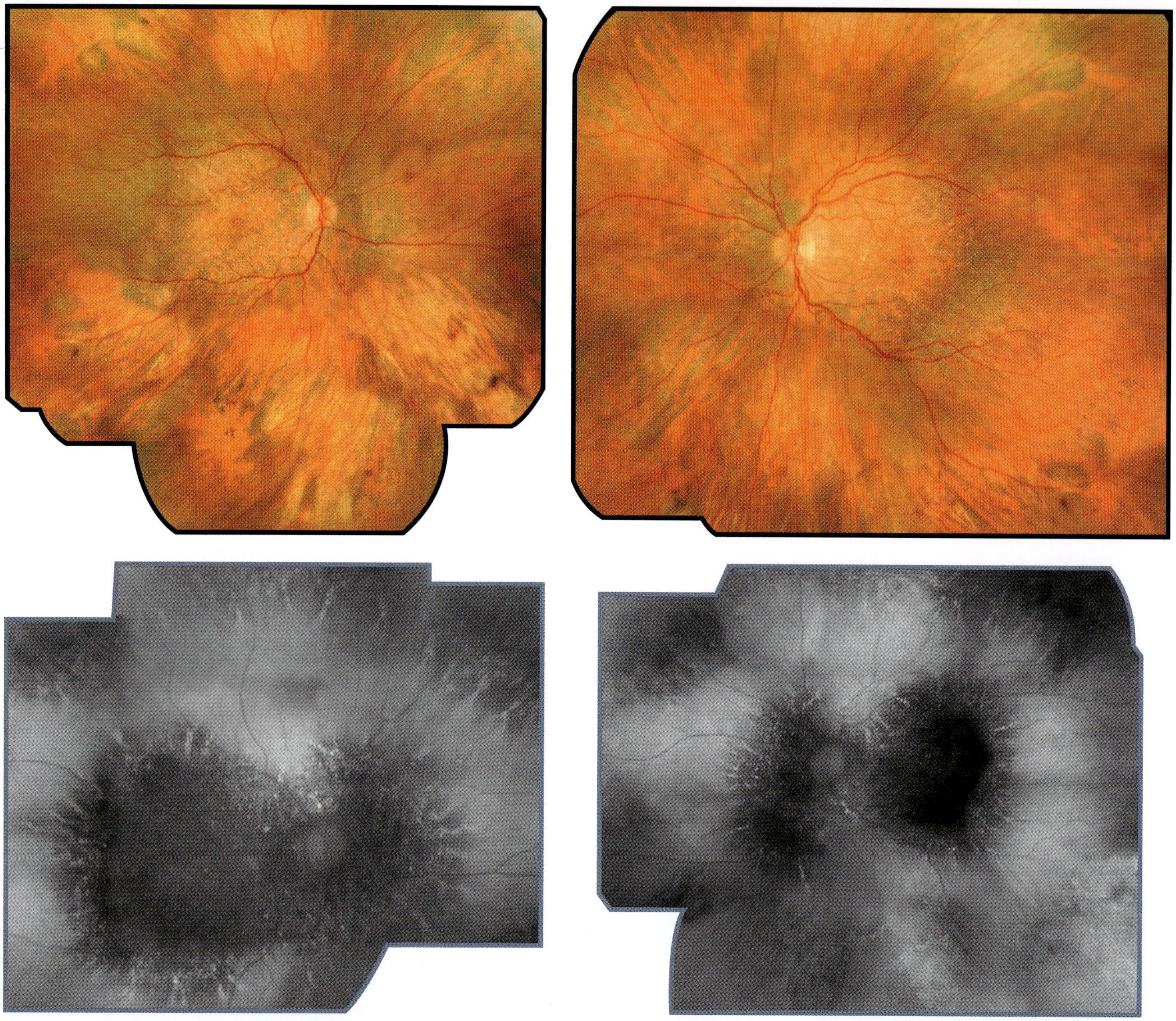

In this patient with Bietti crystalline corneoretinal dystrophy, there are zonal areas of atrophy (and pigment hyperplasia) in the posterior pole and periphery. Fundus autofluorescence demonstrates the atrophic zones more prominently. At its margins are flares of hyperautofluorescence that may represent RPE hypertrophy.

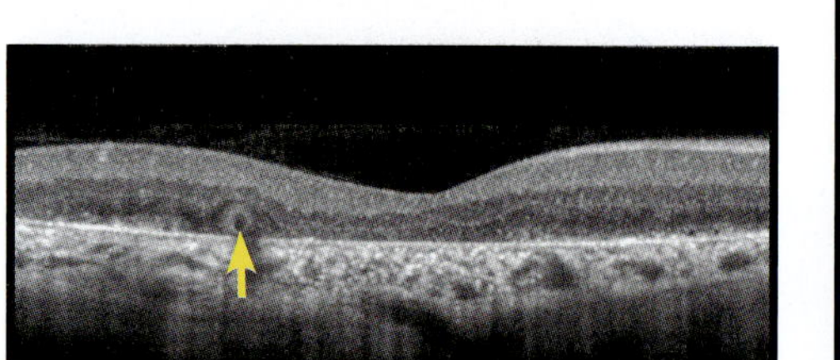

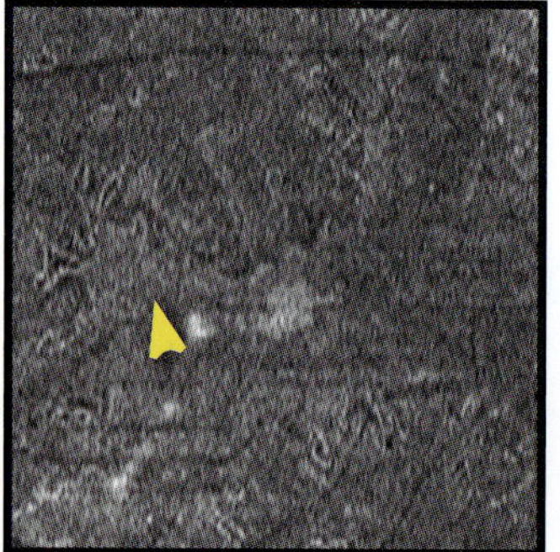

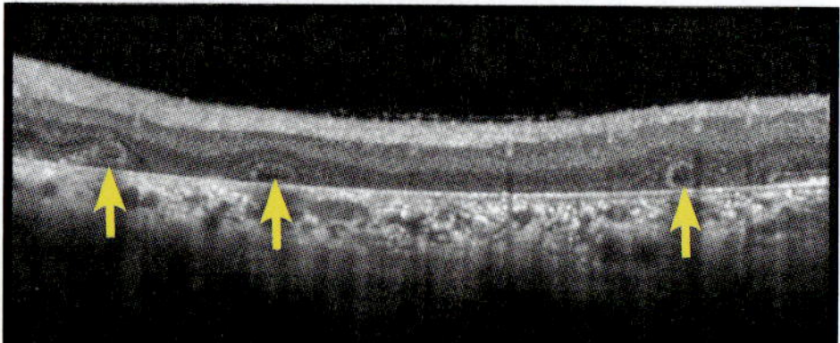

The OCT images from each eye show areas of outer retinal tubular degeneration *(arrows)* associated with diffuse outer macular atrophy. With *en face* OCT, areas of circular and ovoid tubular degeneration are also evident *(arrowhead)*.

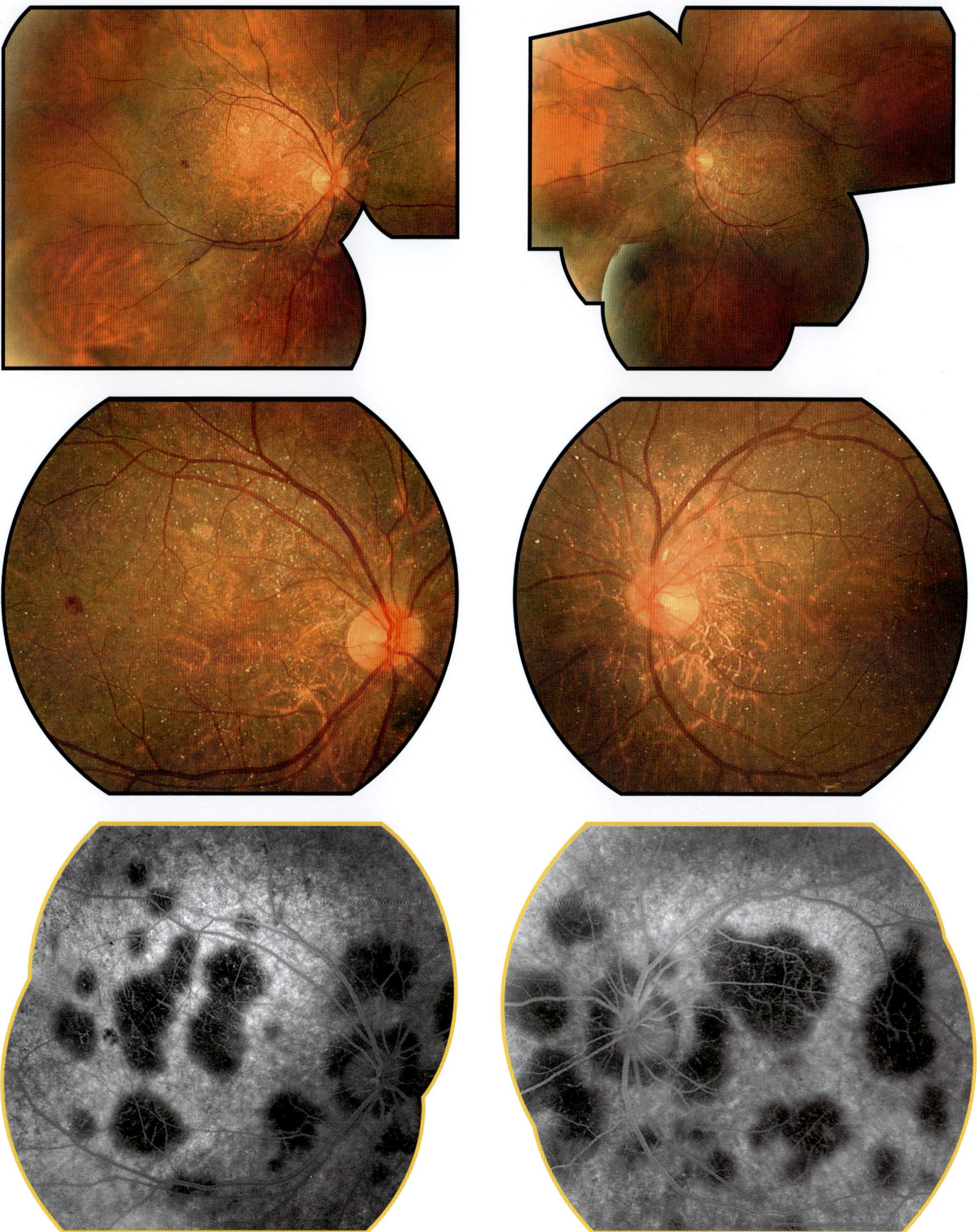

In this patient with Bietti crystalline corneoretinal dystrophy, there are prominent crystals throughout the fundus that are present within and outside the areas of RPE and choroidal atrophy. *Courtesy of Dr. Ketan Laud*

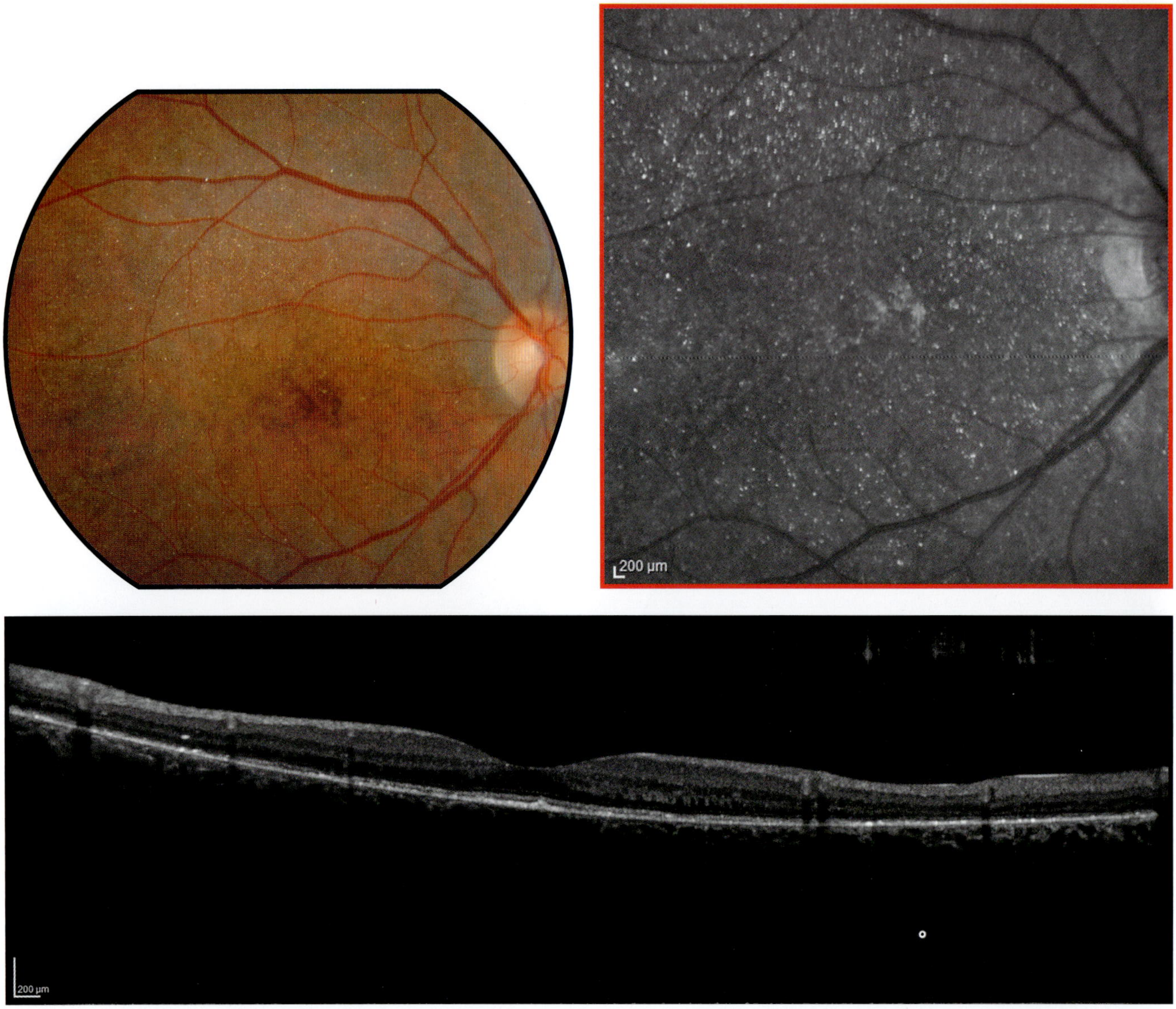

Fundus photo of a patient with Bietti crystalline corneoretinal dystrophy shows crystalline deposits which are highlighted on infrared imaging and can be seen as hyper-reflective deposits on SD-OCT. There is diffuse paramacular ellipsoid loss with SD-OCT. *Images courtesy of Eric Souied, MD*

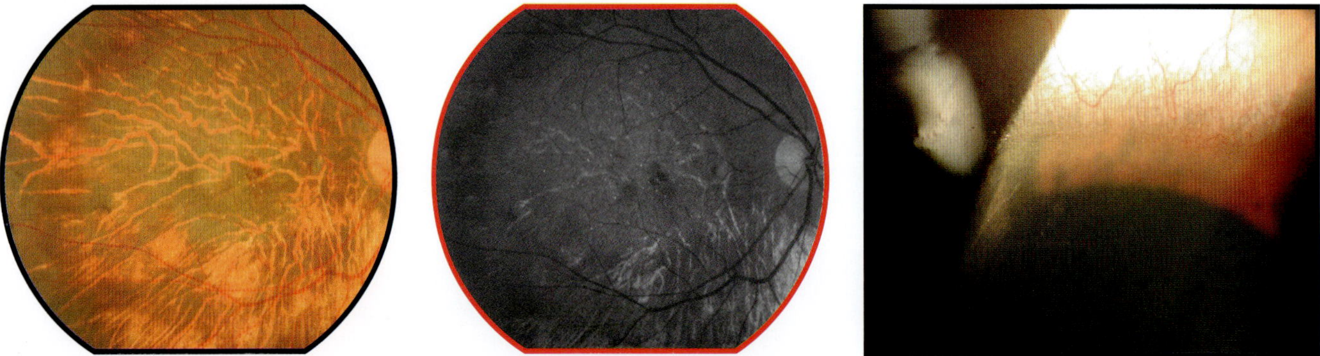

This patient with Bietti crystalline corneoretinal dystrophy has macular atrophy with crystal deposition seen on fundus photography and red-free imaging. The patient also had crystal deposits in the cornea seen here on slit lamp examination *(right)*. *Images courtesy of Eric Souied, MD*

Primary Hyperoxaluria

Primary hyperoxaluria is a rare inborn error of glyoxalate metabolism. There are two types: type I primary hyperoxaluria is caused by a mutation in the gene encoding alanine-glyoxylate aminotransferase (AGXT) located on chromosome 2q36 and type II primary hyperoxaluria is caused by mutation in the glyoxylate reductase/hydroxypyruvate reductase gene (GRHPR) located on chromosome 9cen. This disorder is characterized by continuous, high urinary oxalate excretion with progressive bilateral oxalate urolithiasis, nephrocalcinosis, and chronic renal failure in childhood or early adulthood. Type II is a milder disease and has mostly renal manifestations with no associated ocular findings. In later stages of type I disease, extrarenal deposition of oxalate crystals occurs. Approximately 30% of patients develop a crystalline retinopathy with innumerable discrete yellow refractile flecks that are widely scattered throughout all layers of the retina and RPE and within the retinal vessels. Irregular dense clumps of hypertrophied and hyperplastic RPE as well as fibrous metaplasia, ranging from small ringlets to large geographic plaques, are seen in the macula. Visual acuity can be good even in the presence of advanced maculopathy. Optic atrophy is the most important cause of blindness in these patients. Arteriolar attenuation and secondary choroidal neovascularization may also be seen.

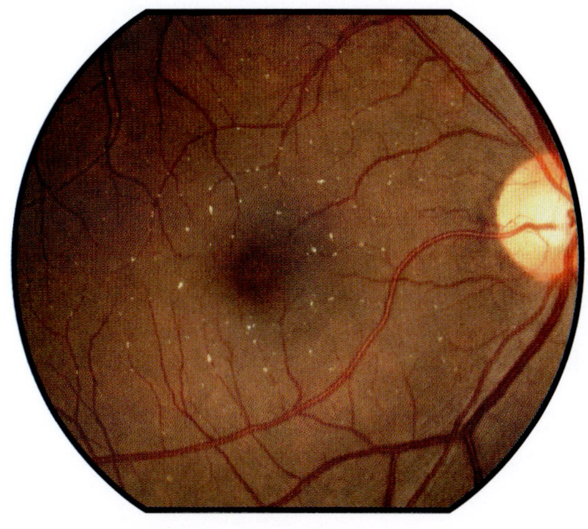
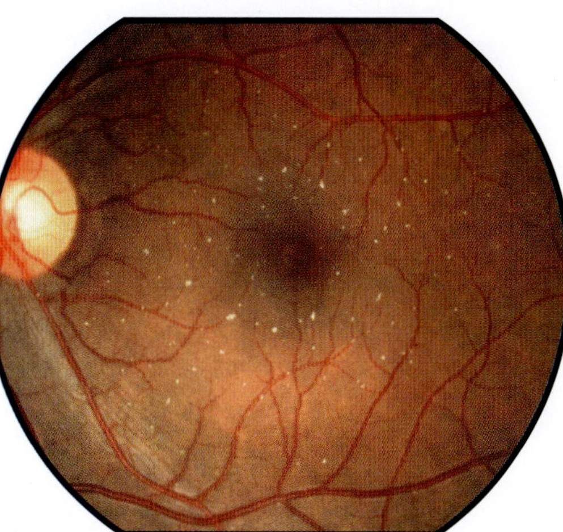

This patient has primary hyperoxaluria with crystalline deposits in the retina. *Courtesy of Michael P. Kelly, CRA*

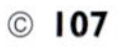
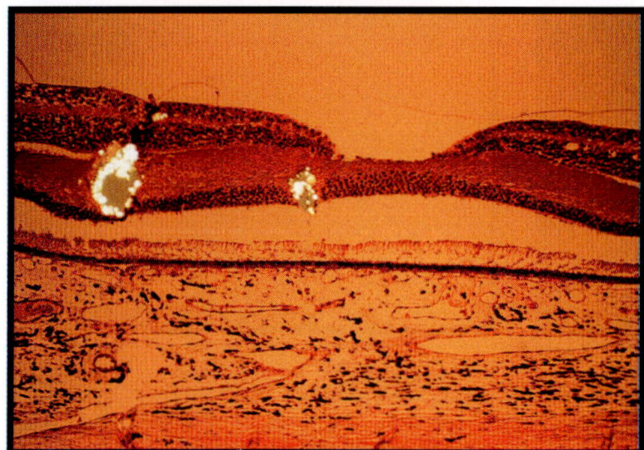
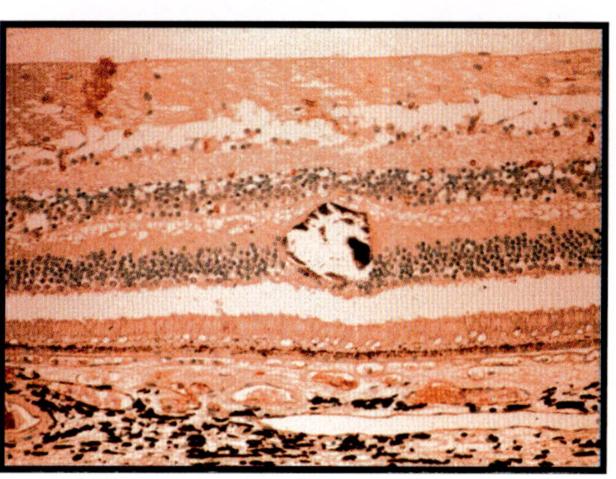

© 107

Oxalate crystals are seen on the histopathological sections within the retina.

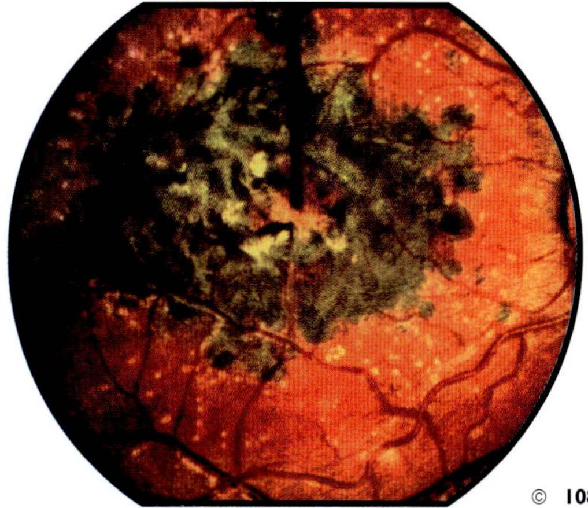

© 108

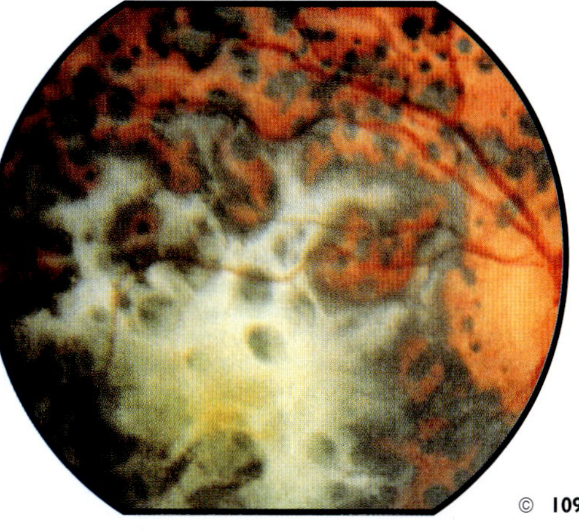

© 109

Primary hyperoxaluria may be associated with pigment epithelial hyperplasia and fibrous scarring, as seen in these two patients.

Cystinosis

Cystinosis is an inherited disorder caused by mutation on chromosome 17p13 in the gene encoding cystinosin, a protein involved in lysosomal cysteine transport. This results in the accumulation of the amino acid cysteine. Cystinosis has been classified as a lysosomal storage disorder on the basis of cytologic and intralysosomal localization of stored cysteine. These patients experience growth retardation, hyperthyroidism, renal tubular and glomerular dysfunction, and Fanconi syndrome, resulting in end stage renal disease requiring renal transplantation by 10 years of age. Abnormal crystals may be found in the conjunctiva, iris, and cornea with crystal deposition beginning in the peripheral superficial corneal stroma and subsequently involving central and deeper stroma. Symptoms of photophobia begin in early childhood. Yellowish mottling of the RPE in the macula with more marked degenerative changes in the periphery are characteristic of cystinosis. Fine yellow, refractile crystalline deposits may be observed on fundus exam in some patients. Histopathologically, intracellular crystals are seen within the RPE and choroid but not in the retina. Ocular non-nephropathic cystinosis, a variant of the classic nephropathic type of cystinosis is also inherited in an autosomal recessive pattern and caused by a mutation in the cystinosin gene. It is characterized by photophobia due to corneal cystine crystals, but does not result in renal disease. Treatment with oral cysteamine can lower tissue levels of cysteine and decrease renal and visual complications of the disease.

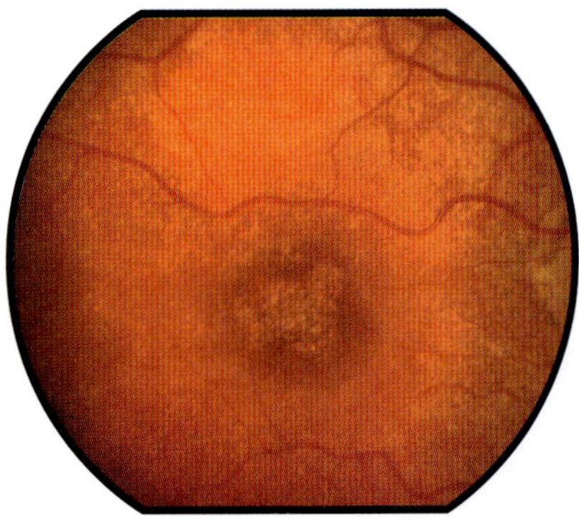
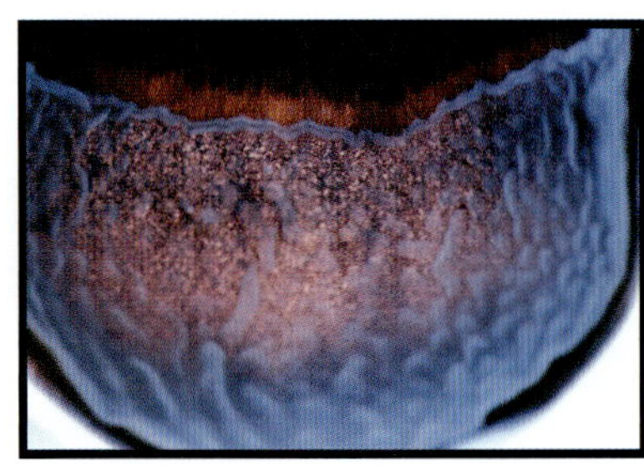
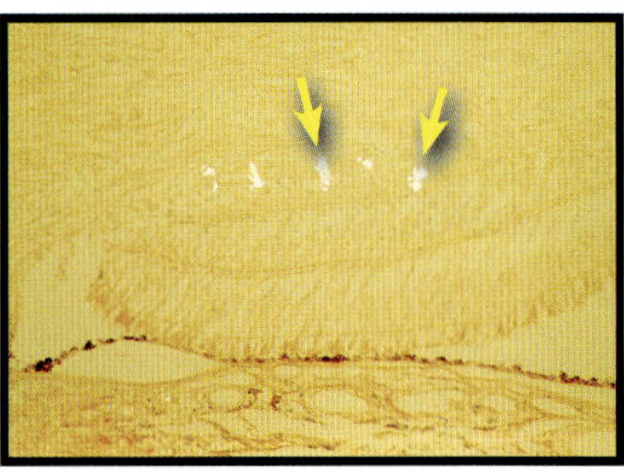

There are crystalline deposits and atrophy in the macular region of this patient with cystinosis. The histopathology shows a pigmentary degenerative change in the fundus with multiple small crystals in the retina *(arrows)*. *Middle and right images courtesy of Dr. V.G. Wong*

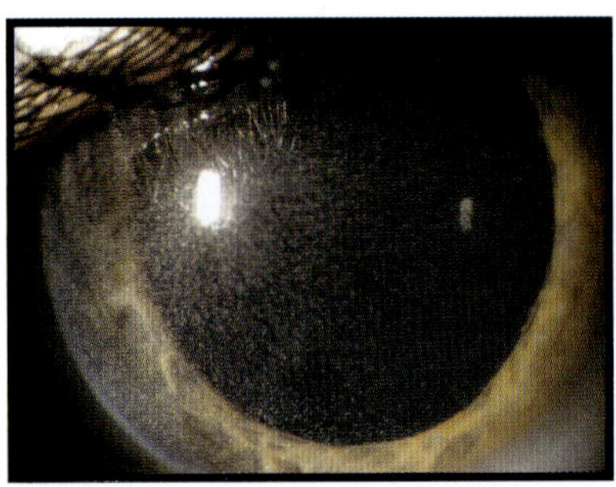
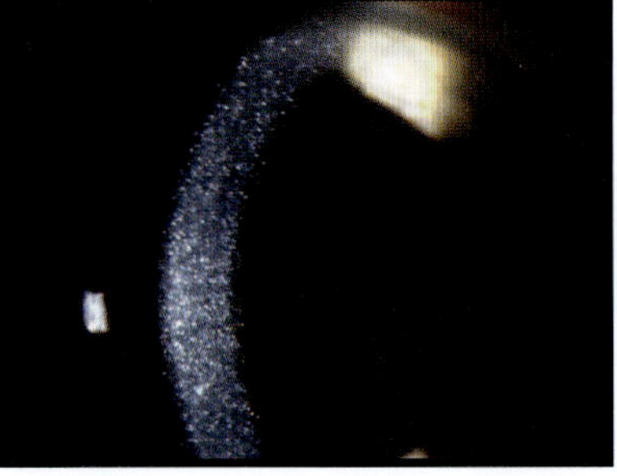
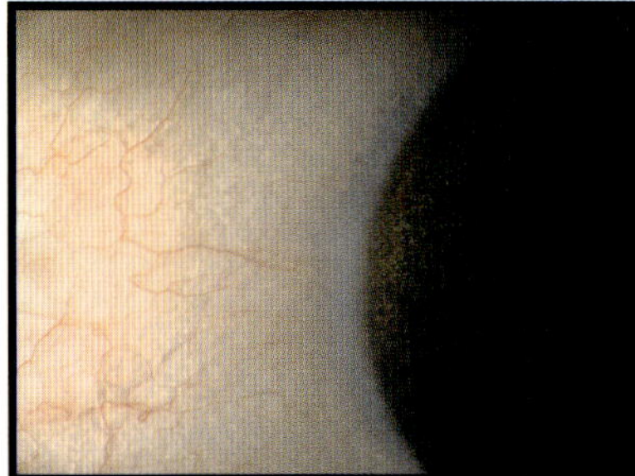

Crystals may be seen in the cornea, as well as the sclera in cystinosis.

In the late stage of cystinosis, pigmentary atrophic degeneration is present, and renal failure is common. The pigmentary degeneration in the peripheral fundus may exist without evidence of crystalline changes. *Courtesy of Dr. V.G. Wong*

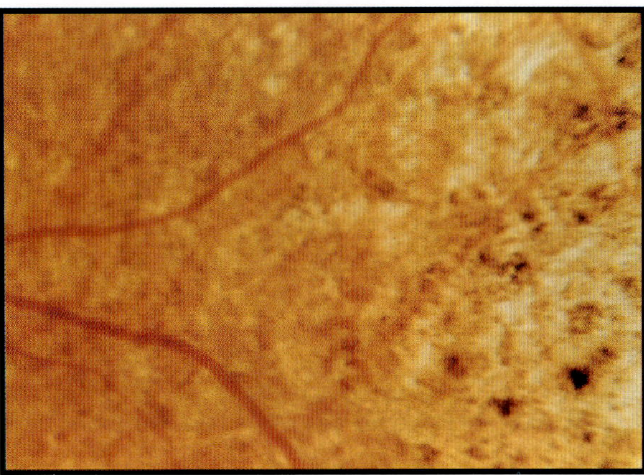
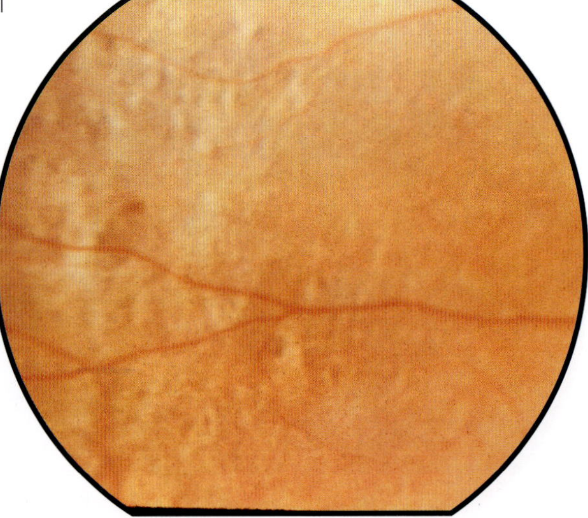

Sjögren–Larsson Syndrome

Sjögren–Larsson syndrome is a rare autosomal recessive disorder caused by mutation in the gene encoding fatty aldehyde dehydrogenase (ALDH3A2), which leads to the accumulation of fatty aldehydes in several tissues. Clinical features include ichthyosis often present at birth, mild to moderate mental retardation, and symmetric spastic paresis involving the lower extremities. Approximately 30–50% of these patients will manifest yellowish pigmentary changes in the central macula with very subtle perifoveal yellow-white crystalline dots. Optical coherence tomography may show hypo-reflective areas representing the crystalline deposits and characteristic thinning of the fovea and inner retinal atrophy.

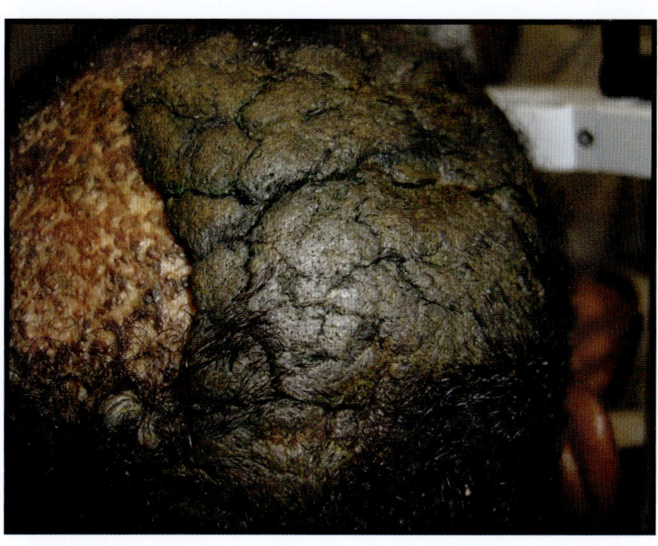

This patient with Sjogren–Larsson syndrome has ichthyosis with scalp involvement.

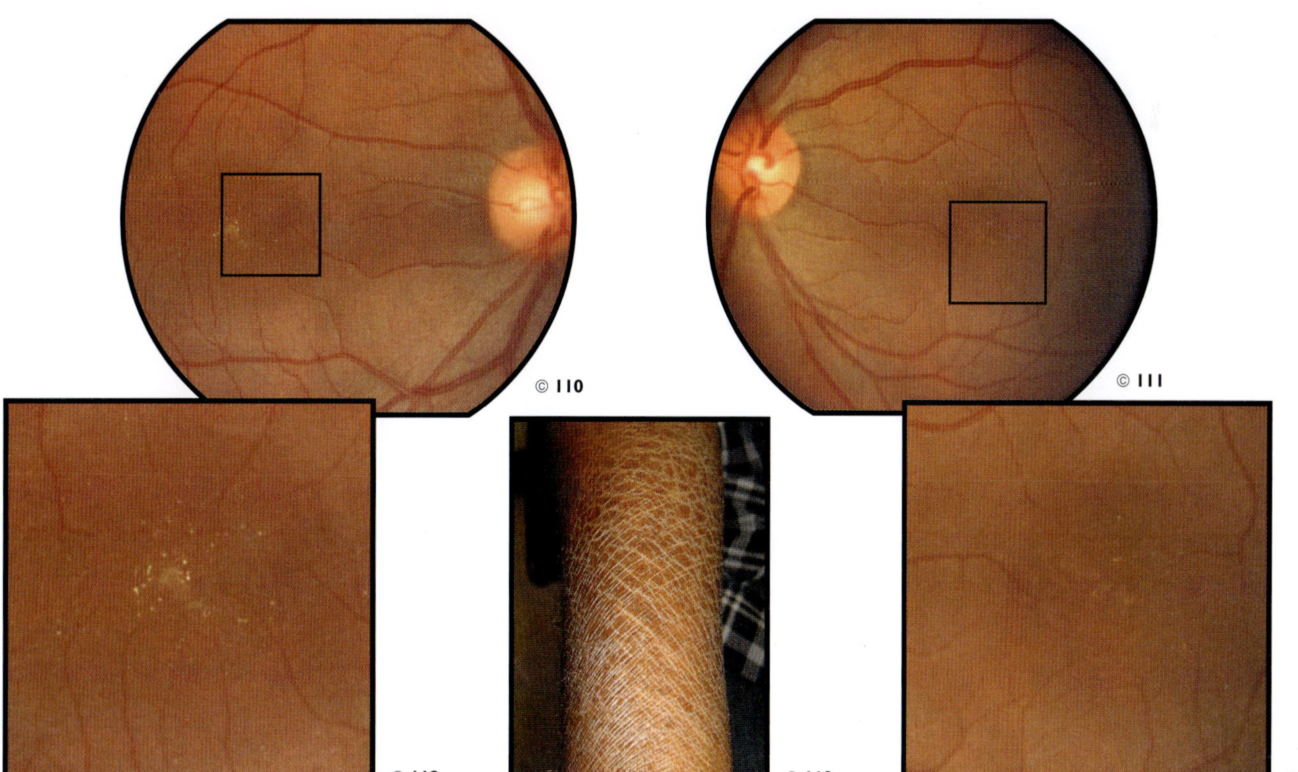

This same patient has a crystalline maculopathy. High magnification photos reveal multifocal crystalline deposits as well as drusenoid changes. Note again the presence of ichthyosis of the skin of the forearm.

Flecked Retinal Syndromes

Flecked retinal syndromes refer to a diverse group of disorders characterized by a widespread uniform density of outer retina or RPE flecks present throughout the fundus. These diseases range from a benign familial disorder without functional deficit to a more severe disorder that is associated with progressive loss of vision, for example, retinitis punctata albescens.

Benign Flecked Retina Syndrome (Benign Familial Flecked Retina)

Benign flecked retina syndrome is an autosomal recessive congenital abnormality that is associated with widespread discrete yellow-white fleck lesions, at the level of the RPE bilaterally, extending to the far periphery, but sparing the macular region. The flecks vary in size from small flecks in the posterior pole to larger more confluent flecks in the periphery and tend to be polygonal in shape. Recently biallelic mutation in the gene PLA2G5 has been associated with this disorder. Visual acuity is typically normal without nyctalopia or delay in dark adaptation and a normal ERG. Fluorescein angiography is within normal limits except for mild, generalized irregular hypofluorescence that does not correspond to the fleck lesions, suggesting a diffuse abnormality of the retinal pigment epithelium. Increased autofluorescence of the flecks suggests that the lesions correspond to an autofluorescent material that may be lipofuscin.

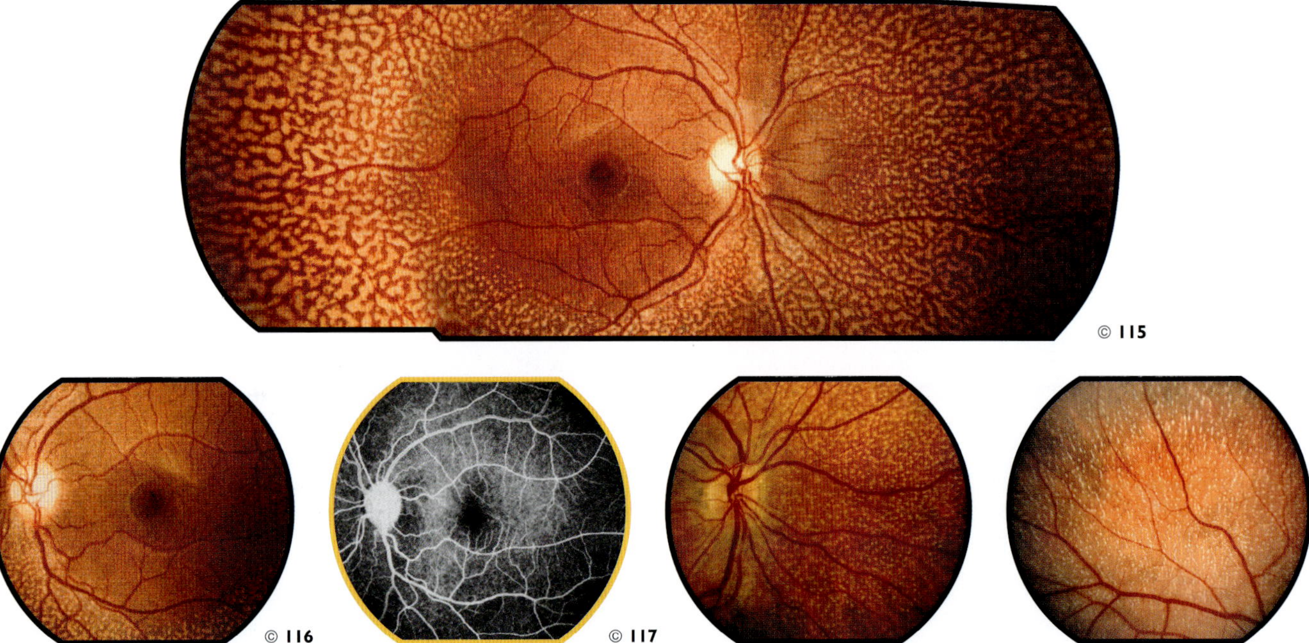

This patient with benign flecked retina syndrome shows white polygonal irregular flecks scattered widely throughout the fundus and did not demonstrate any visual deficit or abnormalities on the ERG. The fluorescein angiogram shows subtle hyperfluorescent window defects corresponding to some of the flecks that have depigmented the RPE. There is no leakage.

This patient with the benign flecked retina syndrome has irregular flecks in the posterior pole and throughout the entire fundus in a diffuse and homogeneous pattern. *Courtesy of Dr. Michael Ober*

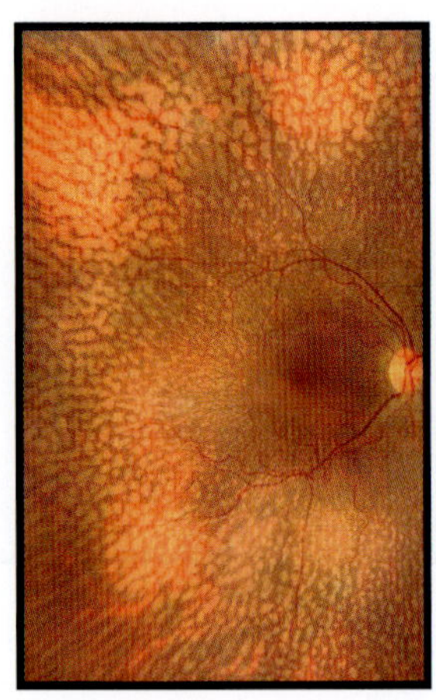

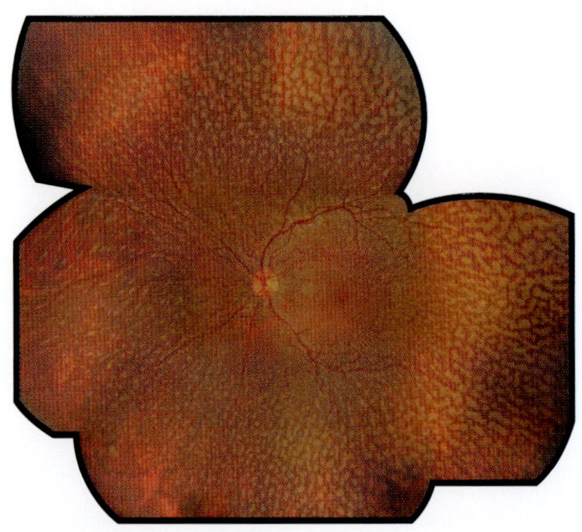

Flecked Retina of Kandori

Flecked retina of Kandori is a rare autosomal recessive disorder in which abnormalities of the RPE are associated with stationary night blindness. Original cases were described in patients from Japan. The fundus changes are characterized by sharply defined, yellowish, irregular flecks of various sizes distributed in the postequatorial fundus and usually sparing the macular region. In some areas, the flecks may coalesce. Areas of RPE atrophy may also be present. The flecks are larger, more irregular, and fewer in number than those seen in fundus albipunctatus.

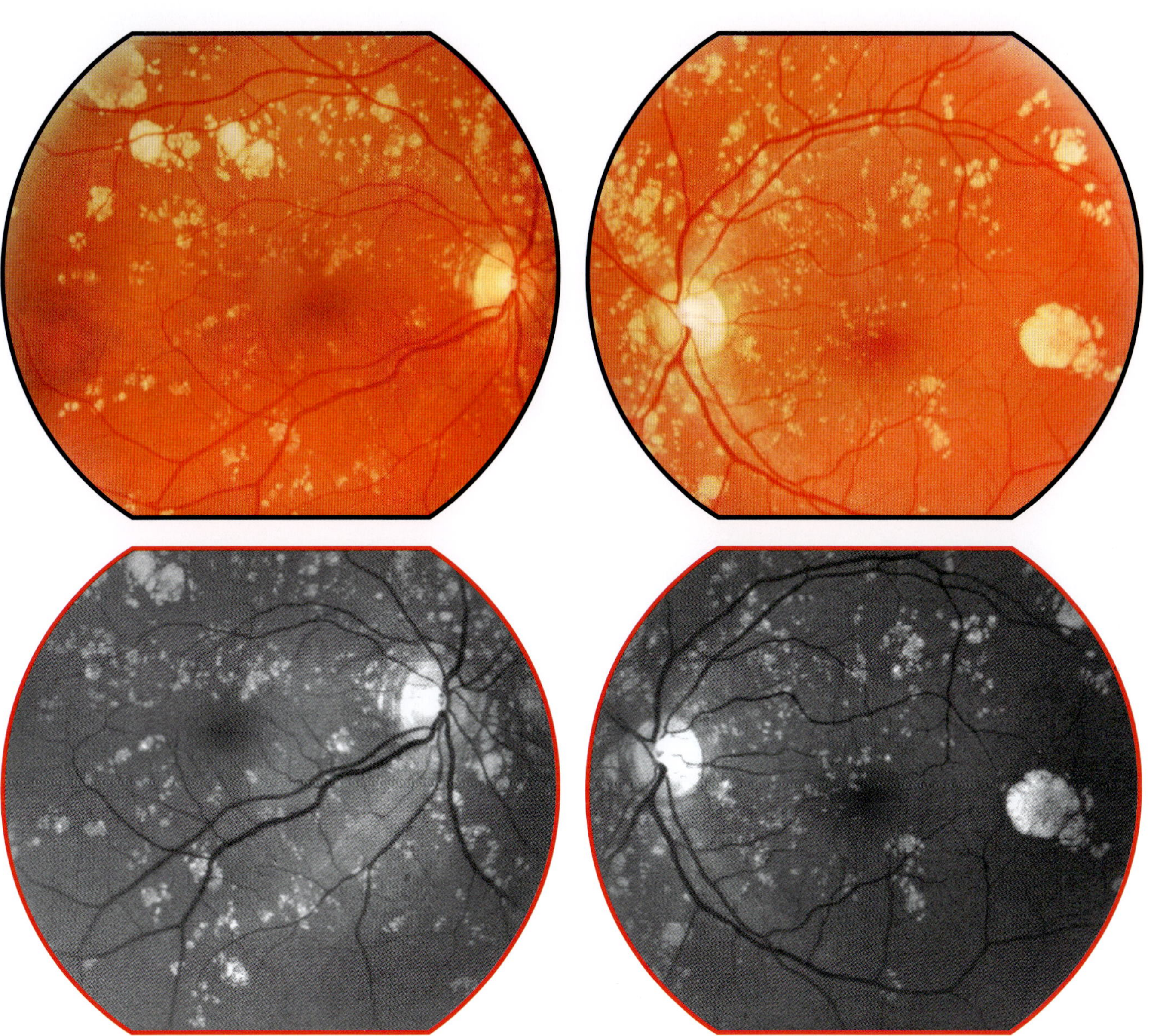

In this patient with flecked retina of Kandori, note the variably sized deposition of flecks scattered throughout the fundus. They may be better appreciated on red-free photography, as noted above. *Courtesy of Dr. Jayme Arana*

Fundus Albipunctatus

Congenital stationary night blindness (CSNB) may present with a diverse phenotypic spectrum including a myopic fundus associated with an electronegative ERG due to disruption of the transmission signal between rods and bipolar ON cells. Fundus albipunctatus is a very interesting form of CSNB that presents with multiple small and discrete nummular yellow-white dots that are regular and monotonous in their uniformity throughout the fundus from the paramacular region to the equator. Both autosomal dominant and recessive inheritance patterns have been described. The disorder is most commonly associated with mutation in the RDH5 gene which encodes retinol dehydrogenase 5, an enzyme needed for proper function of the visual cycle. Rods are predominantly affected and severe prolongation of dark adaptation is evident on ERG. Fundus autofluorescence is diffusely decreased owing to a paucity of lipofuscin accumulation. SD-OCT may show hyper-reflective lesions present in the outer retina.

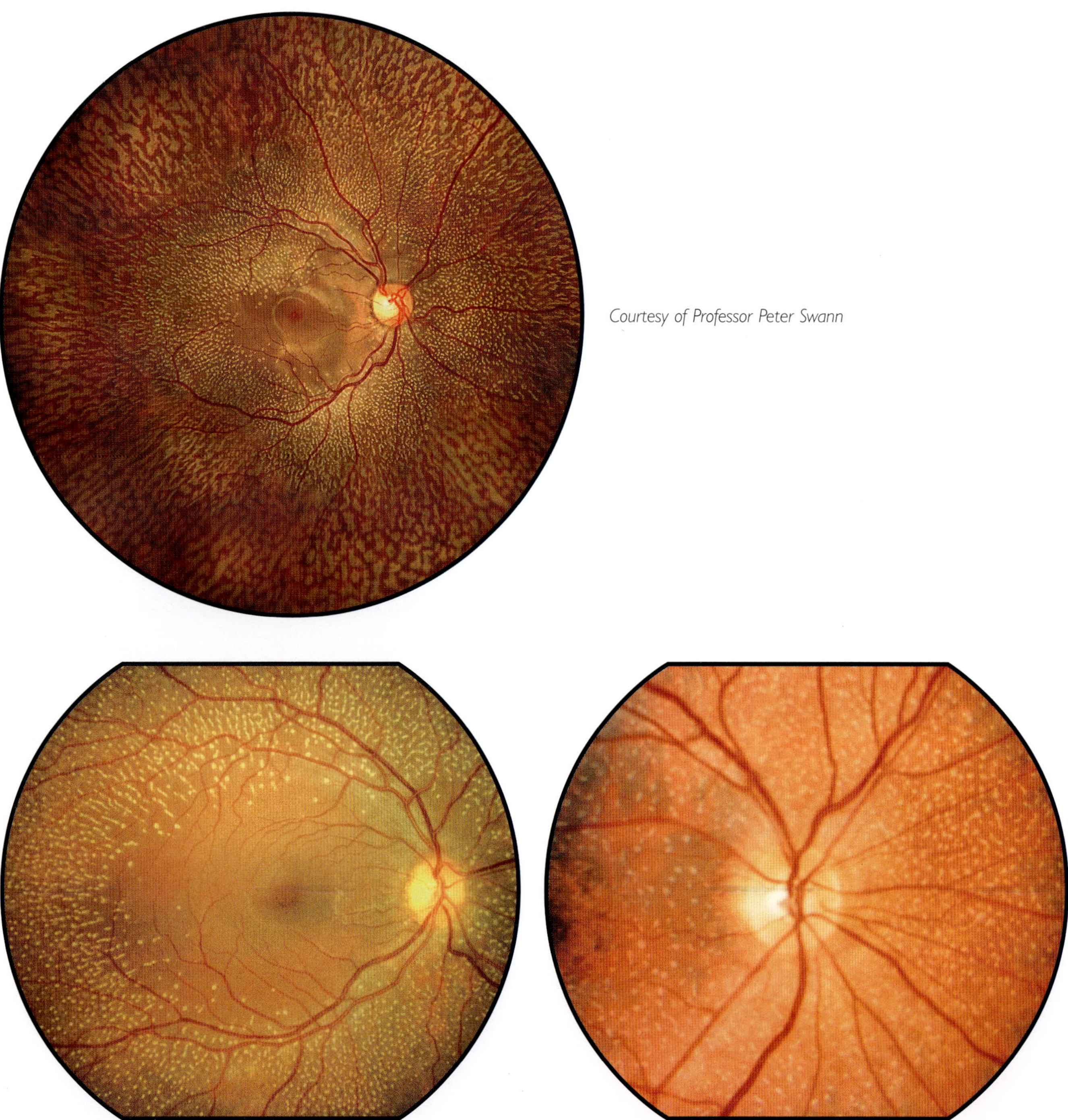

Courtesy of Professor Peter Swann

These 3 cases of fundus albipunctatus show the typical spots throughout the fundus, smaller in the paramacular region and larger in the more peripheral aspects of the fundus. Mild electroretinographic changes were evident in the first patient, but after 3 hours of dark adaptation, the ERG normalized. *Bottom left image courtesy of Dr. Michael Ober, right image courtesy of Drs Sheila Margolis, Ron Carr and I. Siegel*

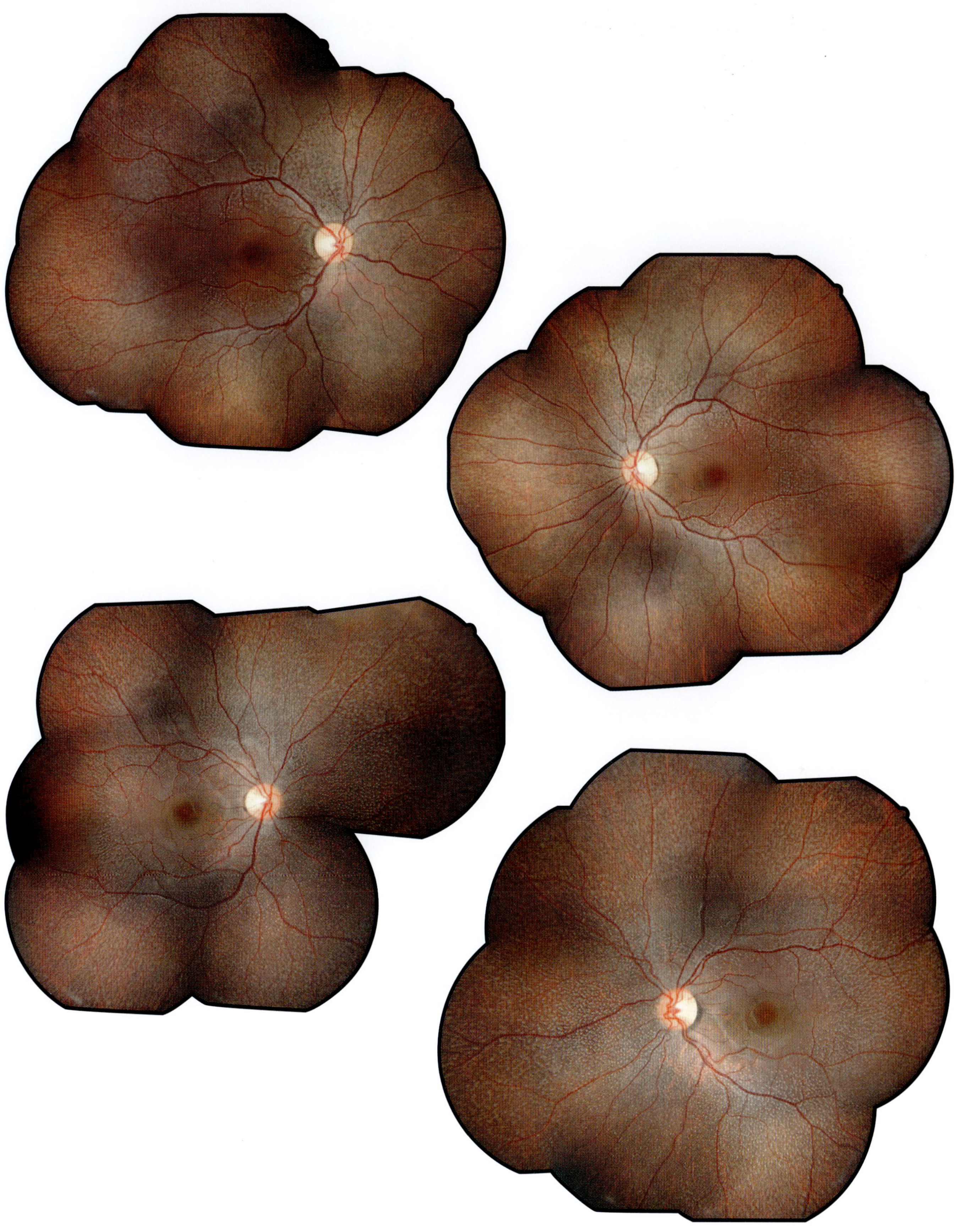

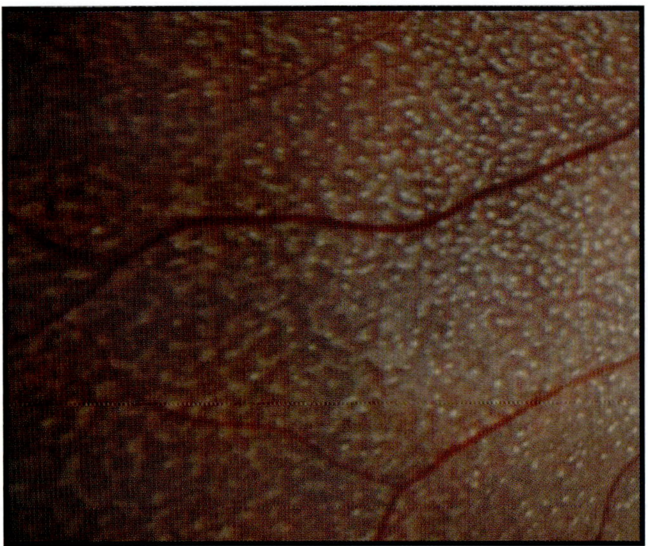

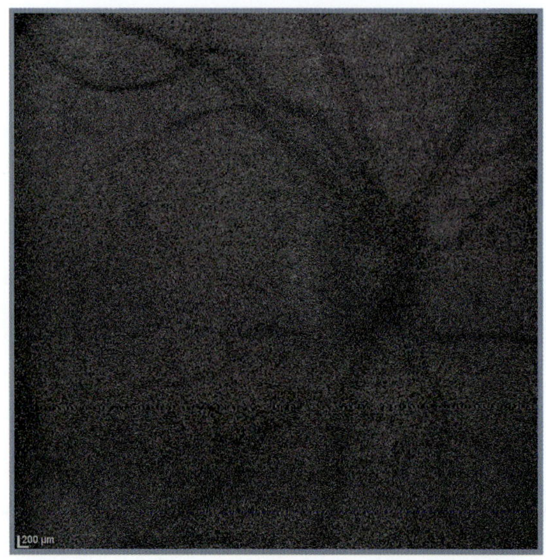

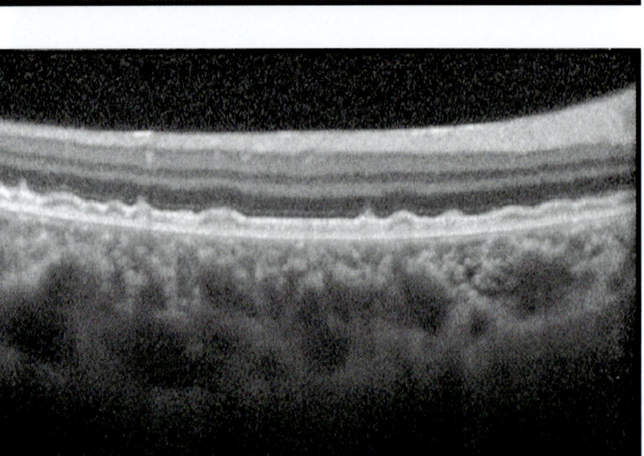

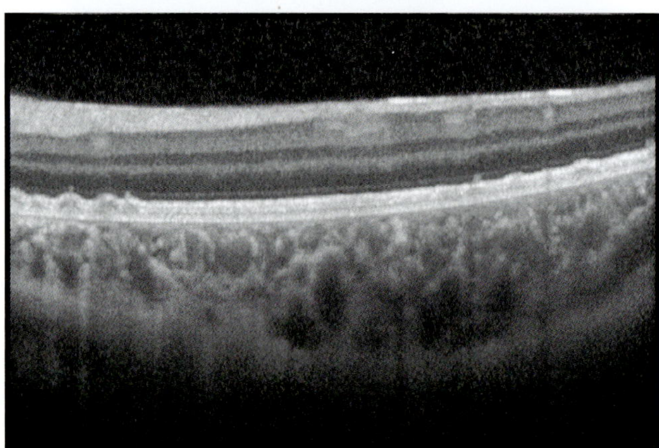

Color photo montages of two siblings with fundus albipunctatus. Autofluorescence imaging of the second sibling shows generalized loss of autofluorescence. Note that the characteristic white spots are drusenoid deposits at the level of the RPE/outer segment junction with SD-OCT analysis. *Images courtesy of Sam Yang, MD*

Oguchi Disease

Oguchi disease, an autosomal recessive form of congenital stationary night blindness, is caused by mutation in the arrestin gene (13q34) or the rhodopsin kinase gene (2q37.1). It is associated with a very characteristic golden brown tapeto-retinal metallic sheen to the fundus. The vessels stand out against the dense RPE changes that obscure the background details of the choroidal vasculature, and the macula appears abnormally dark, in contrast to its surroundings. Abnormally slow dark adaptation is seen in these individuals. The Mizuo–Nakamura phenomenon describes the unusual tapetal sheen that normalizes after prolonged dark adaptation. After exposure to light the retina then slowly reverts to its original metallic color. With prolonged dark adaptation, the initial single flash stimulus can yield a normal rod response, but subsequently the rod response is extinguished until prolonged dark adaptation again takes place. This may be explained by rhodopsin kinase and arrestin, which act one after the other to arrest the phototransduction cascade. However, in these patients, rhodopsin molecules are left in a photoactivated, excited state, and continuously stimulate the phototransduction cascade mimicking the effect of background light. ERG findings in these patients show subnormal rod function that reverses after prolonged dark adaptation. Cone function is generally preserved. Histopathology has revealed, that there are abnormally large cones extending 20° temporal to the disc, shortened rod outer-segments, the presence of an abnormal layer of granular pigment between the photoreceptor outer segments, and the retinal pigment epithelium, as well as an abnormal accumulation of lipofuscin.

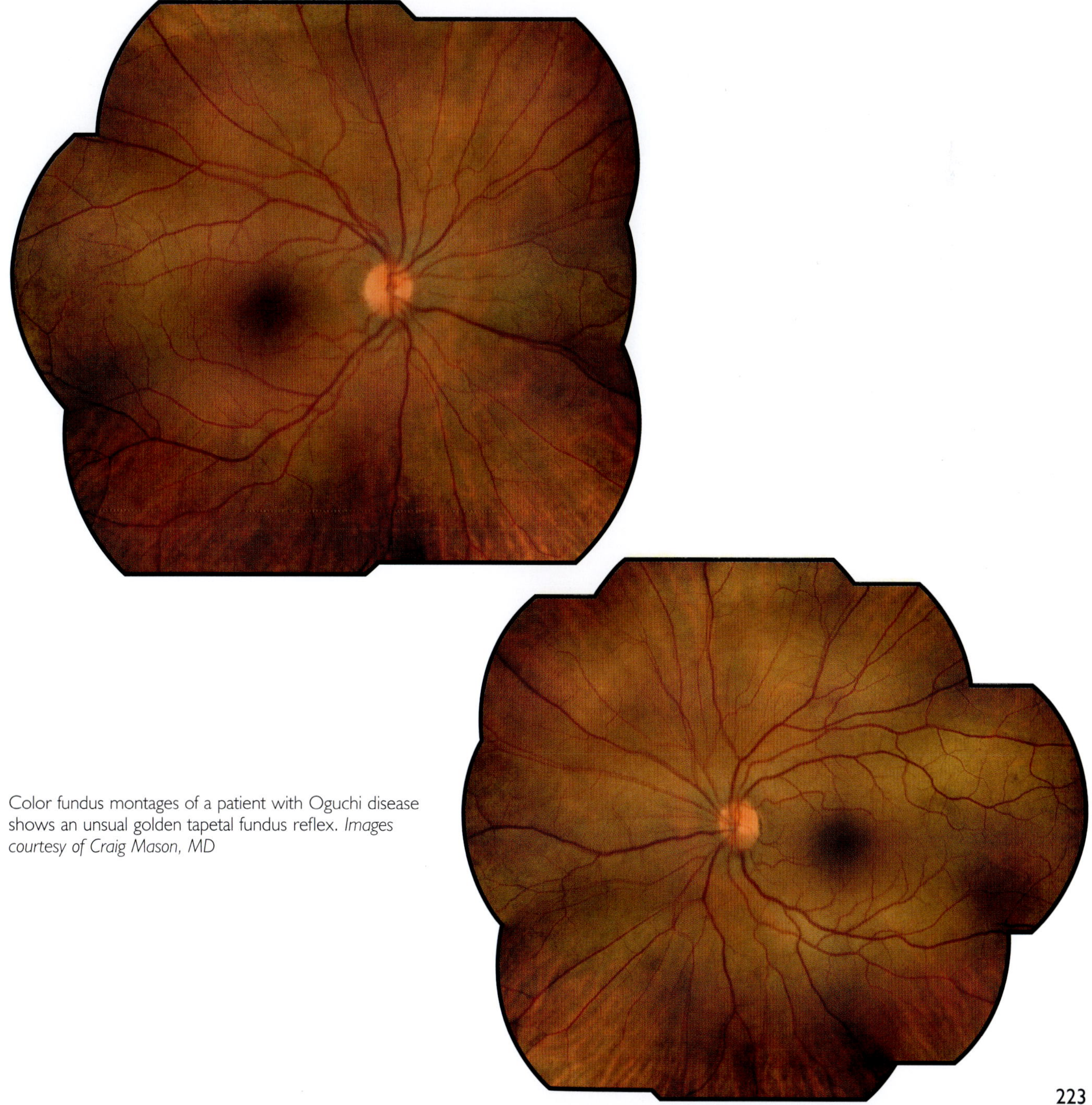

Color fundus montages of a patient with Oguchi disease shows an unsual golden tapetal fundus reflex. *Images courtesy of Craig Mason, MD*

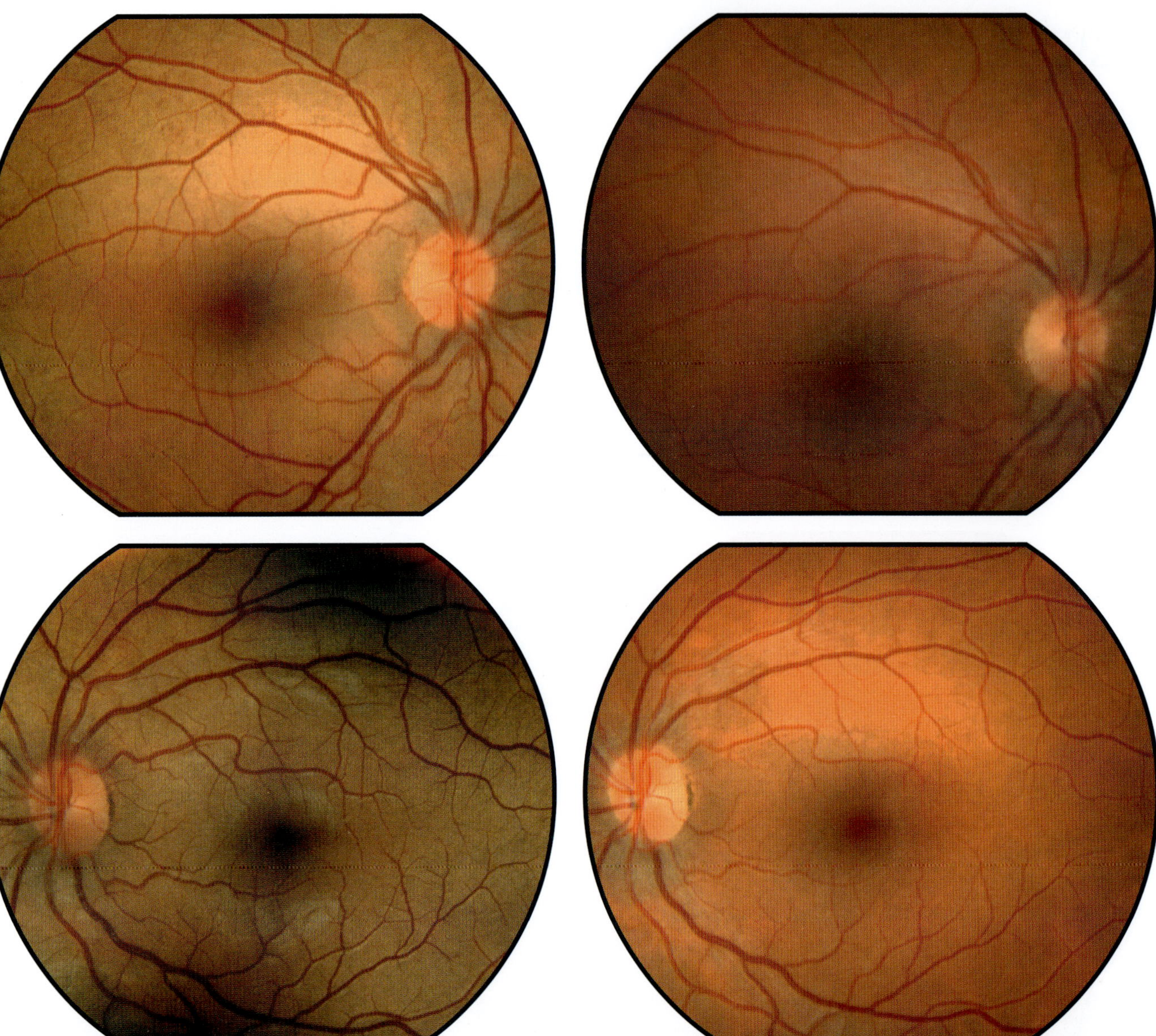

Note the golden tapetal reflex (*left images*) which resolves after 8 hours of dark adaptation (*right images*) in both the right and left eye. This is referred to as the Mizuo–Nakamura phenomenon. *Images courtesy of Craig Mason, MD*

Mizuo–Nakamura Phenomenon

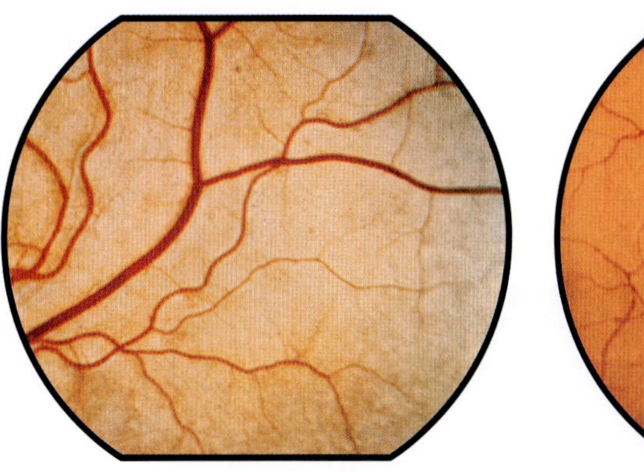

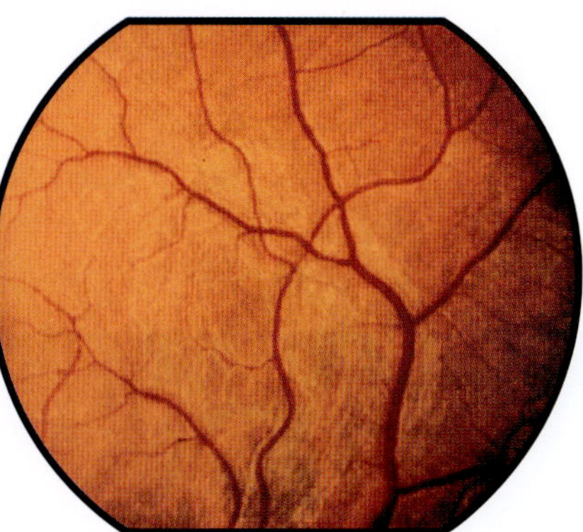

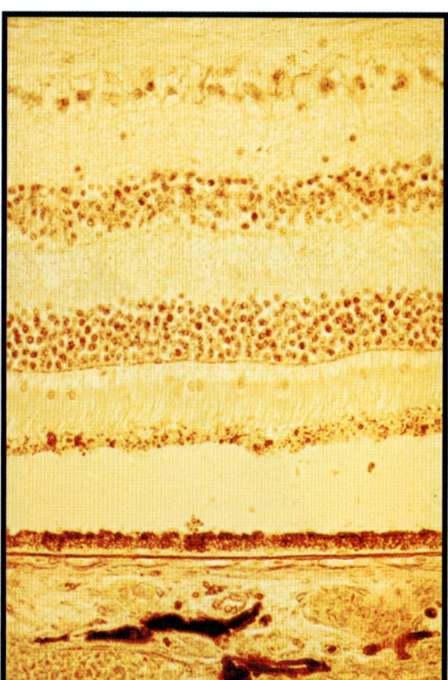

The histopathological findings in Oguchi disease reveal a normal retina, except for the accumulation of pigment between photoreceptors and the retinal pigment epithelium. In this case, there is also migration of the photoreceptor nuclei into the inner segment area. *Courtesy of Dr. Jeffrey Shakin*

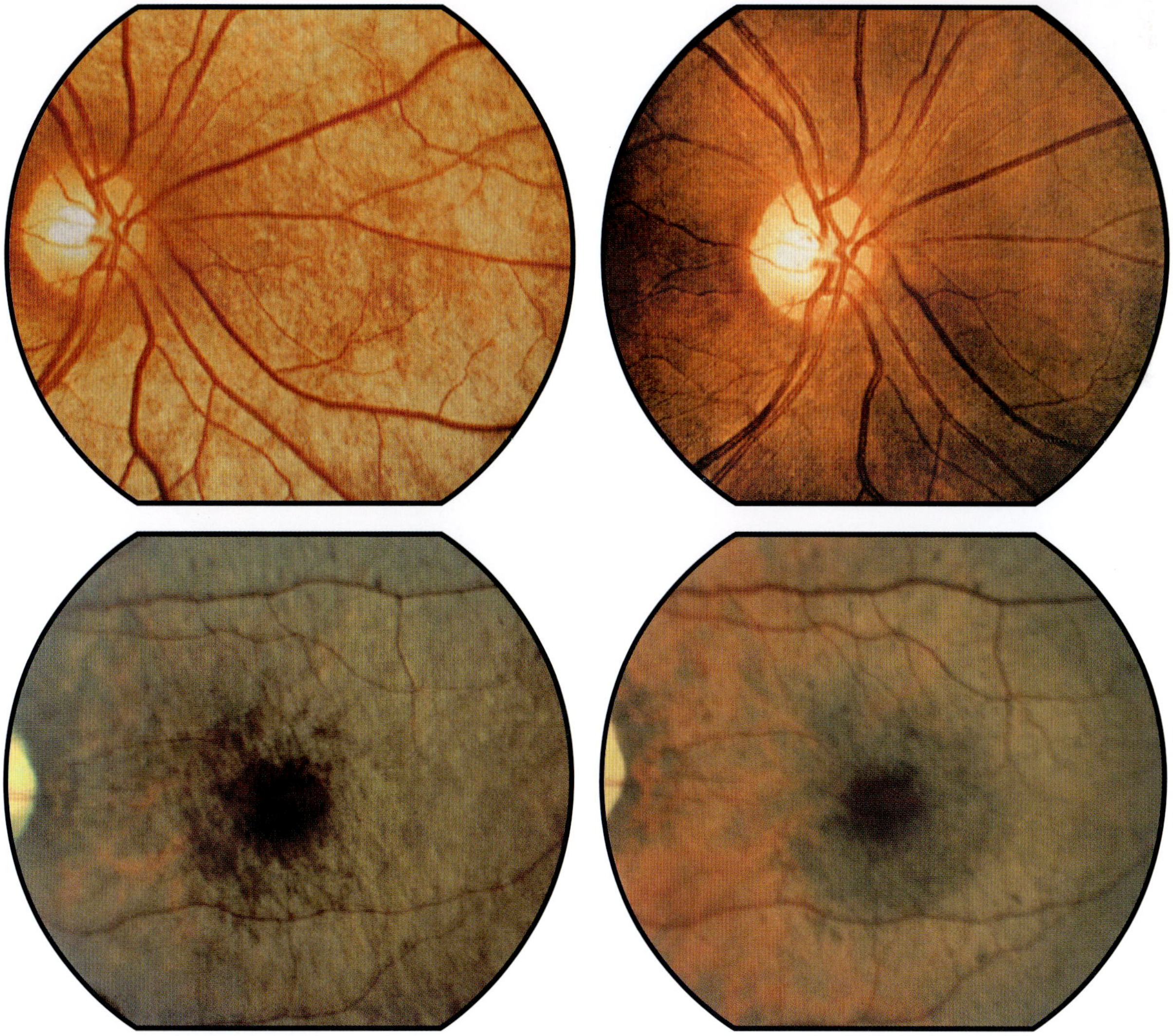

The characteristic ophthalmic features of Oguchi disease are seen in each of these patients. They include a peculiar golden brown sheen of the retina (*left images*) that normalizes with dark adaptation (*right images*) in each case termed the Mizuo–Nakamura phenomenon.

Retinitis Punctata Albescens

Retinitis punctata albescens (RPA) is a subtype of retinitis pigmentosa caused by mutation in the retinaldehyde binding protein 1 gene (RLBP1) and inherited in an autosomal recessive pattern. It is characterized by small white dots (similar to those in fundus albipunctatus) that are scattered throughout the fundus that may or may not be associated with some typical RP findings including peripheral pigment clumping, mild arterial attenuation, and midperipheral chorioretinal atrophy. Involvement of the macula is common. Patients suffer from childhood-onset nyctalopia with later development of progressive paracentral scotoma sometimes in combination with peripheral constriction. ERG findings are consistent with rod–cone dystrophy, often with severe panretinal depression.

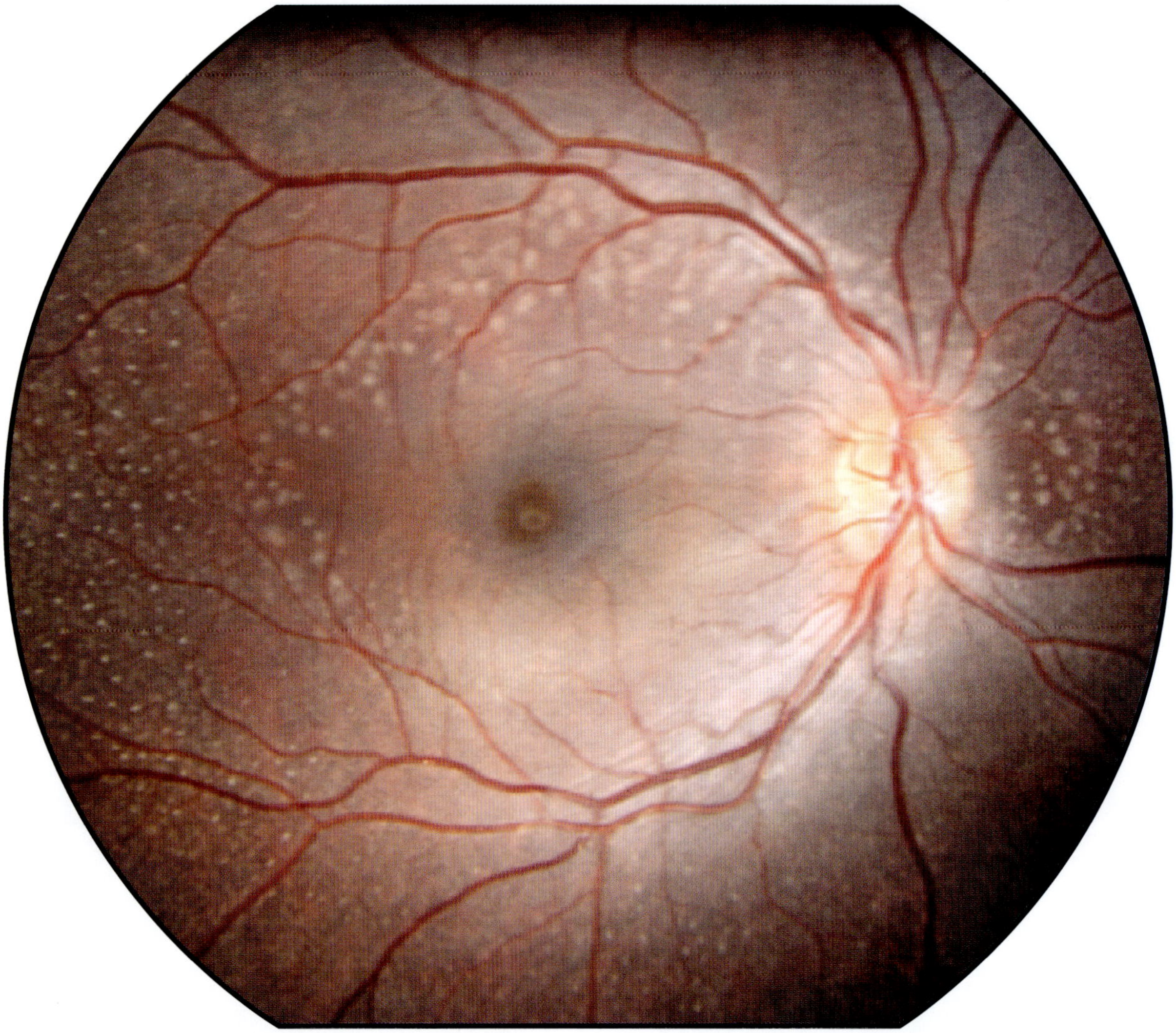

This is a patient with retinitis punctata albescens. Note the scattered spots of variable size surrounding the posterior pole, but also extending into the paramacular region. The typical small lesions in the posterior segment with larger lesions extending toward the periphery, as seen in fundus albipunctatus, are not seen in these patients.

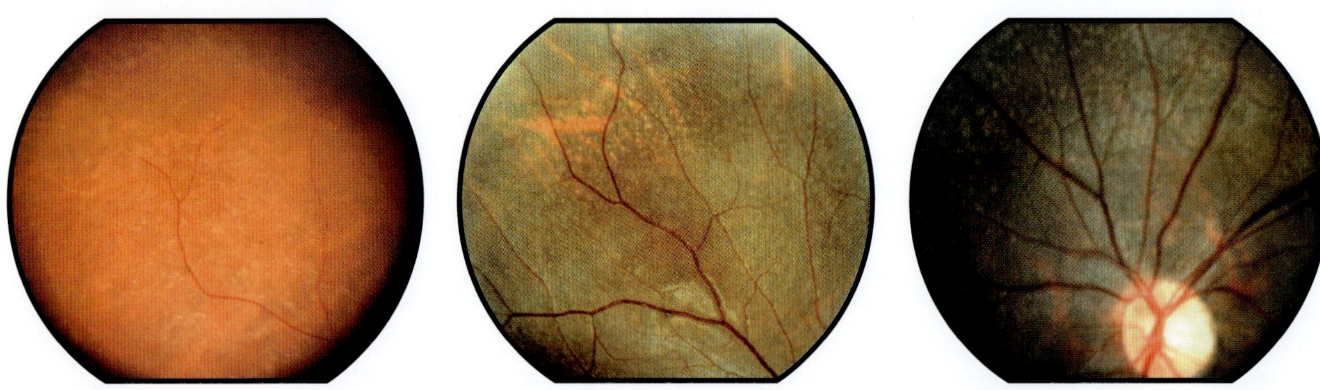

Peripheral lesions are small but discernible in the fundus of retinitis punctata albescens, as seen in these three patients.

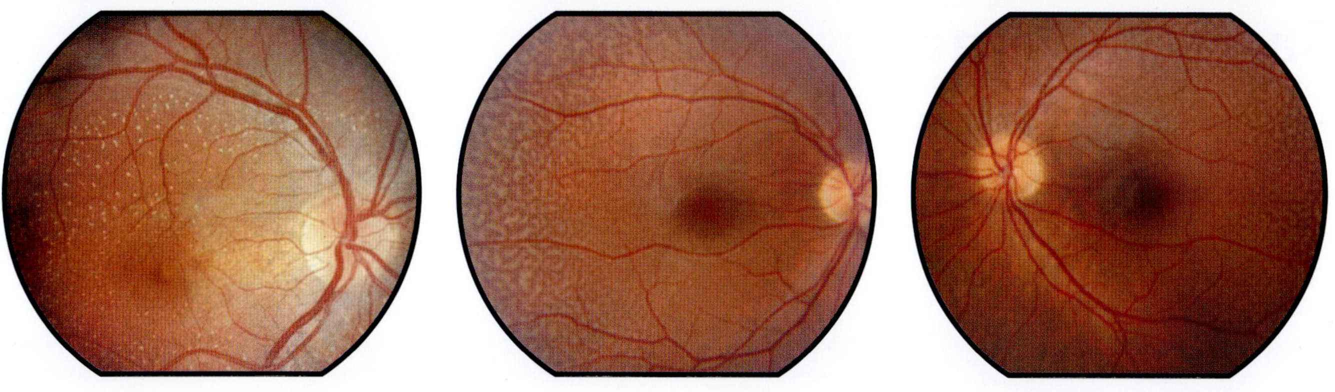

These patients with retinitis punctata albescens have spots in the posterior pole but few in number in the periphery. *Left image courtesy of Dr. Michael Ober, middle and right images courtesy of Dr. Alessandro Iannaccone*

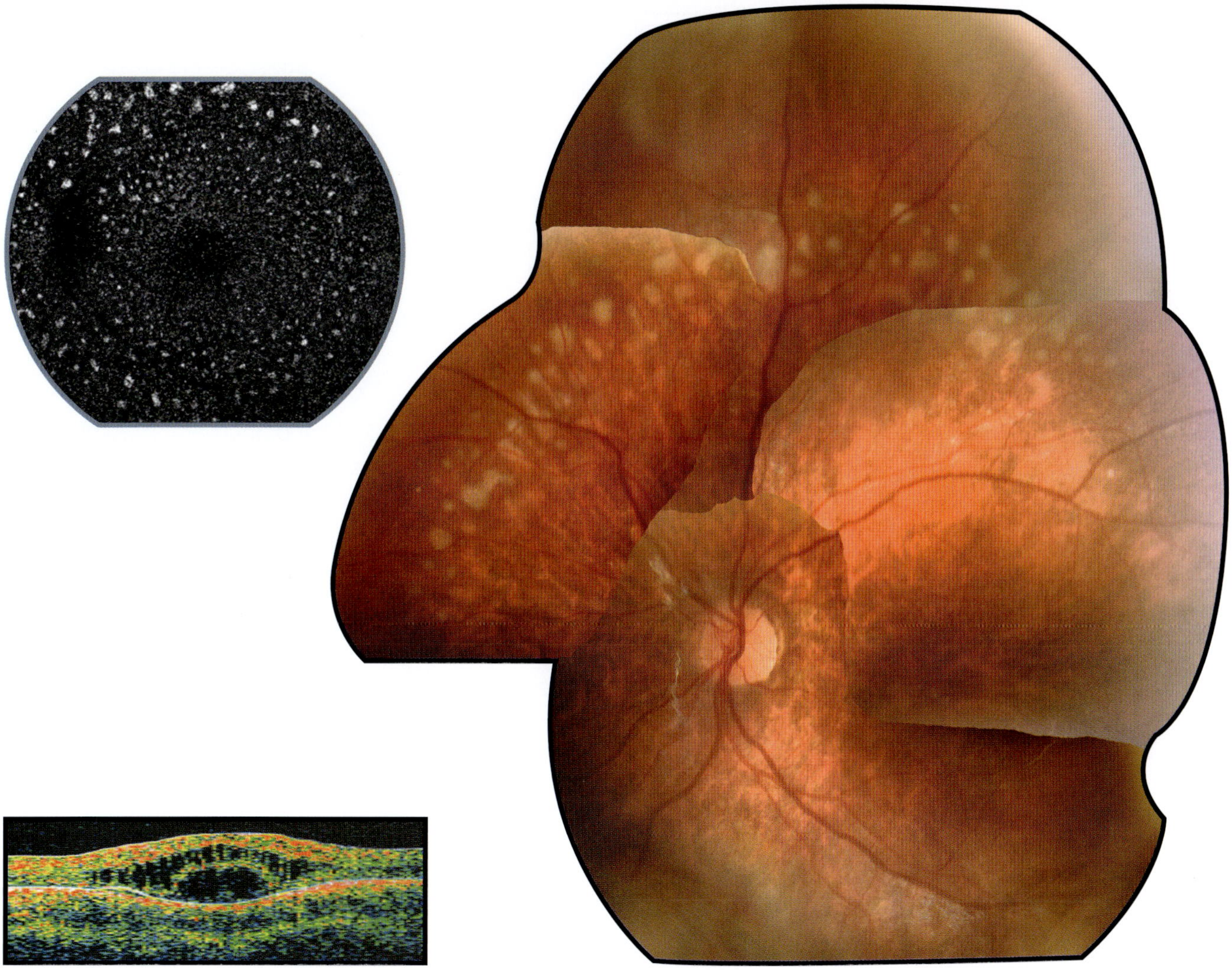

This patient with retinitis punctata albescens has drusenoid-like flecks outside the vascular arcades. There is a wreath of atrophy in the paramacular region and some atrophic degeneration in the fovea. The OCT shows cystic change within the retina and a foveal detachment from edema. The fundus autofluorescence shows hyperfluorescence of the spots which most likely contain a chromophore such as A2E. *Courtesy of Dr. Ulrich Kellner*

Suggested Reading

Stickler Syndrome

Blair, N.P., Albert, D.M., Liberfarb, R.M., et al., 1979. Hereditary progressive arthro-ophthalmopathy of Stickler. Am. J. Ophthalmol. 88, 876–888.

MacRae, M.E., Patel, D.V., Richards, A.J., et al., 2006. Type I Stickler syndrome: a histological and ultrastructural study of an untreated globe. Eye (Lond.) 20, 1061–1067.

Snead, M.P., McNinch, A.M., Poulson, A.V., et al., 2011. Stickler syndrome, ocular-only variants and a key diagnostic role for the ophthalmologist. Eye (Lond.) 25 (11), 1389–1400.

Wagner Syndrome

Brown, D.M., Graemiger, R.A., Hergersberg, M., et al., 1995. Genetic linkage of Wagner disease and erosive vitreoretinopathy to chromosome 5q13–14. Arch. Ophthalmol. 113, 671–675.

Graemiger, R.A., Niemeyer, G., Schneeberger, S.A., et al., 1995. Wagner vitreoretinal degeneration. Follow-up of the original pedigree. Ophthalmology 102, 1830–1839.

Hirose, T., Lee, K.Y., Schepens, C.L., 1973. Wagner's hereditary vitreoretinal degeneration and retinal detachment. Arch. Ophthalmol. 89, 176–185.

Lewis, H., 2003. Peripheral retinal degenerations and the risk of retinal detachment. Am. J. Ophthalmol. 136 (1), 155–160.

Marfan Syndrome

Allen, R.A., Straatsma, B.R., Apt, L., et al., 1967. Ocular manifestations of the Marfan syndrome. Trans. Am. Acad. Ophthalmol. Otolaryngol. 71, 18–38.

Sharma, T., Gopal, L., Shanmugam, M.P., et al., 2002. Retinal detachment in Marfan syndrome: clinical characteristics and surgical outcome. Retina 22, 423–428.

Autosomal Dominant Vitreoretinochoroidopathy

Boon, C.J., Klevering, B.J., Leroy, B.P., et al., 2009. The spectrum of ocular phenotypes caused by mutations in the BEST1 gene. Prog. Retin. Eye Res. 28 (3), 187–205.

Blair, N.P., Goldberg, M.F., Fishman, G.A., et al., 1984. Autosomal dominant vitreoretinochoroidopathy (ADVIRC). Br. J. Ophthalmol. 68, 2–9.

Kaufman, S.J., Goldberg, M.F., Orth, D.H., et al., 1982. Autosomal dominant vitreoretinochoroidopathy. Arch. Ophthalmol. 100, 272–278.

Snowflake Vitreoretinodegeneration

Lee, M.M., Ritter, R. 3rd, Hirose, T., et al., 2003. Snowflake vitreoretinal degeneration: follow-up of the original family. Ophthalmology 110 (12), 2418–2426.

Familial Internal Limiting Membrane Dystrophy

Polk, T.D., Gass, D.M., Green, W.R., et al., 1997. Familial internal limiting membrane dystrophy: a new sheen retinal dystrophy. Arch. Ophthalmol. 115, 878–885.

X-linked Juvenile Retinoschisis

Dubovy, S., Puliafito, C.A., Rosenfeld, P.J., 2009. Macular spectral-domain optical coherence tomography in patients with X linked retinoschisis. Br. J. Ophthalmol. 93 (3), 373–378.

Gieser, E.P., Falls, H.F., 1961. Hereditary retinoschisis. Am. J. Ophthalmol. 51, 1193–1200.

Khandhadia, S., Trump, D., Menon, G., et al., 2011. X-linked retinoschisis maculopathy treated with topical dorzolamide, and relationship to genotype. Eye (Lond.) 25 (7), 922–928.

Mooy, C.M., Van Den Born, L.I., Baarsma, S., et al., 2002. Hereditary X-linked juvenile retinoschisis: a review of the role of Müller cells. Arch. Ophthalmol. 120, 979–984.

Yanoff, M., Kertesz Rahn, E., Zimmerman, L.E., 1968. Histopathology of juvenile retinoschisis. Arch. Ophthalmol. 79, 49–53.

Stellate Nonheriditary Idiopathic Foveomacular Retinoschisis

Ober, M.D., Freund, K.B., Shah, M., et al., 2014. Stellate nonhereditary idiopathic foveomacular retinoschisis. Ophthalmology 121 (7), 1406–1413.

Enhanced S-Cone Syndrome (Goldmann–Favre Syndrome)

Fishman, G.A., Jampol, L.M., Goldberg, M.F., 1976. Diagnostic features of the Favre-Goldmann syndrome. Br. J. Ophthalmol. 60, 345–353.

Hull, S., Arno, G., Sergouniotis, P.I., et al., 2014. Clinical and Molecular Characterization of Enhanced S-Cone Syndrome in Children. JAMA Ophthalmol 132 (11), 1341–1349.

Peyman, G.A., Fishman, G.A., Sanders, D.R., et al., 1977. Histopathology of Goldmann–Favre syndrome obtained by full-thickness eye-wall biopsy. Ann. Ophthalmol. 9, 479–484.

Hereditary or Familial Retinal Artery Tortuosity

Goldberg, M.F., Pollack, I.P., Green, W.R., 1972. Familial retinal arteriolar tortuosity with retinal hemorrhage. Am. J. Ophthalmol. 73, 183–191.

Wells, C.G., Kalina, R.E., 1985. Progressive inherited retinal arteriolar tortuosity with spontaneous retinal hemorrhages. Ophthalmology 92, 1015–1024.

Fabry Disease

Samiy, N., 2008. Ocular features of Fabry disease: diagnosis of a treatable life-threatening disorder. Surv. Ophthalmol. 53 (4), 416–423.

Familial Exudative Vitreoretinopathy

Boldrey, E.E., Egbert, P., Gass, D.M., et al., 1985. The histopathology of familial exudative vitreoretinopathy: a report of two cases. Arch. Ophthalmol. 103, 238–241.

Gow, J., Oliver, G.L., 1971. Familial exudative vitreoretinopathy: an expanded view. Arch. Ophthalmol. 86, 150–155.

Kashani, A.H., Learned, D., Nudleman, E., et al., 2014. High prevalence of peripheral retinal vascular anomalies in family members of patients with familial exudative vitreoretinopathy. Ophthalmology 121 (1), 262–268.

Incontinentia Pigmenti

Bell, W.R., Green, W.R., Goldberg, M.F., 2008. Histopathologic and trypsin digestion studies of the retina in incontinentia pigmenti. Ophthalmology 115, 893–897.

O'Doherty, M., Mc Creery, K., Green, A.J., et al., 2011. Incontinentia pigmenti–ophthalmological observation of a series of cases and review of the literature. Br. J. Ophthalmol. 95 (1), 11–16.

Watzke, R.C., Stevens, T.S., Carney, R.G. Jr., 1976. Retinal vascular changes of incontinentia pigmenti. Arch. Ophthalmol. 94, 743–746.

Norrie Disease

Dickinson, J.L., Sale, M.M., Passmore, A., et al., 2006. Mutations in the NDP gene: contribution to Norrie disease, familial exudative vitreoretinopathy and retinopathy of prematurity. Clin. Exp. Ophthalmol. 34, 682–688.

Drenser, K.A., Fecko, A., Dailey, W., et al., 2007. A characteristic phenotypic retinal appearance in Norrie disease. Retina 27, 243–246.

Parsons, M.A., Curits, D., Blank, C.E., et al., 1992. The ocular pathology of Norrie disease in a fetus of 11 weeks' gestational age. Graefes Arch. Clin. Exp. Ophthalmol. 230, 248–251.

Facioscapulohumeral Muscular Dystrophy

Desai, U.R., Sabates, F.N., 1990. Long-term follow-up of facioscapulohumeral muscular dystrophy and Coats' disease. Am. J. Ophthalmol. 110, 568–569.

Gurwin, E.B., Fitzsimons, R.B., Sehmi, K.S., et al., 1985. Retinal telangiectasis in facioscapulohumeral muscular with deafness. Arch. Ophthalmol. 103, 1695–1700.

Parry–Rhomberg Syndrome

Theodossiadis, P.G., Grigoropoulos, V.G., Emfietzoglou, I., et al., 2008. Parry–Romberg syndrome studied by optical coherence tomography. Ophthalmic Surg. Lasers Imaging 39, 78–80.

Duchenne Muscular Dystrophy

Diago, T., Valls, B., Pulido, J.S., 2010. Coats' disease associated with muscular dystrophy treated with ranibizumab. Eye (Lond.) 24 (7), 1295–1296.

Sigesmund, D.A., Weleber, R.G., Pillers, D.A.M., et al., 1994. Characterization of the ocular phenotype of Duchenne and Becker muscular dystrophy. Ophthalmology 101, 856–865.

Dyskeratosis Congenita

Finzi, A., Morara, M., Pichi, F., et al., 2014. Vitreous hemorrhage secondary to retinal vasculopathy in a patient with dyskeratosis congenita. Int. Ophthalmol. 34 (4), 923–926.

Cohen Syndrome

Chandler, K.E., Biswas, S., Lloyd, I.C., et al., 2002. The ophthalmic findings in Cohen syndrome. Br. J. Ophthalmol. 86, 1395–1398.

Stargardt Disease

Berisha, F., Feke, G.T., Aliyeva, S., et al., 2009. Evaluation of macular abnormalities in Stargardt's disease using optical coherence tomography and scanning laser ophthalmoscope microperimetry. Graefes Arch. Clin. Exp. Ophthalmol. 247, 303–309.

Haji Abdollahi, S., Hirose, T., 2013. Stargardt-Fundus flavimaculatus: recent advancements and treatment. Semin. Ophthalmol. 28 (5–6), 372–376.

Klien, B.A., Krill, A.E., 1967. Fundus flavimaculatus. Clinical, functional and histopathologic observations. Am. J. Ophthalmol. 64, 3–23.

Best Vitelliform Macular Dystrophy

Booij, J.C., Boon, C.J., van Schooneveld, M.J., et al., 2010. Course of visual decline in relation to the Best1 genotype in vitelliform macular dystrophy. Ophthalmology 117 (7), 1415–1422.

O'Gorman, S., Flaherty, W.A., Fishman, G.A., et al., 1988. Histopathologic findings in Best's vitelliform macular dystrophy. Arch. Ophthalmol. 106, 1261–1268.

Querques, G., Zerbib, J., Georges, A., et al., 2014. Multimodal analysis of the progression of Best vitelliform macular dystrophy. Mol. Vis. 20, 575–592.

Autosomal Recessive Bestrophinopathy

Boon, C.J., van den Born, L.I., Visser, L., et al., 2013. Autosomal recessive bestrophinopathy: differential diagnosis and treatment options. Ophthalmology 120 (4), 809–820.

Pattern Dystrophy of the RPE

Marmor, M.F., Byers, B., 1977. Pattern dystrophy of the pigment epithelium. Am. J. Ophthalmol. 84, 32–44.

Watzke, R.C., Folk, J.C., Lang, R.M., 1982. Pattern dystrophy of the retinal pigment epithelium. Ophthalmology 89, 400–406.

Adult-Onset Vitelliform Macular Dystrophy

Fishman, G.A., Trimble, S., Rabb, M.F., et al., 1977. Pseudovitelliform macular degeneration. Arch. Ophthalmol. 95, 73–76.

Butterfly-Shaped Pattern Dystrophy

Zhang, K., Garibaldi, D.C., Li, Y., et al., 2002. Butterfly-shaped pattern dystrophy: a genetic, clinical, and histopathological report. Arch. Ophthalmol. 120 (4), 485–490.

Myotonic Dystrophy 1

Kimizuka, Y., Kiyosawa, M., Tamai, M., et al., 1993. Retinal changes in myotonic dystrophy; clinical follow-up evaluation. Retina 13, 129–135.

Makino, S., Ohkubo, Y., Tampo, H., 2012. Butterfly-shaped pattern dystrophy in myotonic dystrophy. Intern. Med. 51 (16), 2253–2254.

Sjögren Reticular Pattern Dystrophy

Deutman, A.F., Rumke, A.M., 1969. Reticular dystrophy of the retinal pigment epithelium. Dystrophia reticularis laminae pigmentosa retinae of H. Sjögren. Arch. Ophthalmol. 82, 4–9.

Malattia Leventinese

Héon, E., Piguet, B., Munier, F., et al., 1996. Linkage of autosomal dominant radial drusen (malattia leventinese) to chromosome 2p16–21. Arch. Ophthalmol. 114, 193–198.

Sohn, E.H., Wang, K., Thompson, S., et al., 2014. Comparison of drusen and modifying genes in autosomal dominant radial drusen and age-related macular degeneration. Retina 35 (1), 48–57.

Membranoproliferative Glomerulonephritis

D'Souza, Y.B., Jones, C.J., Short, C.D., et al., 2009. Oligosaccharide composition is similar in drusen and dense deposits in membranoproliferative glomerulonephritis type II. Kidney Int. 75 (8), 824–827.

Leys, A., Vanrenterghem, Y., Van Damme, B., et al., 1991. Fundus changes in membranoproliferative glomerulonephritis type II: a fluorescein angiographic study of 23 patients. Graefes Arch. Clin. Exp. Ophthalmol. 229, 406–410.

Ritter, M., Bolz, M., Haidinger, M., et al., 2010. Functional and morphological macular abnormalities in membranoproliferative glomerulonephritis type II. Br. J. Ophthalmol. 94 (8), 1112–1114.

Alport Syndrome

Ahmed, F., Kamae, K.K., Jones, D.J., et al., 2013. Temporal macular thinning associated with X-linked Alport syndrome. JAMA Ophthalmol. 131 (6), 777–782.

Cervantes-Coste, G., Fuentes-Paez, G., Yeshurun, I., et al., 2003. Tapetal-like sheen associated with fleck retinopathy in Alport syndrome. Retina 23, 245–247.

Colville, D.J., Savige, J., 1997. Alport syndrome. A review of the ocular manifestations. Ophthalmic Genet. 18 (4), 161–173.

Sorsby Pseudoinflammatory Fundus Dystrophy

Capon, M.R.C., Marshall, J., Kraft, J.I., et al., 1989. Sorsby's fundus dystrophy: a light and electron microscopic study. Ophthalmology 96, 1769–1777.

Hoskin, A., Sehmi, K., Bird, A.C., 1981. Sorsby's pseudo-inflammatory macular dystrophy. Br. J. Ophthalmol. 65, 859–865.

Sivaprasad, S., Webster, A.R., Egan, C.A., et al., 2008. Clinical course and treatment outcomes of Sorsby fundus dystrophy. Am. J. Ophthalmol. 146, 228–234.

North Carolina Macular Dystrophy

Khurana, R.N., Sun, X., Pearson, E., et al., 2009. A reappraisal of the clinical spectrum of North Carolina macular dystrophy. Ophthalmology 116 (10), 1976–1983.

Small, K.W., Voo, I., Flannery, J., et al., 2001. North Carolina macular dystrophy: clinicopathologic correlation. Trans. Am. Ophthalmol. Soc. 99, 233–237, discussion 237–238.

Stone, E.M., Nichols, B.E., Kimura, A.E., et al., 1994. Clinical features of a Stargardt-like dominant progressive macular dystrophy with genetic linkage to chromosome 6q. Arch. Ophthalmol. 112, 765–772.

Benign Concentric Annular Macular Dystrophy

Van den Biesen, P.R., Deutman, A.F., Pinckers, A.J.L.G., 1985. Evolution of benign concentric annular macular dystrophy. Am. J. Ophthalmol. 100, 73–78.

Deutman, A.F., 1974. Benign concentric annular macular dystrophy. Am. J. Ophthalmol. 78, 384–396.

van Lith-Verhoeven, J.J., Hoyng, C.B., van den Helm, B., et al., 2004. The benign concentric annular macular dystrophy locus maps to 6p12.3–q16. Invest. Ophthalmol. Vis. Sci. 45, 30–35.

Fenestrated Sheen Macular Dystrophy

Daily, M.J., Mets, M.B., 1984. Fenestrated sheen macular dystrophy. Arch. Ophthalmol. 102, 855–856.

O'Donnell, F.E. Jr., Welch, R.B., 1979. Fenestrated sheen macular dystrophy. A new autosomal dominant maculopathy. Arch. Ophthalmol. 97, 1292–1296.

Martinique Crinkled Retinal Pigment Epitheliopathy

Jean-Charles, A., Cohen, S.Y., Merle, H., et al., 2013. Martinique (West Indies) crinkled retinal pigment epitheliopathy: clinical description. Retina 33 (5), 1041–1048.

Cone Dystrophy

Berson, E.L., Gouras, P., Gunkel, R.D., 1968. Progressive cone degeneration, dominantly inherited. Arch. Ophthalmol. 80, 77–83.

Michaelides, M., Hunt, D.M., Moore, A.T., 2004. The cone dysfunction syndromes. Br. J. Ophthalmol. 88 (2), 291–297.

Wang, N.K., Chou, C.L., Lima, L.H., et al., 2009. Fundus autofluorescence in cone dystrophy. Doc. Ophthalmol. 119 (2), 141–144.

Weiss, A.H., Biersdorf, W.R., 1989. Blue cone monochromatism. J. Pediatr. Ophthalmol. Strabismus 26, 218–223.

Occult Macular Dystrophy

Ahn, S.J., Ahn, J., Park, K.H., et al., 2013. Multimodal imaging of occult macular dystrophy. JAMA Ophthalmol. 131 (7), 880–890.

Miyake, Y., Horiguchi, M., Tomita, N., et al., 1996. Occult macular dystrophy. Am. J. Ophthalmol. 122, 644–653.

Wildberger, H., Niemeyer, G., Junghardt, A., 2003. Multifocal electroretinogram (mfERG) in a family with occult macular dystrophy (OMD). Klin. Monatsbl. Augenheilkd 220, 111–115.

Cone-Rod Dystrophies

Thiadens, A.A., Phan, T.M., Zekveld-Vroon, R.C., et al., 2012. Clinical course, genetic etiology, and visual outcome in cone and cone-rod dystrophy. Ophthalmology 119 (4), 819–826.

Jalili Syndrome

Jalili, I.K., 2010. Cone-rod dystrophy and amelogenesis imperfecta (Jalili syndrome): phenotypes and environs. Eye (Lond.) 24 (11), 1659–1668.

Non-Syndromic Retinitis Pigmentosa

Boon, C.J., den Hollander, A.I., Hoyng, C.B., et al., 2008. The spectrum of retinal dystrophies caused by mutations in the peripherin/RDS gene. Prog. Retin. Eye Res. 27 (2), 213–235.

Ferrari, S., Di Iorio, E., Barbaro, V., et al., 2011. Retinitis pigmentosa: genes and disease mechanisms. Curr. Genomics 12 (4), 238–249.

Heckenlively, J.R., 1982. Preserved para-arteriole retinal pigment epithelium (PPRPE) in retinitis pigmentosa. Br. J. Ophthalmol. 66 (1), 26–30.

Salvatore, S., Fishman, G.A., Genead, M.A., 2013. Treatment of cystic macular lesions in hereditary retinal dystrophies. Surv. Ophthalmol. 58 (6), 560–584.

Pigmented Paravenous Retinochoroidal Atrophy

Bozkurt, N., Bavbek, T., Kazokoğlu, H., 1998. Hereditary pigmented paravenous chorioretinal atrophy. Ophthalmic Genet. 19, 99–104.

McKay, G.J., Clarke, S., Davis, J.A., et al., 2005. Pigmented paravenous chorioretinal atrophy is associated with a mutation within the crumbs homolog 1 (CRB1) gene. Invest. Ophthalmol. Vis. Sci. 46, 322–328.

Miller, S.A., Stevens, T.S., Myers, F., et al., 1978. Pigmented paravenous retinochoroidal atrophy. Ann. Ophthalmol. 10, 867–871.

Traboulsi, E.I., Maumenee, I.H., 1986. Hereditary pigmented paravenous chorioretinal atrophy. Arch. Ophthalmol. 104, 1636–1640.

Kearns-Sayre Syndrome

Kearns, T.P., Sayre, G.P., 1958. Retinitis pigmentosa, external ophthalmoplegia, and complete heart block; unusual syndrome with histologic study in one of two cases. Arch. Ophthalmol. 60, 280–289.

Khambatta, S., Nguyen, D.L., Beckman, T.J., et al., 2014. Kearns-Sayre syndrome: a case series of 35 adults and children. Int. J. Gen. Med. 7, 325–332.

Zeviani, M., Moraes, C.T., DiMauro, S., et al., 1988. Deletions of mitochondrial DNA in Kearns- Sayre syndrome. Neurology 38, 1339–1346.

MELAS and MIDD Syndromes

de Laat, P., Smeitink, J.A., Janssen, M.C., et al., 2013. Mitochondrial retinal dystrophy associated with the m.3243A>G mutation. Ophthalmology 120 (12), 2684–2696.

Latkany, P., Ciulla, T.A., Cacchillo, P.F., et al., 1999. Mitochondrial maculopathy: geographic atrophy of the macula in the MELAS associated A to G 3243 mitochondrial DNA point mutation. Am. J. Ophthalmol. 128 (1), 112–114.

Massin, P., Virally-Monod, M., Vialettes, B., et al., 1999. Prevalence of macular pattern dystrophy in maternally inherited diabetes and deafness. GEDIAM Group. Ophthalmology 106, 1821–1827.

Neurogenic Weakness Ataxia and Retinitis Pigmentosa Syndrome

Chowers, I., Lerman-Sagie, T., Elpeleg, O.N., et al., 1999. Cone and rod dysfunction in the NARP syndrome. Br. J. Ophthalmol. 83 (2), 190–193.

Gelfand, J.M., Duncan, J.L., Racine, C.A., et al., 2011. Heterogeneous patterns of tissue injury in NARP syndrome. J. Neurol. 258 (3), 440–448.

Rawle, M.J., Larner, A.J., 2013. NARP Syndrome: A 20-Year Follow-Up. Case Rep. Neurol. 5 (3), 204–207.

Alström Syndrome

Millay, R.H., Weleber, R.G., Heckenlively, J.R., 1986. Ophthalmologic and systemic manifestations of Alström's disease. Am. J. Ophthalmol. 102, 482–490.

Tremblay, F., LaRoche, R.G., Shea, S.E., et al., 1993. Longitudinal study of the early electroretinographic changes in Alström's syndrome. Am. J. Ophthalmol. 115, 657–665.

Bardet–Biedl Syndrome

Green, J.S., Parfrey, P.S., Harnett, J.D., et al., 1989. The cardinal manifestations of Bardet–Biedl syndrome, a form of Laurence–Moon–Biedl syndrome. N. Engl. J. Med. 321, 1002–1009.

Mockel, A., Perdomo, Y., Stutzmann, F., et al., 2011. Retinal dystrophy in Bardet-Biedl syndrome and related syndromic ciliopathies. Prog. Retin. Eye Res. 30 (4), 258–274.

Senior–Loken Syndrome

Ronquillo, C.C., Bernstein, P.S., Baehr, W., 2012. Senior-Loken syndrome: a syndromic form of retinal dystrophy associated with nephronophthisis. Vision Res. 75, 88–97.

Senior, B., Friedmann, A.I., Braudo, J.L., 1961. Juvenile familial nephropathy with tapetoretinal degeneration; a new oculo-renal dystrophy. Am. J. Ophthalmol. 52, 625–633.

Joubert Syndrome

Khan, A.O., Oystreck, D.T., Seidahmed, M.Z., et al., 2008. Ophthalmic features of Joubert syndrome. Ophthalmology 115 (12), 2286–2289.

Sturm, V., Leiba, H., Menke, M.N., et al., 2010. Ophthalmological findings in Joubert syndrome. Eye (Lond.) 24 (2), 222–225.

Jeune Asphyxiating Thoracic Dystrophy

Schmidts, M., Vodopiutz, J., Christou-Savina, S., et al., 2013. Mutations in the gene encoding IFT dynein complex component WDR34 cause Jeune asphyxiating thoracic dystrophy. Am. J. Hum. Genet. 93 (5), 932–944.

Wilson, D.J., Weleber, R.G., Beals, R.K., 1987. Retinal dystrophy in Jeune's syndrome. Arch. Ophthalmol. 105 (5), 651–657.

Usher Syndrome

Boughman, J.A., Vernon, M., Shaver, K.A., 1983. Usher syndrome: definition and estimate of prevalence from two high-risk populations. J. Chronic. Dis. 36, 595–603.

Fishman, G.A., Kumar, A., Joseph, M.E., et al., 1983. Usher's syndrome: ophthalmic and neuro- otologic findings suggesting genetic heterogeneity. Arch. Ophthalmol. 101, 1367–1374.

Sorusch, N., Wunderlich, K., Bauss, K., et al., 2014. Usher syndrome protein network functions in the retina and their relation to other retinal ciliopathies. Adv. Exp. Med. Biol. 801, 527–533.

Adult Refsum Disease

Hansen, E., Bachen, N.K., Flage, T., 1979. Refsum's disease: eye manifestations in a patient treated with low phytol low phytanic acid diet. Acta Ophthalmol. (Copenh) 57, 899–913.

Ruether, K., Baldwin, E., Casteels, M., et al., 2010. Adult Refsum disease: a form of tapetoretinal dystrophy accessible to therapy. Surv. Ophthalmol. 55 (6), 531–538.

Alagille Syndrome

Brodsky, M.C., Cunniff, C., 1993. Ocular anomalies in the Alagille syndrome (arteriohepatic dysplasia). Ophthalmology 100, 1767–1774.

Kim, B.J., Fulton, A.B., 2007. The genetics and ocular findings of Alagille syndrome. Semin. Ophthalmol. 22, 205–210.

Romanchuk, K.G., Judisch, G.F., LaBrecque, D.R., 1981. Ocular findings in arteriohepatic dysplasia (Alagille's syndrome). Can. J. Ophthalmol. 16, 94–99.

Bassen–Korenzweig Syndrome

Chowers, I., Banin, E., Merin, S., et al., 2001. Long-term assessment of combined vitamin A and E treatment for the prevention of retinal degeneration in abetalipoproteinaemia and hypobetalipoproteinaemia patients. Eye (Lond.) 15, 525–530.

Cogan, D.G., Rodrigues, M., Chu, F.C., et al., 1984. Ocular abnormalities in abetalipoproteinemia: a clinicopathologic correlation. Ophthalmology 91, 991–998.

Gouras, P., Carr, R.E., Gunkel, R.D., 1971. Retinitis pigmentosa in abetalipoproteinemia: Effects of vitamin A. Invest. Ophthalmol. 10, 784–793.

Cockayne Syndrome

Levin, P.S., Green, W.R., Victor, D.I., et al., 1983. Histopathology of the eye in Cockayne's syndrome. Arch. Ophthalmol. 101, 1093–1097.

Pearce, W.G., 1972. Ocular and genetic features of Cockayne's syndrome. Can. J. Ophthalmol. 7, 435–444.

Hallervorden–Spatz Disease

Egan, R.A., Weleber, R.G., Hogarth, P., et al., 2005. Neuro-ophthalmologic and electroretinographic findings in pantothenate kinase-associated neurodegeneration (formerly Hallervorden–Spatz syndrome). Am. J. Ophthalmol. 140, 267–274.

Luckenbach, M.W., Green, W.R., Miller, N.R., et al., 1983. Ocular clinicopathologic correlation of Hallervorden–Spatz syndrome with acanthocytosis and pigmentary retinopathy. Am. J. Ophthalmol. 95, 369–382.

Newell, F.W., Johnson, R.O. 2nd, Huttenlocher, P.R., 1979. Pigmentary degeneration of the retina in the

Hallervorden–Spatz syndrome. Am. J. Ophthalmol. 88, 467–471.

Kjellin Syndrome

Farmer, S.G., Longstreth, W.T. Jr., Kalina, R.E., et al., 1985. Fleck retina in Kjellin's syndrome. Am. J. Ophthalmol. 99, 45–50.

Frisch, I.B., Haag, P., Steffen, H., et al., 2002. Kjellin's syndrome: fundus autofluorescence, angiographic, and electrophysiologic findings. Ophthalmology 109, 1484–1491.

Spinocerebellar Ataxia

de Jong, P.T., de Jong, J.G., Jong-Ten Doeschate, J.M., et al., 1980. Olivopontocerebellar atrophy with visual disturbances: an ophthalmologic investigation into four generations. Ophthalmology 87, 793–804.

To, K.W., Adamian, M., Jakobiec, F.A., et al., 1993. Olivopontocerebellar atrophy with retinal degeneration; an electroretinographic and histopathologic investigation. Ophthalmology 100, 15–23.

Vaclavik, V., Borruat, F.X., Ambresin, A., et al., 2013. Novel maculopathy in patients with spinocerebellar ataxia type 1 autofluorescence findings and functional characteristics. JAMA Ophthalmol. 131 (4), 536–538.

Albinism

Falls, H.F., 1951. Sex-linked ocular albinism displaying typical fundus changes in the female heterozygote. Am. J. Ophthalmol. 34 (Pt 2), 41–50.

King, R.A., Lewis, R.A., Townsend, D., et al., 1985. Brown oculocutaneous albinism; clinical, ophthalmological, and biochemical characterization. Ophthalmology 92, 1496–1505.

Mohammad, S., Gottlob, I., Kumar, A., et al., 2011. The functional significance of foveal abnormalities in albinism measured using spectral-domain optical coherence tomography. Ophthalmology 118 (8), 1645–1652.

Nusinowitz, S., Sarraf, D., 2008. Retinal function in X-linked ocular albinism (OA1). Curr. Eye Res. 33, 789–803.

Choroideremia

van Bokhoven, H., van der Hurk, J.A.J.M., Bogerd, L., et al., 1994. Cloning and characterization of the human choroideremia gene. Hum. Mol. Genet. 3, 1041–1046.

Cameron, J.D., Fine, B.S., Shapiro, I., 1987. Histopathologic observations in choroideremia with emphasis on vascular changes of the uveal tract. Ophthalmology 94, 187–196.

Koenekoop, R.K., 2007. Choroideremia is caused by a defective phagocytosis by the RPE of photoreceptor disc membranes, not by an intrinsic photoreceptor defect. Ophthalmic Genet. 28, 185–186.

Syed, R., Sundquist, S.M., Ratnam, K., et al., 2013. High-resolution images of retinal structure in patients with choroideremia. Invest. Ophthalmol. Vis. Sci. 54 (2), 950–961.

Gyrate Atrophy

Akaki, Y., Hotta, Y., Mashima, Y., et al., 1992. A deletion in the ornithine aminotransferase gene in gyrate atrophy. J. Biol. Chem. 267, 12950–12955.

Kaiser-Kupfer, M.I., Caruso, R.C., Valle, D., 1991. Gyrate atrophy of the choroid and retina: long term reduction of ornithine slows retinal degeneration. Arch. Ophthalmol. 109, 1539–1548.

Sergouniotis, P.I., Davidson, A.E., Lenassi, E., et al., 2012. Retinal structure, function, and molecular pathologic features in gyrate atrophy. Ophthalmology 119 (3), 596–605.

Yuan, A., Kaines, A., Jain, A., et al., 2010. Ultra-wide-field and autofluorescence imaging of choroidal dystrophies. Ophthalmic Surg. Lasers Imaging 41 Online, e1–e5.

Late-Onset Retinal Dystrophy

Soumplis, V., Sergouniotis, P.I., Robson, A.G., et al., 2013. Phenotypic findings in C1QTNF5 retinopathy (late-onset retinal degeneration). Acta Ophthalmol. 91 (3), e191–e195.

Central Areolar Choroidal Dystrophy

Ashton, N., 1953. Central areolar choroidal sclerosis: a histopathological study. Br. J. Ophthalmol. 37, 140–147.

Boon, C.J., Klevering, B.J., Cremers, F.P., et al., 2009. Central areolar choroidal dystrophy. Ophthalmology 116, 771–782, 782.e1.

Smailhodzic, D., Fleckenstein, M., Theelen, T., et al., 2011. Central areolar choroidal dystrophy (CACD) and age-related macular degeneration (AMD): differentiating characteristics in multimodal imaging. Invest. Ophthalmol. Vis. Sci. 52 (12), 8908–8918.

Posterior Polar Choroidal Dystrophy

Chen, K.J., Iranmanesh, R., Yannuzzi, L.A., 2005. Peripheral curvilinear pigmentary clumping in posterior polar dystrophy. Retina 25, 947–948.

Bietti Crystalline Corneoretinal Dystrophy

Francois, J., De Laey, J.J., 1978. Bietti's crystalline fundus dystrophy. Ann. Ophthalmol. 10, 709–716.

Halford, S., Liew, G., Mackay, D.S., et al., 2014. Detailed phenotypic and genotypic characterization of Bietti crystalline dystrophy. Ophthalmology 121 (6), 1174–1184.

Wilson, D.J., Weleber, R.G., Klein, M.L., et al., 1989. Bietti's crystalline dystrophy. A clinicopathologic correlative study. Arch. Ophthalmol. 107, 213–221.

Primary Hyperoxaluria

Fielder, A.R., Garner, A., Chambers, T.L., 1980. Ophthalmic manifestations of primary oxalosis. Br. J. Ophthalmol. 64, 782–788.

Small, K.W., Scheinman, J., Klintworth, G.K., 1992. A clinicopathological study of ocular involvement in primary hyperoxaluria type I. Br. J. Ophthalmol. 76, 54–57.

Cystinosis

Kaiser-Kupfer, M.I., Gazzo, M.A., Datiles, M.B., et al., 1990. A randomized placebo-controlled trial of cysteamine eye drops in nephropathic cystinosis. Arch. Ophthalomol. 108, 689–693.

Sanderson, P.O., Kuwabara, T., Stark, W.J., et al., 1974. Cystinosis; a clinical, histopathologic, and ultrastructural study. Arch. Ophthalmol. 91, 270–274.

Tsilou, E.T., Rubin, B.I., Reed, G., et al., 2006. Nephropathic cystinosis: posterior segment manifestations and effects of cysteamine therapy. Ophthalmology 113 (6), 1002–1009.

Sjögren–Larsson Syndrome

Bhallil, S., Chraibi, F., Andalloussi, I.B., et al., 2012. Optical coherence tomography aspect of crystalline macular dystrophy in Sjögren-Larsson syndrome. Int. Ophthalmol. 32 (5), 495–498.

Sjögren, T., Larsson, T., 1957. Oligophrenia in combination with congenital ichthyosis and spastic disorders; a clinical and genetic study. Acta Psychiatr. Neurol. Scand. Suppl. 113, 32–44.

Benign Flecked Retina Syndrome

Sabel Aish, S.F., Dajani, B., 1980. Benign familial fleck retina. Br. J. Ophthalmol. 64, 652–659.

Flecked Retina of Kandori

Kandori, F., 1959. Very rare case of congenital nonprogressive nightblindness with fleck retina. J. Clin. Ophthalmol. (Tokyo) 13, 384–386.

Fundus Albipunctatus

Levy, N.S., Toskes, P.P., 1974. Fundus albipunctatus and vitamin A deficiency. Am. J. Ophthalmol. 78, 926–929.

Nakamura, M., Skalet, J., Miyake, Y., 2003. RDH5 gene mutations and electroretinogram in fundus albipunctatus with or without macular dystrophy: RDH5 mutations and ERG in fundus albipunctatus. Doc. Ophthalmol. 107, 3–11.

Sekiya, K., Nakazawa, M., Ohguro, H., et al., 2003. Long-term fundus changes due to Fundus albipunctatus associated with mutations in the RDH5 gene. Arch. Ophthalmol. 121, 1057–1059.

Oguchi Disease

Dryja, T.P., 2000. Molecular genetics of Oguchi disease, fundus albipunctatus, and other forms of stationary night blindness: LVII Edward Jackson Memorial Lecture. Am. J. Ophthalmol. 130, 547–563.

Kuwakara, Y., Ishihara, K., Akiya, S., 1963. Histopathological and electron microscopic studies of the retina of Oguchi's disease. Acta. Soc. Ophthalmol. Jpn. 67, 1323.

Retinitis Puntacta Albescens

Smith, B.F., Ripps, H., Goodman, G., 1959. Retinitis punctata albescens, a functional and diagnostic evaluation. Arch. Ophthalmol. 61, 93–101.

CHAPTER 3

Pediatrics

A number of retinal abnormalities are limited to the pediatric setting. These include congenital and hereditary abnormalities. While many of these disorders are reviewed in Chapter 2, this pediatric chapter will include those disorders that more typically present in the congenital or infantile stage. Images of pediatric retinal conditions, many of them rare in nature, constitute an essential tool in our armamentarium to educate young pediatric ophthalmologists and retina specialists to more skillfully diagnose and manage these challenging patients. Certain findings represent risk factors for sight-threatening events in their natural course; others may simply affect visual acuity and field.

Congenital Abnormalities

A variety of congenital abnormalities may be seen by the pediatric retinal physician. They include anomalies and abnormalities of the retinal vasculature, the optic nerve, and choroid.

Retinopathy of Prematurity

Retinopathy of prematurity (ROP) is a retinal vascular disorder that affects severely premature babies, resulting from incomplete peripheral vascularization at birth followed by abnormal vascularization in the subsequent weeks to months. Abnormal proliferation of blood vessels can lead to fibrovascular networks that exert traction on the retina and may progress to retinal detachment and blindness in the most advanced cases. There are many risk factors for the development of ROP, which include low birth weight, low gestational age, supplemental oxygen therapy, and a possible genetic component. Screening guidelines vary in different parts of the world based upon the characteristics of the premature population and practice patterns of neonatal intensive care units. In the United States, retinal screening is recommended for all babies weighing 1500 grams and/or born before 30 weeks gestational age. In general, the smaller and more premature the baby, the higher the risk for developing ROP. Treatment in the United States, when deemed necessary, consists of panretinal photocoagulation to the areas of avascular retina; however, ROP regresses without treatment in over 90% of cases. More recently intravitreal anti-VEGF therapy has been suggested as primary treatment or as a supplement to laser therapy. Multiple studies have demonstrated efficacy in inducing regression of neovascularization especially in more advanced disease. However the optimal treatment indications, timing, dosage, and follow-up are yet to be determined and therefore this treatment remains off-label in the United States.

Stage I

In stage I, there is a fine, thin demarcation line between the vascular and avascular region in the peripheral retina. The junction is flat.

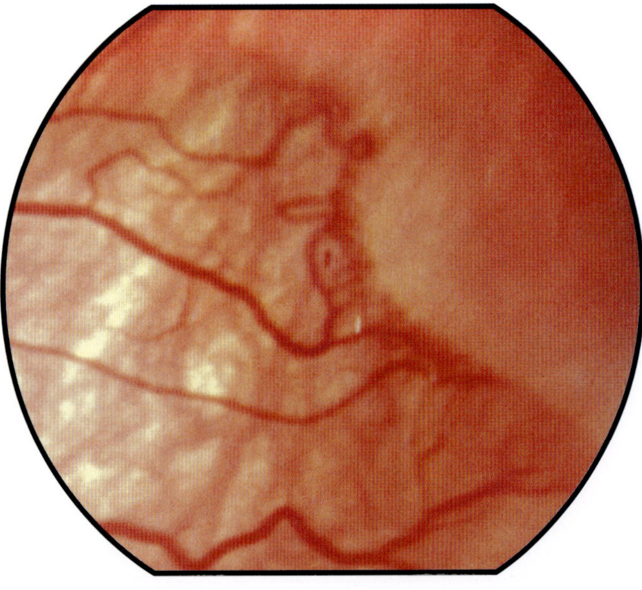

Courtesy of Earl A. Palmer, Casey Eye Institute

Stage II

In stage II, a broad, thick ridge clearly separates the vascular from the avascular retina.

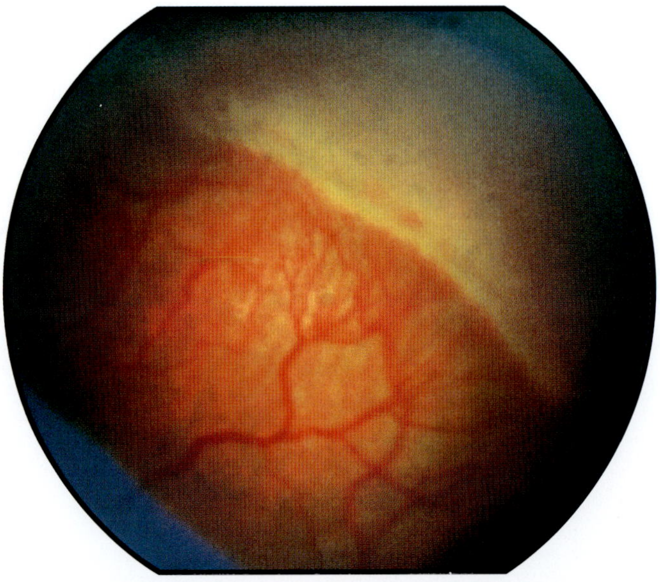

Stage III

In stage III, neovascularization is present on the posterior edge of the ridge, which has an indistinct, velvety appearance and a ragged border.

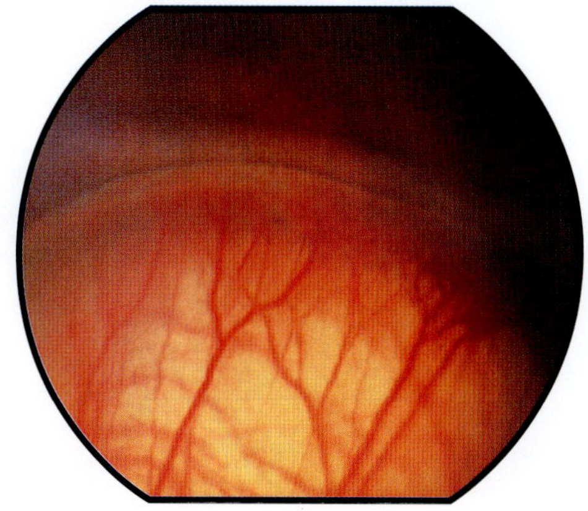

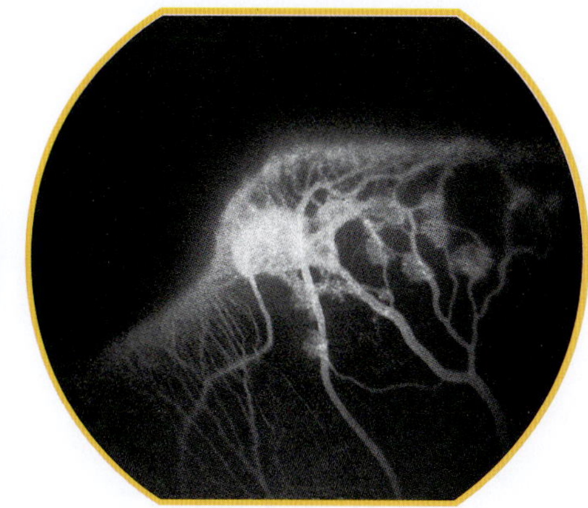

Stage IV-A

In stage IV-A, there is a subtotal retinal detachment beginning at the fibrovascular ridge. The retina is under traction anteriorly, beginning at the ridge, and the fovea is uninvolved. Subretinal fluid may also be seen.

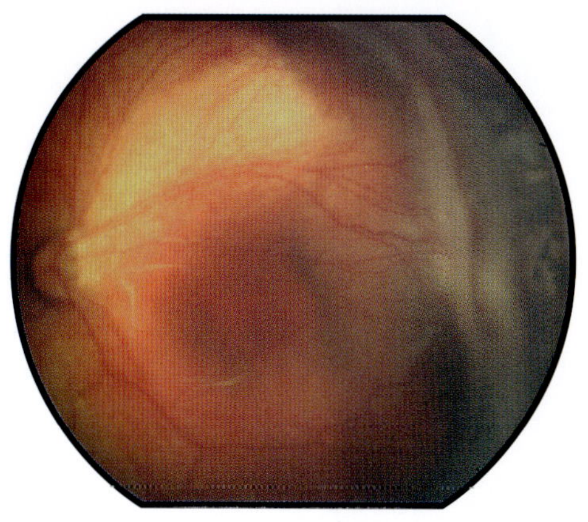

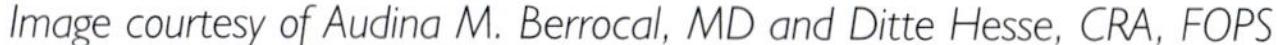

Image courtesy of Audina M. Berrocal, MD and Ditte Hesse, CRA, FOPS

Stage IV-B

In Stage IV-B a subtotal retinal detachment is present but the fovea is involved.

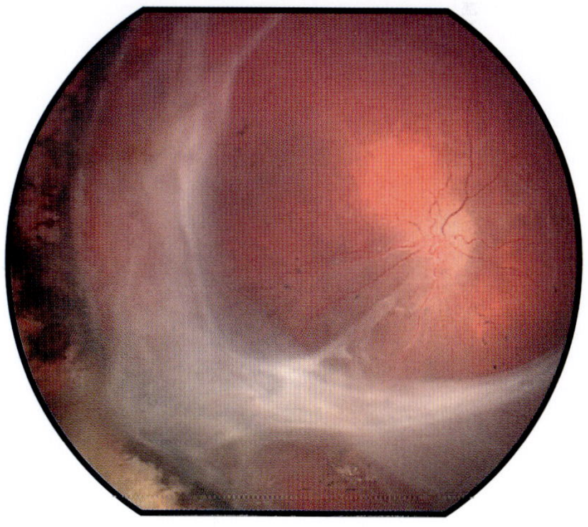

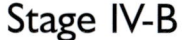

Image courtesy of Audina M. Berrocal, MD and Ditte Hesse, CRA, FOPS

Stage V

In stage V-A, there is a total retinal detachment that may eventually evolve into the shape of an open funnel seen below in the left image. Stage V-B is classified as a closed funnel, seen below in the right image.

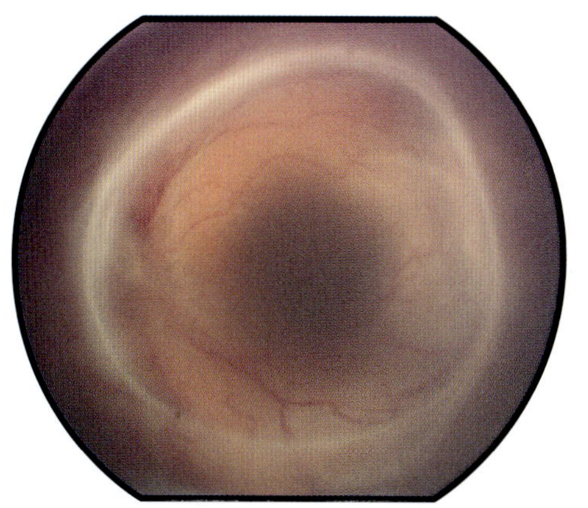

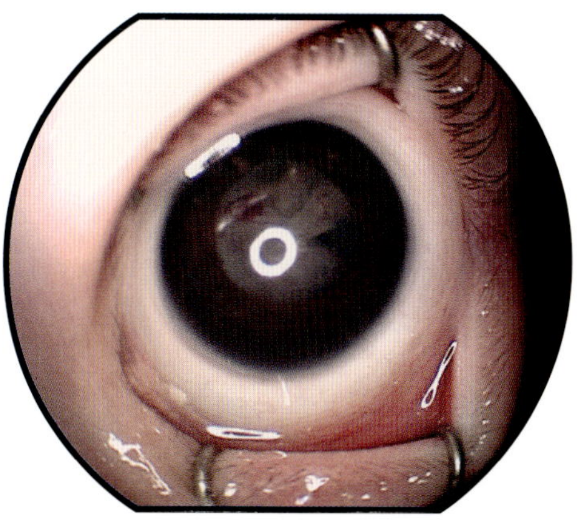

Images courtesy of Audina M. Berrocal, MD and Ditte Hesse, CRA, FOPS

Plus Disease

Plus disease is characterized by arteriolar tortuosity and venous engorgement in the posterior pole and indicates an especially aggressive form of ischemic disease with a poor prognosis and the need for early aggressive treatment. Iris vascular engorgement, pupillary rigidity, and vitreous haze may also be part of this classification; the latter is a poor prognostic finding.

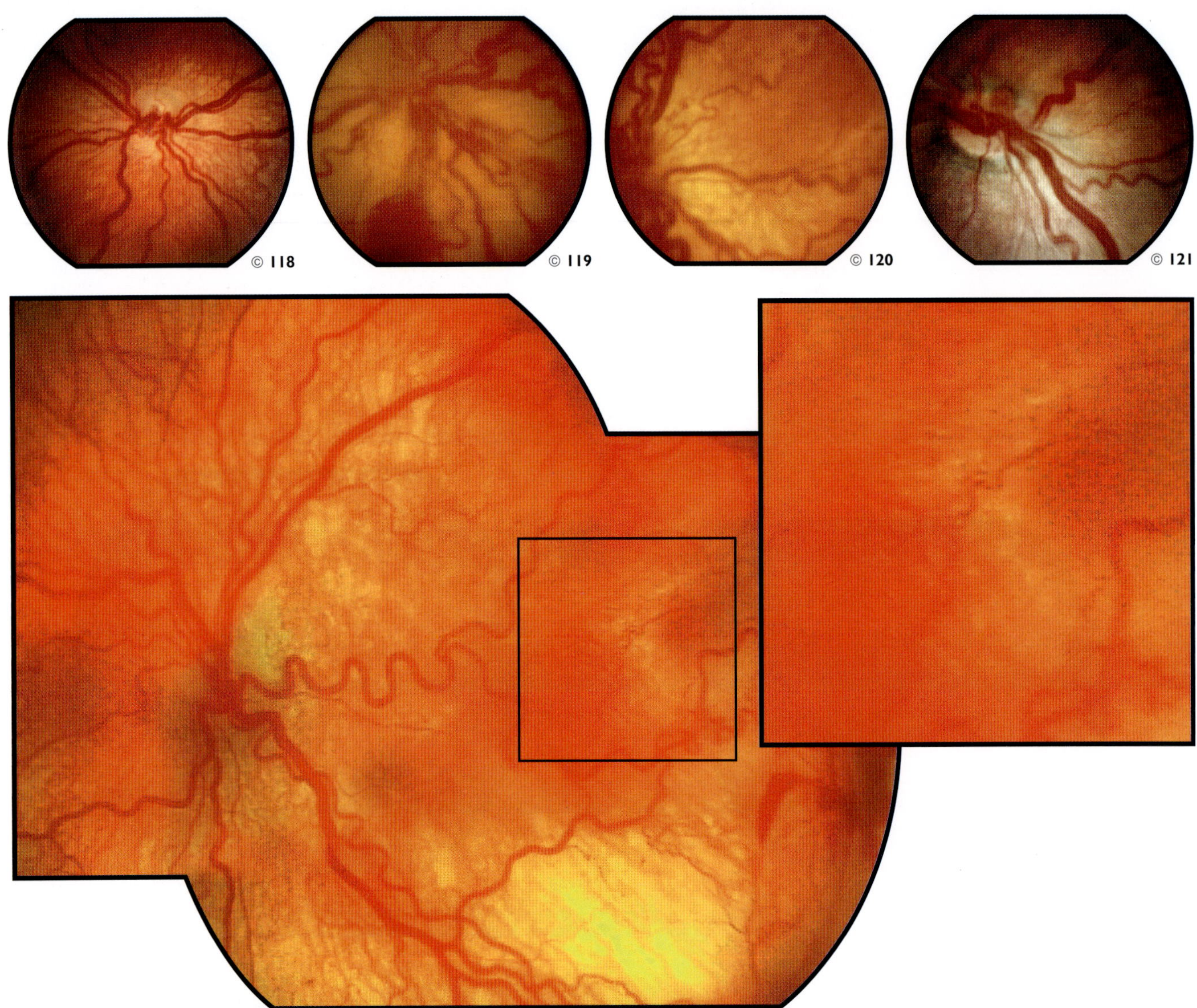

In the case of aggressive posterior ROP, flat neovascularization and pre-retinal hemorrhage are seen around a posterior ridge. Prominently dilated and tortuous retinal vessels (Plus disease) involving all 12 clock hour positions are also seen.

Spectrum of ROP

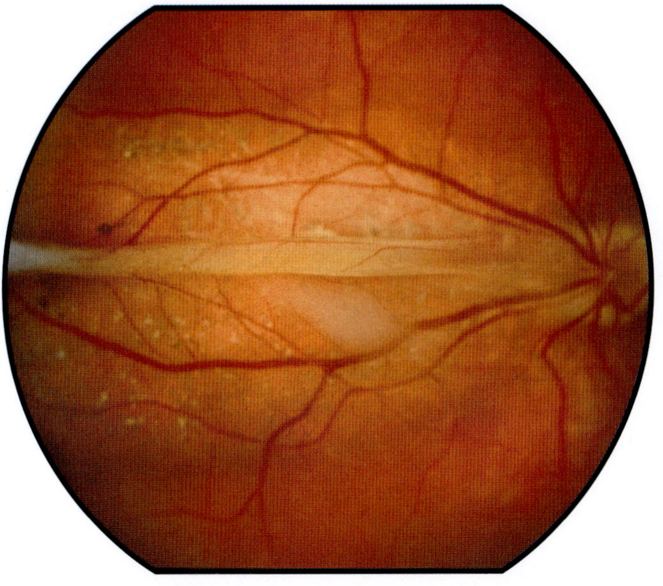

This patient demonstrates the clinical presentation in ROP with advanced severity. There is a large retinal fold and peripheral dragging of the retinal vasculature.

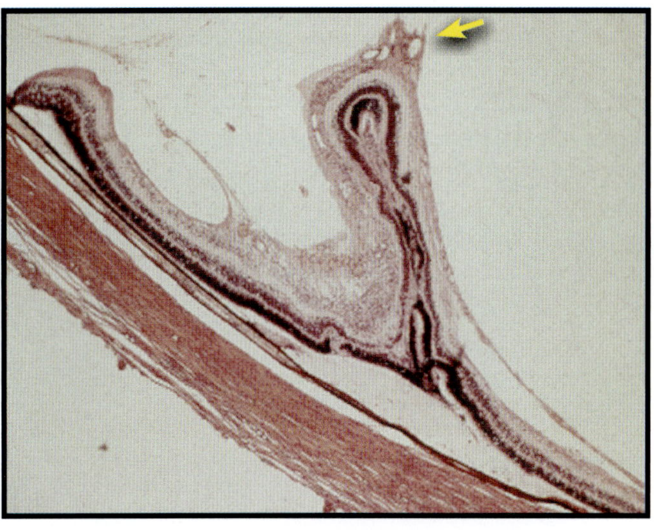

The histopathological image shows the nature of the retinal fold and endothelial proliferation extending into the vitreous *(arrow)*.

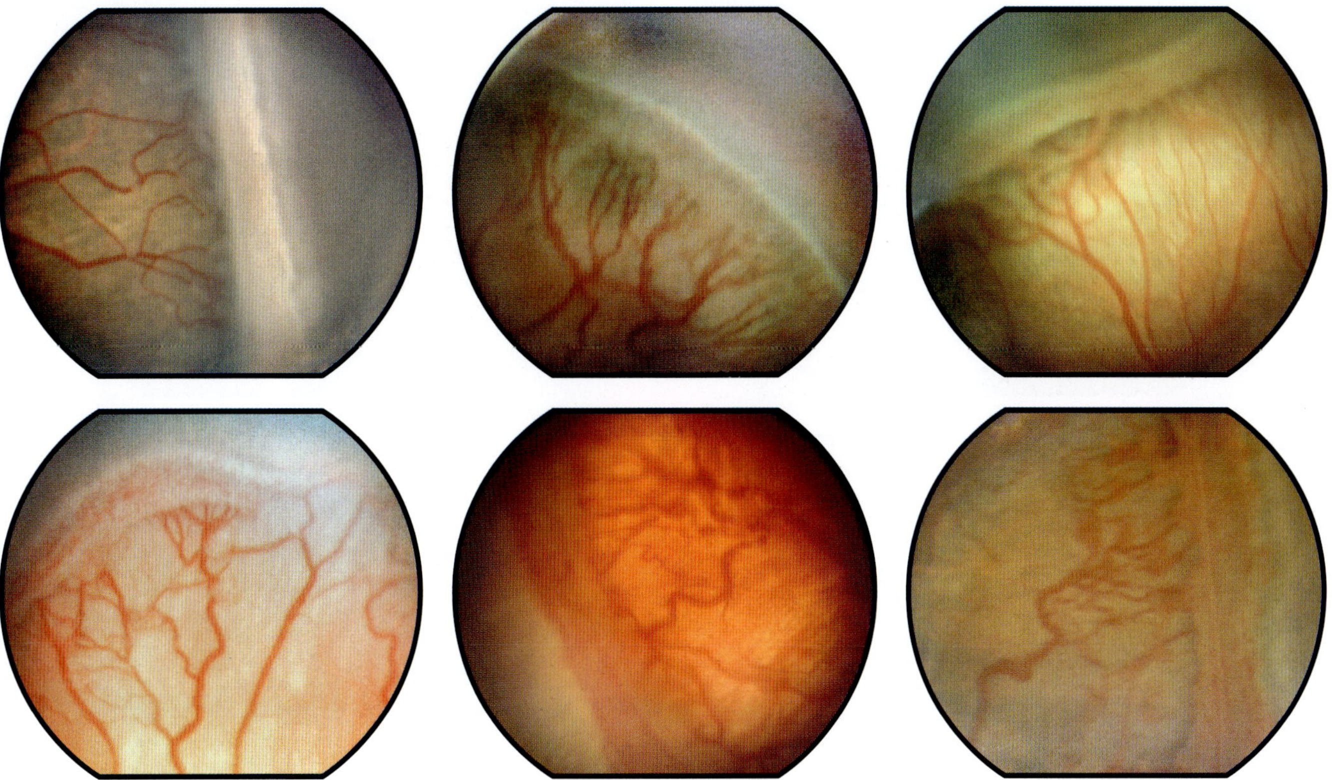

In these patients with ROP there is an elevated ridge of fibrovascular proliferation bordered posteriorly by prominent vessels (Plus disease). There is evidence of nodular, endothelial cell proliferation posterior to the ridge referred to as "popcorn lesions." These lesions may represent isolated tufts of extraretinal fibrovascular proliferation left behind as a ridge regresses more anteriorly, or conversely they may represent nascent fibrovascular proliferation that grow to become confluent with a progressing ridge.

ROP "Popcorn Lesions"

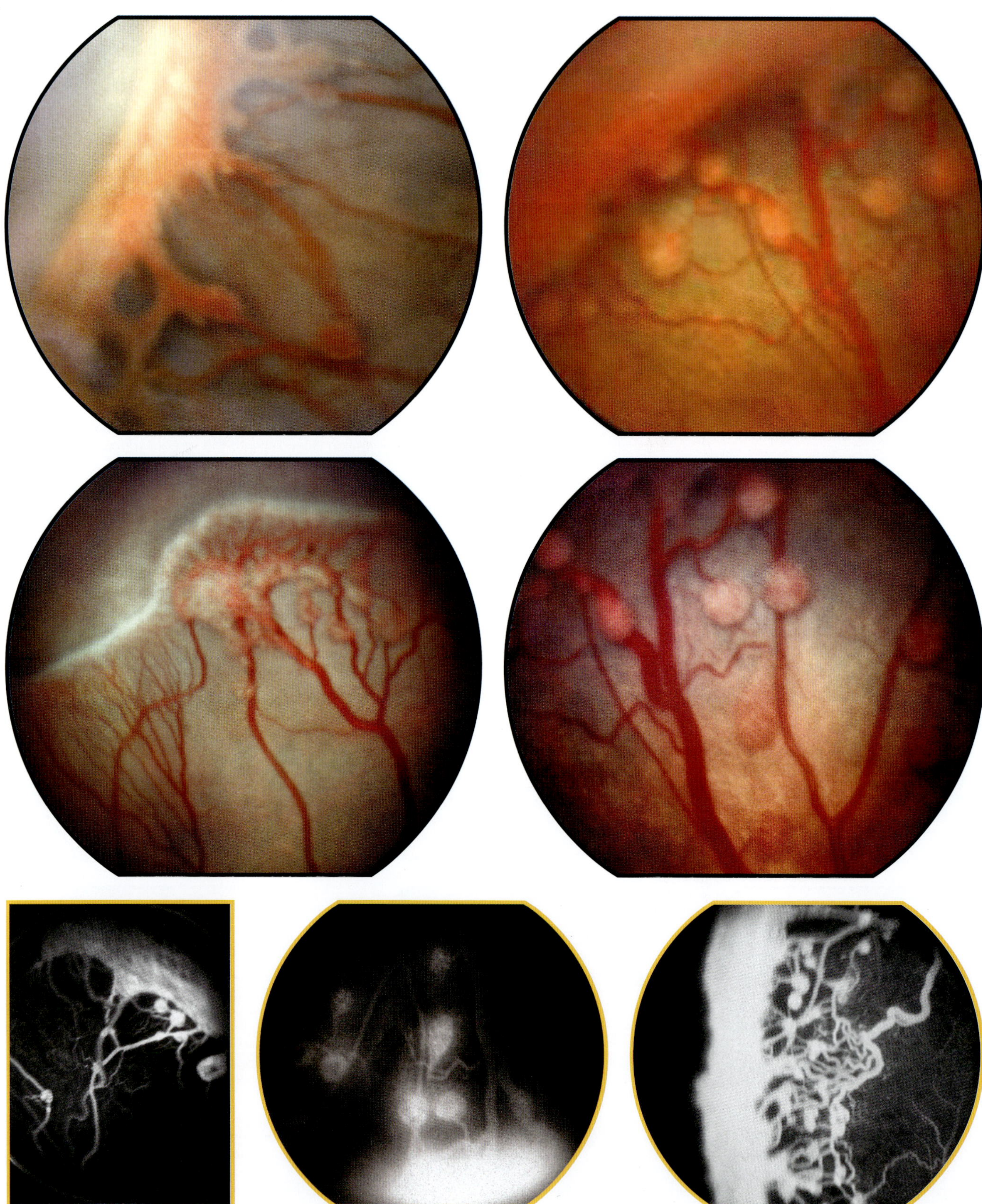

These images demonstrate the so-called "popcorn lesions" or nodular endothelial proliferation that is seen at the posterior ridge of fibrovascular proliferation in ROP. Note that the "popcorn lesions" hyperfluoresce, but do not leak very intensely. The neovascularization at the anterior edge of the vasculopathy does leak intensely, although this active permeability regresses as the fibrovascular proliferation consolidates.

ROP and Fibrous Scarring

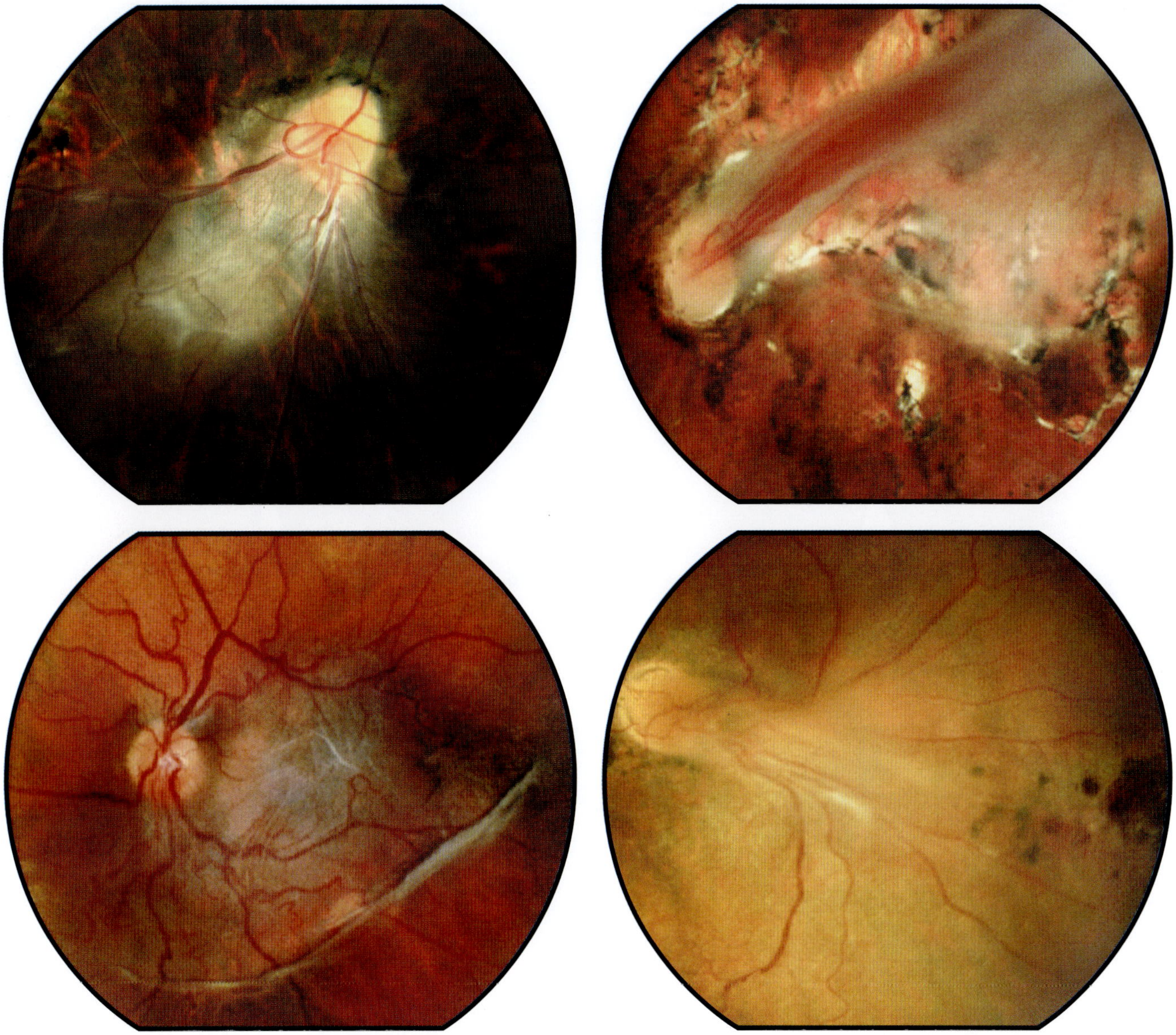

In these 4 cases, there has been extensive peripheral treatment of the ROP with ablative modalities such as photocoagulation and cryotherapy. There is extensive fibrosis in the posterior pole of each eye and the tractional extension of vessels from the nerve to the periphery.

© 122 © 123

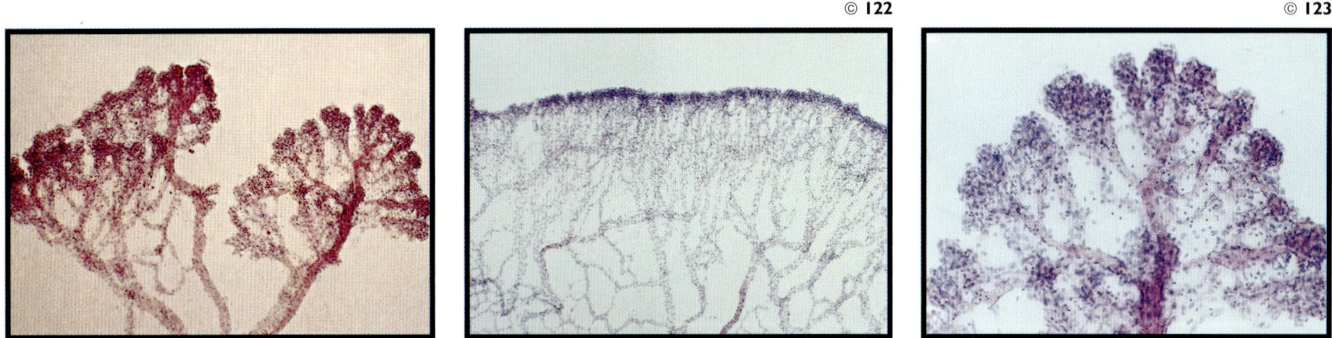

Trypsin digest preparations show intraretinal neovascularization resembling a sea-fan like configuration in ROP.

Persistent Fetal Vasculature Syndrome (Persistent Hyperplastic Primary Vitreous)

During embryogenesis, the developing structures of the eye are fed by the hyaloid artery, which emerges from the optic nerve head and extends to a network of vessels surrounding the lens collectively referred to as the tunica vasculosa lentis. This fetal vascular system typically regresses by apoptotic mechanisms; however, in some patients it fails to involute, resulting in persistent vascular elements in the posterior segment. This is termed persistent fetal vasculature syndrome (PFVS).

PFVS has a spectrum of presentations depending upon the extent of involution of the hyaloid artery and tunica vasculosa lentis. The retrolental fibrovascular tissue may obstruct the visual axis or cause early cataract. Contraction of the hyaloid fibrovascular remnants can lead to recurrent retinal and vitreous hemorrhages and even tractional retinal detachments. PFVS may also be associated with a variable degree of retinal dysplasia, optic nerve hypoplasia, and fibrovascular proliferation.

PFVS is typically unilateral. When bilateral PFVS is present, the possibility of Norrie disease must be ruled out, as it may mimic PFVS, but with more severe hemorrhagic and dysplastic retinal manifestations.

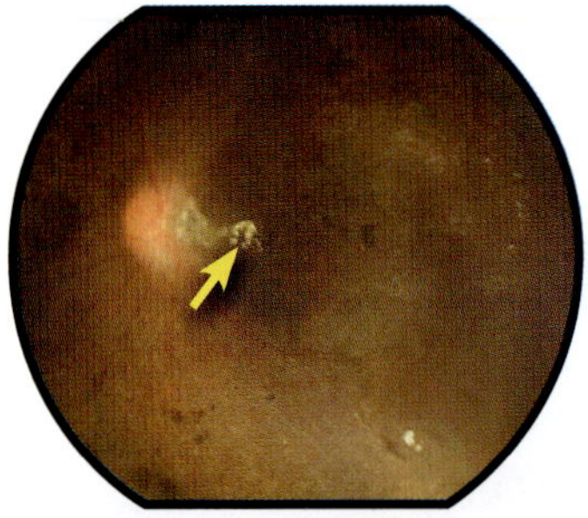
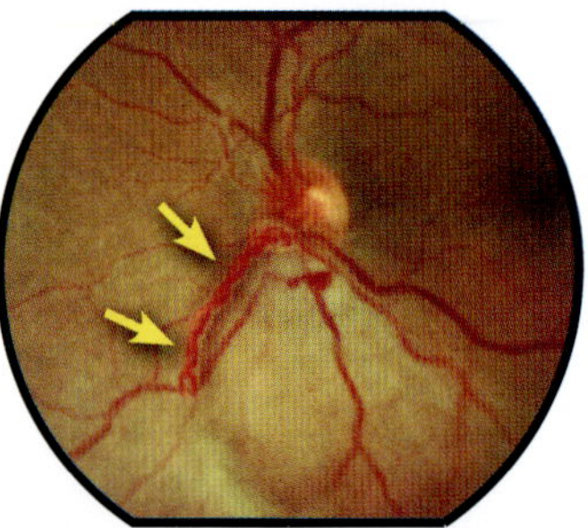
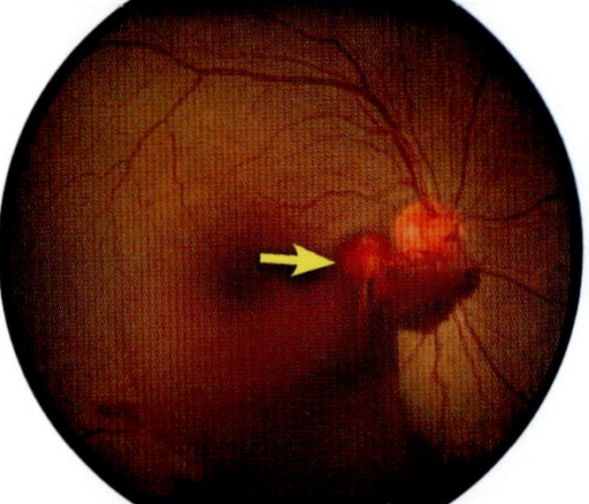
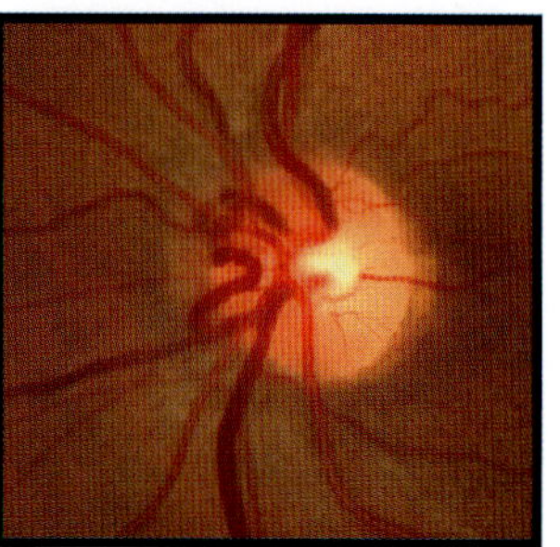

These images show vascular changes at the optic nerve. They represent the proximal portion of the hyaloidal vasculature. On the far left is a tortuous fibrotic remnant *(arrow)*, which is also referred to as a Bergmeister papilla. A prepapillary arteriolar vascular loop is associated with an inferior branch retinal artery occlusion (*arrows, second image*) and associated with vitreous hemorrhage (*arrow, third image*), which can be seen in such congenital vascular loops. The image on the far right is a congenital venular loop, which is less common. *Far left image courtesy of Dr. David Abramson*

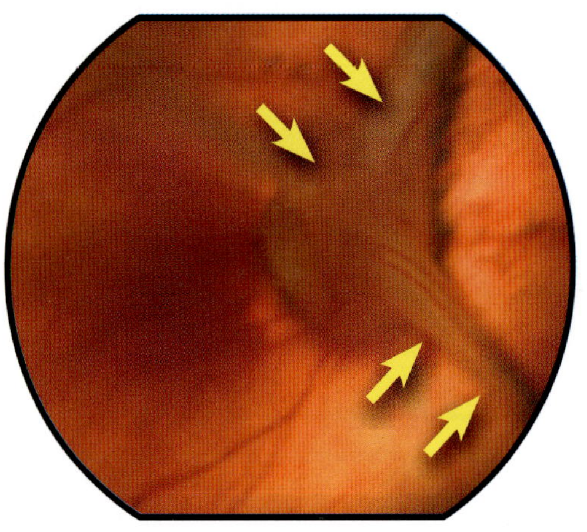
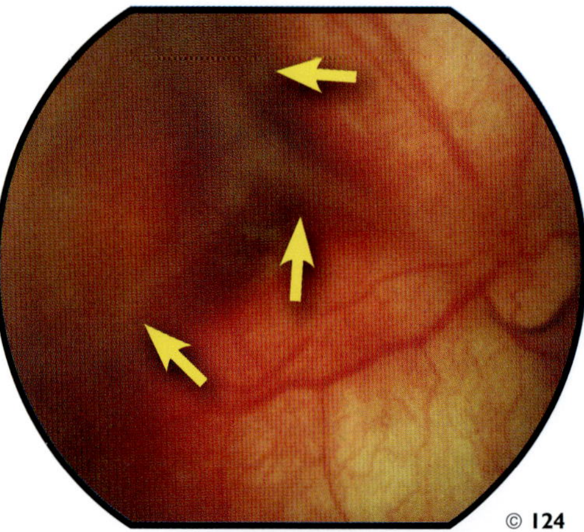

These patients have PFVS with variable degrees of incomplete regression of the posterior hyaloid. A fibrous stalk of vasculature is present in both patients and associated with one or more prominent retinal folds *(left, arrows)*. Bleeding into the vitreous has occurred in the patient on the right *(arrows)*.

© **124**

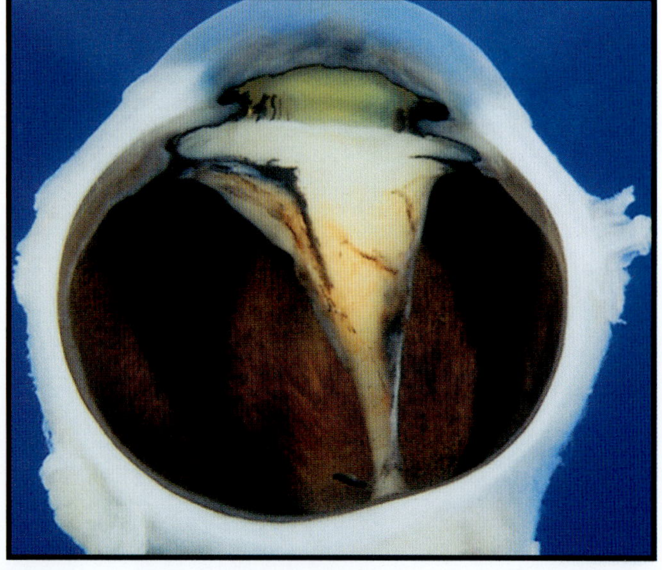

A remnant of the hyaloid vasculature with associated fibrovascular proliferation extends from the optic nerve to the posterior lens capsule in the left eye of this 9-month-old patient with PFVS. *Courtesy of Dr. Mort Goldberg*

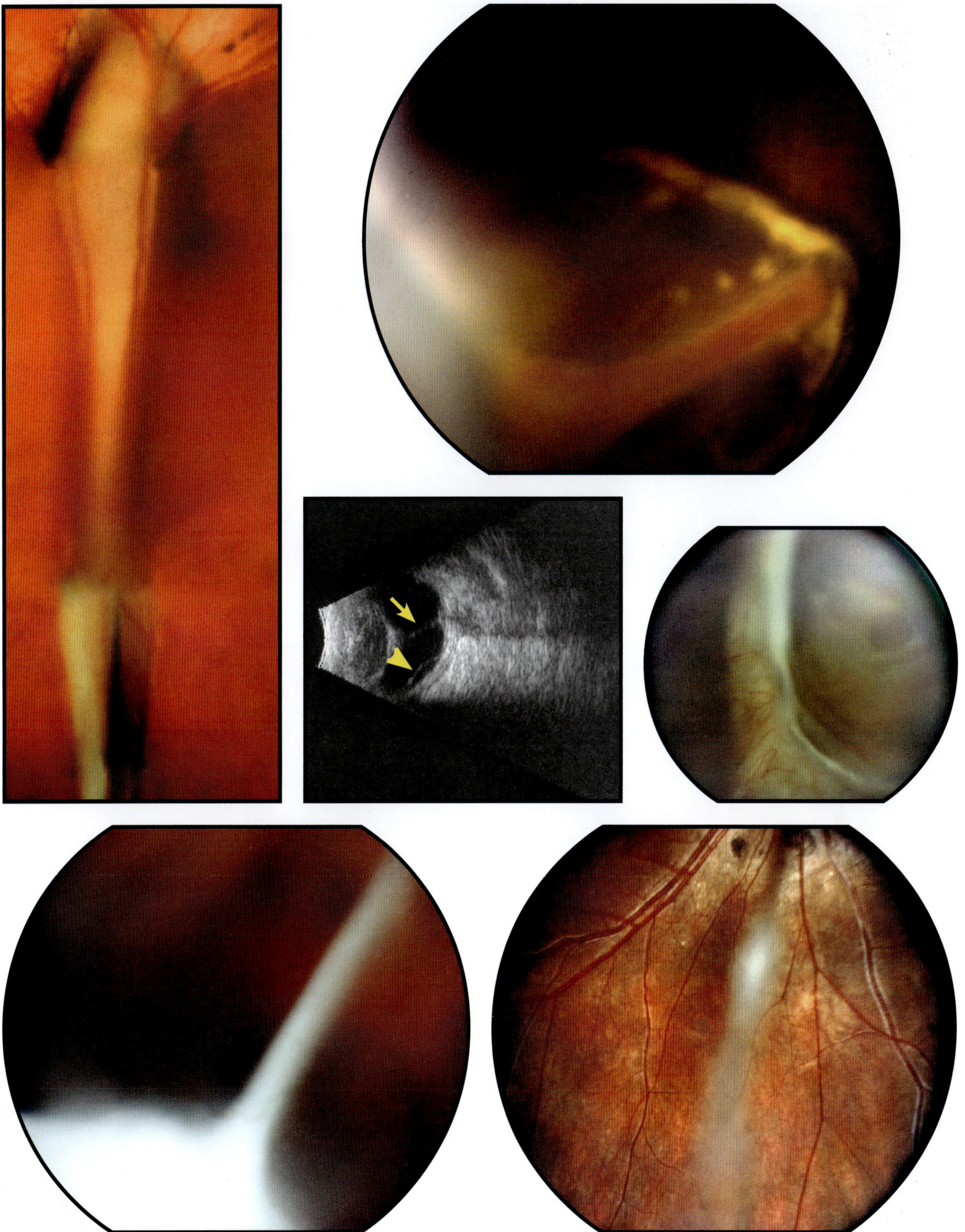

Note the variation in the clinical presentation of the persistent posterior hyaloid. Some clinical cases appear to be primarily associated with dysplastic changes (*middle row, right*). B-scan ultrasonography illustrates the hyaloid artery (*arrow*) and associated tractional retinal detachment (*arrowhead*).

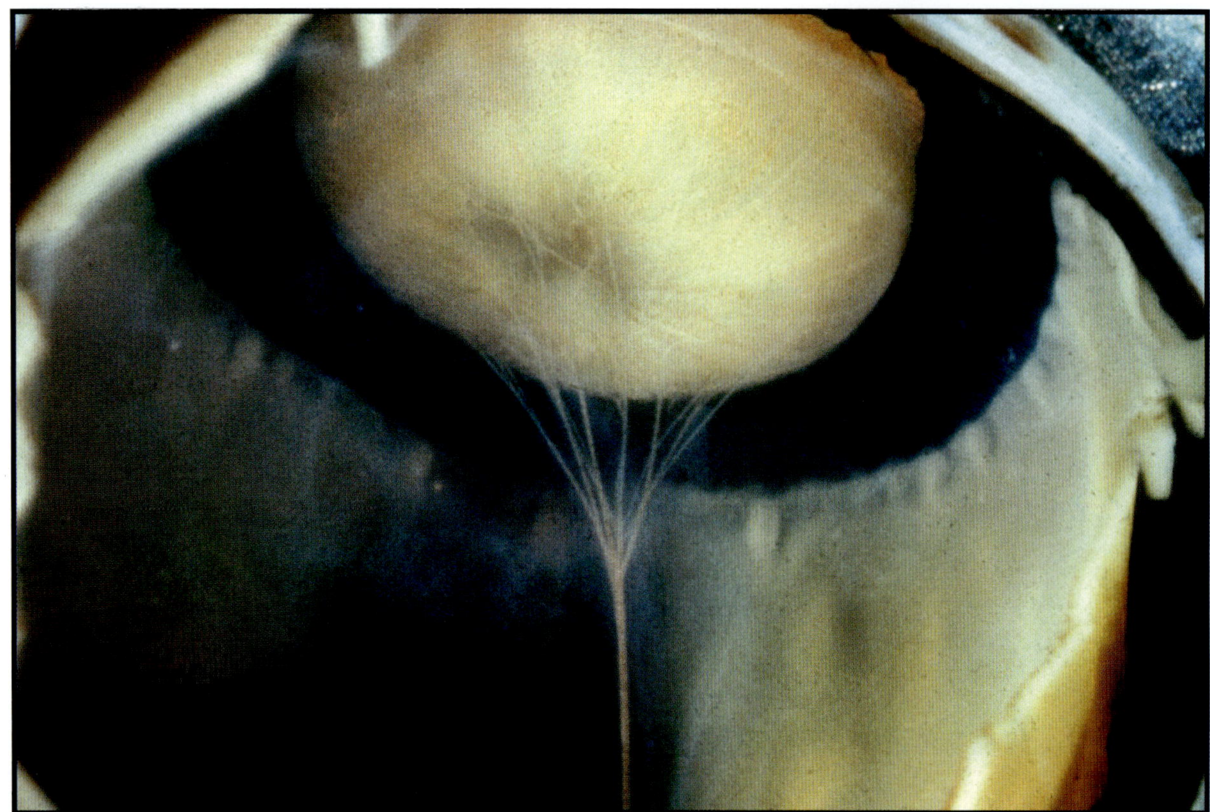

This image shows the delicate persistent tunica vasculosa lentis in communication with the persistent hyaloidal artery. *Courtesy of Dr. Mort Goldberg*

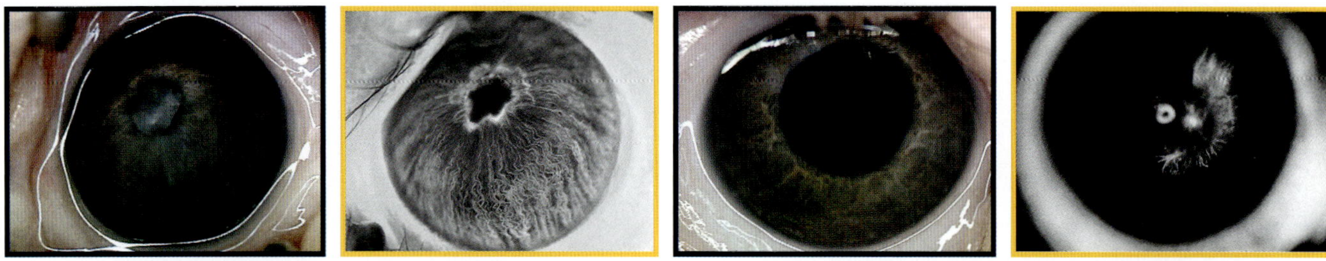

These patients have persistence of the anterior tunica vasculosa lentis, which extends into the margins of the iris and is seen best with fluorescein angiography.

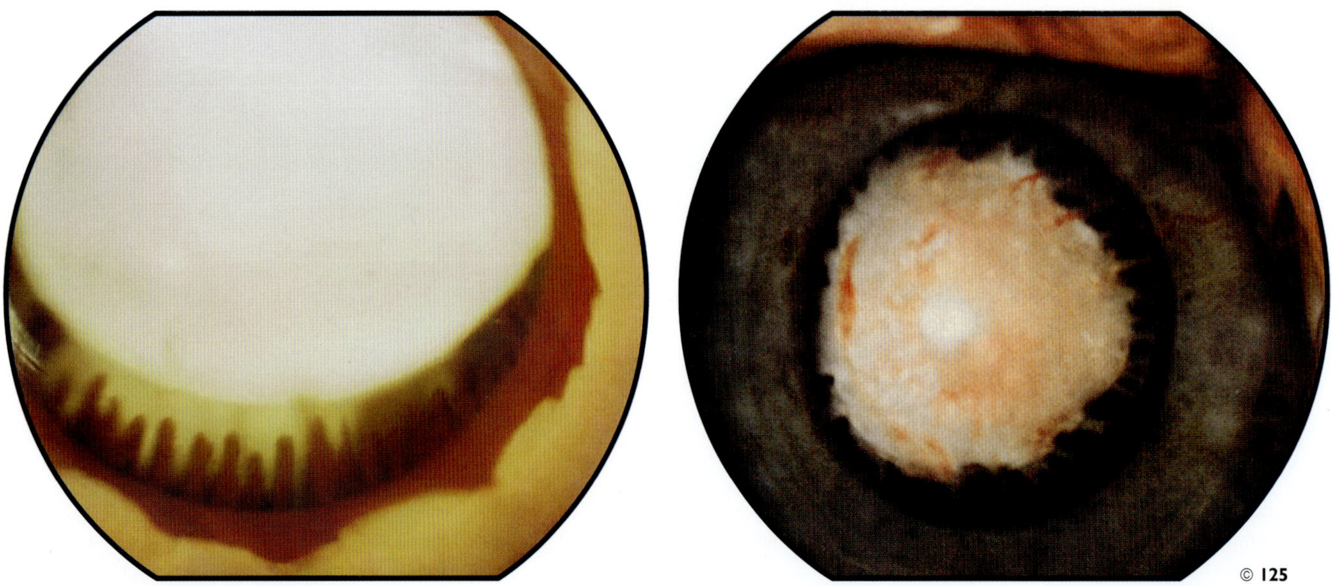

PFVS involving the anterior tunica vasculosa lentis has resulted in dense cataract formation in these two patients. These eyes are microphthalmic as well. *Courtesy of Dr. David Abramson*

Chorioretinal Coloboma

Coloboma may involve many ocular structures including the iris, lens, ciliary body, retina, choroid, or optic nerve and result from incomplete fusion of the embryonic fissure. Chorioretinal coloboma are most often located in the inferonasal quadrant as this is the last sector of the embryonic fissure to close during embryogenesis. Size and location of the coloboma can vary and accordingly visual acuity ranges from normal to no light perception depending upon the extent of the lesion and involvement of the optic nerve and macula. Occasionally, chorioretinal coloboma can produce a white pupil (leukocoria) on ophthalmoscopy that may simulate a mass lesion such as a retinoblastoma. Patients with chorioretinal coloboma are at risk of various complications throughout life including rhegmatogenous retinal detachment and choroidal neovascular membrane formation. Macular schisis and detachment may complicate optic nerve coloboma and other congenital optic disc anomalies and this entity is comprehensively reviewed in Chapter 15. Chorioretinal colobomas may be isolated or can be associated with a number of systemic syndromes including fetal alcohol syndrome, infections (e.g. congenital rubella syndrome), and various genetic syndromes including CHARGE syndrome (coloboma, heart abnormalities, anal atresia, renal abnormalities, genitourinary abnormalities, ear anomalies) associated with CHD7 mutation and papillorenal syndrome (PAX2 mutation), characterized by optic nerve or chorioretinal coloboma in association with congenital kidney disease.

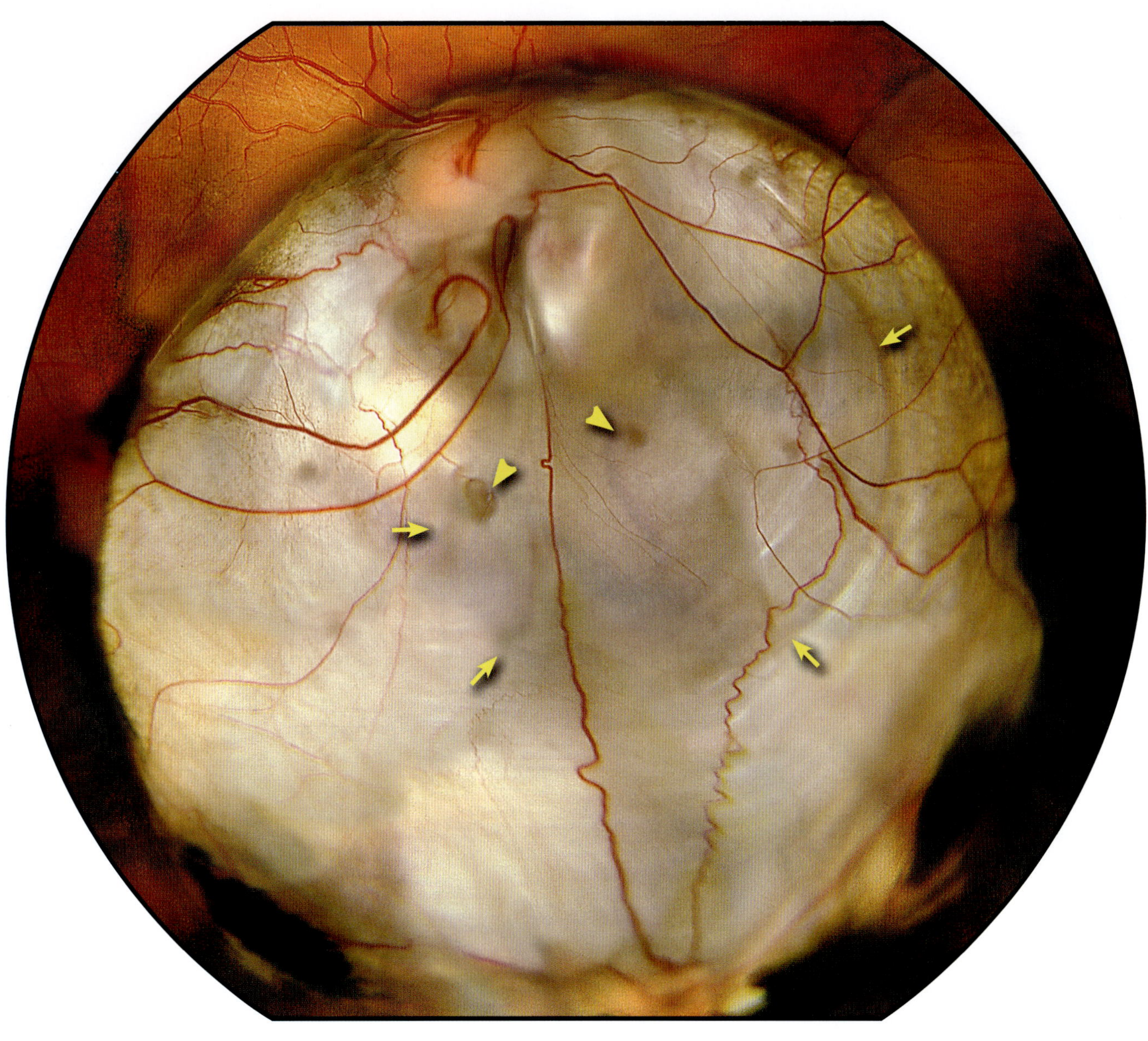

This is a very large coloboma that involves the optic nerve and choroid. There is a staphylomatous abnormality within the central choroidal colobomatous area *(arrows)*. The circular abnormalities within the staphylomatous area *(arrowheads)* may represent tiny fistulous tracks into the retrobulbar area. A child with such a large coloboma may present with leukocoria simulating a retinoblastoma.

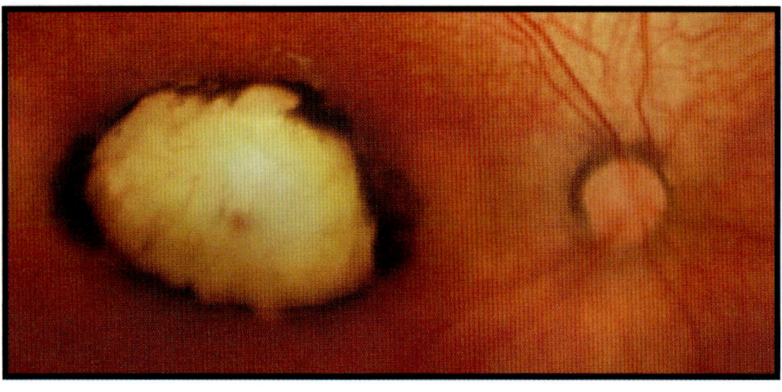
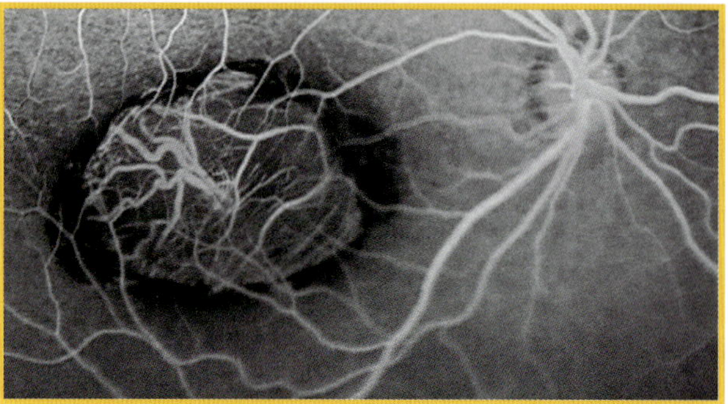

This is a fundus photo and fluorescein angiogram of a macular scar from a 14-month-old boy with congenital toxoplasmosis, which simulates a coloboma. It is excavated, bordered by pigment, and irregular at its edges.

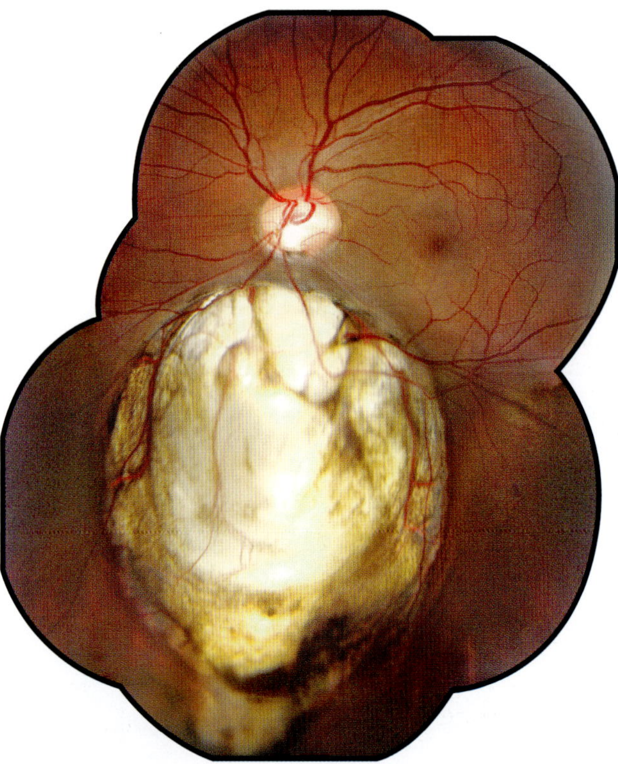
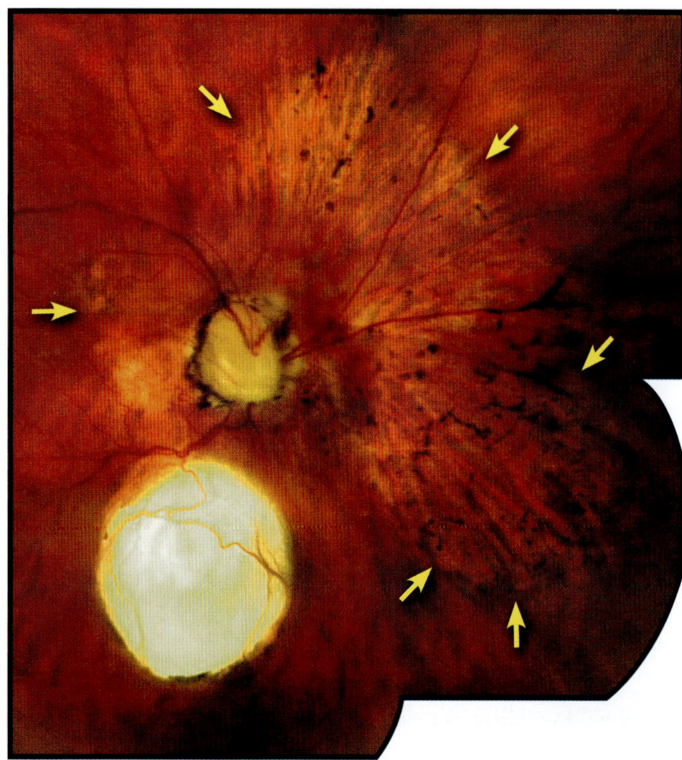

These are two patients with a congenital choroidal coloboma. These are associated with colobomatous changes involving the optic nerve. A zonal area of chorioretinal atrophy and pigment epithelial hyperplasia (*arrows*) is presumed to be the result of an antecedent retinal detachment that has spontaneously resolved. *Courtesy of Ophthalmic Imaging Systems, Inc*

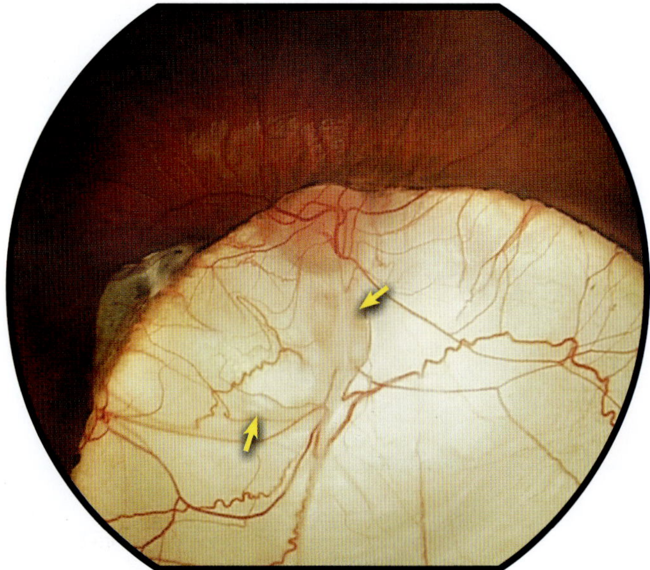

This is a large posterior coloboma encompassing the optic nerve and choroid. There is a fibrous membrane overlying the coloboma (*arrows*). These congenital abnormalities are inferiorly located in the fundus. In addition, the patient harbored an iris coloboma.

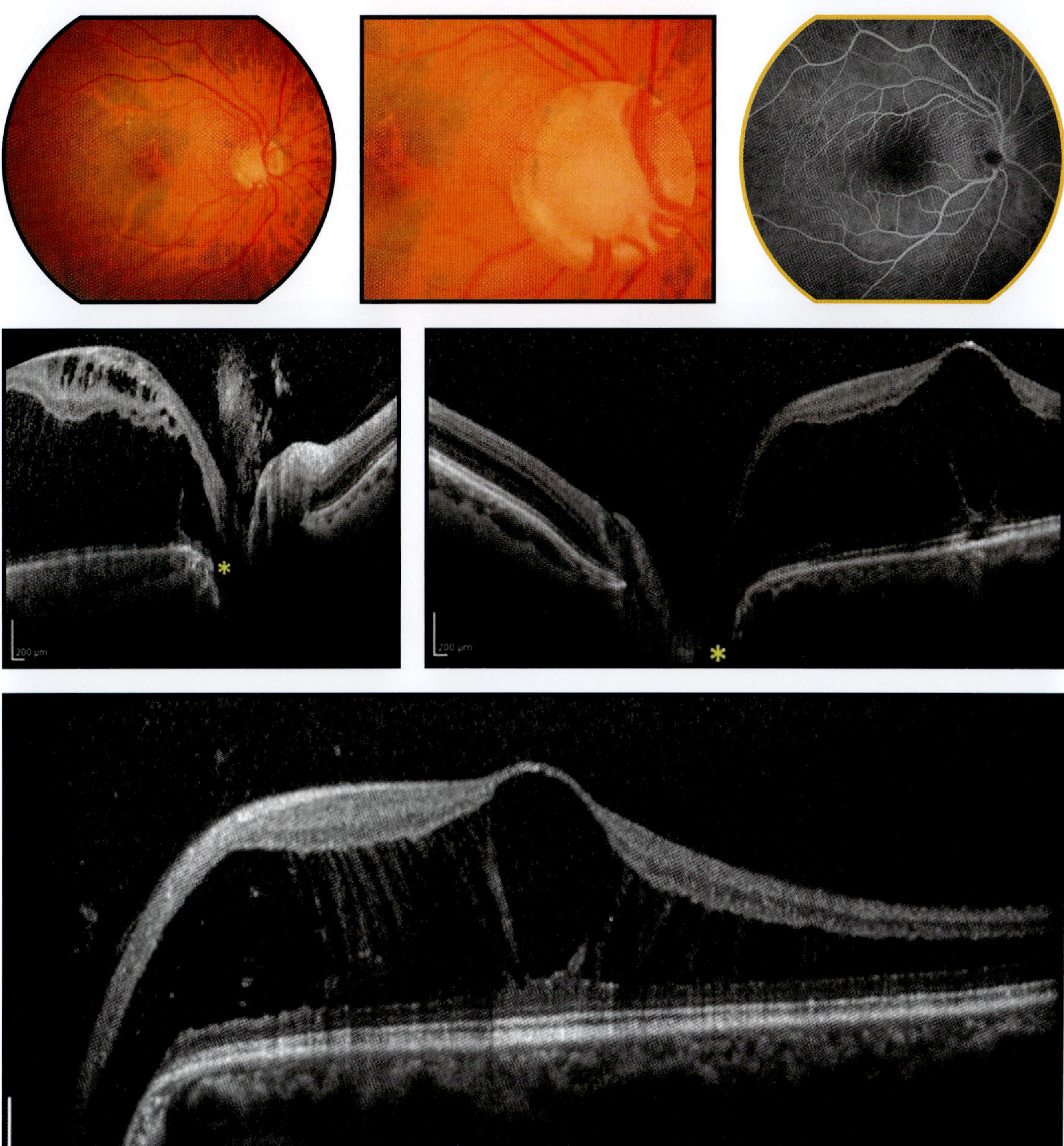

Color fundus photograph of a patient with papillorenal syndrome showing a blunted foveal reflex and inferotemporal optic disc coloboma (versus an optic nerve pit) of the right eye *(top left)* with magnified view of the optic nerve *(top middle)*. Fluorescein angiogram of the right eye highlights the optic nerve coloboma (versus an optic nerve pit) *(top right)*. SD-OCT through the nerve of the right *(middle left)* and left *(middle right)* eyes demonstrates the optic nerve colobomas *(asterisks)* and SD-OCT through the macula *(bottom)* demonstrates retinoschisis. Genetic testing revealed a heterozygotic mutation in the PAX2 gene. The patient also had hearing loss, which can be characteristic of this disorder. *Images courtesy of Ricardo Japiassú, MD*

Congenital Folds

Congenital retinal fold is a rare abnormality consisting of an anomalous fold of retina and associated vessels coursing through the posterior segment from the optic disc to the ora serrata. It is often associated with disorders of the peripheral retinal vasculature such as ROP, familial exudative vitreoretinopathy (FEVR), incontinentia pigmenti, and Norrie disease. It therefore may not represent a separate clinical entity, but instead may exist as part of the spectrum of these diseases. It should, however, be differentiated from a glial mass and from persistent fetal vasculature. In the absence of other ocular disorders and when associated with hyperopia, posterior microphthalmos syndrome should be excluded. Congenital folds are most often found bilaterally and symmetrically and may be associated with visual dysfunction and nystagmus.

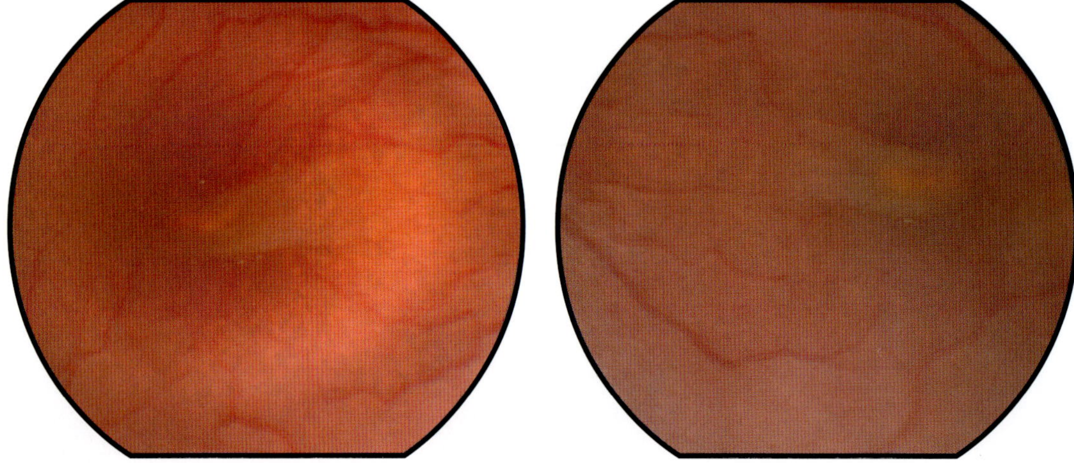

This patient demonstrated 18 diopters of hyperopia in each eye. Posterior microphthalmos and bilateral, symmetric congenital retinal folds in the macular region are illustrated. *Courtesy of Dr. Thomas W. Wilson*

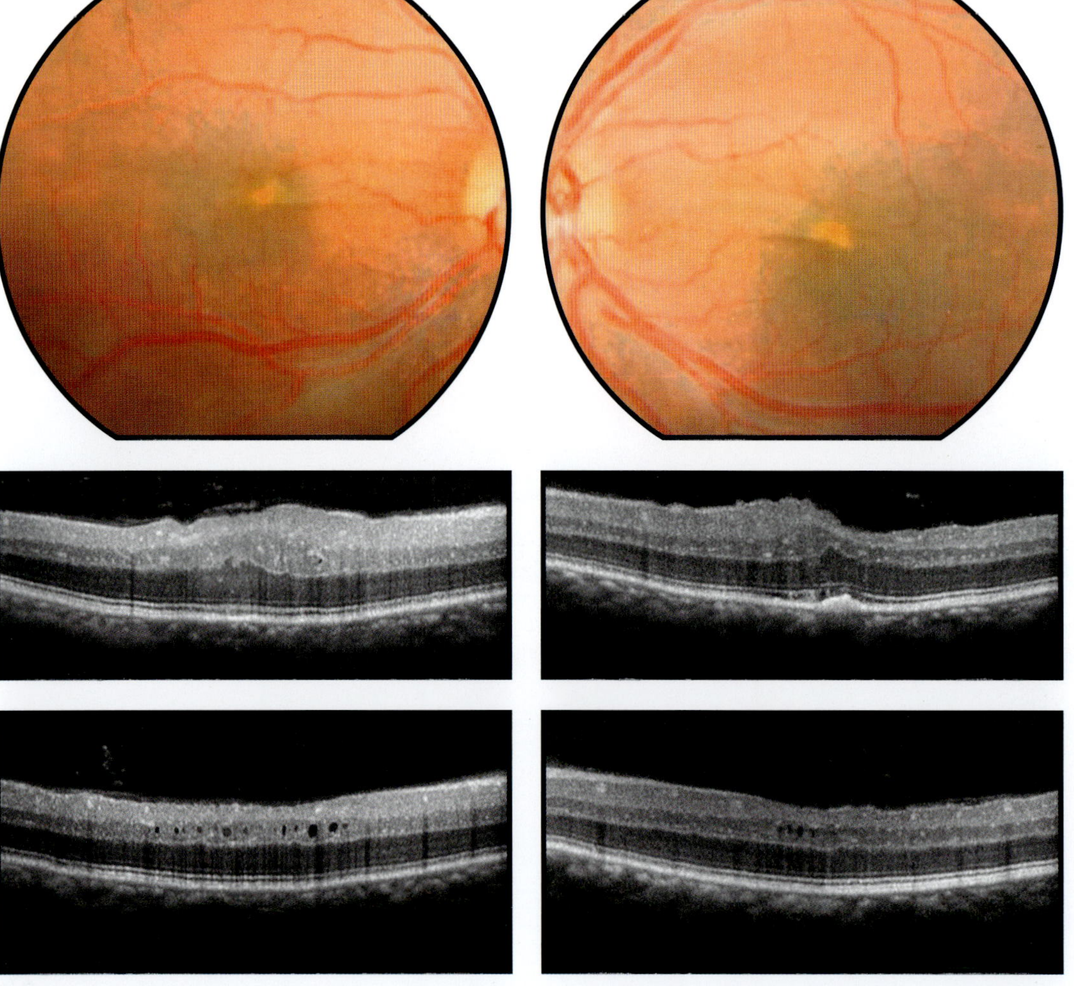

The color fundus photographs of this patient with posterior microphthalmos demonstrates subtle papillomacular folds, an abnormal foveal reflex, and a crowded disc. SD-OCT demonstrates retinal folds and mild cystoid macular edema. Axial length was measured to be 15.44 mm. *Images courtesy of Alan Bird, MD and Philip Hykin, MD*

Phakomatoses

This group of disorders arises due to genetic mutations typically involving tumor suppressor genes that result in the development of benign and/or malignant tumors, which classically involve the brain, skin, and eye. Retinal lesions can be the important clue to the diagnosis of the systemic condition that can be fatal if left untreated. Phakomatoses often present during the pediatric years, although lesions may be acquired during the lifetime of the patient. While many of these retinal lesions are more comprehensively discussed in the oncology chapter (Chapter 8), we will briefly review the salient retinal and systemic features in this chapter as these findings are not entirely uncommon in the pediatric population.

Neurofibromatosis Type I

Neurofibromatosis type I (NFI) is an autosomal dominant disease caused by mutation in the NFI gene on chromosome 17q11.2. NFI occurs in approximately 1 in 3000 live births, and 50% of cases are secondary to spontaneous mutation. The NFI gene normally functions as a tumor suppressor, and mutation leads to abnormal proliferation of multiple neural tissues. Diagnosis is based upon the presence of some combination of axillary or inguinal freckling, optic glioma, Lisch nodules, cutaneous neurofibromas, plexiform neurofibromas, certain osseous lesions, and the presence of a first-degree relative with NFI. The most common ophthalmologic finding is the presence of iris Lisch nodules, which affect nearly all patients by the age of 20 years old. More recently choroidal hamartomas consisting of abnormal proliferations of Schwann cells have been described in 78 to 100% of NFI patients. These lesions are best seen with enhanced depth optical coherence tomography or infrared imaging.

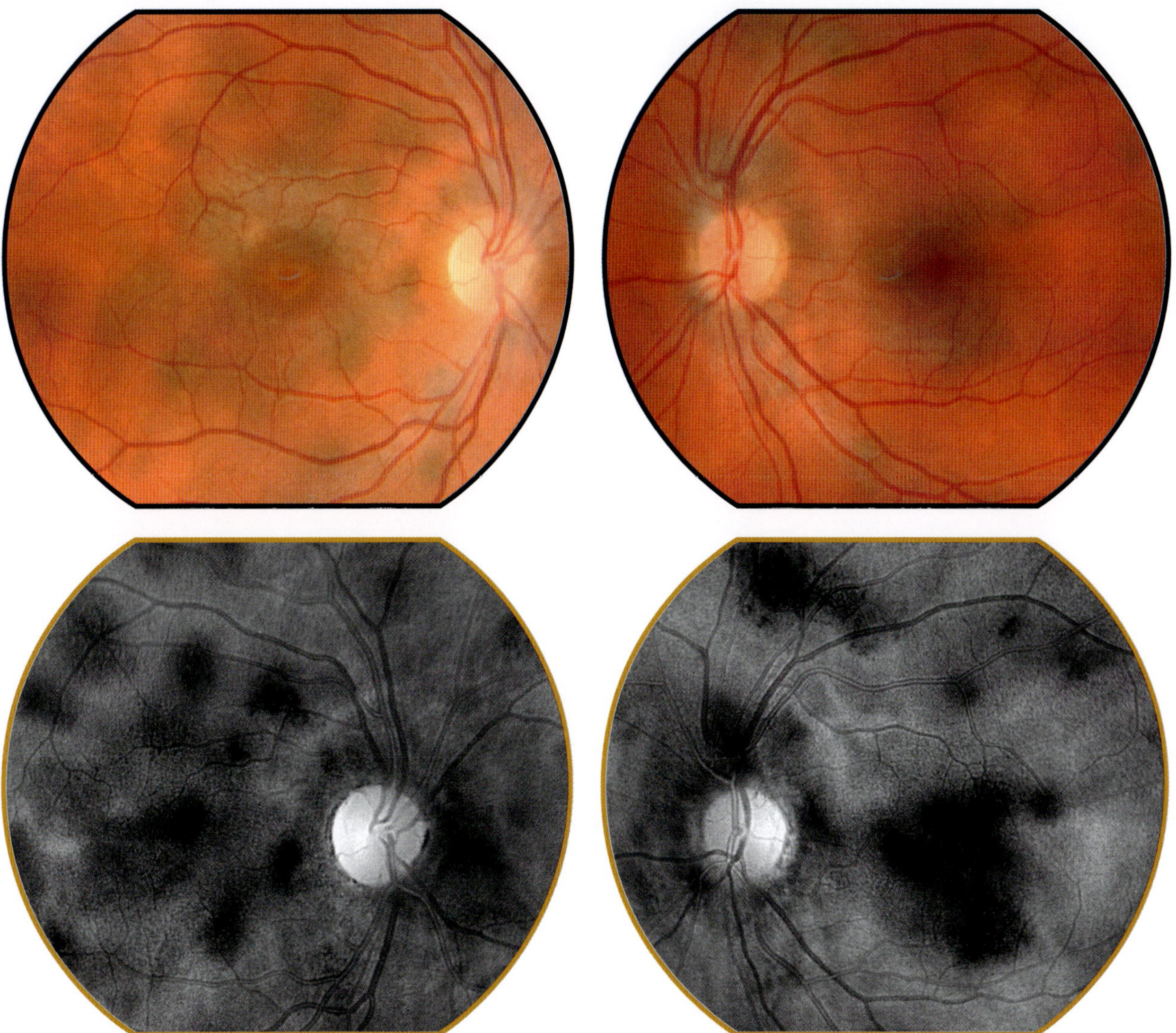

Color fundus photographs of this patient with neurofibromatosis type I shows subtle deep hyperpigmented lesions at the level of the choroid, that are made much more apparent by infrared imaging *(bottom row)*. These lesions represent hamartomatous proliferations of Schwann cells similar in histology to neurofibromata of the skin and Lisch nodules.

Neurofibromatosis Type 2

Neurofibromatosis type 2 is a rare hereditary phakomatosis caused by mutation in the NF2 tumor suppressor gene on chromosome 22. It is inherited in an autosomal dominant manner but approximately 50% of cases result from *de novo* mutations. Clinically, the disease is characterized by bilateral vestibular schwannomas, multiple central nervous system tumors, and several ocular abnormalities, the most frequent of which is posterior subscapular cataract. Posterior manifestations include combined hamartoma of the retina and retinal pigment epithelium and epiretinal membrane (ERM). The ERMs that complicate NF2 may appear similar to the typical ERM of inflammatory etiology, or may have a distinct, scaphoid appearance with edges curled up toward the vitreous. There may be a correlation with the presence of ERM and severity of the systemic disease.

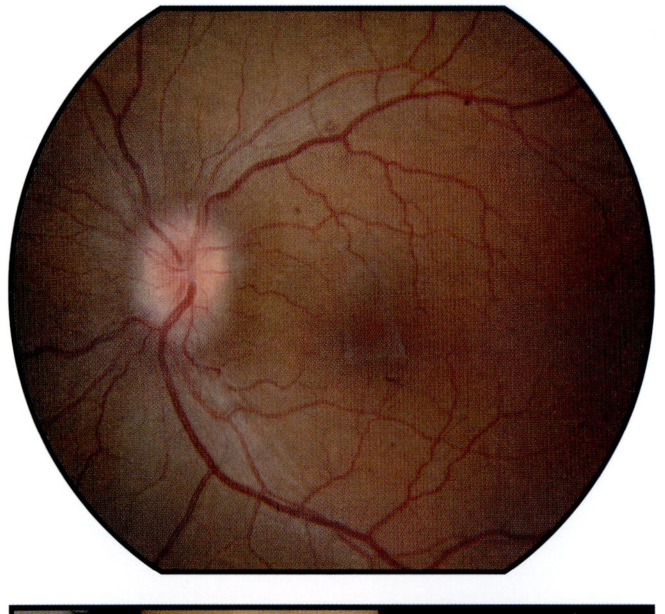

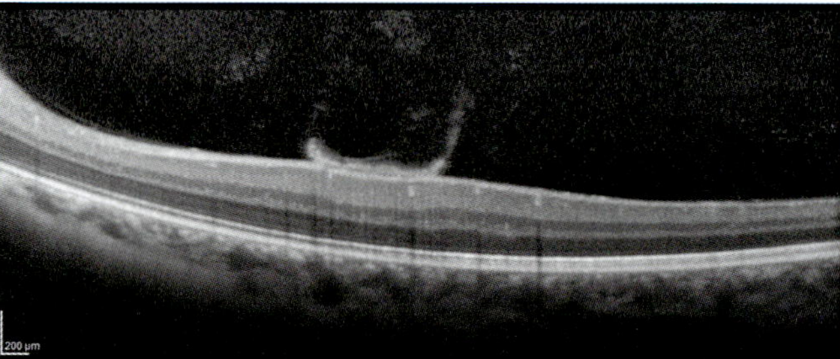

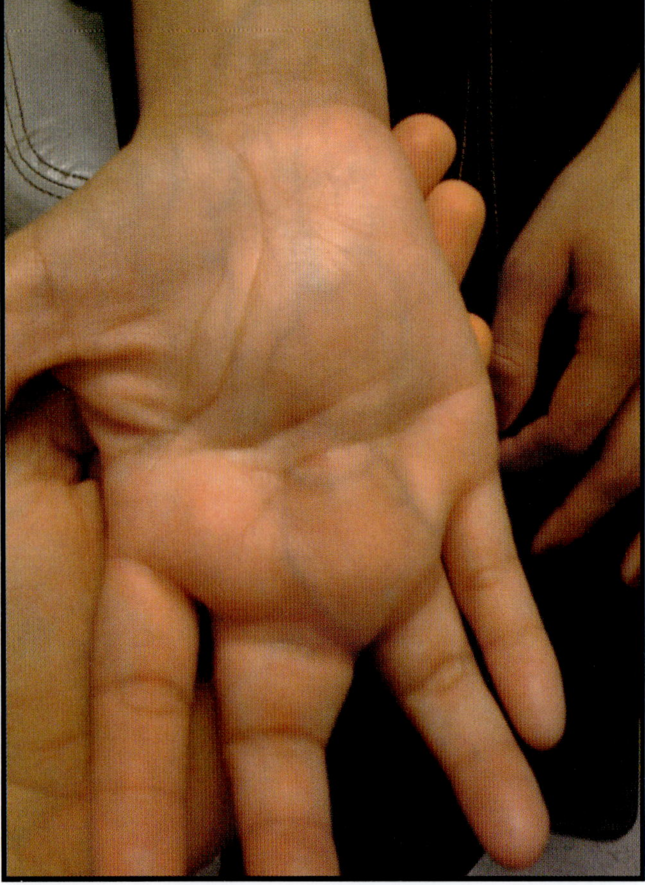

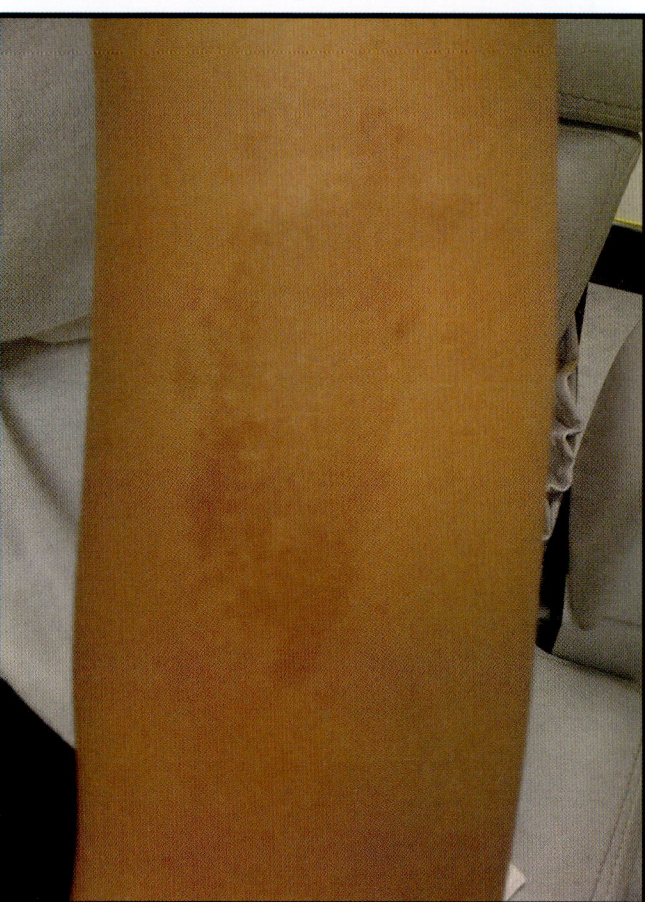

This patient with NF2 was found to have an ERM with the characteristic scaphoid morphology seen in NF2. Color photograph of the patient's hand and lower leg shows a neurofibroma on the palm and a café au lait spot respectively.

Combined Hamartoma of the Retina and RPE

A hamartoma of the retina may present to the pediatric retinal physician with its characteristic vitreoretinal interface disturbance, prominent retinal vessels, and variably reactive pigment epithelium.

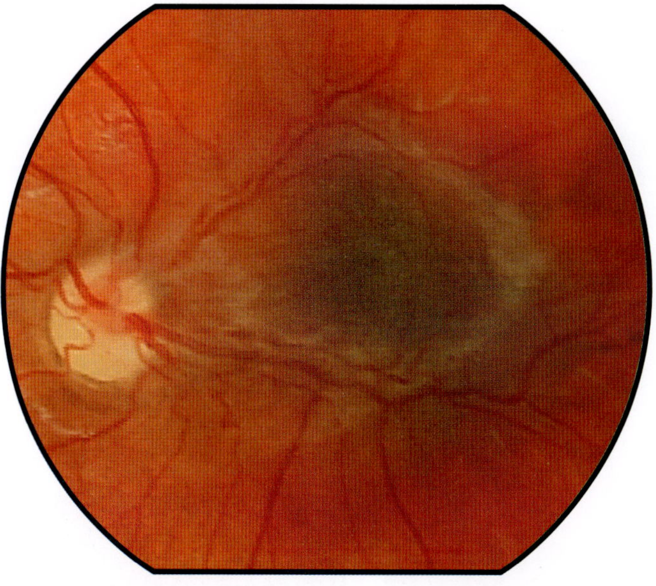

This 17-month-old boy has a characteristic elevated pigmented hamartomatous mass involving both the retina and the retinal pigment epithelium with overlying glial tissue.

Arterial–Venous Malformations (Wyburn Mason Syndrome)

Wyburn Mason syndrome is a rare, nonhereditary phakomatosis consisting of arterial–venous malformations (AVM) of the retina, ipsilateral central nervous system, and face. Retinal angiomas are typically asymptomatic and inert and do not affect vision unless the retinal vascular abnormality is extensive or involves the macula. Rarely leakage and exudation and hemorrhage may develop. Reports of retinal ischemia resulting from retinal arterial shunting exist. Of greater concern are the potential complications of intracranial (typically involving the midbrain) and intraorbital lesions, which if present, may result in compressive optic neuropathy, hemiplegia, or even death from intracranial hemorrhage.

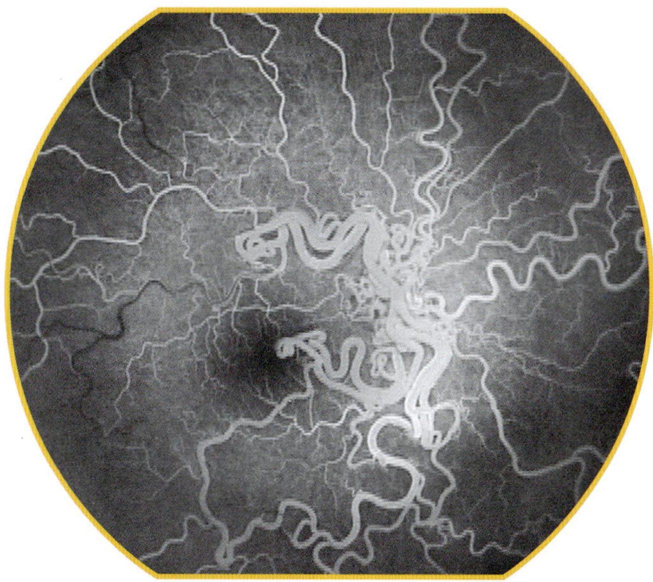

Fluorescein angiography of a patient with Wyburn Mason syndrome demonstrates rapid filling of this type III arteriovenous malformation. No leakage was seen from these vessels in late phases of the study *(not shown)*.

Congenital Retinal Macrovessel

Congenital retinal macrovessel is a rare anomaly of the retinal vasculature characterized by a large aberrant vessel, typically venous, which crosses the horizontal raphe. These are typically asymptomatic, but occasionally complications may develop, which result in decreased vision. These complications include branch retinal vein occlusion, cystoid macular edema, serous retinal detachment, and angioscotoma among others. Although not typically associated with other systemic abnormalities, one case of a coexistent intracranial venous malformation has been described.

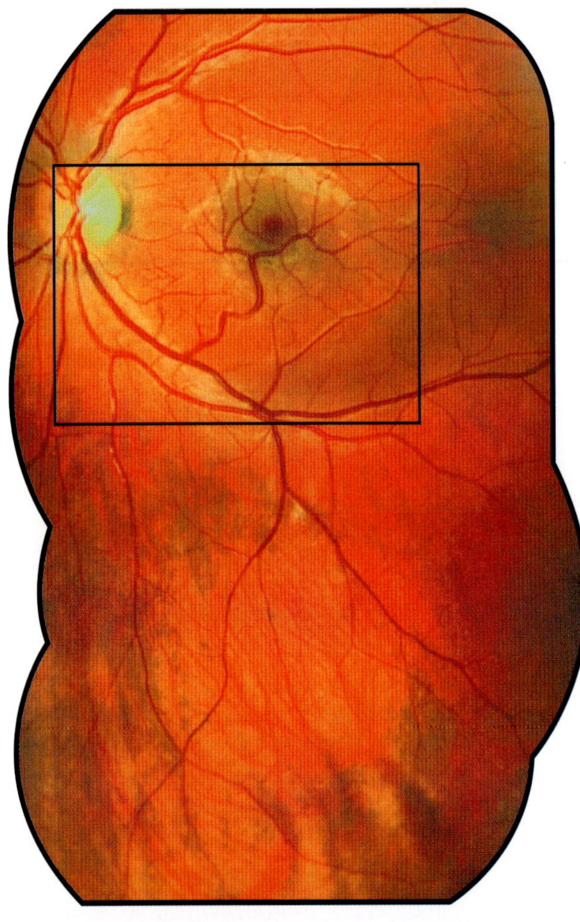

Color fundus montage and high magnification color fundus photograph of a congenital retinal venous macrovessel.

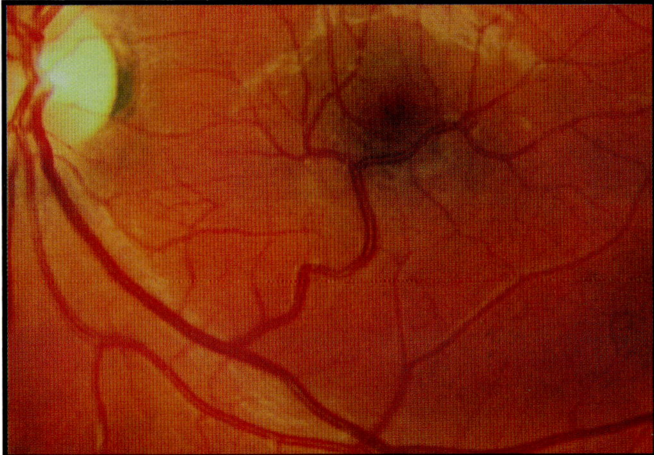

Color fundus photo of a patient with a left-sided congenital retinal venous macrovessel complicated by a small venous tributary occlusion *(arrow)*. Magnetic resonance imaging of the same patient revealed an ipsilateral intracranial congenital venous malformation *(arrow)*.

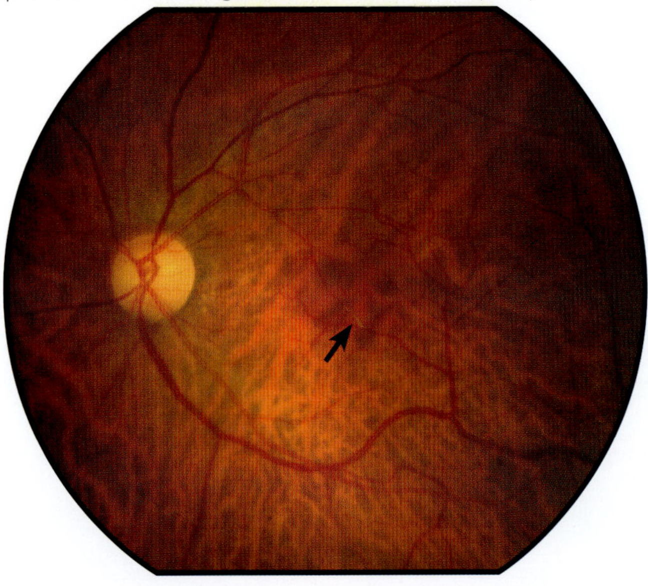

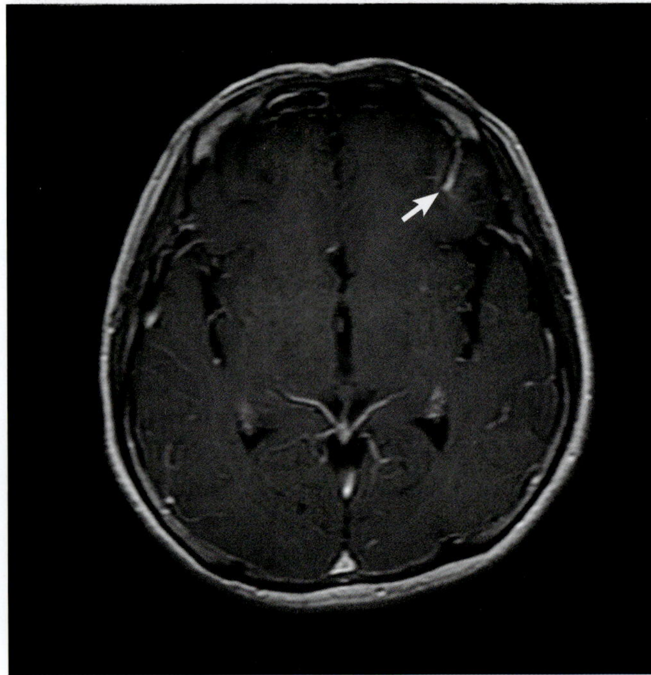

von Hippel–Lindau Syndrome (VHL)

von Hippel–Lindau syndrome is a rare disease caused by mutation in the VHL gene on chromosome 3. The mutation affects HIF1 (hypoxia inducible factor) that functions in the angiogenic cascade upstream from other cytokines such as VEGF. VHL is characterized by the formation of various systemic tumors including CNS hemangioblastoma, renal cell carcinoma, pancreatic cyst, and pheochromocytoma among others. Ocular manifestations include retinal capillary hemangioblastomas, which are hamartomatous vascular lesions. The variable effects these lesions have on vision depends on their location, size, and exudative effects. Recognition of this entity in the pediatric setting has critical implications. Renal cell carcinoma is the most common cause of mortality and systemic management of cerebellar and spinal and renal complications can prevent morbidity and mortality. Retinal hemangioblastoma can progressively grow and lead to severe exudative and blinding complications if left untreated and therefore prophylactic laser and/or cryotherapy can prevent vision loss and blindness. Frequent monitoring for systemic and ocular complications is essential.

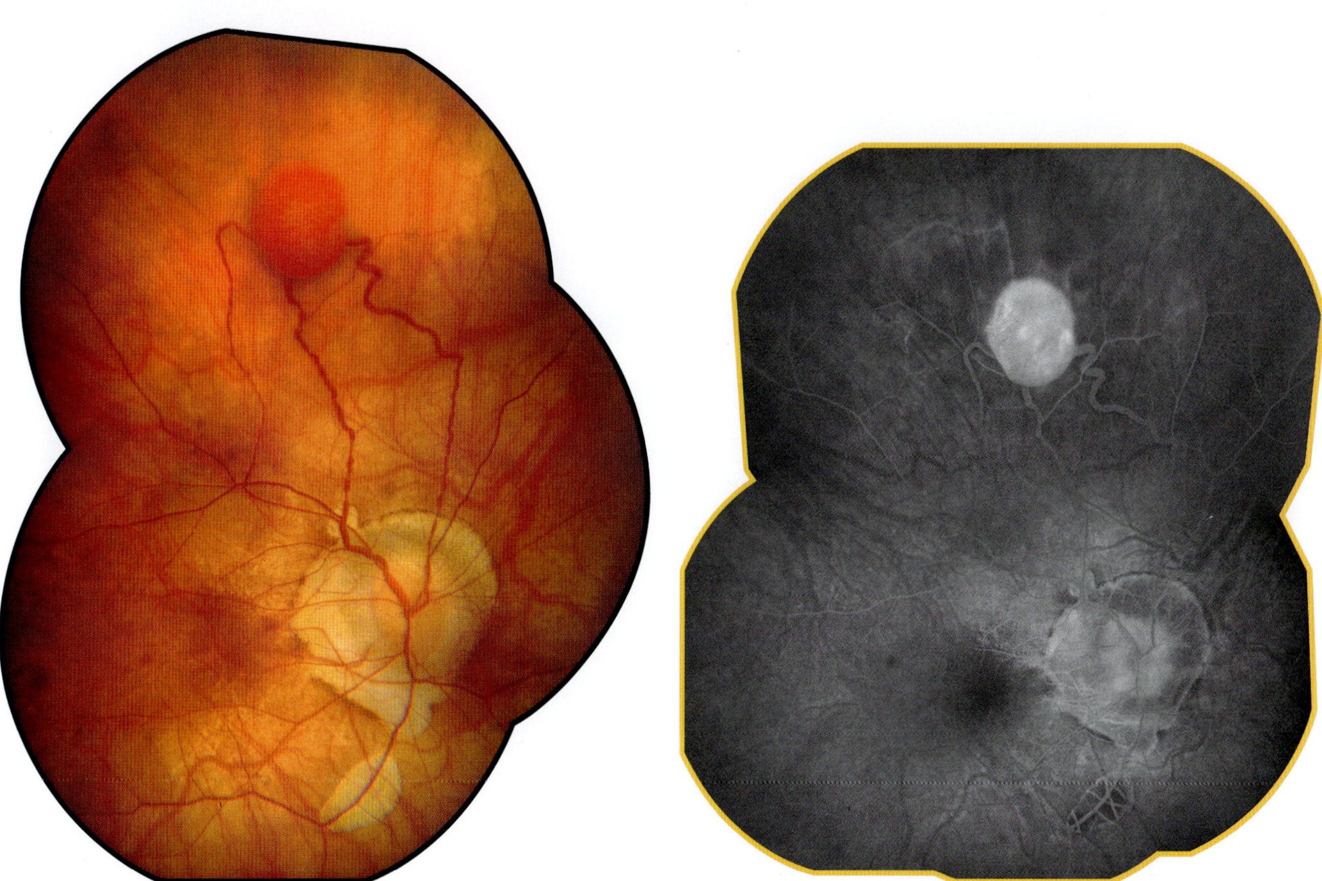

Color fundus photographic montage showing a large sporadic hemangioblastoma with dilated and beaded feeder and draining vessels in this myopic patient. The lesion stains in the late phase of the FA montage.

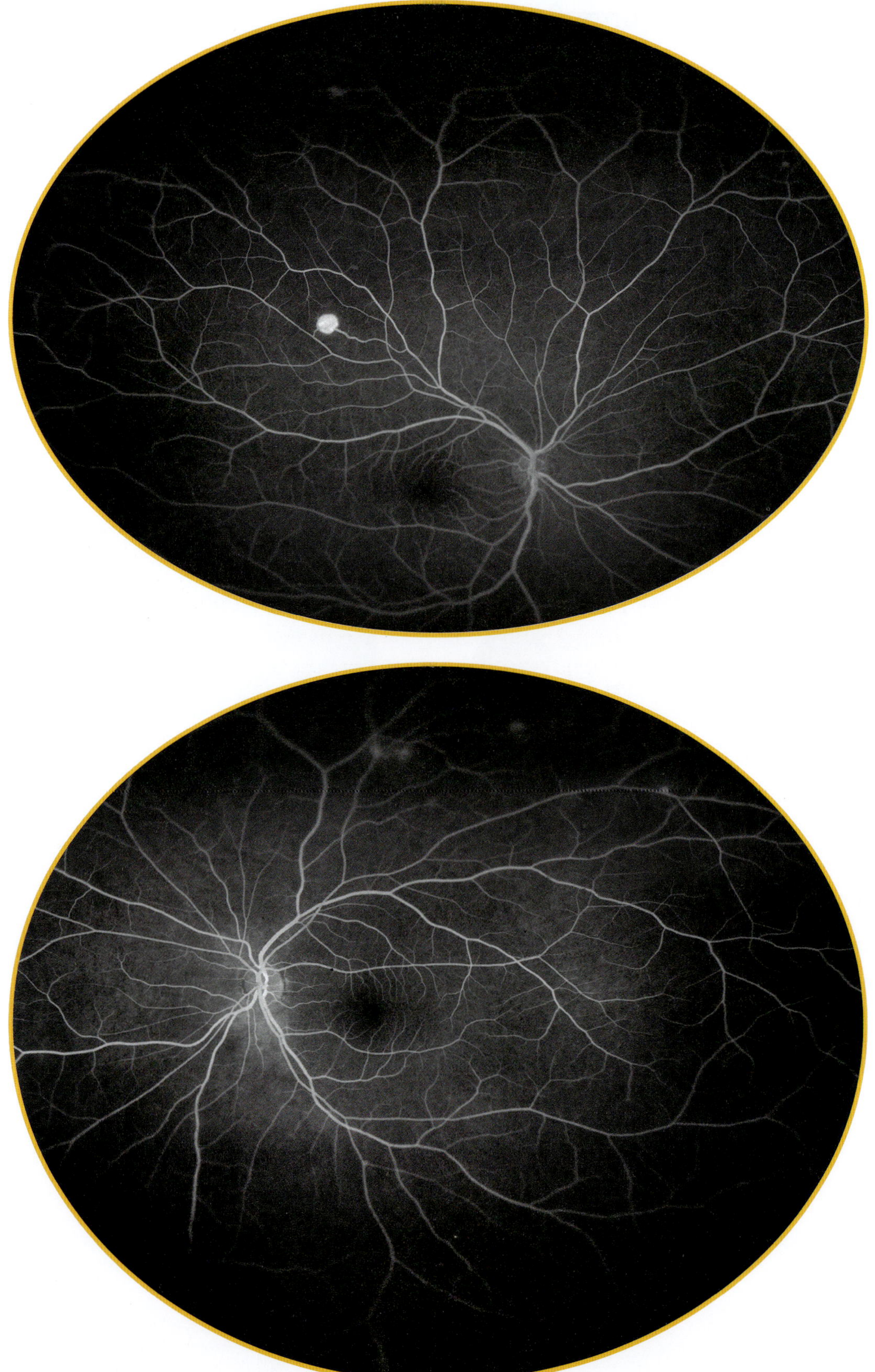

This patient with VHL disease has multiple hemangioblastomas, many of which are small and peripherally located. Wide-field fluorescein angiography in VHL disease may reveal more lesions than can be appreciated on funduscopy or conventional fluorescein angiogram. Note the small superior lesions identified with wide-field imaging in each eye. *Images courtesy of Steven D. Schwartz, MD*

Retinal Cavernous Hemangioma

Retinal cavernous hemangioma is a rare vascular tumor of the retina and appears clinically as multiple aneurysmal dilatations (described as a "cluster of grapes") along the course of a single vein or multiple retinal veins. Fluorescein angiography is characteristic and demonstrates layering of the plasma erythrocytes within the aneurysms. This vascular abnormality is typically inert and benign and sporadic, but can be associated with an autosomal dominant disorder and caused by a KRIT 1 mutation on chromosome 7. In such cases, there may be associated cutaneous, intracranial, or spinal angiomas and therefore these should be excluded. The clinical course of retinal cavernous hemangiomas is nonprogressive but may be rarely complicated by recurrent hyphema, recurrent vitreous hemorrhage, secondary glaucoma, and phthisis.

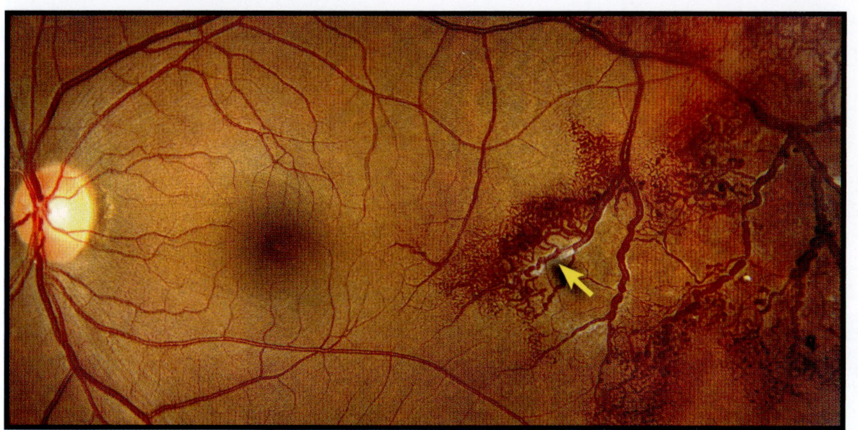

© 126

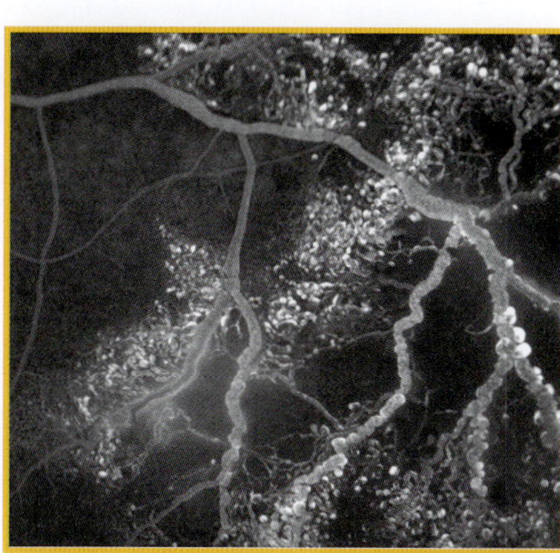

© 127

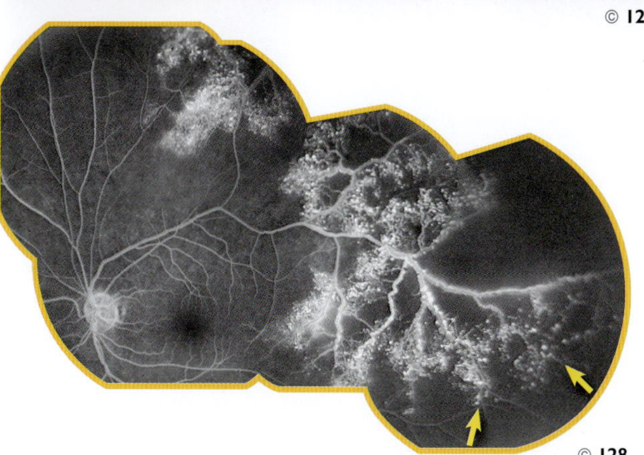

© 128

This patient has a retinal cavernous hemangioma that follows the course of an anomalous retinal macrovessel crossing the horizontal raphe. The fluorescein angiogram shows the distribution of the abnormal venule and the prominent aneurysmal changes along its course. There is also segmental fibrosis or gliosis seen on the color image *(arrow)* and peripheral ischemia and nonperfusion on the fluorescein angiogram montage *(arrows)*, which is atypical of retinal cavernous hemangiomas. The large aneurysmal changes demonstrate plasma erythrocyte layering or "cuffing," but there is no significant leakage, which is characteristic of this vasculopathy.

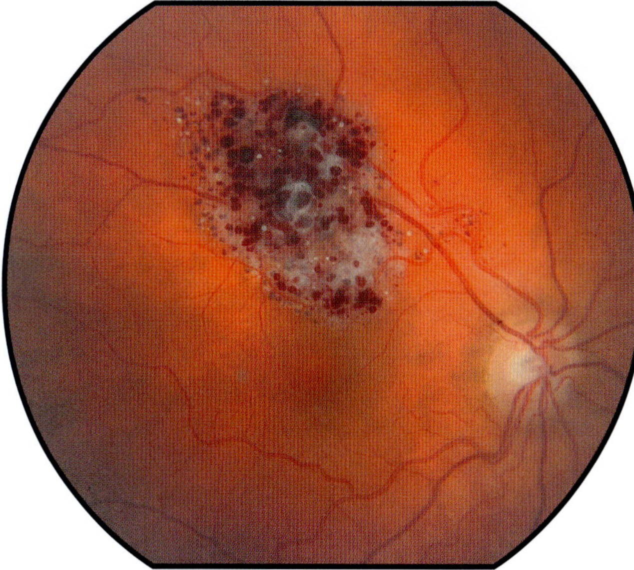

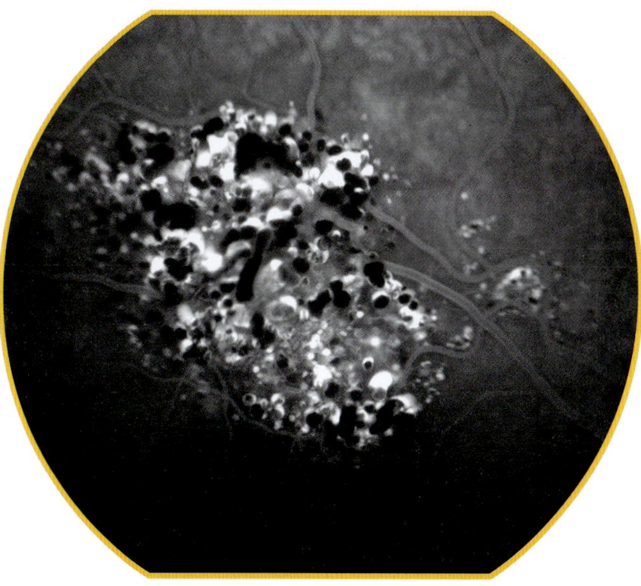

Color fundus photo showing the characteristic "cluster of grapes" appearance. Fluorescein angiogram shows blocking from hemorrhage and characteristic layering within the aneurysms.

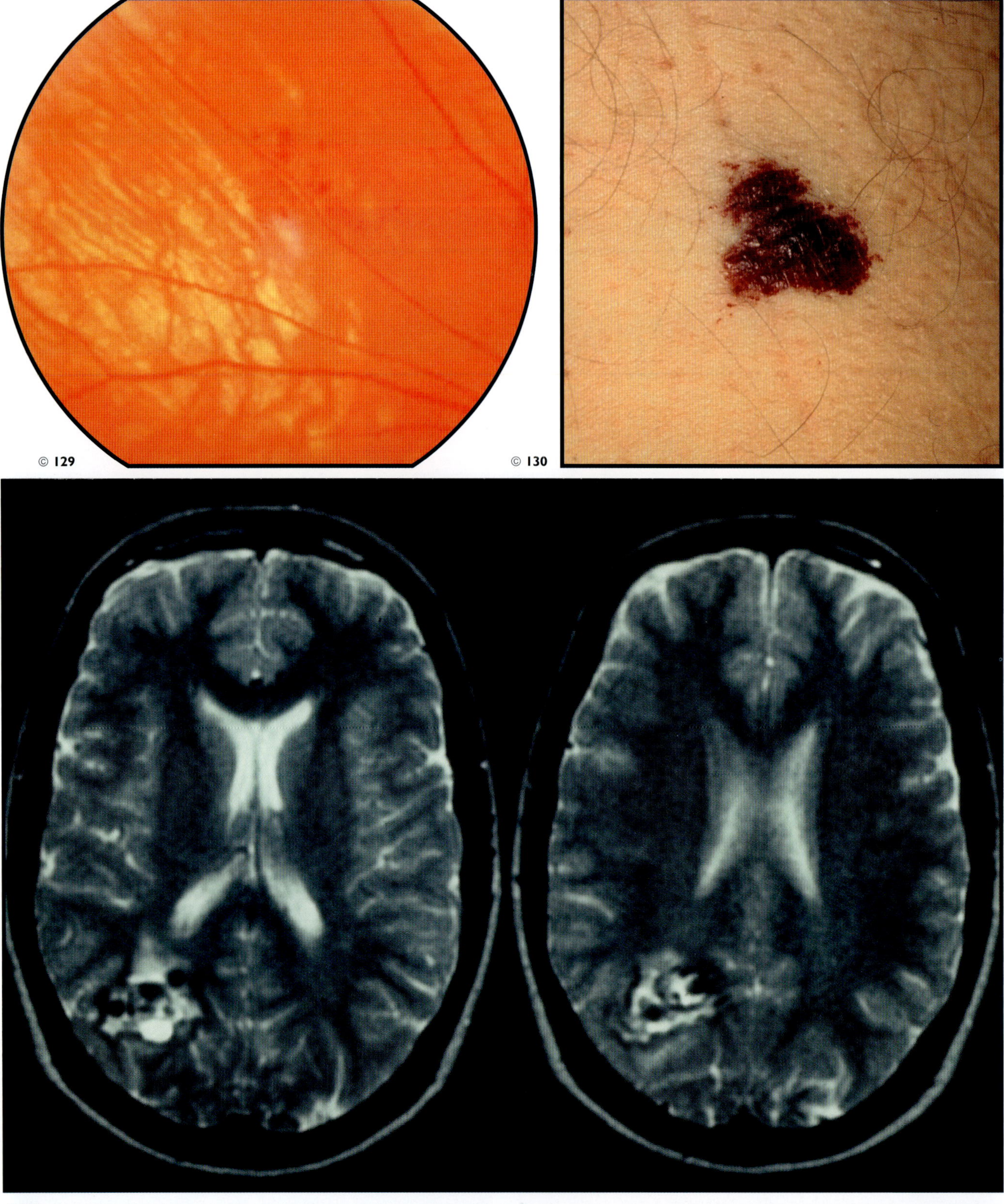

Color fundus photograph of a young male patient with a retinal cavernous hemangioma *(top left)*. Color photograph of the patient's grandfather showing a cutaneous hemangioma *(top right)*. MRI of the patient's aunt revealed a cerebral cavernous hemangioma *(bottom row)*.

Leber Congenital Amaurosis

Leber congenital amaurosis is a genetically and phenotypically diverse group of disorders characterized by a generalized retinal degeneration at birth with a profoundly abnormal or extinguished ERG. The majority of cases are inherited in an autosomal recessive pattern. Mutations in over 20 distinct genes with variable function have been identified thus far, accounting for approximately 70% of cases. The frequency of involved genes varies widely with ethnicity, but the most frequently involved in those of European decent are CEP290, GUCY2D, AIPL1, and RPE65. LCA is considered a nonsyndromic form of retinitis pigmentosa; however, the disease may be associated with mental retardation in up to 20% of cases. Reports of many other associations exist likely owing to the diversity of the disease. These include high hyperopia, skeletal abnormalities, renal disease, and a myriad of neurological abnormalities.

Children with LCA have profound vision loss or even blindness and present with nystagmus at birth or early infancy. The retinal appearance may be normal initially, with variable changes occurring later including vascular attenuation, "salt and pepper" pigmentary changes with para-arteriolar sparing (CRB1 mutation), peripheral bone spicule changes, pigmentary maculopathy and macular coloboma. Other clinical signs may be helpful in making the diagnosis, such as the oculodigital reflex in which children compulsively push on their eyes in order to stimulate a visual response. These children may also exhibit a paradoxical pupillary response with initial pupillary constriction with reduced light. Severe vision impairment persists throughout childhood, resulting in an inability to read or ambulate independently. Total blindness by the third or fourth decade generally occurs.

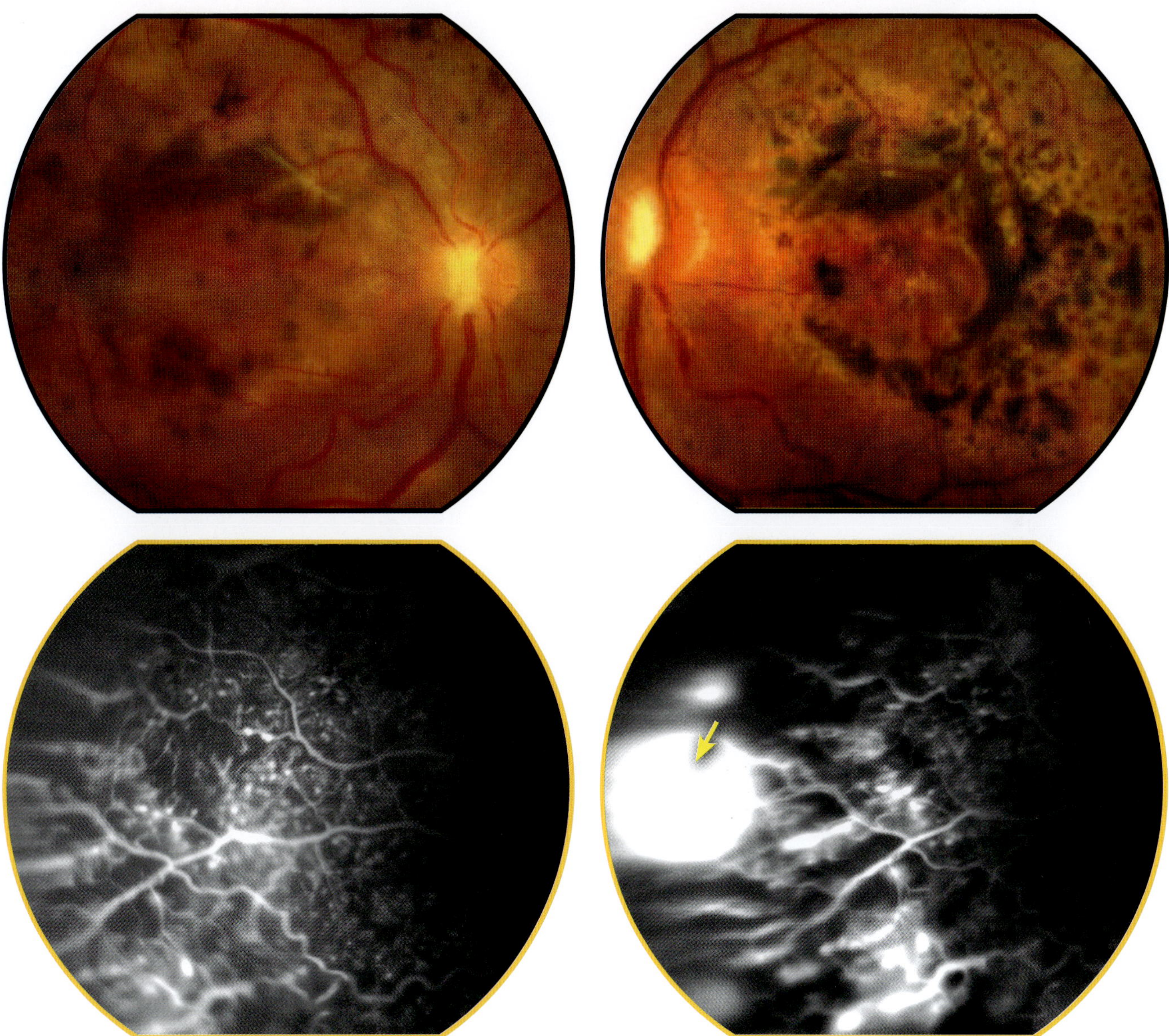

This patient with LCA has a CRB-1 mutation. Note the dense pigment clumping in the posterior fundus surrounding central atrophy. There is widespread pigment epithelial disease noted with fluorescein angiography. Also note the Coats-like aneurysmal changes in the bottom left image with associated leakage, and the vasoproliferative tumor with leakage in the lower right image *(arrow)*. The CRB-1 mutation is also found in patients with retinitis pigmentosa with associated retinal angiomatous proliferation in the fundus and preserved para-arteriolar retinal pigment epithelium.
Courtesy of Dr. Susan Lightman

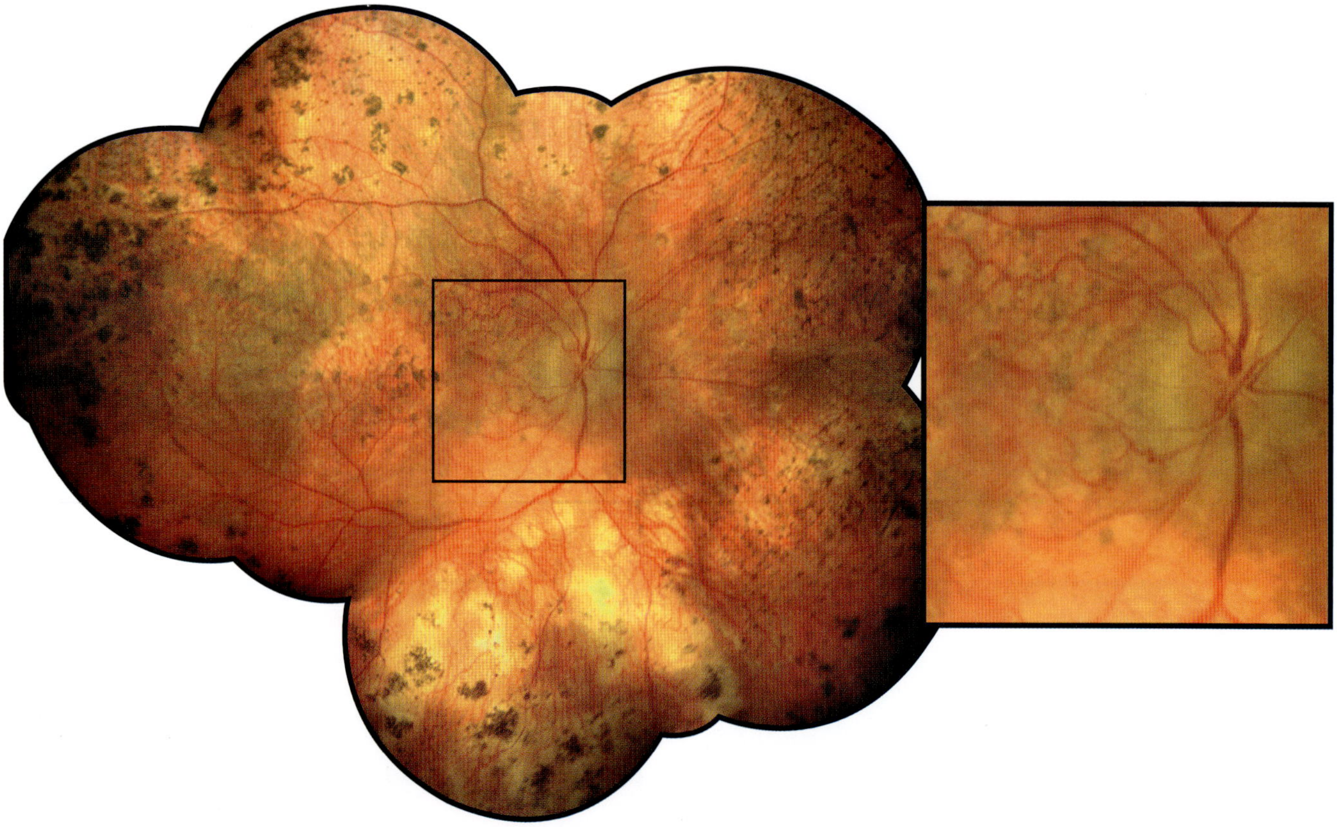

This patient has Leber congenital amaurosis. Note the widespread pigment epithelial degenerative change. There are irregular and nummular pigment epithelial hyperplastic spots in the fundus as well. This patient has a CRB-1 chromosome abnormality. *Courtesy of Dr. Stephen H. Tsang*

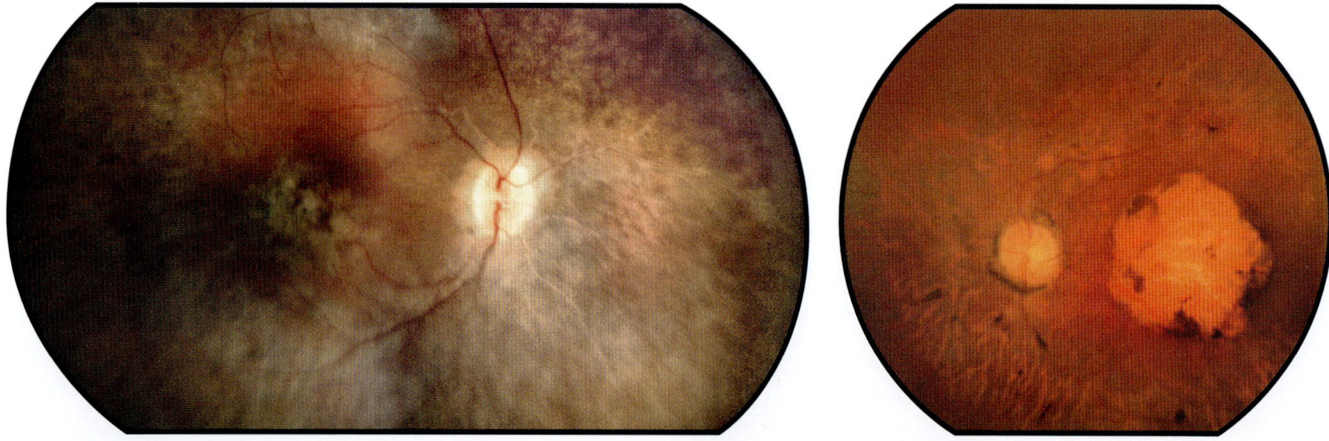

In these patients, the clinical variation in the spectrum of Leber congenital amaurosis is clearly displayed. The patient in the left figure shows widespread degenerative pigment epithelial disease with patchy atrophy and hyperplasia. The same is true for the patient on the right, where there is a more advanced stage of macular atrophy.

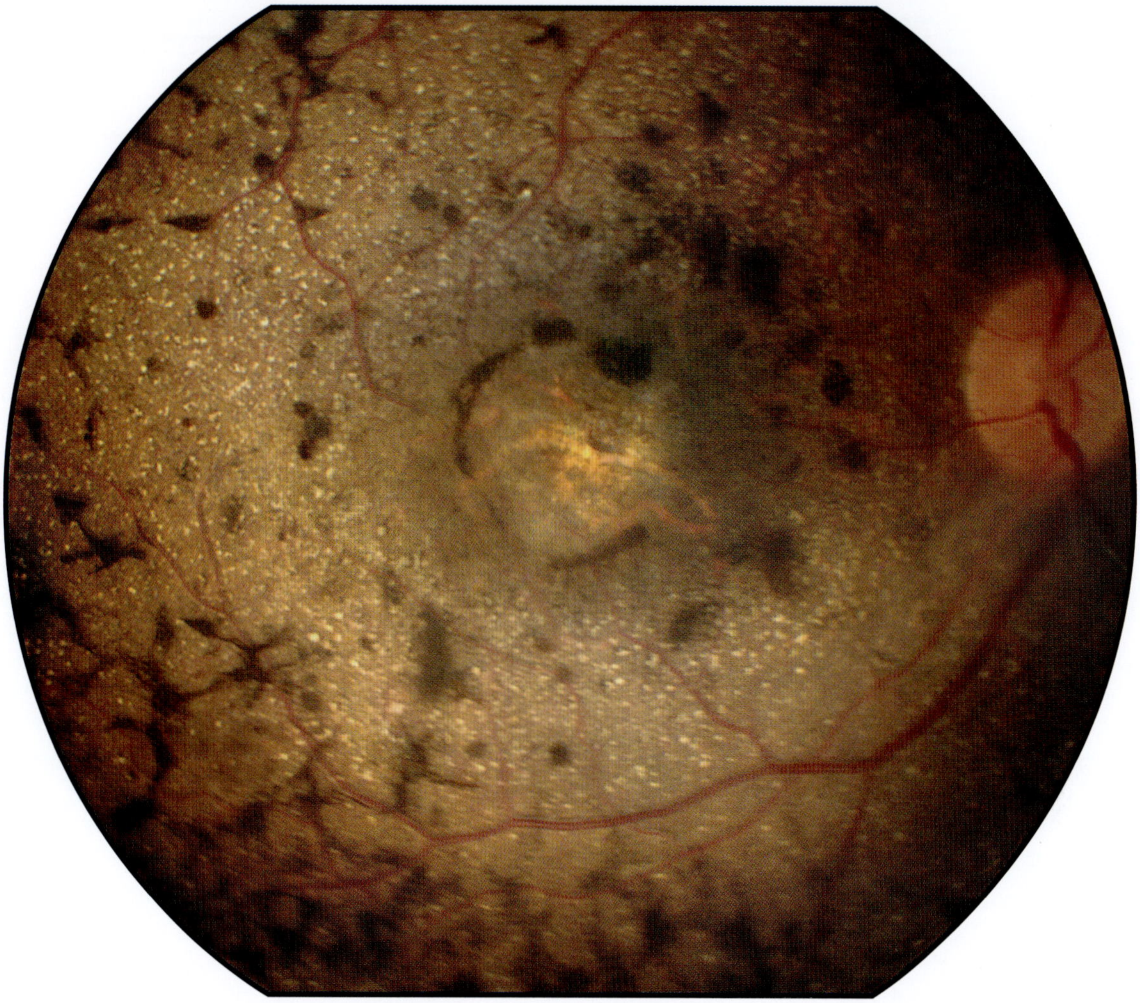

In this patient with Leber congenital amaurosis, there are scattered white dots and an array of pigment epithelial hyperplastic findings, seen as spots and flecks. A circumscribed area of atrophy is seen centrally.

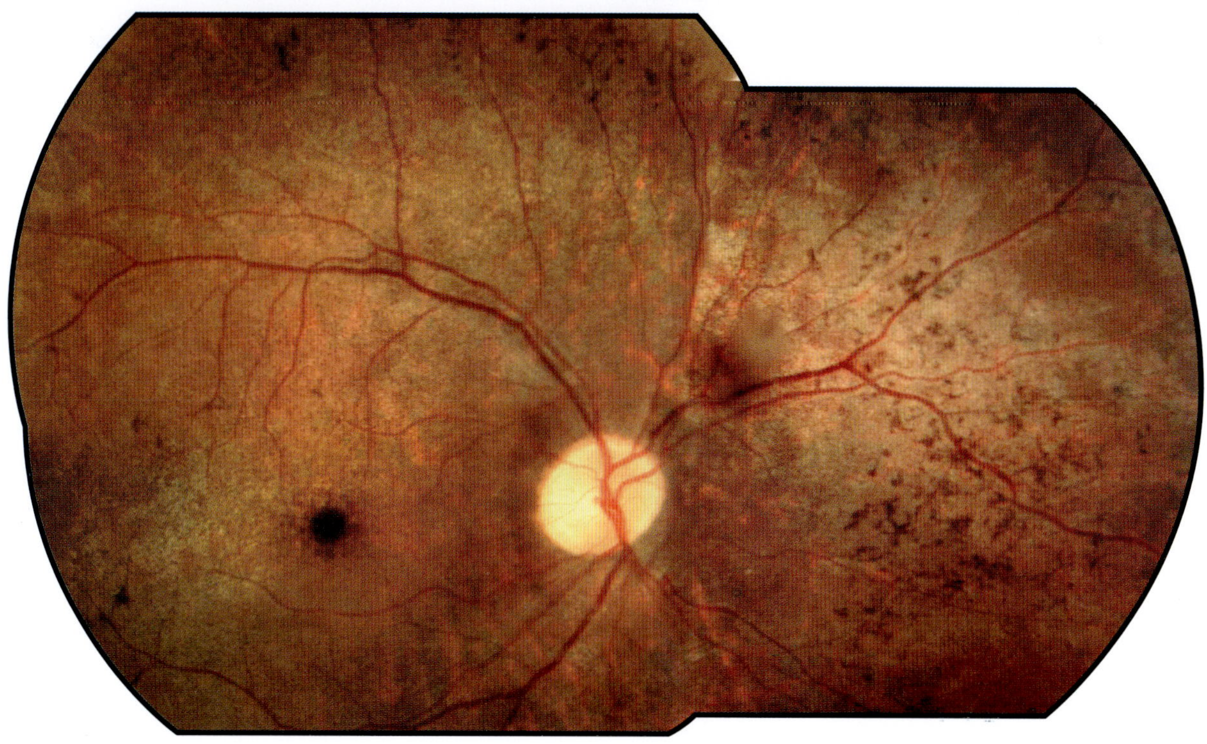

In this patient, there is diffuse atrophy and pigment epithelial hyperplasia. Perifoveal atrophy is also present. *Courtesy of Dr. Robert Henderson*

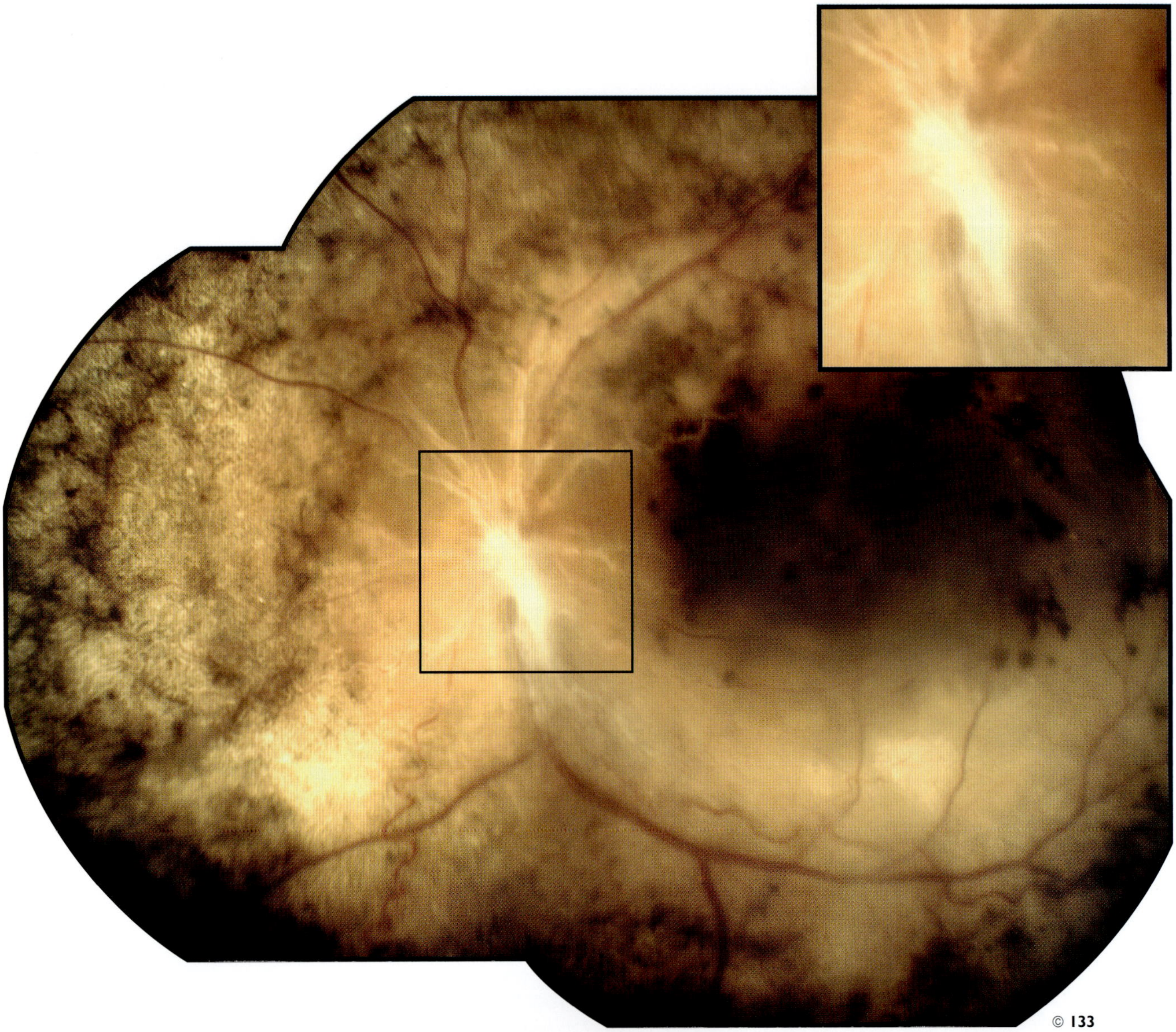

© 132

© 133

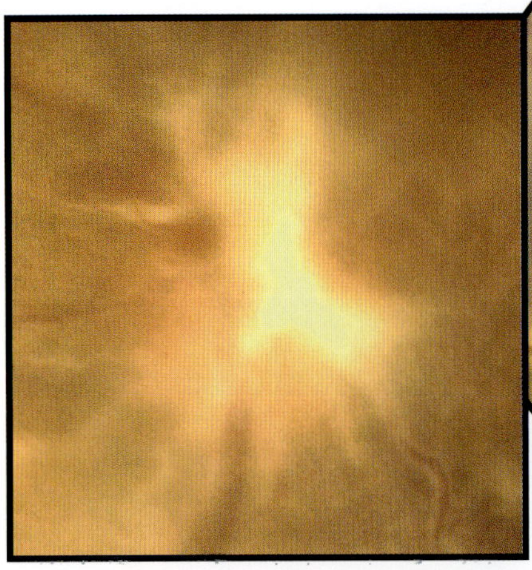

© 134

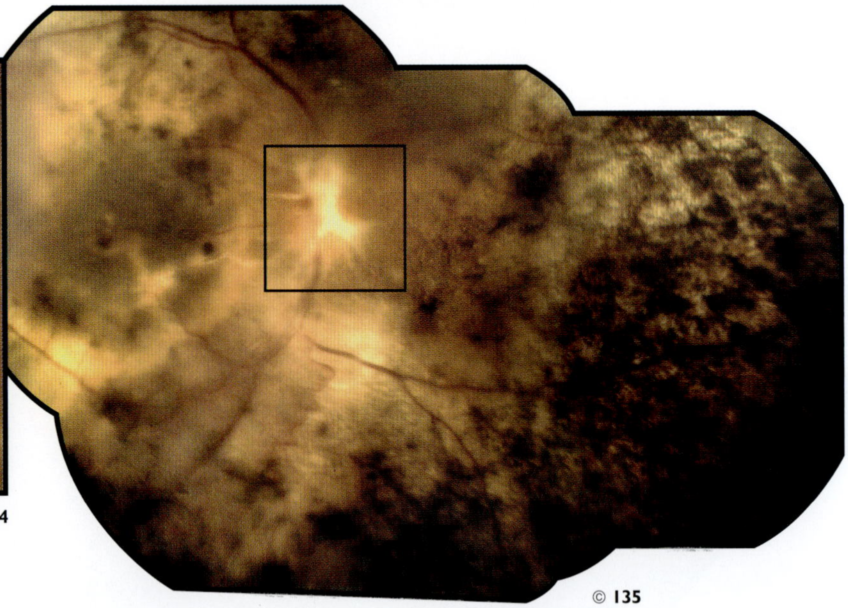

© 135

In this patient with Leber congenital amaurosis, there is widespread vascular sheathing and dense hyperplastic pigmentary degeneration as well as pre-retinal fibrosis focused around the nerve.

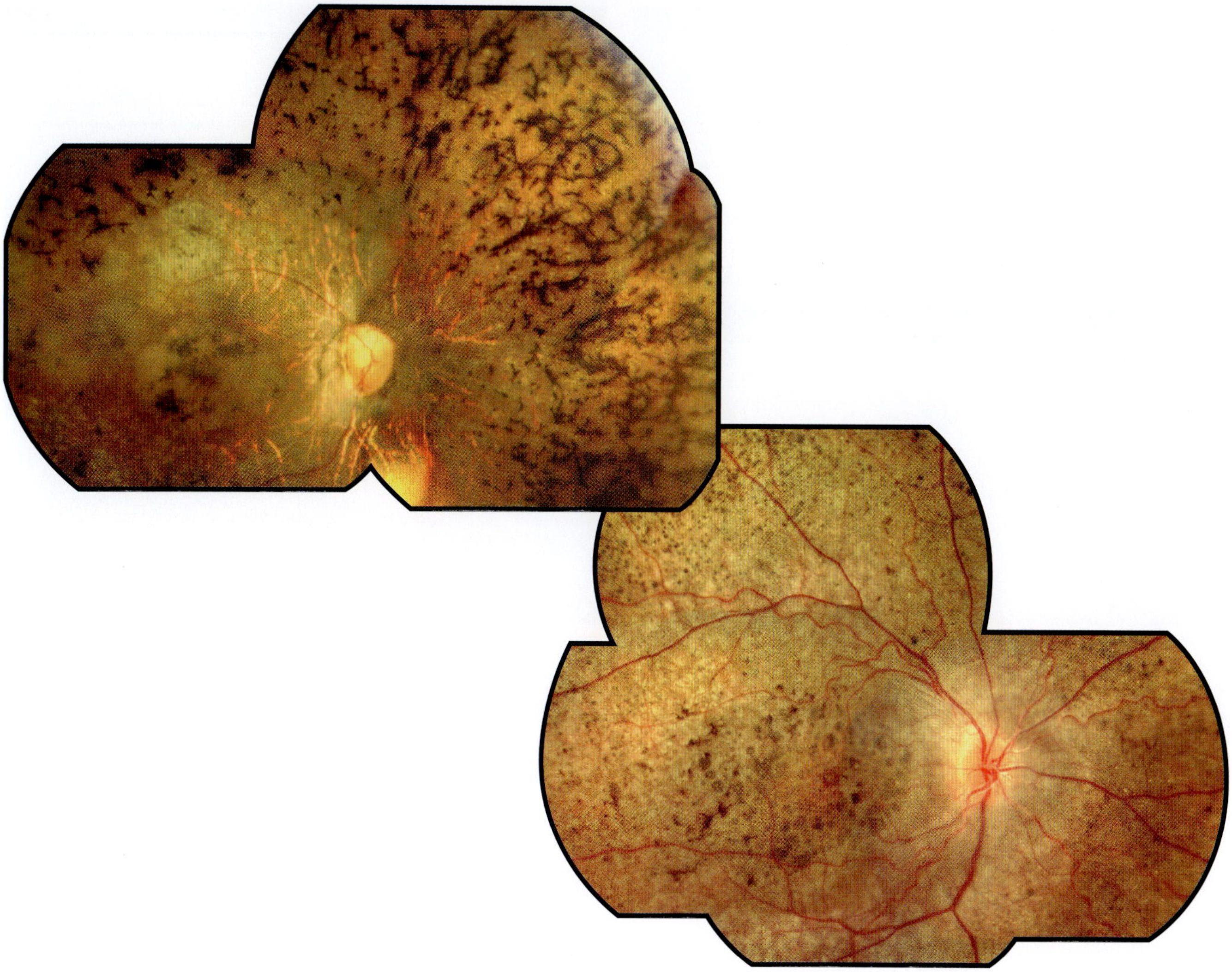

In Leber congenital amaurosis the pigment epithelial hyperplasia may be very pronounced, as seen in these patients. *Images courtesy of Dr. Stephen H. Tsang (left) and Dr. Robert Henderson (right)*

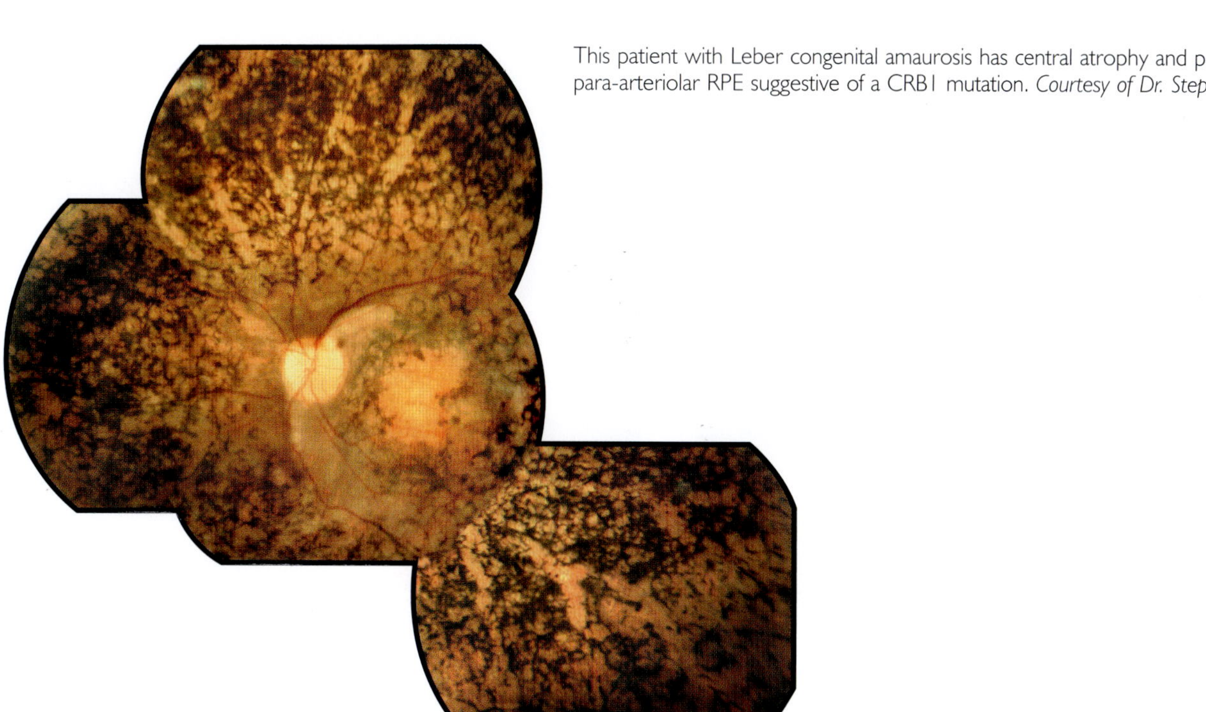

This patient with Leber congenital amaurosis has central atrophy and preserved para-arteriolar RPE suggestive of a CRB1 mutation. *Courtesy of Dr. Stephen H. Tsang*

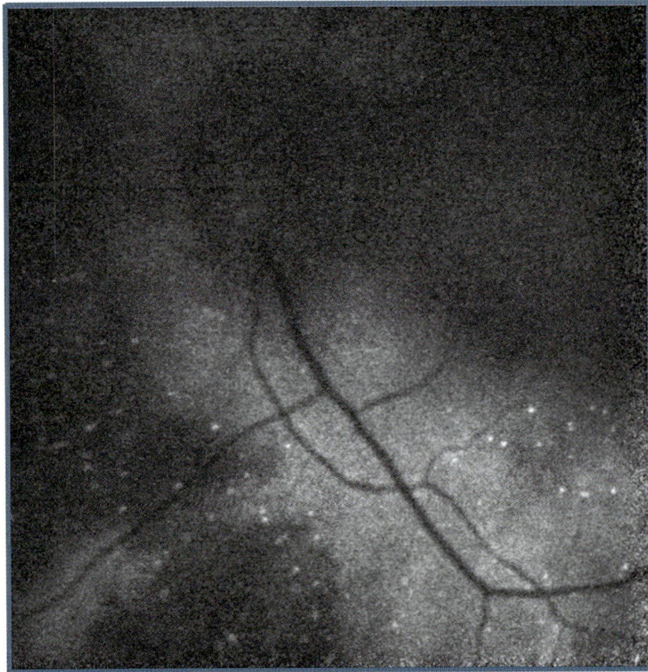

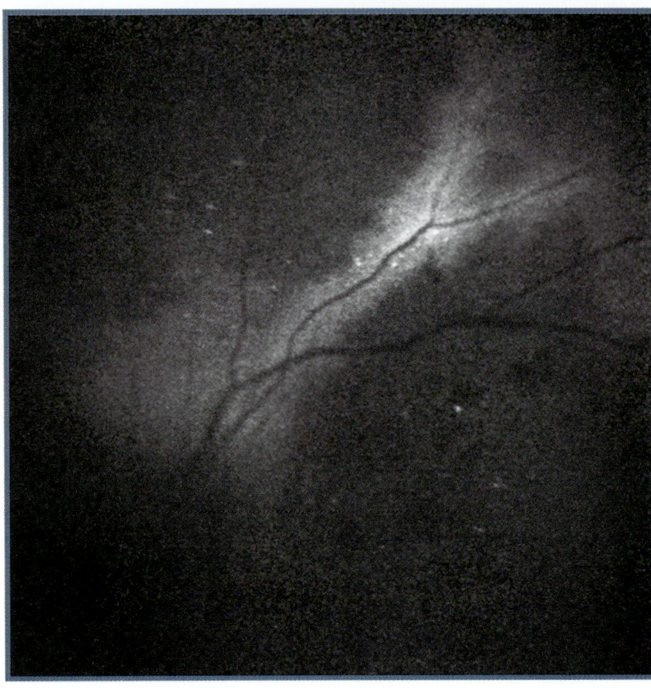

The pattern of para-arteriolar preservation of retinal pigment epithelium is nicely demonstrated in the fundus autofluorescence of a patient with Leber congenital amaurosis. Note that there is hyperautofluorescence surrounding the arterioles in each eye and bordered by huge areas of atrophy represented as hypoautofluorescence. *Courtesy of Dr. Joaquin Tosi*

Pigmented Paravenous Chorioretinal Atrophy

Pigmented paravenous chorioretinal atrophy (PPCRA) is a rare disorder of unknown origin, characterized by atrophy and bony corpuscular pigmentation along the distribution of retinal veins. There may be an associated atrophic disturbance in the macula. The Norrie gene has now been associated with this peculiar abnormality, which may be seen in the pediatric retinal setting. The abnormality has also been associated with the CRB-1 gene.

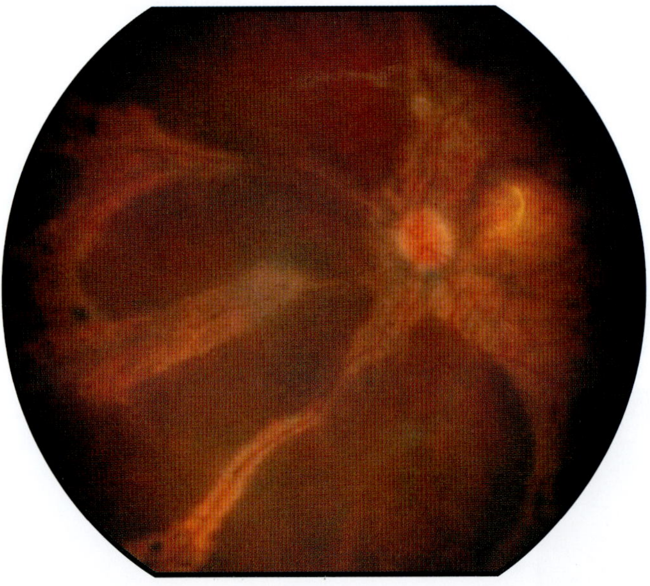

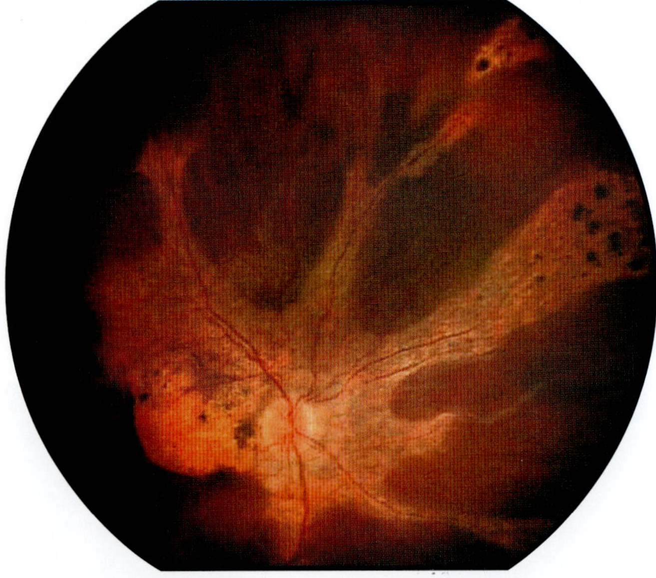

Note the peculiar paravenous atrophy seen in both eyes of this 3-month-old child. The atrophy is more prominent around the disc, but extends into the central macula. *Courtesy of Dr. Scott Brodie*

Aicardi Syndrome

Aicardi syndrome is an X-linked dominant disorder seen in females, lethal in the hemizygous male, with a mutation localized to chromosome Xp22. Infantile spasms, agenesis or dysgenesis of the corpus collusum, and lacunae of chorioretinal atrophy are seen in Aicardi syndrome. Flexion spasms in the infant represent the usual mode of clinical presentation. These patients have mental retardation, microcephaly, generalized seizures, hypotonia, and cortical heterotopia. Fundoscopically variably sized, well-defined, circular, white lacunae with minimal pigmentation at their borders are seen generally clustered around the optic disc. They are bilateral and symmetric in distribution and may be seen in the posterior pole and periphery. These atrophic chorioretinal lesions can be up to two disc diameters in size or more. Histopathologically, the lesions demonstrate areas of depigmentation and deficiency in the RPE and gross choriodal atrophy, likely representing a dysgenesis rather than a progressive dystrophic disorder. Other associated ocular abnormalities include microphthalmia, persistent pupillary membrane, colobomas of the optic nerve and choroid, and glial tissue extending from the optic disc.

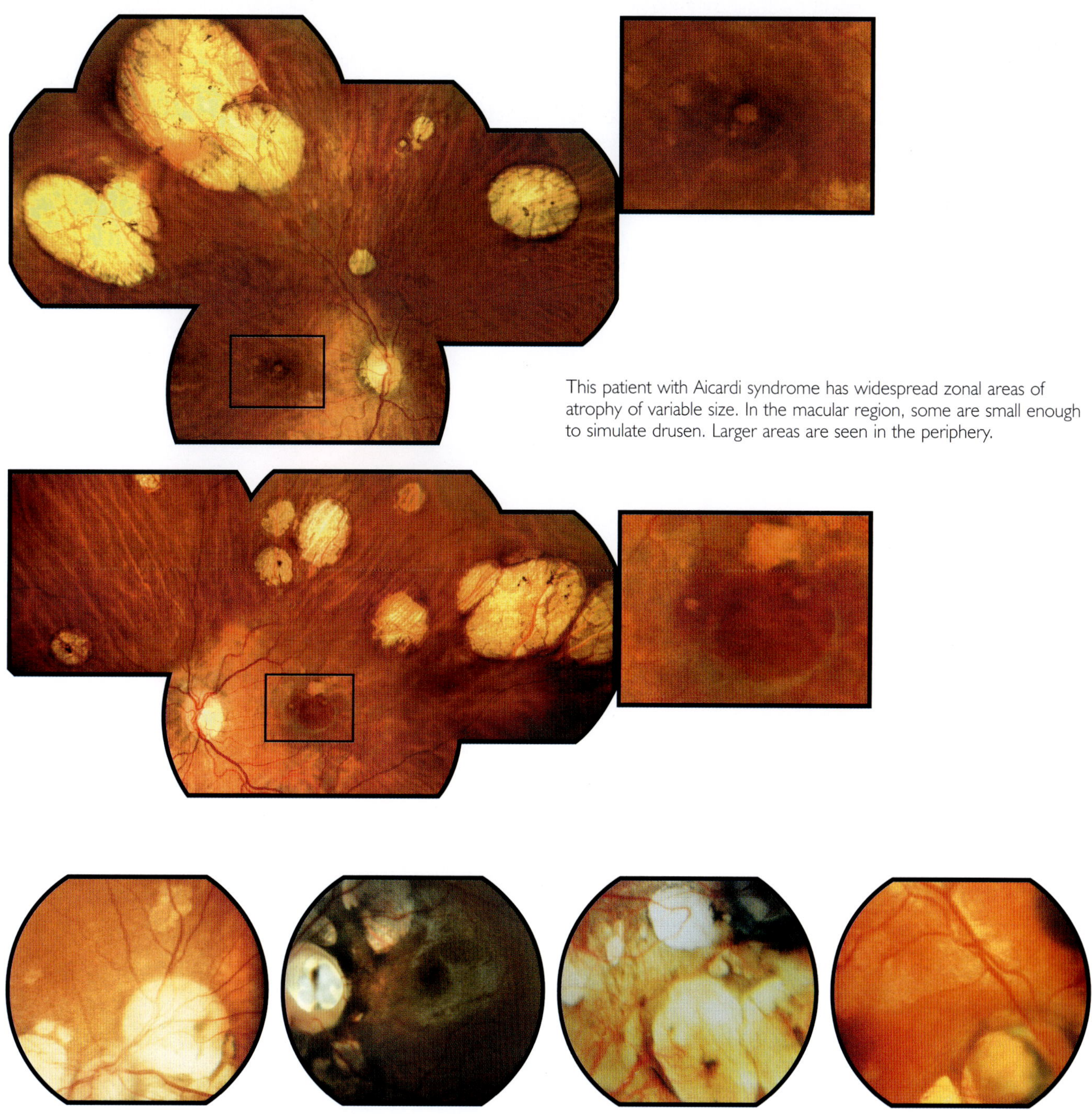

This patient with Aicardi syndrome has widespread zonal areas of atrophy of variable size. In the macular region, some are small enough to simulate drusen. Larger areas are seen in the periphery.

These images demonstrate the variability in the chorioretinal focal areas of atrophy seen in Aicardi syndrome.

This group of systemic disorders is typically the result of an autosomal recessive mutation causing dysfunction of a cellular enzymatic protein leading to lysosomal storage abnormalities and accumulation of mucopolysaccharide, lipid, or other biochemical compounds. These disorders present almost exclusively in the pediatric population as life expectancy tends to be shortened due to systemic complications of the disease and retinal manifestations include various forms of maculopathy or retinitis pigmentosa.

Neuronal Ceroid Lipofuscinoses

The neuronal ceroid lipofuscinoses (CLN) are a group of diseases characterized by the accumulation of PAS- and Sudan black-positive, electron-dense, and autofluorescent granules within the lysosomes of nerve cells. They are most commonly autosomal recessive and collectively represent the most common neurodegenerative diseases of childhood. Affected individuals typically have severe psychomotor deterioration leading to seizures, vision loss, vegetative state, and premature death. Fourteen types of the human CLN disorder have been identified, each with slightly different clinical characteristics and caused by mutation in different defining genes. CLN3 is the most common of these entities, usually appearing between the ages of 4 and 10. It is caused by a mutation in the CLN3 gene. The vision loss is due to retinal degeneration that is remarkable for a "bull's-eye" maculopathy with or without associated wrinkling of the inner limiting membrane, pale optic discs, narrow arterioles, and peripheral pigment abnormalities. In the early stages, there is a diminished electroretinogram (ERG) b-wave and normal electrooculogram (EOG). Later, a non-recordable scotoptic and photoptic ERG can be seen and some studies have demonstrated a severely abnormal EOG. On electron microscopy, the lipoprotein deposits take on characteristic patterns that are used for diagnosis and classification into the subgroups.

Neuronal Ceroid Lipofuscinosis 1 (CLN1, Santavuori–Haltia Disease, Hagberg–Santavuori Disease)

Neuronal CLN1 is an infantile-onset form of CLN caused by a mutation in the gene encoding for palmitoyl-protein thioesterase-1 (PPT1). It usually presents at 8-24 months of age with severe psychomotor deterioration, microcephaly, and blindness. Vascular sheathing and optic atrophy, along with retinal degeneration, are prominent features of this disease.

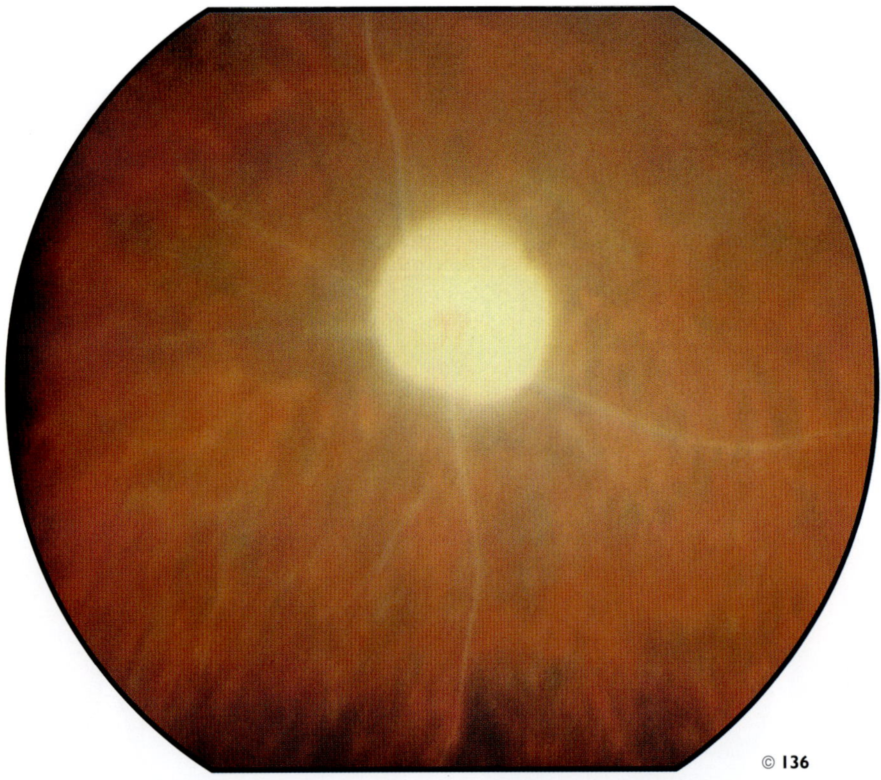

© 136

This patient with neuronal ceroid lipofuscinosis 1 had mental and motor degeneration, ataxia, and hypotonia. The fundus revealed vascular sheathing, retinal degeneration, and severe optic atrophy.

Neuronal Ceroid Lipofuscinosis 2 (CLN2, Jansky–Bielschowsky Disease)

CLN2 is a late infantile-onset form of CLN that presents between 2 and 4 years of age with severe neurological symptoms such as ataxia, loss of speech, regression of developmental milestones, and seizures that precede the visual symptoms. There is rapid progression of the disease resulting in progressive visual loss, coma, and death within a few years.

Neuronal Ceroid Lipofuscinosis 3 (CLN3, Batten Disease, Vogt–Spielmeyer Disease, Spielmeyer–Sjögren Disease)

CLN3 is a juvenile-onset form that presents between the ages of 4 and 8 with advanced visual symptoms that lead to loss of vision over 1–2 years followed by neurodegenerative symptoms. Diffuse retinal atrophy with patchy perifoveal pigmentary changes and a "bull's-eye" maculopathy are noted. Dementia, ataxia, seizures, and vision loss due to generalized rod–cone degeneration occur, with death by age 20. This is the major subgroup of these disorders.

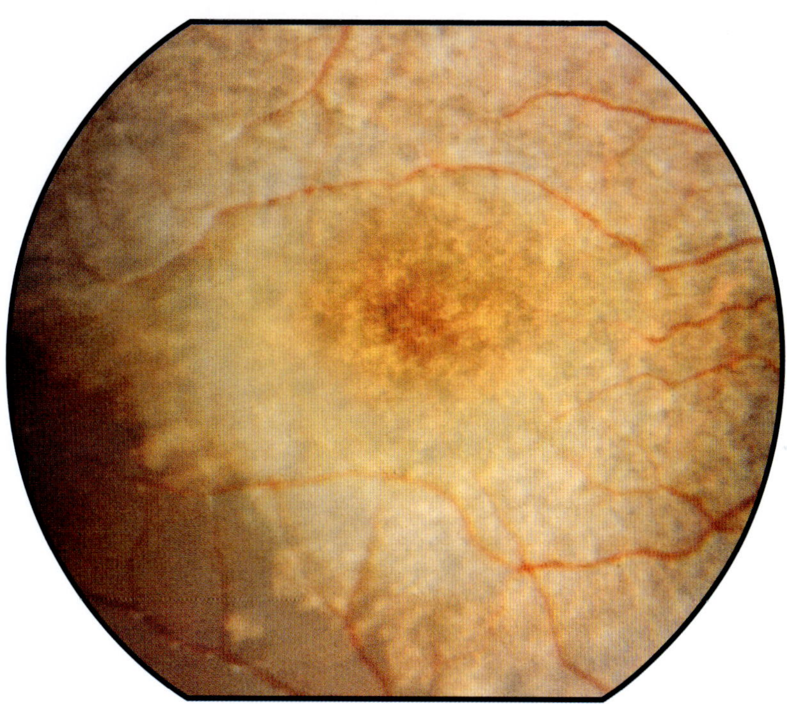

This patient with neuronal ceroid lipofuscinosis 3 demonstrates a diffuse atrophic area with patchy perifoveal pigmentary changes resembling a "bull's-eye" configuration. *Courtesy of Dr. Irene Maumenee*

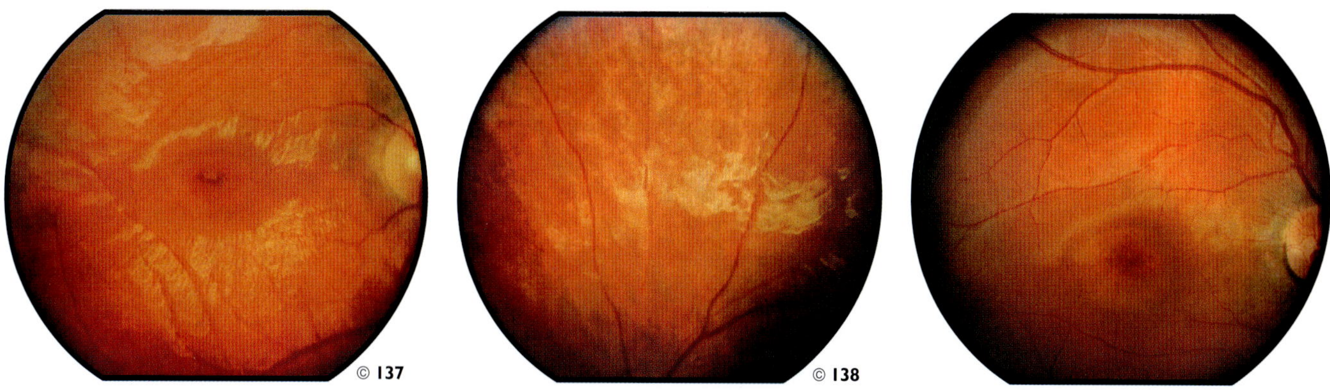

Affected patients may have macular and pigmentary changes, including a "bull's-eye" maculopathy, internal limiting membrane wrinkling, pigmentary changes, and attenuated vessels. *Right image courtesy of Bateman, Lang, Maumenee*

Mucopolysaccharidoses

Mucopolysaccharidoses are a group of inherited lysosomal storage diseases caused by enzyme deficiencies that lead to defective degradation of glycosaminoglycans. Seven distinct clinical types and numerous subtypes have been identified, with Hurler syndrome (MPS IH) being the most severe. All are inherited in an autosomal recessive pattern except Hunter syndrome (MPS II), which is inherited in an X-linked recessive pattern. They share many of the same clinical features, but have varying degrees of severity based on the subtype, which include mental retardation, hearing loss, coarse facies, skeletal abnormalities, dermal melanocytosis, hepatosplenomegaly, cardiorespiratory abnormalities, and variable life expectancy typically with a period of normal development followed by a decline in physical and/or mental function. Diagnosis can be made by a urine test indicating excess mucopolysaccharides with peripheral leukocyte enzyme assays reserved for more definitive diagnosis. Ocular findings include, most commonly, corneal clouding, seen in most subgroups except MPS II, as well as optic atrophy, glaucoma, and pigmentary retinal degeneration of the rod–cone type, with rods more affected than cones. No correlation exists between the ophthalmoscopic appearance and the ERG findings. Retinal vascular attenuation and sheathing may be present, but they are often masked by pigmentary changes in the fundus. Retinal findings are only seen in MPS types I, II, and III due to heparan sulfate accumulation. Histopathologically, fibrillogranular, and membranolamellar inclusions can be seen in the RPE and ganglion cells.

Mucopolysaccharidosis Type I (Hurler, Scheie, and Hurler–Scheie Syndrome; MPS IH, IS, IHS)

MPS I (Hurler, Scheie, and Hurler–Scheie syndrome) results from a deficiency of the enzyme alpha-L-iduronidase mapped to chromosome 4p16.3, which results in the accumulation of both heparan and dermatan sulfate. Children with Hurler syndrome appear normal at birth and develop the characteristic coarse facies over the first years of life. Significant growth retardation, mental retardation, and death occur by the first decade of life. Scheie syndrome has milder systemic manifestations, normal life expectancy, and lacks growth and mental retardation. Corneal clouding is common and progressive, leading to significant photophobia and visual impairment. Crystalline keratopathy may also complicate both subtypes. Retinal degeneration, optic nerve swelling, and glaucoma are also seen.

Mucopolysaccharidosis Type II (Hunter Syndrome A, B; MPS IIA, IIB)

MPS II (Hunter syndrome) is inherited in an X-linked recessive pattern, primarily affecting males, and is caused by a deficiency of iduronate sulfatase on chromosome Xq28, which results in the accumulation of both heparan and dermatan sulfate. There are two subtypes: the infantile form, which resembles Hurler syndrome, and the milder form, which resembles Scheie syndrome. Retinal degeneration is seen, but corneal clouding is not a feature of this subgroup.

Mucopolysaccharidosis Type III (Sanfilippo Syndrome A, B, C, D; MPS IIIA, IIIB, IIIC, IIID)

MPS III (Sanfilippo syndrome) is characterized by severe central nervous system degeneration with progressive dementia, aggressive behavior, hyperactivity, and seizures, but only mild somatic disease including moderately severe claw hand and visceromegaly, and mild or absent skeletal abnormalities. Ocular findings include retinal degeneration with little or no corneal clouding. There are four distinct types of Sanfilippo syndrome, each caused by alteration of a different enzyme leading to impaired degradation and accumulation of heparan sulfate. Minimal clinical difference exists between these four types but symptoms appear most severe and progressive in children with Sanfilippo type A, which is caused by a deficiency in heparan *N*-sulfatase. Sanfilippo B is caused by alpha-*N*-acetylglucosaminidase deficiency, Sanfilippo C is caused by acetyl-coalpha-glucosaminide acetyltransferase deficiency, and Sanfilippo D is caused by deficiency in *N*-acetylglucosamine-6-sulfatase.

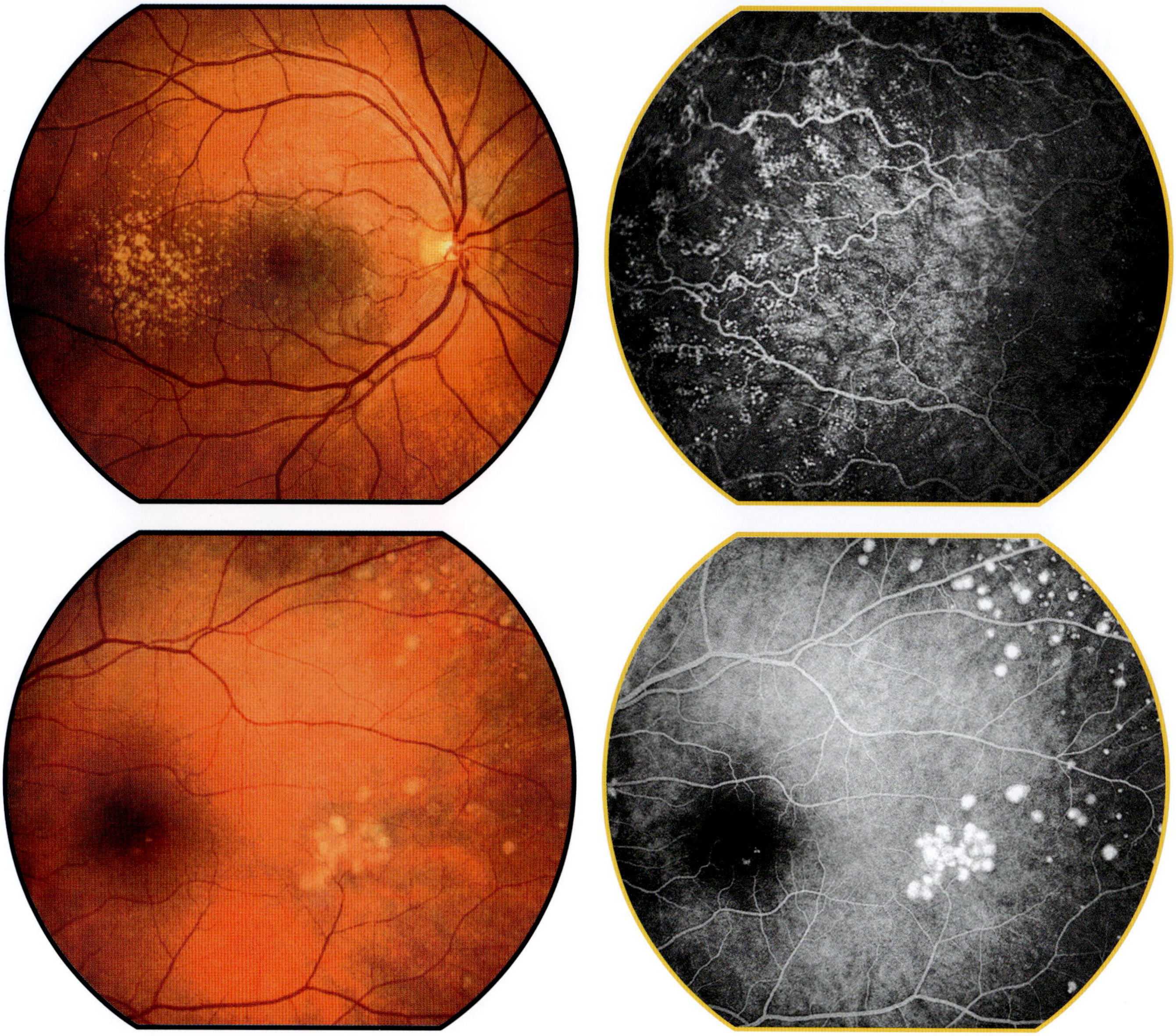

Patients with Hunter syndrome or MPS II often show drusenoid changes in the macula. They may range from small drusen with moderate confluency *(upper two images)* to larger, discrete drusenoid changes in the temporal near-periphery and more peripherally *(lower two images)*.

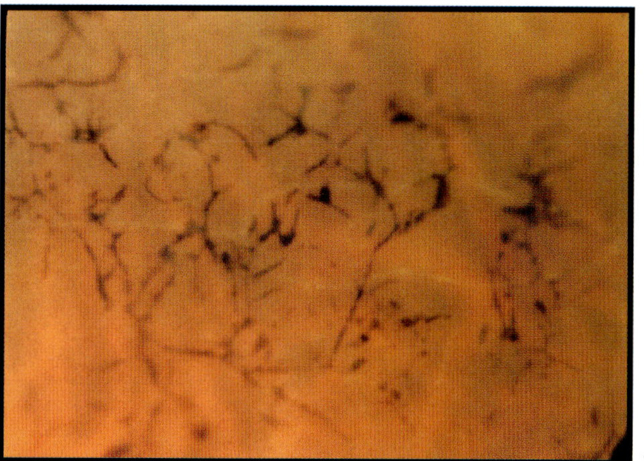

© **139**

This patient with Sanfilippo syndrome or MPS IIIA shows a retinitis pigmentosa-like fundus with hyperplasia of the retinal pigment epithelium and migration of pigment spicules into the retina in a perivascular distribution.

Mucolipidoses

Mucolipidoses are a group of autosomal recessive lysosomal storage disorders that share many clinical features with mucopolysaccharidoses. These disorders are divided into four groups as follows.

Mucolipidosis Type I (ML I, Sialidosis Type I, Sialidosis Type II, Neuraminidase Deficiency, Cherry-Red Spot Myoclonus Syndrome)

ML I is caused by a mutation in the gene encoding neuraminidase, located on chromosome 6p21.3, which results in progressive accumulation of sialidated glycopeptides and oligosaccharides within lysosomes. Symptoms of ML I are either present at birth or develop within the first year of life. In many infants with ML I, excessive swelling throughout the body is noted at birth. These infants are often born with coarse facial features and skeletal malformations and often develop myoclonus and cherry-red spots in the macula. Tremors, ataxia, impaired vision, seizures, hepatosplenomegaly, extreme abdominal swelling, hypotonia, and mental retardation are additional features of this disorder. Most infants with ML I die before the age of 1 year. A more rare form of sialidosis, sialidosis type 1, has an onset of symptoms during the second decade of life and is a milder form of disease. Myoclonus and cherry-red spot within the macula are often the initial features followed by the development of seizures, worsening coordination, and progressive mental deterioration. Histopathologically, enlarged ganglion cells with eosinophilic granular intracytoplasmic material and eccentrically displaced nuclei have been noted in the macular region.

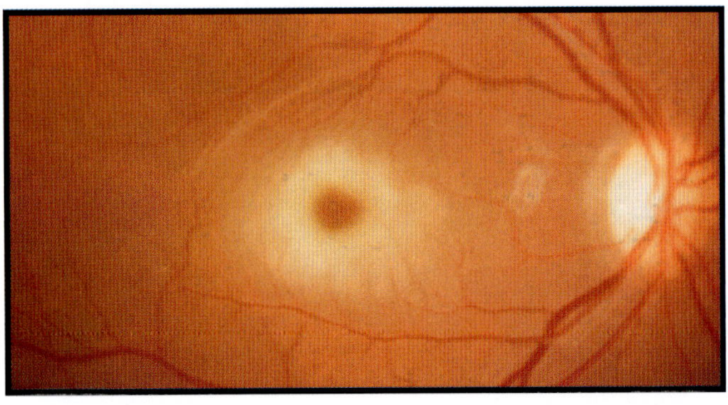

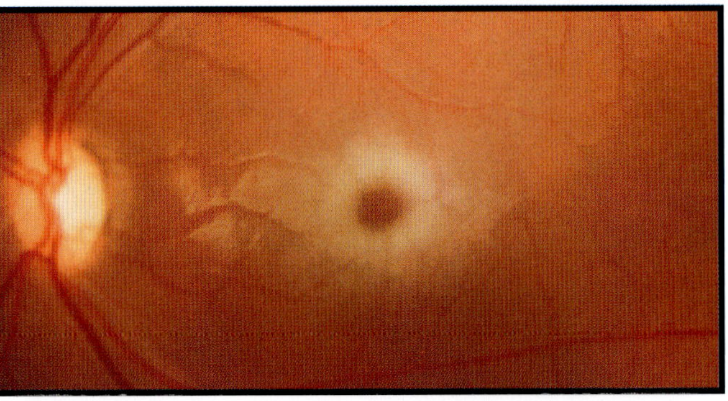

Cherry-red spots are seen in this patient with mucolipidosis type I (specifically sialidosis type II). These changes are also seen in Landing disease (gangliosidosis), Farber disease (disseminated lipogranulomatosis), or metachromatic leukodystrophy. *Courtesy of Dr. Stefanos Kokolakis*

The deposition in this patient with mucolipidosis type I is more extensive, extending into the paramacular area. The fluorescein angiogram shows no evidence of leakage. *Courtesy of Dr. Ken Wald*

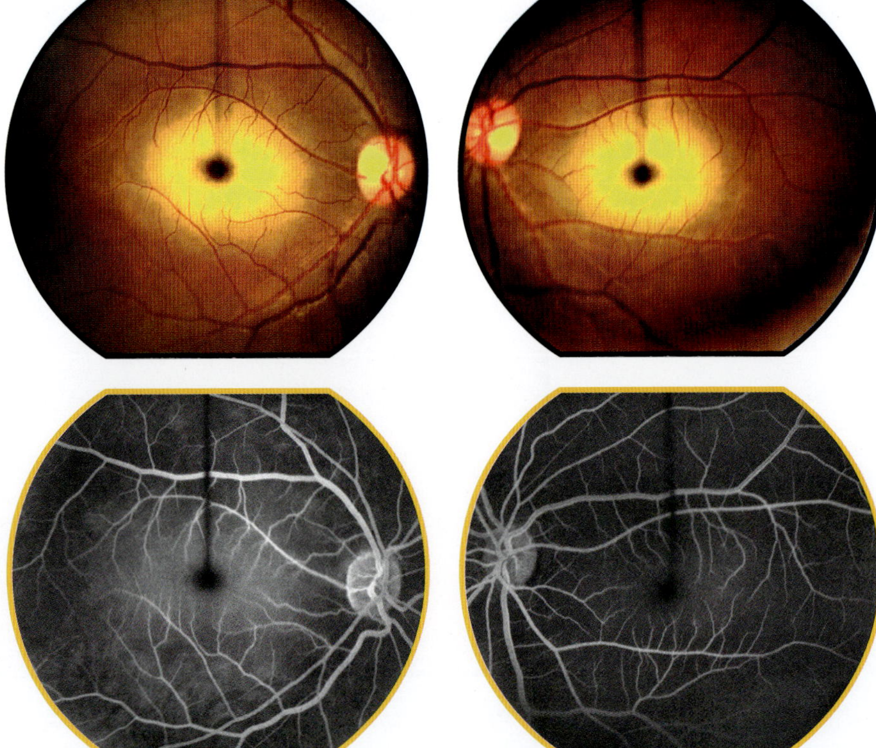

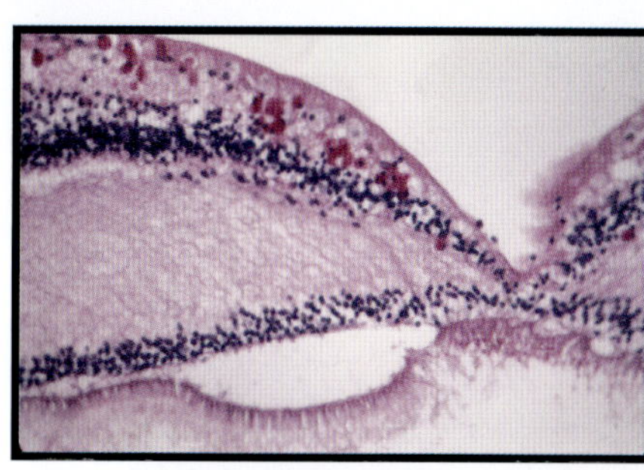

This patient with mucolipidosis type I (specifically sialidosis type II) shows additional storage in the temporal macula. The histopathology shows accumulation of the abnormal molecule in the inner retina.

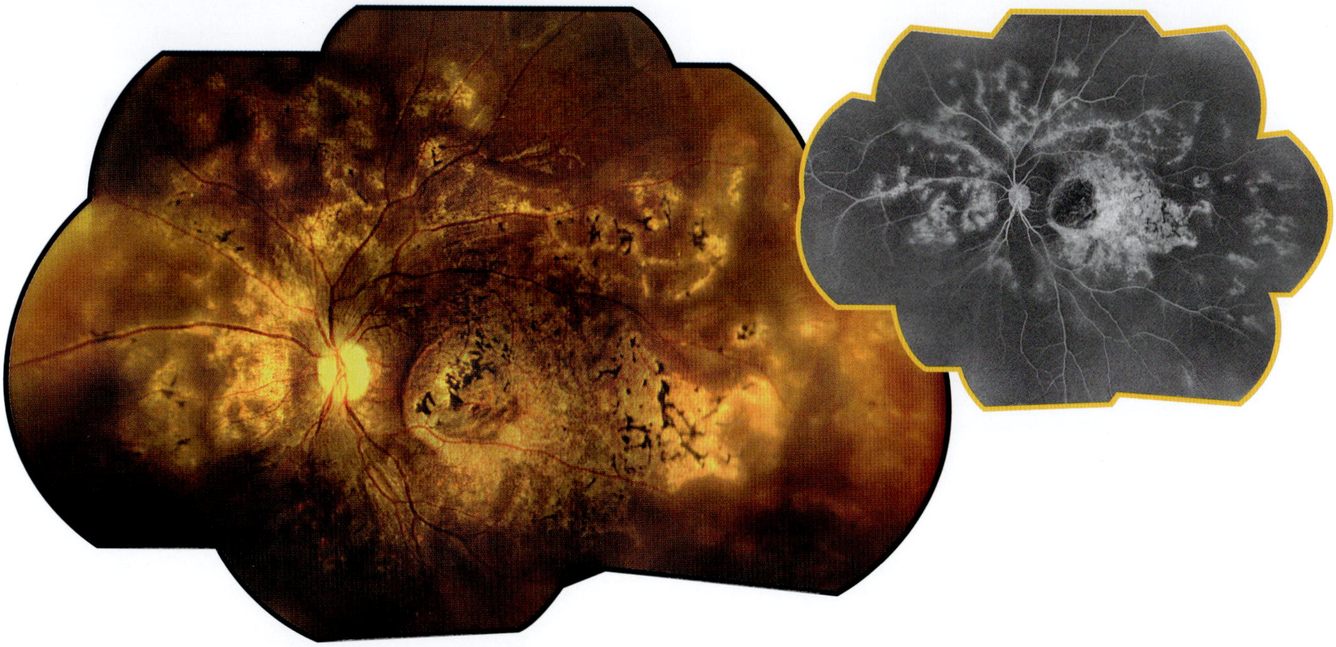

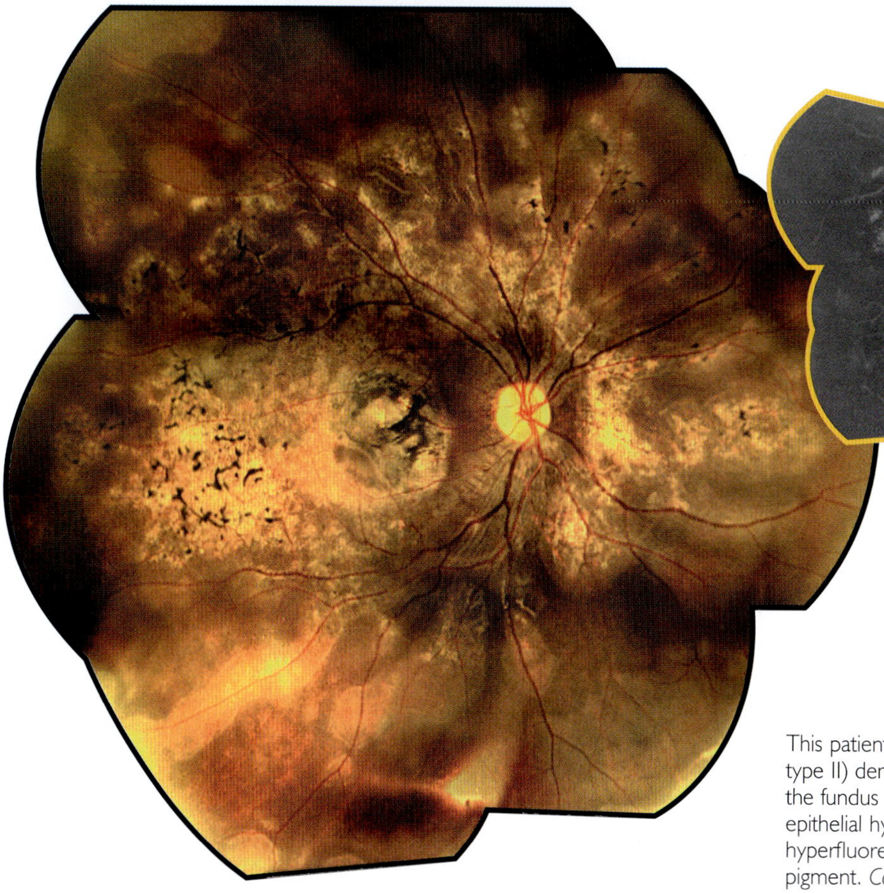

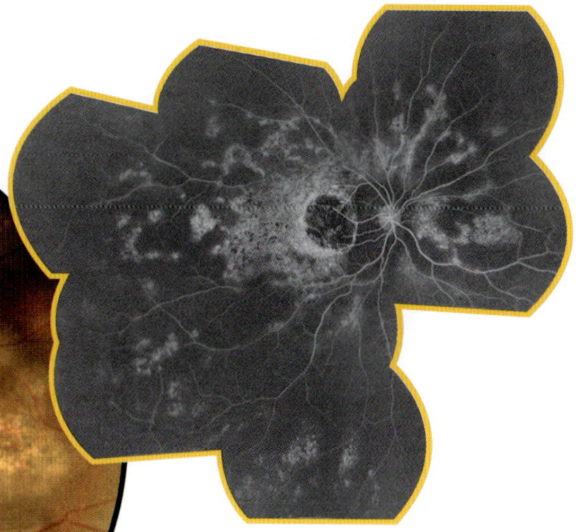

This patient with mucolipidosis type I (specifically sialidosis type II) demonstrates widespread abnormalities throughout the fundus and associated severe atrophy, as well as pigment epithelial hyperplasia. The fluorescein angiogram shows hyperfluorescence in atrophic areas and blockage by the pigment. *Courtesy of Dr. Ken Wald*

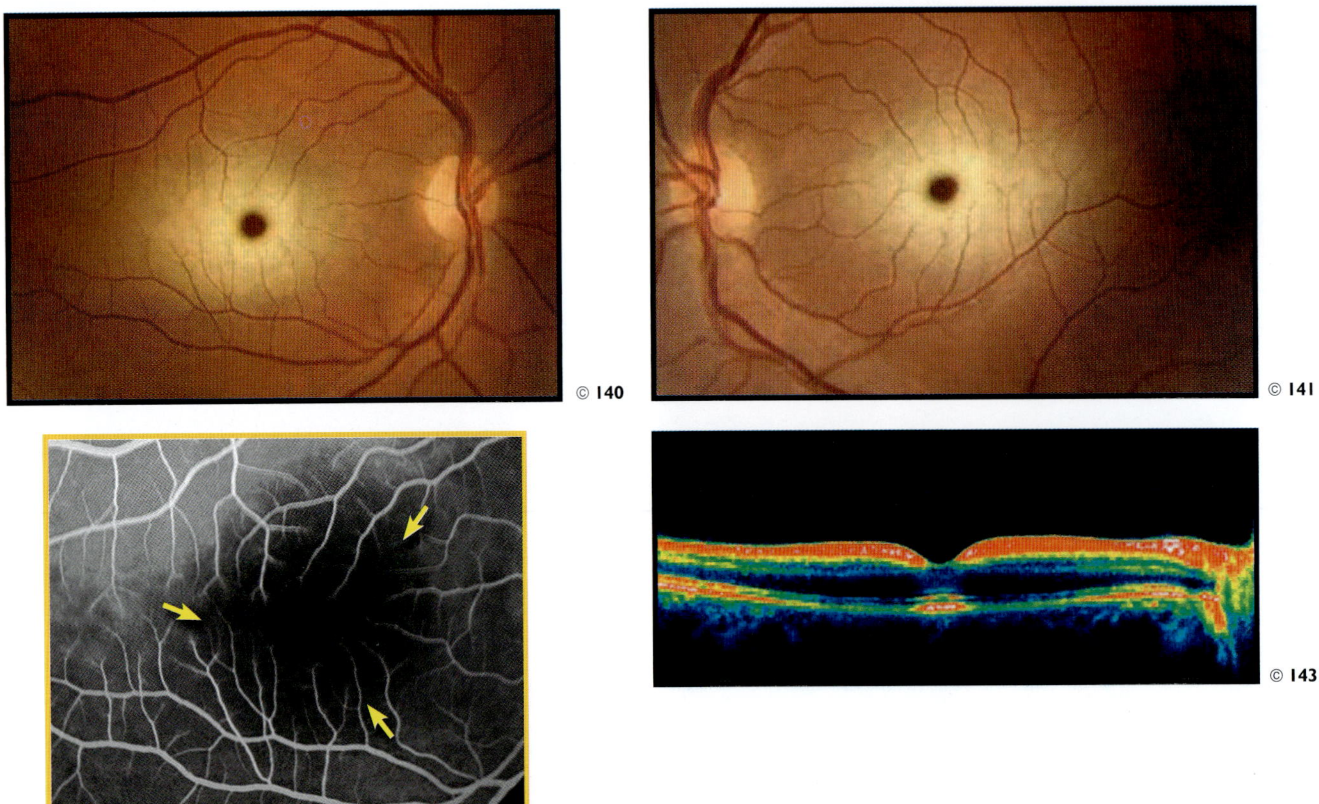

© 140 © 141 © 142 © 143

This patient with mucolipidosis type I (specifically sialidosis type II) has the characteristic cherry-red spot and a mild degree of shadowing on the fluorescein angiogram from blockage of the choriocapillaris *(arrows)*. The OCT demonstrates diffuse hyper-reflectivity of the ganglion cell layer due to severe mucolipid deposition and note the photo reflectance in the fovea due to the absence of any metabolic accumulation in that focal area.

Mucolipidosis Type II (ML II, Inclusion-cell (I-cell) Disease) and Mucolipidosis Type III (ML III, Pseudo-Hurler Polydystrophy)

ML II and ML III are both caused by a mutation in the GNPTAB (alpha/beta-subunits precursor gene of GLcNAc-phosphotransferase) gene (gene locus 12q23.3), with a variant of ML III caused by a GNPTG (gamma subunit) mutation.

Mucolipidosis Type II, Also Referred to as I-Cell Disease

This is so named because carbohydrates, lipids, and proteins accumulate in inclusion bodies. The detection of inclusion bodies in tissues often provides the diagnosis of the disease. It is the most severe form of the mucolipidoses and clinically resembles Hurler syndrome (mucopolysaccharidosis type I).

Mucolipidosis Type III (Pseudo-Hurler Polydystrophy)

ML III is closely related to I-cell disease. Symptoms are often not noticed until the child is 3–5 years of age, are less severe, and progress more slowly. Mental retardation is usually mild or absent. However patients manifest skeletal abnormalities, coarse facial features, short height, and corneal clouding. Posterior segment findings include retinal vascular tortuosity, optic nerve head swelling, and ERM. These individuals may survive until their fourth or fifth decade of life.

Mucolipidosis Type IV (ML IV, Sialolipidosis)

ML IV is caused by a mutation in mucolipin-1 (gene locus 19p13.3-p13.2), a nonselective cation channel, TRPML1. The lysosomal hydrolases in ML IV are normal, in contrast to most other storage diseases. Ocular manifestations include strabismus, corneal clouding, optic nerve pallor, retinal vascular attenuation, and diffuse RPE mottling.

Niemann–Pick Disease (Sphingomyelin Lipidosis)

Niemann–Pick disease is a group of lysosomal storage diseases usually inherited in an autosomal recessive fashion. The three most commonly recognized forms are types A, B, and C. Types A and B are both caused by mutations in the sphingomyelin phosphodiesterase-1 gene (SMPD1), which encodes acid sphingomyelinase (ASM).

Niemann–Pick disease type A occurs in infancy and is characterized by hepatosplenomegaly, jaundice, failure to thrive, and profound neurodegeneration leading to death by age 3 years. Ocular findings include a cherry-red spot in at least 50% of cases, mild corneal clouding, and brown granular discoloration of the anterior lens cortex or capsule. The clinical course is similar to Tay–Sachs disease; however, the visual loss is delayed due to the preservation of ganglion cells resulting in a less well-defined opacification that extends farther into the periphery but persists. Niemann–Pick disease type A occurs more frequently among individuals of Ashkenazi Jewish descent.

Niemann–Pick disease type B is a non-neuropathic form that occurs in all populations. Patients tend to have normal vision, hepatosplenomegaly, and usually survive into adulthood. A macular halo is classically observed.

Niemann–Pick disease type C is caused by mutations in either the NPC1 (~95%) or NPC2 (~5%) gene. The NPC1 gene produces a protein that is located in membranes inside the cell and is involved in the movement of cholesterol and lipids within cells. A deficiency of this protein leads to the abnormal build-up of lipids and cholesterol within cells. The NPC2 gene produces a protein that binds and transports cholesterol, although its exact function is not fully understood. Type C is characterized by onset in childhood with progressive psychomotor deterioration, moderate visceral and central nervous system involvement, vertical ophthalmoplegia, normal vision, and a macular halo similar to that seen in Type B. Type C is usually fatal by age 20.

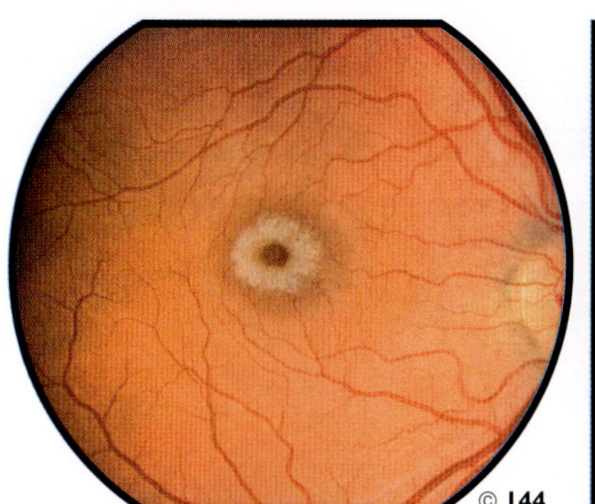

© 144

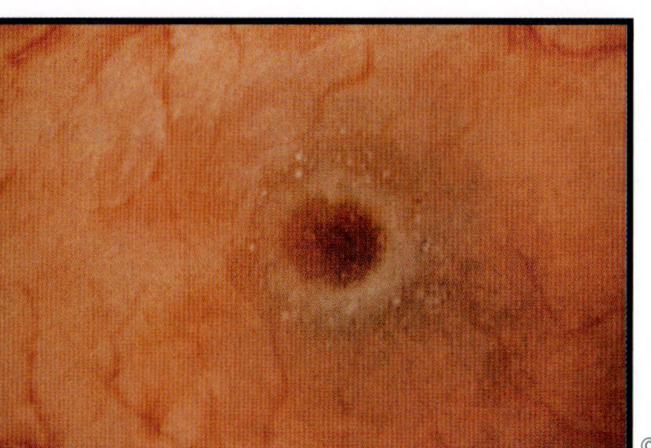

© 145

This patient shows evidence of abnormal inner retinal accumulation of sphingomyelin and cholesterol in the perifoveal region, which causes a cherry-red spot. The photo on the right shows a macular halo, which is a classic presentation of this disorder. There are also multifocal spots produced by the abnormal storage.

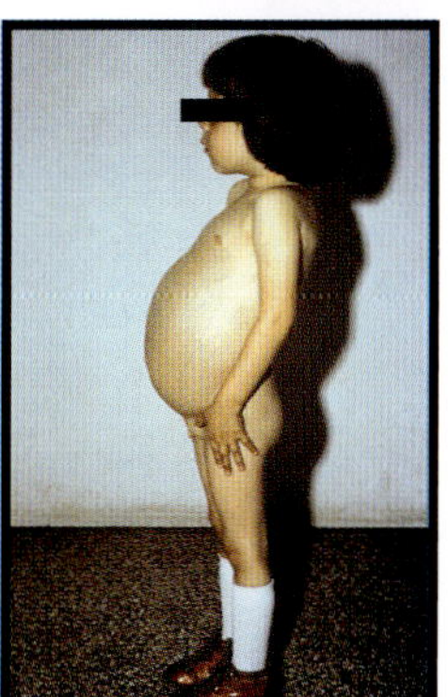

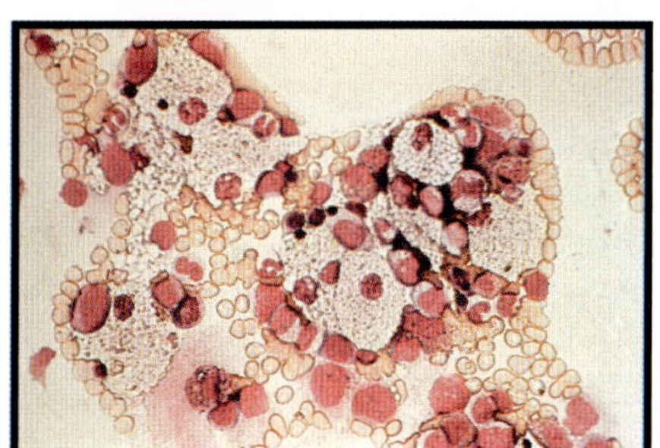

© 146

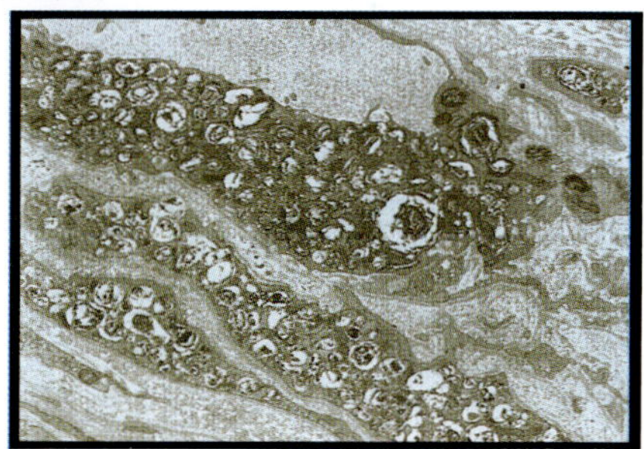

© 147

Sphingomyelin and cholesterol also accumulate in the abdomen, which causes a characteristic distension of the midsection, as seen in this young child. Light microscopy and electron microscopy reveal lipid accumulations in the retina.

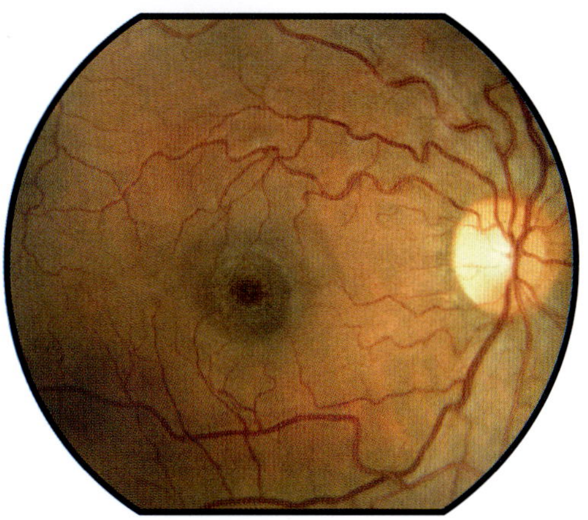

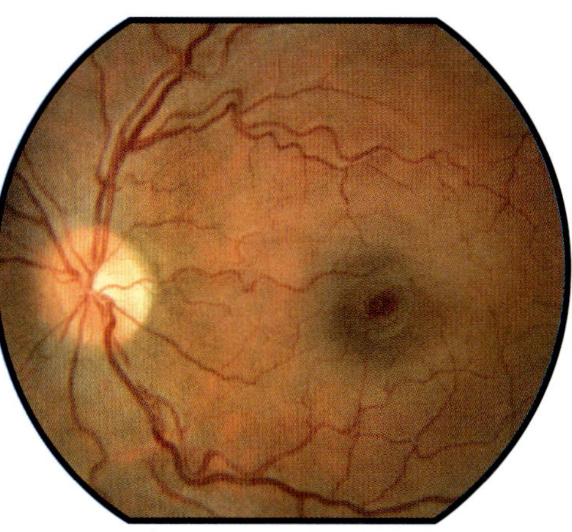

This patient with Niemann–Pick disease has a less prominently evident halo in the perifoveal region with a cherry-red spot.

Tay–Sachs Disease (GM2 Gangliosidosis, Type I)

Tay–Sachs disease is an autosomal recessive, progressive neurodegenerative disorder that begins in infancy. It is caused by a mutation in the alpha subunit of the hexosaminidase A gene (HEXA) that results in the accumulation of ganglioside GM2 in nervous tissue leading to cell damage. Ocular findings include a cherry-red spot caused by a gray-white opacification around the fovea due to lipid-laden ganglion cells. Progressive optic atrophy is also present. Infants with Tay–Sachs disease appear to develop normally for the first 6 months of life. Shortly thereafter they manifest blindness and psychomotor deterioration, resulting in death by 2–3 years of age. Tay–Sachs disease, like Niemann–Pick disease, is more prevalent in the Ashkenazi Jewish population.

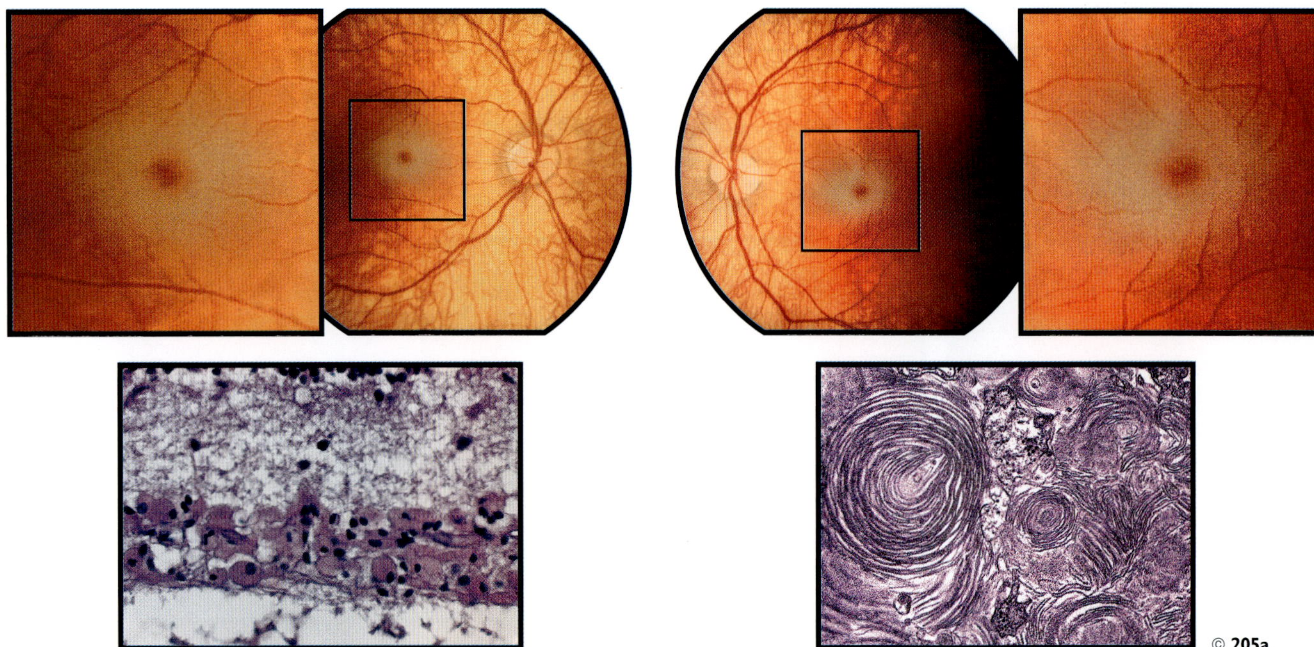

Color photographs are from a patient with Tay-Sachs disease illustrating bilateral cherry-red spots and perifoveal gray-white opacification. There are distended ganglion cells from ganglioside accumulation in the retina *(bottom left)*. The photo on the bottom right demonstrates the accumulation of the ganglioside, forming a multimembranous pattern. *Courtesy of Dr. Albert Aandekerk*

Sandhoff Disease (GM2 Gangliosidosis, Type II)

Sandhoff disease is a rare progressive neurodegenerative disorder that is difficult to clinically distinguish from Tay–Sachs disease but is not limited to the Ashkenazi Jewish population. Sandhoff disease is an autosomal recessive disorder caused by a mutation in the HEXB gene that encodes the beta subunit of hexosaminidase A and B, which results in a deficiency in these lysosomal enzymes. This results in accumulation of ganglioside GM2 in neurons, particularly in the brain and macula, producing a cherry-red spot. Other organs are involved, including the liver, pancreas, and kidney, whereas in Tay–Sachs disease, the material is mainly limited to the central nervous system. Biochemical analysis is used to differentiate these two disorders. Death usually occurs by age 3.

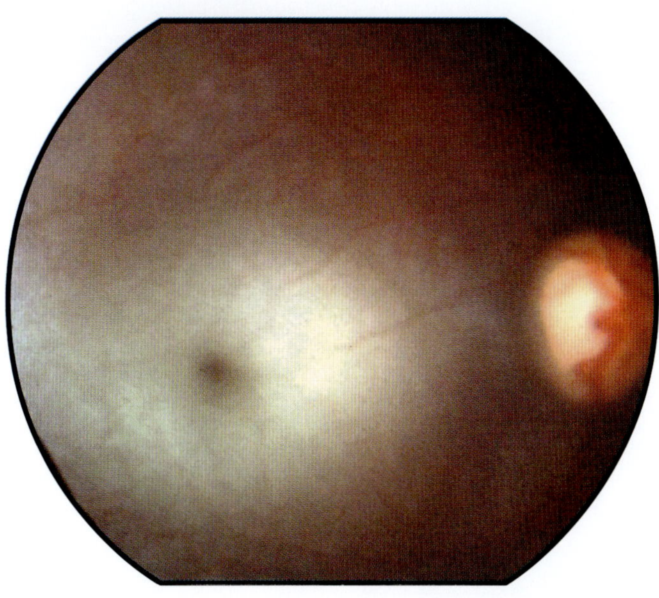

In this patient with Sandhoff disease, deposition of the ganglioside extends around the fovea into the paramacular region. There is still a prominent fovea evident clinically. *Courtesy of Dr. Mark Dailey*

Multiple Sulfatase Deficiency

Multiple sulfatase deficiency is a very rare hereditary lysosomal storage disease caused by mutations in the sulfatase-modifying factor-1 gene leading to a deficiency of arylsulfatases A, B, and C. These deficiencies cause abnormal accumulation of acid mucopolysaccharides in several tissues, and histopathology sections of peripheral nerves show a metachromatic degeneration of myelin. Clinically, the disorder combines features of metachromatic leukodystrophy and mucopolysaccharidosis including facial abnormalities, deafness, hepatosplenomegaly, and skeletal abnormalities. Neurologic deterioration is rapid with progressive mental retardation, dementia, hypertonia, ataxia, spastic quadriplegia, and early death. Ophthalmologic features include optic atrophy and a pigmentary retinopathy.

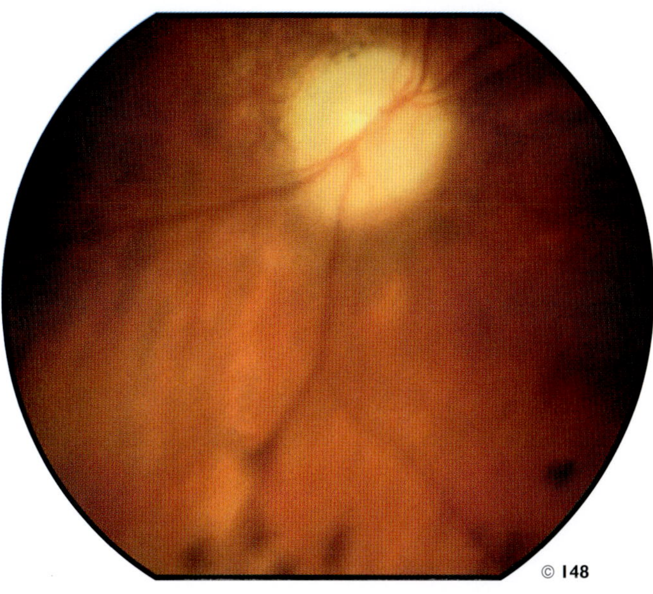

© 148

This patient with multiple sulfatase deficiency had psychomotor retardation, organomegaly, and ichthyosis. Optic atrophy and a pigmentary degeneration were evident in the fundus.

Gaucher Disease

Gaucher disease is the most common of the lysosomal storage diseases. It is an autosomal recessive disorder caused by a deficiency of the enzyme glucocerebrosidase (β-glucosidase), which catalyzes the breakdown of glucocerebroside. Consequently, there is an accumulation of this material in the spleen, liver, lungs, bone marrow, and, sometimes in the central nervous system. Histopathologically, glycolipid-laden macrophages containing "crinkled paper" cytoplasm are seen; these macrophages are known as "Gaucher cells." There are three main subtypes. Type I is non-neuronopathic, the most common and least severe form, which usually presents in childhood with hepatosplenomegaly and pancytopenia. It does not affect the brain. Type II is the acute infantile neuronopathic form, which presents by 3–6 months and causes severe progressive brain damage leading to death often by age 2. Type III is the chronic neuronopathic form that can begin in childhood or adulthood with liver and spleen enlargement and variable neurologic involvement. Ocular manifestations in Gaucher disease include white deposits in the corneal epithelium, anterior-chamber angle, ciliary body, and pupil margin. Scattered, discrete, and variably sized white spots identified in the posterior fundus and located in the superficial retina or on its surface, especially along the inferior vascular arcades, have also been described. These deposits are very nicely appreciated on the surface of the retina with SD OCT imaging. Perimacular grayness may be present, and macular atrophy and increased retinal vascular permeability have been reported in a case with a long-term follow-up.

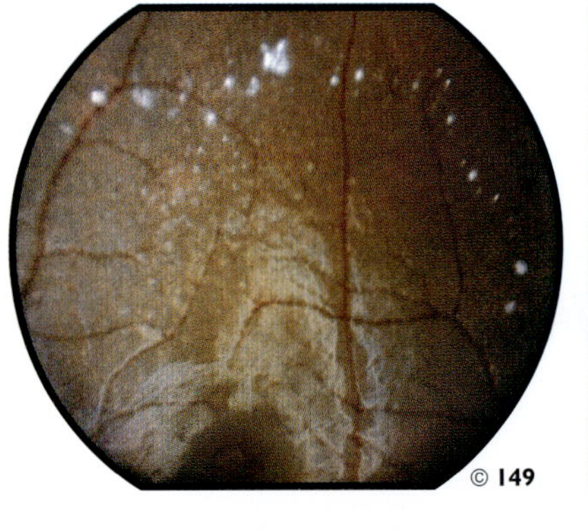
© 149

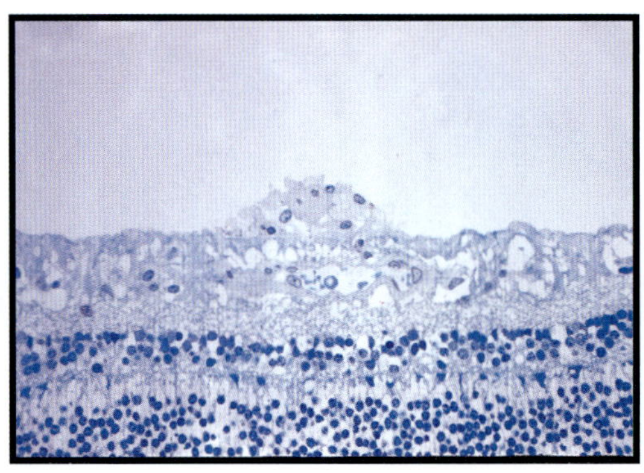
© 150

In this patient with Gaucher disease, there are discrete deposits found in a semicircular pattern surrounding the central macula. The histopathology shows typical deposits of "Gaucher cells" within the inner retina.

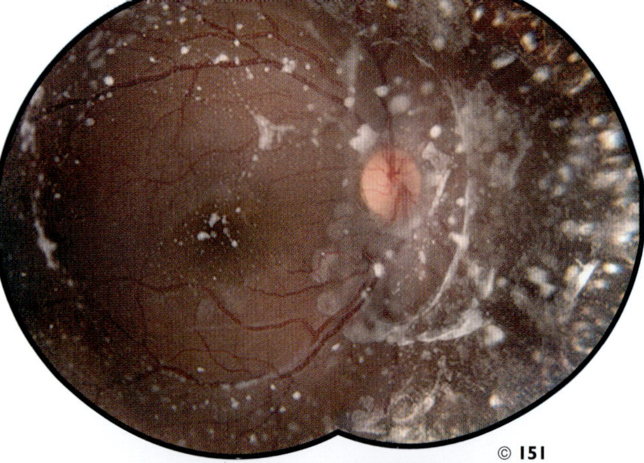
© 151

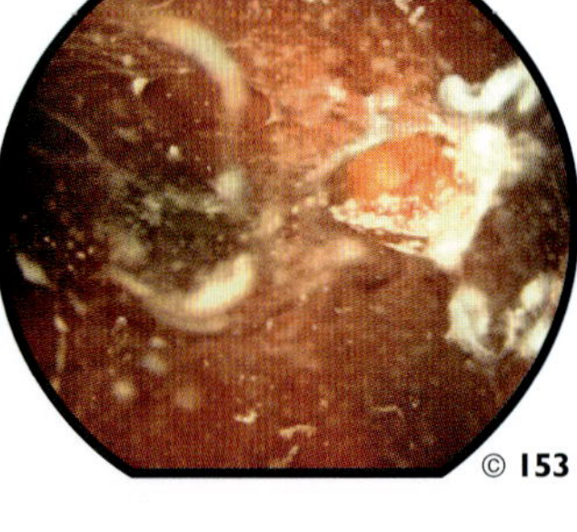
© 153

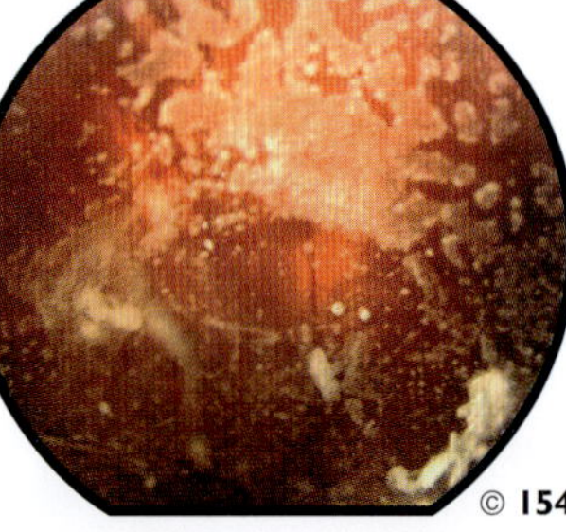
© 154

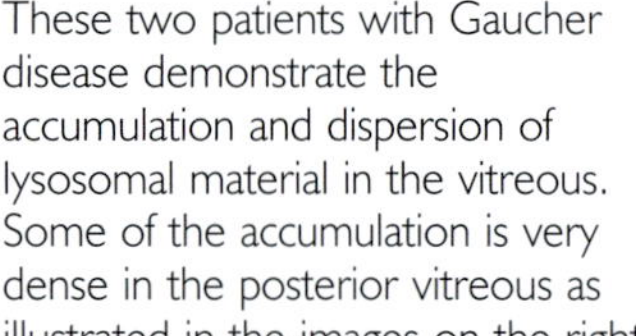
These two patients with Gaucher disease demonstrate the accumulation and dispersion of lysosomal material in the vitreous. Some of the accumulation is very dense in the posterior vitreous as illustrated in the images on the right.

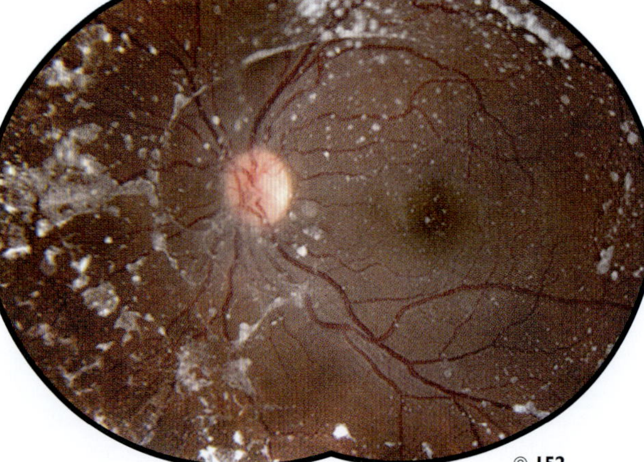
© 152

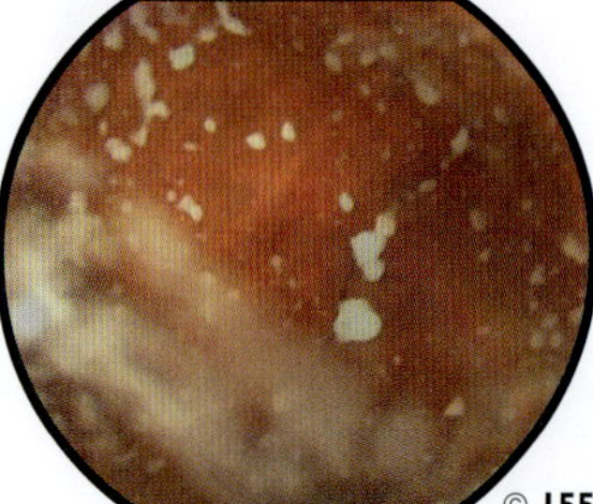
© 155

Female Carrier of Gaucher Disease

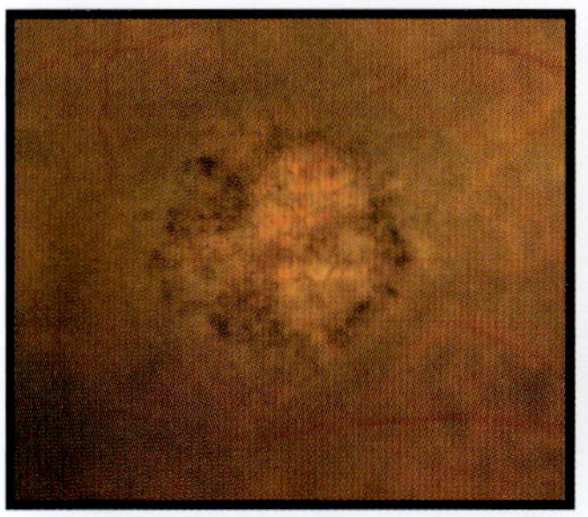
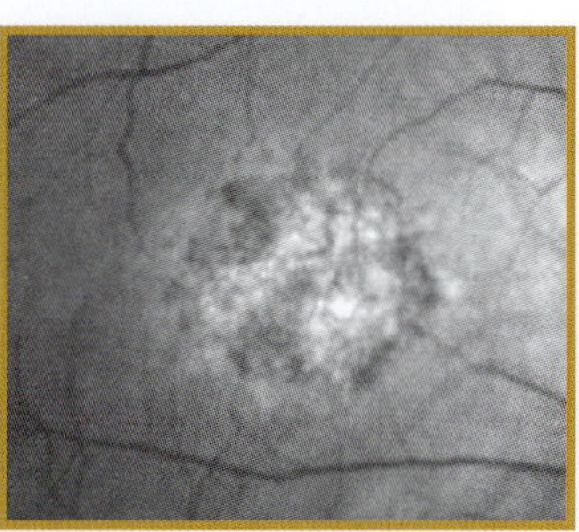
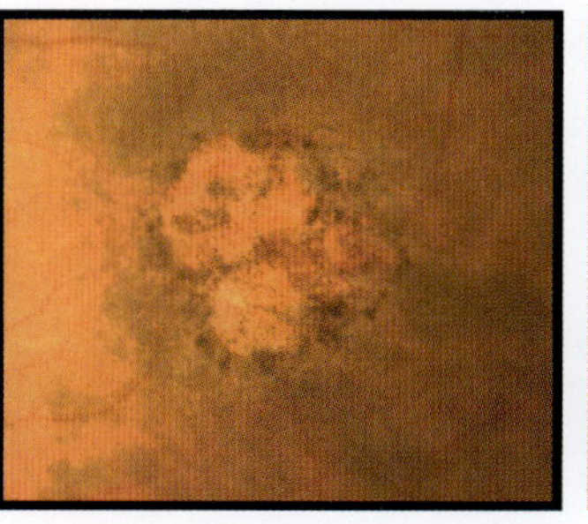
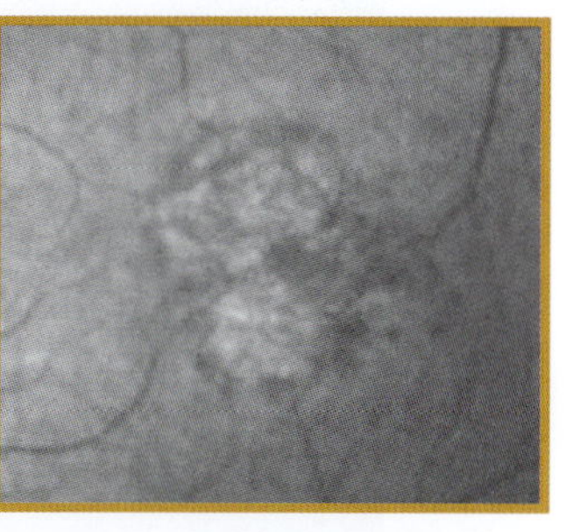

A female carrier of Gaucher disease may demonstrate macular pathology, as is evidenced here in this patient with atrophy and pigment epithelial hyperplasia. There are multifocal dots of inner retinal storage evident on the red-free photographs.

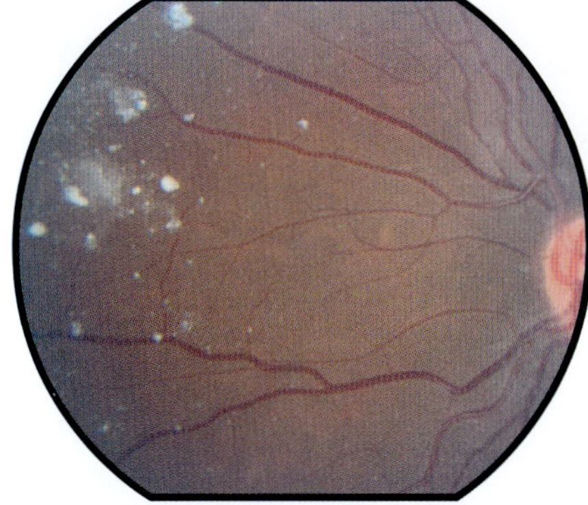
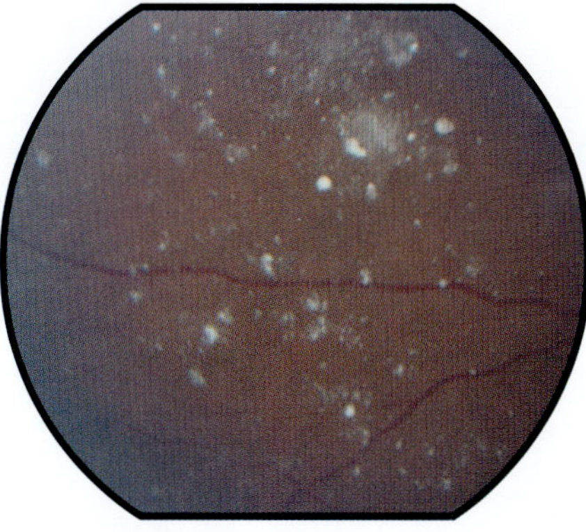
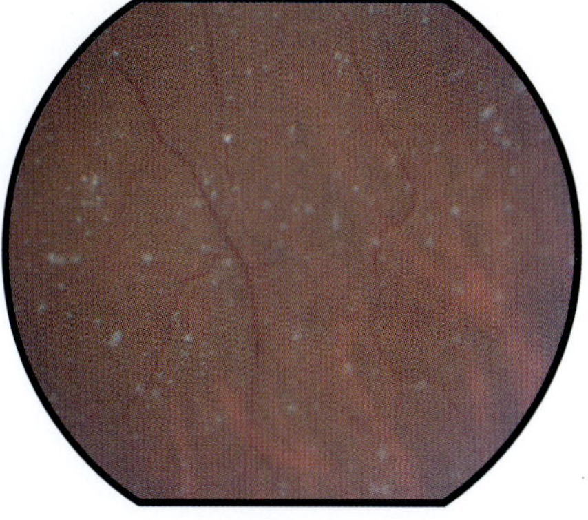

Color fundus photographs of the peripheral retina in this patient with Gaucher disease shows the white, pre-retinal deposits known as Gaucher cells, which are sometimes seen in this disease. *Images courtesy of SriniVas Sadda, MD and Jennifer Hu, MD*

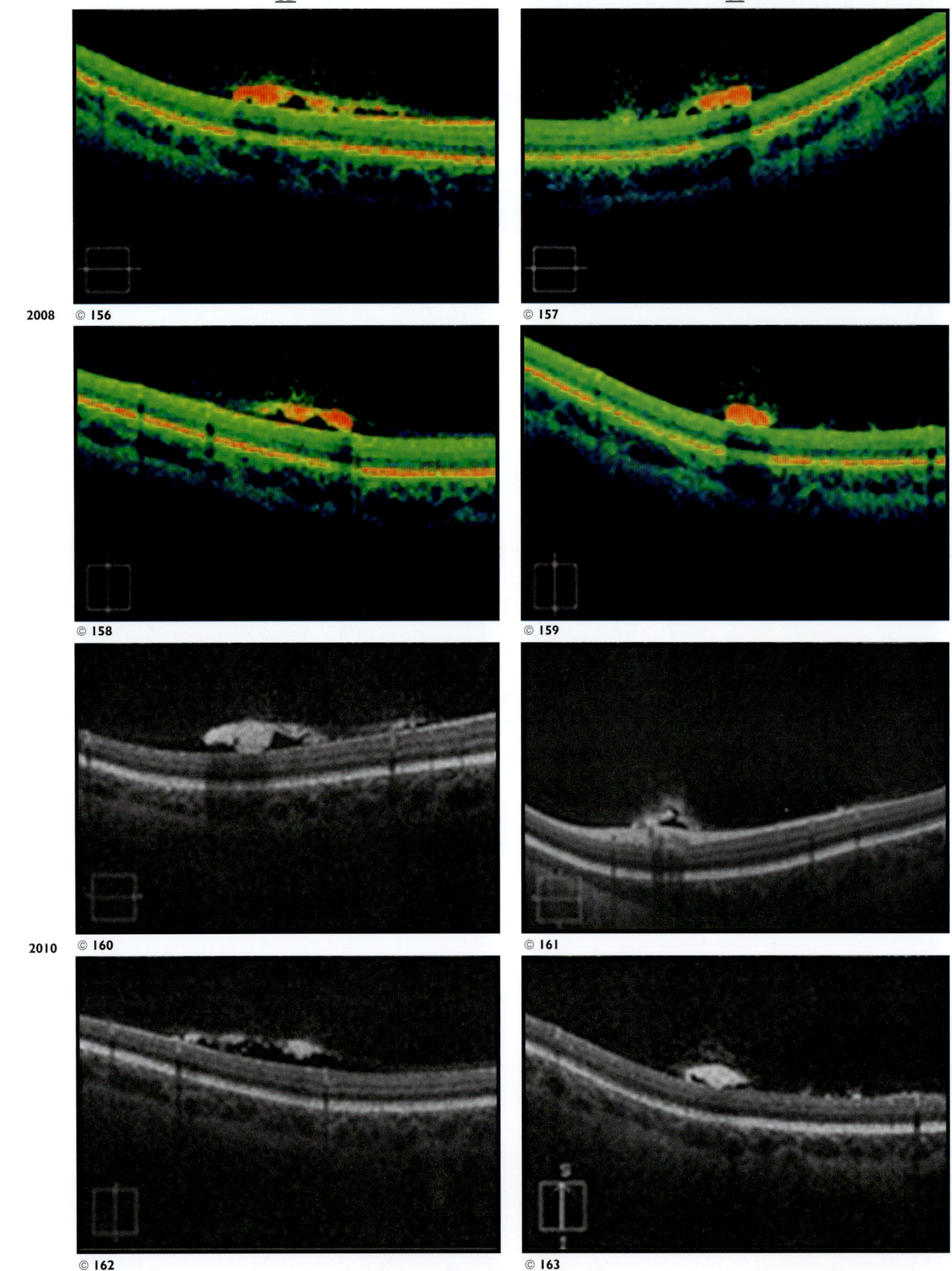

TD-OCT and SD-OCT through the pre-retinal lesions in a patient with Gaucher disease over a 2 year period.

Shaken Baby Syndrome

Shaken baby syndrome is a well-recognized entity in the pediatric retinal setting characterized by pre-retinal, intraretinal, and subretinal hemorrhages that develop because of child abuse. White centered hemorrhages may also be present and other disorders such as leukemia should be excluded. The mechanism of this type of bleeding is likely a result of vitreoretinal traction placing shearing forces on retinal blood vessels during repetitive acceleration and deceleration. Some authors have also proposed that the hemorrhages might result from increased ICP and intrathoracic pressure causing increased venous pressure within the eye. The hemorrhages will spontaneously resolve once intervention to stop the cycle of abuse has taken place. Pre-retinal neovascularization and vitreous hemorrhage may complicate this condition and peripheral laser photocoagulation to ischemic zones may rarely be necessary. Vitrectomy to clear significant vitreous hemorrhage may be considered to prevent amblyopia.

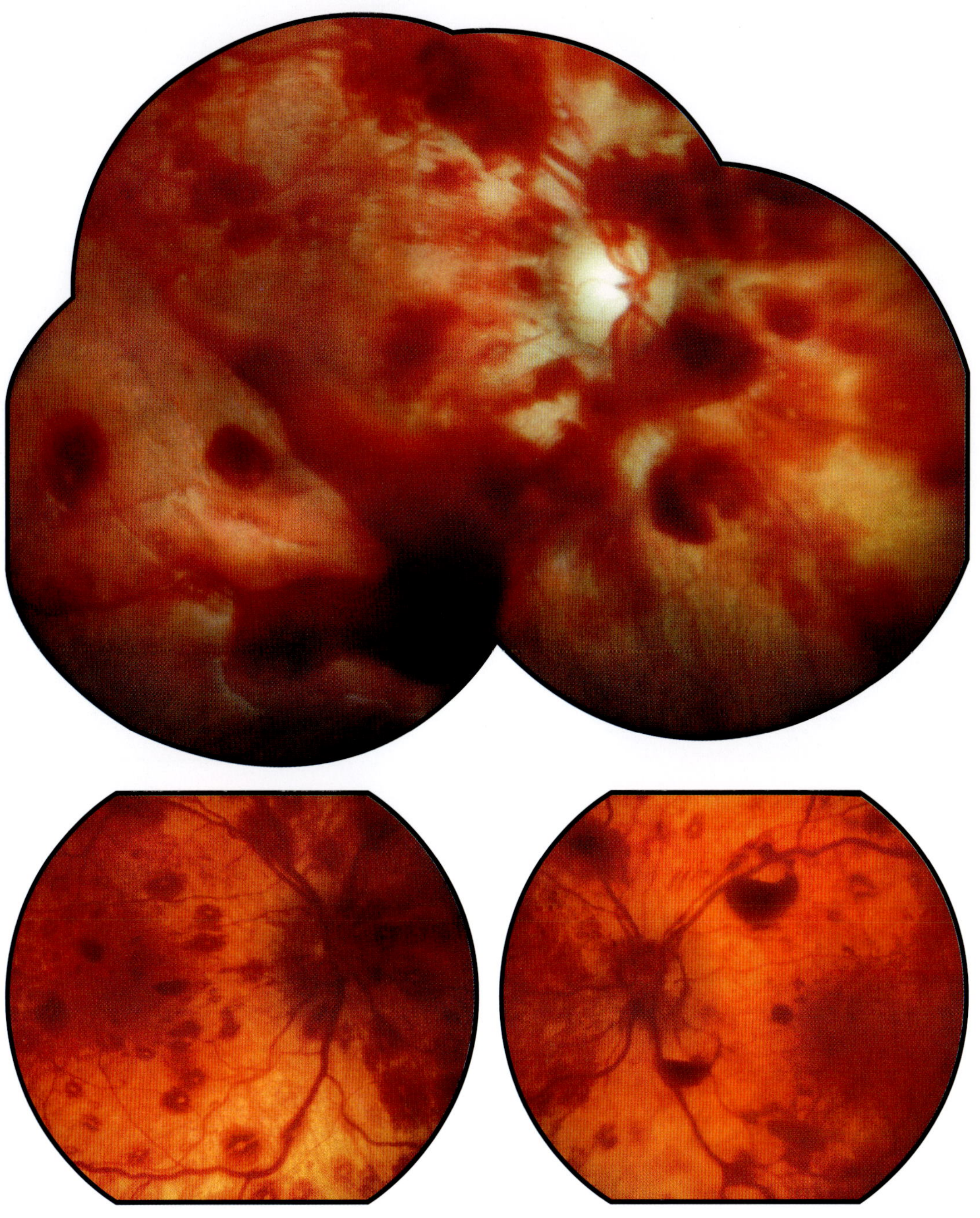

These patients with shaken baby syndrome show severe hemorrhagic complications in the posterior fundus. Note the vitreous hemorrhage in the image above and the white-centered hemorrhages and pre-retinal hemorrhage in the images below. *Bottom row courtesy of Dr. Richard Spaide*

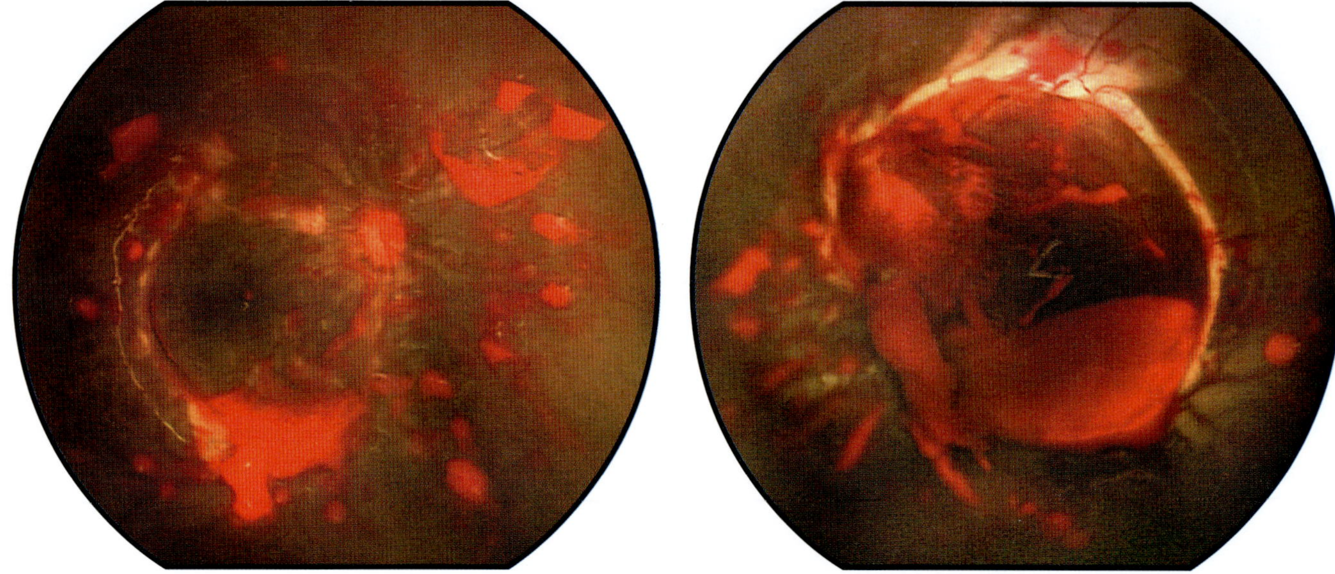

The shaken baby syndrome present in this patient is particularly severe. Pre-retinal hemorrhage has occurred in the vitreous and leveled out near the macula in a boat-shaped configuration in each eye. *Courtesy of Dr. Suzanna Airani*

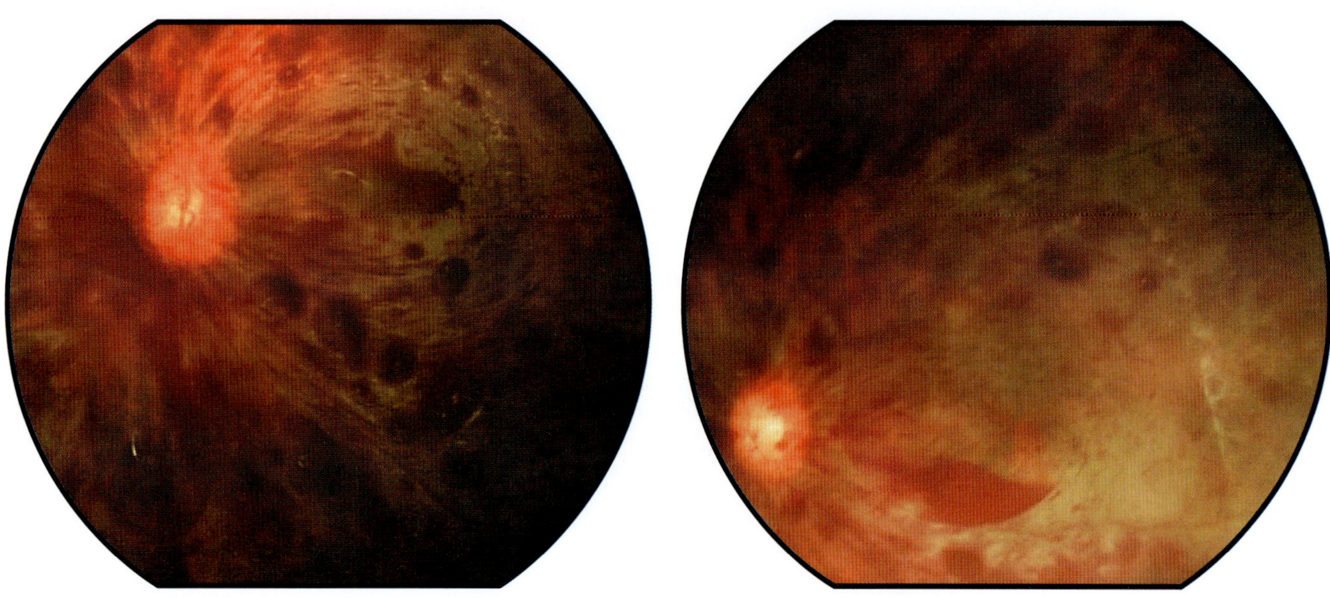

Hemorrhages in multiple layers of the retina are seen in both eyes of this 14-month-old victim of child abuse.

Suggested Reading

Retinopathy of Prematurity

Cryotherapy for Retinopathy of Prematurity Cooperative Group, 2005. Fifteen-year outcomes following threshold retinopathy of prematurity. Final results from the Multicenter Trial of Cryotherapy for Retinopathy of Prematurity. Arch. Ophthalmol. 123, 311–318.

Hellstrom, A., Smith, L.E., Dammann, O., 2013. Retinopathy of prematurity. Lancet 382 (9902), 1445–1457.

Klufas, M.A., Chan, R.V., 2015. Intravitreal anti-VEGF therapy as a treatment for retinopathy of prematurity: what we know after 7 years. J. Pediatr. Ophthalmol. Strabismus 52 (2), 77–84.

Reynolds, J.D., Dobson, V., Quinn, G.E., et al., 2002. Evidence-based screening criteria for retinopathy of prematurity: natural history data from the CRYO-ROP and LIGHT-ROP studies. Arch. Ophthalmol. 120, 1470–1476.

STOP-ROP Multicenter Study Group, 2000. Supplemental therapeutic oxygen for prethreshold retinopathy of prematurity (STOP-ROP), a randomized, controlled trial. I. Primary outcomes. Pediatrics 105, 295–310.

Persistent Fetal Vasculature Syndrome

Ceron, O., Lou, P.L., Kroll, A.J., et al., 2008. The vitreo-retinal manifestations of persistent hyperplasic primary vitreous (PHPV) and their management. Int. Ophthalmol. Clin. 48 (2), 53–62.

Goldberg, M.F., 1997. Persistent fetal vasculature (PFV): an integrated interpretation of signs and symptoms associated with persistent hyperplastic primary vitreous (PHPV). LIV Edward Jackson Memorial Lecture. Am. J. Ophthalmol. 124, 587–626.

Jampol, L.M., 2007. Persistent fetal vasculature. Arch. Ophthalmol. 125, 432.

Congenital Folds

Khairallah, M., Messaoud, R., Zaouali, S., et al., 2002. Posterior segment changes associated with posterior microphthalmos. Ophthalmology 109, 569–574.

Neurofibromatosis Type I

Gallego-Pinazo, R., Sherman, J., Yannuzzi, L.A., et al., 2013. Choroidal lesions in neurofibromatosis detected by multispectral imaging. Retin. Cases Brief Rep. 7 (2), 176–178.

Goktas, S., Sakarya, Y., Ozcimen, M., et al., 2014. Frequency of choroidal abnormalities in pediatric patients with neurofibromatosis type 1. J. Pediatr. Ophthalmol. Strabismus 51 (4), 204–208.

Yasunari, T., Shiraki, K., Hattori, H., et al., 2000. Frequency of choroidal abnormalities in neurofibromatosis type 1. Lancet 356 (9234), 988–992.

Neurofibromatosis Type 2

Grant, E.A., Trzupek, K.M., Reiss, J., et al., 2008. Combined retinal hamartomas leading to the diagnosis of neurofibromatosis type 2. Ophthalmic Genet. 29 (3), 133–138.

Sisk, R.A., Berrocal, A.M., Schefler, A.C., et al., 2010. Epiretinal membranes indicate a severe phenotype of neurofibromatosis type 2. Retina 30 (4 Suppl.), S51–S58.

Combined Hamartoma of the Retina and RPE

Gass, J.D.M., 1973. An unusual hamartoma of the pigment epithelium and retina simulating choroidal melanoma and retinoblastoma. Trans. Am. Ophthalmol. Soc. 71, 171–185.

Schachat, A.P., Shields, J.A., Fine, S.L., et al., 1984. Combined hamartoma of the retina and retinal pigment epithelium. Ophthalmology 91, 1609–1615.

Shields, C.L., Mashayekhi, A., Dai, V.V., et al., 2005. Optical coherence tomography findings of combined hamartoma of the retina and retinal pigment epithelium in 11 patients. Arch. Ophthalmol. 123, 1746–1750.

Wyburn Mason Syndrome

Schmidt, D., Pache, M., Schumacher, M., 2008. The congenital unilateral retinocephalic vascular malformation syndrome (Bonnet–Dechaume–Blanc syndrome or Wyburn–Mason syndrome): review of the literature. Surv. Ophthalmol. 53, 227–249.

Congenital Retinal Macrovessel

de Crecchio, G., Alfieri, M.C., Cennamo, G., et al., 2006. Congenital macular macrovessels. Graefes Arch. Clin. Exp. Ophthalmol. 244, 1183–1187.

von Hippel–Lindau Syndrome

Singh, A.D., Shields, C.L., Shields, J.A., 2001. von Hippel–Lindau disease. Surv. Ophthalmol. 46, 117–142.

Toy, B.C., Agron, E., Nigam, D., et al., 2012. Longitudinal analysis of retinal hemangioblastomatosis and visual function in ocular von Hippel-Lindau disease. Ophthalmology 119 (12), 2622–2630.

Retinal Cavernous Hemangioma

Sarraf, D., Payne, A.M., Kitchen, N.D., et al., 2000. Familial cavernous hemangioma: An expanding ocular spectrum. Arch. Ophthalmol. 118 (7), 969–973.

Shields, J.A., Eagle, R.C. Jr., Ewing, M.Q., et al., 2014. Retinal cavernous hemangioma: fifty-two years of clinical follow-up with clinicopathologic correlation. Retina 34 (6), 1253–1257.

Leber Congenital Amaurosis

Hufnagel, R.B., Ahmed, Z.M., Correa, Z.M., et al., 2012. Gene therapy for Leber congenital amaurosis: advances and future directions. Graefes Arch. Clin. Exp. Ophthalmol. 250 (8), 1117–1128.

Lambert, S.R., Kriss, A., Taylor, D., et al., 1989. Follow-up and diagnostic reappraisal of 75 patients with Leber's congenital amaurosis. Am. J. Ophthalmol. 107, 624–631.

Smith, D., Oestreicher, J., Musarella, M., 1990. Clinical spectrum of Leber's congenital amaurosis in the second to fourth decades of life. Ophthalmology 97, 1156–1161.

Neuronal Ceroid Lipofuscinoses

Hainsworth, D.P., Liu, G.T., Hamm, C.W., et al., 2009. Funduscopic and angiographic appearance in the neuronal ceroid lipofuscinoses. Retina 29 (5), 657–668.

Traboulsi, E.I., Green, W.R., Luchenbach, M.W., et al., 1987. Neuronal ceroid lipofuscinosis; ocular histopathologic and electron microscopic studies in the late infantile, juvenile, and adult forms. Graefes Arch. Clin. Exp. Ophthalmol. 225, 391–402.

Mucopolysaccharidoses

Ashworth, J.L., Biswas, S., Wraith, E., et al., 2006. The ocular features of the mucopolysaccharidoses. Eye (Lond.) 20, 553–563.

Topping, T.M., Kenyon, K.R., Goldberg, M.F., et al., 1971. Ultrastructural ocular pathology of Hunter's syndrome; systemic mucopoly-saccharidosis type II. Arch. Ophthalmol. 86, 164–177.

Yoon, M.K., Chen, R.W., Hedges, T.R. 3rd, et al., 2007. High-speed, ultrahigh resolution optical coherence tomography of the retina in Hunter syndrome. Ophthalmic Surg. Lasers Imaging 38, 423–428.

Mucolipidoses

Pradhan, S.M., Atchaneeyasakul, L.O., Appukuttan, B., et al., 2002. Electronegative electroretinogram in mucolipidosis IV. Arch. Ophthalmol. 120, 45–50.

Smith, J.A., Chan, C.C., Goldin, E., et al., 2002. Noninvasive diagnosis and ophthalmic features of mucolipidosis type IV. Ophthalmology 109, 588–594.

Traboulsi, E.I., Maumenee, I.H., 1986. Ophthalmologic findings in mucolipidosis III (pseudo-Hurler polydystrophy). Am. J. Ophthalmol. 102, 592–597.

Niemann–Pick Disease

McGovern, M.M., Wasserstein, M.P., Aron, A., et al., 2004. Ocular manifestations of Niemann-Pick disease type B. Ophthalmology 111, 1424–1427.

Palmer, M., Green, W.R., Maumenee, I.H., et al., 1985. Niemann-Pick disease type C; ocular histopathologic and electron microscopic studies. Arch. Ophthalmol. 103, 817–822.

Tay–Sachs Disease

Cotlier, E., 1971. Tay-Sachs' retina. Deficiency of acetyl hexosaminidase A. Arch. Ophthalmol. 86, 352–356.

Kivlin, J.D., Sanborn, G.E., Myers, G.G., 1985. The cherry-red spot in Tay-Sachs and other storage diseases. Ann. Neurol. 17, 356–360.

Tay, W., 1881. Symmetrical changes in the region of the yellow spot in each eye of an infant. Trans. Ophthalmol. Soc. UK 1, 55–57.

Sandhoff Disease

Brownstein, S., Carpenter, S., Polomeno, R.C., et al., 1980. Sandhoff's disease (GM2 gangliosidosis type 2). Histopathology and ultrastructure of the eye. Arch. Ophthalmol. 98, 1089–1097.

Sandhoff, K., Andreae, U., Jatzkewitz, H., 1968. Deficient hexozaminidase activity in an exceptional case of Tay–Sachs disease with additional storage of kidney globoside in visceral organs. Life Sci. 7, 283–288.

Multiple Sulfatase Deficiency

Bateman, J.B., Philippart, M., Isenberg, S.J., 1984. Ocular features of multiple sulfatase deficiency and a new variant of metachromatic leukodystrophy. J. Pediatr. Ophthalmol. Strabismus 21, 133–139.

Gaucher Disease

Cogan, D.G., Chu, F.C., Gittinger, J., et al., 1980. Fundal abnormalities of Gaucher's Disease. Arch. Ophthalmol. 98, 2202–2203.

Coussa, R.G., Roos, J.C., Aroichane, M., et al., 2013. Progression of retinal changes in Gaucher disease: a case report. Eye (Lond.) 27 (11), 1331–1333.

Wollstein, G., Elstein, D., Strassman, I., et al., 1999. Preretinal white dots in adult-type Gaucher disease. Retina 19, 570–571.

Shaken Baby Syndrome

Buys, Y.M., Levin, A.V., Enzenauer, R.W., et al., 1992. Retinal findings after head trauma in infants and young children. Ophthalmology 99, 1718–1723.

Morad, Y., Wygnansky-Jaffe, T., Levin, A.V., 2010. Retinal haemorrhage in abusive head trauma. Clin. Experiment. Ophthalmol. 38 (5), 514–520.

CHAPTER 4

Inflammation

Multiple Evanescent White Dot Syndrome (MEWDS)

Multiple evanescent white dot syndrome (MEWDS) is an acute inflammatory disorder in which patients present with unilateral, multiple, small, white spots at the level of the outer retina and retinal pigment epithelium. Patients typically are young, myopic, and female (75%) and present with symptoms of temporal field loss (enlarged blind spot), blurred vision, and photopsia, often following a flu-like illness. The disorder is typically self-limited with visual recovery over a few to several weeks. During the subacute phase white dots in the fovea may impart a granular appearance; old lesions may fade while new lesions develop in other areas. Vitreous cells and a mild papillophlebitis may occur. Fluorescein angiography (FA) shows early hyperfluorescent dots overlying larger spots ("wreath" pattern) corresponding to the white funduscopic lesions. With indocyanine green (ICG) angiography the dots and spots are hypofluorescent and with fundus autofluorescence the spots are hyperfluorescent and in each case more extensive than seen with color fundus photography or FA. With spectral domain optical coherence tomography (OCT) the spots correspond to loss or discontinuity of the inner segment ellipsoid band and the dots correspond to outer retinal hyper-reflective foci; these resolve briskly with resolution of the illness.

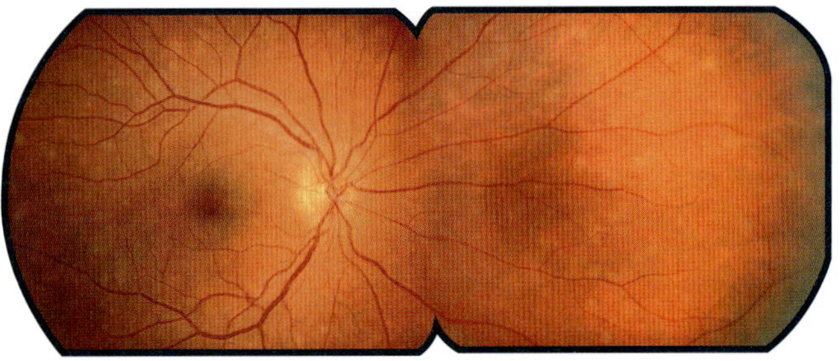
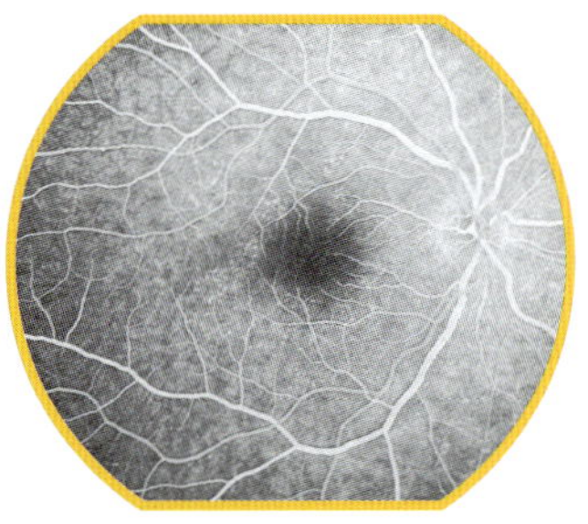
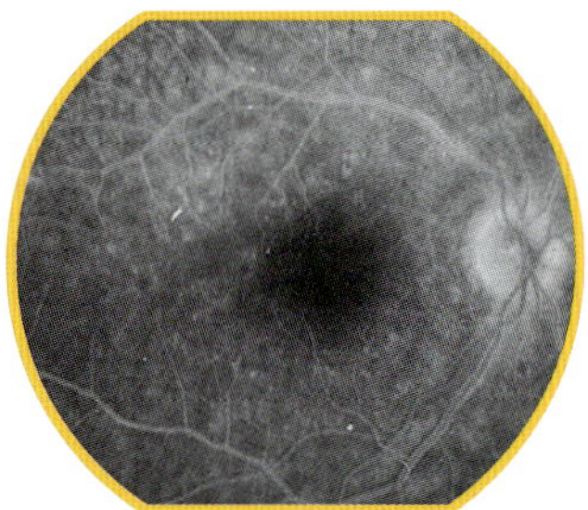

This patient with MEWDS has faint, small whitish lesions characteristic of the white spots noted in this condition. The fluorescein study reveals wreath-like punctate hyperfluorescent spots, which strongly stain in the late study. There is also slight staining of the optic nerve.

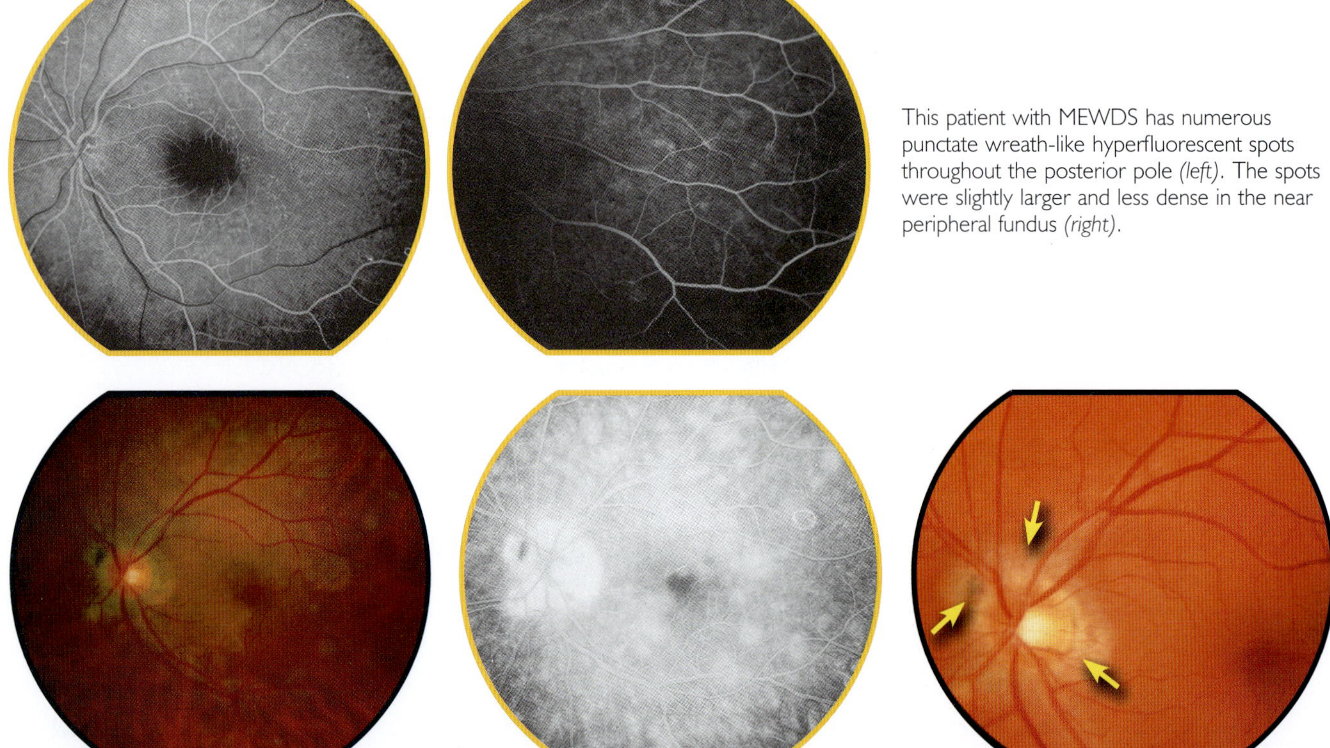

This patient with MEWDS has numerous punctate wreath-like hyperfluorescent spots throughout the posterior pole *(left)*. The spots were slightly larger and less dense in the near peripheral fundus *(right)*.

In this patient with MEWDS, widespread spots are larger and deeper in the fundus, which causes an alteration in the posterior blood ocular barrier, which is evident as leakage on the late-stage fluorescein angiogram. There is disc staining in this patient, a frequent finding in patients with this condition. Peripapillary atrophy and pigmentary disturbance may be seen in some patients *(arrows)*. Three weeks later, there is disappearance of the spots and improvement of the vision. Enlargement of the blind spot is seen after the acute manifestation resolves, as is common in patients with MEWDS; however, in some patients, it may only improve but not disappear completely, such as in this case.

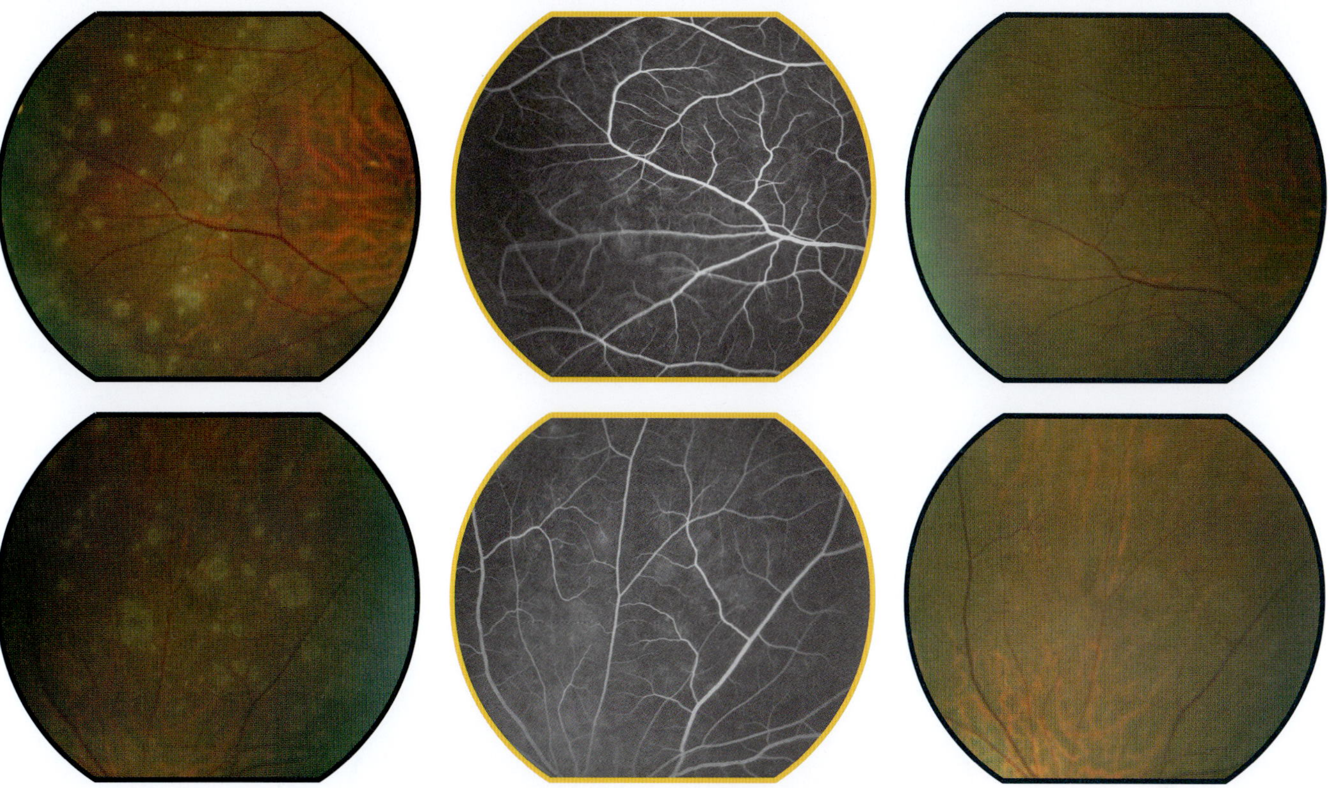

This patient with MEWDS has prominently evident white spots. Note the distribution and variable sizes of the spots temporally *(upper row, left)* and superiorly *(lower row, left)*. The fluorescein angiogram shows punctate and multifocal hyperfluorescence *(middle images)*. Following resolution of the acute process, the fundus clears without any evidence of pigment epithelial or choroidal disturbance.

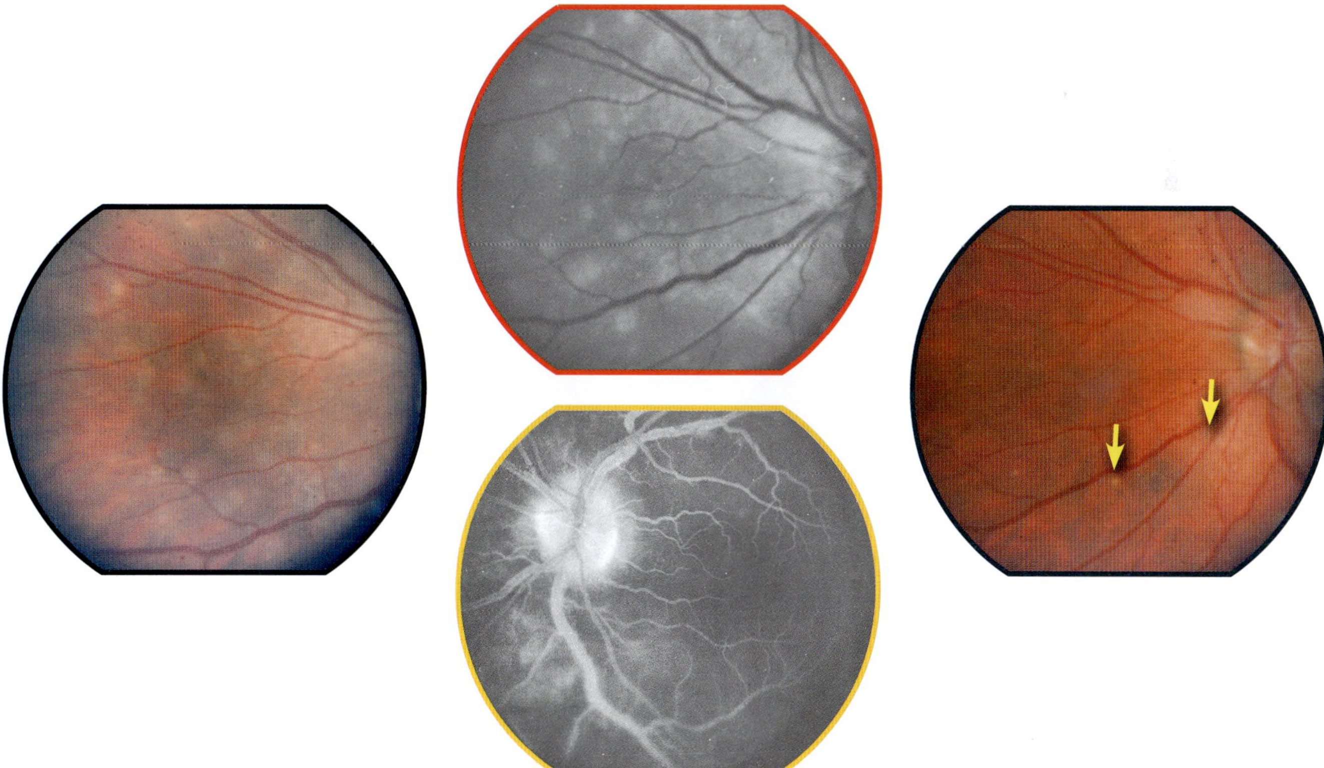

In this patient with MEWDS, spots are predominantly in the nasal posterior pole. They are more prominently evident on the red-free image *(middle upper)*. The fluorescein angiogram shows hyperfluorescence of some of the nasal peripapillary spots, and dilation of veins with some venular staining, and leakage at the optic nerve *(middle lower)*. Following resolution of the acute stage of the disease, there is a notable absence of pigmentary and atrophic chorioretinal abnormalities, except for two atrophic spots, most likely due to the inflammation of the pigment epithelium *(arrows)*. A mild optic neuritis seen in MEWDS may account for the blind spot enlargement.

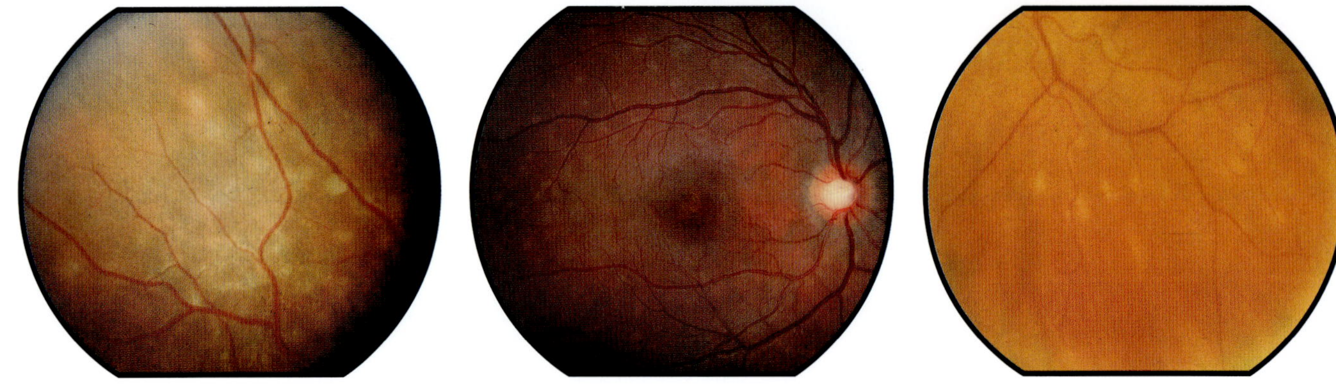

These clinical photographs are examples of the variability of the white spots that are seen in MEWDS. Some are prominently evident as larger nummular retinal abnormalities *(left)*. Some are very faintly evident *(middle)* and, in other cases, there are just a few spots clustered in a small, zonal area *(right)*. New spots may appear as older lesions fade in a few to several days.

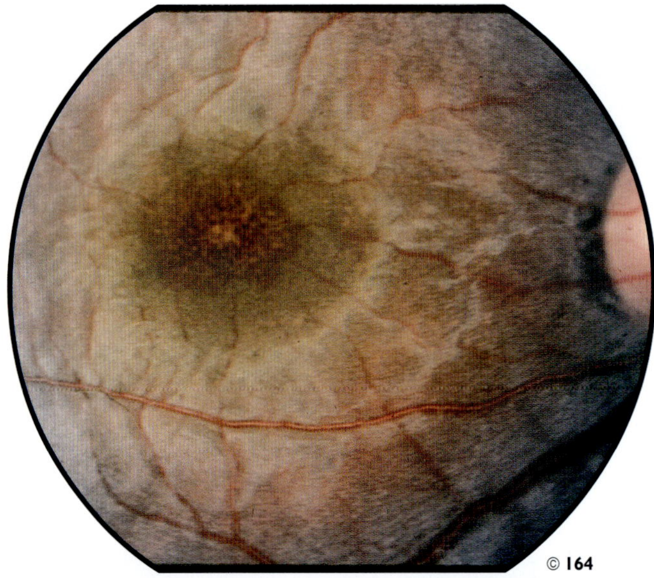

© 164

There is always some degree of associated foveal granularity. In this case the clinical findings are quite prominently evident in a patient of African descent, due to the pigmentation in the fundus. This change of the fovea may persist after the acute manifestations.

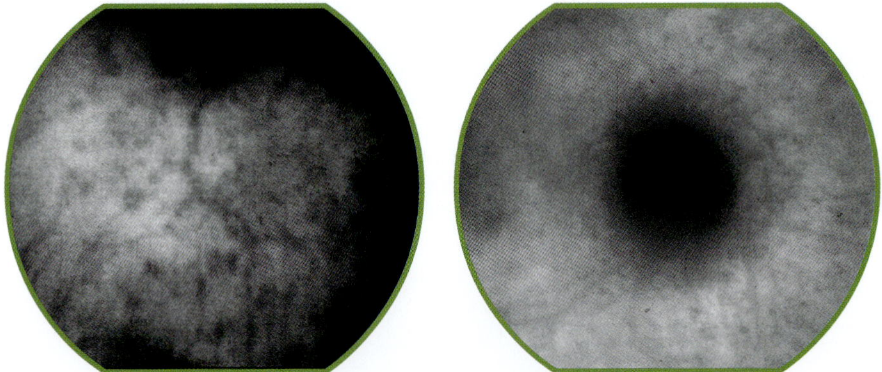

The ICG angiogram generally shows more hypofluorescent spots than clinically evident or seen on the fluorescein study. Surrounding the optic nerve, there is a collarette of hypofluorescent spots with confluency, accounting for enlargement of the blind spot described in these patients *(right image)*.

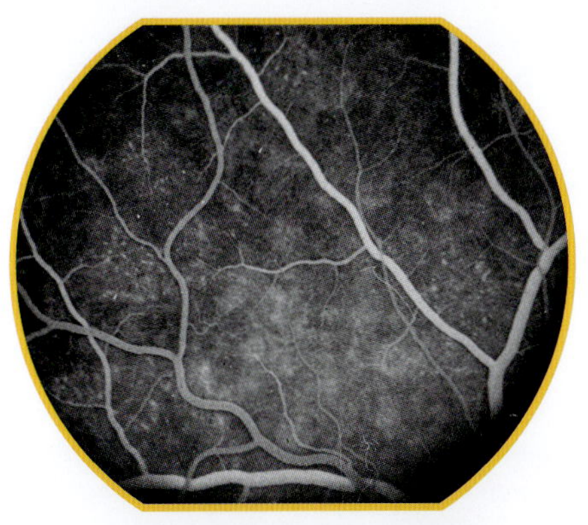

The fluorescein angiogram in this patient with MEWDS shows punctate wreath-like hyperfluorescent dots, some of which overlie larger hyperfluorescent spots. These "dots and spots" reside at the level of the outer retina and ellipsoid, respectively, on the basis of recent *en-face* imaging studies.

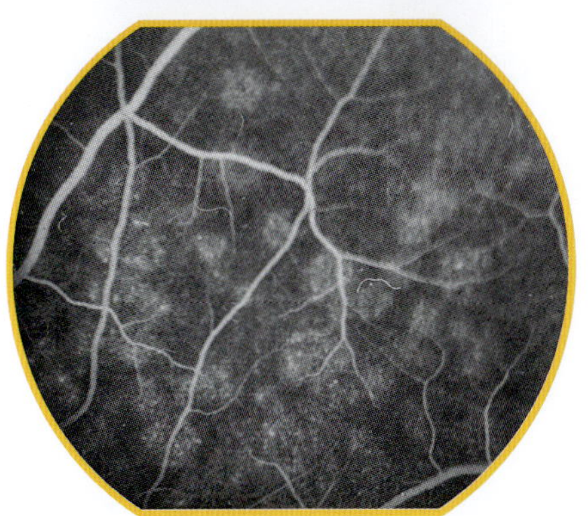

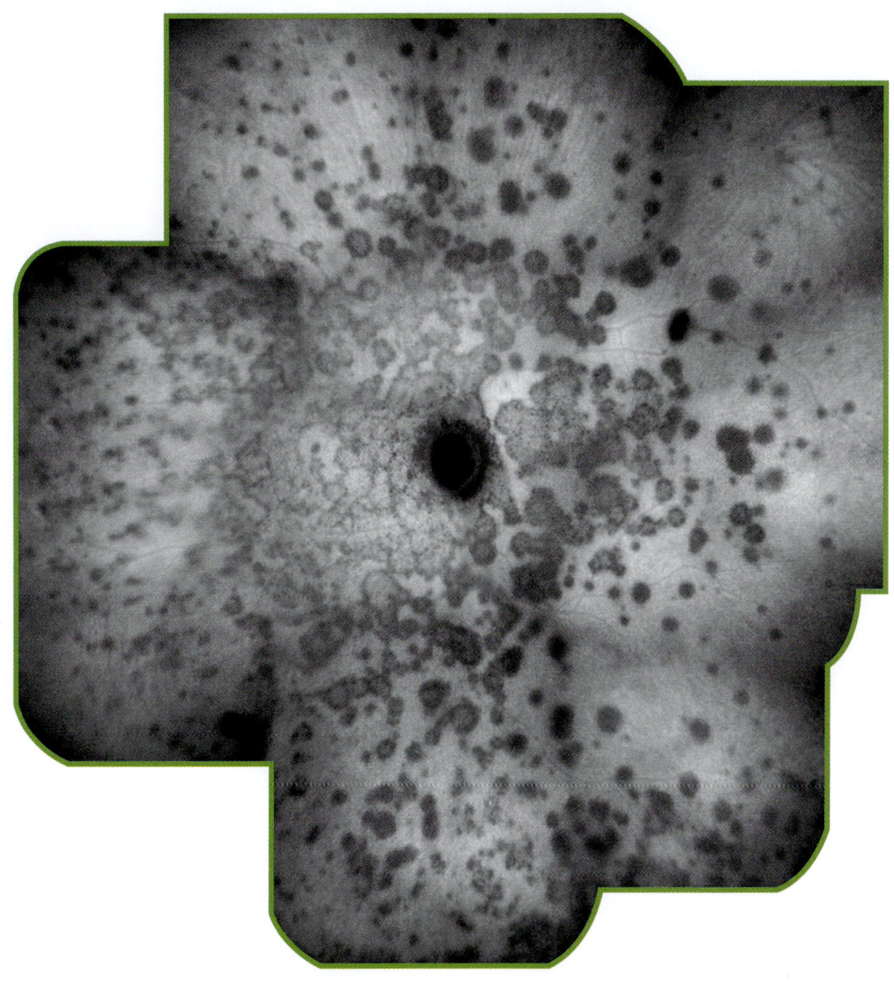

The ICG angiogram of this patient with MEWDS shows numerous deep retinal lesions with some confluence. Involvement of the peripapillary area is associated with blind-spot enlargement.

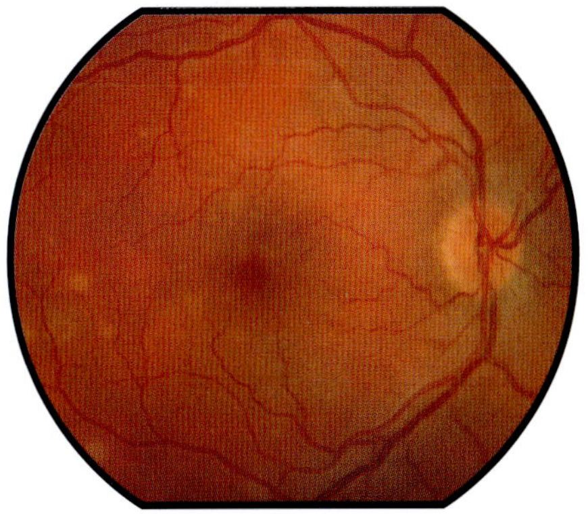

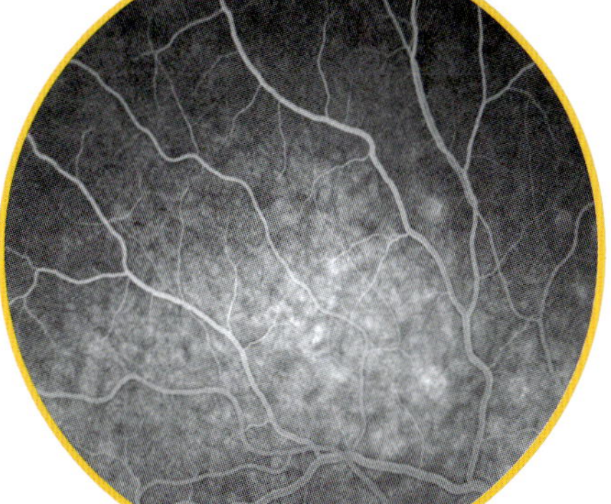

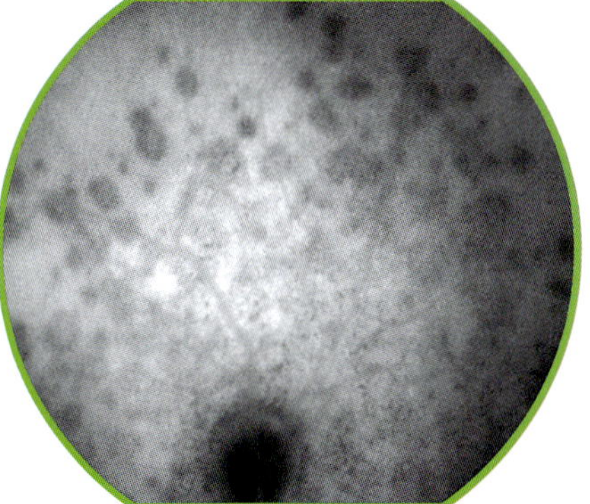

This patient has acute MEWDS with enlargement of the blind spot. There are scattered white spots throughout the posterior fundus with minimal abnormalities noted with FA *(middle)*. A corresponding ICG angiogram *(right)* shows widespread, hypofluorescent spots.

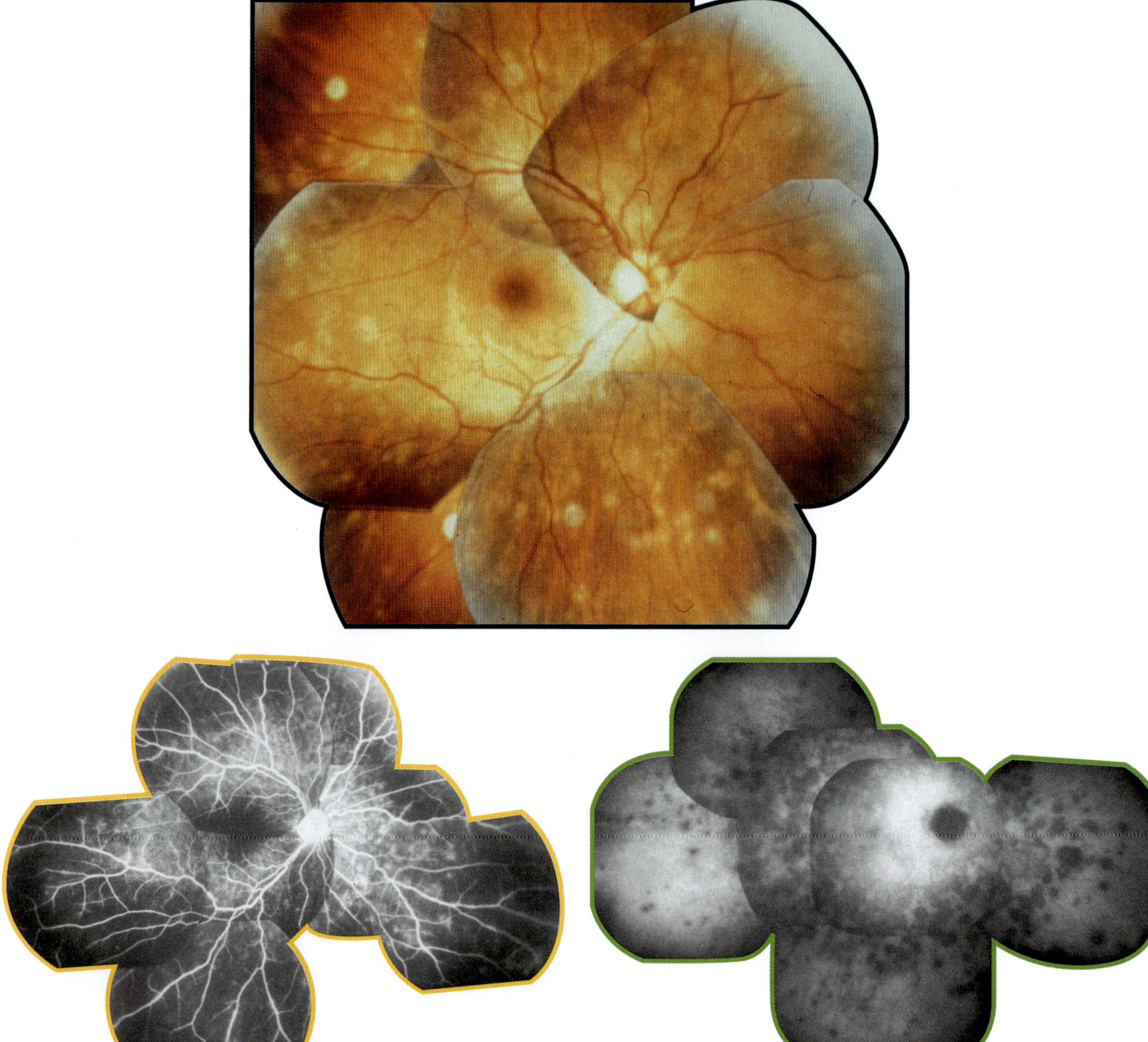

This patient with MEWDS has white spots throughout the fundus. They are larger than the fine dots that are often associated with this disorder. These lesions are hyperfluorescent with fluorescein angiogram (*left*) but are best visualized as hypofluorescent lesions with late phase ICG angiogram (*right*).

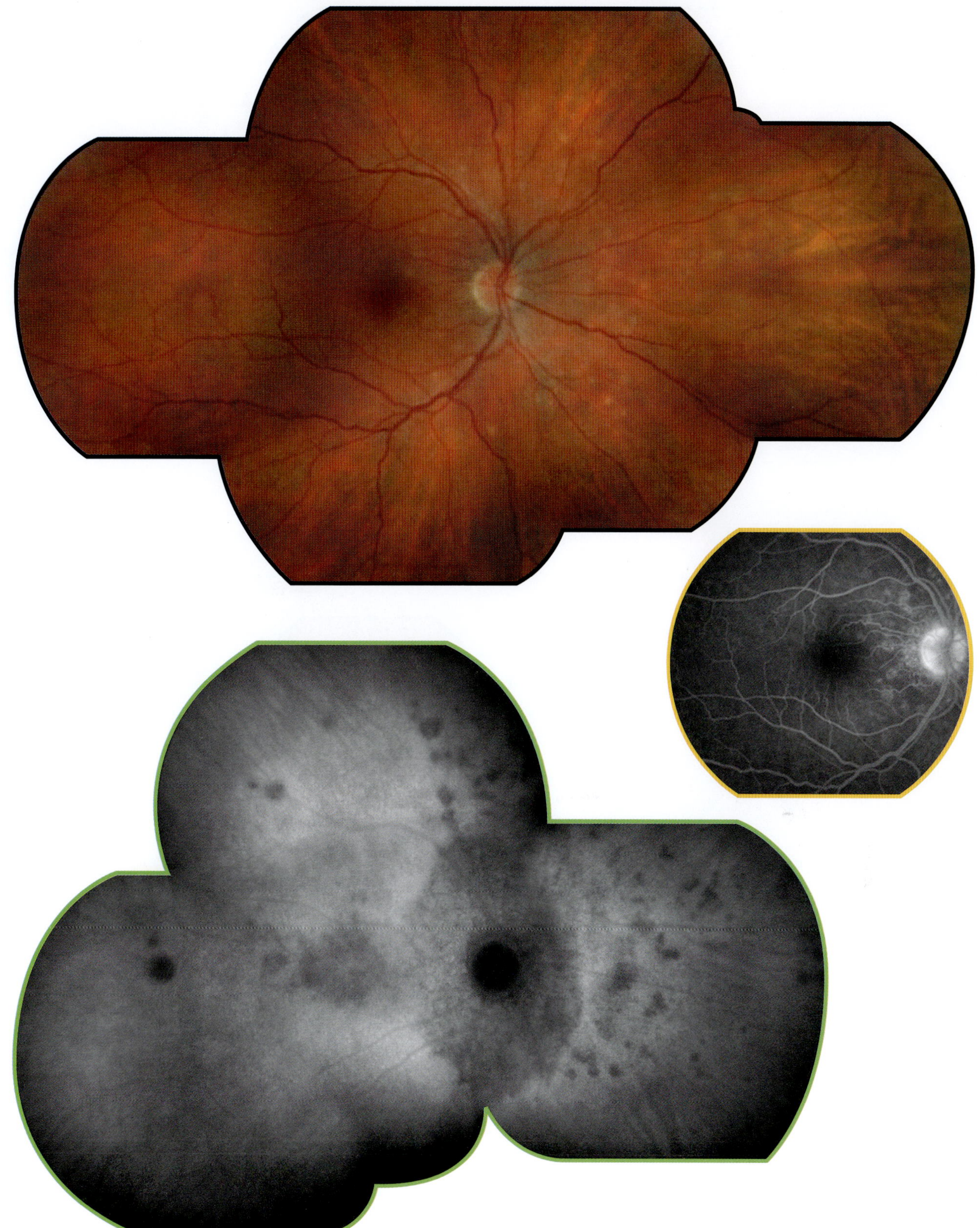

This patient with MEWDS has scattered white lesions throughout the fundus, particularly around the disc and in the nasal periphery. The fluorescein angiogram shows hyperfluorescence of the lesions and staining of the optic disc due to a mild papillitis. The late phase ICG study shows numerous hypofluorescent lesions throughout the fundus and confluent peripapillary hypofluorescence that is very characteristic of MEWDS and correlates with an enlarged blind spot.

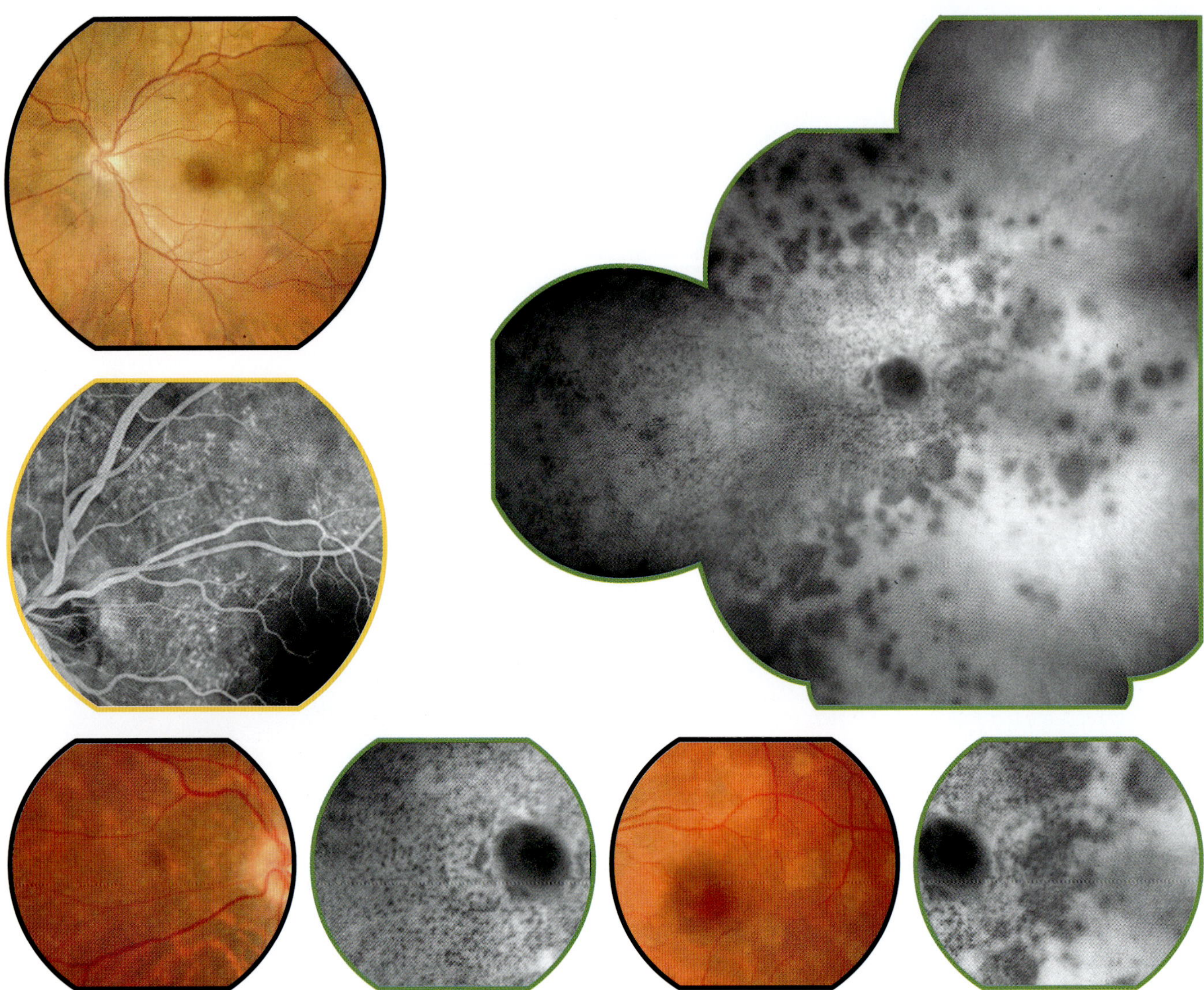

This patient with MEWDS has a variant of the disease, which presents with widespread small lesions or "dots" and deeper lesions or "spots." The clinical photos show numerous white spots. There are larger lesions located in the peripheral fundus. The fluorescein angiogram *(second row)* shows numerous wreath-like hyperfluorescent dots corresponding to the retinal lesions. The late phase ICG angiograms show an increased number of lesions including many dots and more confluent spots *(bottom row, second image and bottom row far right image)*.

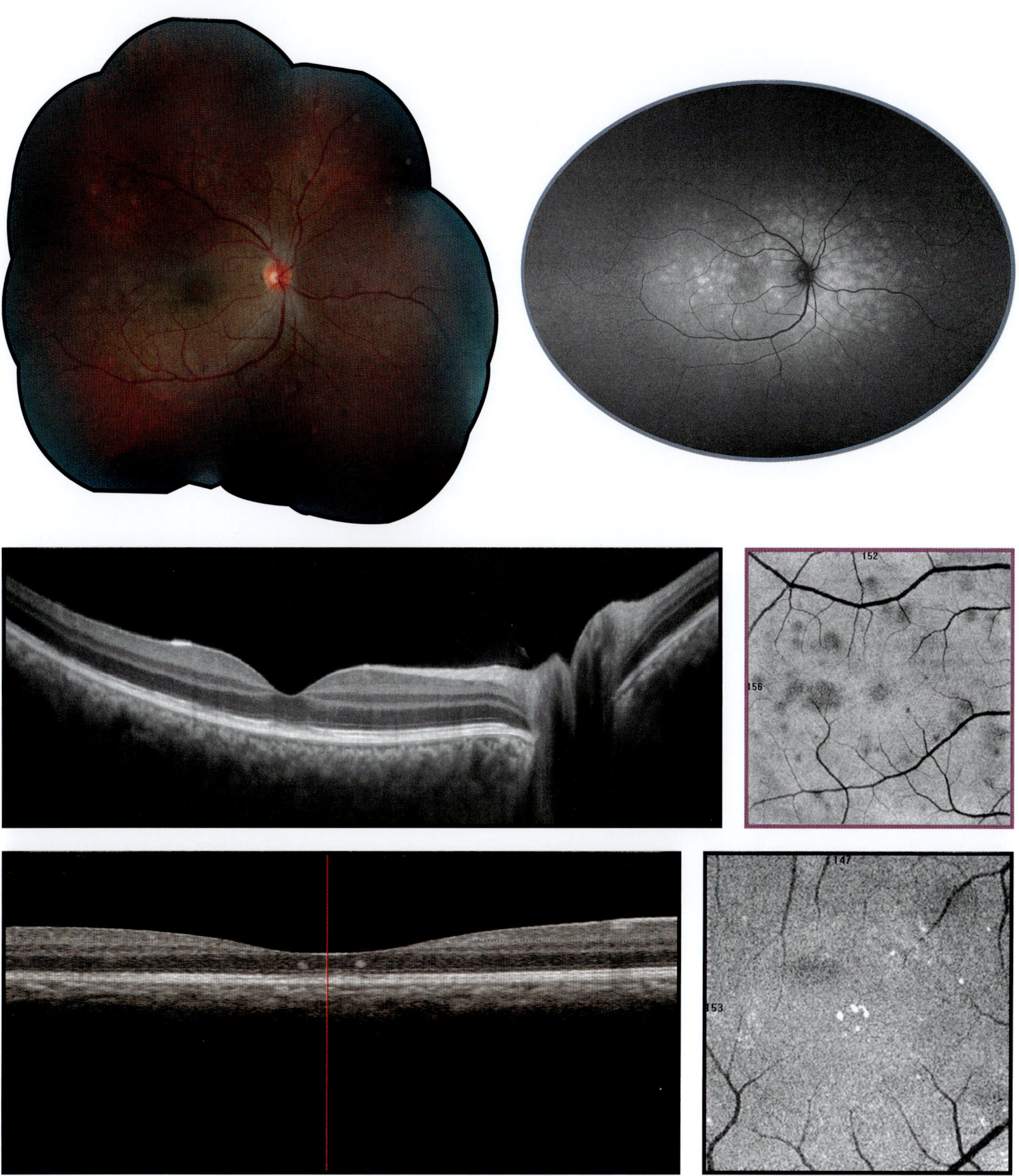

This young male patient presented with photopsias in the right eye. Color fundus montage demonstrates white spots throughout the posterior pole *(top left)*. Widefield fundus autofluorescence shows more hyperfluorescent spots than can be identified on color photography *(top right)*. Spectral domain optical coherence tomography (SD-OCT) illustrates a disrupted ellipsoid zone *(second row, left)*. Recently *en-face* OCT imaging has localized the spots to the ellipsoid level and the dots to the outer nuclear layer. Note loss of the inner segment ellipsoid corresponding to the hyporeflective spots *(second row)* and punctate hyper-reflective foci in the outer nuclear layer (ONL) corresponding to the dots *(third row)*.

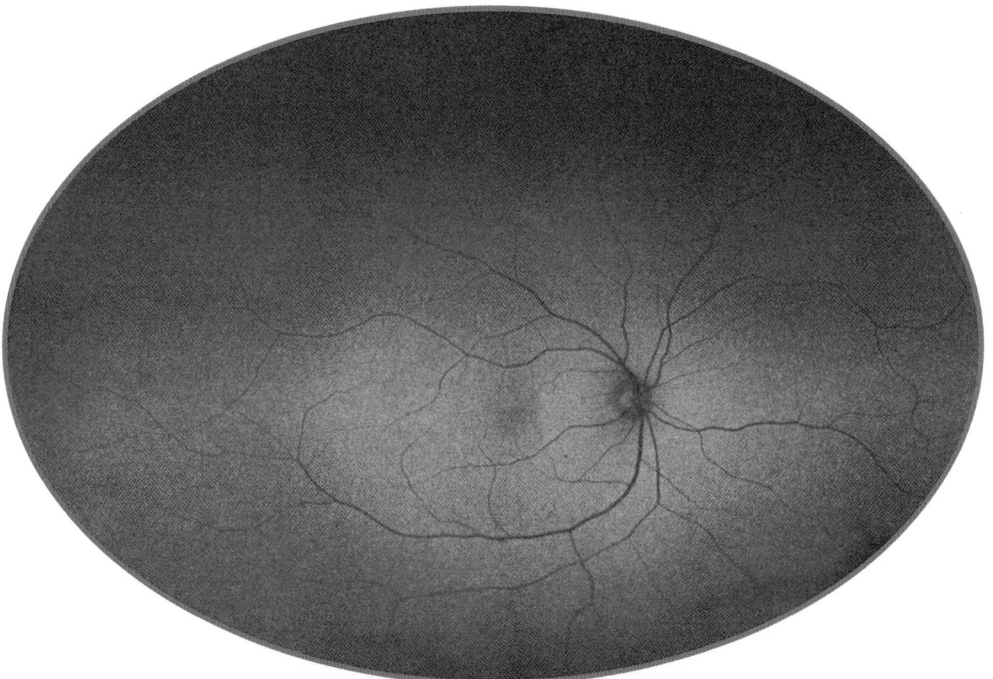

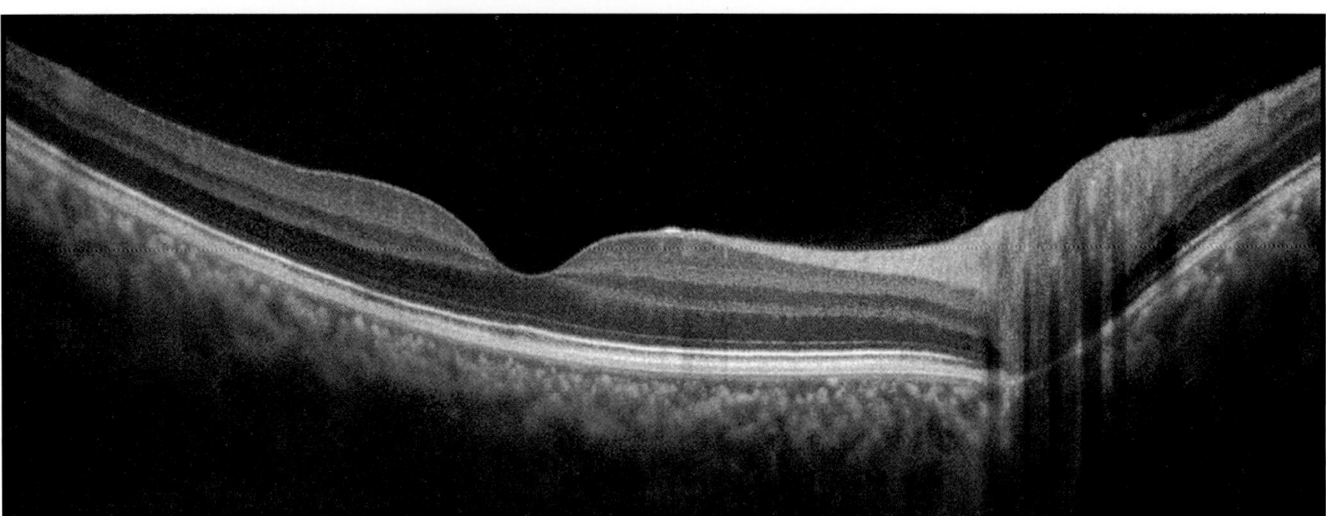

Follow-up autofluorescence *(top)* and SD-OCT *(bottom)* illustrates complete resolution of the hyperautofluorescent spots and normalization of the ellipsoid zone band.

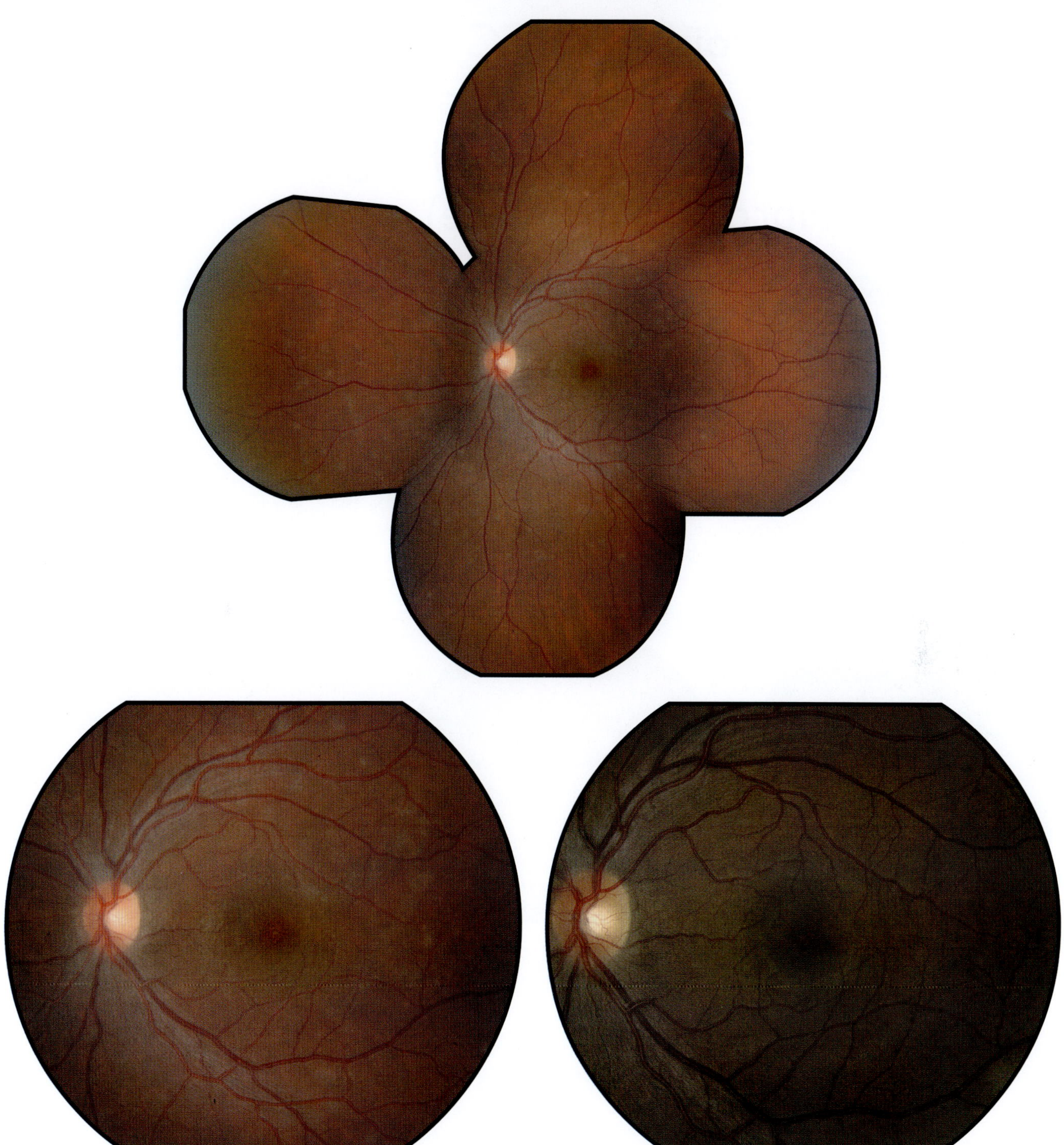

Color fundus montage of this patient with MEWDS illustrates white spots scattered throughout the posterior pole and into the midperiphery. Note the granular appearance of the fovea *(bottom left)*. Follow-up at 6 weeks shows resolution of the white spots and persistent foveal granularity *(bottom right)*.

Multifocal Choroiditis (MFC) (Punctate Inner Choroidopathy (PIC), Multifocal Choroiditis and Panuveitis (MCP), Idiopathic Progressive Subretinal Fibrosis Syndrome)

Punctate inner choroidopathy (PIC) and MFC are related, if not identical, entities. Both tend to affect young females (<75%) who are often myopic. These patients develop focal areas of inflammation in the deep retina and choroid that progress into punched-out, atrophic, and pigmented chorioretinal scars. The acute lesions are typically multiple, bilateral, and yellow-white or grayish in appearance. Occasionally, there may be an overlying neurosensory detachment. When these inflammatory spots are small and confined to the posterior pole with minimal vitreous reaction, the entity is typically referred to as PIC. More diffuse disease with larger lesions and associated panuveitis is referred to as MFC. These eyes may present with peripapillary fibrosis and linear clusters of lesions in the peripheral fundus forming curvilinear or concentric streaks (Schlaegel's line) similar to those seen in the presumed ocular histoplasmosis syndrome (POHS). The presence of uveitis, most commonly anterior and vitreous cells, distinguishes MFC from POHS. Like POHS, both PIC and MFC are frequently associated with secondary choroidal neovascularization (CNV), which can lead to subretinal fibrosis. Rarely, this subretinal fibrosis can be extensive and progressive, in which case it is referred to as the idiopathic progressive subretinal fibrosis syndrome.

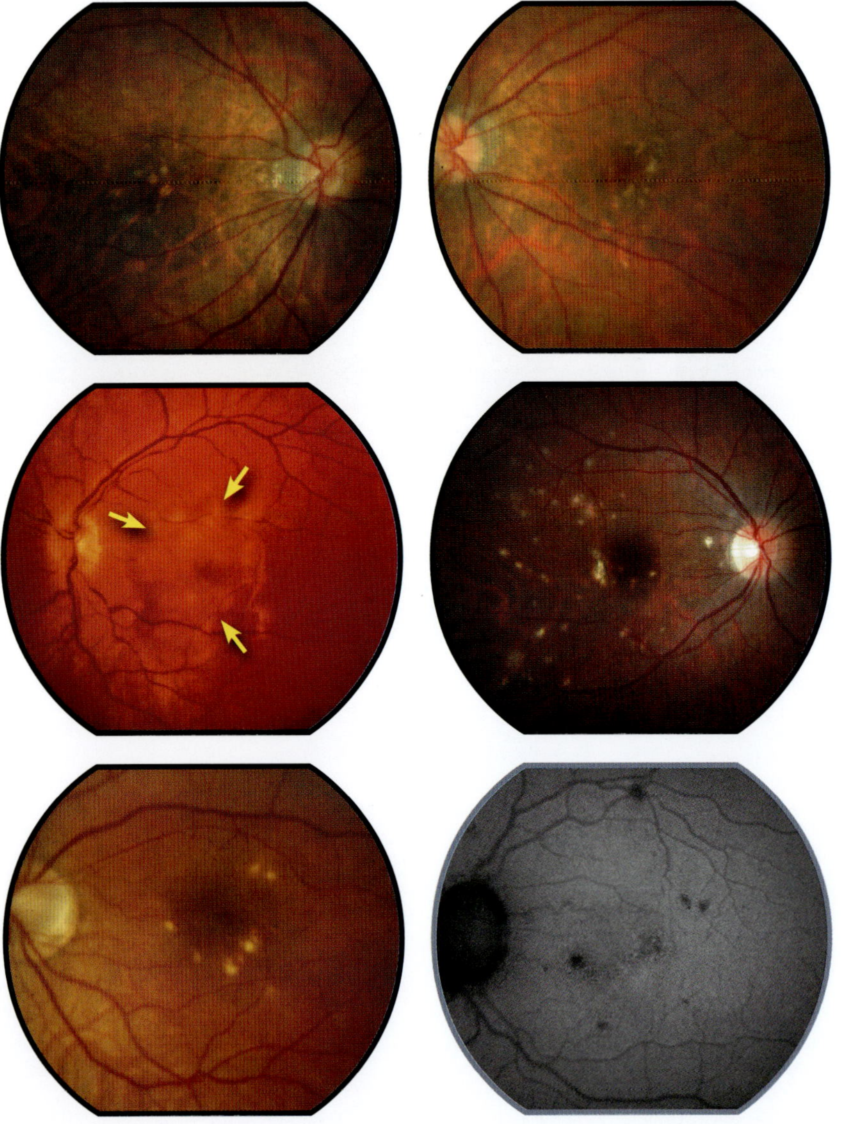

These patients have multiple chorioretinal inflammatory spots in the posterior pole. Sometimes they are associated with cells in the posterior vitreous or even an exudative detachment *(arrows)*. Evidence of previous fibrovascular scarring may be seen in some cases *(middle row, left)*. A more accurate number of the lesions is detectable with fundus autofluorescence *(lower right)*. *Courtesy of Dr. James Folk*

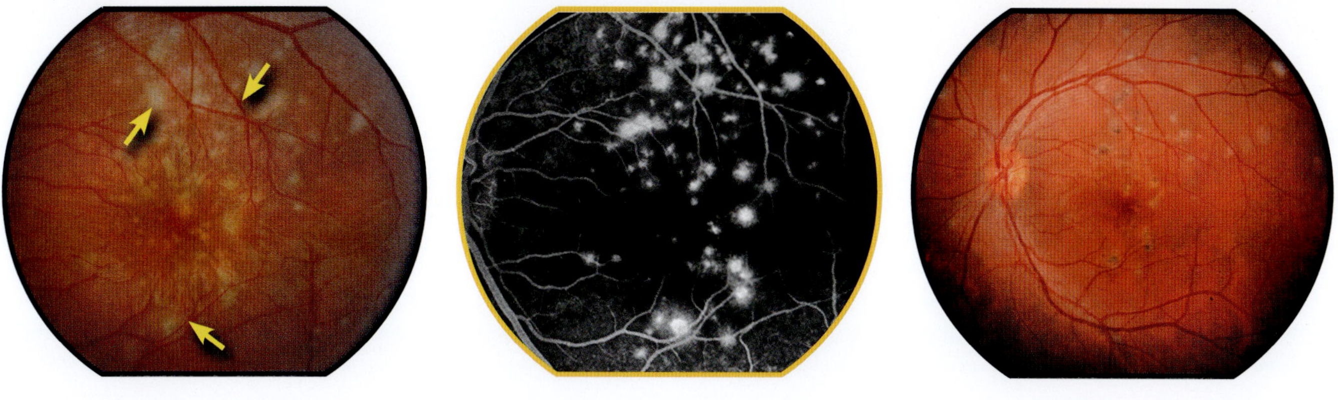

This case demonstrates the acute and resolved forms of MFC in the same patient. Note the whitish lesions in the acute phase *(arrows)* and the more hyperpigmented, well-defined lesions in the healed stage. The fluorescein angiogram shows staining and even leakage of the acute lesions in the posterior pole *(middle image)*.

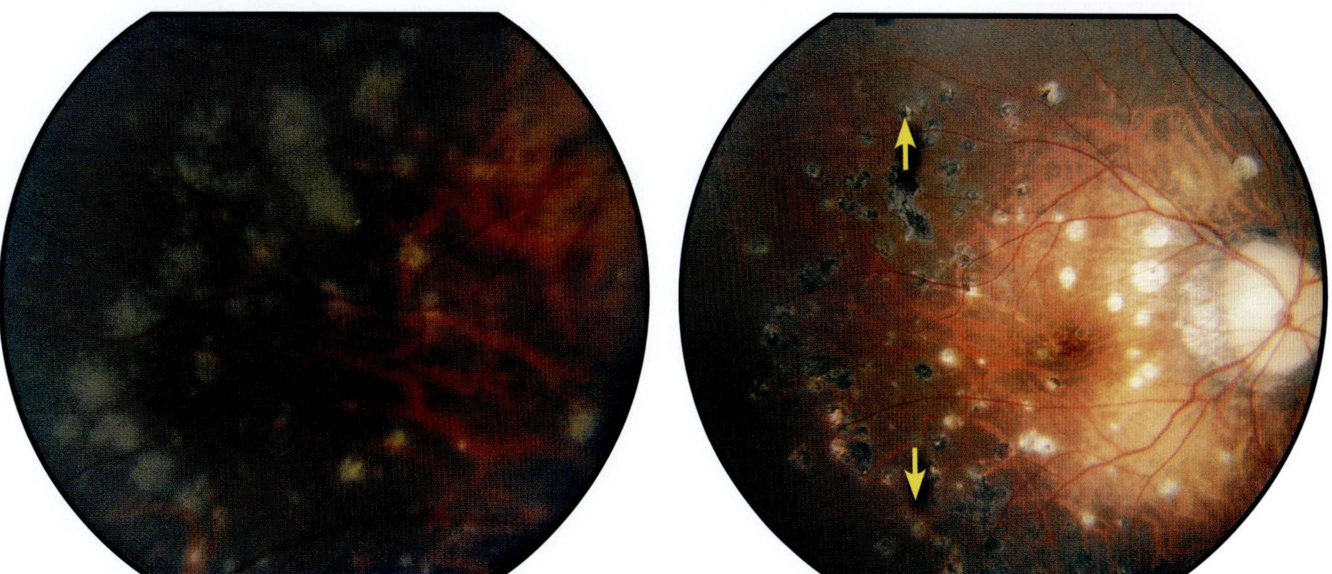

This myopic patient shows the acute lesions of MFC *(left)*. These acute inflammatory lesions resolve into chorioretinal scars upon follow-up *(right, arrows)*. The white atrophic lesions in the posterior pole are present within thinned retina associated with the myopic staphyloma.

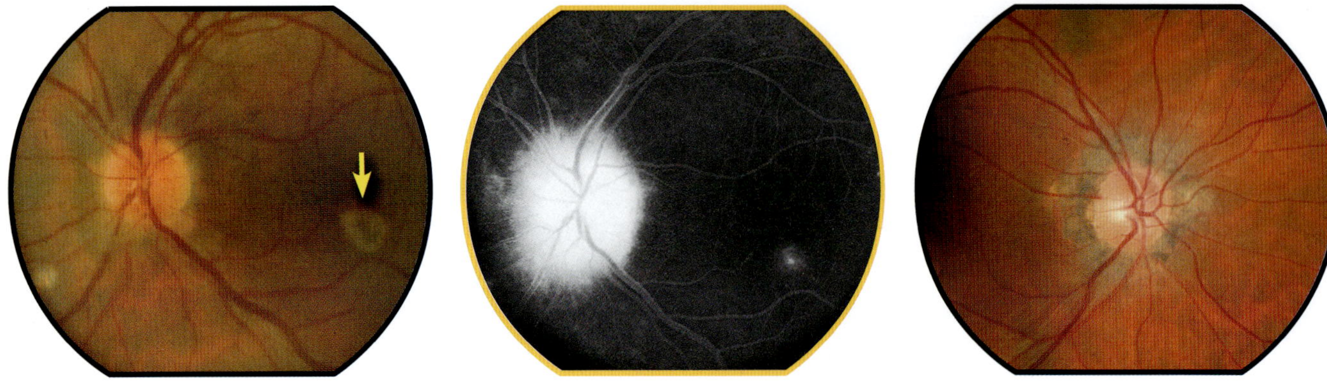

This patient has MFC and secondary CNV *(arrow)*. The fluorescein angiogram shows punctate hyperfluorescence of the CNV inferior to the fovea and optic disc leakage. Optic disc inflammation is an important feature of MFC not associated with presumed ocular histoplasmosis syndrome. The right eye developed peripapillary atrophy and pigmentation following acute inflammation *(right)*.

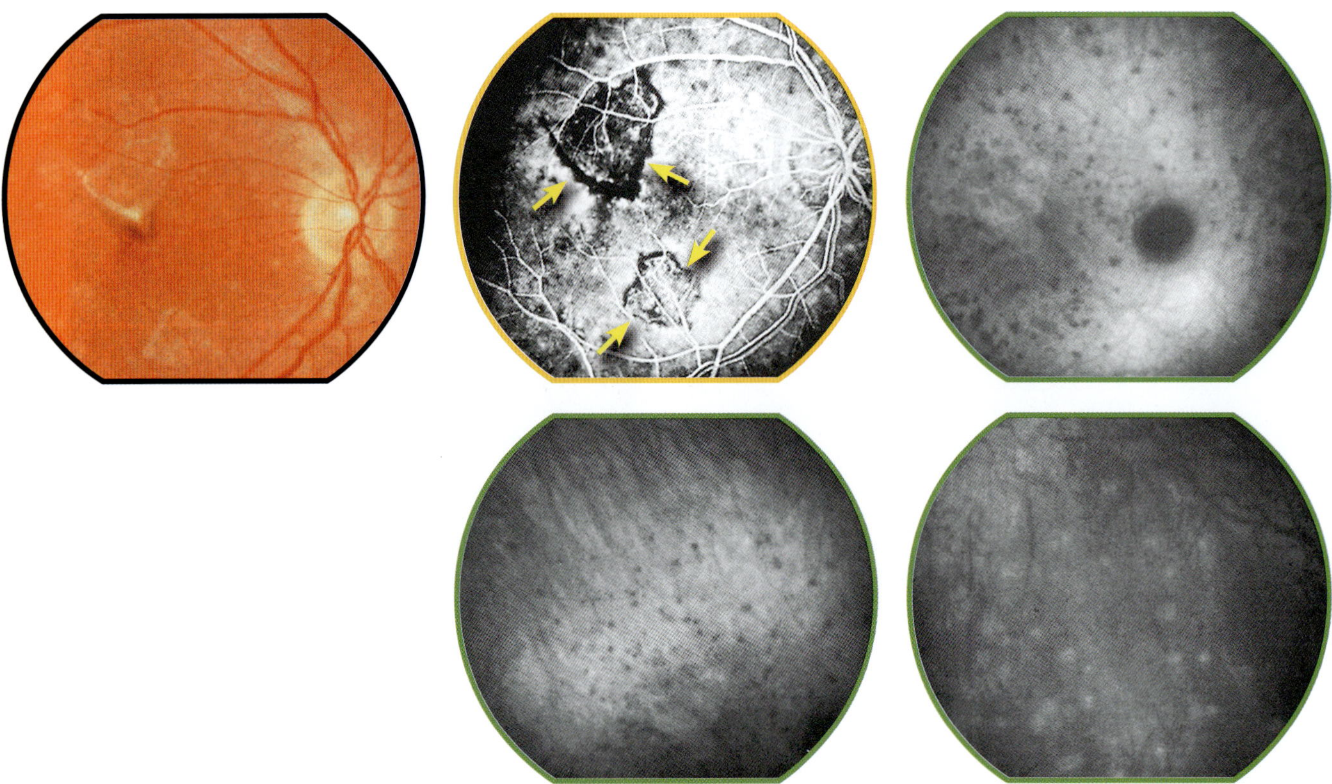

This patient has MFC complicated by active CNV *(arrows)*, noted with color fundus photography and with FA *(left and middle images)*. Note that the 2 neovascular lesions are classic (i.e. type 2) with FA showing an early well-defined lacy appearance and a pigment ring of blockage. An ICG angiogram shows widespread multifocal spots throughout the posterior fundus *(upper right)* and in the periphery multifocal hypofluorescent lesions and more acute hyperfluorescent lesions (*bottom images*) are noted.

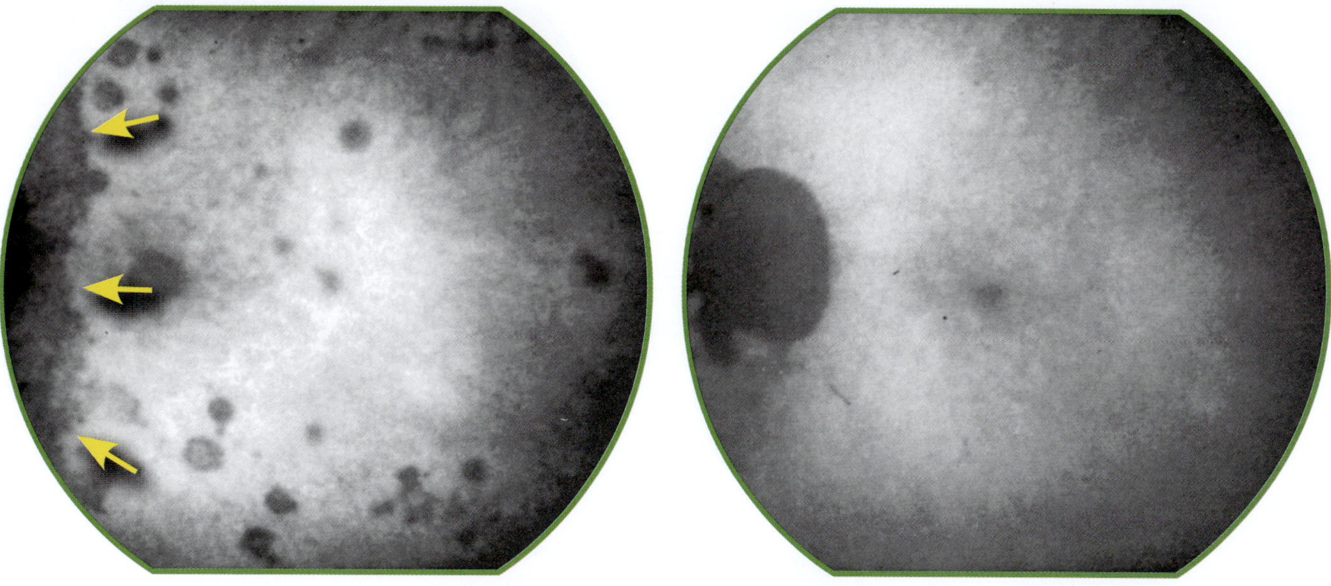

The late-phase ICG study of a patient with active MFC and an enlarged blind spot of the left eye demonstrates multiple large hypofluorescent lesions extending toward the periphery and confluence around the temporal border of the optic nerve *(arrows)*. Oral prednisone therapy was administered for 6 weeks. Another late-phase ICG study 6 months following treatment demonstrates complete resolution of the hypofluorescence in the macula and around the optic nerve. Vitritis and visual field changes also resolved. Pre-existing peripapillary atrophy remains.

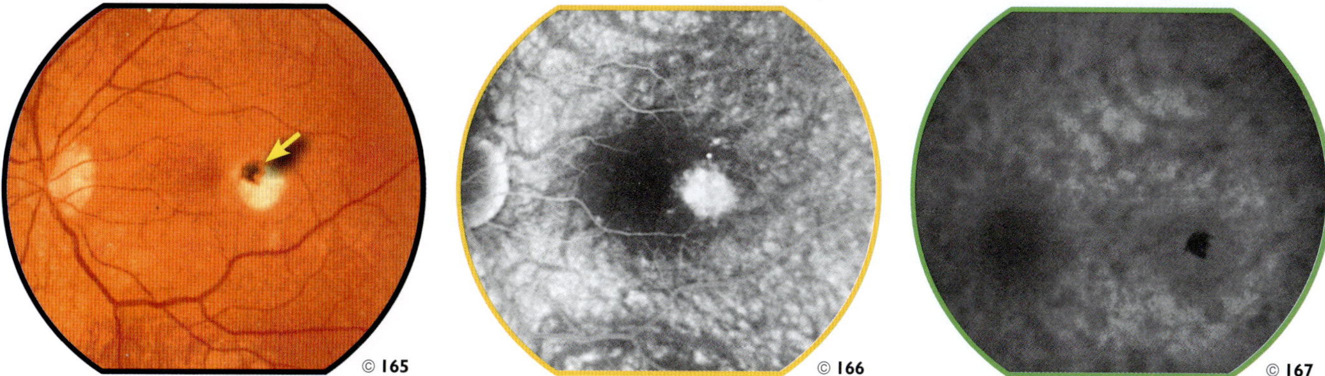

This patient had CNV that was ablated with laser photocoagulation *(arrow)*. He presented 2 years later complaining of an enlarged blind spot in the same left eye. A fluorescein angiogram showed staining of the laser scar and multiple new hypo- and hyperfluorescent spots. The ICG angiogram illustrates hypofluorescence surrounding the nerve and the chorioretinal scar and widespread areas of hypofluorescent lesions in the choroid consistent with recurrent MFC in a patient with a previous episode of MFC. Note the peculiar filamentous extensions around the macular scars, as seen on the angiograms, that are characteristic of MFC. This lesion may be related to hypervascularity induced by the antecedent inflammation.

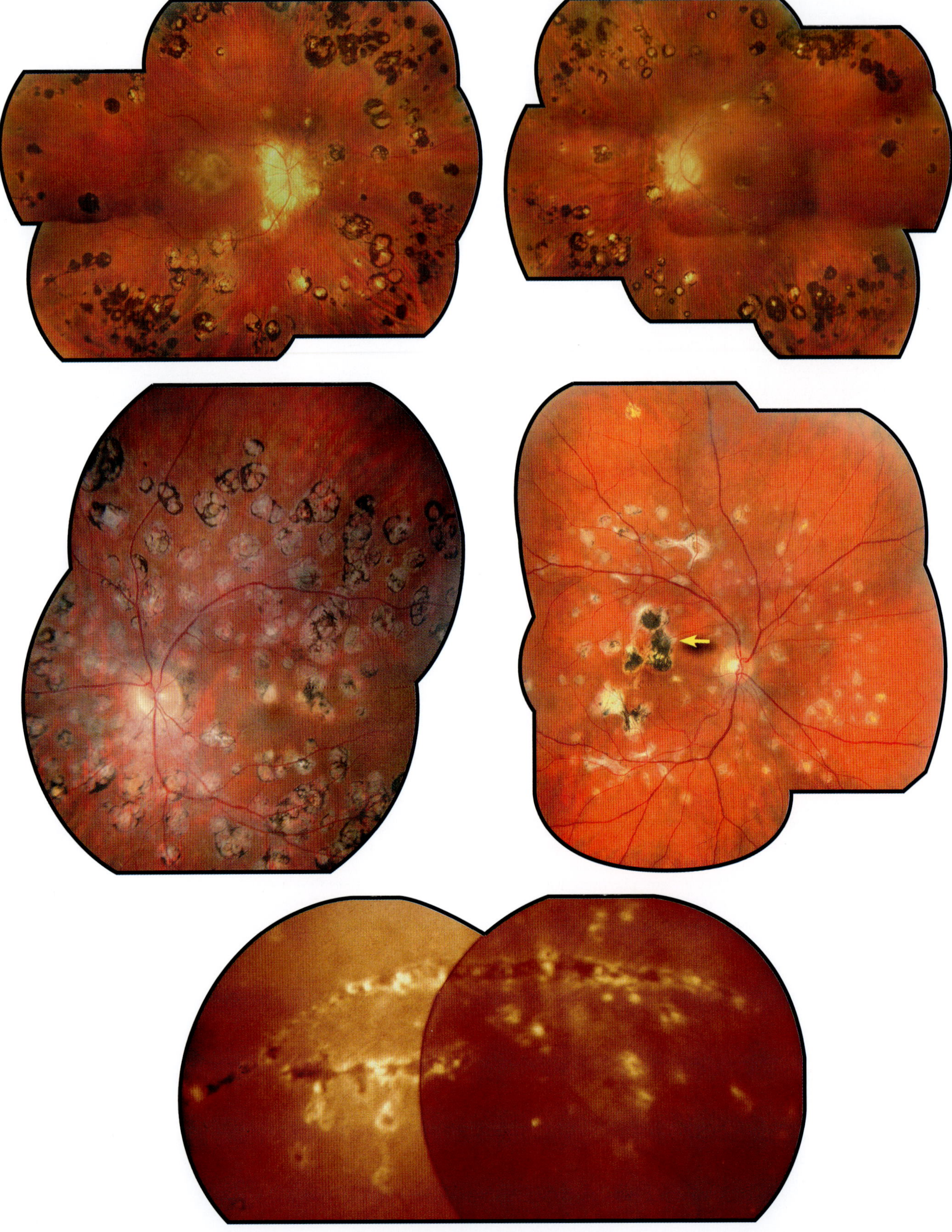

During a quiescent stage of MFC, the fundus may contain numerous chorioretinal scars in the peripheral fundus with a variable distribution. There may be peripapillary atrophy or macular scarring *(arrow)*. Each of these cases had peripapillary atrophy. In the periphery, one or more curvilinear or concentric lines of chorioretinal scars may be appreciated (Schlaegel's line) that are characteristic of MCP and POHS *(lower image)*.

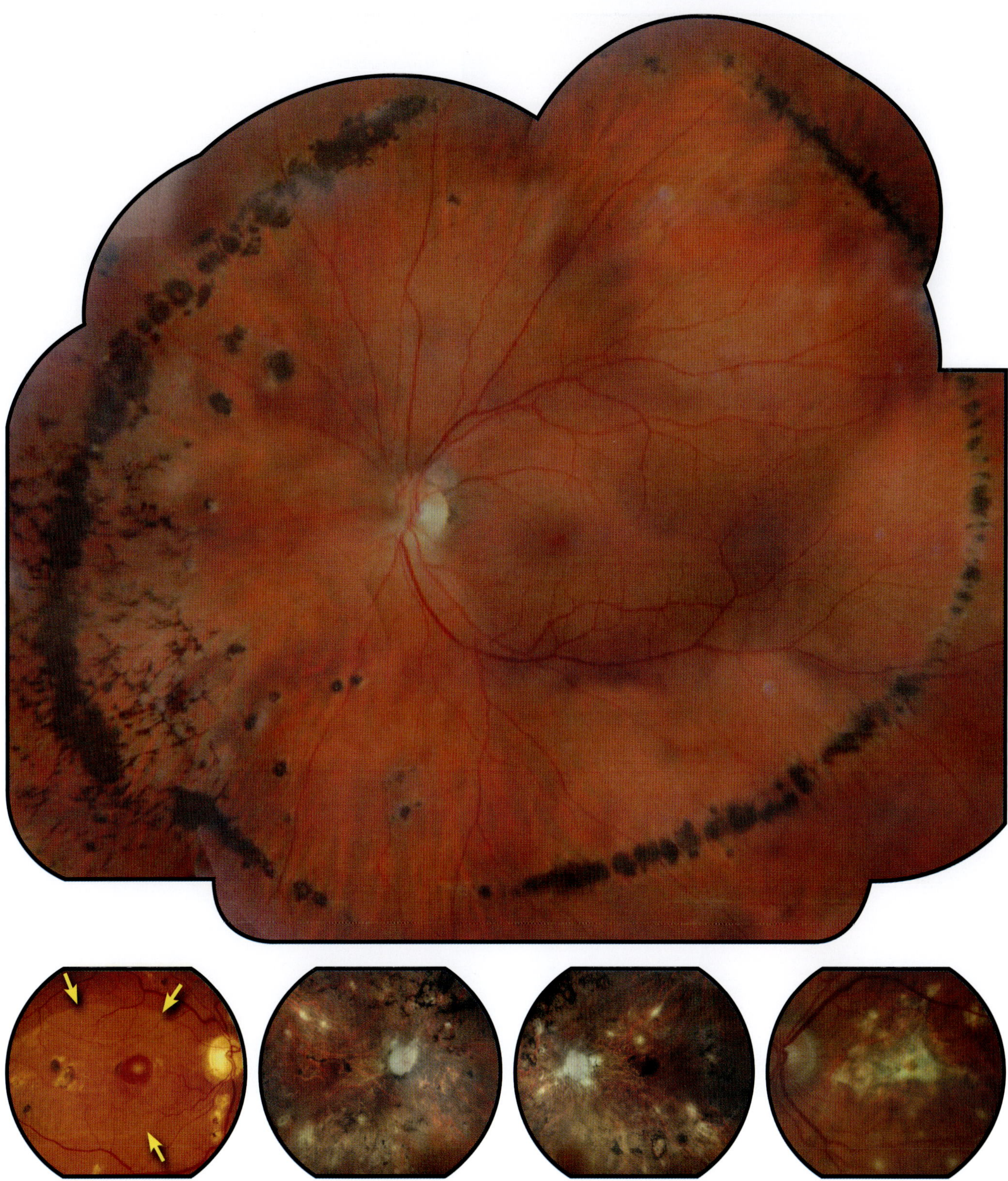

These patients have manifestations of MFC in its quiescent stage. The montage shows concentric pigmentary scars encircling the globe. Note the presence of pigment hyperplasia in the nasal periphery. The photo on the left shows a macular hole with detachment *(arrows)*. This may be the result of vitreoretinal traction. The macular images on the right show fibrovascular scarring due to antecedent CNV.

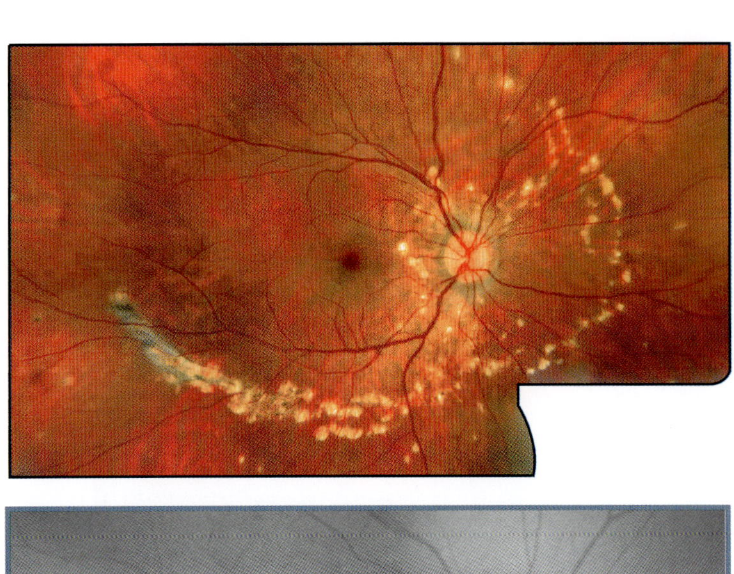

These cases of MFC show the variation in shapes and patterns of the curvilinear or concentric postinflammatory scars referred to as Schlaegel's lines.

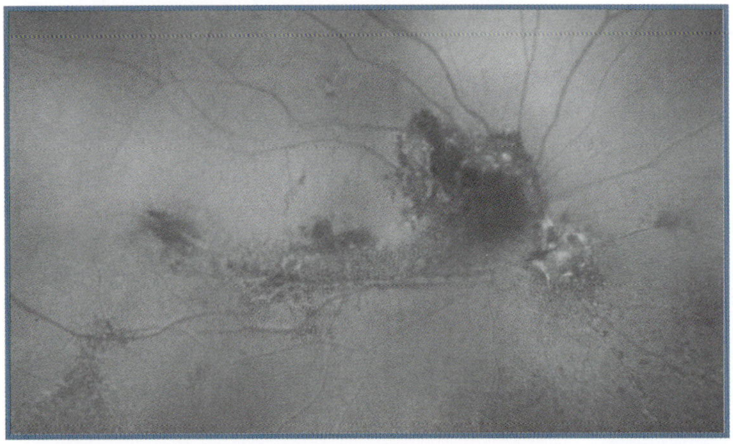

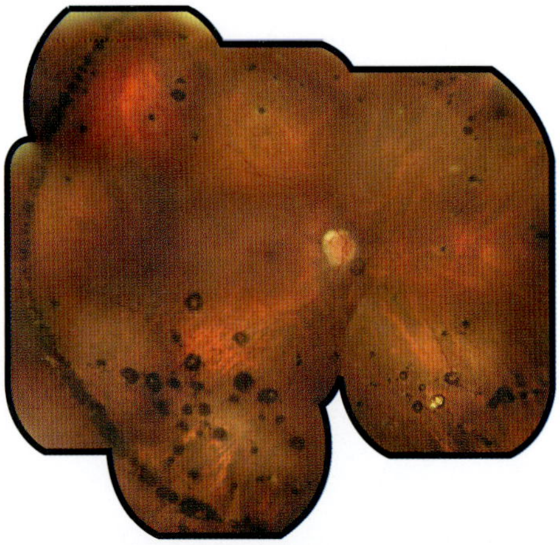

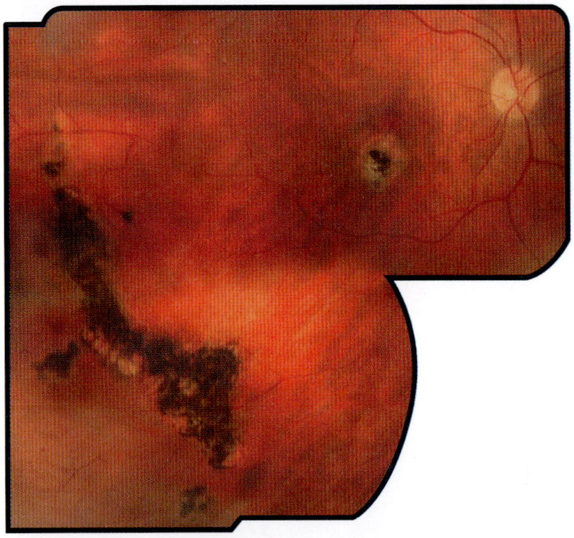

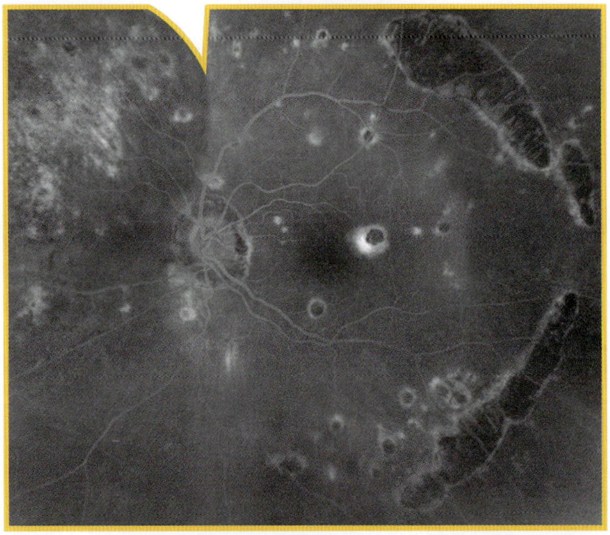

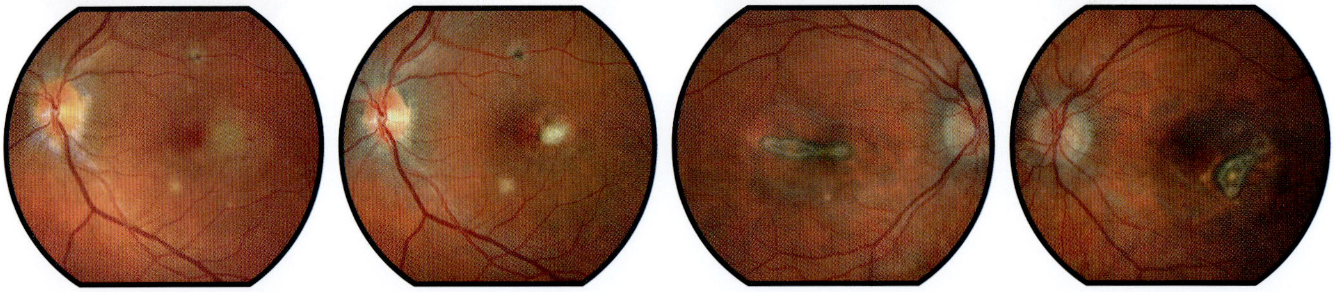

These two patients with MFC demonstrate type 2 neovascularization, the most common subtype in this disorder. A fibrotic scar surrounded by atrophy occurred in the patient on the left following photocoagulation in the left eye. The patient on the right has regressed CNV in each eye with surrounding chorioretinal atrophy.

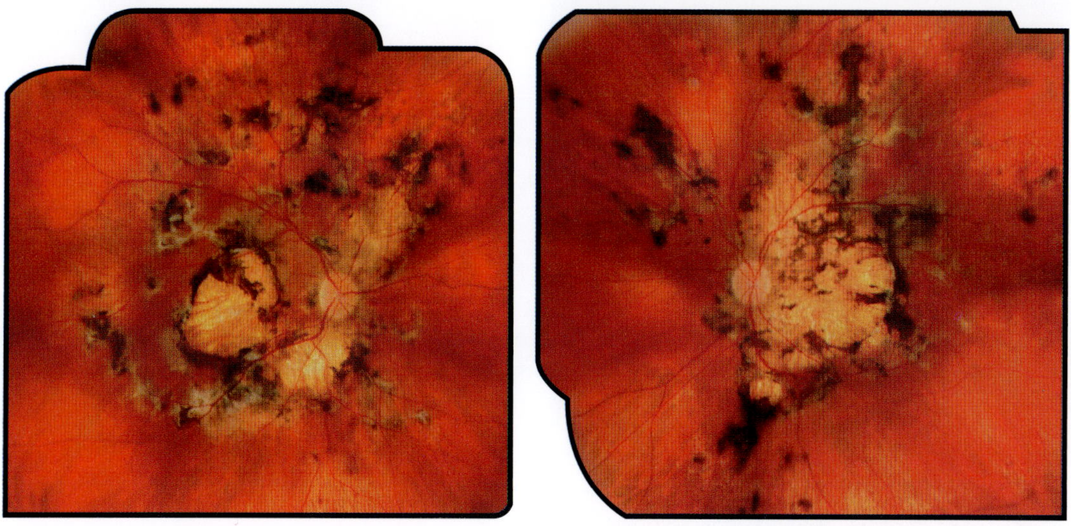

This montage shows MFC in a quiescent stage. There is severe atrophy in the macular region, as well as pigment epithelial hyperplastic and atrophic change from the inflammatory stages of the disease.

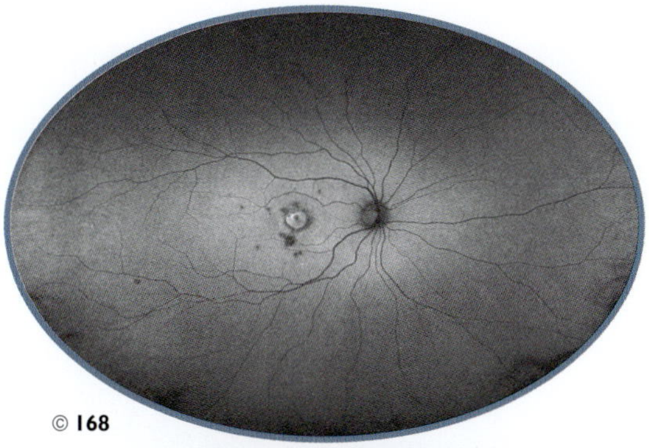

© 168

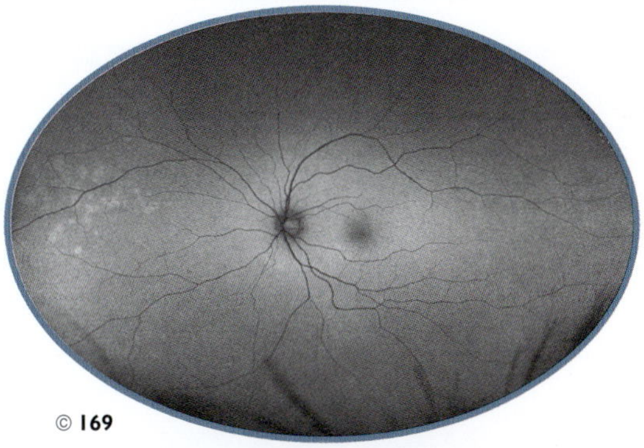

© 169

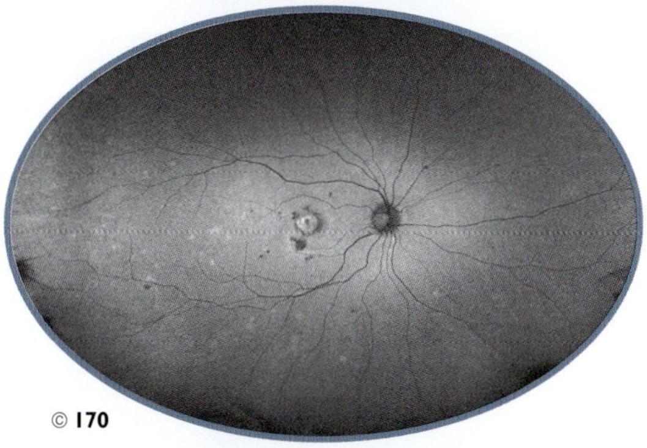

© 170

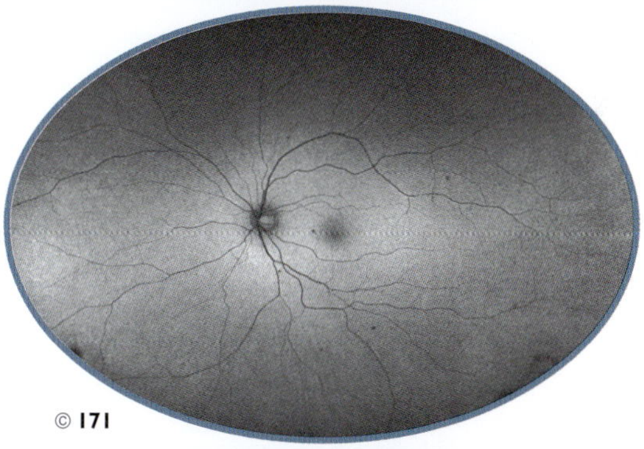

© 171

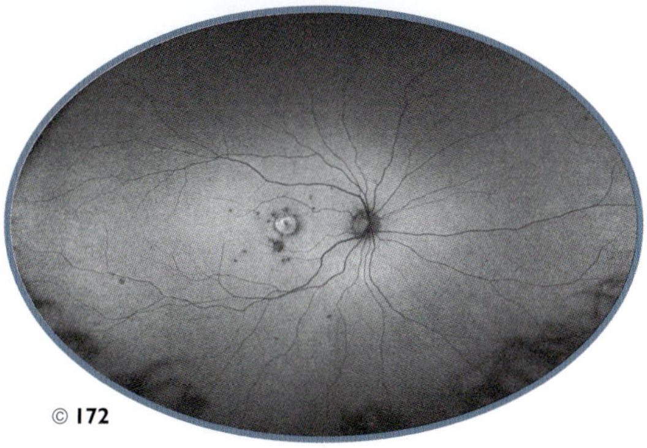

© 172

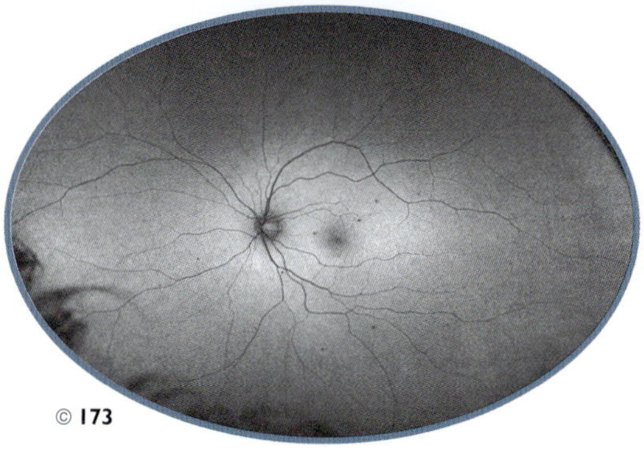

© 173

This young female patient presented with photopsias in the left eye. Widefield autofluorescence illustrates small discreet hyperfluorescent spots in the nasal periphery of the left eye *(top right)* consistent with PIC. She was started on a course of oral NSAIDS and returned 1 month later. The spots are resolved in the left eye *(middle right)*, but new spots appeared in the temporal periphery of the right eye *(middle left)*. After 2 months on NSAIDS she returned again and the spots are resolved in both eyes *(bottom row)*.

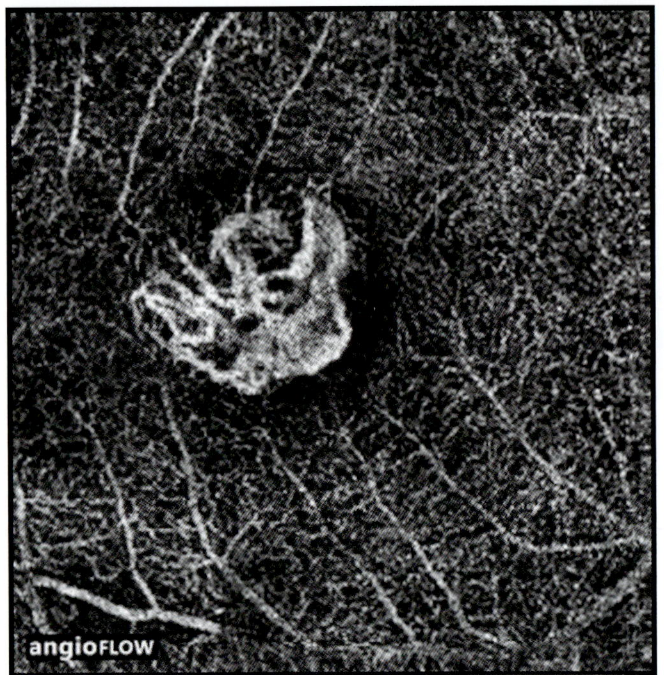

OCT angiography of the right eye of the same patient illustrates a choroidal neovascular membrane in the macula.

© 174

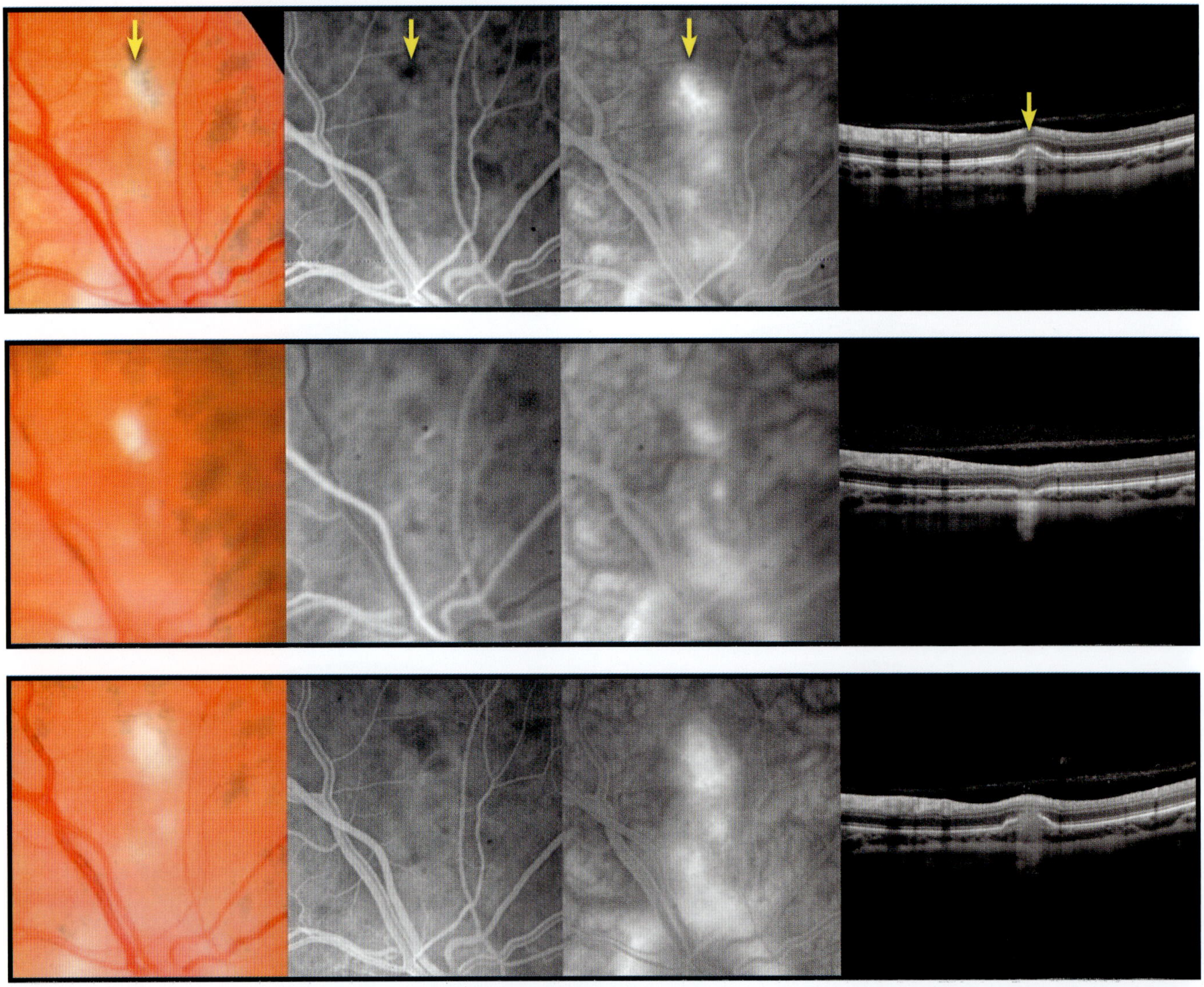

This patient with MFC presented with an acute flare and new choroidal infiltrates *(top row, arrows)*. The lesion blocks in early phase fluorescein angiogram and stains in the late phase *(top row, second and third images)*. SD-OCT illustrates a choroidal infiltrate extending into the outer retina. The patient was initiated on oral steroid therapy with significant improvement *(second row)*. After tapering steroids, however, the infiltrate recurred *(bottom row)*.

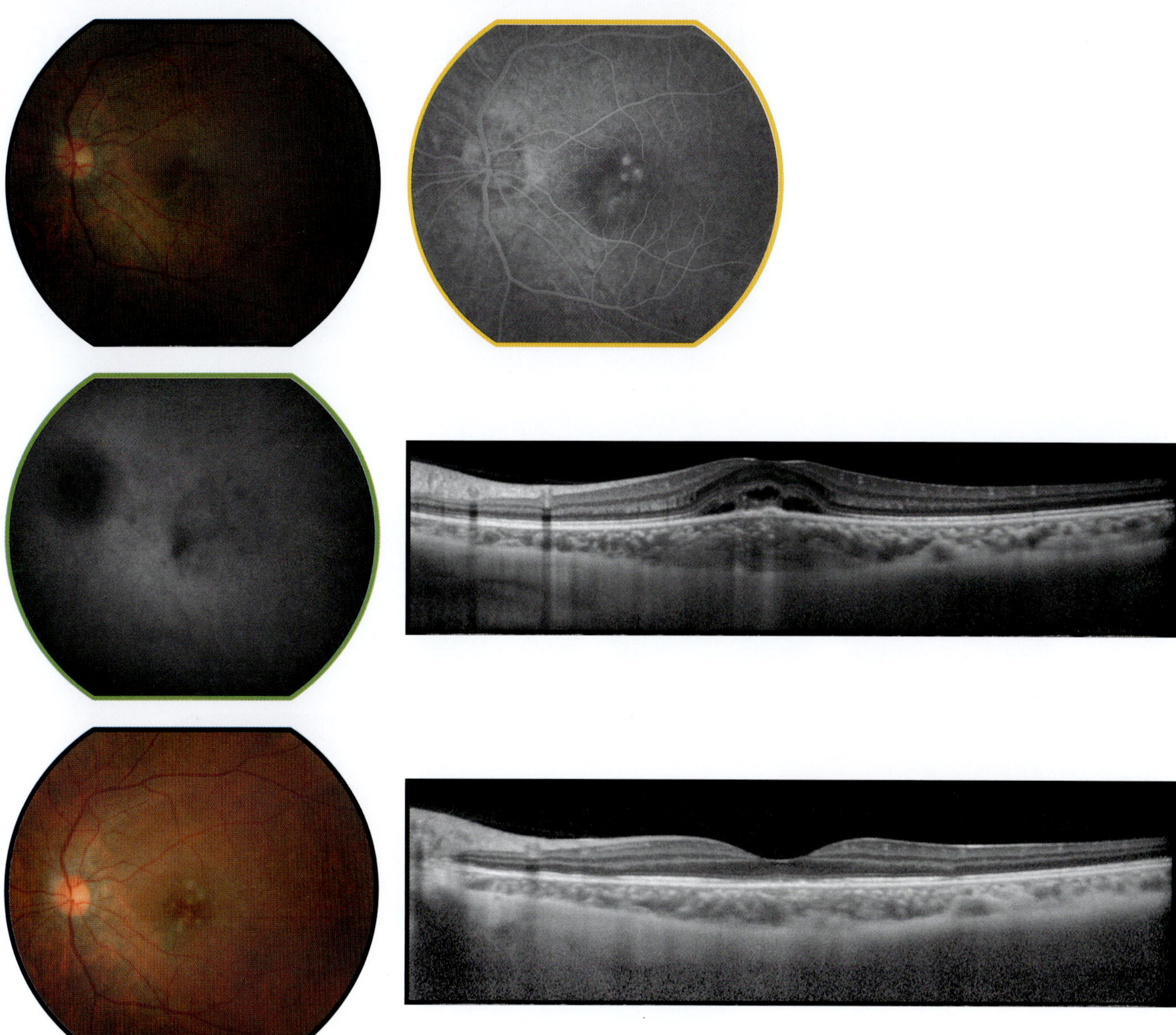

This patient with MFC presented with new infiltrates in the posterior pole well identified with color fundus photography *(top, left)*. The lesions stain late on fluorescein angiogram, and block on ICG angiogram *(top right and second row left)*. SD-OCT at presentation illustrates choroidal infiltrates and thickening with overlying subretinal fluid. Color fundus photos taken 15 days after initiation of treatment show consolidation of the white infiltrates *(bottom left)*. SD-OCT at follow-up shows a significantly reduced choroidal thickness and resolution of the subretinal fluid *(bottom right)*.

Acute Zonal Occult Outer Retinopathy (AZOOR)

Acute zonal occult outer retinopathy (AZOOR) is an idiopathic inflammatory disorder usually affecting young healthy women who develop photopsia and acute progressive visual field loss in one or both eyes due to damage of broad zones of the outer retina. The field abnormality typically begins as enlargement of the blind spot, often described with movements of colors within the scotoma. Funduscopy upon initial presentation may be normal with the exception of mild vitritis. However, in later stages, retinal pigment epithelium (RPE) atrophy, pigment clumping, and arterial attenuation may develop. Approximately one-third of patients develop recurrent disease. Electroretinogram (ERG) testing, autofluorescent imaging, fluorescein and ICG angiography, and OCT localize the abnormality to the photoreceptor–RPE complex. Recently a trizonal appearance on autofluorescence, ICG angiography, and SD-OCT has been described as a defining feature of AZOOR. On SD-OCT this is characterized by normal retina outside of the AZOOR lesion (zone 1) and subretinal drusenoid deposits (zone 2) and RPE and choroidal atrophy (zone 3) within the lesion. On autofluorescence and ICG angiography this trizonal pattern is characterized by a hyperfluorescent line demarcating the AZOOR lesion adjacent to normal retina (zone 1), speckled hyperfluorescence within the AZOOR lesion (zone 2), and hypofluorescence corresponding to choroidal atrophy within the lesion (zone 3).

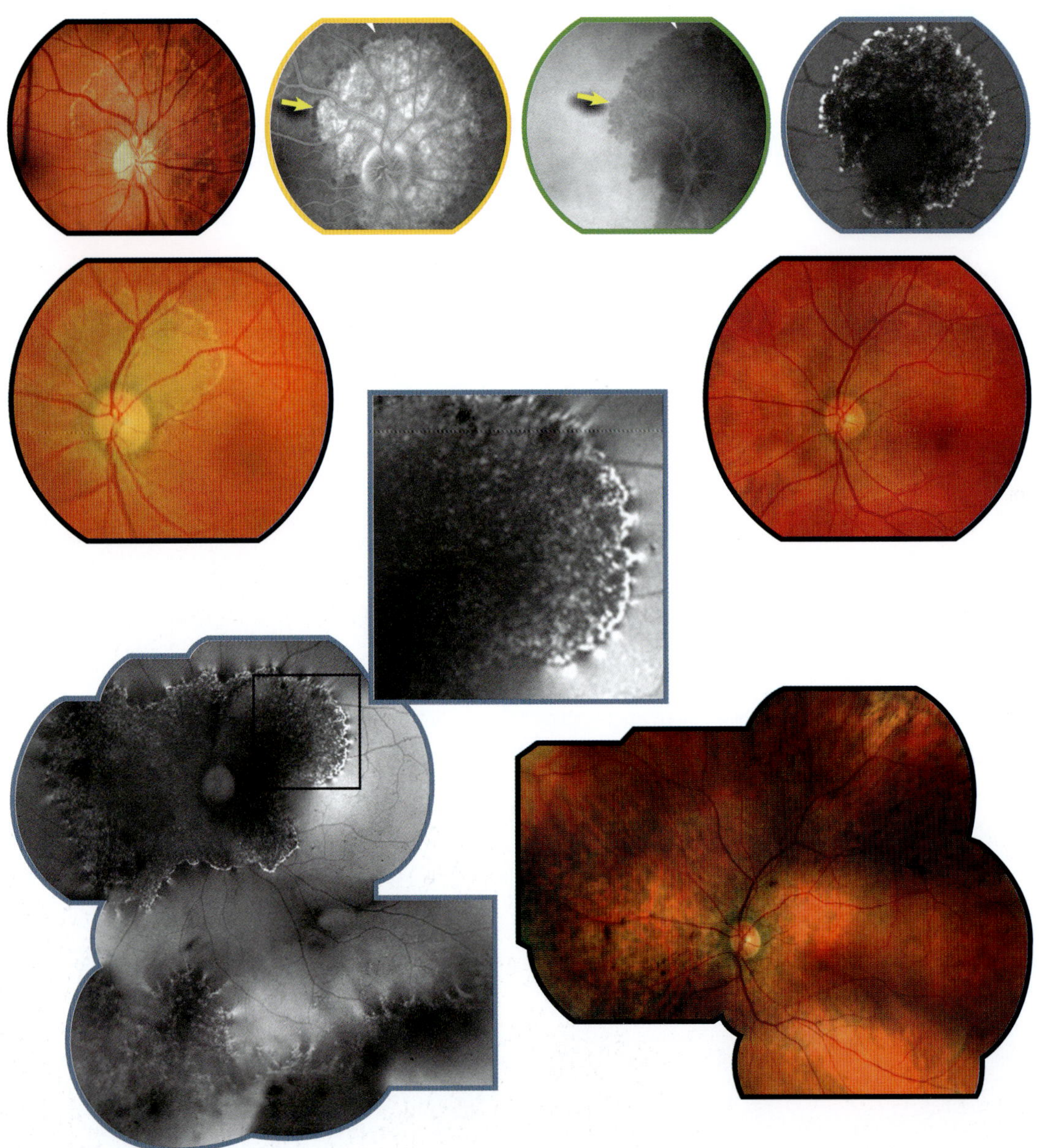

This patient had bilateral AZOOR. The findings were relatively stable in the right eye compared to the left. Note the well-demarcated annular border at the junction between involved and uninvolved retina *(arrows)* in the right eye. The middle row shows the progressive area of peripapillary inflammation in the fellow left eye at baseline and 3 years later. Five years later, there was a large zonal area also noted in the inferior fundus *(bottom row, left)*. Seven years later, there was diffuse atrophic and pigment epithelial degenerative disease in the fundus *(bottom right)*. The fundus autofluorescent montage and magnified image show a characteristic hyperautofluorescent flare at the margins of the zonal defects *(lower left)* and the aforementioned trizonal pattern of disease.

This color montage shows peripapillary AZOOR with a clearly delineated margin bordering the atrophic region with the normal retina. The larger montage shows a well-demarcated inactive nasal region remarkable for atrophy and pigmentation and a large active zone of progressive inflammation extending from the superior macula and bordered by a characteristic outer annular ring *(arrows)*.

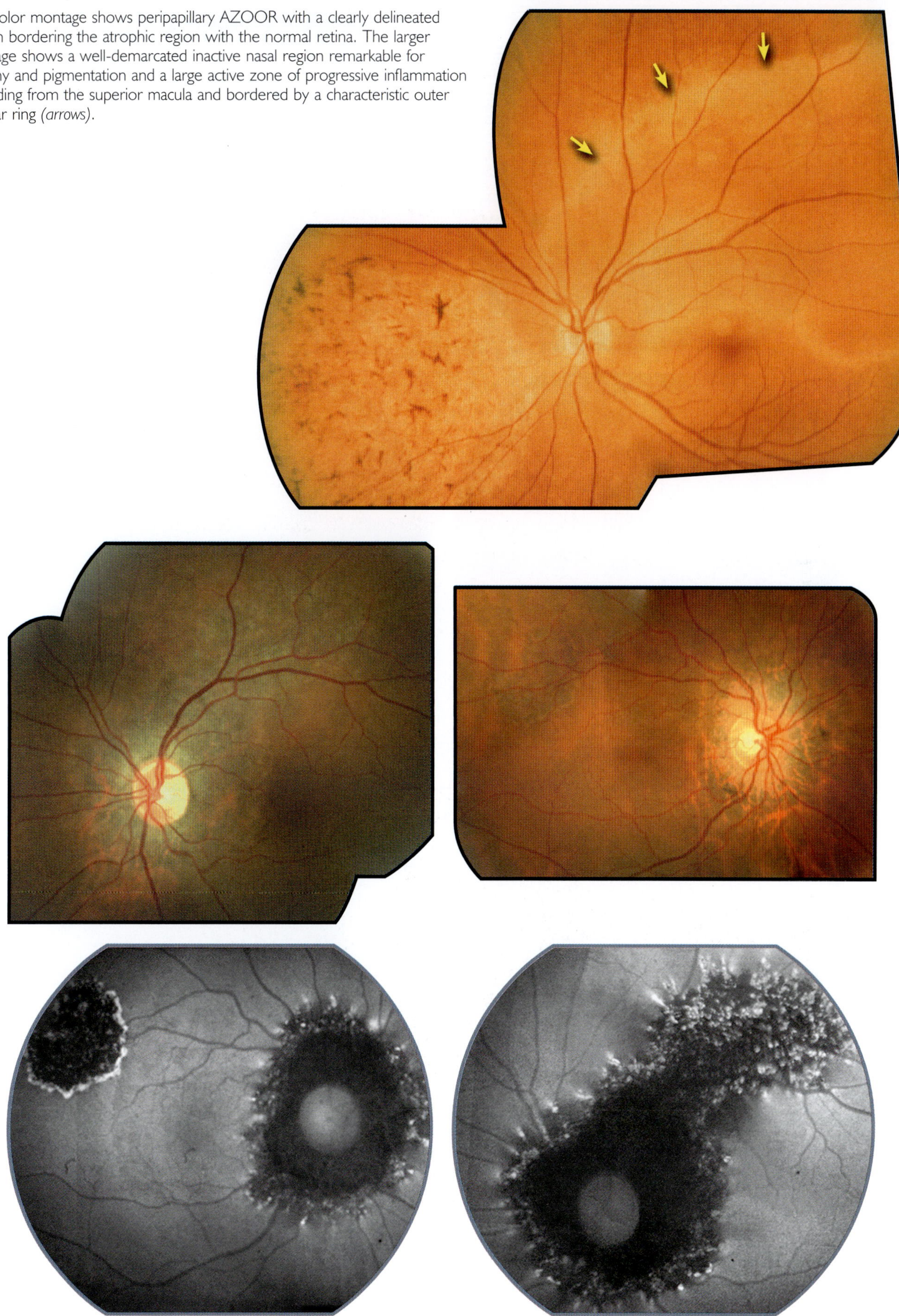

This is an asymptomatic patient that was diagnosed with AZOOR on routine evaluation. When tested, there was field loss corresponding to the multizonal abnormalities. Note the trizonal pattern of involvement with autofluorescence. The margins of the lesion show a flare of hyperautofluorescence typical of AZOOR. As the acute zonal areas become quiescent, the hyperautofluorescent margins become more normal.

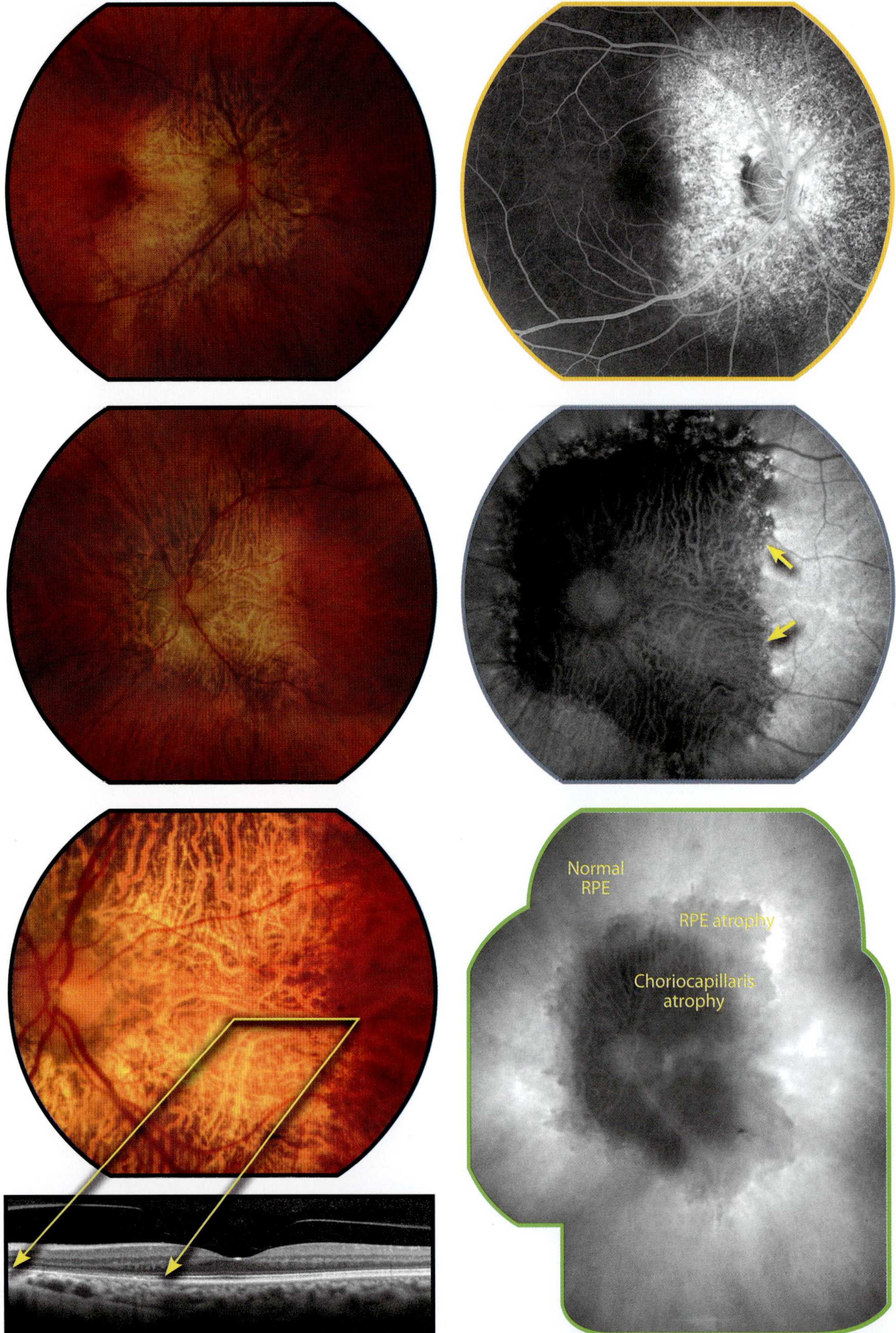

This patient has bilateral symmetric AZOOR. The color photograph of each eye shows peripapillary atrophy. The atrophic area is delineated on OCT imaging by the absence of the inner segment ellipsoid, beginning from the nasal aspect of the fovea *(lower left, arrows)*. The ICG study reveals a trizonal abnormality. The black area corresponds to absence of choriocapillaris and the gray area represents atrophy of the pigment epithelium adjacent to normal RPE. At the border of abnormal and normal pigment epithelium, there may be a distinct area of fundus hyperautofluorescence, which is actually not present in this patient, although flares of hyperautofluorescence extend from the junction between atrophic pigment epithelium and normal pigment epithelium *(arrows, middle row right)*.

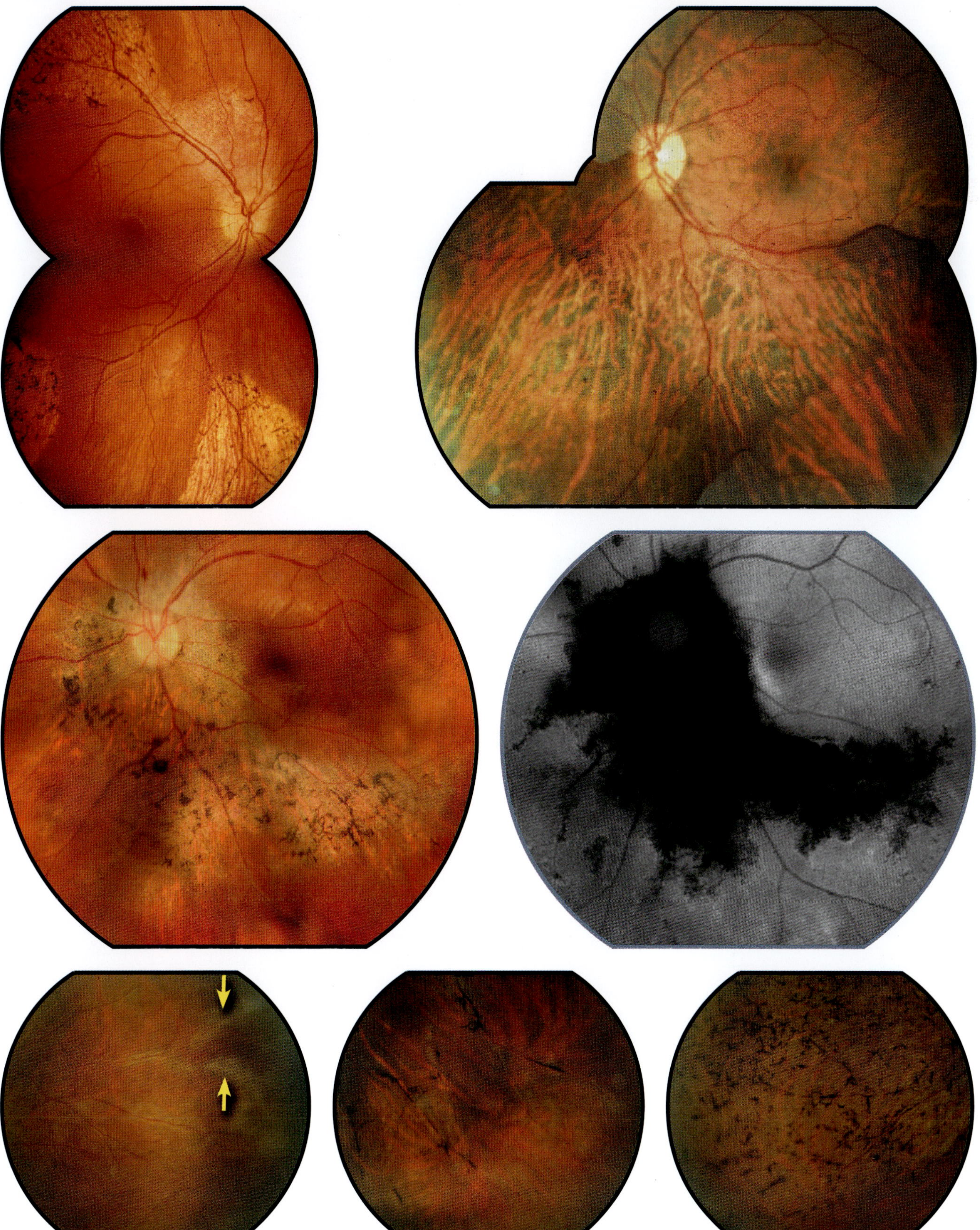

These images show the variability of AZOOR with atrophic zones present at different locations in the fundus. Note the sparing of the fovea associated with good visual acuity in the top row case. The patient in the middle row experienced photopsia and progressive field loss over several years, but then remained stable for the subsequent 11 years. The lower row shows various peripheral changes in AZOOR, including perivascular inflammatory sheathing *(arrows)*, atrophy, and hyperplastic pigment epithelial migration into the retina.

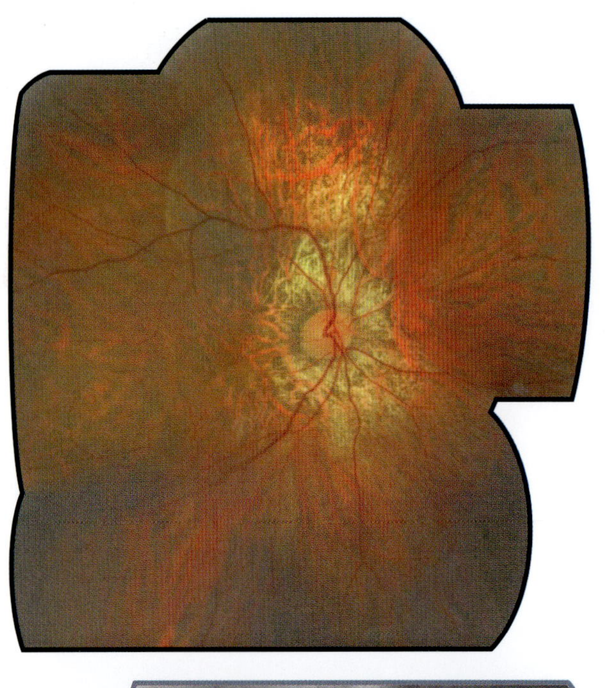

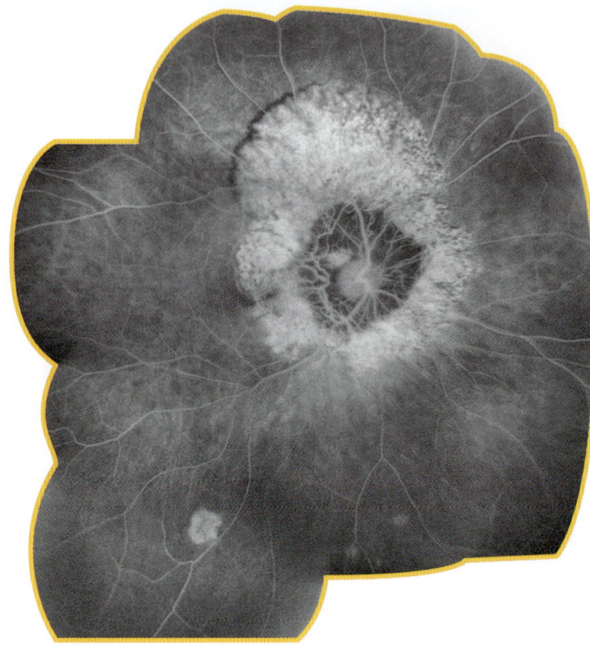

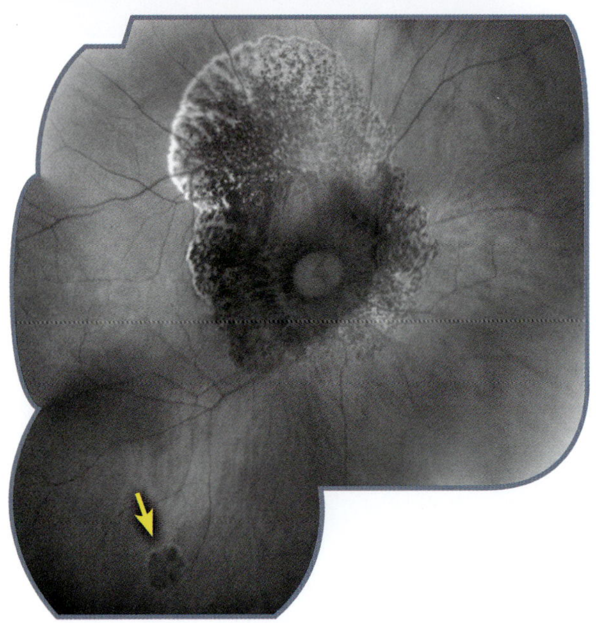

This male patient was first diagnosed with AZOOR at the age of 70. Note the delineating annulus or margin of chorioretinal degeneration superior to the nerve. The high-resolution ICG and autofluorescent montage sharply demarcate the zone of peripapillary degeneration. There is a smaller lesion inferiorly *(arrow)* with an annulus or delineating margin.

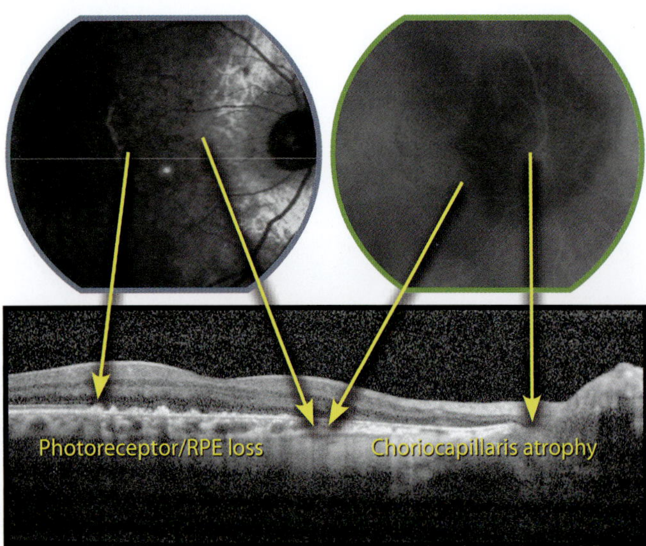

The OCT shows the basis for the trizonal pattern. The following can be seen: choriocapillaris atrophy in the immediate juxtapapillary area; adjacent RPE and photoreceptor degeneration with reticular-like drusenoid deposition; and a contiguous normal photoreceptor–RPE–choriocapillaris complex.

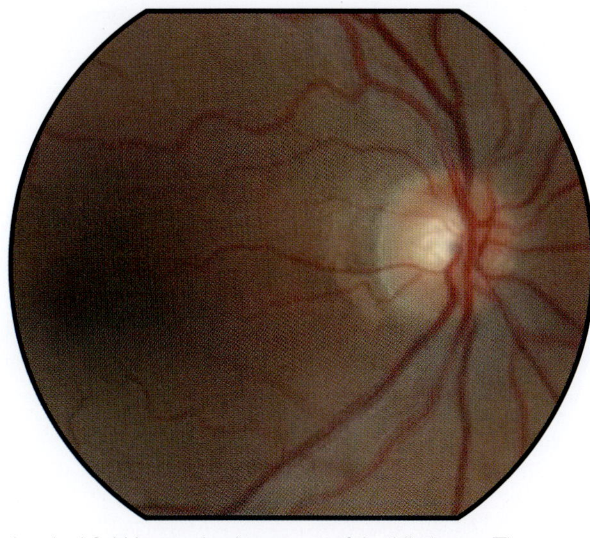

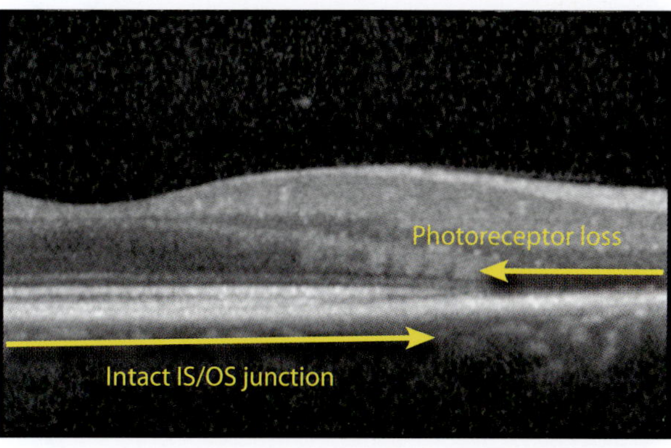

This patient had field loss and enlargement of the blind spot. There were no clinical findings evident. The only abnormality was the high-resolution OCT that showed an absence of photoreceptors, which correlated with the field loss. Note the sharp junction between normal and abnormal inner segment ellipsoid.

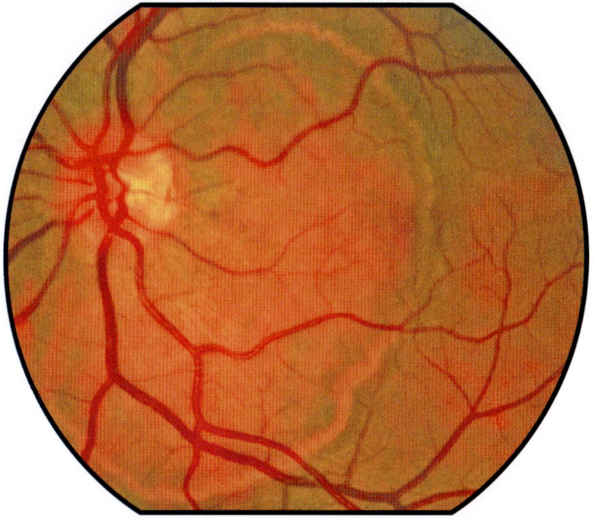

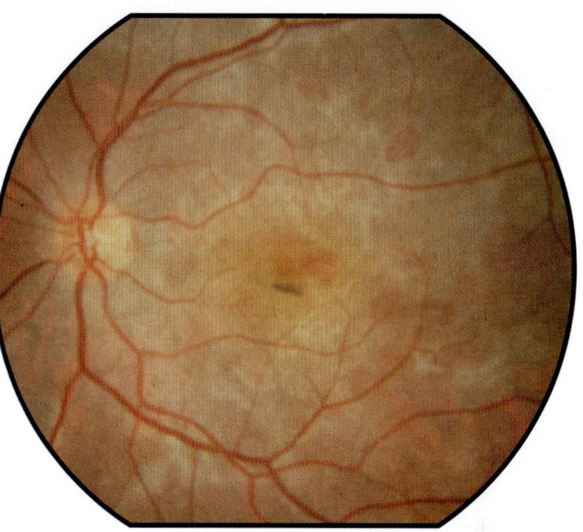

The fundus image at presentation is on the left, and the follow-up image several years later is on the right. This patient with AZOOR experienced diffuse subretinal fibrosis, not the characteristic pigmentation and atrophy, in the affected macula.

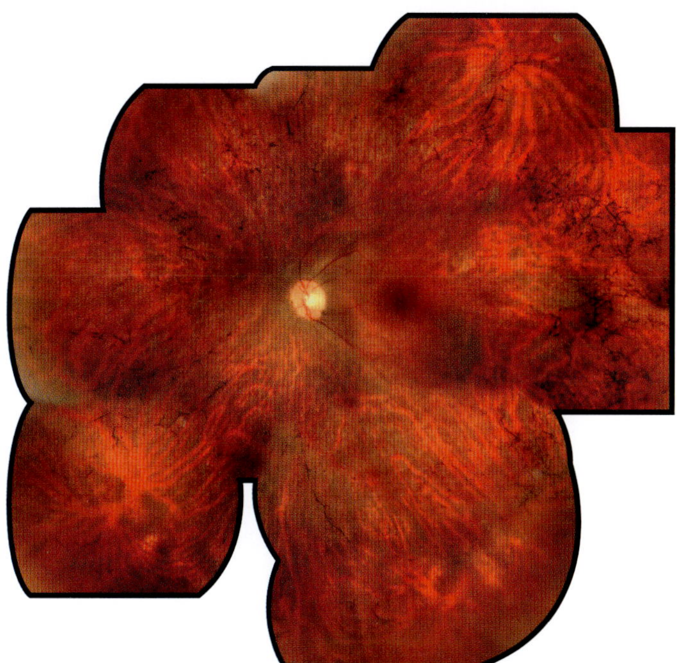

This patient with AZOOR experienced diffuse progressive photoreceptor and pigment epithelial degeneration.

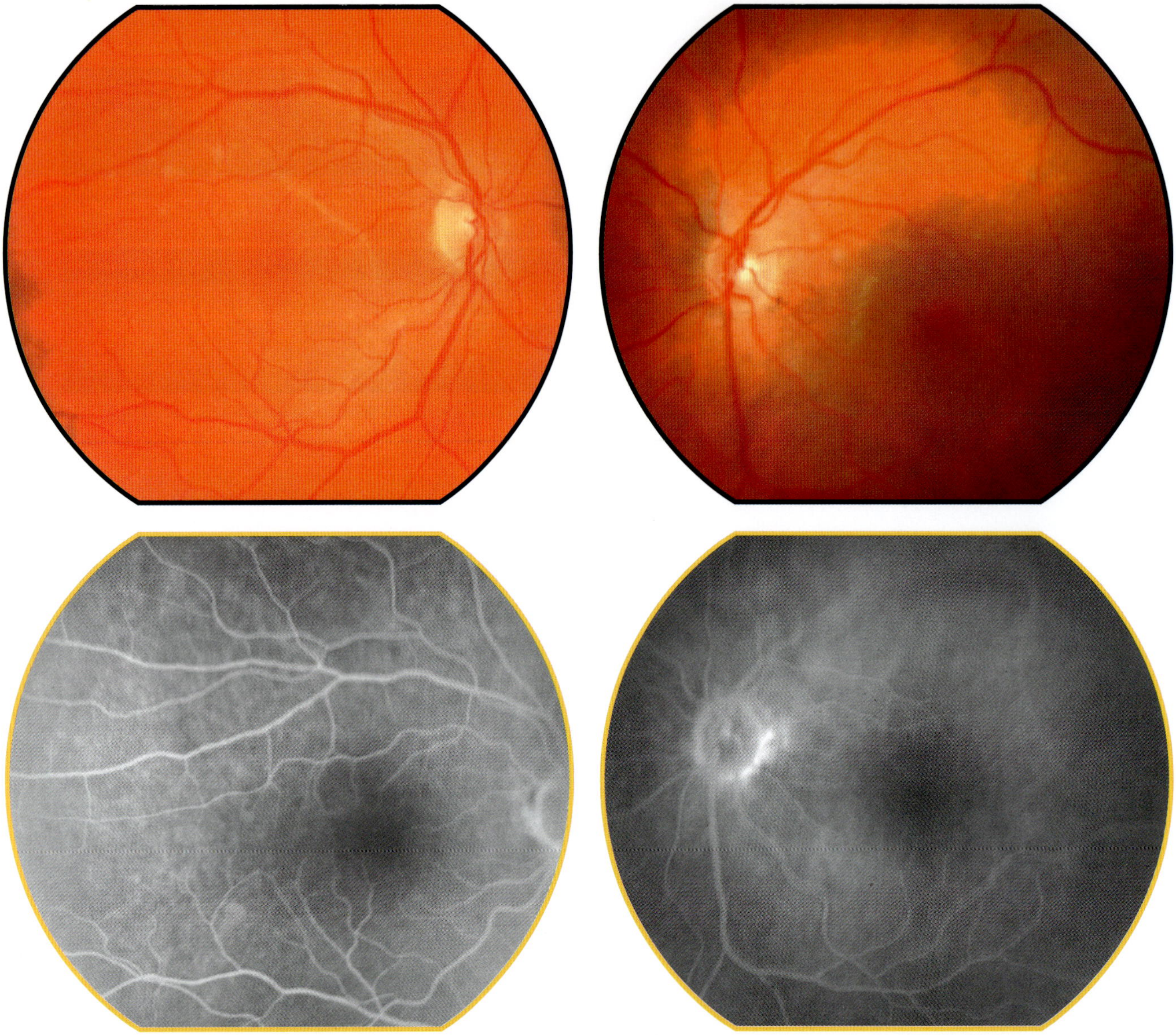

This patient developed recurrent episodes of floaters and blurry vision. Color fundus photos show linear white lines in the parafoveal zones. Late phase fluorescein angiograms *(bottom)* show late hyperfluorescent lesions. The partial annular pattern of the lesions suggested acute annular outer retinopathy, which is a variant of AZOOR. *Images courtesy of Amani Fawzi, MD*

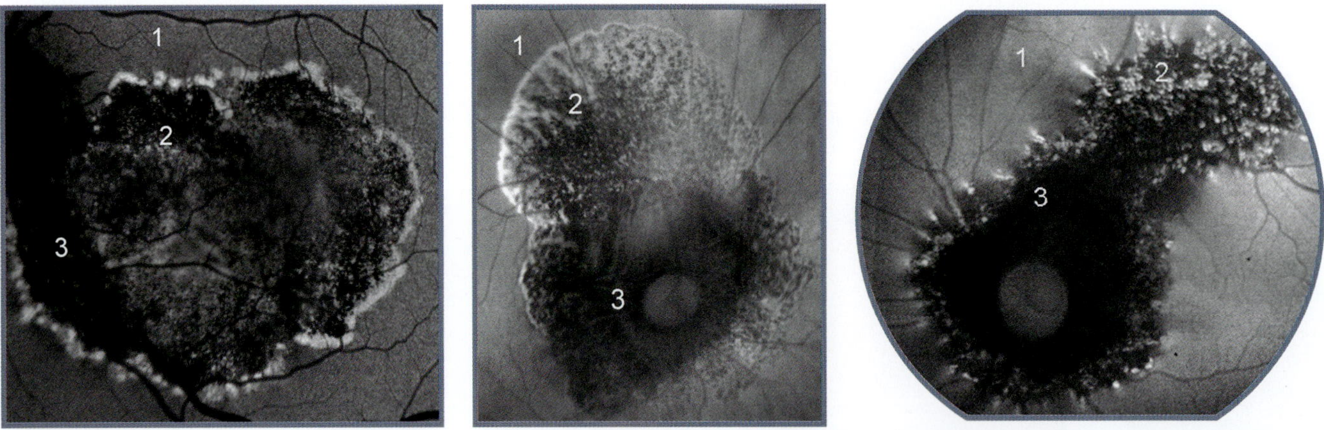

Autofluorescence images of these three patients with AZOOR demonstrate the trizonal pattern characteristic of the disease, as described in the text above.

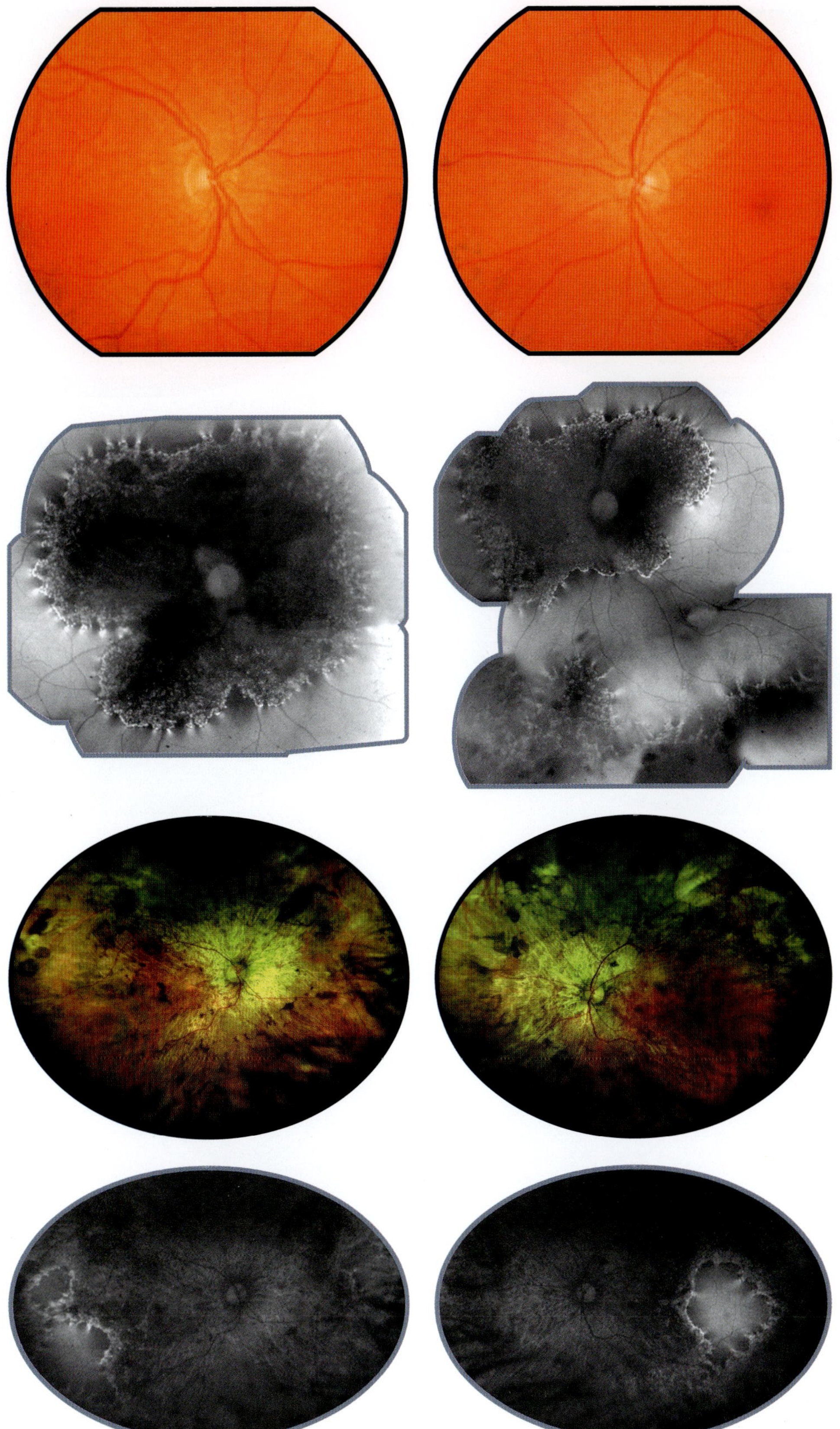

This patient initially presented with creamy, plaque-like peripapillary lesions seen here on color fundus photography *(top row)*. Six years later, autofluorescence imaging demonstrates progression in both eyes and the trizonal autofluorescence pattern characteristic of AZOOR *(second row)*. Progression continued, and 13 years after initial presentation widefield color fundus photos show widespread atrophy of the retina and RPE *(third row)*. Widefield autofluorescence imaging illustrate an island of temporal sparing, but with surrounding active disease demonstrated by the hyperautofluorescent edge adjacent to the remaining unaffected retina *(bottom row)*.

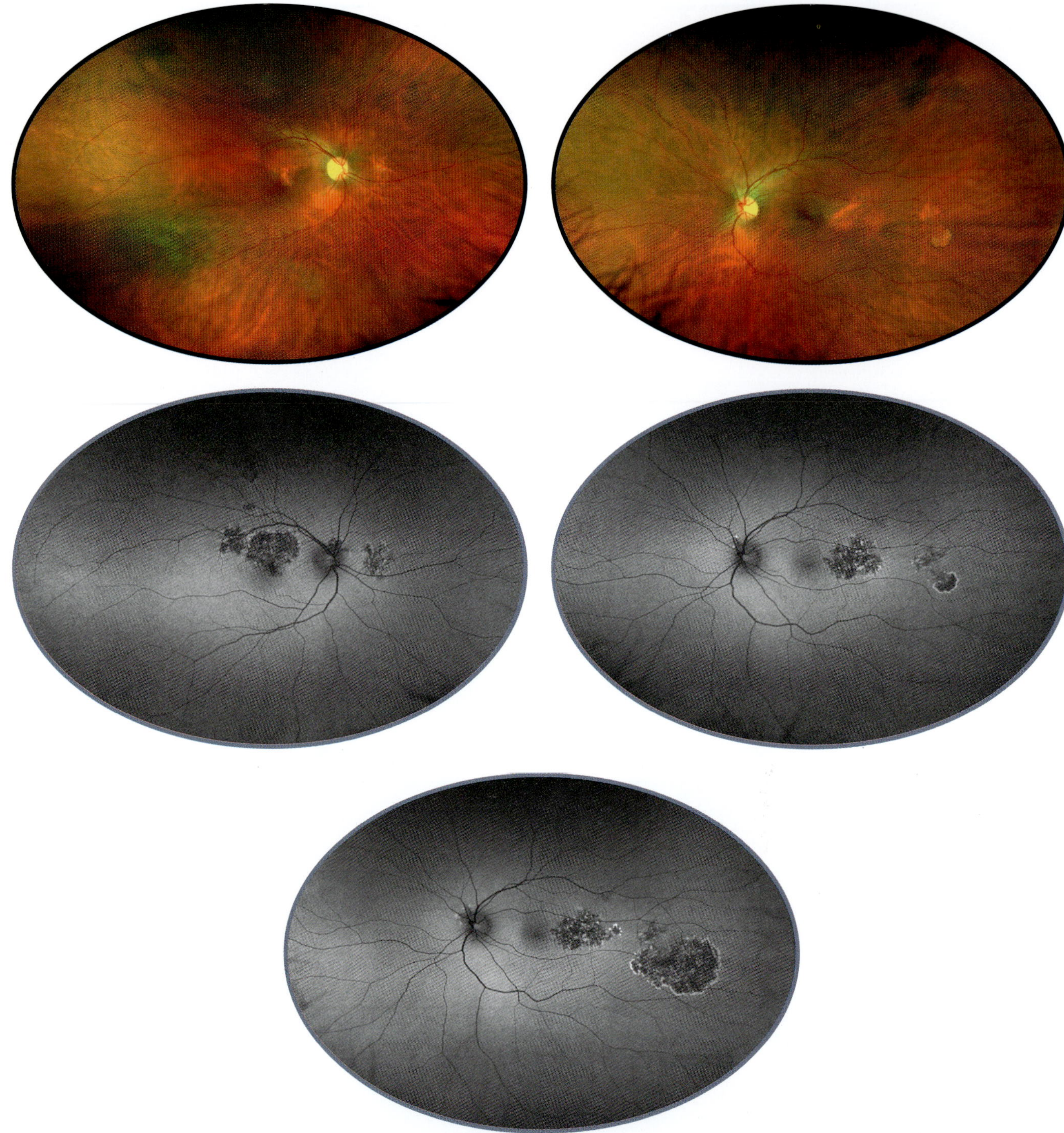

Widefield color photographs of this patient with AZOOR illustrates subtle areas of pigment changes in the posterior poles of both eyes *(top row)*. Widefield autofluorescence demonstrates the typical trizonal pattern in both eyes characteristic of this disease *(second row)*. Follow-up widefield autofluorescence of the left eye 4 months after presentation shows progression of the lesions *(bottom)*.

Acute Posterior Multifocal Placoid Pigment Epitheliopathy (APMPPE)

APMPPE is a syndrome of multiple, plaque-like, creamy lesions at the level of the RPE that typically affects young healthy men and women in the second and third decade of life. Patients develop rapid visual loss that may be associated with central or paracentral scotomas, photopsia, and metamorphopsia. Most cases are bilateral and the second eye is involved within a few days; however, delayed involvement of the second eye by several weeks can occur. Approximately one-third of the patients report a flu-like syndrome, particularly headaches preceding the visual symptoms. The characteristic clinical finding is the presence of multiple, yellow-white, placoid lesions at the level of RPE, located primarily in the posterior pole. New lesions may develop more peripherally. The size of the lesions varies, but they are usually less than one disc diameter. Associated ocular findings include mild vitritis, papillitis, retinal vasculitis, exudative retinal detachment, and retinal neovascularization and hemorrhage. The active lesions begin to resolve within a few days after the onset of the symptoms and are replaced by RPE atrophy and hyperpigmentation. As the old lesions fade, new active lesions may appear. The visual acuity may return to near normal, but patients may experience prolonged recovery associated with persistent scotomas and more uncommonly even severe vision loss. Rarely stroke and even death have been reported due to central nervous system vasculitis.

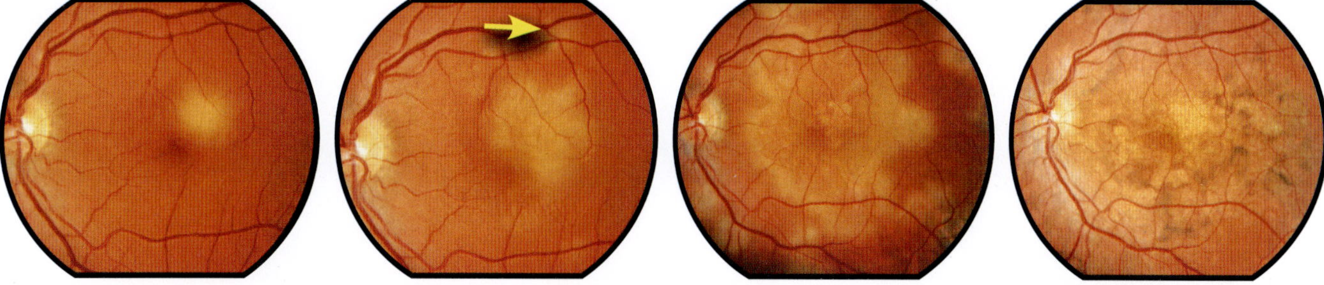

This patient with APMPPE presented with a solitary deep whitish-yellow lesion near the macula. Four days later, the lesion enlarged and a satellite lesion developed *(arrow)*. Two weeks after presentation, there is further progression. Three months after presentation, the resolved lesions appeared atrophic and hyperpigmented.

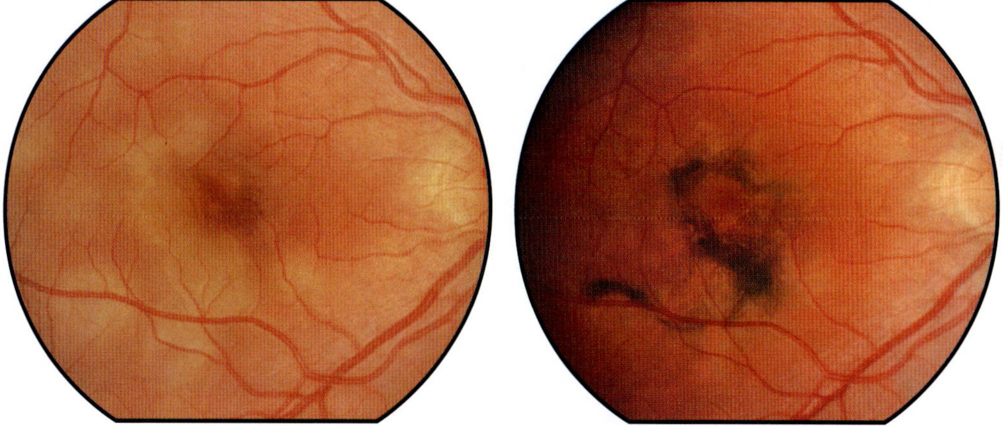

Note the creamy white lesions at the level of the RPE in this patient with APMPPE. Although most cases of APMPPE resolve with a good prognosis, some patients may develop central hyperpigmentation with a poor visual prognosis, as occurred in this case.

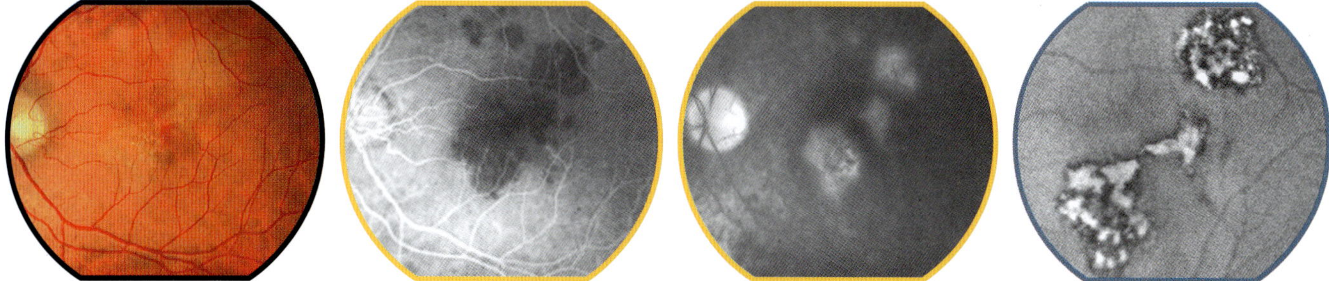

This patient with APMPPE shows a few larger lesions in the posterior pole of the left eye. Note the creamy-colored placoid abnormalities with geographic variation. There are also a few smaller spots in the superior paramacular region. The early fluorescein angiogram shows hypofluorescence from blockage versus a perfusion abnormality of the inner choroid with late staining of the lesions. The fundus autofluorescence shows hyperautofluorescence corresponding to the more recent lesions and hypoautofluorescence matching the healed lesions.

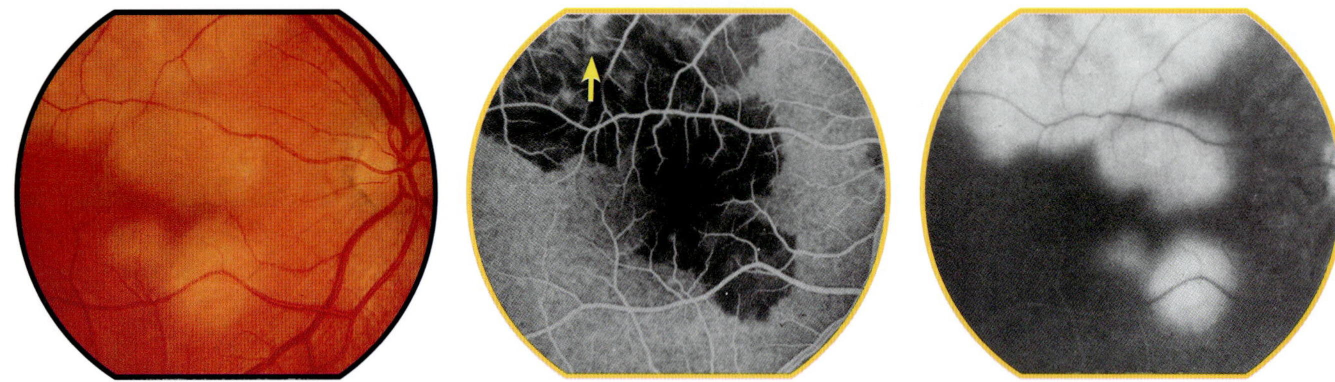

This is a patient with APMPPE and typical fluorescein angiographic (FA) findings of early hypofluorescence and late staining of the lesions. The FA shows visibility of the choroidal circulation in the superior macula, corresponding to window defect or transmitted choroidal fluorescence *(arrow)*. This is a subacute lesion in which the pigment epithelium has become atrophic.

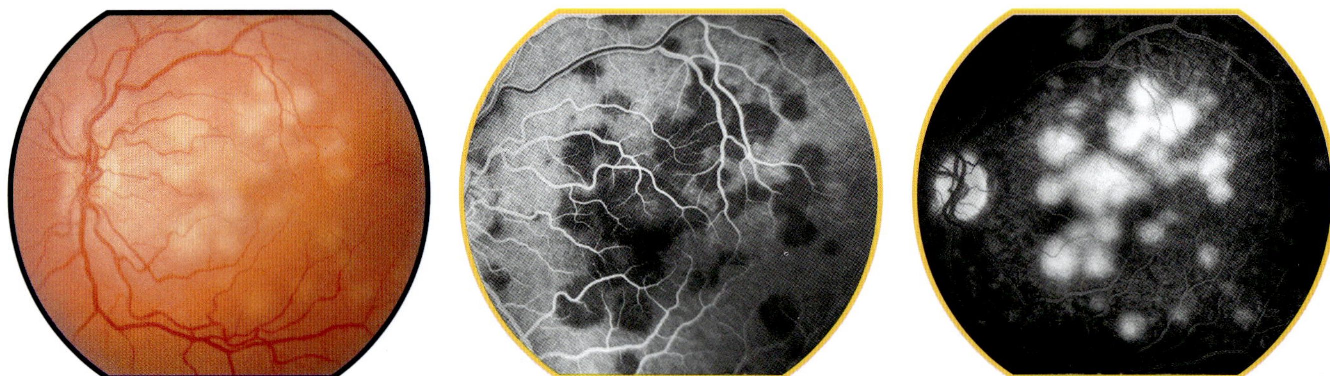

This patient has APMPPE with typical FA findings of early hypofluorescence *(middle)* and late staining *(right)* of the acute lesions. Early hypofluorescence may be attributed to RPE blockage versus choroidal ischemia. More recent evidence with OCT angiography indicates that inner choroidal ischemia is the etiology of APMPPE and related placoid disorders. *Courtesy of Dr. Howard Schatz*

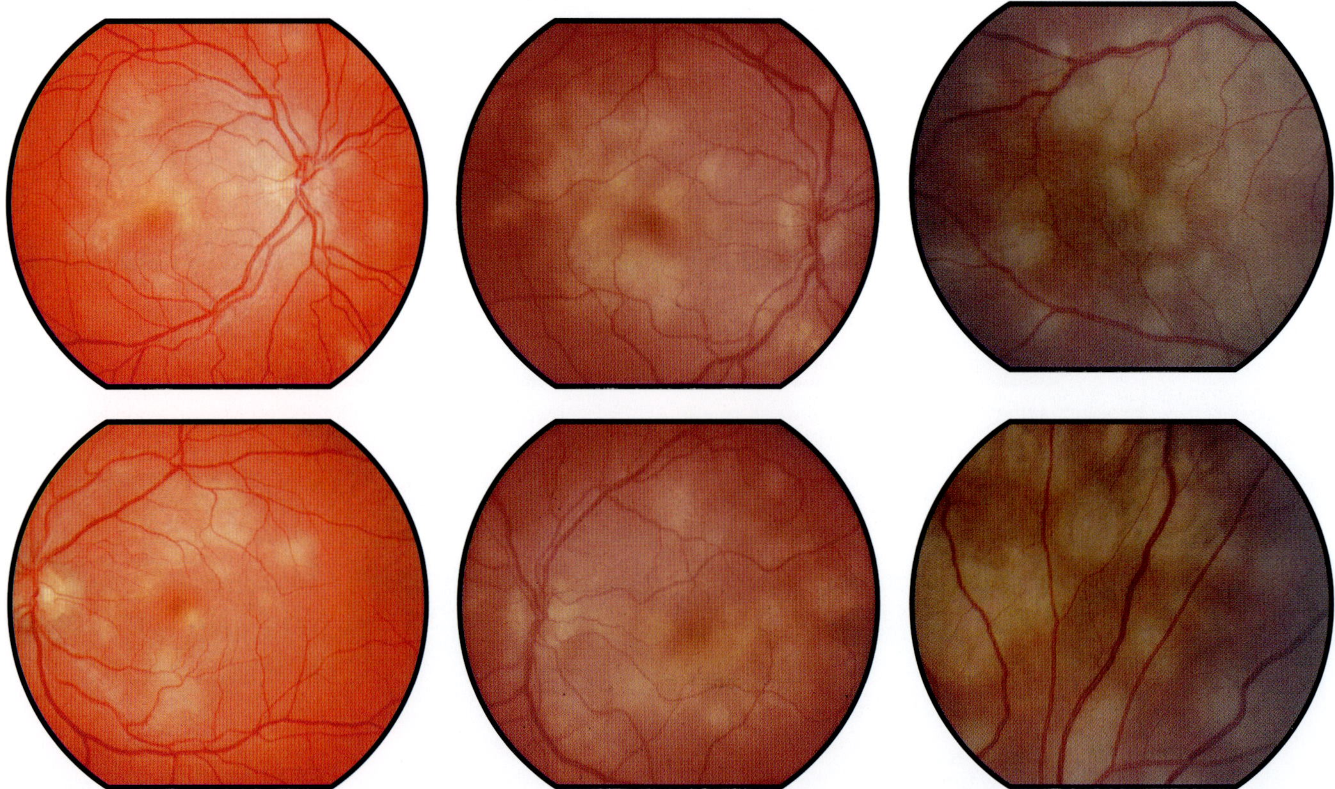

These are additional patients with APMPPE that demonstrate variation in the distribution and confluency of the acute lesions. *Top and lower right images courtesy of Dr. Frank Holz*

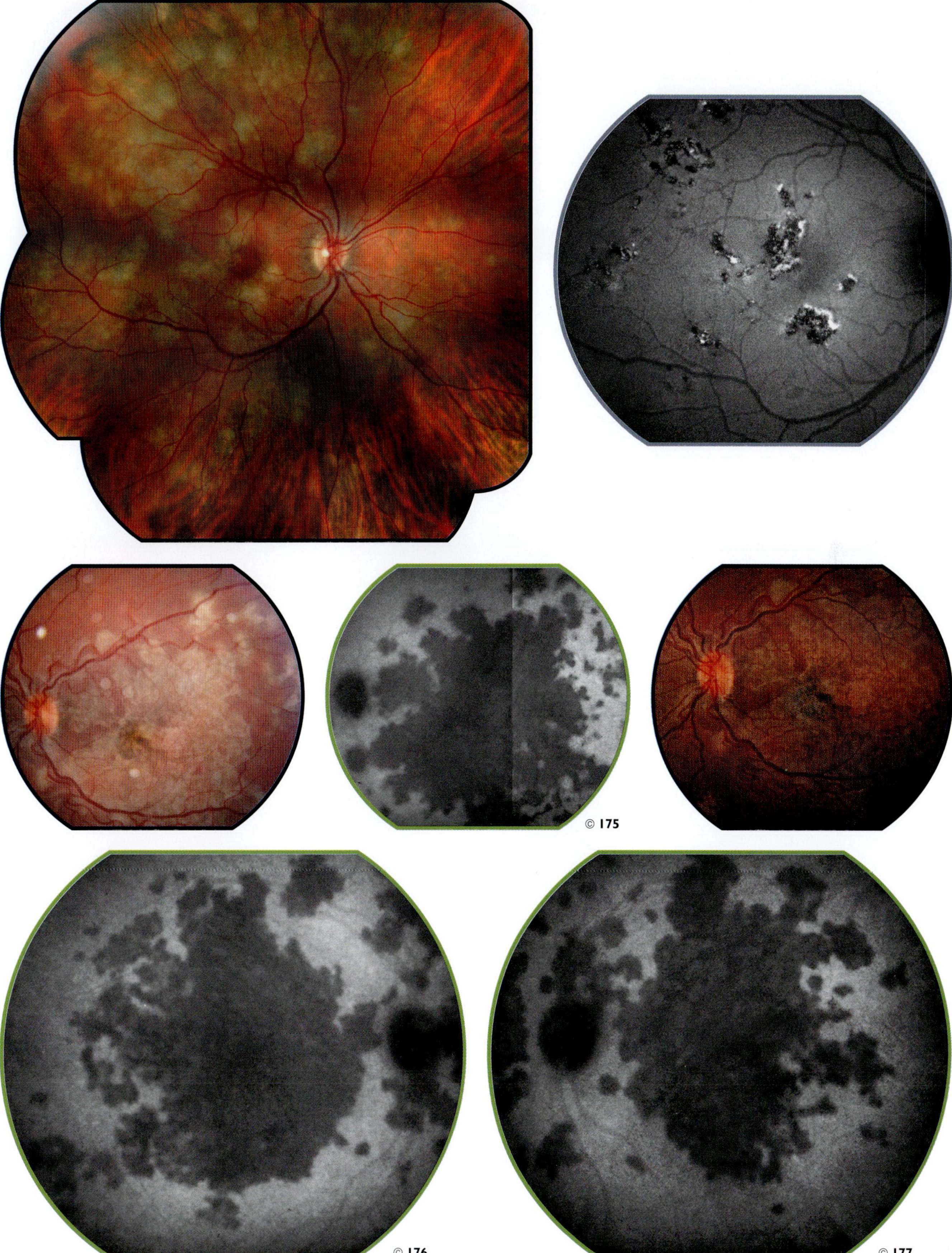

In addition to angiography, fundus autofluorescence *(top right)* may be useful in determining the precise localization and disease activity of the lesions. Montage photography is also helpful to identify all lesions. Atrophy and pigment degeneration may develop and are associated with a poor visual outcome (*middle right*). Note the diffuse lesion acutely involving the macula *(bottom left and right)* and confirmed with ICG angiography.

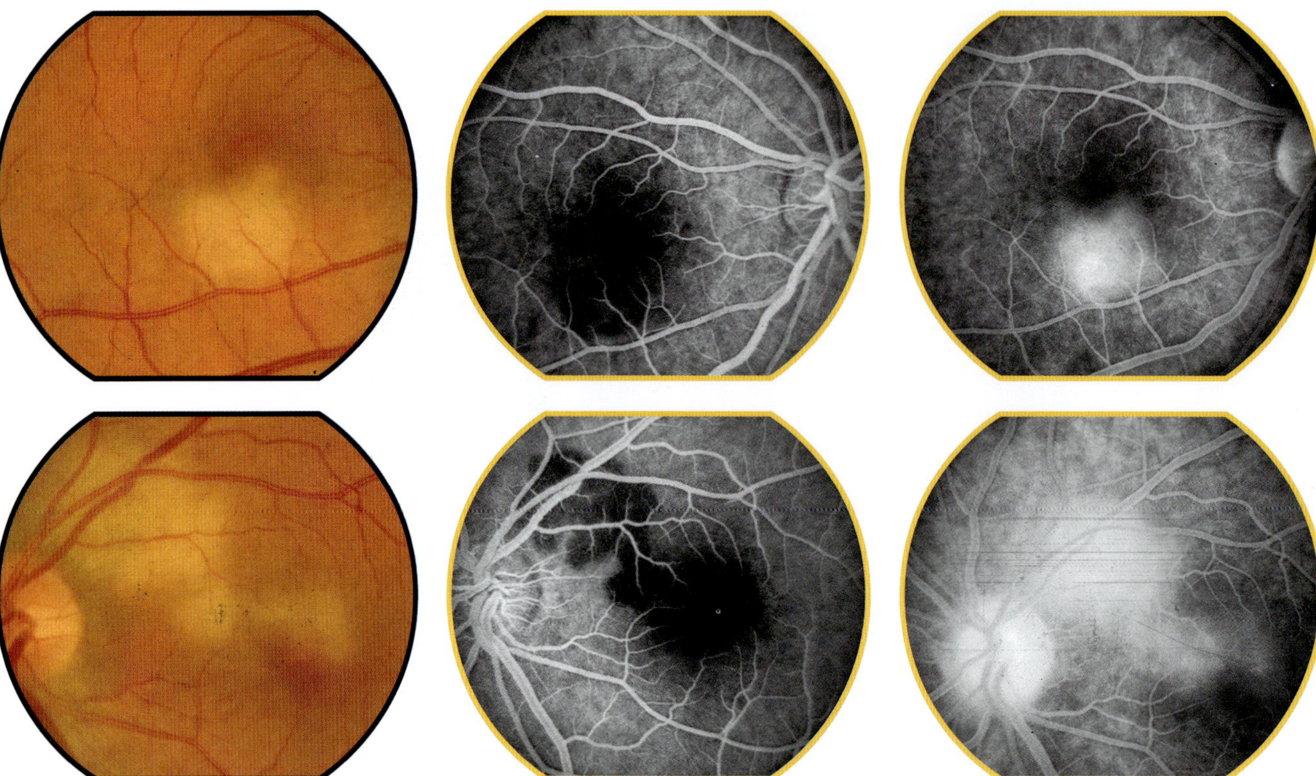

This patient with APMPPE shows acute bilateral geographic macular lesions with a mild papillitis associated with disc staining in the left eye. Spontaneous resolution ensued without recurrence over many years. A presentation such as this must be differentiated from serpiginous choroidopathy, granulomatous disease, and syphilis.

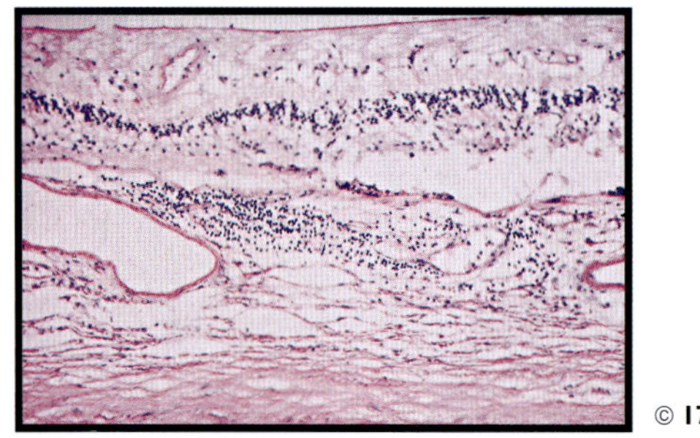

© **178**

The histopathology in this patient who had APMPPE and died of cerebral vasculitis, shows a choroidal granuloma beneath the RPE with focal disruption of the monocellular tissue. The choriocapillaris was spared. Systemically, the patient had granulomatous vasculitis and multinucleated giant cells in the large cerebral arteries.

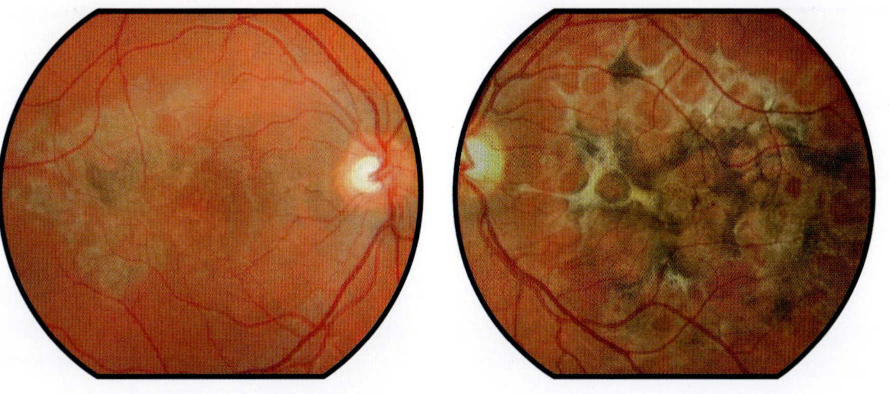

This case of resolved APMPPE shows a variation in the healing process. Comparatively minimal atrophy and sparing of the fovea are noted in the right eye *(left)* while widespread fibrous metaplastic and pigmentary degeneration are identified in the fellow eye. *Courtesy of Dr. Dimitrios Karagiannis*

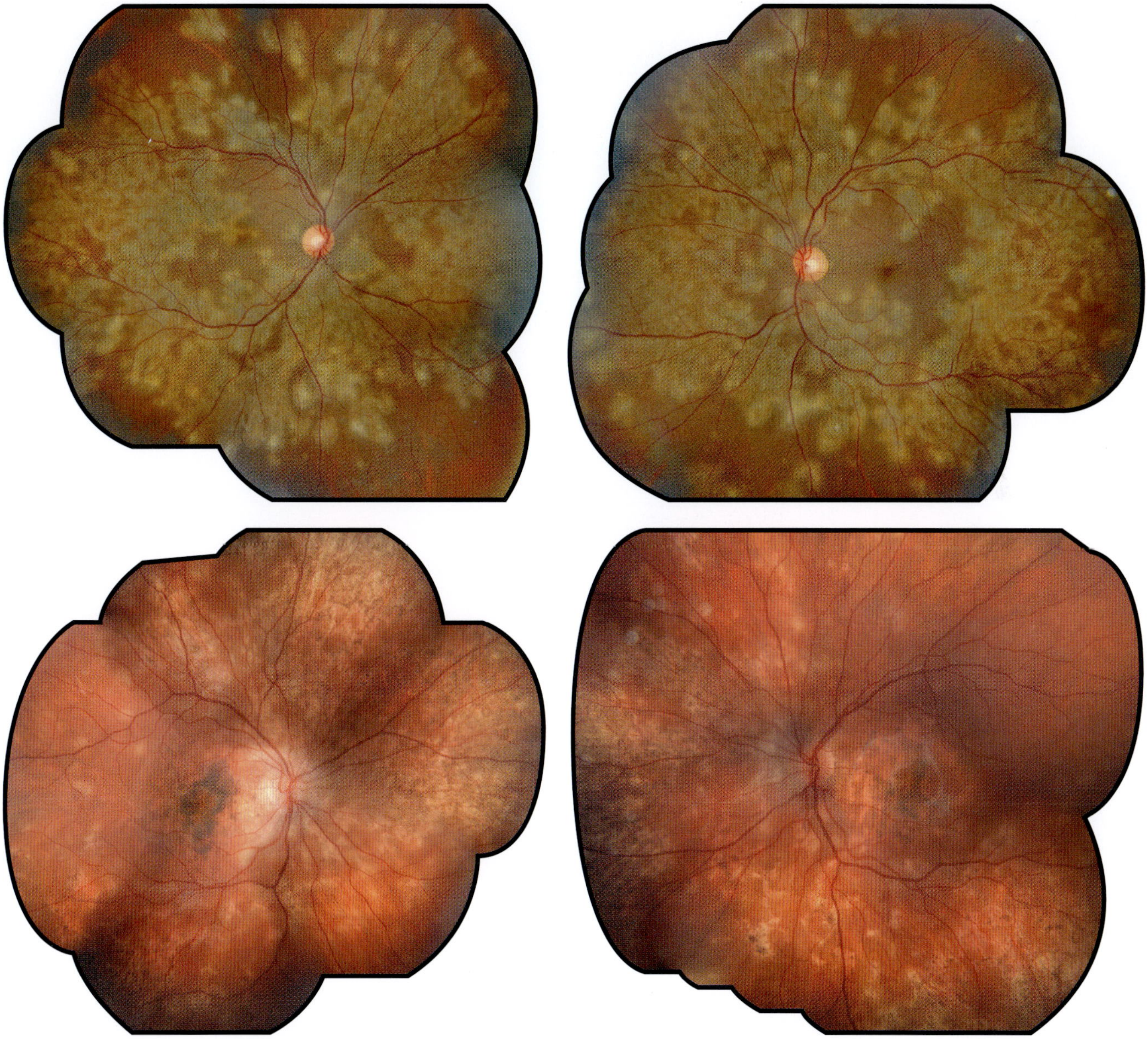

Note the widespread and confluent posterior and peripheral lesions that are acute in the first case *(top row)* and resolved with atrophy and pigmentary scarring in the second case *(bottom row)*. *Bottom row courtesy of Dr. Mark Blumenkranz*

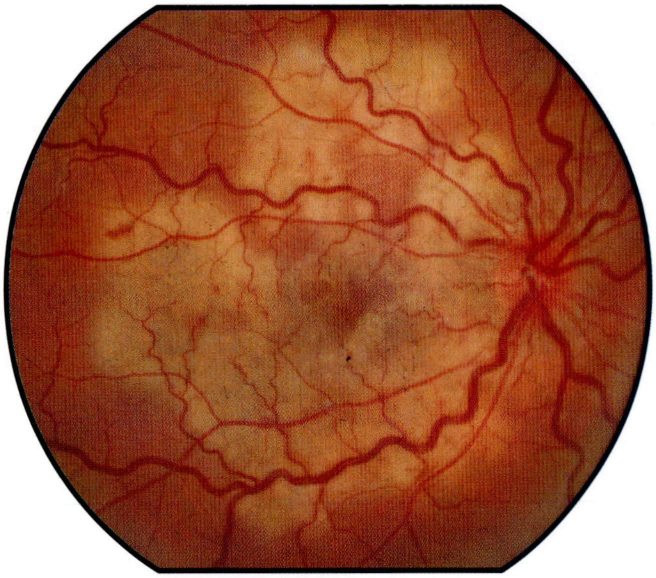

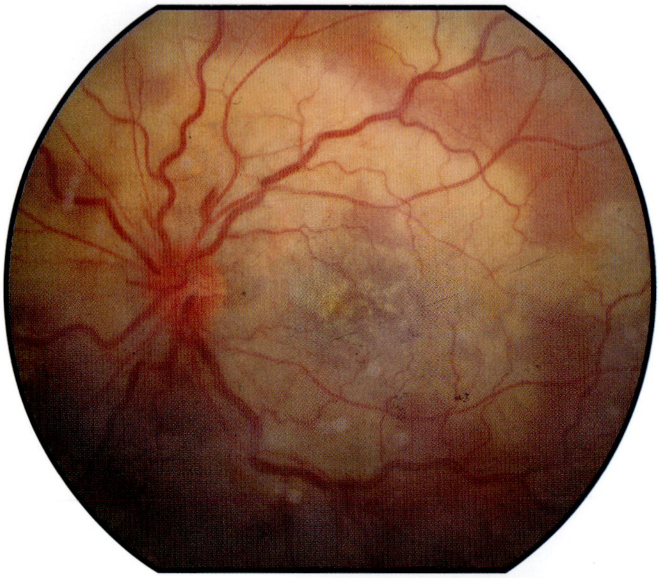

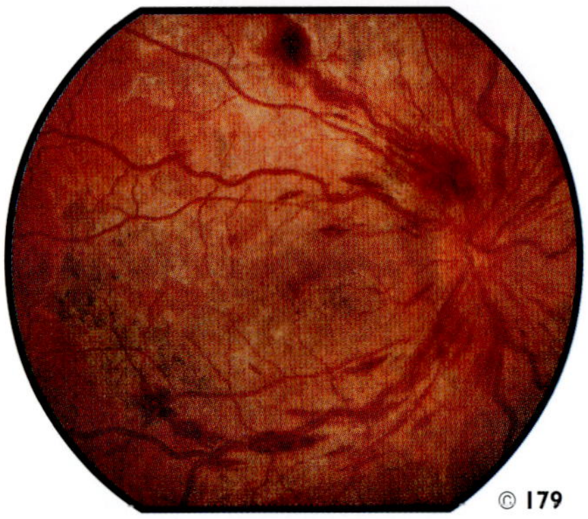

© 179 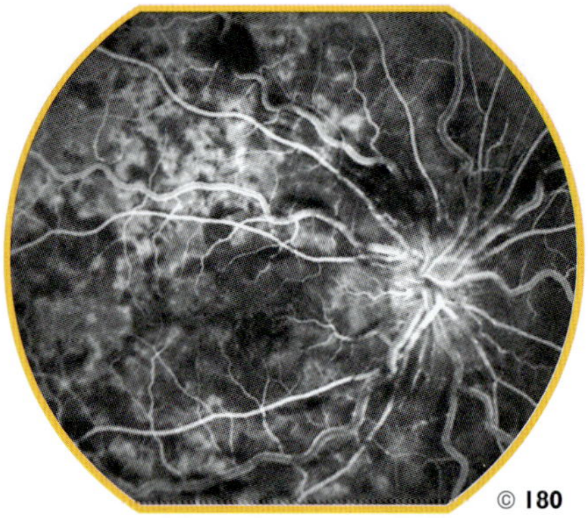 © 180 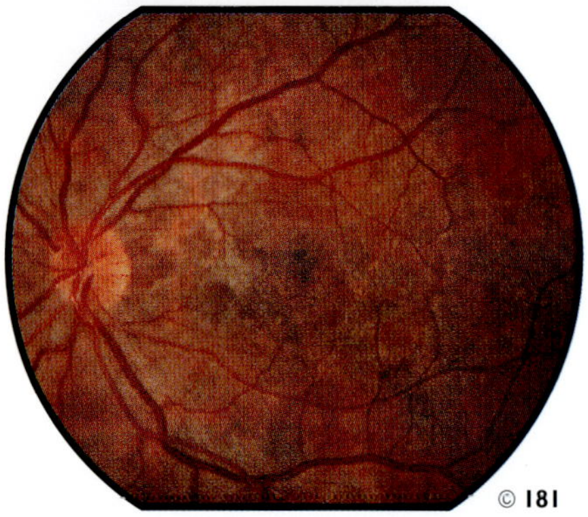 © 181

This patient with APMPPE had associated optic nerve edema and venous stasis bilaterally that was more severe in the right eye. At presentation, there were a few retinal hemorrhages in the left eye during the acute stage of the disease. The right eye then developed frank central retinal vein occlusion (CRVO) with scattered hemorrhages *(bottom left)* throughout the fundus that block on the fluorescein angiogram *(bottom middle)*. The hemorrhages in the left eye resolved with less venous engorgement and tortuosity *(bottom right image)*. This case illustrates CRVO in each eye associated with APMPPE.

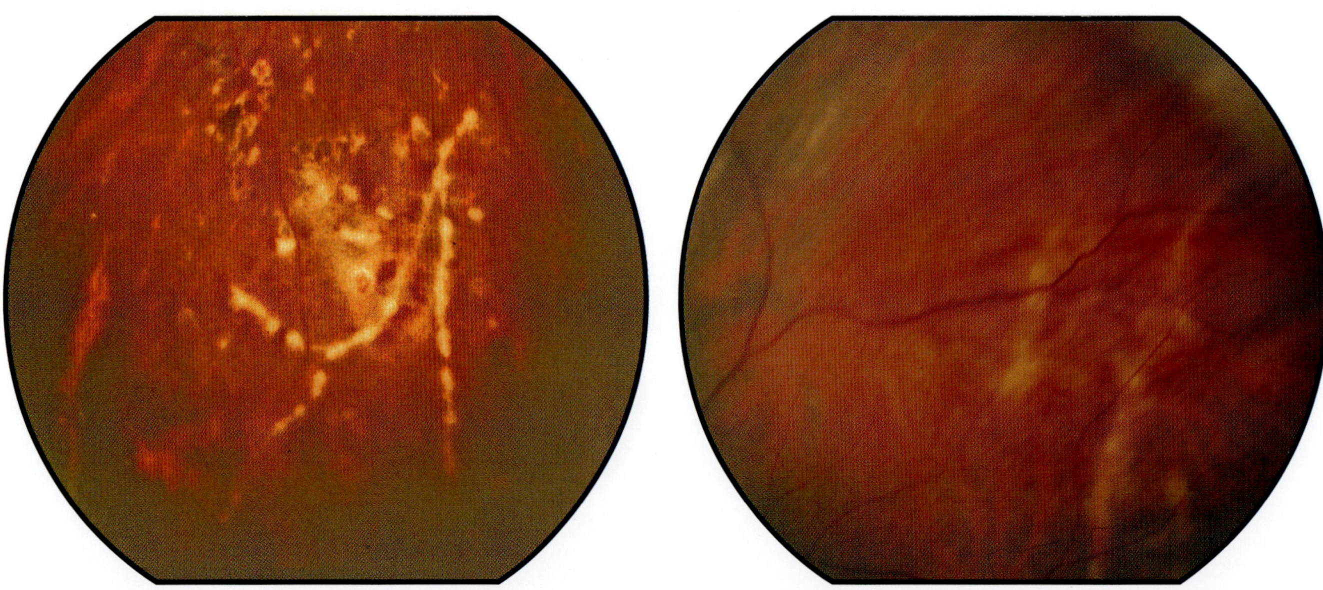

A choroidal segmental inflammatory process may rarely be seen in the peripheral fundus of patients with APMPPE as illustrated here. This segmental choroidal vasculitis may not be coincidental because panvasculitis is known to occur in APMPPE. It may also be indicative of an inflammatory process in the choroid as a primary mechanism for the pathogenesis of the disease.

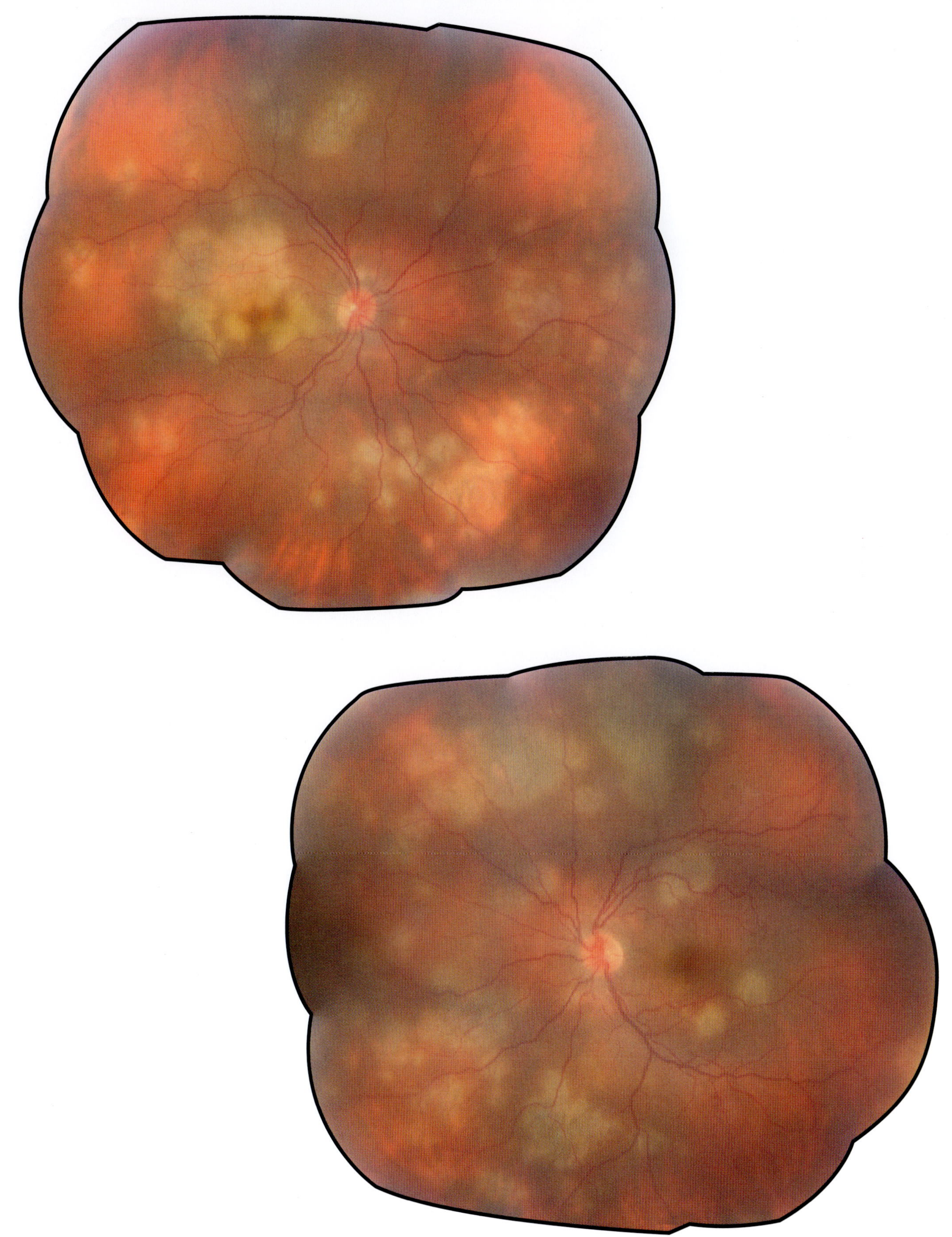

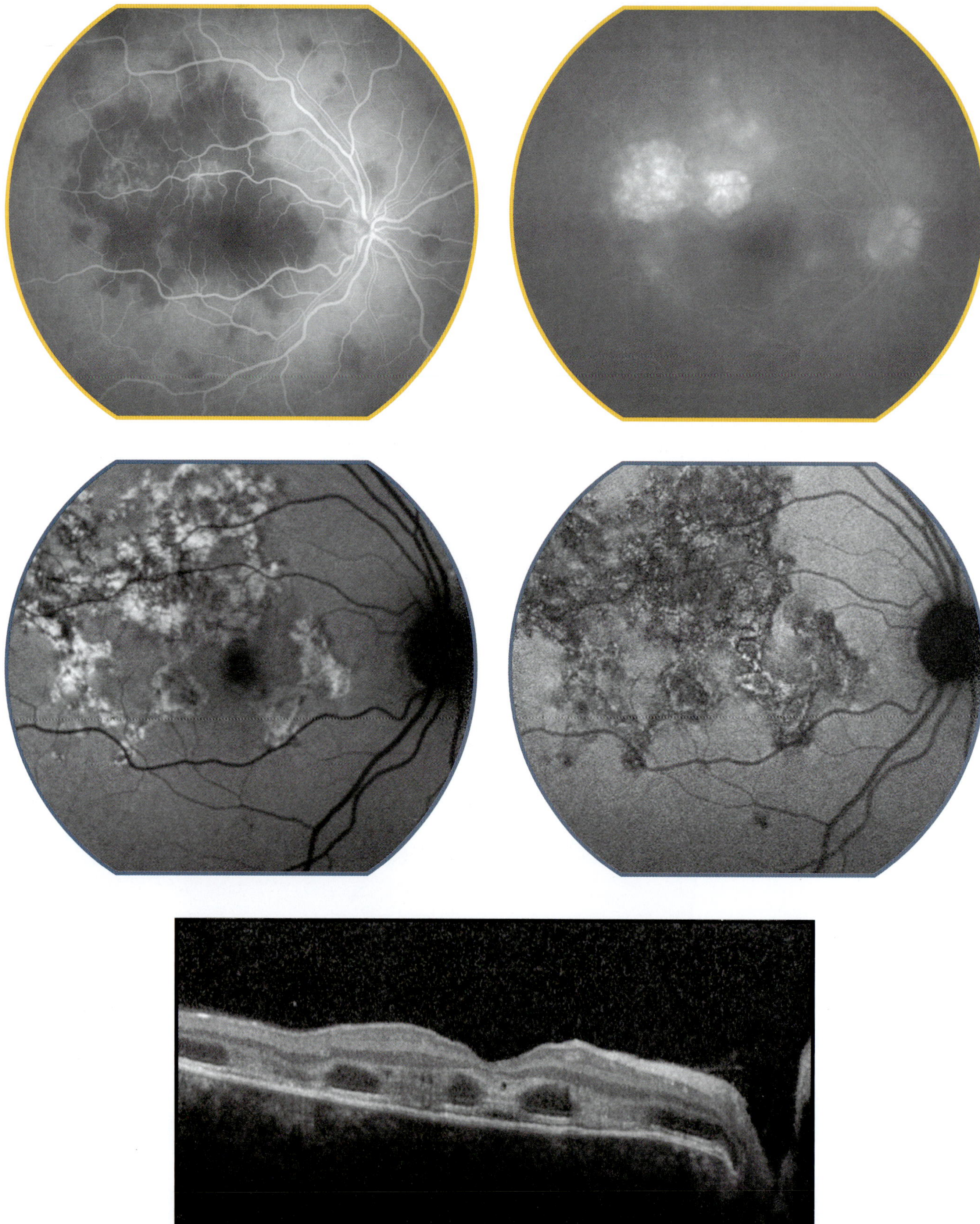

Color fundus montage of this patient with APMPPE illustrates multiple yellow creamy plaque-like lesions scattered throughout the posterior pole and midperiphery of both eyes. Fluorescein angiogram shows early blockage and late staining of the lesions. Autofluorescence of the posterior pole of the right eye at presentation demonstrates hyperautofluorescence of the lesions. Healed lesions at follow-up illustrate hypoautofluorescence. SD-OCT illustrates disruption of the ellipsoid zone and hyperreflective lesions tracking through the outer retina and into the outer plexiform layer of Henle. *Images courtesy of Lee Jampol, MD*

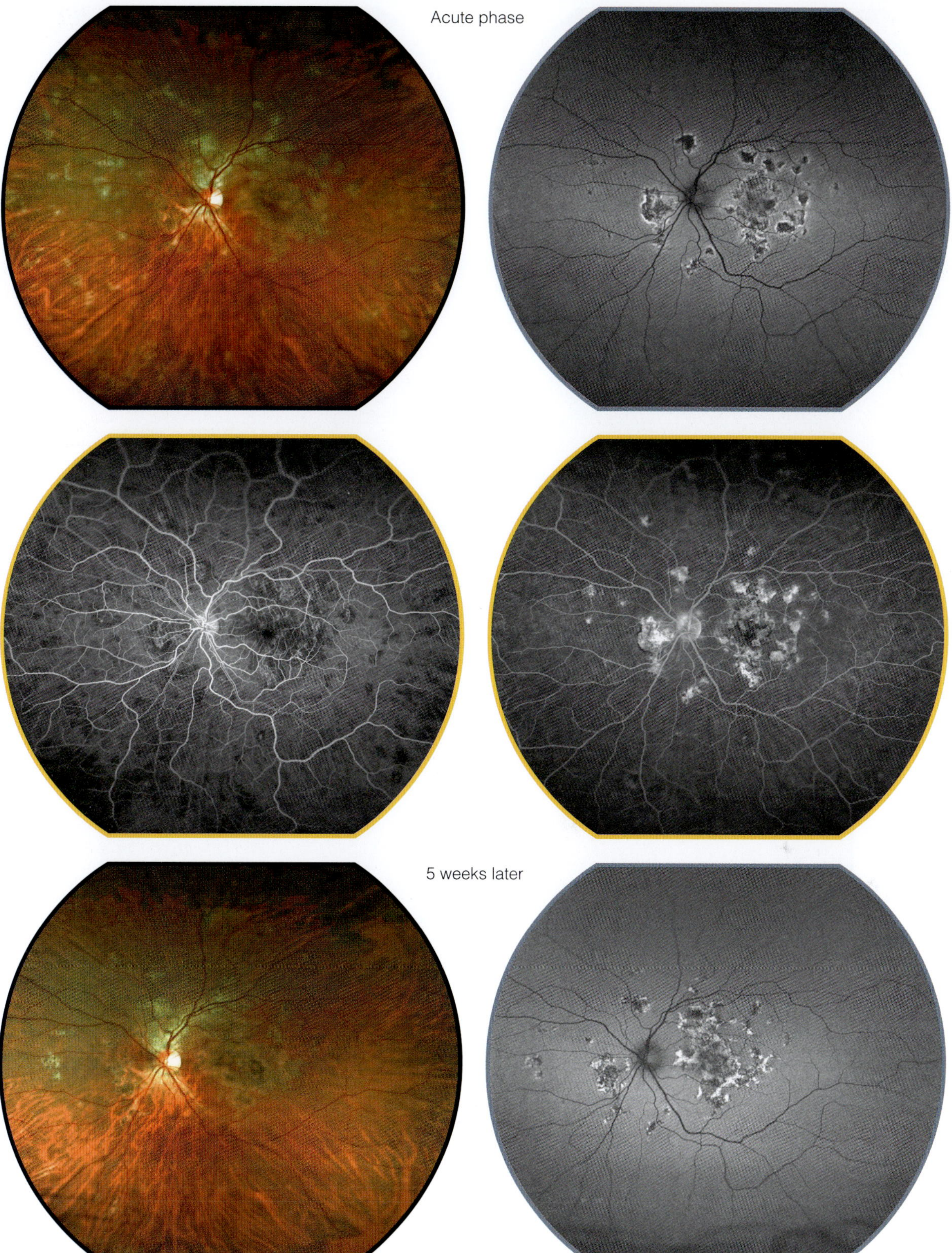

Widefield color fundus photos *(top left)*, widefield fundus autofluorescence *(top right)* and widefield fluorescein angiogram *(middle row)* in this patient with APMPPE demonstrates more lesions than can be detected with fluorescein angiogram versus color and autofluorescence imaging. These lesions block in the early frames of the angiogram and stain in the late phase. The early blocking may be the result of choroidal inflammation, which prevents normal filling of the choroidal vasculature.

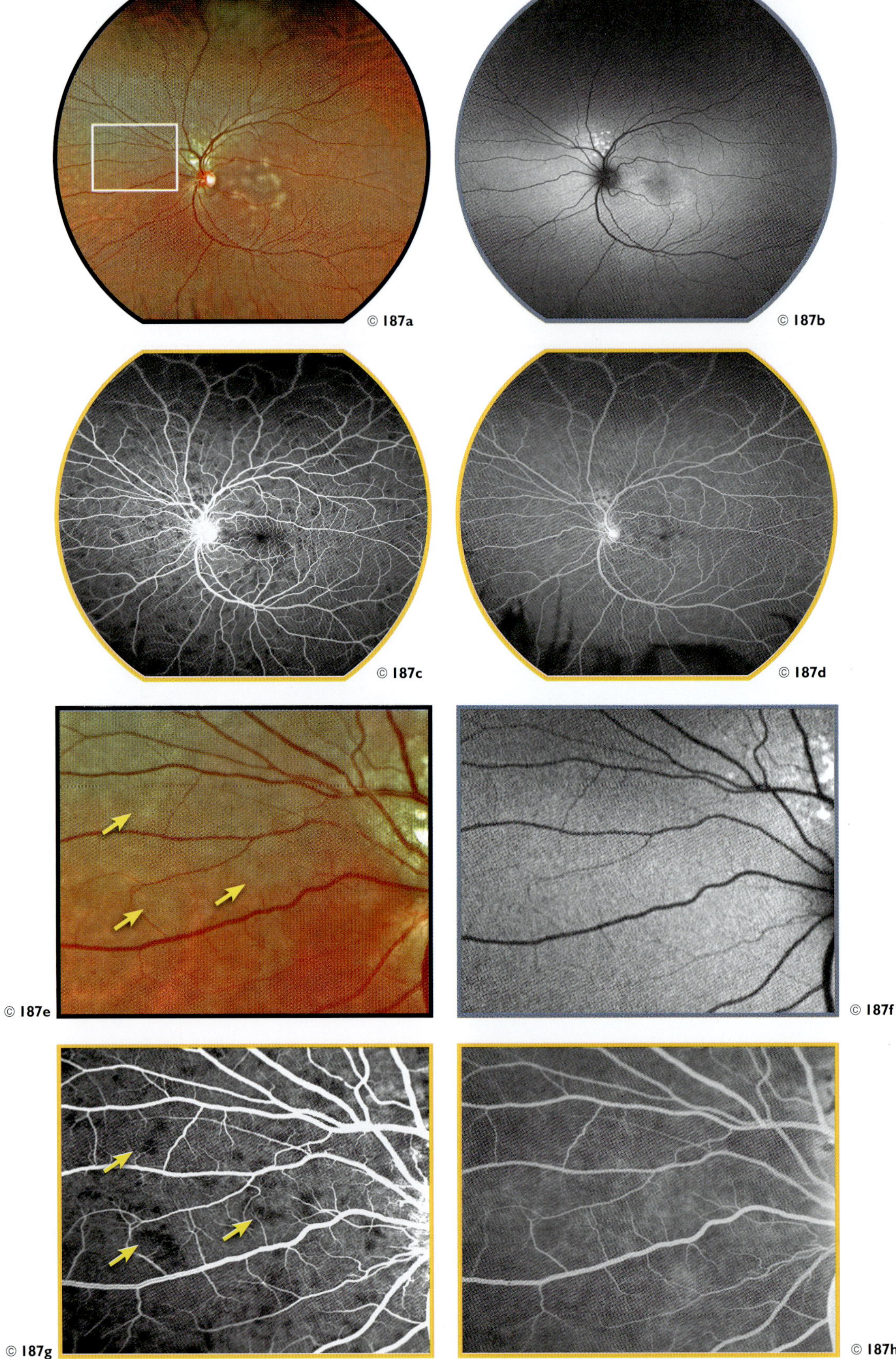

Color fundus photos *(top and third row, left)* autofluorescence *(top and third row, right)* and fluorescein angiogram *(second and bottom rows)* in this patient with APMPPE also demonstrates that more lesions can be seen on fluorescein angiogram than can be seen on autofluorescence, which is likely due to the choroidal location of the lesions. These lesions block in the early frames of the angiogram *(second and bottom row, left)*.

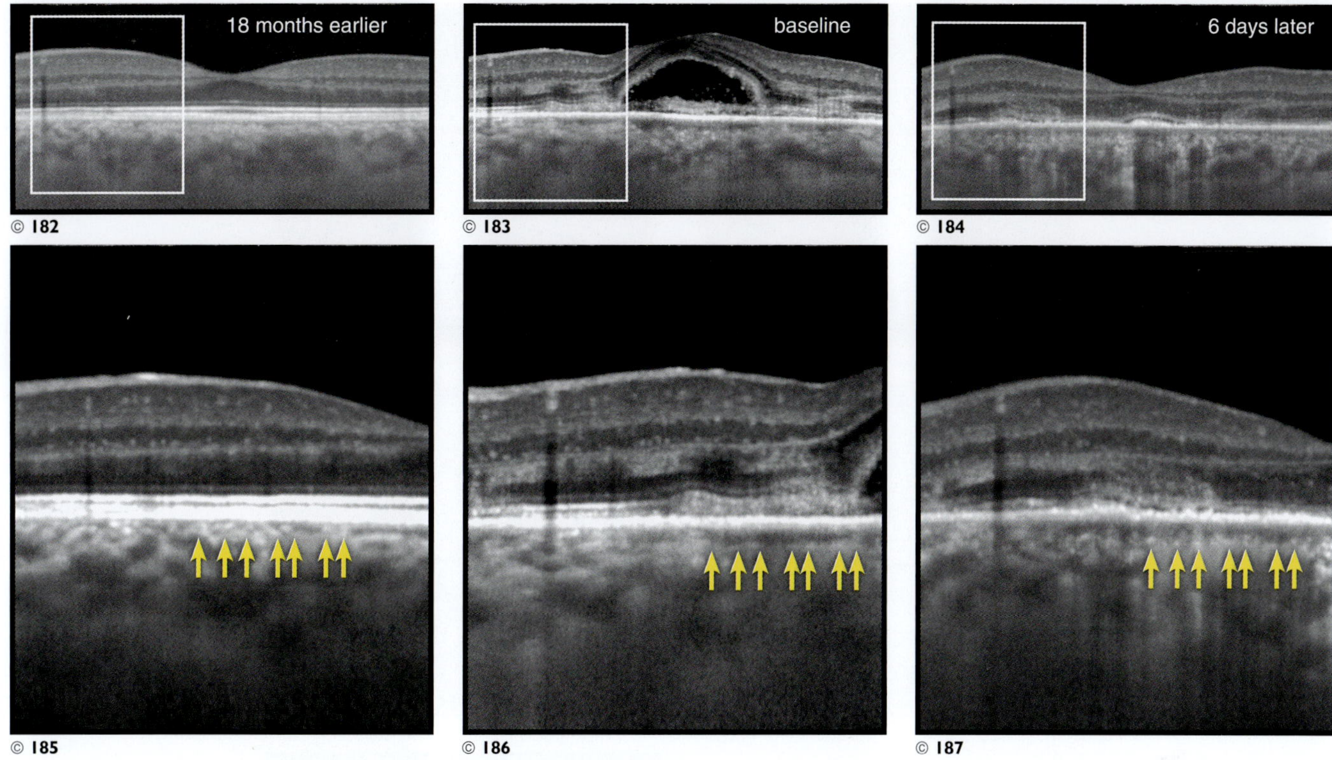

SD-OCT of this patient with APMPPE at 18 months before his acute presentation *(left column)* is essentially normal. The arrows in the bottom left image denote a normal choriocapillaris. The patient then presented with new visual disturbances and SD-OCT revealed hyper-reflective lesions in the outer retina and intraretinal fluid *(middle column)*. Note the thickening of the choriocapillaris that develops 6 days after presentation *(right column)*.

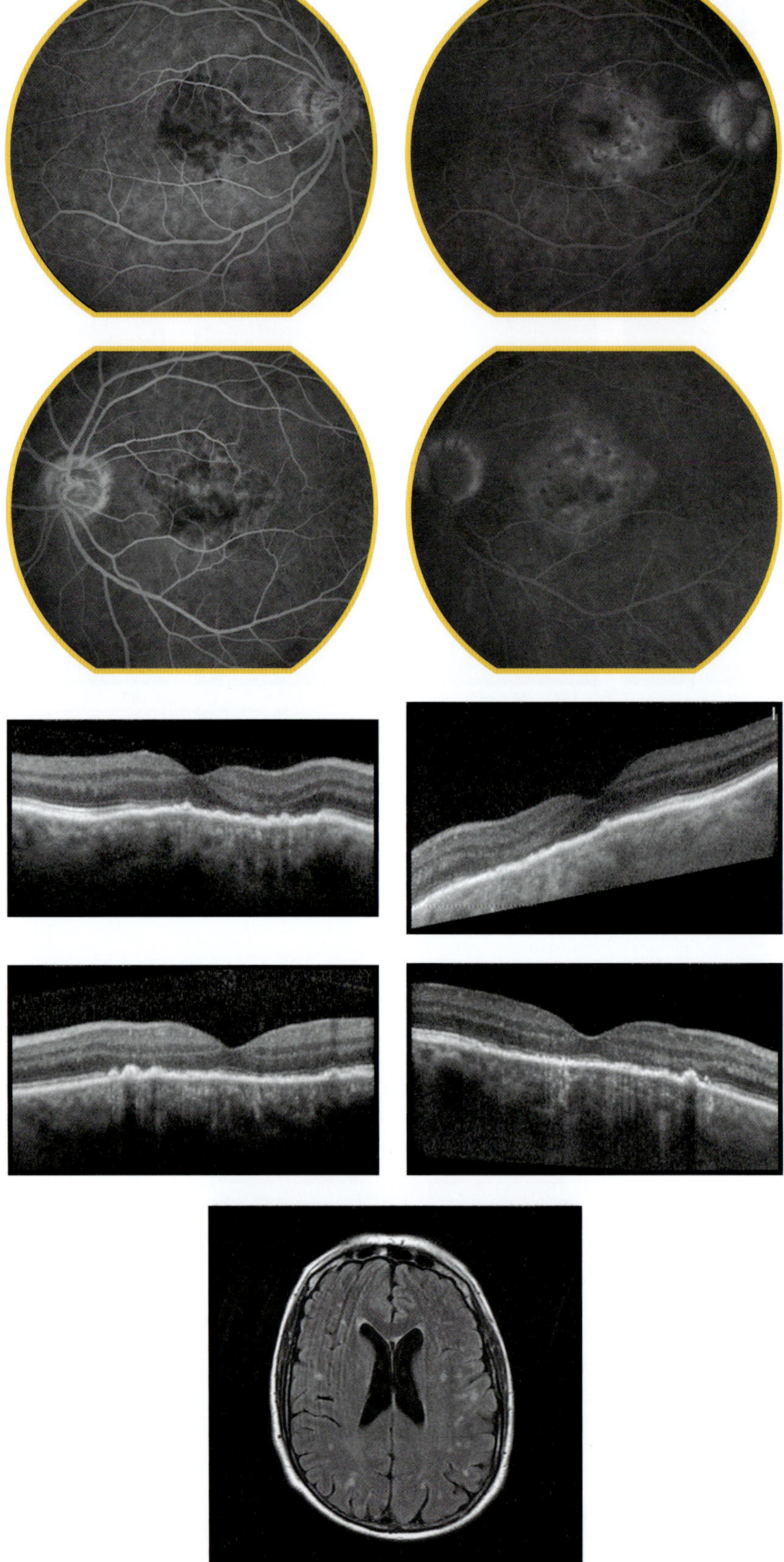

This 68-year-old man presented with eye pain and a floater in his left eye. Fluorescein angiogram of the right and left eyes illustrates macular lesions that block early and stain late *(first and second row)*. SD-OCT images of the right and left eyes show irregular elevations at the level of the RPE with overlying disruption of the ellipsoid band and a thickened choroid. The patient was started on oral steroids but presented to the emergency room complaining of decreased coordination shortly after. MRI of the brain illustrates hyperintense lesions scattered throughout the brain, but was not suggestive of cerebral vasculitis. After initiation of further immunosuppressive therapy his symptoms improved. *Images courtesy of Nicole Benitah, MD*

Serpiginous Choroiditis

Serpiginous choroiditis is a rare, usually bilateral, recurrent inflammatory chorioretinitis that affects middle-aged men or women. It remains an idiopathic entity; however, recently, many reports have demonstrated an association with tuberculosis exposure in some cases. The acute, grayish-white, subretinal lesions typically originate in the peripapillary region and localize to the outer retina, RPE, and choroid. Over time, there is gradual progression away from the nerve in a helicoid or serpiginous manner, often toward the macula. Chronic lesions show pigmentary changes and fibrous atrophy. New lesions often originate from the margin of older lesions as finger-like extensions. Occasionally, the disorder may originate in the macula, in which case it may be referred to as "macular serpiginous." CNV is a common complication of serpiginous choroiditis. A vitritis is seen in approximately one-third of cases. Retinal vasculitis and branch retinal artery and vein occlusions have been reported in some cases.

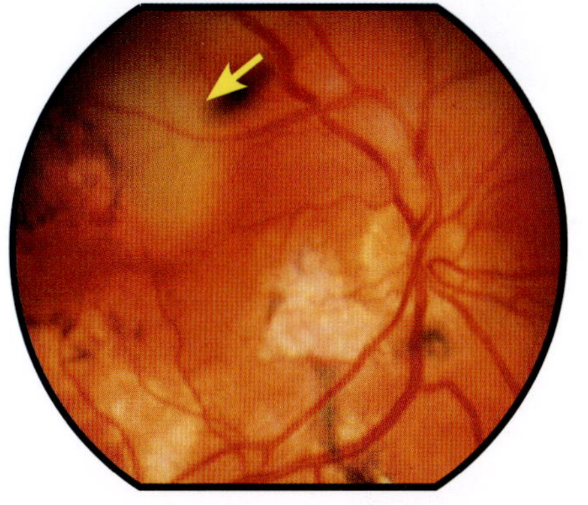

This patient has serpiginous choroidopathy. Note the pigmentary changes consistent with chronic serpiginous disease. Also note the fluffy whitish-yellow lesion superiorly that represents an active recurrence *(arrow)*.

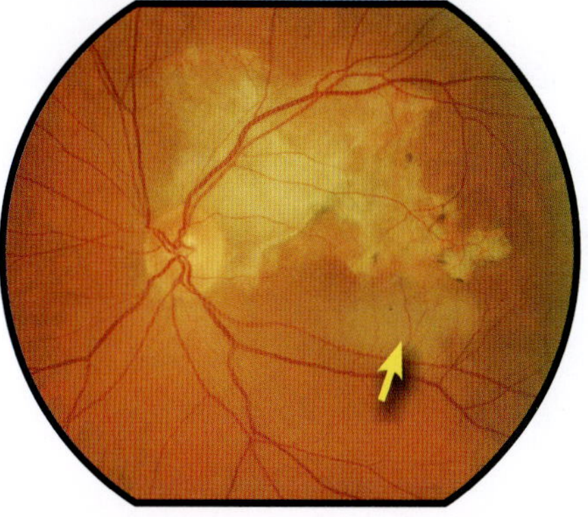

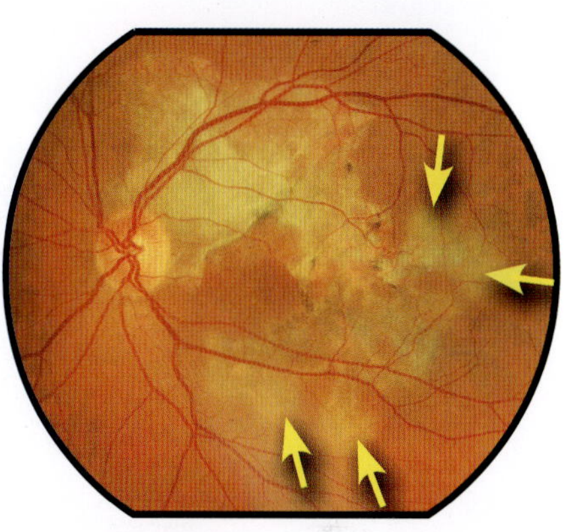

This patient shows atrophy and fibrosis originating from the peripapillary area in a serpiginous-like pattern. Note the acute fluffy white lesion at the inferior border of the lesion *(arrow in the left image)*, which represents a recurrence. Approximately 2 months later, the acute lesion has resolved with atrophy and scarring, and additional acute lesions have developed *(arrows in the right image)*. *Courtesy of Dr. Stuart L. Fine*

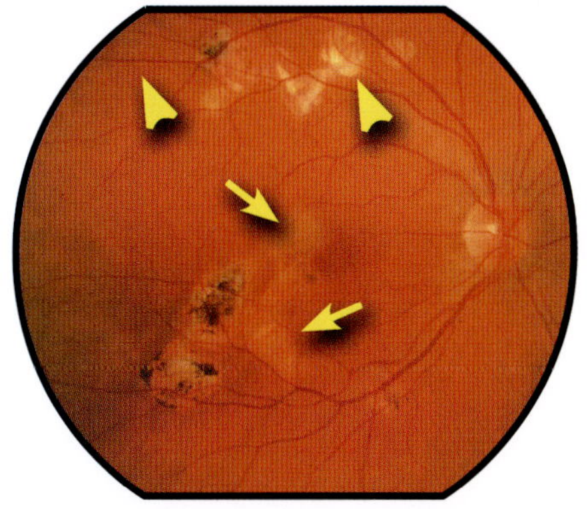

This patient with serpiginous choroidopathy demonstrates an acute lesion *(arrows)* near the central macula. There are multiple foci of chorioretinal scarring. Note the satellite or "skip" lesions *(arrowheads)*, which are common in this disorder.

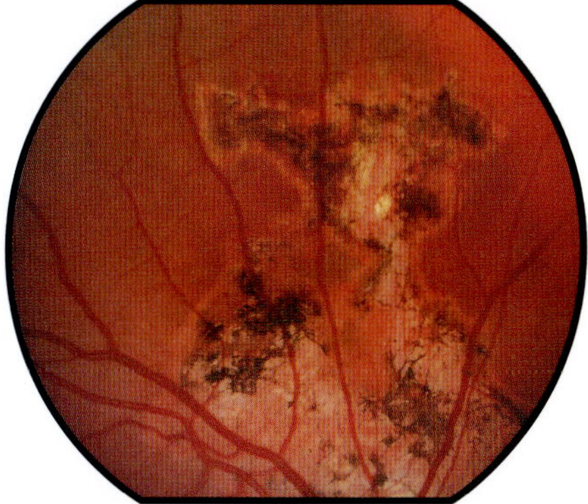

The chronic stage of serpiginous choroidopathy with atrophic and pigmented chorioretinal scars can be seen in this patient. Note that the choroidal vasculature can be observed because of the overlying atrophy.

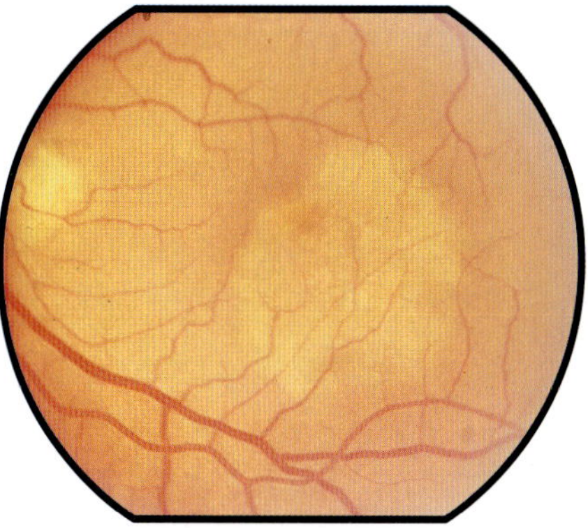

Serpiginous choroidopathy may begin anywhere. This patient has solitary serpiginous choroiditis that started in the macular region (macular serpiginous). *Courtesy of Dr. Maurice Rabb, University of Illinois at Chicago*

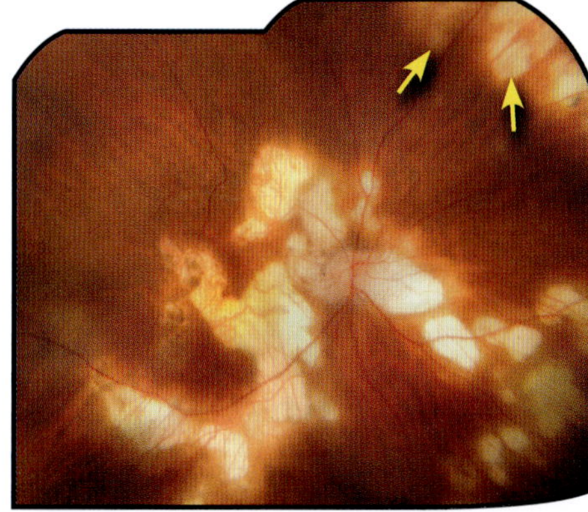

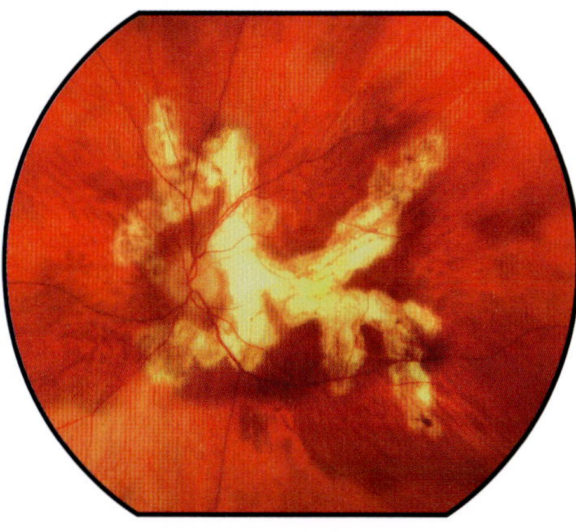

This patient with serpiginous choroidopathy shows the characteristic geographic, progressive, serpiginoid extension of the process from the disc into the macula and beyond in each eye. There are skip lesions in the periphery of the right eye *(left image, arrows)*.

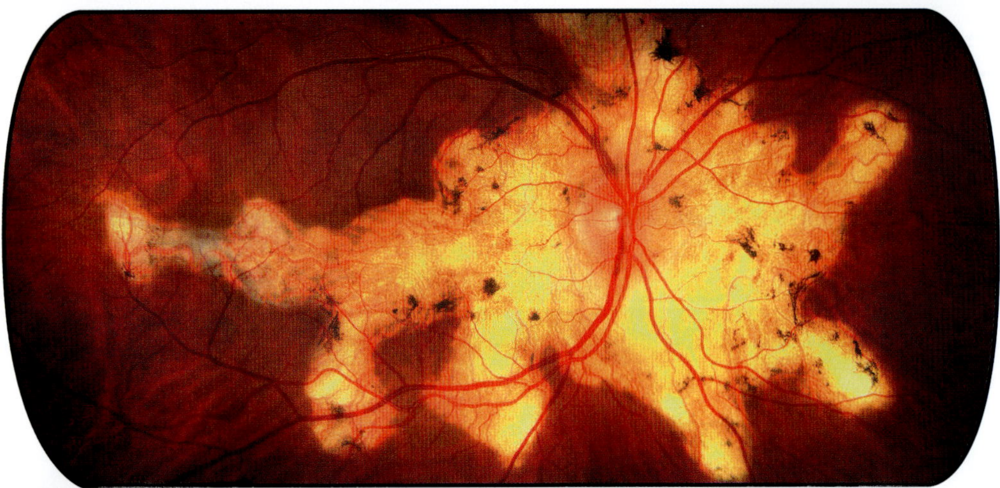

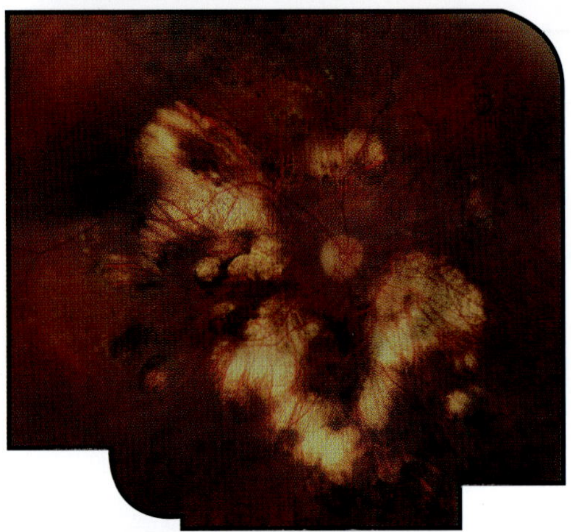

These are two additional patients with serpiginous choroidopathy that show a variation in the geometric pattern, commonly referred to as "jigsaw" in nature.

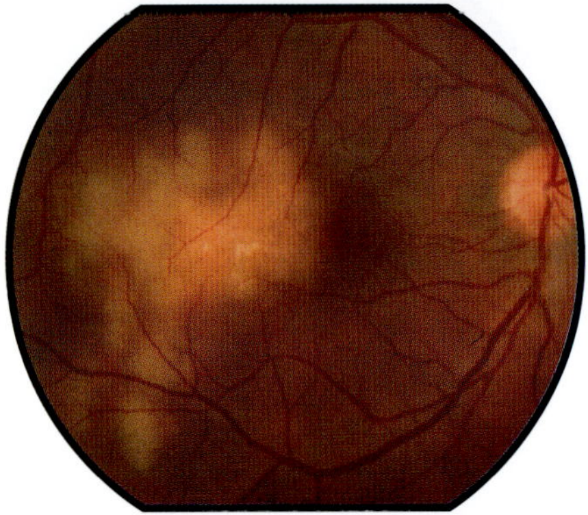

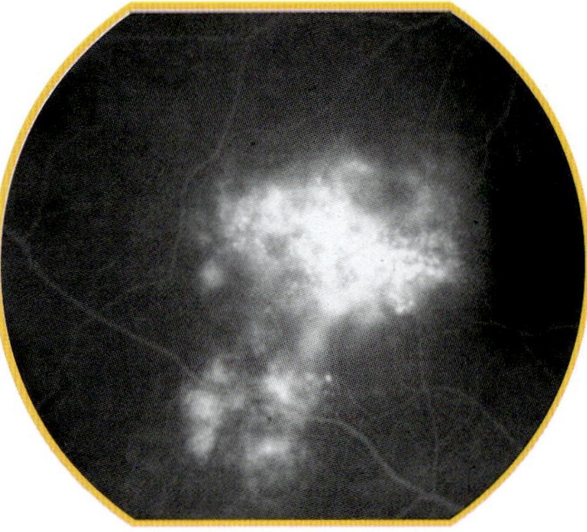

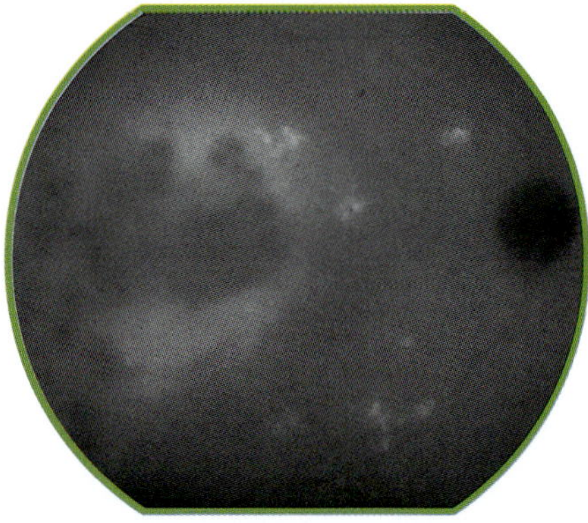

This patient illustrates recurrent serpiginous choroidopathy surrounding a central primary lesion that had healed. The fluorescein angiogram shows staining of the original lesion *(middle)*. An ICG angiogram shows additional multifocal areas of choroidal staining that could represent quiescent lesions *(right)*.

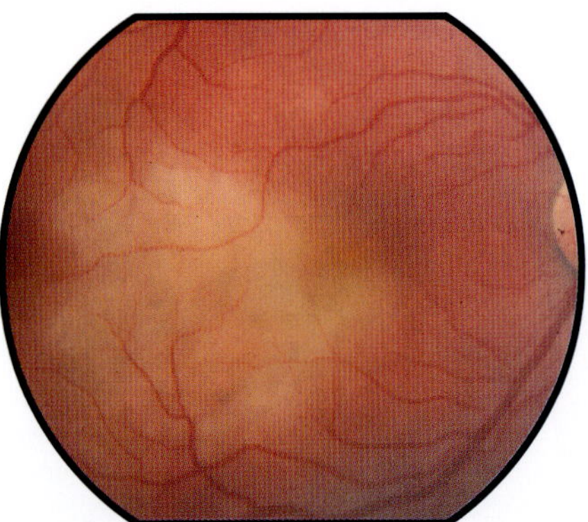

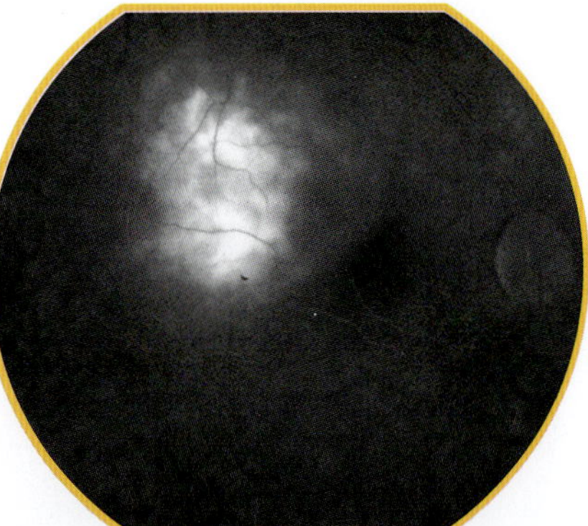

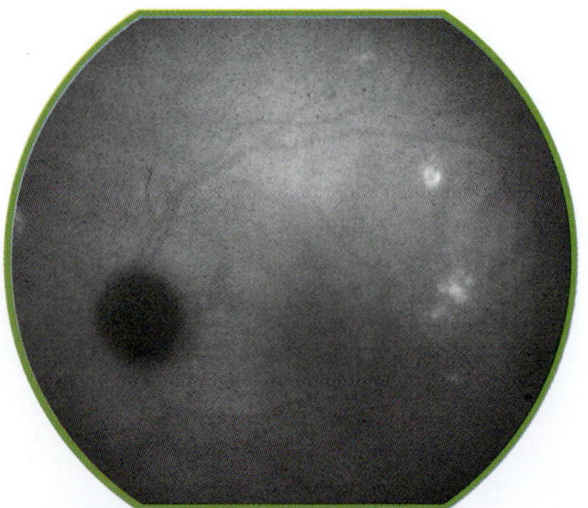

In this patient with acute serpiginous choroidopathy, there is a geographic lesion noted with color fundus photography *(left)* and FA *(middle)*. The ICG study shows additional multifocal areas of staining in the temporal region of the fellow left eye that were not evident clinically or with FA. These foci may represent occult lesions that have not yet become active.

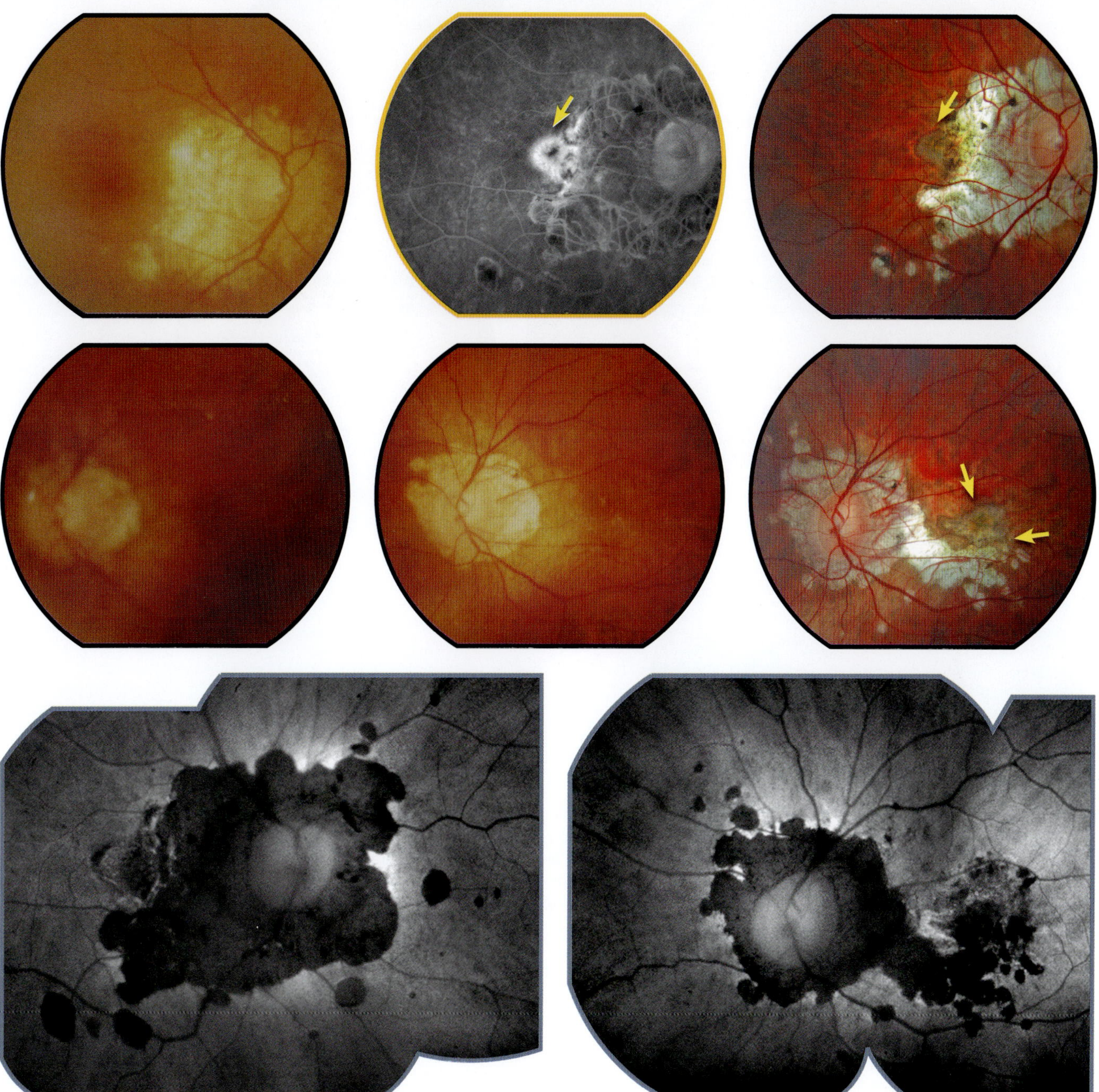

This patient with serpiginous choroidopathy initially showed a peripapillary lesion in each eye. Over a period of several years, he experienced chronic and/or recurrent acute attacks with extension of the serpiginoid atrophy into the macular region of each eye. He subsequently developed secondary CNV *(arrows)* in each eye, which is not uncommon in this disorder. The fundus autofluorescence more clearly delineates the hypofluorescent atrophic pattern and multiple skip lesions throughout the fundus.

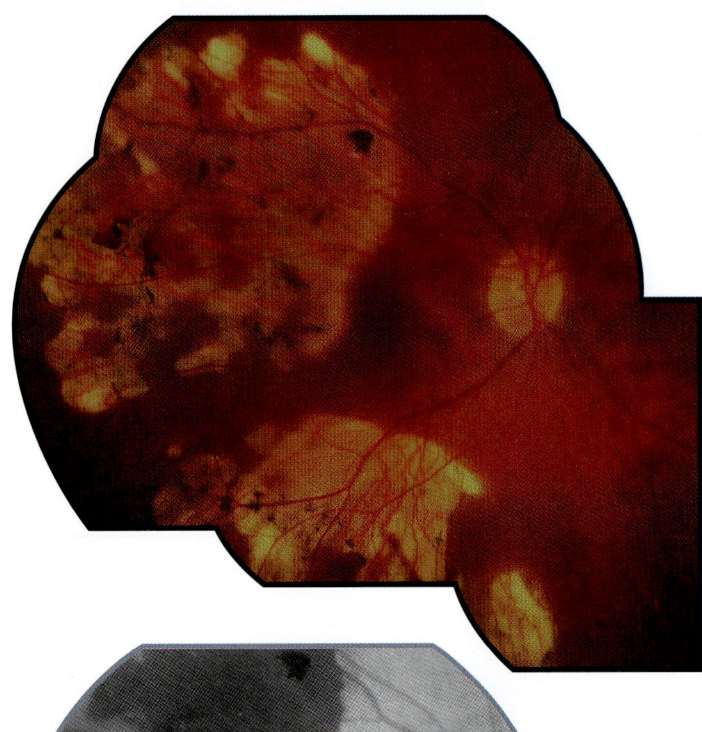

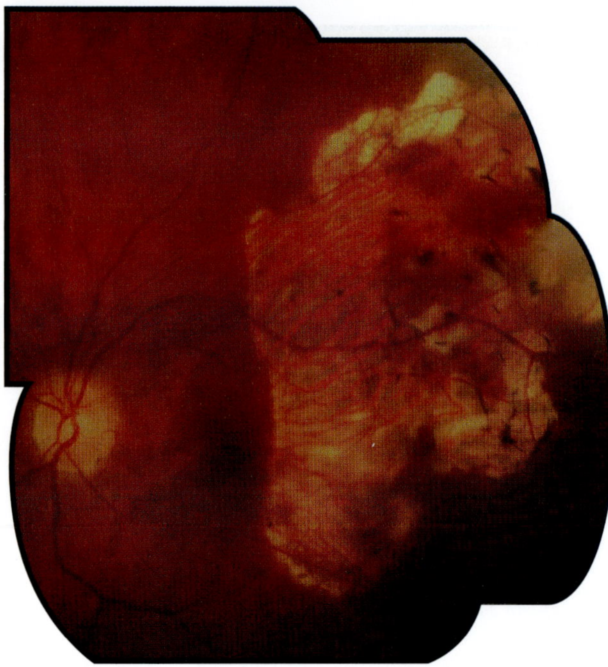

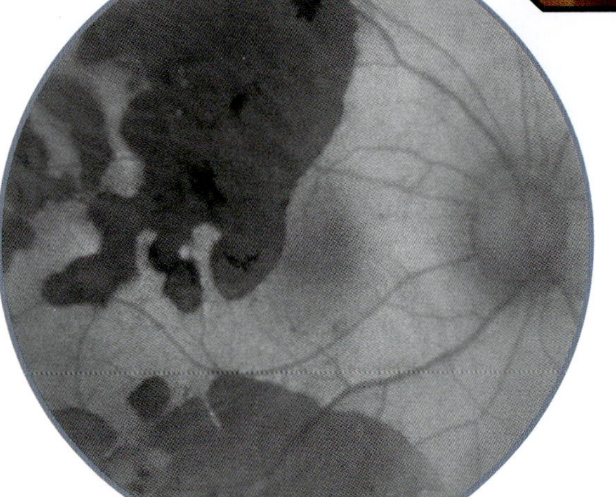

This patient has serpiginous choroidopathy with multiple large atrophic lesions in the right eye and a single substantial atrophic lesion in the left eye. There is fibrous scarring and pigmentary degeneration in each eye. Fundus autofluorescence shows the sharp demarcation line between the hypofluorescent atrophic lesions and normal retina in this disease.

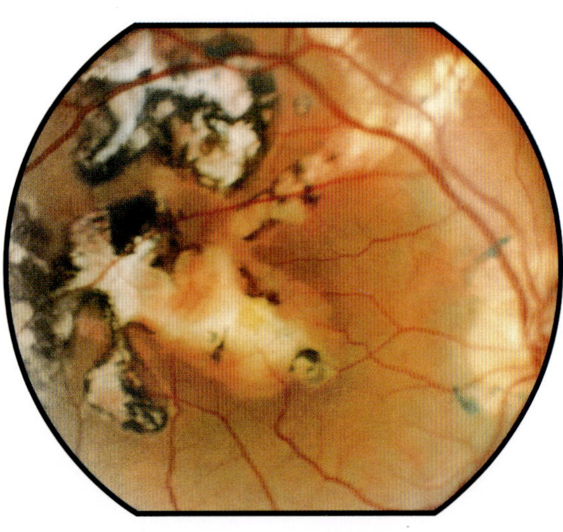

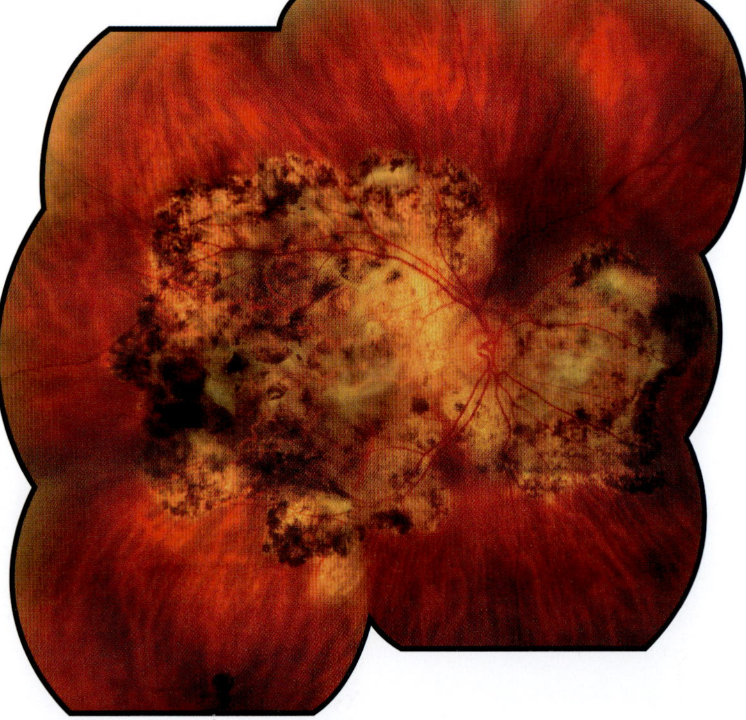

These patients with serpiginous choroidopathy demonstrate the severe pigmentary and atrophic degeneration and fibrous scarring that may occur in this inflammatory disorder.

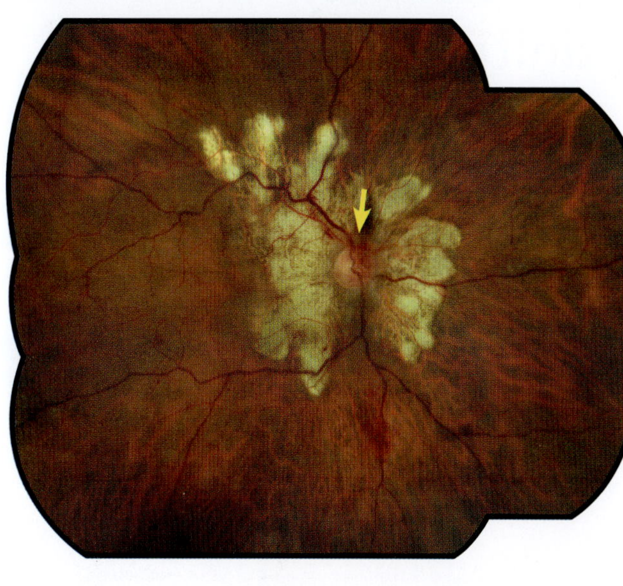

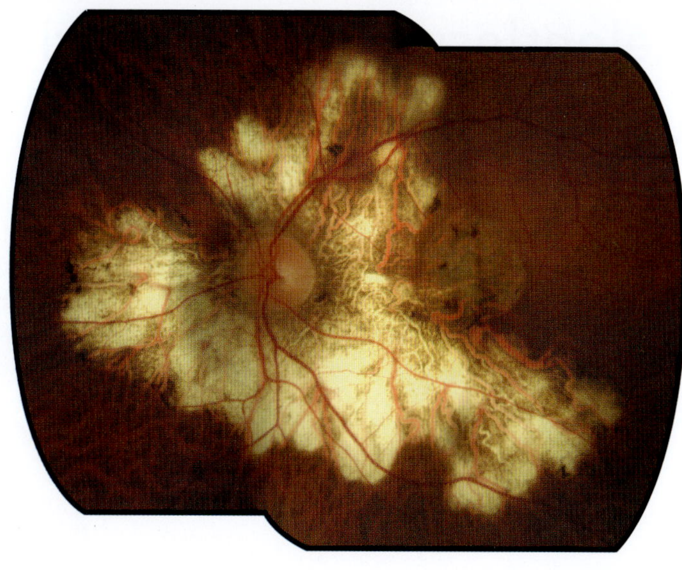

This patient has had serpiginous choroidopathy for 33 years. Progressive atrophy has extended into the fovea of the left eye and is causing severe central vision loss to 20/200. In the right eye, he experienced a sudden change in vision, secondary to CRVO. There are a few scattered hemorrhages throughout the fundus and tortuosity of the retinal veins and hemorrhage over the disc (*arrow*). *Right image courtesy of Dr. Edward Eagan*

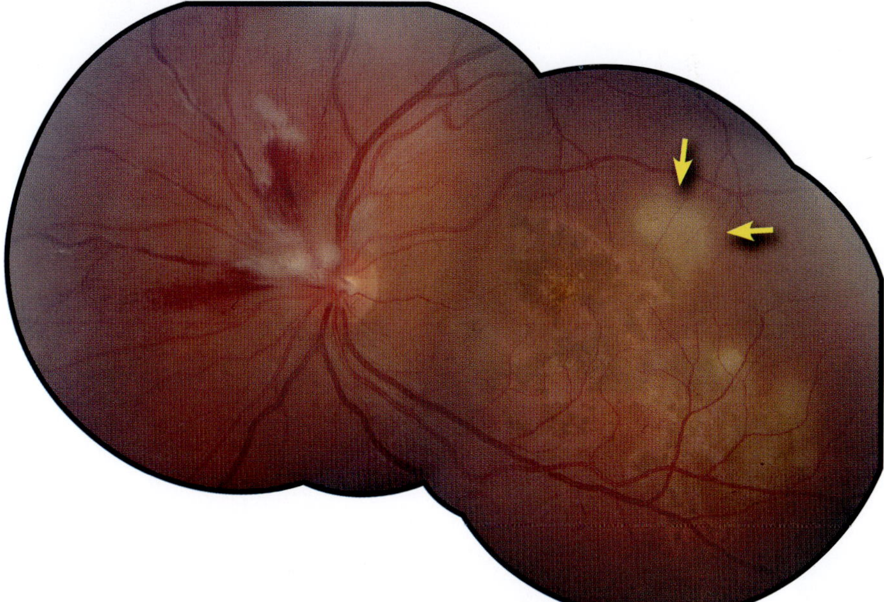

This patient illustrates recurrent serpiginous choroiditis *(arrows)*. Note the associated papillitis, retinal phlebitis, and nasal retinal vein occlusion. Although rare, retinal venous occlusive disease is known to occur in serpiginous choroidopathy, as the subretinal inflammatory process may extend into the retina to produce a focal retinitis and retinal vascular obstruction (not necessarily at an arteriolar-venular crossing). *Courtesy of Dr. George Williams*

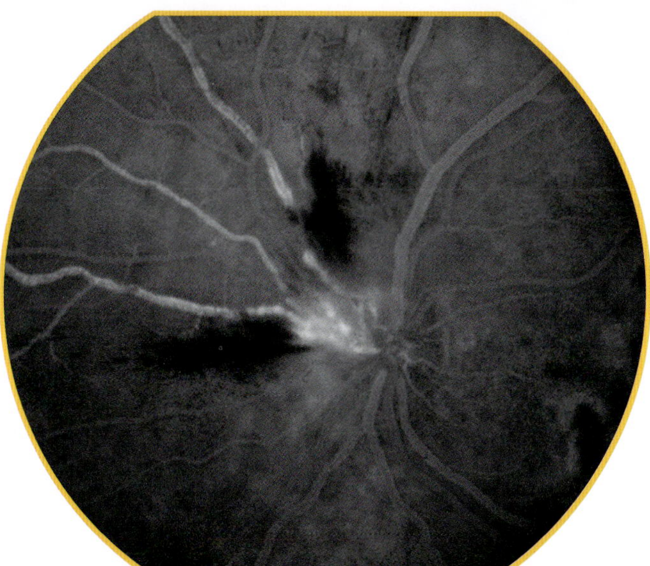

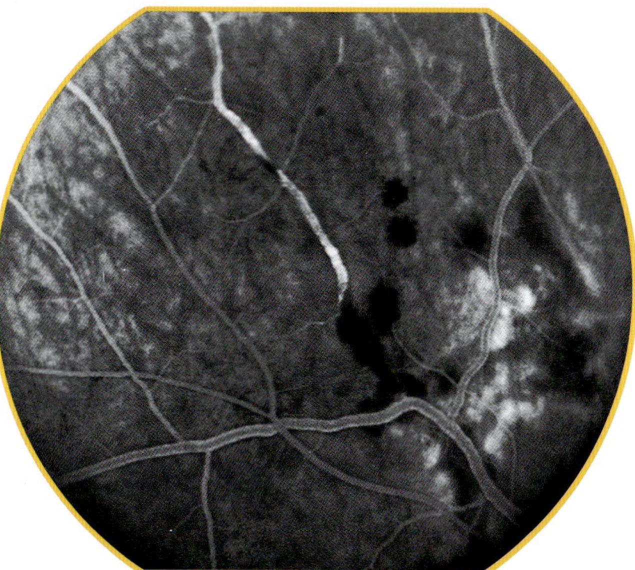

Relentless Placoid Chorioretinitis (Ampiginous Choroiditis)

Relentless placoid chorioretinitis (RPC) is a rare entity in which multiple recurrent inflammatory lesions resembling those seen in APMPPE and serpiginous choroiditis develop, usually in both eyes. Unlike APMPPE, the lesions in RPC continue to expand in size and number with a relentless course over many months. Unlike serpiginous choroiditis, the lesions of RPC are multifocal and eventually involve all areas of the retina, including the area anterior to the equator. Vitritis is commonly seen in RPC. Most patients are between 30 and 50 years of age.

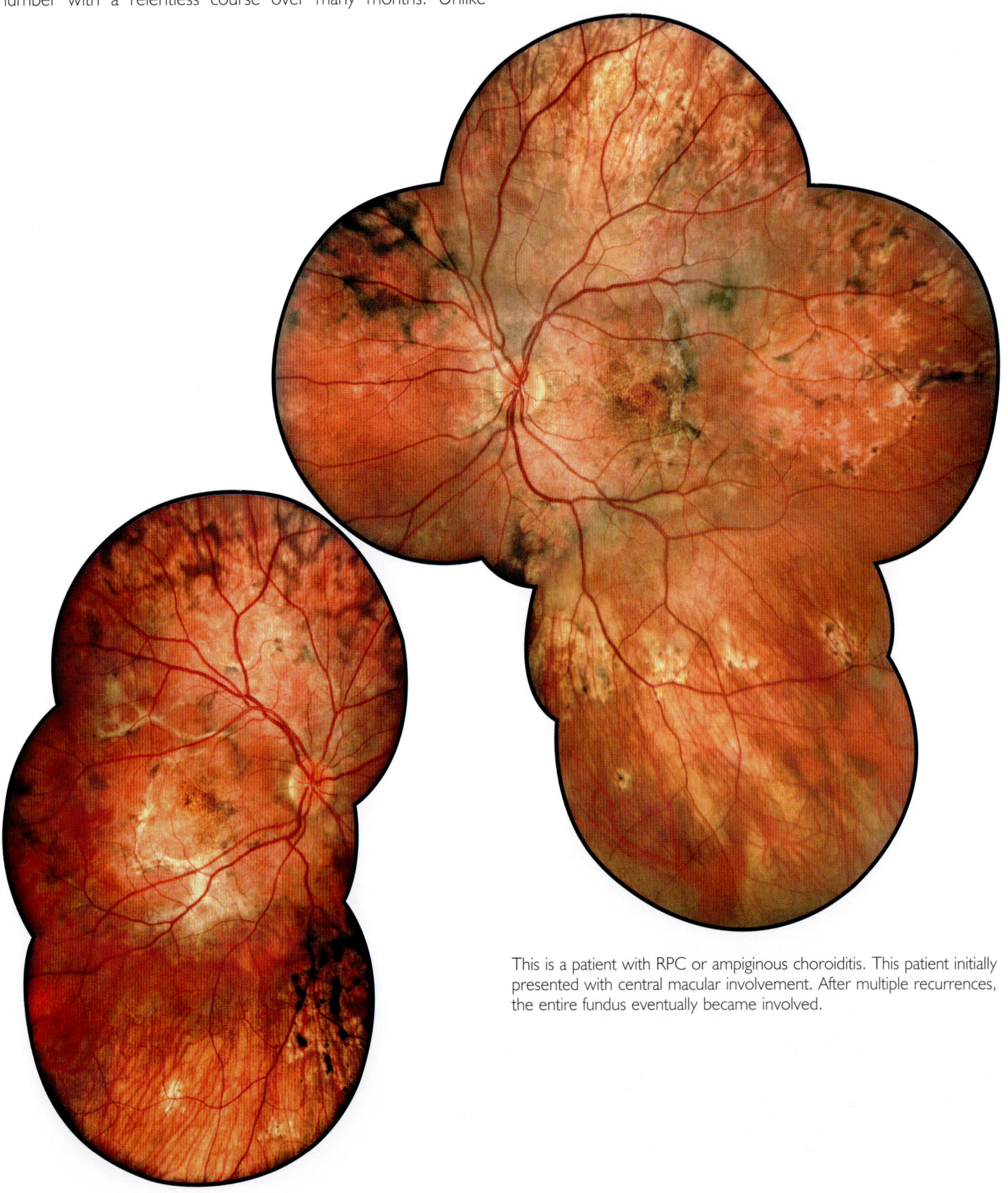

This is a patient with RPC or ampiginous choroiditis. This patient initially presented with central macular involvement. After multiple recurrences, the entire fundus eventually became involved.

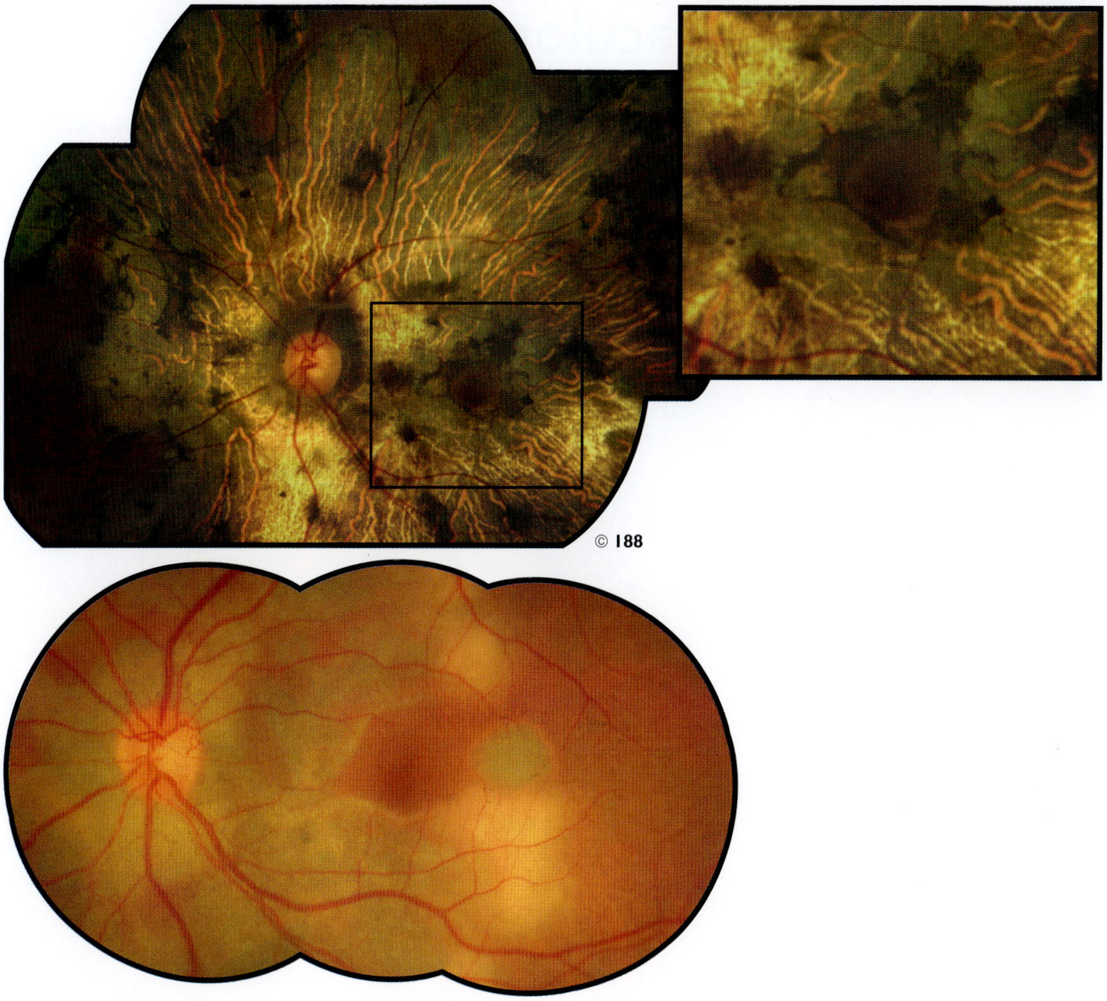

© 188

This patient also had relentless chorioretinitis with peripheral involvement in each eye. Steroids, both oral and periocular, and immunosuppressive agents were unsuccessful at halting the recurrence. Preservation of the central macula persisted for a number of years, before he was lost to follow-up. The bottom row image shows the original acute lesion in the left eye.

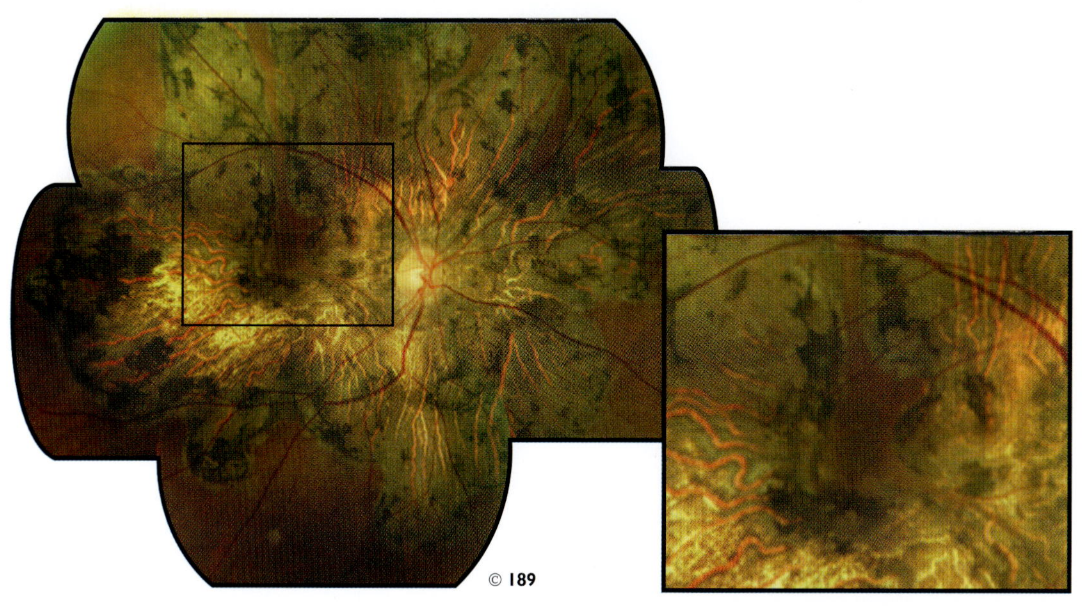

© 189

In this patient with relentless chorioretinitis there is a peculiar sparing of the fovea in each eye.

Persistent Placoid Maculopathy

Persistent placoid maculopathy (PPM) is a rare entity in which central, well-delineated, whitish plaque-like lesions remain active with persistent angiographic hypofluorescence and without resolution for weeks. Like macular serpiginous choroidopathy, the lesions are usually bilateral, but they differ in that they are more symmetric and may remain stable, but active, for extended periods. Unlike macular serpiginous choroidopathy, vision is minimally affected unless complicated by secondary CNV, which is typical in this disease.

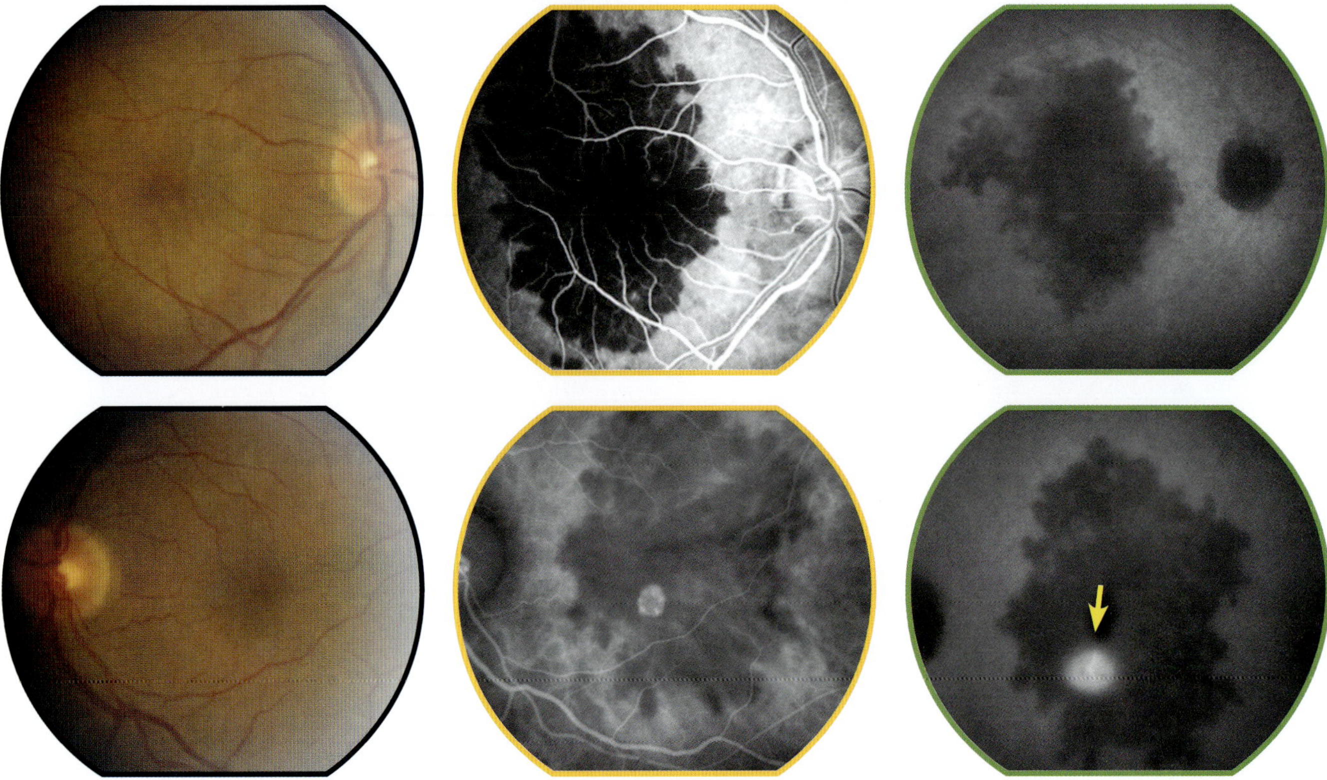

This patient developed bilateral PPM. The lesion in each macula was comparatively small but began to progress circumferentially over a period of several months in a jigsaw fashion as a placoid recurrence surrounding the edges of the initial lesion. The macula itself was flat without evidence of hemorrhage. Eventually, he developed CNV in the left eye, noted here with fluorescein and ICG angiography *(arrow)*.

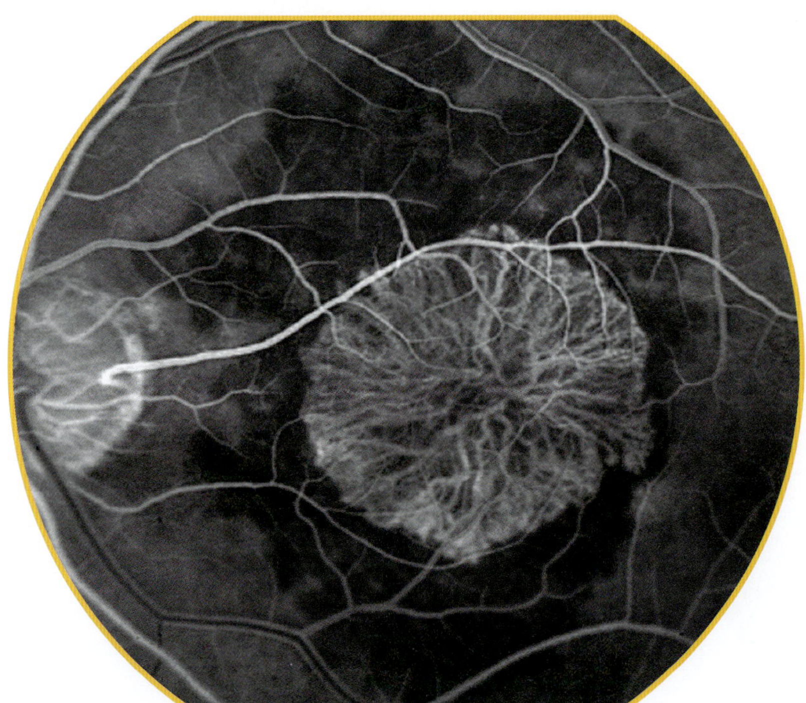

Note the very large and aggressive type 2 neovascular membrane with a classic lacy appearance with FA and an underlying large area of persistent placoid hypofluorescence very characteristic of PPM. *Courtesy of Dr. David Wilson*

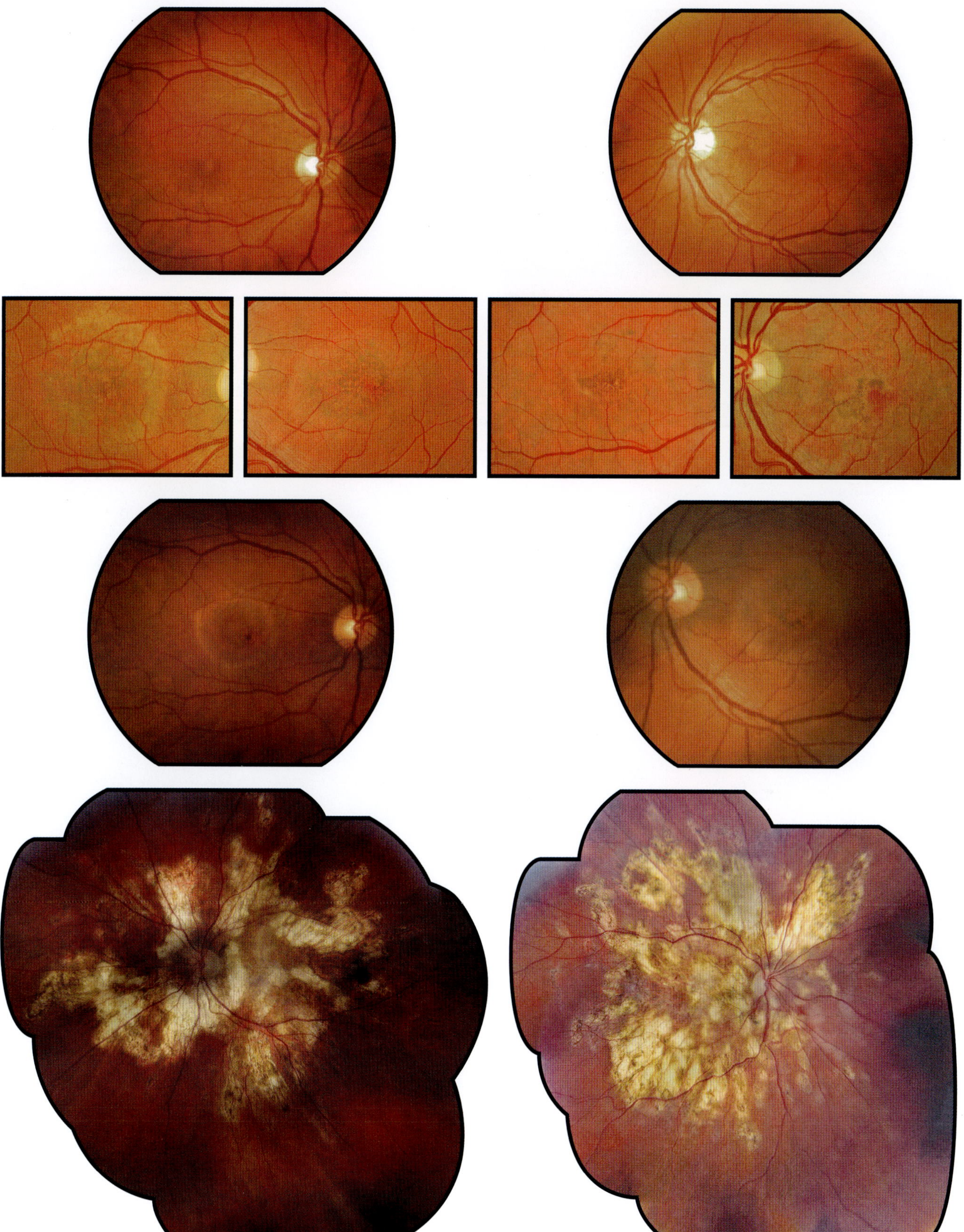

This 30-year-old male developed a visual disturbance with a focal abnormality in the foveal region of each eye. Within several months, the lesion had expanded with a pigment epithelial disturbance surrounded by a ring of creamy infiltration, best identified in the right eye *(second row left two images)*. These changes became complicated by the presence of neovascularization at the fovea *(second row right two images)*. Over a period of several months, there was a placoid pigmentary and atrophic plaque in each eye *(third row)*. Ultimately, the patient experienced chronic and/or recurrent disease that terminated in a jigsaw atrophic and pigmentary pattern, resembling serpiginous choroidopathy. In this very atypical case, a bilateral inflammatory disease presented as a plaque-like bilateral disturbance similar to persistent placoid choroidopathy, but ended with a typical disease pattern as seen in serpiginous choroidopathy. This emphasizes the similarities between the two diseases and the challenge in making an accurate diagnosis in some patients. *Courtesy of Dr. Jim Vander*

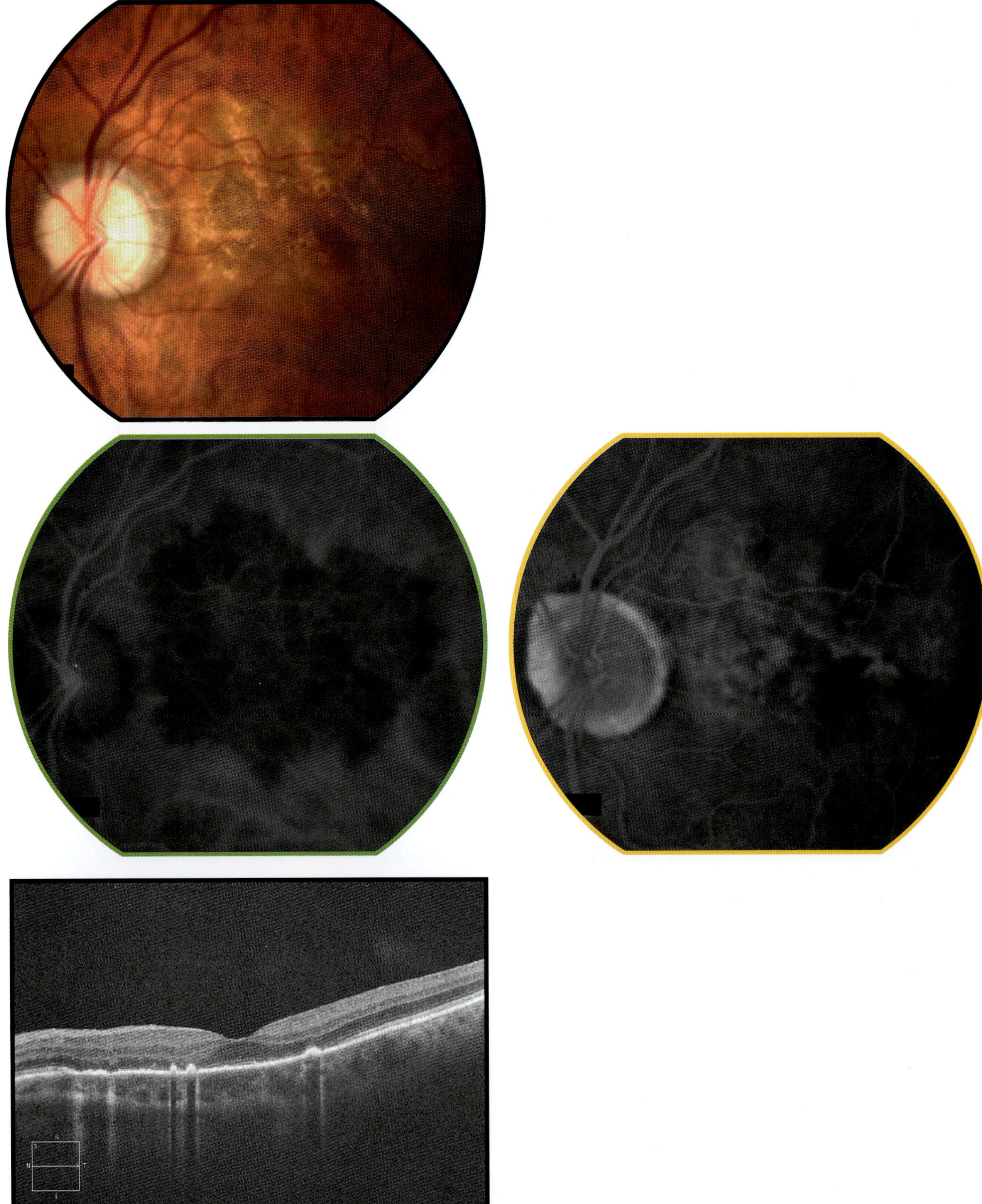

This patient presented with a central scotoma of the left eye. Color fundus photo at the time of presentation *(top)* illustrates a yellow, creamy appearing plaque involving the macula. ICG angiogram at the time of presentation shows a hypofluorescent macular lesion that persisted late into the study *(second row, left)*. Fluorescein angiogram blocks early and stains late *(second row, right)*. SD-OCT at the same time *(third row)* shows an irregularly thickened RPE with patchy ellipsoid loss. The patient had persistent vision loss without resolution of the macular lesion and therefore an intravitreal triamcinolone injection was administered. *Images courtesy of Mark Walsh, MD*

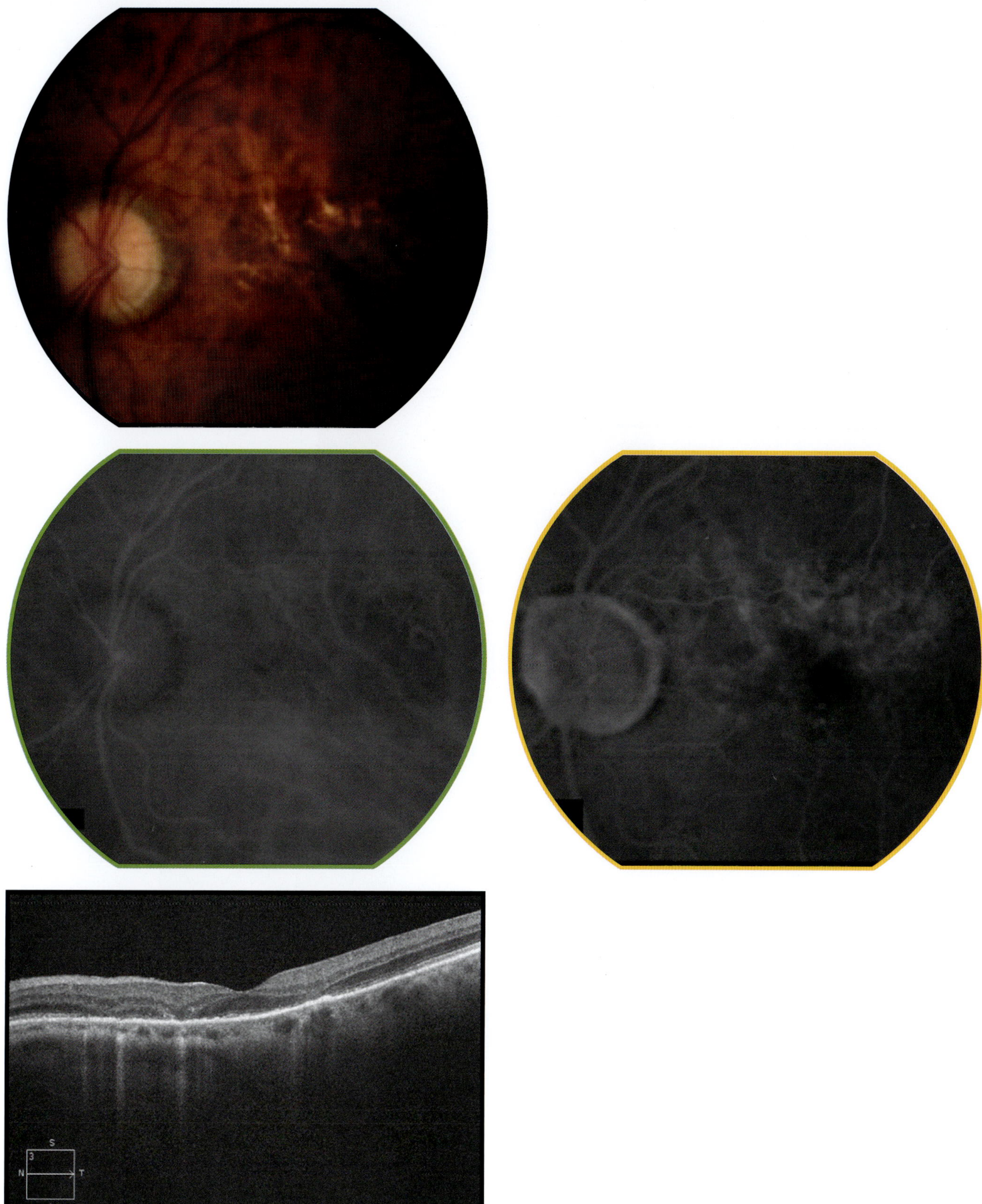

Five months later, visual acuity improved. Color fundus photos at follow-up *(top row)* illustrate more evidence of macular scarring. Note a persistent hypofluorescence with ICG angiography *(second row, left)* consistent with a diagnosis of PPM. There is late staining of the lesion with FA *(second row, right)* and persistent abnormalities at the level of the RPE and inner and outer segments on SD-OCT *(bottom)*. *Images courtesy of Mark Walsh, MD*

Birdshot Chorioretinopathy

Birdshot chorioretinopathy is a rare, chronic, bilateral inflammatory disorder in which multiple cream-colored depigmented lesions are scattered throughout the fundus, mostly in the postequatorial region. Patients are usually healthy men or women in their third to sixth decade of life. Essentially 100% of patients carry a particular variant of human leukocyte antigen (HLA) A29, making this the strongest of any known HLA-disease association. Patients often present with vitreous floaters and reduction of vision especially in low-light conditions, but with minimal discomfort. The characteristic round or ovoid spots localize to the choroid and may often follow the larger choroidal vessels. Patients may have other ocular inflammatory findings including vitritis and optic disc edema. The anterior segment is most often free of significant inflammatory changes though a mild anterior uveitis may be present. Secondary cystoid macular edema related to increased capillary permeability is commonly responsible for vision loss in these patients. Secondary CNV and vitreous hemorrhage due to retinal neovascularization may also occur. Retinal breaks and detachments, as well as posterior subcapsular cataracts are commonly seen. In long-standing disease, there may be widespread chorioretinal atrophy although pigmentary degeneration is atypical.

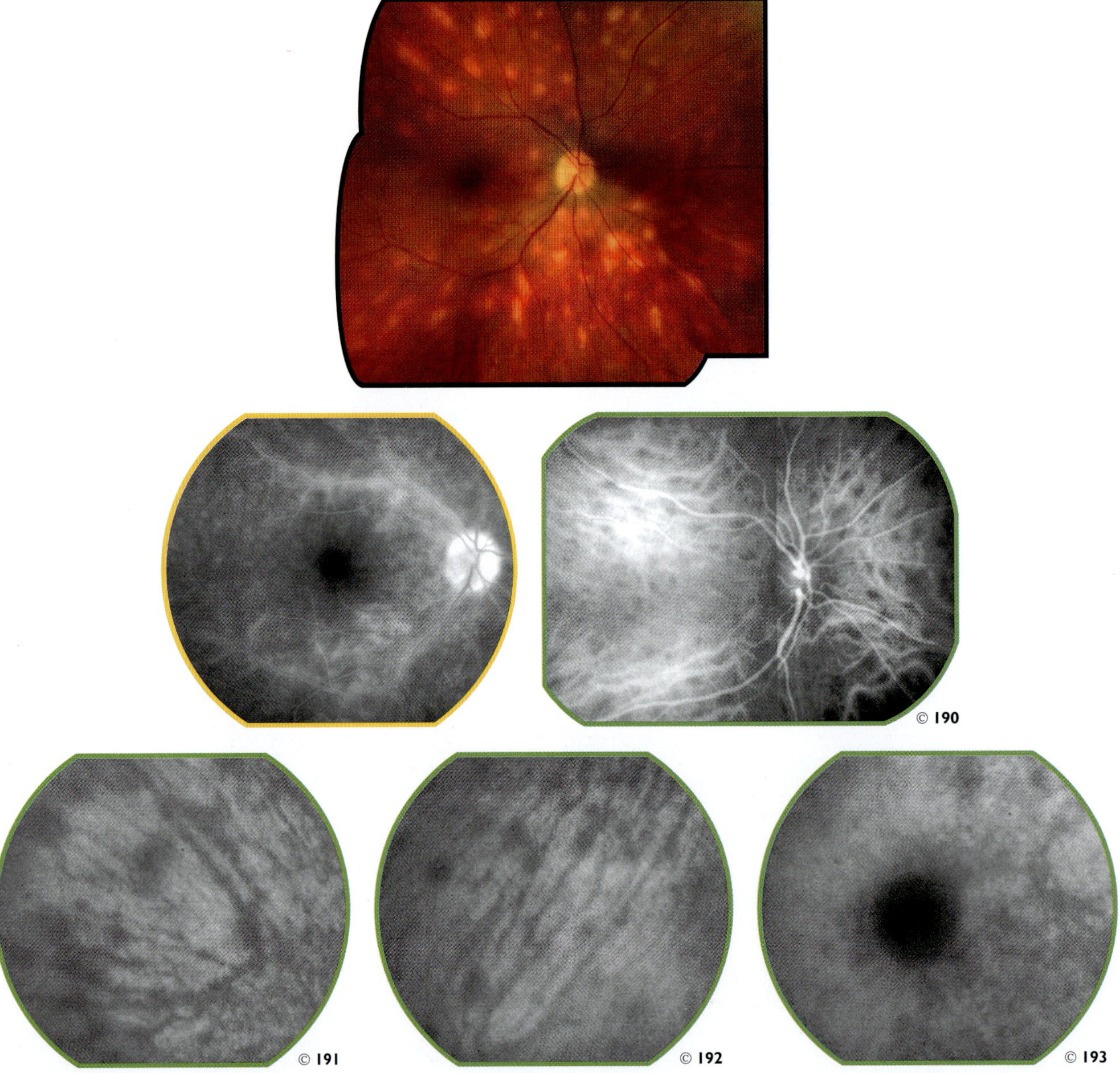

This patient has a birdshot chorioretinopathy with oval, circular and flat areas of depigmentation. Note the absence of associated fibrosis or pigmentary hyperplastic change in these lesions, which is typical. Infiltrates conform to the choroidal circulation, converging on the macula from the periphery. The fluorescein angiogram *(middle left)* illustrates retinal vascular leakage, while the spots faintly stain late in the study. ICG angiography shows numerous choroidal lesions not evident on clinical or fluorescein angiographic examination seen in the same patient *(middle right)*. The periphery also shows scattered lesions, which line up along and adhere to the choroidal vessels (choroidotropic). There is also a peripapillary, irregular cluster of (papillotropic) hypofluorescent spots *(bottom row right)*.

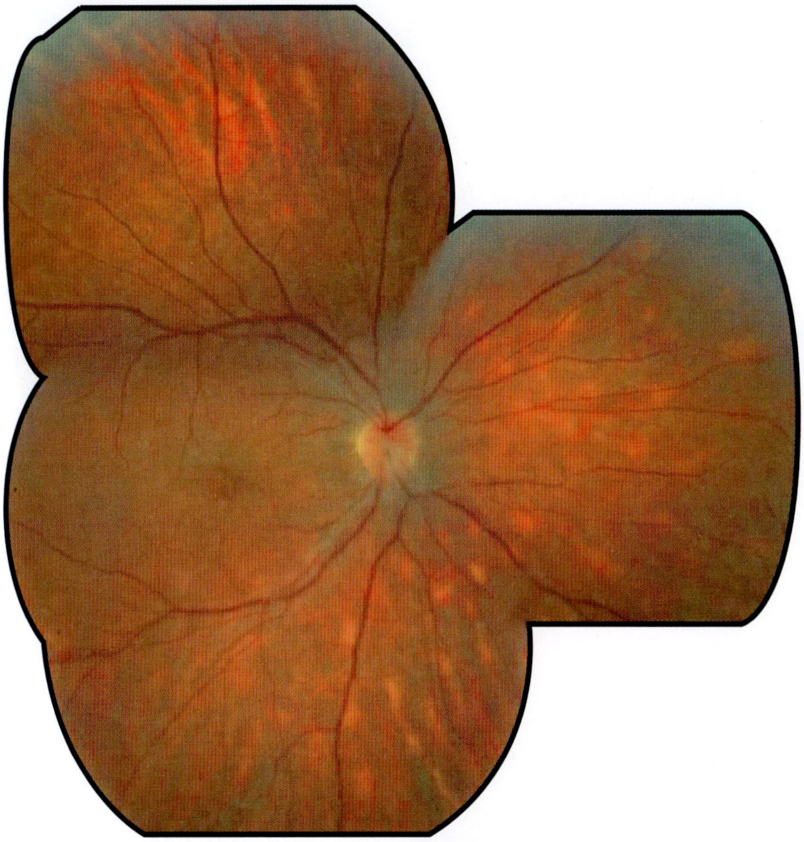

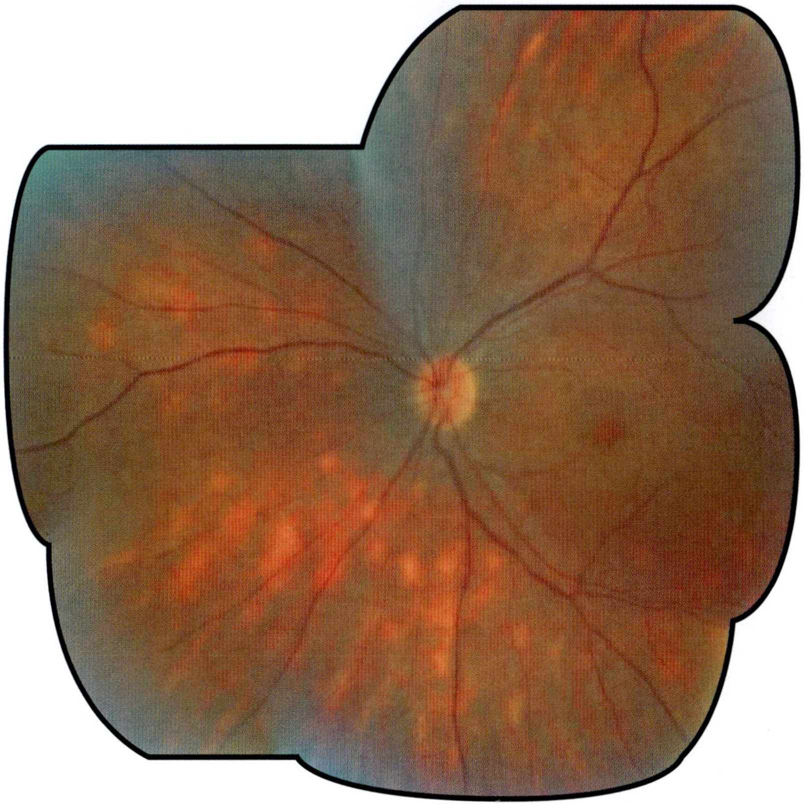

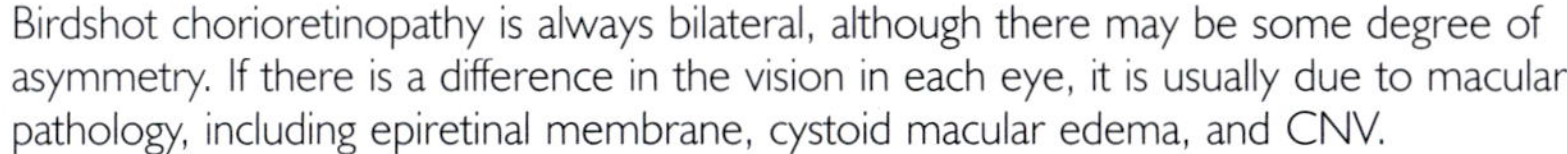

Birdshot chorioretinopathy is always bilateral, although there may be some degree of asymmetry. If there is a difference in the vision in each eye, it is usually due to macular pathology, including epiretinal membrane, cystoid macular edema, and CNV.

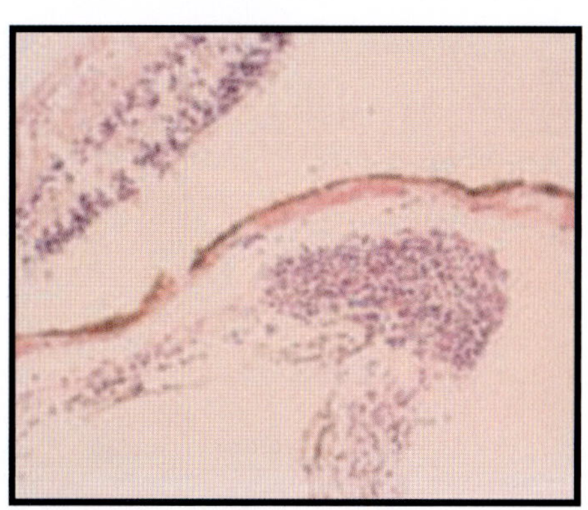

© 194

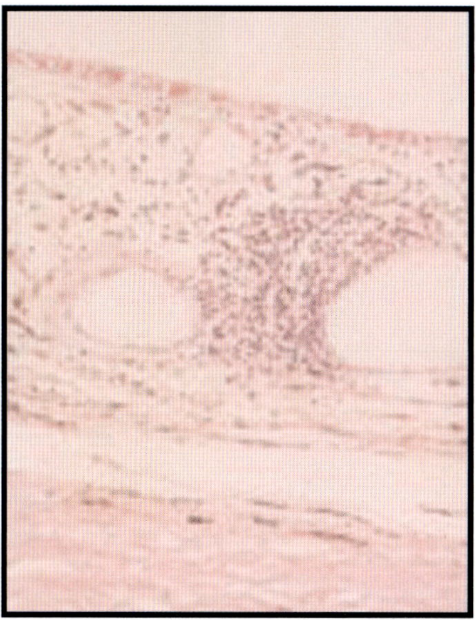

© 195

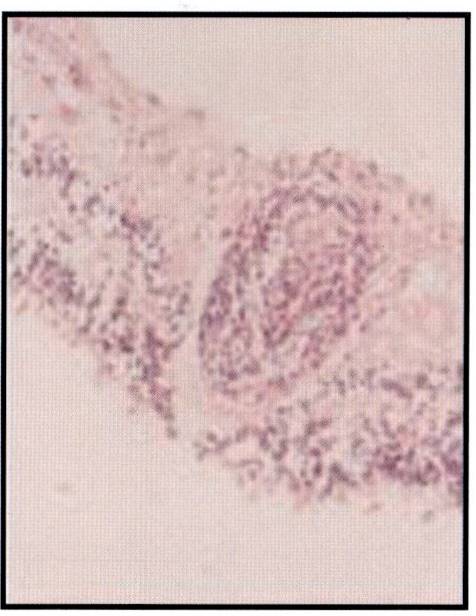

© 196

This patient was diagnosed with birdshot chorioretinopathy and the histopathology shows foci of lymphocytic aggregation in the deep choroid with additional foci in the optic nerve head and along the retinal vasculature without involvement of the RPE and outer retina.

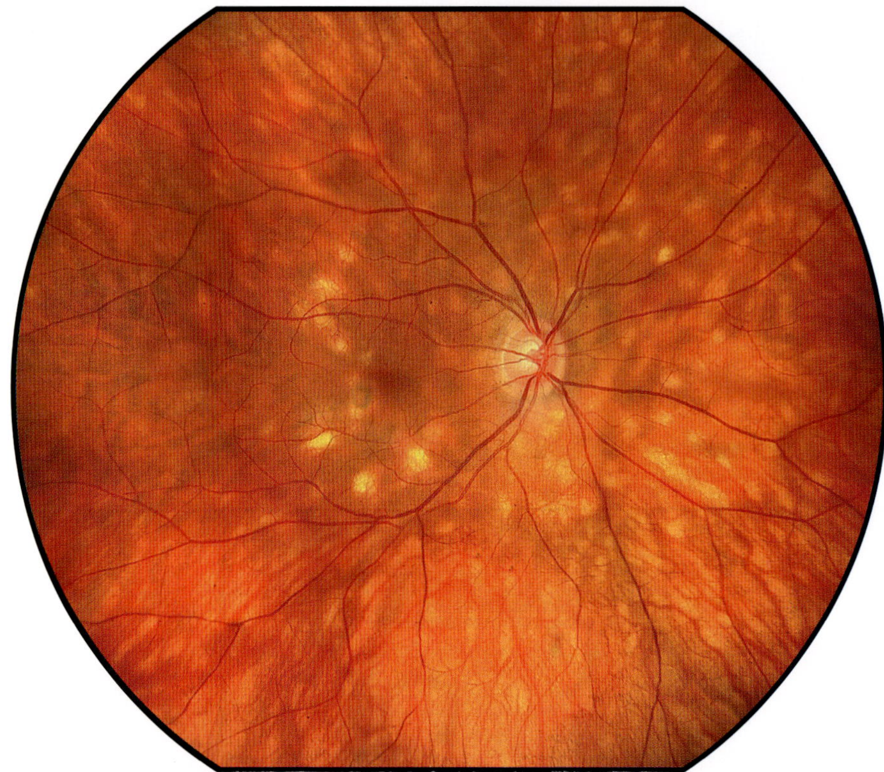

This patient with birdshot chorioretinopathy has begun to develop some confluency of the lesions, forming linear atrophic areas. Diffuse chorioretinal atrophy is a late-onset factor that leads to electroretinographic decline, nyctalopia, and field loss. ERG and formal visual field analysis can be important modalities in order to assess disease progression and response to therapy as progressive vision loss can be insidious.

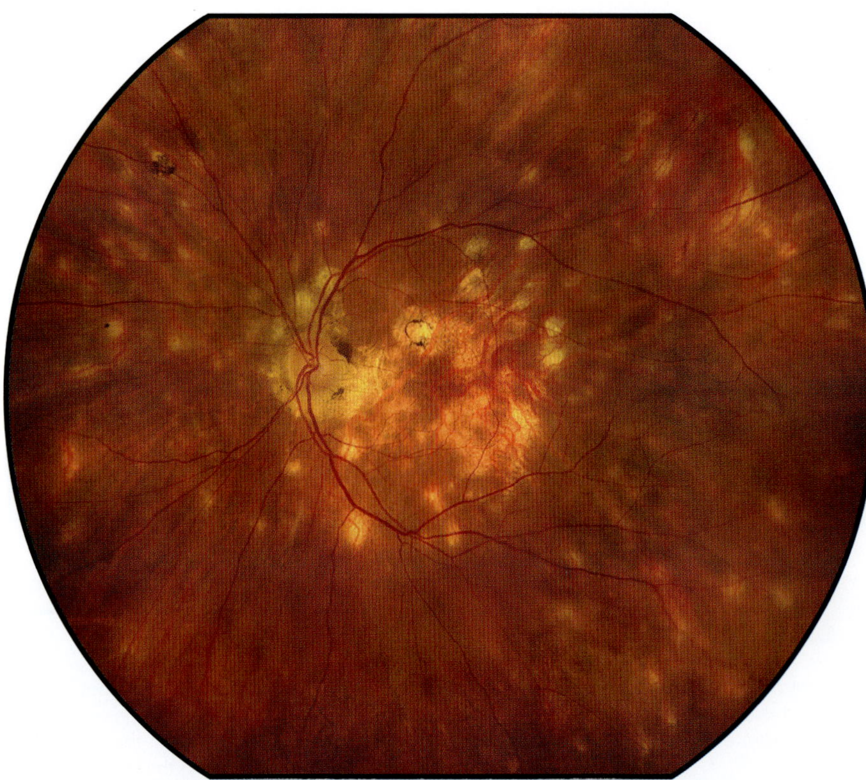

This patient has birdshot chorioretinopathy with chorioretinal atrophic spots that contain pigmentation. This is an atypical presentation that is seen only in long-standing disease or in eyes with concomitant pathology from other disorders. Note the presence of severe macular atrophy.

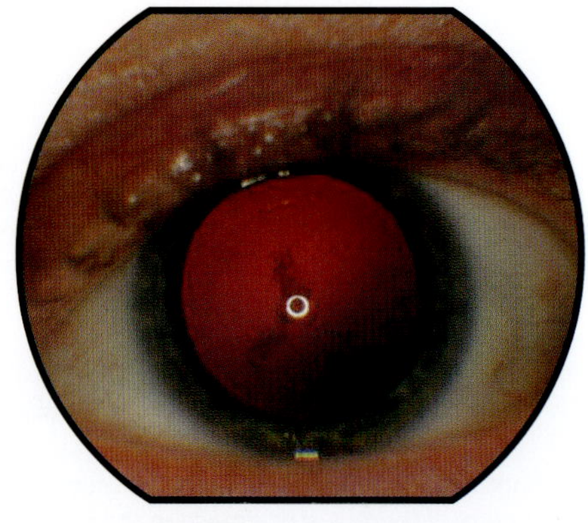

Patients may also lose vision from posterior subcapsular cataract due to inflammation in the vitreous and/or from the treatment, which is generally steroid therapy versus immunosuppressive drugs that are commonly employed to manage this progressive disorder.

Macular Manifestations in Birdshot Chorioretinopathy

Patients may develop numerous macular complications in birdshot chorioretinopathy, including epiretinal membrane, chorioretinal atrophy, CNV, and most commonly, cystoid macular edema.

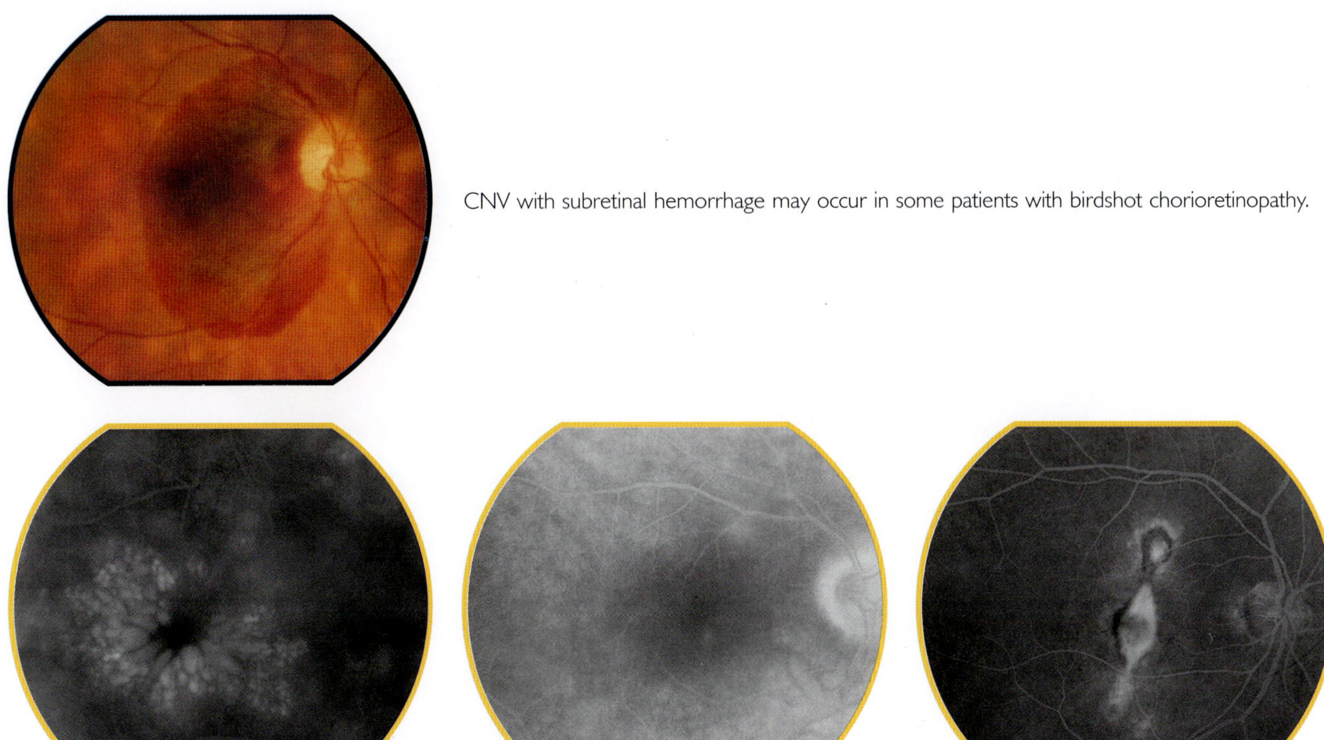

CNV with subretinal hemorrhage may occur in some patients with birdshot chorioretinopathy.

This patient developed petaloid cystoid macular edema with birdshot *(left)*. This is the most visually significant manifestation that affects vision, although epiretinal membrane may actually be more common. Following steroid treatment, there was resolution of the edema and improvement of the vision *(middle)*. The patient on the right developed CNV.

Diseases Simulating Birdshot Chorioretinopathy

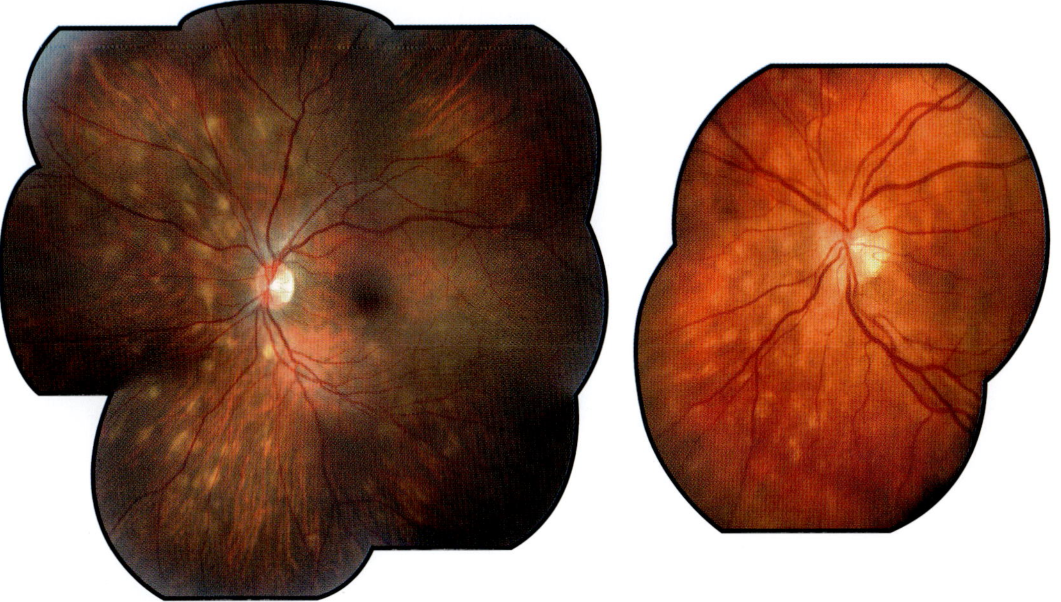

If there is pathology in the fundus that resembles birdshot chorioretinopathy, but the condition is unilateral in nature, it is most likely due to another process. The patient on the left has choroidal infiltrates due to mucosal-associated lymphoid tumor (MALT) infiltration of the left eye or reactive lymphoid hyperplasia with lesions simulating birdshot. In the patient on the right, there are unilateral spots with a choroidotropic pattern in the left eye highly suggestive of birdshot chorioretinopathy. The patient was A29 positive but also was noted to have sarcoidosis.

Birdshot Chorioretinopathy and Chorioretinal Atrophy

Chronic long-standing birdshot chorioretinopathy may lead to severe diffuse atrophy and intervening pigmentary proliferation in the fundus.

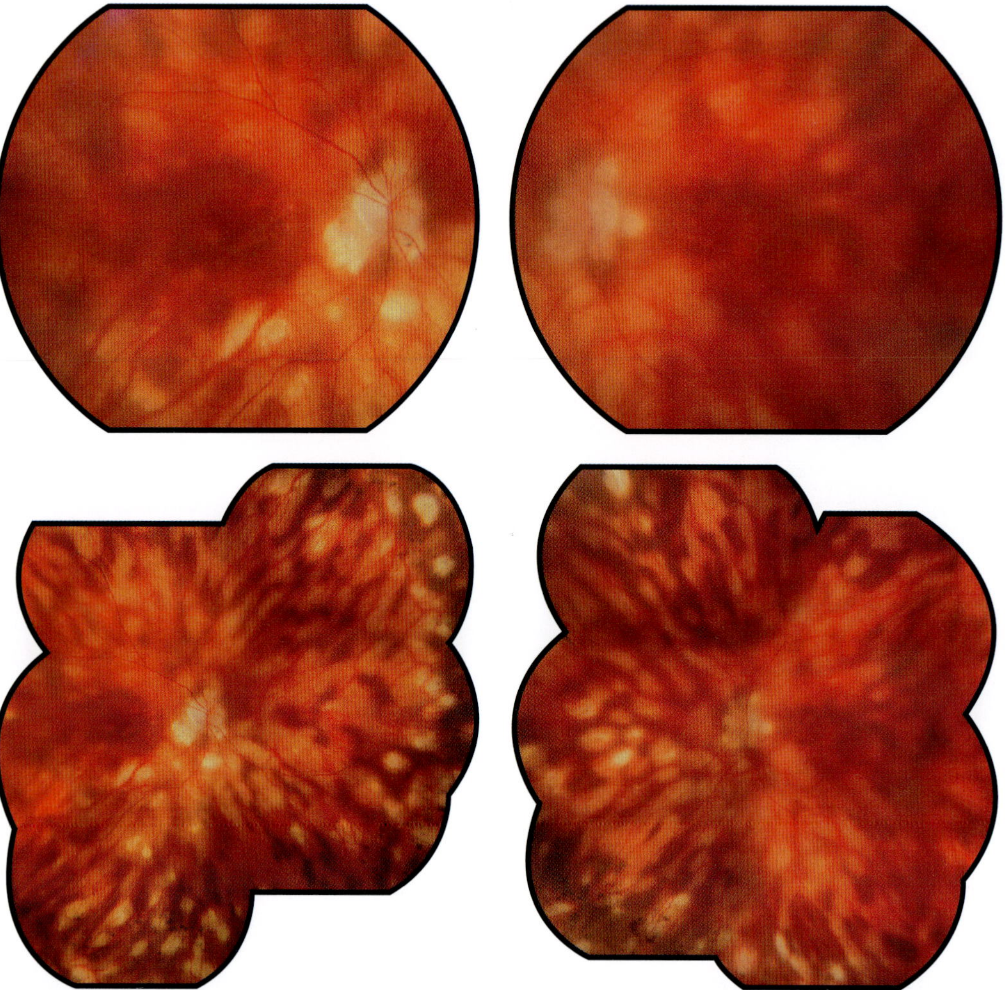

This patient developed birdshot chorioretinopathy with typical spots throughout the fundus of each eye. Cataract formation in the left eye was also present. Over the years, the lesions began to expand, forming confluent atrophy. The patient suffered from nyctalopia and field loss.

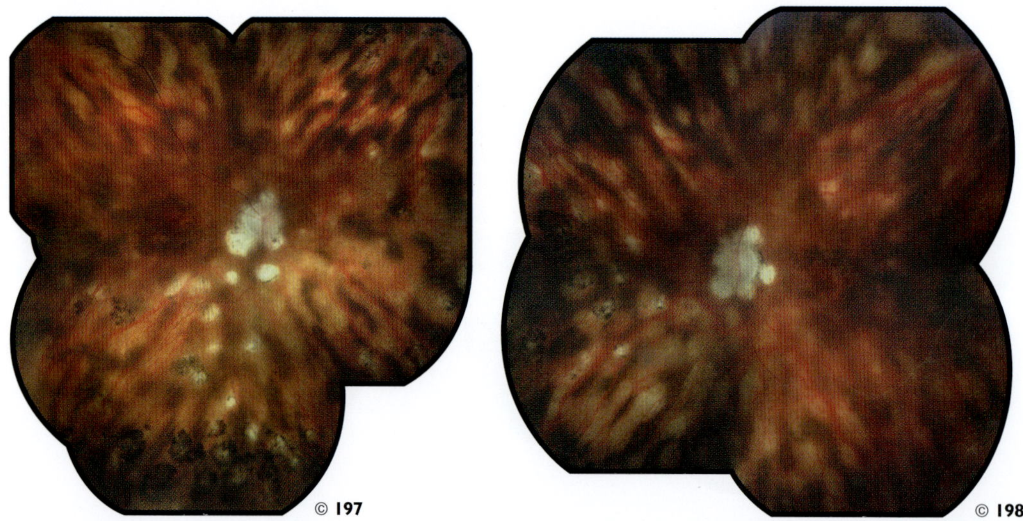

Twenty-six years later, the patient developed widespread chorioretinal atrophy and marked hyperpigmentation, producing a mosaic pattern of the fundus. Pigmentary scarring is uncommon except in long-standing disease, as in this patient. Note the presence of bilateral peripapillary atrophy due to chronic inflammation.

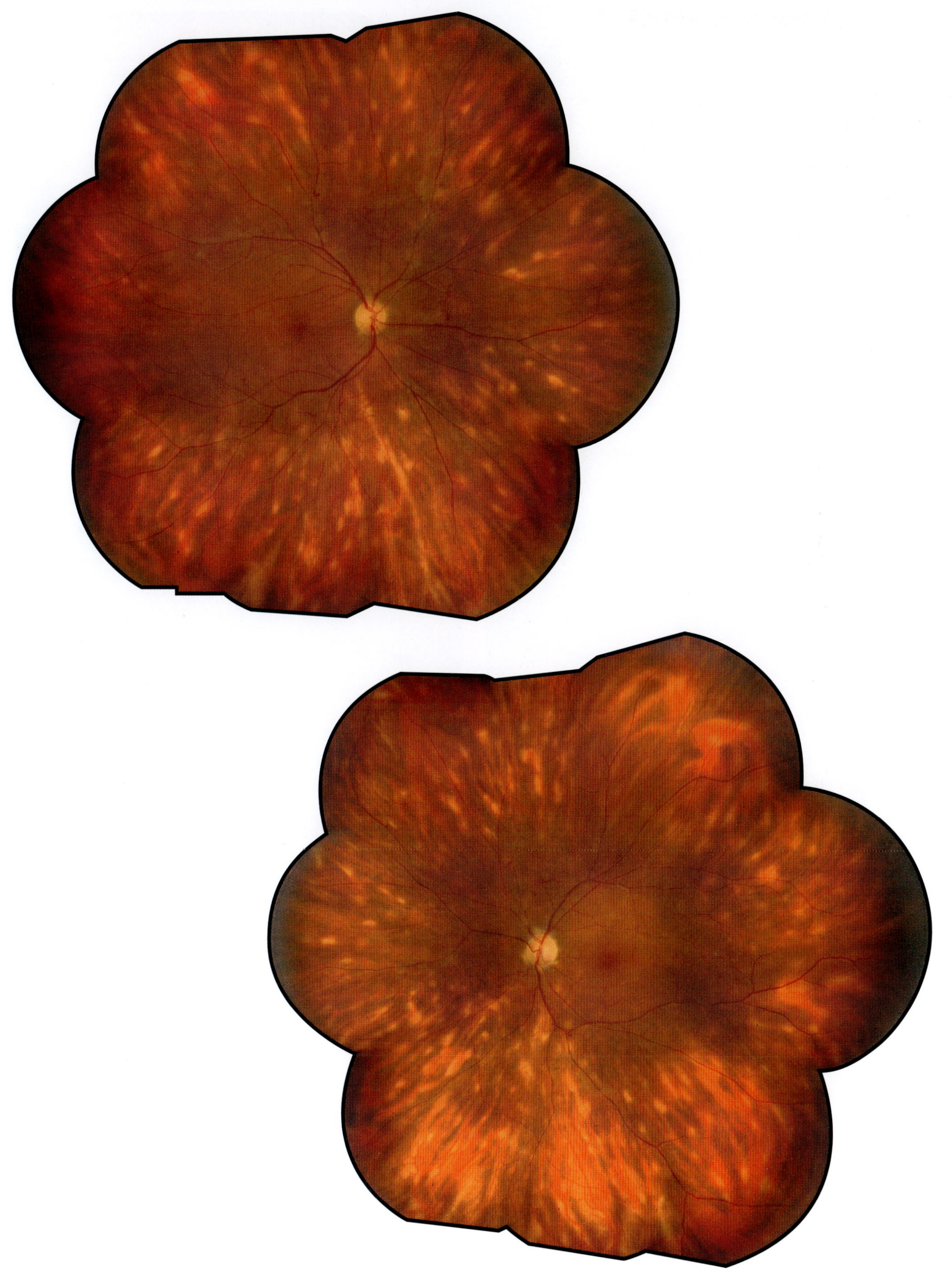

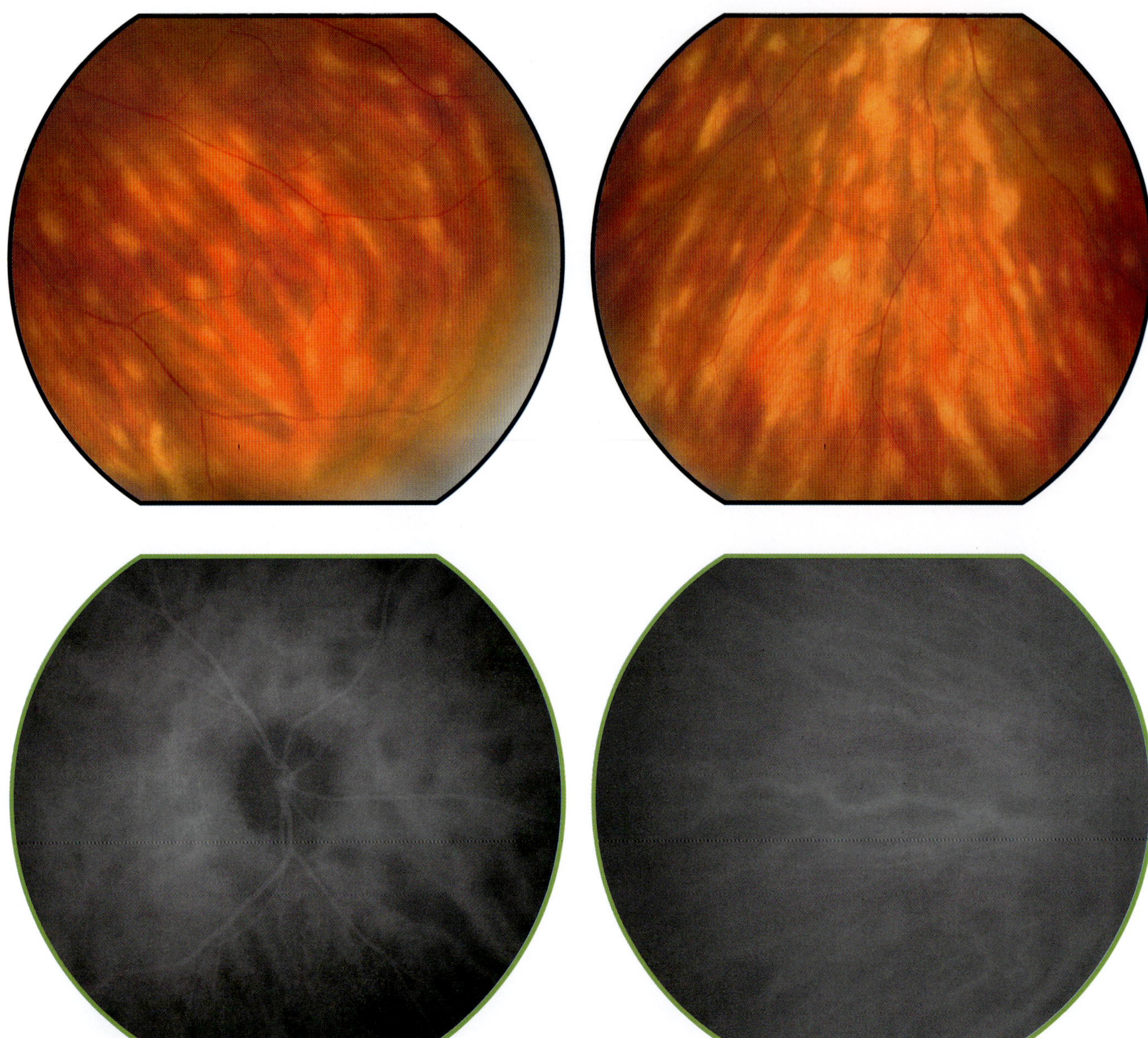

This patient with birdshot chorioretinopathy has multiple deep white spots that can be seen on color fundus montage. These lesions track along the choroidal vasculature, which is highlighted in color fundus images of the periphery and in the ICG angiogram images.

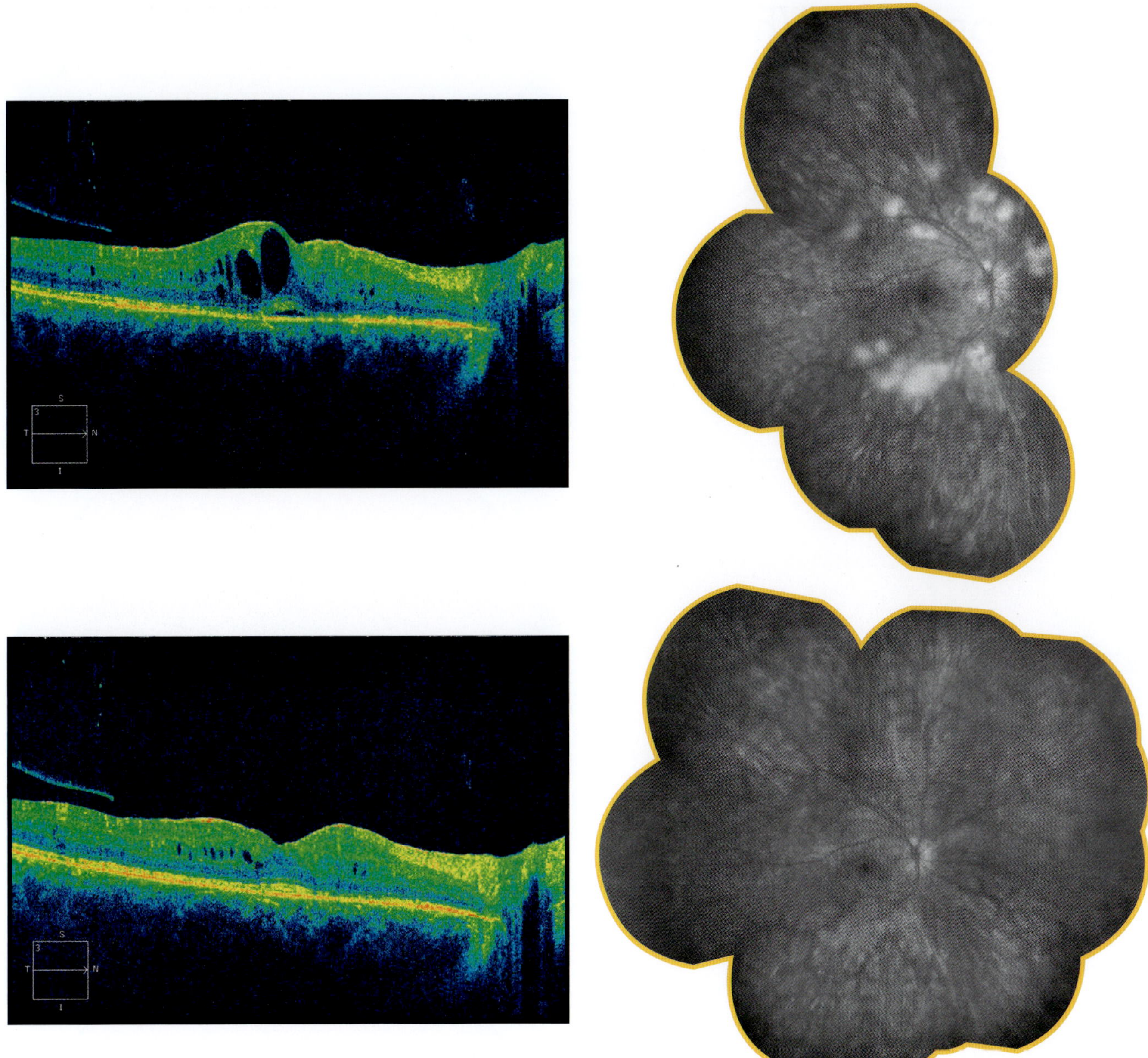

SD-OCT demonstrates cystoid macular edema and patchy loss of the ellipsoid band *(top row, left)*. The patient also developed neovascularization along the major arcades in the right eye, which can be seen on the fluorescein angiogram montage *(top row, right)*. Both the cystoid macular edema and the neovascularization improved following anti-VEGF injections *(bottom row)*.

Overlapping "White Dot" Syndromes

Idiopathic inflammatory disorders involving multifocal white dots or spots in the fundus have been referred to as "white dot" syndromes. These disorders include MEWDS, MFC, acute zonal occult outer retinopathy, APMPPE, birdshot chorioretinopathy, and others. There are known cases in which a patient experiences more than one of these rare diseases, and these combined diseases are referred to as overlapping "white dot" syndromes. The occurrence of an overlapping syndrome suggests common risk factors related to the pathogenesis of the diseases. In general, it has been hypothesized that an inciting infectious agent induces an immune-mediated response in a genetically susceptible individual.

Multiple Evanescent White Dot Syndrome (MEWDS) and Acute Macular Neuroretinopathy (AMN)

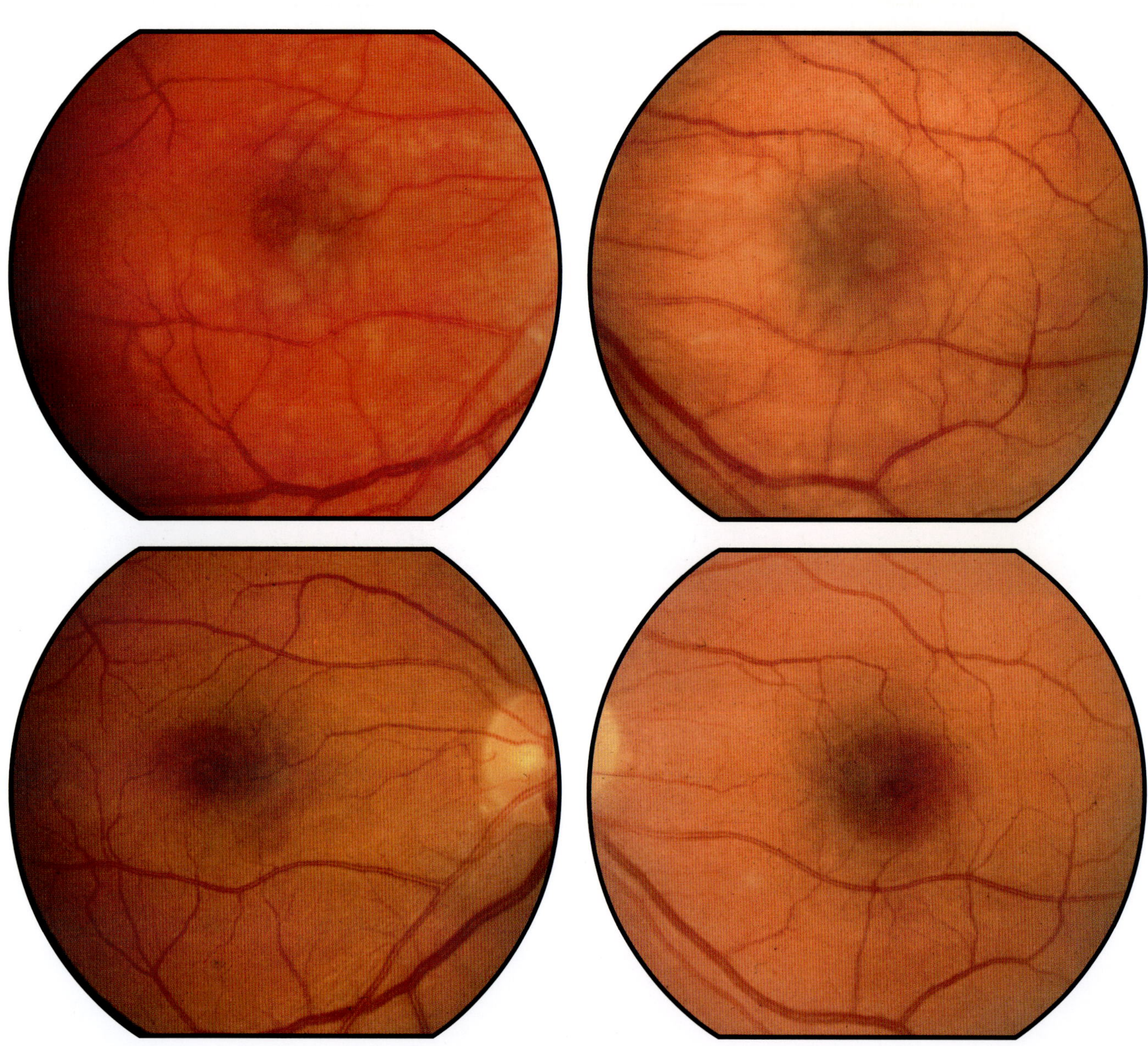

This patient had characteristic findings of MEWDS with photopsia, enlargement of the blind spot and white spots in the fundus of each eye, *(top images)*. Following spontaneous resolution of the white-spot lesions, there was a reddish intraretinal discoloration with a corresponding central field loss in each eye, characteristic of the acute macular neuroretinopathy syndrome.

MEWDS and AZOOR

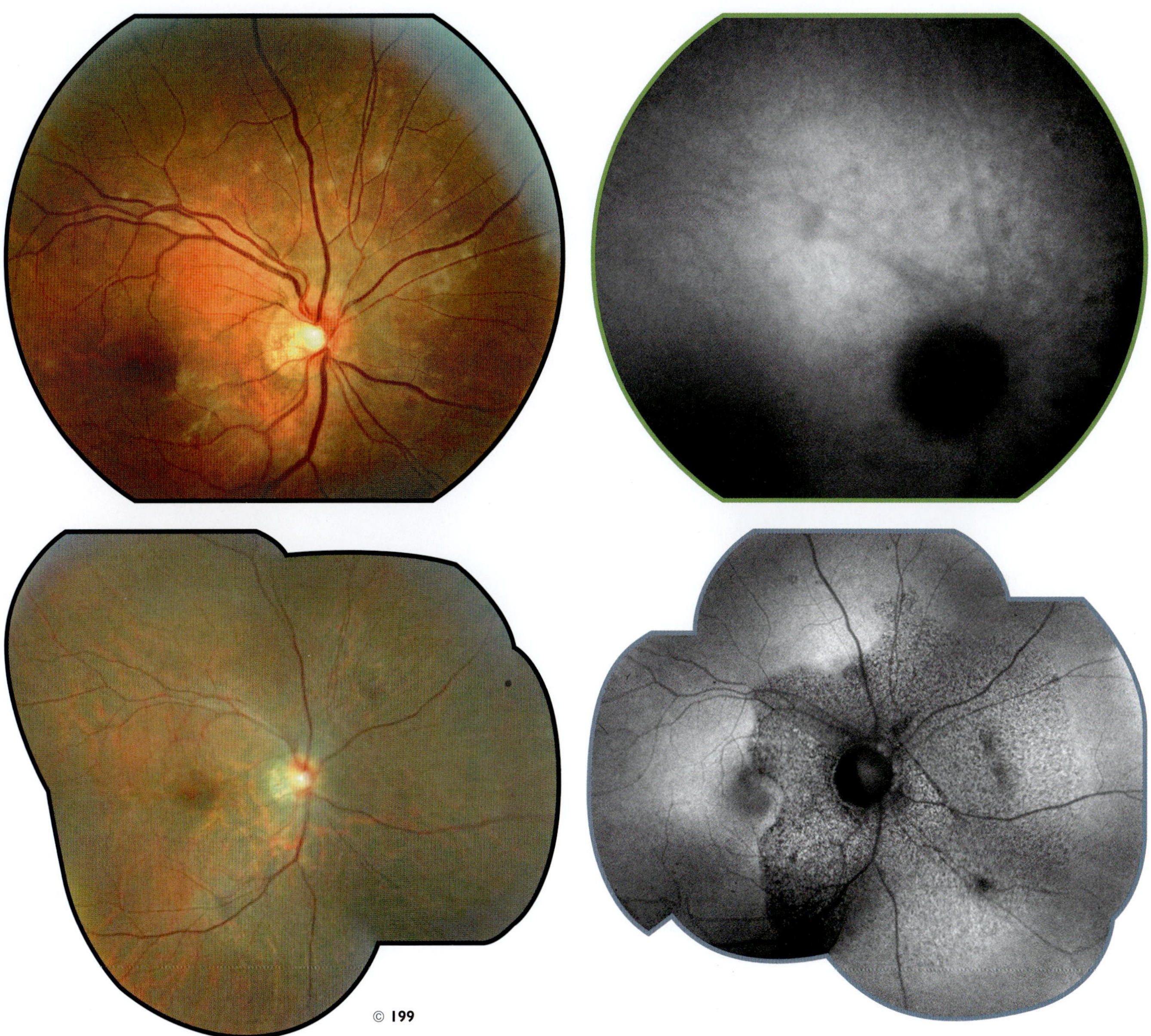

This patient developed acute MEWDS and peripapillary white spots as seen with color fundus photography and ICG angiography *(top row)*. After resolution of the acute lesions, there was progressive peripapillary atrophy extending to the more peripheral fundus consistent with AZOOR. Color fundus photography and fundus autofluorescence montage show progressive peripapillary atrophy with perifoveal sparing that may be seen in AZOOR. The left eye was normal.

MFC and MEWDS

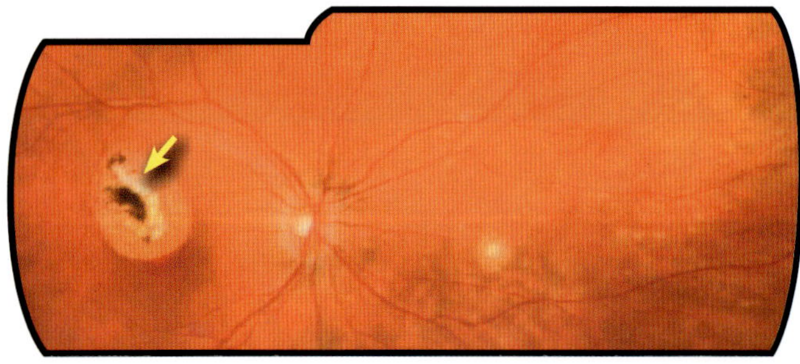

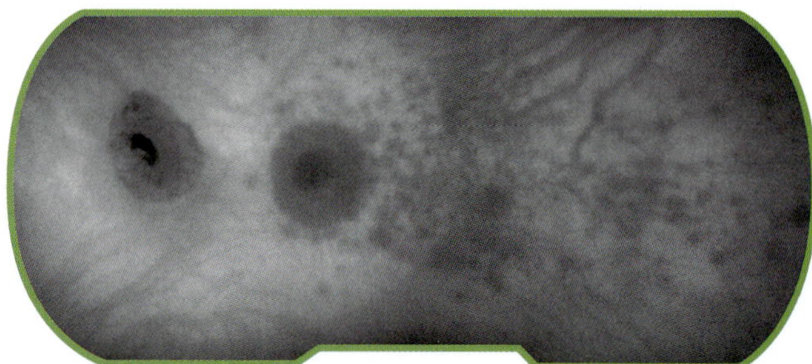

This patient developed macular CNV treated with laser photocoagulation *(arrow)*. Note the chorioretinal lesion in the nasal retina consistent with multifocal chorioretinitis. Three years later, she experienced photopsia and field loss. White spots were seen scattered through the peripapillary region and extending along the horizontal raphe into the nasal periphery corresponding to hypofluorescent lesions with ICG angiography. These spots cleared spontaneously and the blind spot improved suggestive of MEWDS versus recurrent MFC.

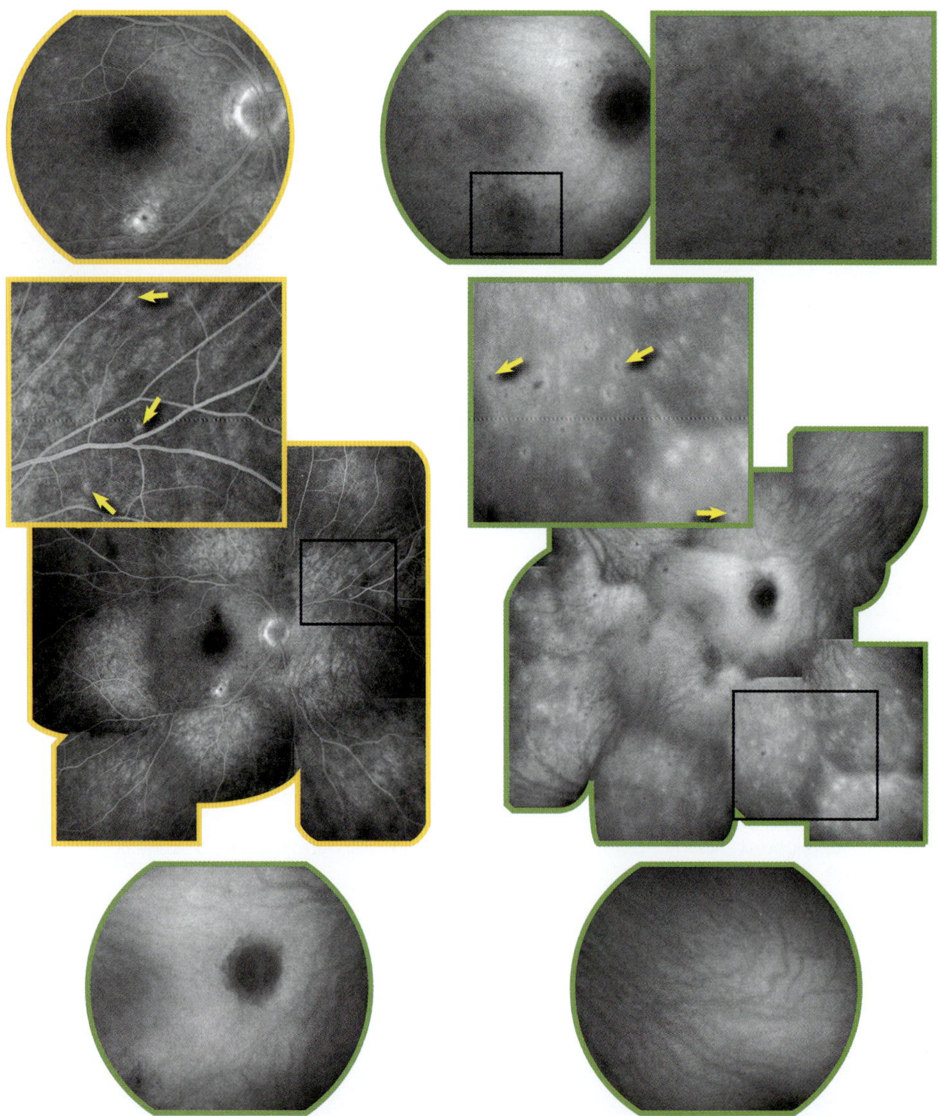

This is a patient with MFC. On the top row, a pre-existing chorioretinital scar is noted with FA. The ICG angiogram (with and without magnification) shows hypofluorescence of the scar in addition to multifocal areas of hypofluorescent dots, which correspond to active choroidal lesions. There is also peripapillary involvement and enlargement of the blind spot. In the middle row, the fluorescein angiogram illustrates few hyperfluorescent spots in the periphery superonasally *(middle row left, arrows)*. In contrast, the ICG angiogram shows an array of numerous inflammatory lesions in the inner choroid. The acute lesions are hyperfluorescent, while the resolving lesions begin to show hypofluorescence in the central portion of the inflammatory abnormality ("target lesion," *arrows*), similar to the macular lesion. The "target" abnormalities are seen in the magnified insets. Following resolution of the acute process, there is clearing of the choroidal lesions on the ICG angiogram *(bottom left and right)*. Recurrent MFC with lesions that do not permanently scar the RPE is the likely explanation as opposed to overlapping MEWDS.

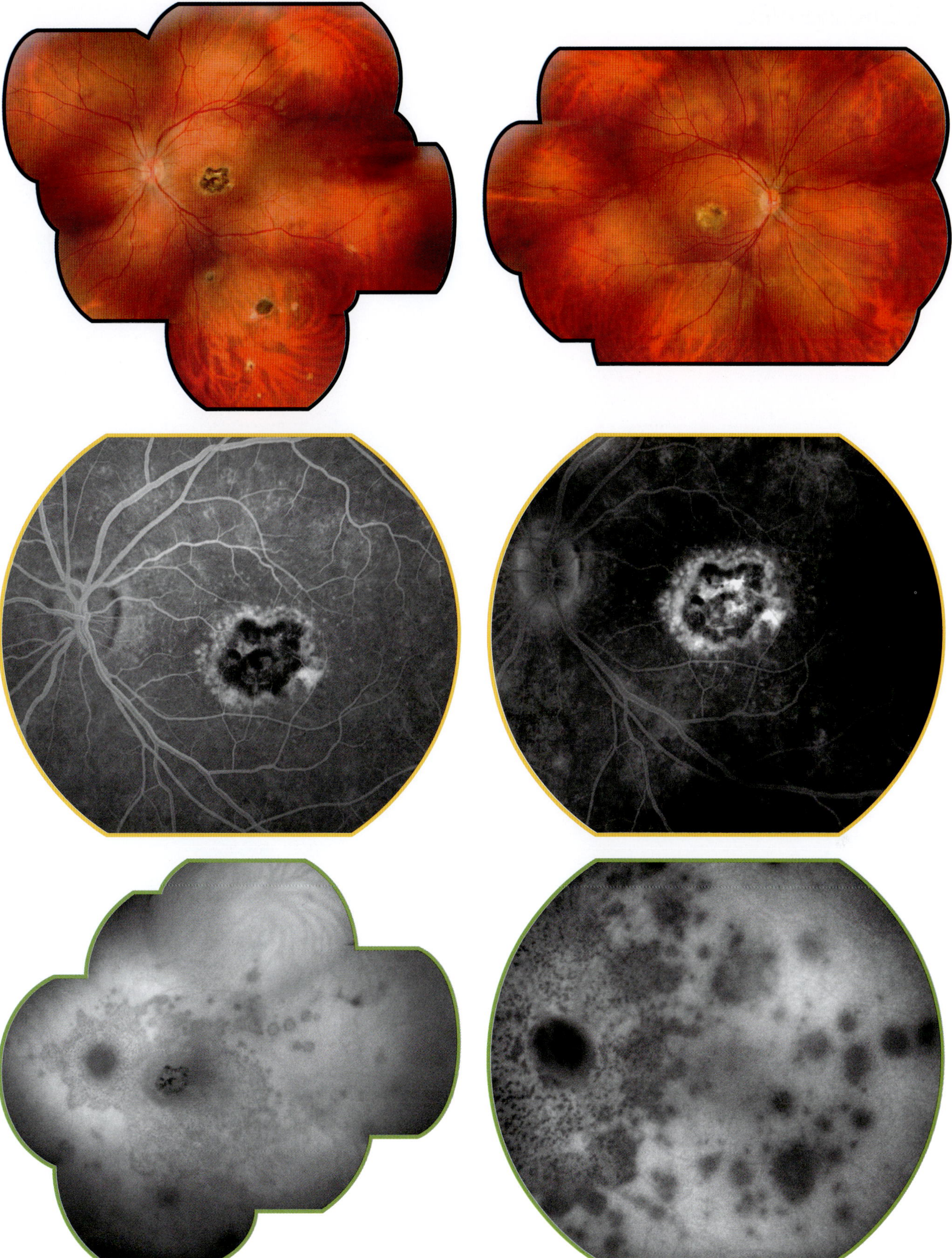

This patient had Best vitelliform macular dystrophy and peripheral fundus lesions, indicative of MFC. There were atrophic and pigmentary lesions in the fundus of the left eye. That eye also developed a more recent visual disturbance and the diagnosis of MEWDS was made. Note the wreath-like hyperfluorescence of the macular lesions on the fluorescein angiogram in the middle row. The lower row shows the ICG with large and small lesions, the so-called "dot and spot" variant of the disease. Smaller lesions are seen at the level of the outer retina overlying larger lesions at the level of the inner segment ellipsoid–pigment epithelium complex. Peripapillary involvement accounted for blind-spot enlargement. All of the acute manifestations resolved spontaneously by 3 months, leaving no lasting effect on her visual acuity or field.

AZOOR and MFC

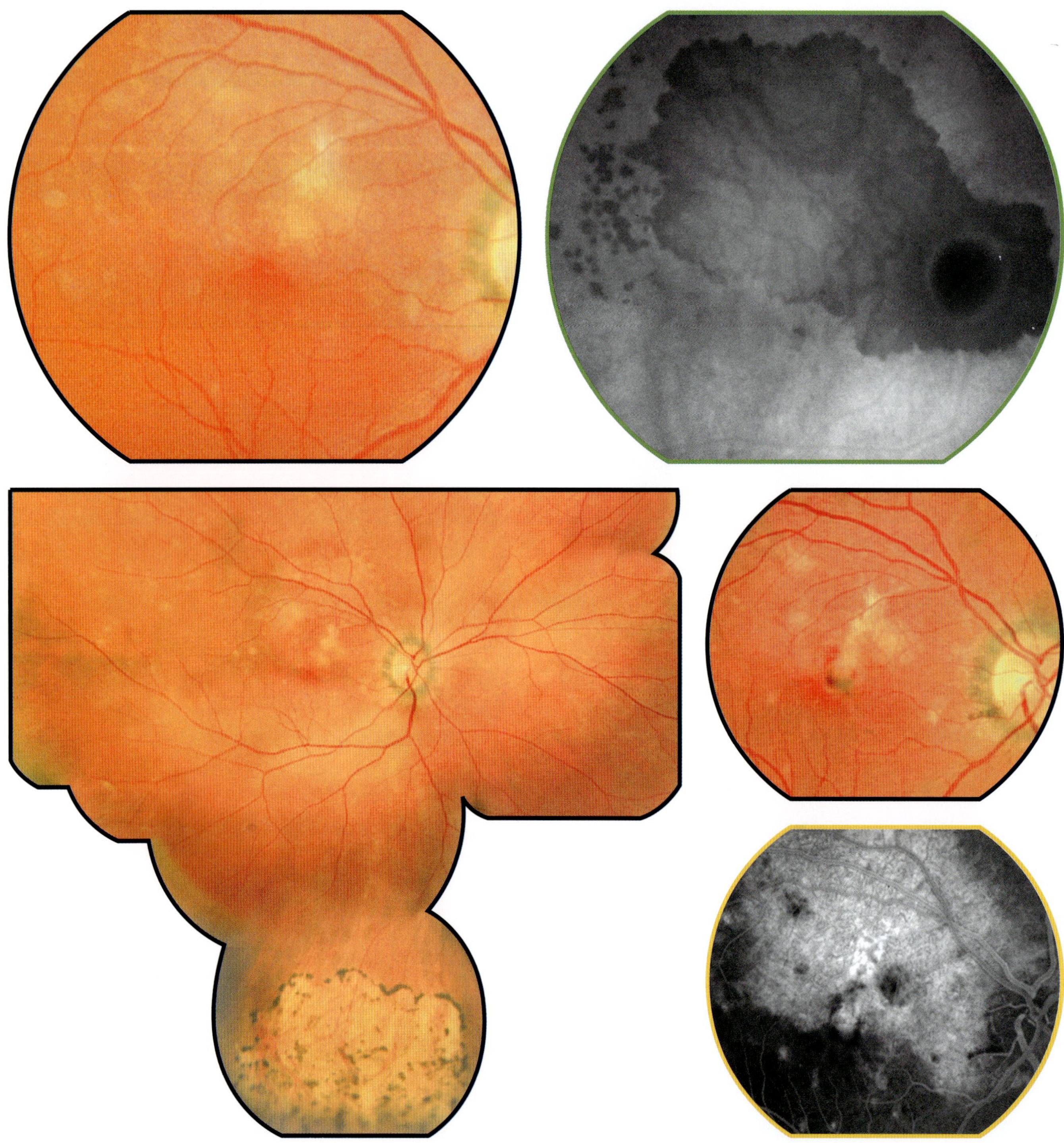

This patient presented with a large zonal defect consisting of peripapillary atrophy, which extended along the superior temporal arcade. This defect can be seen best with ICG angiography *(top right)*. There was a second zonal defect in the inferior fundus (alternatively this may represent atrophic congenital hypertrophy of the RPE or CHRPE), as seen on the montage. Later, this patient developed CNV. Note the multifocal choroidal lesions at the initial presentation and also at the time of CNV development in the right eye.

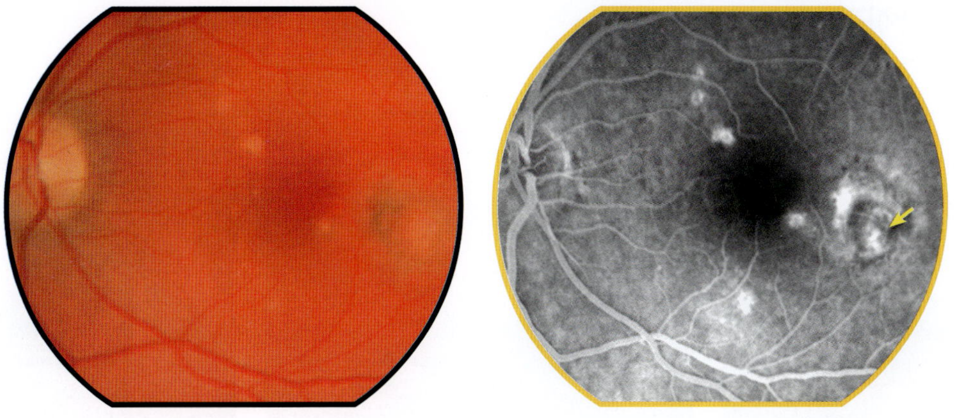

The left eye (same patient as above) had multifocal areas of atrophic chorioretinal scarring. Three years after neovascularization was noted in the right eye, CNV developed in the temporal macula of the left eye *(arrow)*. This is a case of peripapillary zonal atrophy and subsequent CNV associated with MFC. MFC followed by AZOOR may explain the findings in the right eye. Zonal atrophy in a patient with MFC in both eyes, or AZOOR in one eye and MFC in the other, may be an alternative explanation.

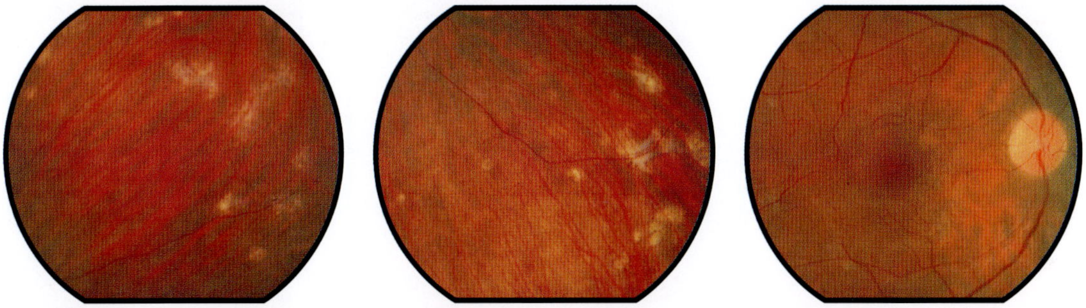

Onset

One year later

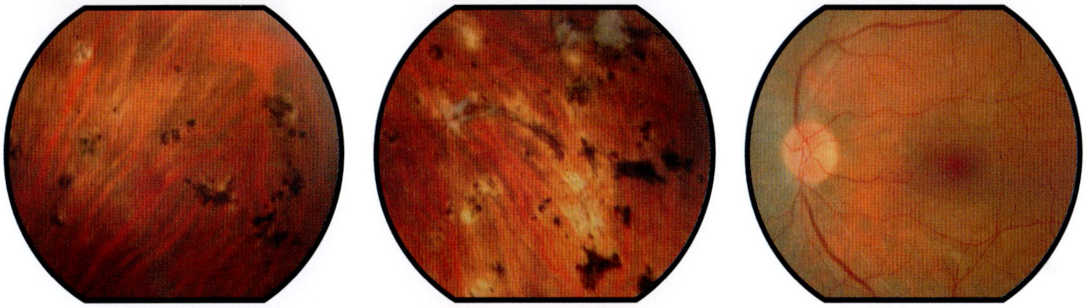

Three months later

One year later

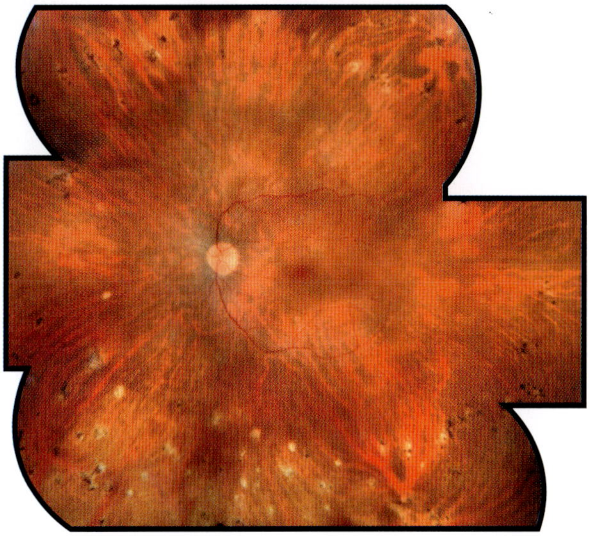

This 24-year-old female with multiple immune-mediated systemic inflammatory diseases experienced photopsia and an enlarged blind spot in each eye. Note the multiple atrophic peripheral chorioretinal lesions in each eye with minimal fibrous metaplasia. She gradually began to experience progressive field loss as the peripheral lesions became more fibrotic and pigmentary in nature. Optic nerve pallor and generalized retinal vascular thinning associated with a nearly extinguished ERG, similar to rod-cone dystrophy, eventually developed. She was diagnosed as AZOOR with MFC, a syndrome once referred to as MFC type 2A by J. Donald Gass.

APMPPE and MEWDS

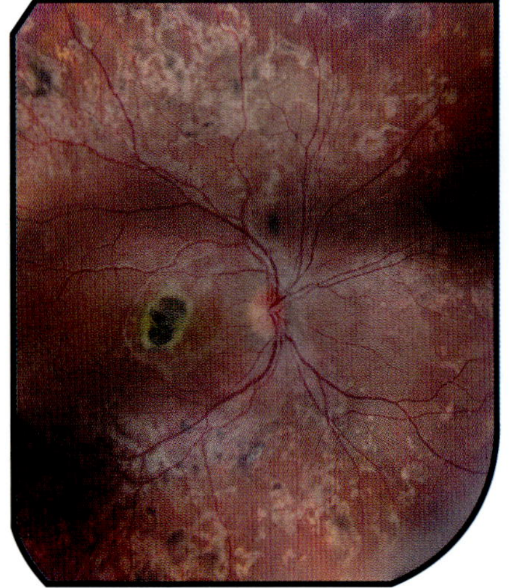

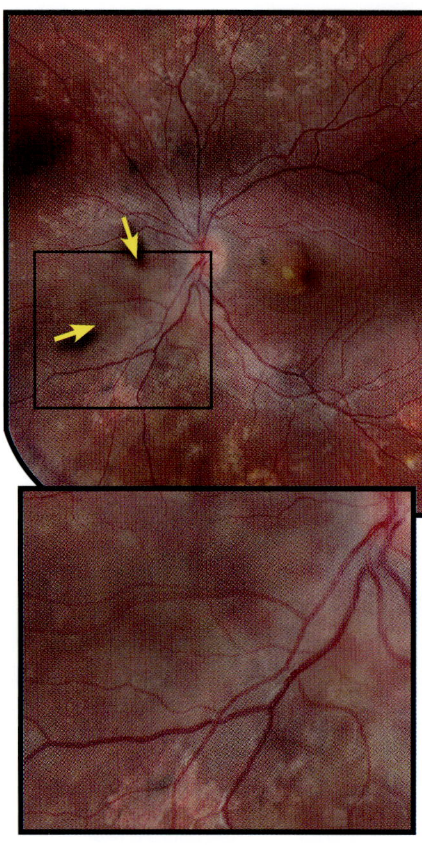

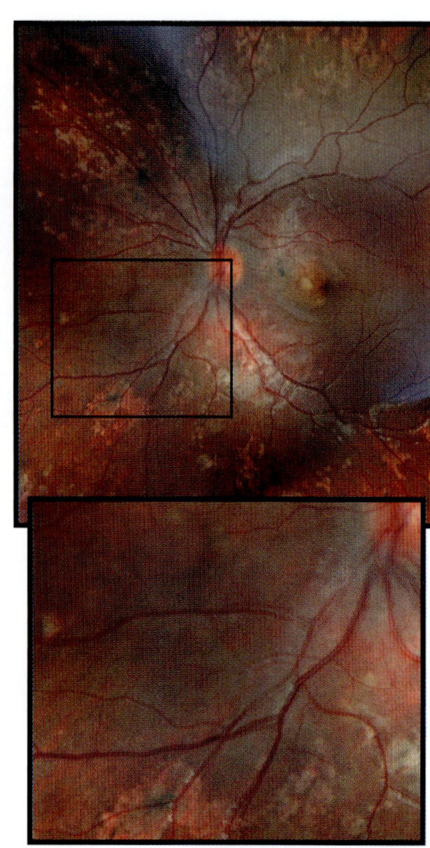

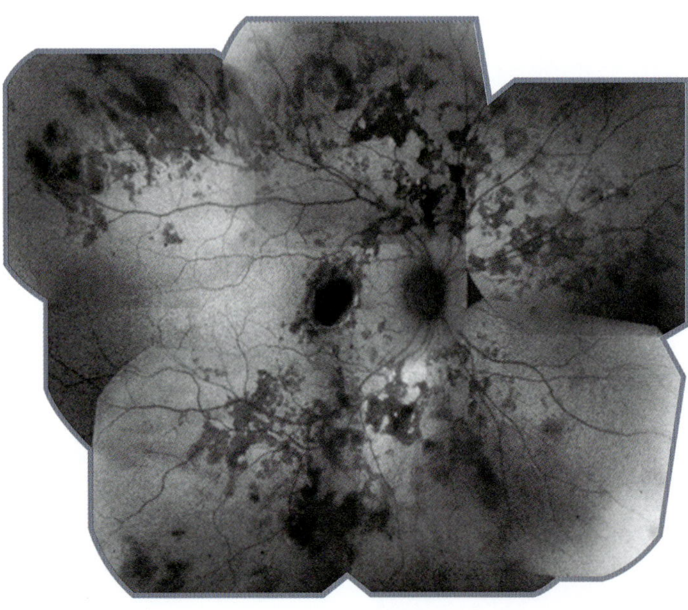

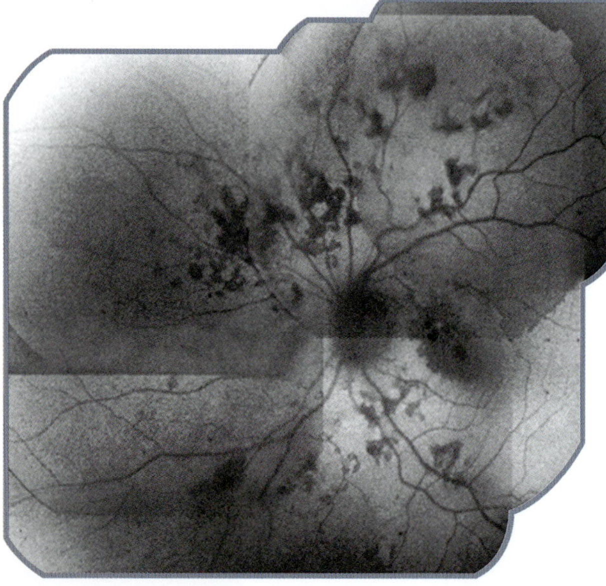

This 9-year-old child experienced a bilateral acute inflammatory disease interpreted as APMPPE in each eye. Three years later, there was a recurrent visual disturbance in the left eye. Multifocal intraretinal spots were evident, consistent with MEWDS *(arrows, top middle image)*. Spontaneous resolution of the lesions occurred without any visual sequelae and without atrophic or pigmentary degeneration *(top right image)*. The fundus autofluorescence shows the typical pattern following APMPPE *(bottom images)*. Note that current research has indicated that while APMPPE is primarily a chorioretinal inflammatory disease, MEWDS is an inflammatory disease at the level of the photoreceptor/RPE complex.

Lymphoma Simulating a "White Dot" Syndrome

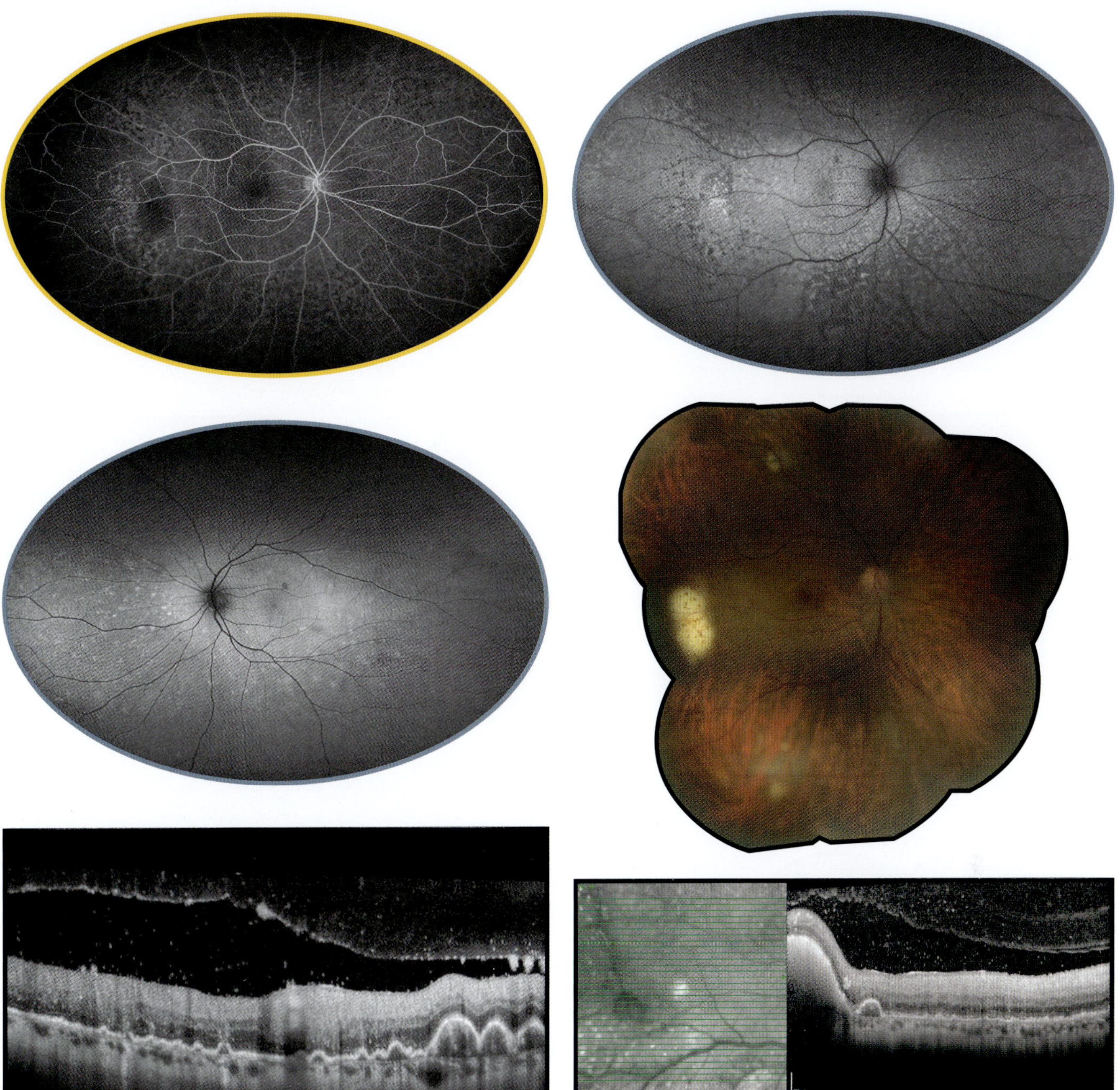

This 52-year-old female presented with a history of photopsias in both eyes for 6 months. Widefield fluorescein angiogram of the right eye *(top left)* illustrates multiple hyperfluorescent and hypofluorescent spots scattered throughout the posterior pole and periphery. The hyperfluorescent lesions are hypoautofluorescent on widefield autofluorescence and the hypofluorescent lesions are hyperautofluorescent *(top row right and second row left)*. Follow-up color fundus photo montage shows a large creamy infiltrate with pigment ("leopard spotting") in the temporal midperiphery *(second row right)*. SD-OCT demonstrates multiple drusenoid pigment epithelial detachments and a "lumpy bumpy" appearance to the RPE *(third row left)*. SD-OCT through one of the infiltrative lesions is shown *(third row right)*. The patient underwent vitreous biopsy, which revealed atypical lymphocytes consistent with intraocular lymphoma. This case demonstrates that lymphoma may masquerade as a white dot syndrome similar to MEWDS. *Images courtesy of Pradeep Prasad, MD*

Pars Planitis

Pars planitis is the term given to idiopathic intermediate uveitis not typically associated with any underlying disease, although this presentation can complicate certain diseases such as multiple sclerosis (MS) and systemic sarcoid. It is a relatively common inflammatory syndrome primarily involving the pars plana and peripheral retina in young adults and children. Pars planitis represents approximately 4-16% of all uveitis. Most studies show no sex, racial, or geographic predilection. The initial presentation may be asymmetric; however, 80% of cases develop bilateral involvement. Patients typically present with vitreous floaters and decrease in vision from vitreous cellular debris or cystoid macular edema. Patients typically do not have pain, photophobia, or severe anterior-segment inflammation. In the posterior segment, vitreous inflammatory debris develops, and may accumulate as a fibrocellular deposition in the inferior vitreous base overlying the pars plana and anterior retina, which is commonly referred to as a "snowbank" lesion. Anterior vitreous infiltrates referred to as "snowballs" may also develop. Optic disc edema, peripheral periphlebitis, peripheral retinal neovascularization, and vitreous hemorrhage may occur. Cystoid macular edema is the most common cause of decreased vision.

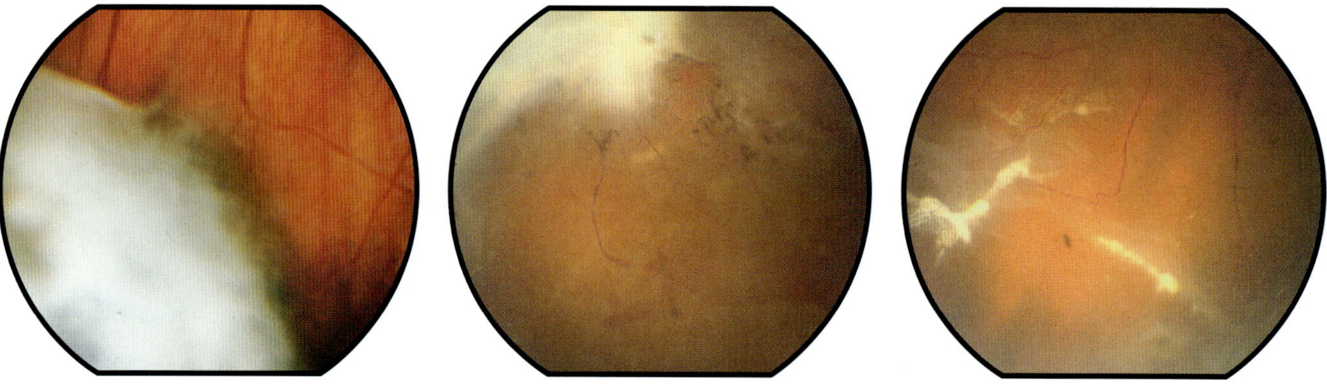

These patients have pars planitis and intermediate uveitis. There is typical accumulation of inflammatory debris peripherally referred to as a "snow bank" lesion *(left and middle image)*. The right image shows white inflammatory debris at the margin of a schisis cavity.

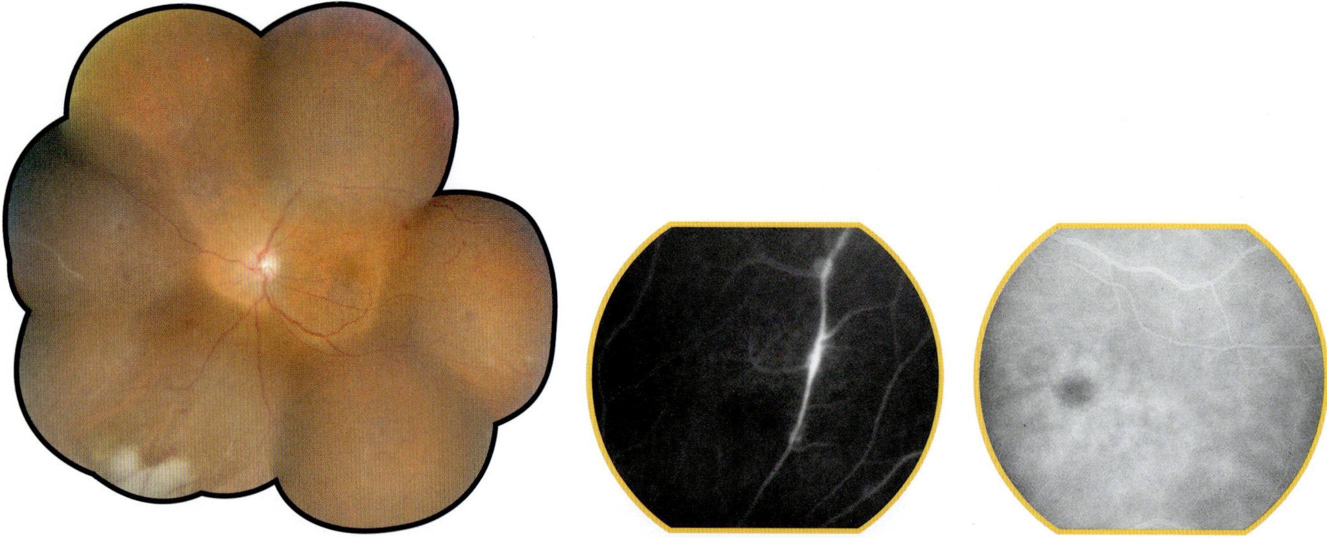

The color montage shows a cloudy vitreous due to cellular infiltration and peripheral inflammatory exudate *(left)*. Macular edema is the principal reason for reduced vision in these patients. Note the presence of diffuse cystoid macular edema affecting the left eye *(right)*. The fluorescein angiogram *(middle)* shows segmental staining of a retinal vein consistent with a retinal phlebitis.

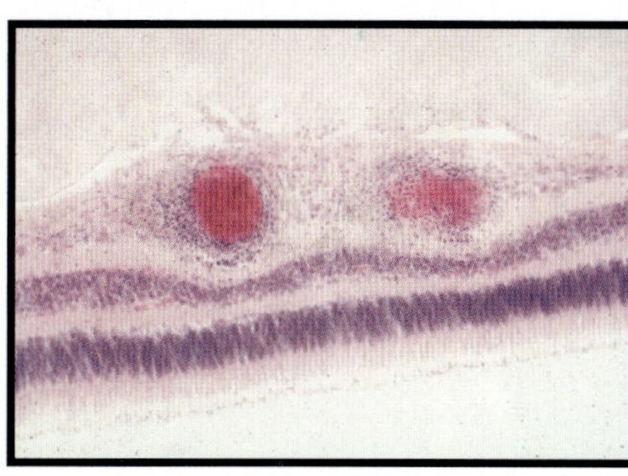

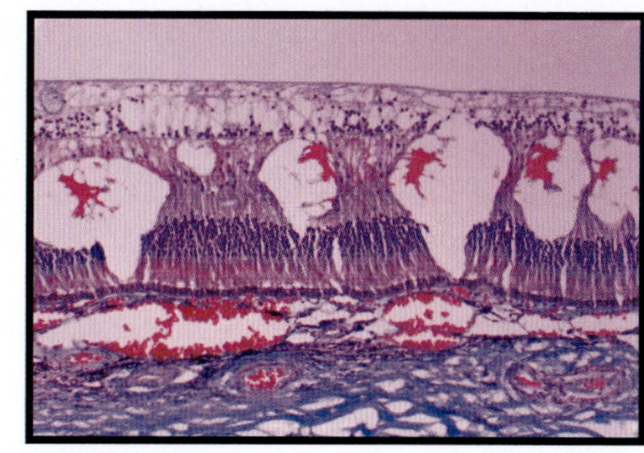

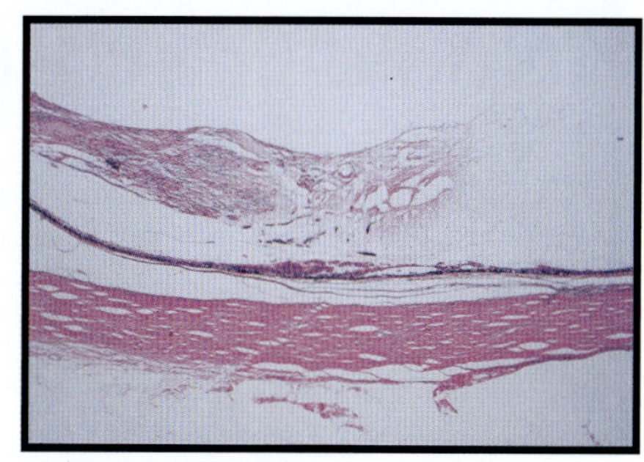

These histopathological illustrations of a patient with intermediate uveitis and pars planitis show retinal phlebitis *(left)*, cystoid macular edema *(middle)*, and "snowbank" lesions composed of collapsed and condensed vitreous with glial cell proliferation and early pre-retinal neovascularization *(right)*.

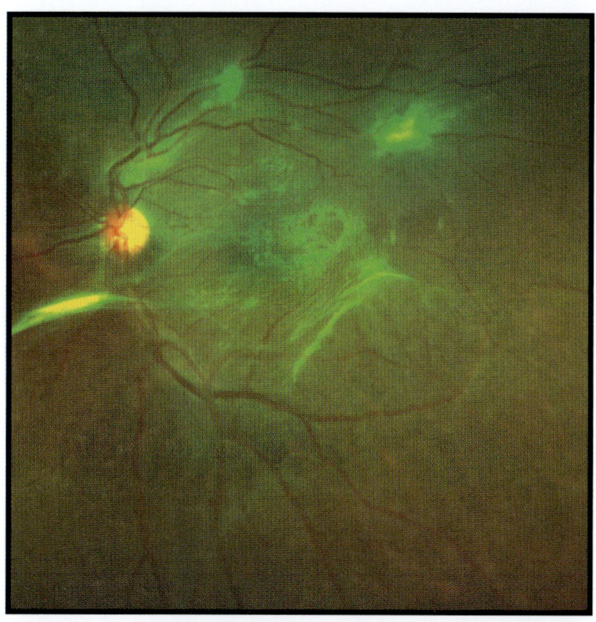

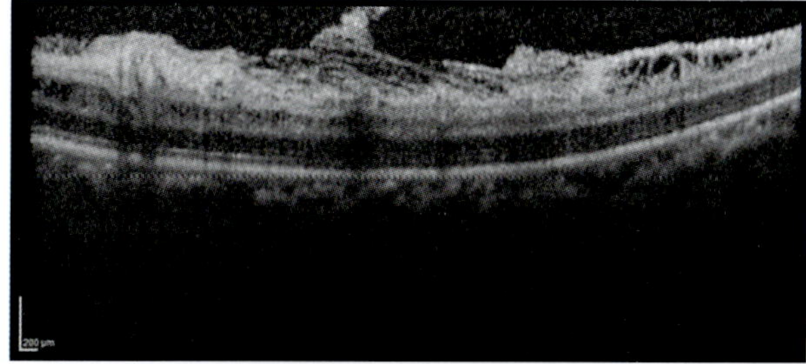

This 38-year-old female with idiopathic pars planitis presented with decreased vision in her left eye for 1 year. A color fundus photograph of the left eye illustrates a hyperemic nerve and SD-OCT shows a dense epiretinal membrane and a severe macular pucker. Widefield fluorescein angiogram demonstrates inferior peripheral non-perfusion with hyperfluorescent areas likely representing neovascularization from pars planitis.

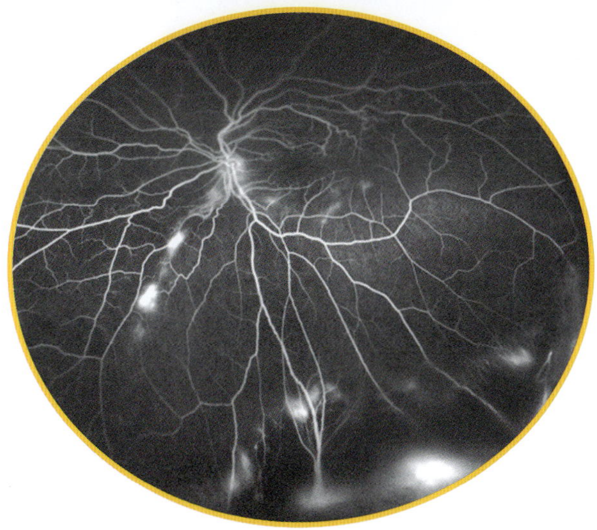

Multiple Sclerosis

Multiple sclerosis (MS) is a chronic demyelinating disease of the central nervous system that may be associated with a number of ocular problems including optic neuritis, internuclear opthalmoplegia, uveitis, and retinal vasculitis. Uveitis has been reported in up to 28.5% of MS patients, with intermediate uveitis being most common, followed by granulomatous anterior uveitis. Peripheral retinal phlebitis may occur in 9-23% of patients with MS. Retinal ischemia with neovascularization and cystoid macular edema have been reported.

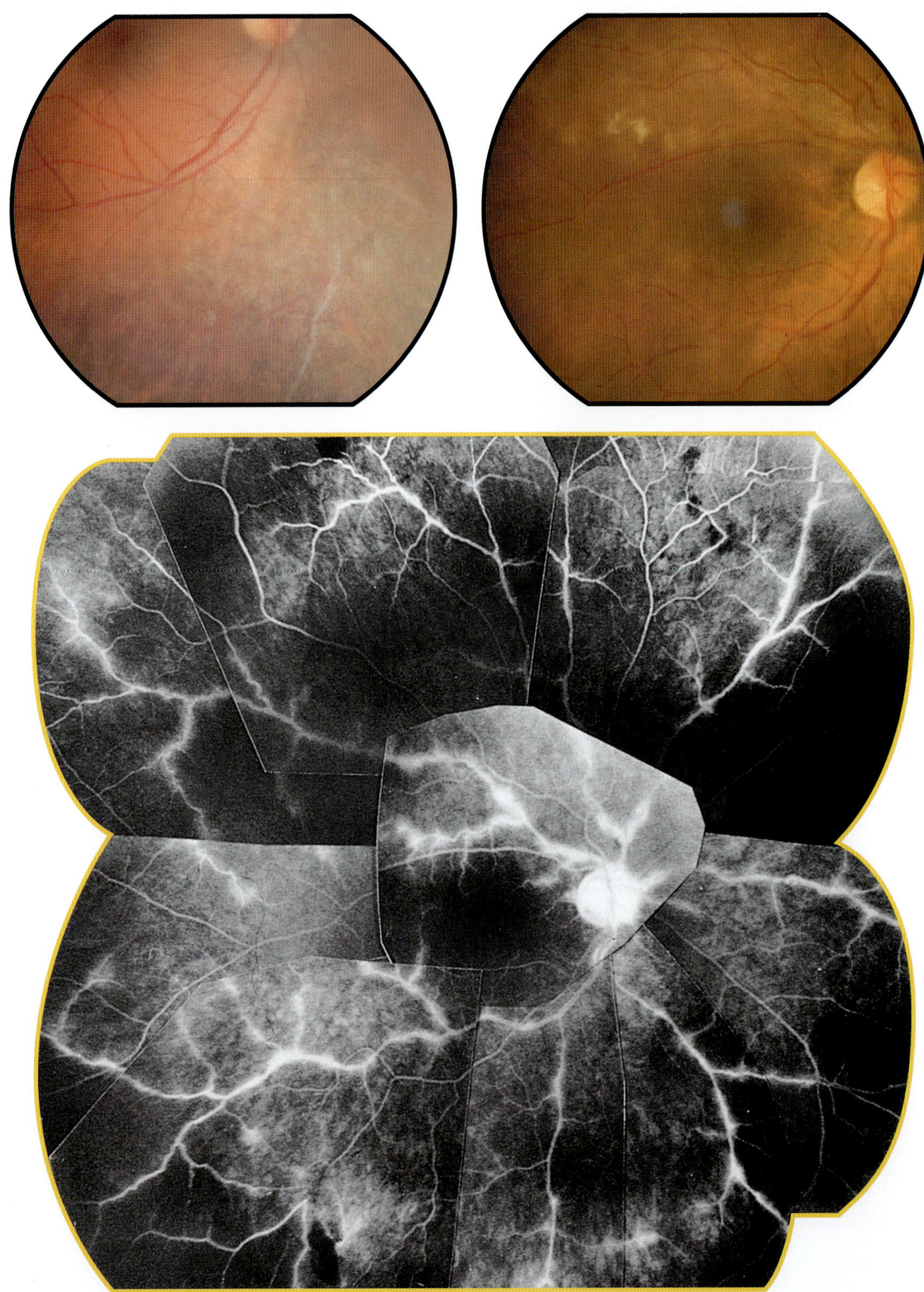

These patients with MS show retinal vascular sheathing *(top left)* and whitish-yellow retinal infiltrates *(top right)*. FA shows retinal venous leakage and phlebitis *(bottom)*. *Courtesy of Dr. Anita Leys*

Behçet Disease

Behçet disease is a chronic systemic disorder characterized by a necrotizing vasculitis affecting multiple organ systems. It is most common in Asia and the Middle East where men are more likely to be affected than women. The disease is much less common in the USA where there is a more equal gender distribution. Non-ocular findings of Behçet disease include oral and genital ulcers, an asymmetric nondestructive large-joint polyarthritis, and a cutaneous vasculitis, which includes erythema nodosum. Ocular findings occur in 68-85% of patients and are usually bilateral. Uveitis and retinal vasculitis are the most common ocular findings. The uveitis is a nongranulomatous iridocyclitis, which occasionally presents as a sterile hypopyon. Posterior-segment findings include vitritis, perivasculitis, retinal arterial and venous vascular occlusion, retinitis, cystoid macular edema, papillitis, and optic atrophy. Secondary complications such as cataract, glaucoma, vitreous hemorrhage, and retinal detachment may occur.

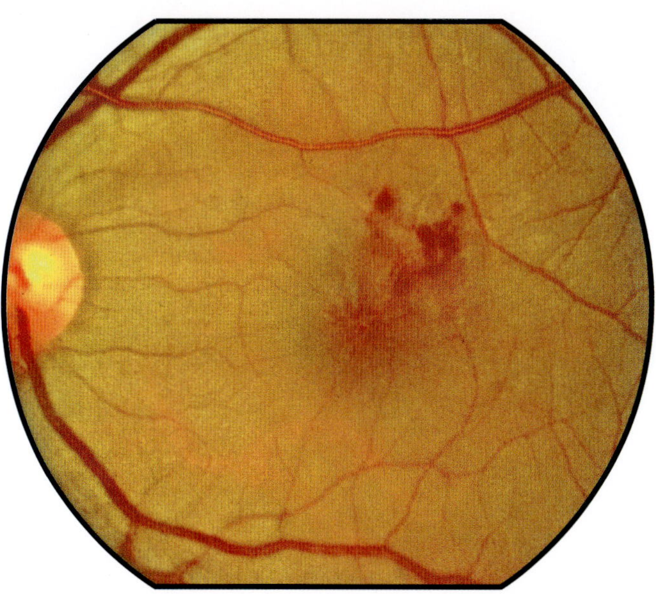

This fundus photograph from a patient with Behçet disease demonstrates a localized retinal vasculitis with focal hemorrhage. *Courtesy of Dr. Douglas A. Jabs*

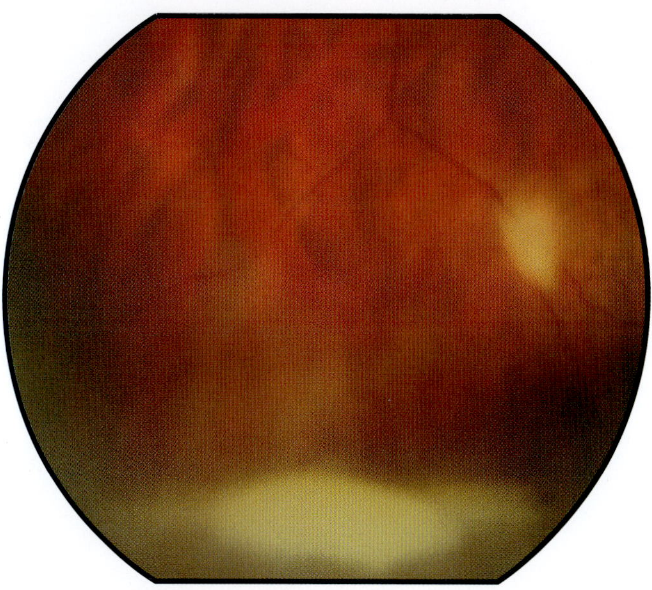

This patient has a "snowbank" in the peripheral fundus secondary to inflammation from Behçet disease. *Courtesy of Dr. Richard Klein*

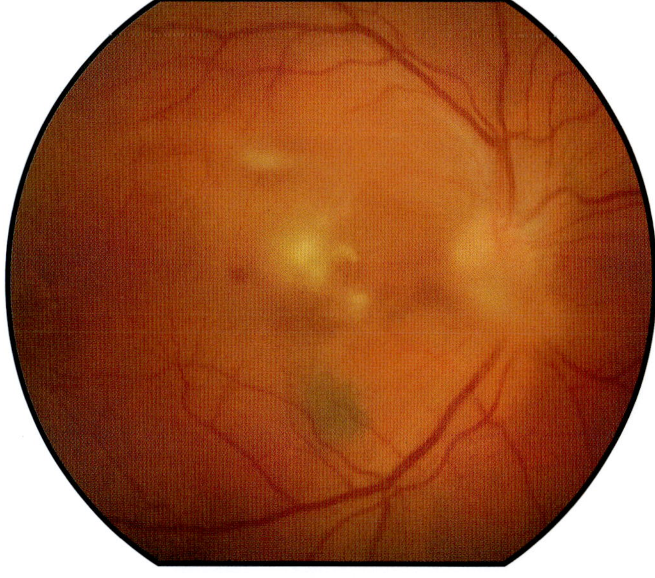

This patient with Behçet disease has a serous detachment of the macula with associated lipid exudates. There is also vitreous opacification, especially near the optic disc. *Courtesy of Dr. Richard Klein*

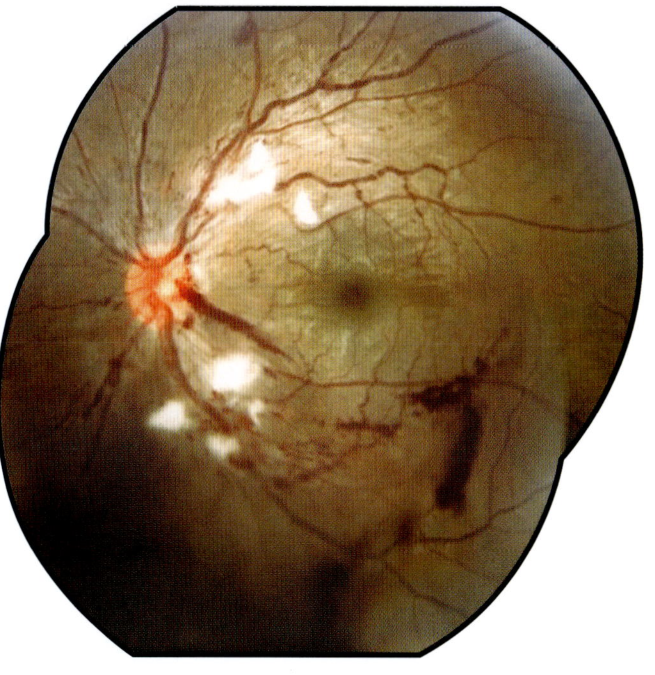

This patient with Behçet disease has retinal hemorrhages and multiple cotton-wool spots.

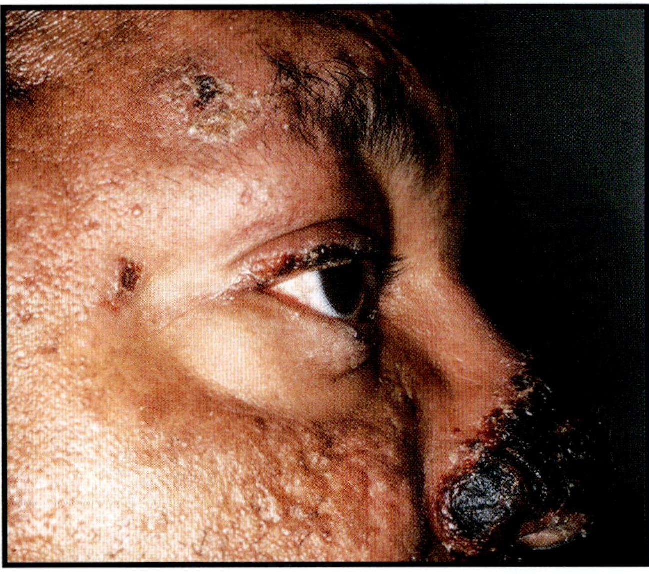

Behçet disease can have numerous systemic manifestations including genital and/or skin ulcers.

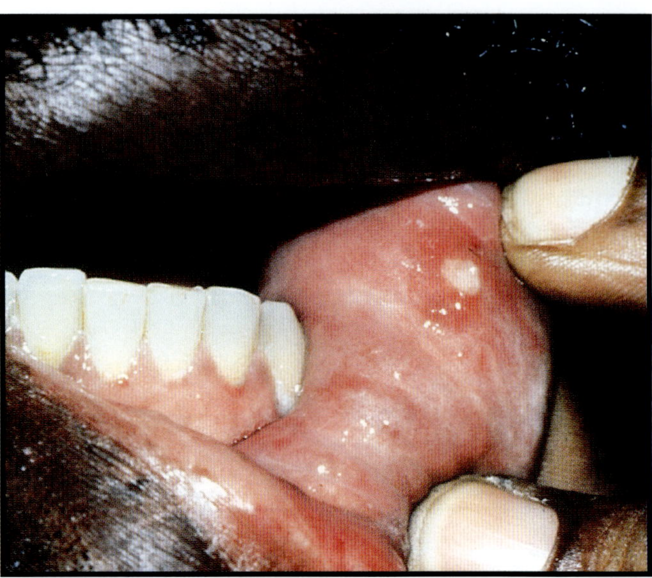

Oral aphthous ulcers may also occur in Behçet disease. *Courtesy of Dr. W. Culbertson*

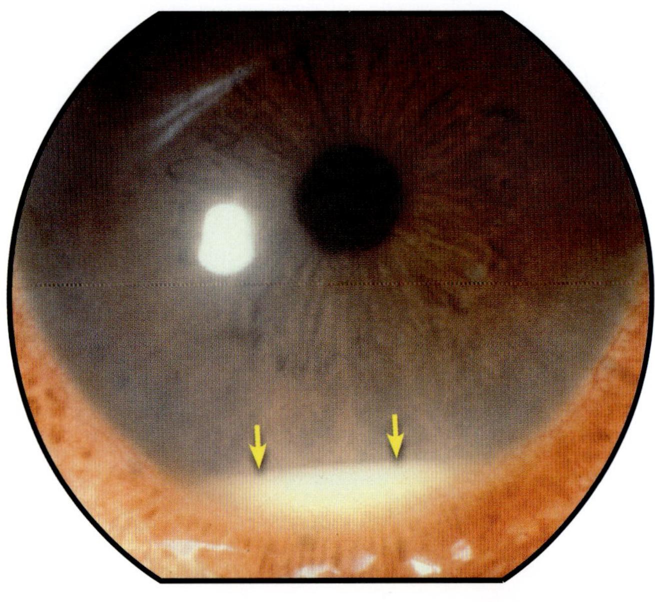

In this patient with Behçet disease, anterior uveitis and a hypopyon *(arrows)* are noted.

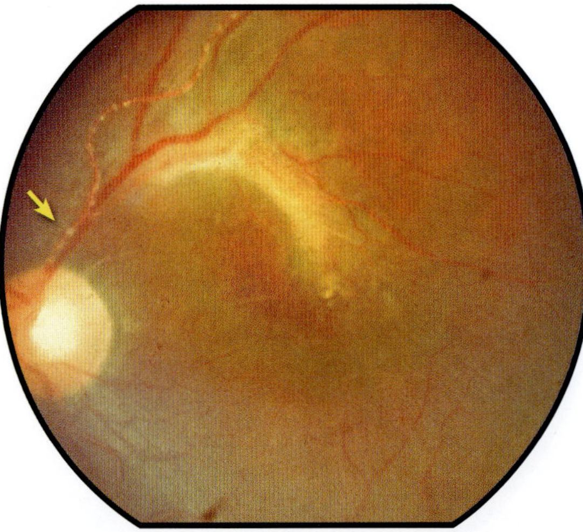

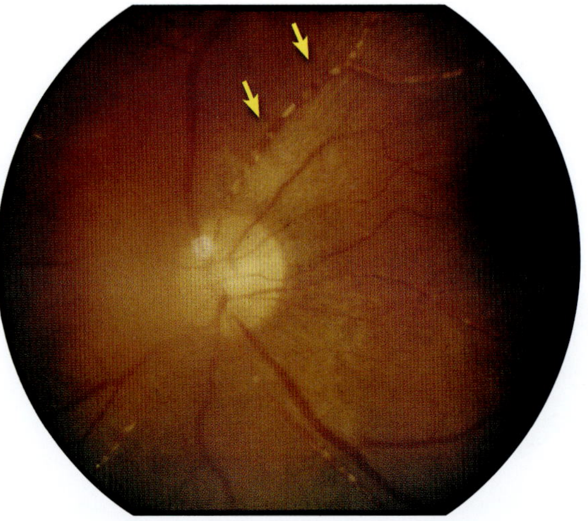

These two patients demonstrate chronic anterior and posterior uveitis from Behçet disease. Note the presence of pre-retinal fibrosis along the macular vessel superior in the left eye *(left image)*. There are also calcific or so-called Kyrieleis plaques along the arteries superior to the disc in each patient *(arrows)*.

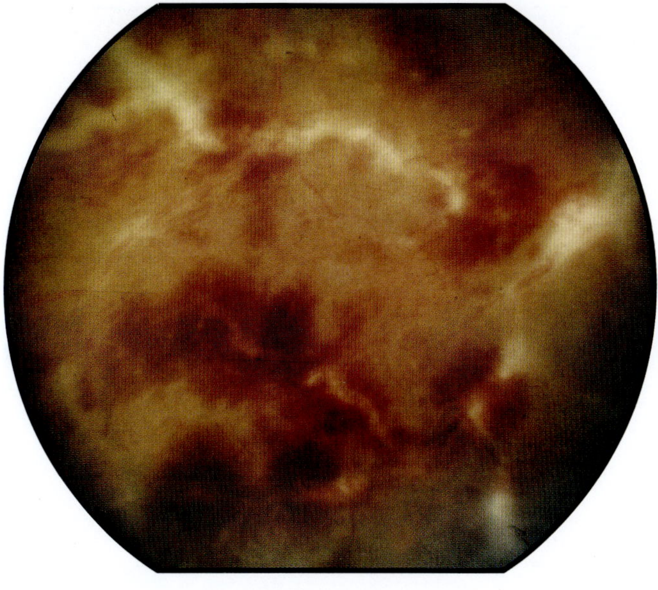

This patient has a severe frosted branch angiitis with hemorrhagic phlebitis, venous occlusive disease, chronic edema, and inflammation from Behçet disease.

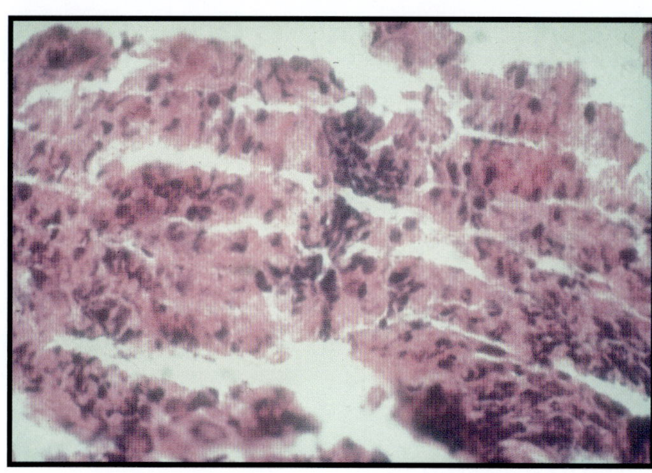

This histopathology specimen shows inflammatory cells, necrosis, and deformed nuclei in Behçet disease.

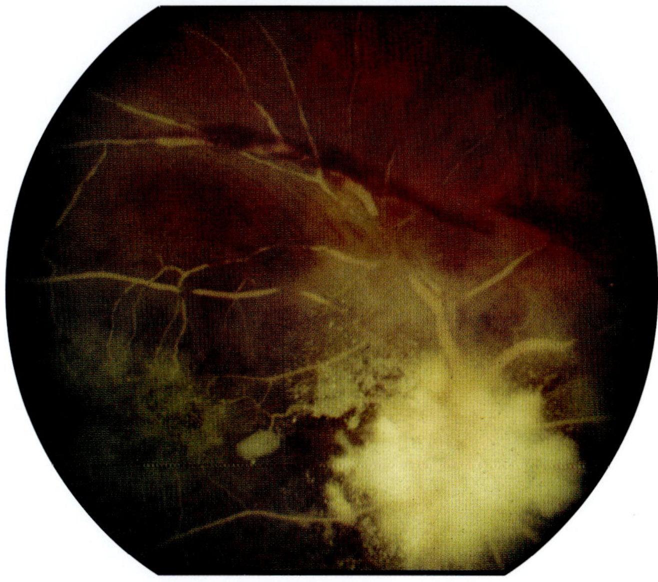

Severe Behçet disease can lead to massive ischemia of the fundus. This patient has a pre-retinal hemorrhage, widespread vasculitis with sheathing and ischemia, and disc edema and pallor.

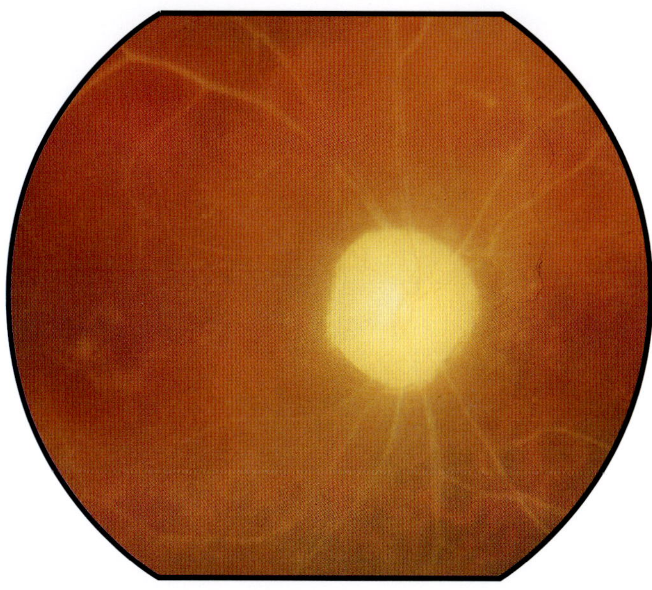

This patient has end-stage Behçet disease in the fundus with optic atrophy and severe sheathing of the retinal vessels. Progressive retinal degeneration due to fulminant retinal vascular ischemia and retinitis warrants aggressive immunotherapy in most cases. *Courtesy of Dr. Leyla Atmaca*

Inflammatory Bowel Disease

Inflammatory bowel disease (IBD) refers to a spectrum of disorders that cause chronic inflammation within the digestive tract. IBD is primarily comprised of two distinct diseases: ulcerative colitis and Crohn's disease. Both of these disorders have extraintestinal manifestations that can affect the eye. The most common ocular manifestations of IBD are episcleritis, scleritis, and uveitis. Uveitis is more common in women than men and may affect up to 17% of IBD patients. Most often this is a recurrent anterior uveitis; however, up to 10% of cases may involve the posterior segment in the form of panuveitis, chorioretinitis, or retinal vasculitis. Retinal vascular occlusions, retinal edema, and serous retinal detachments have all been described. Additionally, ulcerative colitis is associated with the presence of HLA-B27, and therefore these patients are at risk for the ocular complications associated with HLA-B27 disease.

Crohn's Disease

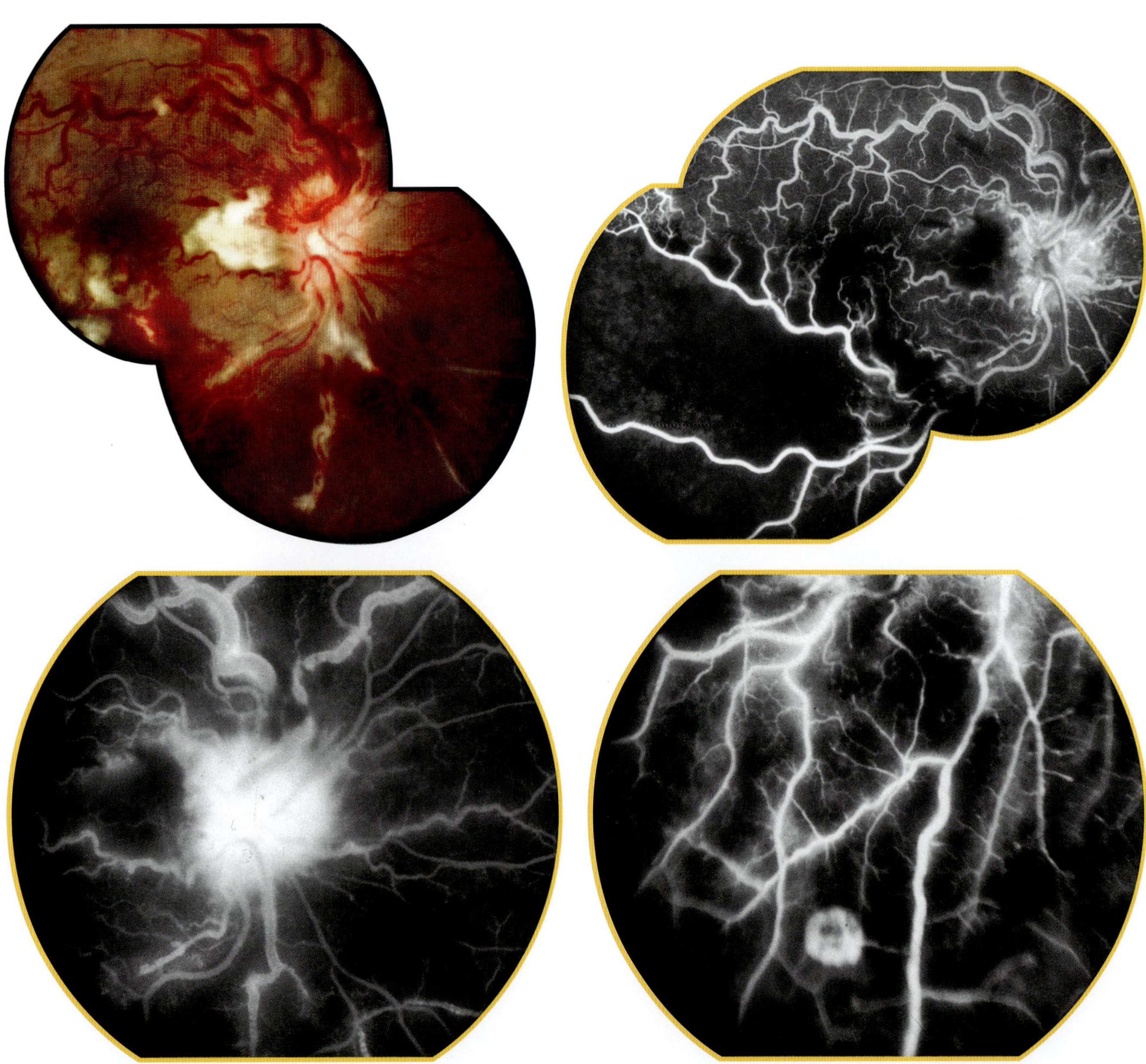

In this patient with Crohn's disease, note the presence of a hemorrhagic retinal vasculitis and possible CRVO complicated by ciliary retinal artery occlusion. The fluorescein angiogram shows severe retinal ischemia and non-perfusion, staining of the retinal vessels, and disc edema. Following therapy, there was resolution of the retinal vascular inflammation and disc edema. *Courtesy of Dr. Jay Duker*

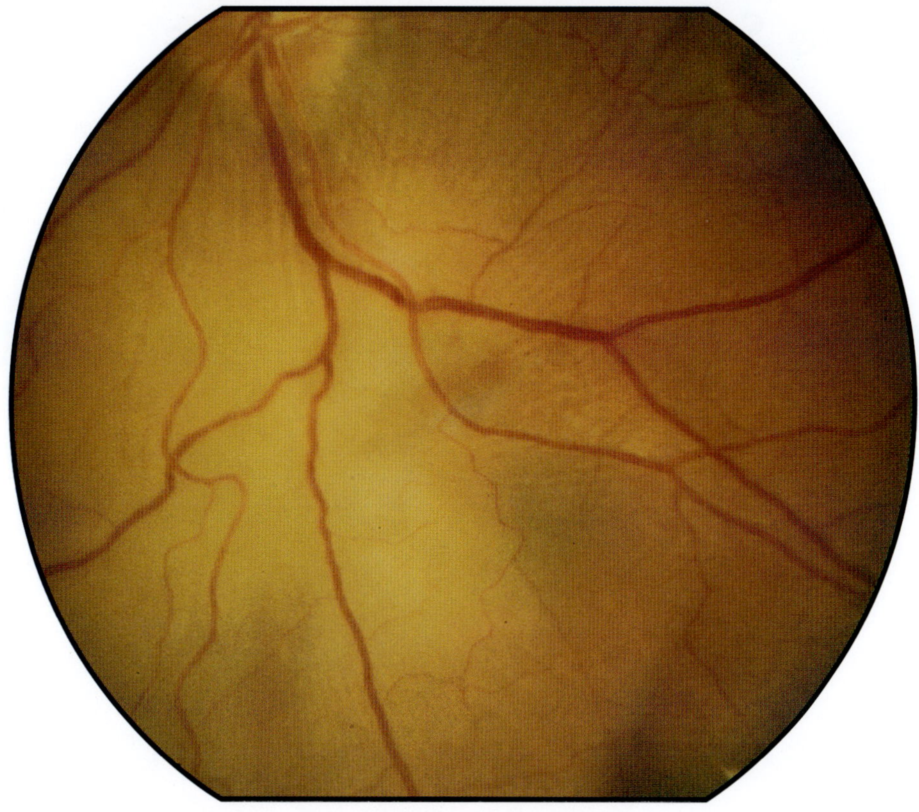

This patient with Crohn's disease developed inferior exudative retinal detachment. It could have been related to the use of corticosteroids, causing a central serous chorioretinopathy-related detachment.

Ulcerative Colitis

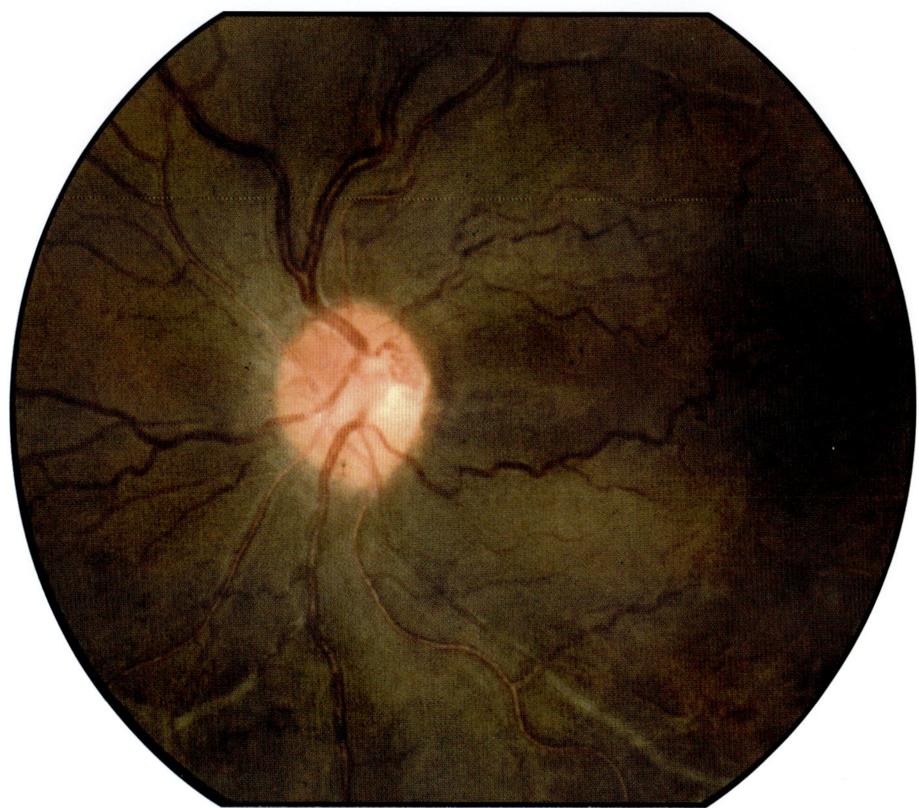

This patient with ulcerative colitis shows widespread retinal vascular ischemic disease that developed during an episode of acute vasculitis. There is sheathing and sclerosis of the retinal vessels, as well as venous occlusive disease with compensatory collateralization.

Seronegative Spondyloarthropathies

The seronegative spondyloarthropathies are a group of inflammatory disorders that involve the axial skeleton in patients who are negative for rheumatoid factor. The prototypical disease is ankylosing spondylitis, but other diseases in the group include reactive arthritis, psoriatic arthritis, and the IBDs. The presence of the HLA complex HLA-B27 is strongly associated with these diseases. There are many ocular manifestations, most commonly anterior uveitis. Posterior segment manifestations may include intermediate uveitis, retinal phlebitis and vascular occlusive disease, macular edema, and disc edema.

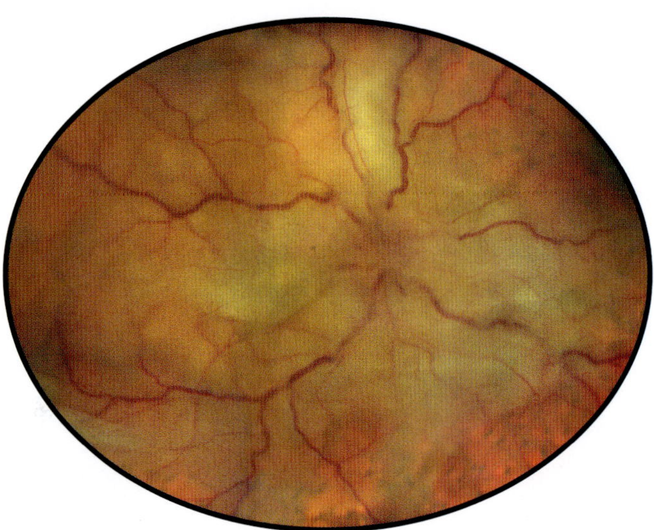

This patient with intermediate uveitis has widespread venous stasis with retinal vascular tortuosity, disc edema, and a turbid exudative retinal detachment. *Courtesy of Dr. A. Edward Maumenee*

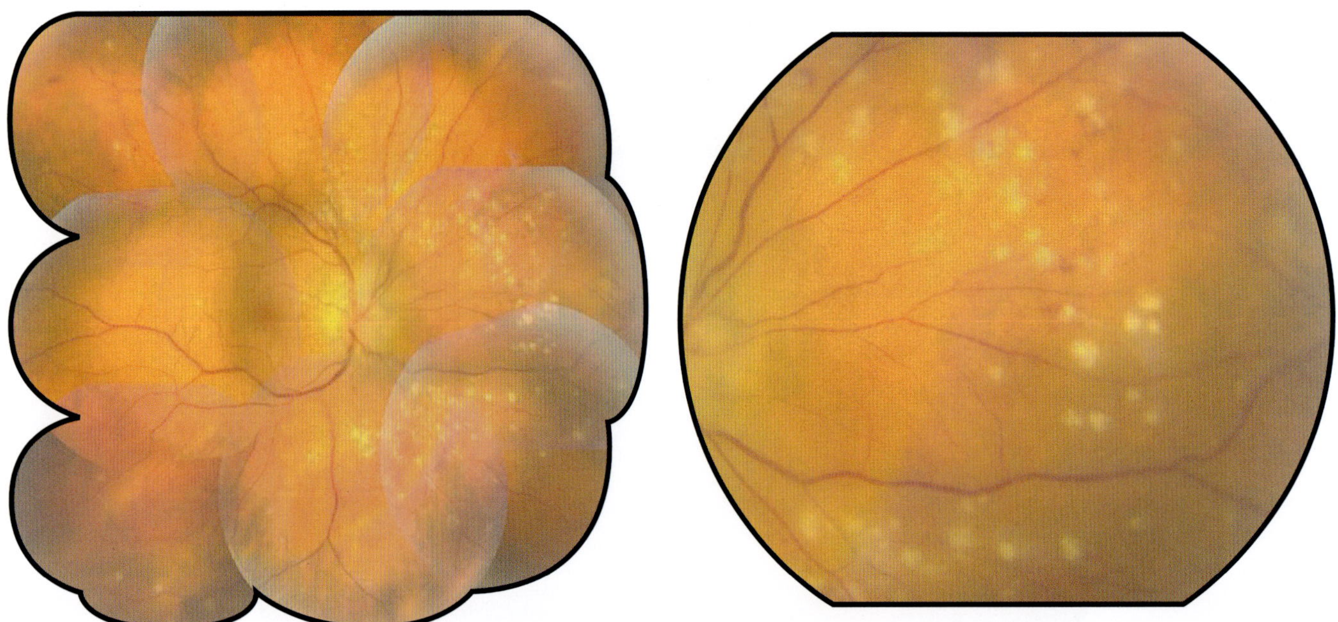

This 61-year-old male with ankylosing spondylitis experienced reduced vision initially from an anterior uveitis. The inflammatory process progressed to become an intermediate uveitis, and he developed chorioretinal infiltrates in the fundus. His medical workup revealed only ankylosing spondylitis. *Courtesy of Dr. Helen Li*

Rheumatological Diseases

Rheumatological diseases are clinical disorders involving joints, soft tissues, and connective tissues. The pathogenesis of these diseases is not well understood, but they are considered to be autoimmune disorders in genetically predisposed individuals. Intraocular manifestations of rheumatological diseases are generally inflammatory and include scleritis, but retinal vascular occlusive complications are more typical. Some rheumatological diseases, such as systemic lupus erythematosus and polyarteritis nodosa, have a marked predilection for retinal vascular occlusive abnormalities. In this atlas, we have included these diseases in the retinal vascular chapter (Chapter 6).

Scleroderma

Scleroderma is a chronic connective tissue disorder characterized by the presence of thickened or hardened skin. The disease can be categorized into two main groups, limited cutaneous or systemic. The limited cutaneous form is frequently associated with CREST syndrome defined as the presence of calcinosis, Raynaud phenomenon, esophageal dysmotility, sclerodactyly, and telangiectasia. Systemic disease is more serious and results in widespread vascular dysfunction and fibrosis of multiple organs. This can lead to pulmonary fibrosis, renal disease, serious systemic hypertension, and even death. Retinal complications associated with scleroderma include macular edema, occlusive retinal vasculitis, sheathing, retinal vascular obstruction, and ischemic retinopathy, which may lead to retinal neovascularization.

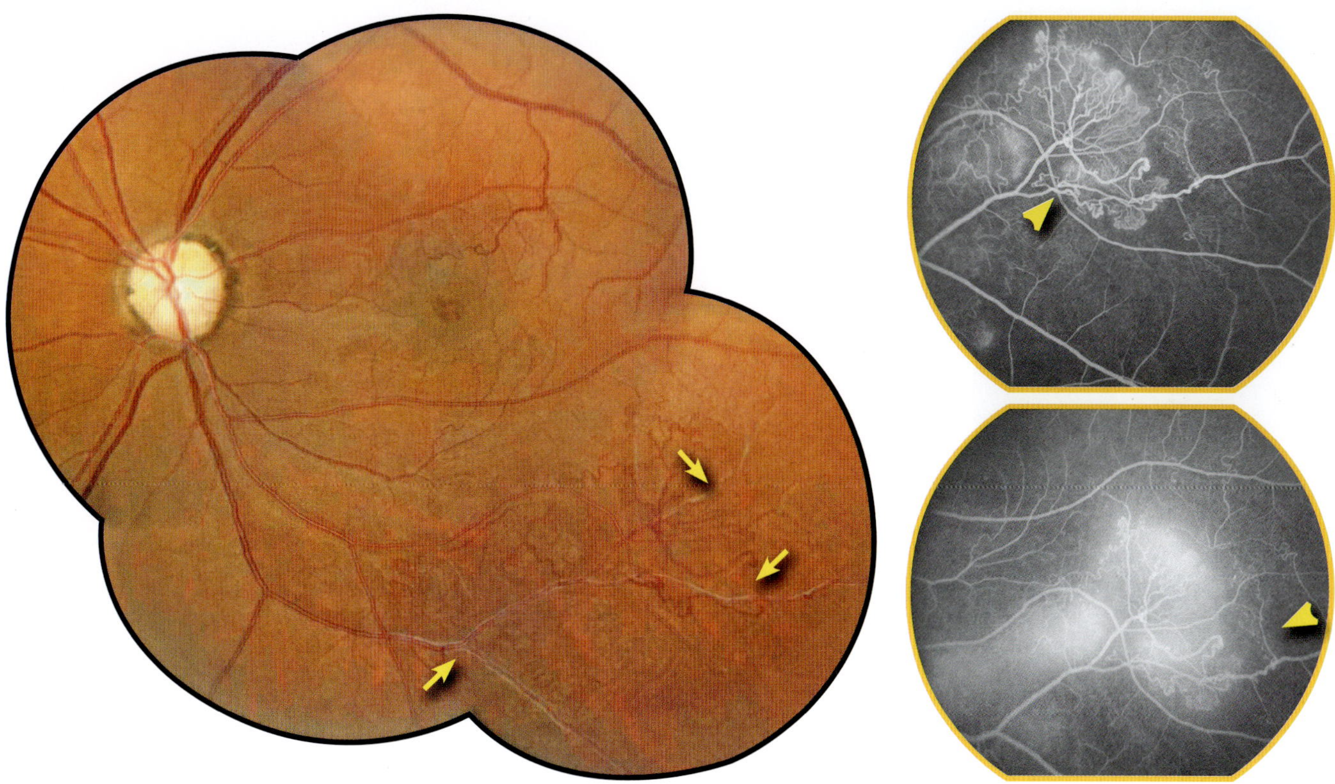

This patient with scleroderma has inferotemporal retinal vascular ischemic disease. Note the sheathed vessels *(arrows)* and the presence of ischemia and neovascularization *(arrowheads)* with FA.

Churg–Strauss Syndrome (Allergic Granulomatosis and Angiitis)

Churg–Strauss Syndrome (CSS) is a rare systemic disease characterized by small-vessel necrotizing vasculitis, eosinophilia, and asthma. The diagnosis is made by the presence of 4 of 6 characteristic features: asthma, more than 10% eosinophils on peripheral smear, neuropathy, pulmonary infiltrates, paranasal sinus abnormalities, and biopsy-confirmed tissue eosinophilia. The vasculitis is associated with a positive P-ANCA. Rarely, the eyes may be involved with reported abnormalities that include amaurosis fugax, branch retinal artery occlusion, ischemic optic neuropathy, uveoscleritis, inflammatory pseudotumor, and cranial nerve palsies.

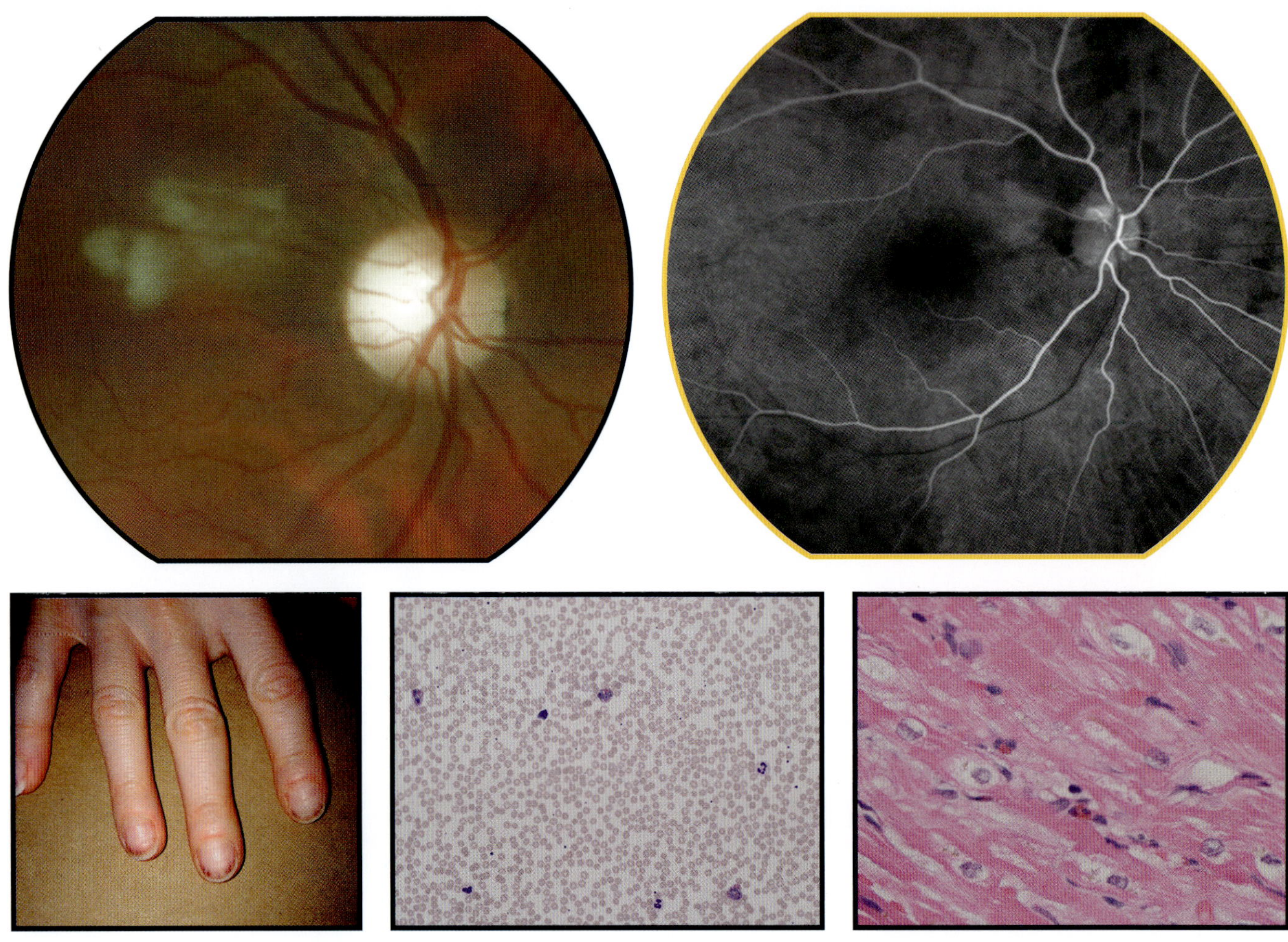

This 30-year-old female was admitted to the cardiology service for congestive heart failure and central scotoma in the right eye. Color fundus photos of the right eye illustrate areas of retinal whitening along the course of a branch retinal artery. Fluorescein angiogram shows the presence of a small branch arterial occlusion. Past medical history was significant for asthma, sinusitis, and sensorimotor axonal neuropathy. Examination of the hands demonstrate splinter hemorrhages of the nail beds *(second row, left)* and a mural thrombus was identified with echocardiogram. Peripheral blood smear shows 39% eosinophils *(second row, middle)*. A biopsy of the endocardium was performed and shows eosinophils extravasated into the cardiac tissue *(second row, right)*. Further radiologic and laboratory workup confirmed the presence of positive P-ANCA and pulmonary infiltrates. The diagnosis of Churg–Strauss was made and the patient was started on immunosuppressive therapy with remarkable improvement.
Images courtesy of Robert W. Wong, MD

Relapsing Polychondritis

Relapsing polychondritis is rare rheumatologic disorder characterized by recurrent inflammation of cartilaginous tissues in the body. The disease has many ocular manifestations that include conjunctivitis, episcleritis, scleritis, peripheral ulcerative keratitis, anterior uveitis, and posterior-segment inflammation. Intermediate uveitis, optic disc edema, retinal vasculitis, vascular occlusion, macular edema, and exudative retinal detachment have all been reported.

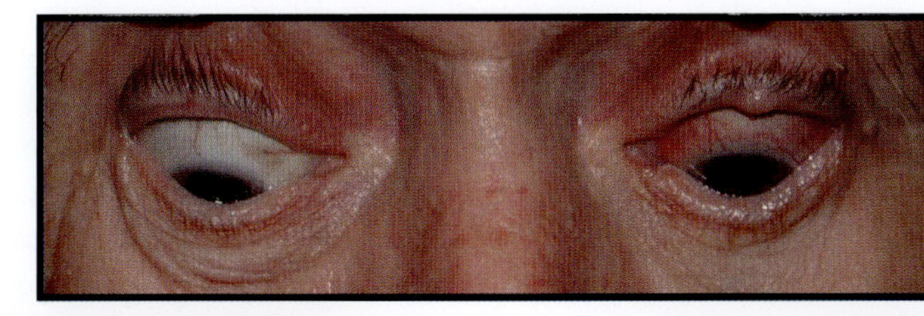

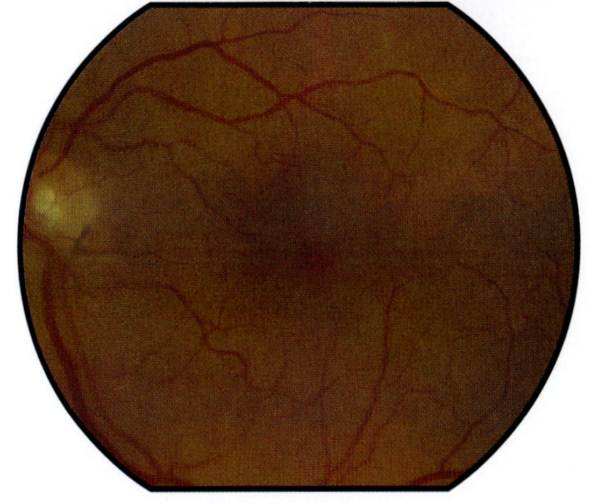

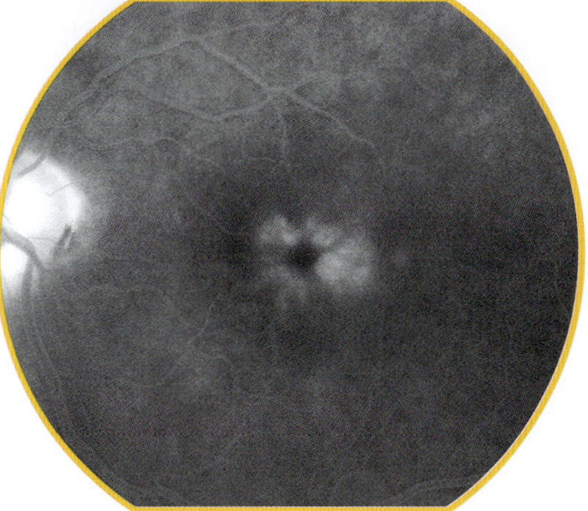

This patient with relapsing polychondritis has anterior scleritis and intermediate uveitis of the left eye. Note the presence of disc staining, and petaloid cystoid macular edema with FA. *Courtesy of Dr. R. S. Dhaliwal*

Adult-Onset Still's Disease

Still's disease is a form of idiopathic juvenile arthritis characterized by spiking fevers and transient rashes. Although Still's disease was first described in children, it is now known to occur less commonly in adults, in whom it is called adult-onset Still's disease (AOSD). AOSD affects men and women equally, usually in the second to third decade of life. Patients with AOSD may develop a retinal microangiopathy, including a Purtscher-like retinopathy.

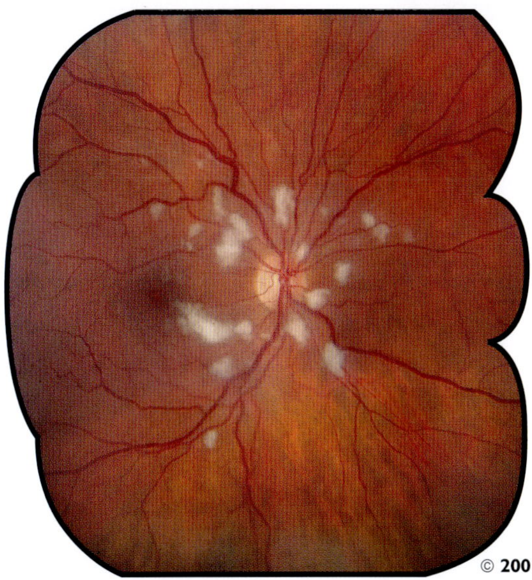

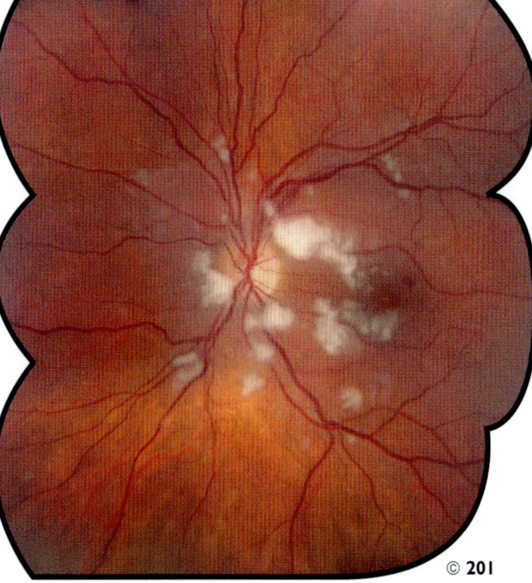

This is a 27-year-old white male with Still's disease who presented with a 3-day history of acute vision loss in each eye. Note the cluster of cotton-wool spots due to capillary ischemia causing axoplasmic stasis in these eyes with Purtscher-like retinopathy.

Idiopathic Retinal Vasculitis, Aneurysms, and Neuroretinitis (IRVAN)

IRVAN is a rare entity diagnosed clinically by the presence of bilateral retinal artery macroaneurysms, retinal vasculitis, and neuroretinitis. The retinal artery macroaneurysms typically appear at the first or second order arterial bifurcations or along the course of the optic nerve-head arterioles. The disease usually presents in the third or fourth decade of life, but has been reported as early as age seven. The disease may be idiopathic but has also been described in association with systemic sarcoid. Visual loss is usually the result of capillary non-perfusion, retinal neovascularization, and/or macular edema or exudation, which may frequently complicate the disorder. While early reports described an often self-limited course, longer follow-up periods have revealed that the disorder may frequently lead to severe bilateral vision loss if left untreated, as a result of progressive retinal ischemia. In these severe cases, vitreous hemorrhage and neovascular glaucoma may even occur. For this reason some authors advocate treatment with panretinal photocoagulation when significant peripheral retinal vascular non-perfusion is first noted on angiography studies.

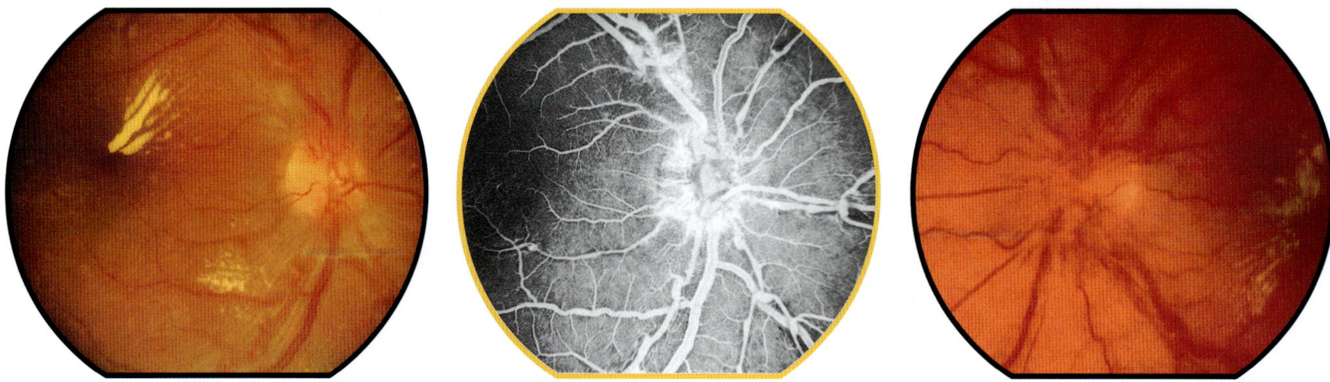

This healthy patient has lipid exudation with a macular star and tortuous vessels secondary to a peculiarly rare syndrome termed bilateral IRVAN. The fluorescein angiogram delineates the multiple macroaneurysms, which are at vessel bifurcations. The findings were similar in both eyes. *Left and middle images courtesy of Johnny Justice*

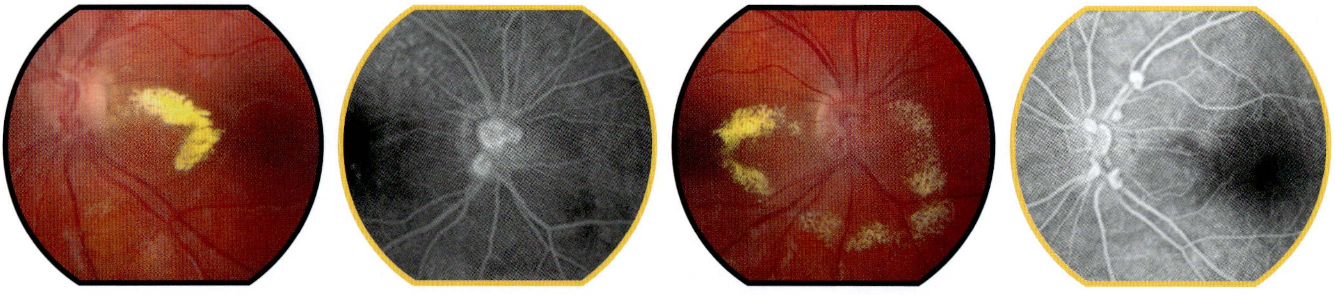

In this patient with IRVAN, the macroaneurysms are predominantly at the nerve head. Lipid deposition is very common from the inflammation and the aneurysmal leakage. The condition was bilateral but symmetric in this 14-year-old boy.

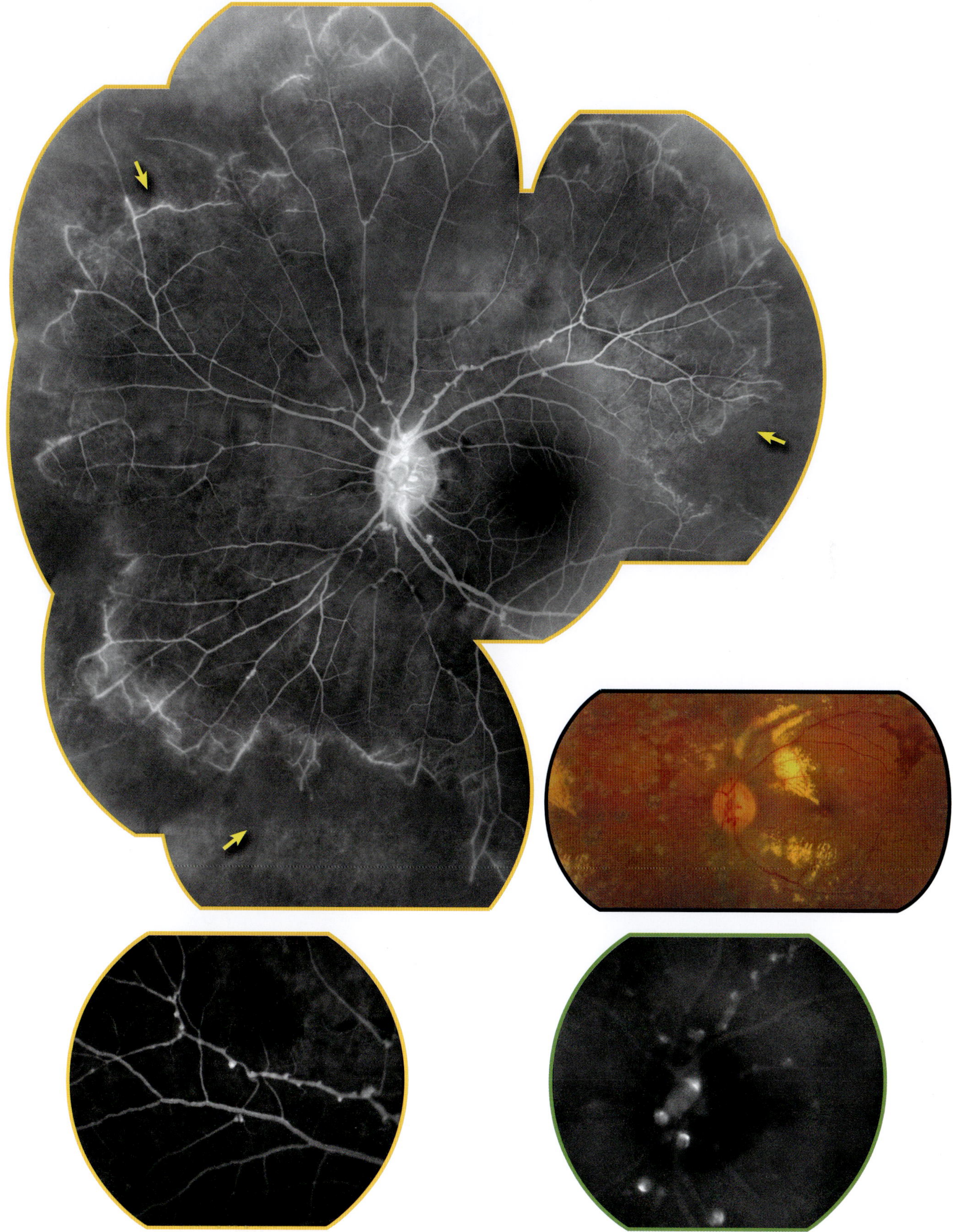

In patients with IRVAN, the peripheral retina should always be examined to exclude ischemia and neovascularization. This patient had lipid in the macula and retinal vascular manifestations of IRVAN clearly evident in the posterior pole. Widefield angiography of the peripheral fundus illustrates severe ischemia or non-perfusion *(arrows)*. The fluorescein and ICG angiograms enhance detection and documentation of the aneurysms *(bottom row)*.

Idiopathic Frosted-Branch Angiitis

Idiopathic frosted-branch angiitis is a rare, usually bilateral, retinal vasculitis occurring in otherwise healthy, immunocompetent patients. Its etiology is unknown; however, it is frequently reported following a multitude of different systemic viral and bacterial infections, and therefore a post-infectious inflammatory reaction has been hypothesized. The age of onset has a bimodal distribution, with peaks in the first and fourth decades of life; however, cases have been reported in individuals as young as 11 months and as old as 80 years. Patients typically present with floaters, photopsias, or a rapid loss of visual acuity, which may be profound. In children, marked sheathing of both the arteries and veins is noted, along with vitritis, optic nerve head edema, and, rarely, exudative retinal detachment. In adults, the sheathing predominantly involves the retinal veins. Vitritis, iritis, and macular edema are commonly seen, and less frequently, papillitis; exudative retinal detachment has not been described. Patients are typically treated with systemic corticosteroids with a recovery to near normal vision over several weeks in most cases. A similar fundus appearance has been reported in association with active cytomegalovirus infection, hematologic malignancies, as well as in specific autoimmune diseases, like systemic lupus erythematosus and sarcoidosis. In these cases, the fundus appearance is considered a clinical sign of the underlying disease, rather than a distinct clinical entity. Accordingly, some authors have proposed reserving the term "idiopathic frosted-branch angiitis" to those patients without a known underlying cause.

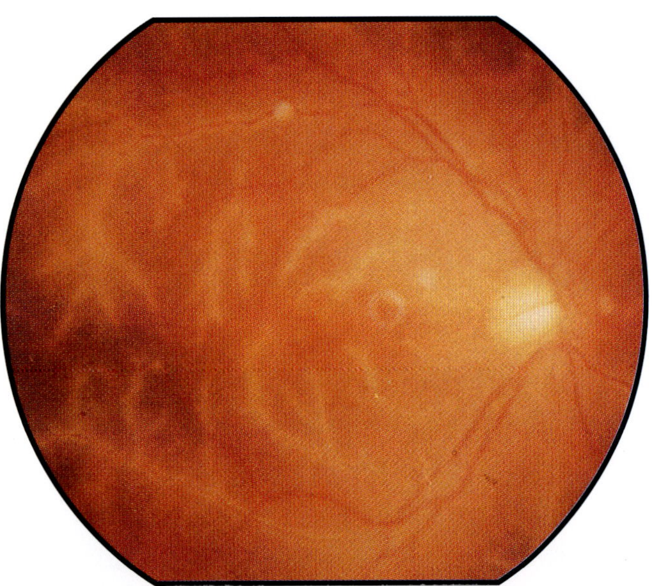

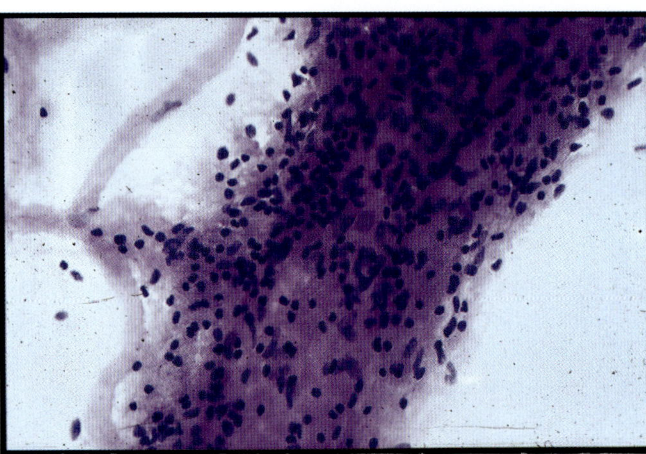

This patient has classic idiopathic frosted-branch angiitis with the deposition of thick white material along the involved vessels. The histopathological specimen demonstrates numerous inflammatory cells in an inflamed vessel, which is presumed to be the mechanism for the frosted appearance.

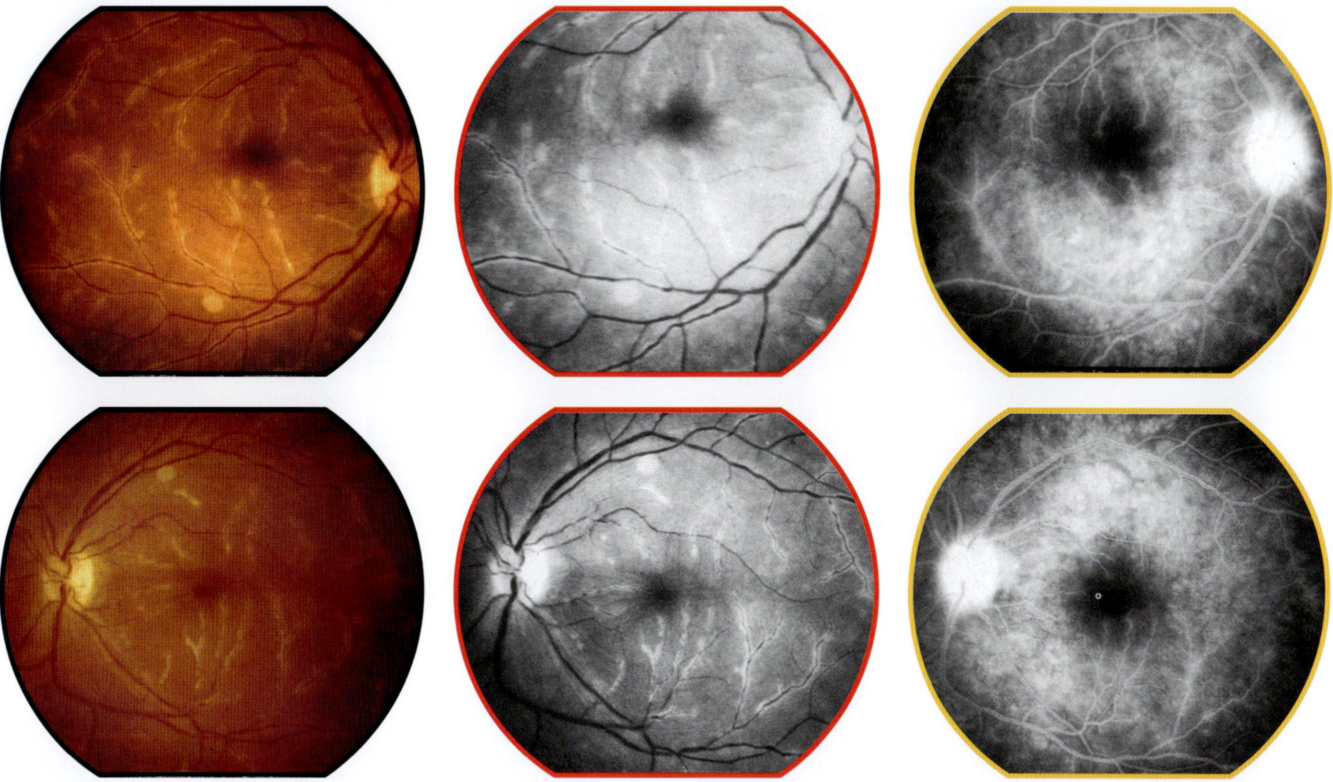

This patient has idiopathic frosted-branch angiitis. There is deposition of inflammatory exudate along the walls of the retinal vessels, predominantly along the veins. The manifestations are more dramatically evident on the red-free photographs *(middle images)*. FA shows staining of the involved vessels and disc leakage.

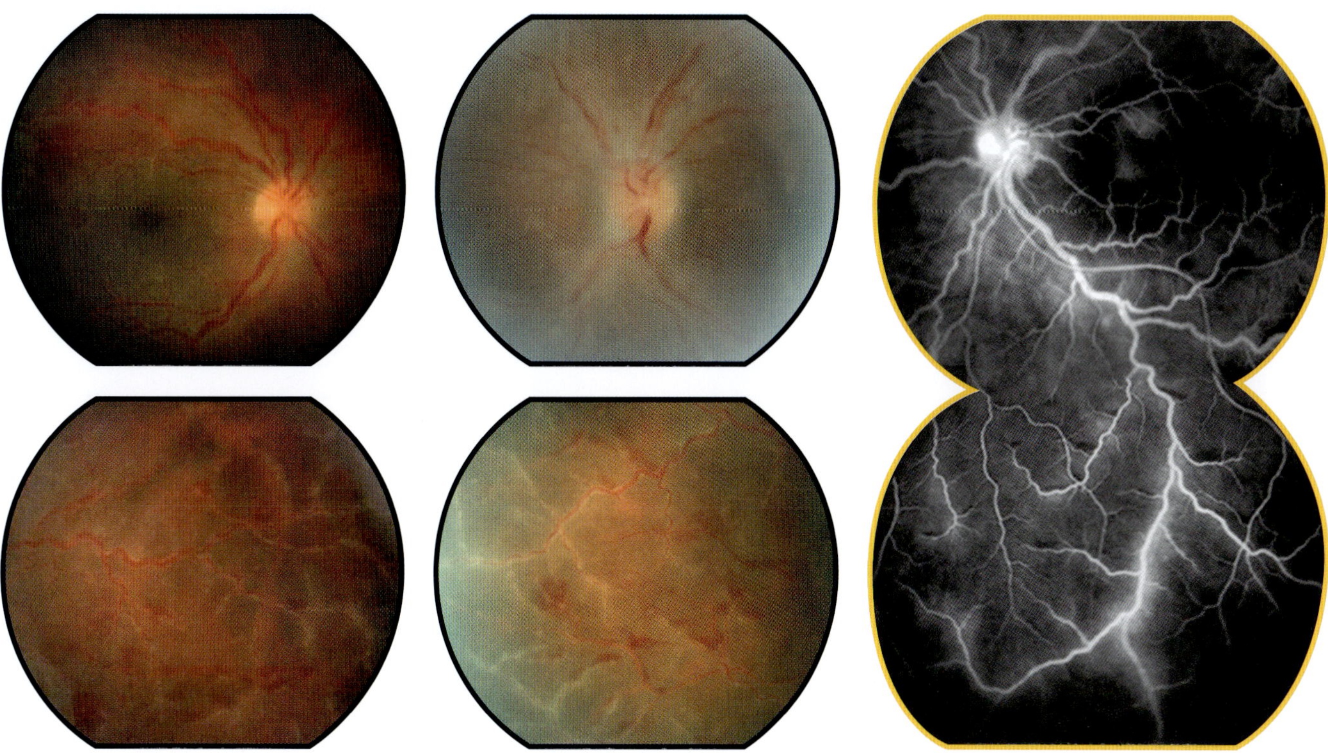

This is an 11-year-old female who experienced bilateral vision loss from idiopathic frosted-branch angiitis. The posterior pole shows disc swelling and macular edema. More peripherally, classic frosted branch angiitis is identified with intervening hemorrhages. Over a period of several months, this patient responded to steroid therapy, and there has been no recurrence for 17 years.

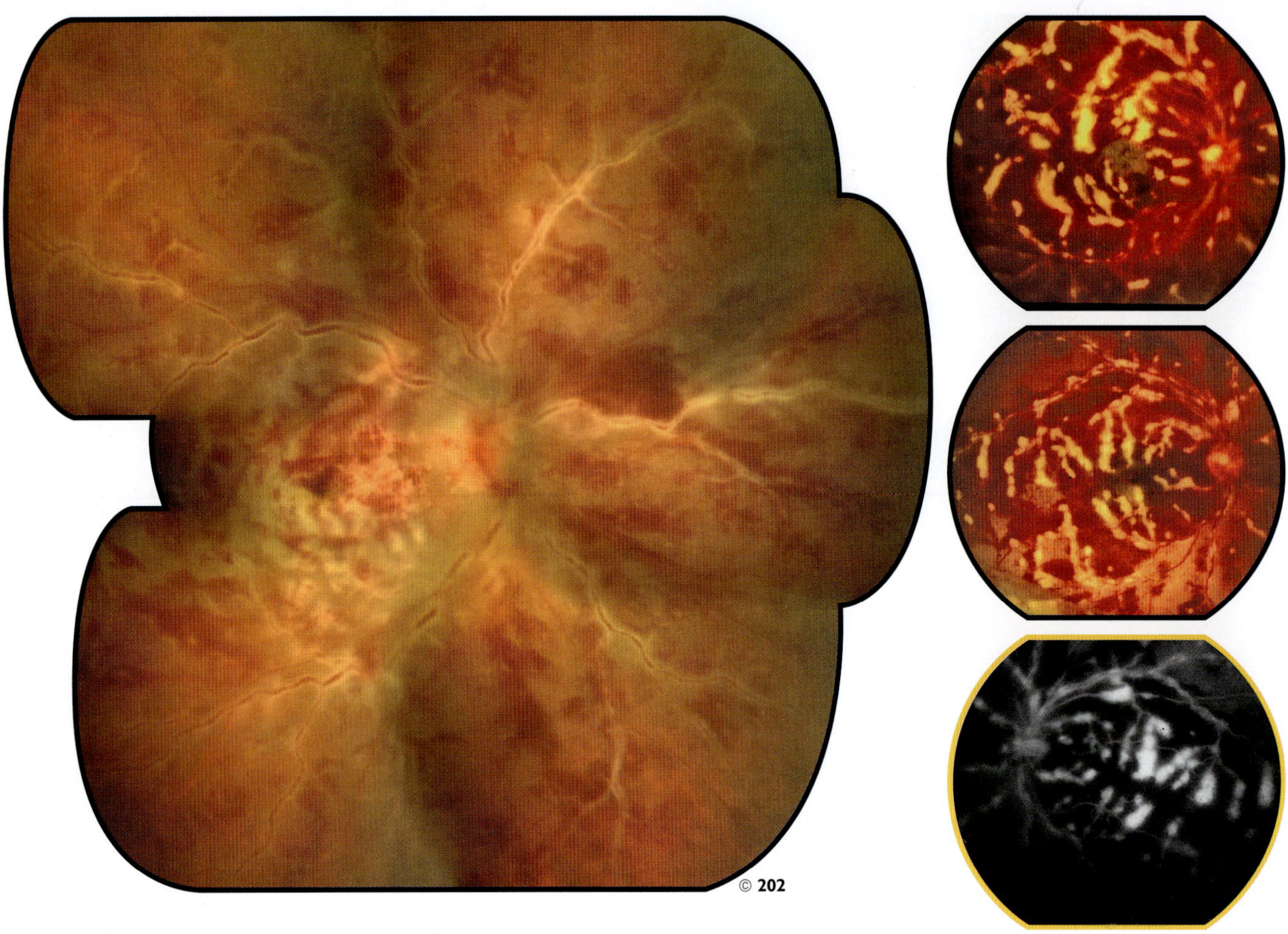

These three patients have idiopathic frosted-branch angiitis with diffuse retinal involvement. There is also severe macular edema, extensive intraretinal and preretinal hemorrhage, and papillitis. There was no systemic abnormality noted after a very extensive medical workup.

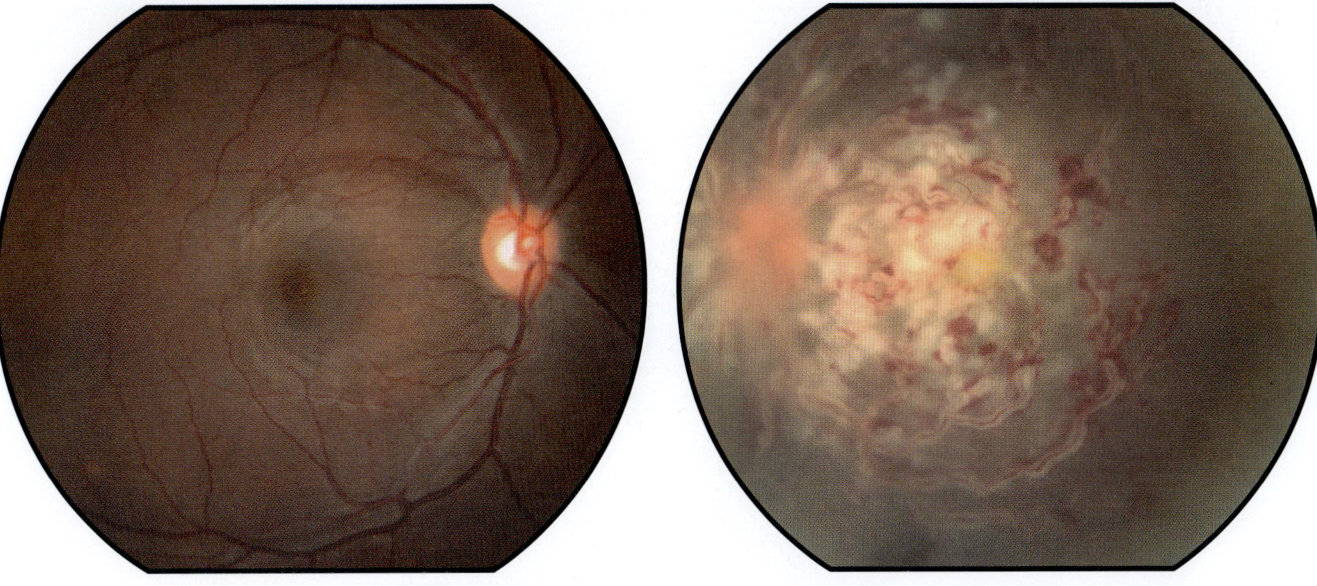

This 29-year-old male developed back pain, an inability to control his left leg, and vision loss in his left eye. Color fundus photos of the right eye were normal on presentation. Color fundus photo of the left eye demonstrates optic nerve hyperemia, intraretinal hemorrhages and sheathing of the vessels in a "frosted-branch" type pattern. *Images courtesy of Mark J. Daily, MD*

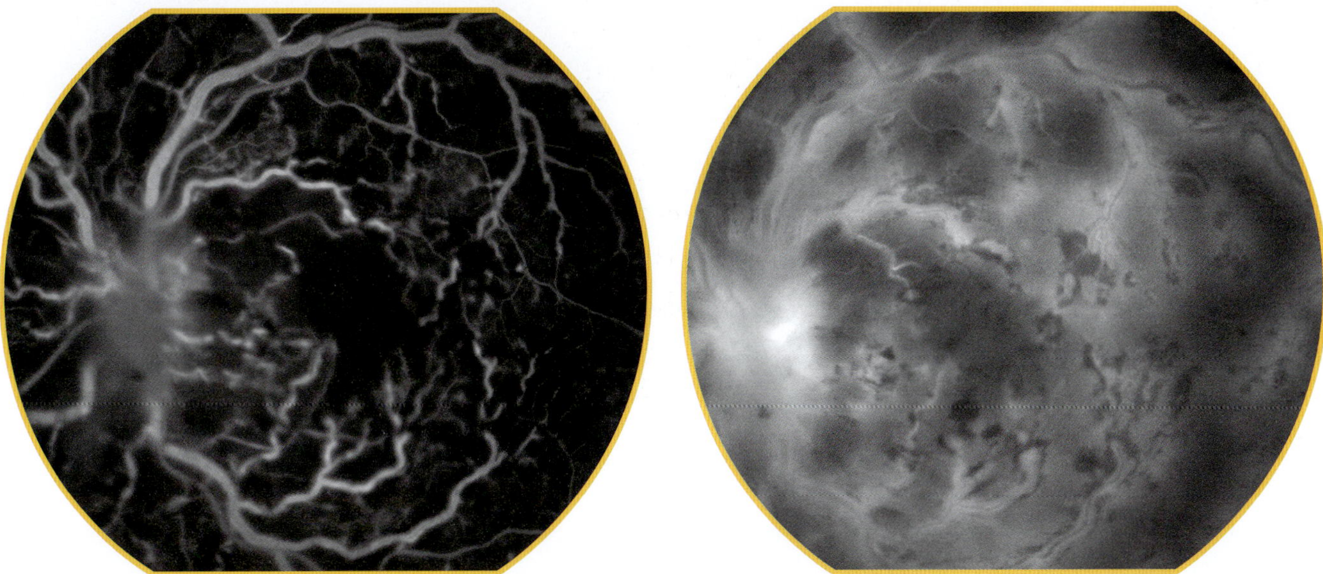

In the same patient, fluorescein angiogram of the left eye on presentation confirms optic disc leakage, blocking of intraretinal hemorrhages, and staining and leakage from the retinal vasculature. *Images courtesy of Mark J. Daily, MD*

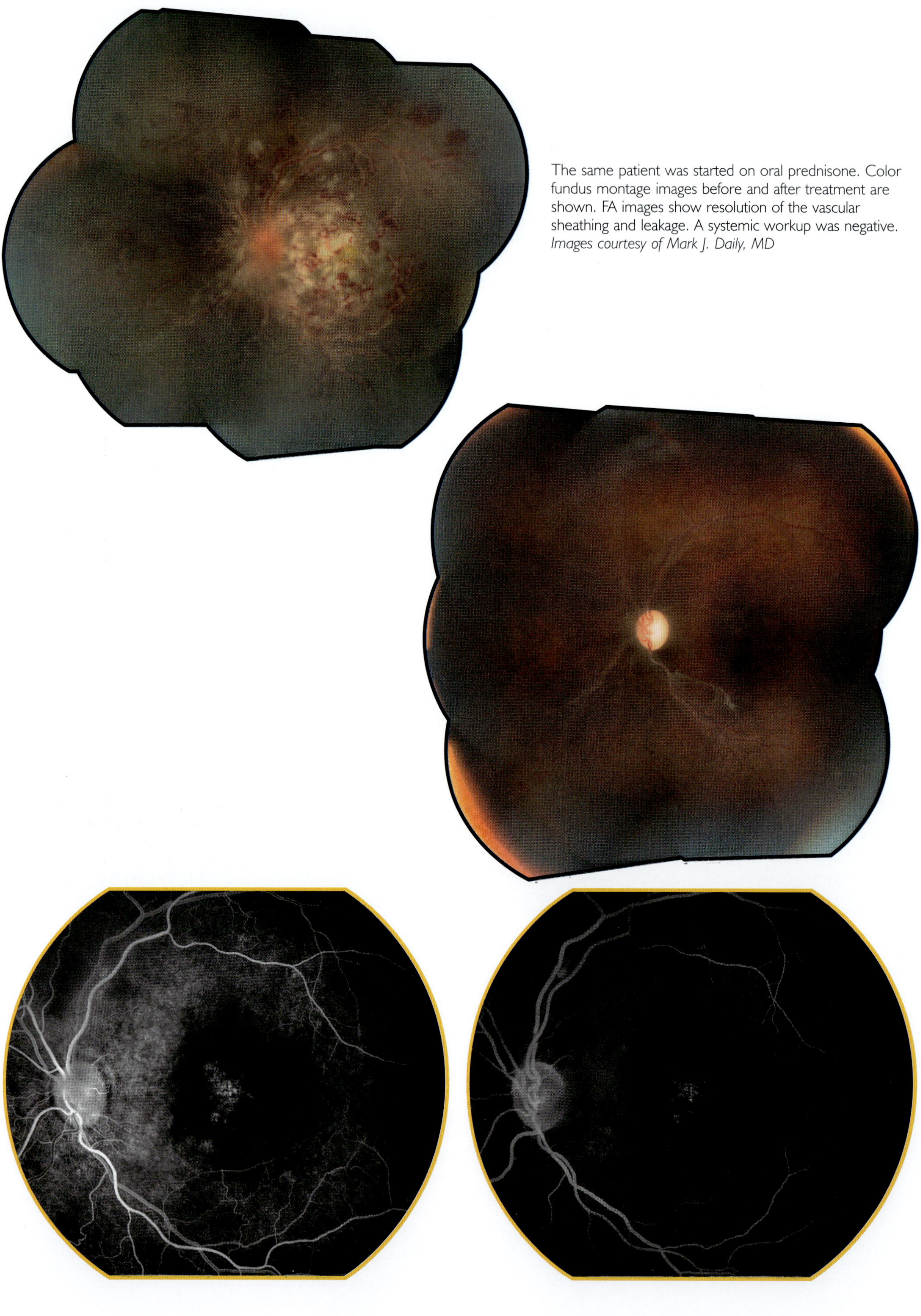

The same patient was started on oral prednisone. Color fundus montage images before and after treatment are shown. FA images show resolution of the vascular sheathing and leakage. A systemic workup was negative. *Images courtesy of Mark J. Daily, MD*

Sarcoidosis

Sarcoidosis is a chronic idiopathic multisystem inflammatory disorder characterized by noncaseating granulomas. Sarcoidosis can involve virtually any organ but typically begins in the lungs and lymph nodes. Sarcoidosis most commonly affects young adults, with women slightly more likely to be affected than men. In the USA, sarcoidosis is more common in people of African descent than in Caucasians, especially in younger patients. Approximately 20% of patients with sarcoidosis have ophthalmic involvement. The findings may be extraocular, and involve the orbit, lacrimal glands, eyelids, and conjunctiva. Intraocular findings of sarcoidosis involve the anterior segment and include a granulomatous anterior uveitis [anterior-chamber cell and flare, mutton-fat keratic precipitates, and (Koeppe) iris nodules], interstitial keratitis, and band kerotopathy. Posterior-segment findings occur in approximately 28% of sarcoidosis patients with ocular involvement. Posterior-segment findings include vitritis (both diffuse and focal, including "snowball" and "string of pearl" opacities), pars planitis, retinal vasculitis (periphlebitis), retinal vascular occlusion, retinal neovascularization, cystoid macular edema, epiretinal membrane, choroidal infiltrates or granulomas, optic disc edema or neovascularization, and optic nerve-head granulomas. The periphlebitis may be focal or diffuse and may have the appearance of "candle wax drippings."

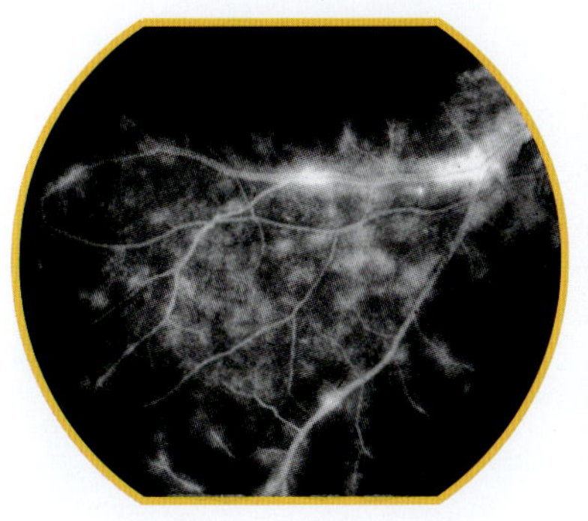

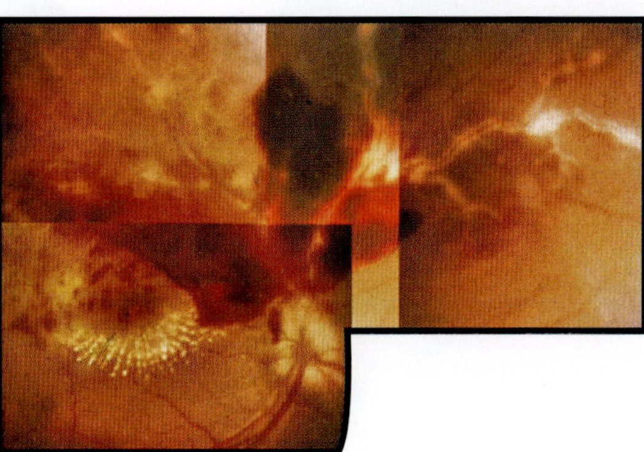

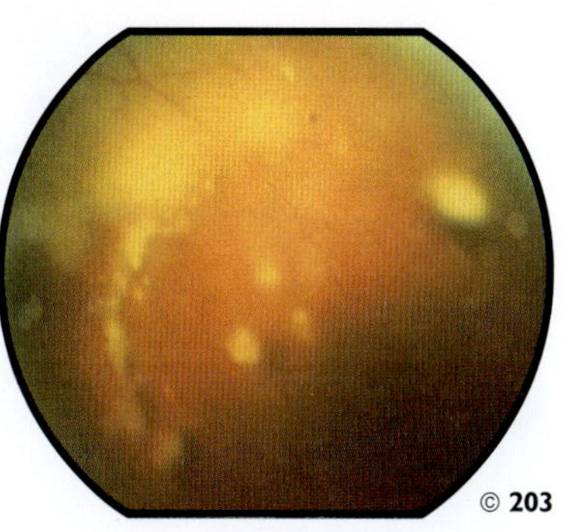

© 203

These patients with sarcoidosis reflect the myriad of changes that may be seen in the fundus. The patient on the left has a retinal periphlebitis identified with FA. In the center, there is evidence of retinal vascular occlusive and inflammatory disease due to sarcoid. Note the exudates within the walls of vessels, producing a "frosted branch" appearance. There is severe hemorrhage and lipid exudation in the macula, and optic disc swelling *(middle)*. The patient on the right shows vitreous inflammation with exudates and infiltrates within the retina and the posterior vitreous.

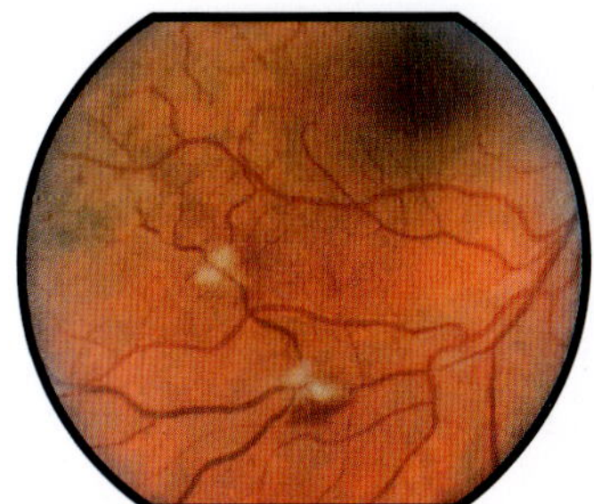

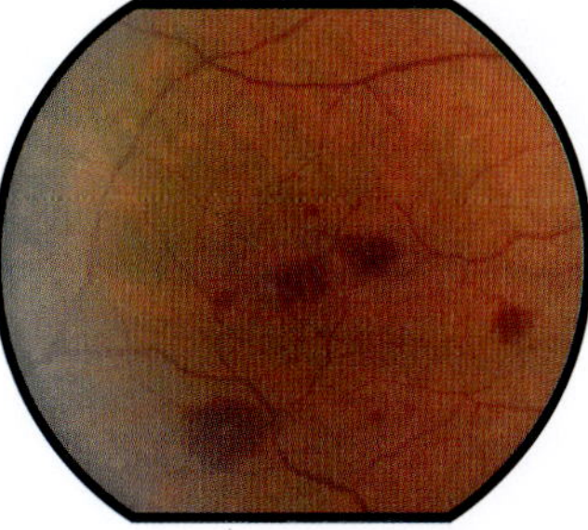

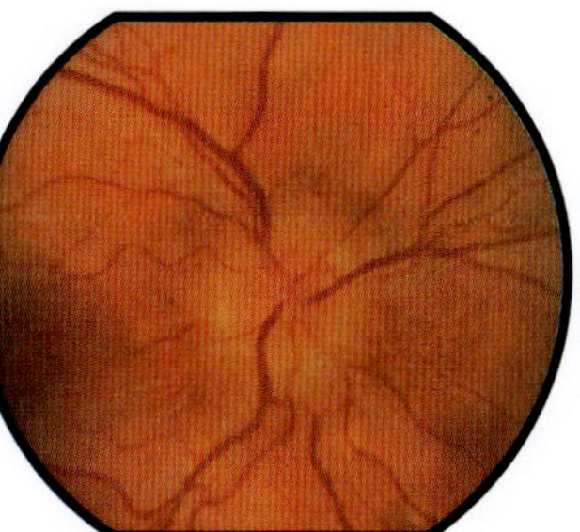

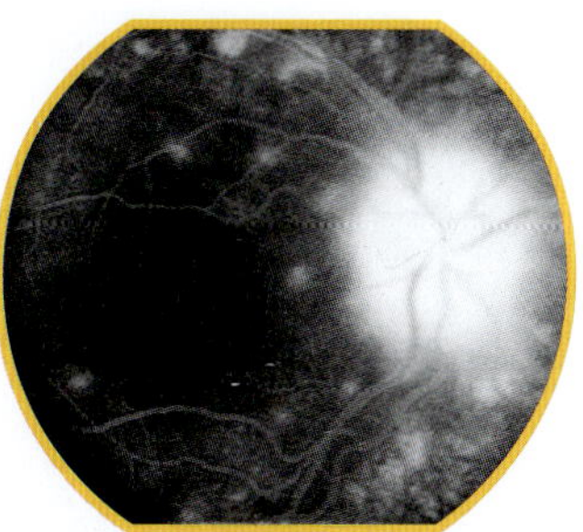

This patient with sarcoidosis (diagnosed by mediastinal biopsy) has a branch retinal vein occlusion. There are several hemorrhages with white centers or Roth spots *(second image)*. Note that the vein occlusion occurs at the site of localized phlebitis rather than at an arteriovenous crossing. There is subtle elevation or swelling of the optic nerve *(third image)*. There are also faintly evident spots at the level of the RPE and inner choroid in the peripapillary region, presumably multifocal granulomas. The fluorescein angiogram study shows leakage of the optic nerve, as well as the peripapillary spots in the choroid.

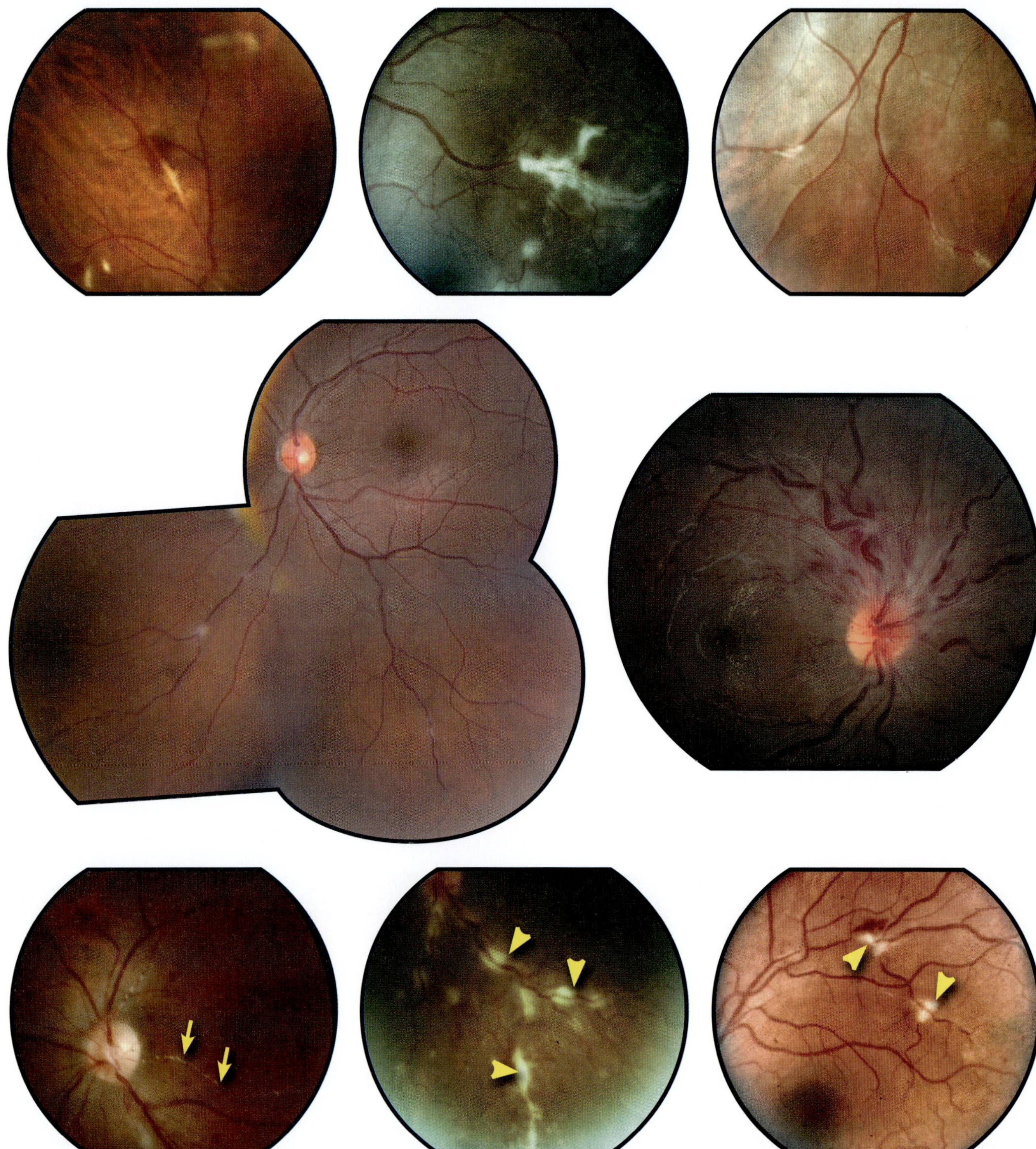

These patients show variations in the clinical spectrum of sarcoid-associated retinal phlebitis. Note the segmental frosted angiitis or so-called "candle wax drippings" *(top and middle rows)*. Axoplasmic debris accumulation *(middle left)*, hemorrhage with inflammatory exudation *(middle right)*, focal phlebitis *(arrowheads)*, and calcific plaques within arterioles or so-called Kyrieleis plaques *(lower row left, arrows)* are also noted.

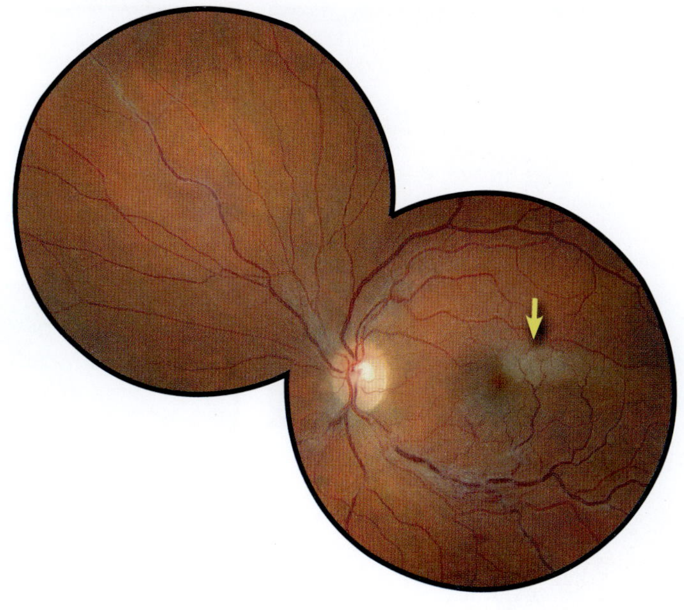

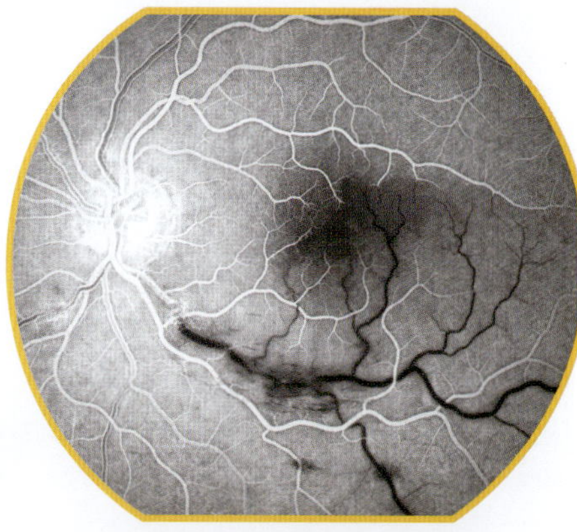

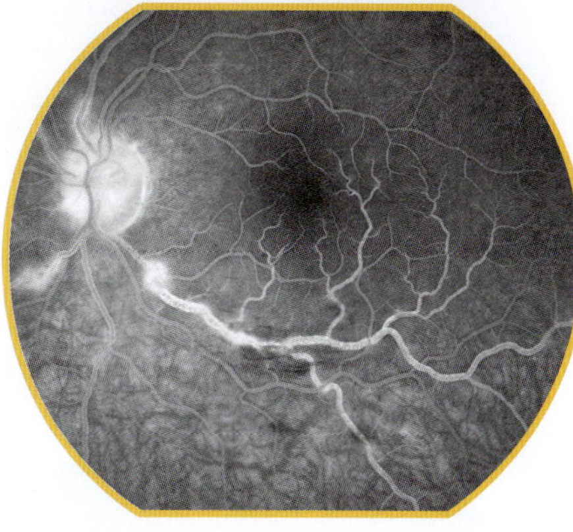

This patient with sarcoidosis has retinal vascular occlusive disease. An arteriolar occlusion is noted as grayish whitening in the superotemporal juxtafoveal area associated with non-perfusion of the arteriole *(arrow)*. Delayed perfusion and late staining of the inferotemporal retinal vein is also evident on the fluorescein angiogram *(right images)*.

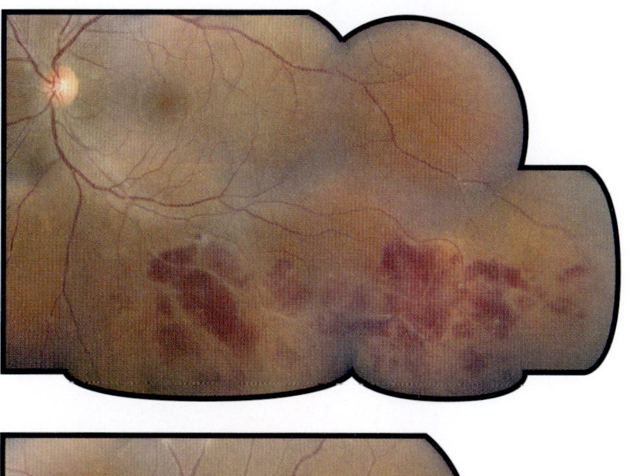

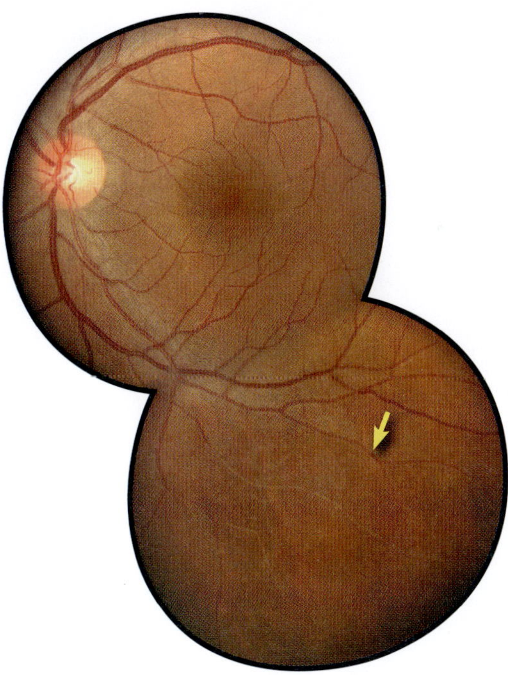

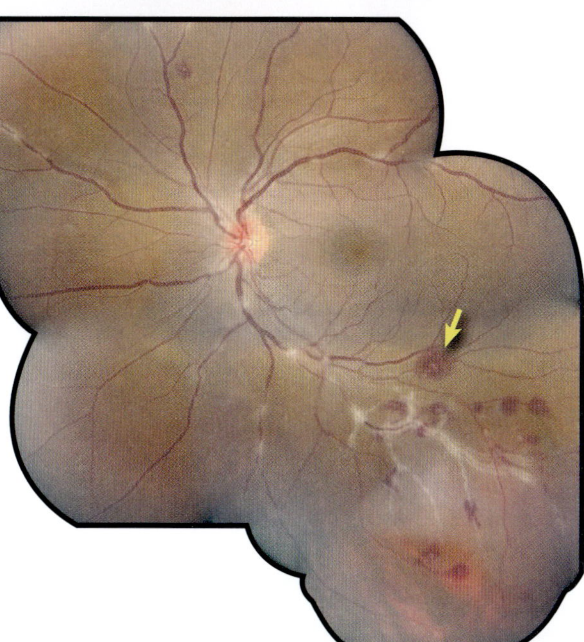

This patient with sarcoidosis has inferotemporal hemorrhagic retinal venous occlusive disease and inflammatory retinal phlebitis *(upper left)*. The inflammation progressed with the development of a frosted appearance in the walls of the involved inferotemporal retinal veins. There was also peripheral hemorrhage, which included a discrete white-centered hemorrhage *(arrow, left)* and peripheral ischemia. Following anti-inflammatory therapy, all of the exudative changes resolved, leaving a legacy of retinal vascular sheathing in the inferotemporal periphery *(above, arrow)*.

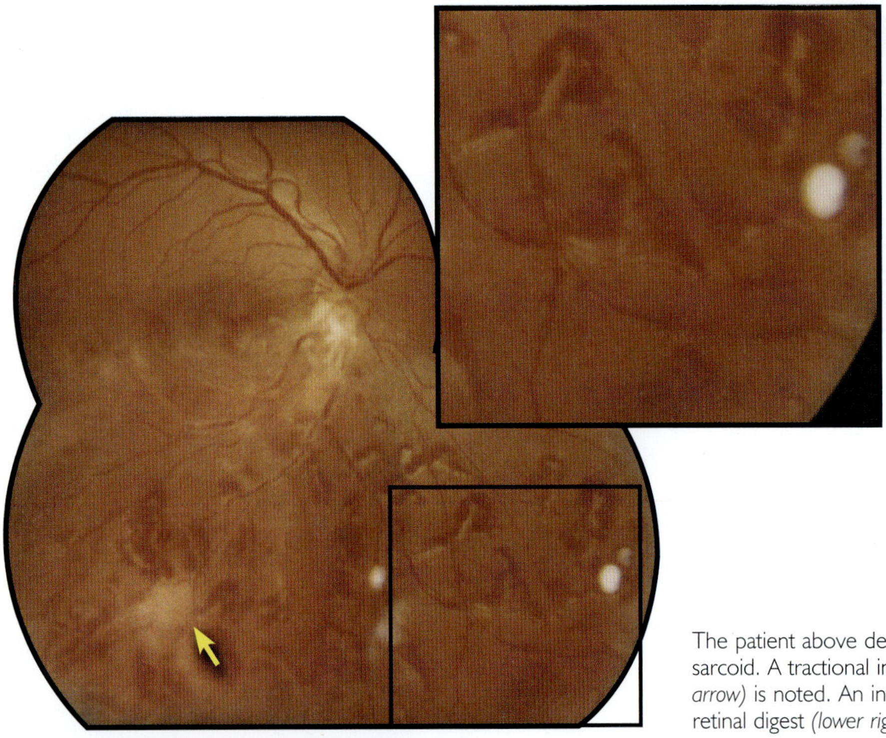

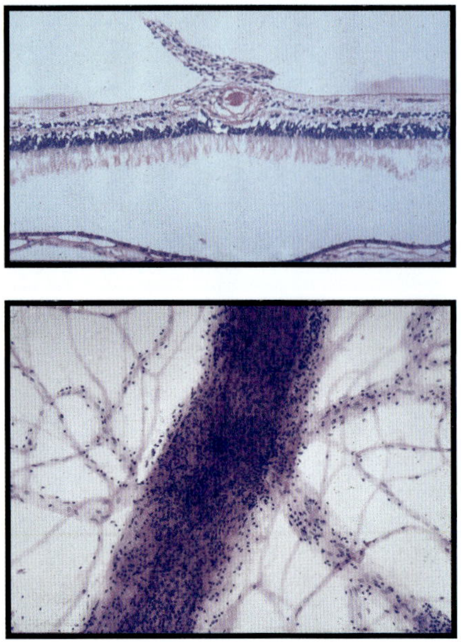

The patient above demonstrates a hemorrhagic retinal vasculitis due to sarcoid. A tractional inflammatory band along a retinal arteriole *(left, arrow)* is noted. An inflammatory cellular infiltration was noted with this retinal digest *(lower right)* in the second patient.

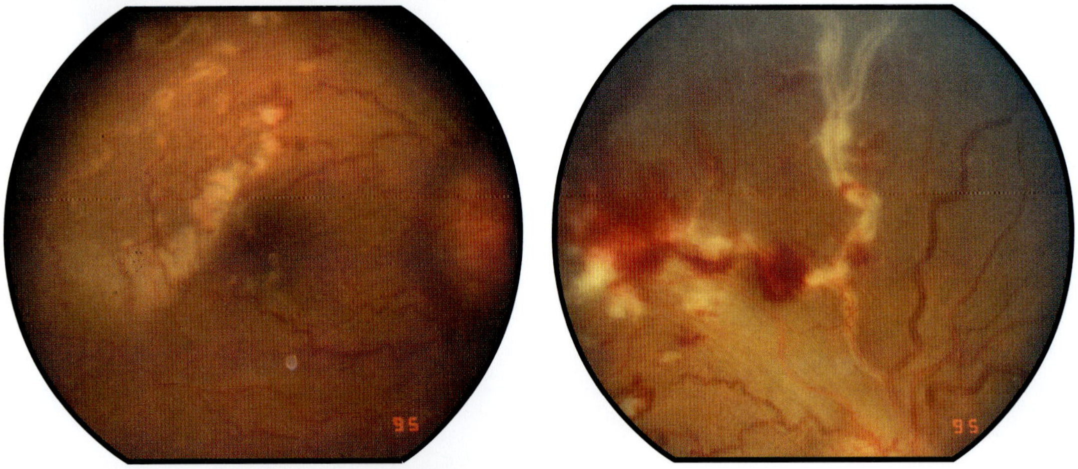

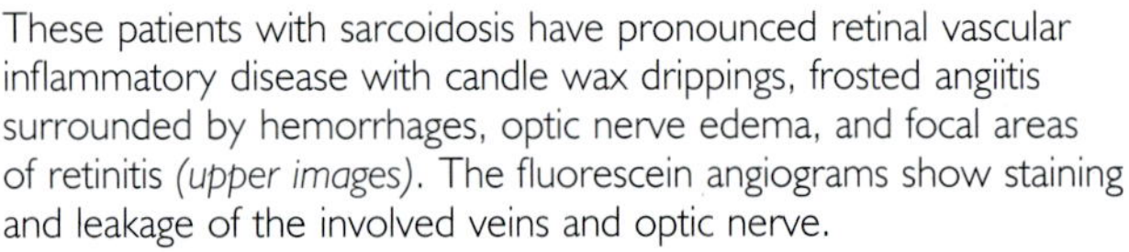

These patients with sarcoidosis have pronounced retinal vascular inflammatory disease with candle wax drippings, frosted angiitis surrounded by hemorrhages, optic nerve edema, and focal areas of retinitis *(upper images)*. The fluorescein angiograms show staining and leakage of the involved veins and optic nerve.

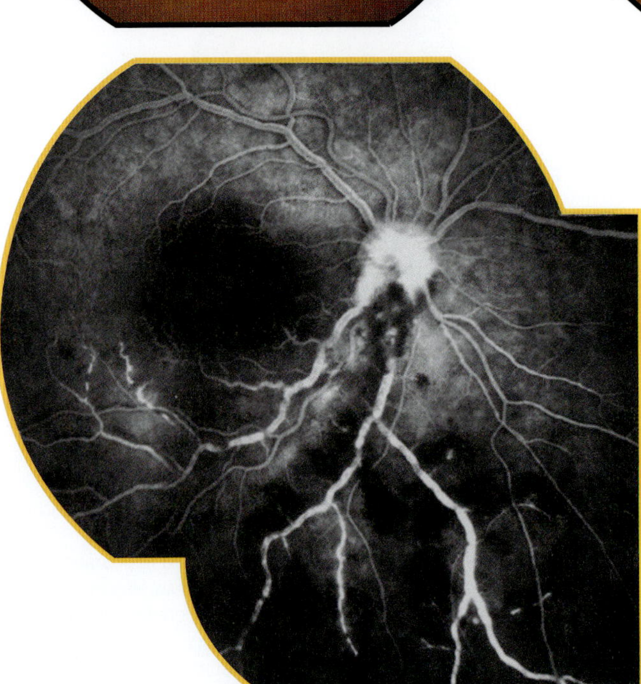

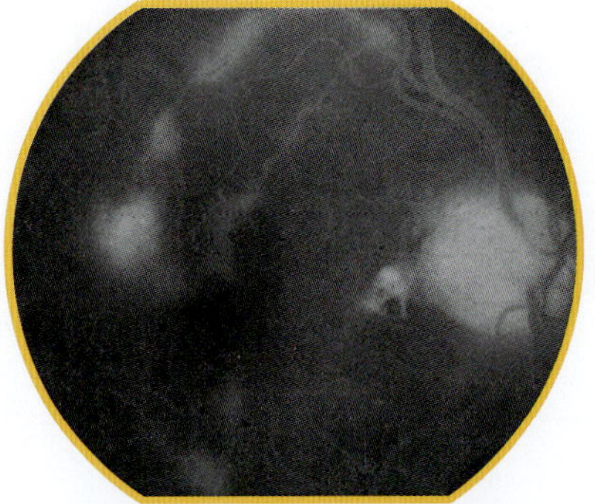

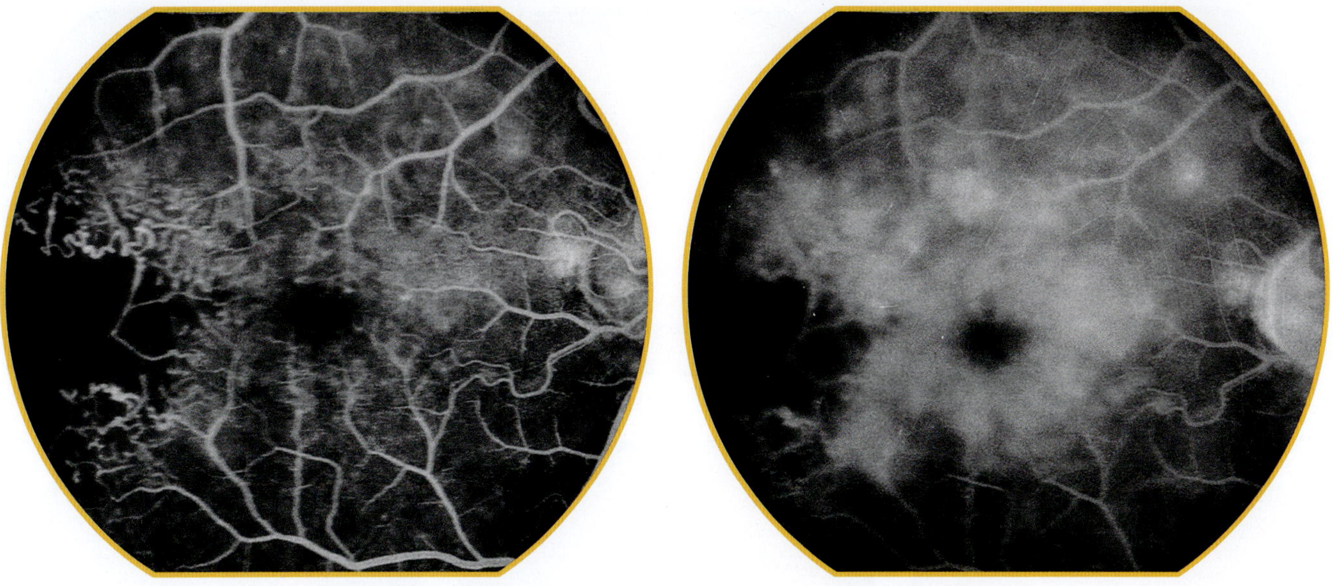

In this patient with sarcoidosis, fluorescein angiography studies illustrate a microangiopathy, including telangiectatic vascular changes, microaneurysms, temporal macular ischemia, and cystoid macular edema and leakage.

© 204

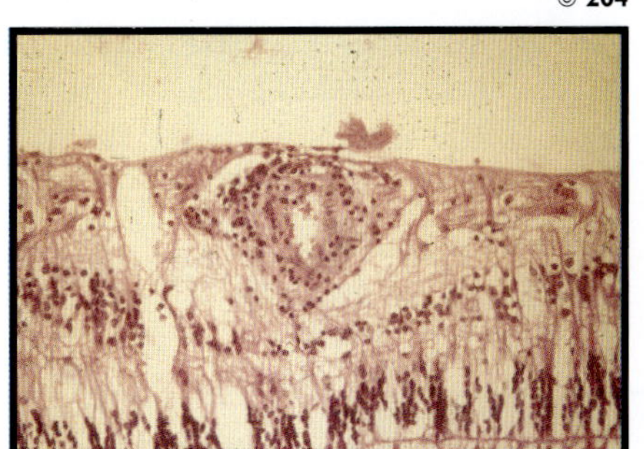

© 205

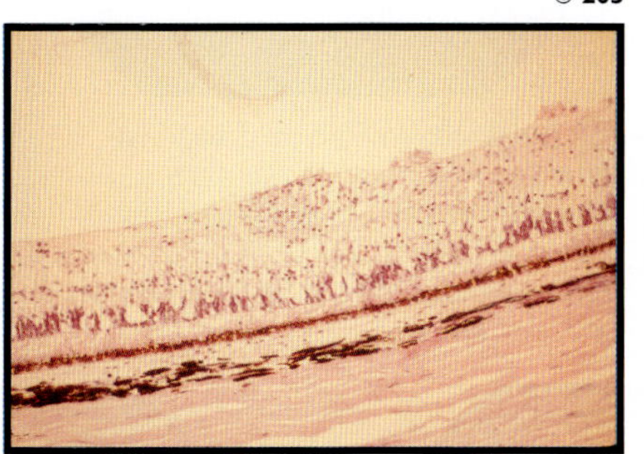

This patient with sarcoidosis illustrates sarcoid granulomas involving the inner surface of the retina. The left image shows a higher power view of the granuloma.

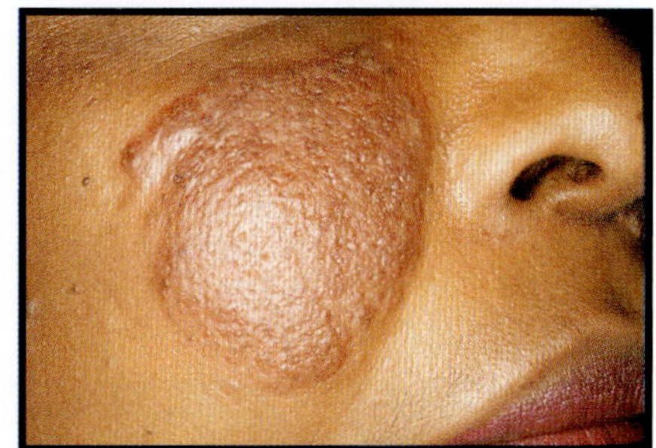

This patient has a sarcoid nodule on the cheek.

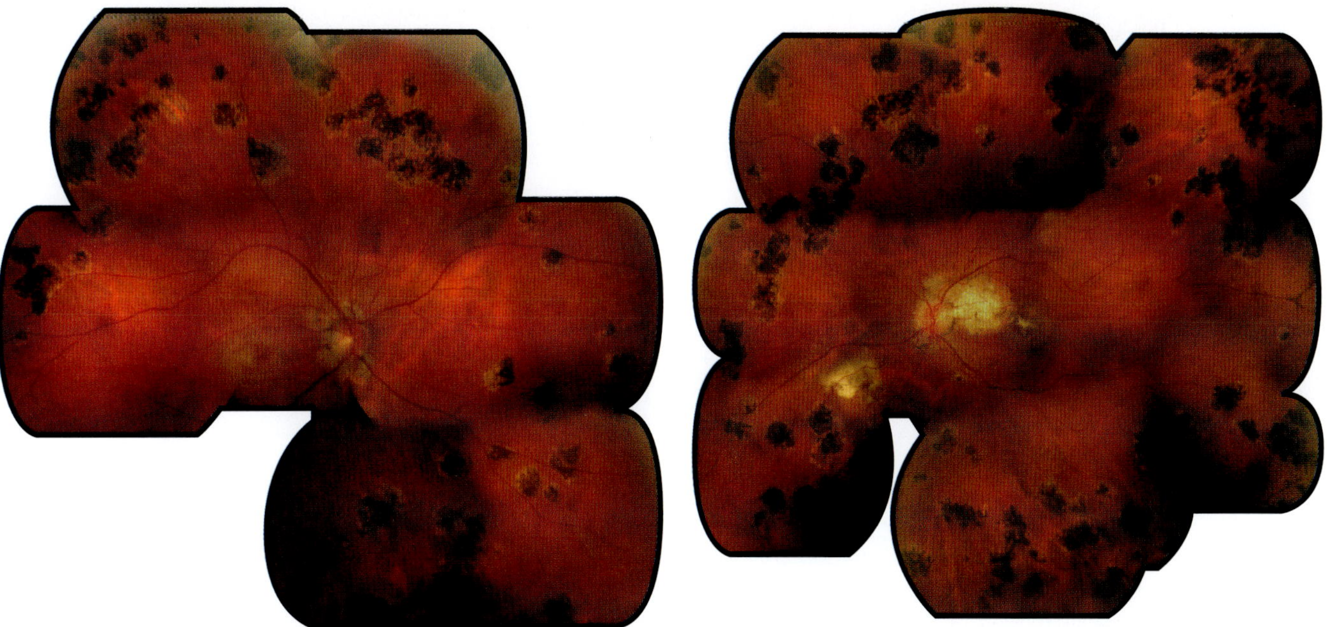

This patient with sarcoidosis had multiple areas of choroiditis, which led to multifocal pigmented chorioretinal scars resembling MFC. Note the atrophy and scarring of the macula of the left eye as well.

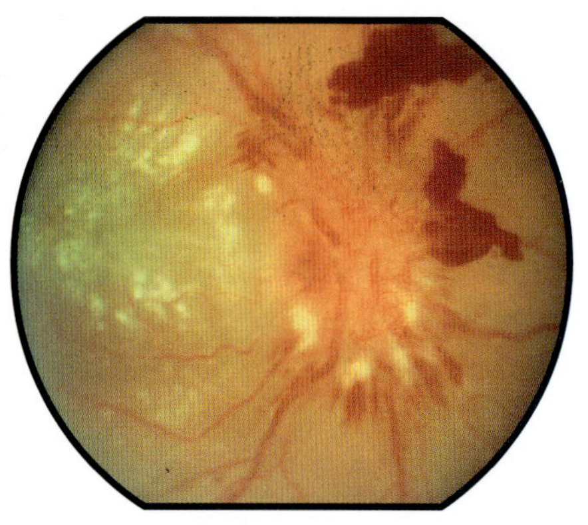
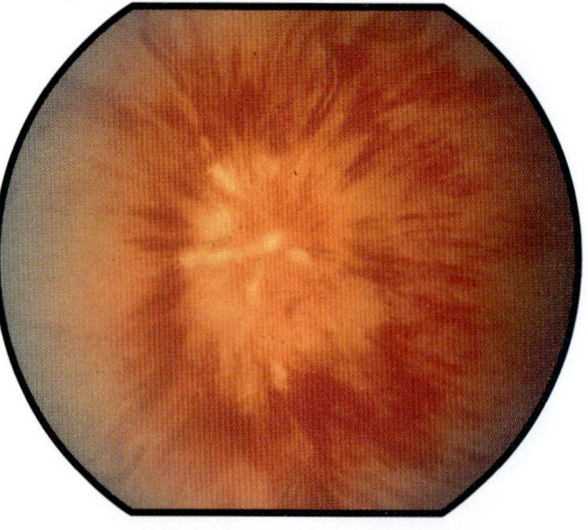
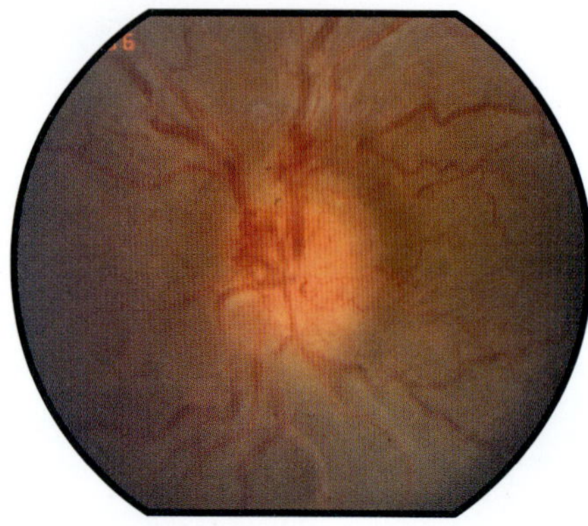

Sarcoidosis can be associated with optic nerve edema and hemorrhage, and leakage into the macula, as seen in these patients with neuroretinitis.

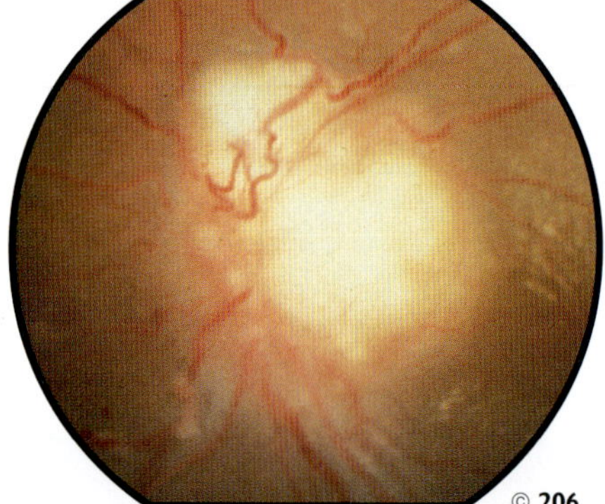

© 206

This case shows an optic nerve mass in a patient with sarcoidosis. Retinal vessels communicate with the granulomatous lesion. Note the candle wax drippings, which are inflammatory plaques along the retinal venules, best identified inferonasal to the nerve.

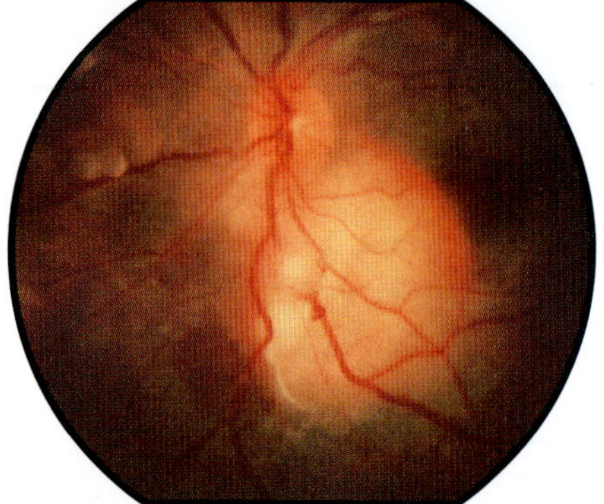

This patient has a choroidal granuloma secondary to sarcoidosis. Note the associated subretinal hemorrhage and serous retinal detachment. Vision was 6/200. This nodule regressed after steroid treatment. *Courtesy of Dr. Rollins Tindell, Jr*

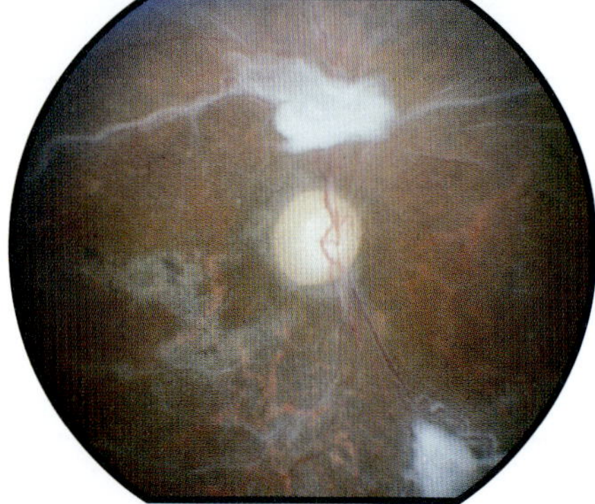

Extensive sheathing of retinal vessels with fibrosis may occur in the end stage of ocular sarcoidosis. Note the presence of optic disc atrophy, severe vascular sheathing and non-perfusion, pre-retinal fibrosis, and retinal pigment epithelial atrophy.

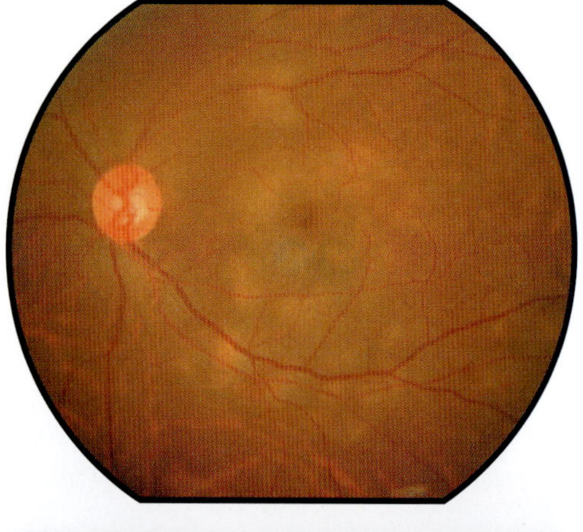
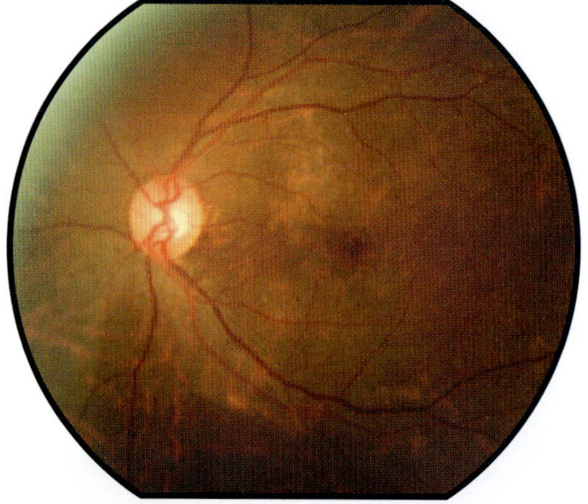
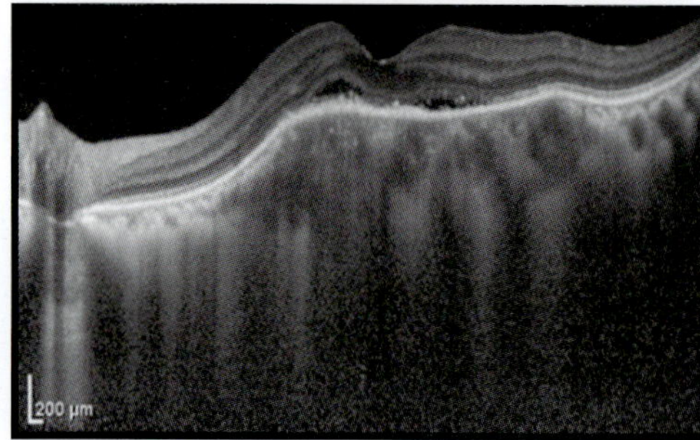

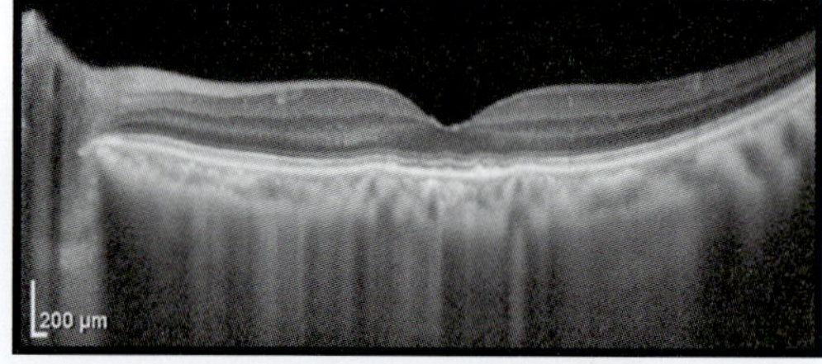

This 66-year-old female with a history of breast cancer presented with decreased vision in the left eye. Color fundus photos illustrate deep creamy yellow choroidal infiltrates involving the posterior pole *(top left)*. SD-OCT through the lesions at presentation show choroidal infiltration and thickening with overlying pockets of subretinal fluid and inner segment ellipsoid disruption. Subsequent workup revealed lung infiltrates and prominent mediastinal lymph nodes. Lymph node biopsy revealed noncaseating granuloma consistent with sarcoid. The patient was started on prednisone and the chorioretinal infiltrates and subretinal fluid resolved *(top right, bottom right)*. *Images courtesy of Sandeep Randhawa, MD*

Vogt–Koyanagi–Harada Syndrome

Vogt–Koyanagi–Harada syndrome (VKH) is an immune-mediated disease affecting melanocyte-containing tissues, including the uvea. VKH tends to affect primarily pigmented races, particularly Asians, Hispanics, and American Indians. In most reports, women are affected more commonly than men. Classically, the disease progresses through a well-defined clinical course consisting of four stages: prodromal, acute uveitic, chronic-recurrent, and convalescent. The prodromal phase is characterized by a nonspecific flu-like illness and patients may even experience headache, neck stiffness, and auditory disturbances, including tinnitus and dysacusis. This is followed by the acute uveitic phase that most often consists of a bilateral granulomatous uveitis and vitritis and thickening of the posterior choroid with multiple areas of exudative retinal detachment. Optic nerve head hyperemia and edema are common at this stage. Later, during the chronic and recurrent stage of the disorder, there are varying degrees of fundus pigmentary alterations, which can mimic MFC or birdshot chorioretinopathy. While the serous retinal detachments will resolve, especially with immunosuppressant therapy, and do not typically recur, a chronic recurrent anterior uveitis may develop and may persist for years. The convalescent phase is characterized predominantly by pigment drop-out including vitiligo, poliosis, and also alopecia. A pale nerve surrounded by red-orange choroidal depigmentation is referred to as "sunset-glow" fundus and is a defining feature of this stage. Cataract, CNV, glaucoma, and optic atrophy may occur in some patients. The ocular inflammation in VKH is typically very responsive to corticosteroids, which may require a gradual taper over many months. Rarely patients will require more aggressive immunosuppressive therapy. Very rarely this disease can be complicated by cerebral vasculitis and even death and neurological consultation may be indicated in some cases.

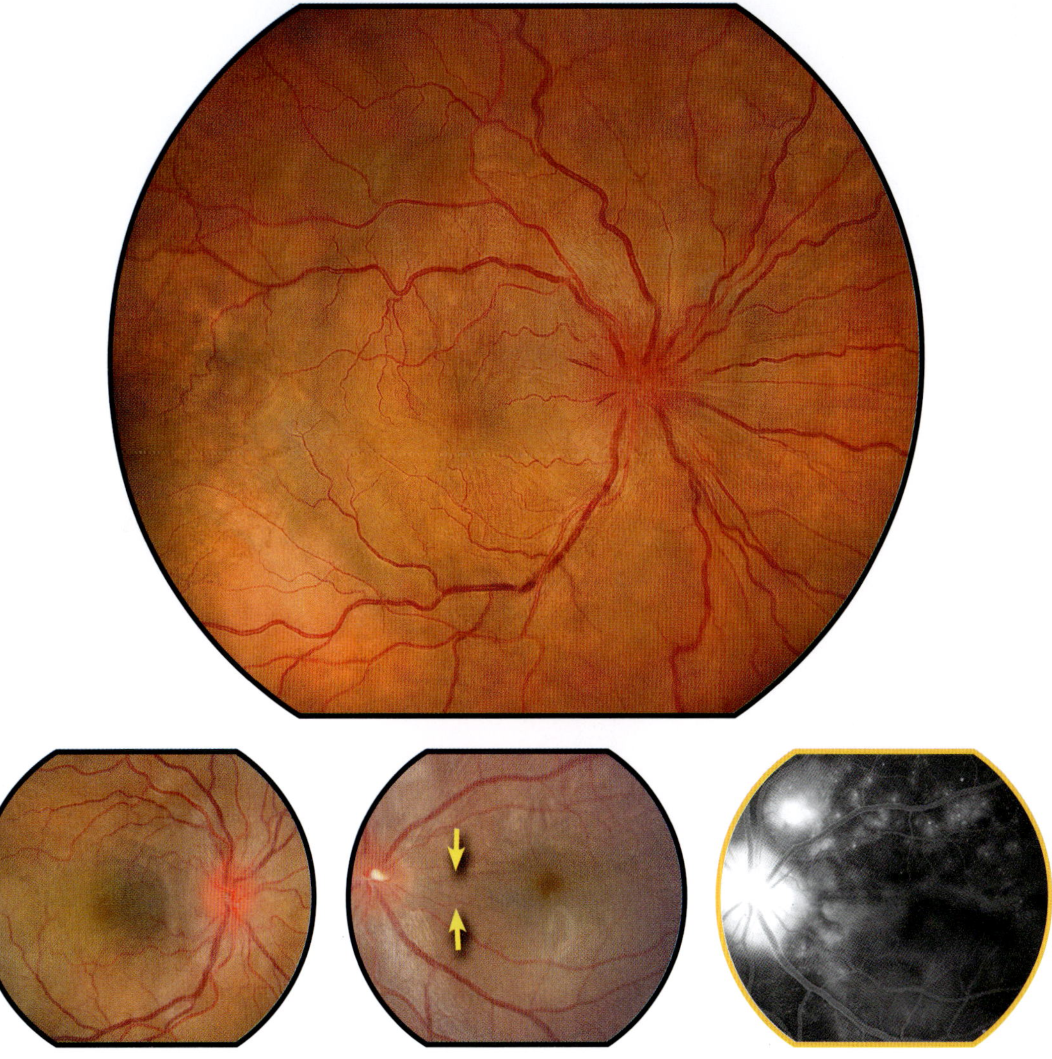

These patients have VKH with multifocal areas of choroiditis, an inflamed disc, retinal vascular engorgement, multiple serous retinal detachments, and multiple pinpoint leaks at the level of the RPE that pool into the subneurosensory retinal space on FA *(right)*. Radiating chorioretinal folds are also very common in this disease and evident in these patients *(arrows)*.

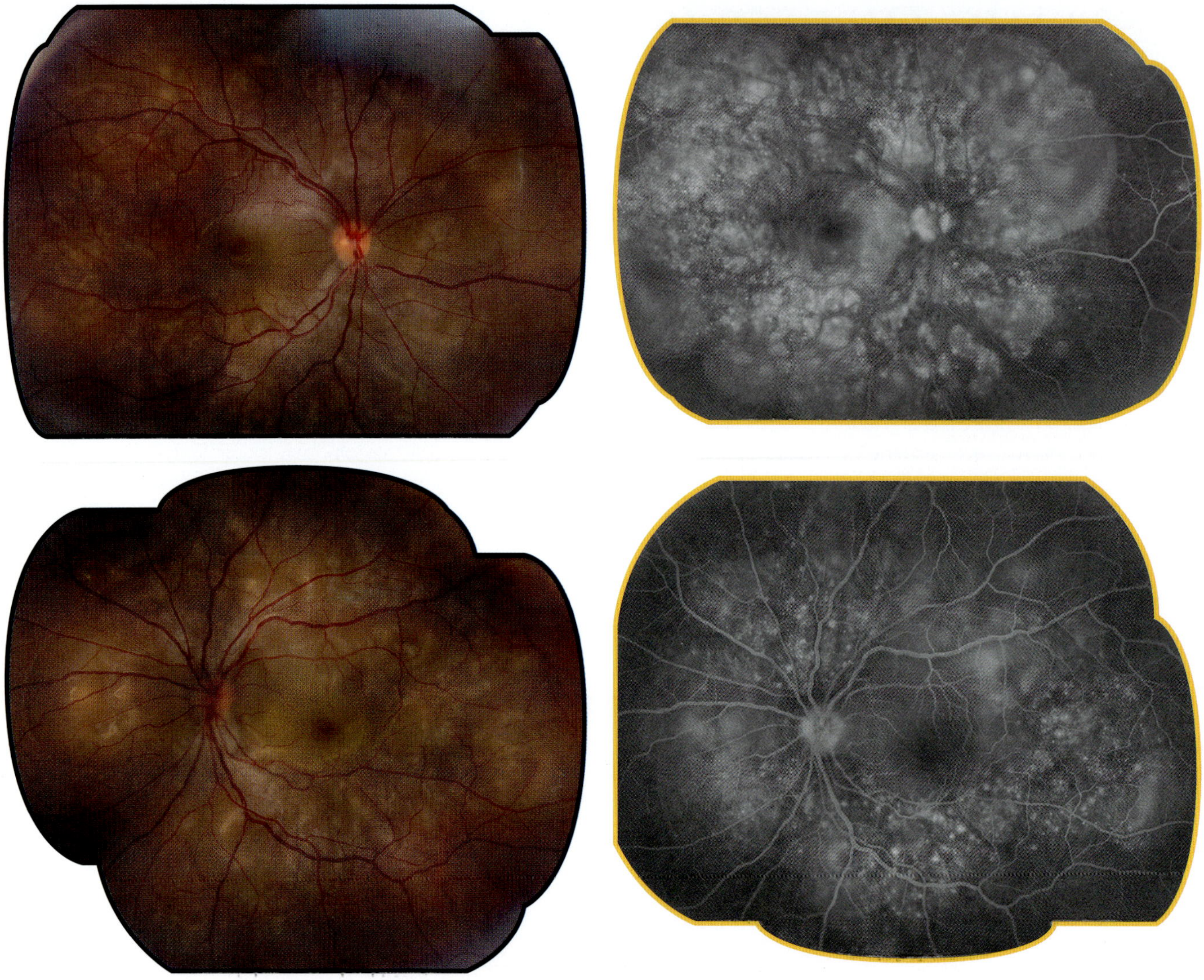

This 32-year-old Hispanic female developed VKH disease with exudative retinal detachments in the posterior pole and periphery of each eye. Multifocal leaks at the level of the RPE demonstrate pooling into the subneurosensory retinal space.

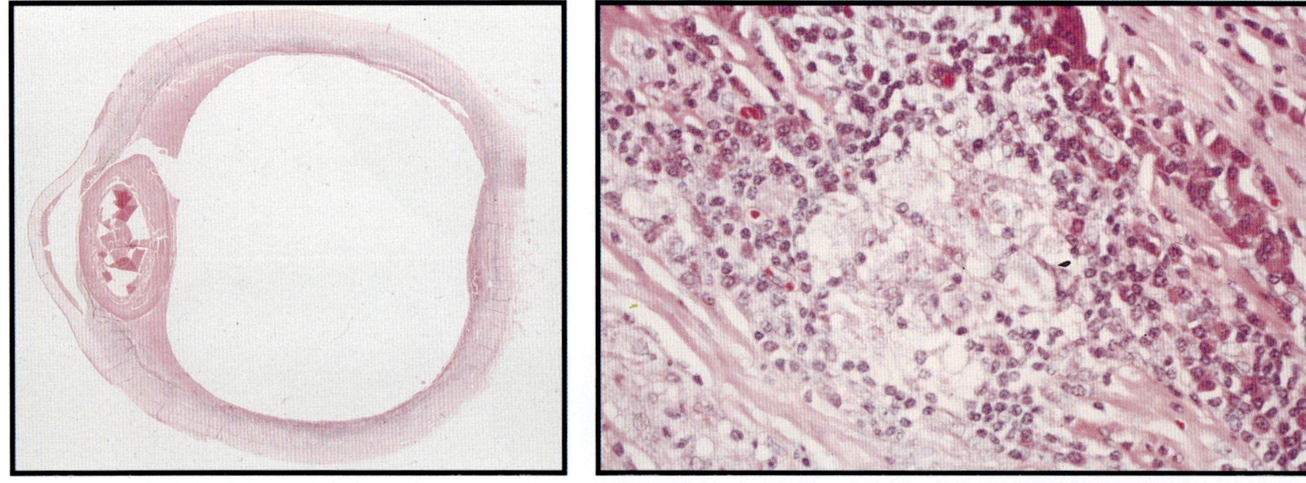

This cross-section of an eye with VKH shows extensive choroidal thickening *(left)*. These histopathological images are from a patient with Harada disease. There is a chronic, granulomatous infiltrate beneath the pigment epithelium.

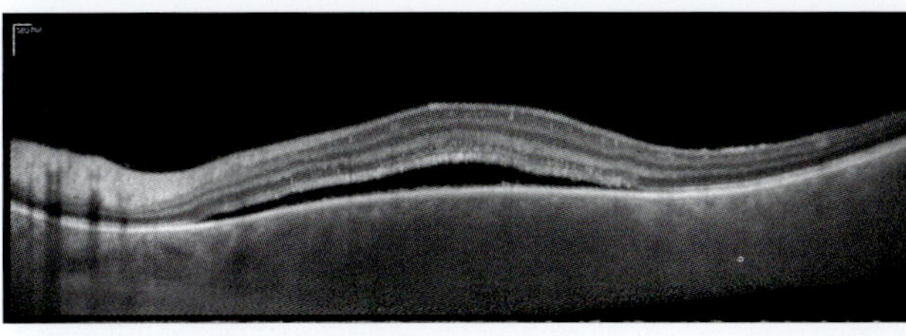
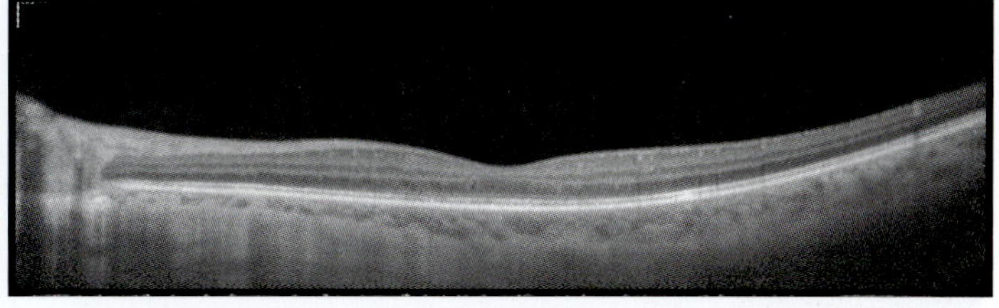

This patient with VKH illustrates serous detachment of the macula. The OCT shows a very thick choroid *(left)* affecting the left eye. Following steroid treatment, there was resolution of the macular detachment and a return of the normal choroidal thickness *(right)*.

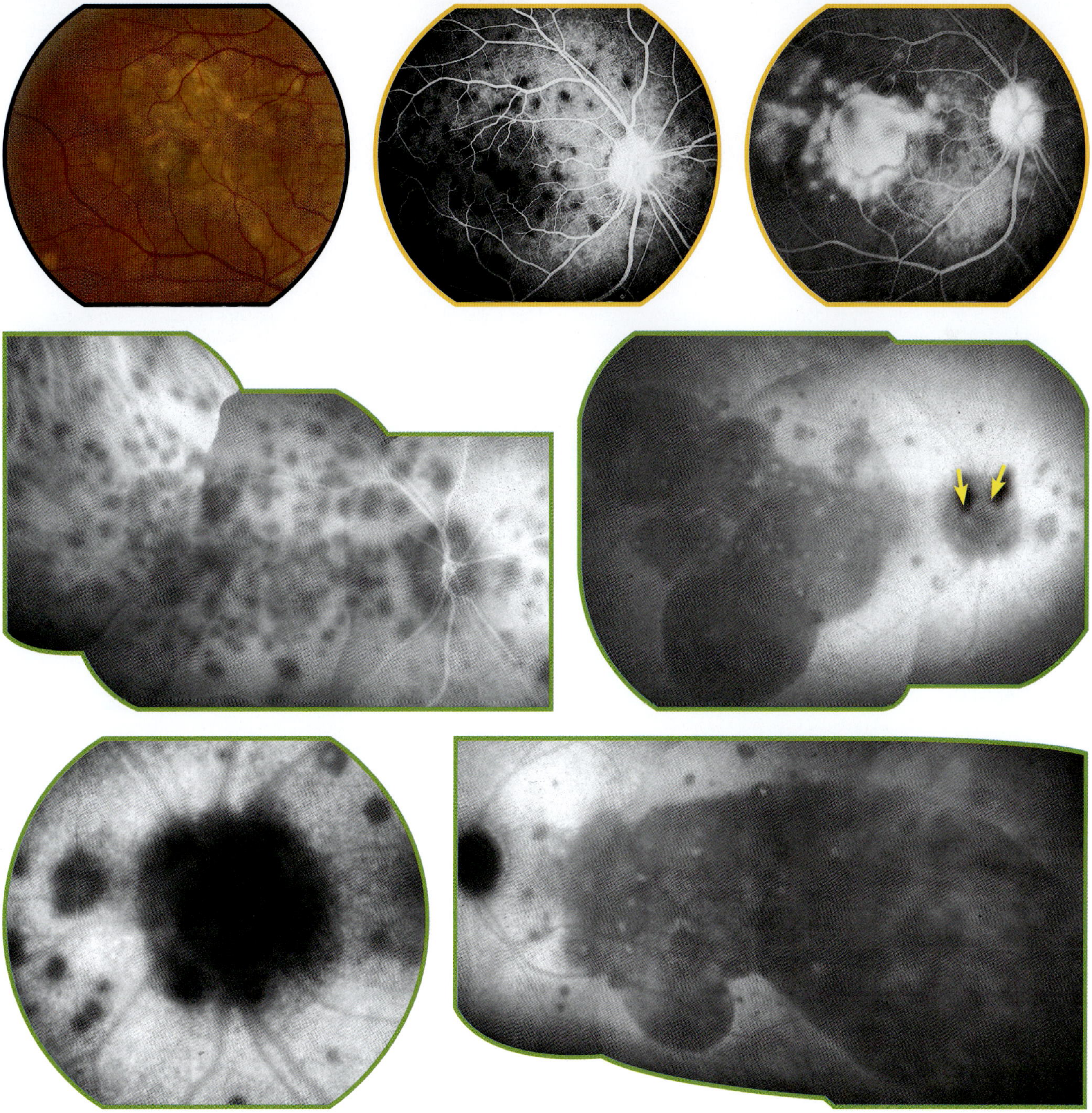

This patient demonstrates multiple neurosensory retinal detachments secondary to VKH. In some patients, multiple yellowish-orange spots beneath the detachments are the most conspicuous clinical feature and are identified in the right eye of this patient. FA findings in this patient demonstrate hypofluorescence at the site of the yellowish-orange spots and pooling of dye into the neurosensory detachments. Intense late staining of the optic nerve or frank leakage is also characteristic of this syndrome. ICG angiography facilitates the identification of the hypofluorescent multifocal granulomatous choroidal lesions seen in this disease. There is also hypofluorescence corresponding to the neurosensory detachments and around the disc *(arrows)*.

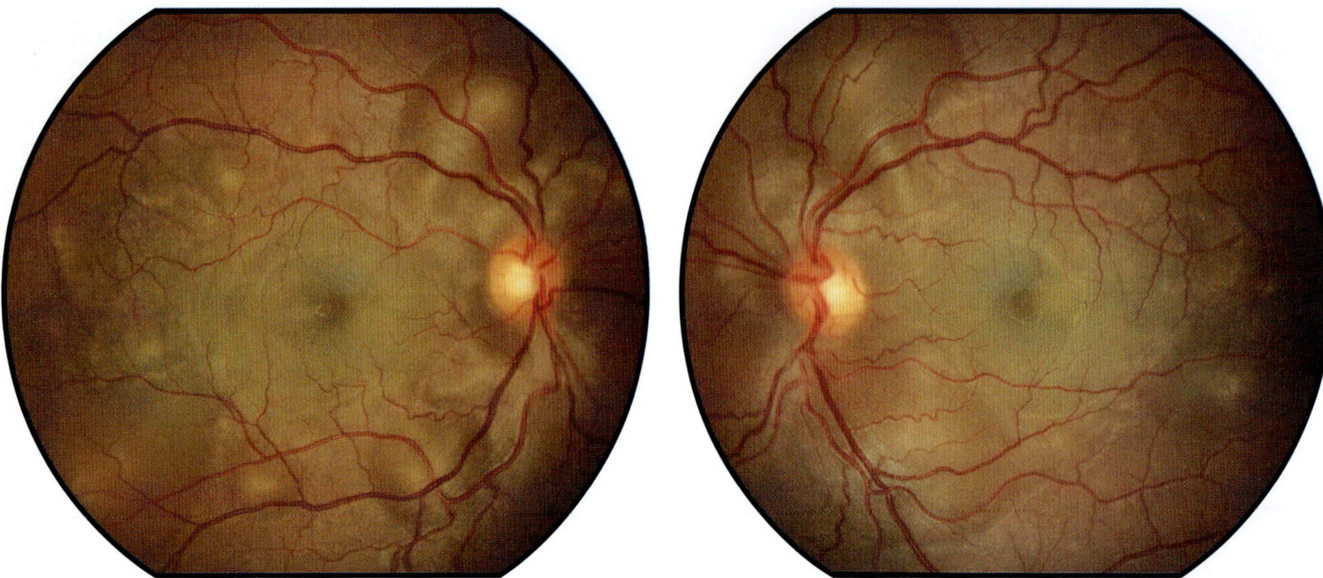

This patient illustrates the classic findings in VKH. There are multiple serous detachments of the neurosensory retina. Note the whitish subretinal spots resembling the Dalen–Fuchs' nodules seen in sympathetic ophthalmia. Mild vitritis and a hyperemic optic disc are also present. Extensive fibrinous subretinal fluid may lead to subretinal scarring. The changes of VKH are due to an exudative choroidopathy and may occur in other inflammatory disorders such as posterior scleritis and sympathetic ophthalmia. The most common cause of an exudative choroidopathy is central serous chorioretinopathy, which can be easily excluded due to the presence of inflammation and the disseminated nature of RPE leaks in VKH. Other causes of an exudative choroidopathy include infiltrative diseases such as leukemia and other systemic conditions including disseminated intravascular coagulopathy, toxemia of pregnancy, lupus choroidopathy, and malignant hypertension. Rarer disorders such as bilateral diffuse uveal melanocytic proliferation (BDUMP) and eosinophilic granuloma can also cause exudative choroidopathy and serous retinal detachment.

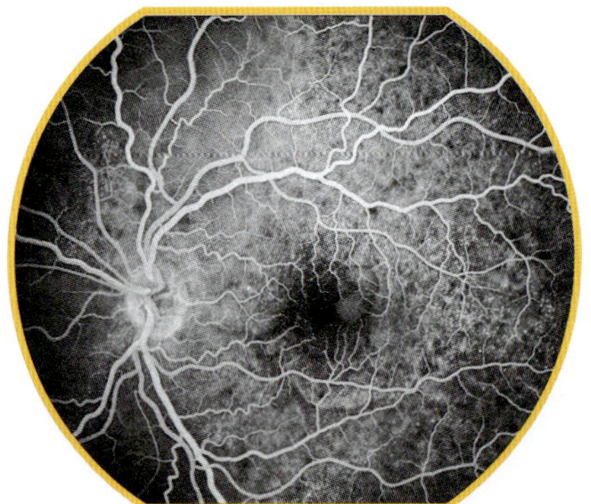

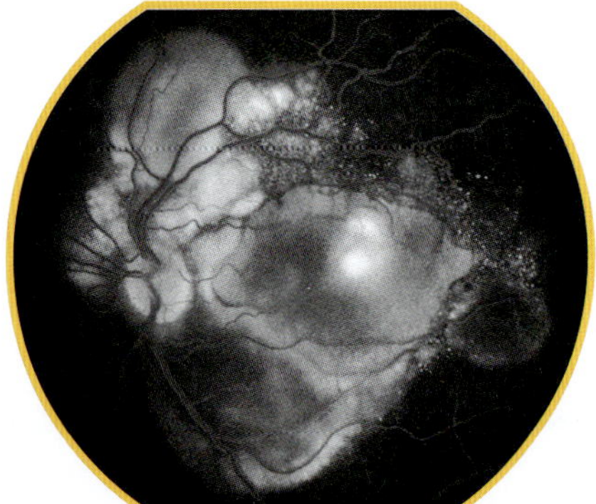

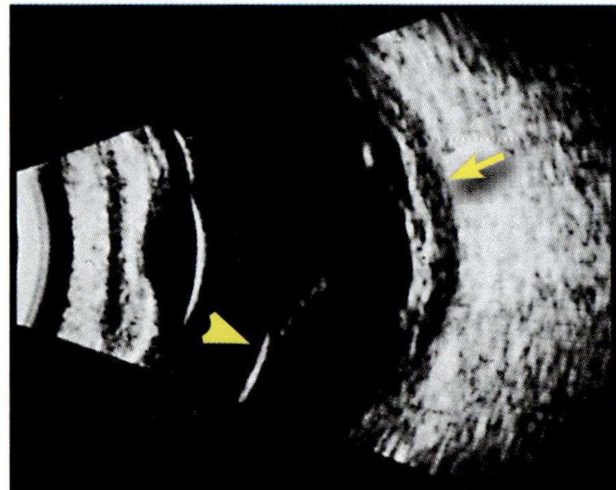

The fluorescein angiogram shows early pinpoint areas of hyperfluorescence *(left)*. These pinpoint leaks pool into serous retinal detachments *(middle)* later in the study. The dye may actually fill the subneurosensory retinal space, giving a fluorescein angiographic impression of a serous pigment epithelial detachment. In central serous chorioretinopathy, fluorescein will delineate or outline the neurosensory detachment and only fill the entire space very late in the study. The ultrasound in this disease shows retinal detachment *(arrowhead)*, and choroidal thickening *(arrow)*.

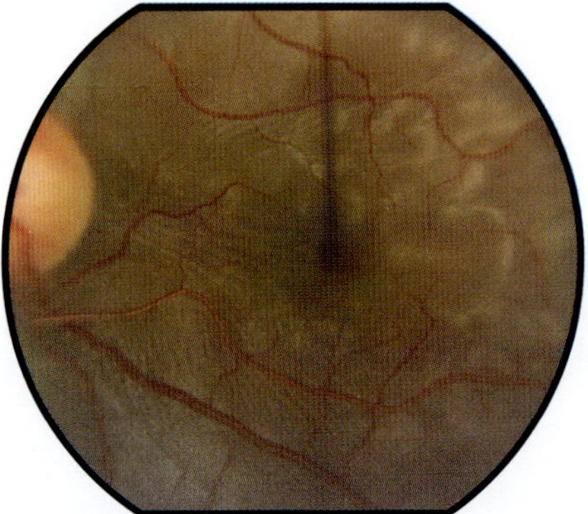

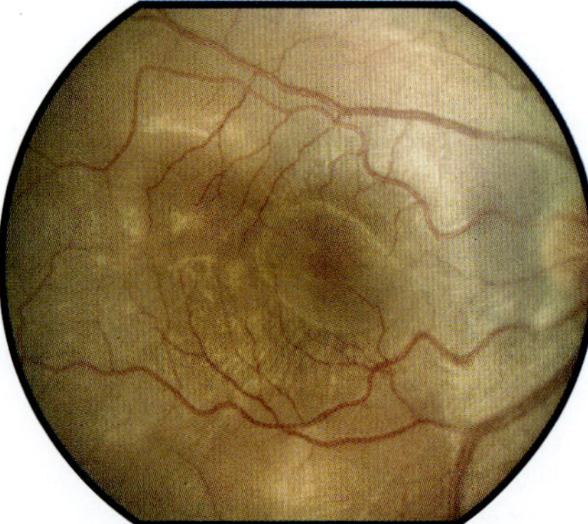

These patients with VKH show diffuse serous macular detachment and associated chorioretinal folds. There is a more proteinaceous exudate at the margins of the detachments, which is also characteristic of the disease.

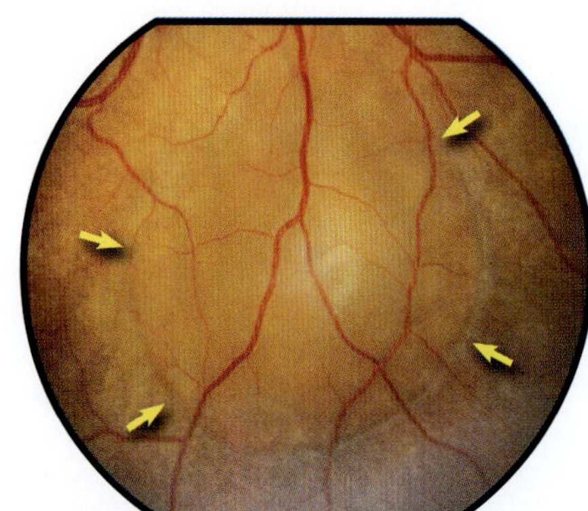

Large dependent detachments may also occur secondary to VKH and gravitate inferiorly, as in this teardrop detachment *(arrows)*.

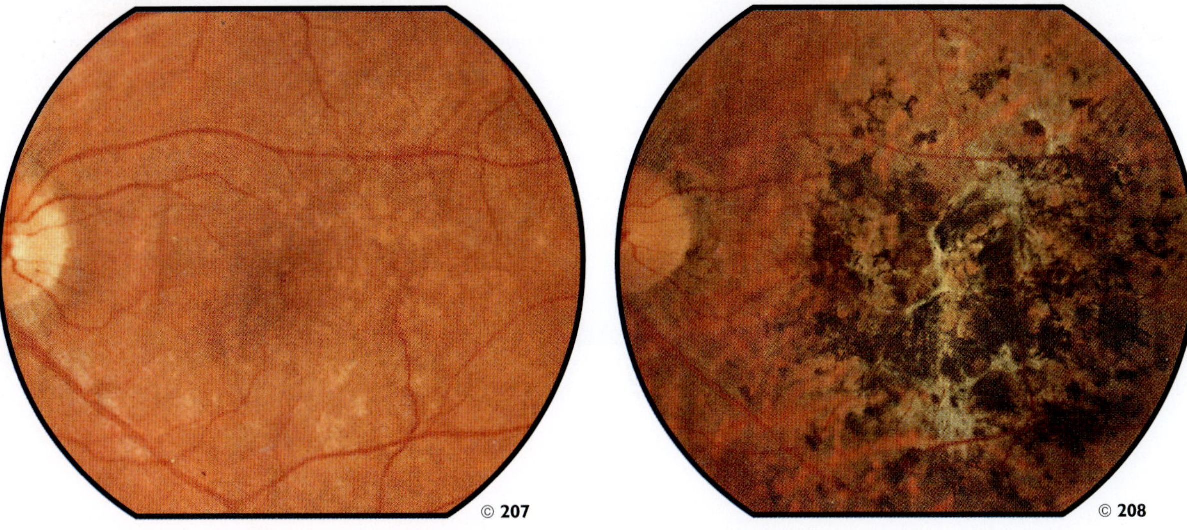

This patient with VKH had an initial acute attack, leaving a legacy of atrophy and pigment epithelial stippling *(left)*. Multiple recurrent attacks eventually led to heavy hyperpigmentation and fibrotic scarring, with severe vision loss *(right)*.

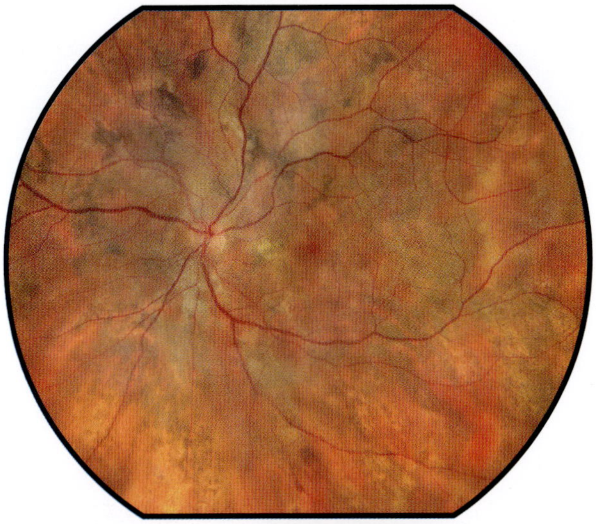

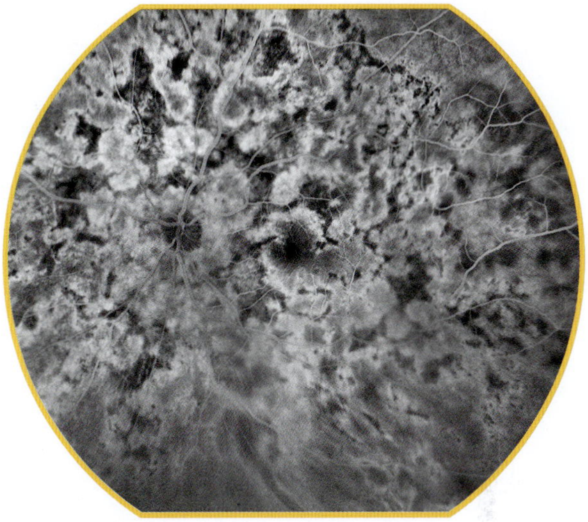

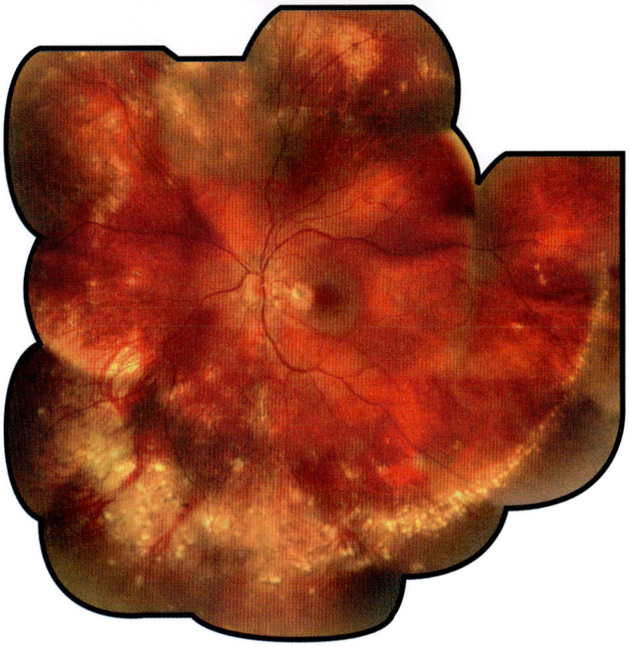

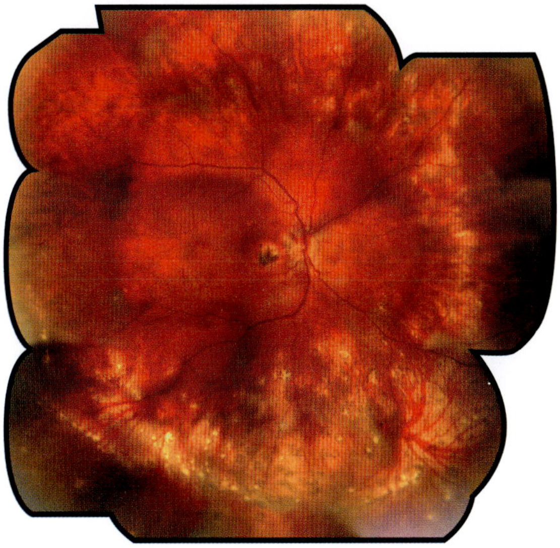

Patients with severe VKH may end up with chronic detachment, leading to atrophy, pigment epithelial hyperplasia, fibrosis, chorioretinal spots, and even peripheral curvilinear tracts, similar to MFC.

© 209

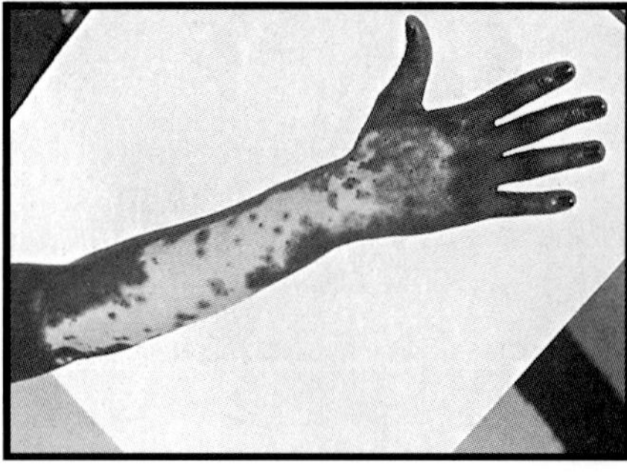

© 210

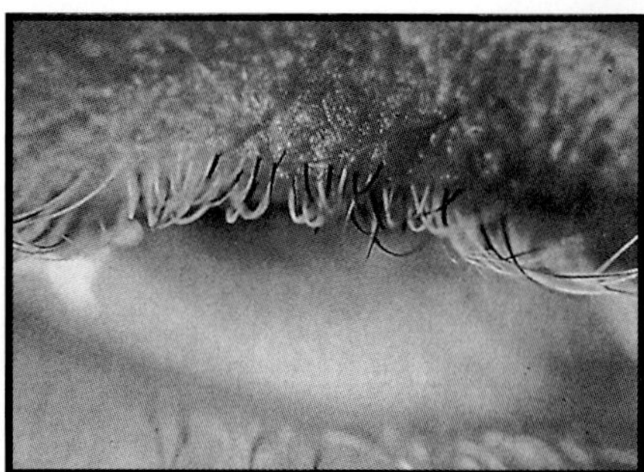

© 211

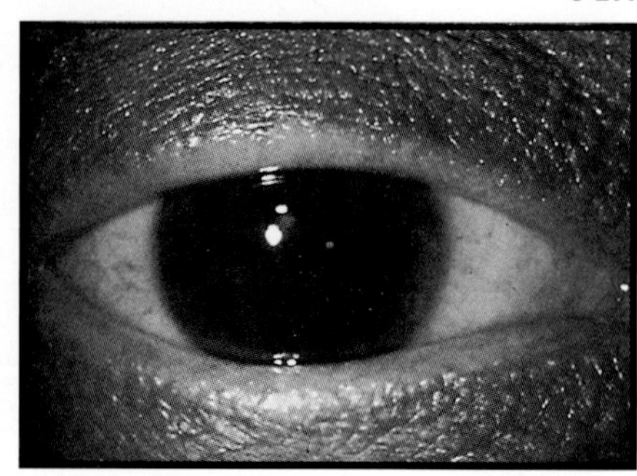

Cutaneous abnormalities are part of the VKH syndrome. Note the vitiligo *(left)*, the poliosis *(middle)*, and the madarosis *(right)*.

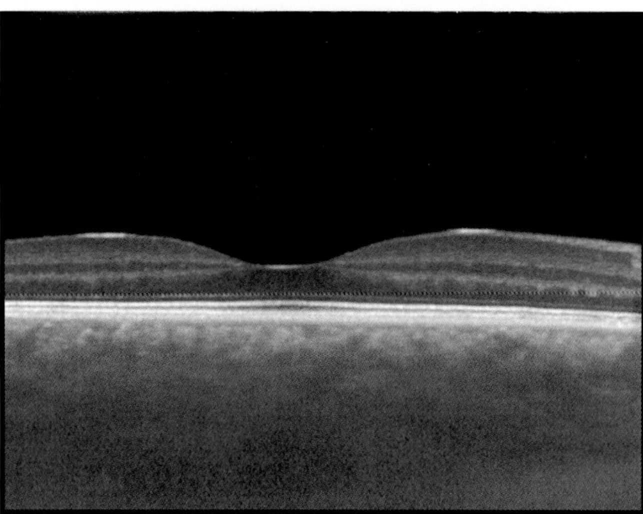

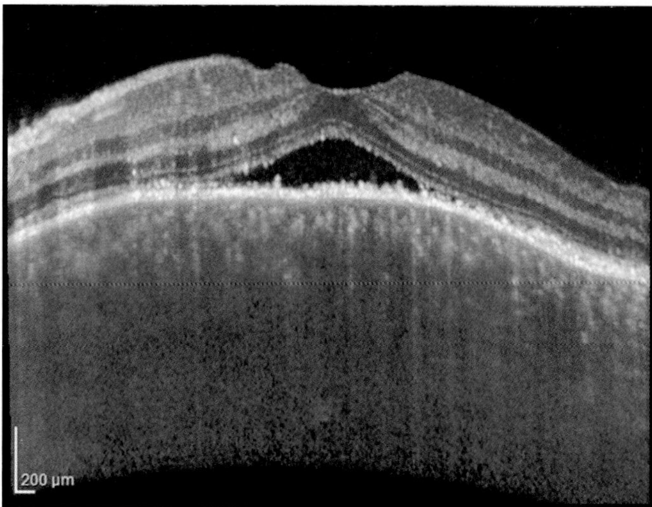

This patient with VKH initially presented with a small serous retinal detachment involving the macula in the left eye. Note the thickened choroid on SD-OCT in both eyes. The patient was started on oral NSAIDs.

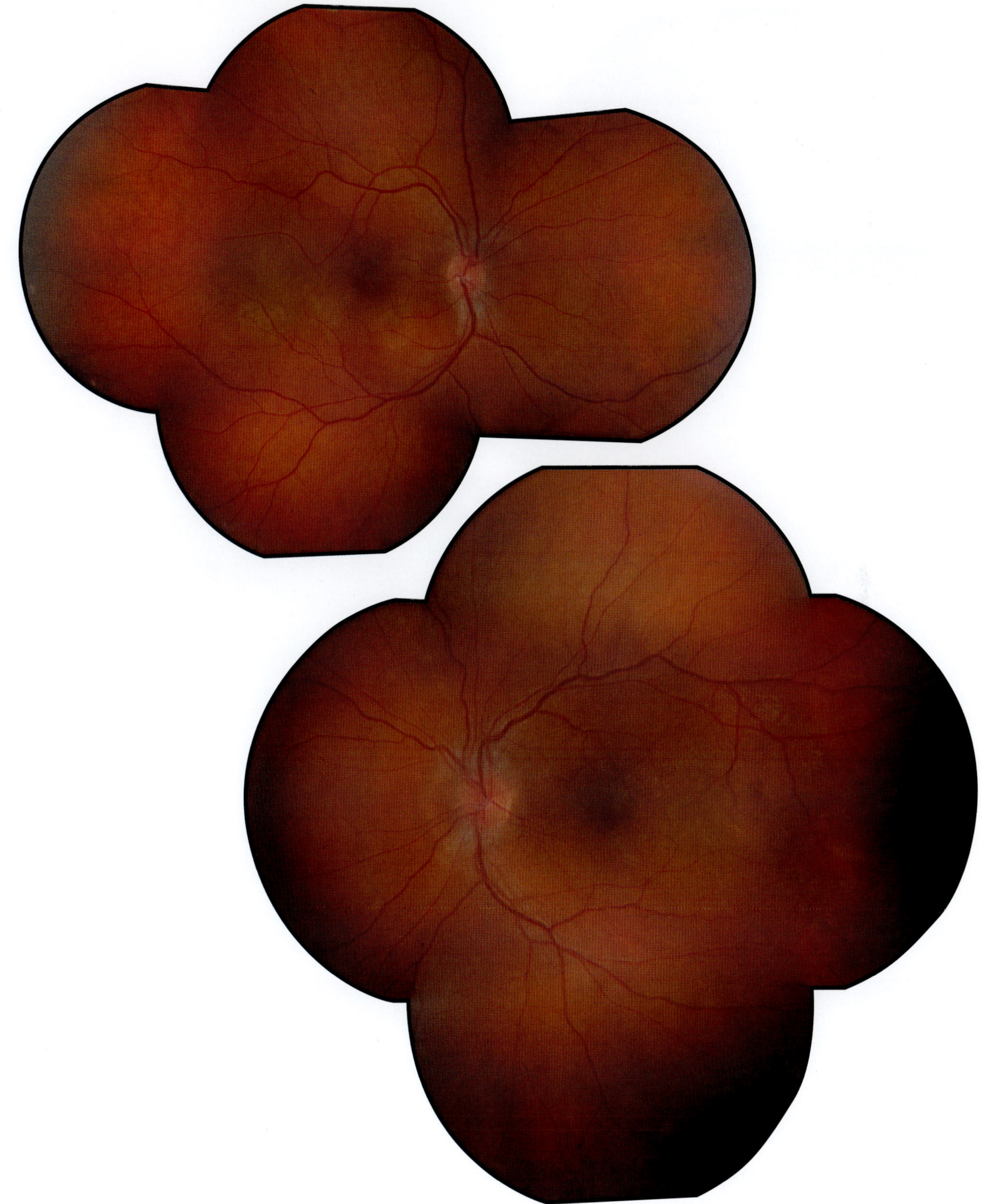

At the two-week follow-up visit, the same patient developed a serous retinal detachment in the right eye and the detachment in the left eye had progressed.

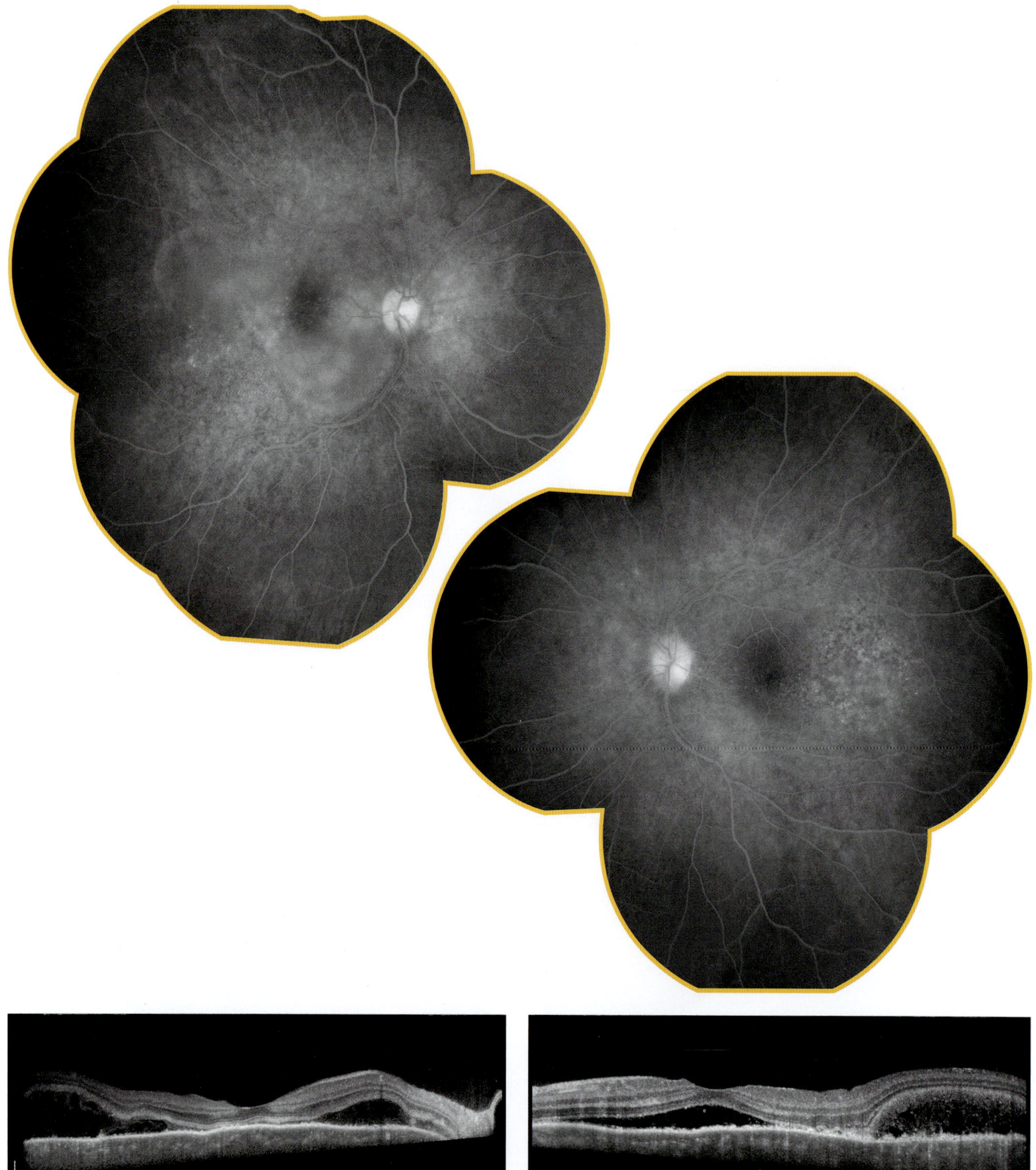

Fluorescein angiogram montage of the right and left eyes shows stippled hyperfluorescence in the macula of both eyes with pooling into the detachments. SD-OCT of the right eye *(bottom left)* and left eye *(bottom right)* demonstrates extensive serous retinal detachments involving the macula of each eye.

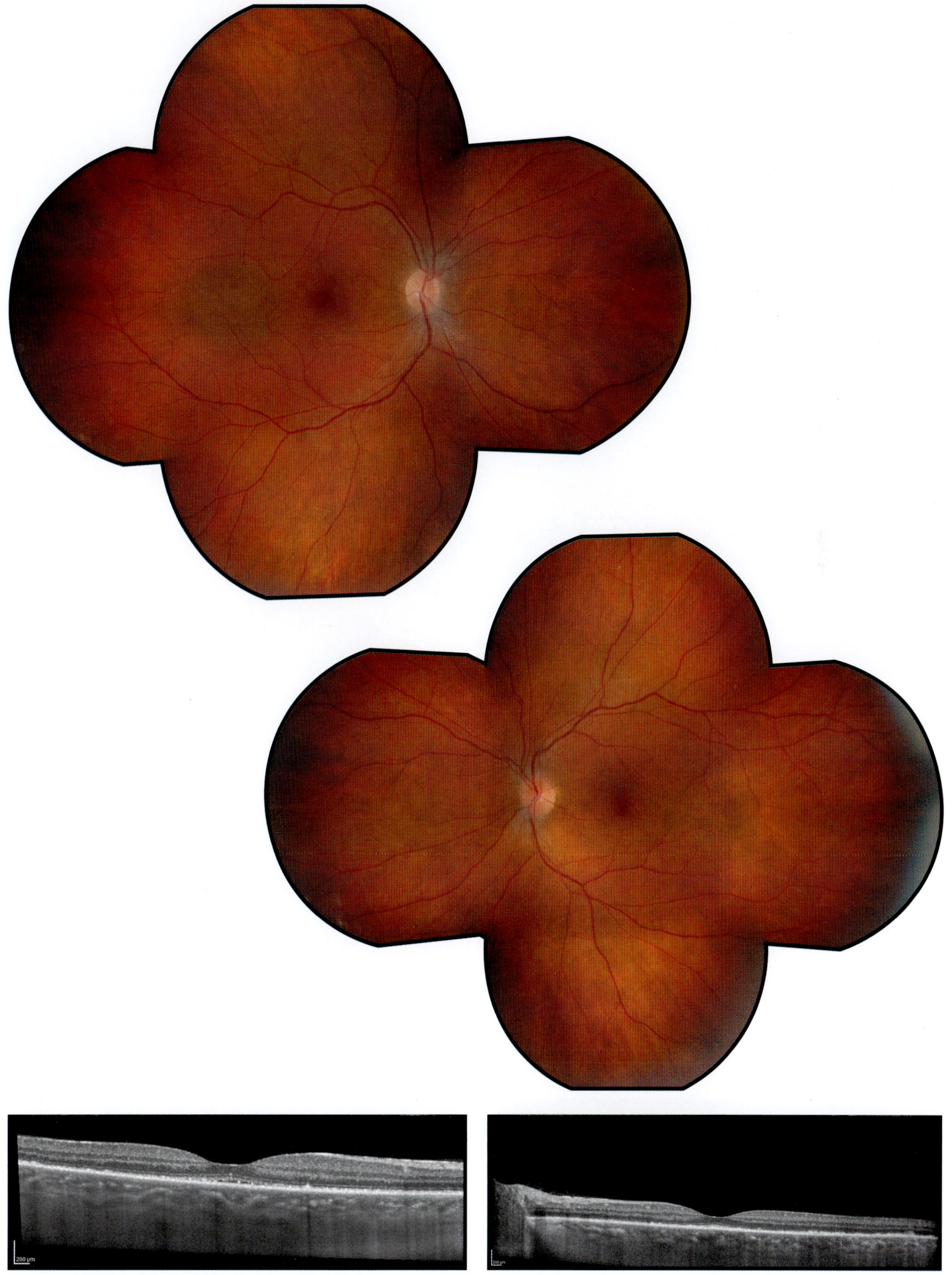

Color fundus photo montage and SD-OCT at one-month follow-up shows resolution of the serous detachments in both eyes and markedly reduced choroidal thickness after steroid therapy was initiated.

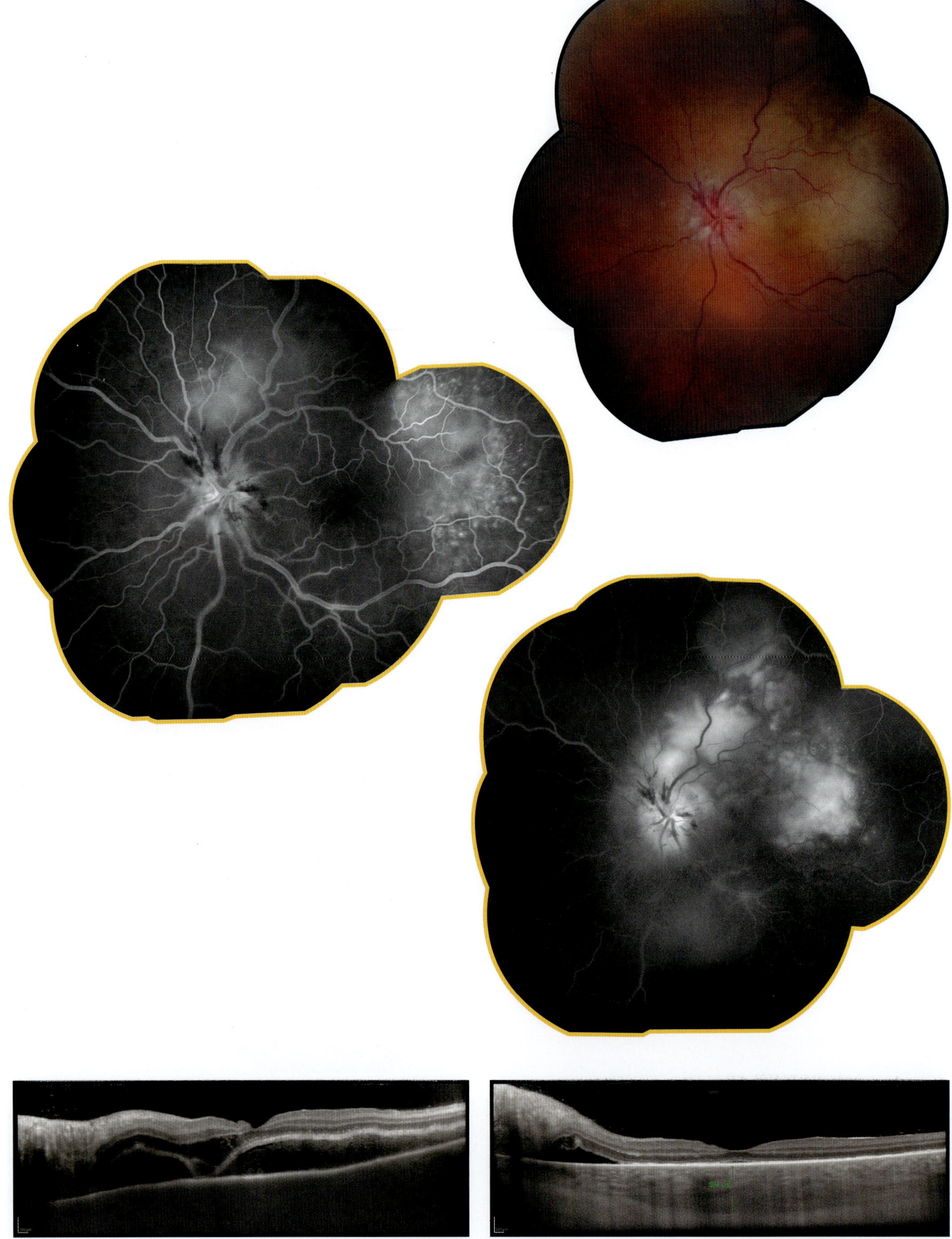

This 32-year-old female presented with decreased vision in her left eye for one week. Color fundus photo montage of the left eye illustrates a hyperemic and swollen nerve with disc hemorrhages and a large exudative retinal detachment. Mid-phase fluorescein angiogram shows stippled hyperfluorescence with late pooling into the exudative retinal detachment. SD-OCT at baseline presentation and follow-up shows sub-neurosensory fluid and a thickened choroid.

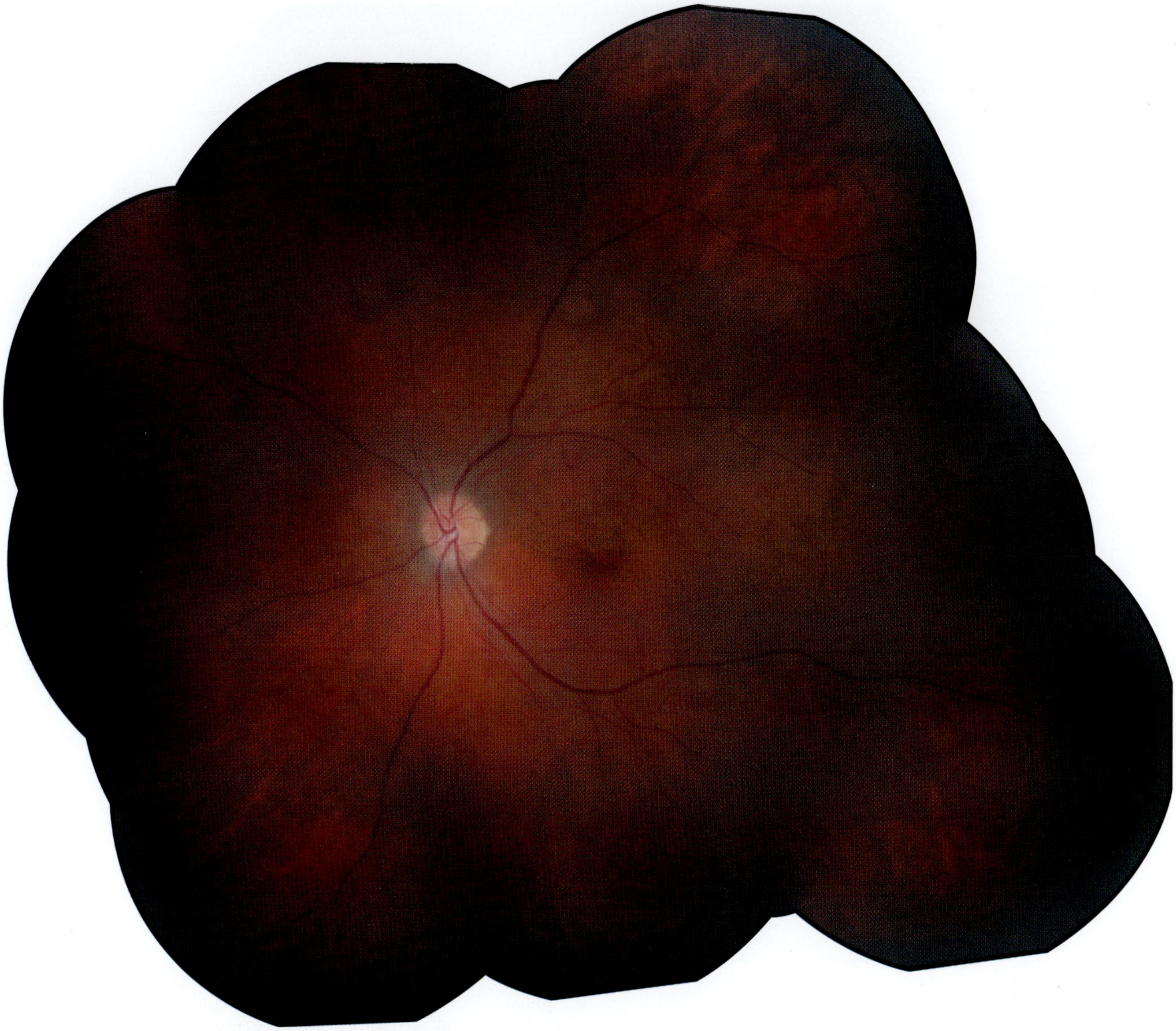

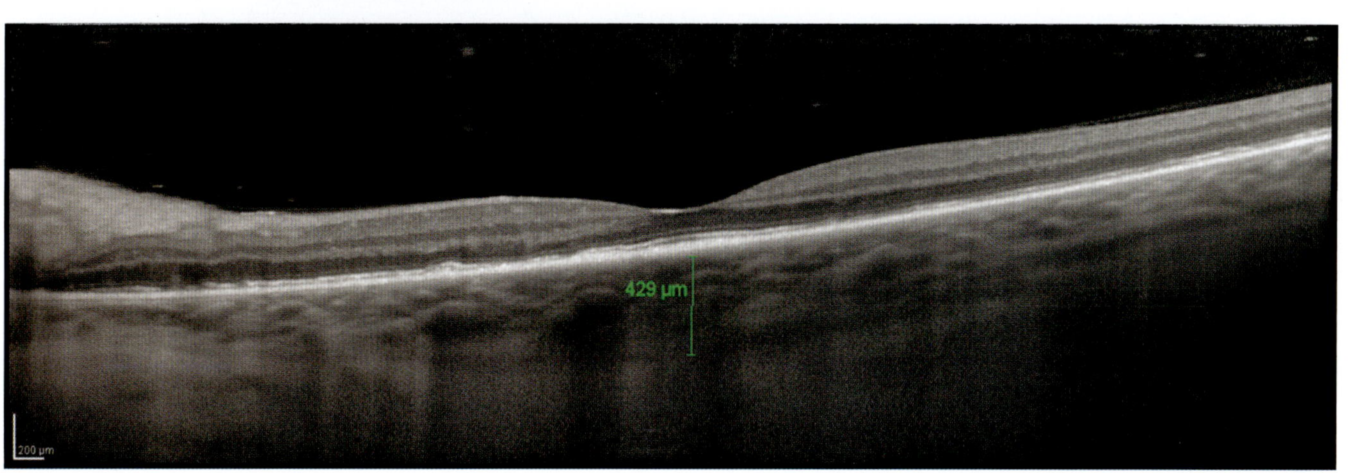
429 µm
200 µm

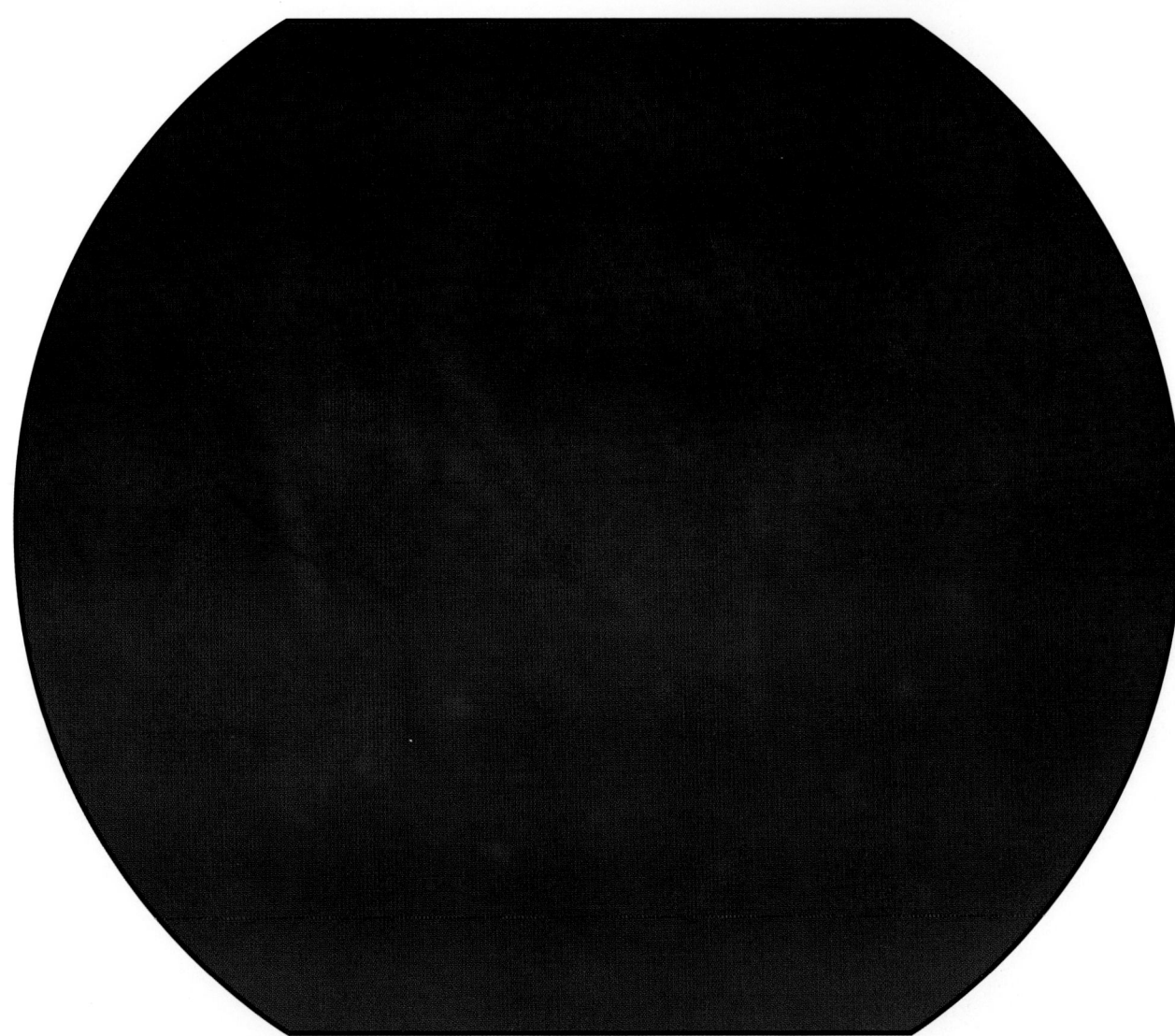

The patient was initiated on systemic steroid therapy. Follow-up color images and SD-OCT show resolution of the exudative detachment, and improvement in the choroidal thickening. Hypopigmented Dalen-Fuchs-like lesions are noted inferiorly following resolution *(bottom)*.

Sympathetic Ophthalmia

Sympathetic ophthalmia is a granulomatous uveitis, which occurs in the fellow eye following accidental or surgical penetrating trauma of one eye. Onset of inflammation in the fellow eye may occur within days to many years following the inciting injury, but typically occurs within the first several months. Patients initially report mild ocular discomfort, blurred vision, photophobia, and loss of accommodation. Ocular findings include anterior chamber cell and flare and keratic precipitates on the corneal endothelium. Posterior segment changes include vitritis, papillitis, and an exudative neurosensory detachment, which may mimic Harada disease. Small yellow-white spots beneath the RPE known as Dalen–Fuchs nodules are characteristic of the disorder. Treatment usually involves the use of corticosteroids or other immunosuppressive agents with varying degrees of success. Enucleation of the inciting eye once inflammation has begun remains controversial.

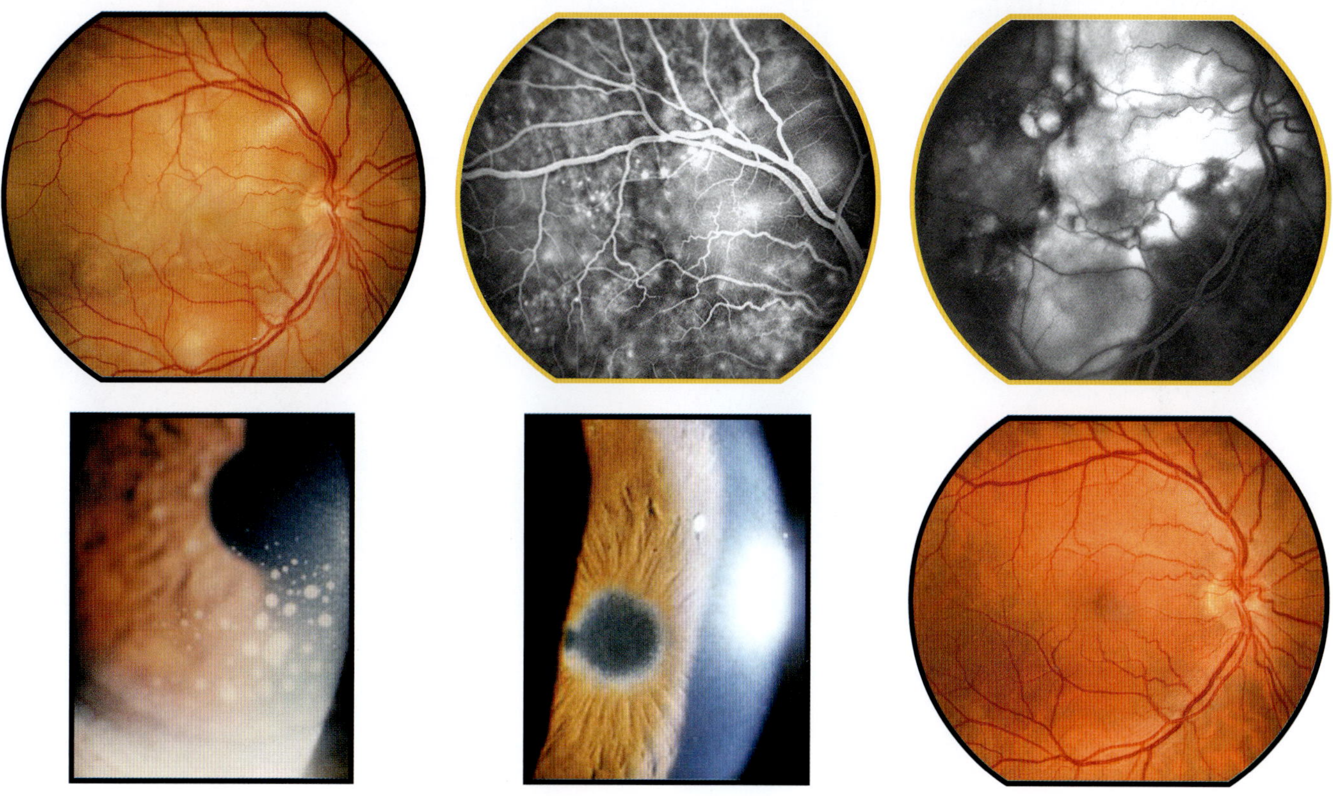

This patient appeared to have Harada disease. Anterior segment photos demonstrate mutton fat granulomatous keratic precipitates and posterior synechiae *(bottom row left and middle)*. Note the bullous neurosensory retinal detachments with stippled late pooling on FA *(top row middle and top row right)*. The patient's condition improved after steroid treatment *(bottom row right)*. Histopathologic study of the fellow eye indicated that the patient actually had sympathetic ophthalmia. *Courtesy of Dr. Thomas Aaberg*

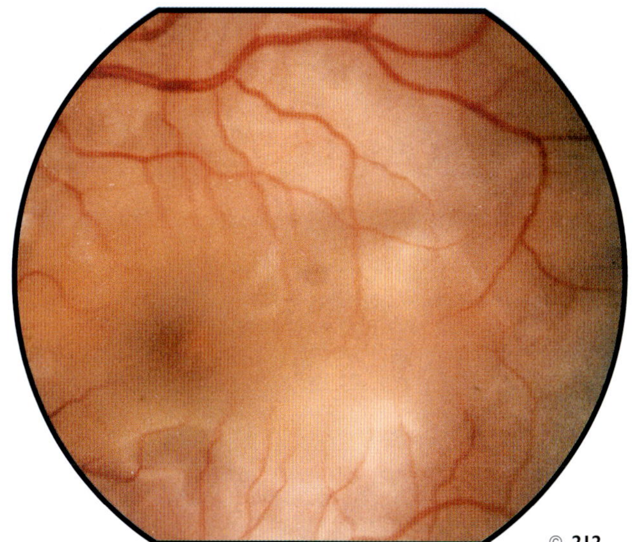

© **212**

Sympathetic ophthalmia may resemble Harada disease with multiple neurosensory retinal detachments forming bullous elevations of the retina. Multiple pinpoint leaks at the level of the RPE account for the overlying exudative detachment. The presumed whitish spots are Dalen–Fuchs nodules.

© 213 © 214 © 215

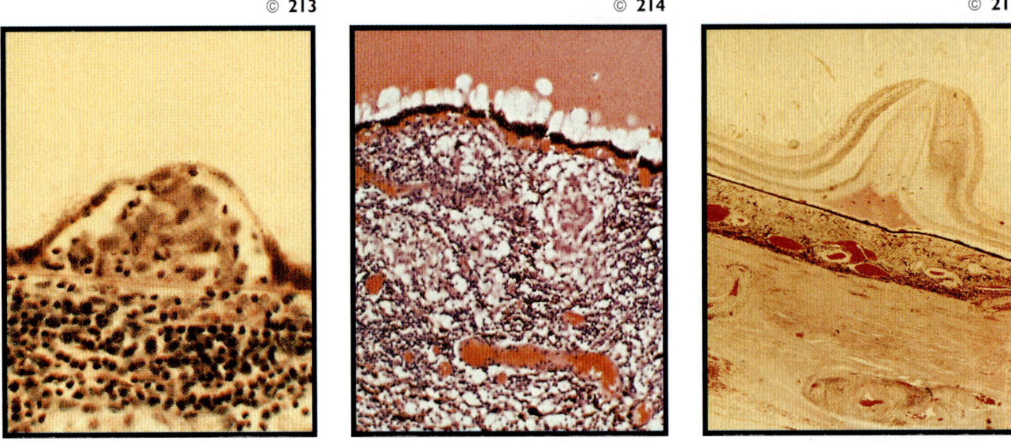

The histopathological images show granulomatous inflammation within the choroid. Note also the sparing of the choriocapillaris and the subretinal fluid *(left)*. The middle image shows serous detachment of the sensory retina as well as inflammatory cells surrounding an emissary blood vessel in the sclera. The image to the far right shows a Dalen–Fuchs nodule. Note the collection of mononuclear cells beneath the attenuated retinal pigment epithelium.

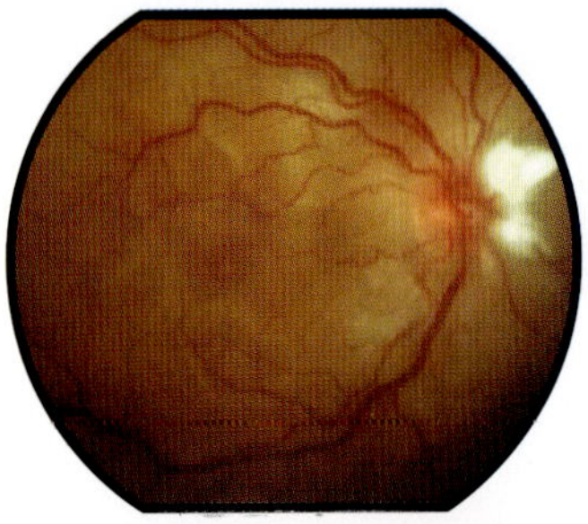

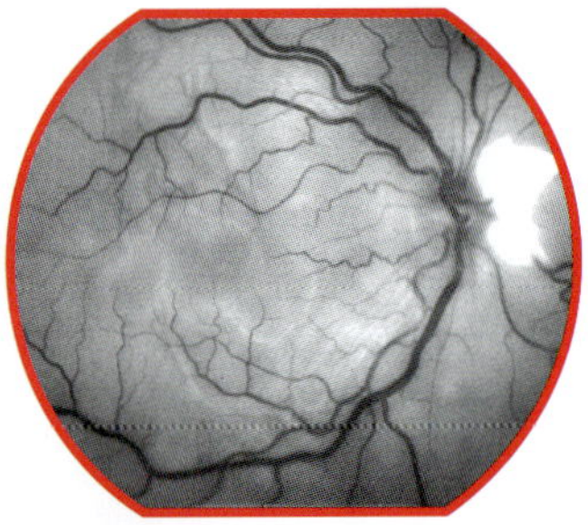

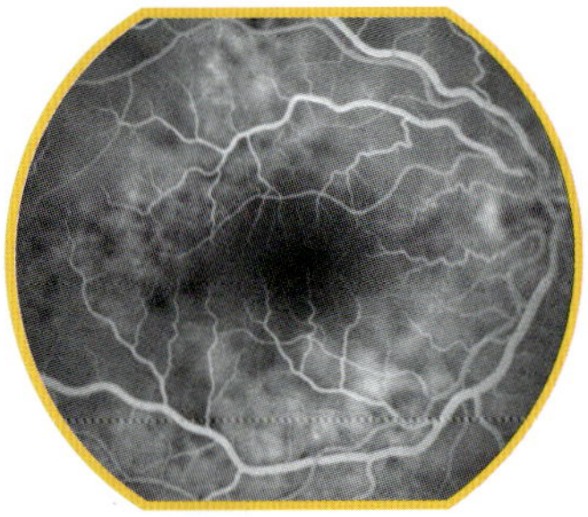

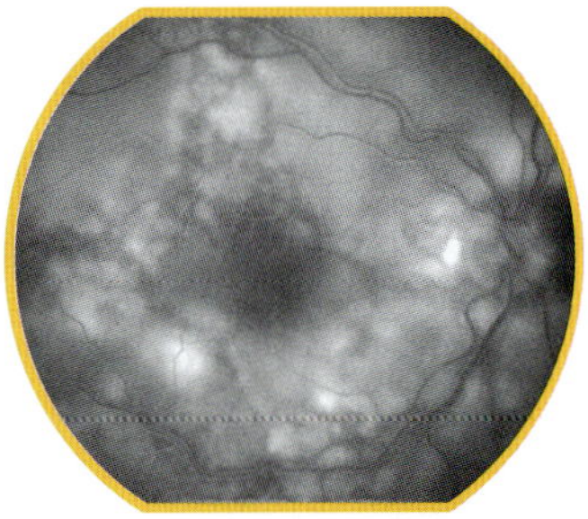

Courtesy of Dr. Hermann Schubert

Note the Harada like serous retinal detachment associated with subretinal leakage in this sympathizing eye.

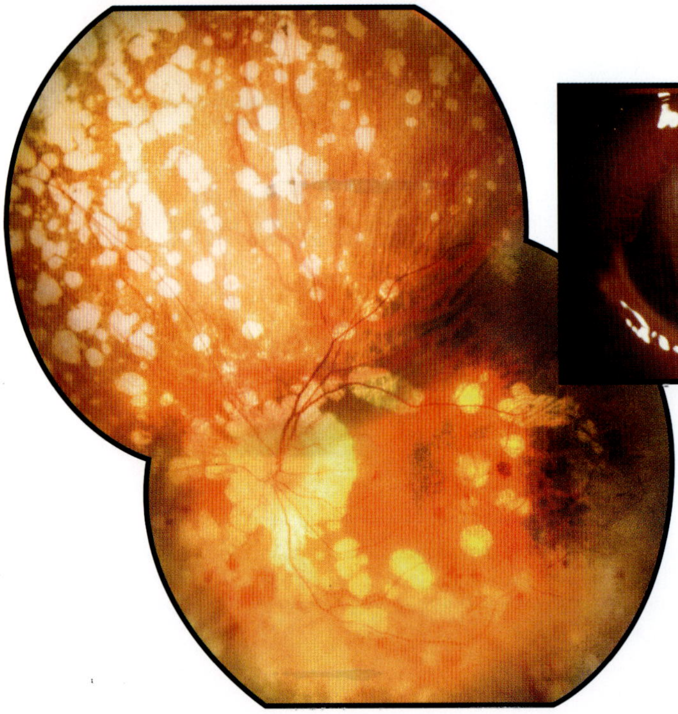

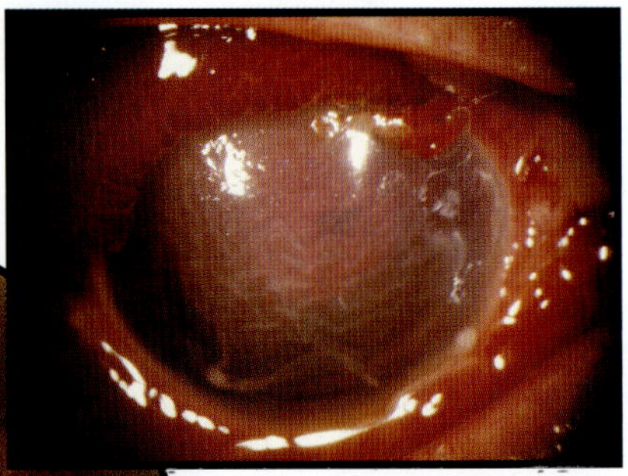

This patient with sympathetic ophthalmia has multifocal areas of fibrinoid necrosis throughout the fundus, as well as multiple neurosensory detachments. The montage shows retinitis pigmentosa-like widespread chorioretinal atrophy and pigmentation similar to MCP. The anterior segment photo shows the traumatized, inciting eye.

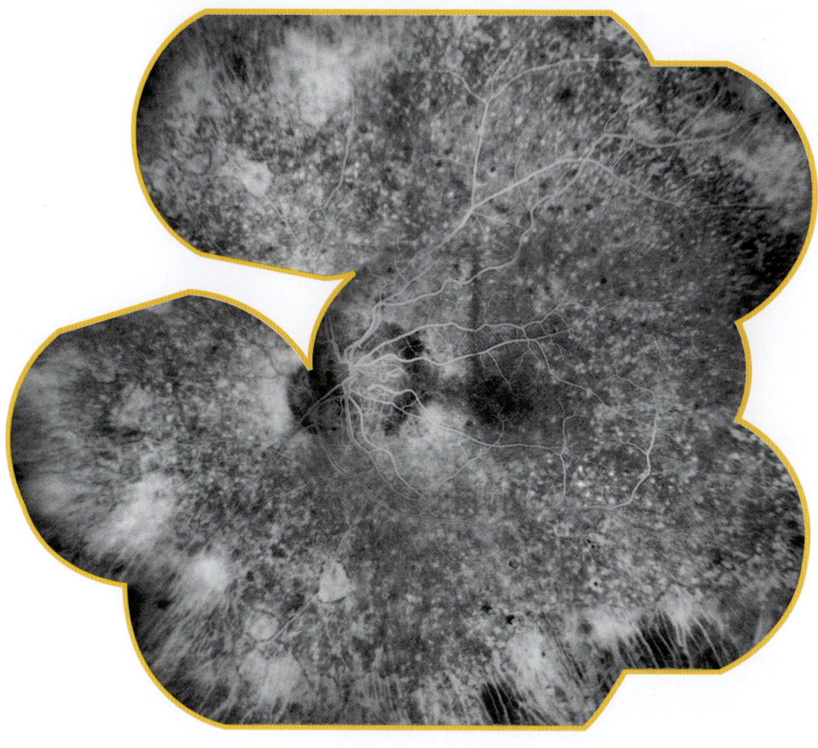

This is a 39-year-old white male with sympathetic ophthalmia. He received steroids with cyclosporine, thermal laser twice, and antivascular endothelial growth factor agents. *Courtesy of Dr. David Fischer*

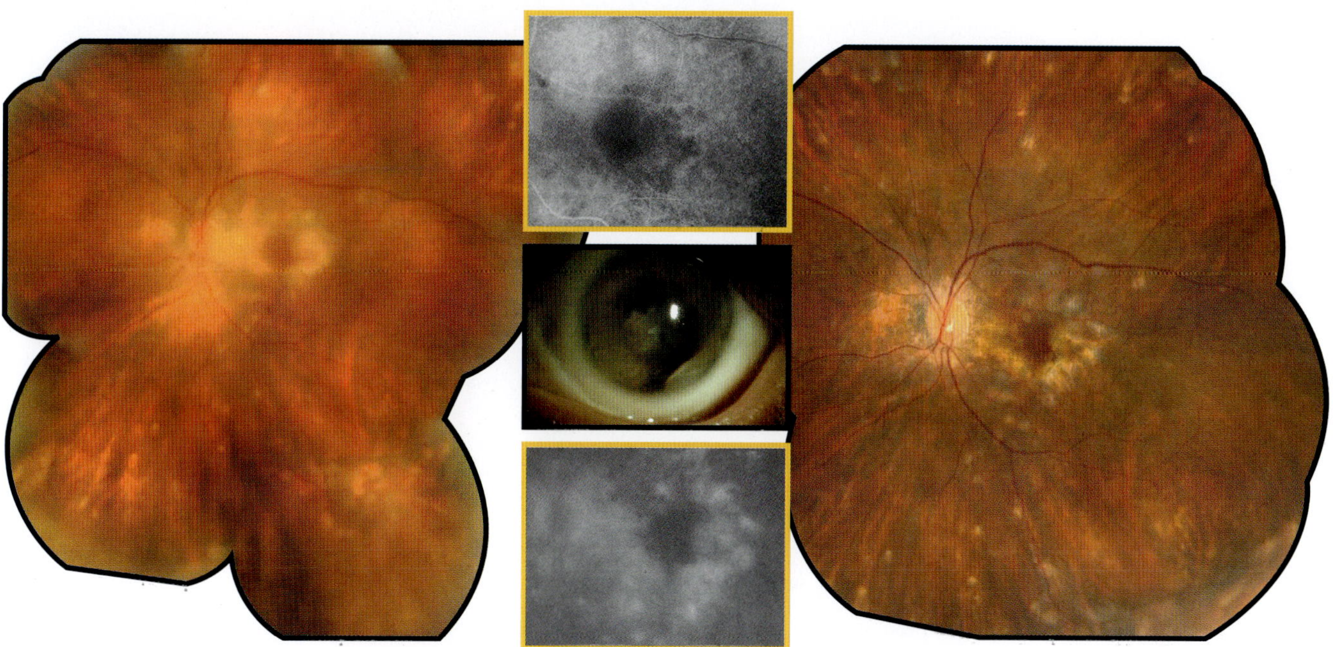

This is a patient who had multiple retinal detachment procedures in the right eye with a very poor outcome. The other eye developed inflammation. After immunosuppressive drugs and an intravitreal injection of triamcinolone, the inflammatory abnormalities eventually cleared, leaving a legacy of paramacular atrophy and multiple peripheral chorioretinitic atrophic spots. These peripheral lesions corresponded to granulomatous inflammation in the inner choroid-pigment epithelium. There were anterior-segment inflammatory changes as well.

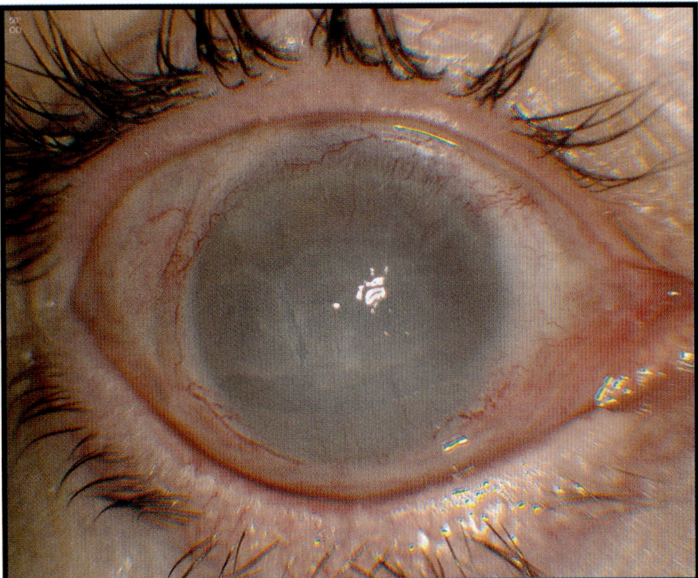

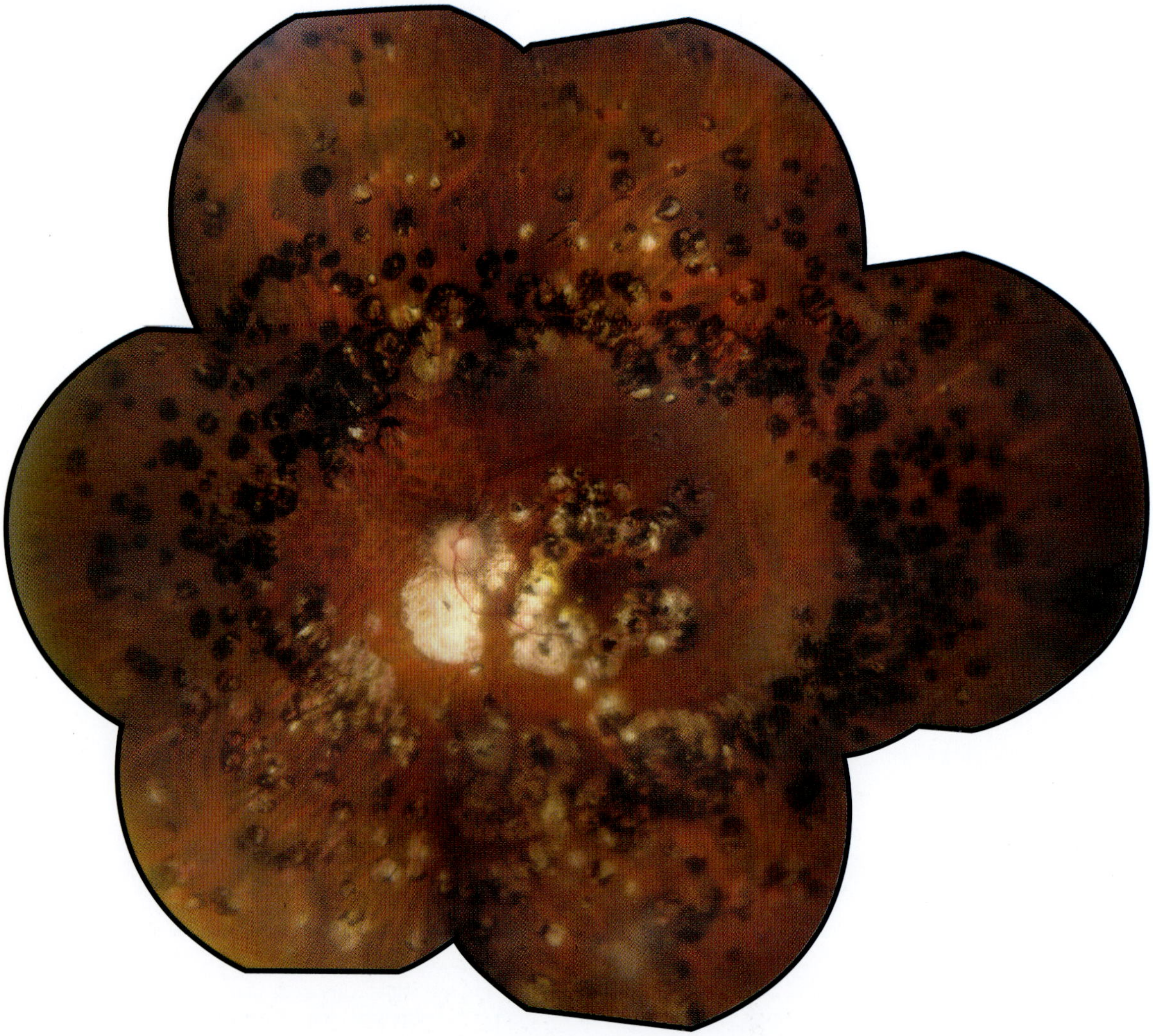

This 42-year-old male had a history of multiple unsuccessful retinal detachment surgeries, including vitrectomy, in the right eye. Anterior segment photo of the right, now phthisical eye is shown above. The patient subsequently developed new floaters in the left eye. Color fundus montage of the left eye illustrates pigmented chorioretinal scarring involving the posterior pole and peripheral retina. The circumferential pattern of lesions is reminiscent of multifocal choroiditis and panuveitis.

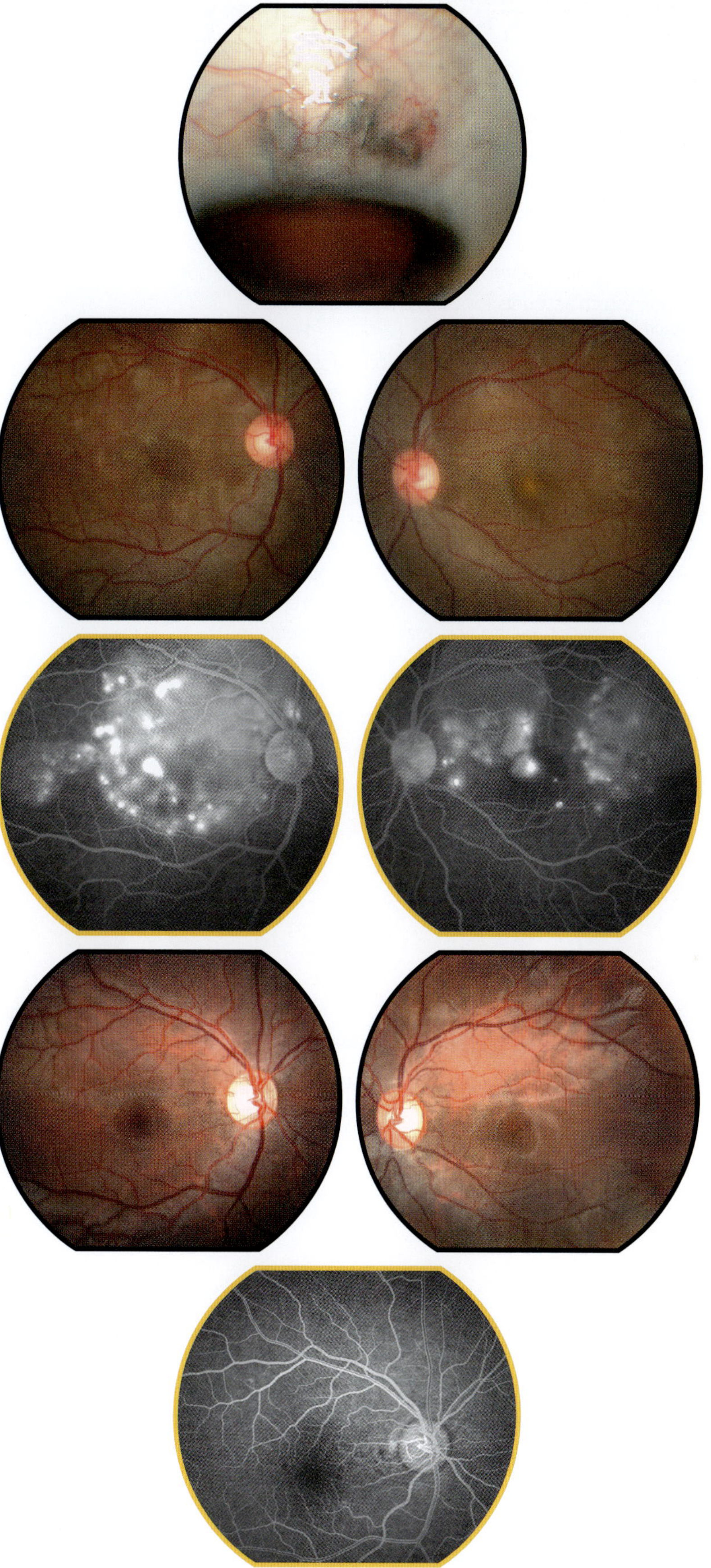

This 16-year-old female suffered a ruptured globe of the right eye and underwent surgical repair. Anterior segment photograph of the traumatized eye is shown *(top row)*. At one-month follow-up, the patient developed a headache and decreased visual acuity to 20/400 OD and counting fingers OS. Color fundus images of the posterior pole illustrates subretinal fluid and neurosensory detachment involving the posterior poles of both eyes *(second row)*. Fluorescein angiogram shows stippled hyperfluorescence with late pooling into the neurosensory detachments *(third row)*. The patient was started on oral steroids. Color fundus photographs and fluorescein angiogram 6 weeks after initiation of steroid therapy show resolution of the detachments and subretinal fluid *(fourth and fifth rows)*. *Images courtesy of Amani Fawzi, MD*

Scleritis

Scleritis refers to inflammation of the sclera, which may be associated with an underlying systemic autoimmune disease. Scleritis is classified as either anterior (diffuse, nodular, or necrotizing with or without inflammation) or posterior, which accounts for only 2-7% of cases. Posterior scleritis is defined as scleral inflammation posterior to the ora serrata, which frequently occurs in association with anterior inflammatory diseases. Involvement of contiguous structures such as the orbit, choroid, retina, and optic disc is common. Patients, usually middle-aged females, typically present with unilateral ocular pain and decreased vision. In approximately 70% of those affected, there is no known systemic disease association. Necrotizing scleritis without inflammation (scleromalacia perforans) is a rare, usually painless, bilateral condition occurring predominantly in elderly females with severe long-standing rheumatoid arthritis. These patients may develop uveitis and macular edema in addition to nonpainful areas of profound scleral thinning with areas of exposed choroid and uveal prolapse that are high risk for traumatic rupture. Thinning may occur posteriorly and cause a staphyloma.

Posterior segment findings include optic disc edema, choroidal folds, exudative retinal detachment, and, occasionally, a well-delineated area of subretinal thickening that simulates a choroidal mass or tumor. Ultrasonography demonstrates scleral and choroidal thickening with fluid beneath Tenon capsule that creates a squaring-off of the interface between the optic nerve and the sclera, known as the "T" sign. Rarely scleritis may be associated with life-threatening autoimmune conditions such as polyangiitis with granulomatosis (previously referred to as Wegener granulomatosis) and therefore patients should be appropriately evaluated upon presentation.

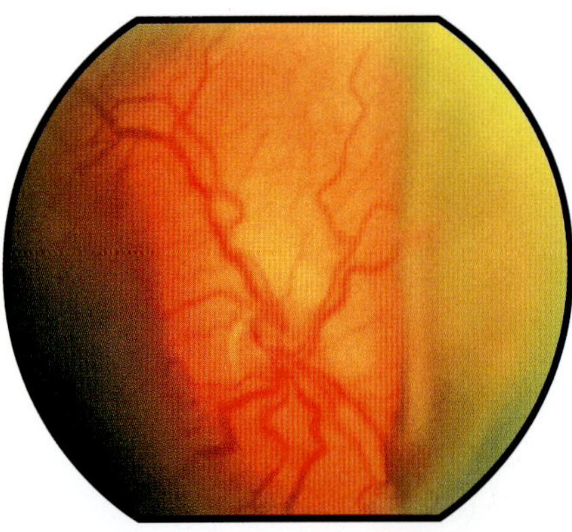

This patient has a choroidal effusion secondary to posterior scleritis.

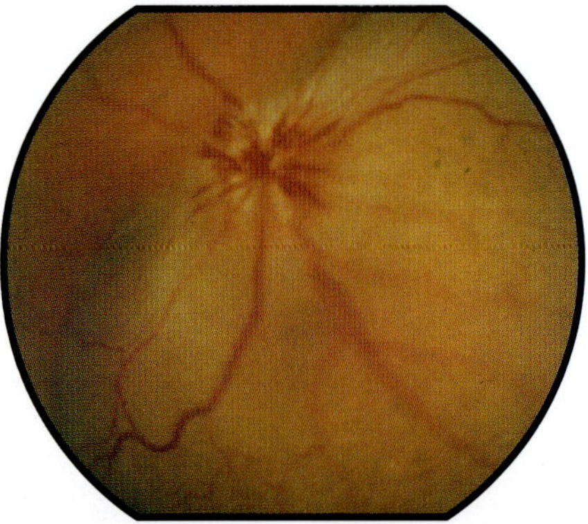

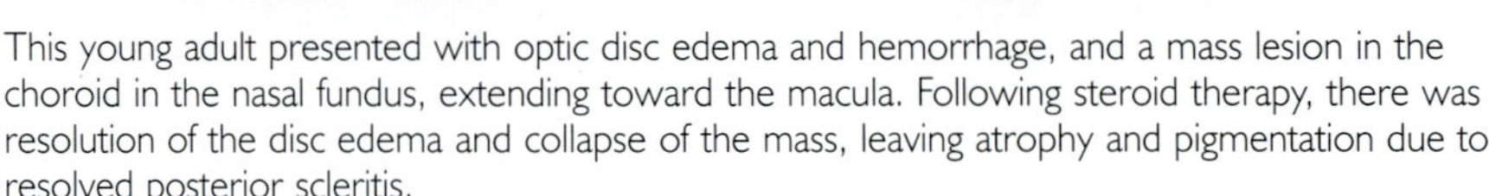

This young adult presented with optic disc edema and hemorrhage, and a mass lesion in the choroid in the nasal fundus, extending toward the macula. Following steroid therapy, there was resolution of the disc edema and collapse of the mass, leaving atrophy and pigmentation due to resolved posterior scleritis.

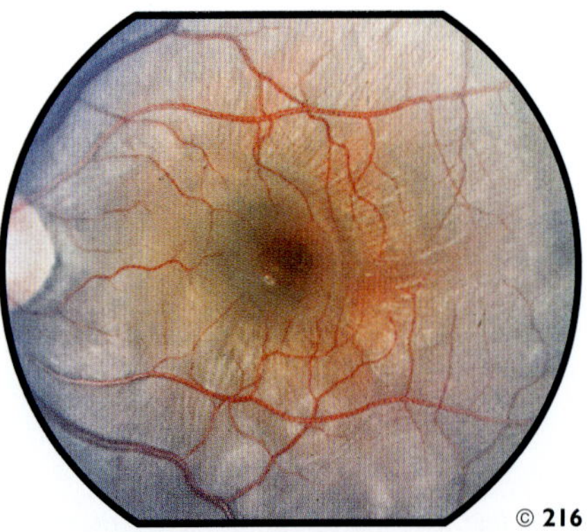

© 216

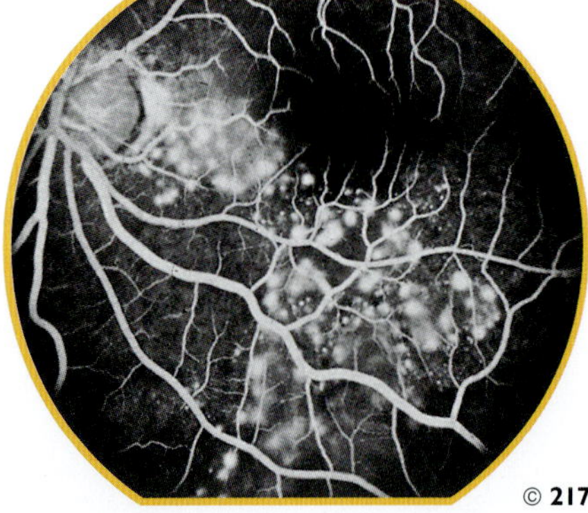

© 217

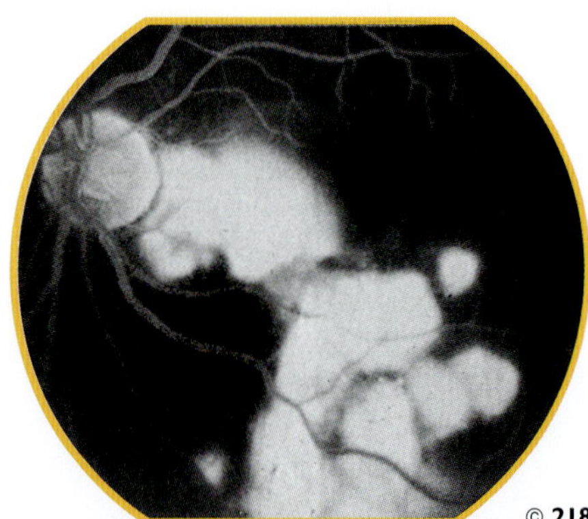

© 218

Scleritis can clinically and angiographically resemble Harada disease with multiple serous retinal detachments, choroidal folds, and punctate leaks at the level of the RPE that pool into the subneurosensory retinal space with FA.

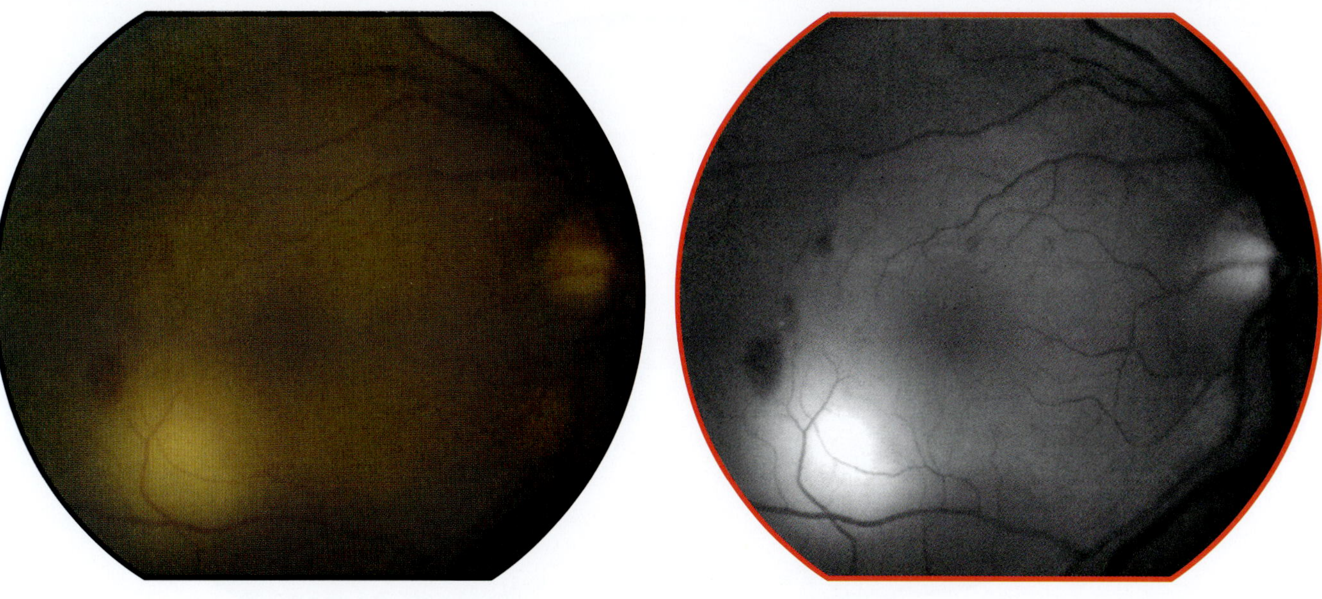

This is a 56-year-old Hispanic female seen as an emergency with a one-week history of headache and right eye pain with movement associated with a yellow-green spot in the center of her vision and symptoms of photopsia in the right eye. Note the focal subretinal granuloma in the inferotemporal paramacular region associated with a spot of hemorrhage and an exudative macular detachment in this patient with posterior scleritis. *Courtesy of Dr. Ramin Sarrafizadeh*

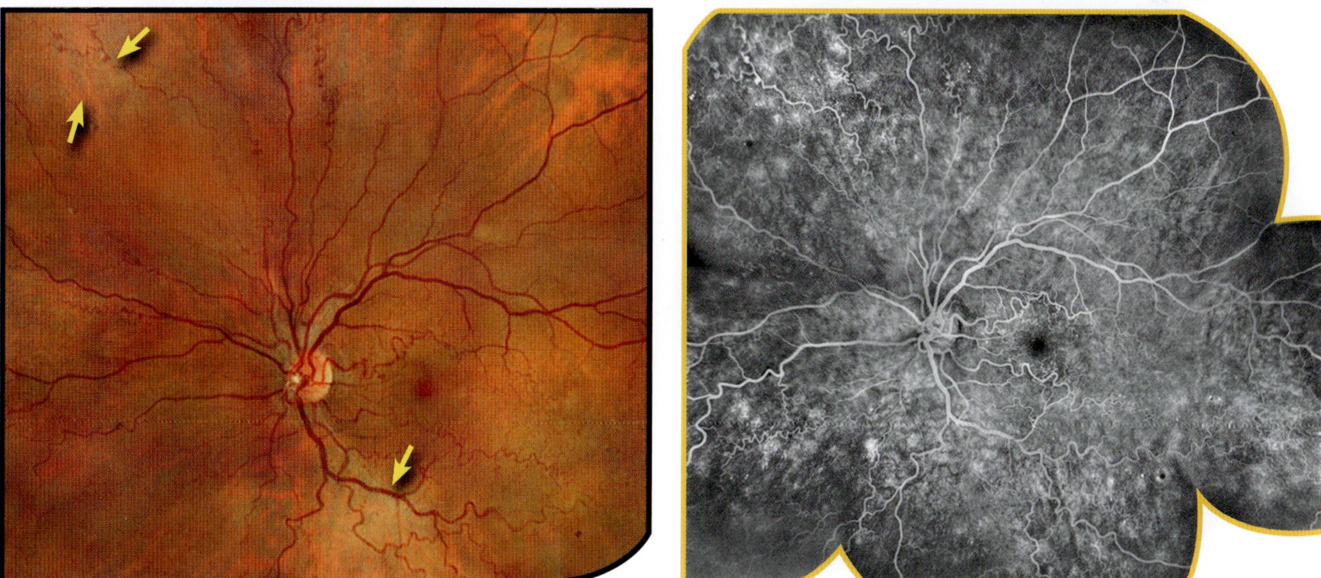

This patient had two focal areas of posterior scleritis: inferior to the disc and superonasal in the peripheral fundus *(arrows)*. There is an associated retinal microangiopathy with microaneurysms and leaking capillaries with the peripheral lesion and a shallow detachment of the neurosensory retina over each lesion.

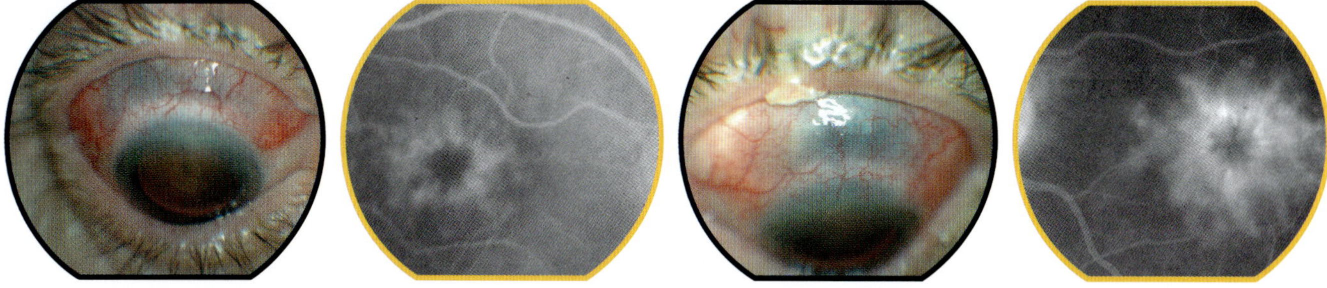

This patient with rheumatoid arthritis has necrotizing scleritis in each eye. Note the presence of petaloid cystoid macular edema in each eye.

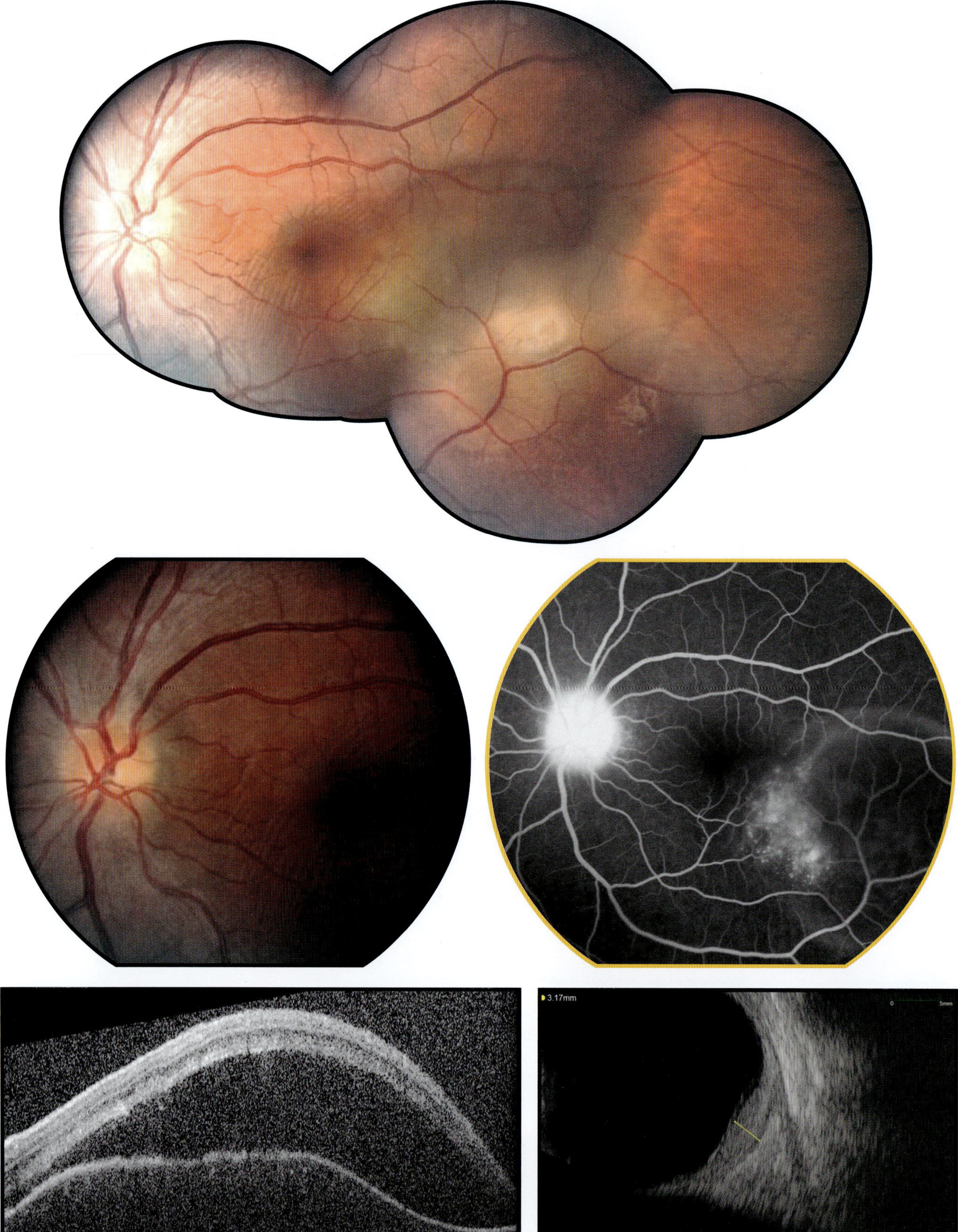

This 23-year-old female patient was referred for a choroidal mass in the left eye. Review of systems was significant for decreased vision in the left eye, headache, and left eye pain worse with lateral gaze. Color fundus photo montage revealed choroidal folds, an apparently solid subretinal elevation with overlying serous retinal detachment *(top)*. Late phase fluorescein angiogram shows a hyperfluorescent optic nerve and stippled hyperfluorescence with pooling into the serous detachment *(second row, right)*. An SD-OCT image taken through the lesion confirmed choroidal elevation with overlying subretinal fluid *(bottom left)*. B-scan ultrasound of the left eye revealed thickening of the posterior sclera with medium to high internal reflectivity *(bottom right)*. A diagnosis of posterior nodular scleritis was made. The patient had remarkable improvement after initiation of oral steroids.

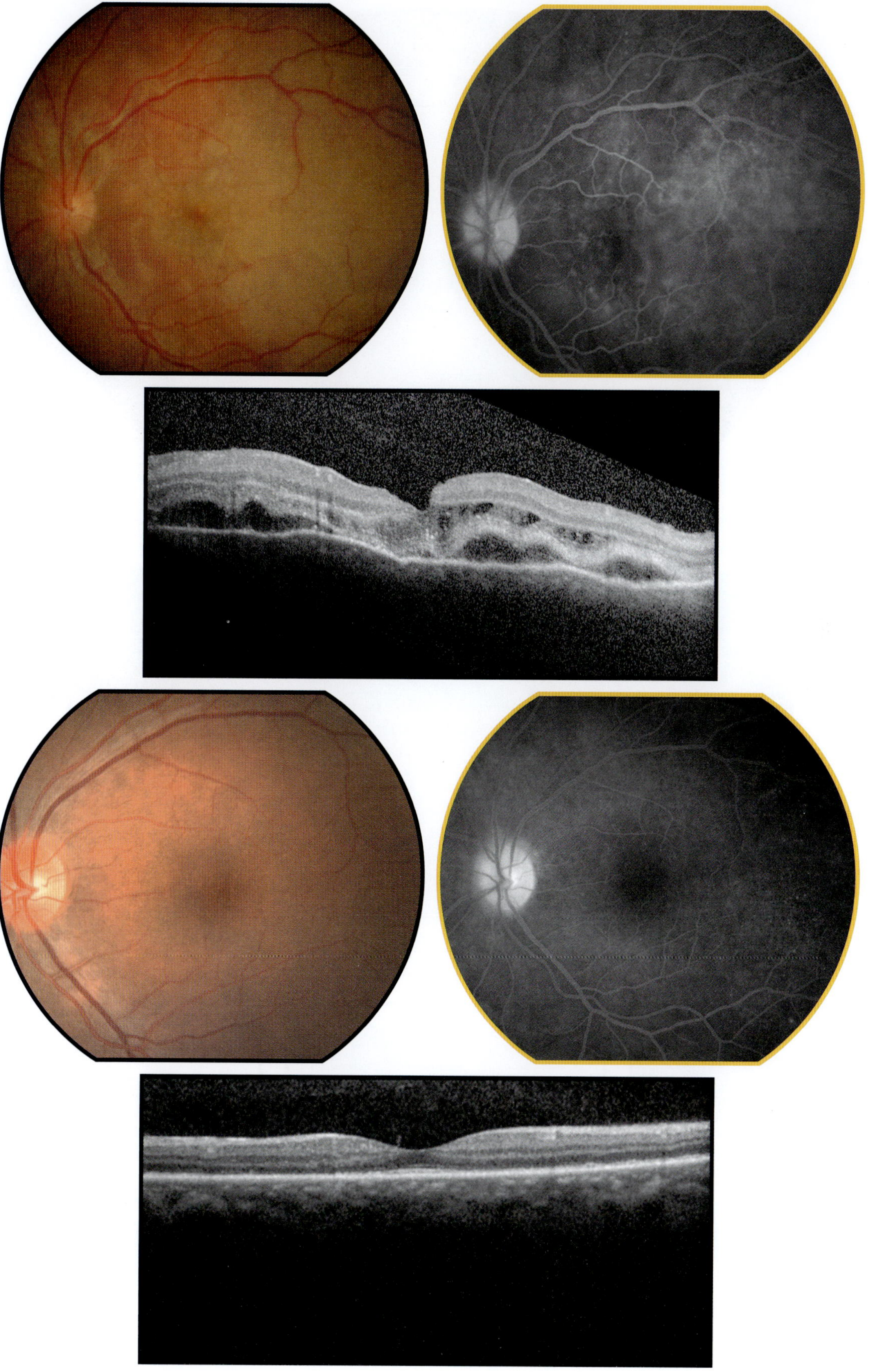

This 38-year-old female presented with pain and decreased vision in the left eye for 3 weeks. Color fundus photograph of the left eye on presentation illustrates subretinal fluid involving the macula and subtle inferior choroidal folds *(top row, left)*. Fluorescein angiogram shows stippled hyperfluorescence with pooling into a serous retinal detachment *(top row, right)*. SD-OCT confirms the presence of subretinal and intraretinal fluid *(second row)*. A diagnosis of posterior scleritis was made and the patient was started on oral steroids. Color fundus photograph *(third row, left)*, fluorescein angiogram *(third row, right)*, and SD-OCT *(bottom row)* taken at one-month follow-up show resolution of the serous retinal detachment. *Images courtesy of Mark J. Daily, MD*

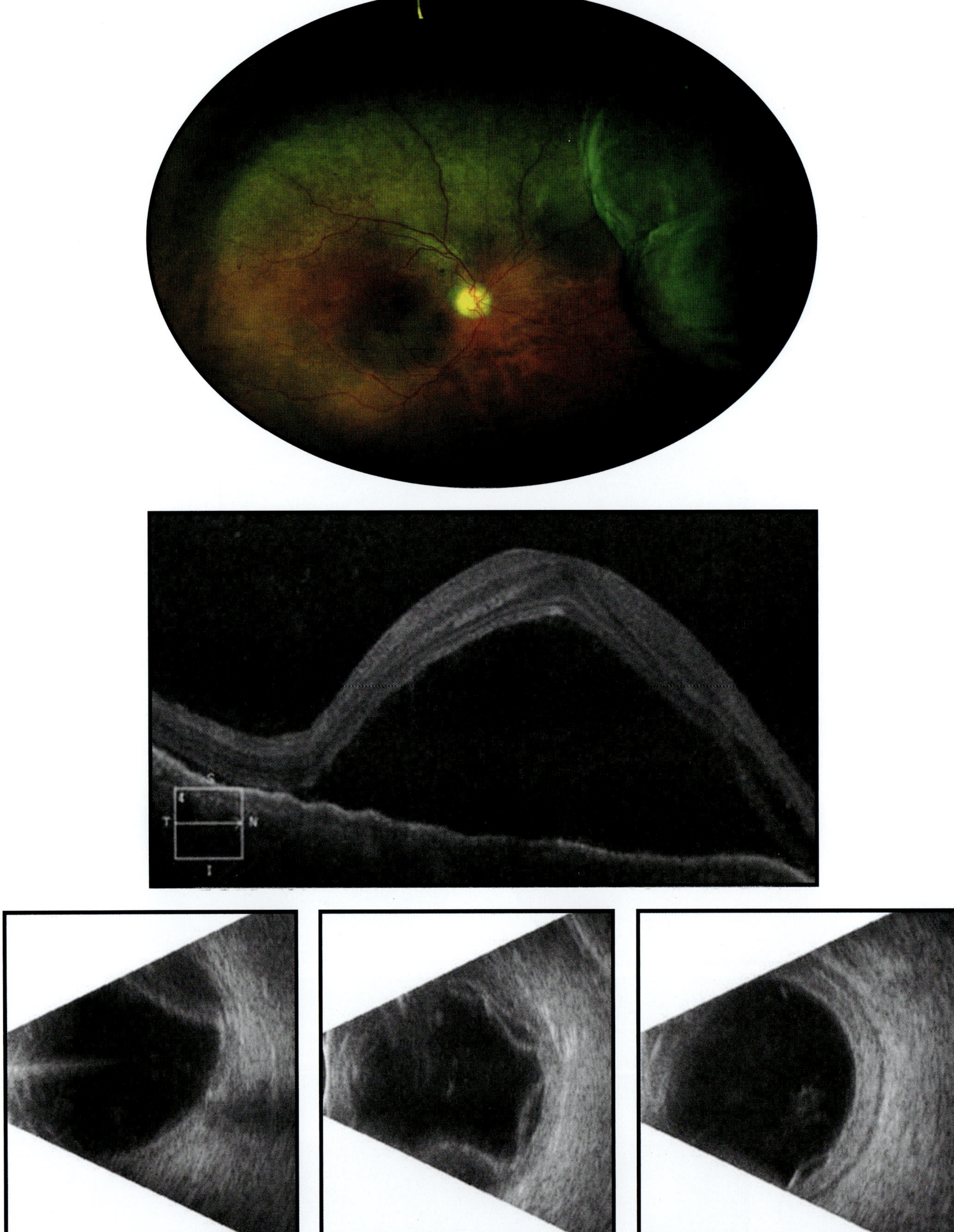

This 78-year-old male presented with blurred vision and painful red right eye for several days. Widefield color fundus photos illustrate a serous retinal detachment involving the macula of the right eye and a solid-appearing mass involving the nasal peripheral retina with overlying subretinal fluid *(top row)*. SD-OCT confirms the presence of a severe exudative macular detachment *(second row)*. B-Scan ultrasound shows sclerochoroidal thickening associated with choroidal and exudative retinal detachment *(third row)*. *Images courtesy of Calvin Mein, MD*

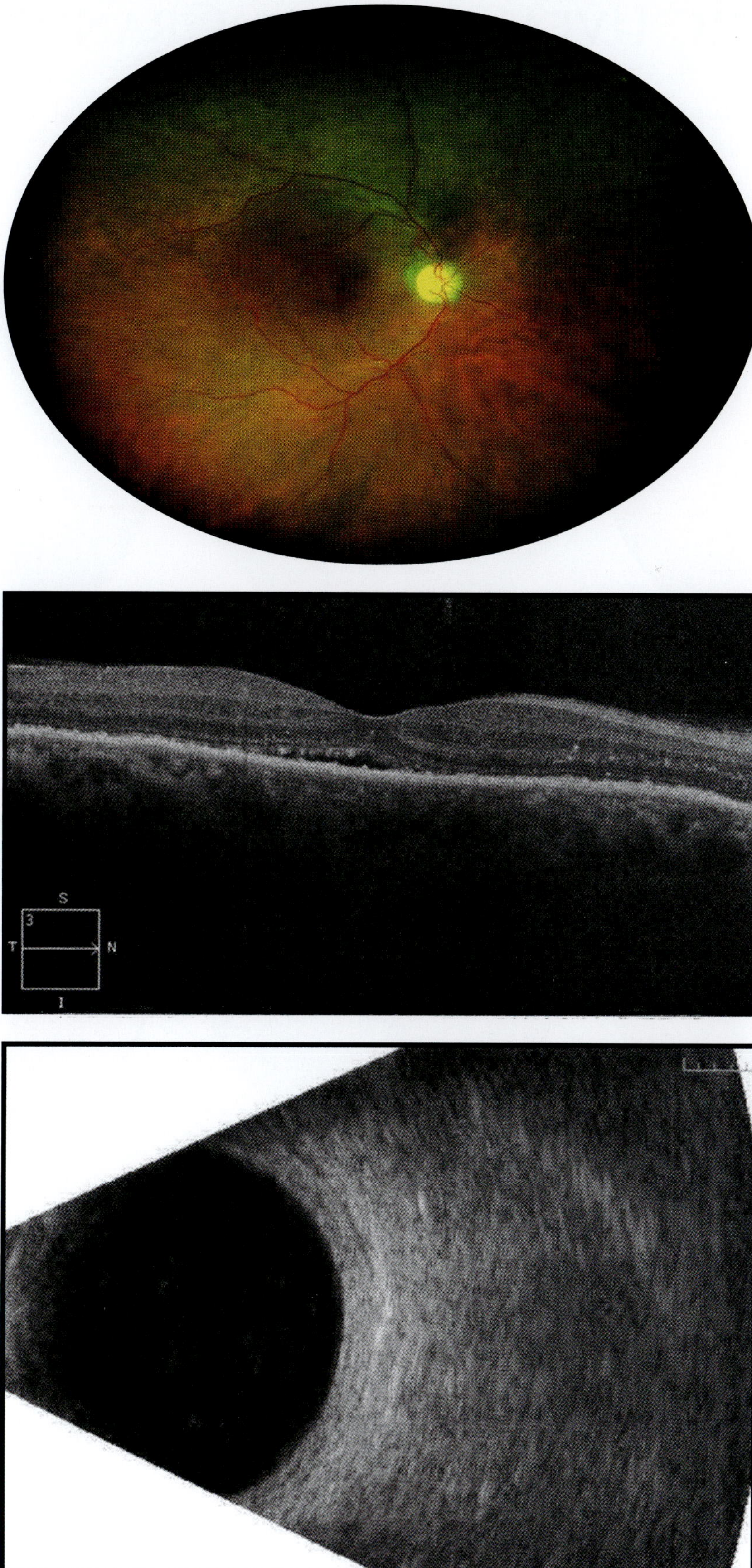

The same patient was started on oral prednisone. Widefield color photography taken at one-week follow-up shows resolution of the sclerochoroidal mass, near resolution of central subretinal fluid with SD-OCT, and normalization of the B-scan ultrasound. *Images courtesy of Calvin Mein, MD*

Idiopathic Uveal Scleral Granuloma

An idiopathic uveal scleral granuloma, also known as solitary helioid granuloma or solitary idiopathic granuloma, is a bright yellow mass lesion of the uveal scleral tissue with overlying retinal vascular changes and sometimes overlying exudative retinal detachment. It is typically an idiopathic inflammatory condition; however, a thorough investigation to rule out underlying inflammatory and infectious diseases such as sarcoidosis and tuberculosis should be undertaken. Once these have been ruled out, it is best managed with systemic steroids.

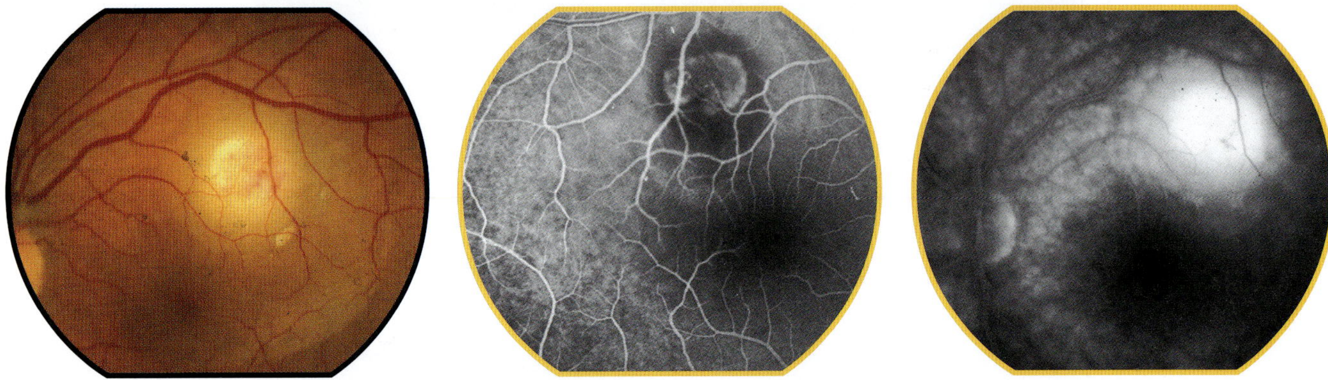

This patient has an idiopathic uveal scleral granuloma with a large turbid serous retinal detachment that extends into the macula. The fluorescein angiogram illustrates CNV overlying the mass with late leakage.

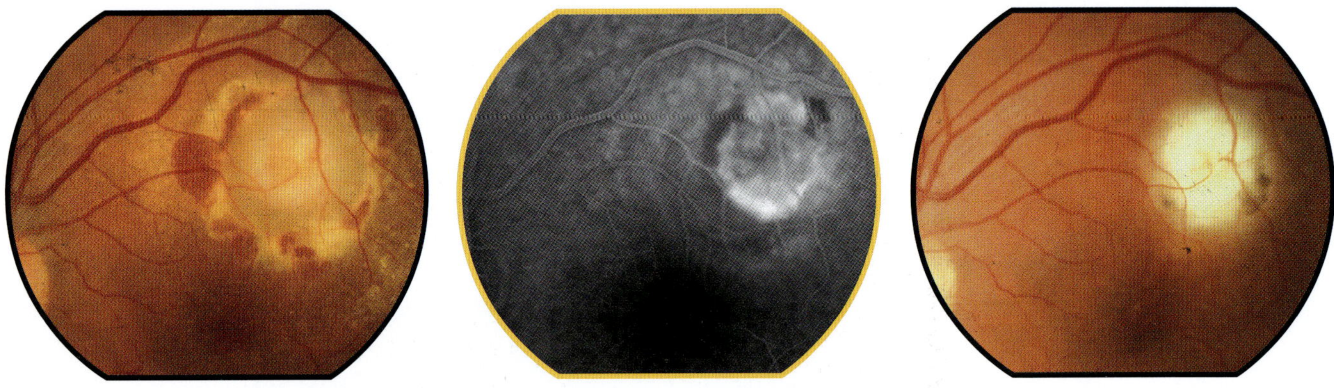

Laser photocoagulation ablation of the neovascular complex was performed, but there was further proliferation of the new vessels with hemorrhage. Steroid treatment was then administered and the granuloma regressed with complete resolution of the serosanguineous detachment and the neovascular membrane *(right)*.

Suggested Reading

Multiple Evanescent White Dot Syndrome

Gross, N.E., Yannuzzi, L.A., Freund, K.B., et al., 2006. Multiple evanescent white dot syndrome. Arch. Ophthalmol. 124, 493–500.

Jampol, L.M., Sieving, P.A., Pugh, D., et al., 1984. Multiple evanescent white dot syndrome. I Clinical findings. Arch. Ophthalmol. 102, 671–674.

Li, D., Kishi, S., 2009. Restored photoreceptor outer segment damage in multiple evanescent white dot syndrome. Ophthalmology 116, 762–770.

Pichi, F., Srvivastava, S.K., Chexal, S., et al., 2016. En face optical coherence tomography and optical coherence tomography angiography of multiple evanesceny white dot syndrome: new insights into pathogenesis. Retina [Epub ahead of print].

Sieving, P.A., Fishman, G.A., Jampol, L.M., et al., 1984. Multiple evanescent white dot syndrome. II. Electrophysiology of the photoreceptors during retinal pigment epithelial disease. Arch. Ophthalmol. 102, 675–679.

Sikorski, B.L., Wojtkowski, M., Kaluzny, J.J., et al., 2008. Correlation of spectral optical coherence tomography with fluorescein and indocyanine green angiography in multiple evanescent white dot syndrome. Br. J. Ophthalmol. 92, 1552–1557.

Multifocal Choroiditis (MFC) (Punctate Inner Choroidopathy (PIC), Multifocal Choroiditis and Panuveitis (MCP), Idiopathic Progressive Subretinal Fibrosis Syndrome)

Dreyer, R.F., Gass, J.D.M., 1984. Multifocal choroiditis and panuveitis: a syndrome that mimics ocular histoplasmosis. Arch. Ophthalmol. 102, 1776–1784.

Gass, J.D.M., Margo, C.E., Levy, M.H., 1996. Progressive subretinal fibrosis and blindness in patients with multifocal granulomatous chorioretinitis. Am. J. Ophthalmol. 122, 76–85.

Haen, S.P., Spaide, R.F., 2008. Fundus autofluorescence in multifocal choroiditis and panuveitis. Am. J. Ophthalmol. 145, 847–853.

Kedhar, S.R., Thorne, J.E., Wittenberg, S., et al., 2007. Multifocal choroiditis with panuveitis and punctate inner choroidopathy: comparison of clinical characteristics at presentation. Retina 27, 1174–1179.

Palestine, A.G., Nussenblatt, R.B., Parver, L.M., et al., 1985. Progressive subretinal fibrosis and uveitis. Br. J. Ophthalmol. 68, 667–673.

Parnell, J.R., Jampol, L.M., Yannuzzi, L.A., et al., 2001. Differentiation between presumed ocular histoplasmosis syndrome and multifocal choroiditis with panuveitis based on morphology of photographed fundus lesions and fluorescein angiography. Arch. Ophthalmol. 119, 208–212.

Slakter, J.S., Giovannini, A., Yannuzzi, L.A., et al., 1997. Indocyanine green angiography of multifocal choroiditis. Ophthalmology 104, 1813–1819.

Spaide, R.F., Yannuzzi, L.A., Freund, K.B., 1991. Linear streaks in multifocal choroiditis and panuveitis. Retina 11, 229–231.

Thorne, J.E., Wittenberg, S., Jabs, D.A., et al., 2006. Multifocal choroiditis with panuveitis incidence of ocular complications and of loss of visual acuity. Ophthalmology 113, 2310–2316.

Watzke, R.C., Packer, A.J., Folk, J.C., et al., 1984. Punctate inner choroidopathy. Am. J. Ophthalmol. 98, 572–584.

Acute Zonal Occult Outer Retinopathy

Fekrat, S., Wilkinson, C.P., Chang, B., et al., 2000. Acute annular outer retinopathy: report of four cases. Am. J. Ophthalmol. 130, 636–644.

Francis, P.J., Marinescu, A., Fitzke, F.W., et al., 2005. Acute zonal occult outer retinopathy: towards a set of diagnostic criteria. Br. J. Ophthalmol. 89, 70–73.

Gass, J.D., 2003. Acute zonal occult outer retinopathy: Donders Lecture: The Netherlands Ophthalmological Society, Maastricht, Holland, June 19, 1992. 1993. Retina 23, 79–97.

Gass, J.D., Agarwal, A., Scott, I.U., 2002. Acute zonal occult outer retinopathy: a long-term follow-up study. Am. J. Ophthalmol. 134, 329–339.

Jacobson, D.M., 1996. Acute zonal occult outer retinopathy and central nervous system inflammation. J. Neuroophthalmol. 16, 172–177.

Li, D., Kishi, S., 2007. Loss of photoreceptor outer segment in acute zonal occult outer retinopathy. Arch. Ophthalmol. 125, 1194–1200.

Mrejen, S., Khan, S., Gallego-Pinazo, R., et al., 2014. Acute zonal occult outer retinopathy: a classification based on multimodal imaging. JAMA Ophthalmol. 132 (9), 1089–1098.

Spaide, R.F., Koizumi, H., Freund, K.B., 2008. Photoreceptor outer segment abnormalities as a cause of blind spot enlargement in acute zonal occult outer retinopathy-complex diseases. Am. J. Ophthalmol. 146, 111–120.

Acute Posterior Multifocal Placoid Pigment Epitheliopathy

Deutman, A.F., Oosterhuis, J.A., Boen-Tan, T.N., et al., 1972. 1545 Acute posterior multifocal placoid pigment epitheliopathy. Pigment epitheliopathy of choriocapillaritis? Br. J. Ophthalmol. 56, 863–874.

Dhaliwal, R.S., Maguire, A.M., Flower, R.W., et al., 1993. Acute posterior multifocal placoid pigment epitheliopathy. An indocyanine green angiographic study. Retina 13, 317–325.

Fishman, G.A., Rabb, M.F., Kaplan, J., 1974. Acute posterior multifocal placoid pigment epitheliopathy. Arch. Ophthalmol. 92, 173–177.

Gass, J.D., 1968. Acute posterior multifocal placoid pigment epitheliopathy. Arch. Ophthalmol. 80, 177–185.

Spaide, R.F., 2006. Autofluorescence imaging of acute posterior multifocal placoid pigment epitheliopathy. Retina 26, 479–482.

Spaide, R.F., Yannuzzi, L.A., Slakter, J., 1991. Choroidal vasculitis in acute posterior multifocal placoid pigment epitheliopathy. Br. J. Ophthalmol. 75, 685–687.

Serpiginous Choroiditis

Cardillo Piccolino, F., Grosso, A., Savini, E., 2009. Fundus autofluorescence in serpiginous choroiditis. Graefes Arch. Clin. Exp. Ophthalmol. 247, 179–185.

Cordero-Coma, M., Benito, M.F., Hernández, A.M., et al., 2008. Serpiginous choroiditis. Ophthalmology 115, 1633.e1–1633.e2.

Giovannini, A., Mariotti, C., Ripa, E., et al., 1996. Indocyanine green angiographic findings in serpiginous choroidopathy. Br. J. Ophthalmol. 80, 536–540.

Mackensen, F., Becker, M.D., Wiehler, U., et al., 2008. QuantiFERON TB-Gold—a new test strengthening long-suspected tuberculous involvement in serpiginous-like choroiditis. Am. J. Ophthalmol. 146, 761–766.

Relentless Placoid Chorioretinitis (Ampiginous Choroiditis)

Amer, R., Florescu, T., 2008. Optical coherence tomography in relentless placoid chorioretinitis. Clin. Experiment. Ophthalmol. 36, 388–390.

Jones, B.E., Jampol, L.M., Yannuzzi, L.A., et al., 2000. Relentless placoid chorioretinitis: a new entity or an unusual variant of serpiginous chorioretinitis? Arch. Ophthalmol. 118, 931–938.

Persistent Placoid Maculopathy

Golchet, P.R., Jampol, L.M., Wilson, D., et al., 2007. Persistent placoid maculopathy: a new clinical entity. Ophthalmology 114, 1530–1540.

Birdshot Chorioretinopathy

Fardeau, C., Herbort, C.P., Kullmann, N., et al., 1999. Indocyanine green angiography in birdshot chorioretinopathy. Ophthalmology 106, 1928–1934.

Fuerst, D.J., Tessler, H.H., Fishman, G.A., et al., 1984. Birdshot retinochoroidopathy. Arch. Ophthalmol. 102, 214–219.

Gaudio, P.A., Kaye, D.B., Crawford, J.B., 2002. Histopathology of birdshot retinochoroidopathy. Br. J. Ophthalmol. 86, 1439–1441.

Koizumi, H., Pozzoni, M.C., Spaide, R.F., 2008. Fundus autofluorescence in birdshot chorioretinopathy. Ophthalmology 115, e15–e20.

Nussenblatt, R.B., Mittal, K.K., Ryan, S., et al., 1982. Birdshot retinochoroidopathy associated with HLA-A29 antigen and immune responsiveness to retinal S-antigen. Am. J. Ophthalmol. 94, 147–158.

Trinh, L., Bodaghi, B., Fardeau, C., et al., 2009. Clinical features, treatment methods, and evolution of birdshot chorioretinopathy in 5 different families. Am. J. Ophthalmol. 147 (6), 1042–1047, 1047.e1.

Pars Planitis

Oruc, S., Duffy, B.F., Mohanakumar, T., et al., 2001. The association of HLA class II with pars planitis. Am. J. Ophthalmol. 131, 657–659.

Tang, W.M., Pulido, J.S., Eckels, D.D., et al., 1997. The association of HLA-DR15 and intermediate uveitis. Am. J. Ophthalmol. 123, 70–75.

Wetzig, R.P., Chen, C.C., Nussenblatt, R.B., et al., 1988. Clinical and immunopathological studies of pars planitis in a family. Br. J. Ophthalmol. 75, 5–10.

Multiple Sclerosis

Birch, M.K., Barbosa, S., Blumhardt, L.D., et al., 1996. Retinal venous sheathing and the blood-retinal barrier in multiple sclerosis. Arch. Ophthalmol. 114, 34–39.

Gordon, L.K., Goldstein, D.A., 2014. Gender and uveitis in patients with multiple sclerosis. J. Ophthalmol. 2014, 565262.

Kerrison, J.B., Flynn, T., Green, W.R., 1994. Retinal pathologic changes in multiple sclerosis. Retina 14, 445–451.

Vine, A.K., 1992. Severe periphlebitis, peripheral retinal ischemia, and preretinal neovascularization in patients with multiple sclerosis. Am. J. Ophthalmol. 113, 28–32.

Behçet Disease

Tugal-Tutkun, I., Onal, S., Altan-Yaycioglu, R., et al., 2004. Uveitis in Behçet disease: an analysis of 880 patients. Am. J. Ophthalmol. 138, 373–380.

Yang, P., Fang, W., Meng, Q., et al., 2008. Clinical features of Chinese patients with Behçet's disease. Ophthalmology 115, 312–318, e4.

Inflammatory Bowel Disease/ Crohn's Disease/Ulcerative Colitis

Ernst, B.B., Lowder, C.Y., Meisler, D.M., et al., 1991. Posterior segment manifestations of inflammatory bowel disease. Ophthalmology 98, 1272–1280.

Ghanchi, F.D., Rembacken, B.J., 2003. Inflammatory bowel disease and the eye. Surv. Ophthalmol. 48 (6), 663–676.

Keyser, B.J., Hass, A.N., 1994. Retinal vascular disease in ulcerative colitis. Am. J. Ophthalmol. 118, 395–396.

Ruby, A.J., Jampol, L.M., 1990. Crohn's disease and retinal vascular disease. Am. J. Ophthalmol. 110, 349–353.

Seronegative Spondyloarthropathies

Zagora, S.L., McCluskey, P., 2014. Ocular manifestations of seronegative spondyloarthropathies. Curr. Opin. Ophthalmol. 25 (6), 495–501.

Scleroderma

Farkas, T.G., Sylvester, V., Archer, D., 1972. The choroidopathy of progressive systemic sclerosis (scleroderma). Am. J. Ophthalmol. 74, 875–886.

Tailor, R., Gupta, A., Herrick, A., et al., 2009. Ocular manifestations of scleroderma. Surv. Ophthalmol. 54, 292–304.

West, R.H., Barnett, A.J., 1979. Ocular involvement in scleroderma. Br. J. Ophthalmol. 63, 845–847.

Churg-Strauss Syndrome (Allergic Granulomatosis and Angiitis)

Takanashi, T., Uchida, S., Arita, M., et al., 2001. Orbital inflammatory pseudotumor and ischemic vasculitis in Churg-Strauss syndrome: report of two cases and review of the literature. Ophthalmology 108 (6), 1129–1133.

Relapsing Polychondritis

Yoo, J.H., Chodosh, J., Dana, R., 2011. Relapsing polychondritis: systemic and ocular manifestations, differential diagnosis, management, and prognosis. Semin. Ophthalmol. 26 (4–5), 261–269.

Adult-Onset Still's Disease

Okwuosa, T.M., Lee, E.W., Starosta, M., et al., 2007. Purtscher-like retinopathy in a patient with adult-onset Still's disease and concurrent thrombotic thrombocytopenic purpura. Arthritis Rheum. 57, 182–185.

Semple, H.C., Landers, M.B. 3rd., Morse, L.S., 1990. Optic disk neovascularization in juvenile rheumatoid arthritis. Am. J. Ophthalmol. 110, 210–212.

Idiopathic Retinal Vasculitis, Aneurysms, and Neuroretinitis

Chang, T.S., Aylward, G.W., Davis, J.L., et al., 1995. Idiopathic retinal vasculitis, aneurysms, and neuro-retinitis. Retinal Vasculitis Study. Ophthalmology 102, 1089–1097.

Samuel, M.A., Equi, R.A., Chang, T.S., et al., 2007. Idiopathic retinitis, vasculitis, aneurysms, and neuroretinitis (IRVAN): new observations and a proposed staging system. Ophthalmology 114, 1526–1529.

Idiopathic Frosted-Branch Angiitis

Kleiner, R.C., 1997. Frosted branch angiitis: clinical syndrome or clinical sign? Retina 17 (5), 370–371.

Walker, S., Iguchi, A., Jones, N.P., 2004. Frosted branch angiitis: a review. Eye (Lond.) 18, 527–533.

Sarcoidosis

Chan, C.C., Wetzig, R.P., Palestine, A.G., et al., 1987. Immunohistopathology of ocular sarcoidosis. Arch. Ophthalmol. 105, 1398–1402.

Jabs, D.A., Johns, C.J., 1986. Ocular involvement in chronic sarcoidosis. Am. J. Ophthalmol. 102, 297–301.

Spalton, D.J., Sanders, M.D., 1981. Fundus changes in histologically confirmed sarcoidosis. Br. J. Ophthalmol. 65, 348–358.

Vogt–Koyanagi–Harada Syndrome

Beniz, J., Forster, D.J., Lean, J.S., et al., 1991. Variations in clinical features of the Vogt–Koyanagi–Harada syndrome. Retina 11, 275–280.

Bouchenaki, N., Herbort, C.P., 2001. The contribution of indocyanine green angiography to the appraisal and management of Vogt–Koyanagi–Harada disease. Ophthalmology 108, 54–64.

Bykhovskaya, I., Thorne, J.E., Kempen, J.H., et al., 2005. Vogt–Koyanagi–Harada disease: clinical outcomes. Am. J. Ophthalmol. 140, 674–678.

da Silva, F.T., Damico, F.M., Marin, M.L., et al., 2009. Revised diagnostic criteria for Vogt–Koyanagi–Harada disease: considerations on the different disease categories. Am. J. Ophthalmol. 147, 339–345, e5.

Perry, H.D., Font, R.L., 1997. Clinical and histopathologic observations in severe Vogt–Koyanagi–Harada syndrome. Am. J. Ophthalmol. 83, 242–254.

Rao, N.A., Marak, G.E., 1983. Sympathetic ophthalmia simulating Vogt–Koyanagi–Harada's disease: a clinico-pathologic study of four cases. Jpn J. Ophthalmol. 27, 506–511.

Scleritis

Akpek, E.K., Thorne, J.E., Qazi, F.A., et al., 2004. Evaluation of patients with scleritis for systemic disease. Ophthalmology 111, 501–506.

Calthorpe, C.M., Watson, P.G., McCartney, A.C., 1988. Posterior scleritis: a clinical and histological survey. Eye (Lond.) 2, 267–277.

McCluskey, P.J., Watson, P.G., Lightman, S., et al., 1999. Posterior scleritis: clinical features, systemic associations, and outcome in a large series of patients. Ophthalmology 106, 2380–2386.

Singh, G., Guthoff, R., Foster, C.S., 1986. Observations on long-term follow-up of posterior scleritis. Am. J. Ophthalmol. 101, 570–575.

Wald, K.J., Spaide, R., Patalano, V.J., et al., 1992. Posterior scleritis in children. Am. J. Ophthalmol. 113, 281–286.

Idiopathic Uveal Scleral Granuloma

Feldman, R.B., Moore, D.M., Hood, C.I., et al., 1985. Solitary eosinophilic granuloma of the lateral orbital wall. Am. J. Ophthalmol. 100, 318–323.

Margo, C., Zimmerman, L.E., 1984. Idiopathic solitary granuloma of the uveal tract. Arch. Ophthalmol. 102, 732–735.

CHAPTER 5

Infection

Viruses
Human Immunodeficiency Virus (HIV) Associated Retinopathy

The most common retinal manifestation of human immunodeficiency virus (HIV) is a retinal microvasculopathy, also known as noninfectious acquired immunodeficiency syndrome (AIDS) retinopathy. This microvasculopathy is characterized by diabetic retinopathy-like findings including cotton-wool spots and retinal hemorrhages or microaneurysms in the posterior pole and/or periphery. Opportunistic infections such as cytomegalovirus (CMV) retinitis, acute retinal necrosis (ARN), and progressive outer retinal necrosis (PORN) are more visually devastating viral retinal infections associated with HIV and require emergent systemic and/or local antiviral therapy. Very rarely HIV can cause a primary retinal infection.

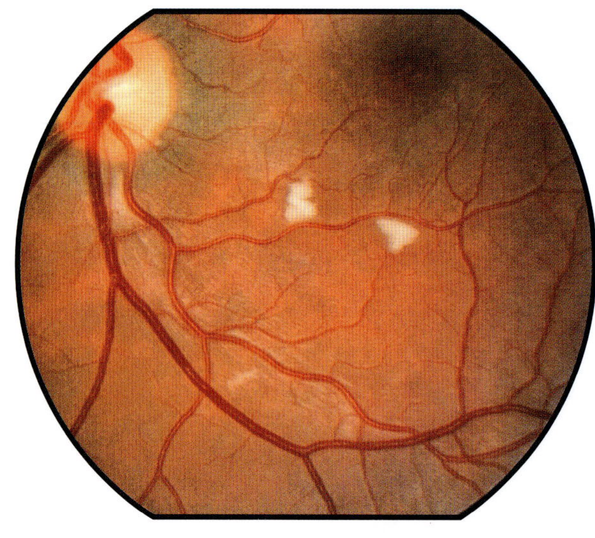

Cotton-wool spots due to noninfectious HIV retinopathy. *Courtesy of Dr. Jay Pepose*

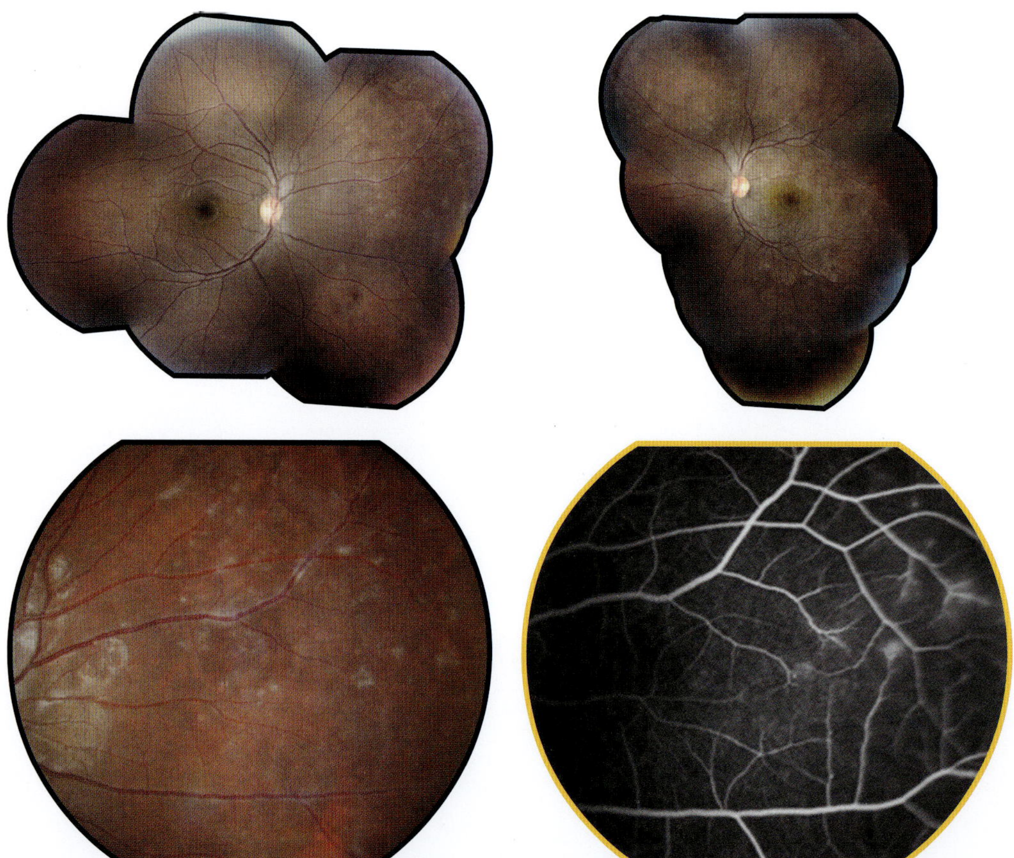

This is an AIDS patient with retinal infiltrates associated with HIV infection. Note the small multifocal white peripheral retinal infiltrates in each eye with staining on the fluorescein angiogram (FA). *Courtesy of Dr. Robin Vora and Dr. Emmett Cunningham*

Cytomegalovirus Retinitis

Cytomegalovirus (CMV) retinitis is the most common ocular opportunistic infection in AIDS and may also occur in other immunocompromised patients, especially in those with CD4 counts under 50/mm^3. In the era of highly active antiretroviral therapy, the immune status of AIDS patients has dramatically improved and opportunistic retina infections such as CMV retinitis are more rarely encountered. Symptoms will vary, as peripheral disease (zone 3) may go unnoticed by patients. Visual changes will be perceived by patients if the infection involves the posterior pole (zone 1). Mild intraocular inflammation in the anterior chamber and vitreous may be present. The classic retinal findings of CMV retinitis include a hemorrhagic retinitis with a sectoral or perivascular distribution.

A "frosted branch angiitis" in areas with and without retinitis may be appreciated. Retinal venous occlusive disease and optic disc neovascularization may complicate the course. Patients should be closely monitored for the eventual development of rhegmatogenous retinal detachment requiring surgical intervention to prevent severe vision loss and blindness.

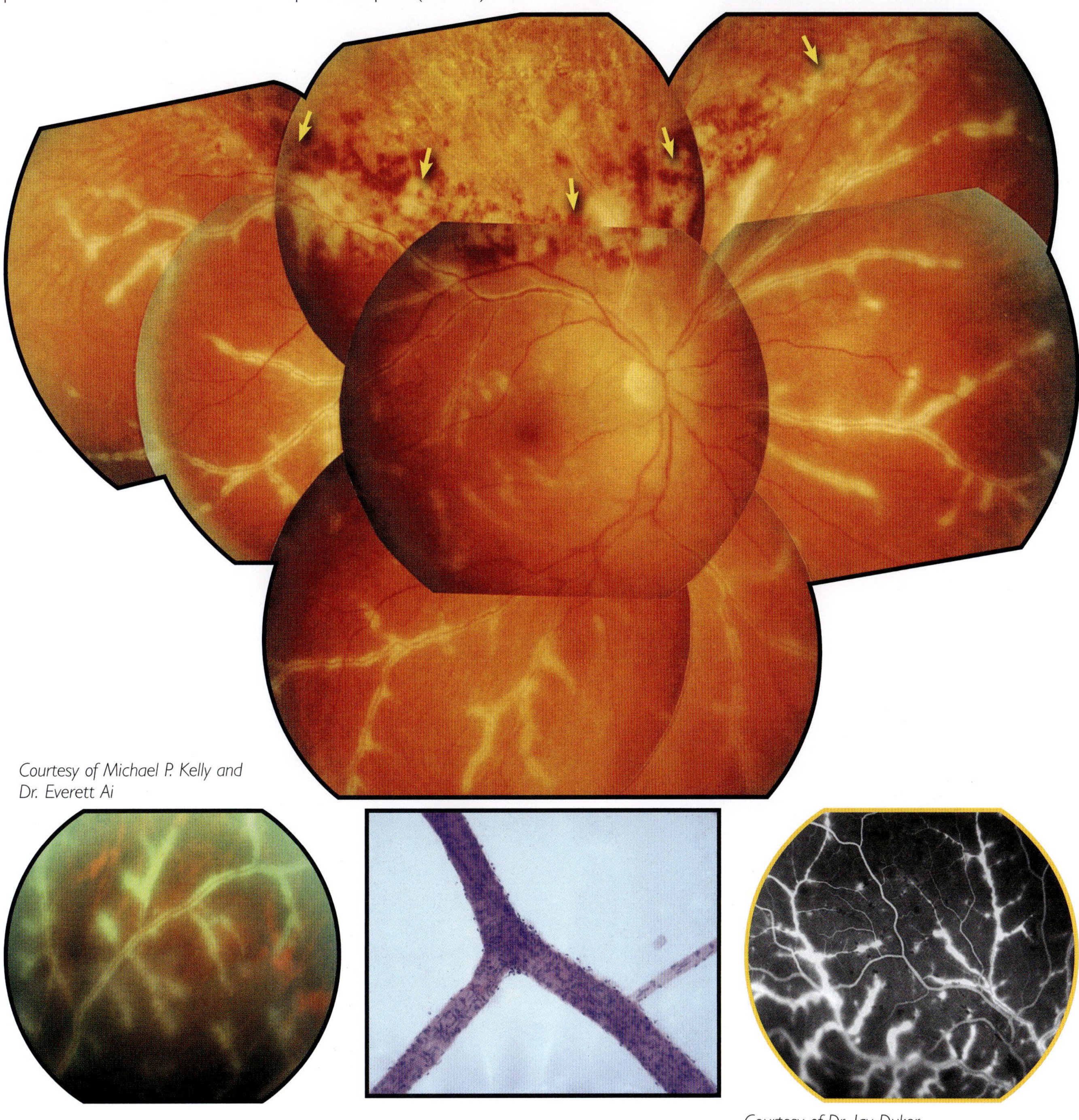

Courtesy of Michael P. Kelly and Dr. Everett Ai

Courtesy of Dr. Jay Duker

These are patients with CMV retinitis. A hemorrhagic retinitis is noted superiorly in the color montage with patch areas of "cheesy" necrosis associated with retinal hemorrhages in a perivascular distribution *(arrows)*. Note the widespread "frosted branch angiitis" pattern throughout the fundus *(top)* and in the peripheral color photograph. The histopathology shows inflammatory cells along the walls of a retinal vessel. The FA shows active staining of the inflamed retinal vessels in a frosted branch angiitis pattern.

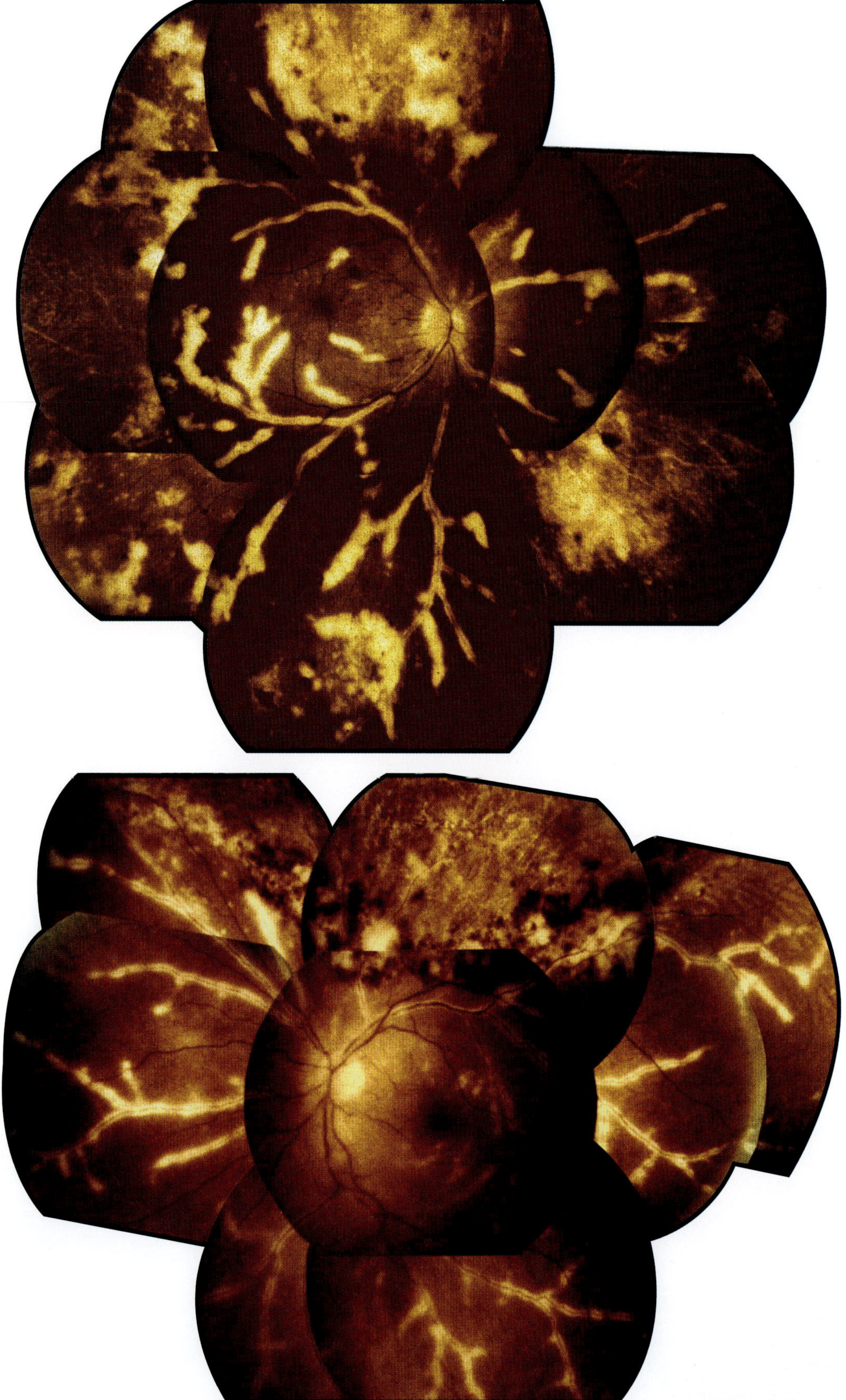

This is a patient with bilateral CMV retinitis. There is a diffuse frosted branch angiitis in both eyes. In the upper image, the right eye shows fibrous opacification of the superior chorioretinal area. In the lower image, the left eye shows a superior zonal region of atrophy from prior infection bordered by hemorrhage from an active necrotizing retinitis. There is involvement, but relative sparing of the paramacular region.

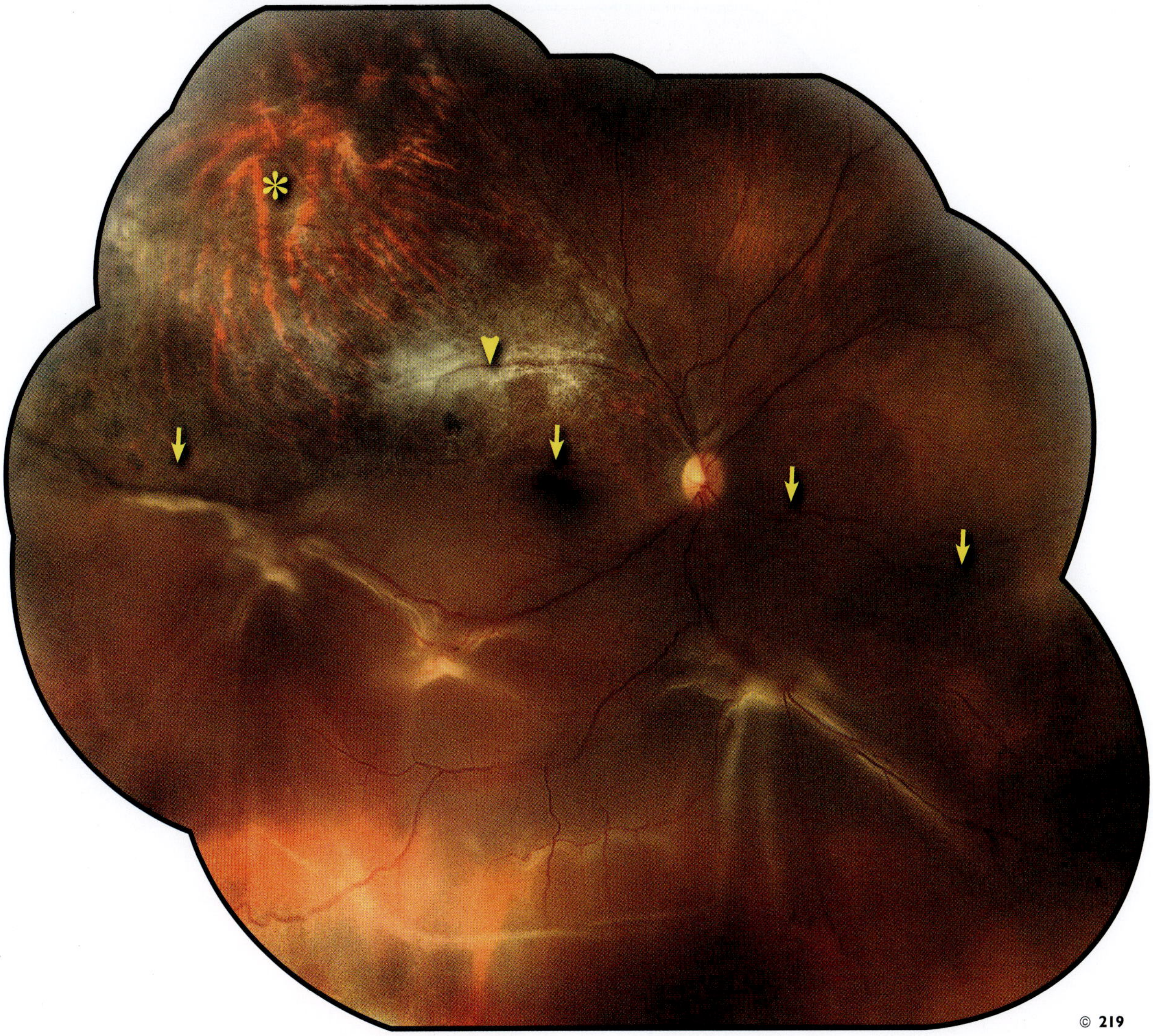

© 219

This patient shows resolving CMV retinitis with zonal atrophy superotemporally *(asterisk)* and active retinitis with opacification of the retina along the superotemporal arcade *(arrowhead)*. There is a hemispheric retinal detachment *(arrows)* in the inferior fundus. Multiple areas of retinal folds and fibrous proliferative vitreoretinopathy have complicated the detachment.

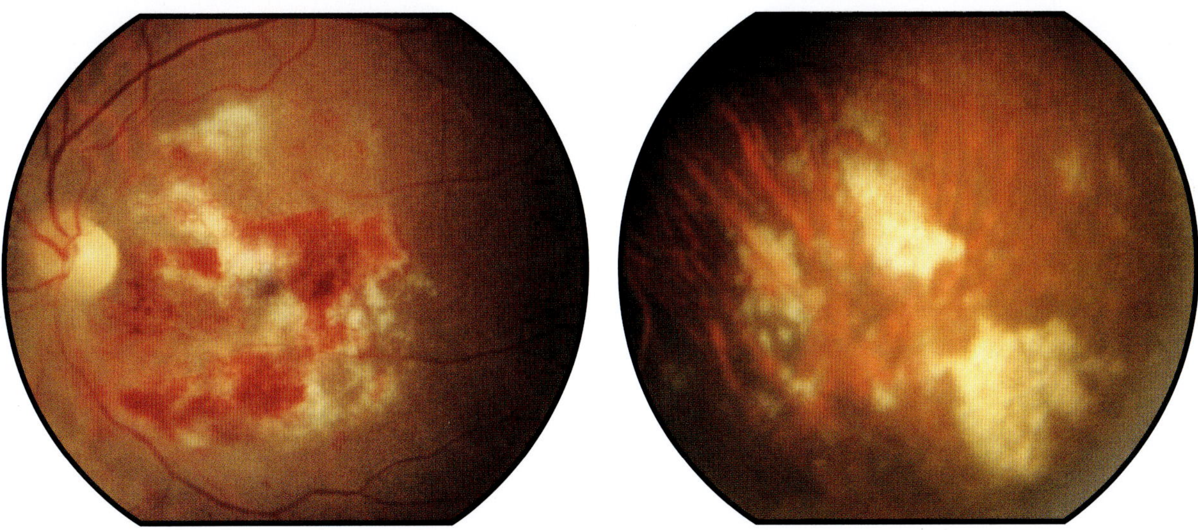

Note the presence of macular CMV retinitis in the left color fundus photograph. The right photograph demonstrates active patches of peripheral retinitis in a different patient.

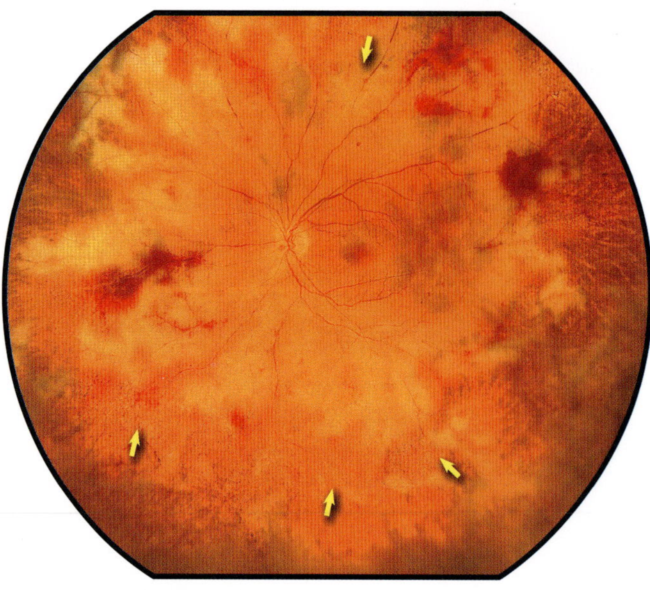

This patient has active CMV retinitis with diffuse perivascular necrosis of the peripheral retina. There are patchy hemorrhages bordering the infected tissue. There is also peripheral retinal atrophy, consistent with healing in areas with previously active infection *(arrows)*.

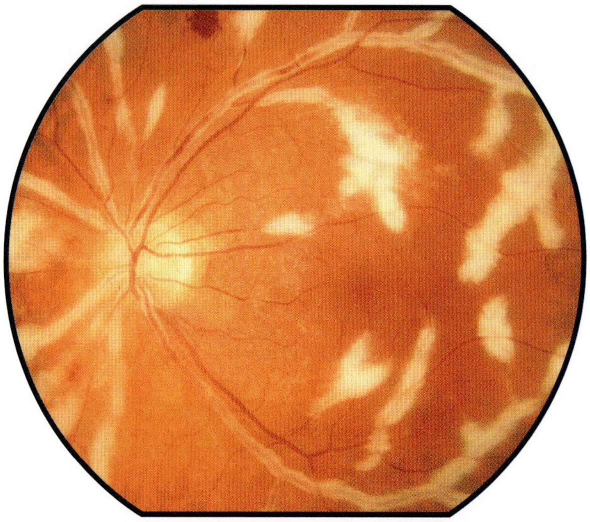

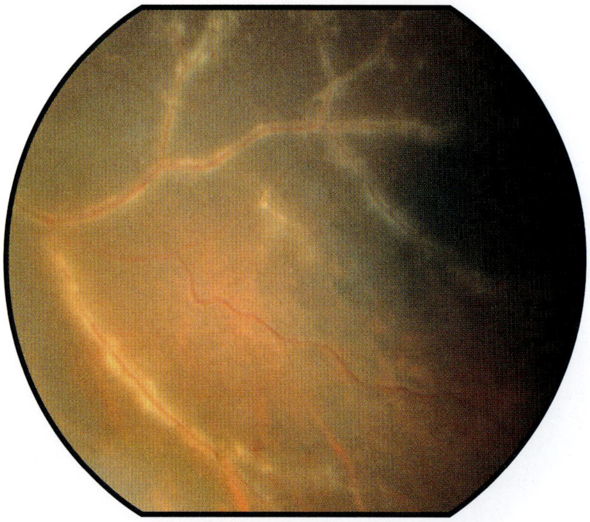

These two patients have frosted branch angiitis secondary to CMV infection. *Upper image courtesy of Michael P. Kelly and Dr. Everett Ai*

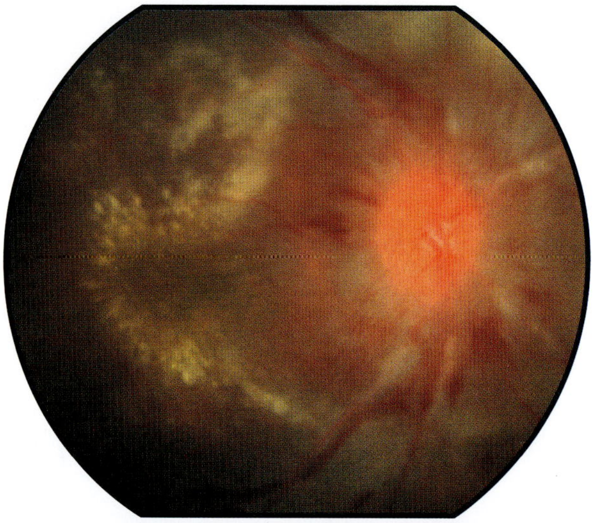

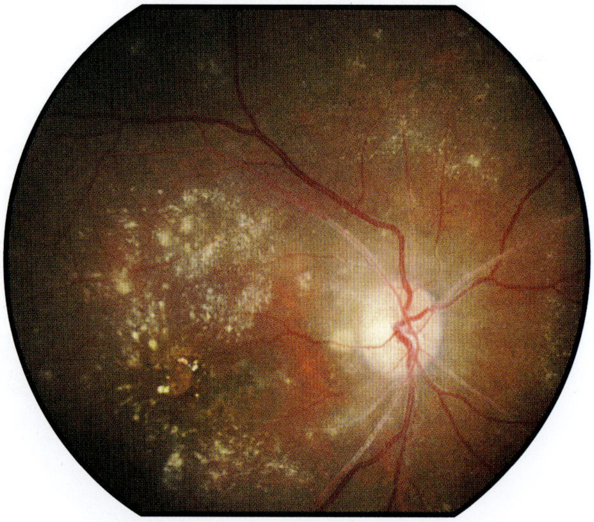

This patient has CMV retinitis and papillitis. Following antiviral medication, there is resolution of the infection, but note the presence of optic atrophy and sheathed retinal vessels and persistent macular exudates. *Courtesy of Dr. Richard Spaide*

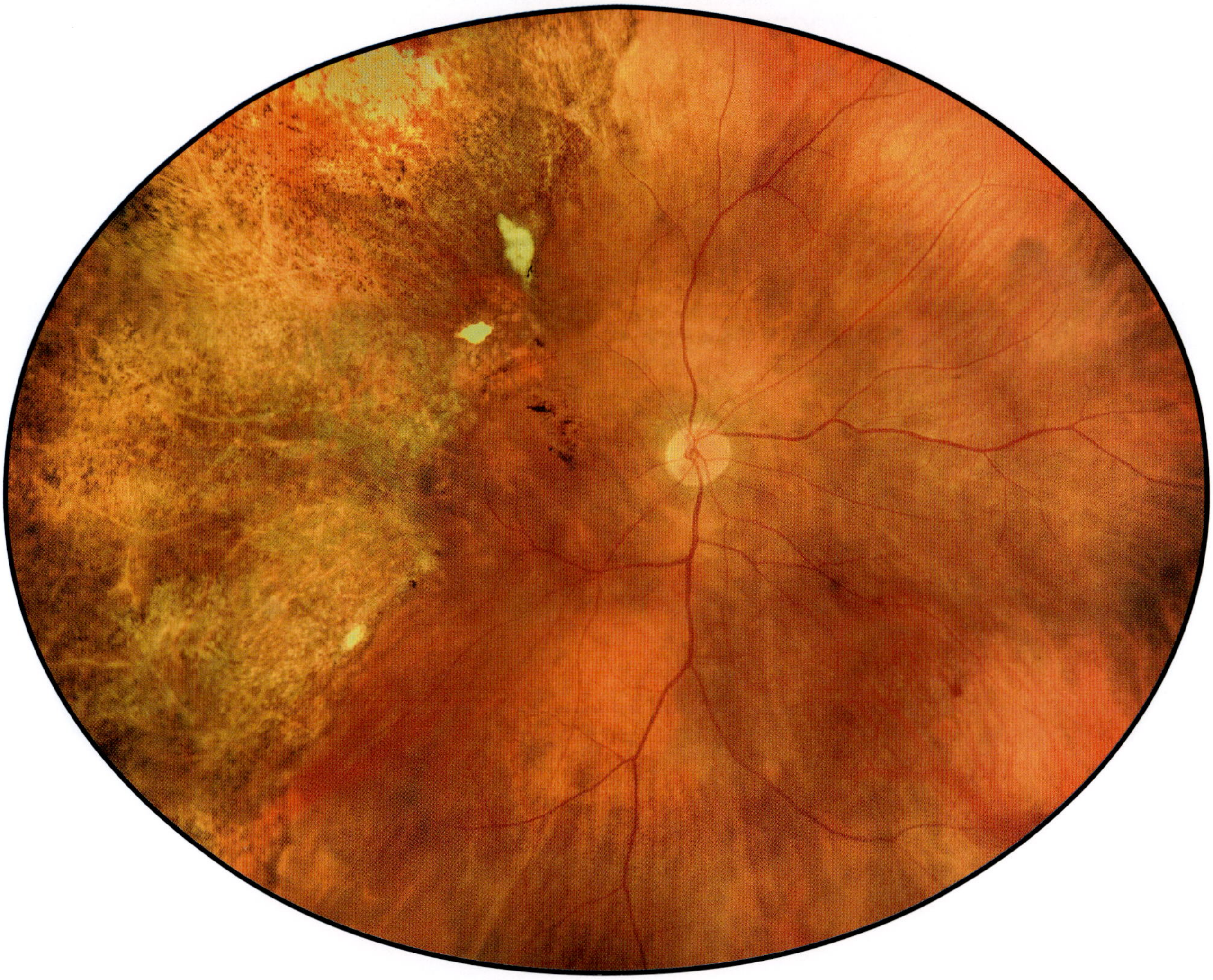

This montage demonstrates a well-demarcated zone of peripheral atrophy in the temporal fundus following CMV retinitis.

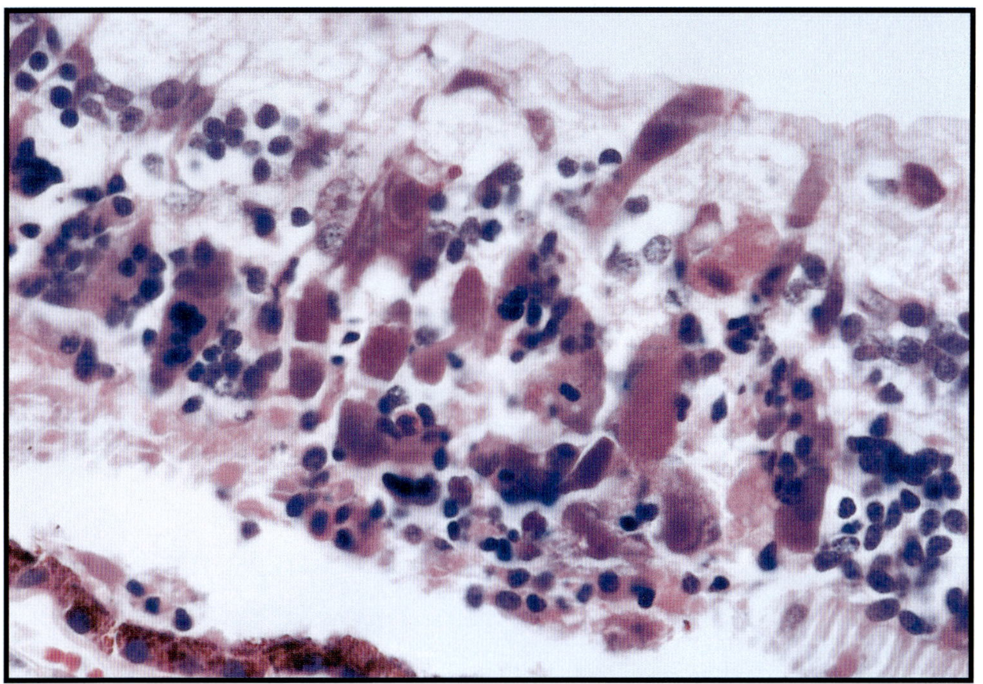

Light microscopy of a case of acute necrotizing retinitis due to CMV shows large cells (neurons) containing eosinophilic intranuclear and intracytoplasmic inclusions.

Acute Retinal Necrosis Syndrome

Acute retinal necrosis (ARN) syndrome can affect immunocompromised or immunocompetent patients and most typically occurs in otherwise healthy individuals. Clinical characteristics include (1) concentric areas of peripheral retinal necrosis with discrete borders; (2) relentless posterior progression of disease or development of new foci in the absence of antiviral therapy; (3) eventual macular involvement in the absence of antiviral therapy; (4) presence of an occlusive obliterative angiopathy; and (5) marked anterior and vitreal inflammation. Optic atrophy and rhegmatogenous retinal detachment due to multiple ragged round retinal tears at the border of resolved disease may complicate the course in a significant number of patients. The etiology of ARN is due to the herpes group of viruses that affect all layers of the retina. Herpes simplex virus type 1 and 2 (HSV-1, HSV-2) and varicella zoster virus (VZV) are the most common causative agents. Patients with HIV or AIDS are at risk for developing ARN following herpes zoster ophthalmicus, even after the skin lesions resolve.

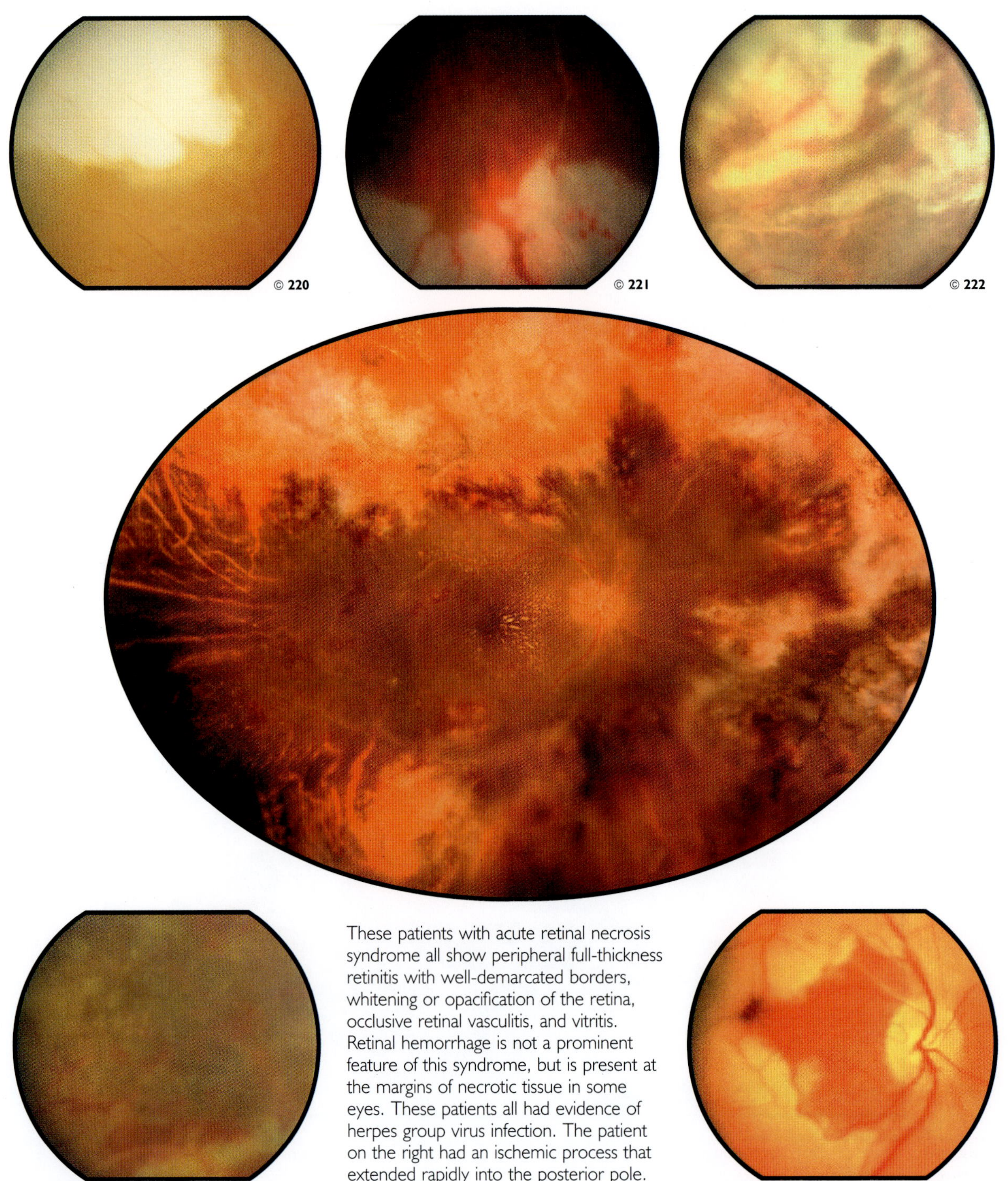

These patients with acute retinal necrosis syndrome all show peripheral full-thickness retinitis with well-demarcated borders, whitening or opacification of the retina, occlusive retinal vasculitis, and vitritis. Retinal hemorrhage is not a prominent feature of this syndrome, but is present at the margins of necrotic tissue in some eyes. These patients all had evidence of herpes group virus infection. The patient on the right had an ischemic process that extended rapidly into the posterior pole.

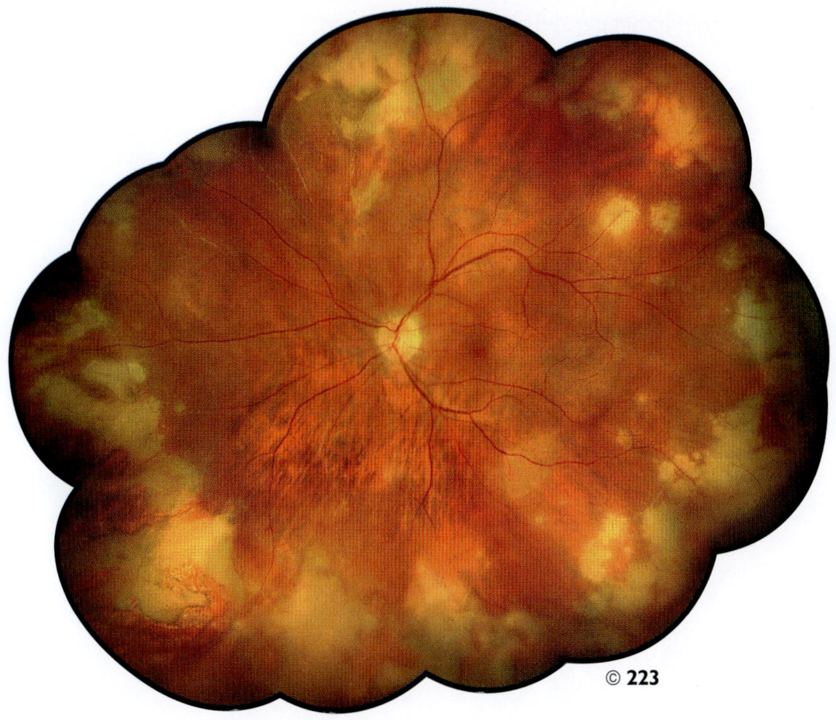

This patient has diffuse peripheral retinal necrosis in a concentric pattern with vitreous inflammation consistent with ARN. Note the absence of retinal hemorrhage that is characteristic of the lesions. The confluent yellow–white appearance with irregular scalloped posterior margins and sharp transition between involved and non-involved portions of the retina is typical. *Courtesy of Dr. Alex Aizman*

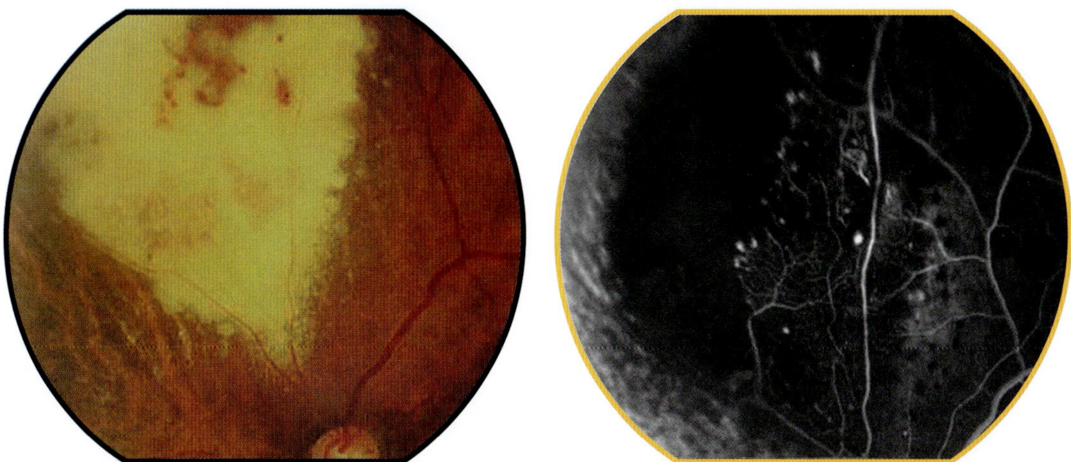

This patient with ARN shows necrotizing retinitis with obliterative angiopathy in the area of retinal infection. FA shows retinal ischemia associated with this necrotizing obliterative angiopathy. *Courtesy of Dr. Tatiana Forofonova*

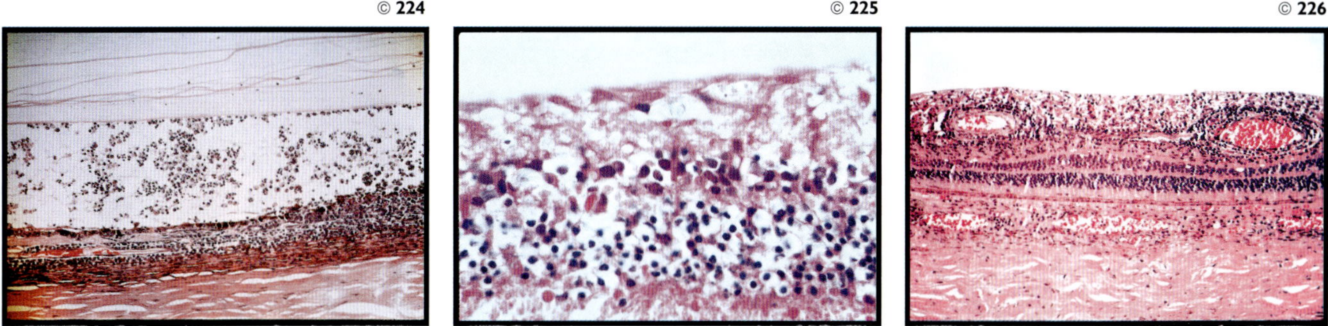

These patients with the ARN syndrome demonstrate eosinophilic intranuclear inclusions *(left and middle image)*. Inflammatory cells can be seen around retinal vessels *(right image)* and are predominantly mononuclear cells. Zones of retinal pigment epithelium (RPE) proliferation and migration underlying thin, necrotic retina are also evident.

Acute Retinal Necrosis Syndrome: Herpes Simplex Type 1

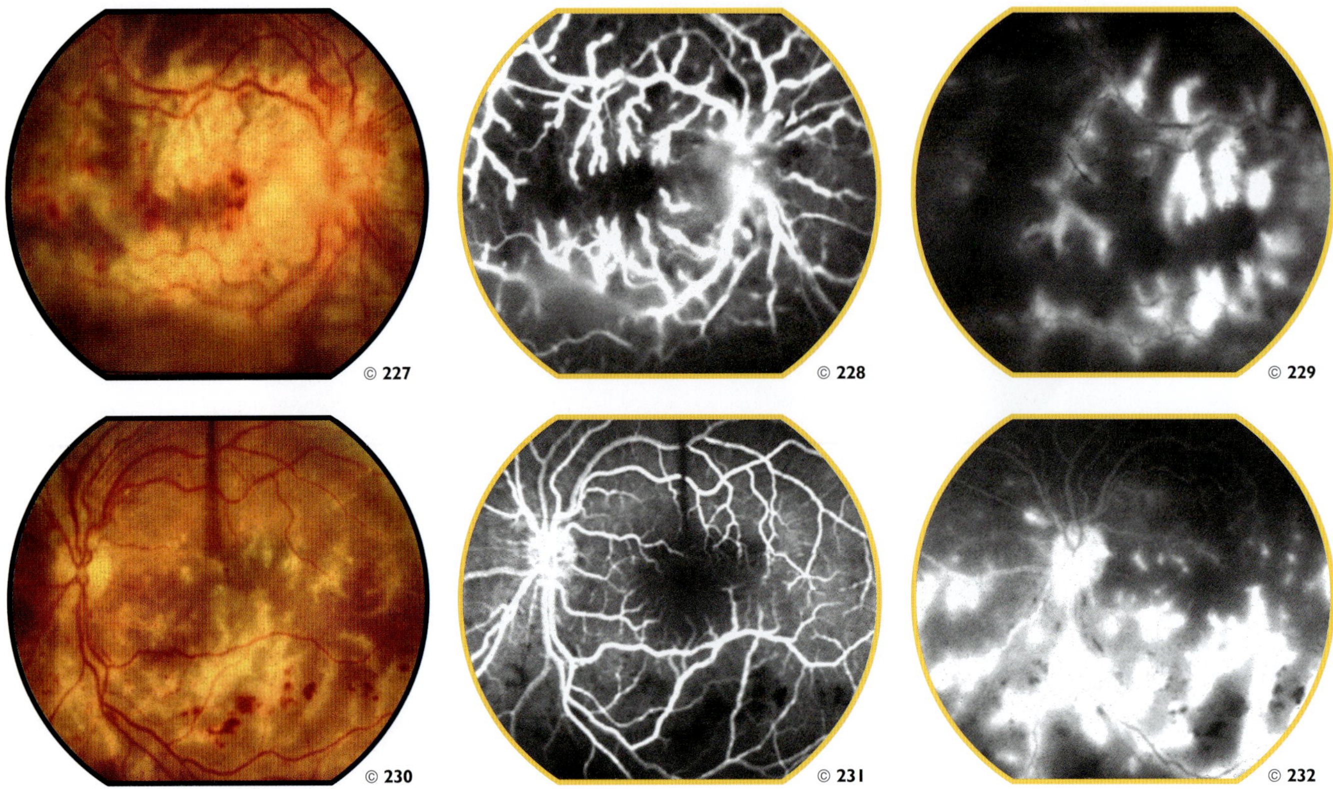

In the ARN syndrome secondary to herpes virus, there are some characteristic, but not pathognomonic changes seen with herpes simplex type 1 versus type 2. In this patient with bilateral ARN due to herpes simplex type 1, there is predominantly a retinitis characterized by inflammatory changes (frosted branch angiitis) around infected vessels.

Acute Retinal Necrosis Syndrome: Herpes Simplex Type 2

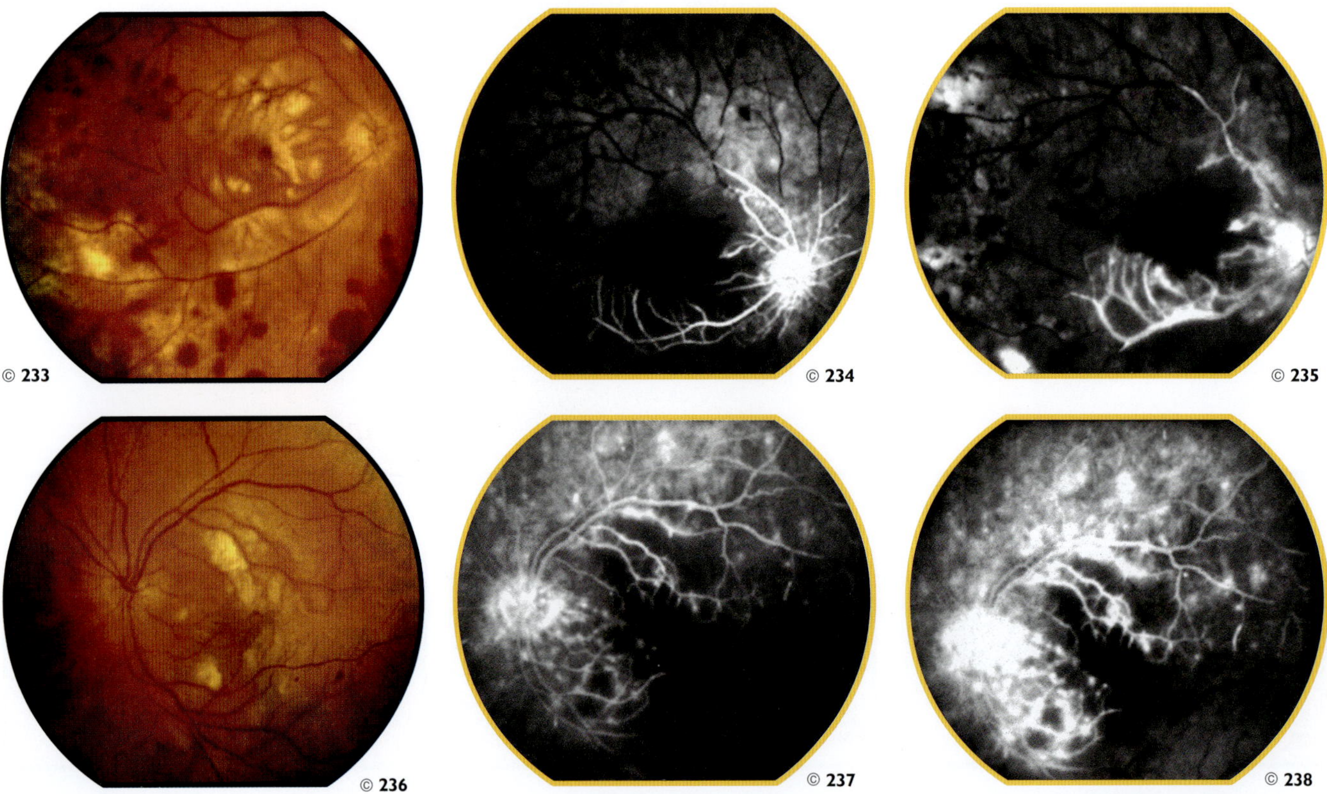

In this patient with bilateral ARN due to herpes simplex type 2 infection, the predominant characteristic is that of ischemia or an obliterative necrotizing vasculitis.

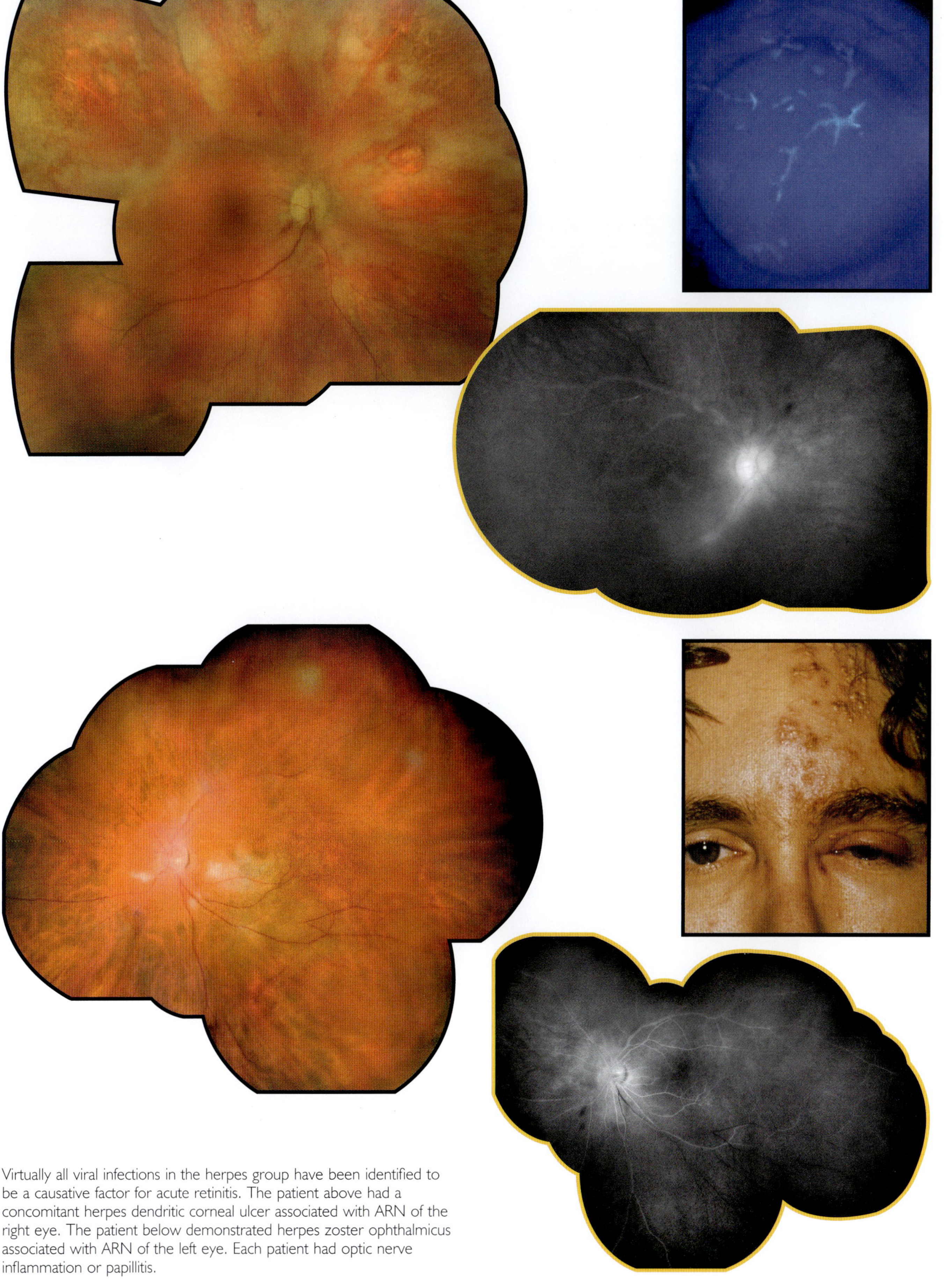

Virtually all viral infections in the herpes group have been identified to be a causative factor for acute retinitis. The patient above had a concomitant herpes dendritic corneal ulcer associated with ARN of the right eye. The patient below demonstrated herpes zoster ophthalmicus associated with ARN of the left eye. Each patient had optic nerve inflammation or papillitis.

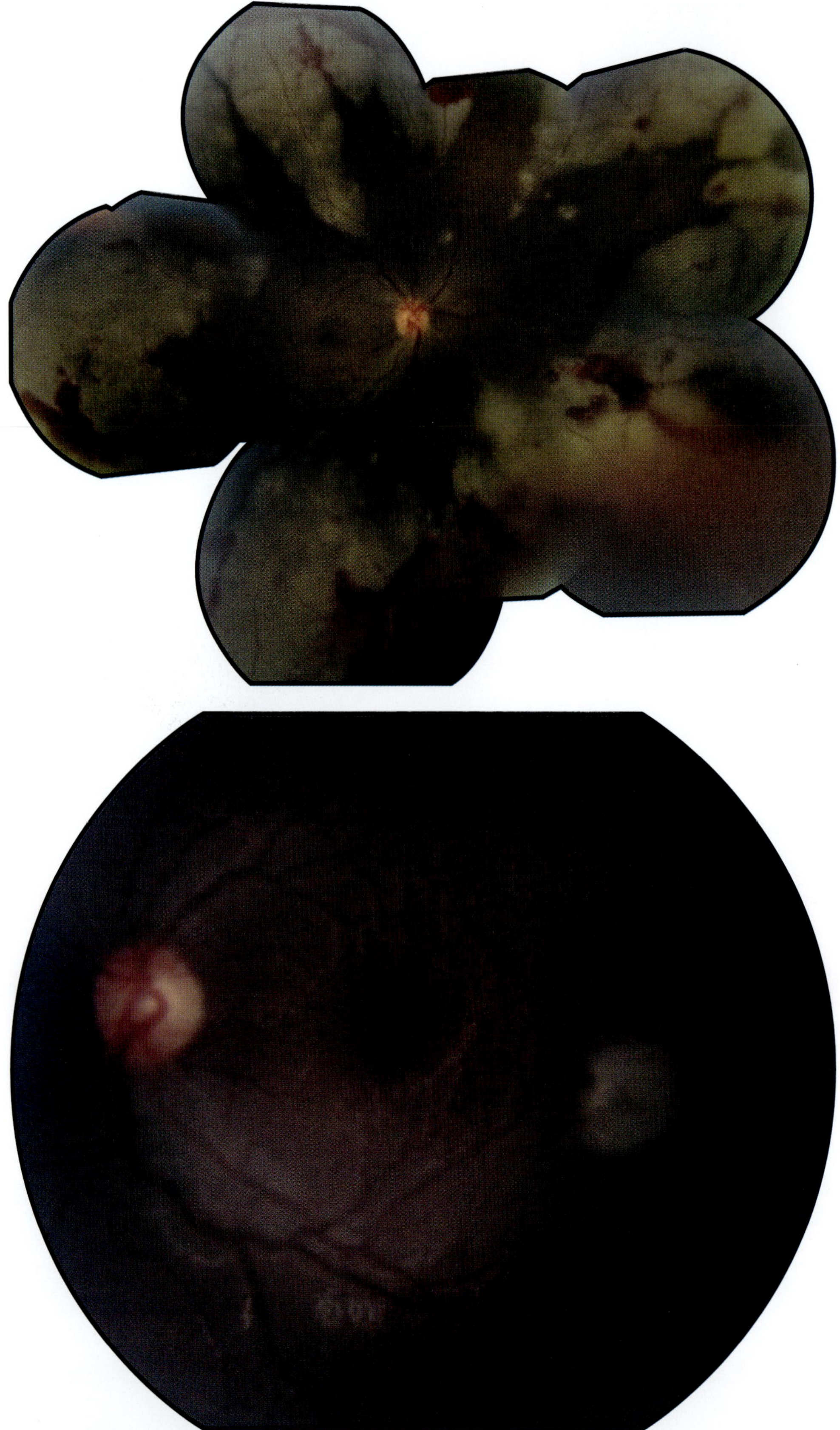

This immunosuppressed patient with hypogammaglobulinemia developed bilateral ARN soon after administration of the Varivax vaccine and while being treated with multiple immunosuppressant therapies. Note the peripheral full-thickness retinal necrosis with retinal hemorrhages in the right eye and focal necrosis in the temporal macula of the left eye. The vaccine strain of herpes zoster was isolated through PCR of a vitreous sample. *Courtesy of Dr. Ashleigh Levinson*

Progressive Outer Retinal Necrosis

Progressive outer retinal necrosis (PORN) is a severe variant of a necrotizing herpetic retinopathy in profoundly immunocompromised patients with CD4 counts less than 5/mm^3. It is believed to be the second most frequent opportunistic retinal infection after CMV retinitis in patients with AIDS. Clinical laboratory evidence suggests that the varicella zoster virus is the causal agent. Early clinical manifestations include patchy deep retinal lesions in the posterior pole and peripheral fundus, unlike ARN, which is typically peripheral in the early stages of disease. These discrete areas of retinal opacification are usually multiple and can range in size from 50 to several thousand microns in diameter. The retinitis is characterized by primary involvement of the outer retina with sparing of the inner retina until later stages of the disease process. The acute lesions progress rapidly, resulting in confluent patches of full-thickness necrosis with minimal or no aqueous or vitreal inflammation. A retinal vasculopathy is not characteristic of PORN. A perivascular lucency thought to represent early removal of necrotic debris or edema can result in a pattern of scarring that has a "cracked-mud" appearance. Optic nerve involvement, including swelling and atrophy, may occur. End-stage PORN leads to retinal detachment and blindness.

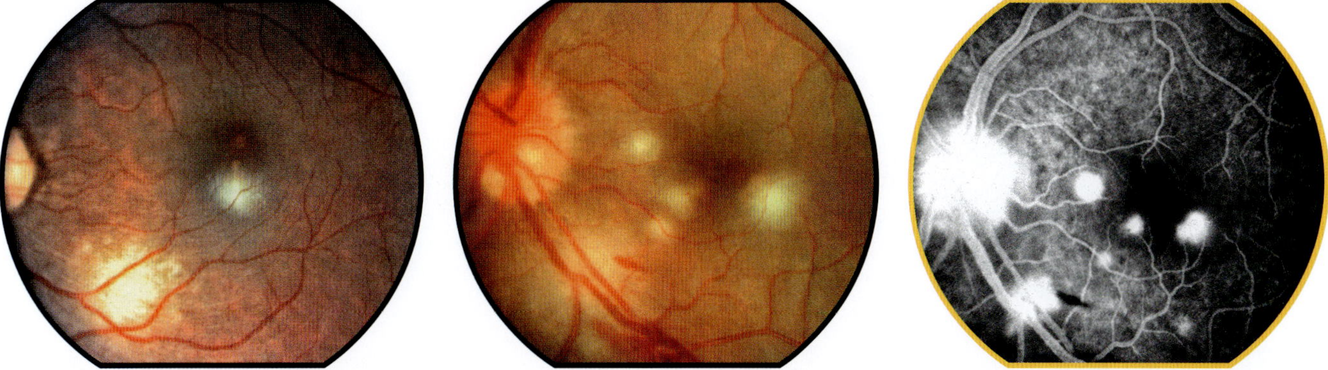

These are patients with PORN with initial focal and multifocal areas of outer retinitis involving the macula. There is leakage seen with FA.

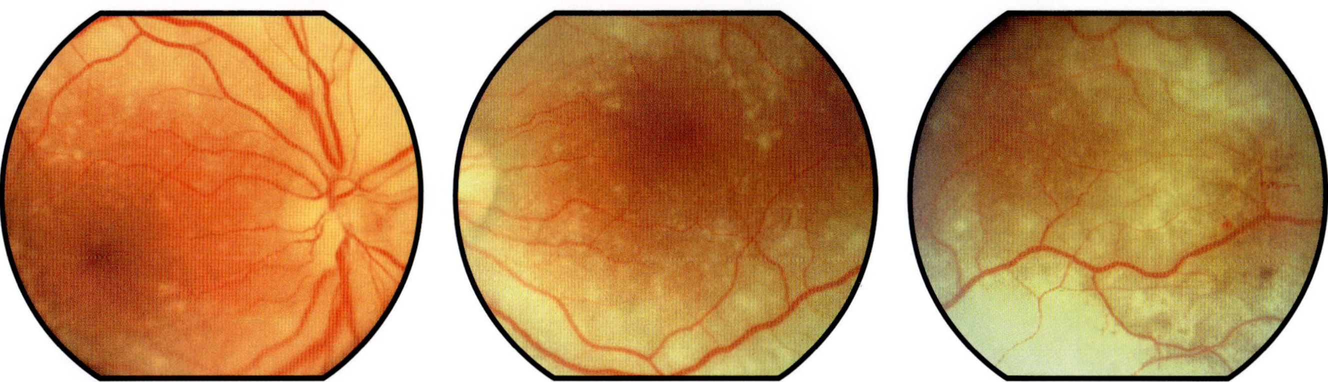

This patient with PORN demonstrates progressive confluency of the outer retinal necrosis. The retinal vessels are seen to be anterior to the outer retinal infection. *Left image courtesy of Dr. Richard Spaide*

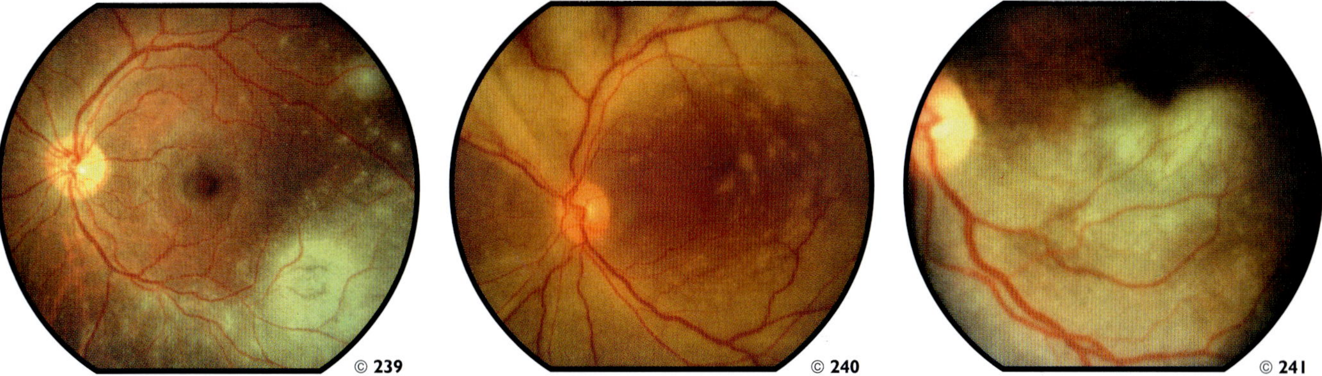

More widespread and diffuse infection is seen as the initial lesion becomes dense and confluent and, in some areas, involves full-thickness retina as in these patients with PORN.

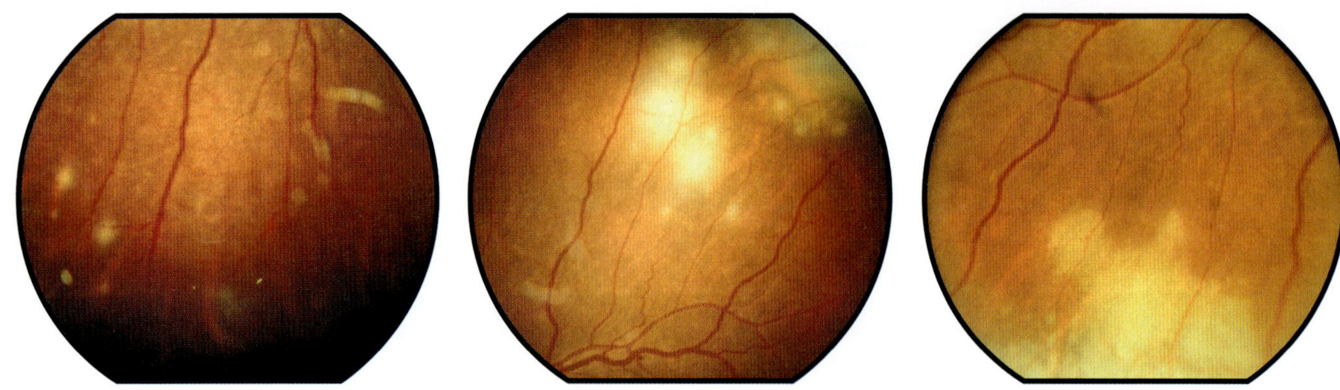

Variable manifestations of multifocal areas of infection with progression in the outer retina are seen in these patients with PORN.

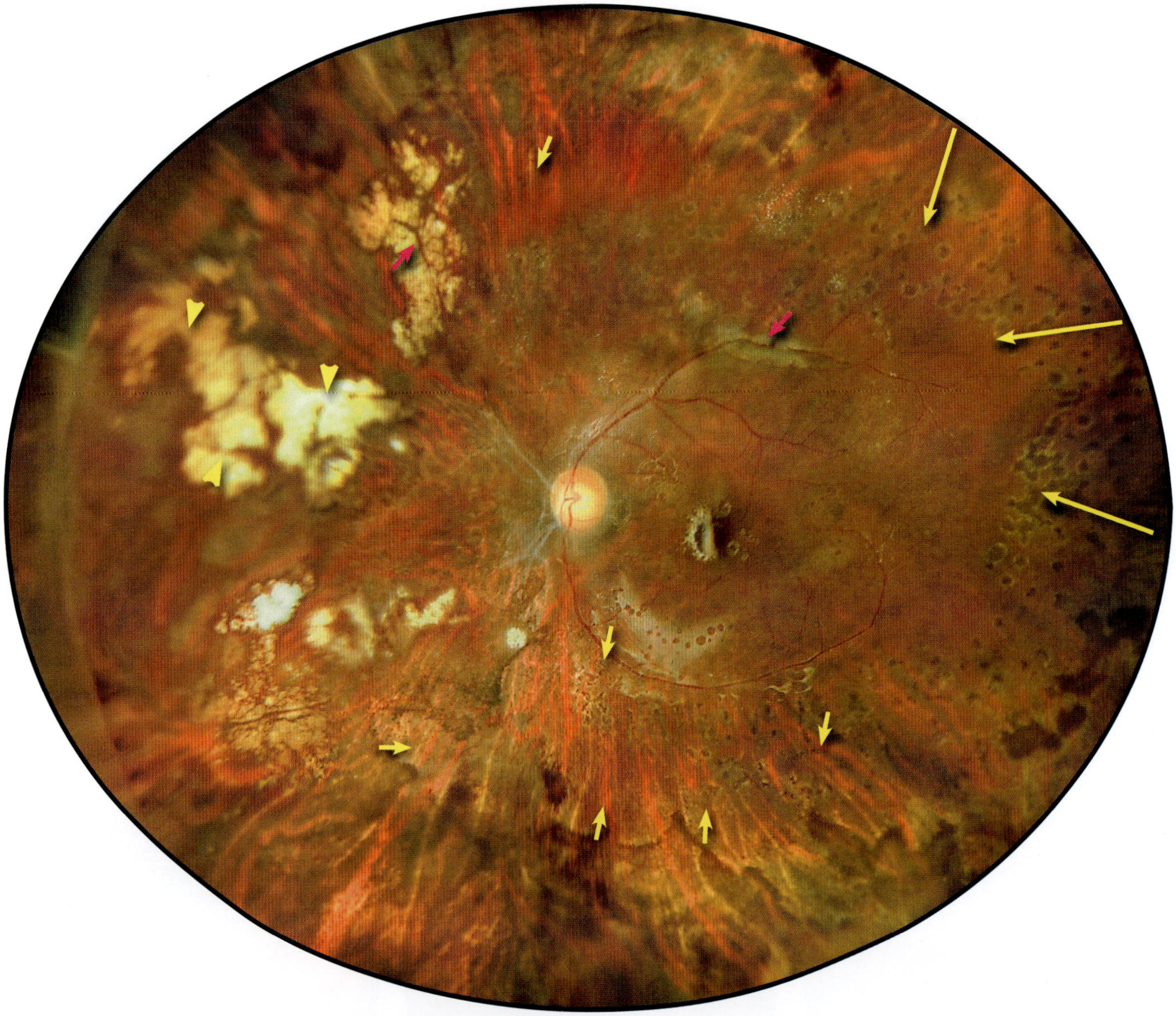

This montage shows a myriad of changes in PORN. First, there are zonal areas of outer retinal and pigment epithelial atrophy in regions of antecedent acute infection *(short arrows)*. Acute infection is also seen elsewhere, particularly in the nasal quadrant *(arrowheads)*. This patient has also been treated with laser photocoagulation in the temporal and superotemporal periphery *(long arrows)*. Marked ischemic changes and sheathing are also noted in the retinal vasculature, particularly in the nasal juxtapapillary region. A "cracked-mud" appearance is seen surrounding some vessels *(pink arrows)*. Presumably this lucency around the vessels is due to resolving necrotic debris or edema.

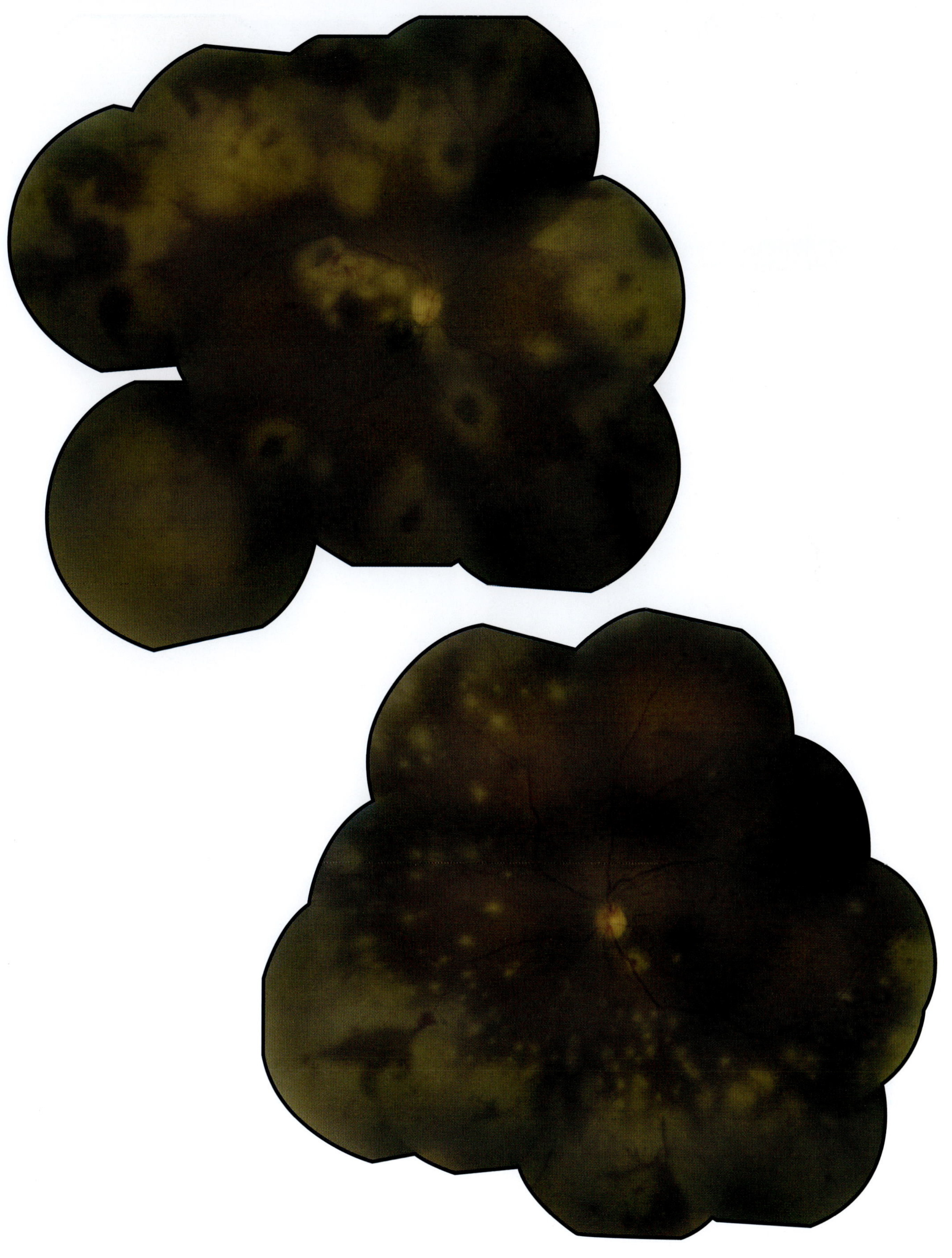

This patient developed bilateral PORN from VZV. Note in the color fundus photos the diffuse peripheral outer retinal whitening with scattered retinal hemorrhages.

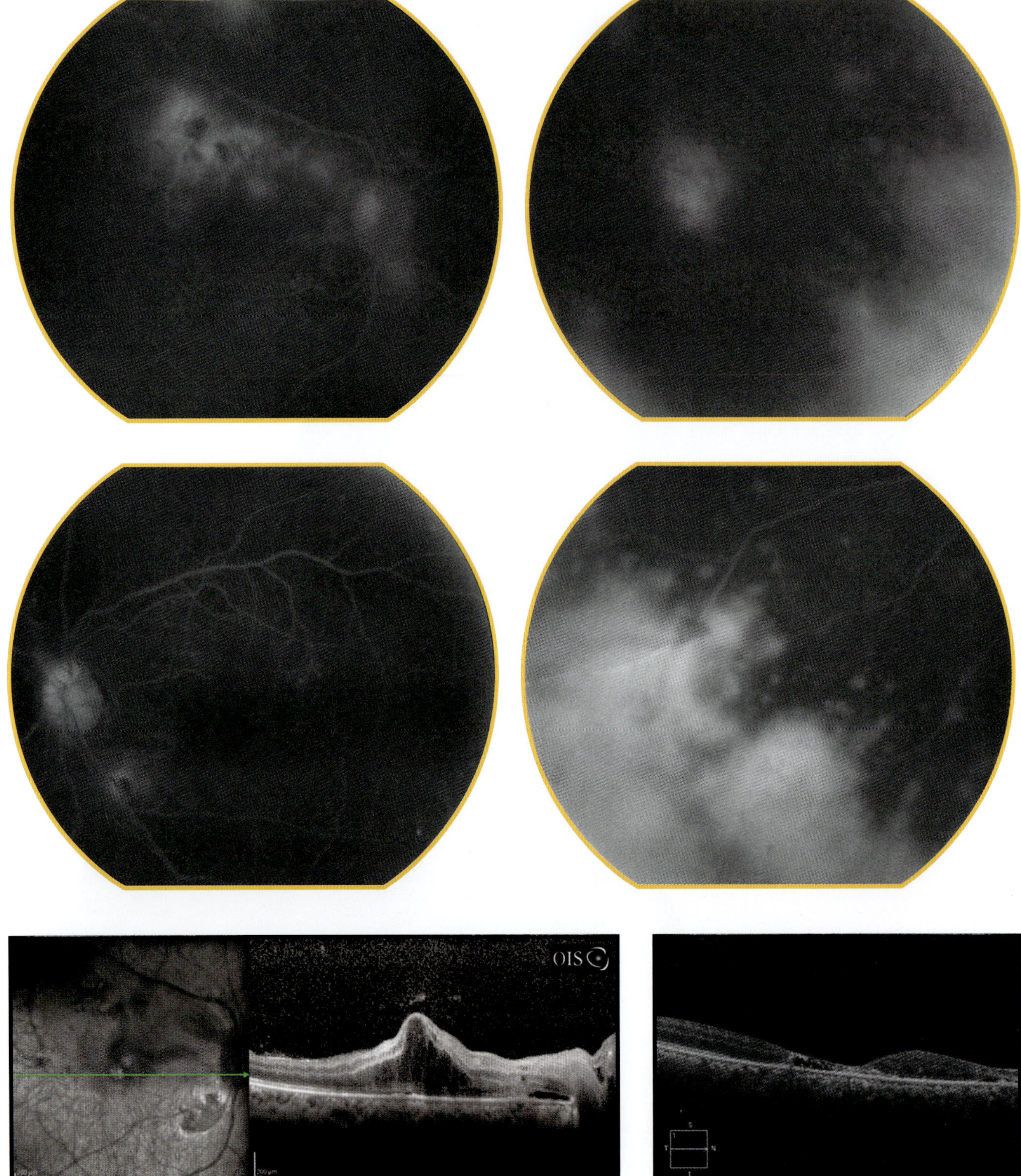

Note on the FA the leakage in the areas of confluent infection both in the macula of the right eye and in the periphery of both eyes. Spectral domain (SD)-OCT of right eye *(bottom left photo)* shows retinitis and cystoid macular edema (CME). SD-OCT after intravenous antiviral treatment *(bottom right photo)* for VZV (patient was PCR positive) shows diffuse retinal atrophy and cavitation with resolution of CME and retinitis. *Courtesy of Dr. Purnima Patel*

Epstein–Barr Virus Retinitis

The Epstein–Barr virus (EBV) may very rarely cause a retinitis that produces whitening of the retina with patterns that have indistinct margins and very minimal hemorrhage and inflammation.

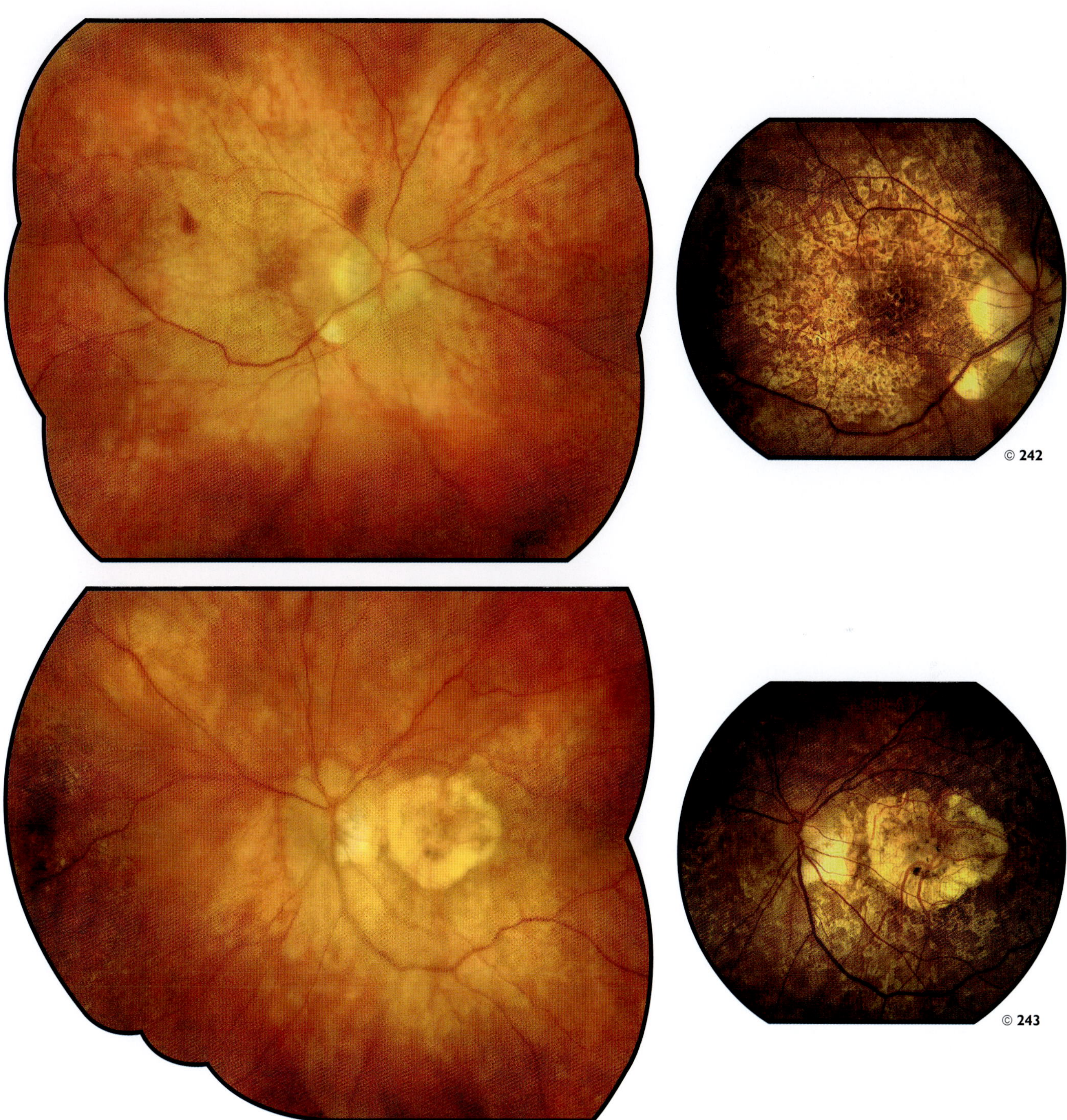

This patient presented with a diffuse retinitis in the posterior pole and periphery of both eyes due to presumed EBV infection (*left images*). After resolution diffuse atrophy and pigment mottling are shown in the posterior pole and periphery of both eyes and a dense atrophic scar is noted in the macula of the left eye (*right images*). *Courtesy of Drs. Stephen Jae Kim and Daniel F. Martin*

Rubeola Virus: Subacute Sclerosing Pancencephalitis (SSPE)

Rubeola virus may very rarely cause a chronic progressive encephalitis and retinitis that affects primarily children and young adults. It is the result of a persistent infection of immune-resistant measles virus (rubeola). A variety of central nervous system (CNS) abnormalities are associated with this infection, and there may be ocular manifestations that can lead to blindness.

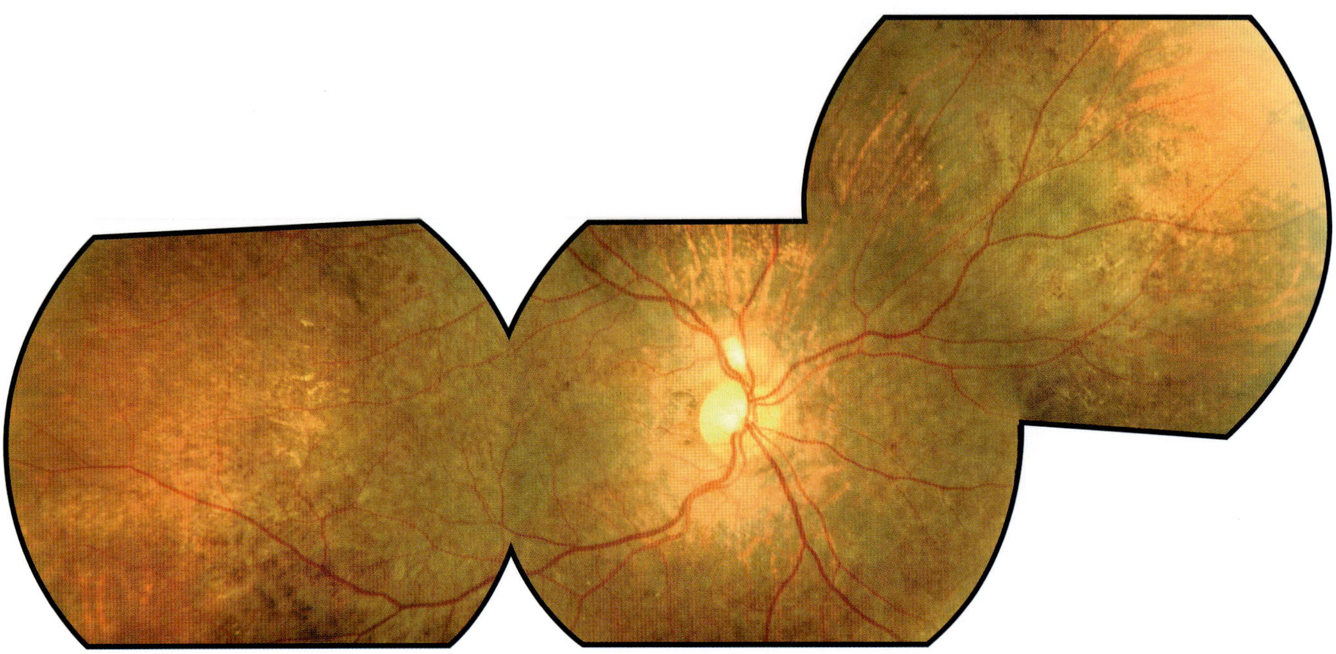

This patient has diffuse atrophy and mottling of the retinal pigment epithelium (RPE) due to SSPE, which was relentlessly progressive.

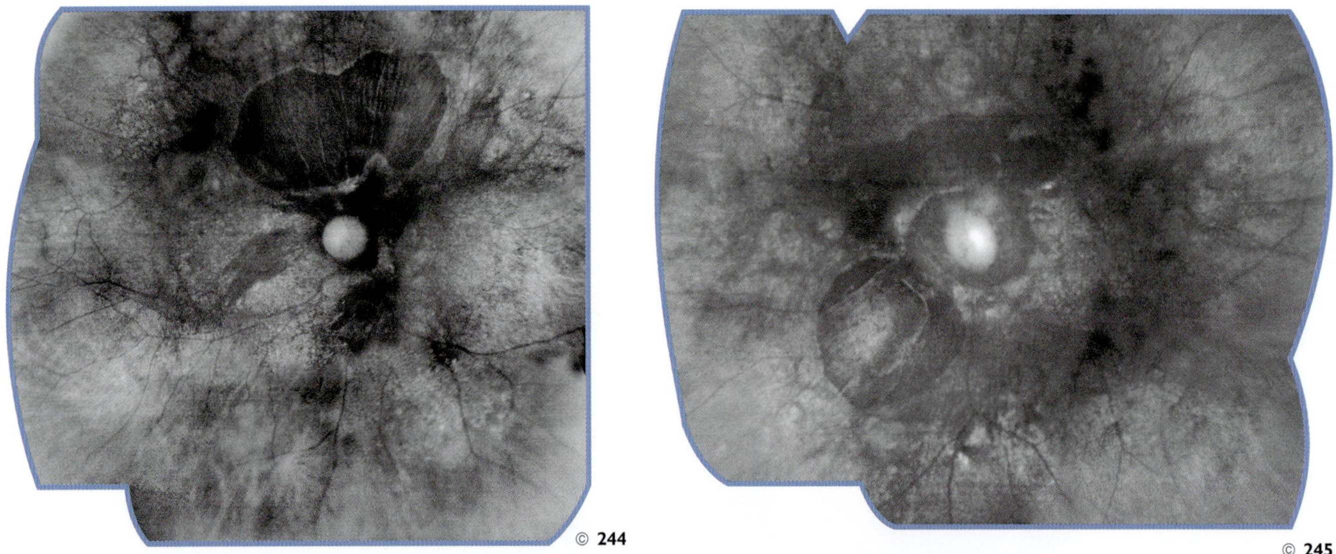

This patient with SSPE experienced a relentless retinitis that left a diffuse pattern of chorioretinal degeneration illustrated with widefield fundus autofluorescence. Large patches of chorioretinal atrophy are seen in both eyes.

Congenital Rubella Syndrome

The congenital rubella syndrome, caused by the rubella virus, may be associated with microphthalmos, congenital cataracts, iris abnormalities, and coloboma formation of various ocular structures. Children born to mothers who contracted rubella in the first trimester of pregnancy are at high risk of deafness and pigmentary retinopathy that consists of patchy RPE atrophy and pigment epithelial mottling and hyperplasia referred to as "salt and pepper" retinopathy. Active ocular inflammation and/or retinitis are not appreciated with this syndrome. In later life, such patients are subject to choroidal neovascularization and disciform scarring of the macula.

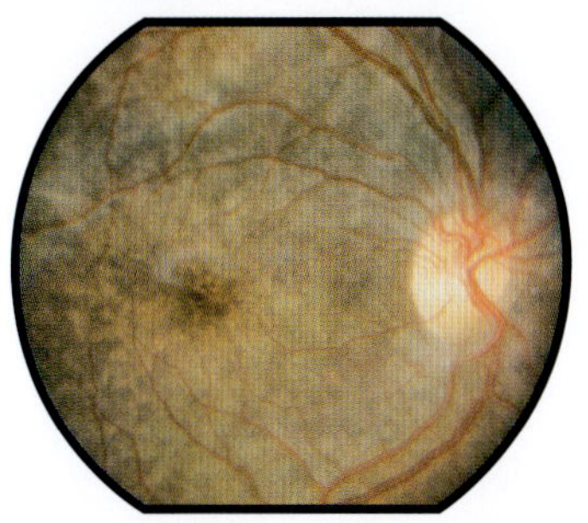

This patient has congenital rubella retinopathy demonstrating patchy RPE atrophy and pigment epithelial mottling and hyperplasia throughout the fundus.

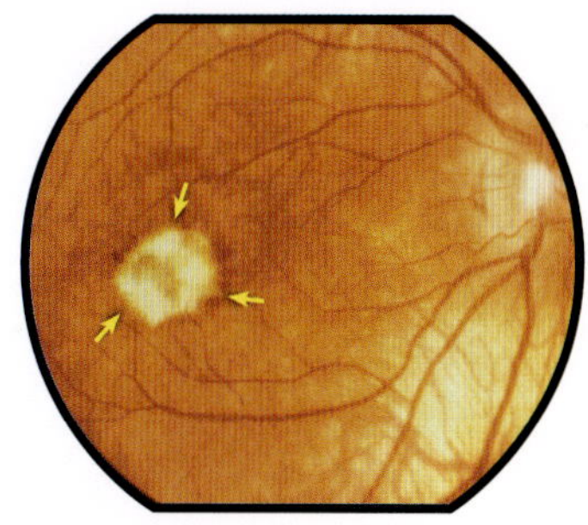

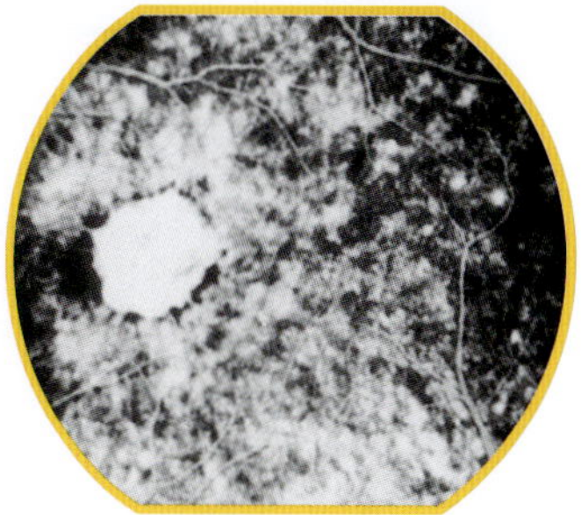

This patient developed secondary choroidal neovascularization in the central macula. The vascular proliferation has evolved to a fibrous disciform scar *(left, arrows)* that stains on the FA.

Coxsackievirus

Acute Retinal Pigment Epitheliitis

Coxsackievirus may be the etiology of infectious diseases of the retina and pigment epithelium with predilection for the central macula. A multifocal perifoveal reaction associated with pigment epithelial changes and macular edema, as well as a papillitis, is a very rare clinical presentation associated with this virus. A more typical association is the acute idiopathic maculopathy (AIM) syndrome, wherein there is increasing evidence of coxsackievirus as an etiological agent.

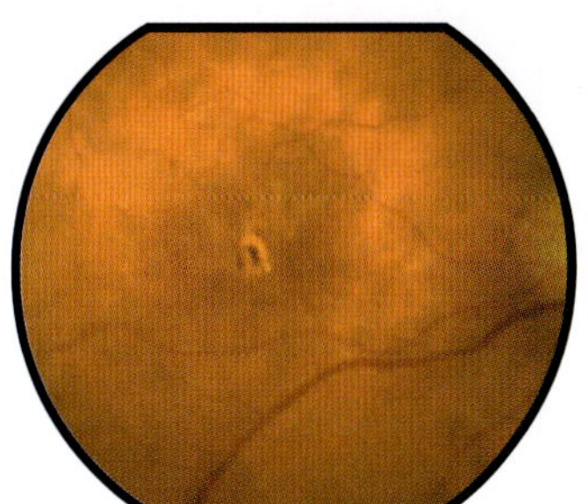

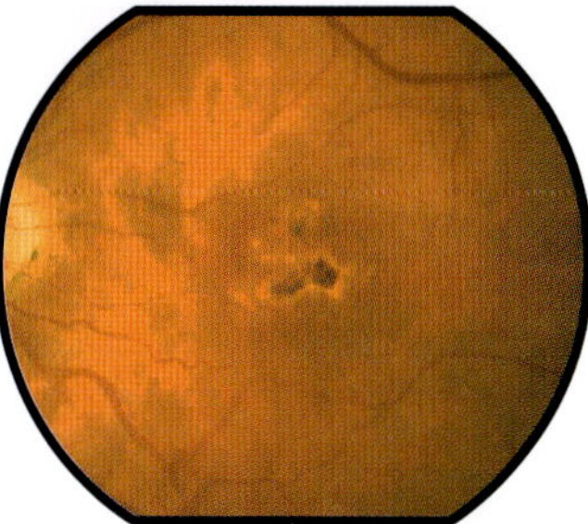

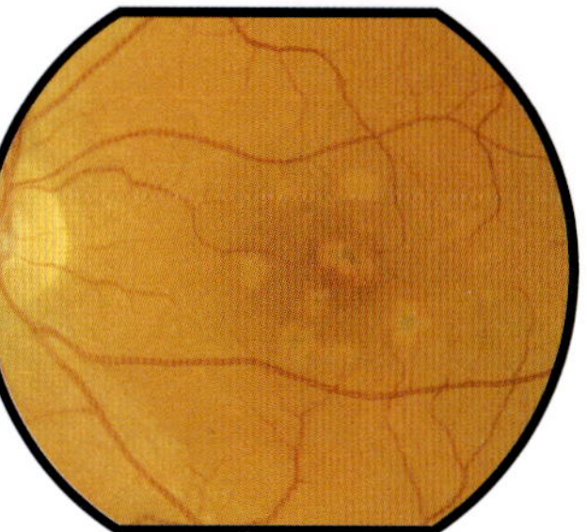

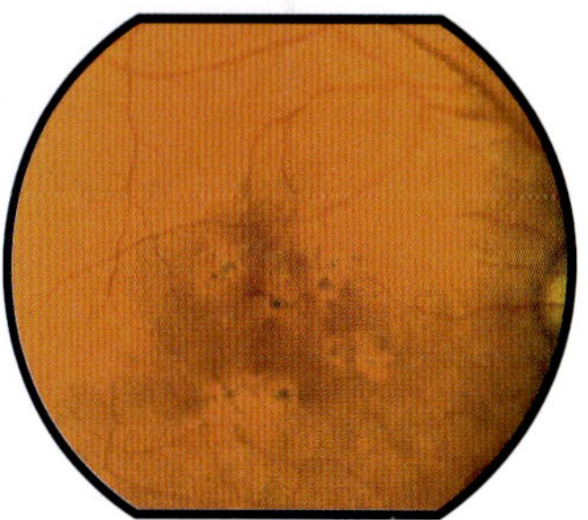

Coxsackievirus has been implicated in a perifoveal pigment epitheliitis, which is a very rare disorder, referred to as Krill disease. Note the pigmentary lesions surrounded by haloes in the macula of each eye in this patient (*left two images*) with an antecedent febrile illness and mouth ulcers (not shown). The two images on the right were unilateral cases. *Two images on left courtesy of Dr. Richard G. Gieser*

Acute Idiopathic Maculopathy

Acute idiopathic maculopathy (AIM) is a rare disorder that affects healthy young adults. Patients present with sudden central vision loss, usually in one eye. Symptoms often follow a viral prodrome, presumed to be coxsackievirus that is the etiology of hand-foot-mouth disease. During the acute phase, a neurosensory detachment overlying a grayish plaque at the level of the RPE is seen, often eccentric to the fovea, which may simulate the appearance of choroidal neovascularization. Associated intraretinal hemorrhages, few vitreous cells, and a mild papillophlebitis may be present and the FA shows rapid and severe subretinal leakage. Most cases resolve spontaneously over several weeks with near-complete recovery of vision. A lasting "bull's-eye" pigment epithelial maculopathy is typically seen following resolution of the acute lesion.

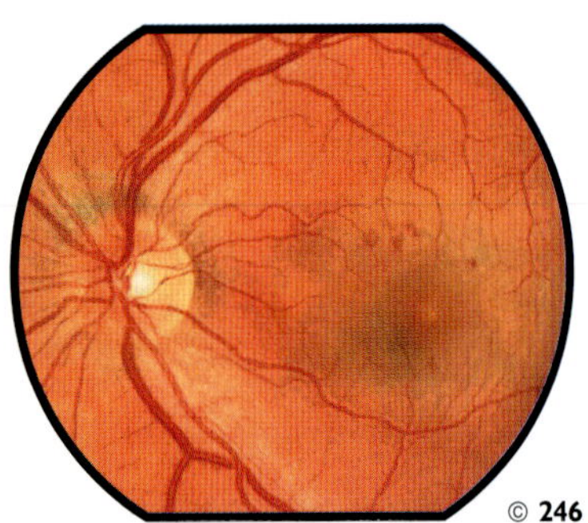

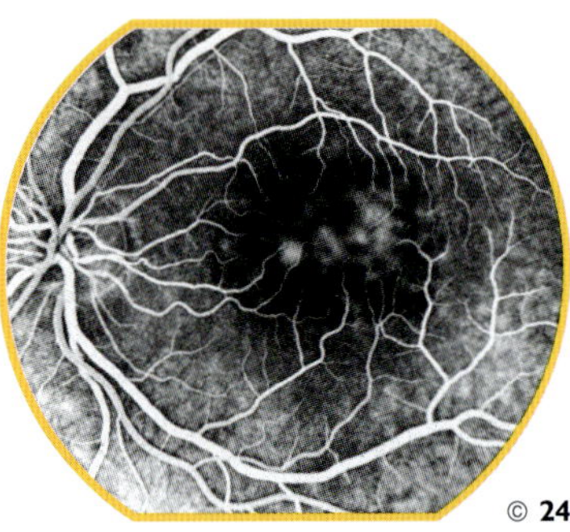

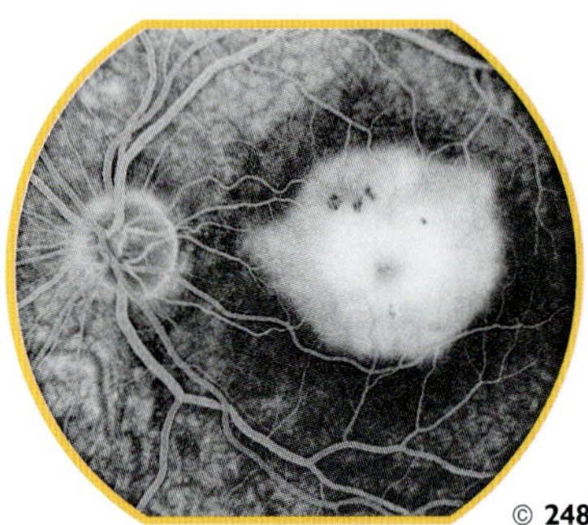

This 45-year-old man with AIM presented with a 3-day history of vision loss. Visual acuity was 20/200. An irregular exudative detachment of the neurosensory retina is noted. There is an area of intraretinal hemorrhage superior to the macula and subfoveal placoid thickening at the level of the RPE. The FA shows early blockage with rapid and severe late leakage into the neurosensory macular detachment. The lesion resolved spontaneously.

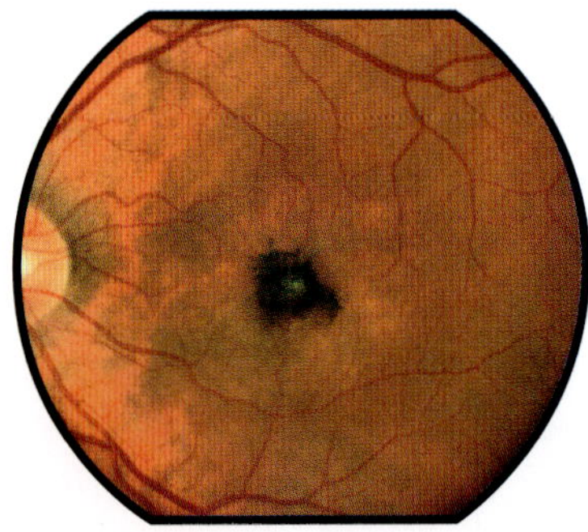

One year later, irregular pigment epithelial hyperpigmentation surrounds a central area of presumed subretinal fibrosis in the foveal region.

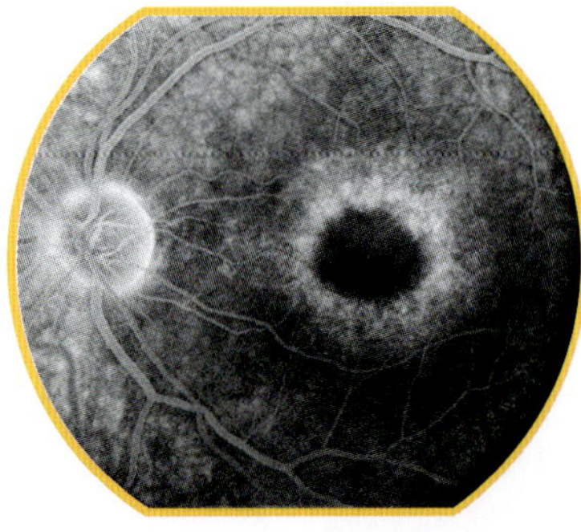

The corresponding FA of the same patient shows a concentric area of RPE atrophy consistent with a "bull's-eye" maculopathy. Visual acuity improved to 20/25.

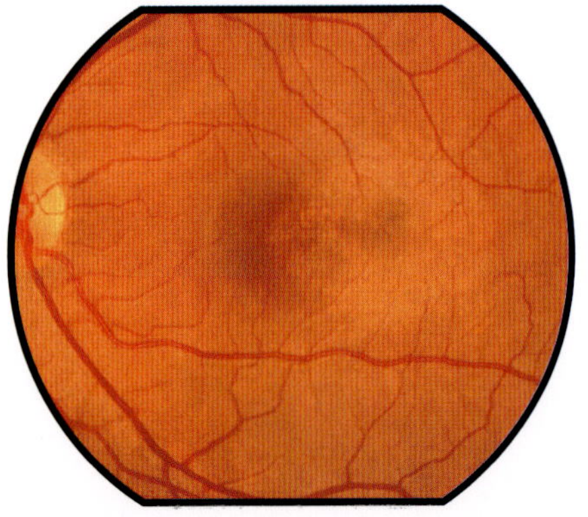

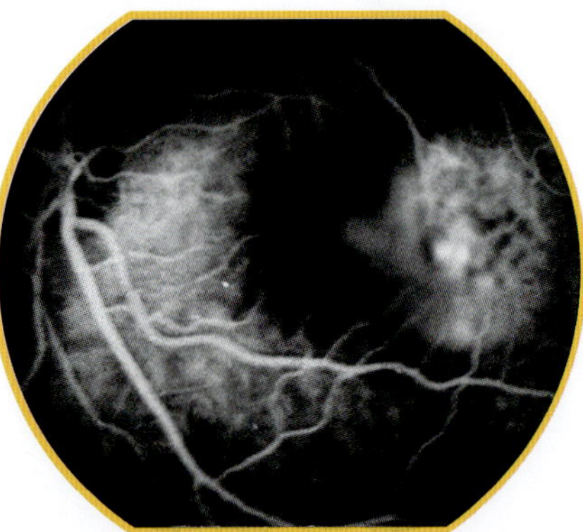

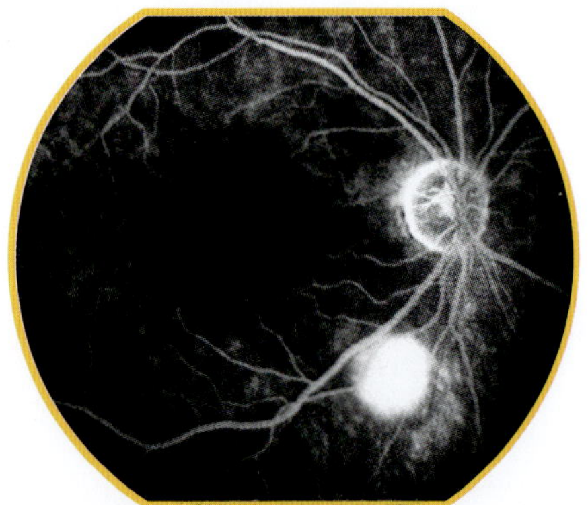

This patient with AIM has an eccentric neurosensory retinal detachment with intraretinal hemorrhages corresponding to multiple focal areas of hypofluorescence on the fluorescein angiogram within the detached area. There is also an underlying placoid area of fluorescence corresponding to flat, inflammatory change at the level of the RPE. There is significant leakage into the neurosensory detachment, which simulates choroidal neovascularization or inflammatory disease. In this patient, there was an additional AIM lesion inferior to the disc *(right image)* in the fellow eye. The patient, whose daughter was afflicted with coxsackievirus infection, experienced a similar febrile, prodromal illness prior to her visual symptoms.

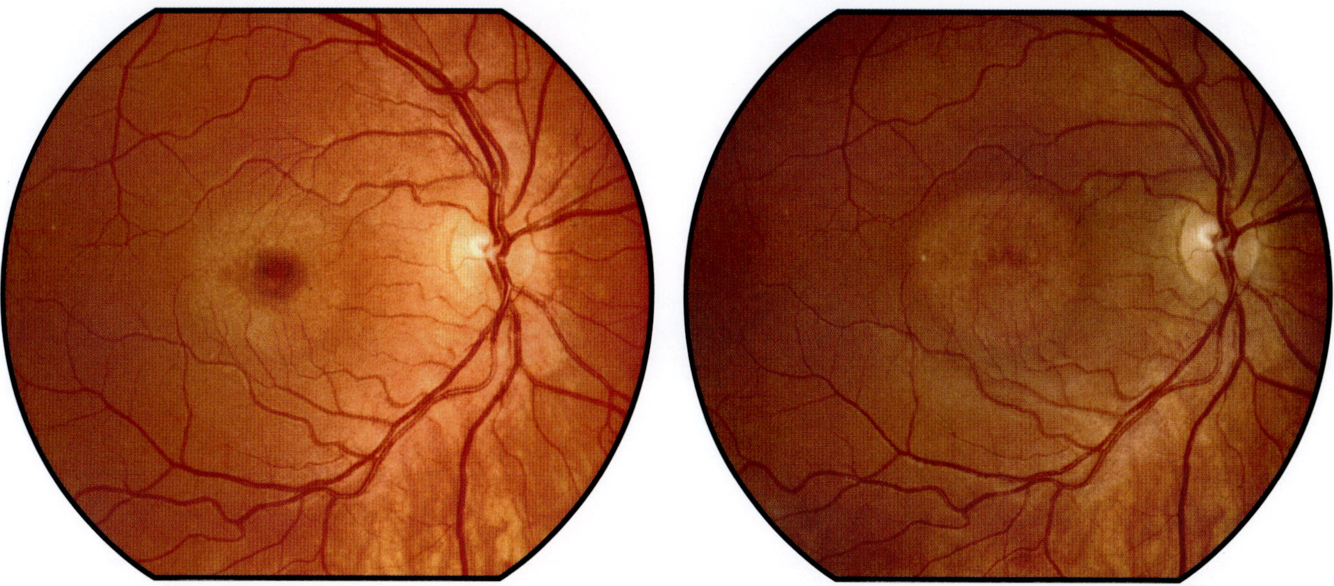

This patient with AIM presentation shows a circumscribed area of detachment of variable size and translucency. This singular manifestation in the fundus was associated with a sudden and profound decline in vision, which recovered spontaneously.

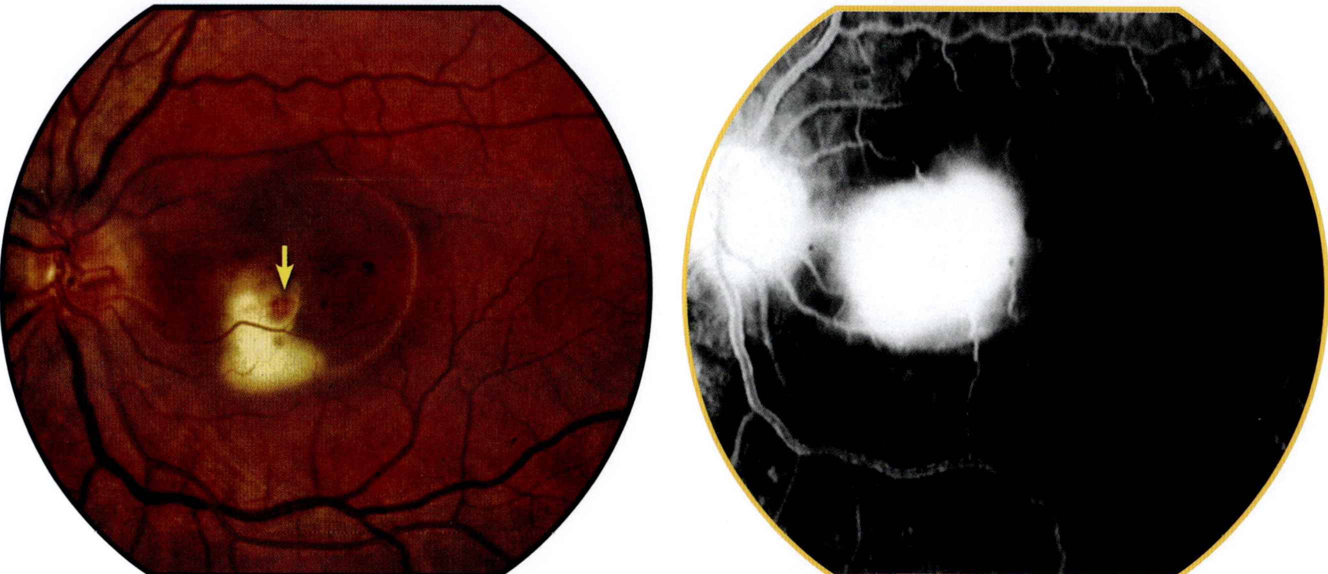

This patient had AIM with a patch of subretinal whitening beneath the neurosensory detachment. Note the associated intraretinal hemorrhage *(arrow)*. Severe subretinal leakage is seen with the FA. The optic nerve was also inflamed, exhibiting late staining on the FA, indicative of a papillitis.

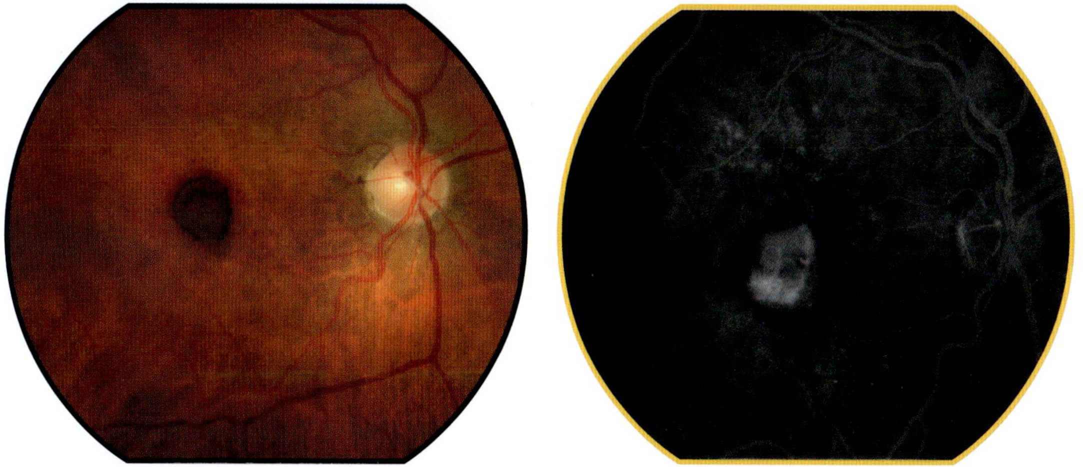

This patient had AIM and, 18 months after resolution of the acute manifestations, developed choroidal neovascularization. The neovascular lesion is bordered by a margin of subretinal hemorrhage, and demonstrates a "classic" appearance with FA (type 2 neovascularization).

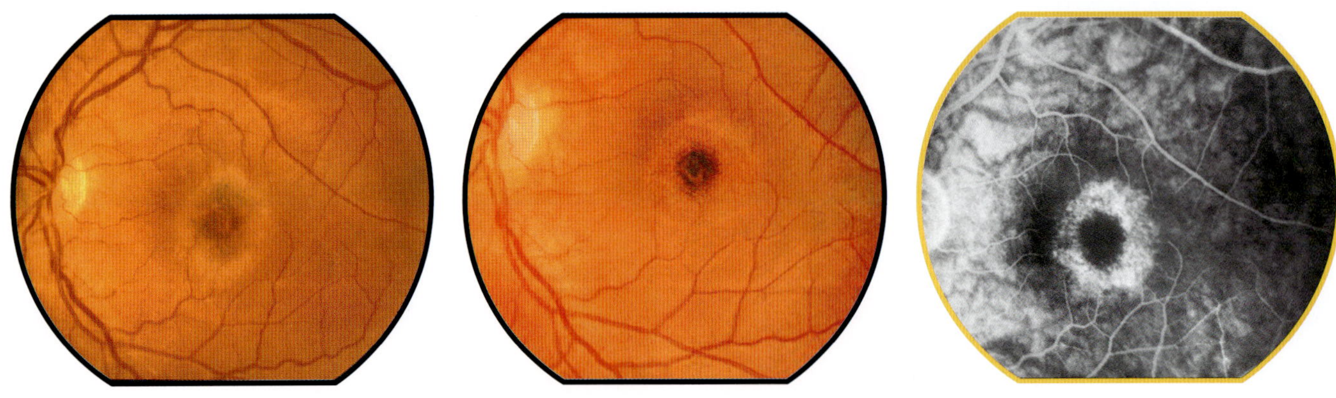

Following resolution of the acute manifestations, AIM patients commonly demonstrate a "bull's-eye" appearance to the macula. Hyperpigmentation is present at the site of the acute placoid subretinal inflammatory lesion. The concentric or "bull's-eye" pattern of atrophy corresponds to the previous macular detachment.

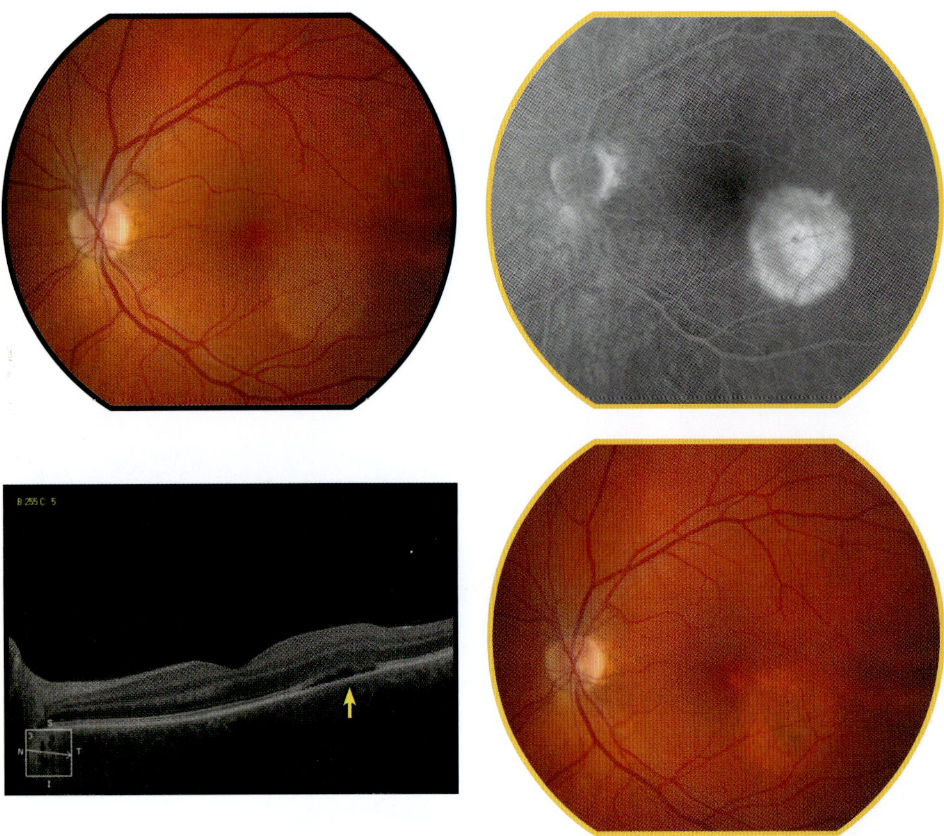

This patient with acute idiopathic maculopathy (AIM) presented with a well-demarcated yellow–white lesion with subtle punctate intraretinal heme and gray central pigment *(top left)*. The FA shows significant pooling within the neurosensory detachment. OCT of the lesion confirms the presence of subretinal fluid *(arrow)*. Eight months after initial presentation, visual acuity was stable at 20/20. The bottom right photo shows RPE hyperpigmentation and depigmentation in a "bull's-eye" pattern with resolution of hemorrhages. *Courtesy of Dr. Yannis Paulus*

Rift Valley Virus

Rift Valley fever is a viral zoonosis that primarily affects animals but also has the capacity to infect humans. The virus is a member of the *Phlebovirus* genus, and it was first identified in the Rift Valley of Kenya. It is transmitted to humans from direct or indirect contact with the blood of an infected animal or the bite of an insect, most commonly the *Aedes* mosquito. Systemic disease, including hemorrhagic fever and meningoencephalitis, may occur. When it affects the eye, there is usually retinal vascular involvement, which may include hemorrhage, vasculitis, and occlusive disease.

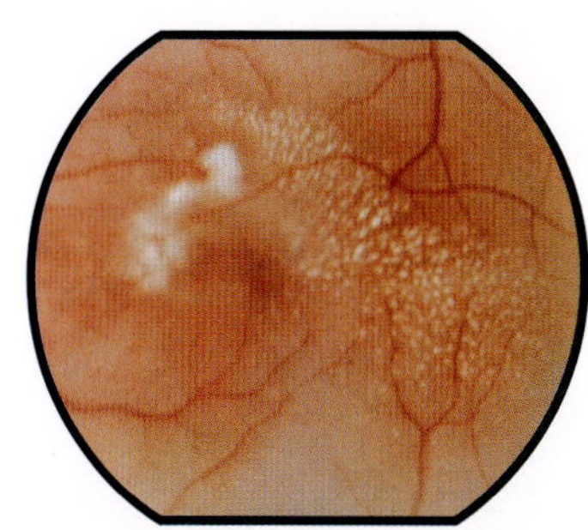

A Rift Valley infection in this patient has produced a retinitis with cotton-wool spots and lipid exudation in a macular star pattern. *Courtesy of Dr. Maurice Luntz*

West Nile Virus

West Nile virus, a member of the flavivirus family, is transmitted by a mosquito and may result in severe systemic, CNS, and ocular manifestations. In the fundus, a vitritis with scattered creamy-yellow circular or round chorioretinal lesions may develop that resembles multifocal choroiditis. As they heal, they leave atrophic areas. Linear scars are characteristic. Retinal hemorrhages and exudates may also be noted.

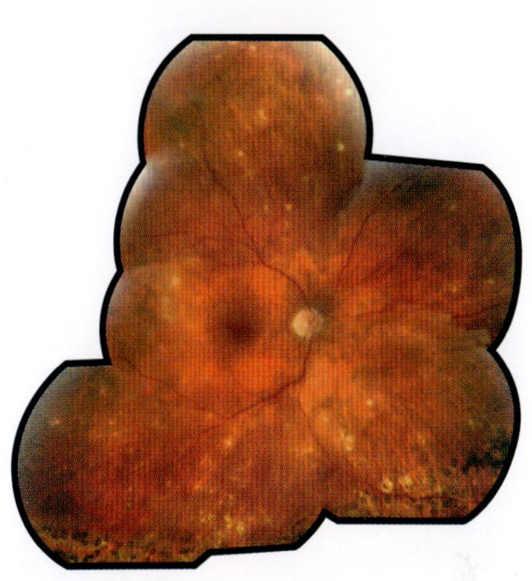

This patient with West Nile virus has diffusely scattered, punched-out multifocal chorioretinal lesions following the acute infection. *Courtesy of Dr. Nicole Hauptman-Siegel*

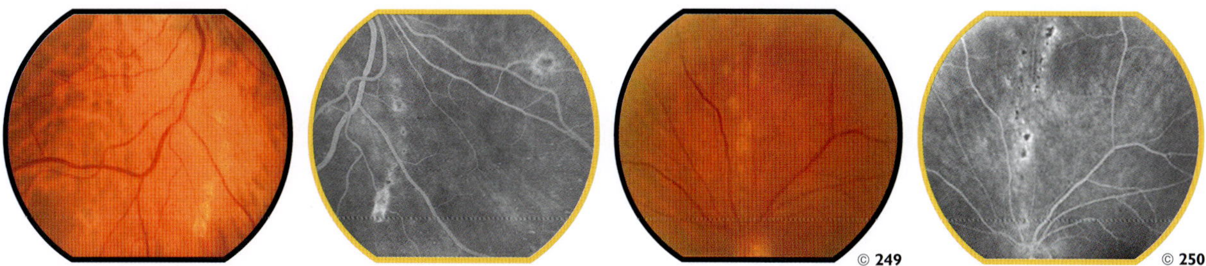

These two patients experienced a West Nile virus systemic illness. Each developed a multifocal curvilinear area of atrophic and pigmentary abnormalities that resemble a multifocal choroiditis. The lesions are actually random and do not follow what appears to be a choroidal vascular pathway. *Left two images courtesy of Dr. Ron Adelman*

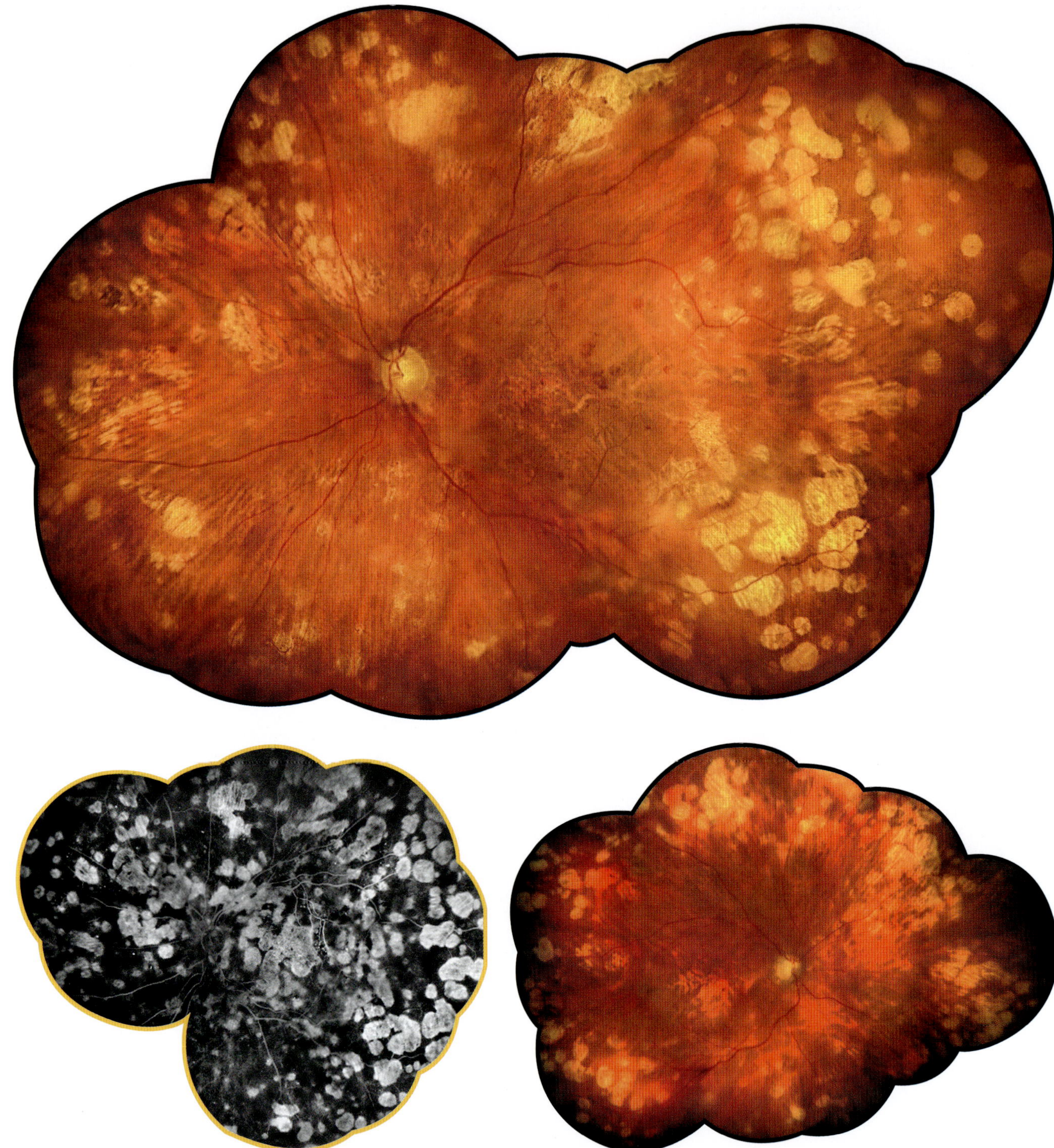

This patient had an acute West Nile virus infection with severe systemic symptoms, which included coma. There was also bilateral ocular involvement. Following the acute infection, which involved the retina, there were multifocal areas of chorioretinal atrophy with some confluency of contiguous lesions. The FA, taken at a later date, shows staining of the many atrophic chorioretinal scars. The random distribution of these lesions resembles multifocal choroiditis without fibrosis or significant hyperpigmentation. The lower right color montage of the fellow eye has similar manifestations. *Courtesy of Dr. Mark Johnson*

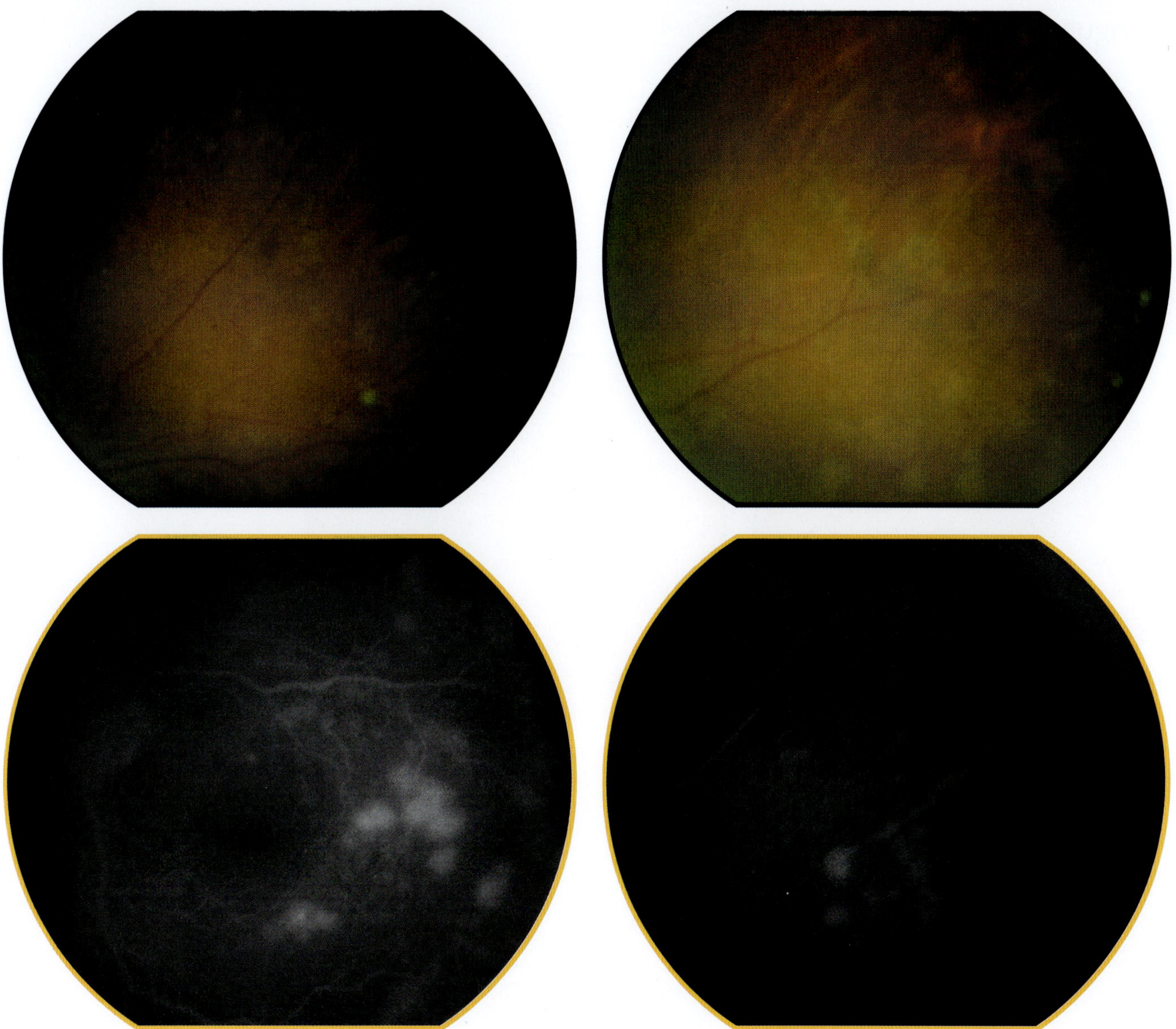

This is a case of West Nile Virus chorioretinitis. The color fundus photos show numerous mid-peripheral cream-colored round chorioretinal lesions (some with a halo configuration) that stain with FA. IgM and IgG antibodies were positive for West Nile Virus. *Courtesy of Dr. Susan Anderson-Nelson*

Dengue Virus Maculopathy

The dengue virus is an RNA virus (of the flavivirus family) with four distinct serotypes that is widespread in tropical climate locales. It causes the clinical disease dengue fever, which is marked by high fevers, joint and bone pain, headache, and rash. In its most severe form victims suffer from dengue hemorrhagic fever, which is characterized by the aforementioned symptoms in addition to thrombocytopenia and often multiorgan failure. Dengue virus can cause a maculopathy associated with blurred vision and/or a scotoma. Fundus findings include macular and/or optic disc edema, retinal hemorrhages, venous sheathing, and yellow subretinal dots. More recently, multimodal imaging findings typical of acute macular neuroretinopathy have been described in these patients. Oral and intravenous steroids are the mainstay of treatment as the pathogenesis is postulated to be immune-mediated.

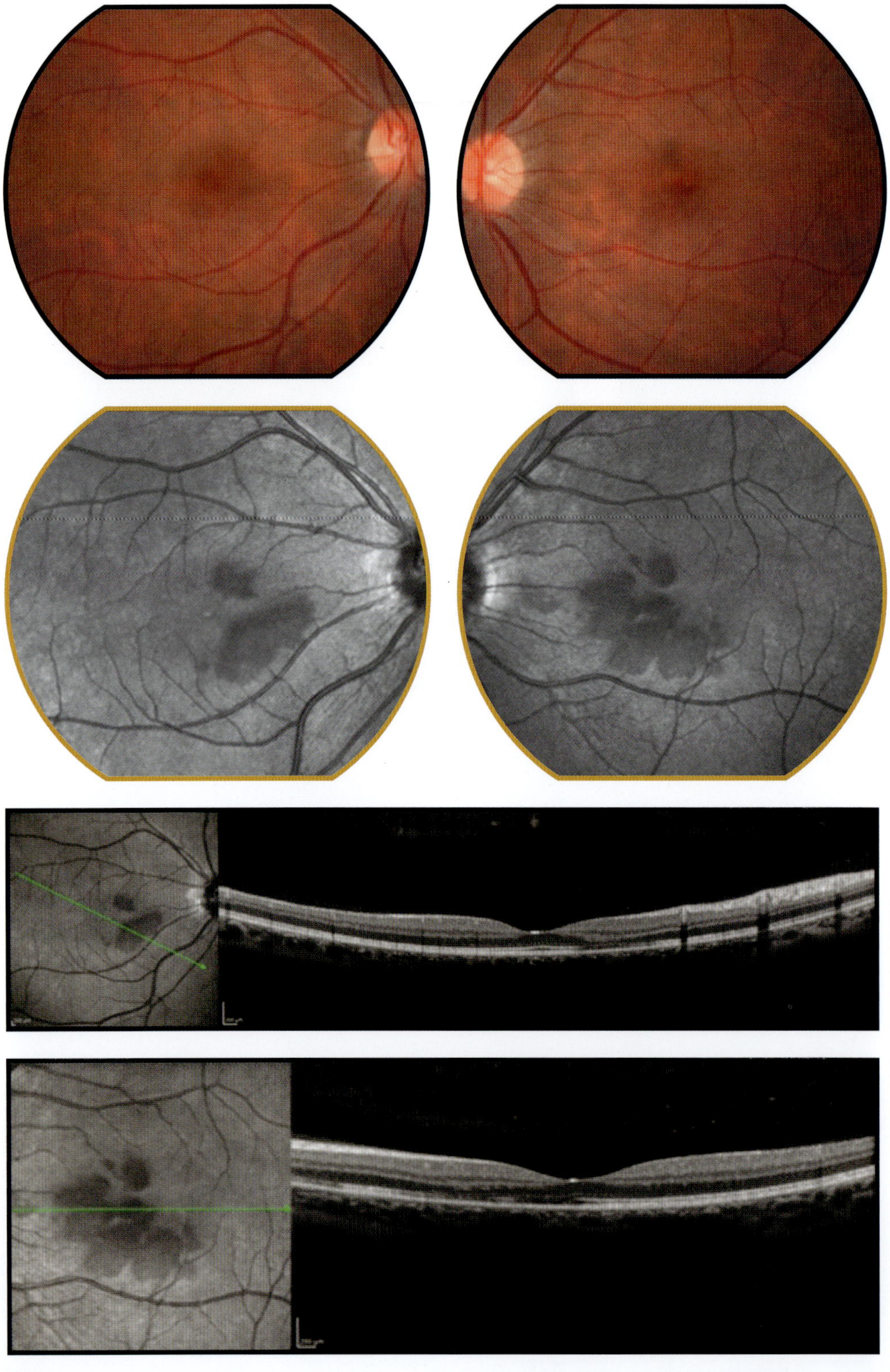

This patient with dengue has normal-appearing fundi in color photos but the infrared images reveal the characteristic hyporeflective paracentral lesions of acute macular neuroretinopathy (AMN). SD-OCT shows loss of the interdigitation zone and attenuation of both the inner segment ellipsoid band and the external limiting membrane (ELM) with corresponding hyper-reflectivity of the Henle layer. Vision improved to 20/30 OU after systemic steroid treatment. *Courtesy of Dr. Eduardo Cunha de Souza and Munk, M.R., Jampol, L.M., Cunha Souza, E., et al., 2016. New associations of classic AMN. Br. J. Ophthalmol. 100(3), 389-394*

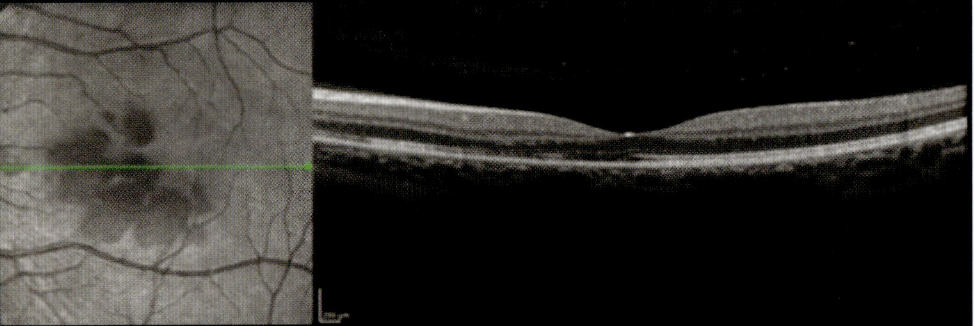

Protozoa

Toxoplasmosis

Toxoplasmosis infection is caused by the obligate intracellular protozoan, *Toxoplasma gondii*. There are two stages of the life cycle of the protozoan found in humans. The tachyzoites, measuring about 6 μm in length, comprise the first stage and the bradyzoites, thousands of which may be contained in cysts measuring up to 200 μm in diameter, comprise the second stage. Toxoplasmosis retinitis is the most common retinal infection and is typically only active in one eye at a time.

In immunocompromised patients, the CNS is the preferred site of infection, with cerebral toxoplasmosis reported in as many as 40% of autopsy eyes. Ocular toxoplasmosis is much less common than cerebral toxoplasmosis, accounting for less than 1% of AIDS-related retinal infections in the USA. Systemic infection with *T. gondii* is most commonly asymptomatic and approximately 500 million people worldwide have antibodies to the organism.

Most toxoplasmosis infections are in otherwise healthy hosts and symptoms are due to reactivation of organisms. Pre-existing chorioretinal scars indicate prior infection. Primarily acquired toxoplasmosis infection of the retina with an absence of pre-existing chorioretinal scars is more typical in AIDS patients. Acute toxoplasmic lesions (primary or reactivated) are focal yellow–white areas of necrotizing retinitis associated with a severe vitritis ("headlight in the fog"). The lesions have fluffy borders with few scattered hemorrhages. Vascular sheathing may be prominent (Kyrieleis plaques).

Congenital Toxoplasmosis Scars

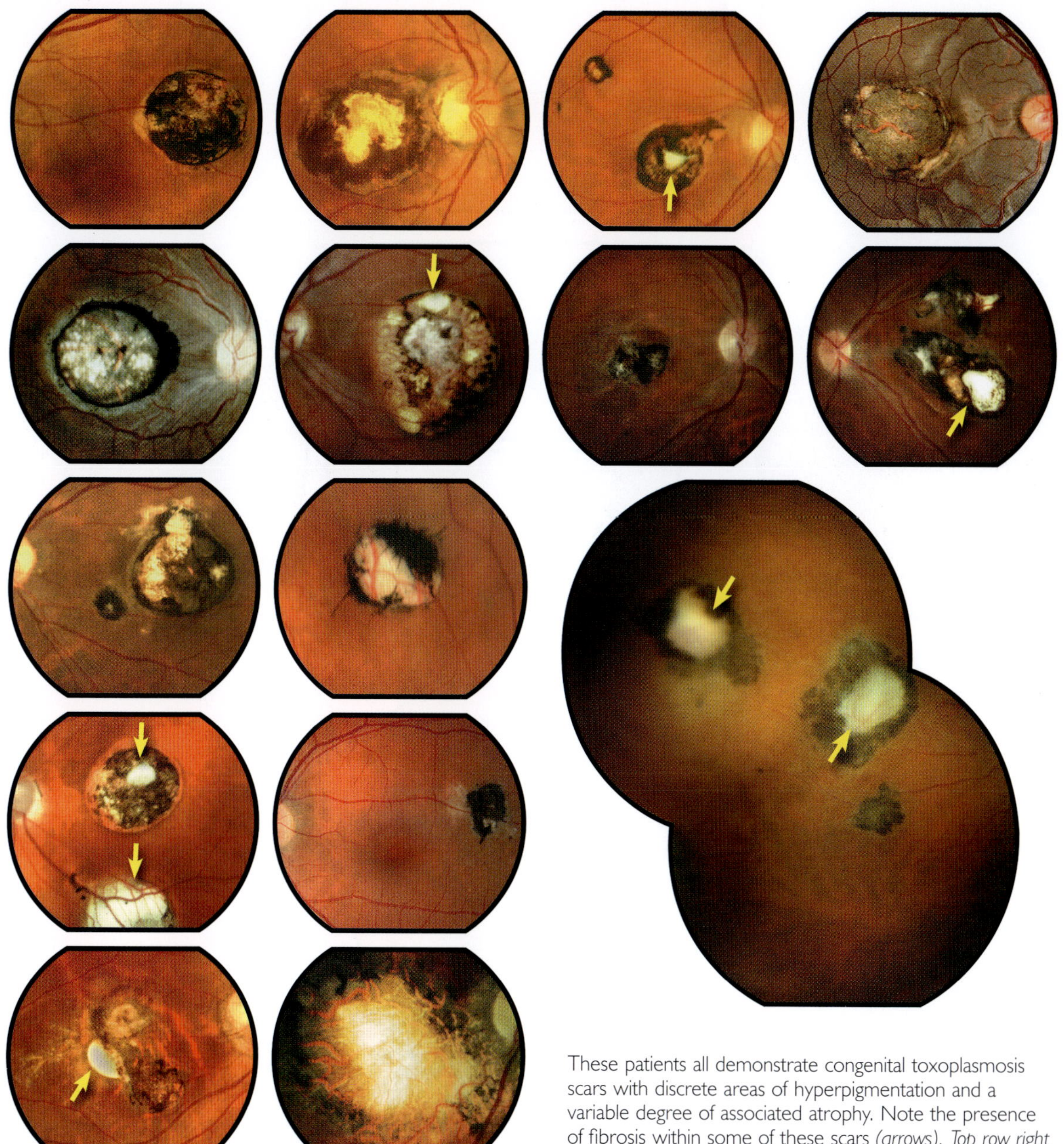

These patients all demonstrate congenital toxoplasmosis scars with discrete areas of hyperpigmentation and a variable degree of associated atrophy. Note the presence of fibrosis within some of these scars *(arrows). Top row right image courtesy of Alan Campbell, CRA*

Acute Toxoplasmic Lesions

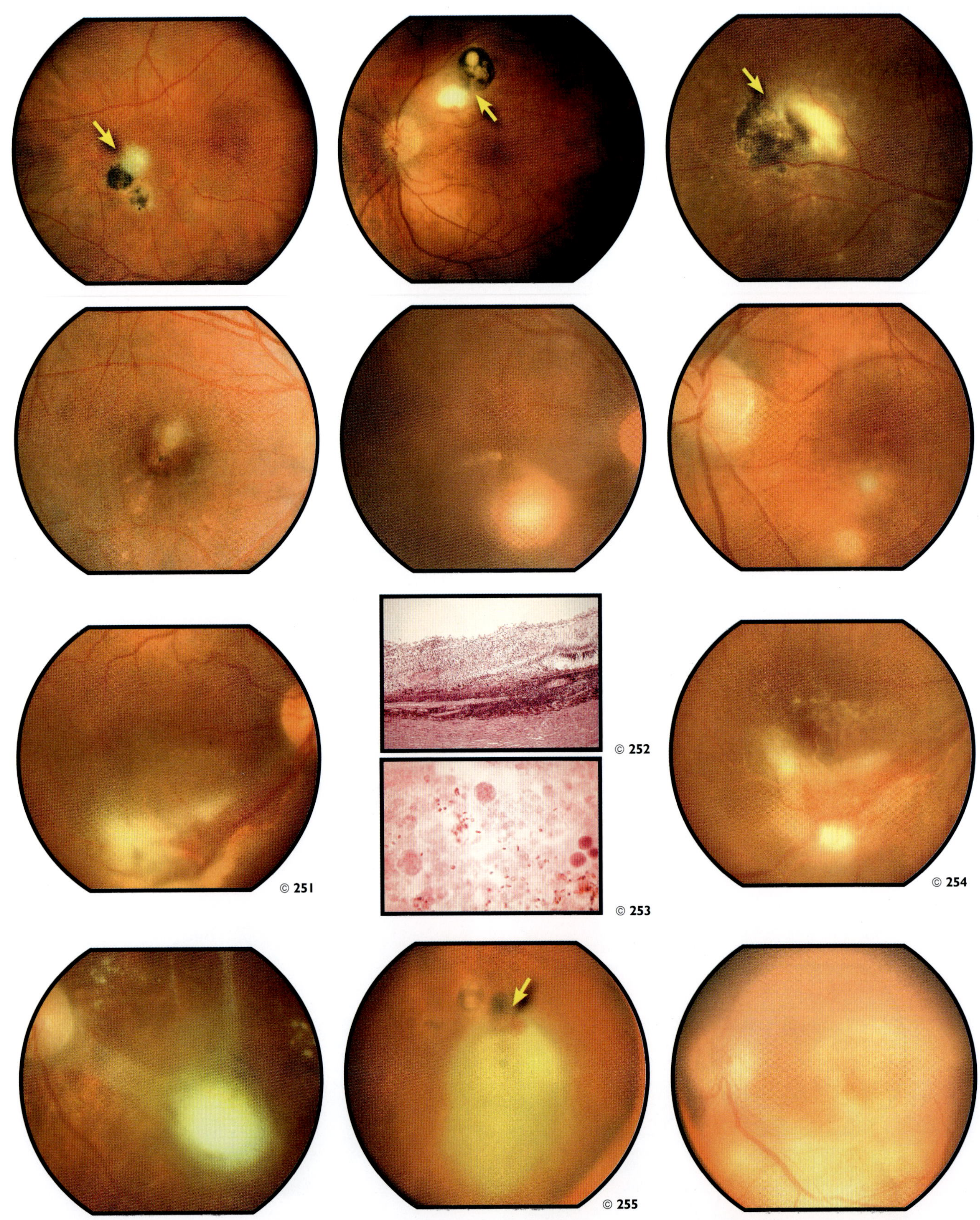

Acute toxoplasmosis presents with a focal yellow–gray inflammatory infiltrate within the retina. Satellite lesions may also be noted. A variable degree of overlying vitreous inflammation is typically present and a papillitis may also be noted. The acute lesions are often seen in contiguity with an old pigmentary scar *(arrows)* indicating reactivated disease.

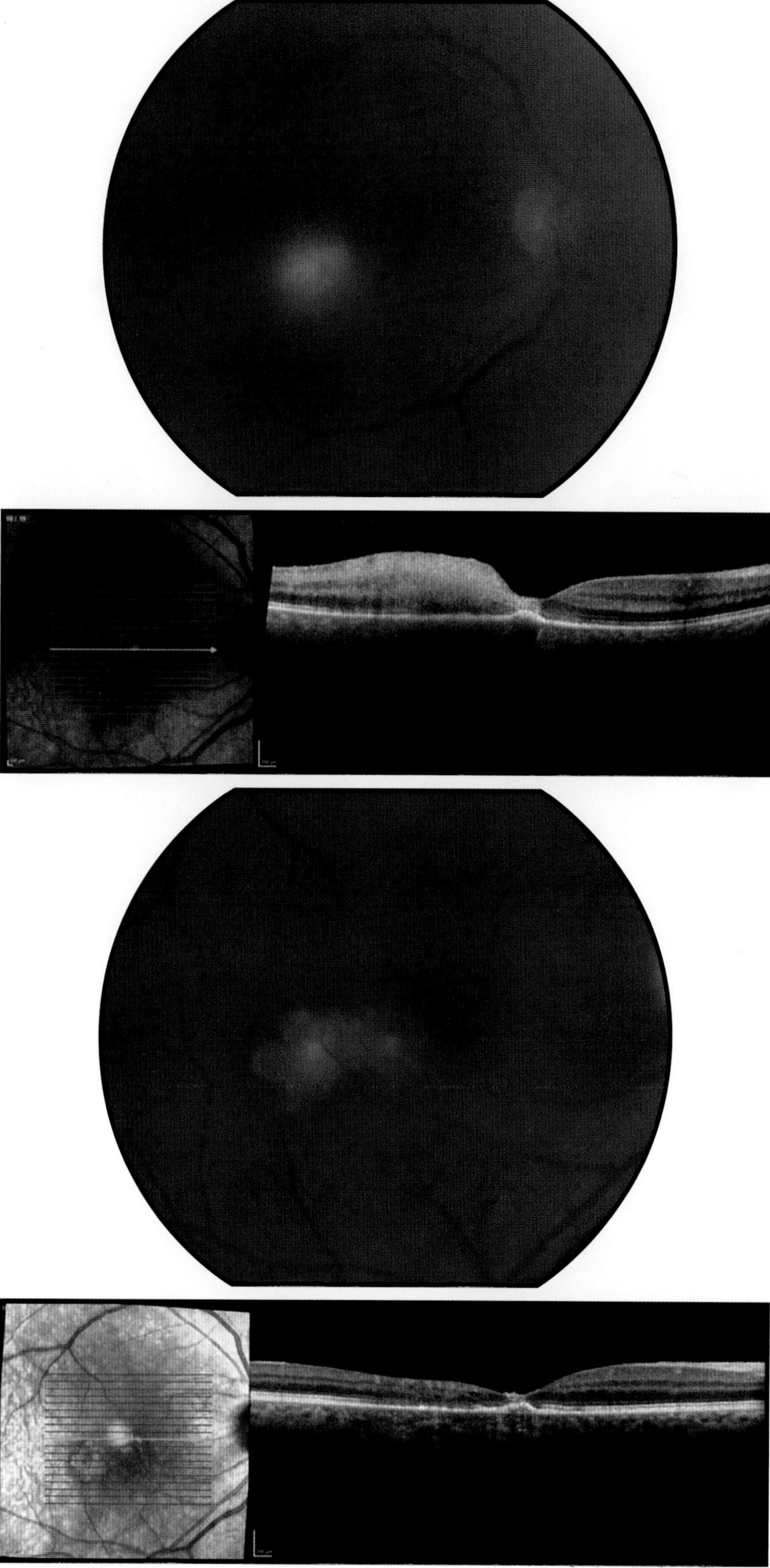

This patient with acute toxoplasmosis presented with iritis and vitritis as well as a cream-colored inflammatory lesion in the macula *(top photo)*. SD-OCT revealed inner retinal opacification. With intravitreal and oral antibiotics as well as oral steroids the vitritis and inner retinitis both resolved.

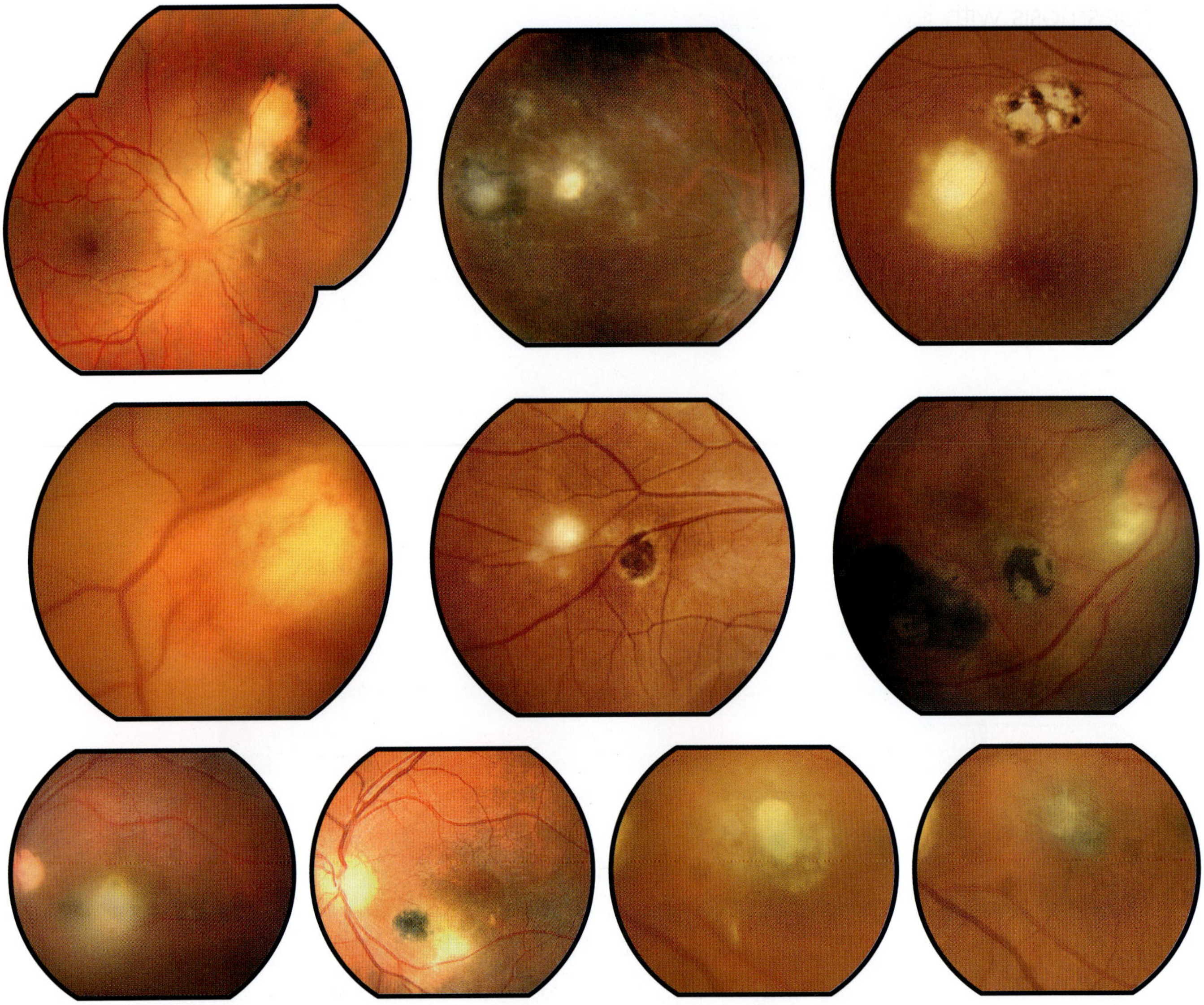

These patients show the variable presentation of an acute toxoplasmosis lesion in the fundus. Note the proximity to chorioretinal pigmentary scars and associated inflammatory activity in the fundus. Conversion from an acute to a healed lesion is appreciated in the two cases in the bottom row. *Top row middle image courtesy of Dr. Emmett Cunningham*

Miliary Toxoplasmosis

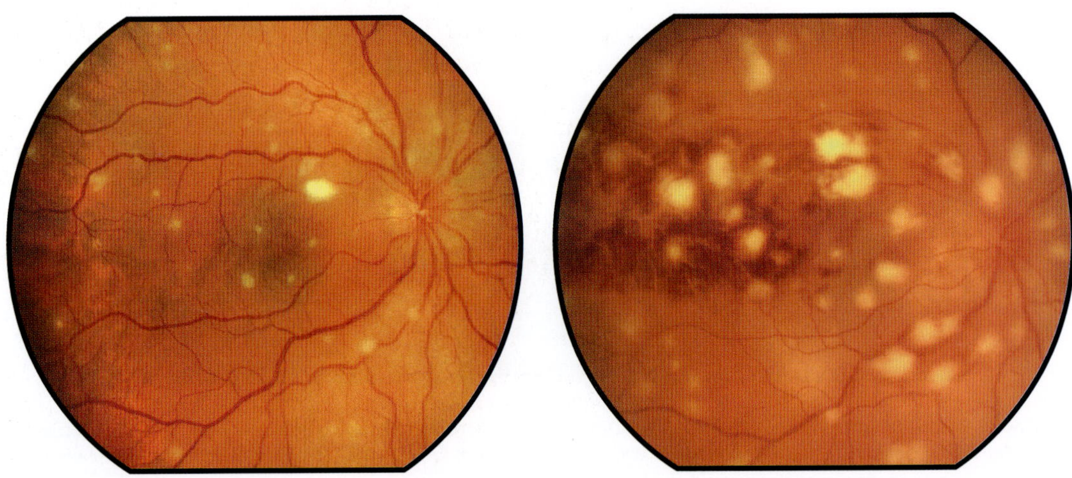

This HIV patient had miliary toxoplasmosis retinitis. Multifocal yellow–white retinitis is seen *(left)*. Macular hemorrhage was noted 5 weeks later due to venous occlusive disease. There were also numerous additional infectious lesions evident at that time. *Courtesy of Dr. William Freeman*

Toxoplasmosis with Kyrieleis Plaques

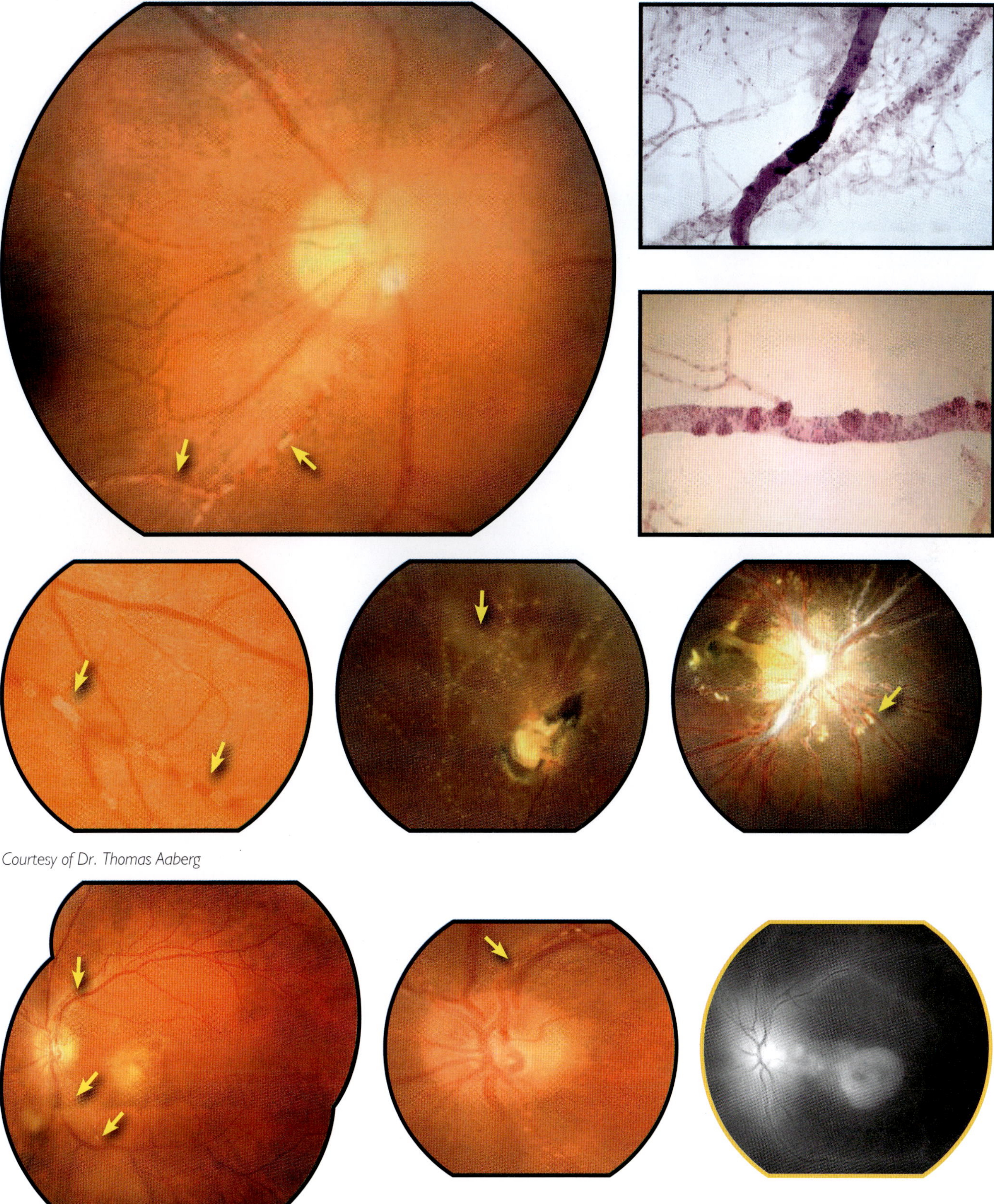

Courtesy of Dr. Thomas Aaberg

Although first described in association with tuberculosis retinitis by Dr. Werner Kyrieleis, calcific plaques on the walls of blood vessels are a well-known complication of toxoplasmosis retinitis. Note the refractile calcific-like lesions *(arrows)* along the course of inflamed vessels in these patients. The noncorrelating histopathology suggests that there are inflammatory cells that aggregate on the walls of the vessels to produce mineralization seen clinically. The bottom images *(left and middle)* show an acute toxoplasmosis lesion with Kyrieleis plaques near the disc. The retinitis is associated with staining of the optic nerve and a neurosensory retinal detachment in the macula, as illustrated in the FA *(bottom right)*. Kyrieleis plaques are also seen in a variety of other infectious, inflammatory, and infiltrative disorders associated with retinal vasculitis. *Bottom row courtesy of Dr. Ketan Laud*

Toxoplasmosis and Choroidal Neovascularization

Patients with toxoplasmosis retinitis may experience a significant decline in vision from recurrent infection or from secondary choroidal neovascularization.

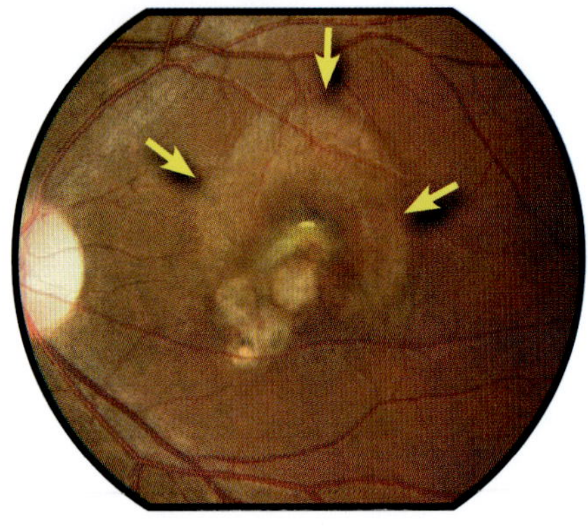
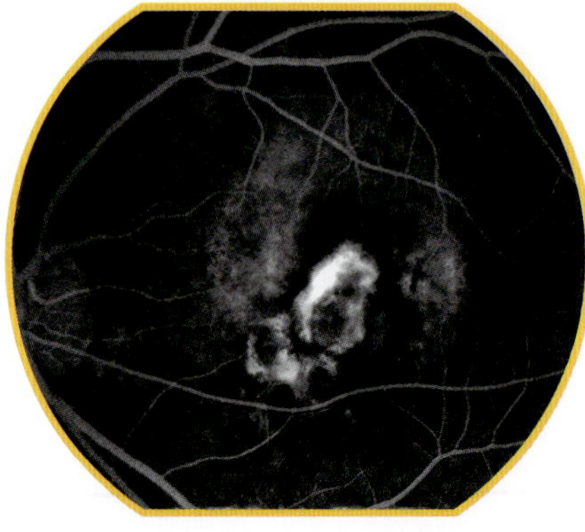
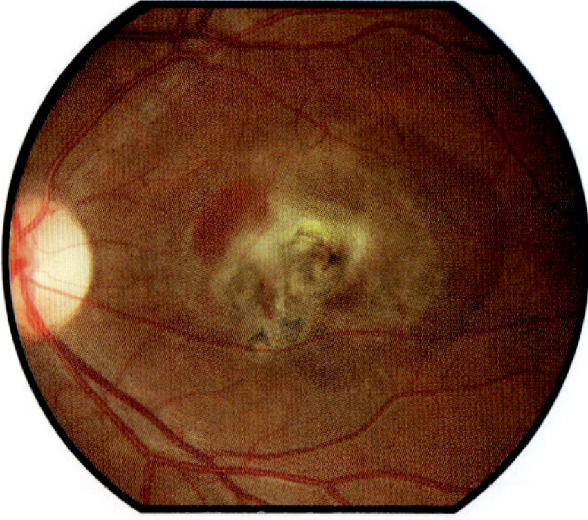

This patient has an acute exudative macular detachment *(arrows)* from choroidal neovascularization, which emerged from the edge of a healed congenital toxoplasmosis scar. The FA shows classic type 2 neovascularization in the central macula, bordered inferiorly by a chorioretinal scar. Unfortunately, there was recurrent neovascularization with subretinal hemorrhage and fluid *(right)*, leading ultimately to a disciform scar. *Right image courtesy of Dr. Alan Berger*

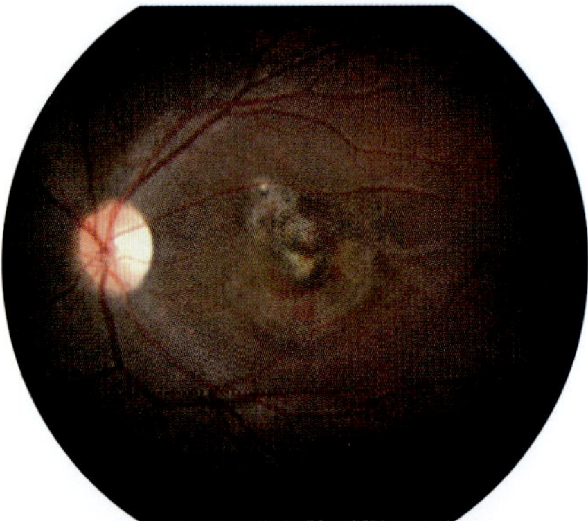
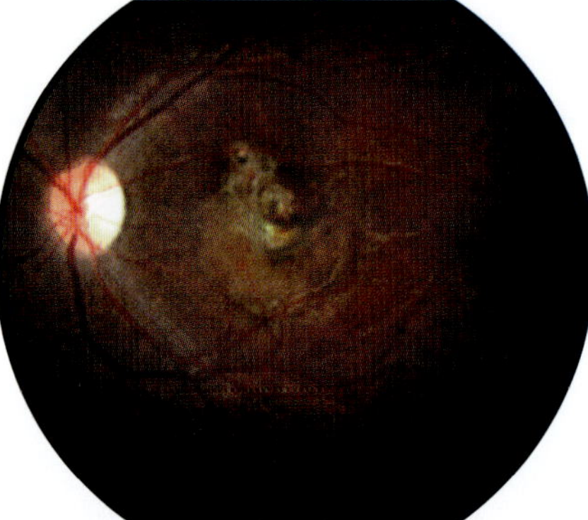

This patient had a congenital toxoplasmosis scar. At the age of 11, she developed acute choroidal neovascularization with subretinal hemorrhage and an exudative macular detachment *(left)*. She was treated with anti-angiogenic therapy, which induced consolidation of the fibrovascular lesion and resolution of the serosanguineous detachment. However, there was a legacy of a macular scar.

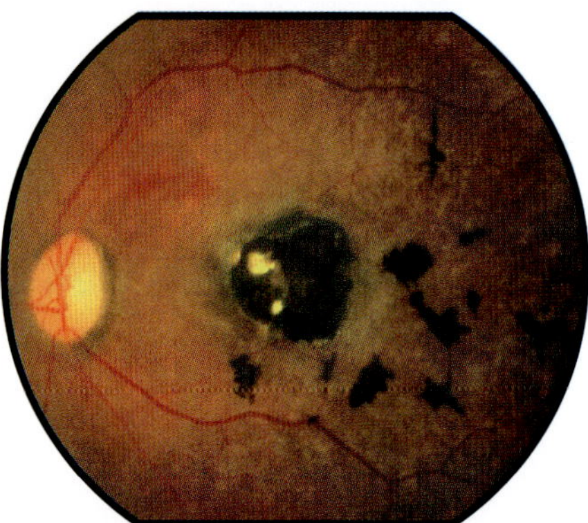

This patient had congenital toxoplasmosis, and she developed choroidal neovascularization at the nasal margin of the scar with serosanguineous detachment.

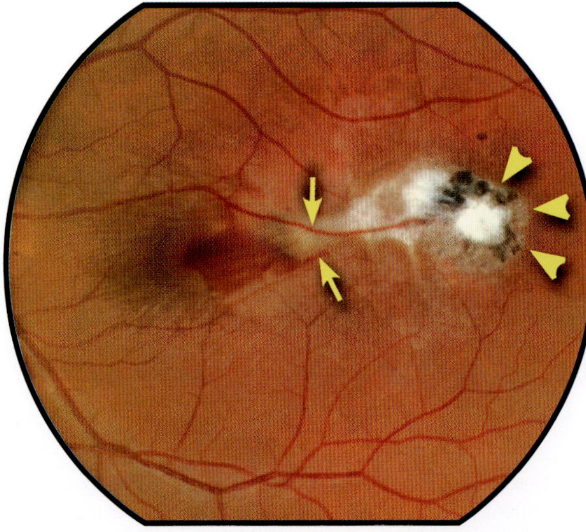
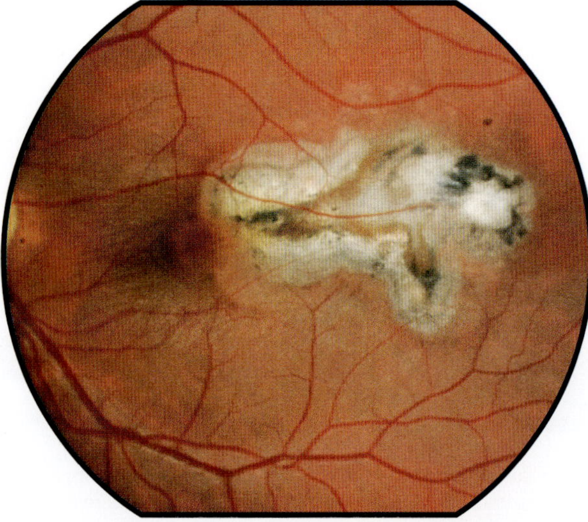

This patient demonstrates an old fibrotic and pigmentary toxoplasmosis scar. There is fibrosis *(arrowheads)* temporal to an occluded vessel, which is surrounded by pigmentation. Choroidal neovascularization (CNV) occurred on the foveal side of the scar *(arrows)* with bleeding into the fovea. Laser treatment was carried out to ablate the neovascular lesion, resulting in obliteration of the membrane and the development of an atrophic scar surrounding the lesion with sparing of the fovea *(right image)*.

Giardiasis

Giardia is a protozoan organism that can cause ocular complications such as pigment epithelial changes in a "salt and pepper" pattern. Giardiasis may also be associated with mild non-specific intraocular inflammation.

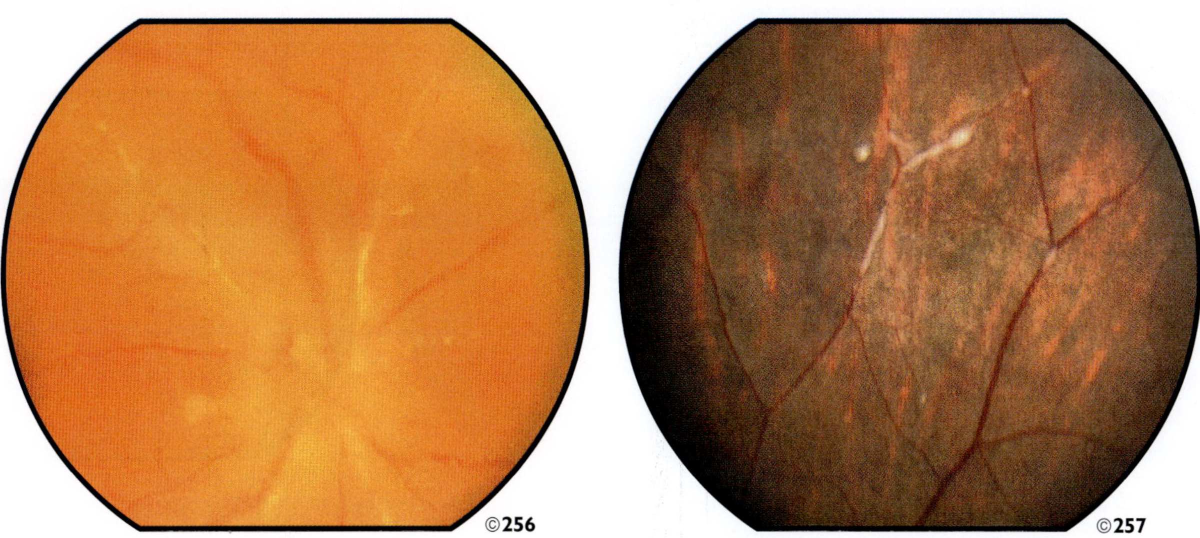

These patients have chronic giardiasis infection and associated retinal vasculitis. Note the presence of sheathing and infiltration of the retinal vessels in each case.

Bacteria

Leprosy

Leprosy or Hansen disease is caused by *Mycobacterium leprae*. Systemic manifestations are the result of nerve damage leading to structural deformities of the hands and feet. Cutaneous scarring, which includes a remarkable leonine appearance of the face, is characteristic of this disease. Ocular manifestations include sclerokeratitis and cataract formation. Retinal manifestations are very rare as the organism prefers infestation of tissues associated with cooler environments.

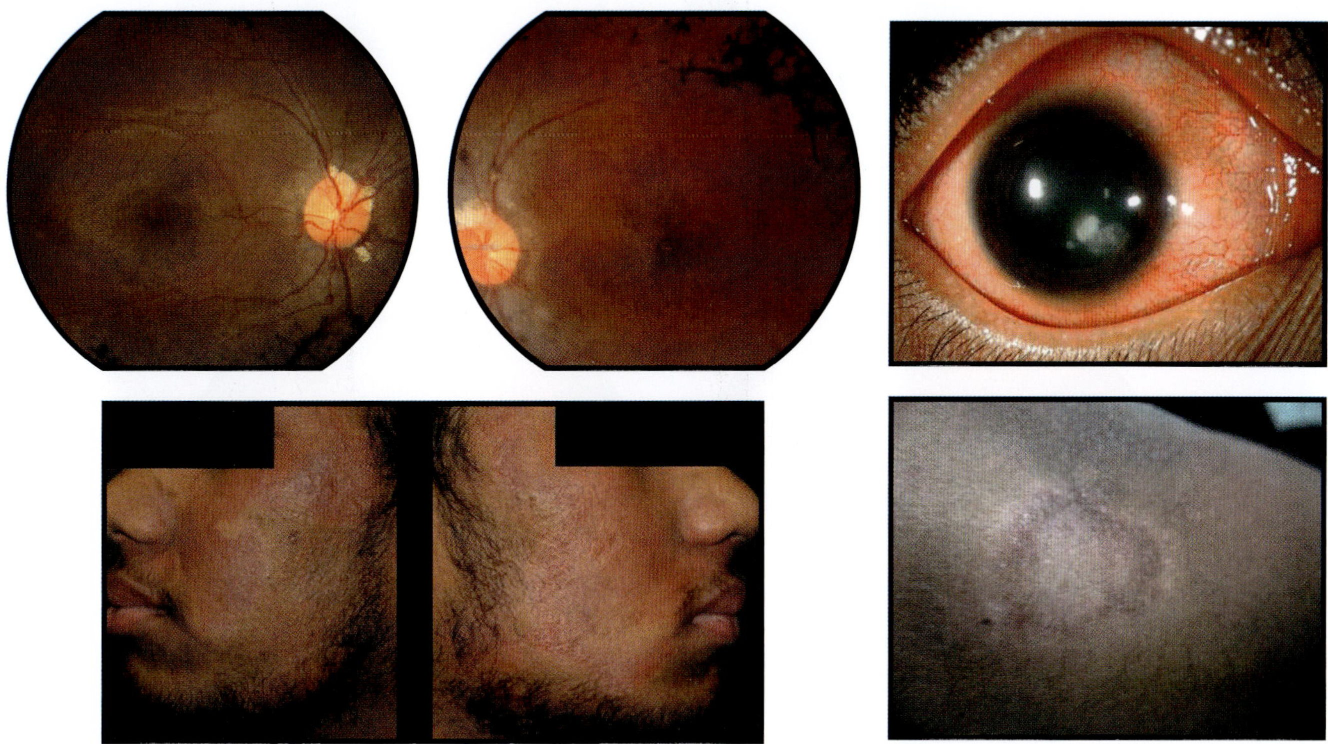

This patient has leprosy with corneal infiltration and multiple cutaneous lesions. An old inactive retinal phlebitis is noted with perivascular retinal atrophy and hyperpigmentation and scarring. *Courtesy of Dr. Karen M. Gehrs*

Tuberculosis

Tuberculosis remains a major cause of morbidity and mortality worldwide. The HIV-infected population accounts for most of the increase in the prevalence of this infection. Choroidal tubercles and tuberculomas are the most common manifestation of ocular tuberculosis. Uveitis, optic neuritis, and retinal vasculitis in the posterior pole and peripheral fundus may also be encountered.

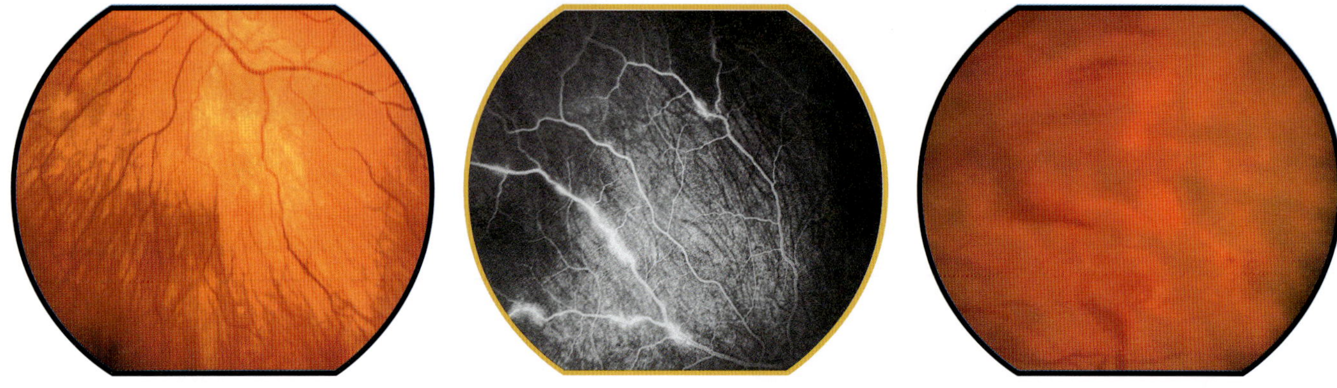

Tuberculosis may produce a retinal vasculitis. Note the evidence of retinal vascular staining and leakage with the FA. Hemorrhages into the vitreous may occur from new blood vessel proliferation *(right image)*.

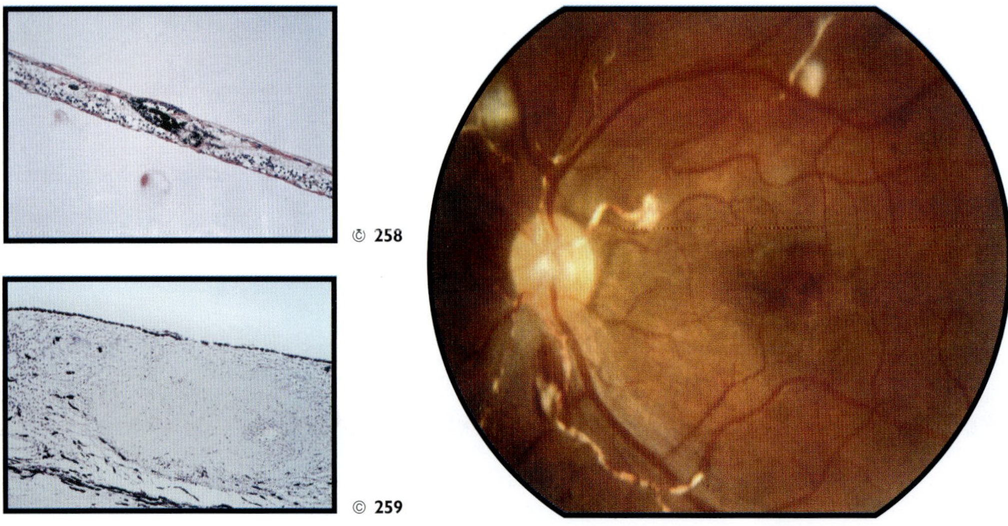

The histopathology images show inflammatory cells in the walls of vessels with associated mineralization. In the right image, we see that there are calcific-like plaques within the walls of the arterioles referred to as Kyrieleis plaques, which are a non-specific change in the retinal vasculature following inflammation or infection.

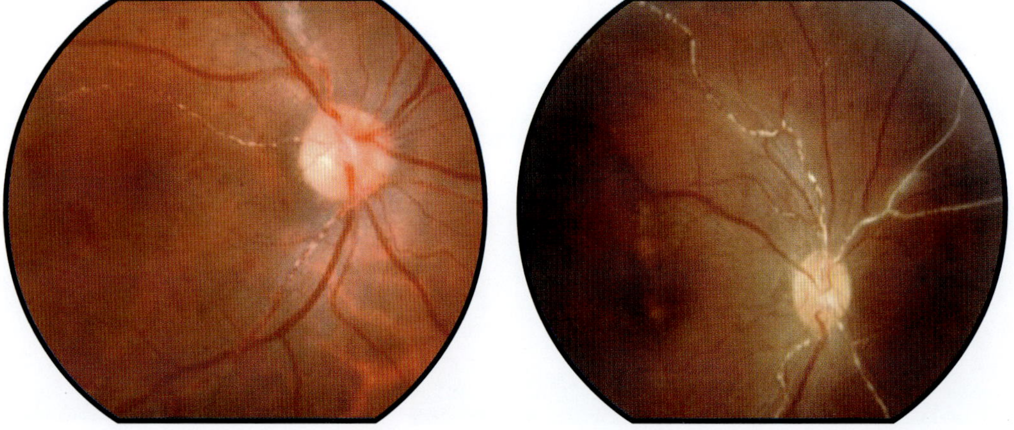

This patient with tuberculosis retinitis has calcific deposition in the walls of the arterioles (Kyrieleis plaques) following acute inflammation. Tuberculosis was the first disease associated with these calcific plaques, as was described by Dr. Werner Kyrieleis. *Courtesy of Dr. Richard Rosen*

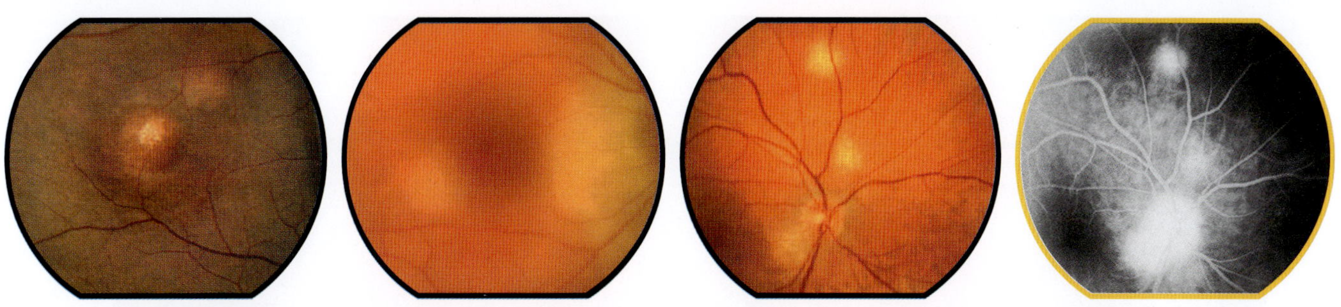

Tuberculosis may present as focal and multifocal choroidal granulomas. Small granulomas are seen in this patient *(left)*. Larger, multifocal lesions are seen with vitreous inflammation in the second case *(second from left)*. The third patient has multifocal chorioretinitis and optic neuritis from tuberculosis. The FA image shows leakage in the retina and optic nerve. *Courtesy of Dr. Richard Spaide*

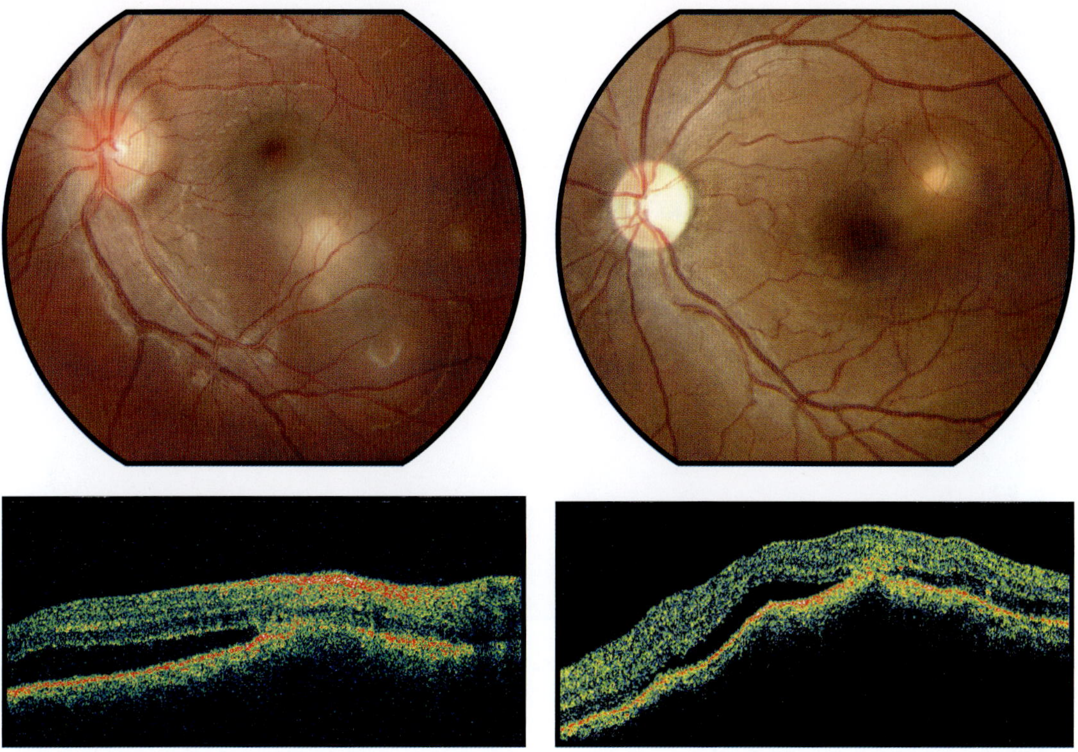

These are two cases of focal tuberculous choroiditis with an overlying localized exudative macular detachment. The OCT images show fibrous adherence between the detached retina and the retinal pigment epithelium and associated subretinal fluid. *Courtesy of Amjad Salman, MS*

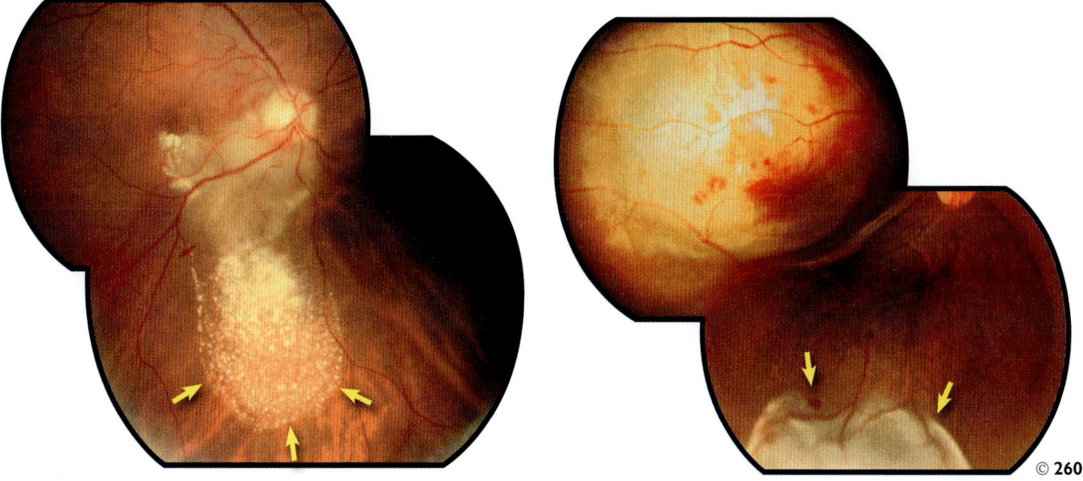

These two patients have choroidal granulomas from tuberculous choroiditis. The granuloma is close to the optic nerve *(left)*. Radial exudate is extending into the macula and a dependent exudative detachment is noted inferiorly *(arrows)*. The second color montage includes images of a large fibrotic choroidal granuloma with active associated hemorrhage. Blood and exudation have gravitated inferiorly to form a dependent detachment *(arrows)*. *Left image courtesy of Dr. Scott Sneed*

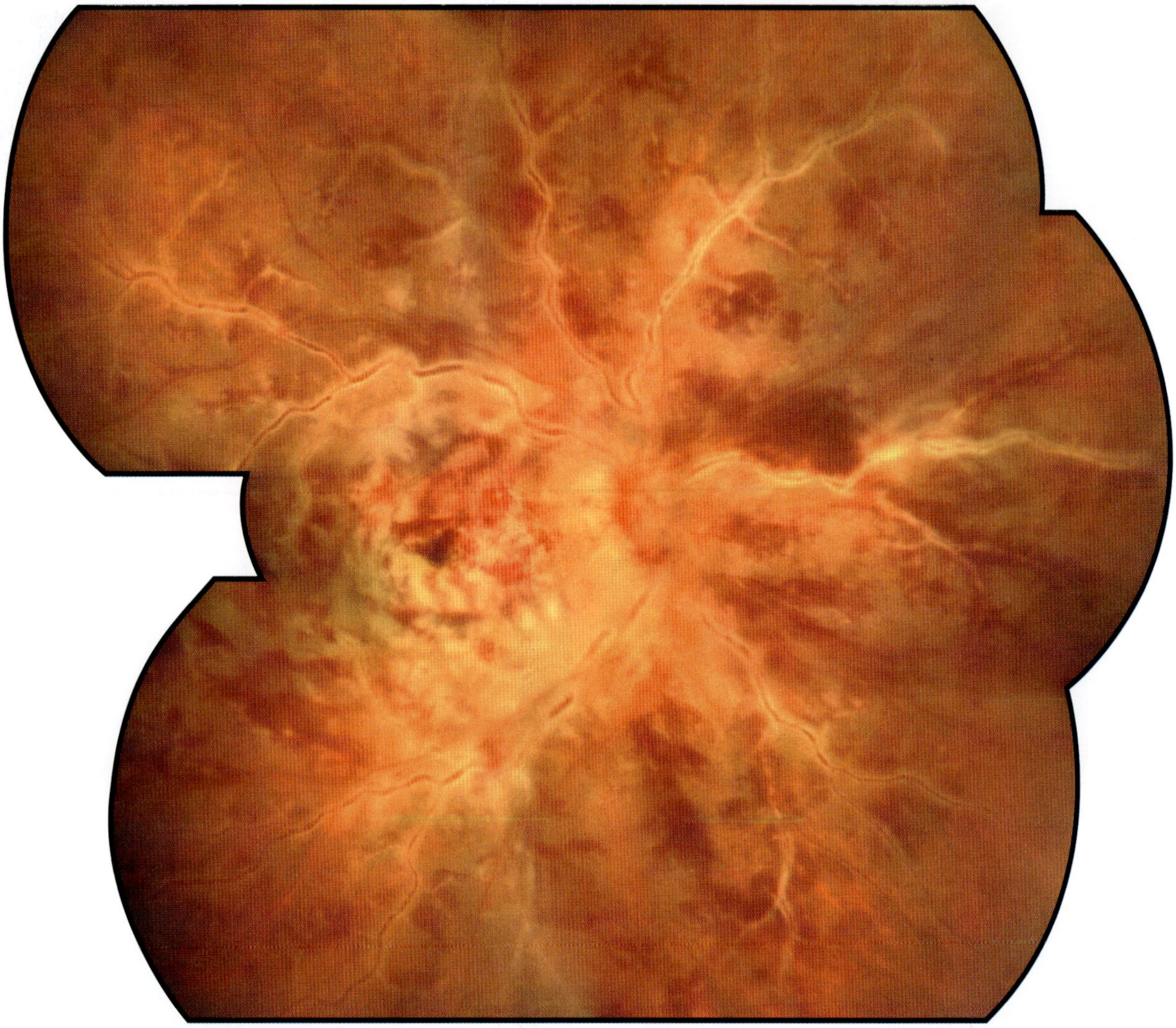

This patient has widespread retinal vascular inflammation with a frosted-branch angiitis presentation, retinal venous occlusive disease with scattered hemorrhages, and optic neuritis from tuberculosis.

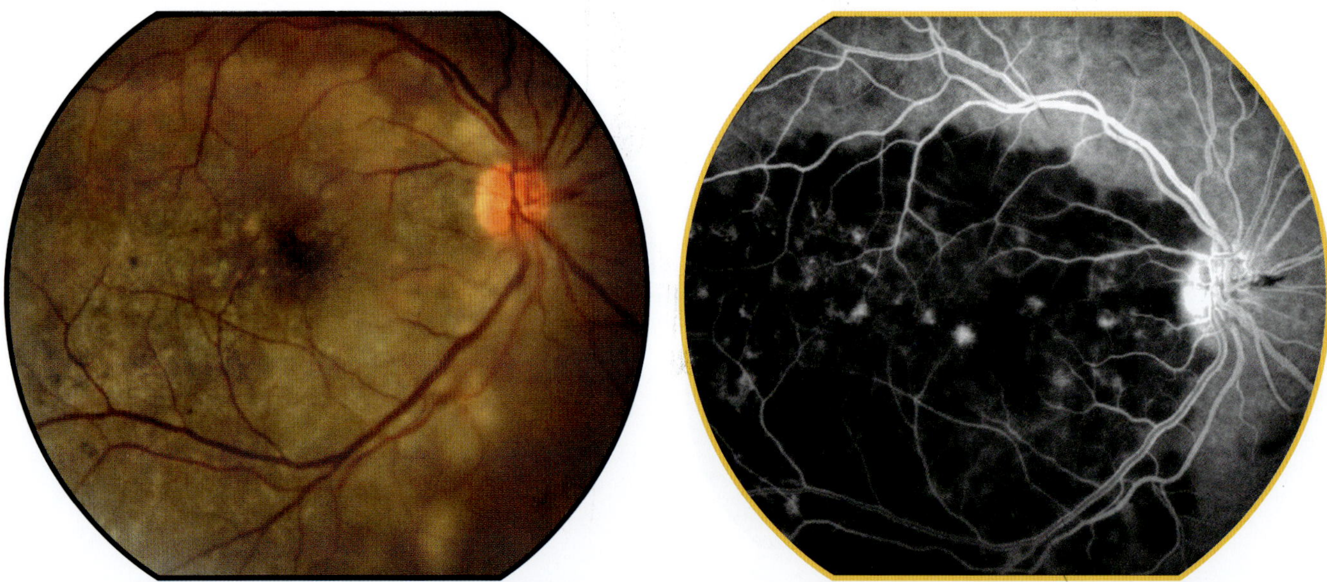

This patient has tuberculosis that resembles a placoid choroidopathy. The FA shows blockage of the choroidal fluorescence with multifocal punctate staining within the acute placoid lesion. This presumed variant of serpiginous choroidopathy with a progressive course resembling relentless placoid chorioretinitis or so-called ampiginous chorioretinopathy is common in India in patients with tuberculosis. *Courtesy of Dr. Benjamin Freilich*

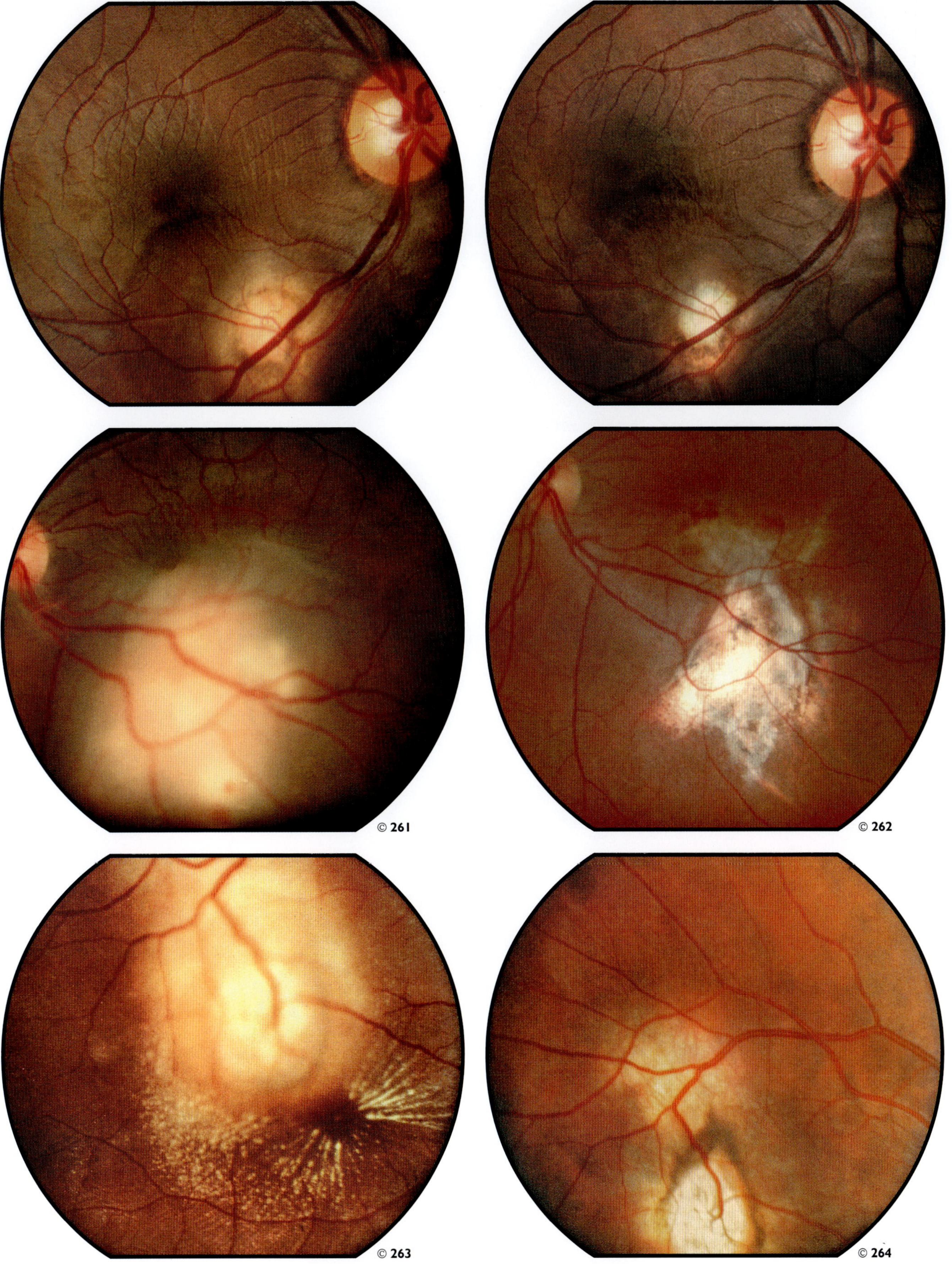

These are three patients with acute choroidal granuloma due to tuberculosis with variable degrees of exudative retinal detachment *(left images)*. Following treatment there was resolution of the exudation and regression of the choroidal granuloma with the development of chorioretinal atrophy and fibrous scarring in each of the three cases *(right images)*.

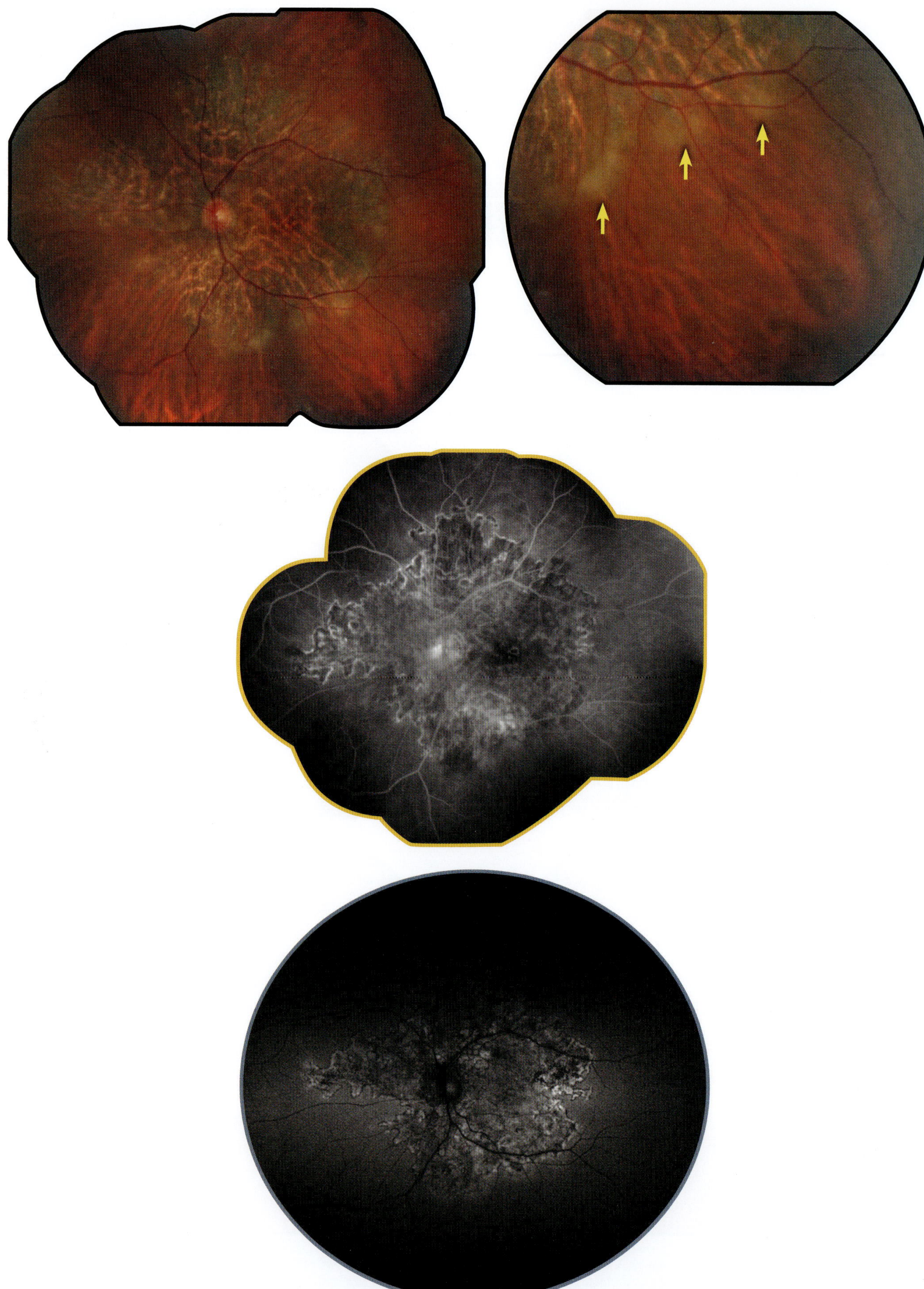

This is a case of tuberculosis presenting as serpiginous choroiditis. The color fundus photographs show a large chorioretinal scar throughout the posterior pole with an active border of yellow-gray subretinal infiltrates *(arrows)*. Mottled fluorescence of the lesion is seen with FA and fundus autofluorescence.

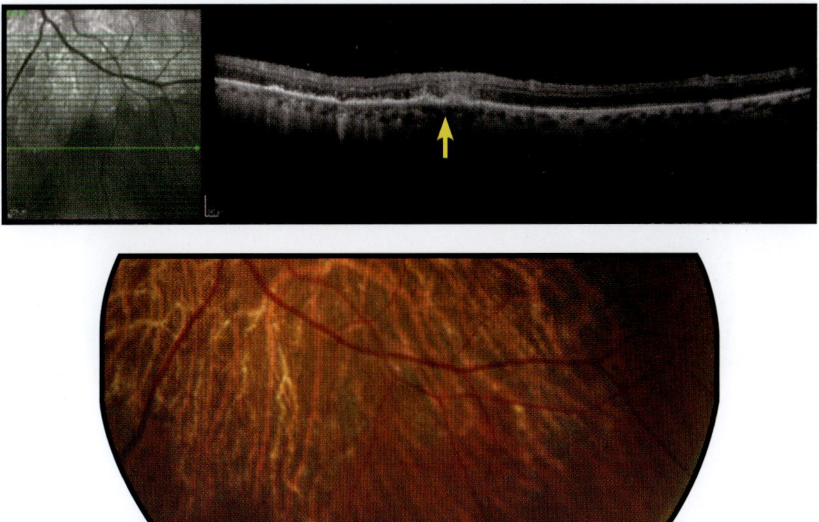

The spectral domain (SD) OCT shows a cross section through the active subretinal infiltrate *(arrow)*. With a regimen of isoniazid, rifampin, ethambutol, and pyrazinamide the chorioretinal infiltrates resolved as seen in the final color fundus image.

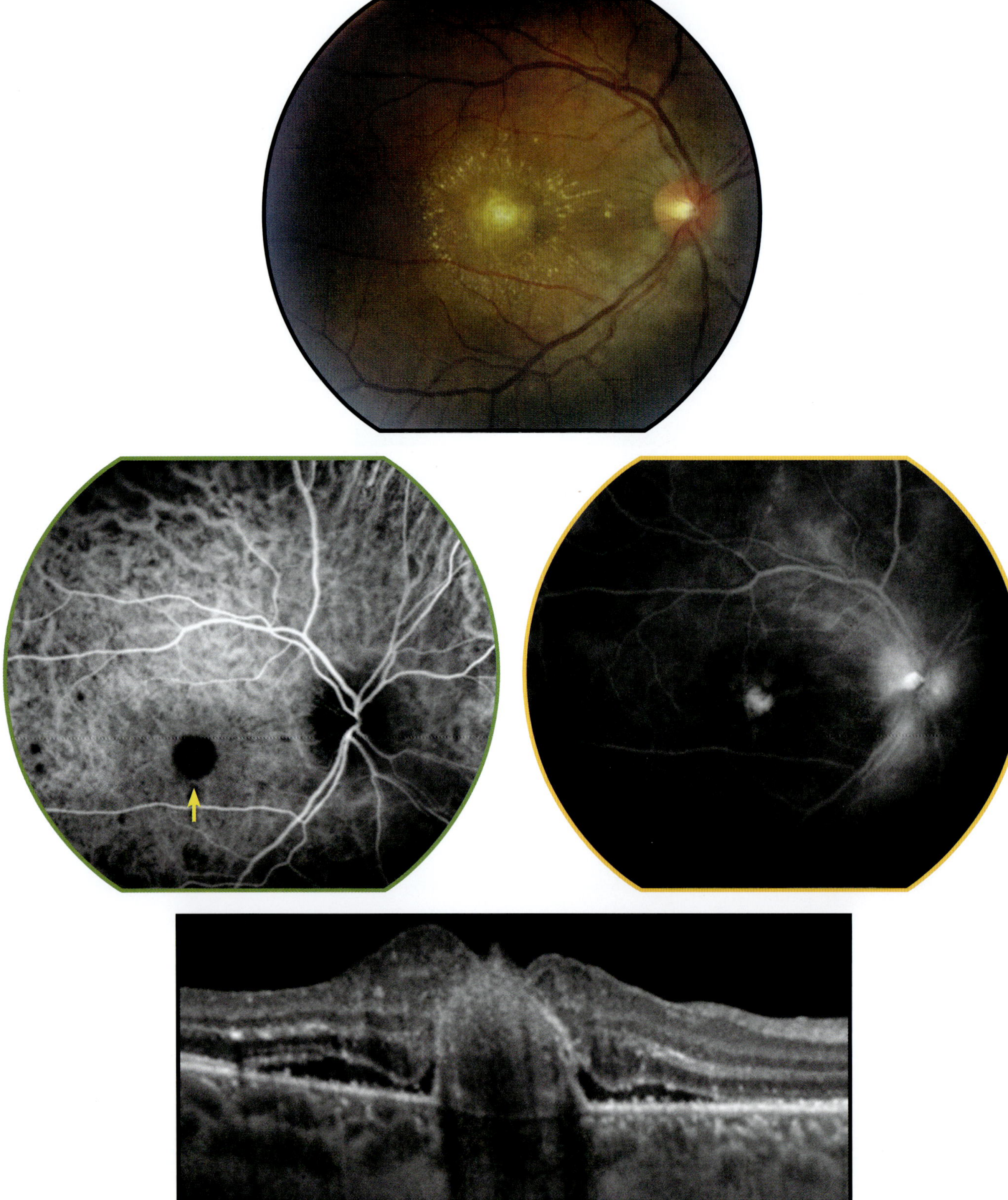

This patient with tuberculosis presented with a macular star, disc hyperemia, and vitreous haze as seen in the color photograph of the right eye *(top)*. Indocyanine green (ICG) angiography reveals a macular choroidal nodule *(arrow)*, and FA shows staining of the nodule and late disc leakage. SD-OCT reveals a large subfoveal choroidal granuloma with associated subretinal fluid. The vision worsened due to noncompliance with medication. *Courtesy of John A. Gonzales, MD*

Nocardiosis

Nocardia is a Gram-positive, rod-shaped bacterium. Some species are pathogenic, producing a wide spectrum of systemic abnormalities, including ocular involvement. The infection occurs by inhalation of the bacteria or through traumatic introduction. A localized granulomatous-like mass lesion, which is yellowish in color, in association with hemorrhage and overlying exudative detachment, may be seen in the fundus. It may also produce an infection in the cornea.

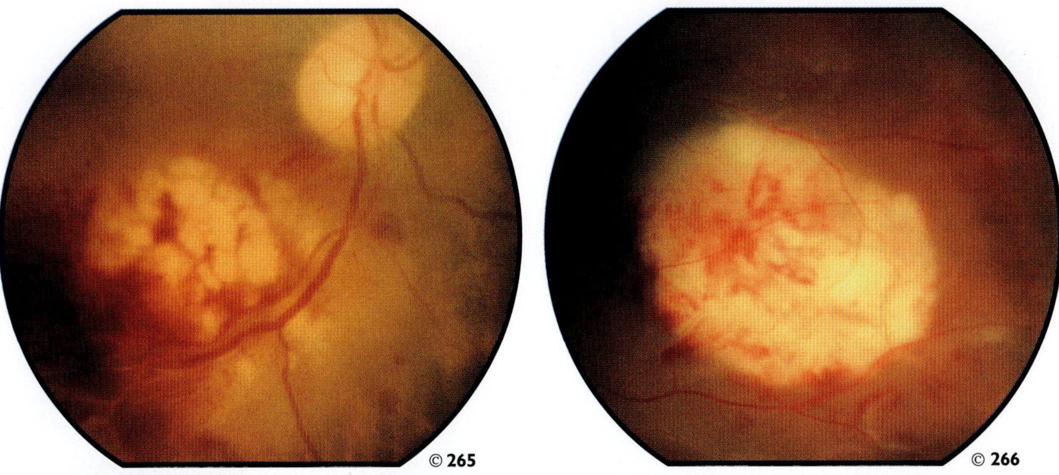

These are acute infiltrative *Nocardia* infectious lesions with extensive hemorrhage due to hematogenous extension through the retinal vasculature.

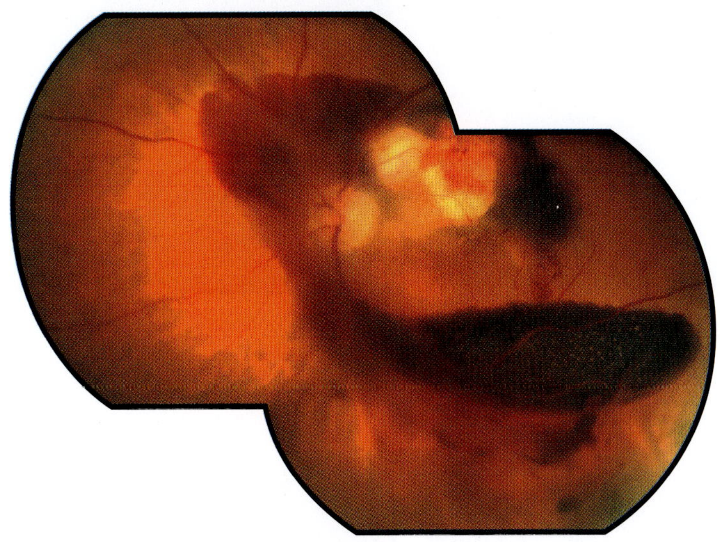

Hemorrhage is seen in this acute *Nocardia* infection at the site of the lesion, but also into the vitreous, forming a subhyaloidal accumulation of blood.

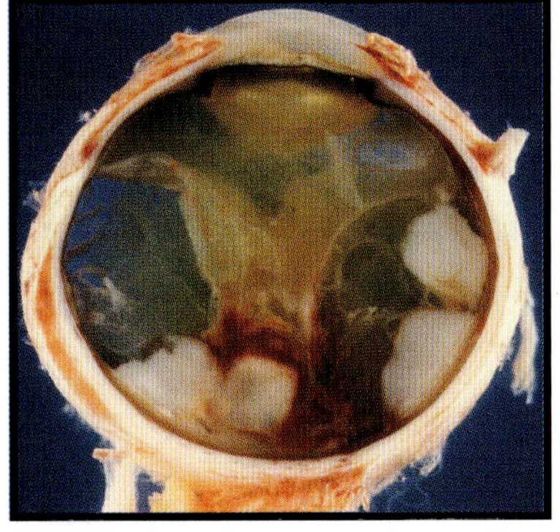

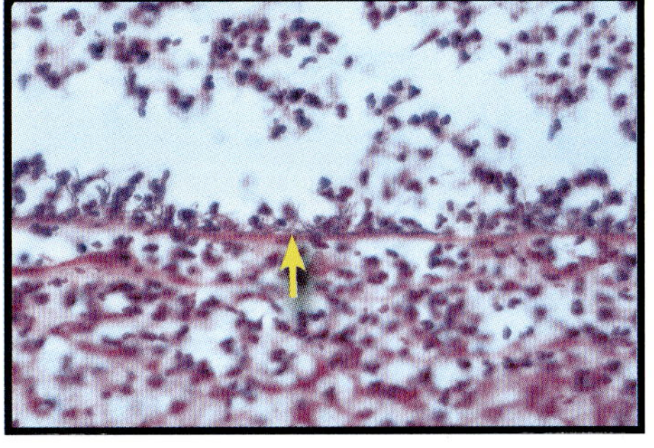

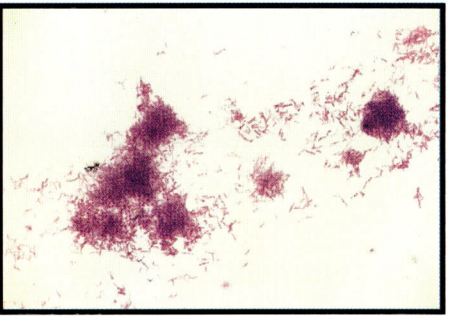

© 267

The gross pathology of an eye with *Nocardia* shows a multifocal amorphous mass lesion with hemorrhage and retinal detachment. The histopathology examination in this case revealed a whitish, subretinal pigment epithelial abscess with organisms located along the inner aspect of Bruch membrane *(arrow). Courtesy of Dr. Ramon LeFont*

A transneedle aspiration biopsy revealed *Nocardia* organisms.

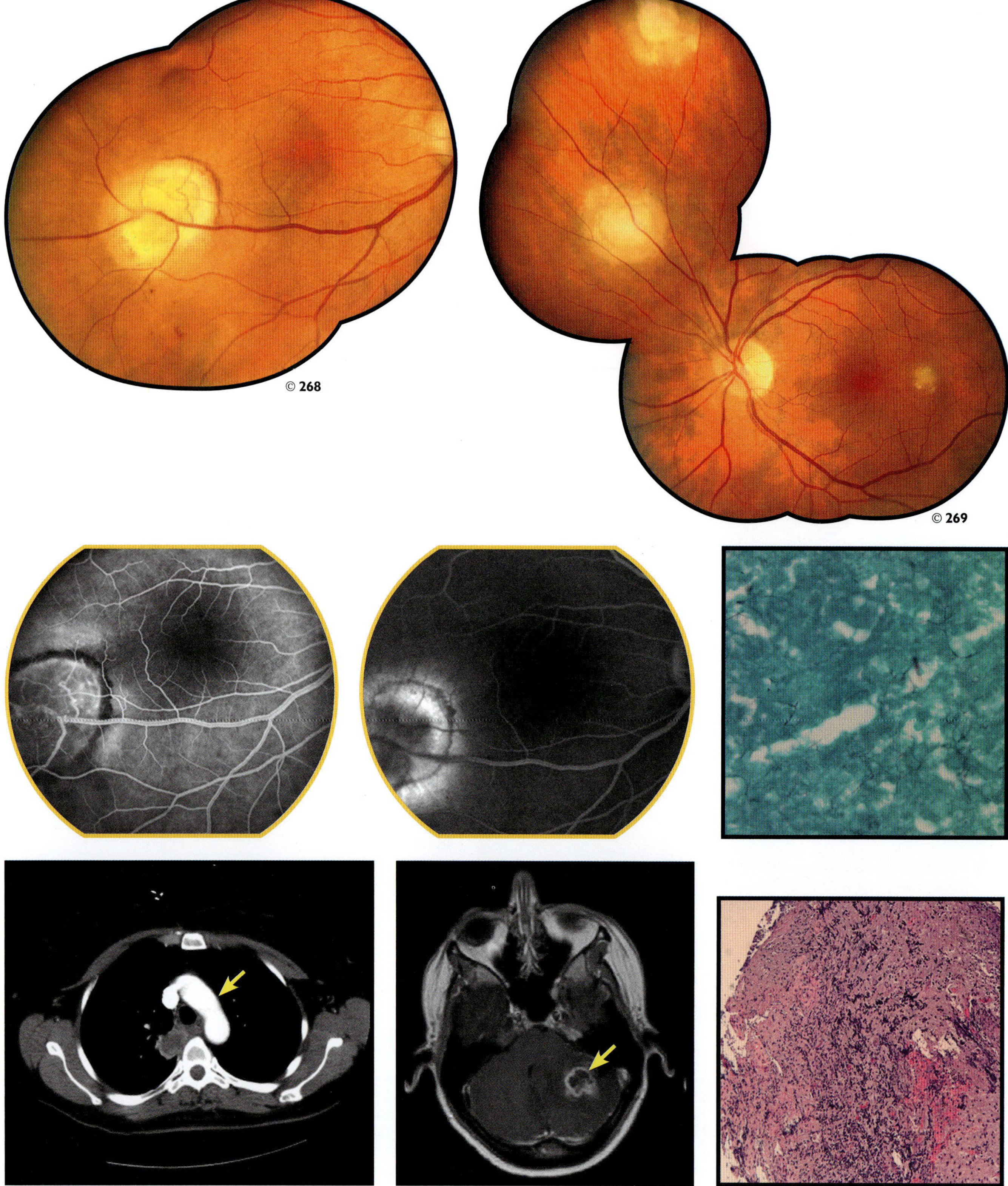

This is a patient with bilateral *Nocardia* granulomatous choroidal lesions. The clinical and FA images of the right eye show a yellow choroidal tumor that is infiltrating the retina and margined by blood and exudative detachment. The FA shows communicating vessels between the retina and choroid in a vascular lesion along the inferior temporal vasculature. In the left eye *(middle row, left)*, the lesions are more peripheral to the central macula. The CT scans show a large *Nocardia* lesion in the thorax and in the brain *(arrows)*. The histopathology shows chronic infection with inflammatory cells and numerous branching Gram-positive filamentous organisms in the subretinal space as well as a neutrophilic and lymphocytic infiltration. *Bottom two rows images courtesy of Dr. Lawrence Singerman*

Whipple Disease

This is a rare systemic infectious disease caused by *Tropheryma whipplei*, a Gram-positive rod bacterium. It is primarily a gastrointestinal disorder, which may affect any part of the body with inflammatory changes. A jejunal biopsy is used to disclose periodic acid–Schiff (PAS)-positive granules in macrophages of the lamina propria. Ocular changes can be bilateral and include an iritis, inflammatory vitreous opacities, panuveitis, and small round, grayish retinal lesions.

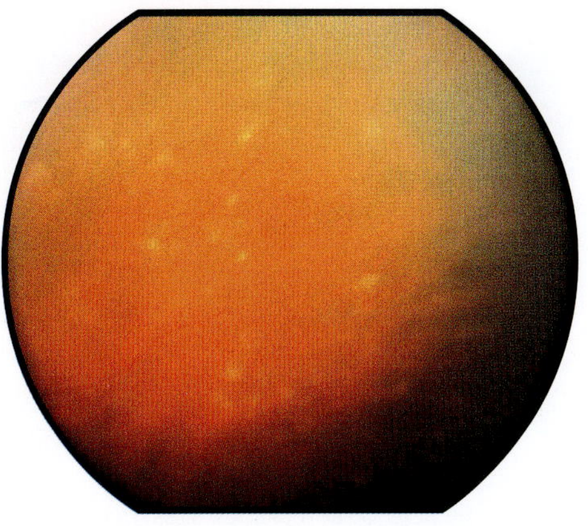

This patient had chronic loss of vision in conjunction with a gastrointestinal disturbance. There is vitreous hypercellularity and multifocal chorioretinal gray–white spots. *Courtesy of Dr. Alan Friedman*

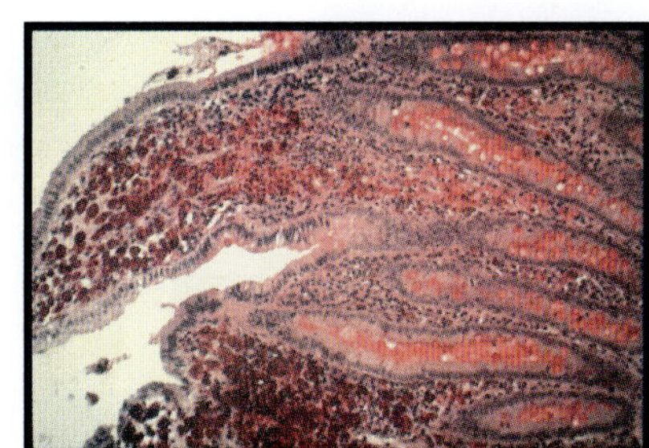

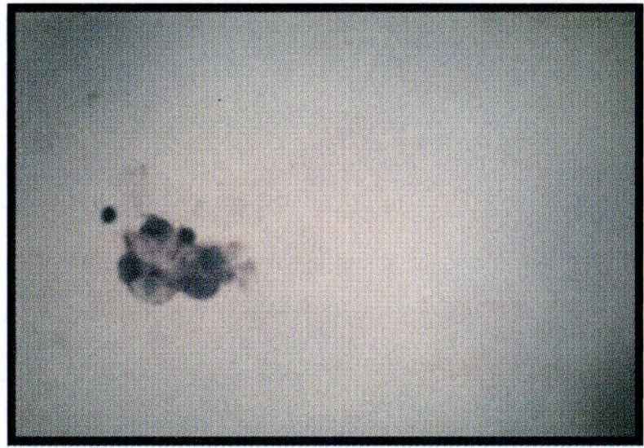

Courtesy of Dr. Alan Friedman

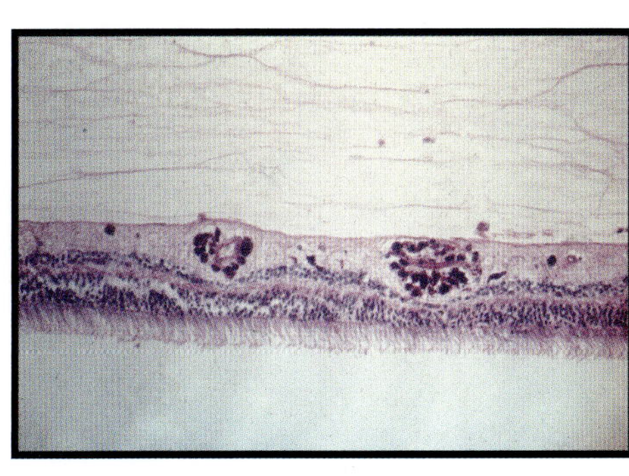

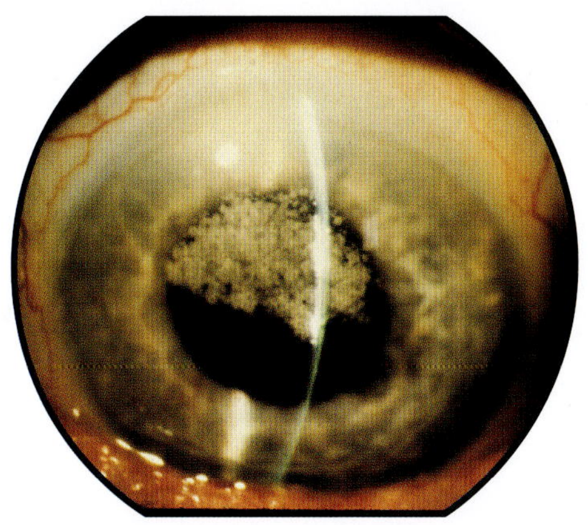

The histopathology of the jejunum shows PAS-positive granules in macrophages in the lamina propria and a typical involved cell with basophilic granules. The anterior segment image on the right shows characteristic anterior vitreous infiltration in a patient with Whipple disease.

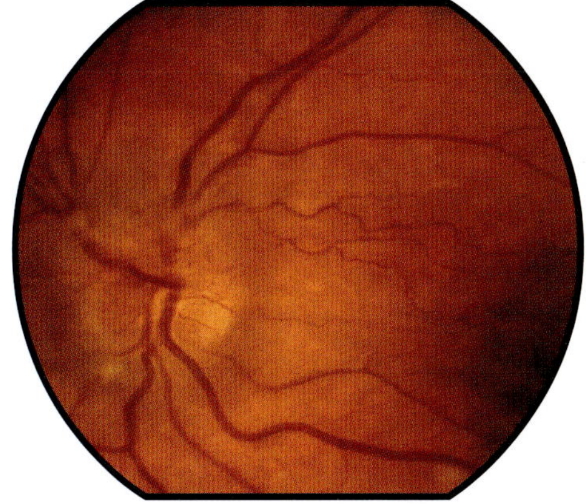

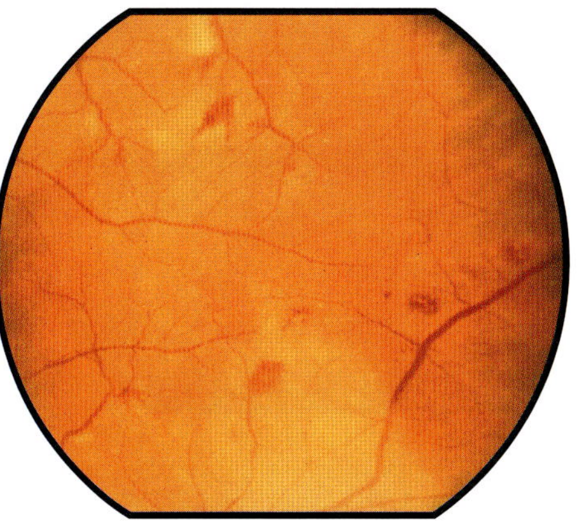

This patient with Whipple disease has a mild retinal vasculitis with optic nerve edema and scattered retinal hemorrhages.

Bartonella: Cat-Scratch Disease

Cat-scratch disease is caused by the Gram-negative rod *Bartonella henselae,* that may produce an array of ocular manifestations in the fundus, which include optic neuritis associated with macular detachment and focal retinitis with or without vascular occlusion. Resolution of the inflammatory lesion with radial or stellate lipid precipitation in the macula (and vitreous) is characteristic of the course of this disease.

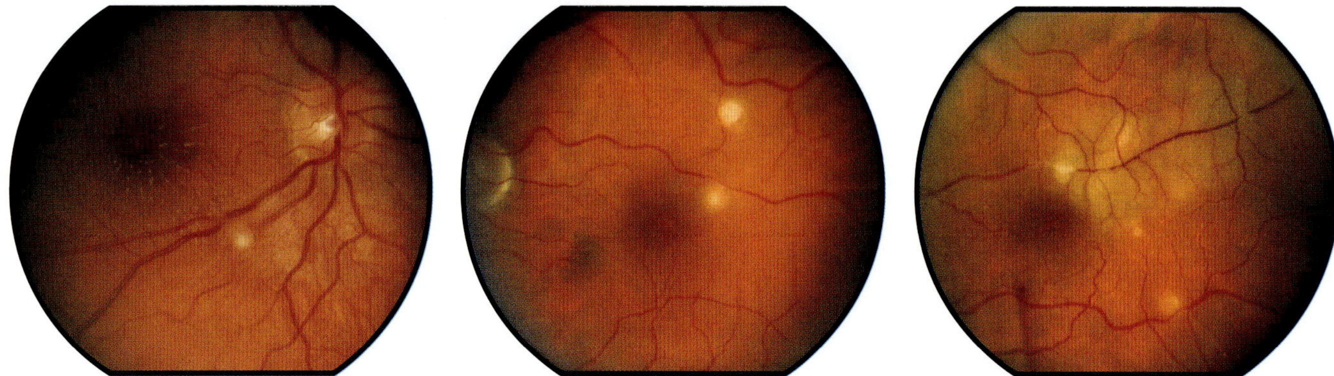

These patients have a focal retinitis from *Bartonella* infection. The retinitis can occur at an arteriole *(left)* or at multifocal sites *(middle)*. A retinal arteriolar occlusion may complicate the focal retinitis, producing whitening of the retina due to obstruction of the vessel *(right)*. *Courtesy of Dr. Emmett Cunningham*

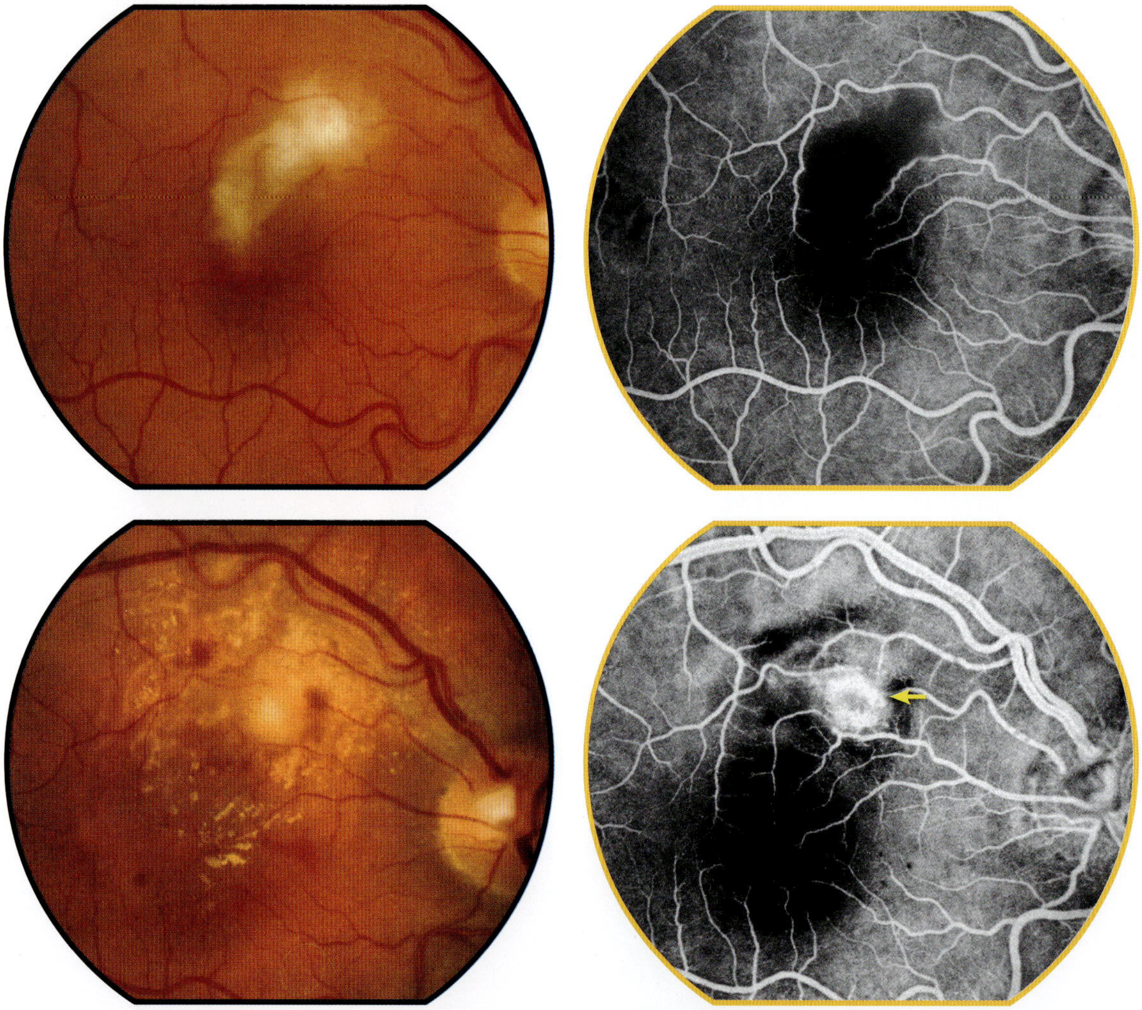

This patient with *Bartonella* had a focal retinitis at an arteriole, resulting in a retinal arteriolar occlusion *(upper left).* The FA shows blockage from the whitening of the retina and non-perfusion *(upper right).* A stellate exudative maculopathy developed. As the process resolved, there was reperfusion but staining of the infectious site on FA *(arrow).* In time, there was resolution of the acute inflammatory and ischemic changes, as well as a reperfusion of the obstructed vessels.

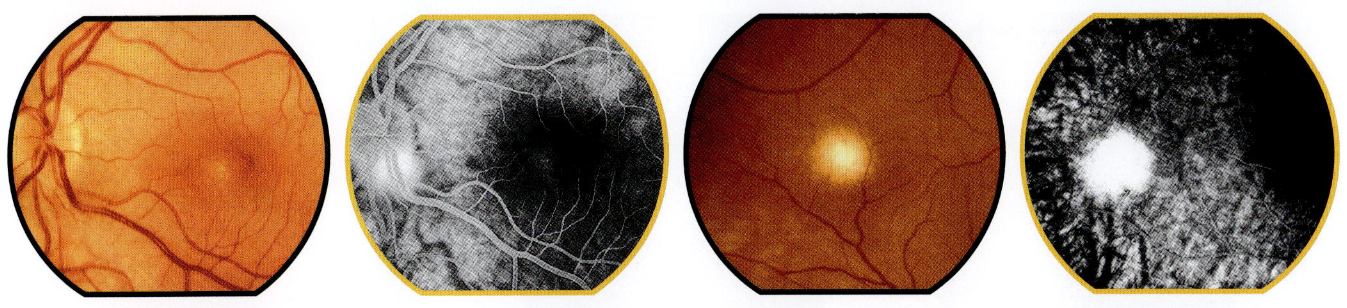

This patient with *Bartonella* had a disturbance of the vision in the left eye. Note that there is mild inflammation of the inferotemporal aspect of the nerve that stains with FA *(second from left)*. In the fellow eye, there is a focal choroidal infectious lesion with exudative detachment. This lesion also stains with FA *(right)*. *Left two images courtesy of Dr. Thomas Aaberg*

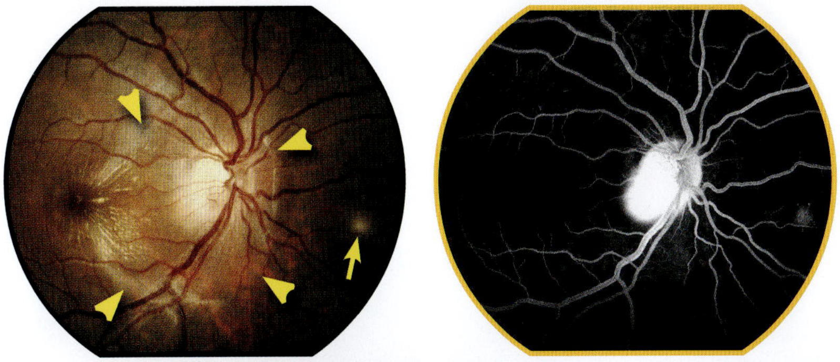

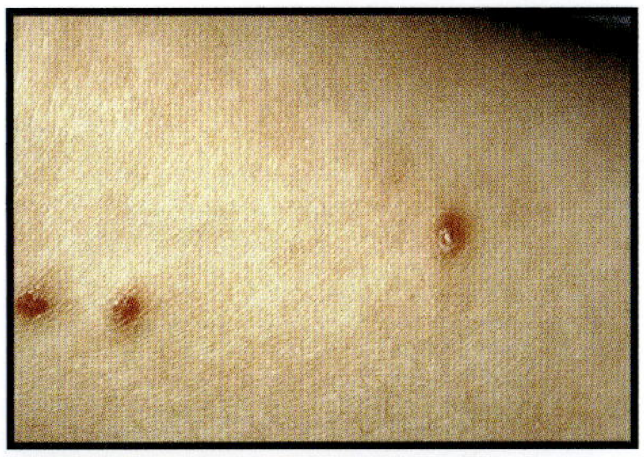

Courtesy of Dr. John Gittenger Jr

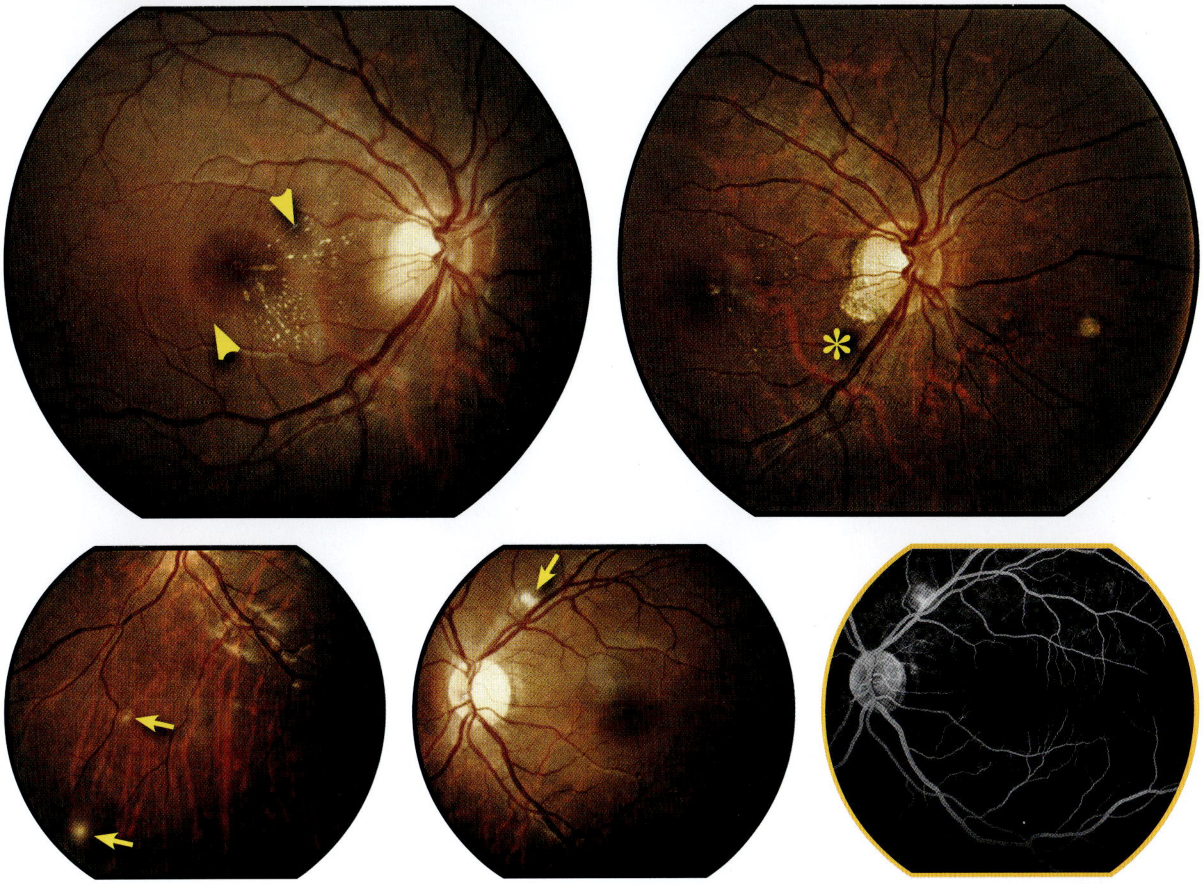

This patient presented with a bilateral *Bartonella* infection. In the right eye, there is a papillitis with a peripapillary exudative detachment and evidence of radial lipid precipitation *(arrowheads, top left)*. The FA shows staining of the optic nerve *(top row, middle)*. A focal retinitis in the nasal juxtapapillary area *(arrow, top left)* that stains with fluorescein was also noted. Over a period of 3 months, there was resolution of the detachment but a mild degree of lipid persisted *(arrowheads, middle row)*. The optic nerve inflammation was associated with subsequent fibrotic change *(asterisk)*. The focal retinitis left a small atrophic scar nasal to the disc. In the fellow left eye, a multifocal retinitis was noted *(arrows, bottom)*. The FA showed staining of the retinal lesions after the acute inflammation resolved. This patient also had multiple skin lesions *(top right)* that appeared vascular in nature. *Courtesy of Dr. J. Arch McNamara*

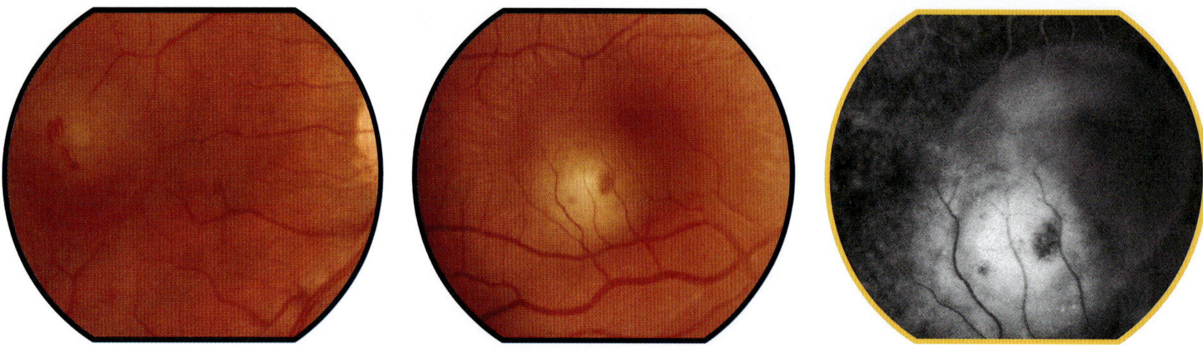

This patient with *Bartonella* infection demonstrates a focal area of choroiditis with spot retinal hemorrhages and exudative detachment of the macula. The lesion and the detachment stain with fluorescein.

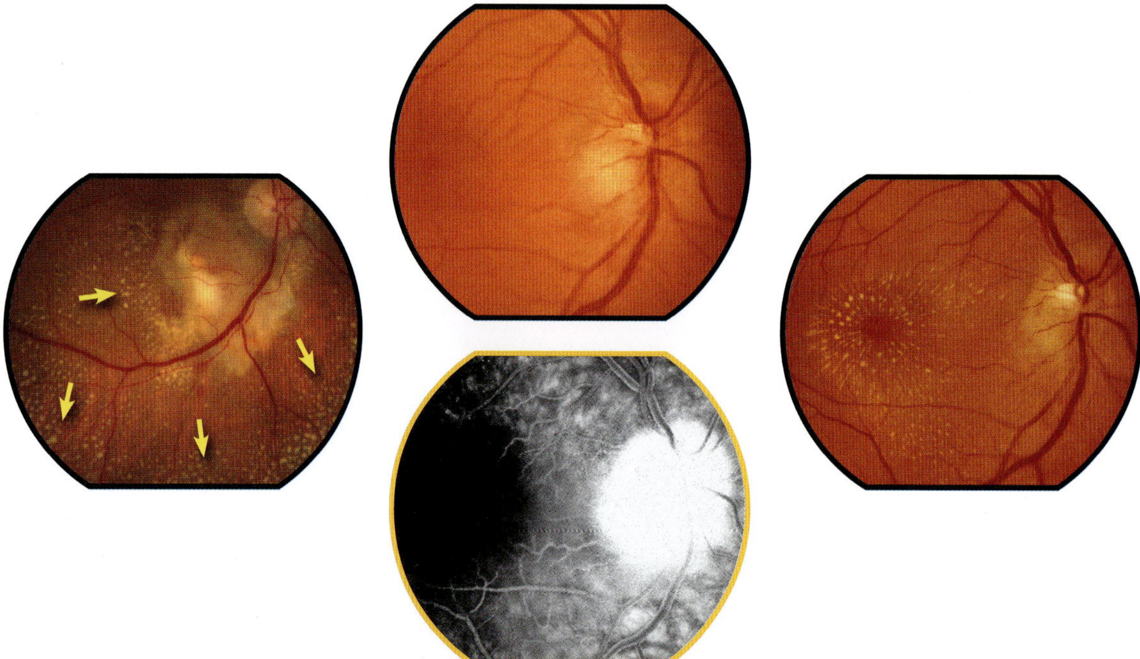

This patient illustrates a focal choroiditis from a *Bartonella* infection. There is an exudative detachment, which has gravitated inferiorly. In its resolving state, lipid precipitation has also diffused into the overlying vitreous as well as the subretinal space *(arrows)*. The second case *(middle and right images)* illustrates an inferotemporal juxtapapillary chorioretinal lesion with diffuse disc leakage on FA and subsequent lipid precipitation with a macular star.

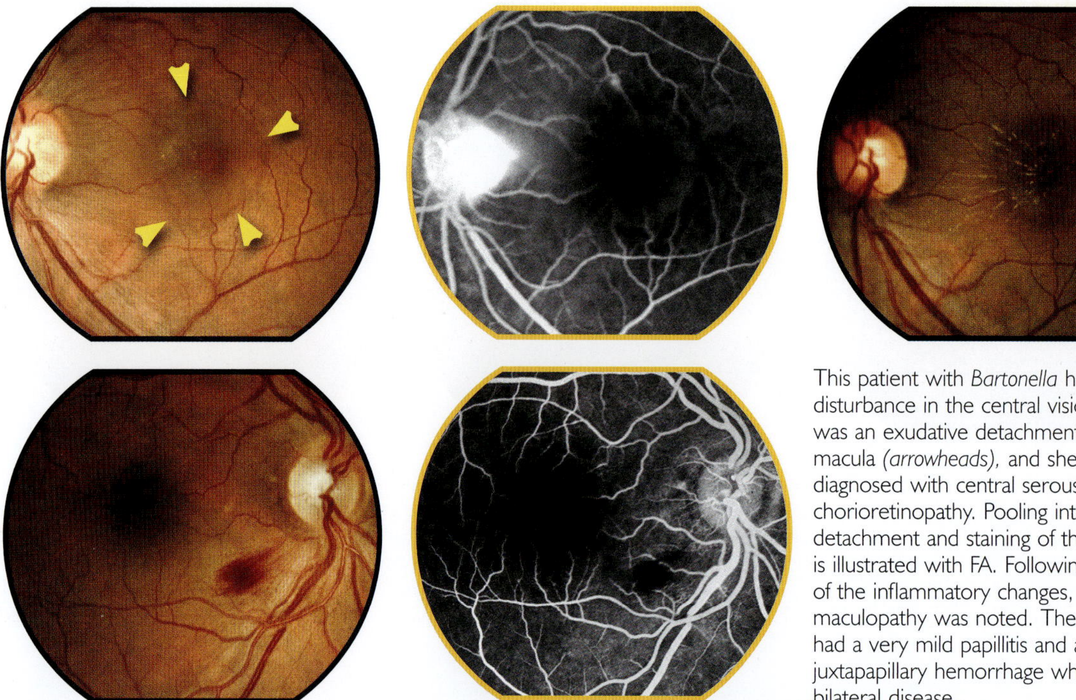

This patient with *Bartonella* had a vague disturbance in the central vision. There was an exudative detachment of the macula *(arrowheads)*, and she was diagnosed with central serous chorioretinopathy. Pooling into the macular detachment and staining of the optic nerve is illustrated with FA. Following resolution of the inflammatory changes, a stellate lipid maculopathy was noted. The fellow eye had a very mild papillitis and a juxtapapillary hemorrhage which indicated bilateral disease.

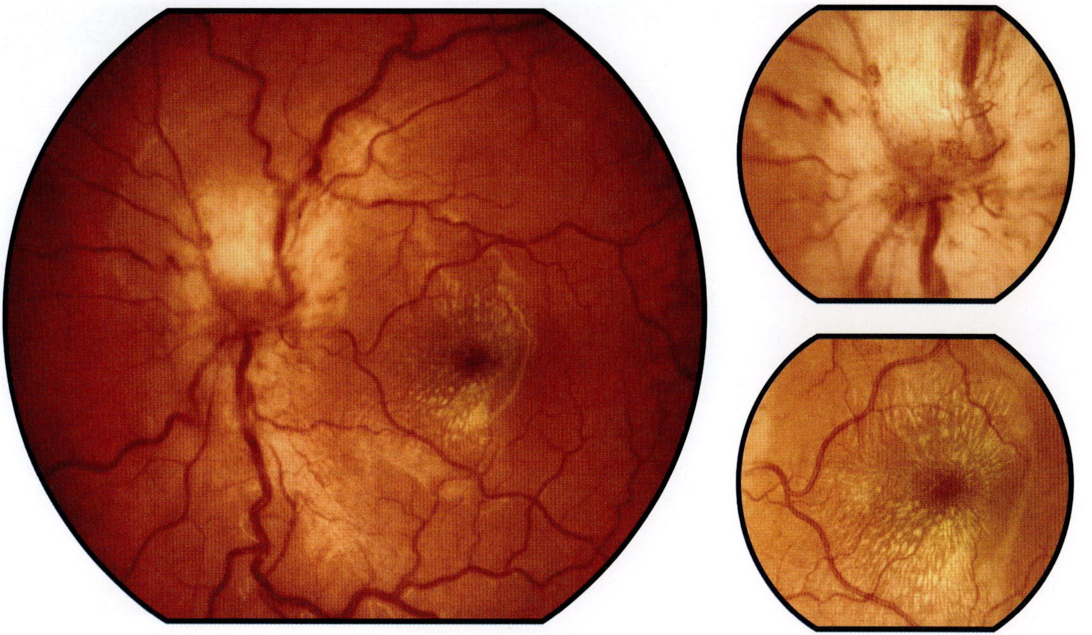

This patient with *Bartonella* had an infection of the nerve and juxtapapillary choroid. As the infection resolved, lipid precipitation in the macula developed *(left and bottom right)*. Typical of the disease, there is a coincidental anomalous retinal vessel. *Left image courtesy of Dr. John M. Gittenger*

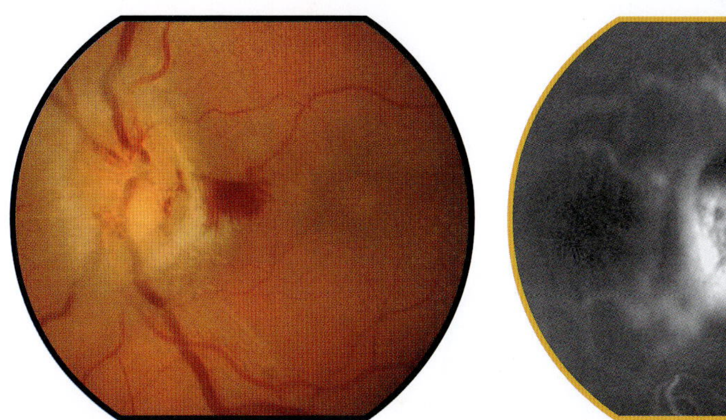

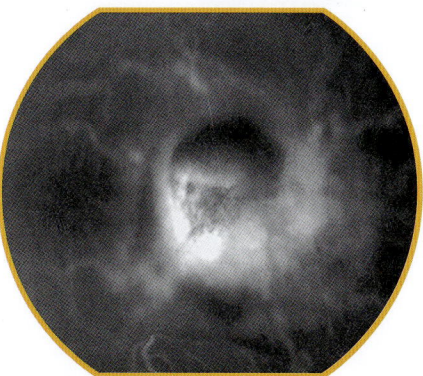

Note the papillitis and juxtapapillary hemorrhage in this patient. There is fluorescein staining and leakage surrounding the optic nerve. *Right image courtesy of Dr. Michael Cooney and Dr. Sunil Srivastava*

The histopathology shows *Bartonella* and associated inflammatory cells.

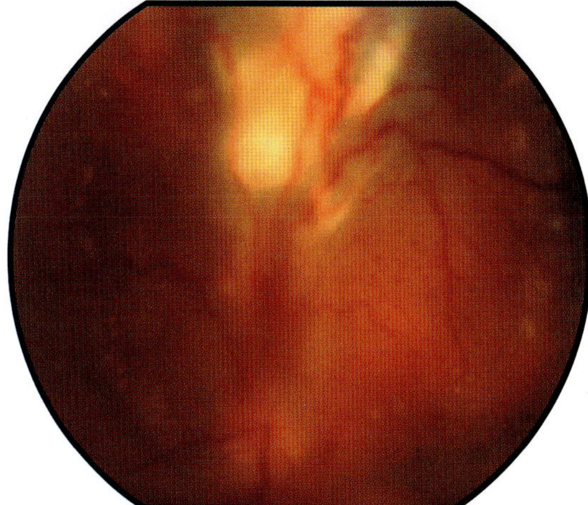

This patient with *Bartonella* infection presented with severe chorioretinal infiltration with overlying retinal vasculitis, hemorrhage, and retinal detachment. Inflammatory cells are noted in the vitreous. *Courtesy of Dr. Mark Hatfield*

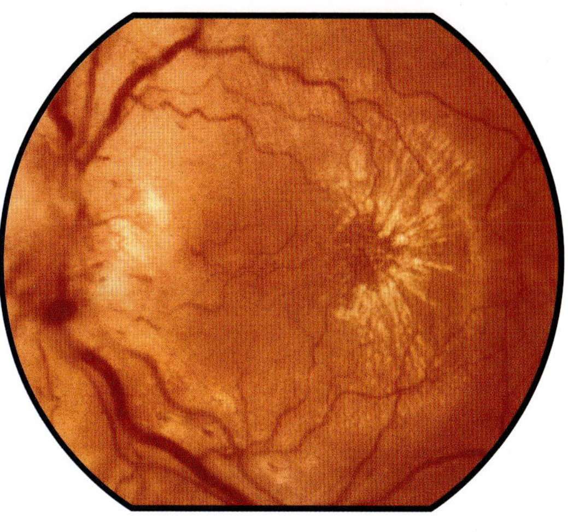

This patient has a resolving *Bartonella* infection with papillitis, peripapillary detachment, and precipitating lipid exudation in a radial pattern in the macula.

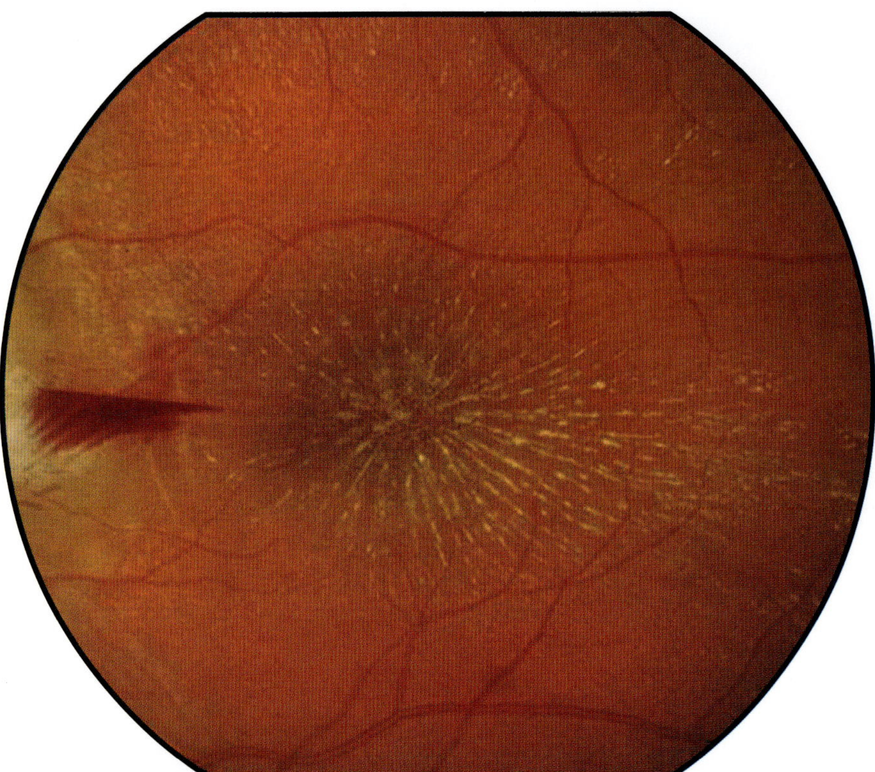

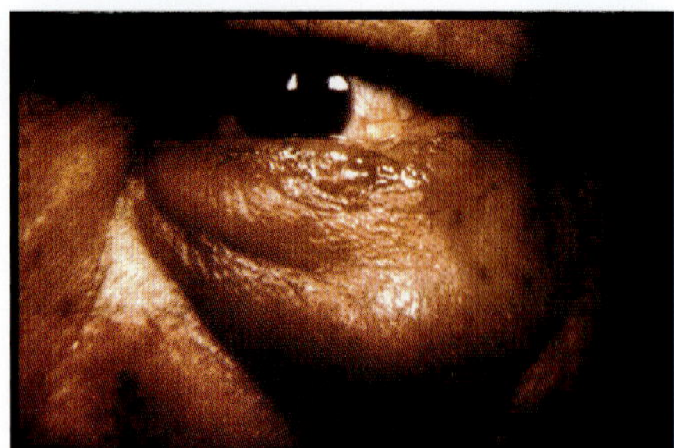

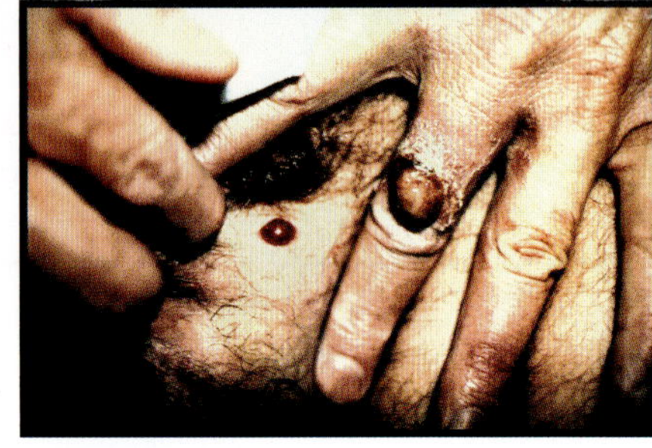

These patients have bacillary granulomatosis, which is seen in patients with AIDS who develop a *Bartonella* infection. *Courtesy of Dr. Murray Meltzer*

The characteristic stellate lipid maculopathy is nicely illustrated in this *Bartonella* patient.

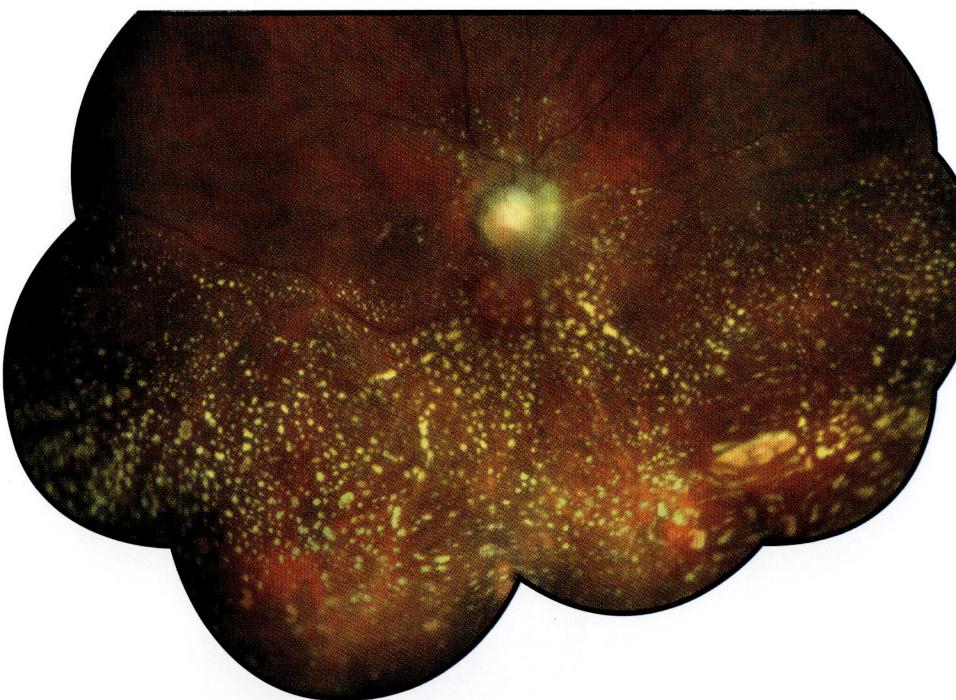

Extensive lipid exudate has precipitated into the inferior vitreous cavity as the inflammatory process has improved in this case of *Bartonella* infection causing optic neuritis. *Courtesy of Ophthalmic Imaging Systems, Inc*

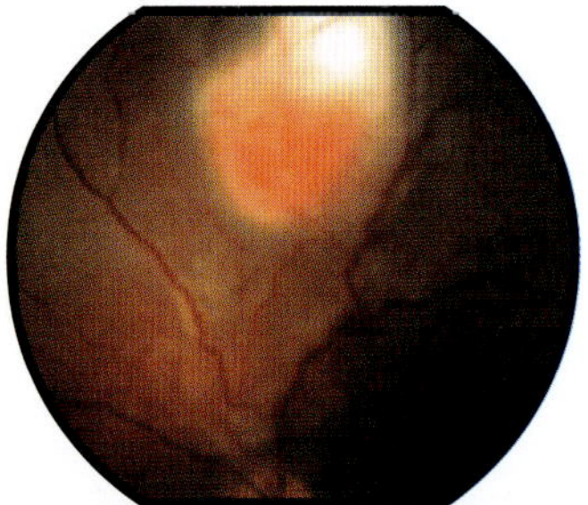

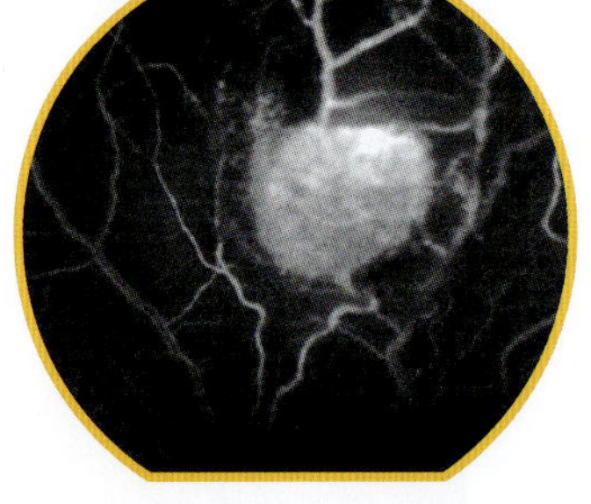

This patient demonstrates reddish orange mass lesion superior to the disc. The FA shows a vascular component to the lesion with late staining and an associated microvasculopathy. This case demonstrates the angiomatous nature of the infectious process in *Bartonella*. *Courtesy of Dr. Mark Hatfield*

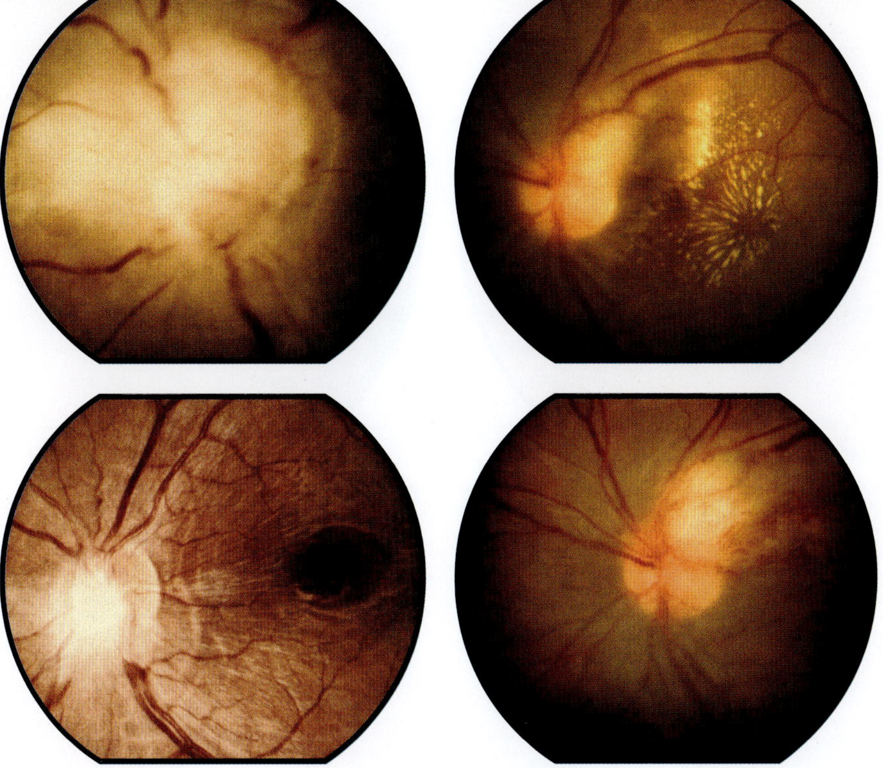

Bartonella infection with an optic neuritis is present in these patients *(top row)*. Note the infiltrated nerve head and the prominent vessels. Stellate lipid maculopathy is seen with resolution of the infection. As the infection continues to resolve, the macular exudate clears, the nerve becomes more discernible and distinct at its margins, and fibrous scarring can develop over the disc *(lower row)*. *Courtesy of Dr. Michael Cooney and Dr. Sunil Srivastava*

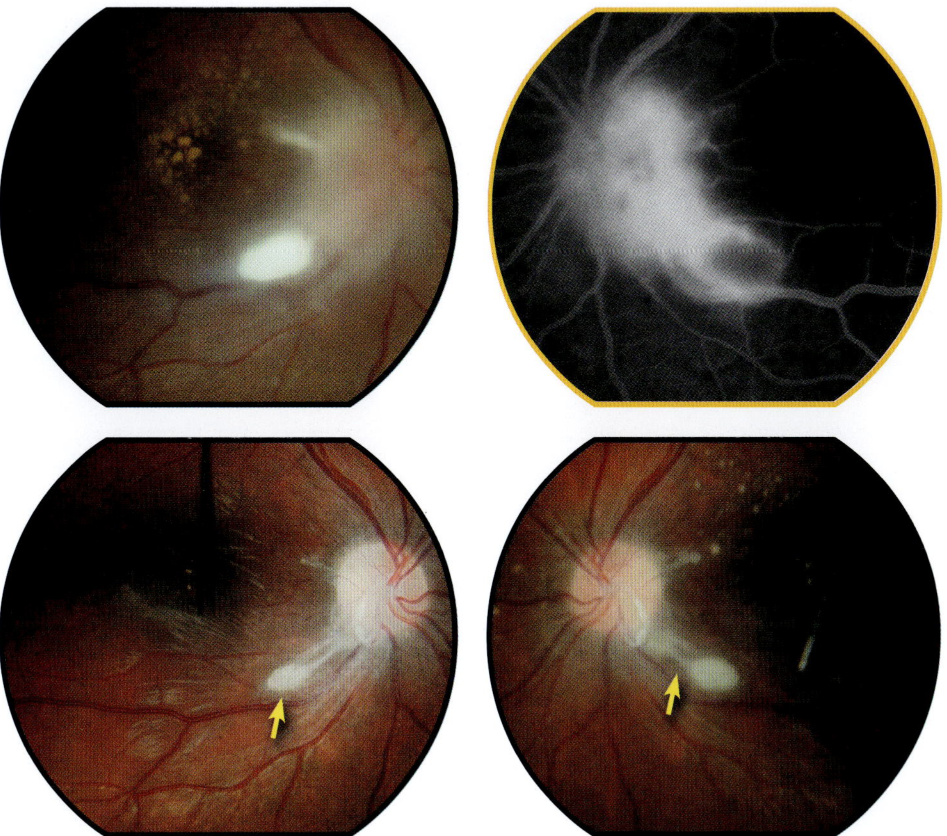

This patient had bilateral *Bartonella* optic neuritis with juxtapapillary choroidal involvement. The FA shows staining of the optic nerve and of the peripapillary retinal vasculature and choroid. As the process resolved, fibrous proliferation around the disc developed and extended into the macular region *(arrows)*. *Courtesy of Dr. Richard Hamilton*

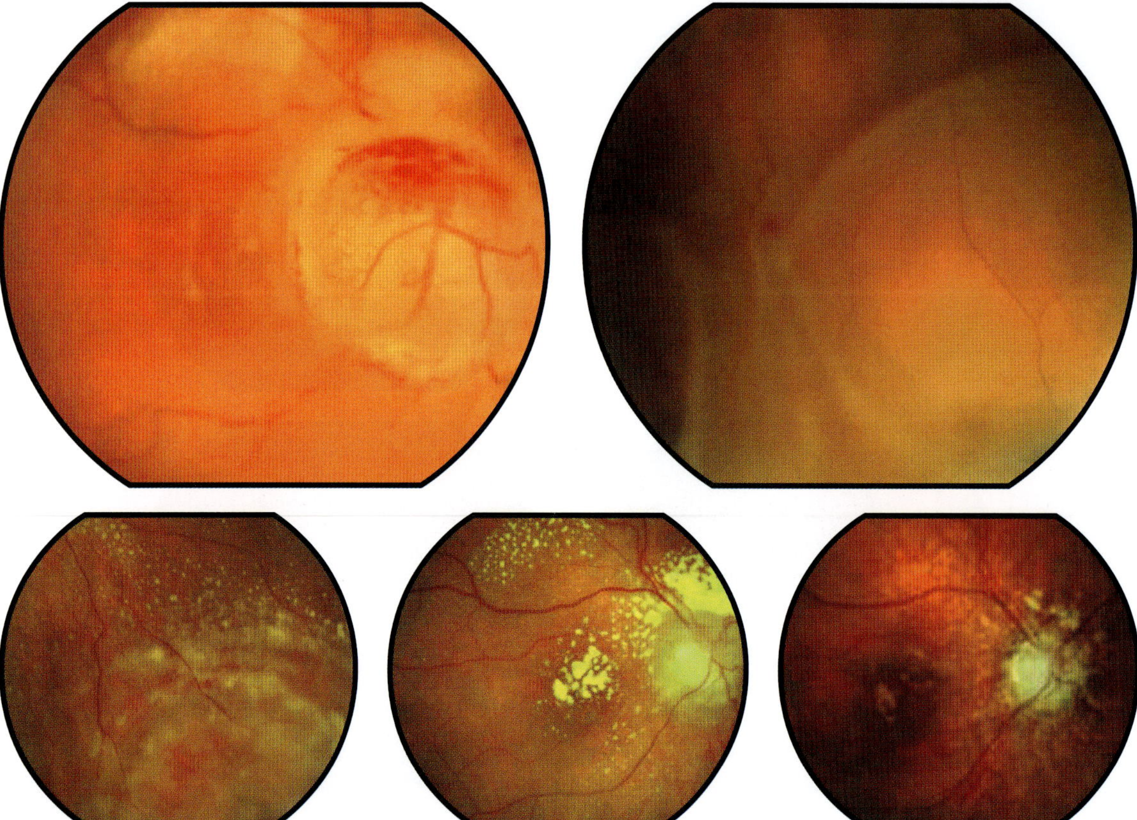

This patient illustrates a mass lesion at the disc with overlying hemorrhage and surrounding exudation from a *Bartonella* infection *(upper left)*. A gravitational exudative retinal detachment was present that was bullous in nature *(upper right)*. Eventually, the detachment began to resolve, taking on a turbid consistency *(lower left)*. In the posterior pole, lipid precipitation in the macula is noted *(lower middle)*. Eventually, the exudate cleared *(lower right)*, but persistent atrophy of the nerve is identified. *Courtesy of Dr. Sunil Srivastava*

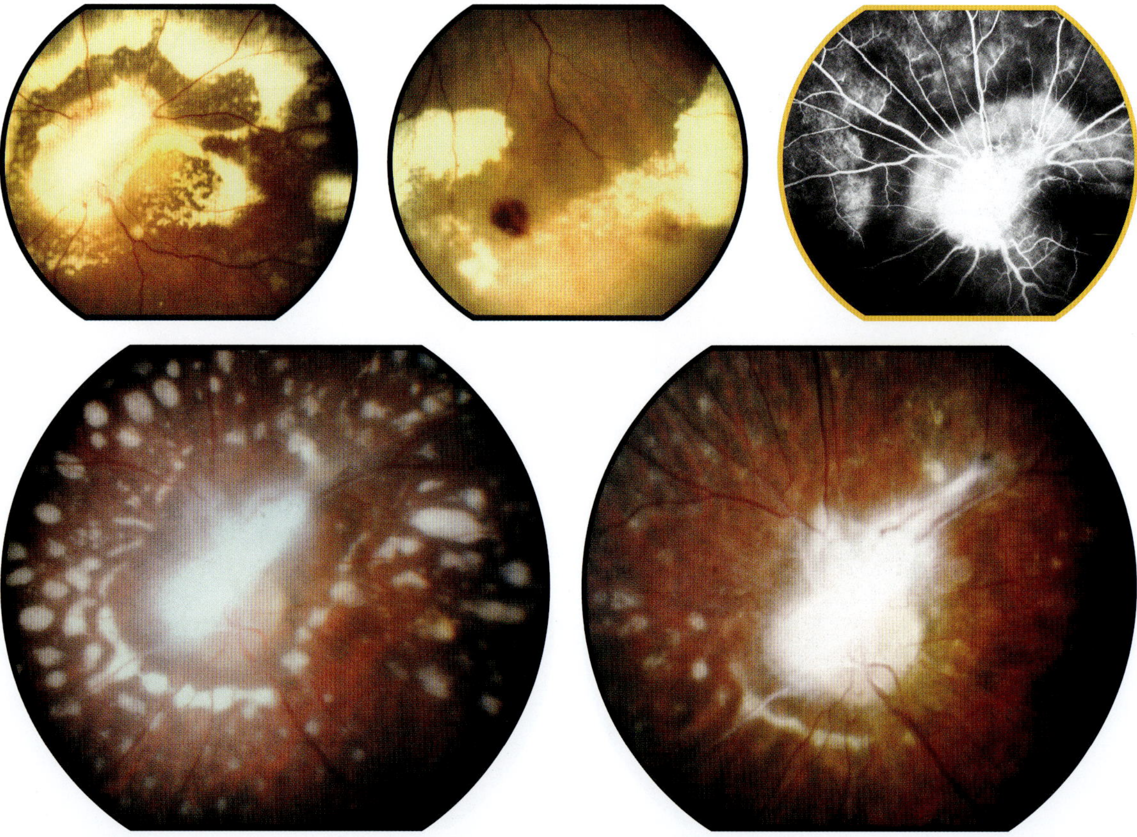

Note the huge mass lesion at the disc with circinate lipid exudation and a dependent retinal detachment in this patient with *Bartonella* infection. With resolution of macular exudation, multifocal areas of lipid globules precipitated into the overlying vitreous. In time, the exudation resolved, but there was fibrous proliferation at and contiguous with the nerve and optic atrophy *(lower right)*.

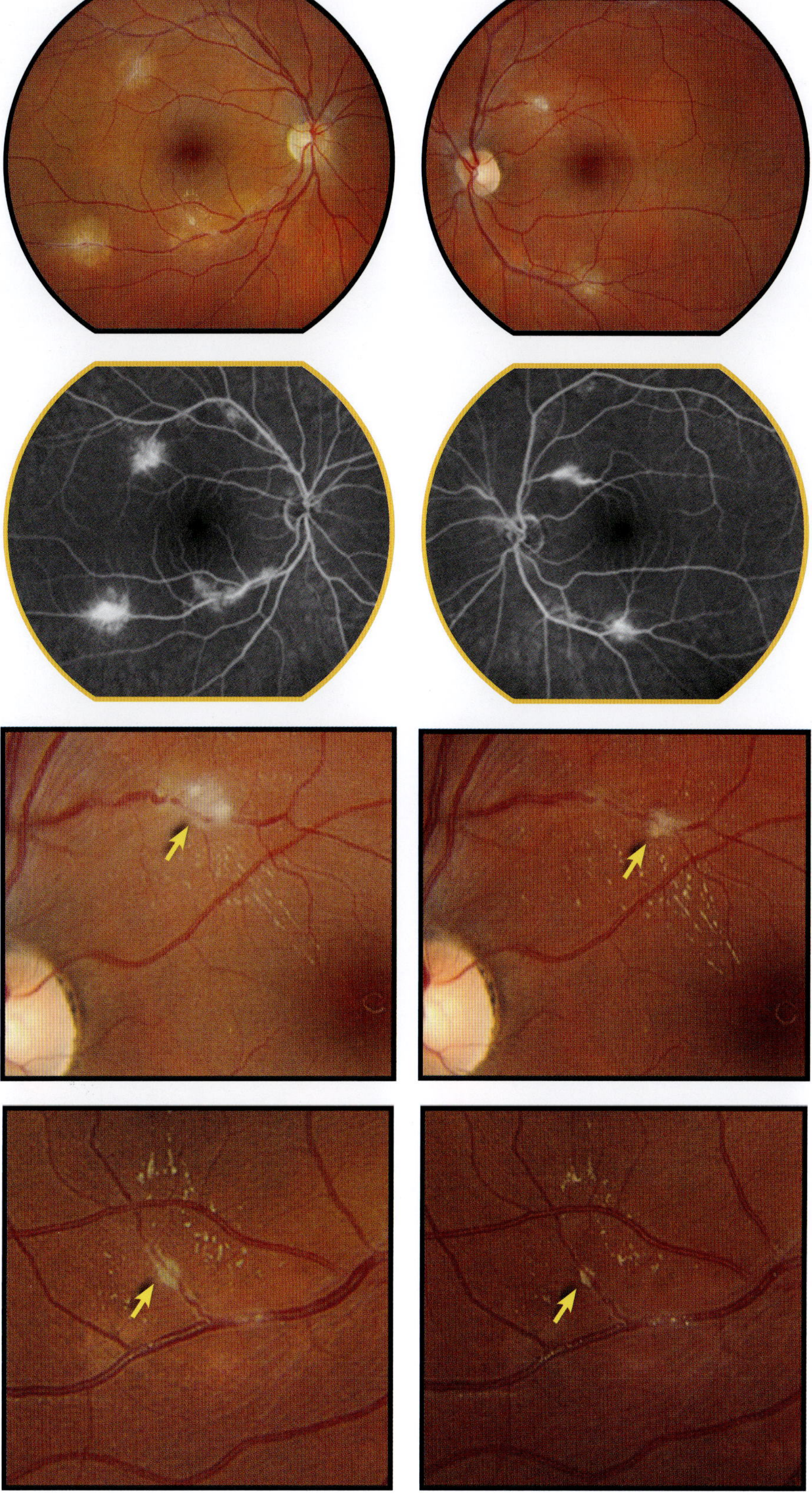

Bilateral focal retinal phlebitis from *Bartonella* is illustrated *(top row)*. FA shows leakage bilaterally in the areas of the phlebitis. High magnification color photos *(third and fourth rows)* show phlebitis *(arrows)* pre- and post-systemic doxycycline therapy *(right photos post treatment). Courtesy of Dr. Emmett T. Cunningham*

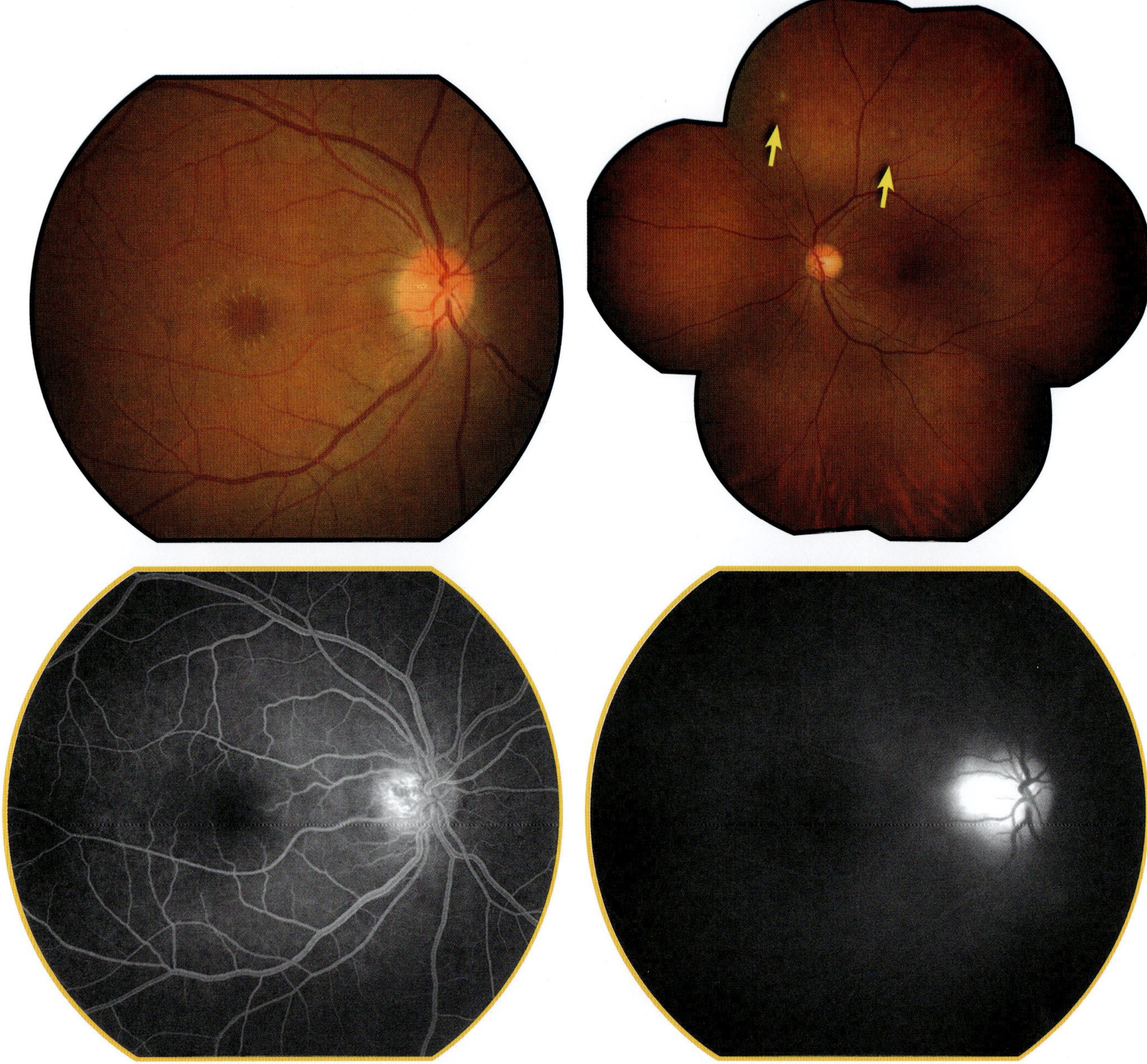

This patient presented with *Bartonella* neuroretinitis of the right eye. The top photo illustrates the characteristic stellate lipid maculopathy or "macular star" along with temporal optic disc edema. The color montage of left eye illustrates several retinal infiltrates in the mid-periphery (*arrows*). FA demonstrates late leakage of the optic disc.

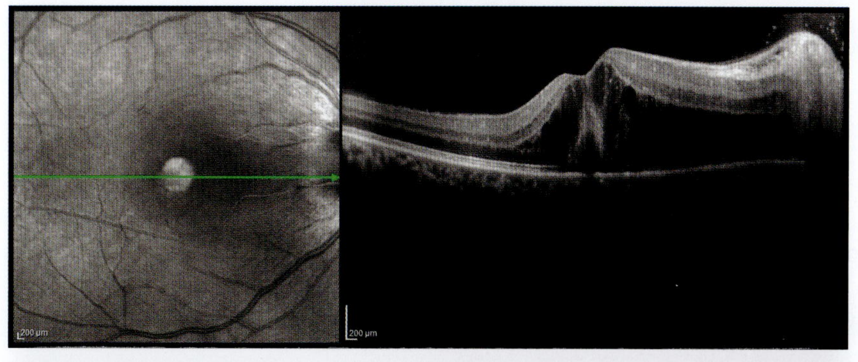

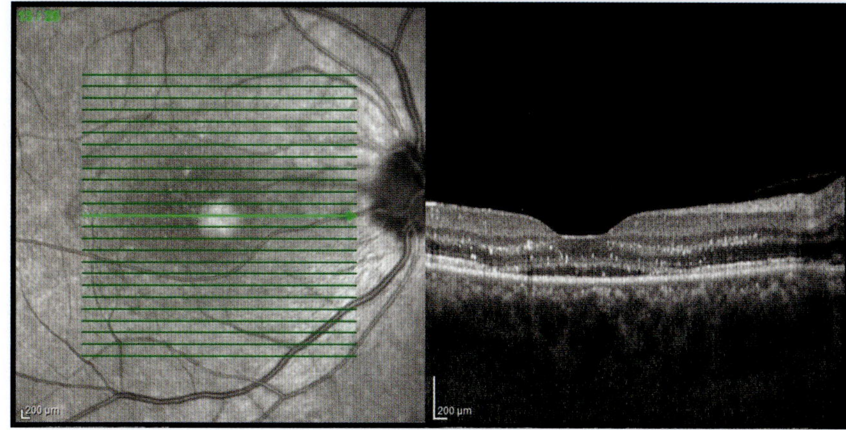

OCT of the macula (*top*), from the same patient, illustrates severe cystoid macular edema (CME). The lipid maculopathy, disc edema, and CME on OCT (*bottom*) significantly improved with systemic antibiotic therapy.

Spirochetes
Syphilis

Syphilis has recently emerged again as a global public health problem. The causative agent of syphilis is *Treponema pallidum*, a member of the family Spirochaetaceae. It is transmitted predominantly through sexual contact but also through blood or contact with an infected lesion. Classic stages include primary, secondary, and tertiary syphilis. The latter may include the neurosyphilis stage.

Ocular syphilis is considered equivalent to neurosyphilis. The posterior segment manifestations include vitritis, retinal vasculitis, focal or placoid outer retinal infiltrate (or acute syphilitic posterior placoid chorioretinitis), multifocal retinitis or superficial retinal infiltrates, and optic neuritis.

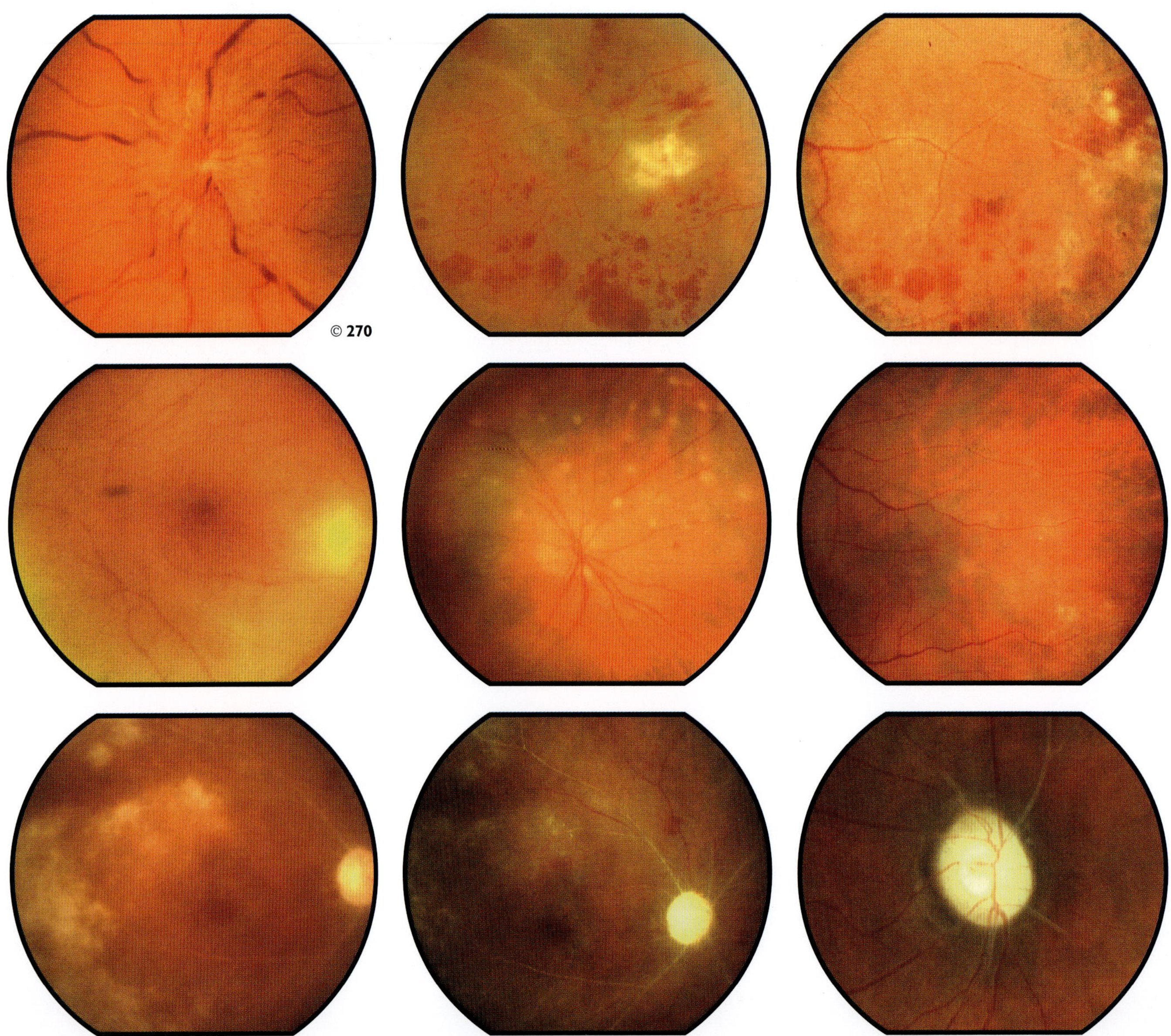

Syphilis can produce a myriad of changes in the fundus, which mimic virtually any inflammatory or infectious disease. Note the presence of phlebitis and papillitis *(top left)*. Retinal and vitreous hemorrhage *(top middle and right)* are also illustrated. Vitritis *(middle left)* and multifocal retinitis *(middle center)*, and a variable degree of retinal opacification and optic atrophy *(lower left)* are all noted in these cases. Note the severe optic atrophy and retinal vascular sheathing seen in these patients presenting with very poor vision *(lower middle and right)*.

Acute Syphilitic Posterior Placoid Chorioretinitis

In syphilis, there may be a zonal area of outer retinitis and pigment epitheliitis.

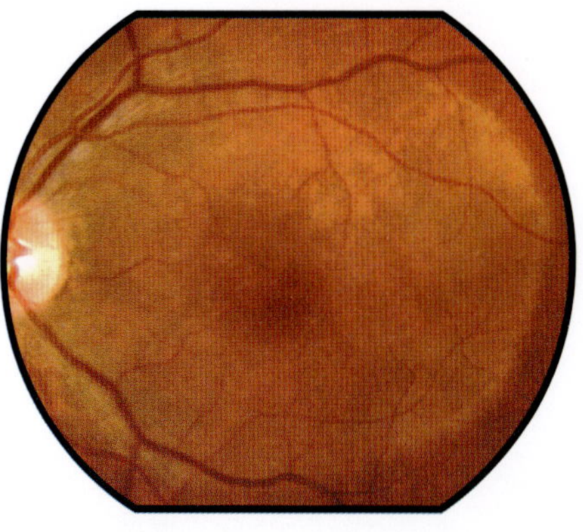
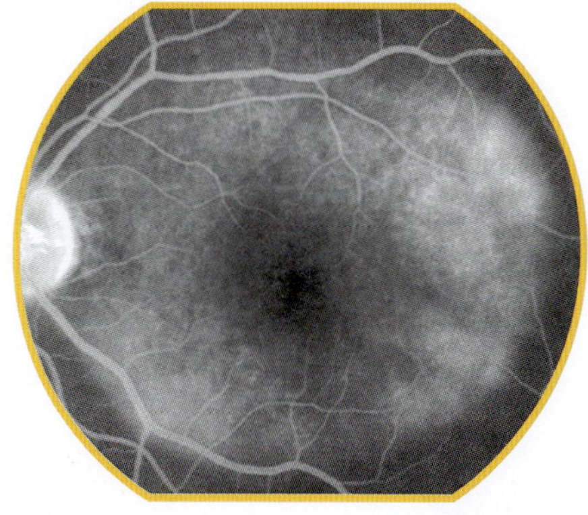
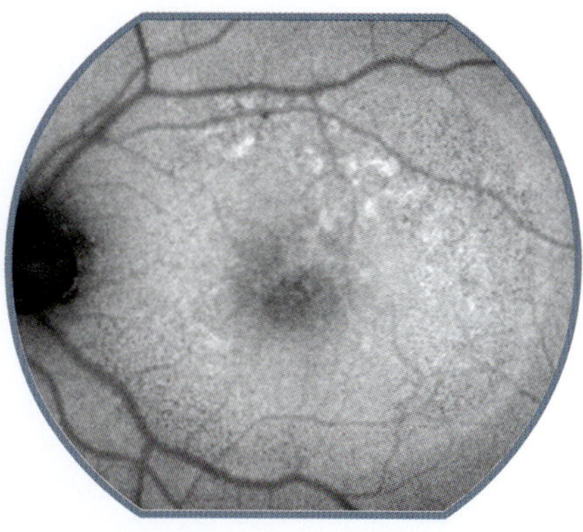

In this patient, there is an outer placoid retinitis (i.e. acute syphilitic posterior placoid chorioretinitis) and pigment epitheliitis. Note the white placoid lesion extending in an ovoid fashion through the fovea. The FA shows staining of the outer retina and pigment epithelium especially at the border of the placoid lesion. The fundus autofluorescence shows patchy hyperautofluorescence from accumulation of cellular debris in the subretinal space and pigment epithelium.

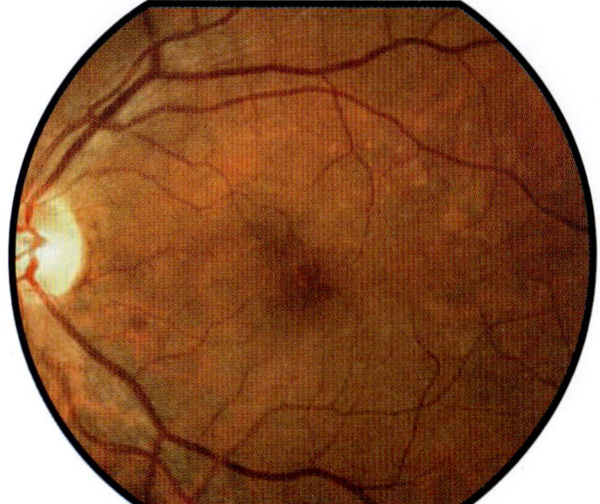
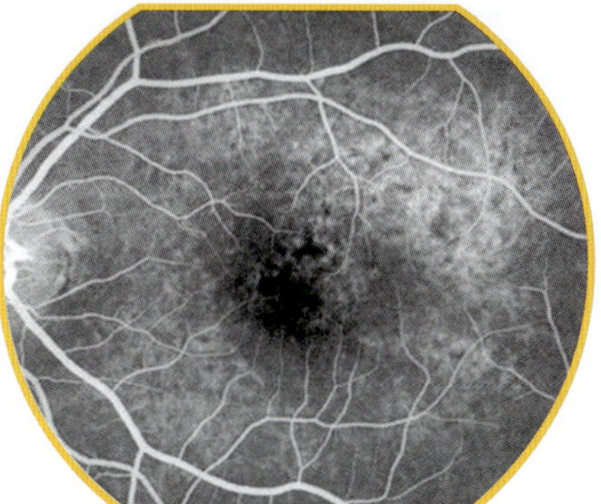
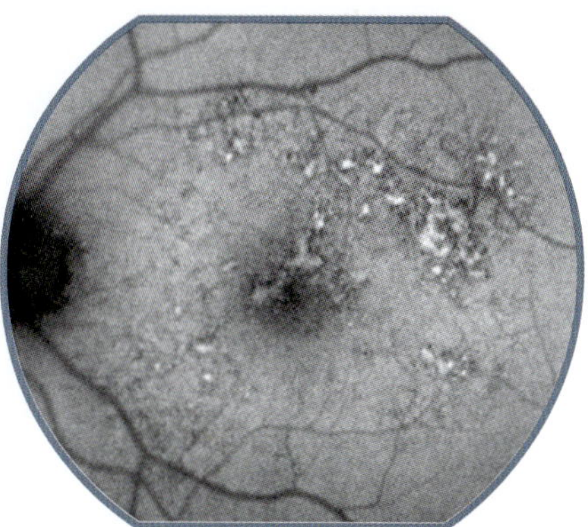

Following treatment, this patient experienced pigment epithelial atrophy and mottling, that is more dramatically evident on the FA. The placoid whitening resolved. The fundus autofluorescence shows irregular hyperautofluorescence, characteristic of the resolving stage of this inflammation. The hyperautofluorescent areas may resolve uneventfully or may become associated with pigment epithelial and photoreceptor atrophy.

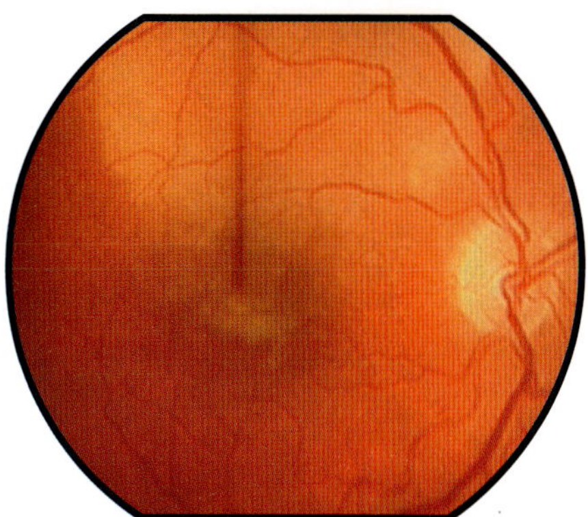
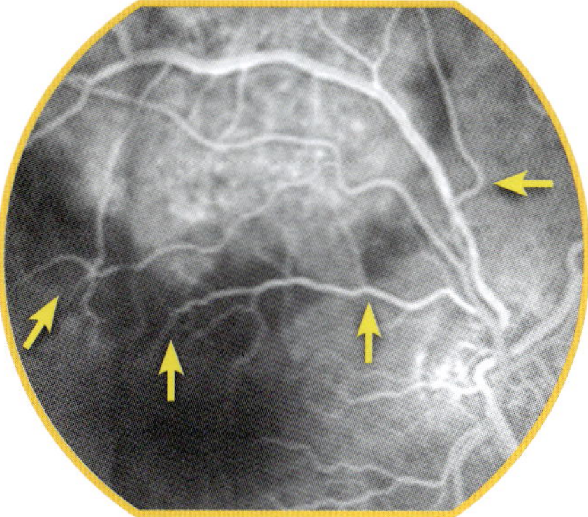
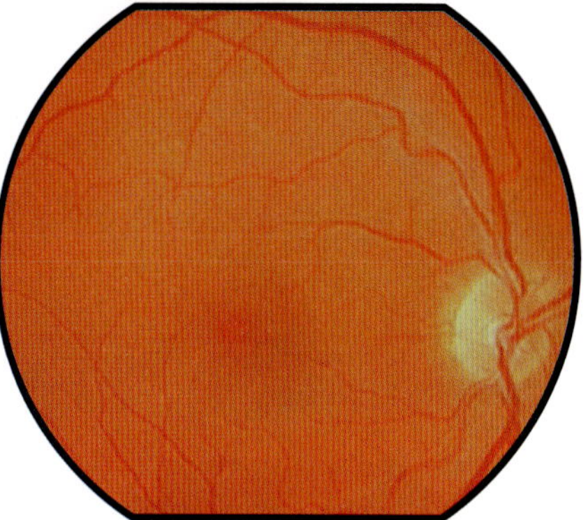

This patient has acute outer placoid retinitis and pigment epitheliitis (i.e. acute syphilitic posterior placoid chorioretinitis) as seen on the left as a zonular area of outer retinal whitening. The FA shows a curvilinear area of hypofluorescence bordering the inferior margin of the placoid lesion *(arrows)* and correlating with exudative detachment of the retina. Following treatment, all of these findings resolved, except for mild pigment epithelial atrophy and mottling in the superior paramacular area. *Courtesy of Dr. Frederick Davidof*

Optic Neuritis

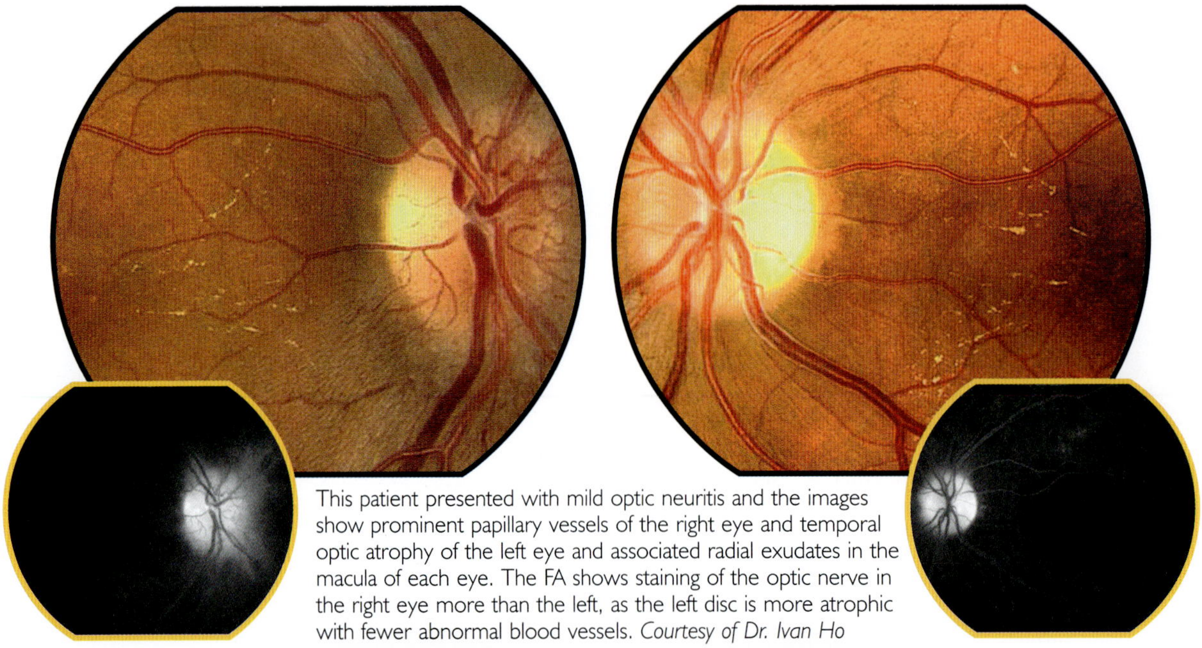

This patient presented with mild optic neuritis and the images show prominent papillary vessels of the right eye and temporal optic atrophy of the left eye and associated radial exudates in the macula of each eye. The FA shows staining of the optic nerve in the right eye more than the left, as the left disc is more atrophic with fewer abnormal blood vessels. *Courtesy of Dr. Ivan Ho*

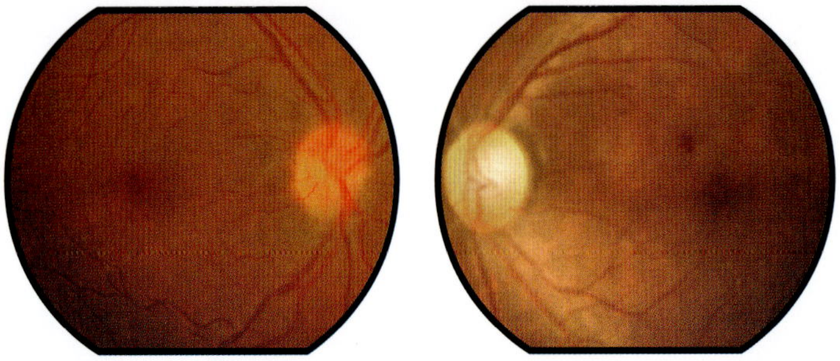

This patient demonstrates mild papillitis in the right eye and optic nerve atrophy in the left eye from chronic inflammation. There is also mild vitreous inflammation bilaterally.

Chorioretinitis

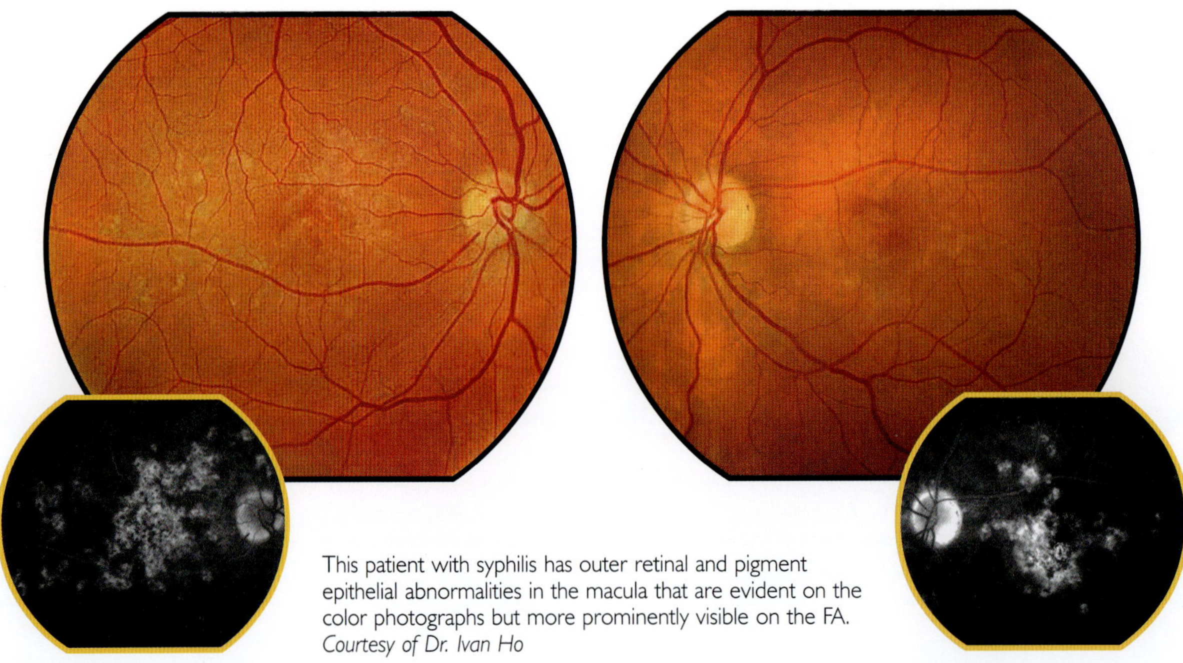

This patient with syphilis has outer retinal and pigment epithelial abnormalities in the macula that are evident on the color photographs but more prominently visible on the FA. *Courtesy of Dr. Ivan Ho*

Vasculitis

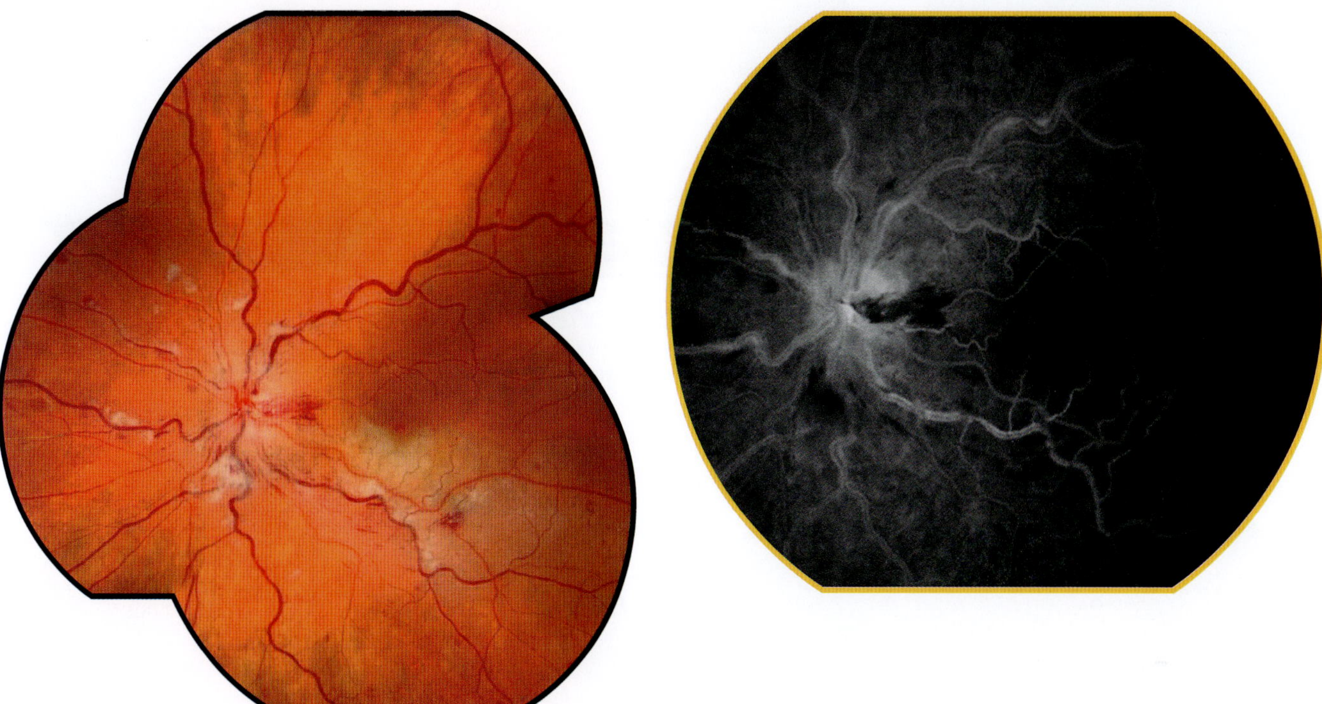

The retinal venous system is remarkably tortuous in this patient with syphilis and retinal phlebitis. Retinal ischemic whitening from an associated arteriolar occlusion is illustrated. Optic nerve edema or papillitis is also noted. *Courtesy of Dr. Ivan Ho*

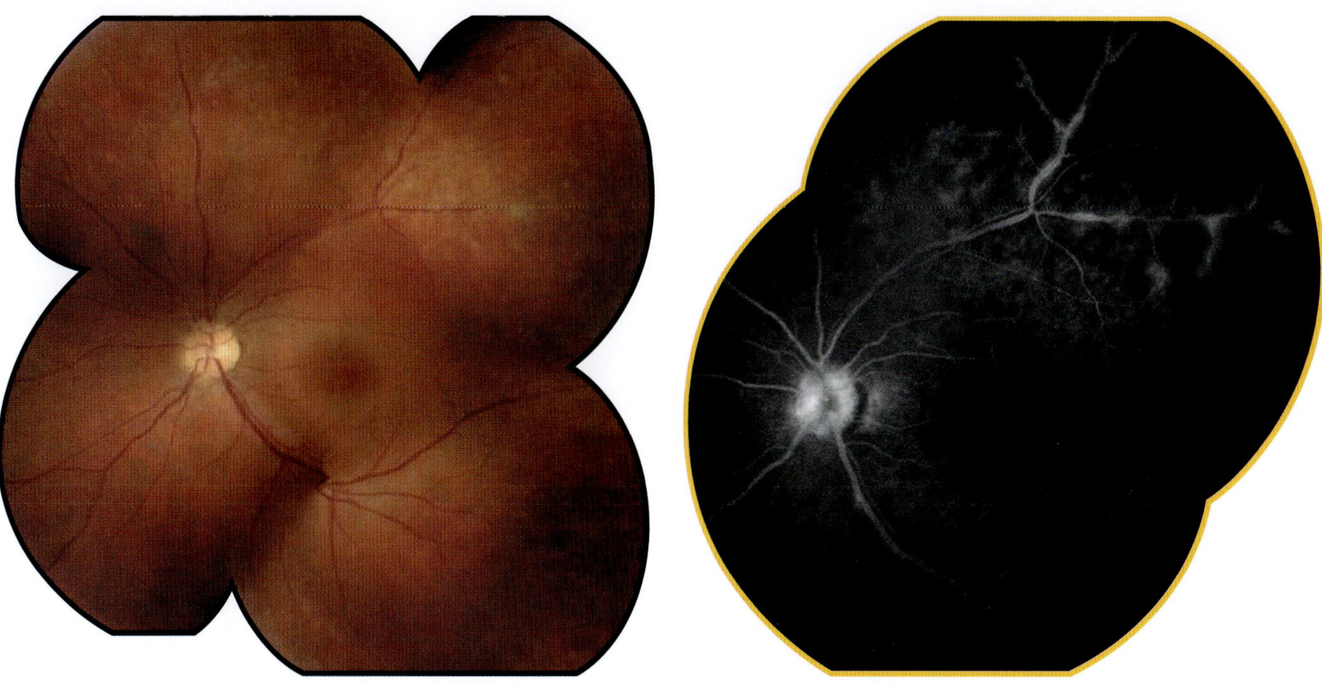

This patient with syphilis has peripheral retinal phlebitis and an optic neuritis of the left eye. Note the staining and leakage of the involved retinal vein superotemporally. *Courtesy of Dr. Ivan Ho*

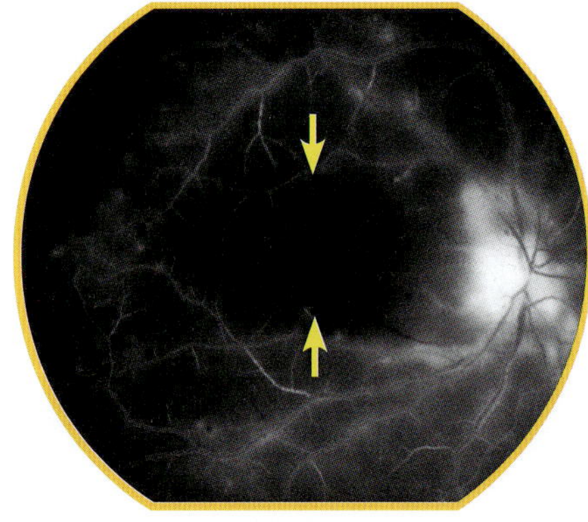

This patient illustrates a papillitis and retinal vasculitis and severe macular ischemia *(arrows)*.

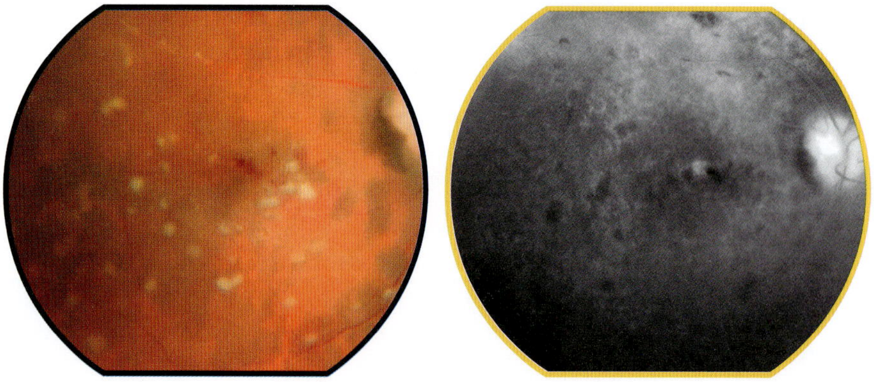

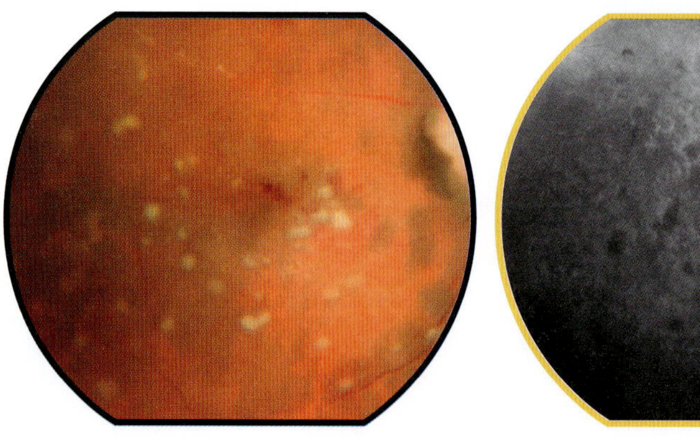

This patient illustrates multifocal retinitis associated with retinal hemorrhage and a mild papillitis due to syphilis infection. These multifocal white inflammatory lesions appear superficial and are very characteristic of a syphilitic retinal infection. *Courtesy of Dr. Ivan Batlle*

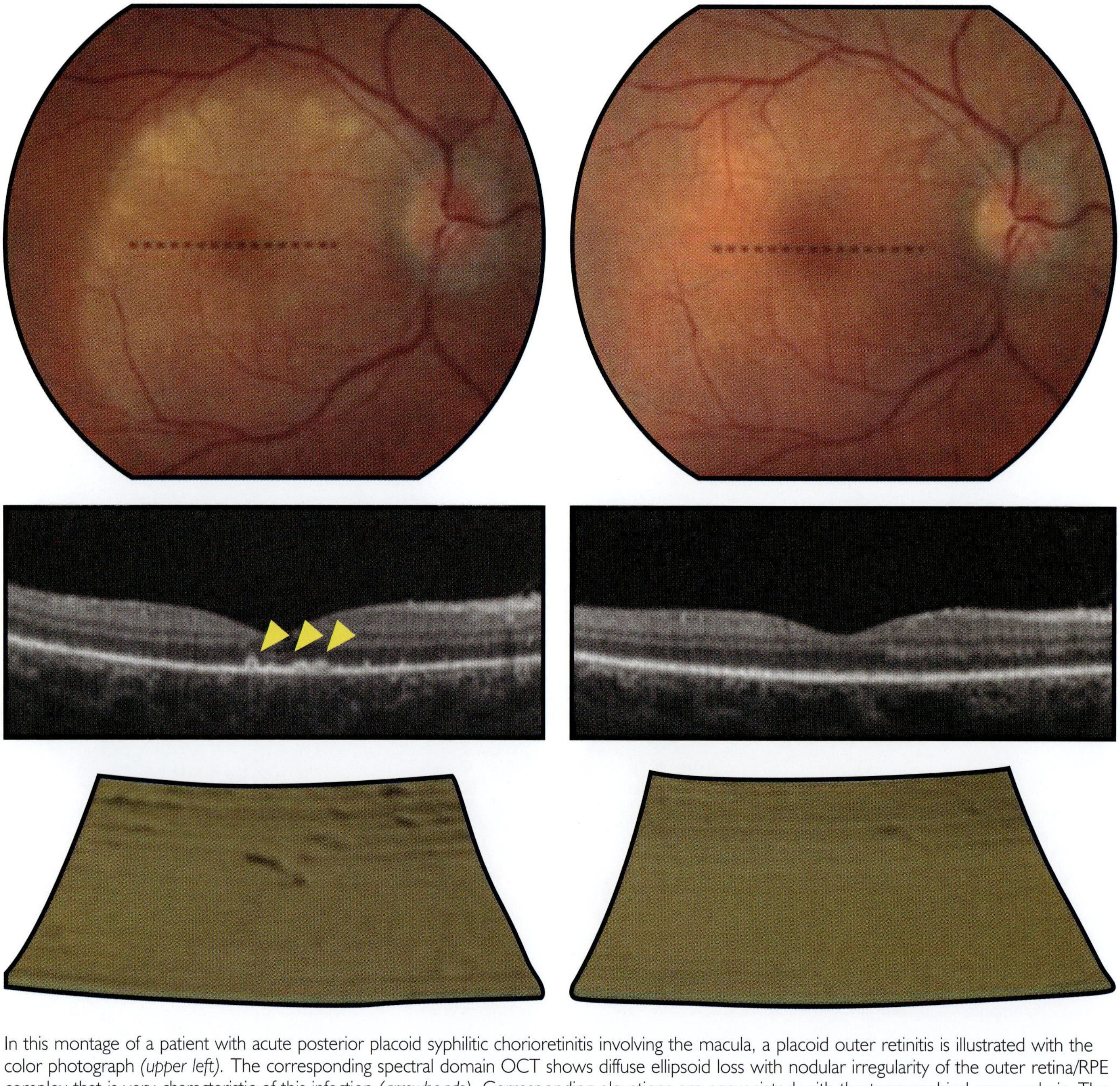

In this montage of a patient with acute posterior placoid syphilitic chorioretinitis involving the macula, a placoid outer retinitis is illustrated with the color photograph *(upper left)*. The corresponding spectral domain OCT shows diffuse ellipsoid loss with nodular irregularity of the outer retina/RPE complex that is very characteristic of this infection *(arrowheads)*. Corresponding elevations are appreciated with the topographical map analysis. The color photograph and OCT and topographic map on the right were taken 30 days after IV penicillin treatment showing resolution of the outer retinal/RPE findings. *Courtesy of Dr. Francesco Pichi*

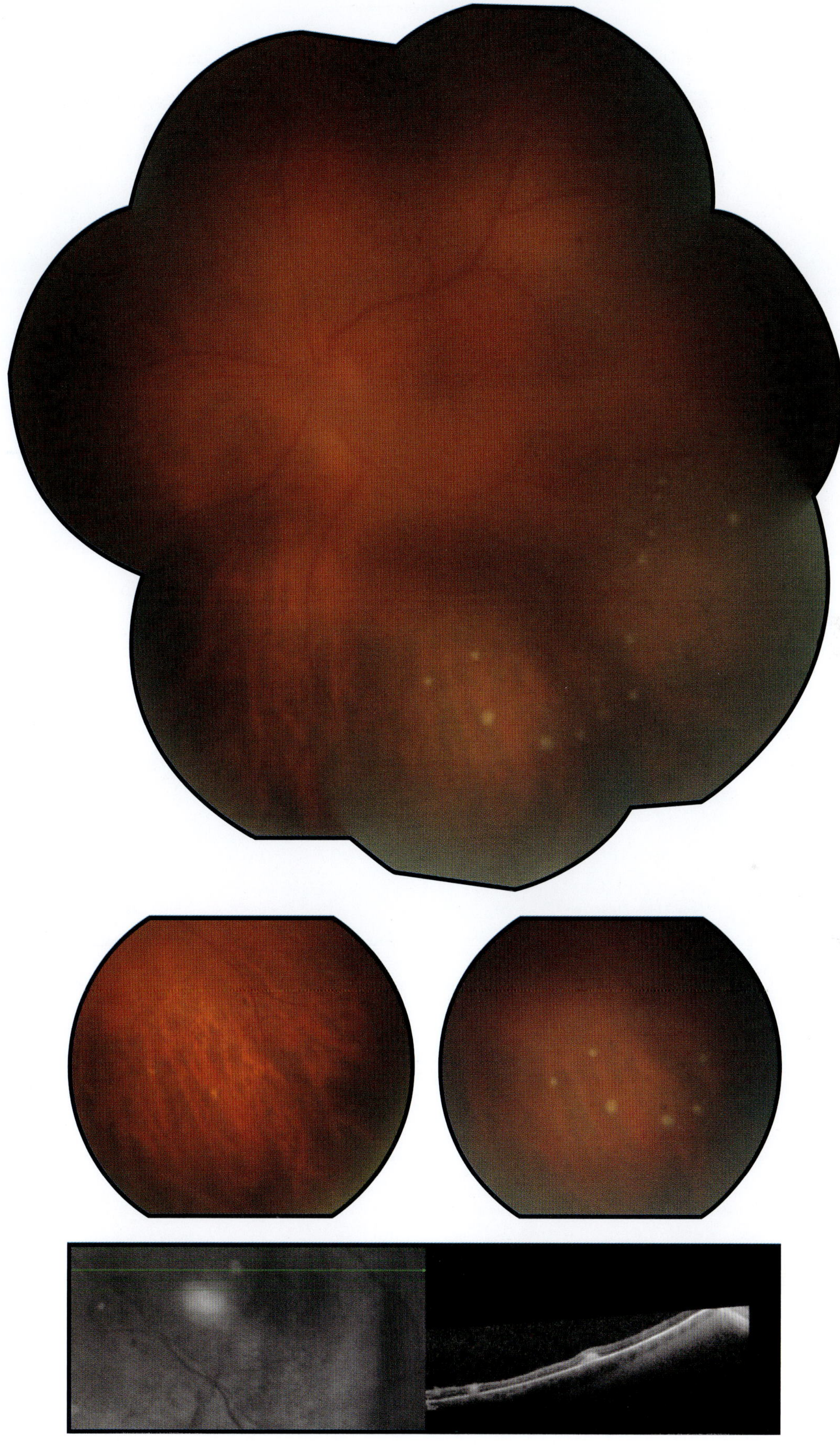

This patient presented with a panuveitis and pathognomonic multifocal retinal infiltrates secondary to syphilis infection. The middle left color fundus photo graph reveals resolution of the vitritis and multifocal retinal infiltrates after a 14-day course of IV penicillin. Spectral domain OCT imaging shows that the superficial-appearing active precipitates are located within the retina. *Courtesy of Curi AL, Sarraf D, Cunningham ET, Jr 2015. Multimodal Imaging of Syphilitic Multifocal Retinitis. Retin Cases Brief Rep. 9, 277-280*

Vitritis

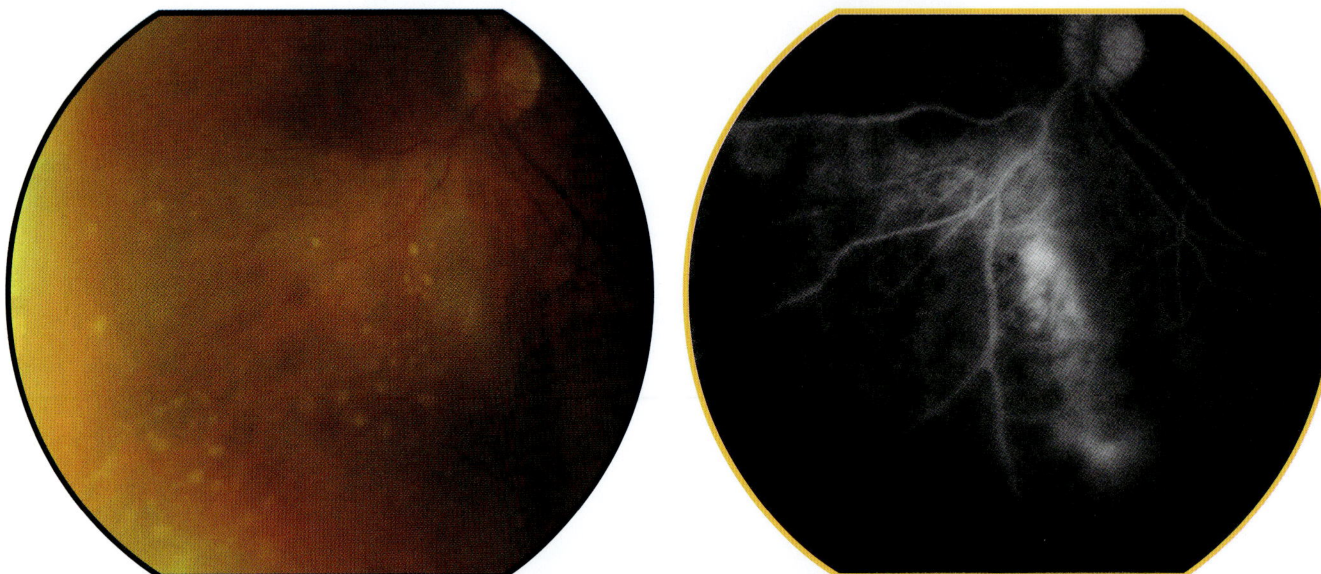

Note the multifocal retinitis associated with a placoid (or triangular) outer retinitis converging toward the posterior pole, best illustrated by the FA, which shows staining of the infected tissue especially at the advancing edge. *Courtesy of Dr. Ivan Ho*

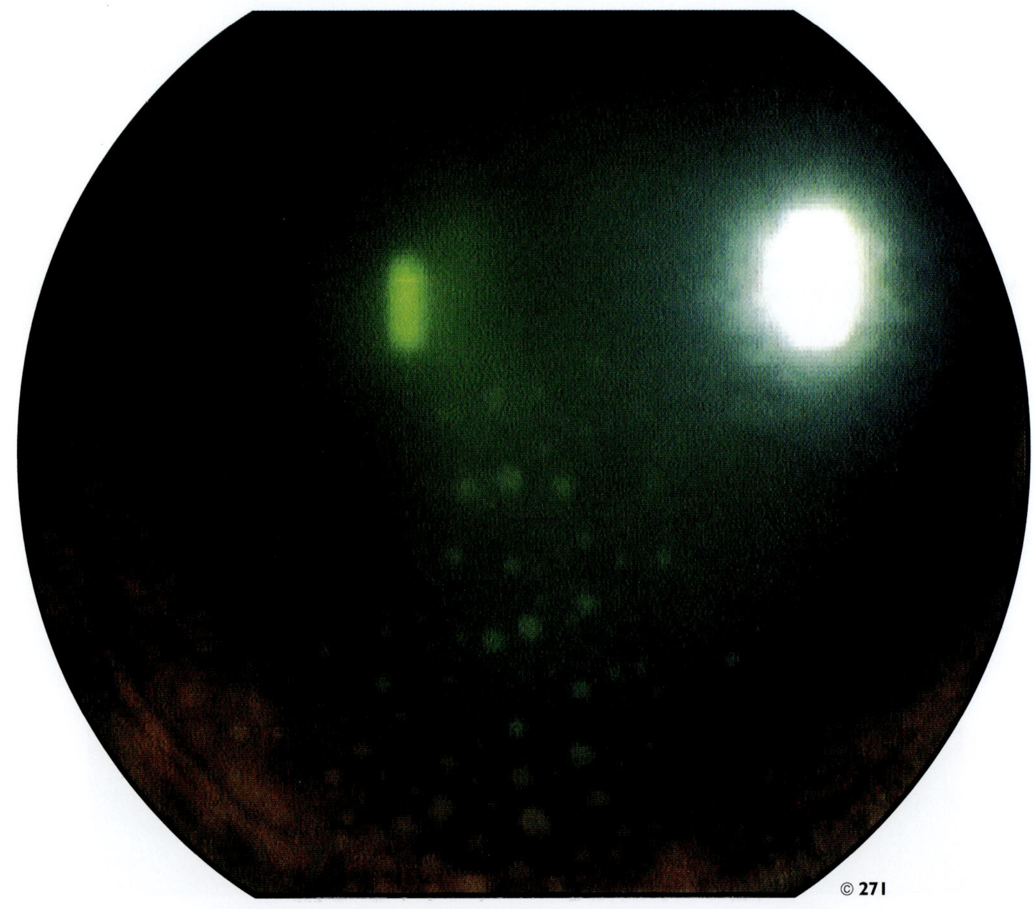

In this patient, there is a granulomatous anterior uveitis with deposits of inflammatory debris on the endothelium of the cornea due to syphilis infection.

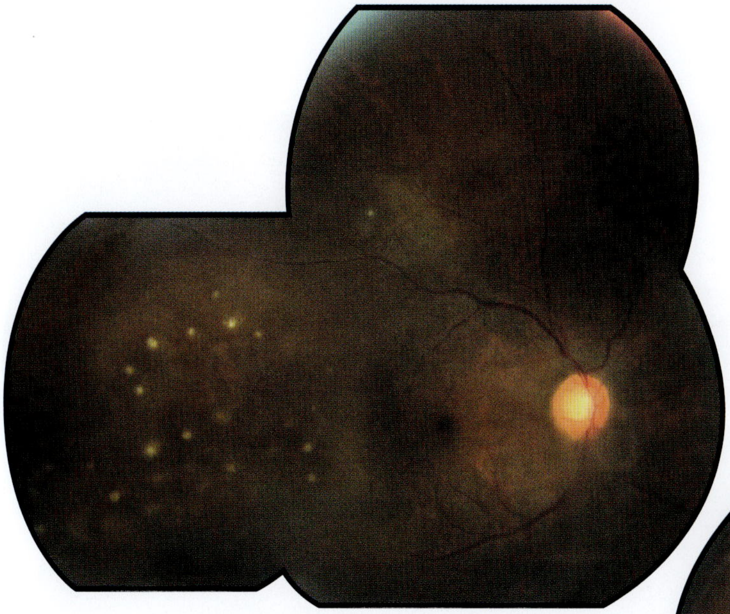

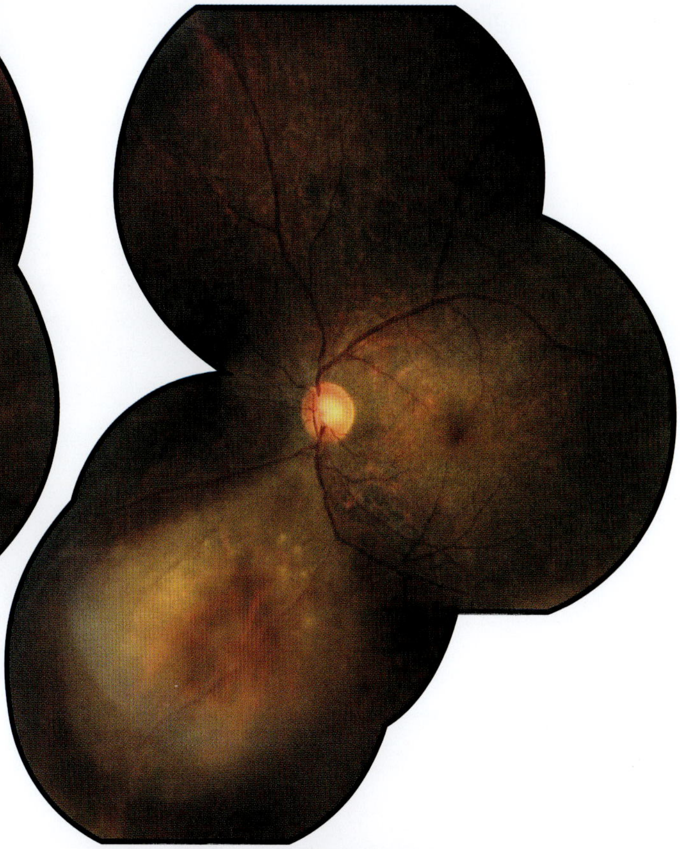

This patient has acute syphilitic placoid chorioretinitis associated with multifocal retinitis in each eye. Bilateral optic neuritis is also present. In the right eye *(upper left image)* there are multifocal retinal infiltrates associated with a placoid retinitis that is characteristic of this disease. Similar changes are seen in the left eye *(above)*.

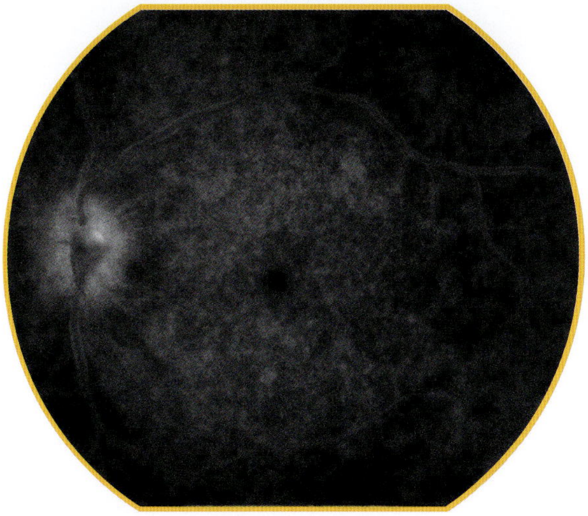

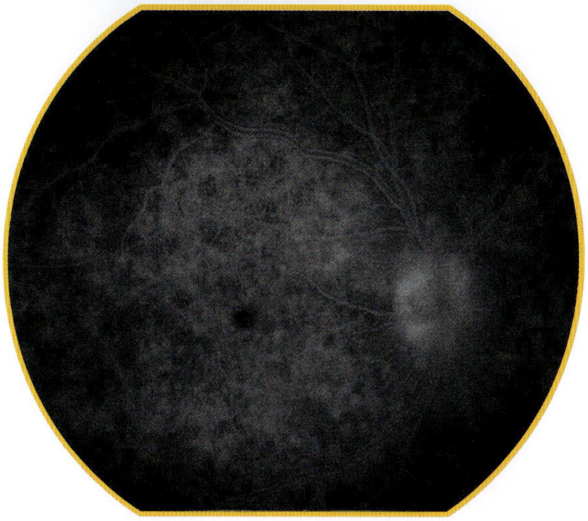

Courtesy of Dr. Daniel Martin and Dr. Sunil Srivastava

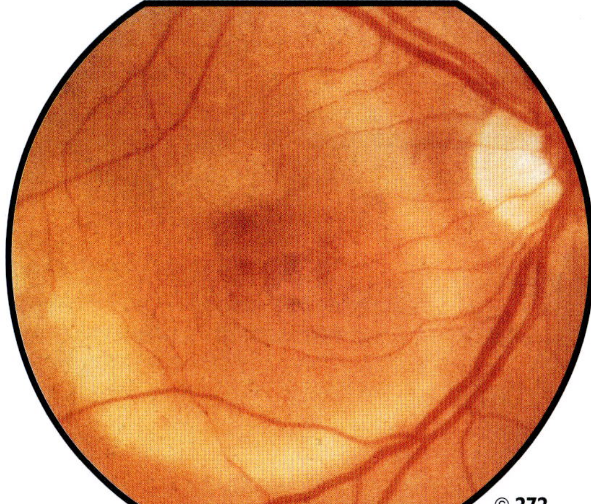

This patient with placoid outer retinitis (i.e. acute syphilitic posterior placoid chorioretinitis) showed gradual clearing centrally in the lesion as the acute infection progressed.

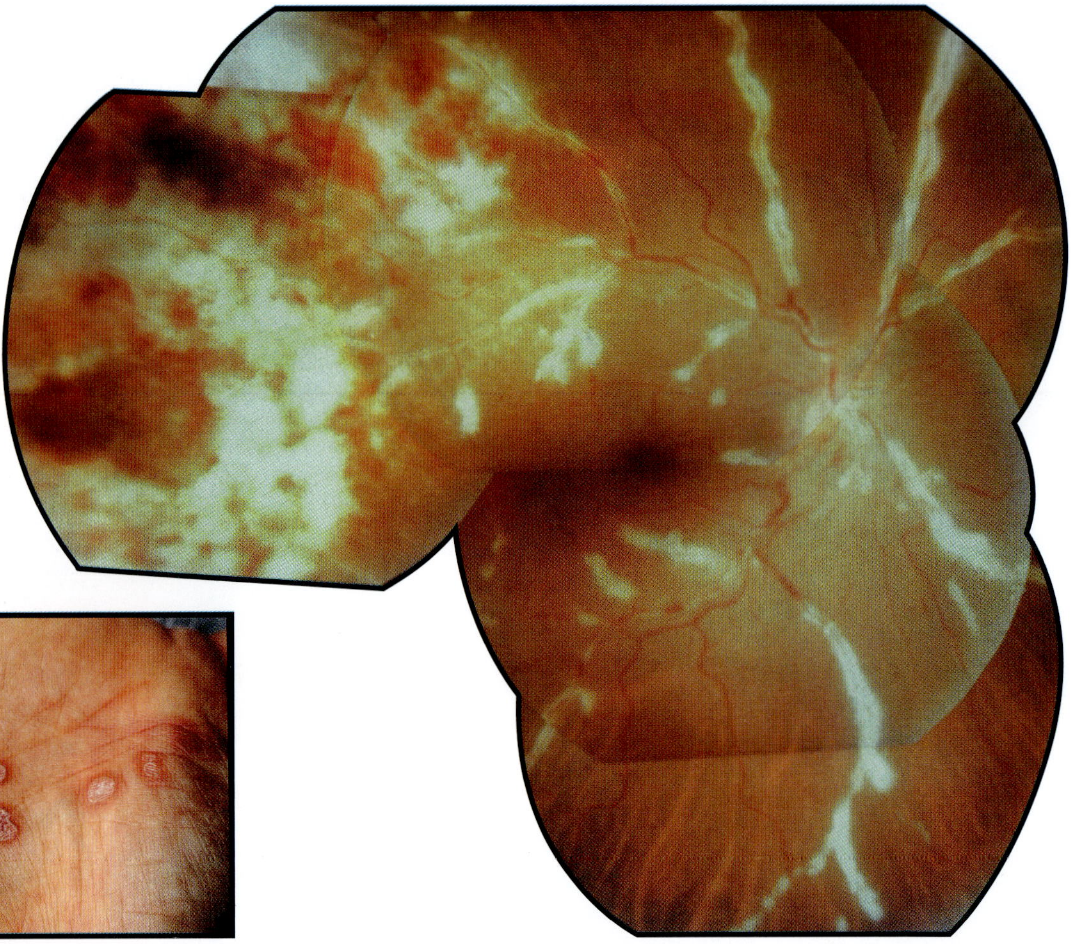

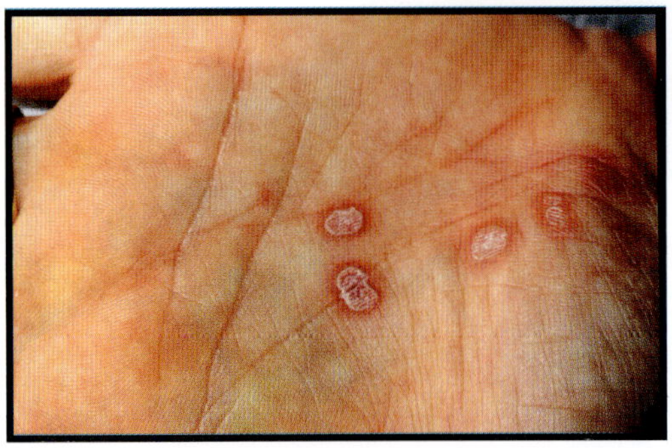

Frosted Angiitis

The palms of this patient with secondary syphilis show the typical chancre lesions. *Courtesy of Dr. R.G. Chenoweth*

This patient with syphilitic retinitis illustrates a frosted branch angiitis. Note the superotemporal area of prominent infection with hemorrhage. *Courtesy of Dr. Stephanie Sugin*

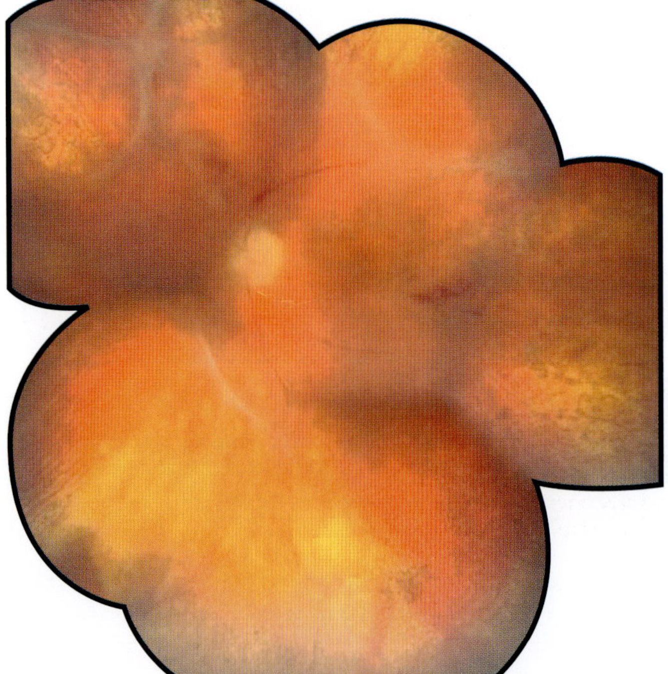

This syphilitic patient has a severe retinitis, which has led to atrophy and fibrosis. A papillitis with optic nerve atrophy is noted. Sheathed retinal vessels and fibrotic proliferation into the vitreous is also identified.

Resolved Chorioretinitis

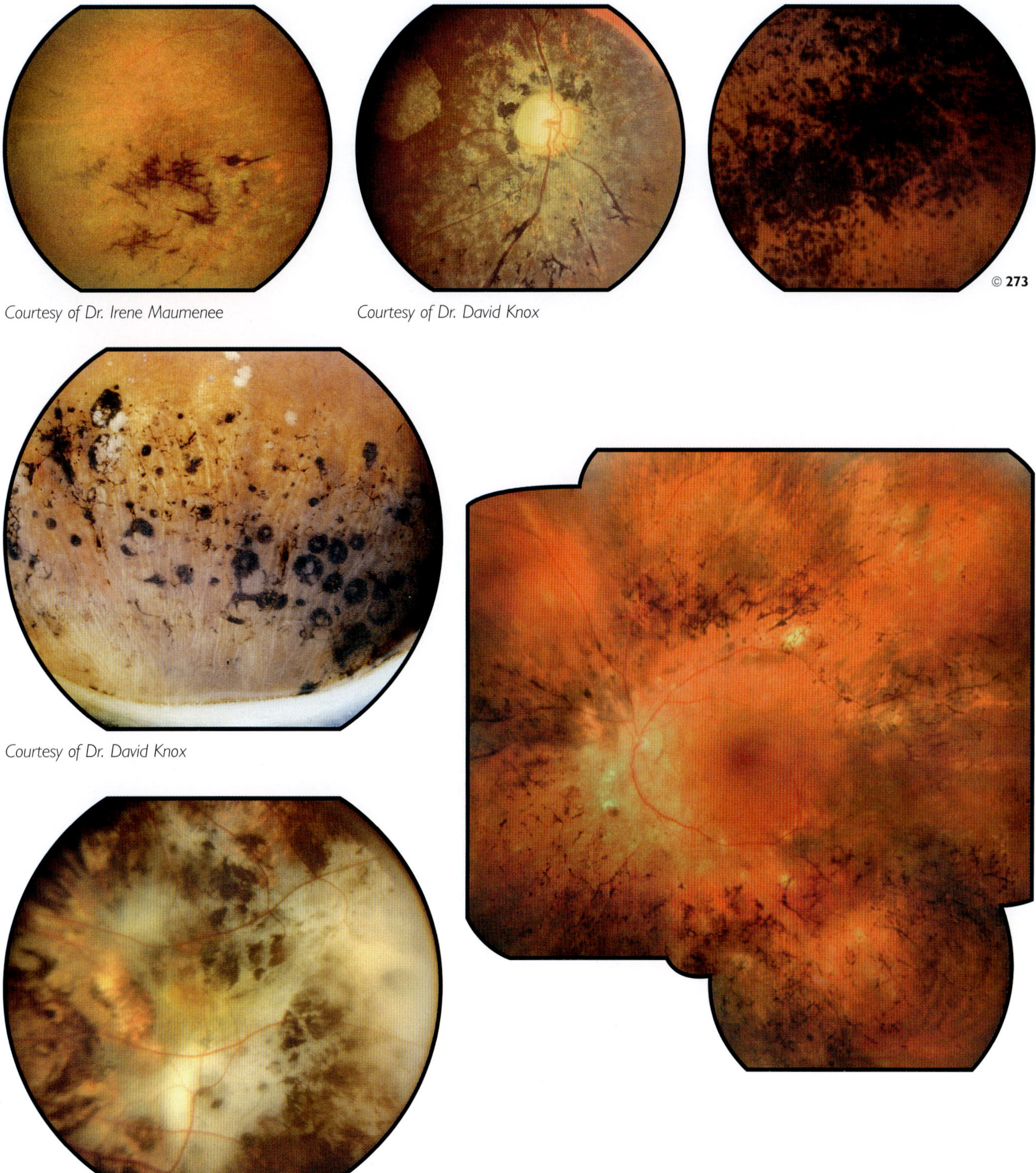

Courtesy of Dr. Irene Maumenee

Courtesy of Dr. David Knox

Courtesy of Dr. David Knox

Following severe acute and diffuse infection, syphilis can be associated with cicatricial changes in the pigment epithelium, retina, and optic nerve. Note the pigment epithelial hyperplastic abnormalities *(top row)*, widespread fibrosis *(bottom left)*, and optic atrophy *(top middle)* present in these multiple syphilitic cases. The pigmentary changes are also evident in the gross specimen *(middle left)*. In the color montage, there is remarkable pigment epithelial hyperplasia and chorioretinal atrophy throughout the fundus, which produces a retinitis pigmentosa-like appearance.

Leptospirosis

Leptospirosis is caused by an unusual bacterium, known as *Leptospira*, which is spiral-shaped and motile. Transmission is through human exposure to water contaminated by uterine fluids or urine. It is commonly seen in tropical climates during monsoon seasons in India, Brazil, and Louisiana in the USA. A severe uveitis may develop. Other ocular associations include papillitis and retinal vasculitis with macular edema.

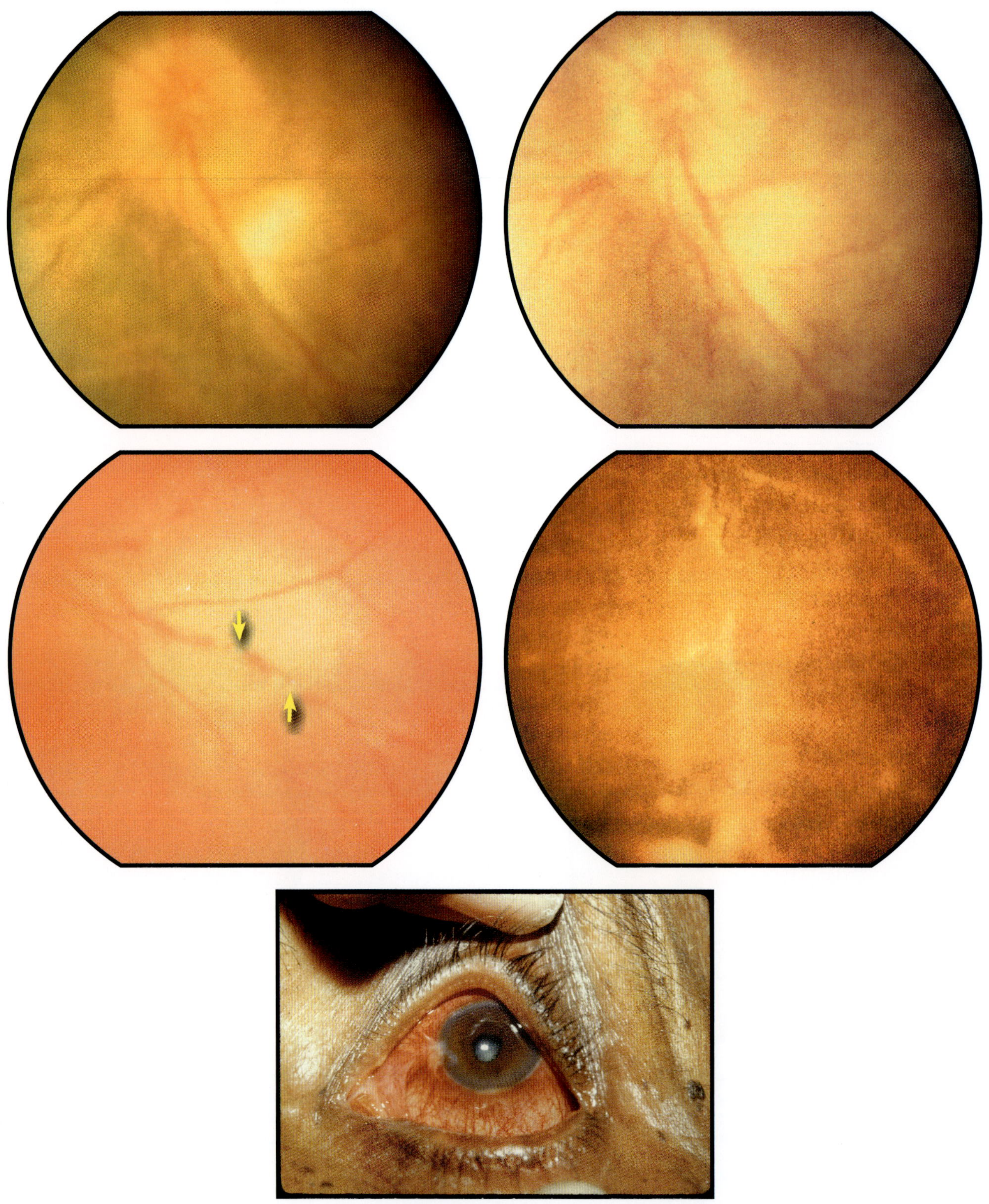

Leptospirosis may produce inflammation throughout the eye, including conjunctivitis and keratitis as seen in this patient. Severe uveitis and calcific deposits in the walls of some vessels (Kyrieleis plaques) *(arrows)* are noted. Papillitis and patchy retinitis are also identified.

Fungi
Candida albicans Chorioretinitis

Candida albicans is one of the most common ocular pathogens that cause fungal endophthalmitis. Exogenous infections of *Candida* may occur after intraocular surgery or penetrating ocular trauma. Endogenous infection may be associated with prolonged systemic antibiotics, general surgical procedures (especially gastrointestinal), hematologic malignancies, poorly controlled diabetes, or indwelling intravenous catheters. The clinical manifestations of endogenous *Candida* infection are variable and include a focal chorioretinitis with cotton-wool infiltrates in the vitreous and an intravitreal abscess, which may present as a chalk-white "puff ball" or a "string of pearls." Retinal hemorrhage often surrounds the focal chorioretinitis, and there may be an associated papillitis, scleritis, or anterior uveitis.

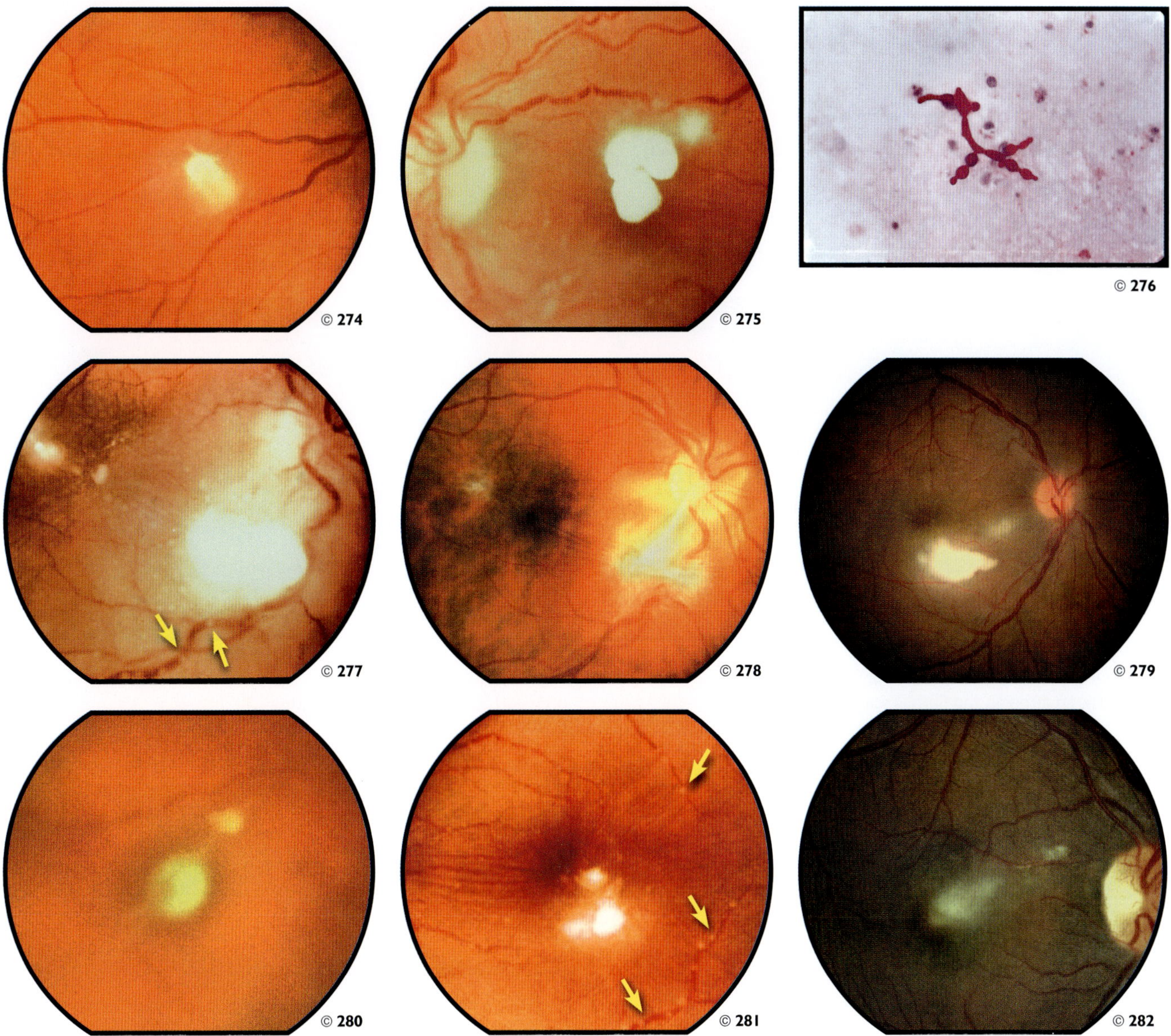

These patients all demonstrate *Candida albicans* chorioretinitis. The light microscopy image illustrates pseudohyphae and budding blastospheres, which are characteristic of *Candida*. The acute lesion may be focal *(upper left)* or multifocal *(upper middle)*. Some confluency exists in larger lesions particularly as seen here *(middle row)*. A papillitis is not uncommon in these patients. Occasionally, a vitreous abscess may be noted *(lower left)* and some of the retinal vessels may demonstrate multifocal areas of mineralization or Kyrieleis plaques *(middle left, arrows and lower middle, arrows)*.

Aspergillosis

Aspergillus fumigatus is a fungus that may produce intraocular complications, including endophthalmitis and chorioretinitis. The organism is widespread in nature and commonly resides in the nose or nasopharynx where infection may develop and spread to the orbit. It may settle in periocular tissue, particularly in elderly patients with debilitating disease. Inflammation in the orbit may induce compression of the optic nerve, causing disc edema, venous engorgement, and even central vascular occlusions. *Aspergillus* may also produce a focal or multifocal infection in the fundus, occasionally with a massive chorioretinitis, that can have a predilection for the macula with associated hemorrhage.

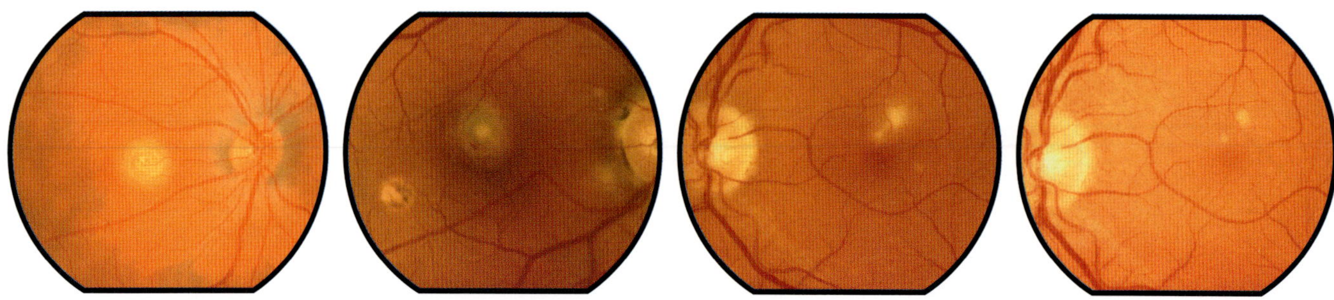

These are examples of *Aspergillus* infection in the eye. The two photographs on the right show mild multifocal infection that resolved following therapy with minimal atrophic scarring in the macula.

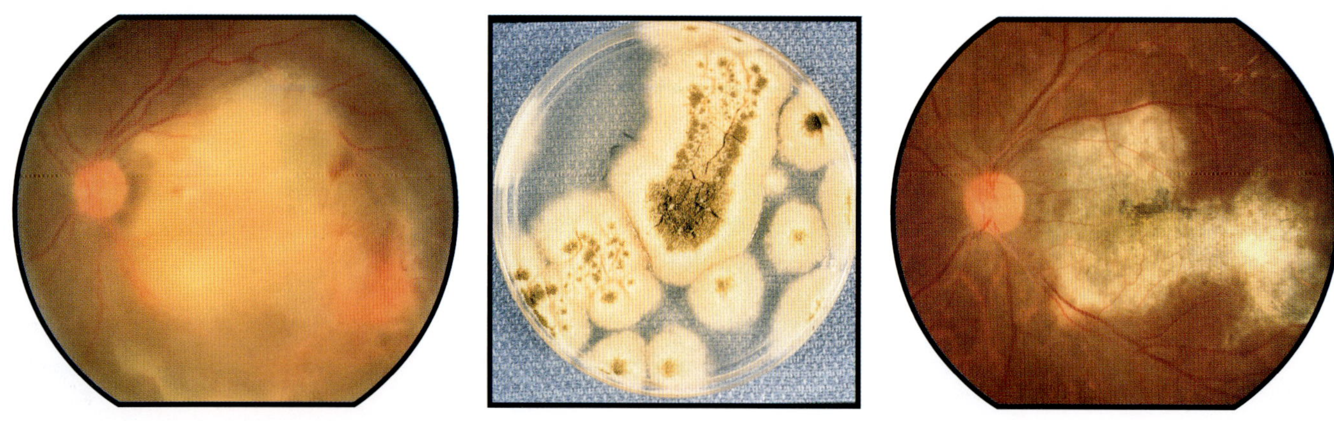

This patient illustrates a severe endophthalmitis due to *Aspergillus* with a large macular abscess. The organisms are evident on the culture. Following vitrectomy, an atrophic and fibrotic scar developed in the central macula region *(right). Courtesy of Dr. Charles Barr*

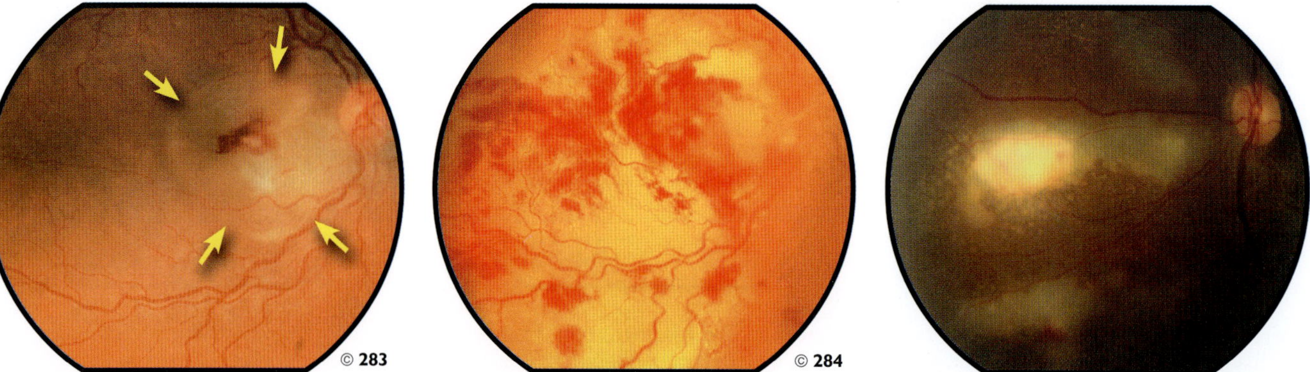

This patient illustrates an *Aspergillus* infection with juxtapapillary inflammation and hemorrhage and detachment in the central macula *(arrows)*. Four days later, the patient's infection progressed extensively with diffuse retinitis, macular hemorrhage, and necrosis. This case illustrates the potentially virulent nature of this fungal organism.

This patient has a multifocal *Aspergillus* infection in the fundus with a nodular area of necrosis at the peripheral aspect of the central lesion.

Cryptococcosis

Cryptococcus neoformans is a round to oval encapsulated yeast with a worldwide distribution, commonly found in high concentrations in pigeon feces. Acquired through the respiratory tract, it is spread hematogenously, with a predilection for the CNS. It is one of the most common life-threatening fungal pathogens in patients with AIDS. A focal chorioretinal lesion may be seen as a mass lesion in the fundus with hemorrhage and necrosis. Involvement of the optic nerve is typical.

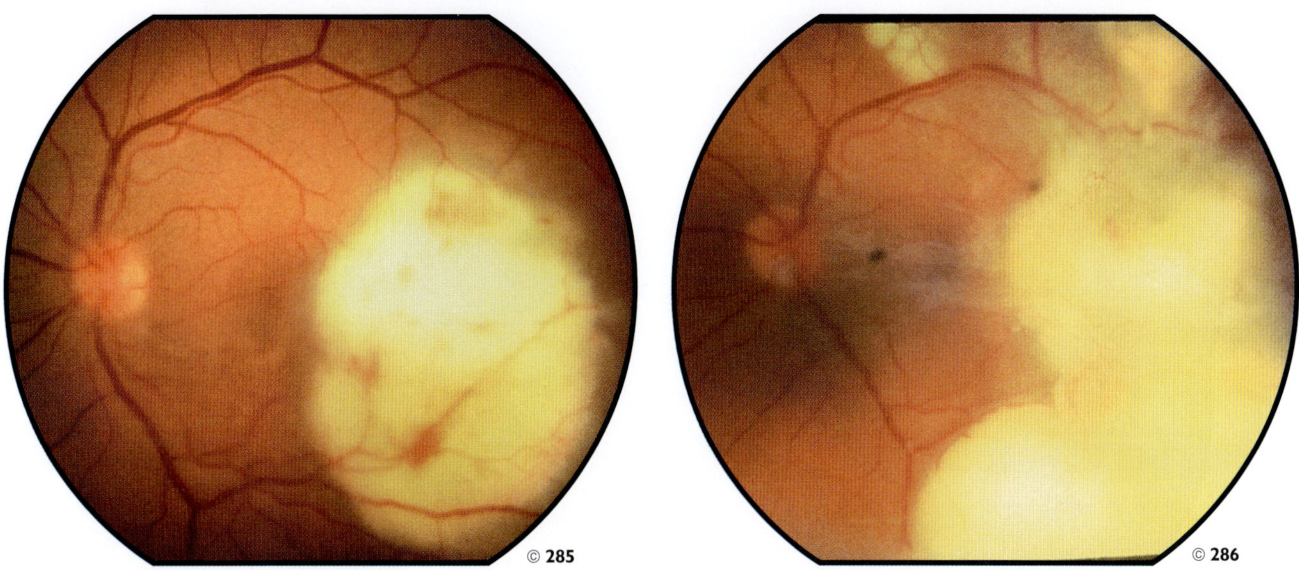

This patient illustrates a singular large *Cryptococcus* chorioretinal mass in the temporal macula. It rapidly progressed to involve the temporal and peripheral fundus and infiltrated through the retina into the vitreous.

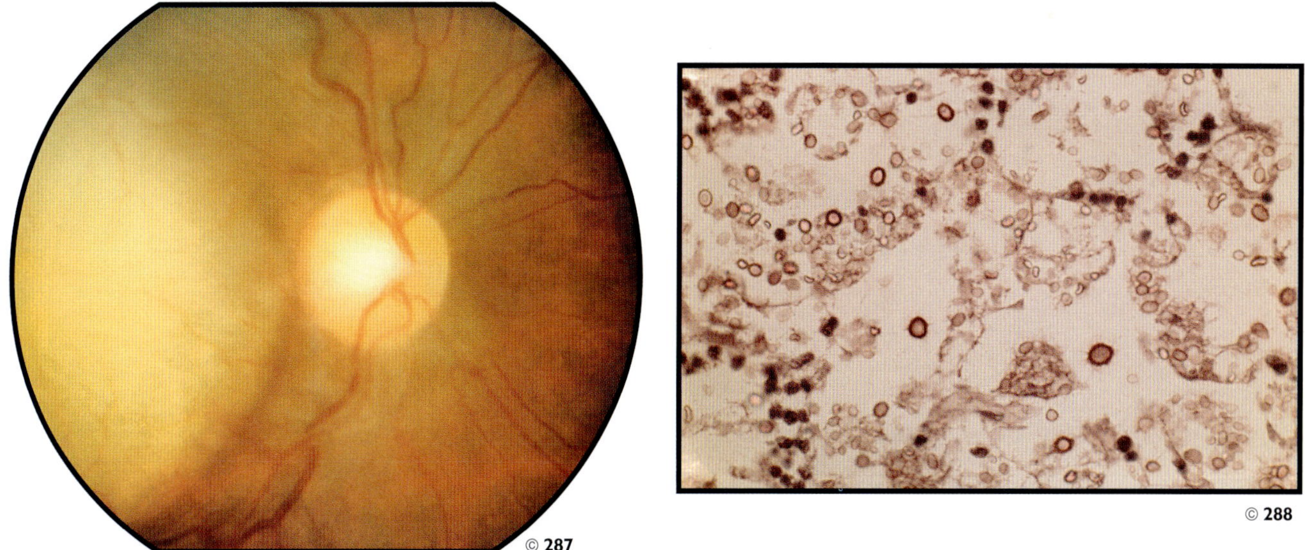

This patient shows a *Cryptococcus* infection that began at the temporal edge of the disc and extended peripherally. There was minimal bleeding, which is typical of this infection *(left)*. Cryptococcal organisms with their characteristic mucopolysaccharide capsule are seen in the histopathological specimen *(right)*.

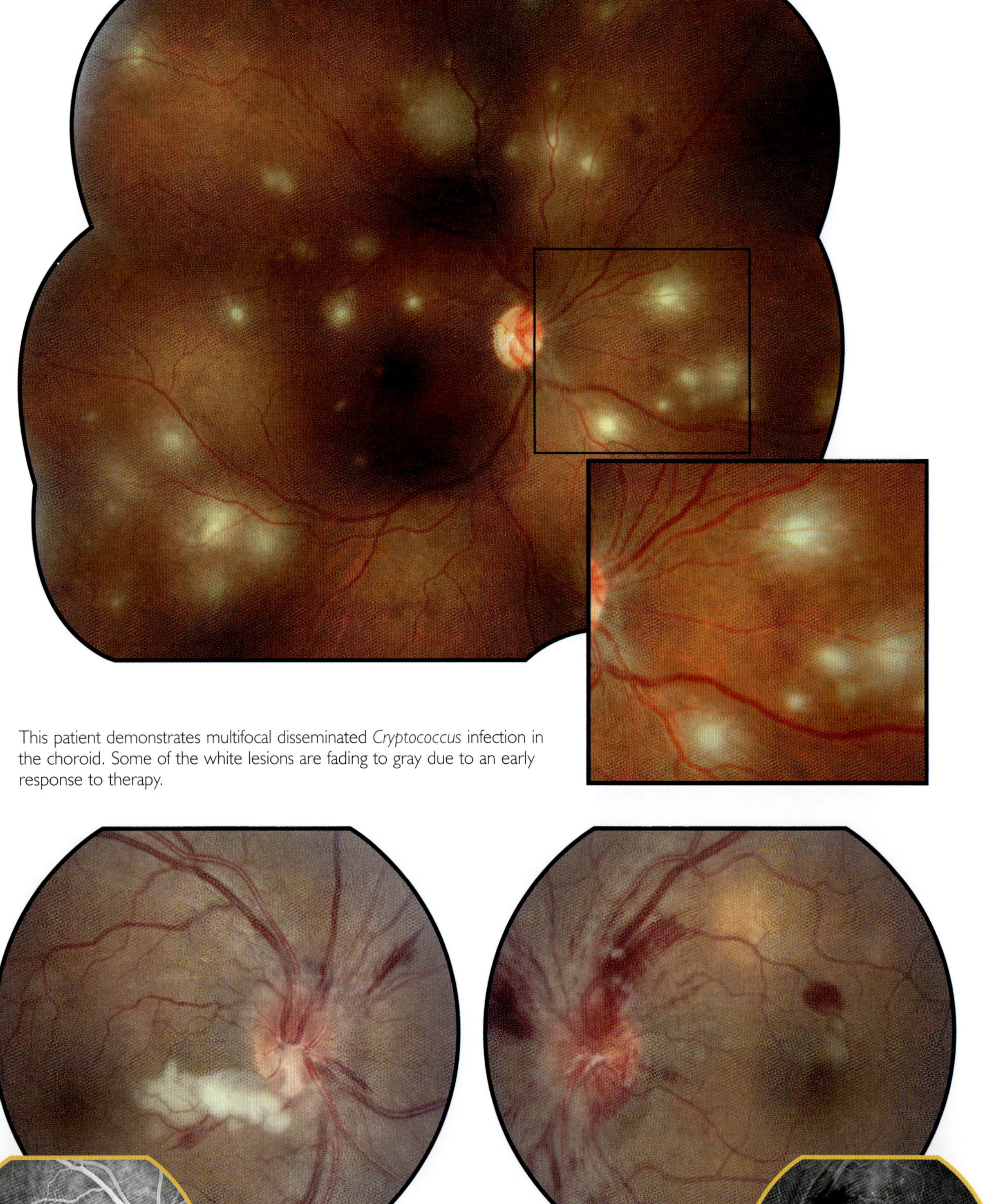

This patient demonstrates multifocal disseminated *Cryptococcus* infection in the choroid. Some of the white lesions are fading to gray due to an early response to therapy.

This patient illustrates bilateral *Cryptococcus* choroiditis and retinitis. Note the retinal whitening of the right eye and the choroidal infiltrate in the left eye and bilateral disc edema with Paton folds in the left eye. FA shows diffuse leakage from both discs and a retinal arteritis in the macula of the right eye. Serum cryptococcal antigen was positive and lumbar puncture showed a positive India-ink stain for *Cryptococcus*. *Courtesy of Dr. SriniVas Sadda*

Presumed Ocular Histoplasmosis Syndrome (POHS)

Histoplasmosis capsulatum is a fungus that is endemic in certain parts of the world, particularly the midwestern and southeastern portion of the USA (Mississippi and Ohio river valley regions). Disseminated mid-peripheral, "punched-out" chorioretinal scars, which are pigmented and atrophic, are typical findings in the absence of uveitis. Peripapillary atrophy is also noted, and eyes are at high risk for the development of choroidal neovascularization in the macula with disciform scarring. Patients are usually in the second or third decade when this disorder, which tends to be bilateral, is first diagnosed. In the adult, the principal problem is not recurrent inflammation, but secondary neovascularization in the macula.

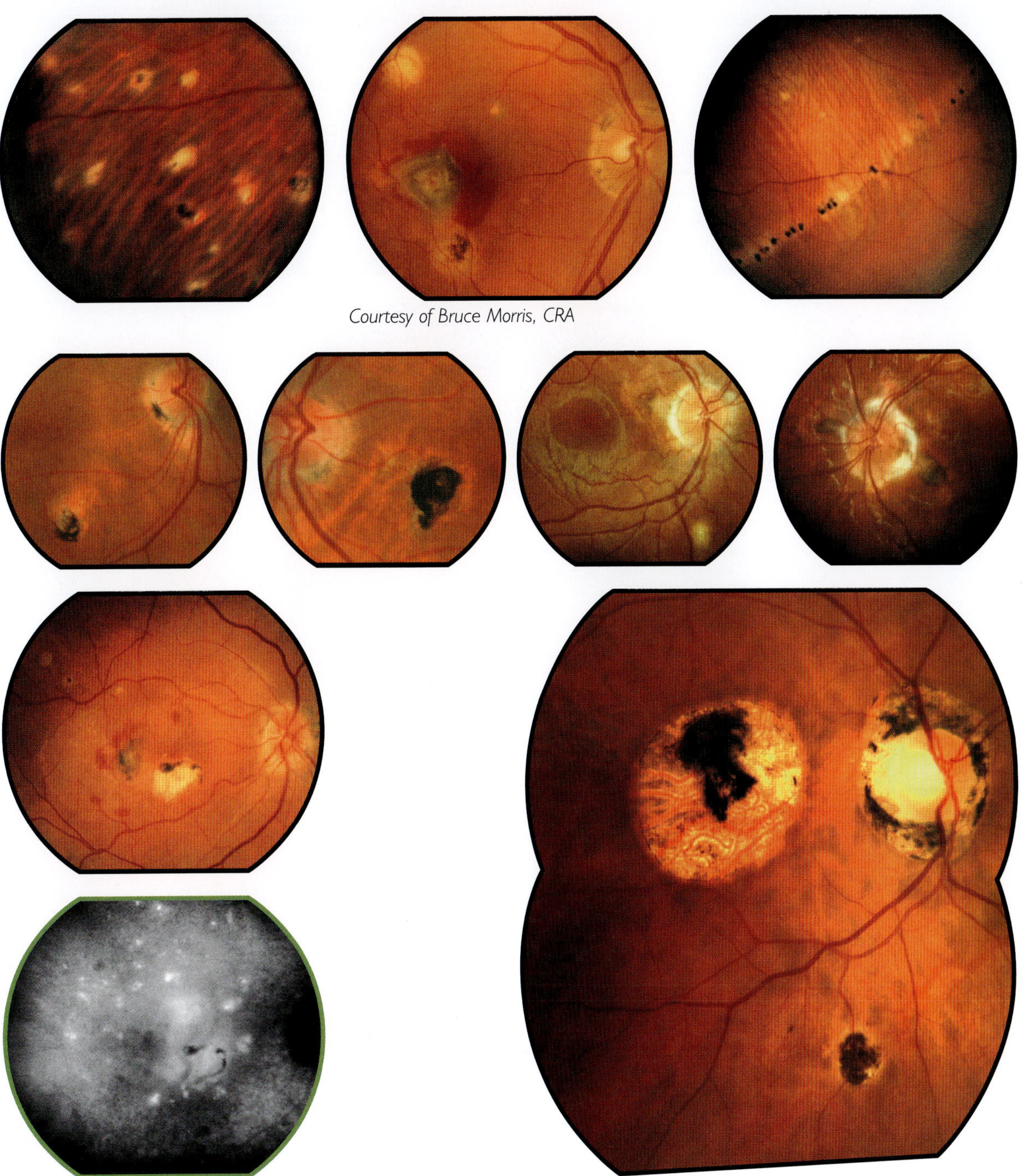

Courtesy of Bruce Morris, CRA

These patients show the typical manifestations of POHS. There are punched out, atrophic, and pigmented chorioretinal scars; peripapillary atrophy; choroidal neovascularization with surrounding hemorrhage *(top row, middle);* and pigmentary and atrophic lesions in the fundus, in a concentric curvilinear pattern, referred to as the Schaelgel sign *(top row, right).* Other manifestations include hyperpigmentation and peripapillary scarring *(second row);* hemorrhagic detachment of the macular from choroidal neovascularization *(third row, left);* staining of chorioretinal scars or so-called "histo spots" on ICG angiography *(bottom row, left);* and atrophy following laser photocoagulation of active choroidal neovascularization *(bottom right). Courtesy of Bruce Morris, CRA*

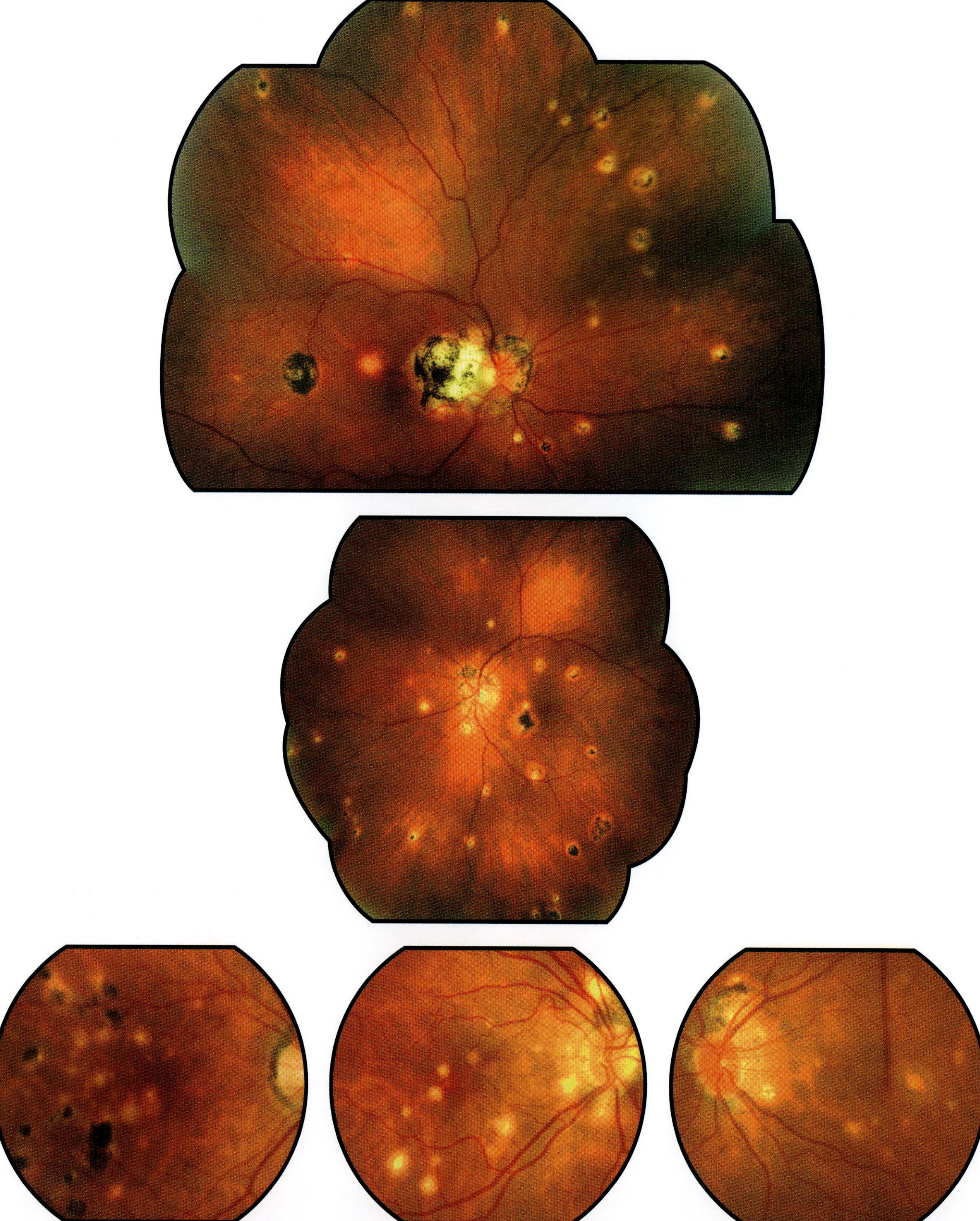

These patients show the morphological variation of the chorioretinal histo spots and peripapillary atrophy seen in POHS. There is also fibrotic and pigment scarring in the macular region from choroidal neovascularization *(top image)*. Punched-out chorioretinal lesions or histo spots may be identified in the periphery and in the central macular area. *Bottom row middle and right images courtesy of Dr. Calvin Mein*

Blastomycosis

Blastomycosis is a chronic granulomatous fungal infection of humans and lower animals caused by the dimorphic fungus *Blastomyces dermatitidis*. This disease is particularly common in the midwestern states of the Mississippi river valley in the USA. Pulmonary and cutaneous manifestations are typical of the disease. Pneumonia and a skin lesion that resembles a verrucous ulcer with heaped-up edges are typical. In the fundus, there may be one or more choroidal granulomas or even a panophthalmitis. A yellow granulomatous lesion of the choroid with an overlying exudative retinal detachment is a typical presentation.

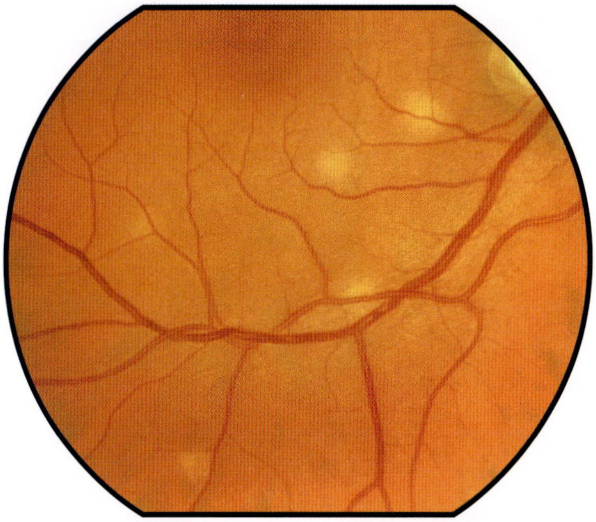

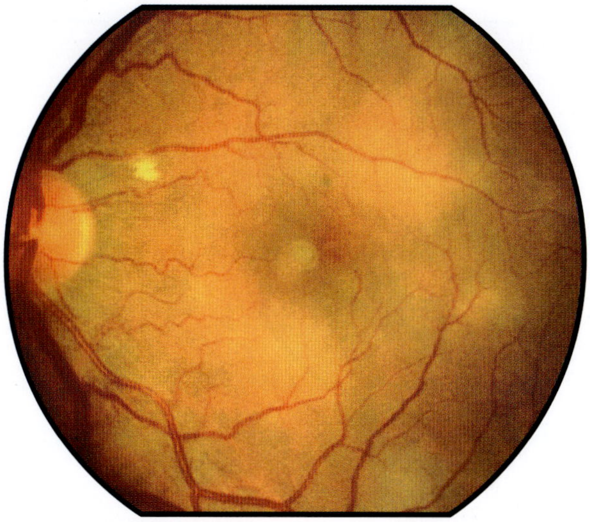

Courtesy of Dr. Froncie Gutman

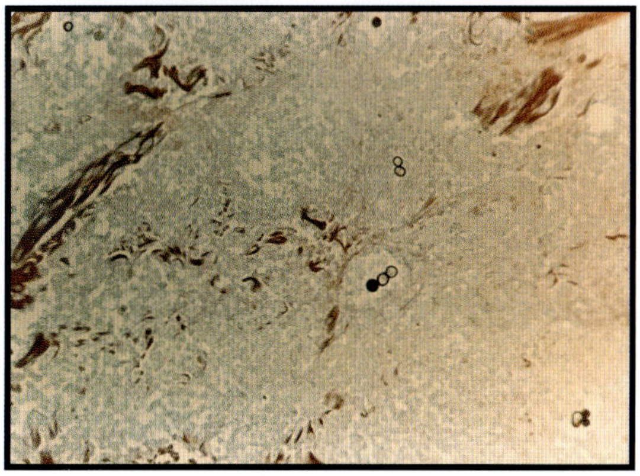

© 289

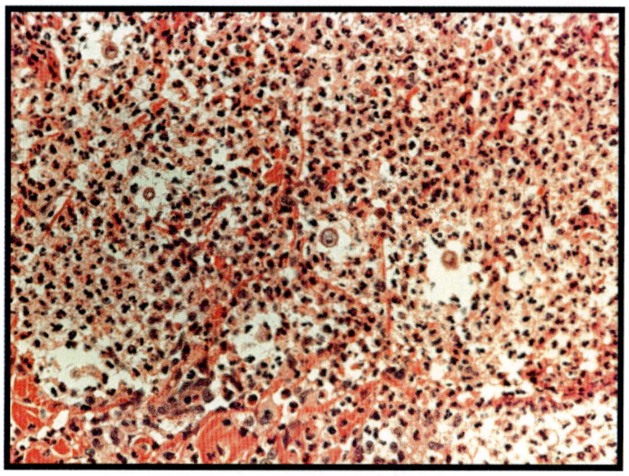

© 290

Scattered choroidal infiltrates are seen in this patient with blastomycosis *(upper left)*. There is more confluency of the lesions in a diffuse-type infiltration in a second patient with blastomycosis *(upper right)*. The histopathology images show granulomatous inflammation and the presence of *Blastomyces* organisms.

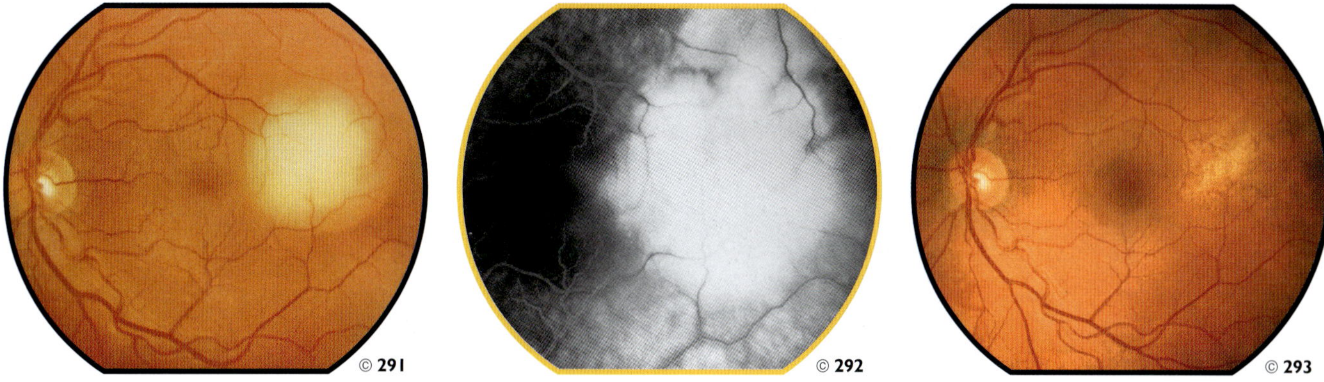

© 291 © 292 © 293

This patient with blastomycosis shows a creamy–yellow choroidal mass lesion in the temporal macula that shows significant staining and leakage with FA. Following treatment, there is regression of the lesion, leaving an atrophic and fibrous scar, surrounded by some pigment epithelial granularity.

Ocular Coccidioidomycosis

Coccidioides immitis is a dimorphic fungus endemic in the arid and semi-arid soils of Central and South America, as well as the southwestern part of the USA. The organism exists in two phases of reproduction. The saprophytic phase resides in soil, its natural habitat, and contains septate hyphae. This phase culminates in the production of thin-walled structures (arthroconidia) that are released into the air and inhaled from airborne dust, thereby initiating infection. Ocular coccidioidomycosis may affect either the anterior or posterior segment of the eye. Multifocal choroiditis or chorioretinitis or even an endophthalmitis may complicate infection with this fungal organism.

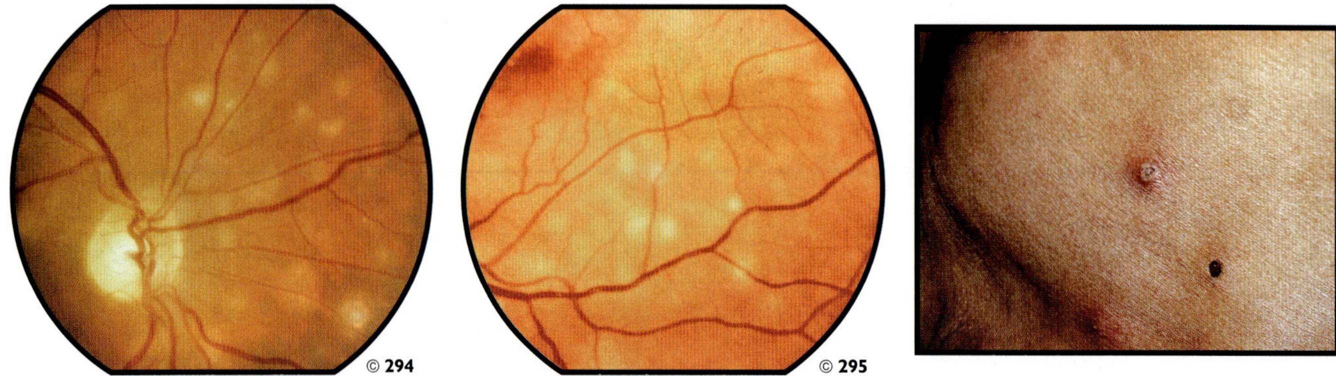

These patients have scattered choroidal lesions in the fundus from *Coccidioides immitis*. The skin lesions show an erythematous, nodular, and umbilicated coccidioidomycosis eruption.

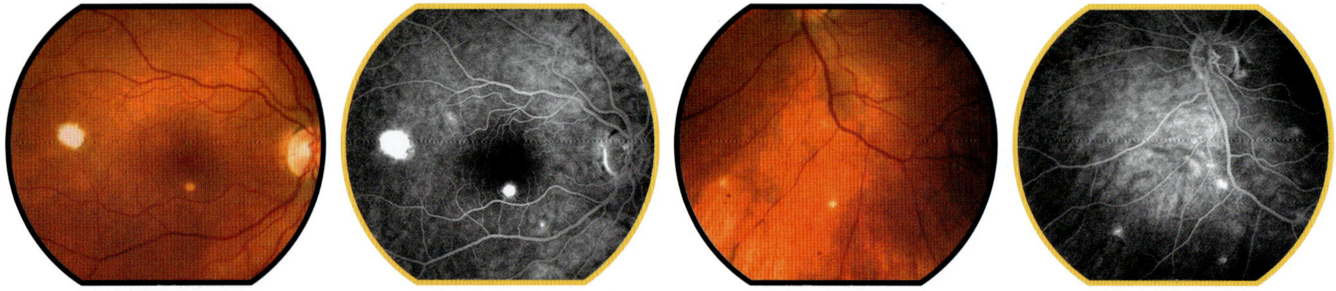

This 42-year-old Caucasian female noticed a blurry spot in her right eye for a few days while she was in hospital. She also had dizziness, lightheadedness, and confusion. She was hospitalized for elevated intracranial pressure. Note that the multifocal choroidal lesions are scattered randomly throughout the fundus in each eye and stain with FA. *Courtesy of Dr. Hua Gao*

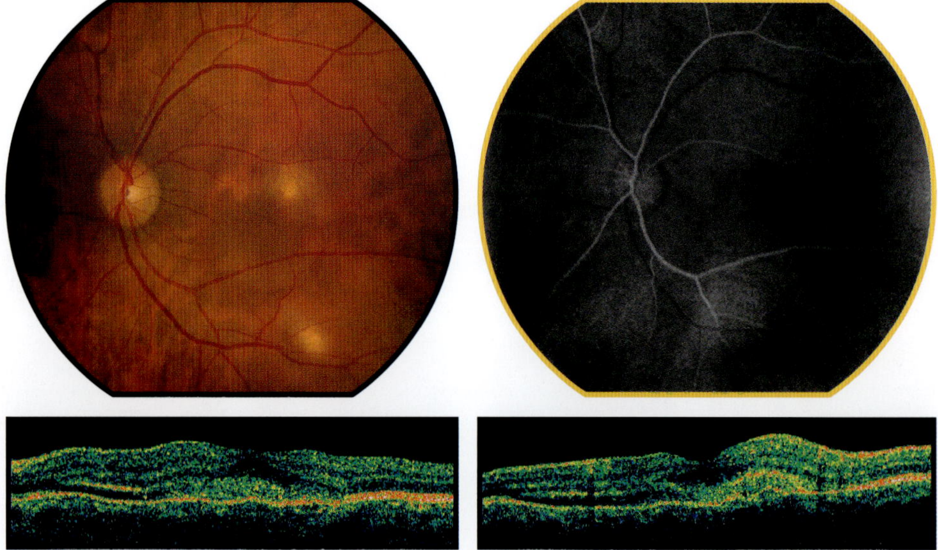

This patient illustrates multifocal choroidal lesions that do not stain with fluorescein in acute stages.There is evidence of choroidal and subretinal involvement with time domain OCT imaging. Adherence of the pigment epithelium to the overlying retina is present. The OCT image shows a subretinal infiltrate with minimal elevation of the neurosensory retina. *Courtesy of Dr. Matthew MacCumber*

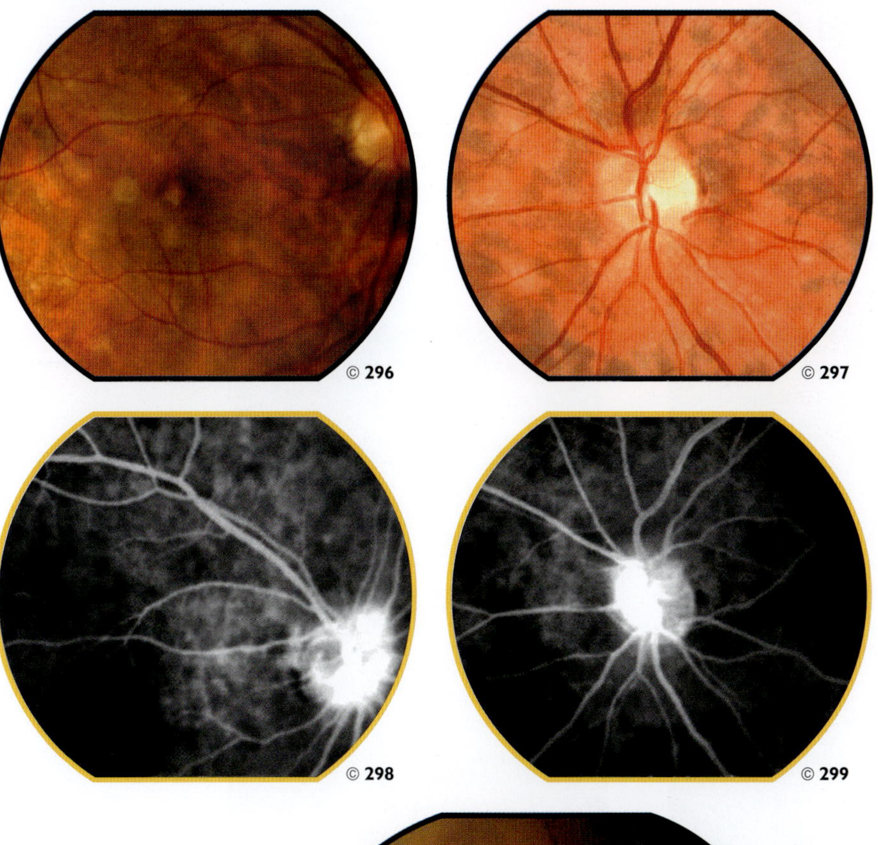

This patient illustrates bilateral coccidioidomycosis with scattered chorioretinitic lesions in both eyes. The FA does not show staining of these lesions; rather, they are hypofluorescent. However, the optic nerve stains in each eye due to an associated papillitis.

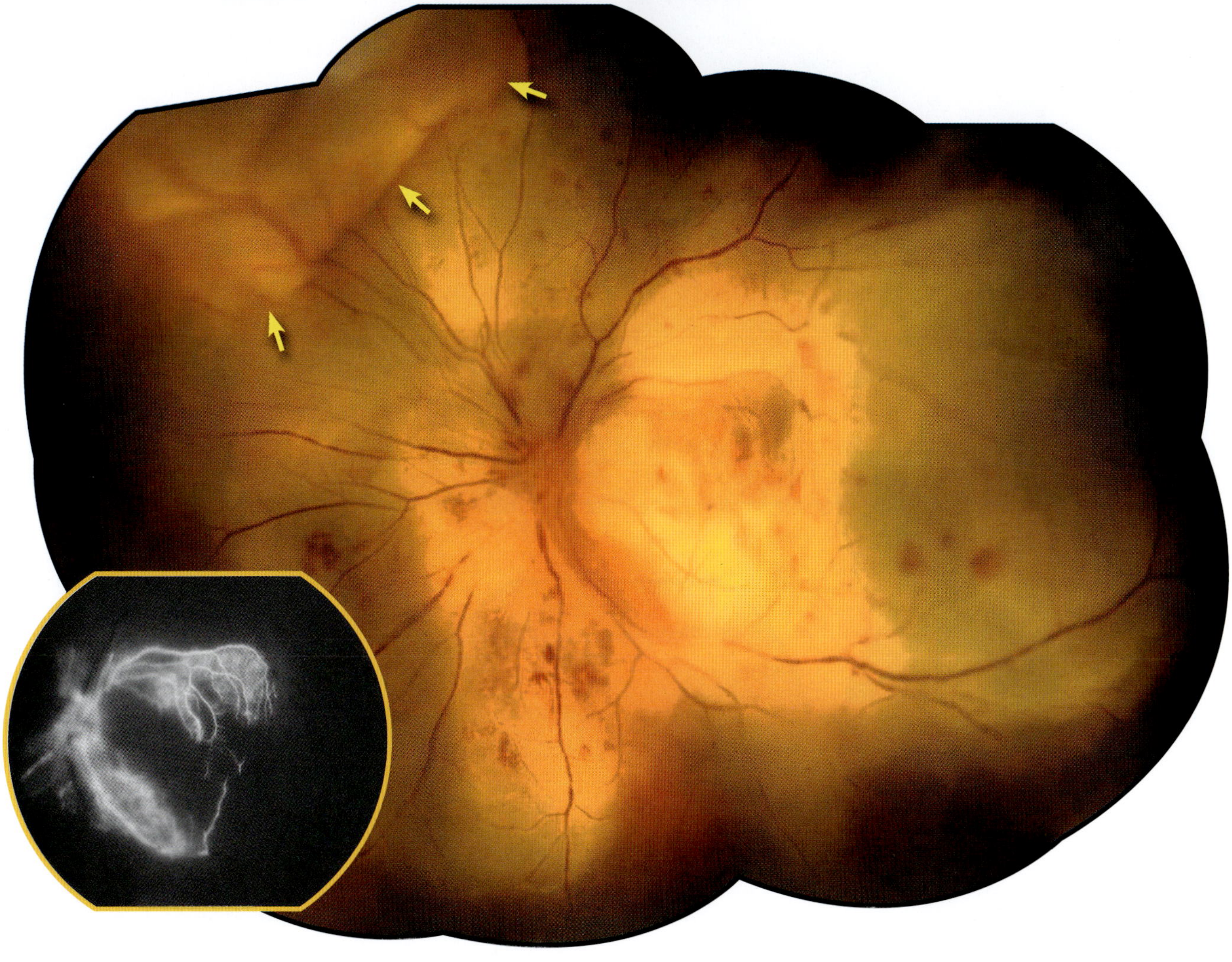

This patient has severe disseminated coccidioidomycosis with a massive area of chorioretinal involvement throughout the posterior and peripheral fundus. There was an associated exudative detachment of the retina evident clinically *(arrows)*. The FA shows severe ischemia and non-perfusion due to a necrotizing, obliterative retinitis and retinal vasculitis. *Courtesy of Dr. Gurav Shah*

Fusarium Keratitis, Vitritis, and Retinal Papillitis

Fusarium is one of the more common fungi that produce a mycotic keratitis. The organism is ubiquitous in air, soil, and organic waste. It may rarely result in an endophthalmitis or a severe uveitis with associated retinal vascular inflammatory changes and optic nerve swelling.

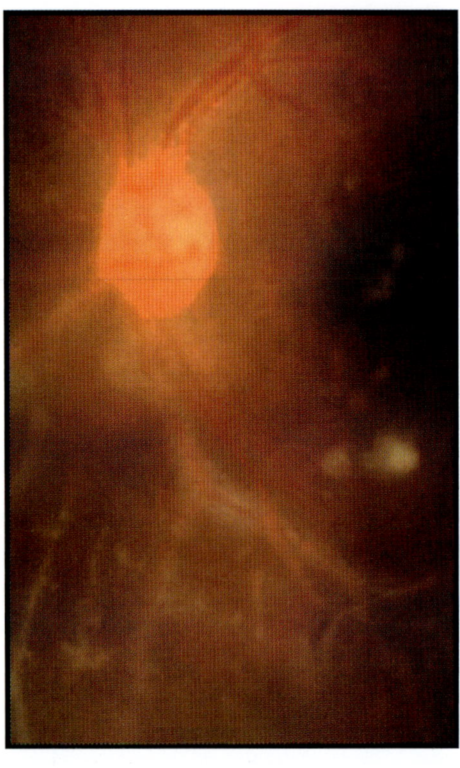

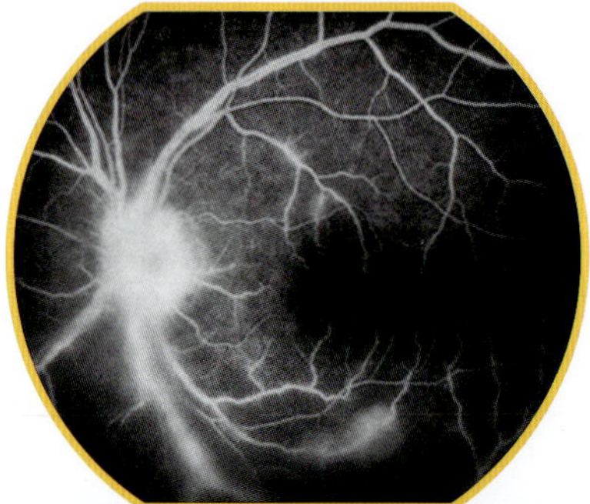

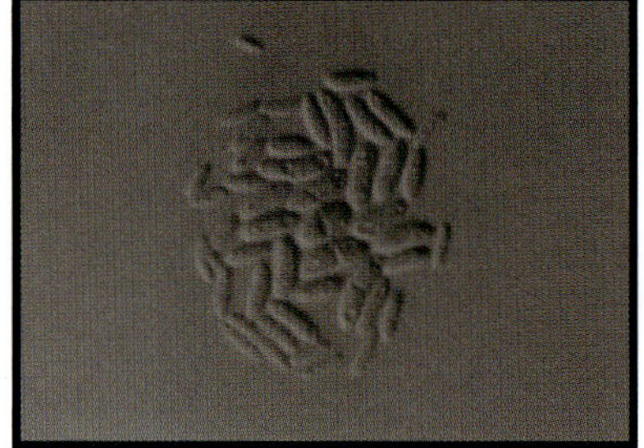

In this patient with *Fusarium* retinal vasculitis and papillitis, a frosted branch angiitis is noted as the inflammatory cells line the involved, infected vessels. There is also staining of these vessels and the optic nerve (i.e. papillitis) with the FA. The bottom right image is impressive and shows the organism in culture. Note the peculiar alignment of the fungus.

Pneumocystis carinii

Pneumocystis carinii pneumonia (PCP) is a rarely encountered systemic opportunistic infection seen in patients with AIDS. The infection most commonly affects the lungs, but extrapulmonary sites include lymph nodes, spleen, liver, bone marrow, small intestine, myocardium, and the choroid. Multifocal choroidal grayish lesions may be seen in the posterior and peripheral fundus. These lesions may slowly enlarge and become round to oval-shaped, eventually resulting in necrosis in the choroid. There is very little associated vitreous inflammation.

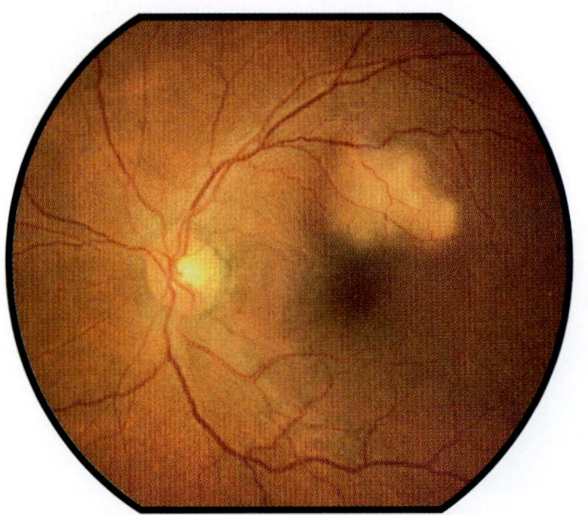

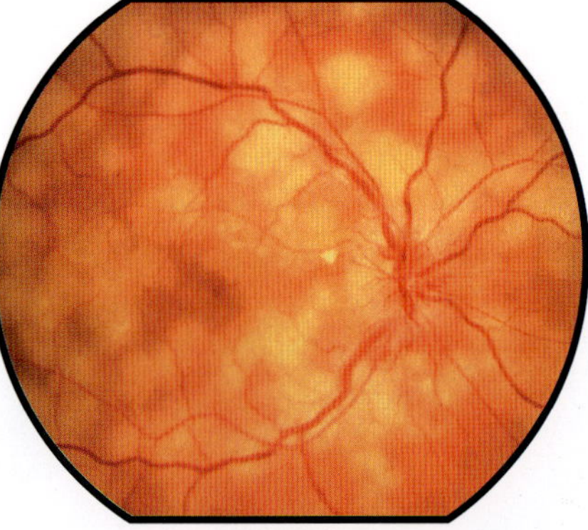

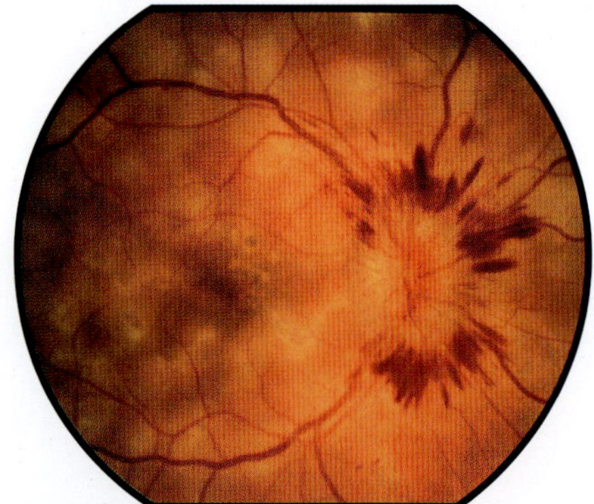

Note the pneumocystis infection illustrated in these patients. Focal *(left)* and widespread lesions throughout the choroid are seen. The inflammatory infiltrates are distributed in the posterior segment in these cases and are very numerous *(middle)*. They may also be present in association with optic nerve edema and hemorrhage *(right)*. *Courtesy of Dr. Murk-Hein Heinemann and Dr. Maria Berrocal*

Nematodes
Cysticercosis

Infestation by *Cysticercus cellulosae,* the larval form of the pork tapeworm *Taenia solium,* is the causative agent for ocular cysticercosis. Ingestion of ova of *Taenia solium* from contaminated food or more infrequently by autoinfection by ingestion of one's own infected feces is the method of transmission in humans. Upon emerging from the egg, the larvae penetrate the intestinal wall and travel via lymphatics and the vascular system to muscles and the CNS. Cysticercosis of the posterior segment is usually seen in the vitreous body or the subretinal space but can also be seen at the nerve.

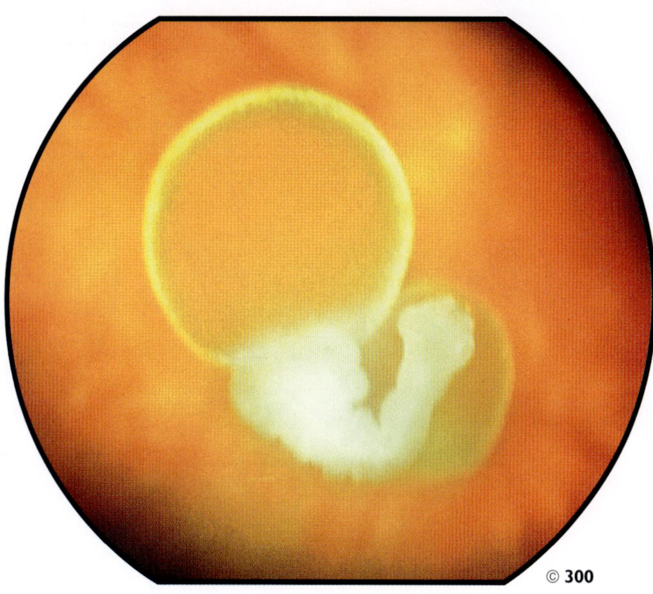

© 300

This case of ocular cysticercosis shows the nematode extending into the vitreous cavity.

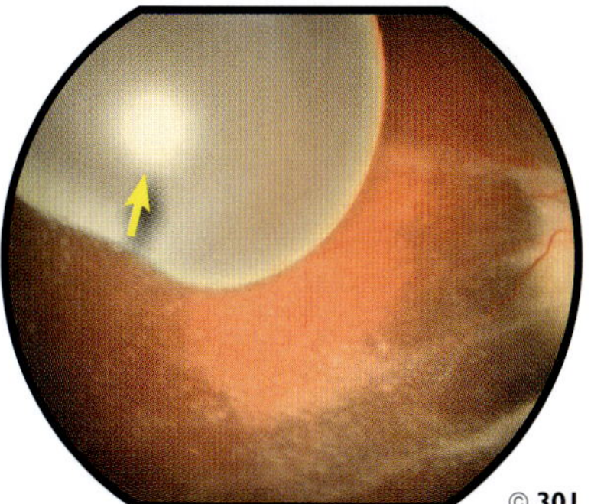

© 301

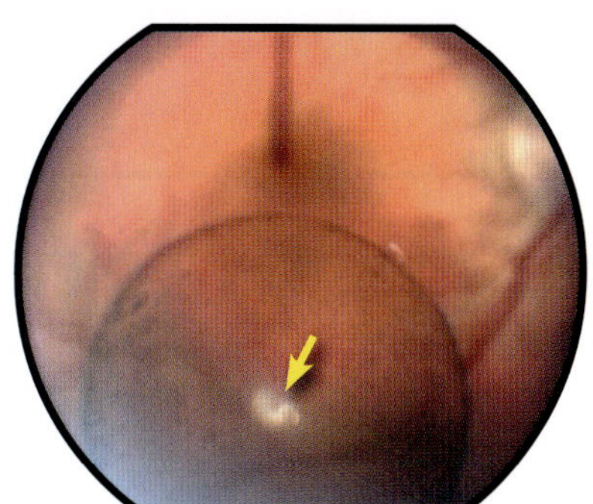

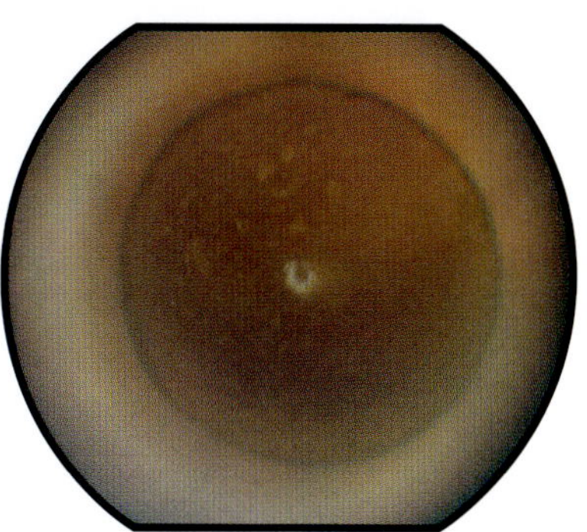

Courtesy of Dr. Veeral Sheth

These two patients have ocular cysticercosis in the vitreous. In the left and middle images, the small organism can be seen within the cystic cavity *(arrows).*

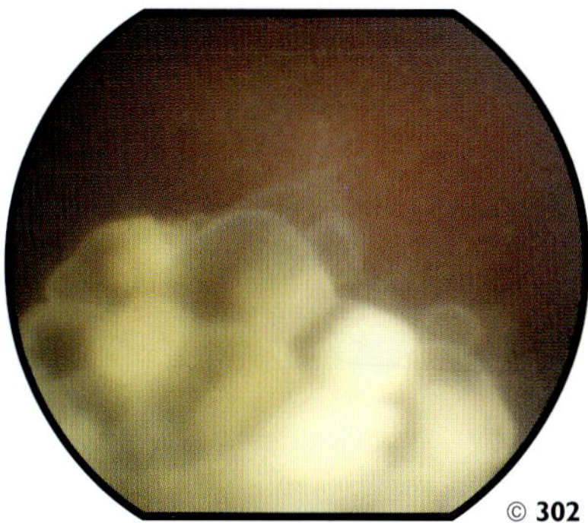

© 302

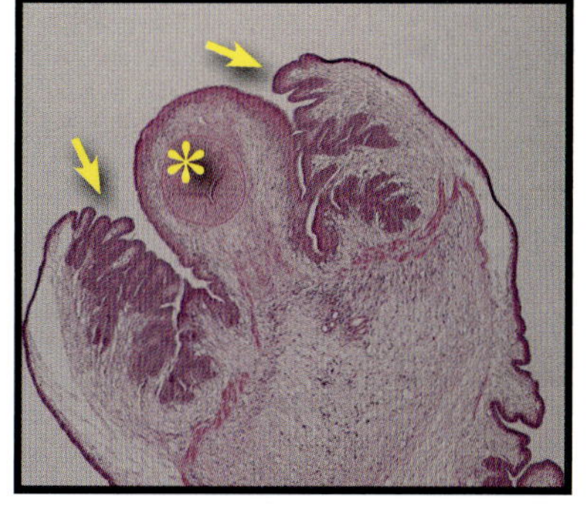

© 303

Cysticercosis is present in the vitreous of this patient. Note the turbid and multi-lobular cystic changes. This organism was excised surgically, revealing the scolex *(asterisk)* and the body *(arrows).*

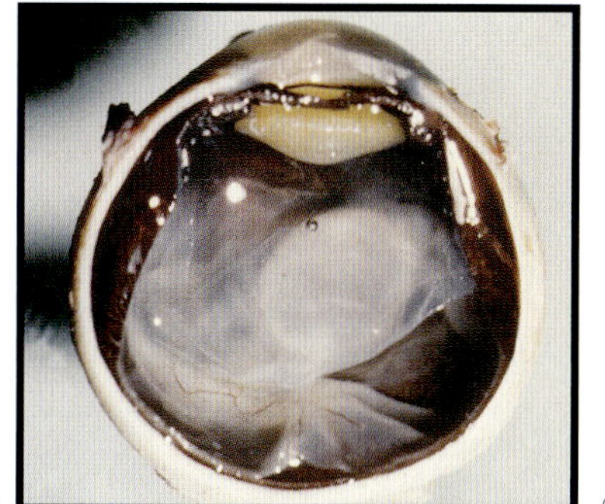

© 304

This is the gross appearance of ocular cysticercosis in the vitreous of a 42-year-old male.

Subretinal Cysticercosis

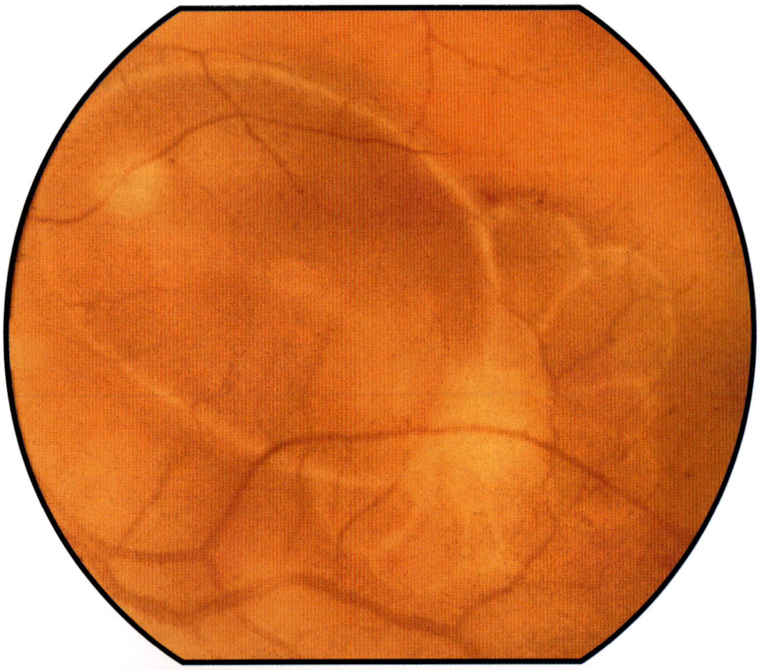

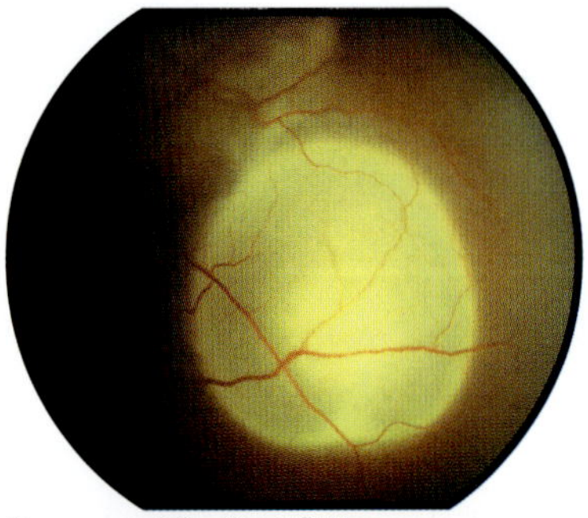

Courtesy of Dr. Yossi Sidikaro

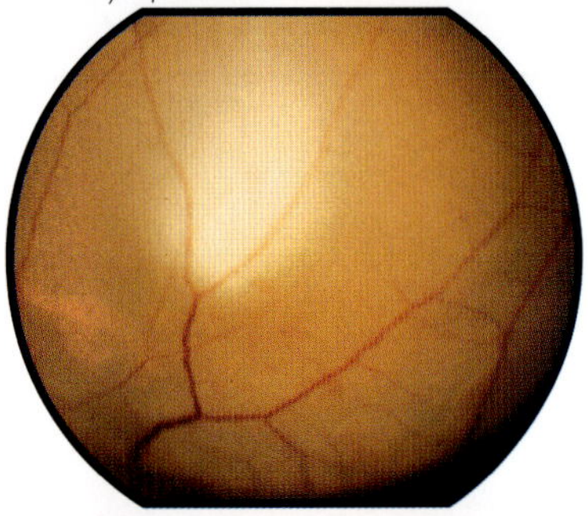

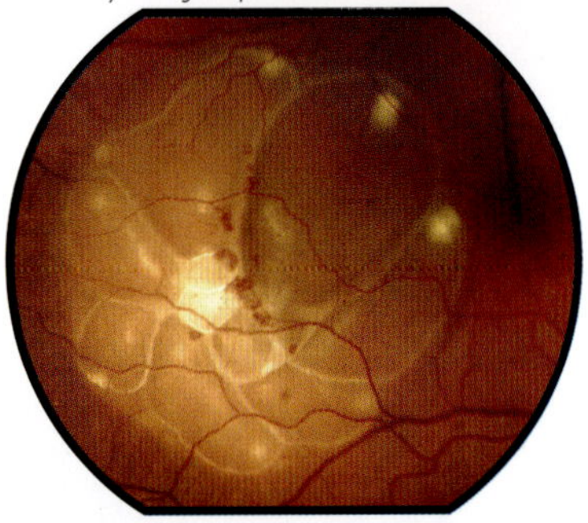

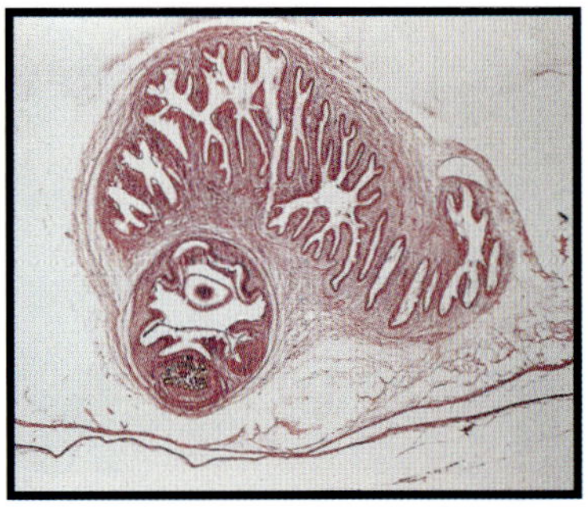

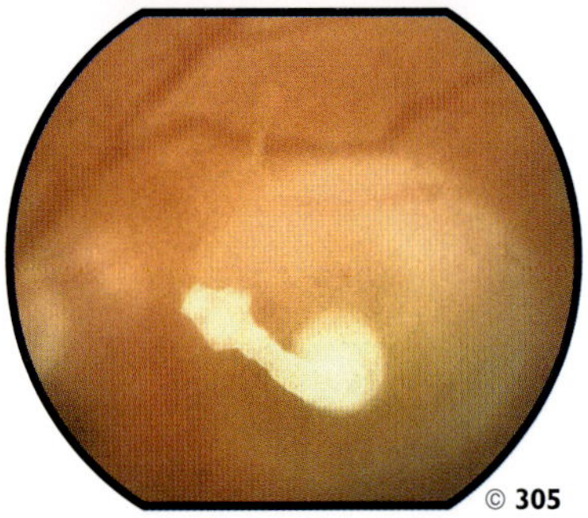

Courtesy Dr. Joesph Olk

© 305

These patients had ocular cysticercosis. Examination revealed the encysted organism under the retina *(top left)*. In another patient, the scolex is emerging from the cystic cavity *(bottom right)*. The histopathology image shows the organism including the cyst wall, the scolex, and the body.

Neural Cysticercosis

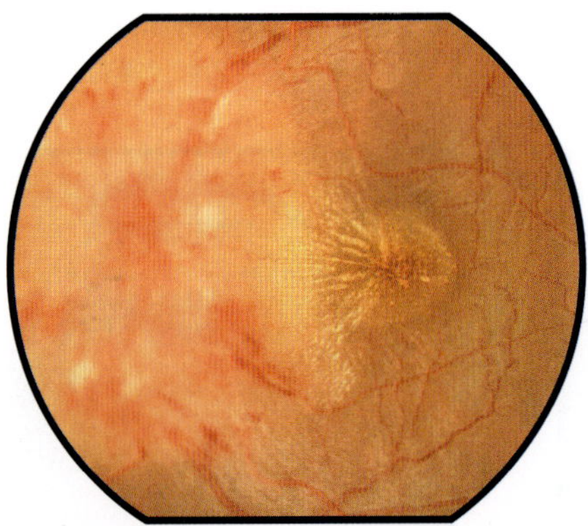

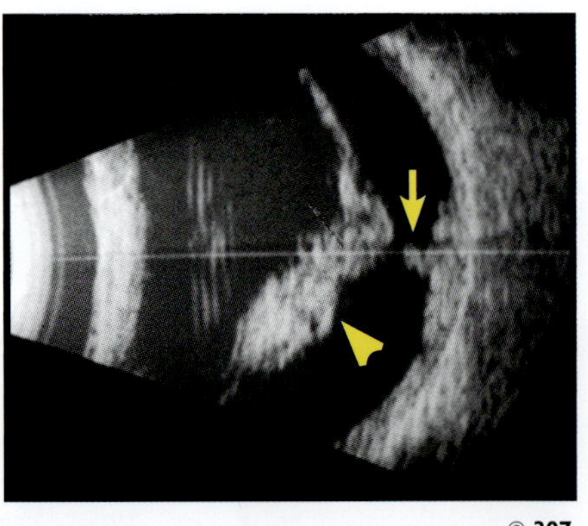

© 307

This is a 20-year-old female with massive optic nerve swelling, radial exudates and macular star, and exudative retinal detachment associated with neural cysticercosis *(left)*. *Courtesy of Rachelle Benner*

Scarring from a patient with cysticercosis due to fibrous proliferation can be seen with ultrasonography on the right *(arrow)*. The scolex of the organism is indicated by the arrow and the arrowhead shows the vitreous fibrotic changes.

Diffuse or Disseminated Unilateral Subacute Neuroretinitis

Diffuse or disseminated unilateral subacute neuroretinitis (DUSN) is a syndrome caused by a nematode that moves around in the subretinal space or vitreous. The precise identification of the nematode is still not resolved. The nematodes range in size from 400 to 2000 μm. The smaller nematode is proposed to be *Ancylostoma caninum*, while the larger nematode has been thought to be *Baylisascaris procyonis*, an intestinal worm of lower carnivores such as raccoons and squirrels. The cardinal symptoms of DUSN include floaters, scotoma, and ocular discomfort. Mild to moderate vitritis, optic disc swelling or atrophy, narrowing of retinal arterioles, and clusters of white inflammatory spots in the deep retina or RPE may be present. In cases with more severe inflammation, focal areas of fibrosis and tractional detachment may occur.

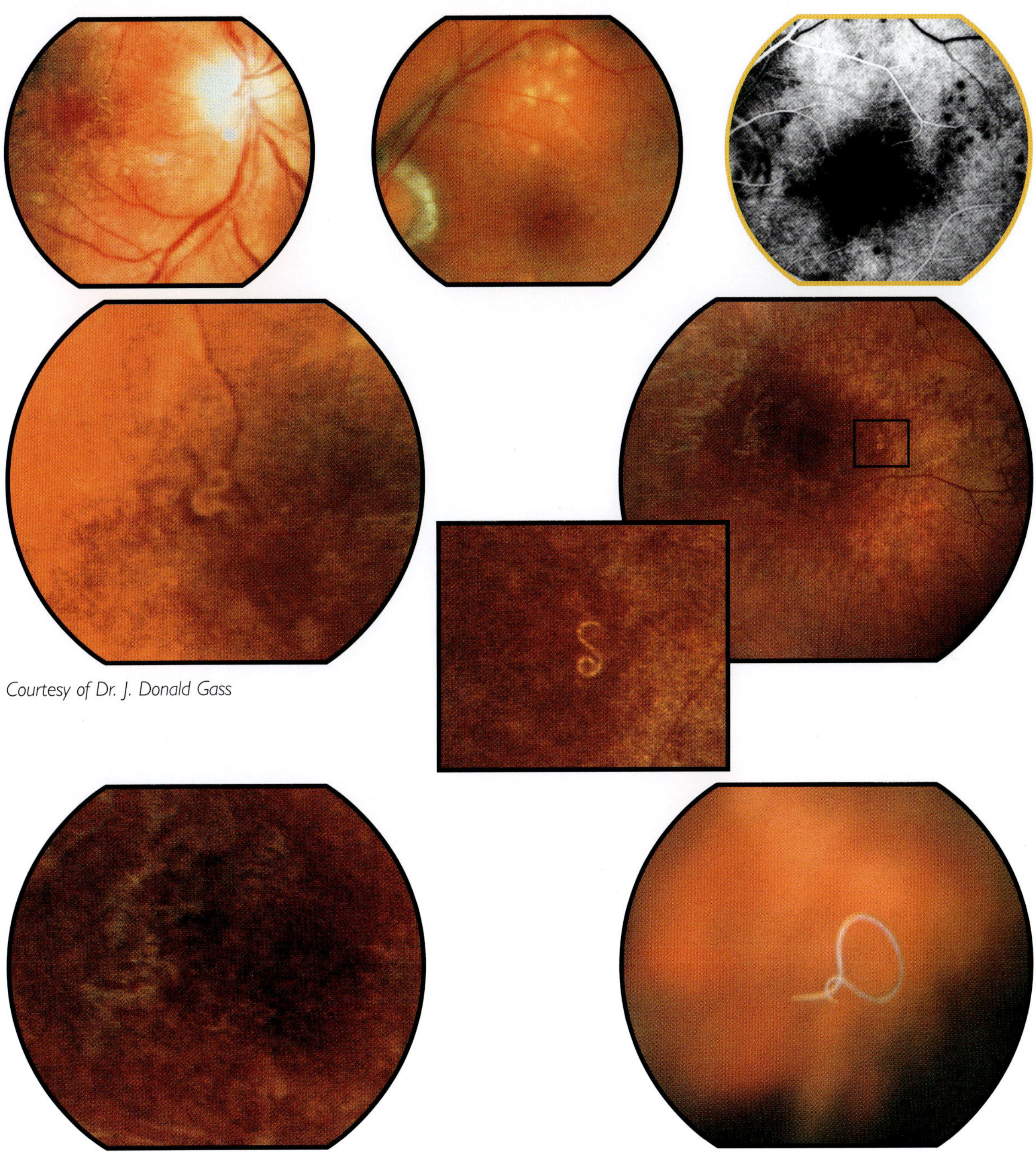

Courtesy of Dr. J. Donald Gass

Courtesy of Dr. Mark Blumenkranz

These are patients with DUSN. The clinical manifestations are typically unilateral with multiple white spots of inflammation, such as those seen in the two upper left photographs. Chorioretinal white spots tend to cluster in distribution. Progressive chorioretinal pigmentary and atrophic degeneration and optic atrophy lead to severe vision loss. Inflammatory infiltrates will block with FA *(upper right)*. Nematodes have a serpentine configuration and may range from 500 to 1500 μm in size and can be seen moving in the vitreous *(lower right)*.

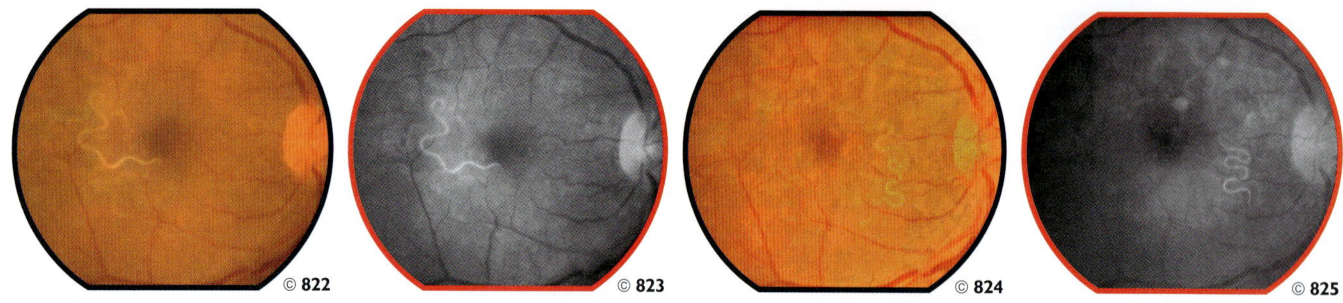

These images of a patient with DUSN demonstrate the elusive and motile worm in the subretinal space. It is one of the larger variants.

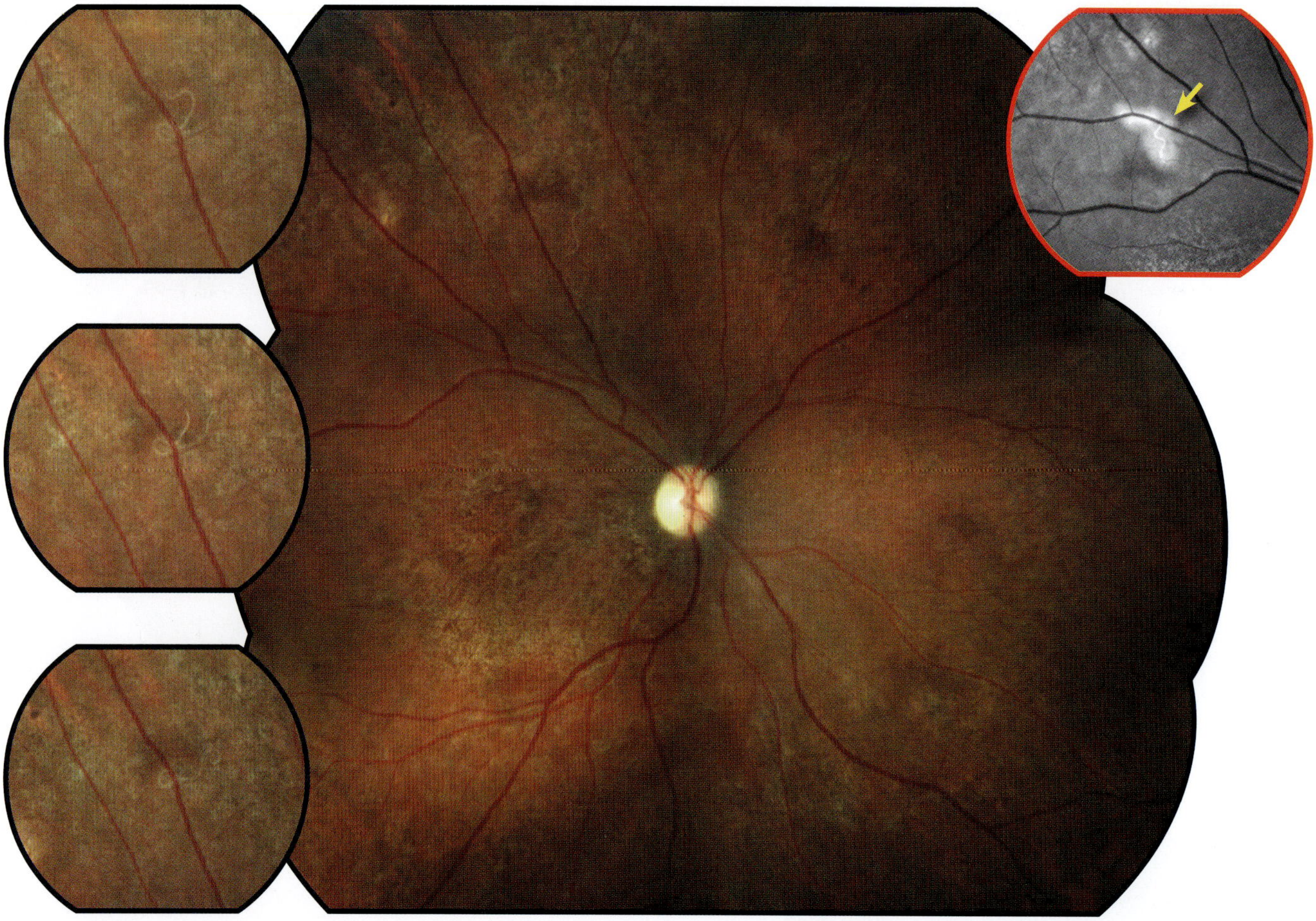

This worm was very elusive. It was finally detected by a motivated retinal fellow at the fundus camera. Its various positions in the subretinal space are noted in the magnified images. A monochromatic photograph shows a white photocoagulation burn applied to destroy the worm. The worm itself may be seen as a silhouette in the intense white photocoagulation lesion *(arrow)*. Widespread pigment epithelium degeneration and atrophy evolved, along with optic atrophy and severe loss of vision in this patient.

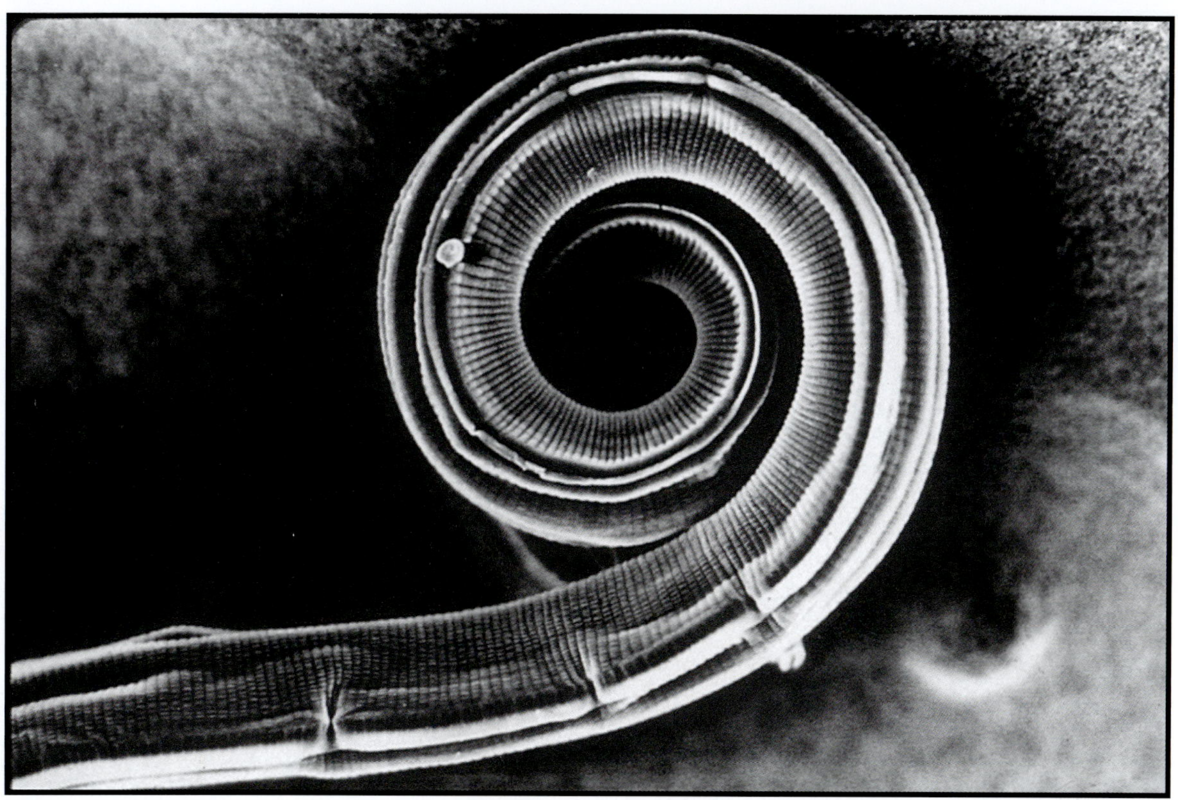

The scanning electron microscope image demonstrates the appearance of this worm, taken after removal from the vitreous. *Courtesy of Dr. Mark Blumenkranz*

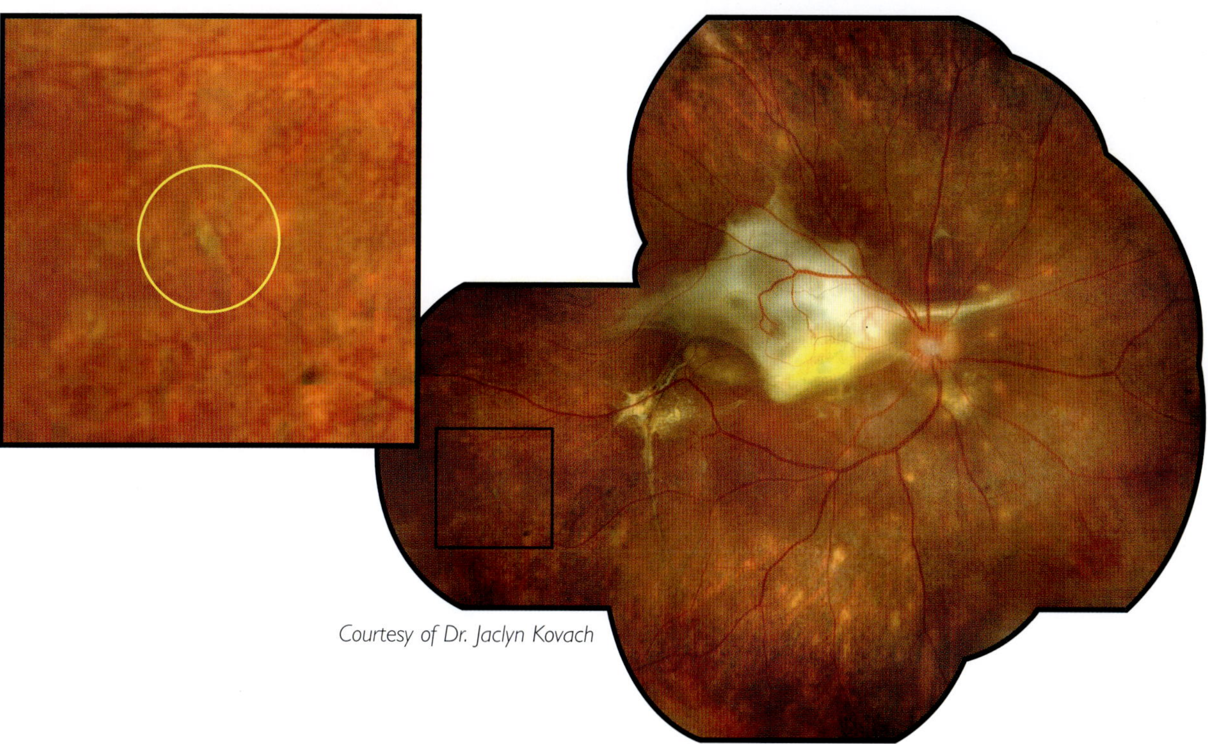

Courtesy of Dr. Jaclyn Kovach

This is a patient with DUSN who presented with extensive unilateral subretinal fibrosis. There are scattered chorioretinal spots, which are also characteristic of the disease. A small worm was seen temporal to the macula *(framed)*.

Toxocariasis

Ocular toxocariasis is due to the roundworm *Toxocara canis*. The natural host of *T. canis* is the dog. Sexual maturation to egg-producing larvae (third stage) occurs only in puppies that become infected by transplacental prenatal transmission. Postnatal acquisition may occur from milk of an infected bitch or by fecal–oral transmission. Transtracheal migration occurs in infected pups and third-stage larvae are coughed up, swallowed, and then mature to sexually differentiated forms in the small intestine. Advanced stage 2 larvae are then shed in the feces. Ocular toxocariasis infection may occur via lymphatic or hematogenous dissemination during initial systemic infection or after late reactivation of dormant larvae inside peripheral tissue. Larvae enter the eye via ciliary, choroidal, or retinal arteries. The nematode larvae is enveloped in an eosinophilic granuloma or abscess, with a central core of eosinophils surrounded by mononuclear cells, histiocytes, epithelioid cells, and occasional giant cells. The condition is predominantly seen in the pediatric population, although there are exceptions. The characteristic findings on ophthalmoscopic examination include (1) peripheral granuloma; (2) posterior pole granuloma; or (3) chronic endophthalmitis. A fibrous or gliotic band with a falciform retinal fold is typically seen between the peripheral granuloma and the optic disc.

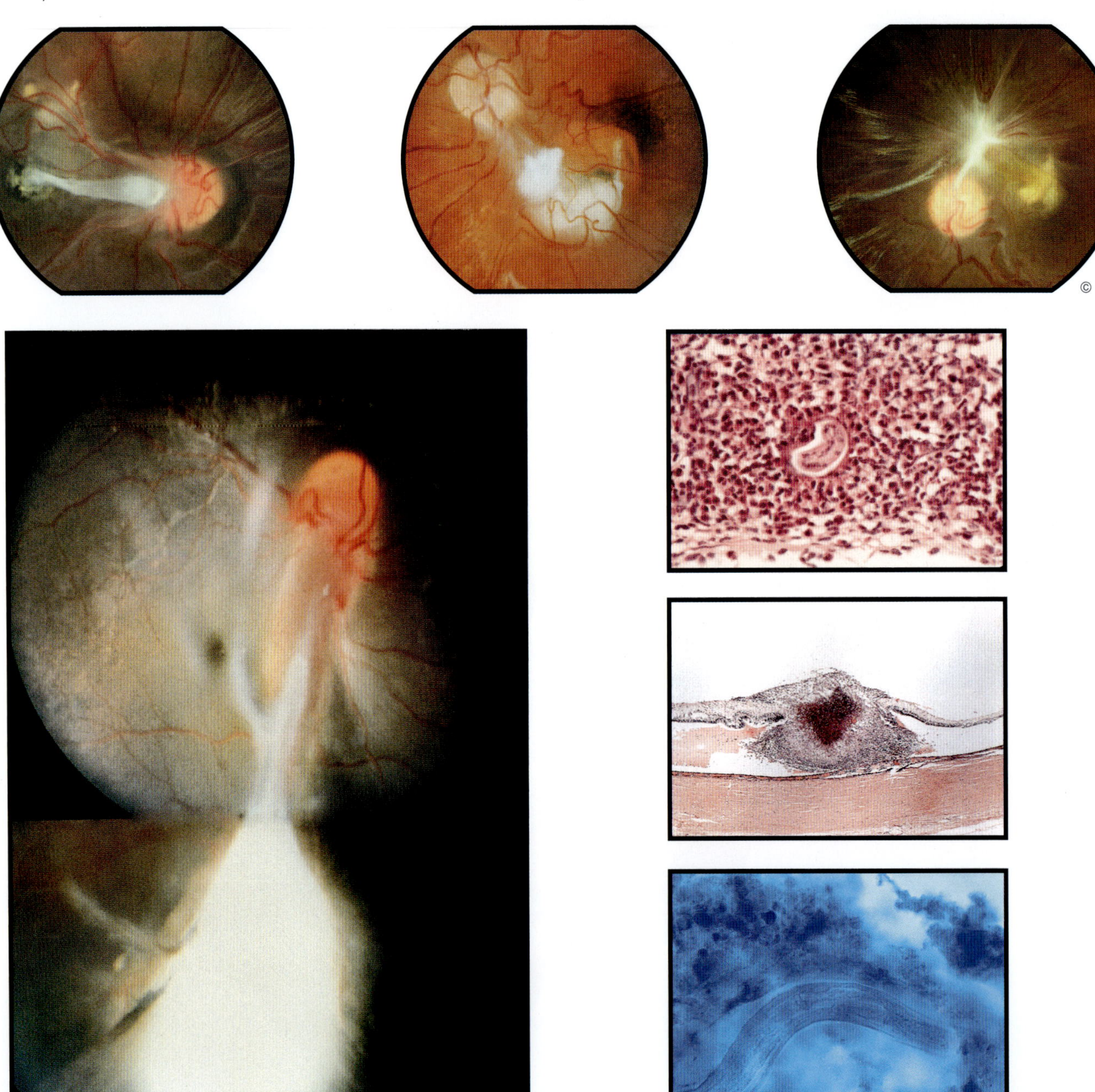

© 308

© 309

These are patients with ocular toxocariasis. There is extensive fibrotic or gliotic change, traction on the macula, and detachment. Dragging of the retinal vasculature from the nerve to the fibrotic scar is very typical. The histology shows the worm in the center of granulomatous inflammation in the subretinal space. The second-stage larvae of the organism are enveloped in an eosinophilic abscess. Clinical pathological correlation revealed an intact *Toxocara* organism. There were numerous neutrophils, epithelioid cells, and multinucleated giant cells surrounding the parasite.

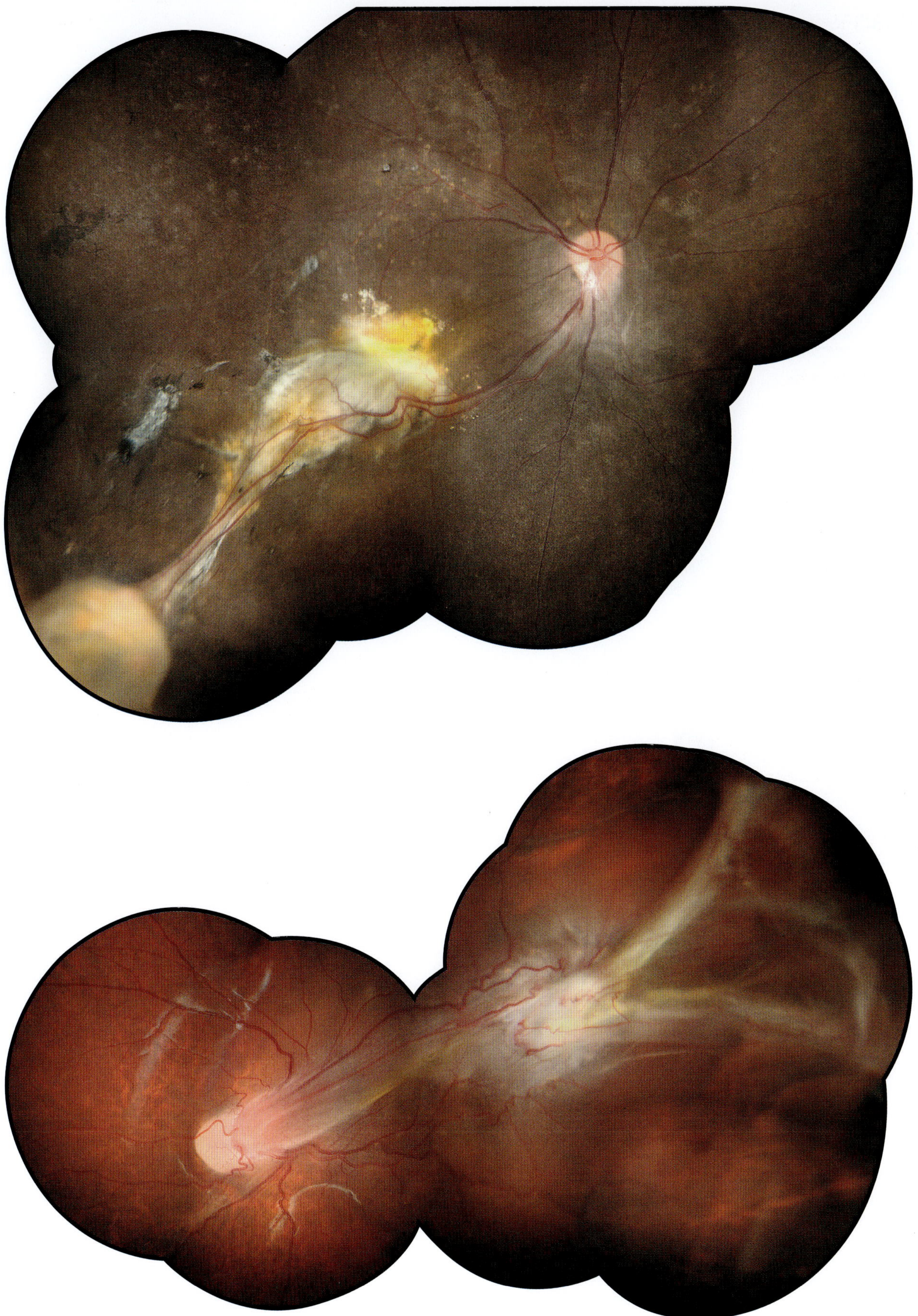

These are two cases of presumed ocular toxocariasis. Note that the vitreoretinal scar travels from the disc to the periphery, where it broadens into a larger fibrotic lesion. Retinal vessels are engaged within the fibrovascular tissue. Localized traction retinal detachment is noted in the second case.

Filariasis

Ocular filariasis is an infectious eye disease caused by a nematode. Species include *Onchocerca volvulus, Loa loa,* and *Wuchereria bancrofti.* Patients can present with a mild to moderate vitritis, optic disc edema, and recurrent outbreaks of multifocal and evanescent white-gray or yellow chorioretinal lesions in the peripheral fundus. The organism can survive up to 4 years in the subretinal space. Optic atrophy and chorioretinal degeneration in addition to secondary glaucoma, cataract, and anterior synechiae can result. The treatment of choice is to photocoagulate the worm, as de-worming pharmacotherapy does not usually eradicate the organism.

Onchocerca volvulus is responsible for a type of human filariasis which is endemic in some areas of Central Africa. The microfilaria are usually found in high numbers in the skin and eye of infected individuals. Abnormalities in the fundus consist of atrophy of the RPE and choroid, optic neuritis, and optic atrophy. The overall appearance of the posterior segment in the eye simulates a generalized rod–cone degeneration.

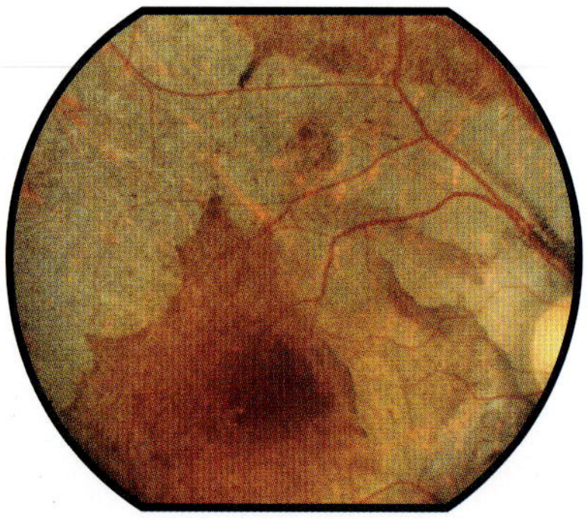

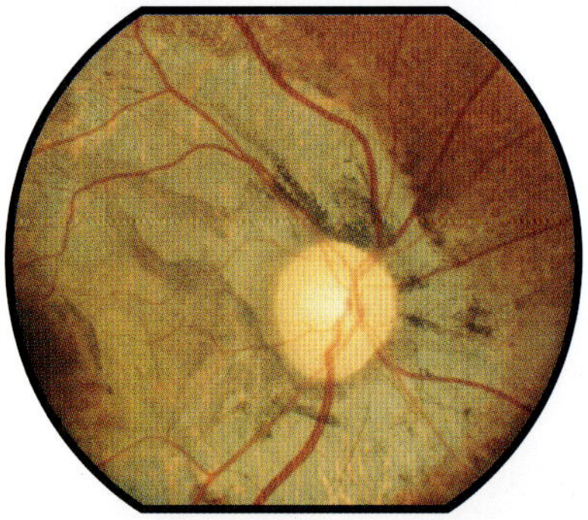

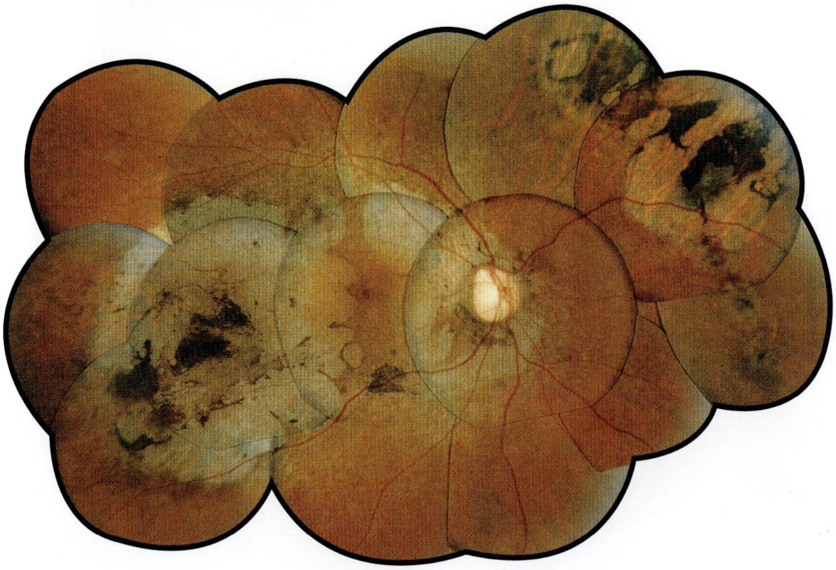

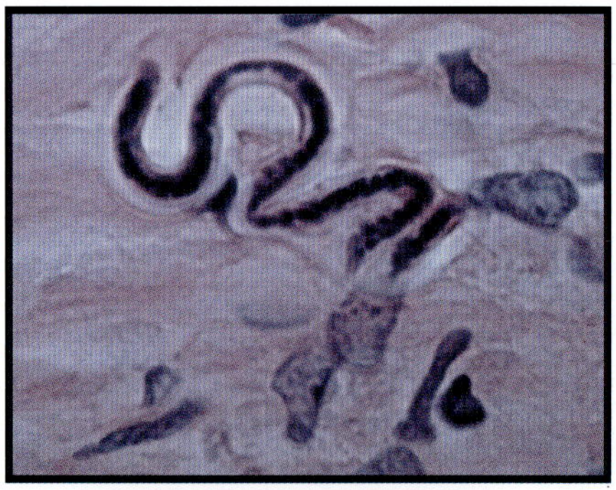

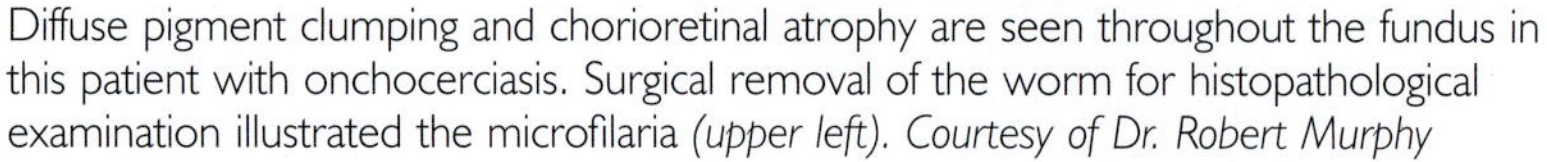

Diffuse pigment clumping and chorioretinal atrophy are seen throughout the fundus in this patient with onchocerciasis. Surgical removal of the worm for histopathological examination illustrated the microfilaria *(upper left). Courtesy of Dr. Robert Murphy*

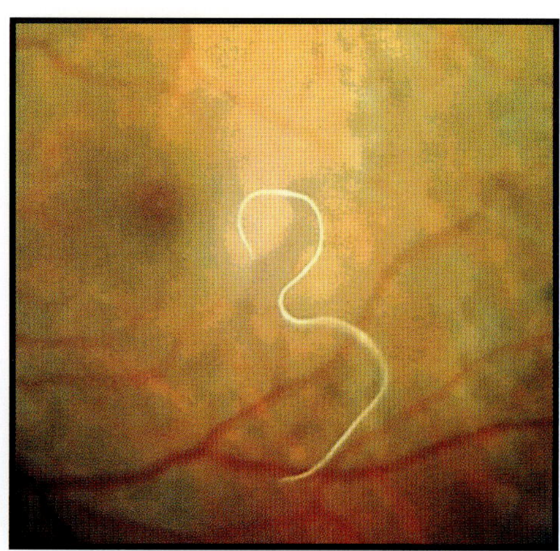

Ocular filariasis due to *Wuchereria bancrofti* may produce a panuveitis. In this eye, this nematode is seen in the vitreous of a 10-year-old girl in India. *Courtesy of Dr. Subina Narang, Government Medical College and Hospital*

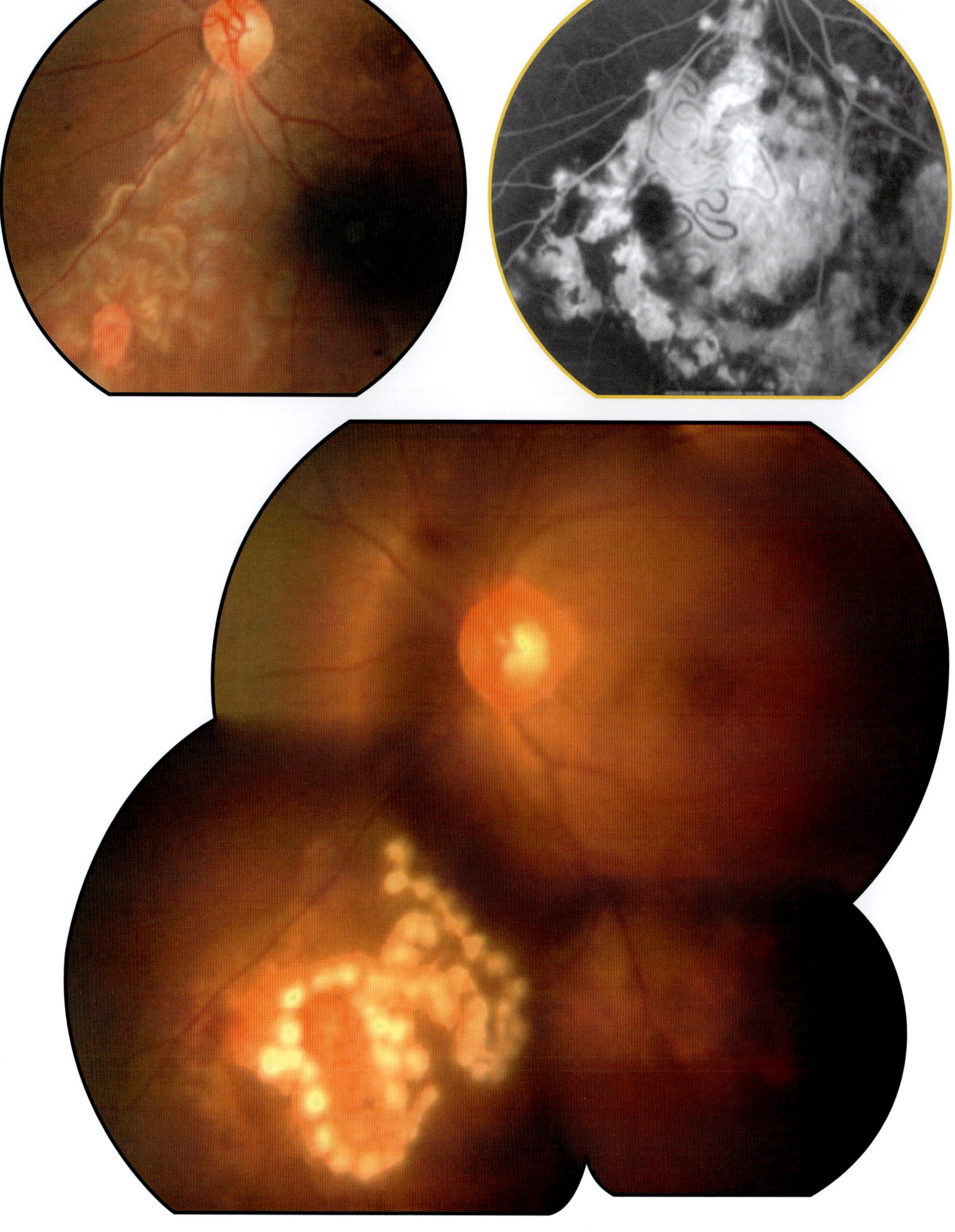

This patient with a presumed filariasis infection presented with multiple worms in the subretinal space inferonasal to the optic disc *(top left)*. FA shows associated diffuse chorioretinal atrophy with late staining. The bottom image shows the treated area of laser photocoagulation. *Courtesy of Dr. Jose Roca*

Alaria Mesocercariae

Alaria species are Diplostomatidae trematodes that live as adults in the small intestine of carnivorous mammals. The snail, the frog, and the third definitive host (carnivores) are involved in their life cycle. Humans become infected by eating intermediate or paratenic hosts containing mesocercariae (e.g. inadequately cooked frogs' legs).

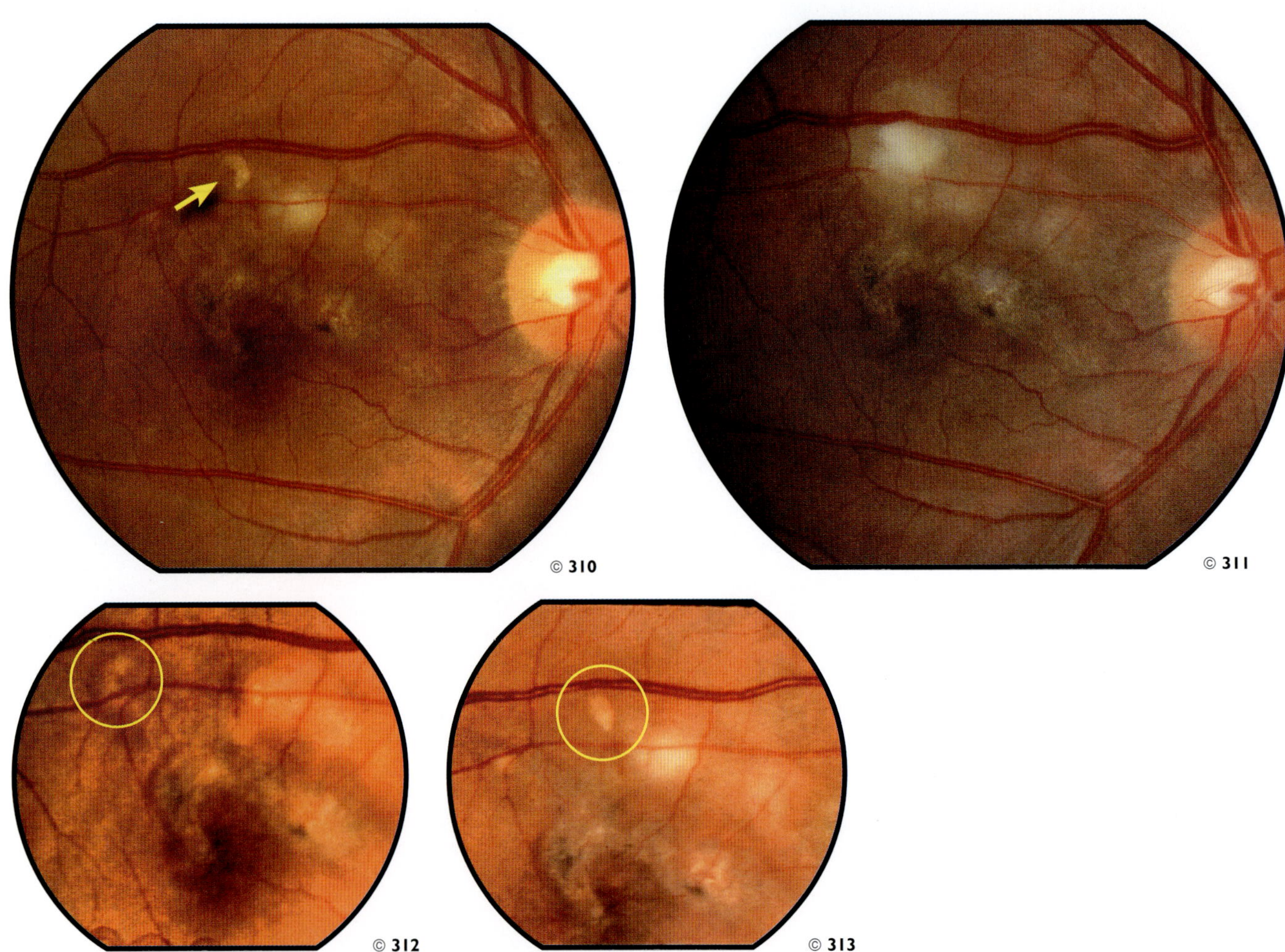

This patient was infected by an *Alaria* worm in the fundus, which was moving *(circles and arrow)*. It was successfully photocoagulated *(upper right image)*. The patient presented with unilateral disease that essentially led to a clinical presentation that was similar to DUSN or even toxocariasis. It was detected by a motivated photographer who noted movement in the fundus.

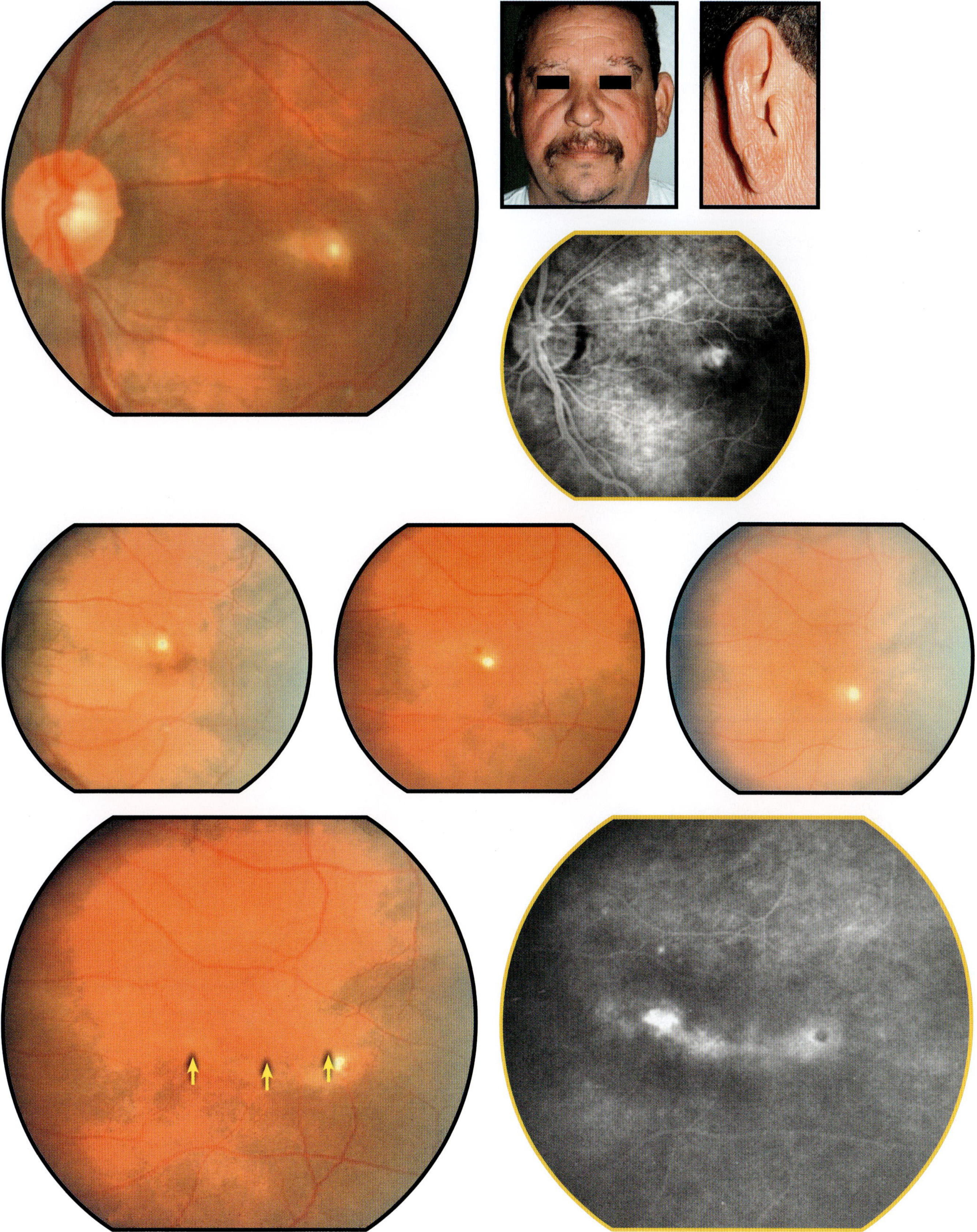

This patient with a history of leprosy *(scant eyebrows and leonine facies, upper right two photos)* presented with a yellow spot in the macula *(top left)* that was noted to have late leakage on FA. The lesion migrated across the macula over a period of 1 week *(middle center photo)* and 1 month *(middle right photo)*. The clinical appearance and pattern of migration were consistent with an *Alaria* infection. The path of migration can be seen in the lower left color photo *(arrows)* and FA *(bottom right)*.

Ophthalmomyiasis

Ophthalmomyiasis is produced by the intraocular invasion into the posterior segment by the larvae of certain flies in the order of Diptera. The larvae of the parasite fly of rodents, *Cuterebra,* may be found in the vitreous, subretinal space, or even in the anterior chamber. The eggs or the larval form of the fly are deposited on the human cornea or conjunctival surface by an adult fly. The larva eventually passes through the sclera to reach the interior of the eye. Within the subretinal space, the larva migrates in a random direction, leaving crisscrossing atrophic tracks in the RPE, a manifestation that is considered to be pathognomonic of the disorder.

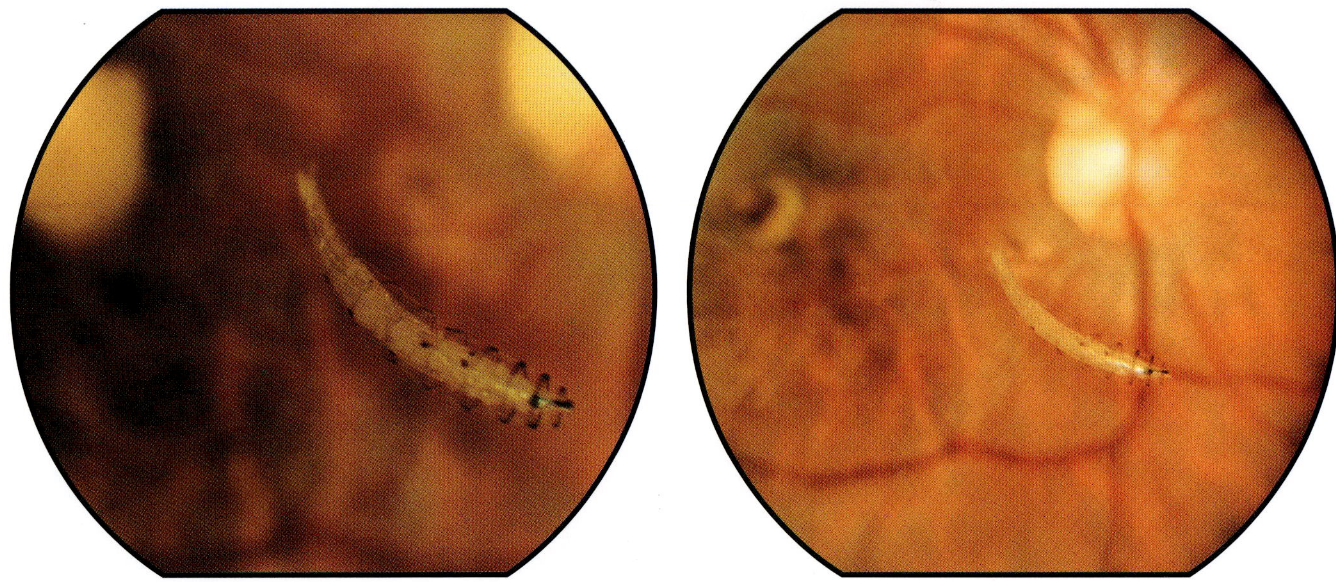

Note the Diptera larva in the vitreous. There is inflammation and pigmentary abnormalities in the macular region. *Courtesy of Kenneth Julian, CRA, FOPS*

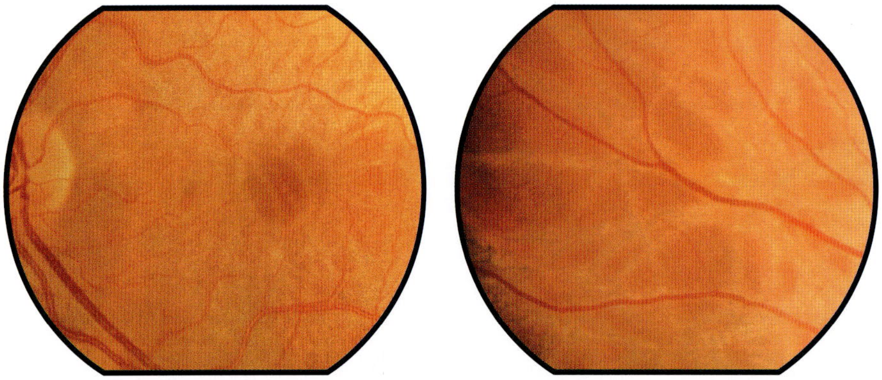

The fundus shows crisscrossing lines of atrophy (parasitic tracks) at the level of the RPE. These can be subtle in a lightly pigmented fundus.

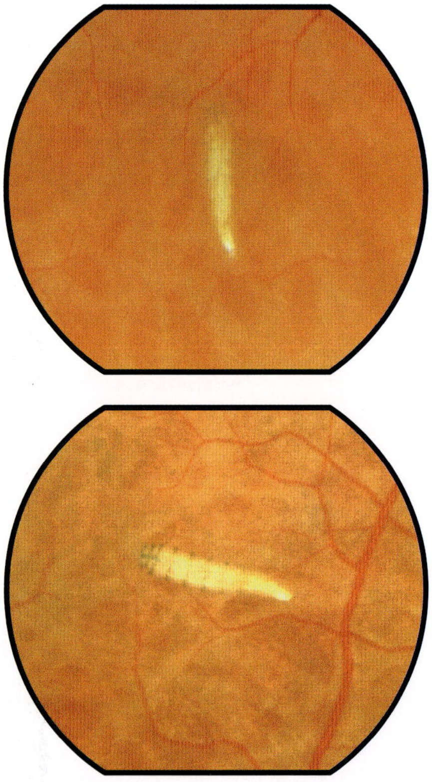

These are two cases demonstrating the larval worm in the vitreous. These patients also have crisscrossing atrophic lines or tracks at the level of the RPE, which are faintly evident.

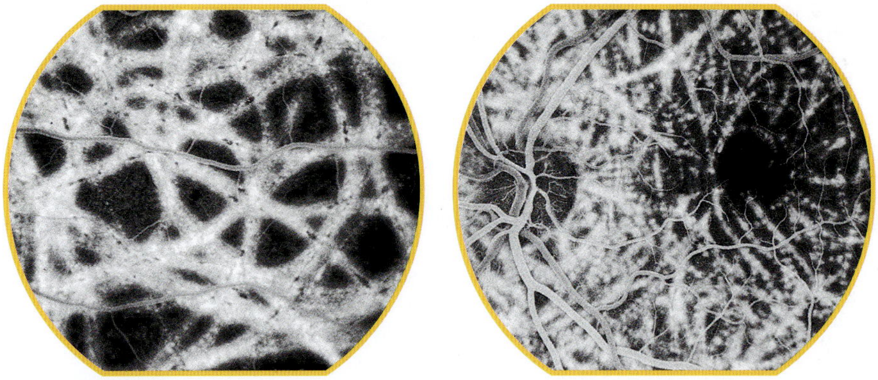

The FA in a chronic case shows numerous crisscrossing lesions or parasitic tracks in the fundus, a pattern that is only associated with ophthalmomyiasis. *Courtesy of Dr. Miriam Ridley*

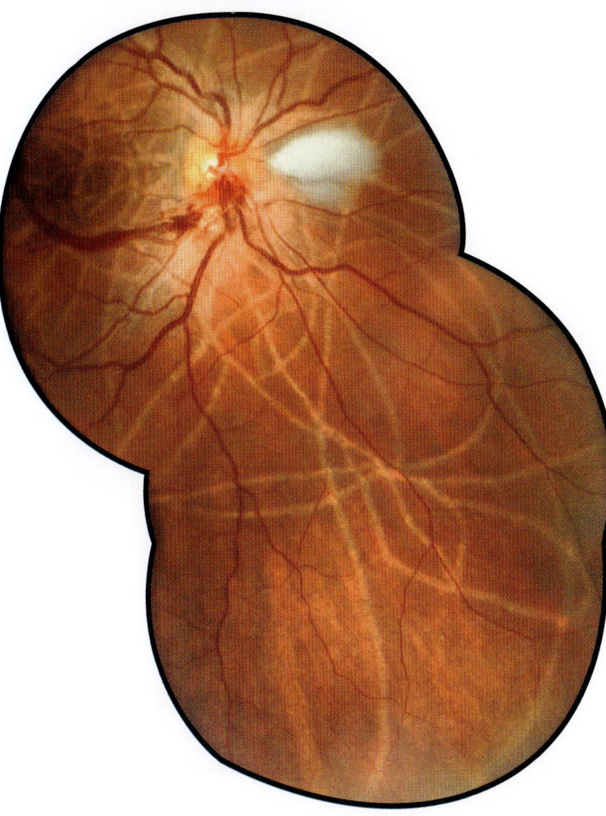

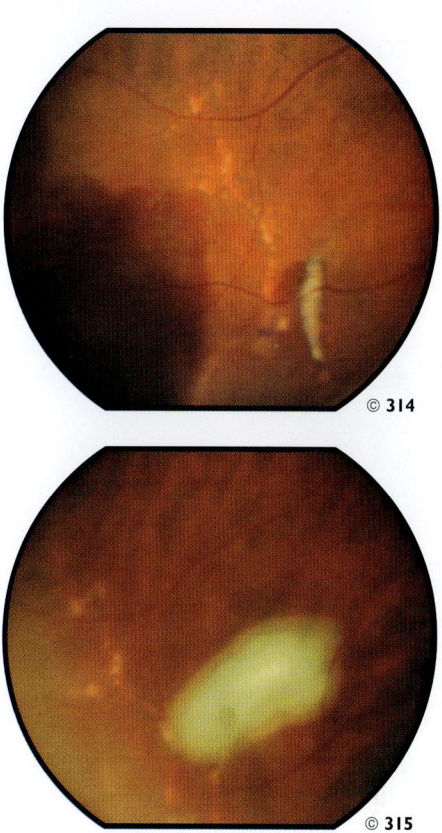

This patient has hemorrhage at the disc, crisscrossing atrophic tracks at the level of the RPE, and a white reaction due to laser ablation of the Diptera larvae.

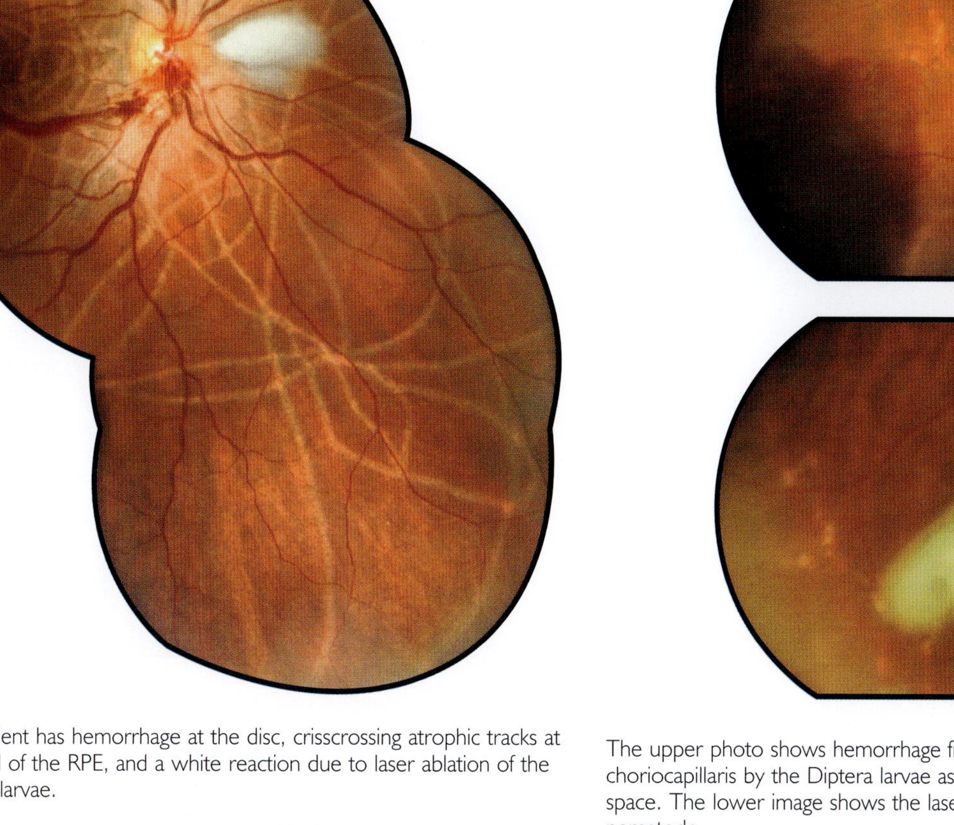

© 314

© 315

The upper photo shows hemorrhage from disturbance of the choriocapillaris by the Diptera larvae as it travels through the subretinal space. The lower image shows the laser reaction after ablation of the nematode.

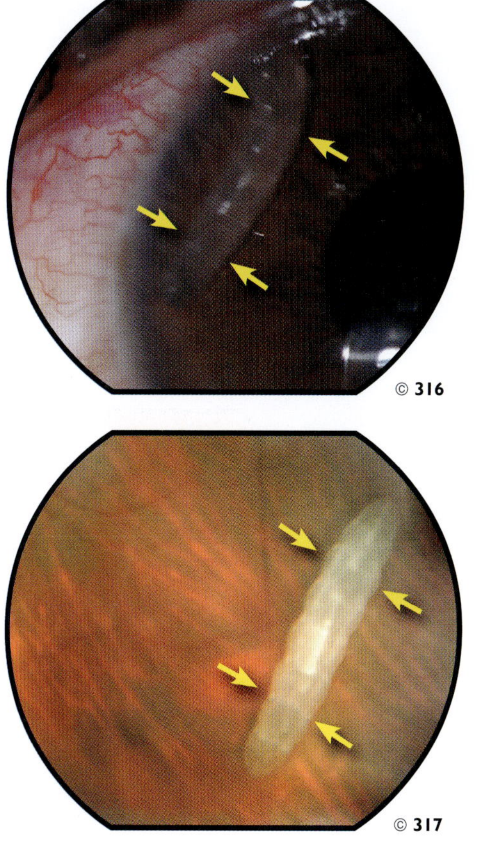

© 316

© 317

These are two patients with ophthalmomyiasis. The larval worm can be present in the anterior chamber *(upper image, arrows)* or the vitreous *(lower image, arrows)*.

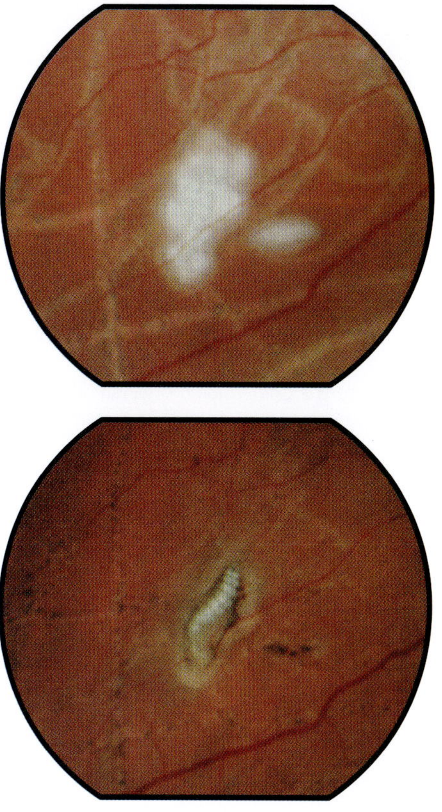

These two images show the photocoagulation reaction after laser ablation of the Diptera larva *(upper image)* with a background of atrophic, crisscrossing pigment epithelial lines or parasitic tracks. The lower image shows the nematode following obliteration by the laser. The silhouette of its structure is evident by a margin of pigmentation.

Gnathostomiasis

Gnathostomiasis is a disease caused by migration and metabolic secretion of the larva of the *Gnathostoma* species. The *Gnathostoma* worm has a distinct head bulb covered by four rows of hooks. The route of entry into the eye is not clear, although the worm may gain access through the retina and choroid, which results in subretinal hemorrhages, retinal scars, and even retinal breaks. A live worm can be found in the anterior chamber or in the vitreous. Associated localized inflammation, retinal hemorrhages and exudates, and even inflammation of the optic nerve may be seen.

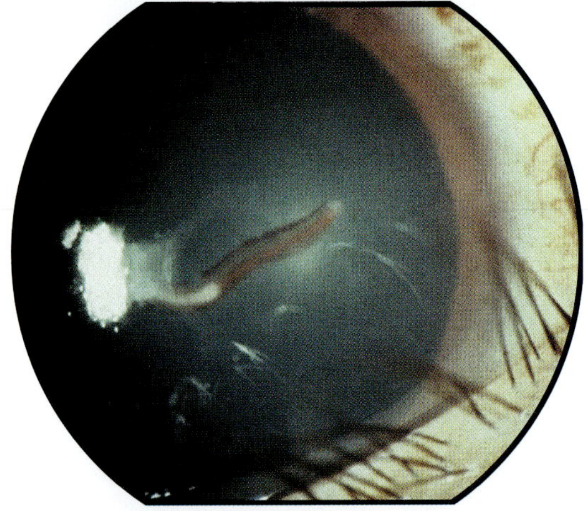

Note the *Gnathostoma* organism in the anterior chamber of this eye.

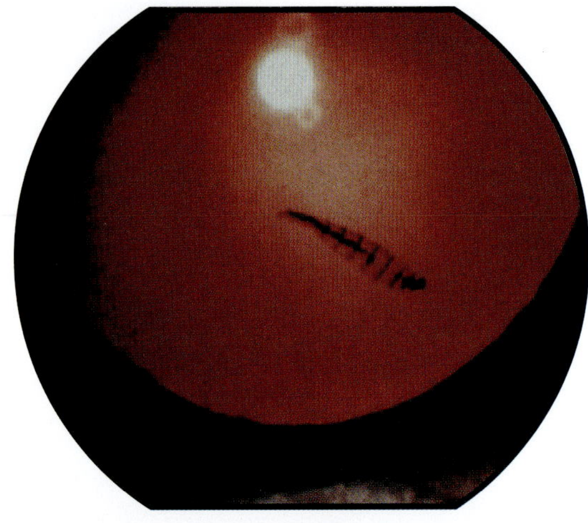

This patient has ophthalmomyiasis simulating gnathostomiasis.

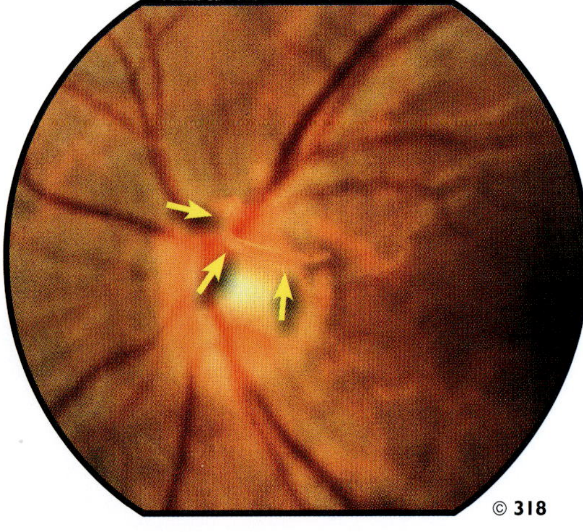

© 318

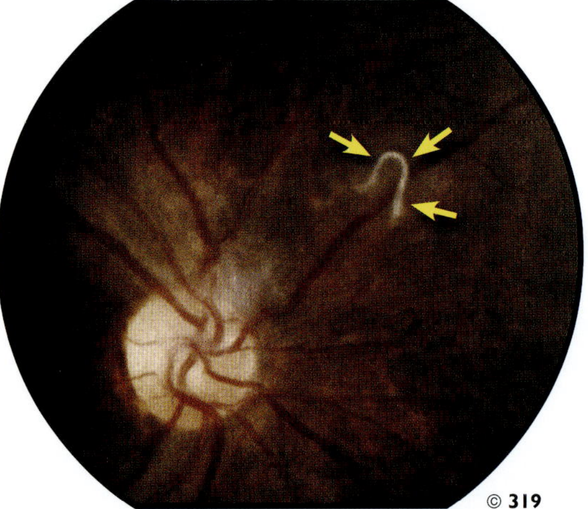

© 319

In these patients, there is a *Gnathostoma* organism in the posterior pole. The images show the nematode overlying the optic nerve and retinal vein and assuming a curvilinear or even an oval configuration *(arrows)*.

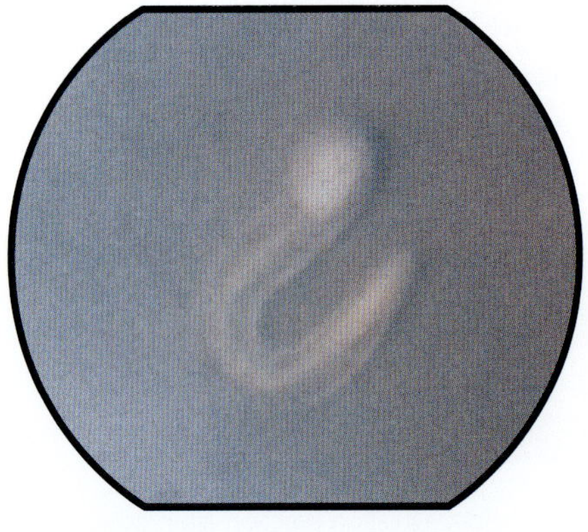

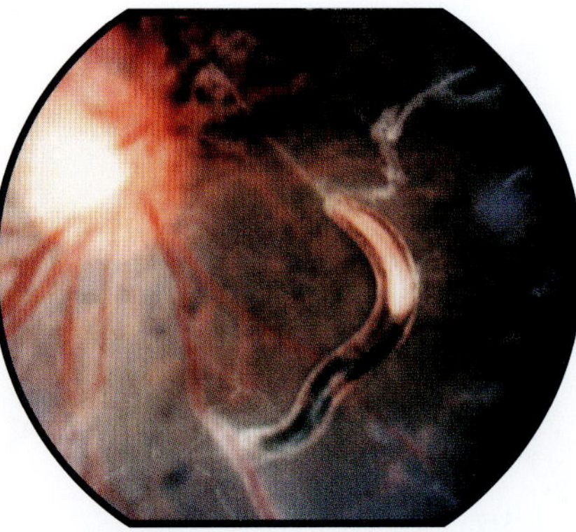

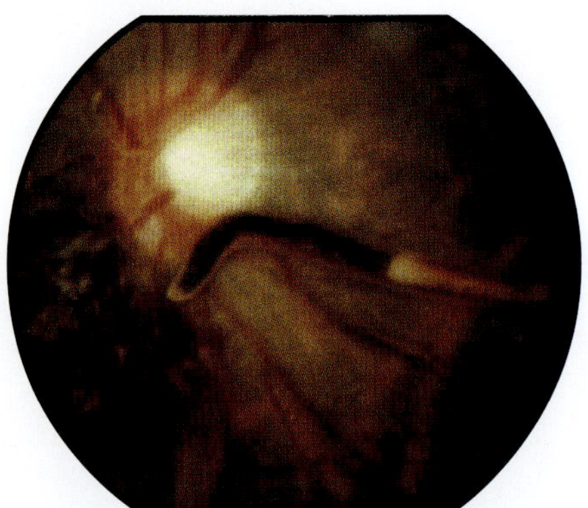

The *Gnathostoma* organism in these patients may be seen in a cloudy vitreous *(left)*, and near the optic nerve, where it induced retinal hemorrhage *(middle and right)*. Blood may be seen in the digestive lumen of the nematode. Waste products may be seen leaving the organism. *Left image courtesy of Dr. Prut Hanutsaha and middle image courtesy of Dr. Charles Mango*

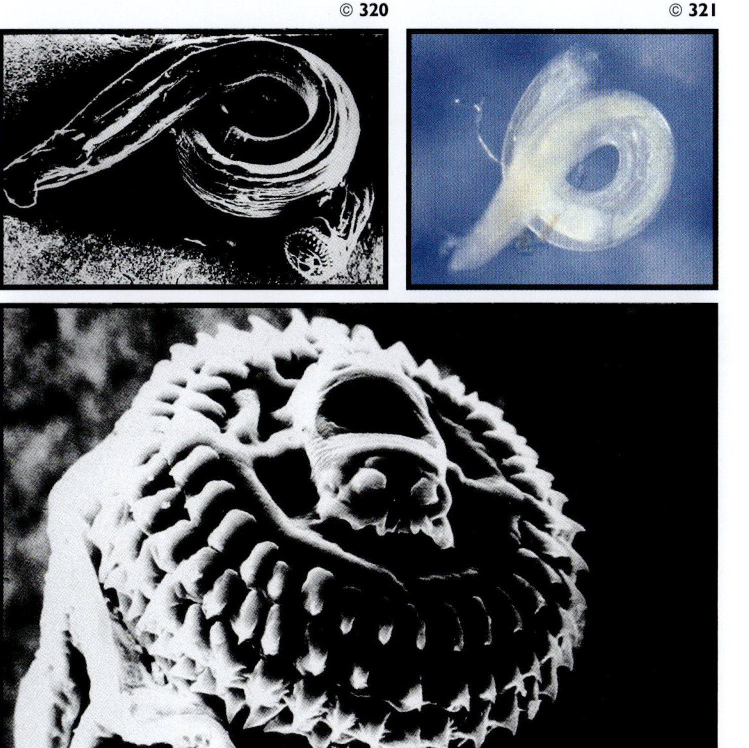

The *Gnathostoma* worm measures 1.5 mm in length and has a knob-like structure at the cephalic end, seen here in the top photographs. Scanning electron micrograph illustrates a segmented head bulb with hooklets. The mouth is located at the head bulb, and it has two lips with sensory papillae.

Angiostrongyliasis

Angiostrongylus cantonensis is the most common cause of eosinophilic meningitis in Southeast Asia. Rats, snails, slugs, and crustaceans are intermediary hosts. Humans are infected by eating raw food such as pila, snails, fish, and crustaceans. Larvae migrate through the circulation to the brain and eye. Ocular manifestations include decreased vision, exophthalmos, and lid swelling. The *Angiostrongylus* worm may be found in the anterior chamber, vitreous, or the subretinal space. Intraocular inflammation, pigment epithelial degenerative abnormalities, and optic nerve edema or pallor may be seen.

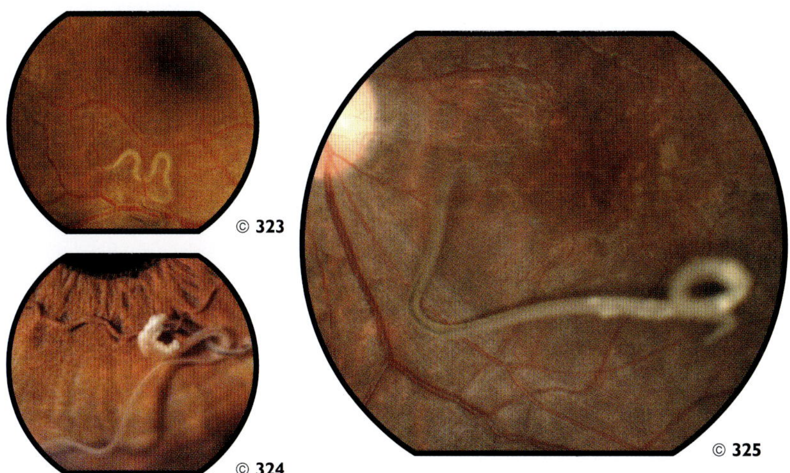

The immature worm is seen in the anterior chamber *(lower left)* and in the vitreous with its head burrowed in the retina *(upper left)*. In the image on the right the worm is identified in both the vitreous and in the subretinal space.

Ascariasis

Porrocaecum heteropterum and *Ascaris lumbricoides* are roundworms that belong to genera of the class Nematoda in the subfamily Ascarididae. Adult worms are found in the stomach and intestine of carnivorous reptiles, birds, and mammals. Thick-shelled eggs are passed in the feces to mature in soil or water to a larval stage that is infective when digested by an intermediate host such as a small mammal. The larvae then infect the final host. Humans are infected by eating raw meat or drinking water contaminated with the egg-bearing feces of a carnivorous final host.

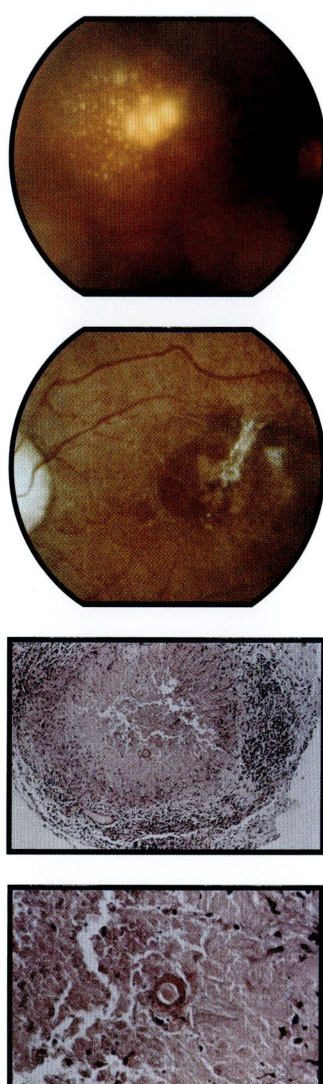

The *Ascaris* worm has induced inflammation in these two patients. In the second color image, optic atrophy and atrophic and pigmentary degeneration of the macula may be seen. The histopathology shows diffuse granulomatous infection with the nematode centrally located, which is most evident on the magnified photograph.

Suggested Reading

HIV Associated Retinopathy

Dunn, J.P., Yamashita, A., Kempen, J.H., et al., 2005. Retinal vascular occlusion in patients infected with human immunodeficiency virus. Retina 25, 759–766.

Faber, D.W., Wiley, C.A., Bergeron-Lynn, G., et al., 1992. Role of human immunodeficiency virus and cytomegalovirus in the pathogenesis of retinitis and retinal vasculopathy in AIDS patients. Invest. Ophthalmol. Vis. Sci. 33, 2345–2353.

Falkenstein, I., Kozak, I., Kayikcioglu, O., et al., 2006. Assessment of retinal function in patients with HIV without infectious retinitis by multifocal electroretinogram and automated perimetry. Retina 26, 928–934.

Freeman, W.R., O'Connor, G.R., 1984. Acquired immune deficiency syndrome retinopathy, Pneumocystis, and cotton-wool spots. Am. J. Ophthalmol. 98, 235–237.

Freeman, W.R., Chen, A., Henderly, D., et al., 1987. Prognostic and systemic significance of non-infectious AIDS associated retinopathy. Invest. Ophthalmol. Vis. Sci. 28, 9.

Goldberg, D.E., Smithen, L.M., Angelilli, A., et al., 2005. HIV-associated retinopathy in the HAART era. Retina 25, 633–649, quiz 682–683.

Gonzalez, C.R., Wiley, C.A., Arevalo, J.F., et al., 1996. Polymerase chain reaction detection of cytomegalovirus and human immunodeficiency virus-1 in the retina of patients with acquired immune deficiency syndrome with and without cotton-wool spots. Retina 16, 305–311.

Holland, G.N., 2008. AIDS and ophthalmology: the first quarter century. Am. J. Ophthalmol. 145, 397–408.

Kuppermann, B.D., Petty, J.G., Richman, D.D., et al., 1992. Cross-sectional prevalence of CMV retinitis in AIDS patients: correlation with CD4 counts. Invest. Ophthalmol. Vis. Sci. 33, 750.

Palestine, A.G., Rodrigues, M.M., Macher, A.M., et al., 1984. Ophthalmic involvement in acquired immune deficiency syndrome. Ophthalmology 91, 1092–1099.

Sadun, A.A., Pepose, J.S., Madigan, M.C., et al., 1995. AIDS-related optic neuropathy: a histological, virological and ultrastructural study. Graefes Arch. Clin. Exp. Ophthalmol. 233, 387–398.

Schuman, J.S., Friedman, A.H., 1983. Retinal manifestations of the acquired immune deficiency syndrome (AIDS): Cytomegalovirus, *Candida albicans*, *Cryptococcus*, toxoplasmosis and *Pneumocystis carinii*. Trans. Ophthalmol. Soc. UK 103, 177–190.

Shah, K.H., Holland, G.N., Yu, F., et al., 2006. Contrast sensitivity and color vision in HIV-infected individuals without infectious retinopathy. Am. J. Ophthalmol. 142, 284–292.

Cytomegalovirus Retinitis

Buchi, E.R., Fitting, P.L., Michel, A.E., 1988. Long-term intravitreal ganciclovir for cytomegalovirus retinitis in a patient with AIDS. Case report. Arch. Ophthalmol. 106, 1349–1350.

D'Amico, D.J., Skolnik, P.R., Kosloff, B.R., et al., 1988. Resolution of cytomegalovirus retinitis with zidovudine therapy. Arch. Ophthalmol. 106, 1168–1169.

Freeman, W.R., Quiceno, J.K., Crapotta, J.A., et al., 1992. Surgical repair of rhegmatogenous retinal detachment in immunosuppressed patients with cytomegalovirus retinitis. Ophthalmology 99, 446–474.

Geier, S.A., Nasemann, J., Klauss, V., et al., 1992. Frosted branch angiitis associated with cytomegalovirus retinitis. Am. J. Ophthalmol. 114, 514–516.

Guyer, Dr, Jabs, D.A., Brant, A.M., et al., 1989. Regression of cytomegalovirus retinitis with zidovudine: a clinicopathologic correlation. Arch. Ophthalmol. 107, 868–874.

Henderly, D.E., Freeman, W.R., Causey, D.M., et al., 1987. Cytomegalovirus retinitis and response to therapy with ganciclovir. Ophthalmology 94, 425–434.

Holland, G.N., Tufail, A., 1995. New therapies for cytomegalovirus retinitis. N. Engl. J. Med. 333, 658–659.

Holland, G.N., Vaudaux, J.D., Shiramizu, K.M., et al., 2008. Characteristics of untreated AIDS-related cytomegalovirus retinitis. II. Findings in the era of highly active antiretroviral therapy (1997 to 2000). Am. J. Ophthalmol. 145, 12–22.

Jabs, D.A., Van Natta, M.L., Thorne, J.E., et al., 2004. Course of cytomegalovirus retinitis in the era of highly active antiretroviral therapy: 2. Second eye involvement and retinal detachment. Ophthalmology 111, 2232–2239.

Marx, J.L., Kapusta, M.A., Patel, S.S., et al., 1996. Use of the ganciclovir implant in the treatment of recurrent cytomegalovirus retinitis. Arch. Ophthalmol. 114, 815–820.

Patel, S.S., Rutzen, A.R., Marx, J.L., et al., 1996. Cytomegalovirus papillitis in patients with acquired immune deficiency syndrome. Visual prognosis of patients treated with ganciclovir and/or foscarnet. Ophthalmology 103, 1476–1482.

Schrier, R.D., Song, M.K., Smith, I.L., et al., 2006. Intraocular viral and immune pathogenesis of immune recovery uveitis in patients with healed cytomegalovirus retinitis. Retina 26, 165–169.

Spaide, R.F., Vitale, A.T., Toth, I.R., et al., 1992. Frosted branch angiitis associated with cytomegalovirus retinitis. Am. J. Ophthalmol. 113, 522–528.

Wren, S.M., Fielder, A.R., Bethell, D., et al., 2004. Cytomegalovirus retinitis in infancy. Eye (Lond.) 18, 389–392.

Acute Retinal Necrosis Syndrome

Almeida, D.R., Chin, E.K., Tarantola, R.M., et al., 2015. Long-term outcomes in patients undergoing vitrectomy for retinal detachment due to viral retinitis. Clin. Ophthalmol. 9, 1307–1314.

Ando, F., Kato, M., Goto, S., et al., 1983. Platelet function in bilateral acute retinal necrosis. Am. J. Ophthalmol. 96, 27–32.

Blair, M.P., Goldstein, D.A., Shapiro, M.J., 2007. Optical coherence tomography of progressive outer retinal necrosis. Retina 27, 1313–1314.

Blumenkranz, M., Clarkson, J., Culbertson, W.W., et al., 1988. Vitrectomy for retinal detachment associated with acute retinal necrosis. Am. J. Ophthalmol. 106, 426–429.

Blumenkranz, M., Clarkson, J., Culbertson, W.W., et al., 1989. Visual results and complications after retinal reattachment in the acute retinal necrosis syndrome. The influence of operative technique. Retina 9, 170–174.

Browning, D.J., Blumenkranz, M.S., Culbertson, W.W., et al., 1987. Association of varicella zoster dermatitis with acute retinal necrosis syndrome. Ophthalmology 94, 602–606.

Ciulla, T.A., Rutledge, B.K., Morley, M.G., et al., 1998. The progressive outer retinal necrosis syndrome: successful treatment with combination antiviral therapy. Ophthalmic Surg. Lasers 29, 198–206.

Culbertson, W.W., Blumenkranz, M.S., Pepose, J.S., et al., 1986. Varicella zoster virus is a cause of the acute retinal necrosis syndrome. Ophthalmology 93, 559–569.

Cunningham, E.T. Jr., Short, G.A., Irvine, A.R., et al., 1996. Acquired immunodeficiency syndrome associated herpes simplex virus retinitis. Clinical description and use of a polymerase chain reaction-based assay as a diagnostic tool. Arch. Ophthalmol. 114, 834–840.

Engstrom, R.J., Holland, G.N., Margolis, T.P., et al., 1994. The progressive outer retinal necrosis syndrome. A variant of necrotizing herpetic retinopathy in patients with AIDS. Ophthalmology 101, 1488–1502.

Freeman, W.R., Thomas, E.L., Rao, N.A., et al., 1986. Demonstration of herpes group virus in acute retinal necrosis syndrome. Am. J. Ophthalmol. 102, 701–709.

Friedlander, S., Rahhal, F.M., Ericson, L., et al., 1996. Optic neuropathy preceding acute retinal necrosis in acquired immunodeficiency syndrome. Arch. Ophthalmol. 114, 1481–1485.

Gain, P., Chiquet, C., Thuret, G., et al., 2002. Herpes simplex virus type 1 encephalitis associated with acute retinal necrosis syndrome in an immunocompetent patient. Acta Ophthalmol. Scand. 80, 546–549.

Gariano, R.F., Berreen, J.P., Cooney, E.L., 2001. Progressive outer retinal necrosis and acute retinal necrosis in fellow eyes of a patient with acquired immunodeficiency syndrome. Am. J. Ophthalmol. 132, 421–423.

Gaynor, B.D., Wade, N.K., Cunningham, E.T. Jr., 2001. Herpes simplex virus type 1 associated acute retinal necrosis following encephalitis. Retina 21, 688–690.

Gonzales, J.A., Levison, A.L., Stewart, J.M., et al., 2012. Retinal necrosis following varicella-zoster vaccination. Arch. Ophthalmol. 130, 1355–1356.

Holland, G.N., 1994. Standard diagnostic criteria for the acute retinal necrosis syndrome. Executive Committee of the American Uveitis Society. Am. J. Ophthalmol. 117, 663–667.

Jabs, D.A., Schachat, A.P., Liss, R., et al., 1987. Presumed varicella zoster retinitis in immunocompromised patients. Retina 7, 9–13.

Kramer, S., Brummer, C., Zierhut, M., 2001. Epstein–Barr virus associated acute retinal necrosis. Br. J. Ophthalmol. 85, 114.

Meffert, S.A., Kertes, P.J., Lim, P., et al., 1997. Successful treatment of progressive outer retinal necrosis using high-dose intravitreal ganciclovir. Retina 17, 560–562.

Pepose, J.S., 1984. Skin test with varicella-zoster virus antigen for ophthalmic herpes zoster. Am. J. Ophthalmol. 98, 825–827.

Pepose, J.S., Flowers, B., Stewart, J.A., et al., 1992. Herpesvirus antibody levels in the etiologic diagnosis of the acute retinal necrosis syndrome. Am. J. Ophthalmol. 113, 248–256.

Perez-Blasquez, E., Traspas, R., Marin, I.M., et al., 1997. Intravitreal ganciclovir treatment in progressive outer retinal necrosis. Am. J. Ophthalmol. 124, 418–421.

Scott, I.U., Luu, K.M., Davis, J.L., 2002. Intravitreal antivirals in the management of patients with acquired immunodeficiency syndrome with progressive outer retinal necrosis. Arch. Ophthalmol. 120, 1219–1222.

Sellitti, T.P., Huang, A.J., Schiffman, J., et al., 1993. Association of herpes zoster ophthalmicus with acquired immunodeficiency syndrome and acute retinal necrosis. Am. J. Ophthalmol. 116, 297–301.

Sergott, R.C., Belmont, J.B., Savino, P.J., et al., 1985. Optic nerve involvement in the acute retinal necrosis syndrome. Arch. Ophthalmol. 103, 1160–1162.

Sergott, R.C., Anand, R., Belmont, J.B., et al., 1989. Acute retinal necrosis neuropathy. Clinical profile and surgical therapy. Arch. Ophthalmol. 107, 692–696.

Spaide, R.F., Martin, D.F., Teich, S.A., et al., 1996. Successful treatment of progressive outer retinal necrosis syndrome. Retina 16, 479–487.

Van Gelder, R.N., Willig, J.L., Holland, G.N., et al., 2001. Herpes simplex virus type 2 as a cause of acute retinal necrosis syndrome in young patients. Ophthalmology 108, 869–876.

Dengue Virus Maculopathy

Bacsal, K., Chee, S., Cheng, C., et al., 2007. Dengue-associated maculopathy. Arch. Ophthalmol. 125, 501–510.

Munk, M.R., Jampol, L.M., Cunha Souza, E., et al., 2016. New associations of classic acute macular neuroretinopathy. Br. J. Ophthalmol. 100 (3), 389–394.

Toxoplasmosis

Abrahams, I.W., Gregerson, D.S., 1982. Longitudinal study of serum antibody responses to retinal antigens in acute ocular toxoplasmosis. Am. J. Ophthalmol. 93, 224–231.

Akstein, R.B., Wilson, L.A., Teutsch, S.M., 1982. Acquired toxoplasmosis. Ophthalmology 89, 1299–1301.

Baarsma, G.S., Luyendijk, L., Kijlstra, A., et al., 1991. Analysis of local antibody production in the vitreous humor of patients with severe uveitis. Am. J. Ophthalmol. 112, 147–150.

Burnett, A.J., Shortt, S.G., Isaac-Renton, J., et al., 1998. Multiple cases of acquired toxoplasmosis retinitis presenting in an outbreak. Ophthalmology 105, 1032–1037.

Chan, C., Palestine, A.G., Li, Q., et al., 1994. Diagnosis of ocular toxoplasmosis by the use of immunocytology and the polymerase chain reaction. Am. J. Ophthalmol. 117, 803–805.

Doft, B.H., Gass, J.D.H., 1985. Punctate outer retinal toxoplasmosis. Arch. Ophthalmol. 103, 1332–1336.

Engstrom, R.E. Jr., Holland, G.N., Nussenblatt, R.B., et al., 1991. Current practices in the management of ocular toxoplasmosis. Am. J. Ophthalmol. 111, 601–610.

Fish, R.H., Hoskins, J.C., Kline, L.B., 1993. Toxoplasmosis neuroretinitis. Ophthalmology 100, 1177–1182.

Folk, J.C., Lobes, L.A., 1984. Presumed toxoplasmic papillitis. Ophthalmology 91, 64–67.

Gilbert, R.E., Stanford, M.R., 2000. Is ocular toxoplasmosis caused by prenatal or postnatal infection? Br. J. Ophthalmol. 84, 224–226.

Holland, G.N., Engstrom, R.E., Glasgow, B.J., et al., 1988. Ocular toxoplasmosis in patients with the acquired immunodeficiency syndrome. Am. J. Ophthalmol. 106, 563–667.

Johnson, M.W., Greven, C.M., Jaffe, G.J., et al., 1997. Atypical, severe toxoplasmic retinochoroiditis in elderly patients. Ophthalmology 104, 48–57.

Mets, M.B., Holfels, E., Boyer, K.M., et al., 1996. Eye manifestations of congenital toxoplasmosis. Am. J. Ophthalmol. 122, 309–324.

Ronday, M.J., Ongkosuwito, J.V., Rothova, A., et al., 1999. Intraocular anti-*Toxoplasma gondii* IgA antibody production in patients with ocular toxoplasmosis. Am. J. Ophthalmol. 127, 294–300.

Silveira, C., Belfort, R. Jr., Burnier, M. Jr., et al., 1988. Acquired toxoplasmic infection as the cause of toxoplasmic retinochoroiditis in families. Am. J. Ophthalmol. 106, 362–364.

Giardiasis

Anderson, M.L., Griffith, D.G., 1985. Intestinal giardiasis associated with ocular inflammation. J. Clin. Gastroenterol. 7, 169–172.

Knox, D.L., King, J. Jr., 1982. Retinal arteritis, iridocyclitis, and giardiasis. Ophthalmology 89, 1303–1308.

Leprosy

Dana, M.R., Hochman, M.A., Viana, M.A., et al., 1994. Ocular manifestations of leprosy in a noninstitutionalized community in the United States. Arch. Ophthalmol. 112, 626–629. Erratum in: Arch Ophthalmol 1995;113: 24.

Johnstone, P.A., George, A.D., Meyers, W.M., 1991. Ocular lesions in leprosy. Ann. Ophthalmol. 23, 297–303.

Michelson, J.B., Roth, A.M., Waring, G.O. 3rd, 1979. Lepromatous iridocyclitis diagnosed by anterior chamber paracentesis. Am. J. Ophthalmol. 88, 674–679.

Nepal, B.P., Shrestha, U.D., 2004. Ocular findings in leprosy patients in Nepal in the era of multidrug therapy. Am. J. Ophthalmol. 137, 888–892.

Tuberculosis

Babu, R.B., Sudharshan, S., Kumarasamy, N., et al., 2006. Ocular tuberculosis in acquired immunodeficiency syndrome. Am. J. Ophthalmol. 142, 413–418.

Bansal, R., Gupta, A., Gupta, V., et al., 2008. Role of anti-tubercular therapy in uveitis with latent/manifest tuberculosis. Am. J. Ophthalmol. 146, 772–779.

Chong, Y.Y., Kodati, S., Kosmin, A., 2007. Ocular tuberculosis. Ann. Ophthalmol. (Skokie) 39, 243–245.

Cimino, L., Herbort, C.P., Aldigeri, R., et al., 2009. Tuberculous uveitis, a resurgent and underdiagnosed disease. Int. Ophthalmol. 29, 67–74.

Daley, C.L., Small, P.M., Schecter, G.F., et al., 1992. An outbreak of tuberculosis with accelerated progression among persons infected with the human immunodeficiency virus. N. Engl. J. Med. 326, 231–235.

Fountain, J.A., Werner, R.B., 1984. Tuberculous retinal vasculitis. Retina 4, 48–50.

Gupta, V., Gupta, A., Arora, S., et al., 2003. Presumed tubercular serpiginouslike choroiditis. Ophthalmology 110, 1744–1749.

Sharma, P.M., Singh, R., Kumar, A., et al., 2003. Choroidal tuberculoma in miliary tuberculosis. Retina 23, 101–104.

Thompson, M.J., Albert, D.M., 2005. Ocular tuberculosis. Arch. Ophthalmol. 123, 844–849.

Nocardiosis

Gregor, R.J., Chong, C.A., Augsburger, J.J., et al., 1989. Endogenous *Nocardia asteroides* subretinal abscess diagnosed by transvitreal fine-needle aspiration biopsy. Retina 9, 118–121.

Phillips, W.B., Shields, C.L., Shields, J.A., et al., 1992. *Nocardia* choroidal abscess. Br. J. Ophthalmol. 76, 694–696.

Rafiei, N., Tabandeh, H., Bhatti, M.T., et al., 2006. Retinal fibrovascular proliferation associated with *Nocardia* subretinal abscess. Eur. J. Ophthalmol. 16, 641–643.

Yin, X., Liang, S., Sun, X., et al., 2007. Ocular nocardiosis: HSP65 gene sequencing for species identification of *Nocardia* spp. Am. J. Ophthalmol. 144, 570–573.

Yu, E., Laughlin, S., Kassel, E.E., et al., 2005. Nocardial endophthalmitis and subretinal abscess: CT and MR imaging features with pathologic correlation: a case report. AJNR Am. J. Neuroradiol. 26, 1220–1222.

Whipple Disease

Nubourgh, I., Vandergheynst, F., Lefebvre, P., et al., 2008. An atypical case of Whipple's disease: case report and review of the literature. Acta Clin. Belg. 63, 107–111.

Relman, D.A., Schmidt, T.M., MacDermott, R.P., et al., 1992. Identification of the uncultured bacillus of Whipple's disease. N. Engl. J. Med. 327, 293–301.

Rickman, L.S., Freeman, W.R., Green, W.R., et al., 1995. Brief report: uveitis caused by *Tropheryma whippelii* (Whipple's bacillus). N. Engl. J. Med. 332, 363–366.

Bartonella: Cat-Scratch Disease

Berguiga, M., Abouzeid, H., Bart, P.A., et al., 2008. Severe occlusive vasculitis as a complication of cat scratch disease. Klin. Monatsbl. Augenheilkd 225, 486–487.

Curi, A.L., Machado, D.O., Heringer, G., et al., 2006. Ocular manifestation of cat-scratch disease in HIV-positive patients. Am. J. Ophthalmol. 141, 400–401.

Gray, A.V., Michels, K.S., Lauer, A.K., et al., 2004. *Bartonella henselae* infection associated with neuroretinitis, central retinal artery and vein occlusion, neovascular glaucoma, and severe vision loss. Am. J. Ophthalmol. 137, 187–189.

Patel, S.J., Petrarca, R., Shah, S.M., et al., 2008. Atypical *Bartonella hensalae* chorioretinitis in an immunocompromised patient. Ocul. Immunol. Inflamm. 16, 45–49.

Roe, R.H., Michael Jumper, J., Fu, A.D., et al., 2008. Ocular *Bartonella* infections. Int. Ophthalmol. Clin. 48, 93–105.

Wimmersberger, Y., Baglivo, E., 2007. *Bartonella henselae* infection presenting as a unilateral acute maculopathy. Klin. Monatsbl. Augenheilkd 224, 311–313.

Syphilis

Anshu, A., Cheng, C.L., Chee, S.P., 2008. Syphilitic uveitis: an Asian perspective. Br. J. Ophthalmol. 92, 594–597.

Browning, D.J., 2000. Posterior segment manifestations of active ocular syphilis, their response to a neurosyphilis regimen of penicillin therapy, and the influence of human immunodeficiency virus status on response. Ophthalmology 107, 2015–2023.

Chao, J.R., Khurana, R.N., Fawzi, A.A., et al., 2006. Syphilis: reemergence of an old adversary. Ophthalmology 113, 2074–2079.

Curi, A.L., Sarraf, D., Cunningham, E.T. Jr., 2015. Multimodal imaging of syphilitic multifocal retinitis. Retin Cases Brief Rep. 9, 277–280.

Díaz-Valle, D., Allen, D.P., Sánchez, A.A., et al., 2005. Simultaneous bilateral exudative retinal detachment and peripheral necrotizing retinitis as presenting manifestations of concurrent HIV and syphilis infection. Ocul. Immunol. Inflamm. 13, 459–462.

Gass, J.D., Braunstein, R.A., Chenoweth, R.G., 1990. Acute syphilitic posterior placoid chorioretinitis. Ophthalmology 97, 1288–1297.

Joseph, A., Rogers, S., Browning, A., et al., 2007. Syphilitic acute posterior placoid chorioretinitis in non-immunocompromised patients. Eye (Lond.) 21, 1114–1119.

Krishnamurthy, R., Cunningham, E.T. Jr., 2008. Atypical presentation of syphilitic uveitis associated with Kyrieleis plaques. Br. J. Ophthalmol. 92, 1152–1153.

Müller, M., Ewert, I., Hansmann, F., et al., 2007. Detection of *Treponema pallidum* in the vitreous by PCR. Br. J. Ophthalmol. 91, 592–595.

Pichi, F., Ciardella, A.P., Cunningham, E.T. Jr., et al., 2014. Spectral domain optical coherence tomography findings in patients with acute syphilitic posterior placoid chorioretinopathy. Retina 34 (2), 373–384.

Reddy, S., Cunningham, E.T. Jr., Spaide, R.F., 2006. Syphilitic retinitis with focal inflammatory accumulations. Ophthalmic Surg. Lasers Imaging 37, 429–431.

Tran, T.H., Cassoux, N., Bodaghi, B., et al., 2005. Syphilitic uveitis in patients infected with human immunodeficiency virus. Graefes Arch. Clin. Exp. Ophthalmol. 243, 863–869.

Westeneng, A.C., Rothova, A., de Boer, J.H., et al., 2007. Infectious uveitis in immunocompromised patients and the diagnostic value of polymerase chain reaction and Goldmann–Witmer coefficient in aqueous analysis. Am. J. Ophthalmol. 144, 781–785.

Pneumocystis carinii

Dugel, P.U., Rao, N.A., Forster, D.J., et al., 1990. Pneumocystis carinii choroiditis after long-term aerosolized pentamidine therapy. Am. J. Ophthalmol. 110, 113–117.

Gupta, A., Hustler, A., Herieka, E., et al., 2010. *Pneumocystis* choroiditis. Eye (Lond.) 24 (1), 178.

Koser, M.W., Jampol, L.M., MacDonell, K., 1990. Treatment of *Pneumocystis carinii* choroidopathy. Arch. Ophthalmol. 108, 1214–1215.

Sneed, S.R., Blodi, C.F., Berger, B.B., et al., 1989. *Pneumocystis carinii* choroiditis in patients receiving inhaled pentamidine. N. Engl. J. Med. 322, 936–937.

Yeh, S., Lam, H.Y., Albini, T.A., et al., 2008. Central retinal vein occlusion in an AIDS patient with presumed *Pneumocystis carinii* pneumonia. Can. J. Ophthalmol. 43, 372–373.

Candida albicans Chorioretinitis

Blumenkranz, M.S., Stevens, D.A., 1980. Therapy of endogenous fungal endophthalmitis: miconazole or amphotericin B for coccidioidal and candidal infection. Arch. Ophthalmol. 98, 1216–1220.

Breit, S.M., Hariprasad, S.M., Mieler, W.F., et al., 2005. Management of endogenous fungal endophthalmitis with voriconazole and caspofungin. Am. J. Ophthalmol. 139, 135–140.

Cantrill, H.L., Rodman, W.P., Ramsay, R.C., et al., 1980. Postpartum *Candida* endophthalmitis. JAMA 243, 1163–1165.

Chakrabarti, A., Shivaprakash, M.R., Singh, R., et al., 2008. Fungal endophthalmitis: fourteen years' experience from a center in India. Retina 28, 1400–1407.

Doft, B.H., Clarkson, J.G., Rebell, G., et al., 1980. Endogenous *Aspergillus* endophthalmitis in drug abusers. Arch. Ophthalmol. 98, 859–862.

Donahue, S.P., Hein, E., Sinatra, R.B., 2003. Ocular involvement in children with candidemia. Am. J. Ophthalmol. 135, 886–887.

Feman, S.S., Nichols, J.C., Chung, S.M., et al., 2002. Endophthalmitis in patients with disseminated fungal disease. Trans. Am. Ophthalmol. Soc. 100, 67–70.

Griffin, J.R., Pettit, T.H., Fishman, L.S., et al., 1973. Blood-borne *Candida* endophthalmitis. A clinical and pathologic study of 21 cases. Arch. Ophthalmol. 89, 450–456.

Kaburaki, T., Takamoto, M., Araki, F., et al., 2010. Endogenous *Candida albicans* infection causing subretinal abscess. Int. Ophthalmol. 30 (2), 203–206.

Khan, F.A., Slain, D., Khakoo, R.A., 2007. *Candida* endophthalmitis: focus on current and future antifungal treatment options. Pharmacotherapy 27, 1711–1721.

Pasqualotto, A.C., Denning, D.W., 2008. New and emerging treatments for fungal infections. J. Antimicrob. Chemother. 61, i19–i30.

Scherer, W.J., Lee, K., 1997. Implications of early systemic therapy on the incidence of endogenous fungal endophthalmitis. Ophthalmology 104, 1593–1598.

Schuman, J.S., Friedman, A.H., 1983. Retinal manifestations of the acquired immune deficiency syndrome (AIDS): cytomegalovirus, *Candida albicans, Cryptococcus*, toxoplasmosis and *Pneumocystis carinii*. Trans. Ophthalmol. Soc. UK 103, 177–190.

Shah, C.P., McKey, J., Spirn, M.J., et al., 2008. Ocular candidiasis: a review. Br. J. Ophthalmol. 92, 466–468.

Weinstein, O., Levy, J., Lifshitz, T., 2007. Recurrent *Candida albicans* endophthalmitis in an immunocompromised host. Can. J. Ophthalmol. 42, 154–155.

Wykoff, C.C., Flynn, H.W. Jr., Miller, D., et al., 2008. Exogenous fungal endophthalmitis: microbiology and clinical outcomes. Ophthalmology 115, 1501–1507.

Yilmaz, S., Ture, M., Maden, A., 2007. Efficacy of intracameral amphotericin B injection in the management of refractory keratomycosis and endophthalmitis. Cornea 26, 398–402.

Aspergillosis

Demicco, D.D., Reichman, R.C., Violette, E.J., et al., 1984. Disseminated aspergillosis presenting with endophthalmitis. A case report and a review of the literature. Cancer 53, 1995–2001.

Doft, B.H., Clarkson, J.G., Rebell, G., et al., 1980. Endogenous *Aspergillus* endophthalmitis in drug abusers. Arch. Ophthalmol. 98, 859–862.

Hunt, K.E., Glasgow, B.J., 1996. *Aspergillus* endophthalmitis. An unrecognized endemic disease in orthotopic liver transplantation. Ophthalmology 103, 757–767.

Jampol, L.M., Dyckman, S., Maniates, V., et al., 1988. Retinal and choroidal infarction from *Aspergillus:* clinical diagnosis and clinicopathologic correlations. Trans. Am. Ophthalmol. Soc. 86, 422–440.

Kramer, M., Kramer, M.R., Blau, H., et al., 2006. Intravitreal voriconazole for the treatment of endogenous *Aspergillus* endophthalmitis. Ophthalmology 113, 1184–1186.

McGuire, T.W., Bullock, J.D., Bullock, J.D. Jr., et al., 1991. Fungal endophthalmitis. An experimental study with a review of 17 human ocular cases. Arch. Ophthalmol. 109, 1289–1296.

Rao, N.A., Hidayat, A.A., 2001. Endogenous mycotic endophthalmitis: variations in clinical and histopathologic changes in candidiasis compared with aspergillosis. Am. J. Ophthalmol. 132, 244–251.

Weishaar, P.D., Flynn, H.W. Jr., Murray, T.G., et al., 1998. Endogenous *Aspergillus* endophthalmitis. Clinical features and treatment outcomes. Ophthalmology 105, 57–65.

Cryptococcosis

Andreola, C., Ribeiro, M.P., de Carli, C.R., et al., 2006. Multifocal choroiditis in disseminated *Cryptococcus neoformans* infection. Am. J. Ophthalmol. 142, 346–348.

Babu, K., Murthy, K.R., Rajagopalan, N., 2008. Primary bilateral multifocal choroiditis as an initial manifestation of disseminated cryptococcosis in a HIV-positive patient. Ocul. Immunol. Inflamm. 16, 191–193.

Carney, M.D., Combs, J.L., Waschler, W., 1990. Cryptococcal choroiditis. Retina 10, 27–32.

Crump, J.R., Elner, S.G., Elner, V.M., et al., 1992. Cryptococcal endophthalmitis: case report and review. Clin. Infect. Dis. 14, 1069–1073.

Henderly, D.E., Liggett, P.E., Rao, N.A., 1987. Cryptococcal chorioretinitis and endophthalmitis. Retina 7, 75–79.

Kestelyn, P., Taelman, H., Bogaerts, J., et al., 1993. Ophthalmic manifestations of infections with *Cryptococcus neoformans* in patients with the acquired immunodeficiency syndrome. Am. J. Ophthalmol. 116, 721–727.

Nakamura, S., Izumikawa, K., Seki, M., et al., 2008. Reversible visual disturbance due to cryptococcal uveitis in a non-HIV individual. Med. Mycol. 46, 367–370.

Histoplasmosis

Adán, A., Navarro, M., Casaroli-Marano, R.P., et al., 2007. Intravitreal bevacizumab as initial treatment for choroidal neovascularization associated with presumed ocular histoplasmosis syndrome. Graefes Arch. Clin. Exp. Ophthalmol. 245, 1873–1875.

Almony, A., Thomas, M.A., Atebara, N.H., et al., 2008. Long-term follow-up of surgical removal of extensive peripapillary choroidal neovascularization in presumed ocular histoplasmosis syndrome. Ophthalmology 115, 540–545.

Bass, E.B., Gilson, M.M., Mangione, C.M., et al., 2008. Surgical removal vs observation for idiopathic or ocular histoplasmosis syndrome-associated subfoveal choroidal neovascularization: Vision Preference Value Scale findings from the randomized SST Group H Trial: SST Report No. 17. Arch. Ophthalmol. 126, 1626–1632.

Bottoni, F.G., Deutman, A.F., Aandekerk, A.L., 1989. Presumed ocular histoplasmosis syndrome and linear streak lesions. Br. J. Ophthalmol. 73, 528–535.

Craig, E.L., Suie, T., 1974. *Histoplasma capsulatum* in human ocular tissue. Arch. Ophthalmol. 91, 285–289.

Gonzales, C.A., Scott, I.U., Chaudhry, N.A., et al., 2000. Endogenous endophthalmitis caused by *Histoplasma capsulatum var. capsulatum:* a case report and literature review. Ophthalmology 107, 725–729.

Klintworth, G.K., Hollingsworth, A.S., Lusman, P.A., et al., 1973. Granulomatous choroiditis in a case of disseminated histoplasmosis. Histologic demonstration of *Histoplasma capsulatum* in choroidal lesions. Arch. Ophthalmol. 90, 45–48.

Schadlu, R., Blinder, K.J., Shah, G.K., et al., 2008. Intravitreal bevacizumab for choroidal neovascularization in ocular histoplasmosis. Am. J. Ophthalmol. 145, 875–878.

Ocular Coccidioidomycosis

Blumenkranz, M.S., Stevens, D.A., 1980. Endogenous coccidioidal endophthalmitis. Ophthalmology 87, 974–984.

Glasgow, B.J., Brown, H.H., Foos, R.Y., 1987. Miliary retinitis in coccidioidomycosis. Am. J. Ophthalmol. 104, 24–27.

Blastomycosis

Font, R.L., Spaulding, A.G., Green, W.R., 1967. Endogenous mycotic panophthalmitis caused by *Blastomyces dermatitidis*. Report of a case and a review of the literature. Arch. Ophthalmol. 77, 217–222.

Gottlieb, J.L., McAllister, I.L., Guttman, F.A., et al., 1995. Choroidal blastomycosis. A report of two cases. Retina 15, 248–252.

Lewis, H., Aaberg, T.M., Fary, D.R., et al., 1988. Latent disseminated blastomycosis with choroidal involvement. Arch. Ophthalmol. 106, 527–530.

Pariseau, B., Lucarelli, M.J., Appen, R.E., 2007. Unilateral *Blastomyces dermatitidis* optic neuropathy case report and systematic literature review. Ophthalmology 114, 2090–2094.

Fusarium Keratitis, Vitritis, and Retinal Papillitis

Alfonso, E.C., 2008. Genotypic identification of *Fusarium* species from ocular sources: comparison to morphologic classification and antifungal sensitivity testing (an AOS thesis). Trans. Am. Ophthalmol. Soc. 106, 227–239.

Bagyalakshmi, R., Therese, K.L., Prasanna, S., et al., 2008. Newer emerging pathogens of ocular non-sporulating molds (NSM) identified by polymerase chain reaction (PCR)-based DNA sequencing technique targeting internal transcribed spacer (ITS) region. Curr. Eye Res. 33, 139–147.

Glasgow, B.J., Engstrom, R.E. Jr., Holland, G.N., et al., 1996. Bilateral endogenous *Fusarium* endophthalmitis associated with acquired immunodeficiency syndrome. Arch. Ophthalmol. 114, 873–877.

Oechsler, R.A., Feilmeier, M.R., Ledee, D.R., et al., 2009. Utility of molecular sequence analysis of the its rRNA region for identification of *Fusarium* spp from ocular sources. Invest. Ophthalmol. Vis. Sci. 50 (5), 2230–2236.

Cysticercosis

Balakrishnan, E., 1961. Bilateral intra-ocular cysticerci. Br. J. Ophthalmol. 45, 150–151.

Danis, P., 1974. Intraocular cysticercus. Arch. Ophthalmol. 91, 238–239.

Hamed, S.A., El-Metaal, H.E., 2007. Unusual presentations of neurocysticercosis. Acta Neurol. Scand. 115, 192–198.

Madigubba, S., Vishwanath, K., Reddy, G., et al., 2007. Changing trends in ocular cysticercosis over two decades: an analysis of 118 surgically excised cysts. Indian J. Med. Microbiol. 25, 214–219.

Venkatesh, R., Ravindran, R.D., Bharathi, B., et al., 2008. Optic nerve cysticercosis. Ophthalmology 115, 2094.

Zinn, K.M., Guillory, S.L., Friedman, A.H., 1980. Removal of intravitreous cysticerci from the surface of the optic nerve head. A pars plana approach. Arch. Ophthalmol. 98, 714–716.

Diffuse or Disseminated Unilateral Subacute Neuroretinitis

de Souza, E.C., Abujamra, S., Nakashima, Y., et al., 1999. Diffuse bilateral subacute neuroretinitis: first patient with documented nematodes in both eyes. Arch. Ophthalmol. 117, 1349–1351.

de Souza, E.C., da Cunha, S.L., Gass, J.D., 1992. Diffuse unilateral subacute neuroretinitis in South America. Arch. Ophthalmol. 110, 1261–1263.

Fox, A.S., Kazacos, K.R., Gould, N.S., et al., 1985. Fatal eosinophilic meningoencephalitis and visceral larva migrans caused by the raccoon ascarid *Baylisascaris procyonis*. N. Engl. J. Med. 312, 1619–1623.

Garcia, C.A., Sabrosa, N.A., Gomes, A.B., et al., 2008. Diffuse unilateral subacute neuroretinitis–DUSN. Int. Ophthalmol. Clin. 48, 119–129.

Gass, J.D.M., 1996. Subretinal migration of a nematode in a patient with diffuse unilateral subacute neuroretinitis. Arch. Ophthalmol. 114, 1526–1527.

Gass, J.D., Gilbert, W.R. Jr., Guerry, R.K., et al., 1978. Diffuse unilateral subacute neuroretinitis. Ophthalmology 85, 521–545.

Mets, M.B., Noble, A.G., Basti, S., et al., 2003. Eye findings of diffuse unilateral subacute neuroretinitis and multiple choroidal infiltrates associated with neural larva migrans due to *Baylisascaris procyonis*. Am. J. Ophthalmol. 135, 888–890.

Vedantham, V., Vats, M.M., Kakade, S.J., et al., 2006. Diffuse unilateral subacute neuroretinitis with unusual findings. Am. J. Ophthalmol. 142, 880–883.

Toxocariasis

Altcheh, J., Nallar, M., Conca, M., et al., 2003. Toxocariasis: clinical and laboratory features in 54 patients. An. Pediatr. (Barc.) 58, 425–431.

Amin, H.I., McDonald, H.R., Han, D.P., et al., 2000. Vitrectomy update for macular traction in ocular toxocariasis. Retina 20, 80–85.

de Visser, L., Rothova, A., de Boer, J.H., et al., 2008. Diagnosis of ocular toxocariasis by establishing intraocular antibody production. Am. J. Ophthalmol. 145, 369–374.

Ellis, G.S. Jr., Pakalnis, V.A., Worley, G., et al., 1986. *Toxocara canis* infestation: clinical and epidemiological associations with seropositivity in kindergarten children. Ophthalmology 93, 1032–1037.

Glickman, L.T., Magnaval, J., 1993. Zoonotic roundworm infections. Infect. Dis. Clin. North Am. 7, 717–732.

Maguire, A.M., Green, W.R., Michels, R.G., et al., 1990. Recovery of intraocular *Toxocara canis* by pars plana vitrectomy. Ophthalmology 97, 675–680.

Pivetti-Pezzi, P., 2009. Ocular toxocariasis. Int. J. Med. Sci. 6, 129–130.

Schantz, P.M., 1994. Of worms, dogs, and human hosts: continuing challenges for veterinarians in prevention of human diseases. J. Am. Vet. Med. Assoc. 204, 1023–1028.

Werner, J.C., Ross, R.D., Green, W.R., et al., 1999. Pars plana vitrectomy and subretinal surgery for ocular toxocariasis. Arch. Ophthalmol. 117, 532–534.

Filariasis

Etya'ale, D., 2008. Onchocerciasis and trachoma control: what has changed in the past two decades? Community Eye Health 21, 43–45.

Gorezis, S., Psilla, M., Asproudis, I., et al., 2006. Intravitreal dirofilariasis: a rare ocular infection. Orbit 25, 57–59.

Gungel, H., Kara, N., Pinarci, E.Y., et al., 2009. An uncommon case with intravitreal worm. Intravitreal *Dirofilaria* infection. Br. J. Ophthalmol. 93, 573–574, 697.

Hopkins, A.D., 2007. Onchocerciasis control: impressive achievements not to be wasted. Can. J. Ophthalmol. 42, 13–15.

Kluxen, G., Hoerauf, A., 2008. The significance of some observations on African ocular onchocerciasis described by Jean Hissette (1888–1965). Bull. Soc. Belge Ophtalmol. 307, 53–58.

Winthrop, K.L., Proaño, R., Oliva, O., et al., 2006. The reliability of anterior segment lesions as indicators of onchocercal eye disease in Guatemala. Am. J. Trop. Med. Hyg. 75, 1058–1062.

Myiasis (Ophthalmomyiasis/Gnathostomiasis/Angiostrongyliasis/*Alaria* Mesocercariae)

Alhady, M., Zabri, K., Chua, C.N., 2008. Ophthalmomyiasis from *Chrysomyia bezziana* (screwworm fly). Med. J. Malaysia 63, 269–270.

Bhattacharjee, H., Das, D., Medhi, J., 2007. Intravitreal gnathostomiasis and review of literature. Retina 27, 67–73.

Funata, M., Custis, P., de la Cruz, Z., et al., 1993. Intraocular gnathostomiasis. Retina 13, 240–244.

McDonald, H.R., Kazacos, K.R., Schatz, H., et al., 1994. Two cases of intraocular infection with *Alaria* mesocercaria (Trematoda). Am. J. Ophthalmol. 117, 447–455.

Price, K.M., Murchison, A.P., Bernardino, C.R., et al., 2007. Ophthalmomyiasis externa caused by *Dermatobia hominis* in Florida. Br. J. Ophthalmol. 91, 695.

Samarasinghe, S., Weerakoon, U., 2007. External ophthalmomyiasis caused by sheep botfly *(Oestrus ovis)* larvae. Ceylon Med. J. 52, 31–32.

Sawanyawisuth, K., Kitthaweesin, K., 2008. Optic neuritis caused by intraocular angiostrongyliasis. Southeast Asian J. Trop. Med. Public Health 39, 1005–1007.

Sharifipour, F., Feghhi, M., 2008. Anterior ophthalmomyiasis interna: an ophthalmic emergency. Arch. Ophthalmol. 126, 1466–1467.

Sinawat, S., Sanguansak, T., Angkawinijwong, T., et al., 2008. Ocular angiostrongyliasis: clinical study of three cases. Eye (Lond.) 22, 1446–1448.5.

CHAPTER 6

Retinal Vascular Disease

Congenital Abnormalities

Congenital retinal vascular abnormalities are uncommon and usually benign. The most frequently encountered congenital abnormality is a large aberrant vessel of arterial or venous origin, known as a macrovessel, located in the posterior pole where it may course through the fovea and cross the horizontal raphe.

Macrovessel

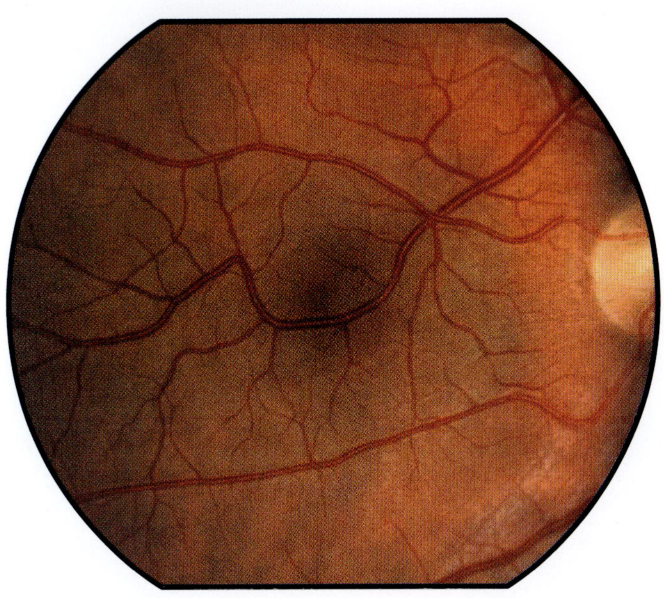

This large retinal macrovessel is an aberrant vein that courses through the fovea and across the horizontal raphe. *Courtesy of Dr. Rama Jager*

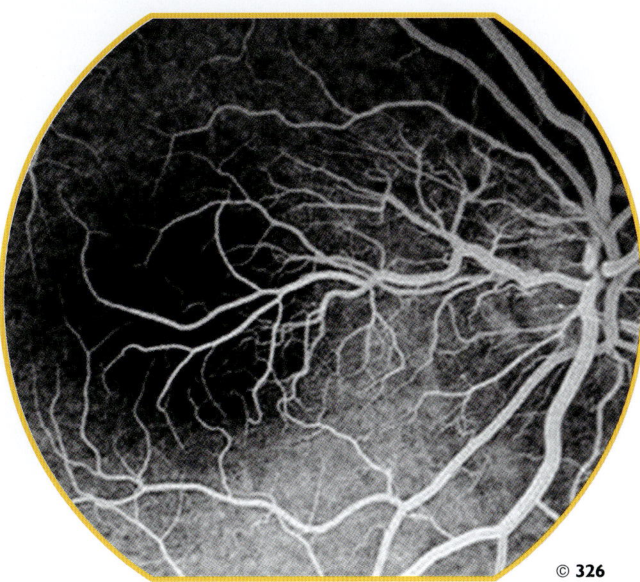

Fluorescein angiography in a different patient reveals a large anomalous venous macrovessel and an abnormal associated capillary plexus. Visual acuity was reduced to 20/40.

Prepapillary Vascular Loop

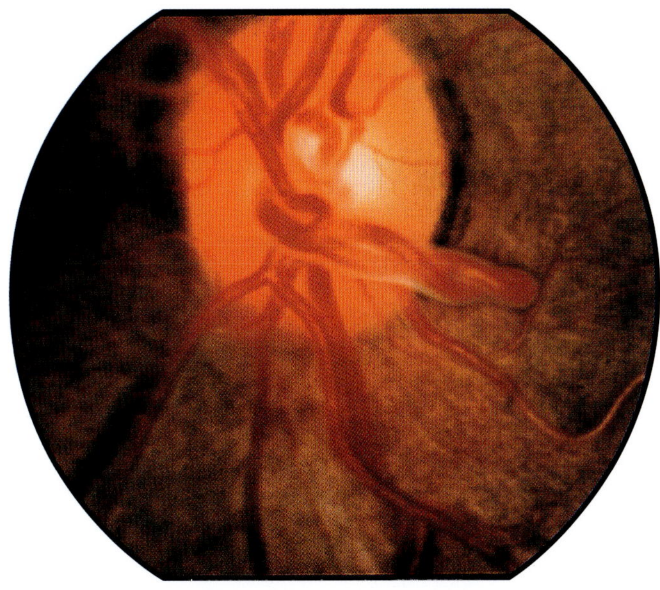

This is an example of a congenital vascular loop that is usually unilateral in asymptomatic patients. Rarely the arteriolar loops can bleed into the vitreous or lead to a branch retinal vein or artery occlusion.

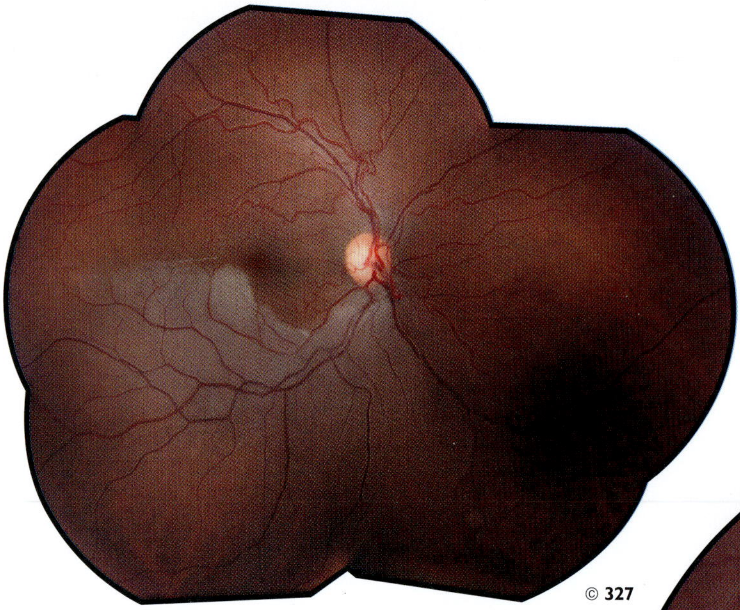

© 327

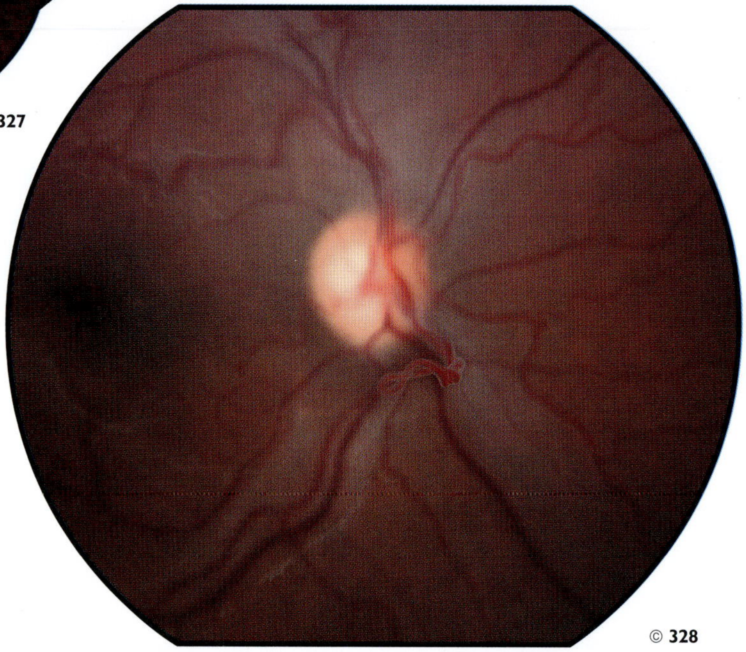

© 328

This 17-year-old otherwise healthy male presented with superior visual field loss in the right eye after sustaining head trauma. Examination revealed an inferior branch retinal artery occlusion (BRAO) *(top)* associated with a congenital vascular loop which had coiled, preventing distal blood flow *(bottom image). Images courtesy of Ehsan Rahimy, MD*

Familial Retinal Arterial Tortuosity

Congenital retinal tortuosity affects the arteries although tortuosity of the retinal veins may also be appreciated. These tortuous vessels are subject to occlusive and hemorrhagic complications.

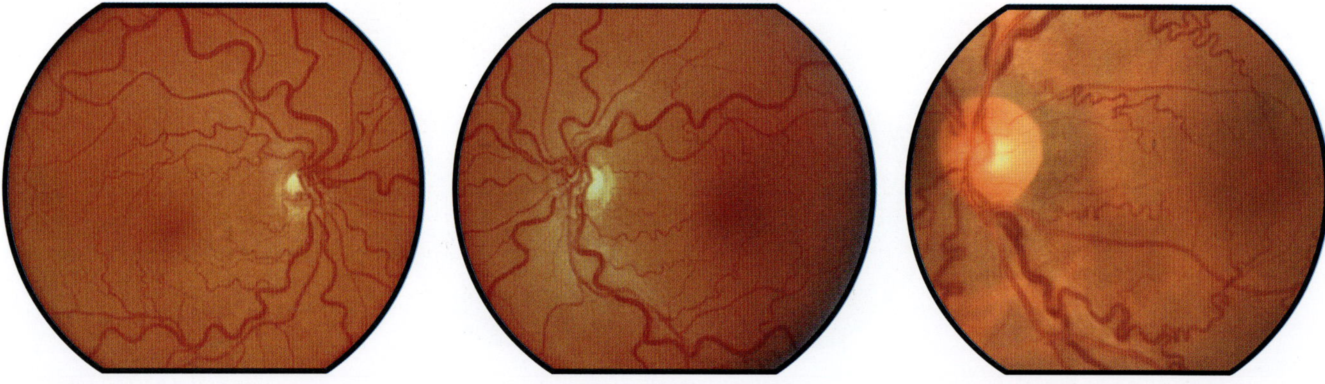

These two patients have familial retinal arterial tortuosity with tortuosity of both the retinal arteries and veins. This disorder occurs bilaterally.

Retinal Arterial Occlusions

Retinal artery obstructive disease includes ophthalmic artery occlusions, central retinal artery occlusions, branch retinal artery occlusions, cilioretinal artery occlusions, and combined arterial and venous obstructions. Cotton-wool spots (CWS) also fit in the broad category of occlusive disease because they represent precapillary arteriolar obstructions of the superficial plexus.

Ophthalmic Artery Occlusion

A patient with an ophthalmic artery occlusion typically presents with no light perception vision. A "cherry red" spot is not present in almost half of these cases because of choroidal insufficiency. Following reperfusion of the obstructed circulation, diffuse retinal pigment epithelium (RPE) abnormalities may develop.

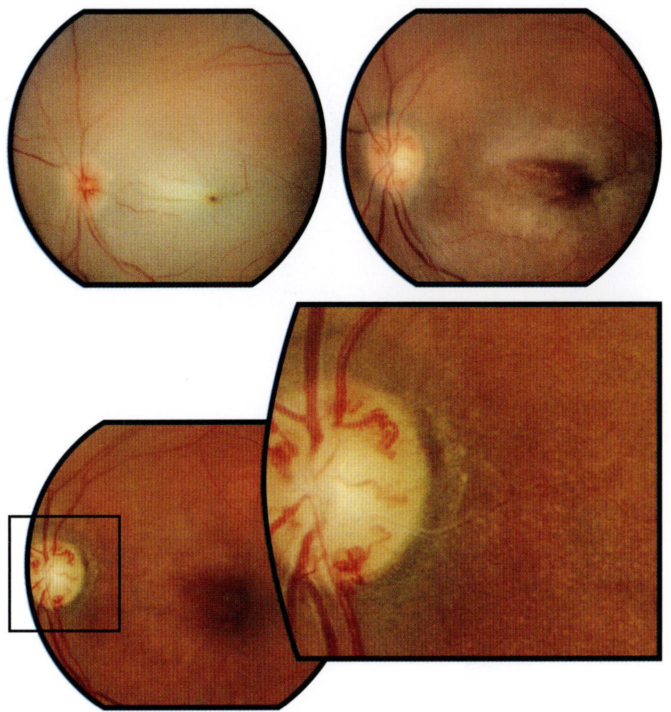

This patient had an ophthalmic artery occlusion. In the acute stage, there is diffuse whitening in the posterior fundus but no "cherry red" spot *(left upper)*. Two months later, the outer retinal ischemia has largely subsided, leaving a reddish-brown discoloration in the foveal region. There is still some perifoveal whitening of the inner retina *(right upper)*. Following resolution of the acute whitening of the retina, the fundus has diffuse RPE changes, decreased retinal vascular caliber, and sheathing irregularities *(lower left)*. Note the compensatory vessels around the circumference of the optic nerve head *(magnified inset),* collaterals between the retinal and ciliary circulations, referred to as Nettleship collaterals.

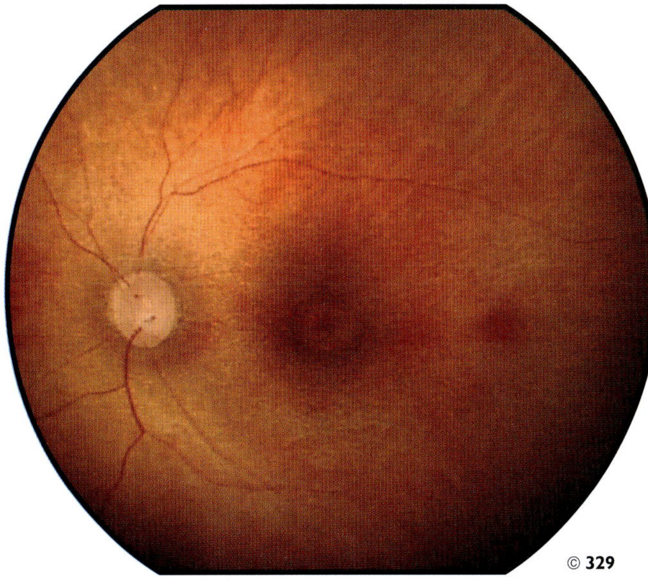

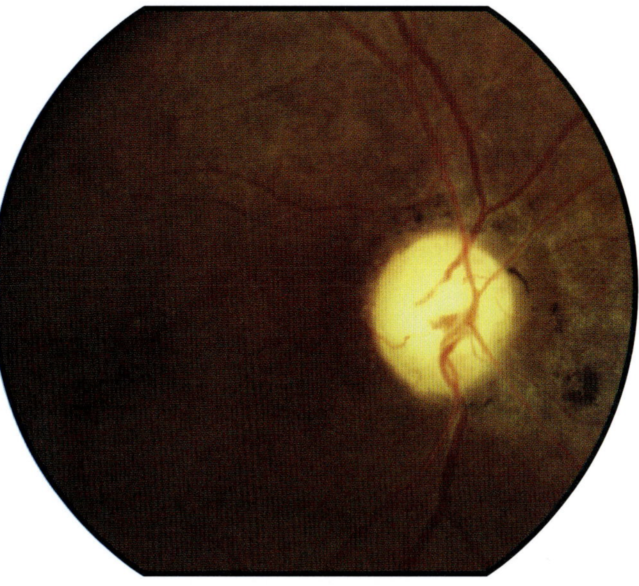

These are two cases of old ophthalmic artery occlusion. There is widespread pigment epithelial atrophy and some granular pigmentation *(left)*. The optic nerve is pale, and the retinal vessels are narrow from the antecedent ischemia. Note the constricted blood vessels, the diffuse pigmentary changes, and the optic atrophy on the right.

Central Retinal Artery Occlusion

Central retinal artery obstructions are most commonly seen in older adults. These patients often have signs of cardiovascular disease. The most common cause is embolism from a carotid artery plaque. In the acute phase there is opacification of the superficial retina except for the fovea in which a "cherry red" spot is present. In some cases, there is segmentation or "boxcarring" of the retinal vasculature.

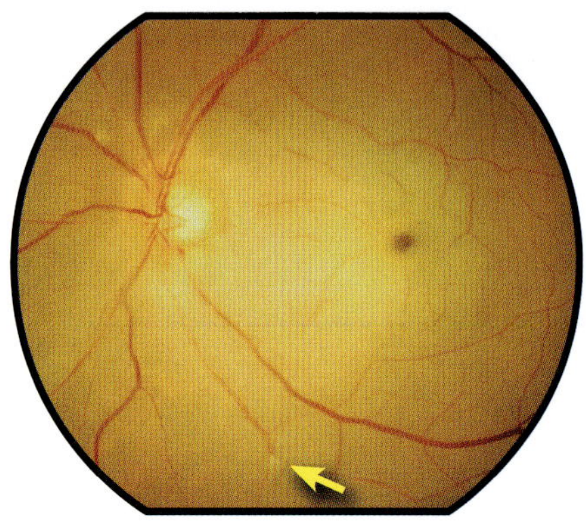

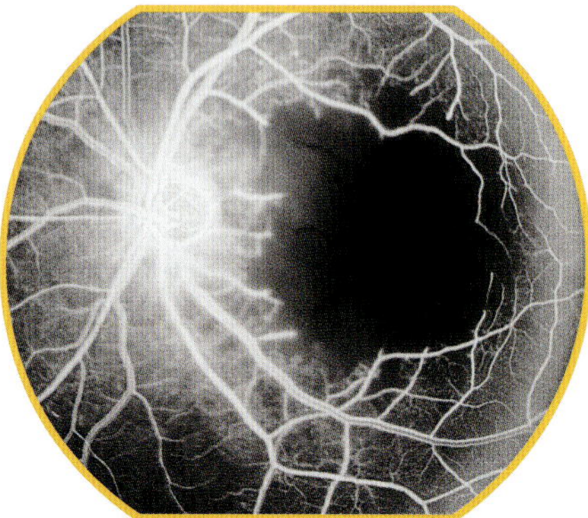

This patient has an acute central retinal artery occlusion with a cherry red spot. Note the plaque inferiorly *(arrow)*. Fluorescein angiogram in this case reveals macular ischemia.

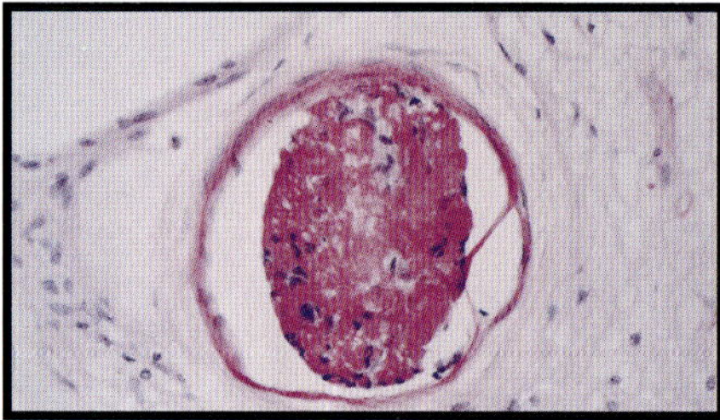

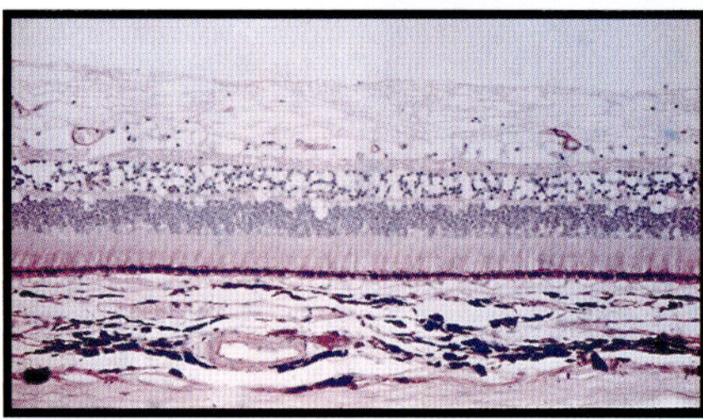

The histopathology shows a recent central retinal artery occlusion with a fresh intravascular thrombus and edema of the inner retinal layers.

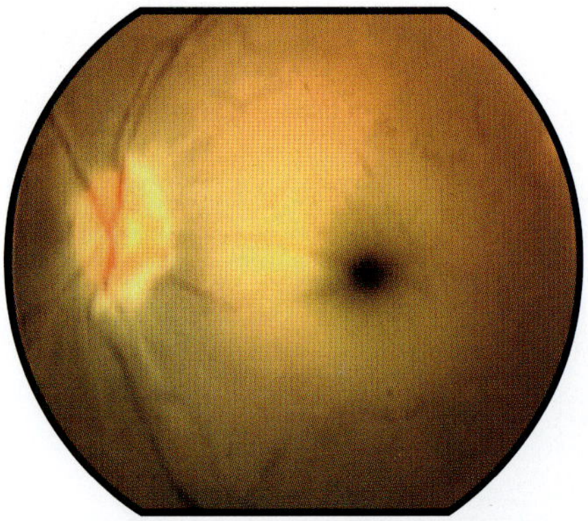

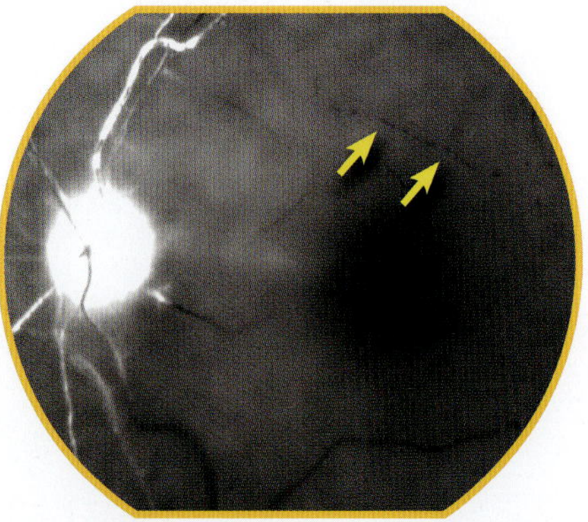

This patient has an acute central retinal artery occlusion with whitening of the retina and a "cherry red" spot. There is severe non-perfusion of the retina with "boxcarring" on the fluorescein angiogram (FA) *(arrows)*. *Courtesy of Dr. Pawan Bhatnagar*

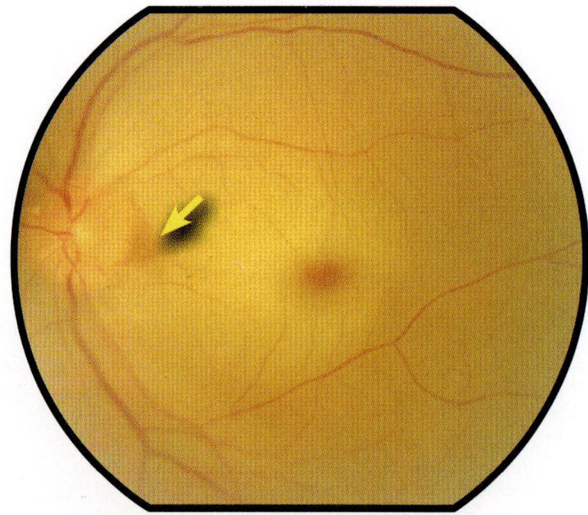

This patient has a central retinal artery occlusion with a "cherry red" spot and retinal whitening. There is very minimal sparing of the temporal peripapillary retina from perfused ciliary vessels *(arrow)*.

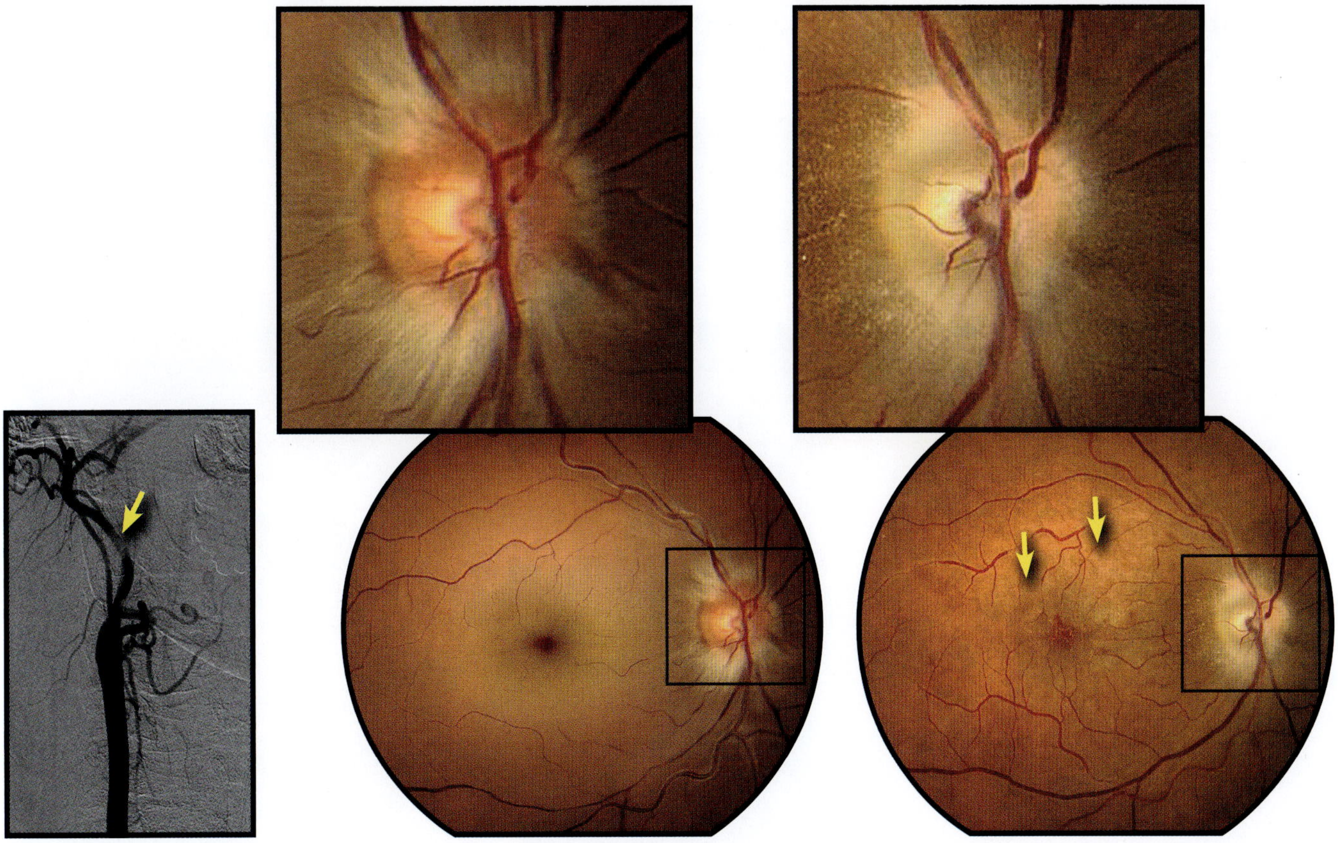

This patient presented with a central retinal artery occlusion with diffuse whitening of the inner retina and a cherry red spot. Note the presence of peripapillary whitening representing axoplasmic stasis. Three weeks later *(right)* most of the whitening has resolved with some persistence in the superior macula *(arrows)*. The optic nerve has become pale and the vision was unimproved. The carotid angiogram *(left)* shows obstruction of the carotid system *(arrow)*. *Courtesy of Dr. Robert Mittra*

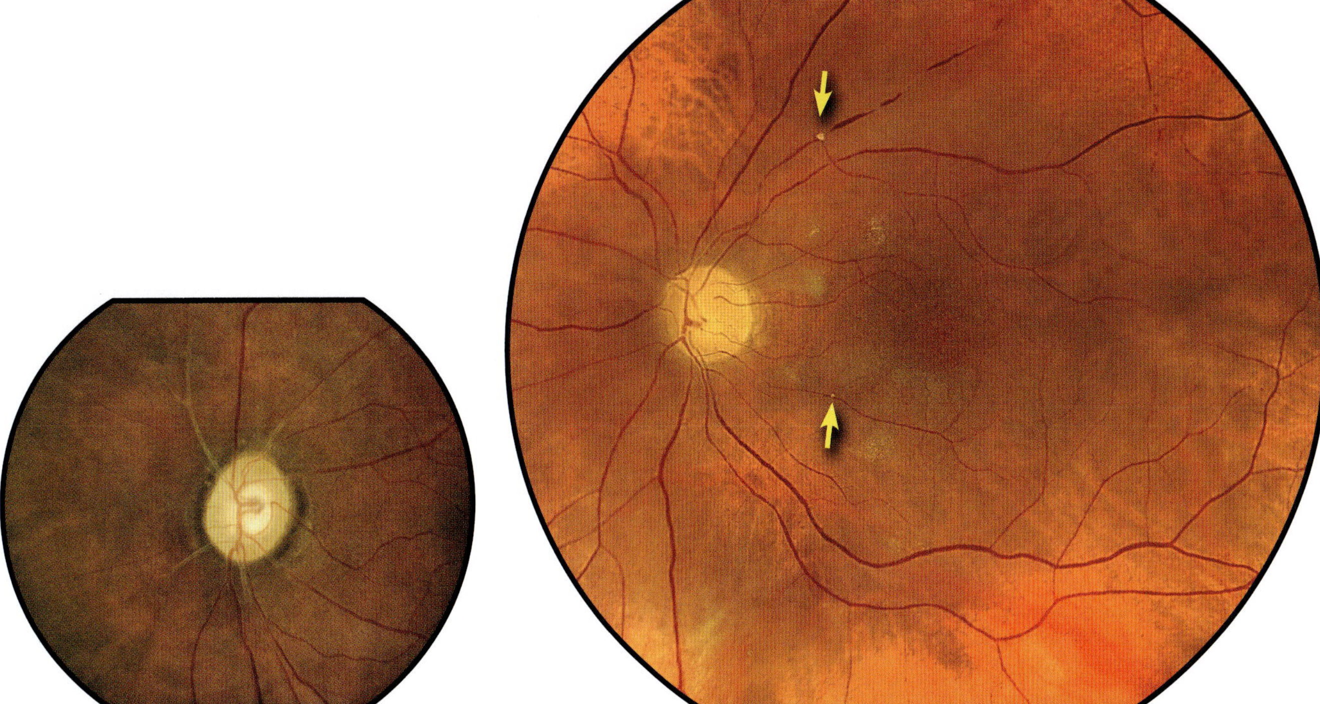

This patient had an old central retinal artery occlusion. There is resultant optic atrophy and peripapillary sheathing of the arteriolar vasculature.

This patient presented with a partial central retinal artery occlusion with multiple CWS. There is boxcarring of the retinal vessels and residual emboli that have passed into the distal vasculature *(arrows)*. The optic nerve is pale.

Central Retinal Artery Occlusion with Sparing of the Ciliary Artery

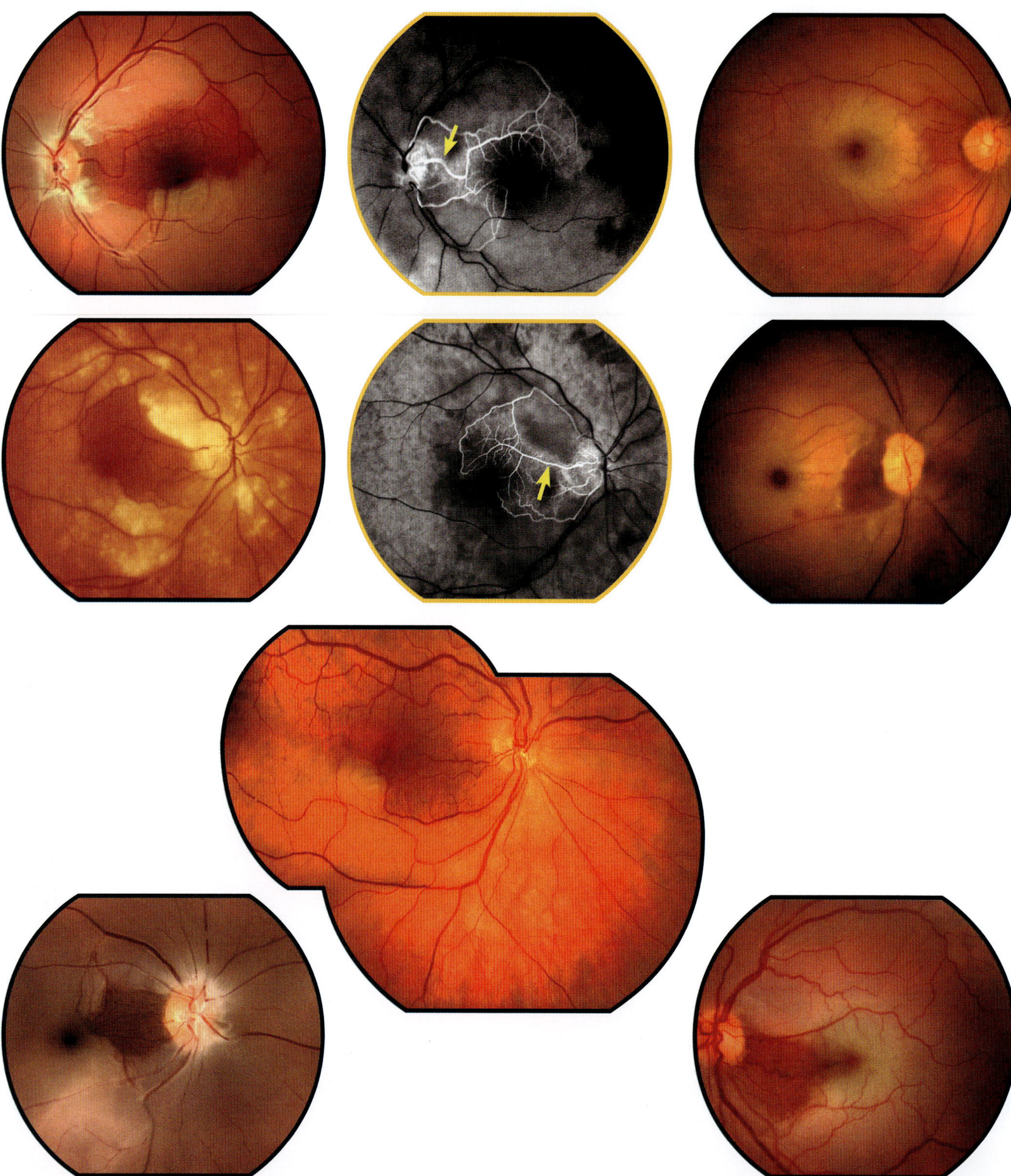

These patients all presented with central retinal artery occlusion with sparing of the ciliary artery. Fluorescein angiography documented persistent perfusion of the ciliary artery, partially sparing the fovea *(arrows)*. Note the presence of retinal venous filling emanating from the ciliary circulation. *Images courtesy of Ophthalmic Imaging Systems, Inc*

Branch Retinal Artery Occlusion

A branch retinal artery obstruction (BRAO) presents with superficial retinal whitening in a geographic distribution of the obstructed arteriole. As is the case for central retinal artery occlusions, most patients have pre-existing cardiovascular disease. The most common cause is embolism from the carotid artery. The absence of a visible intravascular plaque does not necessarily imply a non-embolic cause because plaques may distalize. The visual prognosis is relatively good, unless there is an underlying systemic factor that increases the risk for recurrence.

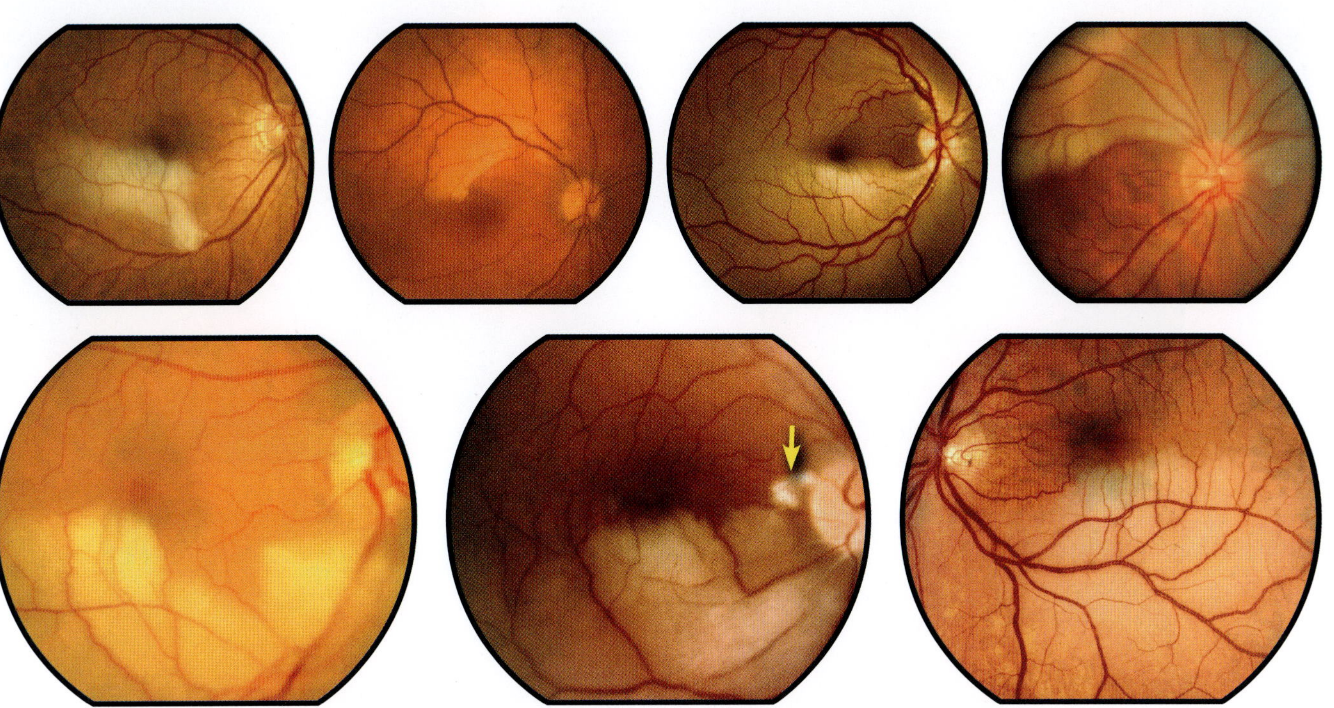

These are examples of acute branch retinal artery occlusions. Note the acute whitening of the inner retina that follows the course of the obstructed vessel. The extent of whitening is dependent on the size of the arteriole. In about one-third of cases, an embolus or plaque on the optic nerve may be identified *(upper right)*. This patient's embolism originated from mitral valve prolapse. There is a cotton-wool spot from superficial capillary occlusion in the lower middle image *(arrow)*.

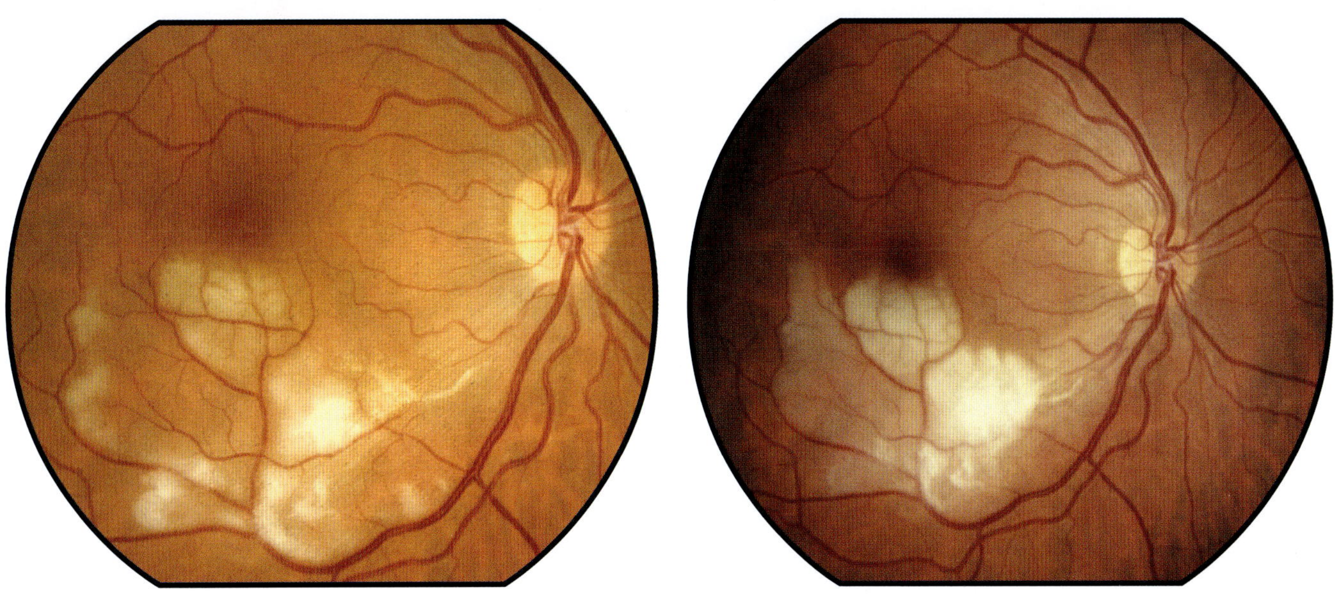

This is a patient with progressive branch retinal artery occlusion. The image on the left was obtained 2 days before the image on the right.

Multiple Branch Artery Occlusions

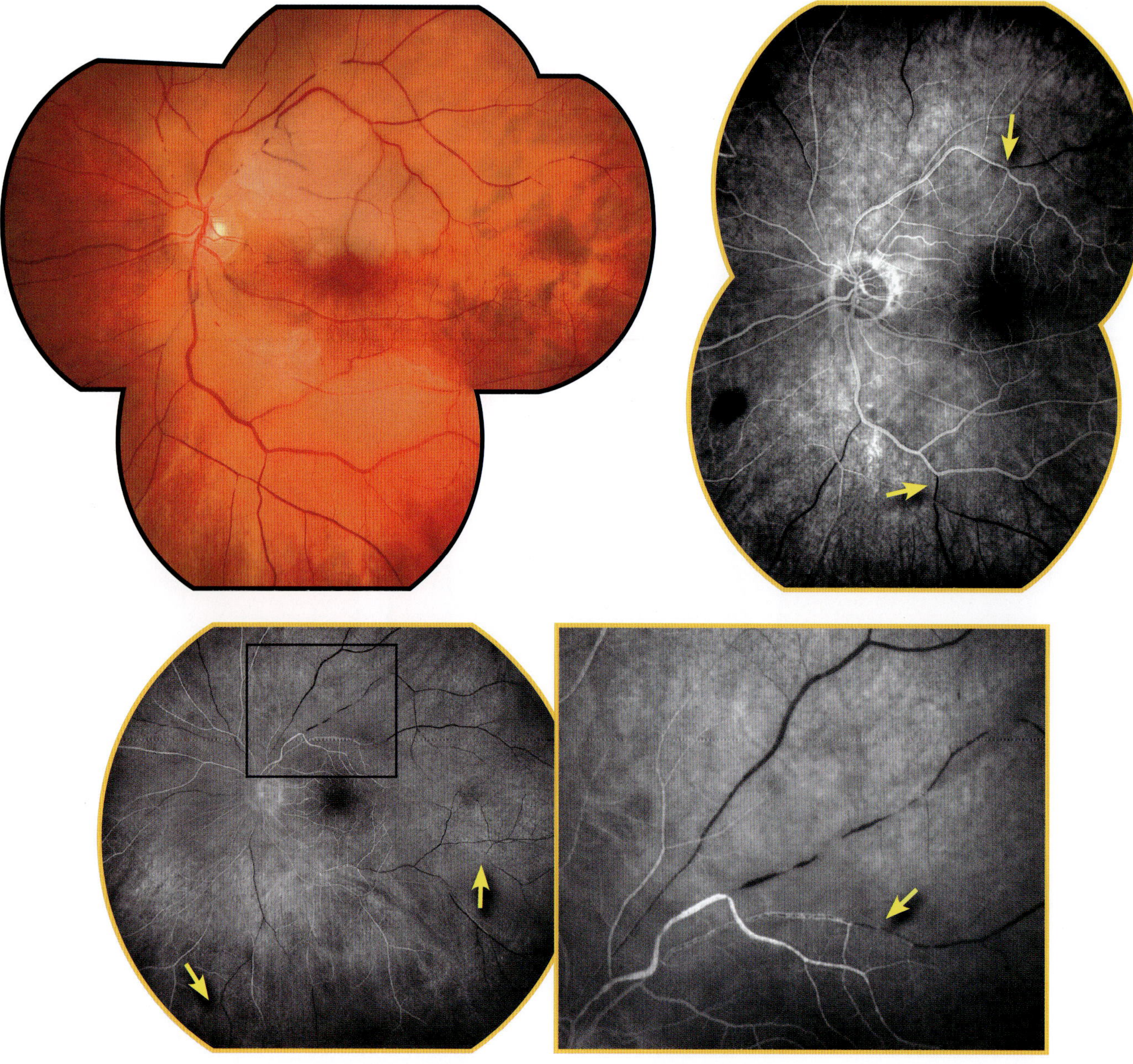

Note the multiple branch retinal artery occlusions in these two patients. The top images are of a patient who experienced embolic disease at the time of cardiac surgery. The bottom images are from a patient with multiple retinal vascular emboli from cardiovascular disease. Note the obstructed sites on the FA *(arrows)*. There is still good perfusion of the central macula.

Recurrent Retinal Artery Occlusions

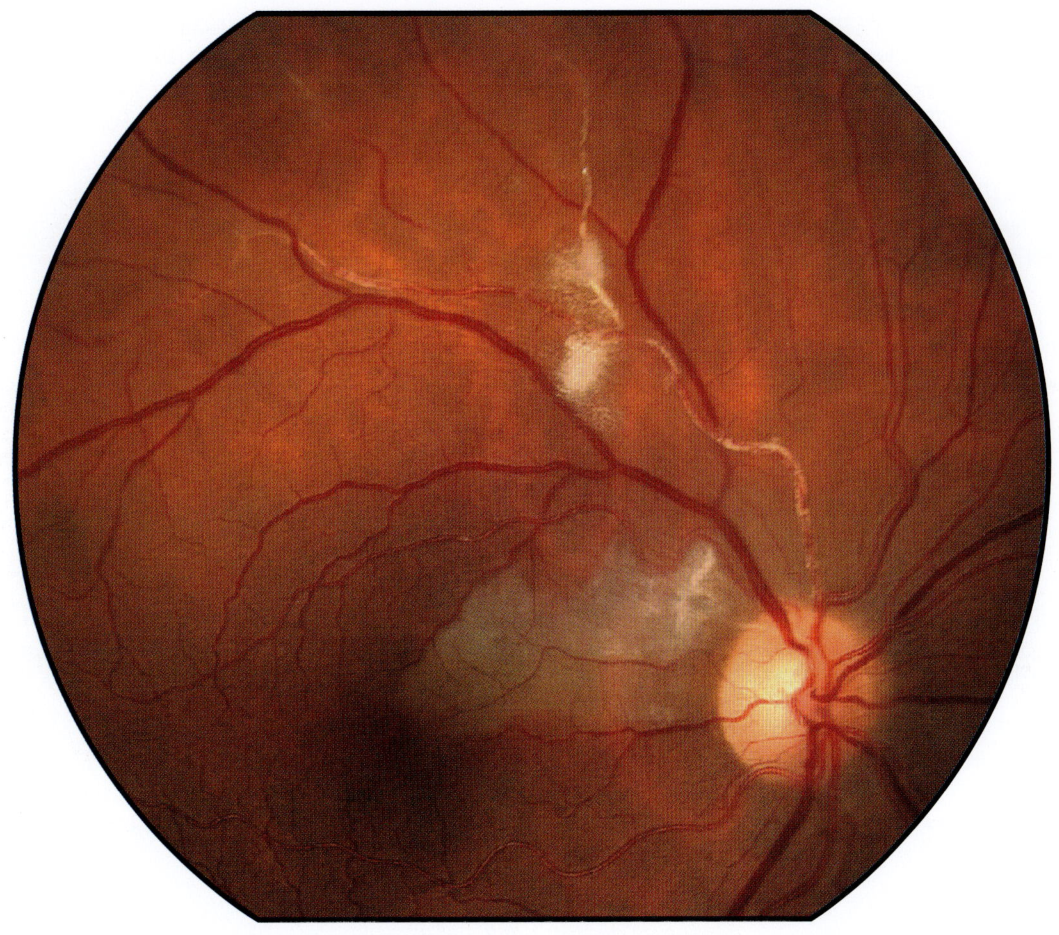

This patient presented with a recurrent branch artery occlusion. An older superotemporal branch occlusion with sheathing and mineralization of the retinal arteriole is present and a more acute branch retinal artery occlusion of the nasal macula is also noted.

Embolus Distalization

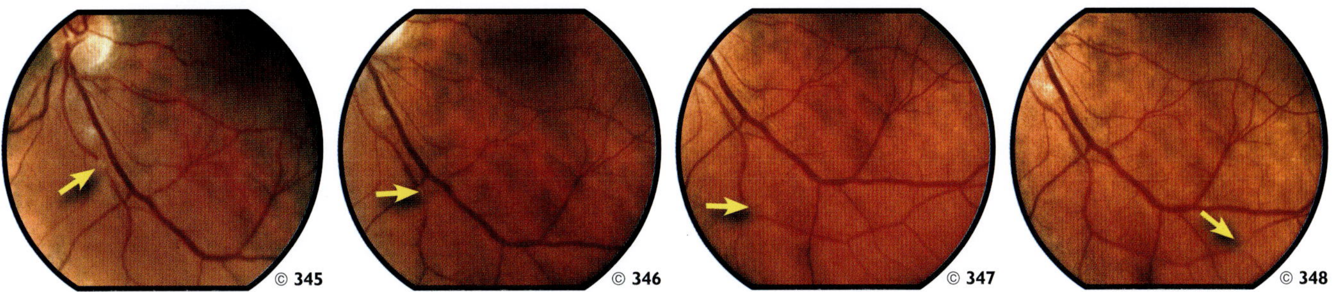

This patient illustrates a retinal vascular embolus first seen at an early bifurcation of the arteriole *(far left image)*. Over the ensuing days, it migrated distally *(arrows)* through the posterior pole to the near peripheral fundus.

PAMM (Paracentral Acute Middle Maculopathy)

Paracentral acute middle maculopathy (PAMM) is a recently described entity with a characteristic band of hyper-reflectivity at the level of the inner nuclear layer on spectral domain optical coherence tomography (SD-OCT). Associated whitening on color fundus photography and hypo-reflectivity with near-infrared reflectance imaging may also be appreciated. Inner nuclear layer (INL) infarction due to ischemia of the deep retinal capillary plexus is the likely etiology. Many ocular and systemic conditions can be associated with PAMM including retinal vein occlusion, retinal artery occlusion, diabetic retinopathy, Purtscher retinopathy, and sickle-cell retinopathy.

PAMM versus CWS

Cotton-wool spot (CWS) is more superficial, chalk white in appearance, and associated with hyper reflectivity at the level of the ganglion cell and nerve fiber layers (with OCT) and due to ischemia or infarction of the superficial retinal capillary plexus.

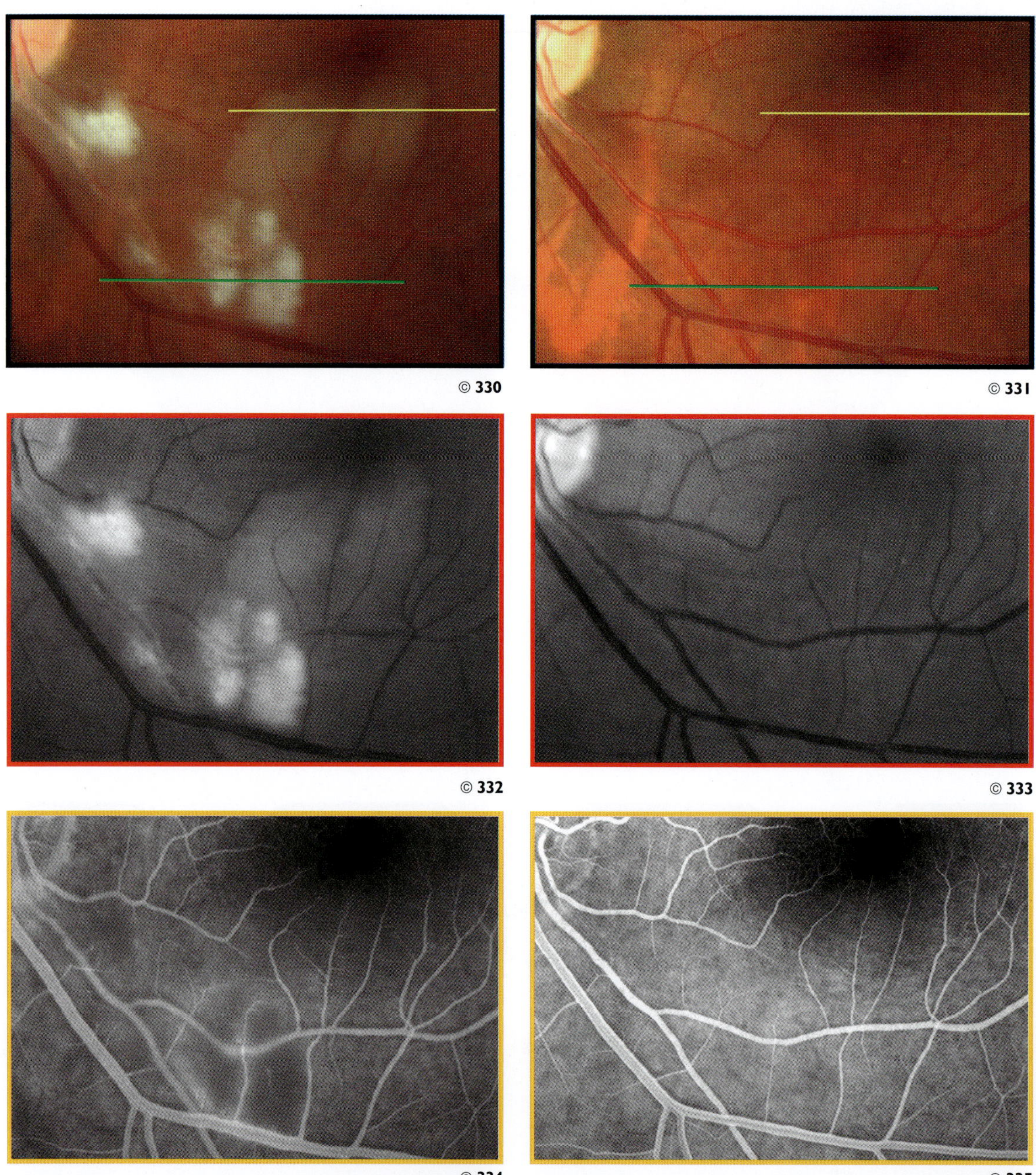

This figure illustrates the difference between a CWS and a PAMM lesion. The images on the right are follow-up images illustrating resolution of the CWS and PAMM lesions. Note the brighter white, and more superficial appearance of the CWS *(top left, green line)* on the color fundus photo compared to the deeper, grayish appearance of the PAMM lesion *(top left, yellow line)*. Red-free images also can highlight this difference with the CWS again appearing bright white compared to the deep gray appearance of the PAMM lesions *(middle left)*. On FA, CWS show hypo-fluorescence, while PAMM lesions appear normal *(bottom left)*.

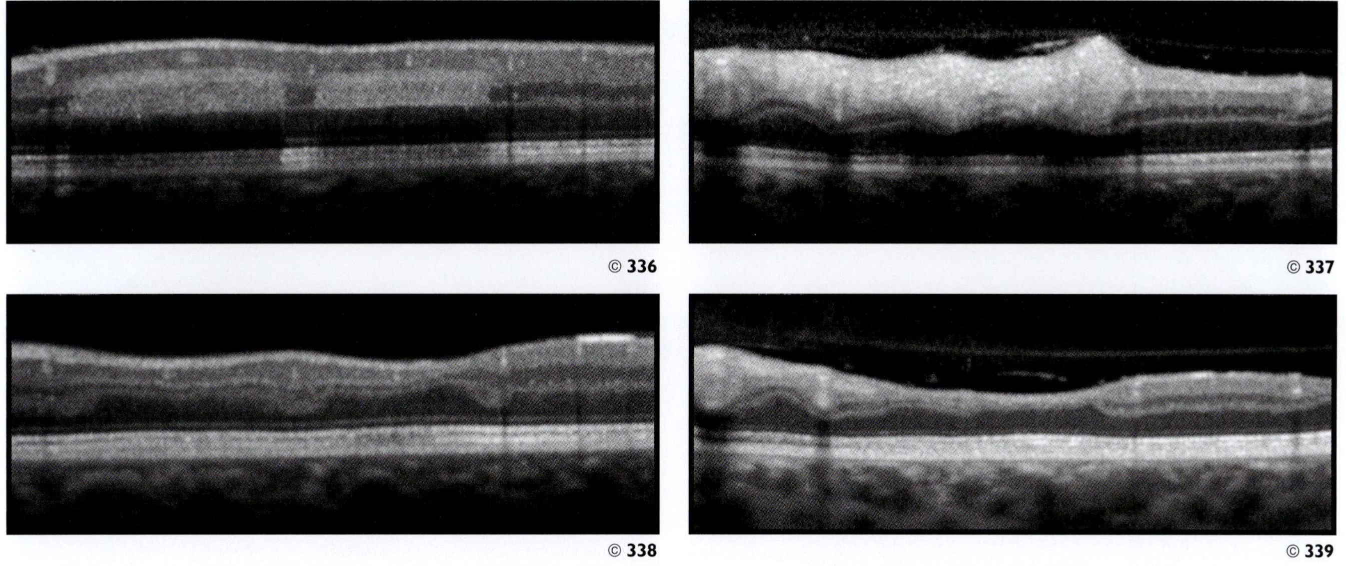

© 336 © 337 © 338 © 339

On spectral domain optical coherence tomography (SD-OCT), PAMM lesions are characterized by hyper-reflectivity in the middle retinal layers in the acute phase *(upper left)* with subsequent thinning of those layers in the chronic phase *(lower left)*. CWS are characterized by hyper-reflectivity and thickening of the NFL and ganglion cell layers in the acute phase *(upper right)* with subsequent thinning of those layers in the chronic phase *(lower right)*.

PAMM Associated with BRAO

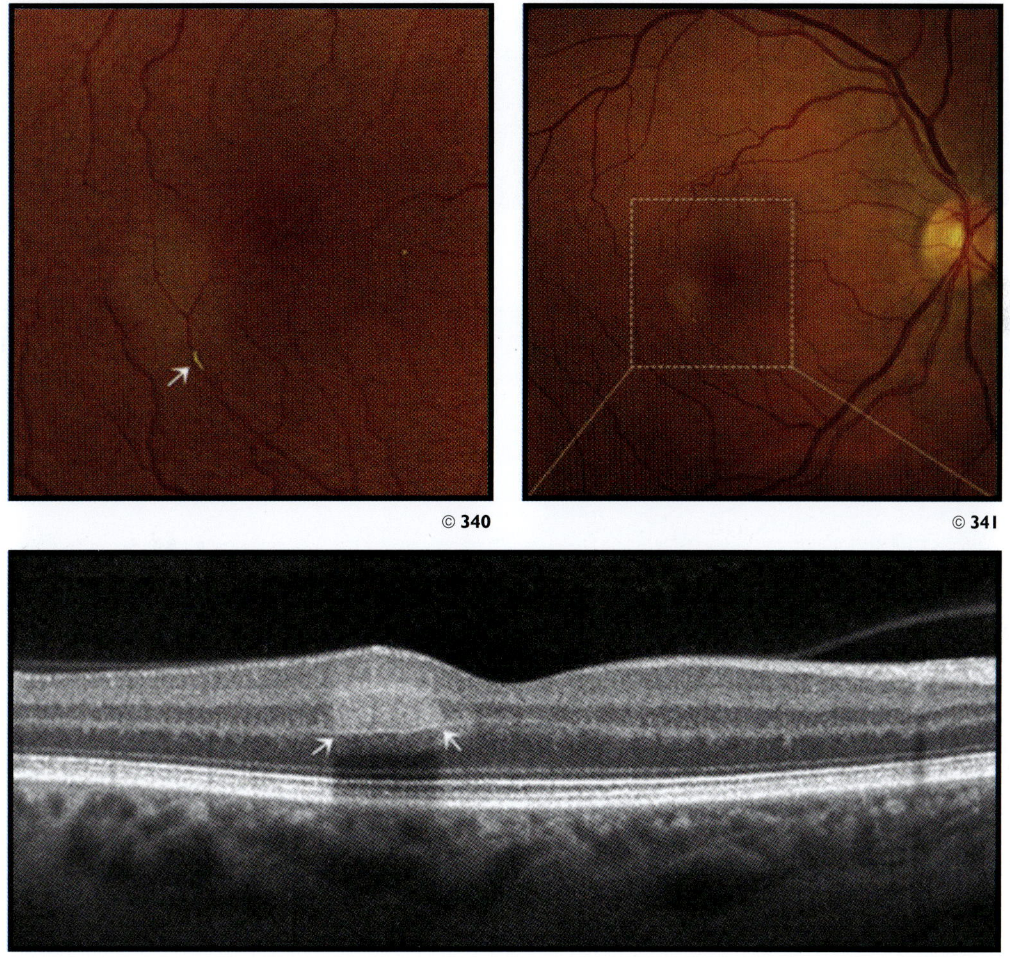

© 340 © 341 © 342

This patient has a small branch artery occlusion in the macula with a visible Hollenhorst plaque *(top left, arrow)* causing a deep gray-white infarct *(top right)*. The corresponding OCT demonstrates PAMM due to ischemia of the deep retinal capillary plexus and infarction of the inner nuclear layer. *Courtesy of Brandon Lujan, MD*

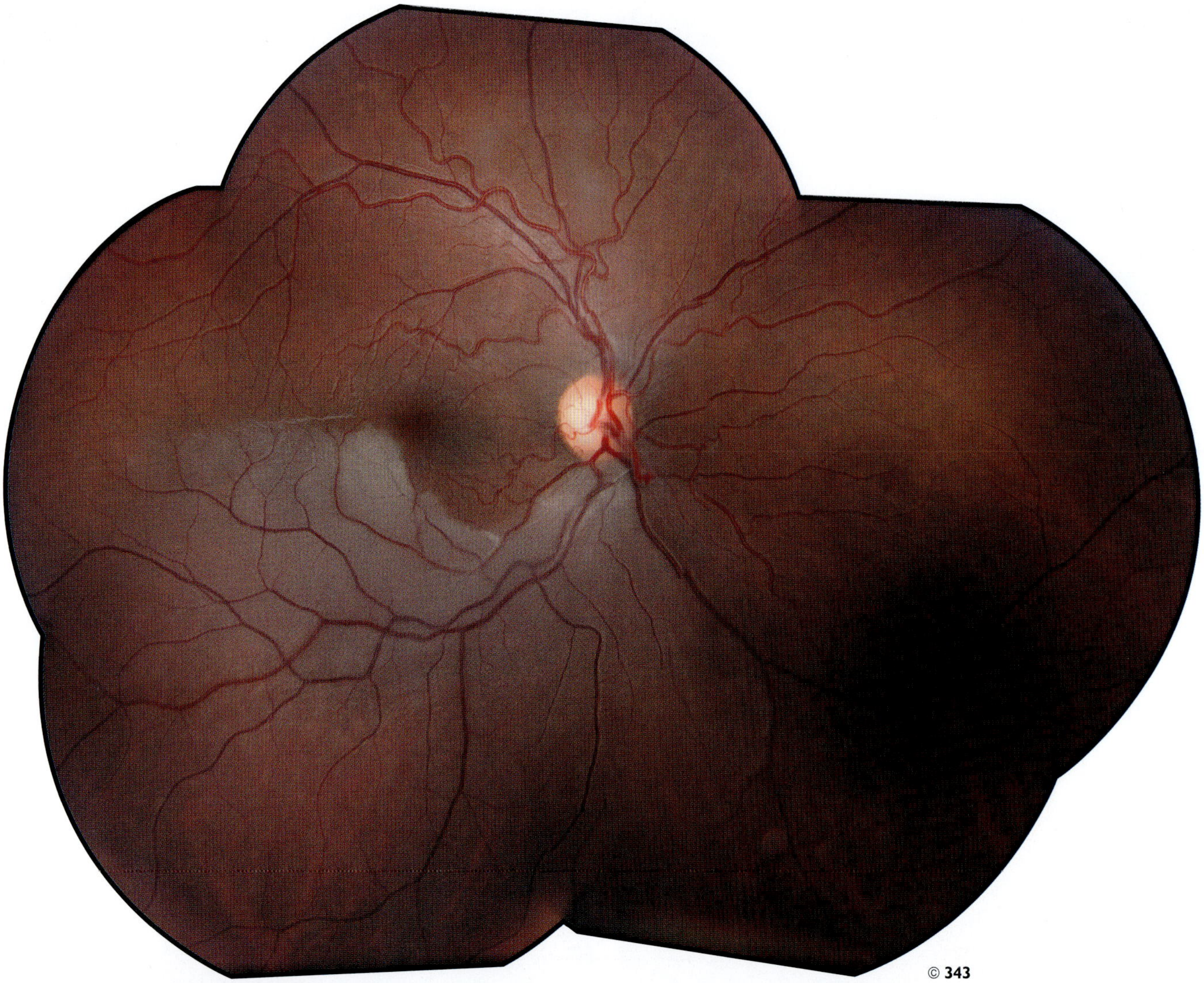

© 343

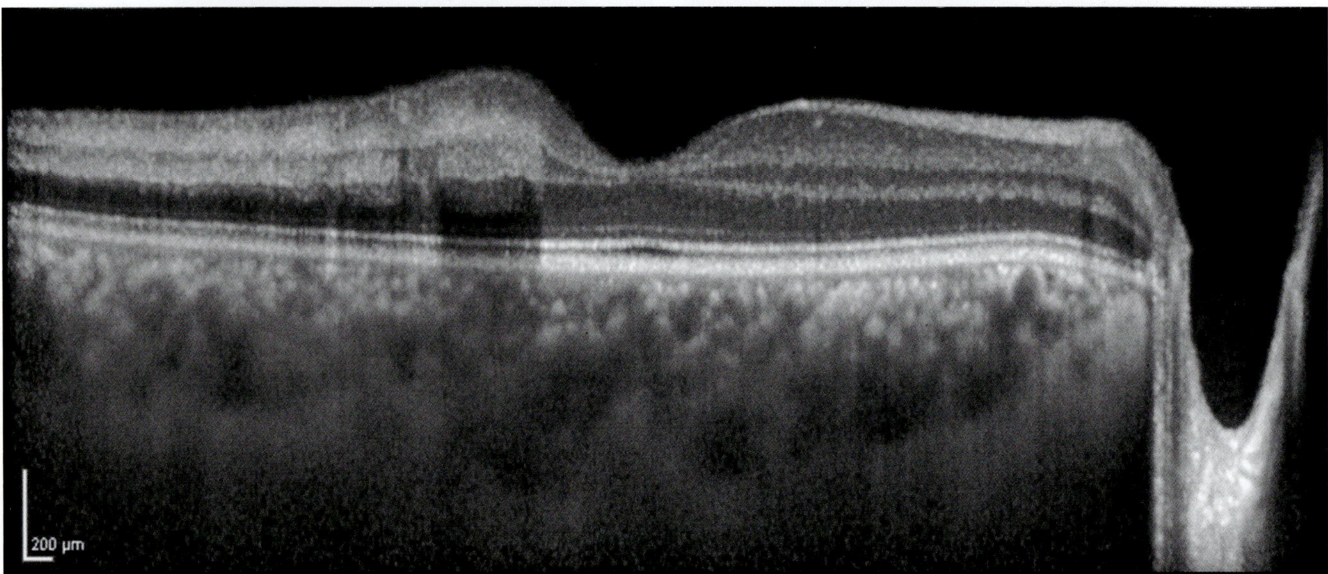

© 344

This patient, described earlier in the "Prepapillary Vascular Loop" section, suffered a BRAO secondary to torsion of a prepapillary vascular loop *(top)*. SD-OCT through the macula reveals diffuse PAMM lesions secondary to ischemia of the deep retinal capillary plexus. *Image courtesy of Ehsan Rahimy, MD*

Cilioretinal Artery Occlusion

Cilioretinal artery occlusions can occur in isolation or in association with giant cell arteritis and central retinal vein occlusion. They generally cause a sudden loss of central vision since these vessels perfuse the central macula. There is acute retinal whitening corresponding to the geographic distribution of the vessel. An FA may show obstruction or delayed perfusion, as in the case below.

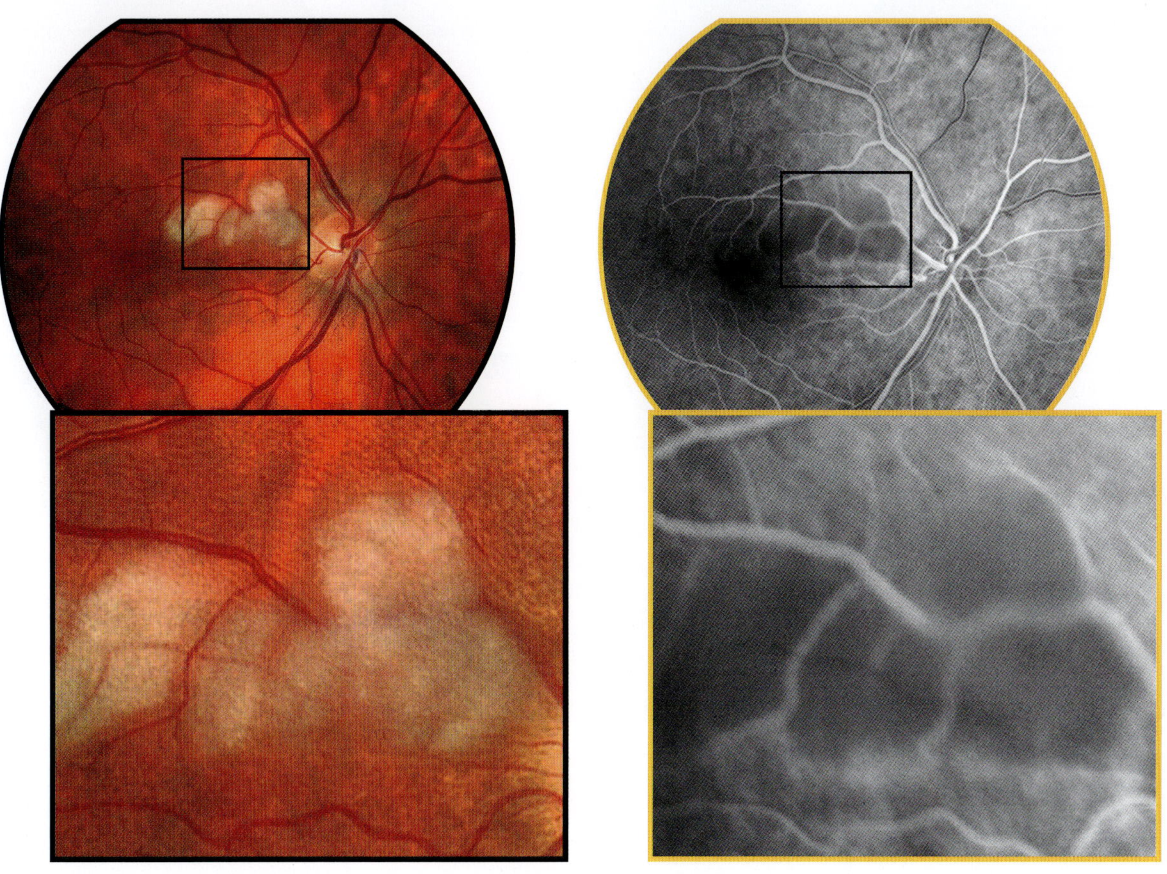

This patient had an occlusion of the superior branch of the cilioretinal artery. Note the ischemic whitening on color fundus photography and the corresponding hypofluorescence with FA.

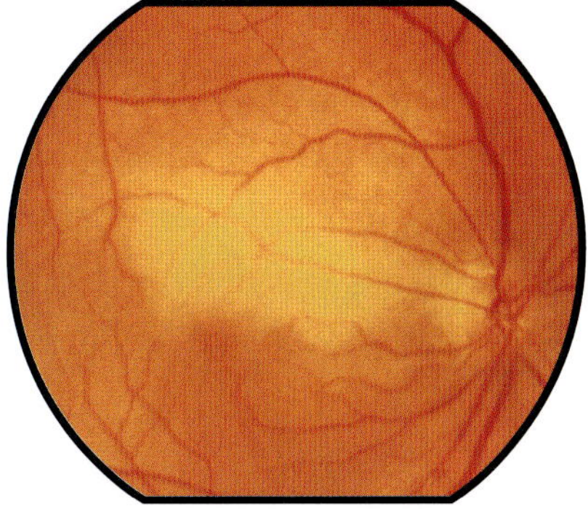

A cilioretinal artery occlusion is noted in this patient with corresponding ischemic whitening in the macula.

Plaques

About one-third of all retinal arteriolar occlusions are noted to be associated with plaques, some of which are glistening or mineralized. They are typically found at bifurcations, but not always. Retinal emboli originate from the carotid artery or the heart.

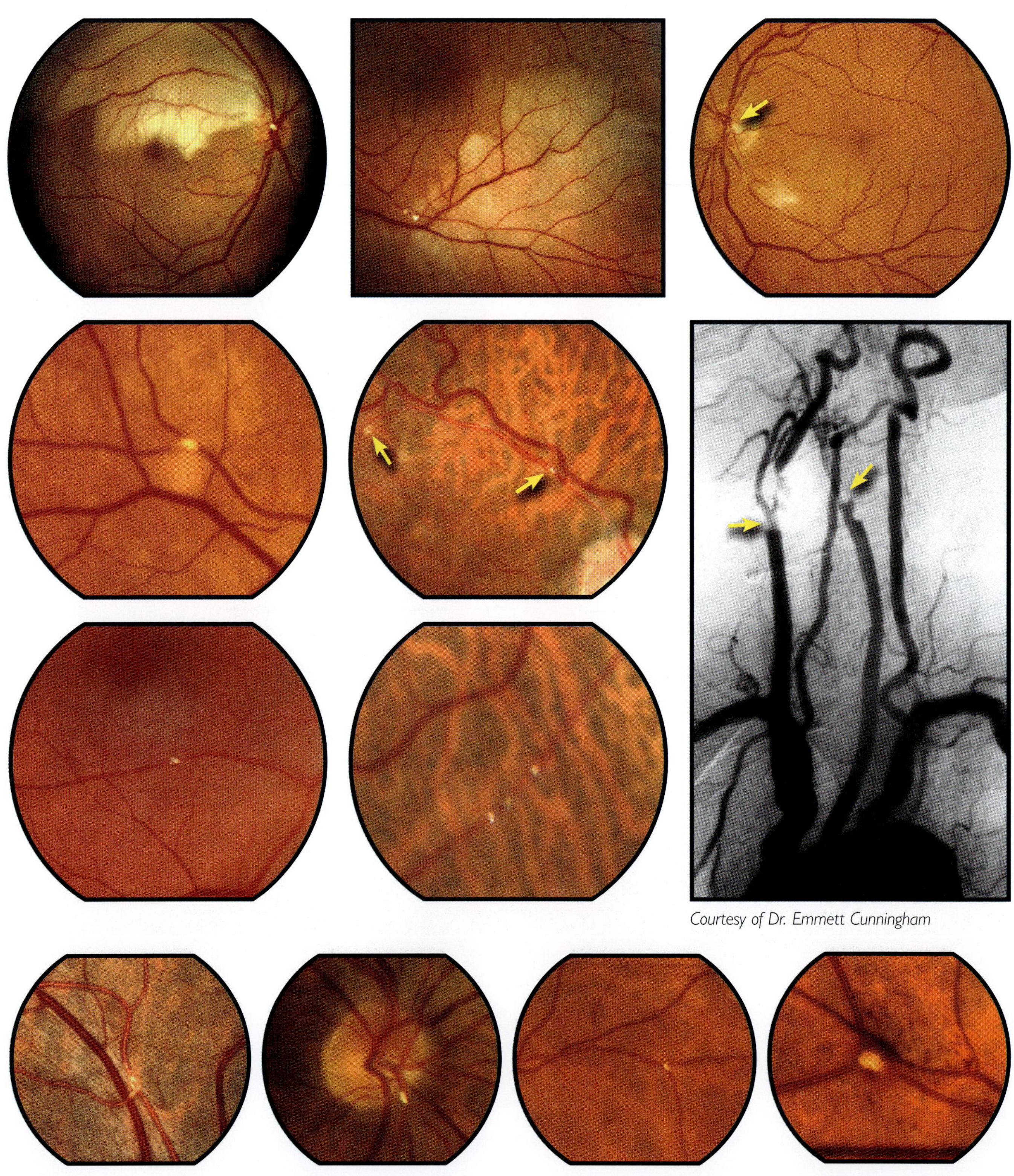

Courtesy of Dr. Emmett Cunningham

Note the multiple cases of branch retinal artery occlusion. Some are acute with ischemic whitening of the retina, whereas others have resolved. Rarely there is hemorrhage surrounding the plaque as noted in the lower right image. The carotid angiogram on the right shows multiple constrictions of the extracranial vessels perfusing the eye *(arrows)*.

Retinal venous occlusion is one of the most common retinal vascular abnormalities in the eye after diabetic retinopathy. Central retinal vein occlusions (CRVO) are usually seen in patients over the age of 50 with other risk factors such as hypertension and diabetes. Younger patients with CRVO should be worked up for hypercoagulable disorders. A central vein occlusion is thought to occur posterior to the lamina cribrosa. There are two forms: non-ischemic versus ischemic retinal venous occlusion. These designations are based on the area of capillary non-perfusion identified with widefield fluorescein angiography and can be predicted by very poor visual acuity or the presence of an afferent papillary defect. Ischemic occlusions can be complicated by vitreous hemorrhage, anterior-segment neovascularization, and neovascular glaucoma. Branch retinal vein occlusions (BRVO) are more common than CRVO. They are typically seen in patients with hypertension or diabetes but may occur without known systemic abnormalities. BRVO develops due to compression of a vein by the artery at an arteriolar-venular crossing encapsulated by a common adventitial sheath.

Central Retinal Vein Occlusion

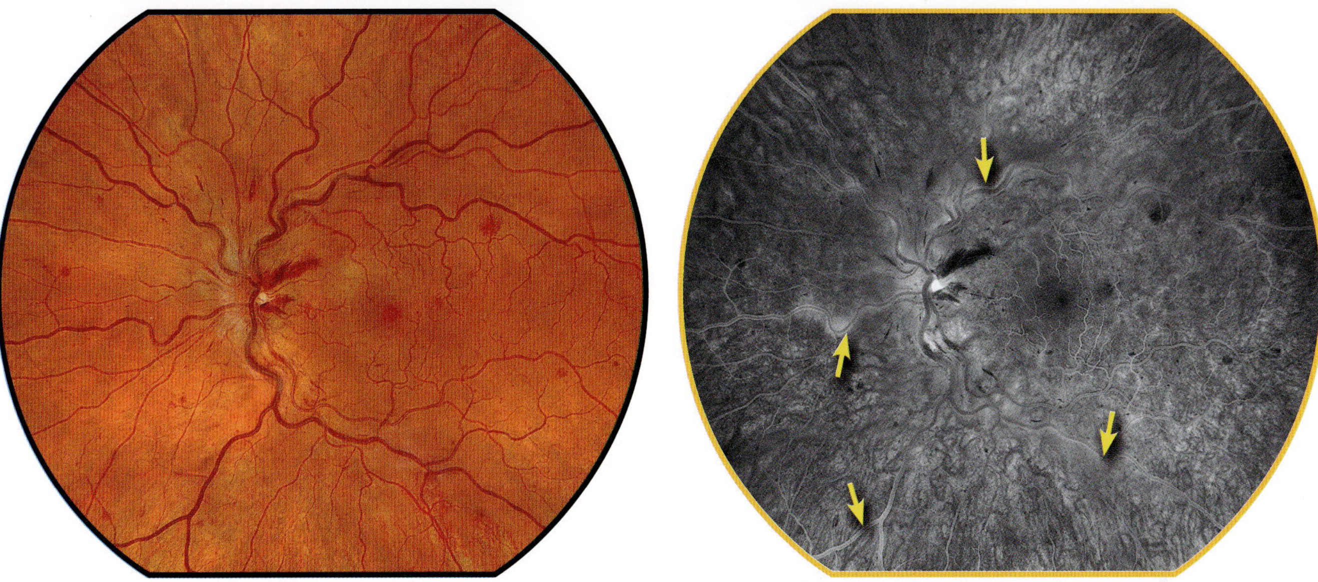

This patient has non-ischemic central venous occlusion with retinal venous tortuosity and few hemorrhages at the disc and in each quadrant of the mid periphery. The FA shows segmental staining of the venules *(arrows)* and minimal leakage at the optic nerve. There is no evidence of significant retinal capillary ischemia or non-perfusion.

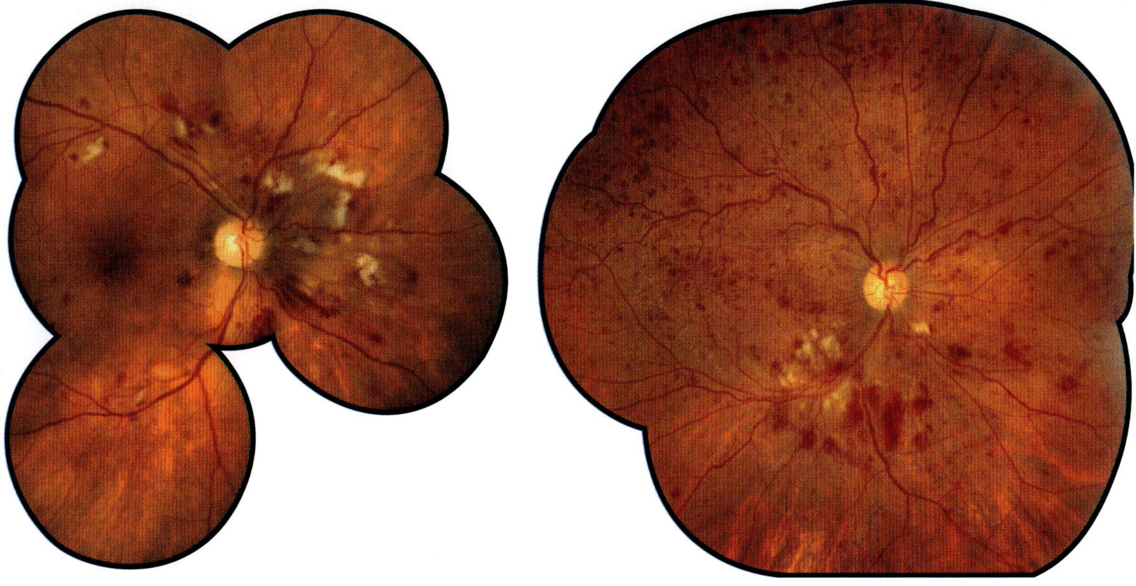

Note these two cases of more severe non-ischemic central venous occlusion with more significant retinal hemorrhage. The retinal hemorrhages are more prominent in the superior hemisphere *(right)*. *Left montage courtesy of Dr. Matthew Benz*

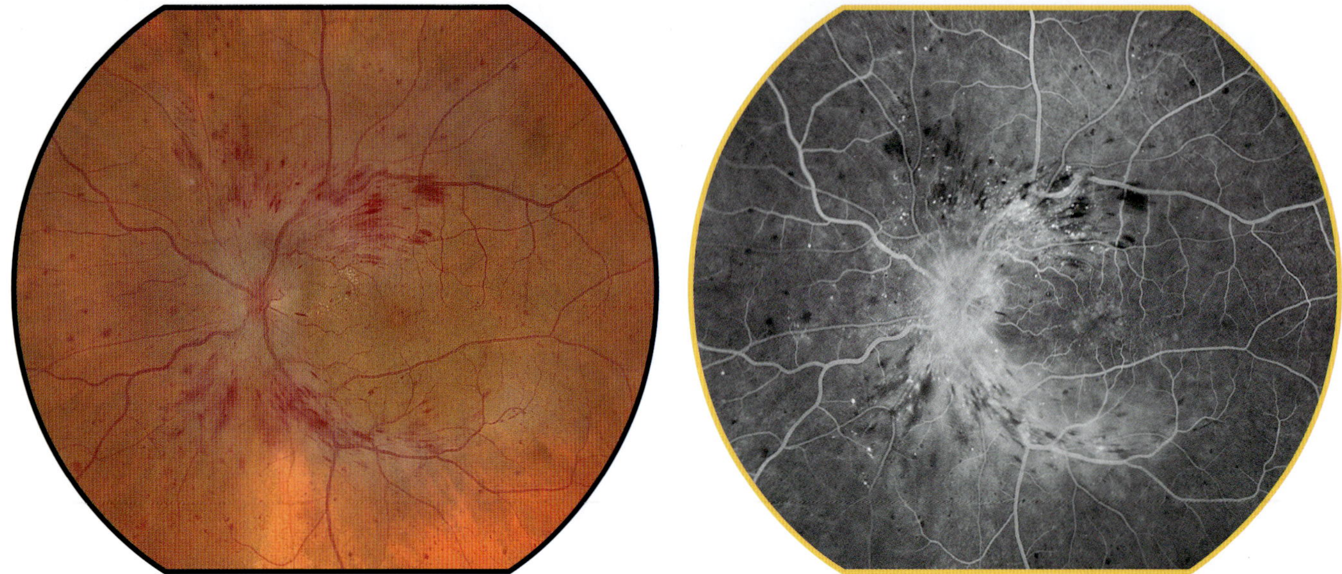

Note the non-ischemic CRVO in this young patient in his 30s, with no history of diabetes or systemic hypertension. There is disc edema, intraretinal hemorrhages and microaneurysms, and no evidence of significant retinal ischemia or non-perfusion with the FA.

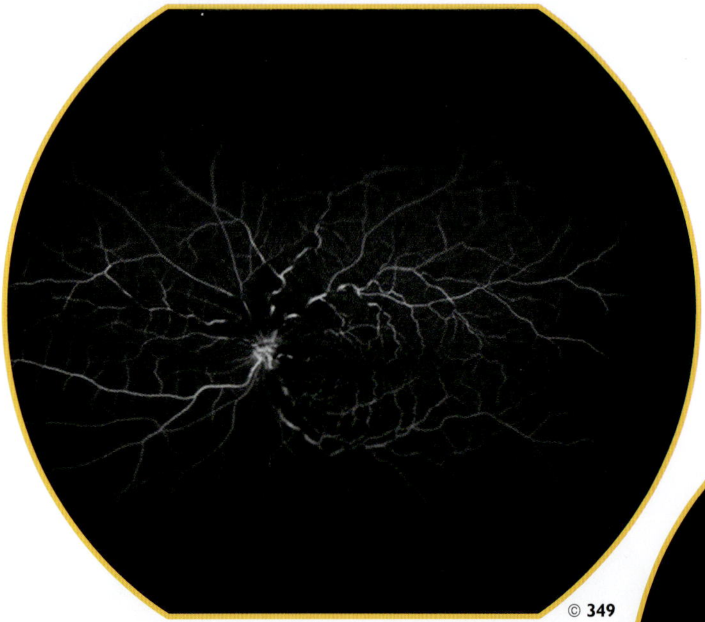

© 349

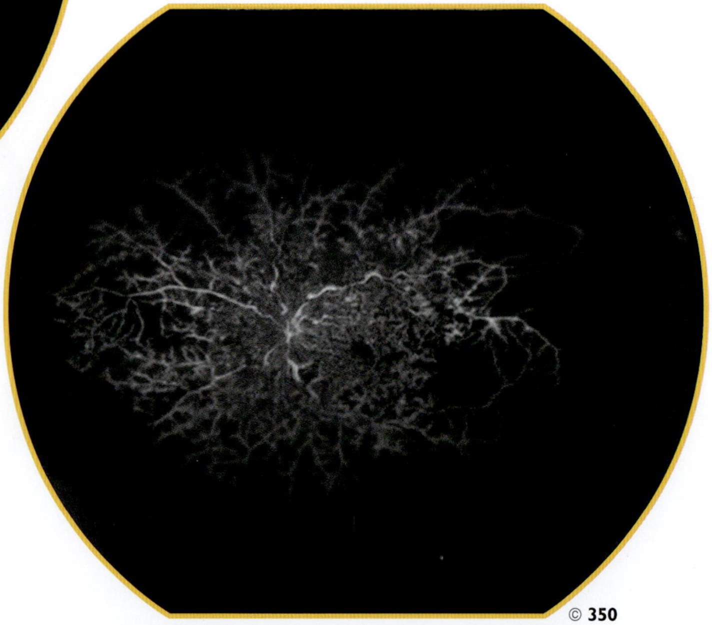

© 350

Ultra widefield angiography of two cases of CRVO is shown. The top image shows patchy blockage from hemorrhage but intact peripheral perfusion. The lower image displays severe capillary non-perfusion.

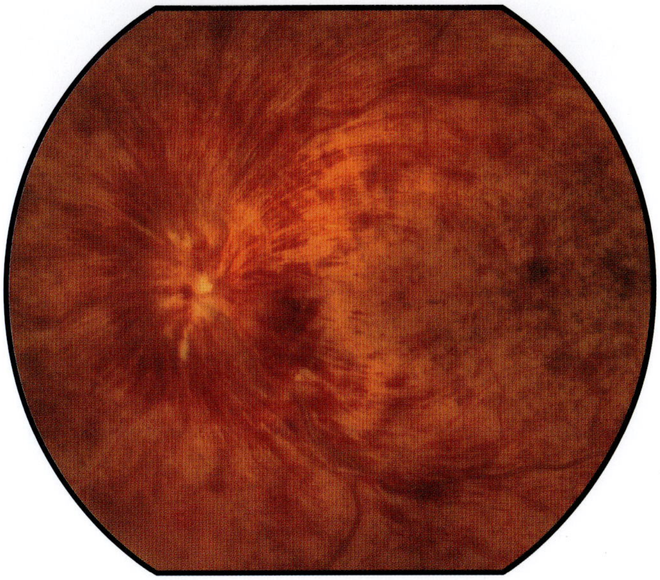

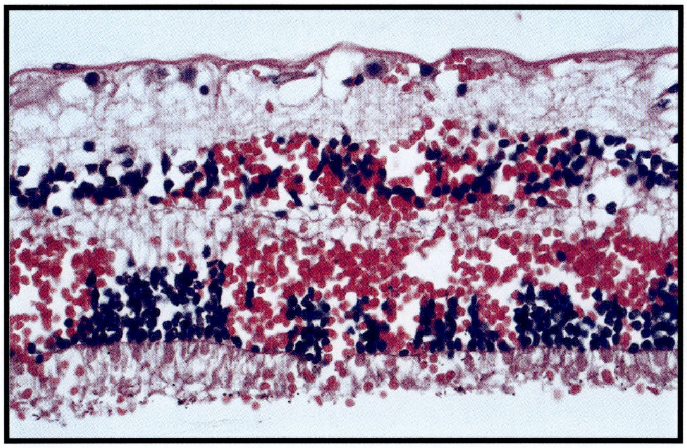

© 351

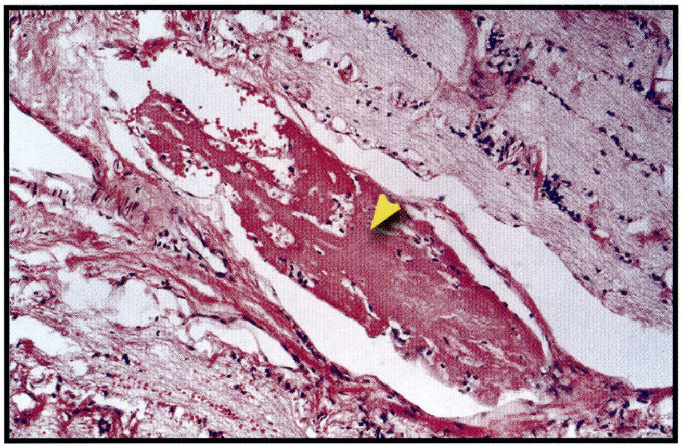

© 352

This is a clinicopathologic correlation of an acute hemorrhagic central retinal vein occlusion within 24 hours. Light microscopy shows marked intraretinal hemorrhage and a fresh thrombus *(arrowhead)* in the central retinal vein at the posterior aspect of the lamina cribrosa.

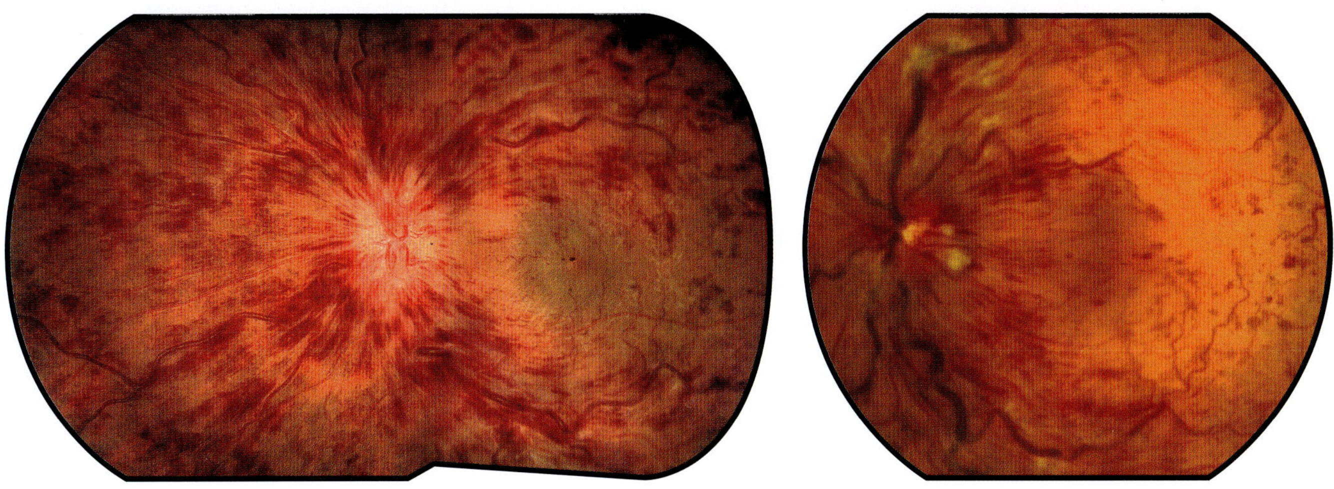

These are two cases of ischemic central retinal vein occlusion. There is marked dilation and tortuosity of the retinal venous system, widespread retinal hemorrhages, and macular edema.

Wyburn–Mason Syndrome and Central Retinal Vein Occlusion

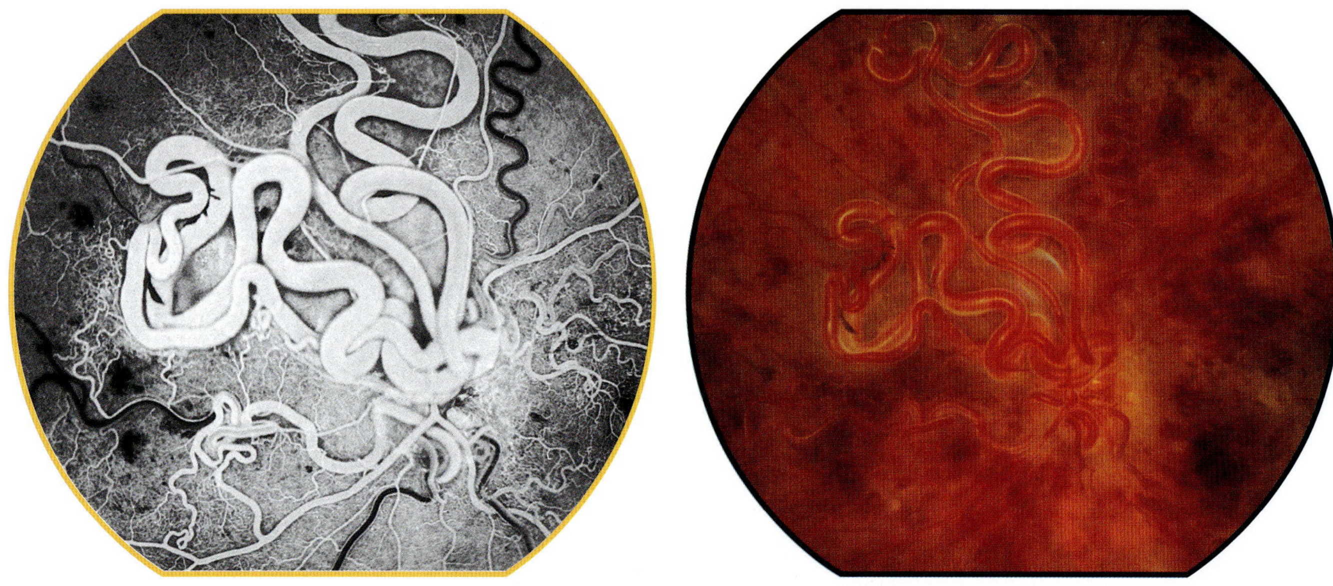

Note the presence of dilated tortuous retinal vessels and arteriolar-venular shunting in this case of Wyburn–Mason syndrome. The FA was taken 3 years prior to development of an acute hemorrhagic central retinal vein occlusion *(right)*. It is not uncommon for these congenital shunts to develop venous occlusive disease and secondary ischemia and neovascularization.

CRVO and Cilioretinal Artery Occlusion

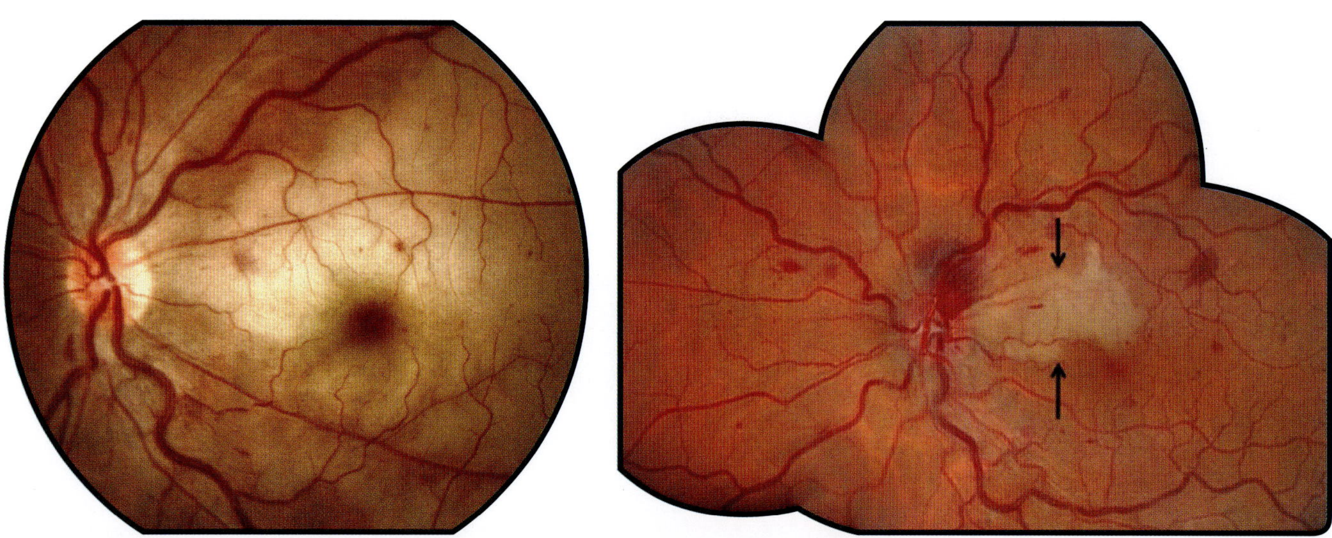

These are examples of non-ischemic CRVO with associated cilioretinal artery occlusions. *Right image courtesy of West Coast Retina*

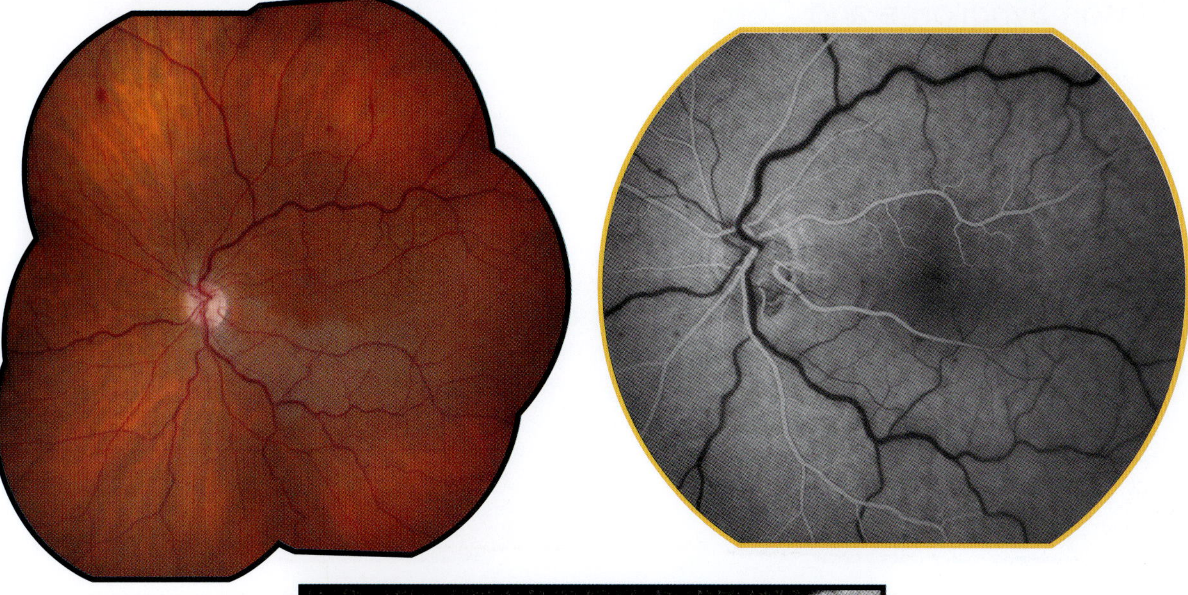

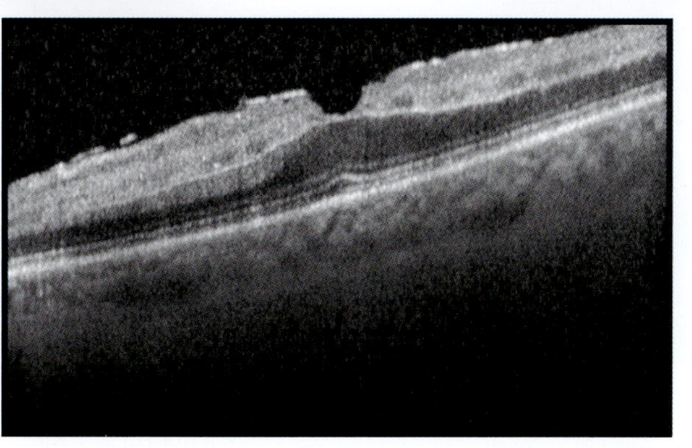

This patient developed a central retinal vein occlusion with cilioretinal artery occlusion. Note the whitening of the inferior macula in the distribution of the cilioretinal artery *(top left)* and the delayed and incomplete filling of the cilioretinal artery on FA taken at 18 s post injection *(top right)*. SD-OCT through the macula illustrates PAMM with hyper-reflective band-like lesions at the level of the inner nuclear layer due to ischemia of the deep retinal capillary plexus.

CRVO and PAMM

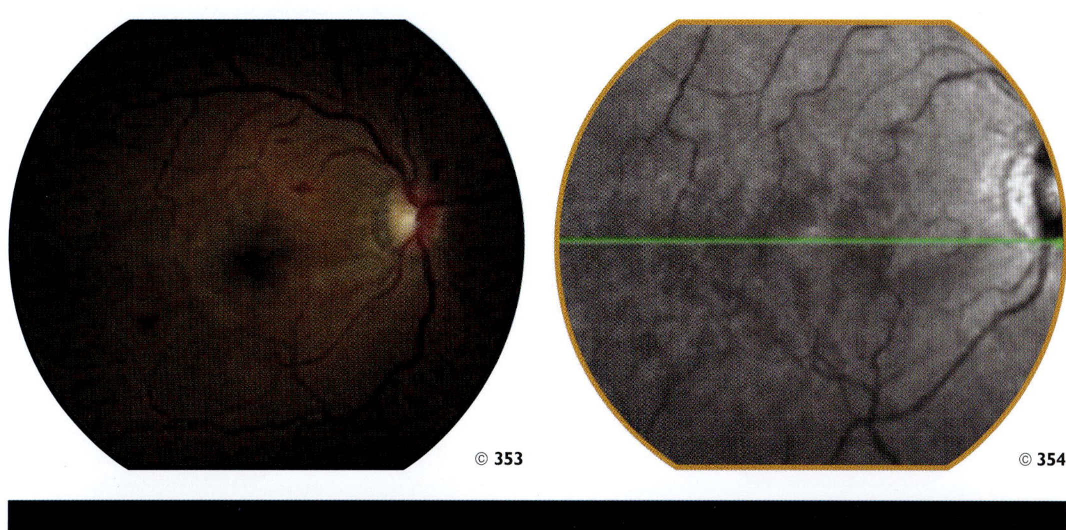

© **353** © **354**

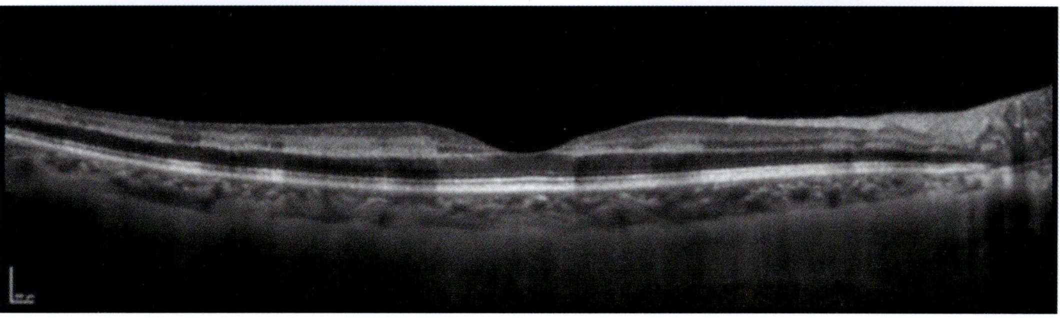

© **355**

This 56-year-old female developed a central retinal vein occlusion with PAMM. Note the engorged venous system with intraretinal hemorrhages and deep gray lesions in the macula *(top left)*. The gray lesions appear dark in a perivenular "fern-like" pattern on near infrared *(top right)* and correspond to hyper-reflective lesions at the level of the inner nuclear layer on SD-OCT *(bottom)*.

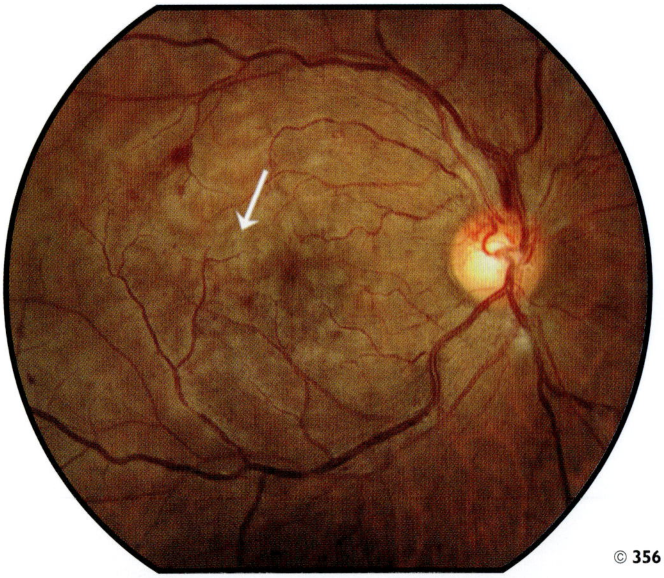

© 356

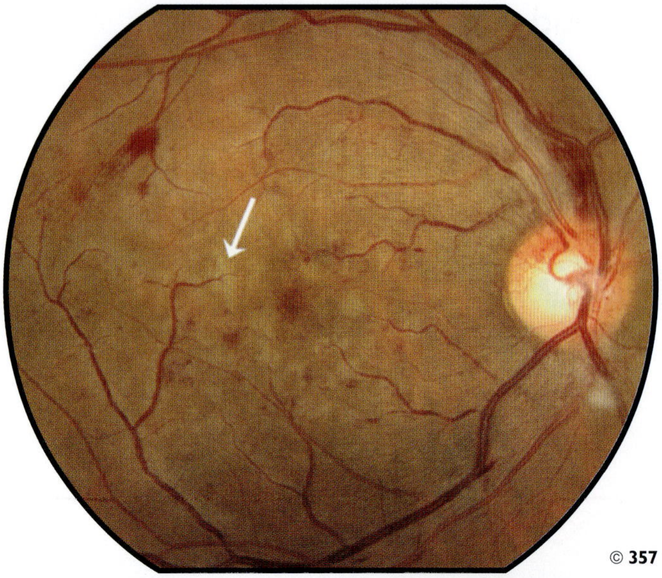

© 357

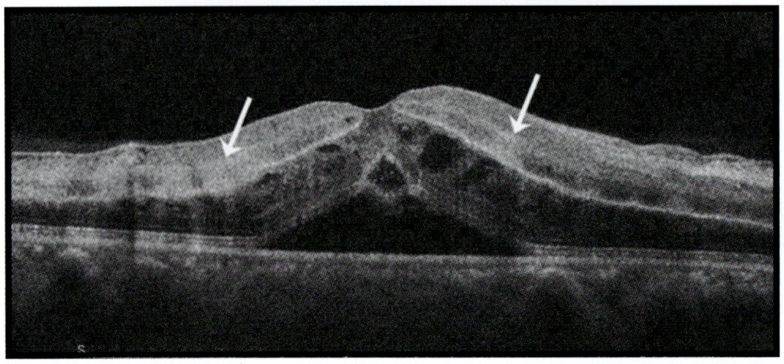

© 358

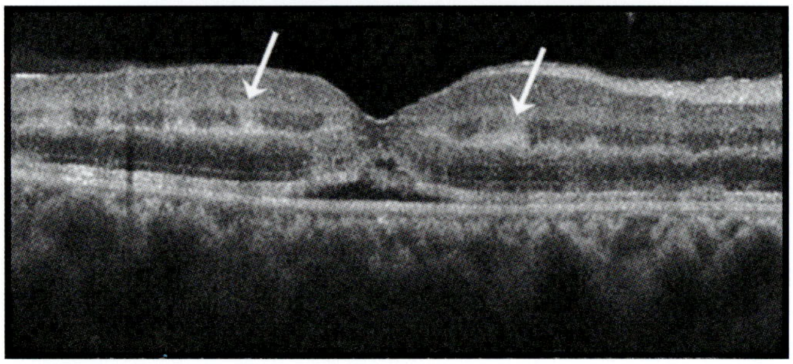

© 359

Note the presence of PAMM *(arrows)* in the color and OCT images *(left)* in this patient with CRVO. The CME is much improved after intravitreal anti-vascular endothelial growth factor (anti-VEGF) therapy (*right,* OCT).

Collateralization

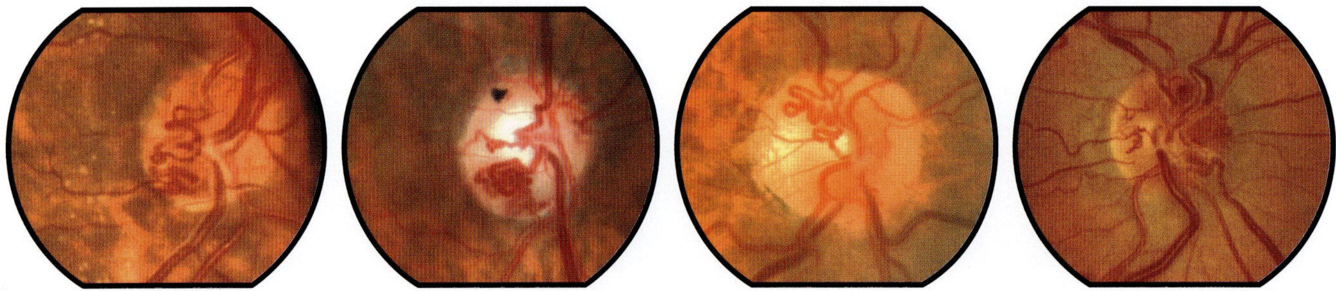

These are four examples of optociliary collaterals that develop in cases of CRVO to bypass the occlusion of the central retinal vein. They are on the venous side of the circulation and do not leak on FA.

Carotid Cavernous Fistula and Central Retinal Vein Occlusion

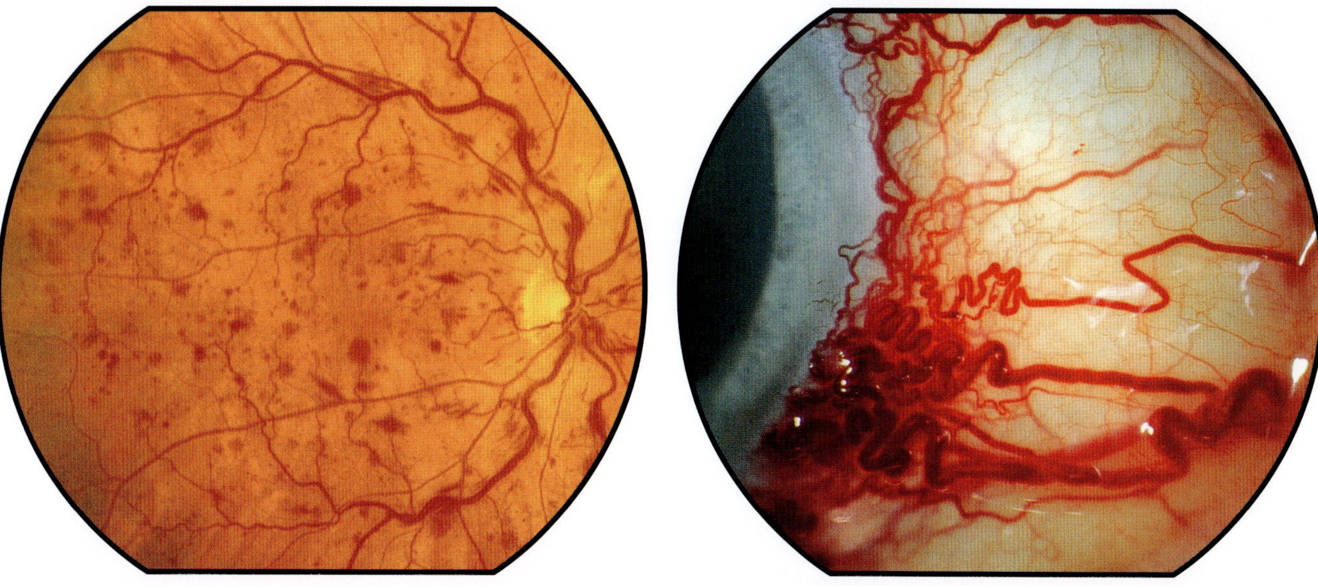

This patient has a CRVO with intraretinal hemorrhages and tortuous vessels and dilated conjunctival vessels due to a carotid cavernous fistula that should be considered in the differential diagnosis of CRVO. *Courtesy of Robert Hammond*

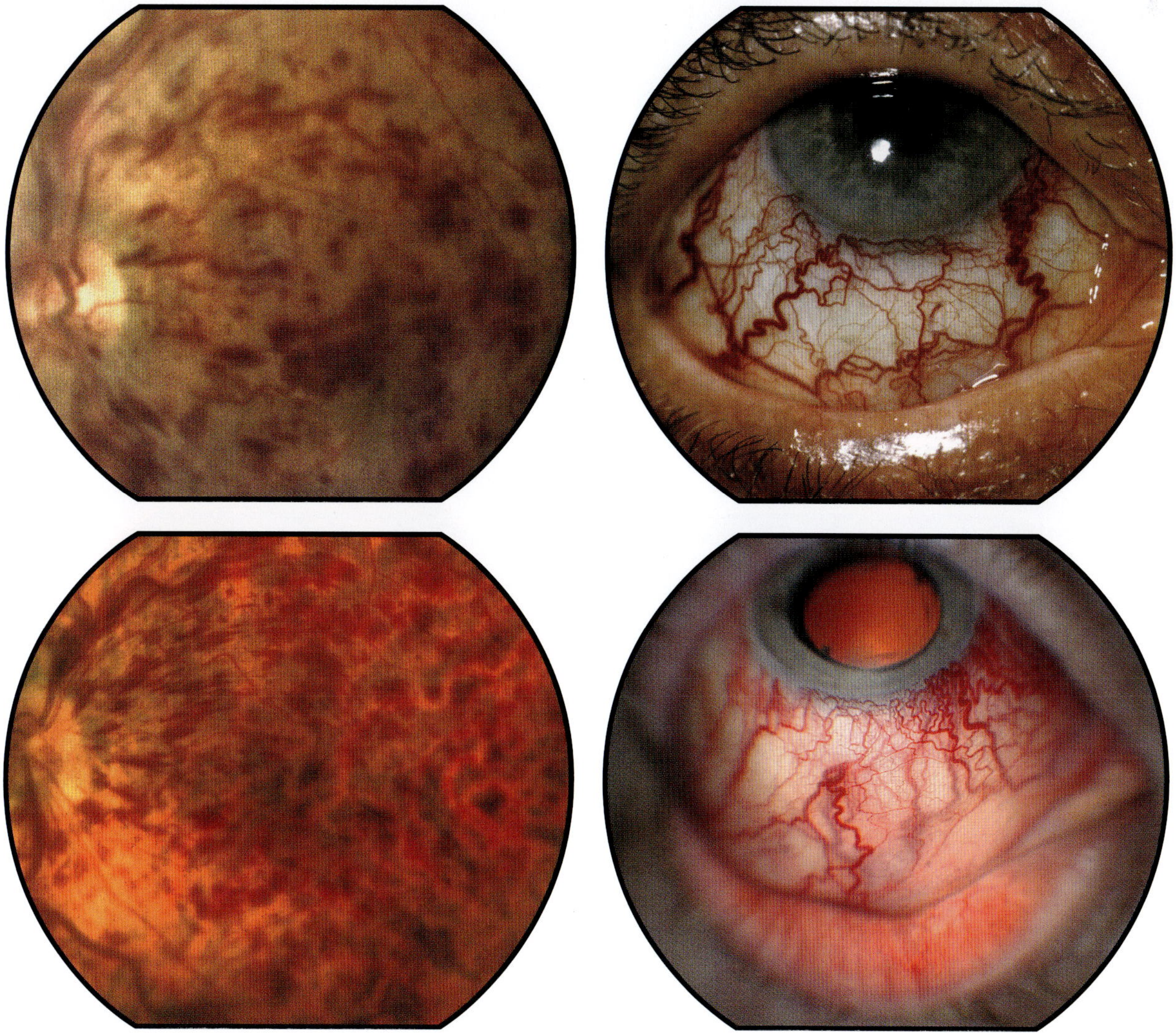

These are two additional cases of CRVO associated with carotid cavernous sinus fistula.

Natural Course

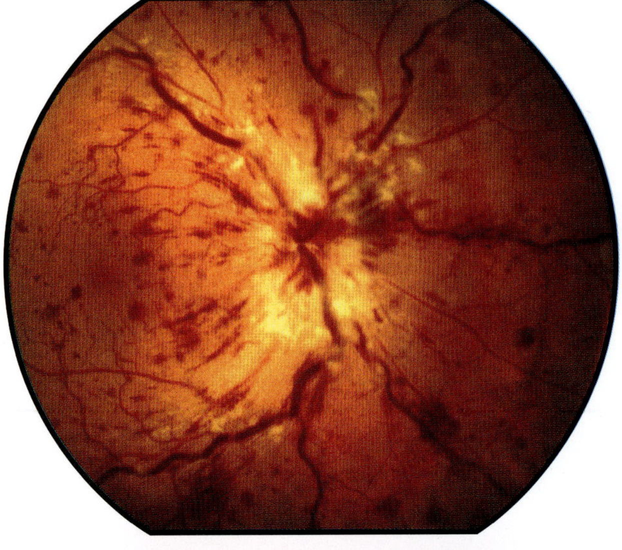

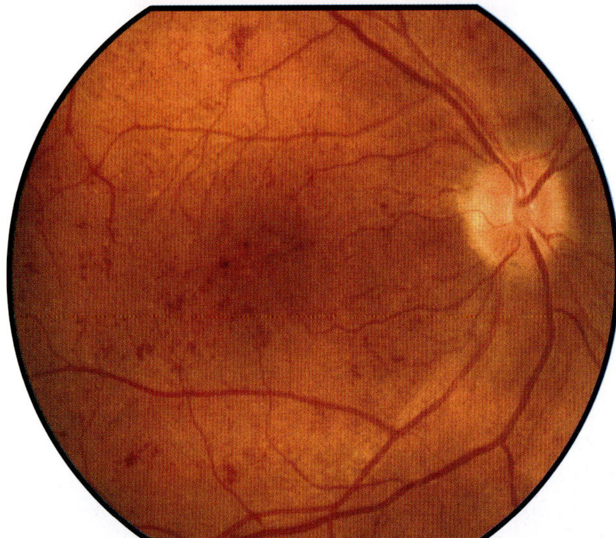

An acute central retinal vein occlusion with severe disc edema and intraretinal hemorrhages is shown *(top)*. There was spontaneous resolution of the obstruction with improvement of vision *(bottom)*.

Treatment: Laser Photocoagulation

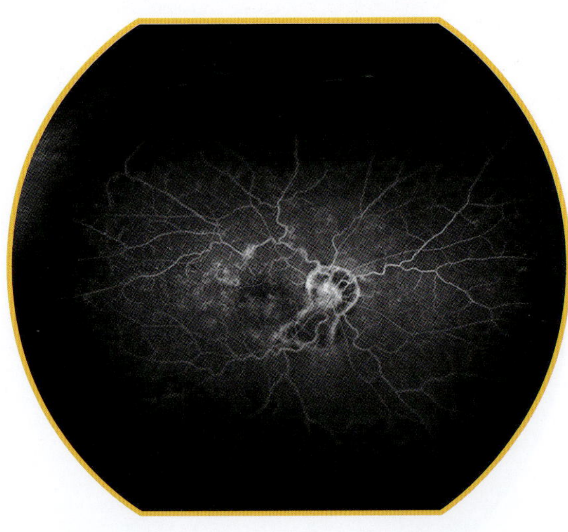

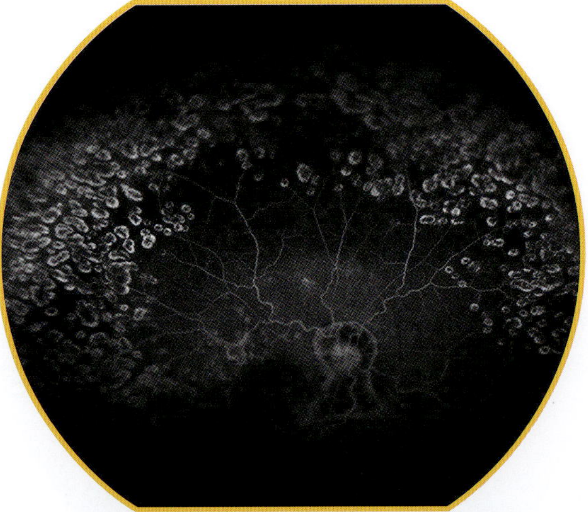

This patient presented with a central retinal vein occlusion with widespread peripheral capillary non-perfusion illustrated with ultra-widefield fluorescein angiography *(left)*. Widefield FA six month after the placement of panretinal photocoagulation (PRP) to ablate the ischemic retina is shown on the right. *Image courtesy of Richard Spaide*

Treatment: Intravitreal Anti-VEGF Therapy

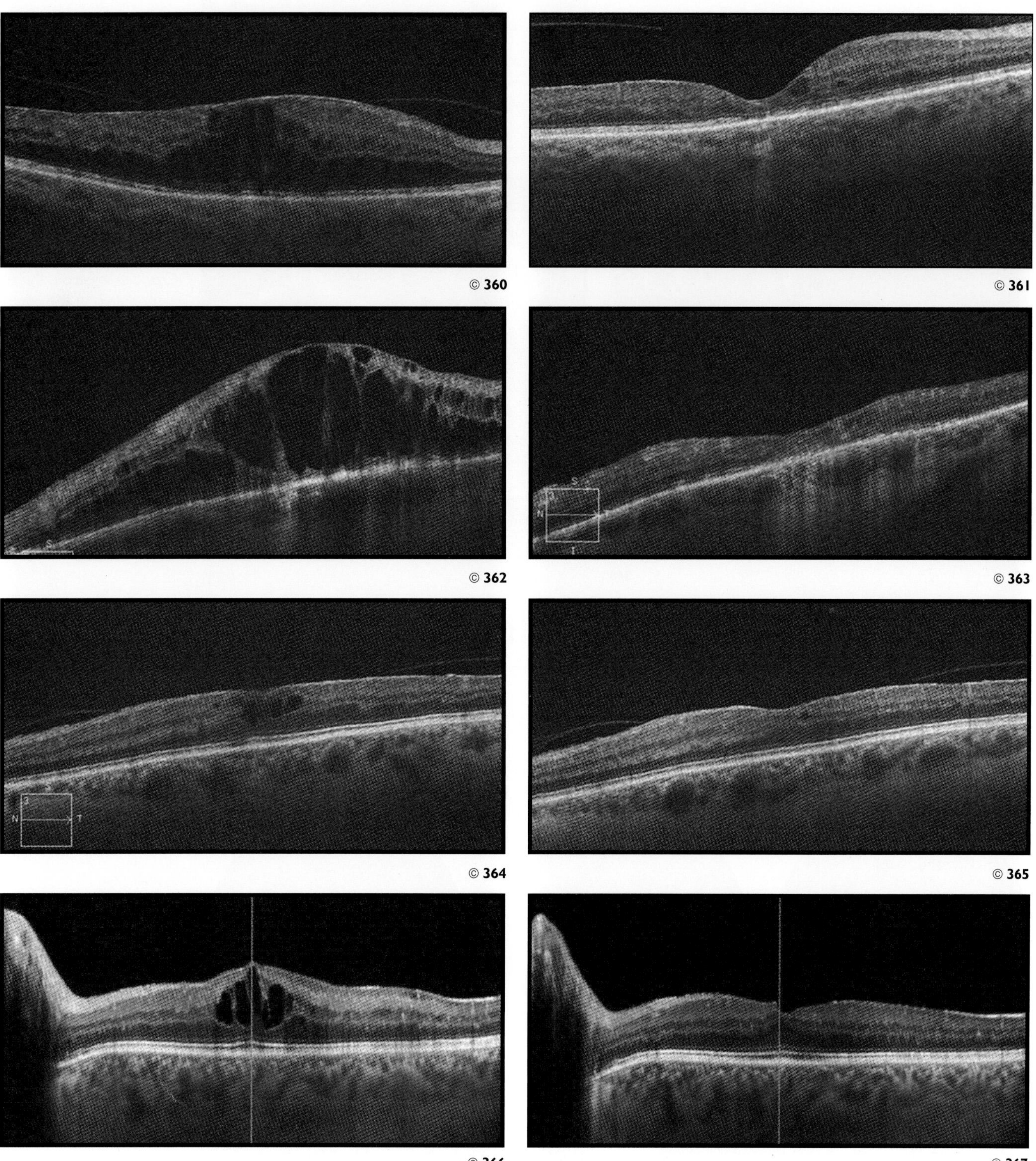

© 360 © 361 © 362 © 363 © 364 © 365 © 366 © 367

Four cases of CRVO complicated by CME are shown with spectral domain OCT prior to treatment *(left images)*. One month after intravitreal anti-VEGF therapy CME is significantly improved in each case *(right images)*.

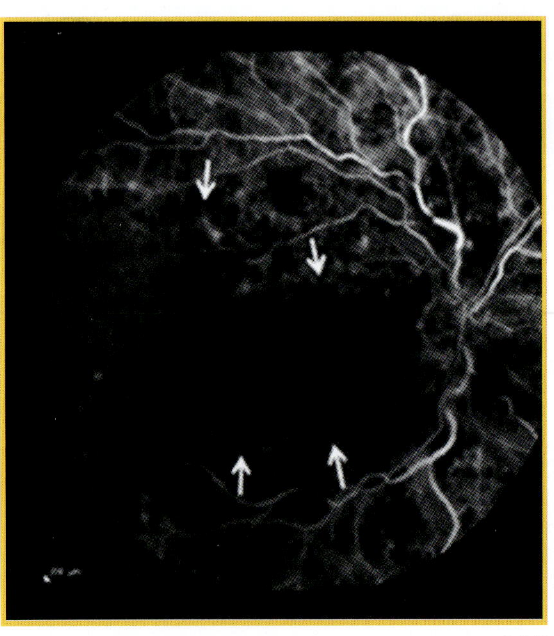

© 368

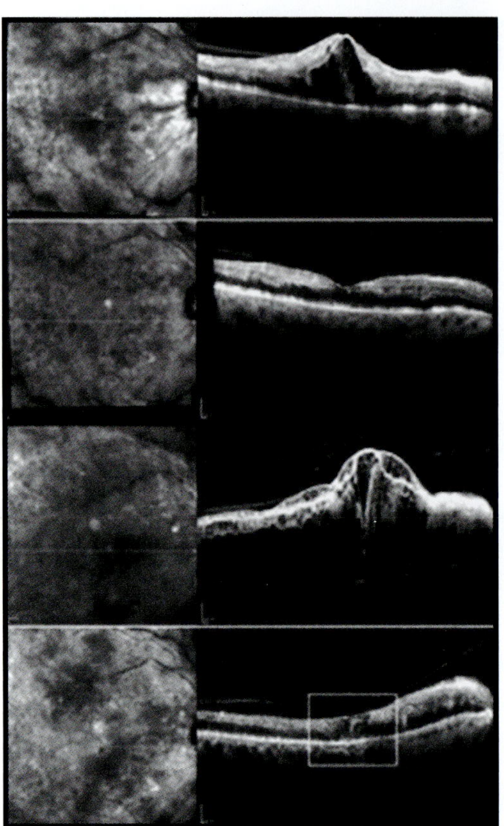

© 369

An ischemic central retinal vein occlusion with macular edema is illustrated. On the left is the FA that shows macular ischemia *(arrows)* and patchy blockage from retinal hemorrhage. The top right OCT shows severe CME at baseline. One month after Ozurdex injection, there is resolution of the edema *(second from top)*, with recurrence 5 months after the injection *(third from top)*. The bottom OCT shows improvement one month after administration of second Ozurdex implant.

Branch Retinal Vein Occlusions

BRVO occurs most frequently in patients with a history of hypertension or diabetes. The occlusion occurs at the site of an arteriole–venous crossing, unless there is a focal inflammatory process in the wall of the vessel. BRVO may be complicated by vitreous hemorrhage, capillary non-perfusion, neovascularization of the disc or retina, fibrous proliferation with traction retinal detachment, and/or macular edema. Recanalization and reperfusion of the vein with compensatory retinal venous to venous collateralization is typical of the chronic phase of the disease. Retinal branch vein occlusions range from small tributary obstructions that become symptomatic when they include the macula to hemispheric occlusions that involve at least half of the fundus.

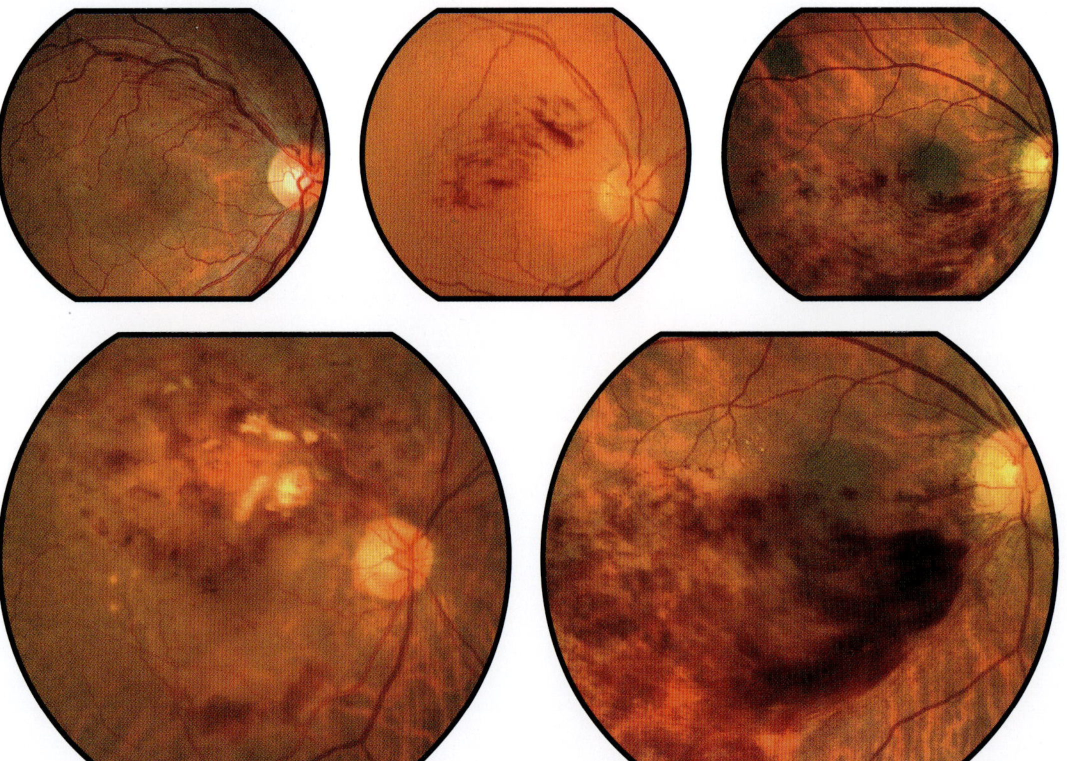

These are examples of patients with BRVO. The top row middle image shows a small macular BRVO that extends into the foveal area. The remaining cases are major BRVOs with quadrantic distribution of edema and hemorrhage.

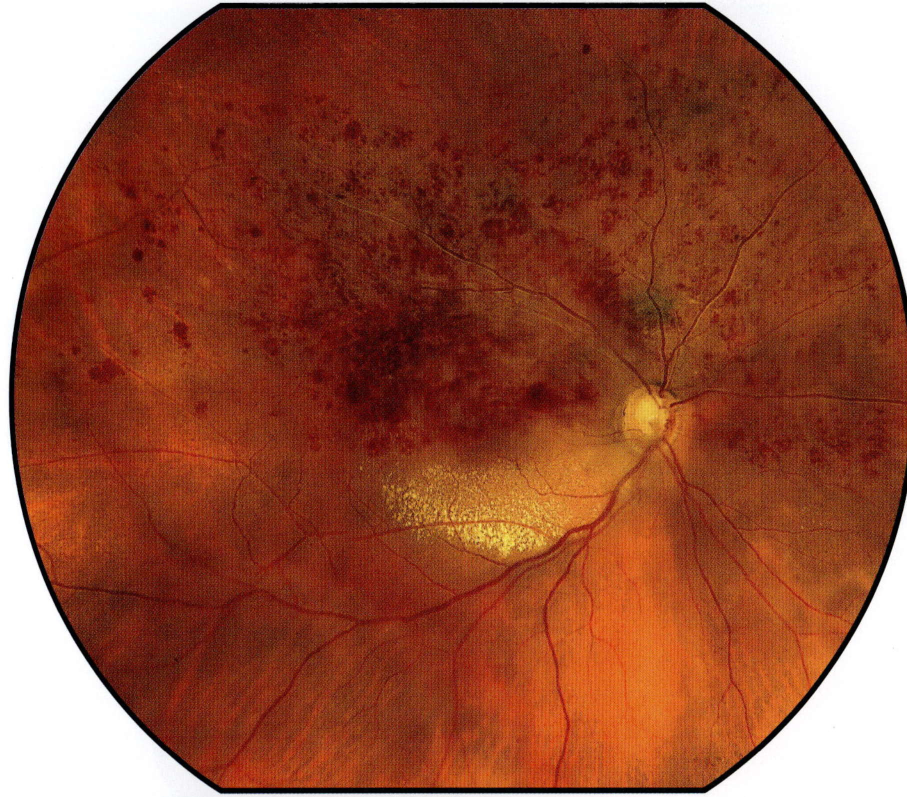

This patient has chronic exudation in the macula with lipid precipitates secondary to hemispheric retinal vein occlusion. *Courtesy of Ophthalmic Imaging Systems, Inc*

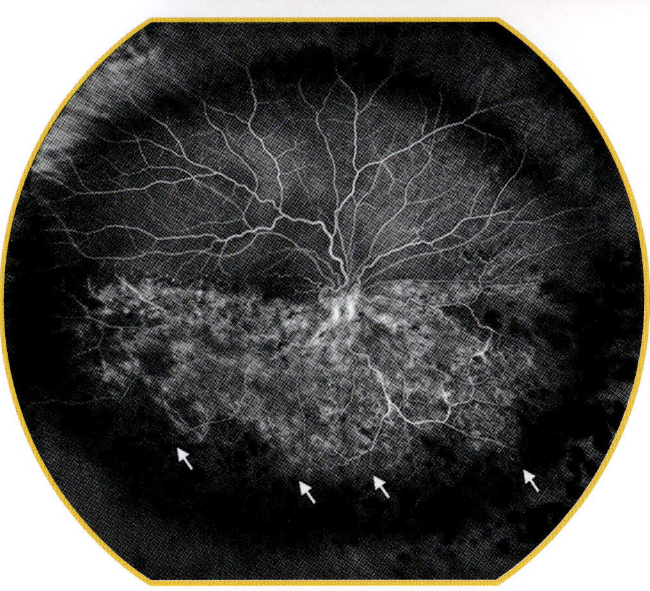

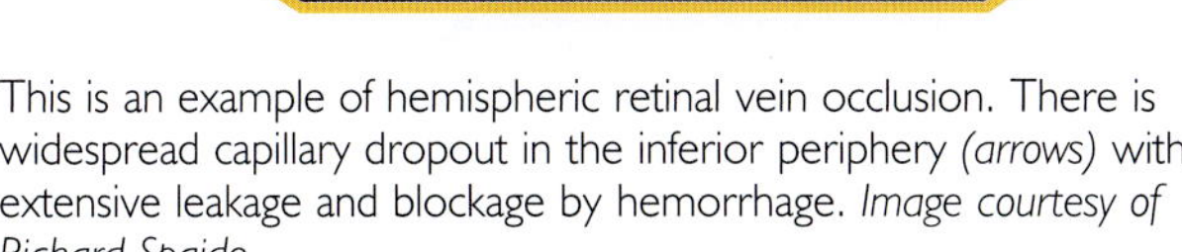

This is an example of hemispheric retinal vein occlusion. There is widespread capillary dropout in the inferior periphery *(arrows)* with extensive leakage and blockage by hemorrhage. *Image courtesy of Richard Spaide*

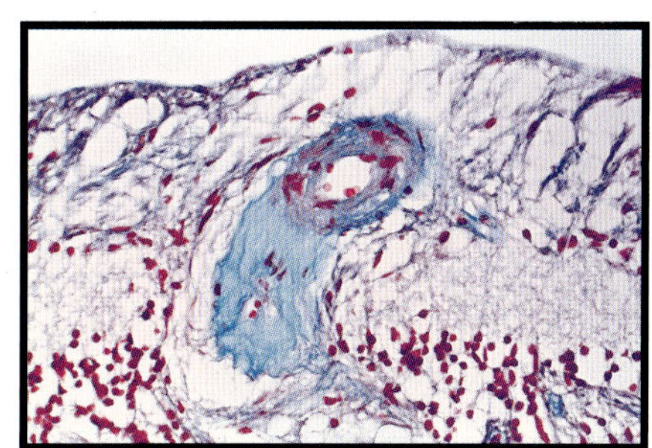

© **370**

This is a histopathology section of a retinal vein occlusion. The area of occlusion reveals a single channel of recanalization of the superotemporal vein as it crosses under the arteriosclerotic artery.

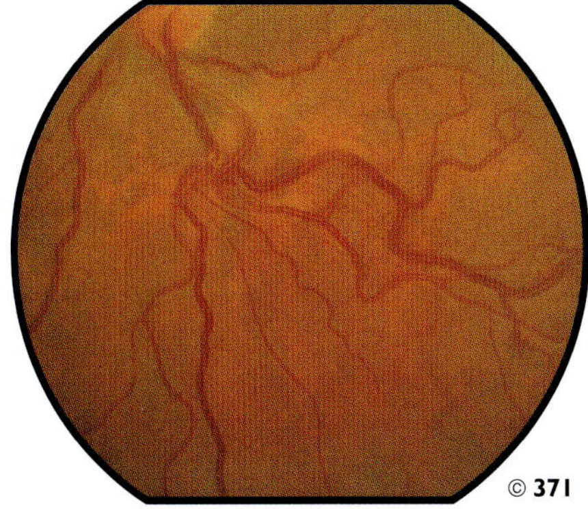

© **371**

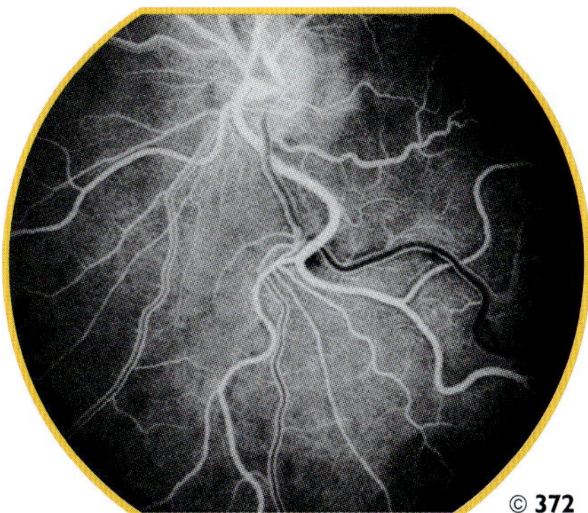

© **372**

An arteriolar-venous crossing abnormality is shown in this patient. It is characterized by prominence of the venule at its proximal segment, a small sentinel hemorrhage at the crossing, and obliteration of the venule at its common sheath with the crossing arteriole. This constellation of findings has been referred to as the pre-thrombotic sign of Bonnet, since some of these patients may progress to an acute BRVO. The FA shows a localized perfusion delay of the compressed retinal vein distal to the arteriolar-venular crossing.

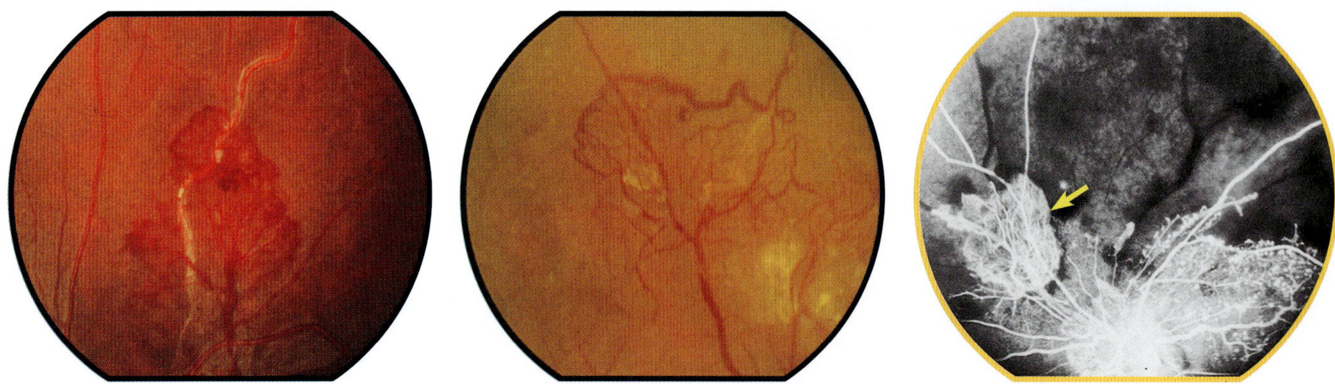

Note the presence of retinal neovascularization associated with BRVO in these three cases. The FA shows peripheral capillary non-perfusion and ischemia and neovascularization *(arrow)*.

Compensatory Collateralization

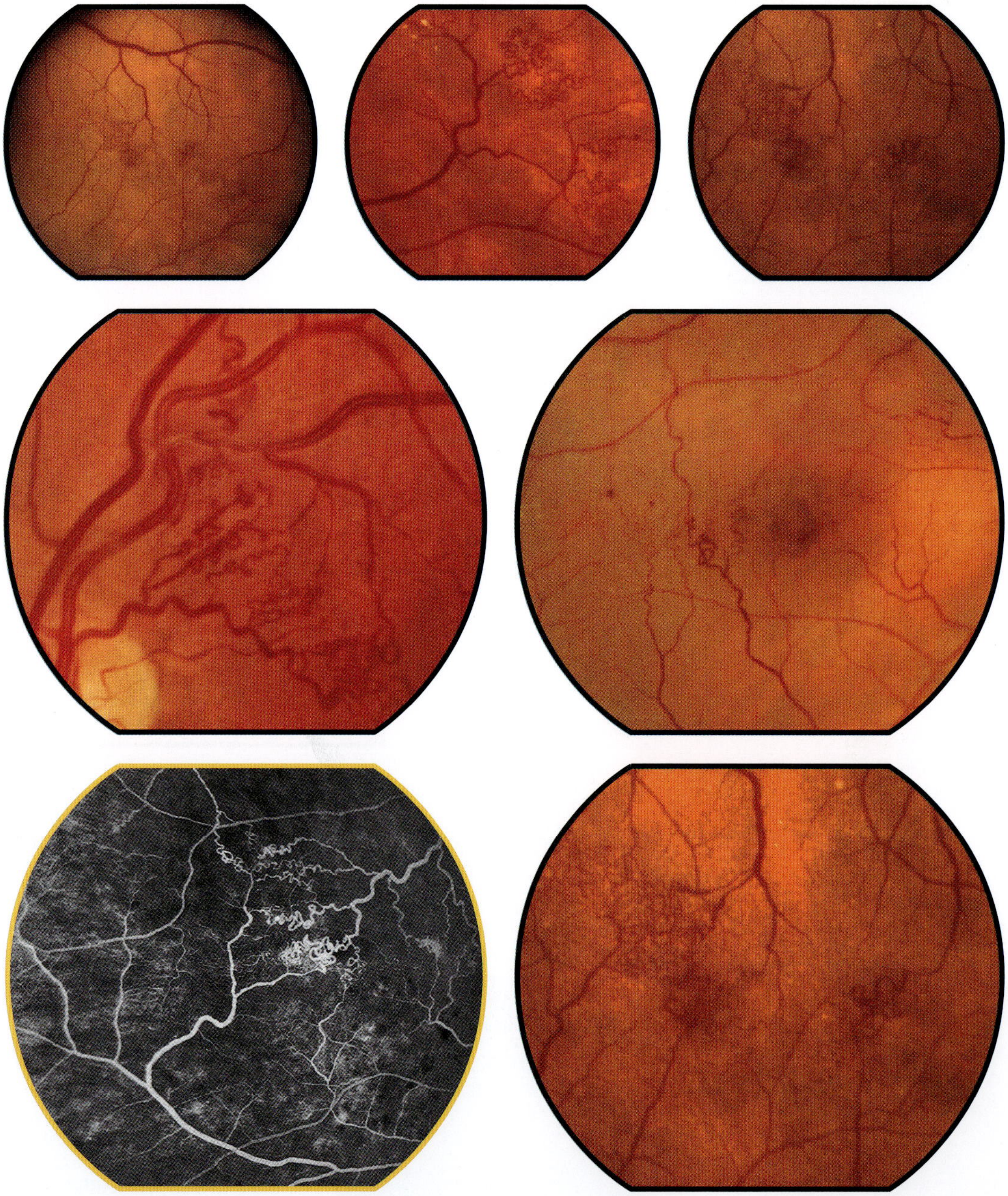

These are patients who have developed collateralization (venous–venous) to compensate for a retinal branch vein occlusion. The collaterals course across the horizontal raphe or bridge the obstructed site or connect to adjacent veins in the far periphery of the fundus. Collaterals do not leak with FA.

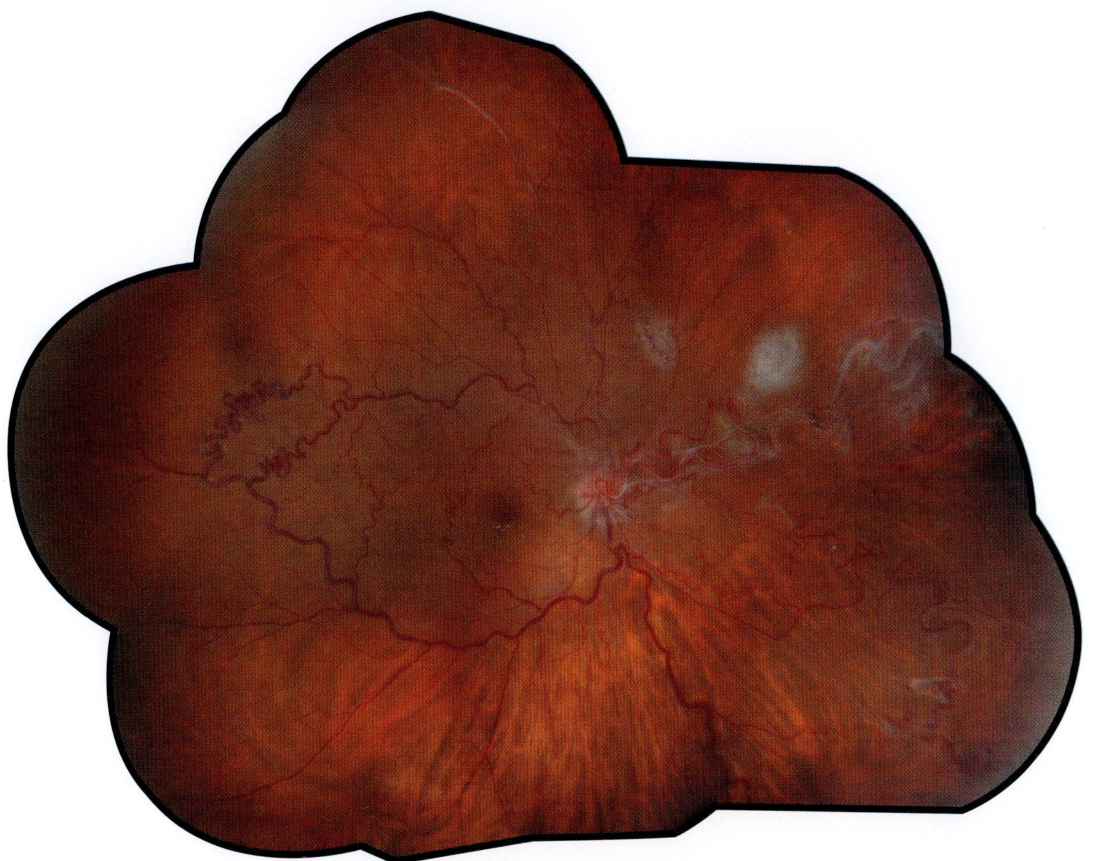

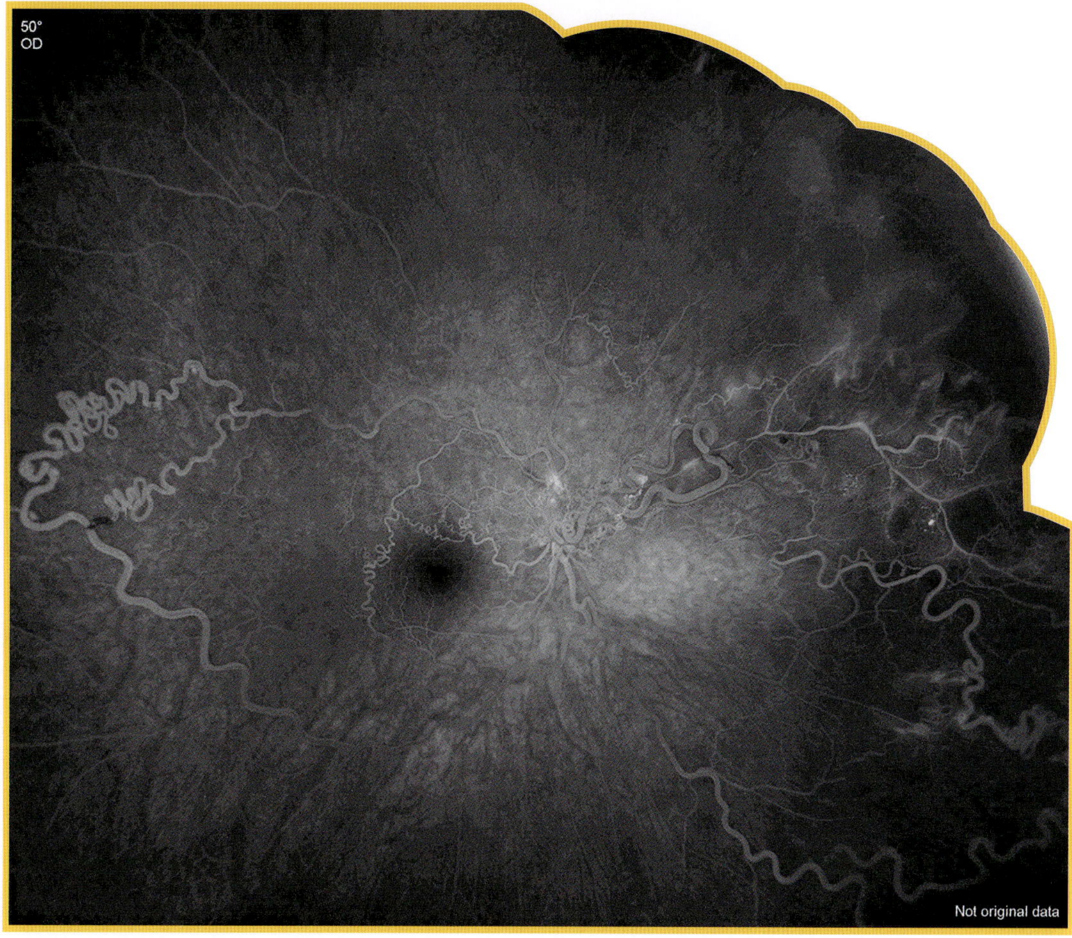

The above color and FA montage demonstrate a case of Wyburn–Mason syndrome with an arteriovenous shunt superonasal off the disc. Note the superotemporal BRVO with prominent collaterals across the temporal raphe.

Treatment: Laser Photocoagulation

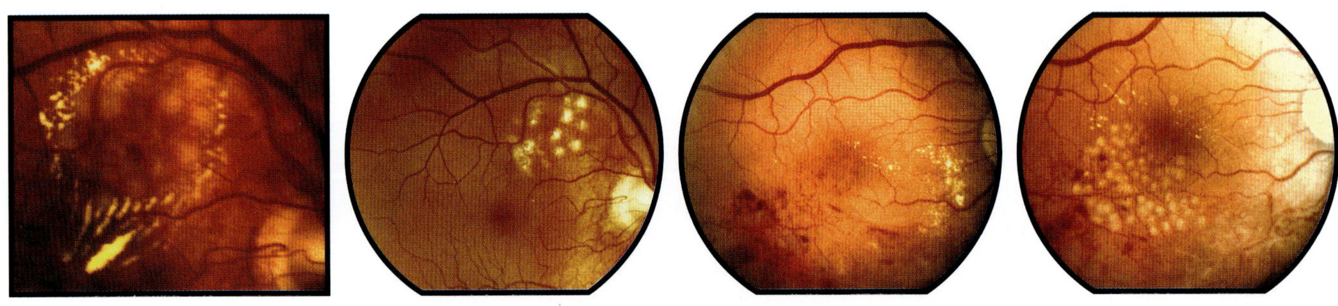

Laser photocoagulation treatment can be used to focally ablate leaking microaneurysms within the zone of the branch vein occlusion *(left)*. Lipid was extending into the fovea and photocoagulation burns gradually induced resolution of the exudation. The patient on the right had chronic diffuse macular edema. A macular grid laser treatment was carried out that resulted in resolution of the central edema and improvement of vision.

Treatment: Intravitreal Pharmacotherapy

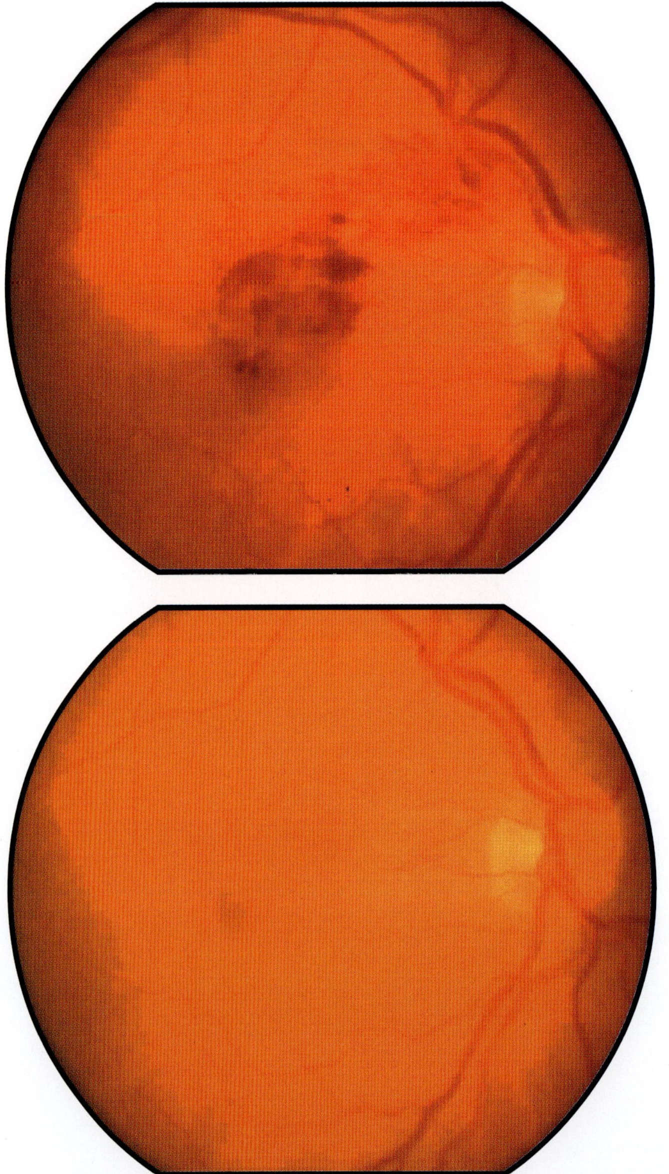

This patient developed a macular BRVO and was treated with intravitreal anti-VEGF therapy with resultant resolution.

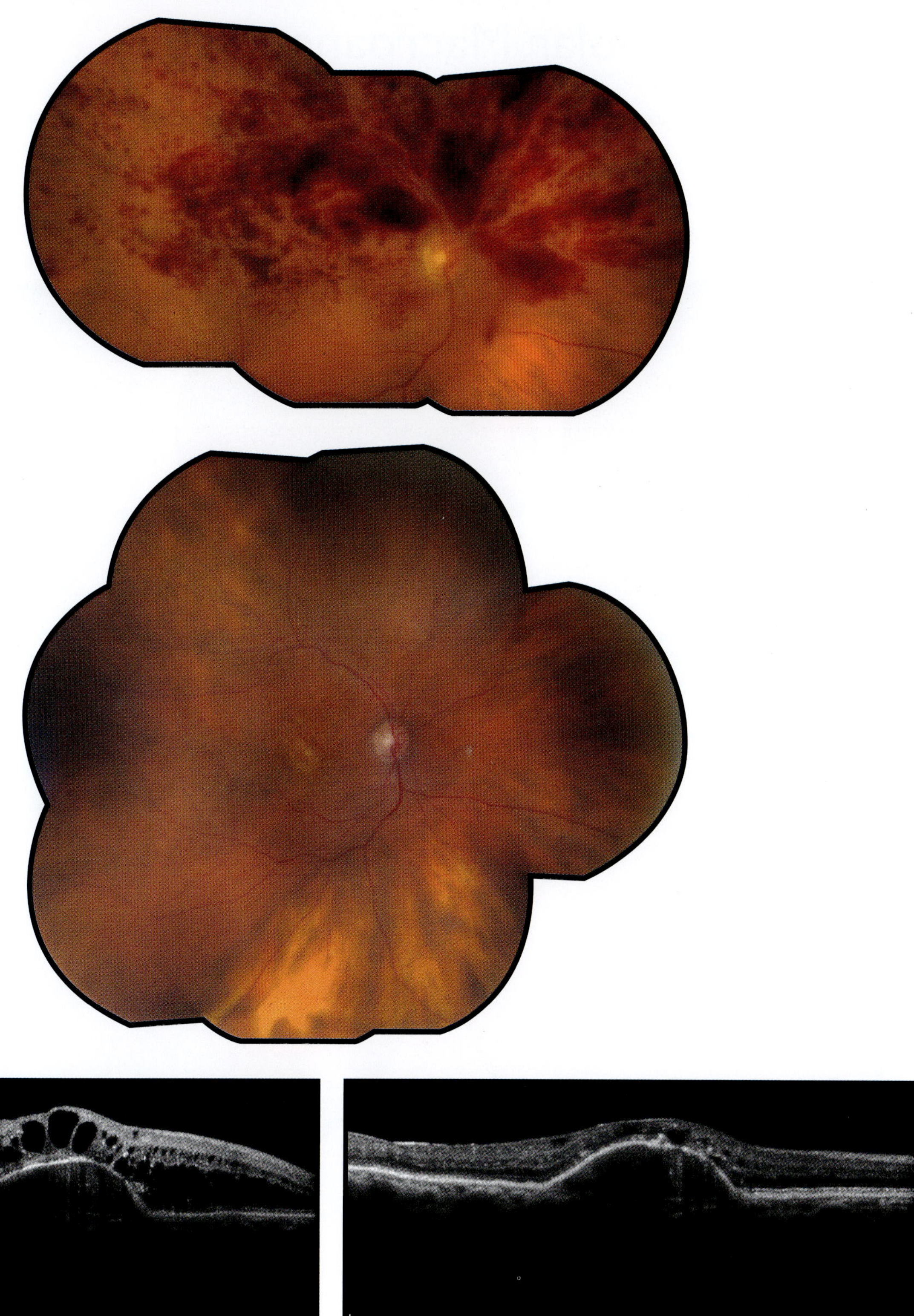

This patient with dry age-related macular degeneration suffered a superior hemispheric retinal vein occlusion, which was treated with intravitreal anti-VEGF therapy. Color fundus montage before *(top)* and after *(second row)* therapy shows marked resolution of the intraretinal hemorrhages, revealing underlying macular drusen. SD-OCT taken at the time of presentation revealed macular edema as well as multiple drusen and a large central drusenoid pigment epithelial detachment (PED) *(third row)*. With anti-VEGF therapy the intraretinal fluid greatly improved *(bottom row)*.

Retinal Arteriolar Macroaneurysm

Retinal arteriolar macroaneurysm is an acquired fusiform or round dilatation that affects a retinal artery within its first three branches from the disc and that occurs typically in the posterior pole. These abnormalities are first observed in the fifth decade of life and are associated with surrounding exudative detachment of the retina, lipid deposition, and hemorrhage beneath, within, and above the retina. Macroaneurysms may be recurrent or multiple, along the course of the same vessel or seen elsewhere at another arteriole in the same eye.

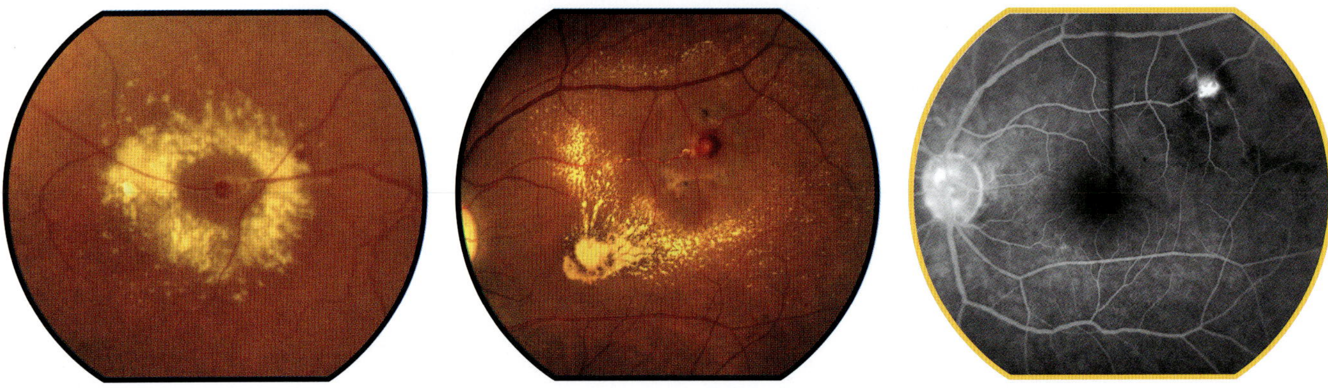

These cases represent retinal arteriolar macroaneurysms. On the left, there is a bilobed aneurysm along the course of the involved arteriole, surrounded by dense circinate lipid exudation. The middle image shows exudative detachment with lipid deposition, which courses to the fovea. On the right is an FA showing aneurysmal staining of the arteriolar macroaneurysm.

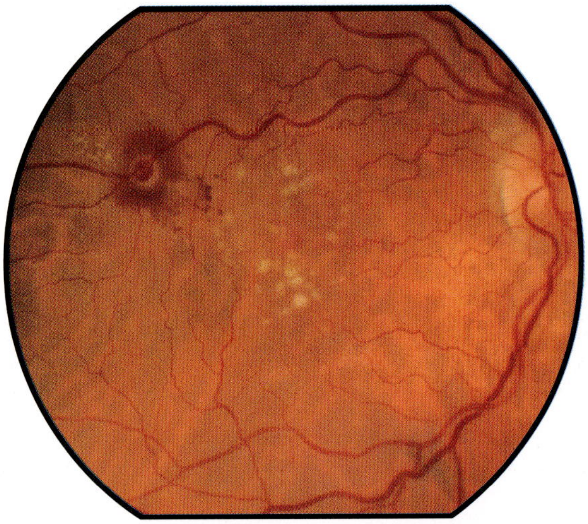

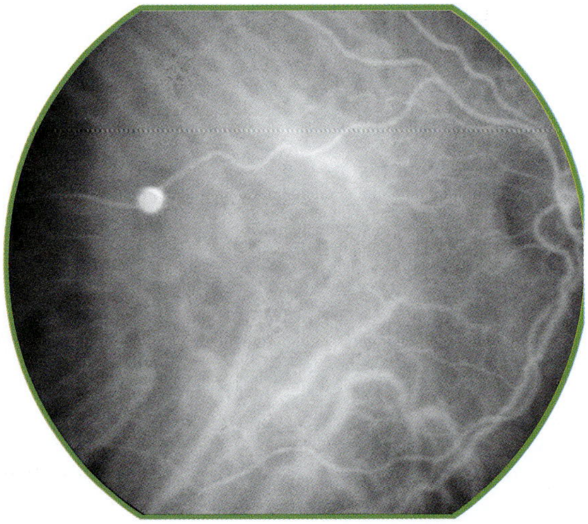

Indocyanine green (ICG) angiography may enhance the detection of a macroaneurysm, particularly if it is partially covered by hemorrhage.

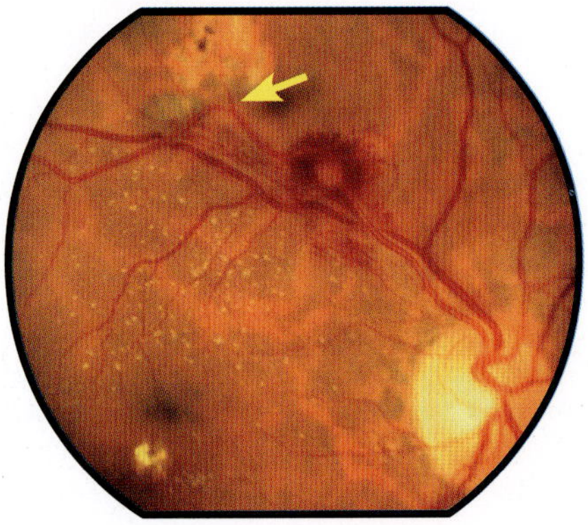

This patient demonstrates that macroaneurysms may be multiple and recurrent. An acute macroaneurysm is seen along the course of the superotemporal arteriole with concentric hemorrhage. An old macroaneurysm that was lasered is noted more distally. Note the atrophic scar and narrowing of the involved vessel *(arrow)*.

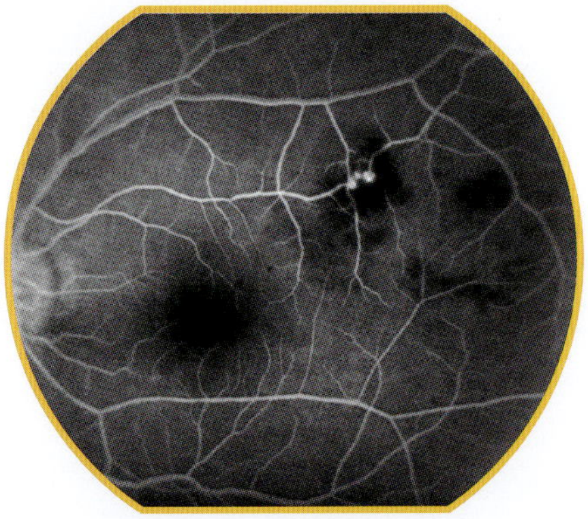

This patient has a bilobed double macroaneurysm along the same vessel with associated hemorrhage and exudation.

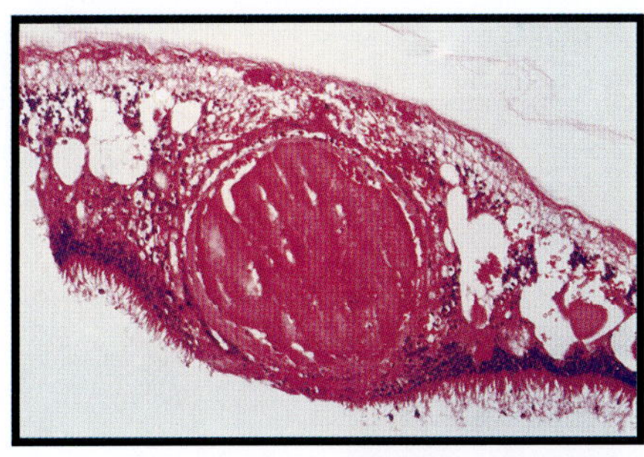

The histopathological specimen shows a thrombosed arteriolar macroaneurysm with retinal hemorrhage and cystic edema within the retina.

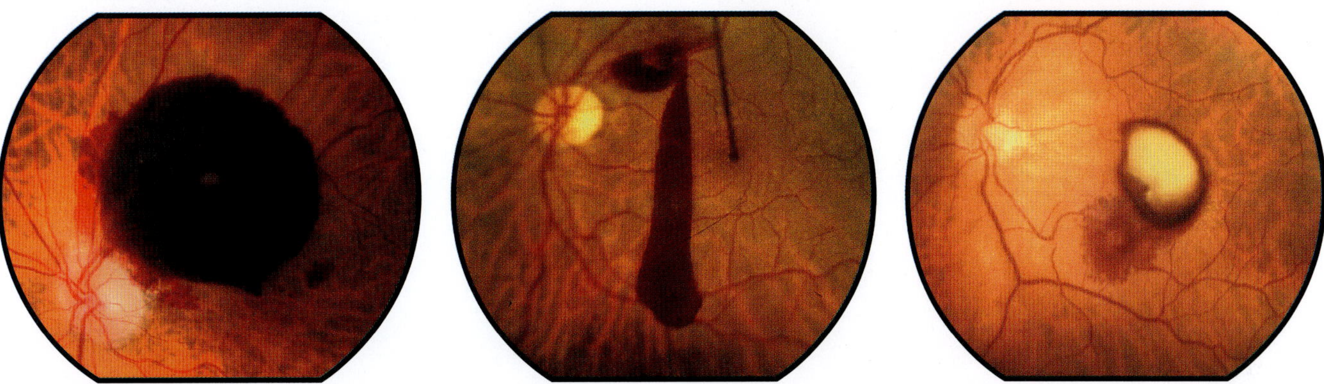

Retinal macroaneurysms may present with pre-retinal, intraretinal, or subretinal hemorrhage. It may form an hourglass configuration with more blood in front of and below than within the retina *(left)*. The bleeding may extend into the vitreous, where it can gravitate inferiorly *(middle)*. As the hemorrhage from a macroaneurysm resolves, it becomes dehemoglobinized with a yellowish color *(right)*.

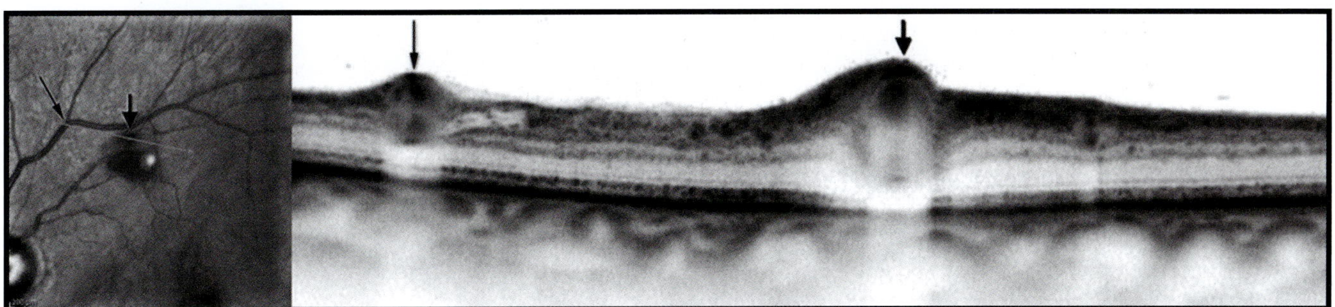

SD-OCT through this macroaneurysm at the superotemporal arcade *(thick arrow)* shows a markedly enlarged vessel contour with mild hemorrhage in the adjacent inner retina. The thin arrow denotes the normal superotemporal arcade vein. *Image courtesy of Anat Loewenstein and David Goldstein*

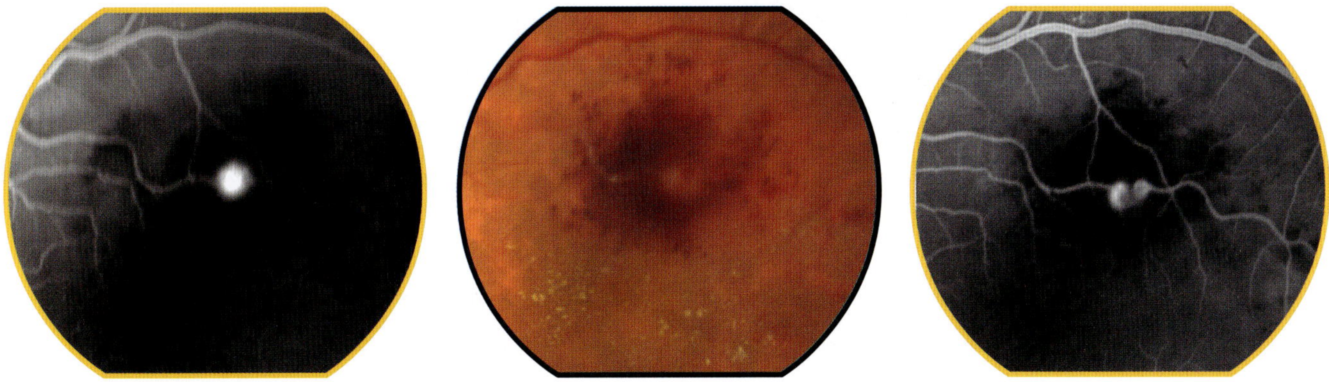

This is a patient with a retinal arteriolar macroaneurysm, as seen on the FA on the left. Following treatment, there was recurrent bleeding *(middle)*. A repeat FA showed regression of the initial lesion but a recurrent macroaneurysm is noted on the nasal side of the original one.

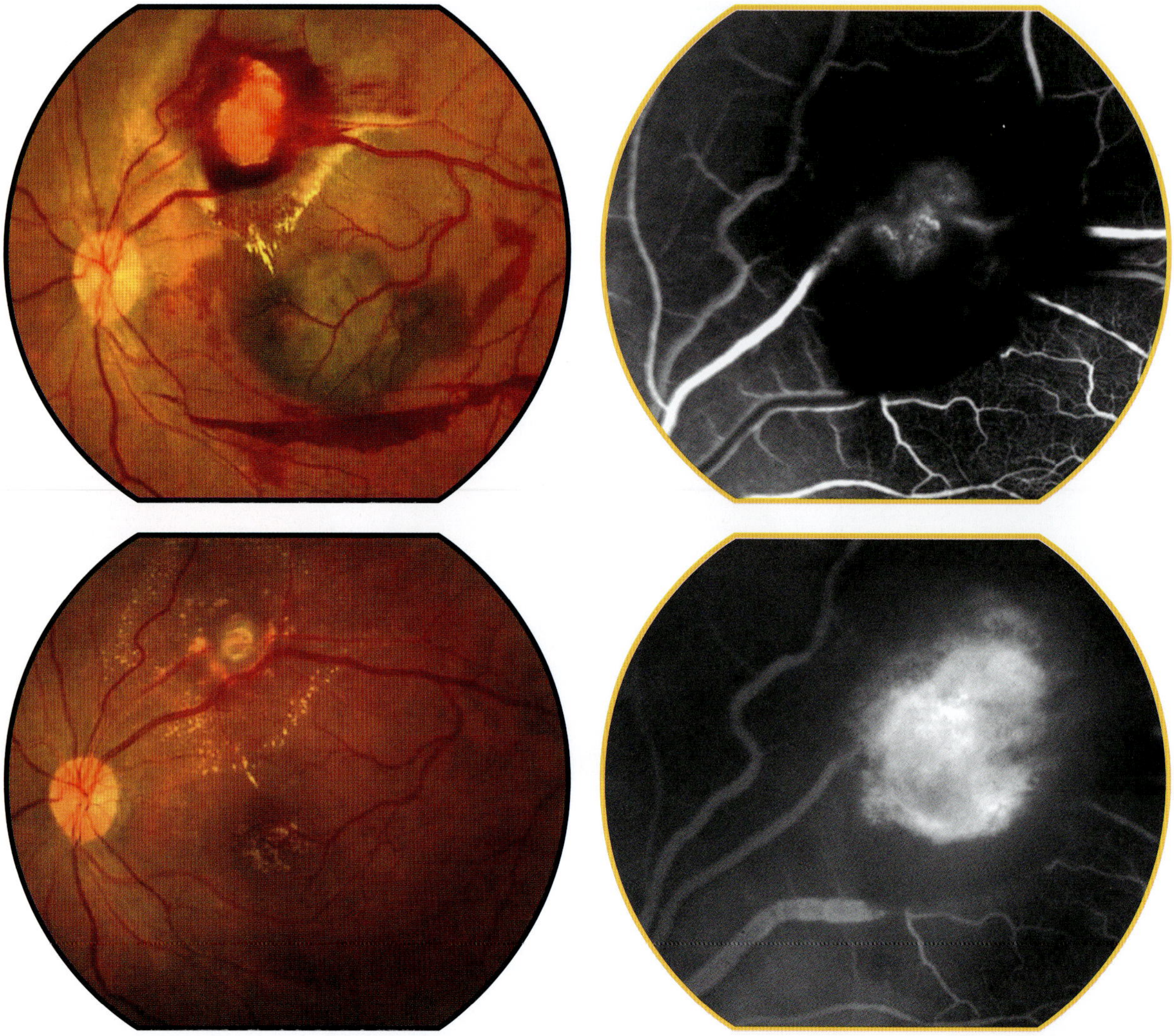

Note the superotemporal hemorrhage that is both pre-retinal and subretinal ("hourglass bleeding"). Central subretinal hemorrhage is also present. There is reactive vascular hyperplasia at the site of the superotemporal macroaneurysm, simulating an angiomatous proliferation that stains with fluorescein angiography. The lower left color image shows spontaneous resolution of the hemorrhage and the retinal arteriolar macroaneurysm, which now has a fibrous capsule. Note the associated large retinal venular macrovessel that extends superotemporally and then inferiorly across the horizontal raphe.

Treatment: Laser

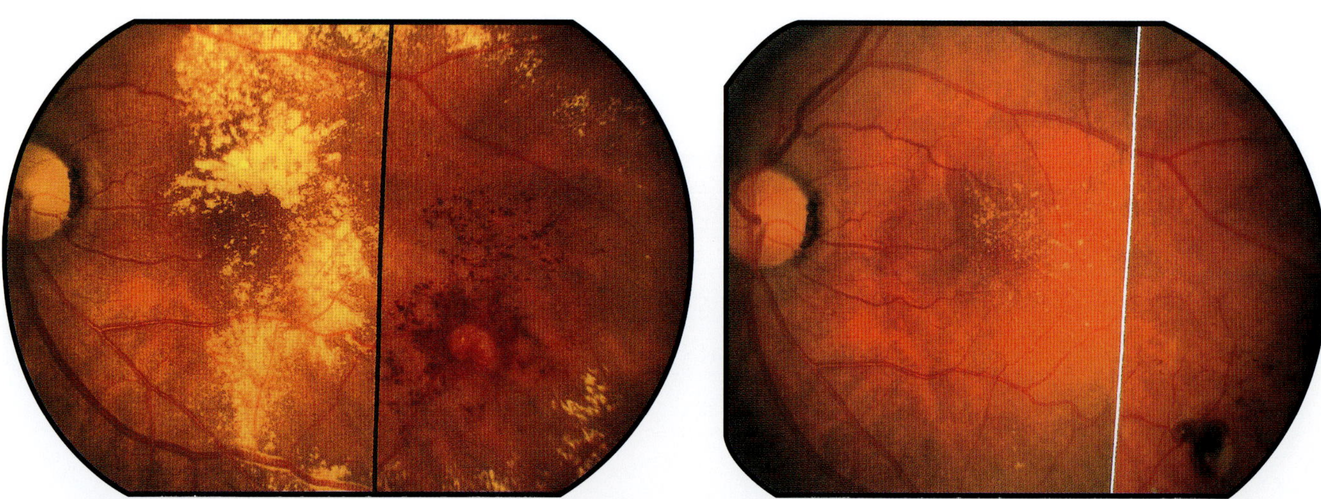

This patient had significant central lipid deposition associated with an inferotemporal retinal arteriolar macroaneurysm. Following focal laser photocoagulation to the macroaneurysm, there was resolution of the exudation over a period of many months. The macroaneurysm regressed to a pigment epithelial hyperplastic scar. *Courtesy of Dr. Maurice Rabb*

Treatment: Anti-VEGF Therapy

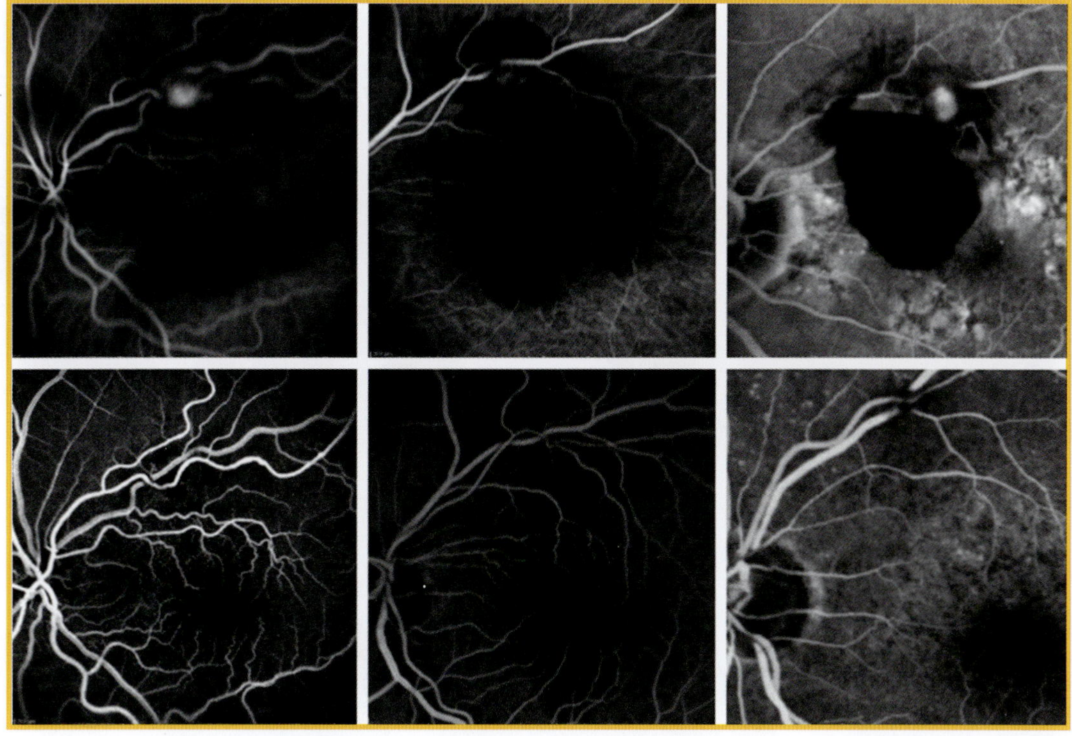

Intravitreal anti-VEGF therapy may be considered to decrease macular edema associated with retinal artery macroaneurysms. Note these three cases of macroaneurysm *(top row)* complicated by hemorrhage. The lower images show resolution of hemorrhage after intravitreal bevacizumab injection in each case that may reflect the natural history of this disorder.

Coats Disease and Macular Telangiectasia Type I (Congenital Telangiectasia, Leber Miliary Aneurysms)

Coats disease is a unilateral disorder with a very high predilection for males and characterized by retinal telangiectasia and lipid exudation. Exudation can be so severe as to cause leukocoria and exudative retinal detachment in young patients. Macular telangiectasia type I is a variant of Coats disease that affects male adults and consists of unilateral dilated and aneurysmal capillaries with associated ischemia and exudation typically limited to the central macular region.

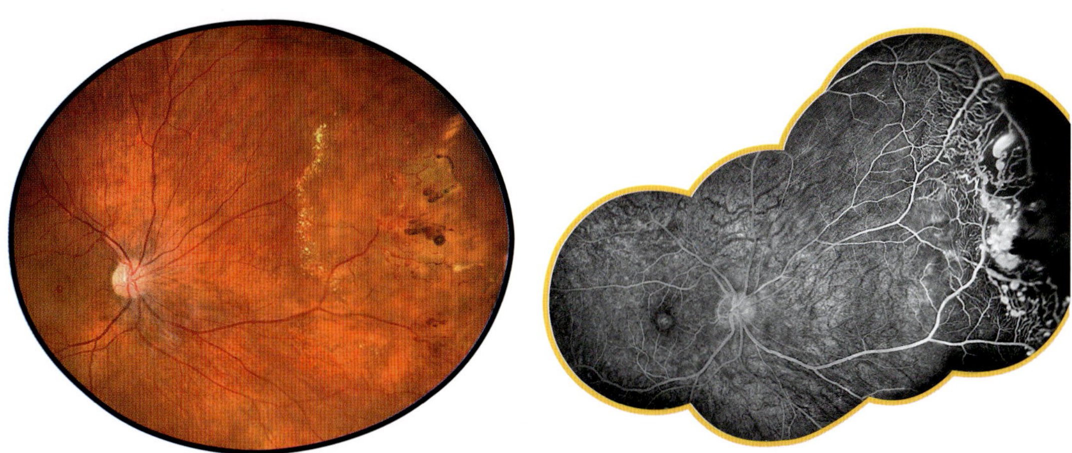

This patient has Coats disease. Peripheral exudative detachment of the nasal retina is noted with lipid deposition at the posterior border. The dilated capillary net is seen posterior to the larger aneurysms. Peripheral to these vascular changes is a zone of ischemia, characteristic of the disorder.

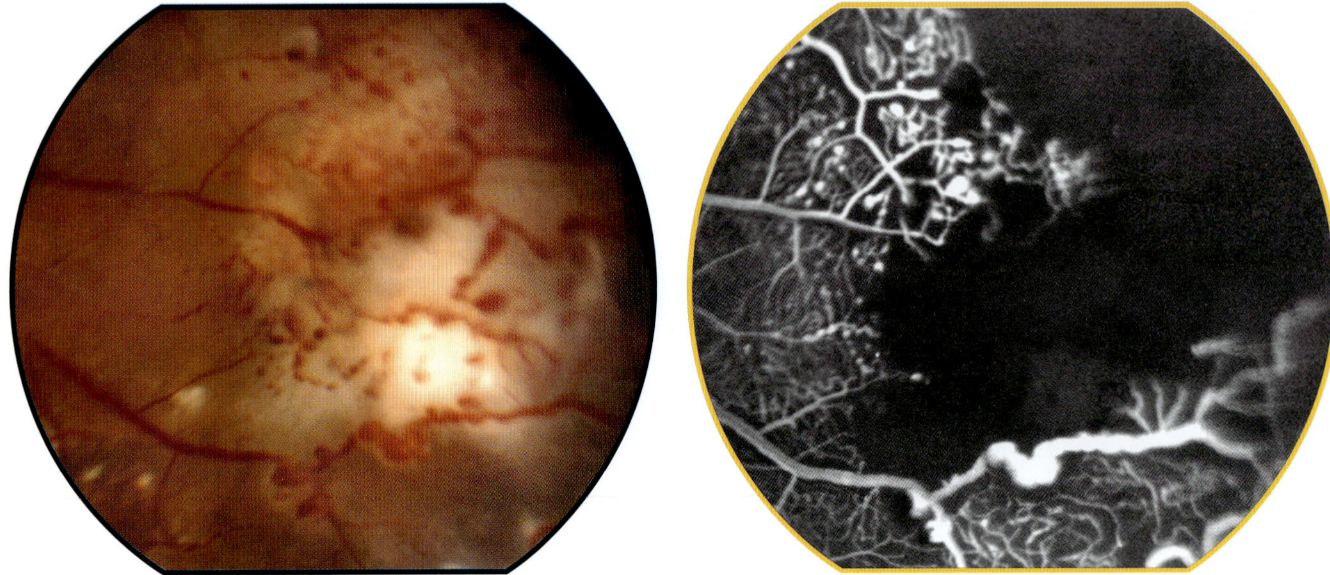

This patient has Coats disease with dilated capillaries and "light bulb" aneurysms, venous macroaneurysms, and peripheral ischemia.

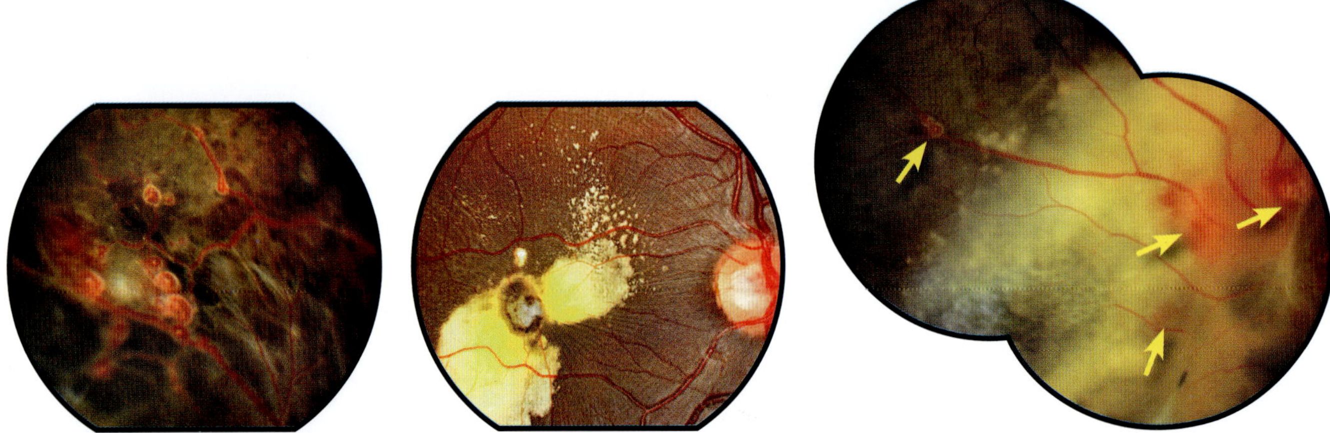

These three patients with Coats disease demonstrate typical manifestations. In the periphery, there are multiple macroaneurysms *(left)*. In the macular region *(middle)*, chronic lipid deposition has resulted in a fibrous pigmented scar at the fovea. The image on the right shows macroaneurysms, which are evident in the periphery, but obscured by dense lipid deposition in the more posterior fundus *(arrows)*.

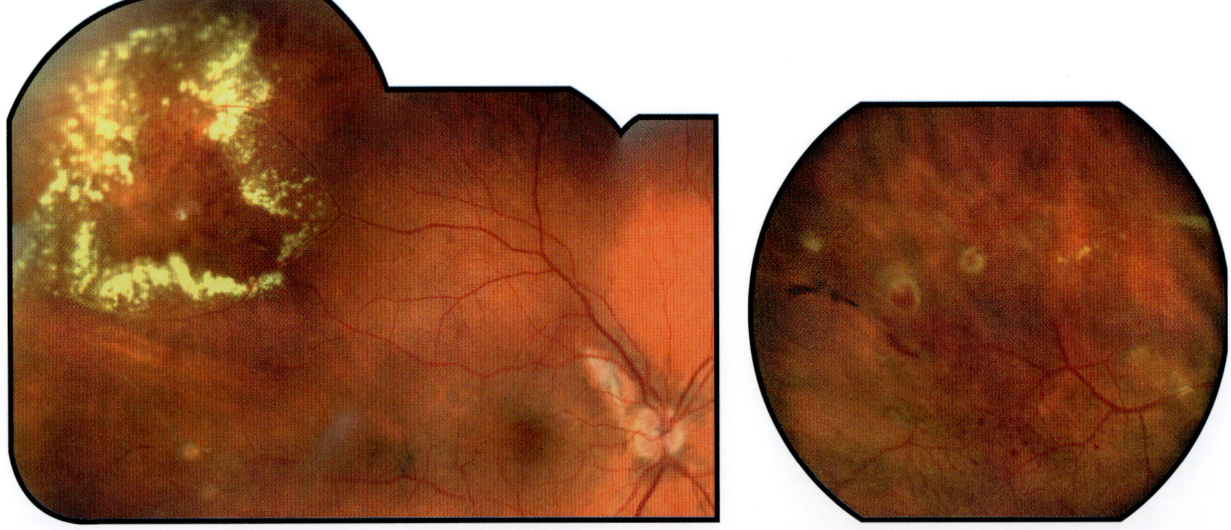

These two patients with Coats disease presented without visual dysfunction. On incidental examination, dilated telangiectatic vessels were noted that were associated with multiple aneurysmal lesions of various sizes. Vascular sheathing peripheral ischemia and a circinate pattern of exudate are present. Note the halo of fibrous proliferation around some of the larger aneurysms. Curiously, neither hemorrhage nor pre-retinal neovascularization is characteristic of this vasculopathy, although vasoproliferative tumors may complicate this disorder.

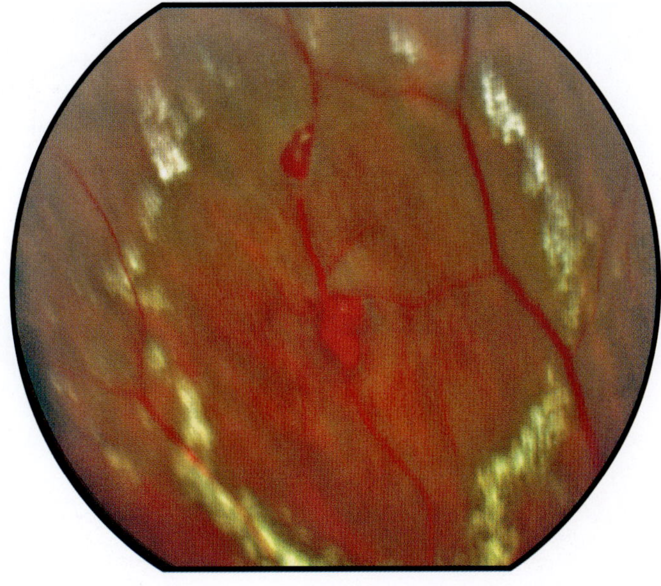

This patient has a zonal area of telangiectatic and aneurysmal lesions due to Coats disease and surrounded by circinate lipid deposition.

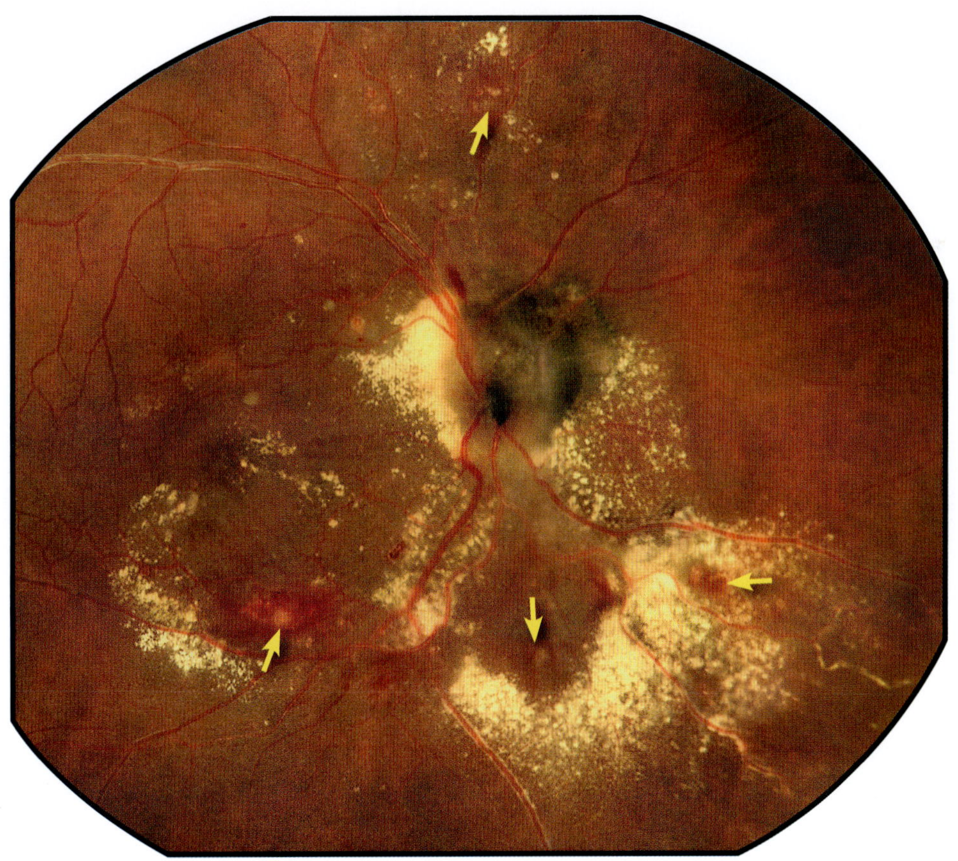

This patient has widespread Coats disease involving the central and peripheral fundus. Macroaneurysms *(arrows)* are seen with associated hemorrhage and widespread circinate lipid deposition. Vascular sheathing is also seen in this patient, which is not uncommon in this disorder. Peripapillary pigmentary scarring was from previous laser photocoagulation treatment.

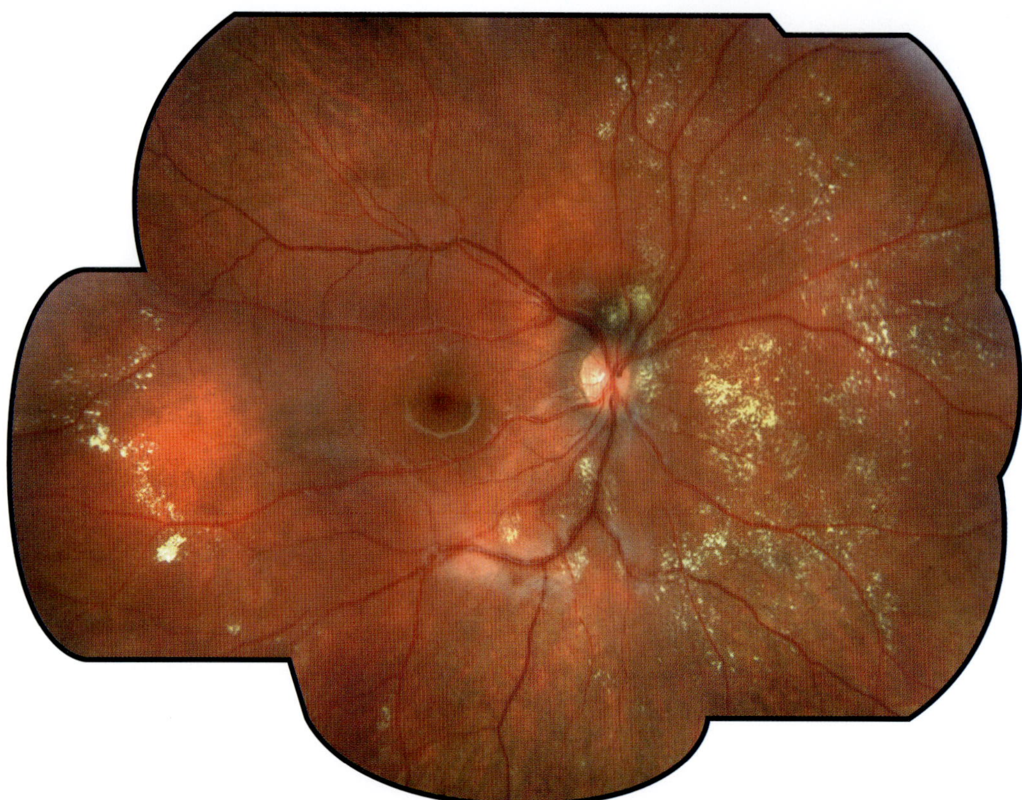

This young patient presented with Coats disease that was incidentally diagnosed. Widespread lipid deposition from telangiectatic vascular abnormalities is evident in the peripheral fundus.

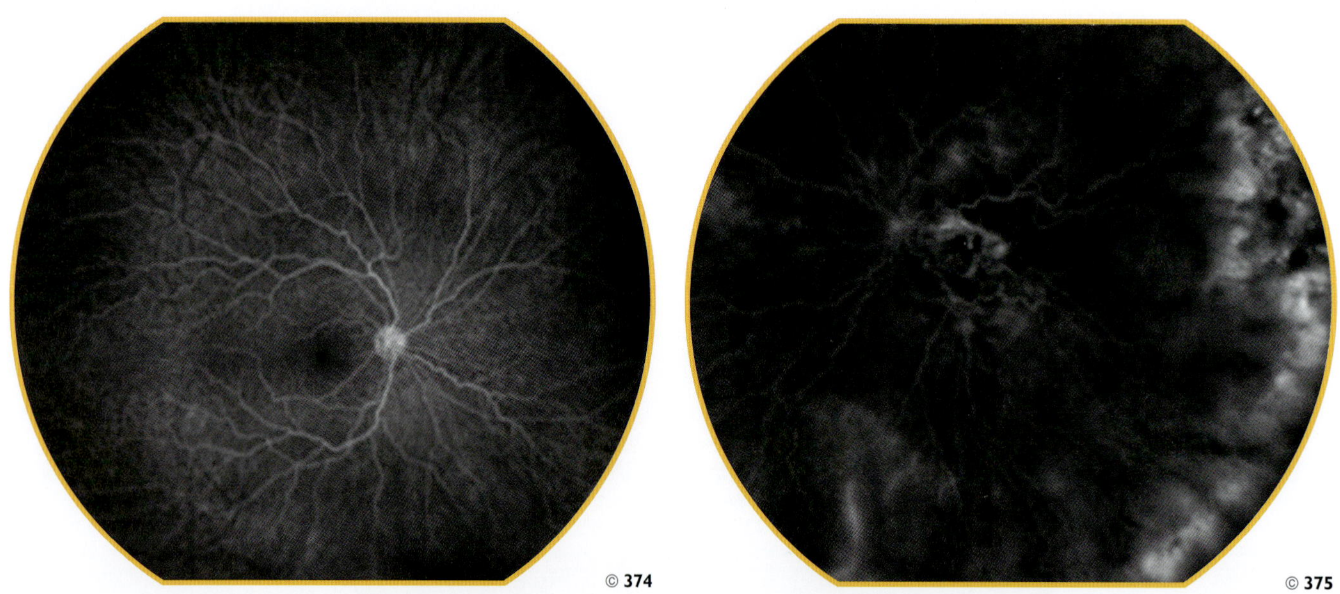

Ultra-widefield fluorescein angiography of this patient with Coats disease shows a normal right eye. The left eye has marked vascular tortuosity, macular edema and exudate. Peripheral capillary telangiectasia with non-perfusion and leakage are also present.

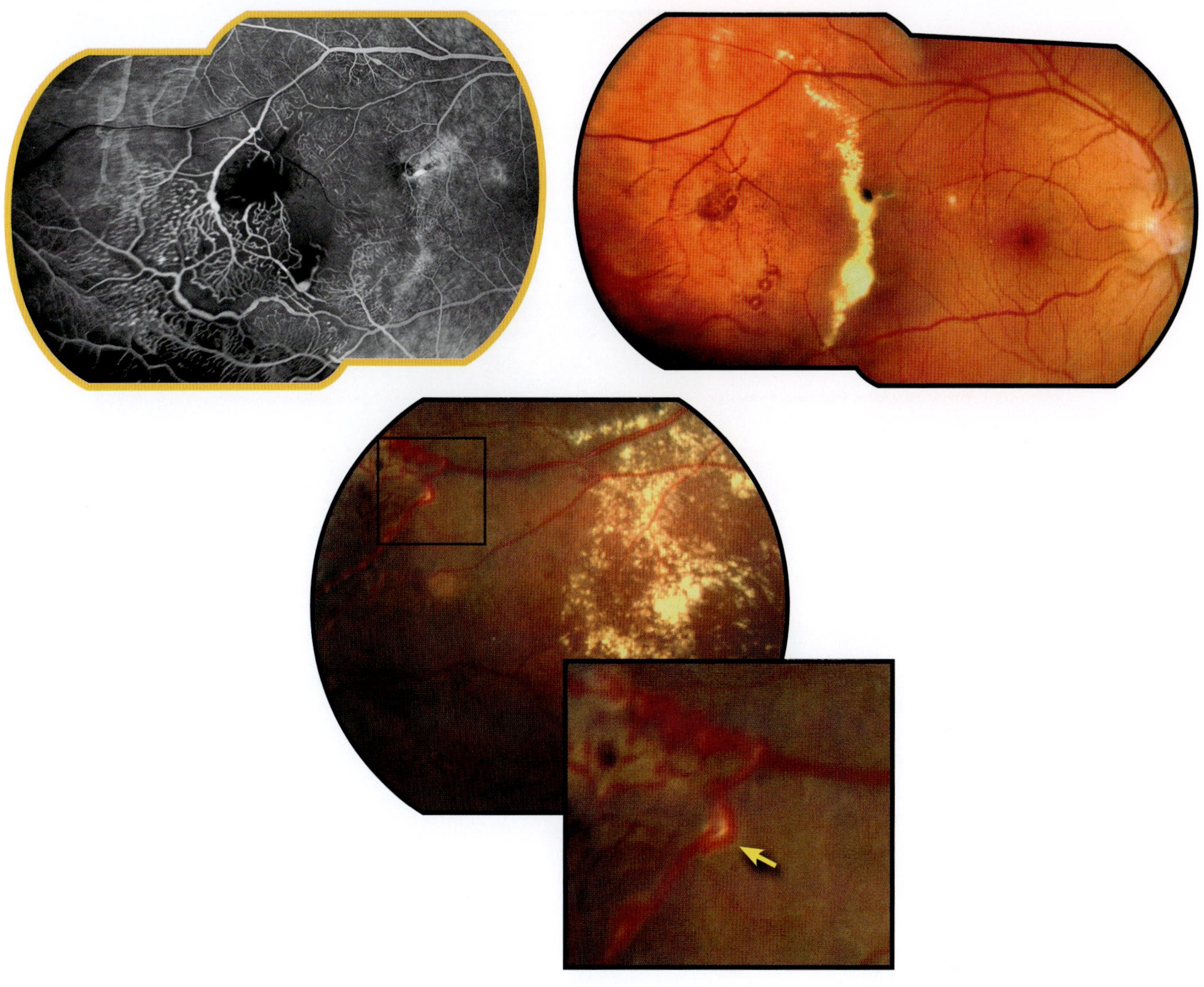

These patients demonstrate the spectrum of clinical findings seen in Coats disease. In the top row, a fringe of lipid deposition is encroaching on the posterior pole and is associated with peripheral telangiectasia. Ischemia, telangiectasia, aneurysmal formation, and leakage are present without pre-retinal hemorrhage or neovascularization, not an unusual finding in this disorder. There is aneurysmal formation on the bottom right image and even a sausage-like swelling of a venule *(arrow)*.

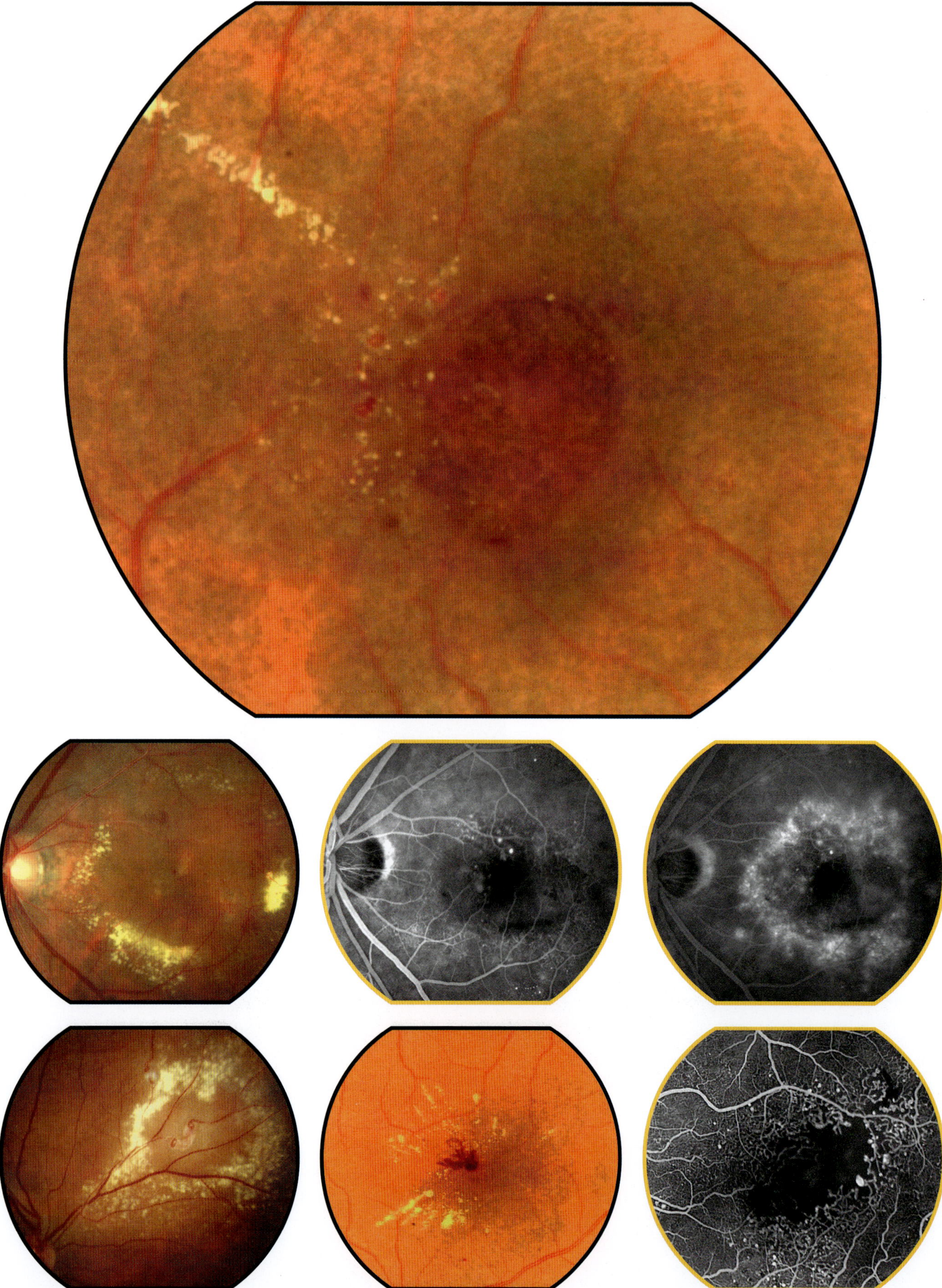

These are patients with macular telangiectasia type 1 or adult-onset Coats disease. The aneurysms can vary in size from small capillaries to macroaneurysms with associated lipid deposition, hemorrhage, ischemia, and leakage. A radial configuration of lipid can be seen, particularly in the central macular area, as shown on the lower middle image.

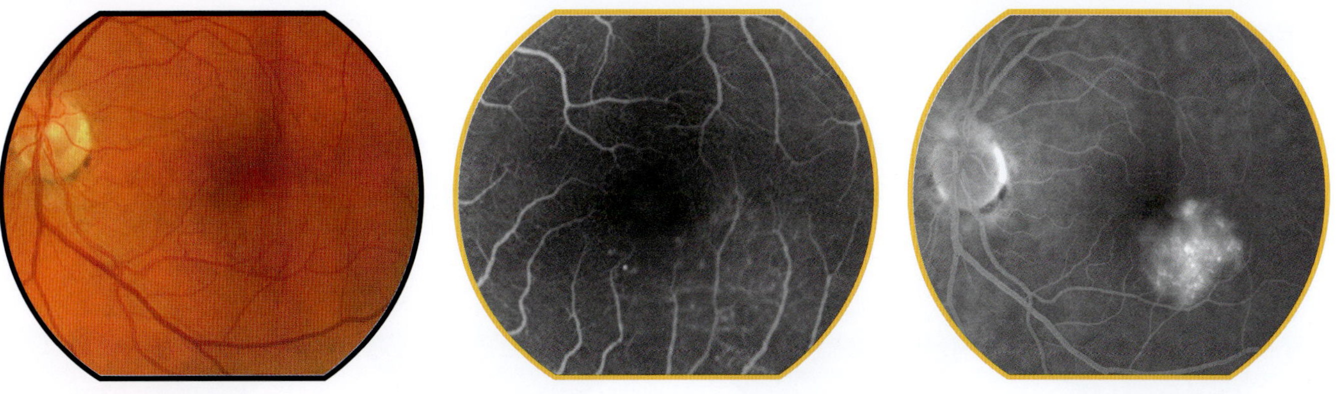

This patient with macular telangiectasia type 1 has prominent capillaries and microaneurysms seen on the early FA *(middle)* with late leakage *(right)* in the juxtafoveal region.

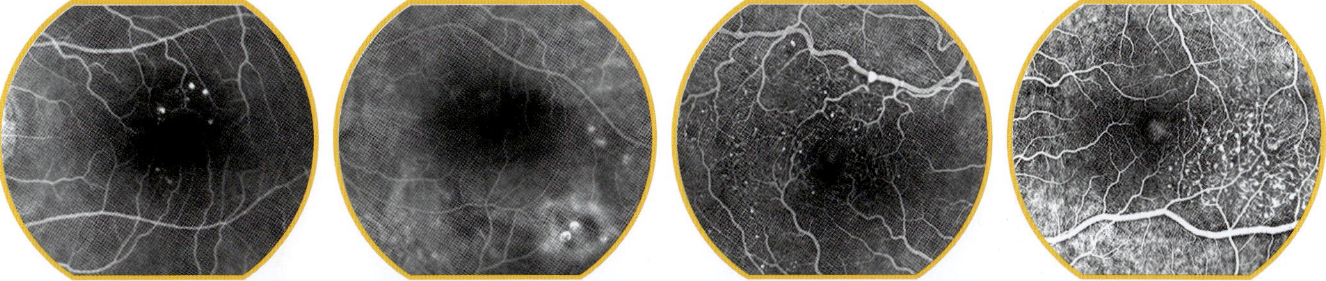

These adult male patients have macular telangiectasia type 1 or adult-onset Coats disease. Note that the unilateral microaneurysms can vary in size, distribution, and density.

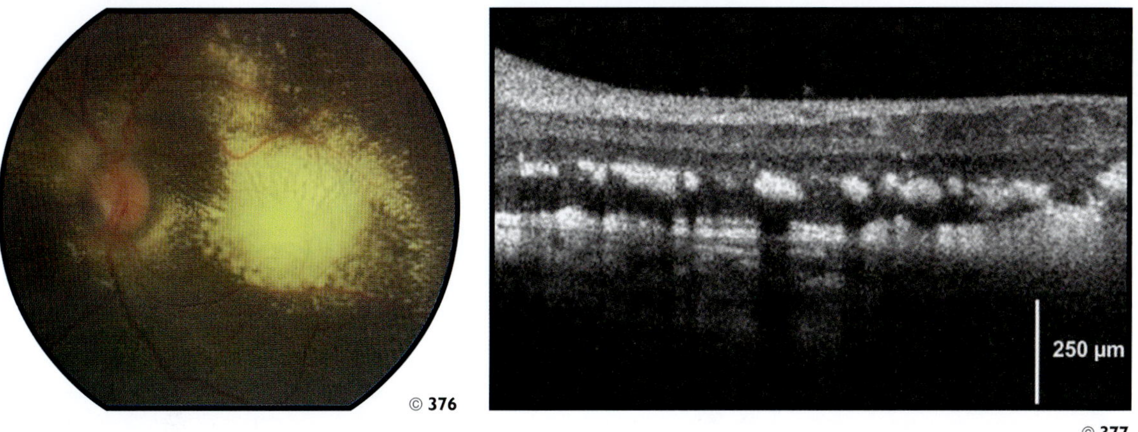

This boy with Coats disease presented with dense subretinal and intraretinal exudation in the macula. Spectral-domain OCT demonstrates hyper-reflective exudates at the level of the outer plexiform layer (immediately beneath the deep retinal capillary plexus) and subretinal exudates temporally.

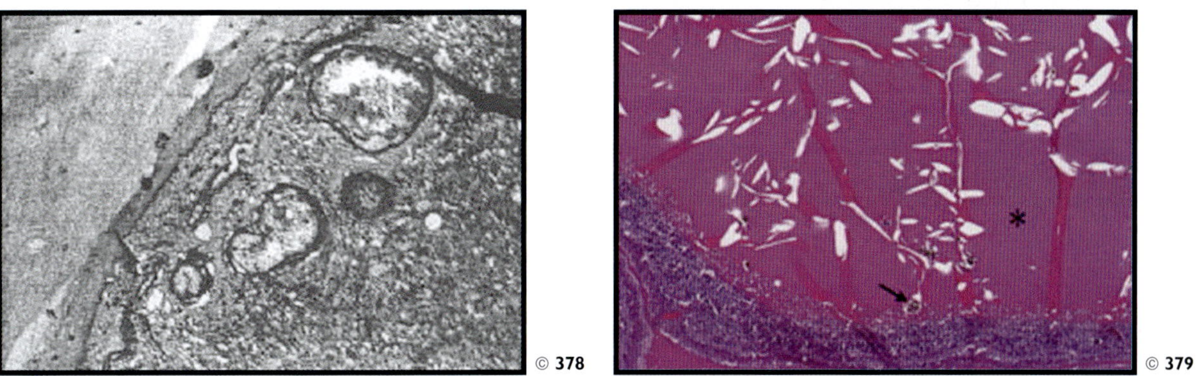

On the left is a histopathological image of macular telangiectasia type 1. Note the large, thin-walled retinal vessels, consisting of both capillaries and arterioles. There are a few endothelial cells and virtually no pericytes. On the right is a specimen from a patient with Coats disease. The subretinal space is filled with cholesterol crystals *(asterisk)* and pigment-laden macrophages *(arrow)*.

Treatment: Laser

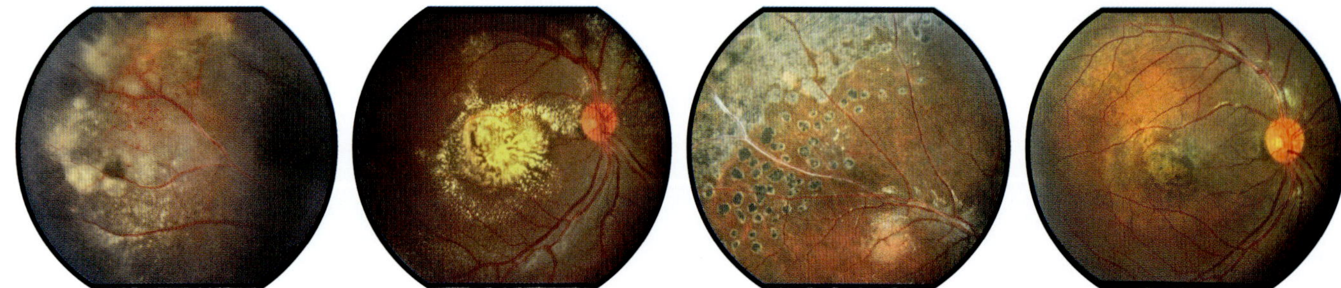

This patient has severe macular lipid exudation secondary to Coats disease in the peripheral part of the fundus. Note the dense lipid in the central macula *(second image)* and the peripheral telangiectasia and aneurysms with associated exudation *(first image)*. Scatter laser treatment was applied to the periphery *(third image)*. Following laser treatment, there was slow but progressive resolution of the lipid in the periphery and in the macula.

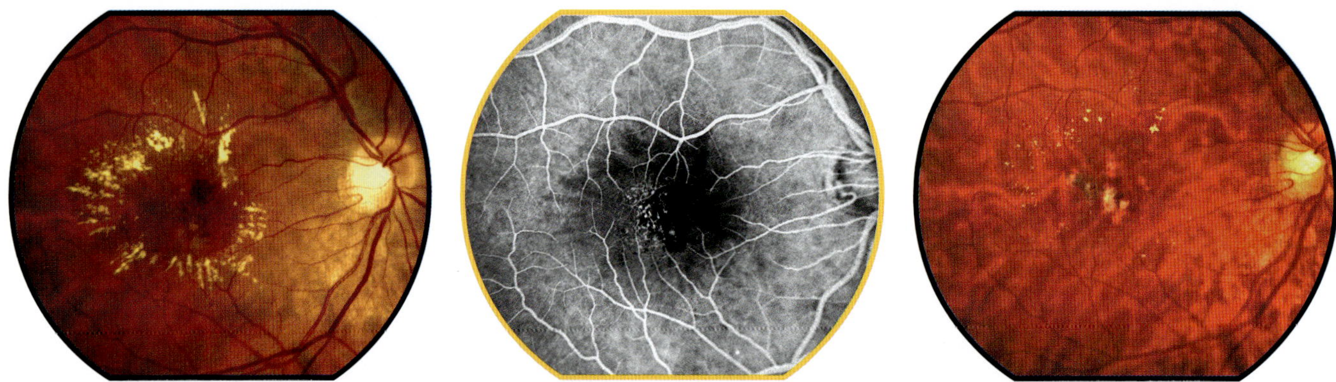

This patient had macular telangiectasia type I with a stellate configuration of circinate lipid deposition surrounding the telangiectatic lesions. A cluster of small microaneurysms were present and noted on the FA. Following focal laser photocoagulation, the exudates resolved with few atrophic scars.

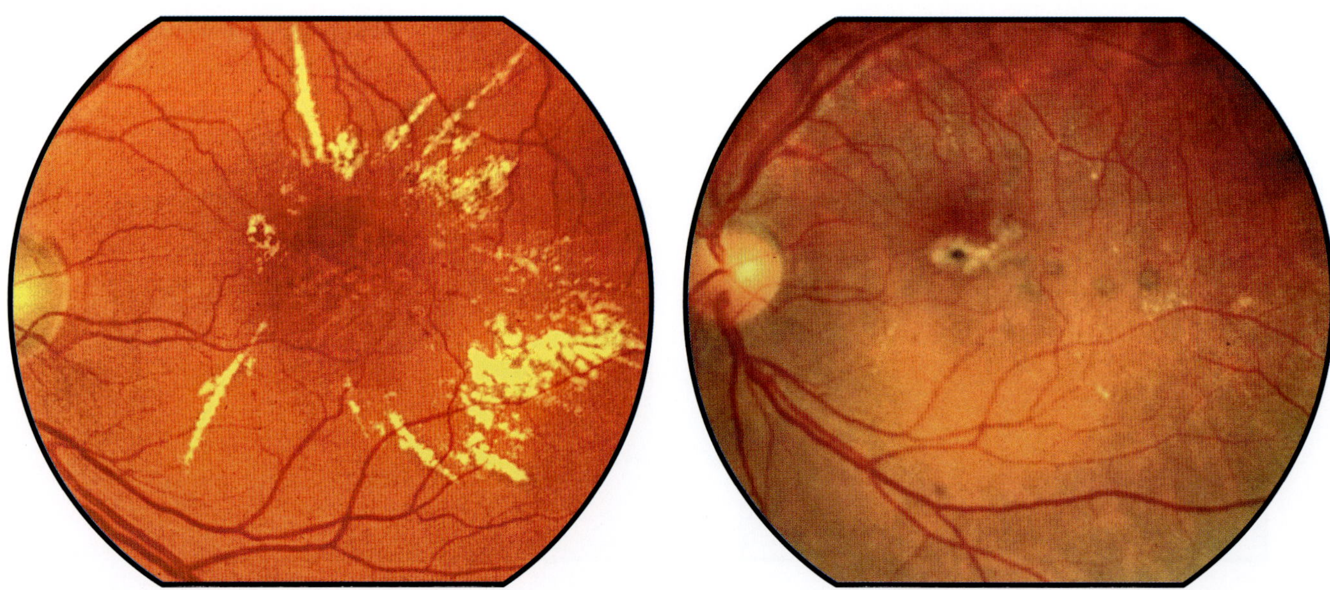

This patient developed macular telangiectasia type I in adulthood. Radial lipid deposition is associated with microaneurysms. Following focal laser photocoagulation, the lipid gradually resolved over several months with few pigmented scars.

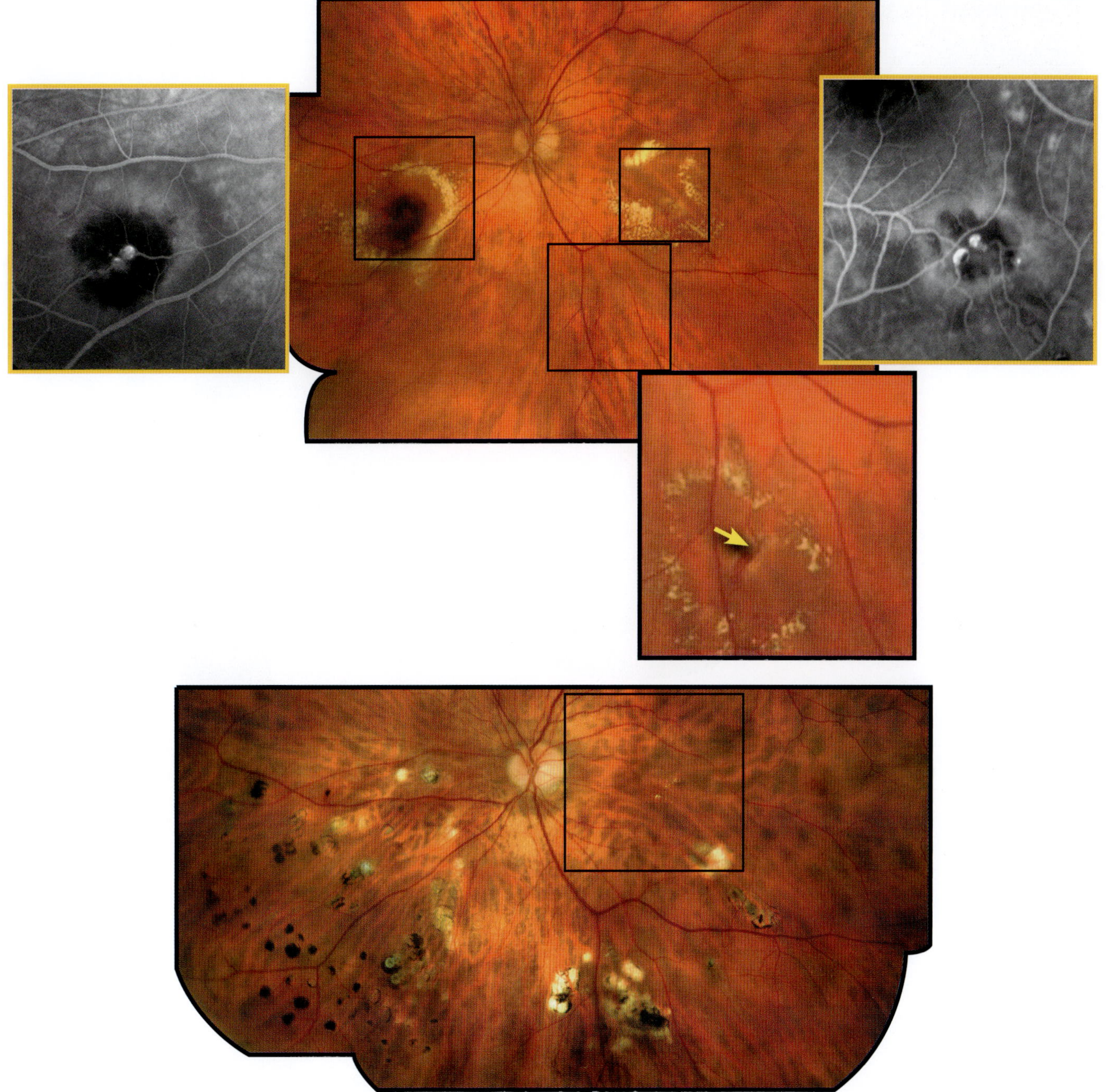

This young adult male presented with telangiectasia involving the macula and inferonasal periphery. The FAs show the aneurysmal lesions. Laser photocoagulation of these areas led to resolution of the exudation. The patient developed a new aneurysmal lesion in the inferior peripheral retina *(arrow, middle color image)*. The lesion was also photocoagulated and the circinate lipid resolved.

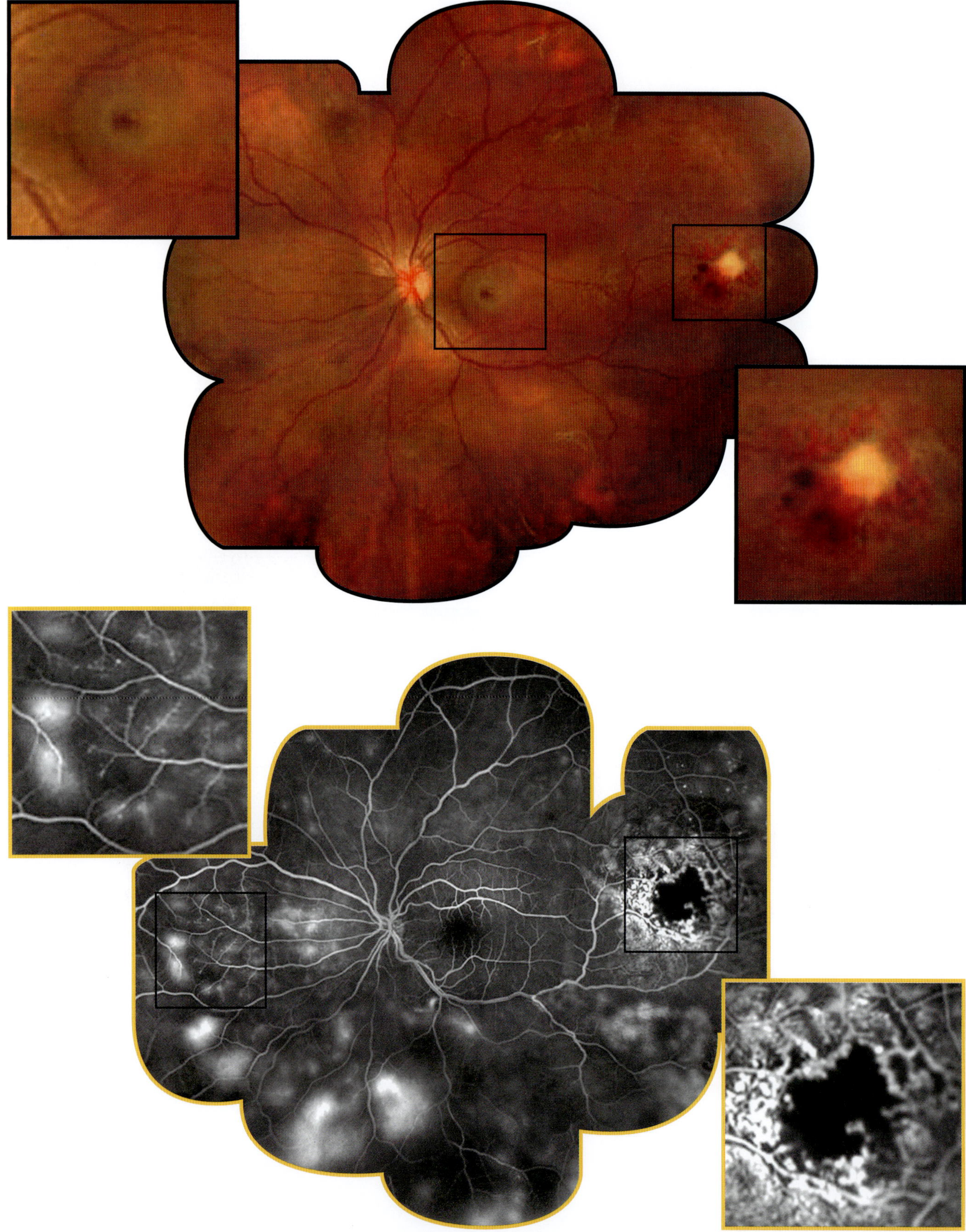

This is a 13-year-old female with Coats disease. There is exudative detachment of the macula, a dependent bullous detachment of the inferior retina, and a focal area of hemorrhage and exudation temporally. The yellowish discoloration may partially represent degenerated blood. The FA shows ischemia and telangiectatic lesions with multiple aneurysms temporally. There is no leakage in the macula where the exudate had pooled in the subneurosensory space. The entire inferior detached retina showed evidence of leakage in areas of dilated capillaries.

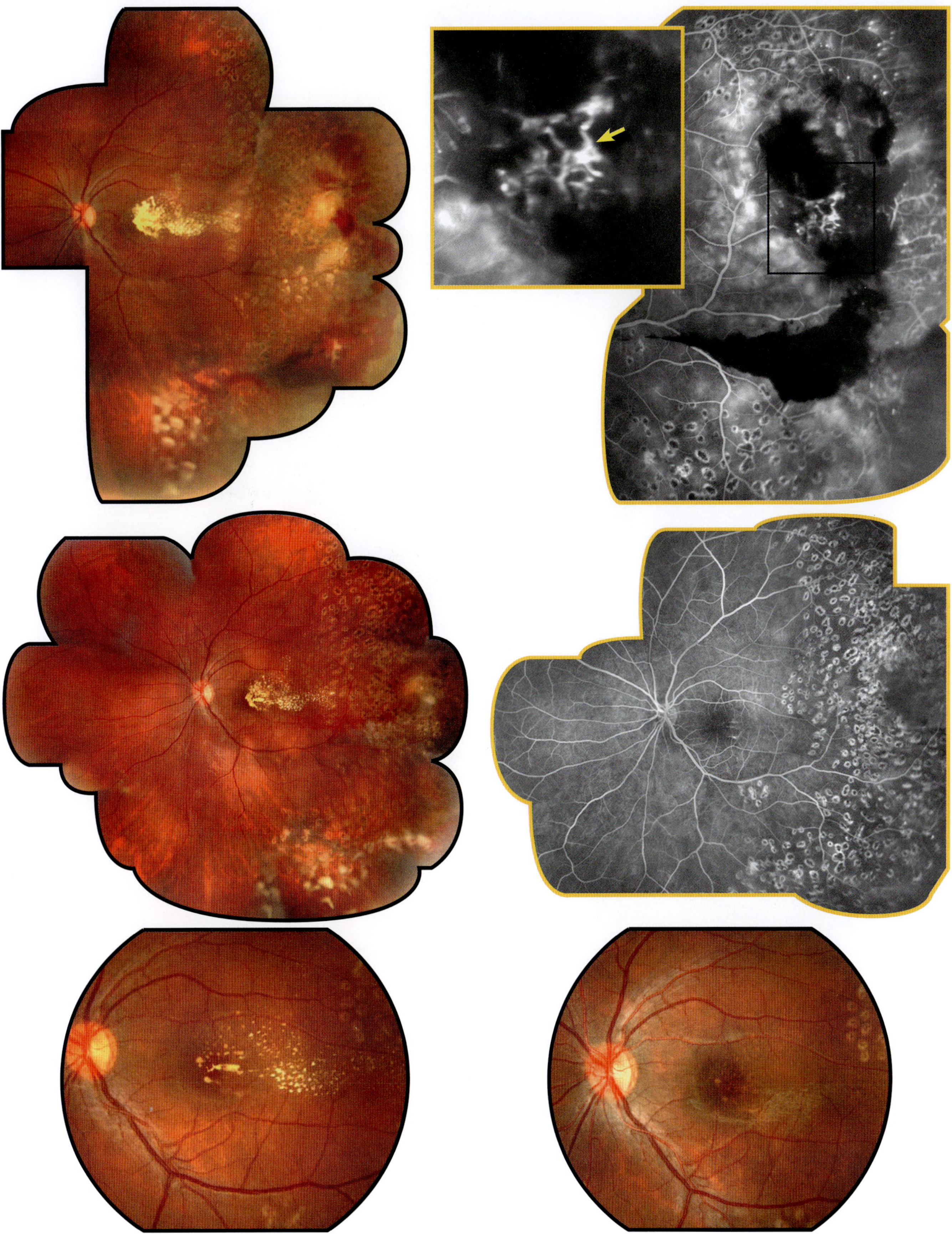

Telangiectatic lesions were directly targeted and lasered in the same patient as above, resulting in the resolution of the inferior detachment but with an increase in macular exudate. Pre-retinal hemorrhage also occurred inferiorly and temporally due to pre-retinal neovascularization *(arrow)*. Additional laser photocoagulation was performed and regression of the neovascularization and resolution of the leakage was noted *(middle row)*. Gradually the lipid in the macular area cleared over a period of 6 months *(lower left)* and 3 years *(lower right)*.

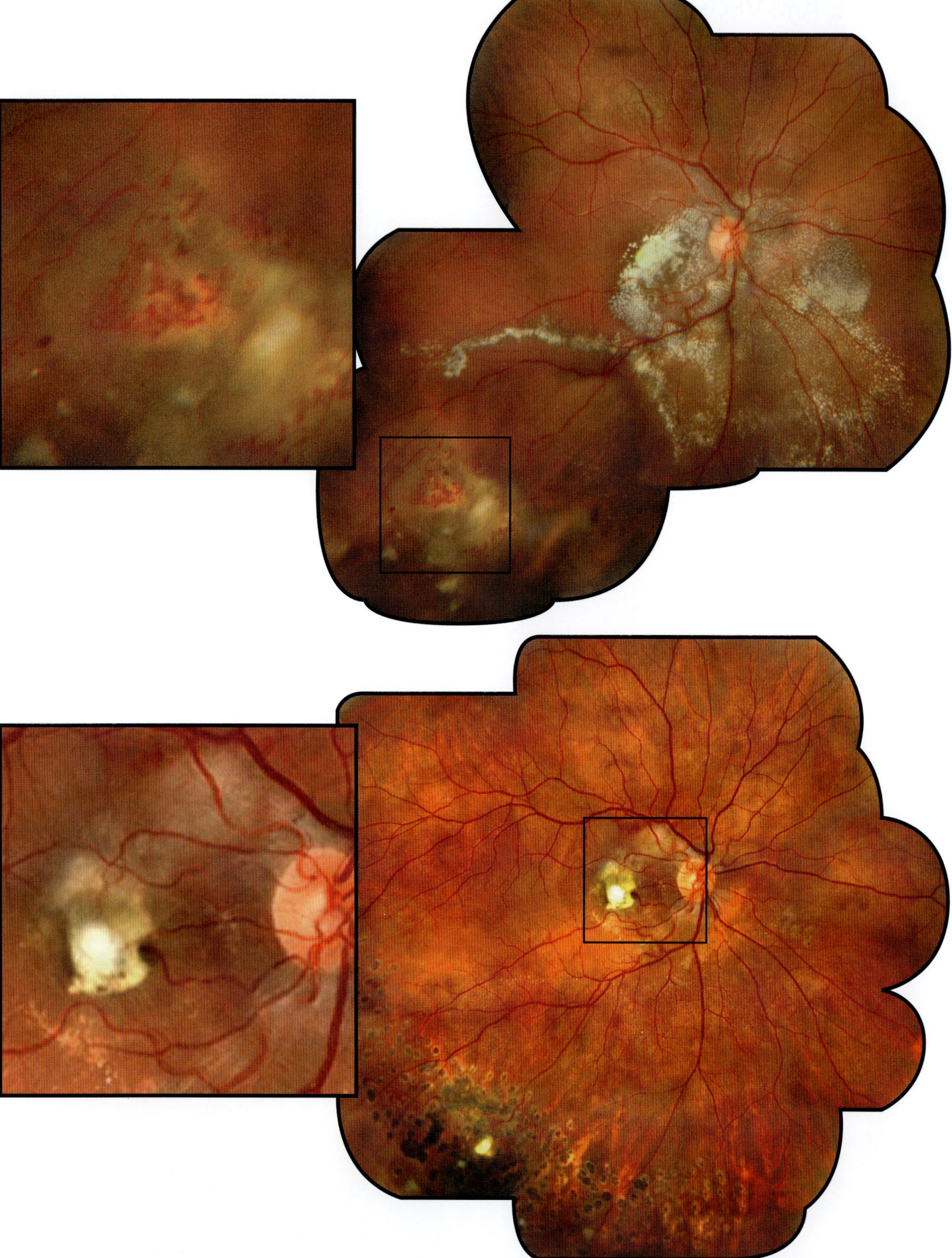

This adult male developed adult Coats disease (i.e., Lebers miliary aneurysms) with telangiectatic vascular disease present inferotemporal in the periphery. There was heavy, dense lipid exudation in the macula. Scatter laser was successful. The detachment resolved but the macula developed a fibrotic scar due to antecedent lipid deposition.

Treatment: Anti-VEGF Therapy

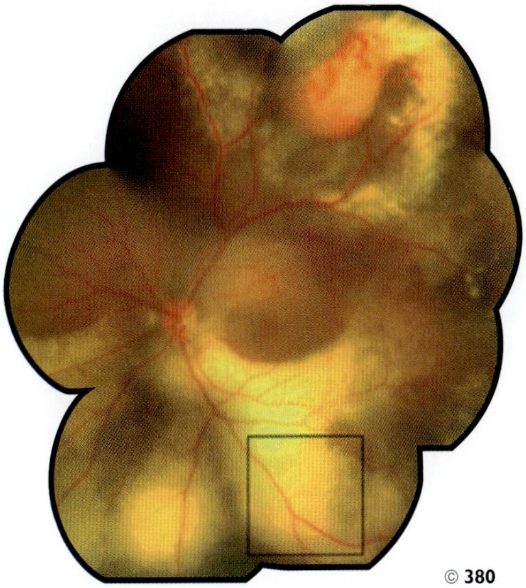

© 380

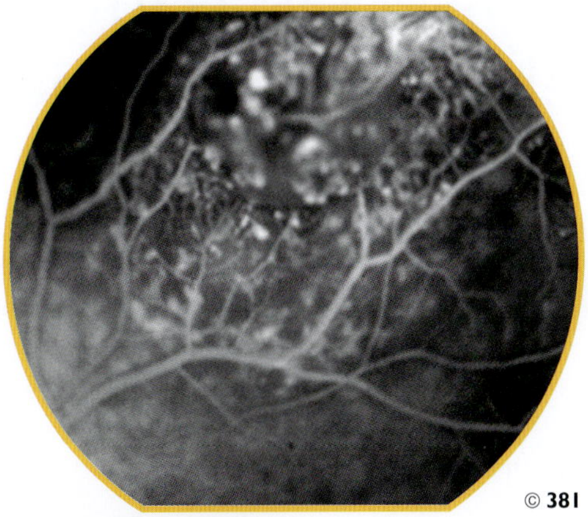

© 381

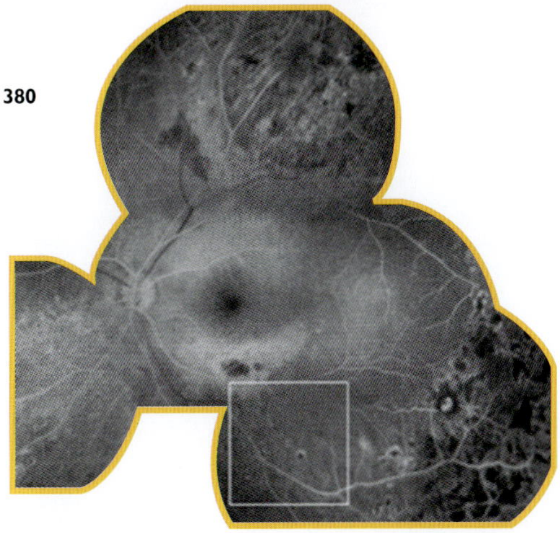

© 382

This case illustrates massive lipid exudation from a vasoproliferative mass (complicating Coats disease) in the superior retina associated with an inferior exudative detachment. Fluorescein angiography *(top right)* shows telangiectatic vessels, aneurysms, and leakage suggestive of Coats and associated with the vasoproliferative tumor. Following laser photocoagulation to the abnormal Coats vessels and after intravitreal bevacizumab injection, the leakage and detachment resolved *(bottom)*.

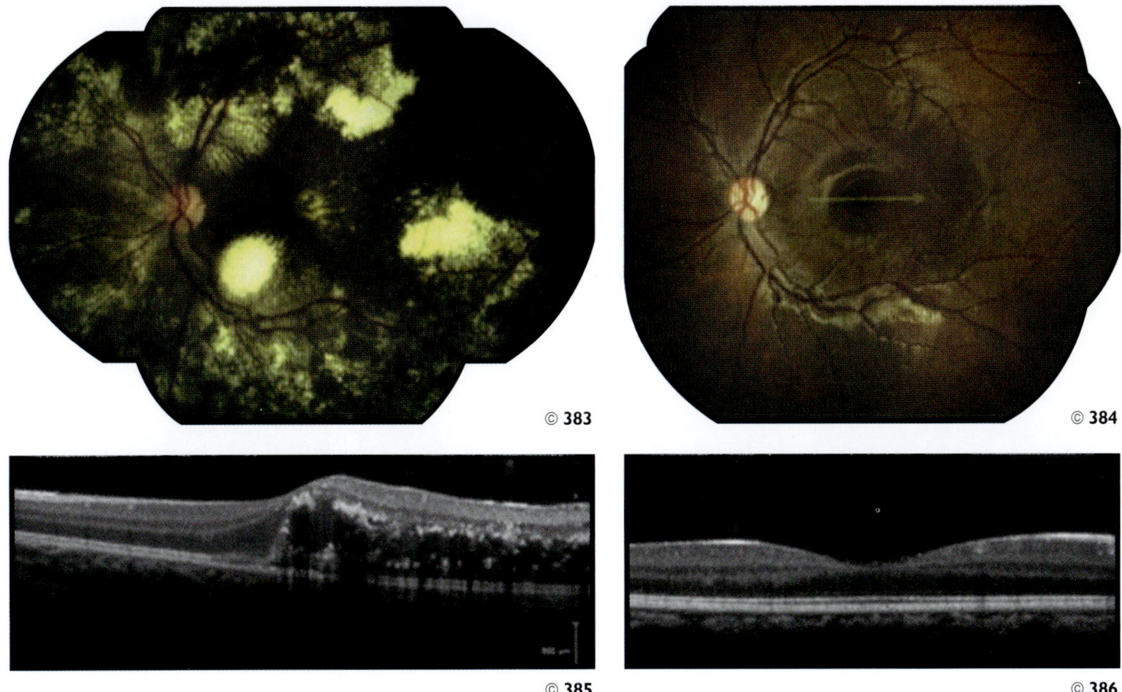

© 383

© 384

© 385

© 386

This patient had diffuse lipid exudation throughout the fundus and involving the macula *(left images)* and associated with cystoid macular edema seen on spectral domain OCT *(bottom left)*. After laser photocoagulation to the leaking vessels and after a single intravitreal bevacizumab injection, the exudates and CME resolved *(right images)*.

Macular Telangiectasia Type 2 (Idiopathic Perifoveal Telangiectasia, Idiopathic Juxtafoveal Telangiectasis Type 2)

Macular telangiectasia type 2 (Mactel type 2) has also been termed idiopathic perifoveal telangiectasia or idiopathic juxtafoveal telangiectasis type 2. It is a slowly progressive bilateral perifoveal disorder with vasculopathic and neurodegenerative features. Although the pathogenesis remains unknown, histologic evidence points to a degeneration of the Müller cells. The earliest findings include loss of the macular pigment, telangiectatic changes in the temporal fovea, and discontinuities in the ellipsoid zone. As the disease progresses, these findings spread circumferentially beyond the temporal fovea with increased leakage, formation of right-angle venules, and further disruption of the retinal architecture with formation of cavitations on OCT. In some instances, intraretinal crystalline deposits and pigmentary changes are present. The vascular changes initially arise in the deep retinal capillary plexus, but in advanced cases, subretinal neovascularization can ensue which can lead to disciform scarring.

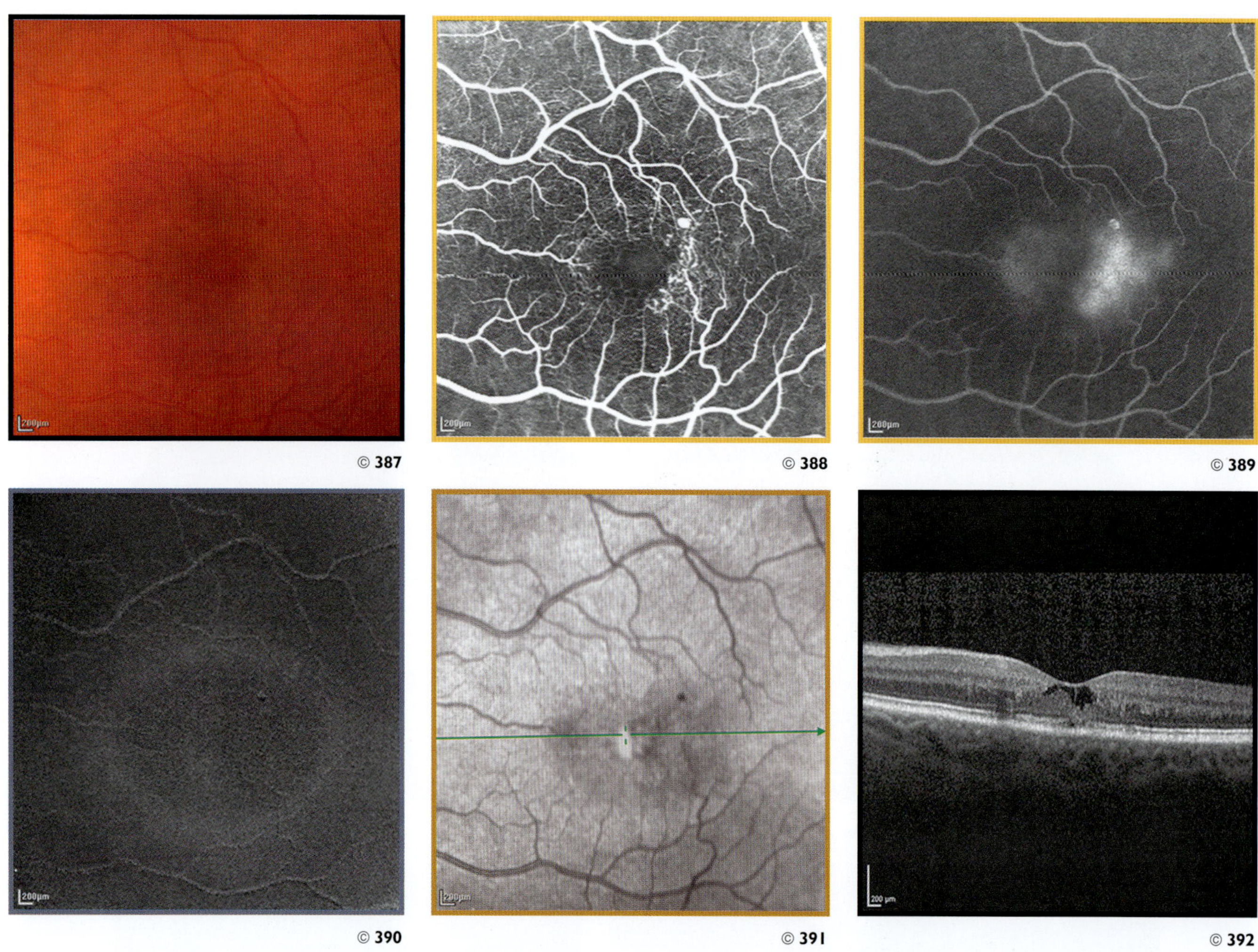

© 387 © 388 © 389 © 390 © 391 © 392

Mactel type 2 has characteristic multimodal imaging findings. The color image shows subtle perifoveal graying. The FA shows dilated telangiectatic capillaries most predominant in the temporal fovea with late hyperfluorescence. The macular pigment is diffusely depleted as seen on dual wavelength autofluorescence. The spectral-domain OCT shows ellipsoid zone loss with an inner retinal cavitary cyst in the retina.

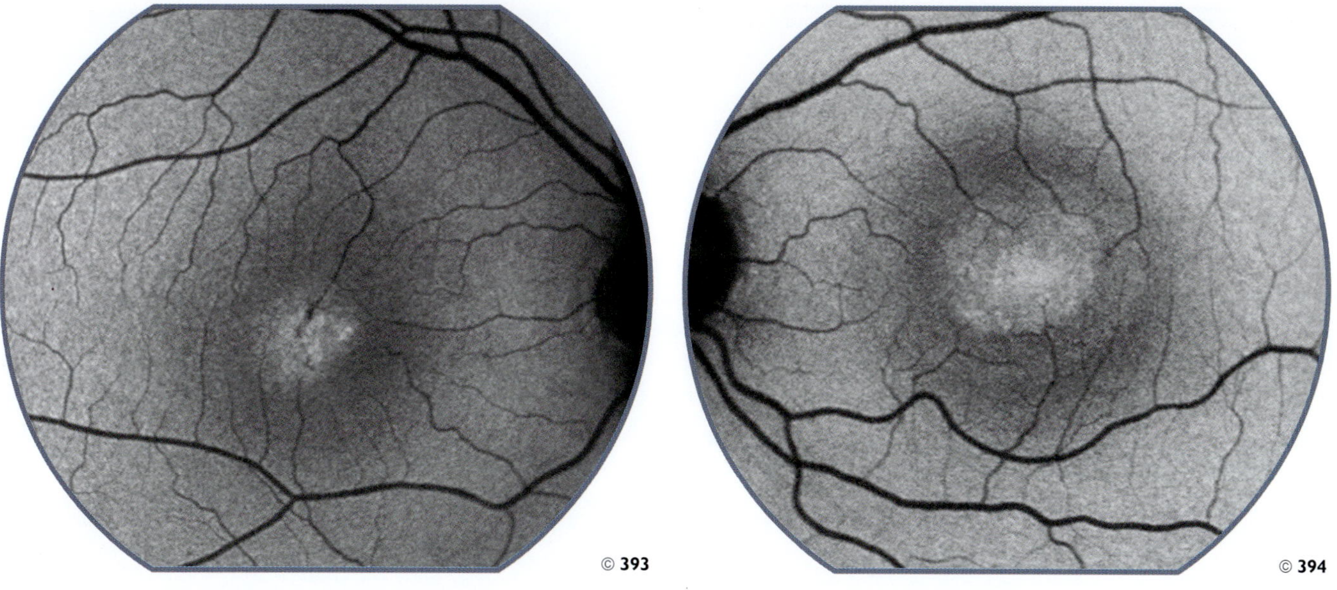

© 393 © 394

These short-wavelength autofluorescence images of patients with Mactel type 2 illustrate the depletion of macular pigment that unmasks the autofluorescence signal of the foveal region.

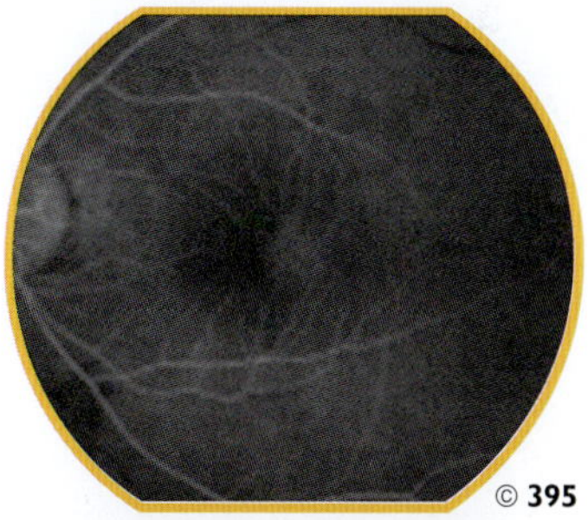

© 395 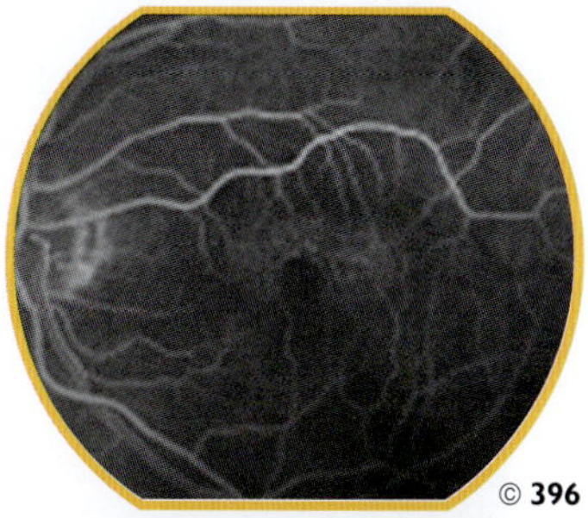 © 396 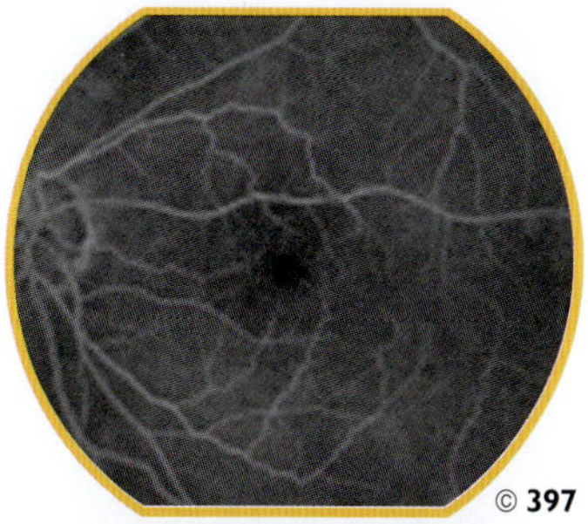 © 397

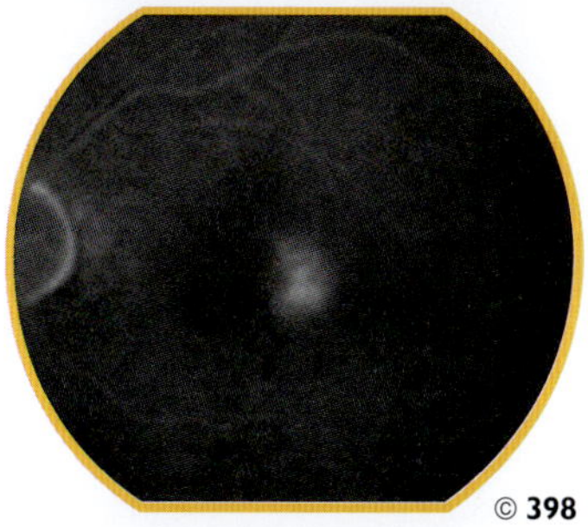

© 398 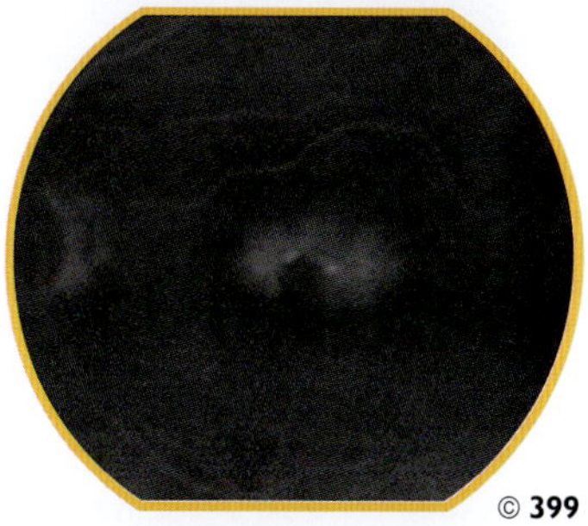 © 399 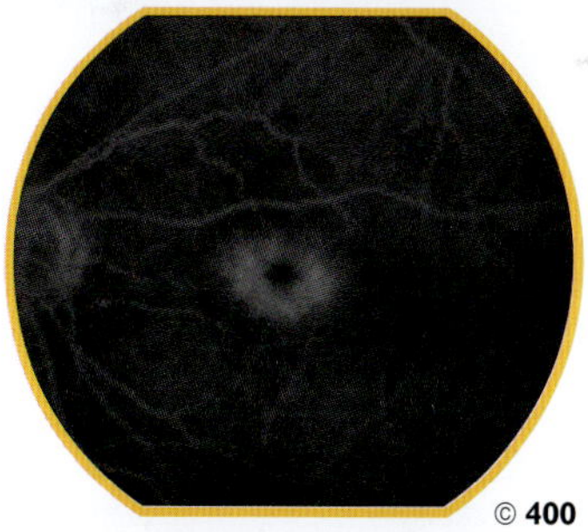 © 400

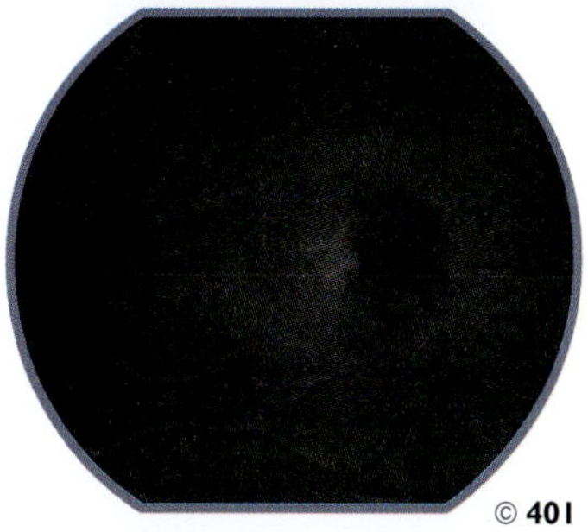

© 401 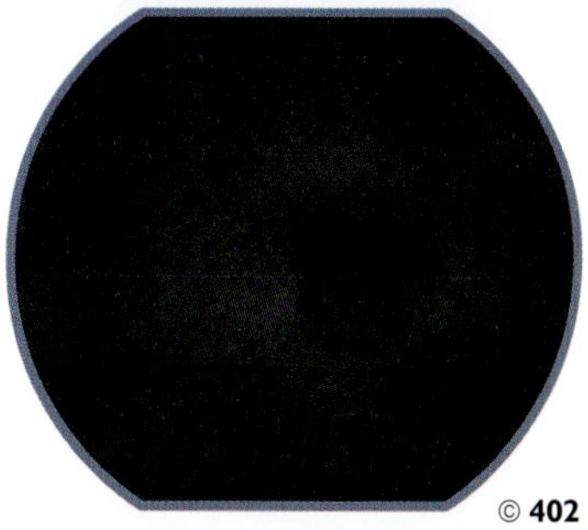 © 402 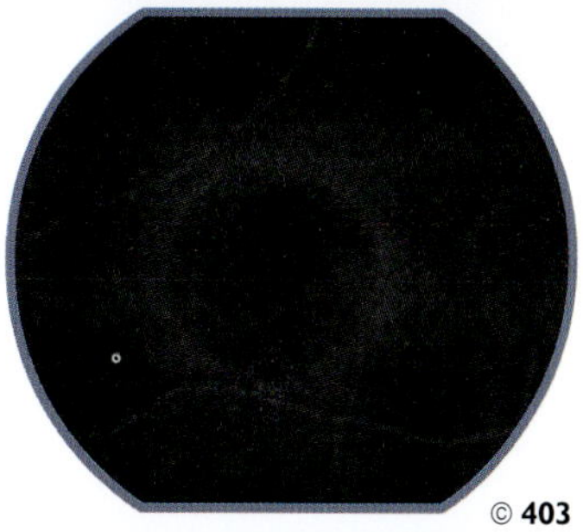 © 403

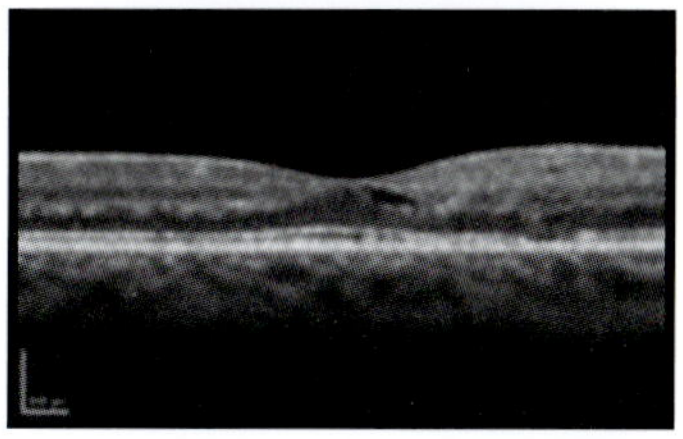

© 404 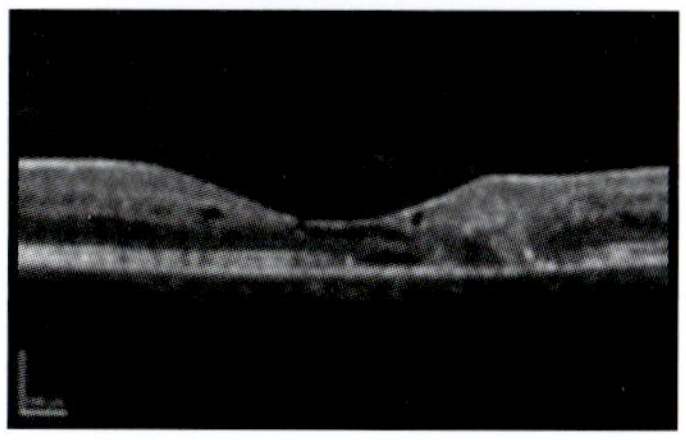 © 405 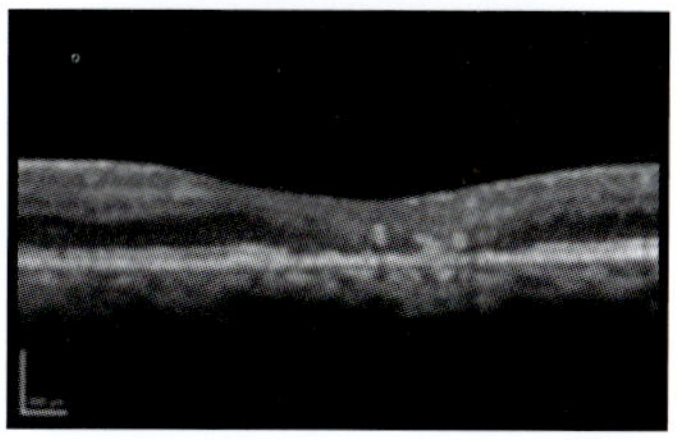 © 406

These images demonstrate the spectrum of disease severity in three separate cases of Mactel type 2. The top two rows show early and late FAs. The third row illustrates dual wavelength autofluorescence and the macular pigment density. The bottom row includes spectral domain OCTs through the fovea. The left column shows a case of early disease with only temporal vascular changes and loss of macular pigment. There is limited ellipsoid zone loss and mild intraretinal cavitation. The middle column is more advanced with both nasal and temporal involvement and more diffuse atrophic and cavitary changes on OCT. The right column is an advanced case with severe outer retinal atrophy but without evidence of subretinal neovascularization.

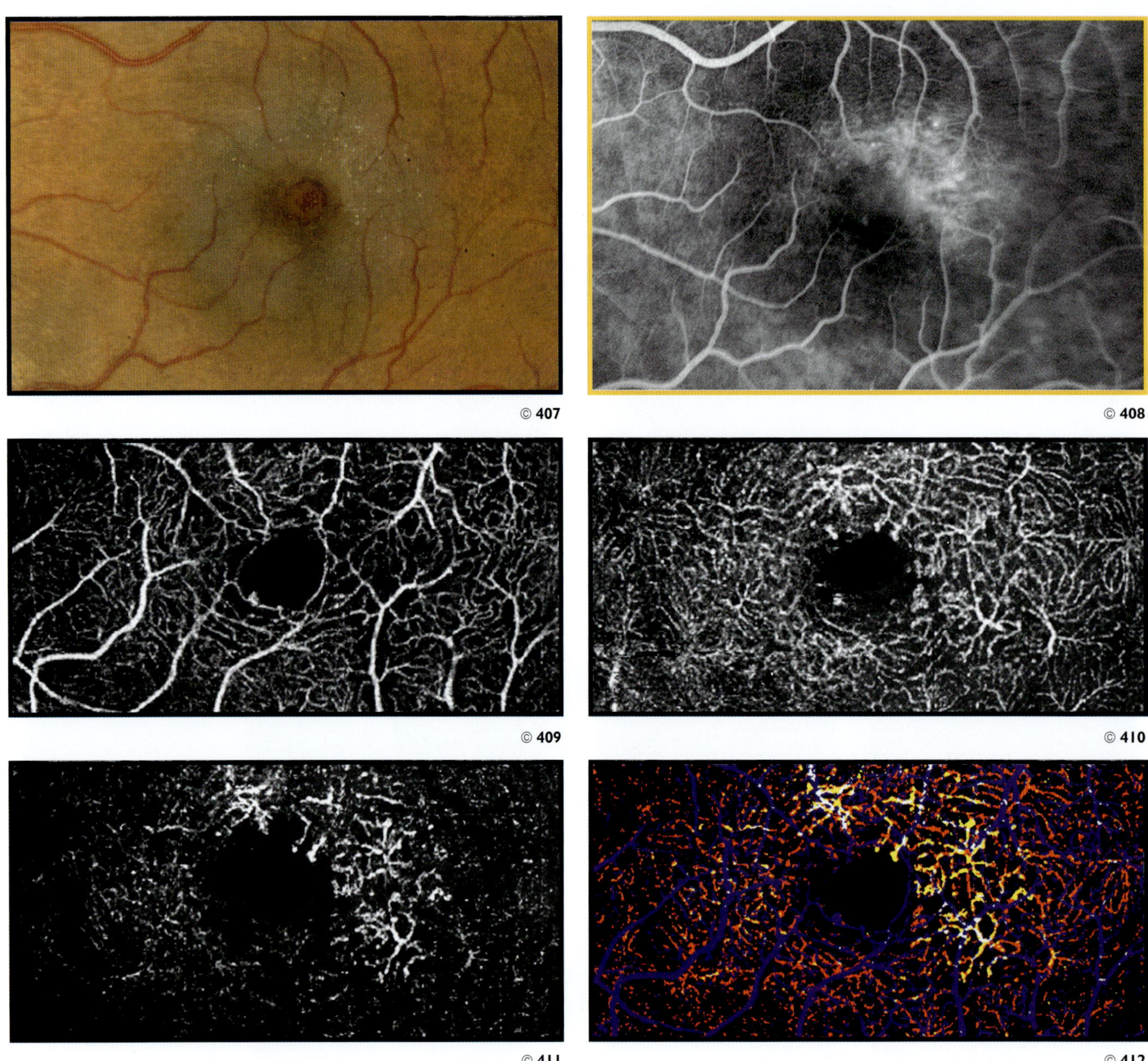

OCT angiography provides enhanced visualization of the abnormal retinal capillaries in Mactel type 2. The color image shows the classic perifoveal graying and crystal deposition. Note the temporal hyperfluorescent staining that blurs the vascular anatomy with fluorescein angiography. OCT angiography of the superficial retinal capillary plexus *(middle left)* in this case is unremarkable but shows a dilated microvascular network with segmentation through the deep capillary plexus (DCP; *middle right and bottom left*). The color montage highlights the abnormal DCP vessels in yellow.

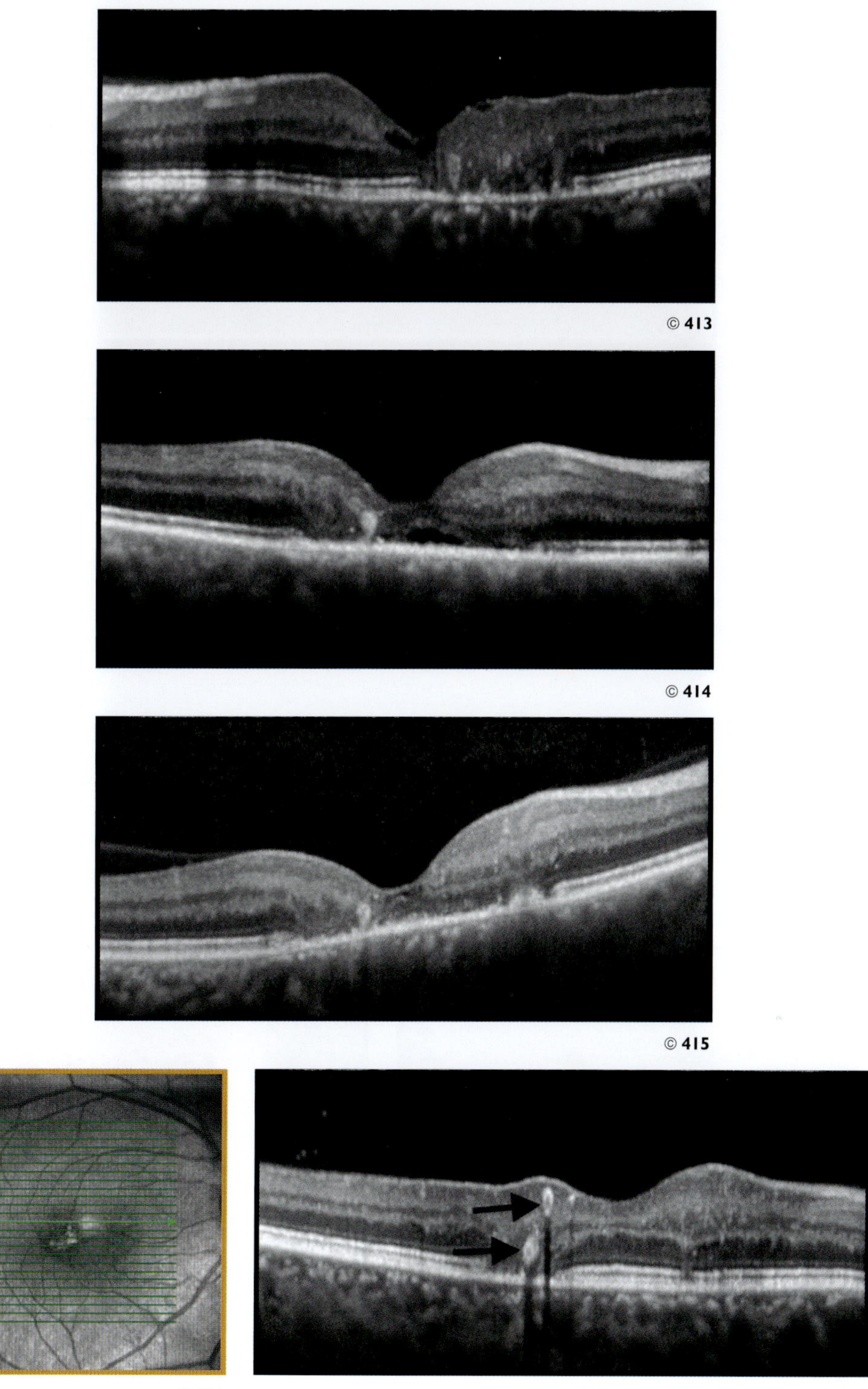

© 413

© 414

© 415

© 416

© 417

SD-OCT illustrates typical alterations seen in Mactel type 2 including outer retinal atrophy and cystic retinal cavitations. The bottom right image illustrates two aneurysmal dilations of vessels in the temporal perifovea *(arrows)*.

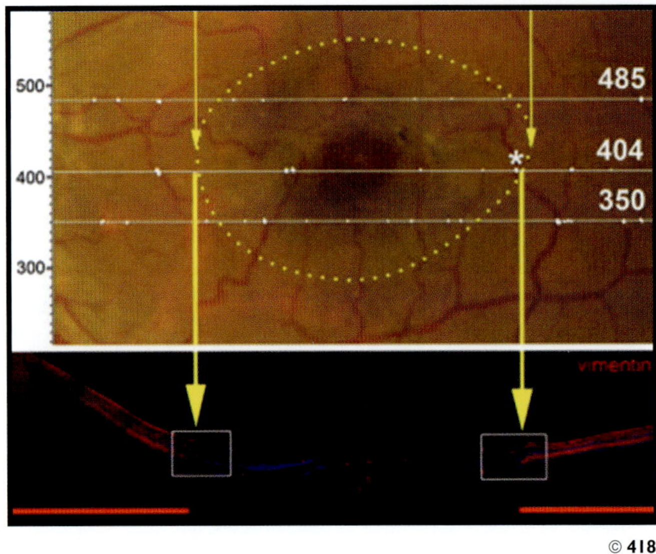

© 418

This is a postmortem clinicopathologic correlation of a patient with Mactel type 2. The color image shows macular pigment depletion and perifoveal pigmentary changes. After histologic processing of the retina, the sections were stained with a vimentin antibody that stains Müller cells. There is notable depletion of the Müller cells in the central affected area.

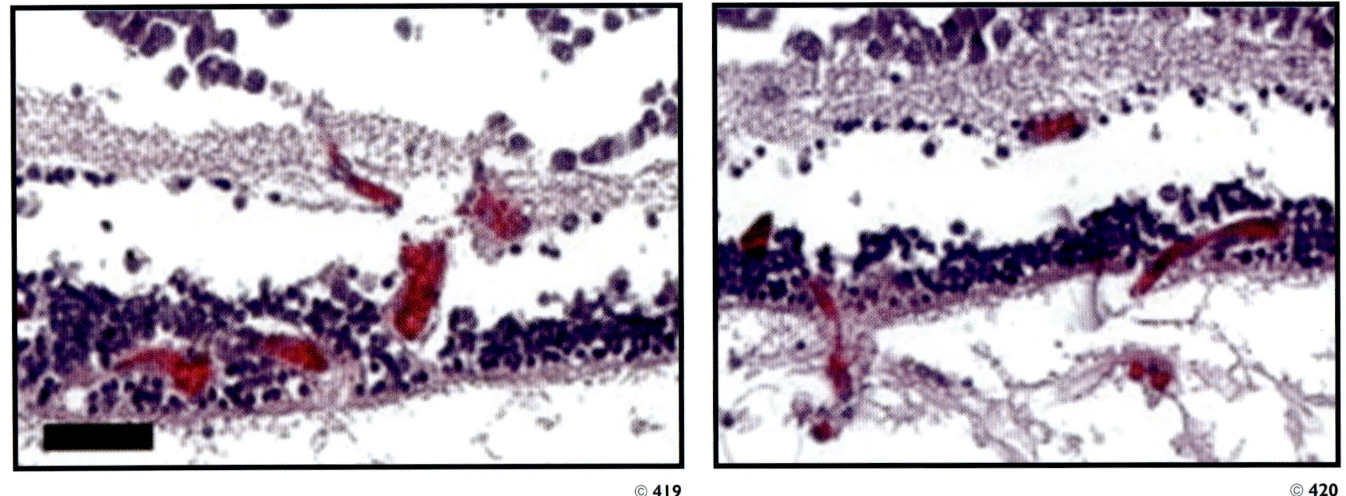

© 419 © 420

This is another postmortem clinicopathologic analysis showing abnormal vessels at the level of the deep capillary plexus.

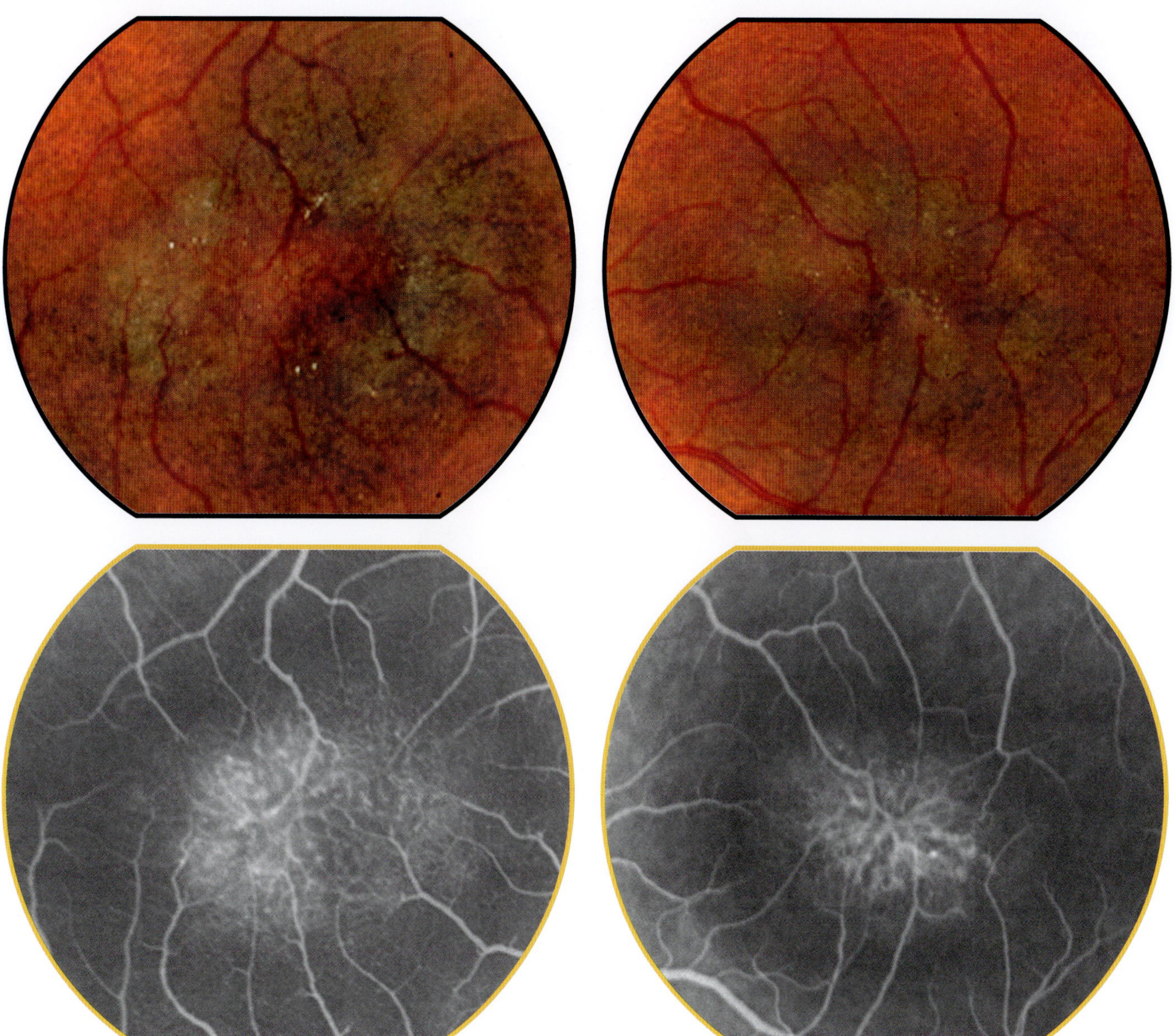

This patient with Mactel type 2 has more advanced disease with vascular abnormalities encompassing the entire foveal area.

Pigment Hyperplasia

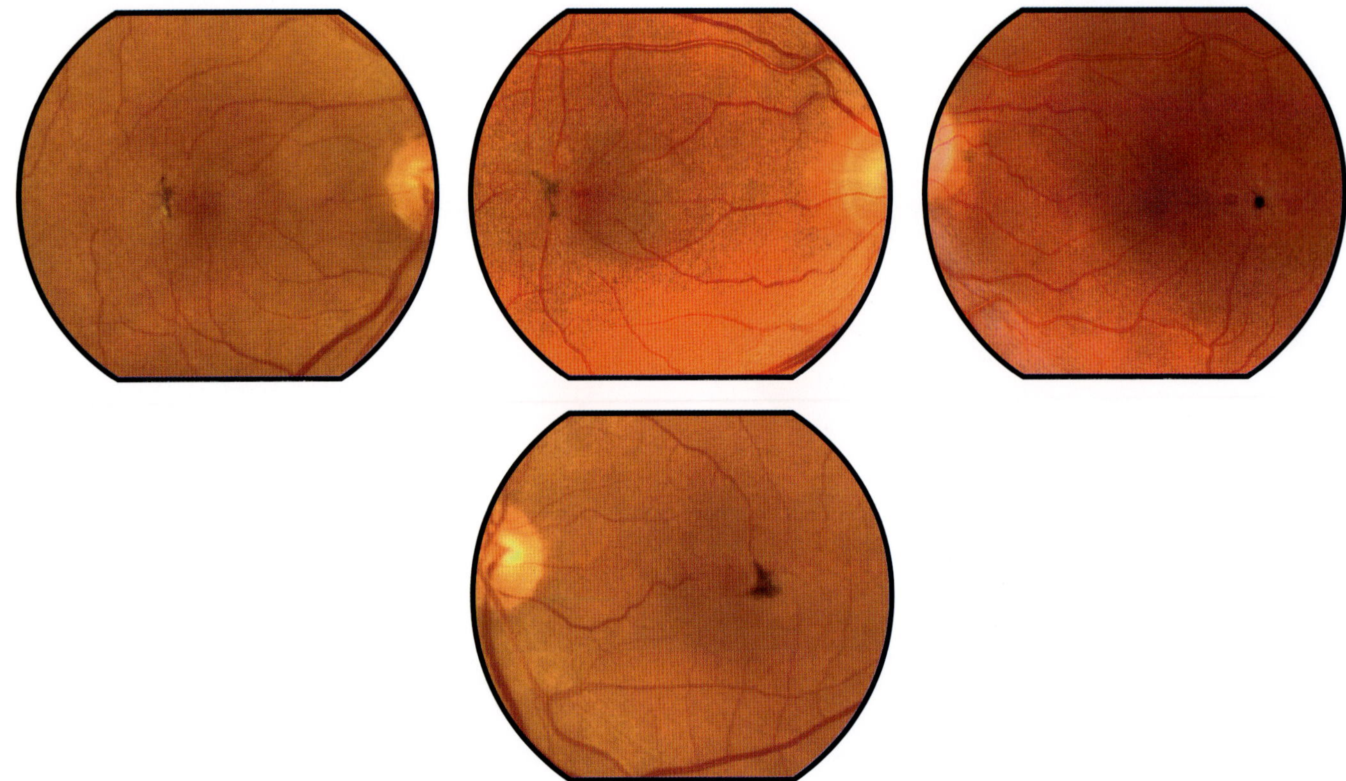

As retinal vessels (e.g., right angle venules) descend from the deep capillary plexus toward the pigment epithelium, reactive pigment epithelial hyperplasia may develop, as seen in these patients with Mactel type 2.

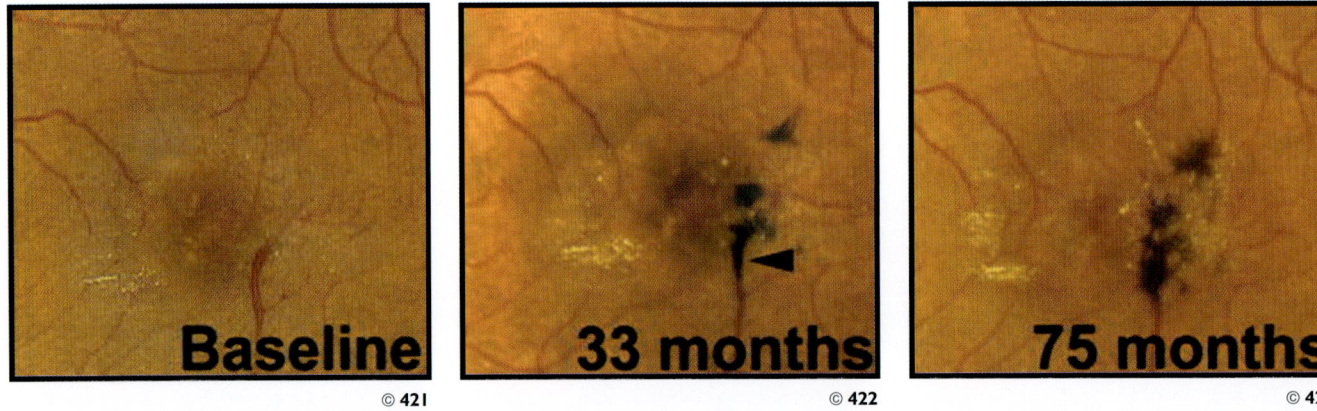

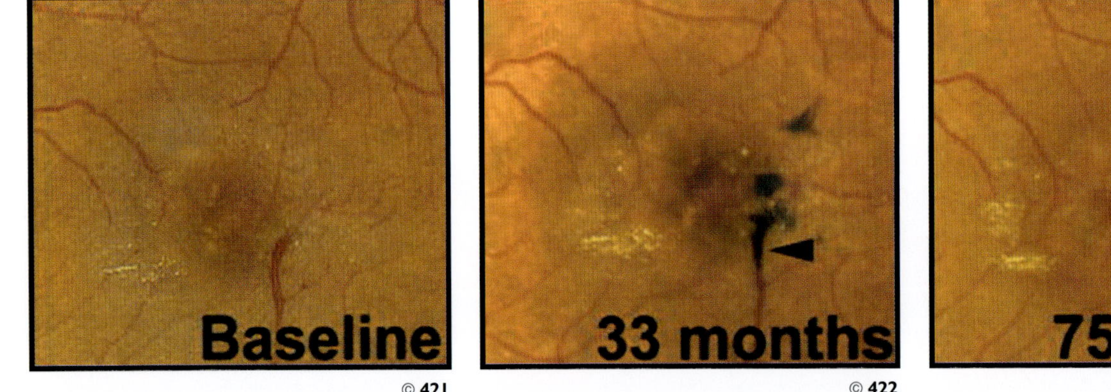

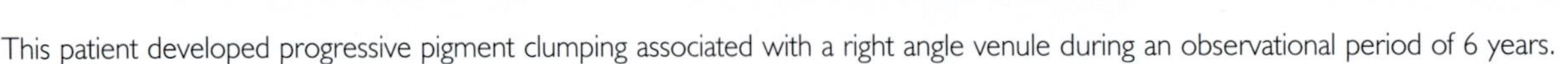

This patient developed progressive pigment clumping associated with a right angle venule during an observational period of 6 years.

Crystals

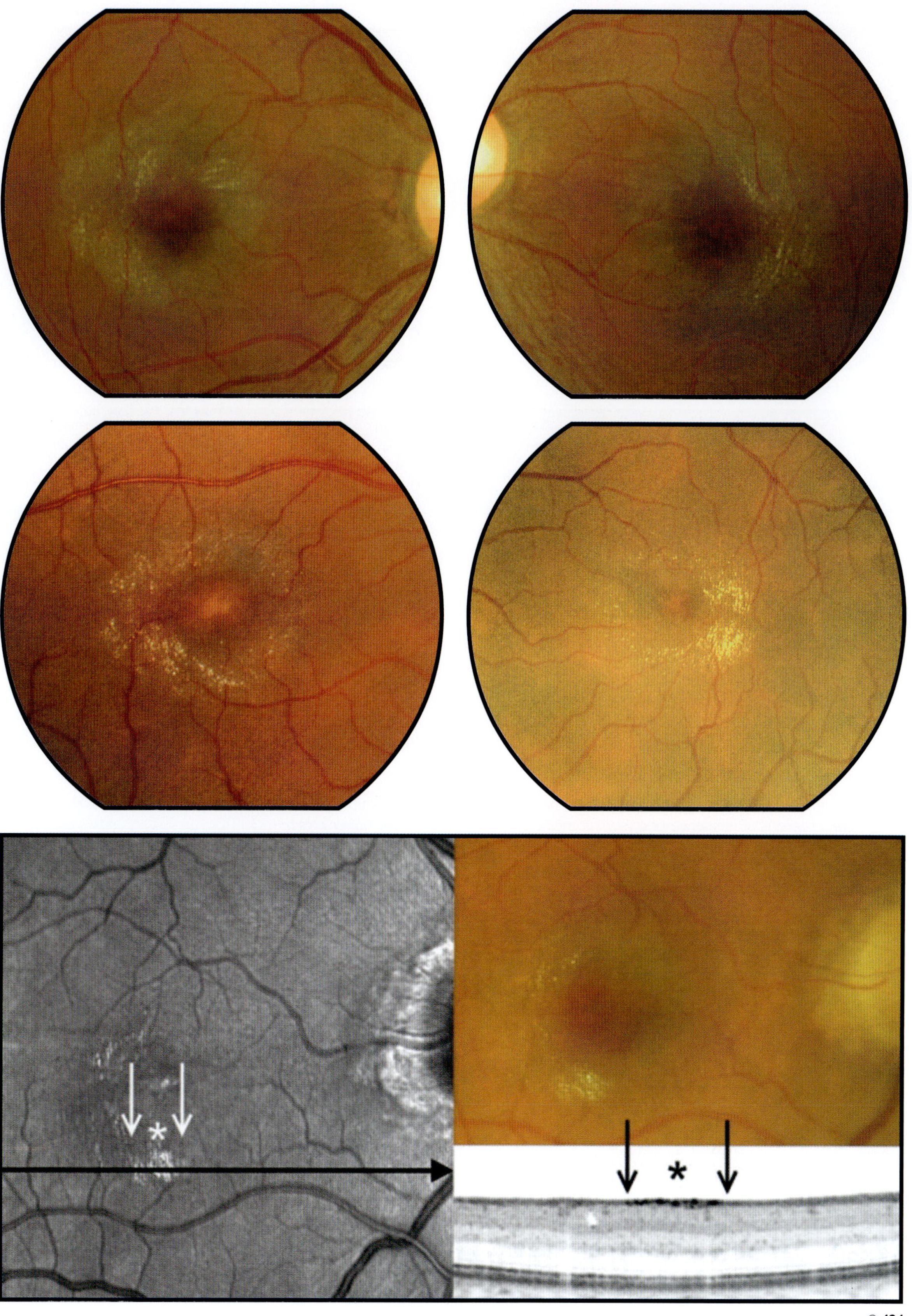

© **424**

These patients with Mactel type 2 illustrate crystalline abnormalities at the level of the vitreoretinal interface. These are generally more prominent in the temporal juxtafoveal region where the process begins. The bottom images illustrate the hyper-reflective crystals on SD-OCT at the level of the internal limiting membrane. *Top row courtesy of Dr. Y. Sato*

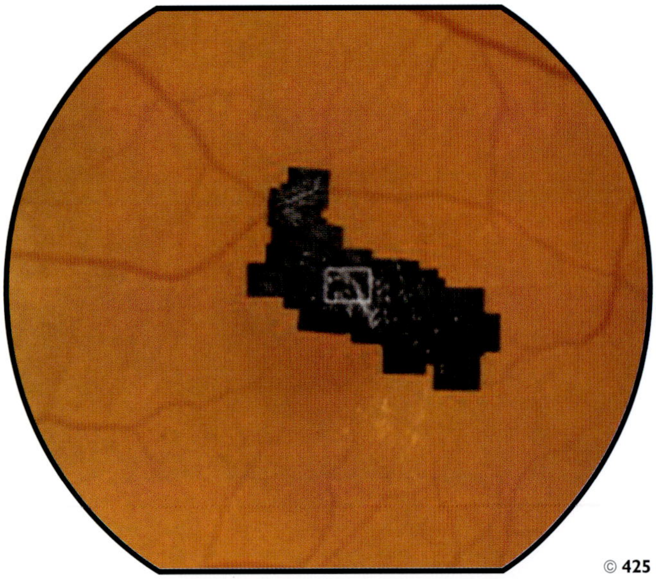

© 425

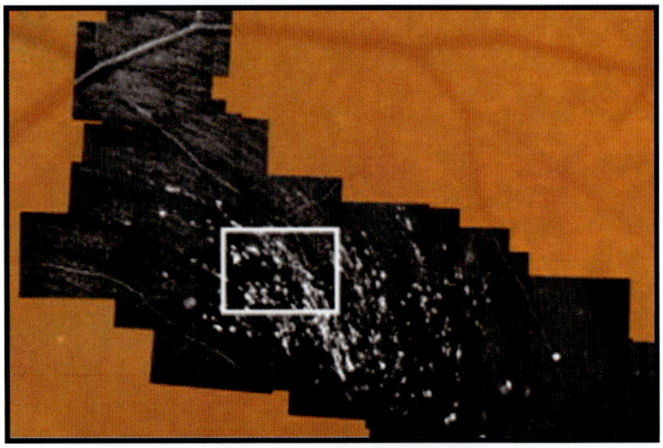

© 426

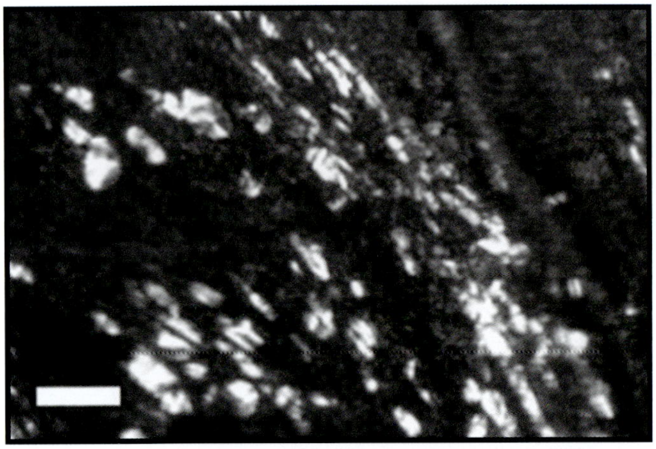

© 427

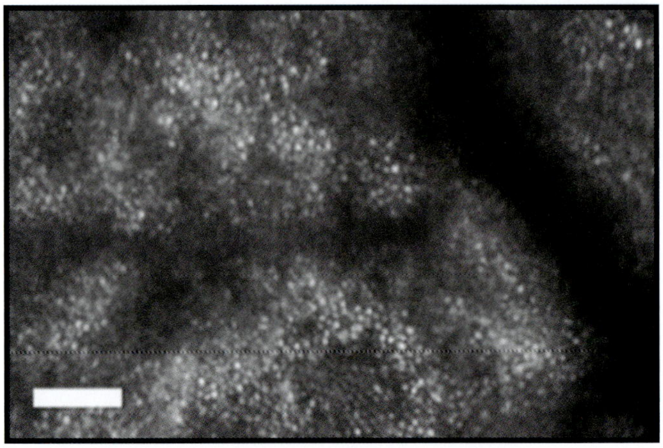

© 428

These are adaptive optics scanning laser ophthalmoscopy images of a patient with Mactel type 2. Note the crystals assume a distribution parallel to the nerve fiber layer. There is no evidence of crystals at the level of the cone mosaic *(lower right)*.

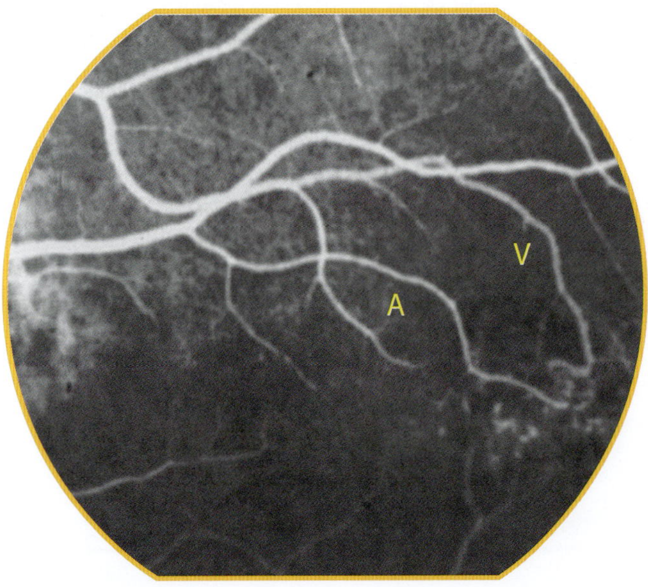

This FA of a patient with mactel type 2 illustrates a prominent perfusing arteriole (A) and draining venule (V) in a looping communication within the retina.

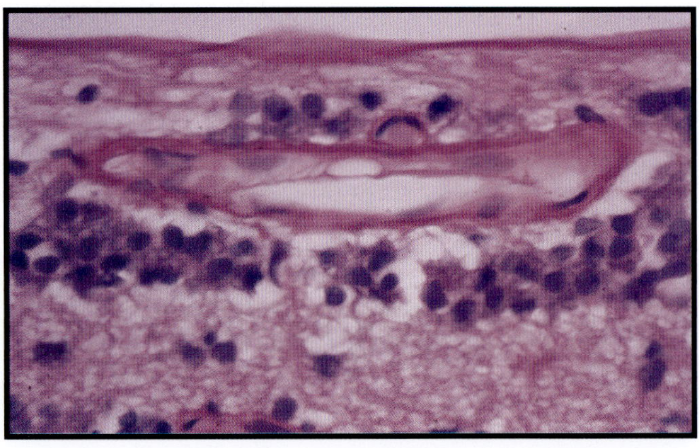

This histopathology specimen of Mactel type 2 shows a large intraretinal venule. There is lamination of the endothelial layers and an increase in basement membrane deposition. Very few endothelial cells are present and pericytes are conspicuously absent.

Subretinal Neovascularization

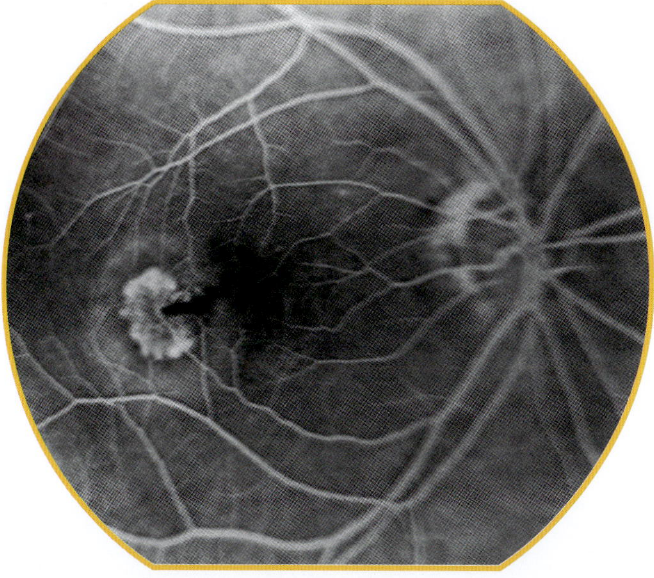

This patient with Mactel type 2 has subretinal neovascularization. The proliferating vessels in the subretinal space are bright compared to the wreath of telangiectatic vessels that forms a halo around the neovascular lesion.

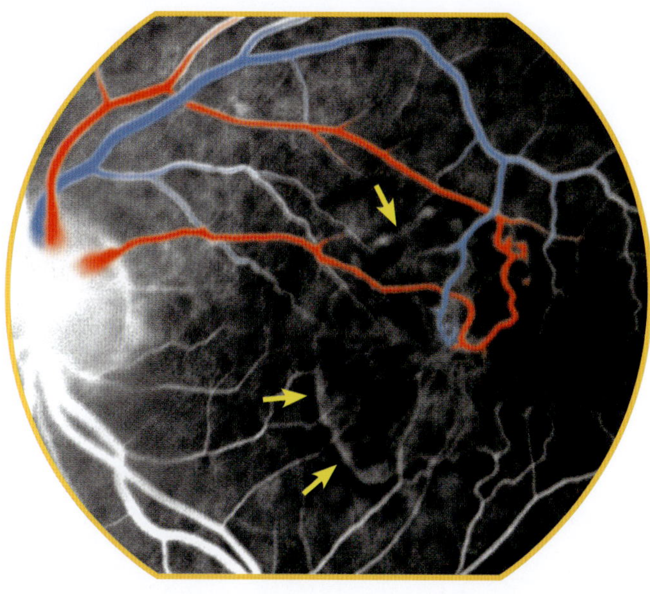

This patient has subretinal neovascularization *(arrows)* that is perfused by two arterioles *(red)* and a venule *(blue)*.

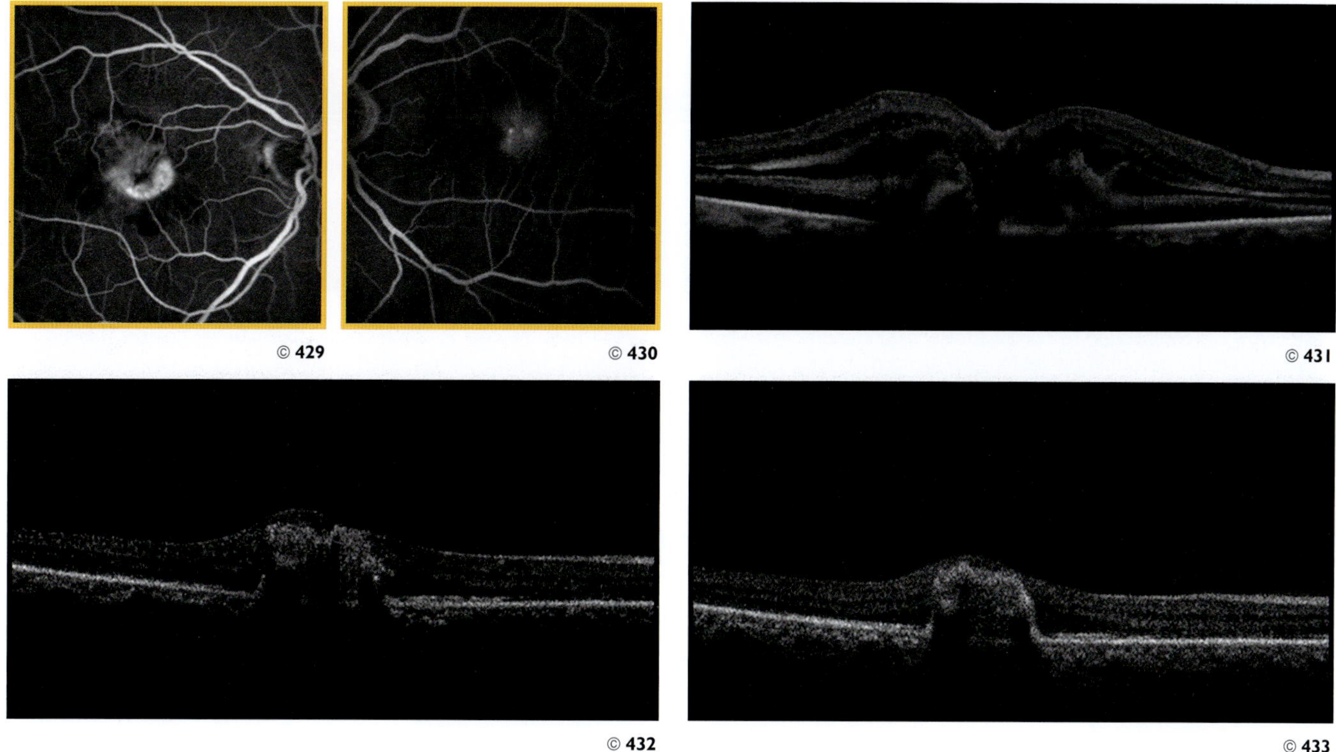

This patient with Mactel type 2 developed subretinal neovascularization in the right eye with leakage and surrounding blocked fluorescence due to hemorrhage. The OCT *(top right)* shows a subfoveal neovascular membrane with associated retinal edema. The bottom OCTs illustrate resolution of the neovascular lesion one month *(bottom left)* and 3 months *(bottom right)* after intravitreal bevacizumab therapy and an associated macular scar.

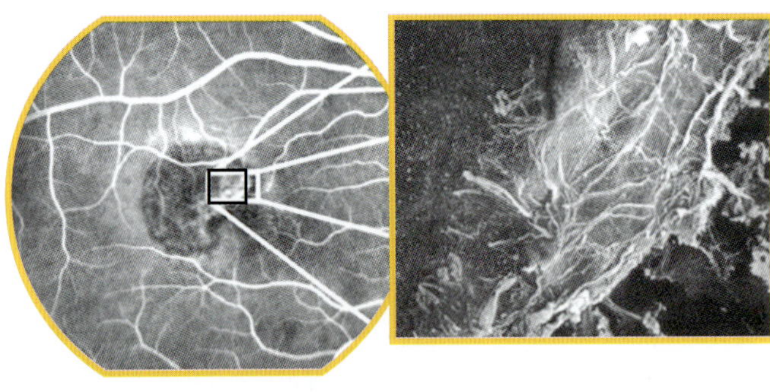

Note the presence of subretinal neovascularization that was excised and studied histopathologically in this patient with Mactel type 2. *Courtesy of Dr. Fred Davidoff*

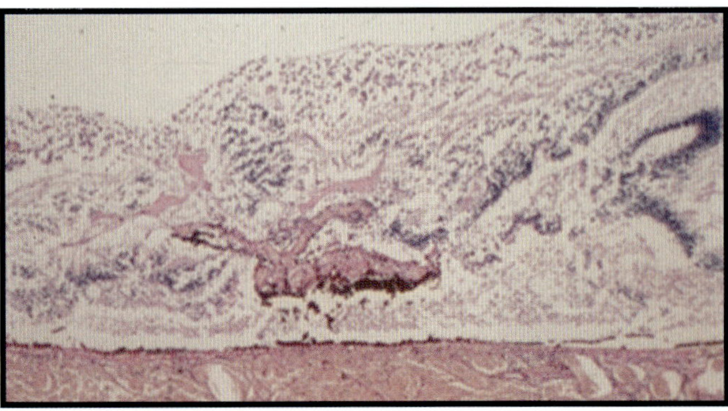

In this histopathological specimen of Mactel type 2, there is extension of the intraretinal vasogenic process throughout all layers of the retina, including the subretinal space. The retinal pigment epithelium is intact.

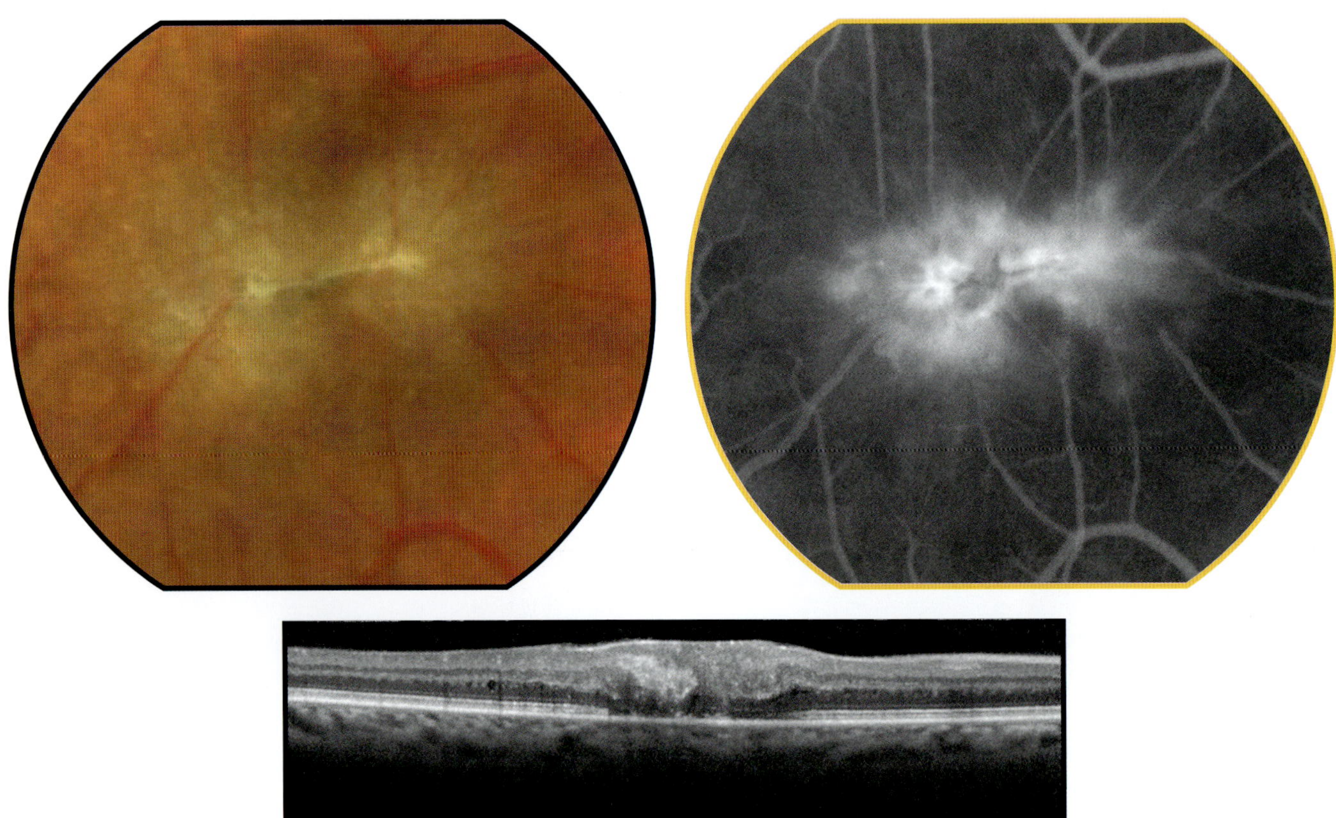

Mactel type 2 is complicated by fibrous proliferation in the retina, which can occur late in the course of the disease. Despite the fibrosis, there is minimal cystic change within the retina, as evidenced on the SD-OCT. The visual acuity was surprisingly good at 20/40.

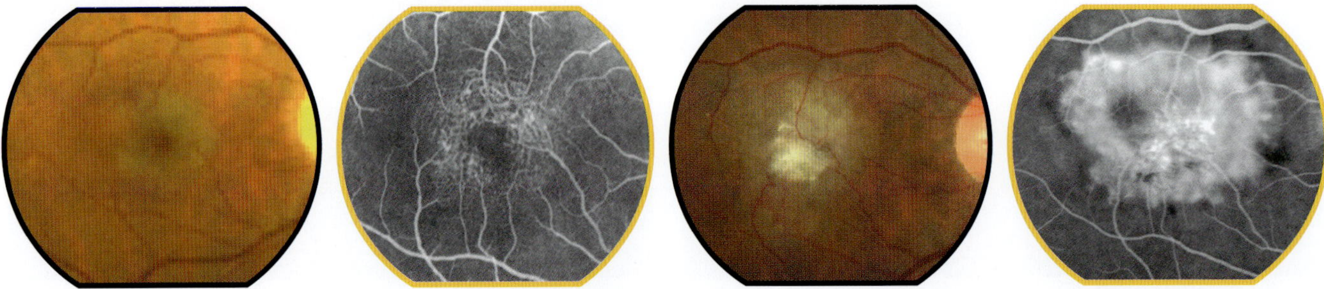

This patient experienced progression through the various stages of Mactel type 2. In the images on the left, the typical early findings of Mactel 2 are illustrated including perifoveal graying and telangiectasia. In the images on the right, the patient has progressed to the proliferative stage. A fibrovascular scar developed 3 years after the initial diagnosis. Note the fibrosis extends from the pre-retinal to the subretinal space with multiple retinal–subretinal anastomoses.

Treatment

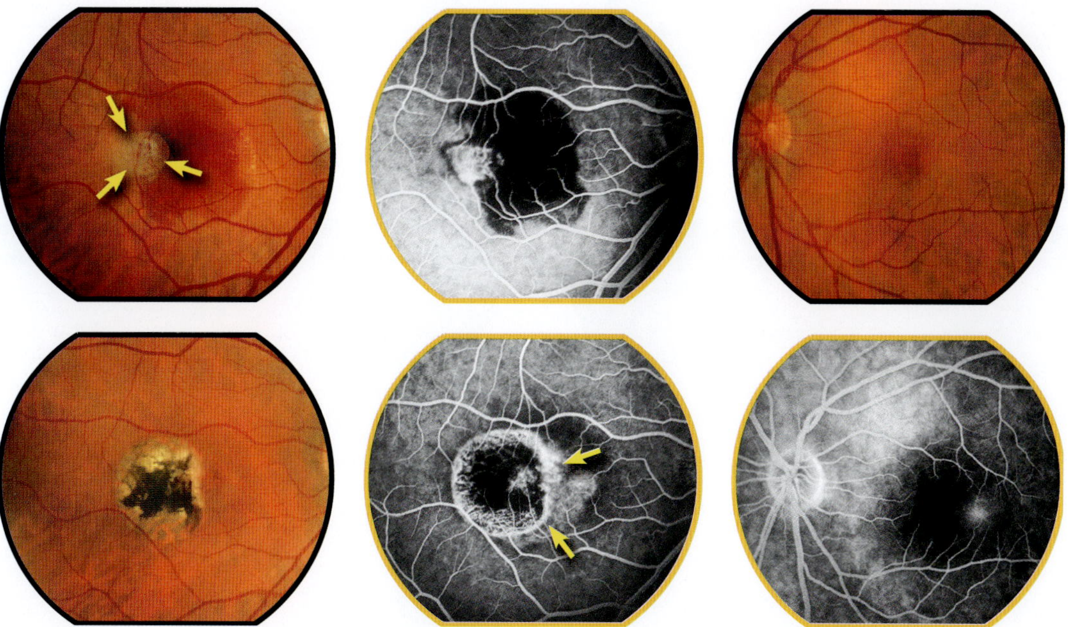

In the past, laser photocoagulation was used to obliterate subretinal neovascularization in patients with Mactel type 2 but this approach has largely been abandoned with the advent of anti-VEGF therapy. This patient presented with macular hemorrhage secondary to subretinal neovascularization *(arrows upper left)* and Mactel type 2. There is a perfusing arteriole and draining venule seen on the FA on the foveal side of the membrane. Laser photocoagulation treatment was carried out to ablate the neovascular complex. A dense pigmented and atrophic scar ensued with central foveal sparing. The FA showed obliteration of the subretinal neovascularization with a concentric rim of staining. Beneath the fovea and beyond, there are telangiectatic changes *(arrows lower middle)*. The fellow eye is shown in the upper right and lower right images. A 12 year follow-up on this patient showed no progression in either eye after the laser photocoagulation treatment.

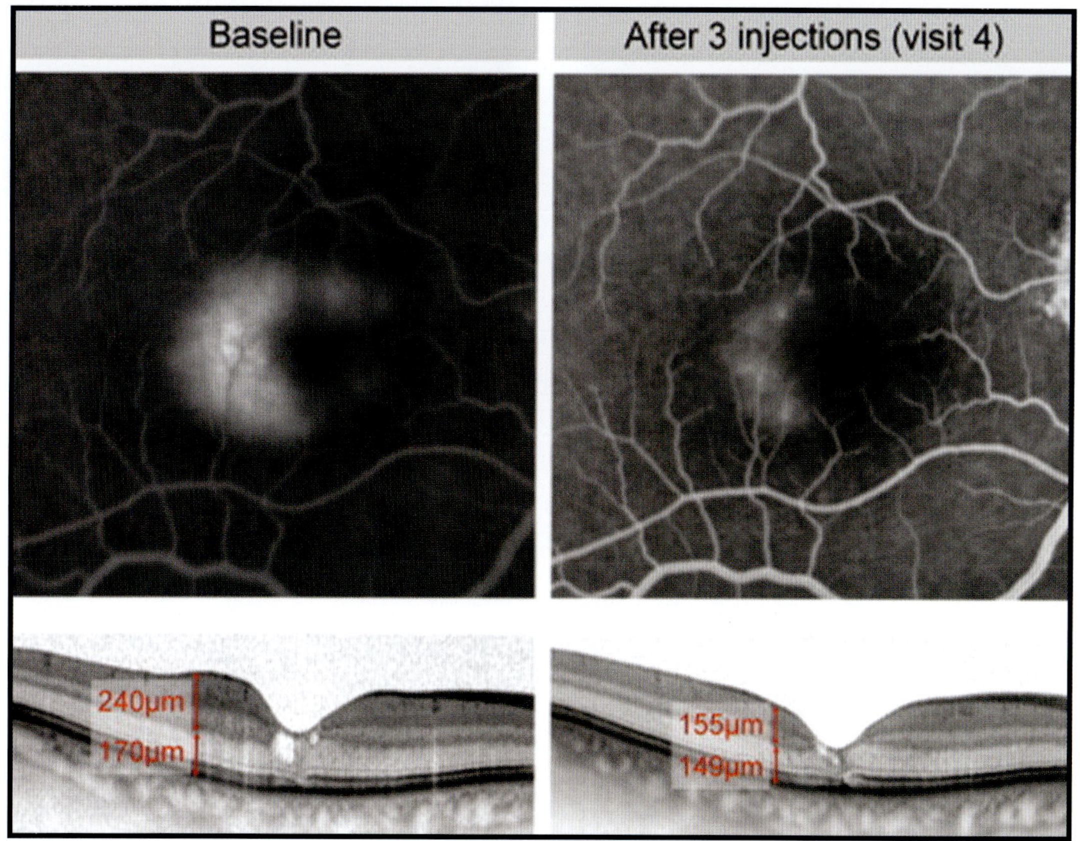

© 434

Intravitreal anti-VEGF therapy has also been attempted to reverse the vascular abnormalities and leakage in the non-proliferative stages of Mactel type 2, but there appears to be no long term functional benefit to VEGF blockade. Here is an example of a patient treated with intravitreal ranibizumab with reduced leakage and decreased retinal thickness after three injections.

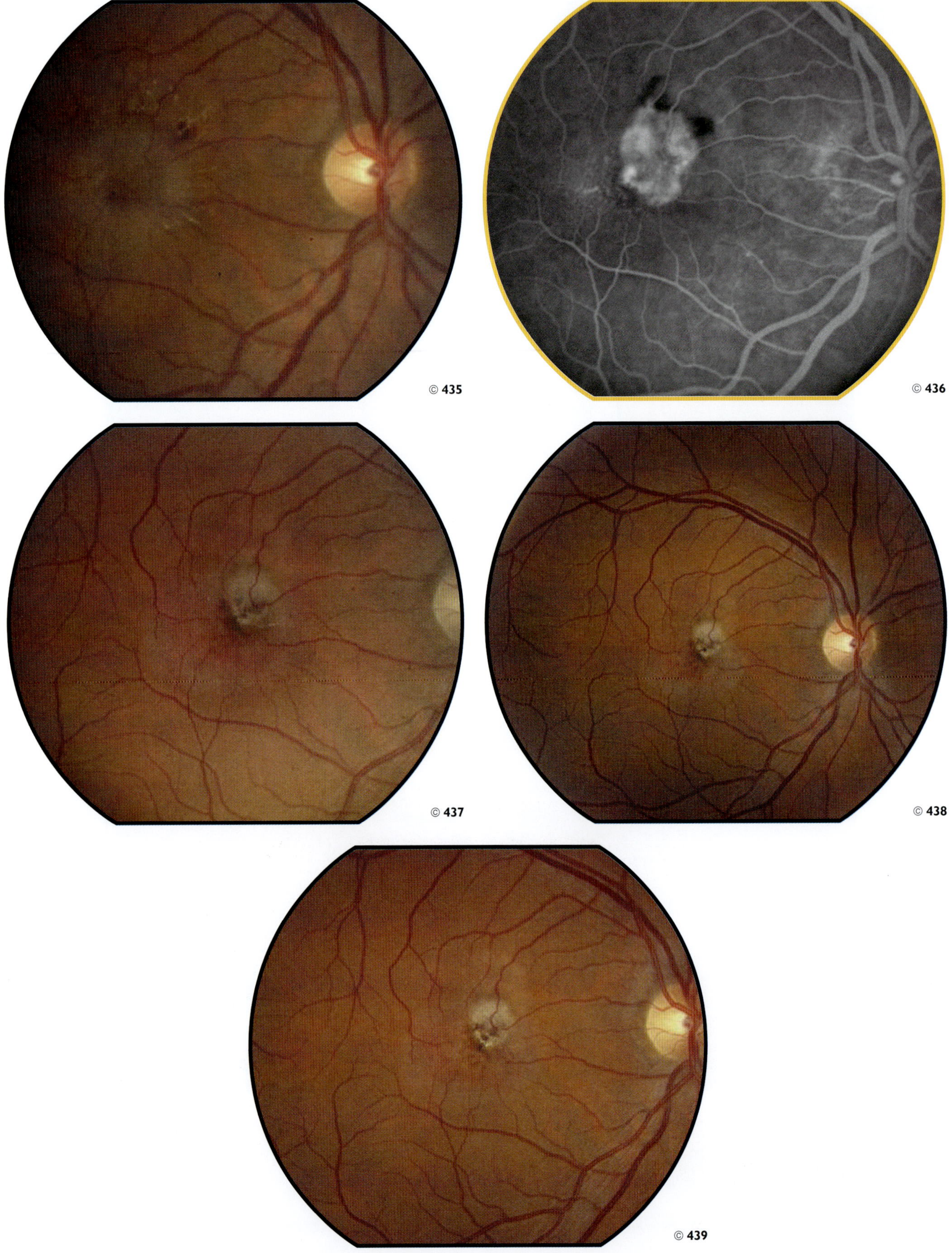

This patient developed subretinal neovascularization in the right eye *(top row)* and received 15 consecutive monthly bevacizumab injections. After 12 months, the exudation resolved and a macular scar developed. After 2 years *(middle right)* and 3 years *(bottom)* the scar stabilized with no evidence of recurrence.

Radiation Retinopathy

Radiation retinopathy may occur from direct radiation treatment of the head, neck, or total body. The retinal abnormalities induced by radiation are similar to the microvascular findings in other diseases such as diabetes, venous occlusive disease, and even primary telangiectatic disorders. Retinal hemorrhages, CWS, perivascular sheathing, macular edema, and neovascularization may develop. In some patients, radiation can induce choroidal and optic nerve complications as well.

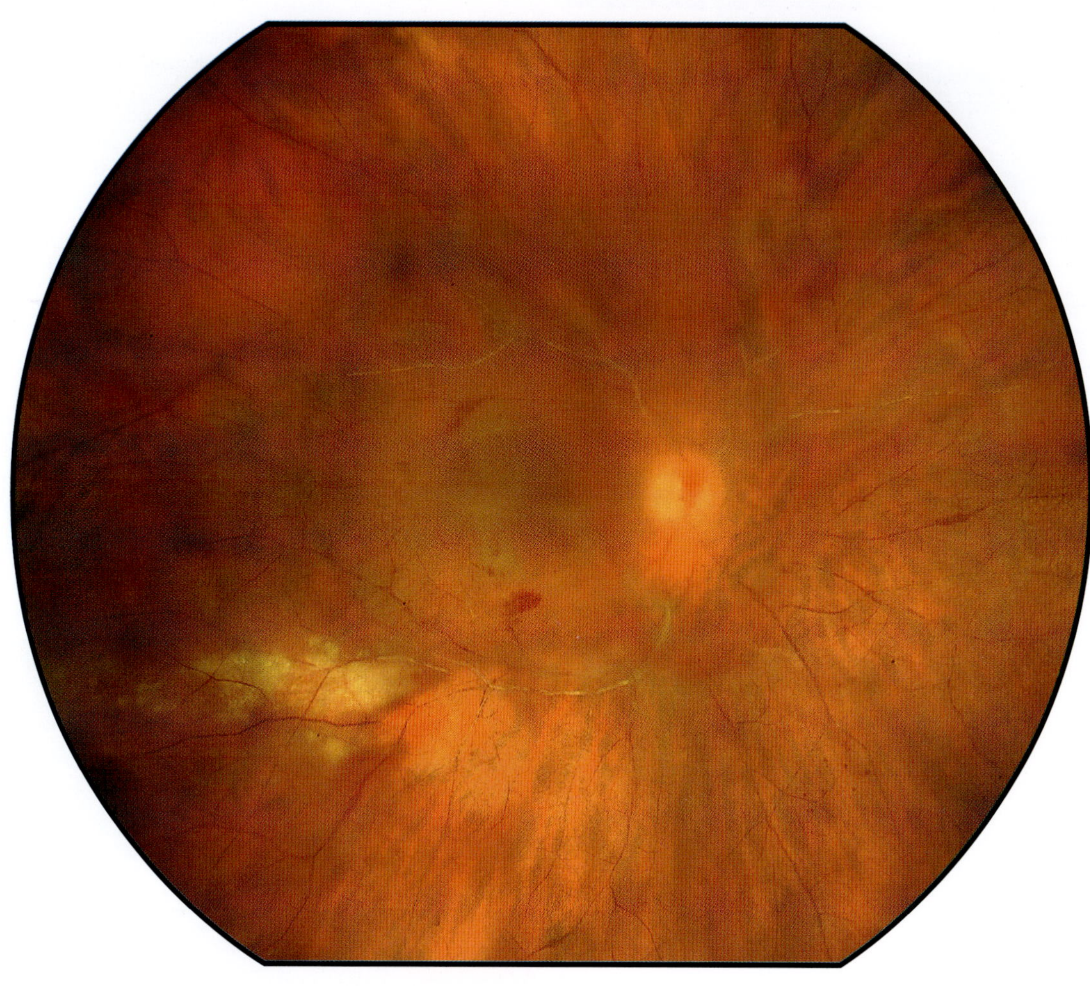

This patient received radiation for a brain tumor. Note the retinal hemorrhages and exudates, sheathed vessels, and telangiectatic and aneurysmal abnormalities. Early optic nerve atrophy may also be present.

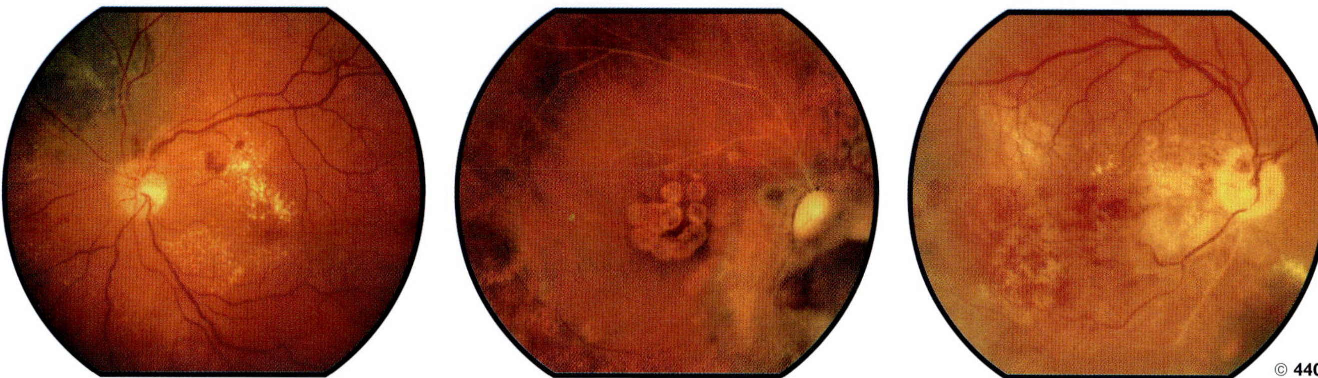

© 440

This patient *(left)* had proton beam irradiation for a choroidal melanoma. Radiation retinopathy with intraretinal hemorrhages, lipid exudation, and macular edema are present. Note the irradiated choroidal melanoma superonasal to the optic disc *(left)*. Note the vascular sheathing secondary to radiation retinopathy *(right)* in this second case. Optic nerve head atrophy is present and a treated choroidal melanoma is noted at the inferonasal border of the nerve. *Courtesy of Dr. Evangelos Gragoudas*

This patient developed a pale optic disc, intraretinal hemorrhages, macular edema, and possible inferotemporal BRVO following proton beam irradiation for a choroidal melanoma. Note the sheathed vessel inferiorly near the irradiated choroidal melanoma.

© 441

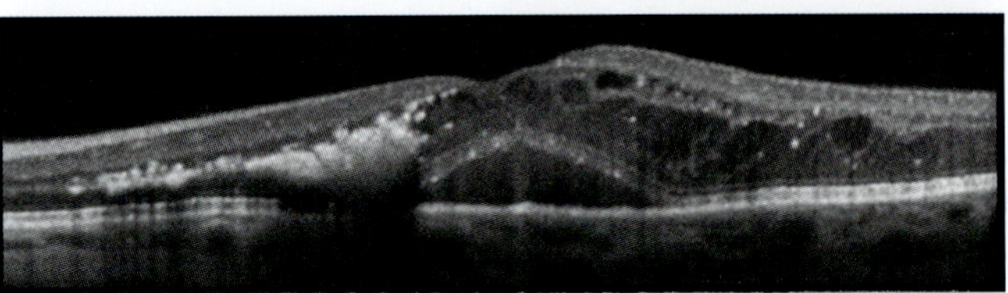

© 442

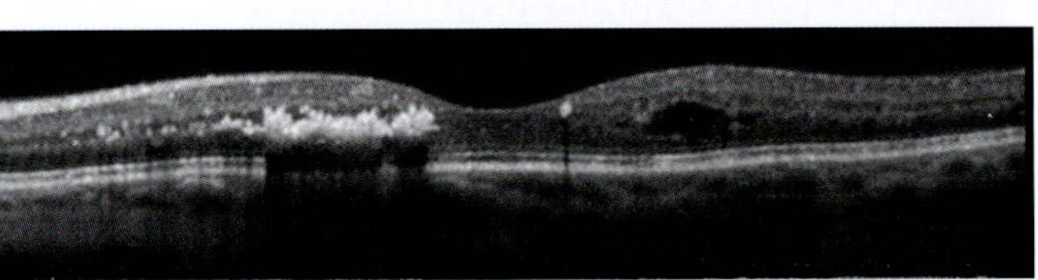

© 443

This patient developed significant macular edema and lipid exudates after receiving plaque brachytherapy for a choroidal melanoma in the temporal periphery of the left eye *(top and middle)*. The lower OCT image shows marked improvement of the edema following one intravitreal injection of bevacizumab, although persistent exudates are still noted at the level of the outer plexiform layer immediately beneath the deep capillary plexus.

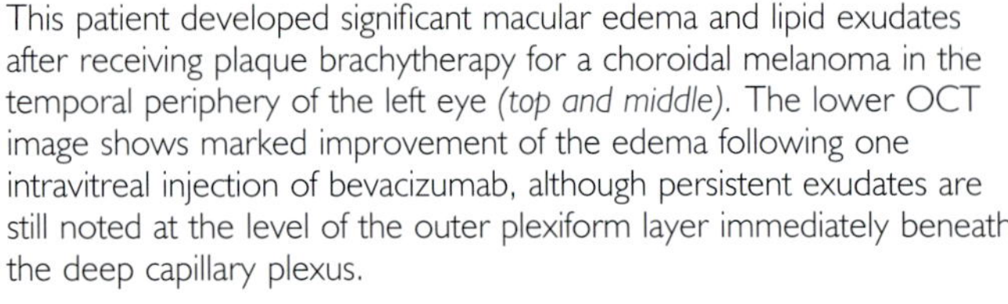

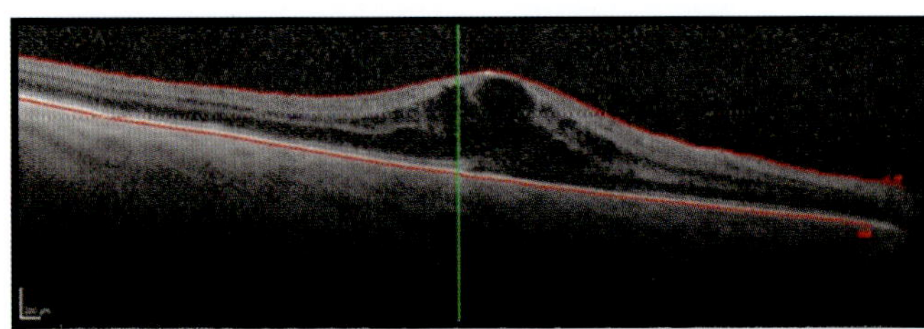

© 444

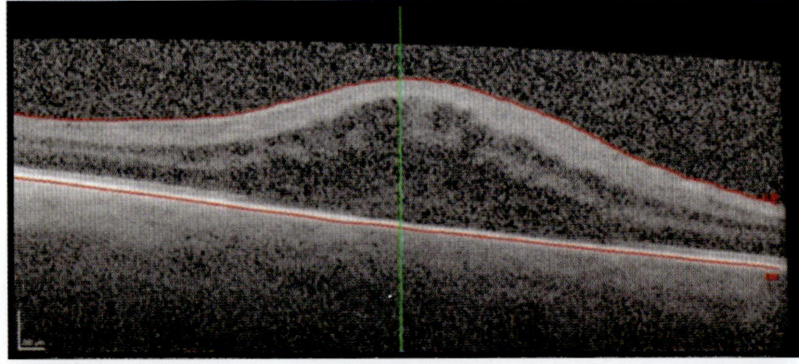

© 445

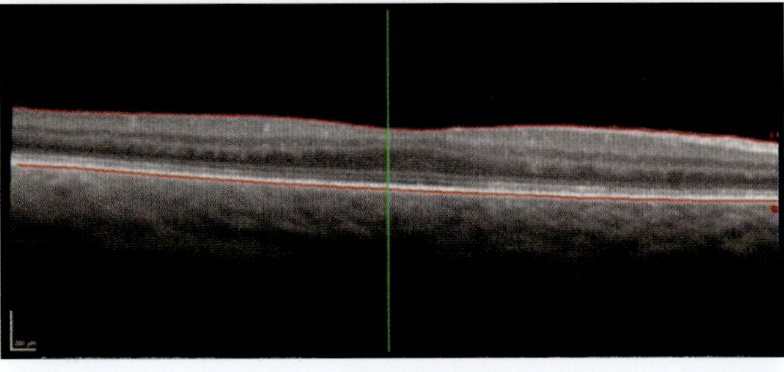

© 446

Note the presence of severe cystoid macular edema in this patient after plaque brachytherapy for uveal melanoma *(top)*. After five months of intravitreal bevacizumab therapy there was no improvement *(middle)*. Following intravitreal triamcinolone therapy, the macular edema resolved and the vision improved *(bottom)*.

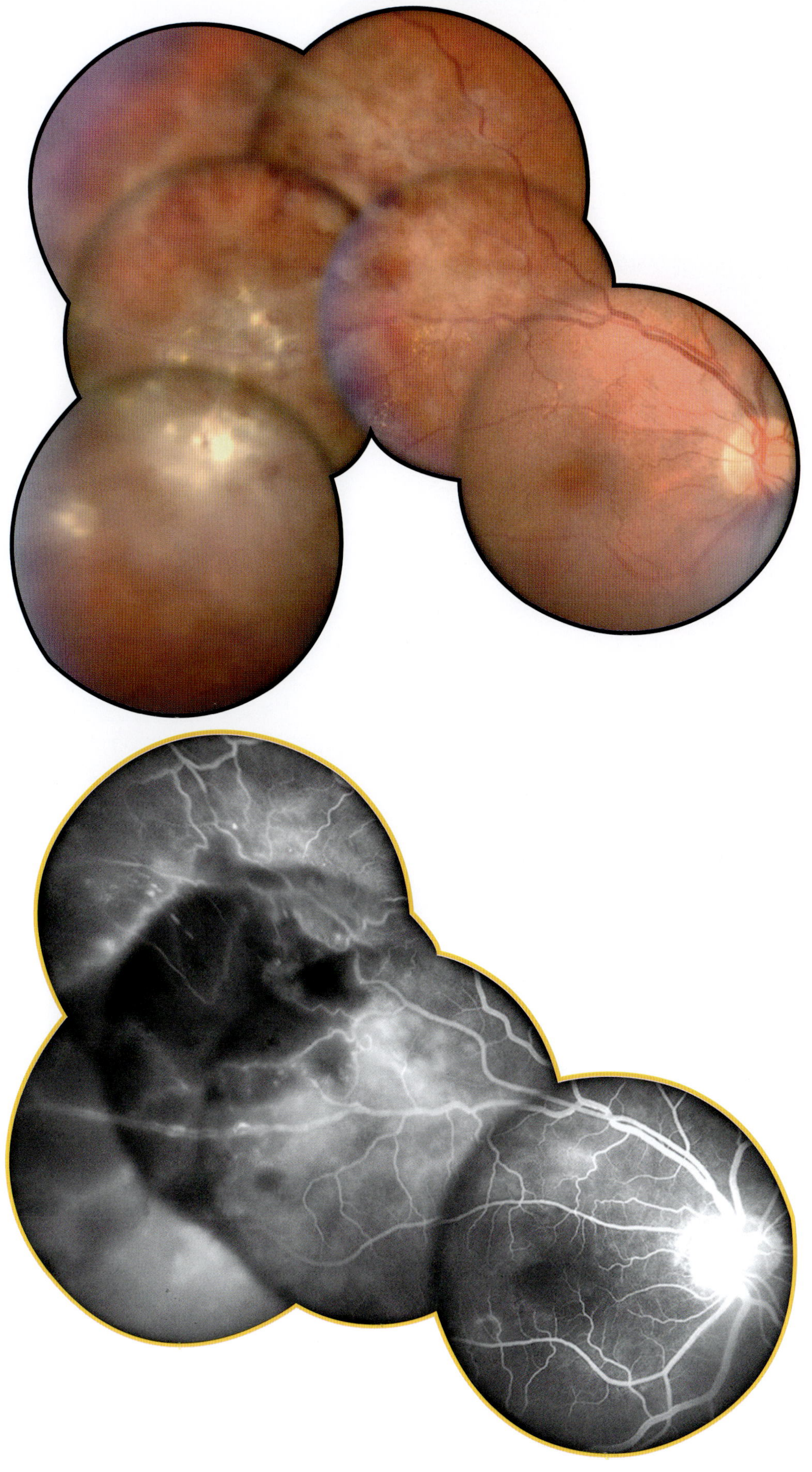

This patient demonstrated severe radiation retinopathy. There is widespread ischemic and exudative disease with a large zonal area of retinal vascular non-perfusion. Leakage of the optic nerve on fluorescein angiography is also present. *Courtesy of Dr. Sanjay Logani*

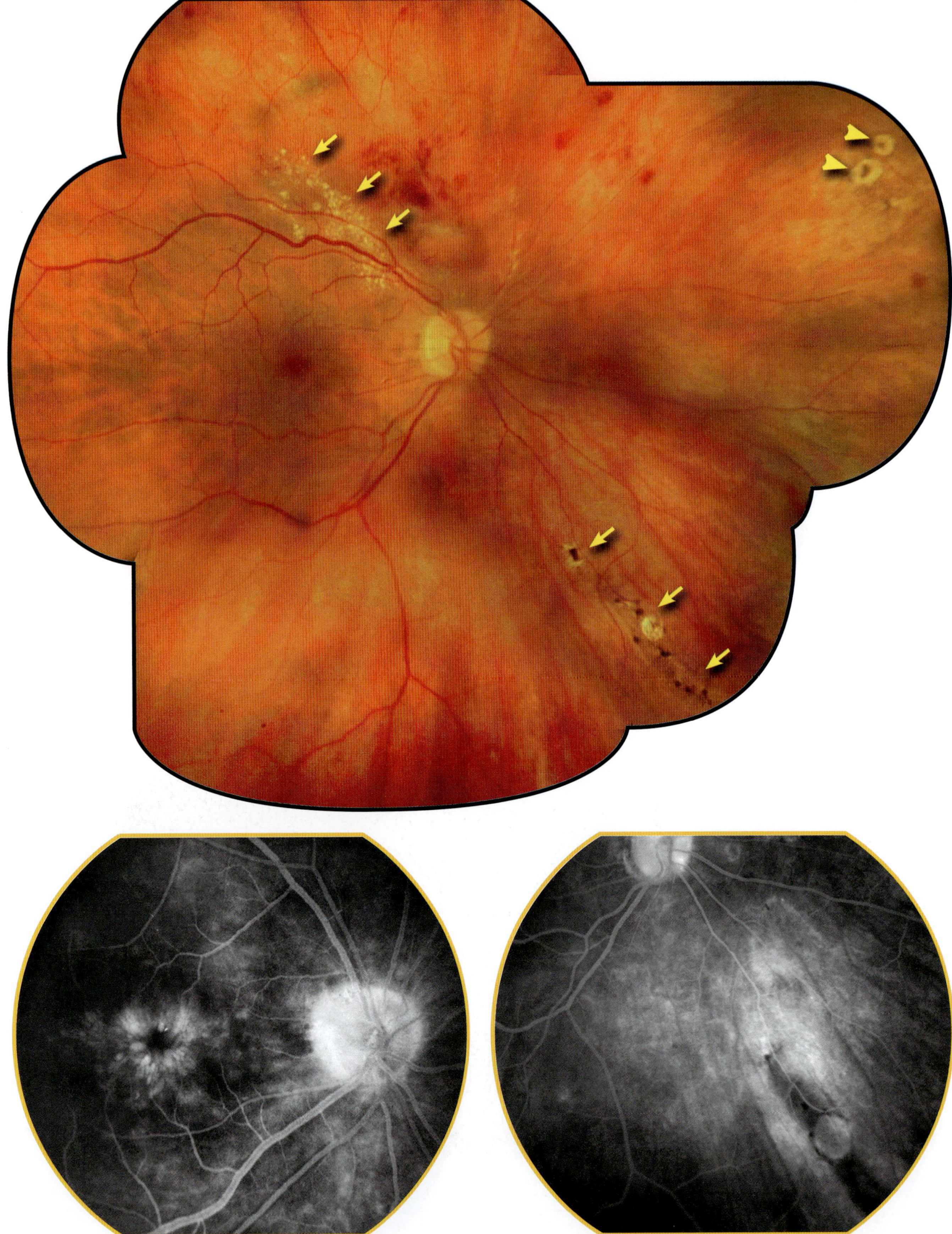

This patient received radiation therapy for sinus malignancy. Thirty years after radiation treatment, the patient began to lose vision due to mild papillitis and macular edema, noted in the FA *(lower left)*. The fundus showed additional abnormalities, including a BRVO along the superotemporal arcade with associated lipid deposition *(upper arrows)*. There are also visible choroidal abnormalities, including a linear atrophic and pigmentary scar or Siegrist streak *(lower arrows)* and Elschnig spots *(arrowheads)*, also seen on the FA *(lower right)*.

Eales Disease (Idiopathic Peripheral Vascular Occlusive Disease)

Eales disease affects the peripheral vasculature, which leads to peripheral non-perfusion and ischemia which can be complicated by pre-retinal neovascularization and vitreous hemorrhage. The spectrum of disease may include perivasculitis or phlebitis, capillary aneurysms, shunt vessels, and macular edema.

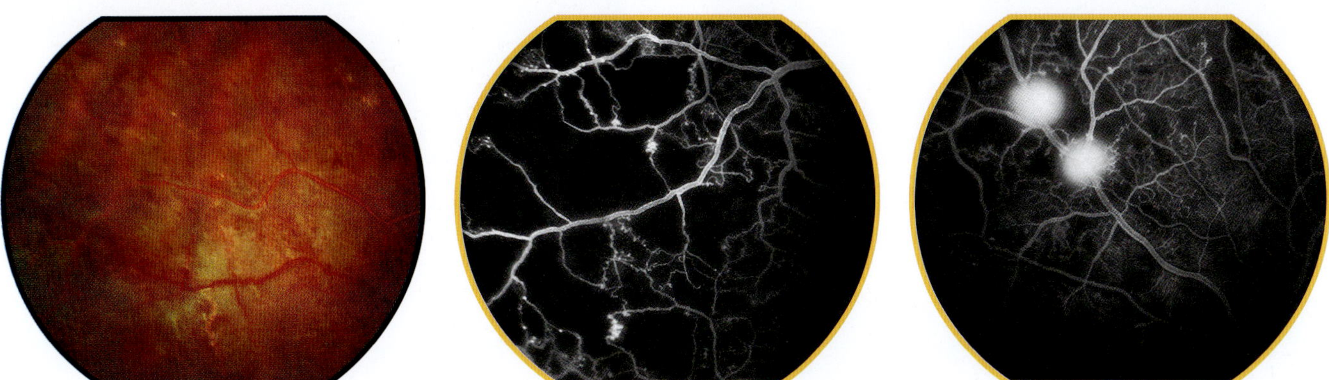

This patient has retinal hemorrhage due to Eales disease with capillary non-perfusion and ischemia and retinal neovascularization demonstrated on the FA. There is no distinct junction between perfused and non-perfused retina, as seen typically in sickle-cell retinopathy.

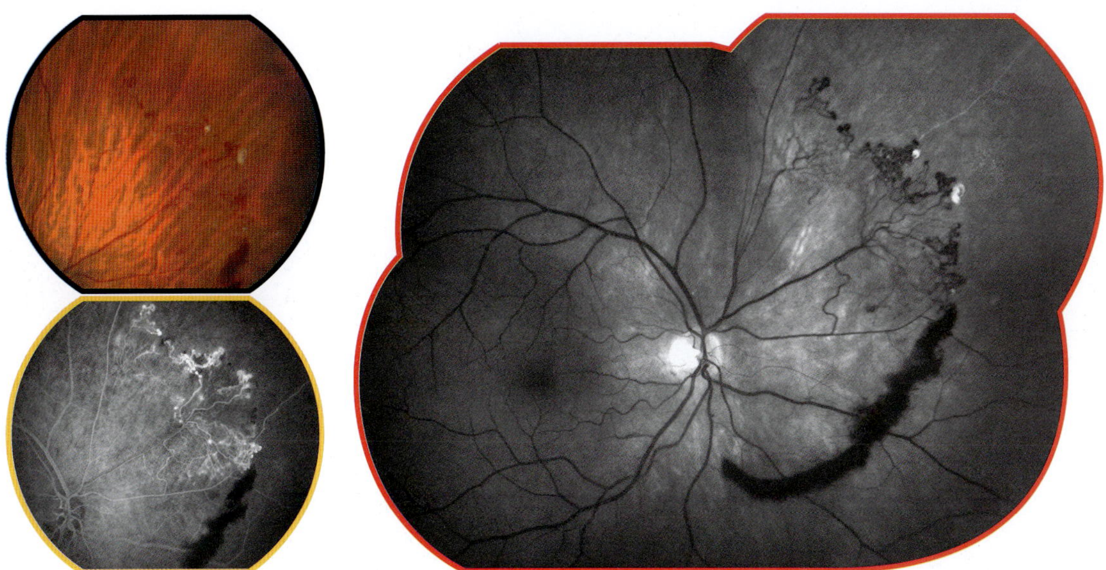

This patient has Eales disease with a ring of nasal retinal neovascularization and pre-retinal hemorrhage. The red-free photograph demonstrates these abnormalities better than the clinical photograph *(upper left)*. The FA *(lower left)* illustrates the neovascularization and peripheral ischemia and non-perfusion.

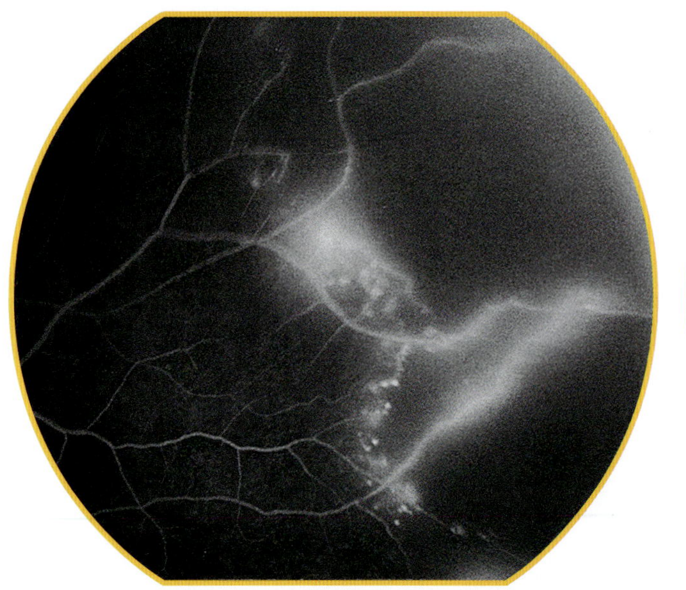

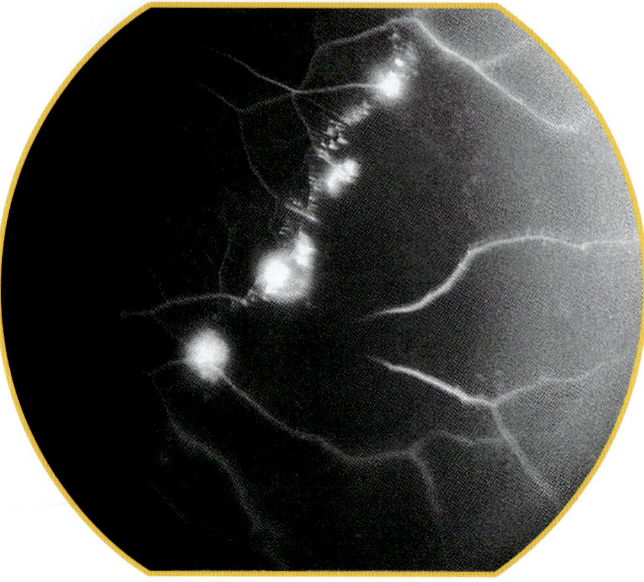

The late-stage angiogram in these two patients with Eales disease shows early retinal neovascularization and peripheral retinal vascular ischemia and non-perfusion. Staining of retinal vessels, not seen in hemoglobinopathies such as sickle-cell retinopathy, is appreciated and may also be seen in proliferative disorders secondary to granulomatous systemic diseases such as sarcoidosis or tuberculosis.

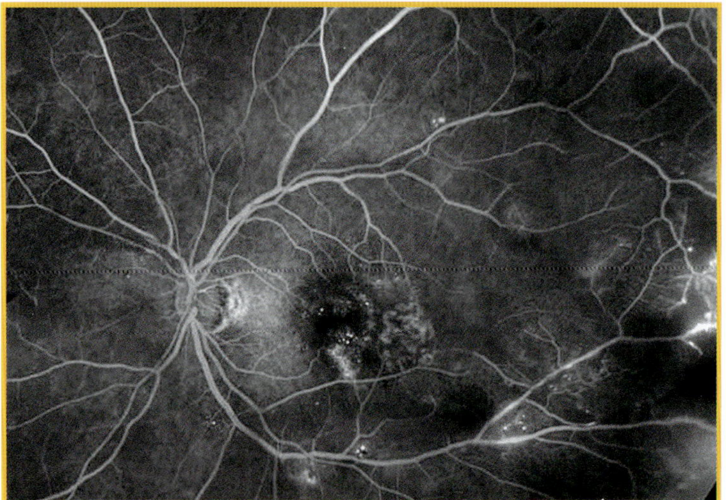

This widefield FA illustrates a case of idiopathic peripheral vascular occlusive disease or Eales disease.

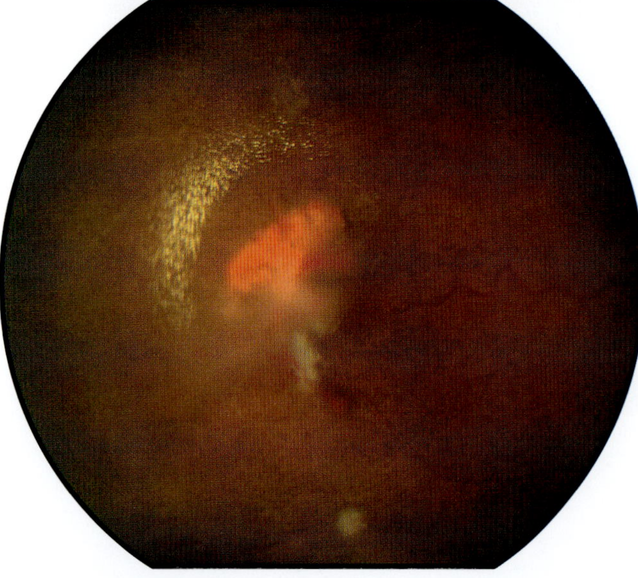

In this case of Eales disease, there is peripheral neovascularization associated with a ring of lipid exudation.

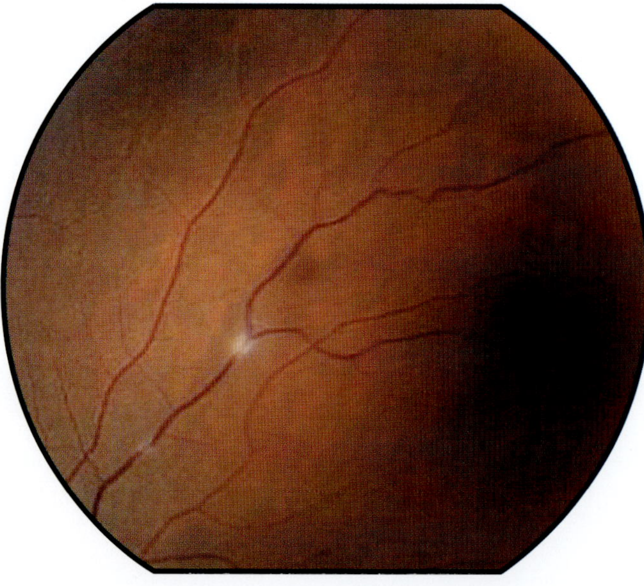

In this case of Eales disease, there is sheathing of the retinal vein suggestive of a multifocal phlebitis. These lesions are similar to the "candle wax drippings" of sarcoid retinal disease. This case may be alternatively classified as an intermediate uveitis with phlebitis. *Courtesy of Dr. Joseph Terry*

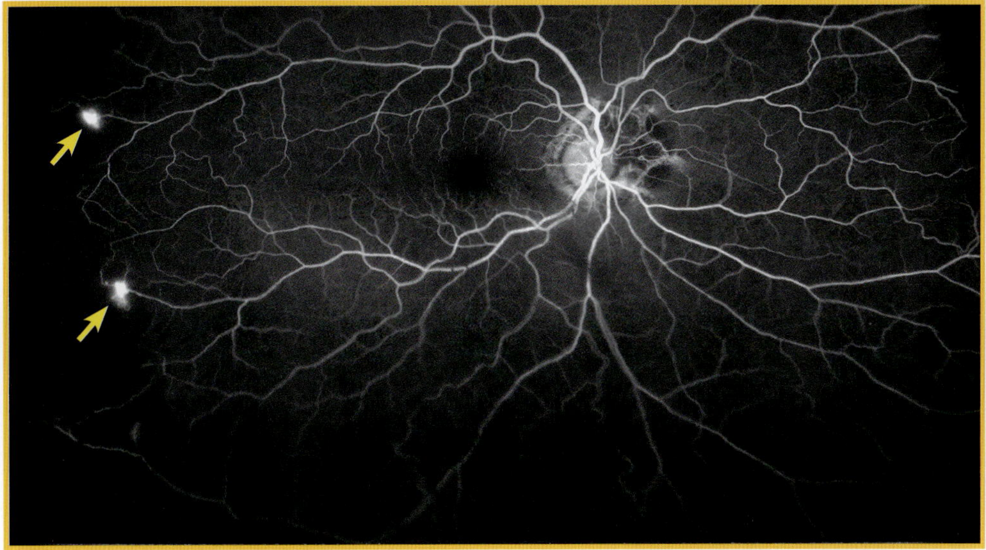

This ultra-widefield FA illustrates peripheral ischemia and non-perfusion and retinal neovascularization *(arrows)* in this patient with idiopathic peripheral vascular occlusive disease or Eales disease.

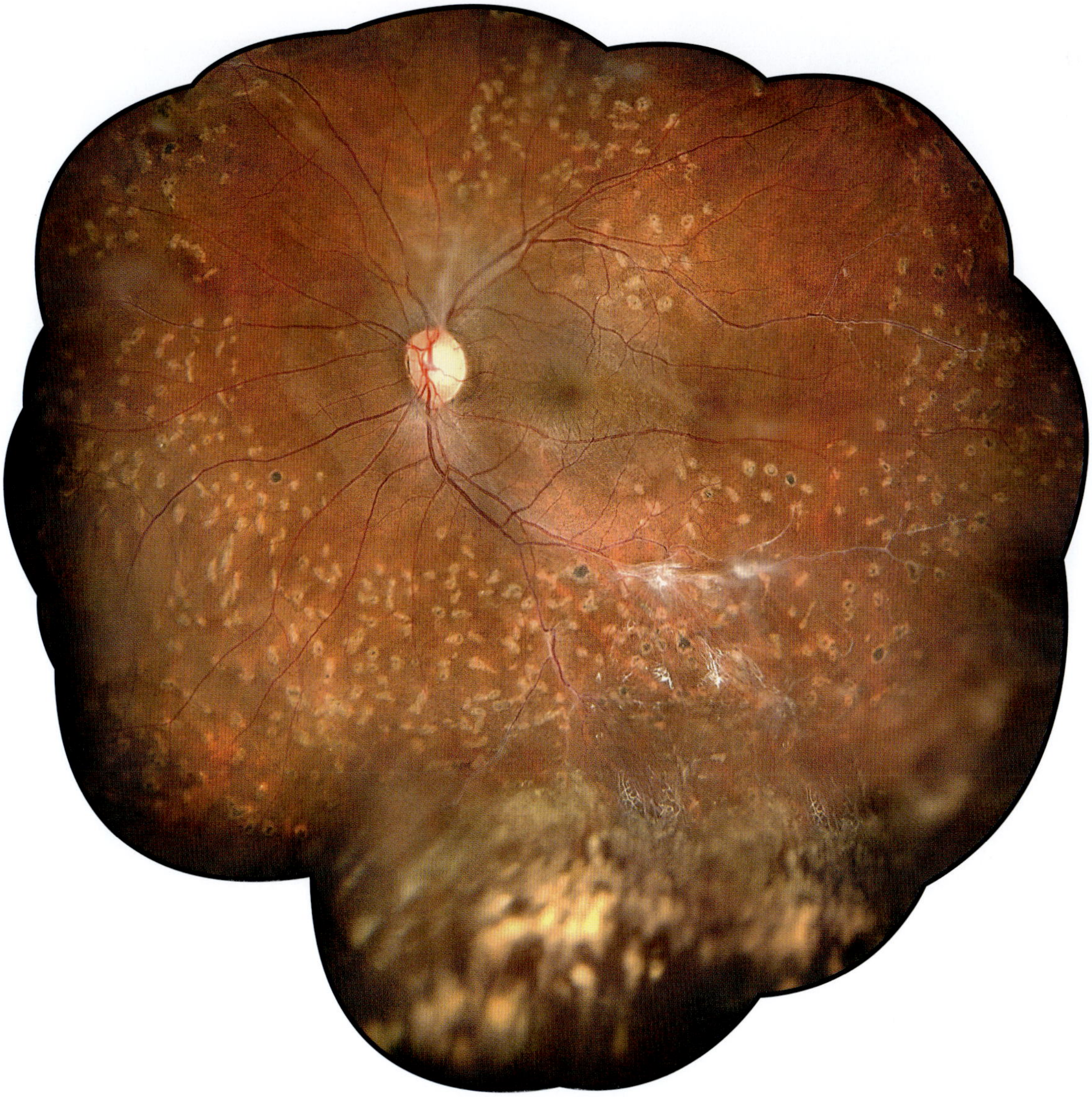

In this patient with idiopathic peripheral vascular occlusive disease (or Eales disease), scatter laser photocoagulation has been administered to treat ischemic retinopathy. Note the presence of resolving inferior vitreous hemorrhage.

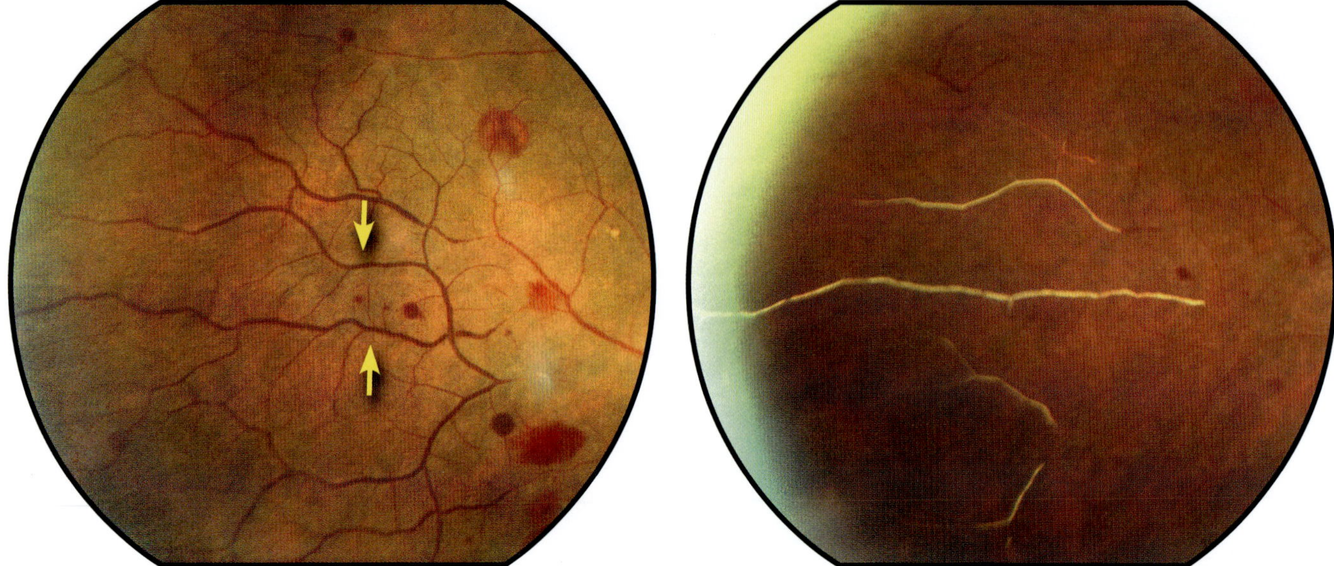

Note the engorged peripheral retinal vessels in this patient with Eales disease *(arrows)*. Few associated retinal hemorrhages are also present *(left)*. Upon follow up, the dilated vessels have assumed a yellowish appearance due to trapped blood that has become dehemoglobinized within the lumen.

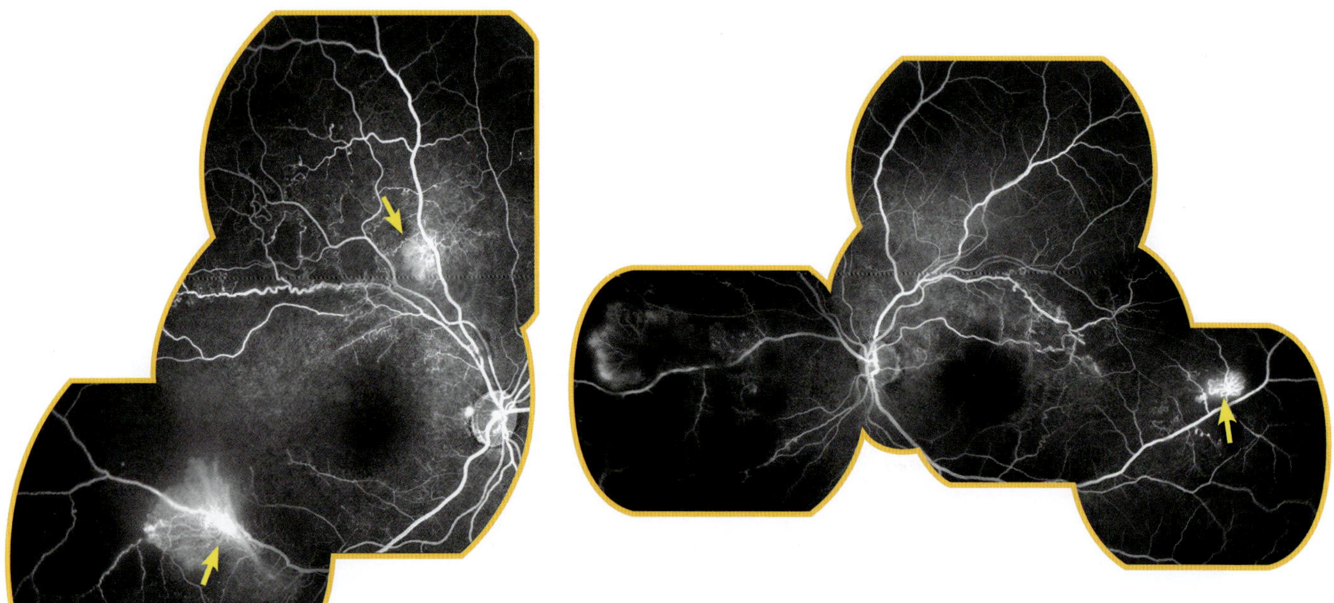

Widefield fluorescein angiography of a patient with Eales disease, which illustrates peripheral ischemia and non-perfusion and retinal neovascularization. The neovascularization in idiopathic peripheral vascular occlusive disease does not necessarily occur at the junction between perfused and non-perfused peripheral retina. It may be present along perfused vessels in the posterior pole and periphery *(arrows)*. *Courtesy of Dr. Irene Barbazetto*

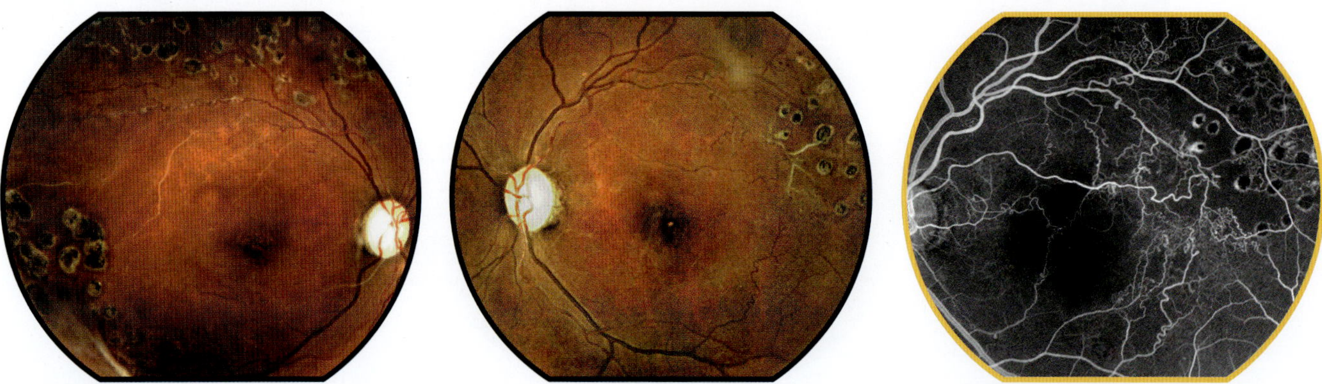

The same patient with Eales disease demonstrated resolved neovascularization with laser photocoagulation therapy. Note the presence of associated optic atrophy. *Courtesy of Dr. Irene Barbazetto*

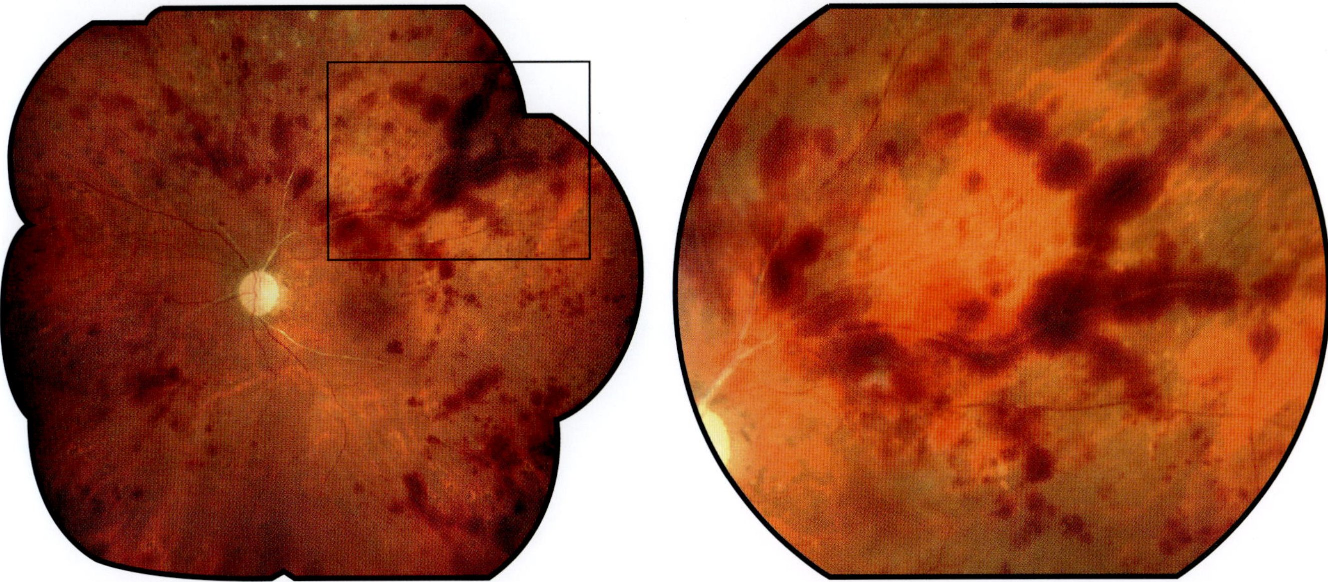

Idiopathic peripheral vascular occlusive disease or Eales disease can be associated with significant retinal hemorrhage as seen in this patient. The magnified image shows presumed ischemia present between the large, irregular branching areas of blood. The optic nerve is pale and peripapillary retinal vessels are sheathed.

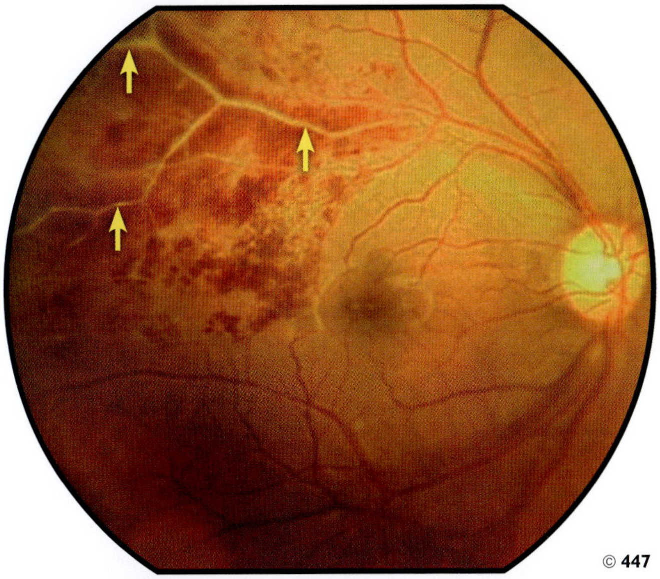

© 447

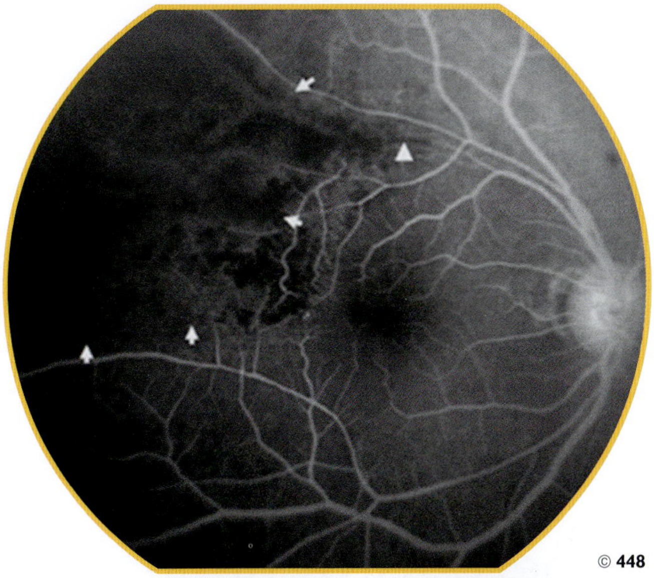

© 448

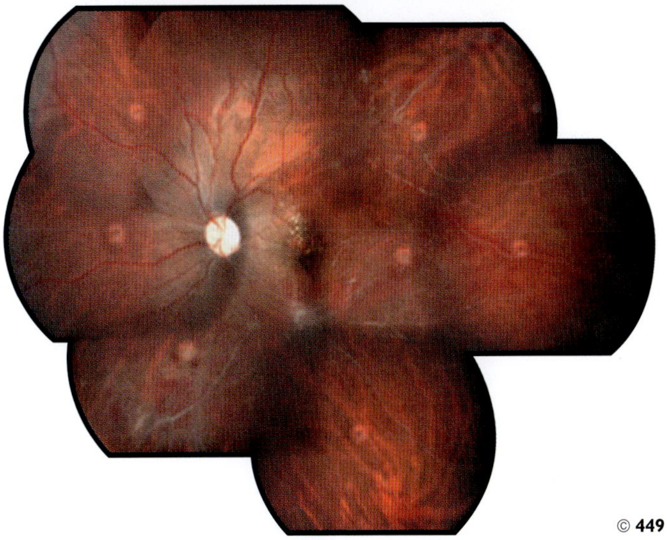

© 449

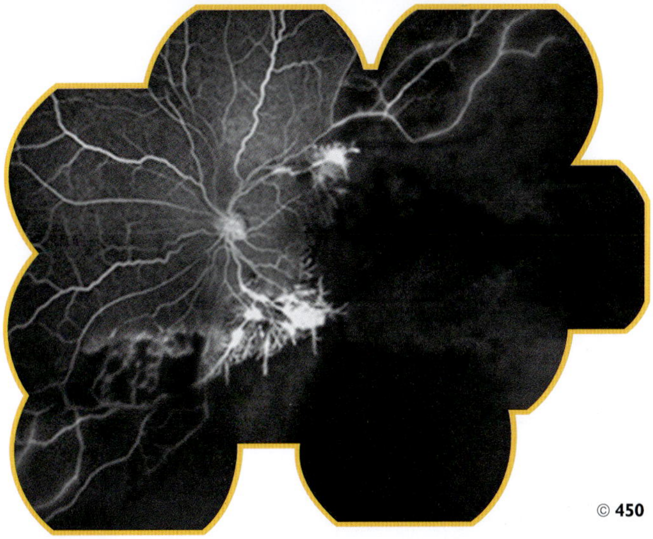

© 450

This patient with Eales disease has bilateral findings typical of the disease. The right eye *(top images)* has an obliterated vessel with a corresponding area of capillary non-perfusion *(arrows, top left and arrowheads, top right)*. The lower widefield montages illustrate several sclerotic vessels in the left eye. The corresponding widefield angiogram reveals a large zone of capillary non-perfusion and adjacent retinal neovascularization.

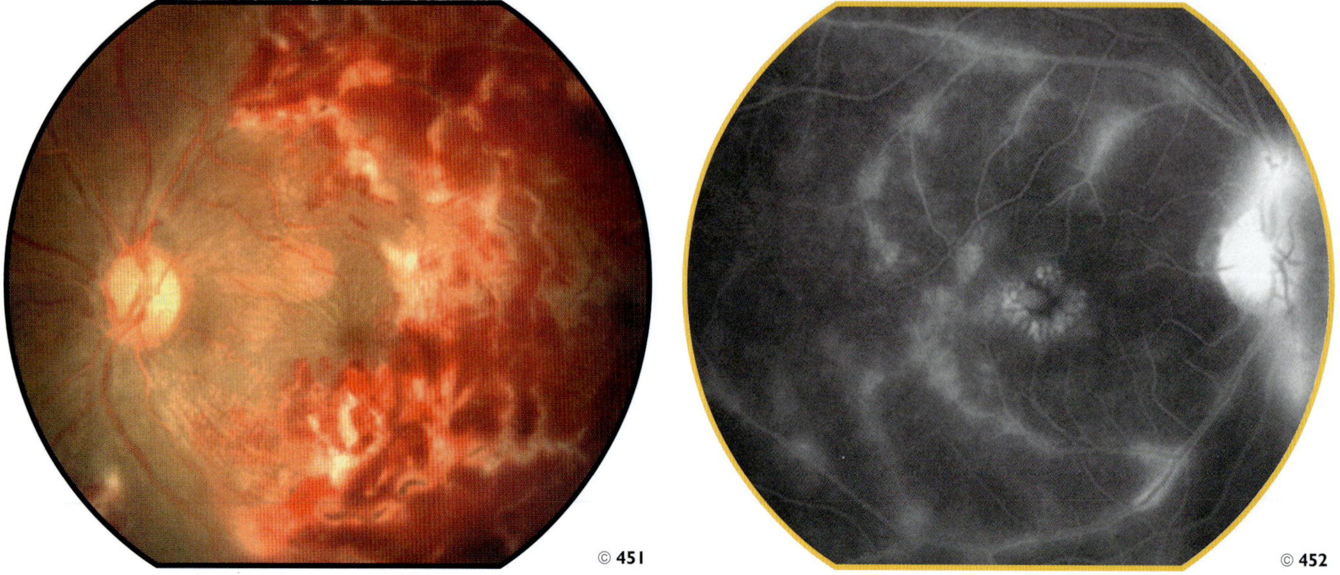

Eales disease can infrequently involve the posterior pole as seen in this patient. Hemorrhagic retinal vasculitis is noted in the left eye. The FA of the right eye shows staining of vessels and cystoid macular edema.

Retinal Vascular Manifestations of Systemic Disease

A number of systemic diseases may be associated with retinal vascular complications. These range from commonly encountered disorders such as systemic hypertension and diabetes to more rarely encountered entities such as those affecting the hematologic or rheumatologic systems. Any systemic disease associated with inflammatory or thrombotic or hemorrhagic findings may cause similar manifestations in the fundus.

Hypertensive Retinopathy

Hypertensive retinopathy is a common retinal vascular abnormality that may be the result of chronic systemic hypertension (Grade 1, 2, and 3) or more acute malignant hypertension (Grade 4). These manifestations may affect the retina, the choroid, and the optic nerve.

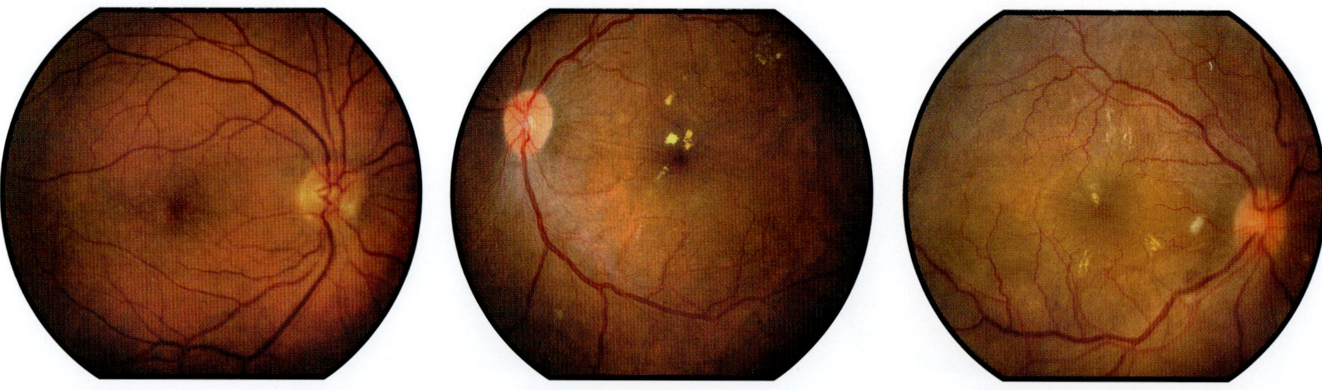

These patients have chronic hypertensive retinopathy with mild retinal venous dilation *(left)*, lipid exudation *(middle)*, and vascular abnormalities including retinal hemorrhages, CWS, and retinal edema *(right)*.

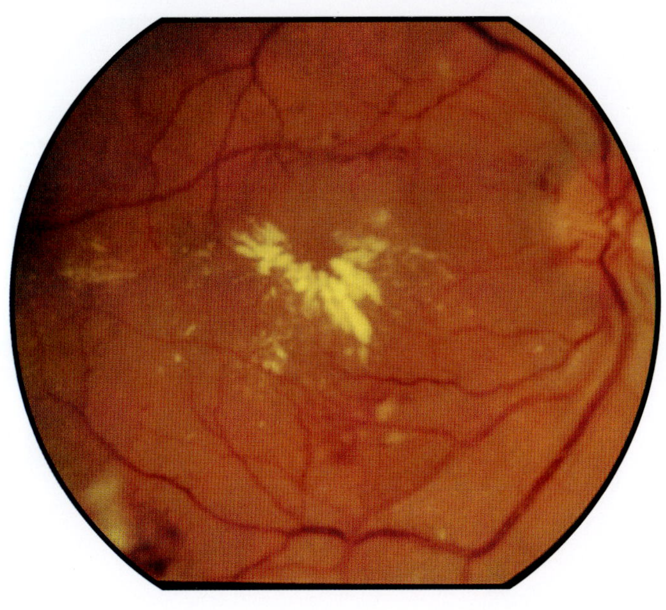

This patient presented with grade 4 hypertensive retinopathy with severe acute elevation of the blood pressure, which caused intraretinal hemorrhages, CWS, lipid exudation ("macular star"), macular edema, and optic nerve edema.

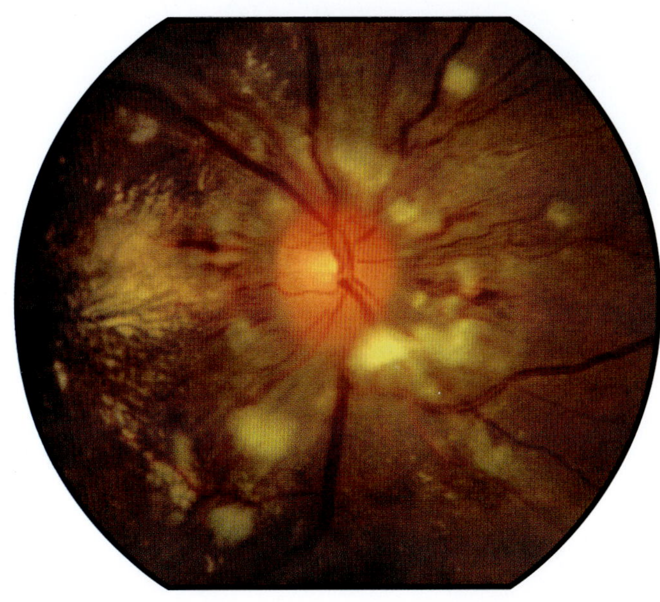

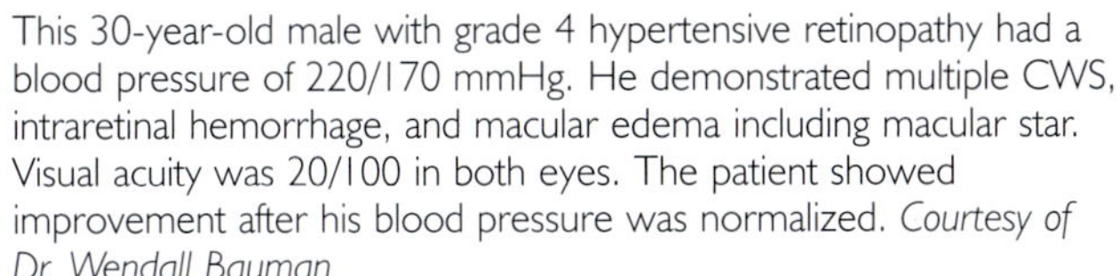

This 30-year-old male with grade 4 hypertensive retinopathy had a blood pressure of 220/170 mmHg. He demonstrated multiple CWS, intraretinal hemorrhage, and macular edema including macular star. Visual acuity was 20/100 in both eyes. The patient showed improvement after his blood pressure was normalized. *Courtesy of Dr. Wendall Bauman*

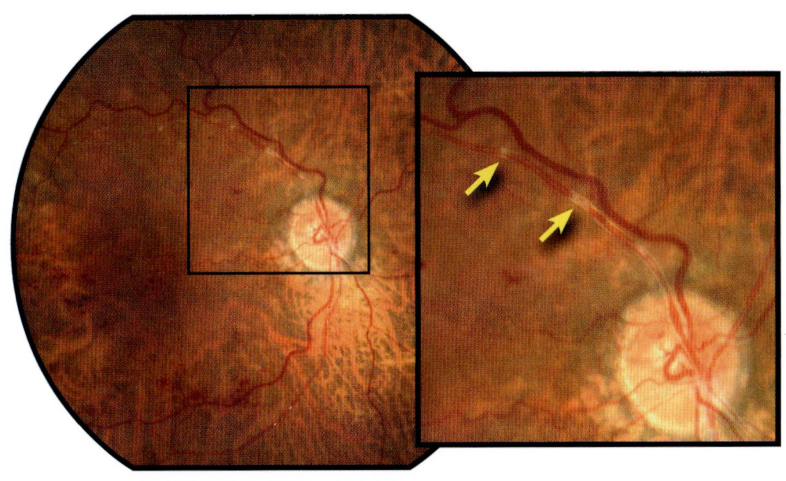

This patient demonstrates chronic systemic hypertension with abnormalities of the arteriolar vasculature. There are focal areas of sheathing, vessel caliber irregularities, arterial-venous crossing defects, and a few retinal hemorrhages. In the inset, note the areas of arteriolar sheathing *(arrows)*. There is also a zone of pallor of the nerve head inferotemporally due to ischemic disease.

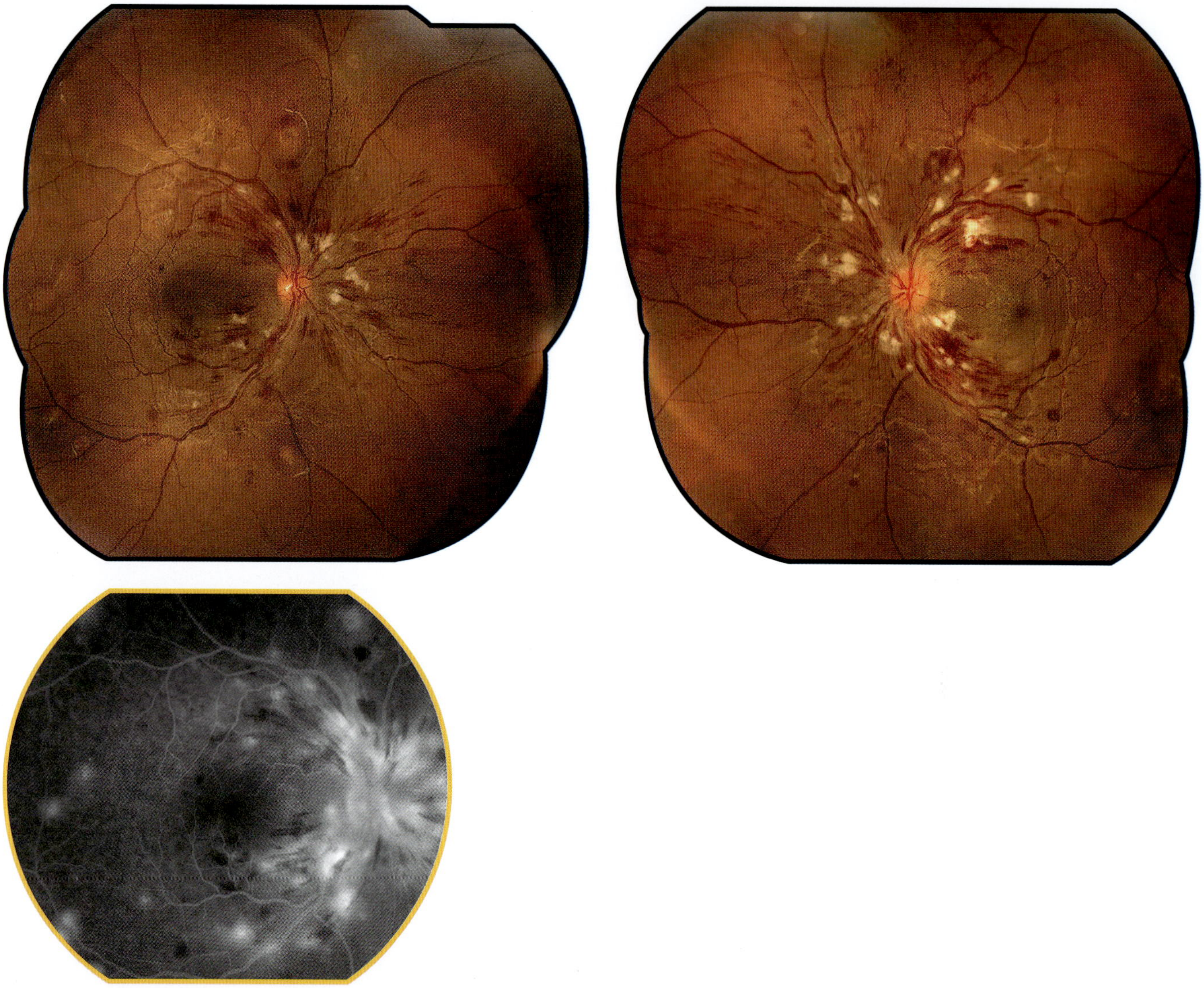

This patient has malignant hypertension and grade 4 hypertensive retinopathy with multiple CWS and retinal hemorrhages scattered throughout the fundus, as well as edema and leakage of the optic nerve on fluorescein angiography. *Courtesy of Dr. Jaclyn Kovach*

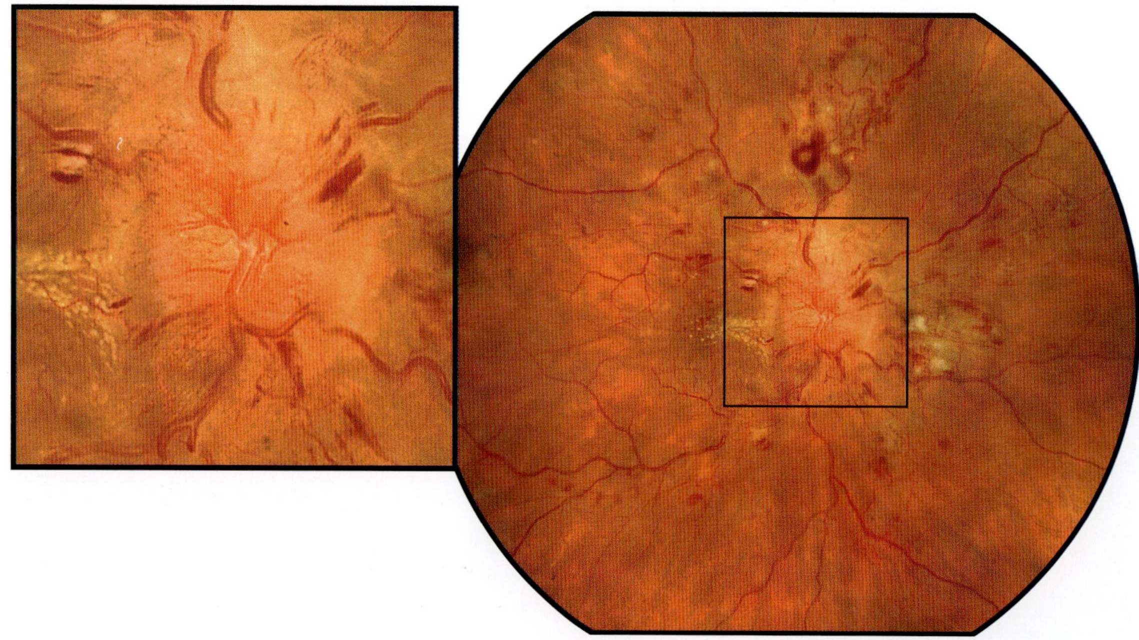

This patient has acute-on-chronic hypertension with associated disc edema. Significant venous tortuosity, arteriolar narrowing, and swelling of the optic nerve are noted.

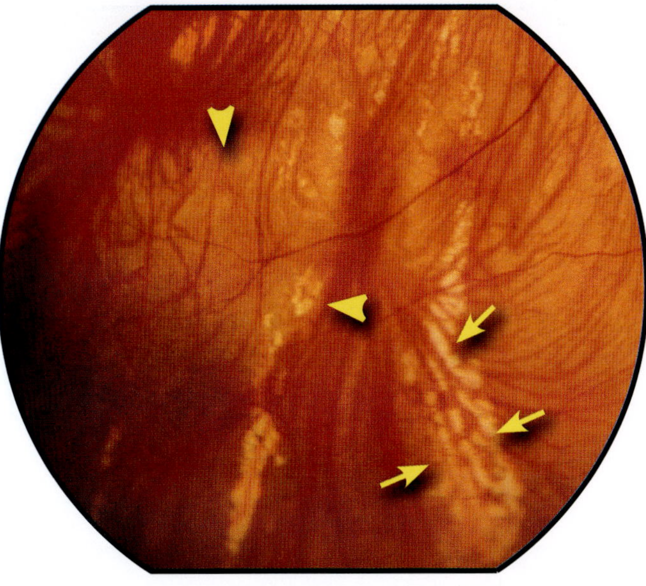

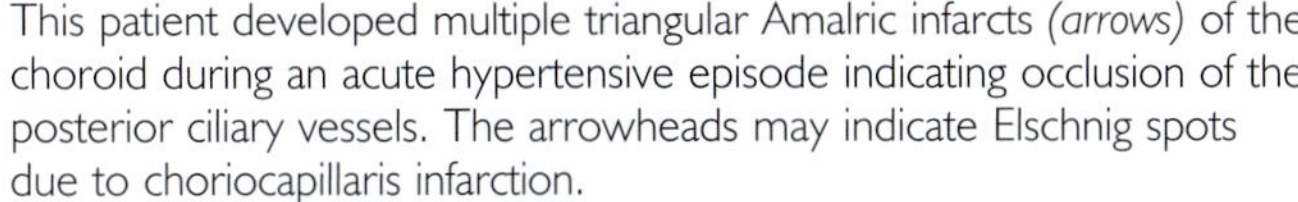

This patient developed multiple triangular Amalric infarcts *(arrows)* of the choroid during an acute hypertensive episode indicating occlusion of the posterior ciliary vessels. The arrowheads may indicate Elschnig spots due to choriocapillaris infarction.

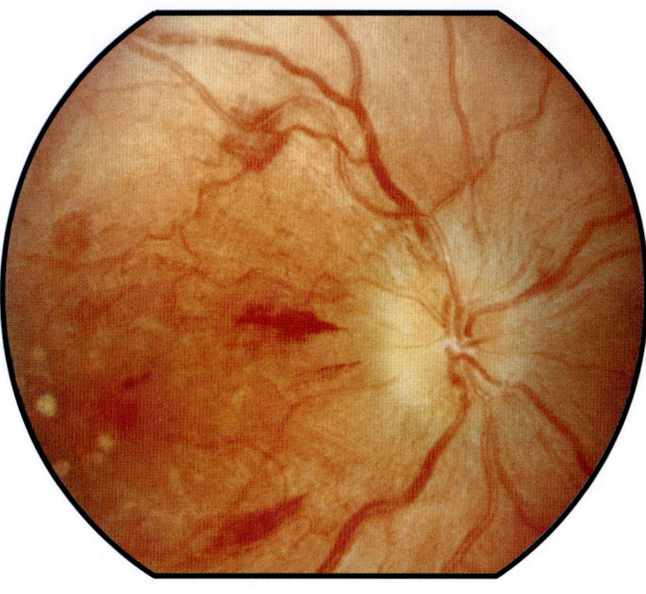

This patient has malignant hypertension and grade 4 hypertensive retinopathy with optic disc edema and flame-shaped nerve fiber layer hemorrhages.

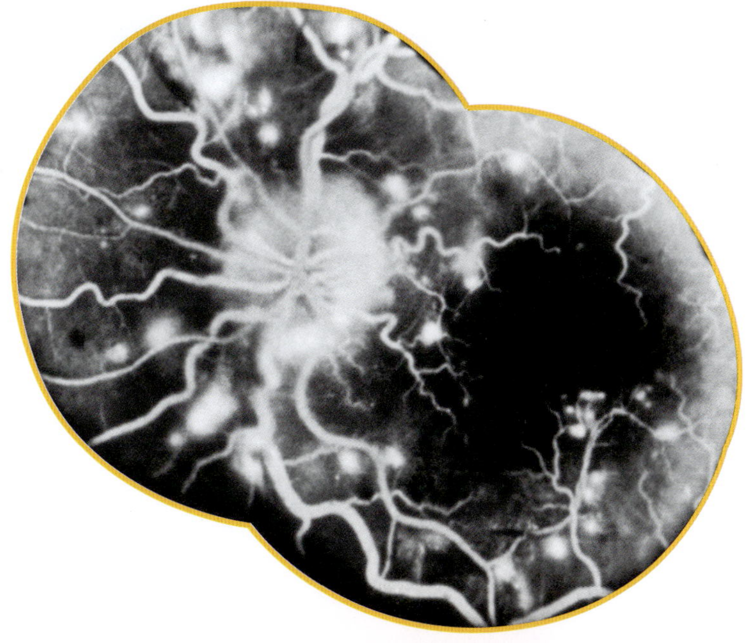

Note the presence of disc edema and leakage in this case of malignant hypertension.

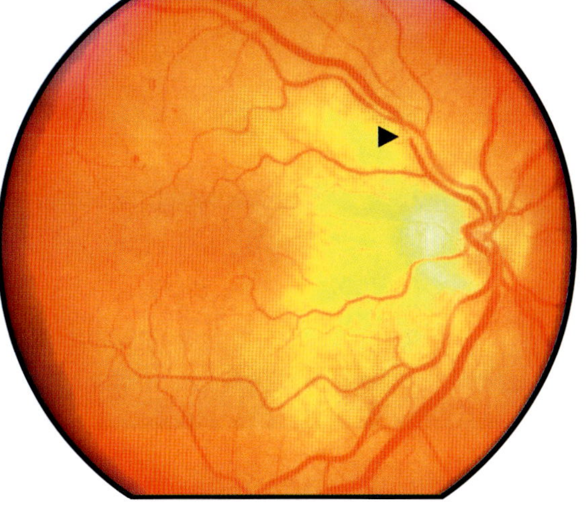

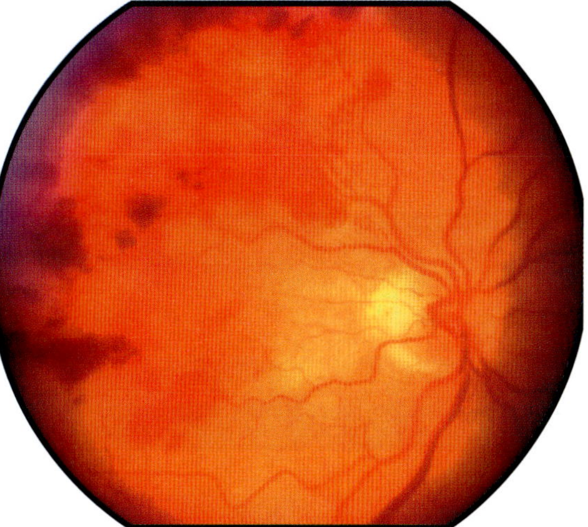

This patient with hypertensive retinopathy showed prominent arteriolar-venous (AV) nicking *(arrowhead)* and subsequently suffered a BRVO of this branch retinal vein.

Diabetic Retinopathy

Diabetic retinopathy is a major cause of blindness in the US and worldwide. It is clinically manifested by a retinal microvasculopathy that is disease duration dependent. Hypertension, renal disease, blood dyscrasias, and hyperlipidemia may all exacerbate retinal disease, but glycemic control is the single most important determinant of disease progression. Hyperglycemia causes progresses microvascular dysfunction leading to aneurysmal changes and ischemia of the retina. The progressive elaboration of VEGF leads to exudation due to breakdown in the inner blood retinal barrier and eventual vasoproliferation. Vitreous hemorrhage, pre-retinal fibrosis, and tractional detachment may complicate retinal neovascularization, leading to severe vision loss and even blindness. While vitreous hemorrhage is the most common cause of blindness, macular edema is the most common cause of moderate vision loss.

Nonproliferative Diabetic Retinopathy

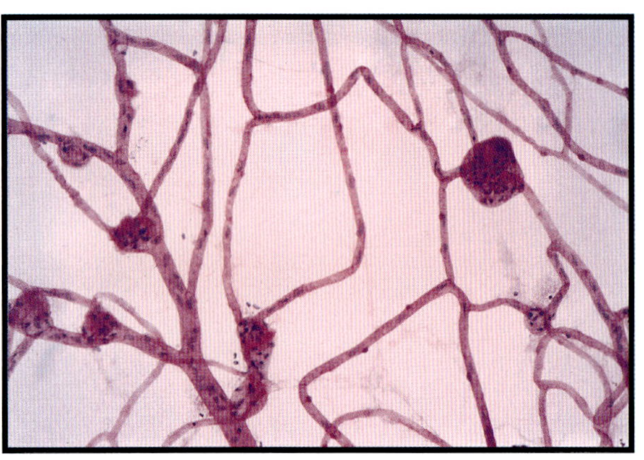

© 453

Trypsin digest in this patient with nonproliferative diabetic retinopathy (NPDR) illustrates the presence of microaneurysms and the absence of pericytes.

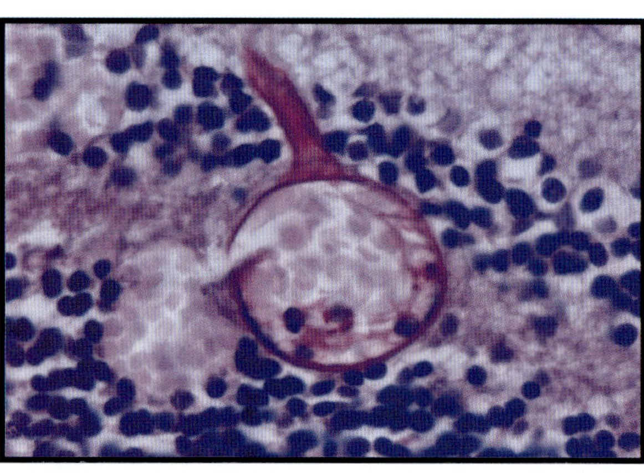

© 454

Capillary microaneurysms are a principal feature of diabetic retinopathy and the first manifestation of retinal disease. Histopathologic examination shows a microaneurysm associated with an area of hemorrhage.

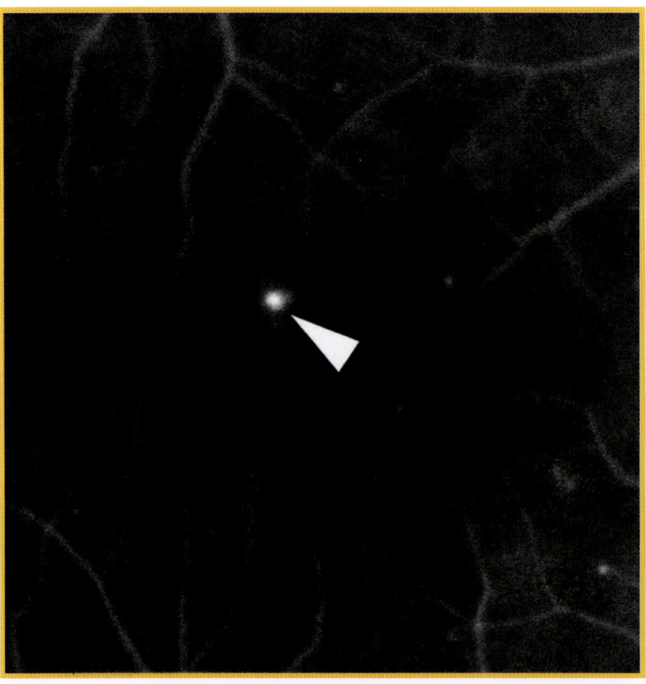

© 455

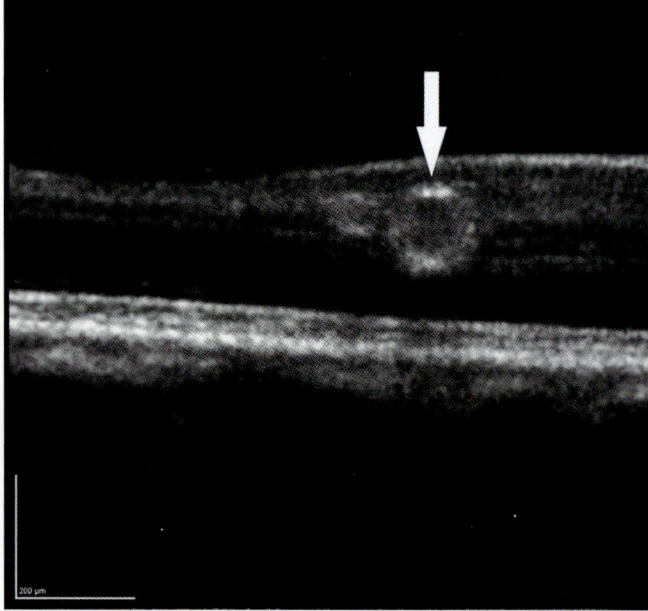

© 456

Microaneurysms appear as hyperfluorescent foci that leak on fluorescein angiography *(arrowhead, left)*. The same microaneurysm on spectral-domain OCT appears as an intraretinal hyper-reflective oval lesion *(arrow, right)*.

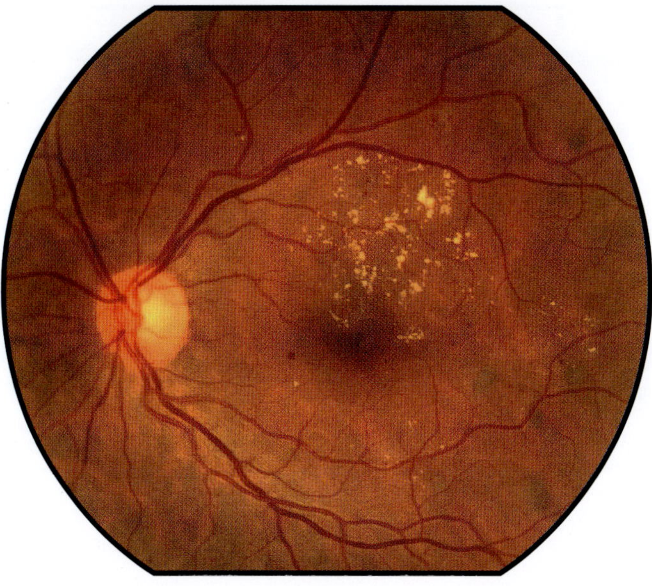

This patient has NPDR with microaneurysms and complicated by clinically significant diabetic macular edema and lipid exudation.

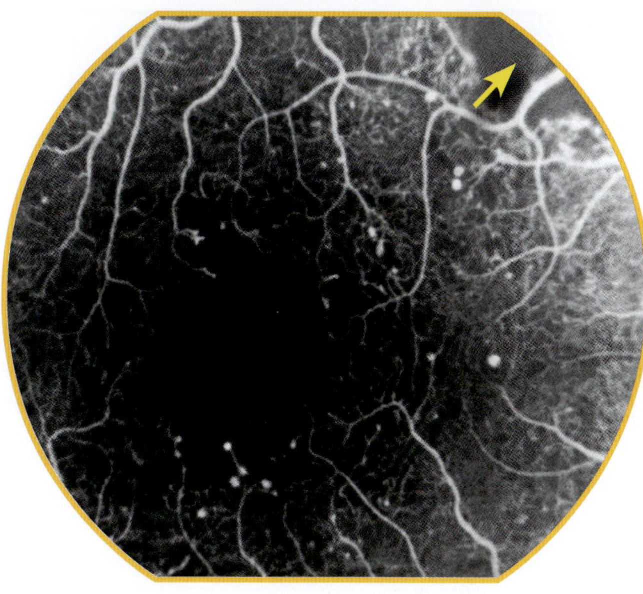

Note the prominent perifoveal microaneurysms and the enlargement of the foveal avascular zone (FAZ) in this FA from a patient with NPDR. Retinal ischemia is also noted superotemporally *(arrow)*.

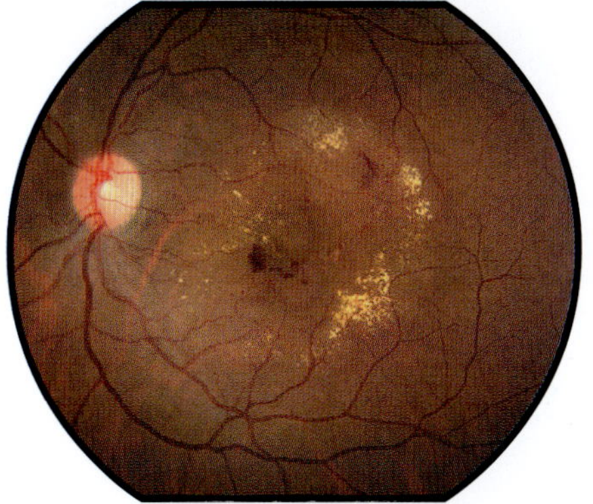

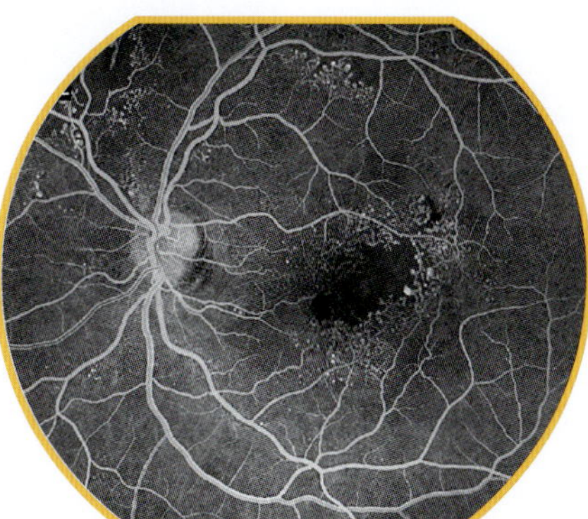

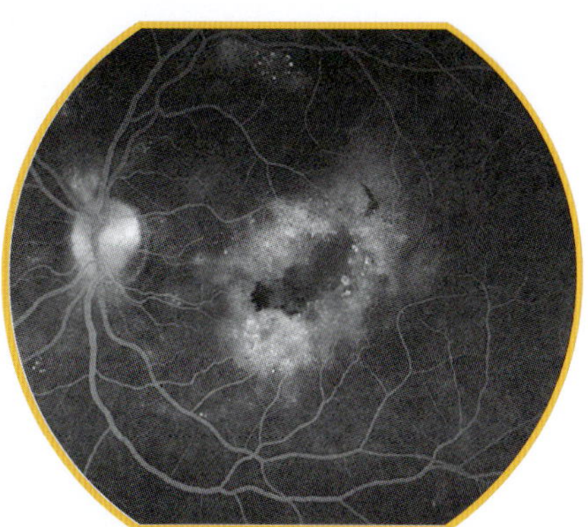

This patient with NPDR and diabetic macular edema demonstrates a lipid maculopathy *(left)*. The FA shows macular ischemia *(middle)* with enlargement of the FAZ and late macular edema *(right)*. Intraretinal microvascular abnormalities may also be appreciated with the FA. *Courtesy of Ophthalmic Imaging Systems, Inc*

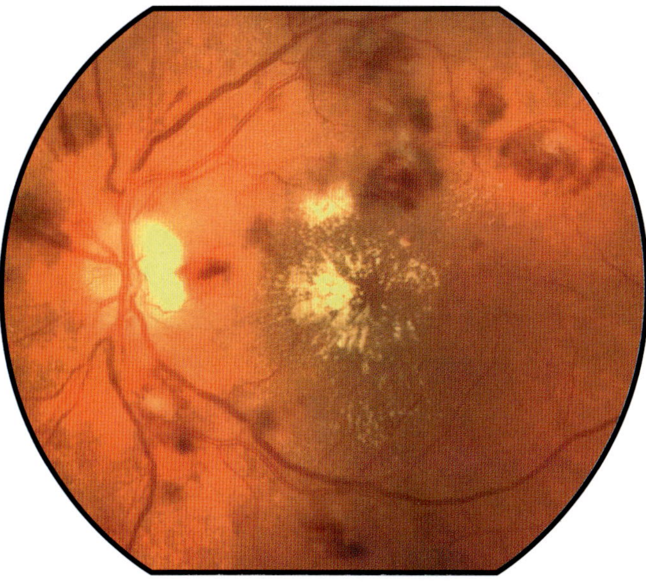

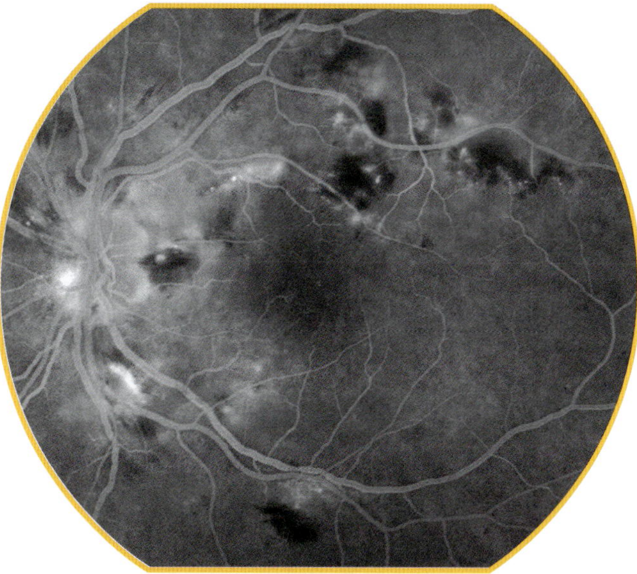

Lipid maculopathy and a macular star are noted in this case of NPDR. Fluorescein angiogram shows blockage from the retinal hemorrhage and leakage from the microaneurysms.

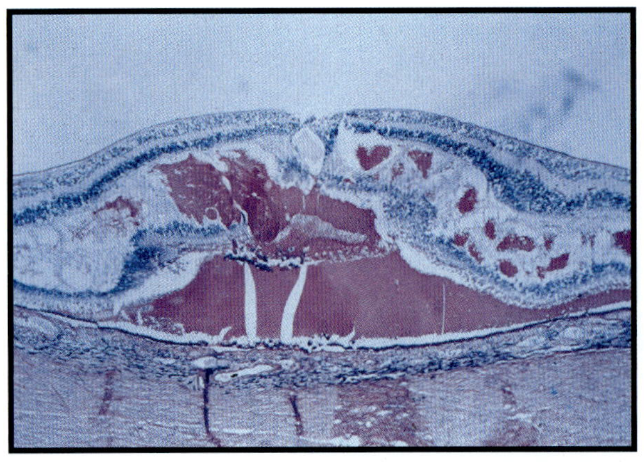

© 457

This histopathologic specimen shows marked diabetic macular edema and subretinal exudation.

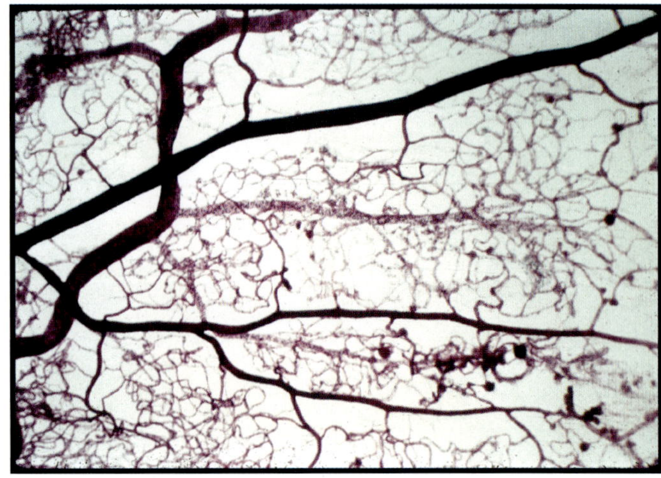

This is a retinal digest of a patient with diabetic retinopathy. Dilated capillaries and microaneurysms can be seen in association with capillary obliteration or non-perfusion.

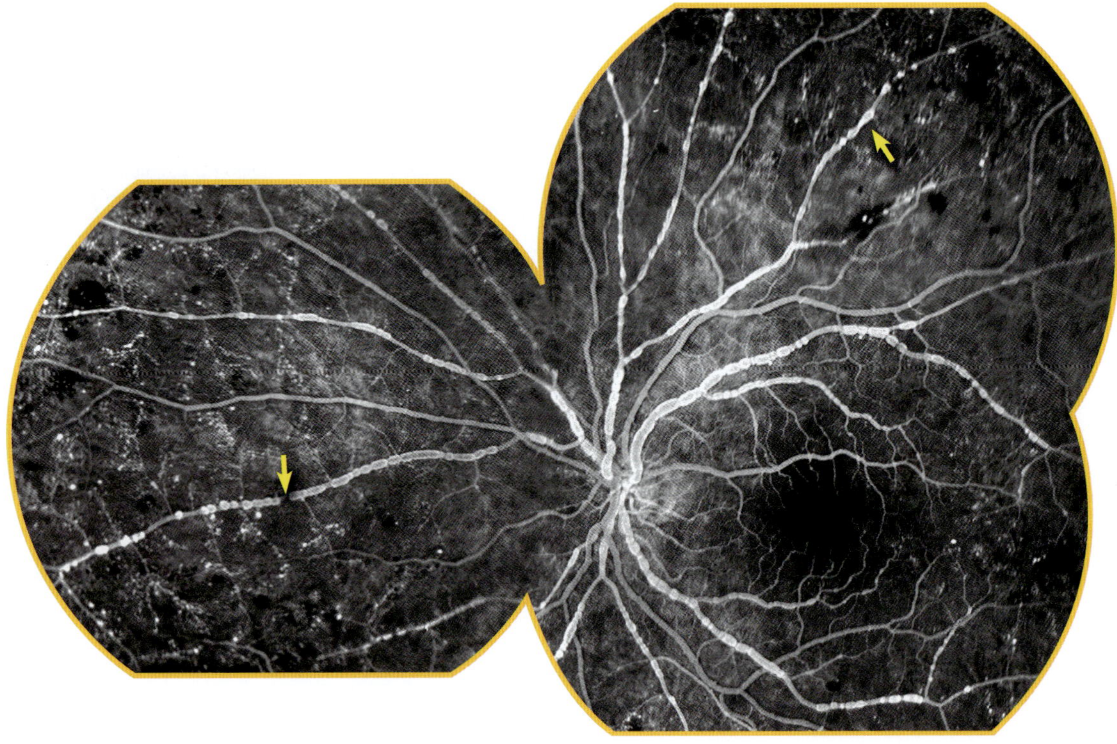

This patient with NPDR has multiple microaneurysms and retinal hemorrhages throughout the fundus and venous beading *(arrows)* and signs of severe NPDR or preproliferative diabetic retinopathy. Patchy peripheral retinal ischemia may also be appreciated.

NPDR can be seen in these patients. On the left, there are two prominent CWS with a large blot hemorrhage. Venous beading is also noted. On the right, the FA in this patient reveals numerous microaneurysms and severe capillary non-perfusion and ischemia.

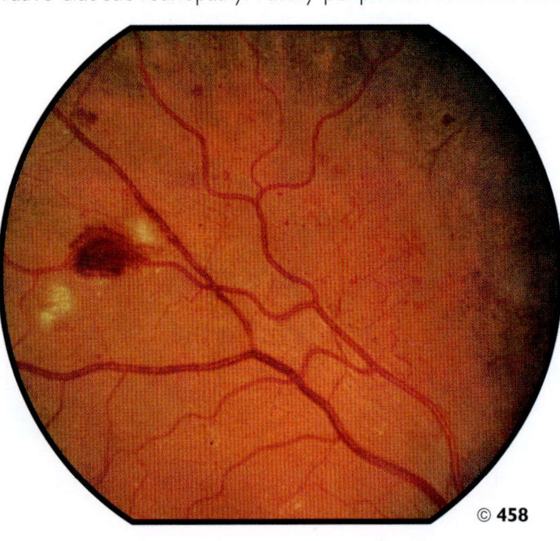

© 458

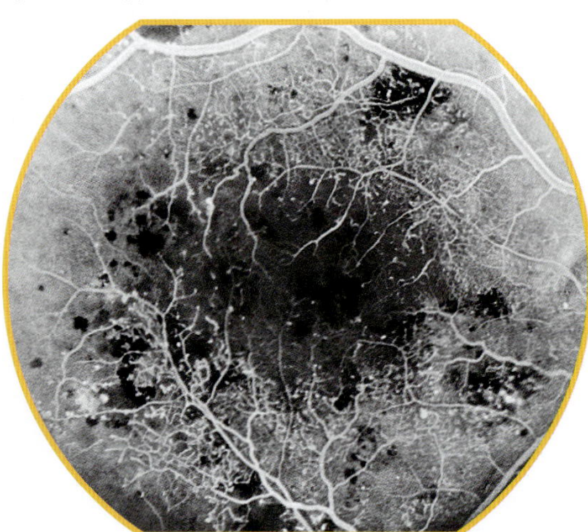

Proliferative Diabetic Retinopathy

Peripheral Ischemia and Neovascularization

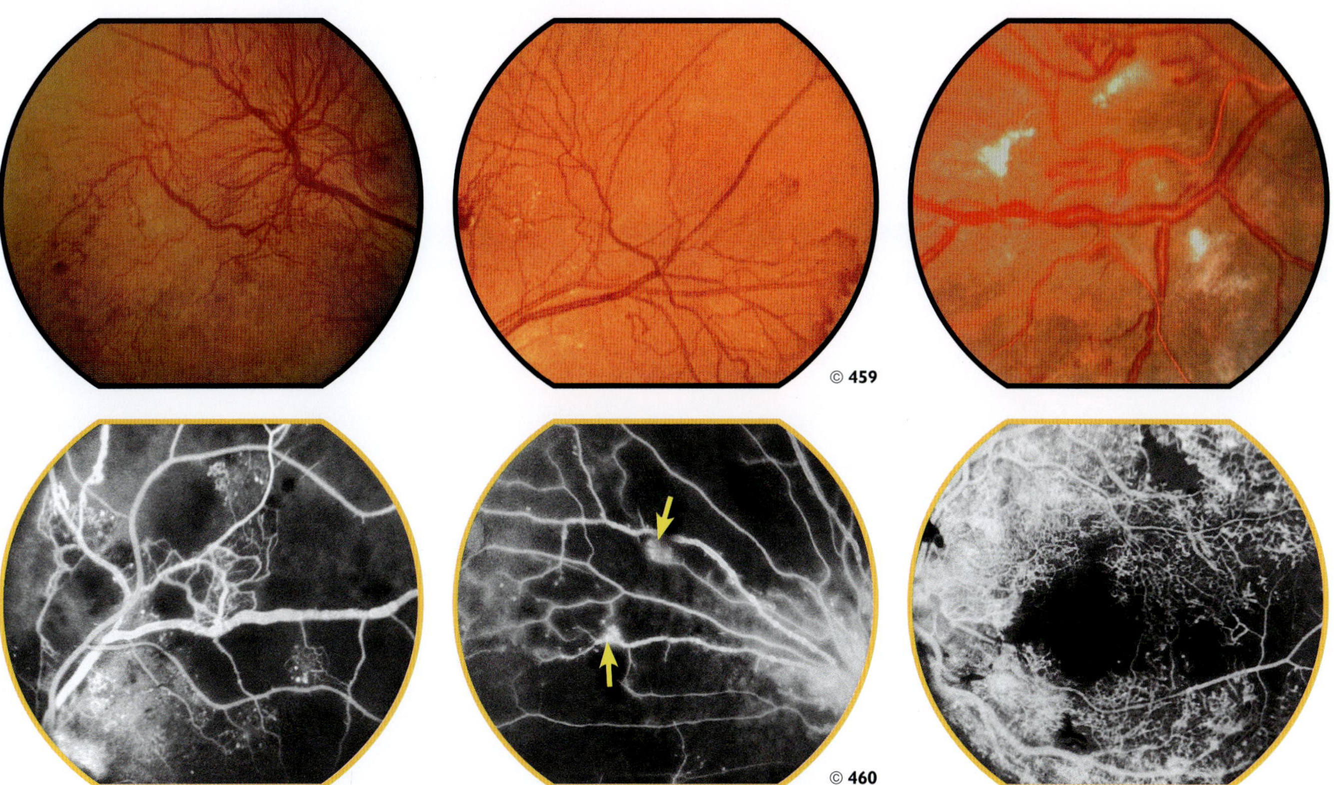

Retinal ischemia leads to pre-retinal neovascularization, as illustrated in these patients. Venous beading is prominent *(top right)*. Frank retinal neovascularization is illustrated *(top left and top middle)* while early pre-retinal neovascularization *(arrows)* and retinal capillary ischemia and non-perfusion are shown in the FA.

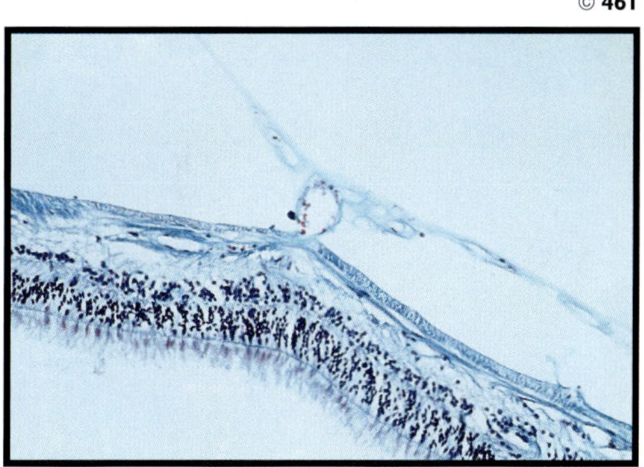

This histopathologic specimen illustrates proliferative diabetic retinopathy and retinal neovascularization that is tethered to the vitreous hyaloid border.

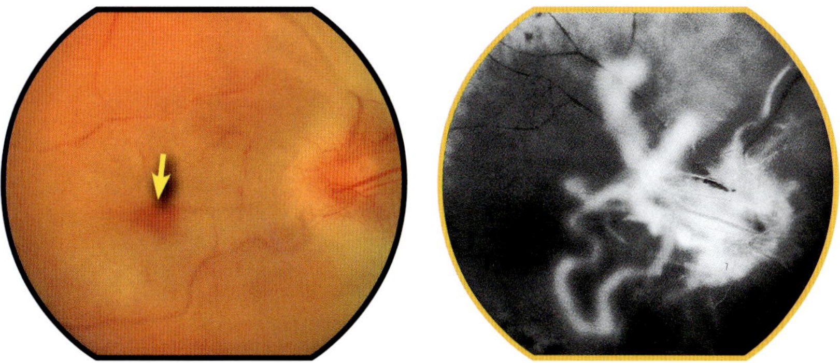

This patient has proliferative diabetic retinopathy, optic disc neovascularization (NVD), and a central retinal artery occlusion. Note the "cherry red" spot *(arrow)*, the perfused area of the ciliary circulation. NVD and disc leakage are illustrated with the FA.

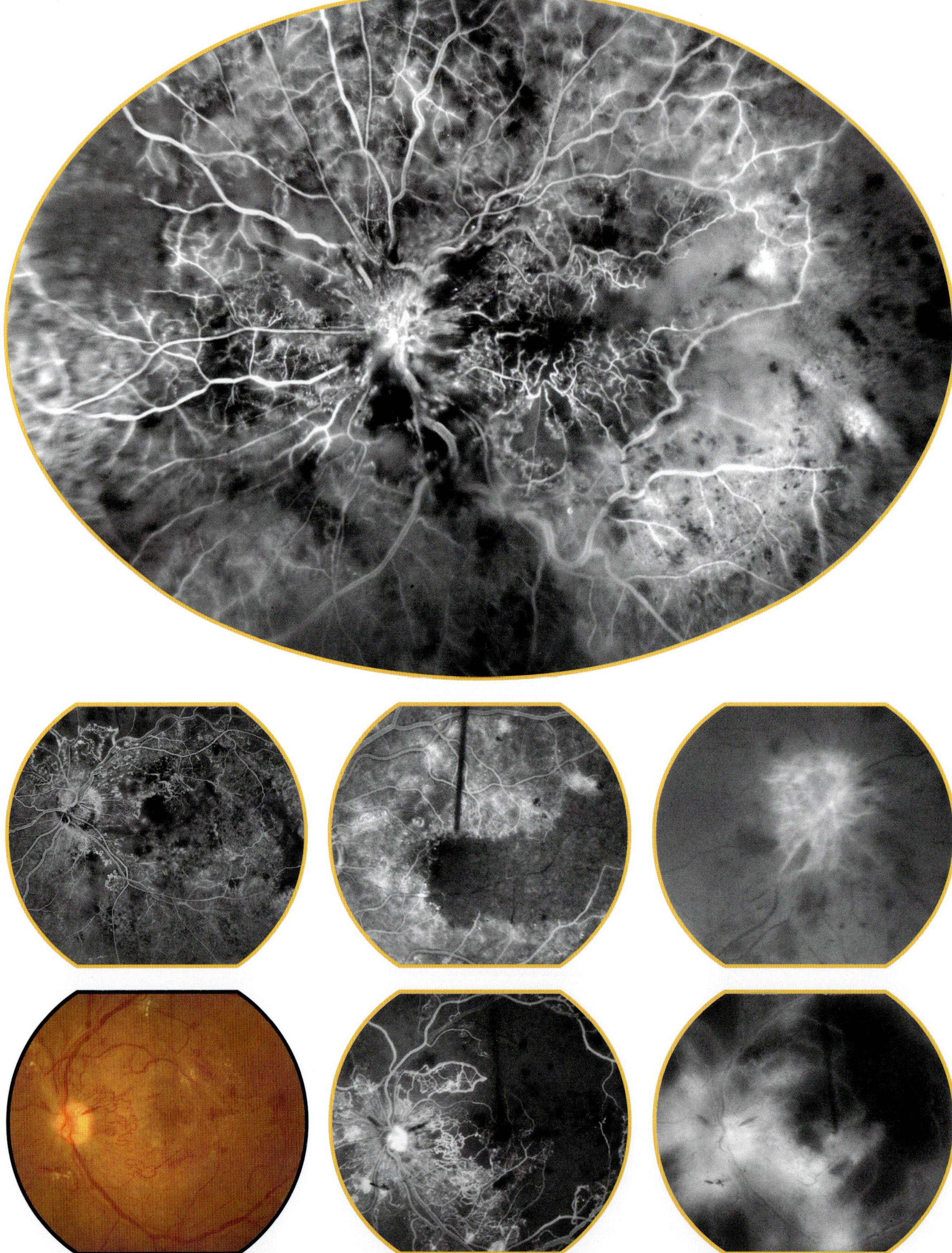

These patients have widespread diabetic microangiopathy and severe ischemia, indicated by the non-perfused areas of the retina. Early neovascularization of the disc and severe macular ischemia and non-perfusion are noted *(middle and lower rows middle)*. Extensive leakage into the retina and vitreous is also noted *(lower row right)*. An infarcted retina with bare perfusion of the nerve *(middle row right)* is illustrated. *Middle row left and center image, and bottom row courtesy of Ophthalmic Imaging Systems, Inc*

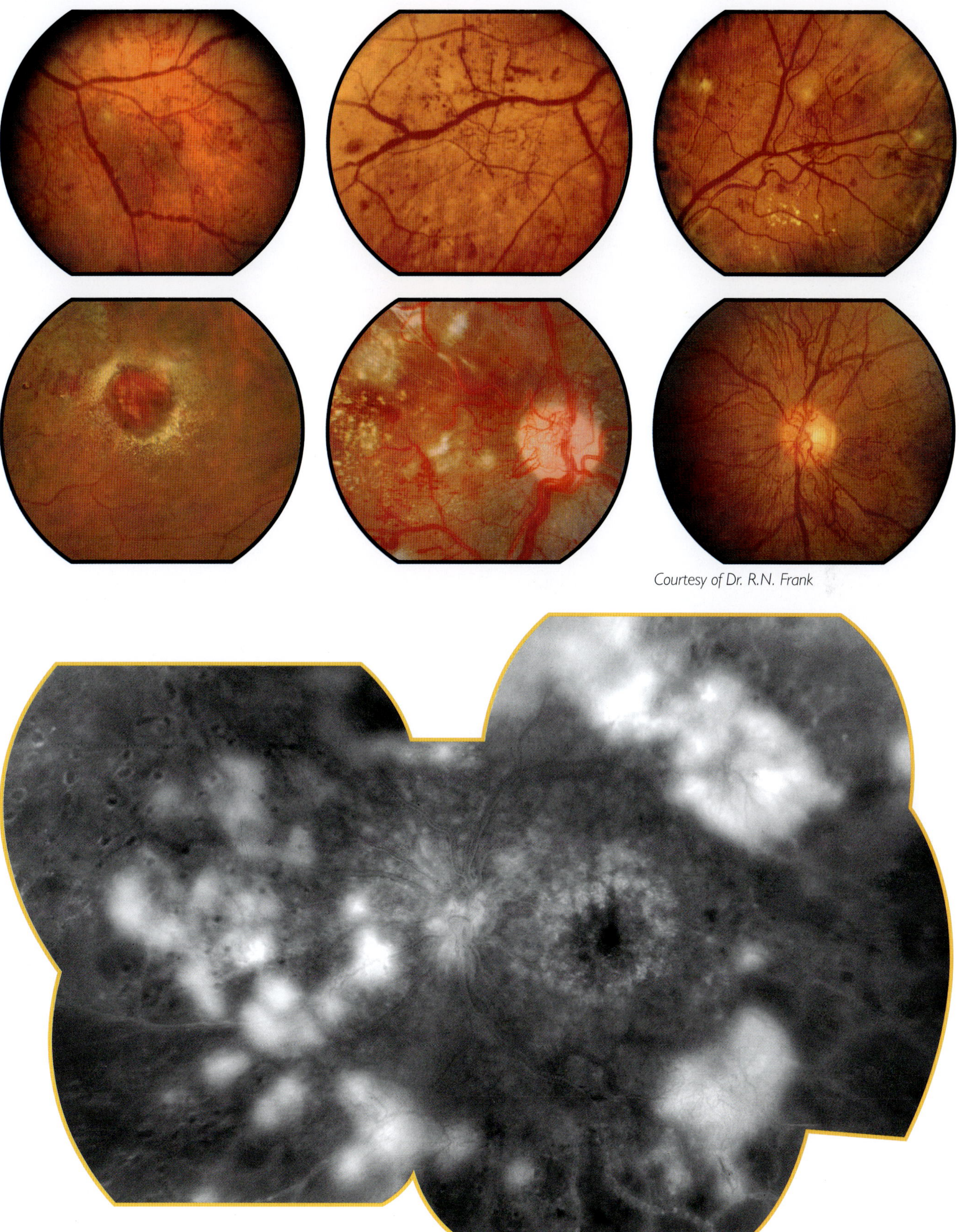

Courtesy of Dr. R.N. Frank

Cases of neovascularization of the disc and retina associated with venous beading are noted in these patients with PDR. NVD is illustrated *(middle and right images from the middle row)*. Note the presence of retinal neovascularization elsewhere (NVE) surrounded by concentric lipid exudation *(middle row left)*. The FA montage shows widespread NVE leaking into the vitreous. Cystoid macular edema and NVD are also present.

Disc Neovascularization

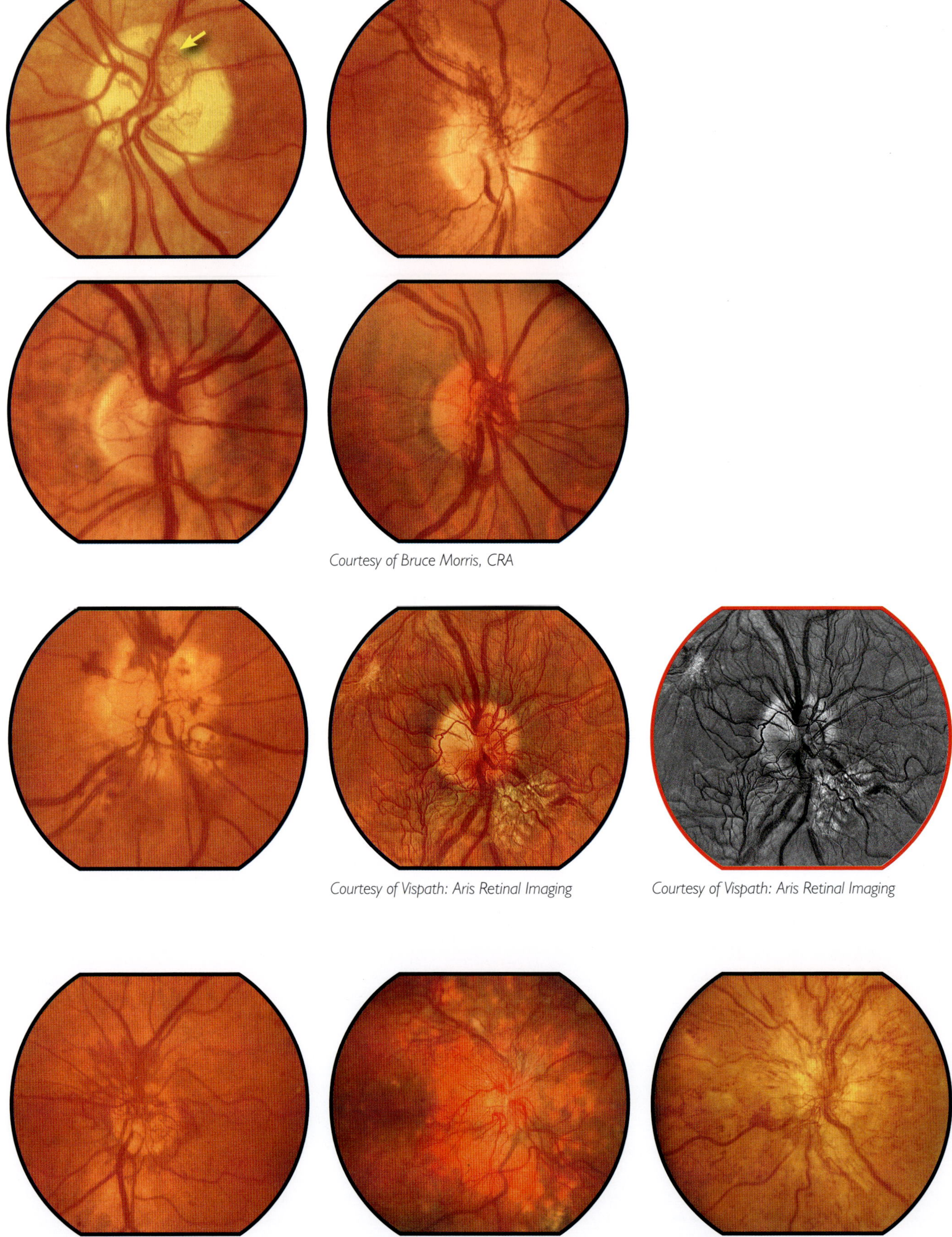

Courtesy of Bruce Morris, CRA

Courtesy of Vispath: Aris Retinal Imaging

Courtesy of Vispath: Aris Retinal Imaging

Note the many illustrations of disc neovascularization ranging from minimal *(arrow)* to severe with peripapillary extension.

Vitreous Hemorrhage

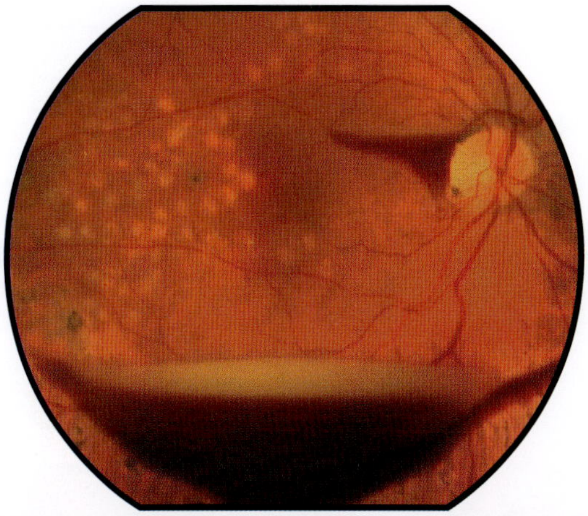

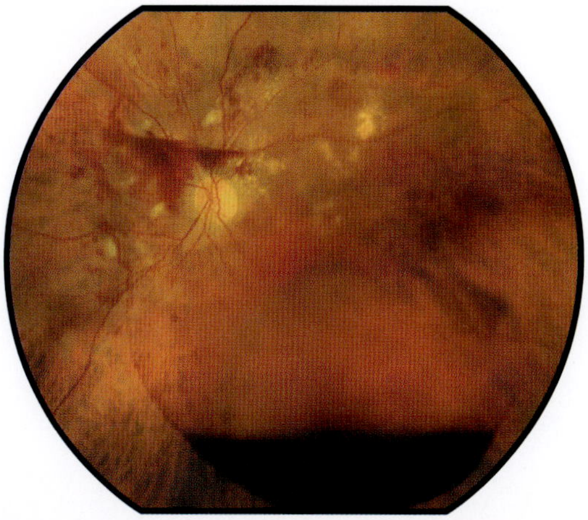

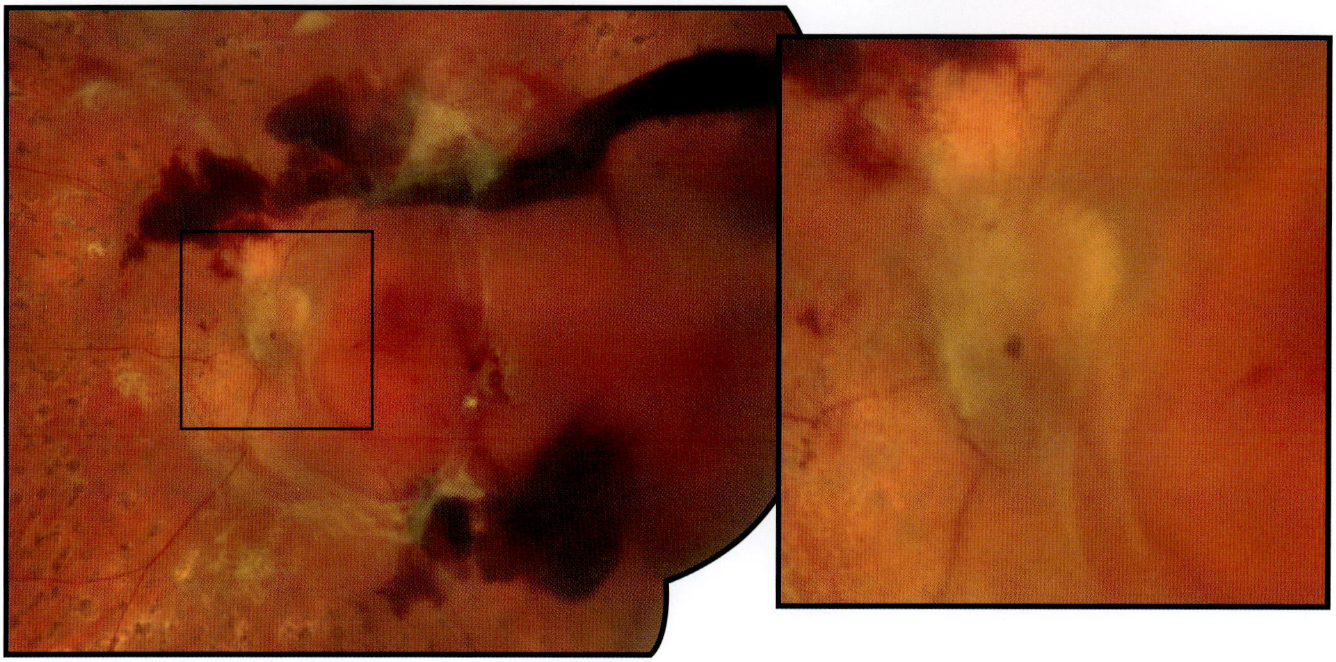

Courtesy of Ophthalmic Imaging Systems, Inc

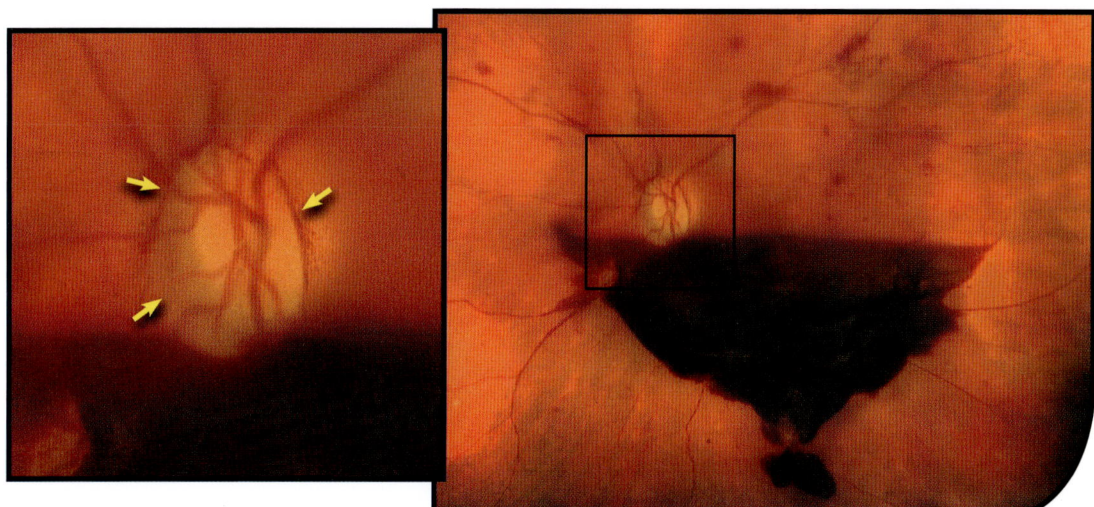

These patients have experienced severe vitreous hemorrhage from disc and retinal neovascularization. Traction caused by the posterior hyaloid may be the cause of these hemorrhages. An incomplete detachment of the vitreous around the nerve is seen in the case on the bottom *(arrows)*.

Fibrous Proliferation

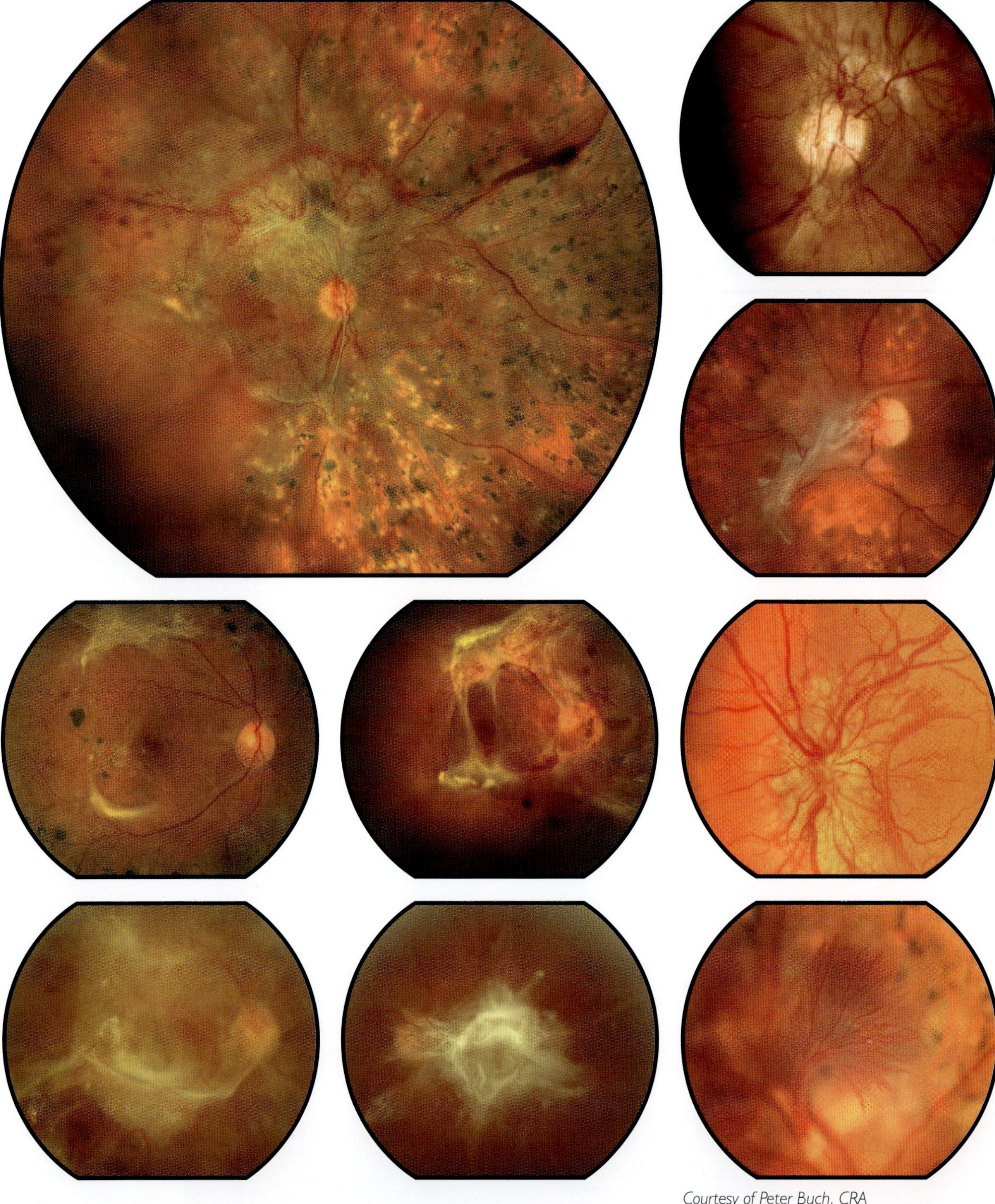

Courtesy of Peter Buch, CRA

Fibrous proliferation may complicate PDR and may induce bleeding and tractional detachment. A circumscribed area of scar formation may not uncommonly encircle the posterior pole.

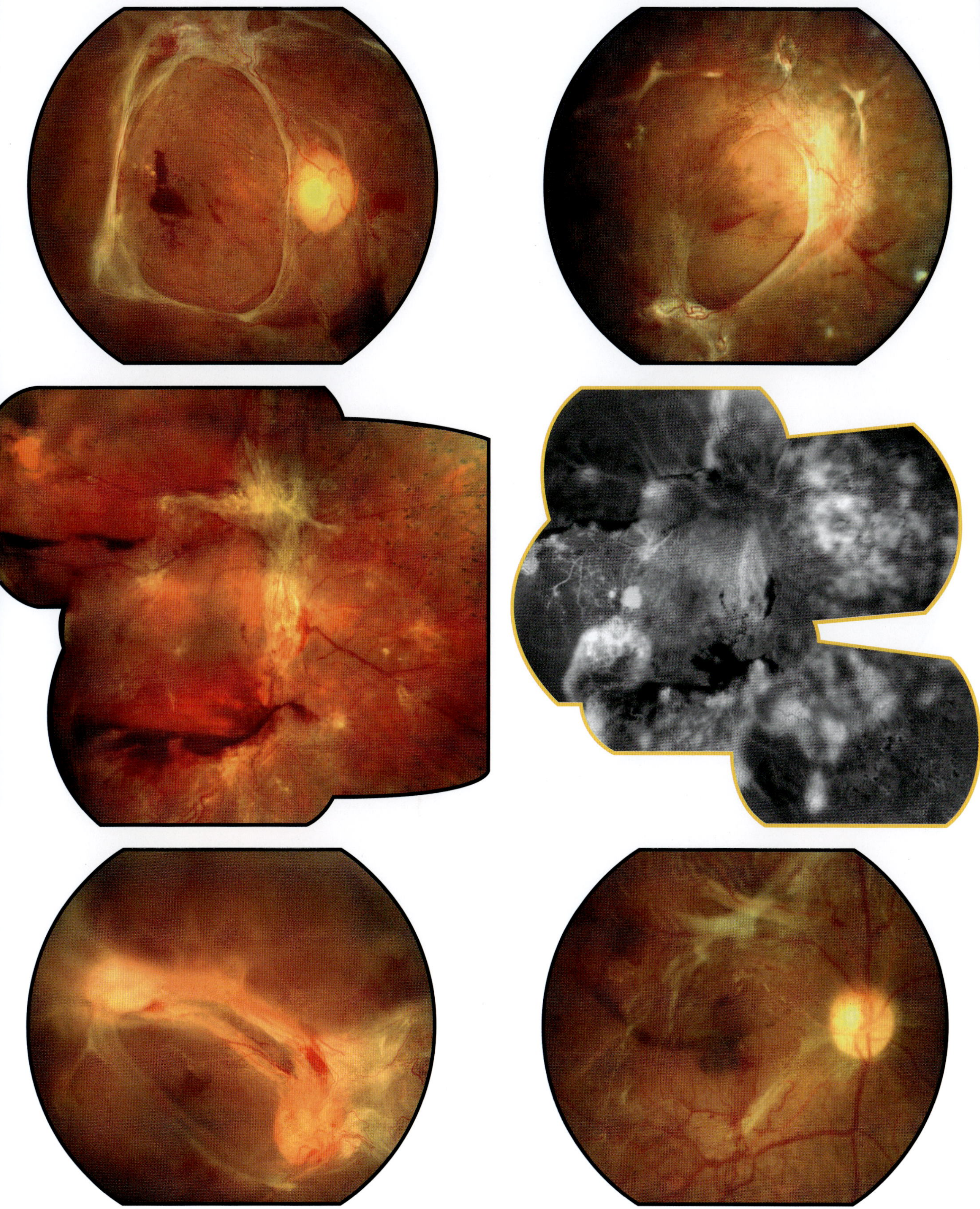

Patients with severe proliferative diabetic retinopathy may have variable severities of fibrous growth. In some instances, the fibrosis may obliterate the view of the optic nerve *(upper right, middle left, and lower left)*. There is active bleeding from the vascular component of these membranes. The FA shows widespread neovascularization and peripheral ischemia.

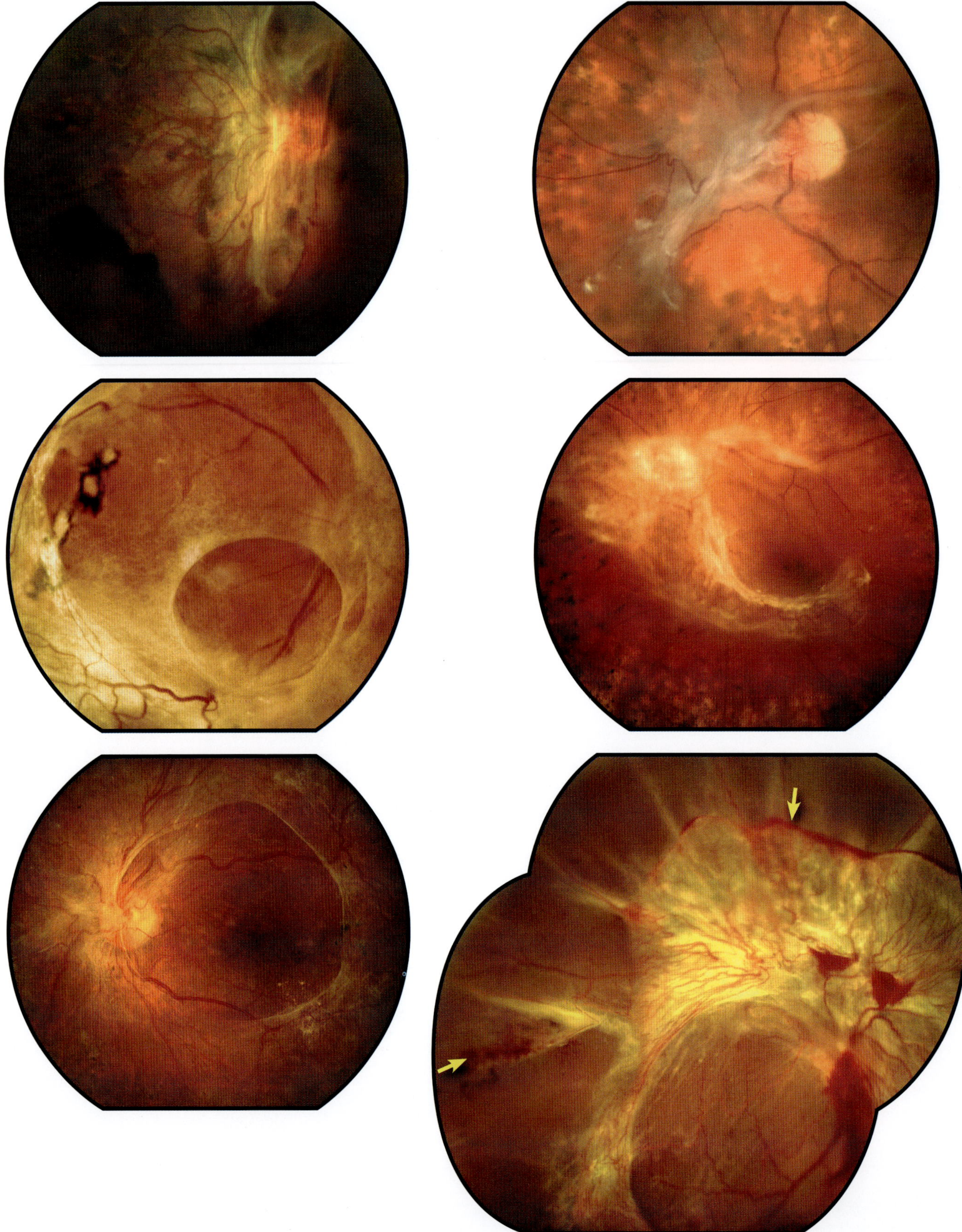

These are examples of fibrous proliferation in PDR. In some instances, it encircles the posterior pole. An ovoid gap may be noted surrounding the paramacular area that may correspond to the precortical vitreous pocket or premacular bursa. The fibrous proliferation may exert traction toward the vitreous causing macular detachment in a "table top" configuration. In some cases, the fibrous tissue has actively proliferating vascular components that cause vitreous bleeding, as seen in the image on the lower right *(arrows)*.

Diabetic Papillopathy

Patients with diabetes may experience diabetic papillopathy that can in some cases be difficult to differentiate from non-arteritic anterior ischemic optic neuropathy (NAION) or NVD. This optic neuropathy may or may not be associated with reduced visual acuity and field loss.

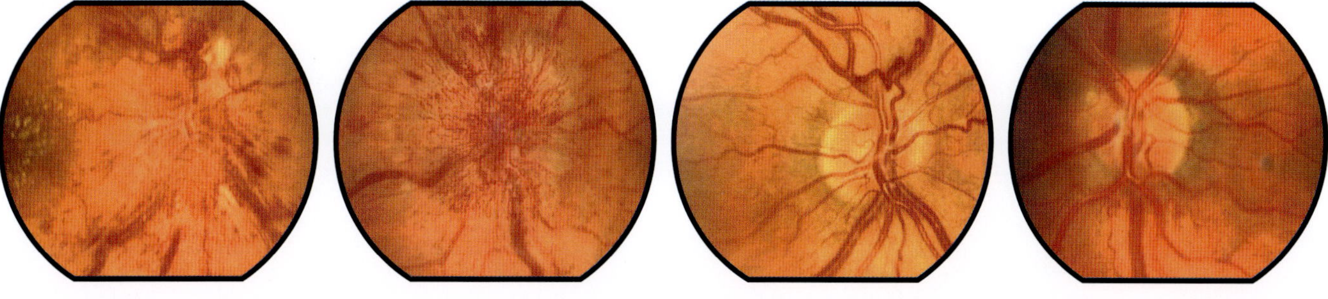

This is a patient with bilateral diabetic papillopathy. Note that the acute manifestations show swelling of the nerve and NVD in the right and left eye *(left images)*. Spontaneous resolution of the optic nerve abnormalities ensued 10 weeks later *(right images)*. *Courtesy of Dr. Sohan Sing-Hayreh*

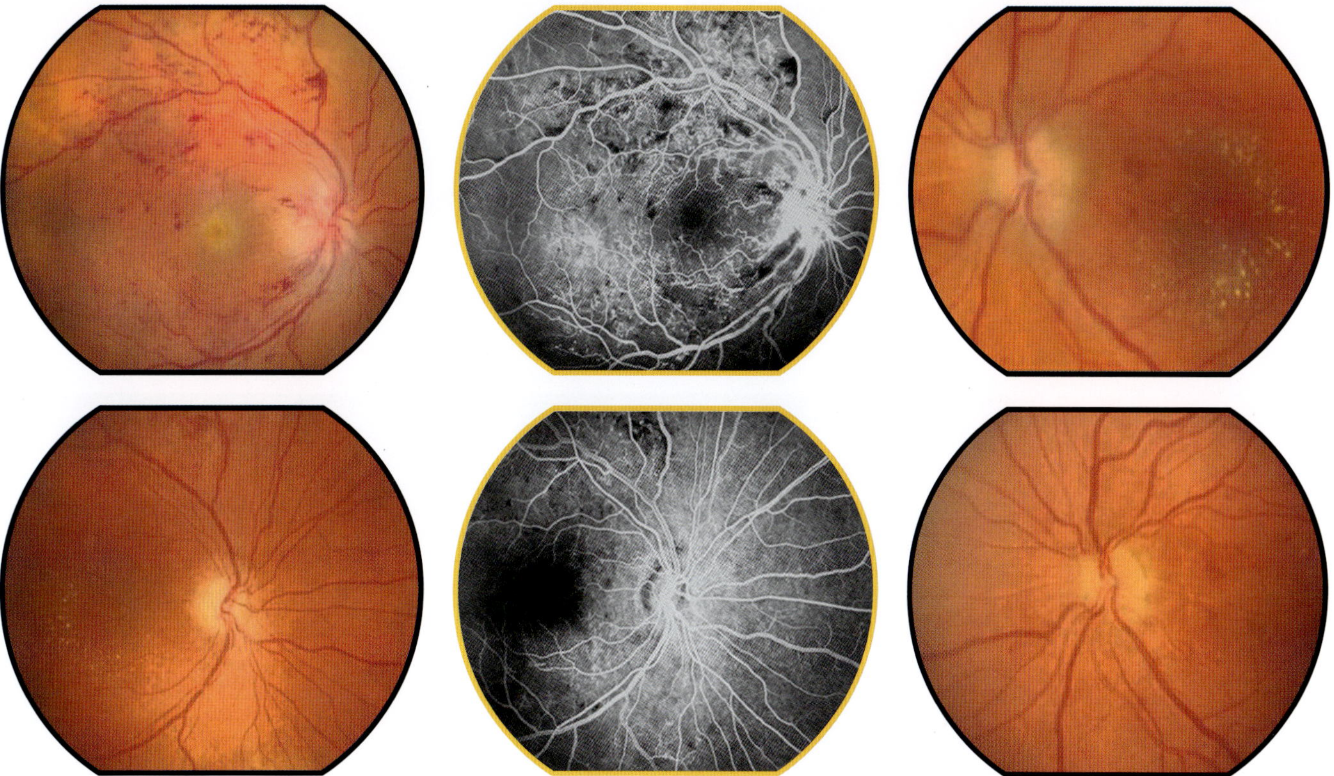

This patient presented with bilateral diabetic papillopathy. There was swelling of the nerve and associated macular edema and severe NPDR *(upper row)*. Ten weeks later, there was spontaneous resolution of the papillopathy in each eye *(lower row)* with subsequent optic atrophy and improvement of the retinopathy, as illustrated in the FA in the lower row, after panretinal laser photocoagulation therapy. *Courtesy of Dr. Sohan Sing-Hayreh*

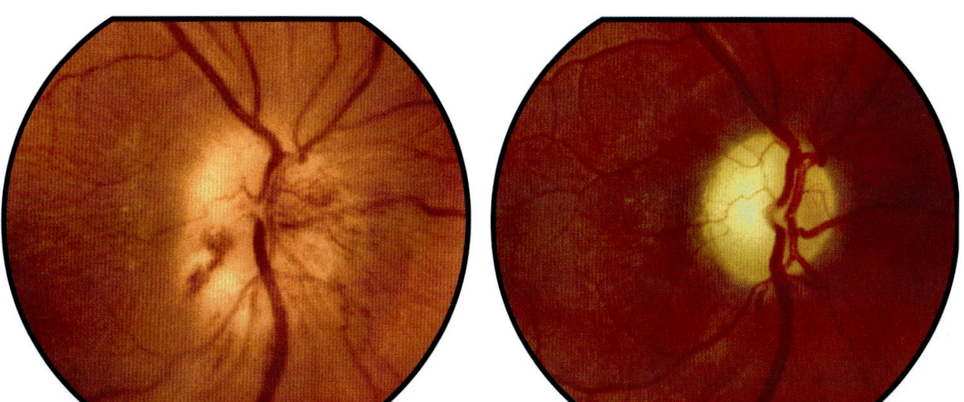

Note the presence of NAION in this patient. There is swelling of the nerve head with associated hemorrhages. Following resolution of the papillopathy, there was resultant optic atrophy *(right)*.

Macular Manifestations of Diabetic Retinopathy

In non-proliferative and proliferative diabetic retinopathy, various macular complications can cause vision loss. Some are manageable with treatment, whereas others are associated with permanent and/or progressive loss of vision.

Macular Edema

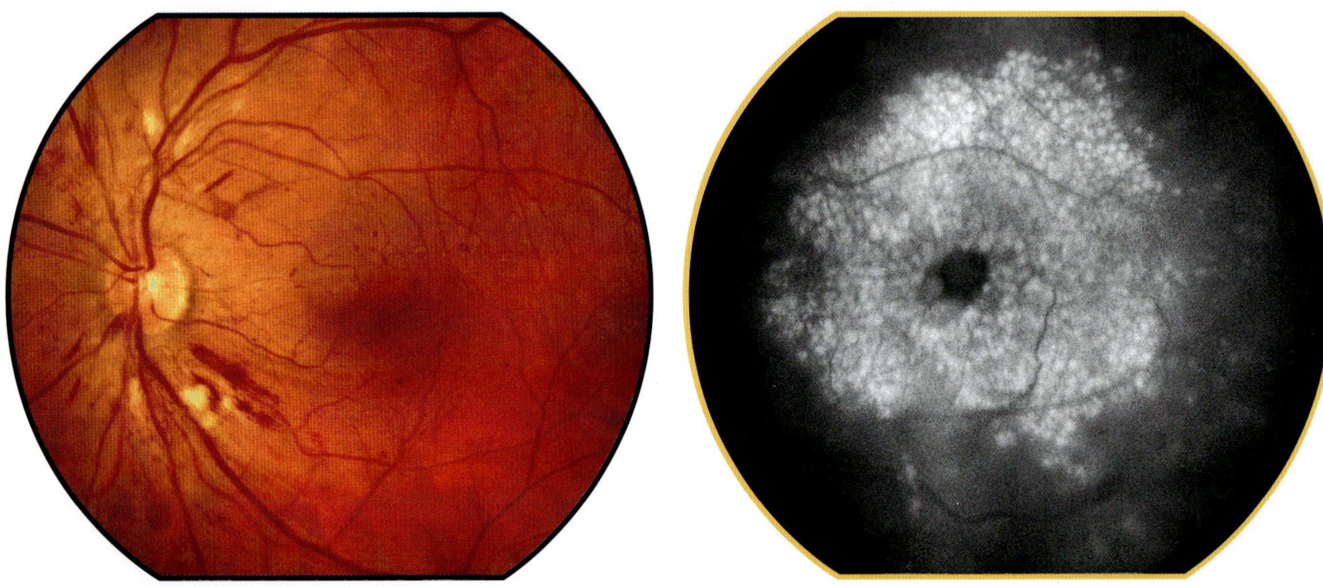

Macular edema is the most common cause of vision impairment in patients with diabetic retinopathy. Microvascular abnormalities such as microaneurysms or telangiectasia or dilated incompetent vessels may leak due to retinal vascular endothelial cell damage and disruption of the inner blood ocular barrier. Note the severe diabetic CME illustrated in the FA. The outer blood-retina barrier at the level of the RPE may also be compromised. Vascular endothelial growth factor is a major contributor to macular edema in diabetics.

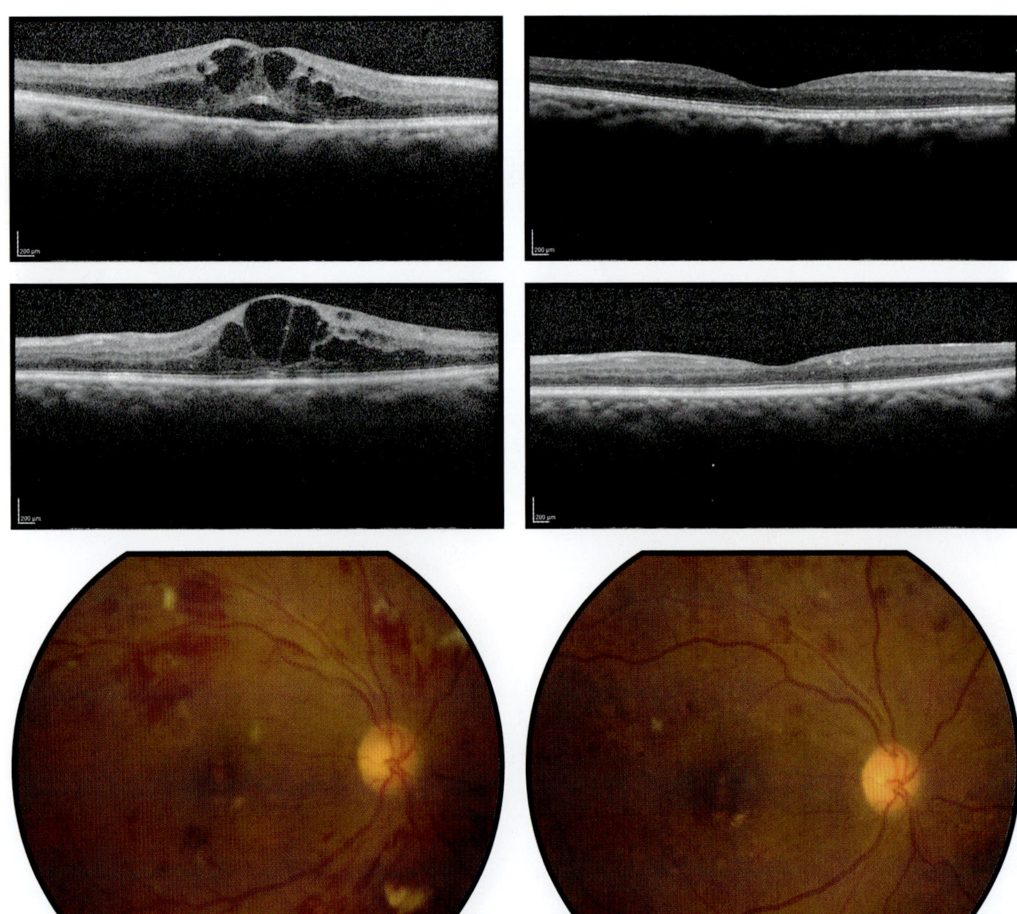

SD-OCT of a patient's right *(top row)* and left *(second row)* eye showing severe diabetic cystoid macular edema at presentation *(left images)*. The patient was treated with anti-VEGF intravitreal injections with resolution of macular edema in each eye *(right images)* as well as significant improvement in intraretinal hemorrhage as shown on the color fundus photos of the right eye *(bottom row)*.

Macular Ischemia

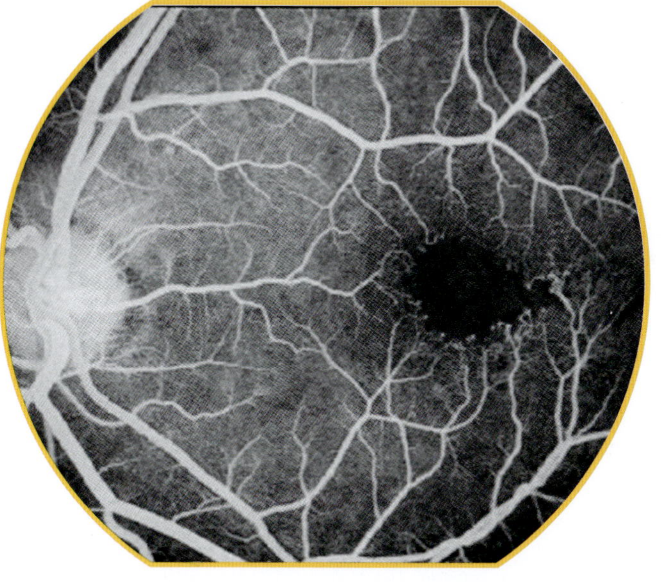

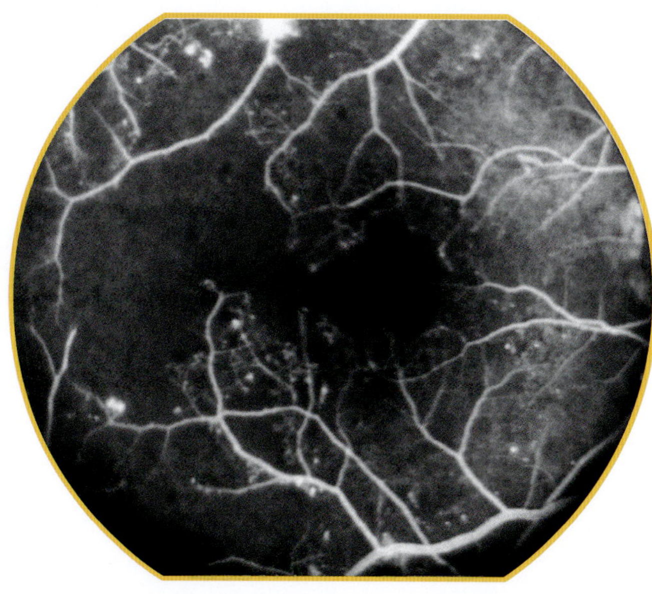

Macular ischemia is another cause of vision loss associated with diabetic retinopathy. Enlargement or pruning of the FAZ is identified in each FA and zones of non-perfusion are shown in the angiogram on the right.

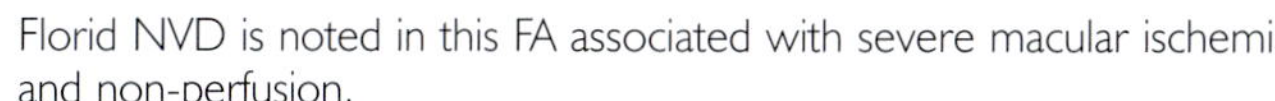

Florid NVD is noted in this FA associated with severe macular ischemia and non-perfusion.

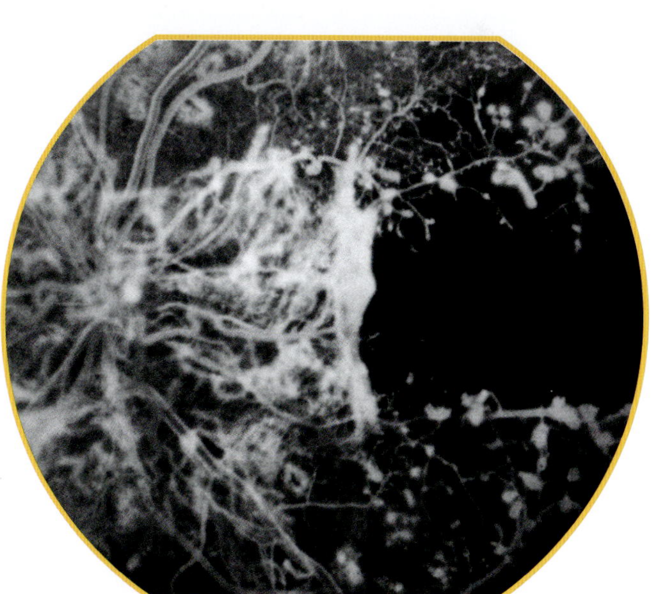

Macular Hole

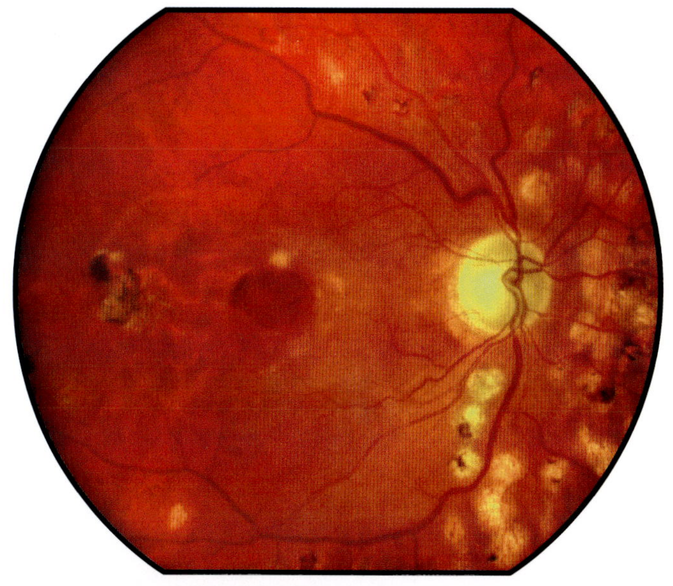

Patients with diabetes can develop macular holes, as seen in this case, due to anterior traction by the vitreous.

Choroidal Neovascularization

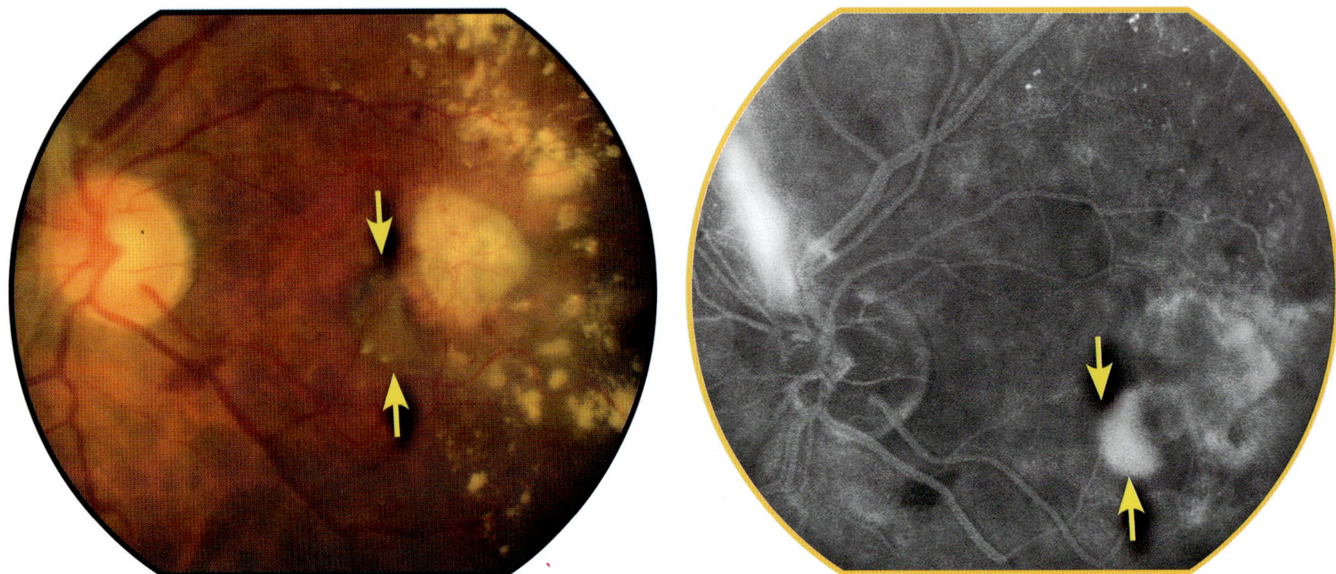

Chronic exudative maculopathy is noted in the color image. A grayish-green choroidal neovascular membrane can be seen adjacent to the fibrotic scar *(arrows)*. Fluorescein angiography illustrates hyperfluorescent leakage of the choroidal neovascularization *(arrows)*. NVD is also present at the superior edge of the disc.

Retinal Hemorrhage

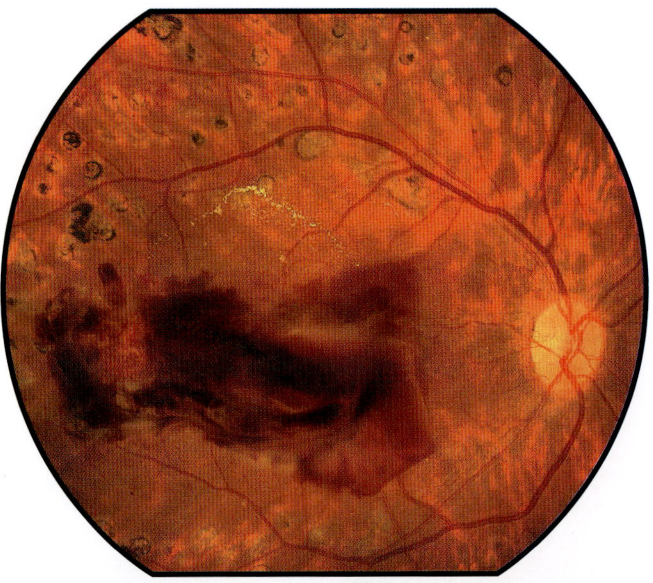

Acute pre-retinal macular hemorrhage may complicate diabetic retinopathy, typically PDR, due to neovascularization and traction, causing sudden vision loss. *Courtesy of Ophthalmic Imaging Systems Inc*

Exudative Lipid Maculopathy

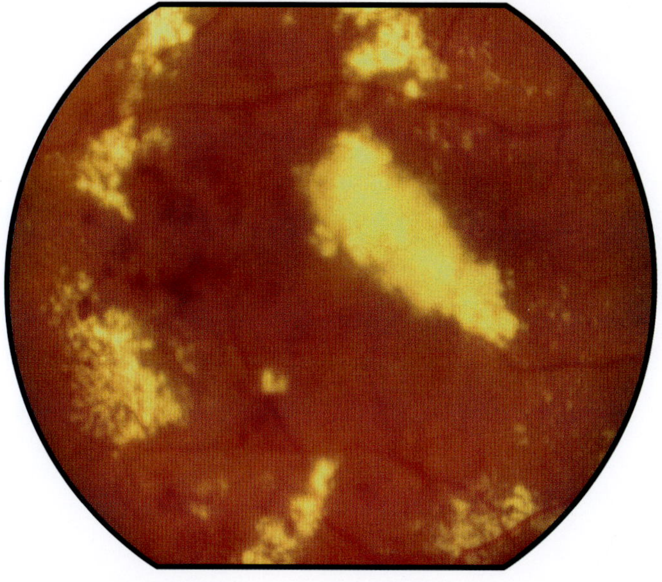

Severe lipid deposition associated with CME can cause permanent vision loss and can progress to cicatricial abnormalities. Systemic lipid profile should be evaluated and optimized.

Macular Scar

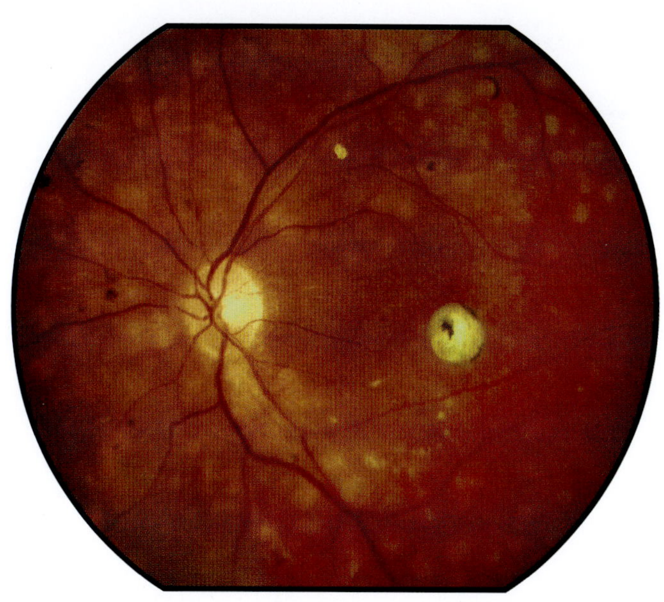

Note the central fibrous scar in this diabetic patient. Diabetic macular scars may result from chronic lipid deposition, fibrovascular proliferation, traction, or hemorrhage.

Exudative Detachment

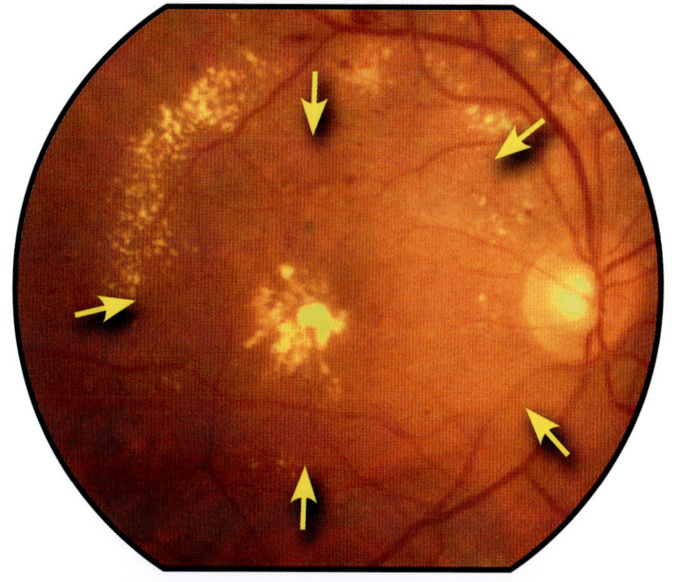

Serous macular detachment *(arrows)* may uncommonly complicate severe diabetic macular edema.

Pre-Retinal Fibrosis

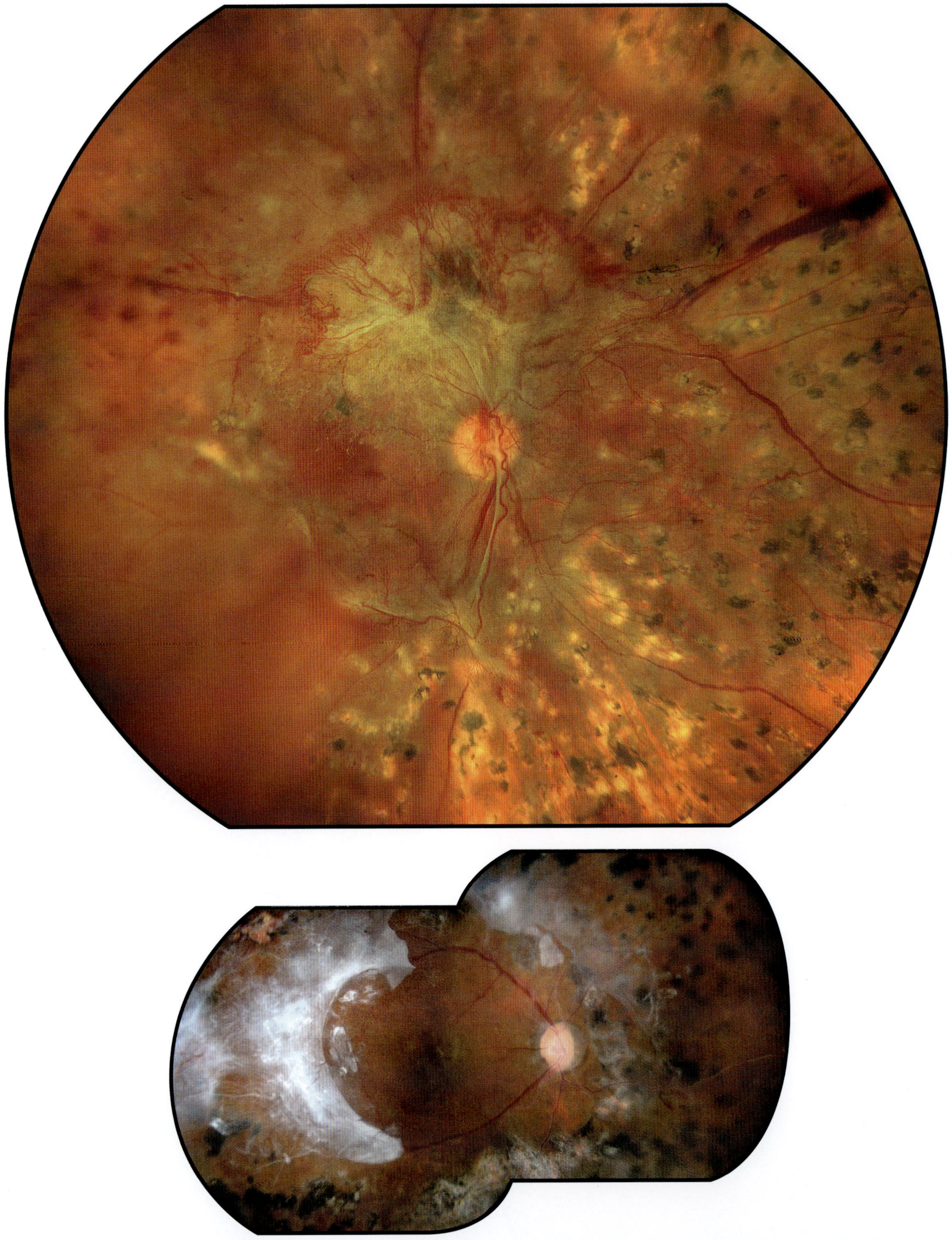

Fibrovascular proliferation leading to vitreous hemorrhage or traction retinal detachment can complicate PDR. In the top image, there is evidence of fibrovascular proliferation and neovascularization with overlying vitreous hemorrhage. A vitrectomy relieved the traction in the bottom image. Considerable fibrosis with traction remains in the temporal macula and peripheral fundus.

Tractional Retinal Detachment

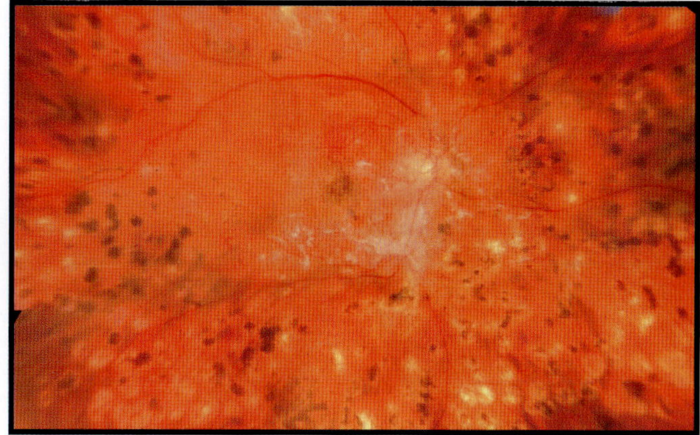

Chronic tractional detachment of the macula developed in this patient with fibrous PDR status post PRP.

Diabetic Retinopathy and Systemic Disease

Diabetic retinopathy can be exacerbated by other systemic disease including hypertension, renal disease, and blood dyscrasias, leading to vision loss.

Hypertension

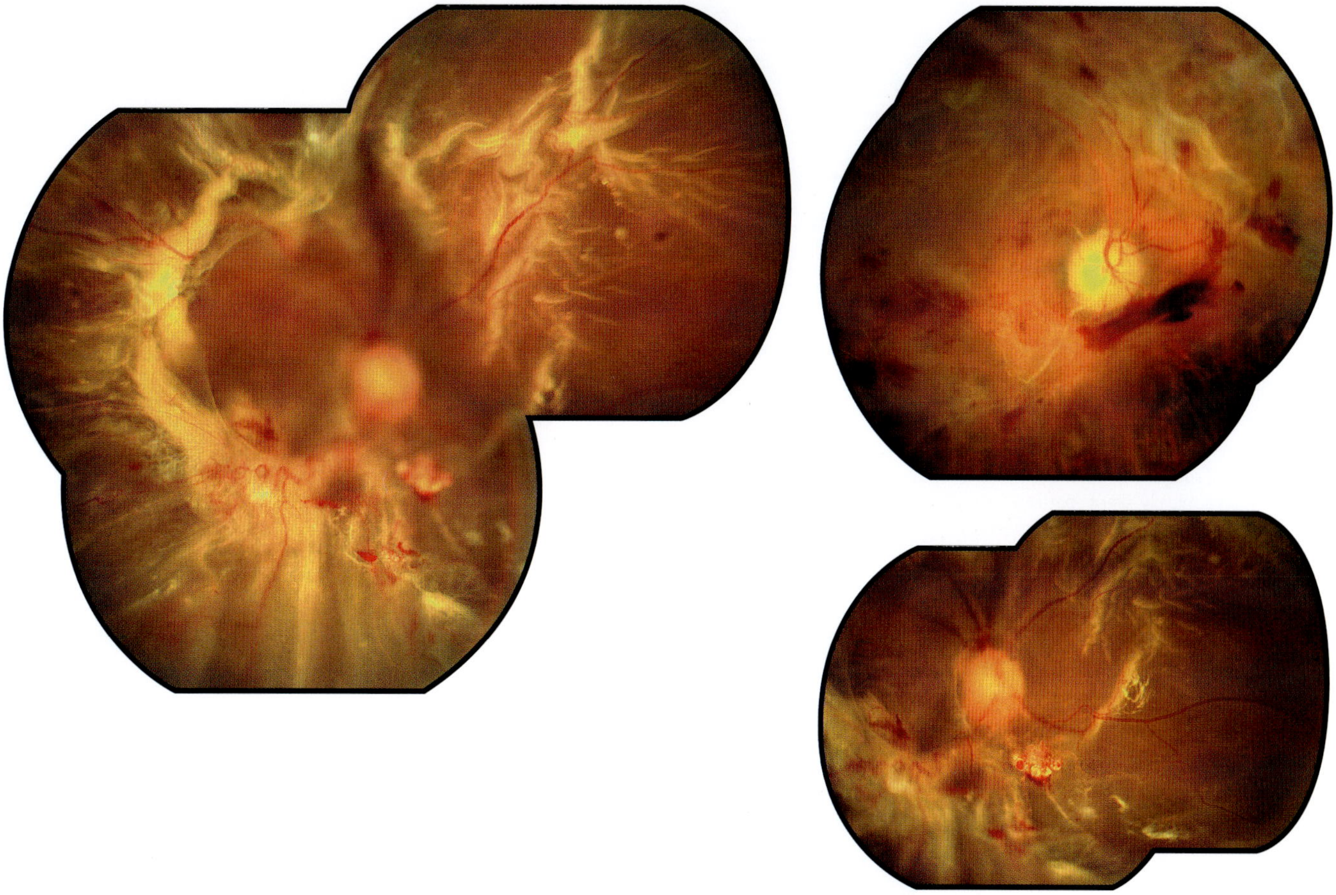

These patients have combined systemic hypertension and proliferative diabetic retinopathy. There is severe fibrovascular proliferation with vitreous hemorrhage and tractional detachment of the retina.

Diabetes and Blood Dyscrasia

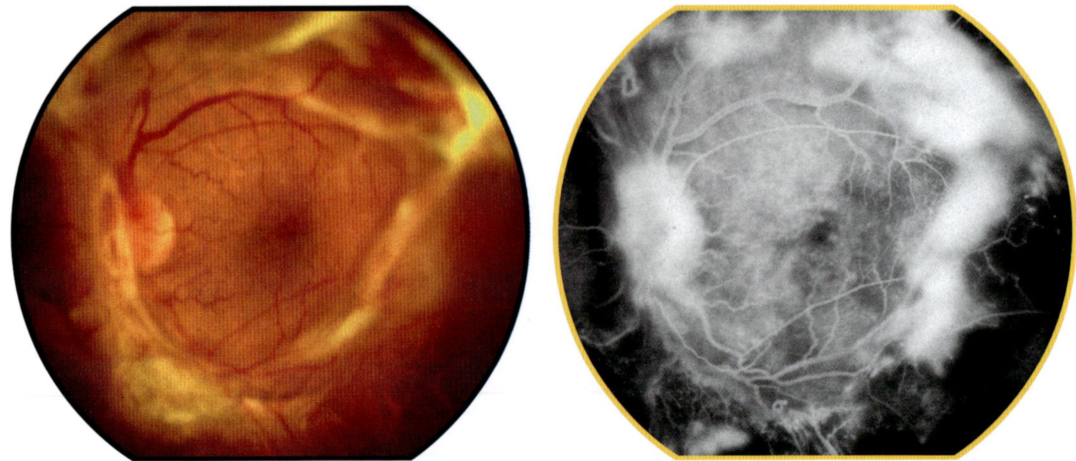

Diabetes and acute leukemia can produce devastating fibrovascular proliferation in a short period of time. This patient was diagnosed as having acute myelogenous leukemia and anemia. There is aggressive neovascularization in the posterior pole, illustrated in the clinical and fluorescein angiographic images. *Courtesy of Dr. Kurt Gitter*

Diabetes and Waldenström Macroglobulinemia

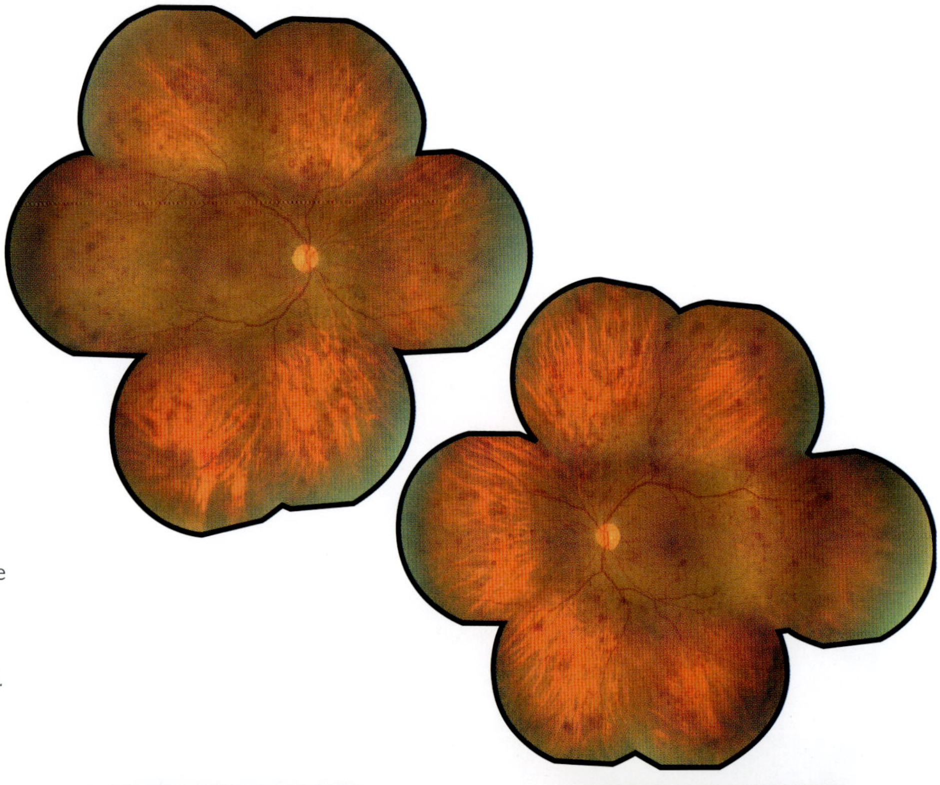

This 60-year-old diabetic presented with decreased vision in both eyes. Funduscopic examination revealed diffuse intraretinal hemorrhages and an engorged venous system illustrated with color fundus montage images of each eye. OCT at the time of presentation revealed serous macular detachments *(images not shown)*, which were angiographically silent *(bottom images)*. The patient was subsequently diagnosed with Waldenström macroglobulinemia.

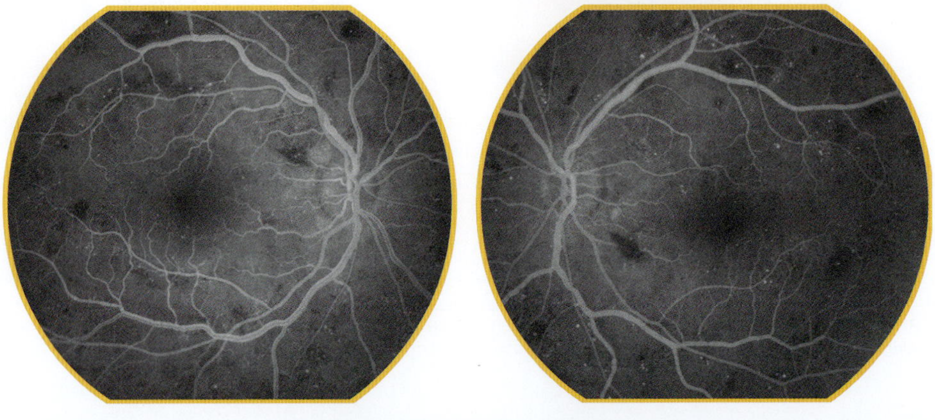

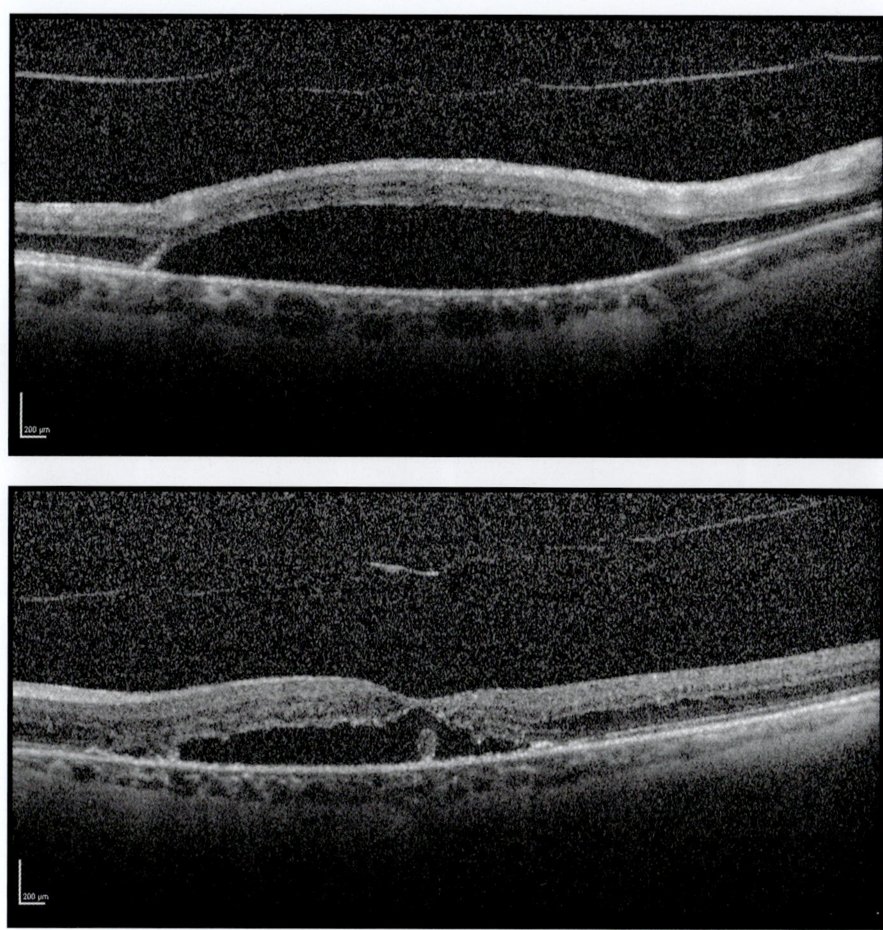

Note the bilateral serous macular detachment in this patient with Waldenström macroglobulinemia.

Lipemia Retinitis

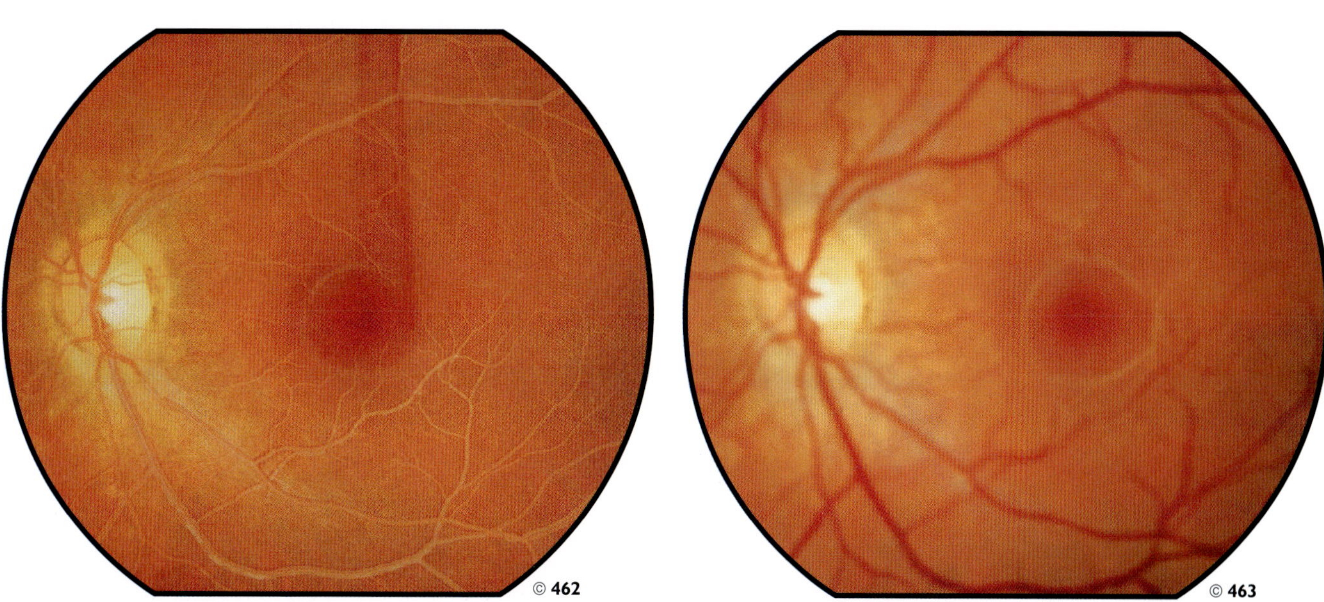

This 9-year-old female with diabetes mellitus had 20/20 vision in both eyes and creamy-white retinal vessels. The background fundus appearance was also lightened. Laboratory findings revealed elevated serum cholesterol, triglycerides, and low-density lipoproteins. Six weeks later, after insulin and lipid lowering therapy, triglyceride levels were lowered and lipemia retinalis resolved *(right image)*.

Treatment: Laser Photocoagulation

Optimization of control of blood pressure and serum glucose are the most important interventional measures in preventing vision loss due to diabetes. Optimizing serum lipid and renal status is also important. Intravitreal administration of anti-angiogenic drugs, laser photocoagulation therapy, pars plana vitrectomy, and combinations of these therapeutic modalities are important in the management of diabetic retinopathy.

Macular Lipid and Edema

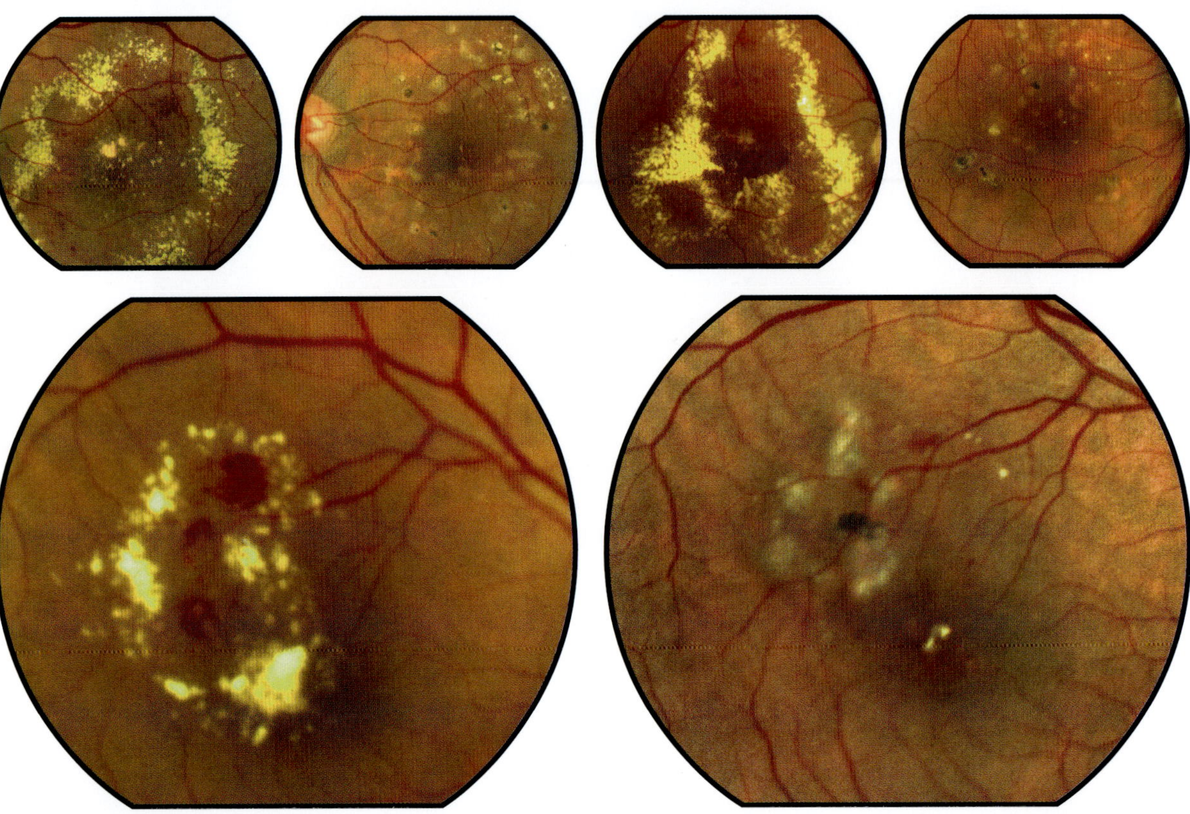

Focal laser photocoagulation may be beneficial in treating diabetic macular edema but has been largely replaced by intravitreal antiangiogenic therapy as the gold standard of care. The left color image of each pair represents the pre-laser clinical state, and the right color image represents the post-laser state, 3-6 months later. Note the resolution of edema and circinate lipid exudates in each of the three cases.

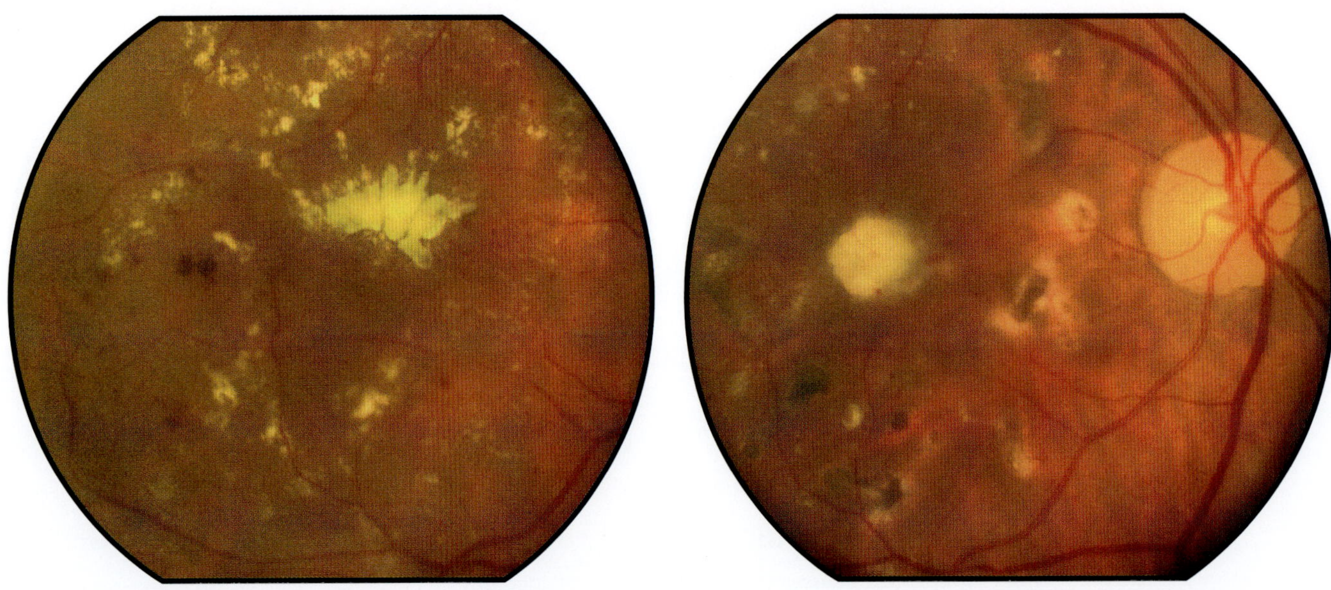

This patient presented with diabetic macular edema and lipid exudation *(left)*. Focal and grid laser photocoagulation was performed with resolution of the edema and lipid. However, a fibrous scar ensued *(right)* due to severe lipid deposition.

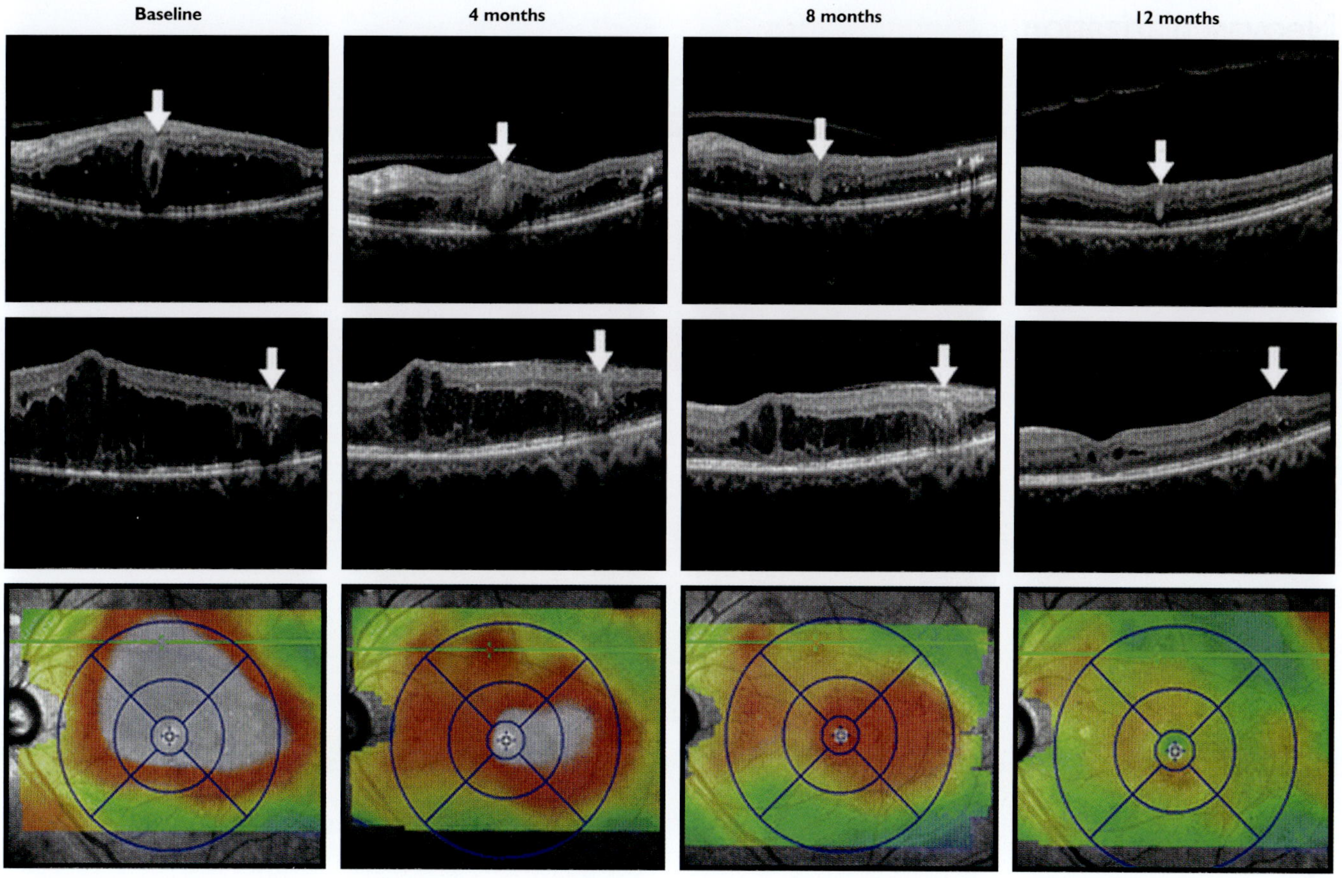

Baseline **4 months** **8 months** **12 months**

© **464**

SD-OCT helped to identify leaking microaneurysms in this patient with diabetic retinopathy *(arrows)*. Focal laser treatment to the aneurysms led to progressive resolution of the cystoid macular edema in this patient.

Retinal Break

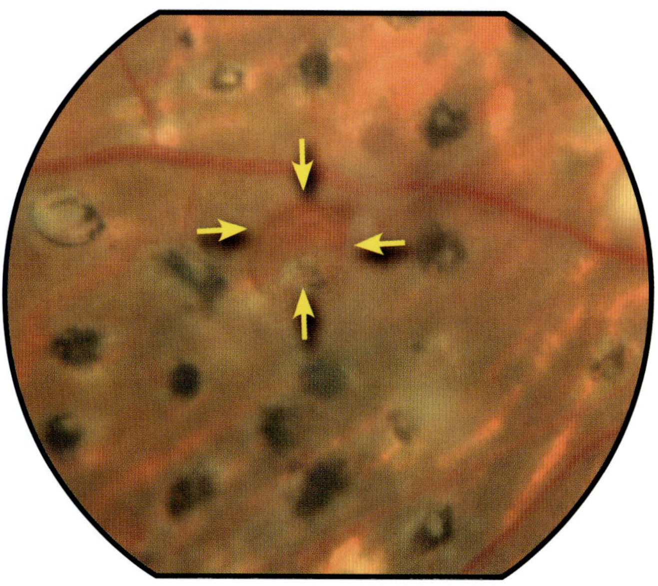

Laser treatment may also be used to barricade retinal breaks, even within an area of previous PRP treatment *(arrows)*. Additional laser was used to encircle a localized retinal tear in this patient with proliferative diabetic retinopathy.

Neovascularization

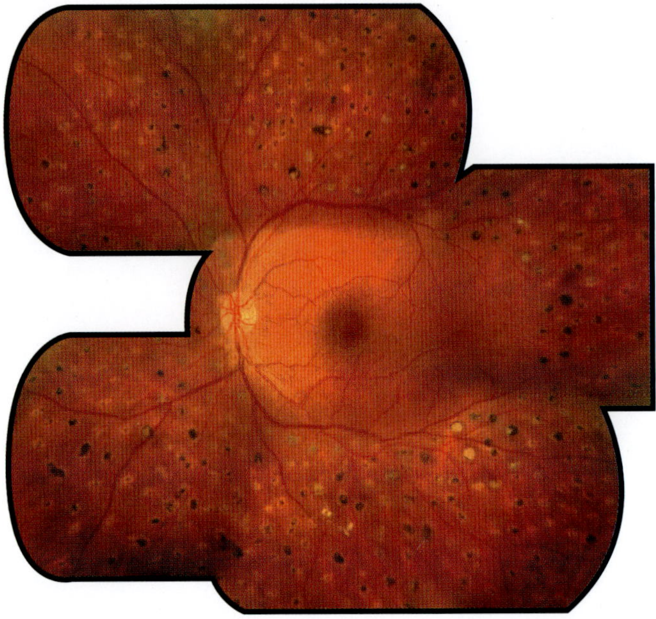

This is a patient who presented with aggressive retinal neovascularization. PRP laser therapy was used to induce regression of the abnormal vessels. The color montage image illustrates the typical pattern of PRP scars.

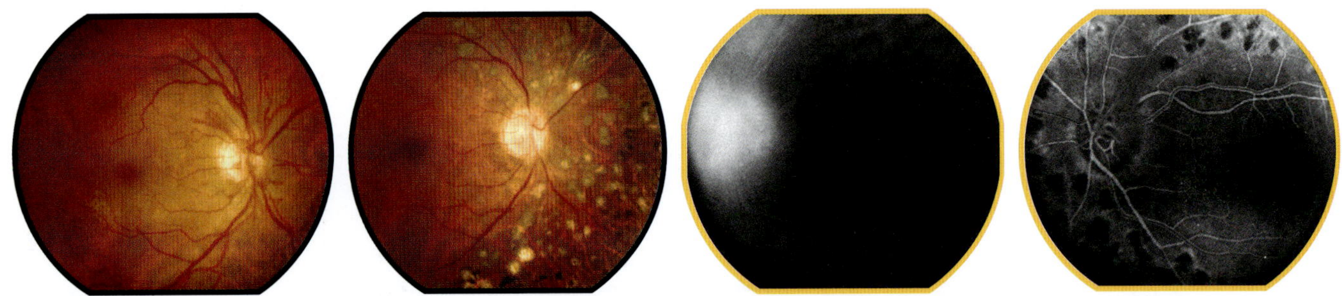

The color image on the left shows pretreatment NVD. Post-treatment regression of NVD is illustrated in the adjacent color image. The two FA images show pretreatment NVD with leakage and regression of the leakage after PRP therapy.

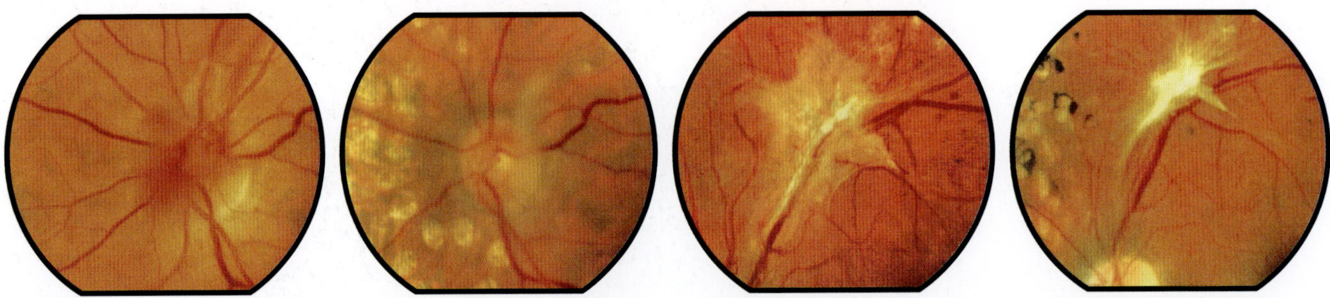

These color images illustrate pre- and post-PRP therapy for proliferative diabetic retinopathy. NVD is seen on the left. Three months later, the neovascularization has regressed and laser photocoagulation scars can be identified *(second from left)*. Fibrous neovascularization (*second from right image*) developed after PRP treatment *(far right)*.

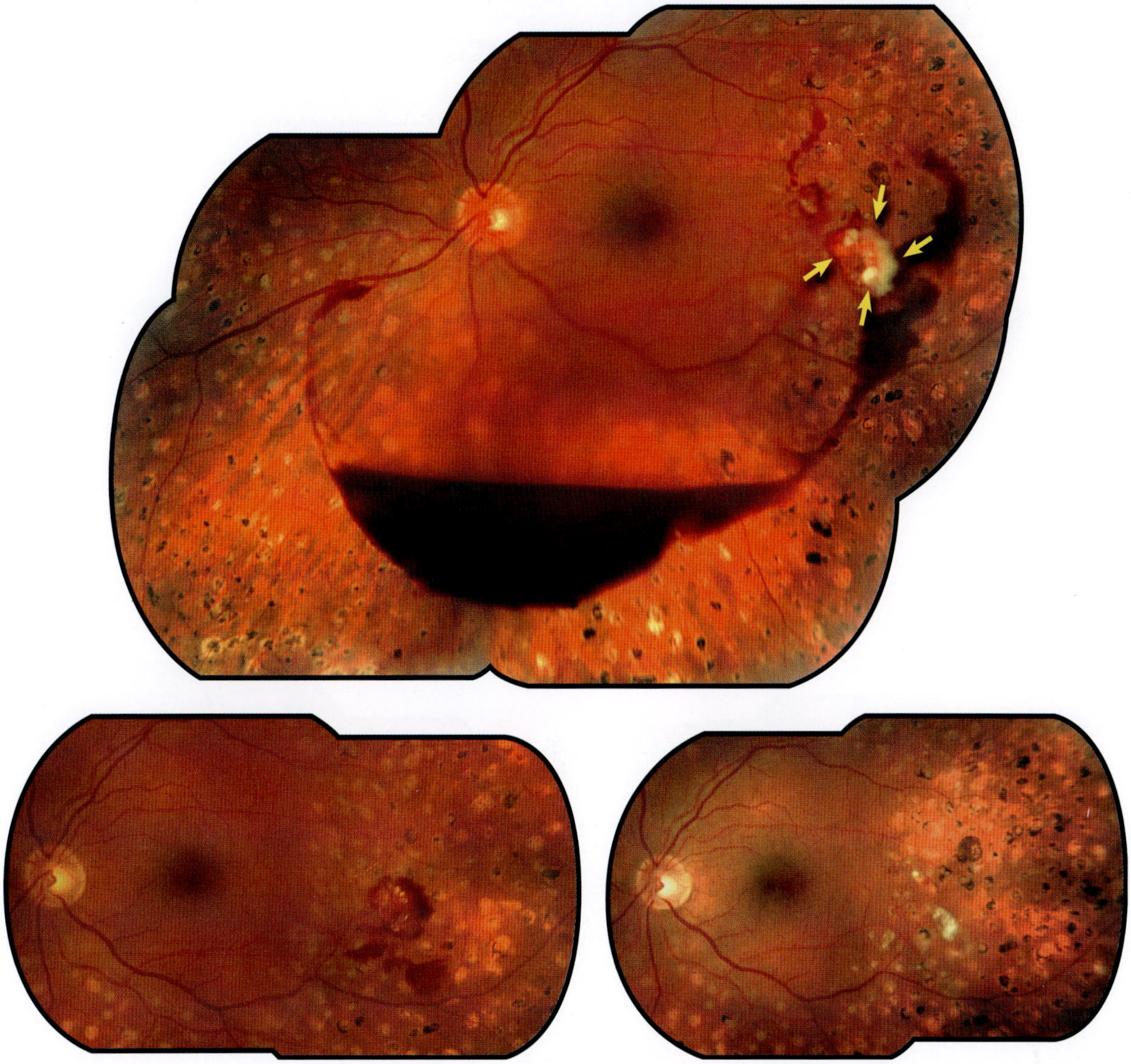

Pre-retinal and vitreous hemorrhage is noted in the color montage above. Additional PRP fill-in therapy was administered because of persistent neovascularization in the temporal macula *(arrows)*. In the lower left image, pre-retinal hemorrhage has improved and early regression of the neovascularization is noted 3 months later. The image on the lower right shows complete regression 2 years after additional photocoagulation treatment.

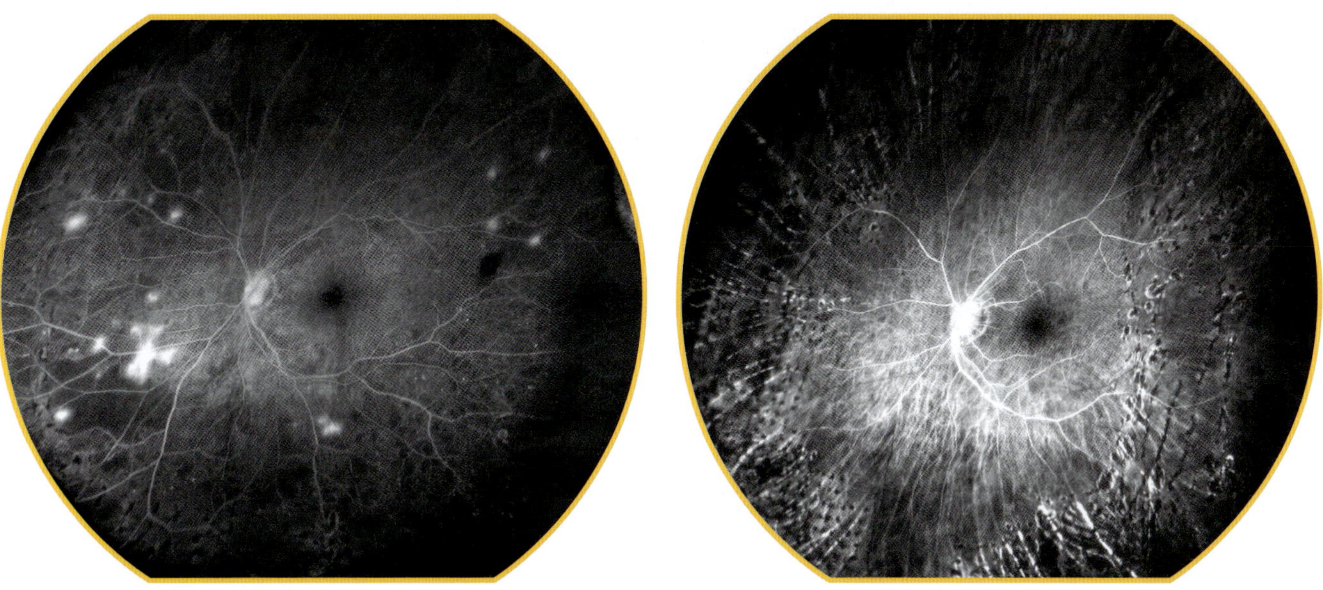

Widefield FA showing neovascularization elsewhere in this patient with proliferative diabetic retinopathy. Following PRP, there is regression of the NVE. *Courtesy of Dr. Mark Blumenkranz*

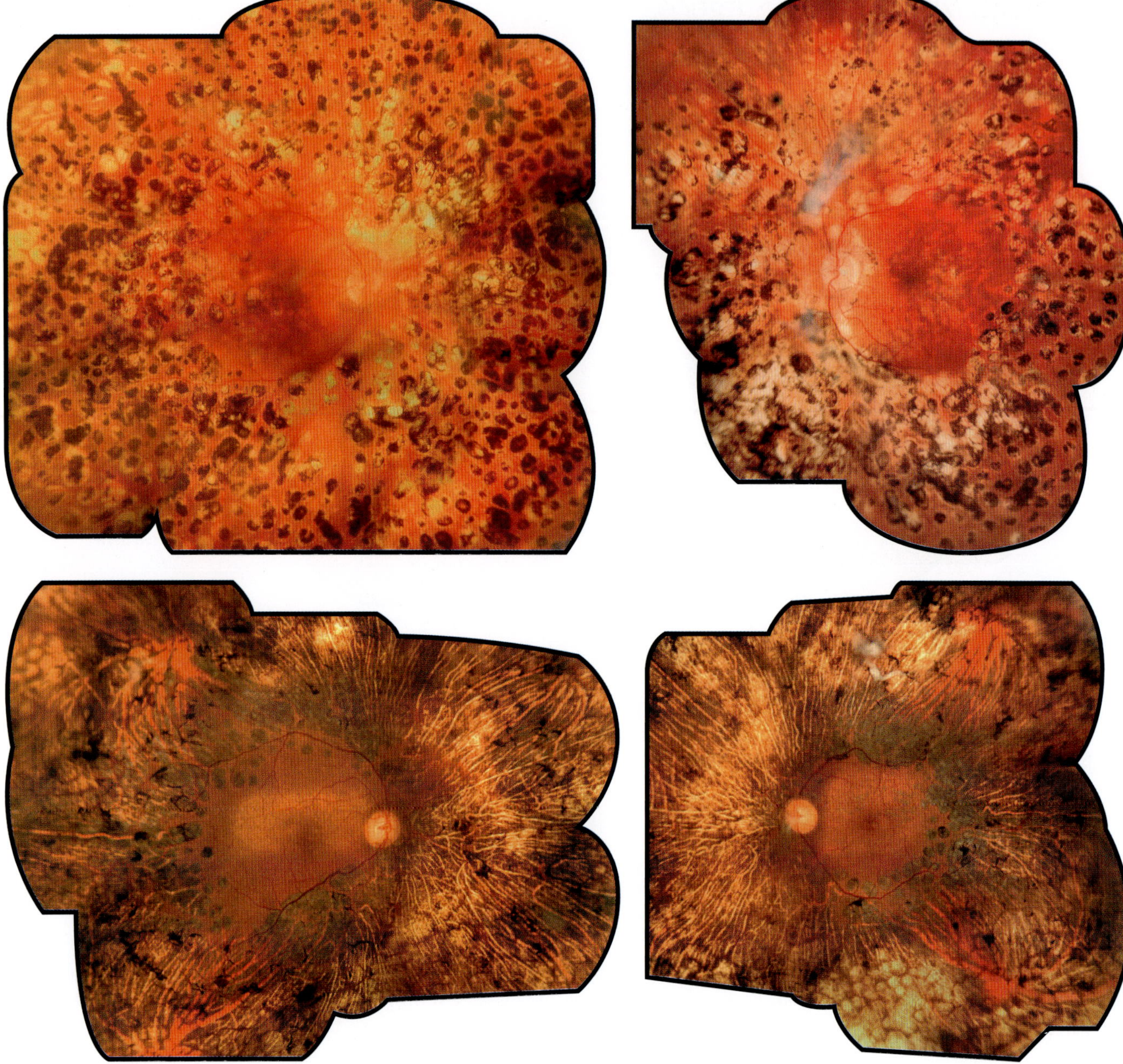

Color montage images of eyes with regressed PDR after PRP therapy. Note the widespread pigmentary and atrophic photocoagulation scars scattered diffusely through the peripheral fundus.

Treatment: Vitreoretinal Surgery

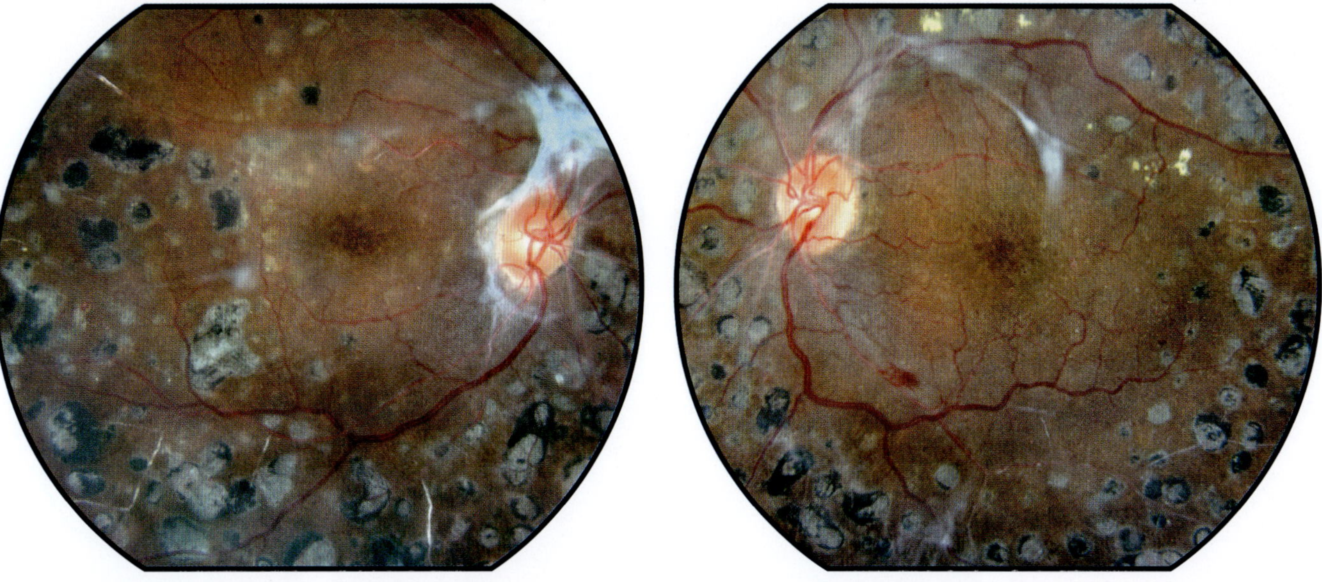

Color images from patient status post combined vitrectomy and endophotocoagulation for active PDR and tractional macular detachment in each eye. Note the remnants of fibrous tissue at the disc and in the posterior pole. The macula is flat in each eye.

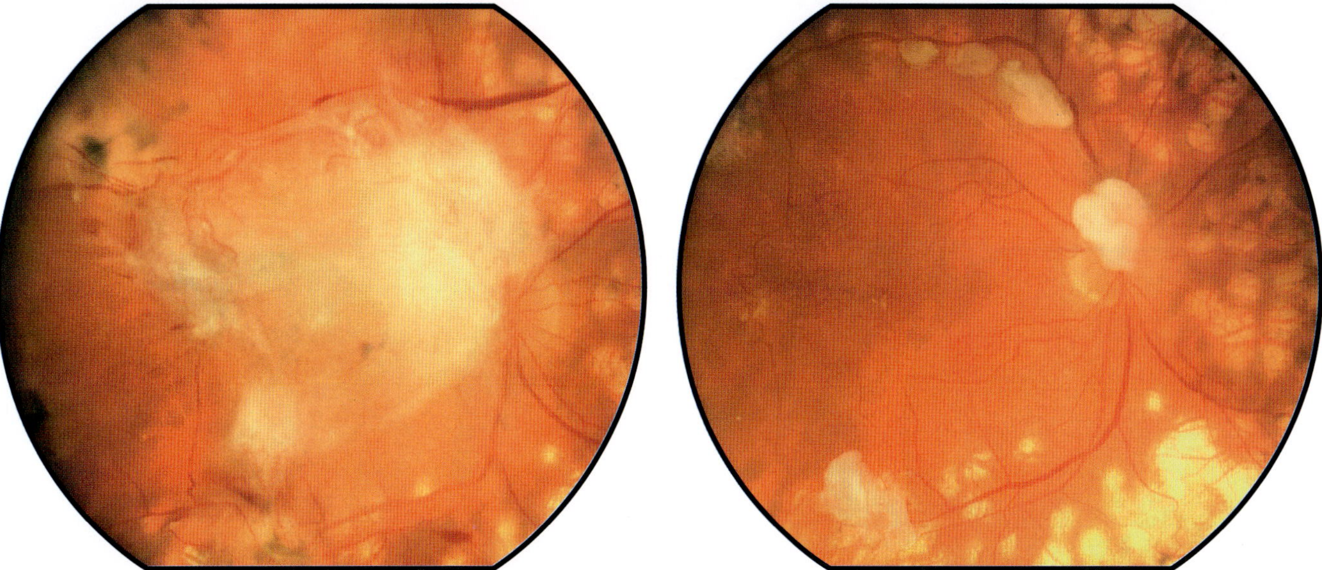

This patient received PRP treatment for active PDR. Fibrous proliferation of the posterior pole ensued *(left)*. Pars plana vitrectomy was performed to remove the fibrous tissue. After surgery the macula was flat and dry, but residual stumps of fibrous tissue along the vascular arcades and at the disc are noted. *Courtesy of Dr. Yale Fisher*

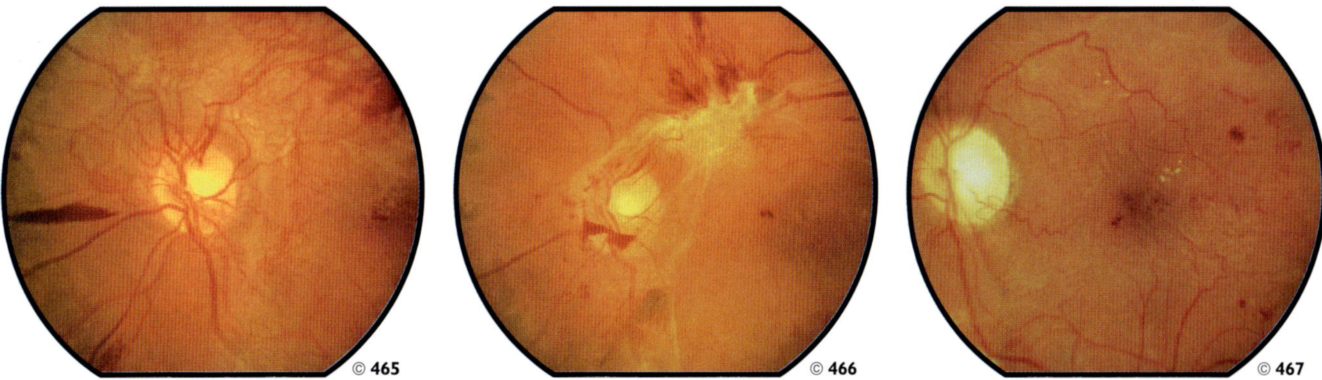

This patient shows severe NVD *(left)*. PRP was performed and the patient experienced a marked decrease in visual acuity. Contraction and consolidation of fibrous tissue caused macular detachment *(middle)*. Vitrectomy was performed with resolution of macular detachment and an improvement of the visual acuity to 20/30 *(right)*.

Treatment: Intravitreal Anti-VEGF Therapy

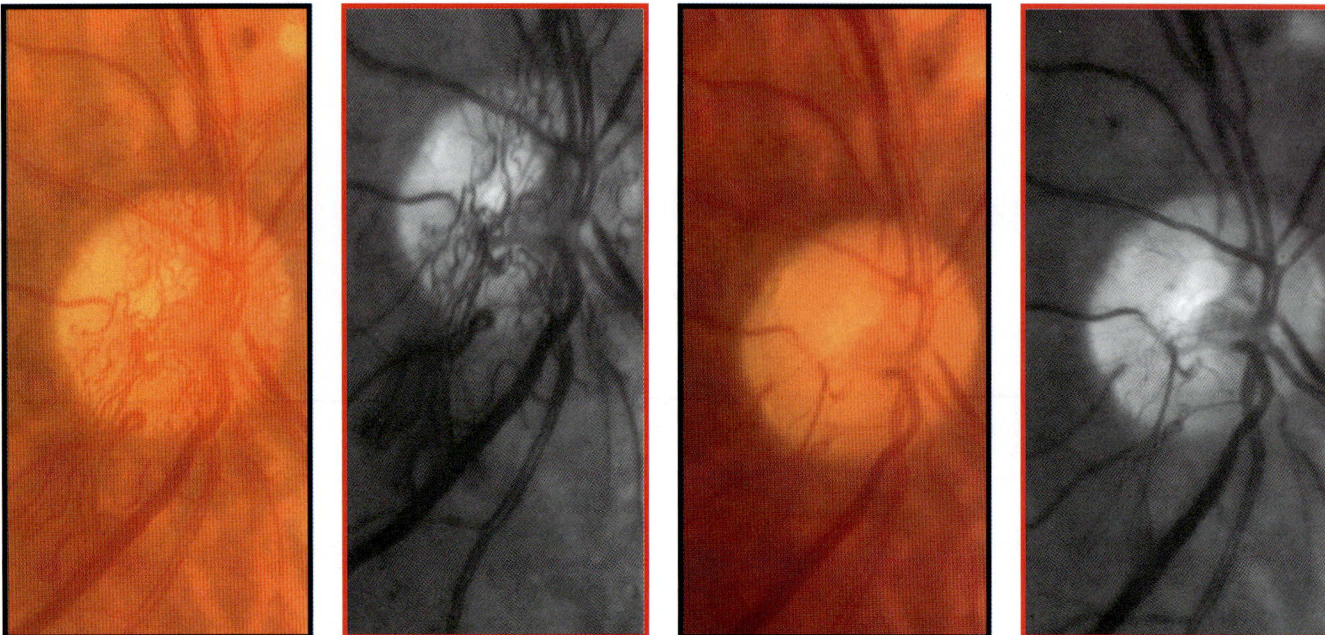

This patient presented with severe NVD *(color, left)*. The neovascularization is better appreciated with red-free photography *(red free, left)*. Following administration of intravitreal bevacizumab, there was dramatic regression of the neovascularization *(color and red-free, right)*. *Courtesy of Dr. Robert Avery*

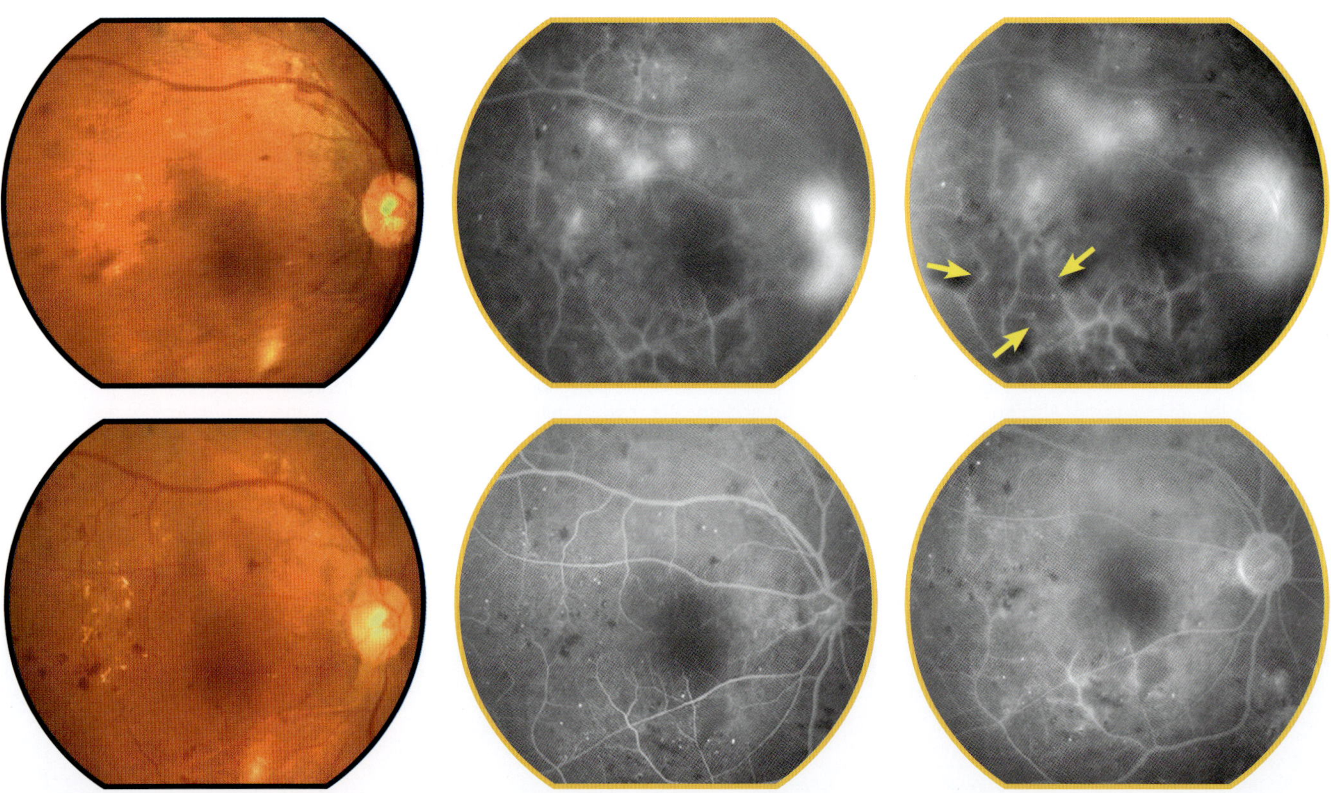

Note the presence of NVD and NVE in this patient *(top row)*. Inferotemporal macular ischemia is also noted *(arrows)*. Following administration of intravitreal bevacizumab *(bottom row)*, there was complete regression of the NVD and NVE. There was also remodeling of the ischemic capillary bed with near complete reperfusion.

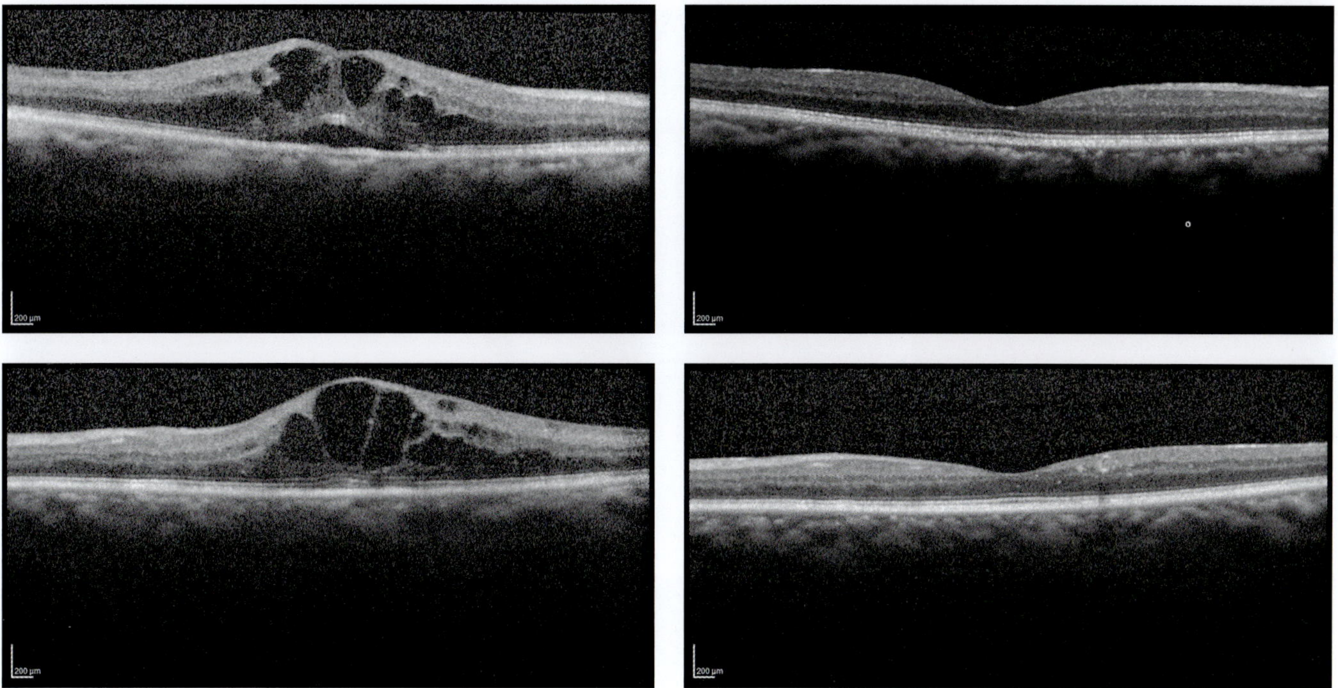

SD-OCT of a patient's right *(top row)* and left *(bottom row)* eye showing severe diabetic cystoid macular edema at presentation *(left images)*. The patient was treated with anti-VEGF intravitreal injections with resolution of macular edema *(right images)*.

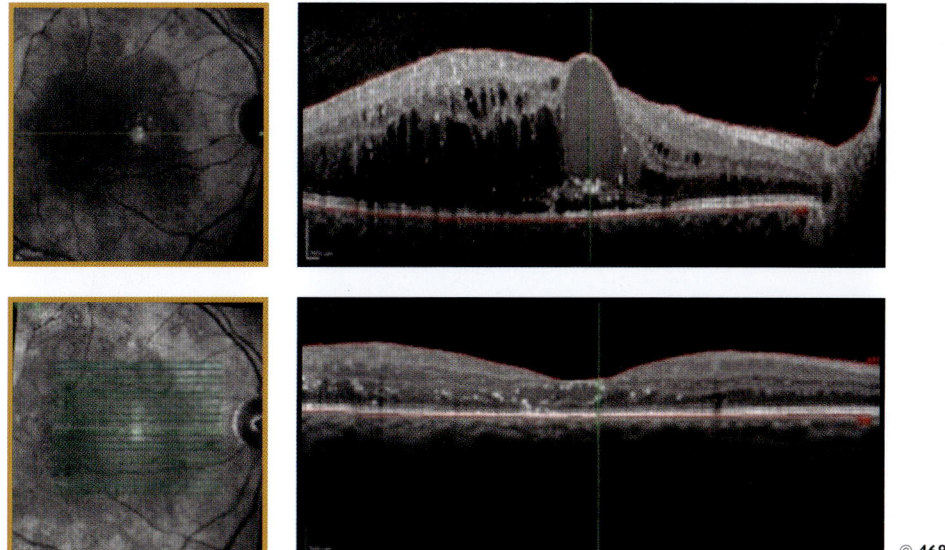

© **468**

This patient has persistent diabetic macular edema following anti-VEGF therapy. Three months after intravitreal dexamethasone injection (Ozurdex), the edema has resolved. There are persistent hyper-reflective foci that likely represent exudates or lipid laden macrophages or microglia.

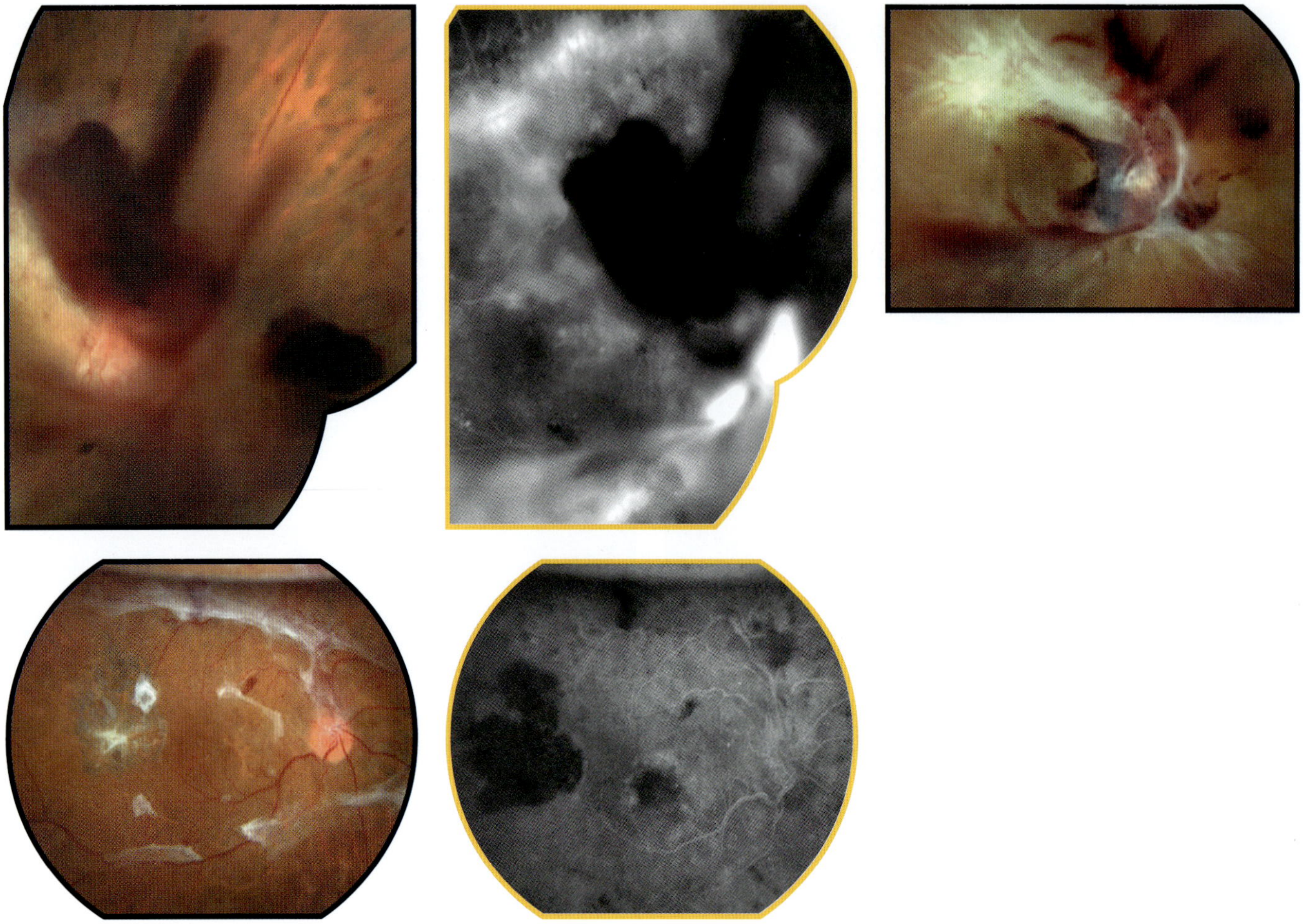

Vitreous hemorrhage and PDR is noted in this patient *(upper row, left)*. The FA shows a ring of neovascularization surrounding the posterior pole *(upper row, middle image)* and blockage from the hemorrhage. Intravitreal bevacizumab was administered and within 10 days actively proliferating neovascularization converted to fibrous stalks of tissue extending into the vitreous *(upper row, right)*. Pars plana vitrectomy was then carried out. After excision of the avascular fibrous tissue, the macular detachment is resolved *(bottom left)* and visual acuity improved to 20/30. The postoperative FA shows resolution of leakage at the disc and in the posterior pole. *Courtesy of Dr. Michael Cooney*

Rubeosis Iridis

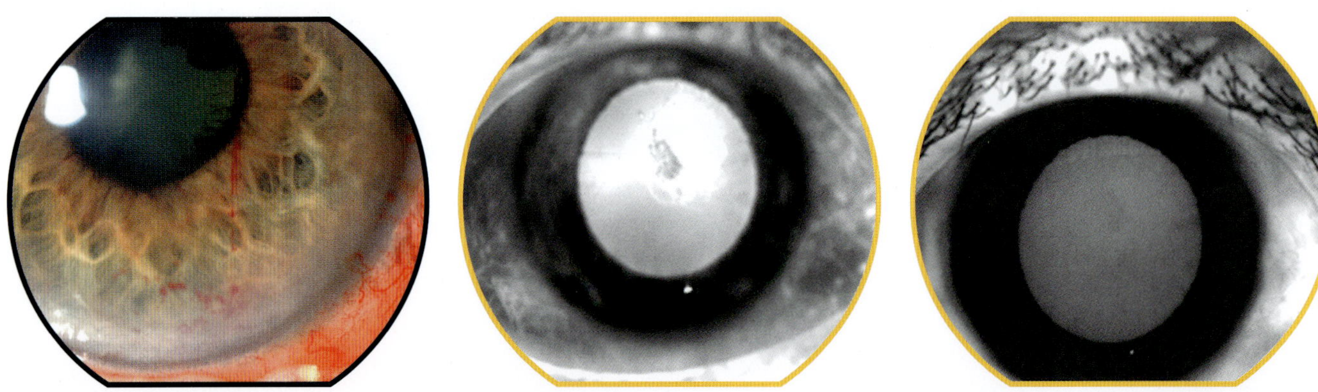

Rubeosis iridis due to retinal vascular ischemia and PDR is noted in this patient. The vessels are noted at the pupillary margin and in the angle *(color photograph)* and associated ectropion uvea is present. The FA shows leakage of these iris vessels *(middle)*. Following one injection of bevacizumab, there is dramatic regression of the neovascularization *(right)*. Leakage on iris fluorescein angiography is resolved following the administration of this drug.

Sickle-Cell Retinopathy

Sickle-cell disease is a spectrum of hemoglobinopathies that cause hemolytic anemia and a systemic vasculopathy. Depending on the inheritance of the specific β-globin polypeptide chain abnormality, various genotypes can arise, including: AS or AC sickle-cell trait, SS or SC sickle-cell disease, and sickle β-thalassemia disease. Those with sickle-cell trait are asymptomatic with no associated morbidity or mortality but may be at greater risk of retinal complications associated with other retinal vascular diseases. Patients with sickle cell disease (SS or SC) experience significant morbidity and even mortality. When exposed to hypoxia, hyperosmolarity, or acidosis, hemoglobin S polymerizes within the erythrocyte and reduces cell pliability. This increases hemolysis and blood viscosity, resulting in vascular occlusion and ischemia. The SC and Sβthal genotypes are most likely to exhibit retinal complications including peripheral retinal vascular ischemia and neovascularization, vitreous hemorrhage, and traction retinal detachment. Nonproliferative sickle-cell retinopathy findings include salmon patch hemorrhages, iridescent spots, and black sunburst scars. A salmon patch is a round retinal hemorrhage. Initially, these hemorrhages are reddish, and later turn salmon in color. Hemosiderin laden macrophages produce the characteristic glistening iridescent spots. Proliferative sickle-cell retinopathy occurs in the peripheral fundus, beginning with an arteriolar occlusion. It is followed by an AV shunt and retinal neovascularization (NV) at the junction between perfused and non-perfused retina. Bleeding into the vitreous (or the sub internal limiting membrane space) may occur. Fibrous NV may develop and induce tractional changes and detachment.

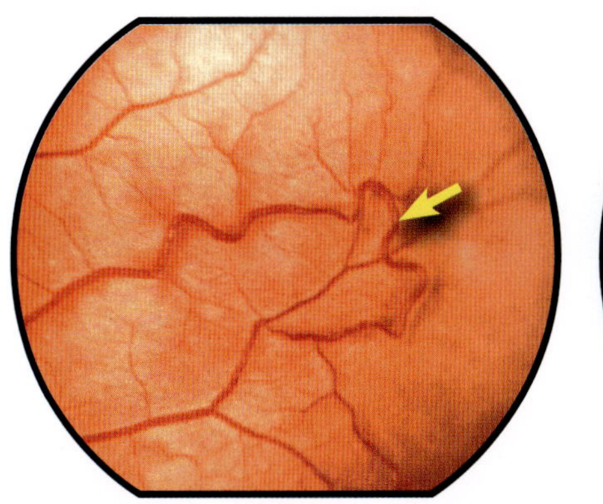
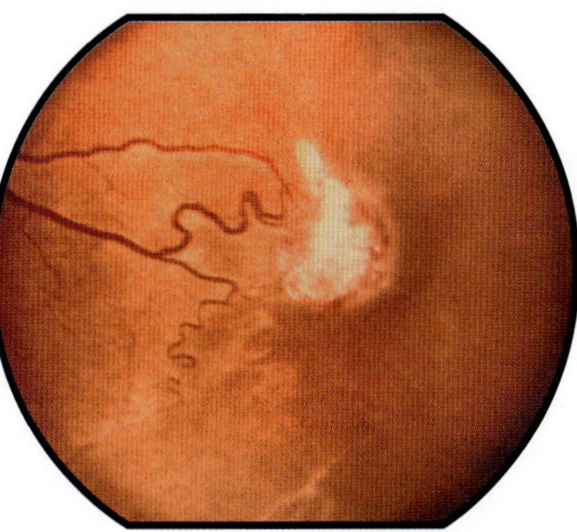
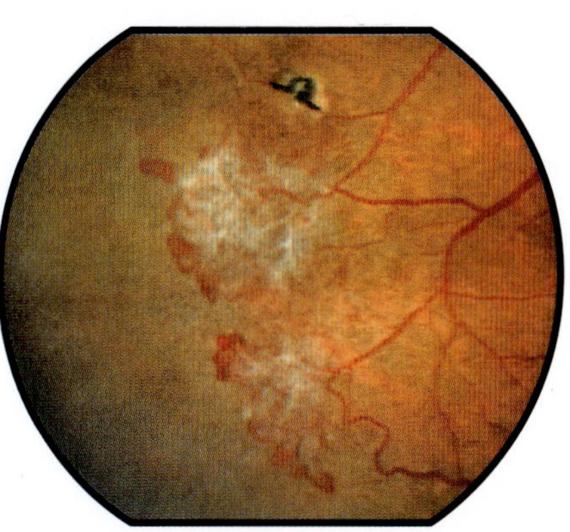

These are patients with peripheral retinal vascular ischemia and NV due to sickle-cell retinopathy. The image on the left shows an arteriovenous shunt at the junction between perfused and non-perfused retina *(arrow)*. The middle and right images show peripheral retinal NV with a significant fibrotic component. The edge of the abnormal vascular bed on the non-perfused side of the retina shows actively proliferating buds of NV.

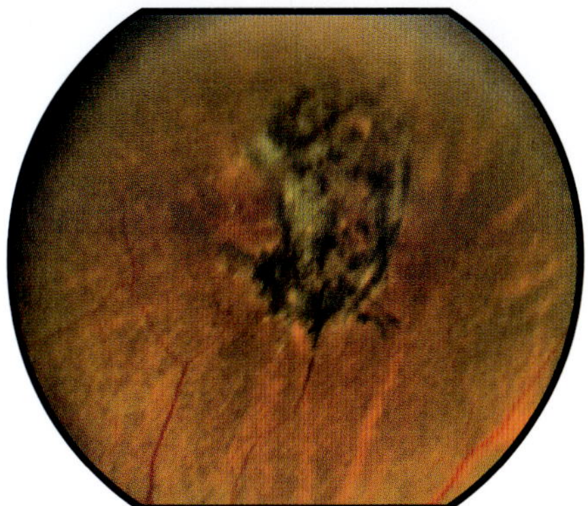
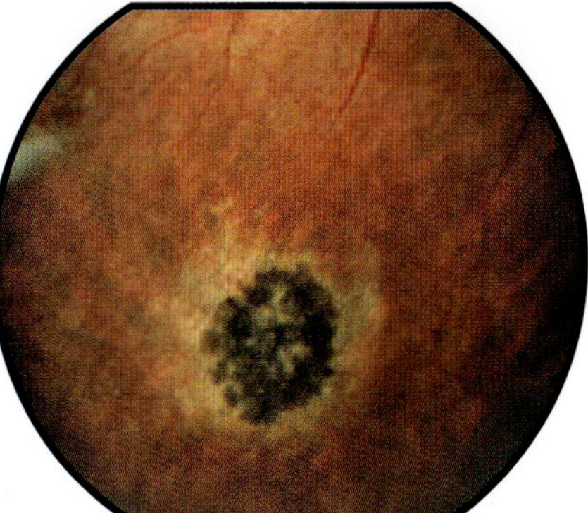
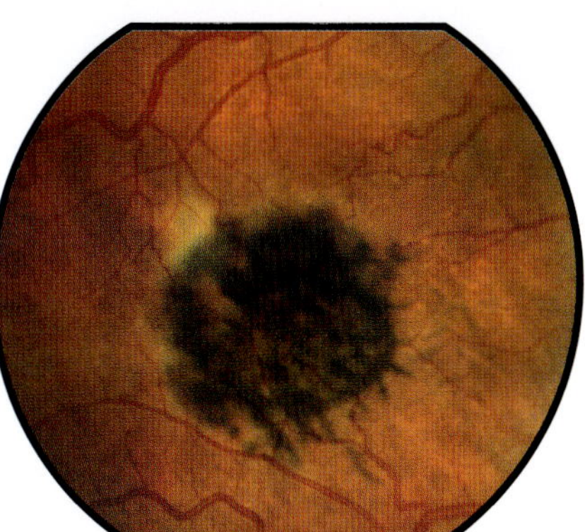

Black sunburst lesions are resorbed subretinal hemorrhages with secondary retinal pigment epithelial hypertrophy and hyperplasia.

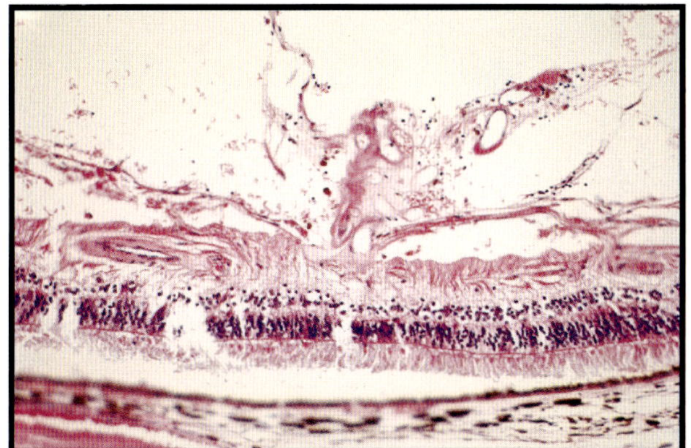

A histopathological section of a patient with sickle-cell retinopathy shows pre-retinal NV. There is a discontinuity of the internal limiting membrane due to the extension of vessels into the vitreous. Fibroglial tissue, few lymphocytes, and numerous sickled erythrocytes are present near the sea fan *(upper part of image)*.

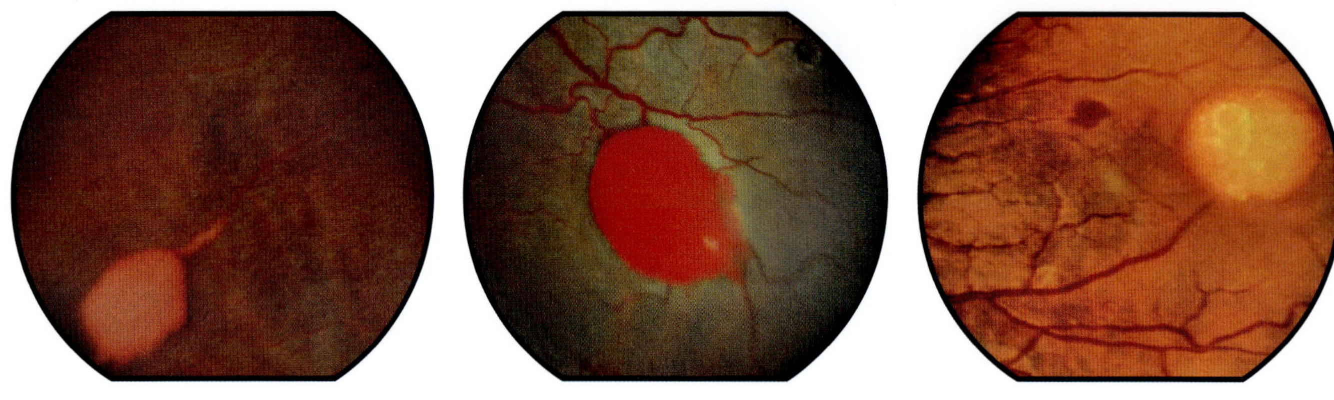

These images illustrate salmon-patch retinal hemorrhages.

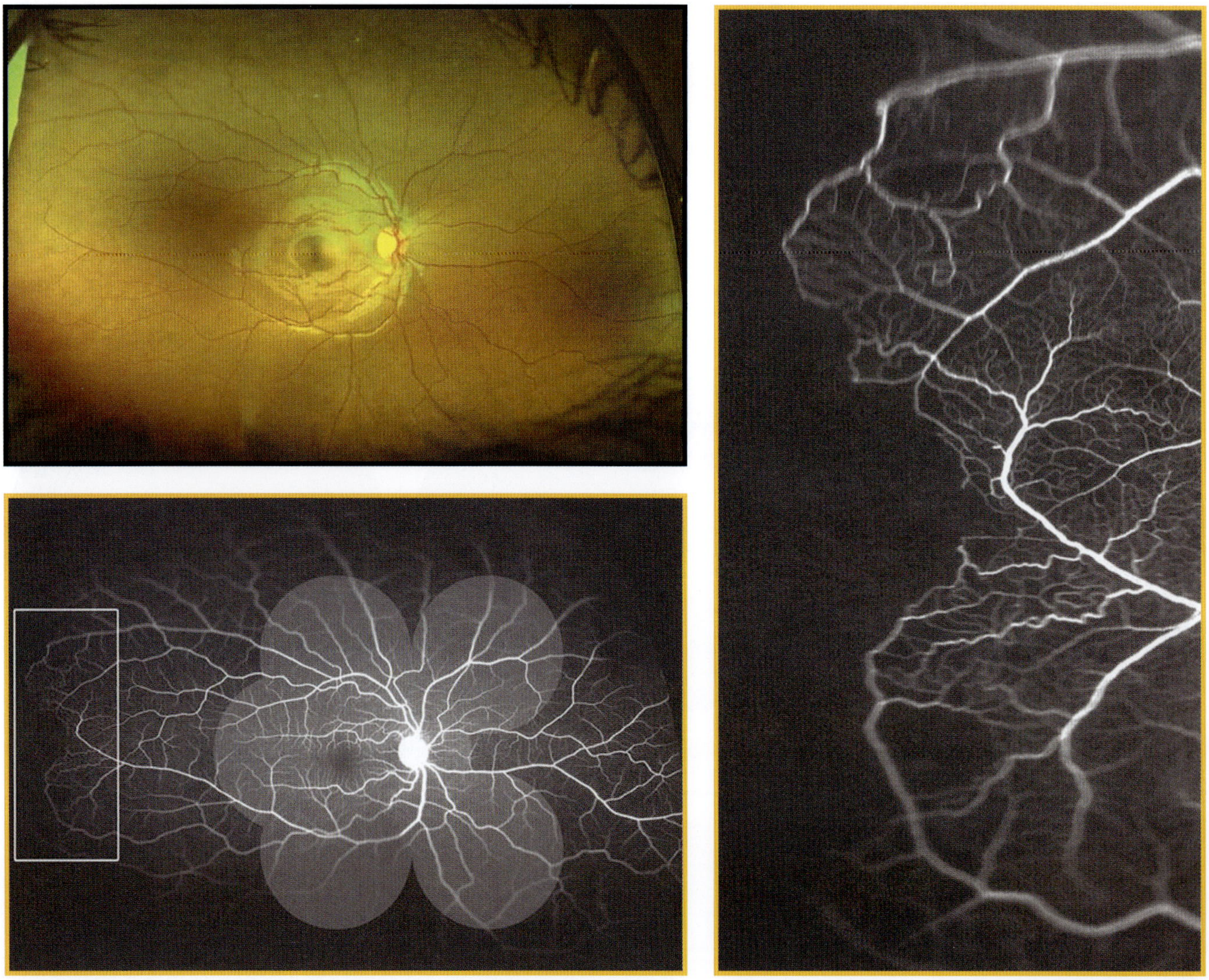

© 470

This is a 10-year-old girl with SC disease. Her widefield fundus photograph is unremarkable *(upper left)*. Widefield angiography reveals large areas of capillary ischemia and non-perfusion in the periphery well beyond the standard seven fields *(shaded area)*. On the right is a magnified view of the boxed area showing arteriovenous anastomosis at the junction of perfused and non-perfused retina.

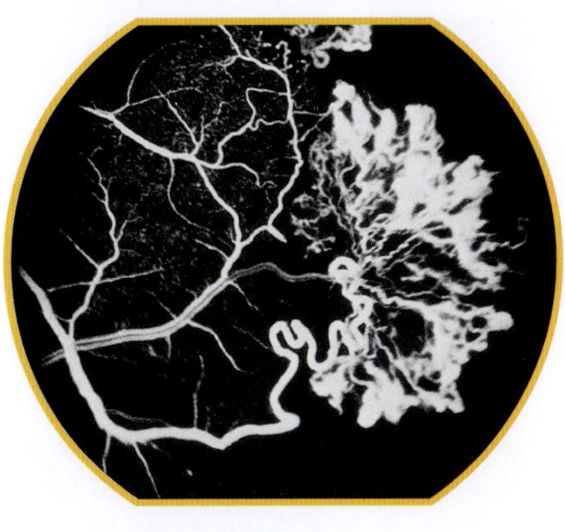
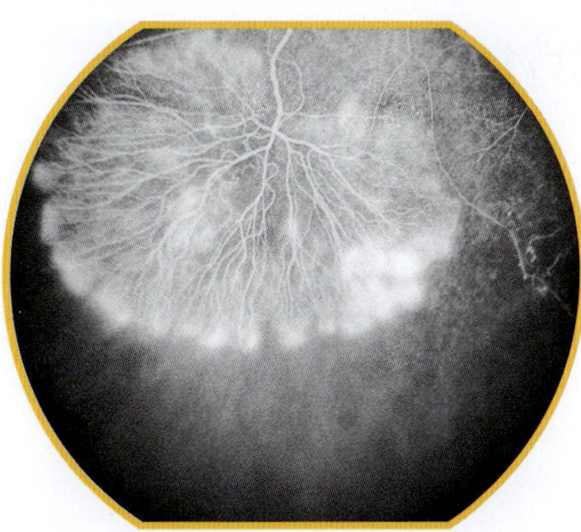
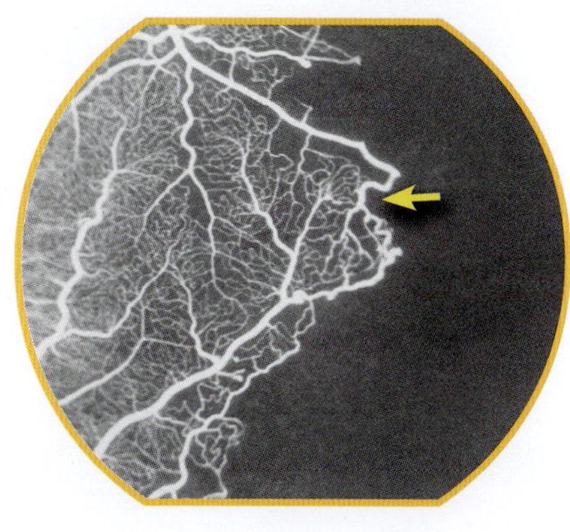

Note the fluorescein angiographic presence of characteristic NV in a sea-fan pattern in proliferative sickle cell retinopathy *(left and middle)*. These abnormal vessels proliferate at a discrete junction between perfused and non-perfused retina. The FA image on the right shows an arteriolar-venular anastomosis *(arrow)* at the junction between perfused and non-perfused retina. Arteriolar infarction can be followed by arteriolar-venular anastomosis and pre-retinal NV.

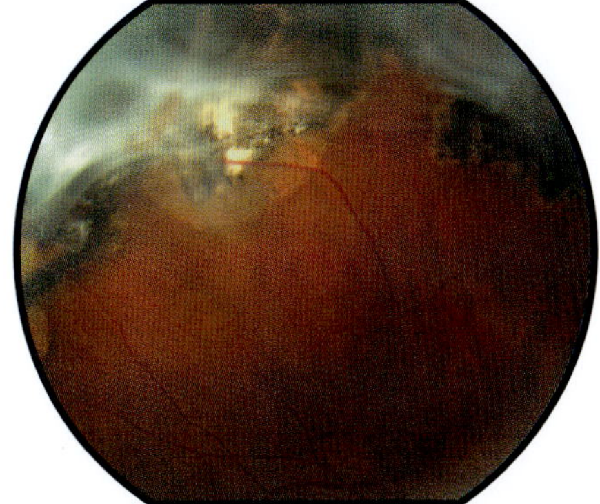
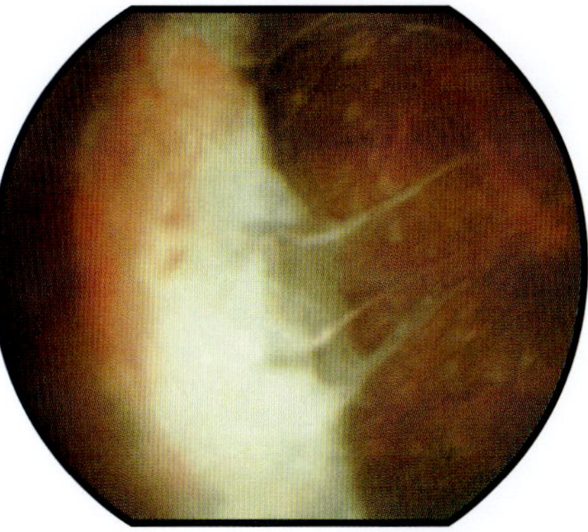
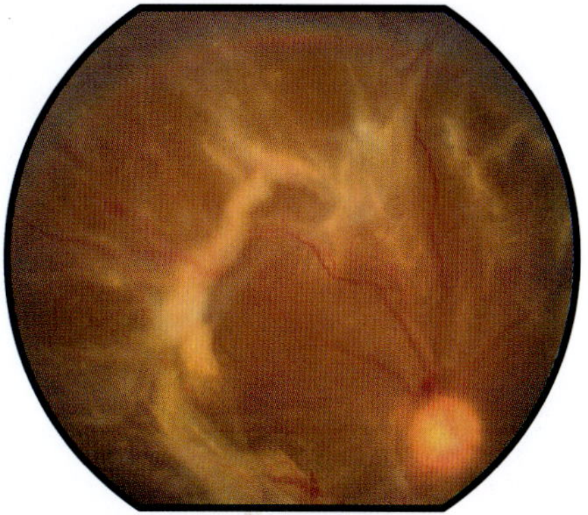

Peripheral retinal NV in sickle-cell retinopathy may result in hemorrhage, fibrosis, vitreoretinal traction, and tractional retinal detachment. Even a rhegmatogenous detachment may occur. Note the severe fibrous proliferation limited to the periphery in the two color images *(left and middle)*. Pre-retinal fibrosis extends to the posterior pole and is associated with traction retinal detachment *(right color image)*. Laser treatment was carried out in an attempt to induce infarction and regression of the neovascularized complex *(left)*. The NV may autoinfarct, which induces a spontaneous fibrous avascular lesion.

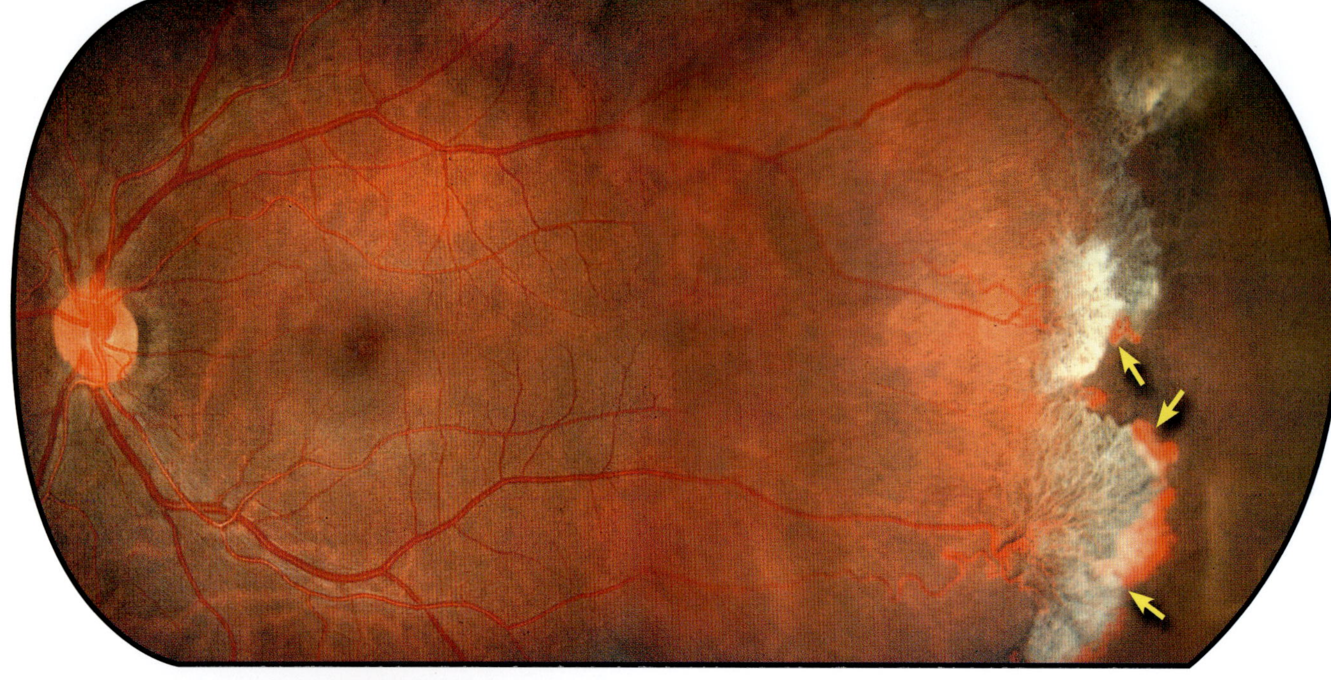

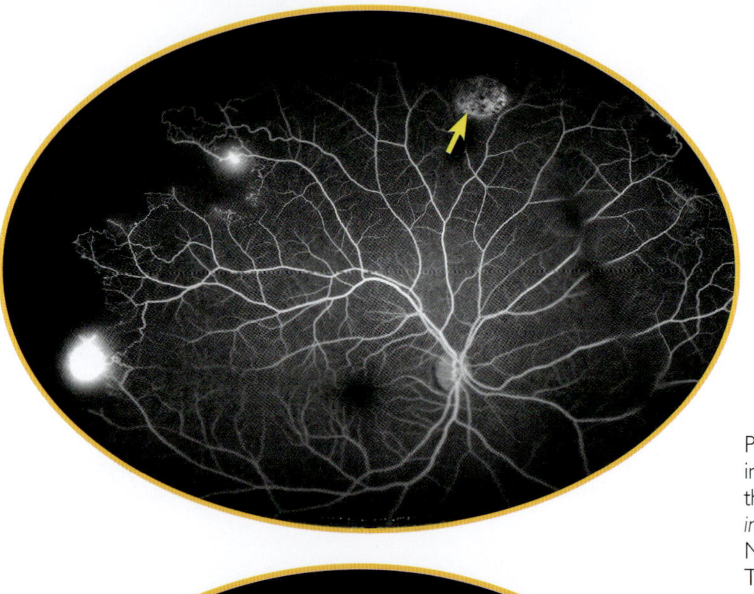

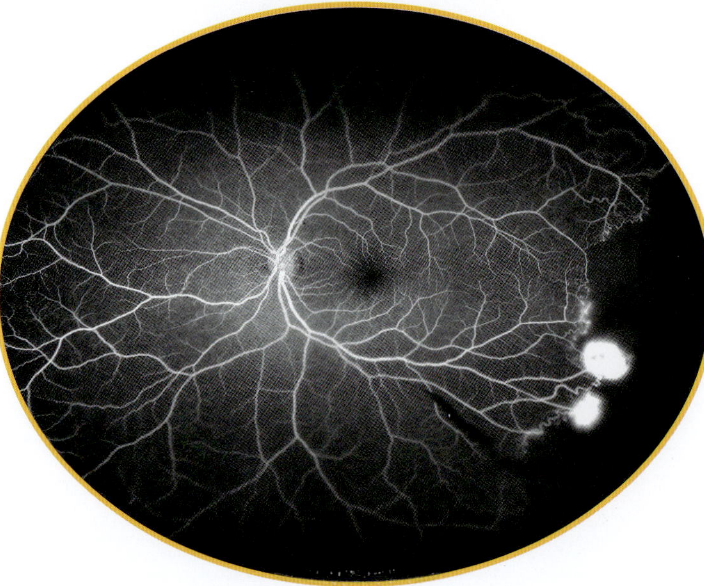

Proliferative sickle-cell retinopathy with fibrovascular NV is noted in the color montage. An active neovascular fringe is present at the junction between perfused and non-perfused retina *(top image, arrows)*. The widefield FA in another sickle patient shows NV at the junction between perfused and non-perfused retina. There is an autoinfarcted area in the middle image *(arrow)* with staining of a pigment epithelial scar. *Images courtesy of Michael P. Kelly, CRA*

Macular Manifestations

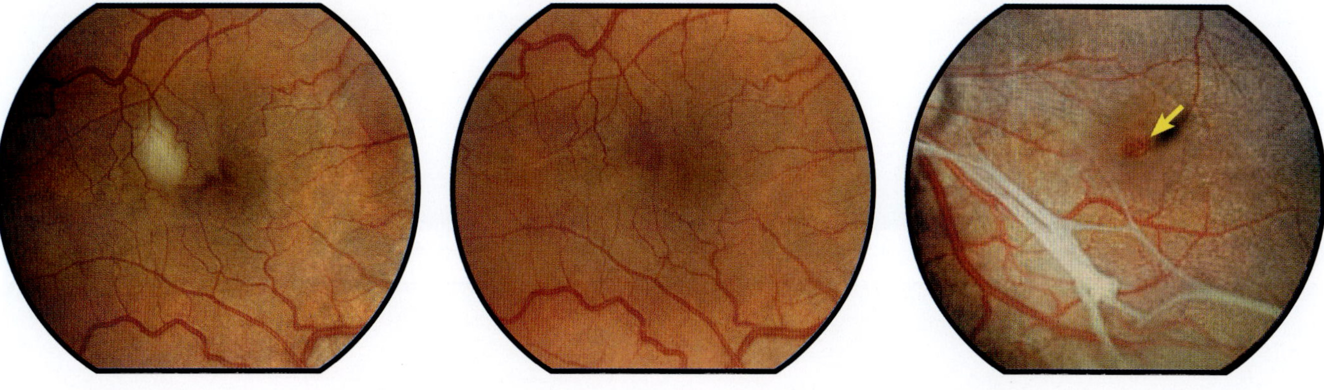

A myriad of retinal vascular abnormalities can be seen in the posterior segment in sickle-cell retinopathy. A large CWS is seen on the color image *(left)*. With resolution there is the characteristic sign of inner retinal depression *(middle)*. The right image shows fibrosis with macular traction and a small macular hole *(arrow)*.

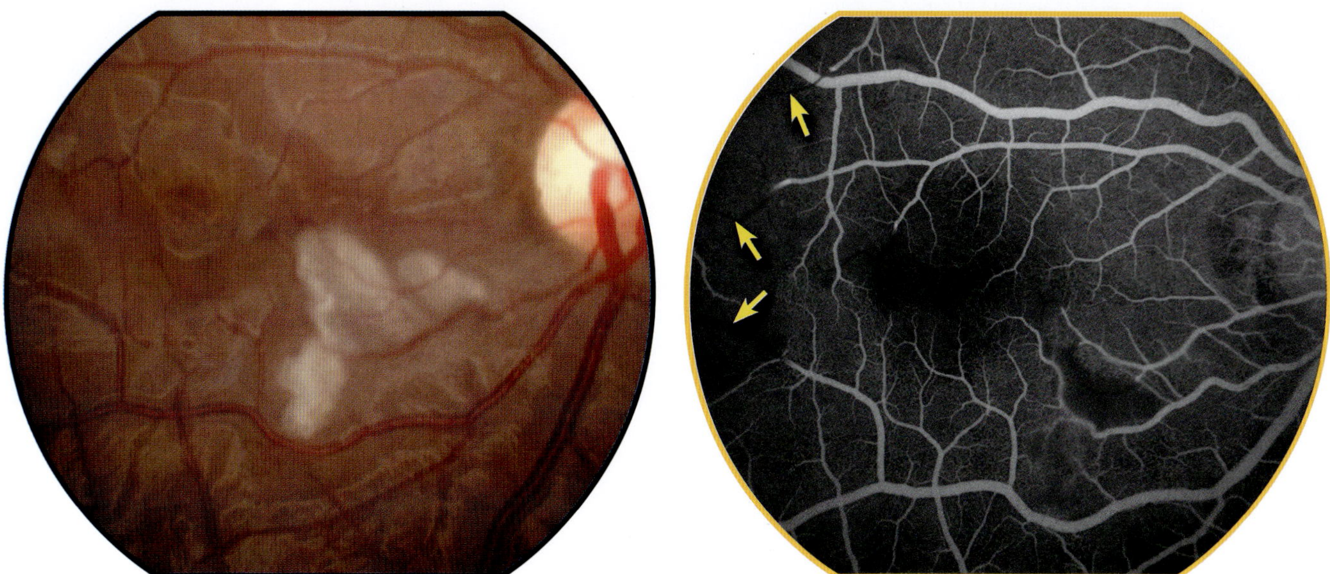

A large inner retinal infarct or large CWS is illustrated *(right)* with capillary ischemia shown on the corresponding FA. More peripheral vessels are also obstructed *(arrows)*.

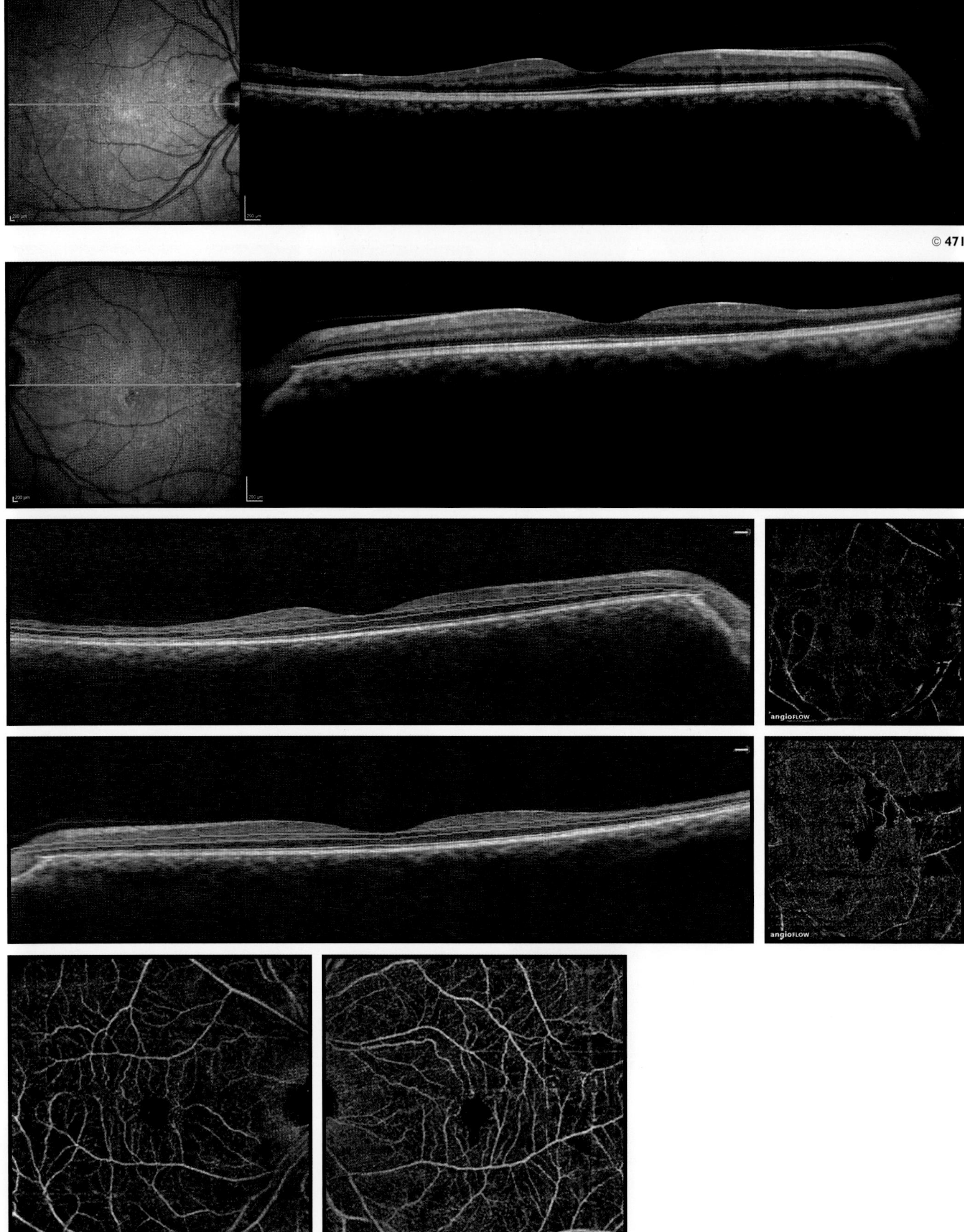

SD-OCT of this patient with sickle cell retinopathy shows inner retinal atrophy of the temporal macula, a finding common in sickle cell maculopathy *(first and second rows, and third and fourth row left images)*. OCT angiography segmented at the level of the deep plexus of the same patient showed more significant flow reduction in the deep retinal capillary plexus *(third and fourth row right images)* versus the superficial capillary plexus *(bottom row). Bottom images courtesy of Dr. Irena Tsui, MD*

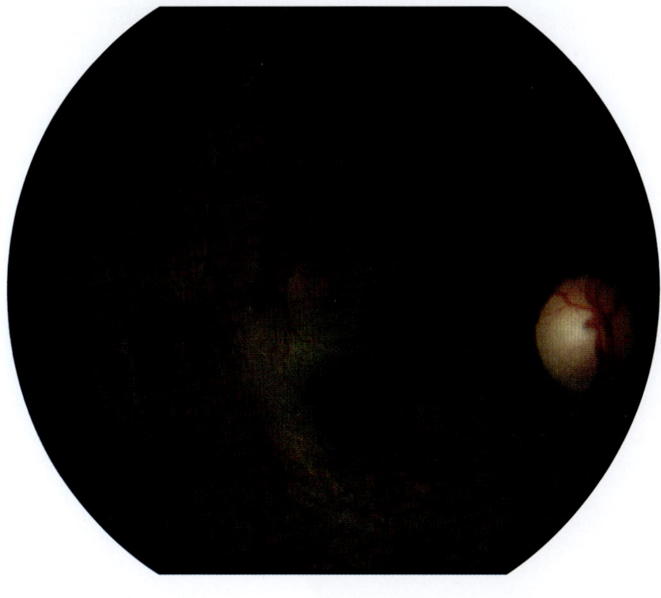

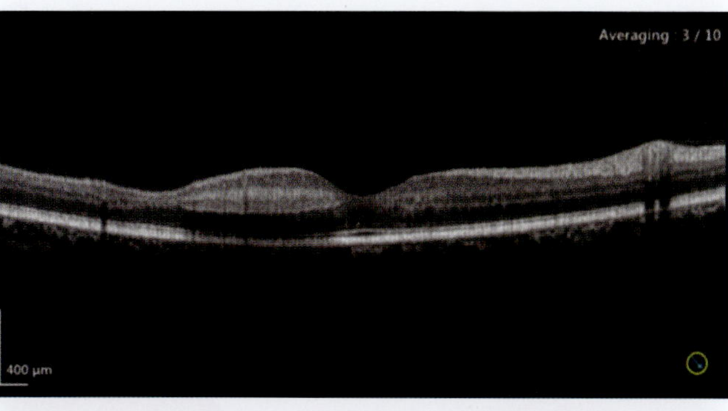

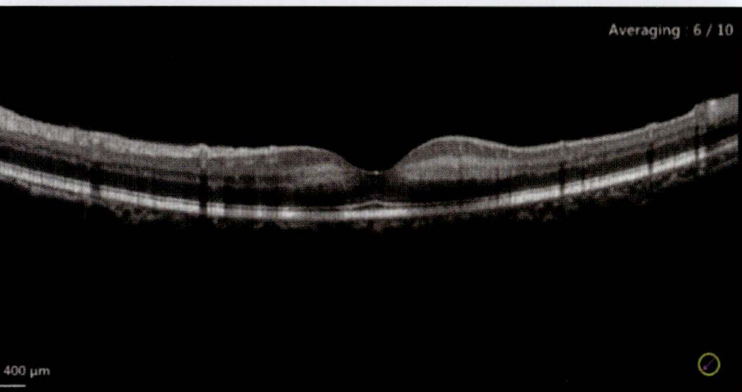

Color fundus photograph of the right eye of a patient with sickle cell retinopathy showing a deep gray retinal infarct temporal to the fovea of the right eye. Corresponding SD-OCT illustrated hyper-reflective band like lesions within the INL consistent with PAMM due to INL infarction. *Images courtesy of Suzanne Yzer*

Detachment

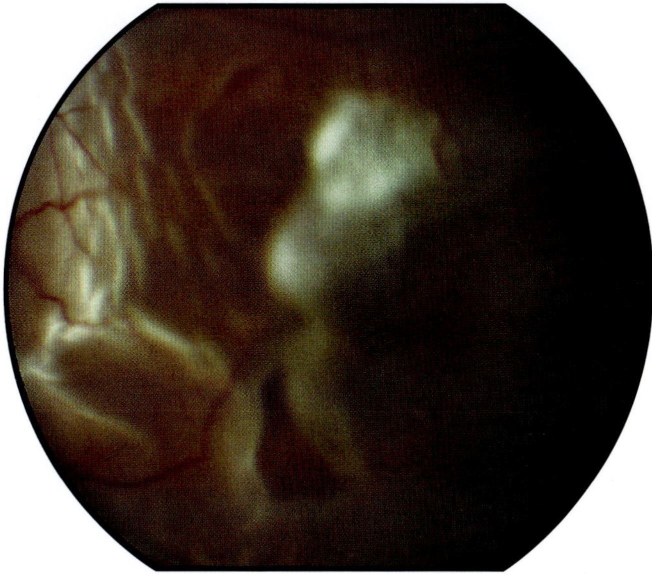

Peripheral rhegmatogenous retinal detachment can be a complication of sickle-cell retinopathy. Note the retinal detachment is associated with fish-mouth retinal tears and retinal folds and early proliferative vitreoretinopathy.

Hyperlipidemia

Severe hyperlipidemia may produce lipemia retinalis, a disorder that is associated with extremely high triglyceride levels exceeding 2000 mg/dL. As the triglyceride levels approach 4000 or higher there is progressive creamy coloration of the vessels in the posterior pole (as well as the periphery) and the fundus may assume a salmon-colored appearance. Lipemia retinalis may be associated with retinal vascular abnormalities, such as BRVO and lipid exudation causing decreased visual acuity.

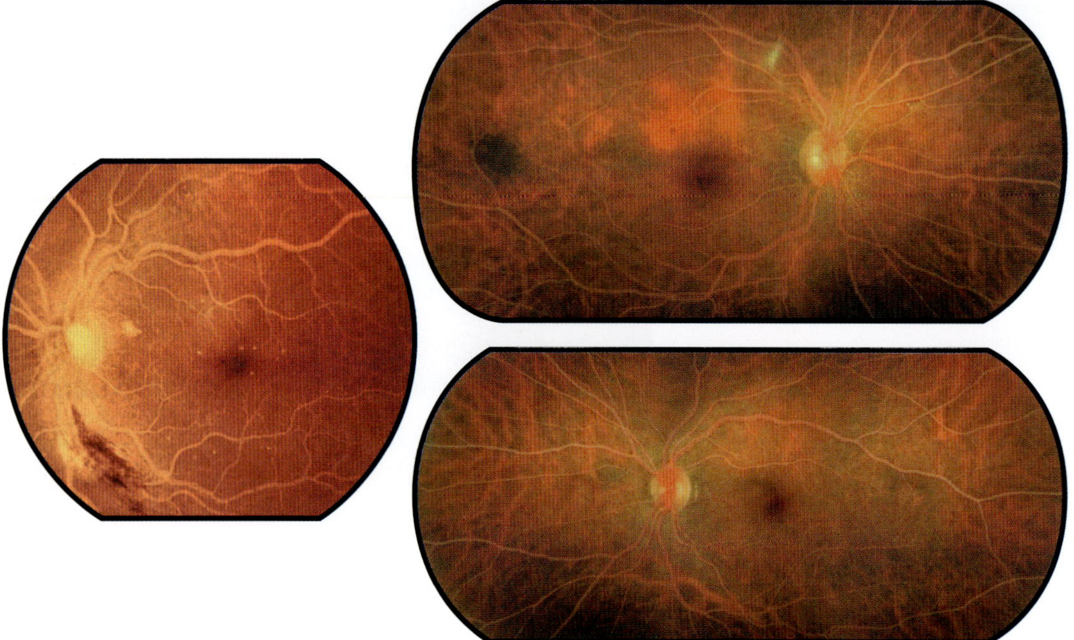

These two patients have lipemia retinalis with markedly elevated triglyceride levels. The discoloration of the retinal vasculature makes it difficult to differentiate arteries from veins. Note the retinal hemorrhages along the course of the inferotemporal retinal vessels consistent with an associated BRVO *(left)*. *Courtesy of Scott Oliver*

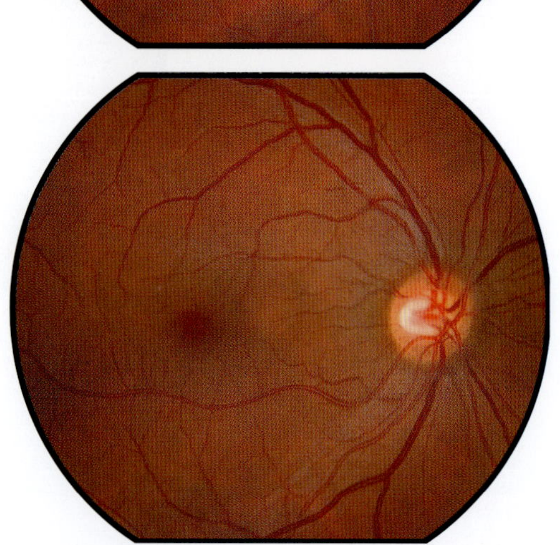

Note the normalization of the fundus appearance with reduction of the high serum triglyceride levels in this patient who presented with lipemia retinalis. *Images courtesy of Michael Fikhman, MD*

Ocular Ischemic Syndrome

Ocular ischemic syndrome is a retinal vascular disorder, previously referred to as venous stasis retinopathy, which is the result of carotid artery insufficiency. It occurs generally after the age of 50 in individuals with significant stenosis of the carotid artery system. It may be unilateral or bilateral. Cardinal retinal signs include retinal venous dilation (but not tortuosity) with scattered midperipheral microaneurysms and dot and blot hemorrhages. Venous beading and associated peripheral ischemia is typical. Vision loss may be the result of macular edema, retinal NV, vitreous hemorrhage, and/or rubeosis iridis. Delayed perfusion of the retinal and choroidal circulation, macular edema, and disc staining are seen with fluorescein angiography. Opposite of a central retinal vein occlusion, the central venous pressure is remarkably reduced.

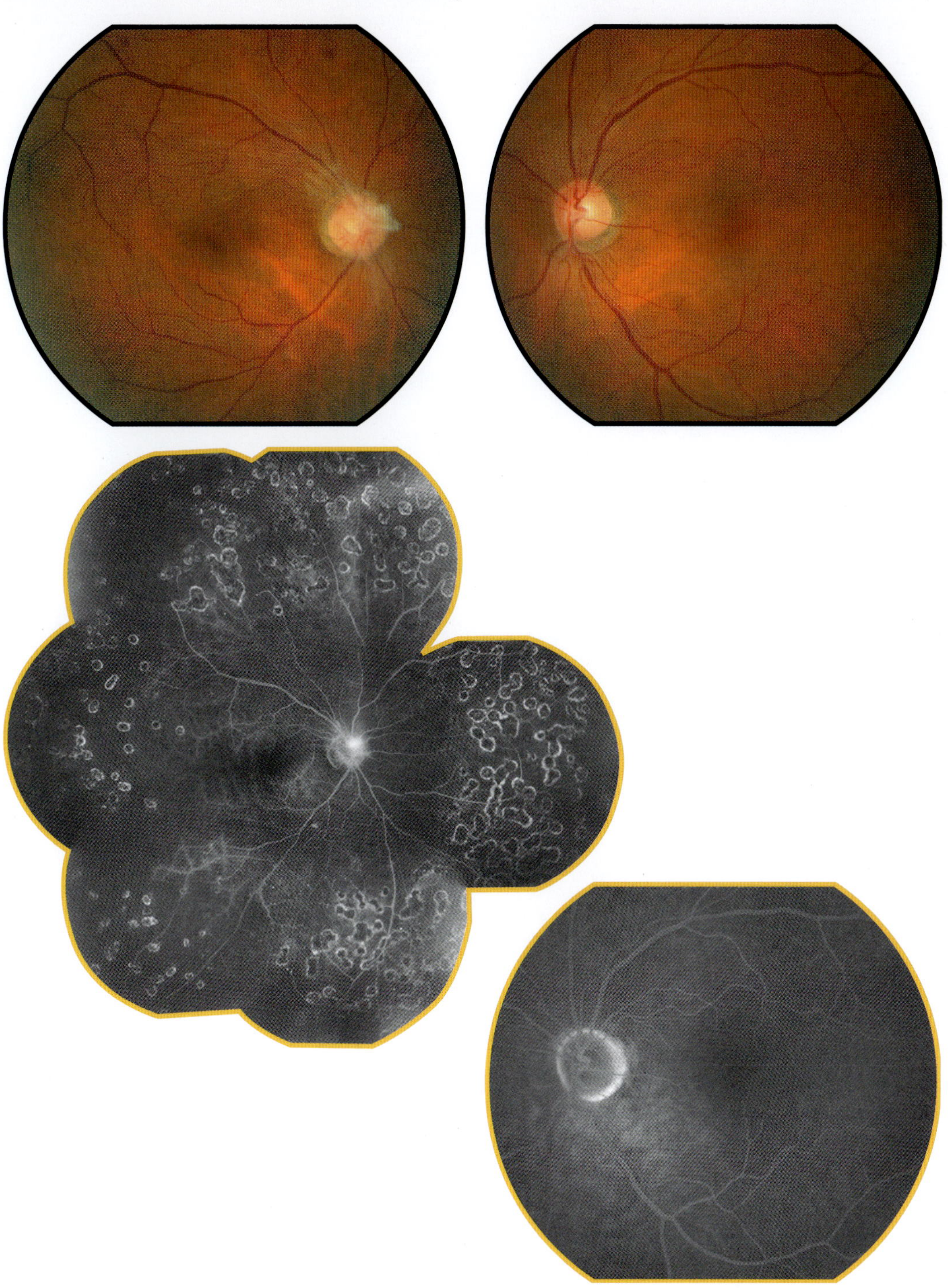

Color fundus photographs of this patient with diabetes illustrates asymmetric retinopathy with fibrovascular neovascularization of the disc (NVD) and midperipheral intraretinal hemorrhages on the right side. Color fundus photography is normal on the left. Fluorescein angiography shows delayed filling of the arterioles, NVD, peripheral non-perfusion and late staining of the retinal venous system on the right. Staining of PRP scars is also noted. FA was normal on the left. Carotid ultrasonography confirmed the diagnosis of ocular ischemic syndrome secondary to severe right-sided carotid occlusive disease.

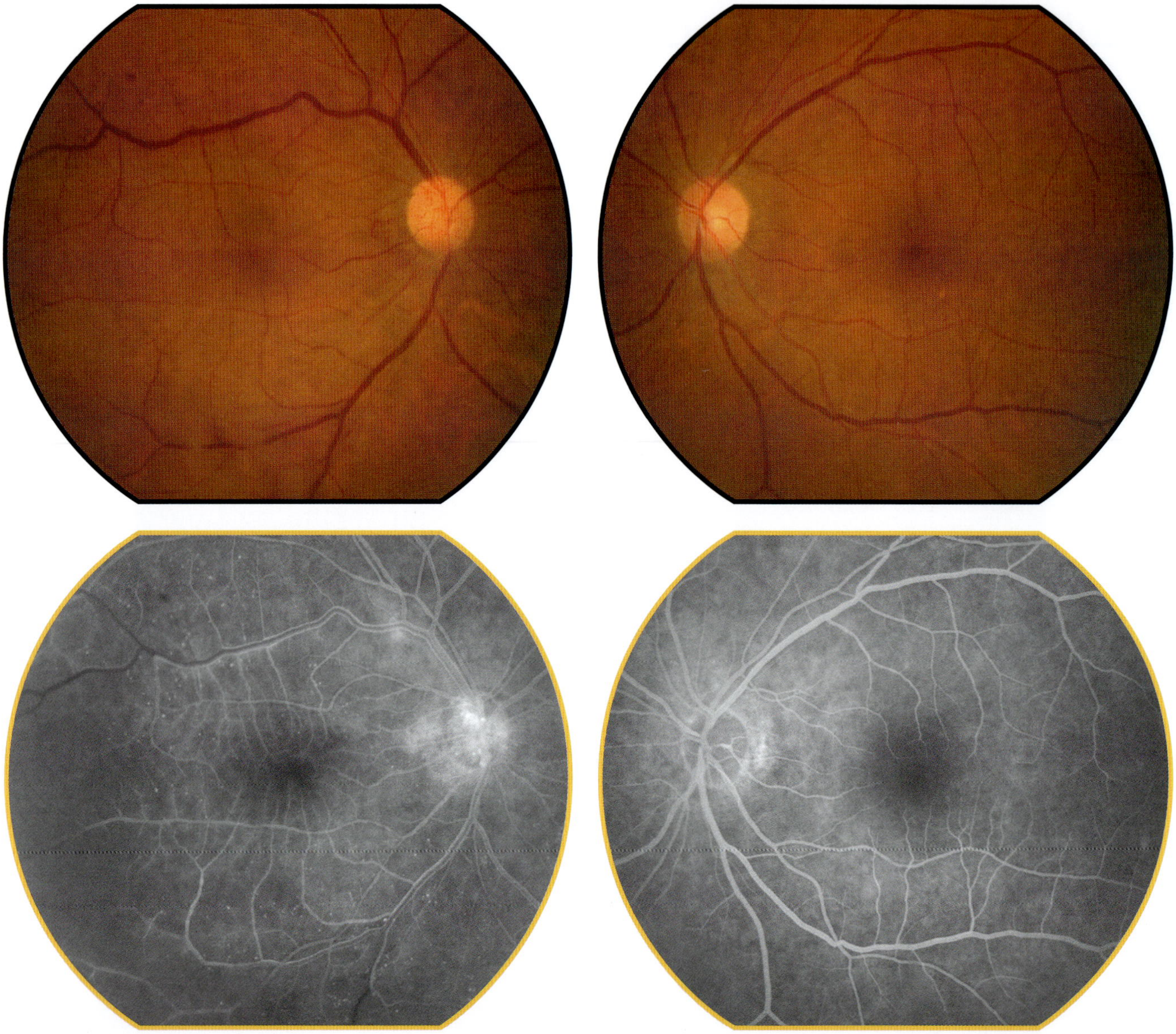

This patient with diabetes and right-sided carotid occlusive disease presented with asymmetric retinopathy. Note the presence of NVD on the right side associated with midperipheral hemorrhages. FA confirmed the presence of NVD and delayed arteriovenous filling. Color fundus photography and angiography were normal in the left eye.

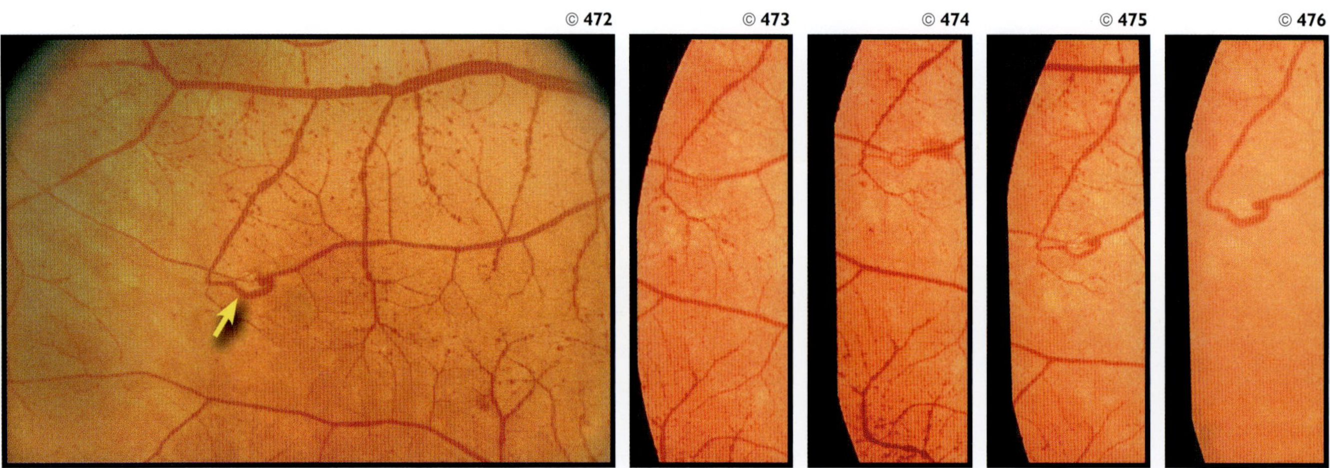

Note the retinal vascular caliber irregularities, including dilatation and venous beading in this patient with ocular ischemic syndrome and carotid disease. Multiple microaneurysms are present and a vascular shunt is noted between the retinal arterial and venous circulations *(arrow)*. Note the development of this shunt over time *(right)*.

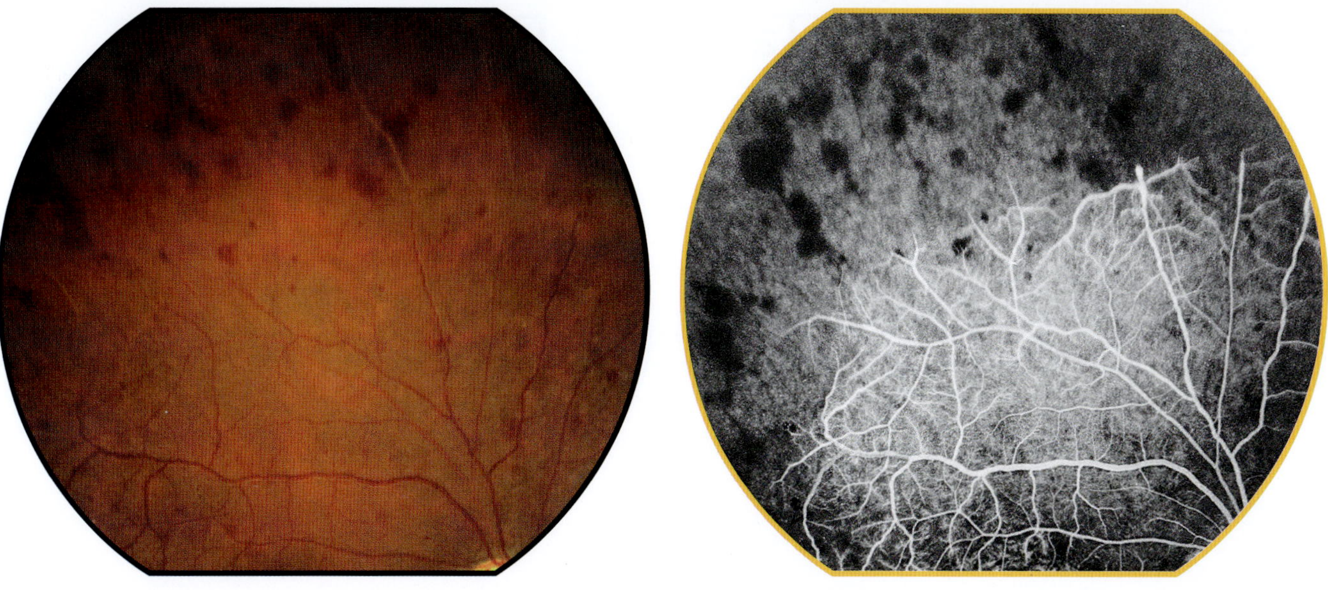

This patient presented with severe carotid artery disease. Note the multiple midperipheral dot and blot hemorrhages and the presence of capillary non-perfusion. The presence of the hemorrhages in the ischemic area implies antecedent capillary perfusion.

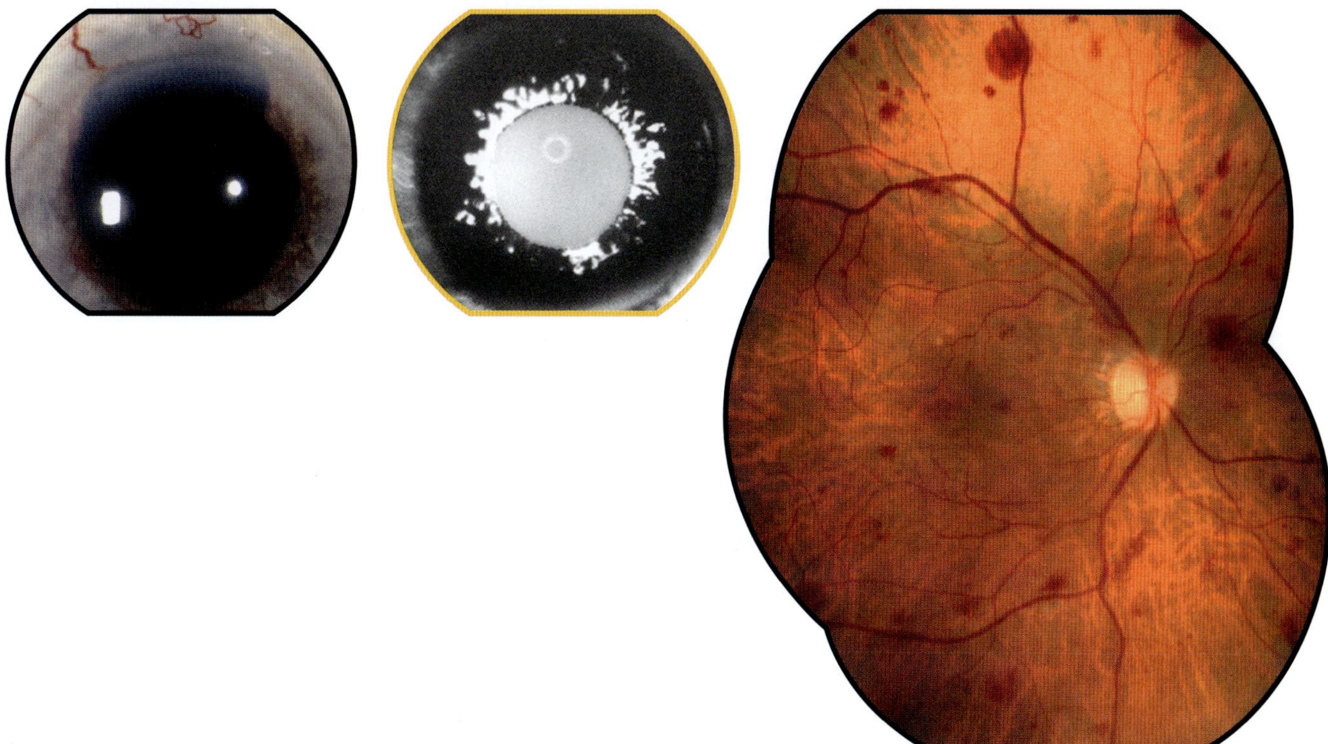

This patient presented with midperipheral blot hemorrhages due to carotid occlusive disease and ocular ischemic syndrome *(right)*. Note that the retinal veins are dilated but not tortuous. The eye developed rubeosis iridis and neovascular glaucoma. Neovascularization is identified at the pupillary margin on the color photograph *(left)*. In another patient, an FA demonstrates iris NV due to ocular ischemic syndrome *(middle)*.

Takayasu Arteritis (Takayasu Disease)

Takayasu arteritis or Takayasu disease is a chronic vascular inflammatory disorder of large blood vessels including the aorta and its branches, and seen most commonly in young Asian women. The disorder presents between the ages of 10 and 30 years and cool, pulseless extremities are the classic systemic finding. Elevated blood pressure can be a complicating factor in this systemic disorder. Steroids and immunosuppressive agents may be necessary to control the progressive nature of the disease and the various systemic complications. In the eye, Takayasu arteritis may present as ocular ischemic syndrome with widespread microaneurysms, retinal vascular occlusions and looping anastomotic connections, and even retinal NV.

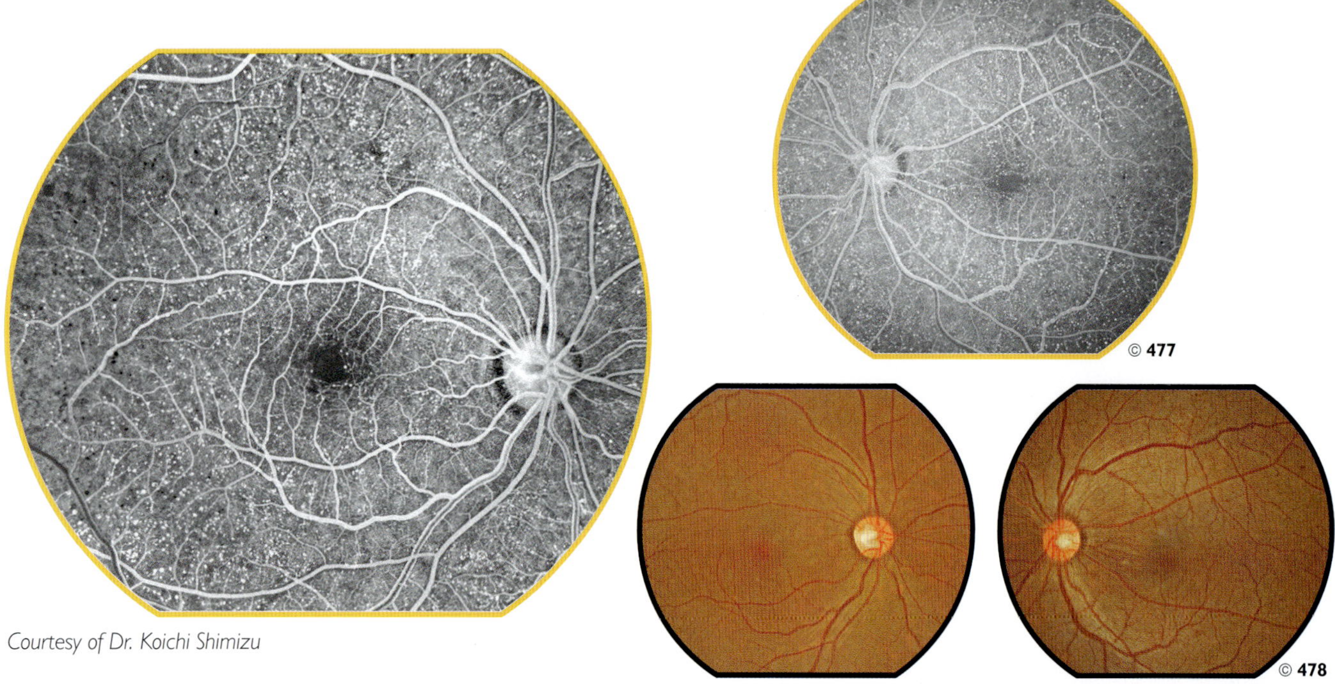

Courtesy of Dr. Koichi Shimizu

© 477

© 478

This patient with Takayasu arteritis has widespread microaneurysm formation without significant large-vessel disease, best illustrated with the FA of each eye.

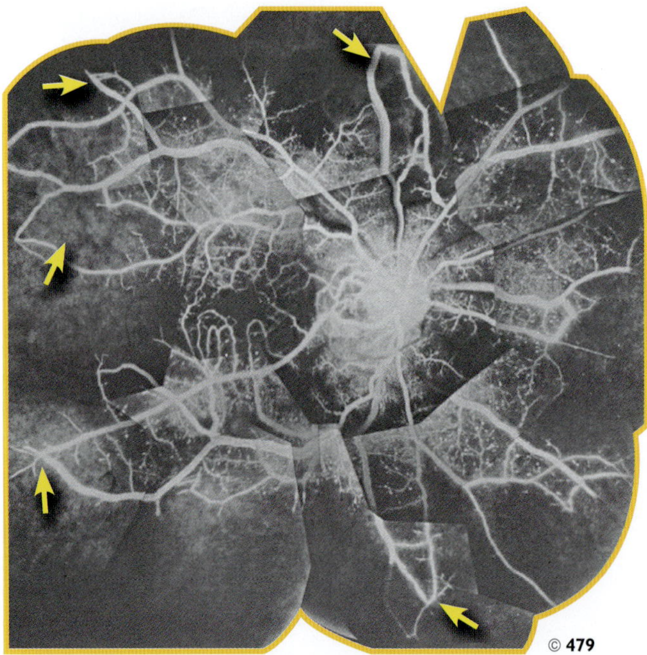

© 479

FA montage of another patient with Takayasu arteritis illustrates diffuse peripheral retinal ischemia. Numerous arteriovenous shunts are noted *(arrows)*.

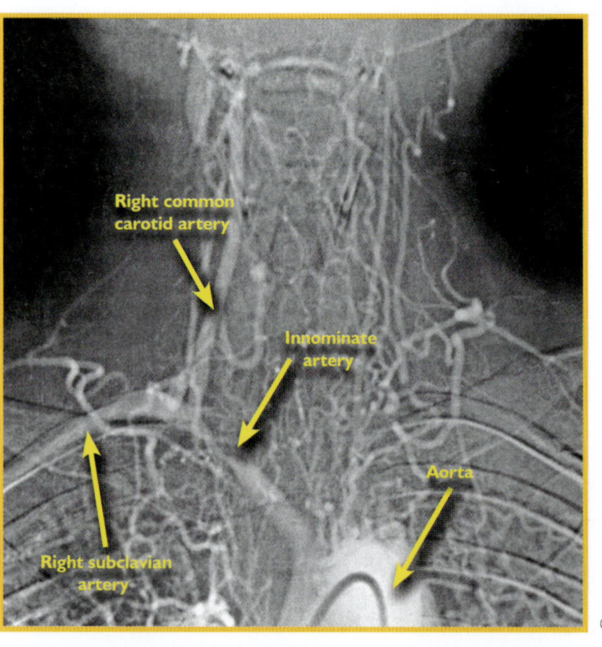

© 480

This is an angiogram of the large vessels coming from the heart through the neck. There is severe stenosis of the innominate artery *(arrow)*. The left carotid artery and the subclavian artery are not seen due to thrombosis in this patient with Takayasu arteritis.

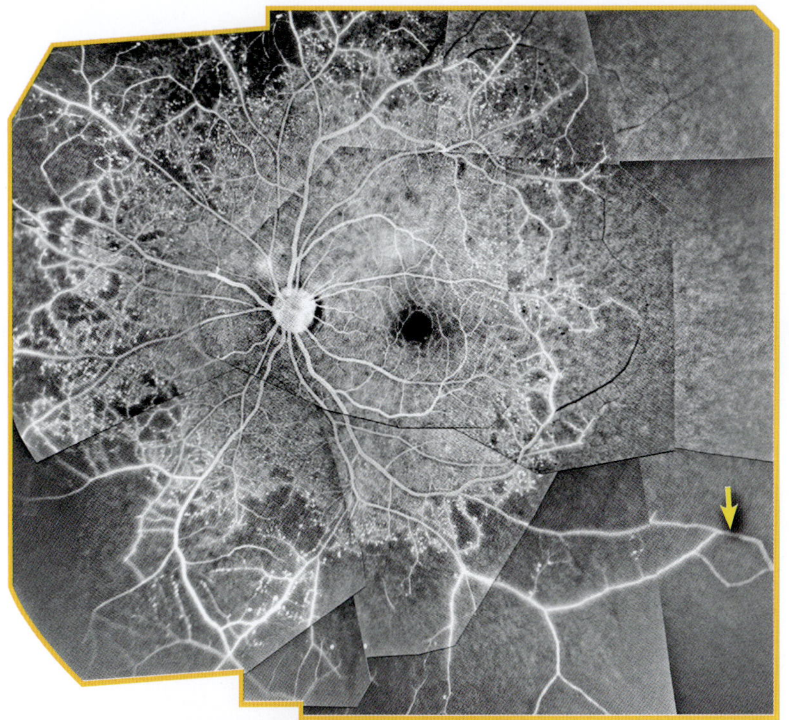

In this patient with severe Takayasu arteritis there is perfusion of the posterior pole but widespread peripheral retinal ischemia and non-perfusion is present. An arteriovenous shunt is noted in the periphery *(arrow)*. *Courtesy of Dr. Koichi Shimizu*

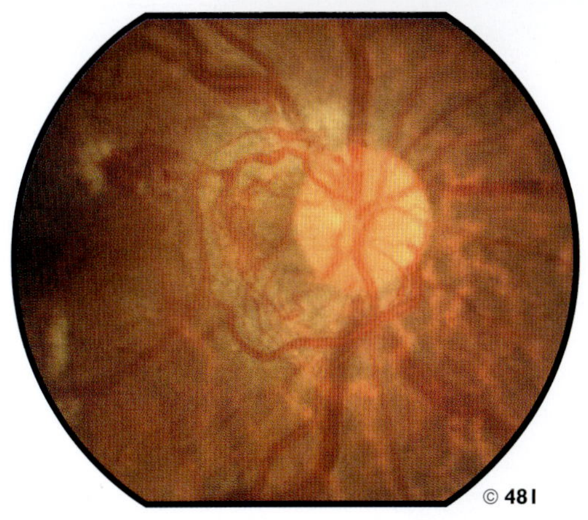

© 481

In another patient with Takayasu disease, severe NV of the disc is noted. A large looping shunt vessel is seen in the epipapillary region secondary to significant retinal ischemia.

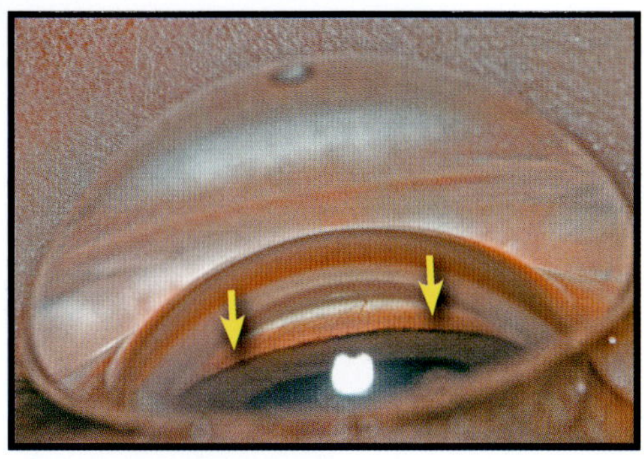

Significant posterior-segment ischemia has led to rubeosis iridis *(arrows)* and neovascular glaucoma in this patient with Takayasu disease. *Courtesy of Dr. Koichi Shimizu*

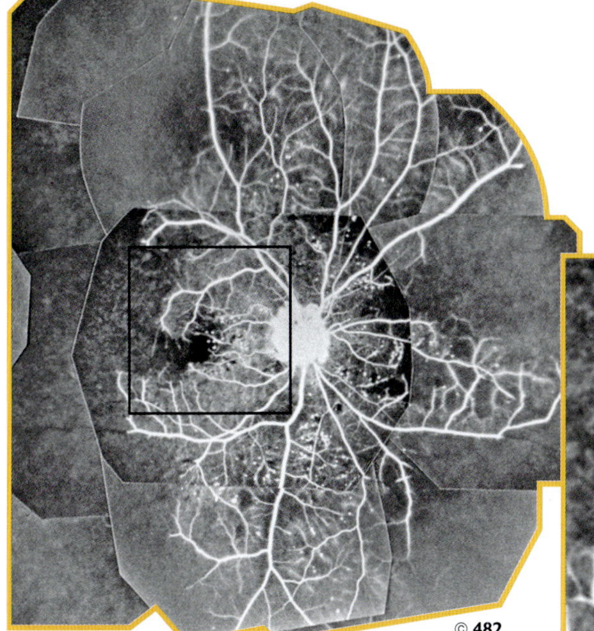

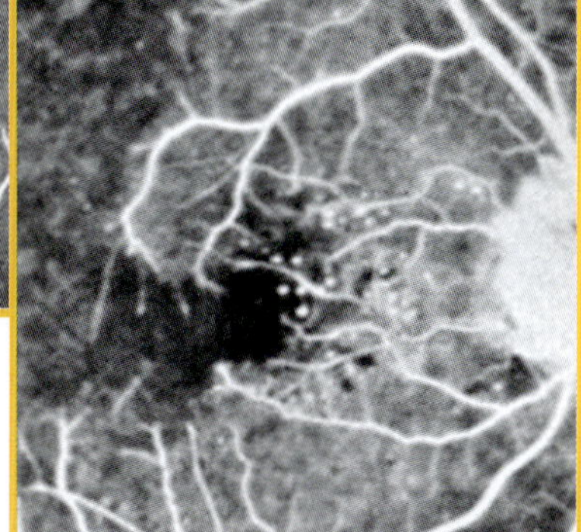

© 482

This patient has severe peripheral retinal ischemia and non-perfusion and macular ischemia with an enlarged FAZ due to Takayasu disease.

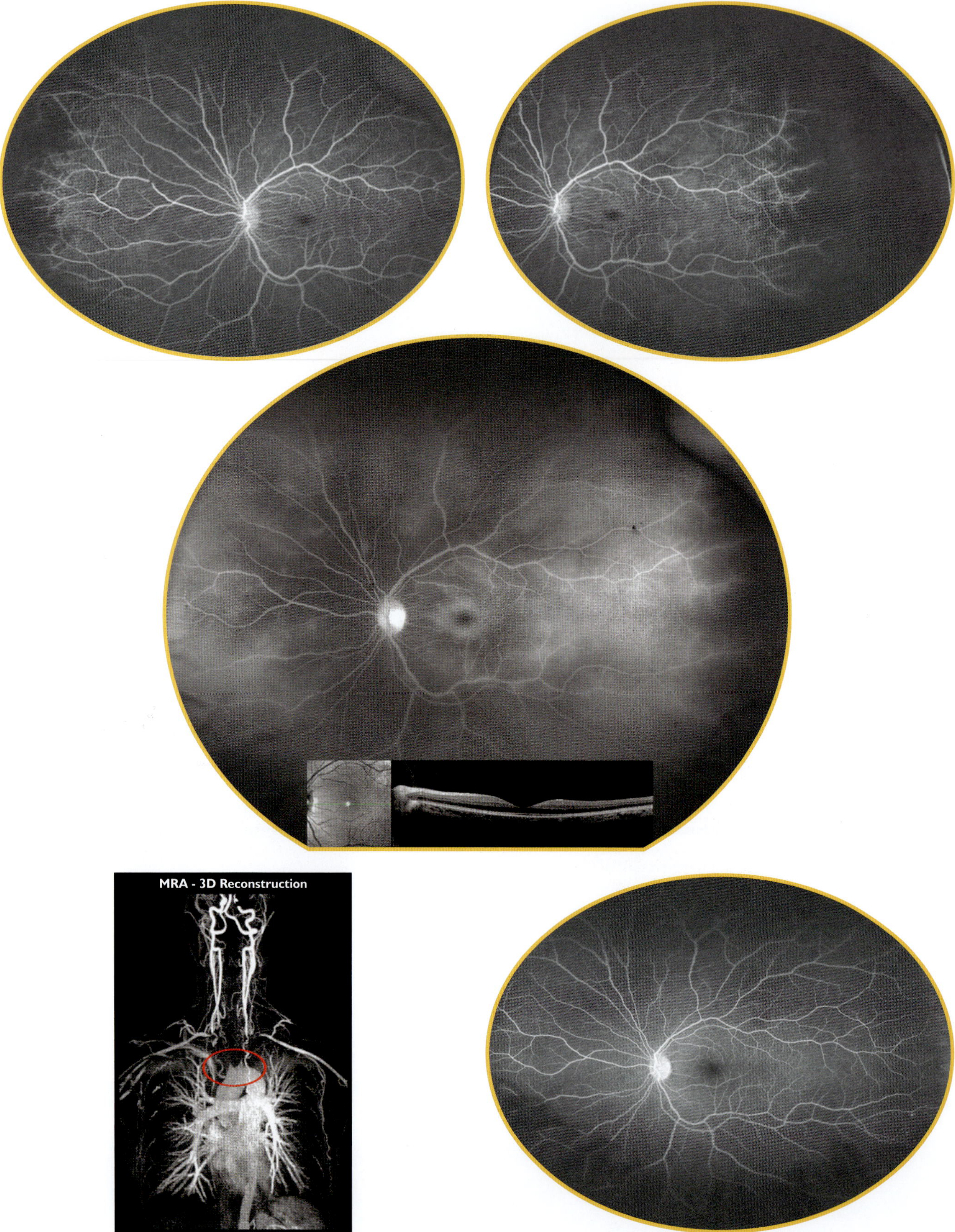

This young African-American woman with Takayasu arteritis illustrates peripheral retinal microaneurysms associated with remarkable peripheral capillary non-perfusion and ischemia with ultra-widefield angiography. Late frame angiogram demonstrates diffuse angiographic leakage, but there was no cystoid macular edema on SD-OCT. A magnetic resonance angiogram shows marked stenosis of the proximal supra-aortic branches. Five months following surgical revascularization, there was dramatic resolution of the capillary ischemia and leakage and only a few residual microaneurysms are noted. *Images courtesy of Steven D. Schwartz, MD*

Polycythemia Vera

Polycythemia vera is a chronic myeloproliferative disorder associated with increased production of blood cells by the bone marrow. The elevated red and white blood cell counts lead to hyperviscosity and retinal vascular occlusive disease.

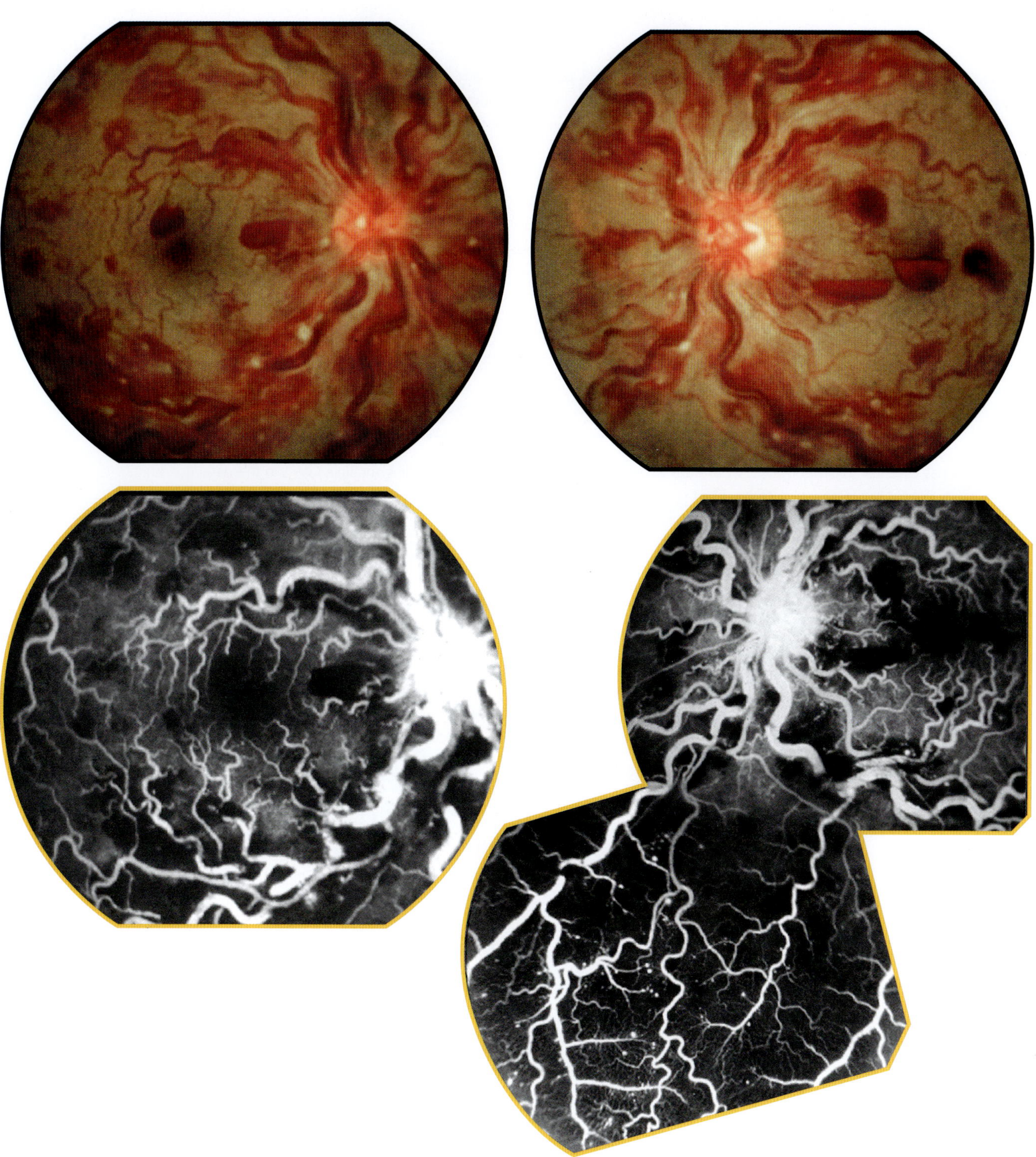

This patient demonstrates hyperviscosity syndrome from polycythemia vera. Bilateral disc edema with retinal venous tortuosity and associated retinal microaneurysms are illustrated on the FA associated with widespread pre-retinal, intraretinal, and even subretinal hemorrhage.

Essential Thrombocytosis

Essential thrombocytosis or essential thrombocythemia is a chronic myeloproliferative disorder associated with a high platelet count. The prothrombotic state leads to vascular occlusive disease and ischemic retinopathy.

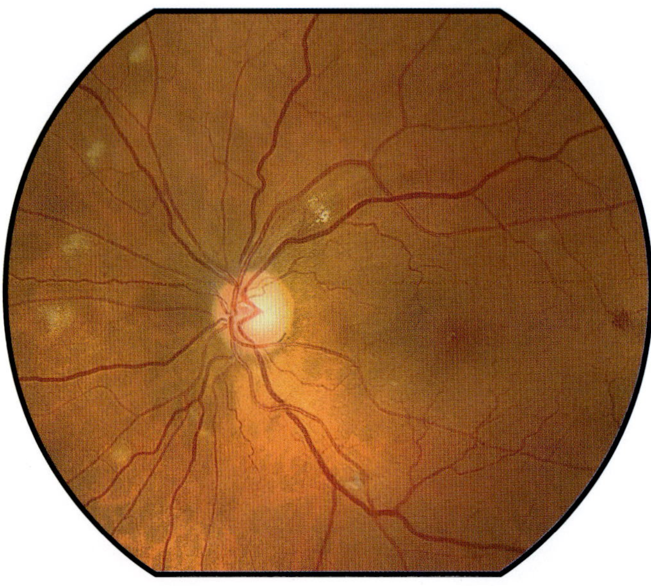

This patient has essential thrombocytosis. There are ischemic changes in the fundus including multiple CWS in the nasal quadrant.

Hyperviscosity Syndrome from Leukemia

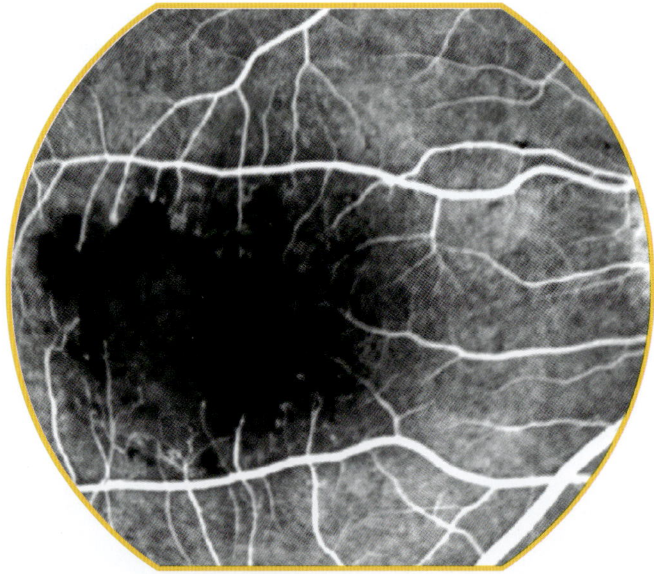

Hyperviscosity syndrome may also be caused by white blood cells. Macular ischemia is noted in this case of leukemia. *Courtesy of Dr. Richard Spaide*

Waldenström Macroglobulinemia

Waldenström macroglobulinemia is the result of a clonal B lymphocyte proliferation, which causes monoclonal IgM immunogammopathy. Hyperviscocity syndrome can complicate this disorder and is associated with venous sludging, which causes intraretinal hemorrhages, microaneurysms, retinal venous engorgement and tortuosity. Peripheral capillary non-perfusion can also be observed. Bilateral serous macular detachment with intraretinal fluid without evidence of leakage on angiography ("silent FA") is a characteristic finding. Many hypothesize that IgM in the subretinal space results in an osmotic gradient that draws fluid into the subretinal compartment.

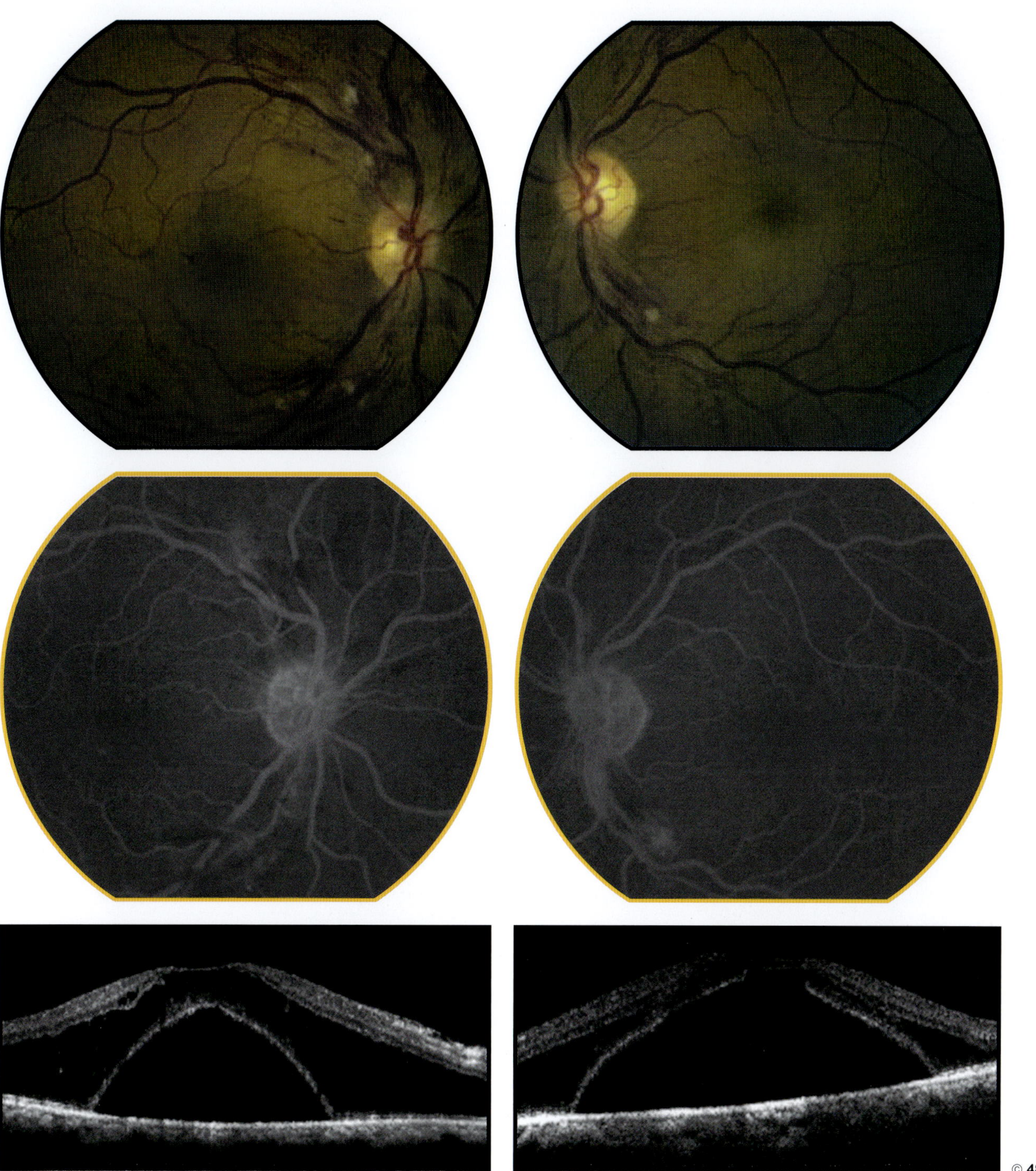

This patient with Waldenström macroglobulinemia and hyperviscosity syndrome presented with bilateral intraretinal hemorrhages, CWS, and macular detachment associated with retinal venous tortuosity *(top row)*. Late FA illustrates scattered microaneurysms and blockage from retinal hemorrhage but no significant leakage in the central macula *(middle row)*. The SD-OCT images however show the characteristic serous macular detachment associated with intraretinal fluid in each eye *(bottom row)*.

Multiple Myeloma

Multiple myeloma is characterized by the clonal proliferation of malignant plasma cells forming plasmacytomas at multiple organ sites. A protein electrophoresis of the blood or urine may show the presence of a monoclonal band, most commonly IgG. There can be associated hypercalcemia, renal insufficiency, anemia, and bone lesions. The retinal manifestations include hyperviscosity retinopathy with hemorrhage and occlusive complications and serous macular detachment as seen with Waldenström macroglobulinemia.

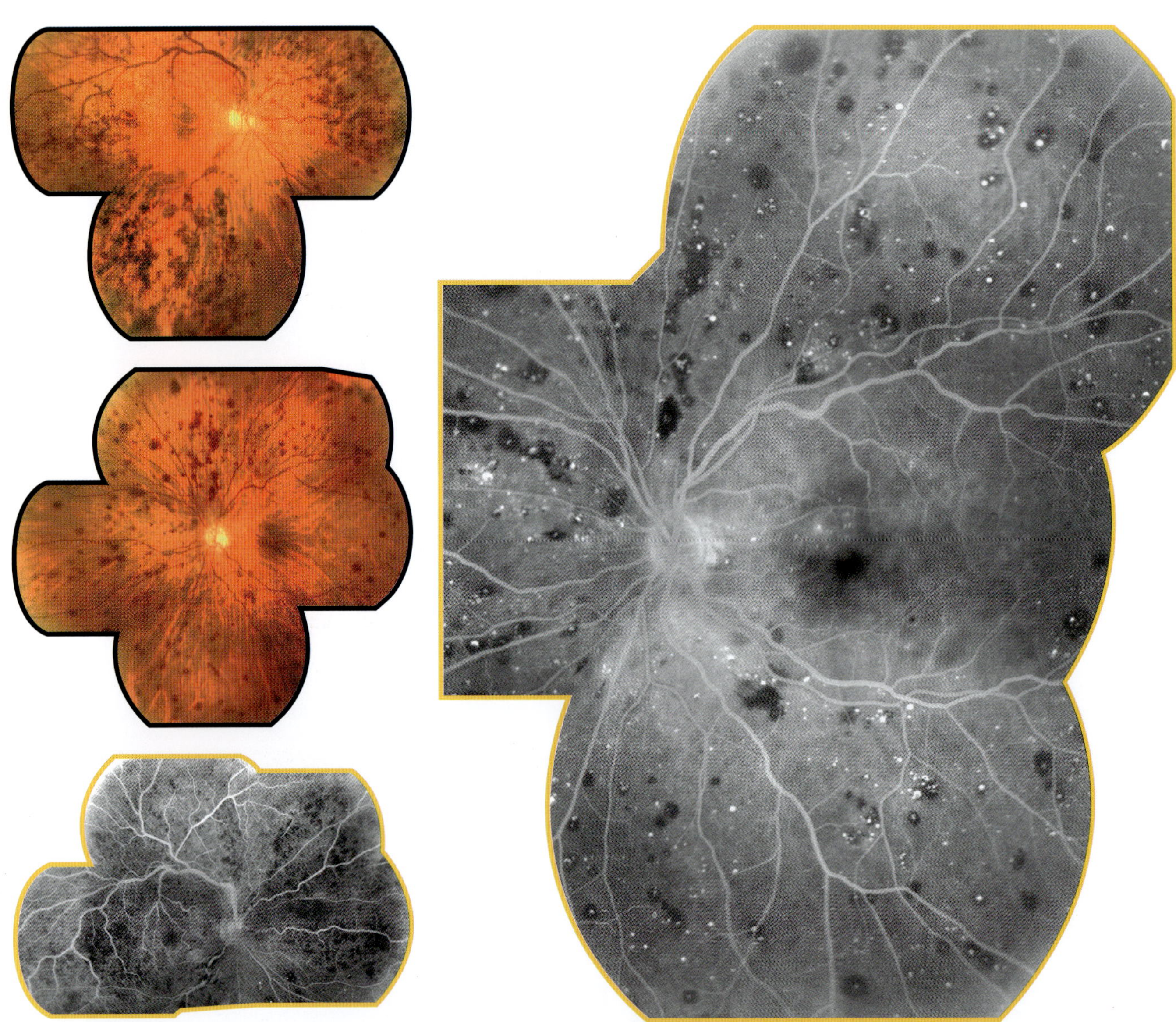

This patient has multiple myeloma. There are scattered retinal hemorrhages and numerous microaneurysms throughout the fundus.

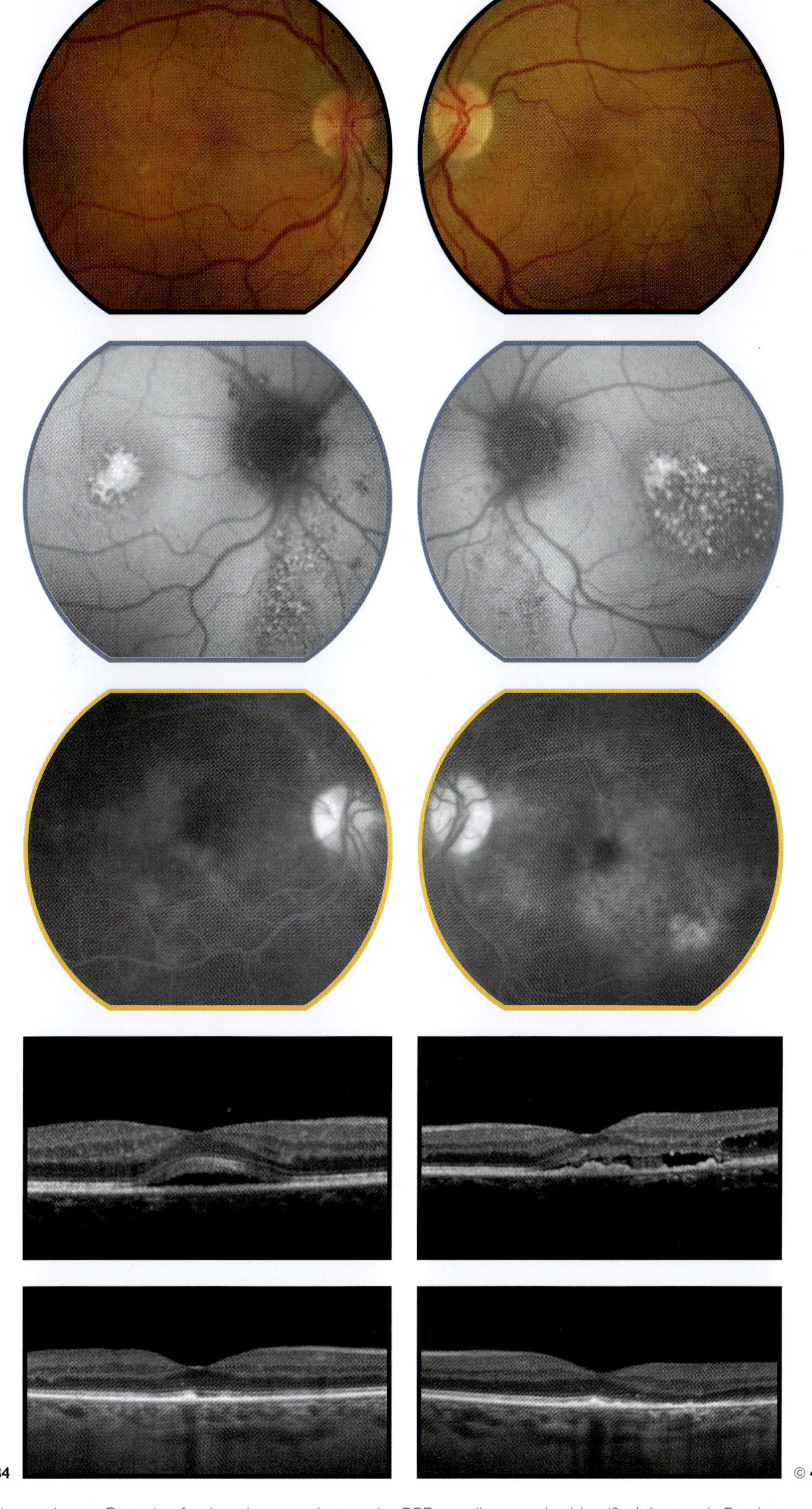

This patient has multiple myeloma. On color fundus photography, patchy RPE mottling may be identified *(top row)*. Fundus autofluorescence illustrates hyperautofluorescent macular lesions associated with granular stippling *(second row)*. Gravitational tracts can be seen inferior to the disc in both eyes. FA shows diffuse macular edema *(third row)*. SD-OCT illustrates serous macular detachments with subretinal vitelliform material *(fourth row)*. Resolution of the macular detachments is noted after treatment with chemotherapy *(bottom row)*.

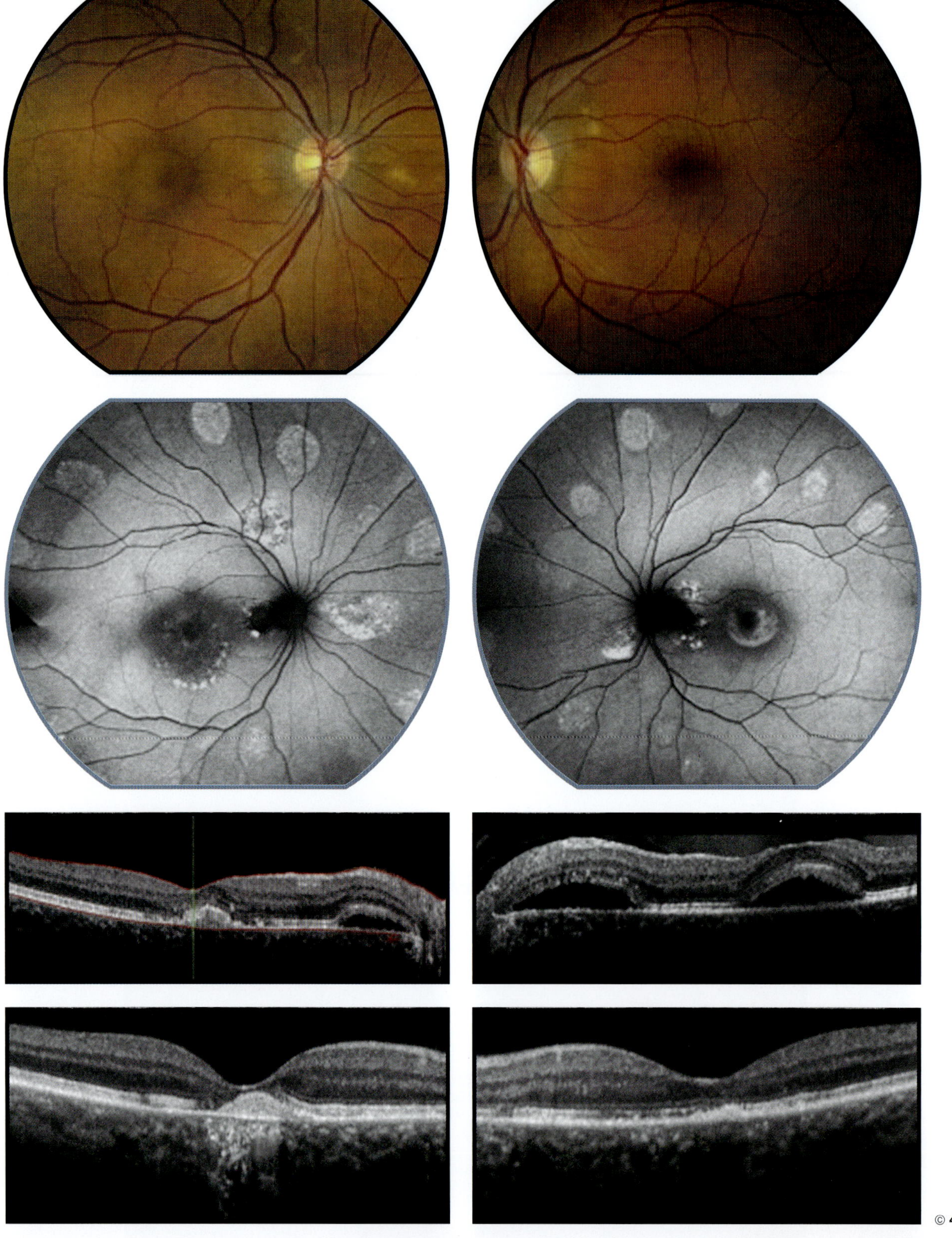

This patient with multiple myeloma illustrates multiple vitelliform detachments in both eyes. Color fundus photography is remarkable for scattered yellow subretinal lesions in the posterior pole and mid-periphery *(top row)*. The subretinal lesions are hyperautofluorescent due to the presence of lipofuscin, consistent with an acquired vitelliform retinopathy *(second row)*. The OCT illustrates serous macular detachment with subretinal vitelliform lesions in both eyes *(third row)*. After receiving a bone marrow transplant, the subretinal fluid and serous detachments resolved with residual subretinal fibrosis in the right eye.

Hypereosinophilic Syndrome

Hypereosinophilic syndrome is a myeloproliferative disorder characterized by persistent peripheral eosinophilia in association with target-organ damage. It must be differentiated from secondary eosinophilia, which is due to another underlying disease process such as malignancy, and familial eosinophilia, which is an autosomal-dominant disorder.

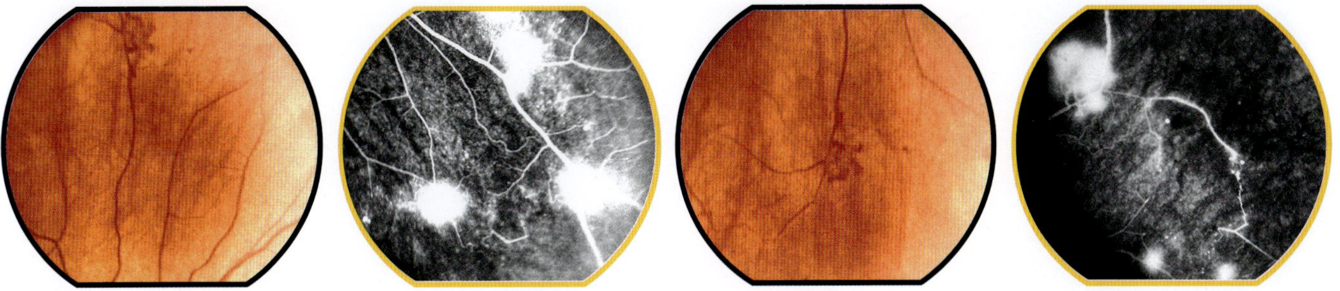

This patient has hypereosinophilic syndrome associated with a hypercoagulable state complicated by bilateral peripheral retinal ischemia and non-perfusion and retinal NV.

Polyneuropathy, Organomegaly, Endocrinopathy, Monoclonal Gammopathy, Skin Changes (POEMS Syndrome)

POEMS syndrome is a rare paraneoplastic disorder secondary to a plasma cell dyscrasia. There is multiorgan system involvement with peripheral polyneuropathy as a common feature. Fundus changes include optic disc edema and cystoid macular edema. Retinal venous occlusive disease may also occur.

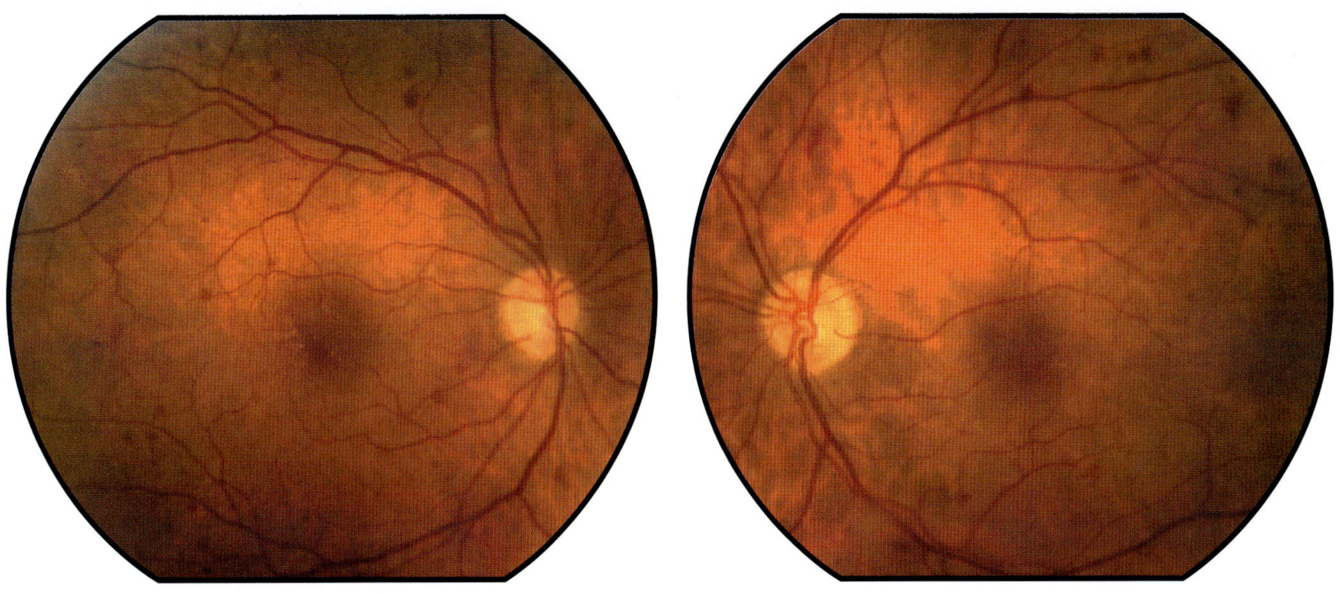

This patient with POEMS syndrome shows bilateral retinal venous occlusive disease with mild disc edema. *Courtesy of Dr. Joseph Maguire*

Hyperhomocysteinemia

Hyperhomocysteinemia is characterized by a hypercoagulable state due to high levels of homocysteine. It has been associated with ischemic heart disease, pulmonary embolism, and other thrombotic events. Ocular manifestations include retinal arterial or venous occlusive disease.

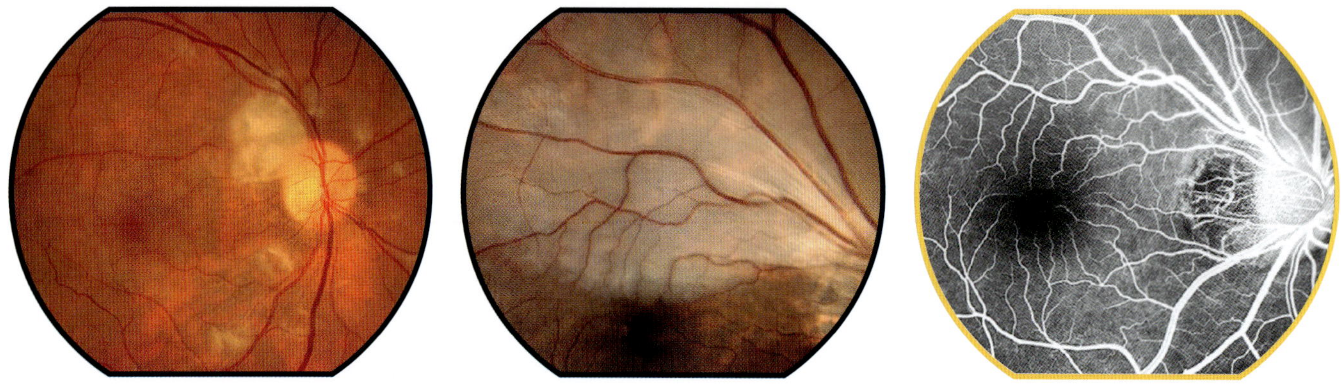

These two patients have hyperhomocysteinemia. Note the CWS in the patient on the left. A branch retinal artery occlusion is illustrated in the second patient *(middle)*. The BRAO resolved promptly with therapy as evidenced in the subsequent FA that showed normal perfusion *(right)*.

Protein C and Protein S Deficiency

Retinal vascular occlusive disease may develop as a result of various abnormalities in the coagulation cascade. Protein C and S are anticoagulation factors, the levels or activity of which can be significantly reduced due to rare genetic mutations leading to a hypercoagulable state.

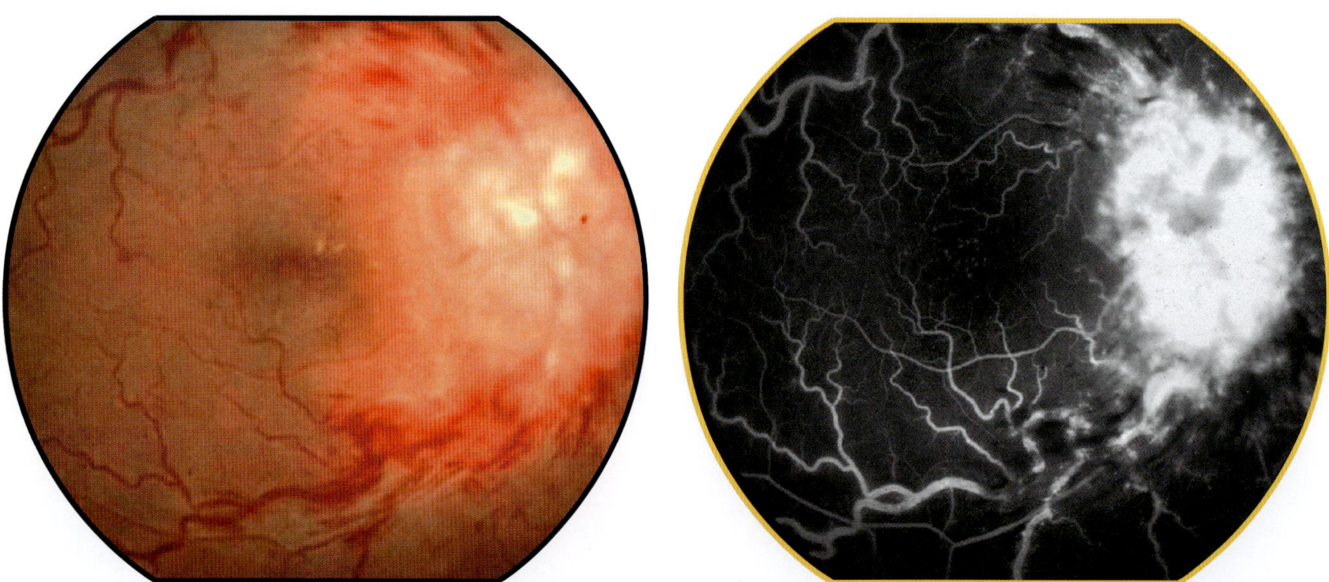

This patient with protein C deficiency illustrates a CRVO with retinal hemorrhages and disc edema and leakage. *Courtesy of Dr. Wendall Bauman*

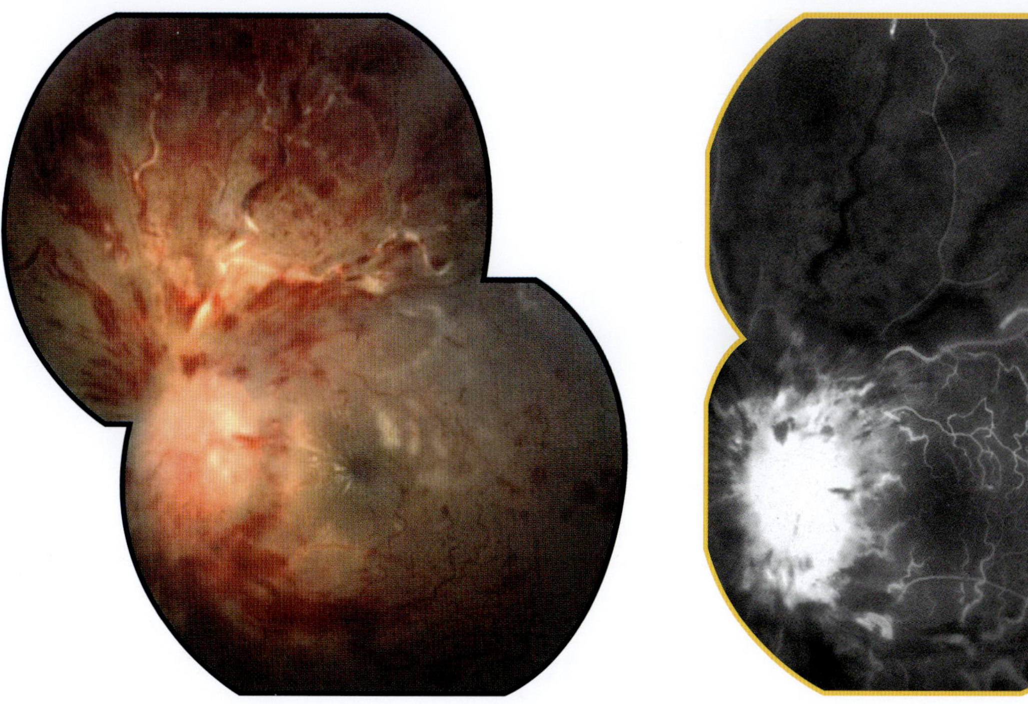

Hemorrhagic retinal vein occlusion is noted in this patient with protein C deficiency. The FA shows disc leakage and widespread retinal ischemia and non-perfusion in the left eye *(lower right)*. *Courtesy of Dr. Jay Duker*

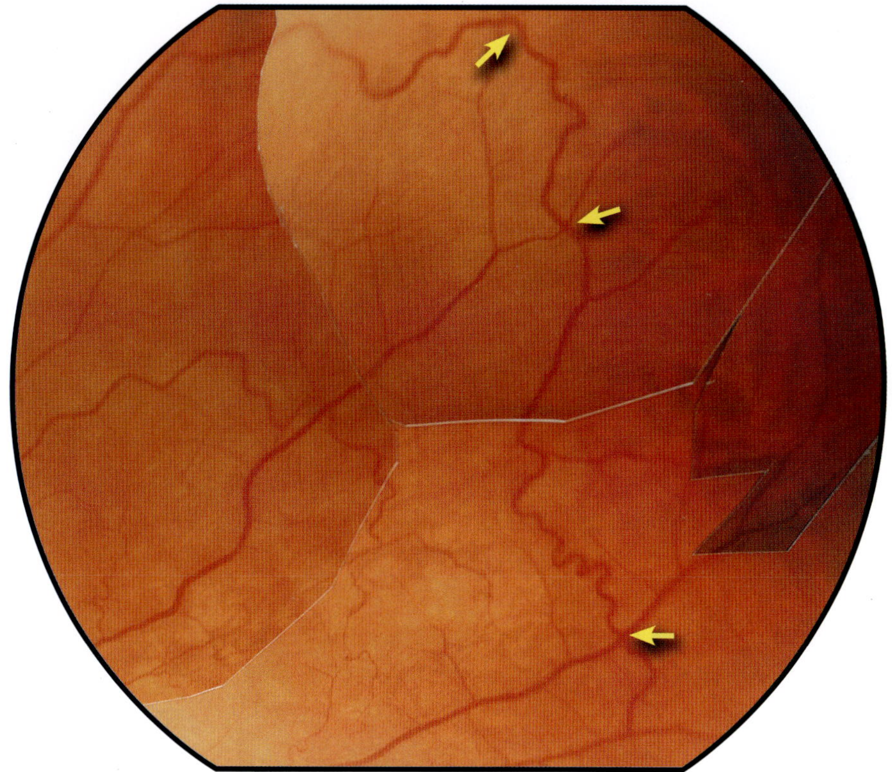

This patient with protein C deficiency illustrates an arterial-to-arterial anastomosis *(arrows)* following peripheral retinal arterial occlusive disease.

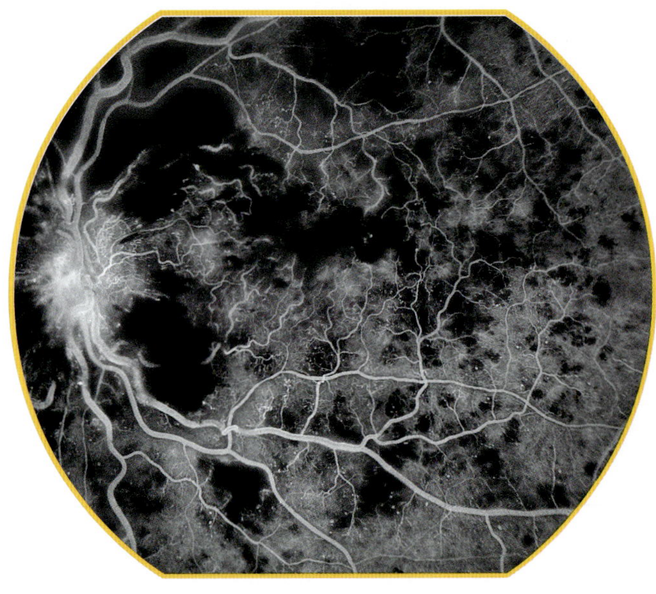

Note the presence of CRVO with retinal hemorrhages and disc edema in this patient with protein S deficiency.

Antithrombin III Deficiency

Antithrombin III is an anticoagulant protein, the deficiency of which can lead to thrombotic events of the heart, the peripheral veins, and the retinal vasculature.

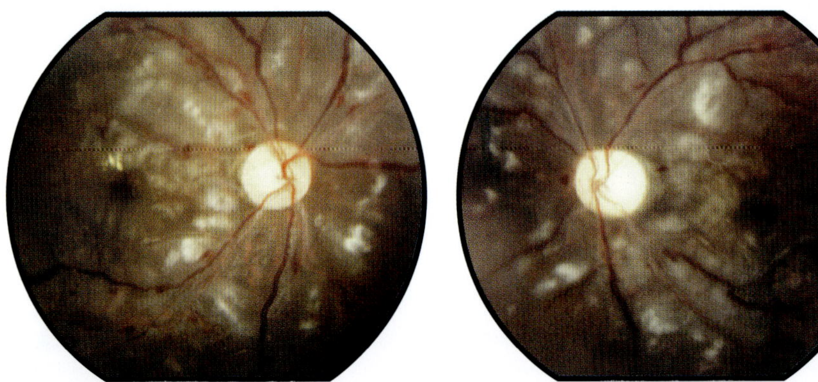

Multiple CWS are noted in this patient with antithrombin III deficiency. Arteriolar narrowing and optic nerve pallor are also identified.

Factor V Leiden

Factor V Leiden is the most common genetic mutation associated with thrombophilia. The risk of venous thrombosis is increased 5- to 10-fold for heterozygotes and as high as 50- to 100-fold for homozygotes and is a rare cause of retinal venous occlusion.

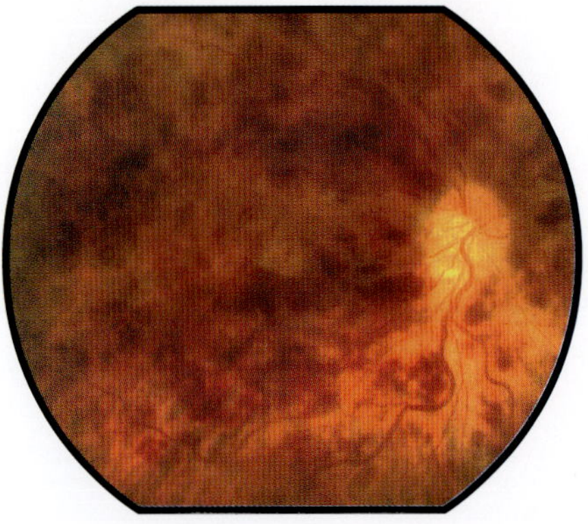

Note the hemorrhagic CRVO in this patient with factor V Leiden and deep vein thrombosis.

Thrombotic Thrombocytopenic Purpura

Thrombotic thrombocytopenic purpura (TTP) is a rare disorder that causes a microangiopathic hemolytic anemia and thrombocytopenia. Neurological abnormalities and end-organ damage may ensue. As seen in other microangiopathic hemolytic anemias, TTP is caused by spontaneous aggregation of platelets and activation of coagulation in small blood vessels. The pathogenesis involves a deficiency or inhibition of the enzyme ADAMTS13. Other thrombotic microangiopathies can be mediated by complement, Shiga toxin (hemolytic uremic syndrome), and medications.

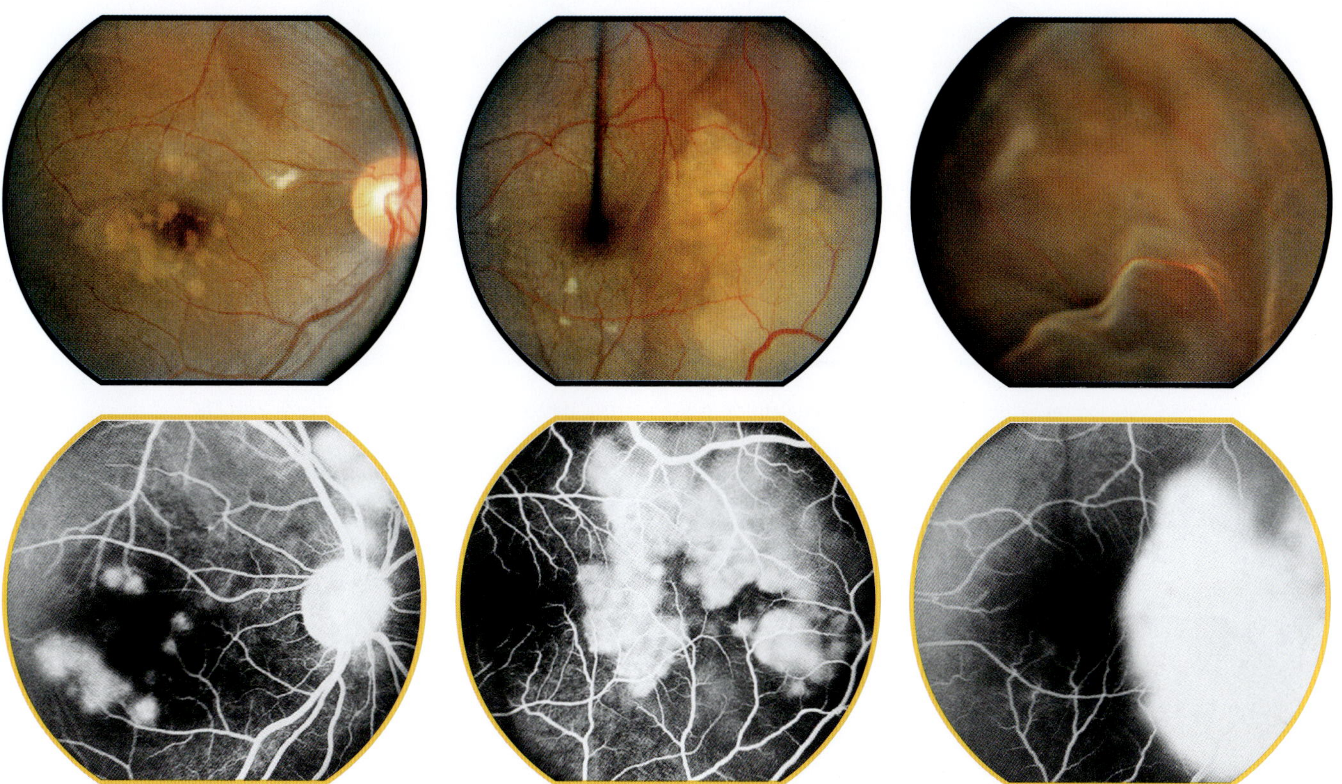

This 32-year-old male presented with a history of fatigue, fainting, disorientation, palpitations, hematemesis, and decreased vision. Serous macular detachment with subretinal exudation is illustrated in each eye. Inferiorly, undulating retinal folds associated with a peripheral detachment are evident. The FAs illustrate multifocal subretinal leakage with pooling into the exudative retinal detachment in each eye. Patients with TTP develop anemia, thrombocytopenia, and neurologic abnormalities due to thrombotic occlusion of the blood vessels. *Courtesy of Dr. Richard Spaide*

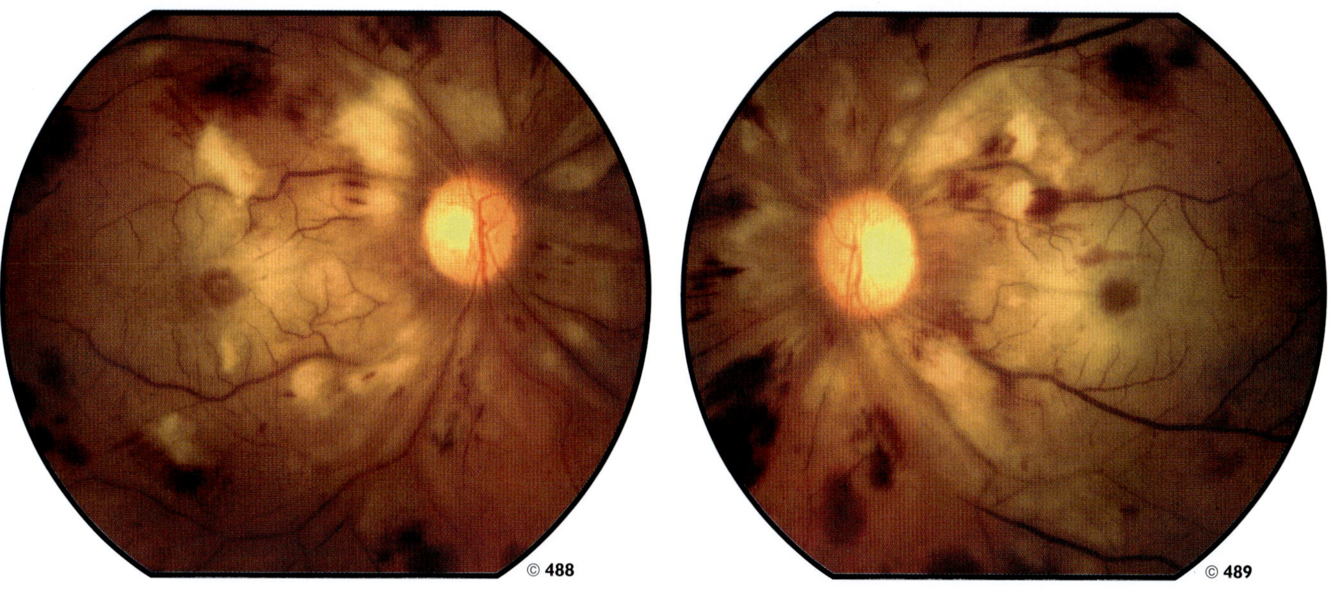

Multiple CWS in the macula associated with retinal hemorrhages in the posterior pole and periphery due to vascular occlusion are identified in this patient with TTP.

Disseminated Intravascular Coagulation

Disseminated intravascular coagulation (DIC) is a pathological activation of coagulation mechanisms in response to a variety of disease states. It leads to extensive microvascular thrombosis and hemorrhage. DIC may be caused by malignancy, abruptio placentae, trauma, burns, or sepsis. Ischemic, exudative, and hemorrhagic complications of the retina and choroid may be identified in patients with this disorder.

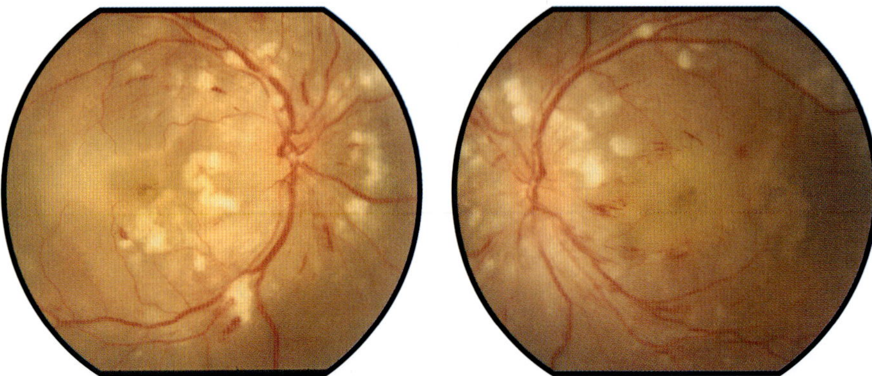

Note the multiple CWS and retinal hemorrhages associated with exudative macular detachment in these two patients with DIC.

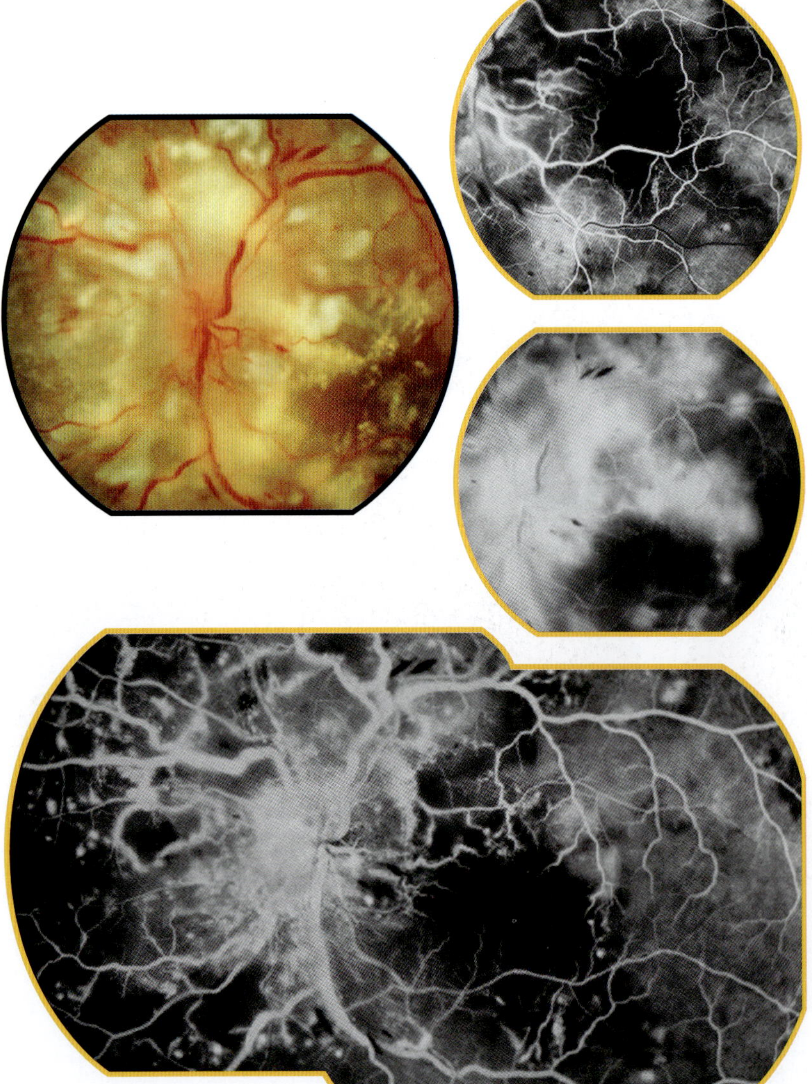

Widespread retinal ischemia and leakage are illustrated in this patient with DIC. Multiple foci of leakage at the level of the retinal pigment epithelium (FA montage) may also be identified consistent with a choroidopathy.

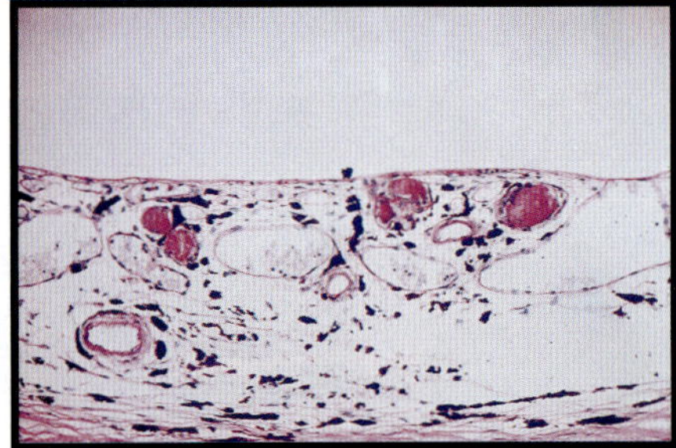

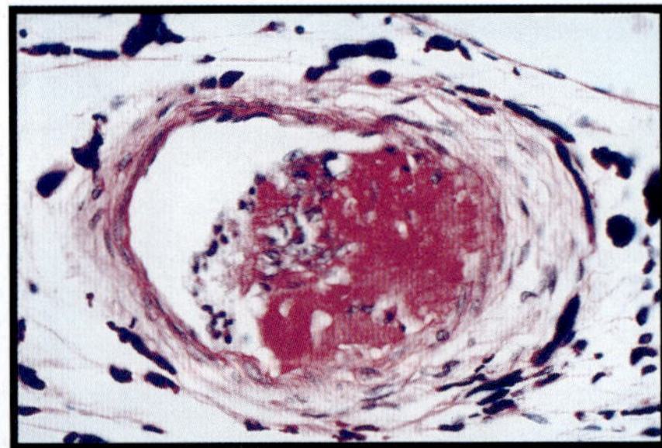

These are histopathologic specimens of a patient with DIC. Note the thrombotic material in the vasculature.

Systemic Lupus Erythematosus

Systemic lupus erythematosus (SLE) is a chronic autoimmune disease that can affect many organ systems, typically the skin, joints, kidneys, heart, lungs, liver, blood vessels, and nervous system. The end-organ dysfunction is thought to be due to immune complex deposition and complement activation. SLE is more common in women and African-Americans. Retinal vasculitis causing retinal hemorrhages, CWS, and vaso-occlusive complications may occur in this disorder. Lupus choroidopathy, less common than lupus retinopathy, may cause exudative retinal detachment and is usually associated with systemic vascular disease such as hypertension due to lupus nephritis.

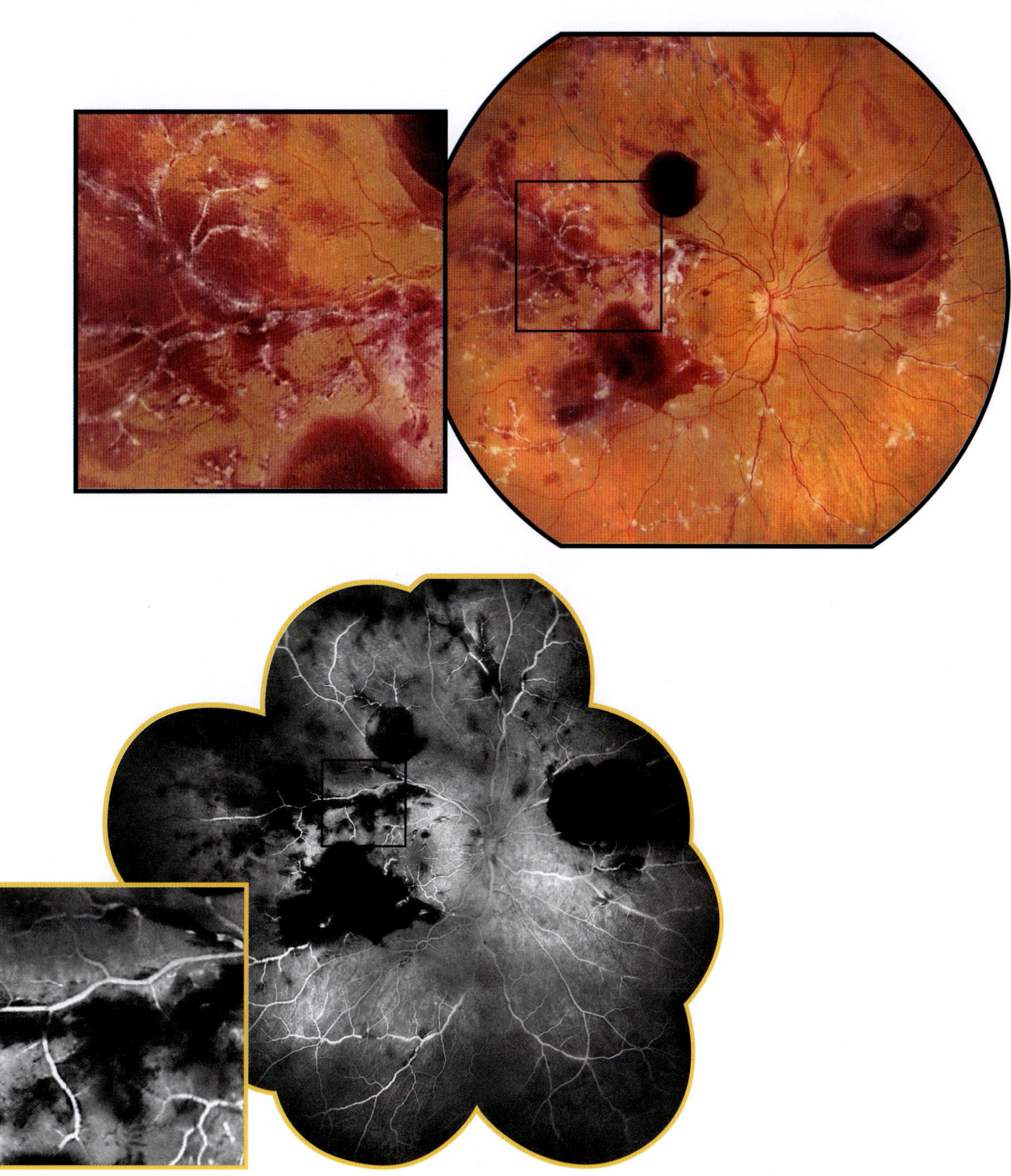

This patient had SLE. Note the pre-retinal, intraretinal, and subretinal hemorrhages. Frosted branch angiitis is also illustrated *(top inset)*. The FA shows severe peripheral retinal vascular ischemia and non-perfusion *(bottom inset)*.

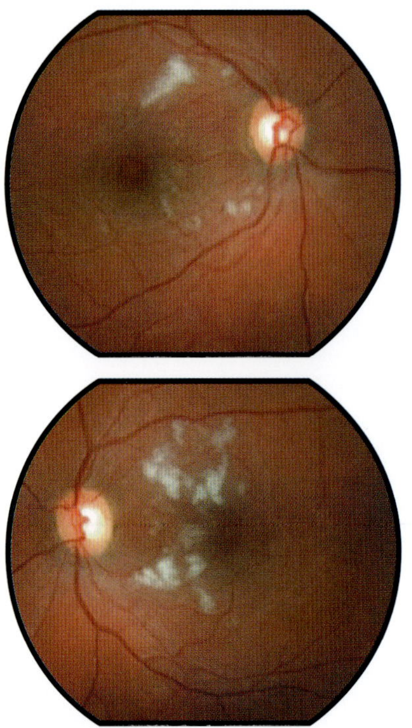

CWS is a typical finding of lupus retinopathy. Note the Purtscher-like retinopathy in each eye in this SLE patient. *Courtesy of Dr. Millie Fell*

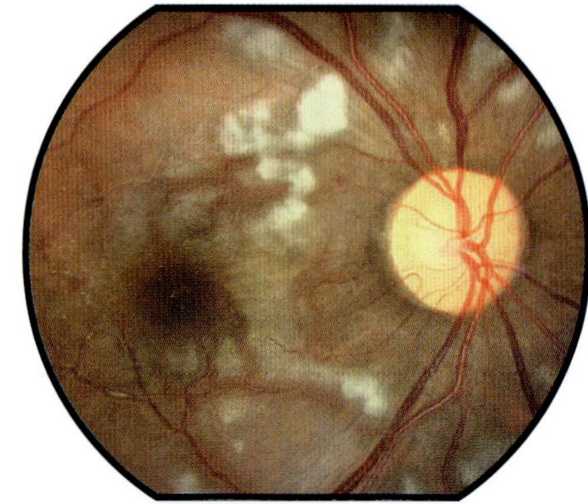

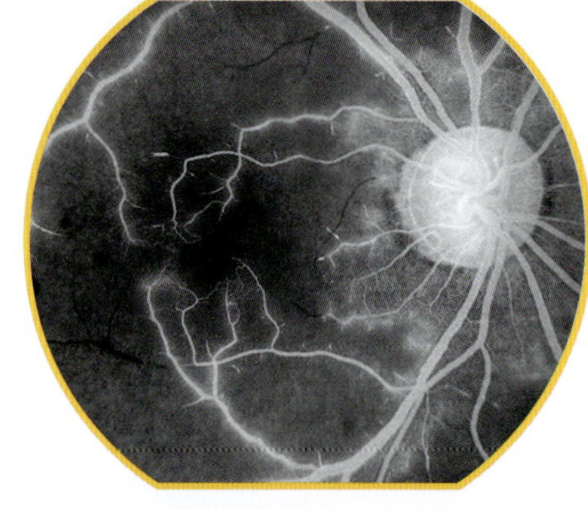

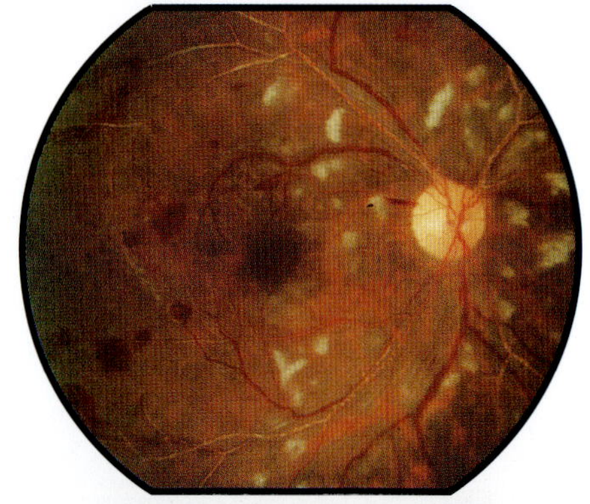

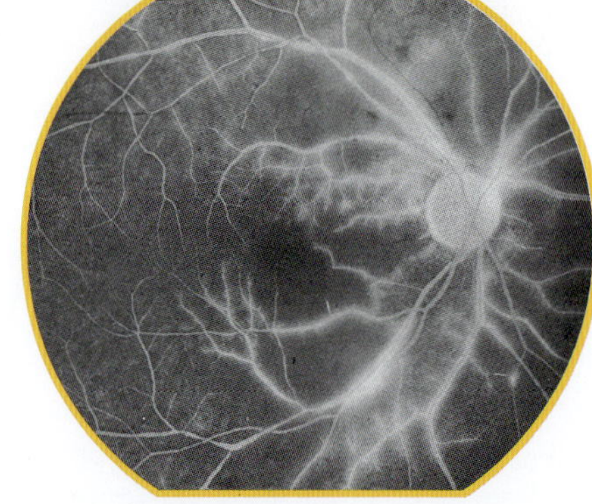

Macular ischemia and non-perfusion associated with CWS and retinal hemorrhages are illustrated in these two SLE patients.

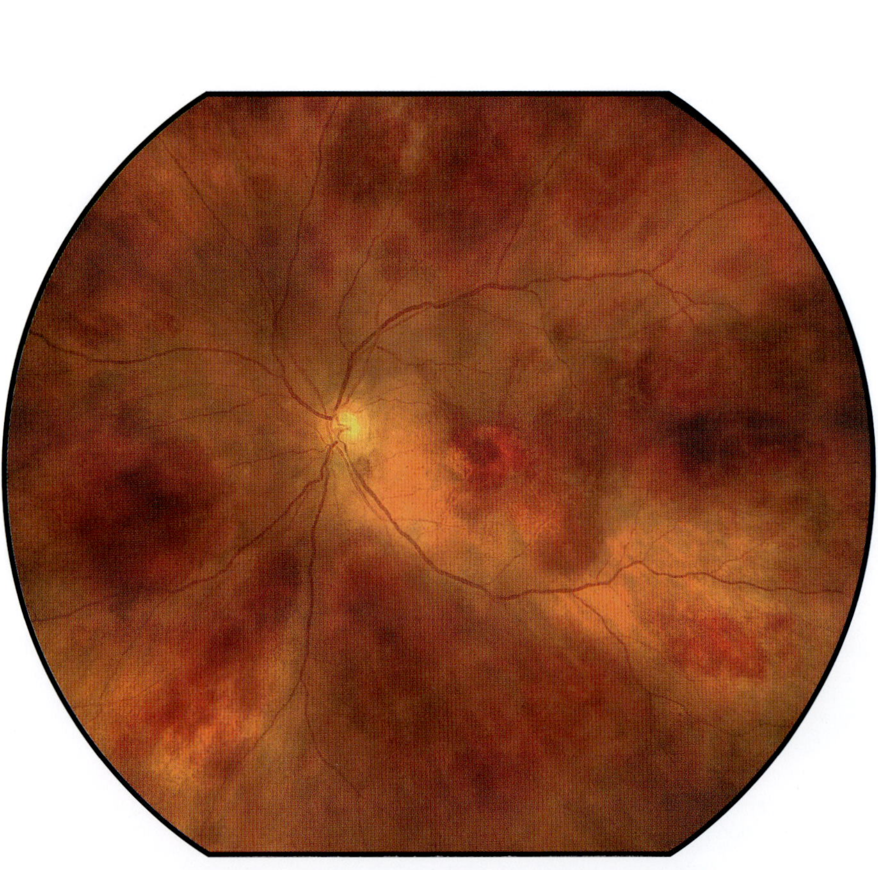

Diffuse retinal hemorrhage is illustrated in this SLE patient likely the result of retinal vasculitis and/or a vaso-occlusive complication.

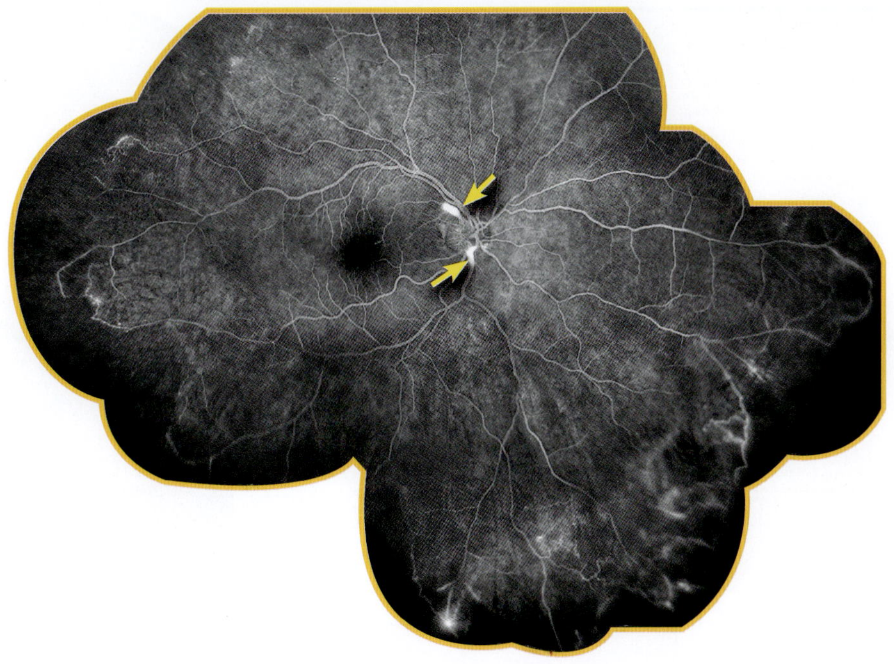

The widefield FA of this SLE patient shows peripheral retinal ischemia, shunting vessels, and early NV in the periphery and at the disc *(arrows)*.

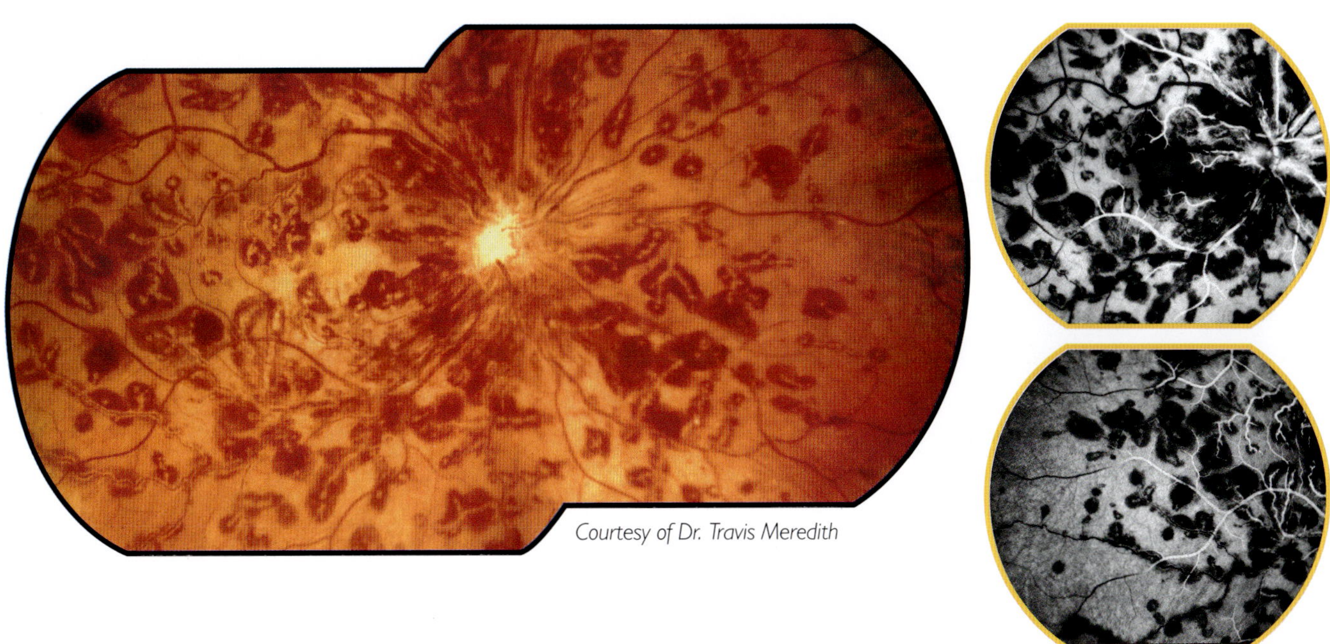

Courtesy of Dr. Travis Meredith

Hemorrhagic retinal vasculitis is noted in this lupus patient. Blockage from the blood and associated retinal vascular ischemia and nonperfusion are illustrated with the two FA images.

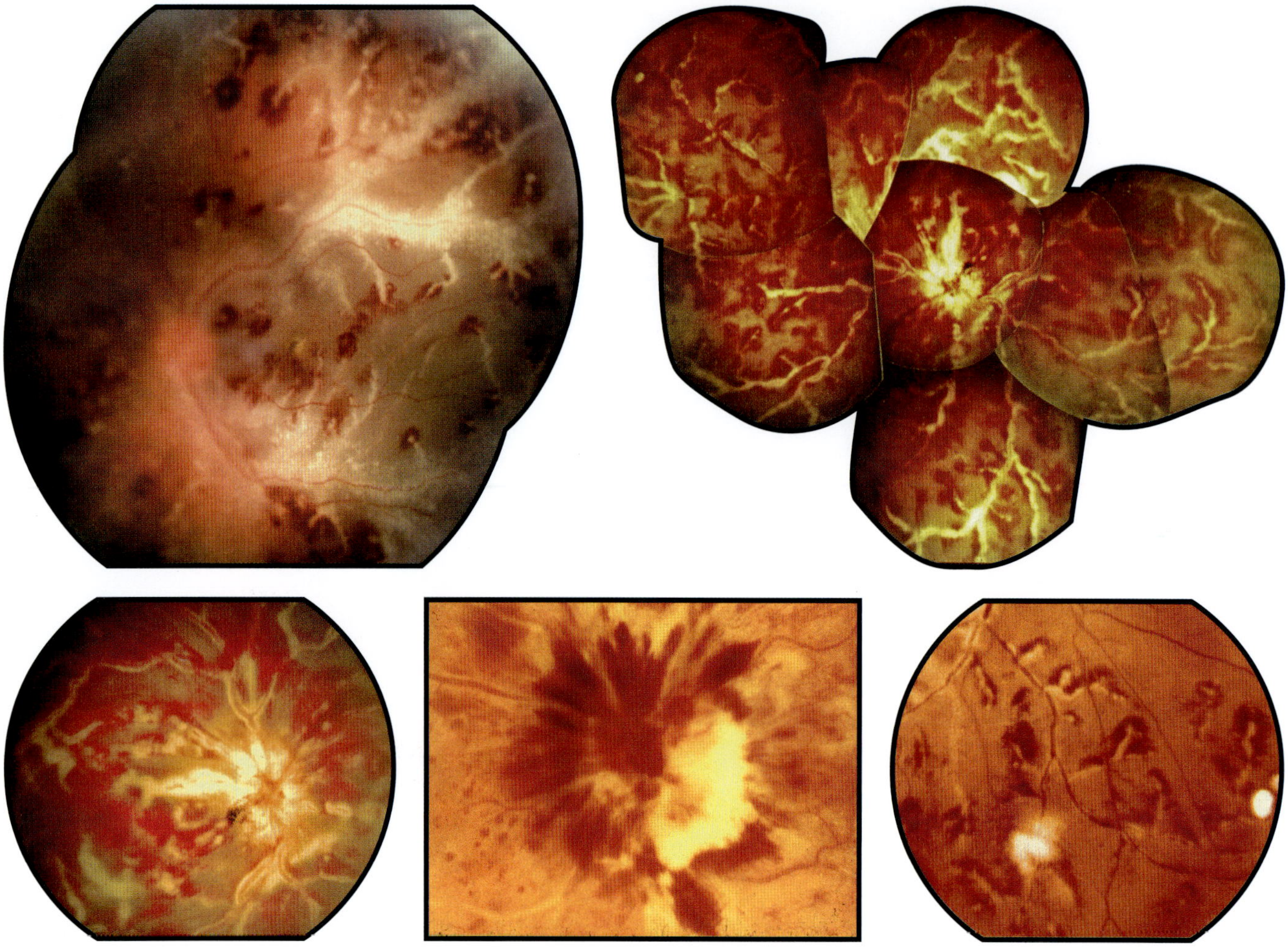

These patients illustrate lupus retinopathy. Hemorrhagic retinal vasculitis and disc edema are shown. A frosted branch angiitis is notable in each case.

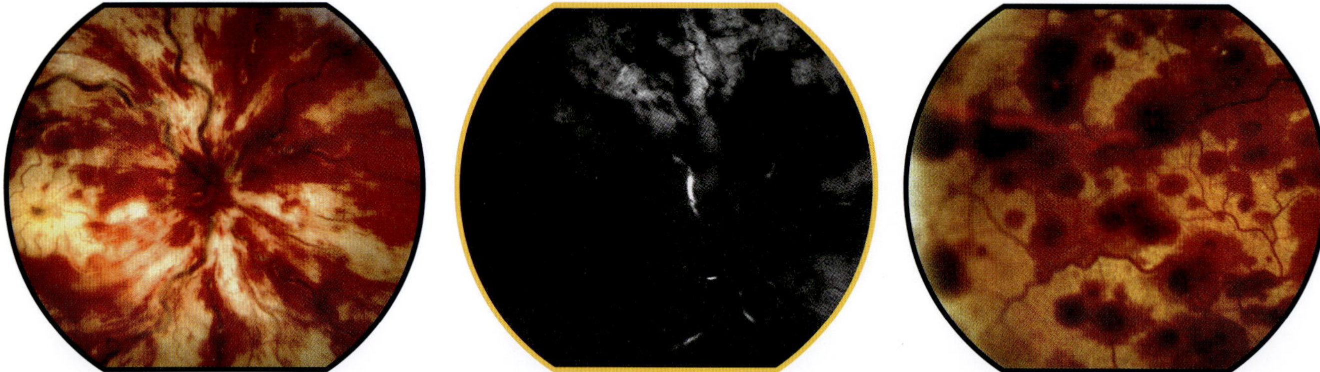

An ischemic hemorrhagic retinal vasculitis is illustrated in this young patient with SLE. Note the blockage from blood and the severe retinal vascular non-perfusion with the FA. *Courtesy of Dr. Lee Jampol*

This patient also has a hemorrhagic fundus from SLE.

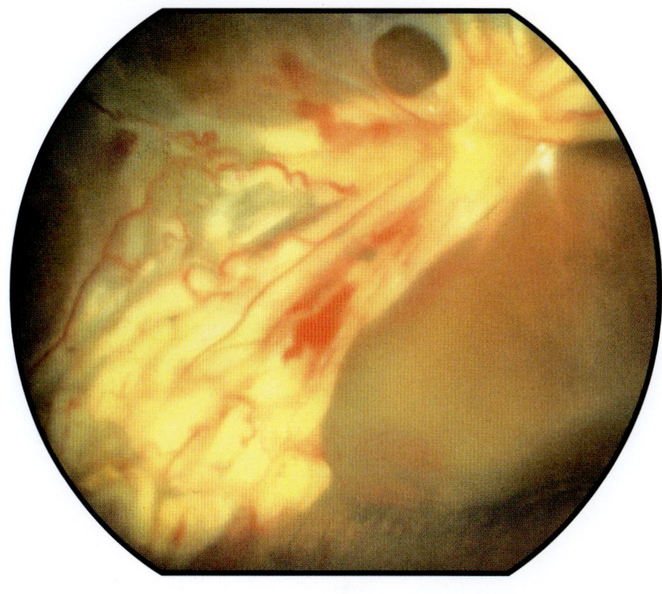

Extensive fibrovascular proliferation with vitreous hemorrhage, retinal traction, and a retinal break are noted in this SLE patient.

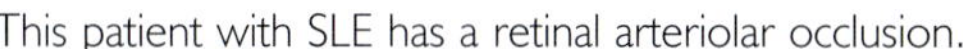

This patient with SLE has a retinal arteriolar occlusion.

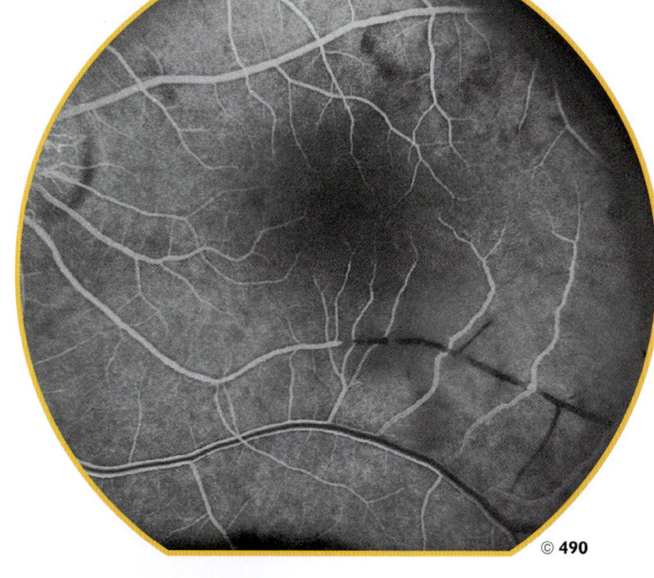

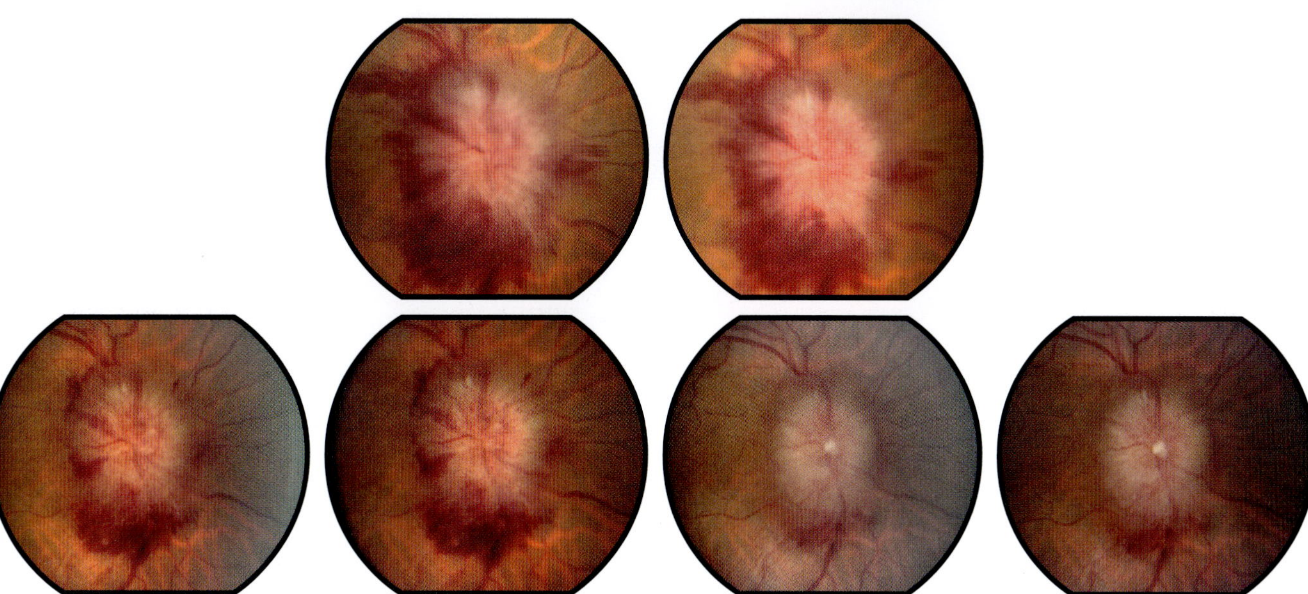

This patient with SLE has bilateral optic neuritis. These photographs represent stereo images of the disc, which is elevated with surrounding hemorrhage *(top row)*. Within 1 week, there was slow but remarkable resolution of the edema and blood *(bottom left)*. By 1 month the edema persisted, but most of the blood had resolved *(bottom right)*.

Lupus Choroidopathy

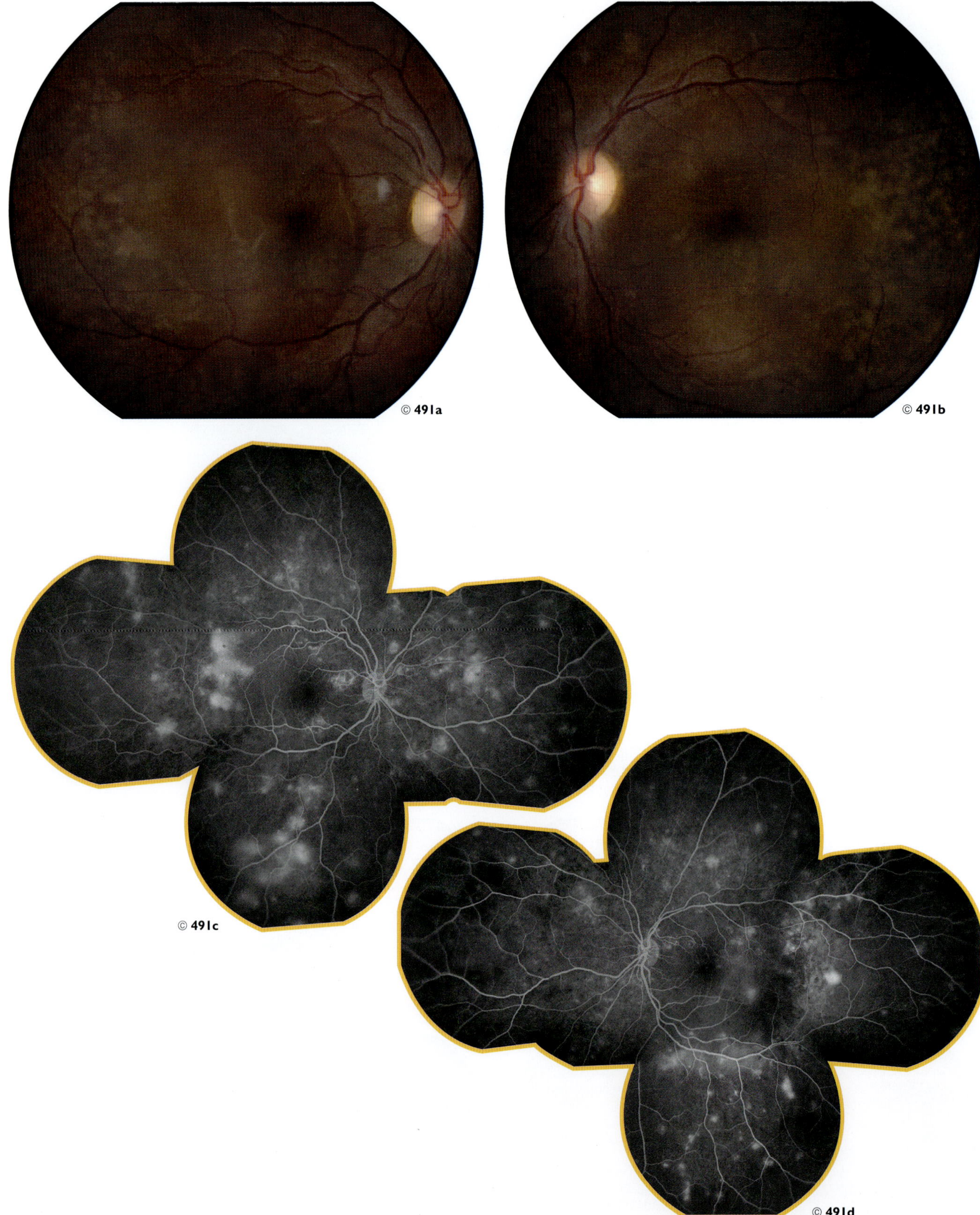

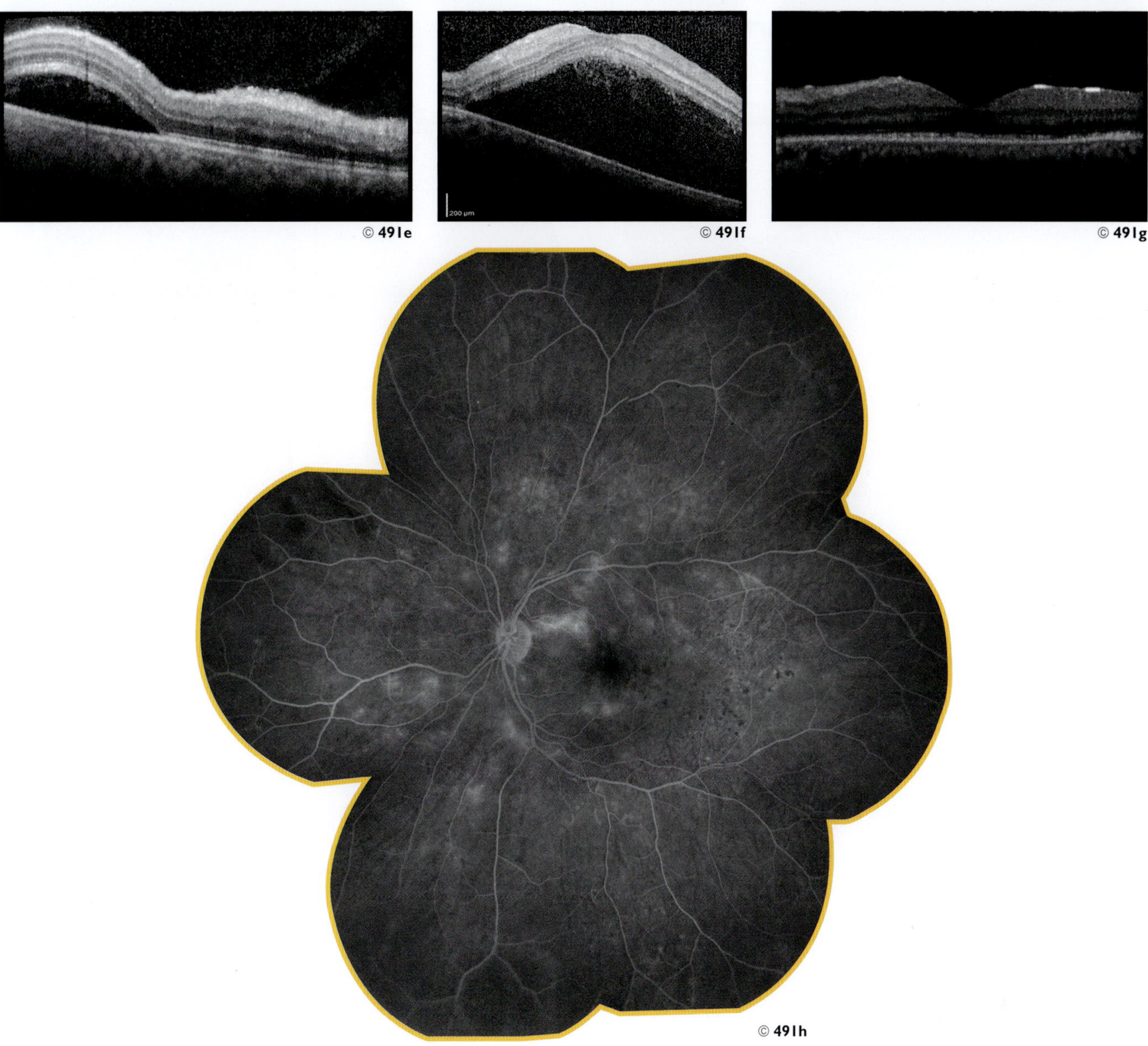

© 491e © 491f © 491g

© 491h

This patient presented with lupus choroidopathy in association with lupus glomerulonephritis and uncontrolled hypertension. Bilateral exudative macular detachment associated with CWS and Elschnig spots (temporal macula of each eye) are illustrated in the color photos. The FA montages show patchy choroidal ischemia and multifocal subretinal hyperfluorescent foci that leak (Elschnig spots). The OCT images confirm the presence of serous macular detachment in each eye. After normalization of blood pressure and administration of rituximab and corticosteroid therapy, the macular detachments resolved (right OCT) with a dramatic improvement in the visual acuity. Multiple pigmented Elschnig spots *(bottom row)* in the temporal macula and peripheral Siegrist streaks *(inferior)* are illustrated in the FA montage *(bottom row)* of the left eye.

Lupus and Malignant Hypertension

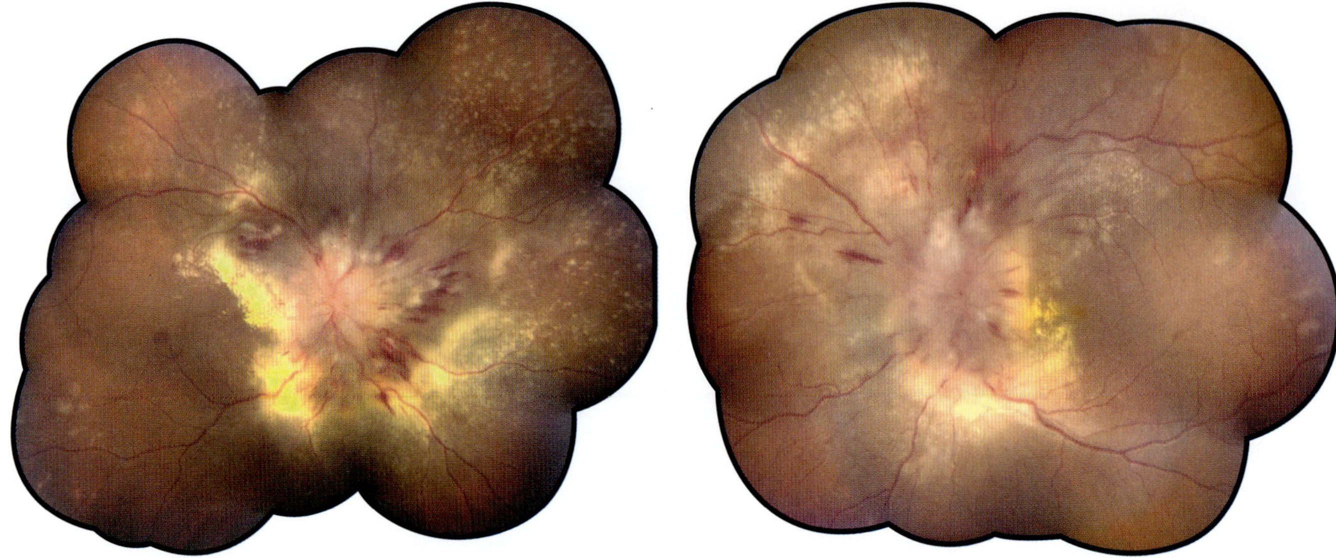

This patient has SLE and malignant hypertension. Severe disc edema associated with peripapillary lipid exudate and flame-shaped retinal hemorrhages are shown. *Courtesy of Dr. Theodore Lin*

Giant Cell Arteritis (Temporal Arteritis)

Giant cell arteritis or temporal arteritis is an inflammatory vasculitis of the large and medium sized arteries. It is associated with sudden occlusive disease affecting branches of the carotid artery. It is seen more frequently in females than males at a ratio of 3 : 1 with a mean age of onset of 70 years. Occlusion of the ophthalmic or central retinal artery or arteritic anterior ischemic optic neuropathy can cause acute blindness in this disease. Prompt diagnosis and emergent treatment is critical to prevent permanent vision loss.

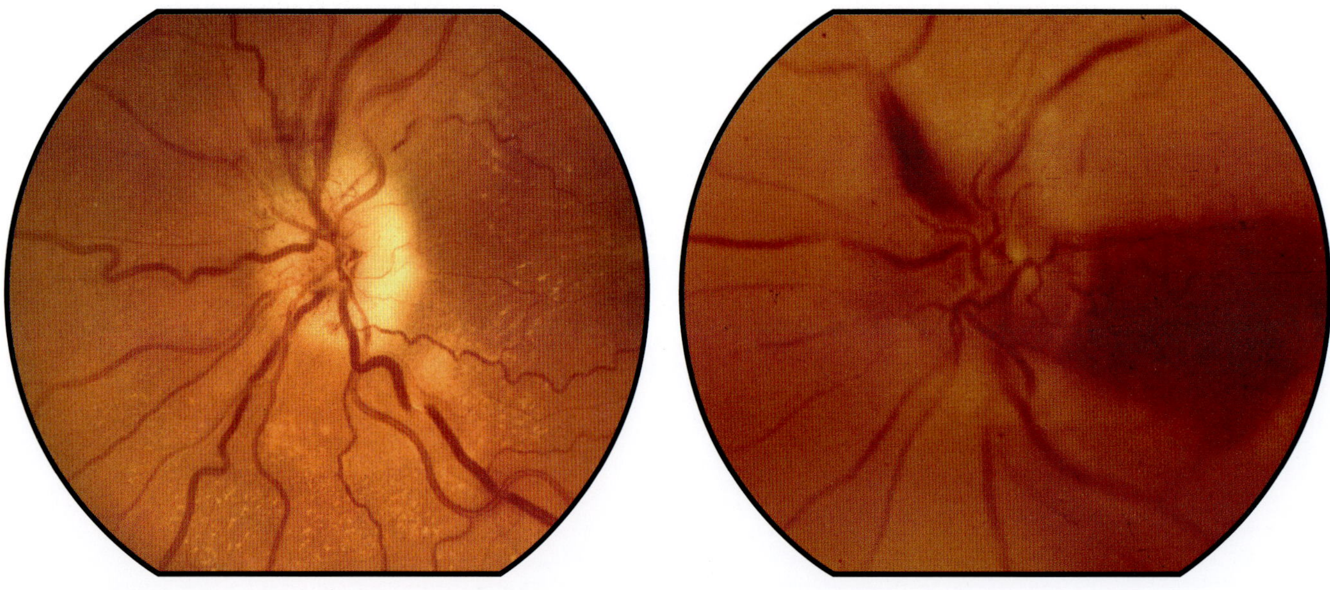

Arteritic anterior ischemic optic neuropathy in two patients with giant-cell arteritis is illustrated. Edema and pallor of the optic disc is shown in each case. Optic disc hemorrhage is also noted in the right color photograph.

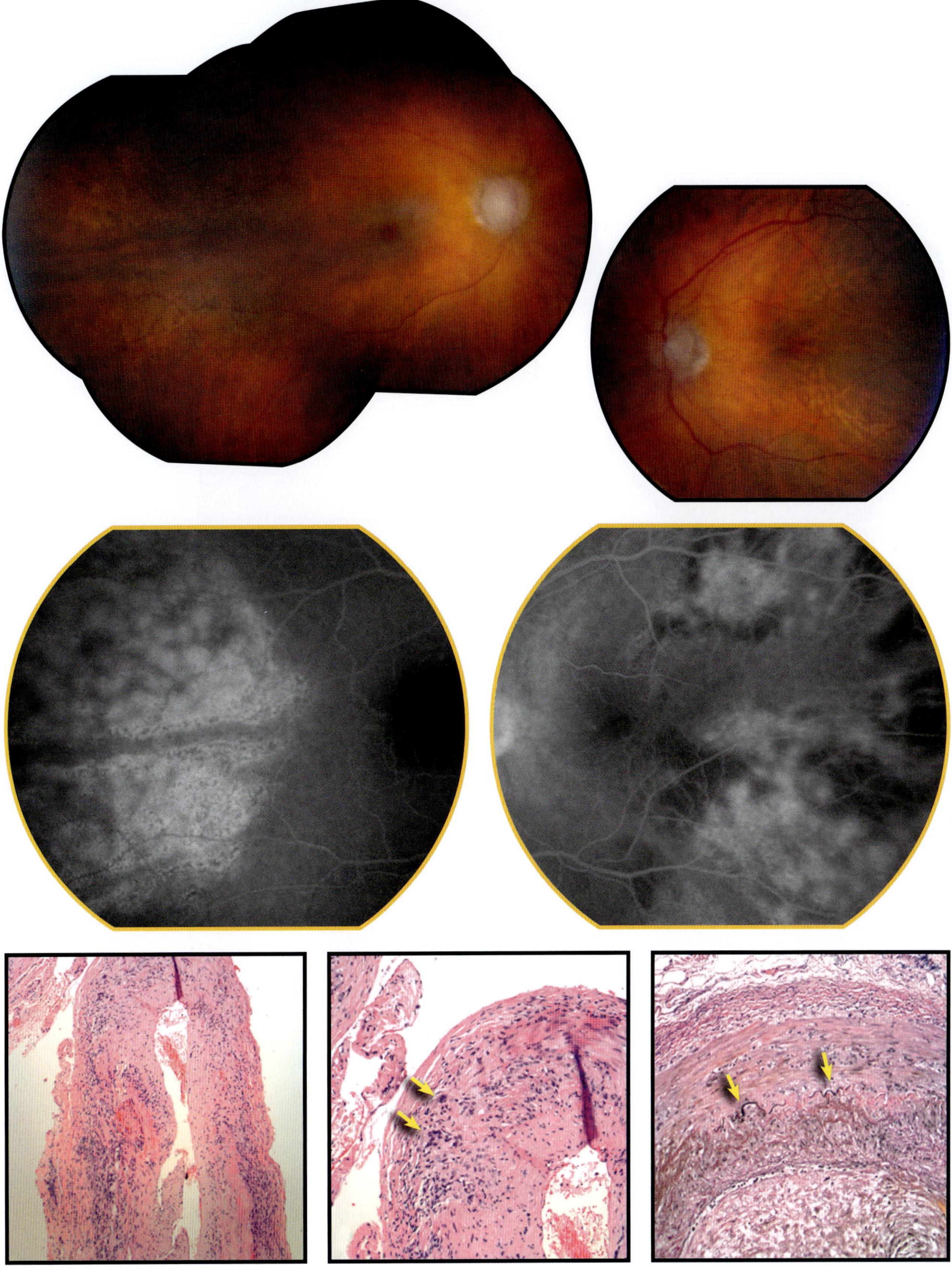

© 491

This elderly female with giant cell arteritis presented with bilateral arteritic anterior ischemic optic neuropathy, central retinal artery occlusion in the right eye, and bilateral choroidal infarctions. Color fundus montage of the right eye shows grayish discoloration of the central and temporal macula with a cherry red spot. Color photo of the left eye shows abnormal grayish appearance in the temporal macula. On late fluorescein angiography, these choroidal infarctions cause staining in a triangular distribution consistent with the triangular sign of Amalric *(middle row)*. Histopathological analysis of the temporal artery biopsy in the patient revealed widespread infiltration of the vessel wall by inflammatory cells *(lower left image)*, multinucleated giant cells *(arrow, lower middle image)*, and widespread loss of the internal elastic lamina with only two small segments remaining *(arrows, lower right image)*.

Polyarteritis Nodosa

Polyarteritis nodosa is a necrotizing vasculitis of small- and medium-sized vessels most commonly affecting the skin, joints, peripheral nerves, gastrointestinal tract, and kidneys. Ocular involvement is rare but can include retinal vascular occlusion, choroidal infarction, and ischemic optic neuropathy.

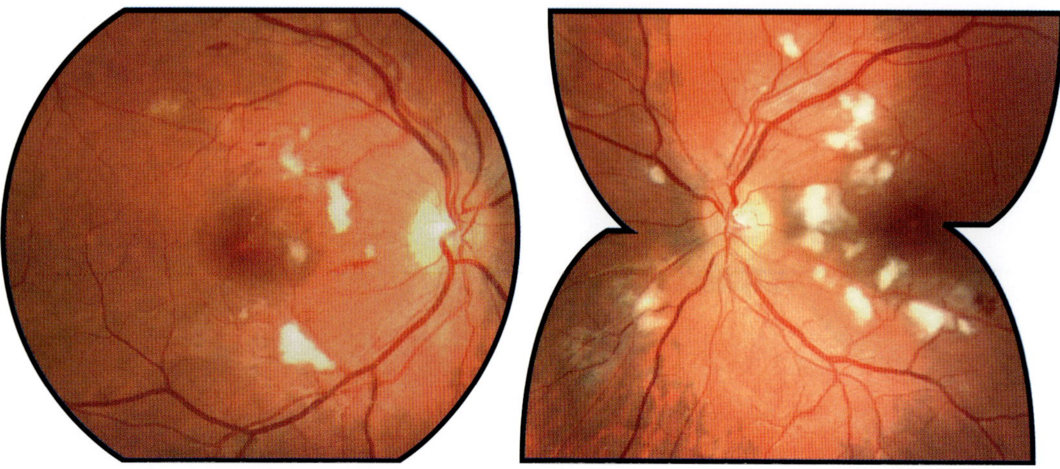

This patient has polyarteritis nodosa with multiple CWS in each eye resembling a Purtscher-like retinopathy.

Churg–Strauss Syndrome

Churg–Strauss syndrome is a systemic necrotizing vasculitis characterized by eosinophilia, asthma, pulmonary infiltrates, peripheral neuropathy, and sinusitis. This small- and medium-sized vasculitis may be complicated by retinal vascular occlusive disease with secondary NV.

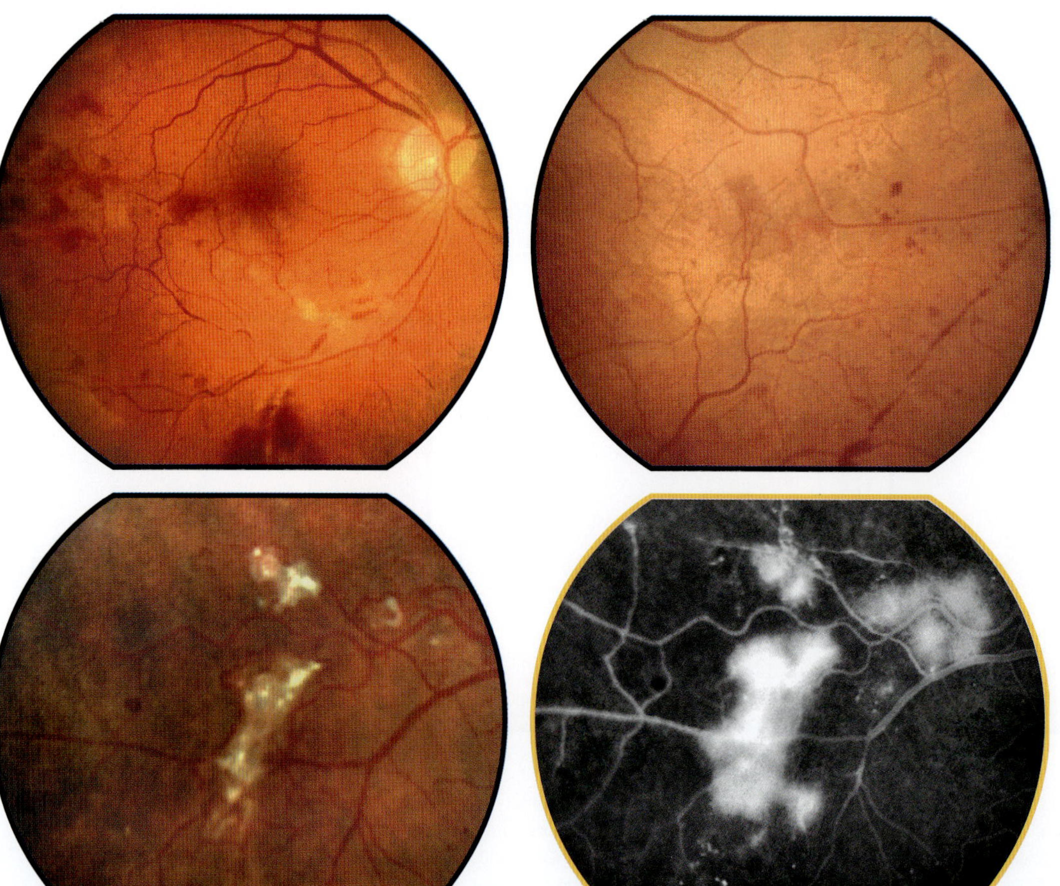

These patients have Churg–Strauss syndrome. Note the scattered retinal hemorrhages and CWS. Retinal NV is illustrated in the color photograph and FA *(bottom)*.

Dermatomyositis

Dermatomyositis is an inflammatory connective tissue disorder characterized by symmetric proximal muscle weakness, a heliotrope rash over the eyelids, and Gottron papules over bony prominences. Dermatomyositis may overlap with other autoimmune diseases such as SLE or scleroderma and can be complicated by a retinal vasculitis.

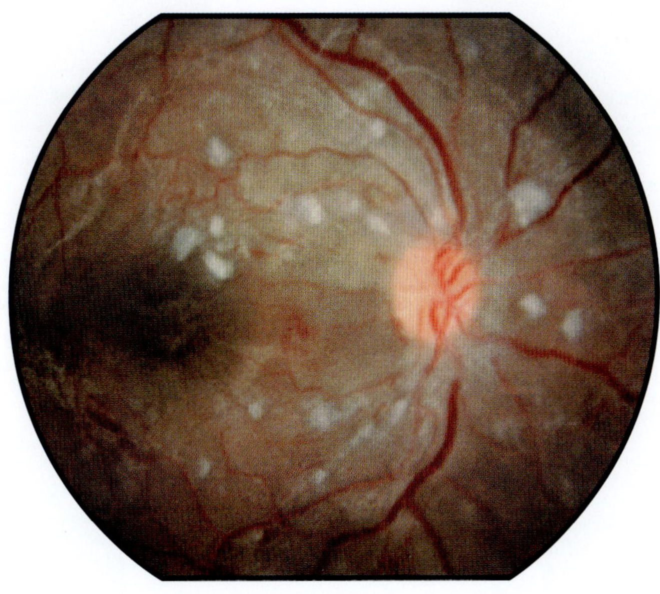

Multiple CWS and retinal hemorrhages are noted in this patient with dermatomyositis and polyarteritis nodosa.

Granulomatosis with Polyangiitis (Wegener's Granulomatosis)

Granulomatosis with polyangiitis (Wegener's granulomatosis) is a systemic granulomatous vasculitis associated with necrotizing granulomas of the upper and lower respiratory tracts and glomerulonephritis. Rare retinal complications include macular edema, retinitis, occlusive disease, and exudative retinal detachment.

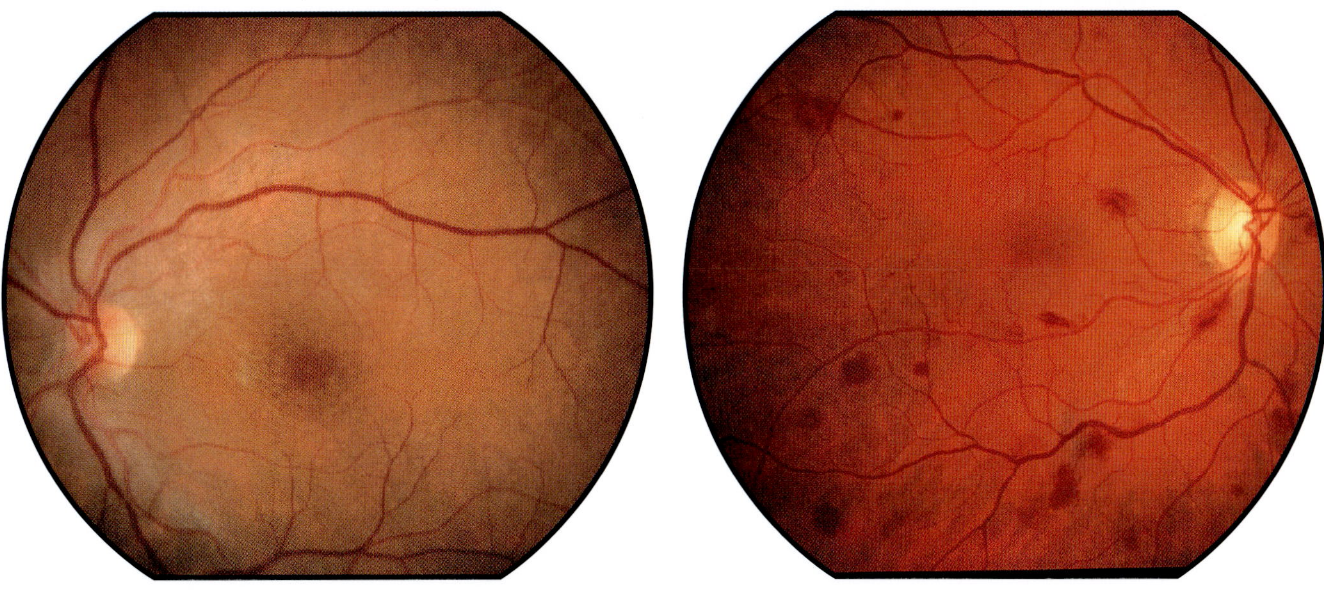

Epiretinal membrane and CME is noted in this patient with Wegener's granulomatosis *(left)*. Non-ischemic central retinal vein occlusion *(right)* is illustrated in a second patient *(right)*.

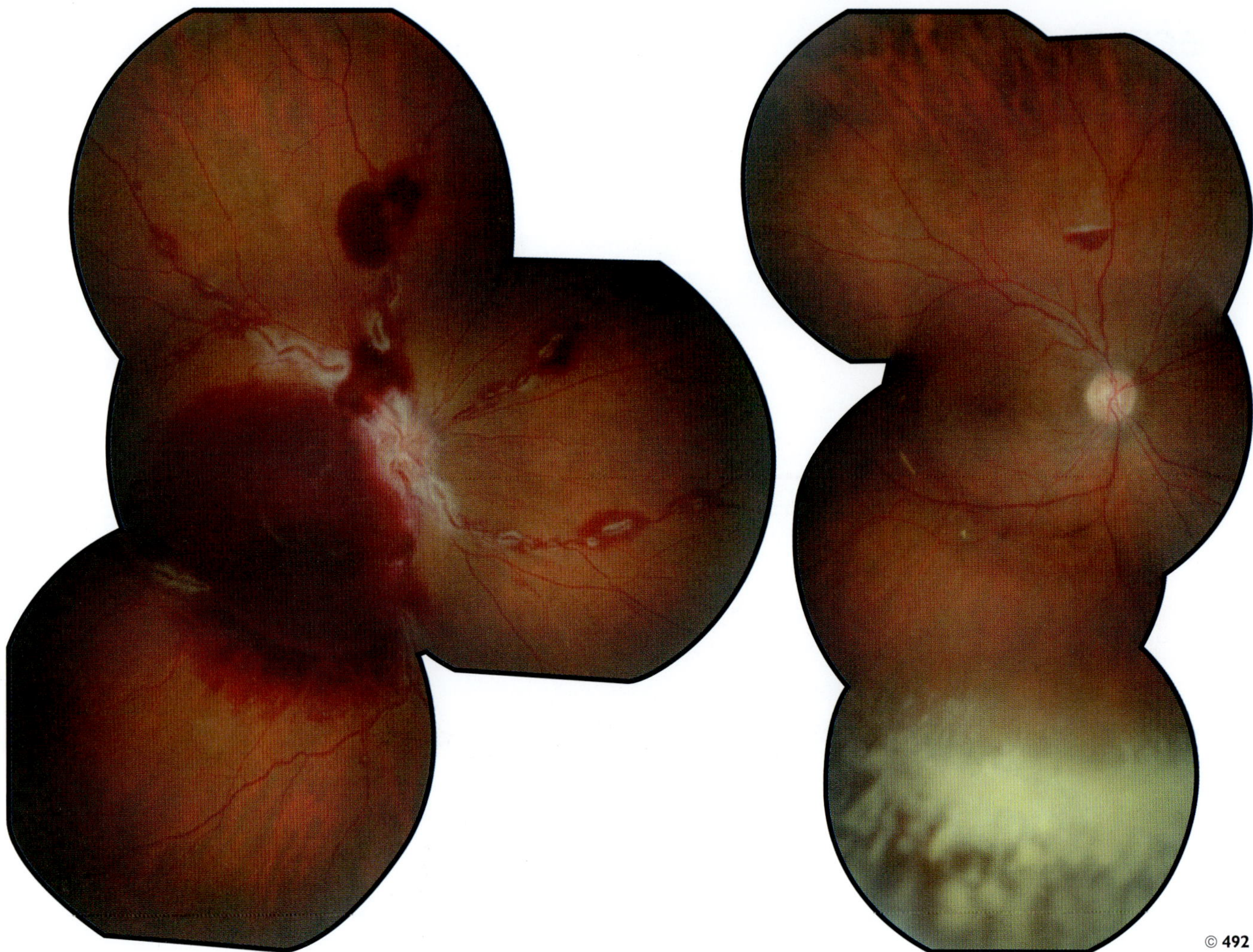

This patient with Wegener's granulomatosis presented with severe pre-macular and retinal hemorrhage associated with a retinal vasculitis *(left)*. Three months after treatment with intravenous corticosteroids and cyclophosphamide, the retinal hemorrhage and angiitis resolved. Dehemoglobinized vitreous hemorrhage is noted inferiorly *(right)*.

Weber–Christian Disease (Nodular Panniculitis)

Weber–Christian disease or nodular panniculitis is a skin disorder that features recurrent inflammation in the cutaneous fat. Recurrent crops of erythematous, sometimes tender, subcutaneous nodules may arise in the disease. It may also affect the bone marrow, lung, heart, intestinal tract, spleen, and kidney. Circulating immune complexes have been noted in some patients. Optic nerve and choroidal involvement may rarely complicate this systemic disorder.

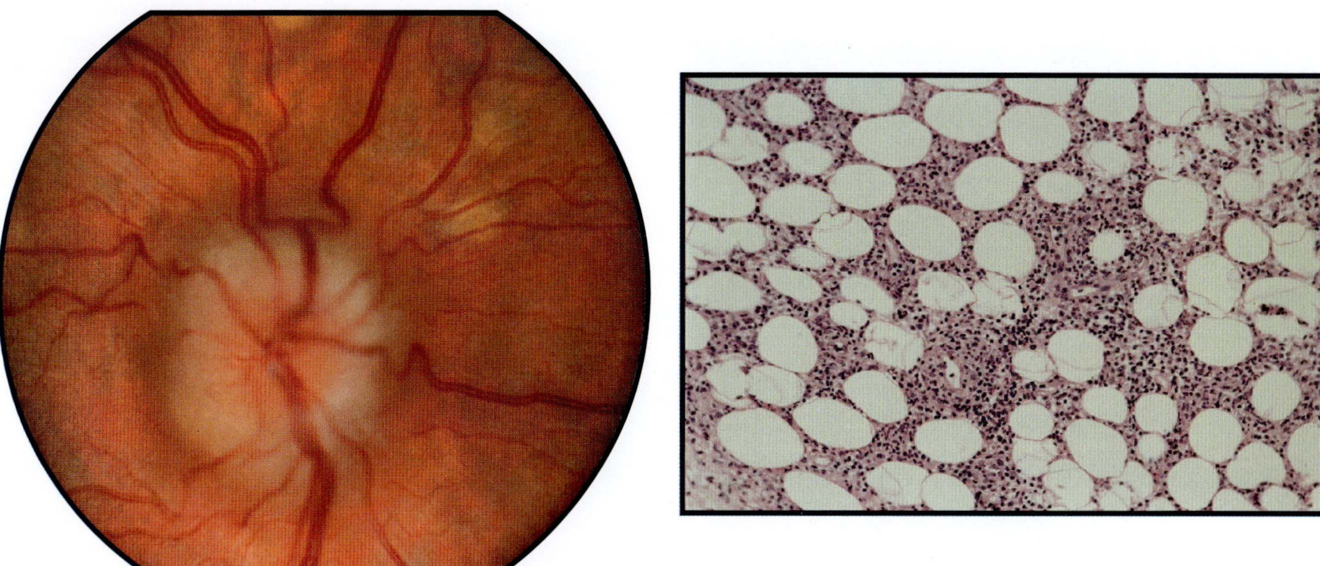

This patient with Weber–Christian disease has yellowish white subretinal lesions and optic disc edema *(left)*. Biopsy was consistent with a histiocytic panniculitis *(right)*.

Systemic Sclerosis

Systemic sclerosis is a connective tissue disorder that leads to progressive fibrosis of target organs. It usually affects the skin and blood vessels, as well as the digestive tract, heart, and lungs. Central retinal artery and vein occlusion may rarely complicate this disease.

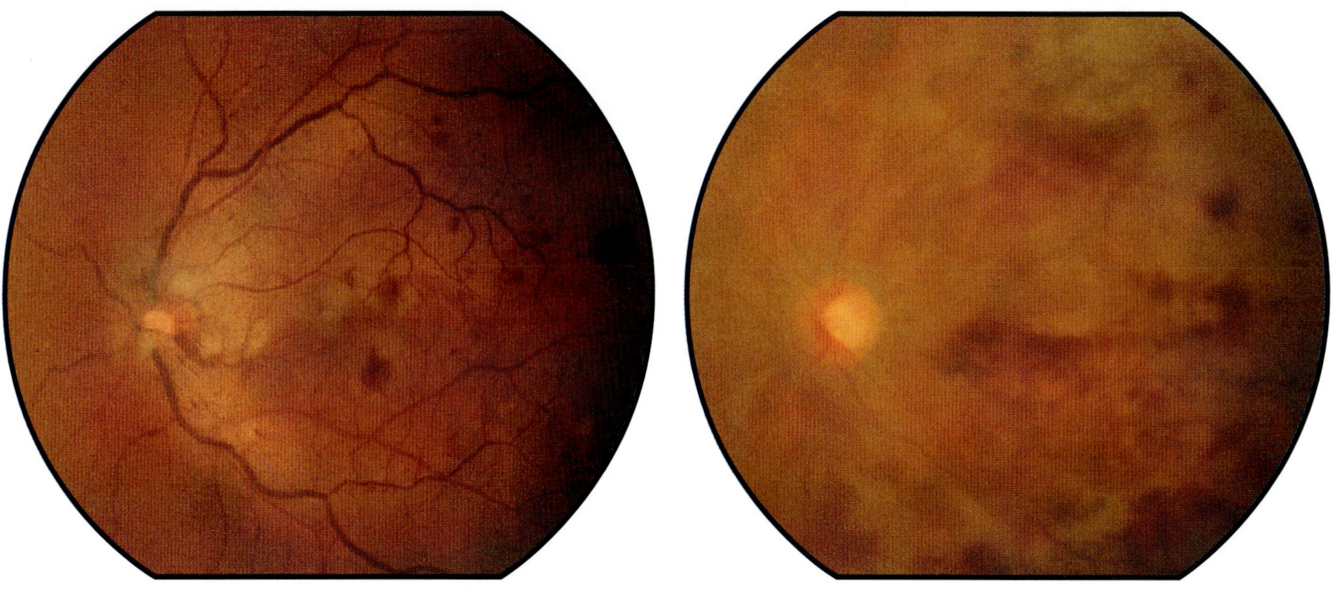

This 60-year-old female with scleroderma developed combined central retinal artery and vein occlusions. Note the progressive retinal hemorrhage and ischemic retinal whitening of the left eye. *Courtesy of Dr. John Sorenson*

Antiphospholipid Antibody Syndrome (Hughes Syndrome)

The antiphospholipid antibody syndrome, also known as Hughes syndrome, is a disorder characterized by the presence of antibodies and associated with either arterial or venous occlusion. The three primary antibodies associated with the disorder are (1) anticardiolipin antibody, (2) the lupus anticoagulant, and (3) anti-β2 glycoprotein-1 antibody. Secondary antiphospholipid antibody syndrome refers to those patients who have an underlying autoimmune disorder versus primary antiphospholipid antibody syndrome in those who do not. Approximately 30% of patients with SLE will develop an antiphospholipid antibody syndrome. The exact mechanism by which these antibodies induce a hypercoagulable state is not known.

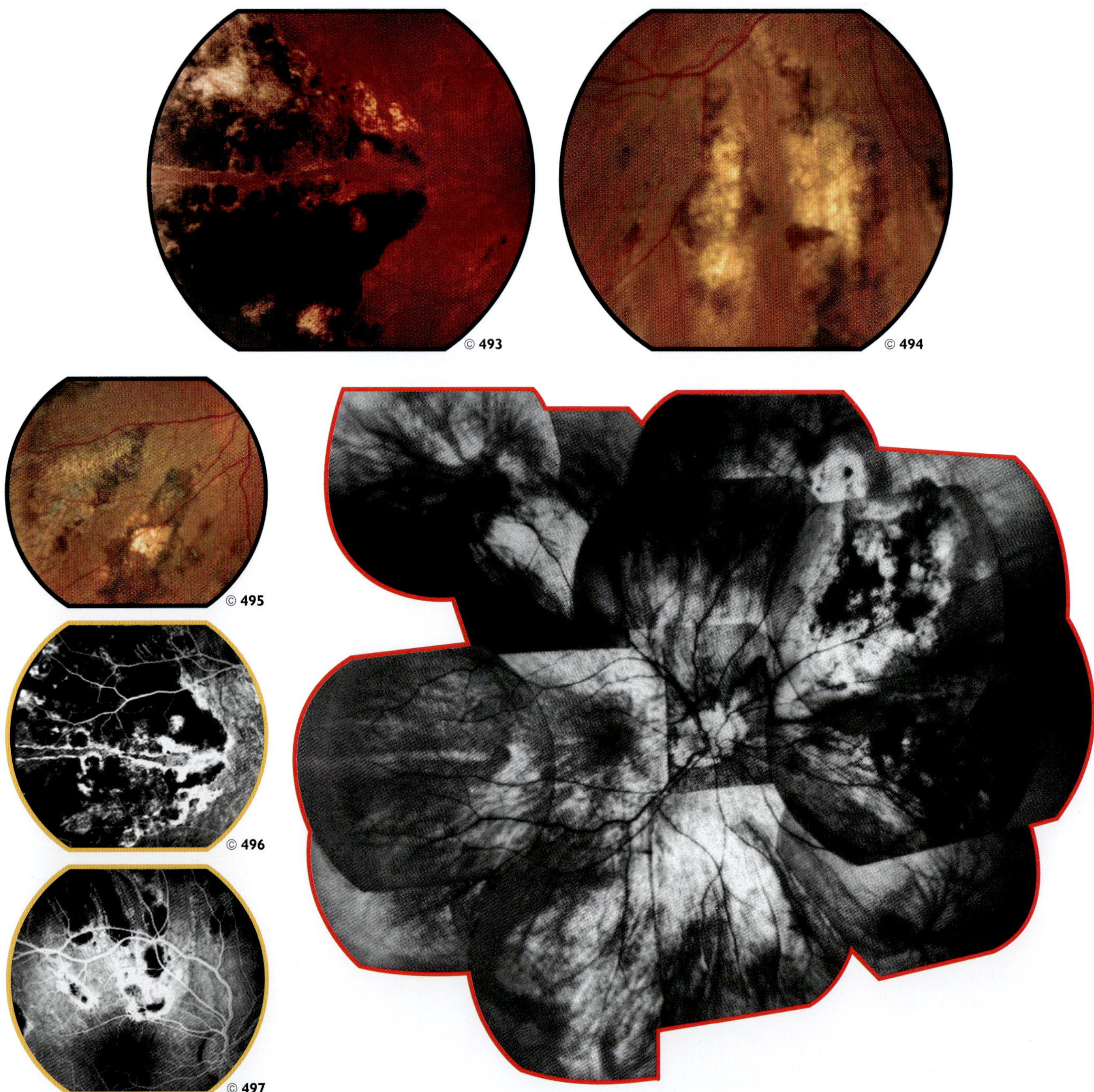

This patient has antiphospholipid antibody syndrome with widespread choroidal vascular occlusive disease. Note the many triangular infarctions of Amalric. The FAs *(lower left)* and red-free montage *(lower right)* show absence of perfusion in the choroid and blockage (due to pigment scarring) associated with the old triangular choroidal infarcts.

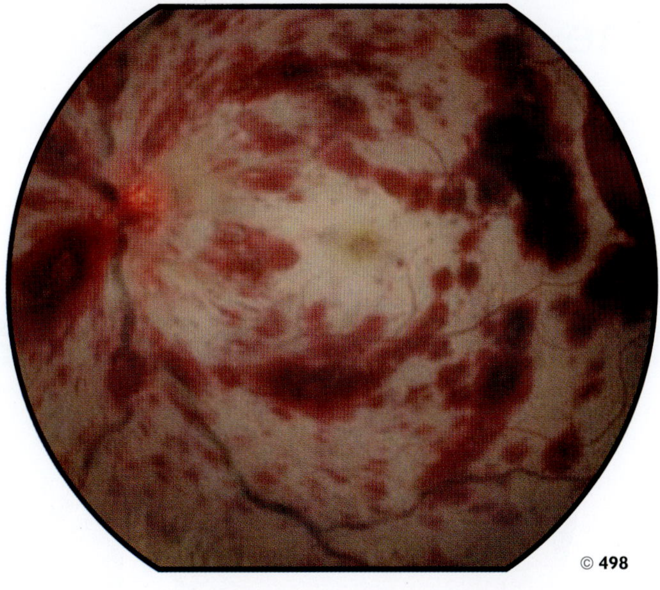

Combined central retinal vein occlusion (CRVO) and central retinal artery occlusion (CRAO) is illustrated in this systemic lupus erythematosus (SLE) patient with secondary antiphospholipid syndrome. Note the presence of retinal venous tortuosity, diffuse retinal hemorrhage, and macular ischemia with a cherry red spot. She tested positive for anticardiolipin antibodies.

Cardiac Myxomas

Cardiac myxomas are the most common benign tumor of the heart, usually arising in the left atrium. Fragments of these tumors can embolize to the retinal and choroidal circulations.

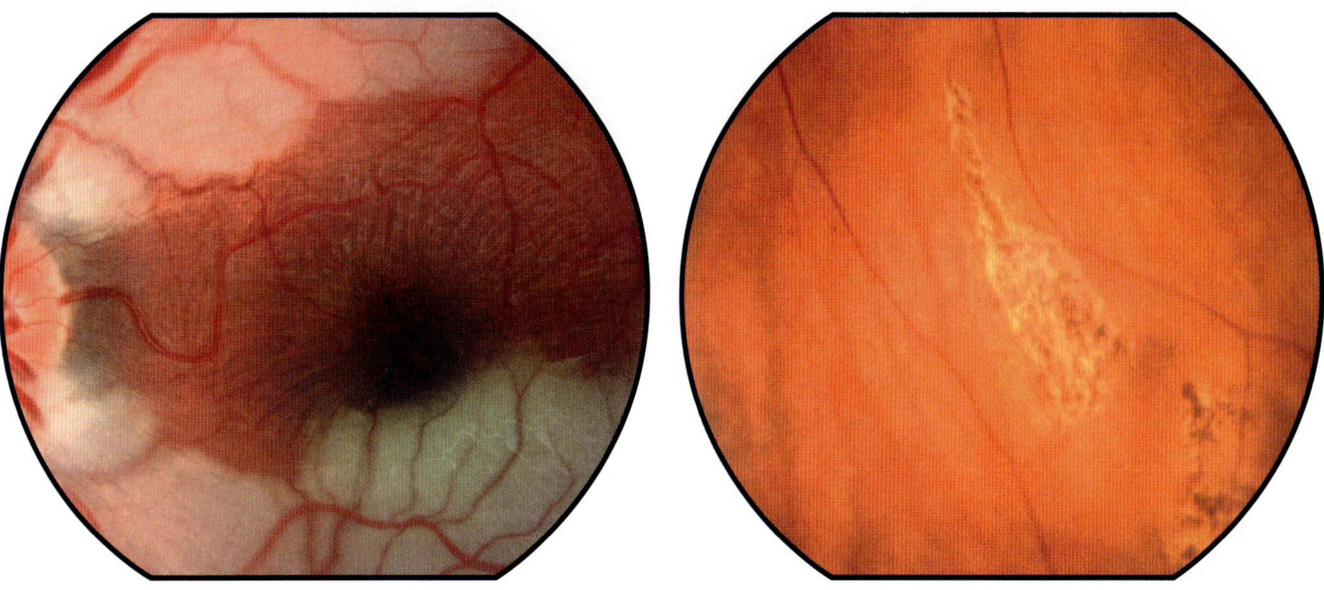

These two patients presented with a cardiac myxoma, each in the left atrium. Note the multiple acute BRAOs on the left color image and the old triangular Amalric choroidal infarct on the right color image. *Courtesy of Dr. Richard Spaide*

Susac Syndrome

Susac syndrome is a systemic microvascular occlusive disease causing hearing loss and impaired vision. Small infarcts of the corpus callosum are pathognomonic. Hearing loss of lower-pitched frequencies is also a characteristic finding. Ocular manifestations include bilateral recurrent branch retinal artery occlusions. The etiology is unknown, but there is evidence to suggest an autoimmune vasculitis.

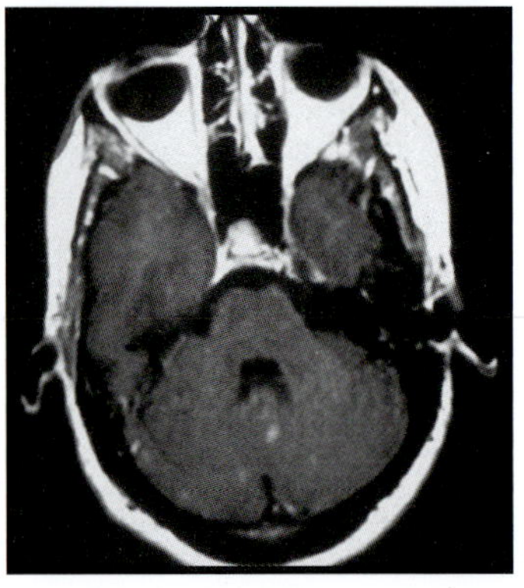

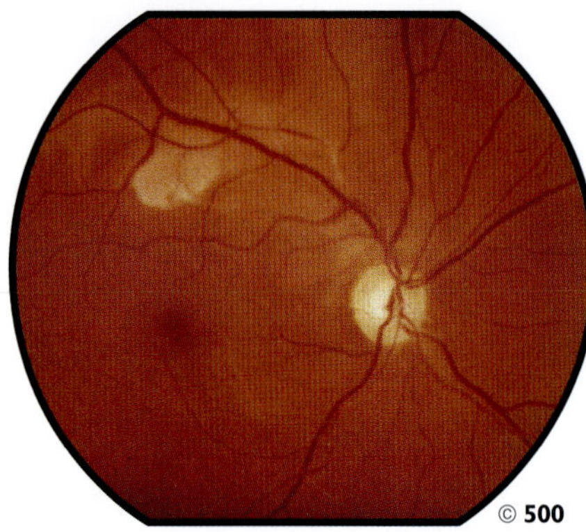

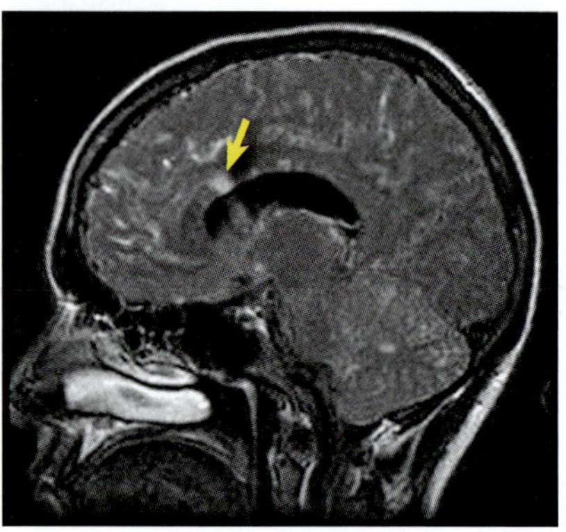

This patient has Susac syndrome. A superotemporal branch retinal arteriolar occlusion is noted on the color photograph. The brain scan shows multiple infarcts of the brain *(left)* with involvement of the corpus callosum *(arrow right)*.

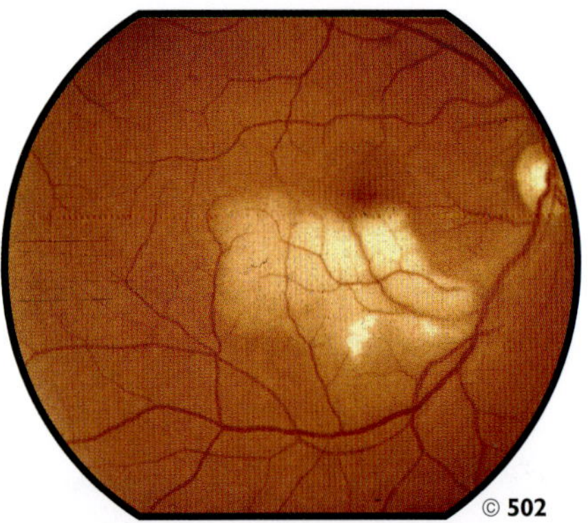

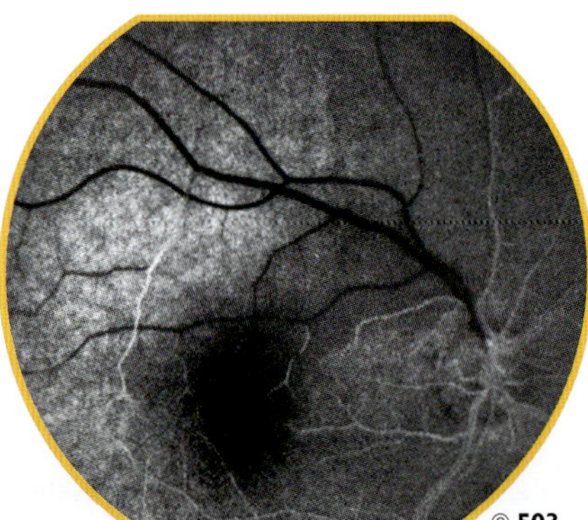

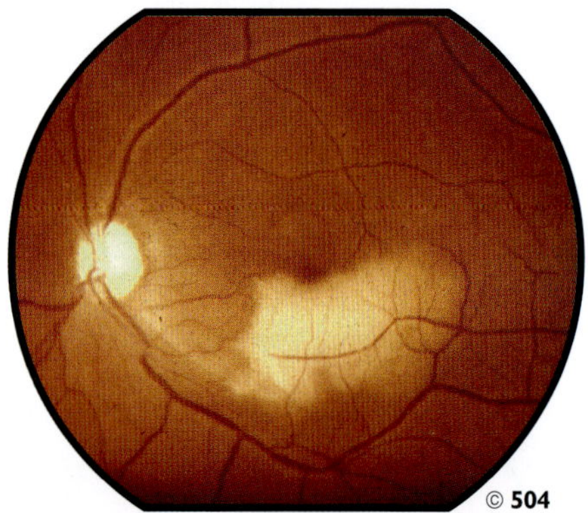

Nine months later, the patient presented with bilateral recurrent BRAO. The FA illustrates non-perfusion in the occluded retinal artery.

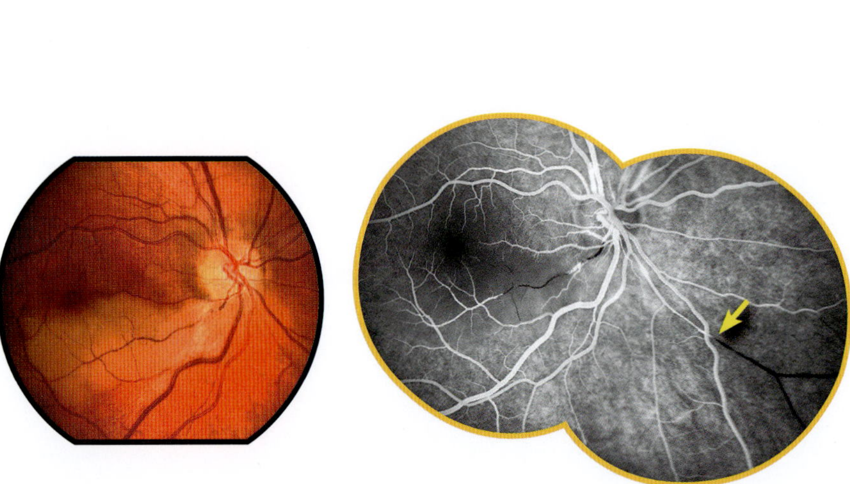

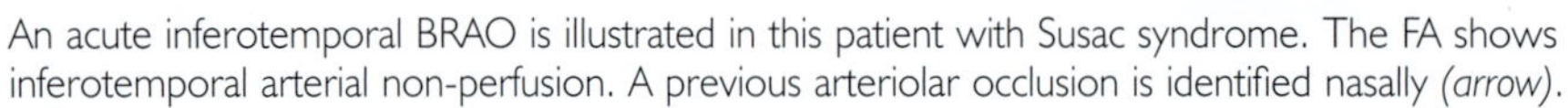

An acute inferotemporal BRAO is illustrated in this patient with Susac syndrome. The FA shows inferotemporal arterial non-perfusion. A previous arteriolar occlusion is identified nasally *(arrow)*.

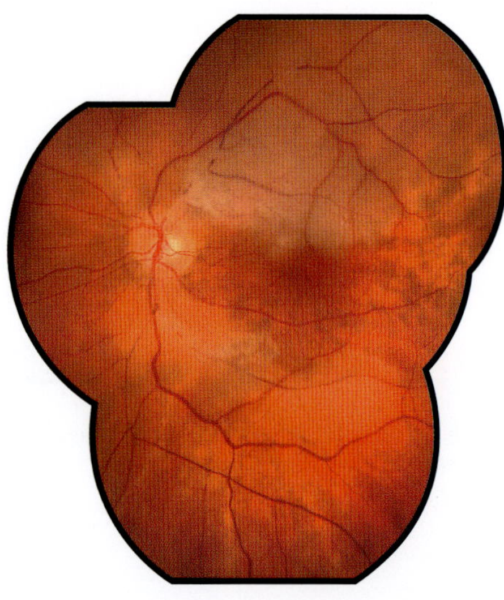

This patient presented with two retinal artery occlusions, superotemporal and inferotemporal, due to Susac syndrome.

Purtscher Retinopathy

Purtscher retinopathy is a hemorrhagic and vascular occlusive disorder caused via several mechanisms. Severe trauma to the head or the long bones or blunt thoracic injury may result in retinal capillary ischemia evidenced by multiple CWS in the posterior pole. A Purtscher-like retinopathy is also described in association with acute pancreatitis, fat embolization, amniotic fluid embolization, and vasculitic diseases.

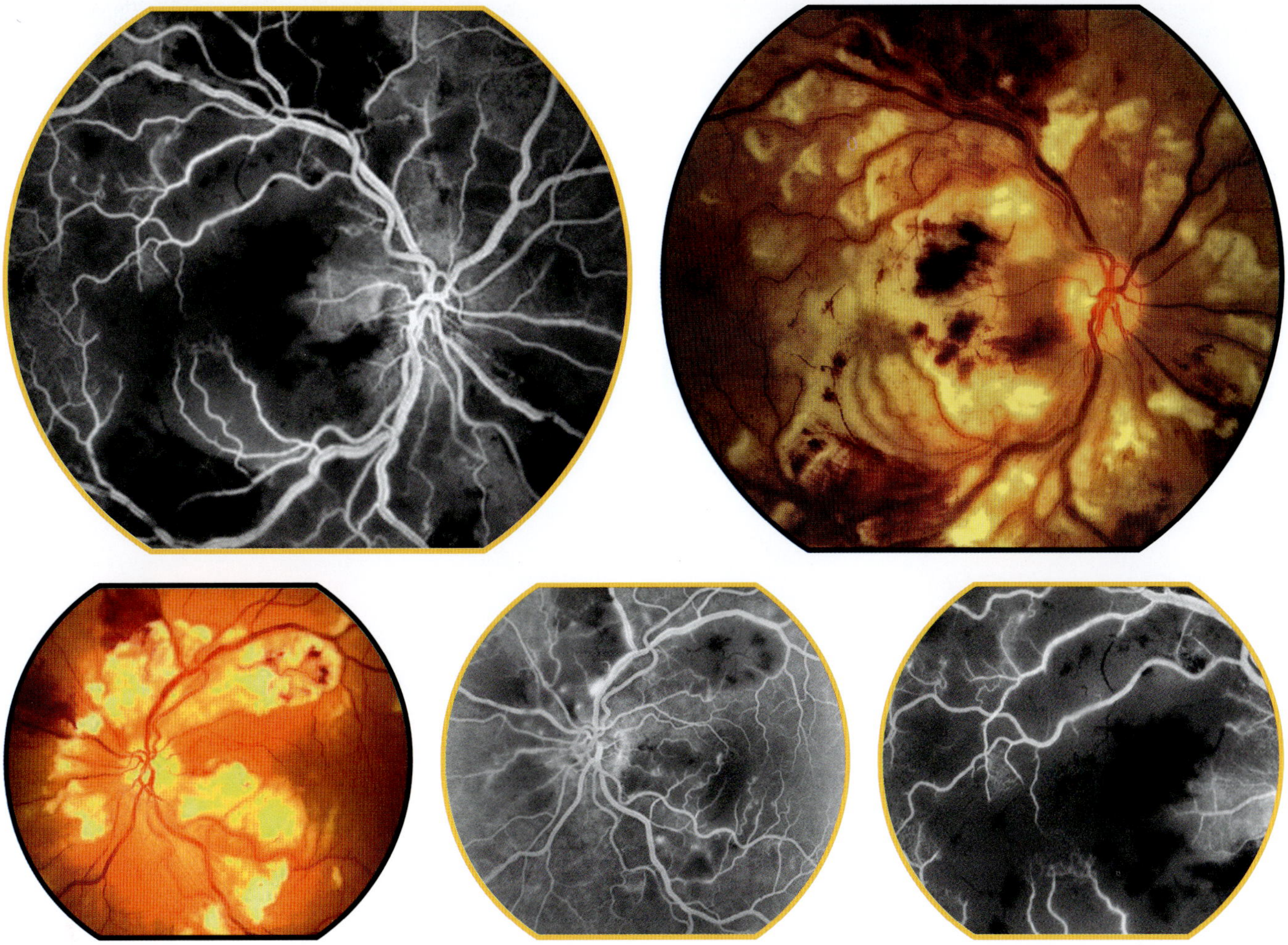

This patient with severe alcoholic pancreatitis presented with acute Purtscher retinopathy. Note the CWS, the retinal hemorrhages, and the severe ischemia and non-perfusion on the FA. *Courtesy of Dr. Murray J. Erasmus*

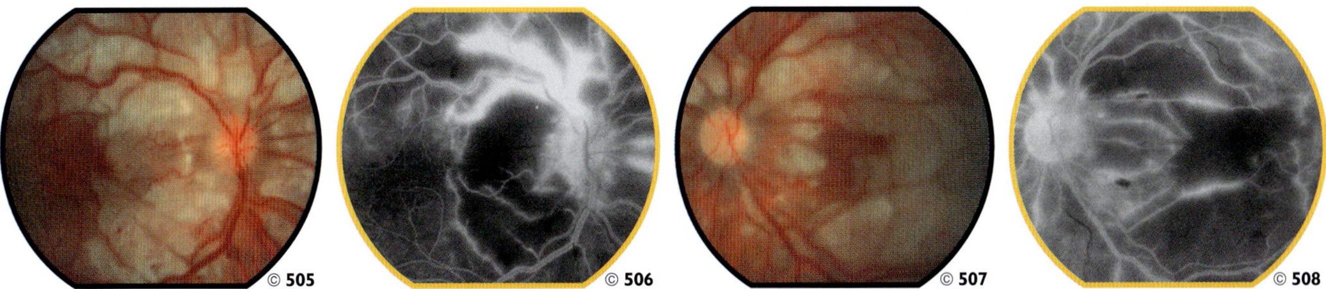

This patient was receiving multiple medications for treatment of HIV. There was an adverse reaction to the drugs and a Purtscher retinopathy resulted. Multiple confluent CWS and macular ischemia and non-perfusion are noted in each eye, with associated retinal vascular staining.

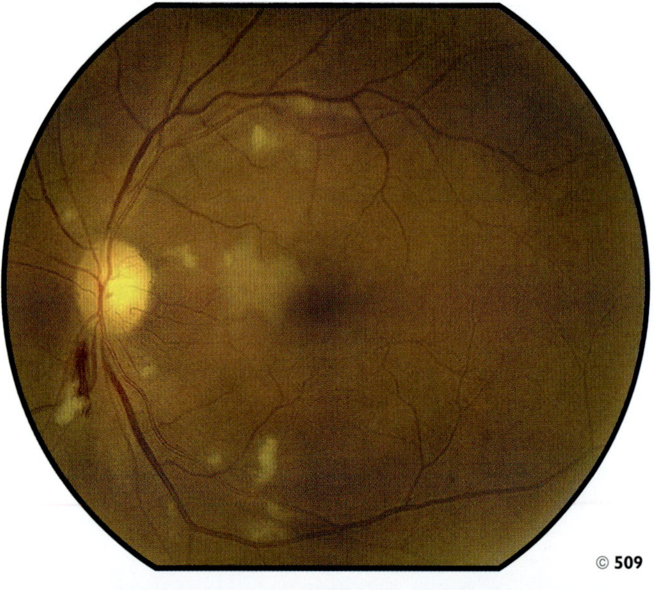

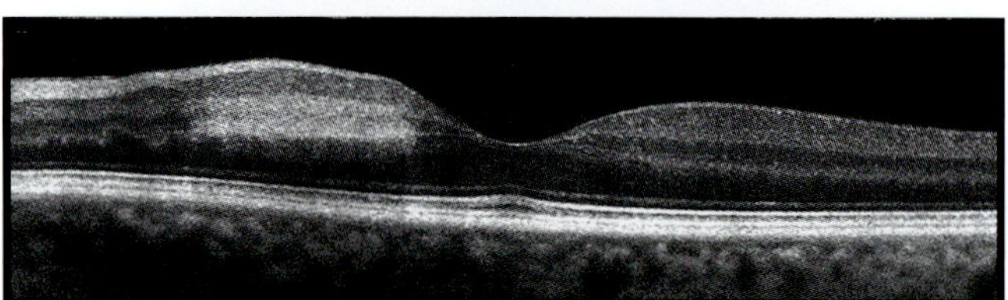

This patient with metastatic pancreatic cancer presented with bilateral Purtscher-like retinopathy. CWS indicating superficial capillary ischemia are seen along the arcades and in a peripapillary distribution. Adjacent to the fovea is a deeper polygonal zone of whitening referred to as Purtscher flecken. These Purtscher flecken correspond to a band-like zone of hyper-reflectivity at the level of the inner nuclear layer on spectral domain OCT referred to as PAMM or paracentral acute middle maculopathy. PAMM can be associated with a wide spectrum of retinal vascular diseases.

Pregnancy

Various choroidal or retinal complications of pregnancy have been described that include central serous chorioretinopathy, choroidal NV, exudative retinal detachment and choroidopathy (e.g., Elschnig spots), Purtscher-like retinopathy, and exacerbation of pre-existing conditions such as diabetic retinopathy. Rarely existing lesions such as uveal melanocytic proliferation and even choroidal osteoma have been reported to grow during pregnancy.

Central Serous Chorioretinopathy

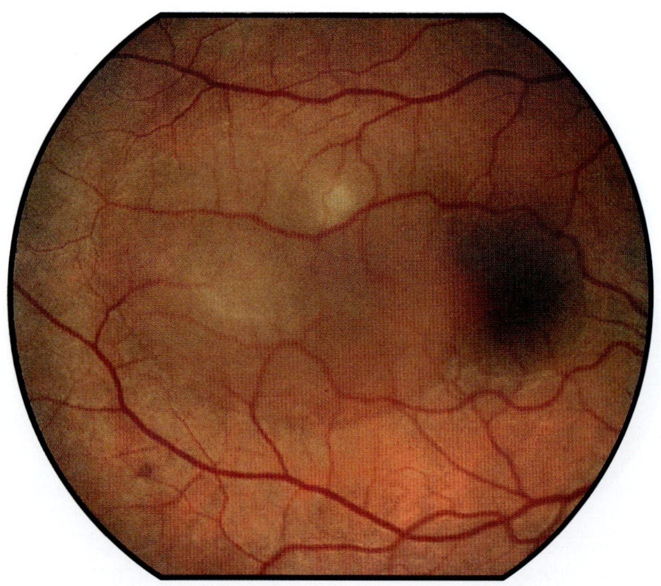

Note the presence of serous macular detachment due to central serous chorioretinopathy in this pregnant patient. There is a greater incidence of fibrin associated with central serous chorioretinopathy (CSCR) in pregnant patients as is illustrated (superotemporal to the fovea) in this case.

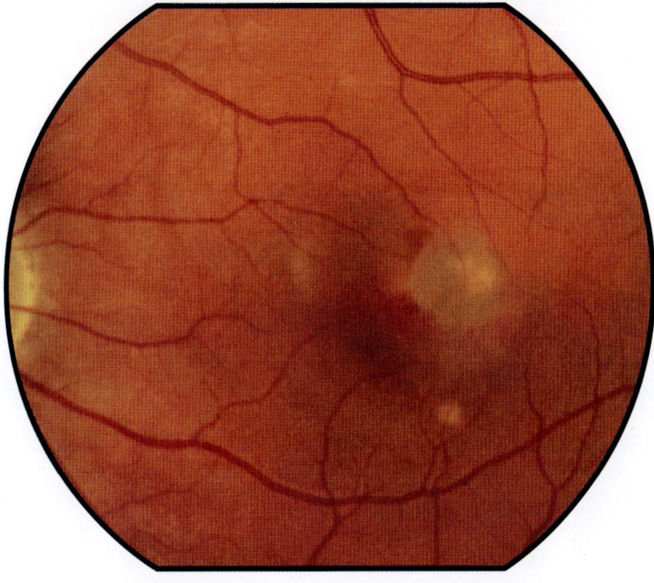

This pregnant patient developed subretinal fluid and hemorrhage and a gray-green membrane consistent with choroidal NV. It is unclear if pregnancy is a risk factor for choroidal NV.

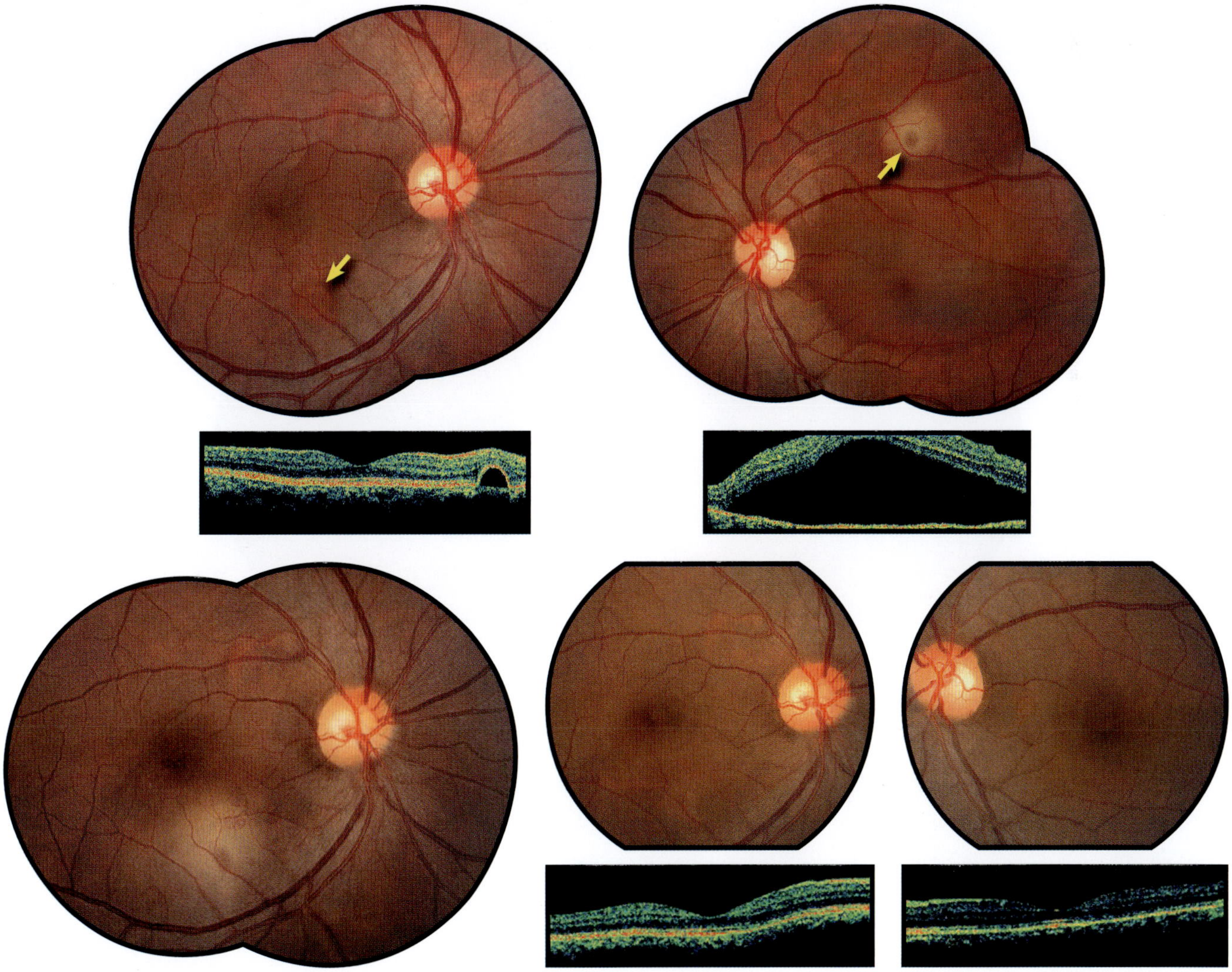

An exudative detachment of the macula is illustrated in the left eye and a serous PED is shown in the right eye *(upper left image, arrow)* in this 23-year-old pregnant female. Time domain OCT confirmed the presence of a PED. Note the presence of fibrin near the superotemporal arcade *(upper right image, arrow)*. The OCT confirmed a serous macular detachment. One month later, active CSCR with subretinal fluid and fibrin developed in the right eye *(lower left image)*. Two months after delivery, the macular detachments and fibrin resolved spontaneously in each eye.

Preeclampsia

Toxemia of pregnancy or preeclampsia is characterized by hypertension and signs of end-organ damage, such as proteinuria, renal failure, neurological abnormalities, pulmonary edema, hepatic dysfunction, and thrombocytopenia. Preeclampsia may progress to eclampsia with the development of tonic-clonic seizures. Patients with underlying thrombophilic diseases such as antiphospholipid syndrome are at higher risk for developing preeclampsia and eclampsia. Up to 40% of women with preeclampsia may develop visual symptoms. Ocular complications include serous macular detachment due to choroidopathy, Purtscher-like retinopathy, and retinal hemorrhage.

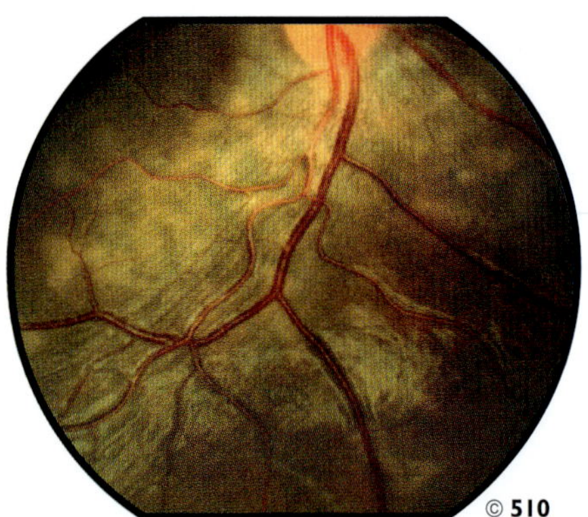

This patient illustrates a neurosensory retinal detachment with white-yellow Elschnig spots due to toxemia of pregnancy.

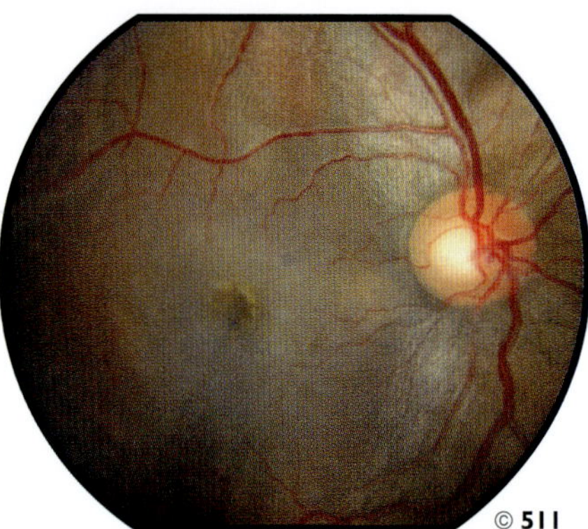

Exudative retinal detachment with barely detectable white spots at the level of the retinal pigment epithelium is noted in this patient with toxemia of pregnancy.

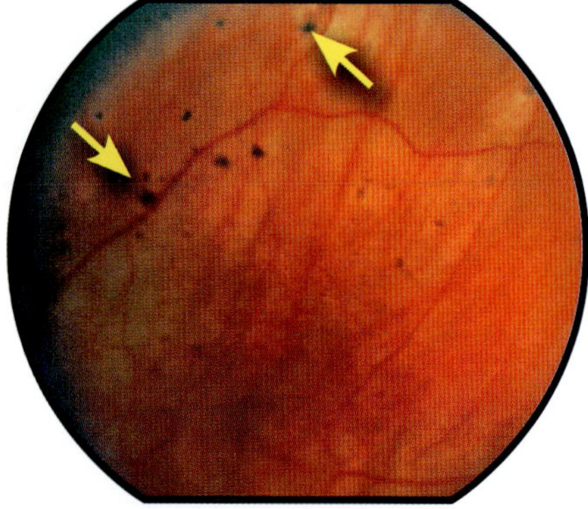

Multiple pigmented spots with a vasculotropic choroidal orientation, referred to as Elschnig spots *(arrows)*, are noted in this patient. When associated with atrophic or pigmented linear lines, they are called Siegrist streaks and are indicative of anterior choroidal ischemia that can be identified in patients with toxemia of pregnancy. *Courtesy of Dr. Lee Jampol*

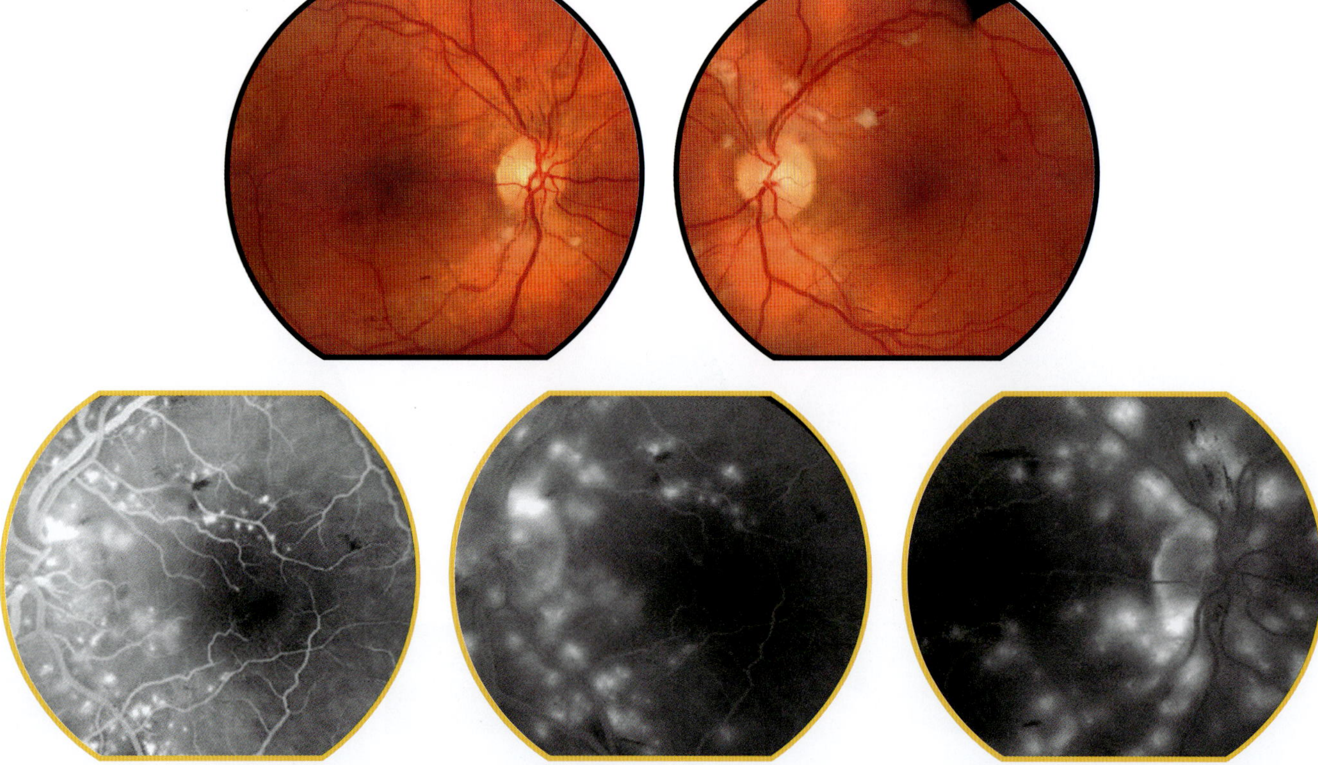

Retinal hemorrhages and CWS associated with serous macular detachment are illustrated *(upper row)* in this pregnant patient. FA shows multifocal subretinal leaks (Elschnig spots) with pooling into the subneurosensory retinal detachment of both eyes. *Courtesy of Dr. Joseph Maguire and Dr. Justis Ehlers*

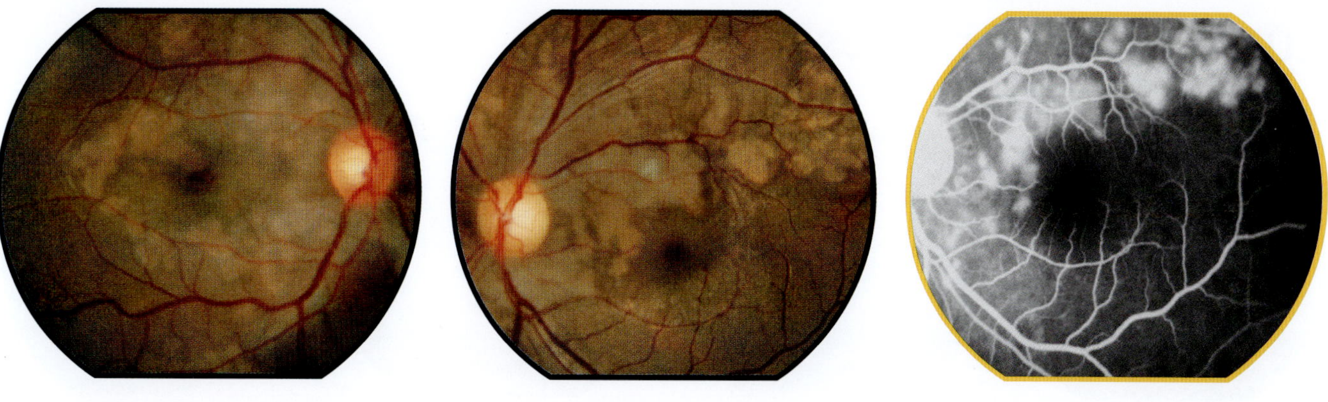

This patient with toxemia noted acute loss of vision in both eyes after delivery. Bilateral exudative macular detachment associated with yellow-white deposits at the level of the retinal pigment epithelium are illustrated. FA performed after delivery illustrates multiple subretinal foci of leakage consistent with pregnancy induced choroidopathy. *Left and middle images courtesy of Dr. Gaetano Barile; right image courtesy of Dr. Gaetano Barile and Mr. José Martinez*

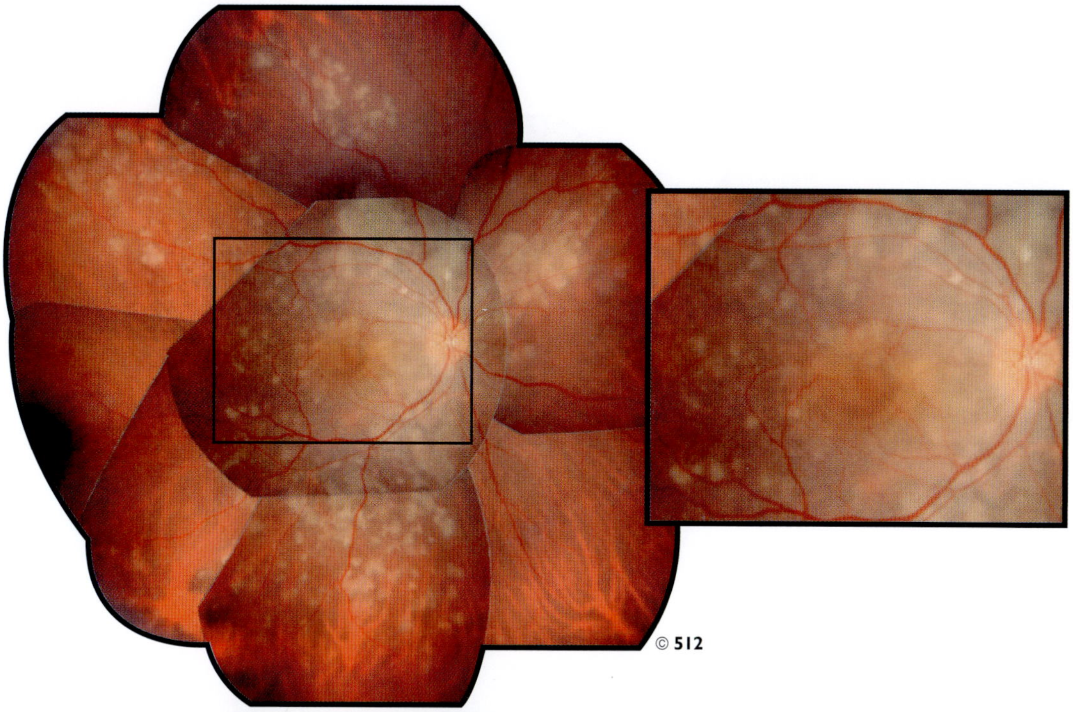

© 512

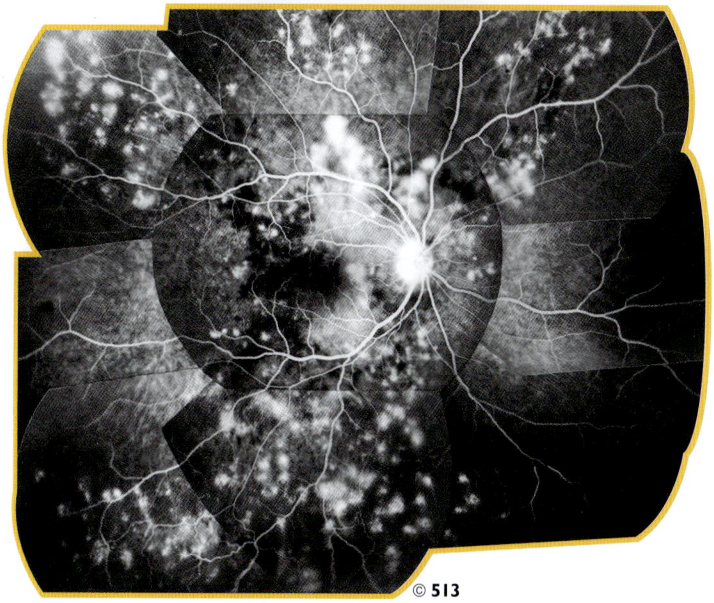

© 513

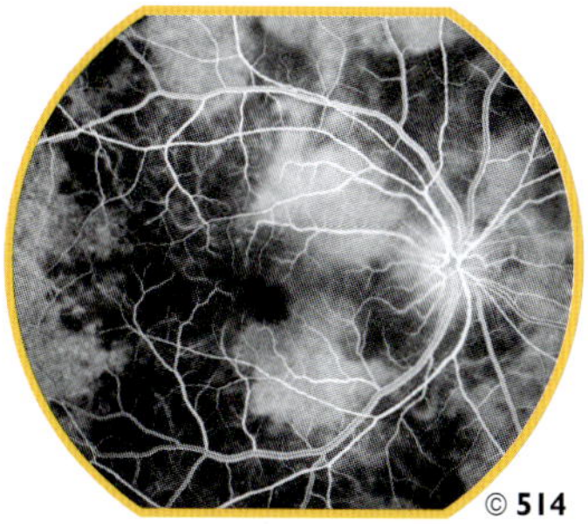

© 514

Clinical findings in this preeclampsia patient include turbid exudative macular detachment and multifocal subretinal Elschnig spots. The early FA *(lower right)* shows a delay in choriocapillaris perfusion due to choroidal ischemia. The late stage FA montage *(lower left)* illustrates multifocal foci of subretinal leakage (Elschnig spots) throughout the entire fundus with pooling into the subneurosensory retinal space.

Lupus Erythematosus

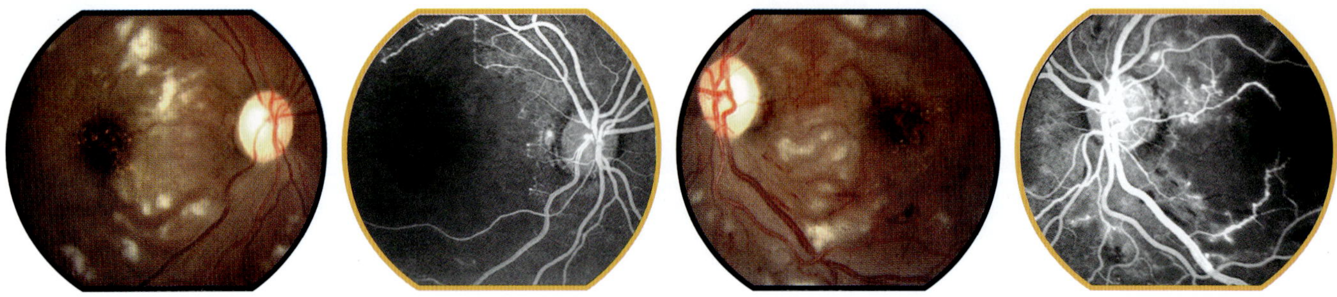

Note the multiple CWS and retinal hemorrhages associated with macular ischemia and non-perfusion in this pregnant patient with lupus erythematosus. The combined thrombotic state of these two diseases may have led to these ocular complications. *Courtesy of Dr. Emmett Cunningham*

Protein S Deficiency

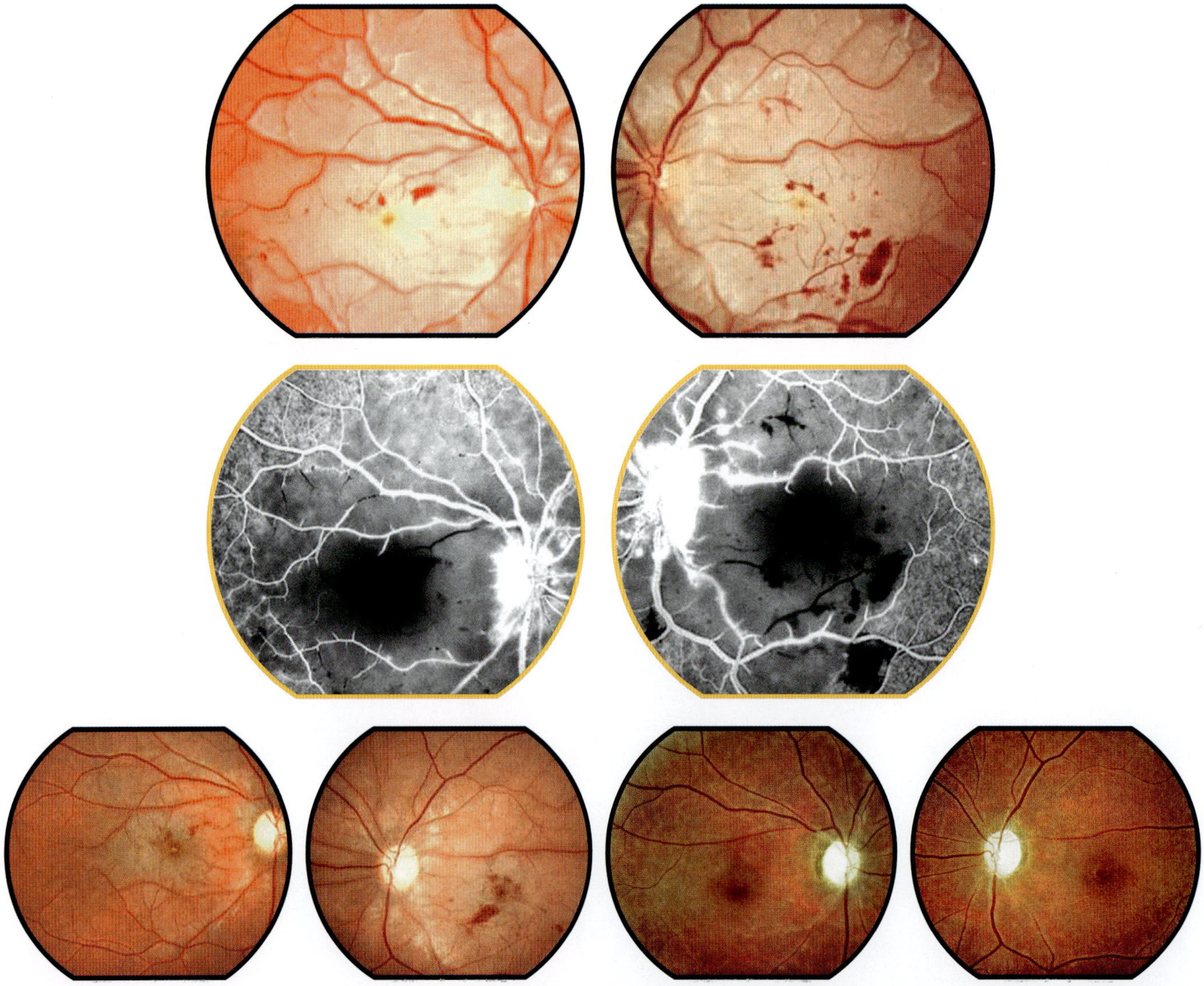

Severe macular infarction is illustrated in this pregnant patient with coexistent protein S deficiency. There is diffuse whitening of the posterior pole with a few scattered retinal hemorrhages. The FA shows severe macular ischemia and non-perfusion and disc leakage in each eye. After 2 months, the whitening has improved *(lower left images)* with some residual hemorrhages. After 4 months, macular whitening has resolved but note the presence of optic atrophy and generalized retinal arteriolar narrowing *(lower two right images)* associated with minimal vision recovery.

Iatrogenic Embolization

Inadvertent embolization of material through the branches of the ophthalmic artery can produce disseminated retinal and choroidal occlusive disease. This has been reported with cosmetic facial fillers and various other cosmetic agents or with embolization of intracranial fistulas.

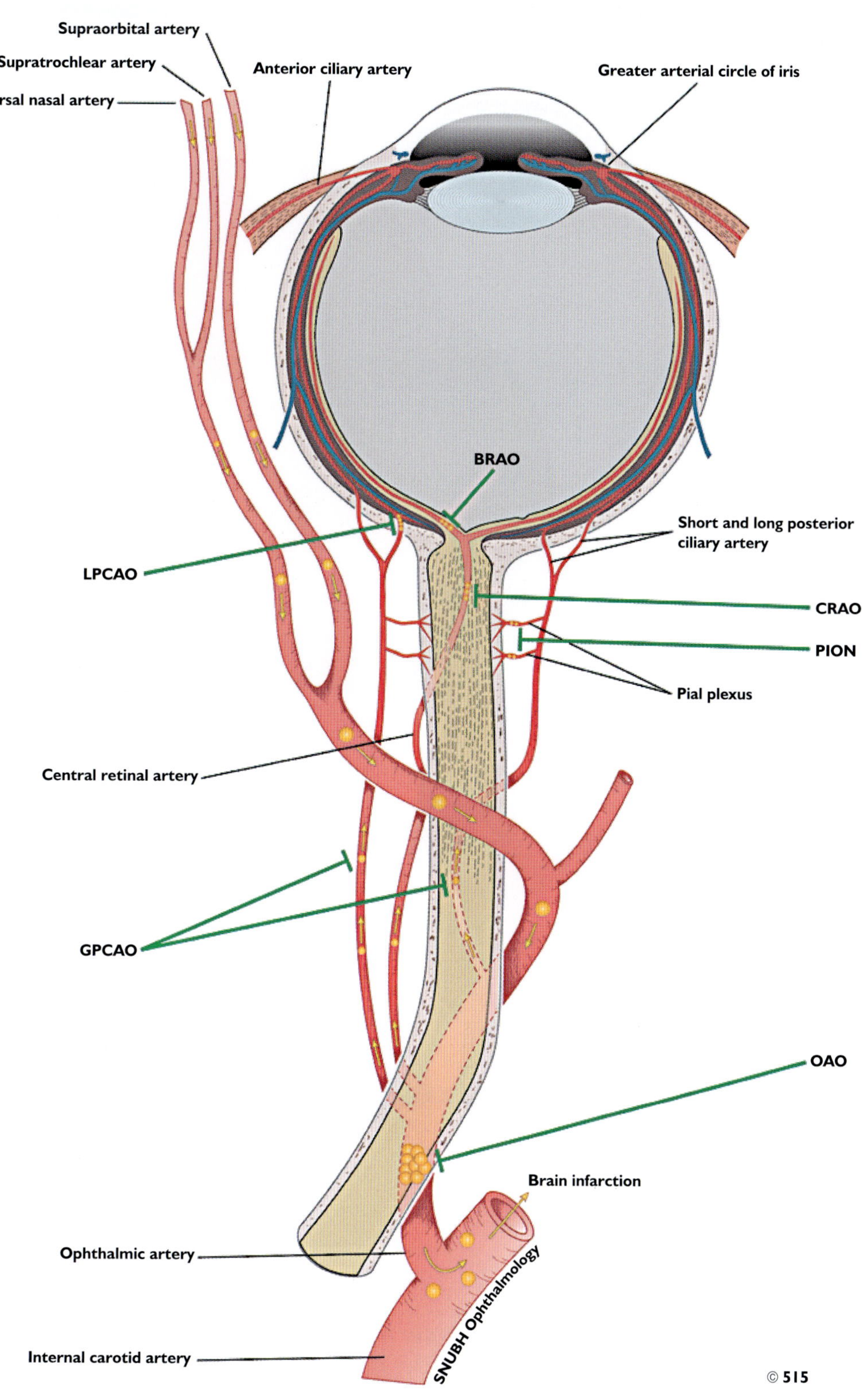

This schematic details the possible entry points by which cosmetic facial filler injections can enter and obstruct the retinal or choroidal vasculature and the brain. It is postulated that the force of injection can cause retrograde flow from superficial arteries into more proximal arteries such as the ophthalmic artery. Green lines indicate potential obstruction points: OAO, ophthalmic artery occlusion; GPCAO, generalized posterior ciliary artery occlusion; PION, posterior ischemic optic neuropathy; CRAO, central retinal artery occlusion; LPCAO, localized posterior ciliary artery occlusion; and BRAO, branch retinal artery occlusion.

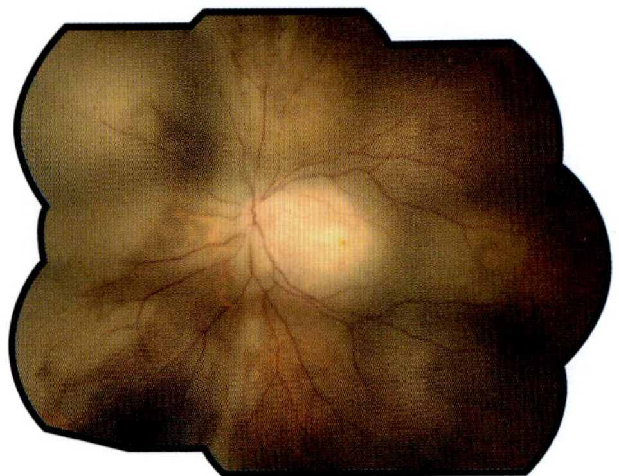

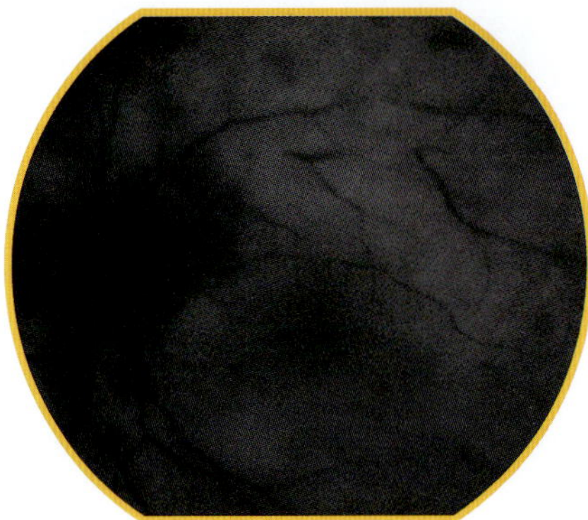

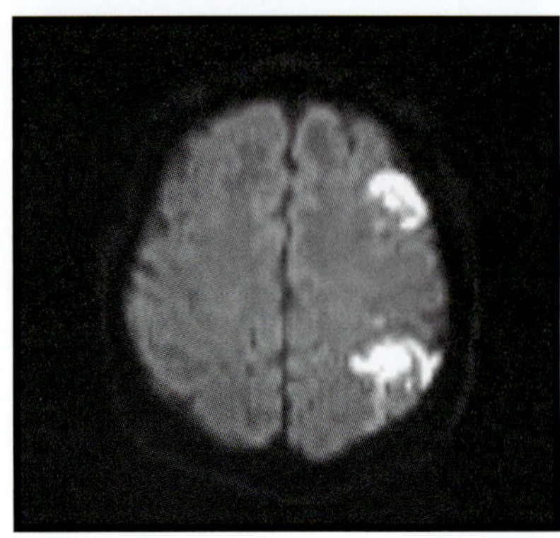

© 516

This patient presented with patchy diffuse retinal whitening of the left eye after autologous fat injection into the glabella and nasolabial fold. A late FA shows dramatic retinal and choroidal perfusion deficit *(middle image)*. This patient also experienced acute multifocal infarcts to the branches of the left middle cerebral artery on diffusion-weighted MRI *(right image)*.

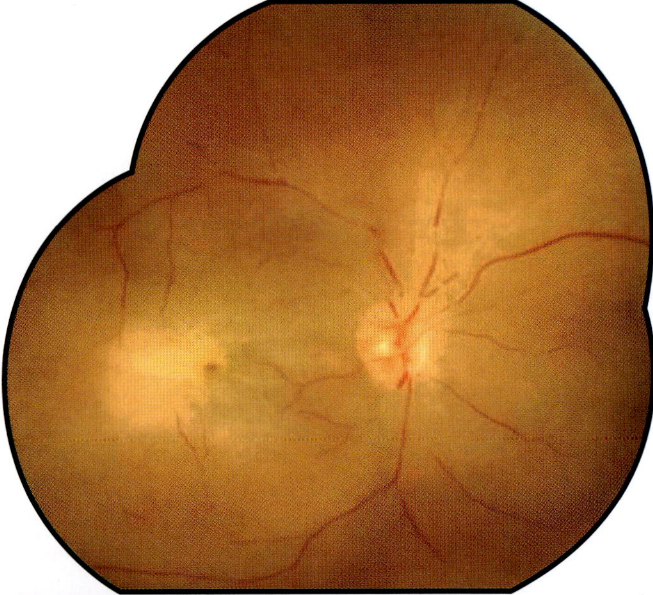

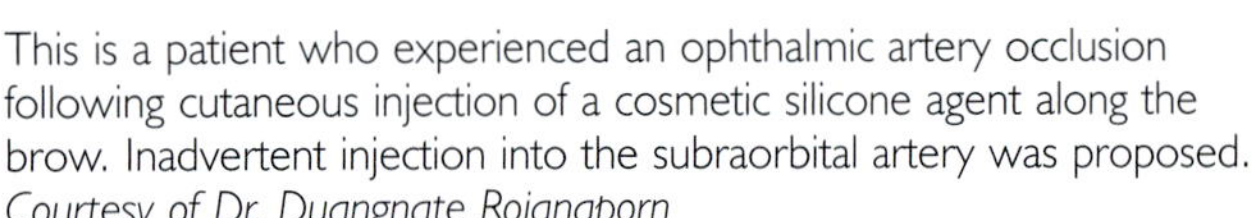

This is a patient who experienced an ophthalmic artery occlusion following cutaneous injection of a cosmetic silicone agent along the brow. Inadvertent injection into the subraorbital artery was proposed. *Courtesy of Dr. Duangnate Rojanaporn*

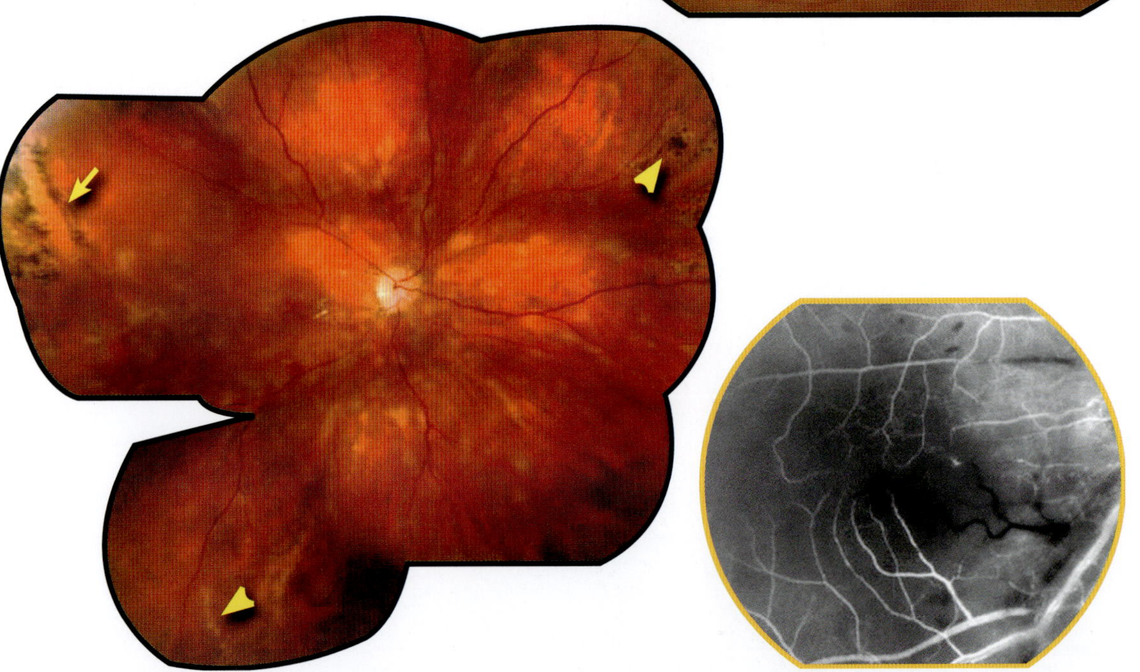

This patient was diagnosed with an intracranial fistula. An attempt to embolize the fistula with *N-butyl* cyanoacrylate and a liquid polymer, Onyx, produced retinal and choroidal vascular occlusive disease. The color montage shows triangular Amalric occlusions of the choroid *(arrow)* and linear Siegrist lines and Elschnig spots *(arrowheads)*, indicative of choroidal infarction. The FA shows occlusion of the inferotemporal and superotemporal retinal arterioles. *Courtesy of Dr. Lee Jampol*

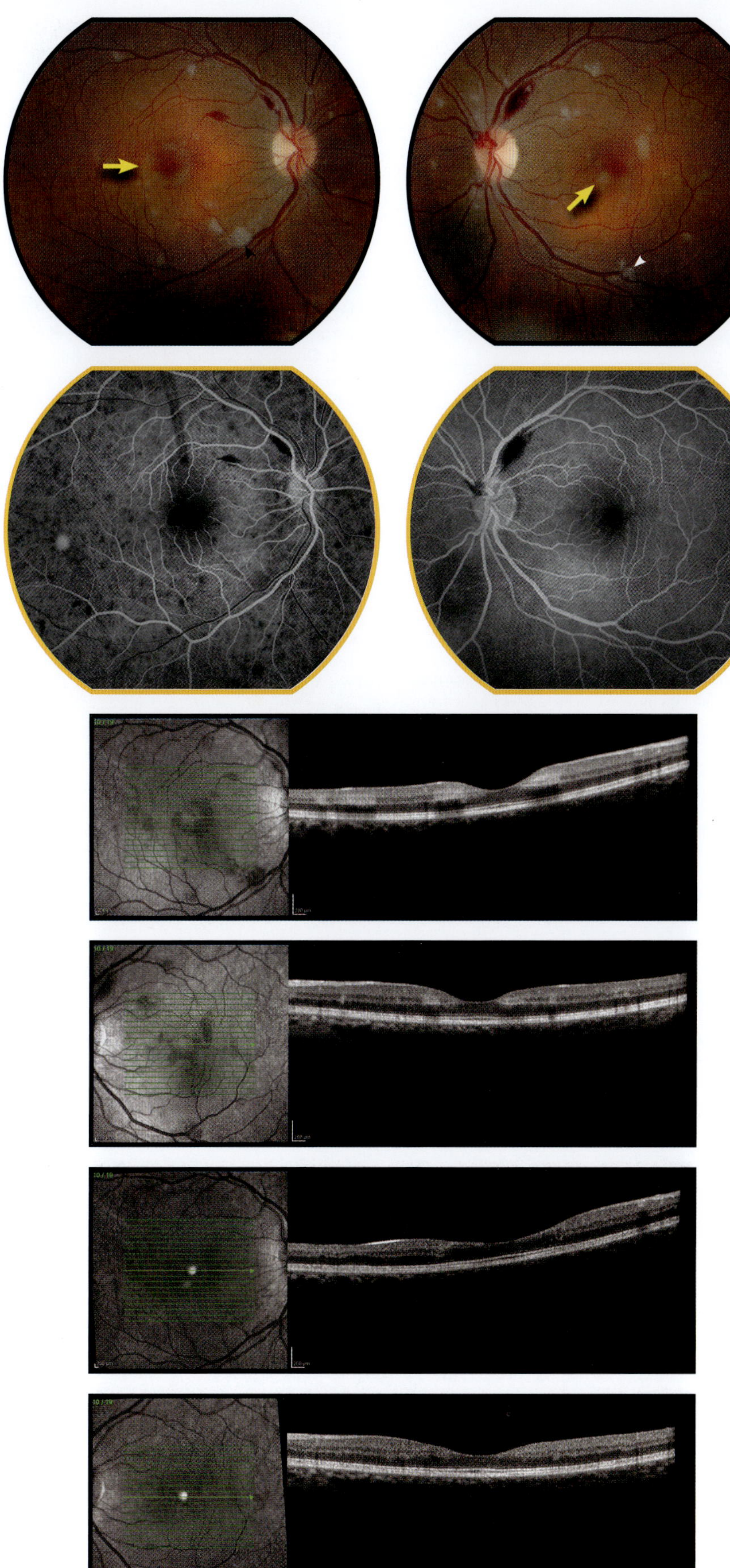

This previously healthy 35-year-old woman underwent cosmetic PMMA injections into the gluteus maximus muscle and five days later developed headache, fever, body aches, and decreased vision. Color fundus photographs of the right and left eyes illustrate multiple inner retinal infarcts or CWS *(arrowheads)* and middle retinal infarcts or PAMM *(arrows)* and intraretinal hemorrhages. Early phase FA shows scattered choroidal perfusion defects especially in the right eye *(second row)*. Hyper-reflective discrete lesions of the inner nuclear layer on SD-OCT were consistent with PAMM. Repeat OCT on follow up showed incremental resolution of these lesions with resultant atrophy of the inner nuclear layer. *Images courtesy of Dr. Azdeh Khatibi*

Suggested Reading

Macrovessel

de Crecchio, G., Alfieri, M.C., Cennamo, G., et al., 2006. Congenital macular macrovessels. Graefes Arch. Clin. Exp. Ophthalmol. 244 (9), 1183–1187.

Jager, R.D., Timothy, N.H., Coney, J.M., et al., 2005. Congenital retinal macrovessel. Retina 25, 538–540.

Petropoulos, I.K., Petkou, D., Theoulakis, P.E., et al., 2008. Congenital retinal macrovessels: description of three cases and review of the literature. Klin. Monatsbl. Augenheilkd 225, 469–472.

Retinal Tortuosity

See Hereditary Chorioretinal Dystrophies Section for Suggested Reading.

Prepapillary Vascular Loop

Mireskandari, K., Aclimandos, W.A., 2001. Probably the longest prepapillary loop in the world. Retina 21 (4), 393–395.

Retinal Artery Occlusions

Augsburger, J.J., Magargal, L.E., 1980. Visual prognosis following treatment of acute retinal artery obstruction. Br. J. Ophthalmol. 64, 913–917.

Biousse, V., Calvetti, O., Bruce, B.B., et al., 2007. Thrombolysis for central retinal artery occlusion. J. Neuroophthalmol. 27, 215–230.

Brown, G.C., Magargal, L.E., 1988. The ocular ischemic syndrome. Clinical, fluorescein angiographic and carotid angiographic features. Int. Ophthalmol. 11, 239–251.

Brown, G.C., Moffat, K., Cruess, A.F., et al., 1983. Cilioretinal artery obstruction. Retina 3, 182–187.

Brown, G.C., Shields, J.A., 1979. Cilioretinal arteries and retinal arterial occlusion. Arch. Ophthalmol. 97, 84–92.

Chapin, J., Carlson, K., Christos, P.J., et al., 2015. Risk factors and treatment strategies in patients with retinal vascular occlusions. Clin. Appl. Thromb. Hemost 21 (7), 672–677.

Dunlap, A.B., Kosmorsky, G.S., Kashyap, V.S., 2007. The fate of patients with retinal artery occlusion and Hollenhorst plaque. J. Vasc. Surg. 46, 1125–1129.

Hayreh, S.S., Podhajsky, P.A., Zimmerman, M.B., 2009. Retinal artery occlusion: associated systemic and ophthalmic abnormalities. Ophthalmology 116 (10), 1928–1936.

Justice, J. Jr., Lehmann, R.P., 1976. Cilioretinal arteries. A study based on review of stereo fundus photographs and fluorescein angiographic findings. Arch. Ophthalmol. 94, 1355–1358.

Klein, R., Klein, B.E.K., Moss, S.E., et al., 2003. Retinal emboli and cardiovascular disease. The Beaver Dam Eye Study. Arch. Ophthalmol. 121, 1446–1451.

Schatz, H., Fong, A.O., McDonald, H.R., et al., 1991. Cilioretinal artery occlusion in young adults with central retinal vein occlusion. Ophthalmology 98, 594–601.

Yu, S., Pang, C.E., Gong, Y., et al., 2015. The spectrum of superficial and deep capillary ischemia in retinal artery occlusion. Am. J. Ophthalmol. 159 (1), 53–63, e1–e2.

PAMM versus CWS

Chen, X., Rahimy, E., Sergott, R.C., et al., 2015. Spectrum of retinal vascular diseases associated with paracentral acute middle maculopathy. Am. J. Ophthalmol. 160 (1), 26–34, e1.

Rahimy, E., Sarraf, D., 2014. Paracentral acute middle maculopathy spectral-domain optical coherence tomography feature of deep capillary ischemia. Curr. Opin. Ophthalmol. 25 (3), 207–212.

Rahimy, E., Sarraf, D., Dollin, M.L., et al., 2014. Paracentral acute middle maculopathy in nonischemic central retinal vein occlusion. Am. J. Ophthalmol. 158 (2), 372–380.

Sarraf, D., Rahimy, E., Fawzi, A.A., et al., 2013. Paracentral acute middle maculopathy: a new variant of acute macular neuroretinopathy associated with retinal capillary ischemia. JAMA Ophthalmol. 131 (10), 1275–1287.

Yu, S., Pang, C.E., Gong, Y., et al., 2015. The spectrum of superficial and deep capillary ischemia in retinal artery occlusion. Am. J. Ophthalmol. 159 (1), 53–63, e1–e2.

Yu, S., Wang, F., Pang, C.E., et al., 2014. Multimodal imaging findings in retinal deep capillary ischemia. Retina 34 (4), 636–646.

Retinal Venous Occlusions

Branch Vein Occlusion Study Group, 1984. Argon laser photocoagulation for macular edema in branch vein occlusion. Am. J. Ophthalmol. 98, 271–282.

Christoffersen, N.L.B., Larsen, M., 1999. Pathophysiology and hemodynamics of branch retinal vein occlusion. Ophthalmology 106, 2054–2062.

Cugati, S., Wang, J.J., Rochtchina, E., et al., 2006. Ten-year incidence of retinal vein occlusion in an older population: the Blue Mountains Eye Study. Arch. Ophthalmol. 124, 726–732.

Elman, M.J., Bhatt, A.K., Quinlan, P.M., et al., 1990. The risk for systemic vascular diseases and mortality in patients with central retinal vein occlusion. Ophthalmology 97, 1543–1548.

Epstein, D.L., Algvere, P.V., von Wendt, G., et al., 2012. Bevacizumab for macular edema in central retinal vein occlusion: a prospective, randomized, double-masked clinical study. Ophthalmology 119 (6), 1184–1189.

Eye Disease Case-Control Study Group, 1993. Risk factors for branch retinal vein occlusion. Am. J. Ophthalmol. 116, 286–296.

Green, W., Chan, C., Hutchins, G., et al., 1981. Central retinal vein occlusions: a prospective histopathologic study of 29 eyes in 28 cases. Retina 1, 27–55.

Hayreh, S.S., Fraterrigo, L., Jonas, J., 2008. Central retinal vein occlusion associated with cilioretinal artery occlusion. Retina 28, 581–594.

Hayreh, S.S., Zimmerman, M.B., 2015. Fundus changes in central retinal vein occlusion. Retina 35 (1), 29–42.

Heier, J.S., Clark, W.L., Boyer, D.S., et al., 2014. Intravitreal aflibercept injection for macular edema due to central retinal vein occlusion: two-year results from the COPERNICUS study. Ophthalmology 121 (7), 1414–1420.

Ip, M.S., Gottlieb, J.L., Kahana, A., et al., 2004. Intravitreal triamcinolone for the treatment of macular edema associated with central retinal vein occlusion. Arch. Ophthalmol. 122, 1131–1136.

Klein, R., Klein, B.E., Moss, S.E., et al., 2000. The epidemiology of retinal vein occlusion: the Beaver Dam Eye Study. Trans. Am. Ophthalmol. Soc. 98, 133–141, discussion 41–43.

Kuppermann, B.D., Haller, J.A., Bandello, F., et al., 2014. Onset and duration of visual acuity improvement after dexamethasone intravitreal implant in eyes with macular edema due to retinal vein occlusion. Retina 34 (9), 1743–1749.

Lahey, J.M., Tunc, M., Kearney, J., et al., 2002. Laboratory evaluation of hypercoagulable states in patients with central retinal vein occlusion who are less than 56 years of age. Ophthalmology 109, 126–131.

Ogura, Y., Roider, J., Korobelnik, J.F., et al., 2014. Intravitreal aflibercept for macular edema secondary to central retinal vein occlusion: 18-month results of the phase 3 GALILEO study. Am. J. Ophthalmol. 158 (5), 1032–1038.

Prasad, P.S., Oliver, S.C., Coffee, R.E., et al., 2010. Ultra wide-field angiographic characteristics of branch retinal and hemicentral retinal vein occlusion. Ophthalmology 117 (4), 780–784.

Rahimy, E., Sarraf, D., Dollin, M.L., et al., 2014. Paracentral acute middle maculopathy in nonischemic central retinal vein occlusion. Am. J. Ophthalmol. 158 (2), 372–380.

Ramchandran, R.S., Fekrat, S., Stinnett, S.S., et al., 2008. Fluocinolone acetonide sustained drug delivery device for chronic central retinal vein occlusion: 12-month results. Am. J. Ophthalmol. 146, 285–291.

Spaide, R.F., 2013. Prospective study of peripheral panretinal photocoagulation of areas of nonperfusion in central retinal vein occlusion. Retina 33 (1), 56–62.

The Eye Disease Case-Control Study Group, 1996. Risk factors for central retinal vein occlusion. Arch. Ophthalmol. 114, 545–554.

Tsui, I., Kaines, A., Havunjian, M.A., et al., 2011. Ischemic index and neovascularization in central retinal vein occlusion. Retina 31 (1), 105–110.

Retinal Arteriolar Macroaneurysm

Goldenberg, D., Soiberman, U., Loewenstein, A., et al., 2012. Heidelberg spectral-domain optical coherence tomographic findings in retinal artery macroaneurysm. Retina 32 (5), 990–995.

Pichi, F., Morara, M., Torrazza, C., et al., 2013. Intravitreal bevacizumab for macular complications from retinal arterial macroaneurysms. Am. J. Ophthalmol. 155 (2), 287–294.

Robertson, D.M., 1973. Macroaneurysms of the retinal arteries. Trans. Am. Acad. Ophthalmol. Otolaryngol. 77, 55–67.

Coats Disease and Macular Telangiectasia Type I (Congenital Telangiectasia, Leber Miliary Aneurysms)

Chang, M., McLean, I.W., Merritt, J.C., 1984. Coats' disease: a study of 62 histologically confirmed cases. J. Pediatr. Ophthalmol. Strabismus 21, 163–168.

Pauleikhoff, D., Kruger, K., Heinriech, T., et al., 1988. Epidemiologic features and therapeutic results in Coats' disease. Invest. Ophthalmol. Vis. Sci. 29, 335.

Reese, A.B., 1956. Telangiectasis of the retina and Coats' disease. Am. J. Ophthalmol. 42, 1–8, 215–218.

Sigler, E.J., Randolph, J.C., Calzada, J.I., et al., 2014. Current management of Coats disease. Surv. Ophthalmol. 59 (1), 30–46.

Takayama, K., Ooto, S., Tamura, H., et al., 2010. Intravitreal bevacizumab for type 1 idiopathic macular telangiectasia. Eye (Lond.) 24 (9), 1492–1497.

Macular Telangiectasia Type 2 (Idiopathic Perifoveal Telangiectasia, Idiopathic Juxtafoveal Telangiectasis Type 2)

Balaskas, K., Leung, I., Sallo, F.B., et al., 2014. Associations between autofluorescence abnormalities and visual acuity in idiopathic macular telangiectasia type 2: MacTel project report number 5. Retina 34 (8), 1630–1636.

Charbel Issa, P., Finger, R.P., Kruse, K., et al., 2011. Monthly ranibizumab for nonproliferative macular telangiectasia type 2: a 12-month prospective study. Am. J. Ophthalmol. 151 (5), 876–886, e1.

Charbel Issa, P., Helb, H.M., Holz, F.G., et al., 2008. Correlation of macular function with retinal thickness in nonproliferative type 2 idiopathic macular telangiectasia. Am. J. Ophthalmol. 145, 169–175.

Chew, E., Gillies, M., Bird, A., 2006. Macular telangiectasia: a simplified classification. Arch. Ophthalmol. 124, 573–574.

Engelbert, M., Yannuzzi, L.A., 2012. Idiopathic macular telangiectasia type 2: the progressive vasculopathy. Eur. J. Ophthalmol. doi:10.5301/ejo.5000163; [Epub ahead of print]; 2012 Nov 6:0.

Gass, J.D.M., Blodi, B.A., 1993. Idiopathic juxtafoveolar retinal telangiectasis: update of classification and follow-up study. Ophthalmology 100, 1536–1546.

Gass, J.D., Oyakawa, R.T., 1982. Idiopathic juxtafoveolar retinal telangiectasis. Arch. Ophthalmol. 100, 769–780.

Narayanan, R., Chhablani, J., Sinha, M., et al., 2012. Efficacy of anti-vascular endothelial growth factor therapy in subretinal neovascularization secondary to macular telangiectasia type 2. Retina 32 (10), 2001–2005.

Powner, M.B., Gillies, M.C., Zhu, M., et al., 2013. Loss of Müller's cells and photoreceptors in macular telangiectasia type 2. Ophthalmology 120 (11), 2344–2352.

Sallo, F.B., Leung, I., Clemons, T.E., et al. on behalf of the MACTEL Study group, 2015. Multimodal imaging in type 2 idiopathic macular telangiectasia. Retina 35 (4), 742–749.

Sallo, F.B., Leung, I., Chung, M., et al., 2011. Retinal crystals in type 2 idiopathic macular telangiectasia. Ophthalmology 118 (12), 2461–2467.

Wu, L., Evans, T., Arevalo, J.F., 2013. Idiopathic macular telangiectasia type 2 (idiopathic juxtafoveolar retinal telangiectasis type 2A, Mac Tel 2). Surv. Ophthalmol. 58 (6), 536–559.

Yannuzzi, L.A., Bardal, A.M., Freund, K.B., et al., 2006. Idiopathic macular telangiectasia. Arch. Ophthalmol. 124, 450–460.

Radiation Retinopathy

Avery, R.B., Diener-West, M., Reynolds, S.M., et al., 2008. Histopathologic characteristics of choroidal melanoma in eyes enucleated after iodine 125 brachytherapy in the collaborative ocular melanoma study. Arch. Ophthalmol. 126, 207–212.

Conway, R.M., Poothullil, A.M., Daftari, I.K., et al., 2006. Estimates of ocular and visual retention following treatment of extra-large uveal melanomas by proton beam radiotherapy. Arch. Ophthalmol. 124, 838–843.

Finger, P.T., Chin, K., 2007. Anti-vascular endothelial growth factor bevacizumab (Avastin) for radiation retinopathy. Arch. Ophthalmol. 125, 751–756.

Grimm, S.A., Yahalom, J., Abrey, L.E., et al., 2006. Retinopathy in survivors of primary central nervous system lymphoma. Neurology 67, 2060–2062.

Groenewald, C., Konstantinidis, L., Damato, B., 2013. Effects of radiotherapy on uveal melanomas and adjacent tissues. Eye (Lond.) 27 (2), 163–171.

Kinyoun, J.L., Lawrence, B.S., Barlow, W.E., 1996. Proliferative radiation retinopathy. Arch. Ophthalmol. 114, 1097–1100.

Shah, N.V., Houston, S.K., Markoe, A., et al., 2013. Combination therapy with triamcinolone acetonide and bevacizumab for the treatment of severe radiation maculopathy in patients with posterior uveal melanoma. Clin. Ophthalmol. 7, 1877–1882.

Eales Disease (Idiopathic Peripheral Vascular Occlusive Disease)

Das, T., Pathengay, A., Hussain, N., et al., 2010. Eales' disease: diagnosis and management. Eye (Lond.) 24 (3), 472–482.

Hypertensive Retinopathy

Ashton, N., 1969. Pathological and ultrastructural aspect of the cotton-wool spot. Proc. R. Soc. Med. 62, 1271–1276.

Duncan, B.B., Wong, T.Y., Tyroler, H.A., et al., 2002. Hypertensive retinopathy and incident coronary heart disease in high risk men. Br. J. Ophthalmol. 86, 1002–1006.

Wong, T.Y., Shankar, A., Klein, R., et al., 2004. Prospective cohort study of retinal vessel diameters and risk of hypertension. Br. Med. J. 329, 79.

Diabetic Retinopathy

Aiello, L.P., Avery, R.L., Arrigg, P.G., et al., 1994. Vascular endothelial growth factor in ocular fluid of patients with diabetic retinopathy and other retinal disorders. N. Engl. J. Med. 331, 1480–1487.

Brown, D.M., Nguyen, Q.D., Marcus, D.M., et al., 2013. Long-term outcomes of ranibizumab therapy for diabetic macular edema: the 36-month results from two phase III trials: RISE and RIDE. Ophthalmology 120, 2013–2022.

Chew, E.Y., Klein, M.L., Murphy, R.P., et al., 1995. Effects of aspirin on vitreous/preretinal hemorrhage in patients with diabetes mellitus. ETDRS report no. 20. Arch. Ophthalmol. 113, 52–55.

Chew, E.Y., Mills, J.L., Metzger, B.E., et al., 1995. Metabolic control and progression of retinopathy. The Diabetes in Early Pregnancy Study. National Institute of Child Health and Human Development Diabetes in Early Pregnancy Study. Diabetes Care 18, 631–637.

Cogan, D., Toussaint, D., Kuwabara, T., 1961. Retinal vascular patterns. IV. Diabetic retinopathy. Arch. Ophthalmol. 66, 366–378.

Cogan, D.G., Toussaint, D., Kuwabara, T., 1961. Retinal vascular patterns. IV. Diabetic retinopathy. Arch. Ophthalmol. 66, 366–378.

Davis, M., Fisher, M., Gangnon, R., et al., 1998. Risk factors for high-risk proliferative diabetic retinopathy and severe visual loss: Early Treatment of Diabetic Retinopathy Study report no. 18. Invest. Ophthalmol. Vis. Sci. 39, 233–252.

Davis, M.D., Fisher, M.R., Gangnon, R.E., et al., 1998. Risk factors for high-risk proliferative diabetic retinopathy and severe visual loss. ETDRS report no. 18. Invest. Ophthalmol. Vis. Sci. 39, 233–252.

DCCT Research Group, 1993. The effect of intensive treatment of diabetes in the development and progression of long-term complications in insulin-dependent diabetes. N. Engl. J. Med. 329, 977–986.

deBustros, S., Thompson, J., Michels, R., et al., 1987. Vitrectomy for progressive proliferative diabetic retinopathy. Arch. Ophthalmol. 105, 196–199.

deVenecia, G., Davis, M., Engerman, R., 1976. Clinicopathologic correlations in diabetic retinopathy. I. Histology and fluorescein angiography of microaneurysms. Arch. Ophthalmol. 94, 1766–1773.

Diabetes Control and Complications Trial Research Group, 1996. Perspectives in diabetes: the relationship of glycemic exposure (HbAlc) to the risk of development and progression of retinopathy in the Diabetes Control and Complications Trial. Diabetes 44, 968–983.

Diabetes Control and Complications Trial Research Group, 1998. Early worsening of diabetic retinopathy in the diabetes control and complications trial. Arch. Ophthalmol. 116, 874–886.

Diabetic Retinopathy Clinical Research Network (DRCR.net), 2009. Three-year follow-up of a randomized trial comparing focal/grid photocoagulation and intravitreal triamcinolone for diabetic macular edema. Arch. Ophthalmol. 127, 245–251.

Diabetic Retinopathy Study Research Group, 1978. Photocoagulation treatment of proliferative diabetic retinopathy. DRS report no 2. Ophthalmology 85, 82–105.

Diabetic Retinopathy Study Research Group, 1981. Photocoagulation treatment of proliferative diabetic retinopathy: clinical application of Diabetic Retinopathy Study (DRS) findings. DRS report number 8. Ophthalmology 88, 583–600.

Diabetic Retinopathy Vitrectomy Study Research Group, 1988. Early vitrectomy for severe proliferative diabetic retinopathy in eyes with useful vision: results of a randomized trial, Diabetic

Retinopathy Vitrectomy Study report no. 3. Ophthalmology 95, 1307–1320.

Diabetic Retinopathy Vitrectomy Study Research Group, 1988. Early vitrectomy for severe proliferative diabetic retinopathy in eyes with useful vision: clinical application of results of a randomized trial. Diabetic Retinopathy Study report no. 4. Ophthalmology 95, 1321–1334.

Diabetic Retinopathy Vitrectomy Study Research Group, 1990. Early vitrectomy for severe vitreous hemorrhage in diabetic retinopathy: four-year results of a randomized trial. Diabetic Retinopathy Study report no. 5. Arch. Ophthalmol. 108, 958–964.

Du, Y., Smith, M.A., Miller, C.M., et al., 2002. Diabetes-induced nitrative stress in the retina, and correction by aminoguanidine. J. Neurochem. 80, 771–779.

Early Treatment Diabetic Retinopathy Study Research Group, 1995. Photocoagulation for diabetic macular edema: relationship of treatment effect to fluorescein angiographic and other retinal characteristics at baseline. ETDRS report no. 19. Arch. Ophthalmol. 113, 1144–1155.

Frank, R.N., Amin, R., Kennedy, A., et al., 1997. An aldose reductase inhibitor and aminoguanidine prevent vascular endothelial growth factor expression in rats with long-term galactosemia. Arch. Ophthalmol. 115, 136–147.

Gillies, M.C., Lim, L.L., Campain, A., et al., 2014. A randomized clinical trial of intravitreal bevacizumab versus intravitreal dexamethasone for diabetic macular edema: the BEVORDEX study. Ophthalmology 121 (12), 2473–2481.

Klein, R., Klein, B.E.K., Moss, S.E., et al., 1984. The Wisconsin Epidemiologic Study of Diabetic Retinopathy. IV. Diabetic macular edema. Ophthalmology 91, 1464–1474.

Klein, R., Klein, B.E., Moss, S.E., et al., 1998. The Wisconsin Epidemiologic Study of Diabetic Retinopathy: XVII. The 14-year incidence and progression of diabetic retinopathy and associated risk factors in type 1 diabetes. Ophthalmology 105, 1801–1815.

Kuppermann, B.D., Blumenkranz, M.S., Haller, J.A., et al., 2007. Randomized controlled study of an intravitreous dexamethasone drug delivery system in patients with persistent macular edema. Arch. Ophthalmol. 125, 309–317.

Martidis, A., Duker, J.S., Greenberg, P.B., et al., 2002. Intravitreal triamcinolone for refractory diabetic macular edema. Ophthalmology 109, 920–927.

Massin, P., Audren, F., Haouchine, B., et al., 2004. Intravitreal triamcinolone acetonide for diabetic diffuse macular edema. Ophthalmology 111, 218–225.

Muraoka, K., Shimizu, K., 1984. Intraretinal neovascularization in diabetic retinopathy. Ophthalmology 91, 1440–1446.

Nguyen, Q.D., Tatlipinar, S., Shah, S.M., et al., 2006. Vascular endothelial growth factor is a critical stimulus for diabetic macular edema. Am. J. Ophthalmol. 142, 961–969.

The Diabetes Control and Complications Trial/ Epidemiology of Diabetes Intervention and Complications Study Research Group, 2002. Effects of intensive therapy on the microvascular complications of type 1 diabetes mellitus. JAMA 287, 2563–2569.

The Diabetes Control and Complications Trial Research Group, 2000. Effect of pregnancy on the microvascular complications. Diabetes Care 23, 1084–1091.

The Eye Disease Prevalence Research Group, 2004. The prevalence of diabetic retinopathy among adults in the United States. Arch. Ophthalmol. 122, 552–563.

UK Prospective Diabetes Study Group, 1998. Tight blood pressure control and risk of macrovascular and microvascular complications in type 2 diabetes. UKPDS 38. Br. Med. J. 317, 703–713.

UK Prospective Diabetes Study (UKPDS) Group, 1998. Intensive blood-glucose control with sulphonylureas or insulin compared with conventional treatment and risk of complications in patients with type 2 diabetes (UKPDS 33). Lancet 352, 837–853.

Vander, J.F., Duker, J.S., Benson, W.E., et al., 1991. Long-term stability and visual outcome after favorable initial response of proliferative diabetic retinopathy to panretinal photocoagulation. Ophthalmology 98, 1575–1579.

White, N.H., Sun, W., Cleary, P.A., et al., 2008. Prolonged effect of intensive therapy on the risk of retinopathy complications in patients with type 1 diabetes mellitus: 10 years after the Diabetes Control and Complications Trial. Arch. Ophthalmol. 126, 1707–1715.

Yanoff, M., 1966. Diabetic retinopathy. N. Engl. J. Med. 274, 1344–1349.

Sickle-Cell Retinopathy

Cho, M., Kiss, S., 2011. Detection and monitoring of sickle cell retinopathy using ultra wide-field color photography and fluorescein angiography. Retina 31 (4), 738–747.

Downes, S.M., Hambleton, I.R., Chuang, E.L., et al., 2005. Incidence and natural history of proliferative sickle cell retinopathy: observations from a cohort study. Ophthalmology 112 (11), 1869–1875.

Elagouz, M., Jyothi, S., Gupta, B., et al., 2010. Sickle cell disease and the eye: old and new concepts. Surv. Ophthalmol. 55 (4), 359–377.

Goldbaum, M.H., Peyman, G.A., Nagpal, K.C., et al., 1976. Vitrectomy in sickling retinopathy: report of five cases. Ophthalmic Surg. 7, 92–102.

Lim, J.I., 2012. Ophthalmic manifestations of sickle cell disease: update of the latest findings. Curr. Opin. Ophthalmol. 23 (6), 533–536.

Witkin, A.J., Rogers, A.H., Ko, T.H., et al., 2006. Optical coherence tomography demonstration of macular infarction in sickle cell retinopathy. Arch. Ophthalmol. 124, 746–747.

Hyperlipidemia

Orlin, C., Lee, K., Jampol, L.M., et al., 1988. Retinal arteriolar changes in patients with hyperlipidemias. Retina 8, 6–9.

Sassa, Y., Matsui, K., Yoshikawa, N., et al., 2005. Lipemia retinalis: low-density lipoprotein apheresis improved the appearance of retinal vessels in a patient with type 5 hyperlipoproteinemia. Retina 25, 803–804.

Shah, G.K., Sharma, S., Walsh, A., 2001. Lipemia retinalis. Ophthalmic Surg. Lasers 32, 77–78.

Ocular Ischemic Syndrome

Amselem, L., Montero, J., Diaz-Llopis, M., et al., 2007. Intravitreal bevacizumab (Avastin) injection in ocular ischemic syndrome. Am. J. Ophthalmol. 144, 122–124.

Chuah, J.L., Ghosh, Y.K., Richards, D., et al., 2006. Ocular ischaemic syndrome: a medical emergency. Lancet 367, 1370.

Costa, V.P., Kuzniec, S., Molnar, L.J., et al., 1999. The effects of carotid endarterectomy on the retrobulbar circulation of patients with severe occlusive carotid artery disease. An investigation by color Doppler imaging. Ophthalmology 106, 306–310.

Mendrinos, E., Machinis, T.G., Pournaras, C.J., 2010. Ocular ischemic syndrome. Surv. Ophthalmol. 55 (1), 2–34.

Takayasu Arteritis (Takayasu Disease)

Chun, Y.S., Park, S.J., Park, I.K., et al., 2001. The clinical and ocular manifestations of Takayasu arteritis. Retina 21, 132–140.

Fraga, A., Medina, F., 2002. Takayasu's arteritis. Curr. Rheum. Rep. 4, 30–38.

Peter, J., David, S., Danda, D., et al., 2011. Ocular manifestations of Takayasu arteritis: a cross-sectional study. Retina 31 (6), 1170–1178.

Polycythemia Vera

Krishnan, R., Goverdhan, S., Lochhead, J., 2009. Peripheral retinal neovascularization associated with polycythemia rubra vera. Jpn J. Ophthalmol. 53 (2), 188–189.

Essential Thrombocythemia

Imasawa, M., Iijima, H., 2002. Multiple retinal vein occlusions in essential thrombocythemia. Am. J. Ophthalmol. 133, 152–155.

Yoshizumi, M.O., Townsend-Pico, W., 1996. Essential thrombocythemia and central retinal vein occlusion with neovascular glaucoma. Am. J. Ophthalmol. 121, 728–730.

Hyperviscosity Syndrome from Leukemia

Davies, C.E., Whitelocke, R.A., Agrawal, S., 2008. Retinal complications associated with hyperviscosity in chronic lymphocytic leukaemia. Intern. Med. J. 38, 140.

Duke, J.R., Wilkinson, C.P., Sigelman, S., 1968. Retinal microaneurysms in leukaemia. Br. J. Ophthalmol. 52, 368–374.

Mansour, A.M., Arevalo, J.F., Badal, J., et al., 2014. Paraproteinemic maculopathy. Ophthalmology 121 (10), 1925–1932.

Waldenström Macroglobulinemia

Ackerman, A.L., 1962. The ocular manifestations of Waldenstrom's macroglobulinemia and its treatment. Arch. Ophthalmol. 67, 701–707.

Baker, P.S., Garg, S.J., Fineman, M.S., et al., 2013. Serous macular detachment in Waldenström macroglobulinemia: a report of four cases. Am. J. Ophthalmol. 155 (3), 448–455.

Koutsandrea, C., Kotsolis, A., Georgalas, I., et al., 2010. Peripheral capillary non-perfusion in asymptomatic Waldenström's macroglobulinemia. BMC Ophthalmol. 10, 30.

Saffra, N., Rakhamimov, A., Solomon, W.B., et al., 2013. Monoclonal gammopathy of undetermined significance maculopathy. Can. J. Ophthalmol. 48 (6), e168–e170.

Multiple Myeloma

Fung, S., Selva, D., Leibovitch, I., et al., 2005. Ophthalmic manifestations of multiple myeloma. Ophthalmologica 219, 43–48.

Khan, J.M., McBain, V., Santiago, C., et al., 2010. Bilateral 'vitelliform-like' macular lesions in a patient with multiple myeloma. BMJ Case Rep. 2010.

Priluck, J.C., Chalam, K.V., Grover, S., 2012. Spectral-domain optical coherence tomography of Roth spots in multiple myeloma. Eye (Lond.) 26 (12), 1588–1589.

Rusu, I.M., Mrejen, S., Engelbert, M., et al., 2014. Immunogammopathies and acquired vitelliform detachments: a report of four cases. Am. J. Ophthalmol. 157 (3), 648–657, e1.

Hypereosinophilic Syndrome

Bozkir, N., Stern, G.A., 1992. Ocular manifestations of the idiopathic hypereosinophilic syndrome. Am. J. Ophthalmol. 113, 456–458.

Chaine, G., Davies, J., Kohner, E.M., et al., 1982. Ophthalmologic abnormalities in the hypereosinophilic syndrome. Ophthalmology 89, 1348–1356.

Gupta, O.P., Zegere, E., Maguire, J.I., 2009. Purtscher-like retinopathy associated with primary hypereosinophilic syndrome. Retin. Cases Brief Rep. 3 (2), 193–196.

Polyneuropathy, Organomegaly, Endocrinopathy, Monoclonal Gamnopathy (POEMS Syndrome)

Kaushik, M., Pulido, J.S., Abreu, R., et al., 2011. Ocular findings in patients with polyneuropathy, organomegaly, endocrinopathy, monoclonal gammopathy, and skin changes syndrome. Ophthalmology 118 (4), 778–782.

Hyperhomocysteinemia

Chua, B., Kifley, A., Wong, T.Y., et al., 2006. Homocysteine and retinal emboli: the Blue Mountains Eye Study. Am. J. Ophthalmol. 142, 322–324.

Di Crecchio, L., Parodi, M.B., Sanguinetti, G., et al., 2004. Hyperhomocysteinemia and the methylenetetrahydrofolate reductase 677C-T mutation in patients under 50 years of age affected by central retinal vein occlusion. Ophthalmology 111, 940–945.

Parodi, M.B., Di Crecchio, L., 2003. Hyperhomocysteinemia in central retinal vein occlusion in young adults. Semin. Ophthalmol. 18, 154–159.

Vine, A.K., 2000. Hyperhomocysteinemia: a risk factor for central retinal vein occlusion. Am. J. Ophthalmol. 129, 640–644.

Wright, A.D., Martin, N., Dodson, P.M., 2008. Homocysteine, folates, and the eye. Eye (Lond.) 22, 989–993.

Protein C and Protein S Deficiency

Cassels-Brown, A., Minford, A.M., Chatfield, S.L., et al., 1994. Ophthalmic manifestations of neonatal protein C deficiency. Br. J. Ophthalmol. 78, 486–487.

Churchill, A.J., Gallagher, M.J., Bradbury, J.A., et al., 2001. Clinical manifestations of protein C deficiency: a spectrum within one family. Br. J. Ophthalmol. 85, 241–242.

Hattenbach, L.O., Beeg, T., Kreuz, W., et al., 1999. Ophthalmic manifestation of congenital protein C deficiency. J. AAPOS 3, 188–190.

Greven, C.M., Weaver, R.G., Owen, J., et al., 1991. Protein S deficiency and bilateral branch retinal artery occlusion. Ophthalmology 98, 33–34.

Mintz-Hittner, H.A., Miyashiro, M.J., Knight-Nanan, D.M., et al., 1999. Vitreoretinal findings similar to retinopathy of prematurity in infants with compound heterozygous protein S deficiency. Ophthalmology 106, 1525–1530.

Vela, J.I., Diaz-Cascajosa, J., Crespi, J., et al., 2007. Protein S deficiency and retinal arteriolar occlusion in pregnancy. Eur. J. Ophthalmol. 17, 1004–1006.

Antithrombin III Deficiency

Acheson, J.F., Sanders, M.D., 1994. Coagulation abnormalities in ischaemic optic neuropathy. Eye (Lond.) 8 (Pt 1), 89–92.

Tekeli, O., Gürsel, E., Buyurgan, H., 1999. Protein C, protein S and antithrombin III deficiencies in retinal vein occlusion. Acta Ophthalmol. Scand. 77, 628–630.

Factor V Leiden

Czerlanis, C., Jay, W.M., Nand, S., 2008. Inherited thrombophilia and the eye. Semin. Ophthalmol. 23, 111–119.

Johnson, T.M., El-Defrawy, S., Hodge, W.G., et al., 2001. Prevalence of factor V Leiden and activated protein C resistance in central retinal vein occlusion. Retina 21, 161–166.

Nagy, V., Steiber, Z., Takacs, L., et al., 2006. Trombophilic screening for nonarteritic anterior ischemic optic neuropathy. Graefes Arch. Clin. Exp. Ophthalmol. 244, 3–8.

Weger, M., Renner, W., Pinter, O., et al., 2003. Role of factor V Leiden and prothrombin 20210A in patients with retinal artery occlusion. Eye (Lond.) 17, 731–734.

Thrombotic Thrombocytopenic Purpura

George, J.N., Nester, C.M., 2014. Syndromes of thrombotic microangiopathy. N. Engl. J. Med. 371 (7), 654–666.

Titah, C., Abisror, N., Affortit, A., et al., 2014. Bilateral serous detachment of retina: an unusual mode of revelation of thrombotic thrombocytopenic purpura of favorable outcome with plasma exchange. Graefes Arch. Clin. Exp. Ophthalmol. 252 (1), 181–183.

Disseminated Intravascular Coagulopathy

Cogan, D.G., 1975. Ocular involvement in disseminated intravascular coagulopathy. Arch. Ophthalmol. 93, 1–8.

Cogan, D.G., 1976. Fibrin clots in the choriocapillaris and serous detachment of the retina. Ophthalmologica 172, 298–307.

Systemic Lupus Erythematosus

Gold, D.H., Morris, D.A., Henkind, P., 1972. Ocular findings in systemic lupus erythematosus. Br. J. Ophthalmol. 56, 800–804.

Graham, E.M., Spalton, D.J., Barnard, R.O., et al., 1985. Cerebral and retinal vascular changes in systemic lupus erythematosus. Ophthalmology 92, 444–448.

Jabs, D.A., Hanneken, A.M., Schachat, A.P., et al., 1988. Choroidopathy in systemic lupus erythematosus. Arch. Ophthalmol. 106, 230–234.

Kleiner, R.C., Nigerian, L.V., Schattten, S., et al., 1989. Vaso-occlusive retinopathy associated with anti phospholipid antibodies (lupus anticoagulant retinopathy). Ophthalmology 96, 896–904.

Maumenee, A.E., 1940. Retinal lesions in lupus erythematosus. Am. J. Ophthamol. 23, 971–981.

Rosove, M.H., Brewer, P.M.C., 1992. Antiphospholipid thrombosis: clinical course after the first thrombotic event in 70 patients. Ann. Intern. Med. 117, 303–308.

Wu, C., Dai, R., Dong, F., et al., 2014. Purtscher-like retinopathy in systemic lupus erythematosus. Am. J. Ophthalmol. 158 (6), 1335–1341.

Yen, Y.C., Weng, S.F., Chen, H.A., et al., 2013. Risk of retinal vein occlusion in patients with systemic lupus erythematosus: a population-based cohort study. Br. J. Ophthalmol. 97 (9), 1192–1196.

Giant Cell Arteritis (Temporal Arteritis)

Cullen, J.F., Coleiro, J.A., 1976. Ophthalmic complications of giant cell arteritis. Surv. Ophthalmol. 20, 247–260.

Kansu, T., Corbett, J.J., Savino, P., et al., 1977. Giant cell arteritis with normal sedimentation rate. Arch. Neurol. 34, 624–625.

Lie, J.T., 1990. Illustrated histopathologic classification criteria for selected vasculitis syndromes. Arthritis Rheum. 33, 1074–1087.

McDonnell, P.J., Moore, G.W., Miller, N.R., et al., 1986. Temporal arteritis: a clinicopathologic study. Ophthalmology 93, 518–530.

McLeod, D., Kohner, E.M., Marshall, J., 1978. Fundus signs in temporal arteritis. Br. J. Ophthalmol. 62, 591–594.

Polyarteritis Nodosa

Akova, Y.A., Jabbur, N.S., Foster, C.S., 1993. Ocular presentation of polyarteritis nodosa. Clinical course and management with steroid and cytotoxic therapy. Ophthalmology 100, 1775–1781.

Gaynon, I.E., Asbury, M.K., 1943. Ocular findings in a case of periarteritis nodosa. Am. J. Ophthalmol. 26, 1072–1076.

Goar, E.L., Smith, L.S., 1952. Polyarteritis nodosa of the eye. Am. J. Ophthalmol. 35, 1619–1625.

Hsu, C.T., Kerrison, J.B., Miller, N.R., et al., 2001. Choroidal infarction, anterior ischemic optic neuropathy, and central retinal artery occlusion from polyarteritis nodosa. Retina 21 (4), 348–351.

Churg–Strauss Syndrome

Cooper, B.J., Bacal, E., Patterson, R., 1978. Allergic angiitis and granulomatosis. Arch. Intern. Med. 138, 367–374.

Miesler, D.M., Stock, E.L., Wertz, R.D., et al., 1981. Conjunctival inflammation and amyloidosisin allergic granulomatosis and angiitis (Churg–Strauss syndrome). Am. J. Ophthalmol. 91, 216–219.

Takanashi, T., Uchida, S., Arita, M., et al., 2001. Orbital inflammatory pseudotumor and ischemic vasculitis in Churg–Strauss syndrome: report of two cases and review of the literature. Ophthalmology 108, 1129–1133.

Dermatomyocytis

Bruce, G.M., 1938. Retinitis in deramatomyositis. Trans. Am. Ophthalmol. Soc. 36, 282–303.

Yan, Y., Shen, X., 2013. Purtscher-like retinopathy associated with dermatomyositis. BMC Ophthalmol. 13, 36.

Granulomatosis with Polyangiitis (Wegner's Granulomatosis)

Androudi, S., Dastiridou, A., Symeonidis, C., et al., 2013. Retinal vasculitis in rheumatic diseases: an unseen burden. Clin. Rheumatol. 32 (1), 7–13.

Bullen, C.L., Liesegang, T.J., McDonald, T.J., et al., 1983. Ocular complications of Wegener's granulomatosis. Ophthalmology 90, 279–290.

Iida, T., Spaide, R.F., Kantor, J., 2002. Retinal and choroidal arterial occlusion in Wegener's granulomatosis. Am. J. Ophthalmol. 133 (1), 151–152.

Straatsma, B.R., 1957. Ocular manifestations of Wegener's granulomatosis. Am. J. Ophthalmol. 44, 789–799.

Tarabishy, A.B., Schulte, M., Papaliodis, G.N., et al., 2010. Wegener's granulomatosis: clinical manifestations, differential diagnosis, and management of ocular and systemic disease. Surv. Ophthalmol. 55 (5), 429–444.

Systemic Sclerosis

Busquets, J., Lee, Y., Santamarina, L., et al., 2013. Acute retinal artery occlusion in systemic sclerosis: a rare manifestation of systemic sclerosis fibroproliferative vasculopathy. Semin. Arthritis Rheum. 43 (2), 204–208.

See INFLAMMATION for other Suggested Reading.

Antiphospholipid Antibody Syndrome (Hughes Syndrome)

Hong-Kee, N., Mei-Fong, C., Azhany, Y., et al., 2014. Antiphospholipid syndrome in lupus retinopathy. Clin. Ophthalmol. 8, 2359–2363.

Cardiac Myxomas and Chorioretinal Occlusions

Cogan, D.G., Wray, S.H., 1975. Vascular occlusions in the eye from cardiac myxomas. Am. J. Ophthalmol. 80, 396–403.

Jampol, L.M., Wong, A.S., Albert, D.M., 1973. Atrial myxoma and central retinal artery occlusion. Am. J. Ophthalmol. 75, 242–249.

Porrini, G., Scassellati-Sforzolini, B., Mariotti, C., et al., 2000. Plurifocal cilioretinal occlusion as the presenting symptom of cardiac myxoma. Retina 20 (5), 550–552.

Susac Syndrome

Dörr, J., Krautwald, S., Wildemann, B., et al., 2013. Characteristics of Susac syndrome: a review of all reported cases. Nat. Rev. Neurol. 9 (6), 307–316.

Egan, R.A., Ha Nguyen, T., Gass, J.D., et al., 2003. Retinal arterial wall plaques in Susac syndrome. Am. J. Ophthalmol. 135 (4), 483–486.

Martinet, N., Fardeau, C., Adam, R., et al., 2007. Fluorescein and indocyanine green angiographies in Susac syndrome. Retina 27 (9), 1238–1242.

Purtscher Retinopathy

Axer-Sieger, R., Hod, M., Fink-Cohen, S., et al., 1996. Diabetic retinopathy during pregnancy. Ophthalmology 103, 1815.

Bedrossian, R.H., 1974. Central serous retinopathy and pregnancy. Am. J. Ophthalmol. 78, 152.

Coady, P.A., Cunningham, E.T. Jr., Vora, R.A., et al., 2015. Spectral domain optical coherence tomography findings in eyes with acute ischaemic retinal whitening. Br. J. Ophthalmol. 99 (5), 586–592.

Errera, M.H., Kohly, R.P., da Cruz, L., 2013. Pregnancy-associated retinal diseases and their management. Surv. Ophthalmol. 58 (2), 127–142.

Lazzeri, S., Figus, M., Nardi, M., et al., 2013. Iatrogenic retinal artery occlusion caused by cosmetic facial filler injections. Am. J. Ophthalmol. 155 (2), 407–408.

Lin, P., Hahn, P., Fekrat, S., 2012. Peripheral retinal vascular leakage demonstrated by ultra-widefield fluorescein angiography in preeclampsia with HELLP syndrome. Retina 32 (8), 1689–1690.

Park, S.W., Woo, S.J., Park, K.H., et al., 2012. Iatrogenic retinal artery occlusion caused by cosmetic facial filler injections. Am. J. Ophthalmol. 154 (4), 653–662, e1.

See TRAUMATIC CHORIORETINOPATHY and INFLAMMATION for further Suggested Reading.

Shaikh, S., Ruby, A.J., Piotrowski, M., 2003. Pre-eclampsia related chorioretinopathy with Purtscher's-like findings and macular ischemia. Retina 23, 247–250.

CHAPTER 7

Degeneration

Vitreous Synchisis and Syneresis

Vitreous degeneration is a physiologic process that occurs with age and may be accelerated in eyes with longer axial length. As the vitreous degenerates, there is liquefaction of the vitreous gel, known as "synchisis," resulting in small pockets of liquefied vitreous within the firmer vitreous. This leads to destabilization of the vitreous and promotes its collapse, known as "syneresis." The boundaries between each liquefied pocket and the vitreous gel may form speckled opacifications that may later manifest as symptomatic floaters. These vitreous opacities may become visible to patients and appear as spots, strings, or cobwebs, in the absence of a posterior vitreous detachment (PVD). There are four grades of physiologic vitreous degeneration as documented with swept-source OCT (SS-OCT).

© 517 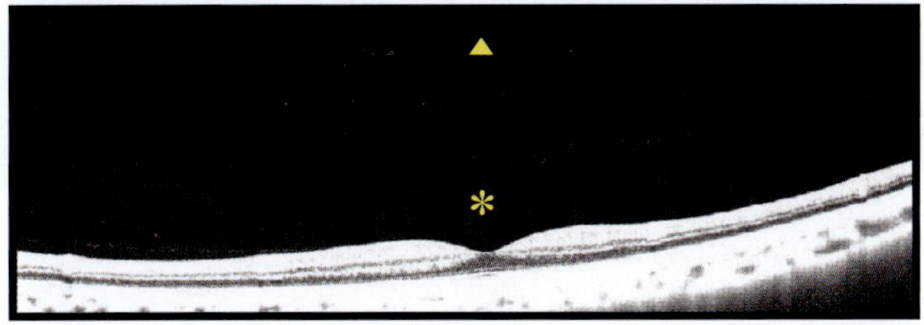

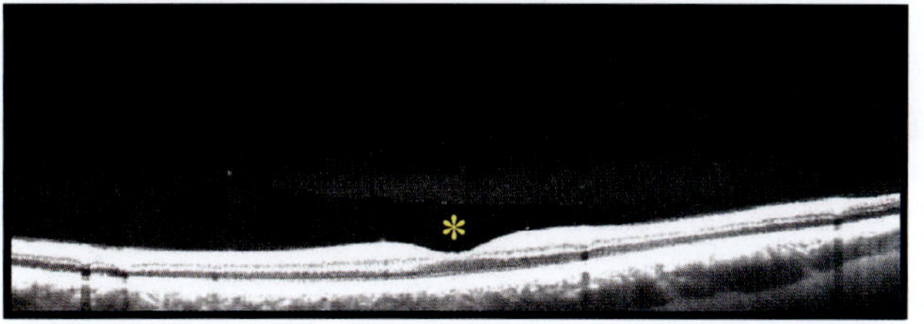 © 518

In Grade 0, there is the presence of a premacular bursa *(asterisk)* with or without a central lacuna *(triangle)*.

© 519 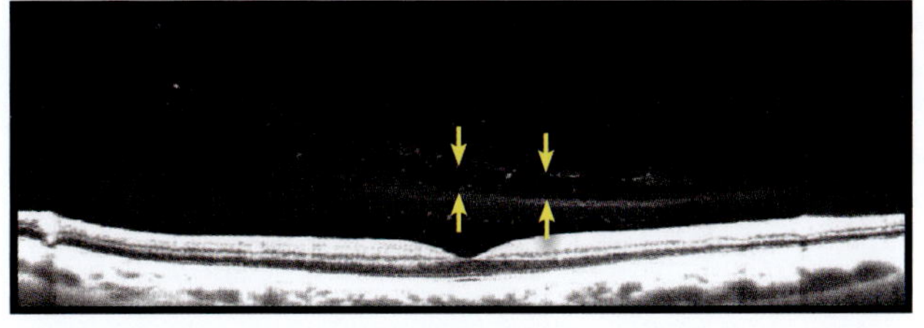

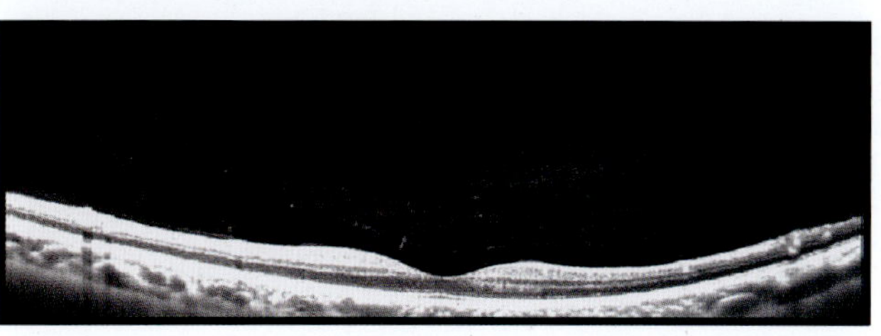 © 520

In Grade 1, there is the presence of a neighboring shallow space without a connection to the premacular bursa, with increased speckled hyperreflectivity along the boundaries of this shallow space *(arrows)*.

© 521 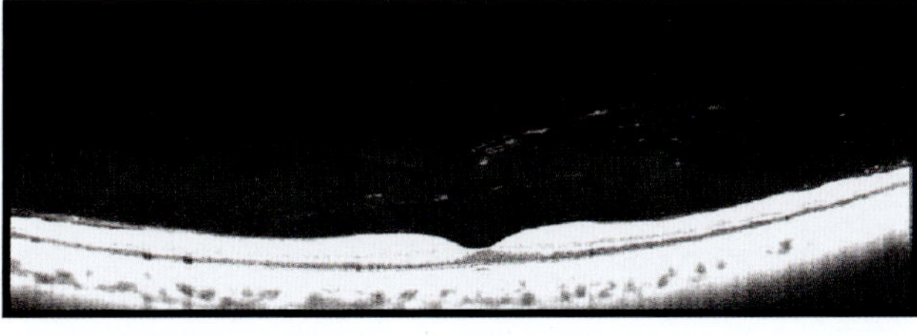

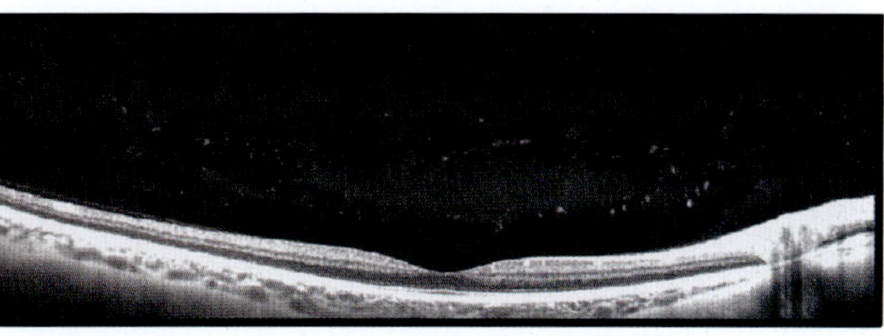 © 522

In Grade 2, there is a connection between these shallow spaces to the premacular bursa.

© 523 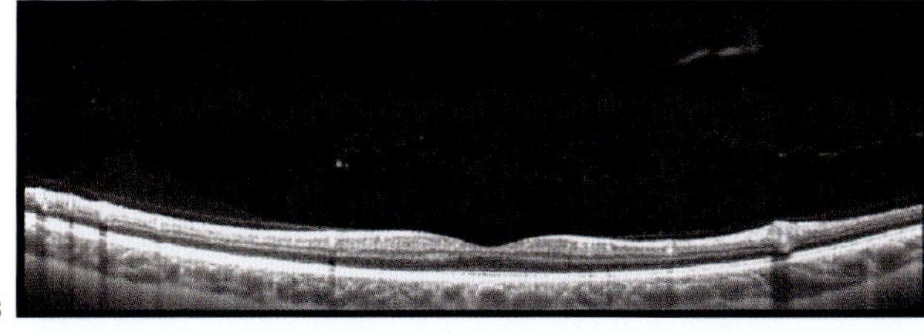

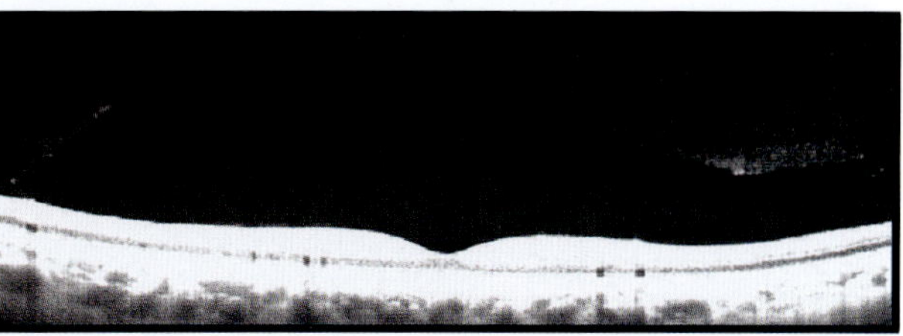 © 524

In Grade 3, there is a connection to a large neighboring space or central lacuna.

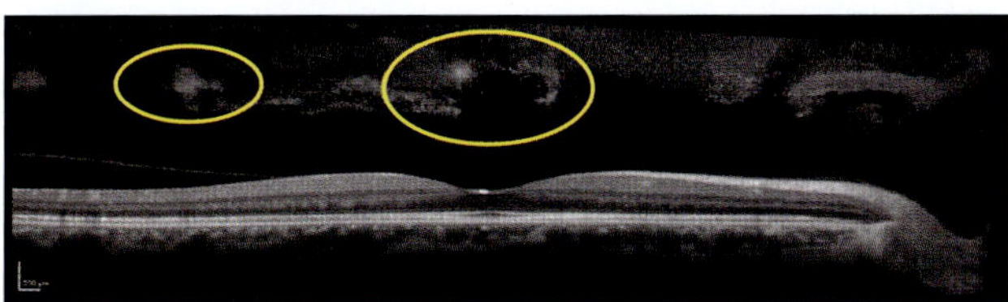

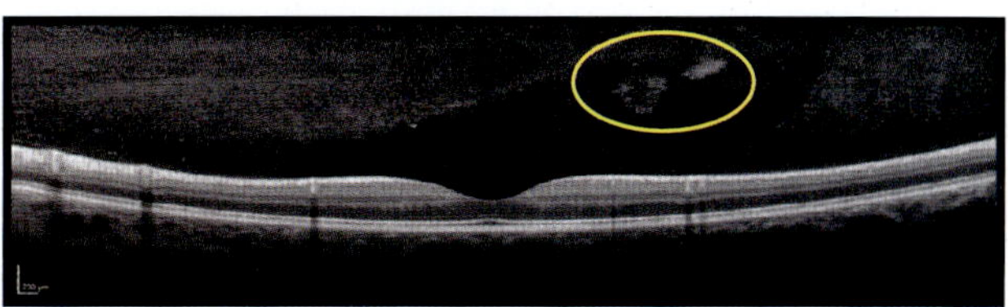

Vitreous opacities *(circles)* may be seen with enhanced vitreous imaging OCT (EVI-OCT) or SS-OCT in patients with symptomatic floaters without a complete PVD. *Images courtesy of Dr. Michael Engelbert*

Posterior Vitreous Detachment

Posterior vitreous detachment (PVD) is a common consequence of aging that occurs with vitreous degeneration. As the vitreous body shrinks with syneresis, there is separation of the vitreous cortex or posterior hyaloid from the retina. PVD may also result from traumatic eye injury or inflammatory diseases, or be induced surgically. The process of PVD may occur in stages beginning with perimacular and perifoveal PVD, followed by vitreofoveal separation with or without a break in the posterior wall of the premacular bursa and, finally, separation of the vitreous from the optic disc. Gel liquefaction without concurrent dehiscence at the vitreoretinal interface leads to anomalous PVD and its complications.

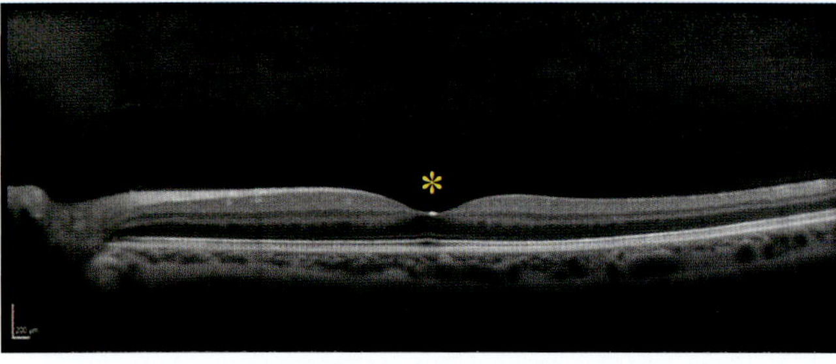

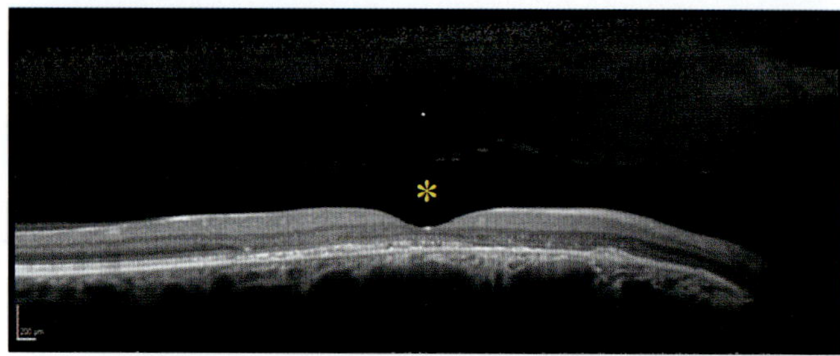

Before a PVD occurs, there is complete vitreous attachment (stage 0). EVI-OCT or SS-OCT shows the posterior hyaloid or cortical vitreous attached to the retina in all areas, with visualization of the premacular bursa *(asterisk)* and pre-optic nerve head space (area of Martegiani). The anterior wall of the premacular bursa may show speckled hyper-reflectivity and should not be misinterpreted as the posterior hyaloid *(right)*.

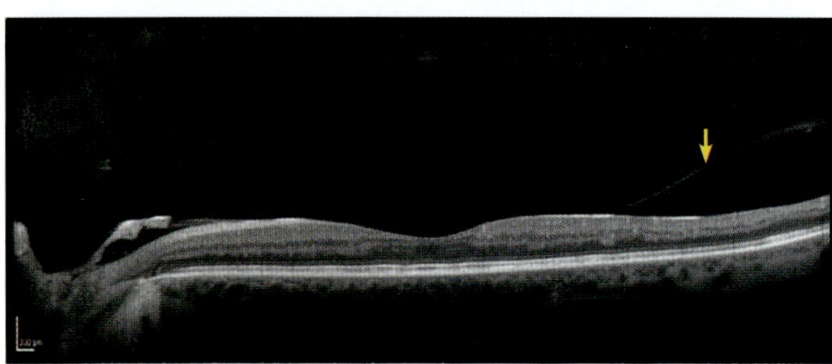

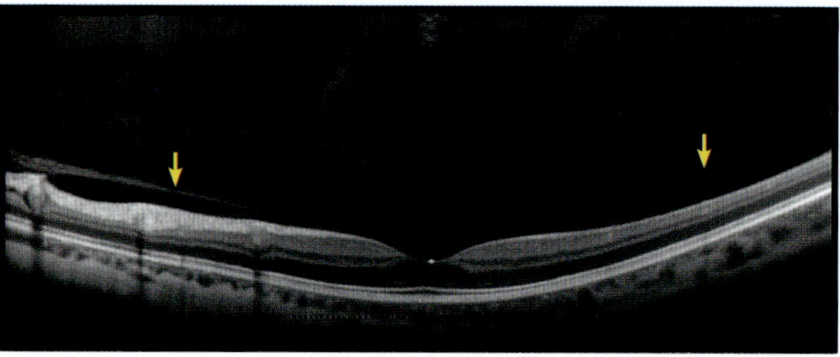

© **525**

PVD begins with focal perimacular PVD (stage 1) where the posterior hyaloid *(arrows)* detaches in one area *(left)* and progresses to a perifoveal PVD (stage 2) where the posterior hyaloid is detached in both nasal and temporal quadrants, with vitreofoveal adhesion and persistent attachment at the optic disc.

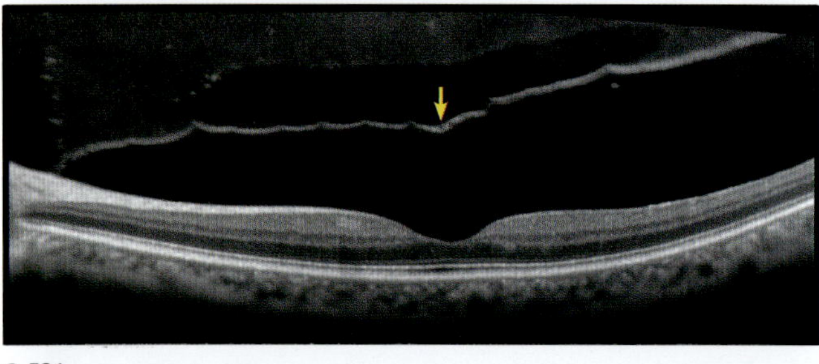

© **526**

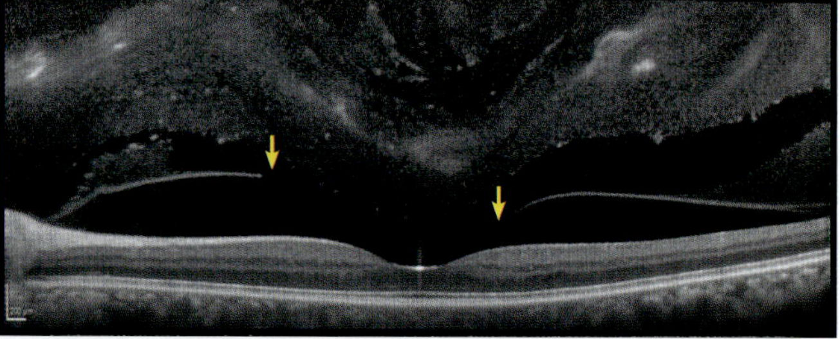

© **527**

With vitreofoveal separation (stage 3), the posterior wall of the premacular bursa *(arrows)* may remain intact (stage 3A, *left image*) or ruptured (stage 3B, *right image*). There is persistent attachment of the vitreous at the optic disc at this stage.

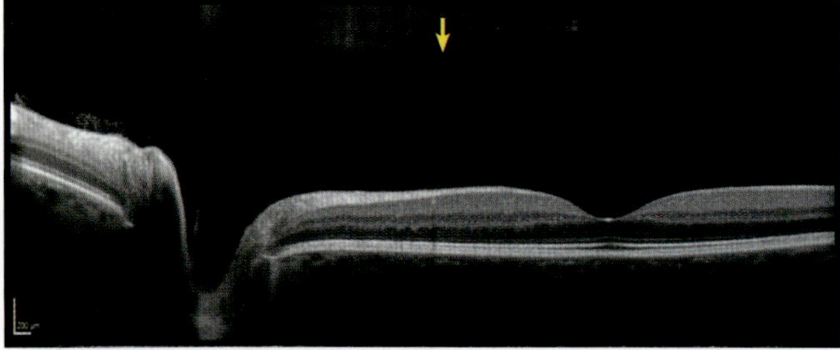

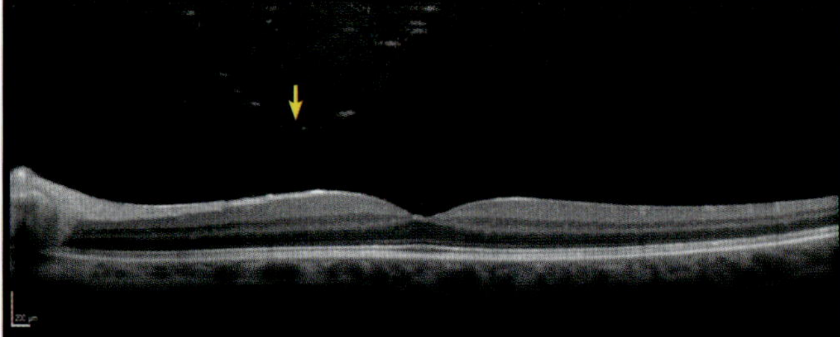

With complete separation of the vitreous at the optic disc (stage 4), the area above the retina appears optically empty and the posterior hyaloid *(arrows)* may be visible. *Images courtesy of Dr. Michael Engelbert*

With complete separation of the vitreous from the optic disc, a Weiss ring corresponding to the site of previous attachment to the optic disc may appear as a symptomatic ring-shaped floater. The Weiss ring may take many forms as shown here or may be fragmented during the process of vitreous separation.

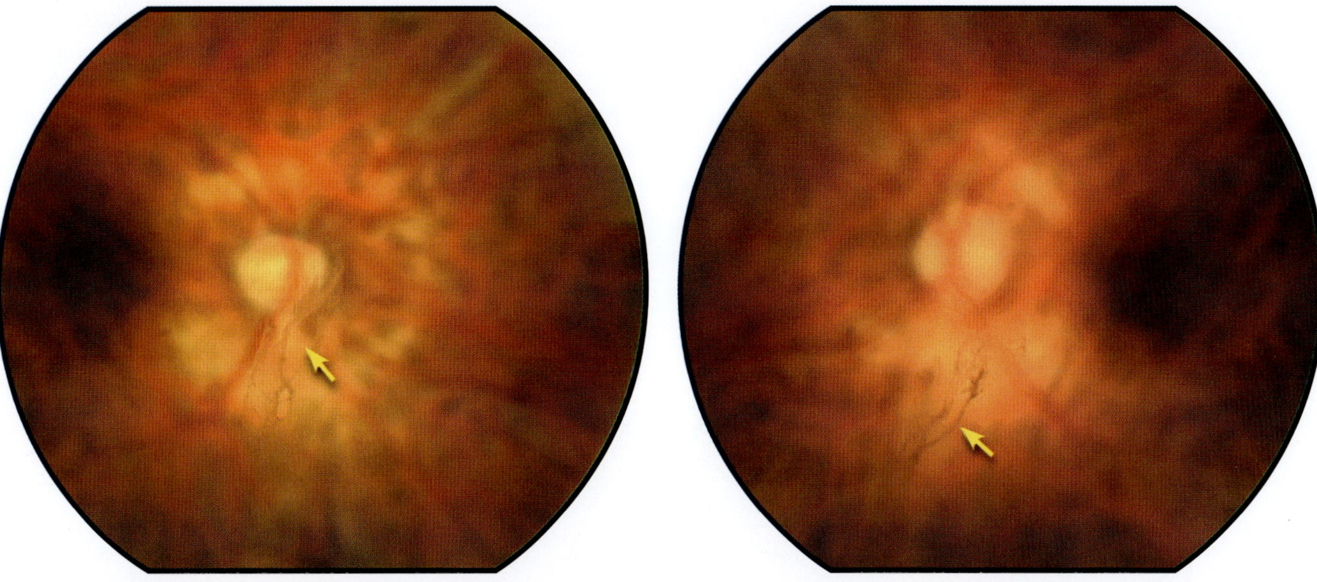

This patient has Weiss rings in both eyes (*arrows*). Standard non-widefield photography focusing on the Weiss ring reveals a "figure of eight" Weiss ring in the right eye and an elliptical Weiss ring in the left eye. The retina is out of focus with non-widefield imaging.

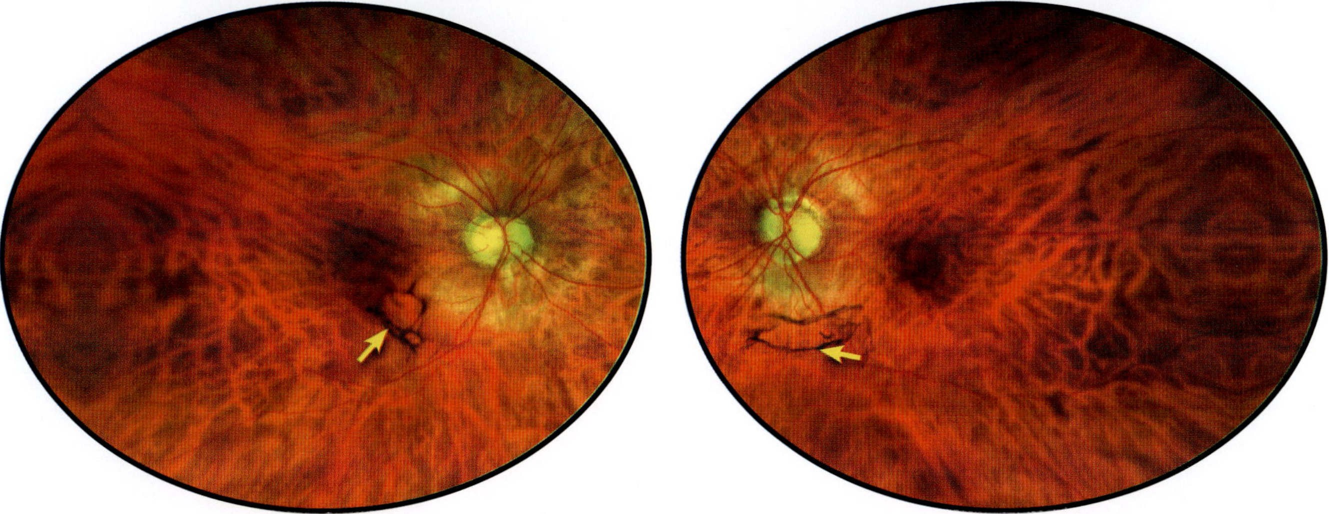

The same patient was imaged with the ultra-widefield system. Notice how ultra-widefield imaging is able to capture the Weiss ring (*arrows*) with the retina still in focus.

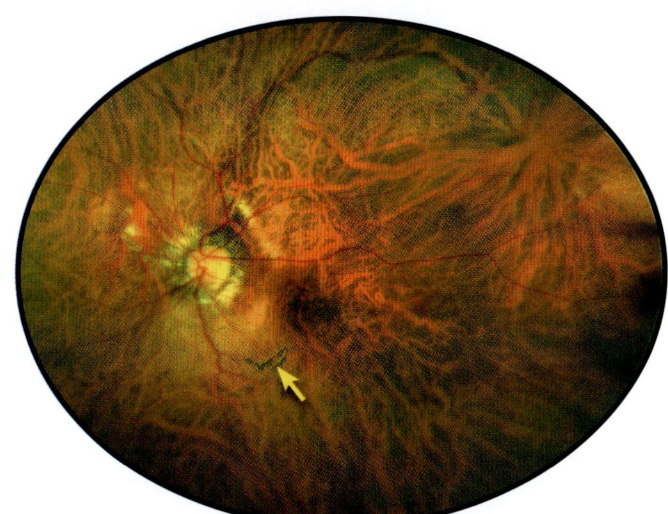

This patient has a PVD with a visible Weiss ring (*arrow*) and parts of the separated vitreous seen in the inferior vitreous cavity.

Asteroid Hyalosis

Asteroid hyalosis is a degenerative condition of the vitreous with a prevalence of 1.2% in adults. It is found to be more frequent with aging, with 0.2% prevalence in 43- to 54-year-old and 2.9% in 75- to 86-year-old patients. Multiple small white deposits that typically have a refractile appearance, which resemble stars (or asteroids) shining in the clear night sky, form in the vitreous. The etiology of asteroid hyalosis is still unknown. There may be an association with diabetes mellitus, hyperlipidemia, atherosclerosis, and hypertension. The asteroid bodies are mostly composed of hydroxyapatite and phospholipids. Asteroid hyalosis is unilateral in 75-90% of cases. Typically, the disorder does not produce symptoms or a reduction in visual acuity. Occasionally, patients may express symptomatic floaters. Treatment is rarely necessary, but, in highly symptomatic cases or when necessary for visualization of the fundus, a vitrectomy may be indicated.

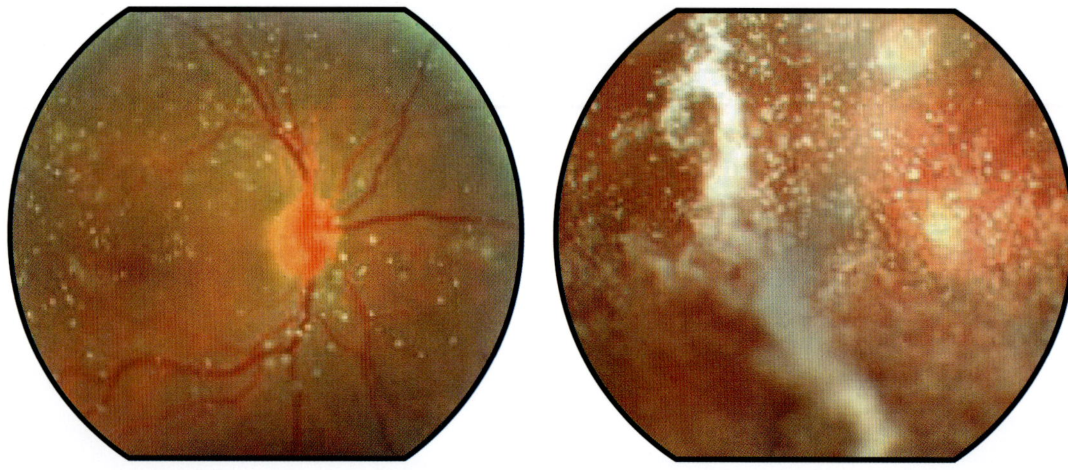

These patients have varying degrees of asteroid hyalosis. Small asteroid bodies are seen in the patient on the left. In the patient on the right, there is a more dense aggregation of the asteroid bodies, which have coalesced into rope-like bands. The asteroid bodies are located in the posterior and mid-vitreous cavity in this case.

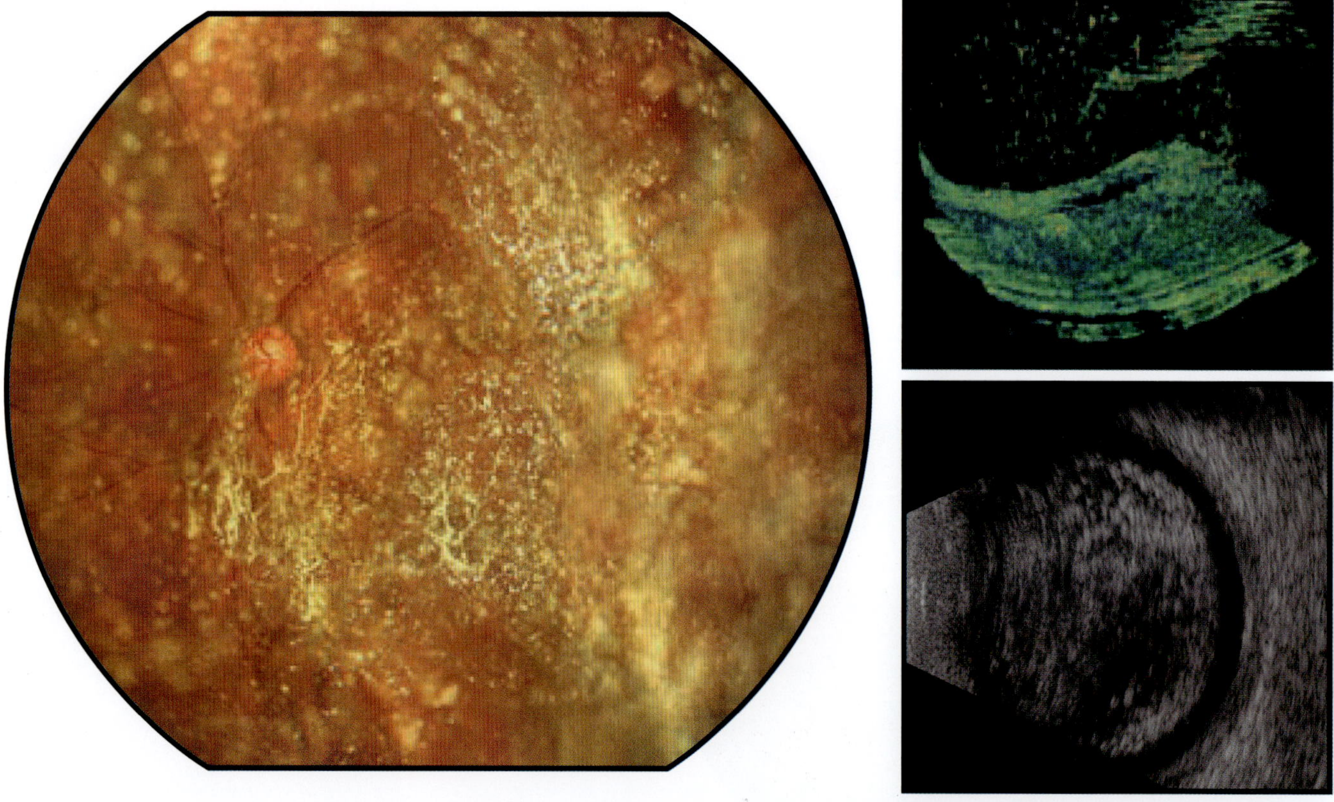

This color photograph shows an extensive degree of asteroid bodies filling the vitreous cavity. Visual acuity can be surprisingly good, even with this degree of vitreous opacification. The 3-D OCT image shows reflectance of cords and flecks of asteroid bodies. B-Scan ultrasonography shows intense reflectivity of the asteroid bodies and a characteristic acoustically clear zone anterior to the retina. *Ultrasound image courtesy of Dr. Yale Fisher*

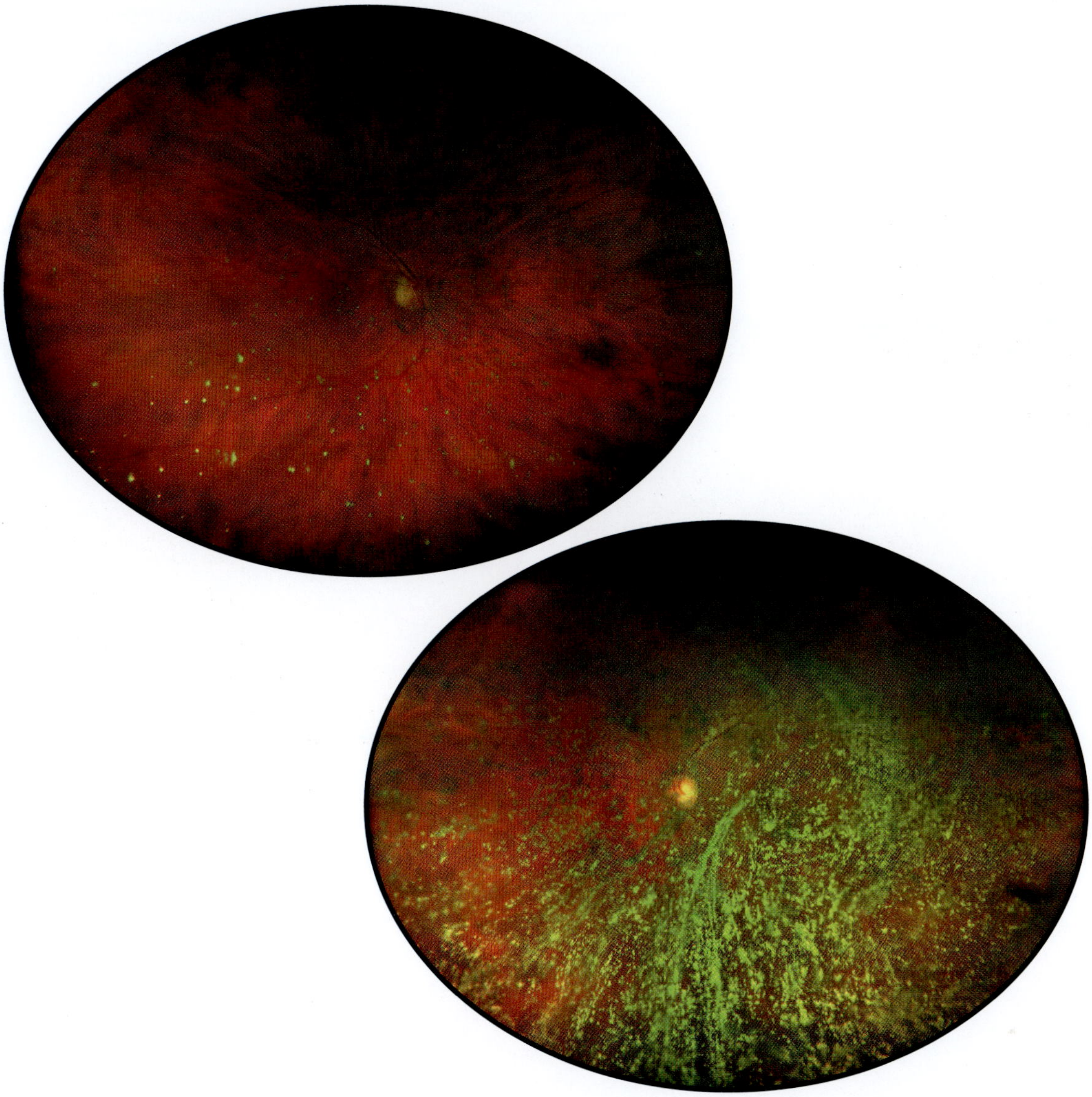

Ultra-widefield imaging shows the full extent of asteroid bodies within the vitreous, ranging from scattering of asteroid bodies *(top)* to dense flecks and cords of asteroid bodies *(bottom)*. The patient on the right has a visual acuity of 20/30.

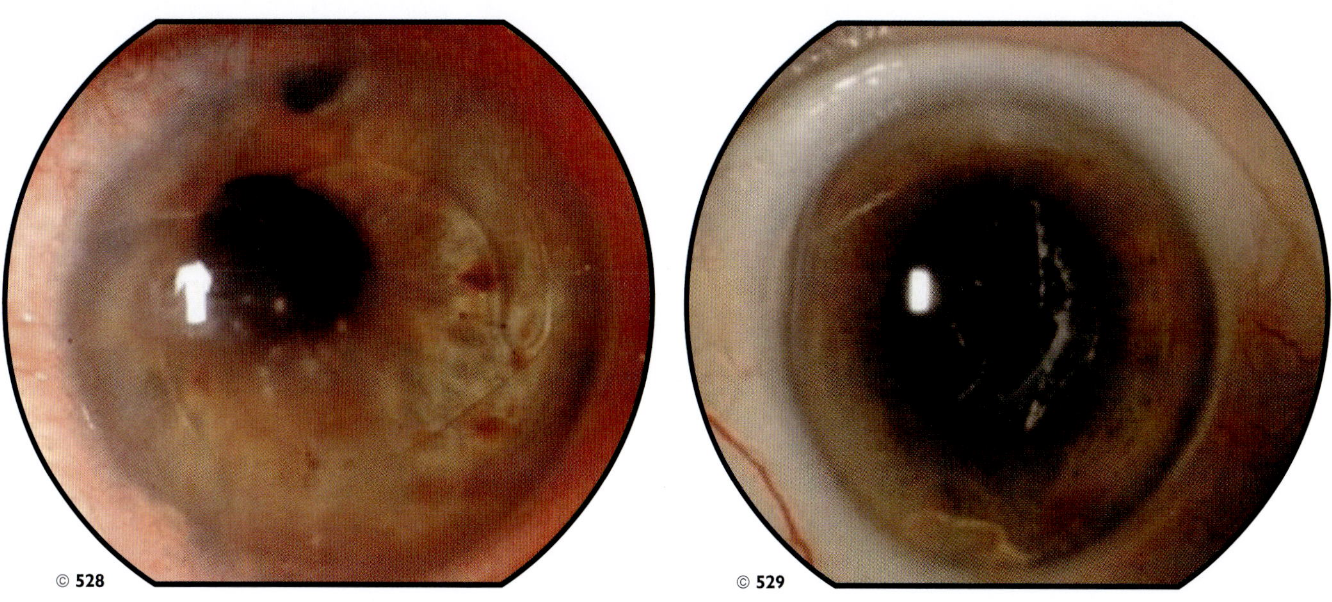

Asteroid bodies may infrequently prolapse into the anterior chamber after cataract surgery and masquerade as iris metastasis. *Images courtesy of Dr. Carol Shields*

Asteroid hyalosis should be differentiated from synchisis scintillans or cholesterosis bulbi, which is an extremely rare accumulation of cholesterol crystals in liquefied vitreous that tend to settle or gravitate inferiorly, causing a snow globe effect. Because synchisis scintillans is an end-stage degenerative condition that occurs in eyes with extensive inflammation, hemorrhage, or trauma, it is usually not visible clinically and more commonly diagnosed after enucleation by the pathologist.

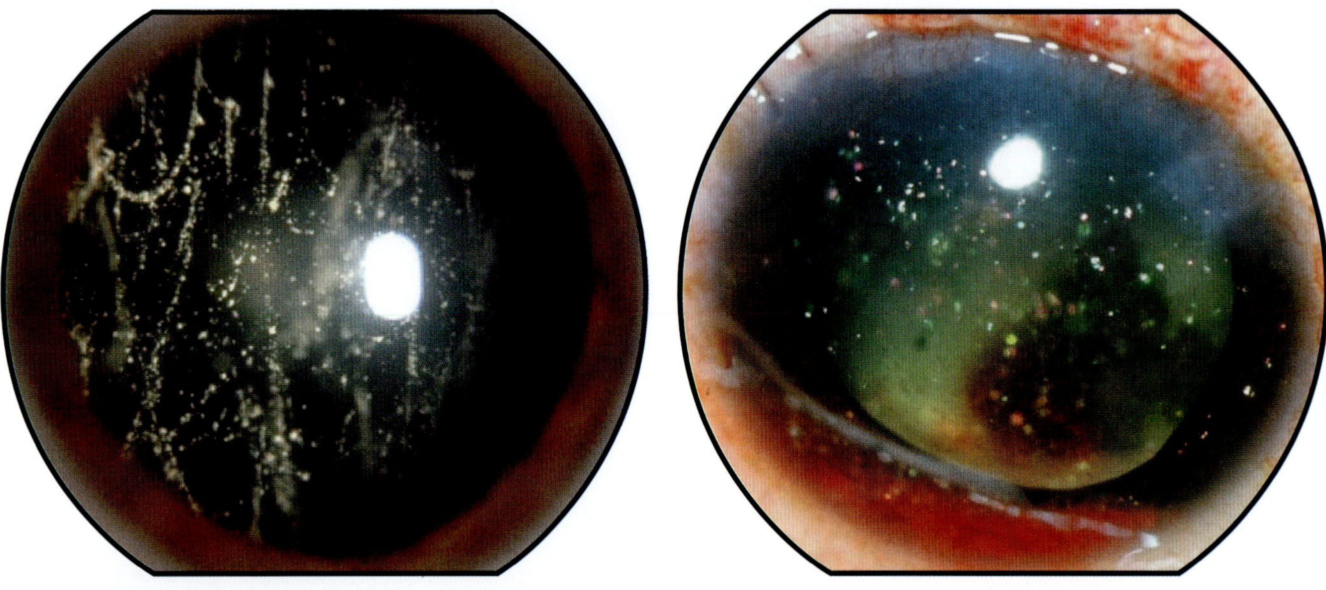

Asteroid bodies are typically adherent to the vitreous framework *(left image)*, while the cholesterol crystals in synchisis scintillans are not *(right image)*.

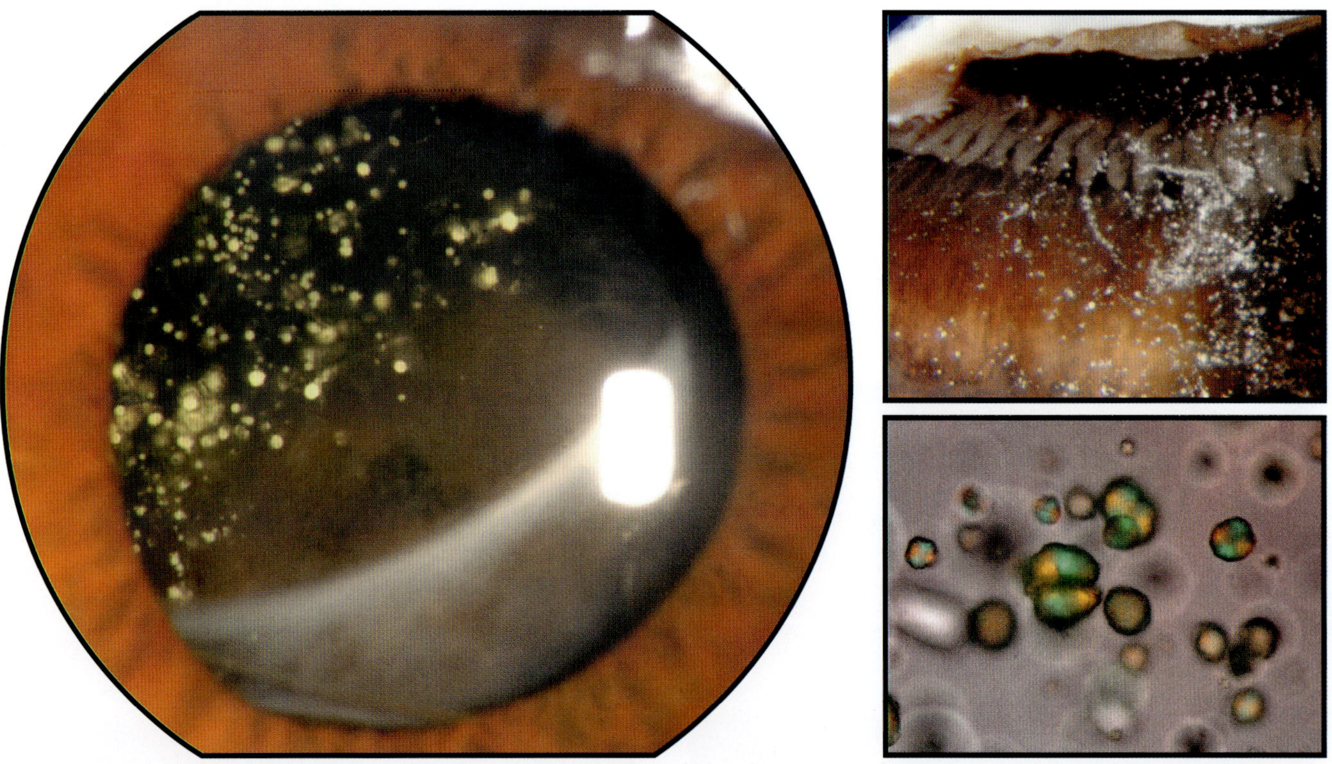

Histopathology of this patient with asteroid bodies shows chalky white spherules with characteristic Maltese cross birefringence under polarized light. *Images courtesy of Dr. Ralph Eagle*

Vitreous Amyloidosis

Amyloidosis encompasses a group of disorders characterized by extracellular deposition of amyloid proteins in various organs and tissues of the body. At least 24 different proteins are known to be amyloidogenic; however, the most common forms are immunoglobulin light-chain (AL protein) in primary amyloidosis and serum amyloid A (AA protein) seen in chronic inflammatory diseases. Amyloid proteins consist of insoluble fibrillar aggregates arranged in a characteristic beta-pleated sheet configuration, which is responsible for the ability to bind Congo red and show birefringence in polarized light. Amyloidosis of the vitreous is a rare condition that may be primary, acquired, or familial in nature. It is more often related to familial amyloid polyneuropathy (FAP); however, it may very rarely occur sporadically.

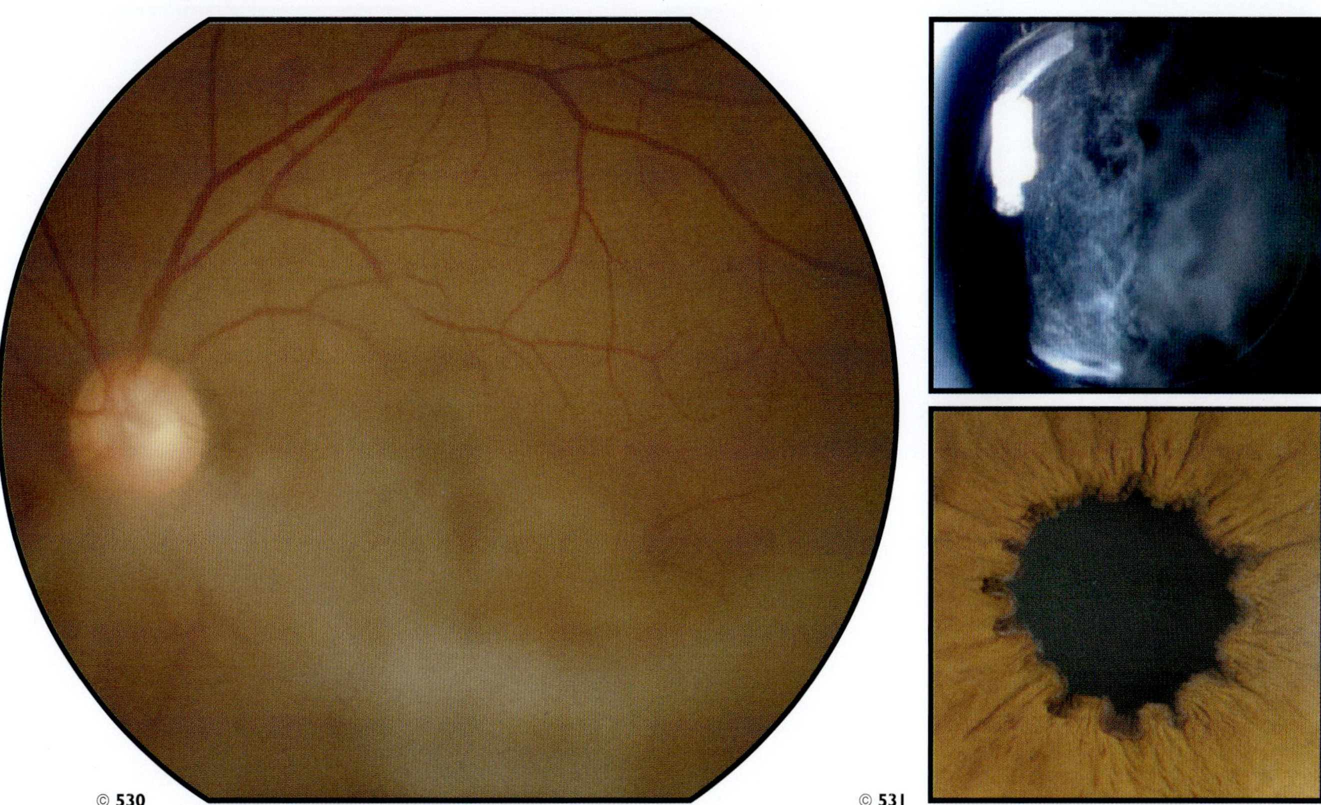

© 530 © 531

Vitreous amyloidosis may be seen as opacities in the vitreous cavity, retrolental "cobweb" opacities *(top right image)*, or as amyloid deposits causing irregularity at the pupillary border *(bottom right image). Images courtesy of Dr. Stanley Chang (top right) and Dr. Ryuhei Hara (left and bottom right)*

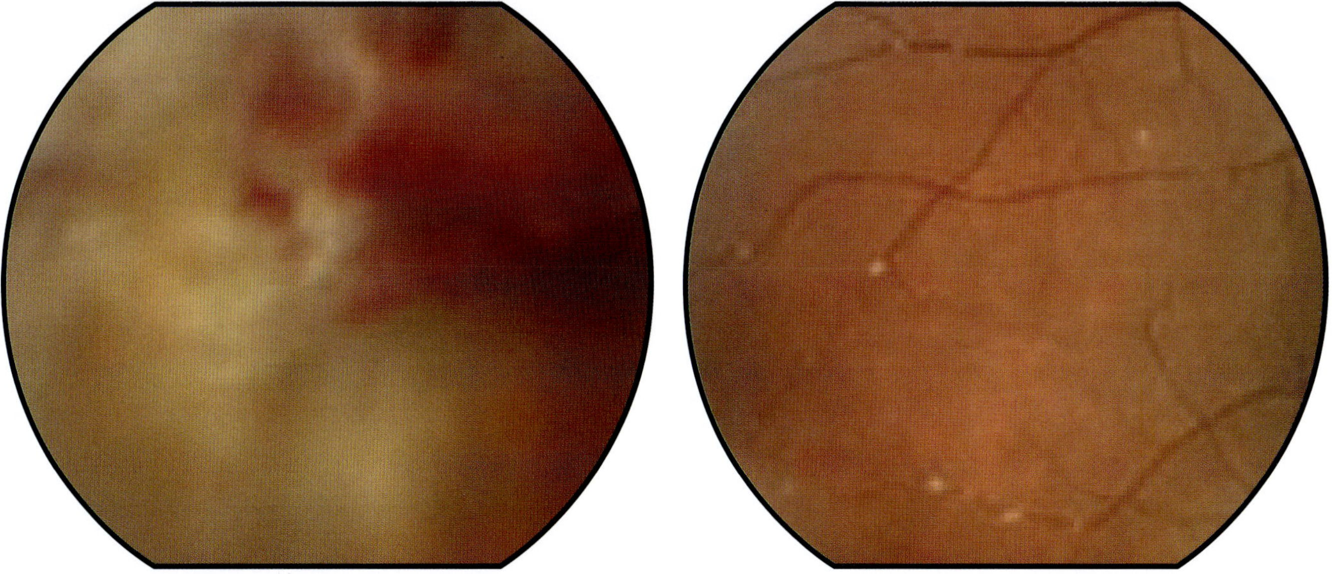

Vitreous amyloidosis may be associated with neovascularization and vitreous hemorrhage due to involvement of the retina. In such cases, vitrectomy and pan-retinal photocoagulation are indicated, although recurrence may occur. Post-vitrectomy photograph reveals peripheral yellow-white amyloid deposits around the retinal blood vessels. *Images courtesy of Dr. Anita Agarwal*

Familial amyloid polyneuropathies (FAPs) are rare forms of amyloidosis associated with amyloid accumulation in the vitreous. FAPs are inherited in an autosomal dominant fashion with variable penetrance and are caused by mutation in the transthyretin (TTR) gene at locus 18q11.2-q12.1. Involvement of the vitreous is usually seen in association with systemic amyloidosis and clinical features including peripheral neuropathy, renal dysfunction, and cardiomyopathy. Amyloid deposition in the vitreous appears as diffuse whitish gray or yellowish material having a "cobweb" or "cotton-wool" appearance. Other fundus findings include perivascular deposits, superficial retinal gray-white deposits, and small vessel occlusions with associated angiographic filling delays on both fluorescein and indocyanine green angiography. Vitreous amyloidosis should be considered in the differential diagnosis of any vitreous opacification or haze. Diagnosis relies on clinical suspicion and staining of vitreous biopsy specimens with Congo red dye. Vitrectomy remains the treatment of choice for symptomatic vitreous opacification.

This is a 43-year-old healthy male who noted floaters in both eyes. There was obscuration of the fundus with amorphous debris in the vitreous. Fluorescein angiography showed hyperfluorescence from the retinal vasculature *(bottom left)*. Six months later, despite the use of topical and periocular steroids, the vitreous haze progressed to form a "cobweb" appearance *(bottom right)*.

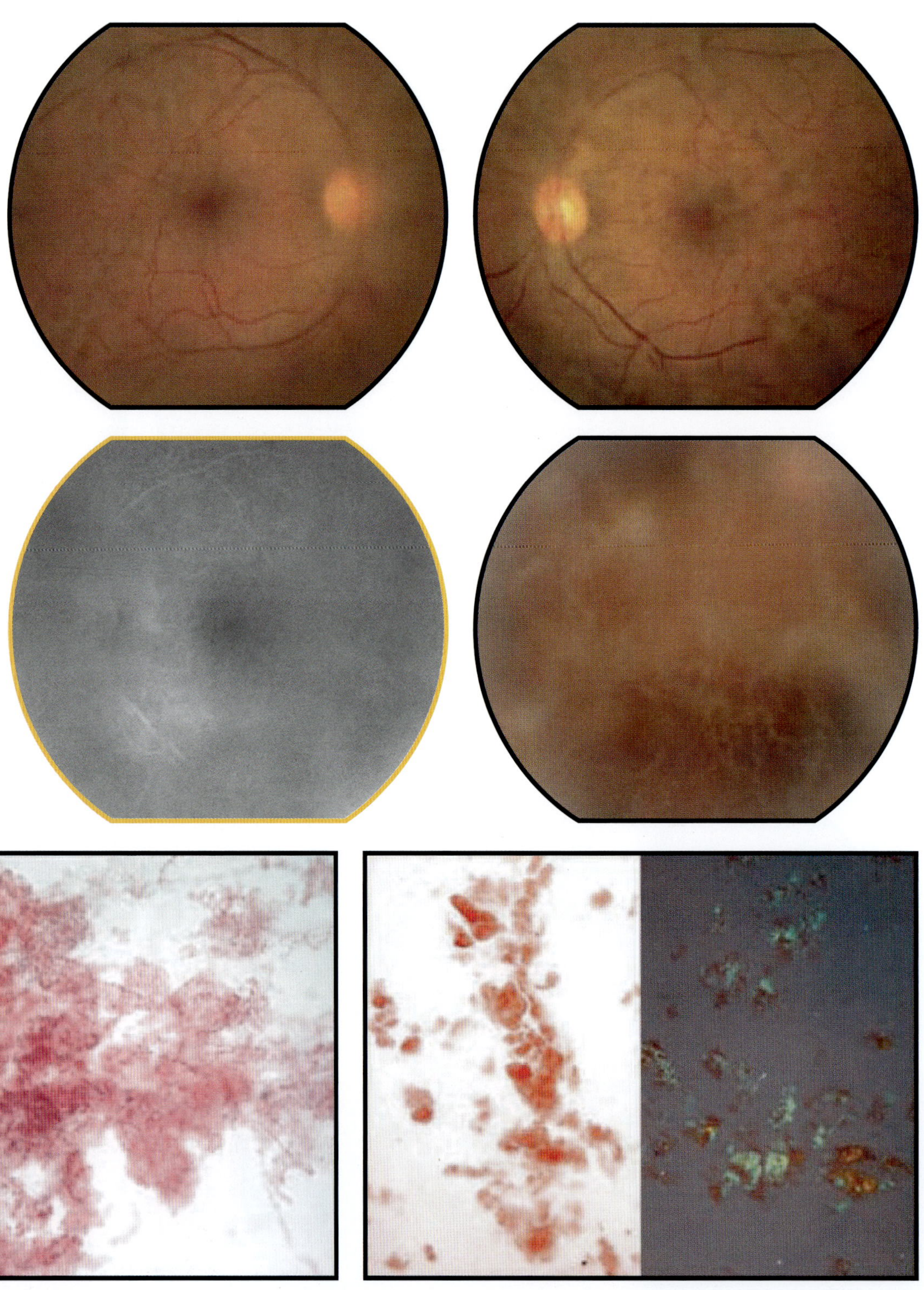

A vitreous biopsy stained with hematoxylin and eosin revealed a large amount of eosinophilic material but no evidence of a cellular infiltration such as lymphocytes *(left)*. The Congo red stain showed the presence of amyloid, which was accentuated on examination with polarization *(right)*.

Vitreous Cyst

Intravitreal cysts are rare ocular curiosities that are usually found incidentally on routine ophthalmological examination. Patients may be asymptomatic or may complain of floaters or transient visual blurring. Vitreous cysts may be classified as congenital or acquired. Congenital cysts are thought to be associated with remnant hyaloid vessels and are usually nonpigmented, smooth, sessile, or pedunculated. Congenital cysts are typically located anterior to the optic disc, and may have limited movement due to vitreous strands attached to the optic disc. Acquired cysts are found in degenerative or inflammatory diseases including retinitis pigmentosa, choroidal atrophy, retinal detachment, retinoschisis, parasitic uveitis, nematode endophthalmitis, and trauma. They are usually pigmented and thought to arise from the degeneration of a ciliary body adenoma breaking into the vitreous cavity or a vitreous reaction to underlying retinal and choroidal degeneration. Vitreous cysts are benign and may be observed without treatment. Symptomatic cysts may be treated with laser photocystotomy or pars plana vitrectomy with cyst excision.

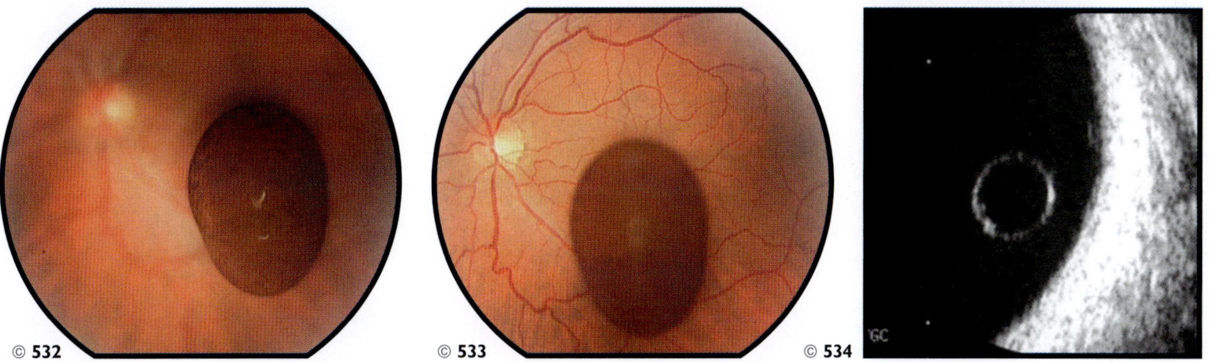

This patient has a free-floating, translucent, smooth, brown-pigmented cyst in the vitreous cavity. Ultrasound shows a spherical hypoechogenic mass with thin hyper-reflective edges that is freely mobile in the posterior vitreous and not attached to any other ocular structures. *Images courtesy of Dr. Noel Padron-Perez*

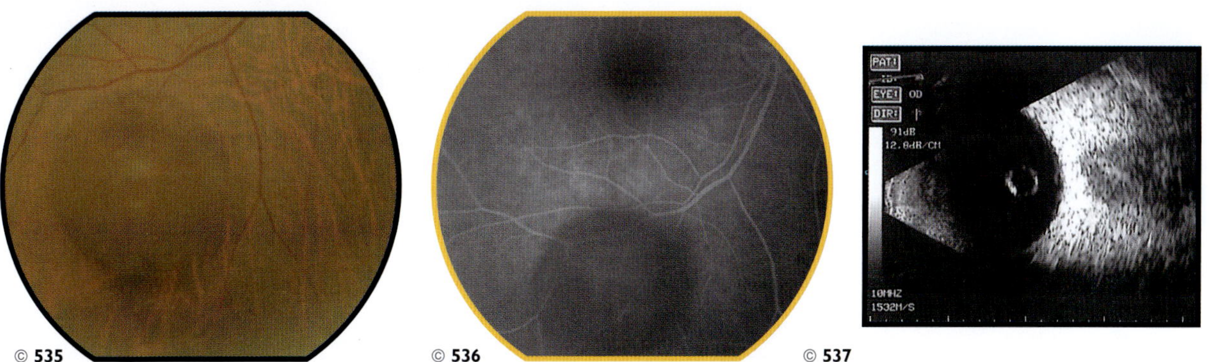

This 50-year-old patient presented with floaters in his right eye. Color photograph shows a smooth, free-floating, vitreous cyst in the inferior fundus. Fluorescein angiography shows a circular area of hypofluorescence due to pre-retinal masking effect and no vascularity of the cyst itself. Ultrasound image shows a free-floating cyst in the posterior vitreous. *Images courtesy of Dr. Yasin Toklu*

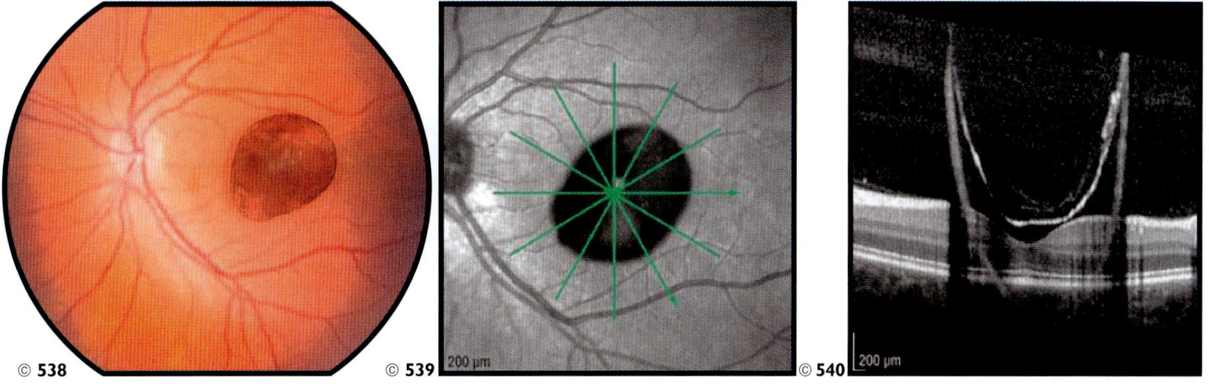

This patient has a free-floating vitreous cyst with some pigmentation. Spectral-domain OCT shows the cyst located over the macula. *Images courtesy of Dr. Shani Reich*

Angioid Streaks

Angioid streaks are visible, irregular crack-like dehiscences in Bruch membrane that are associated with atrophic degeneration of the overlying retinal pigment epithelium. Knapp coined the term "angioid streaks" because their appearance resembles retinal vasculature. Angioid streaks are most commonly associated with pseudoxanthoma elasticum, although they may also be associated with Paget disease of the bone, Ehler–Danlos syndrome, sickle cell or thalassemia hemoglobinopathies, acromegaly, and diabetes mellitus. Patients with angioid streaks are generally asymptomatic, unless they develop complications such as traumatic Bruch membrane rupture or macular choroidal neovascularization (CNV).

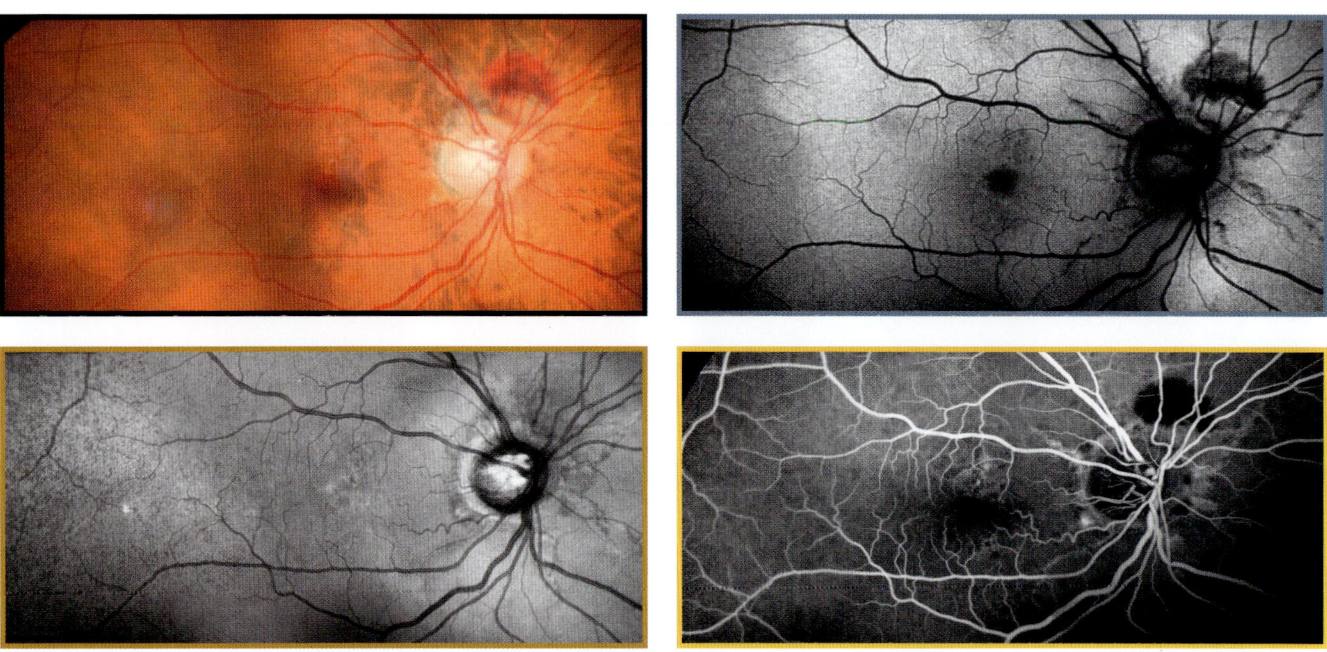

This patient with thalassemia has angioid streaks, *peau d'orange,* and peripapillary CNV. The angioid streaks are best seen with fundus autofluorescence and near-infrared reflectance as radiating dark lines around the disc. The *peau d'orange* is visualized best with near-infrared reflectance, which allows the transition zone between calcified and noncalcified Bruch membrane to be appreciated. With fluorescein angiography, angioid streaks are seen as bright hyperfluorescent lines around the disc.

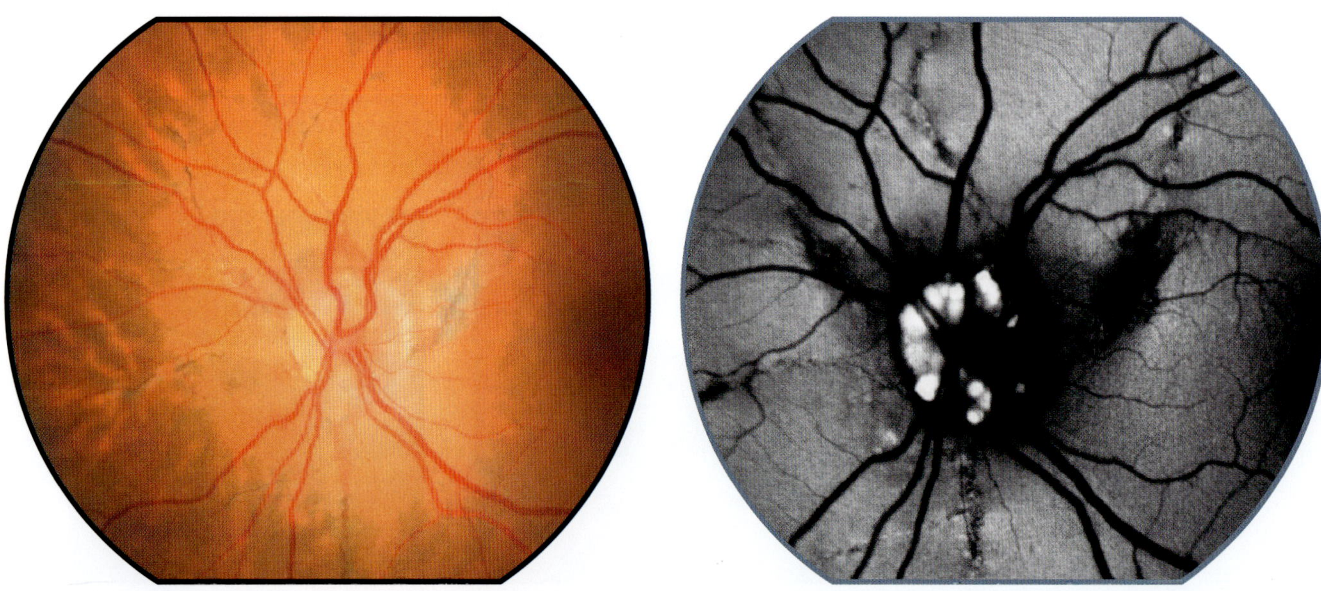

This patient with thalassemia has angioid streaks and optic disc drusen. The optic disc drusen are hyperautofluorescent with fundus autofluorescence. *Images courtesy of Dr. Francesca Viola and Dr. Giulio Barteselli*

Pseudoxanthoma Elasticum

Pseudoxanthoma elasticum (PXE) is an autosomal recessive multi-system disorder associated with dermatologic, gastrointestinal, cardiovascular, and ocular findings. PXE has been associated with mutations in the ABCC6 gene at chromosome 16p13.1. Characteristic skin changes typically affect the neck, axilla, and other flexural areas. Fundus findings include angioid streaks, a reticular macular dystrophy, a speckled appearance temporal to the macula known as *peau d'orange,* optic nerve head drusen, comet-like peripheral crystalline bodies, and peripheral RPE atrophic spots. An exudative detachment with yellowish and clear exudate between the ellipsoid zone and the retinal pigment epithelium may produce an acquired vitelliform lesion in PXE. CNV occurs in 72-86% of eyes and is often bilateral. Treatment of CNV in PXE using thermal laser photocoagulation or verteporfin photodynamic therapy is frequently complicated by recurrences and poor visual outcomes. Recently, intravitreal injections of anti-vascular endothelial growth factor drugs have shown promise in treating these patients.

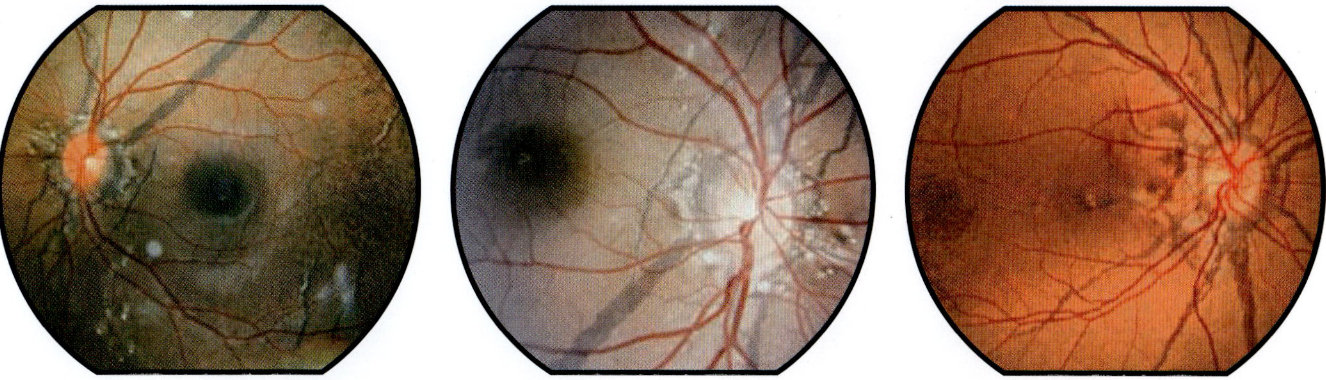

Angioid streaks appear as red, brown, or orange lines representing breaks in Bruch membrane and typically radiate out from the optic nerve in an irregular pattern, which can simulate the appearance of retinal blood vessels. Angioid streaks are not believed to be present at birth but are seen in 90% of PXE patients. Angioid streaks can traverse the macular region, often without a decrease in visual acuity.

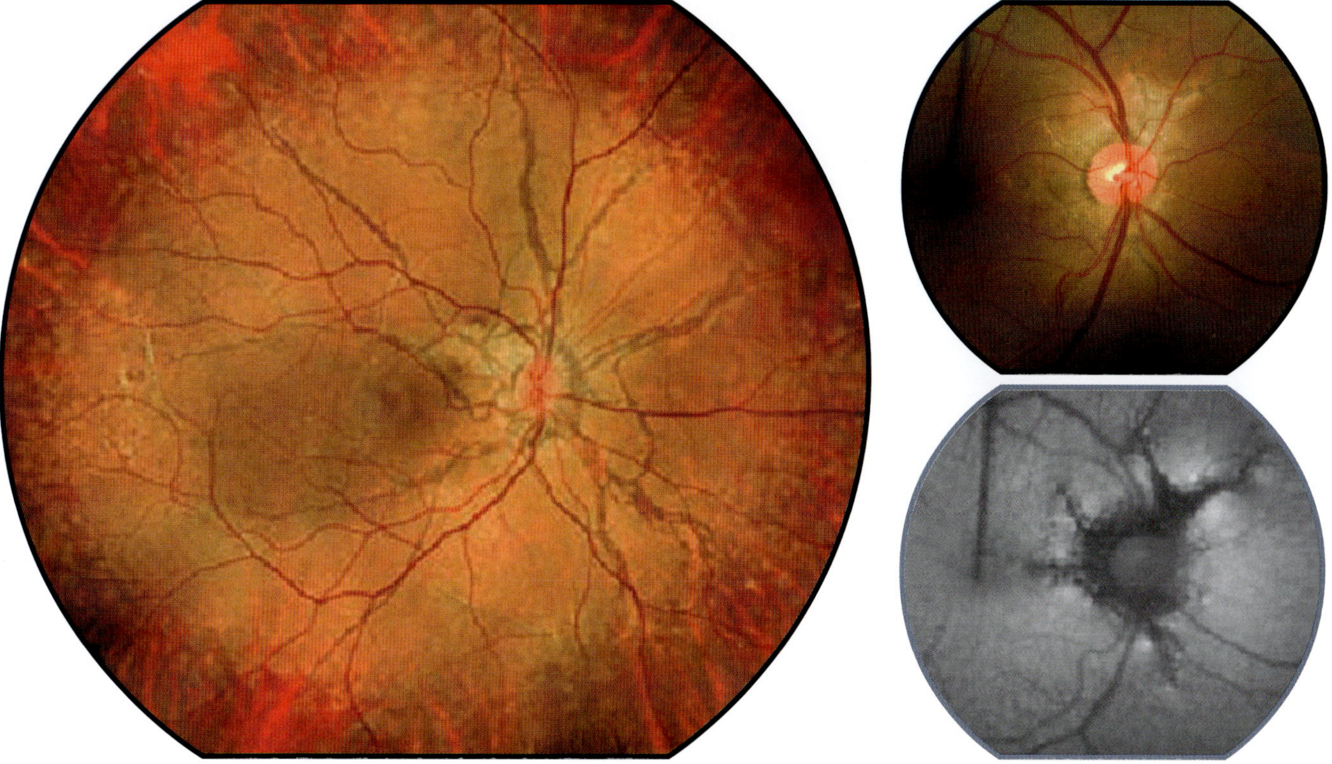

These patients have peripapillary atrophy and angioid streaks that emerge from the edge of the atrophy and course radially into the near and midperiphery, sometimes through the fovea itself. Fundus autofluorescence may display angioid streaks as hypoautofluorescent lines that are sometimes undetectable on clinical examination *(lower right image).*

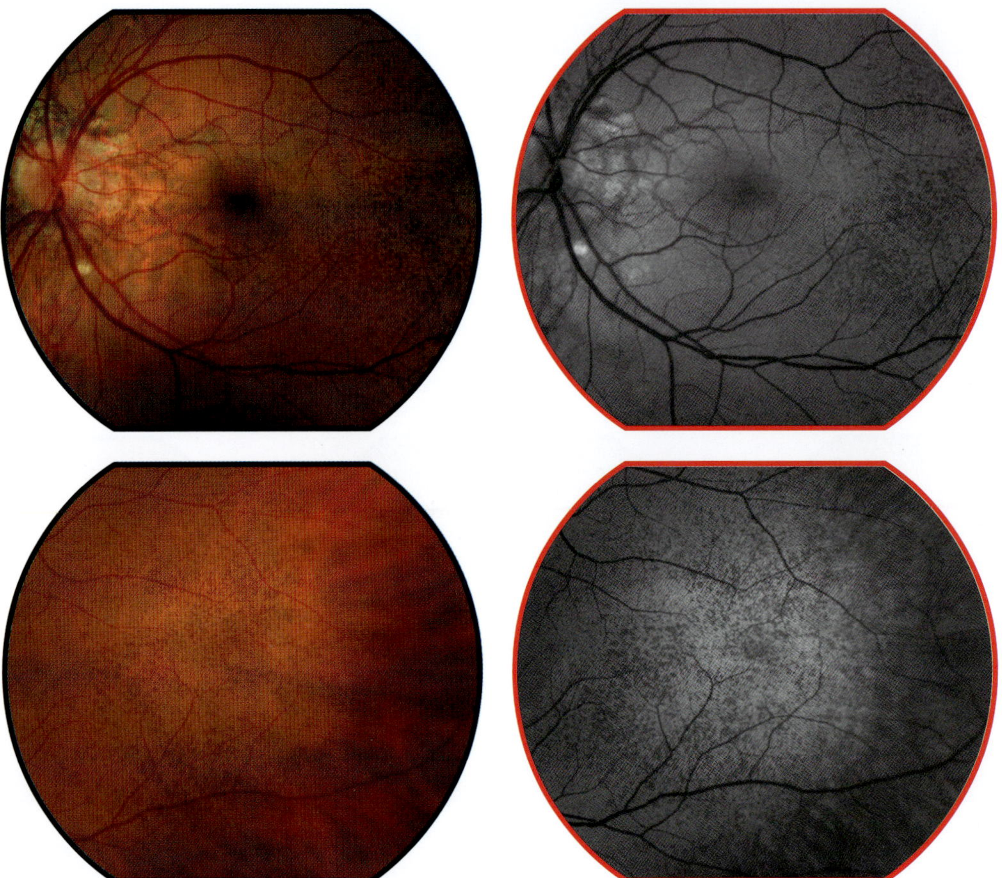

Peau d'orange or yellow mottling at the level of the retinal pigment epithelium begins in the macular region and, as atrophy ensues, extends more temporally. The macular lesions disappear with aging and are seen more temporally over time. This patient has angioid streaks and temporal *peau d'orange* that may be accentuated with red free photography *(right images)*.

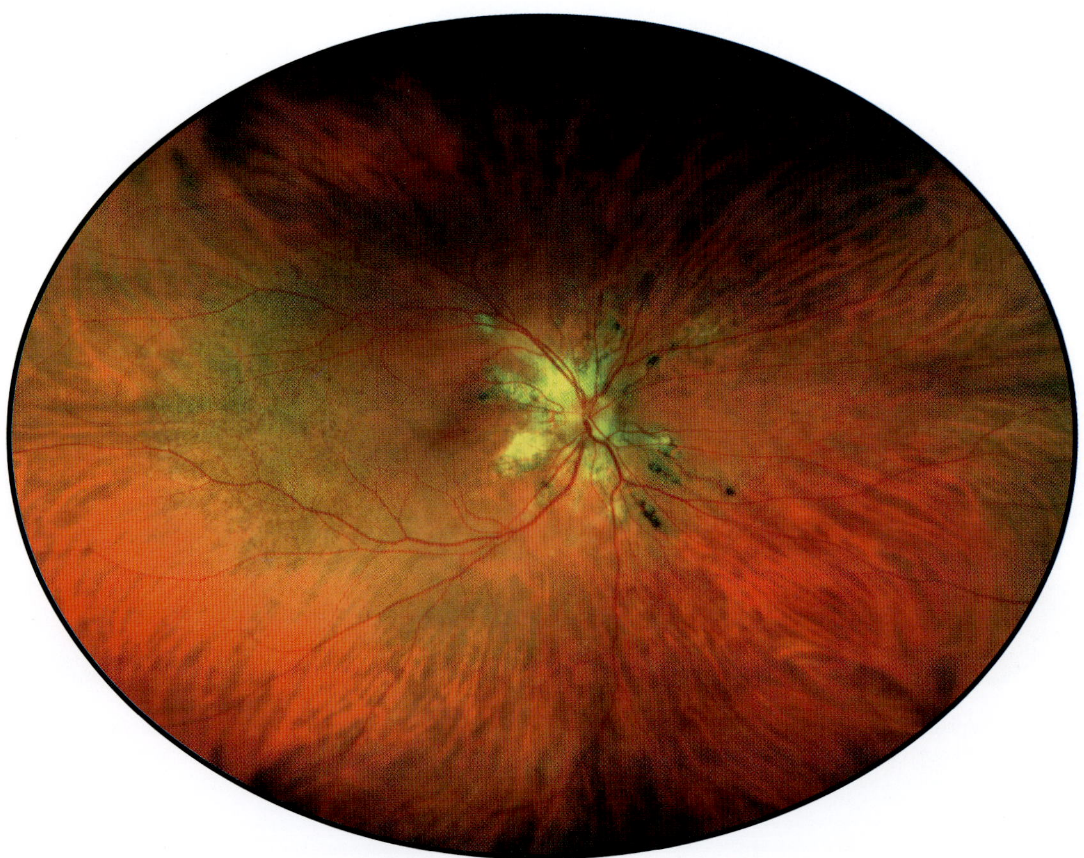

Ultra-widefield photograph demonstrates the full extent of *peau d'orange*.

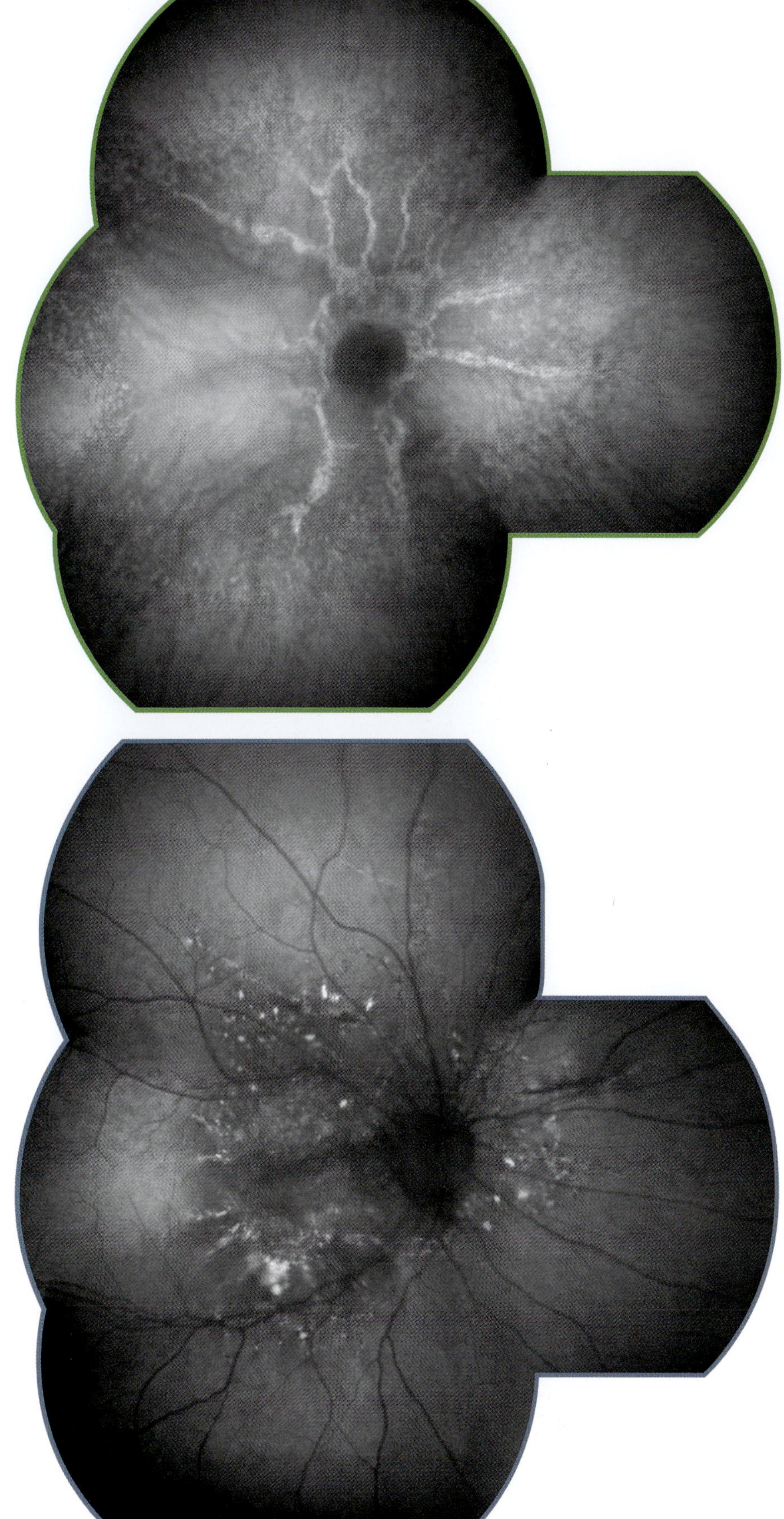

Late phase ICGA demonstrates angioid streaks well and frequently delineates the streaks better than fundus autofluorescence imaging. In this case of PXE, hyperfluorescence is also seen to correlate to sites of *peau d'orange* in the periphery.

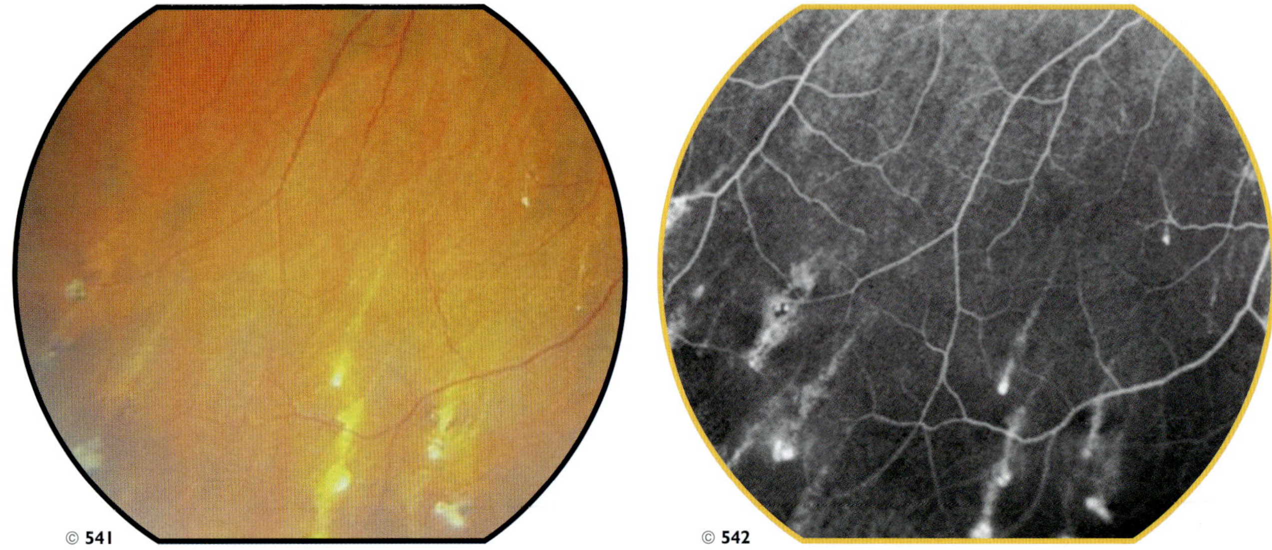

© 541 © 542

Crystalline bodies with or without comet tails may occur in the peripheral fundus and may represent calcified lesions. These lesions appear as solitary, subretinal, nodular, white bodies with or without a tapering white tail pointing toward the optic disc. There may be atrophic RPE changes and pigmentation at the margin of this finding. Sometimes, a spray of comets may be observed, creating the appearance of a "meteor shower." *Images courtesy of Dr. Martin Gliem*

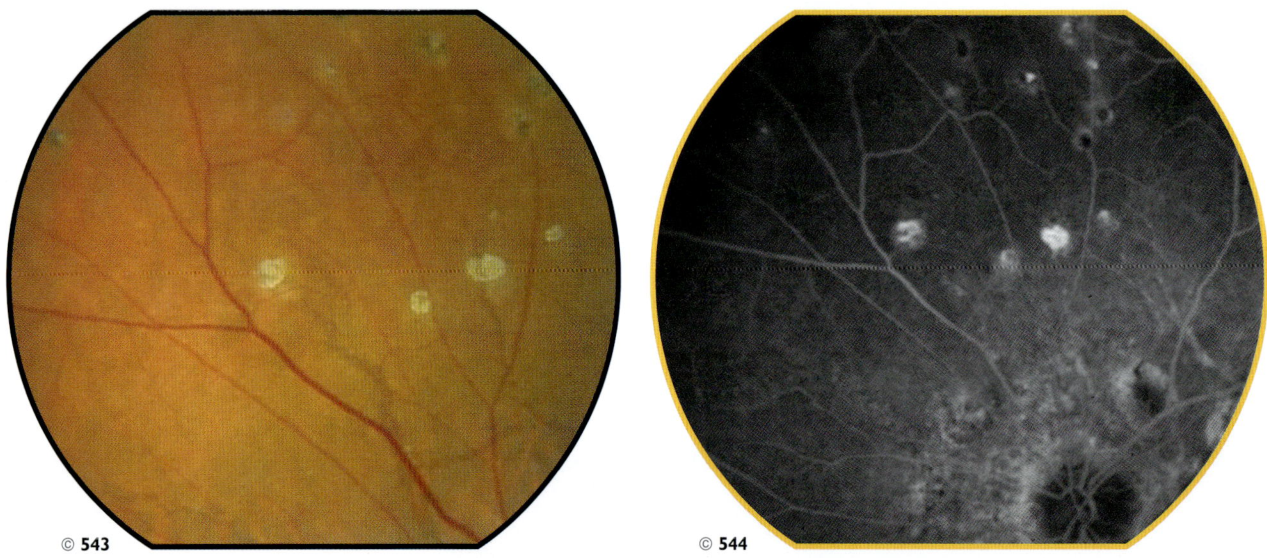

© 543 © 544

Focal atrophic RPE lesions, appearing as small, round, yellow, slightly pink or discretely punched-out white scars with varying amounts of pigment, may occur in the peripheral fundus and have been referred to as "salmon spots." *Images courtesy of Dr. Martin Gliem*

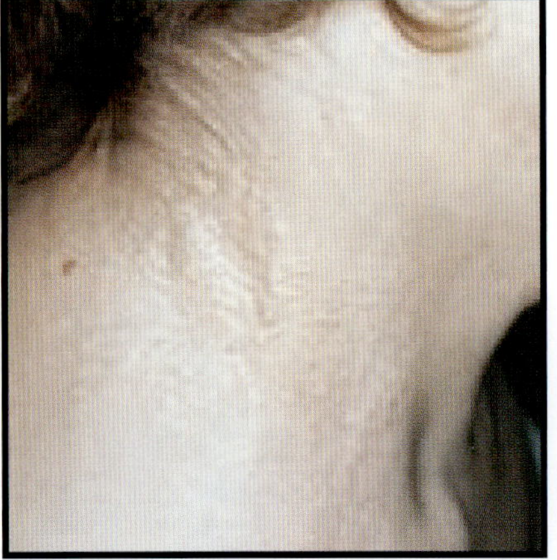

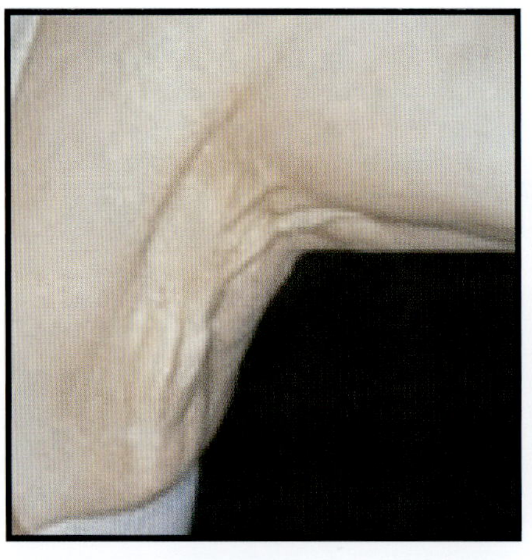

The characteristic systemic findings of pseudoxanthoma elasticum include skin changes (plucked chicken-like appearance). Gastrointestinal and cardiac abnormalities may also be associated with this condition. *Images courtesy of Dr. Mark Lebwohl*

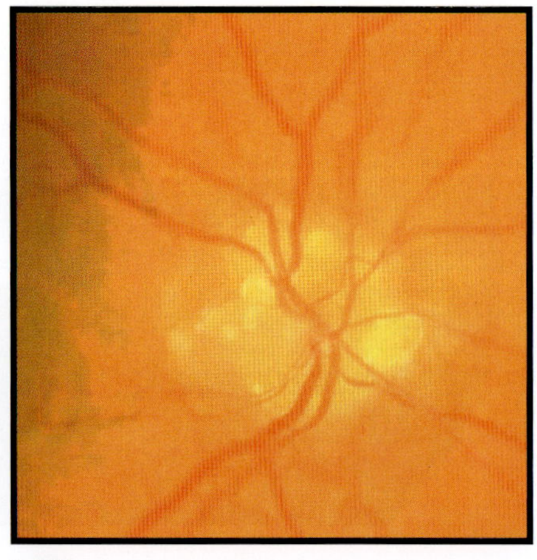

© 545

Optic disc drusen is commonly associated with PXE. *Courtesy of Dr. Martin Gliem*

Pattern Dystrophy

A "pattern dystrophy-like" change of the macula may develop bilaterally in approximately 65% of patients with PXE and may manifest as any of the 5 subclasses of pattern dystrophy, including reticular dystrophy, fundus pulverulentus, fundus flavimaculatus, butterfly-shaped dystrophy, and vitelliform dystrophy. The pattern dystrophy-like appearance may be a combination of any of the 5 subclasses and may progress from one type to another over time. Because this condition is unrelated to the autosomal dominantly inherited pattern dystrophy first described by Sjögren, the continued use of the term "pattern dystrophy" in PXE is controversial. Clinically, it is important to recognize that PXE may appear with pattern dystrophy-like changes especially in cases in which angioid streaks are very subtle.

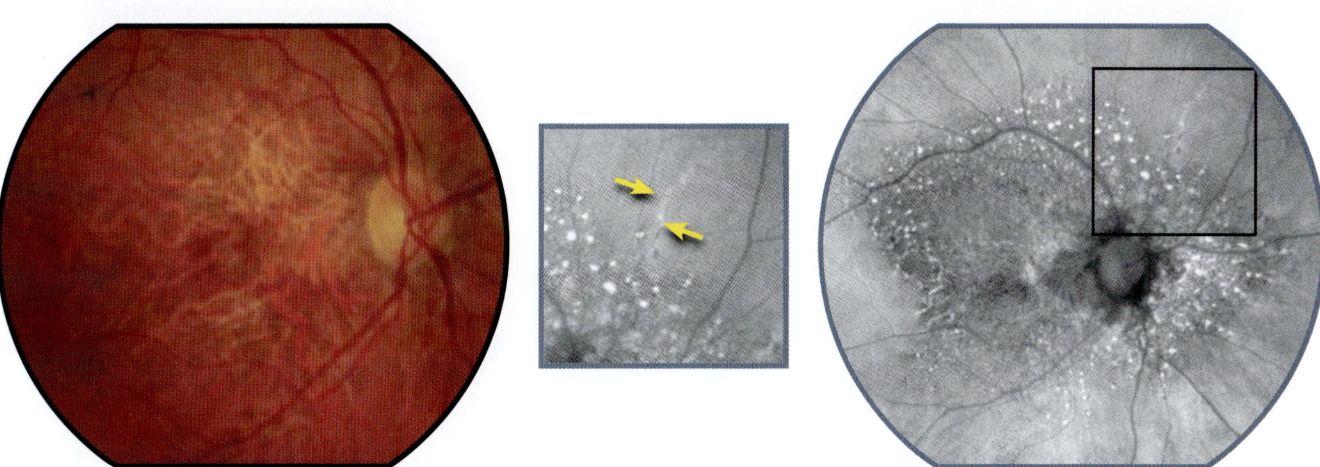

This patient with PXE has no demonstrable streaks on clinical examination, although there is a suggestion of atrophy in the macula. Fundus autofluorescence shows a pattern dystrophy surrounding the posterior pole with peripapillary atrophy and minimal macular atrophy. The inset shows that there is an angioid streak peripheral to the pattern abnormality *(arrows)*. Streaks may not be evident in an eye that has developed diffuse atrophy. PXE in this case is associated with a pattern dystrophy without sparing of the peripapillary area.

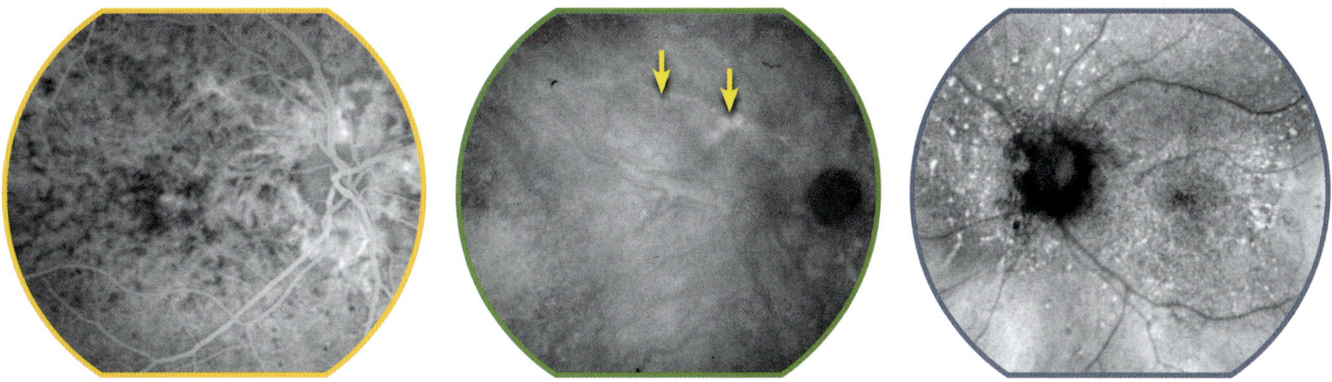

The fluorescein angiogram of the same patient shows multifocal areas of hypofluorescence corresponding to the hyperfluorescence seen on fundus autofluorescence (inverse phenomenon). These nummular areas of pigment epithelial hyperplasia are characteristic but not pathognomonic of PXE. The streaks in the posterior pole are more obvious *(arrows)* with ICG angiography. There is hypoautofluorescence in the central macula of the left eye *(right image)* where there is a scar evident clinically. The fundus autofluorescence shows a similar pattern abnormality with peripapillary atrophy, as seen in the right eye.

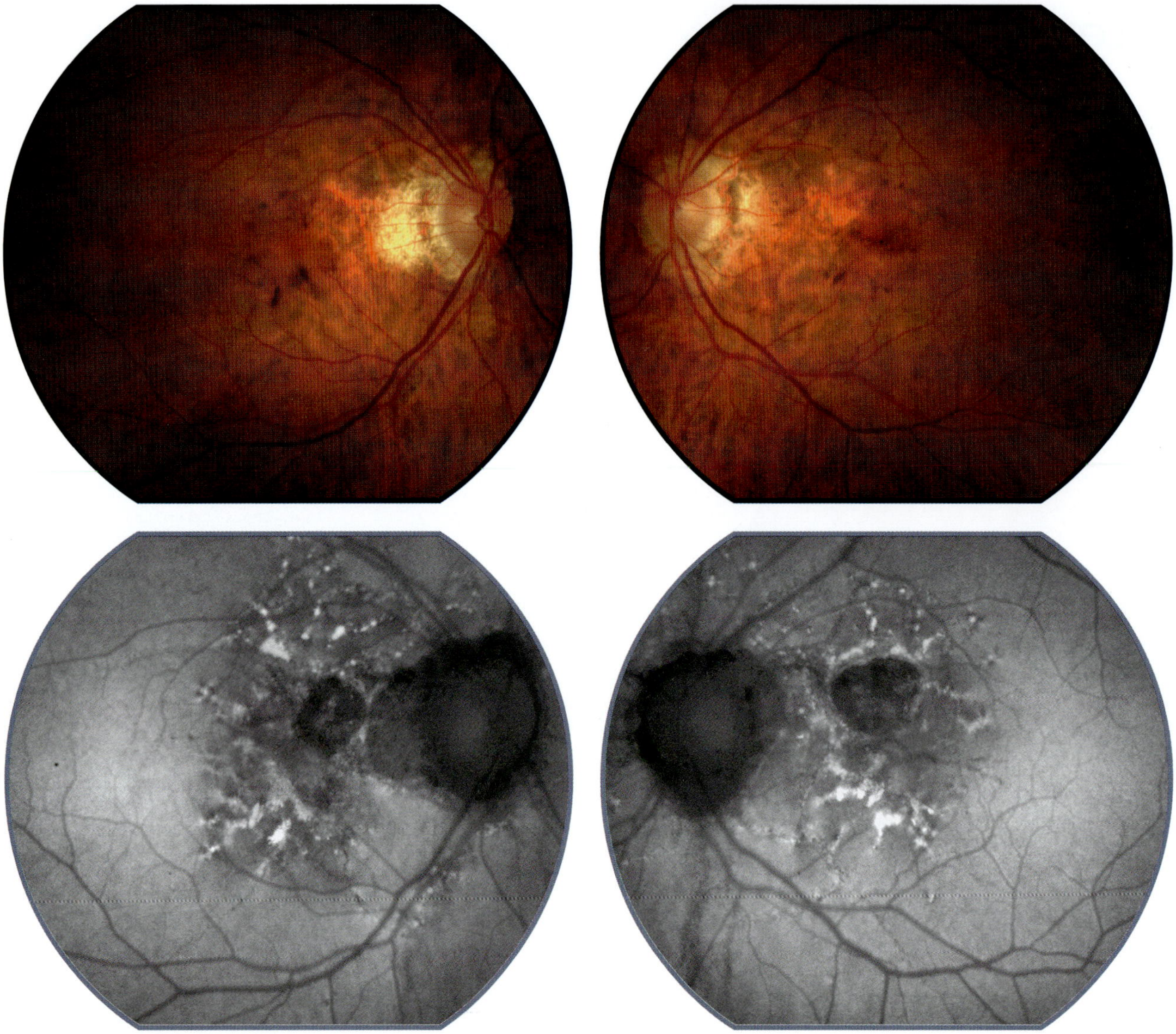

This patient with PXE has atrophy in the posterior pole and a pattern dystrophy-like change on fundus autofluorescence. Note the central as well as peripapillary atrophy in both eyes.

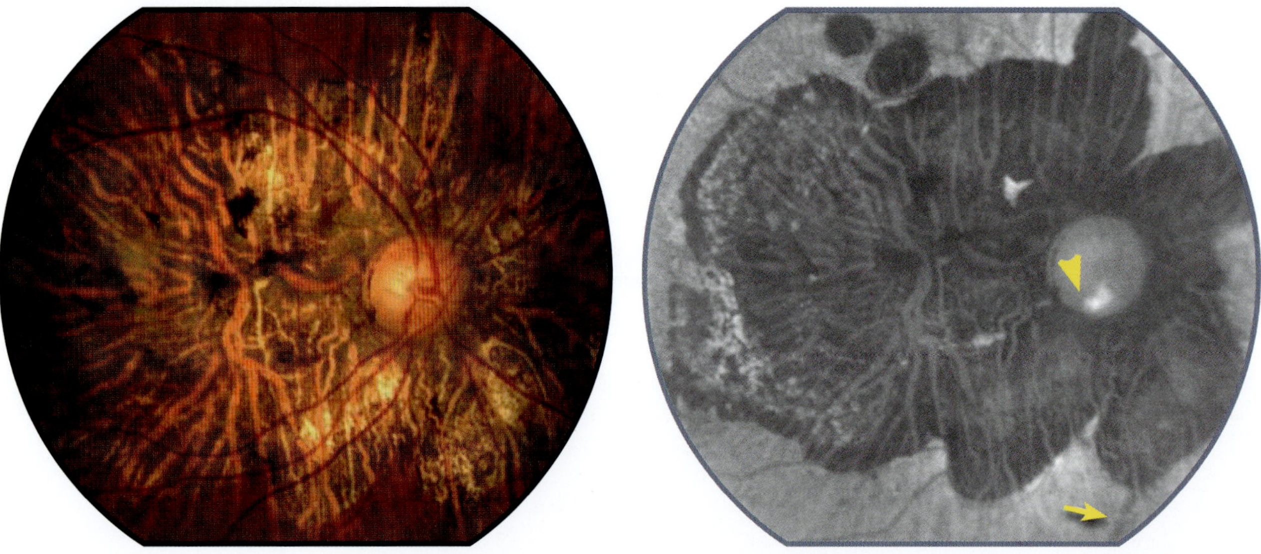

This patient with PXE shows extensive atrophy throughout the posterior pole with hyperpigmentation *(left image)*. Angioid streaks are evident in the near periphery, anterior to the central atrophy *(arrow)*. Note the focal area of hyperautofluorescence on the disc. This corresponds to optic nerve head drusen *(arrowhead)*. Fundus autofluorescence is helpful to detect angioid streaks beyond central atrophy and optic nerve head drusen in PXE.

Subretinal Fluid and Acquired Vitelliform Lesions

Subretinal fluid unrelated to choroidal neovascularization (CNV) may occur in patients with PXE. Subretinal fluid may be found in eyes with no detectable neovascularization or in areas of the fundus remote from neovascular tissue. This form of subretinal fluid is clinically more subtle than the exudation seen with neovascular tissue. The subretinal fluid is thought to accumulate due to RPE dysfunction preceding RPE cell death. It is typically stable over time and shows no change with intravitreal anti-VEGF therapy.

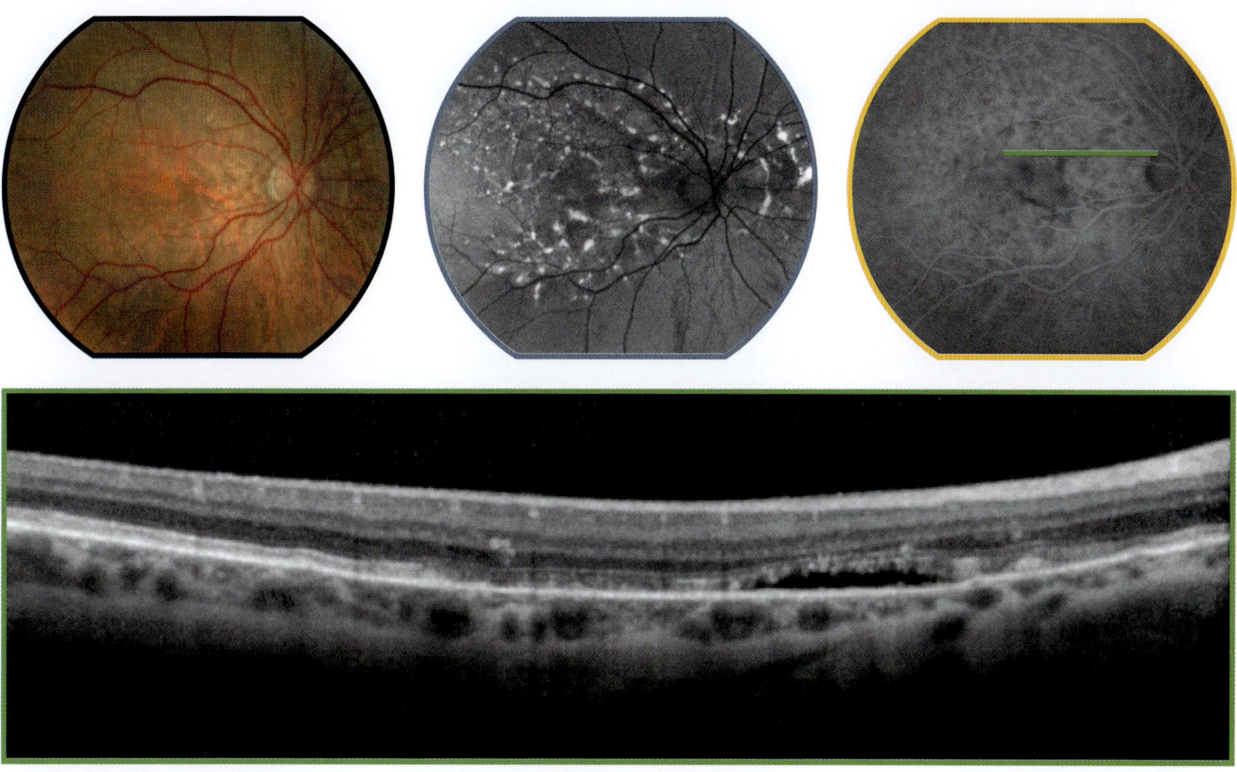

This patient with pattern dystrophy-like changes in the macula, as seen in color photographs and fundus autofluorescence was found to have subretinal fluid on OCT. Fluorescein angiography showed no active leakage and no evidence of CNV.

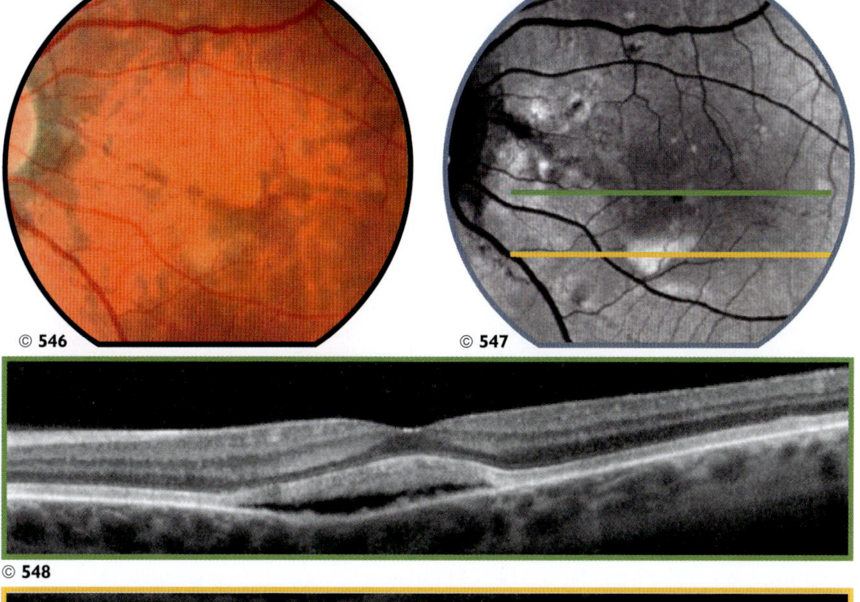

© 546

© 547

© 548

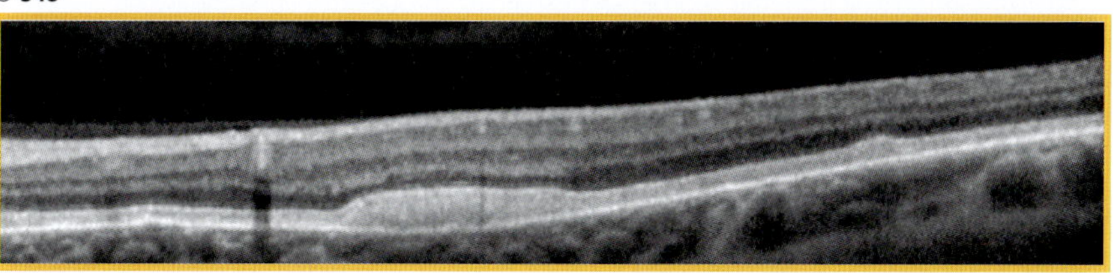

© 549

This color photograph and corresponding fundus autofluorescence shows a localized yellowish material that is hyperautofluorescent. Corresponding OCT shows an acquired vitelliform lesion with fluid accumulating between the ellipsoid zone and the retinal pigment epithelium. PXE is one of the numerous abnormalities that may cause an acquired vitelliform lesion. The acquired vitelliform lesion may occur with or without subretinal fluid and in the absence of CNV. However, there is risk of CNV given the nature of PXE.

Choroidal Neovascularization

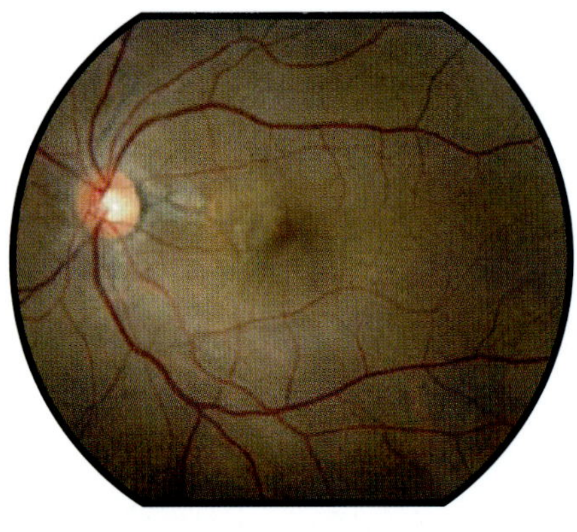
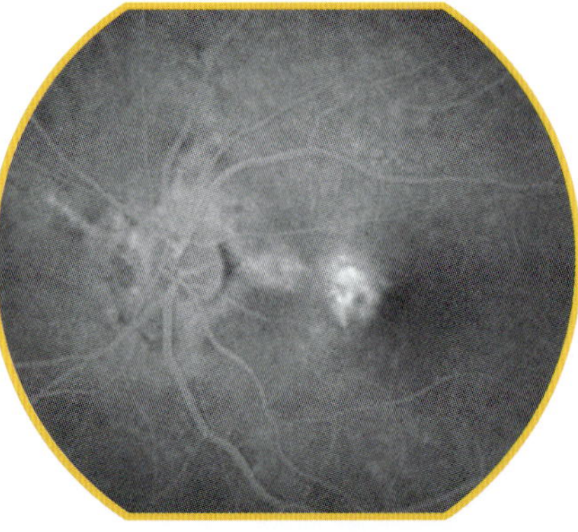
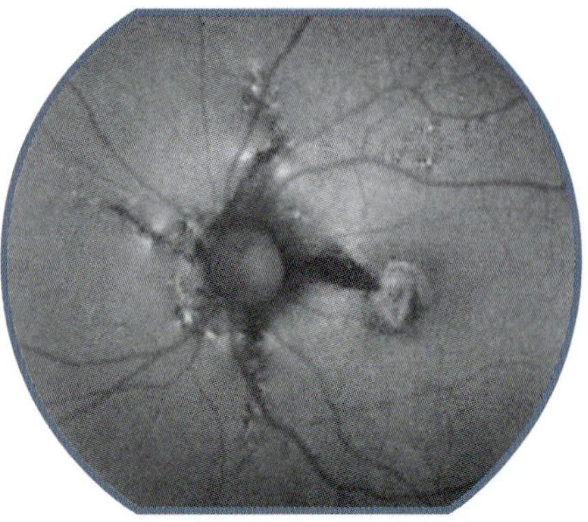

Patients with PXE are at high risk for developing CNV. An estimated 72-86% of patients with angioid streaks may develop CNV. The pathologic new vessels are nearly always type 2 (subretinal), and typically originate from the angioid streaks. Their origin from the streaks is not always visible with fluorescein angiography, but it is more apparent with fundus autofluorescence and/or ICG angiography. In this case, there is subfoveal CNV. Treatment with intravitreal anti-vascular endothelial growth factor therapy will lead to consolidation and regression of the CNV.

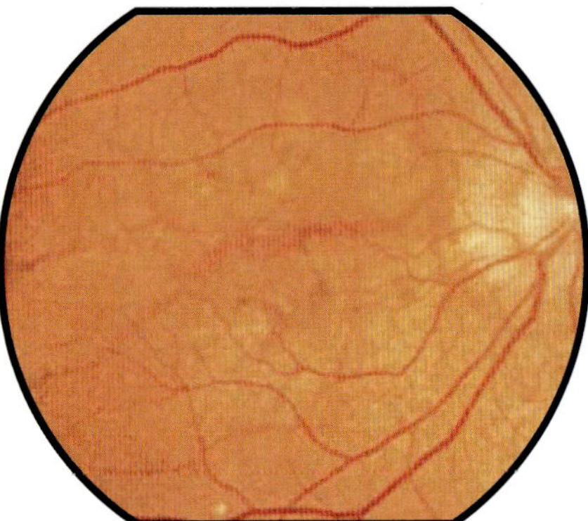
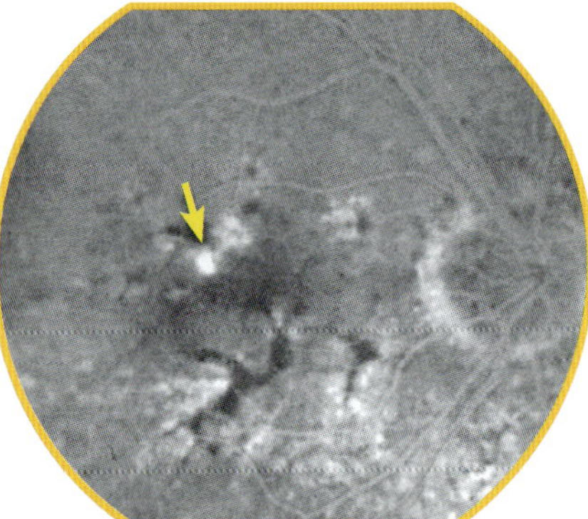
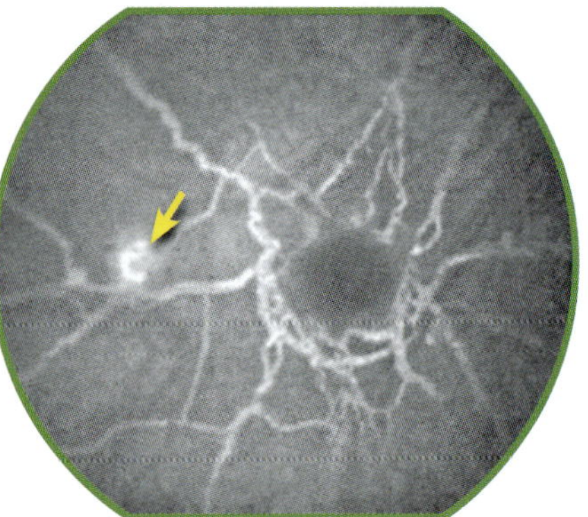

This patient with PXE has angioid streaks and subretinal exudation secondary to CNV. The late-phase fluorescein study shows focal hyperfluorescence corresponding to type 2 neovascularization *(arrow, middle image)*. Some irregular areas of hyperfluorescence and hypofluorescence are consistent with RPE abnormalities, but the angioid streaks are not well visualized on the fluorescein study. The late-phase ICG study demonstrates focal leakage corresponding to CNV *(arrow, right image)*. The radiating irregular hyperfluorescent lines represent the angioid streaks. The CNV is generally noted to occur along the course of one of the angioid streaks.

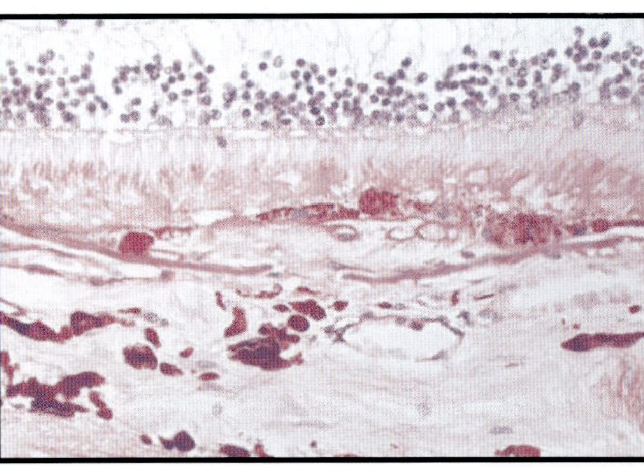
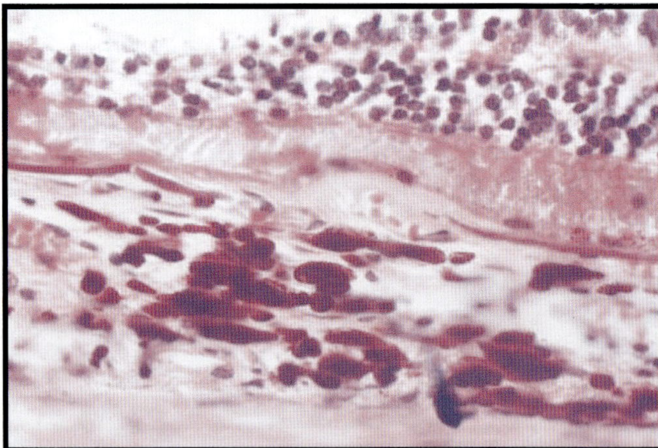

This histopathological specimen of PXE shows fibrovascular tissue originating from the choroid and extending through defects in the Bruch membrane and the overlying retinal pigment epithelium.

Trauma

Patients with PXE are susceptible to intraocular hemorrhages secondary to traumatic rupture of the RPE, Bruch membrane, and choroid. This could be the result of an intrinsic weakness of the Bruch membrane or an associated clotting abnormality in PXE. Patients may present with subretinal or intraretinal hemorrhages overlying the rupture line, which often develop concentric to the disc or, less frequently, in a radial pattern. In time, the hemorrhages clear and may leave a fibrotic scar. The area with the break in the Bruch membrane is at high risk for CNV.

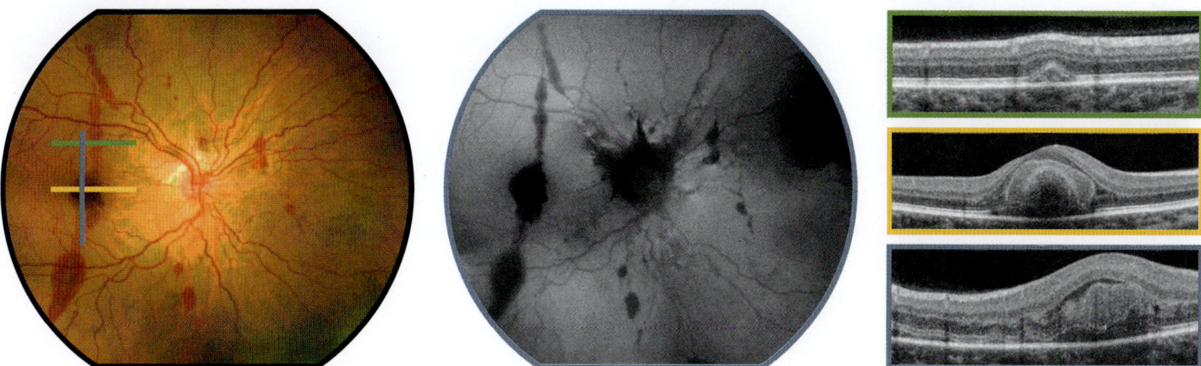

This patient experienced blunt trauma to the right eye from a tennis ball. OCT reveals no visible break in Bruch membrane or choroid. Note that in addition to subretinal hemorrhages, intraretinal hemorrhages may also occur in the outer nuclear layer. *Images courtesy of Dr. Roberto Gallego-Pinazo*

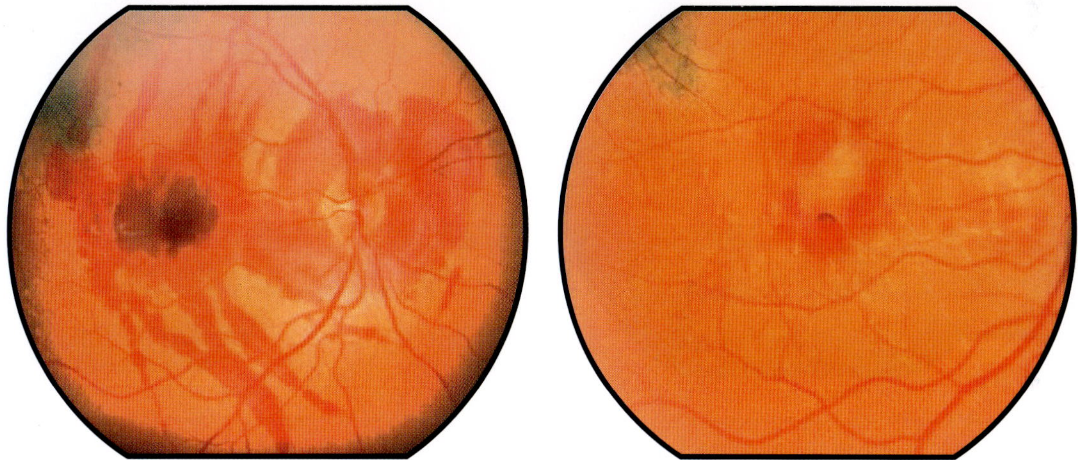

This patient with PXE presented with subretinal hemorrhage in the macular region and around the optic nerve. The blood spontaneously resolved and multiple angioid streaks were revealed. Note that while the *peau d'orange* appearance could be seen temporal to the macula, the angioid streaks were initially obscured by hemorrhage. Later, residual subretinal blood surrounded a localized area of CNV. The *peau d'orange* appearance is not seen in areas of atrophy.

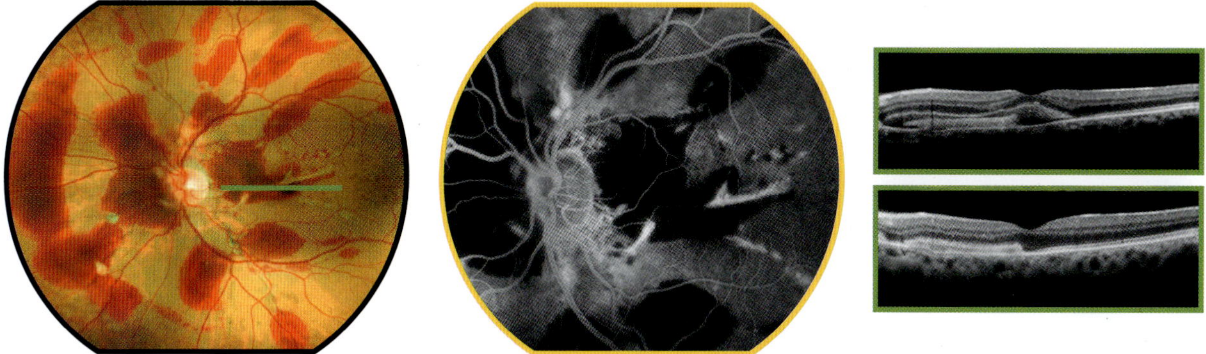

This patient experienced blunt ocular trauma. Note the widespread subretinal hemorrhages with foveal involvement. Fluorescein angiography shows hypofluorescence due to blockage from the hemorrhages and hyperfluorescence due to type 2 neovascularization originating from traumatic ruptures in the macula. OCT *(top right image)* shows hyper-reflective material consistent with type 2 neovascularization and overlying subretinal hemorrhage with a visible break in Bruch membrane. OCT of the same area 3 months later *(bottom right image)* shows resolution of the subretinal hemorrhage but persistence of fibrovascular tissue.

Fibrous Scarring

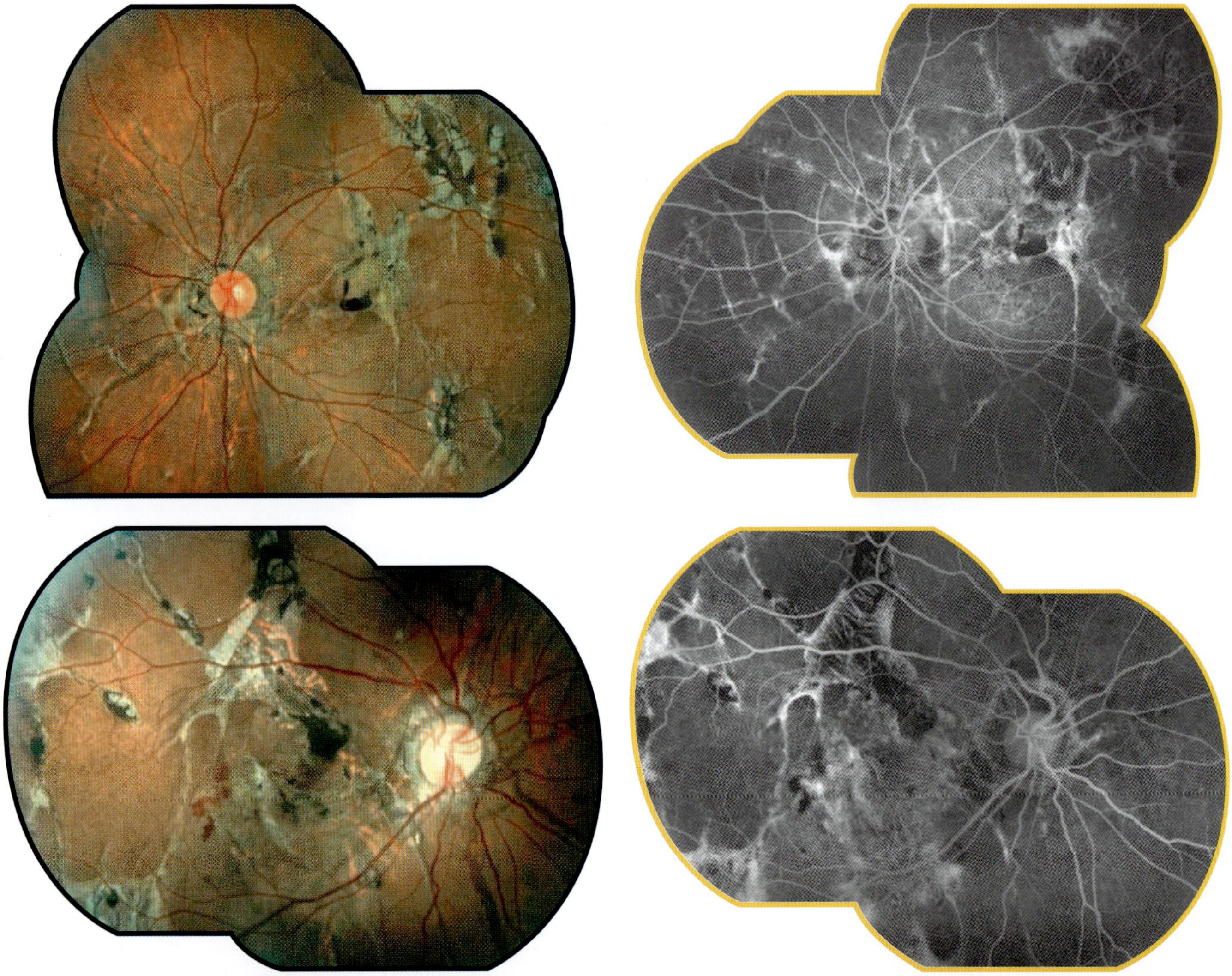

These two patients with PXE experienced severe ocular trauma. Note the widespread choroidal ruptures in conjunction with angioid streaks. There is fibrotic scarring, which is seen as staining on the fluorescein angiogram. There is also considerable pigment epithelial hyperplasia, which is characteristic of eyes with increased fundus pigmentation.

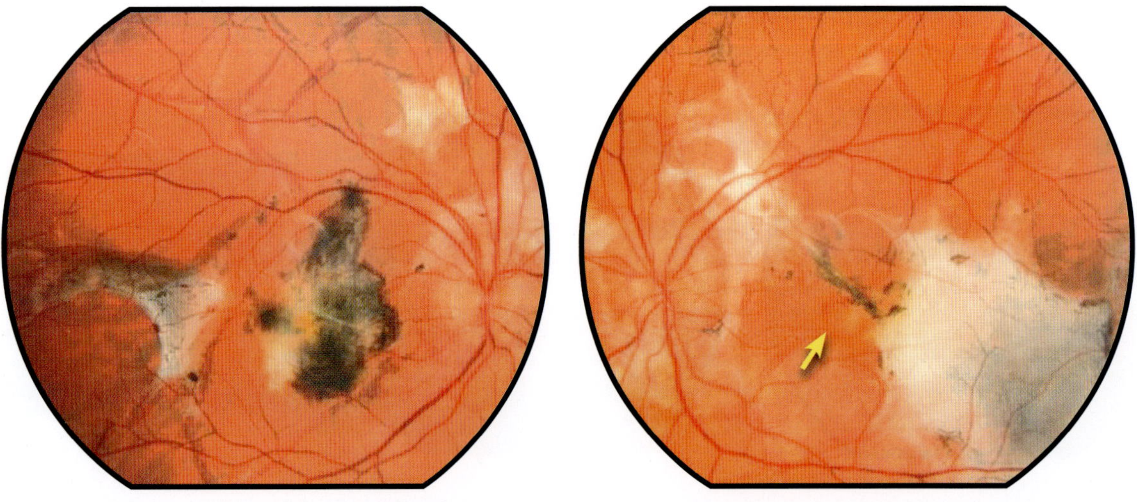

In PXE patients, prior to the availability of intravitreal anti-VEGF therapy, disciform scarring commonly occurred in eyes that developed CNV. This patient with multiple angioid streaks shows extensive scarring from CNV *(left image)*. Another patient with angioid streaks and PXE developed a large disciform scar *(right image)*. Note that the scarring is more fibrotic inferotemporally. In addition, a small area of active CNV with subretinal hemorrhage is present inferior to an island of fibrosis that connects the two larger areas of scarring (*arrow*).

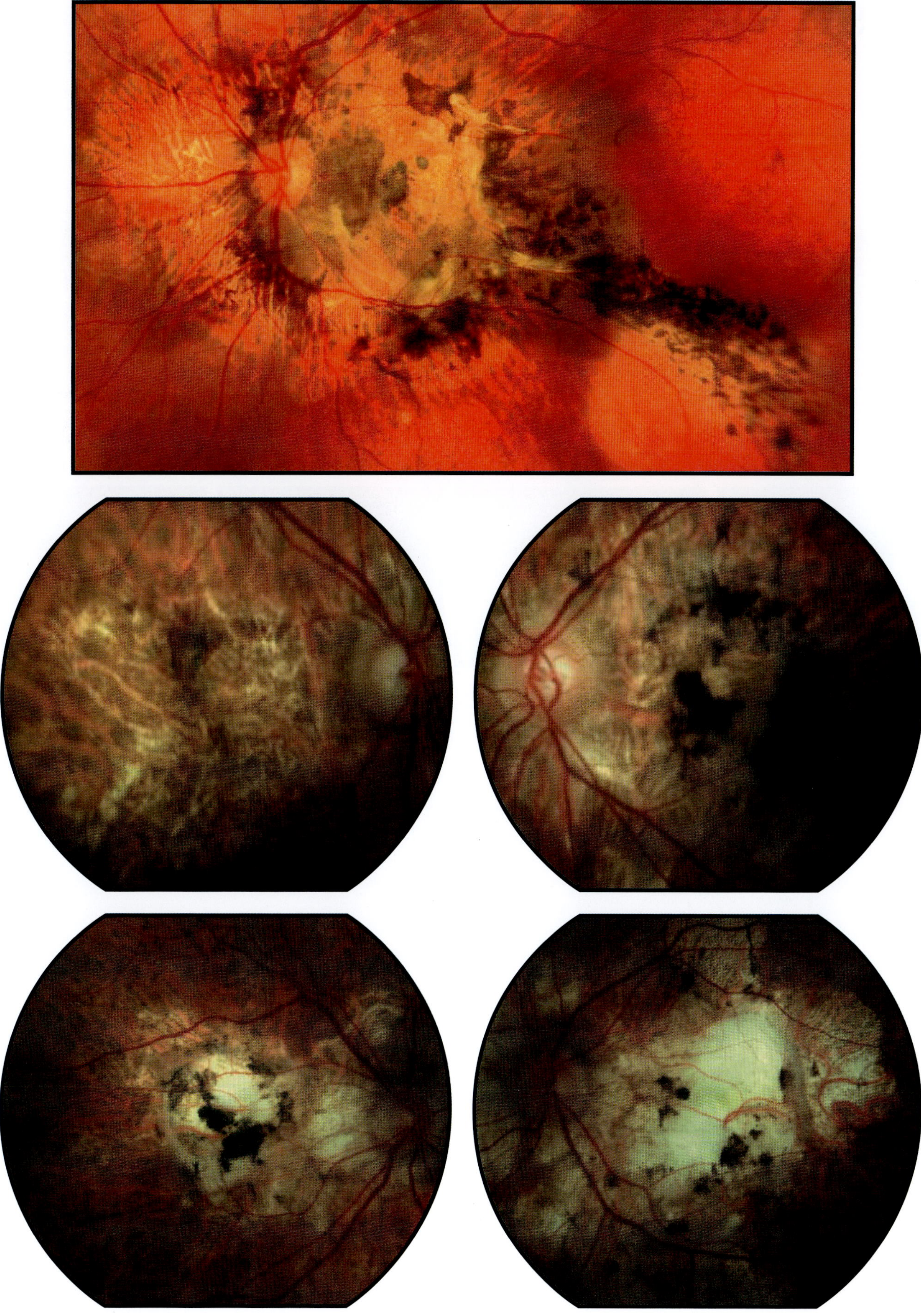

Severe fibrovascular scarring with pigmentation and atrophy may occur as a result of the natural course of this diffuse neovascular maculopathy.

Pathologic Myopia

Pathologic or degenerative myopia is a leading cause of visual impairment worldwide. It is most common in Asia where the prevalence may be more than 10% in certain populations. Although there is no standardized definition, the commonly used criteria include spherical refractive error in excess of –6 D and axial length of greater than 26.5 mm. This entity has been linked to genetic, environmental, and socioeconomic risk factors.

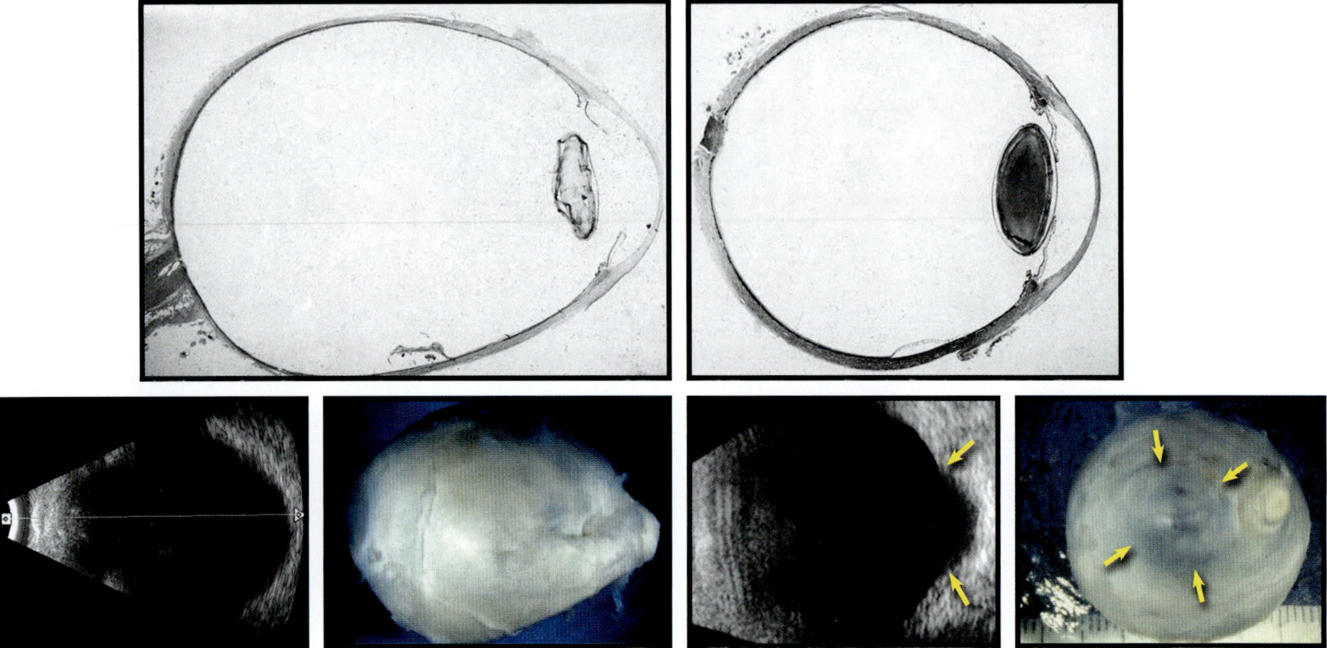

Histological sections of two globes show the difference in size and shape between a pathologically myopic eye *(top left)* and an emmetropic eye *(top right)*. Pathologic myopia may be due to elongation with or without staphylomas (outpouchings of the globe). Ultrasound and pathological specimens of the same eye demonstrate simple elongation *(bottom left two images)* and elongation with a staphyloma *(bottom right two images)*. Arrows demarcate the margins of the staphyloma.

Myopic macular degeneration, often associated with a posterior staphyloma, consists of progressive thinning of the retinal pigment epithelium and choroid, fine yellowish-white breaks in Bruch membrane known as lacquer cracks, subretinal hemorrhages, and secondary CNV. Additional ocular findings in pathologic myopia include macular hole, macular retinoschisis, vitreoretinal interface disturbances, premature PVD, peripheral retinal degeneration, retinal detachment, cataract, and normal-tension glaucoma.

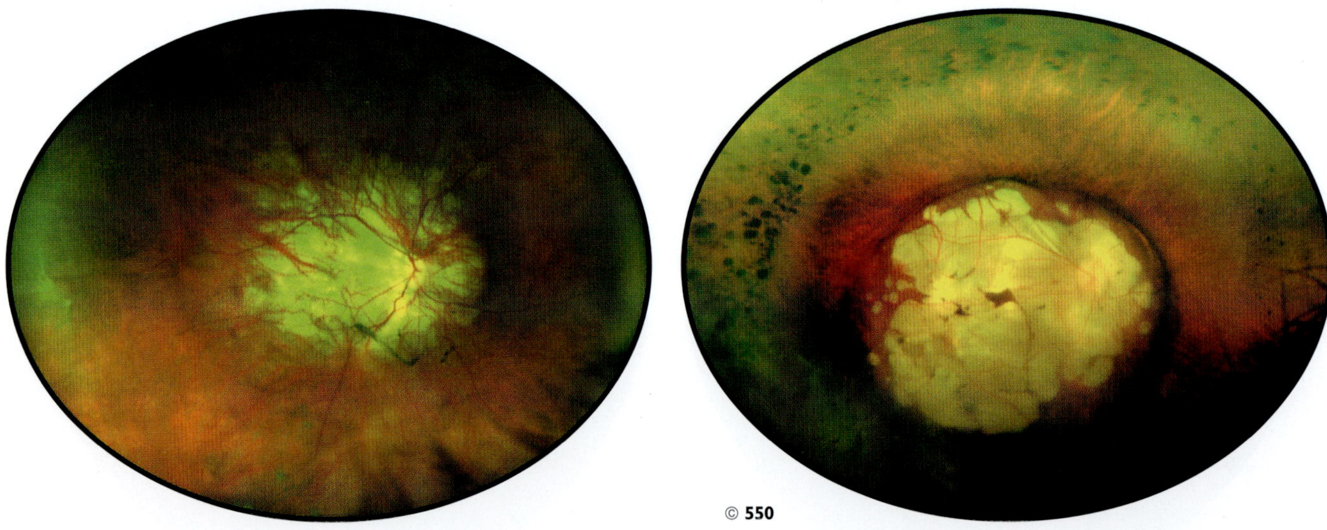

© **550**

The patient on the left has a diffuse staphyloma associated with choroidal thinning and prominent choroidal vessels posteriorly. Fragments of a Weiss ring and vitreous floaters related to a PVD can be seen in the inferior vitreous cavity. The patient on the right is a –34 D myopic male with a well-defined posterior staphyloma associated with chorioretinal atrophy and peripheral pigmentary degeneration.

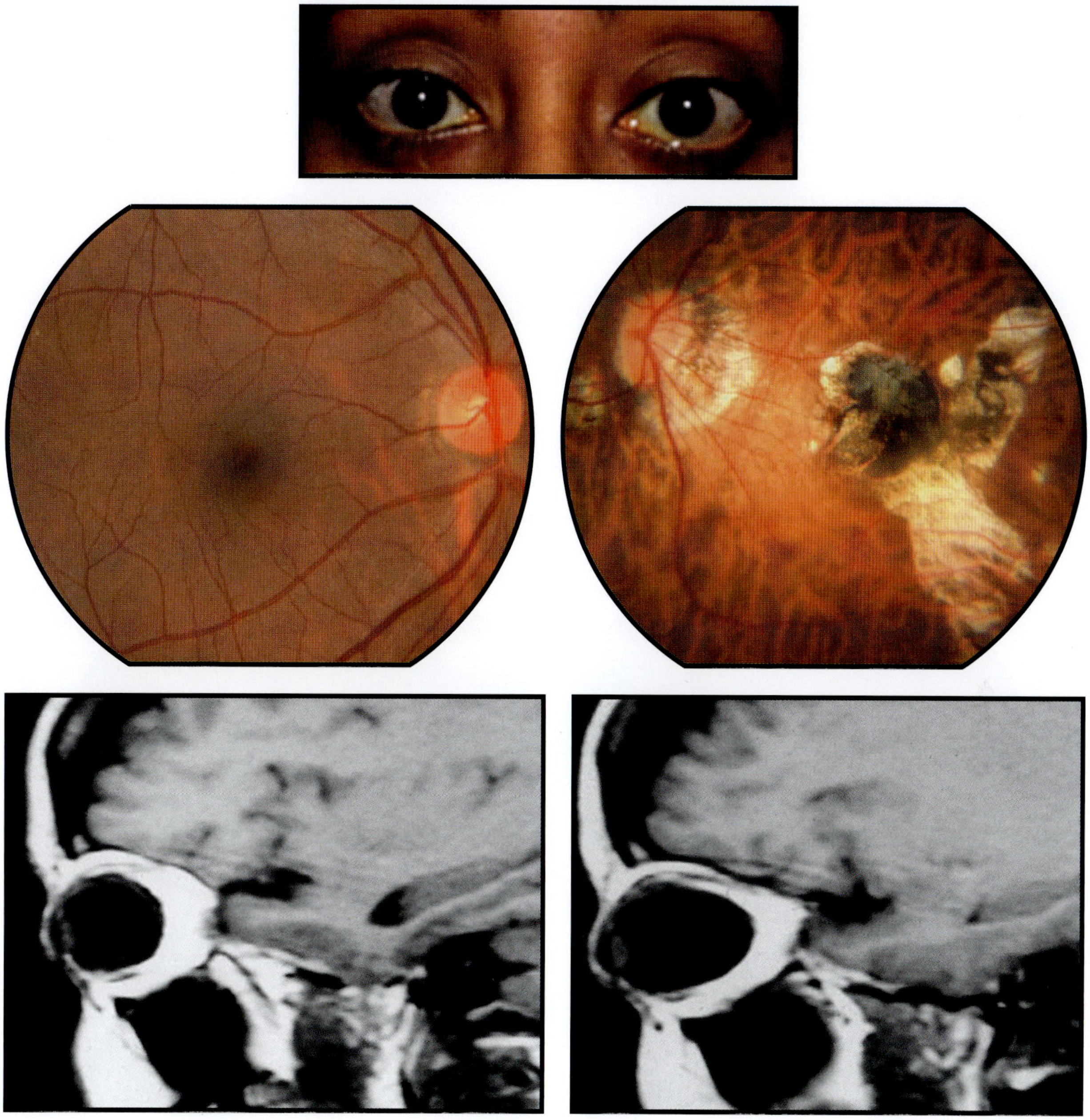

This patient has a high degree of anisometropia with pathologic myopia in her left eye only. There is pseudoexophthalmos of the left eye due to axial elongation of the globe. Note the differences on the clinical photographs of the posterior segments. The right eye is emmetropic with a normal fundus appearance whereas the left eye has RPE thinning and atrophy in addition to a focal area of hyperpigmentation and fibrous proliferation known as a Fuchs spot. MRI scans show the difference in the size and shape of the globes, normal in the right eye *(left image)* and elongated in the pathologically myopic left eye *(right image)*. *Images courtesy of Dr. Jerry Sherman*

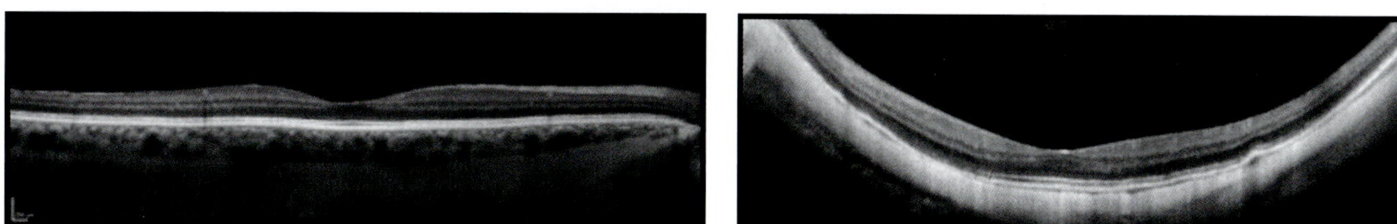

This patient has extreme anisometropia as demonstrated with SD-OCT imaging. Notice the relatively normal choroidal thickness in the right eye and severe choroidal thinning in the left eye, also known as leptochoroid. Leptochoroid, defined as extreme choroidal thinning to less than 20 microns at the subfoveal region, can be compatible with good visual acuity in some patients with high myopia.

Staphyloma

Staphyloma is defined as an outpouching of the ocular wall, the radius of which is less than the surrounding curvature of the globe. The number and location of staphylomas may vary in each eye. Curtin's original classification of staphyloma subtypes used ophthalmoscopic findings and was based on the morphology of irregularities within the staphyloma. However, the advent of OCT imaging has allowed precise visualization of all staphylomatous irregularities within the globe and has resulted in the formulation of a new classification that is based on the morphology of the outermost border of the staphyloma. Staphylomas are now divided into five subtypes.

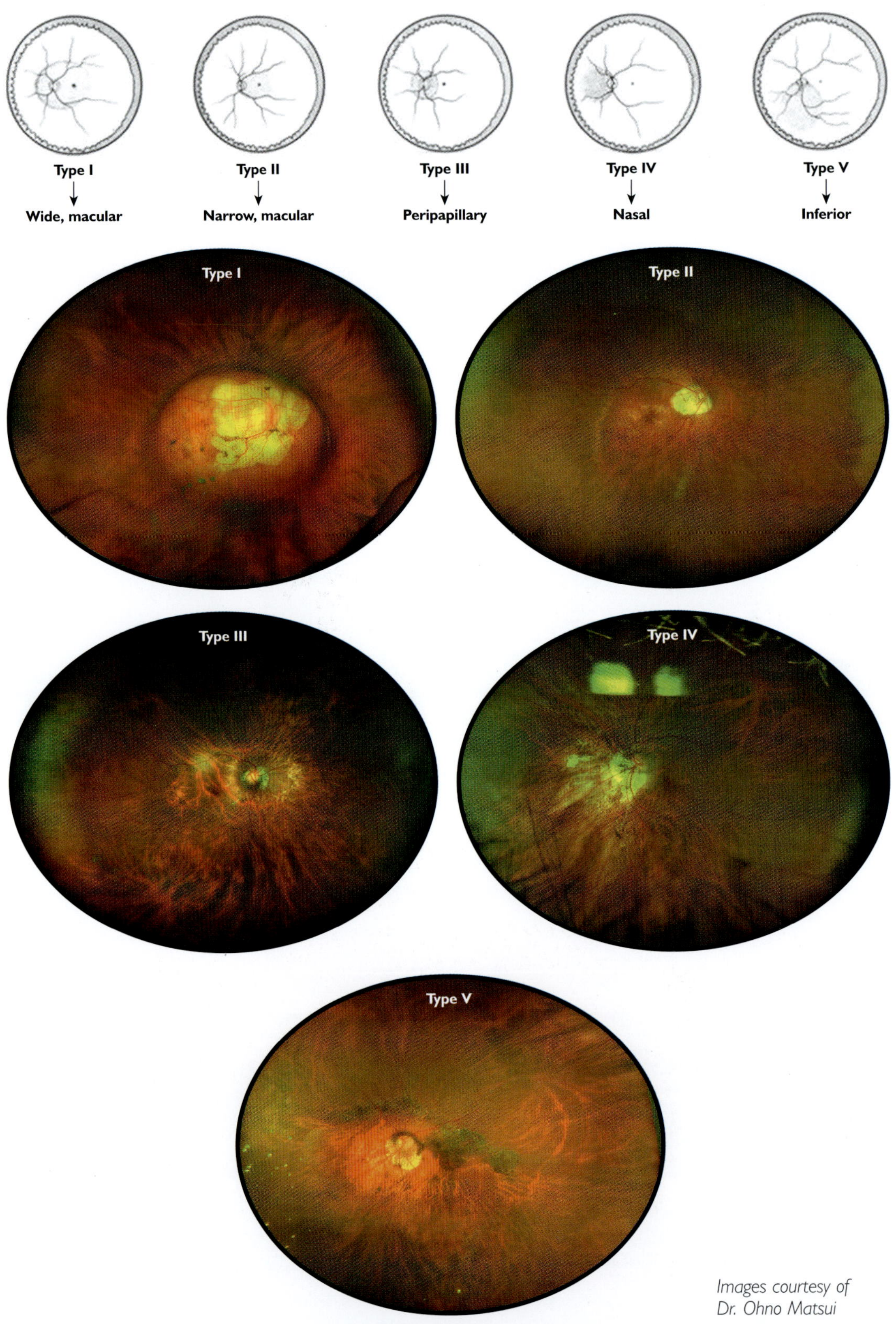

Images courtesy of Dr. Ohno Matsui

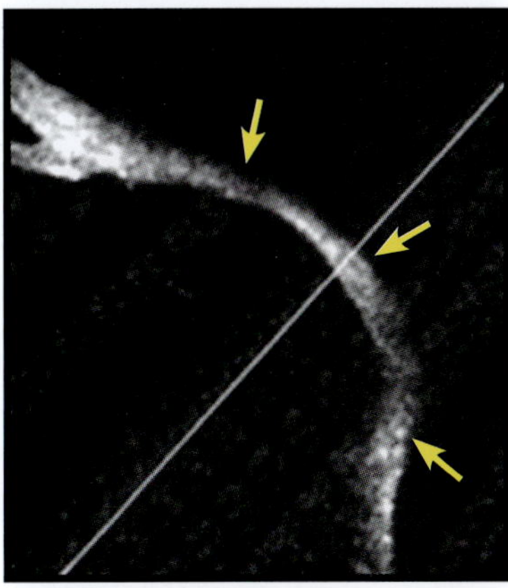

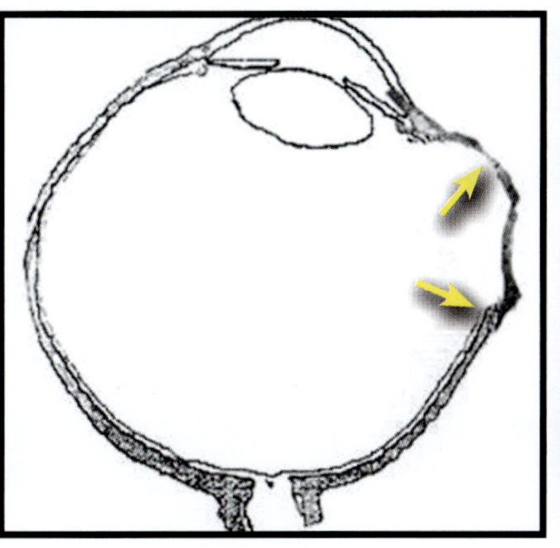

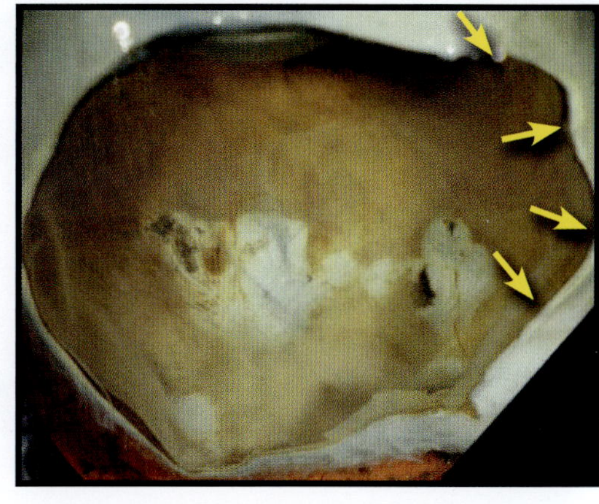

A staphyloma may also occur more anteriorly in the globe. Note the ultrasound *(left image)*, the pathological specimen *(right image)*, and the schematic drawing *(middle image)*, which illustrate the location of this anterior staphyloma *(arrows)*. Eyes such as these are at risk of penetration during retrobulbar injection if the physician is unaware of the presence of such a staphyloma.

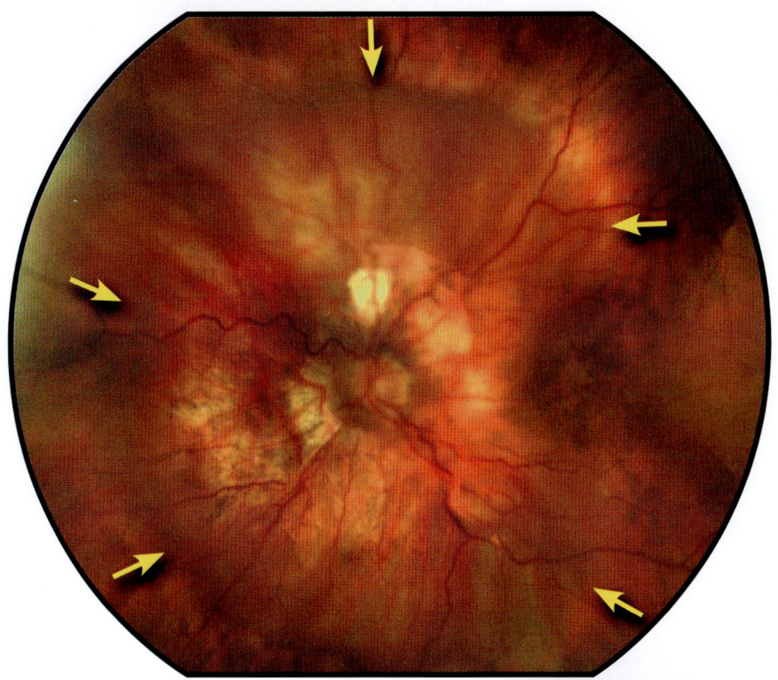

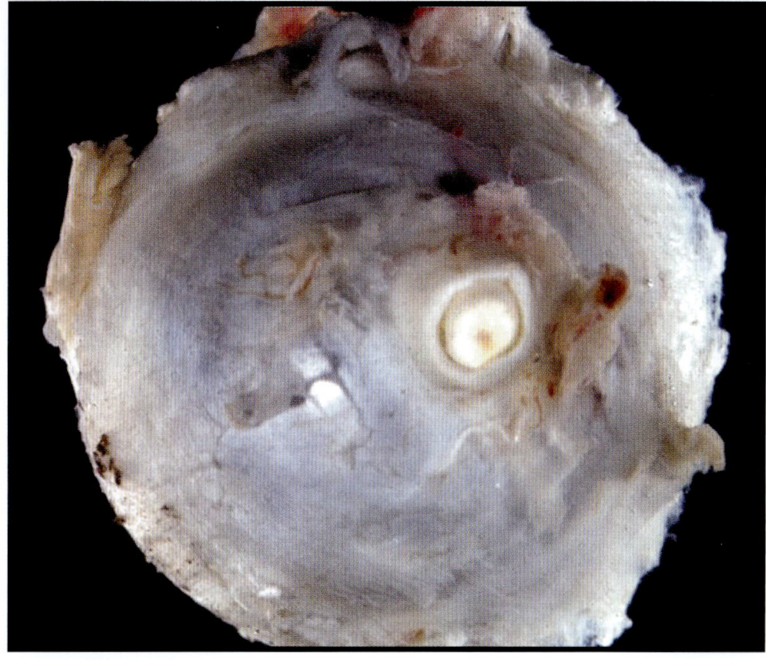

This Type I staphyloma involves the posterior pole *(arrows)*. The post mortem specimen *(right image)* is from a patient with pathologic myopia and shows a similar posterior staphyloma.

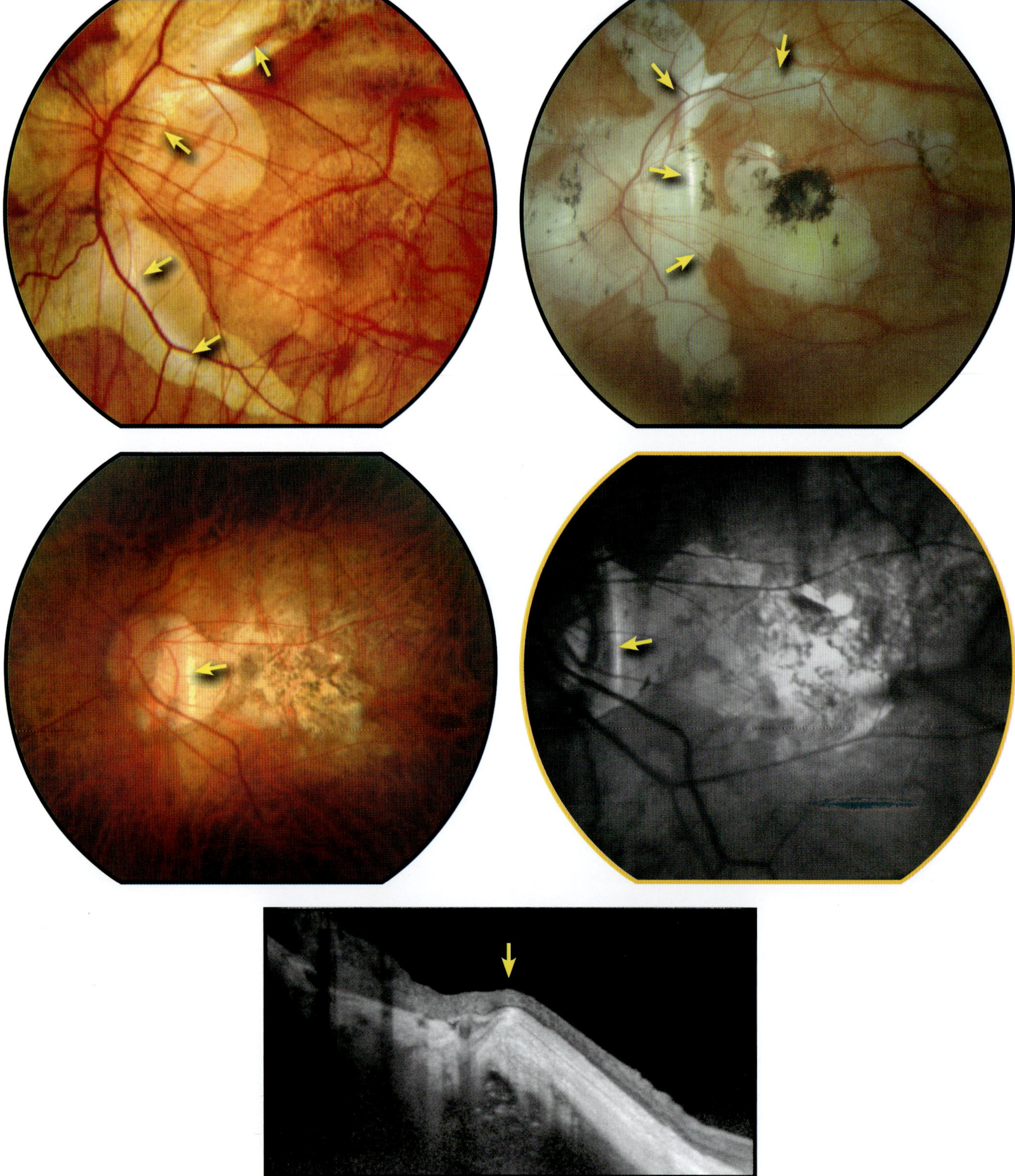

These images show a Type II staphyloma that begins in the temporal juxtapapillary area and extends through the macula. There is RPE atrophy along the temporal vasculature *(top images)*. Notice the bright myopic ridge seen at areas of atrophy that corresponds to the margin of the staphyloma *(middle left image, arrow)*. The bright myopic ridge appears as a hyper-reflective line on both near-infrared reflectance and OCT imaging and corresponds to the sharp angulation of the sclera *(middle right and bottom images)*.

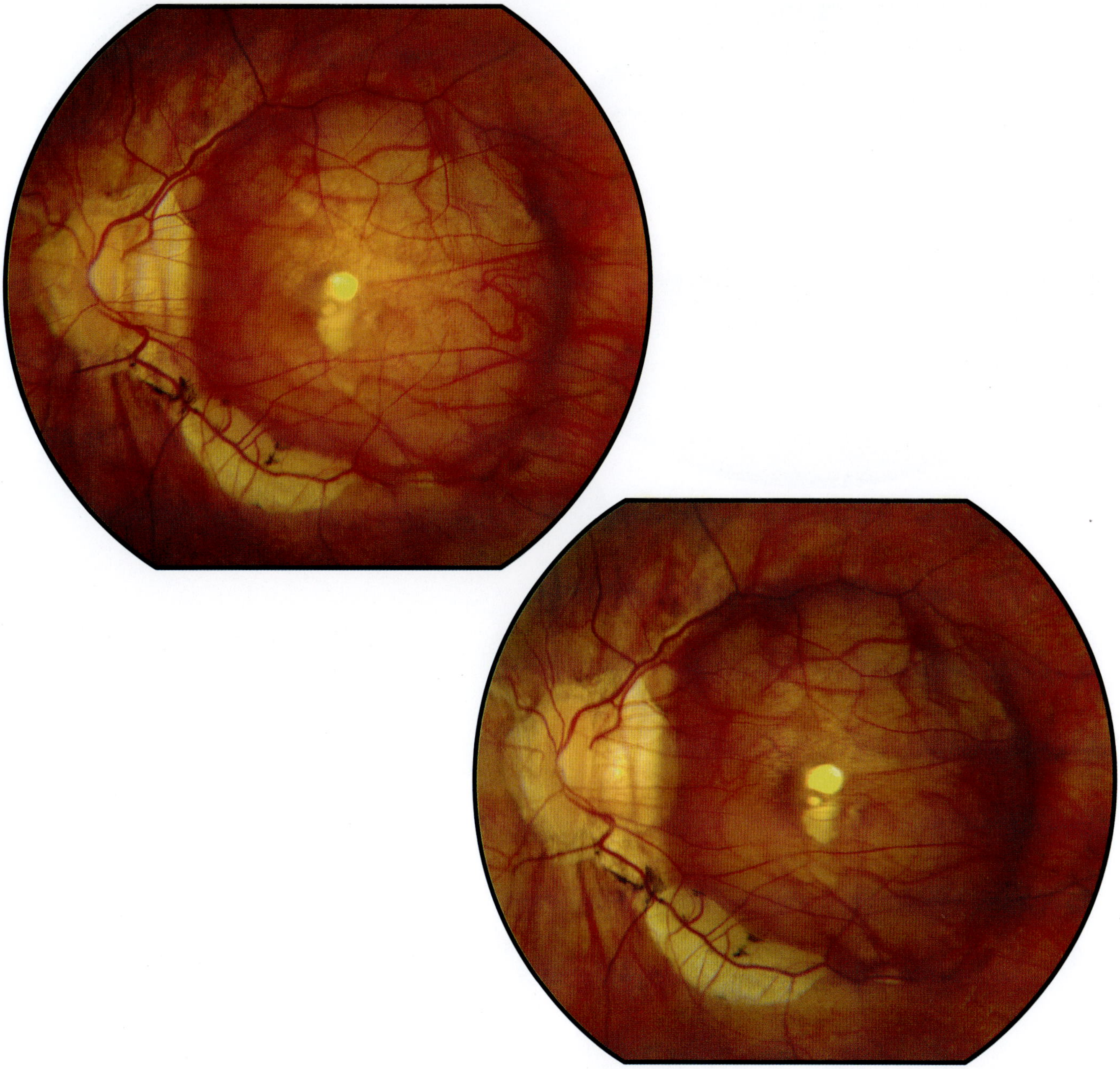

These images are a stereo pair showing an eye with pathologic myopia manifesting a Type II staphyloma involving most of the macula. There is a zone of atrophy along the inferior temporal vasculature that may represent a pigment epithelial tear.

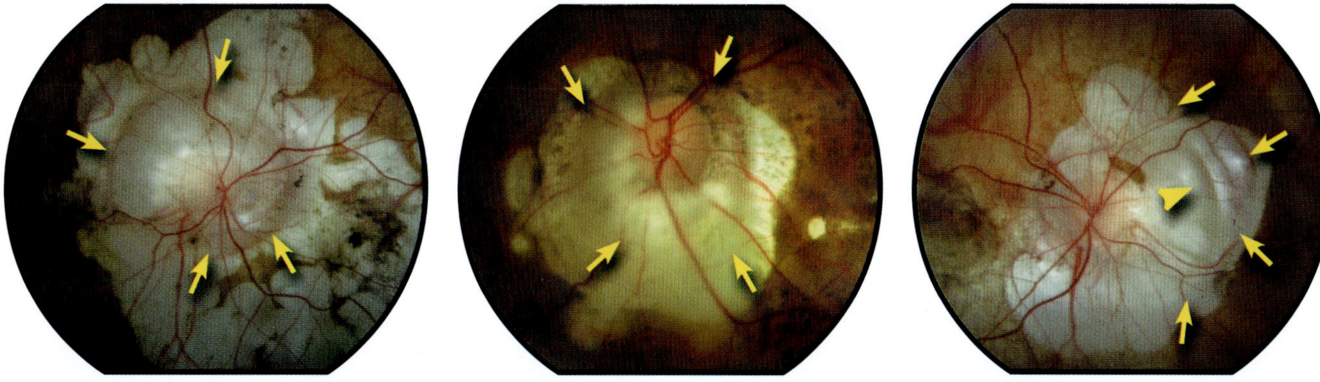

These three patients have Type III posterior staphylomas with bulges surrounding the nerve. The bright myopic ridges help to demarcate the edge of the staphyloma *(arrows)*. The image on the right shows undulating folds within the staphyloma *(arrowhead)*, most probably due to progressive elongation within the bulge of the staphyloma. *Images courtesy of Marian McVicker*

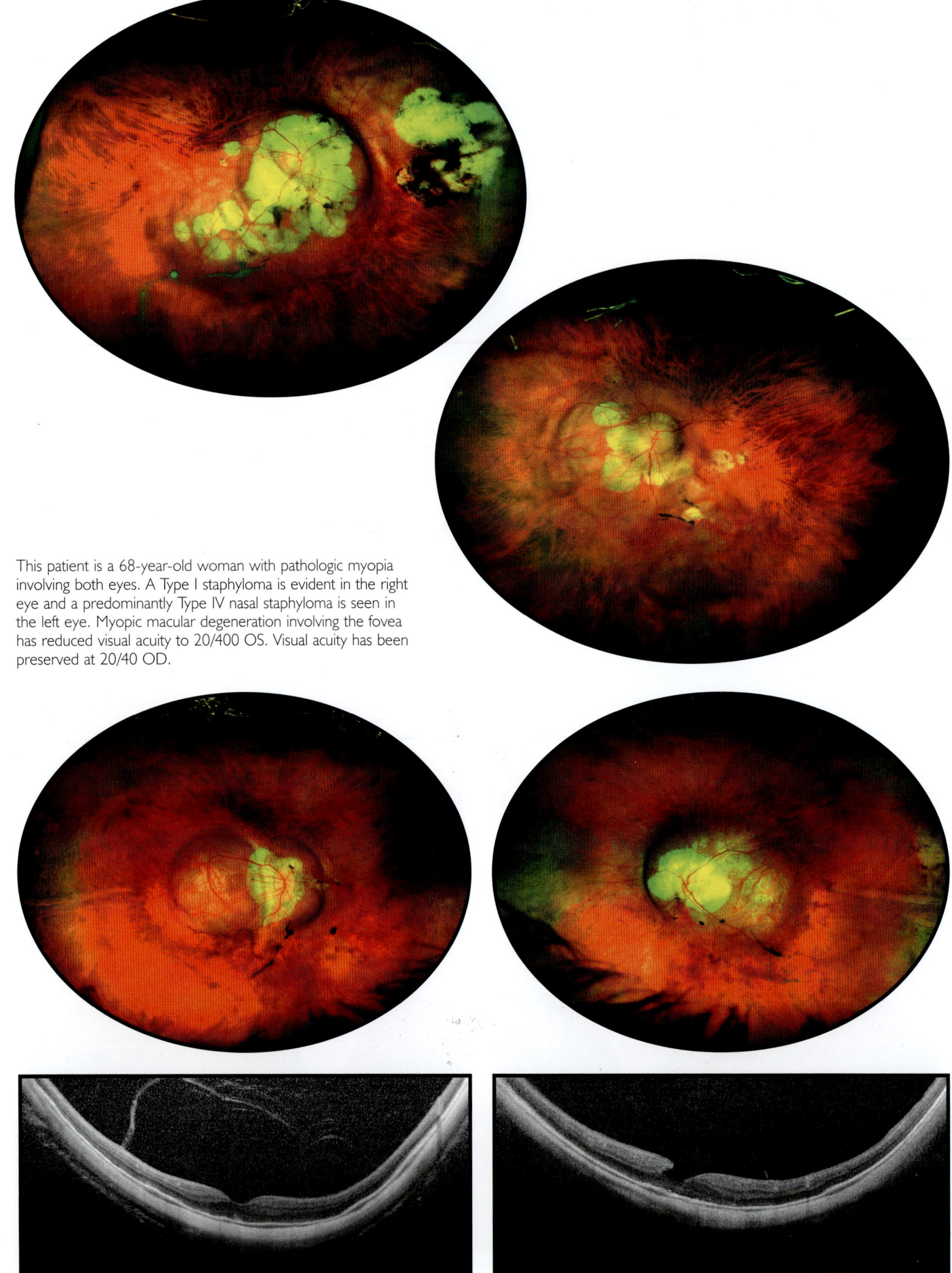

This patient is a 68-year-old woman with pathologic myopia involving both eyes. A Type I staphyloma is evident in the right eye and a predominantly Type IV nasal staphyloma is seen in the left eye. Myopic macular degeneration involving the fovea has reduced visual acuity to 20/400 OS. Visual acuity has been preserved at 20/40 OD.

This patient is a 63-year-old female with a Type II staphyloma in the right eye and a Type I staphyloma in the left eye. A lamellar macular hole is evident in the left eye on spectral domain optical coherence tomography imaging. Visual acuity is 20/30 OU.

Radial Tracts and Myopic Staphyloma

A linear or leaf-like emanation that arises from the posterior edge of the staphyloma is seen in approximately 8% of eyes with a myopic posterior staphyloma. As illustrated in the case below, these tracts *(yellow arrows)* demonstrate clinical features that are comparable to descending tracts in central serous chorioretinopathy; however, they commonly have an anti-gravity orientation. They are proposed to represent sites of previous or existing serous retinal detachment due to RPE injury at the abrupt edge of the staphyloma. The changes in globe curvature are best appreciated on three-dimensional MRI images. OCT images of these regions often demonstrate outer retinal and RPE disruption. (The orientation and site of OCT imaging is represented by the blue arrow.)

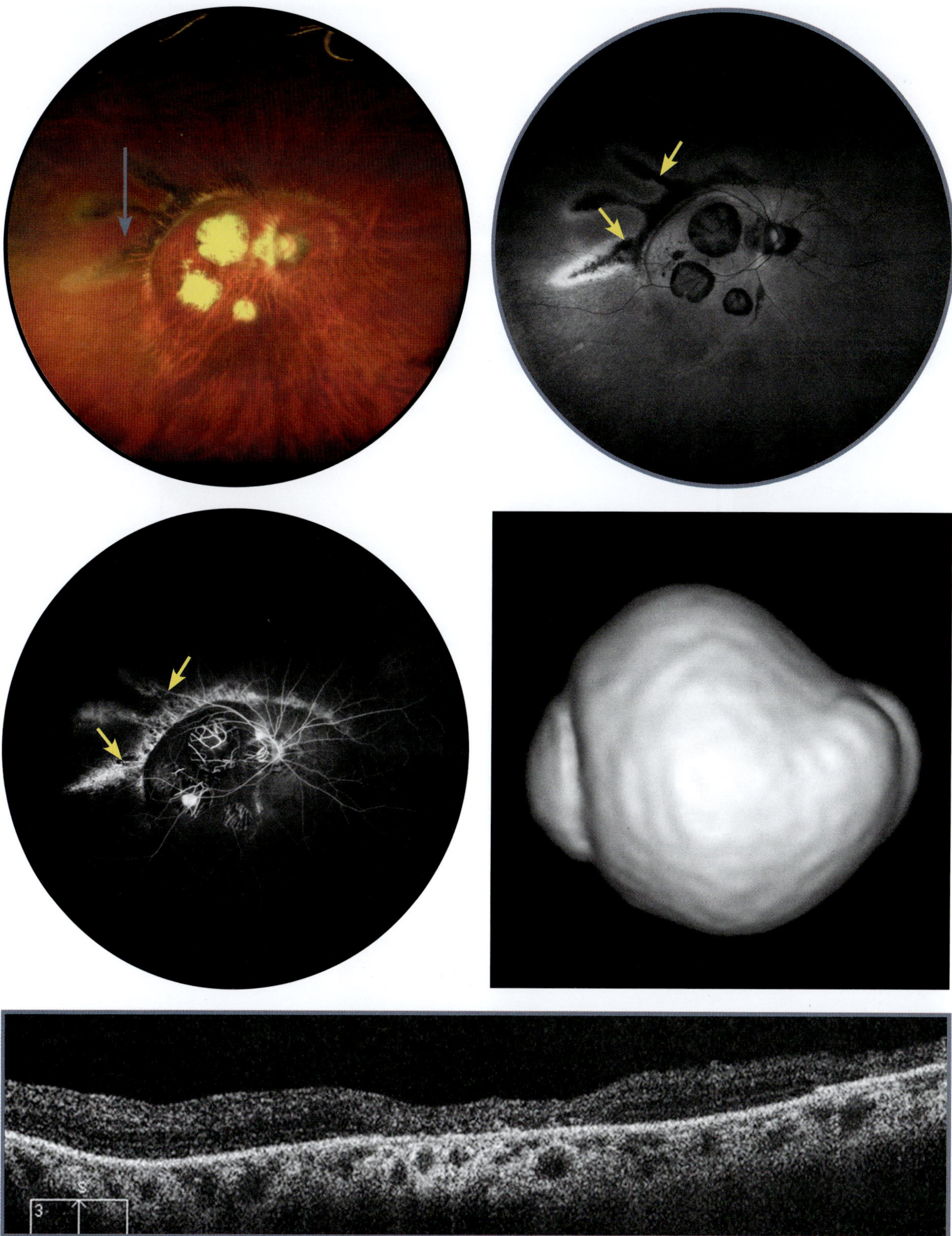

Images courtesy of Dr. Ohno Matsui

Dome-Shaped Macula

Dome-shaped macula (DSM) is a morphological feature recently described using OCT. This entity is characterized by an inward convexity of the macula that, in the majority of cases, is associated with high myopia, but can also be found in eyes with hypermetropia, inherited retinal dystrophies, and central serous chorioretinopathy. The cause is unknown although it is postulated to be related to a localized increase in scleral thickness in the area of the DSM and could be due to the process of ocular expansion in myopia. Macular complications of DSM include CNV in 12% of eyes. Localized serous macular detachment without CNV is found in up to 44% of eyes at the top of the DSM, possibly due to choroidal outflow obstruction by a thick sclera and/or abrupt changes in choroidal thickness. Extrafoveal schisis is found in 18%; however, foveal schisis is uncommon suggesting that DSM may be protective against the development of foveal schisis.

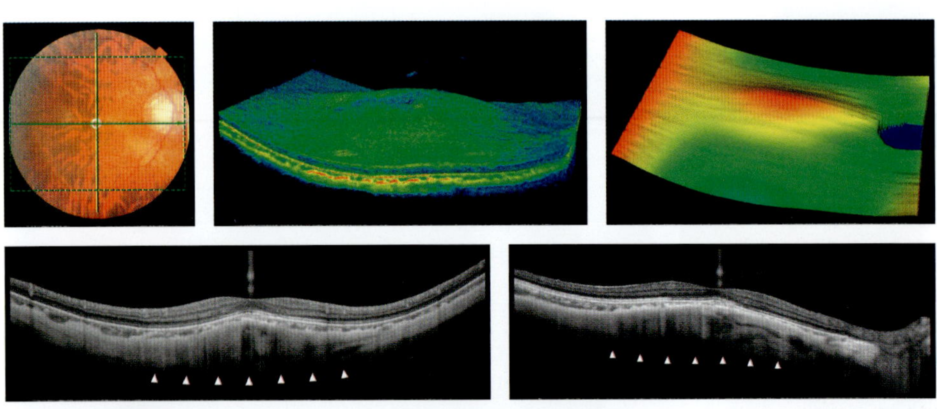

OCT imaging with three-dimensional reconstruction shows the macular bulge of DSM and demonstrates that persistence of a nearly normal scleral thickness at the macular region and scleral-choroidal thinning of the surrounding staphyloma cause the inner protrusion of the macula. *Images courtesy Dr. Ohno Matsui*

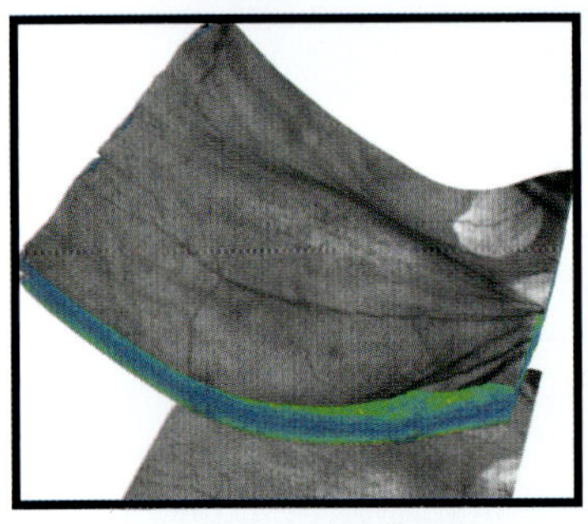

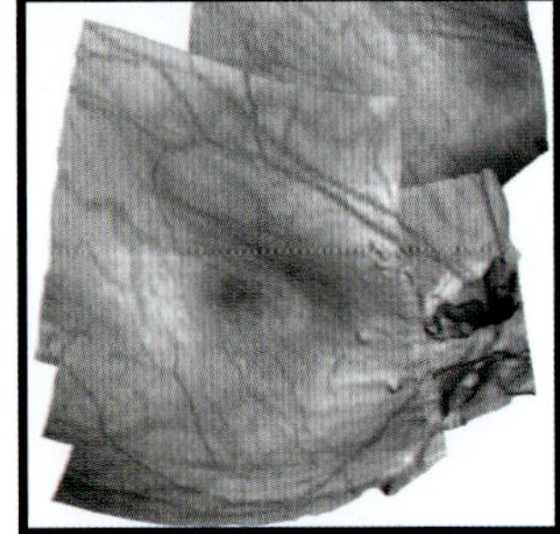

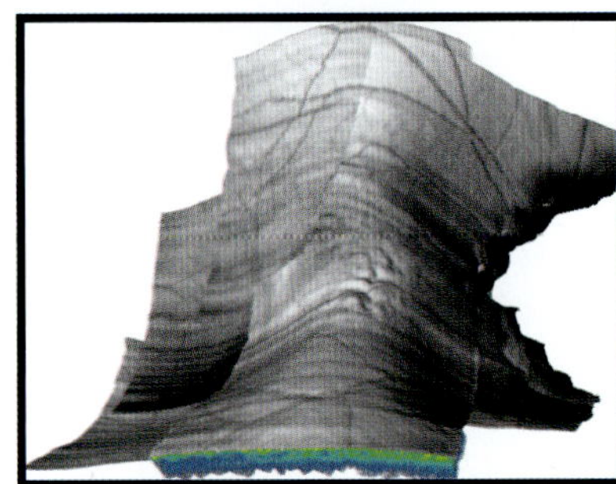

© **551**

The dome of DSM is most commonly horizontal-oval in shape *(left image)*, but may assume a round *(middle image)* or vertical-oval shape *(right image)*. The diagnosis may be easily missed if OCT scans are not done in both horizontal and vertical directions.

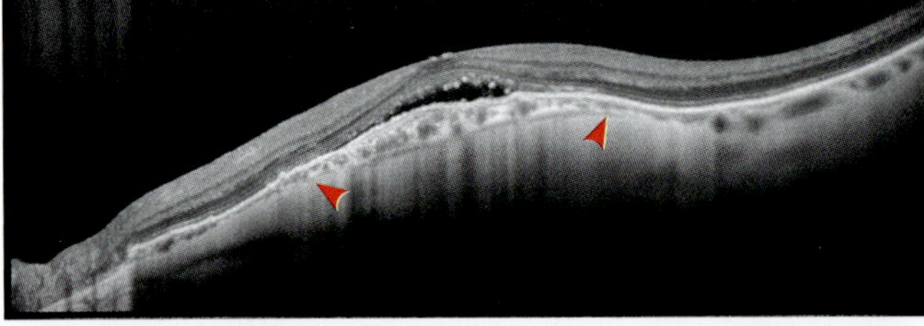

Serous retinal detachment, without CNV can be associated with DSM *(left image)*. Notice how the choroidal thickness changes abruptly at the borders of the dome *(arrows)*, possibly contributing to choroidal outflow obstruction.

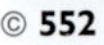

© **552**

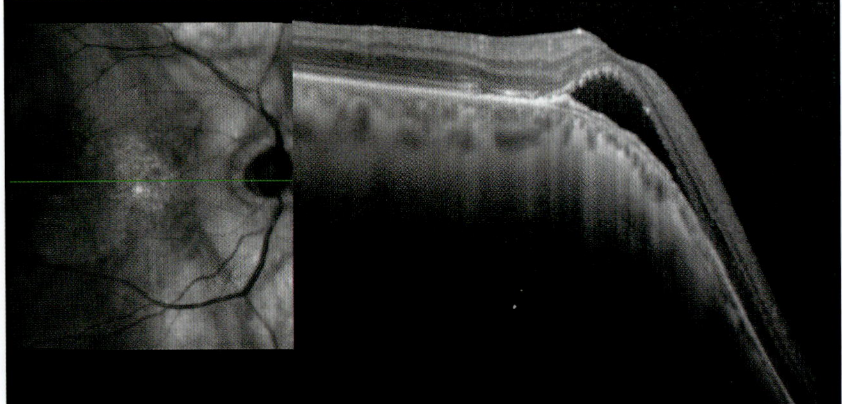

Similar OCT findings may be seen at the superior edge of the inferior staphyloma in the tilted disc syndrome. *Images courtesy of Dr. Suzanne Yzer*

Myopic Macular Degeneration

Patients with pathologic myopia may develop severe vision loss from retinal atrophy and CNV. These changes commonly occur in the central macula within a posterior staphyloma. The atrophy progresses insidiously whereas the neovascularization and resulting disciform scarring may produce sudden loss of central vision.

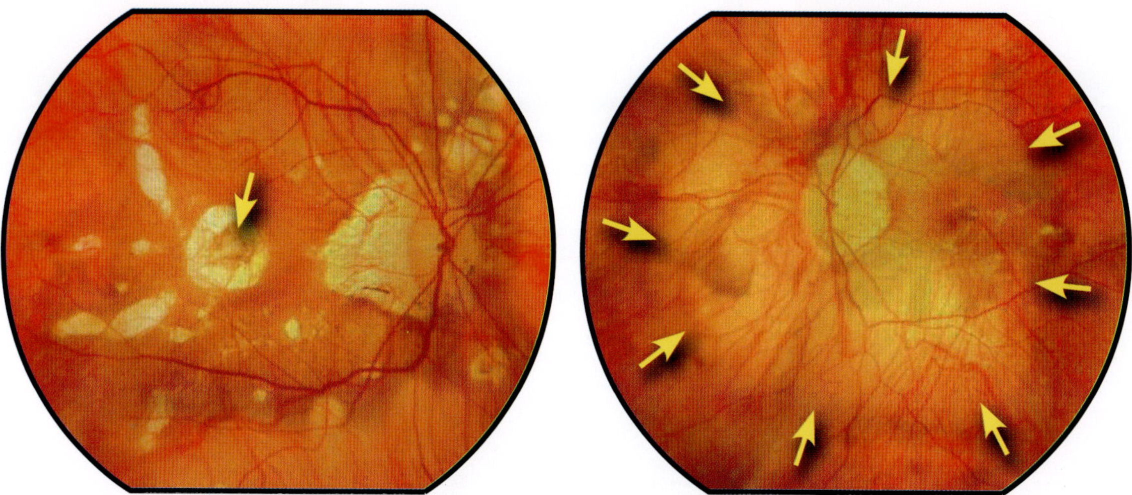

This patient has bilateral pathologic myopia with multifocal atrophy. A disciform scar *(left image, arrow)* is seen with surrounding atrophy in the right eye. Diffuse RPE hypopigmentation is apparent in the left eye within the staphyloma *(right image, arrows)*.

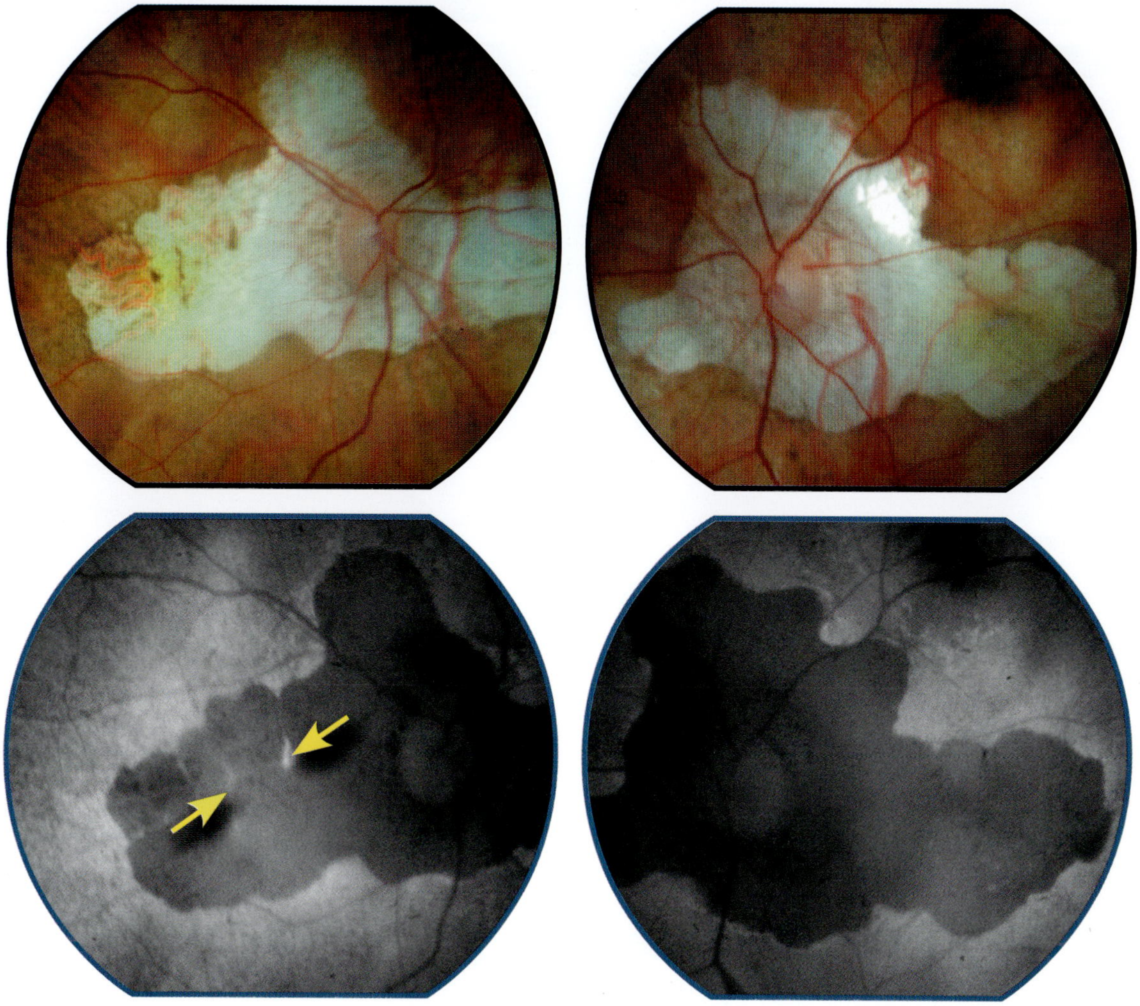

Fundus autofluorescence is useful in delineating the degree of atrophy, as illustrated in this patient. In the right eye there are two islands of preservation in the central macula *(arrows)*, accounting for a slightly better acuity compared to the left eye.

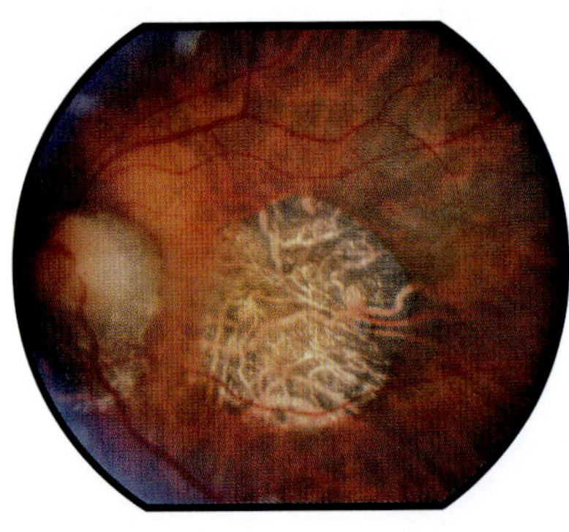
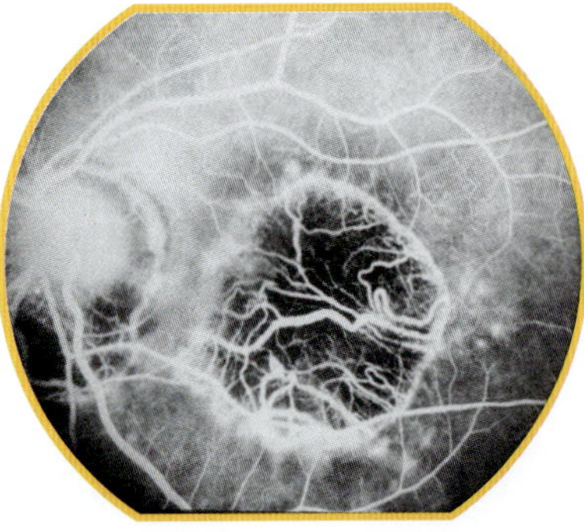
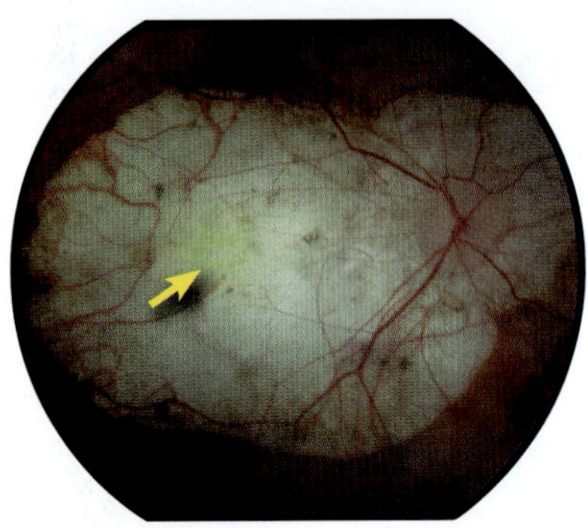

Geographic atrophy in pathologic myopia may be limited to the posterior pole *(left and middle images)* or diffusely involve the peripapillary area and central macula *(right image)*. The right image also shows some yellowish discoloration from macular luteal pigment *(arrow)* and pronounced atrophy of the choriocapillaris and the retinal pigment epithelium.

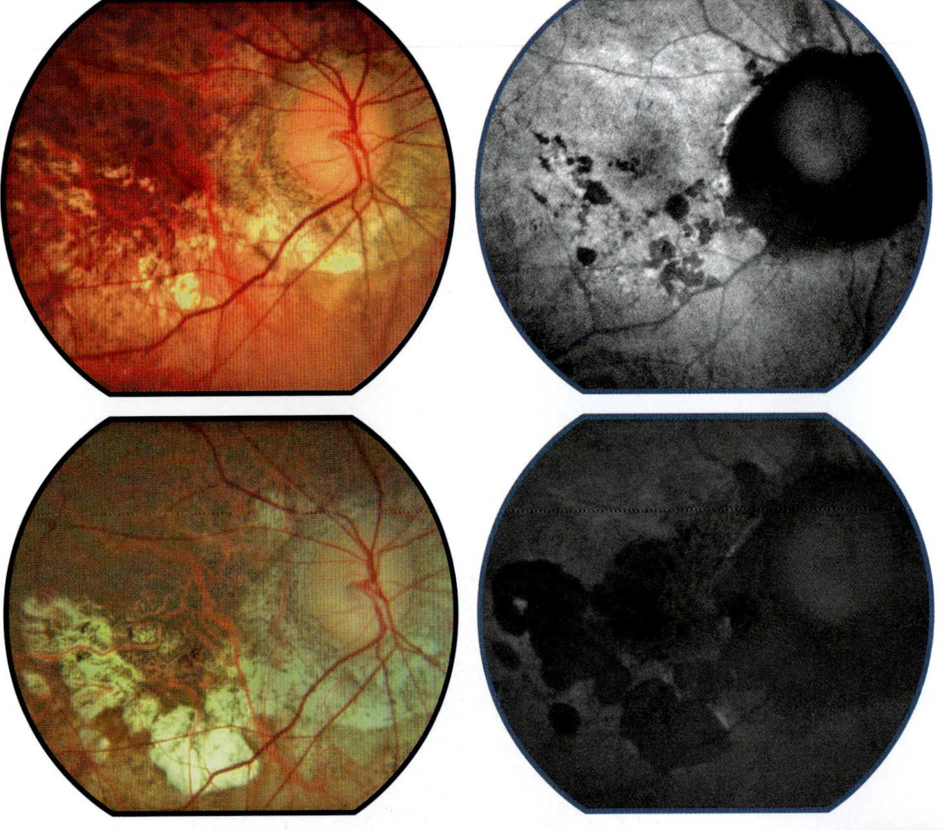

Progressive atrophy in a patient with pathologic myopia can be monitored with fundus autofluorescence imaging. The top two images show the early stages of atrophy (visual acuity 20/50). Eighteen months later *(bottom two images)* visual acuity fell to 20/100 due to the progressive enlargement of the areas of atrophy.

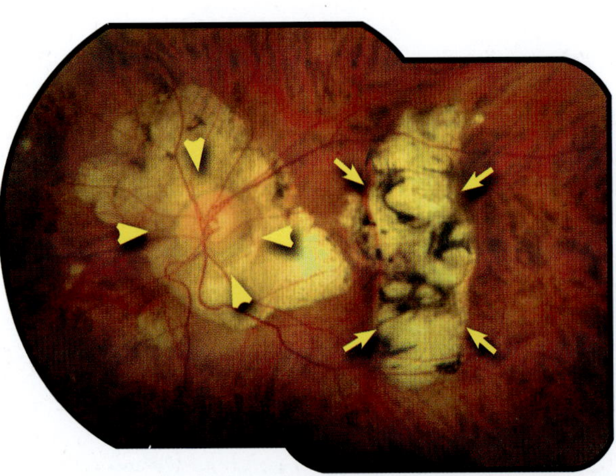

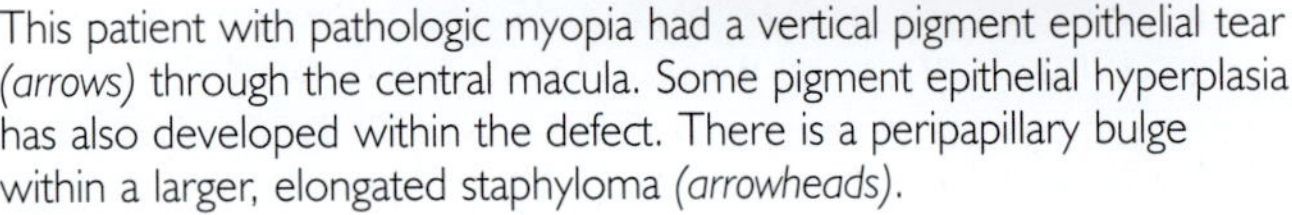

This patient with pathologic myopia had a vertical pigment epithelial tear *(arrows)* through the central macula. Some pigment epithelial hyperplasia has also developed within the defect. There is a peripapillary bulge within a larger, elongated staphyloma *(arrowheads)*.

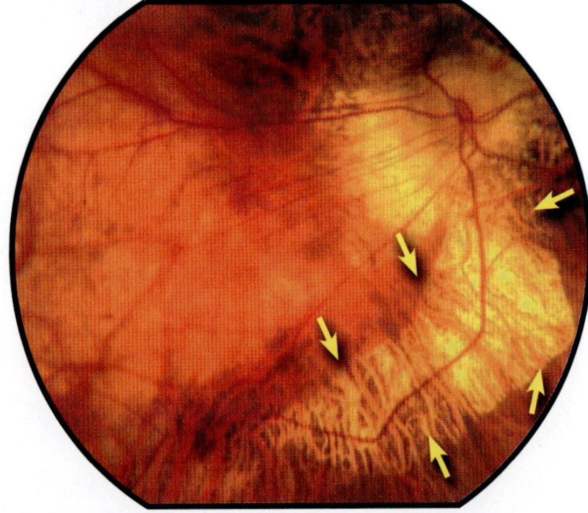

This patient has a pigment epithelial tear *(arrows)* related to a posterior staphyloma. A well-delineated margin of atrophy is seen along the inferior vascular arcade. The tear exposes the choroidal circulation. Tears such as this are probably more common in eyes with pathologic myopia than previously recognized.

Myopic Retinoschisis

Myopic retinoschisis, also known as myopic traction maculopathy, is characterized by retinoschisis of the posterior retina and occurs in 9-34% of highly myopic patients with posterior staphyloma. The pathogenesis is multifactorial involving tangential traction of the inner retina, rigidity of the internal limiting membrane (ILM), thinning of the retina, traction of retinal vessels, and progression of posterior staphyloma. The natural course in a majority of patients can be considered as generally stable with some patients progressing to macular hole formation with or without retinal detachment. Treatment usually involves vitrectomy with ILM peeling and gas tamponade. Although recurrences of myopic retinoschisis may occur, outcomes following repeat vitrectomy can still be favorable.

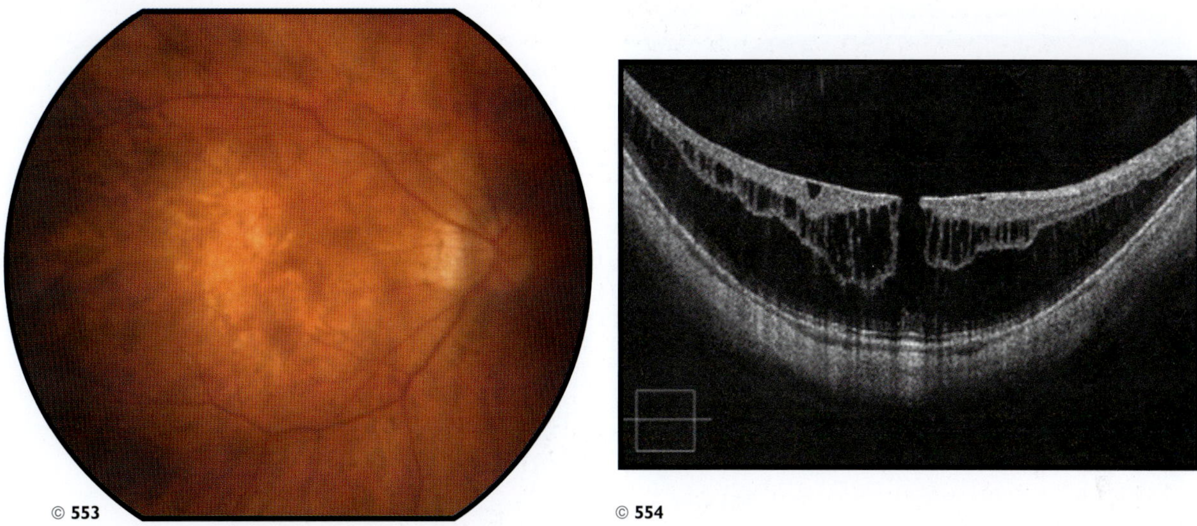

© 553 © 554

This patient has pathologic myopia with a posterior staphyloma, a myopic conus, and a tilted optic disc. OCT image shows myopic retinoschisis with an epiretinal membrane but without a full thickness macular hole or retinal detachment.

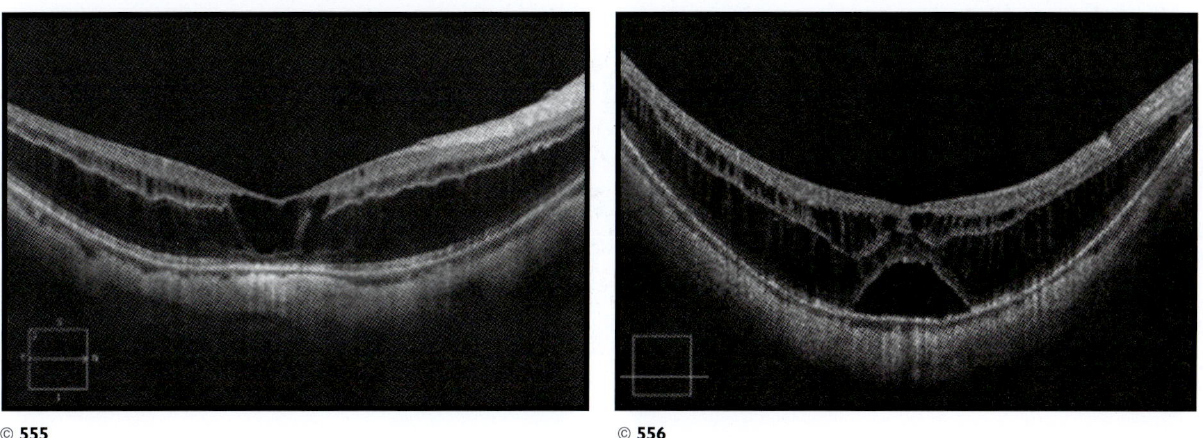

© 555 © 556

These two patients have myopic retinoschisis. The right image shows a subfoveal ellipsoid layer defect with subretinal fluid. *Images courtesy of Dr. Stanley Chang*

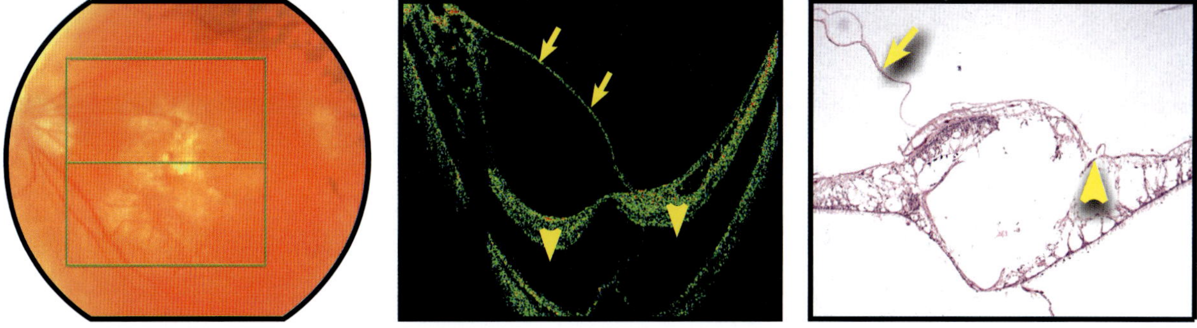

This patient has pathologic myopia with vitreous traction from persistent cortical vitreous *(arrows)*, myopic retinoschisis *(arrowheads)*, and a foveal detachment. Many of these changes are only appreciated on OCT *(middle image)*. The histopathologic specimen *(right image)* shows a large cystic cavity within the retina and Müller cells delineating less prominent schisis changes. Tractional schisis changes may be seen anywhere in the fundus of the pathologic myopic eye but is most common within the staphyloma.

Lacquer Cracks

Lacquer cracks refer to breaks in the RPE-Bruch membrane complex and have a prevalence of 4-9% in highly myopic eyes. Choroidal and scleral stretching, due to increasing axial length, is the postulated mechanism for these lesions. They are more commonly seen in the posterior pole within the posterior staphyloma, but can also be found in the mid-peripheral or peripheral retina. Lacquer cracks may be precursors to myopic CNV and patchy chorioretinal atrophy. They may also be associated with subretinal hemorrhage, in the absence of CNV, due to bleeding from the choriocapillaris.

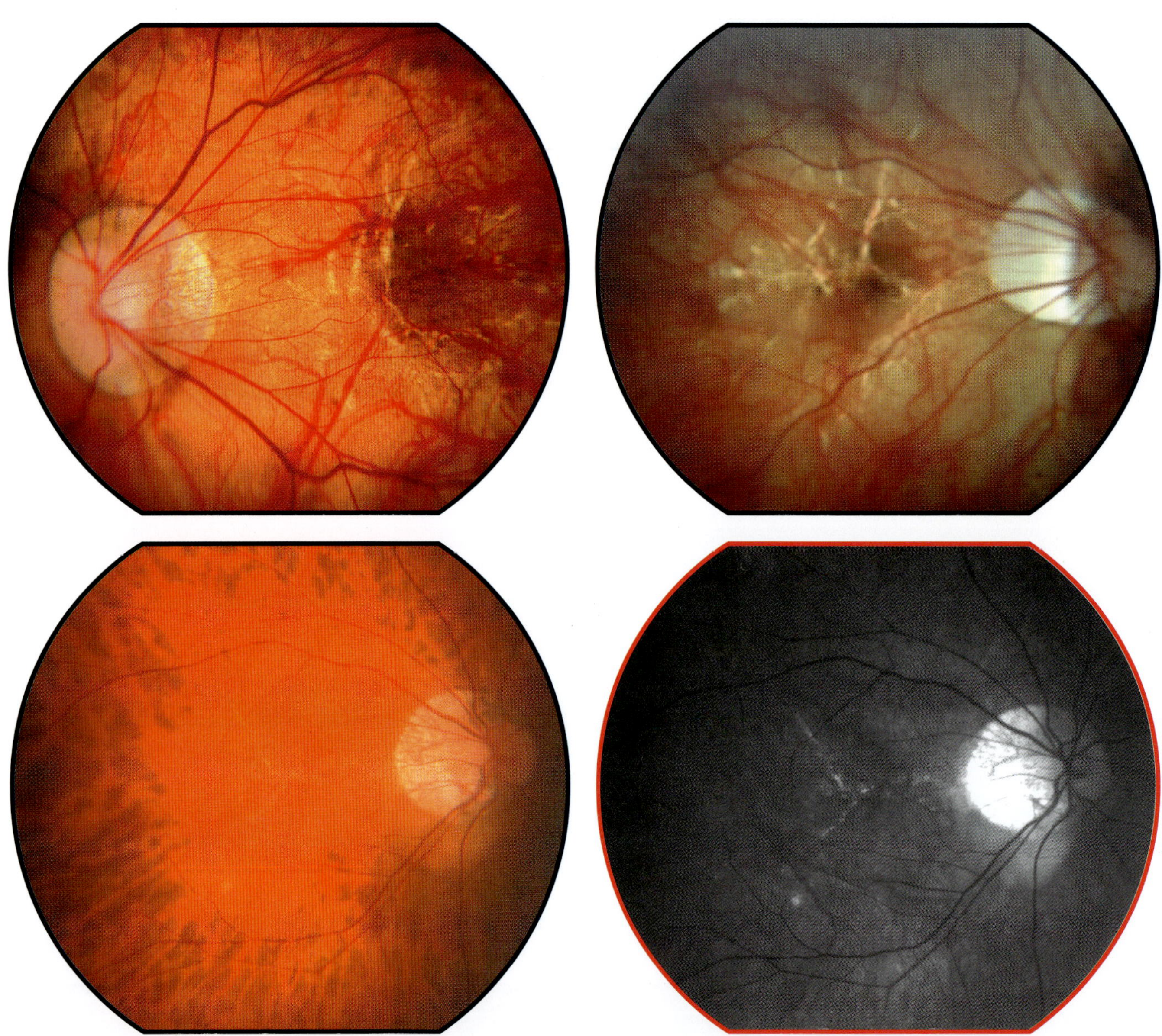

Lacquer cracks appear as pale, yellowish-white, radiating lines. Lacquer cracks may be distributed in a pattern that is concentric to the optic nerve, in a random pattern, or in a pattern that is dictated by the morphological structure of the staphyloma. They appear white on red-free photographs *(right bottom image)*.

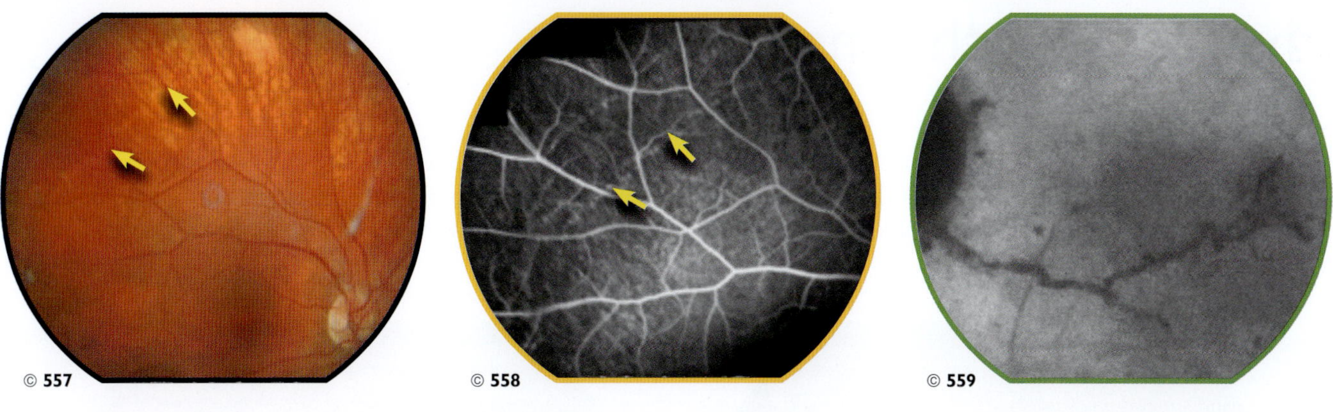

Lacquer cracks may be difficult to see with fluorescein angiography because of relative preservation of the retinal pigment epithelium. When they do appear, they are hyperfluorescent *(middle image, arrows)*. Lacquer cracks are more evident with ICG angiography *(right image)* and appear as dark hypofluorescent irregular lines, which distinguish them from bright hyperfluorescent angioid streaks. *Images courtesy of Dr. Irene Pecorella*

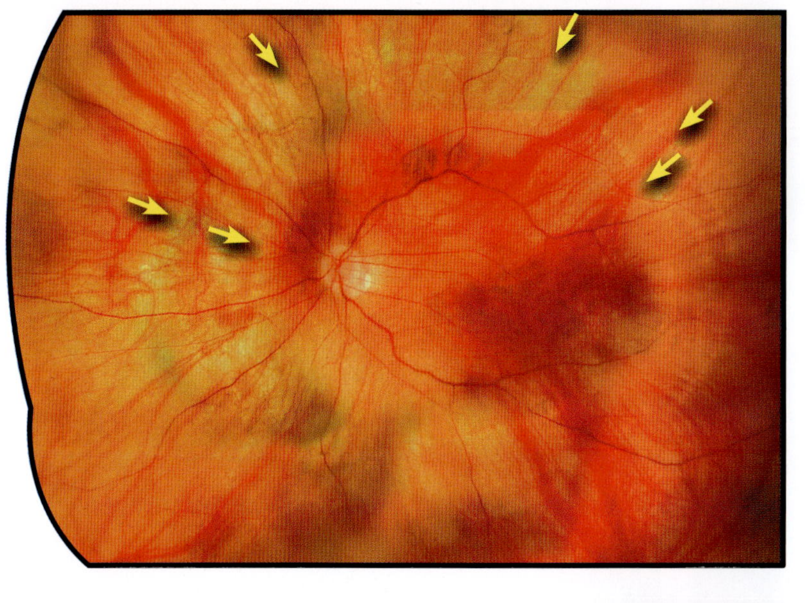

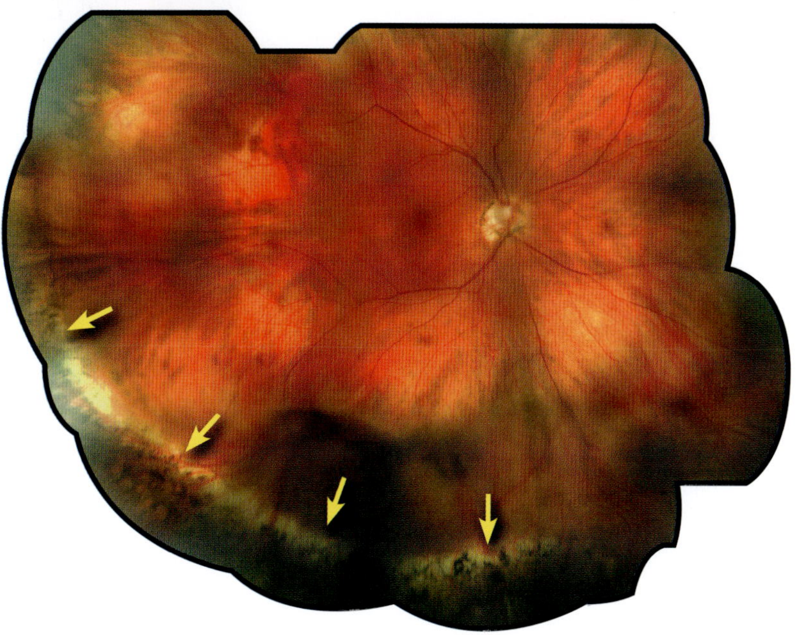

Lacquer cracks may occur anywhere in the posterior segment in the pathologic myopic eye, but they are usually confined to the posterior staphyloma. If a severely myopic eye is simply elongated without a specific staphyloma or bulge, the cracks may be concentric, surrounding the posterior macular region *(arrows top image)*, or in the peripheral retina *(arrows bottom image)*.

Myopic Stretch Lines

Myopic stretch lines are irregular, branching lines found in the posterior fundus of highly myopic eyes and should be differentiated from lacquer cracks. Myopic stretch lines appear hypofluorescent with ICG angiography similar to lacquer cracks. They can be distinguished however by their pigmented brown appearance on ophthalmoscopy, hyperautofluorescence with fundus autofluorescence, and hypofluorescence on fluorescein angiography. Myopic stretch lines are thought to represent retinal pigment epithelium under stress and may be precursors to lacquer cracks.

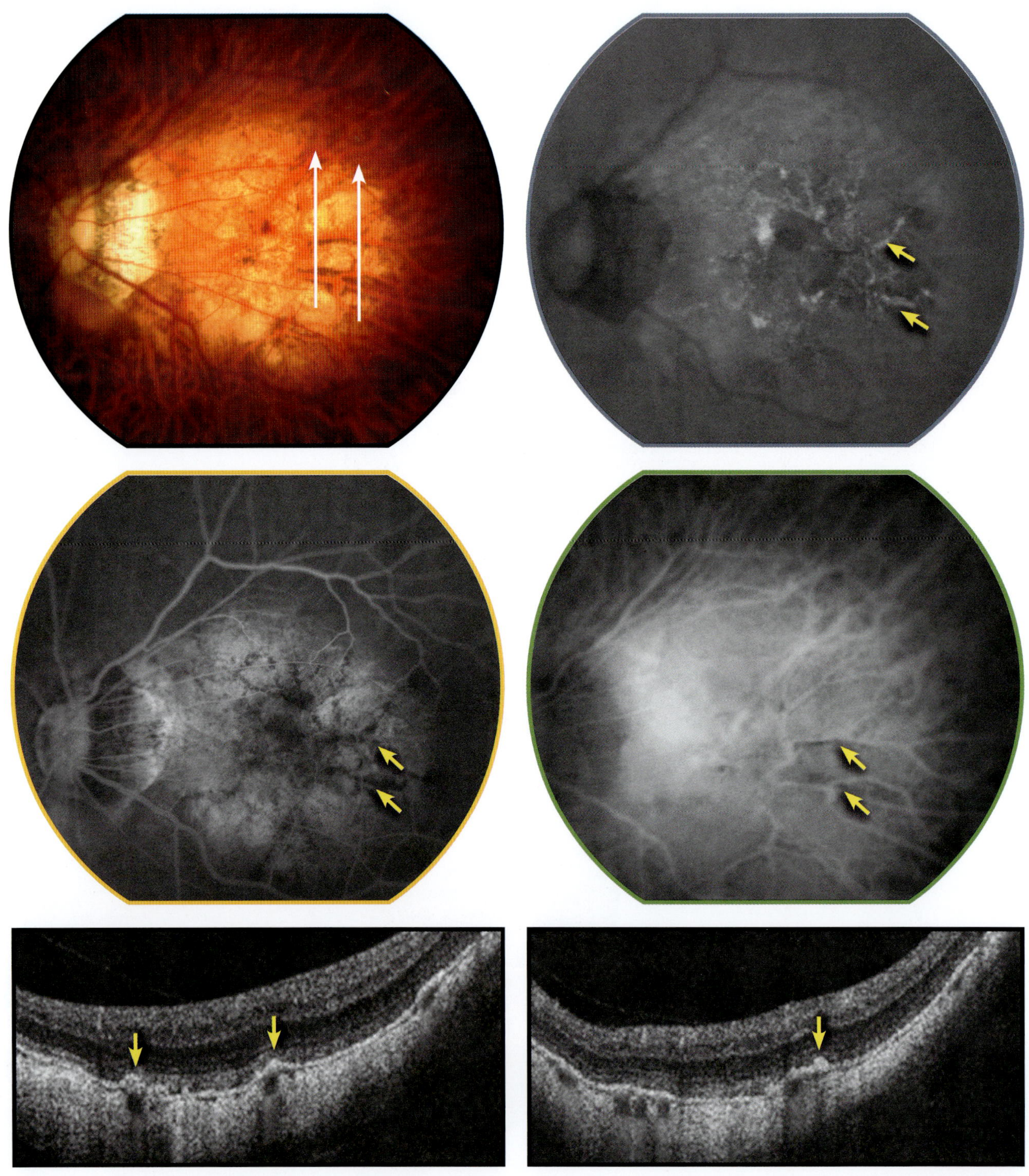

In this patient, myopic stretch lines are seen as brown, pigmented lines running along the large choroidal vessels *(yellow arrows)*. They are most evident on fundus autofluorescence as hyperautofluorescent lines. They appear as hypofluorescent linear lines on both fluorescein and ICG angiography. OCT imaging shows irregular clumping of retinal pigment epithelial cells on and around the large choroidal vessels. (Yellow arrows indicate the site of myopic stretch lines on each imaging modality. Regions imaged with OCT are shown by white arrows on the color picture.)
Images courtesy of Dr. Ohno Matsui

Subretinal Hemorrhages

Patients with pathologic myopia may experience subretinal hemorrhages either from CNV or due to extension of the posterior staphyloma with bleeding from the choriocapillaris. Both types of hemorrhages often coincide with lacquer cracks.

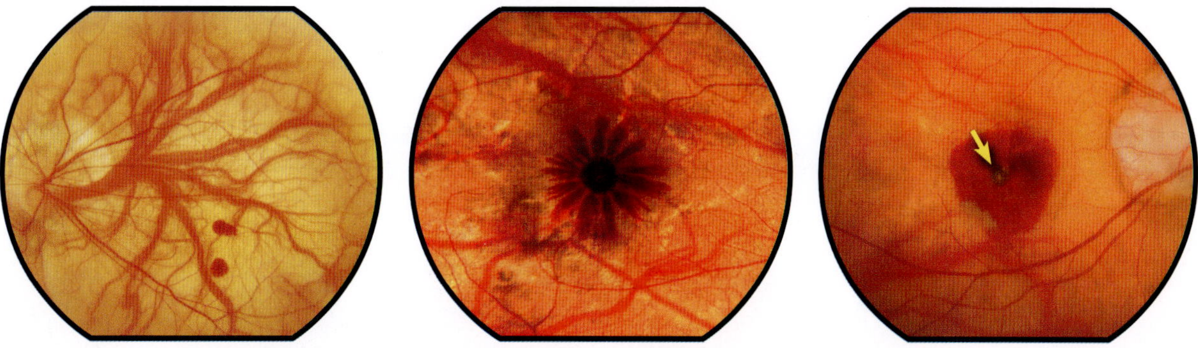

Pathologic myopia and subretinal hemorrhage in three patients. The hemorrhages proved to be non-neovascular in nature in the first two patients *(left and middle image)*. Hemorrhage in the last patient *(right image)* was due to a focal area of CNV *(arrow)*.

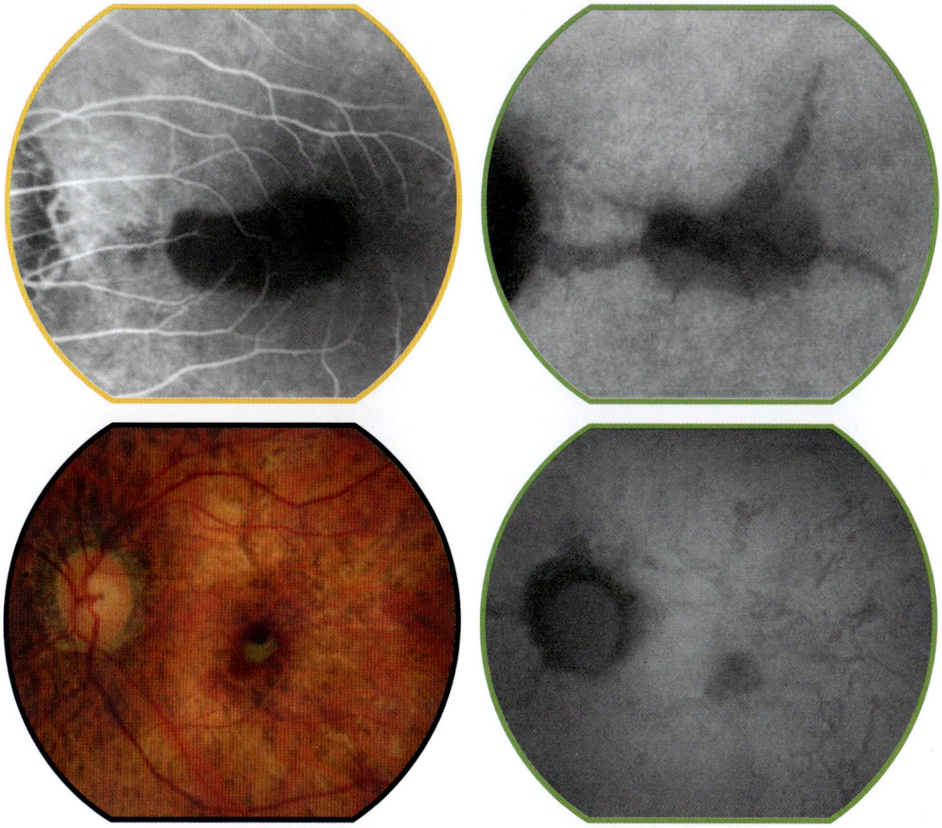

Two different patients with pathologic myopia and subretinal hemorrhage that were suspected of having CNV. In the first patient *(top row)* the fluorescein angiogram shows blocked fluorescence and the ICG angiogram shows lacquer cracks and no CNV. Similar findings were present in the second patient *(bottom row)*. These cases illustrate the usefulness of ICG angiography for excluding CNV when there is an overlying hemorrhage.

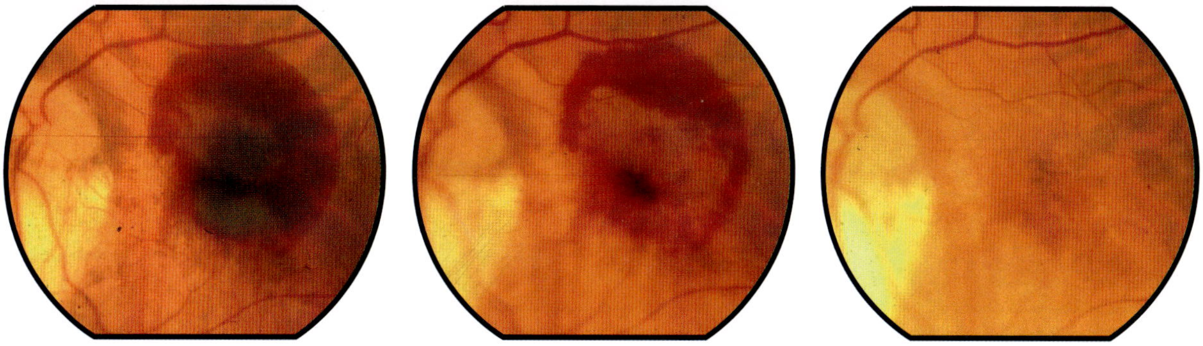

Variably sized subretinal hemorrhages may resolve spontaneously in pathologic myopia. They are not always due to CNV, as can be seen here where the hemorrhage resolved without leaving a Fuchs spot.

Choroidal Neovascularization

The prevalence of myopic CNV in pathologic myopia is between 5-11% and is bilateral in approximately 15% of patients. Features associated with an increased risk of myopic CNV include lacquer cracks, patchy atrophy, thinning of the choriocapillaris and choroid, and CNV in the fellow eye. Type 2 neovascularization is the most common manifestation of proliferating choroidal vessels in myopic macular degeneration. The neovascularized membrane is usually pigmented and is often seen in association with a margin of hemorrhage. It usually develops at a discernible lacquer crack, although this is sometimes not evident clinically. As the CNV regresses, a fibrous pigmented scar sometimes referred to as Fuchs spot, or Forster-Fuchs spot, may form and eventually become surrounded by atrophy. Importantly, myopic CNV must be distinguished from other forms of CNV, in particular, multifocal choroiditis or punctate inner choroidopathy, which tend to occur in myopes as well.

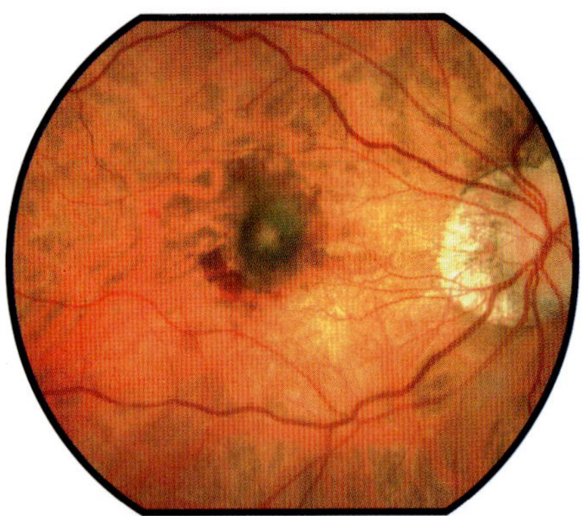
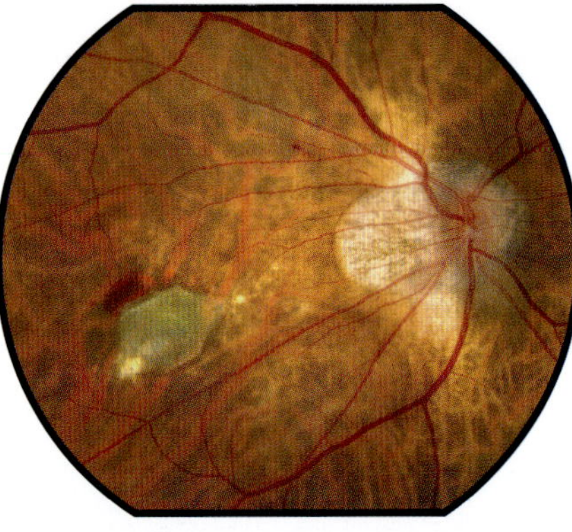
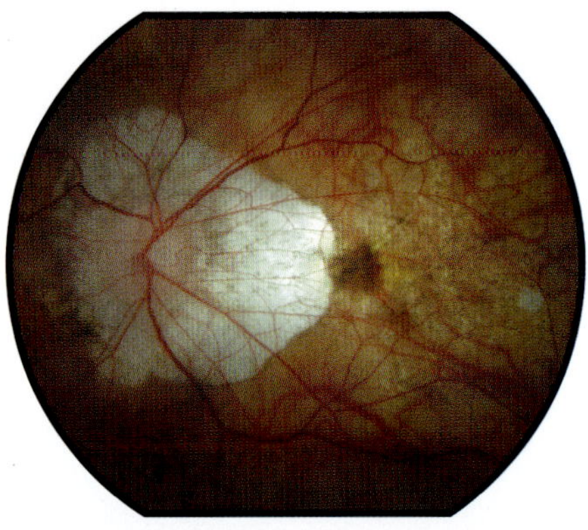

These patients have CNV secondary to pathologic myopia. The CNV may appear pigmented *(left image)* or "dirty gray" *(middle image)* and is often associated with hemorrhage. Neovascular growth commonly extends into the perfused choriocapillaris area rather than into the region of atrophy *(right image)*.

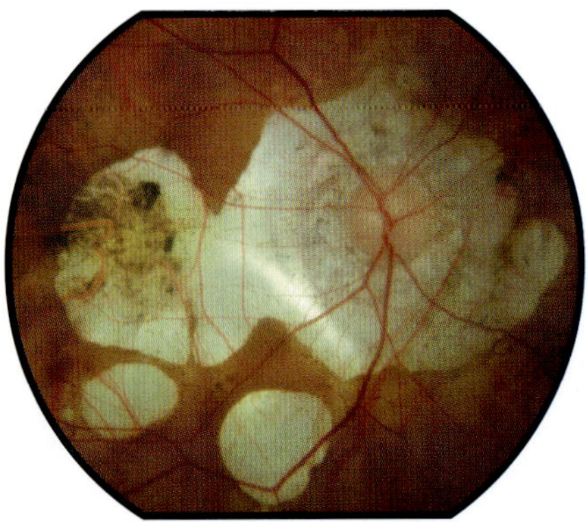
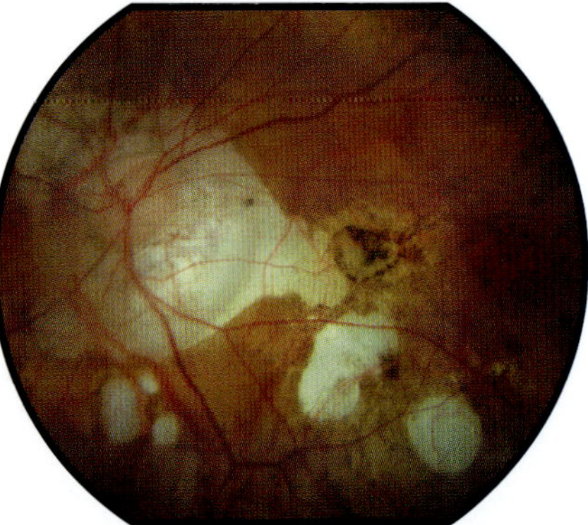
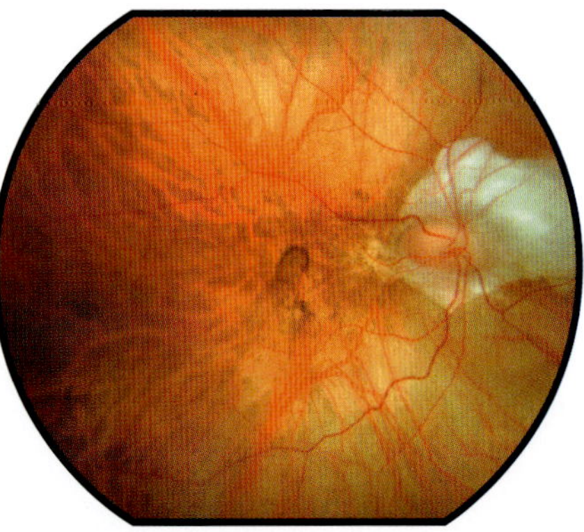

As the neovascularization evolves, it may be detected as a discrete pigmentary and fibrotic membrane *(left and middle images)*. The pigmentation may take the form of a "ring" surrounding the neovascular tissue and recurrence may occur at the area where the ring is incomplete *(right image)*. Retinal pigment epithelial hyperplasia is responsible for the pigmented appearance surrounding an involuted neovascular membrane, also known as a Fuchs spot.

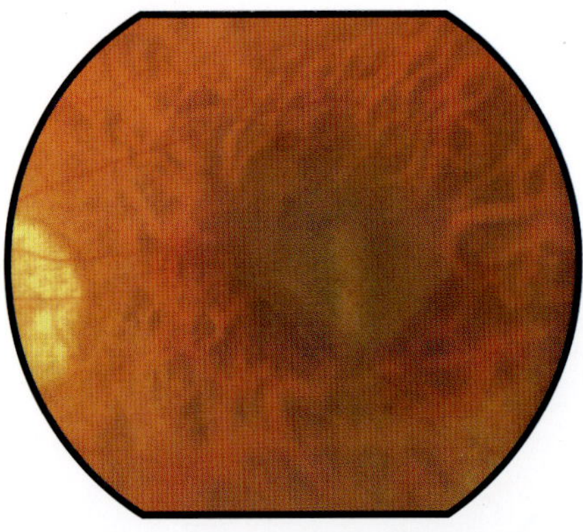
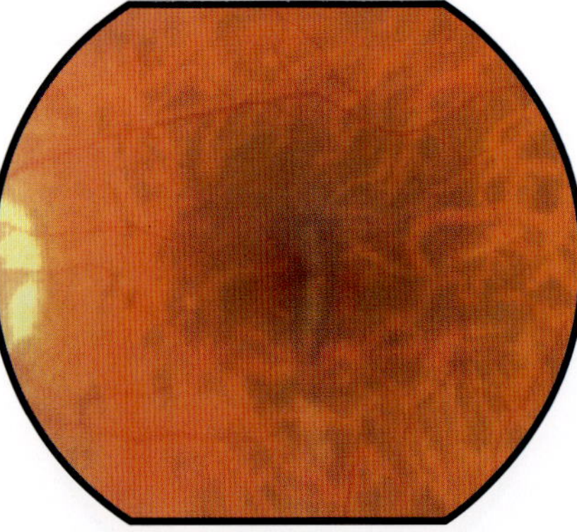
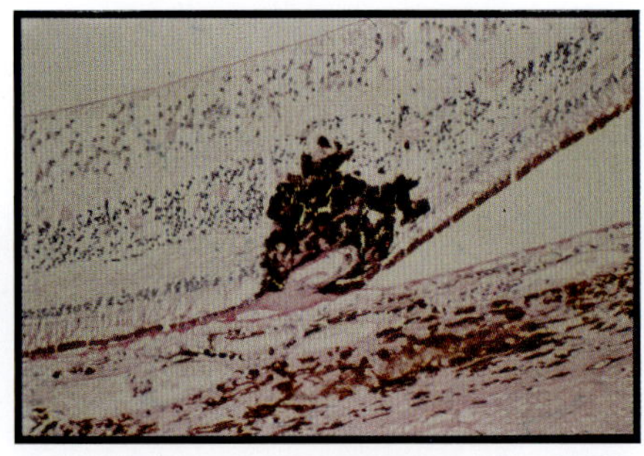

© **630a**

In this case, a lacquer crack is oriented vertically and there is CNV and hemorrhage at its edges. When the exudative detachment resolves, pigment epithelial hyperplasia is seen bordering the edges *(middle image)*. The histopathological specimen shows the appearance of a Fuchs spot near the fovea with neovascular tissue surrounded by hyperplastic retinal pigment epithelium.

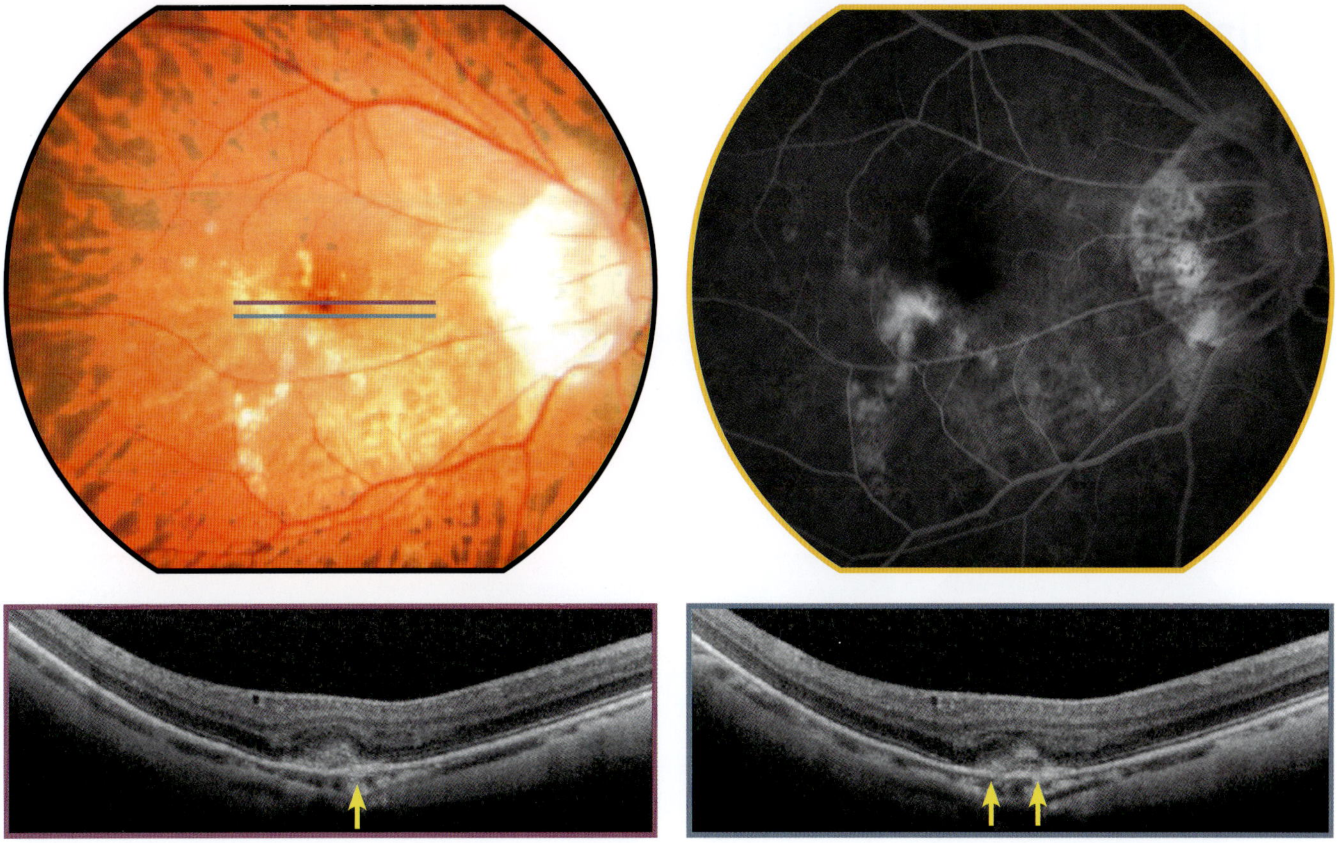

This patient with prominent lacquer cracks developed type 2 neovascularization that showed intense hyperfluorescence on fluorescein angiography. Spectral-domain OCT showed neovascular tissue above the retinal pigment epithelium penetrating through visible cracks in Bruch membrane *(arrows)*.

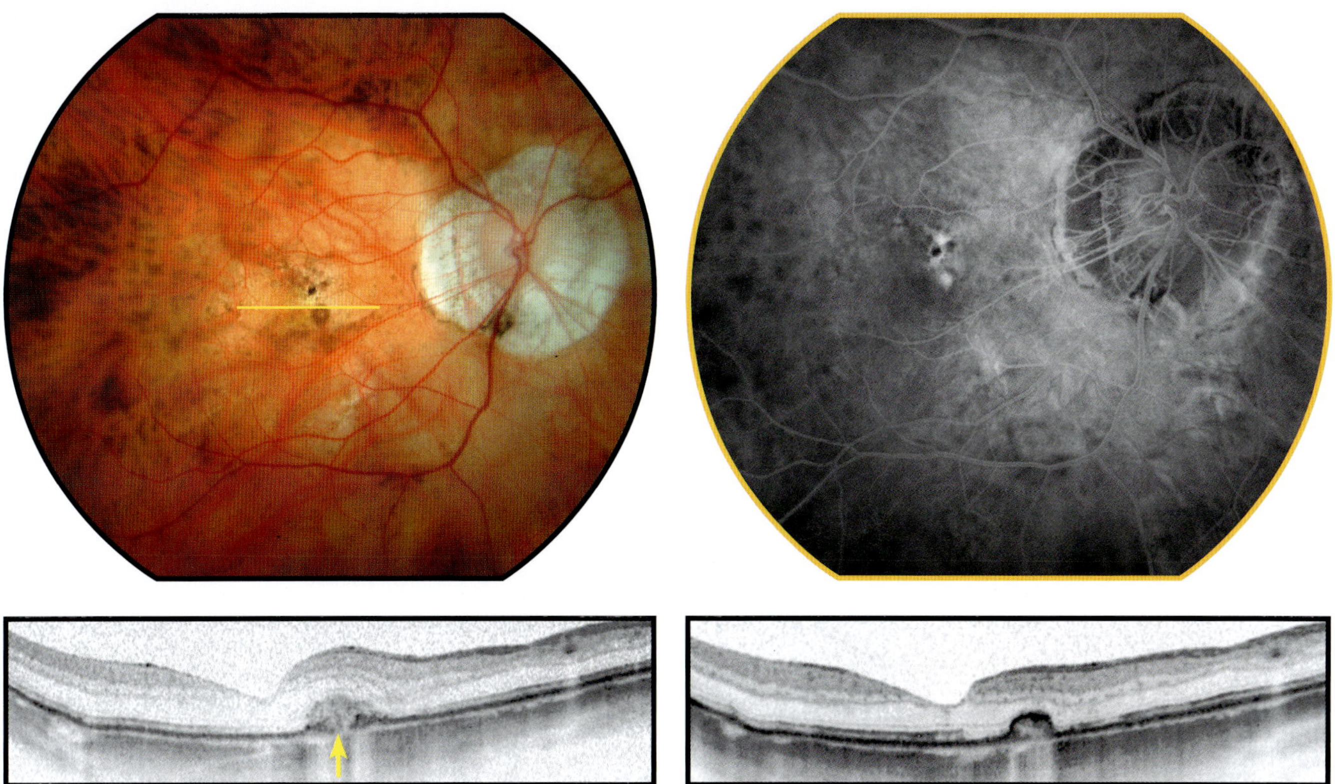

Spectral domain OCT (white on black) illustrates type 2 neovascularization that originates from a break in Bruch membrane *(arrow)*. One month after treatment with an intravitreal anti-vascular endothelial growth factor agent, the neovascular tissue becomes surrounded by hyperplastic retinal pigment epithelium.

Multifocal Choroiditis

Multifocal choroiditis (MFC) can be difficult to distinguish from myopic CNV and commonly occurs in young to middle-aged, myopic women.

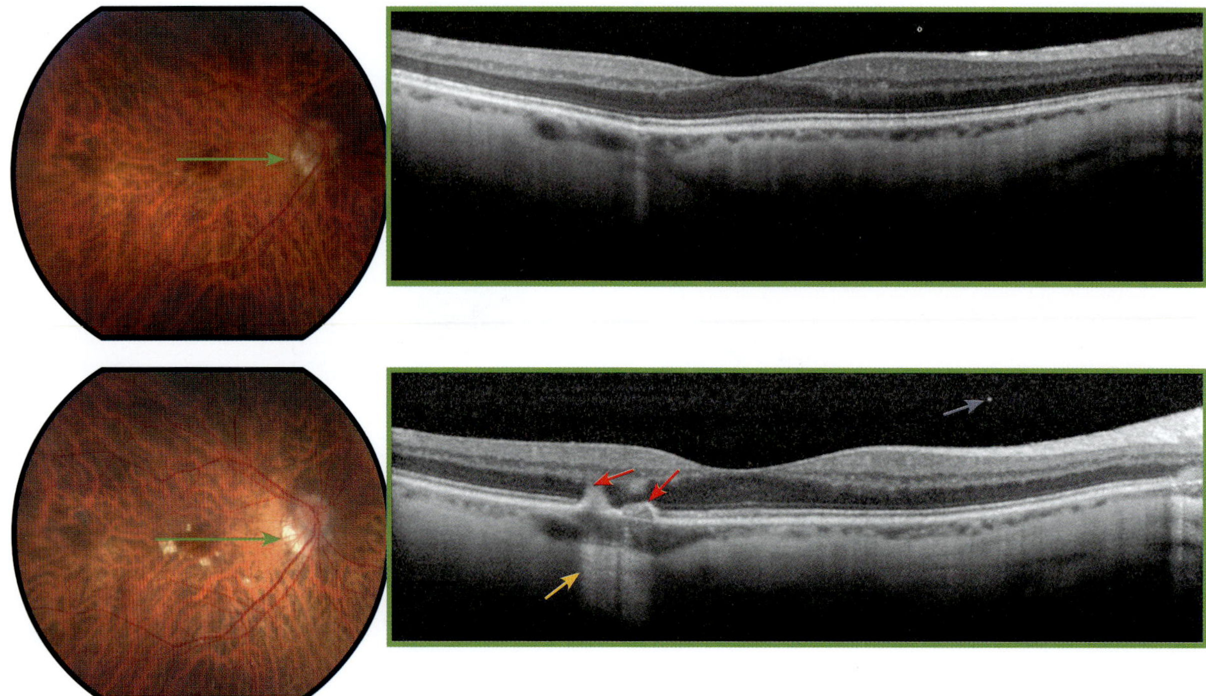

This female presented with myopic macular degeneration *(top row)* and developed new yellow–white lesions two months later *(bottom row)*. With spectral-domain OCT, the lesions appear hyper-reflective and are located between the retinal pigment epithelium (RPE) and Bruch membrane *(red arrows)*. In MFC, the hyper-reflective material may erode through the RPE toward the inner retina and appear as finger-like projections. This is known as the "pitch-fork" sign. These lesions are associated with underlying choroidal thickening and hypertransmission *(yellow arrow)*. Vitreous cells *(blue arrow)* are also suggestive of an inflammatory process.

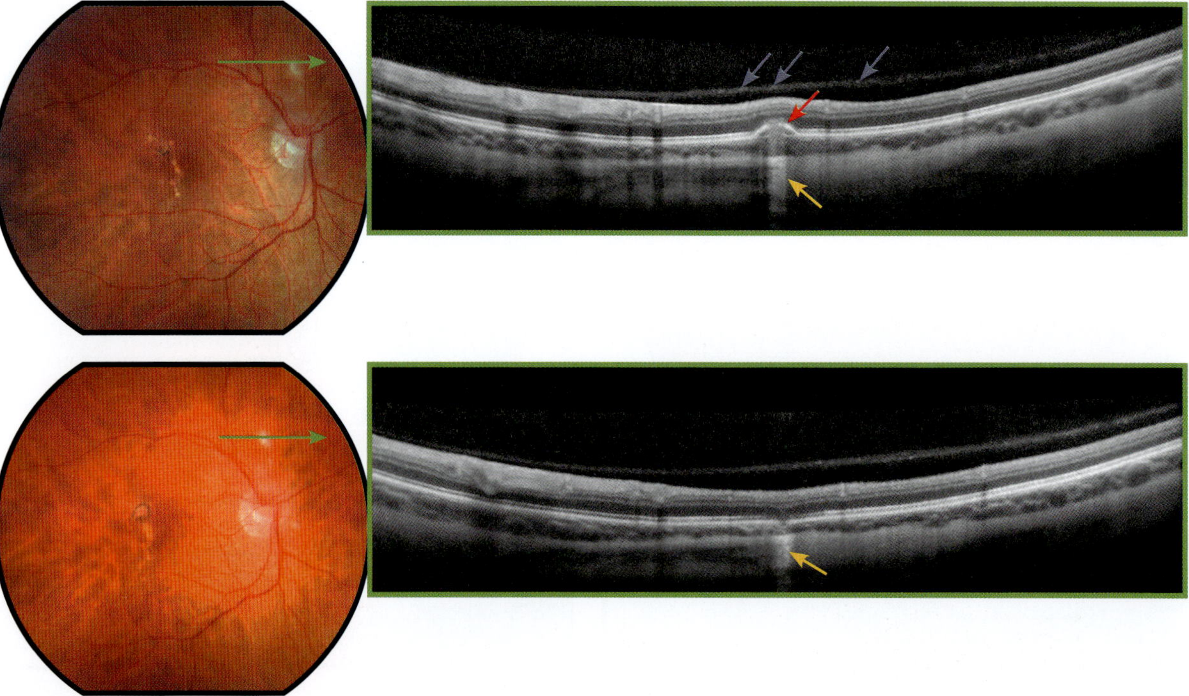

A 32-year-old female previously diagnosed with myopic CNV developed a new yellow–white lesion superior to the optic nerve *(top row)*. Spectral-domain OCT showed sub-RPE material *(red arrow)* associated with underlying choroidal thickening and hypertransmission *(yellow arrows)*. Vitreous cells were also observed *(blue arrows)*. Two years later *(bottom row)*, the lesion appears atrophic. SD-OCT shows resolution of the sub-RPE material. However the hypertransmission remains *(yellow arrow)*.

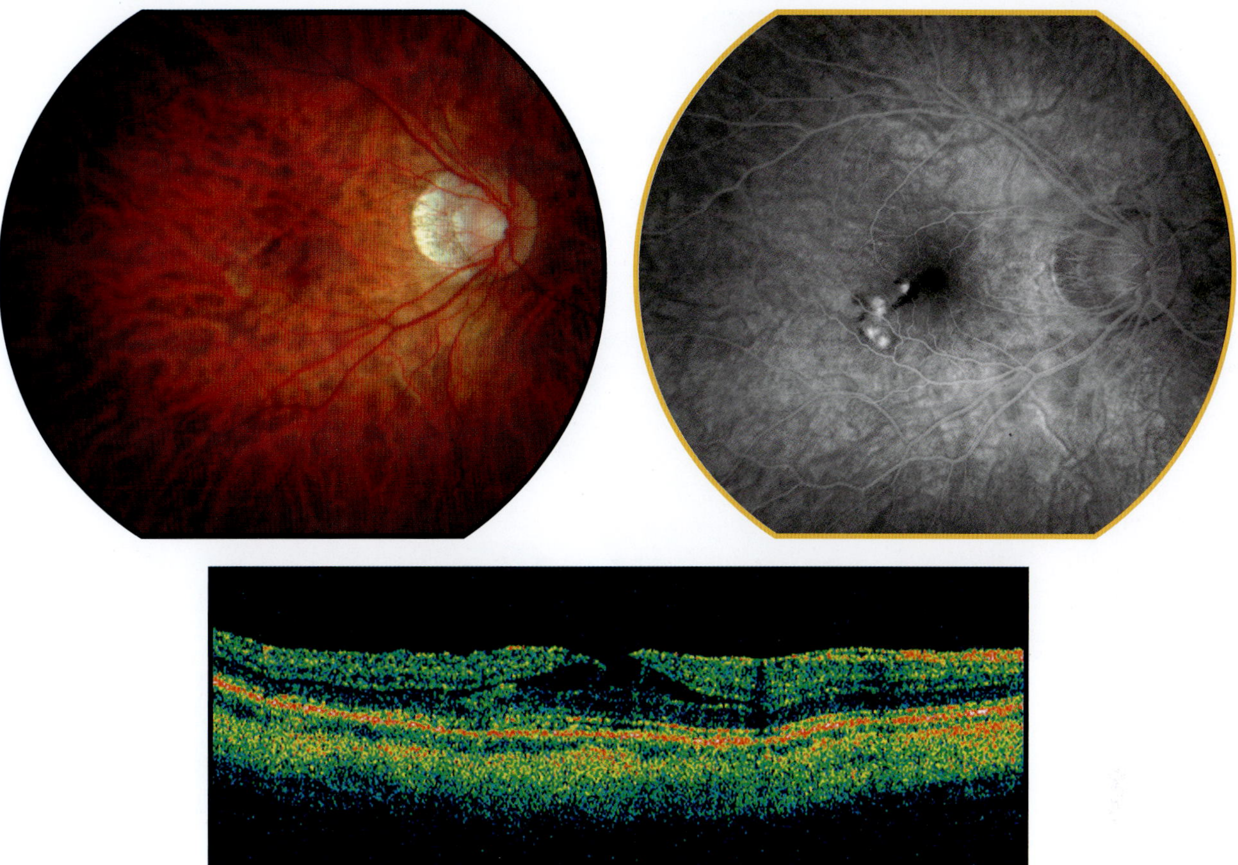

This 36-year-old myopic female was initially diagnosed and treated for myopic CNV in her right eye. There was type 2 neovascularization associated with hemorrhage at the margins which showed early hyperfluorescence on fluorescein angiography.

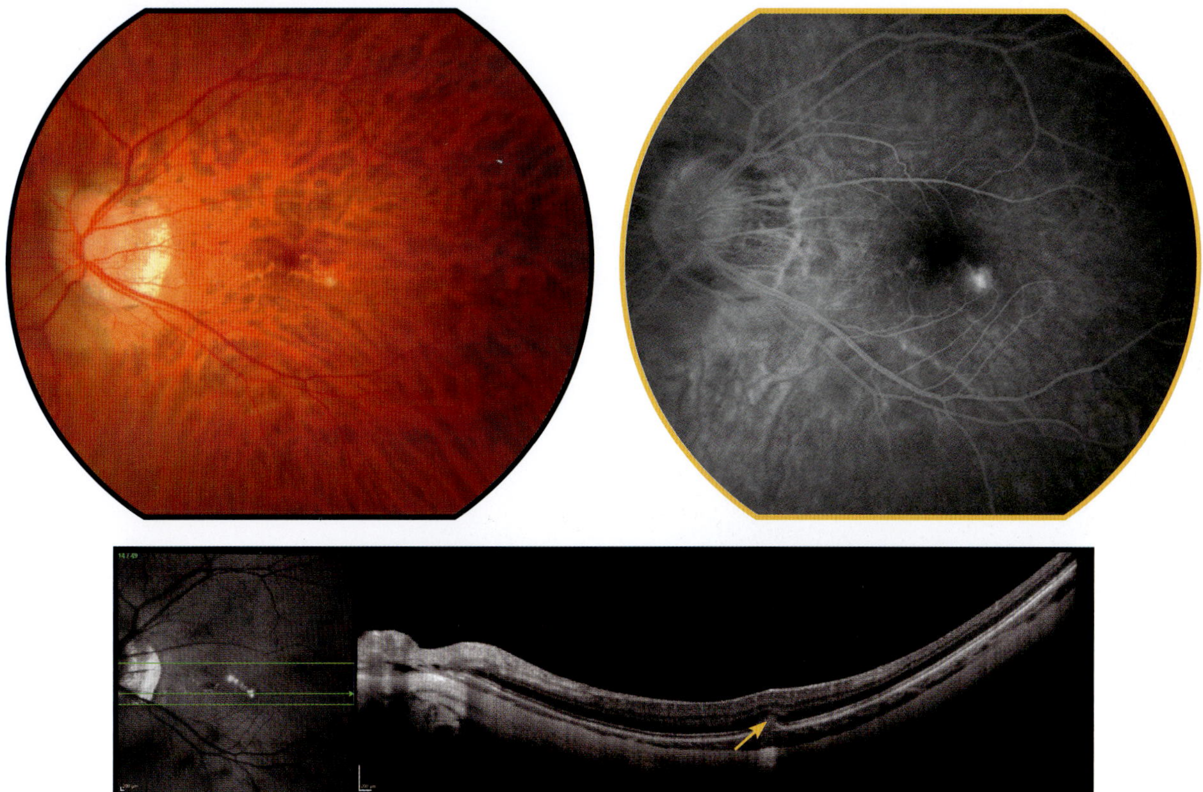

Six years later, the same patient developed a new yellow–white lesion in her left eye. The lesion is situated adjacent to a lacquer crack and shows early hyperfluorescence on fluorescein angiography. However, SD-OCT shows characteristic features of an inflammatory lesion that include hyper-reflective sub-RPE material and underlying hypertransmission *(arrow)*.

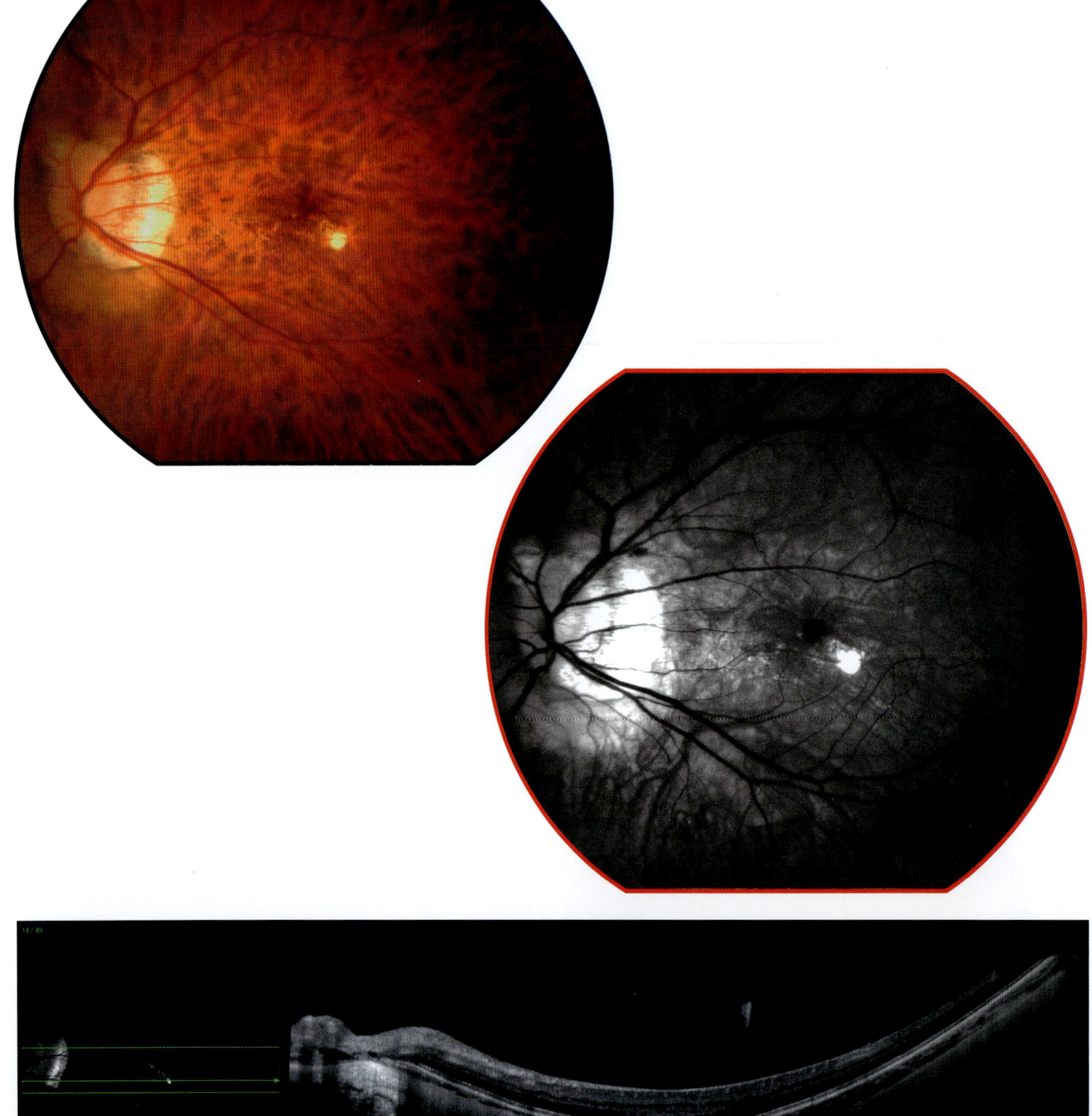

With time, a punched-out atrophic lesion characteristic of multifocal choroiditis developed. SD-OCT shows atrophy of the RPE and outer retina with hypertransmission *(arrow)*.

Peripapillary Choroidal Thickening and Cavitation

Eyes with pathologic myopia often have characteristic morphological changes involving the optic nerve head and peripapillary tissue. Myopic conus is a term used to define the presence of a tilted optic disc and scleral crescent. Less commonly, optic disc abnormalities such as macrodiscs and acquired optic nerve pits may also be seen in pathological myopia. Peripapillary choroidal thickening and cavitation is a more recently described finding that is seen in 5% of eyes with pathologic myopia and may rarely be complicated by macular retinal detachment and visual field defects. It may also masquerade as a flecked retina. This finding has also been called peripapillary intrachoroidal cavitation although cavitation is not always present.

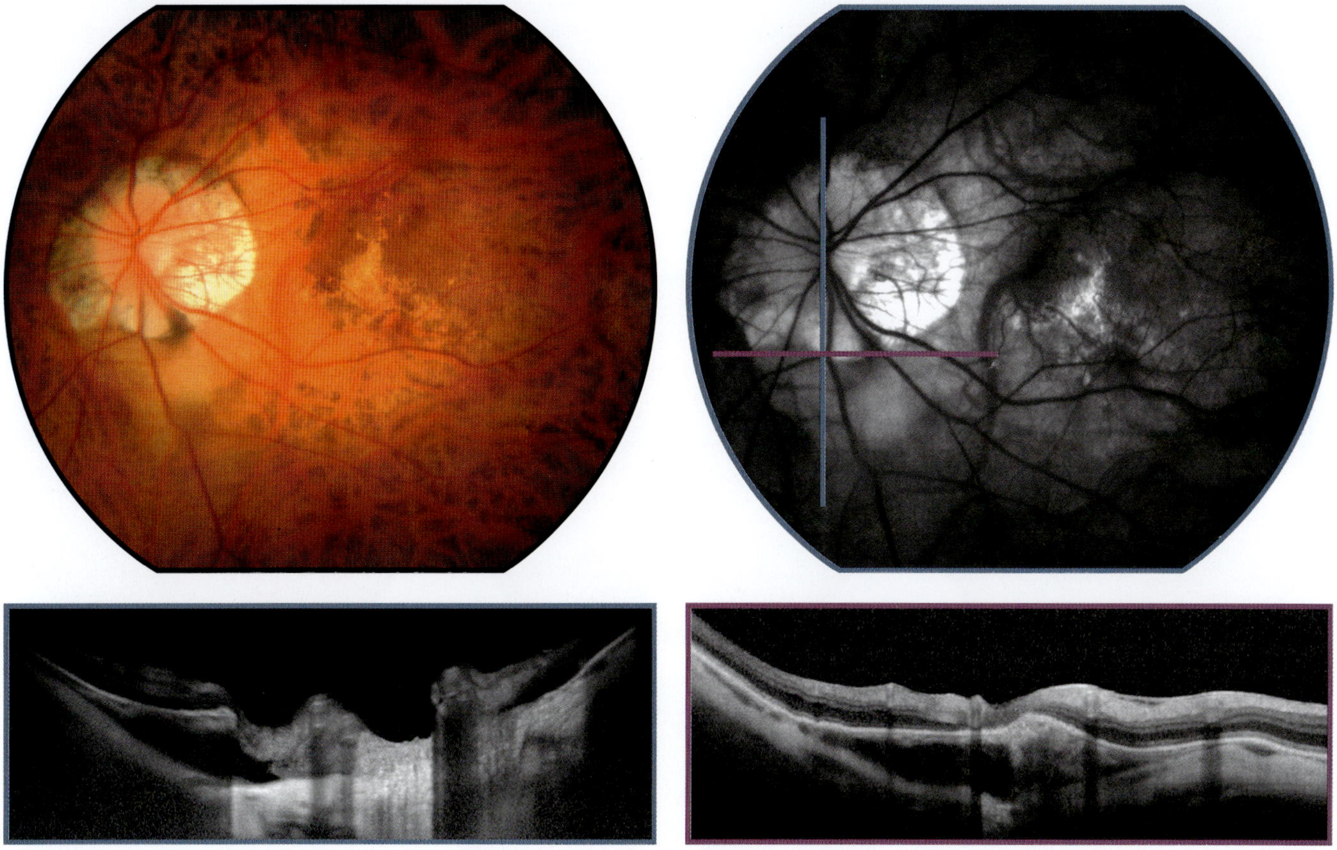

Peripapillary choroidal thickening and cavitation appears as a well-circumscribed yellow-orange lesion and is usually found inferior to the myopic conus. Spectral-domain OCT on horizontal and vertical cuts reveal the choroidal thickening and cavitation.

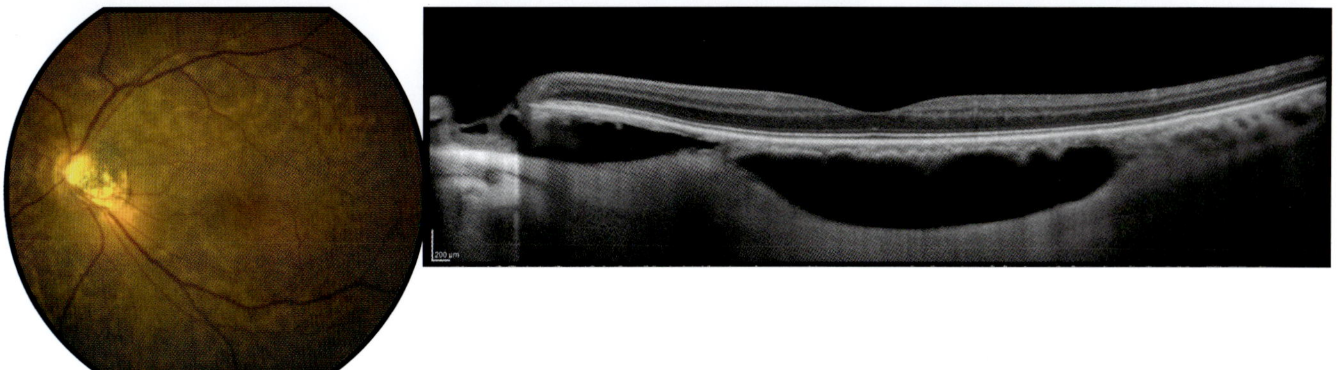

Peripapillary choroidal thickening and cavitation may be unilateral and may extend temporally to masquerade as a flecked retina. *Images courtesy of Dr. James Palmer*

AGE-RELATED MACULAR DEGENERATION

Age-related macular degeneration (AMD) is the leading cause of irreversible legal blindness (20/200 or worse), affecting 10–13% of adults over 65 years of age in North America, Europe, Australia, and Asia. In the USA it is estimated that more than 8 million individuals are affected in one or both eyes by the intermediate and/or advanced forms of AMD. In individuals over the age of 75, the incidence is approximately 30%. Risk factors for AMD include age, female sex, cigarette smoking, cardiovascular disease, obesity, systemic hypertension, and hypercholesterolemia. Dietary factors such as a high fat intake and low consumption of dark green leafy vegetables and fruits have been linked to an increased risk of AMD. Data regarding intake of omega-3 polyunsaturated fatty acids, degree of sunlight exposure, and levels of ocular melanin are conflicting. More recently, several genetic associations have been identified, the most important being allelic variants in the gene encoding for complement factor H (CFH) and age-related macular susceptibility 2 (ARMS2). Although AMD is more accurately described as a spectrum of diseases, it has traditionally been divided into two major subtypes: non-neovascular or "dry" AMD, and neovascular or "wet" AMD.

Non-neovascular AMD: Eyes with drusen, macular pigmentary alterations, non-neovascular pigment epithelial detachments (PEDs), and atrophy of the retinal pigment epithelium (RPE) and choroid.

Neovascular AMD: Eyes with neovascularization, which are further subdivided into type 1, 2, and 3 neovascularization.

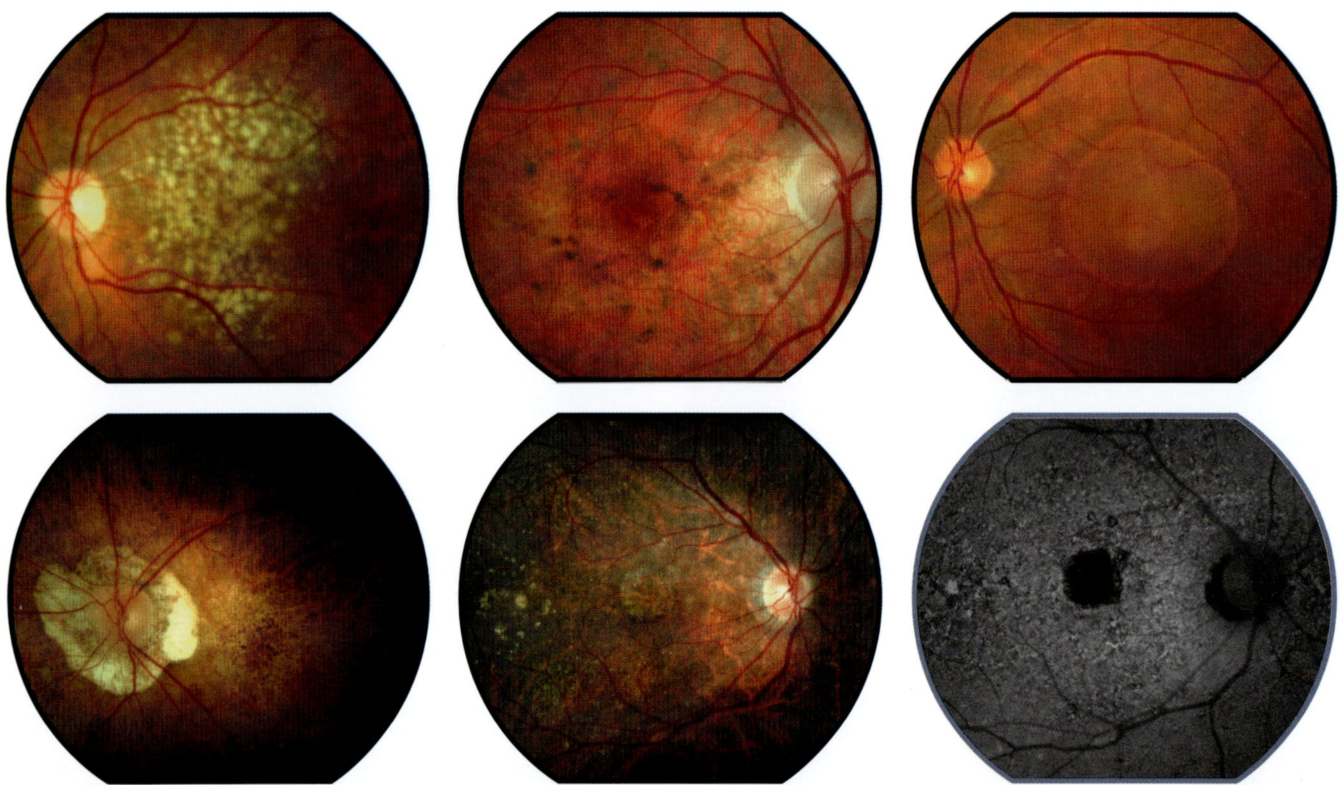

These images show the spectrum of non-neovascular AMD including drusen *(top left)*, macular pigmentary changes *(top middle)*, non-neovascular PED *(top right)*, age-related choroidal atrophy *(bottom left)*, and geographic atrophy *(bottom middle and right)*.

Non-neovascular AMD

Drusen

Drusen are the hallmark clinicopathologic feature of non-neovascular AMD, which is also characterized by alterations of the RPE, including RPE hyperplasia, PED, and RPE atrophy. RPE atrophy associated with choroidal atrophy in well-delineated areas larger than 175 μm is generally termed geographic atrophy. Various types of drusen have been described, including small or hard drusen, large or soft drusen, basal laminar or cuticular drusen, mineralized or calcified drusen, and reticular pseudodrusen. Certain types of drusen and RPE changes may present an increased risk of progression to neovascular AMD.

Drusen size is important in the evaluation of AMD. Small drusen, also termed drupelets or hard drusen, are defined as less than 63 μm in size and appear as small yellow-white lesions with distinct borders located at the level of the Bruch membrane. Medium-sized drusen are 63–124 μm in size. Large drusen, also termed soft drusen, are 125 μm or greater in size and often have indistinct borders. They may coalesce with adjacent large drusen to form a drusenoid PED, which is generally considered to be 350 μm or greater in size.

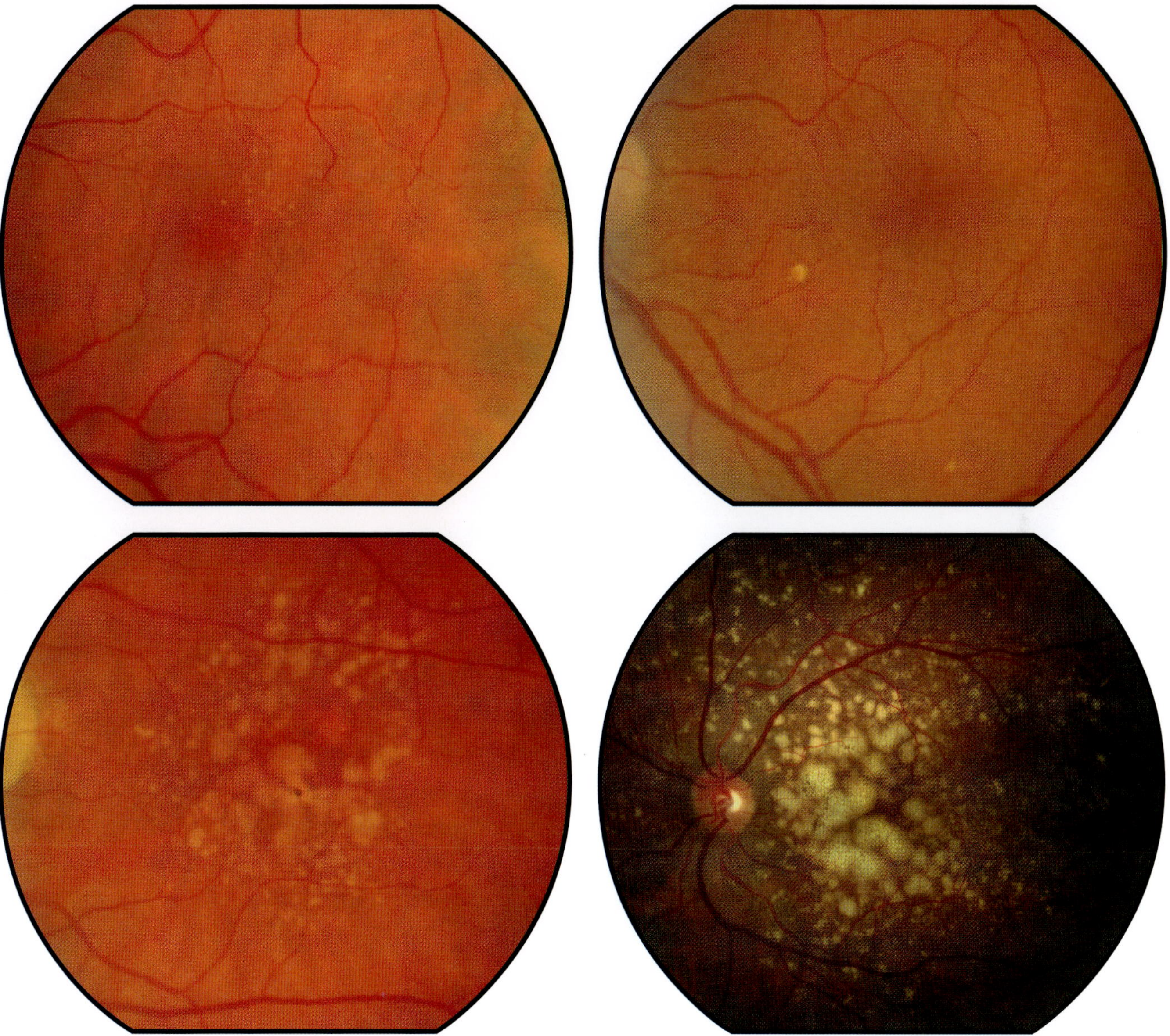

These patients have non-neovascular AMD with a variety of drusenoid changes. The patient on the upper left has a cluster of small drusen. The upper right image shows a single large druse. The lower left image shows variably sized medium and large drusen. The two bottom images show how large drusen may coalesce to form drusenoid PEDs.

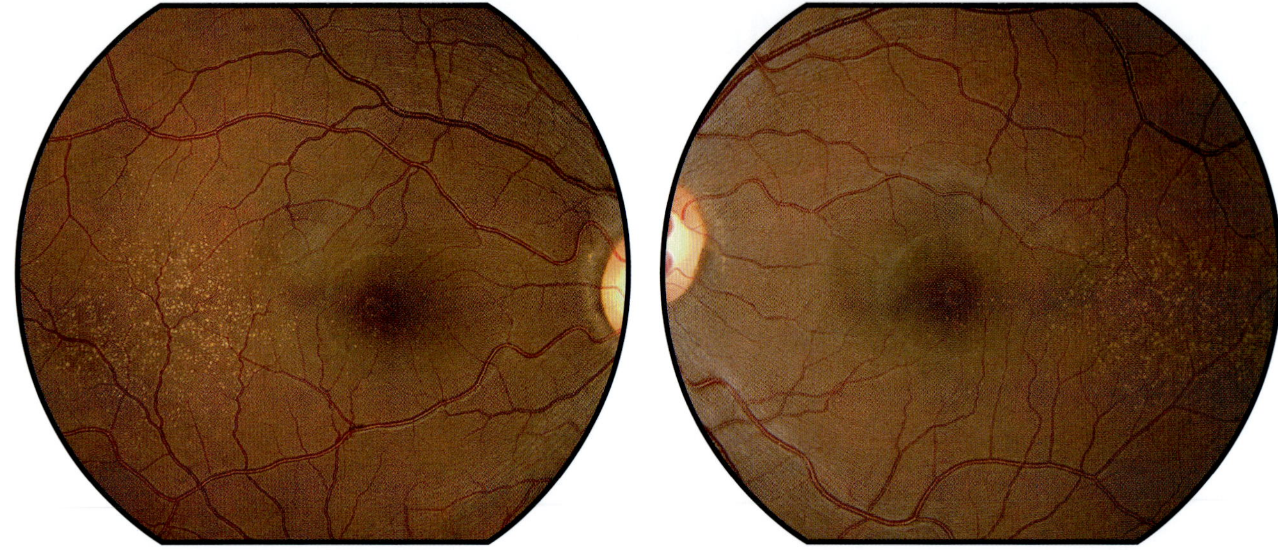

This patient has bilateral symmetric small or hard drusen, predominantly in the temporal macula. These lesions represent minimal risk of progression to the advanced forms of AMD.

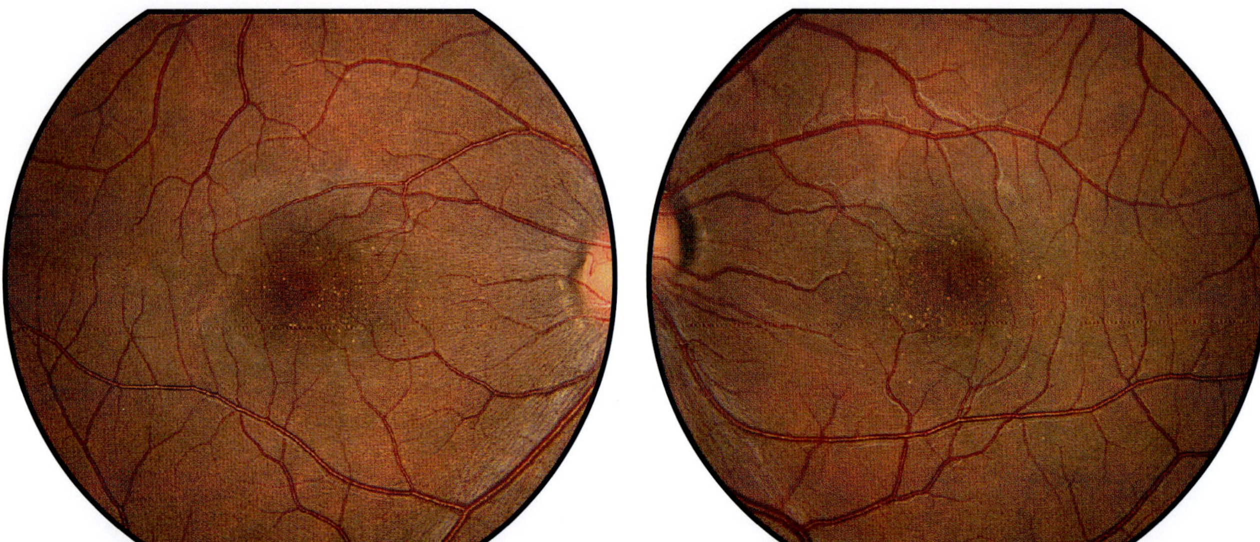

The fundus changes in this patient with small drusen have remained stable over 25 years of follow-up.

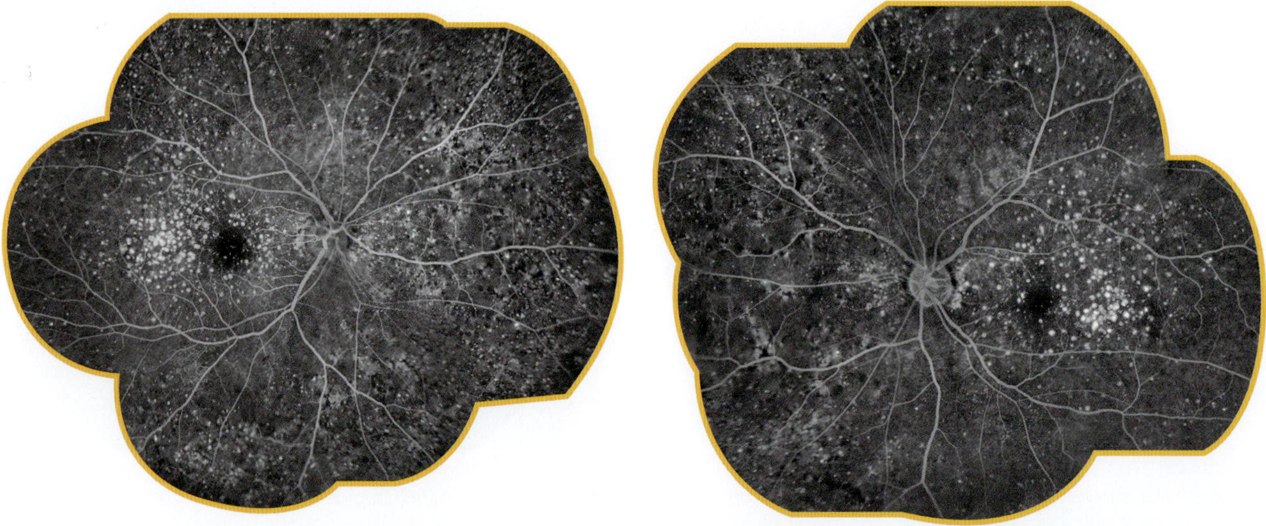

This patient has bilateral small drusen scattered throughout the posterior pole and peripheral fundus. With fluorescein angiography, drusen of this type show early hyperfluorescence or "window defect" from thinning of the pigment epithelium and an intact choriocapillaris. There is symmetry of the drusen involvement and relative sparing of the central macula.

This is a patient with widespread drusen, most of which are small. The drusen extend beyond the central paramacular region and the vascular arcades into the near peripheral retina.

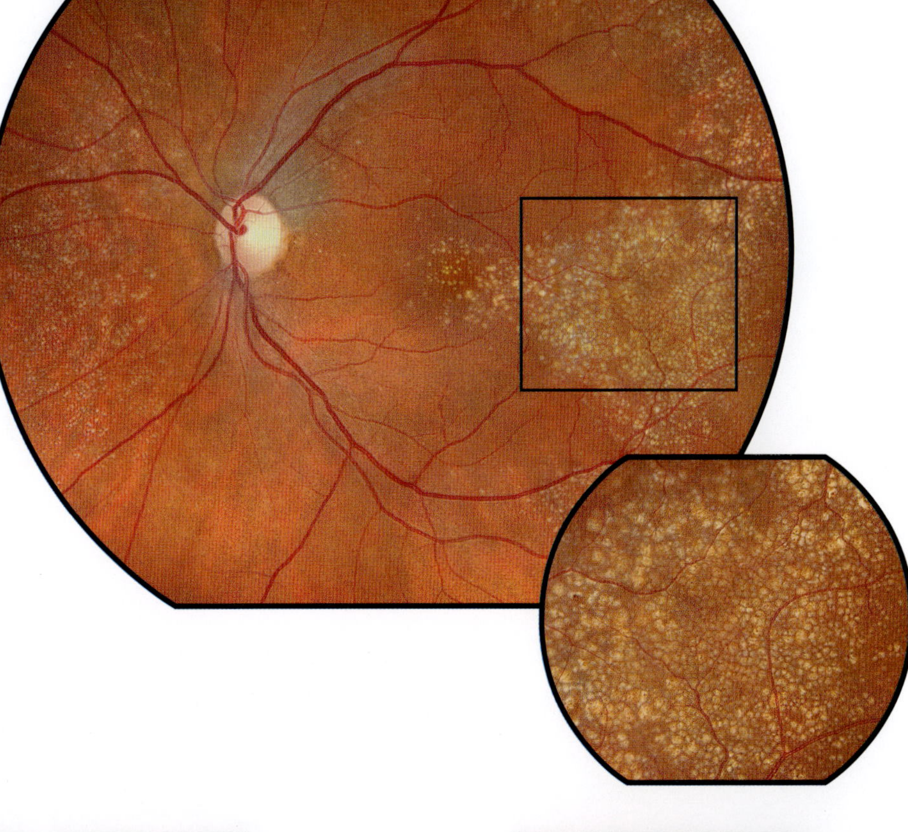

This patient has bilateral large drusen distributed in a symmetric pattern that largely spares the fovea where there are just a few small drusen. Patients with foveal sparing may retain good central vision throughout their lifetime. The natural course of drusen in most patients is toward bilaterality and symmetry.

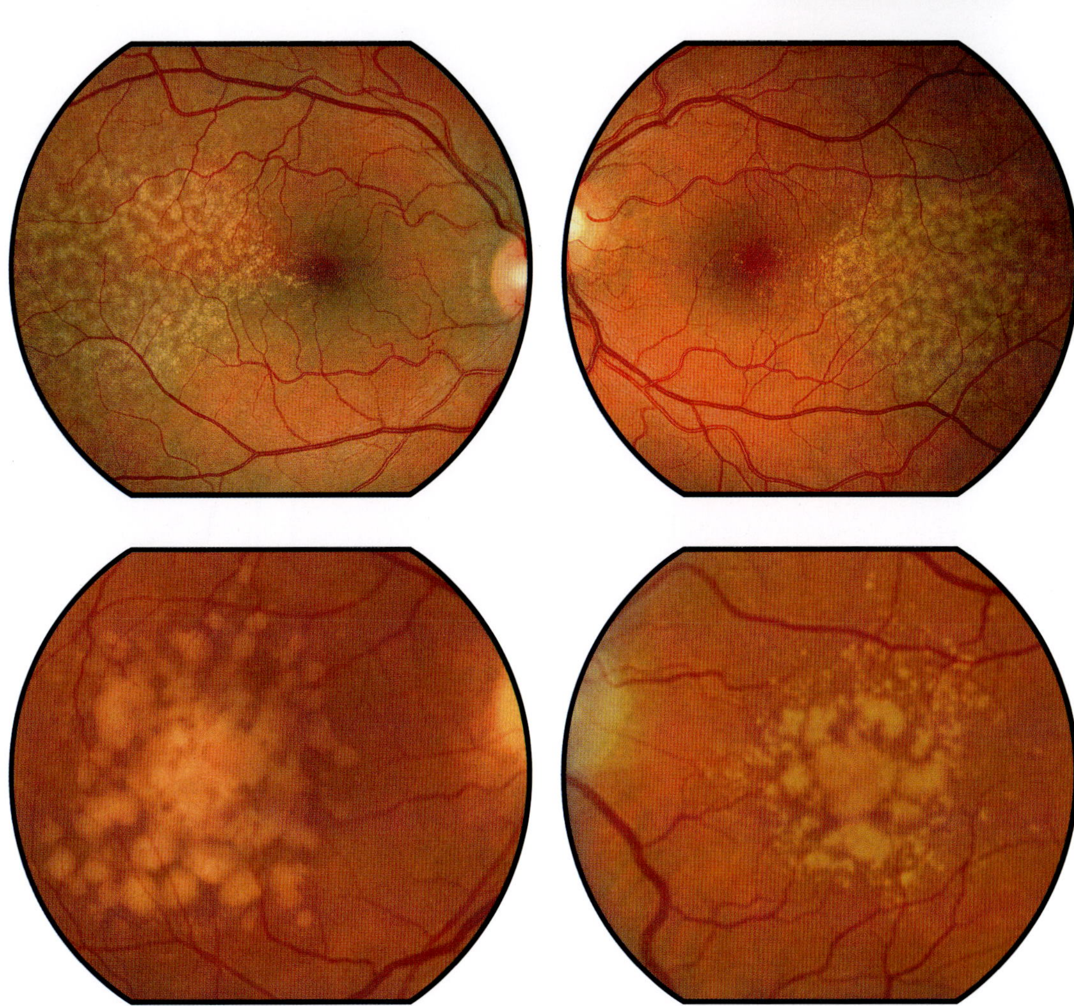

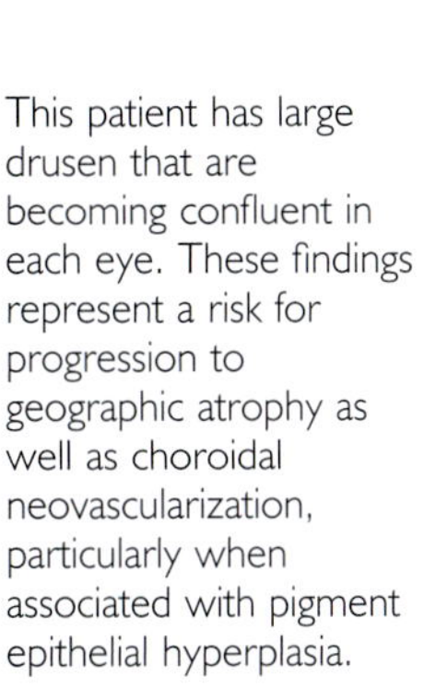

This patient has large drusen that are becoming confluent in each eye. These findings represent a risk for progression to geographic atrophy as well as choroidal neovascularization, particularly when associated with pigment epithelial hyperplasia.

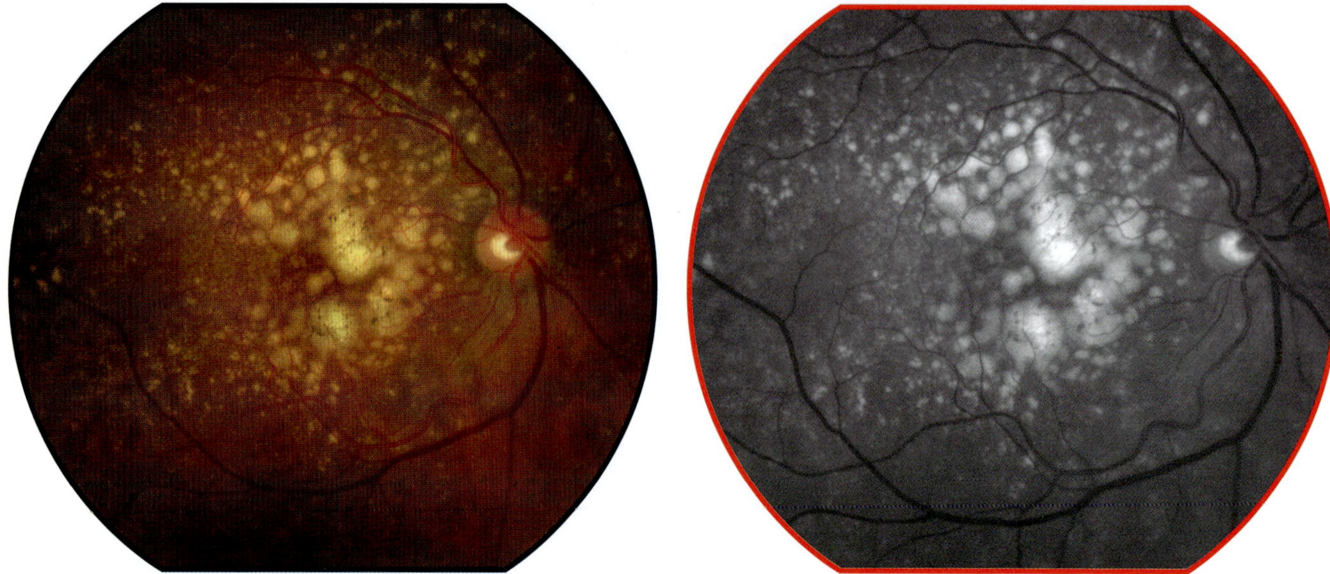

This patient has scattered drusen throughout the fundus, consisting of a mixture of small, medium, and large drusen, which are well shown with red-free photography.

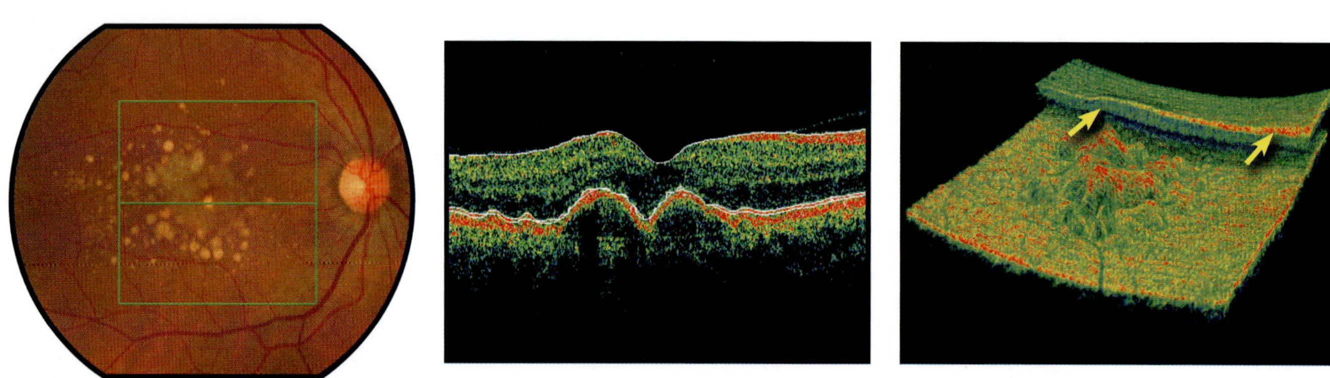

This patient has variably sized drusen with confluency near the fovea. The OCT shows dome-like elevations of the pigment epithelium that are essentially small drusenoid PEDs. The three-dimensional OCT displays the elevations of the pigment epithelium beneath the neurosensory retina, which has been removed with image processing *(arrows)*.

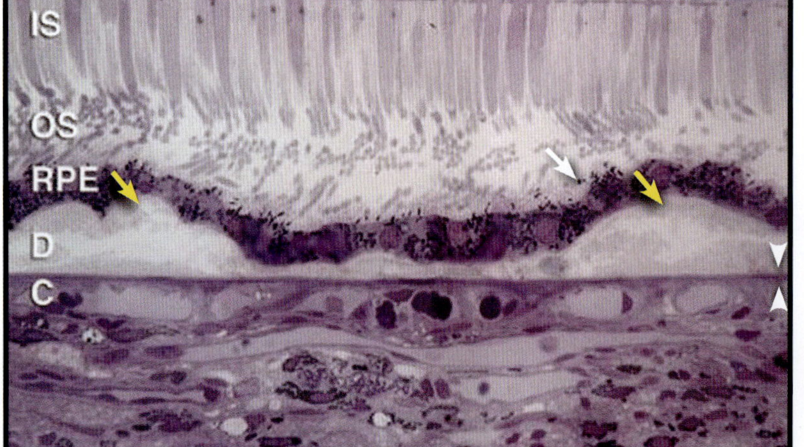

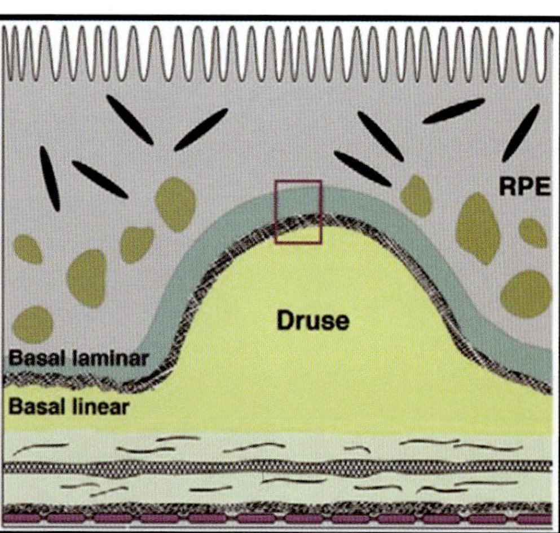

Drusen *(D)* are related to a diffuse thickening of the inner aspect of the Bruch membrane *(arrowheads)*, known as basal linear deposits. This histologic section shows two drusen *(yellow arrows)* connected by basal linear deposit. Drusen contain lipoprotein-derived debris and lipid pools. There is elevation but minimal change to the RPE morphology *(white arrow)*. Basal linear deposit should be differentiated from basal laminar deposit, which is located above the basal lamina of the RPE, as shown in the schematic. *C*, choroid; *IS*, inner segment of photoreceptors; *OS*, outer segment of photoreceptors. *Images courtesy of Dr. Christine Curcio*

Drusen with Pigmentary Abnormalities

Pigmentary abnormalities including hyperpigmentation and hypopigmentation may occur in association with drusen in non-neovascular AMD. These changes are risk factors for progression to atrophic and neovascular disease. Geographic atrophy is often preceded by the appearance of hyperpigmentation overlying confluent drusen, followed by regression of drusen and pigment and the appearance of hypopigmentation.

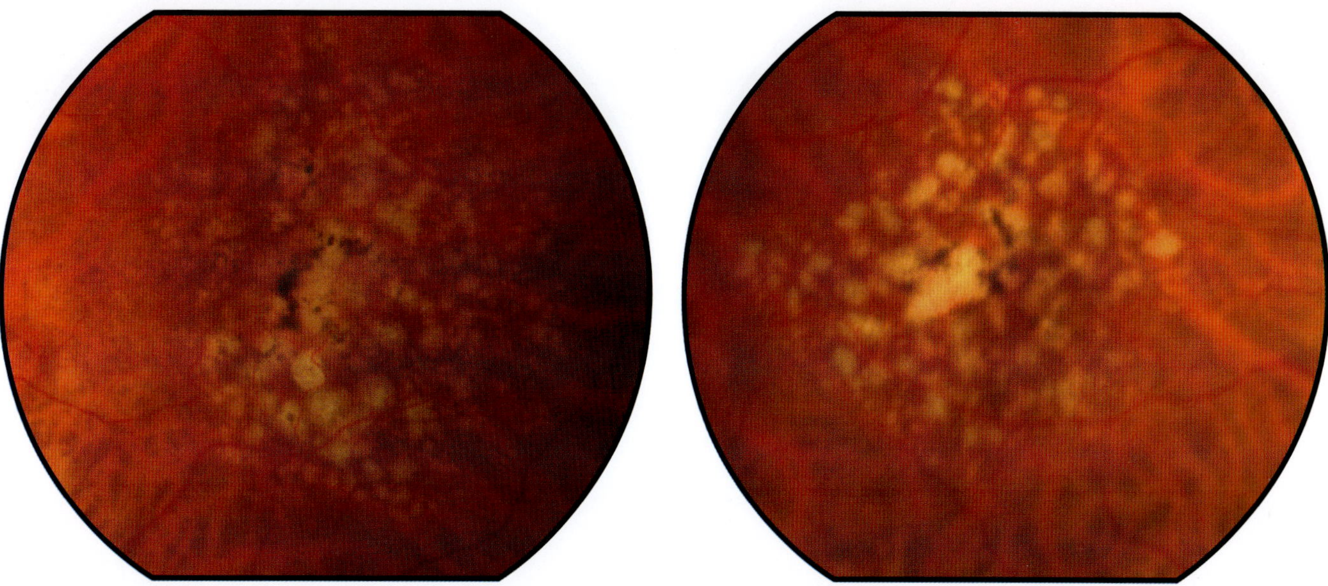

These patients demonstrate a variable degree of pigmentary change associated with drusen. Pigment epithelial hyperplasia is seen overlying confluent drusen.

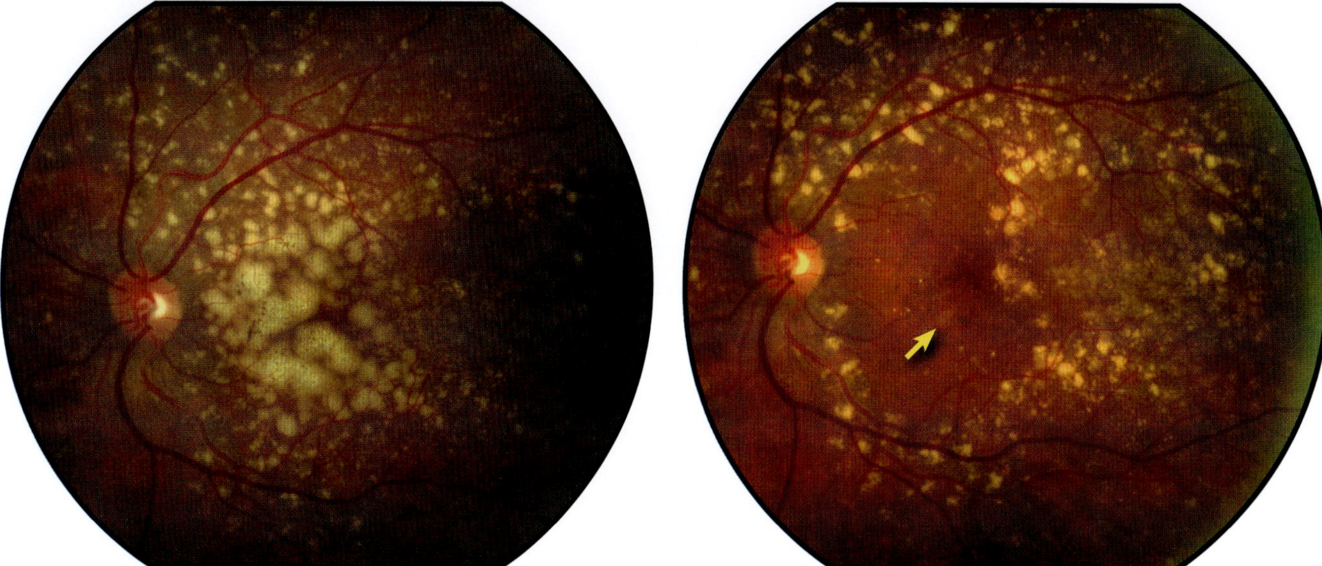

This patient presented with confluent drusen and hyperpigmentation *(left image)* and demonstrated regression of these findings over a course of 4 years *(right)*. An area of hypopigmentation is seen inferior to the fovea *(arrow)*.

A classification system for risk of AMD progression based on fundus lesions including drusen and pigmentary changes, assessed within two disc diameters of the fovea in persons older than 55 years, was proposed as follows:

Classification of AMD	Definition
No apparent aging changes	No drusen and no AMD pigmentary abnormalities
Normal aging changes	Only small drusen (drupelets) and no AMD pigmentary abnormalities
Early AMD	Medium drusen and no AMD pigmentary abnormalities
Intermediate AMD	Large drusen and/or any AMD pigmentary abnormalities
Late AMD	Neovascular AMD and/or any geographic atrophy

Drusen with Refractile Deposits

Drusen may be associated with the appearance of refractile deposits, particularly in relation to regressing drusen at sites of future geographic atrophy. These refractile deposits presumably represent calcification or lipid mineralization of residual lipophilic material within chronic drusen that have not been removed by macrophages.

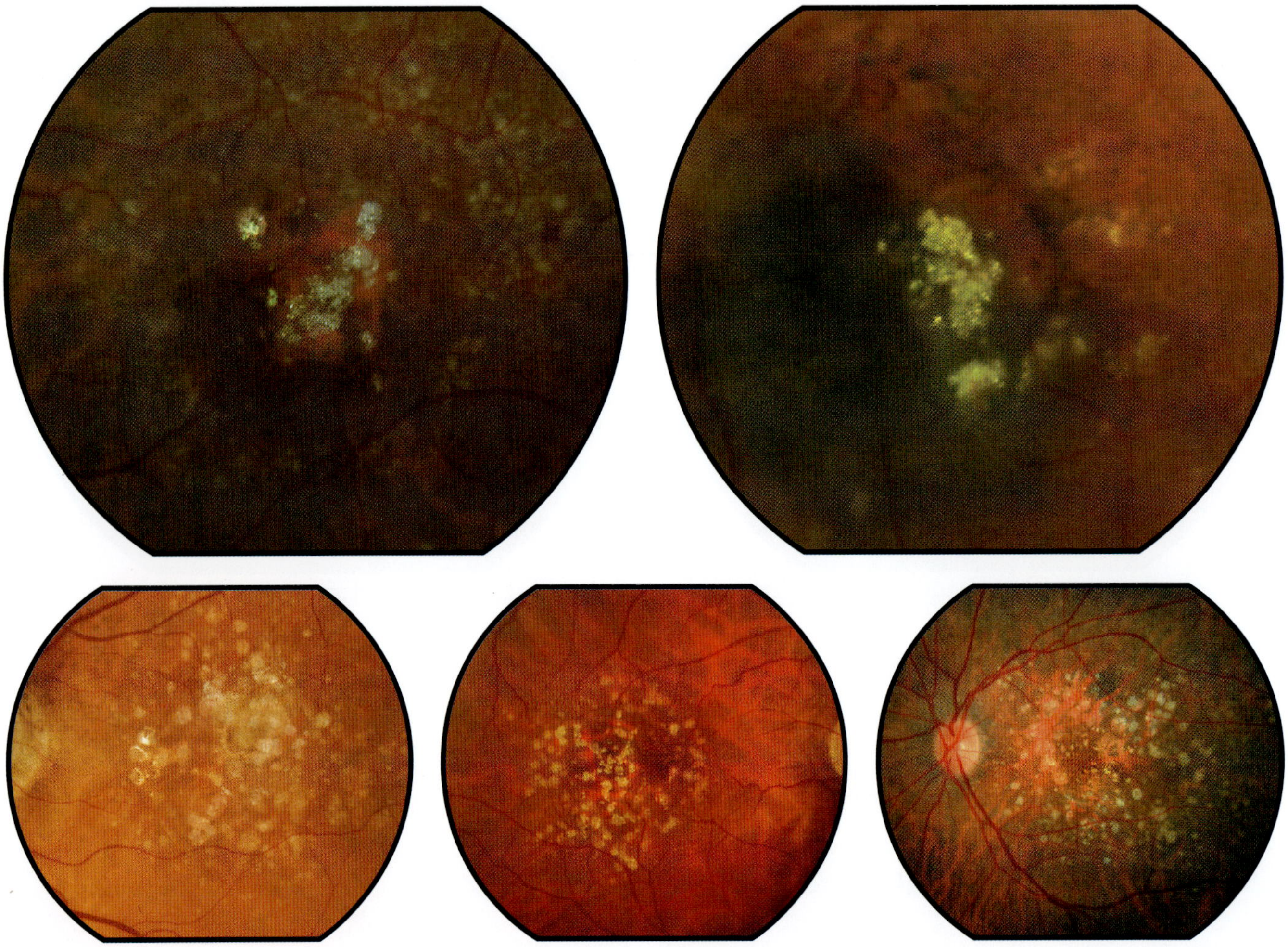

These patients demonstrate typical refractile deposits that contain material that strongly reflects light to produce a glistening appearance.

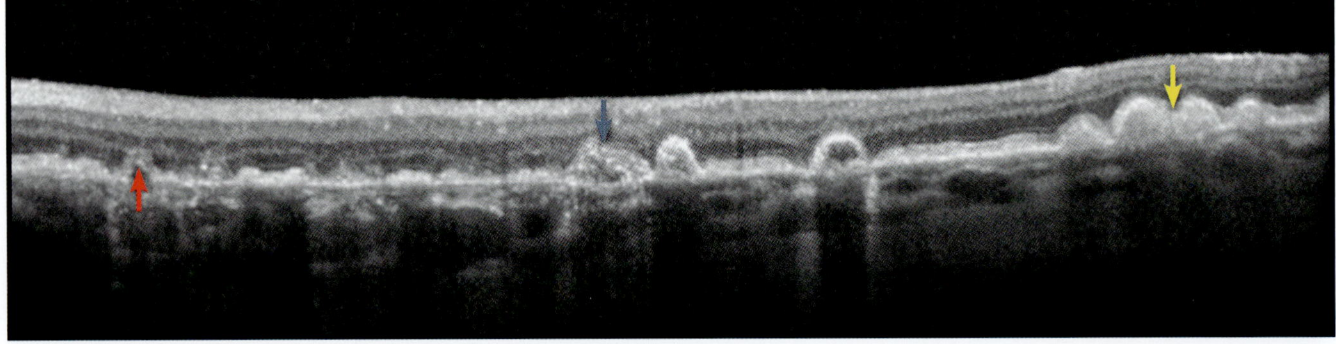

This spectral-domain OCT shows that drusen with refractile deposits may contain hyper-reflective dots *(red and blue arrows)* compared with drusen without refractile deposits *(yellow arrow)*.

Unilateral Drusen

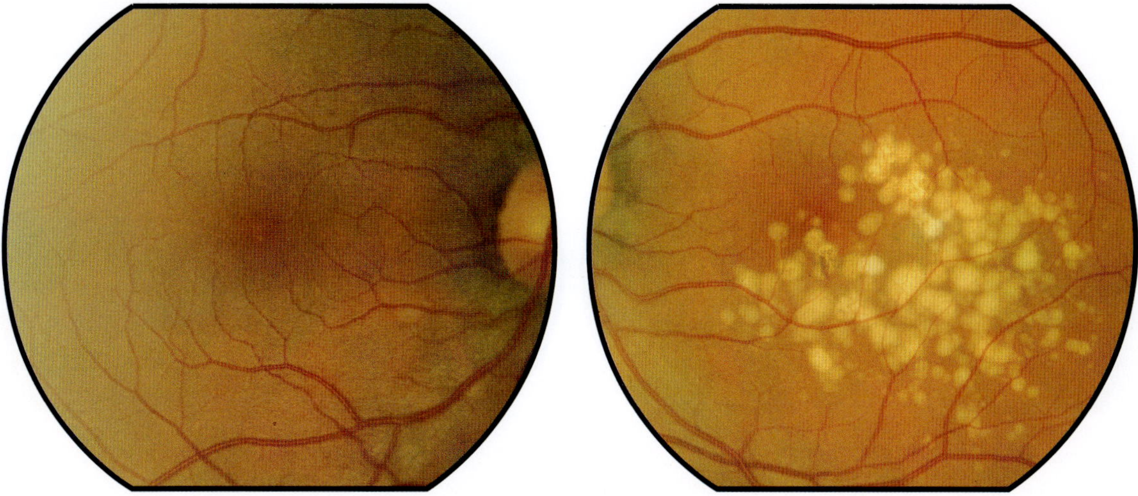

Drusen are usually bilateral and symmetric. However, in this case, marked asymmetry of the drusen can be seen with virtually no changes in one eye *(left image)* and multiple large drusen in the fellow eye *(right image)*. This patient was followed for more than 2 decades without any significant change in the appearance of the fundi.

Peripheral Drusen

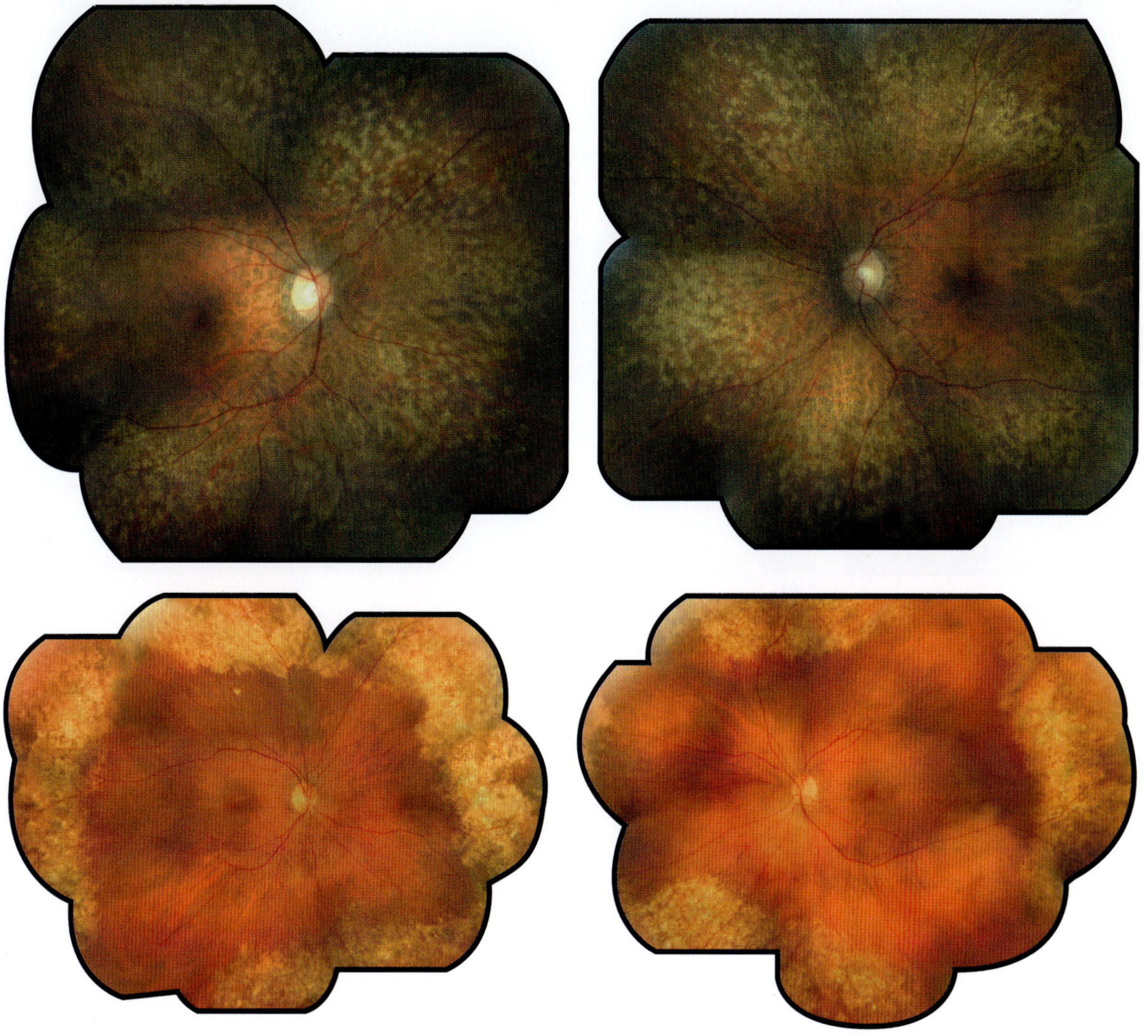

Drusen may occur in the peripheral fundus and can be very extensive in nature. These patients have relative sparing of the posterior pole and do not necessarily have high risk for central vision loss unless drusenoid changes develop in the central macula. More precise characterization of these drusen is possible with multimodal imaging including near-infrared reflectance, fundus autofluorescence, and high-resolution OCT.

Spontaneous Resolution of Drusen

Drusen formation and resorption are dynamic processes that can occur simultaneously in the natural course of AMD. When spontaneous regression of large drusen occurs, it is often followed by progression to geographic atrophy.

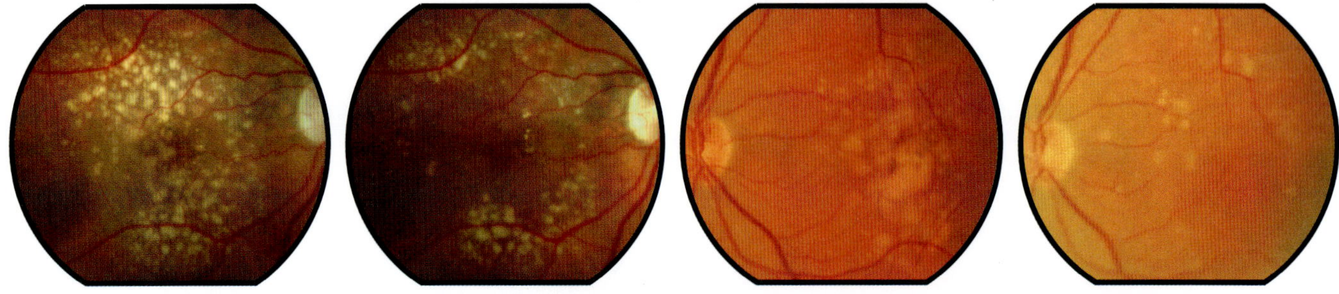

These patients show resolution of drusen without the appearance of geographic atrophy. The photographs with drusen regression were taken approximately 2 years *(left)* and 3.5 years *(right)* after the initial photographs.

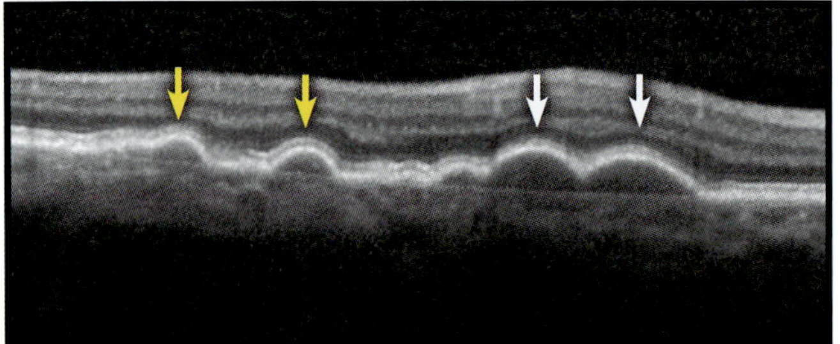

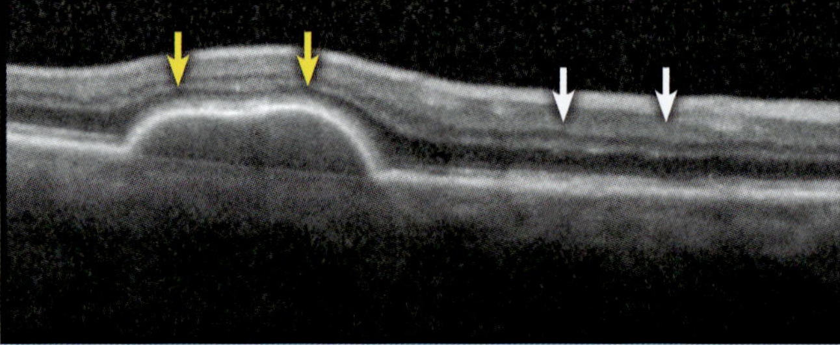

These two OCTs are successive serial eye-tracked scans taken 5 years apart. Note how the two small drusen on the left have coalesced to form a drusenoid PED *(yellow arrows)*, while the two drusen on the right have regressed without atrophy *(white arrows)*.

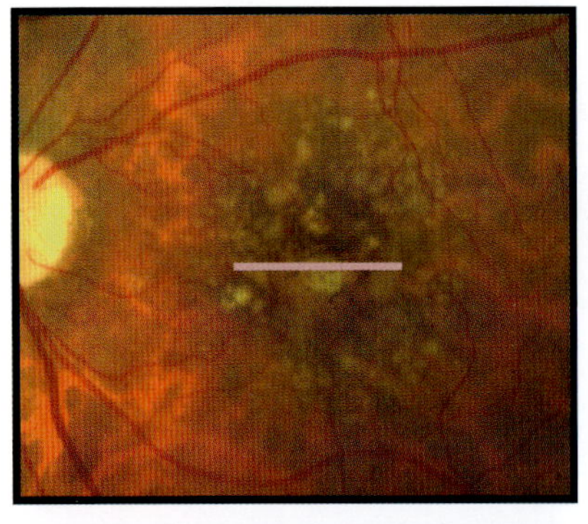

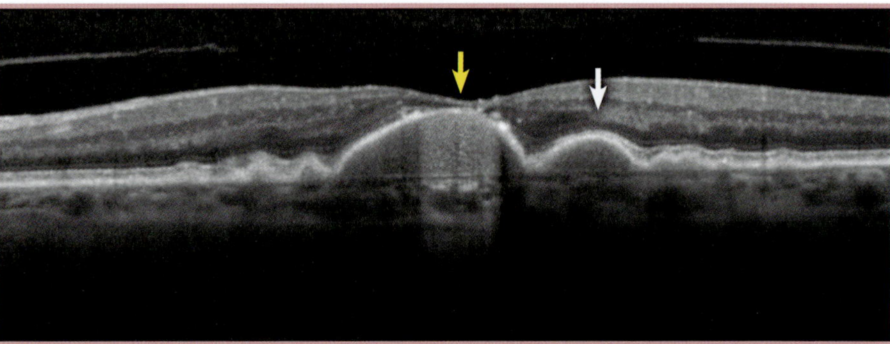

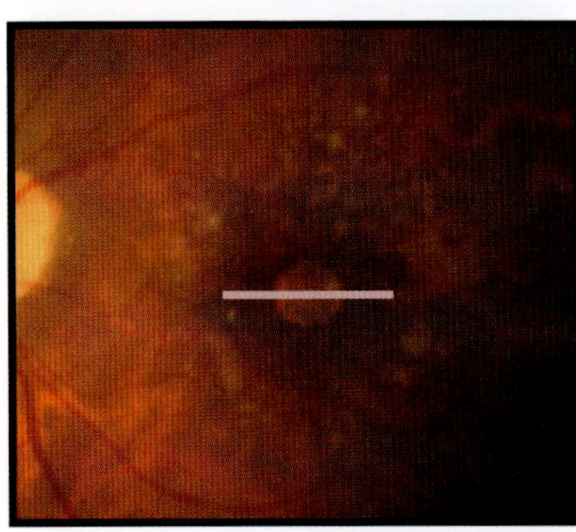

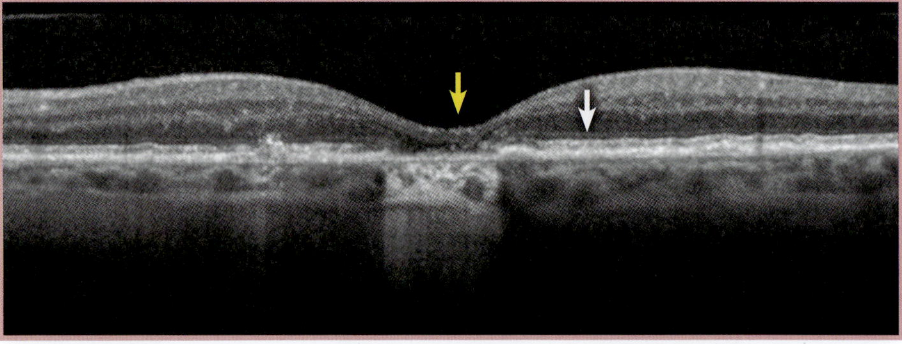

This patient with large drusen and a central drusenoid PED in the macula showed spontaneous regression of drusen, resulting in geographic atrophy centrally *(yellow arrow)* but an absence of atrophy in an adjacent area located more temporally *(white arrow)*. Spectral domain OCT imaging *(top)* shows that photoreceptor loss and retinal pigment epithelial changes including thinning, migration, and clumping were present prior to flattening of the drusenoid PED. These changes associated with a vertical hyper-reflective "column" within the drusenoid PED related to transmission of light through defective tissue (hypertransmission) and may be predictive of the subsequent occurrence of geographic atrophy. There is no observable disruption of the RPE overlying the drusen that resolved without atrophy.

Cuticular Drusen

Cuticular drusen (sometimes referred to as basal laminar drusen) appear as numerous, uniform, round, yellow-white punctate accumulations under the RPE in a densely packed arrangement. They are typically 50–75 μm in diameter and usually present between 40 and 60 years of age. With fluorescein angiography, they demonstrate a classic "starry-sky" or "milky-way" pattern of multiple pinpoint early hyperfluorescent dots against a dark background. These pinpoint dots appear hypoautofluorescent with a ring of hyperautofluorescence on fundus autofluorescence, attributed to the thinning of RPE overlying the apex of the druse, produced by its protrusion into the RPE. This can be appreciated with OCT imaging, which shows a characteristic "sawtooth" pattern. Eyes with cuticular drusen may develop acquired vitelliform lesions. These eyes may also develop large drusen later in their course and are then at a higher risk for developing choroidal neovascularization.

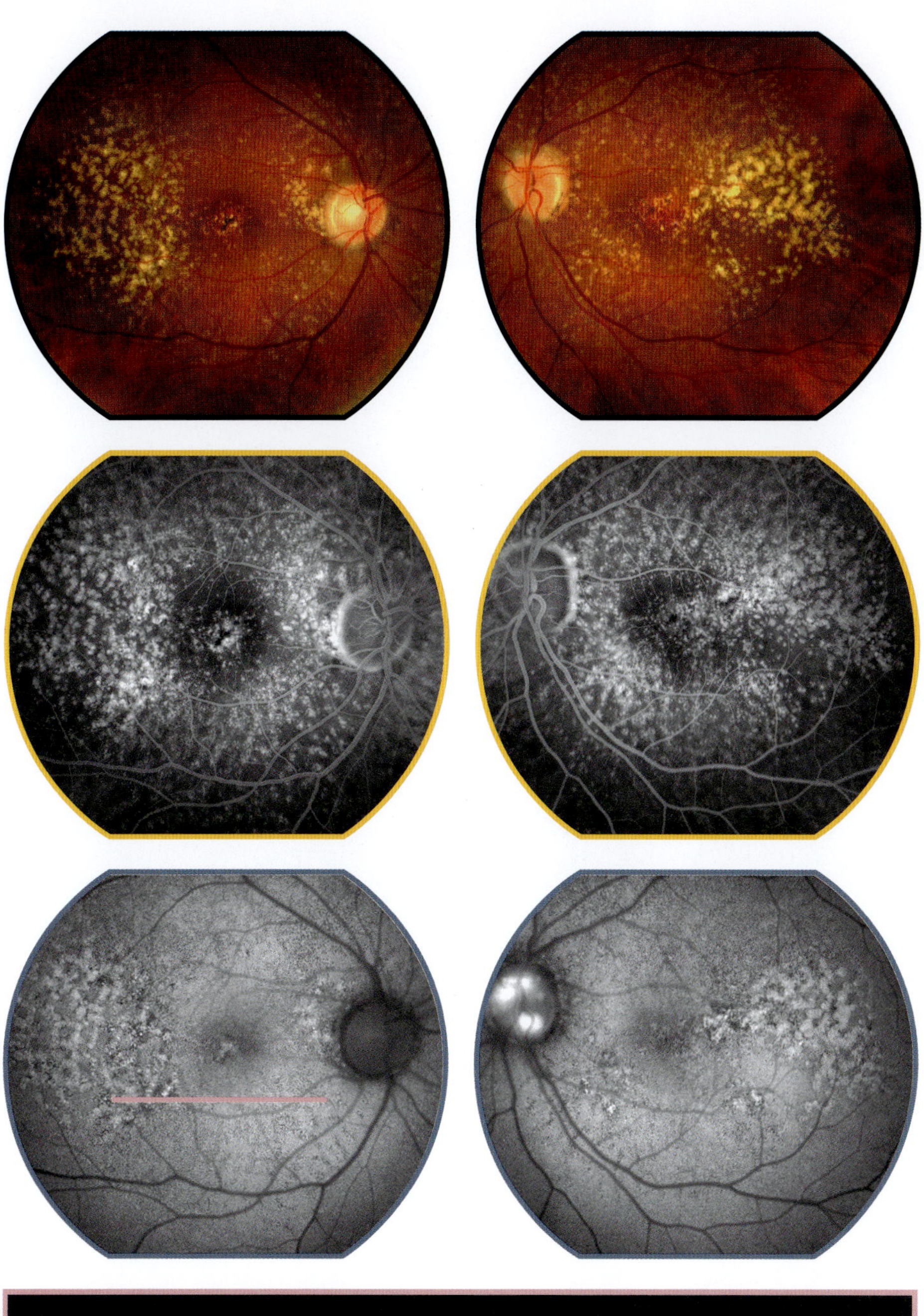

This patient has widespread cuticular drusen and large drusen in the temporal macula. Fluorescein angiography shows a starry-sky appearance, and fundus autofluorescence shows a myriad of hypoautofluorescent dots with a ring of hyperautofluorescence. OCT of the right eye shows a classic sawtooth appearance of the cuticular drusen nasal to the fovea *(yellow arrows)* and dome-like RPE elevations of large drusen temporally *(white arrows)*. Optic disc drusen is also seen in the left eye of this case. Currently, there is no known association between optic disc drusen and cuticular drusen.

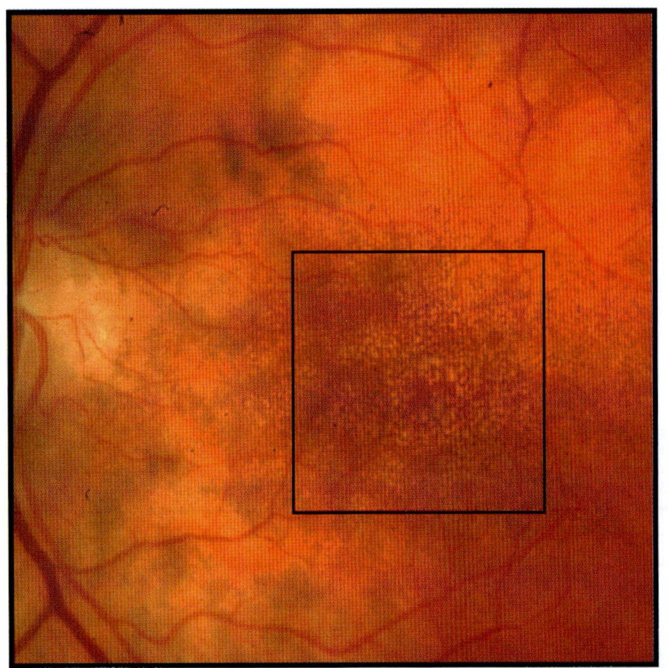

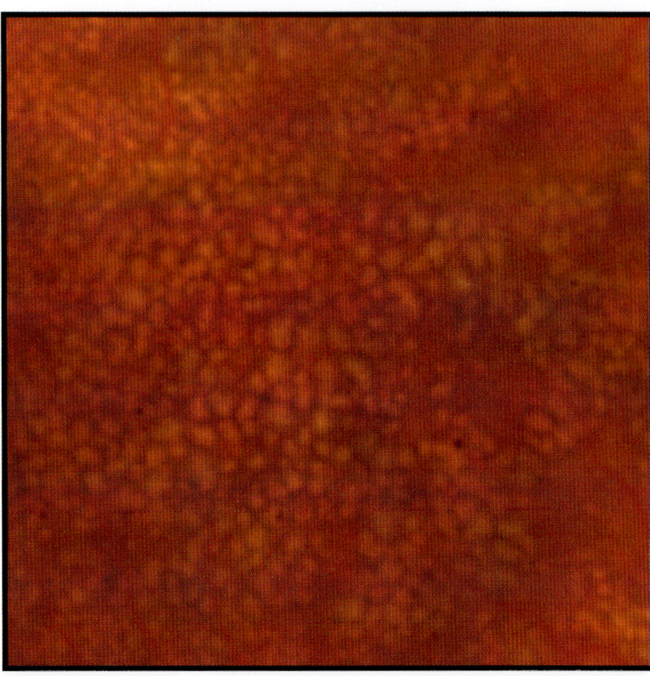

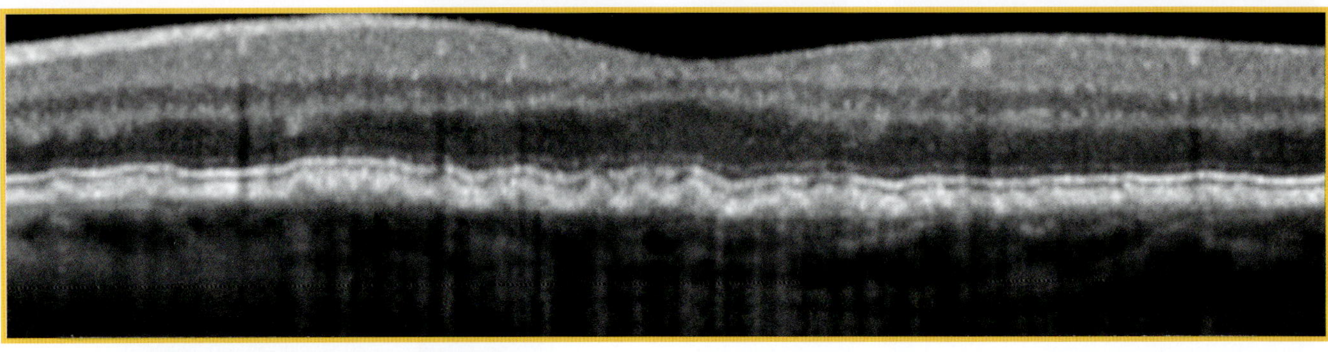

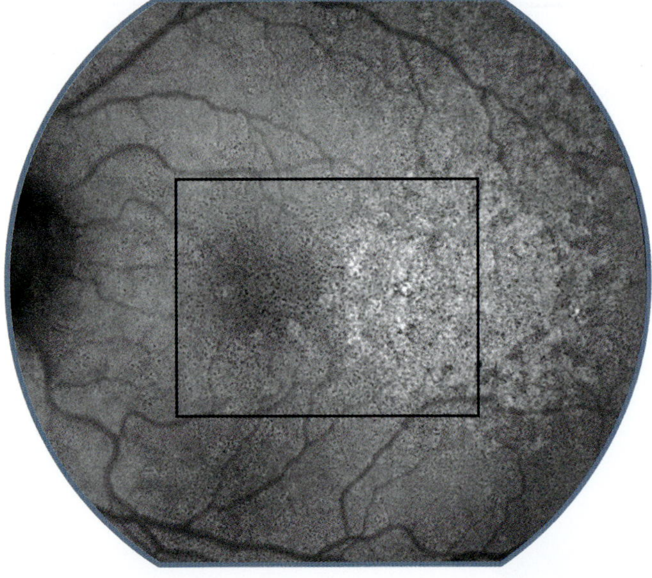

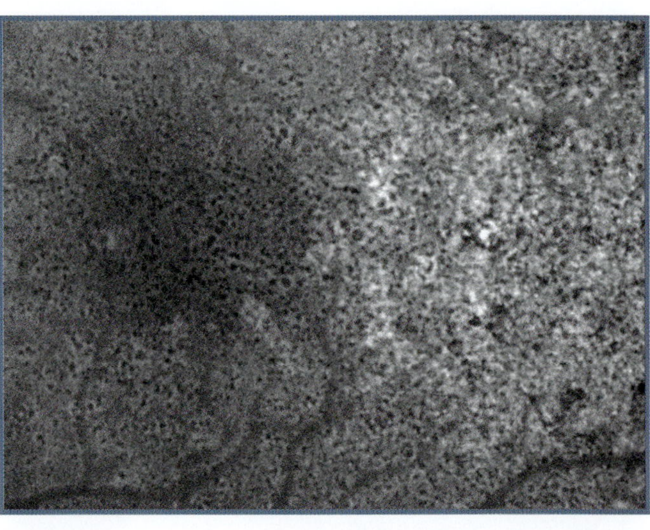

These patients have cuticular drusen involving the fovea. OCT imaging shows the sawtooth appearance of multiple protrusions into the overlying RPE band. Note the thinning of the RPE over the apex of cuticular drusen. With fundus autofluorescence, cuticular drusen are evident as dots of hypoautofluorescence surrounded by a ring of hyperautofluorescence.

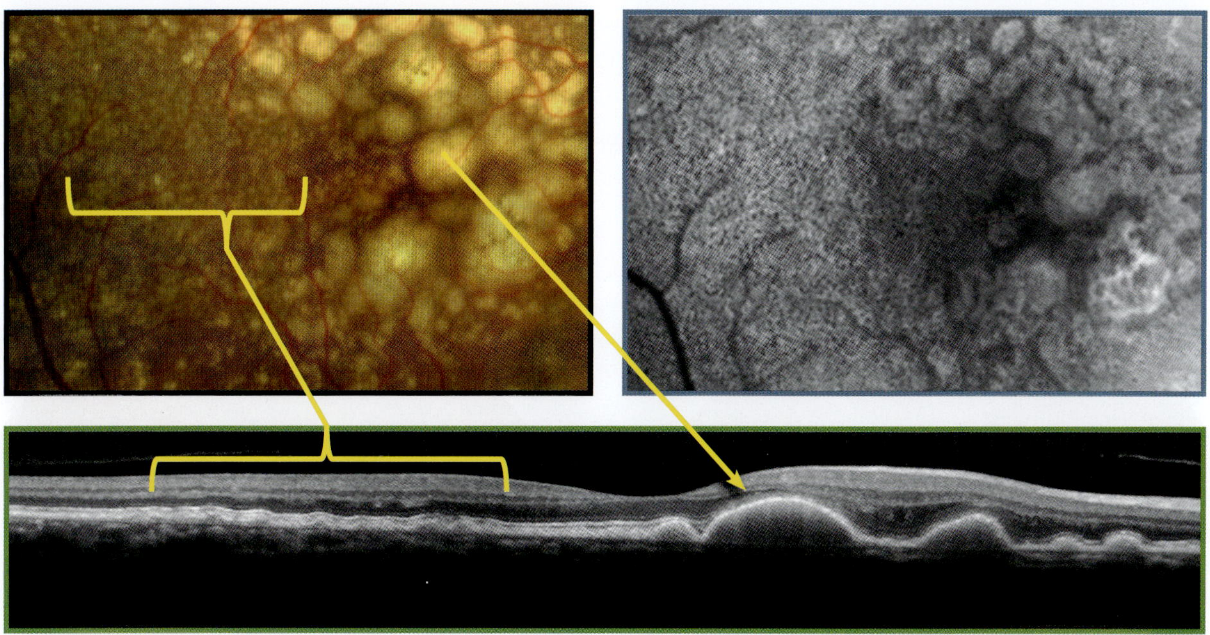

This patient demonstrates a mixture of cuticular and large drusen in the macula. This patient is at risk of developing an acquired vitelliform lesion, choroidal neovascularization, and atrophy.

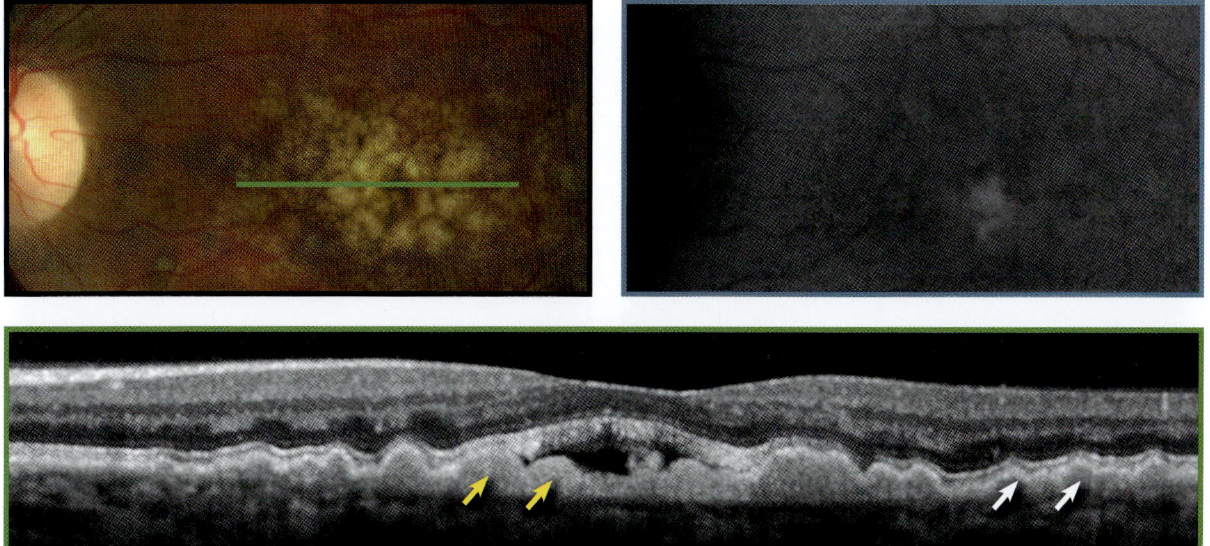

This patient has both widespread cuticular drusen and large drusen. Fundus autofluorescence shows dots of hypoautofluorescence characteristic of cuticular drusen. The OCT shows large drusen *(yellow arrows)* and subretinal fluid within an acquired vitelliform lesion. A sawtooth pattern *(white arrows)*, corresponding to cuticular drusen, is seen temporally.

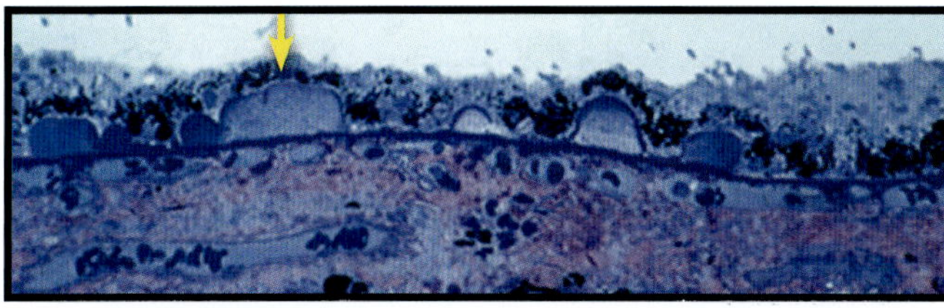

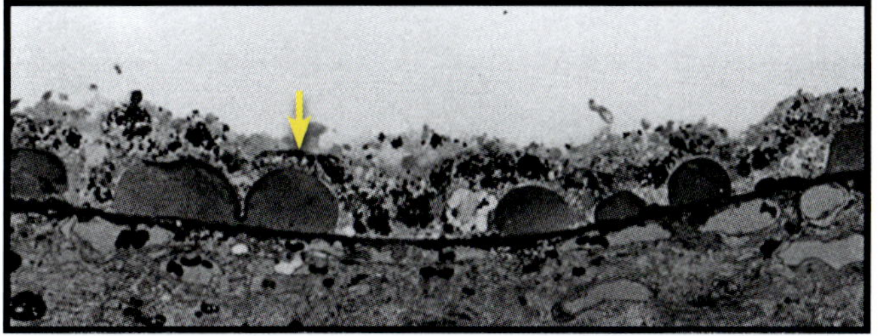

Light microscopy *(top image)* and electron microscopy *(bottom image)* of cuticular drusen showing numerous ovoid accumulations protruding into the overlying RPE monolayer, creating thinning of the RPE at the apex *(arrow)* and thickening of RPE at the base between each druse. *Images courtesy of Dr. John Sarks*

Large Colloid Drusen

Large colloid drusen (LCD) are an uncommon subtype of early onset drusen with a female preponderance. The mean age at diagnosis is 35 years. Similar to soft drusen, LCD are localized in the subretinal pigment epithelial space, but they are much larger and have a mean diameter of approximately 400 microns. They may occur in isolation or demonstrate confluence and are most often present bilaterally. There are limited data regarding the long-term course of LCD, but they are not known to be associated with atrophy or neovascularization. The genetics of LCD also remain to be clarified, but it has not been shown to have a clear inheritance pattern.

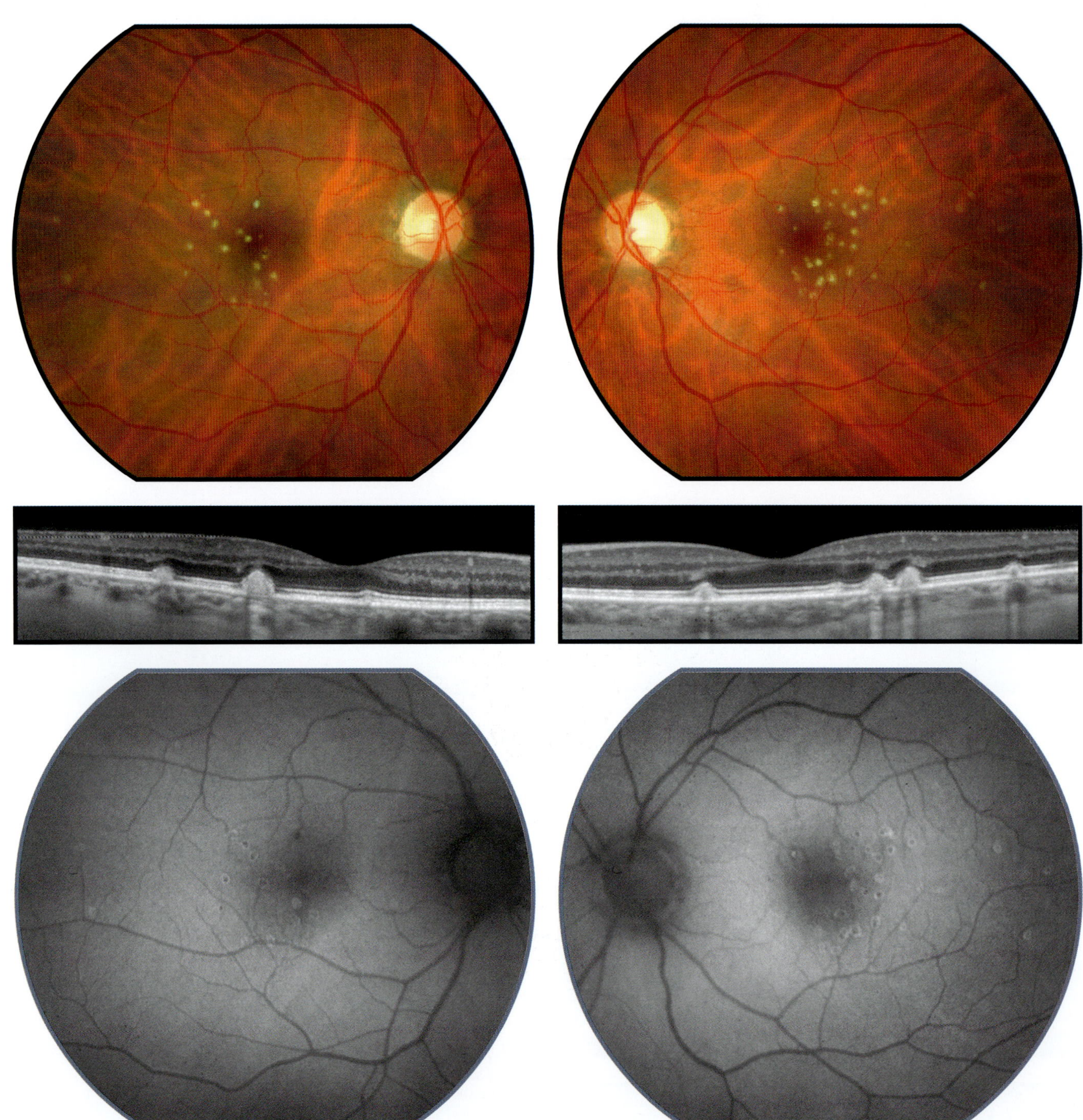

An asymptomatic 49-year-old female with large bilateral drusen predominantly localized to the temporal parafovea. OCT demonstrates homogenous, hyper-reflective lesions in the subretinal pigment epithelial space. Colloidal drusen are hyperautofluorescent on fundus autofluorescence imaging, as shown.

Reticular Pseudodrusen

Reticular pseudodrusen describes an interlacing pattern of yellow-white subretinal material that appears whiter than typical drusen. This material is best visualized with red-free, blue-light, and near-infrared reflectance imaging and may be missed with fluorescein angiography. Reticular pseudodrusen are easily seen in pseudophakic patients in whom there is greater transmission of blue light to the fundus. Reticular pseudodrusen first appear in the superior outer macula and may progress to involve the periphery and central macula. They are associated with a higher risk of type 2 neovascularization than are other types of drusen. The OCT appearance of reticular pseudodrusen is known as subretinal drusenoid deposits.

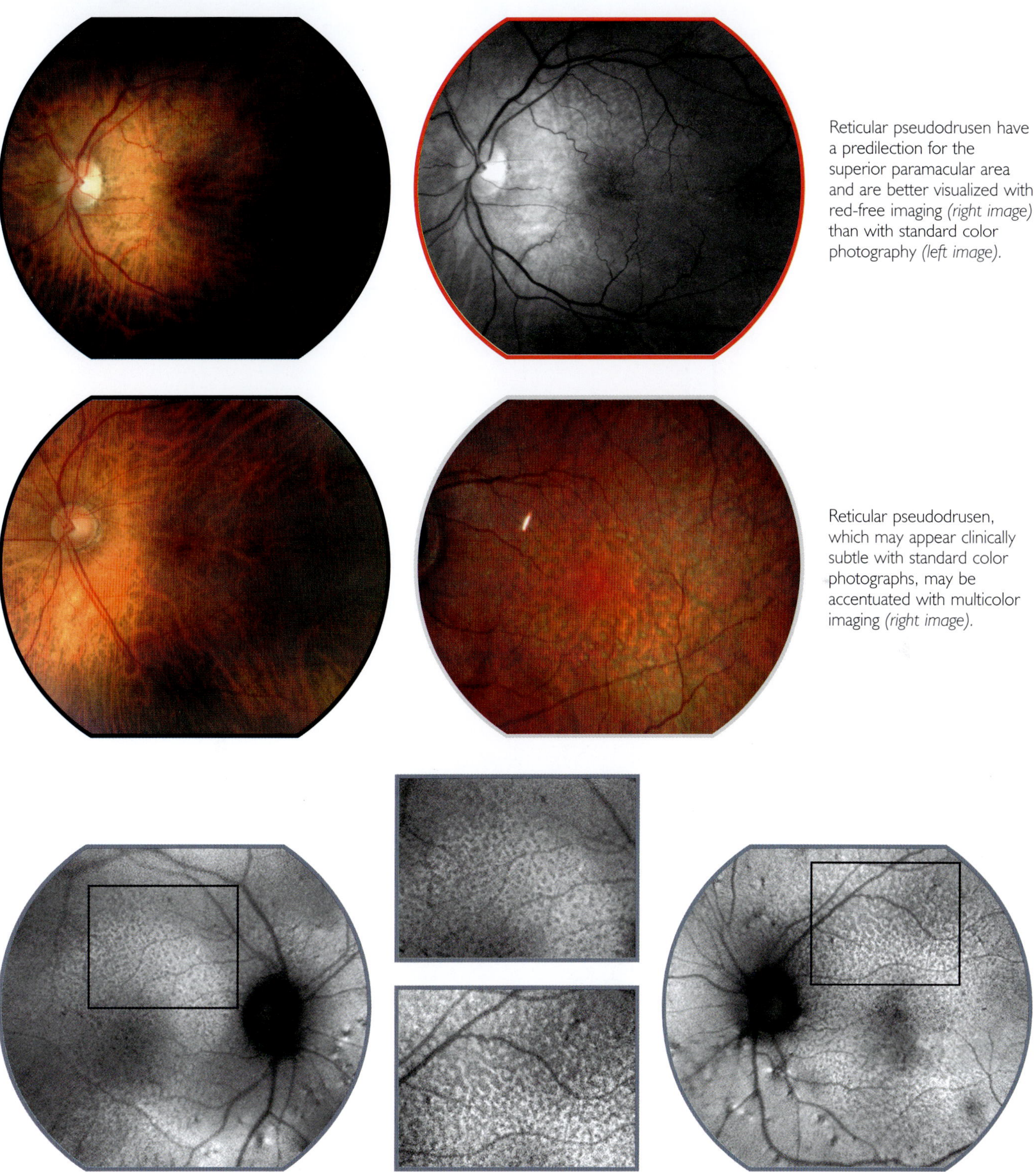

Reticular pseudodrusen have a predilection for the superior paramacular area and are better visualized with red-free imaging *(right image)* than with standard color photography *(left image)*.

Reticular pseudodrusen, which may appear clinically subtle with standard color photographs, may be accentuated with multicolor imaging *(right image)*.

This patient has reticular pseudodrusen throughout the central fundus and beyond. The fundus autofluorescence shows dots of hypoautofluorescence surrounded by a reticular pattern of hyperautofluorescence.

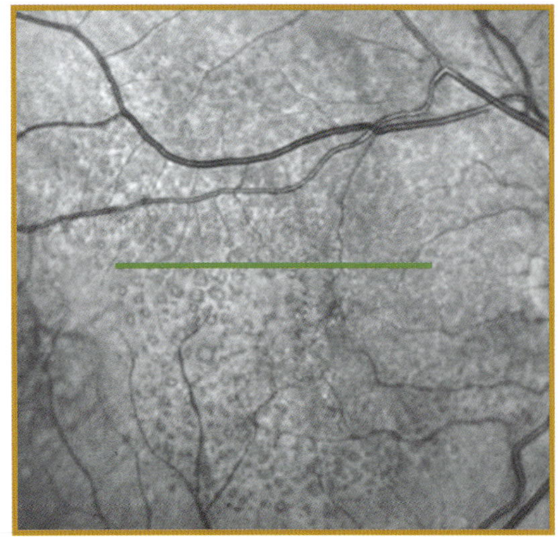

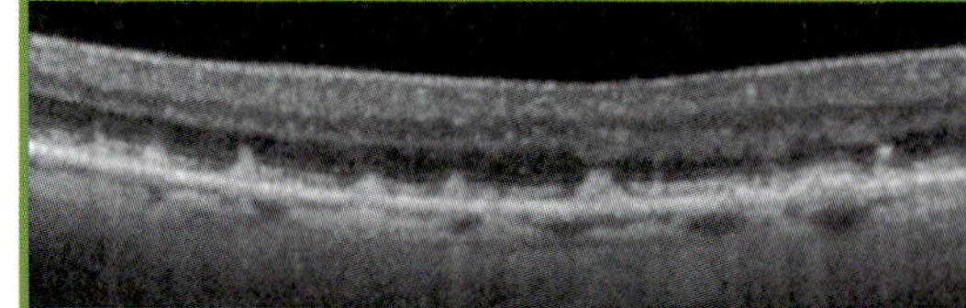

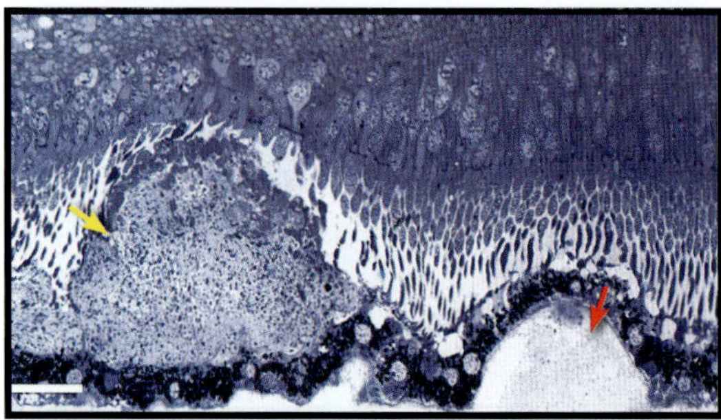

With near-infrared reflectance, reticular pseudodrusen appears as a doughnut pattern with a hyper-reflective center and dark halo. OCT imaging shows the subretinal drusenoid deposits situated above the RPE band of varying shapes and thicknesses that may breach the external limiting membrane. Histology shows the subretinal drusenoid deposit *(yellow arrow)* above the RPE, in contrast to the adjacent soft druse that is below the RPE *(red arrow)*.

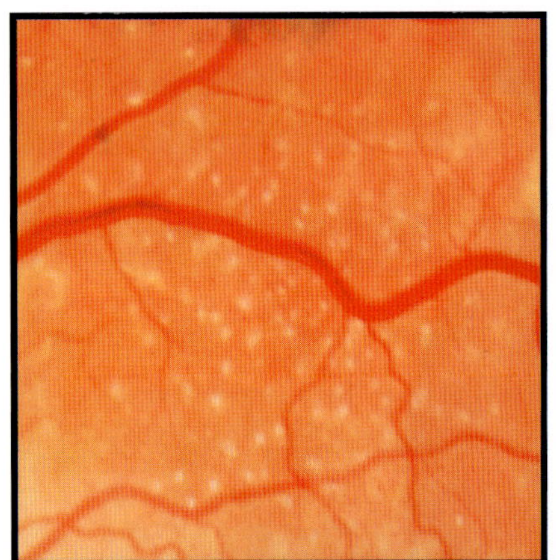

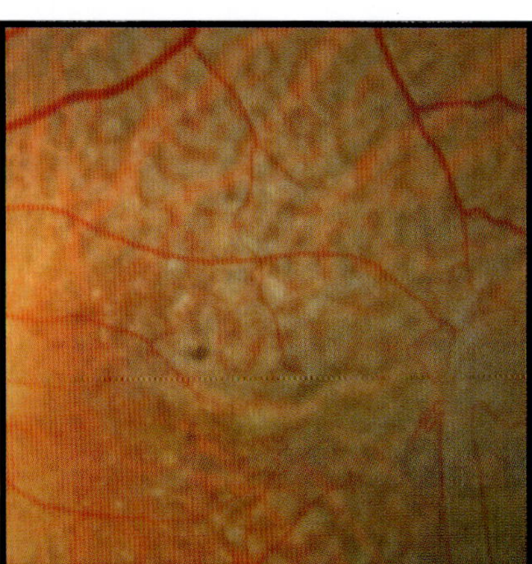

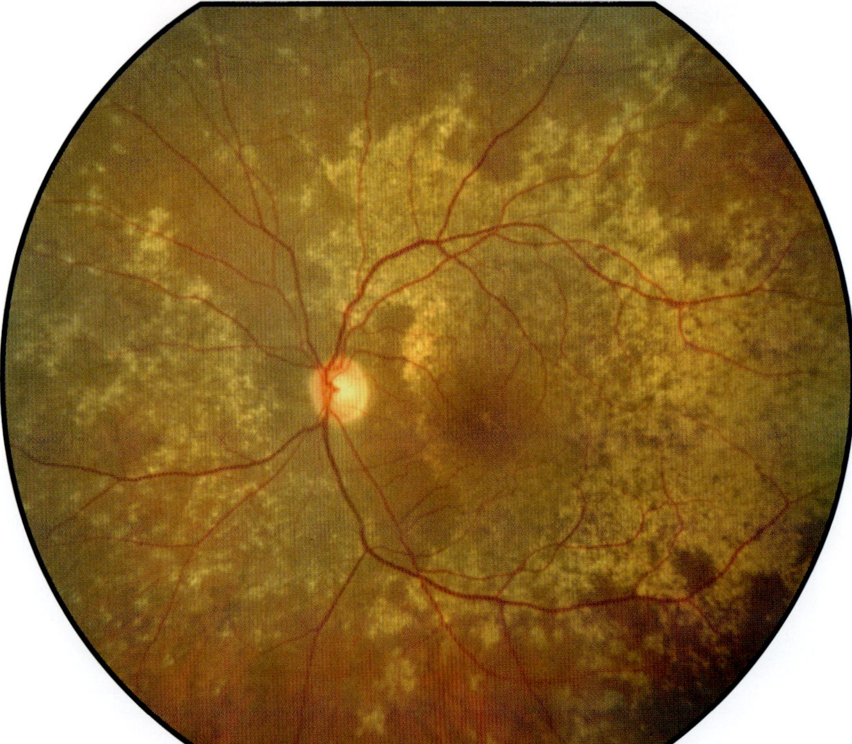

Reticular pseudodrusen may appear in three different forms: dot pseudodrusen, which are more apparent with near-infrared reflectance than color photography *(top left image)*; ribbon pseudodrusen, which are more apparent on color photography than near-infrared reflectance *(top right image)*; and, less commonly, peripheral reticular pseudodrusen, which appear as yellow globules located peripheral to the perifoveal region *(bottom image)*.

Pigment Epithelial Detachment

Pigment epithelial detachment (PED) is a separation of the RPE from the underlying Bruch membrane and occurs in both non-neovascular and neovascular AMD. The classification of PEDs can be divided into drusenoid, serous, vascularized, or mixed categories. Drusenoid PEDs are primarily a feature of non-neovascular AMD. Serous PEDs may occur in the absence of clinically or angiographically detectable neovascularization, although some may be associated with neovascular AMD. Vascularized PEDs are associated with type 1 neovascularization and are discussed in greater detail in the neovascular AMD portion of this chapter.

Drusenoid PED

A drusenoid PED is a high-risk form of non-neovascular AMD that develops in association with large confluent drusen. Although most commonly related to AMD, drusenoid PEDs may also occur in other retinal disorders with AMD-like findings such as malattia leventinese, cuticular drusen, the maculopathy associated with membranoproliferative glomerulonephritis type 2, and overlying choroidal nevi. There is no established size criterion to distinguish large drusen from drusenoid PEDs, although the Age-Related Eye Disease Study has defined a drusenoid PED as measuring 350 μm or greater.

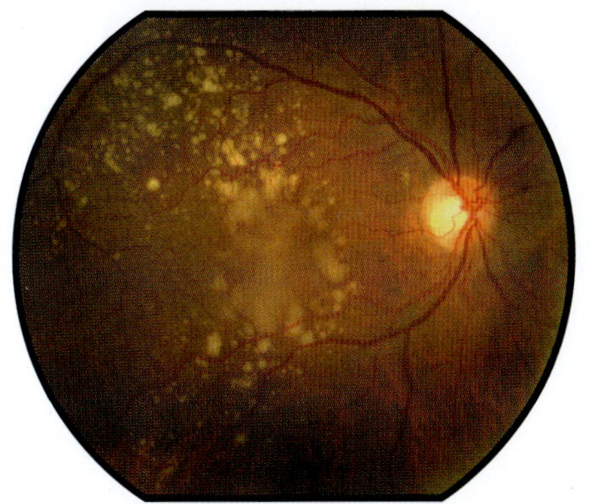
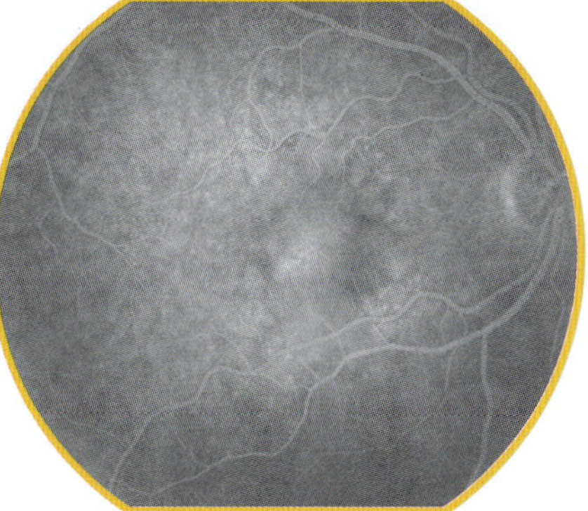
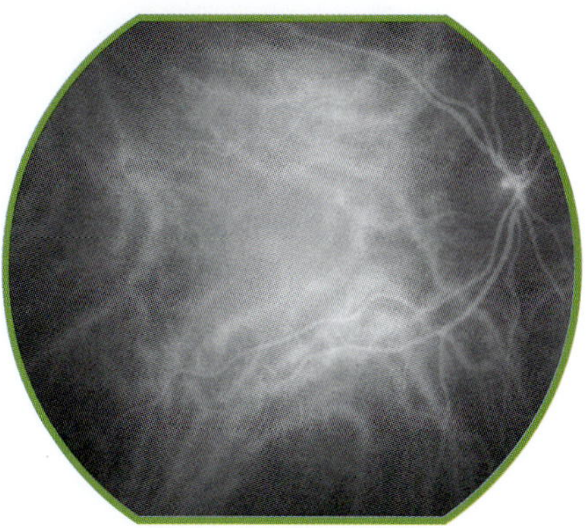

Drusenoid PEDs appear as well-circumscribed yellow elevations of the RPE in the macula and are often surrounded by large soft drusen. Fluorescein angiography of drusenoid PEDs shows a mild hyperfluorescence without leakage, while ICG angiography shows isofluorescence or slight hypofluorescence due to a blocking effect.

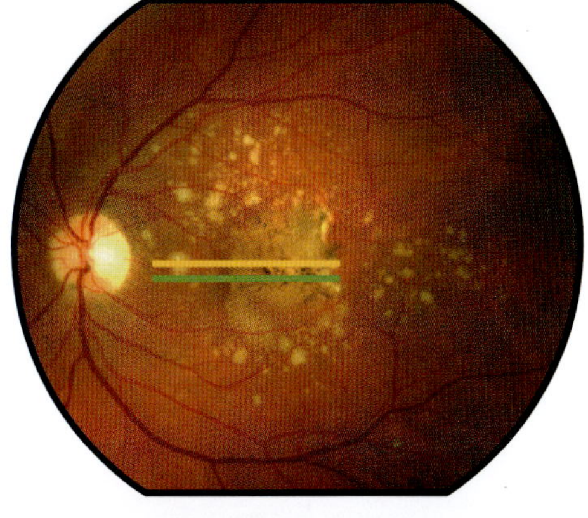
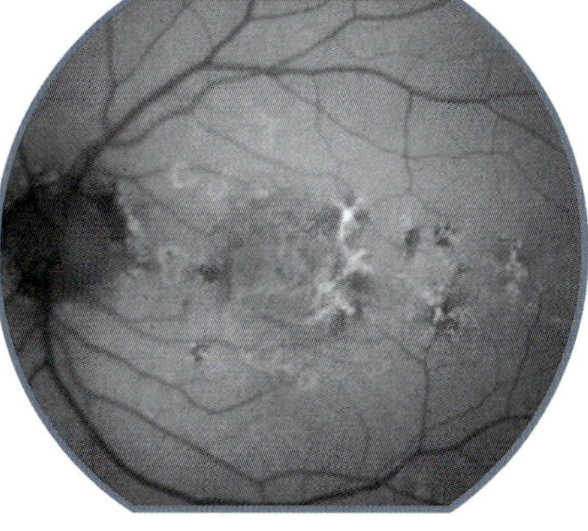
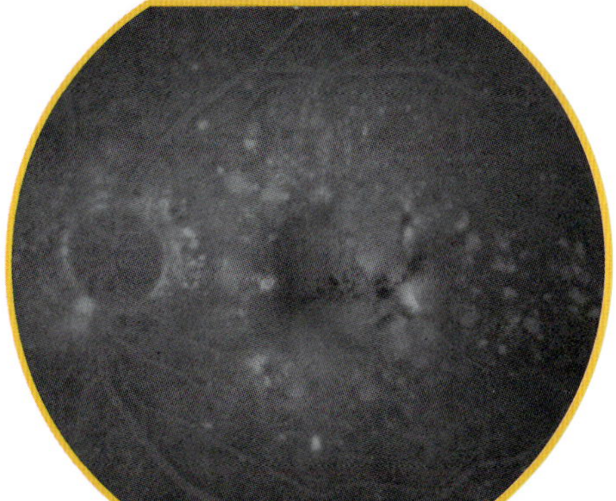
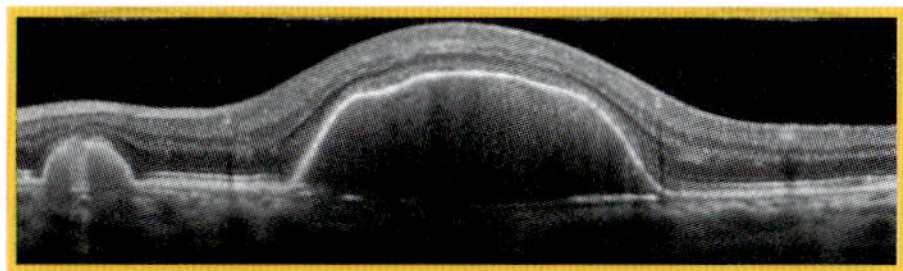
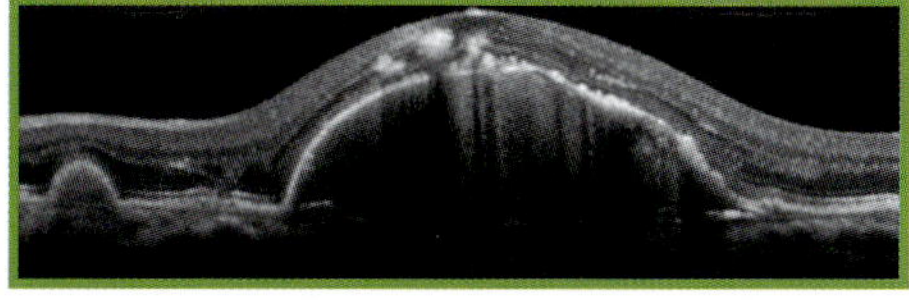

A stellate pattern of hyperpigmentation often gradually appears on the surface of larger drusenoid PEDs. On fundus autofluorescence imaging the drusenoid PED appears relatively isoautofluorescent, while pigmentary changes within it can appear hyperautofluorescent. On fluorescein angiography the pigment changes appear hypofluorescent. OCT shows a dense homogenous and slightly hyper-reflective sub-RPE content with intraretinal pigment migration overlying the dome of the PED.

Drusenoid PED Variants

Drusenoid PEDs may be associated with overlying subretinal fluid or an acquired vitelliform lesion. When subretinal fluid is present, ICG angiography is particularly helpful in excluding the presence of neovascular tissue. The precise mechanism for the development of subretinal fluid or vitelliform material is unclear but is likely to be related to RPE dysfunction that results in the accumulation of shed outer segments and RPE granules in the subretinal space.

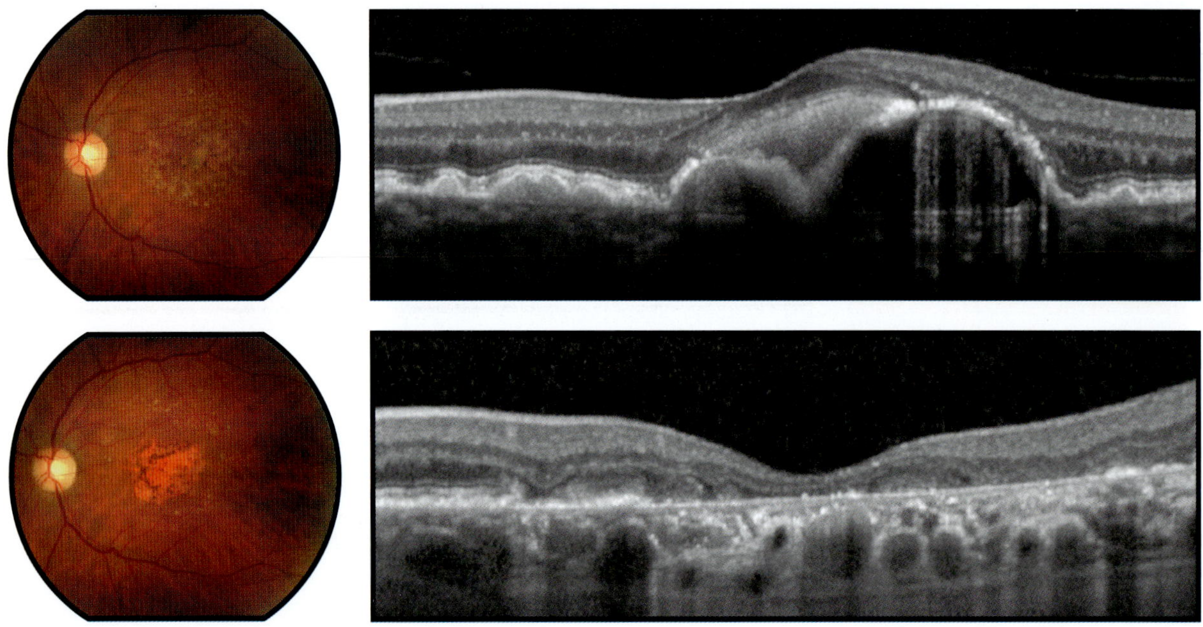

These images show a drusenoid PED with an overlying acquired vitelliform lesion that resolves completely over 4 years *(bottom images)*, leaving a legacy of geographic RPE atrophy and loss of the outer retina.

Mixed Drusenoid and Serous PED

A drusenoid PED may evolve into a mixed PED with a serous component. With high-resolution OCT, the base of the drusenoid material is often seen to be apposed to the Bruch membrane. Over time, the shape and defining contours of drusen commonly remain stable despite the development of an overlying hyporeflective, serous component. The development of a serous component does not necessarily indicate neovascular transformation.

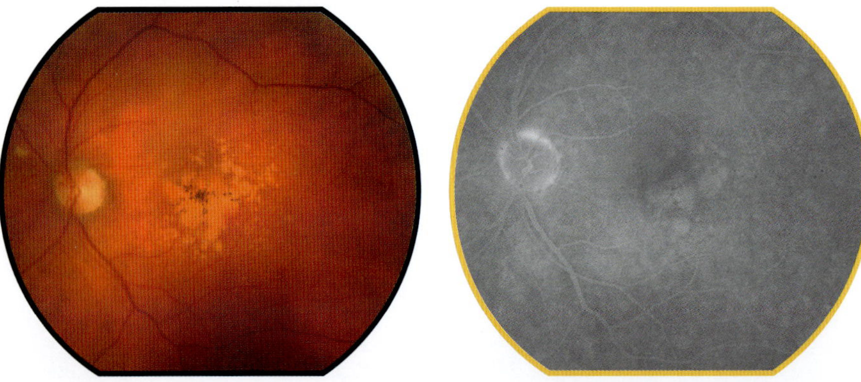

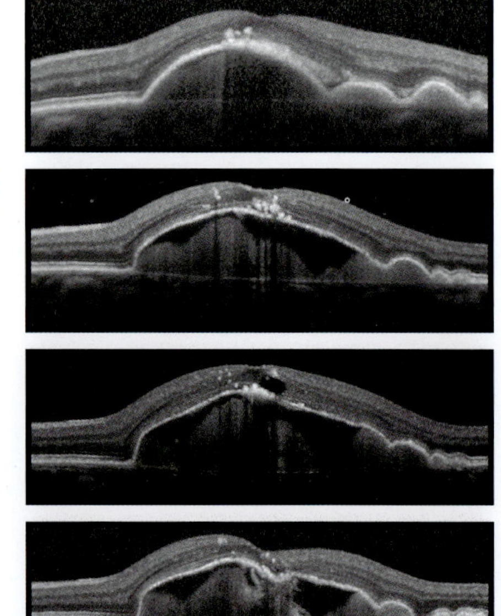

This patient had a drusenoid PED that became mixed with a serous component over 2 years. The drusenoid material remained adherent to the Bruch membrane and retained its original shape *(OCT image in second row)*. Two years later, there is a visible break in the RPE at the apex of the PED with resultant intraretinal cystic changes *(image in third row)*. Neovascularization was absent. The cystic changes resolved spontaneously with collapse of the apex of the PED *(bottom image)*.

Serous PED

Serous PEDs are clear or yellow-orange, circular, or ovoid elevations of the RPE with sharply demarcated borders. They occur most commonly in central serous chorioretinopathy (CSC) and AMD. Although serous PEDs are typically associated with neovascular AMD, only ~1% of patients with neovascular AMD present with a serous PED, while 30% present with a vascularized PED.

With fluorescein angiography, serous PEDs show characteristic intense early hyperfluorescence and progressive rapid pooling within the well-defined sub-RPE space. The intense hyperfluorescent staining in the late phase makes it difficult to differentiate a serous PED from a vascularized PED on fluorescein angiography alone, in which case indocyanine green angiography may be useful.

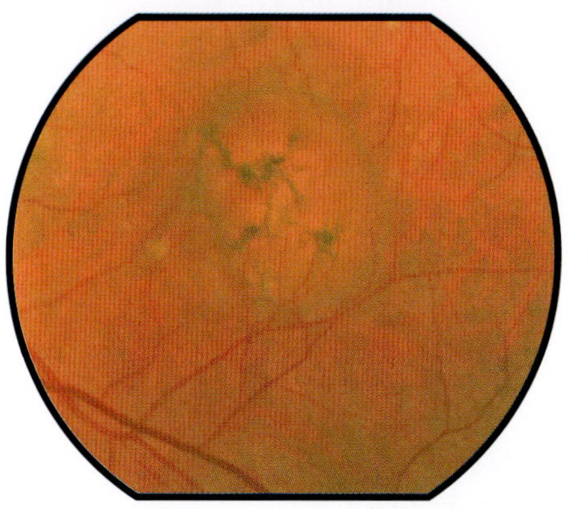
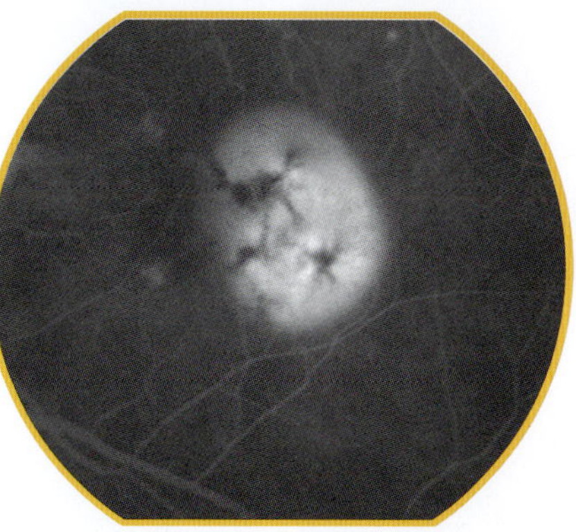
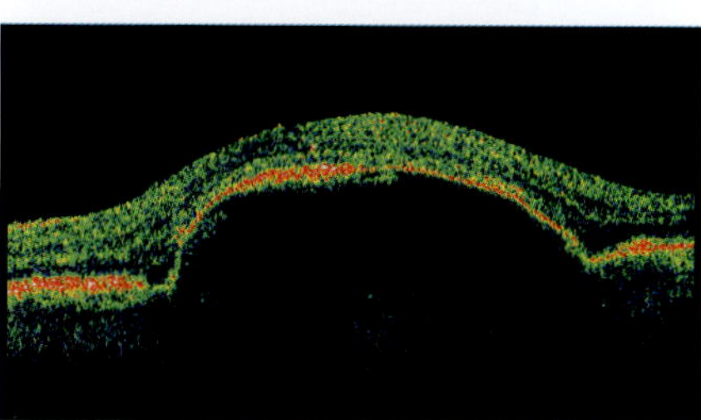

Patients may develop a serous PED with or without other manifestations of non-neovascular AMD. This patient has a discrete PED with chronic pigment epithelial hyperplastic changes. There is no neurosensory detachment, blood, lipid, or other evidence of neovascularization. This is essentially a chronic serous PED. If there are no AMD changes and the patient is below the age of 50, the most common etiology for serous PED is CSC. A serous PED, with subsequent neurosensory detachment, is the hallmark feature of CSC.

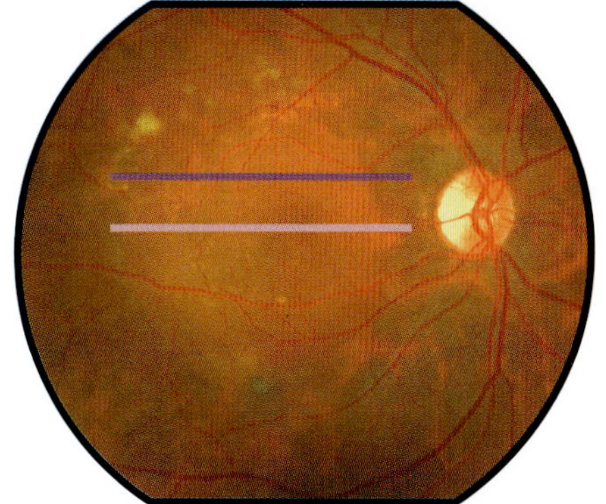
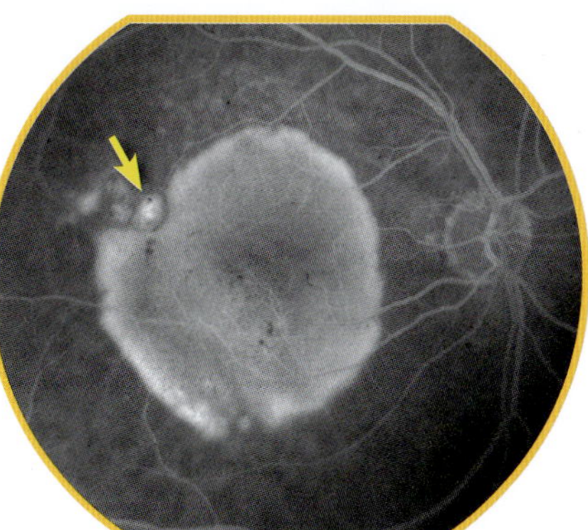
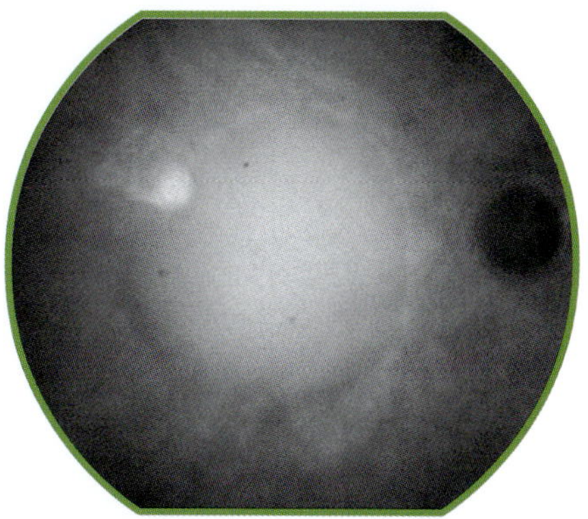

The presence of a hyperfluorescent notch *(arrow)* on fluorescein angiography at the edge of a serous PED may indicate the presence of neovascular tissue or polypoidal lesions. ICG angiography is particularly useful because the PED is typically hypofluorescent and late leakage from neovascularization will be more easily revealed than with fluorescein angiography.

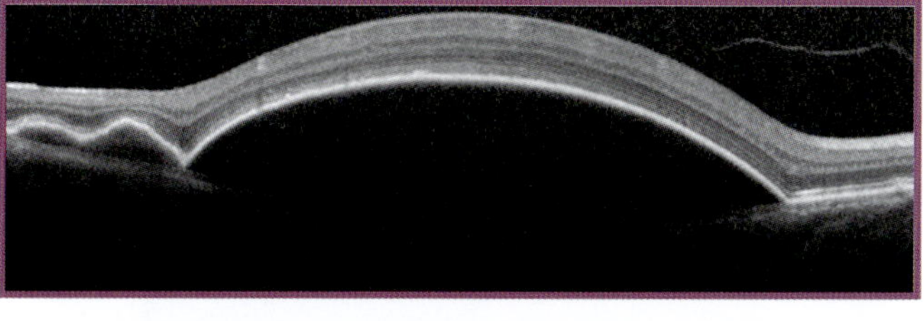
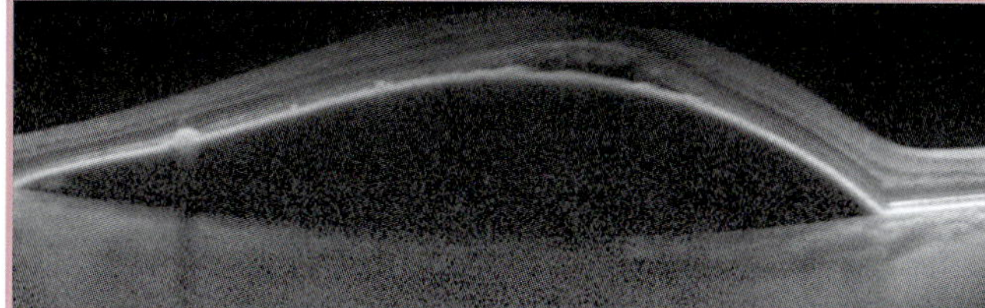
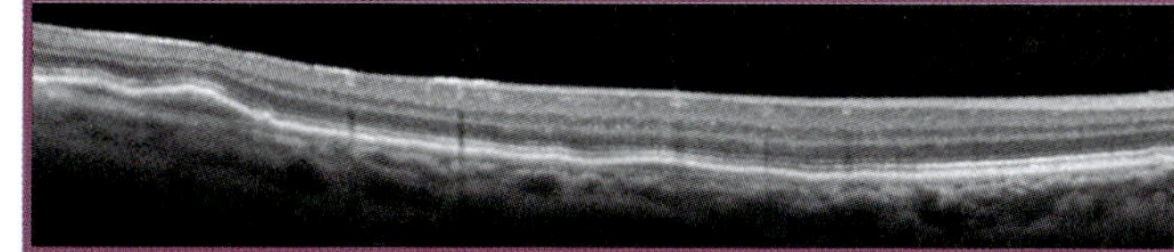
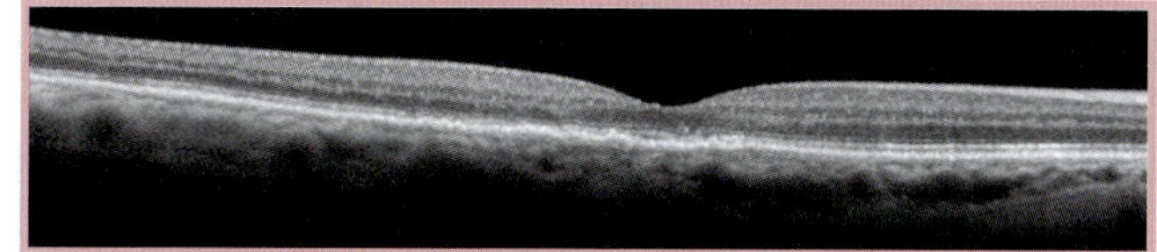

OCT showing the serous PED at the level of the notch and fovea *(top images)*. Three months after treatment with photodynamic therapy and intravitreal aflibercept there is complete resolution *(bottom images)*. The patient had dramatic visual improvement from 20/100 to 20/25.

Serous PED Variants

Serous PEDs may be associated with overlying subretinal fluid and acquired vitelliform lesions. Subretinal fluid may occur in the absence of neovascularization. These findings may be mistaken for a vascularized PED with an overlying exudative detachment. It may be reasonable to observe a serous PED with overlying vitelliform material because intravitreal antivascular endothelial growth factor (anti-VEGF) agents typically do not resolve these findings. Spontaneous resolution may occur with some resultant loss of vision due to outer retinal and RPE atrophy.

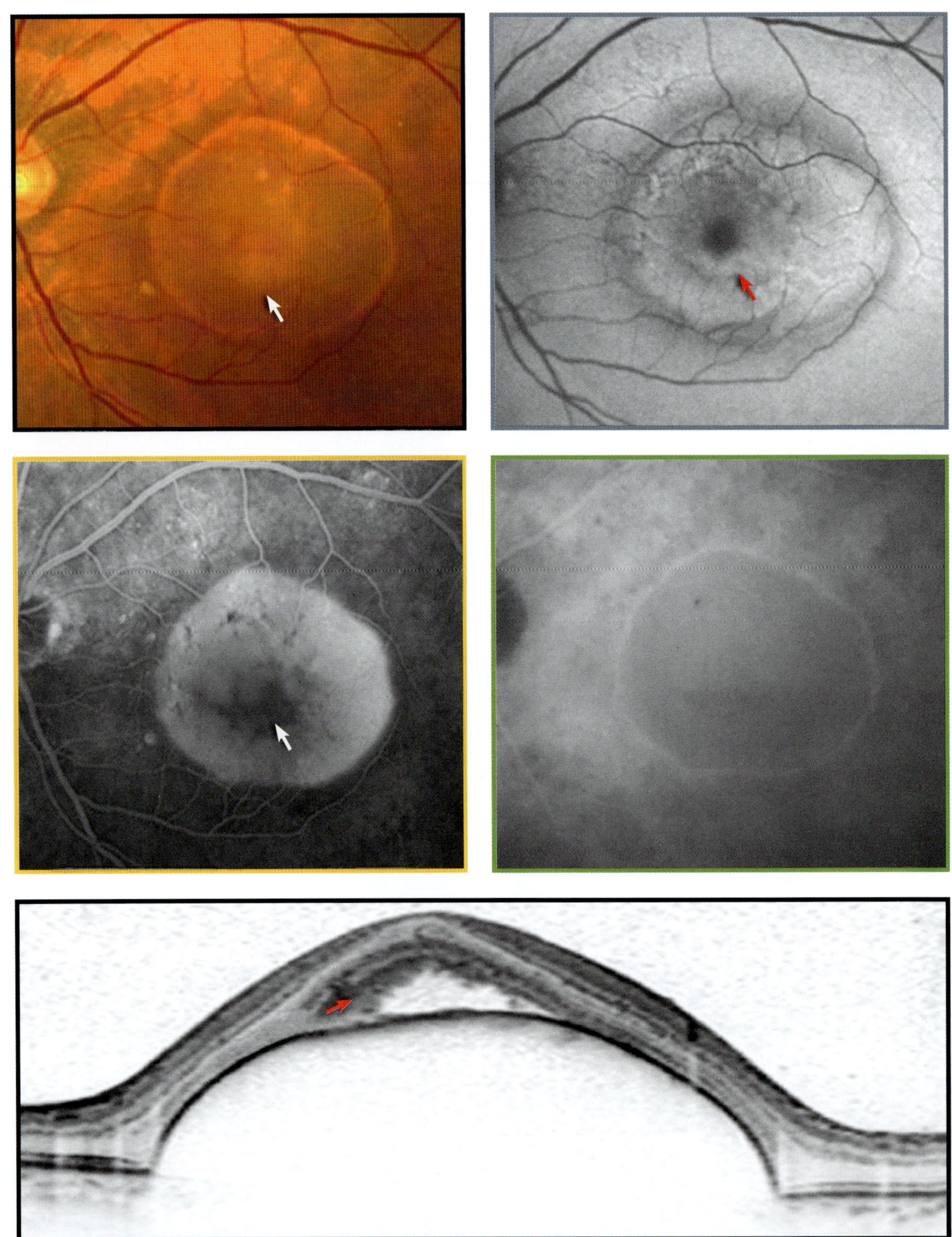

This patient has a large serous RPE detachment with an overlying acquired vitelliform lesion that appears yellow clinically *(arrow)*. On fundus autofluorescence the vitelliform lesion appears hyperautofluorescent, while on fluorescein angiography it is hypofluorescent. Indocyanine green angiography shows no choroidal neovascularization. Spectral-domain OCT shows hyper-reflective vitelliform material beneath the ellipsoid zone and subretinal fluid overlying the serous PED. *Images courtesy of Masaaki Saito*

Acquired Vitelliform Lesions

Acquired vitelliform lesions (AVLs) are accumulations of yellow material in the subretinal space that may occur in association with a variety of entities, including adult-onset foveomacular dystrophy, large drusen or PEDs in non-neovascular AMD, cuticular drusen, reticular pseudodrusen, central serous chorioretinopathy, vitreomacular traction, and pseudoxanthoma elasticum. AVLs were so termed to avoid confusion with the vitelliform lesions that occur in Best vitellifom macular dystrophy. AVLs are typically round yellow lesions that exhibit intense hyperautofluorescence on fundus autofluorescence imaging. This material is believed to contain variable amounts of lipofuscin, melanofuscin granules in macrophages, and extracellular material derived from photoreceptor outer segment discs that accumulate in the subretinal space due to RPE dysfunction or loss of apposition between the photoreceptor tips and the apical surface of the RPE.

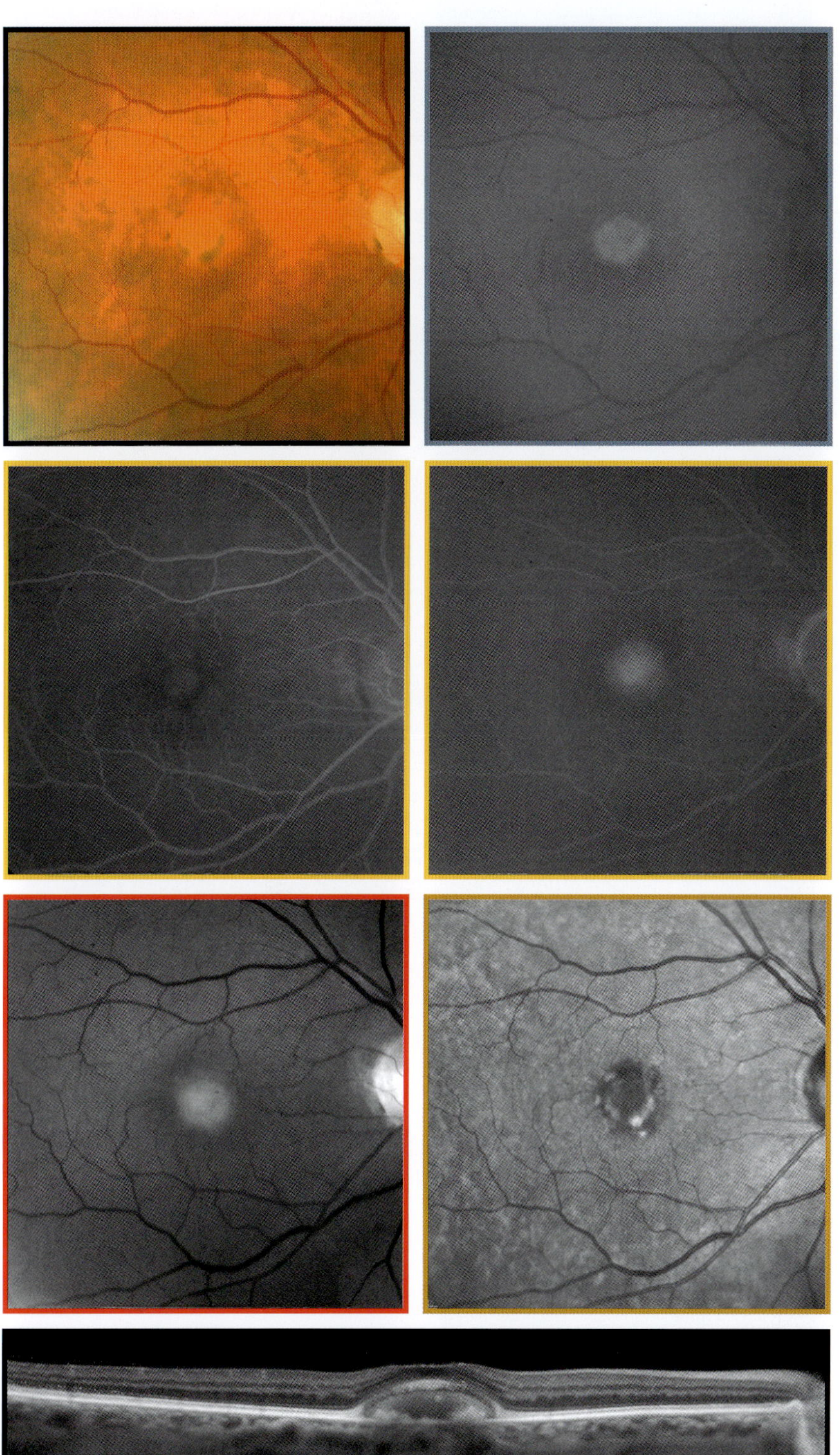

This patient has bilateral acquired vitelliform lesions but only the multimodal imaging features of the right eye are presented. AVLs are intensely hyperautofluorescent and stain in the late frames of FA. Accumulation of vitelliform material occurs in the subretinal space as seen on SD-OCT. In the absence of other features of AMD, the diagnosis of adult-onset foveomacular dystrophy should be considered.

Acquired Vitelliform Lesions in Drusen and PED

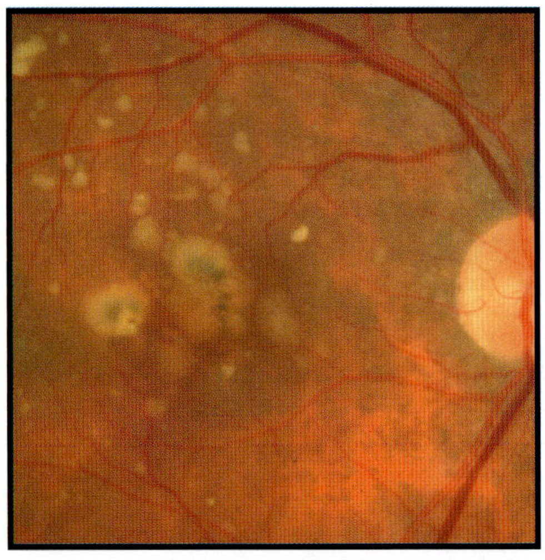

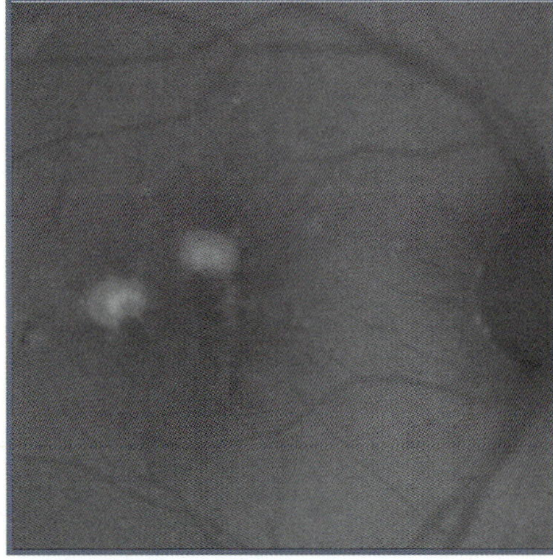

This patient has confluent soft drusen in the center of the macula with overlying vitelliform material that is hyperautofluorescent on fundus autofluorescence imaging. An OCT scan through the fovea shows the hyper-reflective vitelliform material overlying the large drusen *(arrow)*.

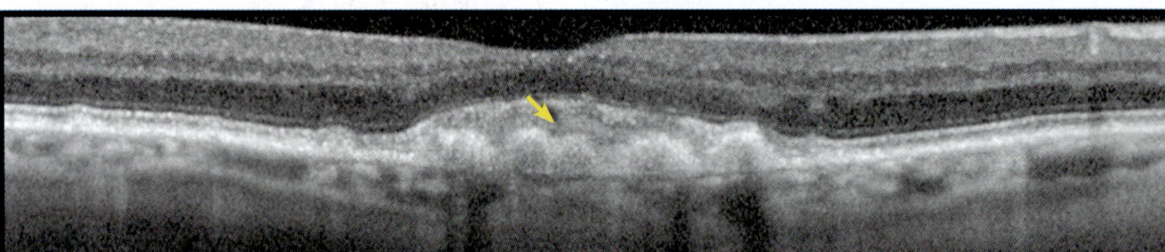

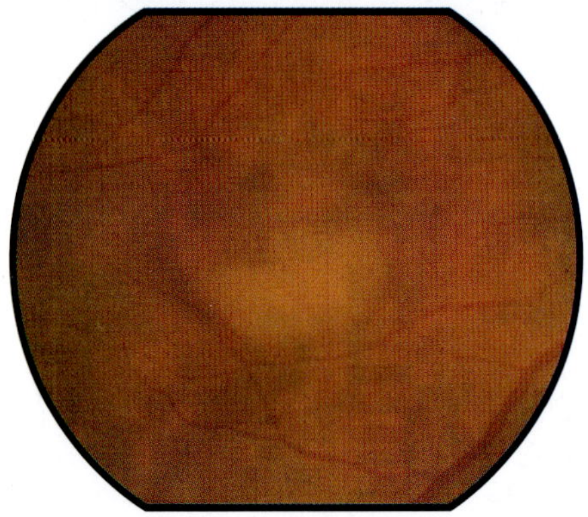

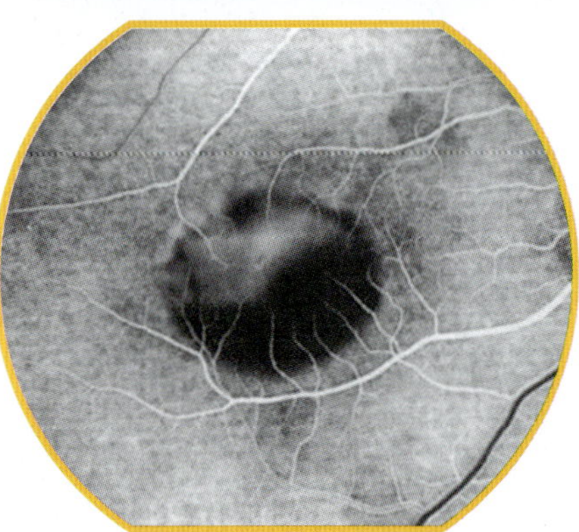

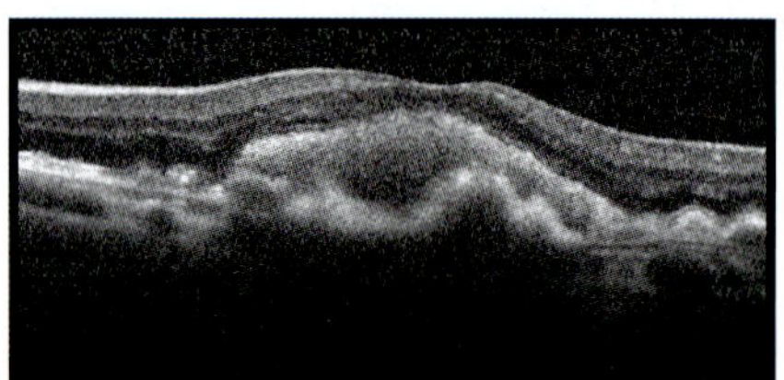

This patient has a long-standing AVL. The subretinal fluid is clear superiorly and exposes the RPE. Fluorescein leakage into the subretinal space is evident. The OCT through the fovea demonstrates the hyper-reflective vitelliform material, some thinning of the overlying retina, and irregular drusenoid elevations of the RPE beneath the vitelliform material.

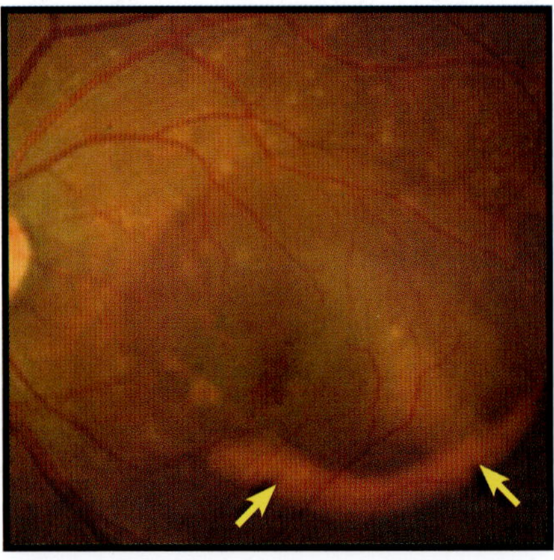

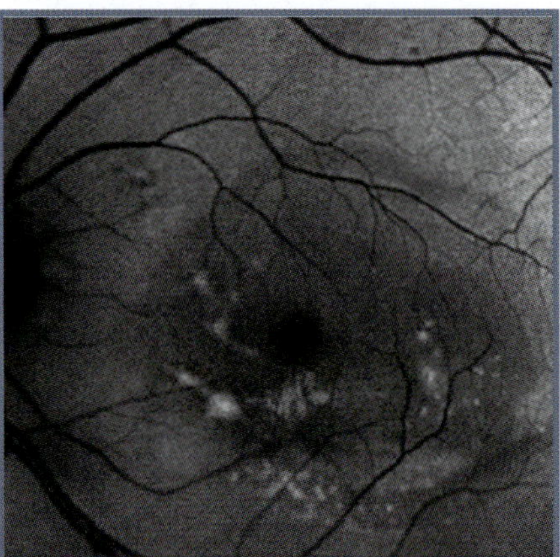

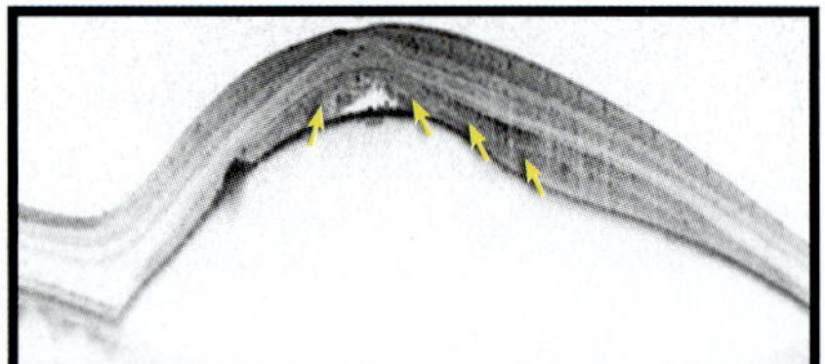

This patient has a large serous PED with an overlying acquired vitelliform lesion. Most of the vitelliform material has gravitated inferiorly in the subretinal space *(arrows)*. Fundus autofluorescence shows multiple hyperautofluorescent foci within the gravitating vitelliform material. OCT shows some residual hyper-reflective vitelliform material over the dome of the PED. *Images courtesy of Masaaki Saito*

Acquired Vitelliform Lesions in Cuticular Drusen

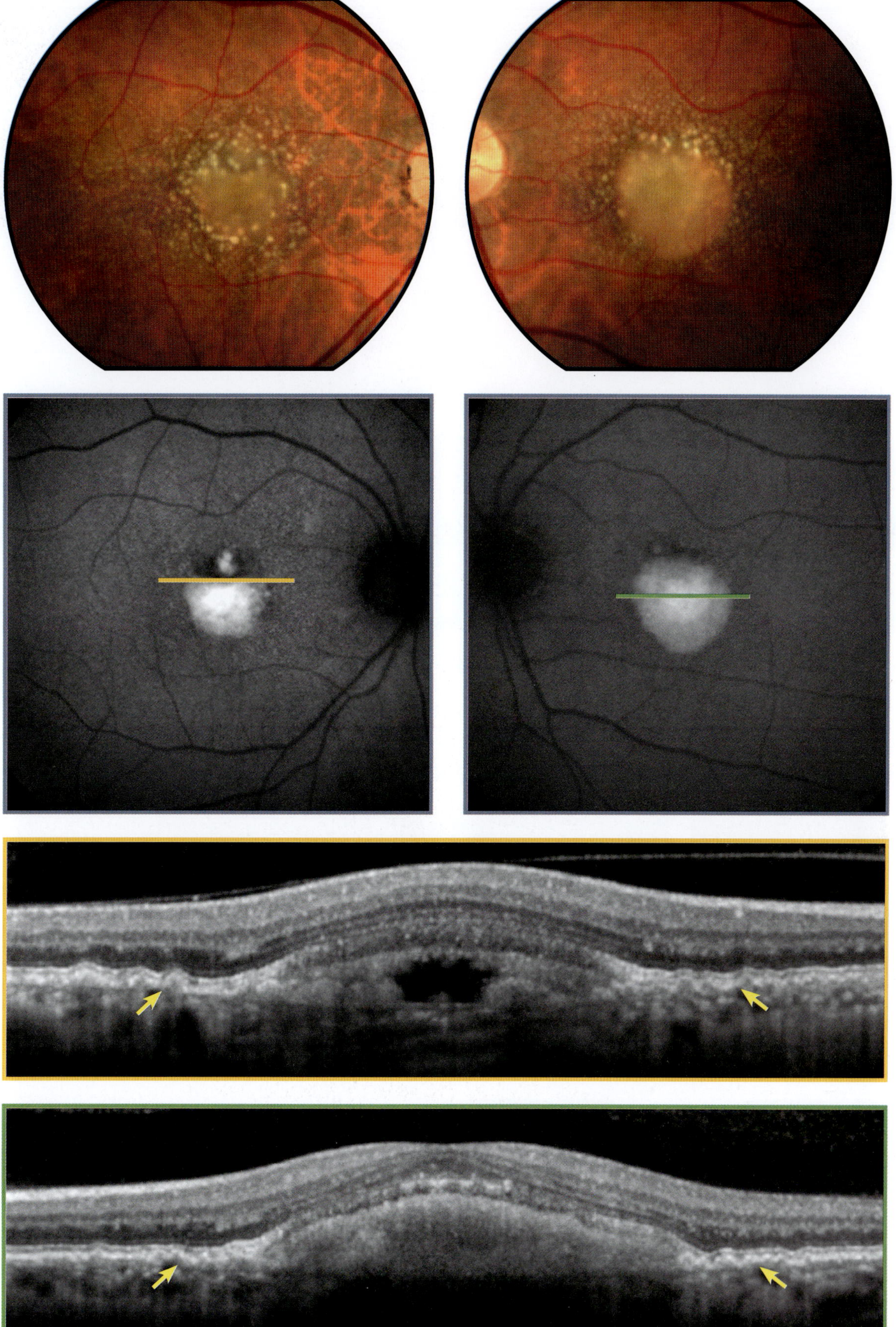

Acquired vitelliform lesions may occur in association with cuticular drusen. OCT imaging shows both subretinal fluid and hyper-reflective vitelliform material in the subretinal space. The characteristic "sawtooth" OCT appearance of cuticular drusen is clearly evident on either side of the vitelliform lesion *(arrows)*.

Acquired Vitelliform Lesions in Reticular Pseudodrusen

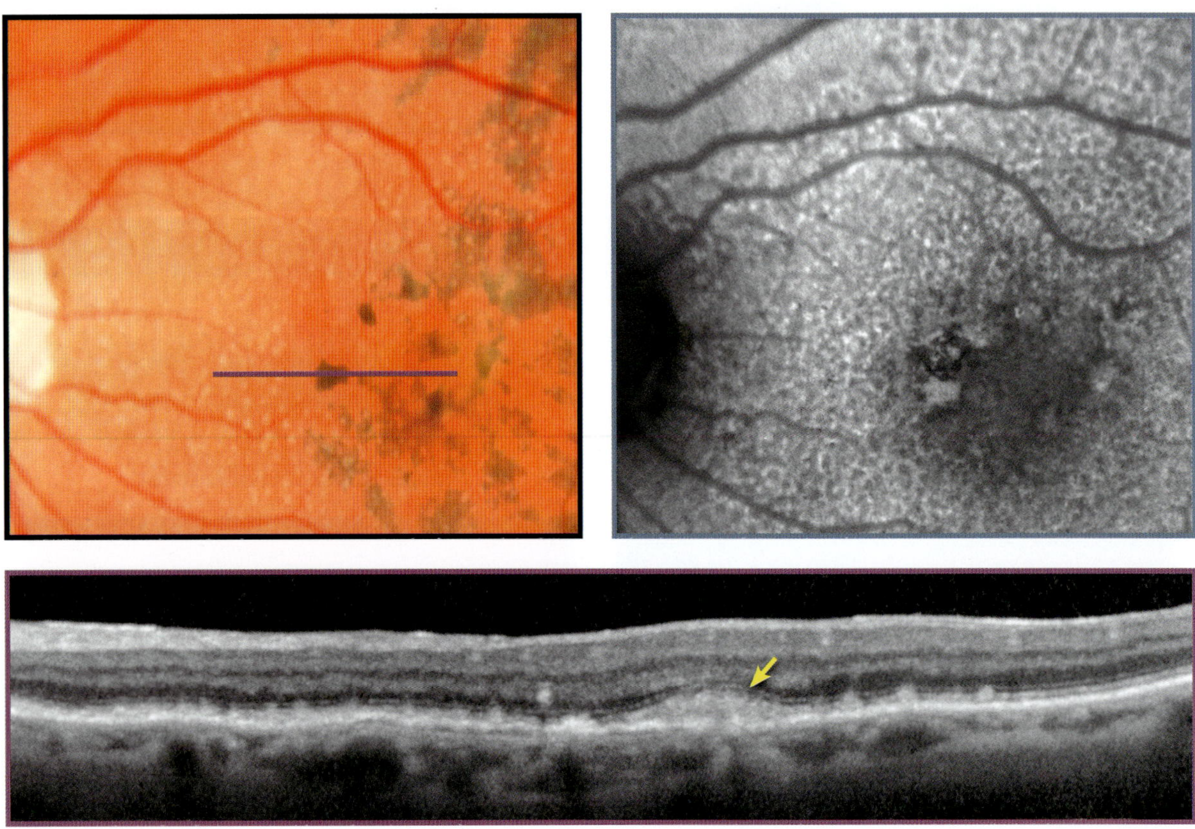

This patient has an acquired vitelliform lesion associated with reticular pseudodrusen. On fundus autofluorescence imaging, reticular pseudodrusen appear as dots of hypoautofluorescence surrounded by a reticular pattern of hyperautofluorescence. OCT shows subretinal hyper-reflective vitelliform material *(arrow)* bordered on either side by subretinal drusenoid deposits that are visible above the RPE. *Images courtesy of Dr. Richard Spaide*

Acquired Vitelliform Lesions in Non-AMD Entities

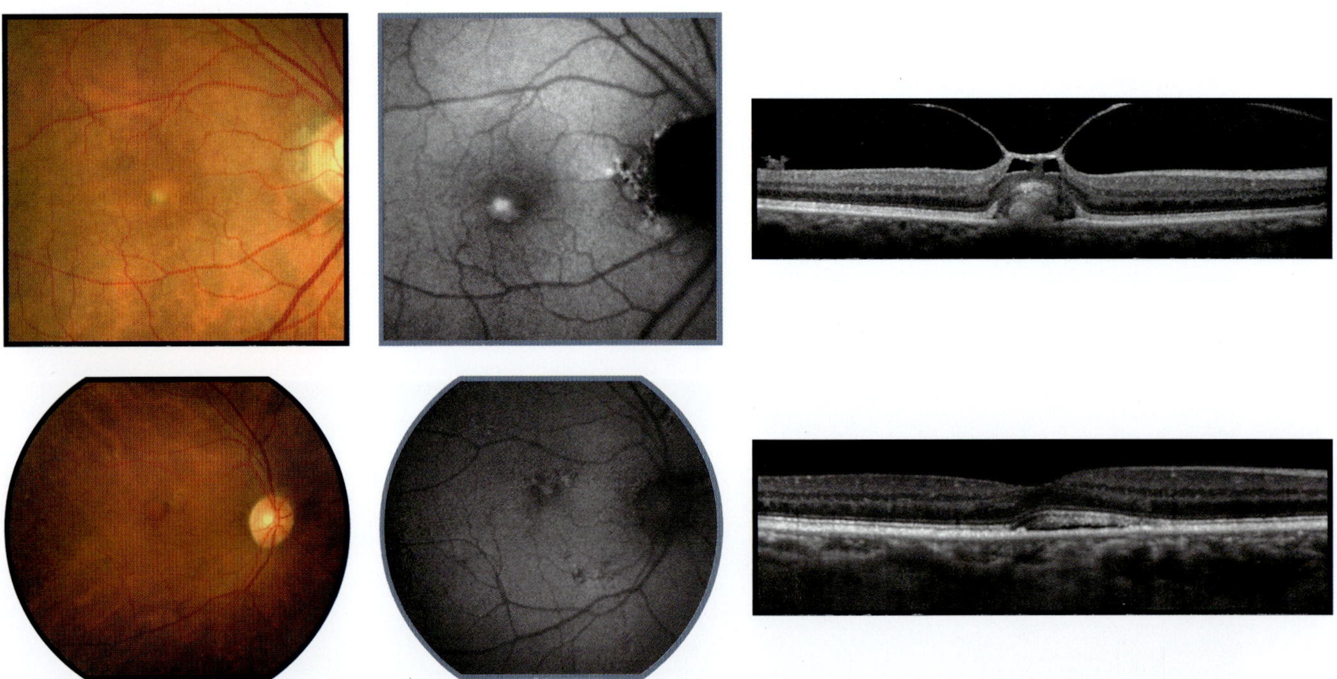

Acquired vitelliform lesions can occur in association with vitreomacular traction *(top row)* and central serous chorioretinopathy *(bottom row)*. In such cases, the loss of apposition between the photoreceptor tips and the apical surface of the RPE may be the primary mechanism of AVL formation.

Natural Course of Acquired Vitelliform Lesions

The natural course of an acquired vitelliform lesion is highly variable. Histopathologic studies have revealed varying degrees of RPE attenuation/loss, intraretinal migration of pigment-laden cells, and thinning of the outer nuclear layer with varying degrees of outer segment thinning and loss. Following resolution of an acquired vitelliform lesion, visual recovery may be limited by a legacy of persistent pigmentation, atrophy, and fibrous metaplasia. Eyes with acquired vitelliform lesions are also at risk of developing choroidal neovascularization.

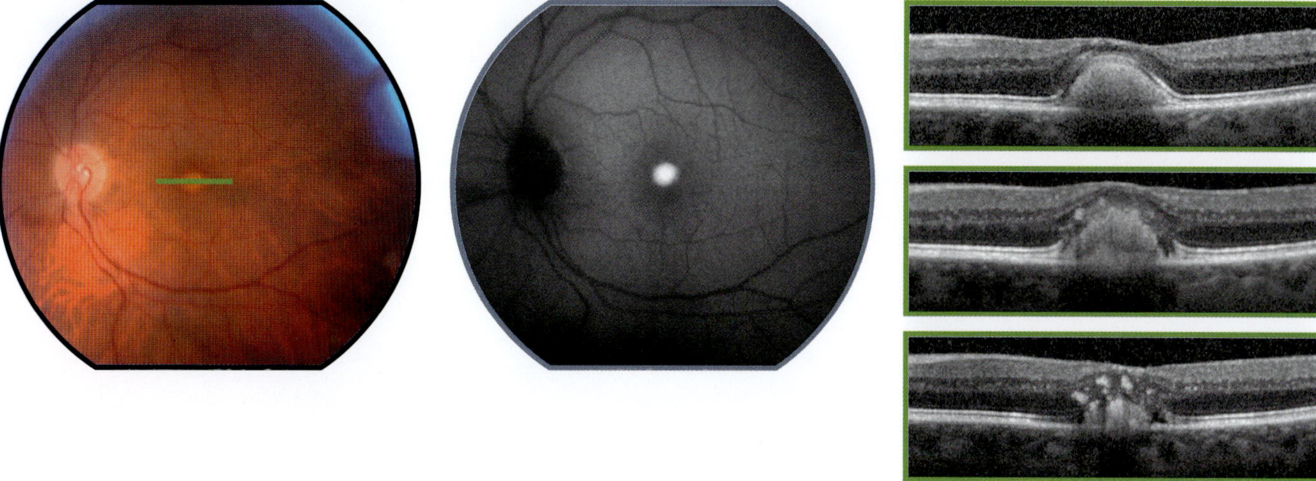

Spectral-domain OCT of this acquired vitelliform lesion demonstrated time-dependent intraretinal migration of hyperreflective material. OCT images at baseline *(top image)*, 3 years *(middle image)*, and 5 years *(bottom image)* are provided.

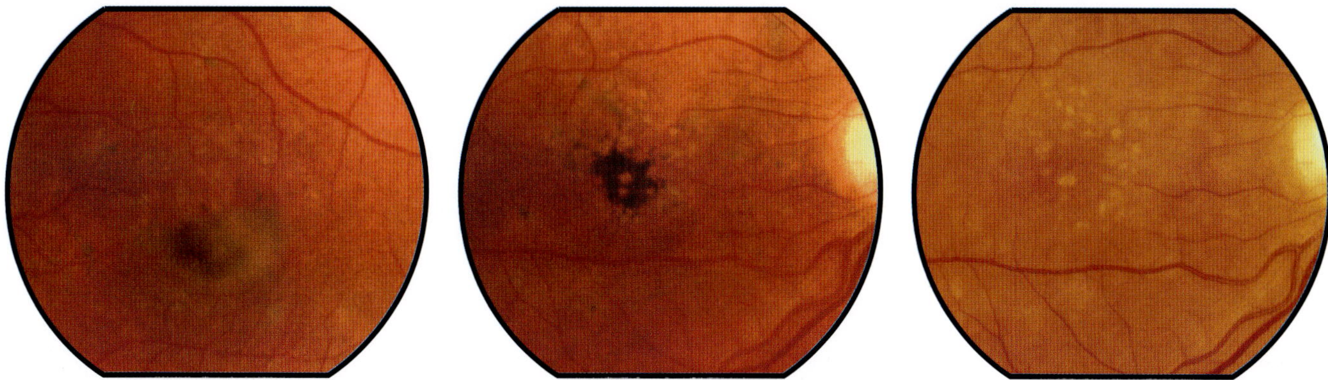

This patient had an acquired vitelliform lesion with a marked degree of intraretinal pigmentation *(left image)*. In the fellow eye, resolution of a neurosensory detachment due to an acquired vitelliform lesion resulted in the formation of a pigment epithelial hyperplastic figure in the central macula *(middle image)*. One year later there was spontaneous resolution of the hyperplastic figure, leaving only a cluster of soft drusen *(right image)*.

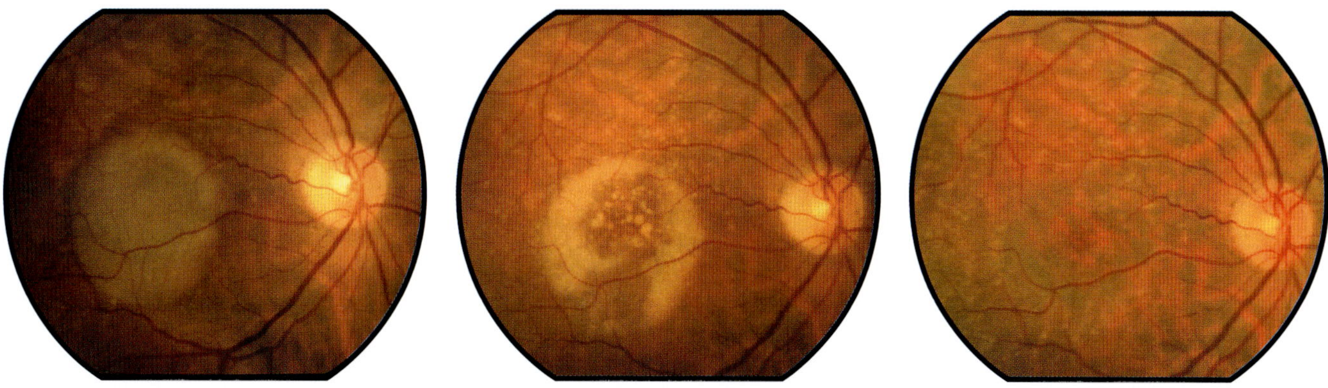

In this patient, an acquired vitelliform lesion remained stable during the initial period of observation *(left image)* after which the vitelliform material began to resolve *(middle image)*. When completely resolved, there was excellent visual recovery despite patchy perifoveal pigment epithelial atrophy *(right image)*.

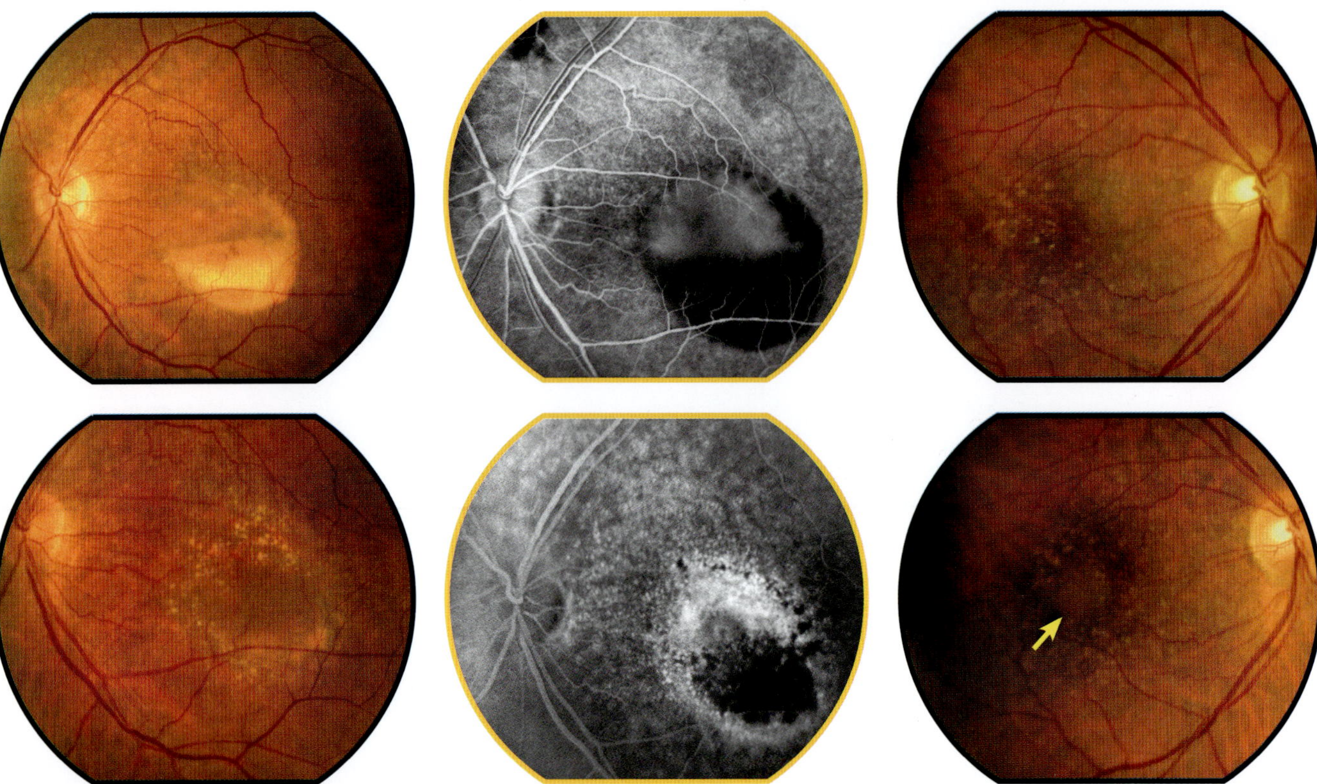

On initial presentation *(top images)* this patient had a large acquired vitelliform lesion in the left eye with a pseudohypopyon line. Small drusen and cuticular drusen were also seen in both eyes. Two and a half years later *(bottom images)* there was resolution of the acquired vitelliform lesion in the left eye and a new small acquired vitelliform lesion in the right eye *(arrow)*.

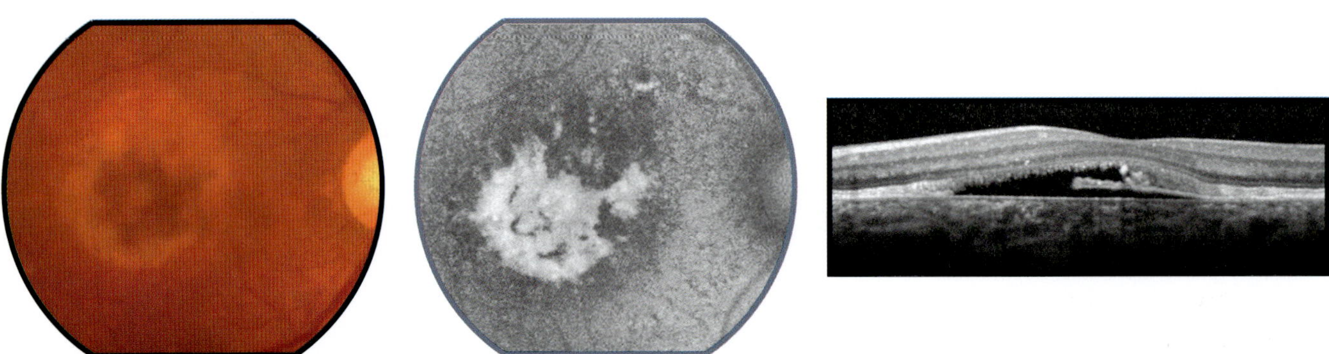

This patient had a long-standing acquired vitelliform lesion. There is fundus hyperautofluorescence at this site and a shallow neurosensory detachment. The visual acuity is still good (20/50) due to partial preservation of the outer retina.

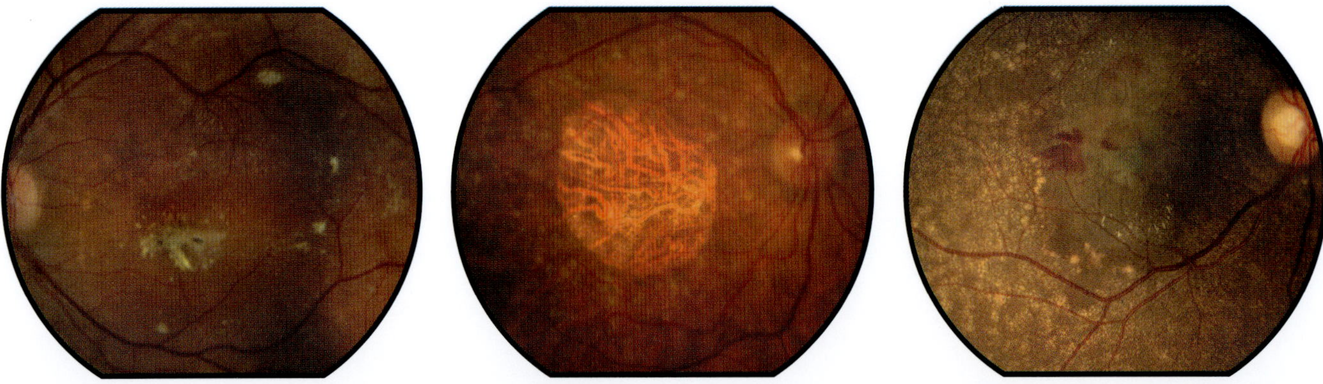

Patients may develop fibrous metaplasia *(left image)* or atrophy *(middle image)* after resolution of the acquired vitelliform lesion. Patients with acquired vitelliform lesions are also at risk of developing choroidal neovascularization. The right image shows subretinal hemorrhage indicative of neovascularization in a patient with a resolving acquired vitelliform lesion.

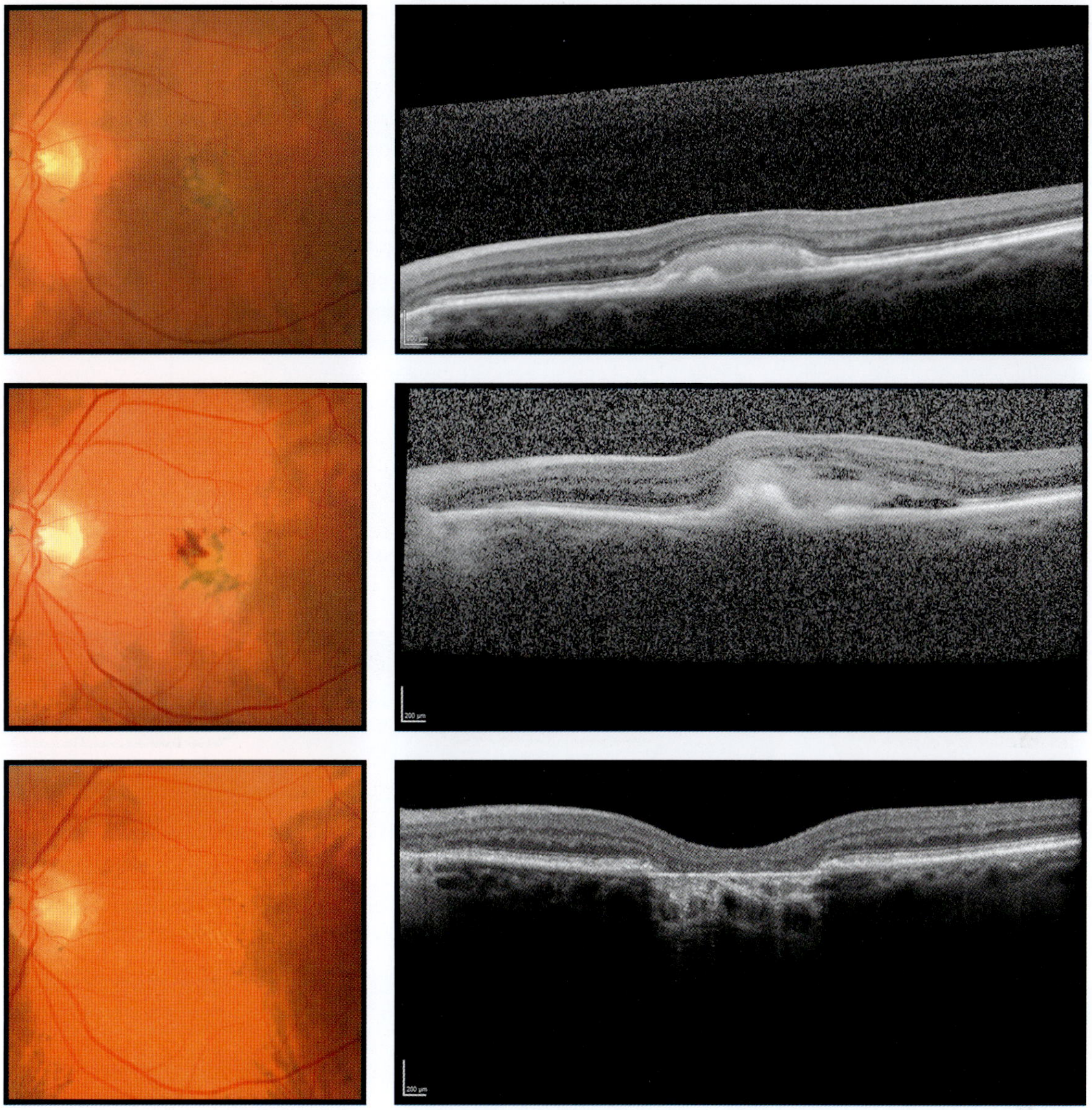

In this patient an acquired vitelliform lesion was identified at baseline examination *(top row)*. Two years later *(middle row)* there was consolidation of vitelliform material and the development of neovascularization, as evidenced by hemorrhage on the nasal margin of the lesion and subretinal fluid on OCT. Elevation of the RPE, suggestive of type 1 neovascularization, is also seen on OCT. Treatment with intravitreal anti-VEGF therapy resulted in reabsorption of the vitelliform material and the development of atrophy within 6 months *(bottom row)*.

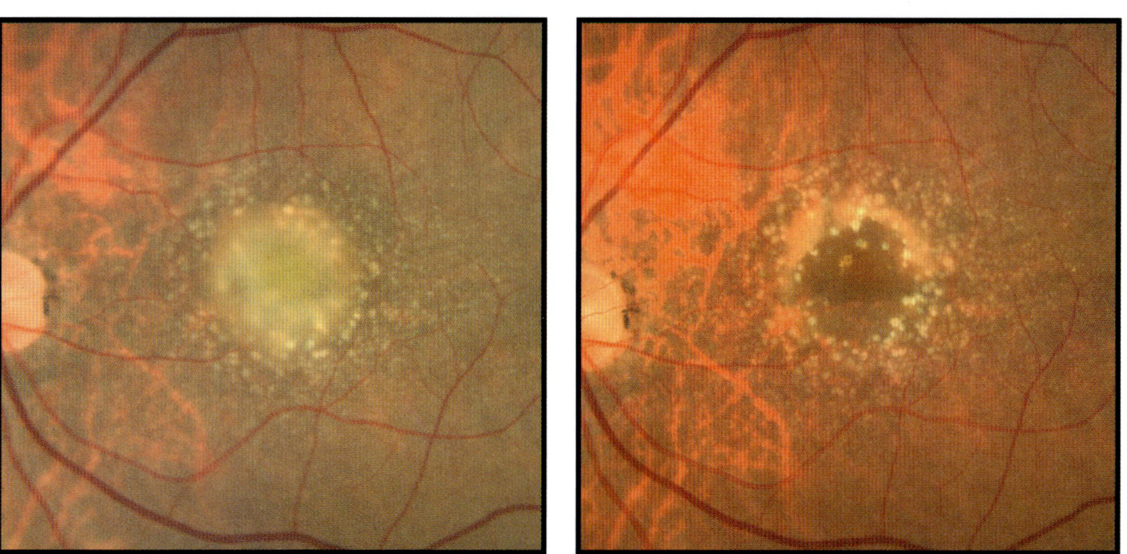

This patient with cuticular drusen and an acquired vitelliform lesion progressed to atrophy over 4 years. The natural course of this lesion was not complicated by neovascularization.

Geographic Atrophy

The current definition of geographic atrophy denotes areas of RPE and choriocapillaris loss that are 175 μm or greater in diameter. The definition of geographic atrophy is currently being revised to incorporate the findings of imaging modalities such as SD-OCT and fundus autofluorescence. Areas of geographic atrophy are often round or oval with a predilection for the central macula. Geographic atrophy may be preceded by focal pigmentary abnormalities and reticular pseudodrusen or may follow regression of large drusen, PED, or acquired vitelliform lesions. The larger choroidal vessels are often visible within the lesion due to loss of overlying RPE and the superficial choroidal layers. Fundus autofluorescence is the best way to document the state of the RPE in atrophic macular disease. Areas of absent RPE and overlying photoreceptors appear hypoautofluorescent with this imaging technique. These areas of geographic atrophy may show a margin of hyperautofluorescence that may indicate cells that are at risk for becoming atrophic in the future. With fluorescein angiography, early well-delineated hyperfluorescence, representing a window defect, is typically apparent. If there is choriocapillaris atrophy, only large choroidal vessels will be seen coursing through the atrophic zone in the early stages of the study. Late staining of visible sclera with a silhouette of the larger choroidal vessels may be seen when the fluorescein dye is no longer in the circulation.

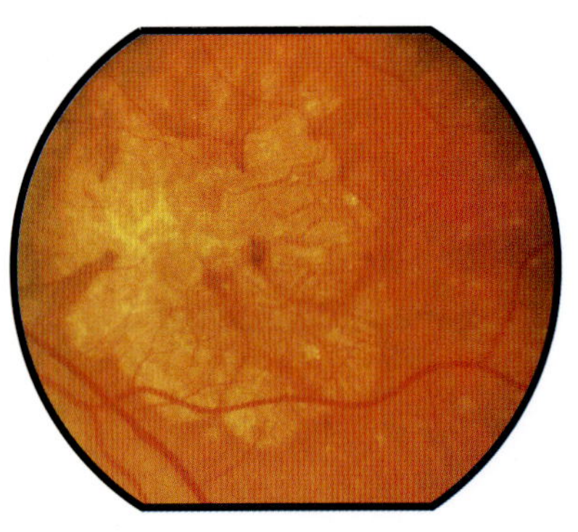
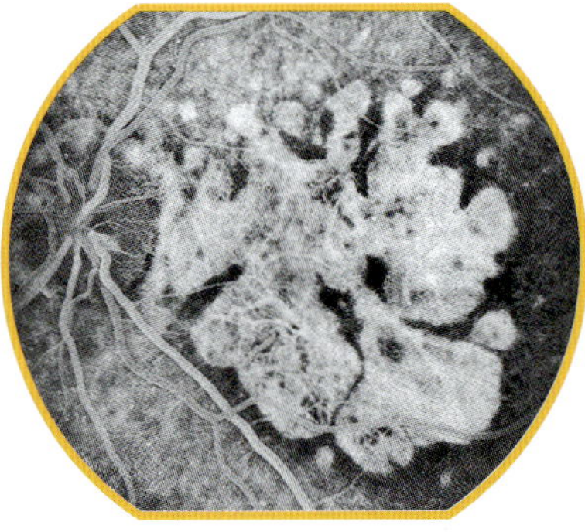
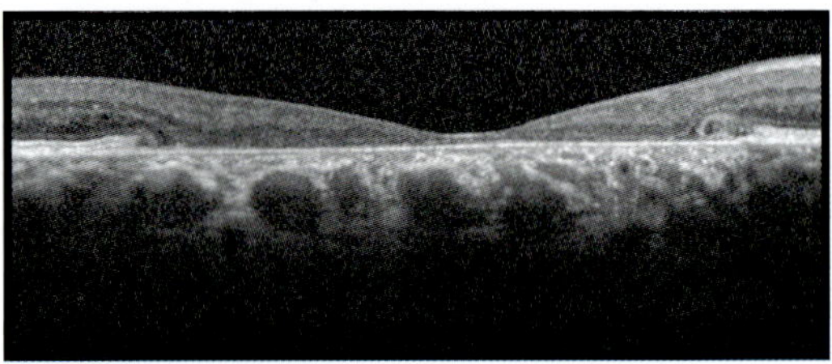

Geographic atrophy is typically considered part of the non-neovascular spectrum of age-related macular degeneration, but it may also occur in eyes with choroidal neovascularization in areas noncontiguous with the neovascular lesion. Retinal pigment epithelial atrophy can be seen, corresponding to window defects on fluorescein angiography and areas of outer retinal thinning due to photoreceptor and RPE loss on OCT *(right image)*.

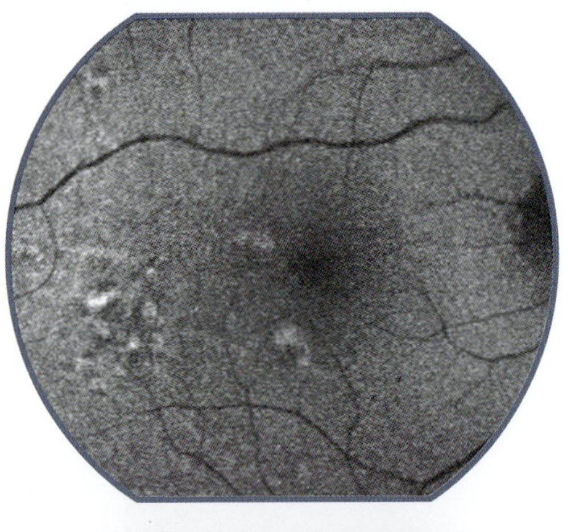
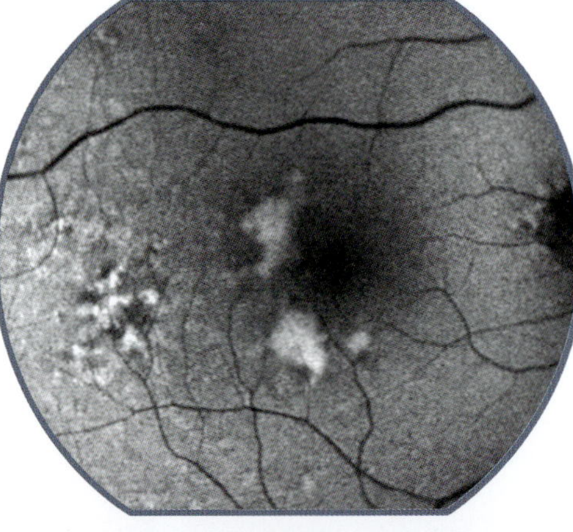

This patient demonstrates an area of increasing hyperautofluorescence over a period of 2½ years that is likely attributed to an increase in RPE lipofuscin. The cells within this area are at risk of atrophy.

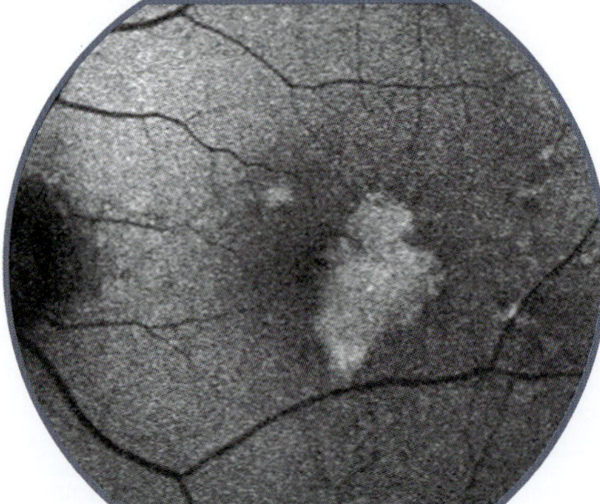
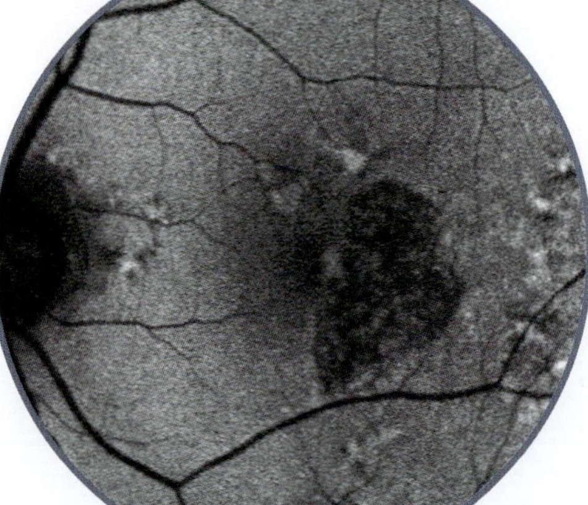

This patient demonstrates an area of hyperautofluorescence that later became hypoautofluorescent due to geographic atrophy.

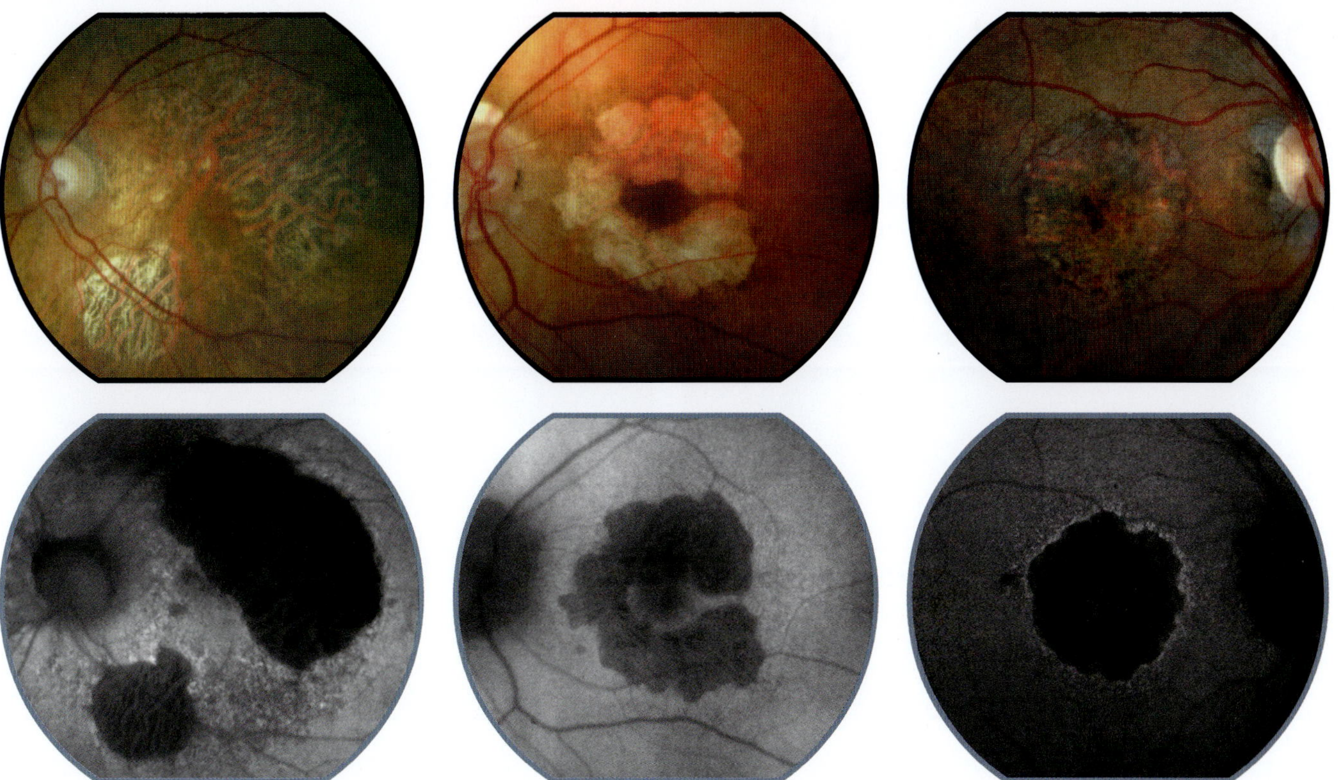

Patients with geographic atrophy may show varying paterns of zonal and multizonal hypoautofluorescence. Geographic atrophy in AMD may be associated with severe vision loss when there is foveal involvement. There may be areas of hyperautofluorescence surrounding the perimeter of these atrophic zones due to RPE cells that are accumulating excessive lipofuscin and/or multilayering of these cells *(bottom right image)*. These marginal areas of hyperautofluorescence are believed to be at risk of progressive atrophy. Fundus autofluorescence may, in some cases, detect central areas of RPE and photoreceptor preservation, accounting for good visual acuity due to foveal preservation *(bottom middle image)*.

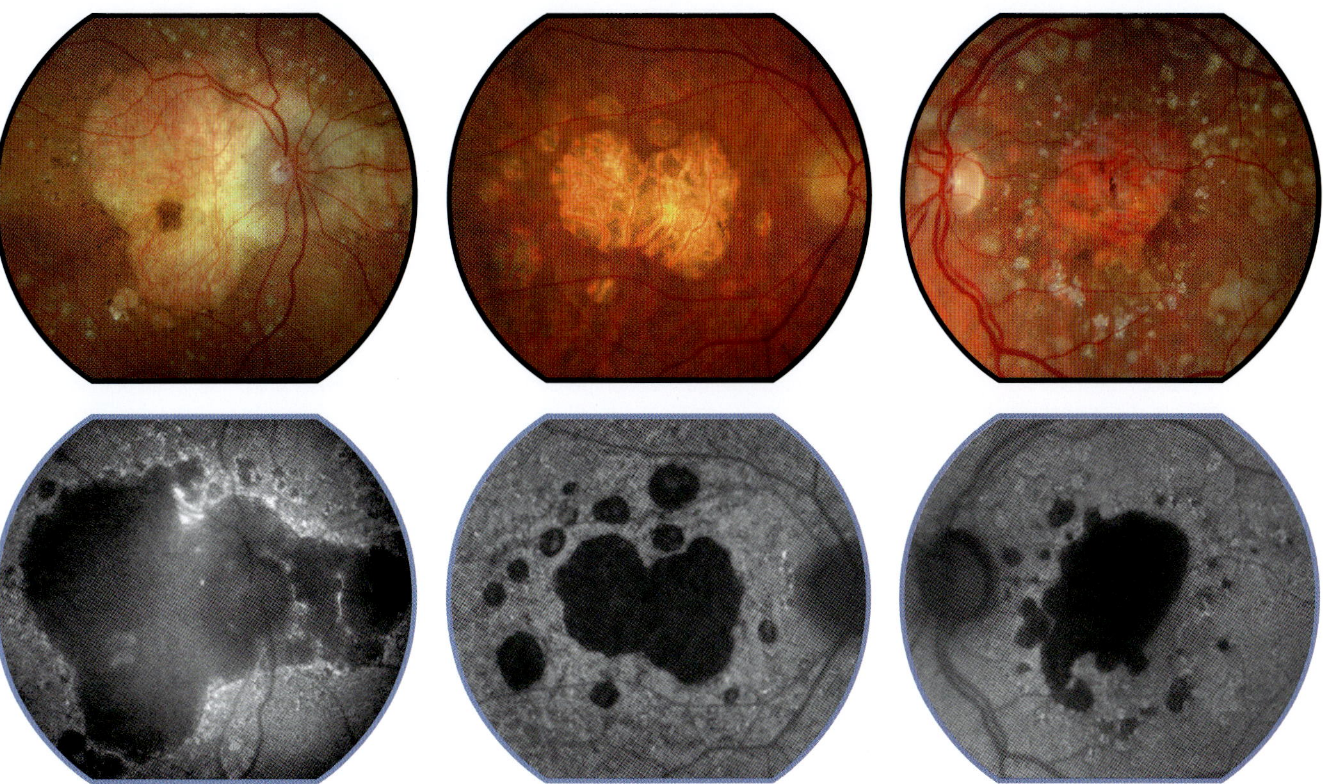

In severe cases of geographic atrophy, the atrophic areas may extend beyond the macula, optic disc, and temporal vascular arcades. These eyes show central geographic atrophy, multifocal areas of atrophy, and a granular pigment epithelial appearance, which indicates cells at risk for progression to atrophy.

Outer Retinal Tubulation

Outer retinal tubulation (ORT) is a distinctive spectral-domain OCT finding of a thick hyper-reflective band surrounding a branching hyporeflective cavity, all within the outer nuclear layer. ORT occurs commonly in advanced age-related macular degeneration over areas of degenerate or absent pigment epithelium. It has been found to occur also in other degenerative retinal disorders, including acute zonal occult outer retinopathy, retinitis pigmentosa, Stargardt disease, gyrate atrophy, choroideremia, and Bietti crystalline dystrophy. Although the pathogenesis is not completely understood, ORT contains degenerate photoreceptors and enveloping Müller cells and is thought to be a sign of photoreceptor cell survival in regions of outer retinal injury. It is important to recognize ORT because it can be easily misinterpreted as cystic fluid, with misleading implications for therapy.

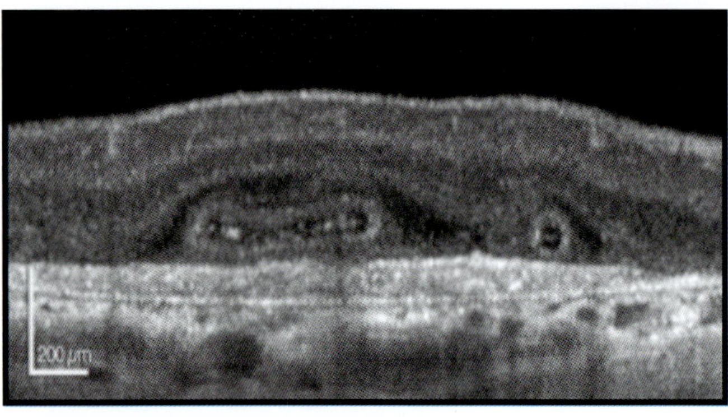

© 561

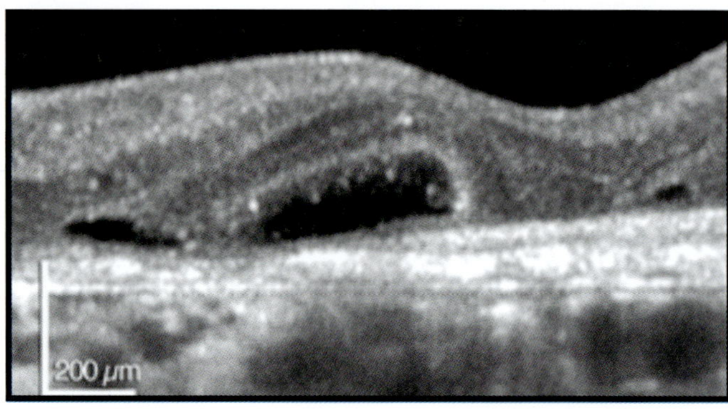

© 562

ORT may appear in varying shapes and sizes in cross-sectional OCT imaging. The left image shows an ovoid and circular ORT within the outer nuclear layer. They are both in a closed configuration, as opposed to an open configuration *(right image)* where there is discontinuity of the hyper-reflective band surrounding the cavity.

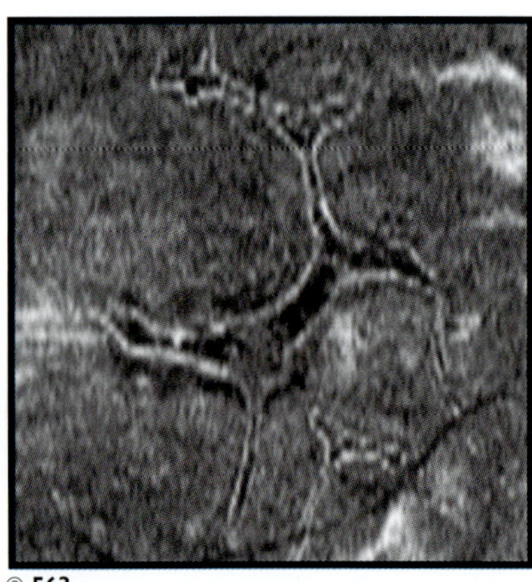

© 563

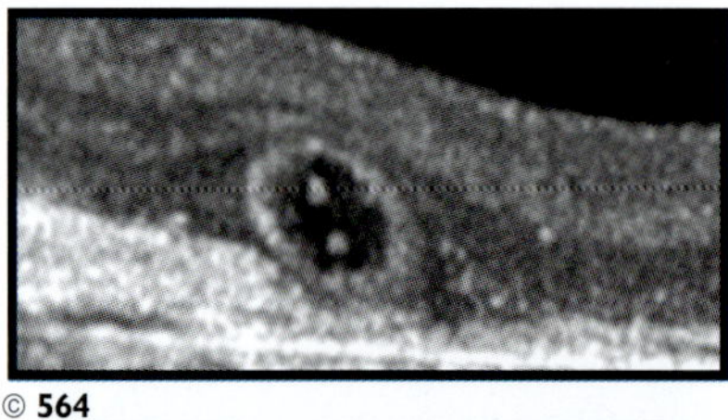

© 564

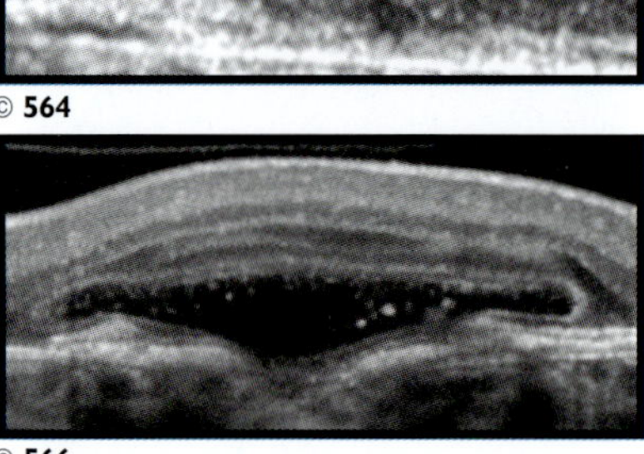

© 566

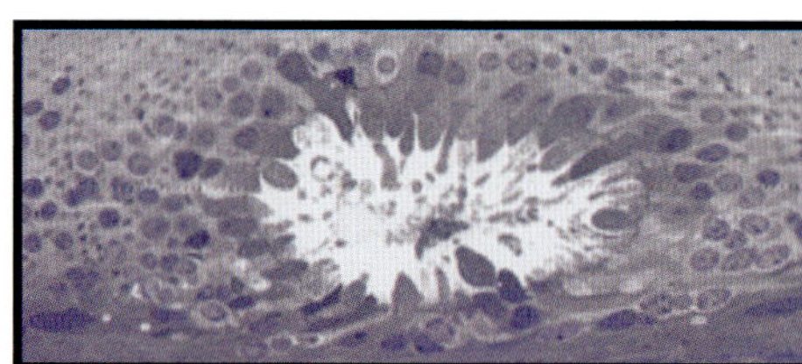

© 565

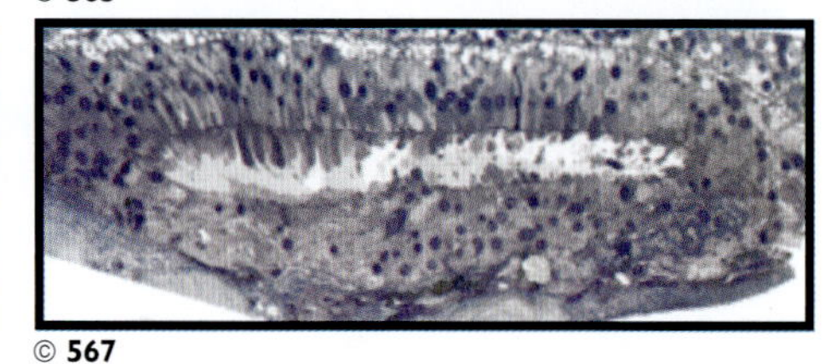

© 567

The branching patterns of ORT are best seen with *en face* OCT imaging *(left image)*. The SD-OCT appearance of a closed, circular ORT *(top row, middle)* and open, ovoid ORT *(bottom row, middle)* correlates well with histology, which shows that ORT is comprised of radially oriented cone and Müller cells. Histology identifies four ORT phases, depending on the contents of the ORT lumen, including the nascent phase when both inner and outer segments are still present within the lumen, mature phase when there are only inner segments present, degenerate phase when there are remnant or absent inner segments, and end stage when there are only Müller cells present. *Histology images courtesy of Dr. Christine Curcio*

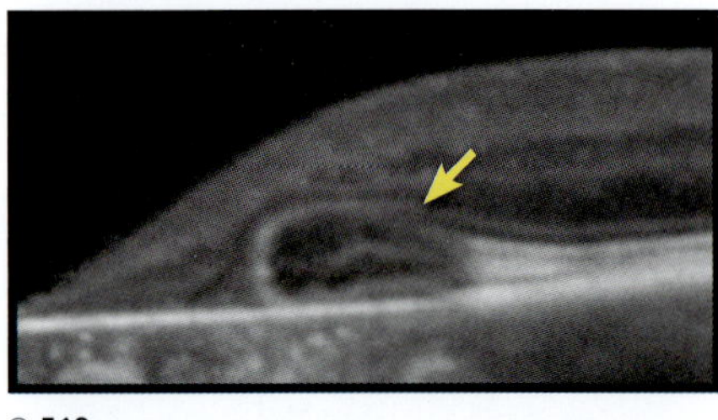

© 568

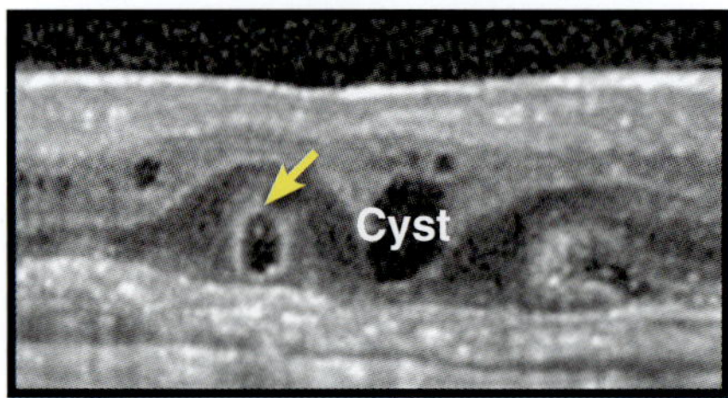

© 569

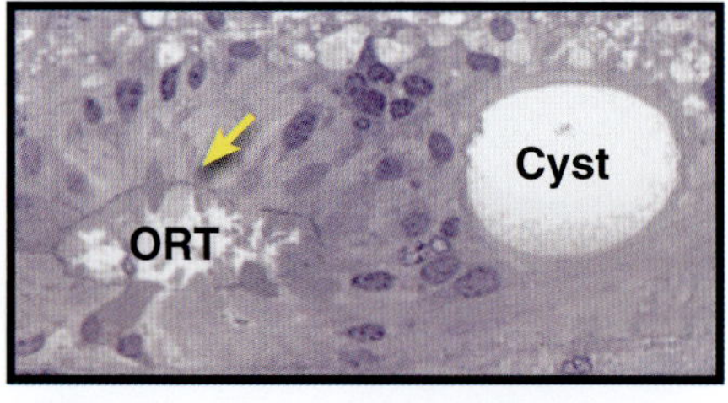

© 570

A "free edge" for the photoreceptors to "scroll" is usually necessary for the formation of ORT. The hyper-reflective border seen on SD-OCT always includes the external limiting membrane *(arrow)* and may include the inner segment ellipsoid as it retracts back to the external limiting membrane as the photoreceptors degenerate *(left image)*. The SD-OCT *(middle image)* and a corresponding histology image *(right image)* show the difference between ORT with the hyper-reflective appearance of the external limiting membrane *(arrows)* and a cystic fluid-filled space adjacent to it that lacks this hyper-reflective border. *Histology images courtesy of Dr. Christine Curcio*

Age-Related Choroidal Atrophy

With the advent of enhanced depth imaging OCT (EDI-OCT), visualization and characterization of the choroid including choroidal thickness measurements can be achieved. There is a growing recognition that age-related macular degeneration can involve atrophy of the choroidal layers in addition to the retinal layers. Although choroidal thickness is known to decrease with age, patients with age-related choroidal atrophy (ARCA) have an accelerated loss of choroidal thickness over time. These patients can have normal fundus autofluorescence imaging implying a relatively normal RPE in contrast to eyes with geographic atrophy. ARCA is characterized by global thinning of the choroid, also now known as a leptochoroid, with rarefied choroidal vessels and loss of pigmentation in the choroid. These eyes often have reticular pseudodrusen and nummular clumps of pigment hyperplasia. These patients appear to be at higher risk for glaucoma.

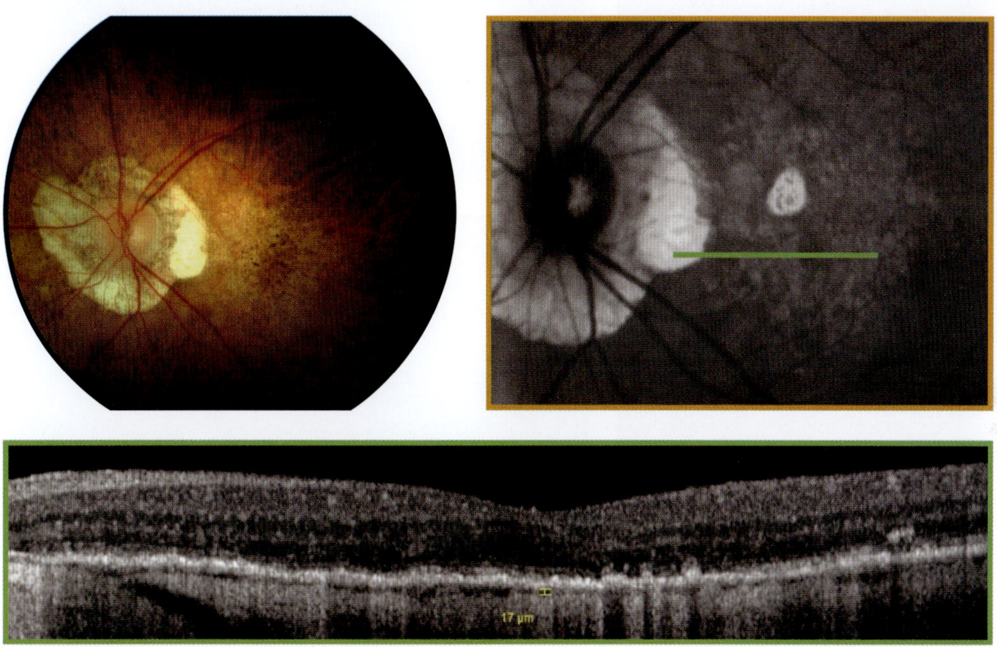

This patient with ARCA has macular pigmentation with intervening areas of depigmentation and a paucity of visible choroidal vessels on color fundus photography and near-infrared reflectance imaging. SD-OCT demonstrates a leptochoroid with a subfoveal choroidal thickness of 17 µm.

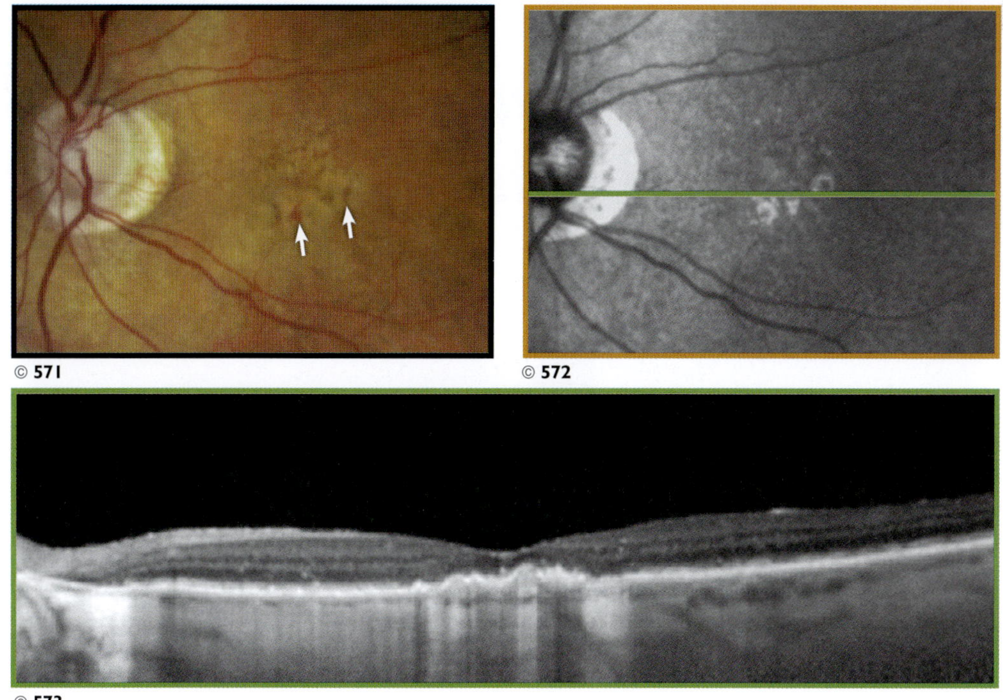

This patient has ARCA with a subretinal hemorrhage *(arrows)* indicative of neovascularization. Near-infrared reflectance imaging shows reticular pseudodrusen in the posterior pole, and EDI-OCT imaging shows RPE elevation and a thin choroid.

Outer Retinal Corrugations

Outer retinal corrugations are a recently described SD-OCT finding of curvilinear, undulating, hyper-reflective material above the Bruch membrane that occurs within areas of macular atrophy. It was first observed in eyes with geographic atrophy and was thought to represent residual sub-RPE deposits and regressing drusen. Subsequently, it has also been noted to occur in areas of choroidal neovascularization. Histologically, outer retinal corrugations are consistent with the rippled layer of basal laminar deposits that persist in areas of RPE atrophy. It has been proposed that outer retinal corrugations form following the loss of the RPE and basal linear deposit, leaving behind a wrinkled sheet of persistent basal laminar deposit.

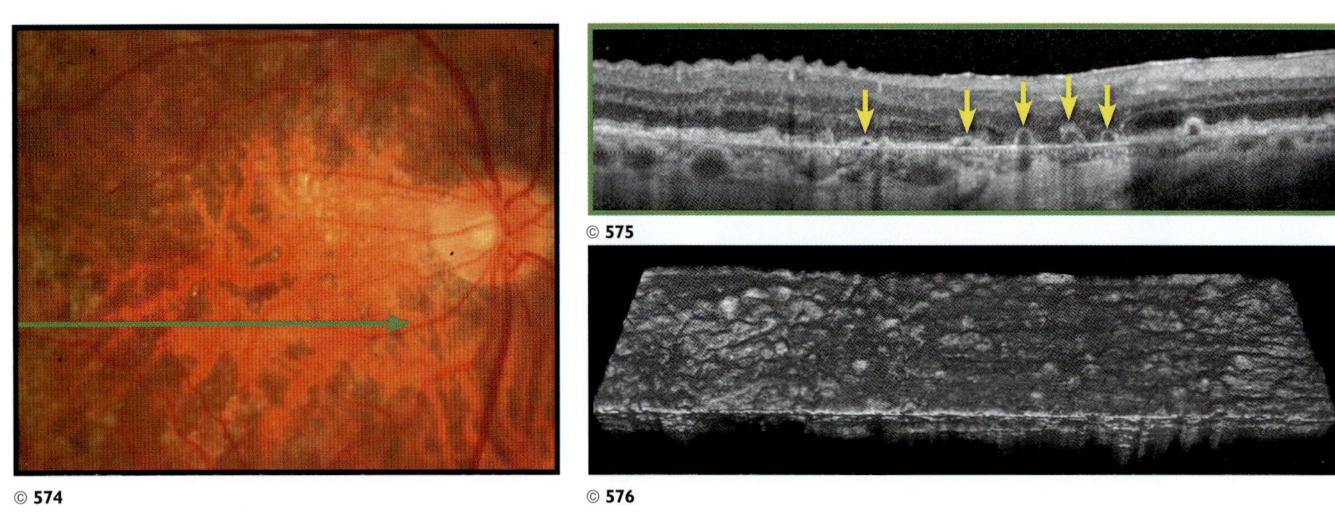

© 575

© 574

© 576

This patient with geographic atrophy shows outer retinal corrugations *(arrows)* on SD-OCT imaging. They appear as undulating hyper-reflective material above the Bruch membrane. A surface volume-rendered OCT image *(bottom right)* demonstrates the topological characteristics of outer retinal corrugations. (The orientation and site where the OCT image was acquired is denoted by a green arrow.)

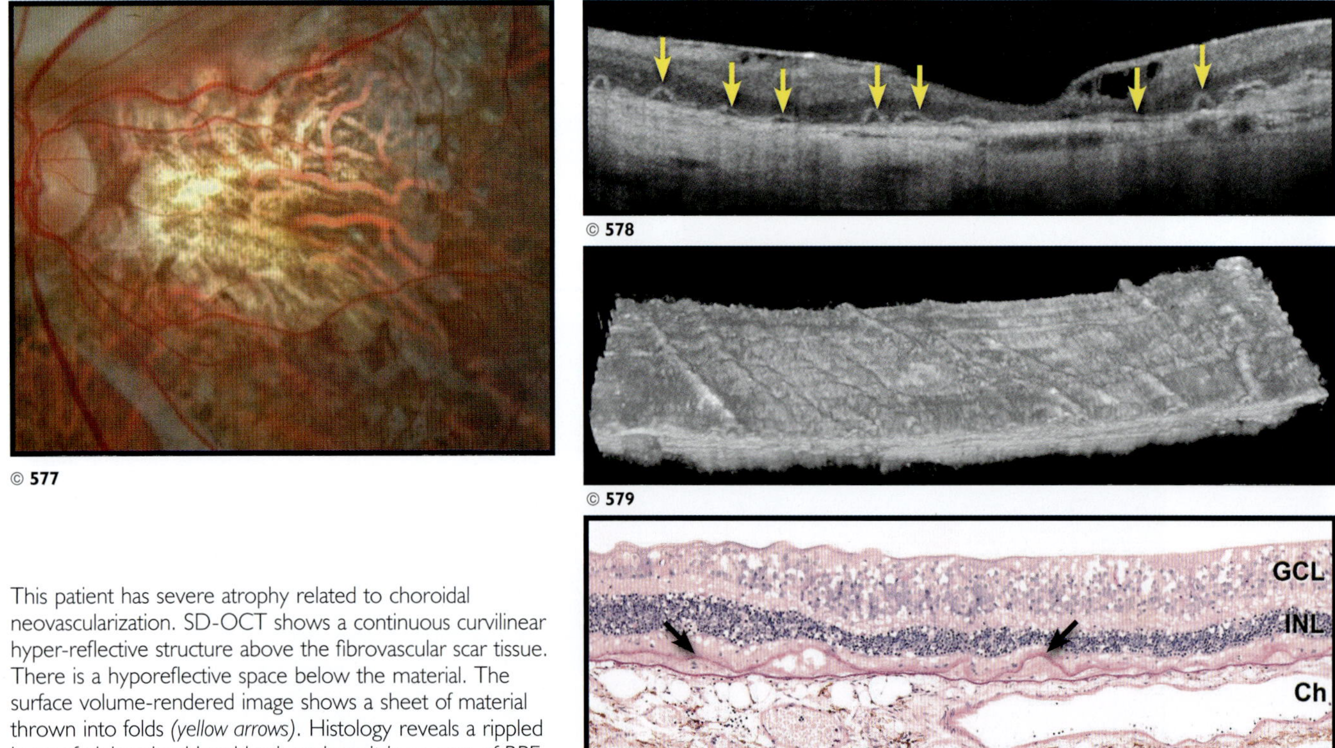

© 578

© 577

© 579

© 580

This patient has severe atrophy related to choroidal neovascularization. SD-OCT shows a continuous curvilinear hyper-reflective structure above the fibrovascular scar tissue. There is a hyporeflective space below the material. The surface volume-rendered image shows a sheet of material thrown into folds *(yellow arrows)*. Histology reveals a rippled layer of pink-stained basal laminar deposit in an area of RPE atrophy *(black arrows)*.

Neovascular Age-Related Macular Degeneration

Neovascular AMD is characterized by the presence of choroidal and/or intraretinal neovascularization with associated serous and hemorrhagic complications. The classification of choroidal neovascularization (CNV) is complex and has traditionally been based on fluorescein angiographic interpretation. However, the broader application of indocyanine green (ICG) angiography, fundus autofluorescence, and OCT have facilitated a greater understanding of the anatomic relationships involved in the neovascular process. This in turn has led to the formulation of an anatomically based classification that was originally described by Dr. J. Donald M. Gass. Based on his interpretations of the histopathologic and fluorescein angiographic characteristics of CNV, Gass suggested that neovascularization proliferating under the RPE was less distinct at its margins, less permeable, and less actively proliferating than other types of neovascularization. He referred to this entity as type 1 neovascularization. With fluorescein angiography, type 1 neovascularization will usually show a poorly defined or "occult" CNV pattern. Fibrovascular PED or flatter irregular elevations of the RPE will also manifest as stippled hyperfluorescent dots with indistinct margins on fluorescein angiography. Gass described a second form, type 2 neovascularization, in which choroidal vessels have penetrated the basement membrane–RPE complex gaining access to the subretinal space. Type 2 neovascularization actively proliferates beneath the neurosensory retina and demonstrates a well-defined or "classic" pattern of fluorescence on fluorescein angiography. One sees early, well-demarcated intense leakage that is associated with dye pooling in the subneurosensory and intraretinal spaces. The leakage typically becomes more intensely fluorescent during the recirculation phase of the angiogram. More recently, a third anatomic subtype of neovascularization in AMD has been described that is associated with proliferation of new vessels within the retina itself and is referred to as type 3 neovascularization. It is sometimes also referred to as retinal angiomatous proliferation. The intraretinal neovascularization occurs in conjunction with a compensatory telangiectatic response that is typified by perfusing arterioles, draining venules, and the eventual formation of anastomoses between the intraretinal proliferation and sub-RPE neovascularization. Type 3 neovascularization may, in some cases, have an initiating or simultaneous choroidal component, but the main feature is active proliferation within neurosensory retina. Another form of neovascularization is polypoidal choroidal vasculopathy (PCV), which is considered a variant of type 1 neovascularization because it resides in the subpigment epithelial space. With PCV, there may be a branching type 1 neovascular network with terminal aneurysmal changes (polyps).

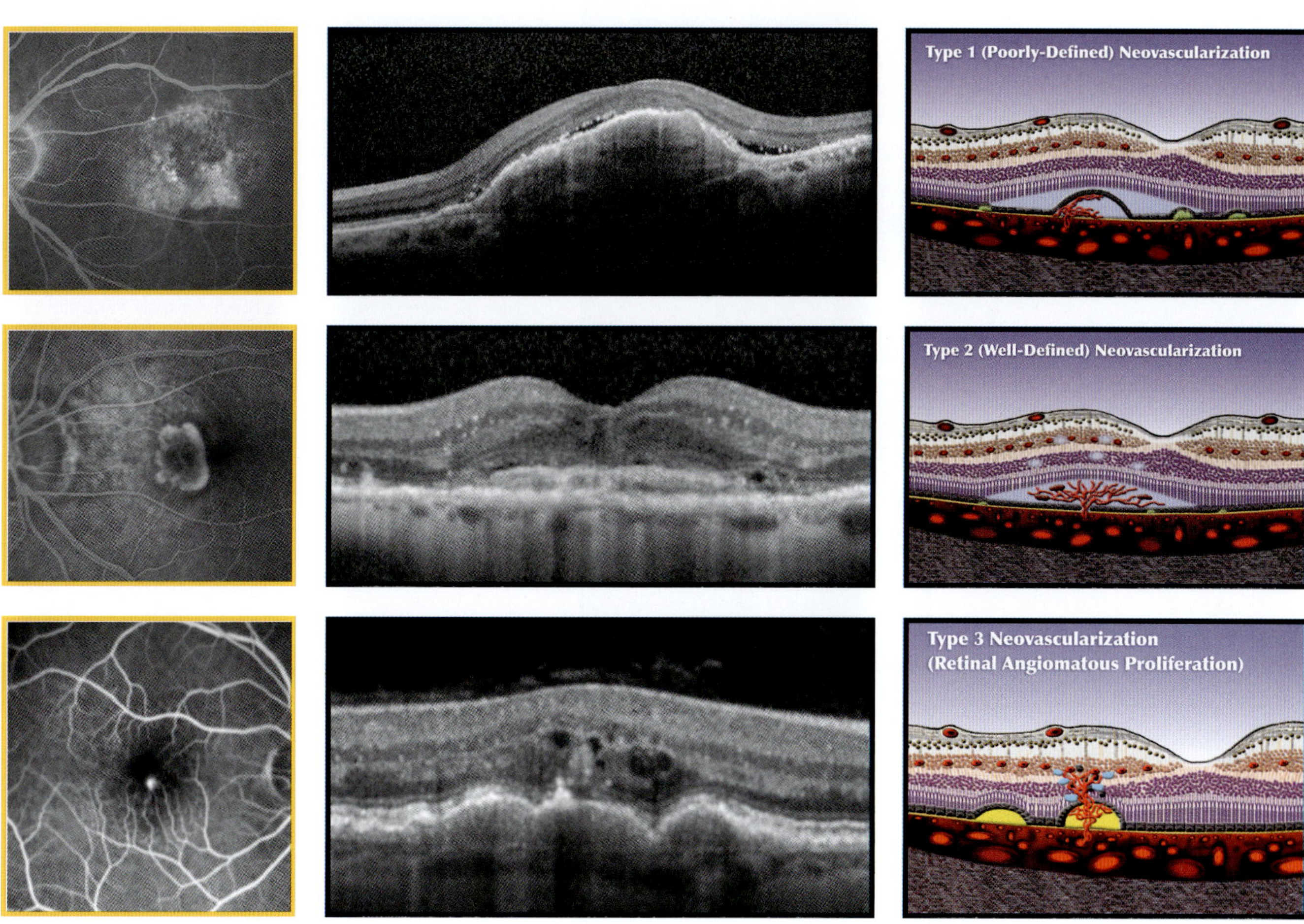

The relative frequency of neovascular subtypes in newly diagnosed neovascular AMD in white patients is approximately 40% type 1 *(top row)*, 9% type 2 *(middle row)*, 34% type 3 *(bottom row)*, and 17% mixed.

Optical Coherence Tomography Angiography of Neovascularization

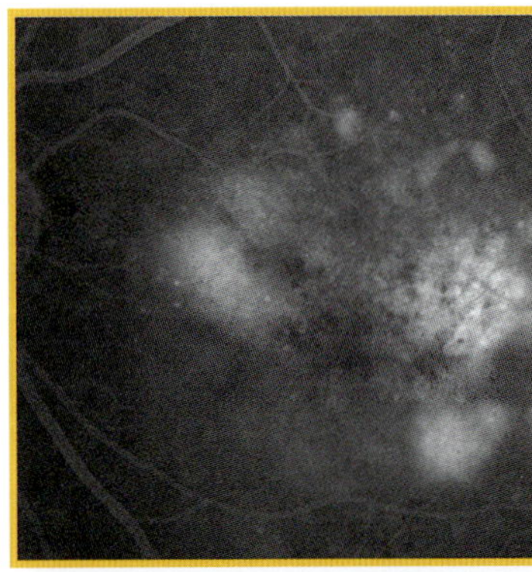

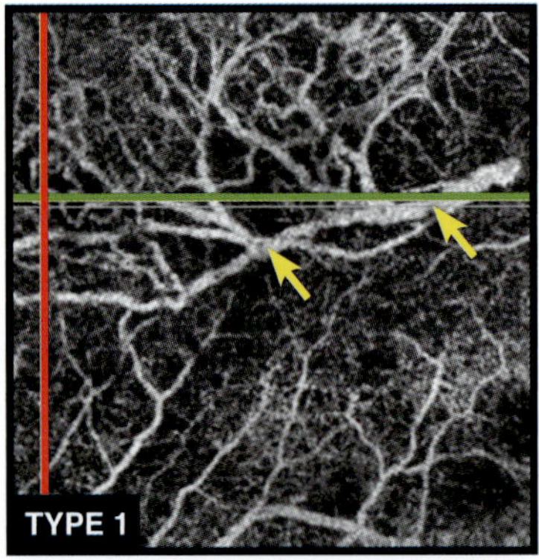

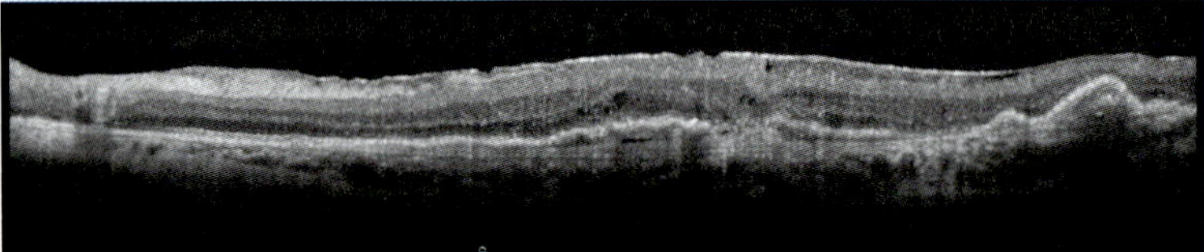

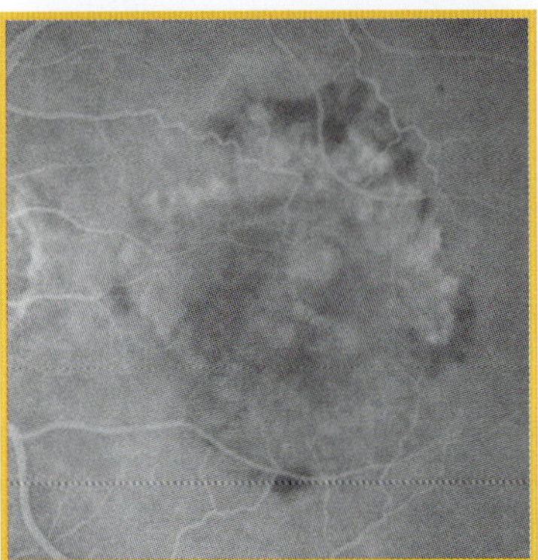

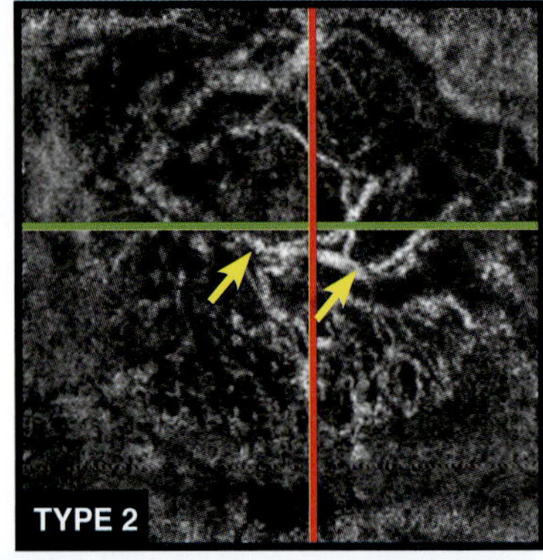

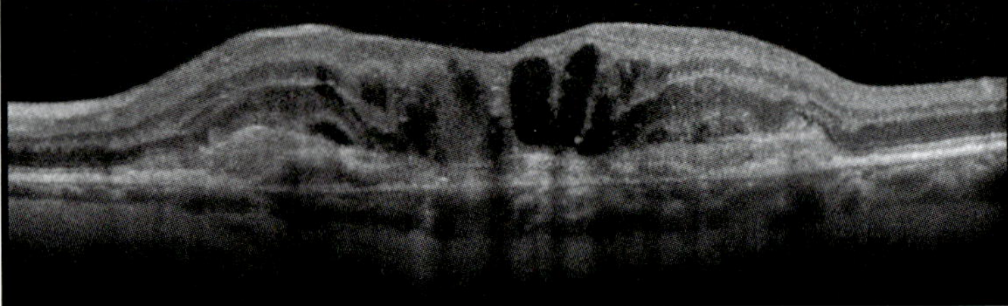

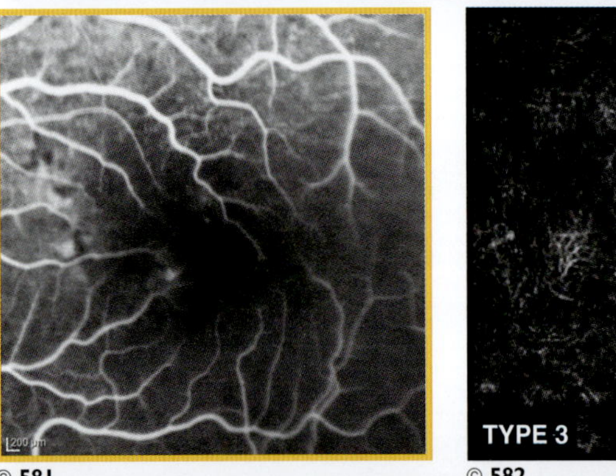

© 581

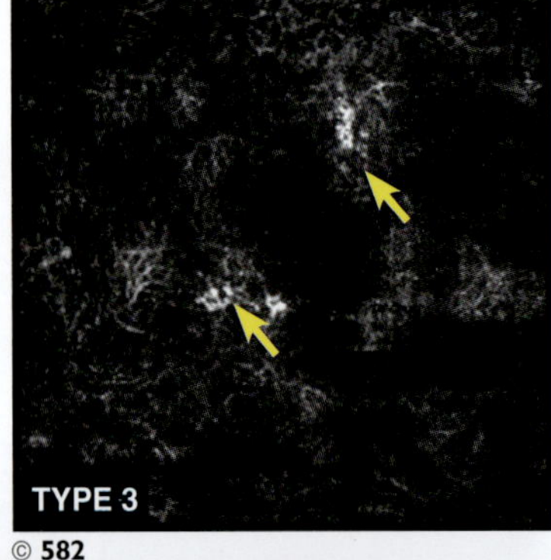

© 582

© 583

Optical coherence tomography angiography (OCTA) is a relatively new, non-contact technique that permits dyeless visualization of the retinal and choroidal circulation. OCTA uses flow characteristics within a defined volume of tissue to reconstruct an image of the vascular network. Because it allows selective visualization of vasculature relative to retinal depth, it is particularly suited for studying the morphology and spatial relationships of different subtypes of neovascularization. FA, OCTA, and structural OCT characteristics of type 1, 2, and 3 neovascularization are provided. The field of view of OCTA is typically 3 × 3 mm and is therefore smaller than most fluorescein angiograms. The intersection of red and green crosshairs on OCTA represents the central fovea. Note the large caliber trunk-like vessels *(yellow arrows)* below the RPE in type 1 and above the RPE in type 2 neovascularization. Type 3 neovascularization is chararacterized by focal points of increased signal intensity in the deep retinal capillary plexus, providing evidence to support a predominantly intraretinal origin for this neovascular subtype.

Type I Neovascularization

Type I neovascularization originates from the choroid and extends under the RPE. Subsequent detachments of the RPE and overlying retina may eventually occur. This form of neovascularization is poorly delineated with fluorescein angiography and stains in the late stages with irregular margins.

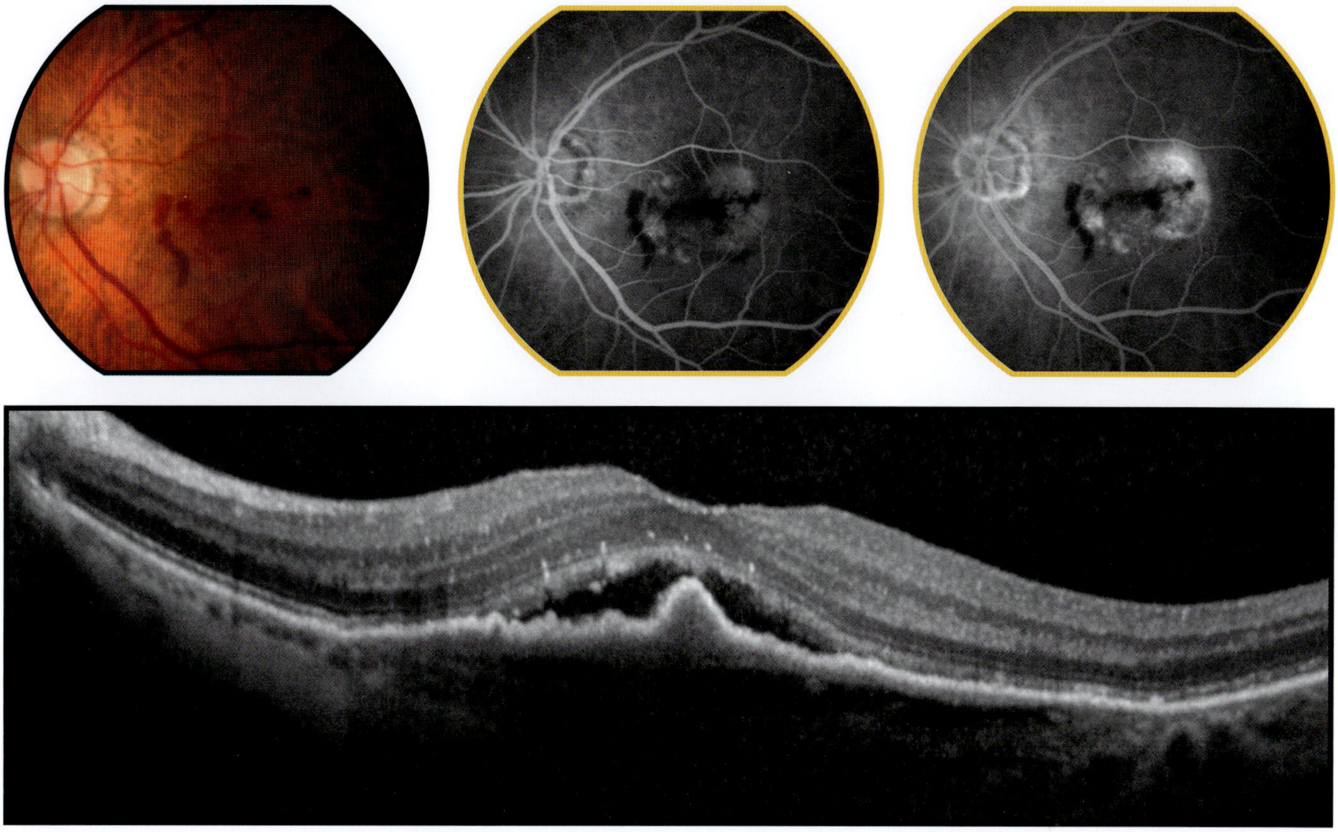

This is an example of type I neovascularization. There is a vascularized PED with secondary elevation of the overlying retina and subretinal hemorrhage. Early in the fluorescein angiogram, there is an indistinct area of subpigment epithelial staining *(top row, middle image)*. In the late stage of the angiogram, there is staining of the subpigment epithelial neovascular complex and leakage into the neurosensory detachment *(top row, right image)*. The OCT shows that neovascularization is confined to the subpigment epithelial space with an overlying area of subretinal fluid. The vascularized PED may appear irregular in height and shape, as shown here. There may be varying degrees of sub-RPE hyper-reflective material comprised of neovascular tissue, exudation and hemorrhage.

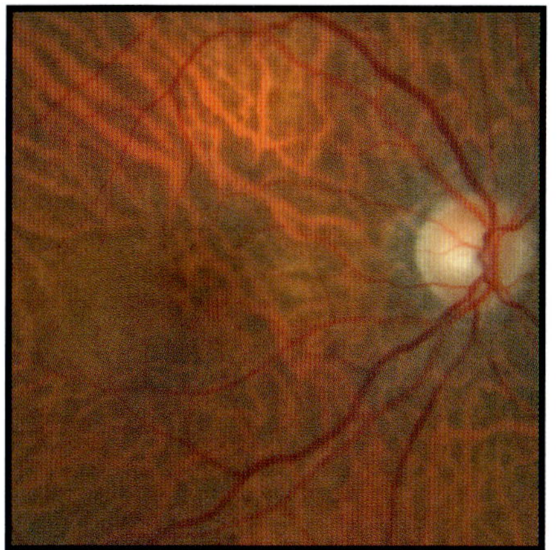

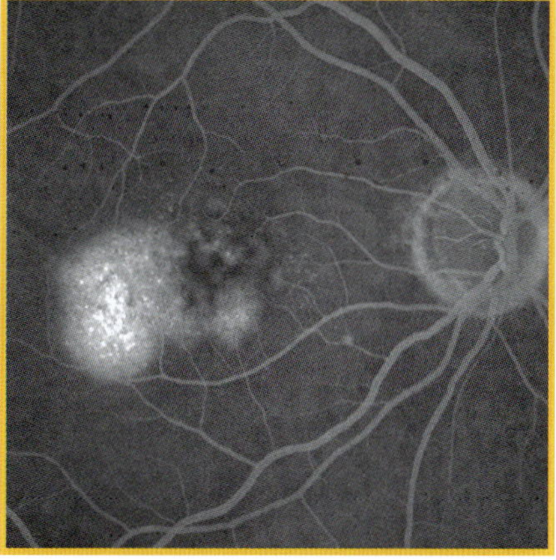

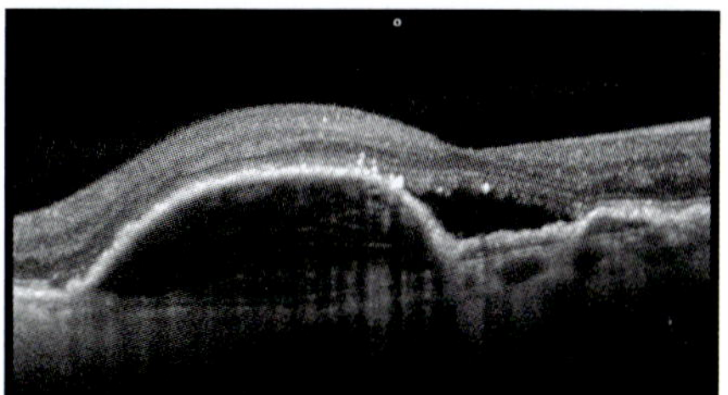

A vascularized PED may also appear as a smooth and well-circumscribed PED with a flattened or notched border. The latter is a sign of hidden or "occult" neovascularization. This color fundus photograph shows a smooth and well-circumscribed yellow-orange PED that demonstrates late staining on fluorescein angiography. The OCT shows a vascularized PED with heterogeneous sub-RPE signals and subretinal fluid.

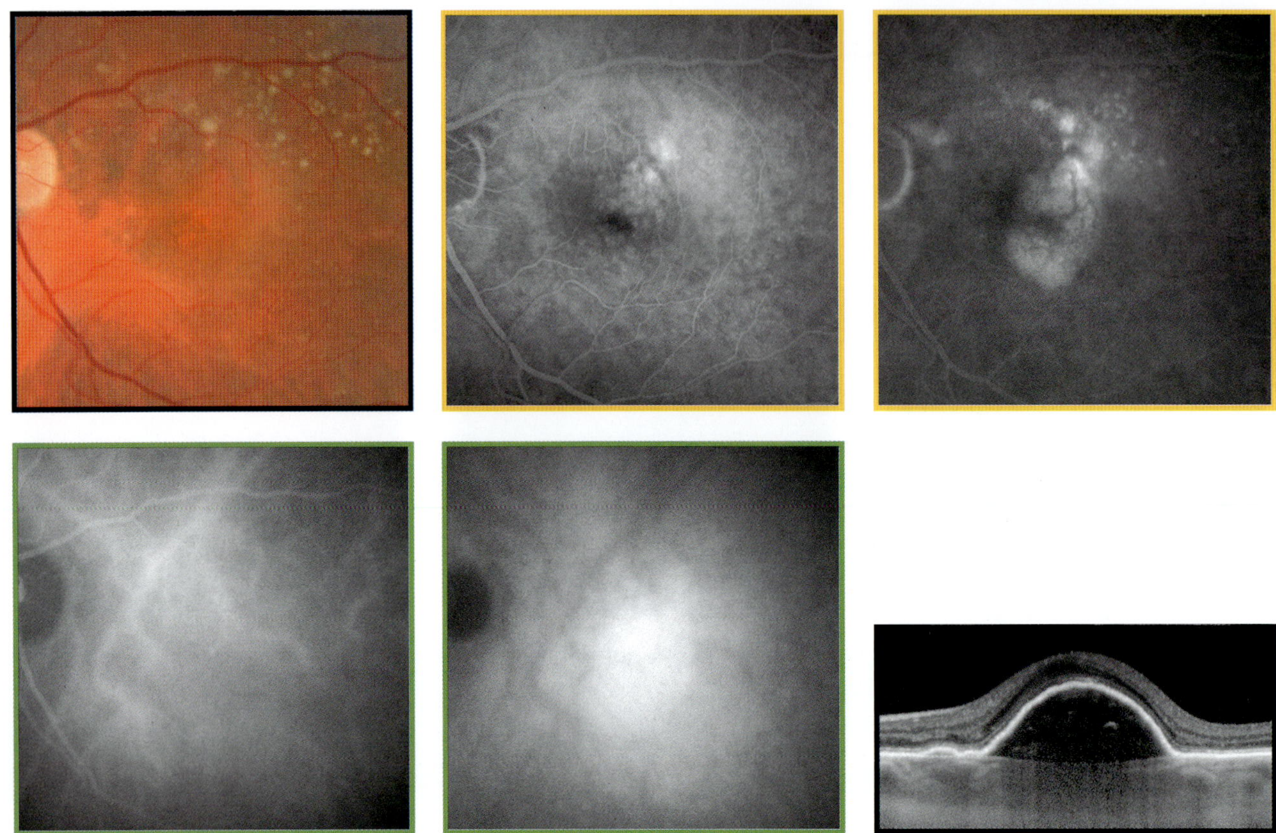

This vascularized PED appears as a smooth and well-circumscribed yellow-orange elevation of the RPE on color fundus photography. Fluorescein angiography reveals minimal stippled and irregular hyperfluorescence in the early phase and staining of the fibrovascular PED with areas of leakage in the later phases, consistent with the appearance of a so-called occult choroidal neovascular membrane. Indocyanine green angiography does not demonstrate a clear delineation of the neovascular complex in the early phase but reveals a well-defined area of hyperfluorescence, referred to as a "plaque," in the late phase. The OCT shows a dome-shaped elevation of the RPE with sub-RPE heterogeneous signals consistent with a vascularized PED.

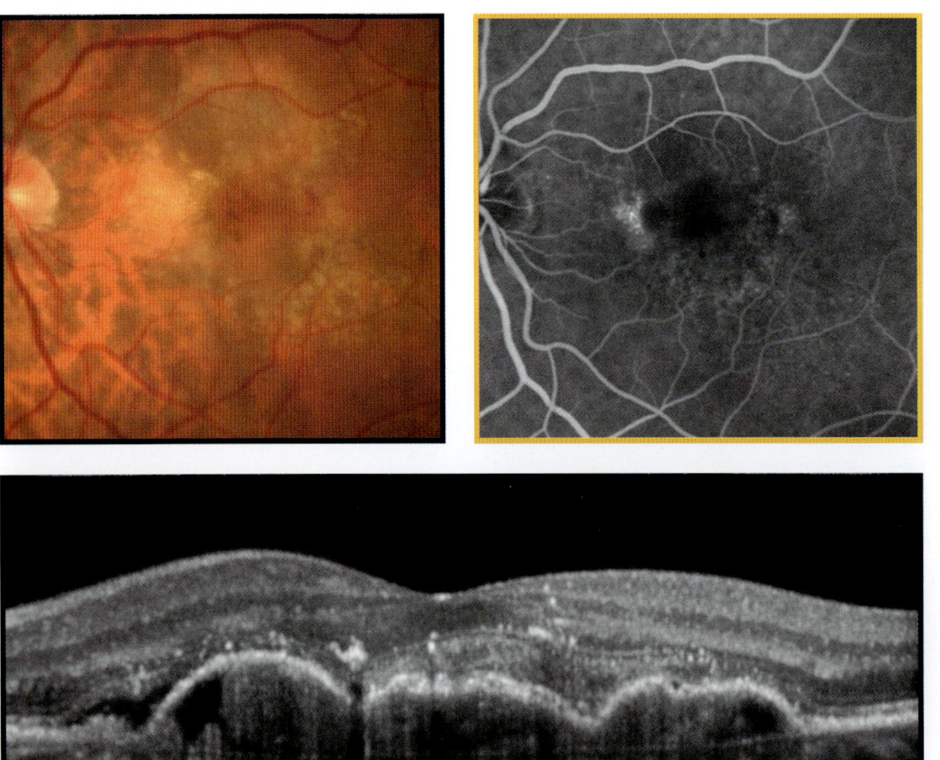

Vascularized PEDs may occur with a mixture of serous, drusenoid, and vascularized components. Fluorescein angiography reveals irregular stippled areas of leakage in the late phase, and OCT shows elevation of the pigment epithelium and subretinal fluid and exudation. The sub-RPE material may be a mixture of serous, drusenoid, and vascular components.

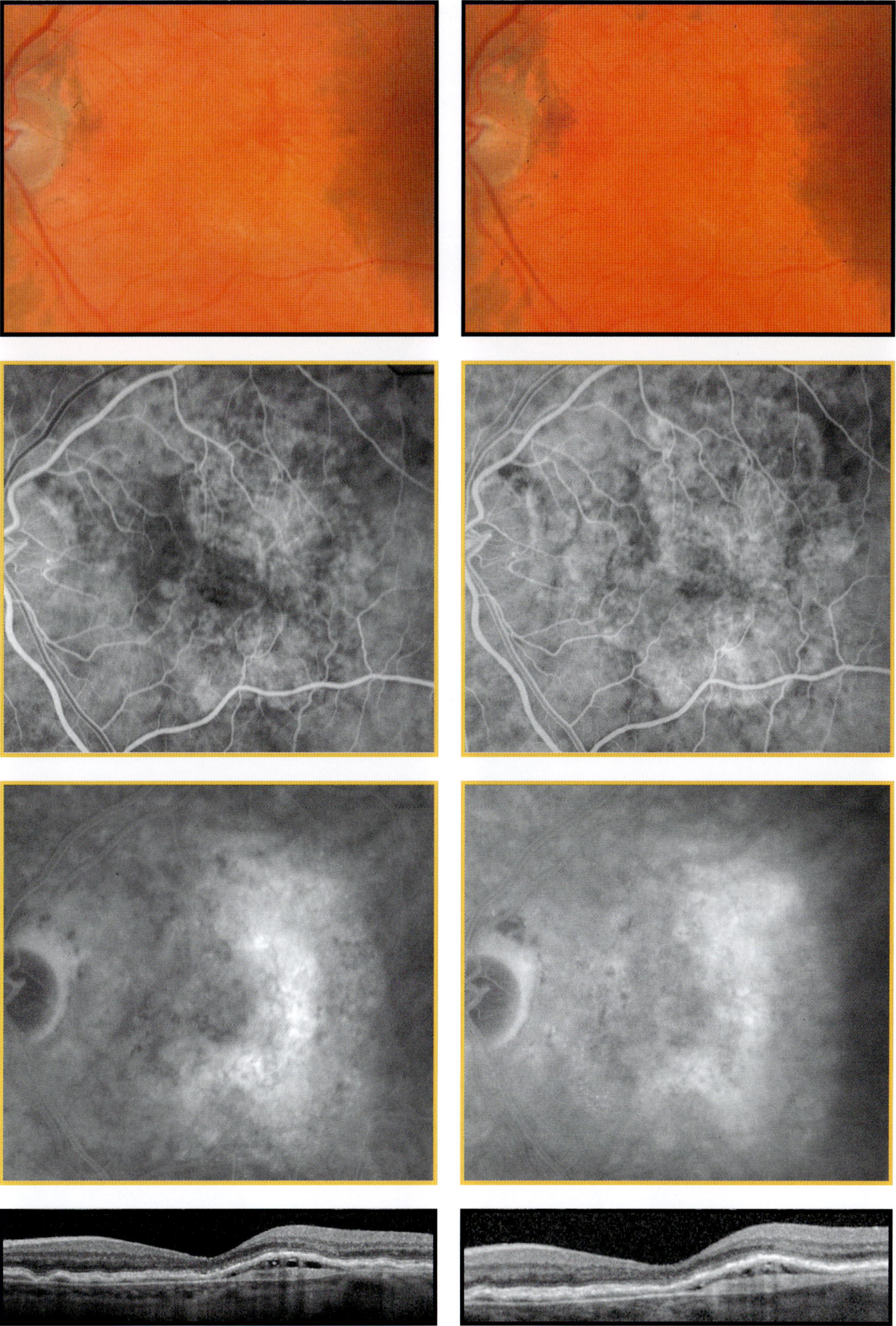

The long-standing, vascularized PED of this patient followed a relatively benign course over 6 years without treatment. Color photograph shows pigment mottling and hypopigmentation with no evidence of lipid or hemorrhage *(top left image)*, which was largely unchanged 6 years later *(top right image)*. Fluorescein angiography shows a somewhat atypical pattern for a type 1 lesion with the neovascularization appearing well delineated due to depigmentation of the overlying RPE *(second row)*. The late images show ill-defined late staining *(third row)*. There has been slow growth of the type 1 lesion over the 6 year interval. Spectral-domain OCT taken on presentation shows a vascularized PED with preserved outer retinal architecture and no evidence of subretinal fluid or exudation *(bottom left image)*. There is an organized lamellar scar noted within the sub-PED compartment. Six years later, the SD-OCT remains largely unchanged *(bottom right image)*. Visual acuity is still 20/30.

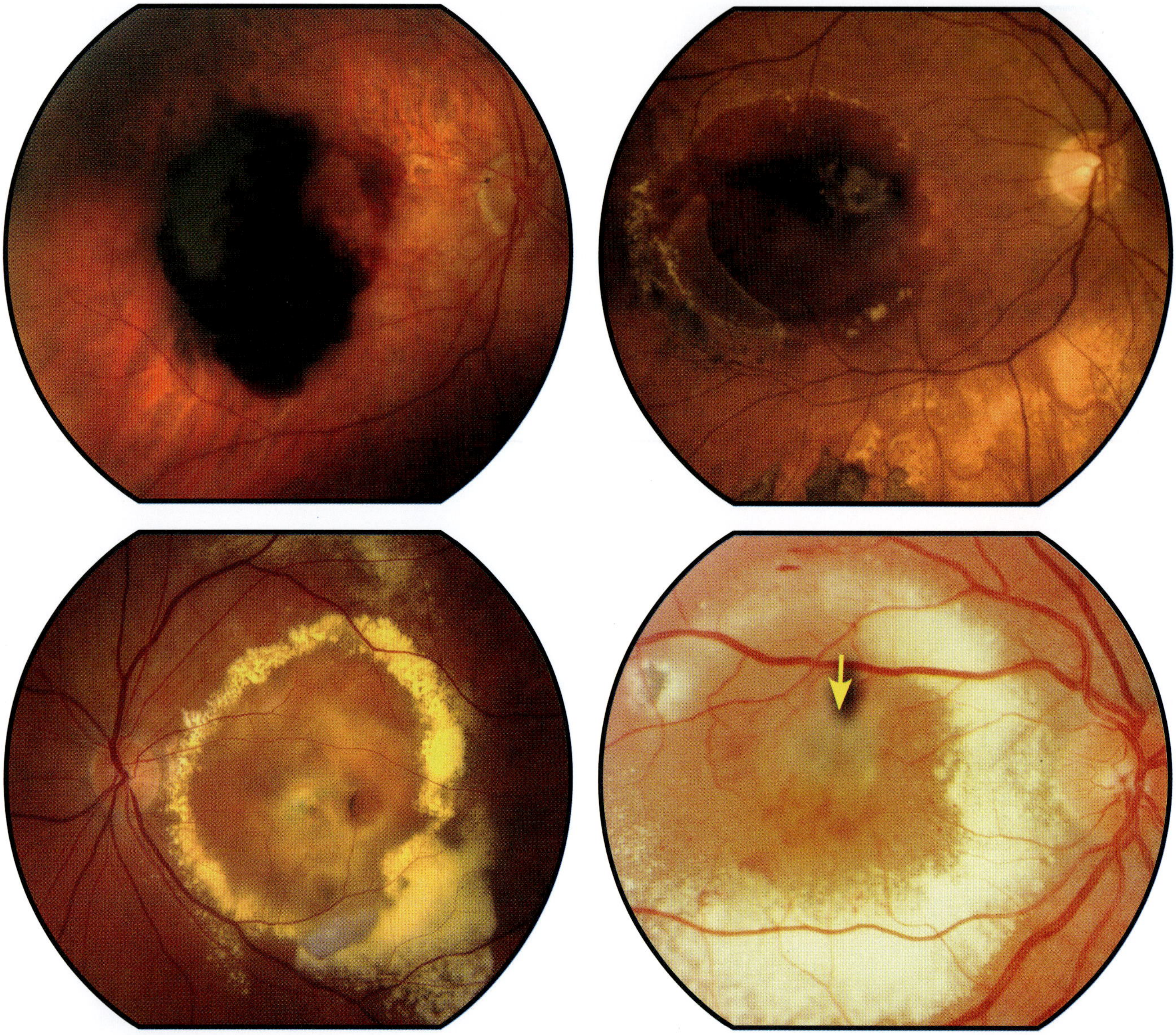

A vascularized detachment of the pigment epithelium may be hemorrhagic *(top images)*, exudative *(bottom images)*, or both. A grayish choroidal neovascular membrane *(arrow)* is seen within the exudate. Early in the exudative process, subretinal fluid, hemorrhage, and lipid may be seen. Generally, the degree of lipid exudation relates to the chronicity of the lesion, the nature of the vascular components, and possibly also the systemic level of serum lipids. *Bottom left image courtesy of Ophthalmic Imaging Systems, Inc.*

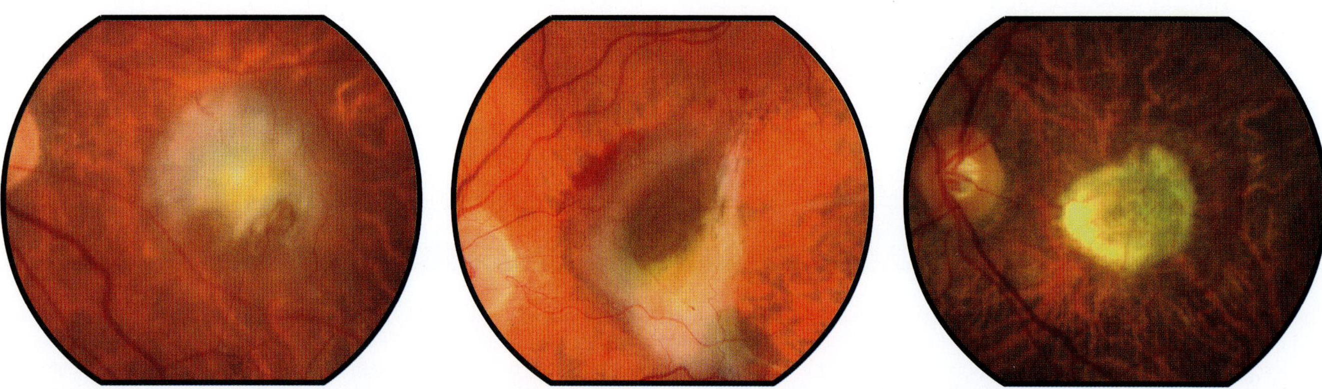

Vascularized PEDs may eventually become fibrotic. In these patients, there is predominantly serous exudation *(left image)*, a combined hemorrhagic and fibrotic vascularized PED *(middle image)*, and a fibrotic vascularized PED or disciform scar *(right image)*. *Left image courtesy of Ophthalmic Imaging Systems, Inc.*

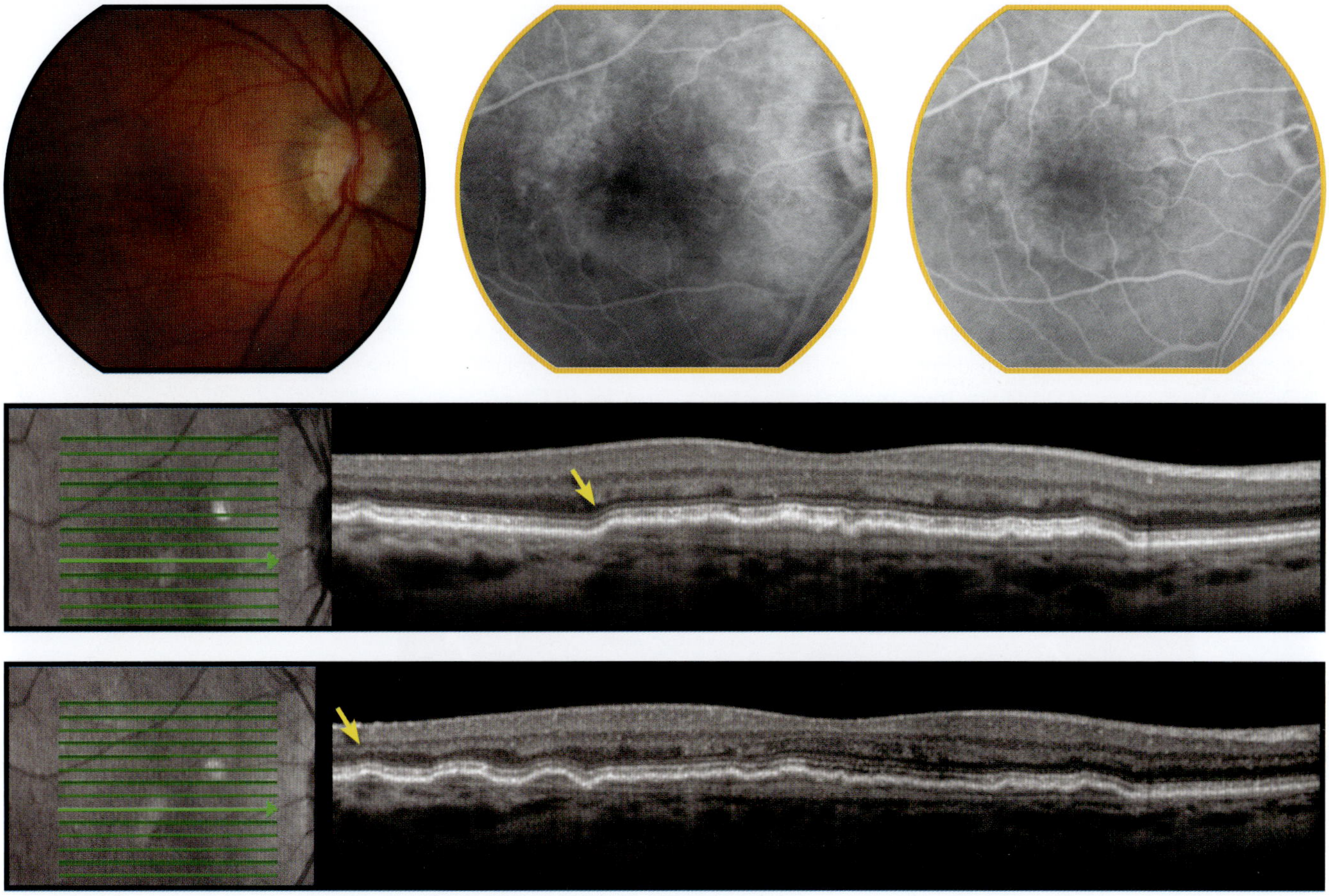

Type I neovascularization may develop years before any clinical evidence of exudation. The color fundus photograph shows no evidence of subretinal hemorrhage or exudation. Fluorescein angiography taken at presentation shows an ill-defined quiescent area of hyperfluorescent staining *(top middle image)*, which has not significantly changed in size after 3 years *(top right image)*. There is minimal angiographic leakage from the neovascular tissue. SD-OCT images show that the area of type I neovascular tissue has grown on its temporal edge *(arrows)* when the OCT from presentation is compared with the more recent image 3 years later *(bottom row image)*.

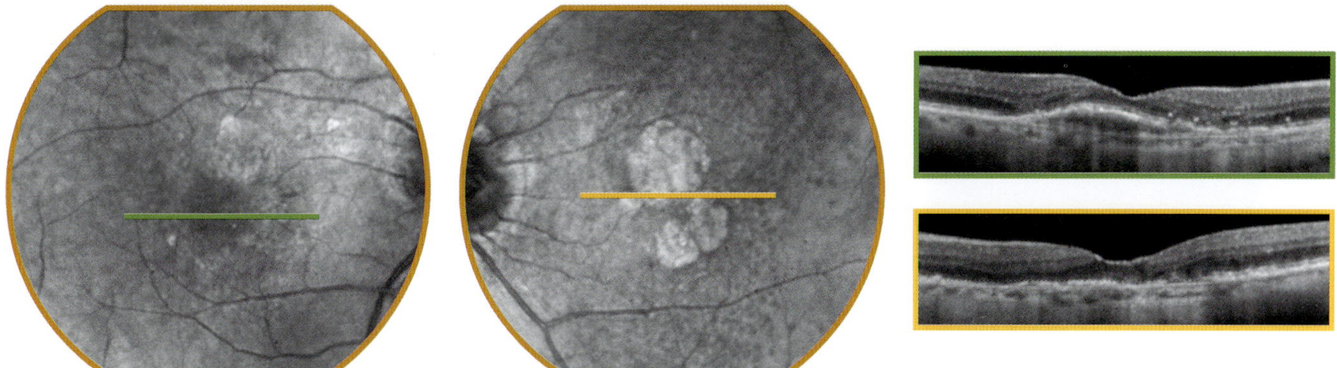

Although the clinical course is variable, type I neovascular lesions tend to behave less aggressively than type 2 and type 3 lesions, which are more likely to be associated with rapid loss of vision and active exudation. In addition, eyes with type I neovascular tissue appear to be more resistant to the occurrence of geographic atrophy when compared with the non-neovascular fellow eye in the same patient. These near-infrared reflectance images taken from the same patient show an absence of geographic atrophy in the right eye and a large central patch of geographic atrophy in the left eye. The corresponding OCT through the fovea of the right eye shows type I neovascularization (vascularized PED). This eye has been receiving intravitreal anti-VEGF therapy under a "treat-and-extend" regimen for 5 years. The OCT through the fovea in the left eye shows areas of outer retinal thinning and photoreceptor and RPE loss within areas of atrophy.

Vascularized PED variants

The advent of spectral-domain optical coherence tomography has permitted detailed characterization of vascularized PEDs, thus enhancing our understanding about the pathophysiology and natural course of these lesions.

Multilayered PED

Eyes with chronic fibrovascular PEDs receiving serial anti-VEGF therapy may demonstrate organized layers of hyper-reflective bands between the RPE monolayer and Bruch membrane. This appearance on SD-OCT has been described as a "multi-layered PED." It has been proposed that these multi-layered lamellar bands are comprised of fibrocellular tissue with contractile properties. They are typically organized in a spindle-shaped configuration. With continuous treatment, many patients with chronic multi-layered PEDs retain good long-term visual acuity and are at lower risk for RPE tears.

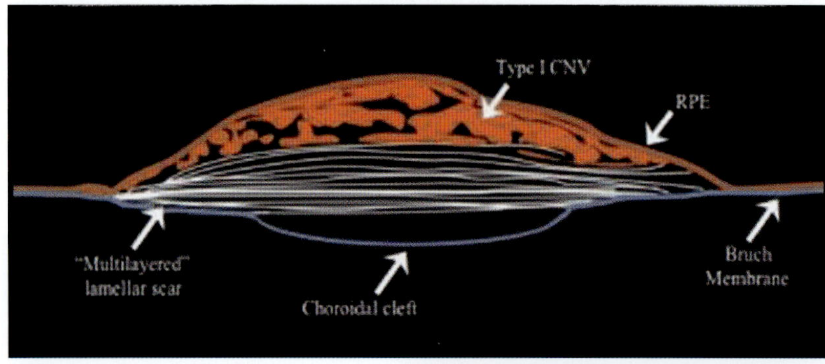

© 584

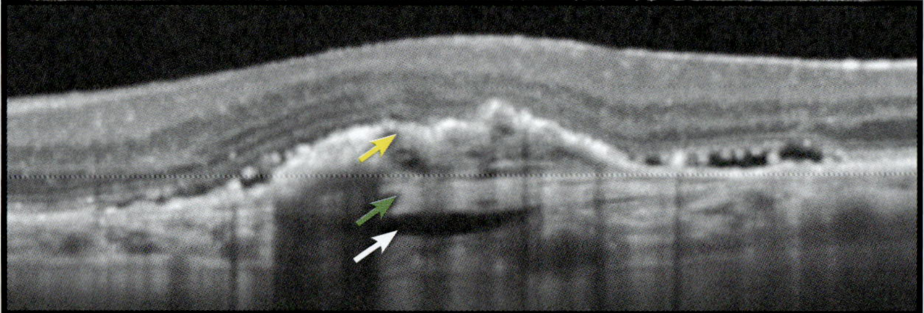

Schematic diagram and SD-OCT correlate of a multilayered PED showing (1) a characteristic fusiform complex of highly organized, layered, lamellar hyper-reflective bands *(green arrow)*; (2) an overlying vascular network *(yellow arrow)*; and (3) an underlying hyporeflective space, termed the pre-choroidal cleft, representing contraction, exudation, or both *(white arrow)*.

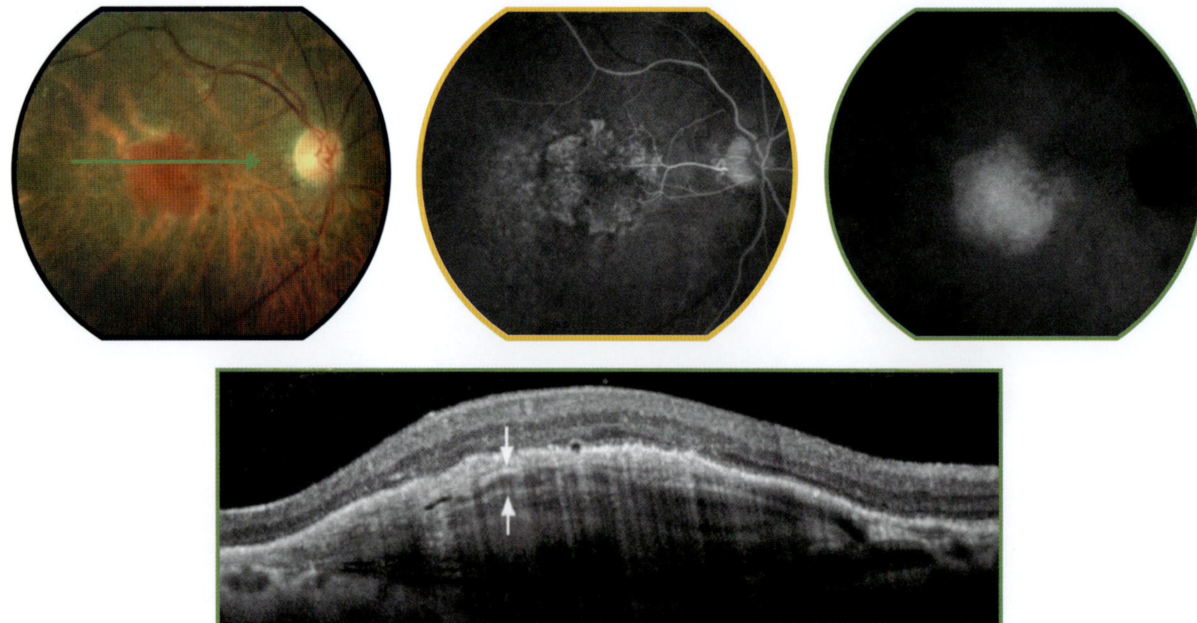

Color fundus photography shows a vascularized PED with a red hue that could be attributed to engorgement of the neovascular complex within the sub-RPE compartment. Fluorescein and indocyanine green angiography show a hyperfluorescent plaque consistent with type 1 neovascular tissue. Corresponding SD-OCT imaging shows a spindle-shaped complex of hyper-reflective bands deep to the RPE within the fibrovascular PED. Beneath the RPE, a heterogeneous, enlarged vascular network *(arrows)* is seen. Underlying the multi-layered lamellar structure, a hyporeflective pre-choroidal cleft is present, separating the neovascular tissue complex from the Bruch membrane.

The "onion sign"

The "onion sign" is a characteristic SD-OCT appearance where hyper-reflective curvilinear bands are organized in a lamellar pattern within a vascularized PED. These bands correlate clinically with sites of sub-RPE lipid exudation and correlate histologically with sites where cholesterol clefts have formed.

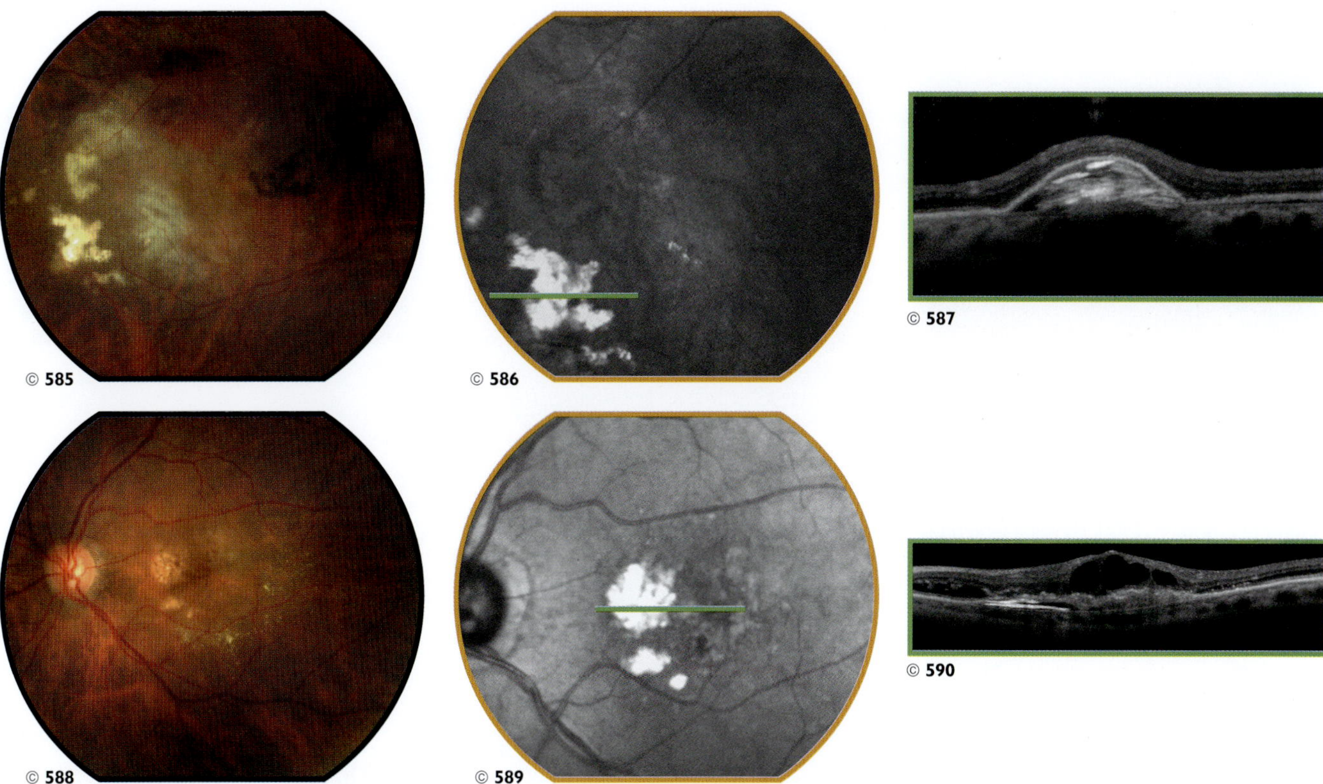

These patients with neovascular AMD and PED have a yellow refractile lesion on color fundus photography that corresponds to a hyper-reflective lesion on near-infrared reflectance imaging. SD-OCT through these lesions reveals hyper-reflective lines.

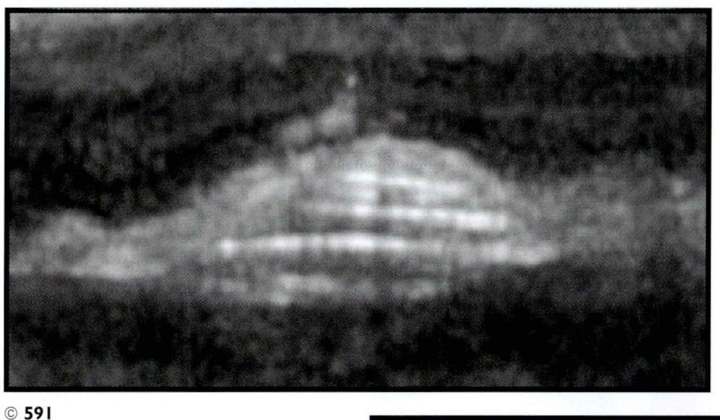

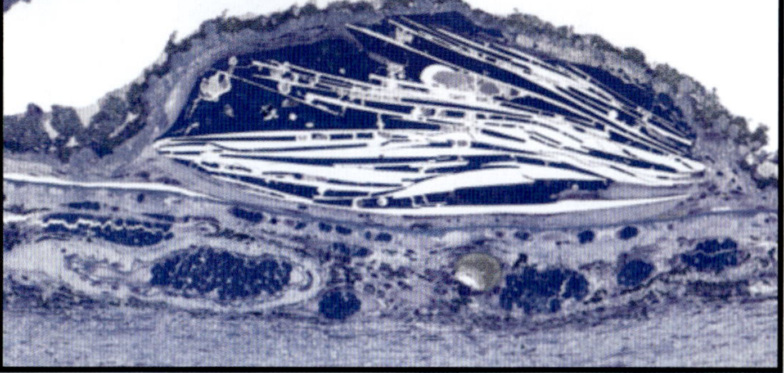

The configuration of hyper-reflective planes on SD-OCT images correlates with the pattern of cholesterol clefts seen on histological specimens. Cholesterol clefts form following the extraction of cholesterol crystals during post-mortem tissue processing. Clinically, cholesterol crystals represent precipitation of lipid during the exudative process.

Retinal Pigment Epithelium Tears

RPE tears can complicate the natural history of fibrovascular PEDs in neovascular AMD. The risk of RPE tear is known to be 5–17% greater in those receiving anti-VEGF therapy. RPE tears may be large and visually catastrophic, but they may also be compatible with preserved central vision when they are small or occur eccentrically. A grading system, based on the measurement of the greatest linear diameter of the RPE tear, was developed to predict visual and anatomic outcomes.

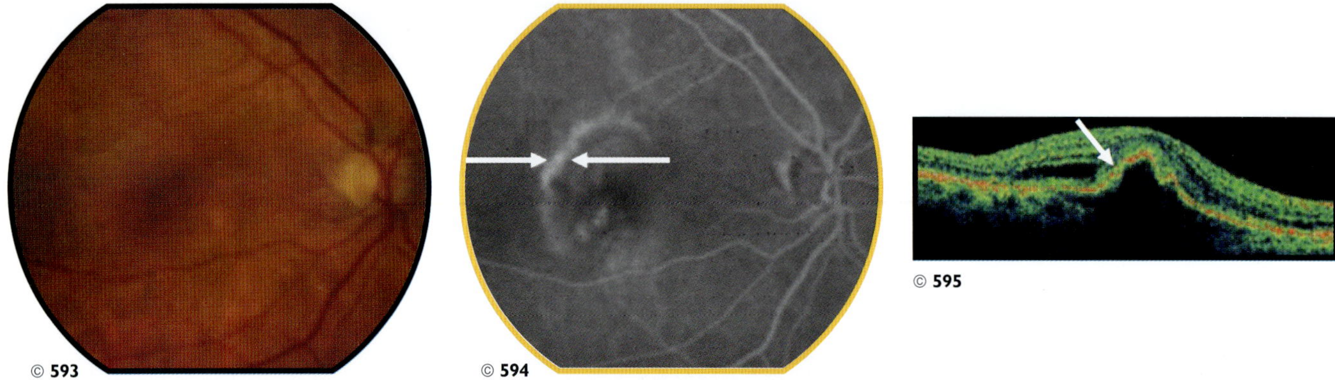

Grade 1 RPE tear—greatest linear diameter less than 200 μm. Fluorescein angiography shows a subtle thin early hyperfluorescent ring at the edge of the PED *(arrows)*. OCT shows a tented up or irregular PED with a microscopic point-like defect at the level of the RPE *(arrow)*. Low-grade RPE tears have better visual outcomes and better response to anti-VEGF therapy than large tears. Small RPE tears may progress to a higher grade tear over time.

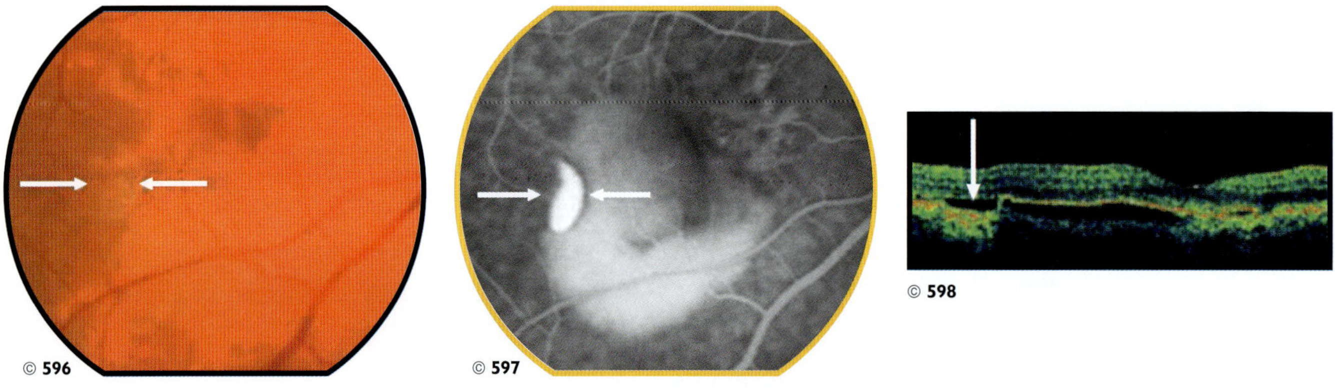

Grade 2 RPE tear—between 200 μm and 1 disc-diameter. Fluorescein angiography shows an oval window defect with late staining of surrounding tissue. There is hypofluorescence along the margin of the tear due to blockage by the scrolled RPE edge. OCT shows a visible defect in the RPE.

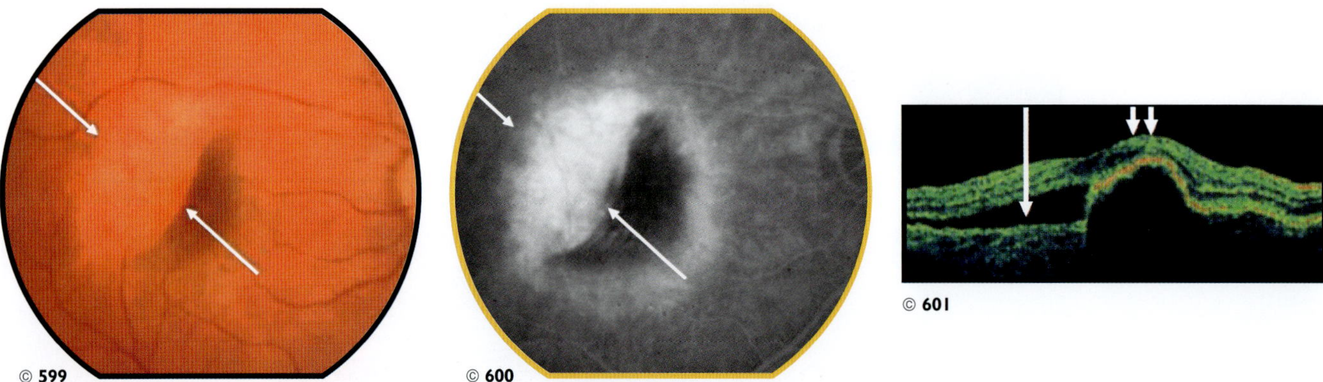

Grade 3 RPE tear—larger than 1 disc-diameter. Fluorescein angiography shows a large crescent-shaped transmission defect with an adjacent patch of hypofluorescence due to blockage. Irregular radiating folds are also present. OCT shows a large RPE defect adjacent to a thickened and irregular PED.

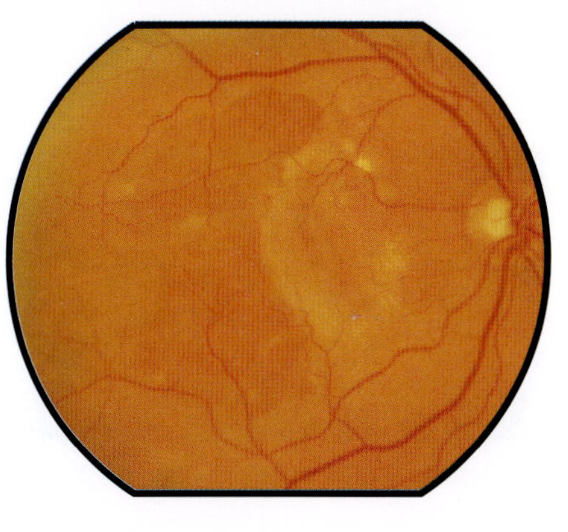
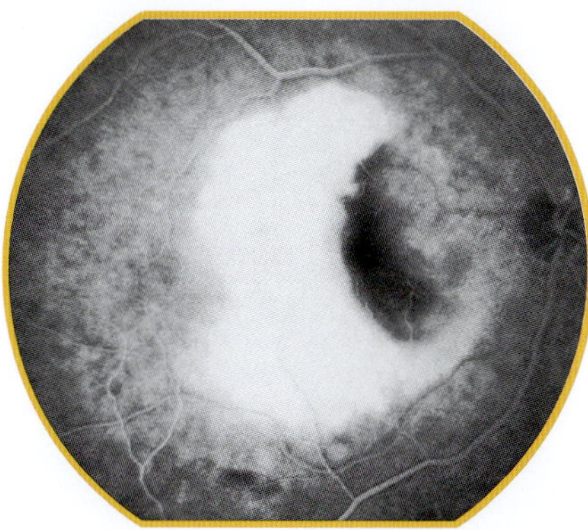
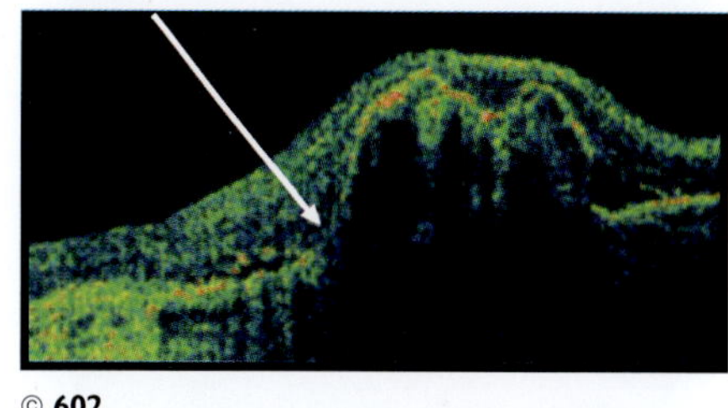

© 602

Grade 4 RPE tear—grade 3 tear that involves the fovea. This patient has a large semilunar RPE rip in the temporal macula with consolidation of the retracting pigment epithelium nasally. Grade 4 tears have a very poor visual prognosis with or without anti-VEGF therapy.

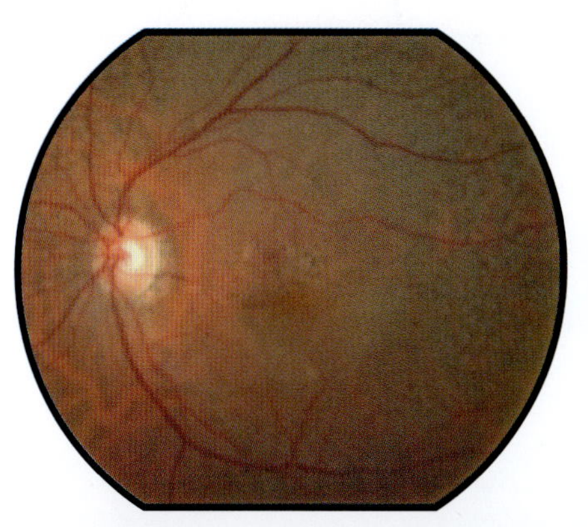
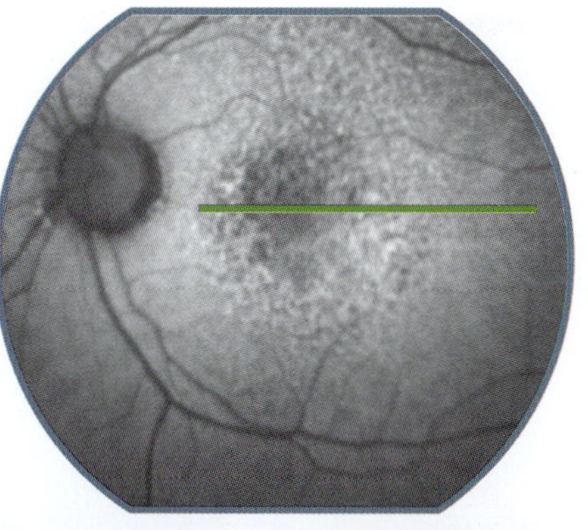
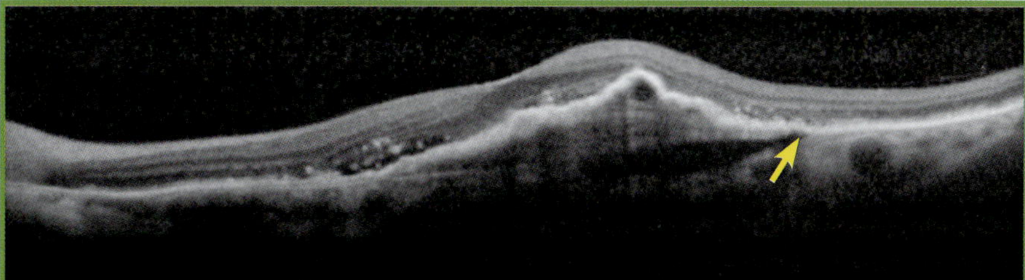
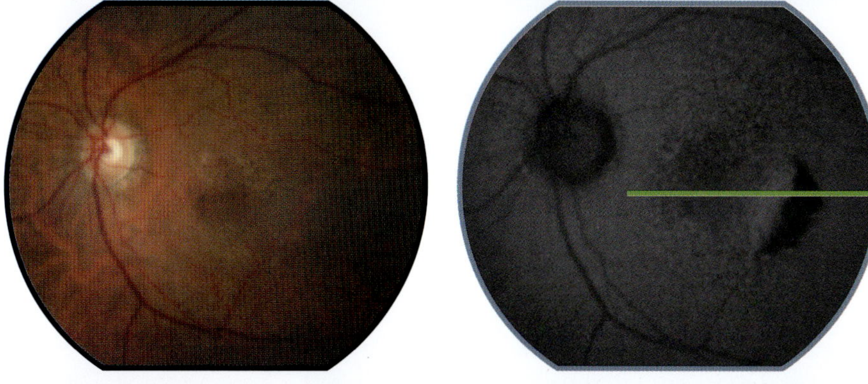
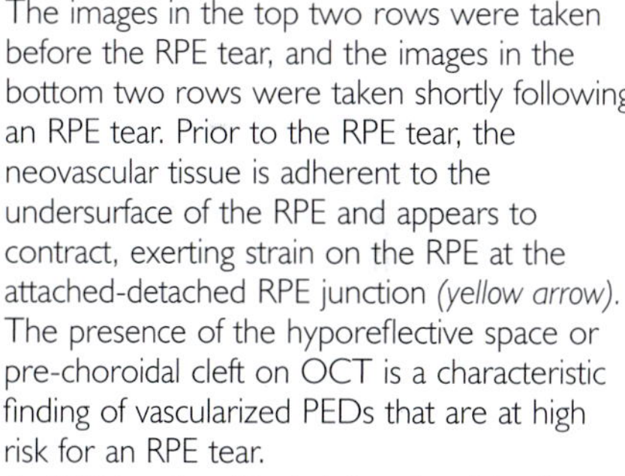
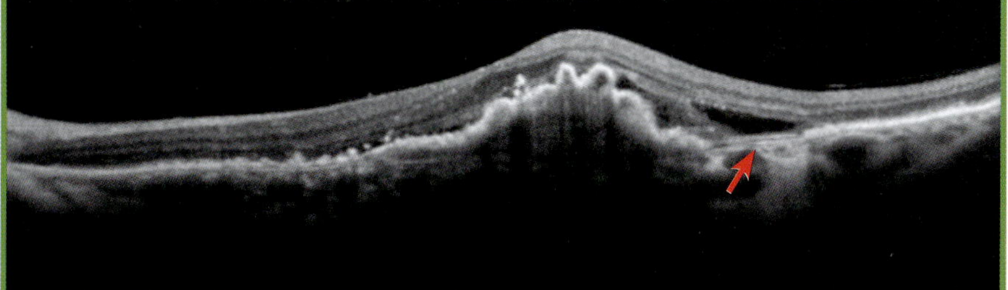

The images in the top two rows were taken before the RPE tear, and the images in the bottom two rows were taken shortly following an RPE tear. Prior to the RPE tear, the neovascular tissue is adherent to the undersurface of the RPE and appears to contract, exerting strain on the RPE at the attached-detached RPE junction *(yellow arrow)*. The presence of the hyporeflective space or pre-choroidal cleft on OCT is a characteristic finding of vascularized PEDs that are at high risk for an RPE tear.
An RPE tear is evident at the site of traction on the subsequent visit *(red arrow)*. Scrolled RPE at the apex of the PED is also evident on OCT. The site of RPE tear is hypoautofluorescent on fundus autofluorescence imaging, and the scrolled RPE is hyperautofluorescent.

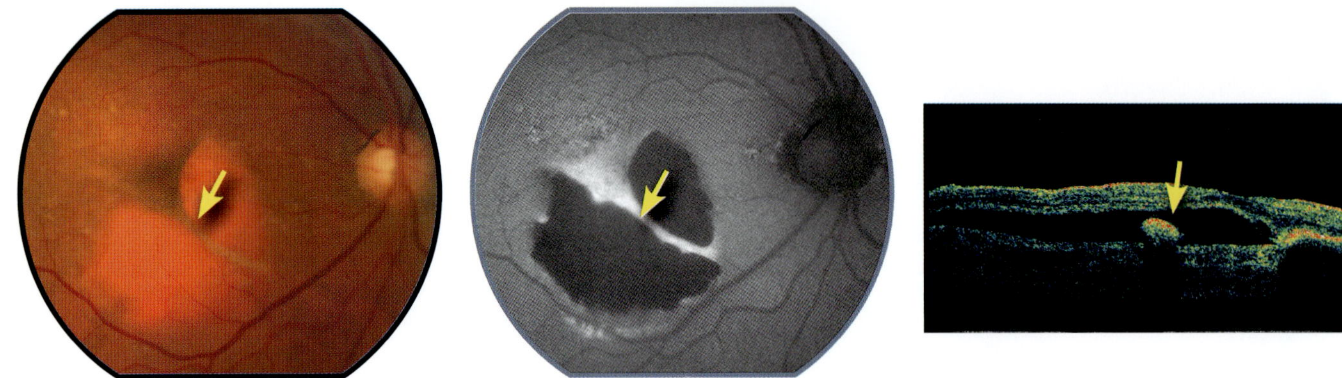

This patient had an unusual bilobed tear of the pigment epithelium. There is a bridging flap of preserved pigment epithelium extending across the defect. There is pigment epithelial hyperpigmentation due to consolidation of that tissue layer. The OCT image shows a nodular area of pigment epithelium, corresponding to the bridging tissue *(arrow)*, with an absence of RPE on either side. Fundus autofluorescence shows hypoautofluorescence in the area of denuded pigment epithelium and hyperautofluorescence of the bridging tissue of coiled and retracted pigment epithelium.

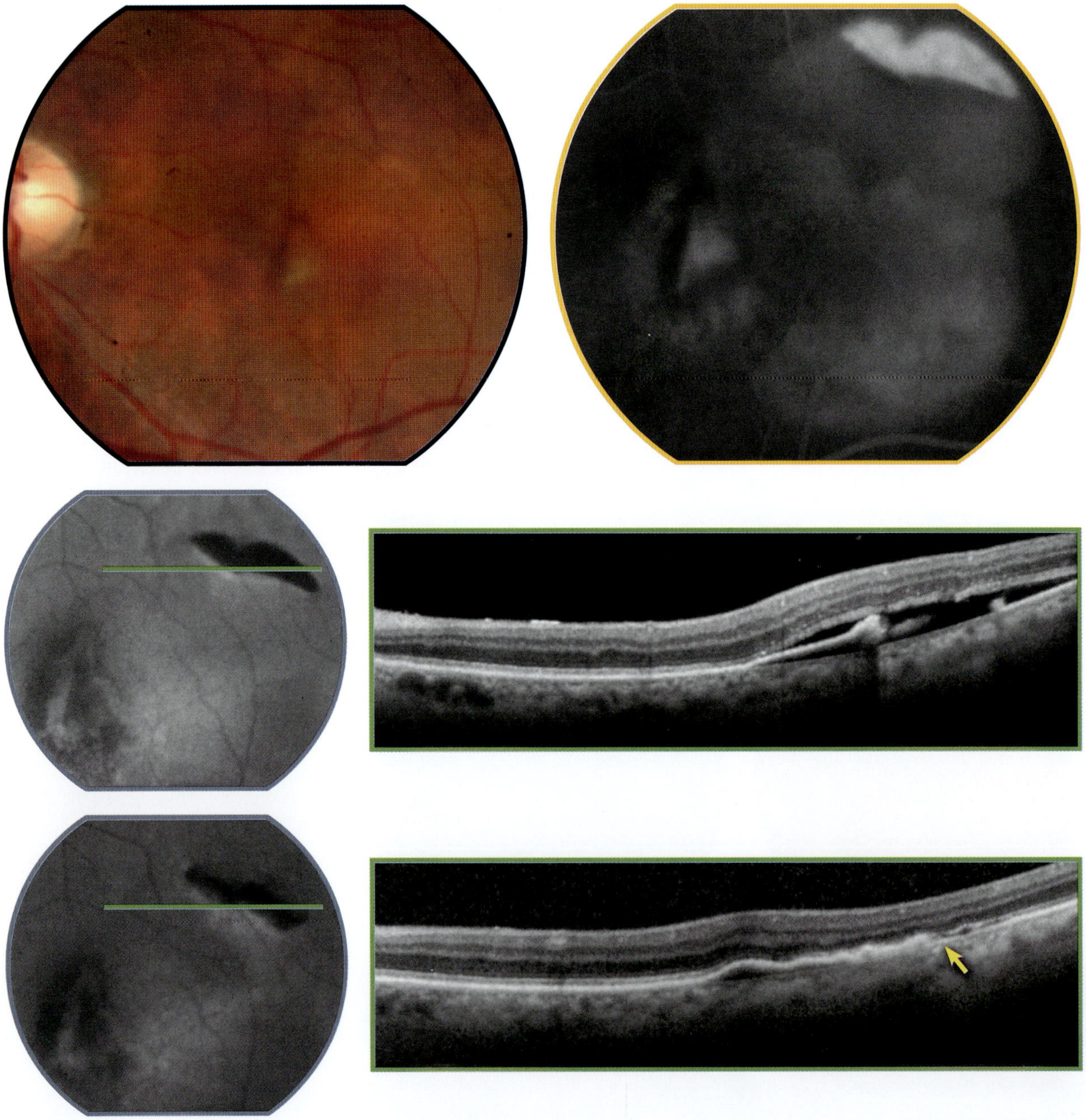

The color fundus photograph and fluorescein angiogram show an RPE tear at its onset. The fundus autofluorescence and SD-OCT at presentation *(middle row)* and 6 months after continued anti-VEGF therapy *(bottom row)* are shown. As seen here, some RPE tears undergo RPE resurfacing due to RPE migration or repopulation *(arrow)*.

Polypoidal Choroidal Vasculopathy

Polypoidal choroidal vasculopathy (PCV) is now recognized as a form of type I neovascularization because the polyps appear to originate from neovascular tissue above the Bruch membrane rather than from the inner choroid, as was originally described. PCV has also been called the posterior uveal bleeding syndrome and multiple recurrent serosanguinous retinal PED syndrome. It was originally described as a distinct entity occurring predominantly in African-American and Asian individuals between 50 and 65 years of age who lacked other typical AMD clinical findings (drusen and pigmentary abnormalities). There is increasing evidence to suggest that PCV is associated with choroidal abnormalities such as increased thickness, hyperpermeability, and pachyvessels. The genetics of PCV are unresolved. Type I neovascularization with polyps, in the absence of other phenotypic and demographic features characteristic of PCV, is commonly referred to as polypoidal neovascularization.

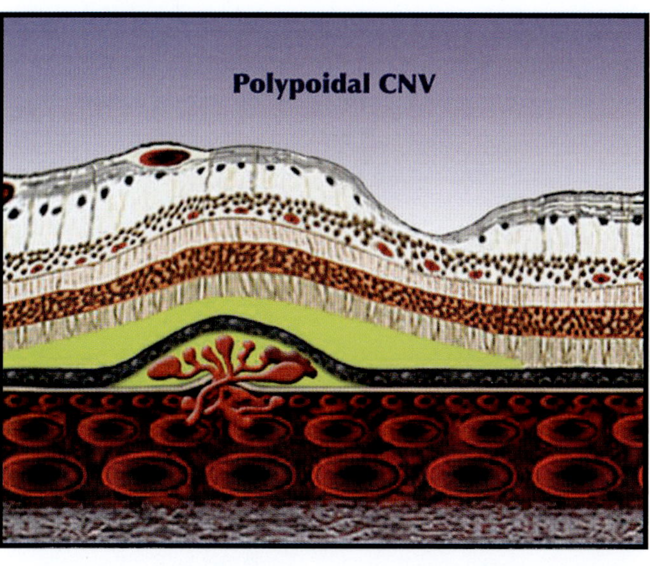

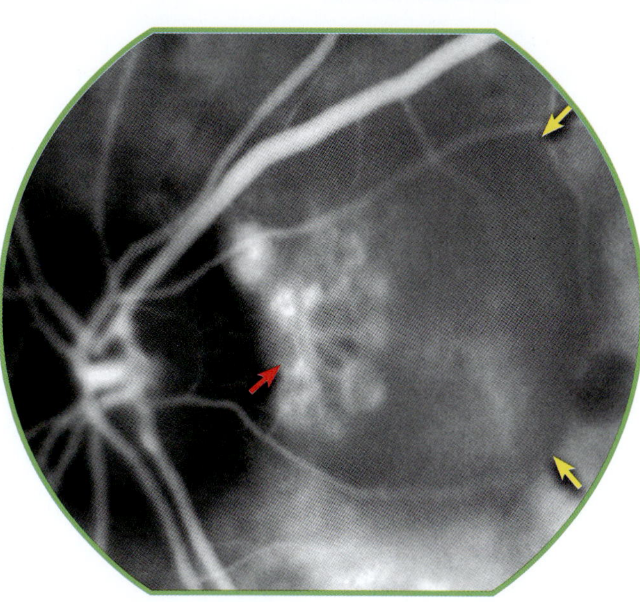

The schematic drawing *(left panel)* illustrates a polypoidal vascular abnormality beneath a detachment of the pigment epithelium, characteristic of type I neovascularization. ICG angiography is superior to FA for imaging PCV, as the near-infrared excitatory and fluorescent wavelengths used for ICG angiography penetrate deeper into the fundus through the RPE and the serosanguinous complications. There is evidence of a hypofluorescent PED *(yellow arrows)* and a branching vascular network, terminating in aneurysmal dilatations or polyps in the sub-RPE space *(red arrow)*.

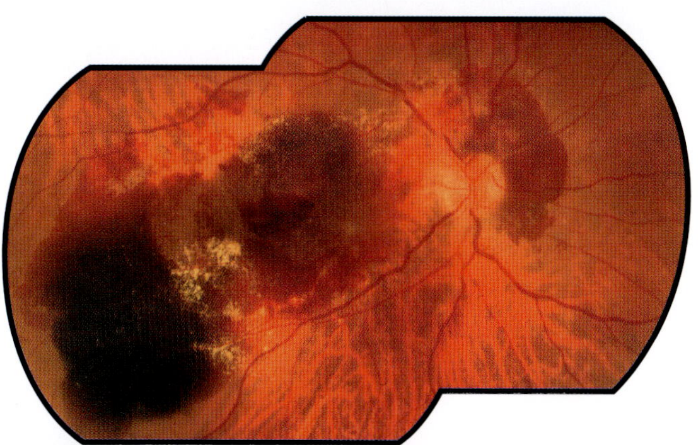

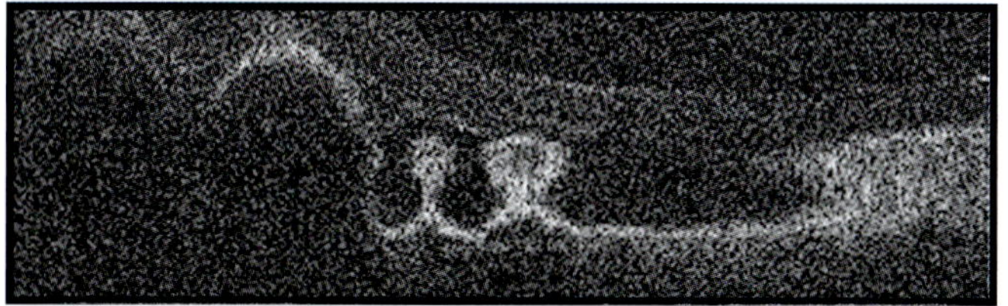

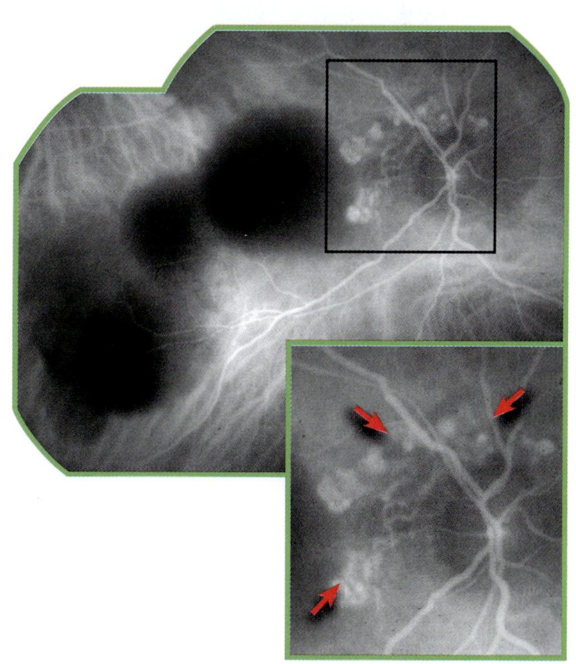

Large hemorrhagic detachments of the pigment epithelium and neurosensory retina are characteristic of PCV, particularly in patients with systemic hypertension. ICG angiography on the right shows a branching vascular network with polypoidal elements in the peripapillary region *(arrows)*. OCT shows circular polypoidal lesions or, in this case, a "dumbbell" appearance of the RPE due to anterior protrusions of subpigment epithelial neovascular tissue.

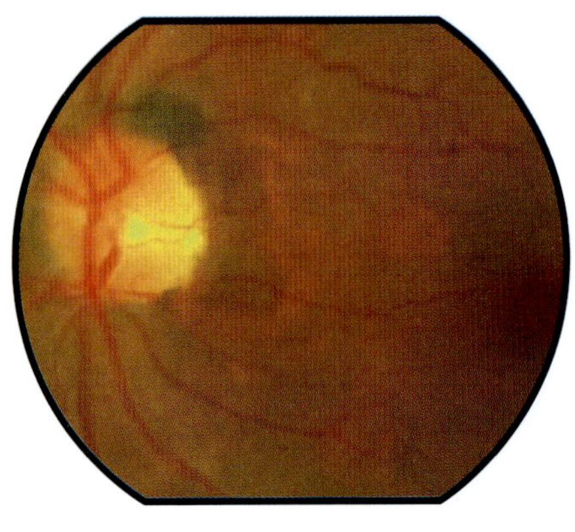

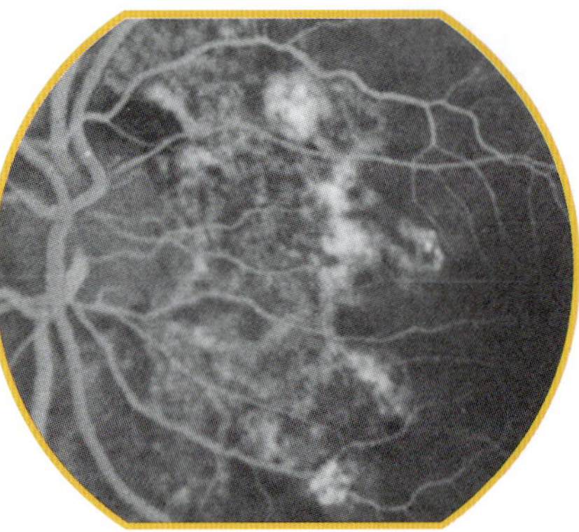

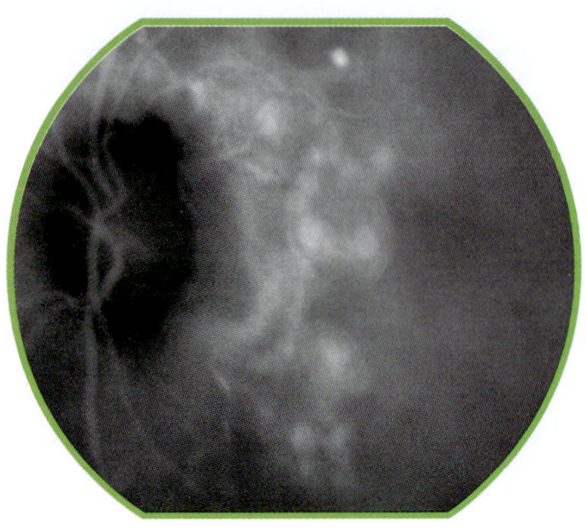

This patient is an African-American female with peripapillary PCV. The typical branching pattern, ending in aneurysmal dilations, is evident through the overlying depigmented RPE. Fluorescein angiography shows an area of hyperfluorescence corresponding to the vascular abnormality *(middle image)*, but the ICG angiogram clearly delineates all the features of the polypoidal lesions.

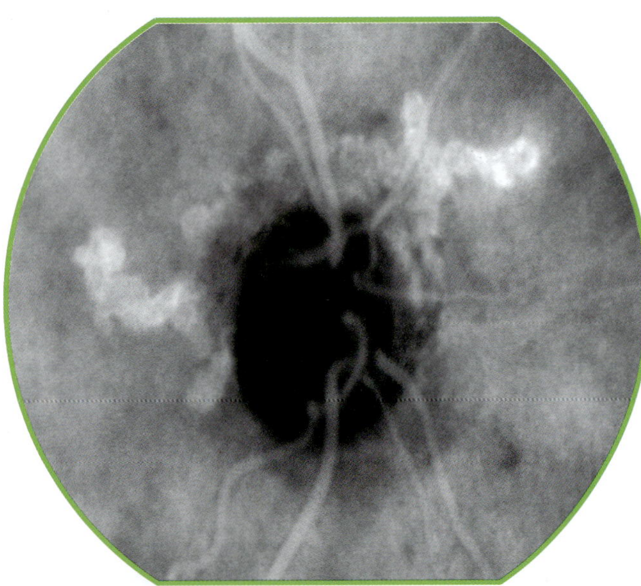

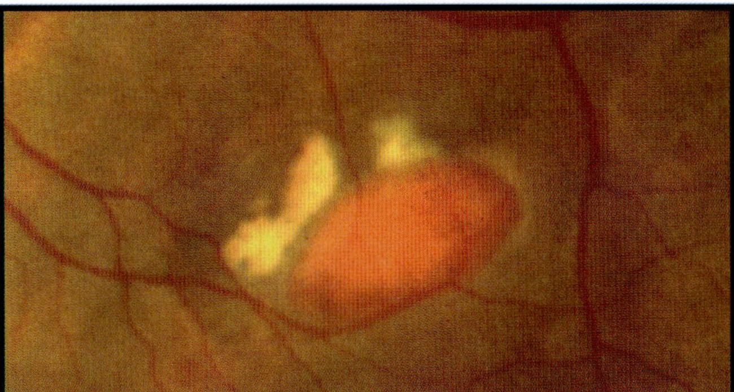

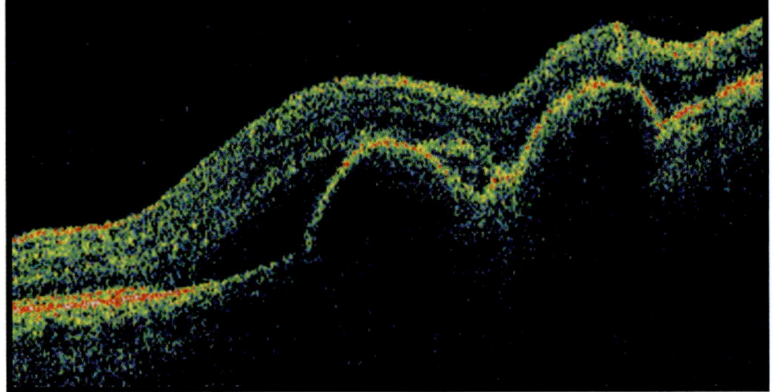

In the USA, PCV is more common in African-American patients than in Caucasian patients and often involves the peripapillary area, rather than the central macular region. The polypoidal lesions may appear orange, simulating a hemangioma, and may have a border of lipid deposition *(top right image)*. The OCT *(bottom right image)* shows multiple PEDs with an overlying neurosensory detachment. In some cases, a "double layer" of reflectance may be seen corresponding to the polyp.

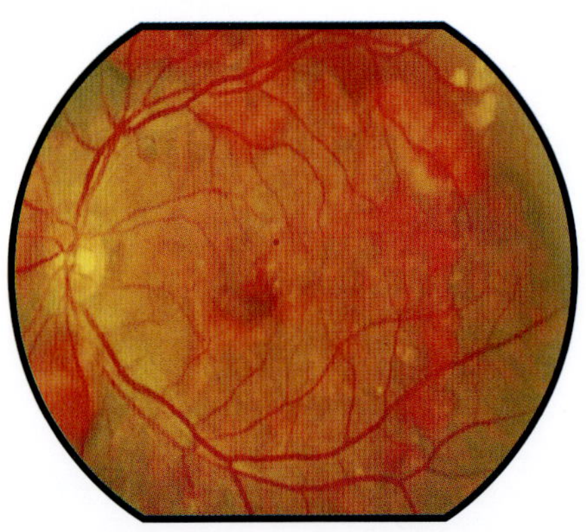

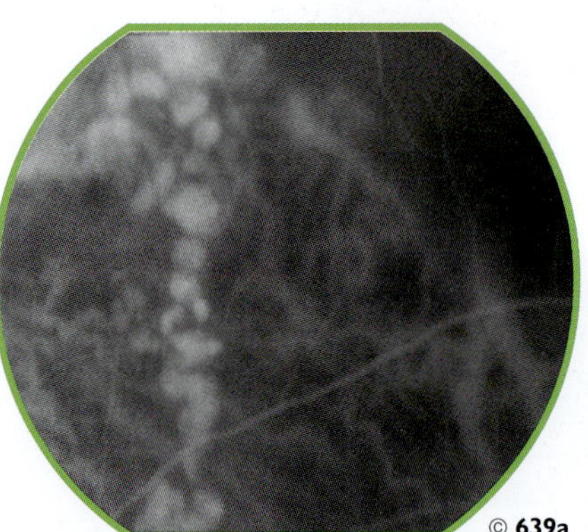

© 639a

© 821

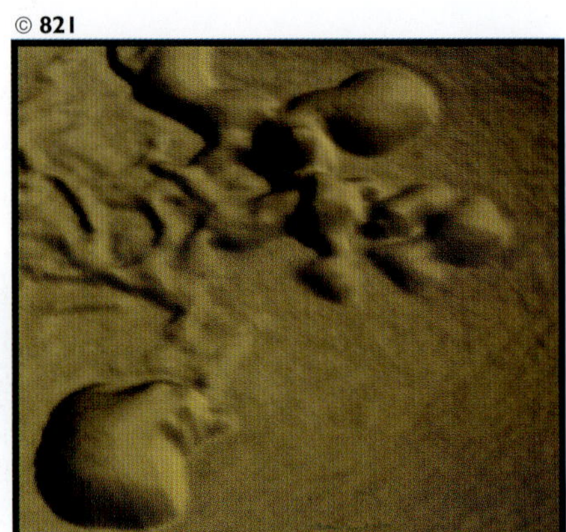

This patient is Japanese with a widespread area of PCV in the central macula. There is vertical alignment of vascular polypoidal lesions, seen best with ICG angiography *(middle image)*. PCV is fairly common in Japanese and Southeast Asian patients in whom central macular involvement is not unusual. The *en face* OCT shows blister-like elevations corresponding to the branching vascular network, PEDs, and the polyps themselves.

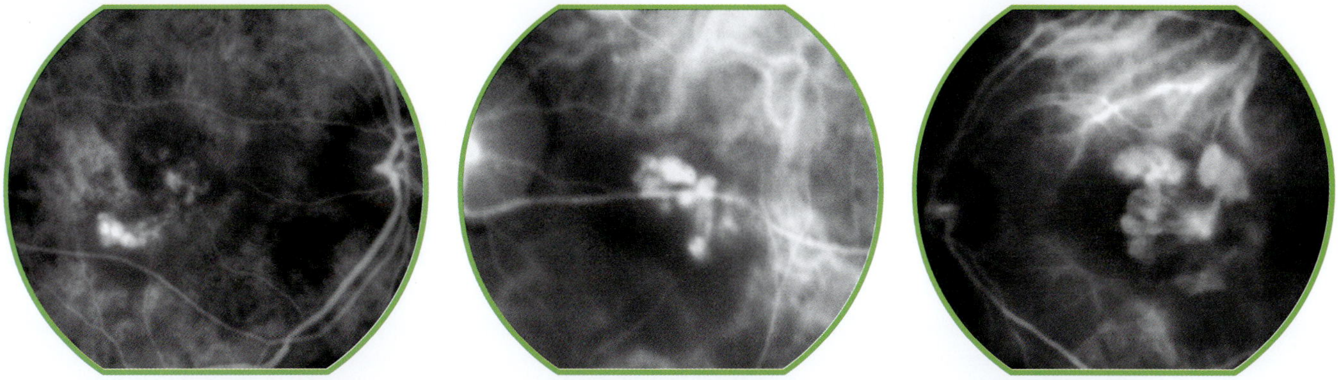

The polypoidal lesions may vary in size and number. These three patients have central polypoidal lesions of varying sizes.

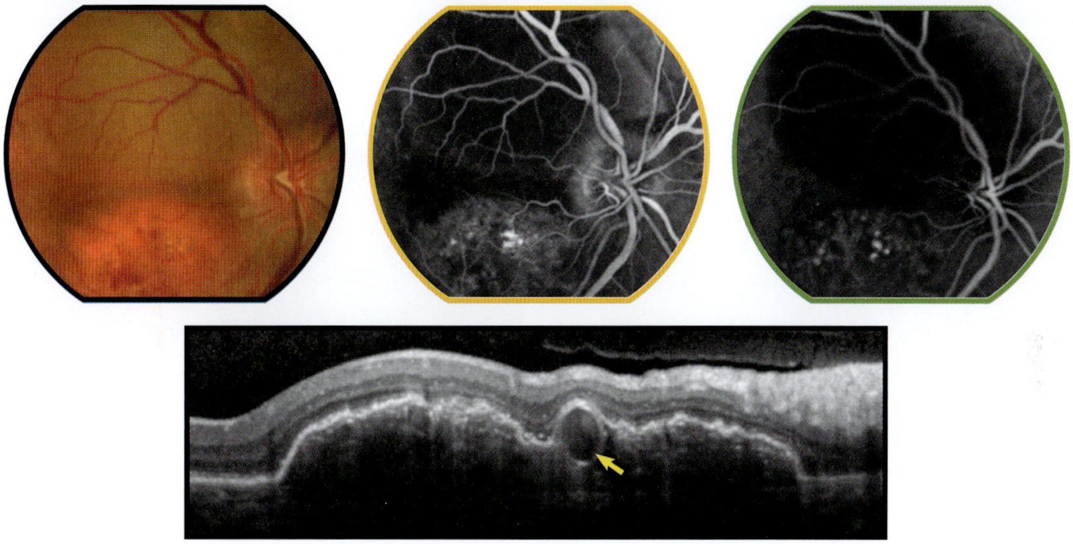

This patient has an orange-red lesion on the color fundus photograph associated with subretinal hemorrhage and a serous PED. The fluorescein angiogram shows hyperfluorescence in the area of a type 1 neovascular membrane and a well-defined serous PED above it. The ICG angiogram shows discrete hyperfluorescent polyps within the type 1 neovascular tissue and a separate hypofluorescent area corresponding to adjacent serous PED. Spectral-domain OCT reveals heterogeneous reflective patterns within the vascularized PED. A well-defined ovoid lesion *(arrow)* is a cross-sectional view of one of the polyps. The polyps are typically found just beneath the RPE within a type 1 lesion above the Bruch membrane and not in the choroid below.

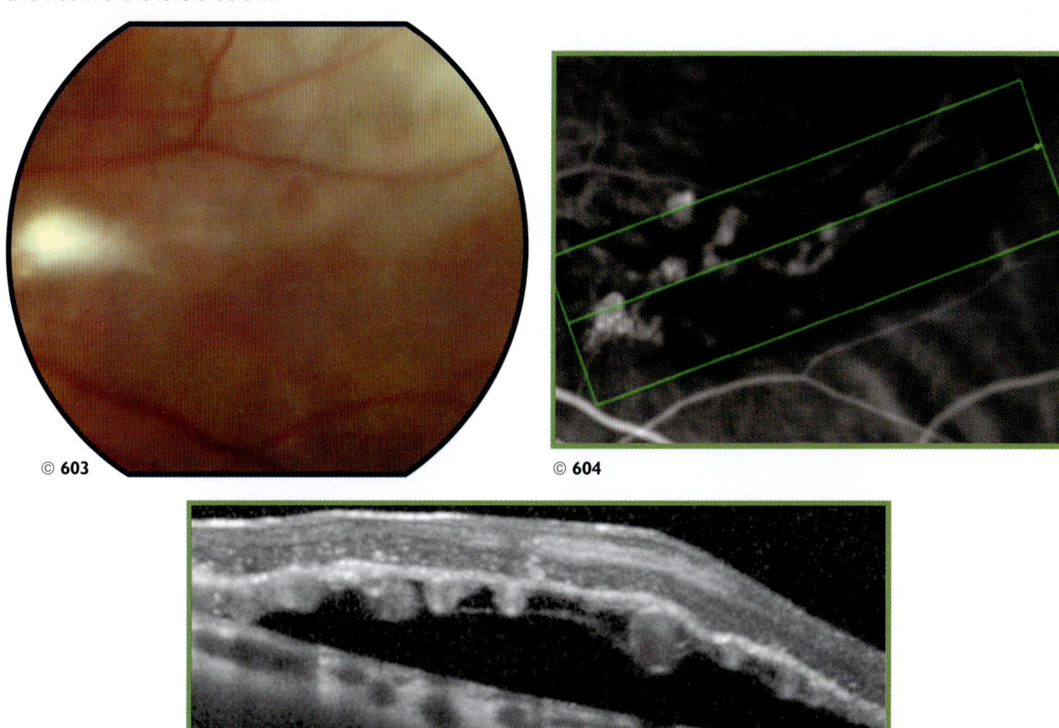

Polypoidal lesions that appear as a string of orange-red lesions on color fundus photography may correspond to a branching vascular network that is best seen on ICG angiography. The polypoidal lesions may be adherent to the undersurface of the RPE and form a "string of pearls" appearance on SD-OCT imaging.

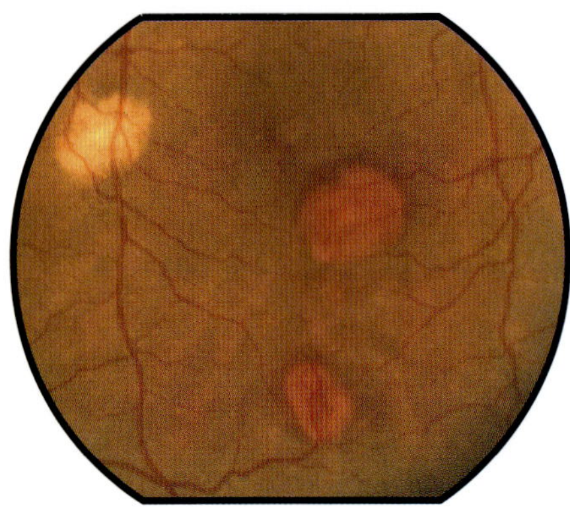

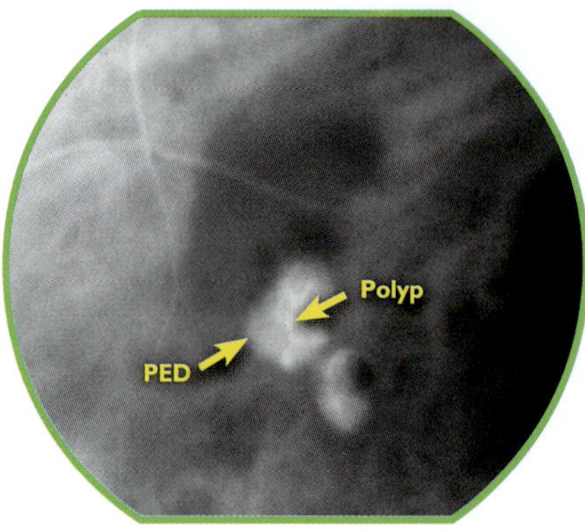

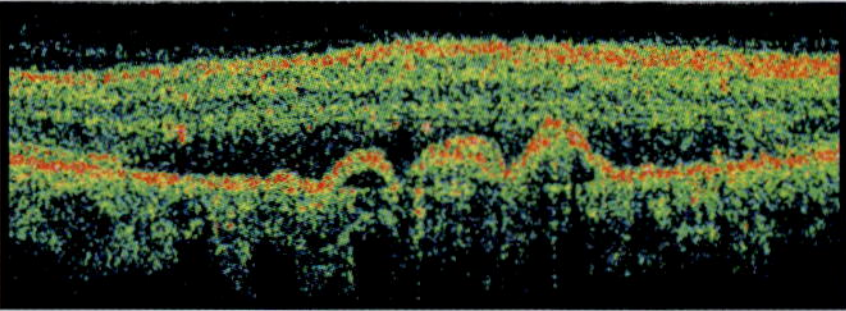

Polypoidal lesions may appear as orange PEDs *(left image)*; however, ICG angiography will reveal the polypoidal vascular abnormality beneath the RPE, which may stain due to leakage *(middle image)*. OCT shows multiple humpback elevations of the PED and reflectance beneath it from the vascular elements *(right image)*.

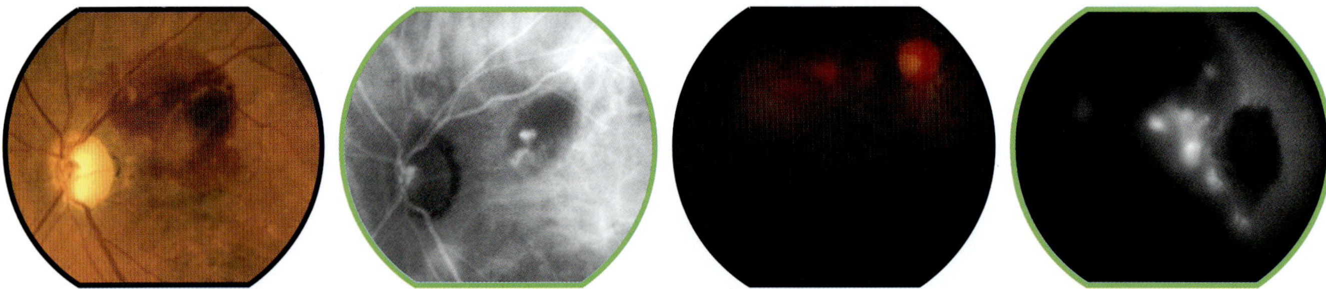

Polypoidal lesions may not be evident clinically, because they may be masked by overlying serosanguineous complications. On color photography, severe subretinal and/or vitreous hemorrhages *(third image from left)* may obscure the nature of the vascular abnormality, but the cluster of peripapillary PCV is often demonstrated well on ICG angiography *(right image)*.

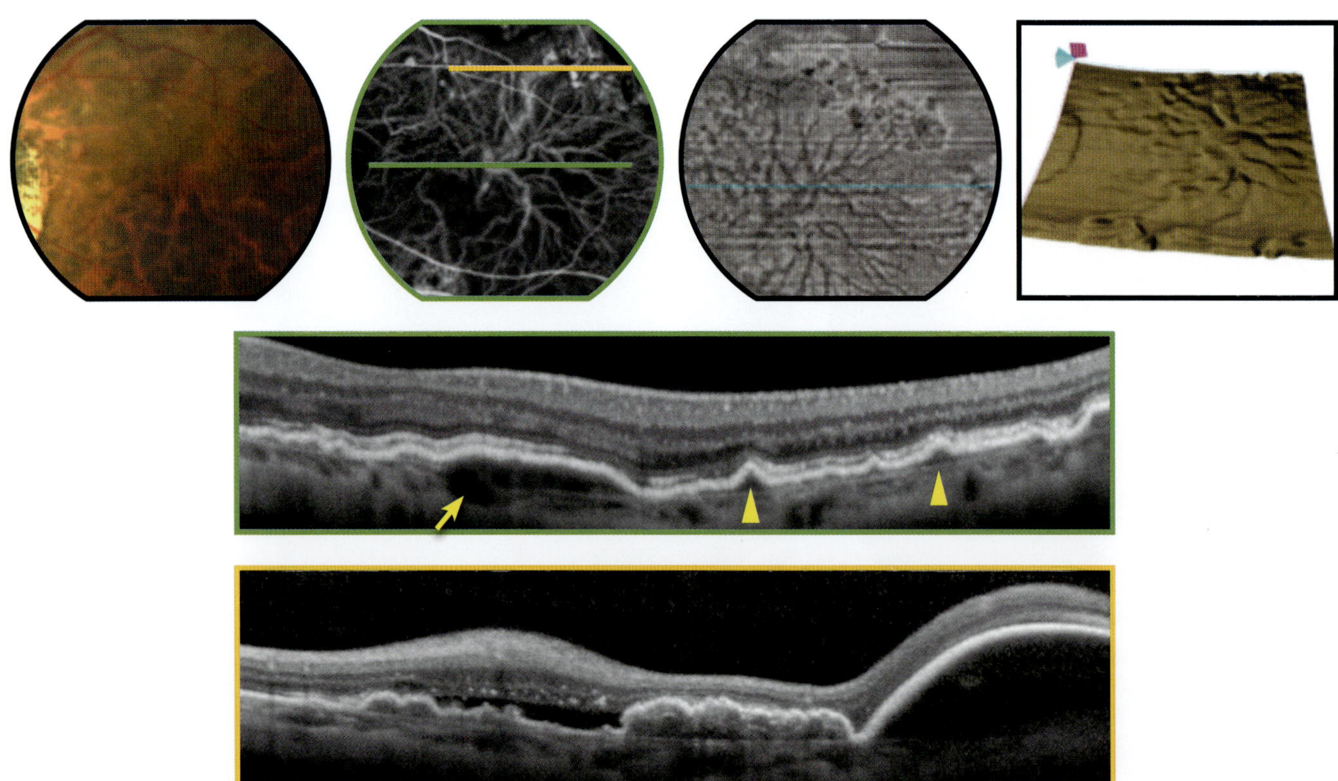

The color fundus photograph and ICG angiogram show a large neovascular network in the central macula that connects to a cluster of polypoidal lesions superotemporally. SD-OCT demonstrates a branching vascular network that lies entirely above the Bruch membrane *(arrow)* causing multiple elevations of the RPE, the so-called double-layer sign *(arrowheads)*. SD-OCT through the polypoidal lesion shows humpback elevations of the RPE with heterogeneous reflectance beneath it from the polypoidal vascular elements.

Natural Course

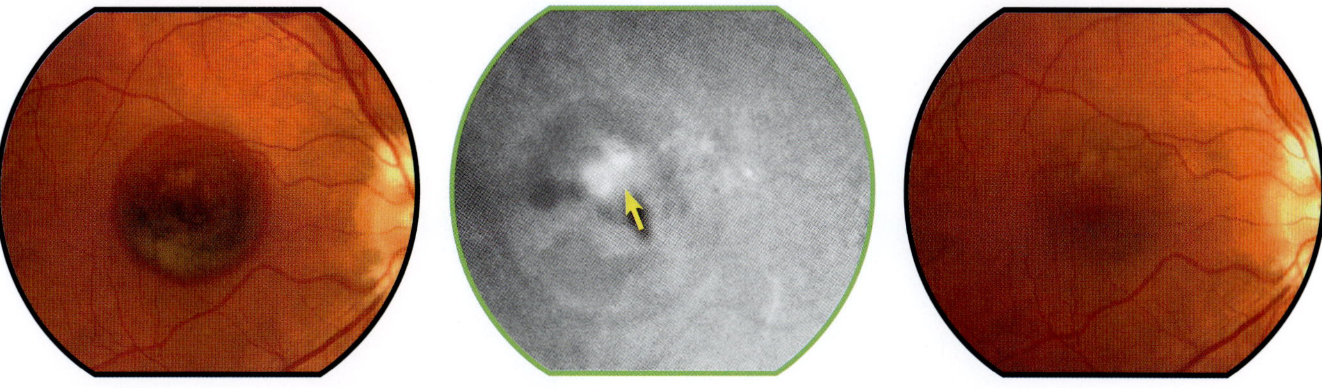

The natural course of polypoidal NV is highly variable. This young adult female Caucasian patient experienced bleeding in the central macula *(left image)*. The ICG image shows leaking polypoidal lesions *(arrow)* in conjunction with hypofluorescence from blood. Following several weeks of observation, there was complete clearing of the subretinal hemorrhage *(right image)*.

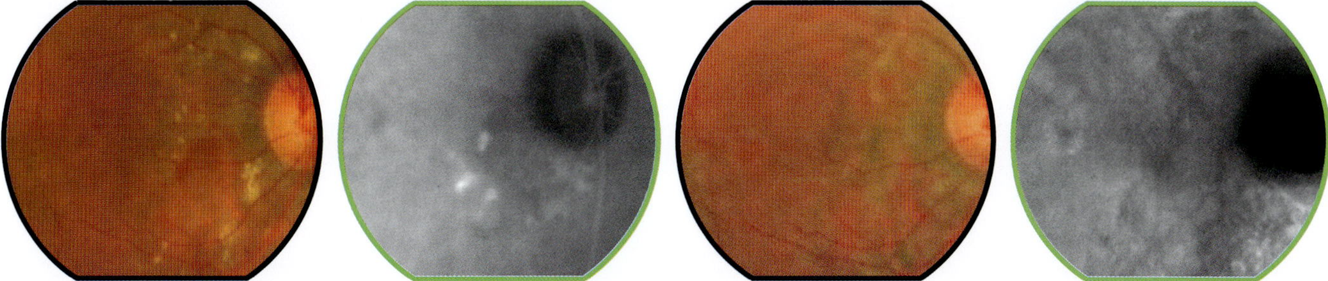

This patient had a cluster of small polypoidal lesions near the optic nerve *(left two images)*. After 5 months of observation, the serosanguineous complications resolved *(right two images)* and there was virtually no evidence of the pre-existing polypoidal abnormalities. Autoinfarction of the lesion is believed to be part of the natural course of polypoidal NV in a small percentage of patients.

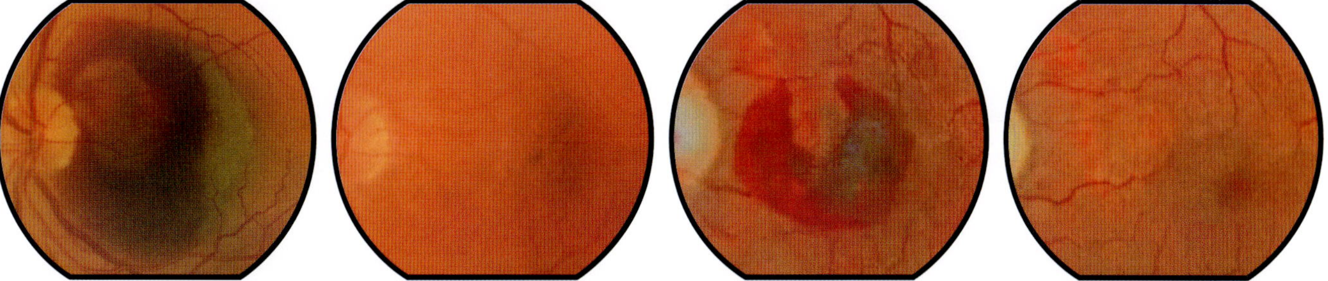

Some patients with polypoidal NV fare better than those with other forms of neovascular AMD. These two patients presented with subretinal hemorrhage that entered into the subfoveal area and threatened the fovea. After several months, the bleeding cleared spontaneously. (Presenting and final images for patient 1 are shown as the left two images and that for patient 2 are shown as the right two images.)

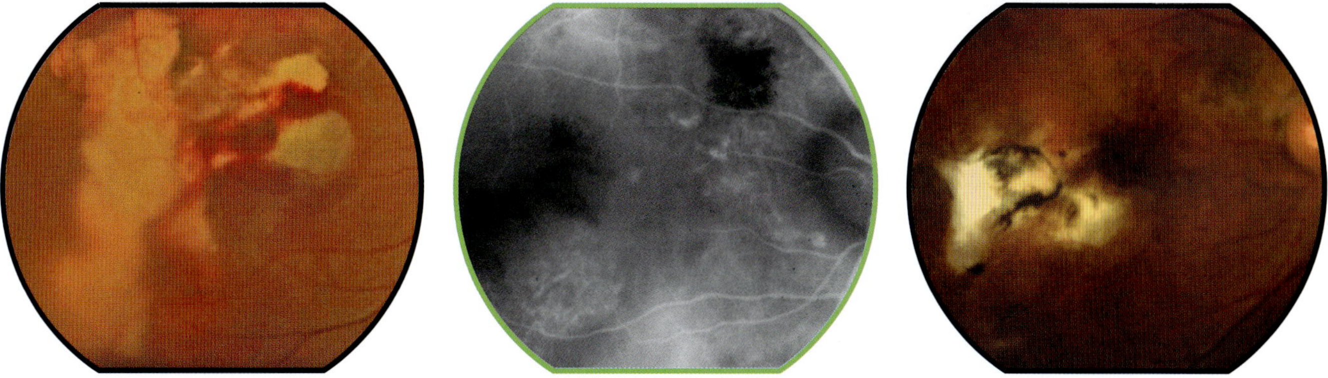

This African-American patient had polypoidal NV with active components in the papillomacular bundle. The vascular abnormality was larger than expected when imaged with ICG angiography. She experienced resolution of the serosanguineous detachment over a period of 14 months. There is residual scarring in the macula, most of which preceded the recent bleeding.

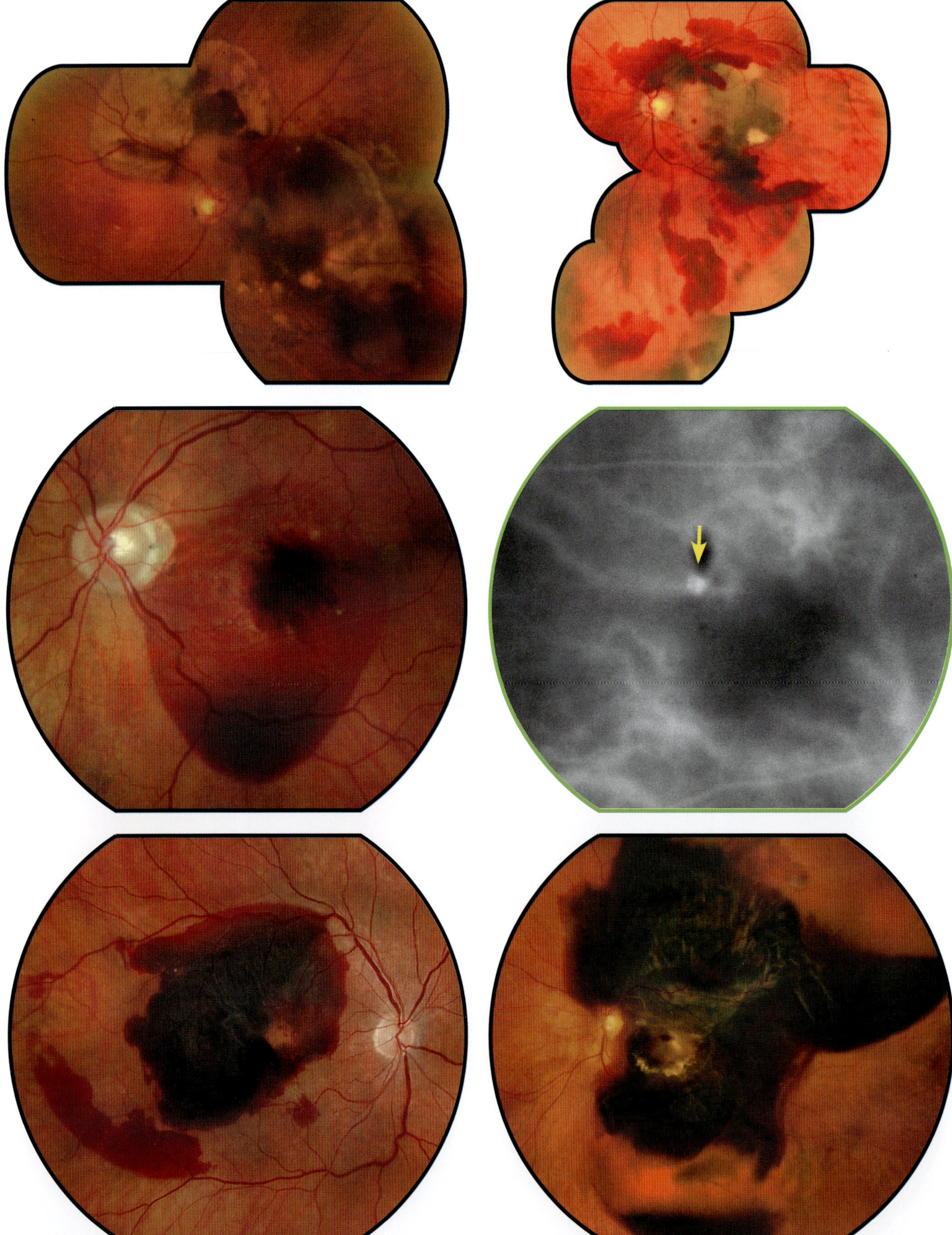

These adult Caucasian male patients have large hemorrhagic detachments secondary to polypoidal NV. Note the gravitating hemorrhage *(top right)* in the posterior pole. The fellow eye had a similar event *(top left)*, except there was sparing of the central macula. The middle photographs show a large central hemorrhage from what appears to be a singular polypoidal lesion *(arrow)*. This is not uncommon in patients who are taking anticoagulants or who have severe systemic hypertension. The two bottom images represent severe hemorrhagic detachments in Caucasian patients without associated soft drusen. Patients with polypoidal NV may present without drusen in either eye, unlike typical type 1 or type 2 neovascularization in AMD.

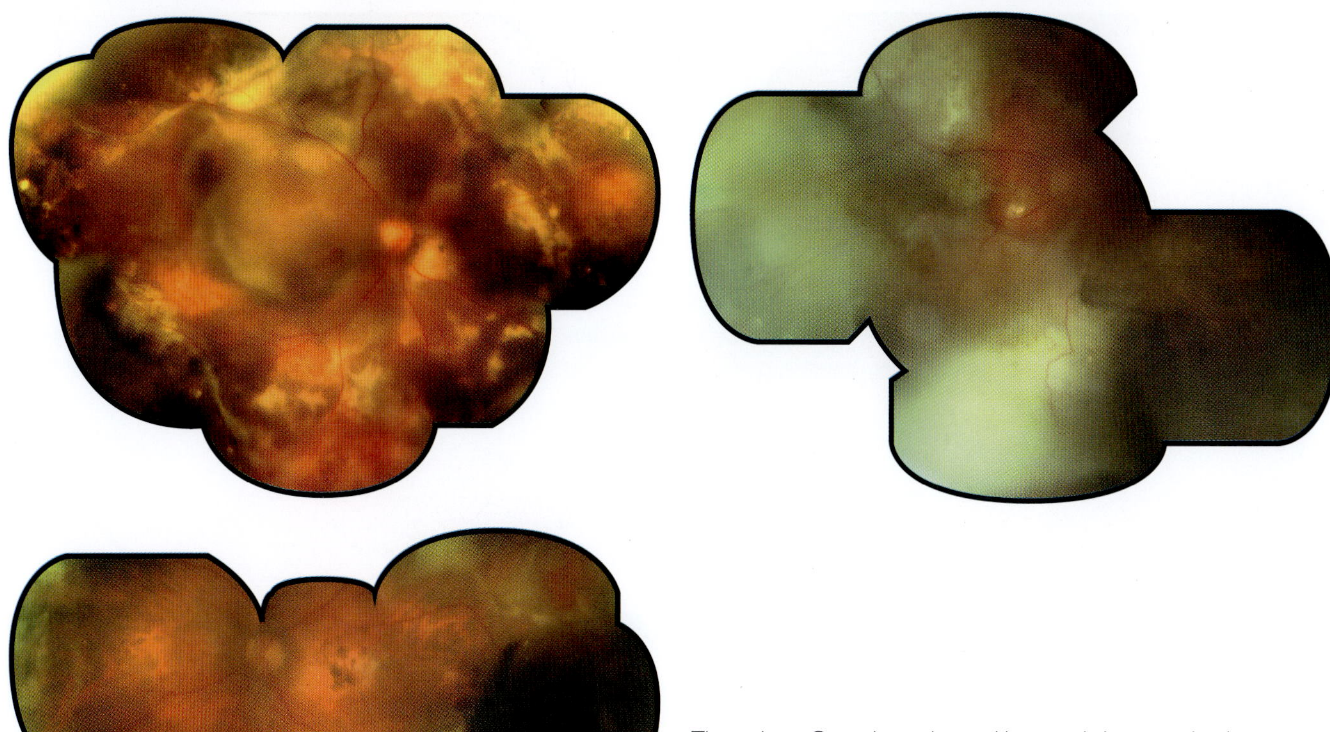

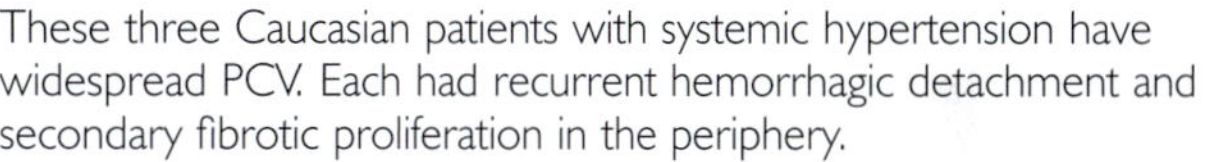

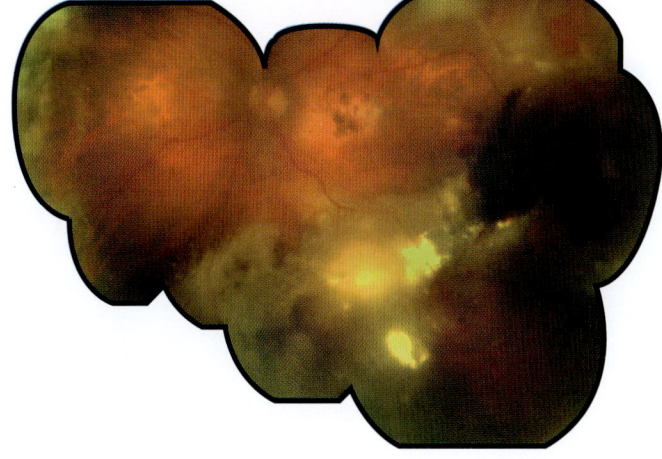

These three Caucasian patients with systemic hypertension have widespread PCV. Each had recurrent hemorrhagic detachment and secondary fibrotic proliferation in the periphery.

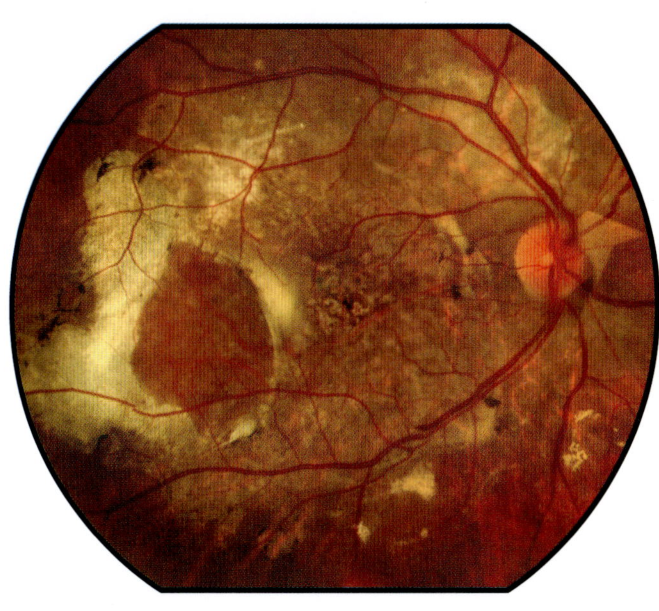

Long-standing, diffuse PCV may result in widespread atrophy, pigment degeneration, fibrosis, and disciform scarring. At this stage of PCV, the disciform scarring seen is indistinguishable from any other form of neovascularization.

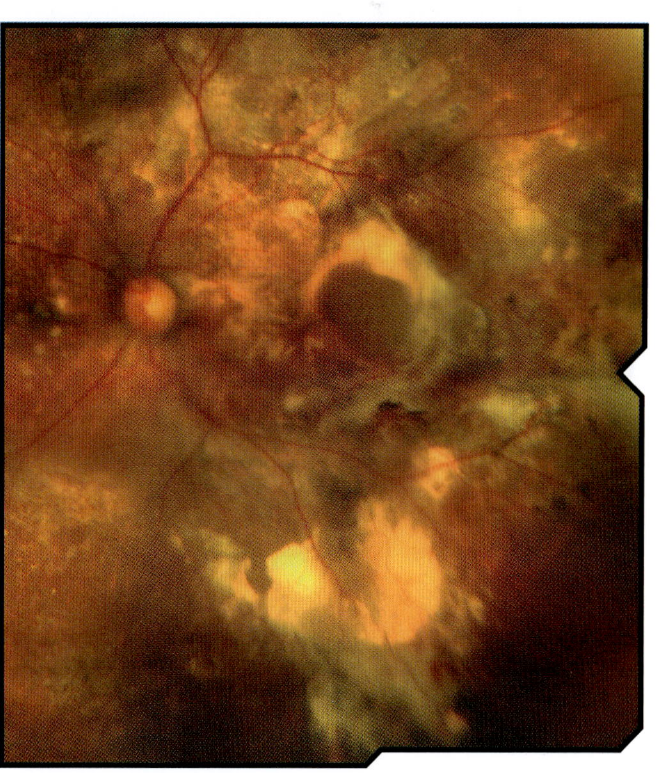

Global detachments have occurred in PCV, leading to rubeosis iridis and requiring enucleation. Note the widespread scarring in this patient.

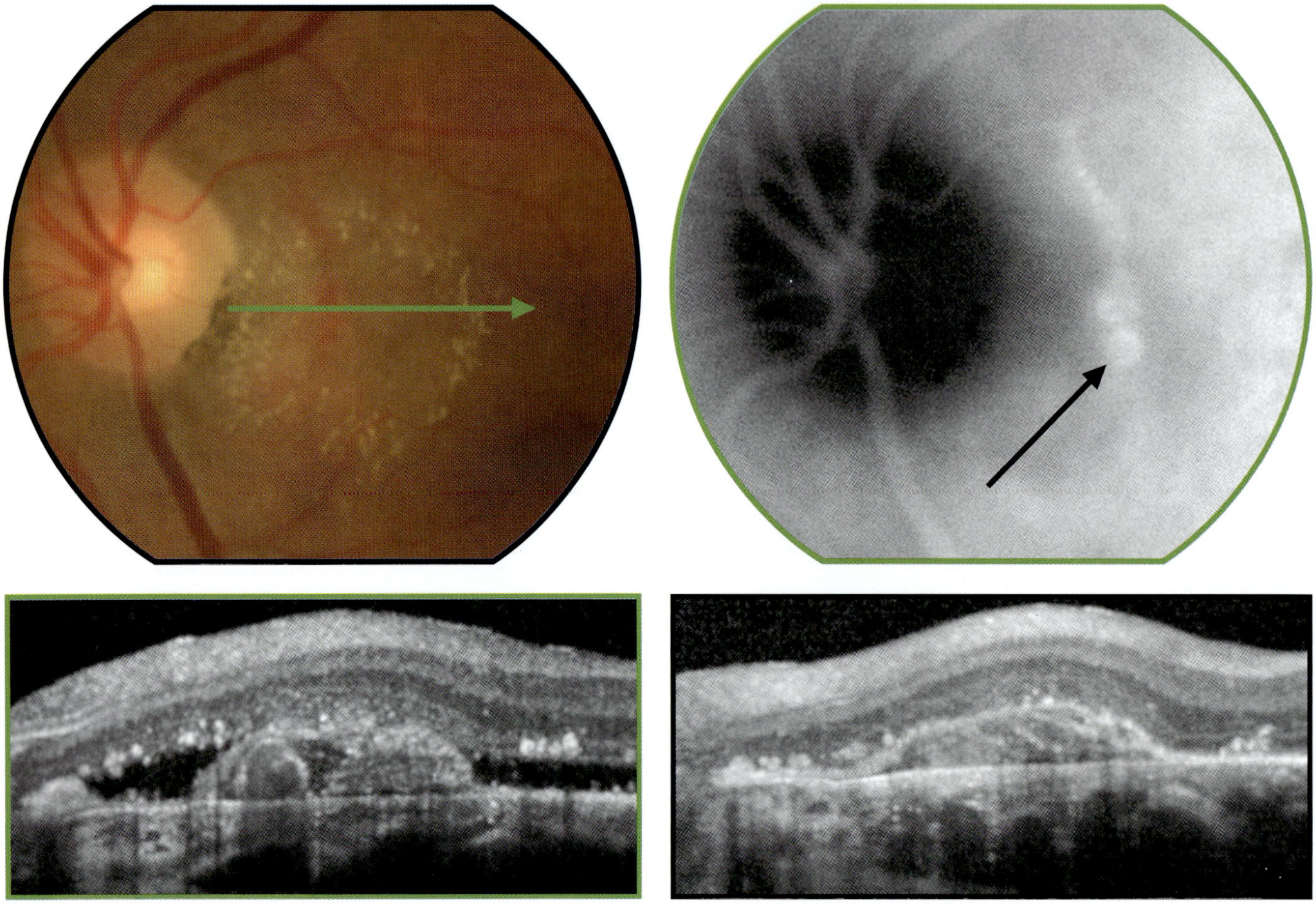

This patient with PCV had orange-red lesions with a circinate ring of lipid exudation on color fundus photography and hyperfluorescent polypoidal lesions on ICG angiography *(black arrow)*. SD-OCT imaging shows a circular polypoidal element within the sub-RPE neovascular complex and multiple intraretinal hyper-reflective foci corresponding to lipid exudation *(bottom left image)*. Light thermal laser photocoagulation was performed under ICG guidance. After treatment, there was regression of polypoidal elements, as demonstrated by SD-OCT imaging *(bottom right image)*.

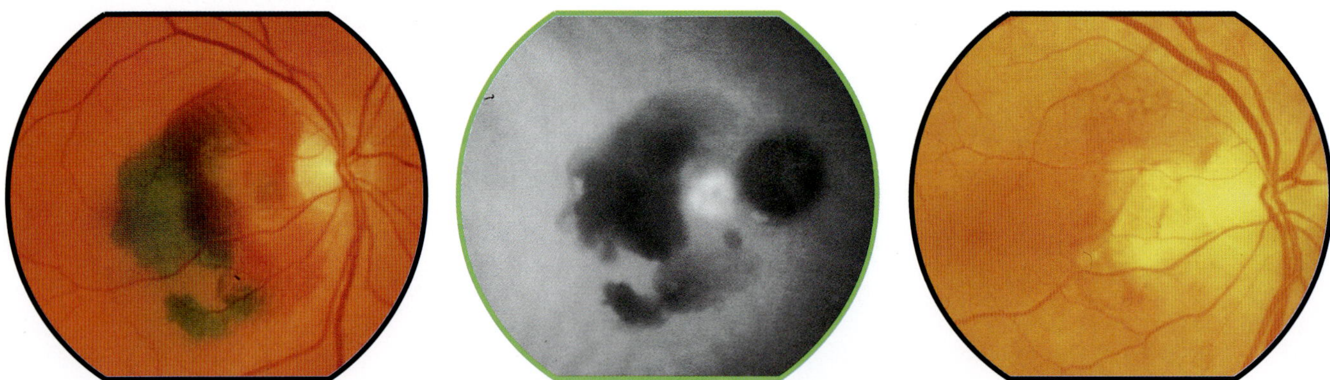

This patient had subretinal hemorrhage involving the fovea with an acute drop in vision to 20/200. The ICG angiogram shows a focal, well-defined lesion. This area was photocoagulated using ICG guidance with resolution of the subretinal hemorrhage and neovascularization. This resulted in a dramatic improvement in visual acuity to 20/30.

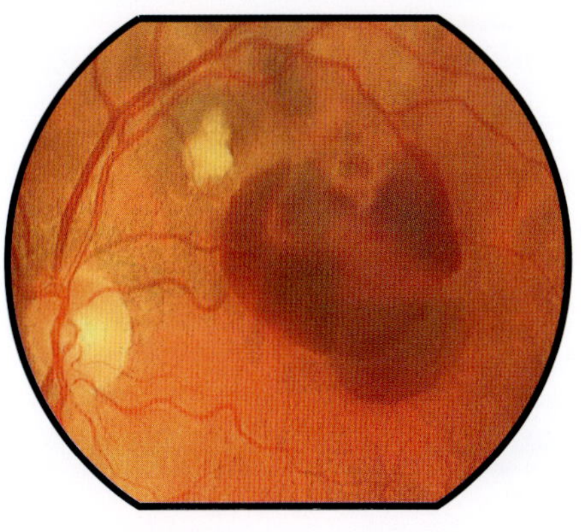
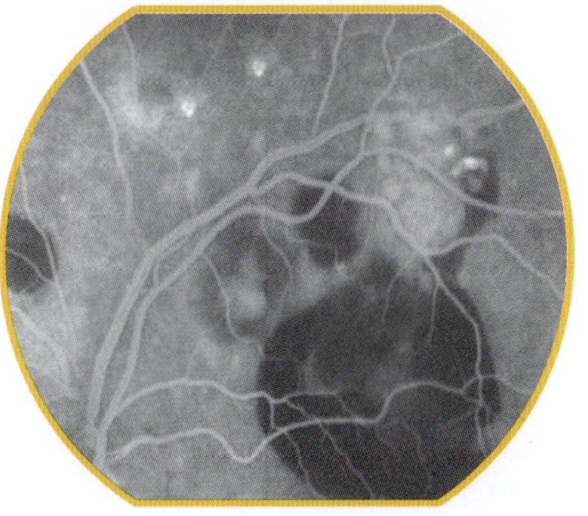
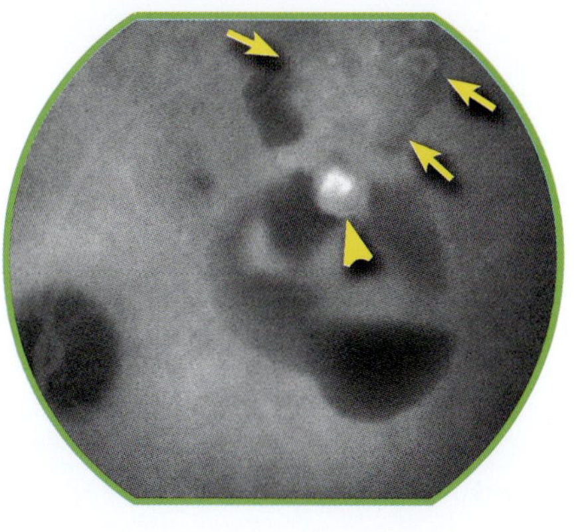

This patient experienced a hemorrhagic detachment. There was a PED that was not imaged clearly with fluorescein angiography *(middle)*. Multiple hyperfluorescent spots were indicative of polypoidal NV. The ICG angiogram showed a distinct active polypoidal lesion *(arrowhead)*. A more widespread polypoidal abnormality was evident superior to the active polypoidal component *(arrows)*.

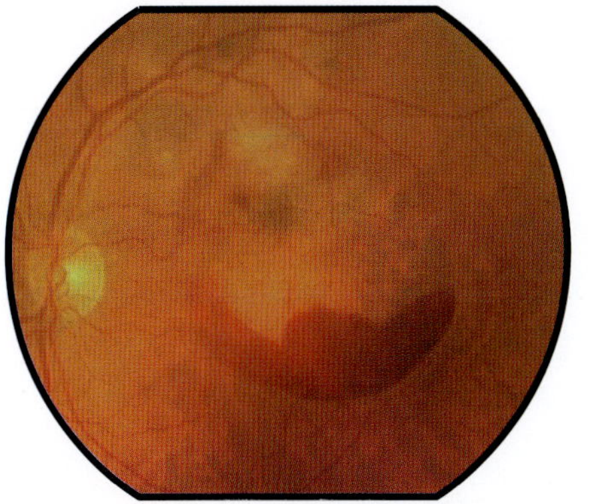
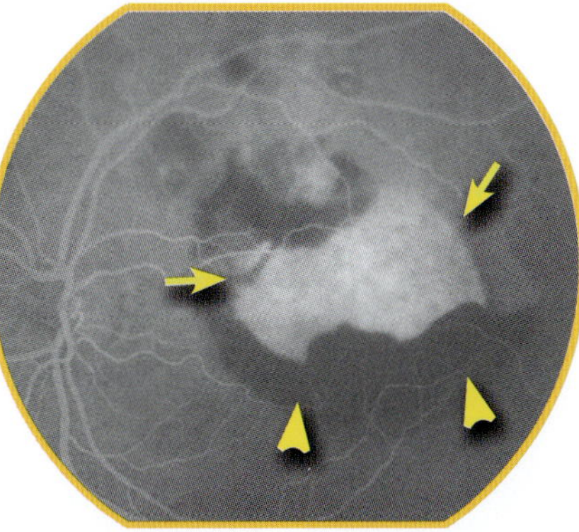
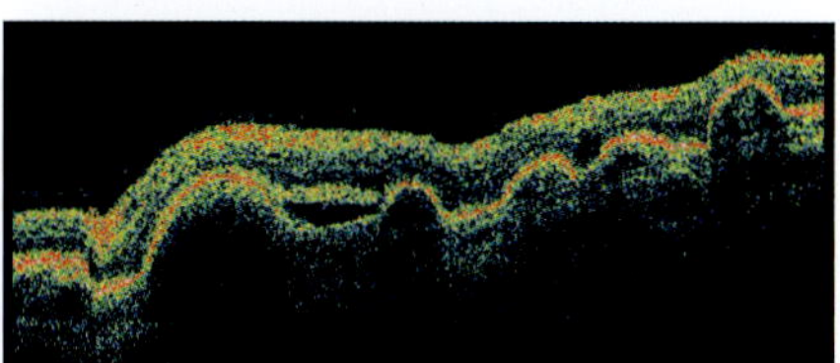
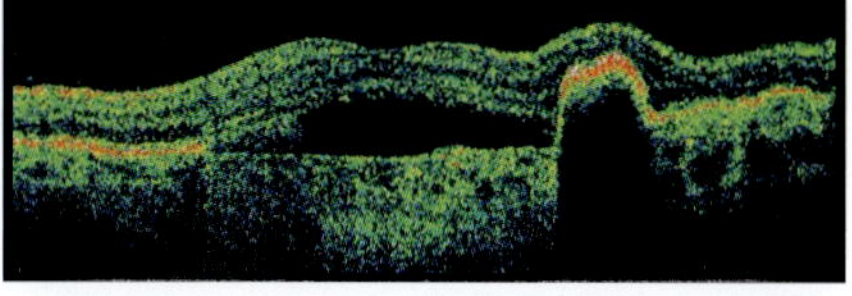

Thermal laser treatment was carried out on the active polypoidal lesion. The patient had resolution of the PED, but 3 months later, he experienced a large pigment epithelial tear *(arrows)* with hemorrhage *(arrowheads)*. The fluorescein angiogram demonstrated the denuded pigment epithelium, which was consolidating and contracting superiorly in the direction of the PCV abnormality. The pre-treatment OCT *(top right image)* showed multiple humpback PEDs and a shallow neurosensory detachment, consistent with PCV. The post-treatment OCT *(bottom right image)* showed a discontinuity in the pigment epithelium beneath a neurosensory detachment; a vertical, marginal elevation to the pigment epithelium characteristic of a pigment epithelial tear; and consolidation of the PCV.

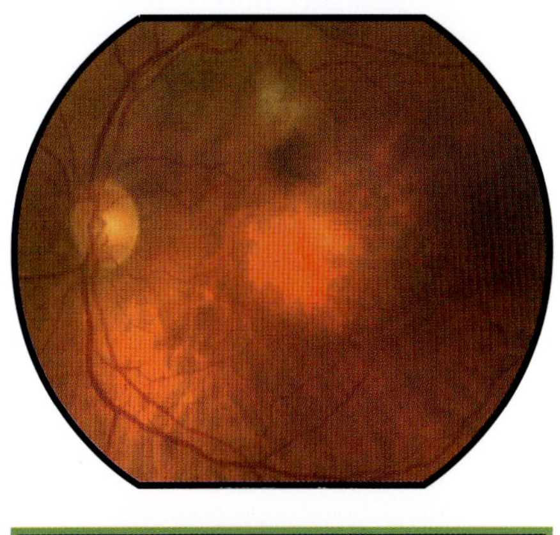
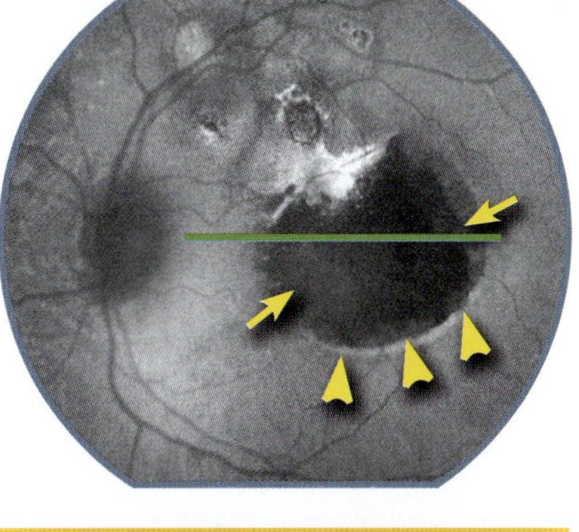
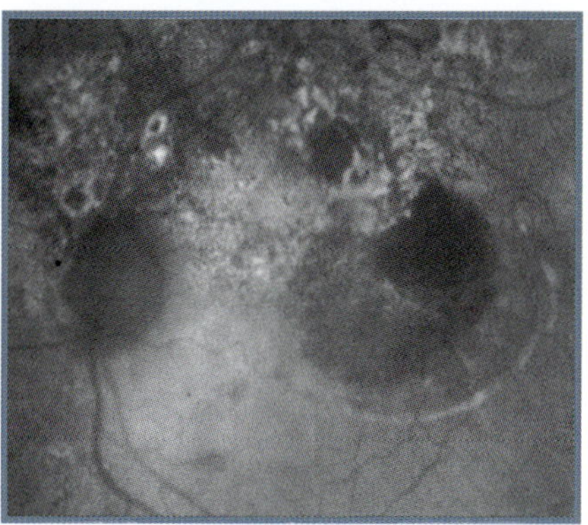
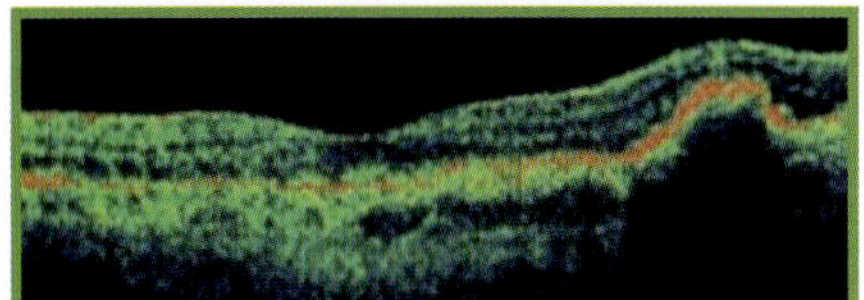
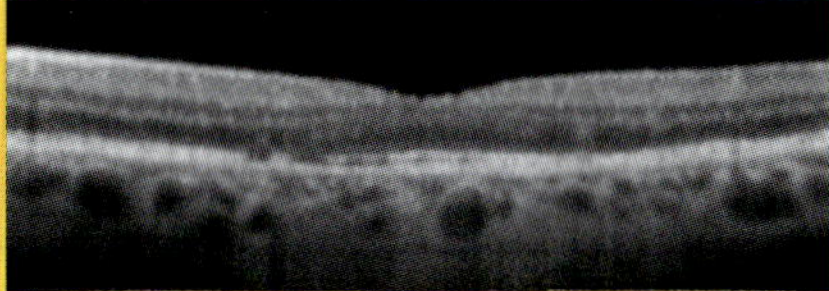

Six months later, the regenerated epithelium was devoid of pigment and showed a relatively pale central macula. However, the visual acuity returned to 20/30. Fundus autofluorescence at 6 months *(top middle image)* delineated the absence of the pigment epithelium, which was now devoid of lipofuscin and appeared hypoautofluorescent. There was consolidation of the choroidal vascular abnormalities superiorly with fundus hyperautofluorescence at the margin of the pigment epithelium *(arrows)*.The edge of the rip showed an annulus of fundus hyperautofluorescence most likely due to a coiled reduplication or fold of the tear *(arrowheads)*. The OCT at 6 months *(bottom left image)* showed reflectance, representing reconstitution of the pigment epithelium. Fundus autofluorescence and OCT 6 years later *(top and bottom right images)* shows resurfacing and reconstitution of the RPE. *All images courtesy of Dr. John Sorenson*

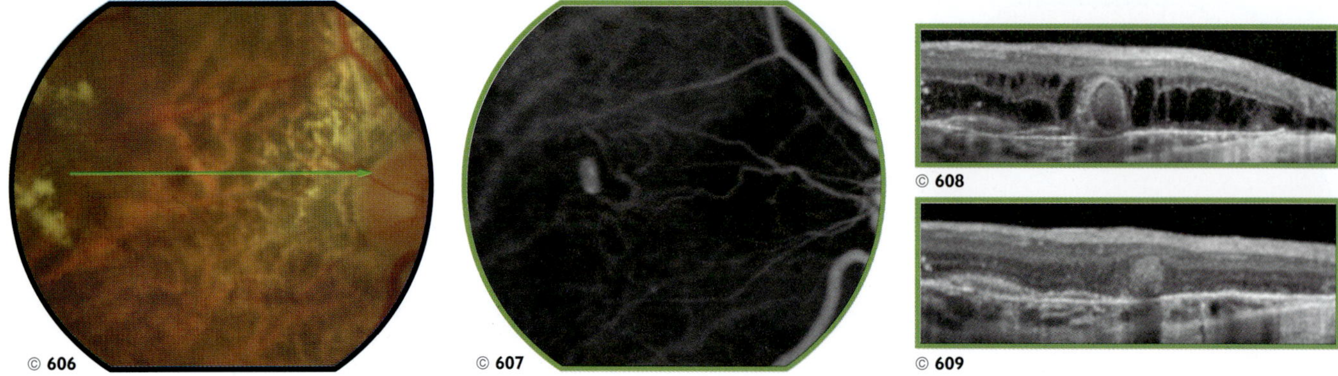

This patient with PCV received verteporfin photodynamic therapy (PDT). SD-OCT shows an ovoid polypoidal structure before treatment *(top right image)* that has regressed and consolidated after treatment *(bottom right image)*. Recently, there have been studies that demonstrate benefits of using adjunctive intravitreal anti-VEGF therapy before the use of PDT in hopes of decreasing the upregulation of vascular endothelial growth factor that occurs following PDT.

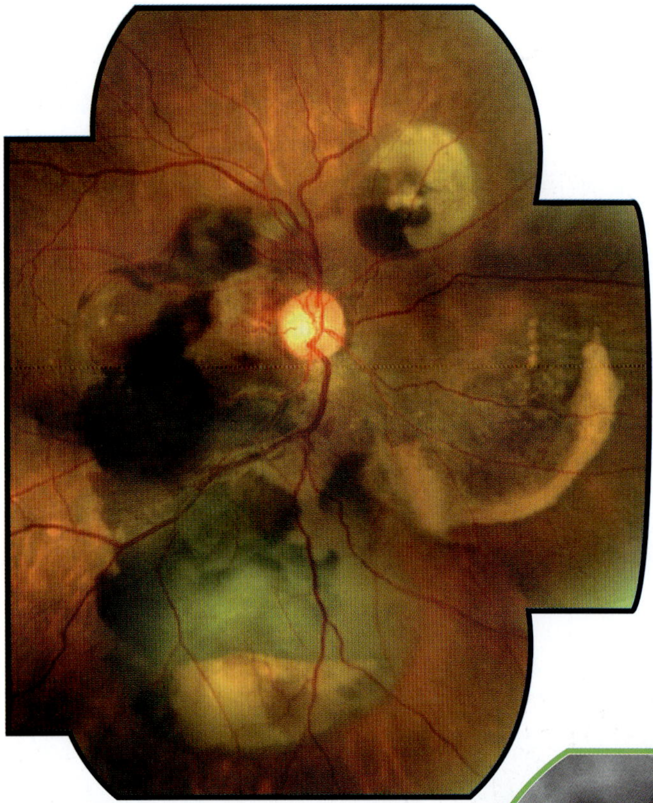

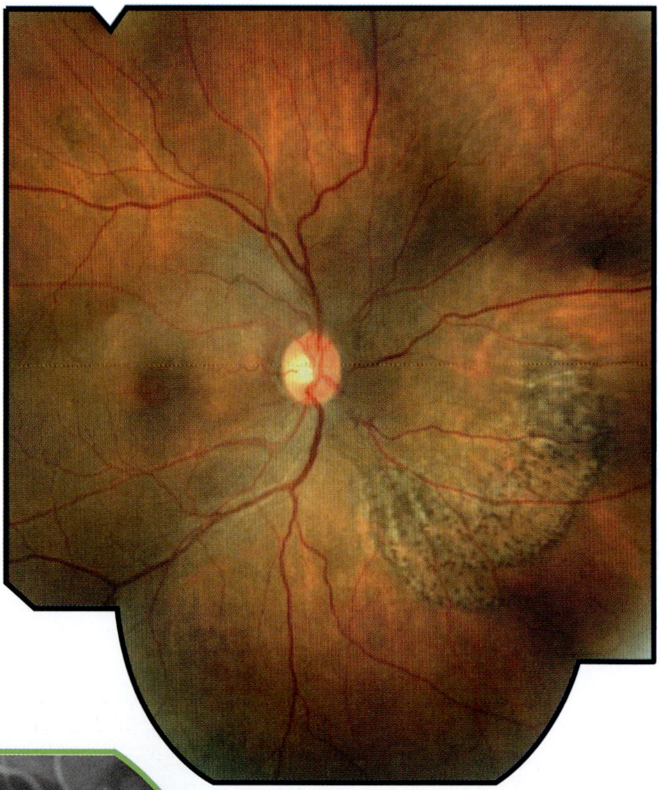

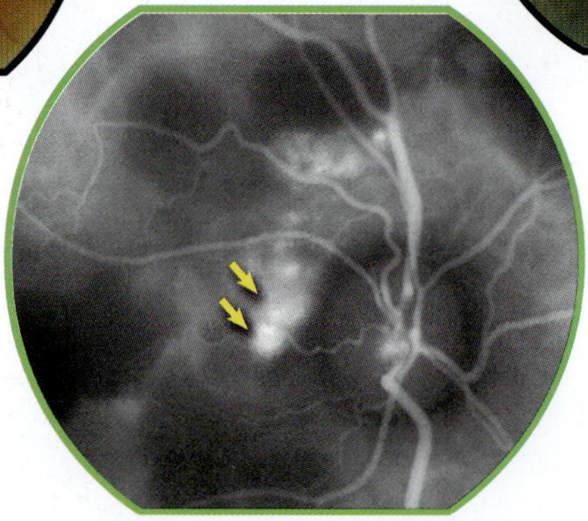

This patient had a massive hemorrhagic detachment from polypoidal NV. The ICG angiogram shows polypoidal lesions near the disc *(arrows)*. Photodynamic therapy was carried out to the active leaking and bleeding polypoidal lesions. Four months later, there was complete resolution of the blood *(right image)*. Only a legacy of pigment epithelial hyperplasia and atrophy from the antecedent blood was evident.

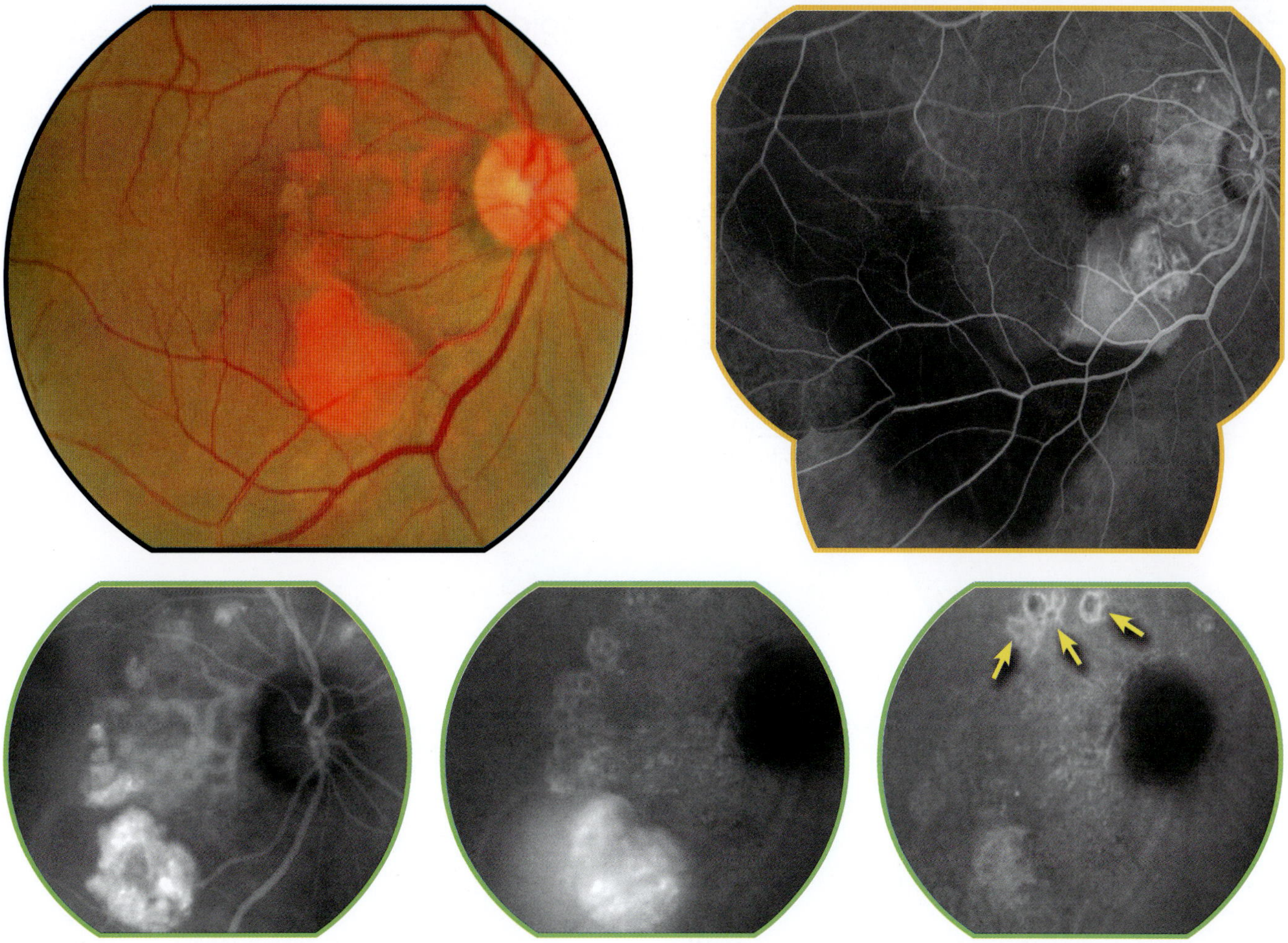

This African-American patient had a huge polypoidal choroidal vascular abnormality in the papillomacular bundle and peripapillary region of the right eye. The fluorescein angiogram documented leakage and bleeding that encircled the posterior pole. The ICG study showed the polypoidal lesion plus a cluster of polyps in the subpigment epithelial space *(bottom left image)*. In the late stage of the angiogram, the polyps leaked beneath the detached pigment epithelium *(bottom center image)*. Over a period of 18 months, the neovascularization regressed and only small inactive polypoidal components were evident superiorly *(arrows)*. The remaining branching vascular network has regressed and is only barely evident in the late stage angiogram *(bottom right image)*.

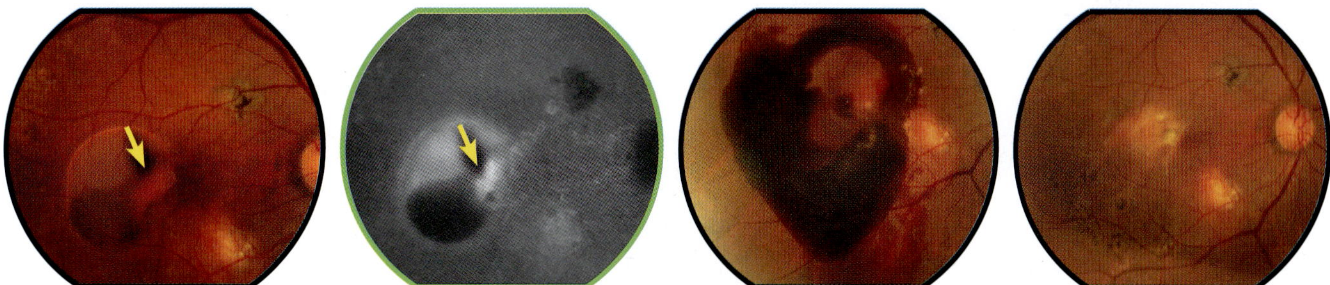

Several years later, the patient experienced recurrent active polypoidal neovascularization near the fovea. Note the leaking and bleeding polypoidal lesions *(arrows)*. He was initially observed without treatment, but 2 months later he experienced a severe hemorrhage. The active polypoidal lesions were then treated with photodynamic therapy, resulting in total clearing of the blood and exudate with recovery of vision. *Images courtesy of Dr. Richard Spaide*

Polypoidal Choroidal Vasculopathy and Polypoidal Neovascularization

New anatomical information concerning the choroid derived from state-of-the-art OCT devices has allowed refinement of the PCV phenotype. PCV was a term that was originally used to define any neovascular lesion that demonstrated polypoidal morphological changes; however, there is increasing evidence to suggest that PCV is a distinct entity that occurs in the setting of pachychoroid. PCV, central serous chorioretinopathy, and pachychoroid pigment epitheliopathy are frequently associated with the pachychoroid phenotype and it is thought that these conditions represent a continuum of the same pathologic process. In contrast to PCV, polypoidal neovascularization is a new term that is being used to define neovascular lesions that demonstrate polypoidal morphological changes without pachychoroid features.

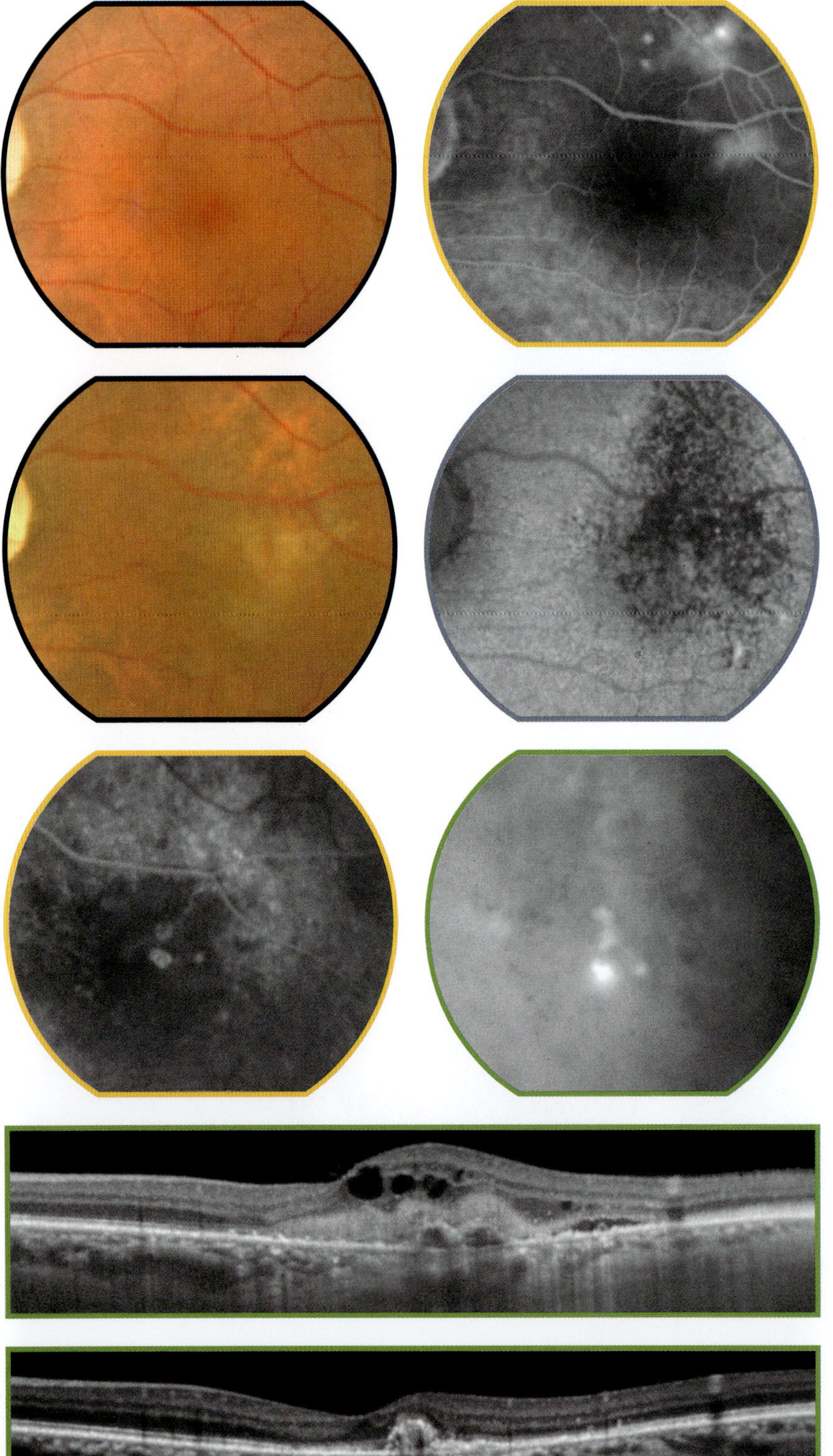

This patient had classic central serous chorioretinopathy 13 years prior with a serous detachment and multifocal areas of leakage on fluorescein angiography *(top row images)*. Thirteen years later *(second row)*, the patient developed orange circular lesions surrounded by yellow exudation consistent with neovascularization. Fundus autofluorescence imaging demonstrated granular hyperautofluorescence and hypoautofluorescence changes in areas of chronic subretinal fluid. High magnification of the fluorescein and ICG angiogram at this stage shows characteristic polypoidal lesions *(third row)*. SD-OCT imaging shows the branching vascular network with two humpback elevations of the RPE consistent with polypoidal elements. There is subretinal hyper-reflective exudation and cystoid macular edema consistent with active neovascularization. After treatment with intravitreal anti-VEGF therapy, there is resolution of the exudative changes and a remnant dome-shaped elevation of the polypoidal lesion.

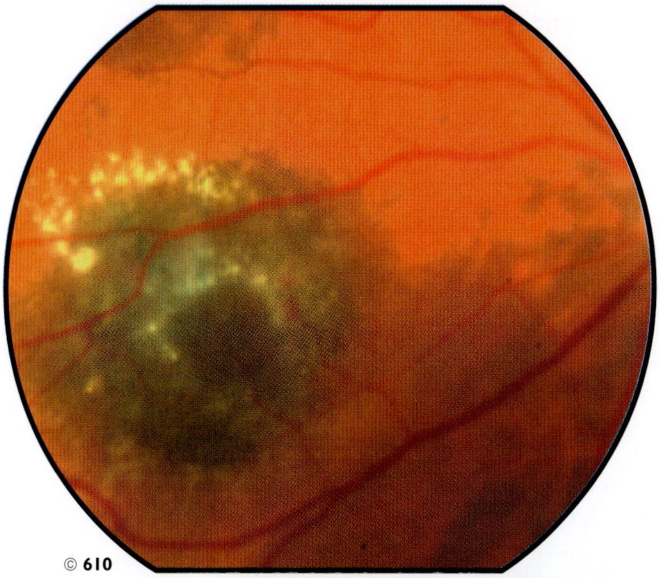

© 610

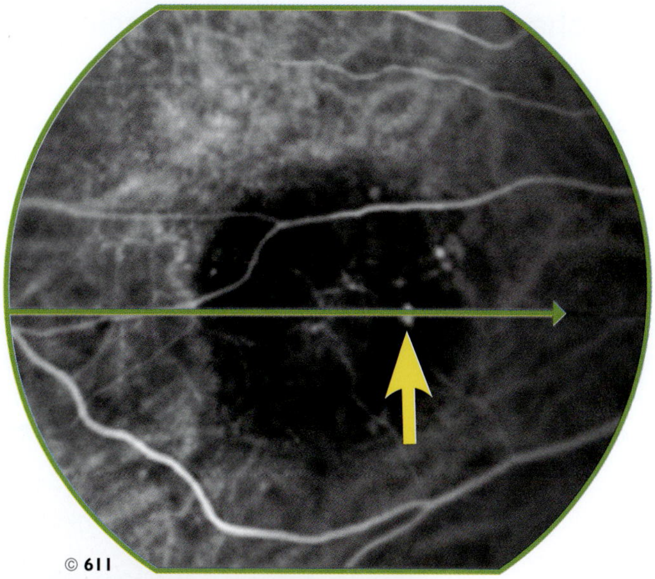

© 611

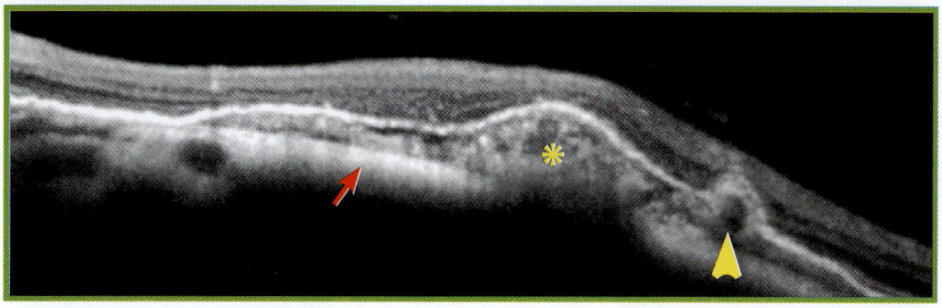

© 612

This patient has a choroidal nevus with overlying type 1 neovascularization. The ICG angiogram shows an area of blocked hypofluorescence due to a nevus and a hyperfluorescent "hot spot" consistent with a polypoidal lesion *(yellow arrow)* overlying it. SD-OCT shows the hyper-reflective border of the nevus causing shadowing of the underlying choroid and sclera *(red arrow)*, an overlying type 1 neovascular complex *(asterisk)*, and a circular polypoidal lesion elevating the RPE *(arrowhead)*. This lesion is defined as polypoidal neovascularization.

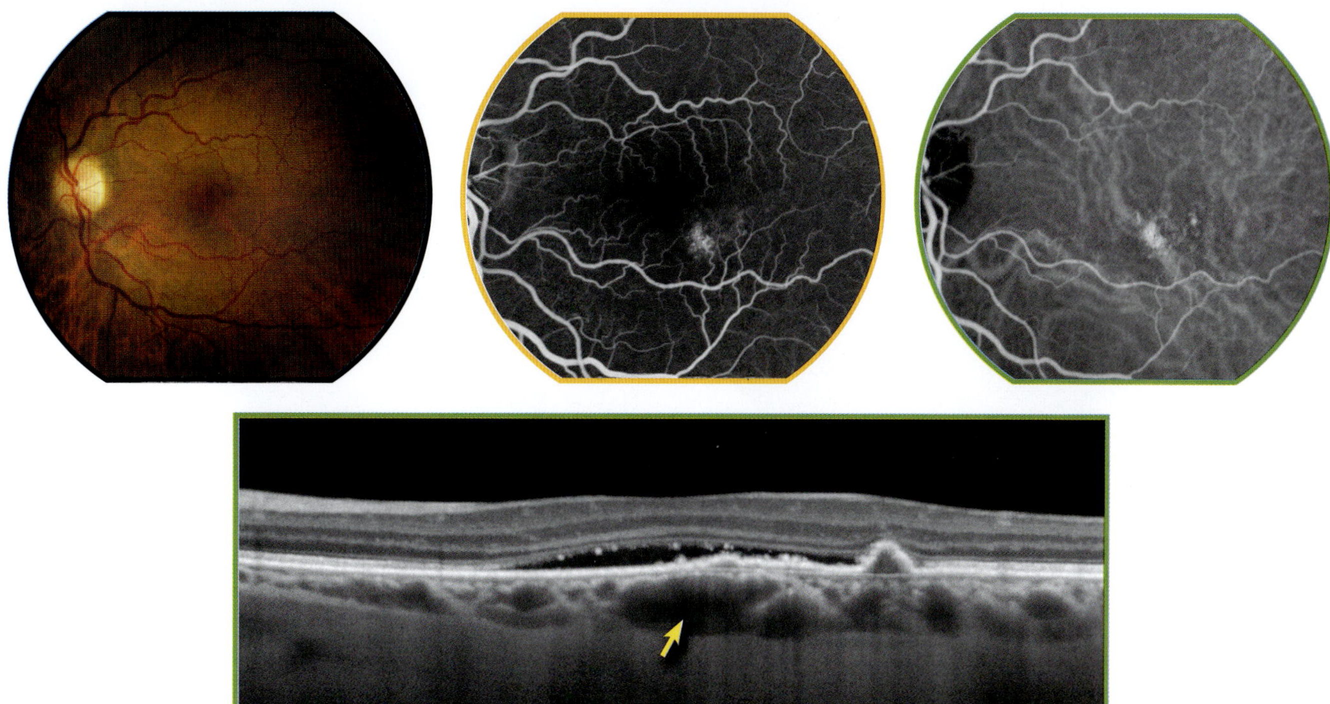

This patient has pachychoroid neovasculopathy. Color image shows a localized area of choroidal thickening in the central macula evident by reduced number of fundus tessellation. Note the lack of other degenerative changes such as drusen or myopic findings. Fluorescein angiography shows hyperfluorescent leakage consistent with neovascularization, and ICG angiography shows a hyperfluorescent "hot spot" consistent with polypoidal lesions. SD-OCT reveals localized choroidal thickening with a large dilated choroidal vessel *(arrow)* underlying the type 1 neovascular complex, which includes a dome-shaped elevation consistent with a polypoidal element. This lesion falls within the definition of PCV.

Peripheral Exudative Hemorrhagic Chorioretinopathy

Peripheral exudative hemorrhagic chorioretinopathy (PEHCR), also called extramacular or peripheral disciform disease, is a peripheral mass lesion that forms after subretinal or sub-RPE hemorrhage. Hemorrhage is almost always due to peripheral choroidal neovascularization, and the pigmented appearance of PEHCR may be confused with choroidal melanoma. Polyps are commonly identified at sites of hemorrhage in PEHCR, and there is growing evidence to suggest that PEHCR is a subgroup of polypoidal choroidal neovascularization that preferentially involves the peripheral retina. Due to involvement of peripheral retina, PEHCR typically has a favorable prognosis and can generally be observed. When hemorrhage is progressive or threatening the fovea, laser therapy, photodynamic therapy, intravitreal anti-VEGF therapy, and, rarely, surgical intervention should be considered.

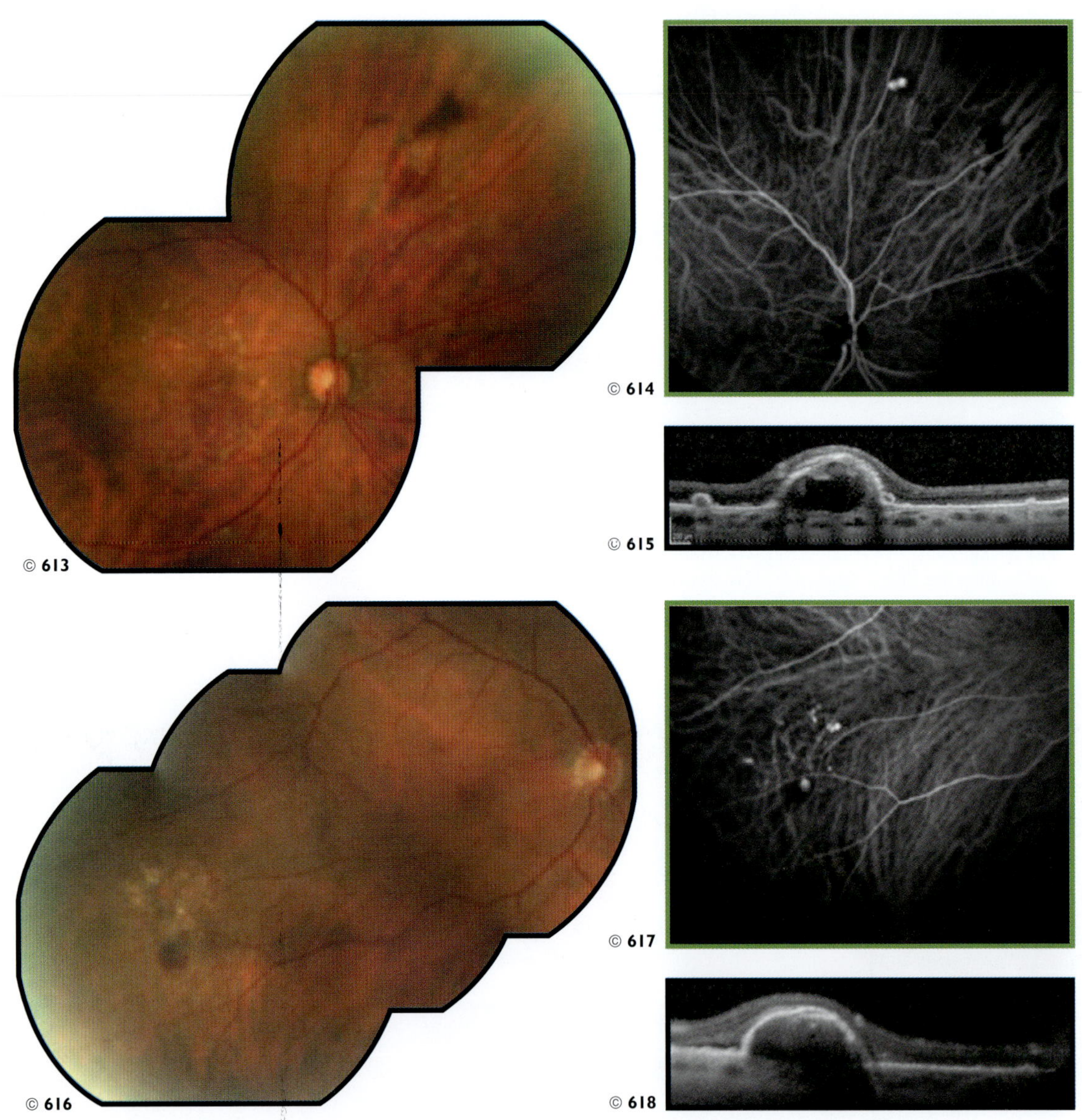

Both these patients demonstrate peripheral exudative hemorrhagic chorioretinopathy due to peripheral polypoidal lesions. On ICG angiography the polypoidal lesions appear circular and hyperfluorescent. SD-OCT imaging shows the sub-RPE neovascular complex with polypoidal elements in each case.

Type 2 Neovascularization

Type 2 neovascularization is neovascular tissue that has penetrated the RPE–Bruch membrane complex and is proliferating in the subretinal space above the RPE monolayer. It may be seen as a well-defined or "classic" early vascular pattern on fluorescein angiography with late leakage as the dye permeates the overlying retina and subretinal space. Pure type 2 neovascular lesions occur in only about 10% of newly diagnosed neovascular AMD cases, but type 2 is the most common lesion type in other maculopathies including pathological myopia, multifocal choroiditis, and pseudoxanthoma elasticum with angioid streaks.

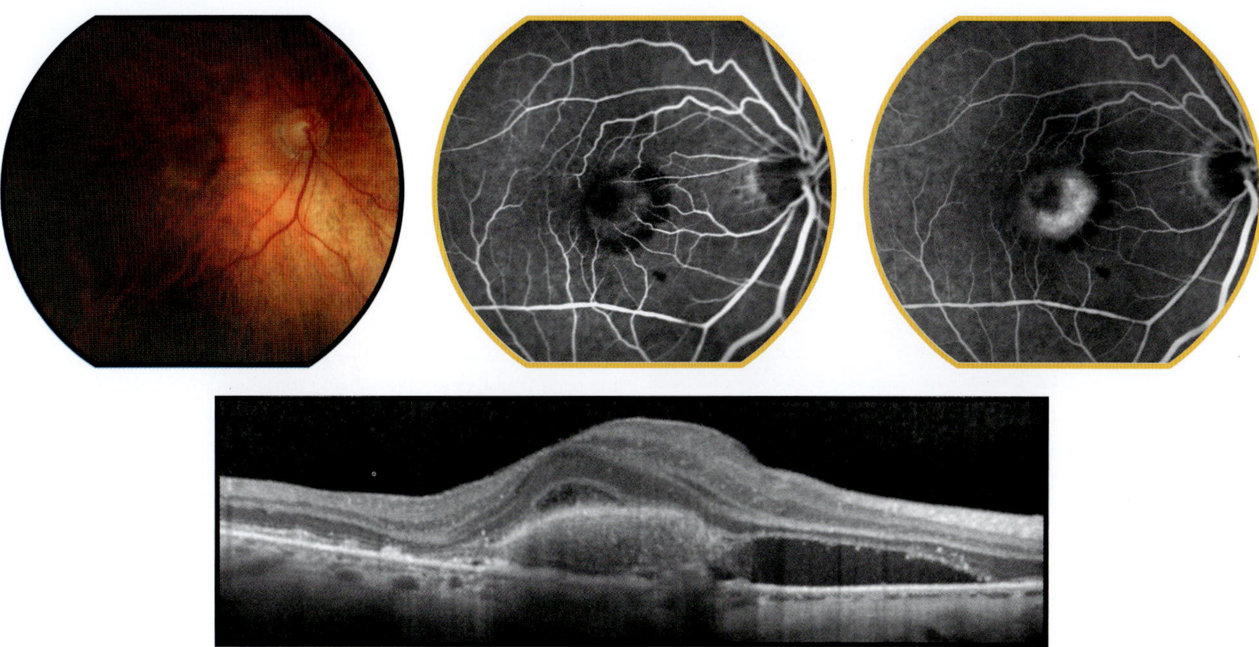

This is an example of type 2 neovascularization with subretinal hemorrhage. The fluorescein angiogram in the early phase shows a well-demarcated hyperfluorescent lesion surrounded by a ring of blocked hypofluorescence *(top middle image)*. In the late phase, there is active leakage with less distinct margins. SD-OCT shows a neovascular complex emanating through a break in the RPE and lying above the RPE with other subretinal hyper-reflective material from hemorrhage and exudation.

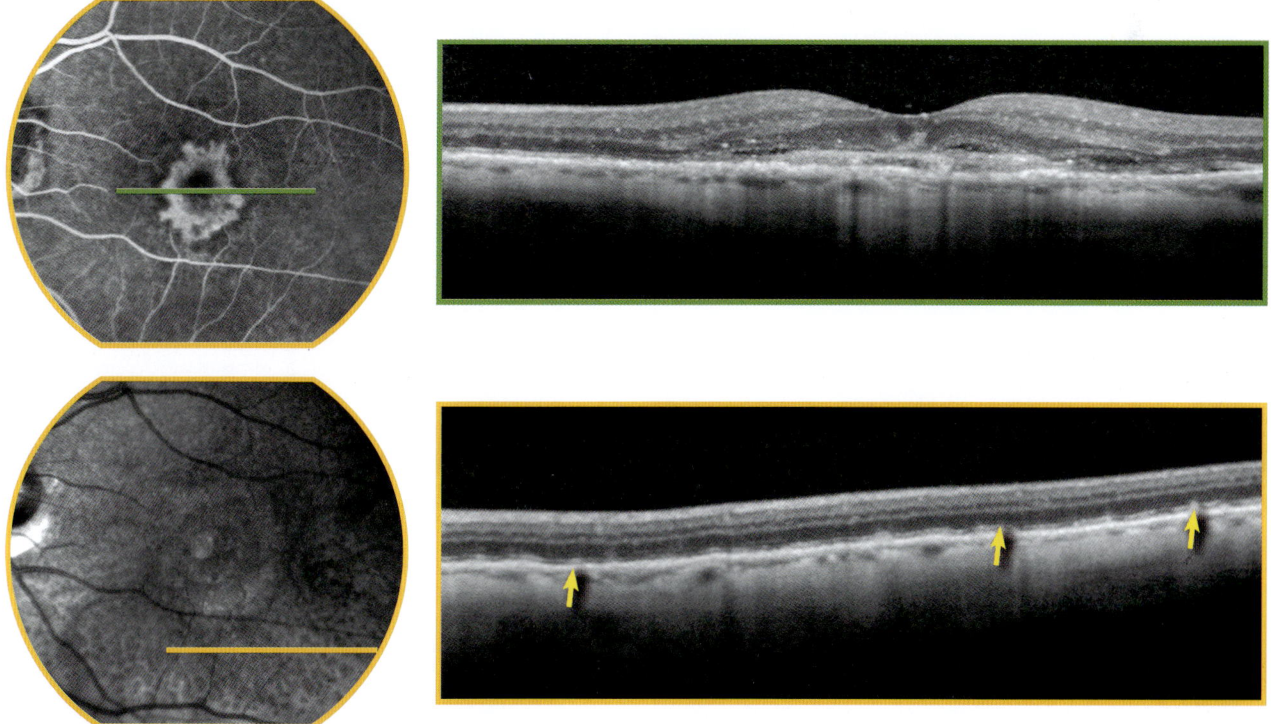

Type 2 neovascularization can occur in eyes with choroidal thinning and reticular pseudodrusen (subretinal drusenoid deposits), as shown in this patient. The reticular pseudodrusen are visualized best with near-infrared reflectance and SD-OCT imaging *(arrows)*.

Type 3 Neovascularization

Type 3 neovascularization, previously referred to as retinal angiomatous proliferation or retinal choroidal anastomosis, is intraretinal neovascularization that occurs in neovascular AMD. There remains considerable debate regarding the origins of type 3 neovascularization and whether it arises from the retinal circulation or the choroidal circulation. With the advent of SD-OCT imaging it has been shown that drusenoid PED, intraretinal pigment migration, and focal outer retinal atrophy commonly precede the development of type 3 vessels. Type 3 lesions are typically associated with prominent intraretinal edema and rarely subretinal fluid, in contrast to type 1 or type 2 neovascularization. Type 3 lesions tend to regress rapidly following anti-VEGF therapy, with no resultant fibrosis, making these lesions highly amenable to early detection and treatment. Type 3 lesions have a high rate of second eye involvement (close to 100% by 3 years).

Vasogenic sequence *(left)*

It has been proposed that type 3 neovascularization arises within a zone of outer retinal thinning and hypoxia where VEGF is upregulated. These changes are likely due to a combination of factors, including the presence of a drusenoid PED, relatively thinner choroid, and migrated RPE cells *(top image)*. Local VEGF production imparts an angiogenic stimulus for the growth of type 3 vessels from the deep capillary plexus *(second image)*. The intraretinal vessels may extend through the disrupted RPE into the sub-RPE space, and the lesion leaks intraretinal fluid *(third image)* followed by sub-RPE fluid, which may result in a serous PED *(fourth image)*. Finally, the intraretinal vessels may extend to the superficial capillary plexus, and the lesion may develop more extensive intraretinal hemorrhage and exudation *(fifth image)*.

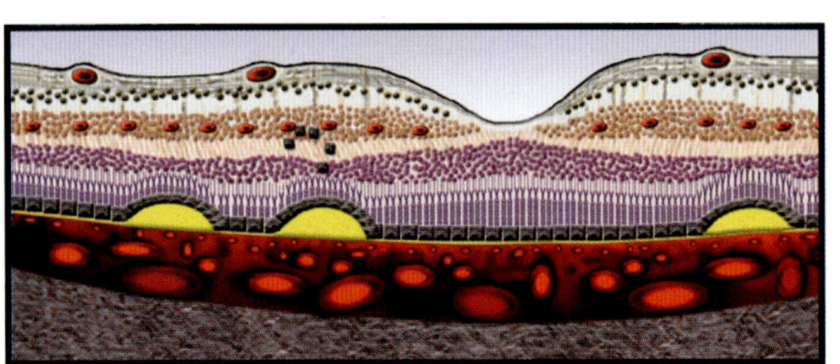

© 619

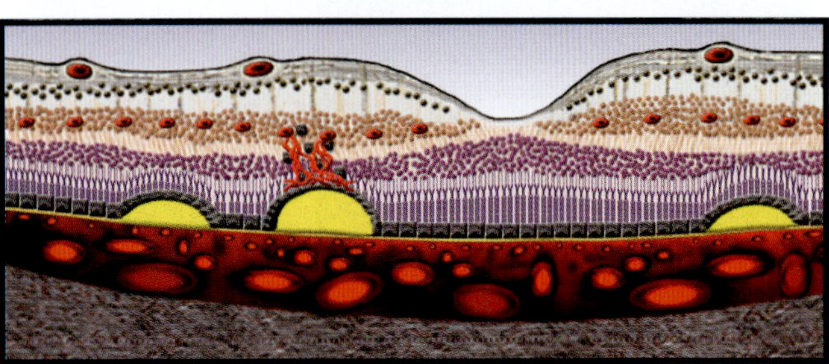

© 620

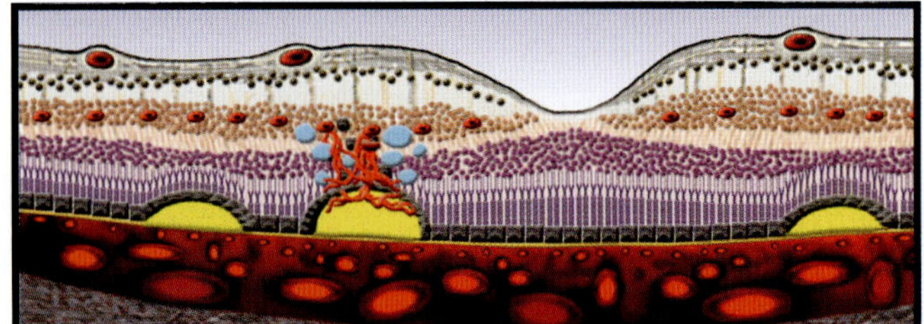

© 621

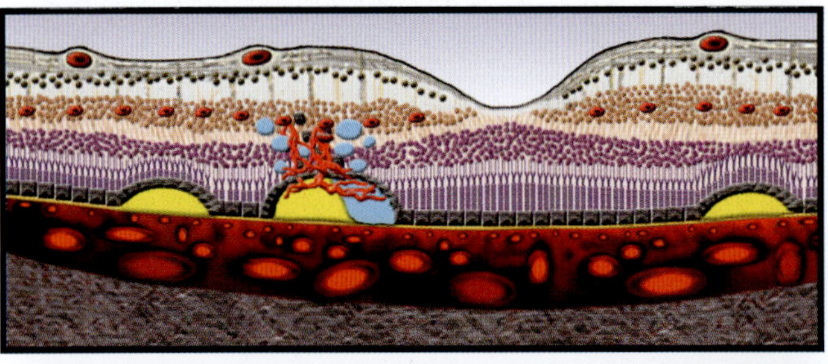

© 622

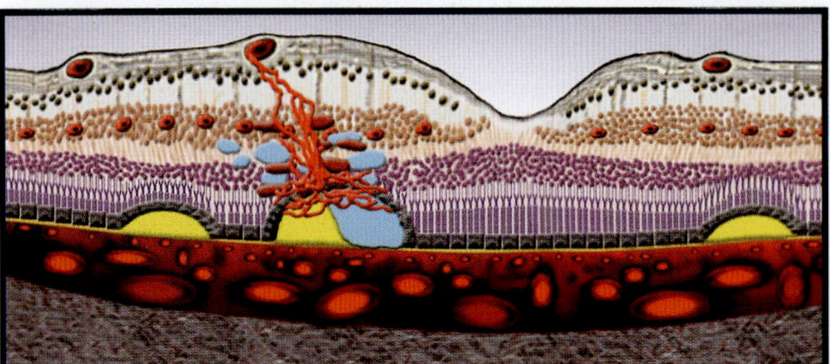

© 624

Alternative hypothesis *(below)*

An alternative hypothesis is that type 3 vessels arise from "occult" type 1 neovascular vessels present beneath the retinal pigment epithelium. This theory hypothesizes that neovascular vessels penetrate the pigment epithelium to enter the retina and produce a similar series of findings.

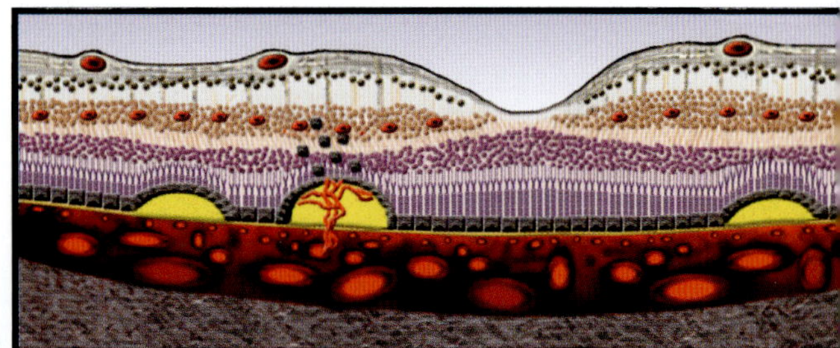

© 623

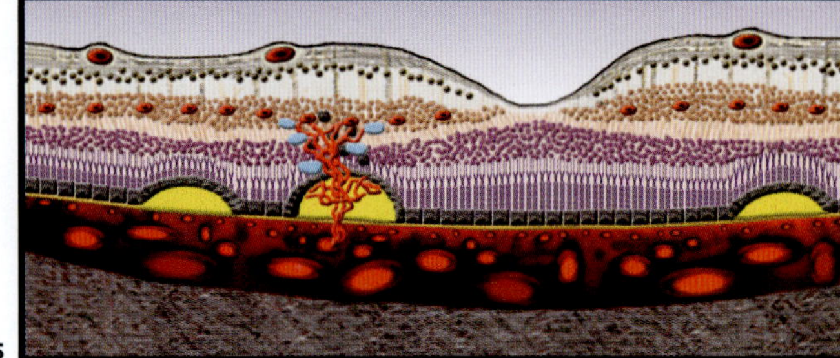

© 625

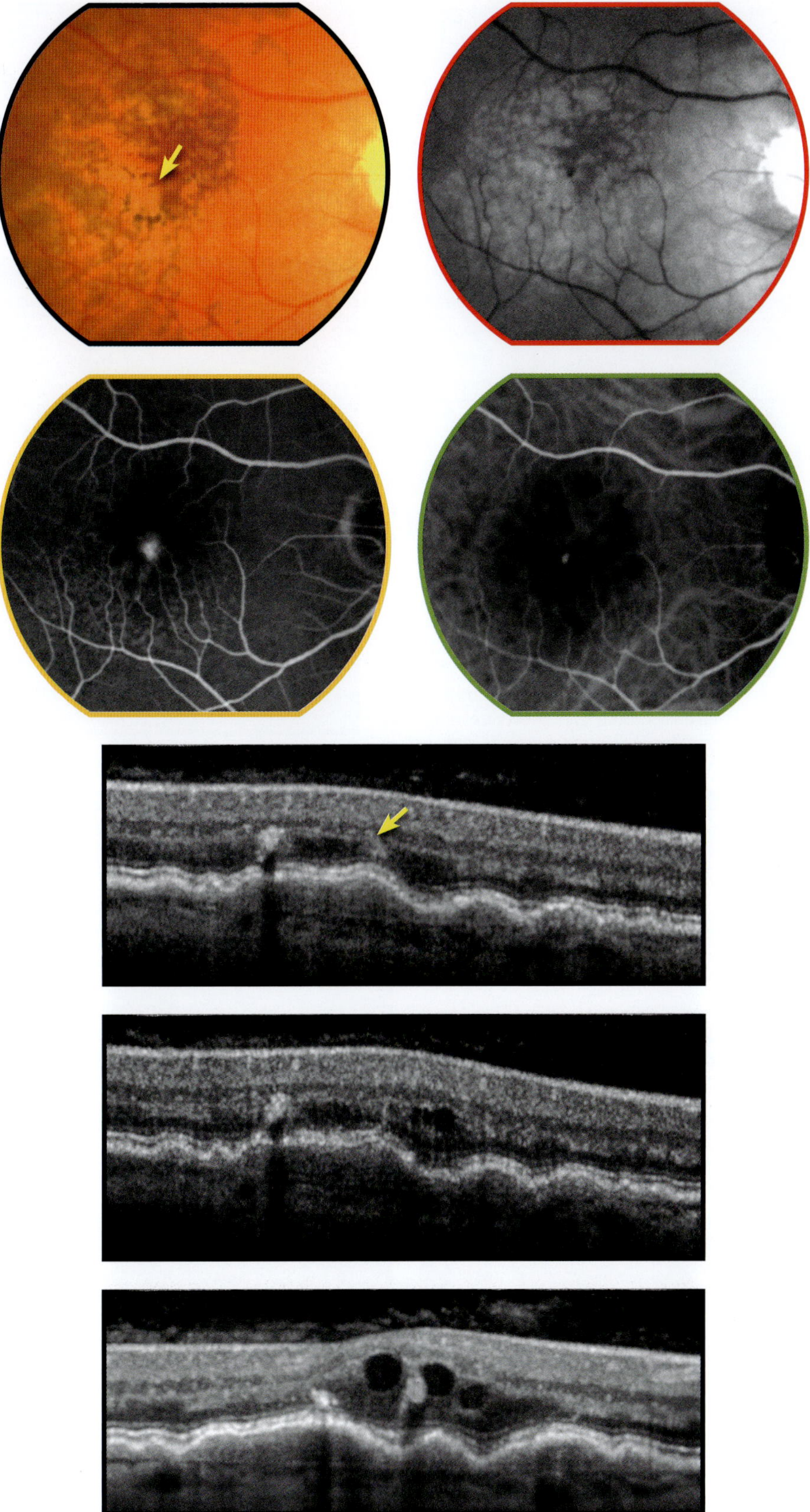

This patient has a small retinal hemorrhage *(arrow)* with surrounding drusen that can be visualized better on red-free photography. Fluorescein angiography shows a well-defined area of early hyperfluorescence that could be easily misinterpreted as a small type 2 lesion. ICG angiography shows a focal area of hyperfluorescence or so-called "hot spot" representing the type 3 neovascularization. Sequential SD-OCT shows the progression of changes at the area of the type 3 vessels. The first OCT *(third row)* shows an intraretinal hyper-reflective lesion *(arrow)* at the level of the outer plexiform layer representing RPE cells or early type 3 vessels overlying a drusenoid PED. The second OCT *(fourth row)* shows development of intraretinal fluid around the area of early type 3 vessels. The third OCT *(fifth row)* shows increasing intraretinal fluid associated with the growing intraretinal type 3 lesion.

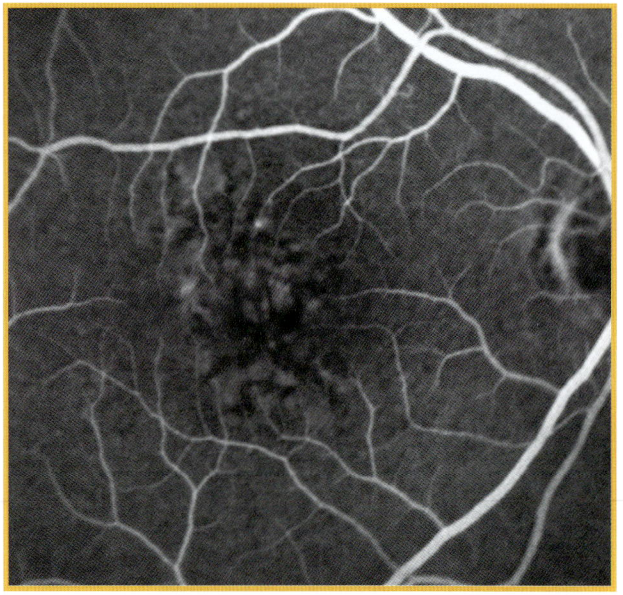

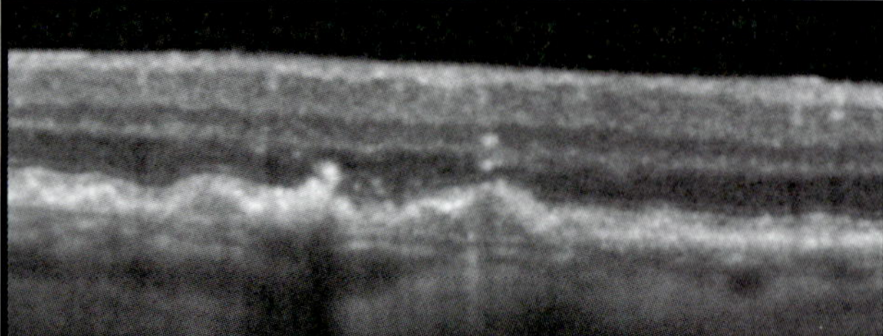

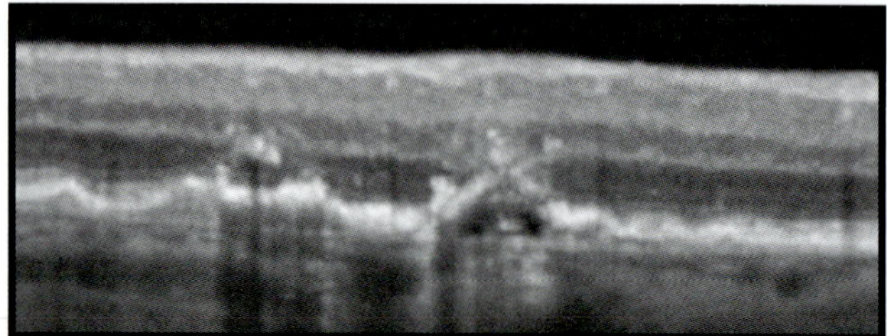

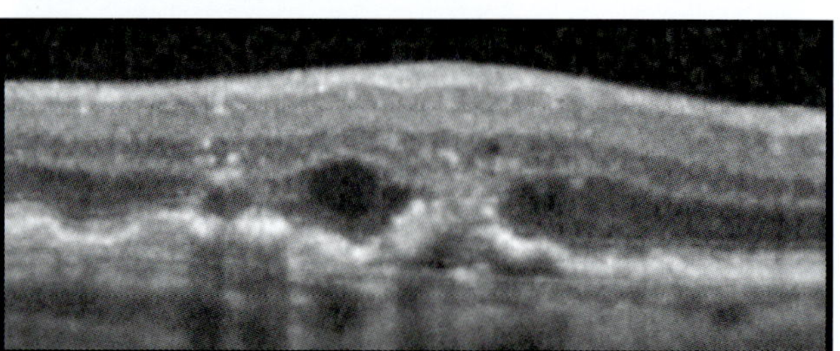

This fluorescein angiogram shows focal leakage at the site of early type 3 neovascularization in a patient with surrounding macular drusen. The initial OCT shows corresponding reflectance within the retina at the level of the outer and inner nuclear layers overlying a drusenoid PED *(top right image)*. The second OCT taken 10 months later shows enlargement of the underlying PED and development of a serous component within the PED *(middle right image)*. The third OCT taken 1 month later shows development of intraretinal cystic fluid around the type 3 lesion *(bottom right image)*.

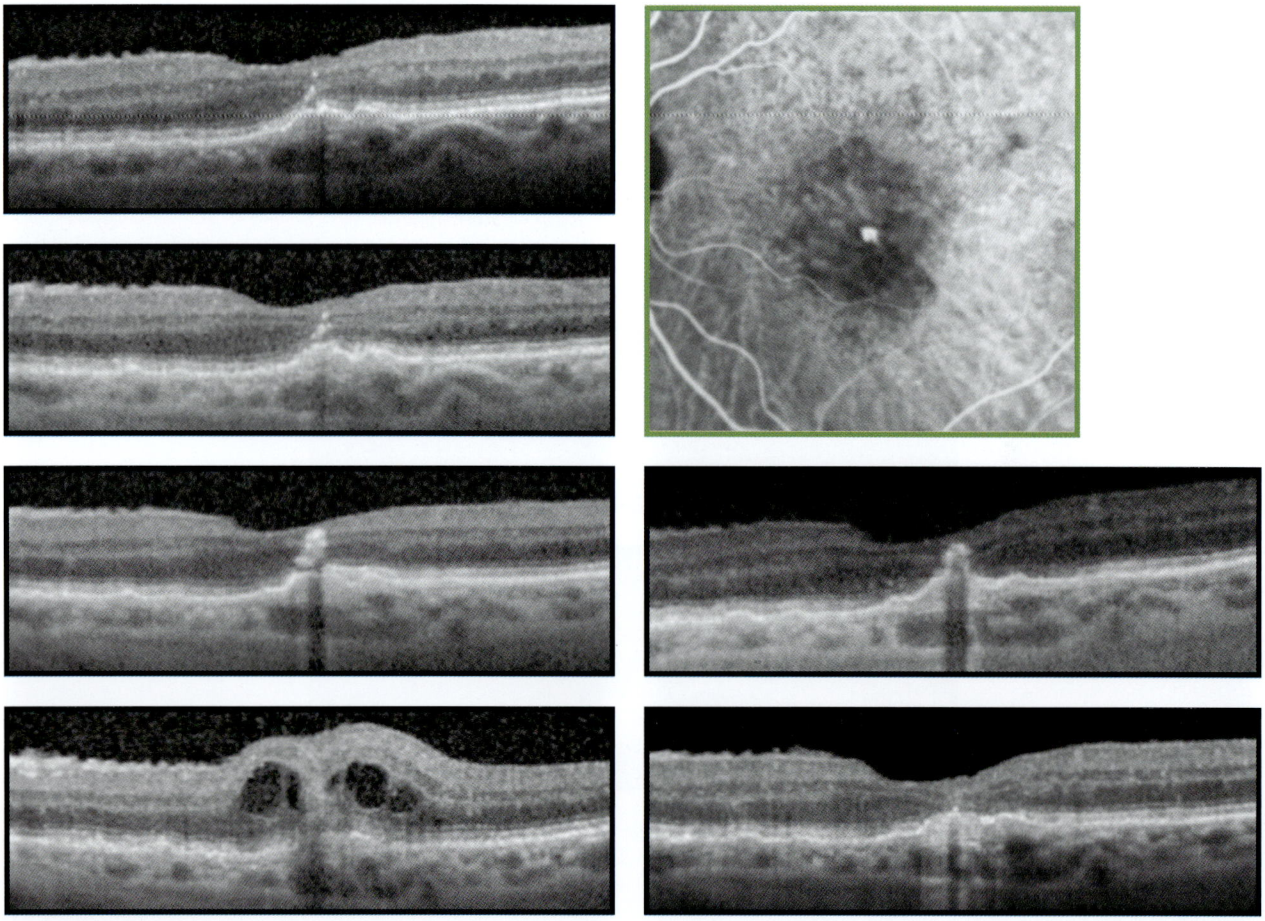

Sequential SD-OCT demonstrates the growth of a type 3 precursor lesion over a drusenoid PED. The first OCT *(top left image)* shows punctate hyper-reflectivity overlying an intact external limiting membrane that enlarged 2 months later *(left, second image from top)* and grew further 6 months later *(left, third image from top)*. OCT taken 2 months later *(bottom left image)* shows development of intraretinal fluid associated with a hot spot observed on ICG angiography *(top right image)*. Treatment with intravitreal anti-VEGF therapy resulted in resolution of the cystoid macular edema *(middle right image)* with regression and collapse of the type 3 lesion *(bottom right image)*.

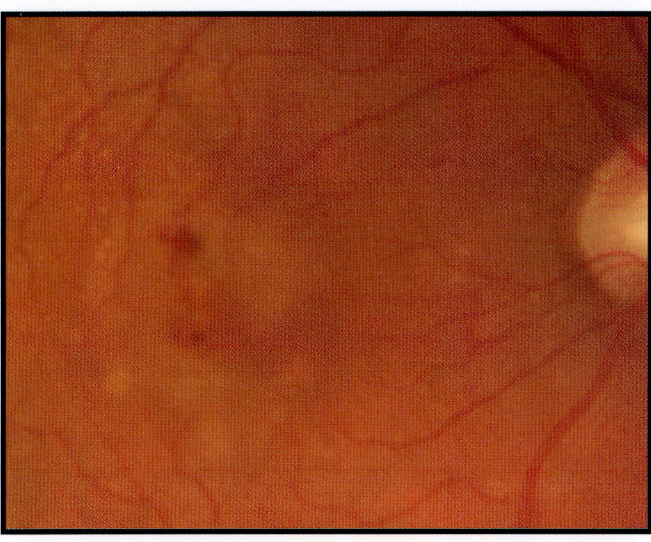

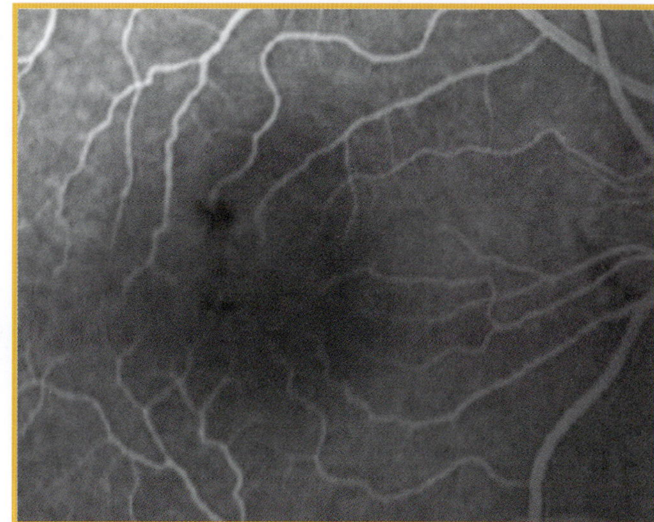

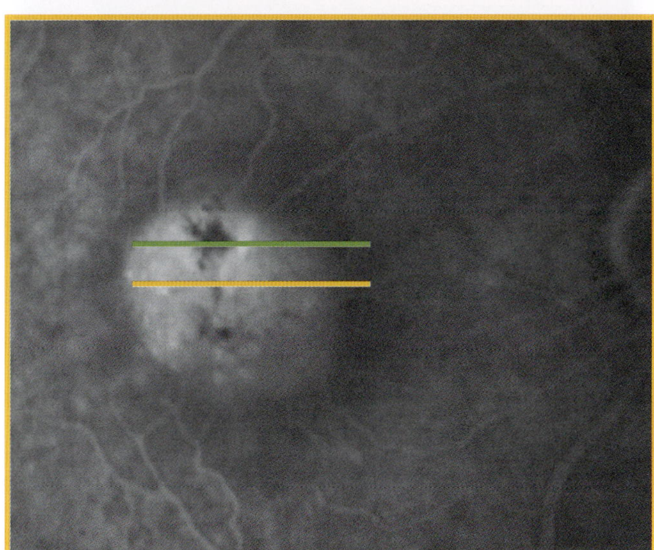

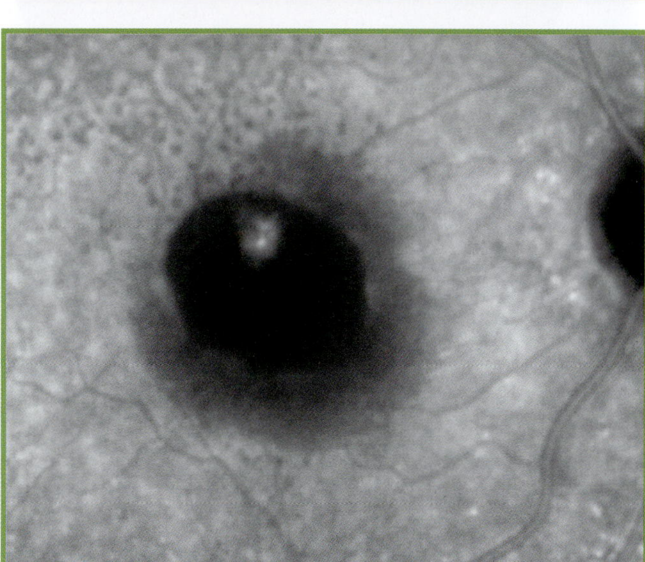

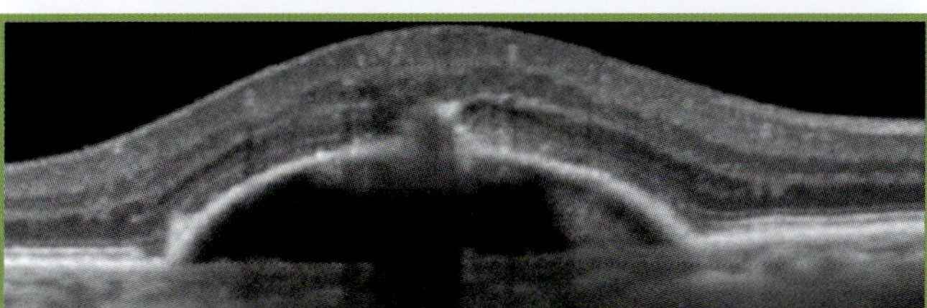

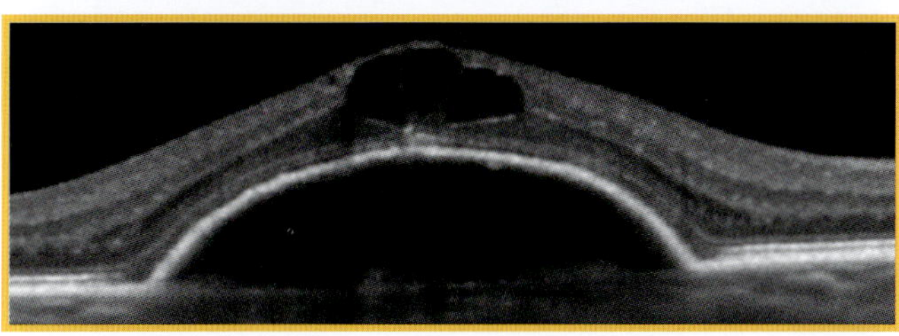

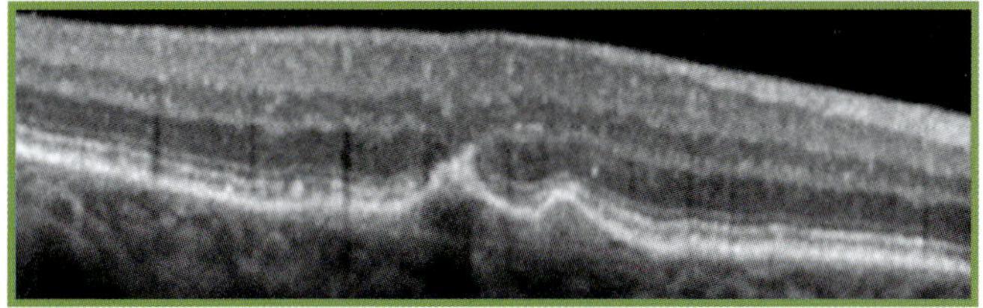

This patient has type 3 neovascularization overlying a large mixed serous/drusenoid PED. Color image *(top row left)* shows a central PED with overlying hemorrhage and adjacent drusen. Early fluorescein angiography *(top row right)* shows diffuse hypofluorescence at the site of the PED and blocked fluorescence at the areas of hemorrhage. Late fluorescein angiography *(second row left)* shows an area of leakage superiorly and pooling within the PED. ICG angiography *(second row right)* shows an area of focal leakage from type 3 neovascularization and the presence of reticular pseudodrusen in the superotemporal macula. Initial OCT *(third row)* shows a large type 3 lesion at the apex of the PED with amorphous material within the PED representing drusenoid material. An adjacent OCT line scan *(fourth row)* shows large intraretinal cystoid spaces. After treatment with a single injection of intravitreal anti-VEGF therapy, there was collapse of the PED with persistent drusenoid deposits and photoreceptor loss at the site of the type 3 vessels *(bottom row)*.

Disciform Scarring

Patients with end-stage neovascular AMD may develop disciform scarring from any type of neovascularization. Often, the type of neovascularization responsible for the fibrosis and scarring is indistinguishable. Some people use the term "fibrovascular scarring" instead of disciform scarring.

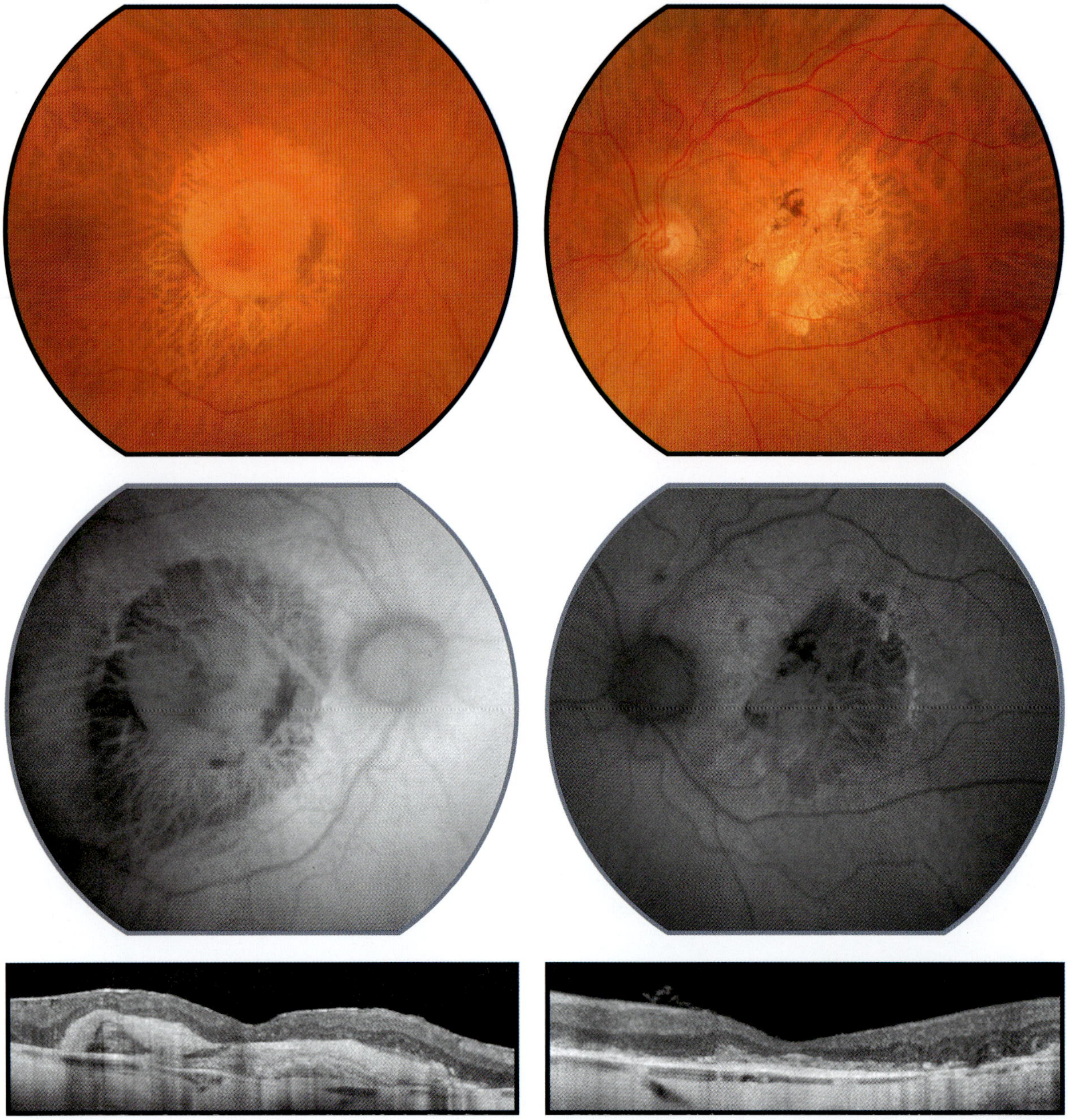

This patient has bilateral neovascular AMD that resulted in chronic fibrosis and disciform scarring. On SD-OCT, fibrotic tissue overlying areas of choroidal and RPE atrophy is seen to be more extensive in the right eye than the left eye.

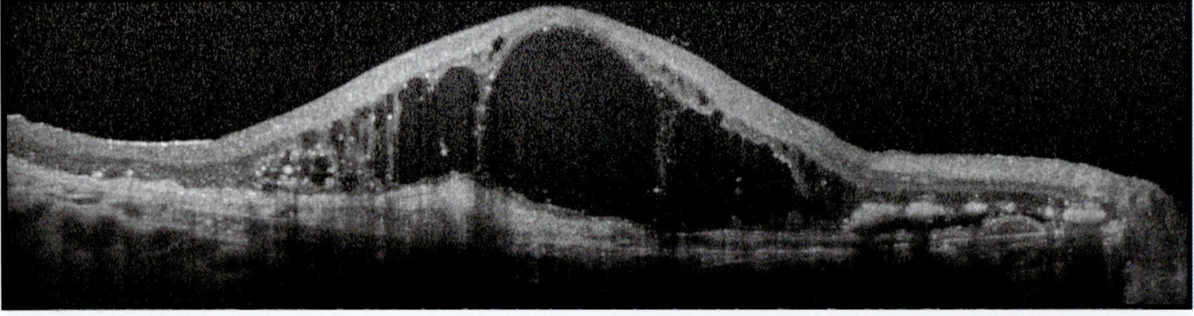

In some eyes, such as the one above, chronic exudation with prominent intraretinal fluid may occur at sites of atrophy and disciform scarring. These findings may be mistaken for subretinal fluid on clinical examination.

Idiopathic Choroidal Neovascularization

Idiopathic choroidal neovascularization is a term used to define choroidal neovascularization in young patients who do not manifest any clinical features that predispose to this complication. Some of these patients may subsequently develop inflammatory chorioretinal disease such as multifocal choroiditis/punctate inner choroidopathy or multiple evanescent white-dot syndrome in the ipsilateral or contralateral eye. In these cases, the neovascularization is usually type 2. With the advent of enhanced depth imaging OCT it is becoming evident that some cases diagnosed with idiopathic choroidal neovascularization may actually have pachychoroid neovasculopathy, a distinct entity associated with increased choroidal thickness, choroidal hyperpermeability, and large choroidal vessel dilatation. In such cases, the neovascularization is usually type 1 and may even progress to polypoidal choroidal vasculopathy in later life.

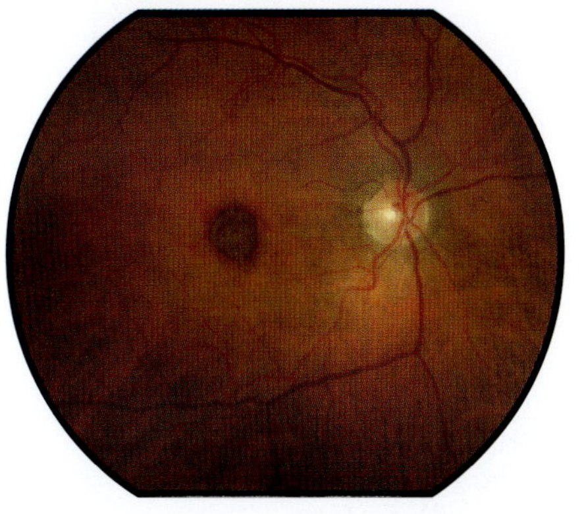
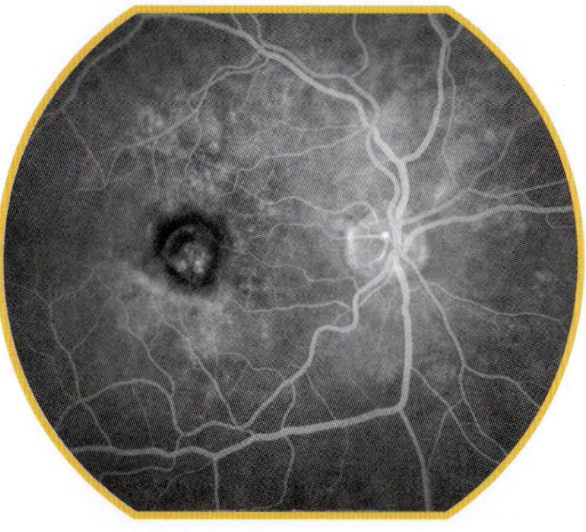
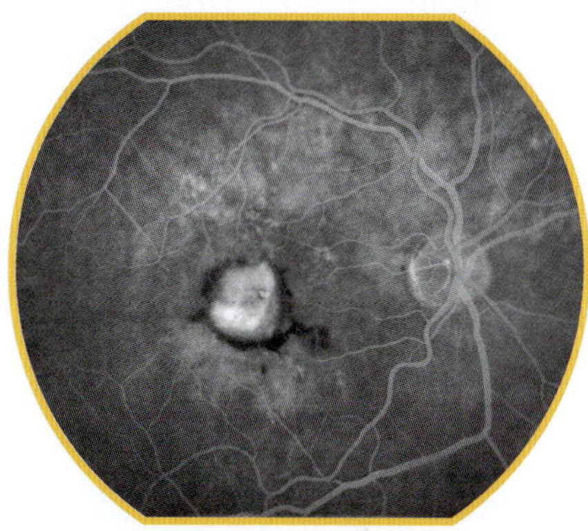

This patient presented with a change in central vision in the right eye. There was choroidal neovascularization and hemorrhage in the subfoveal area. The fluorescein angiogram showed type 2 neovascularization, which was well demarcated in the early stage of the study and leaked into the subneurosensory retinal space in the late frame *(right)*. This patient developed more typical findings of multifocal choroiditis several years later.

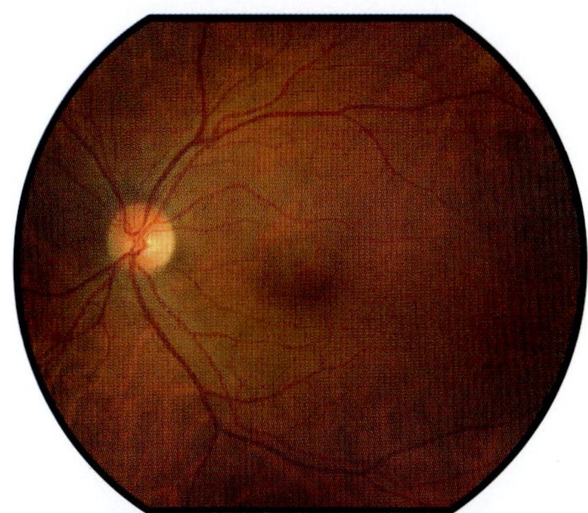
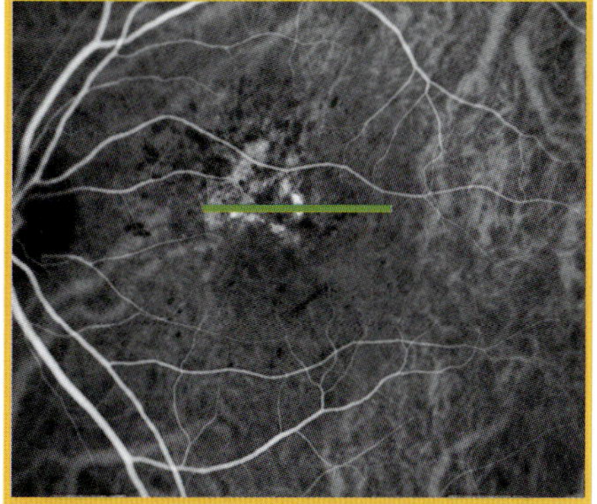
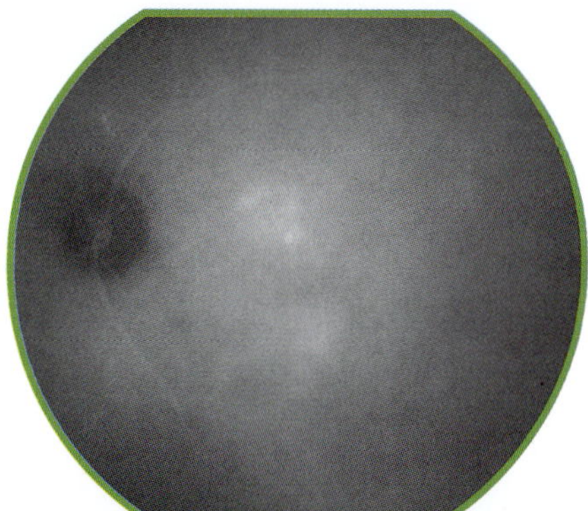
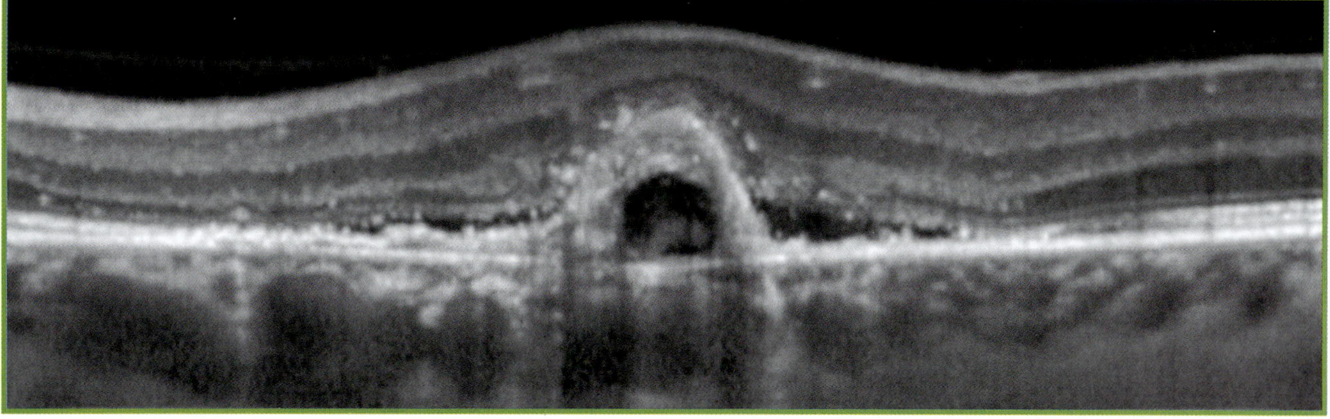

This patient was initially given the diagnosis of idiopathic choroidal neovascularization. The color image shows reduced fundus tessellation and the absence of drusen and other degenerative changes. Fluorescein angiography revealed hyperfluorescent leakage consistent with type 1 neovascularization. ICG angiography showed choroidal hyperpermeability in the area of leakage. SD-OCT showed a type 1 neovascular complex with an ovoid polypoidal element overlying a localized area of choroidal thickening and choroidal vessel dilatation. The patient has polypoidal choroidal vasculopathy.

Suggested Reading

Arnold, J.J., Sarks, J.P., Killingsworth, M.C., et al., 2003. Adult vitelliform macular degeneration: a clinicopathological study. Eye (Lond.) 17, 717–726.

Balaratnasingam, C., Lee, W.K., Koizumi, H., et al., 2016. Polypoidal choroidal vasculopathy: a distinct disease or manifestation of many? Retina 36 (1), 1–8.

Barteselli, G., Dell'arti, L., Finger, R.P., et al., 2014. The spectrum of ocular alterations in patients with β-thalassemia syndromes suggests a pathology similar to pseudoxanthoma elasticum. Ophthalmology 121 (3), 709–718.

Bhatnagar, P., Freund, K.B., Spaide, R.F., et al., 2007. Intravitreal bevacizumab for the management of choroidal neovascularization in pseudoxanthoma elasticum. Retina 27, 897–902.

Boon, C.J., Jeroen Klevering, B., Keunen, J.E., et al., 2008. Fundus autofluorescence imaging of retinal dystrophies. Vision Res. 48 (26), 2569–2577.

Boon, C.J., den Hollander, A.I., Hoyng, C.B., et al., 2008. The spectrum of retinal dystrophies caused by mutations in the peripherin/RDS gene. Prog. Retin. Eye Res. 27 (2), 213–235.

Boon, C.J., van de Ven, J.P., Hoyng, C.B., et al., 2013. Cuticular drusen: stars in the sky. Prog. Retin. Eye Res. 37, 90–113.

Bressler, N.M., Munoz, B., Maguire, M.G., et al., 1995. Five-year incidence and disappearance of drusen and retinal pigment epithelial abnormalities. Waterman study. Arch. Ophthalmol. 113 (3), 301–308.

Bruè, C., Mariotti, C., De Franco, E., et al., 2012. Pigmented free-floating posterior vitreous cyst. Case Rep. Ophthalmol. Med. 2012, 470289.

Caillaux, V., Gaucher, D., Gualino, V., et al., 2013. Morphologic characterization of dome-shaped macula in myopic eyes with serous macular detachment. Am. J. Ophthalmol. 156 (5), 958–967.

Cukras, C., Agrón, E., Klein, M.L., et al., 2010. Natural history of drusenoid pigment epithelial detachment in age-related macular degeneration: Age-Related Eye Disease Study Report No. 28. Ophthalmology 117 (3), 489–499.

Dansingani, K.K., Naysan, J., Freund, K.B., 2015. En face OCT angiography demonstrates flow in early type 3 neovascularization (retinal angiomatous proliferation). Eye (Lond.) 29 (5), 703–706.

de Carlo, T.E., Bonini Filho, M.A., Chin, A.T., et al., 2015. Spectral-domain optical coherence tomography angiography of choroidal neovascularization. Ophthalmology 122 (6), 1228–1238.

Dreyer, R., Green, W.R., 1978. Pathology of angioid streaks. Trans. Penn. Acad. Ophthalmol. Otolaryngol. 31, 158–167.

Ellabban, A.A., Tsujikawa, A., Muraoka, Y., et al., 2014. Dome-shaped macular configuration: longitudinal changes in the sclera and choroid by swept-source optical coherence tomography over two years. Am. J. Ophthalmol. 158 (5), 1062–1070.

Ferris, F.L. 3rd, Wilkinson, C.P., Bird, A., et al., 2013. Clinical classification of age-related macular degeneration. Ophthalmology 120 (4), 844–851.

Freund, K.B., Zweifel, S.A., Engelbert, M., 2010. Do we need a new classification for choroidal neovascularization in age-related macular degeneration? Retina 30 (9), 1333–1349.

Freund, K.B., Ho, I.V., Barbazetto, I.A., et al., 2008. Type 3 neovascularization: the expanded spectrum of retinal angiomatous proliferation. Retina 28 (2), 201–211.

Freund, K.B., Laud, K., Lima, L.H., et al., 2011. Acquired Vitelliform Lesions: correlation of clinical findings and multiple imaging analyses. Retina 31 (1), 13–25.

Freund, K.B., Mukkamala, S.K., Cooney, M.J., 2011. Peripapillary choroidal thickening and cavitation. Arch. Ophthalmol. 129 (8), 1096–1097.

Agarwal, A. (Ed.), 2012. Gass' Atlas of Macular Diseases, fifth ed. Saunders.

Gass, J.D., Jallow, S., Davis, B., 1985. Adult vitelliform macular detachment occurring in patients with basal laminar drusen. Am. J. Ophthalmol. 99 (4), 445–459.

Gliem, M., Zaeytijd, J.D., Finger, R.P., et al., 2013. An update on the ocular phenotype in patients with pseudoxanthoma elasticum. Front. Genet. 4, 14.

Goldberg, N., Freund, K.B., 2012. Progression of an acquired vitelliform lesion to a full-thickness macular hole documented by eye-tracked spectral-domain optical coherence tomography. Arch. Ophthalmol. 130 (9), 1221–1223.

Goldman, D.R., Freund, K.B., McCannel, C.A., et al., 2013. Peripheral polypoidal choroidal vasculopathy as a cause of peripheral exudative hemorrhagic chorioretinopathy: a report of 10 eyes. Retina 33 (1), 48–55.

Grossniklaus, H.E., Green, W.R., 1992. Pathologic findings in pathologic myopia. Retina 12, 127–133.

Hamada, S., Jain, S., Sivagnanavel, V., et al., 2006. Drusen classification in bilateral drusen and fellow eye of exudative age-related macular degeneration. Eye (Lond.) 20, 199–202.

Hariri, A., Nittala, M.G., Sadda, S.R., 2015. Outer retinal tubulation as a predictor of the enlargement amount of geographic atrophy in age-related macular degeneration. Ophthalmology 122 (2), 407–413.

Holz, F.G., Strauss, E.C., Schmitz-Valckenberg, S., et al., 2014. Geographic atrophy: clinical features and potential therapeutic approaches. Ophthalmology 121 (5), 1079–1091.

Hu, X., Plomp, A.S., van Soest, S., et al., 2003. Pseudoxanthoma elasticum: a clinical, histopathological, and molecular update. Surv. Ophthalmol. 48, 424–438.

Imamura, Y., Engelbert, M., Iida, T., et al., 2010. Polypoidal choroidal vasculopathy: a review. Surv. Ophthalmol. 55 (6), 501–515.

Ishida, T., Moriyama, M., Tanaka, Y., et al., 2015. Radial tracts emanating from staphyloma edge in eyes with pathologic myopia. Ophthalmology 122 (1), 215–216.

Johnson, D.A., Yannuzzi, L.A., Shakin, J.L., et al., 1998. Lacquer cracks following laser treatment of choroidal neovascularization in pathologic myopia. Retina 18, 118–124.

Jung, J.J., Chen, C.Y., Mrejen, S., et al., 2014. The incidence of neovascular subtypes in newly diagnosed neovascular age-related macular degeneration. Am. J. Ophthalmol. 158 (4), 769–779.

Klein, M.L., Ferris, F.L. 3rd, Armstrong, J., et al., 2008. Retinal precursors and the development of geographic atrophy in age-related macular degeneration. Ophthalmology 115, 1026–1031.

Klein, R., Cruickshanks, K.J., Nash, S.D., et al., 2010. The prevalence of age-related macular degeneration and associated risk factors. Arch. Ophthalmol. 128 (6), 750–758.

Lengyel, I., Csutak, A., Florea, D., et al., 2015. A population-based ultra-widefield digital image grading study for age-related macular degeneration-like lesions at the peripheral retina. Ophthalmology 122 (7), 1340–1347.

Liang, I.C., Shimada, N., Tanaka, Y., et al., 2015. Comparison of clinical features in highly myopic eyes with and without a dome-shaped macula. Ophthalmology 122 (8), 1591–1600.

Litts, K.M., Messinger, J.D., Dellatorre, K., et al., 2015. Clinicopathological correlation of outer retinal tubulation in age-related macular degeneration. JAMA Ophthalmol. 133 (5), 609–612.

Malagola, R., Pecorella, I., Teodori, C., et al., 2006. Peripheral lacquer cracks as an early finding in pathological myopia. Arch. Ophthalmol. 124 (12), 1783–1784.

Mantel, I., Schalenbourg, A., Zografos, L., 2012. Peripheral exudative hemorrhagic chorioretinopathy: polypoidal choroidal vasculopathy and hemodynamic modifications. Am. J. Ophthalmol. 153 (5), 910–922.

Mieler, W.F., Williams, D.F., Levin, M., 1988. Vitreous amyloidosis. Case report. Arch. Ophthalmol. 106, 881–883.

Milch, F.A., Yannuzi, L.A., Rudick, A.J., 1987. Pathologic myopia and subretinal hemorrhages. Ophthalmology 94, 117.

Moss, S.E., Klein, R., Klein, B.E., 2001. Asteroid hyalosis in a population: the Beaver Dam eye study. Am. J. Ophthalmol. 132, 70–75.

Mrejen, S., Sarraf, D., Mukkamala, S.K., et al., 2013. Multimodal imaging of pigment epithelial detachment: a guide to evaluation. Retina 33 (9), 1735–1762.

Neelam, K., Cheung, C.M., Ohno-Matsui, K., et al., 2012. Choroidal neovascularization in pathological myopia. Prog. Retin. Eye Res. 31 (5), 495–525.

Ohno-Matsui, K., 2014. Proposed classification of posterior staphylomas based on analyses of eye shape by three-dimensional magnetic resonance imaging and wide-field fundus imaging. Ophthalmology 121 (9), 1798–1809.

Ohno-Matsui, K., Akiba, M., Moriyama, M., et al., 2012. Intrachoroidal cavitation in macular area of eyes with pathologic myopia. Am. J. Ophthalmol. 154 (2), 382–393.

Ohno-Matsui, K., Kawasaki, R., Jonas, J.B., et al., 2015. International photographic classification and grading system for myopic maculopathy. Am. J. Ophthalmol. 159 (5), 877–883.

Ooto, S., Vongkulsiri, S., Sato, T., et al., 2014. Outer retinal corrugations in age-related macular degeneration. JAMA Ophthalmol. 132 (7), 806–813.

Pang, C.E., Freund, K.B., Engelbert, M., 2014. Enhanced vitreous imaging technique with spectral-domain optical coherence tomography for evaluation of posterior vitreous detachment. JAMA Ophthalmol. 132 (9), 1148–1150.

Pang, C.E., Schaal, K.B., Engelbert, M., 2015. Association of prevascular vitreous fissures and cisterns with vitreous degeneration as assessed by swept source optical coherence tomography. Retina 35 (9), 1875–1882.

Pece, A., Yannuzzi, L., Sannace, C., et al., 2000. Chorioretinal involvement in primary systemic nonfamilial amyloidosis. Am. J. Ophthalmol. 130, 250–253.

Querques, G., Souied, E.H., Freund, K.B., 2013. Multimodal imaging of early stage 1 type 3 neovascularization with simultaneous eye-tracked spectral-domain optical coherence tomography and high-speed real-time angiography. Retina 33 (9), 1881–1887.

Rahimy, E., Freund, K.B., Larsen, M., et al., 2014. Multilayered pigment epithelial detachment in neovascular age-related macular degeneration. Retina 34 (7), 1289–1295.

Rudolf, M., Clark, M.E., Chimento, M.F., et al., 2008. Prevalence and morphology of druse types in the macula and periphery of eyes with age-related maculopathy. Invest. Ophthalmol. Vis. Sci. 49, 1200–1209.

Russell, S.R., Mullins, R.F., Schneider, B.L., et al., 2000. Location, substructure, and composition of basal laminar drusen compared with drusen associated with aging and age-related macular degeneration. Am. J. Ophthalmol. 129, 205–214.

Saito, M., Iida, T., Freund, K.B., et al., 2014. Clinical findings of acquired vitelliform lesions associated with retinal pigment epithelial detachments. Am. J. Ophthalmol. 157 (2), 355–365.

Sarks, S., Cherepanoff, S., Killingsworth, M., et al., 2007. Relationship of basal laminar deposit and membranous debris to the clinical presentation of early age-related macular degeneration. Invest. Ophthalmol. Vis. Sci. 48, 968–977.

Sarraf, D., Reddy, S., Chiang, A., et al., 2010. A new grading system for retinal pigment epithelial tears. Retina 30 (7), 1039–1045.

Sawa, M., Ober, M.D., Freund, K.B., et al., 2006. Fundus autofluorescence in patients with pseudoxanthoma elasticum. Ophthalmology 113, 814–820.

Schmitz-Valckenberg, S., Bindewald-Wittich, A., Dolar-Szczasny, J., et al., 2006. Correlation between the area of increased autofluorescence surrounding geographic atrophy and disease progression in patients with AMD. Invest. Ophthalmol. Vis. Sci. 47 (6), 2648–2654.

Sepúlveda, G., Chang, S., Freund, K.B., et al., 2014. Late recurrence of myopic foveoschisis after successful repair with primary vitrectomy and incomplete membrane peeling. Retina 34 (9), 1841–1847.

Shah, V.P., Shah, S.A., Mrejen, S., et al., 2014. Subretinal hyperreflective exudation associated with neovascular age-related macular degeneration. Retina 34 (7), 1281–1288.

Shields, C.L., Romanelli-Gobbi, M., Lally, S.E., et al., 2012. Vitreous asteroid hyalosis prolapse into the anterior chamber simulating iris metastasis. Middle East Afr. J. Ophthalmol. 19 (3), 346–348.

Shinohara, K., Moriyama, M., Shimada, N., et al., 2014. Myopic stretch lines: linear lesions in fundus of eyes with pathologic myopia that differ from lacquer cracks. Retina 34 (3), 461–469.

Spaide, R., Donsoff, R., Lam, D.L., et al., 2002. Treatment of polypoidal choroidal vasculopathy with photodynamic therapy. Retina 22, 529–535.

Spaide, R.F., Curcio, C.A., 2010. Drusen characterization with multimodal imaging. Retina 30 (9), 1441–1454.

Spaide, R.F., Noble, K., Morgan, A., et al., 2006. Vitelliform macular dystrophy. Ophthalmology 113, 1392–1400.

Spaide, R.F., Yannuzzi, L.A., Slakter, J.S., et al., 1995. Indocyanine green videoangiography of idiopathic chroidal vasculopathy. Retina 15, 100–110.

Spaide, R.F., Yannuzzi, L.A., Slakter, J.S., et al., 1997. The expanding clinical spectrum of idiopathic choroidal vasculopathy. Arch. Ophthalmol. 115, 478–485.

Spaide, R.F., 2015. Optical coherence tomography angiography signs of vascular abnormalization with antiangiogenic therapy for choroidal neovascularization. Am. J. Ophthalmol. 160 (1), 6–16.

Spaide, R.F., Akiba, M., Ohno-Matsui, K., 2012. Evaluation of peripapillary intrachoroidal cavitation with swept source and enhanced depth imaging optical coherence tomography. Retina 32 (6), 1037–1044.

Spaide, R.F., 2009. Age-related choroidal atrophy. Am. J. Ophthalmol. 147 (5), 801–810.

Suzuki, M., Curcio, C.A., Mullins, R.F., et al., 2015. Refractile drusen: clinical imaging and candidate histology. Retina 35 (5), 859–865.

Toklu, Y., Raza, S., Cakmak, H.B., et al., 2013. Free-floating vitreous cyst in an adult male. Korean J. Ophthalmol. 27 (6), 463–465.

Wang, J.J., Foran, S., Smith, W., et al., 2003. Risk of age-related macular degeneration in eyes with macular drusen or hyperpigmentation: the Blue Mountains Eye Study cohort. Arch. Ophthalmol. 121, 658–663.

Yannuzzi, L., Nogueira, F., Spaide, F., et al., 1998. Idiopathic polypoidal choroidal vasculopathy. Arch. Ophthalmol. 116, 382–384.

Yannuzzi, L.A., Freund, K.B., Goldbaum, M., et al., 2000. Polypoidal choroidal vasculopathy masquerading as central serous chorioretinopathy. Ophthalmology 107, 767–777.

Yannuzzi, L.A., Freund, K.B., Takahashi, B.S., 2008. Review of retinal angiomatous proliferation or type 3 neovascularization. Retina 28, 375–384.

Yannuzzi, L.A., Negrao, S., Iida, T., et al., 2001. Retinal angiomatous proliferation in age-related macular degeneration. Retina 21, 416–434.

Yannuzzi, L.A., Sorenson, J.A., Spaide, R.F., et al., 1990. Idiopathic polypoidal choroidal vasculopathy. Retina 10, 1–8.

Yannuzzi, L.A., Wong, D., Scassellati-Sforzolini, B., et al., 1999. Polypoidal choroidal vasculopathy and neovascularized age-related macular degeneration. Arch. Ophthalmol. 117, 1503–1510.

Zweifel, S.A., Imamura, Y., Freund, K.B., et al., 2011. Multimodal fundus imaging of pseudoxanthoma elasticum. Retina 31 (3), 482–491.

Zweifel, S.A., Imamura, Y., Spaide, T.C., et al., 2010. Prevalence and significance of subretinal drusenoid deposits (reticular pseudodrusen) in age-related macular degeneration. Ophthalmology 117 (9), 1775–1781.

Zweifel, S.A., Spaide, R.F., Curcio, C.A., et al., 2010. Reticular pseudodrusen are subretinal drusenoid deposits. Ophthalmology 117 (2), 303–312.

Zweifel, S.A., Spaide, R.F., Yannuzzi, L.A., 2011. Acquired vitelliform detachment in patients with subretinal drusenoid deposits (reticular pseudodrusen). Retina 31 (2), 229–234.

CHAPTER 8

Oncology

Pediatric Mass Lesions of the Fundus

Idiopathic Granuloma
An idiopathic granuloma of the disc or choroid may be seen rarely in the fundus. This is an idiopathic granuloma at the nerve, which was first diagnosed in childhood and followed without change over a number of years.

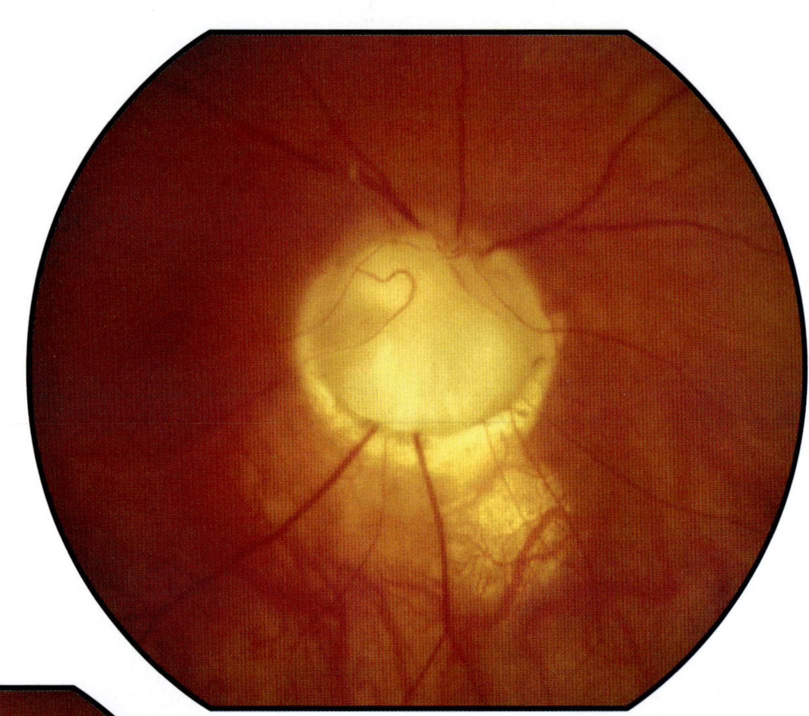

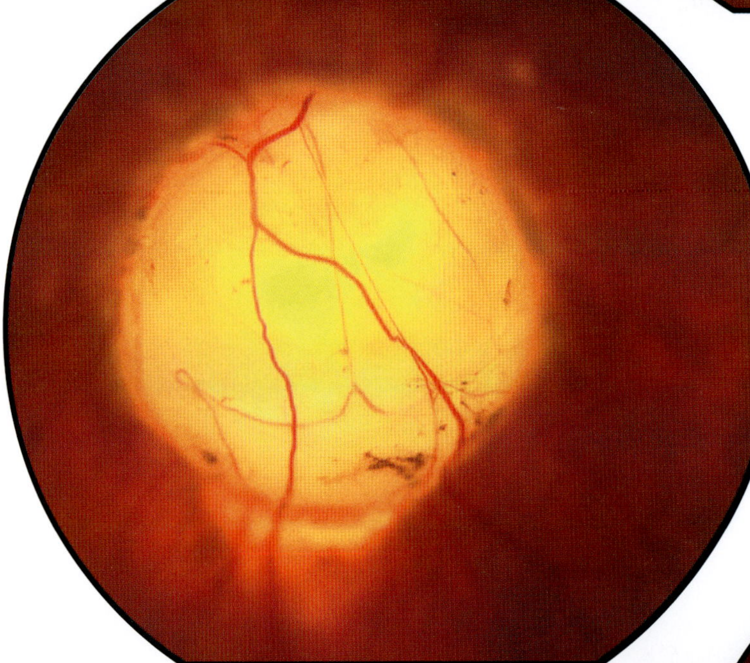

Benign Fibrous Histiocytoma Benign fibrous histiocytoma may be seen in the orbit and rarely in the uveal tract. Diagnosis is sometimes only possible through needle biopsy or enucleation. This approach should only be taken if the lesion shows progression. This patient was diagnosed with idiopathic uveal granuloma until further growth necessitated a needle biopsy that showed histiocytoma.

Juvenile Xanthogranuloma Juvenile xanthogranuloma is a rare, benign histiocytic disorder. Most patients also present with a skin disease characterized by reddish-brown nodular cutaneous changes or papules. Generally, a biopsy is needed to make a definitive diagnosis. Ultrasonography of the eye is often helpful to identify the lesion.

Retinoblastoma

Retinoblastoma is the most common intraocular malignancy of childhood. This malignancy affects approximately 250 to 300 children in the USA each year and about 7000 children worldwide. If detected while the tumor is contained within the eye, survival is excellent. Risks for metastases include optic nerve invasion, choroidal invasion, scleral invasion, anterior chamber invasion, and orbital invasion. In developed nations such as North America, Europe, and Japan, survival is 95%-97% whereas in developing regions, the survival is poorer at approximately 80% in Latin America, 60% in Asia, and 30% in Africa. Poor survival is generally related to advanced disease with late presentation for medical care.

Retinoblastoma classically presents with features of leukocoria or strabismus. Clinical features vary depending upon the extent of tumor and degree of delay in diagnosis. In the USA, most children manifest leukocoria, strabismus, or poor visual acuity. In developing countries, particularly in remote regions of Asia and Africa, features of buphthalmos, proptosis, and leukocoria are common. Efforts are underway internationally to educate clinicians, nurses, patients, and the general populations for detection of retinoblastoma.

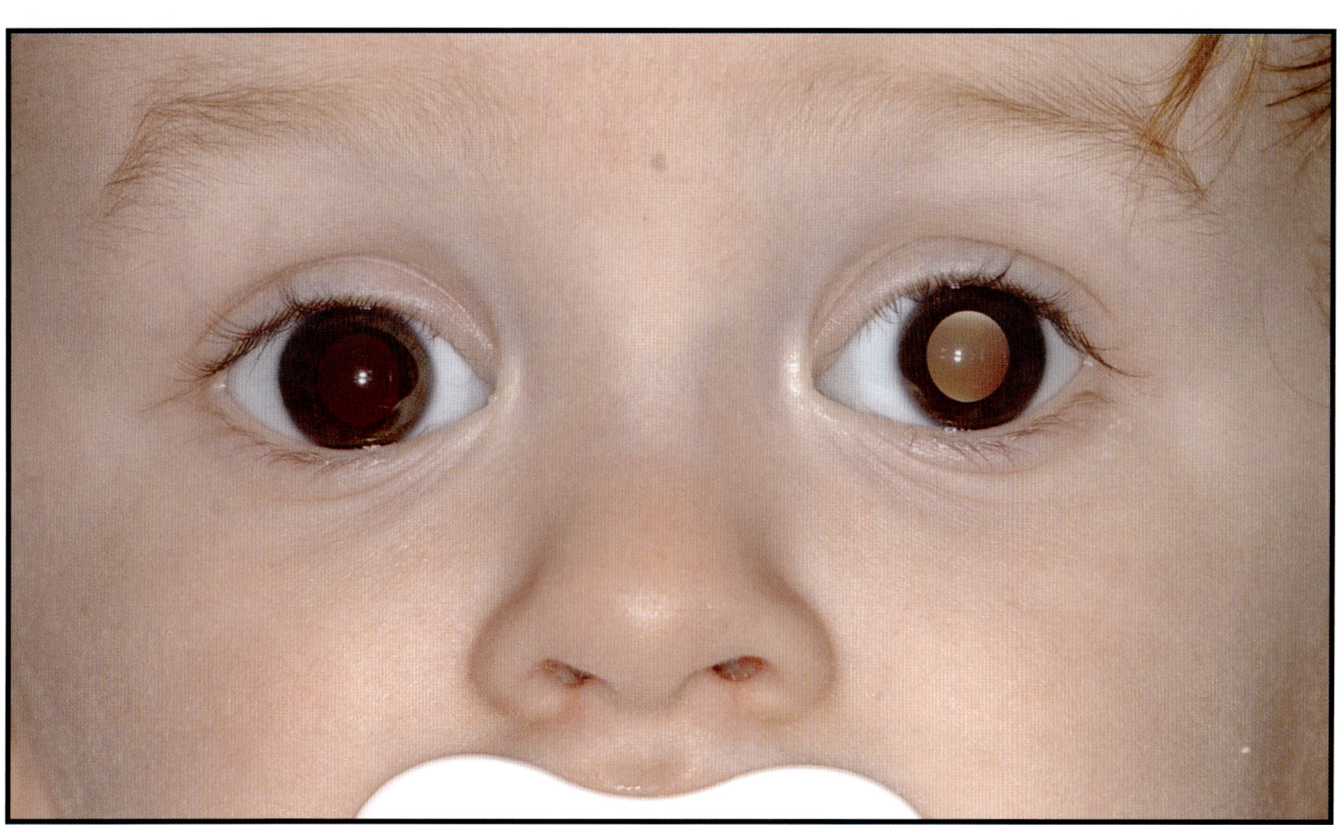

The most common presenting features of retinoblastoma are leukocoria and strabismus, as shown here.

Retinoblastoma Classification

There have been several classifications proposed for intraocular retinoblastoma including the Reese Ellsworth Classification, Essen Classification, Philadelphia Classification, and, most recently, the International Classification of Retinoblastoma. The International Classification of Retinoblastoma is practical and specifically applicable for chemotherapy outcomes, as it has been found predictive of treatment success following intravenous chemotherapy.

The International Classification of Retinoblastoma		
Group	**Philadelphia version**	**Los Angeles version**
A	Rb ≤ 3 mm	Rb ≤ 3 mm, at least 3 mm from the foveola and 1.5 mm from optic nerve. No seeding.
B	Rb > 3 mm or • Macular location or • Juxtapapillary location [< 1.5 mm to disc] or • SRF present	Eyes with no vitreous or subretinal seeding and retinal tumors of any size or location not included in group A. Small cuff of subretinal fluid ≤ 5 mm from tumor margin
C	Rb with • SRS ≤3 mm from Rb or • VS ≤ 3 mm from Rb	Eyes with focal vitreous or subretinal seeding and discrete tumor of any size or location. Seeding must be local, fine, and limited so as to be theoretically treatable with a radioactive plaque. Up to one quadrant subretinal fluid may be present.
D	Rb with • SRS >3 mm from Rb or • VS > 3 mm from Rb	Eyes with diffuse vitreous or subretinal seeding and/or massive, nondiscrete endophytic or exophytic disease. Seeding more extensive than Group C. Retinal detachment > 1 quadrant.
E	Rb with • Size >50% of globe or • Neovascular glaucoma or • Opaque media or • Invasion of optic nerve, choroid, sclera, orbit, anterior chamber	Massive Rb with anatomic or functional destruction of the eye with one or more of the following • Neovascular glaucoma • Massive intraocular hemorrhage • Aseptic orbital cellulitis • Tumor anterior to anterior vitreous face • Tumor touching lens • Diffuse infiltrating tumor • Phthisis or pre-phthisis

Rb, retinoblastoma; SRF, subretinal fluid; SRS, subretinal seeds; VS, vitreous seeds.

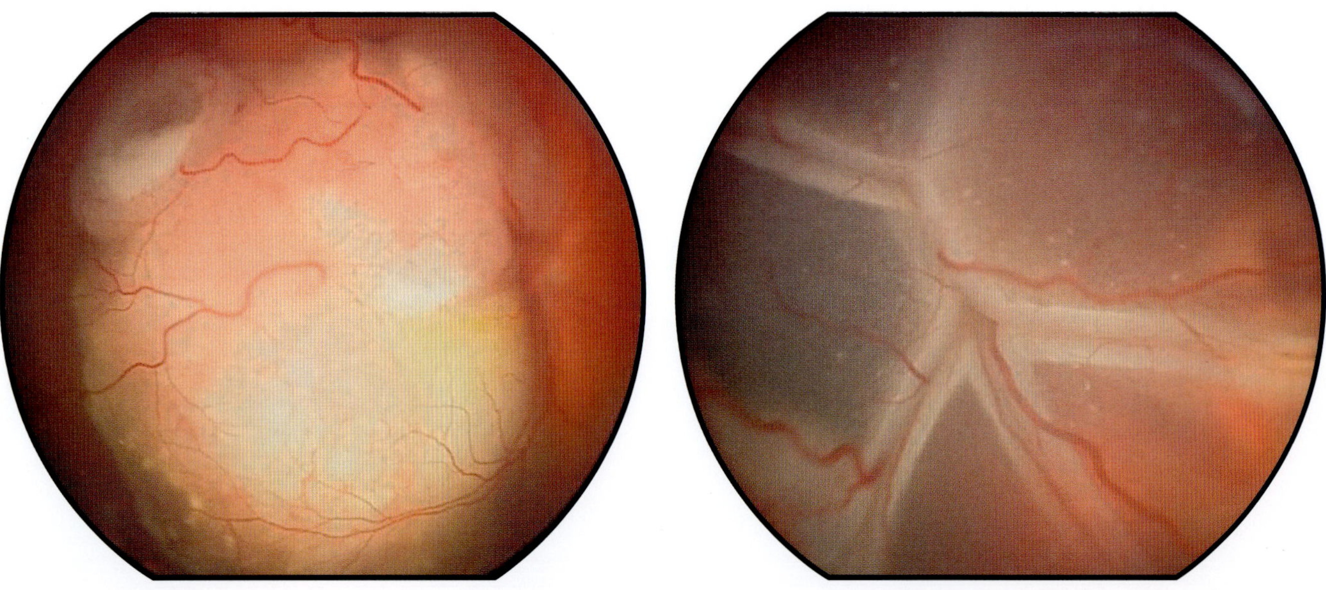

One-year-old child with bilateral retinoblastoma classified as group D in the right eye and group E in the left eye.

International Classification of Retinoblastoma

Group A Retinoblastoma

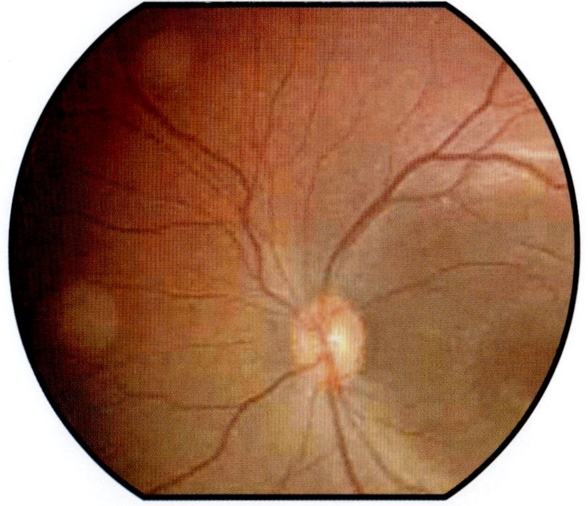

Small extramacular tumor less than 3 mm in diameter. A small retinoblastoma appears as an intraretinal, transparent, or gray lesion, with minimal vascularity.

Group B Retinoblastoma

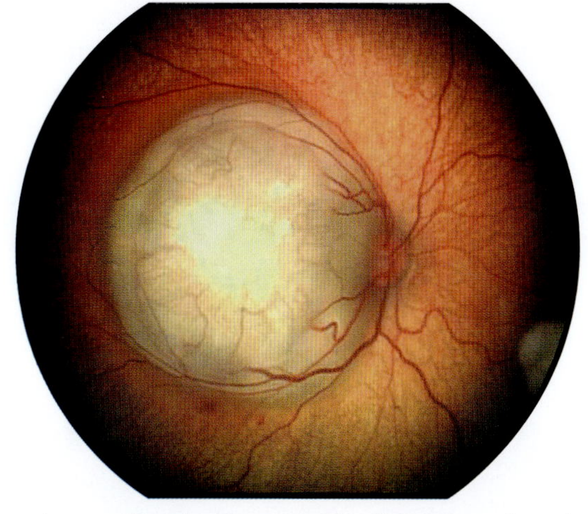

Medium-size macular retinoblastoma with subtle surrounding subretinal fluid. Slightly larger tumors are less transparent and appear solid white, with feeding vessels.

Group C Retinoblastoma

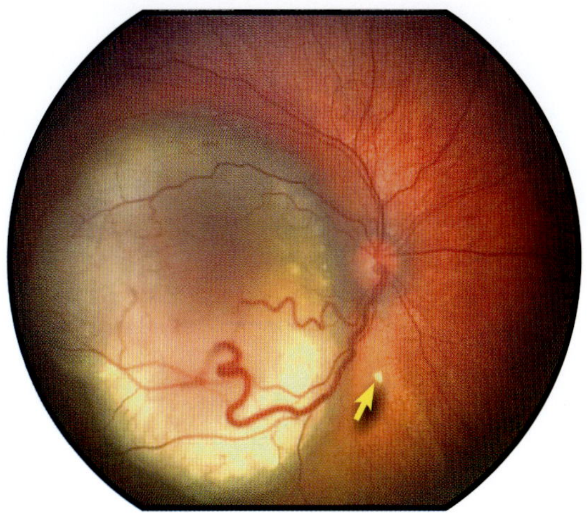

Larger retinoblastoma with localized subretinal seeds *(arrow)*, demonstrating dilated tortuous retinal arteries and veins as well as intralesional calcification.

Group D Retinoblastoma

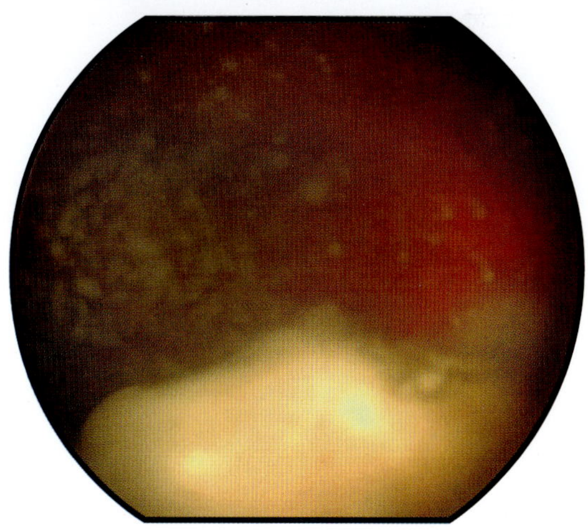

Large retinoblastoma with extensive, diffuse vitreous, and subretinal seeds remote from the tumor.

Group E Retinoblastoma

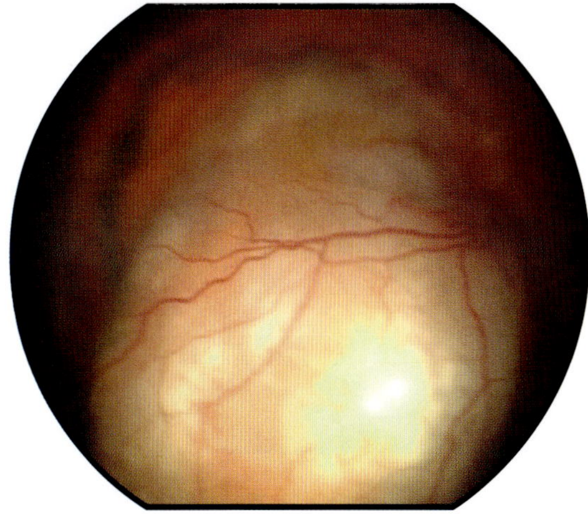

Extensive exophytic/endophytic retinoblastoma with solid mass of 14 mm thickness and involving >50% of the globe.

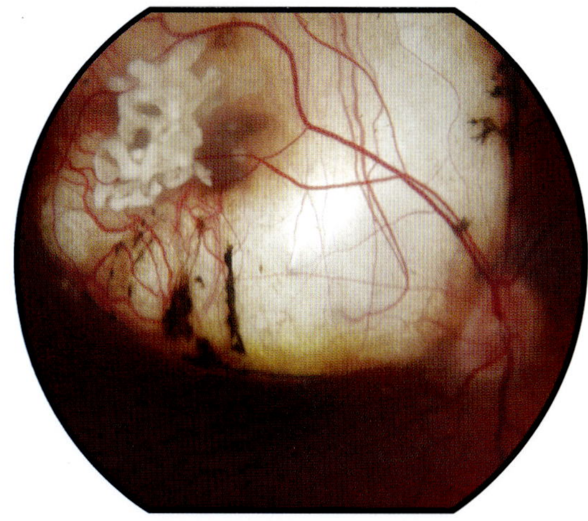

Spontaneously regressed retinoblastoma (retinocytoma) is not categorized by the International Classification of Retinoblastoma.

Retinoblastoma Growth Patterns

Characteristic clinical features of a yellow-white retinal mass often with surrounding subretinal fluid, subretinal seeding, and vitreous seeding establish the diagnosis of retinoblastoma. Retinoblastoma can demonstrate three growth patterns including exophytic, endophytic, and diffuse infiltrating patterns. In some instances, the tumor displays spontaneous arrest or regression of growth, also known as retinoma and retinocytoma, believed to represent a benign form of retinoblastoma.

The diagnosis is established based on clinical features alone. Despite classic manifestations, retinoblastoma can also display a spectrum of unusual features that overlap with other conditions (pseudoretinoblastomas) that can lead to diagnostic confusion. Accurate clinical diagnosis of retinoblastoma is important to avoid mistreatment. The leading simulators of retinoblastoma include Coats disease, persistent fetal vasculature (PFV), vitreous hemorrhage, toxocariasis, and familial exudative vitreoretinopathy.

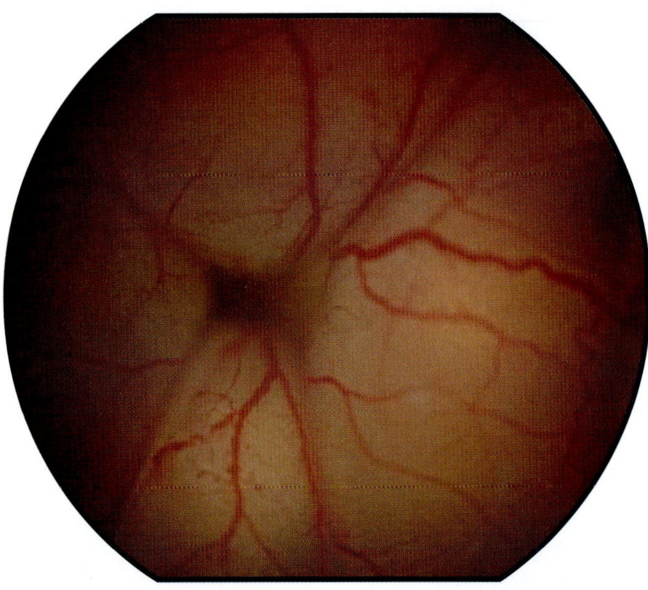

Exophytic retinoblastoma showing a prominent retinal detachment and underlying tumor, resembling Coats disease.

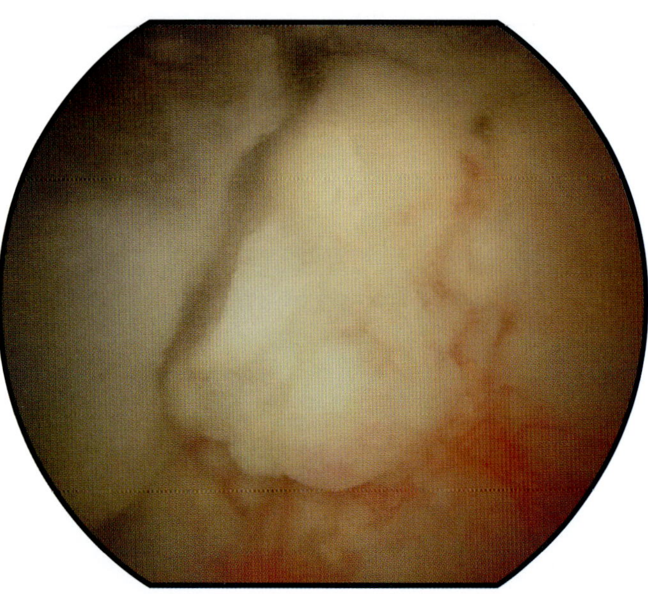

Endophytic retinoblastoma showing prominent vitreous seeding from the underlying tumor, resembling endophthalmitis.

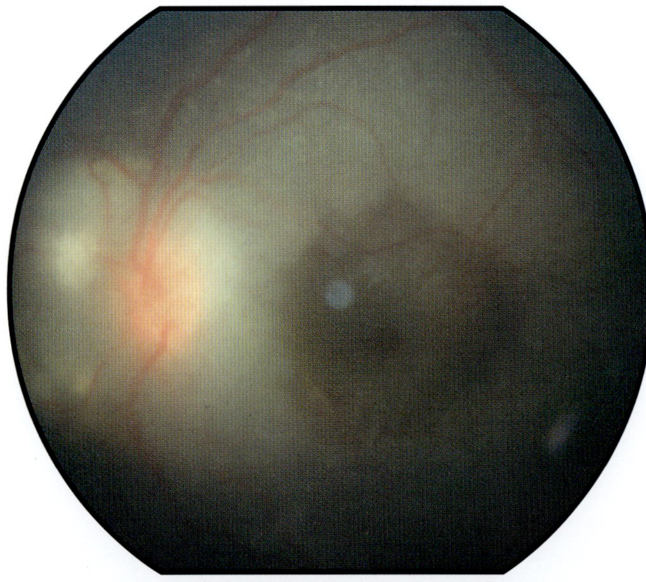

Diffuse infiltrating retinoblastoma with flat growth within the retina and minimal tumor mass, resembling uveitis.

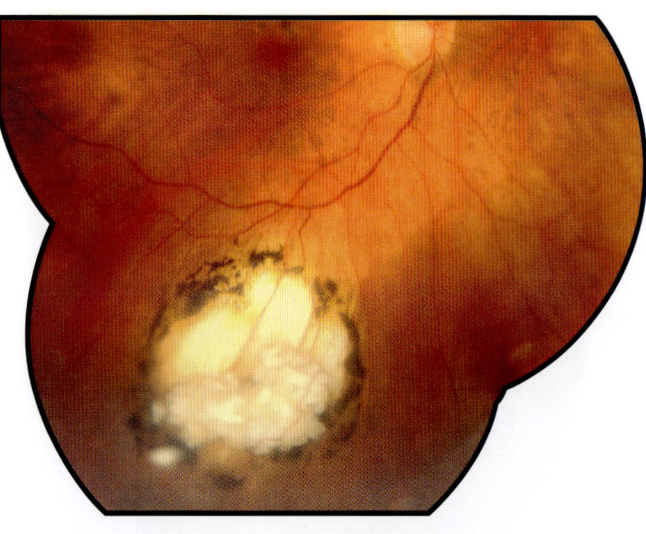

Retinocytoma (spontaneously regressed retinoblastoma) presenting as a small calcified scar with surrounding retinal pigment epithelial atrophy and hyperplasia.

Retinoblastoma Variations

Retinoblastoma can present with several phenotypic variations. The tumor typically appears as an obvious white retinal mass within or underlying the retina. However, on occasion, it can remain hidden behind a cloud of soft white clumped vitreous seeds. Retinoblastoma is a friable tumor with a tendency to produce seeding as it enlarges. Some retinoblastomas display subretinal fluid and subretinal seeds, while others present with vitreous hemorrhage and seeding. The seeding can be extensive, with each seed at risk to produce a solid mass if untreated. Following treatment, retinoblastoma shows regression into one of 5 regression patterns. These include type 0 with tumor disappearance, type I with a completely calcified scar, type II with a noncalcified scar, type III with a partially calcified scar, and type IV with an atrophic chorioretinal scar.

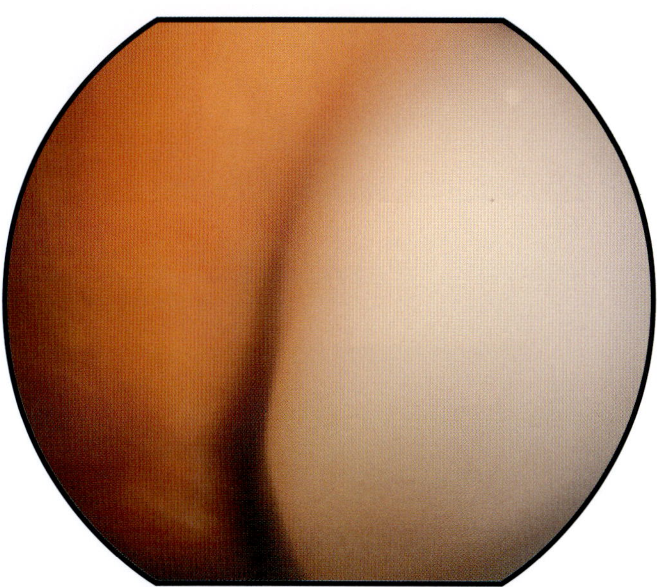

Large retinoblastoma with a solid amorphous mass in the vitreous cavity.

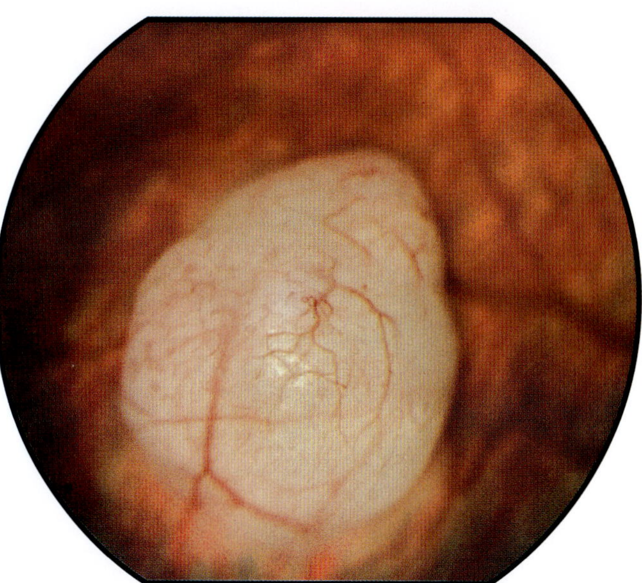

Small retinoblastoma with prominent vascularity.

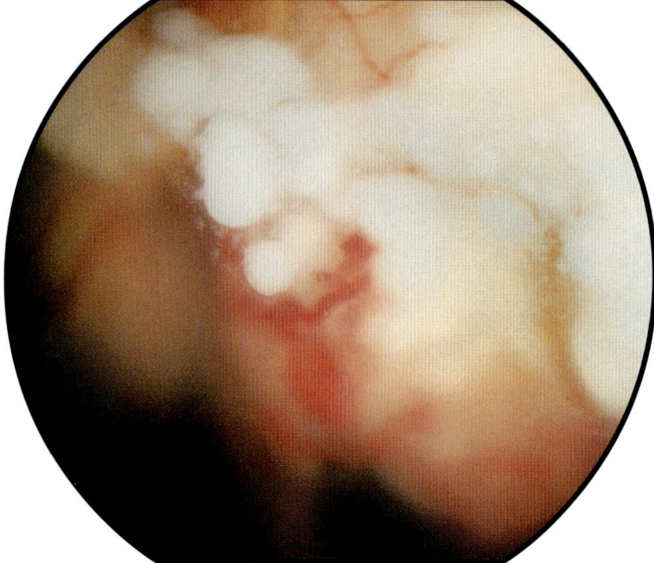

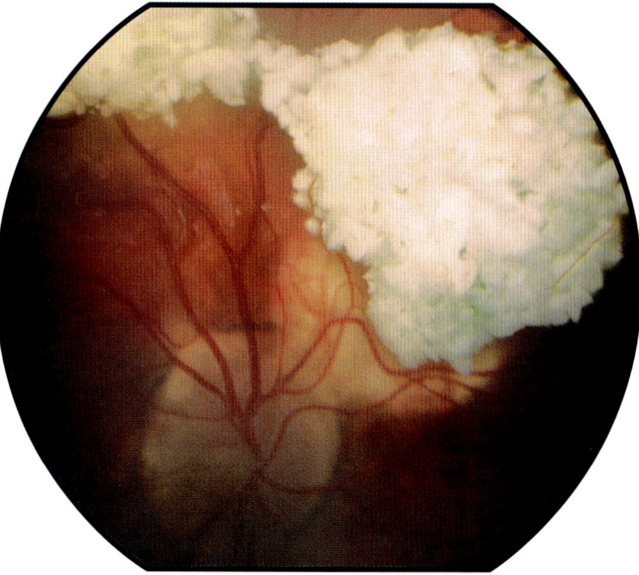

Following treatment, retinoblastoma demonstrates type III regression (*left image*) with calcified and noncalcified components. The right image shows type I regression with a completely calcified mass.

Retinoblastoma Diagnostic Testing

Patients with suspected retinoblastoma require a careful clinical history and examination and often a variety of ancillary diagnostic studies, such as fluorescein angiography, ultrasonography, optical coherence tomography (OCT), and MRI or CT scans.

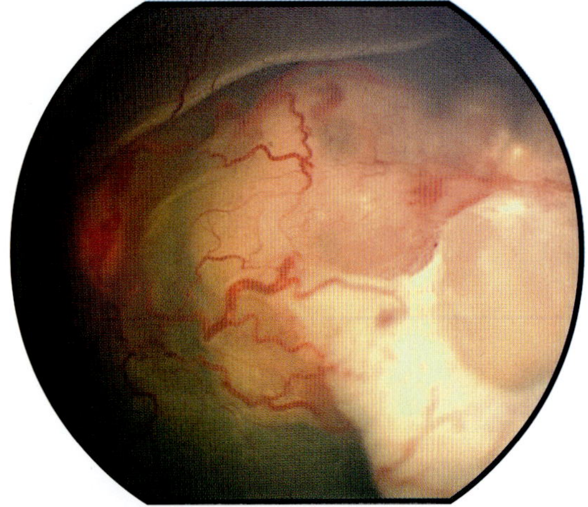

Exophytic retinoblastoma with retinal detachment.

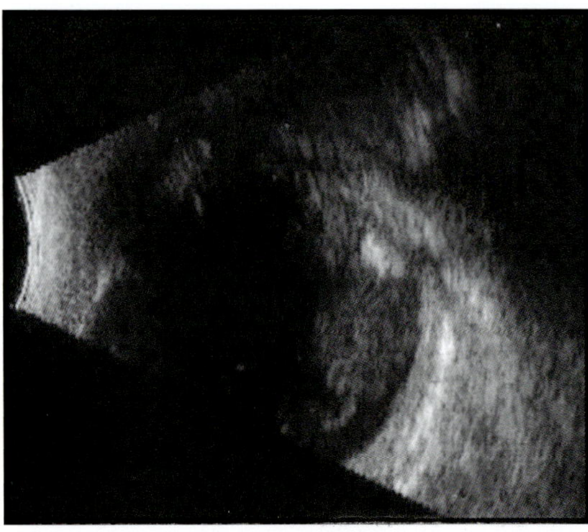

Ocular ultrasonography shows deep calcification and orbital shadowing of the retinoblastoma.

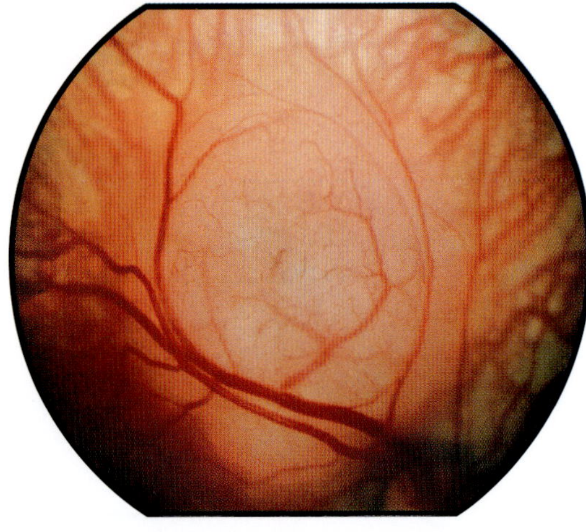

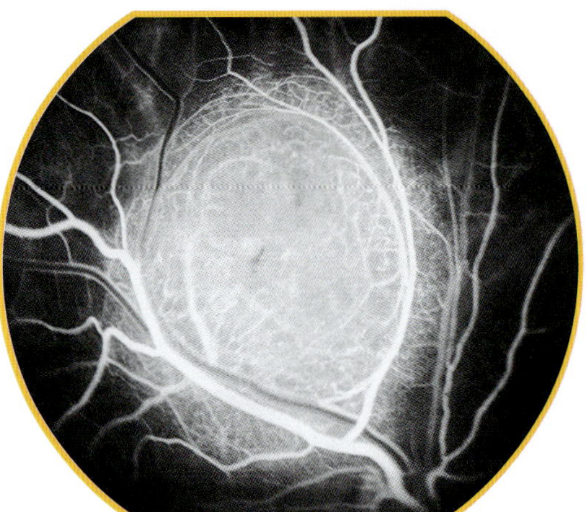

Retinoblastoma can sometimes be confined to the retina and subretinal space, as demonstrated in this 8-year-old white male. Hypervascularity of the tumor is demonstrated on the fluorescein angiogram (*right image*).

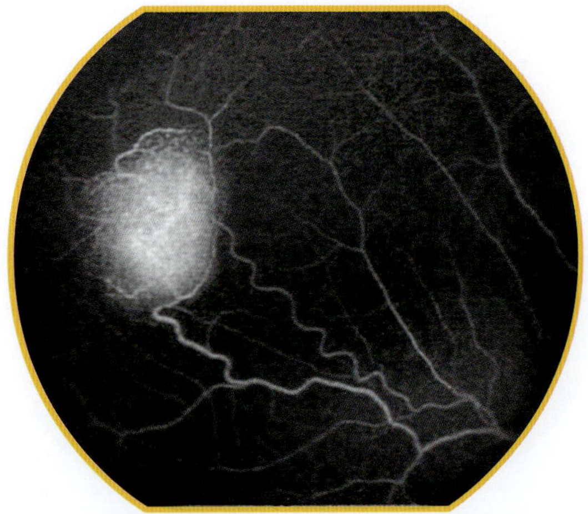

Another patient with hypervascularity on fluorescein angiography.

Retinoblastoma Features

Retinoblastoma features can be variable. There is often a delay in the diagnosis of retinoblastoma until the child reaches an experienced ophthalmologist. Approximately 20% of children with retinoblastoma display iris neovascularization. There is frequently subretinal and vitreous seeding and occasionally anterior chamber seeding.

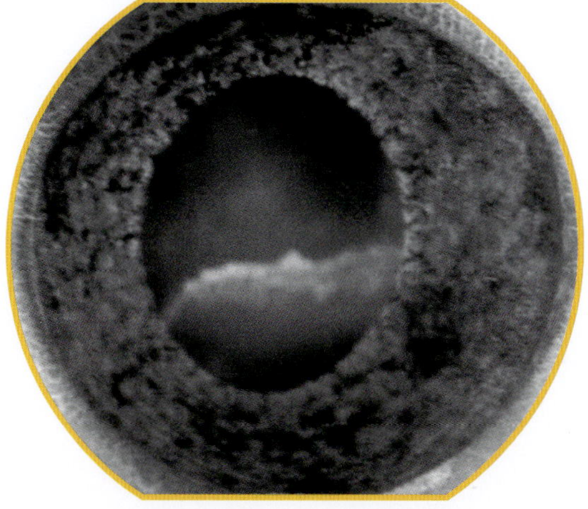

Fluorescein angiography of the iris show diffuse iris neovascularization in an eye with advanced retinoblastoma with total retinal detachment.

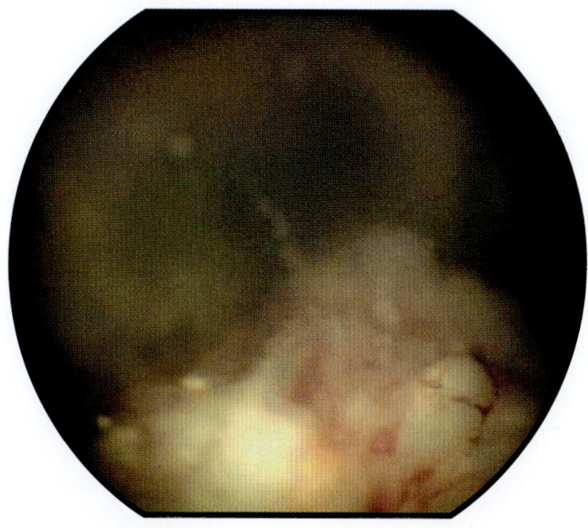

Endophytic growth pattern with mild vitreous hemorrhage can often resemble endophthalmitis.

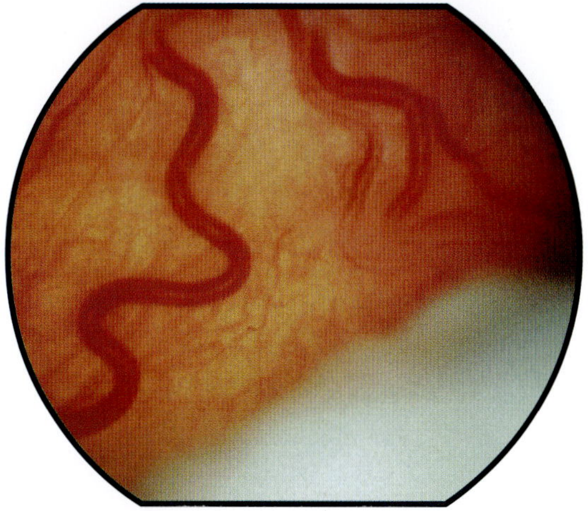

Retinoblastomas are generally fed by dilated, tortuous, retinal arterioles and drained by dilated venules.

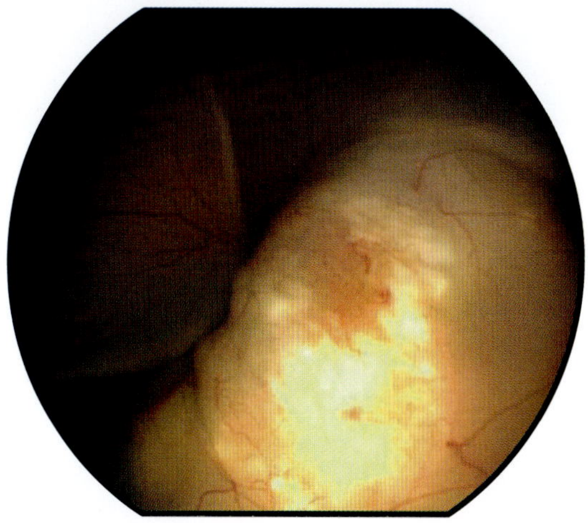

Exophytic growth pattern can also resemble Coats disease.

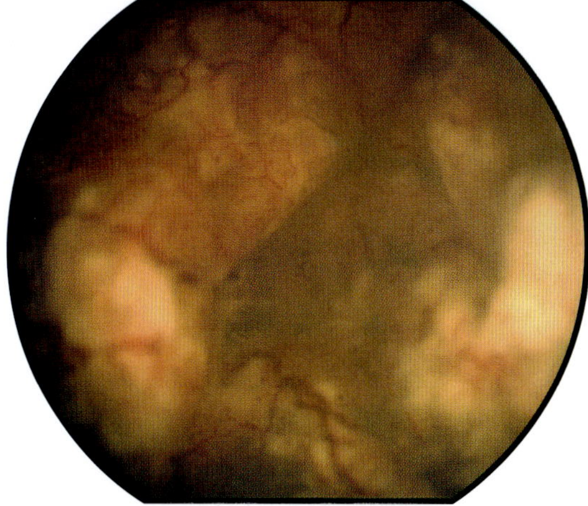

A diffuse growth pattern of retinoblastoma, may resemble acute inflammation or chronic uveitis.

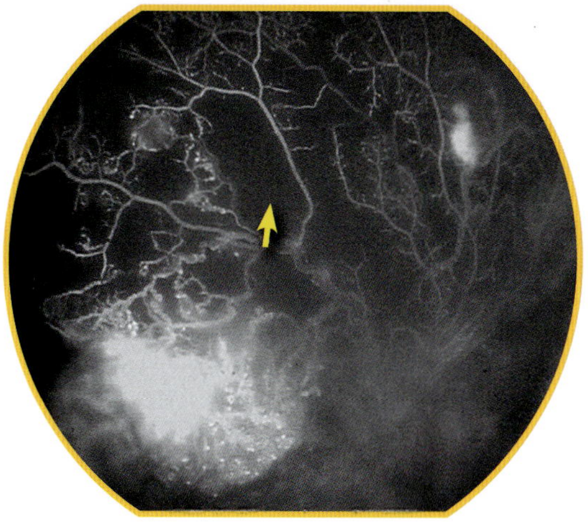

Diffuse growth pattern shows poor perfusion *(arrow)* at the site of intraretinal tumor on fluorescein angiography.

Regression of Retinoblastoma Following Plaque Radiotherapy

A retinoblastoma that is localized to approximately 18 mm or less in basal dimension and 10 mm or less in thickness is suitable for plaque radiotherapy. However, many of these eyes are first treated with chemotherapy with plaque radiotherapy being reserved for tumor recurrence. Properly designed and placed plaque radiotherapy can provide long-term tumor control in 95% of cases. Achieving this high control rate depends on proper tumor selection and precision in radiotherapy application.

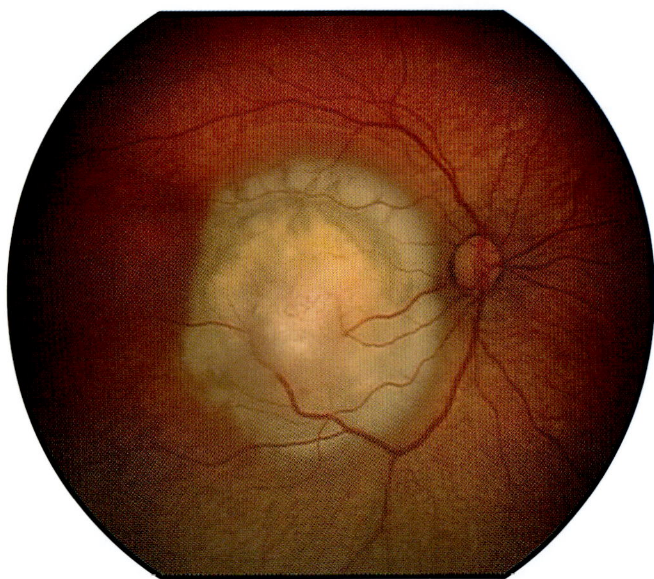

Retinoblastoma before plaque radiotherapy.

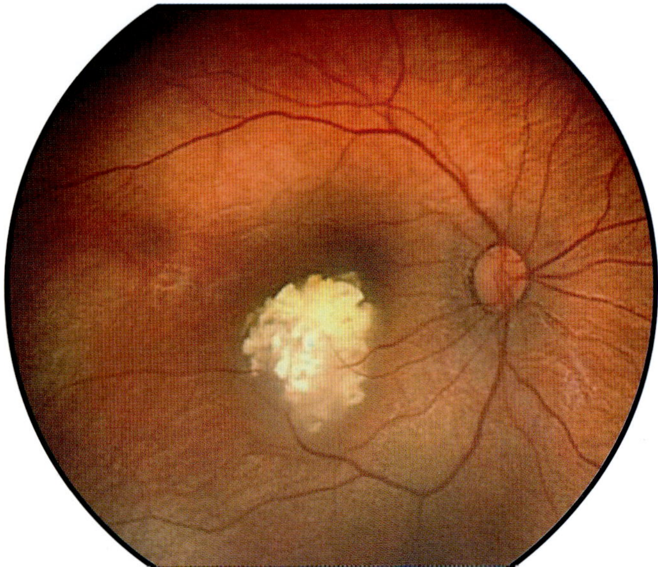

After plaque radiotherapy.

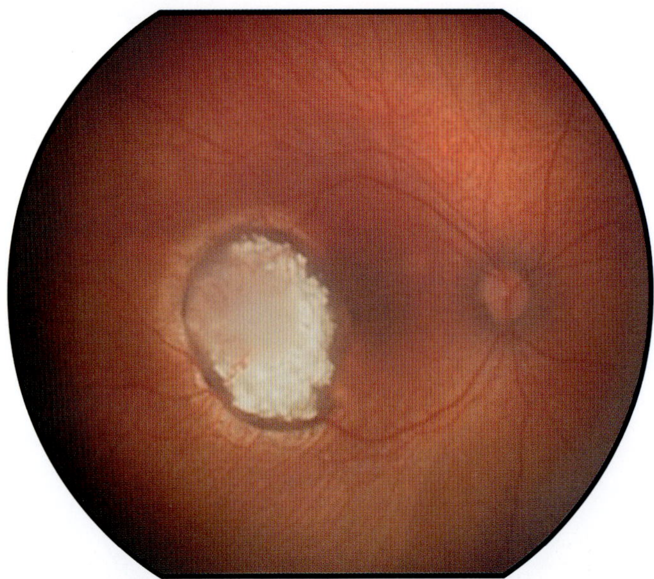

Gelatinous retinoblastoma recurrence after chemoreduction.

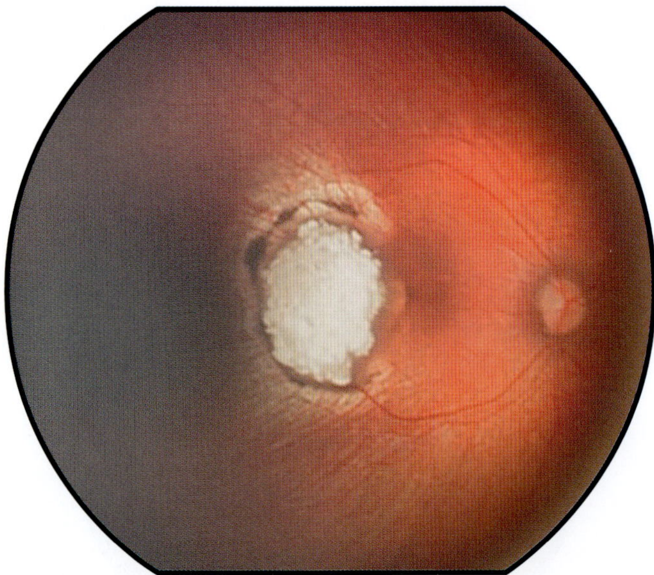

After plaque radiotherapy, tumor has regressed.

Regression of Retinoblastoma Following Intravenous Chemotherapy

Chemoreduction is a method of decreasing tumor size so that it can be treated with a more conservative method. Eyes that would have undergone enucleation or external-beam radiation in the past are now being managed successfully with chemoreduction, often in conjunction with definitive management such as radioactive plaques, thermal therapy, or cryotherapy. Based on the International Classification of Retinoblastoma, this therapy is successful with avoidance of enucleation and external beam radiotherapy in eyes with Group A (100%), Group B (93%), Group C (90%), Group D (47%), and Group E (23%) disease. Addition of intra-arterial chemotherapy and/or intravitreal chemotherapy has increased salvage of Groups D and E eyes.

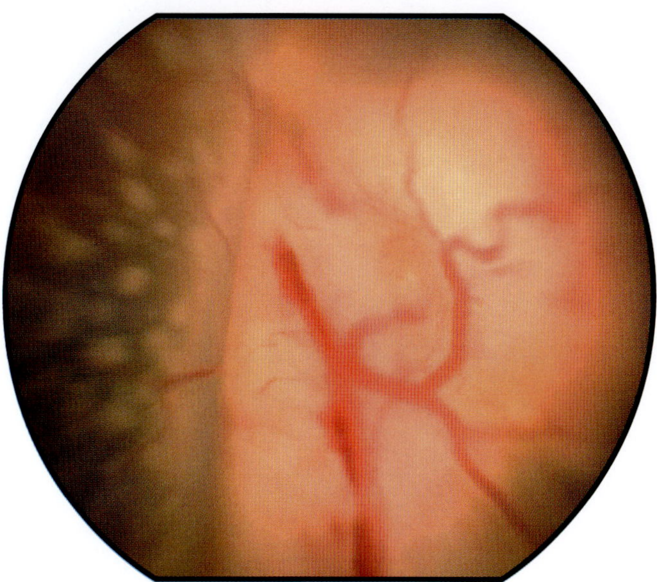

Retinoblastoma (Group E) before chemoreduction.

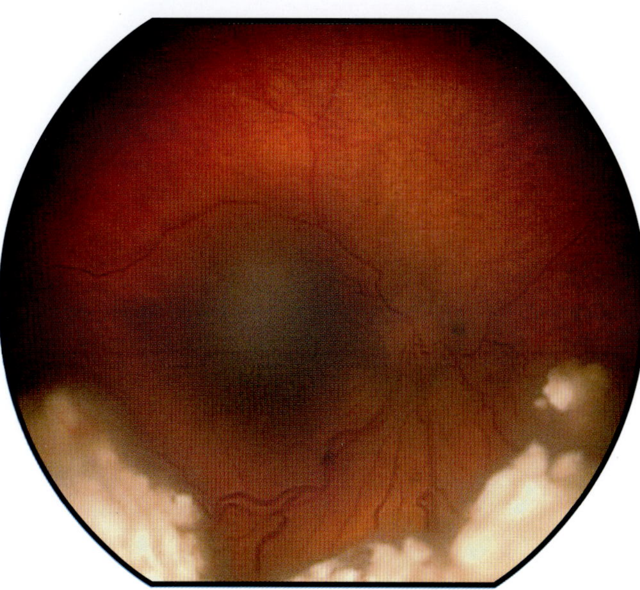

After chemoreduction there is tumor regression with macular sparing.

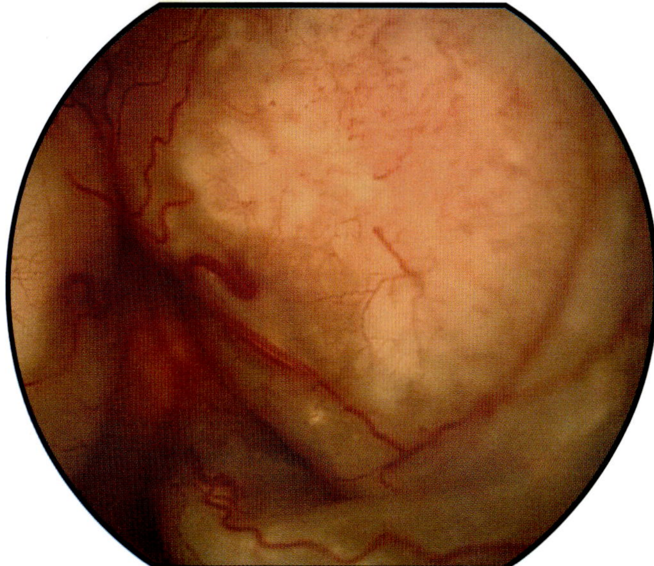

Retinoblastoma (Group D) with a massive tumor before chemoreduction.

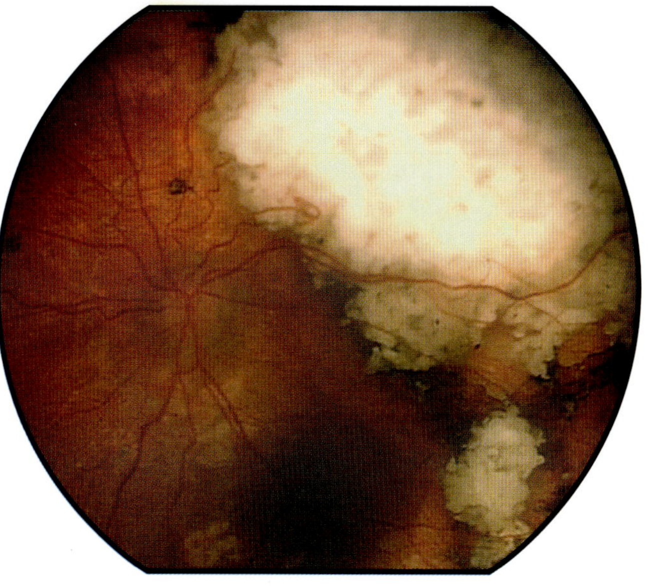

After chemoreduction, there is tumor regression and marked calcification in the macula.

Regression of Retinoblastoma Following Intra-arterial Chemotherapy

Retinoblastoma can be managed with targeted intra-arterial chemotherapy using a neurosurgical technique of ophthalmic artery catheterization with injection of a tiny dose of melphalan, topotecan, and/or carboplatin. The results are impressive. In general, 3 to 5 sessions are necessary for tumor control, but some eyes respond completely to 1 or 2 sessions. This therapy can be toxic to the retinal vasculature with immediate or incipient sclerosis of vessels, leading to vision loss.

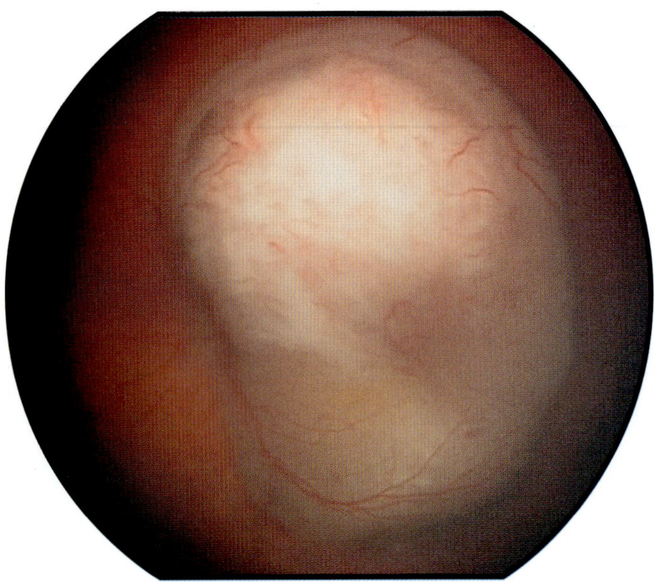

Retinoblastoma (Group C) before intra-arterial chemotherapy.

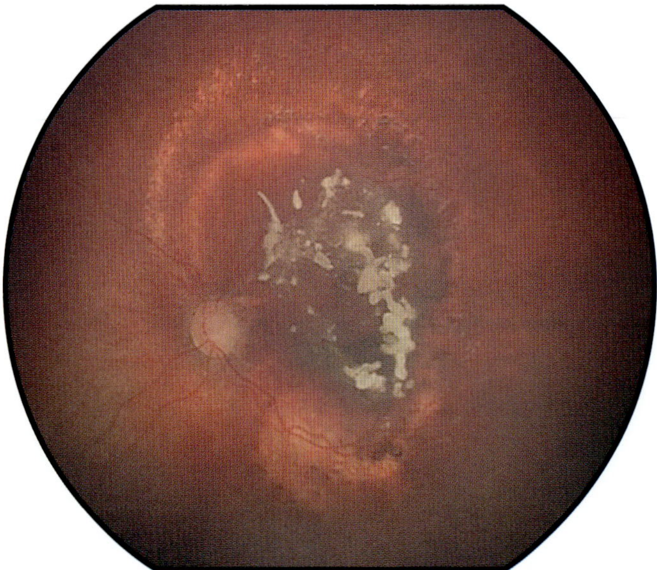

After 2 cycles of intra-arterial chemotherapy using melphalan there is complete tumor regression.

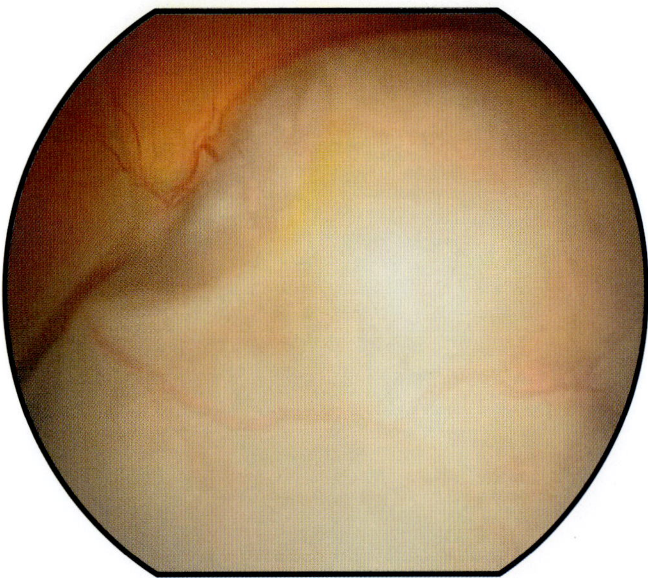

Retinoblastoma (Group D) before intra-arterial chemotherapy.

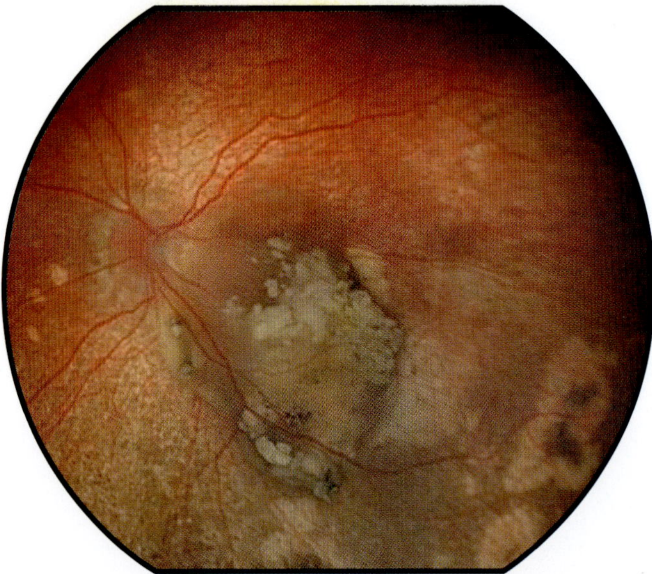

After 3 cycles of intra-arterial chemotherapy using melphalan there is complete tumor regression and surrounding retinal pigment epithelial alterations.

Management of Retinoblastoma with Enucleation

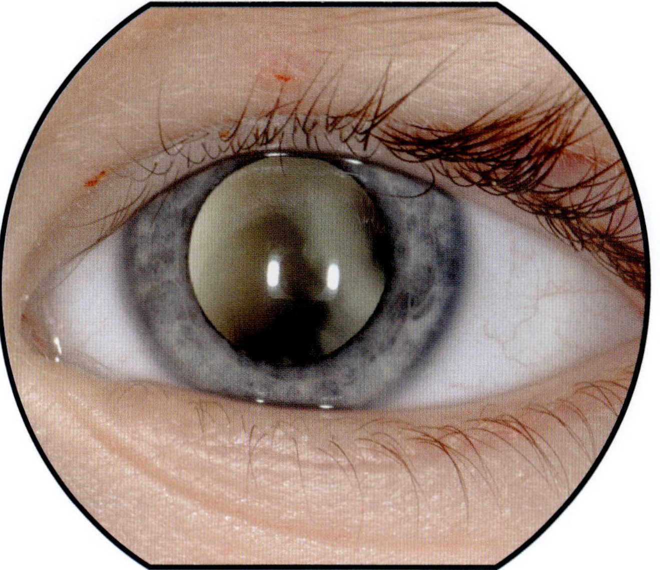

Unilateral leukocoria from retinoblastoma.

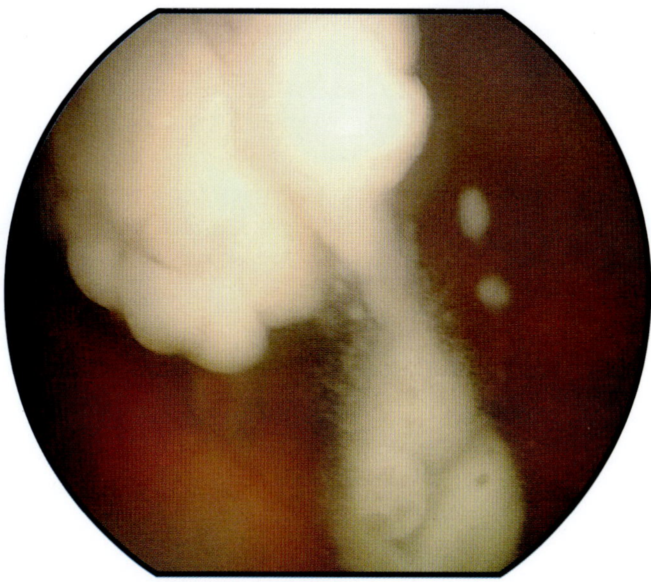

Large endophytic Group D unilateral sporadic retinoblastoma with extensive vitreous seeding.

Gross pathology *(right)* shows the white retinal tumor with extensive vitreous seeding.

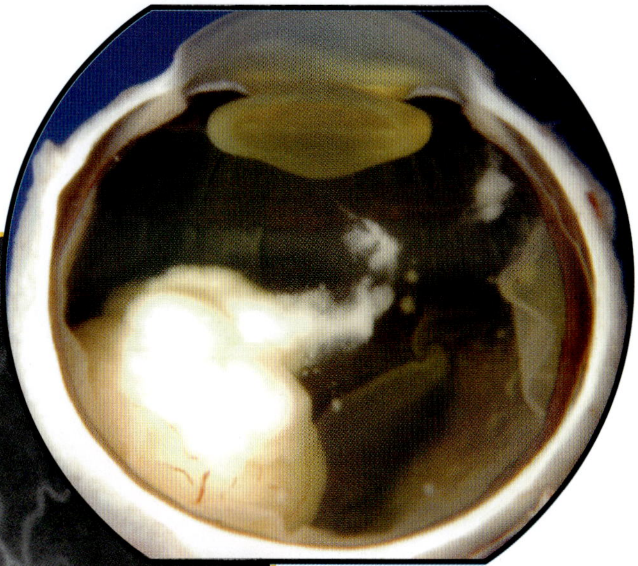

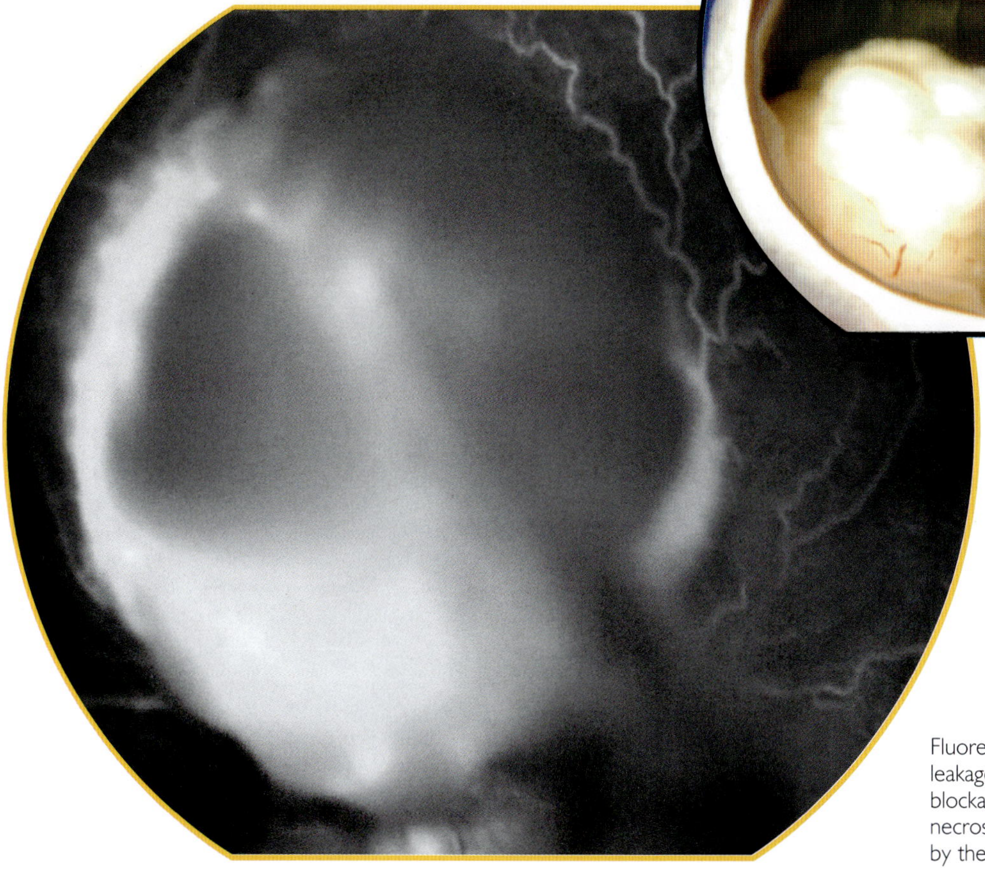

Fluorescein angiography shows vascular leakage within the malignancy and encircling blockage from overlying seeding and tumor necrosis. Retinal vessels have been infiltrated by the tumor mass.

Retinoblastoma Pathology

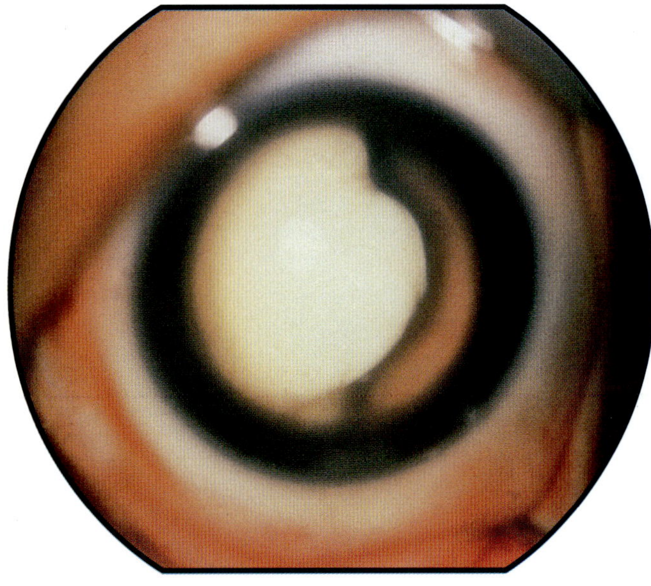

Transpupillary examination reveals a white fundus lesion.

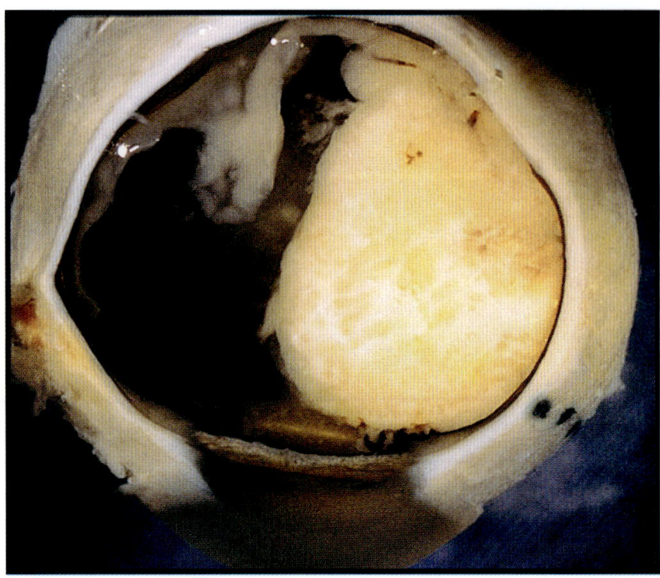

Following enucleation, sectioned globe showed retinoblastoma.

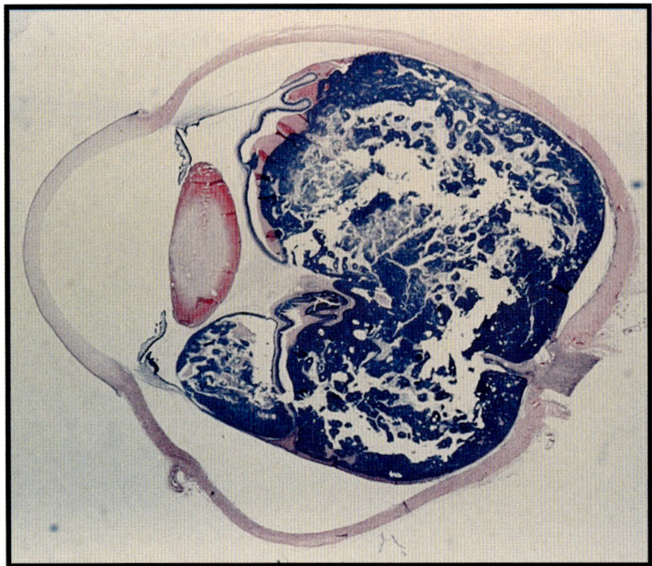

Low-power microscopy shows that retinoblastoma filled most of the intraocular contents. *Courtesy of Dr. Irene Maumenee*

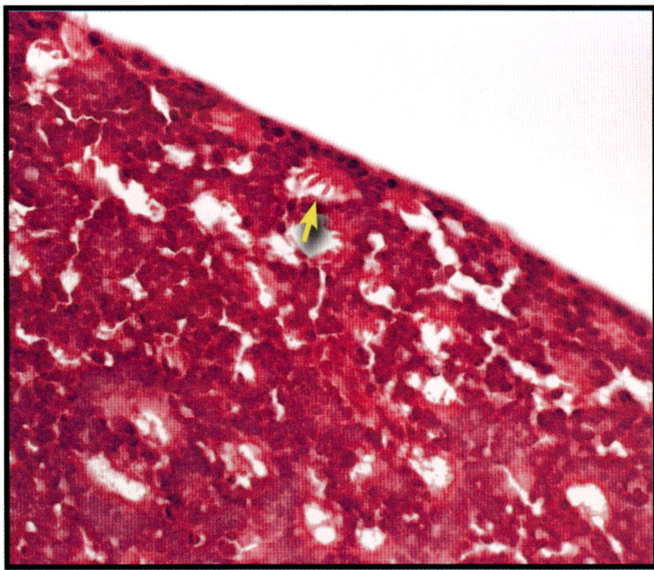

Flexner–Wintersteiner rosettes and fleurettes *(arrow)* are present. They are characteristic of retinoblastoma, but occasionally they are seen in other ophthalmic tumors such as medulloepithelioma. The fleurette is slightly eosinophilic and composed of tumor cells with pear-shaped eosinophilic processes that project through a fenestrated membrane.

Retinoblastoma Pathology—High Risk for Metastasis

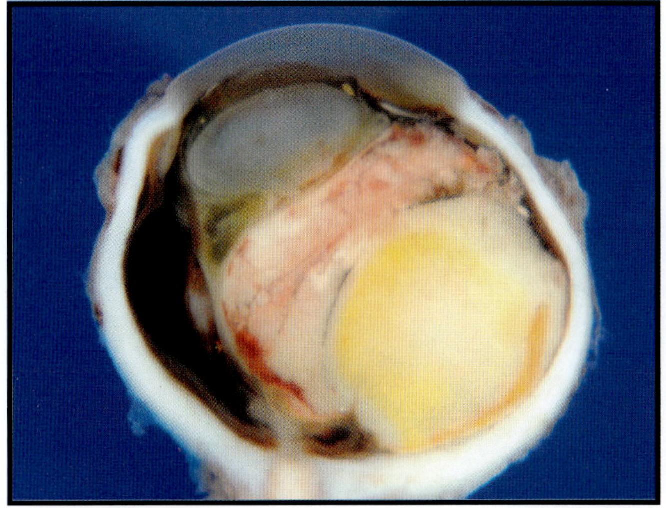

Enucleated globe from a child with retinoblastoma and suspected choroidal invasion.

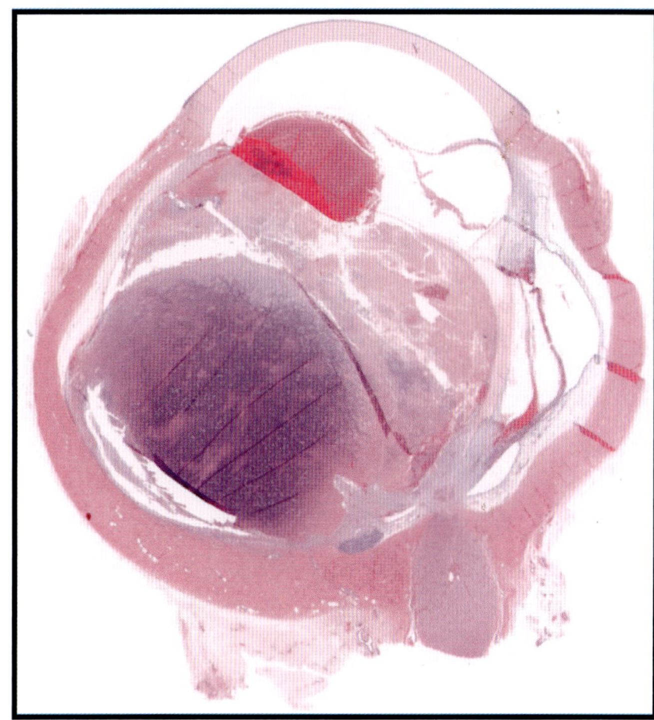

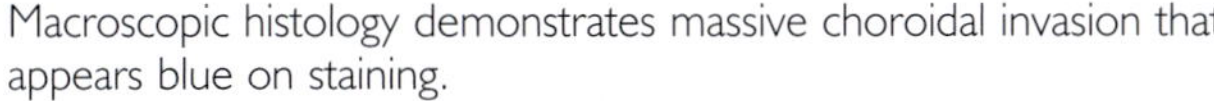

Macroscopic histology demonstrates massive choroidal invasion that appears blue on staining.

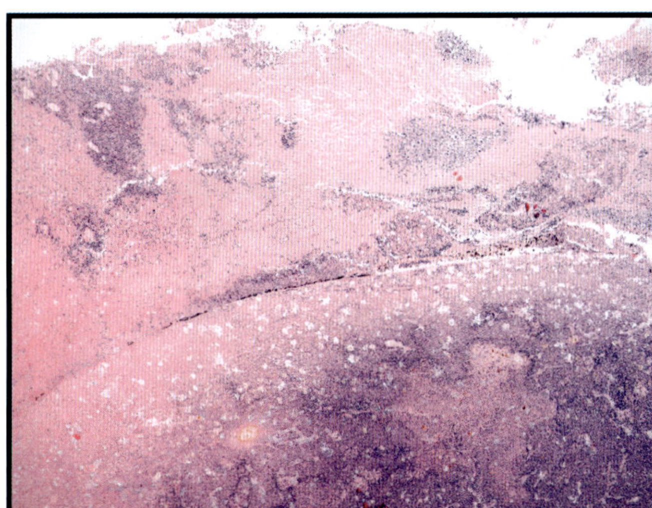

Necrotic retinoblastoma with residual tumor in retina and massive, partially necrotic tumor deep to Bruch membrane, seen as a dark line running horizontally through the specimen.

Teratoma

Congenital intraocular teratoma may be seen in an otherwise healthy, full-term newborn, and may be associated with additional cystic tumors involving other parts of the body. The large amorphous mass or masses in the fundus can resemble a retinoblastoma. The lesion may be associated with minimal angiographic change and there are cystic changes on B-scan ultrasonography, findings that are not typical of retinoblastoma.

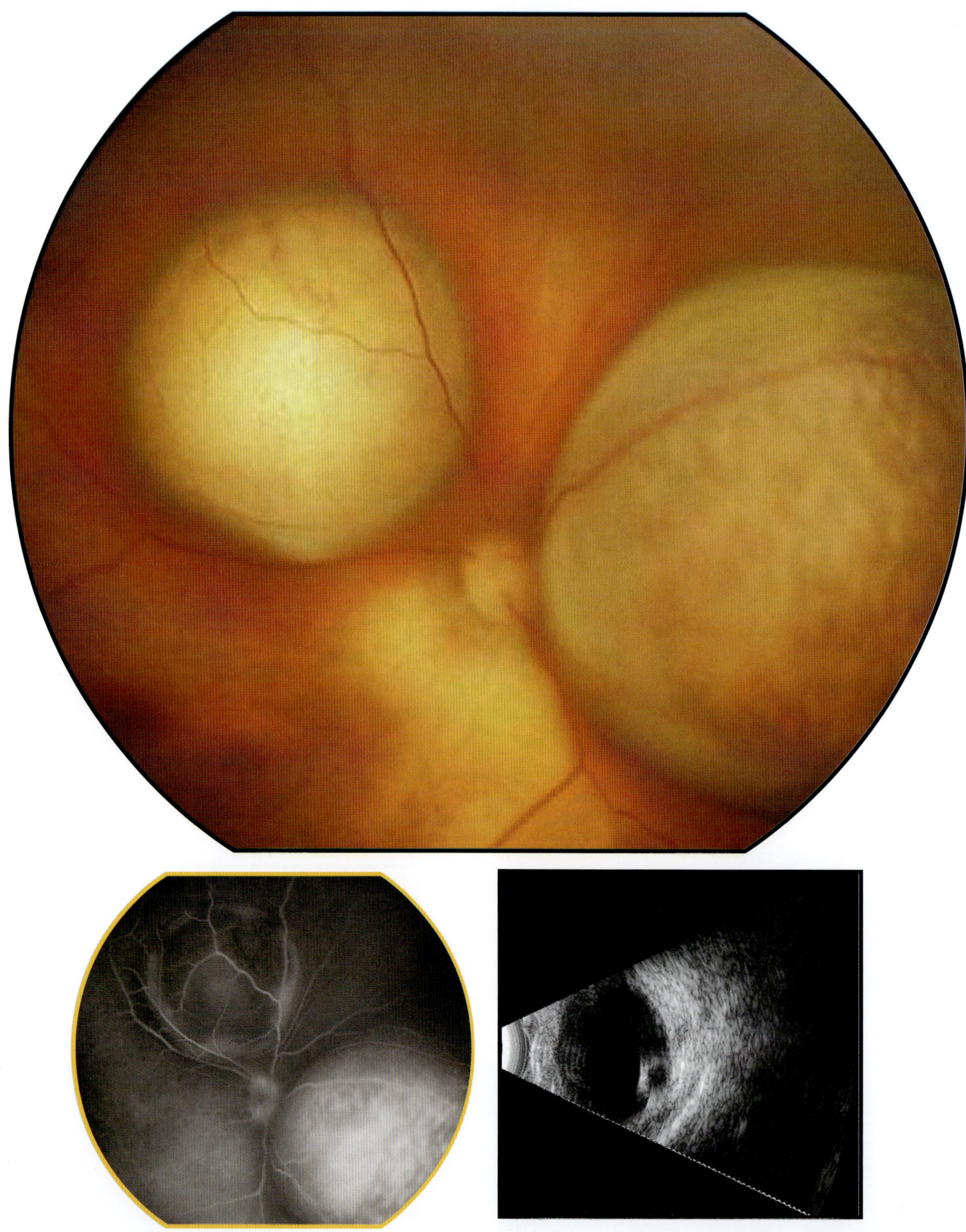

This child had two large dome-shaped cystic masses that resembled a retinoblastoma. The fluorescein angiogram shows minimal retinal vascular alterations. The cystic nature is evident with B-scan ultrasonography. The patient also had a sacral teratoma. *Courtesy of Dr. David Abramson*

Klippel–Trenaunay–Weber Syndrome

Klippel–Trenaunay–Weber syndrome is a rare congenital abnormality of blood vessels and soft tissue. Malformations of the skin and abnormalities of the venous system, lymphatic system, and limbs due to hypertrophy of soft tissue and bone may be seen in this disorder. Ocular vascular abnormalities may be seen, including port-wine stains (nevus flammeus), diffuse choroidal hemangioma, and retinal vascular malformations.

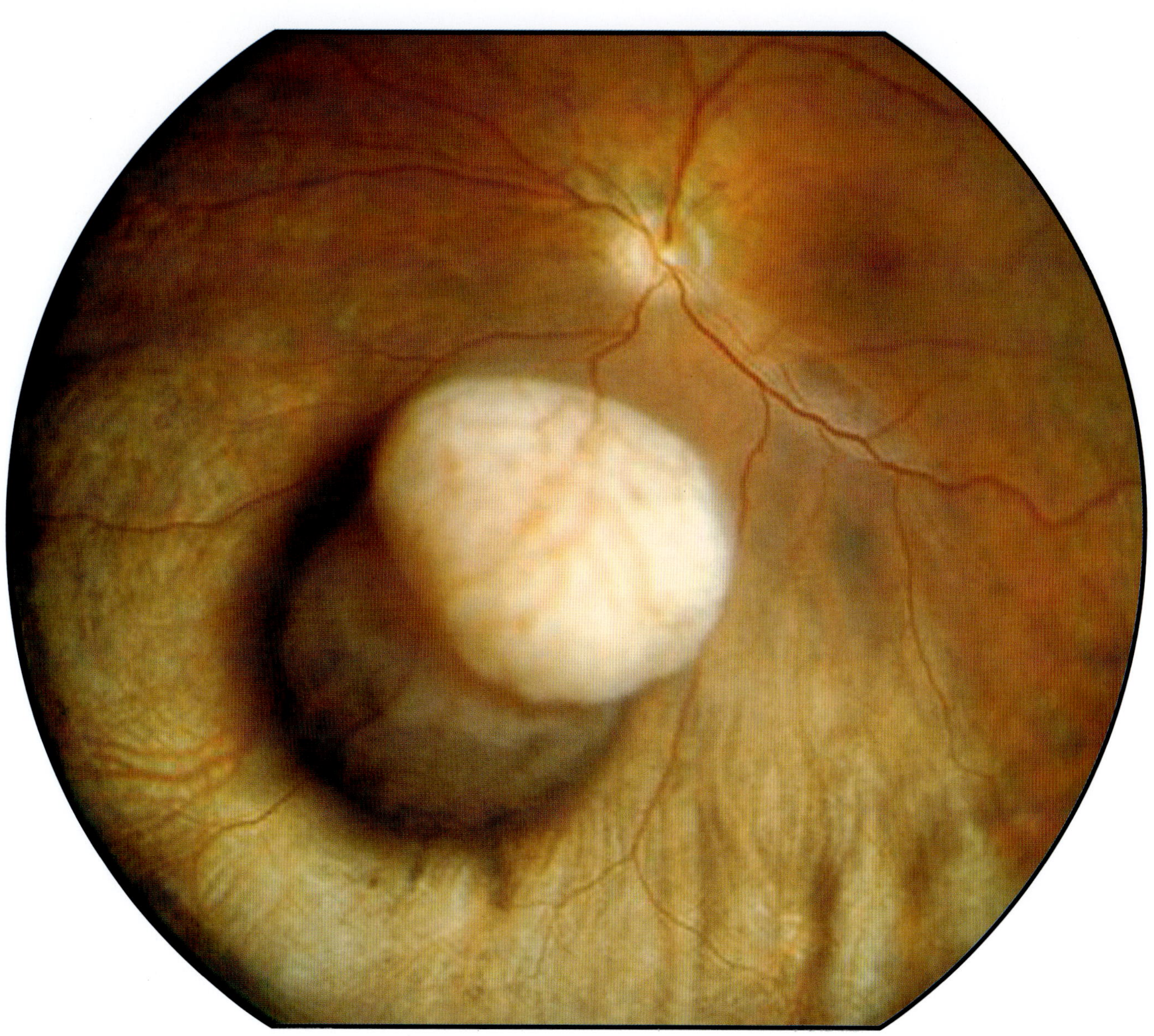

In this patient with Klippel–Trenaunay–Weber syndrome, there was a malignant melanoma. The base is melanotic whereas the mushroom-like extension into the vitreous is amelanotic. Retinal vascular tortuosity and diffuse choroidal hemangioma are more common fundus abnormalities seen in this entity.

Medulloepithelioma

Medulloepithelioma is a congenital tumor that arises from the nonpigmented ciliary epithelium. It can be benign or malignant. It grows slowly in the first few years of life and manifests around age 4 years as a visible mass. Related features include lens coloboma, neovascularization of the iris, and secondary glaucoma. A small medulloepithelioma in the ciliary body is usually asymptomatic and difficult to detect clinically. A larger lesion appears as an amelanotic white-to-pink, often cystic, mass that may be associated with subluxation of the lens.

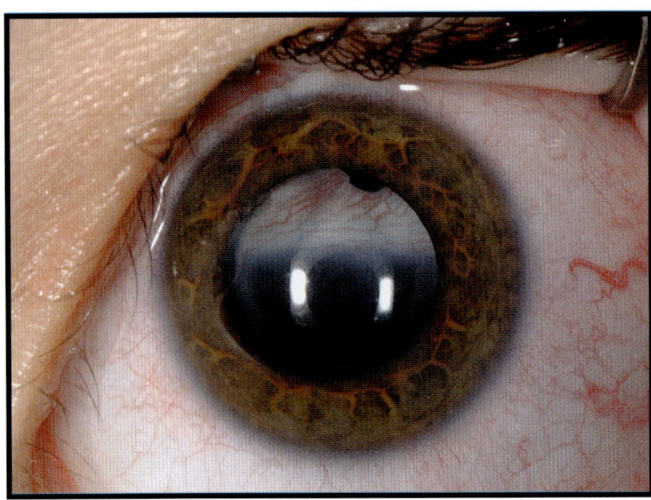

Medulloepithelioma of the nonpigmented ciliary epithelium with a vascular cyclitic membrane. The white ciliary body mass with prominent intrinsic vascularity is noted superiorly behind the clear lens.

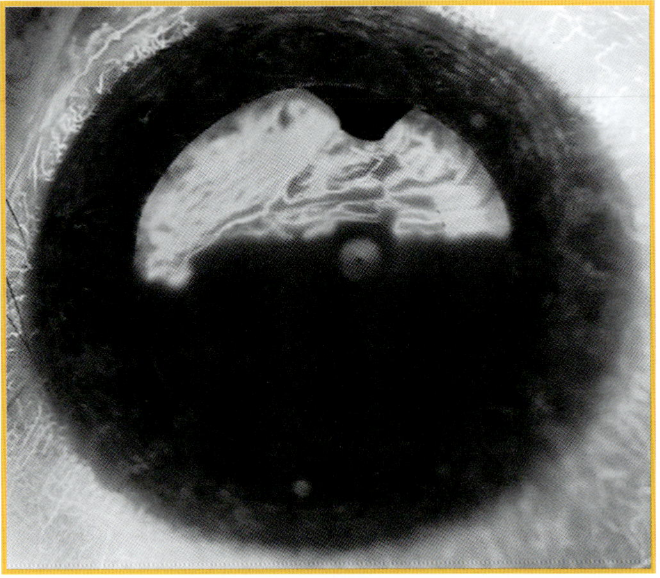

Fluorescein angiography confirms the tumor vascularity. Blockage by dragged pigment epithelium superiorly is visible.

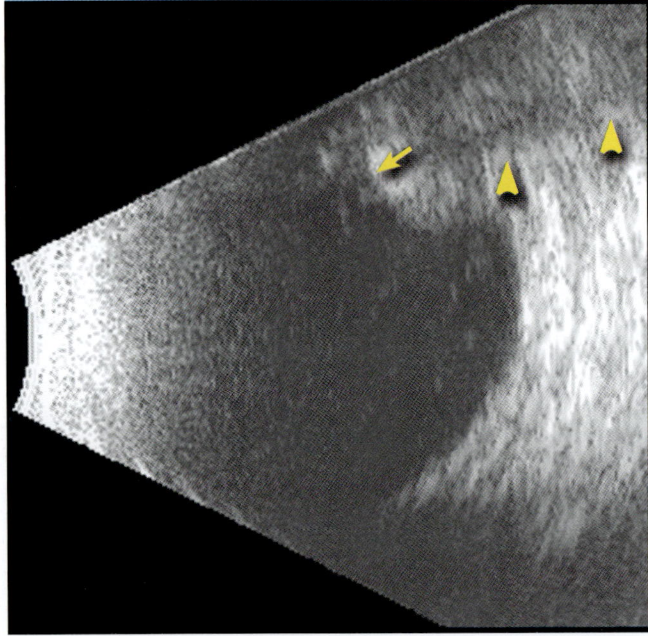

Ocular ultrasonography shows the ciliary body with highly reflective echoes in its apex *(arrow)* and deep shadowing *(arrowheads)*.

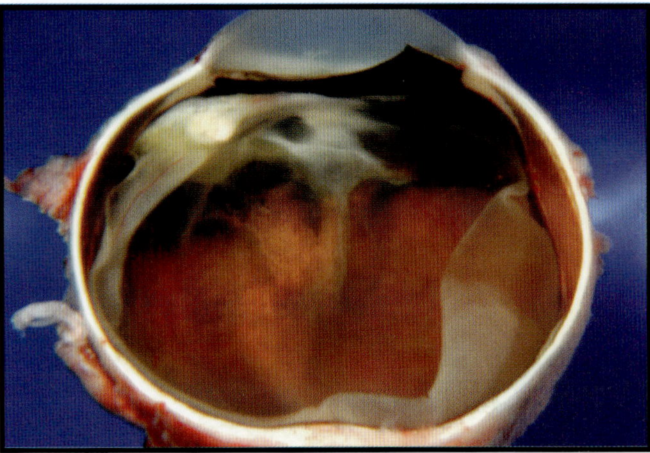

Following enucleation, the medulloepithelioma with fibrosis is seen. Note the extensive tumor growth along the hyaloid interface anteriorly behind the lens and posteriorly along the retina.

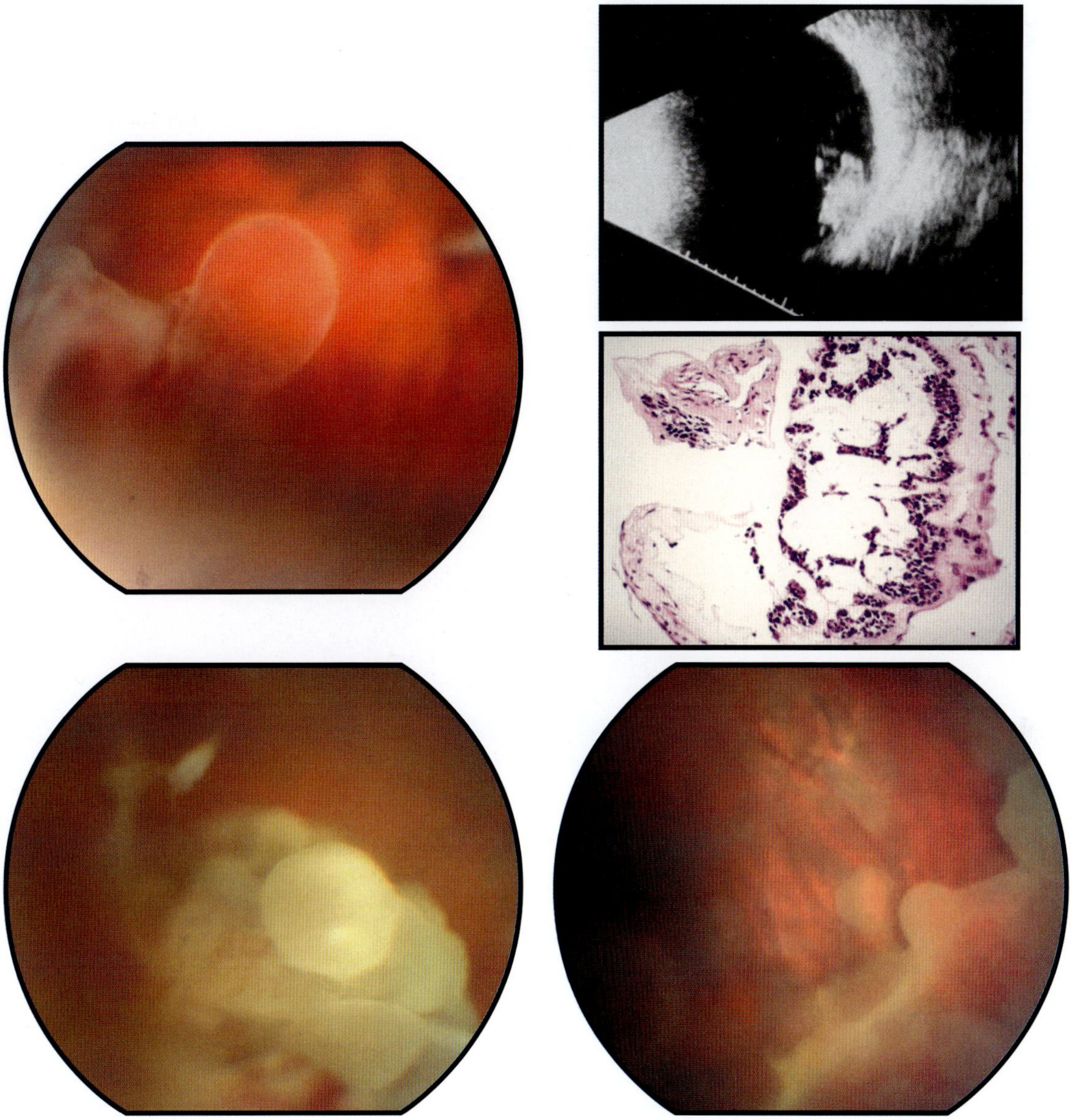

This is a 28-year-old female who complained of floaters. The peripheral fundus examination showed polycystic changes in the vitreous. Ultrasonography showed high reflectance of the mass with reactive changes in surrounding vitreous. The pathology showed medulloepithelioma. Histologically there were multilayered sheaths and cords of poorly differentiated neuroepithelial cells that appeared similar to embryonic retina and ciliary epithelium.

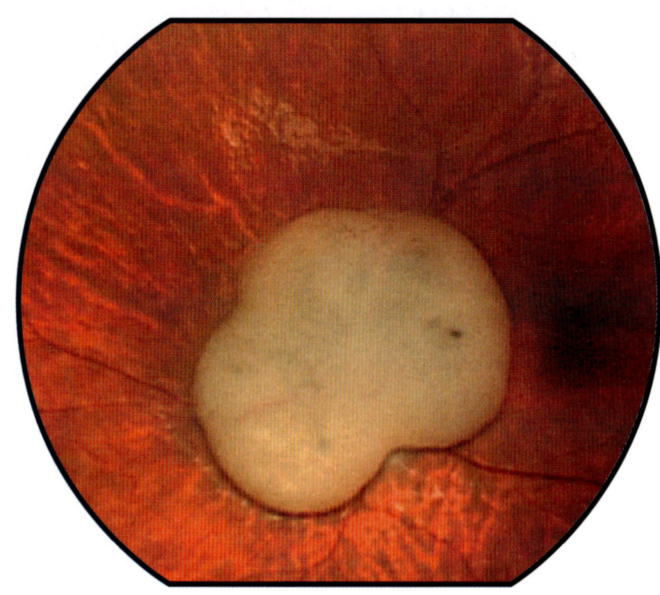

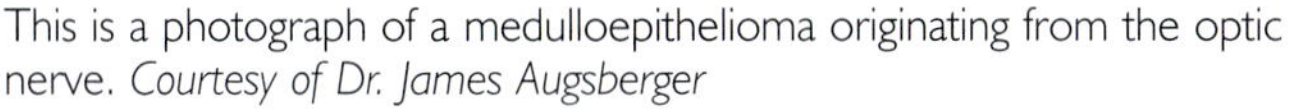

This is a photograph of a medulloepithelioma originating from the optic nerve. *Courtesy of Dr. James Augsberger*

Retinal Astrocytic Hamartoma

Retinal astrocytic hamartoma is a tumor of glial origin and can be found in patients with tuberous sclerosis or neurofibromatosis. In some instances it occurs as a sporadic condition. Astrocytic hamartoma tends to develop in the nerve fiber layer and can cause slight traction with minimal if any dilation of the retinal vessels. Small retinal astrocytic hamartomas can be extremely subtle, appearing as an ill-defined translucent thickening of the nerve fiber layer. Slightly larger tumors become more opaque and appear as sessile white lesions at the level of the nerve fiber layer of the retina. The lesion often contains characteristic dense yellow, refractile calcification that resembles fish eggs or tapioca.

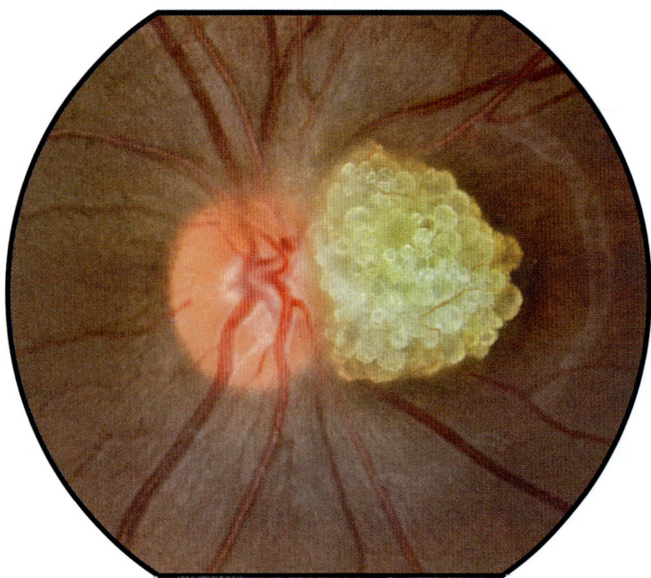

Astrocytic hamartoma touching the optic disc with calcified nodules.

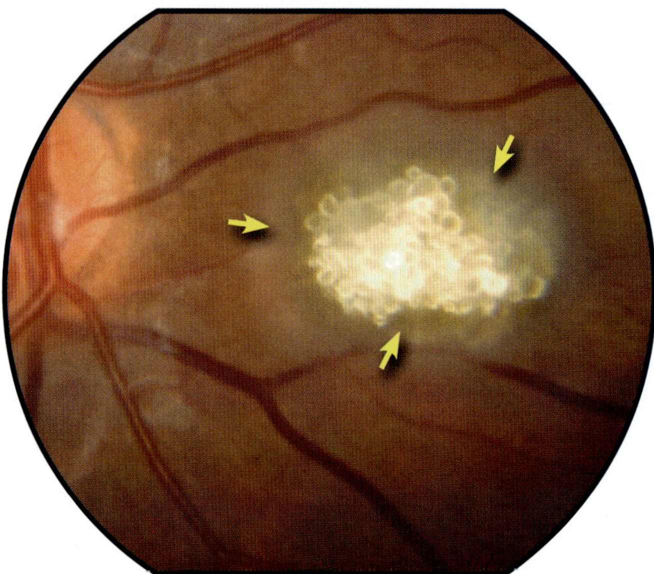

Astrocytic hamartoma with central calcified and peripheral noncalcified zones *(arrows)*.

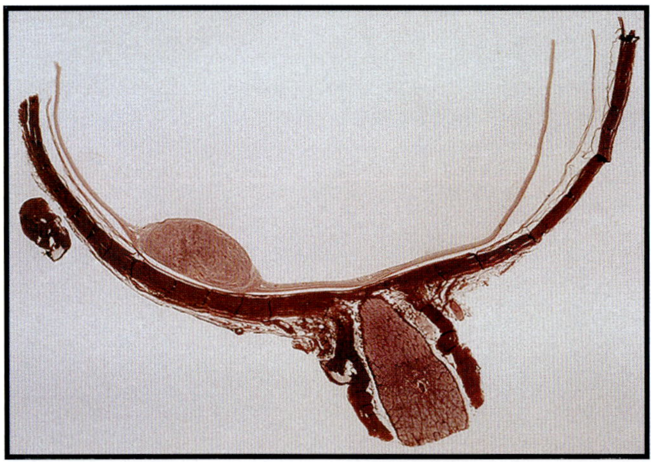

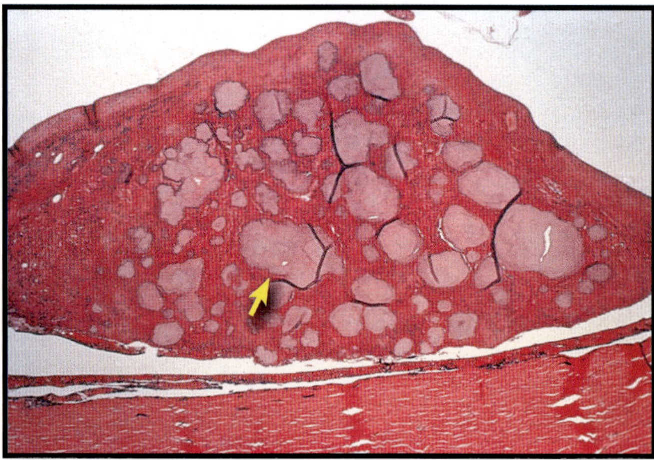

Gross macroscopic appearance of an enucleated specimen is shown in the left image. Histopathologically, the typical noncalcified retinal astrocytic hamartoma appears as a slightly eosinophilic lesion, arising from the nerve fiber layer of the retina. It is composed of well-differentiated, elongated fibrous astrocytes with lightly eosinophilic cytoplasm and round-to-oval nuclei. When calcified, spindle-shaped cells are seen within areas of calcification *(arrow, right image)*. The more calcified tumors show fossilization and peculiar round, basophilic laminated changes resembling corpora arenacea. *Courtesy of Dr. Sergio Cunha*

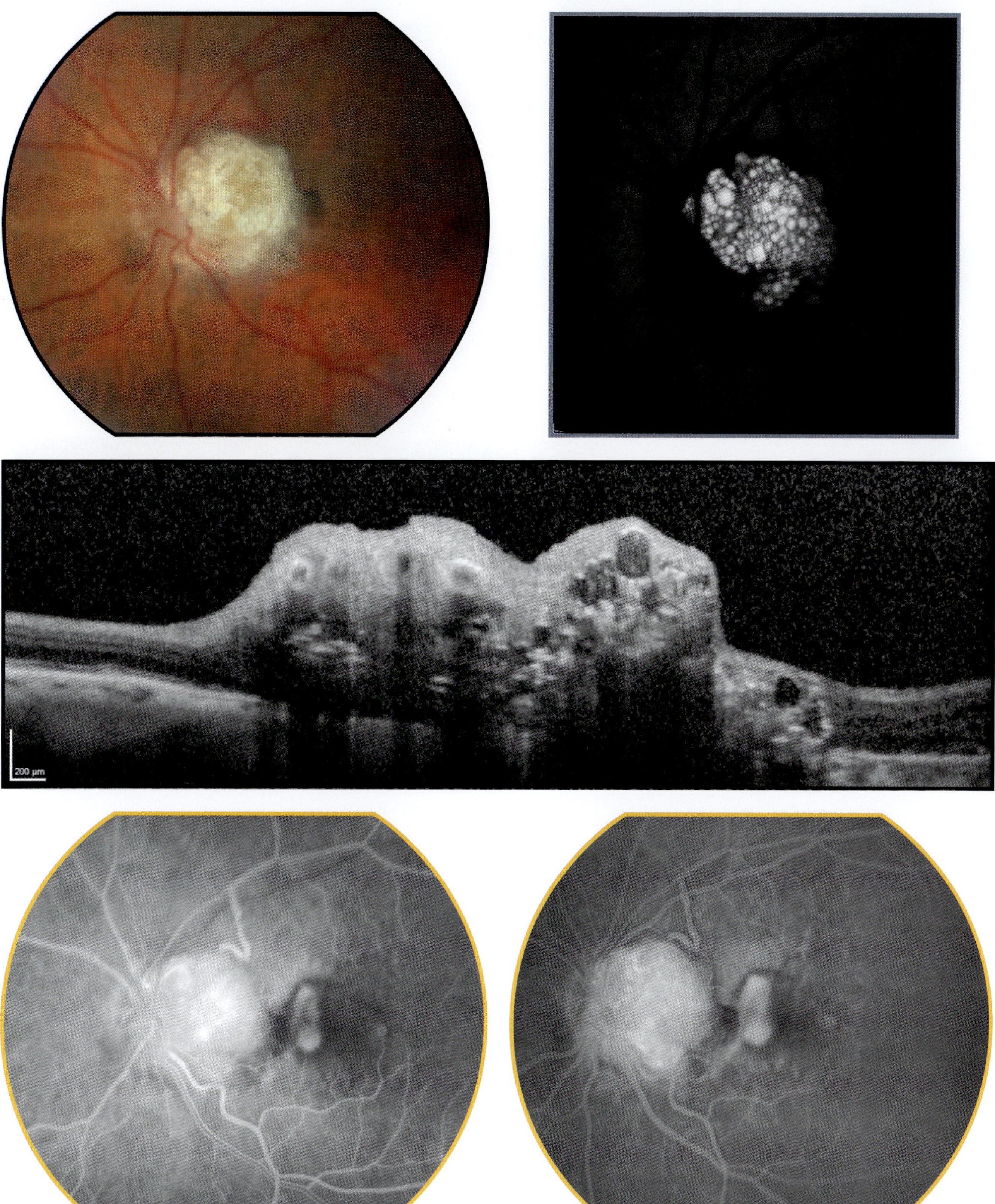

Calcified astrocytic hamartoma of the optic nerve head in an 87-year-old female. Prominent hyper-autofluorescence is seen within the lesion *(top right panel)*. Spectral domain OCT through the lesion demonstrates transition from normal retina to a hyper-reflective intraretinal mass with loss of anatomical organization and posterior optical shadowing. Note the "moth eaten" optically empty spaces representing calcification. This patient developed type 2 neovascularization at the temporal edge of the tumor as seen on fluorescein angiography. Choroidal neovascularization is rarely associated with astrocytic hamartoma.

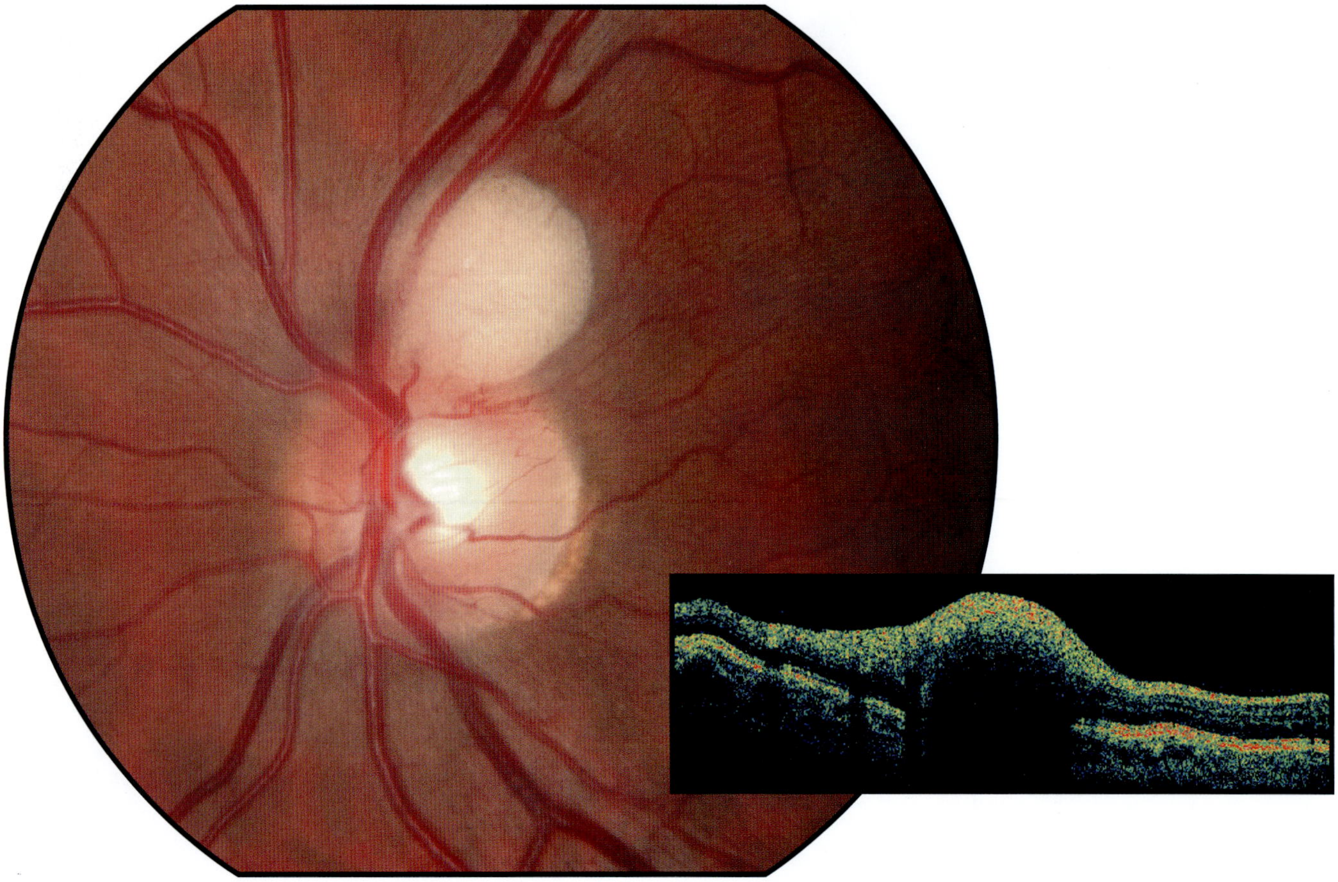

Noncalcified retinal astrocytic hamartoma in a 38-year-old male. The mass involves the nerve fiber layer and overrides retinal vessels. Time domain OCT shows transition from normal retina to a dense intraretinal mass with loss of retinal organization. There is an absence of the "moth eaten" appearance on OCT that is seen with calcified lesions.

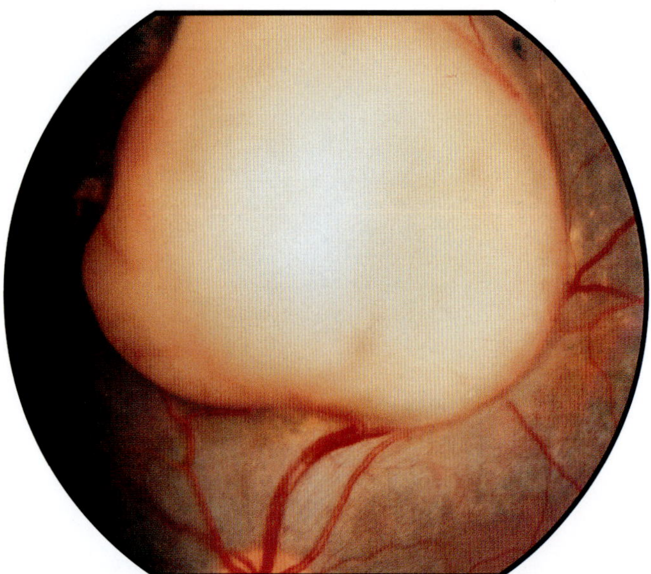

An astrocytic hamartoma can occur as an isolated lesion in a patient without tuberous sclerosis. This elevated, white–yellow mass was arising from the retina without calcification. *Courtesy of Dr. Sergio Cunha*

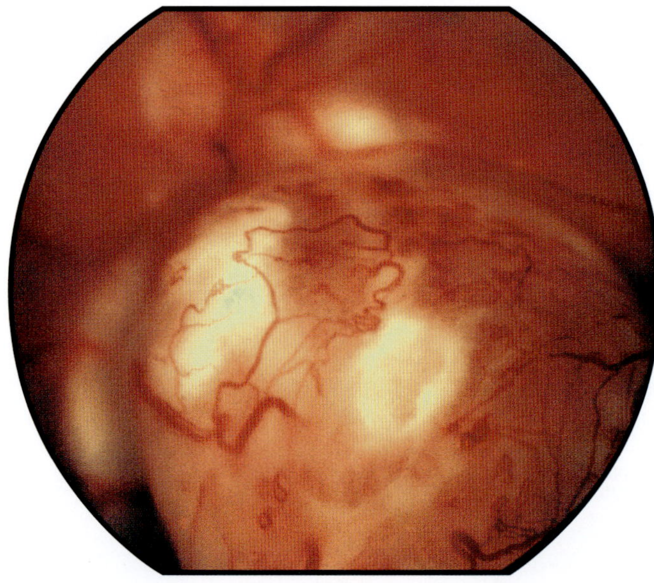

This patient did not have tuberous sclerosis and manifested a white–yellow vascular retinal mass. Histopathology revealed astrocytic hamartoma. *Courtesy of Dr. Robert Ramsay*

Acquired Retinal Astrocytoma

Retinal astrocytoma is an acquired tumor that presents in mid-life or younger, classically in the peripapillary or perimacular region. This form of glial tumor is not related to tuberous sclerosis complex. In contrast to the retina astrocytic hamartoma, this tumor is not typically calcified and it behaves in a more aggressive fashion, demonstrating progressive enlargement, exudation, and retinal detachment, occasionally leading to loss of the eye. Retinal astrocytoma can produce vitreous seeding.

Management of acquired retinal astrocytoma can be difficult as this tumor can be resistant to treatment. Several reports have documented success with the application of 1 or 2 treatments of verteporfin photodynamic therapy. Additionally, plaque radiotherapy can be beneficial in some cases.

Retinal astrocytoma with extensive localized vitreous seeding and prominent feeding vessels.

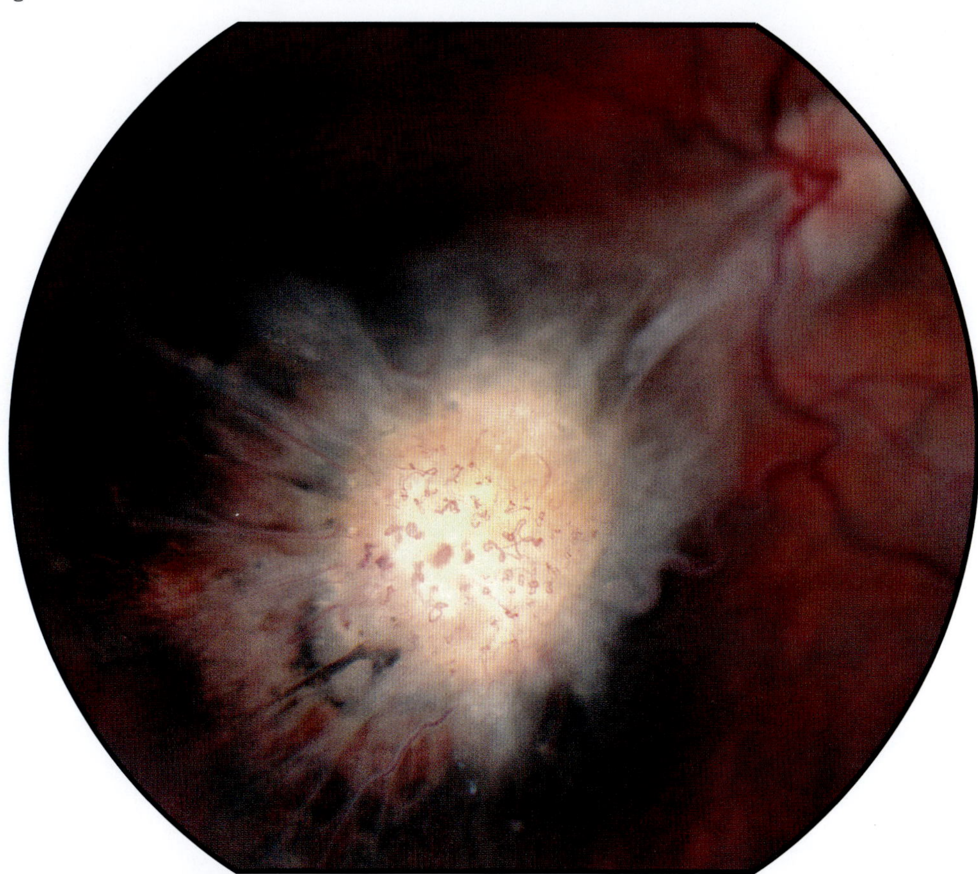

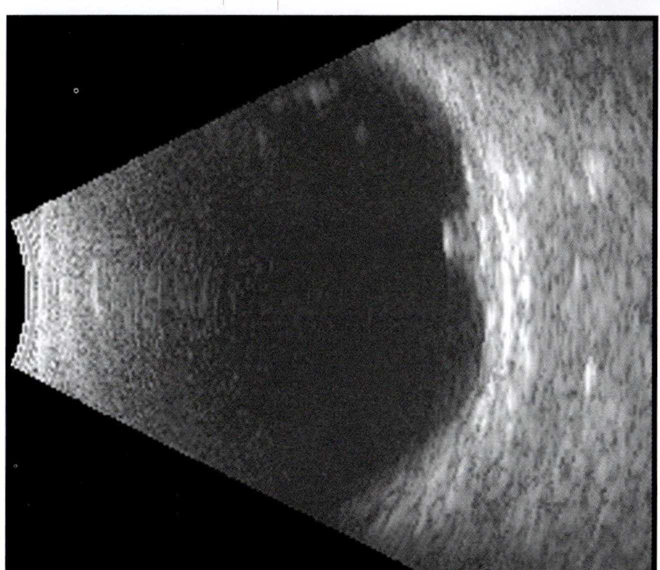

Ultrasonography reveals a noncalcified retinal mass.

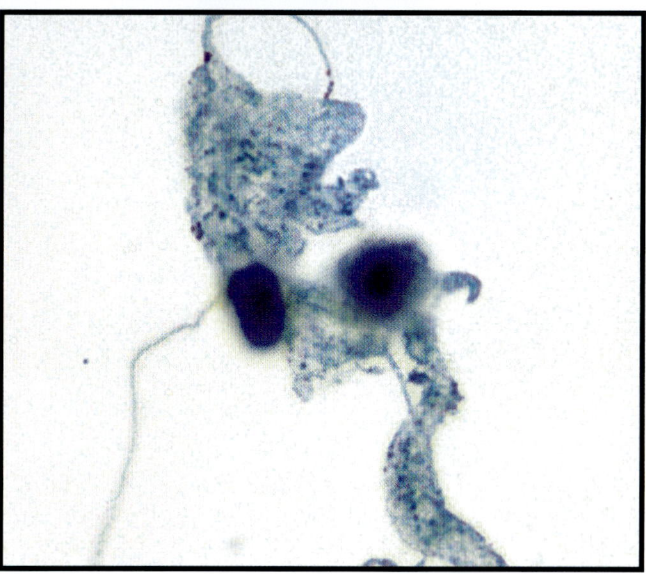

Cytopathology from fine-needle aspiration biopsy shows benign, spindle shaped glial cells, consistent with astrocytoma.

Retinal Acquired Astrocytoma with Exudative Retinopathy

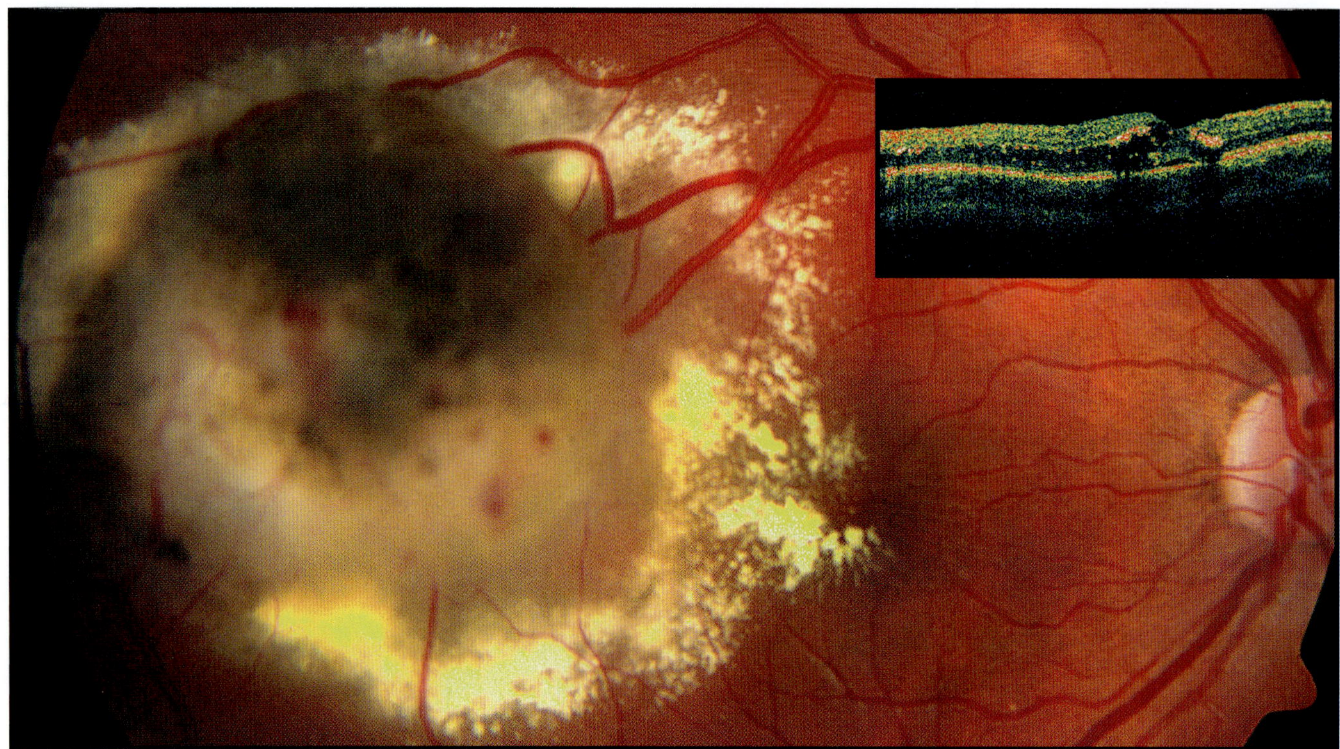

Retinal acquired astrocytoma with surrounding retinal exudation and visual acuity loss to 20/70. Time domain OCT shows intraretinal edema.

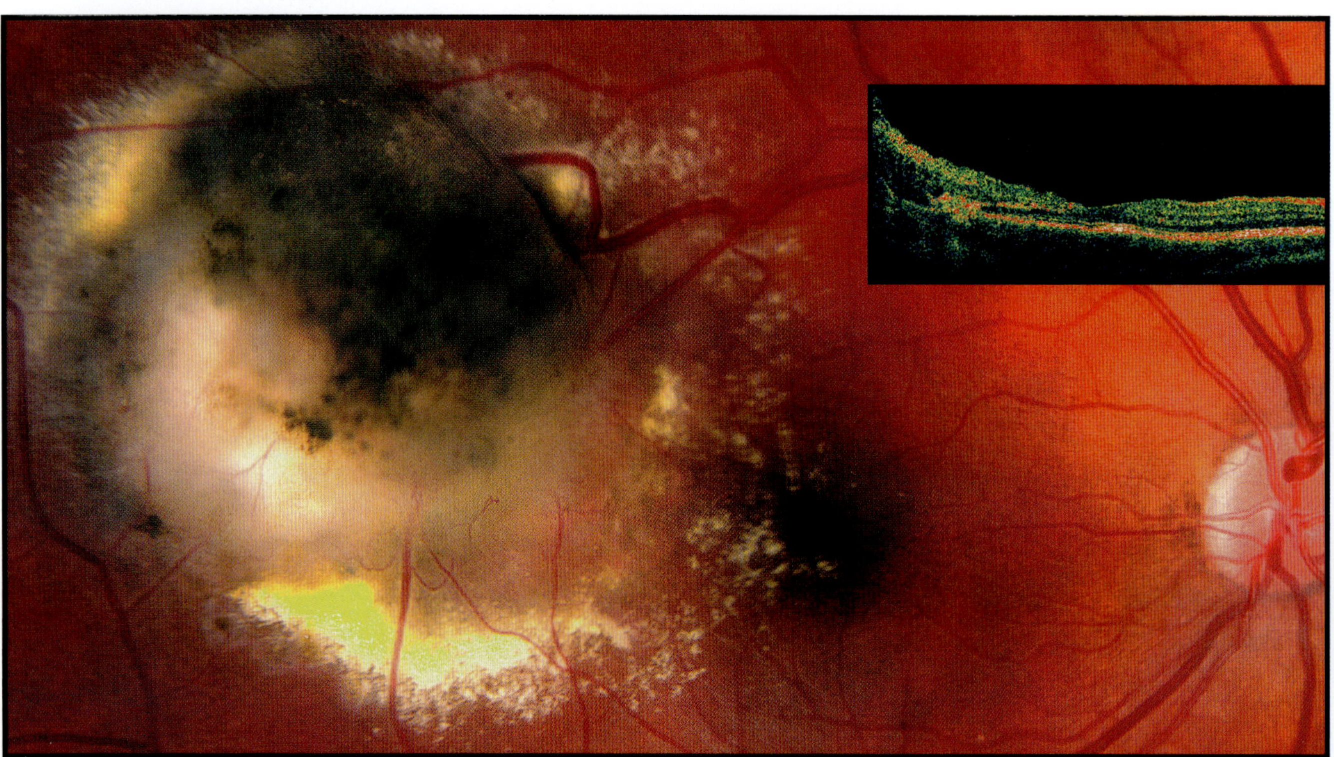

Following photodynamic therapy, the mass showed a slight reduction in size, and the visual acuity improved to 20/30 with partial resolution of the exudation. Time domain OCT shows partial resolution of foveal edema.

Retinal Hemangioblastoma (Capillary Hemangioma)

Retinal hemangioblastoma is a reddish-orange, vascular tumor that can be unifocal or multifocal and occurs as a unilateral or bilateral condition. This tumor is most commonly diagnosed in children or young adults. Hemangioblastoma can involve the macula, equator or peripheral retina and less commonly is found at the optic disc. This tumor is recognized by the markedly dilated and tortuous feeding artery and draining vein. Hemangioblastoma can remain quiescent without visual disturbance or it can appear active and produce subretinal fluid and exudation, intraretinal edema and exudation, and epiretinal membrane with vitreoretinal traction. In some cases, peripheral hemangioblastoma can produce remote macular edema and exudation, leading to poor visual acuity. Retinal hemangioblastoma is comprised of stromal tumor cells that produce vascular endothelial growth factor (VEGF), leading to the development of a highly vascular mass.

Retinal hemangioblastoma can occur as a sporadic tumor or as part of the von Hippel–Lindau disease. Patients with two or more hemangioblastomas are classified as having von Hippel–Lindau disease. Those with only one hemangioblastoma carry a 50% risk for von Hippel–Lindau disease if they are young (<10 years old) compared to a low risk <10% if they are older (>40 years old). All patients with retinal hemangioblastoma should have genetic testing for von Hippel–Lindau disease and should be monitored lifelong for related brain and visceral tumors.

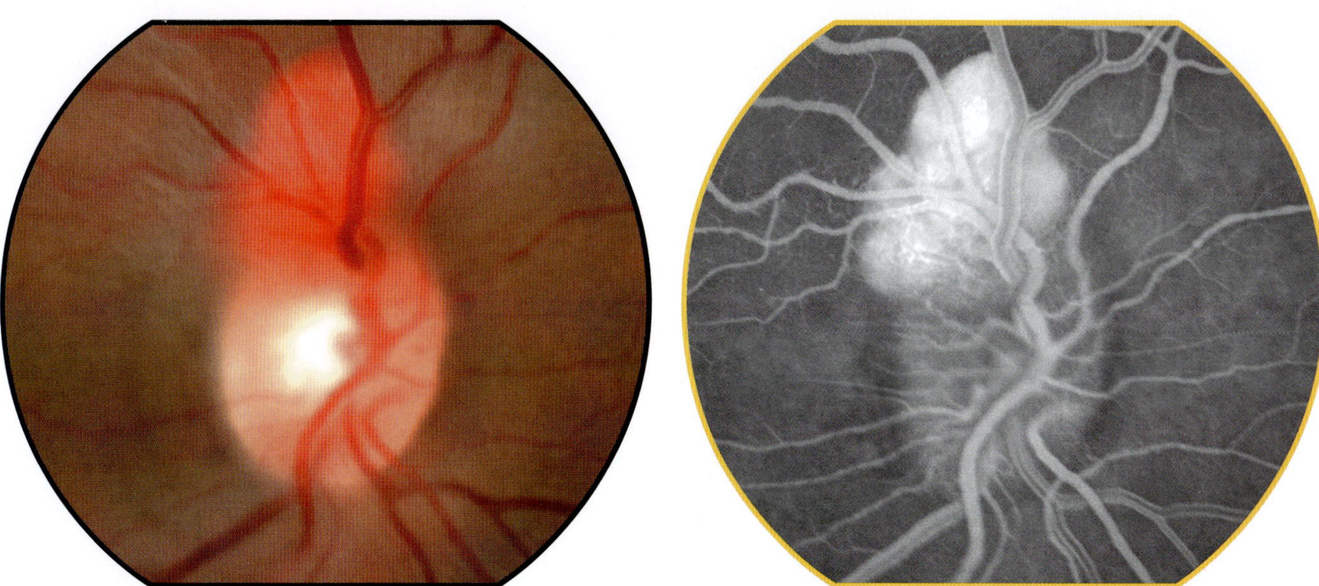

Sporadic retinal hemangioblastoma showing prominent vascular filling on fluorescein angiograpraphy. *Courtesy of Dr. Michael Cooney*

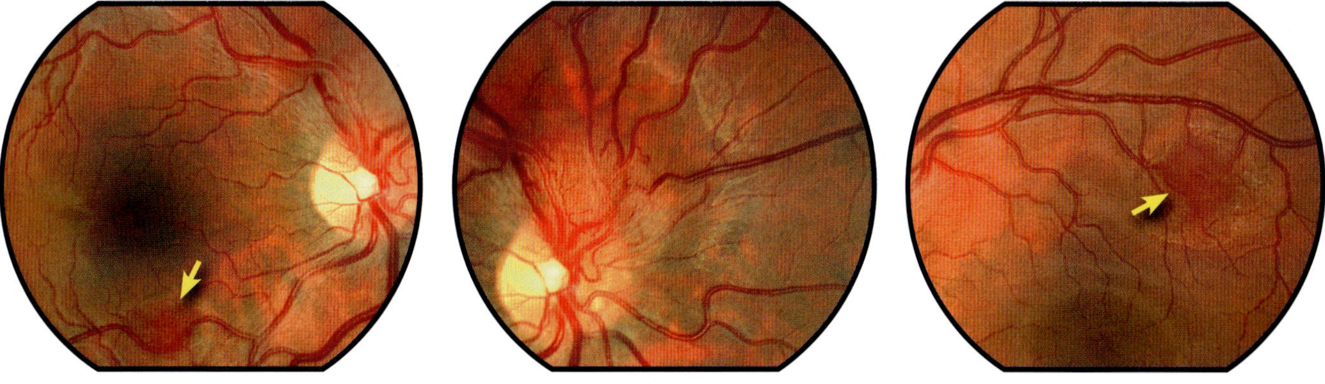

Small retinal hemangioblastomas *(arrows)* are noted in this patient with von Hippel–Lindau disease. *Courtesy of Dr. Eric Holz*

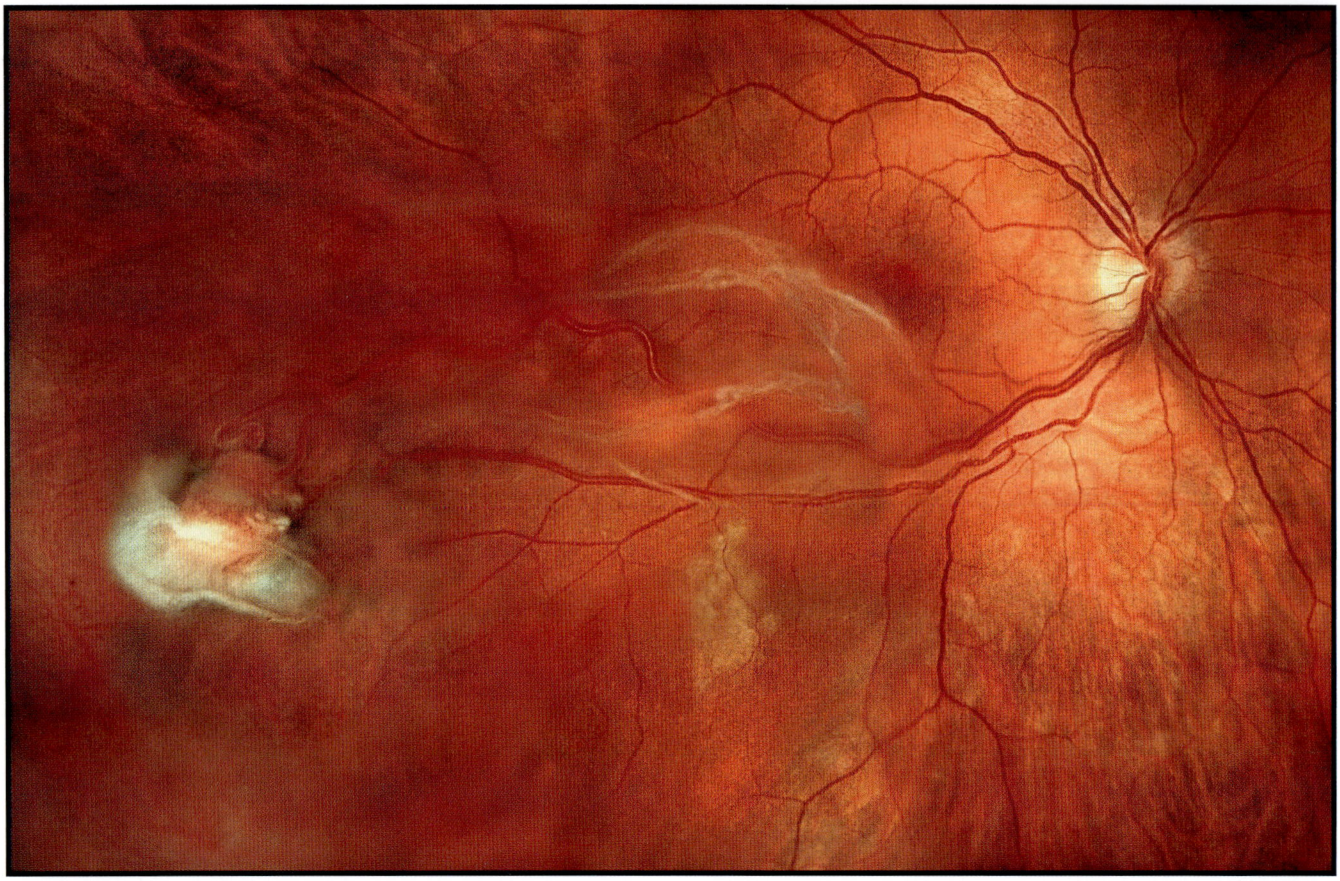

Peripheral retinal hemangioblastoma with remote epiretinal macular fibrosis. There is exudative and tractional retinal detachment. Note the large, tortuous perfusing arterioles and draining venules leading to this hemangioblastoma. *Courtesy of Dr. Mark Johnson*

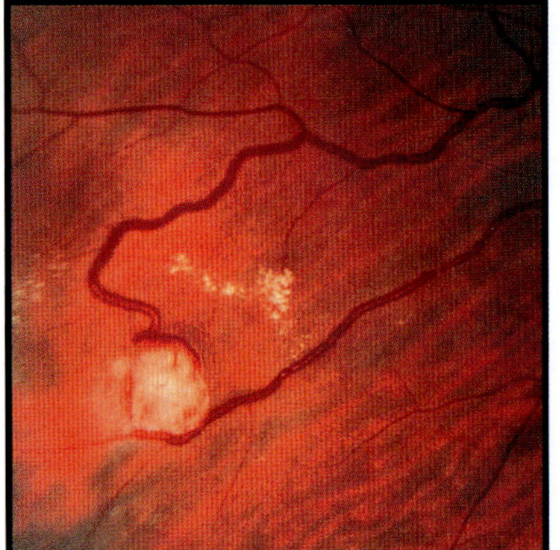

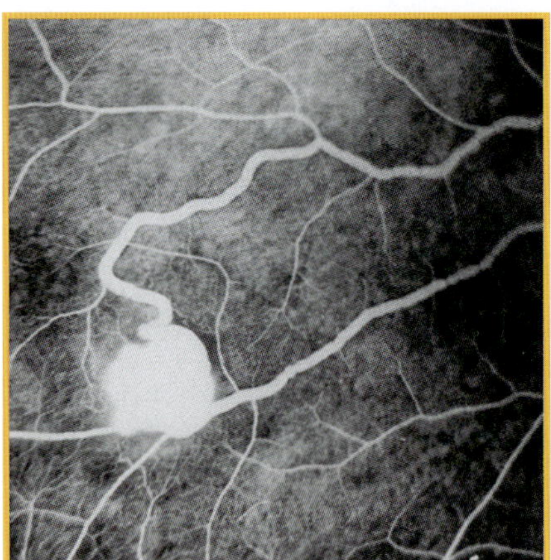

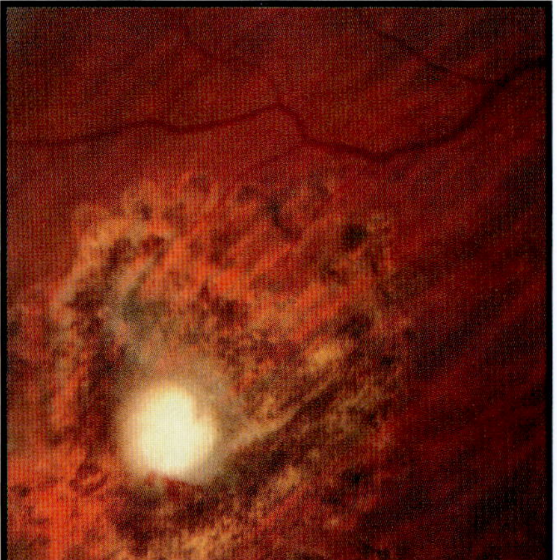

Dilated and tortuous feeding vessels are evident in this small capillary hemangioblastoma. Usually, the draining vessel is larger than the feeding vessel. The fluorescein angiogram shows the hyperfluorescent vascular tumor with its feeding and draining vessels. The patient was treated with laser photocoagulation with regression of the lesion *(right)*.

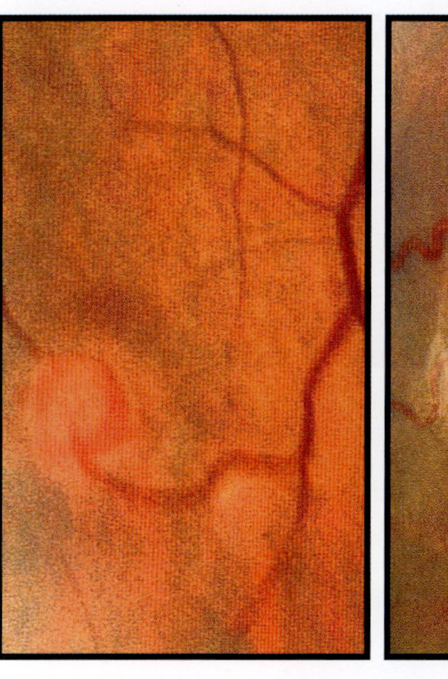
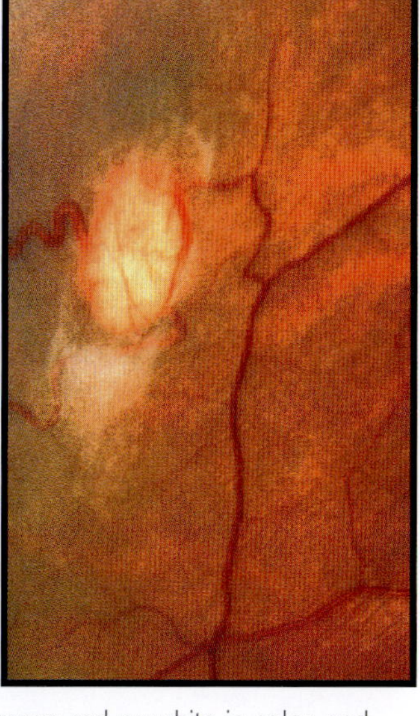

Retinal hemangioblastomas can be orange-red or white in color, and can vary in size from small to large. As they mature, elements of fibrosis evolve.

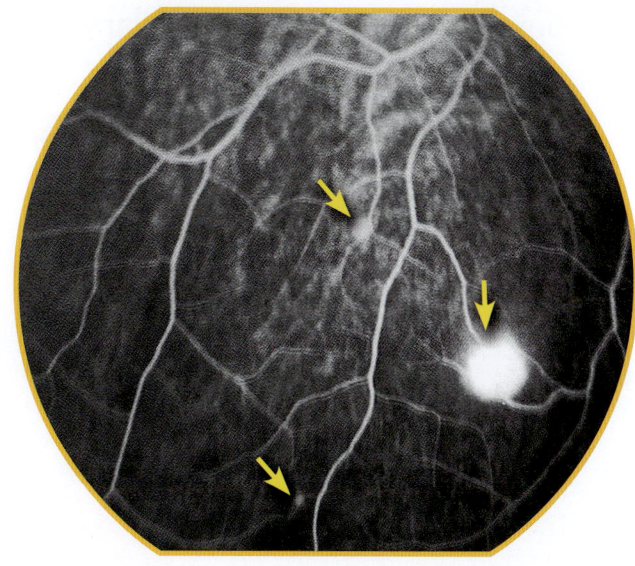

Multiple hemangioblastomas can be demonstrated by fluorescein angiography, as in this case in which three hyperfluorescent hemangioblastomas are noted *(arrows)*.

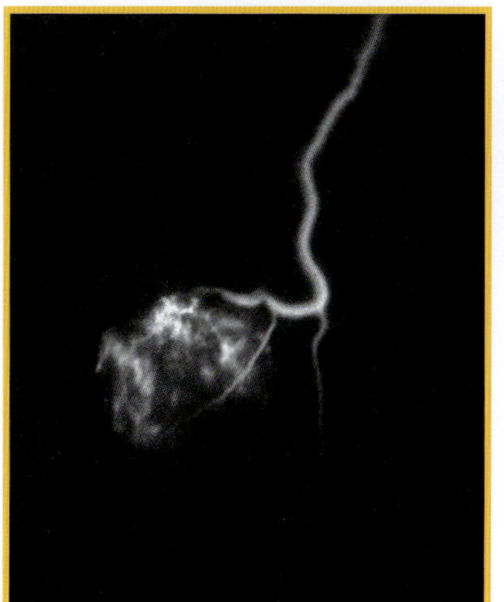
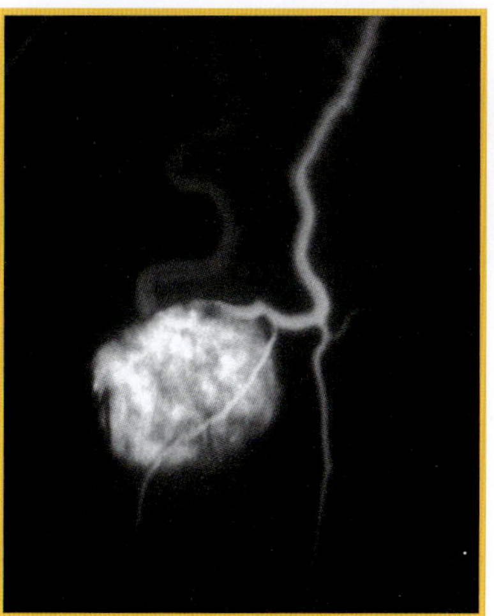
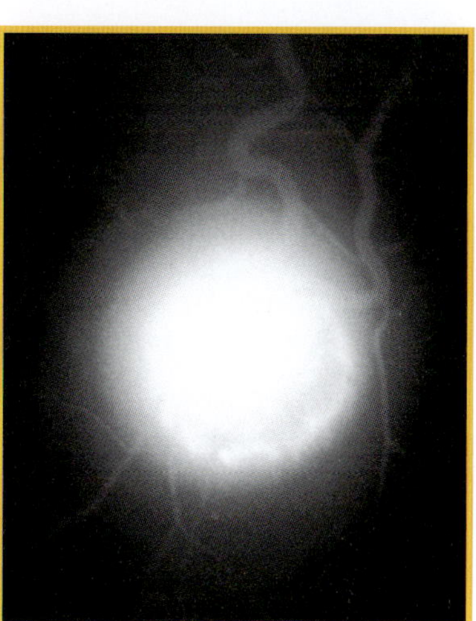

The fluorescein angiography sequence shows the dilated and tortuous peripheral perfusing arterioles and the appearance of a draining venule in this hemangioblastoma. There is extensive late leakage from the tumor vessels *(right)*.

© 626

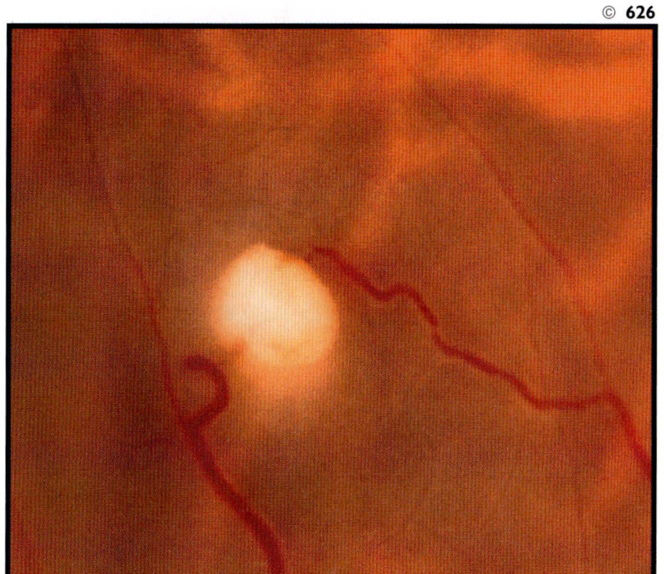

Clinical appearance of a hemangioblastoma from a patient with von Hippel–Lindau disease. The hemangioma has dilated and slightly tortuous feeding and draining blood vessels.

© 627

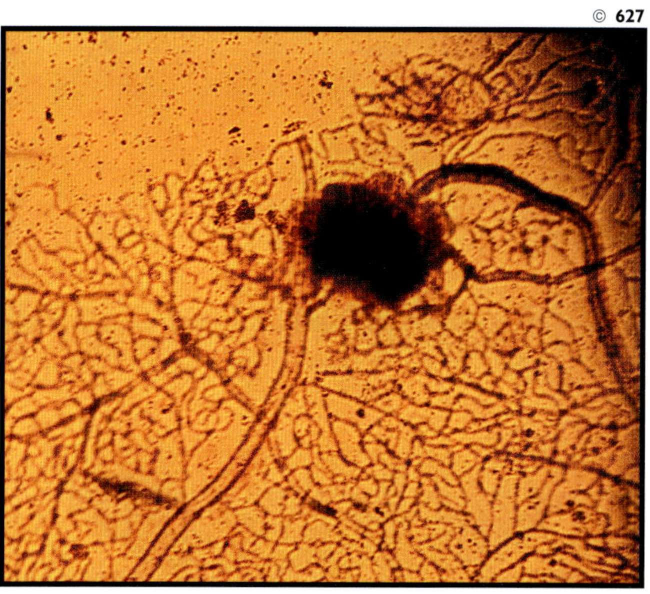

A trypsan digest preparation of a similar case shows a small retinal hemangioblastoma and its related vessels.

Obvious Endophytic Juxtapapillary Retinal Hemangioblastoma

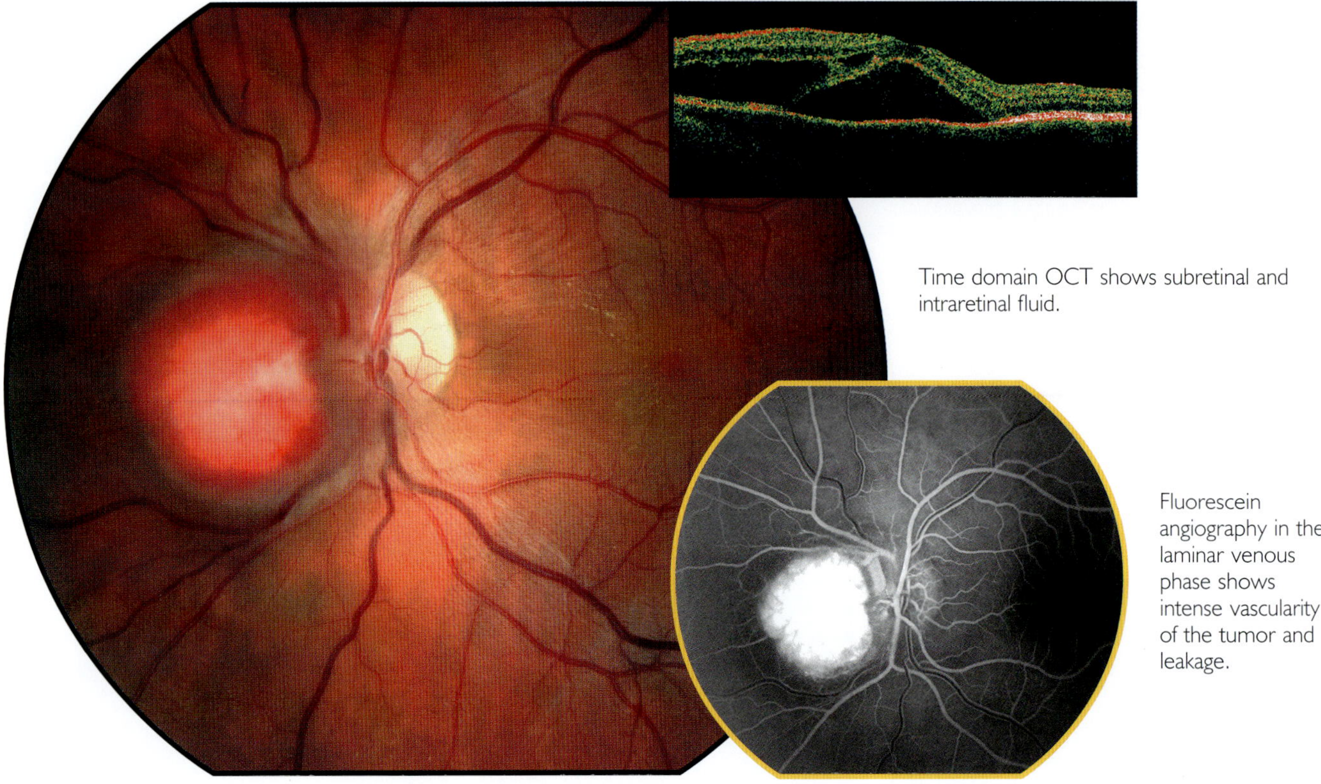

Time domain OCT shows subretinal and intraretinal fluid.

Fluorescein angiography in the laminar venous phase shows intense vascularity of the tumor and leakage.

Retinal hemangioblastoma at the nasal margin of the optic disc results in macular edema and subfoveal fluid.

Subtle Intraretinal Juxtapapillary Retinal Hemangioblastoma

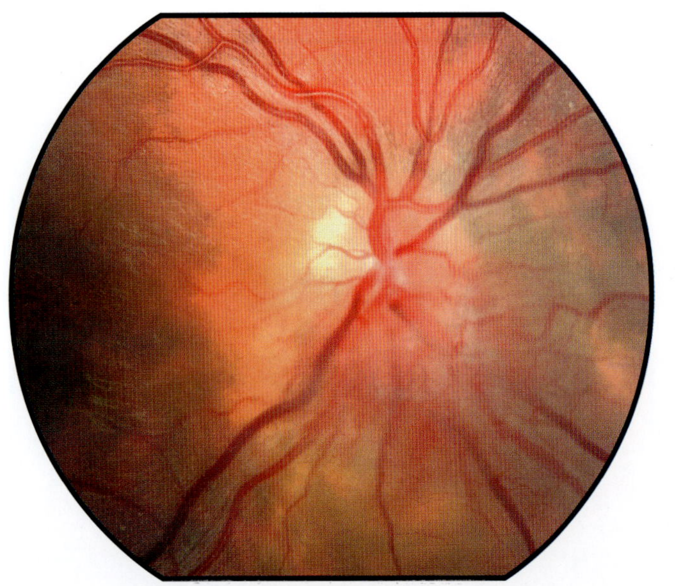

The intraretinal reddish-orange mass obscures the inferior margin of the optic disc and produces slight macular exudation and retinal striae.

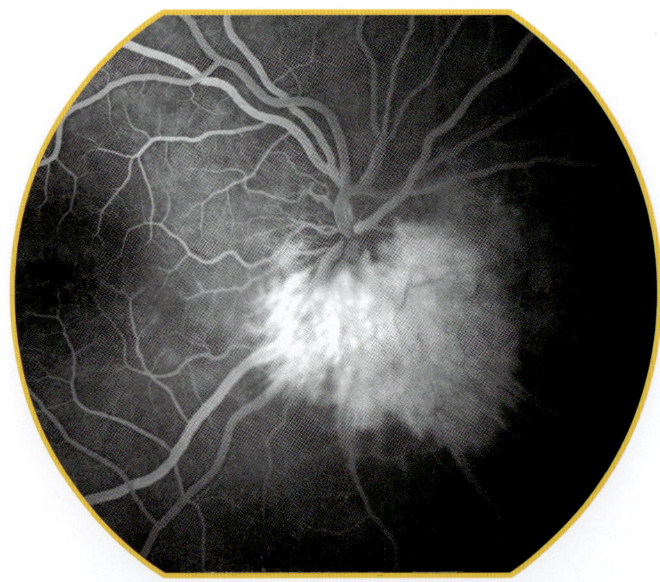

Fluorescein angiography shows intense hyperfluorescent vascularity of the tumor.

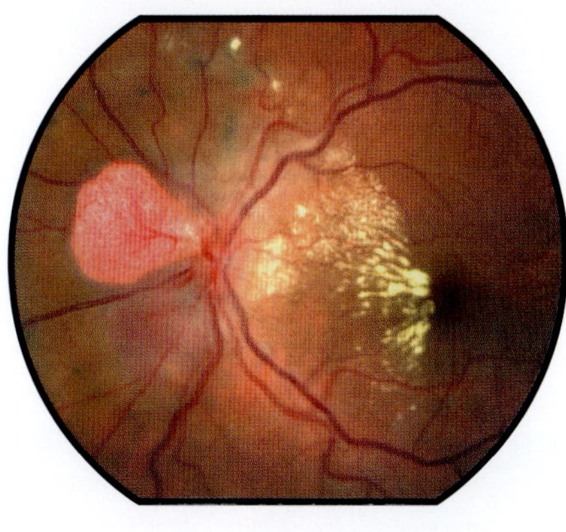

This nodular vascular tumor overhangs the nasal portion of the optic disc. Note the subretinal fluid and macular exudation.

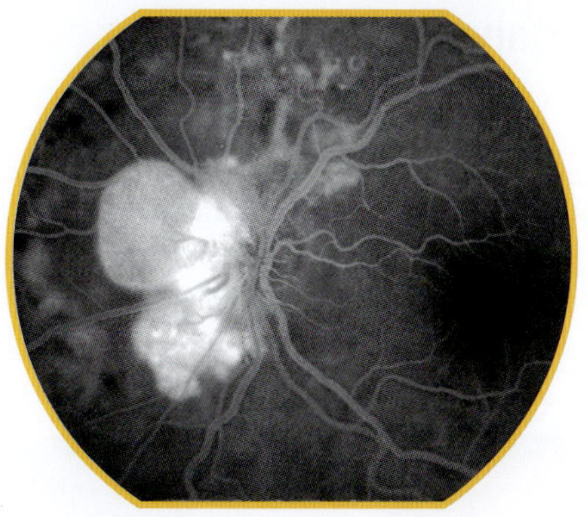

Fluorescein angiography shows the intense vascularity and staining of the mass as well as surrounding vascular leakage.

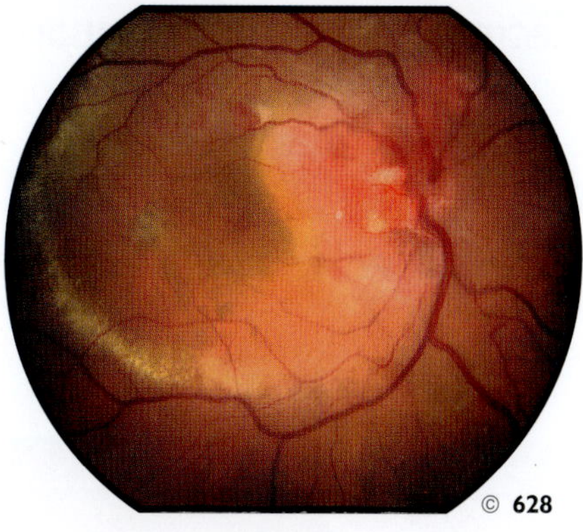

© 628

In this patient, a retinal hemangioblastoma involving the optic disc is associated with an exudative detachment of the macula. The margin of the macula is also fringed with lipid deposition.

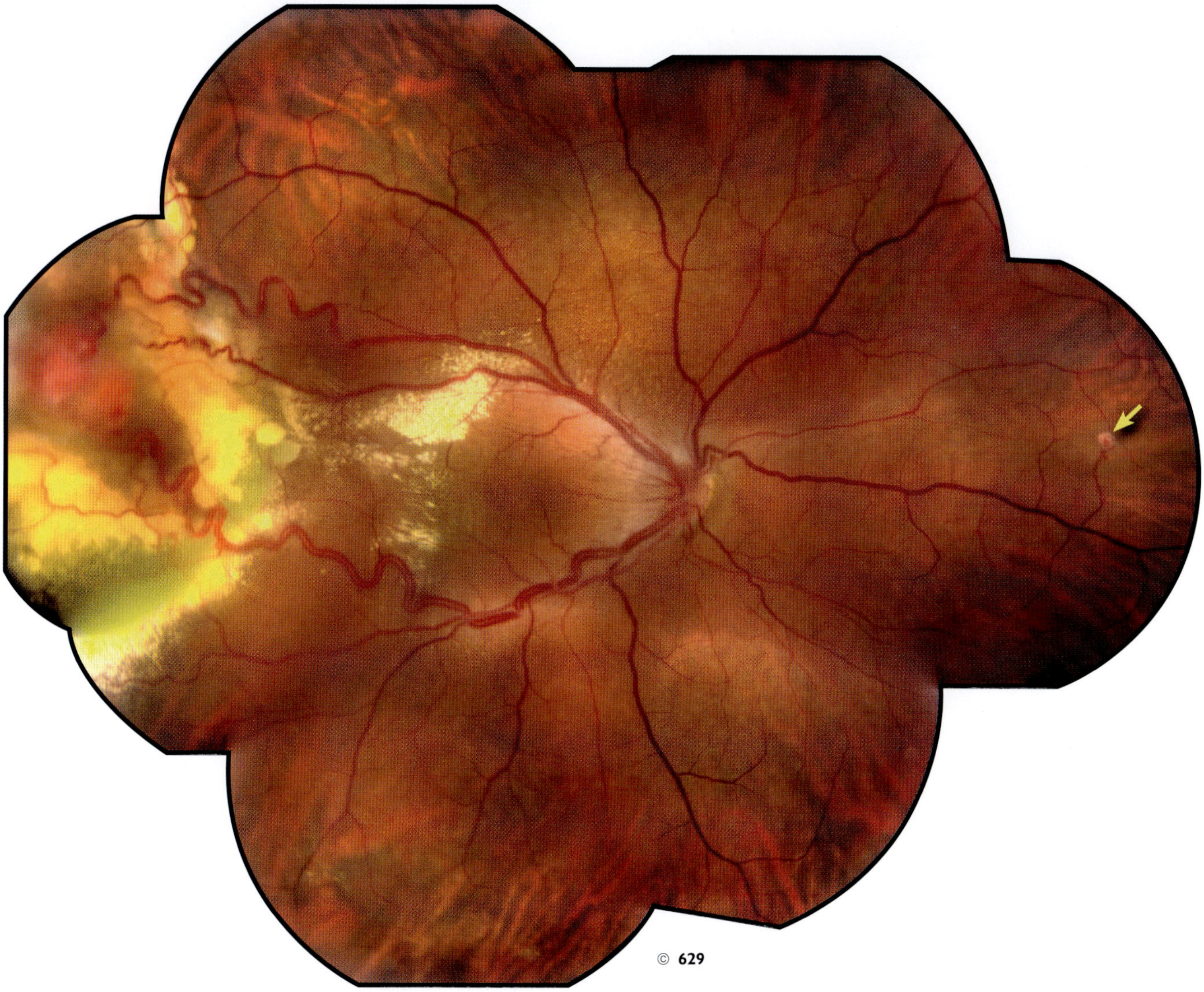

© 629

This patient with von Hippel–Lindau disease has multiple retinal hemangioblastomas in the right eye. The large temporal tumor is surrounded by detachment and exudation that extends into the macula. There are multiple perfusing arterioles and venules. These vessels become dilated and tortuous to accommodate the high flow of blood to the vascular tumor. Note the tiny hemangioblastoma *(arrow)* in the nasal periphery.

Retinal Hemangioblastoma Management

The management of retinal hemangioblastoma depends on the tumor size and location and related features of subretinal fluid and exudation. A pinpoint tumor can be ablated directly with laser photocoagulation whereas a small tumor (<3 mm) can be treated with laser photocoagulation to surround the tumor and close the feeding artery. Medium size tumors (3-6 mm) are managed with photodynamic therapy if located post-equatorially and cryotherapy if located anterior to the equator. Larger tumors (>6 mm) require plaque radiotherapy or vitrectomy with internal resection and silicone tamponade. The use of anti-VEGF medications can be beneficial to reduce subretinal fluid and intraretinal edema but show little effect on the tumor.

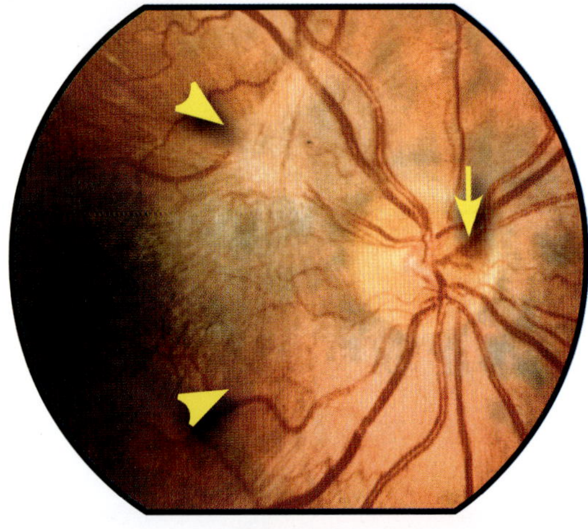
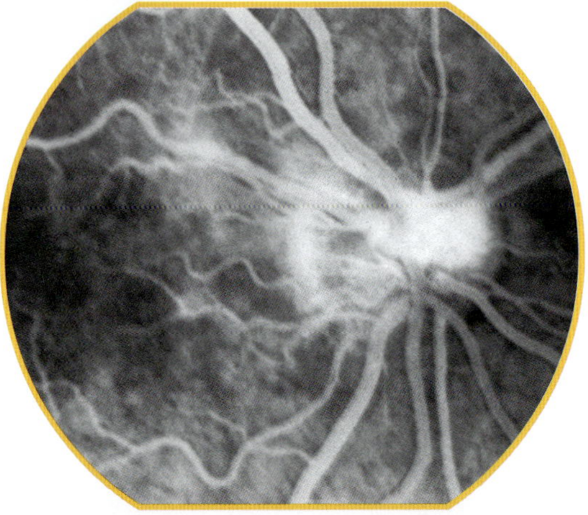

Small hemangioblastoma on the nasal aspect of the optic disc *(arrow)*. There is associated fibrous proliferation in the papillomacular bundle *(arrowheads)*. The fluorescein angiogram shows leakage on the nasal aspect of the disc.

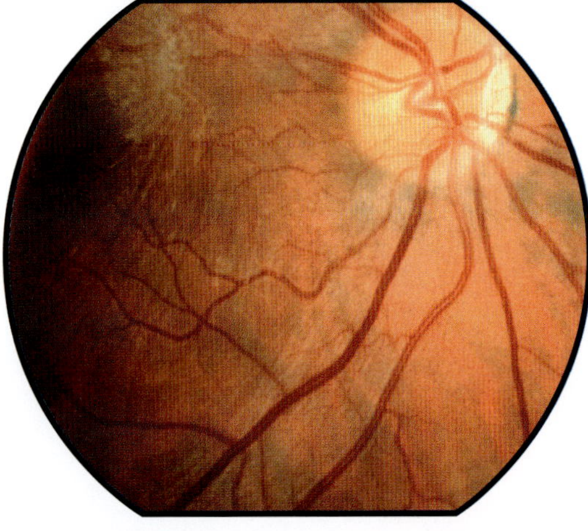
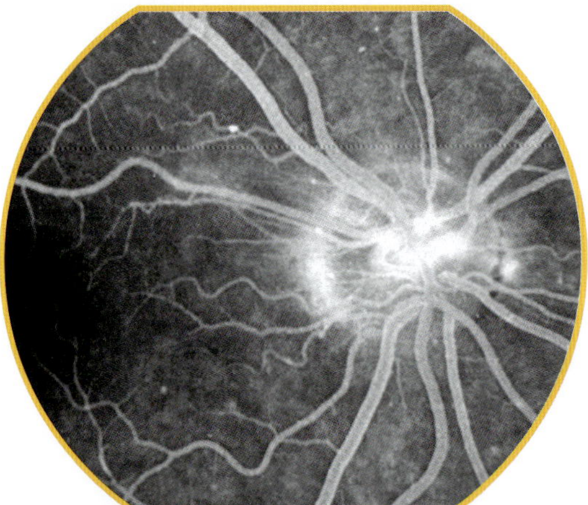

Treatment of the above case with vitrectomy and laser photocoagulation (with yellow dye laser) resulted in a marked reduction in tumor size and left a legacy of minimal residual macular fibrosis. On fluorescein angiography there is only minimal staining of residual reactive vessels in the central portion of the optic nerve head.

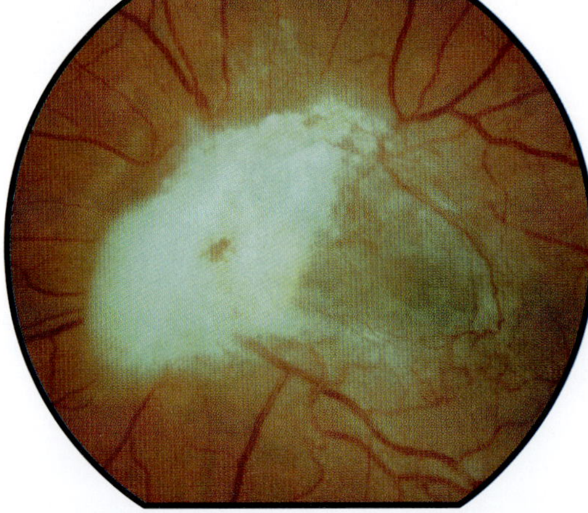
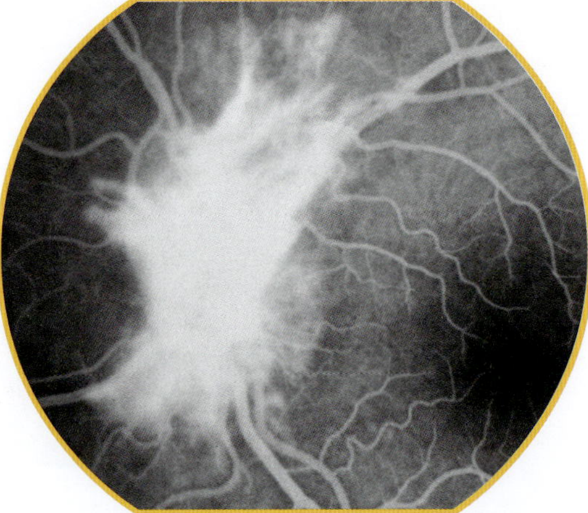

In this patient with retinal hemangioblastoma and von Hippel–Lindau disease there is massive fibrous proliferation at the nerve and secondary detachment of the macula. The fluorescein angiogram shows extensive staining of the optic nerve head.

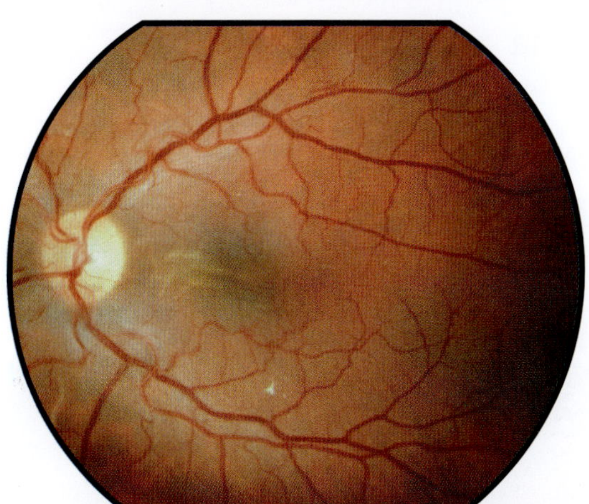

Following pars plana vitrectomy for the tumor described in the previous page, there is elimination of the fibrovascular proliferation and restoration of the optic nerve and retinal vasculature. *Courtesy of Dr. Emily Chew*

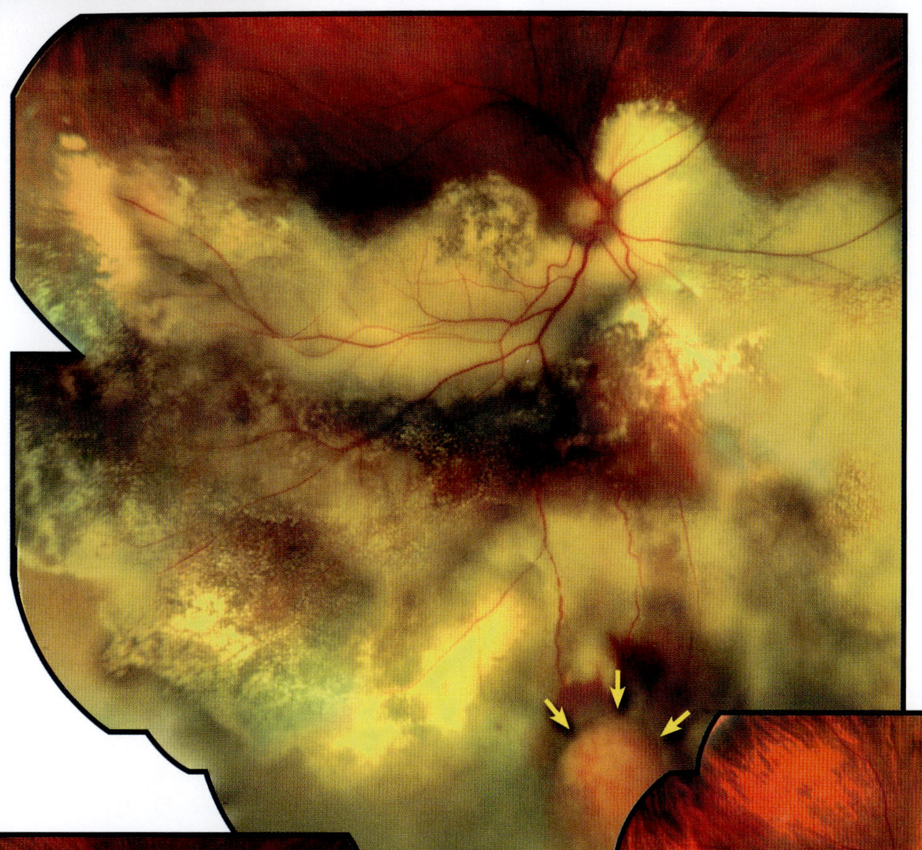

Months after multiple indocyanine green (ICG)-enhanced transpupillary thermotherapy (TTT) treatments *(image above)*, the tumor has consolidated and become fibrotic. There is still residual lipid in the posterior fundus.

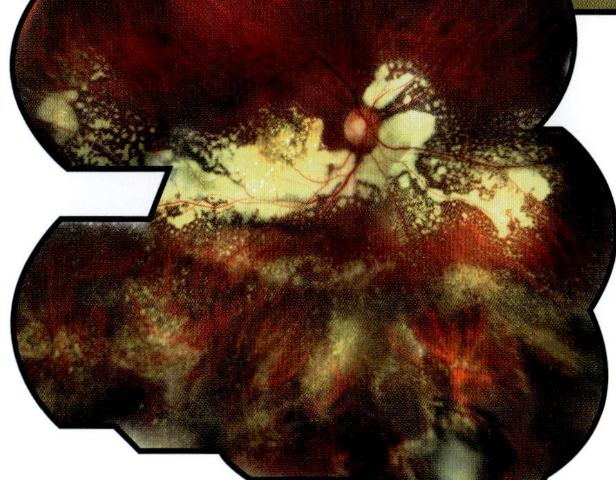

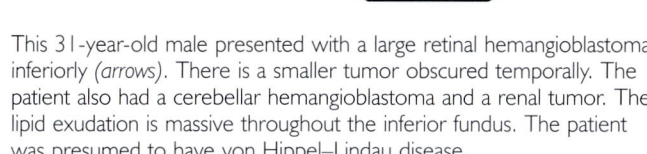

This 31-year-old male presented with a large retinal hemangioblastoma inferiorly *(arrows)*. There is a smaller tumor obscured temporally. The patient also had a cerebellar hemangioblastoma and a renal tumor. The lipid exudation is massive throughout the inferior fundus. The patient was presumed to have von Hippel–Lindau disease.

More than 18 months later *(right image)*, there is total resolution of the lipid, but there is a fibrovascular scar at the site of the lesion and multiple fibrotic scars in the macula. *Courtesy of Dr. Enrico Bertelli*

Endophytic Juxtapapillary Retinal Hemangioblastoma

Endophytic retinal hemangioblastomas can be associated with exudative retinal detachment, vitreous hemorrhage, and lipid exudation, as seen here *(left image)*.

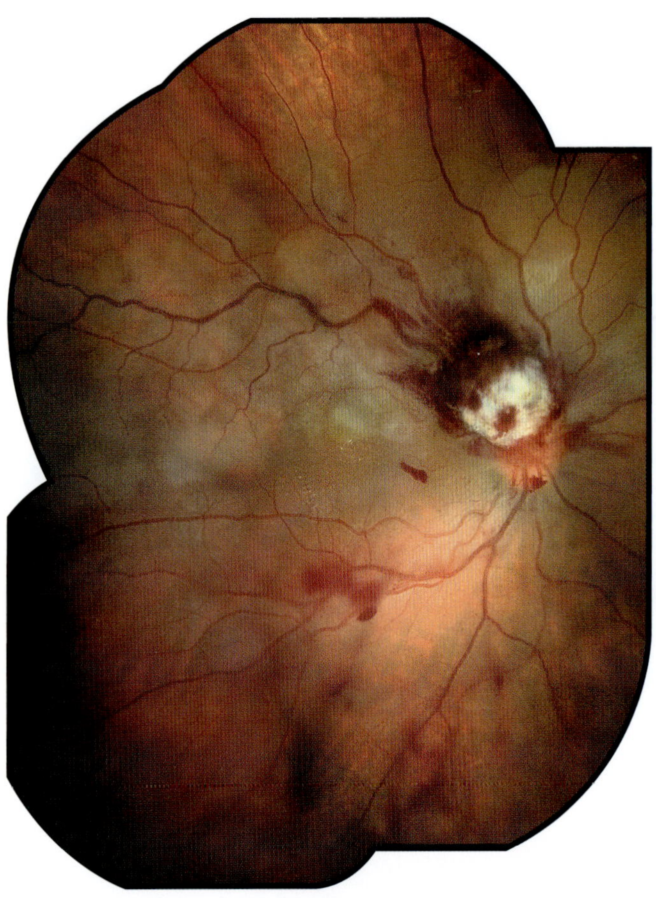

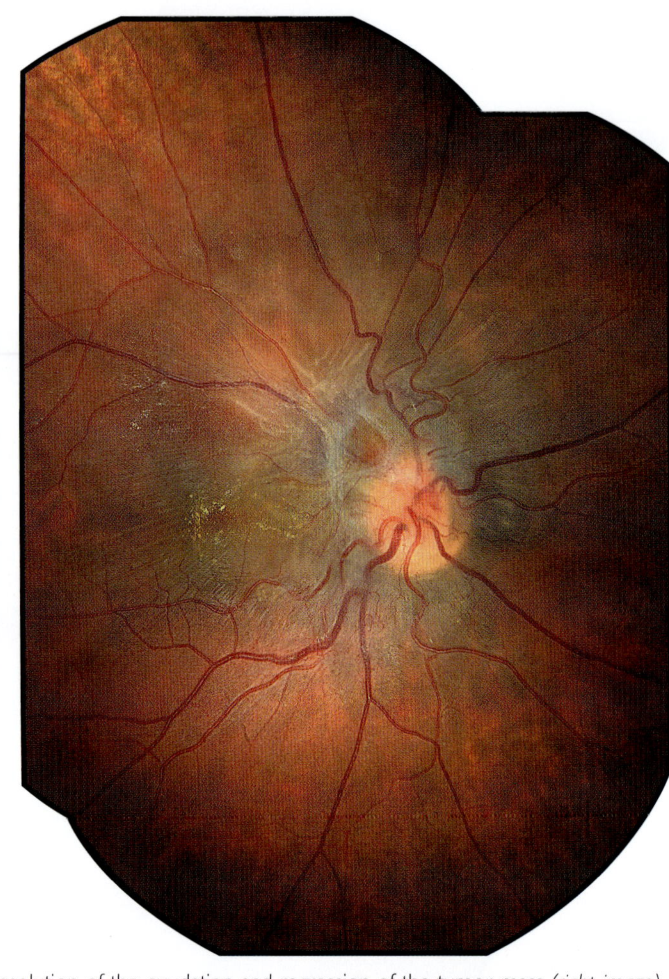

Following treatment with transpupillary thermotherapy there is dramatic resolution of the exudation and regression of the tumor mass *(right image)*. There is also extensive pre-retinal fibrosis. *Courtesy of Dr. Mark Johnson*

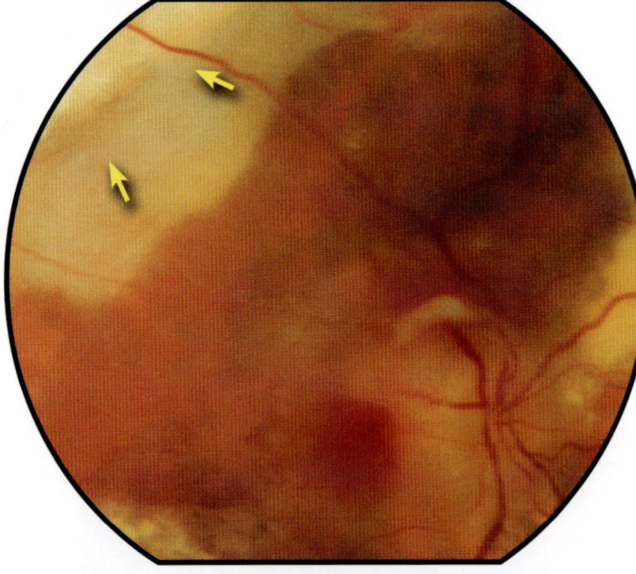

Massive subretinal exudation can occur even with small retinal hemangioblastomas. This patient had a poorly defined hemangioblastoma of the optic disc with endophytic and exophytic growth. Old exudation with fibrous metaplasia is noted superotemporally *(arrows)*.

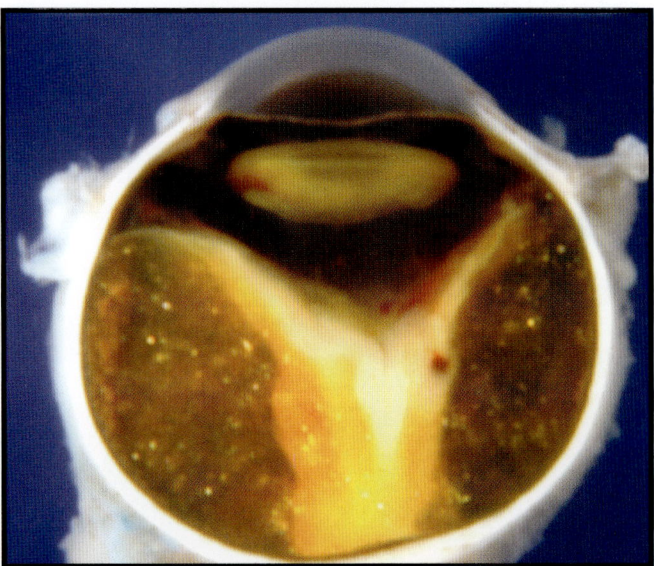

This eye was enucleated due to painful neovascular glaucoma related to an optic disc hemangioblastoma, which caused a total exudative retinal detachment.

Hemangioblastoma with Extensive Fibrosis

Fibrovascular proliferation can occur with extensive exudation, leading to retinal detachment. Some fibrovascular proliferation can be indistinguishable from the hemangioblastoma itself. Note the dilated fine preretinal vessels over the optic disc surrounded by exudative detachment. Vitrectomy was successful in removing the fibrovascular proliferation and reattaching the retina in this case. Removal of the fibrosis was uneventful. This eye also had peripheral hemangioblastomas treated with laser and subsequently developed new lesions 2 years after the vitrectomy.

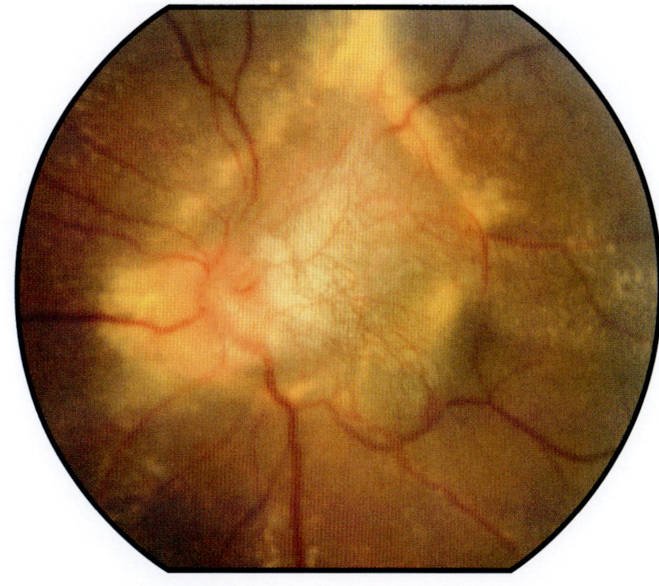

Courtesy of Dr. Yale Fisher

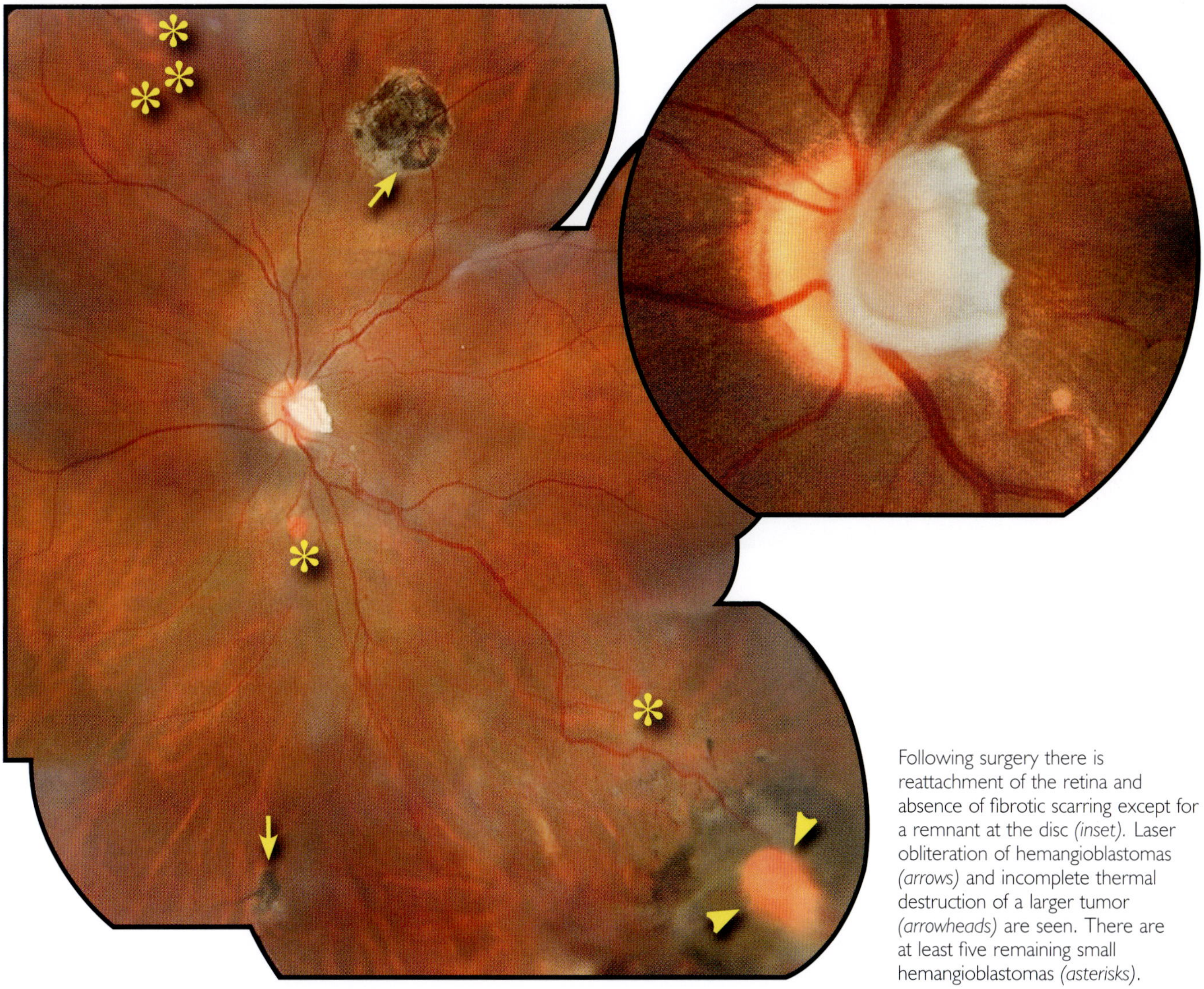

Following surgery there is reattachment of the retina and absence of fibrotic scarring except for a remnant at the disc *(inset)*. Laser obliteration of hemangioblastomas *(arrows)* and incomplete thermal destruction of a larger tumor *(arrowheads)* are seen. There are at least five remaining small hemangioblastomas *(asterisks)*.

Retinal Cavernous Hemangioma

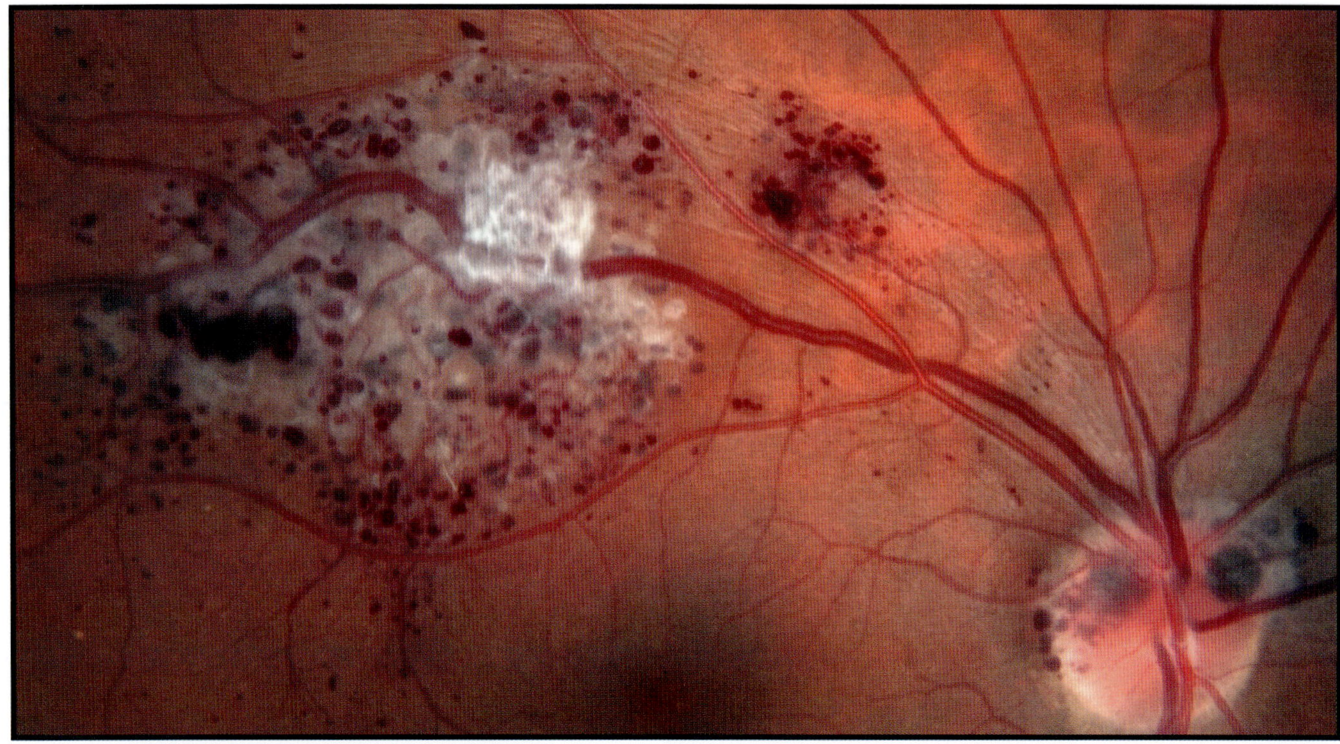

The retinal cavernous hemangioma is a dark, reddish-blue, low flow vascular tumor. Occasionally it can rupture and produce vitreous hemorrhage. Some cases are associated with the KRIT1/CCM1 mutation in which there are cavernous hemangiomas of the retina, brain, and skin. Clinically, a cavernous hemangioma appears as a cluster of dark intraretinal venular aneurysms. Pigment epithelial proliferation may darken some areas and fibrous proliferation may lighten other areas of the lesion. These tumors classically do not leak, but they may occasionally bleed into the vitreous.

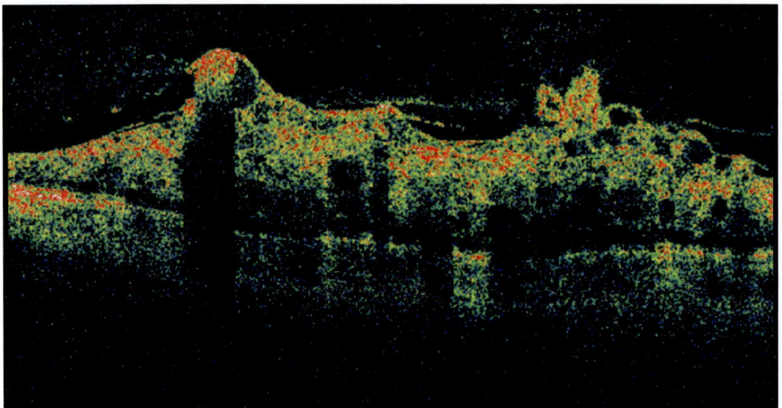

OCT displays the round cavitary intraretinal structures of this vascular tumor.

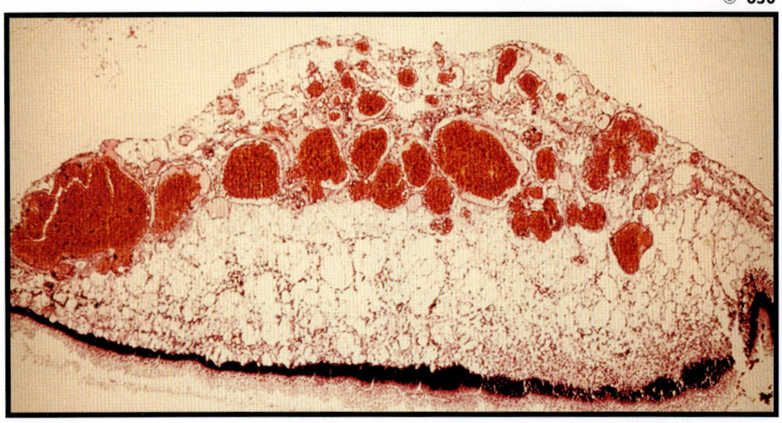

Histopathology of a cavernous hemangioma. Note the thin walls of the cavernous hemangioma that represents a risk for vitreous hemorrhage. The retina is also greatly thickened by edema. Large, normal-appearing blood vessels are seen in the inner retinal layers.

Variations in Presentation

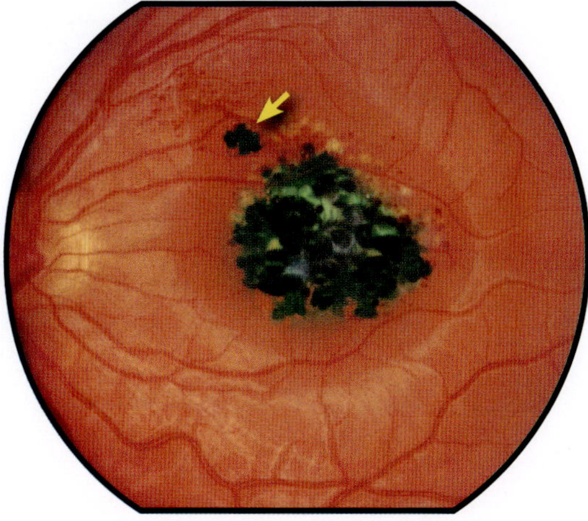

A cavernous hemangioma may resemble a cluster of grapes. Vascular dilation and a purplish vascular configuration can be noted. The cavernous vessels vary in size. Note the small lesions superonasally *(arrow)* and larger lesions centrally. Some of the large lesions reveal a plasma-erythrocyte interface. Pigment epithelial hyperplasia is also noted within the central clump of cavernous vessels.

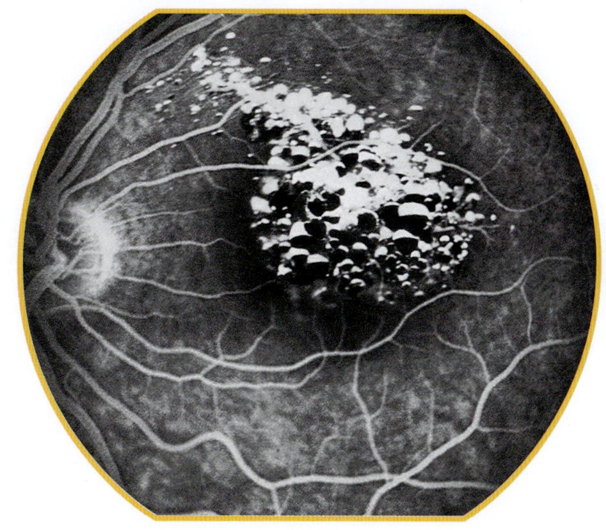

The characteristic filling pattern of a cavernous hemangioma can be demonstrated by fluorescein angiography. The vessels are on the venous side of the circulation; they show a plasma-erythrocyte interface but no leakage. *Courtesy of Ross Jarrett*

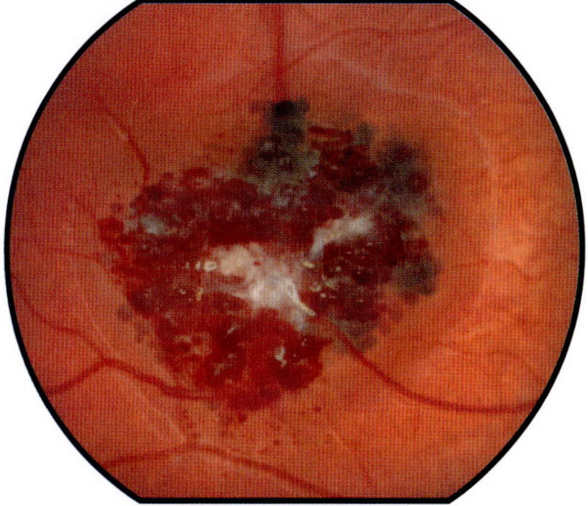

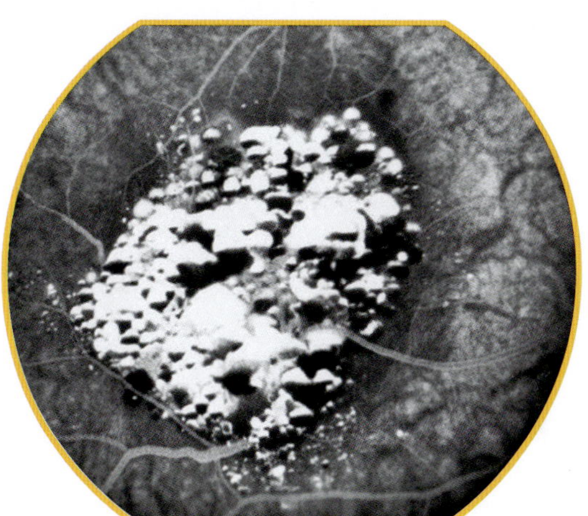

This cavernous hemangioma has variable pigmentation and an element of fibrosis. The fluorescein angiogram shows filling of the lesion except where there is erythrocyte aggregation.

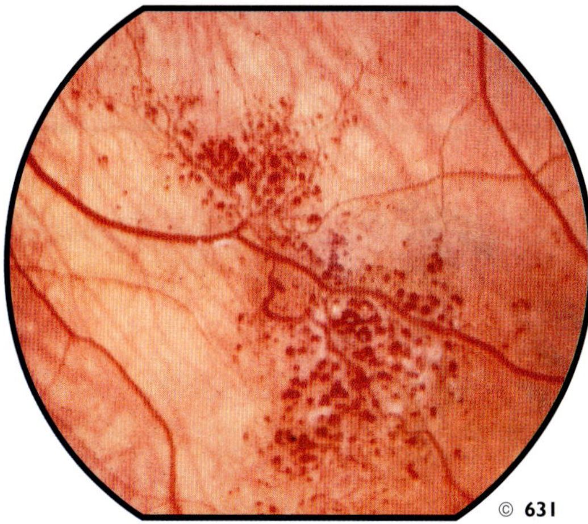

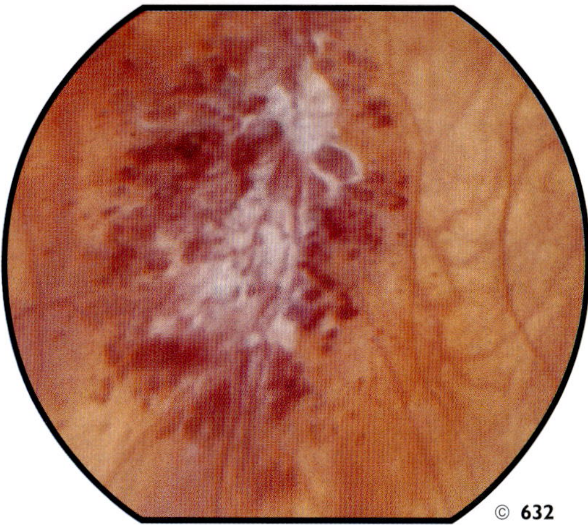

This is a 10-year-old female with bilateral retinal cavernous hemangiomas. Her mother also has a cavernous hemangioma in one eye. Note the extensive fibrosis that is seen in some cases.

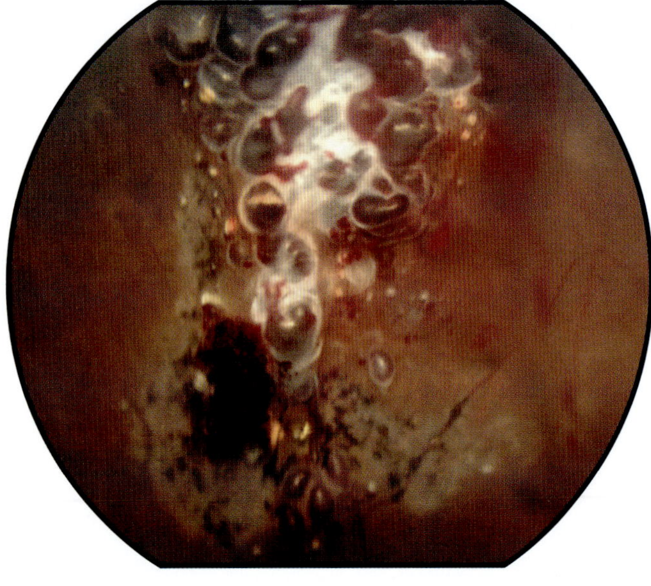

This patient has unusually large, sausage-like, aneurysmal dilatations with deep purple blood in the larger lesions connected by fibrous proliferation.

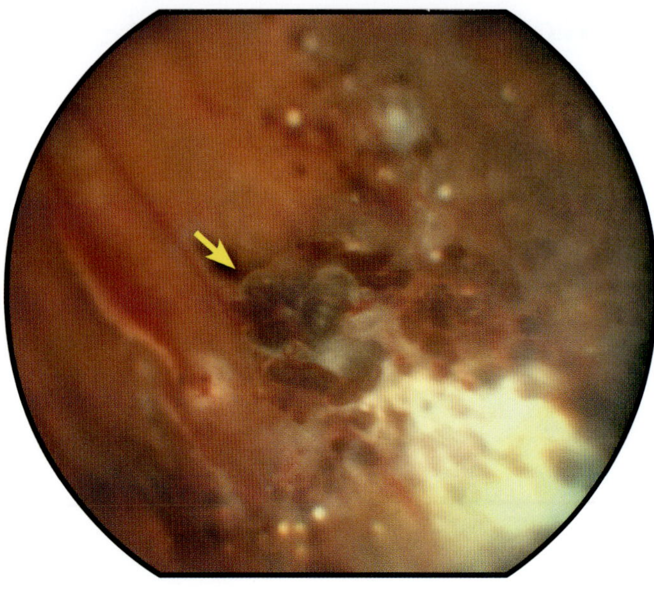

This cavernous hemangioma has a large purple vascular coalescing change centrally *(arrow)*. This may be due to pigment epithelial hyperplasia and/or trapped or slow flow of venous blood in the larger saccular portion of the mass. There is also a chain of scattered smaller lesions and an element of fibrosis.

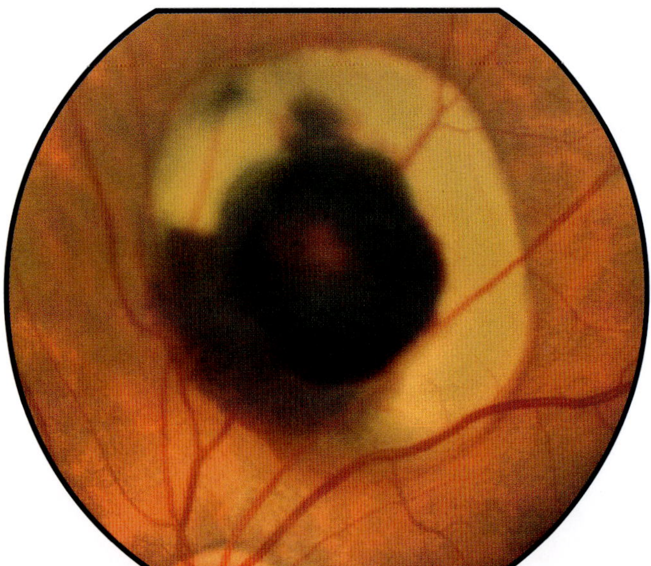

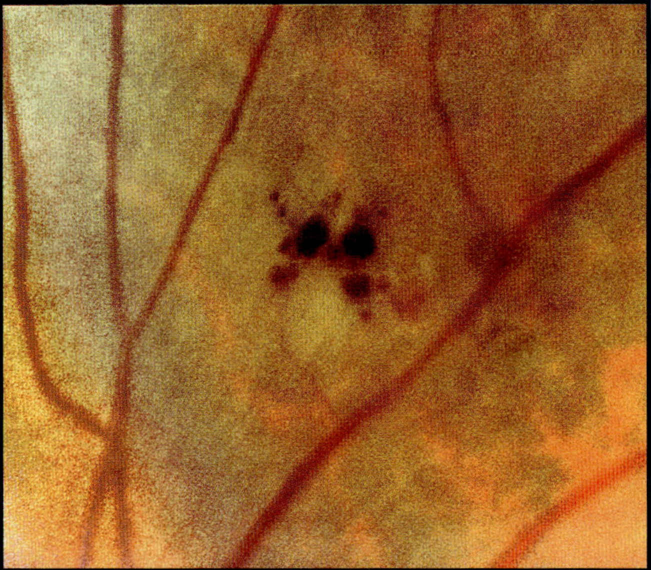

This patient presented with preretinal, intraretinal, and subretinal hemorrhage, which resembles the bleeding pattern seen with retinal arteriolar macroaneurysm *(left image)*. A cavernous hemangioma of the retina was seen after the hemorrhage resolved *(right image)*. This cavernous hemangioma has lesions of variable size with elements of pigmentation and fibrosis.

Retinal Racemose Hemangioma

Retinal racemose hemangioma is a congenital vascular malformation in which some or all of the retinal vessels are dilated, often to the point that the arterial system cannot be distinguished from the venous system. If the hemangioma is extrafoveal, visual acuity can be normal, but, for those eyes with foveal involvement, visual acuity is typically poor. This tumor can be associated with the Wyburn–Mason syndrome in which similar racemose hemangiomas are found in the midbrain, which can lead to stroke, and in the mandible, which can potentially cause profuse bleeding during dental work. These vessels are at risk for venous obstruction, retinal ischemia, and neovascularization.

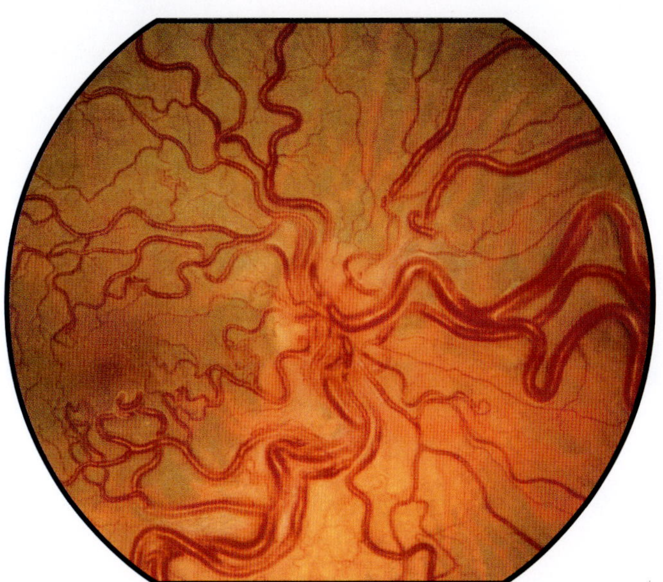

Tortuosity and dilatation of the normal vessels as well as malformed vessels may be noted. Variably sized arteriovenous (AV) communications are demonstrated in this eye.

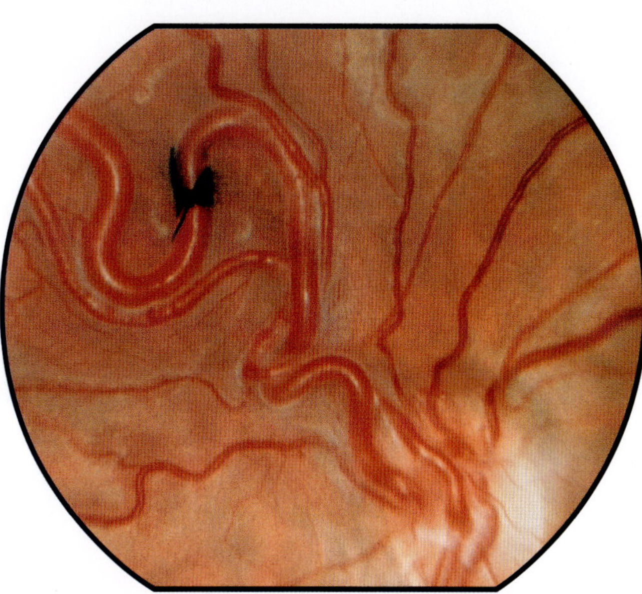

Pigmentation can sometimes be observed around the abnormal vessels in this disorder. *Courtesy of Drs. Ross Jarrett and Neil J. Okun*

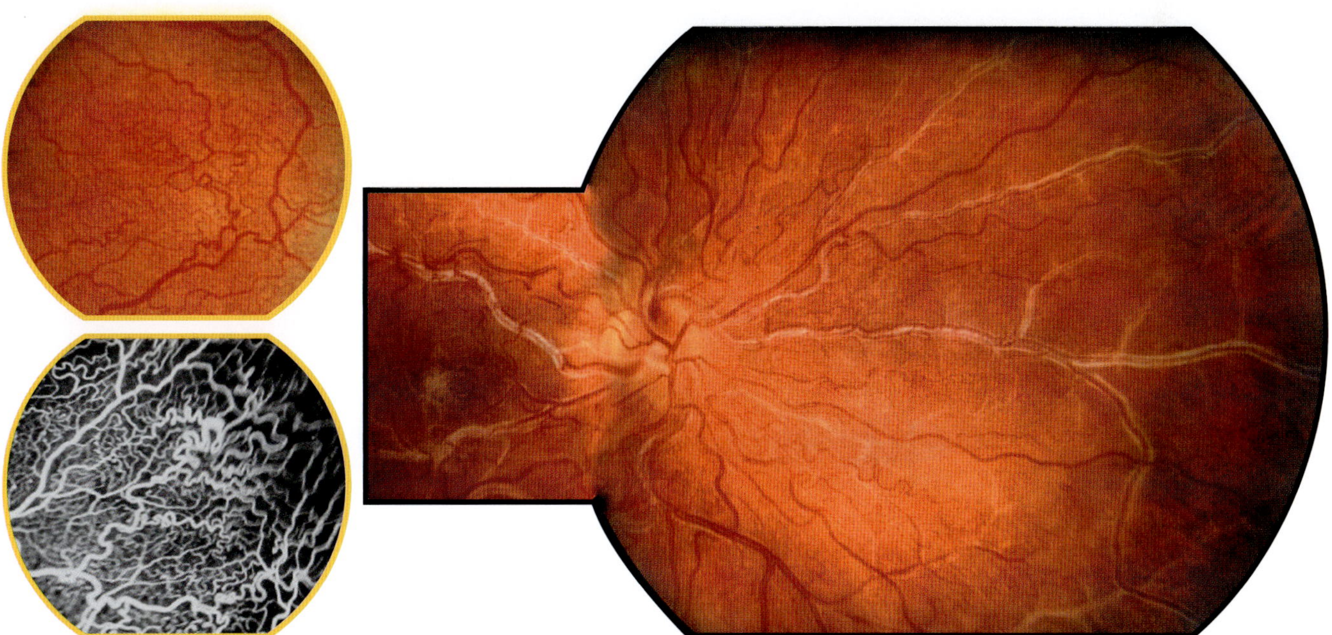

This patient has numerous small capillary shunts evident on the color photograph above. The fluorescein angiogram demonstrates a complex of capillaries that is much more dense and tortuous than that seen in more typical racemose hemangiomas.

In this case of diffuse racemose hemangioma, there are widespread retinal vascular abnormalities, which include multiple shunt vessels, sheathing, tortuosity, and numerous anomalous perfusion patterns throughout the fundus.

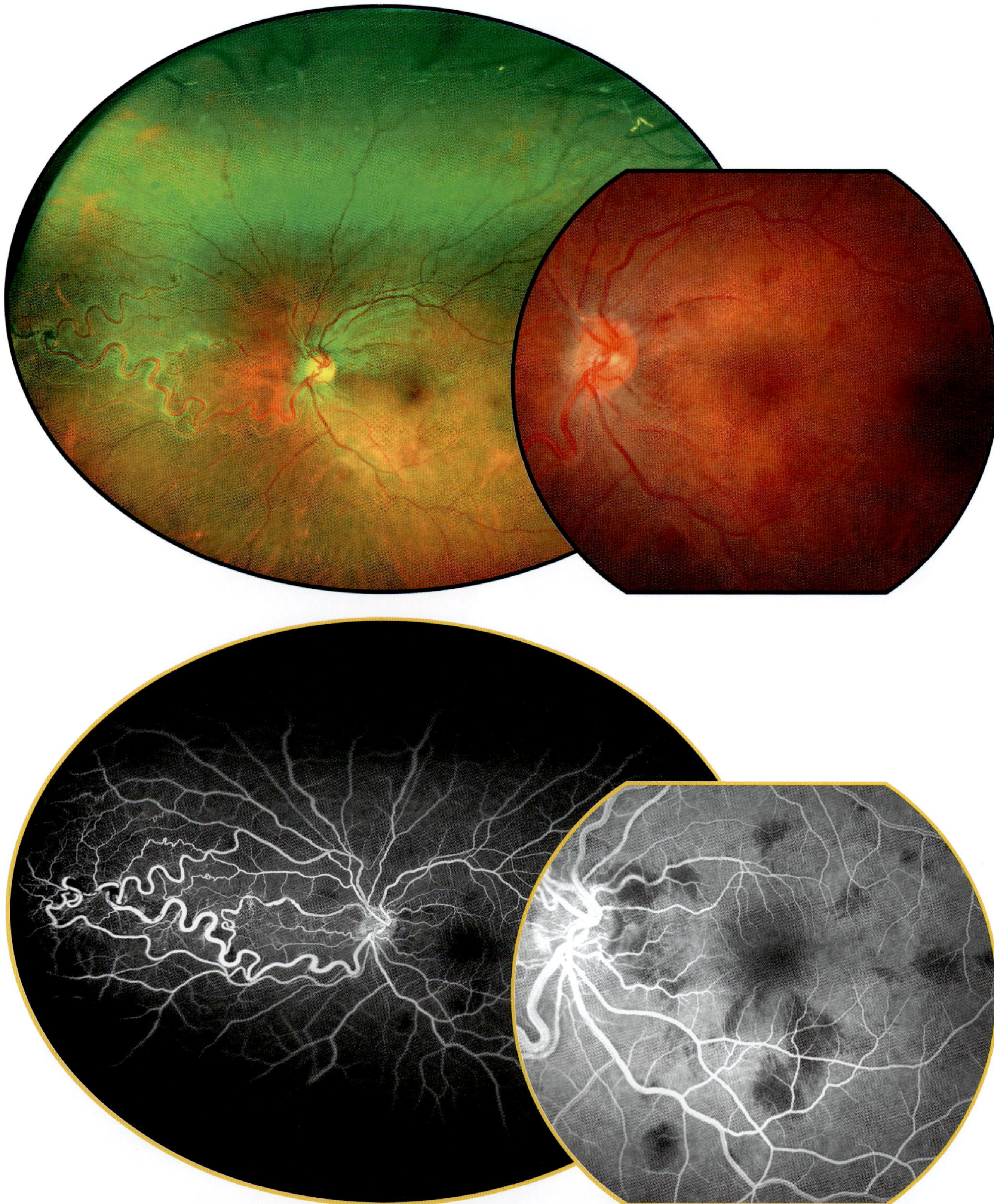

A 27-year-old female with a racemose hemangioma involving the nasal retinal vessels. This lesion is associated with a retinal vein occlusion characterized by large retinal hemorrhages involving all four retinal quadrants and the macula.

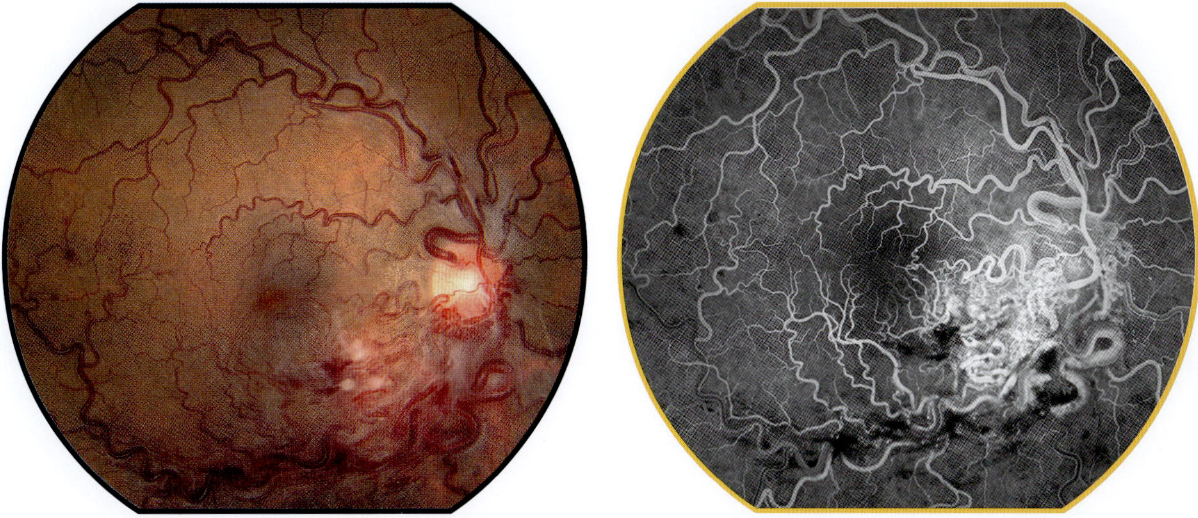

This patient has a diffuse racemose hemangioma associated with an inferior hemispheric retinal vein occlusion. Patients with racemose hemangioma are at risk for vascular occlusions and subsequent proliferative disease. *Courtesy of Dr. Eric van Kujik*

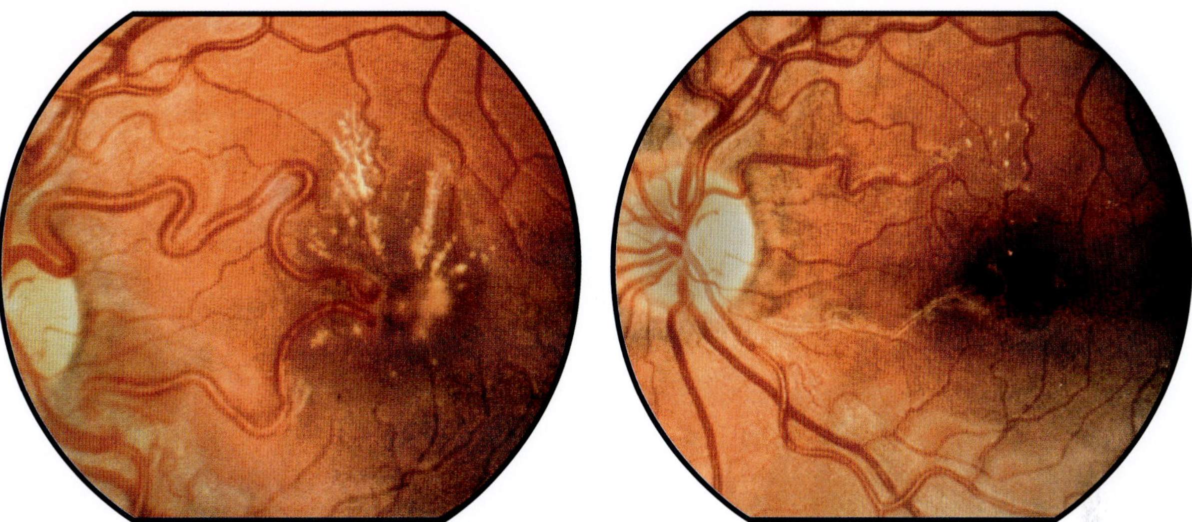

Racemose hemangiomas can show spontaneous regression and then recurrence, as seen in this case with a 17 year follow-up. The patient initially presented with racemose hemangioma and macular edema. Vascular occlusion of the inferior vessel resulted in sheathing, non-perfusion, and resolution of the exudation.

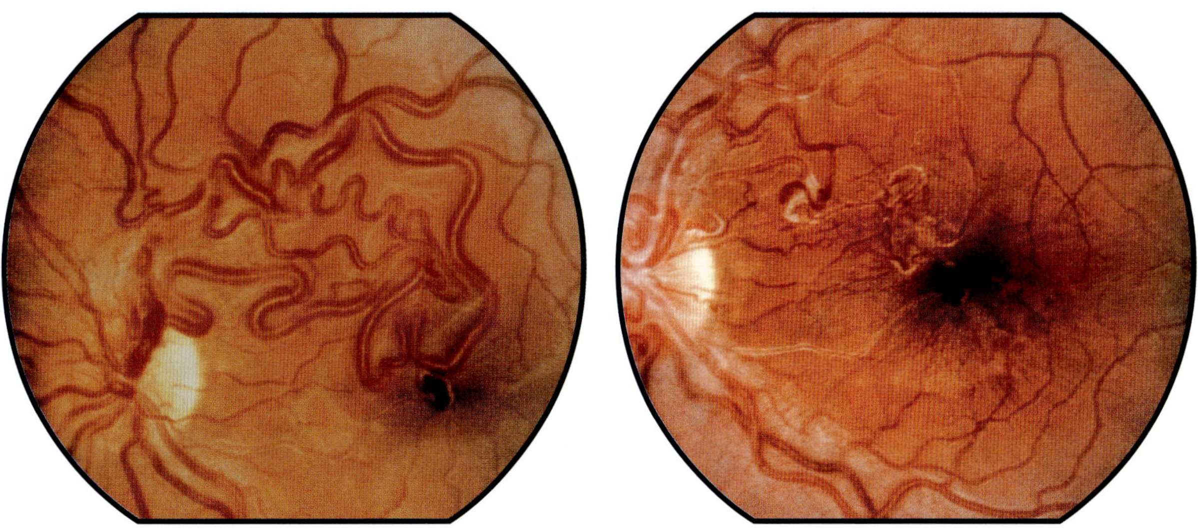

A new AV anastomosis appeared. A hairpin loop is seen connecting the AV segments. There was a subsequent obstruction of the AV anastomosis with closure of the AV communication, and resolution of the edema, and remodeling of the circulation. *Courtesy of Dr. Achim Wessing*

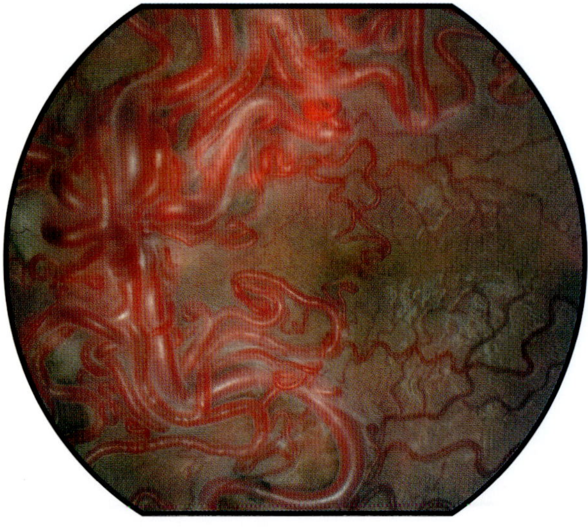

Close-up photograph depicting a racemose hemangioma in the macular and optic disc region. Note that arteries are indistinguishable from veins.

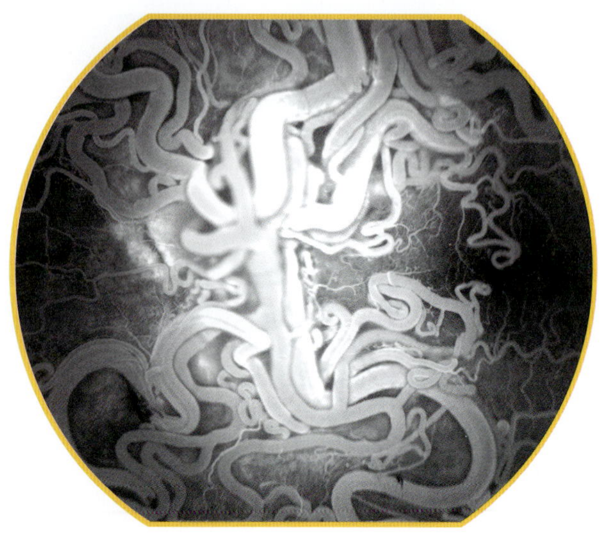

Fluorescein angiography revealing the rapid filling of the vascular tree, but no leakage.

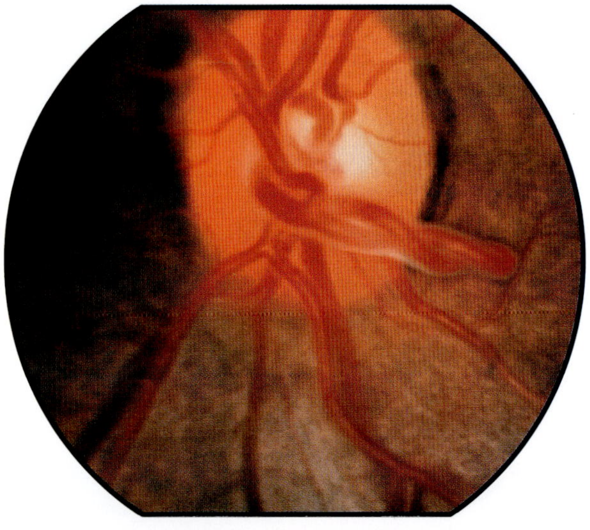

Congenital AV shunt vessels, as seen in this patient at the optic disc, may be a forme fruste of the condition or a Persistent Fetal Vasculature.

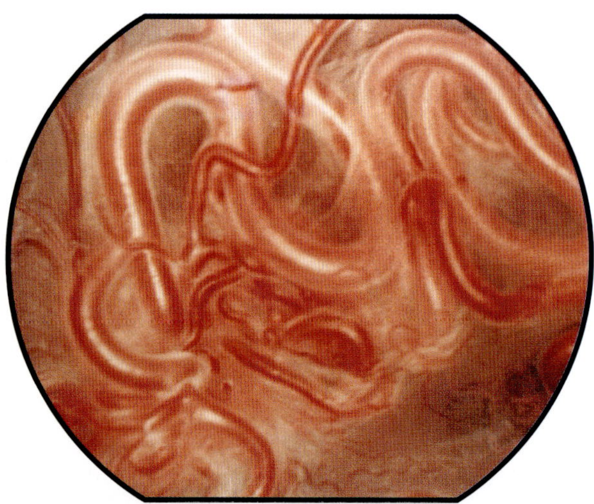

Patients with the Wyburn–Mason syndrome can have large retinal AV malformations. Lesions like this have been referred to as a "bag of worms."

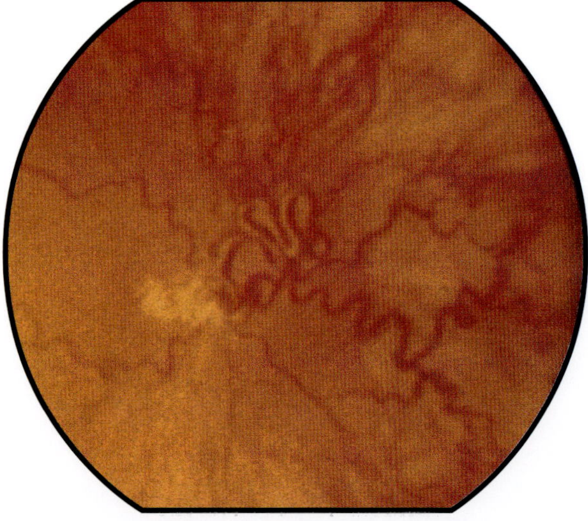

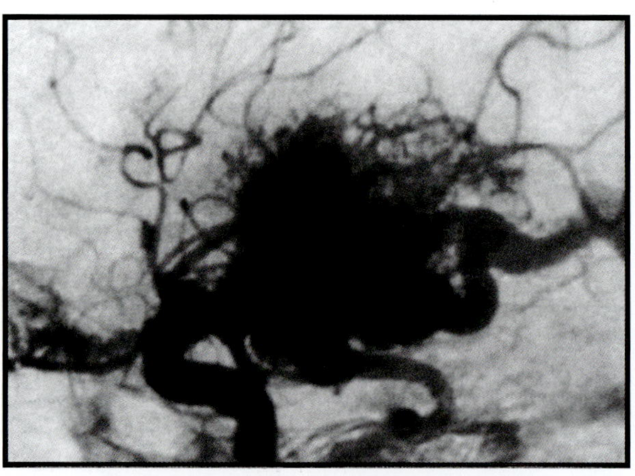

This is a patient with Wyburn–Mason syndrome involving the right fundus *(left)* and an intracranial vascular malformation seen with cerebral angiography *(right)*. *Courtesy of Dr. James Augsberger*

This eye with racemose hemangioma developed peripheral ischemia and neovascularization *(arrow)*. Laser treatment was used to treat peripheral ischemia. Retinal vascular occlusive disease with vascular sheathing, secondary neovascularization, and multiple stages of vascular remodeling are not uncommon with a racemose hemangioma.

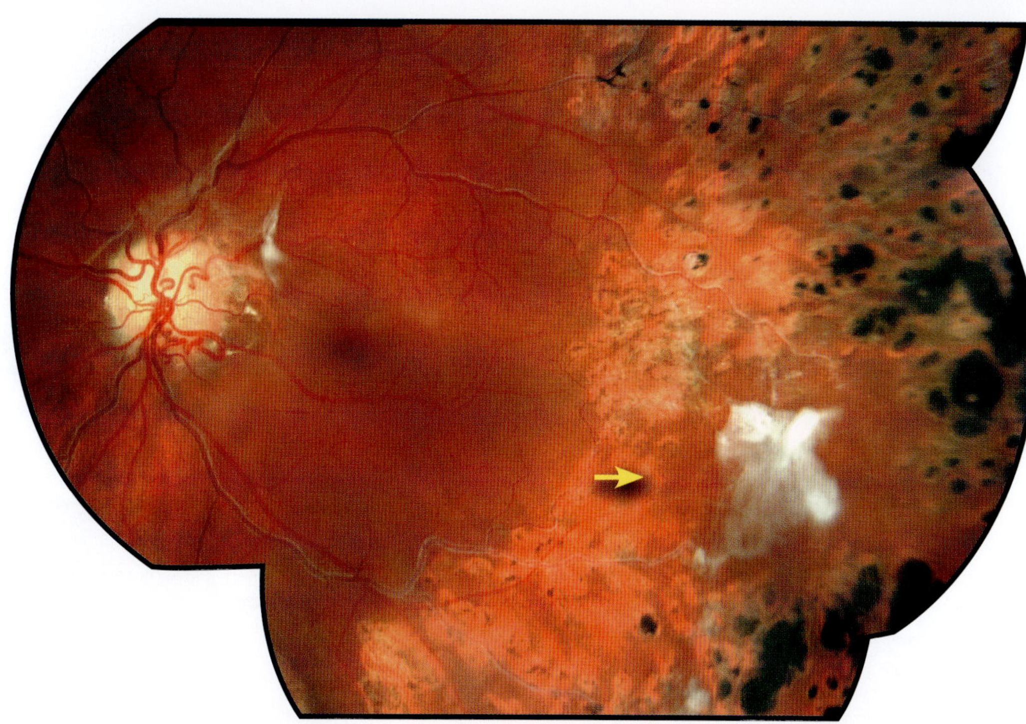

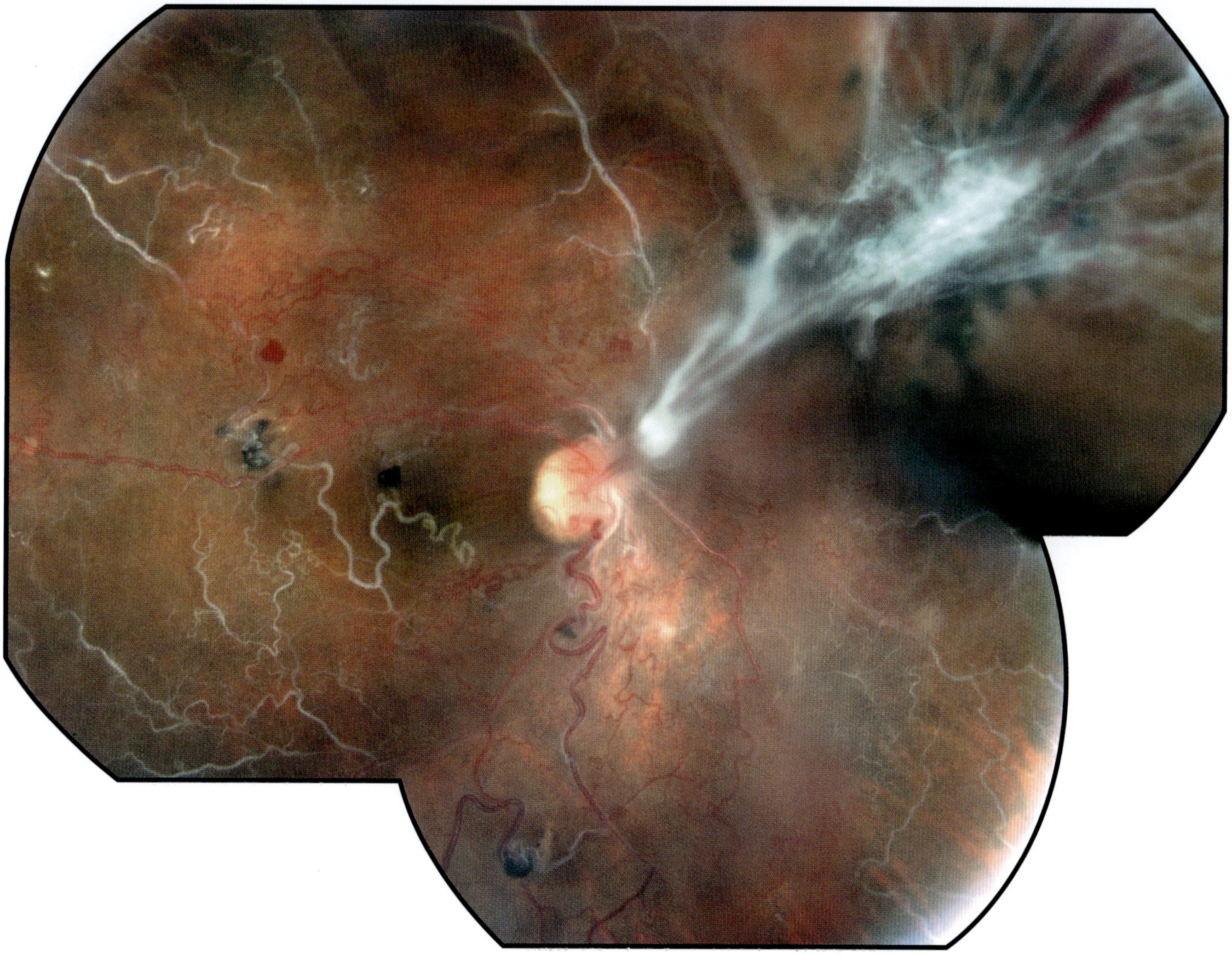

In this case there was extensive occlusive disease, large capillary aneurysms, secondary compensatory vascular tortuosity, ischemia, neovascularization, and fibrous proliferation simulating retinal findings sometimes seen with neurofibromatosis type 2.

Retinal Vasoproliferative Tumor

The retinal vasoproliferative tumor is a vascular mass typically located in the periphery of the fundus near the ora serrata in middle aged and older patients. This benign tumor can produce intraretinal and subretinal exudation, subretinal fluid, cystoid macular edema, and epiretinal membrane leading to poor visual acuity. Even though the retinal vasoproliferative tumor appears clinically similar to the retinal hemangioblastoma (capillary hemangioma), there are some notable differences in that the feeding and draining vessels are minimally dilated, the exudation tends to start at the tumor and extend posteriorly, and it is not associated with von Hippel–Lindau disease. The retinal vasoproliferative tumor is idiopathic in 80% of cases and secondary to previous retinal insults in 20% of cases. The most common conditions leading to vasoproliferative tumor include pars planitis, retinitis pigmentosa, and inflammatory or traumatic conditions that cause retinal and retinal pigment epithelial disturbance. Rarely, a retinal reattachment procedure that involves drainage may result in a vasoproliferative mass lesion.

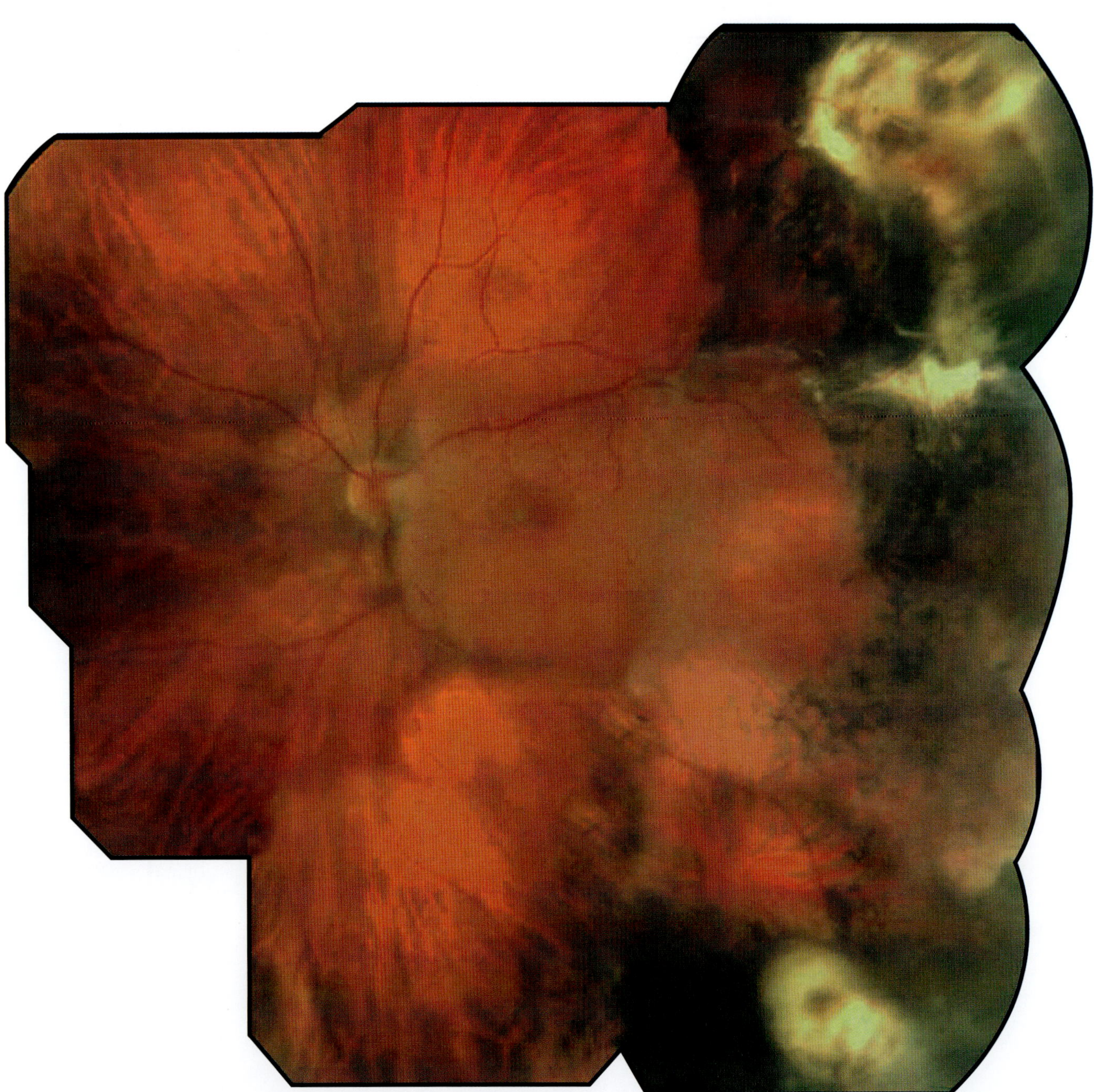

Retinal vasoproliferative tumor with regressing and actively leaking vessels, fibrosis, and hyperpigmentation.

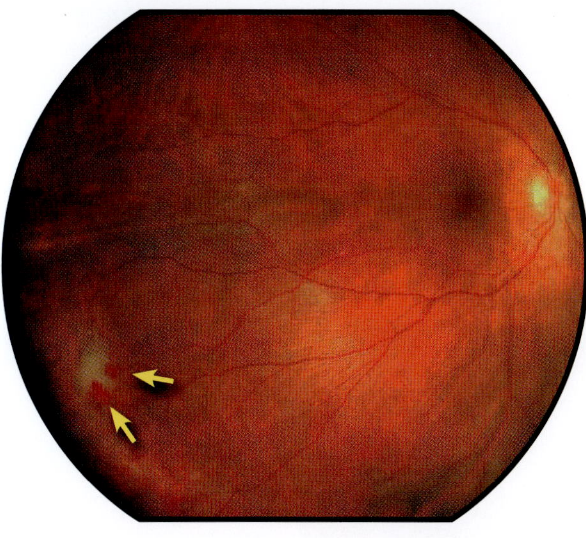

Subtle vasoproliferative tumor *(arrows)* in the inferotemporal ora serrata region with surrounding exudation. This is the most common site for these tumors.

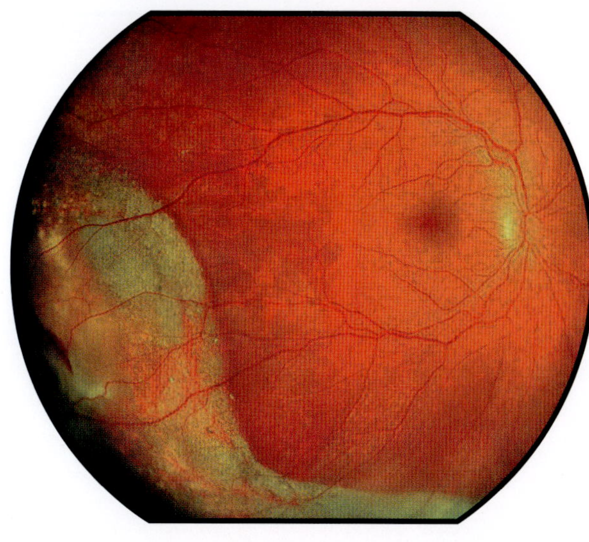

Ill-defined vasoproliferative tumor at the inferotemporal ora serrata with moderate subretinal exudation and retinal hemorrhage.

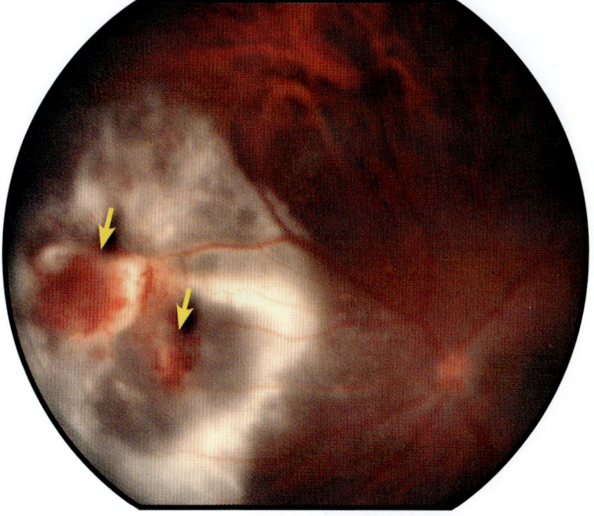

More advanced vasoproliferative tumor at the nasal ora serrata in the left eye. Note the associated subretinal fluid, exudation, fibrosis, and retinal hemorrhage *(arrows)*.

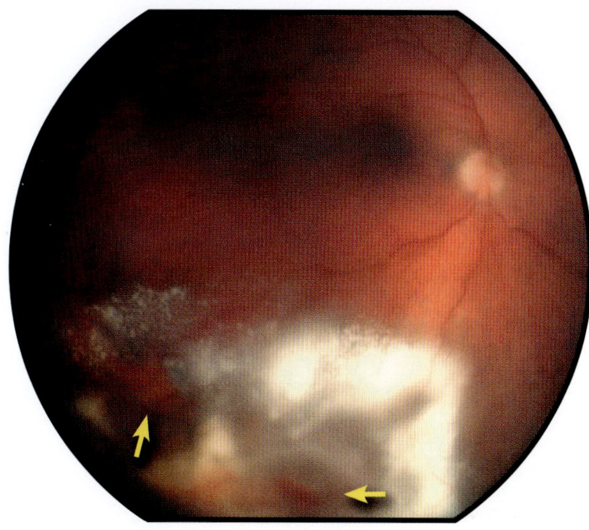

Two tumors *(arrows)* and surrounding exudative retinal detachment are obscured by a cloudy vitreous. The view is hazy due to exudation in the vitreous, as well as tumor-induced posterior subcapsular cataract.

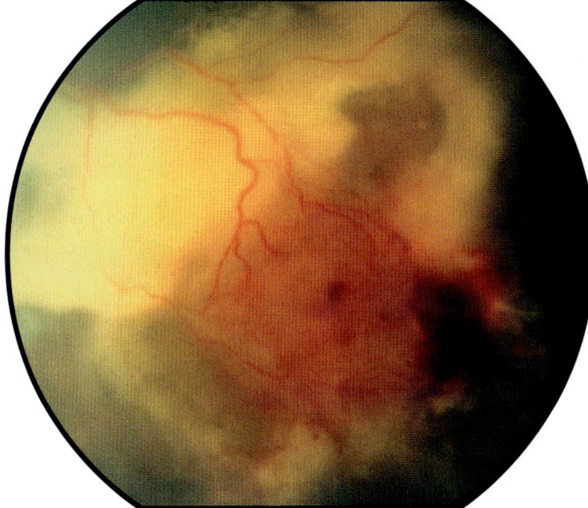

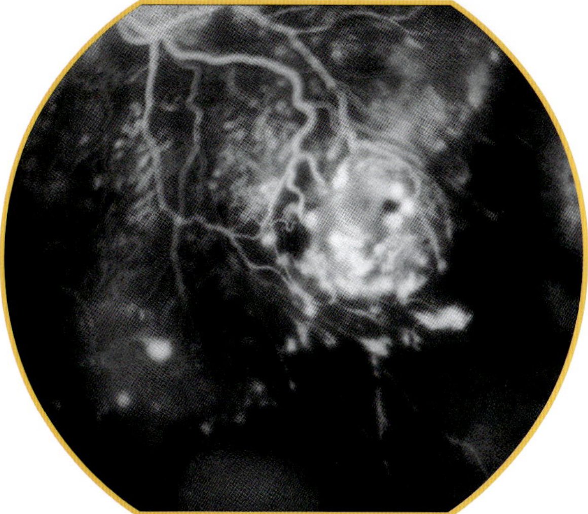

A retinal vasoproliferative tumor is associated with extensive lipid and exudative detachment. There is also hemorrhage but no markedly prominent perfusing or draining vessels.

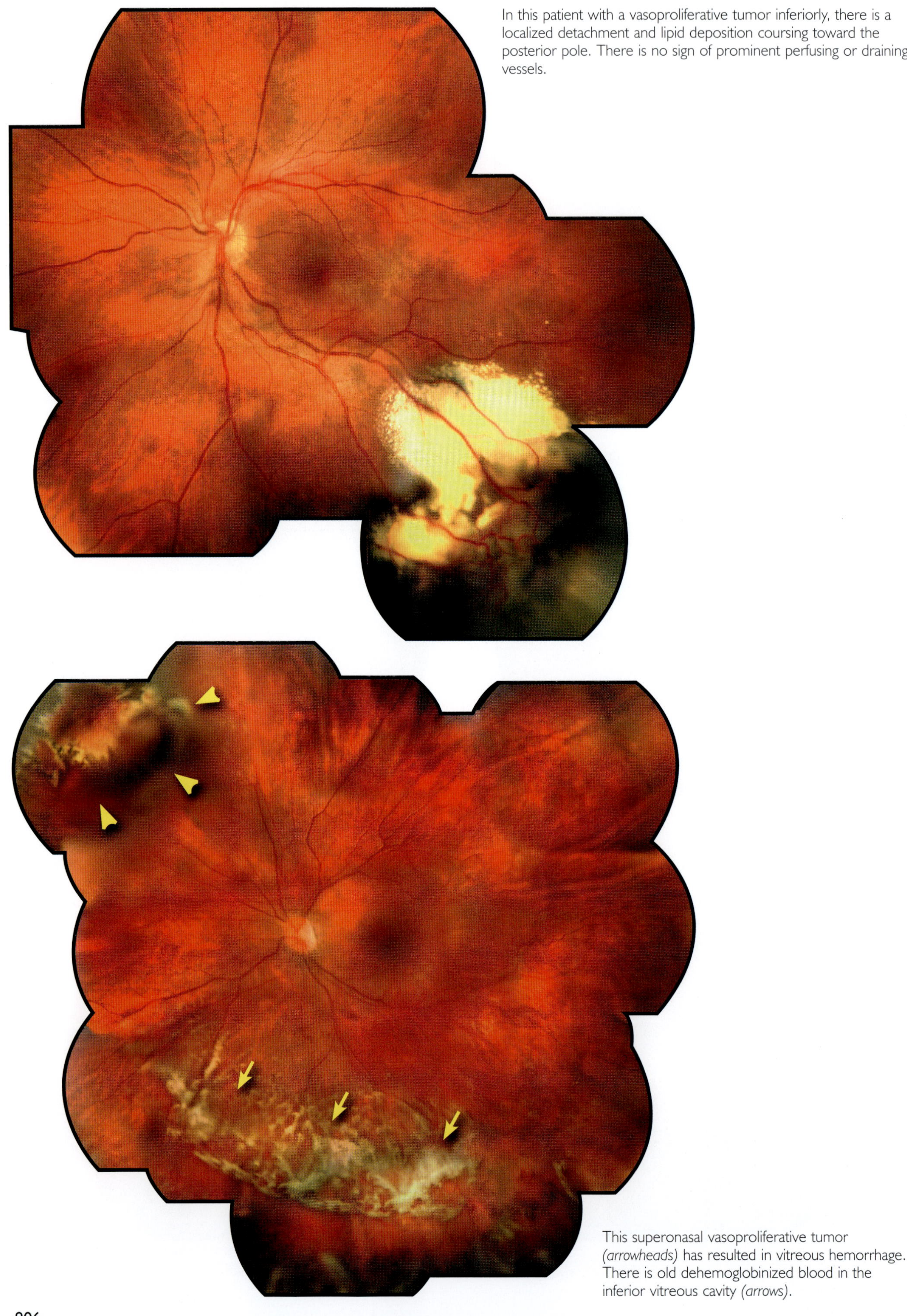

In this patient with a vasoproliferative tumor inferiorly, there is a localized detachment and lipid deposition coursing toward the posterior pole. There is no sign of prominent perfusing or draining vessels.

This superonasal vasoproliferative tumor *(arrowheads)* has resulted in vitreous hemorrhage. There is old dehemoglobinized blood in the inferior vitreous cavity *(arrows)*.

Retinal Vasoproliferative Tumor in Retinitis Pigmentosa

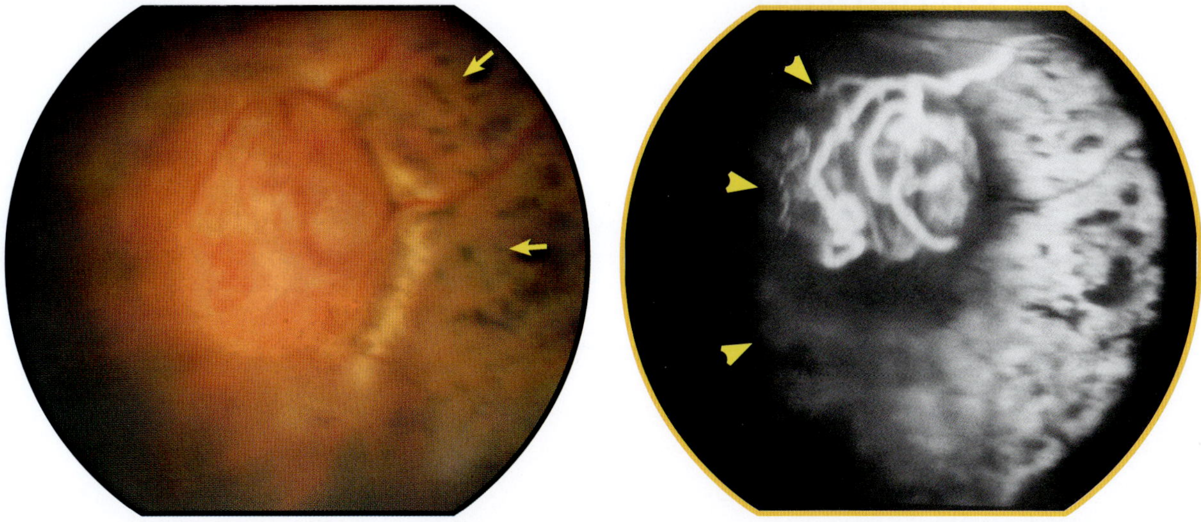

This retinal vasoproliferative tumor with lipid deposition and localized detachment was found in a patient with retinitis pigmentosa. Note the pigmentary retinopathy *(arrows)* and peripheral ischemia *(arrowheads)* anterior to the tumor. The phenotype of Retinitis Pigmentosa that is characterized by Coats-like exudative vasculopathy is sometimes associated with mutations in the Crumbs Homologue 1 (CRB1) gene.

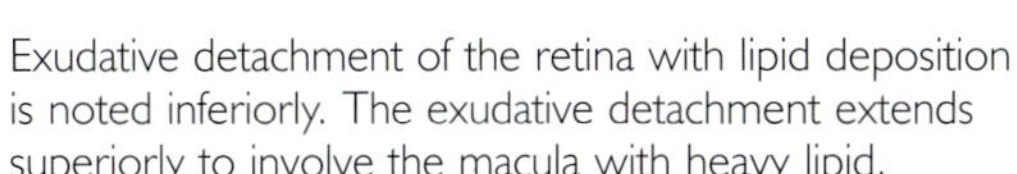

Exudative detachment of the retina with lipid deposition is noted inferiorly. The exudative detachment extends superiorly to involve the macula with heavy lipid.

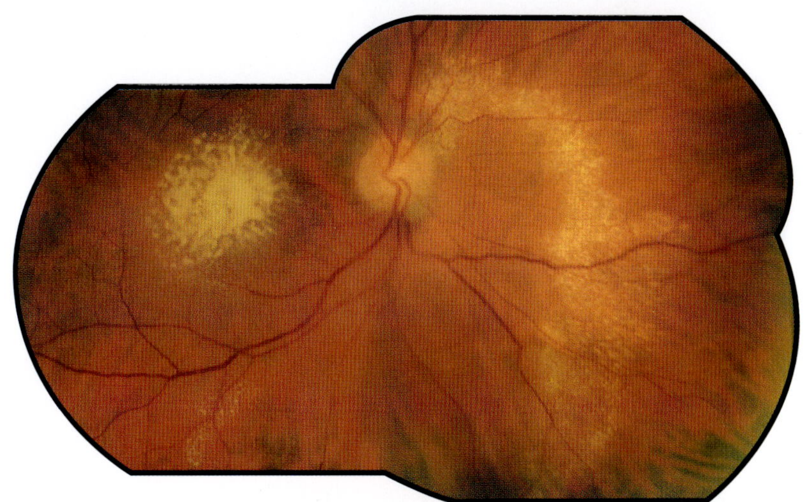

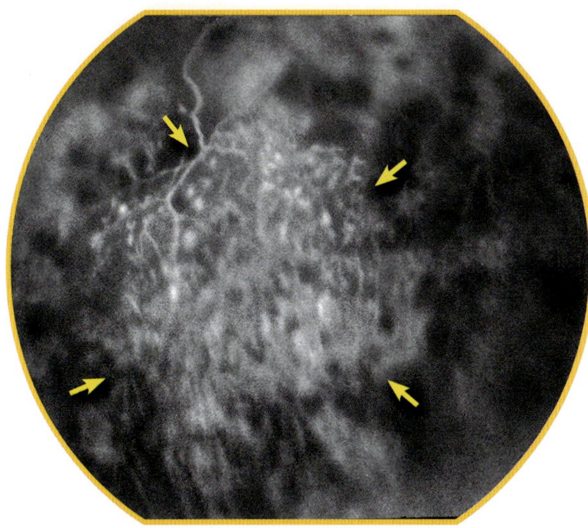

The fluorescein angiogram shows the extensive capillary abnormalities within the tumor *(arrows)*. This patient is a carrier of retinitis pigmentosa.

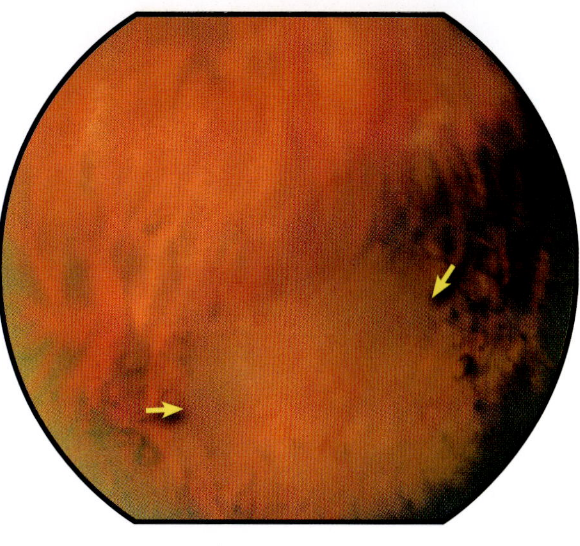

A vascularized gray-pink mass is barely visible within a zone of peripheral pigmentary degeneration *(arrows)*.

Combined Hamartoma of the Retina and Retinal Pigment Epithelium

A combined hamartoma of the retina and retinal pigment epithelium (RPE) is a presumed congenital intraocular tumor usually located adjacent to the nerve head but occasionally in the macular region and less commonly in the periphery. These tumors consist of thickened glial and fibrotic tissue with varying degrees of pigmentation and often occur in the presence of contraction at the inner retinal surface. OCT of these lesions shows tractional retinal distortion in a sawtooth or folded pattern. Rarely, retinal exudation or hemorrhage or alterations in vision secondary to spontaneous release of the epiretinal membrane occur. These lesions can rarely be multiple and can be seen in association with neurofibromatosis type 2.

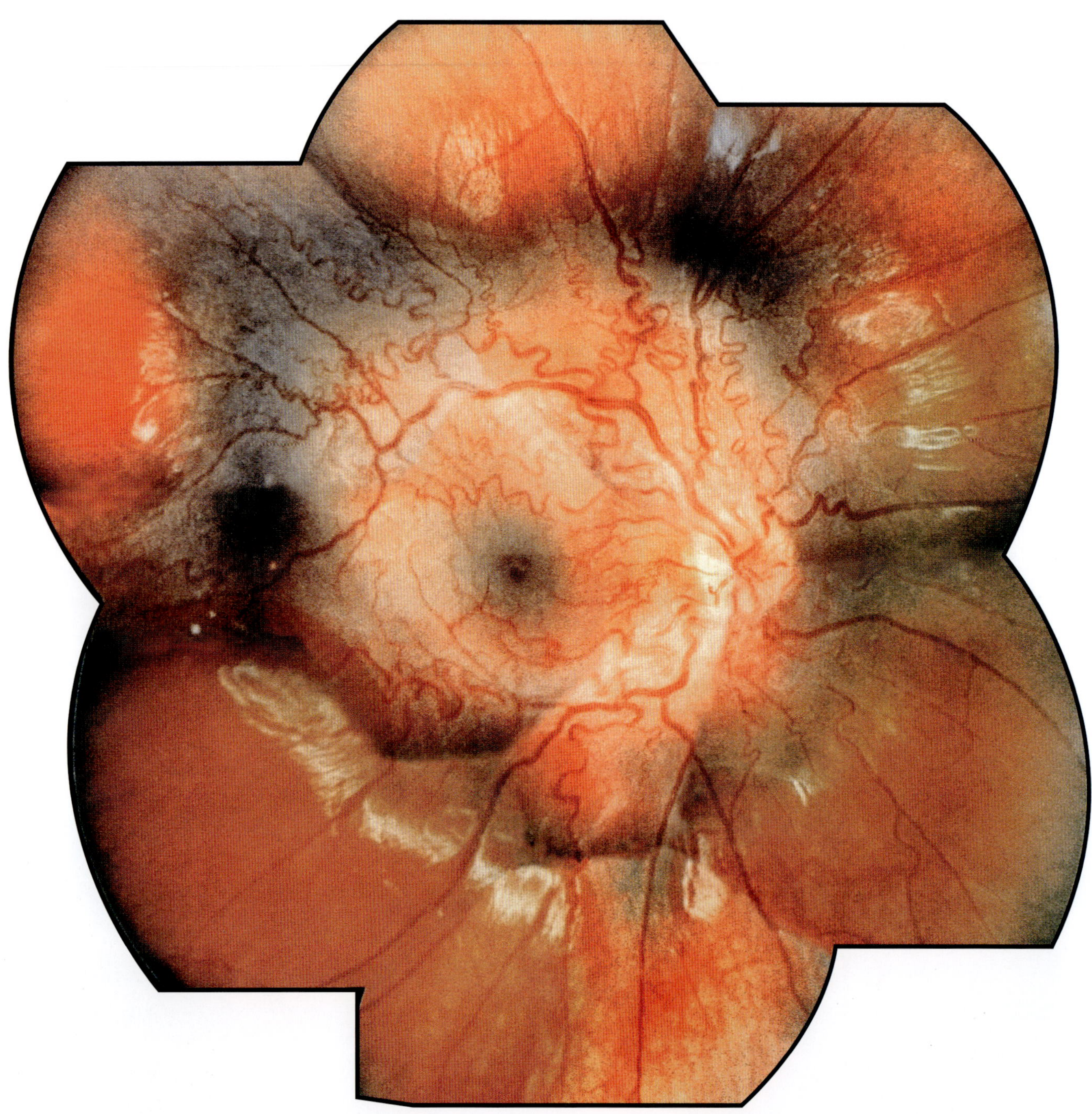

This patient has an extensive combined hamartoma of the retina and RPE with hyperpigmentation and marked vascular tortuosity. *Courtesy of Dr. Edward B. McLean*

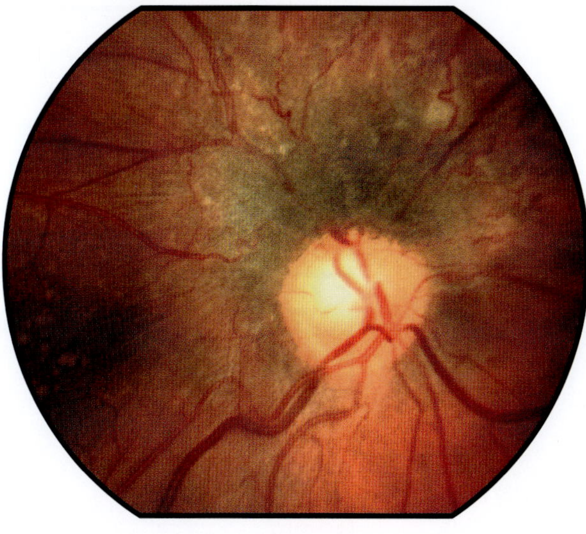

Hyperpigmentation, thought to be a secondary manifestation, may be more marked in some cases. In this particular case, epiretinal membranes, retinal vessel tortuosity, and hyperpigmentation are demonstrated.

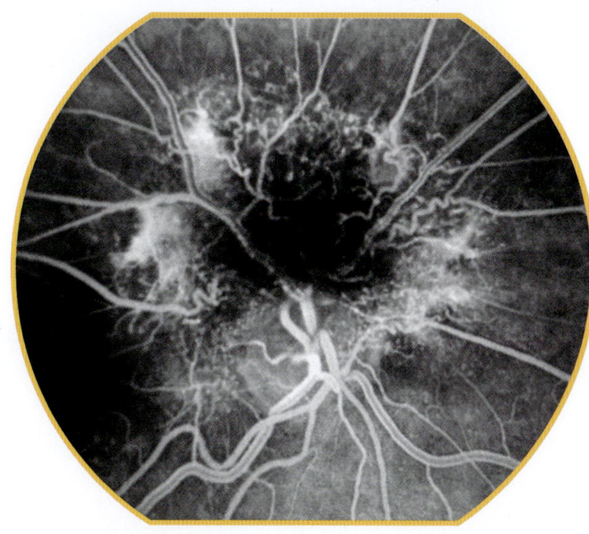

The fluorescein angiogram illustrates the tortuosity of the vessels. The uncomplicated case does not show vascular staining.

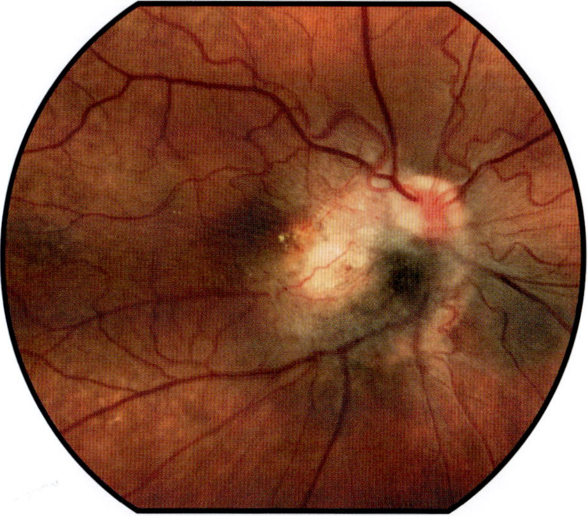

Typical combined hamartoma at the disc. *Courtesy of Dr. Alan Kimura*

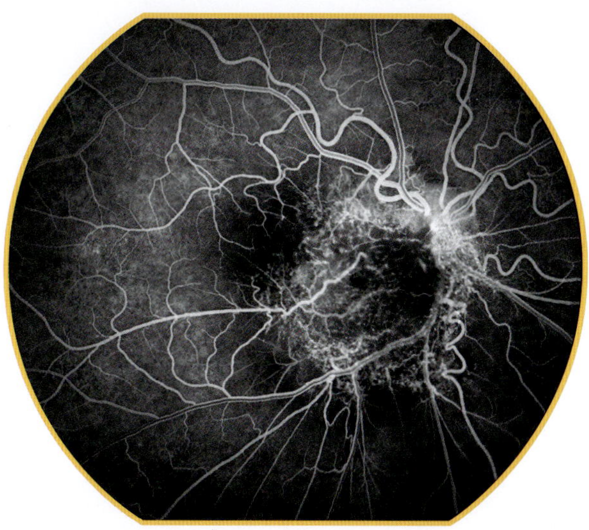

The fluorescein angiogram demonstrates the macular vascular abnormalities.

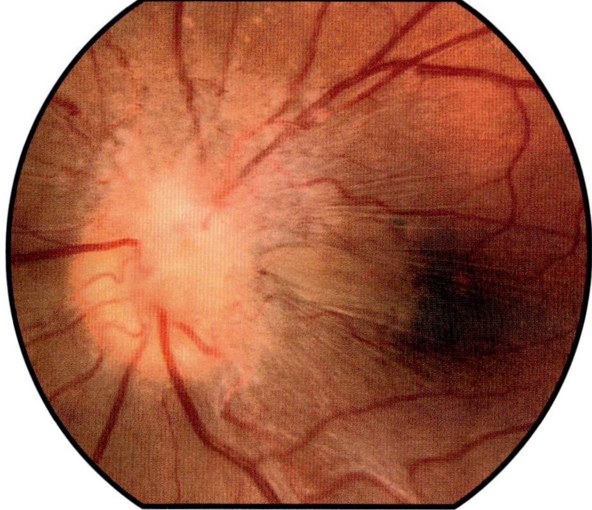

Traction on the retina from the hamartoma without prominent pigmentation can sometimes occur. In some cases, this traction can lead to retinal detachment.

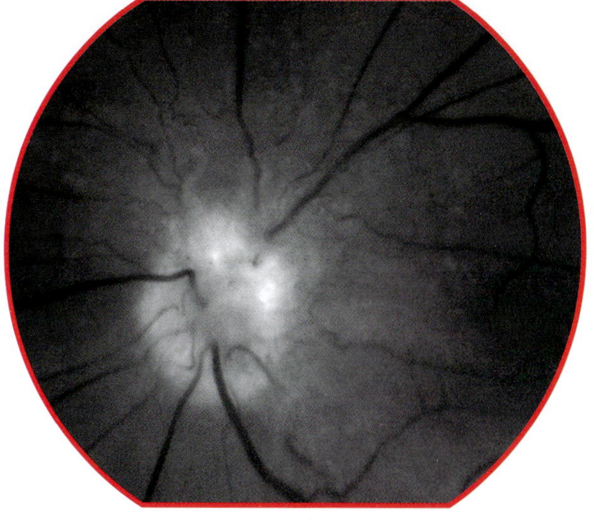

The red-free photograph highlights the vitreoretinal interface disturbance.

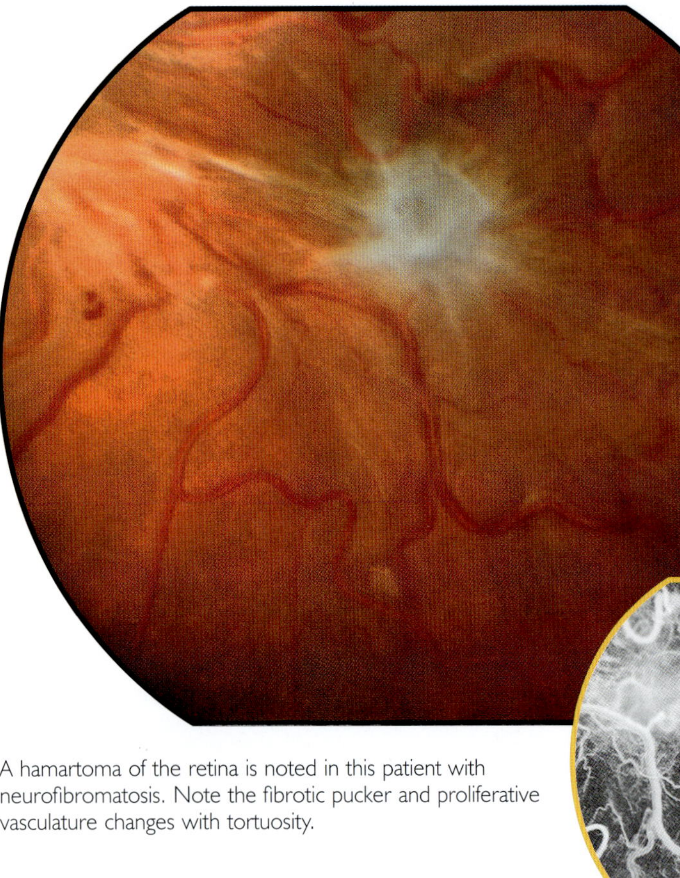

A hamartoma of the retina is noted in this patient with neurofibromatosis. Note the fibrotic pucker and proliferative vasculature changes with tortuosity.

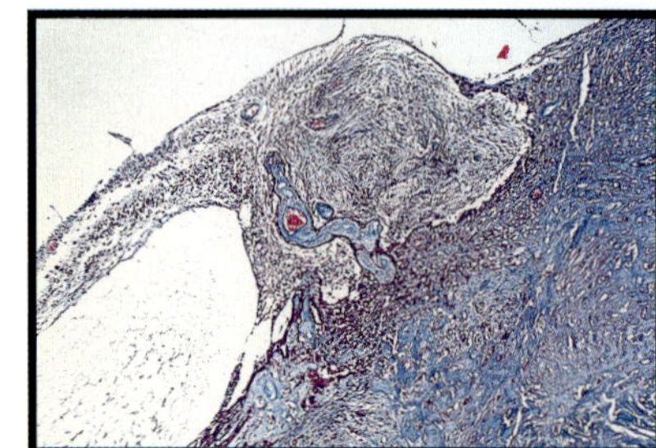

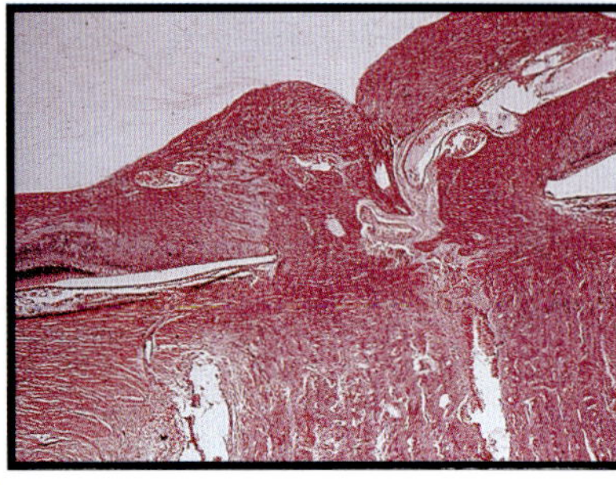

These hamartomas involve the optic nerve head. Both are from patients with neurofibromatosis.

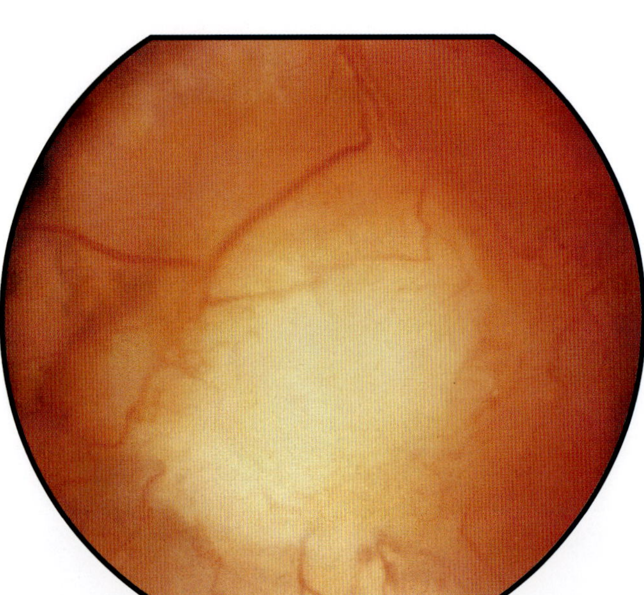

This 39-year-old white female had a nonpigmented hamartoma of the retina and RPE.

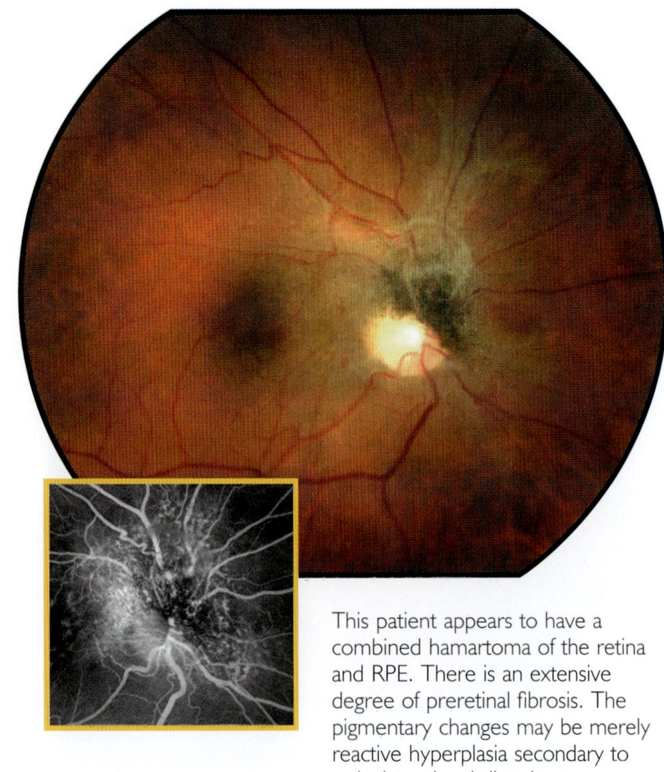

This patient appears to have a combined hamartoma of the retina and RPE. There is an extensive degree of preretinal fibrosis. The pigmentary changes may be merely reactive hyperplasia secondary to retinal tractional disturbances.
Courtesy of Dr. Martin Schwartz

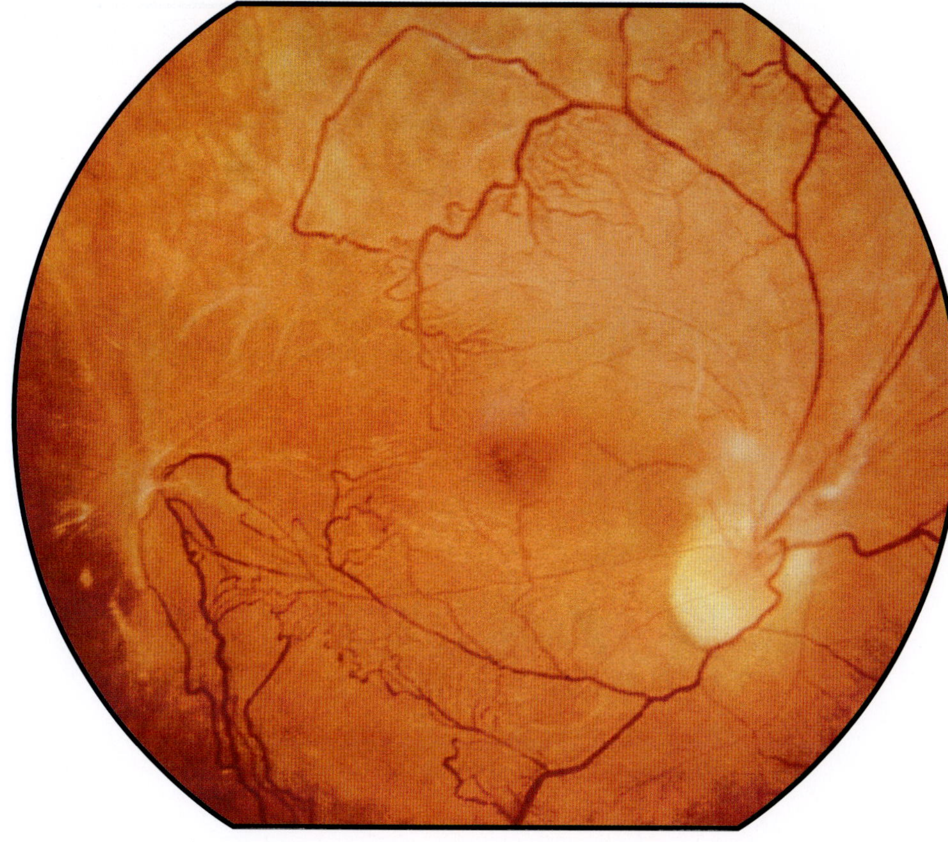

Patients with neurofibromatosis type 2 can have diffuse retinal involvement including astrocytic hamartomas of the retina and peripheral retinal vascular occlusions. A loop of AV anastomosis is noted with obliteration of the arteries and veins in the retina. The temporal retina has widespread ischemia and preretinal neovascularization. Note the islands of nonperfused retina that are present in the posterior pole extending toward the center of the macula.

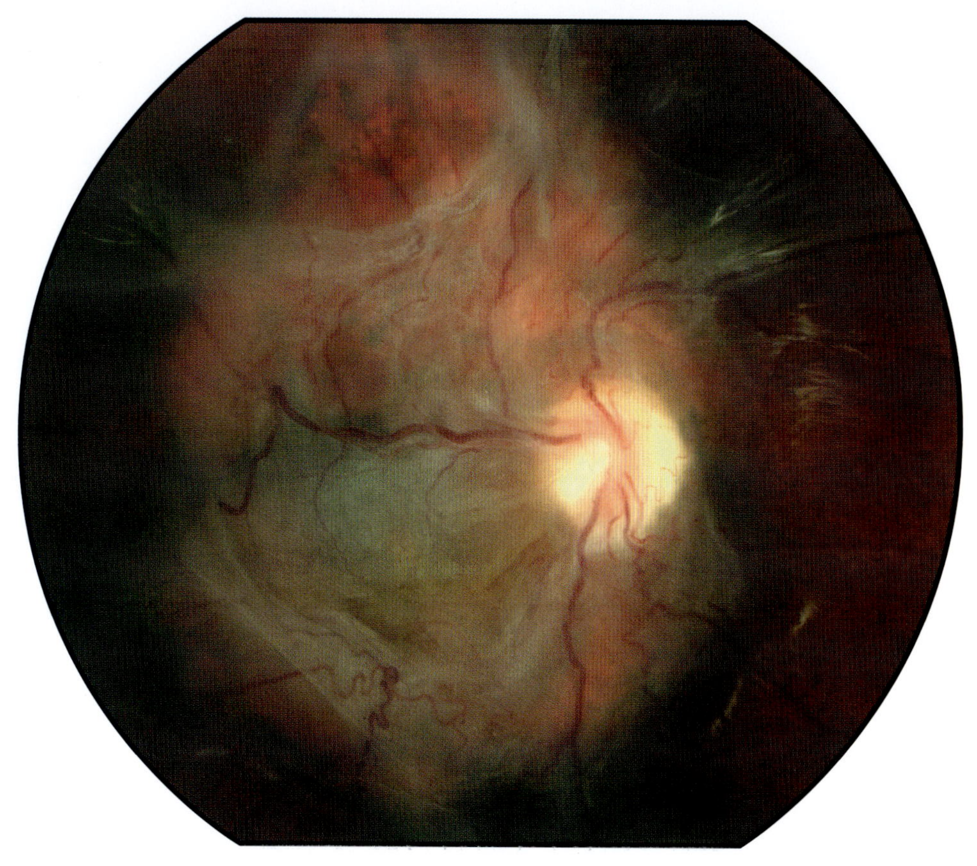

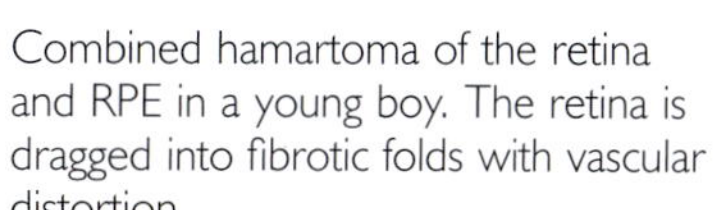

Combined hamartoma of the retina and RPE in a young boy. The retina is dragged into fibrotic folds with vascular distortion.

This temporal macular combined hamartoma of the retina and RPE is in a 14-year-old girl with visual acuity of 20/100. Montage fundus photography shows the gray-green retinal mass with radiating striae and retinal dragging.

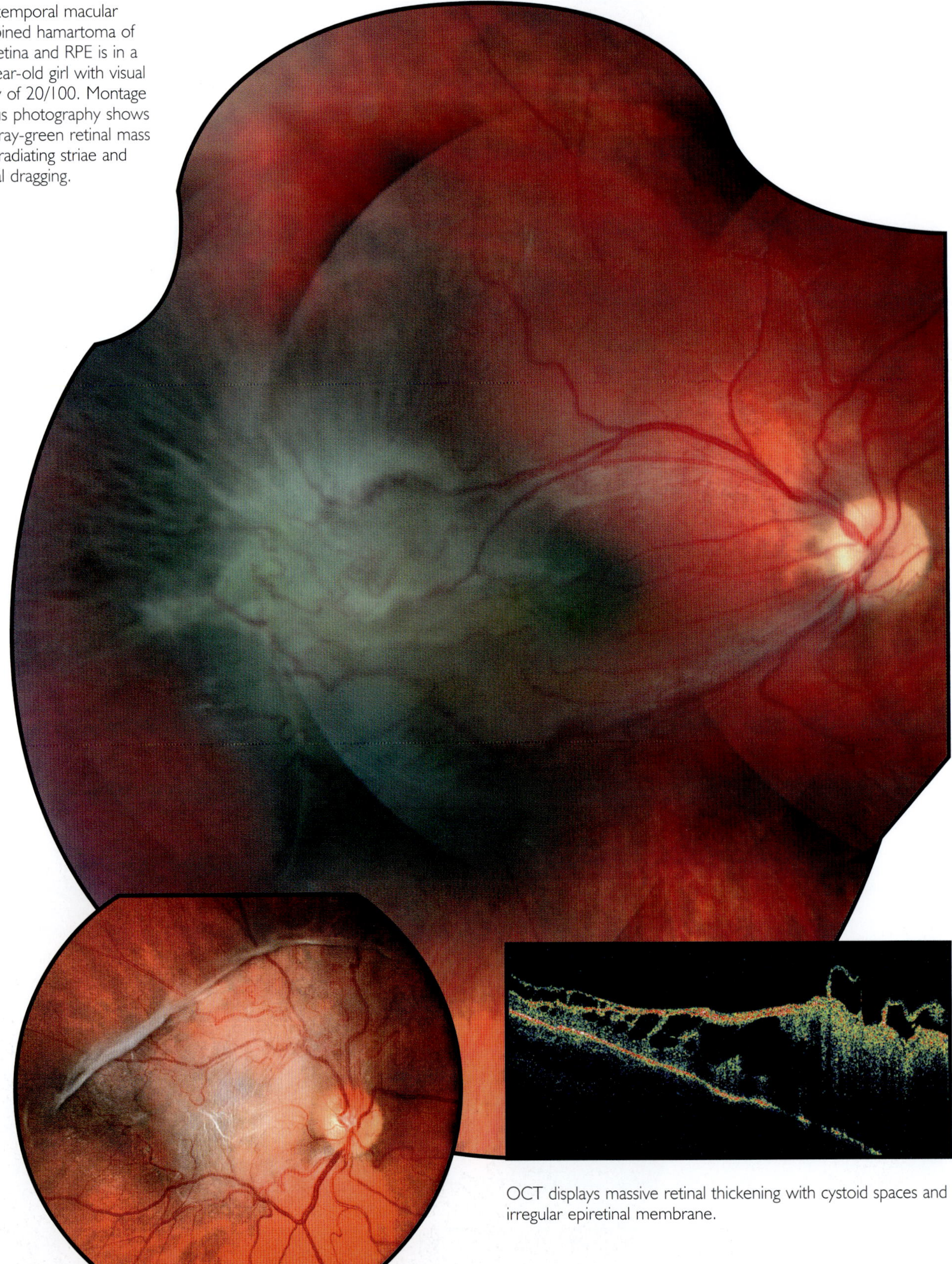

OCT displays massive retinal thickening with cystoid spaces and irregular epiretinal membrane.

This patient with a combined hamartoma has a significant degree of fibrous proliferation overlying a relatively non-pigmented lesion. *Courtesy of Dr. Jeffrey Shakin*

Neurofibromatosis Type 2

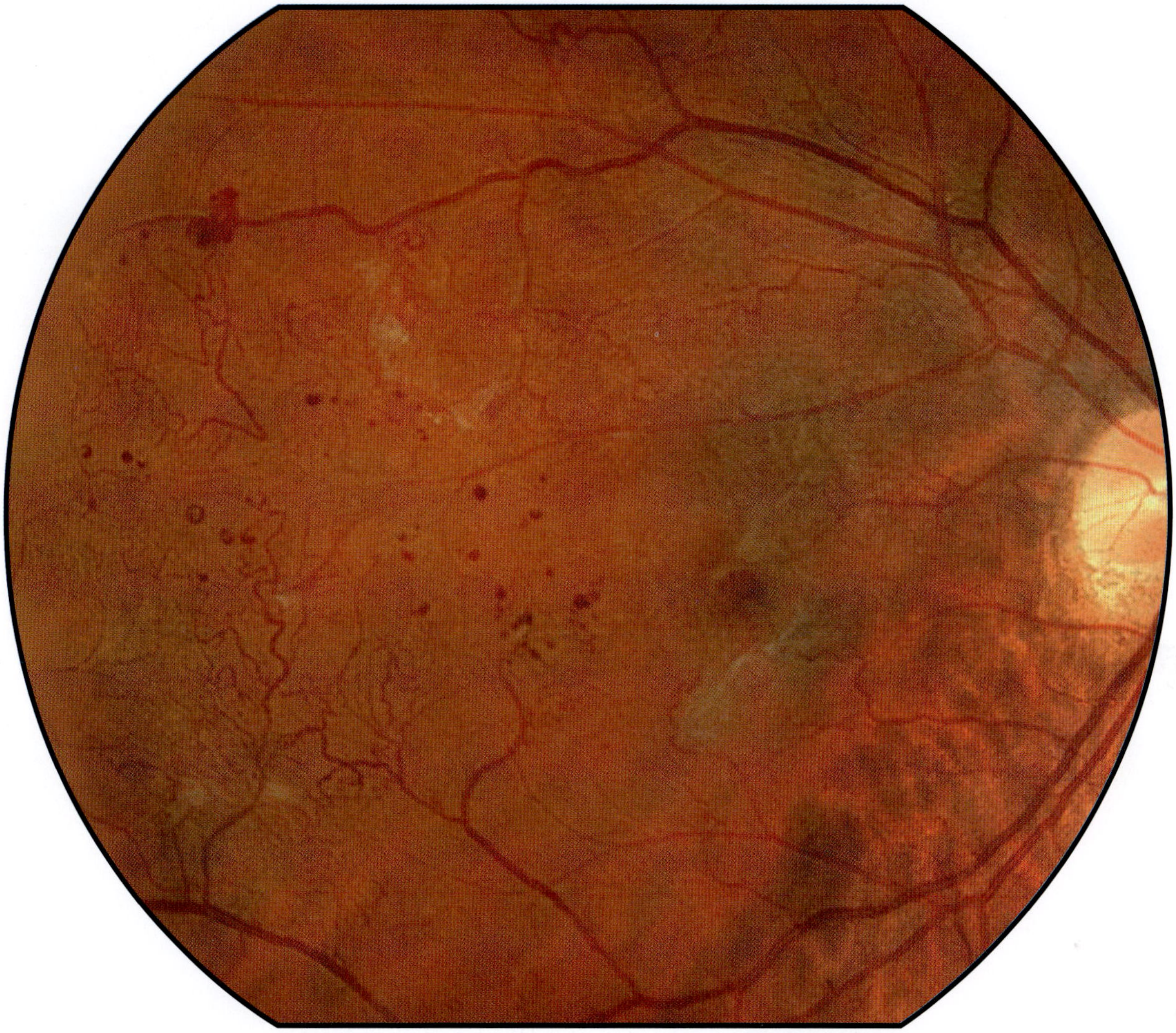

Note the corkscrew vessels and large capillary aneurysms in this patient with neurofibromatosis type 2.

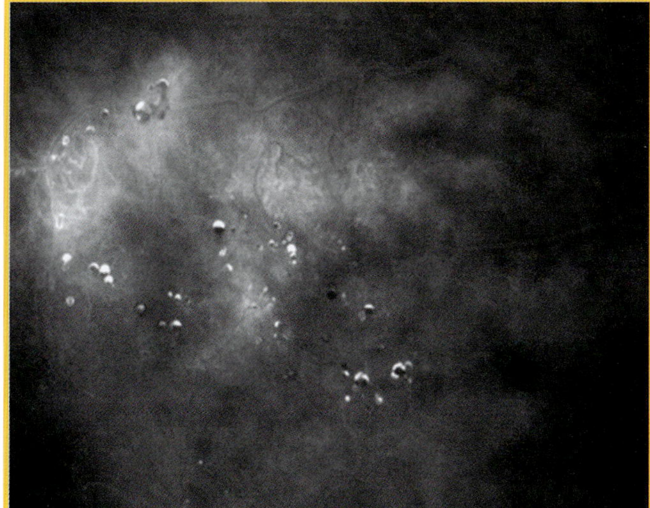

Plasma erythrocyte interface changes are evident at large macro/microaneurysms. *Courtesy of Dr. Paulus de Jong*

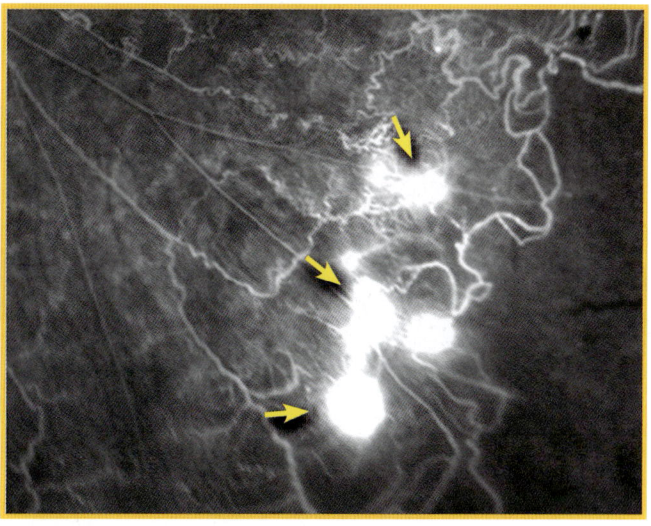

Peripheral retinal ischemia and neovascularization *(arrows)* are evident in this patient. *Courtesy of Dr. Paulus de Jong*

Enhanced Depth Imaging Optical Coherence Tomography of Combined Hamartoma

Combined hamartoma can show two patterns on enhanced depth imaging optical coherence tomography (EDI-OCT), which include sawtooth (mini-peak) and folded (maxi-peak). The type of pattern depends on the degree and chronicity of vitreoretinal traction.

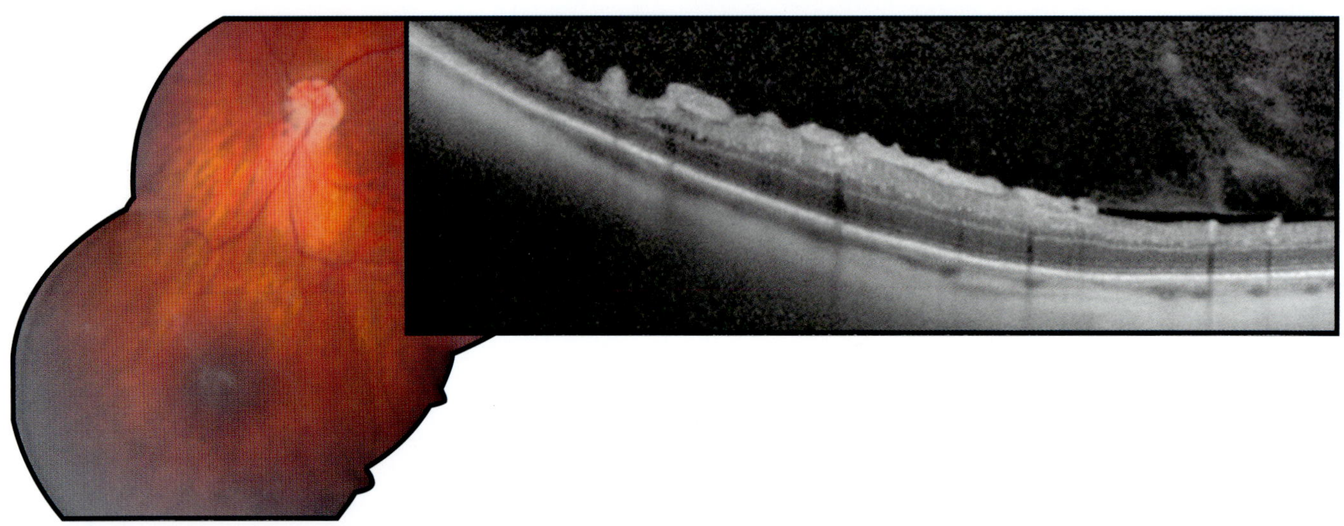

Small peripheral combined hamartoma with sawtooth (mini-peak) pattern.

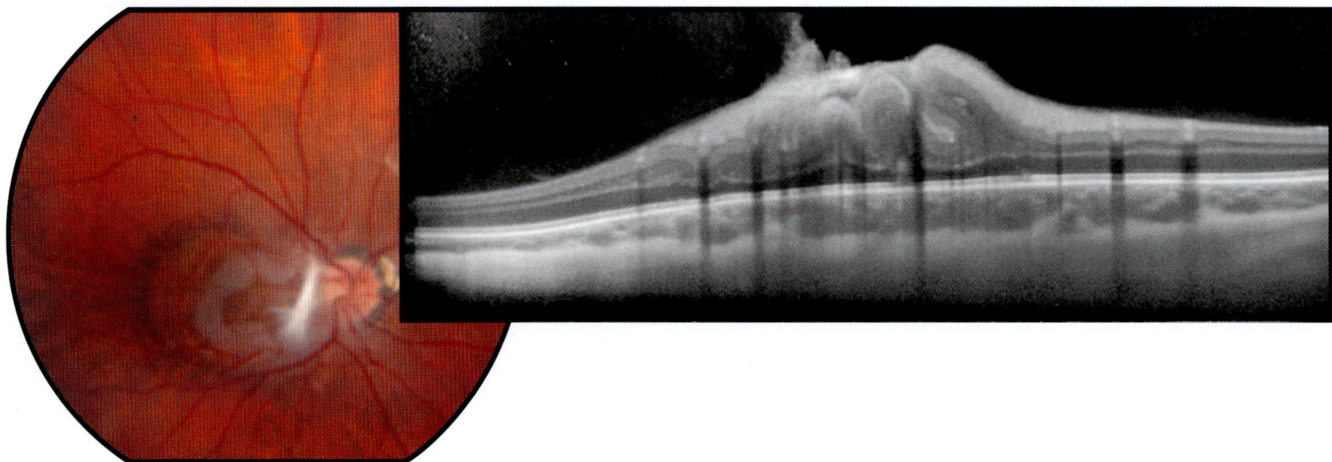

Juxtapapillary combined hamartoma with folded (maxi-peak) pattern.

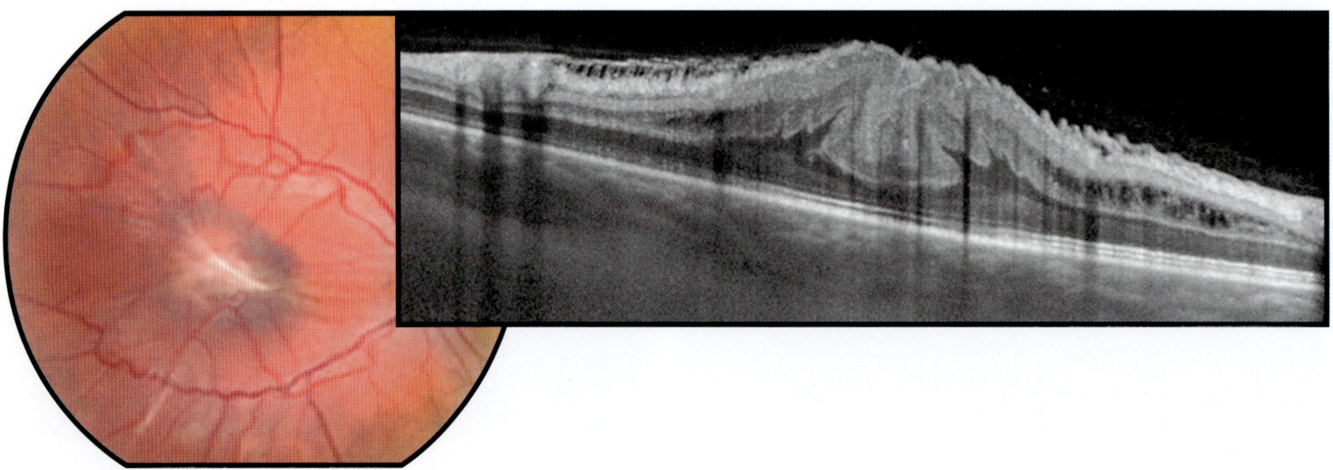

Macular combined hamartoma with both sawtooth and folded configuration.

Congenital Hypertrophy of the Retinal Pigment Epithelium (CHRPE)

CHRPE is a flat pigmented lesion arising deep to the retina, typically in the peripheral fundus. It is often discovered coincidentally on ocular examination as most patients are without related symptoms. CHRPE can display clinical features that resemble those of choroidal nevus or choroidal melanoma. Most clinicians regard CHRPE as a stable, unchanging lesion with little risk. However, slow documented enlargement of CHRPE has been found in over 80% of cases. In addition, in rare instances, CHRPE can produce a nodule of epithelioma (adenoma/adenocarcinoma) of the RPE.

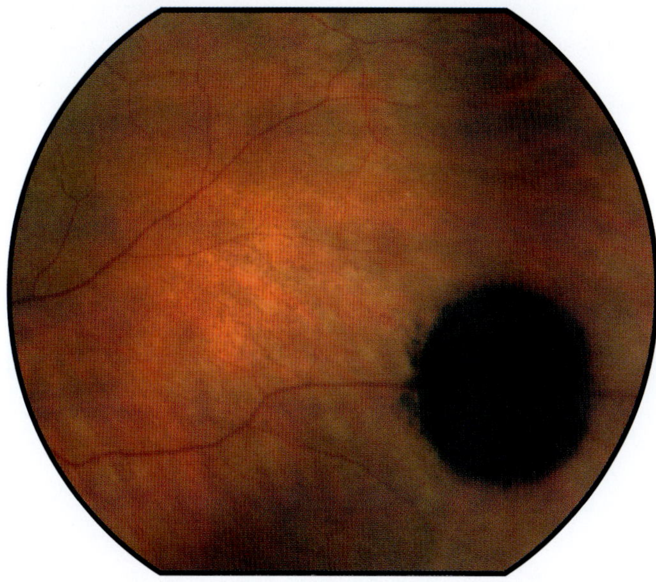

Heavily pigmented CHRPE lesion.

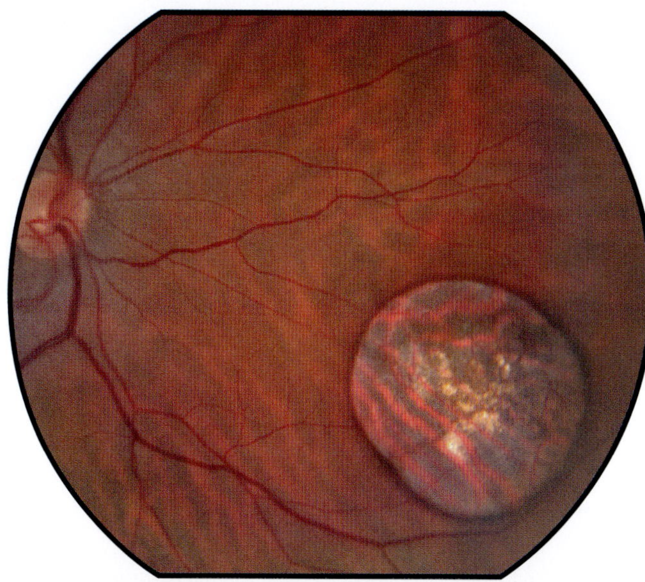

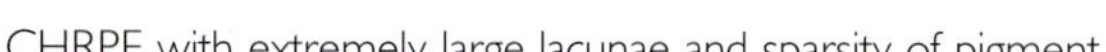

CHRPE with extremely large lacunae and sparsity of pigment.

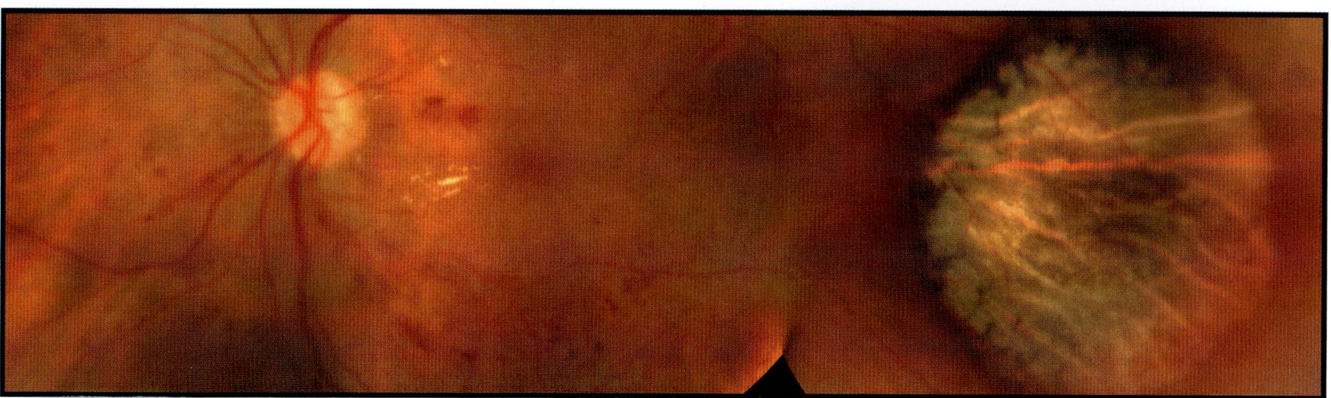

Large CHRPE amelanotic lesion in a patient with diabetic retinopathy.

CHRPE in the Macula

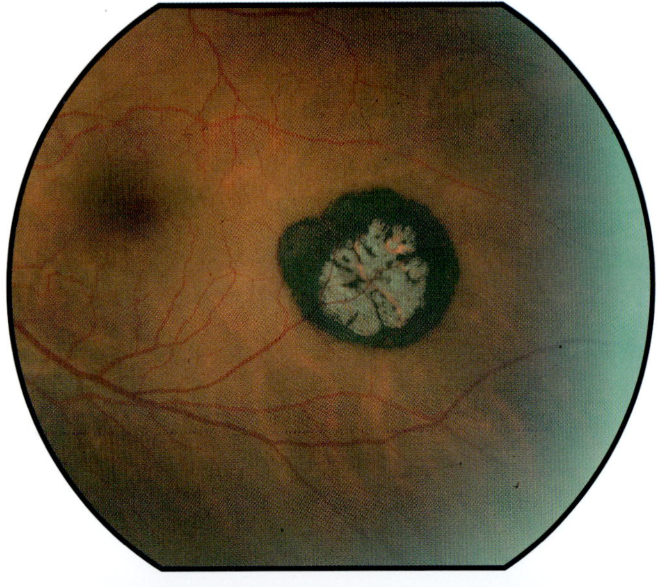

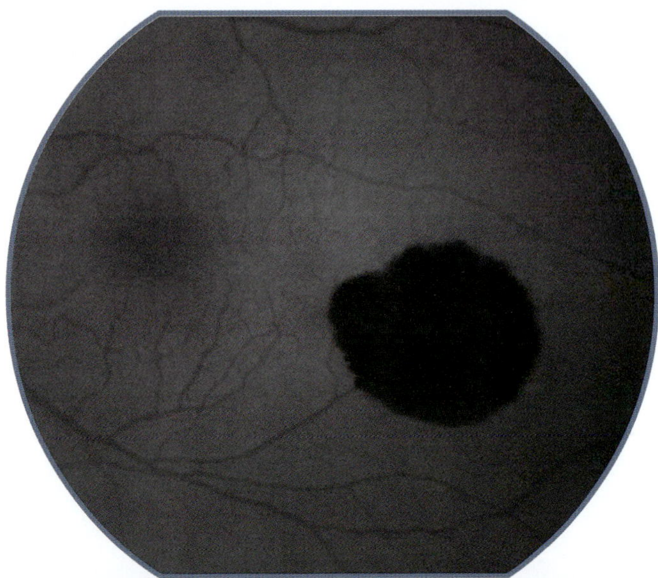

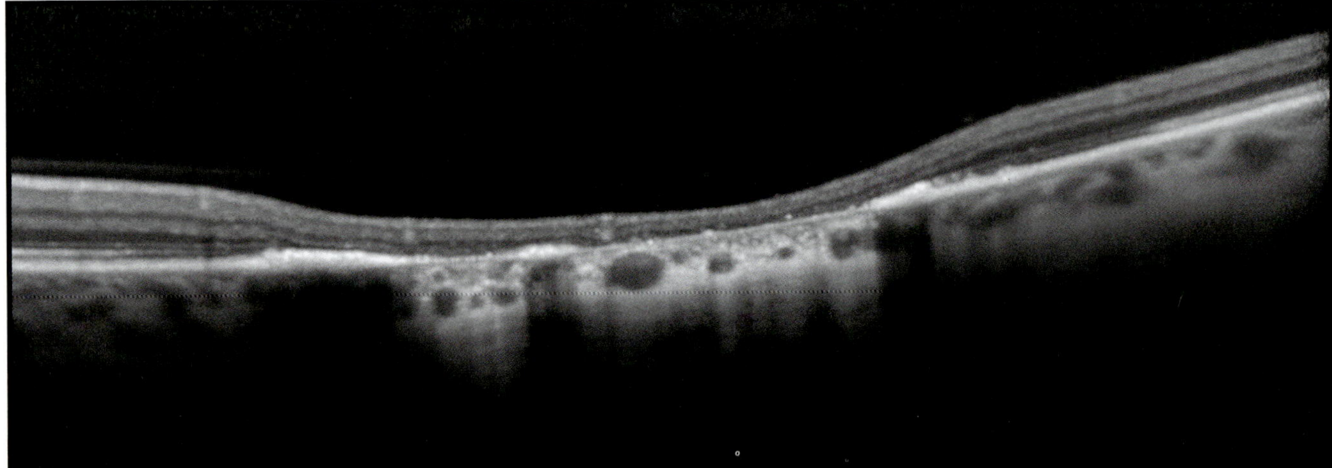

Paramacular CHRPE with crisp margins and lacunae demonstrating complete hypoautofluorescence on fundus autofluorescence. The OCT demonstrates overlying vitreous detachment and a relatively normal underlying choroid. The CHRPE is visualized as areas of mildly thickened RPE. There is outer retinal atrophy with photoreceptor loss. Note that the lacunae transmit light.

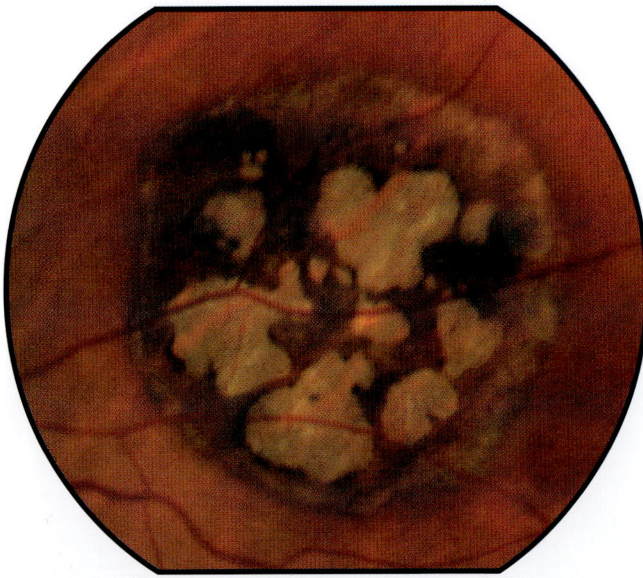

This CHRPE lesion had typical lacunae of RPE atrophy.

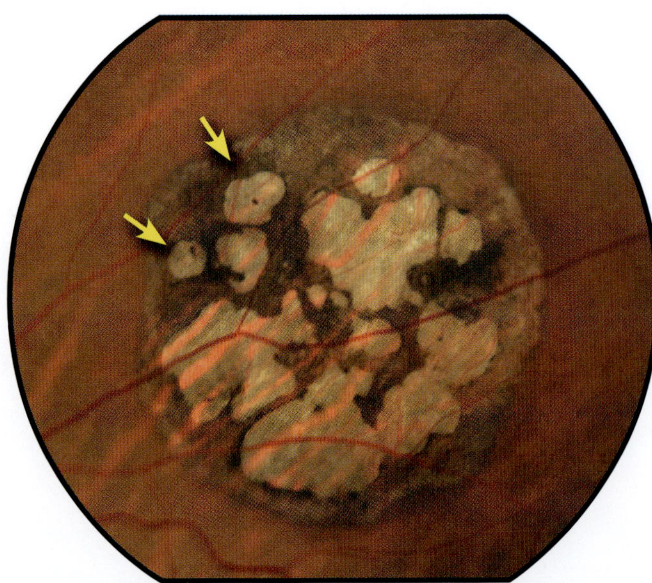

Two years later, there was progressive enlargement of the zonal atrophy *(arrows)*.

Spectrum of CHRPE

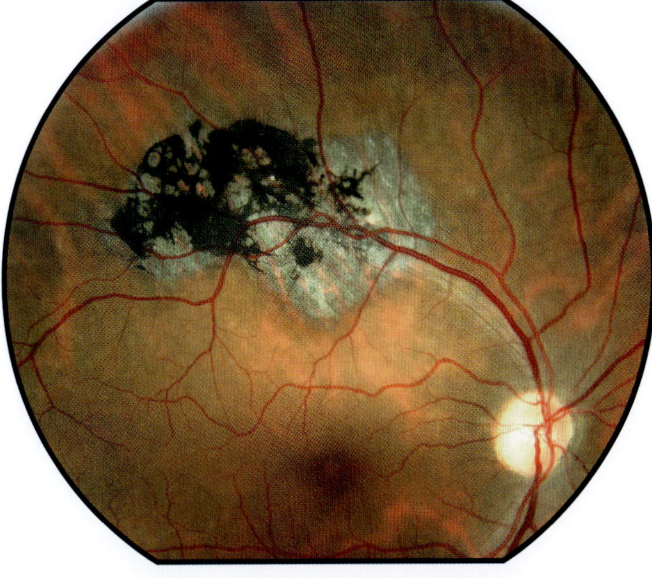

An irregular CHRPE lesion with variable pigmentation and atrophy.

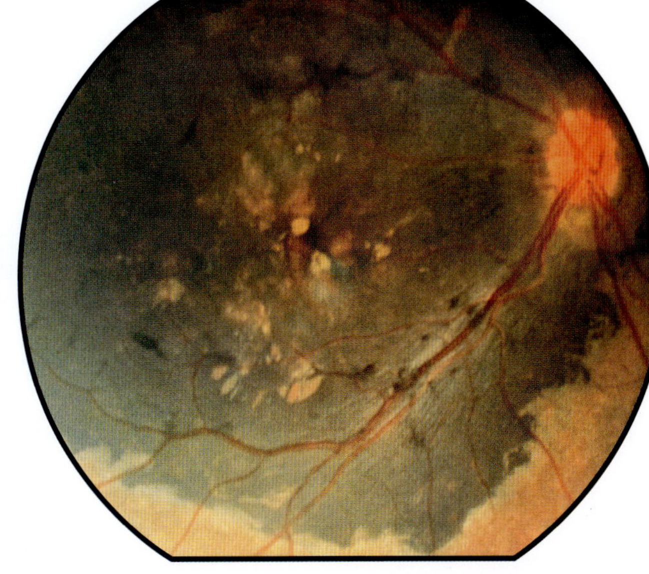

Hypertrophy of the RPE may sometimes be more diffuse and involve the macular region. A characteristic of RPE hypertrophy is a surrounding halo of atrophy, as demonstrated in this case. These lesions often appear singular as a flat roundish area of variable pigmentation. *Courtesy of Dr. Evangelos Gragoudas*

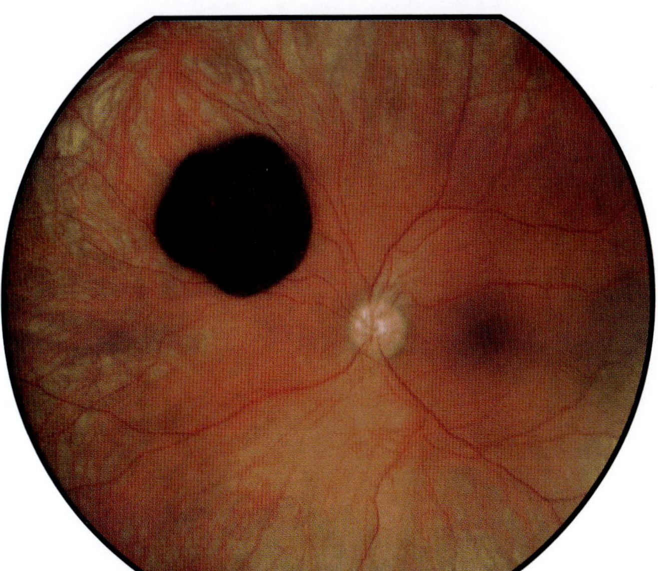

Flat pigmented CHRPE with pinpoint lacunae in a lightly colored fundus.

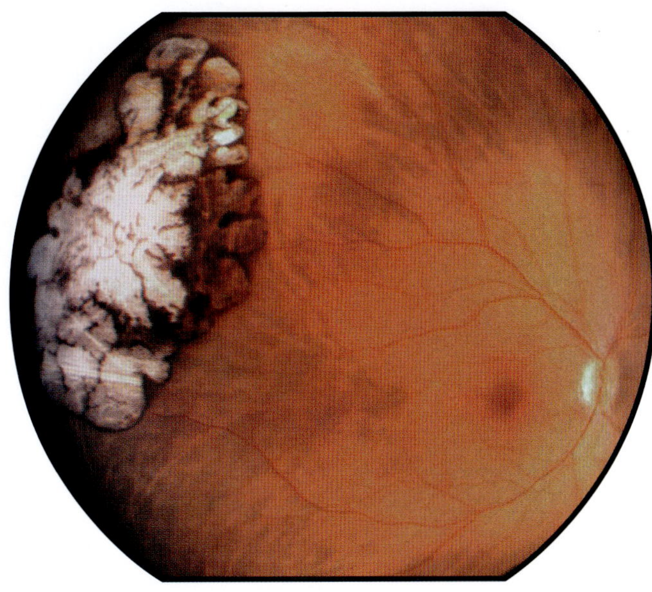

Peripheral CHRPE with large lacunae.

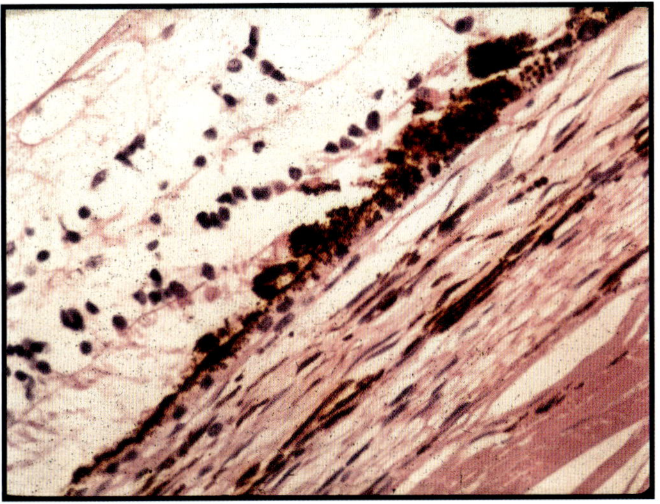

This histological section of congenital hypertrophy of the RPE shows tall, darkly pigmented retinal pigment epithelial cells. In some instances, there may be a loss of the outer and inner segments of the photoreceptors. A depigmented layer at the margin of the RPE cells corresponds to the halo commonly seen around the lesion.

Multifocal CHRPE (Bear Tracks)

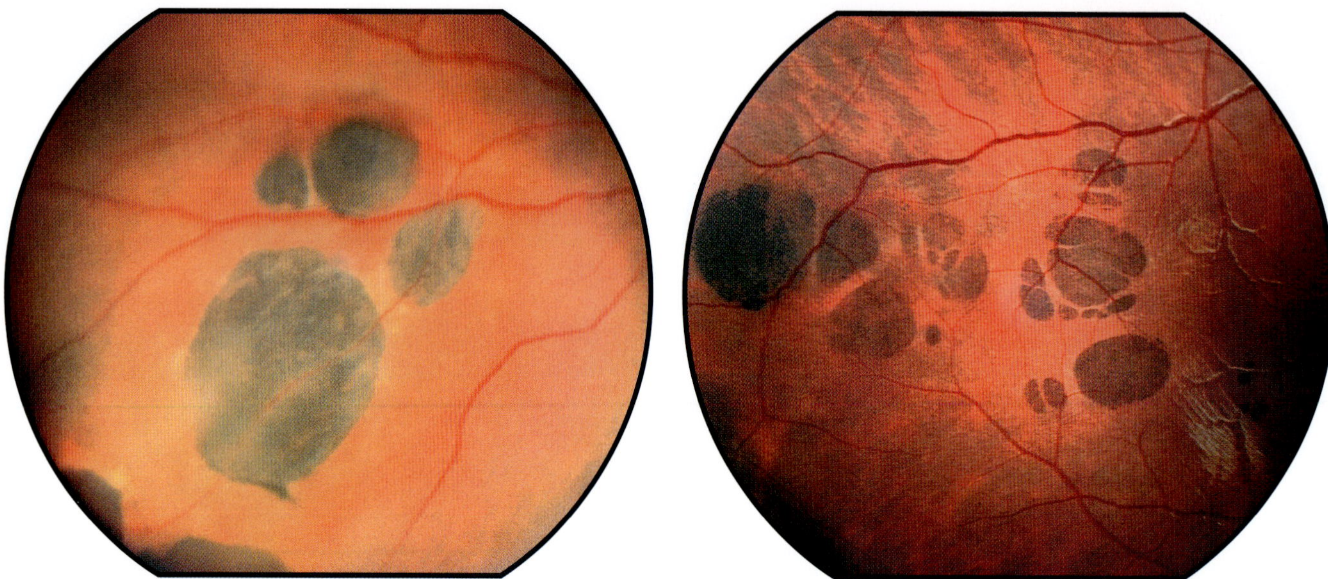

Bear tracks, congenital hypertrophy of the RPE, and grouped pigmentation are different terms for congenital lesions of the RPE. Flat large areas of hyperpigmentation are seen on clinical examination.

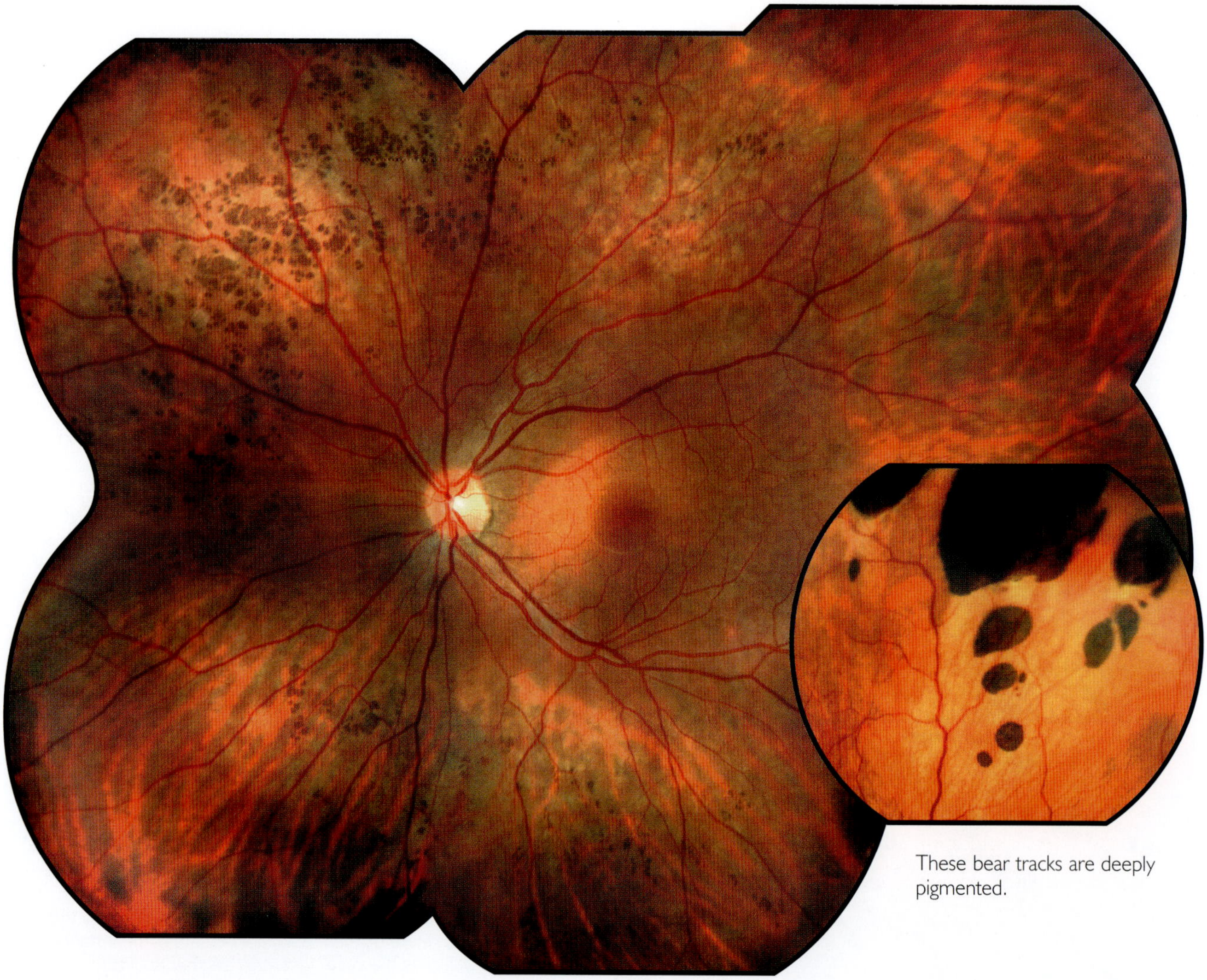

These bear tracks are deeply pigmented.

Widespread bear tracks in the fundus.

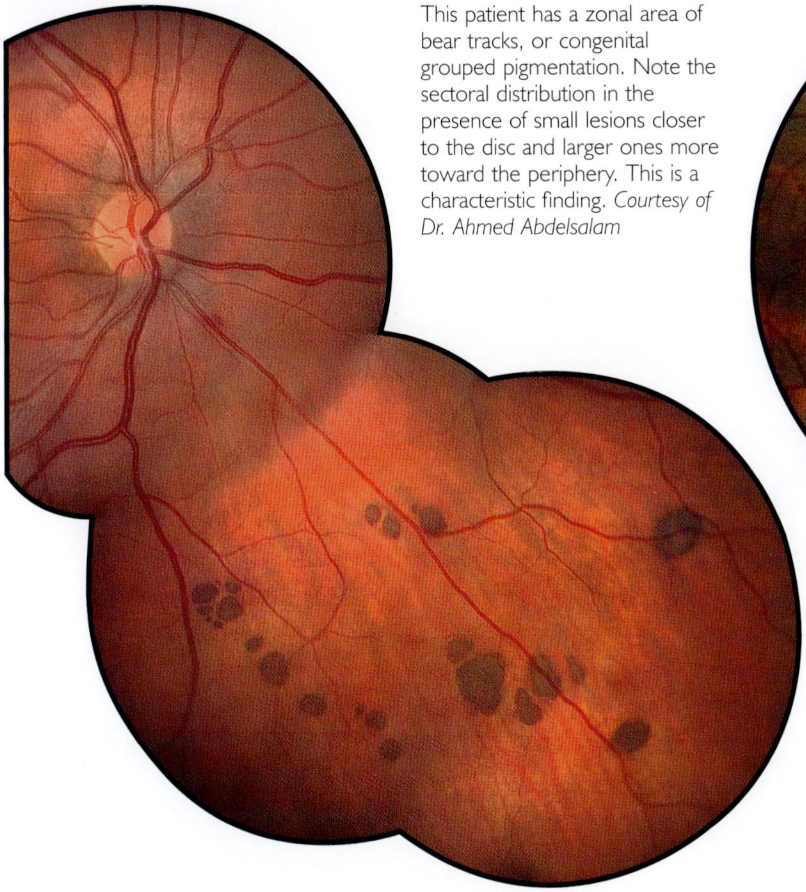

This patient has a zonal area of bear tracks, or congenital grouped pigmentation. Note the sectoral distribution in the presence of small lesions closer to the disc and larger ones more toward the periphery. This is a characteristic finding. *Courtesy of Dr. Ahmed Abdelsalam*

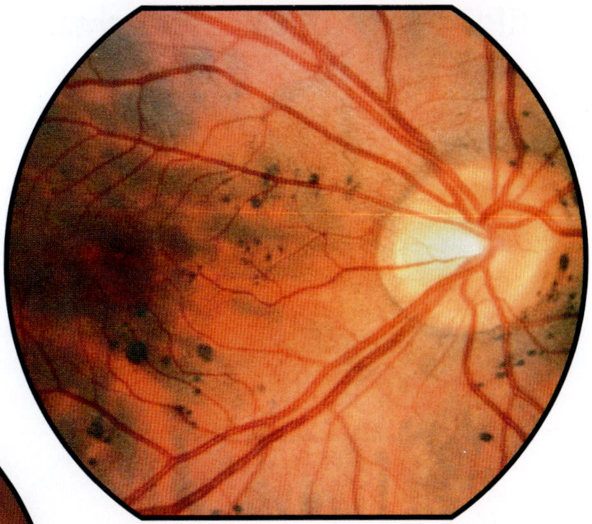

The bear tracks may be multiple in nature and can sometimes be observed around the macular and/or peripapillary region. However, usually they are peripheral in location.

Polar Bear Tracks

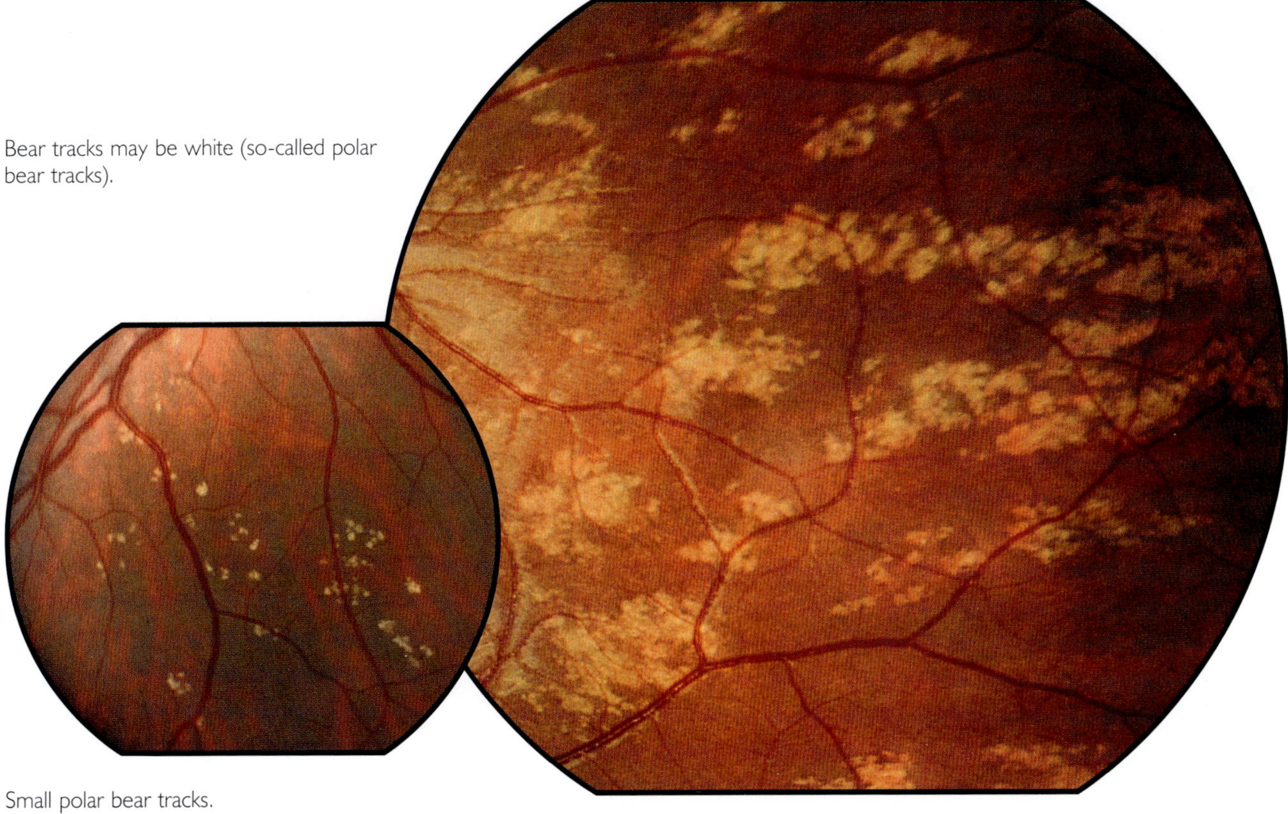

Bear tracks may be white (so-called polar bear tracks).

Small polar bear tracks.

CHRPE with Nodular Adenoma/Adenocarcinoma (Epithelioma)

The CHRPE lesion can occasionally be the origin of an adenoma or adenocarcinoma. Such lesions have a limited growth potential and no tendency to metastasize. Histopathologically, they can be vacuolated, tubular, or mixed. The tumor cells are large and polyhedral in nature with a predominantly apical concentration of pigment. Treatment ranges from observation to local resection with or without plaque radiotherapy.

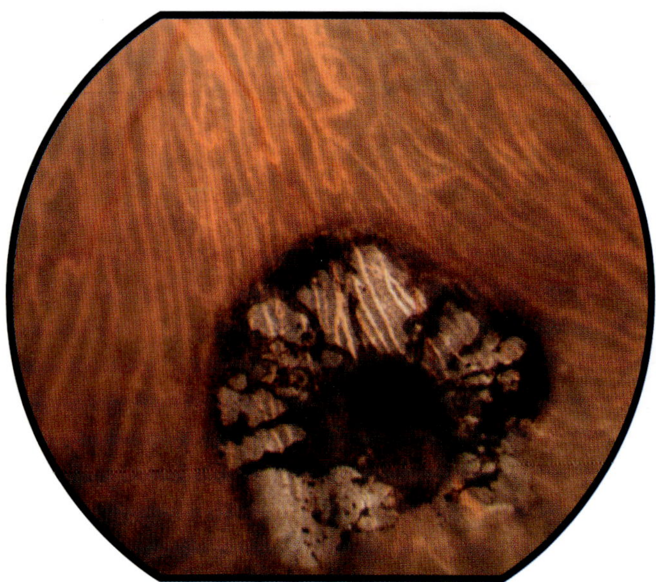

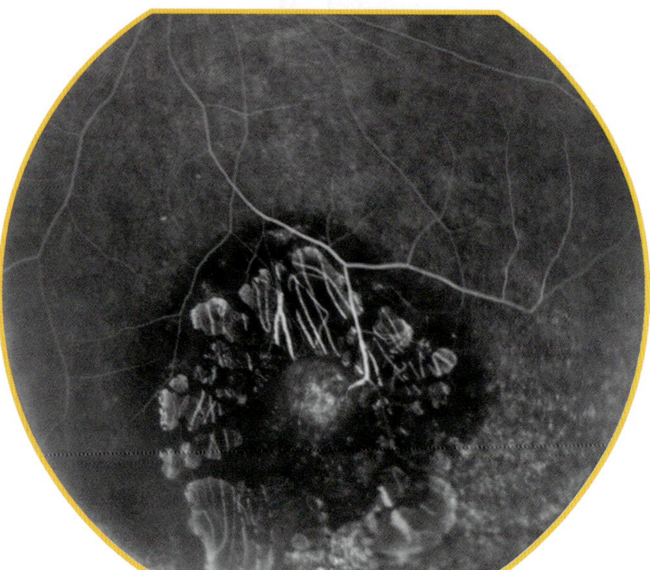

Peripheral CHRPE with central nodule thickening surrounded by lacunae. Fluorescein angiography shows slight fluorescence of the central nodule with a feeding artery and surrounding window defects through the lacunae.

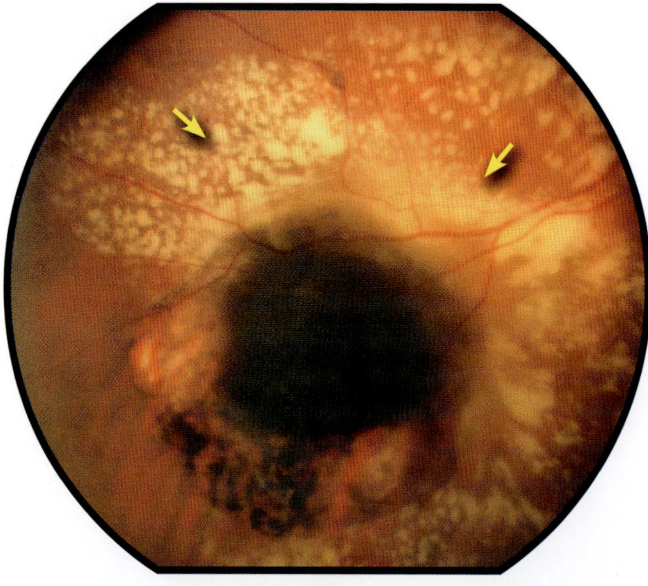

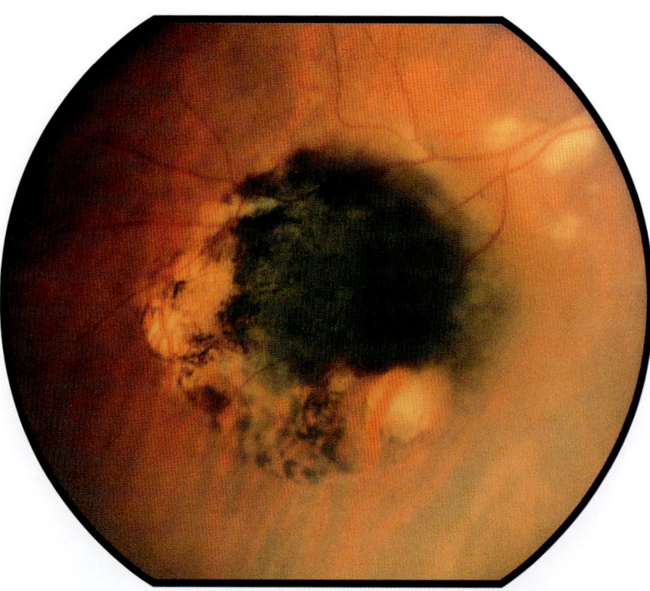

Rarely, choroidal neovascularization secondary to RPE hypertrophy may be noted, as demonstrated in this case with massive lipid exudation *(arrows)*. After laser treatment the exudation regressed and the detachment resolved. *Courtesy of Dr. Mort Rosenthal*

Pigmented Ocular Fundus Lesions with Familial Adenomatous Polyposis

Patients with familial adenomatous polyposis (FAP) can manifest findings in the eye consisting of darkly pigmented, slightly irregular lesions at the level of the RPE. These lesions superficially resemble classic congenital hypertrophy of the RPE, but they are generally multifocal, more irregular and with a "fish tail" configuration, often with areas of depigmentation. These lesions can be used as a marker to identify family members at risk for familial adenomatous polyposis and Gardner syndrome, which is FAP plus several extra-colonic tumors.

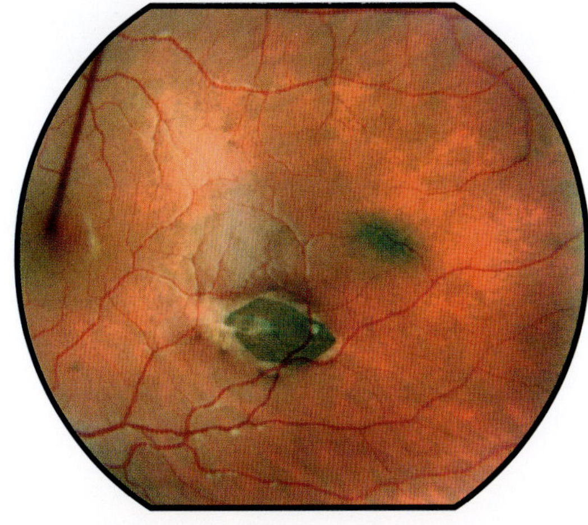

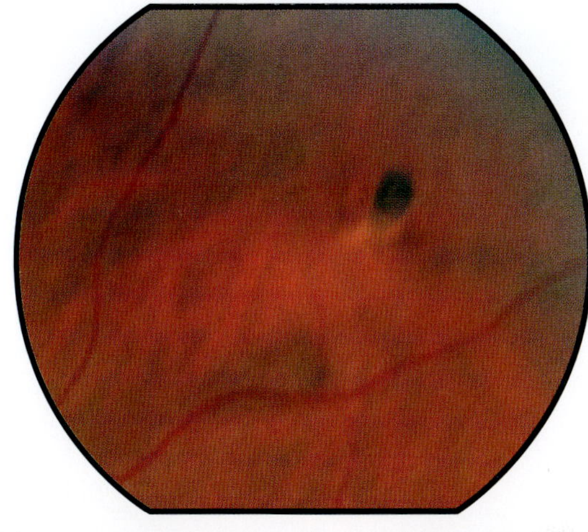

These are two typical CHRPE-like lesions seen in Gardner syndrome. Each has an annulus of atrophy with a tail of depigmentation of the pigment epithelium extending from it.

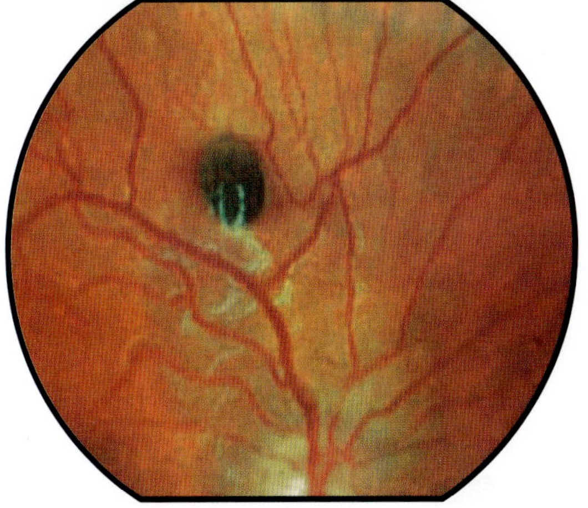

Small pigmented CHRPE-like lesion with thin halo in a young woman with FAP. *Courtesy of Dr. Miguel Materin*

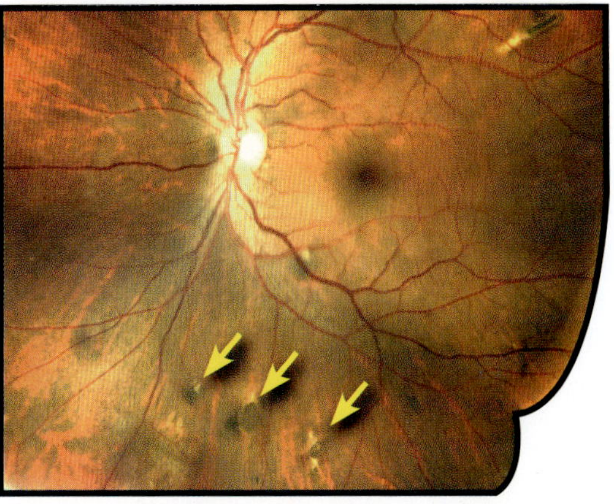

This patient has multiple CHRPE-like lesions in Gardner syndrome. Some are very characteristic, with the "fish tail" configuration *(arrows)*, but there are variable changes in the others. *Courtesy of Deborah Brown*

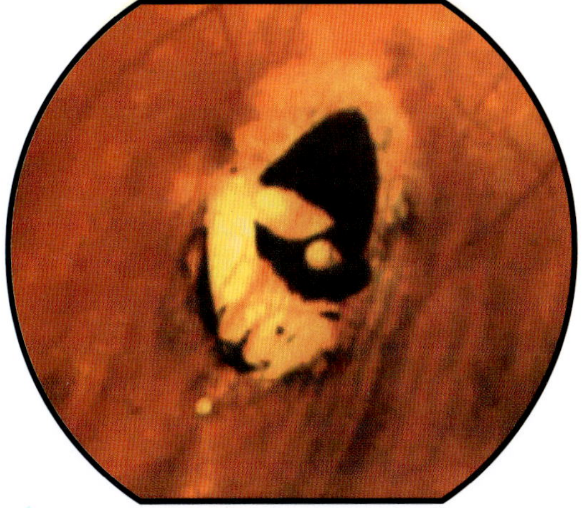

Irregular, partially depigmented CHRPE-like lesion in a patient with FAP.

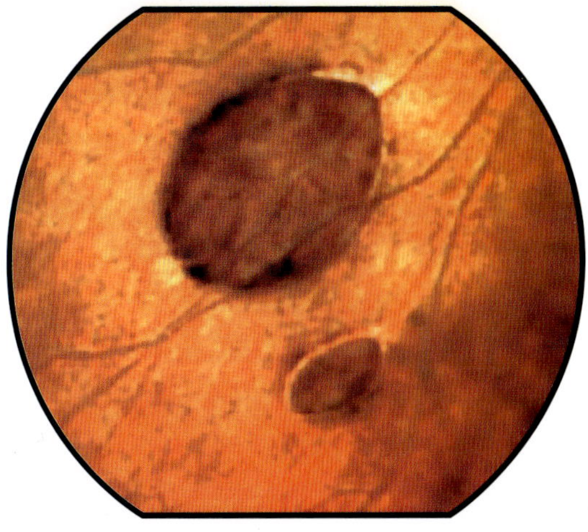

Two pigmented CHRPE-like lesions with depigmented halo and "fish tail" of depigmentation in a patient with FAP.

Congenital Simple Hamartoma of the Retinal Pigment Epithelium

Congenital simple hamartoma of the RPE is a dark black benign tumor located in the macular region, often immediately adjacent to the foveola. It appears like a black ink spot involving full-thickness retina. Fine retinal traction can be noted surrounding the mass. Often there are slightly dilated feeding and draining retinal vessels. This tumor usually remains stable.

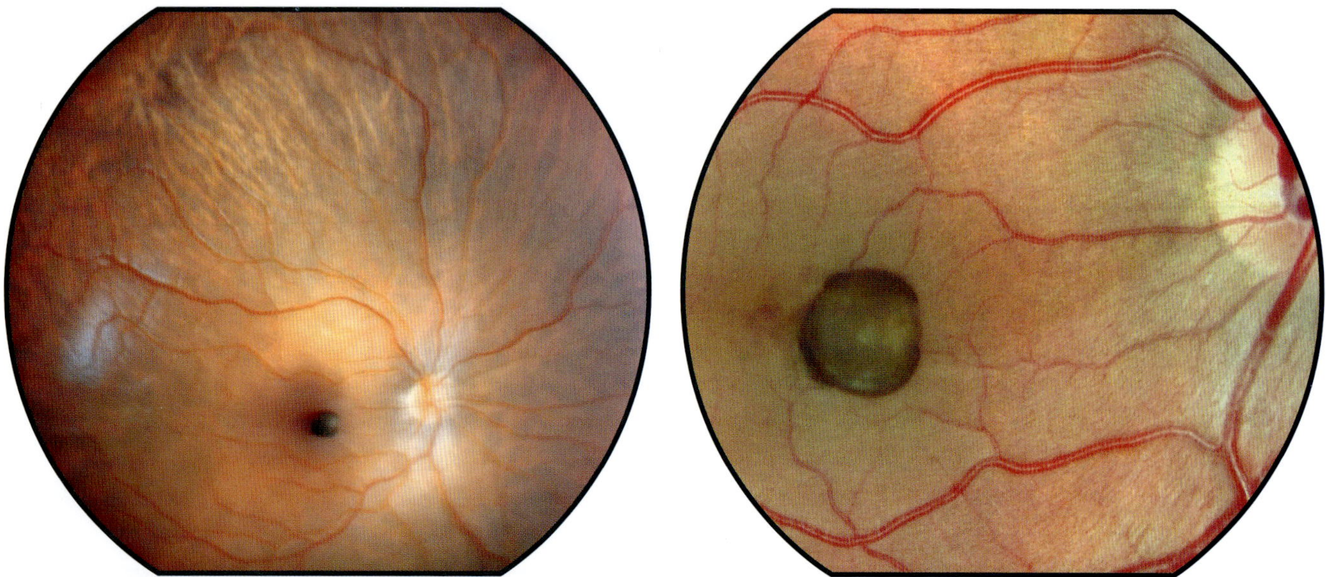

Congenital simple hamartoma in a 12-year-old asymptomatic girl. Wide-angle image showing the circumscribed dark black mass in the fovea. With higher magnification, the abruptly elevated pigmented retinal mass is approximately 200 μm from the foveola. The tumor involves the full-thickness retina with minimal protrusion into the vitreous.

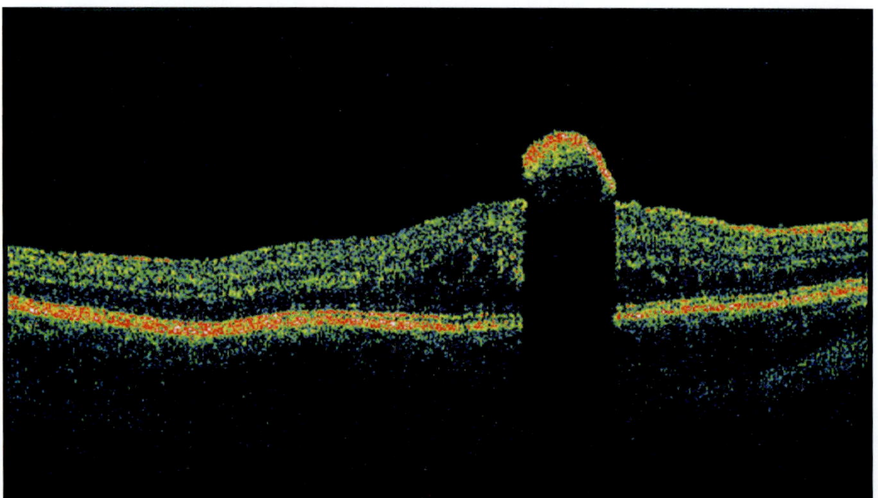

Time domain OCT of the above patient demonstrates an abruptly elevated mass with crisp shadowing of deeper structures.

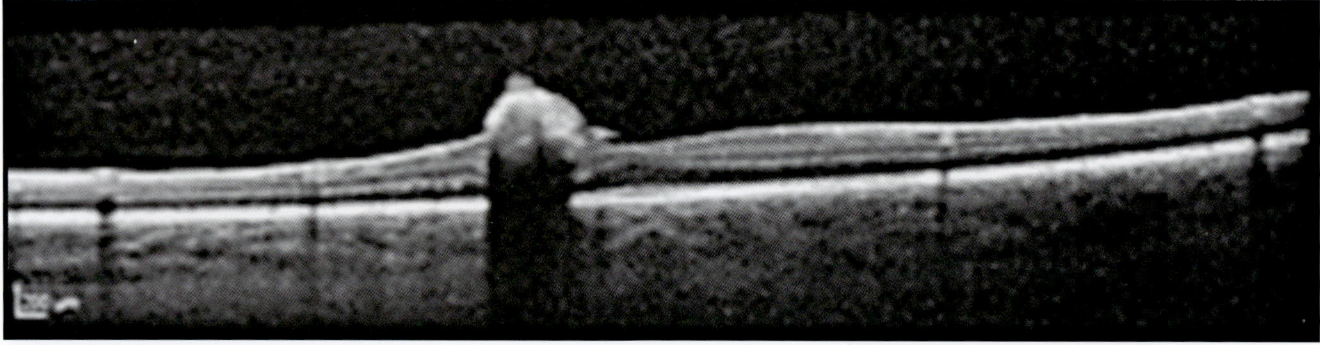

Spectral domain OCT in another case depicts the full thickness retinal mass with abrupt shadowing and no disturbance of adjacent tissue.

Adenoma/Adenocarcinoma (Epithelioma) of the Retinal Pigment Epithelium

Retinal pigment epithelium adenoma and adenocarcinoma are rare. They typically manifest as a dark nodule arising from the pigment epithelium and surrounded by subretinal fluid. Unlike choroidal melanoma, they tend to produce retinal exudation, display a retinal feeding artery and draining vein, and can cause remote epiretinal membrane and macular edema.

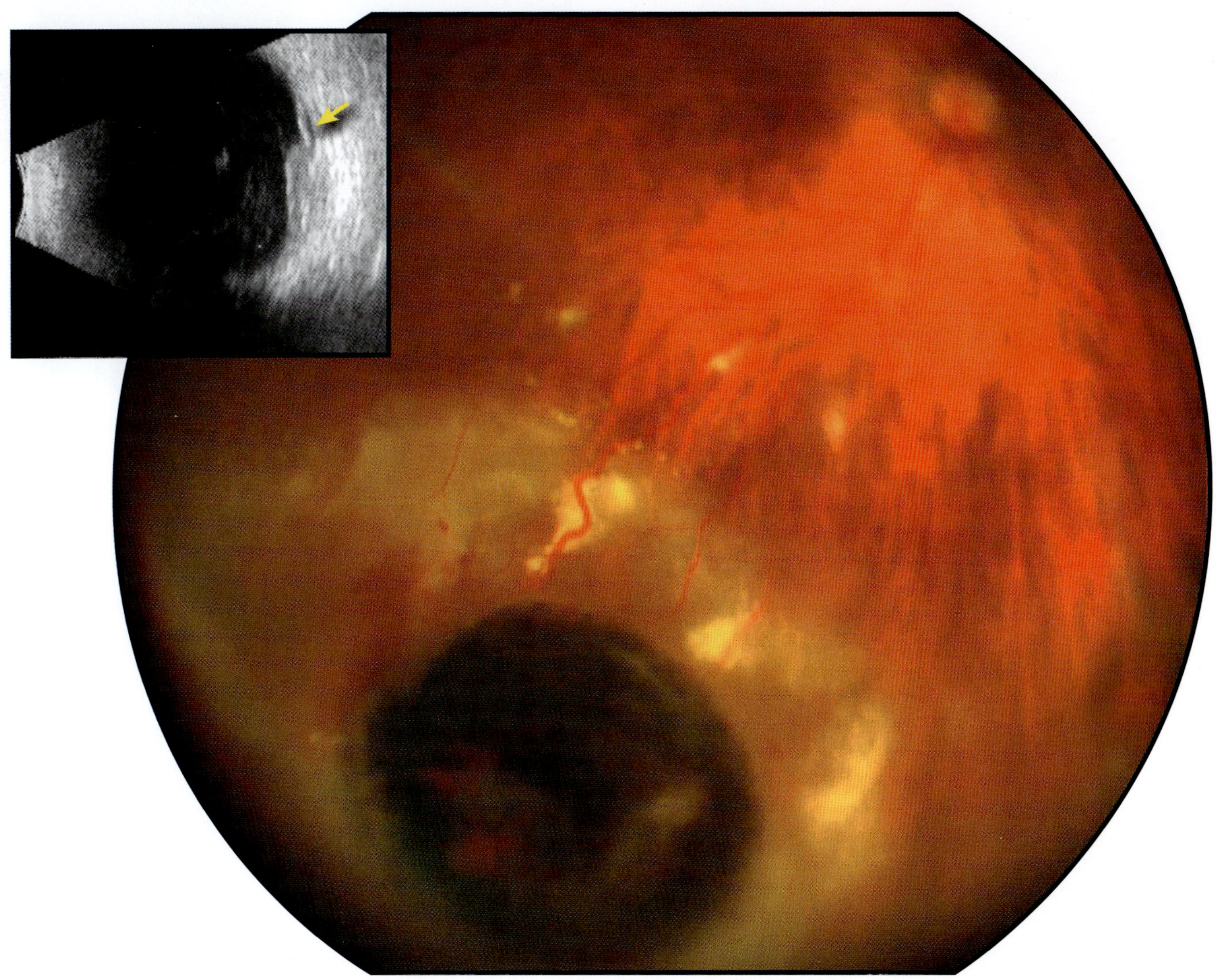

Benign epithelioma of the RPE in a 54-year-old female. Wide-angle imaging shows the darkly pigmented nodular mass of the RPE draping the overlying retina and producing surrounding subretinal fluid with exudation. There are slightly dilated and tortuous feeding and draining vessels. The ocular ultrasonography *(top)* shows the echogenic mass with shallow subretinal fluid *(arrow)* and overlying vitreous debris.

Torpedo Maculopathy of the Retinal Pigment Epithelium

Torpedo maculopathy is a circumscribed, congenital lesion of the RPE and outer retina. As the name suggests, it typically occurs at the macula. It is often unilateral with the long axis oriented horizontally. The nasal tip of the lesion typically points toward the fovea. Segments of the lesion may be hyperpigmented.

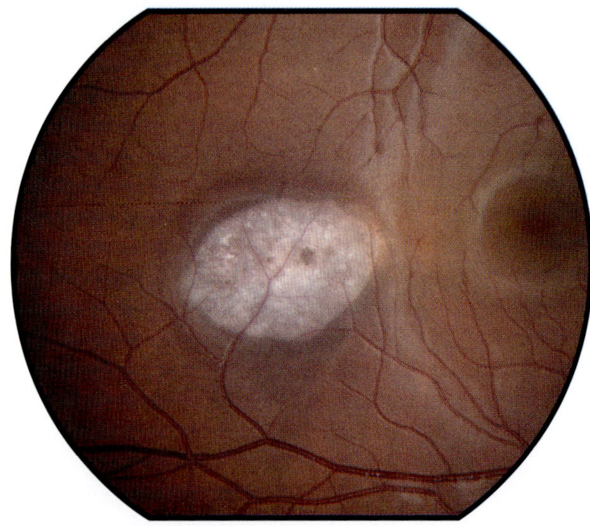

A longstanding amelanotic lesion involving the temporal margin of the macula.

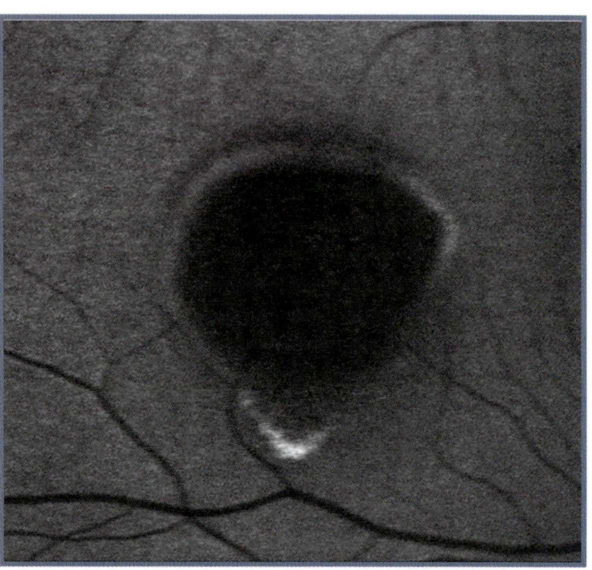

Fundus autofluorescence demonstrates a halo of hyperautofluorescence with the remainder of the lesion being hypoautofluorescent.

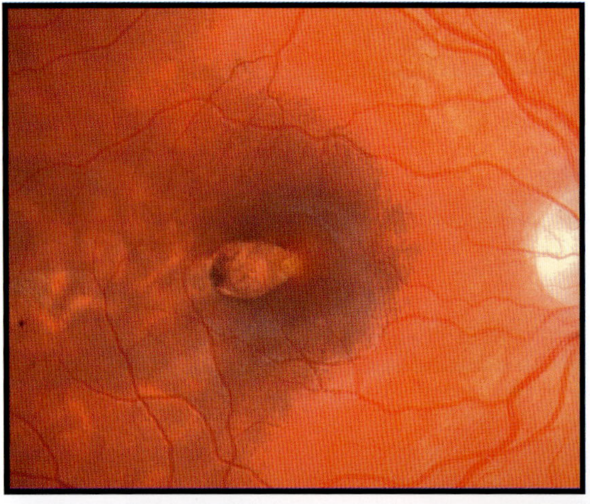

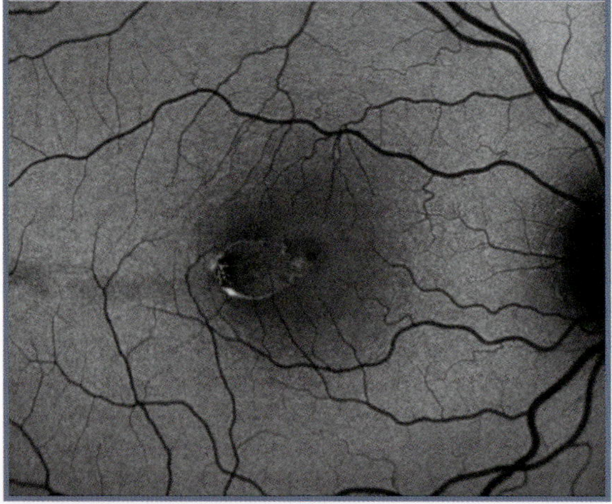

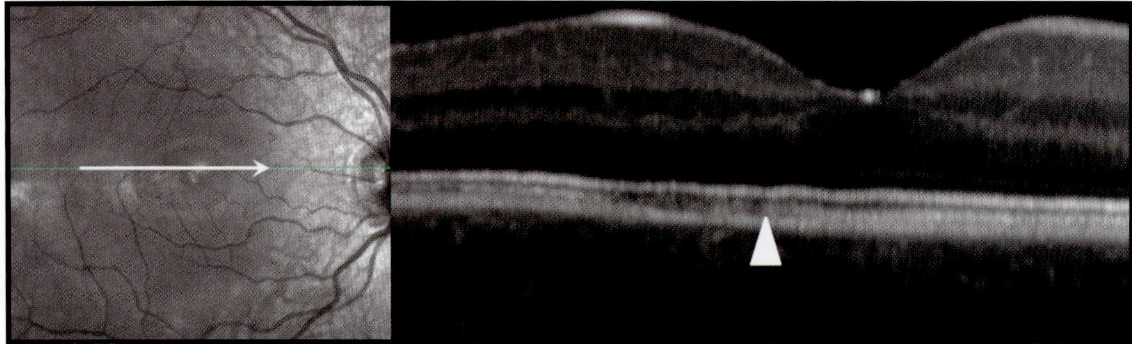

Another patient with torpedo maculopathy demonstrates the typical color fundus and fundus autofluorescence findings. Hyperpigmentation is seen at the temporal margin of the lesion. SD-OCT imaging of the hypopigmented region demonstrates attenuation of the photoreceptor outer segment tips and thinning of the RPE *(white arrowhead). Courtesy of Dr. S Tsang*

Unilateral Dysgenesis of the Retinal Pigment Epithelium

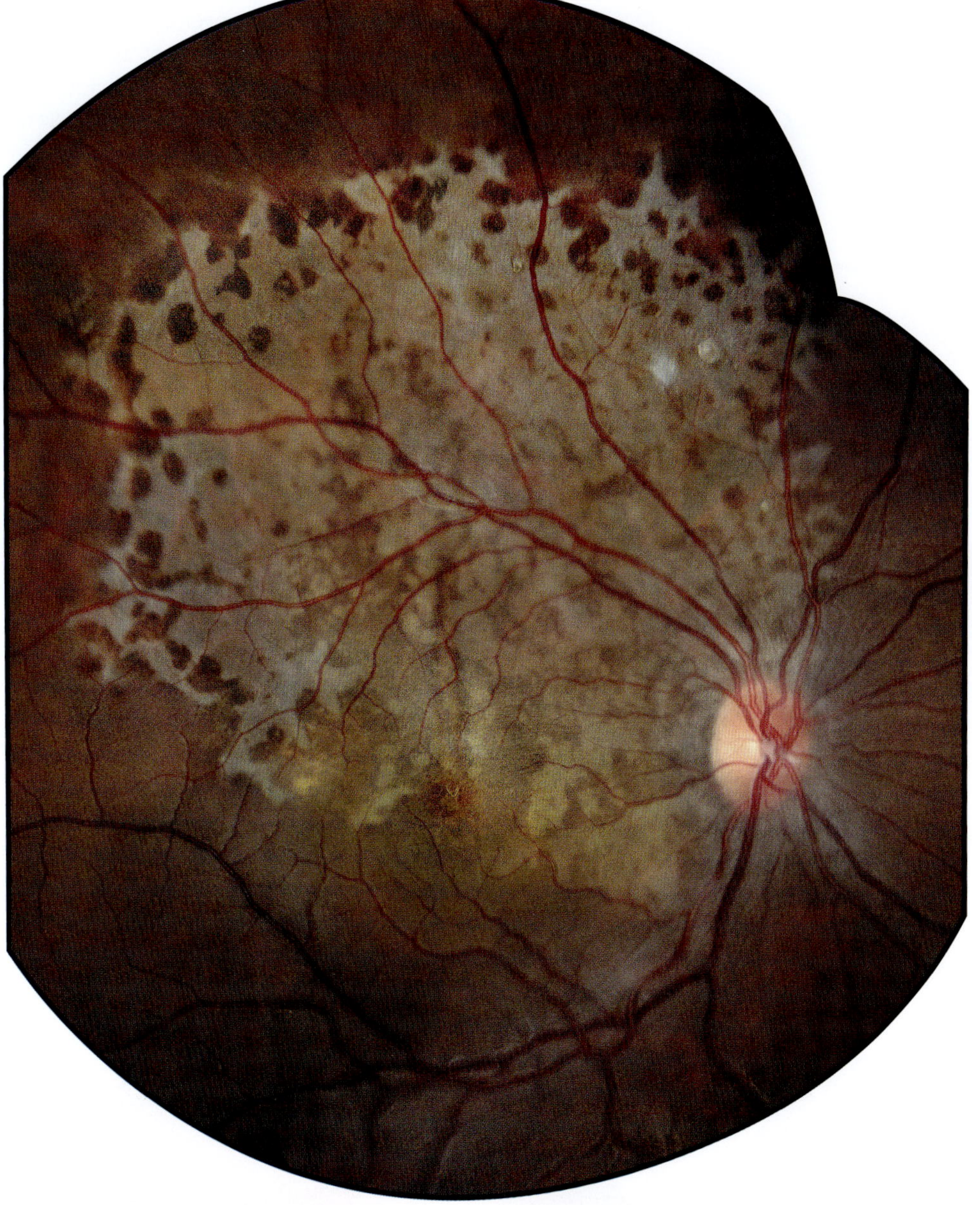

Unilateral dysgenesis of the RPE is a rare and poorly understood condition. It typically occurs in young and middle-aged adults and has a pathognomonic scalloped appearance to the margin of the lesion. "Leopard-spot" changes are commonly seen within the lesion. Complications of this entity include retinal detachment, choroidal neovascularization and epiretinal fibrosis. *Image courtesy of Dr. A Fung*

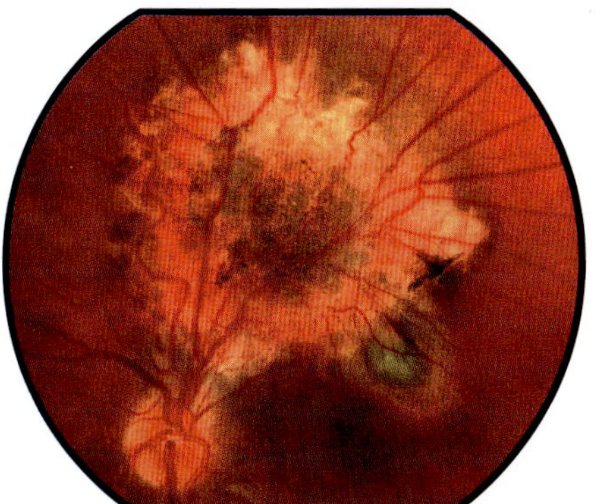

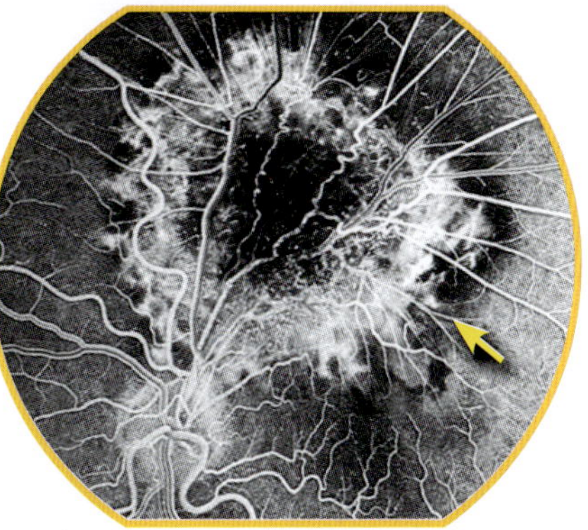

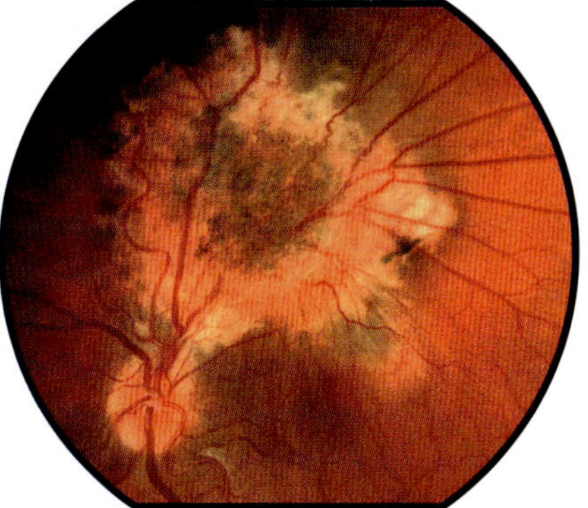

RPE dysgenesis with secondary choroidal neovascularization (CNV). There are retinal vascular irregularities in association with an epiretinal membrane. The lesion may be confused with a combined hamartoma of the retina and RPE. The CNV is clearly evident on the angiogram *(arrow)*. Regression of CNV is seen to occur after laser treatment.

Choroidal Nevus

It is estimated that approximately 6% of adult Caucasians have a choroidal nevus. This tumor appears as a brown, tan, or yellow mass in the choroid, with an oval or round shape. Features of the overlying RPE such as atrophy, hyperplasia, fibrous metaplasia, osseous metaplasia, and drusen imply a chronic nevus. Features such as subretinal fluid or overlying orange pigment imply an active mass and could represent a small choroidal melanoma. Growth of choroidal nevus into melanoma is estimated to occur at a rate of 1/8000 cases. Risk factors for growth of choroidal nevus to melanoma can be remembered with the mnemonic **T**o **F**ind **S**mall **O**cular **M**elanoma, representing Thickness over 2 mm, Subretinal Fluid, Symptoms, Orange pigment, and Margin of tumor within 3 mm of the optic disc. Patients with 3 or more risk factors have 50% or greater risk for transformation of the tumor into melanoma.

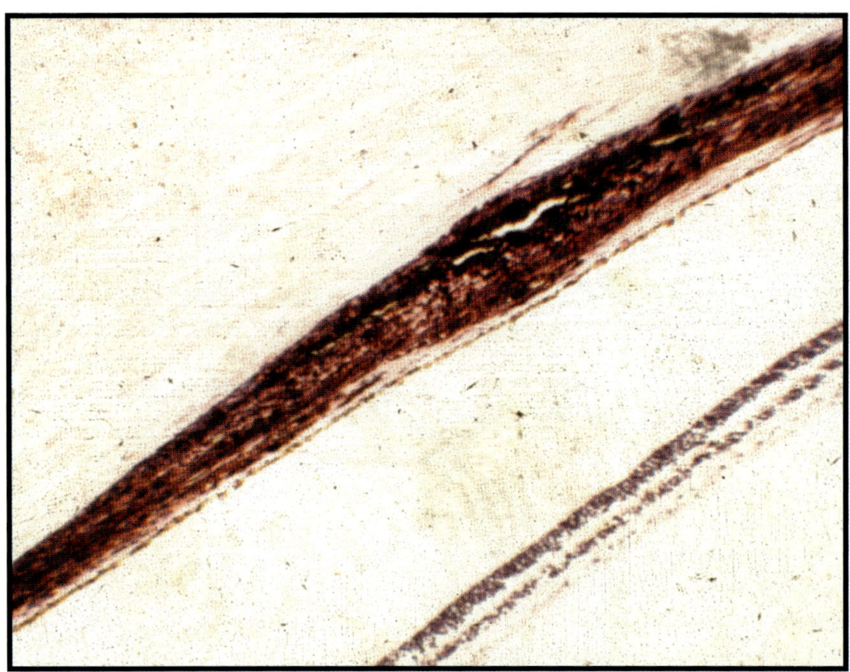

Note the pigmentary cellular thickening of the choroidal nevus in this histopathological specimen.

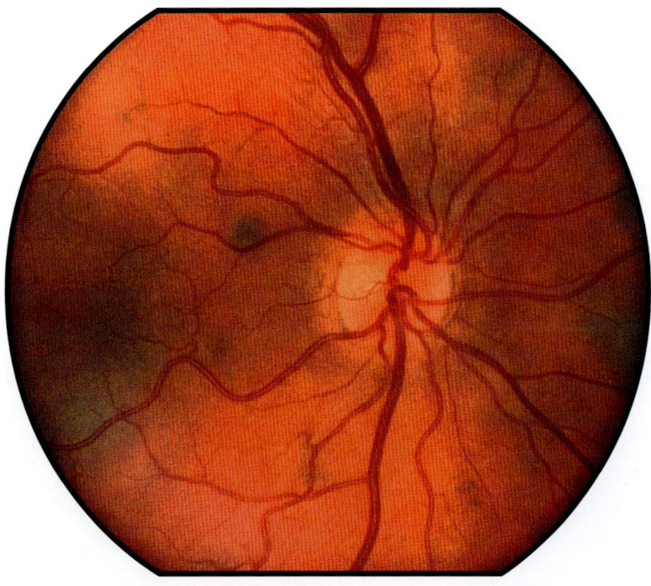

This patient with neurofibromatosis has multiple nevi in the fundus, also known as melanotic hamartomas.

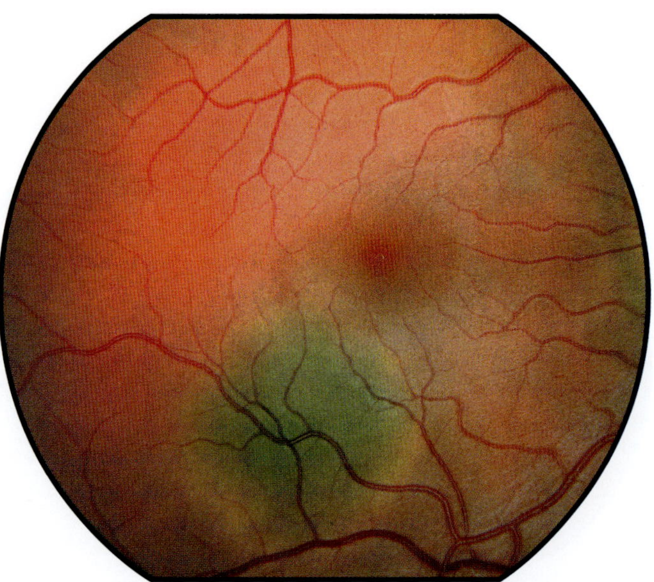

A choroidal nevus with central pigmentation and surrounding amelanotic halo.

The Clinical Spectrum of Choroidal Nevus

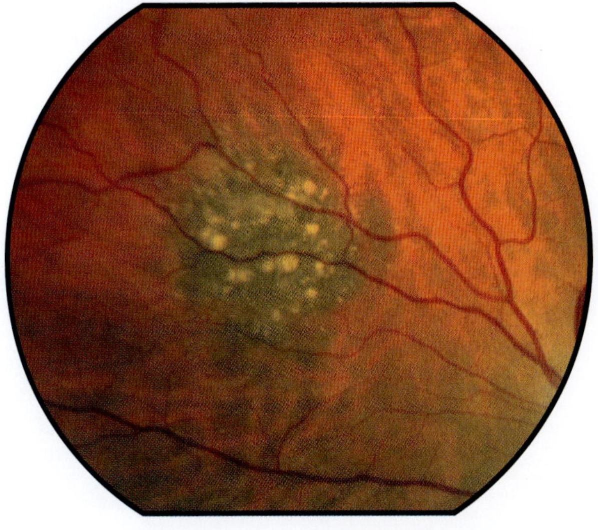

Pigmented choroidal nevus with overlying drusen.

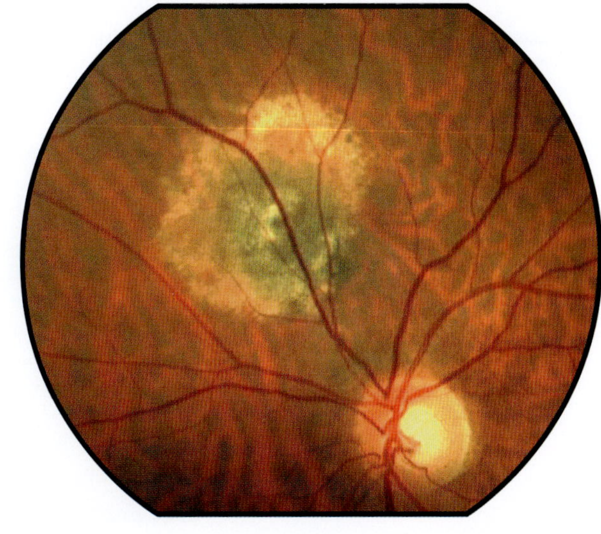

Pigmented choroidal nevus with overlying drusen and retinal pigment epithelial atrophy.

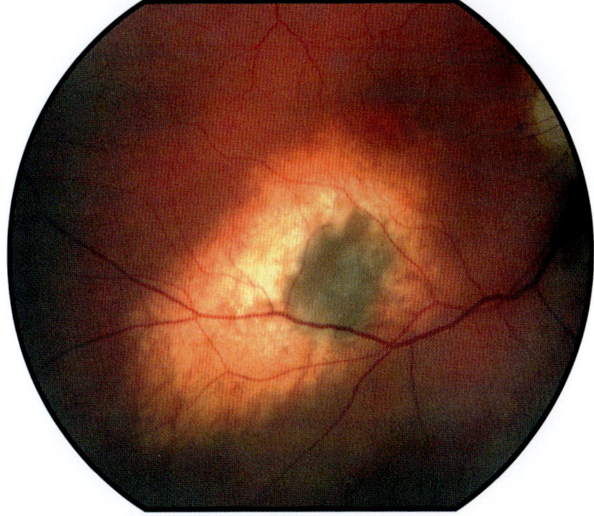

This is a predominantly amelanotic choroidal nevus with central irregular pigmentation.

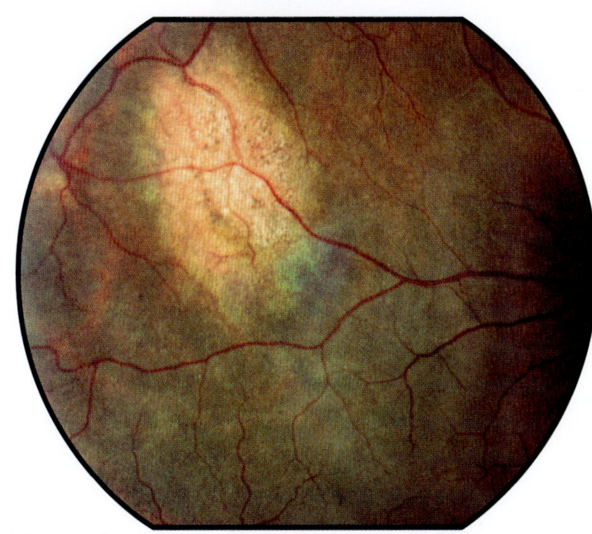

This is a purely amelanotic nevus.

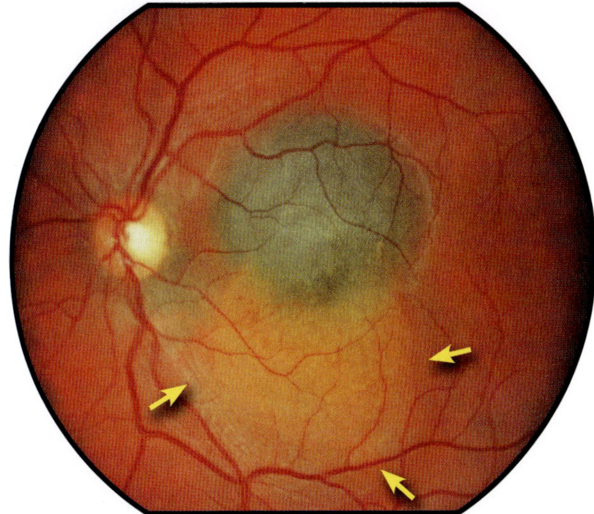

Serous detachments *(arrows)* are seen associated with nevi in this case.

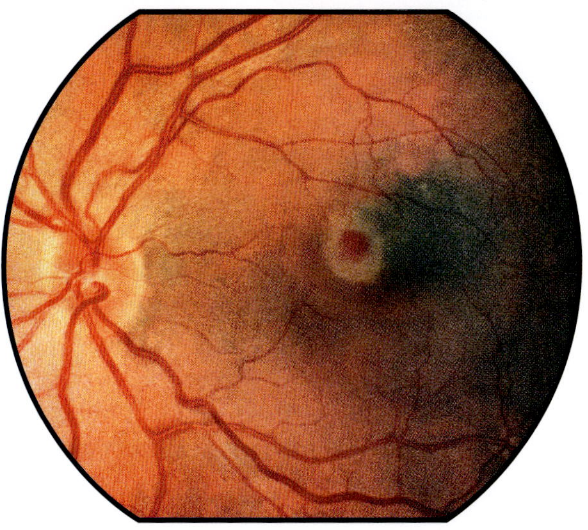

This patient presented with choroidal neovascularization and secondary subretinal exudate and hemorrhage. The neovascularization was treated with laser photocoagulation.

Ocular Melanocytosis

Ocular melanocytosis, oculodermal melanocytosis, and isolated choroidal melanocytosis are causes of choroidal hyperpigmentation. Unlike the former mentioned diseases, isolated choroidal melanocytosis is not associated with pigmentation of other ocular or periocular structures.

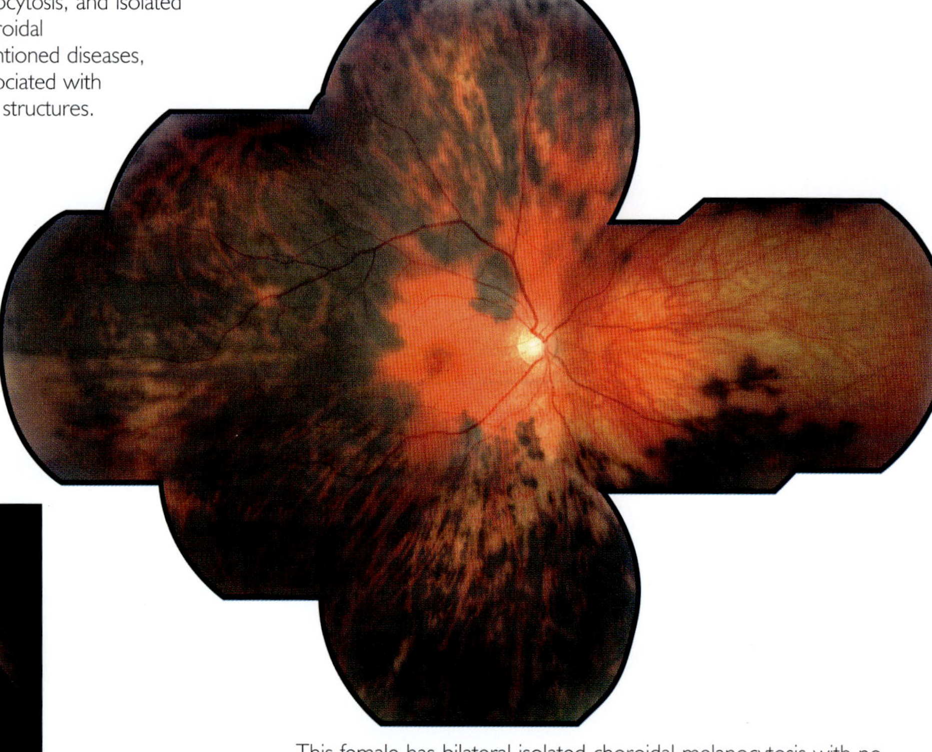

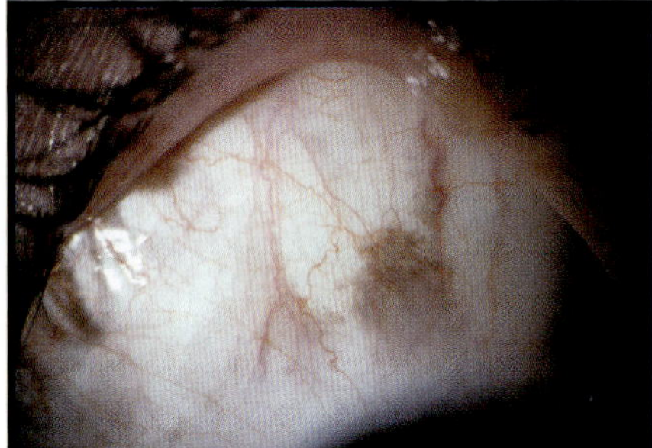

This female has bilateral isolated choroidal melanocytosis with no pigmentation of the sclera or periocular skin. The gaps in pigmentation and sparing of pigmentary change along some choroidal vessels could be confused with choroidal vitiligo.

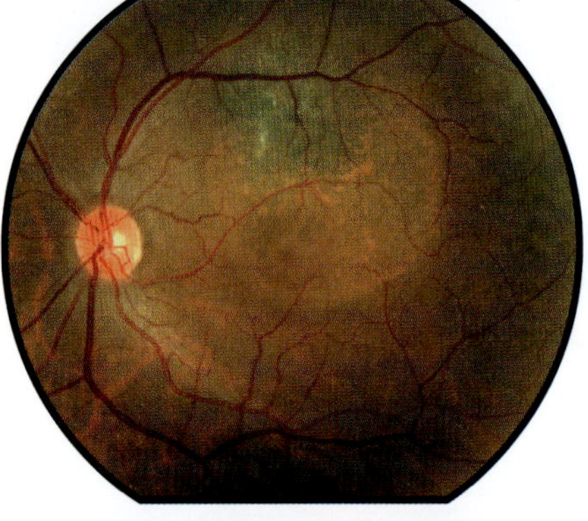

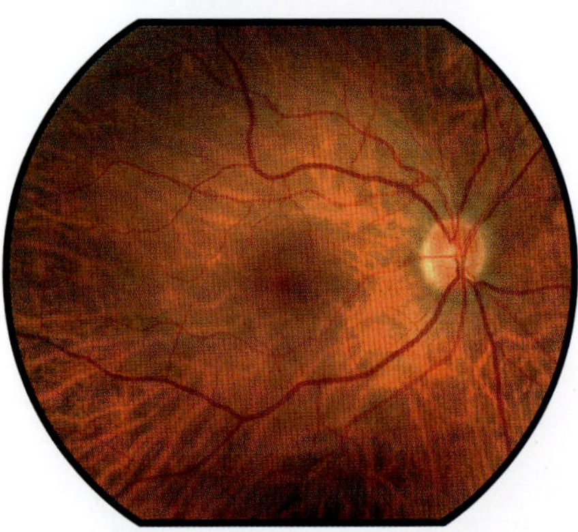

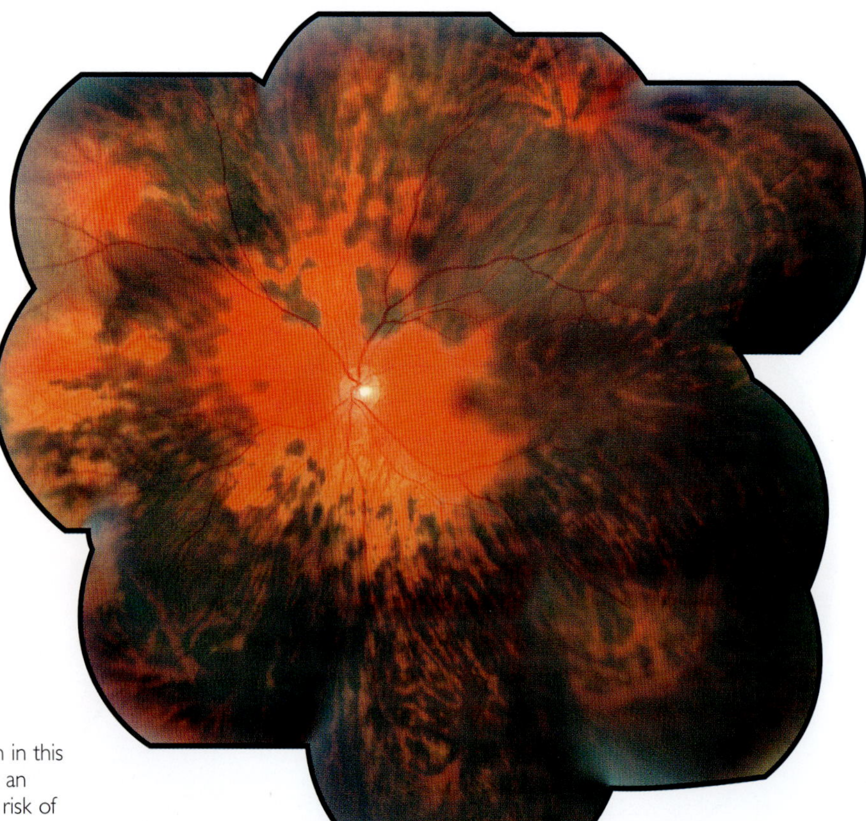

Typical ocular melanocytosis is associated with pigmentation on the lids, sclera, or choroid, as seen in this external image of the left eye *(top)*. The fundus has an abnormal degree of pigmentation and an increased risk of ocular melanoma. The right eye of this patient has a normal background color *(bottom)*.

Optical Coherence Tomography of Retinal Pigment Epithelial Abnormalities Overlying Choroidal Nevus

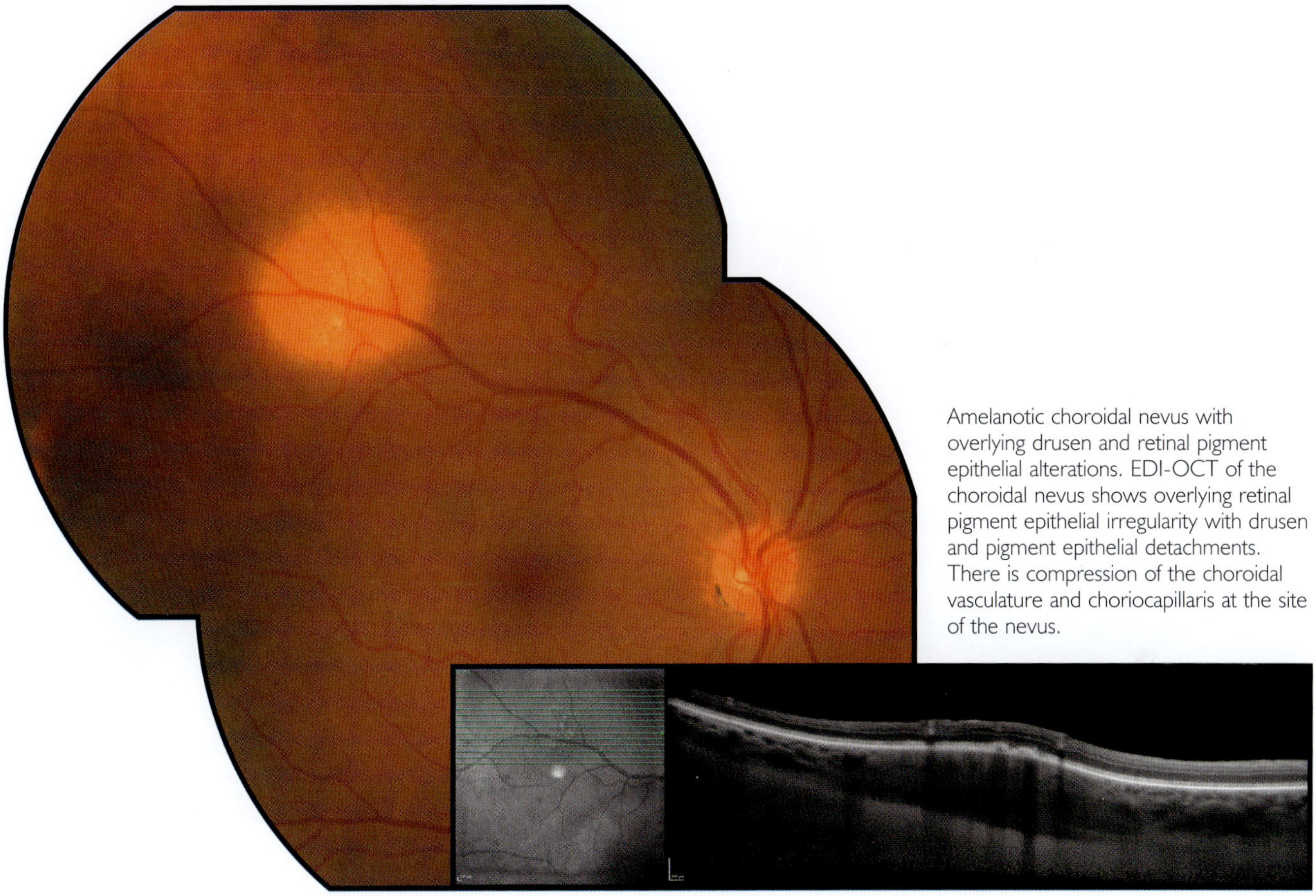

Amelanotic choroidal nevus with overlying drusen and retinal pigment epithelial alterations. EDI-OCT of the choroidal nevus shows overlying retinal pigment epithelial irregularity with drusen and pigment epithelial detachments. There is compression of the choroidal vasculature and choriocapillaris at the site of the nevus.

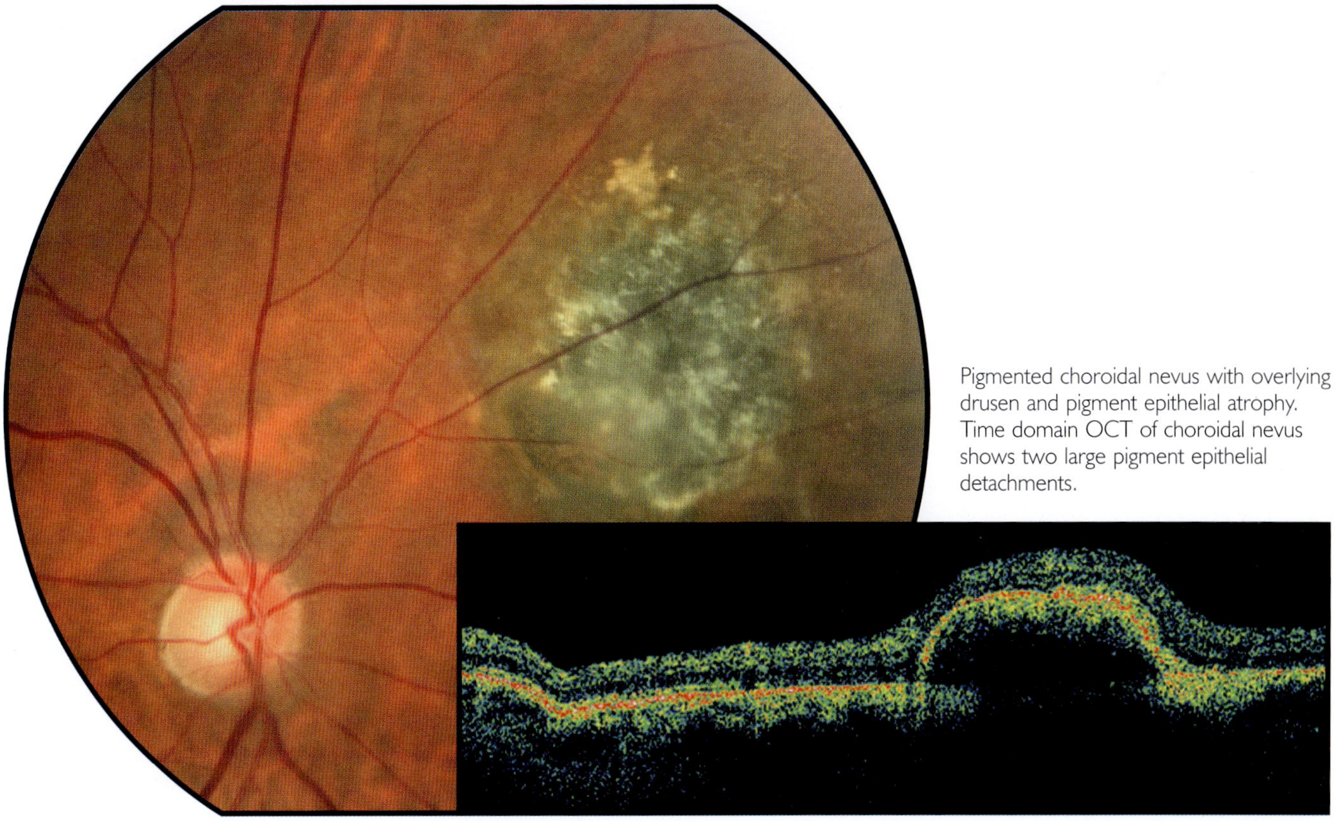

Pigmented choroidal nevus with overlying drusen and pigment epithelial atrophy. Time domain OCT of choroidal nevus shows two large pigment epithelial detachments.

Optical Coherence Tomography of Retinal Pigment Epithelial Abnormalities Overlying Choroidal Nevus

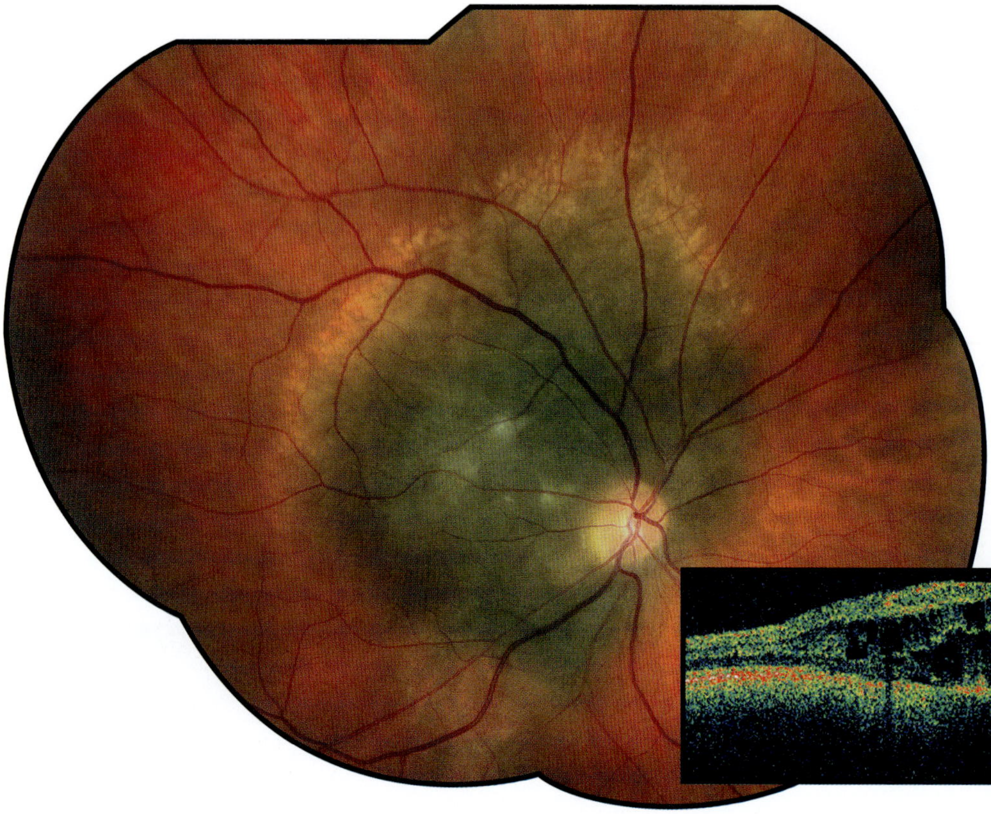

Pigmented juxtapapillary choroidal nevus with overlying retinal pigment epithelial atrophy and fibrosis as well as drusen. Time domain OCT shows intraretinal cystic degeneration overlying the choroidal nevus.

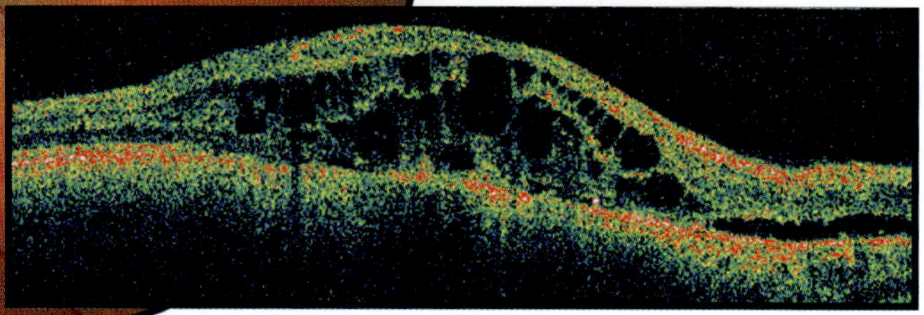

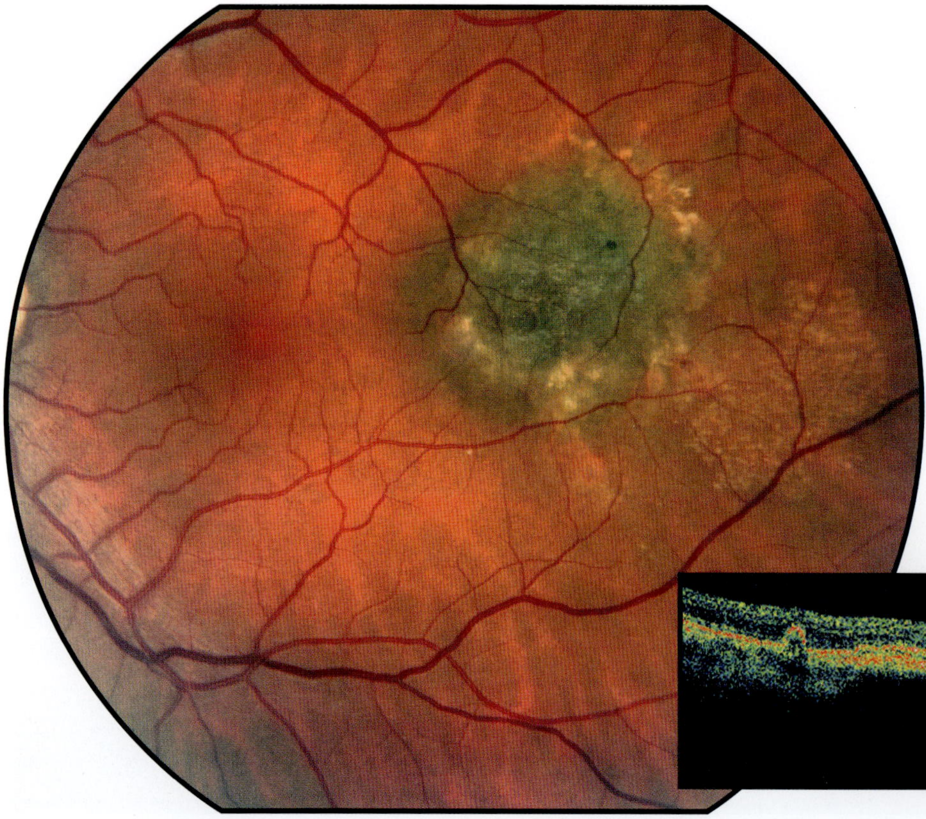

Perimacular choroidal nevus with overlying drusen. Time domain OCT shows overlying drusen and retinal thinning with photoreceptor loss at the site of the optically dense nevus.

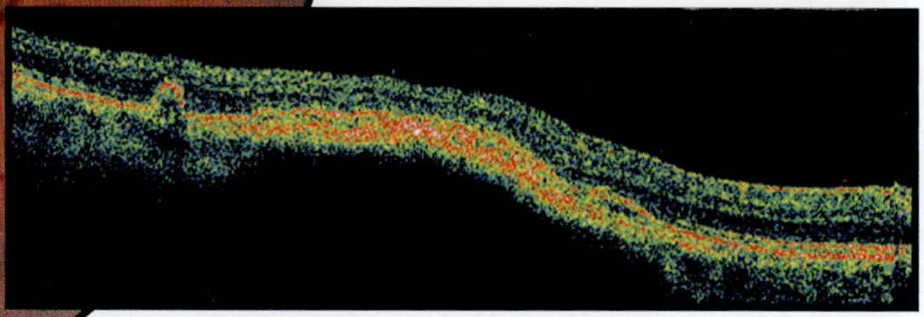

Spectral Domain Optical Coherence Tomography of Choroidal Nevus

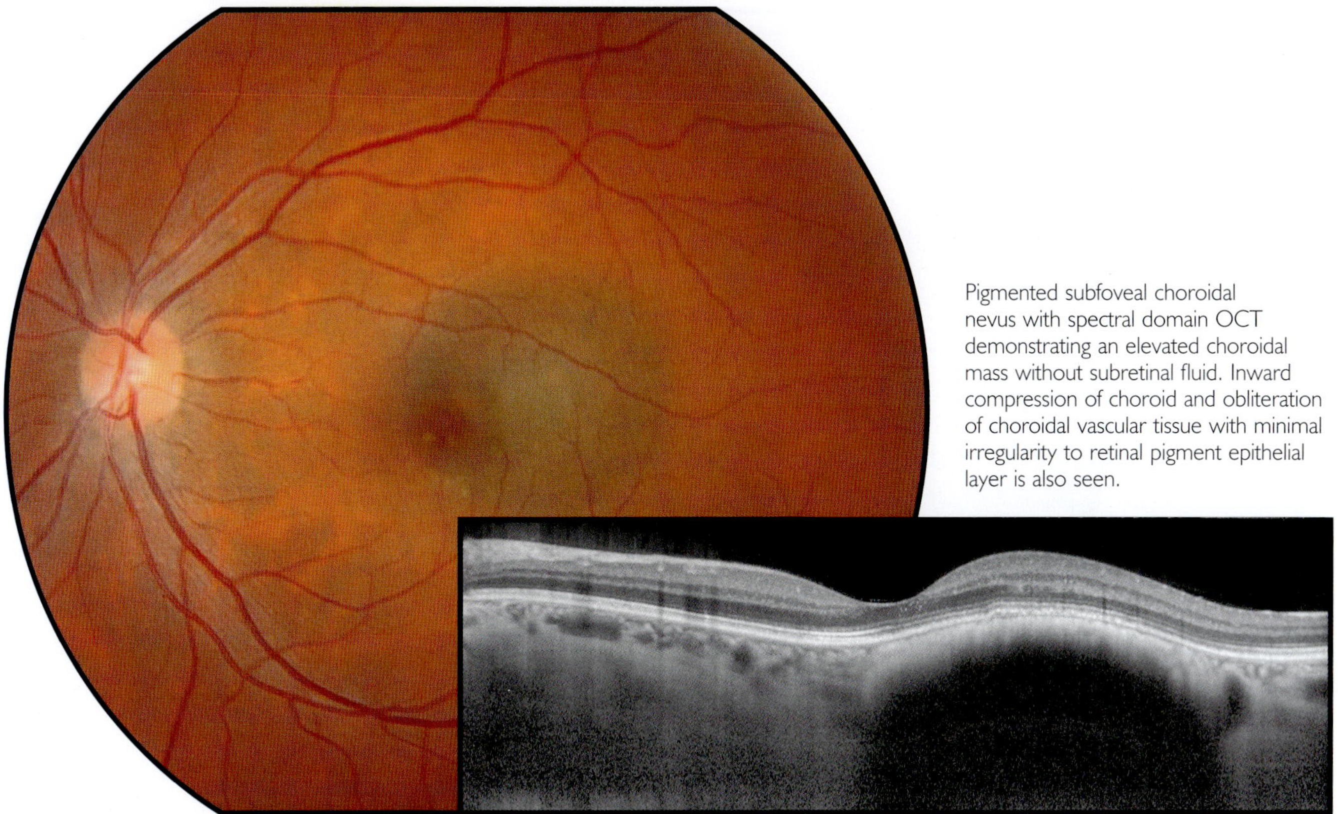

Pigmented subfoveal choroidal nevus with spectral domain OCT demonstrating an elevated choroidal mass without subretinal fluid. Inward compression of choroid and obliteration of choroidal vascular tissue with minimal irregularity to retinal pigment epithelial layer is also seen.

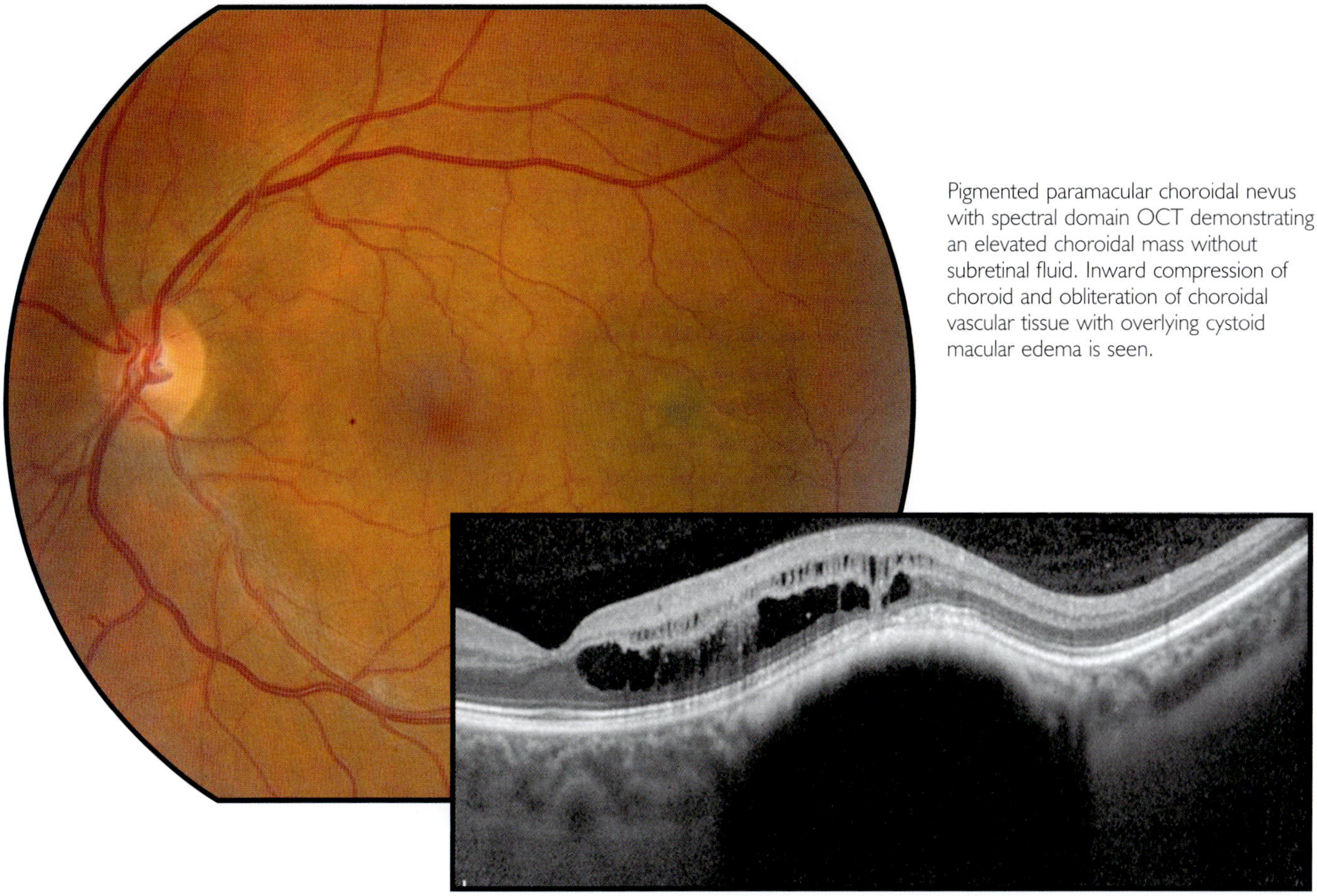

Pigmented paramacular choroidal nevus with spectral domain OCT demonstrating an elevated choroidal mass without subretinal fluid. Inward compression of choroid and obliteration of choroidal vascular tissue with overlying cystoid macular edema is seen.

Suspicious Giant Choroidal Nevus

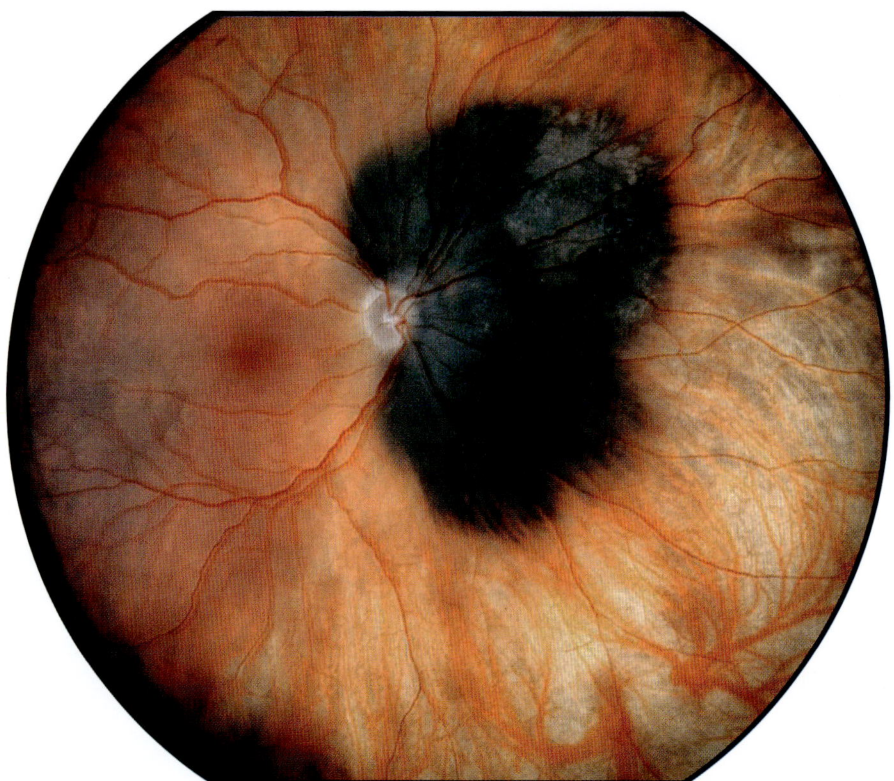

Giant choroidal nevus with overlying retinal pigment epithelial fibrosis that has remained stable for 10 years of photographically documented follow-up. This mass was classified as suspicious due to the feathery margins and was followed closely.

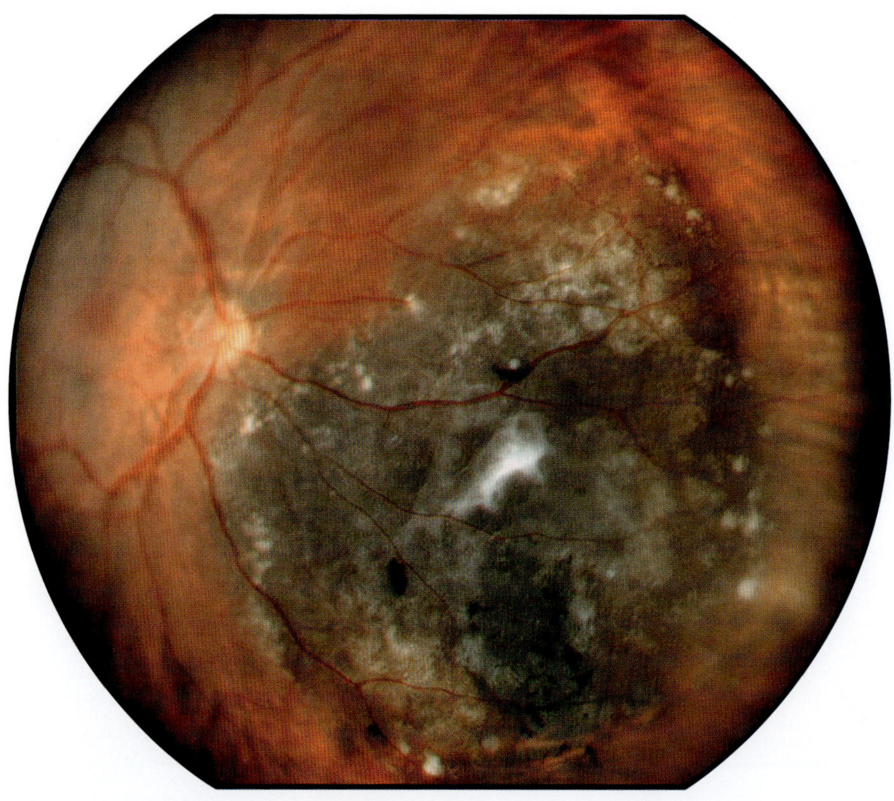

A chronic giant choroidal nevus with extensive overlying drusen and retinal pigment epithelial fibrosis, metaplasia and atrophy that has remained stable for over 20 years of photographically documented follow-up.

Growth of Choroidal Nevus into Choroidal Melanoma

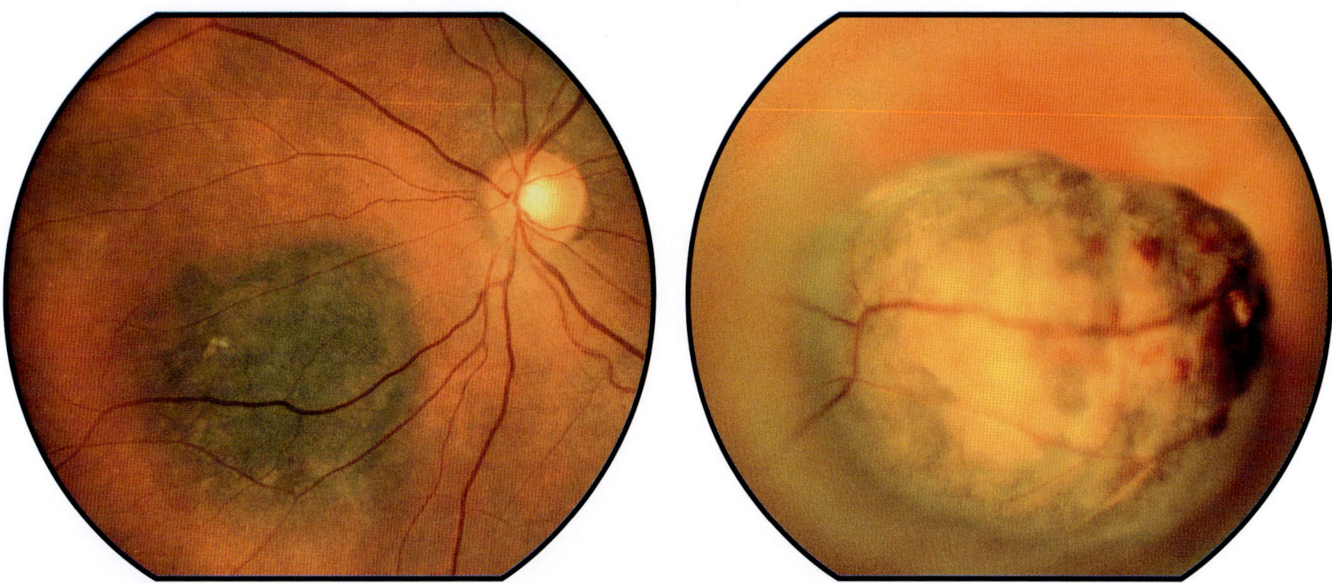

Choroidal nevi must be carefully followed since they can undergo transformation into malignant choroidal melanoma, as in this case in which the patient was followed every 6 months for 11 years. The choroidal nevus *(left)* appeared flat only a few months before its transformation into an elevated malignant choroidal melanoma *(right)*. *Courtesy of Dr. Yale Fisher*

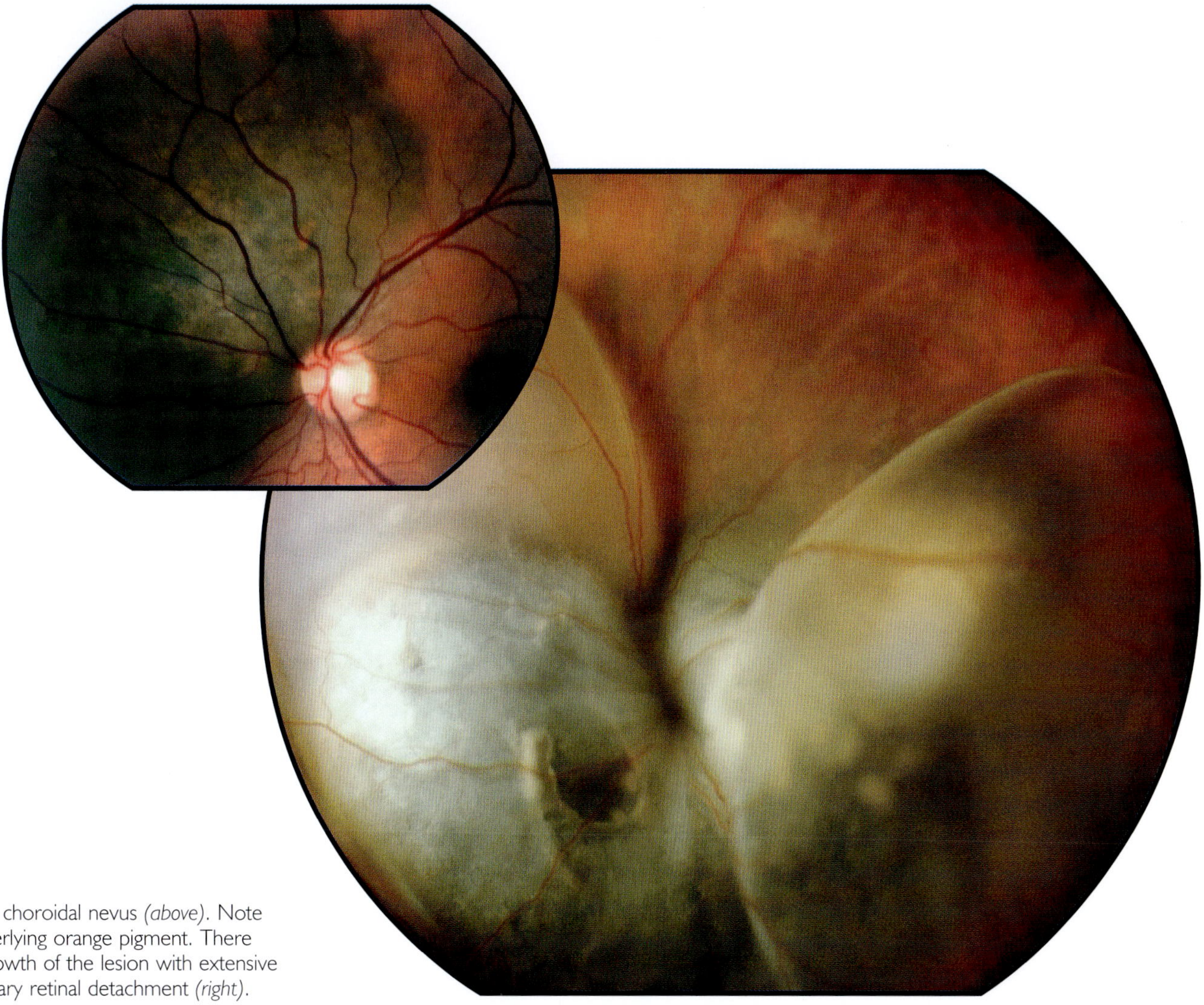

A large choroidal nevus *(above)*. Note the overlying orange pigment. There was growth of the lesion with extensive secondary retinal detachment *(right)*.

Choroidal Melanoma

Choroidal melanoma is classified into small (<3 mm thickness), medium (3.1-8 mm thickness), and large (>8 mm thickness). The melanoma appears as a pigmented or nonpigmented mass, often with overlying subretinal fluid. The tumor can assume a dome-shaped, mushroom-shaped, or diffuse (flat) growth pattern. On ultrasonography, melanoma is usually acoustically hollow with B-scan and shows low internal reflectivity with A-scan. Fluorescein angiography shows a double circulation pattern with vascularity within the tumor and in the overlying retina.

Choroidal Melanoma: Morphological Variations

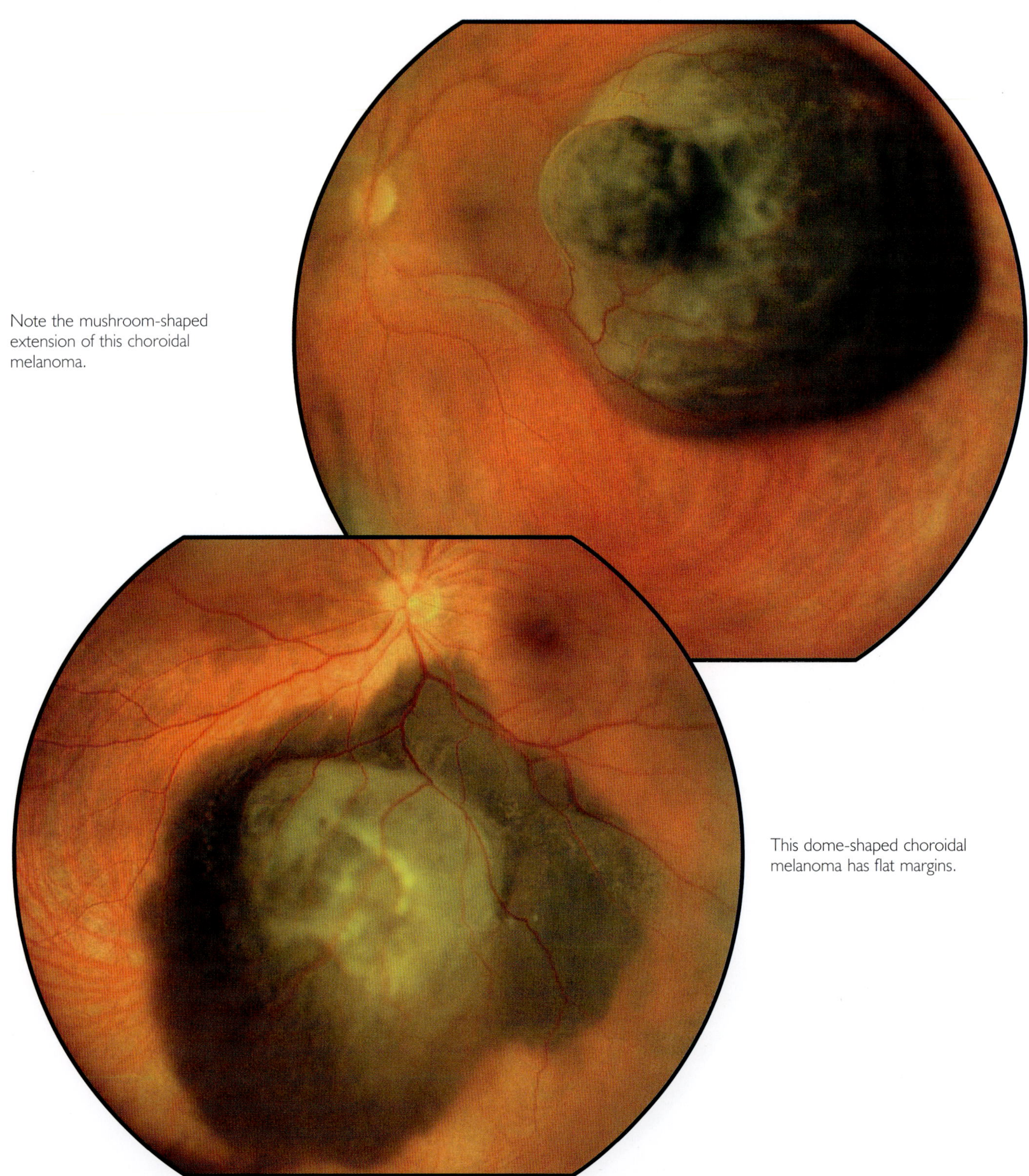

Note the mushroom-shaped extension of this choroidal melanoma.

This dome-shaped choroidal melanoma has flat margins.

American Joint Commission on Cancer (AJCC) Clinical Classification of Posterior Uveal Melanoma (7th edition)

American Joint Commission on Cancer (AJCC) 7th Edition Classification of Uveal Melanoma (Ciliary Body and Choroidal Melanoma) Into Four Tumor (T) Categories Defined by Tumor Thickness and Basal Diameter							
Melanoma thickness (mm)	Category						
>15	4	4	4	4	4	4	4
12.1-15	3	3	3	3	3	4	4
9.1-12	3	3	3	3	3	3	4
6.1-9	2	2	2	2	3	3	4
3.1-6	1	1	1	2	2	3	4
≤3	1	1	1	1	2	2	4
	≤3	3.1-6	6.1-9	9.1-12	12.1-15	15.1-18	>18
	Melanoma basal diameter (mm)						

Step 1—The melanoma is sized using the AJCC classification of tumor size category.

Posterior Uveal Melanoma Category Based on AJCC 7th Edition Classification	
Primary tumor (T)	
T1	Tumor base <3 to 9 mm with thickness ≤6 mm Tumor base 9.1 to 12 mm with thickness ≤3 mm
T1a	T1 tumor without ciliary body involvement and extraocular extension
T1b	T1 tumor with ciliary body involvement
T1c	T1 tumor without ciliary body involvement but with extraocular extension ≤5 mm in diameter
T1d	T1 tumor with ciliary body involvement and extraocular extension ≤5 mm in diameter
T2	Tumor base <9 mm with thickness 6 to 9 mm Tumor base 9.1 to 12 mm with thickness 3.1 to 9 mm Tumor base 12.1 to 15 mm with thickness ≤6 mm Tumor base 15.1 to 18 mm with thickness ≤3 mm
T2a	T2 tumor without ciliary body involvement and extraocular extension
T2b	T2 tumor with ciliary body involvement
T2c	T2 tumor without ciliary body involvement but with extraocular extension ≤5 mm in diameter
T2d	T2 tumor with ciliary body involvement and extraocular extension ≤5 mm in diameter
T3	Tumor base 3.1 to 9 mm with thickness 9.1 to 12 mm Tumor base 9.1 to 12 mm with thickness 9.1 to 15 mm Tumor base 12.1 to 15 mm with thickness 6.1 to 15 mm Tumor base 15.1 to 18 mm with thickness 3.1 to 12 mm
T3a	T3 tumor without ciliary body involvement and extraocular extension
T3b	T3 tumor with ciliary body involvement
T3c	T3 tumor without ciliary body involvement but with extraocular extension ≤5 mm in diameter
T3d	T3 tumor with ciliary body involvement and extraocular extension ≤5 mm in diameter

Continued

Primary tumor (T)	
T4	Tumor base 12.1 to 15 mm with thickness >15 mm Tumor base 15.1 to 18 mm with thickness >12 mm Tumor base >18 mm with any thickness
T4a	T4 tumor without ciliary body involvement and extraocular extension
T4b	T4 tumor with ciliary body involvement
T4c	T4 tumor without ciliary body involvement but with extraocular extension ≤5 mm in diameter
T4d	T4 tumor with ciliary body involvement and extraocular extension ≤5 mm in diameter
T4e	Any tumor size with extraocular extension > 5 mm in diameter

Step 2—The melanoma is categorized into a, b, c, d, or e subsets.

Ciliary Body and Choroidal Melanoma Staging Based on AJCC 7th Edition Classification			
Tumor staging	**Primary tumor (T)**	**Regional lymph node (N)**	**Distant metastasis (M)**
Stage I	T1a	N0	M0
Stage II	T1b-d, T2a-b, T3a	N0	M0
Stage IIA	T1b-d, T2a	N0	M0
Stage IIB	T2b, T3a	N0	M0
Stage III	T2c-d, T3b-d, T4a-c	N0	M0
Stage IIIA	T2c-d, T3b-c, T4a	N0	M0
Stage IIIB	T3d, T4b-c	N0	M0
Stage IIIC	T4d-e	N0	M0
Stage IV	Any T	N1	M0
	Any T	Any N	M1

Step 3—The melanoma is entered into appropriate stage. This is used to predict prognosis.

Choroidal Melanoma Size Variations

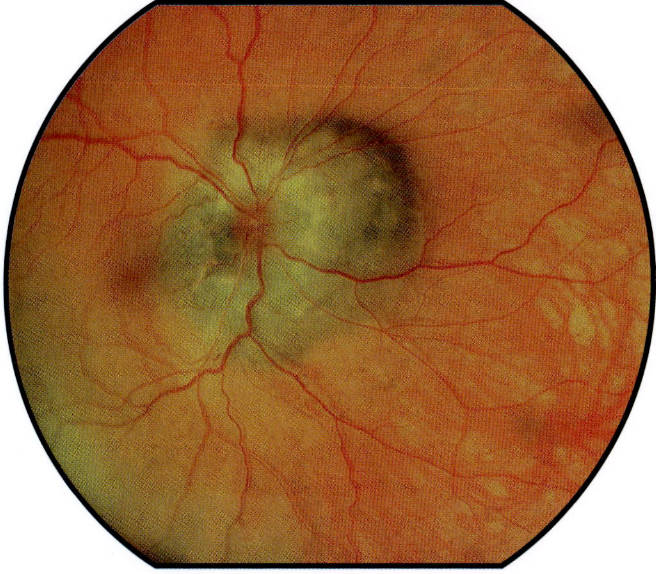

Small circumpapillary choroidal melanoma.

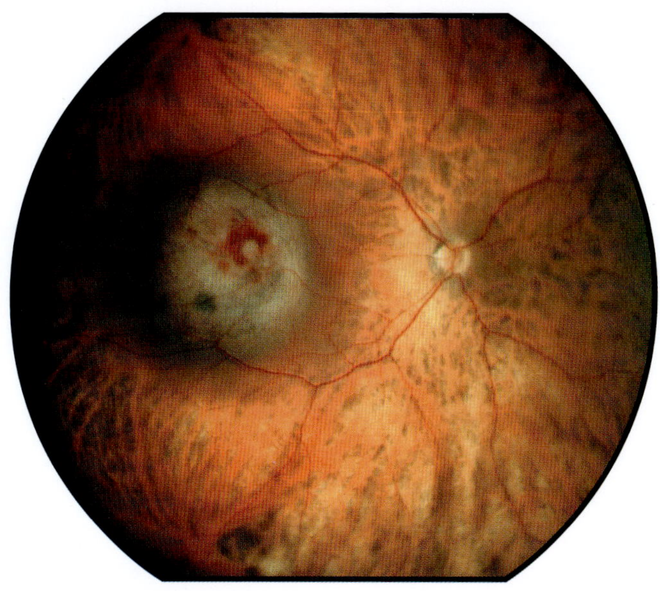

Medium choroidal melanoma.

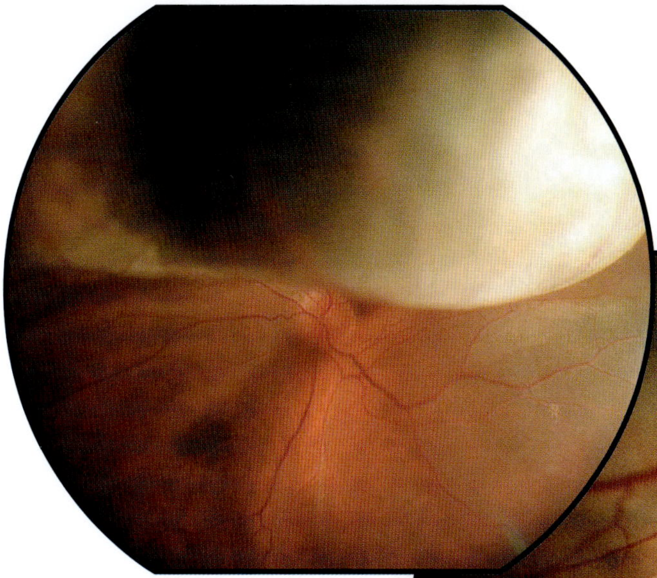

Large choroidal melanoma with associated retinal detachment *(left)*.

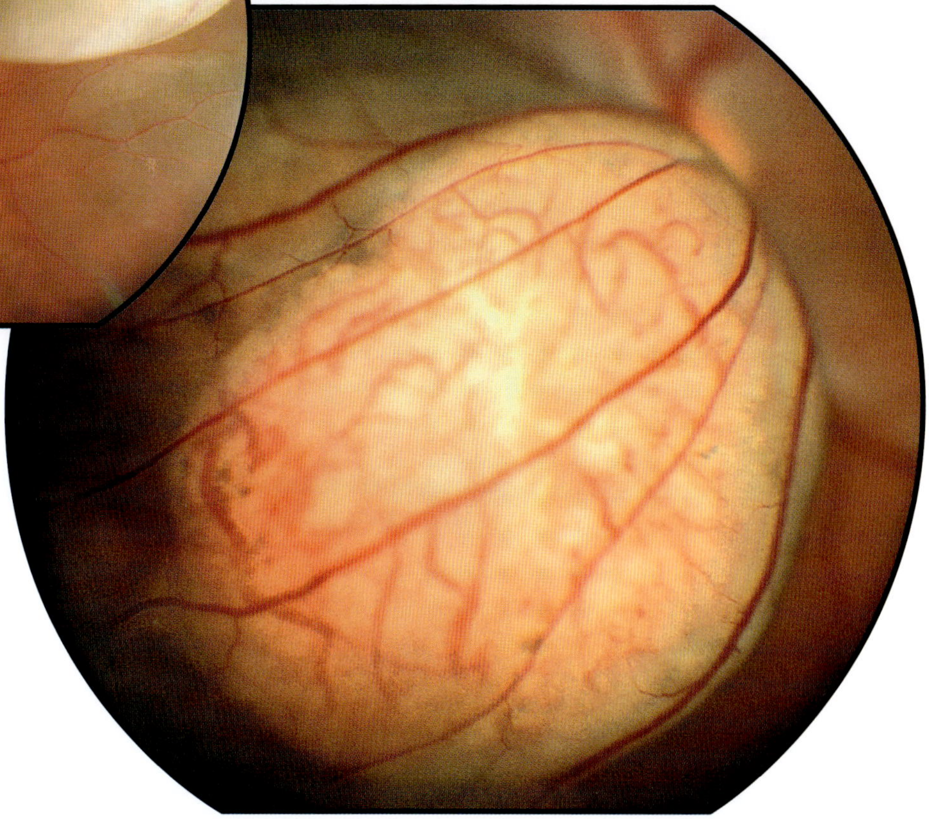

Large choroidal melanoma that is mostly amelanotic and extensively vascularized with secondary detachment *(right)*.

Choroidal Melanoma with Pigmentary Variations

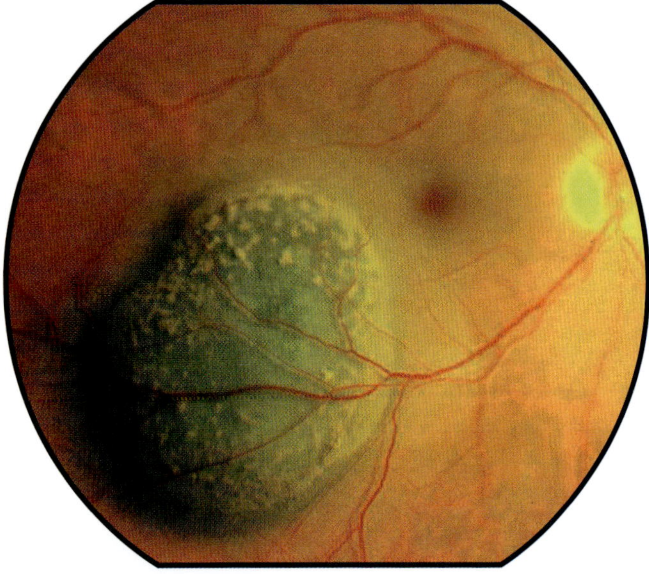

Pigmented choroidal melanoma. Note the overlying orange pigment and surrounding subretinal fluid.

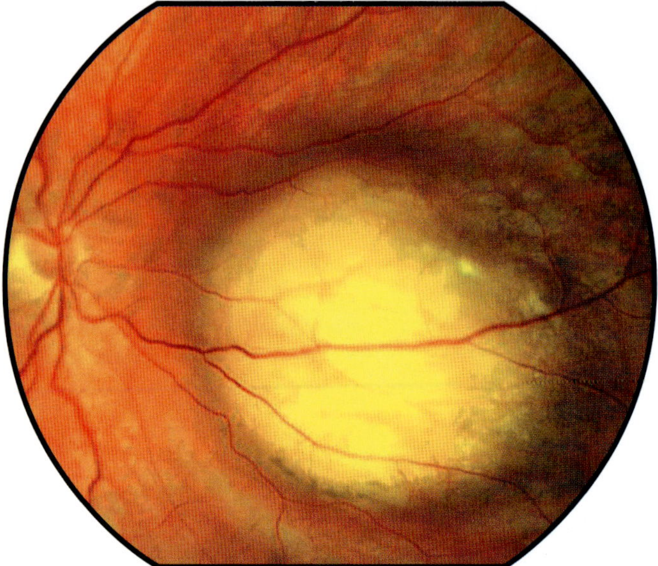

Amelanotic choroidal melanoma.

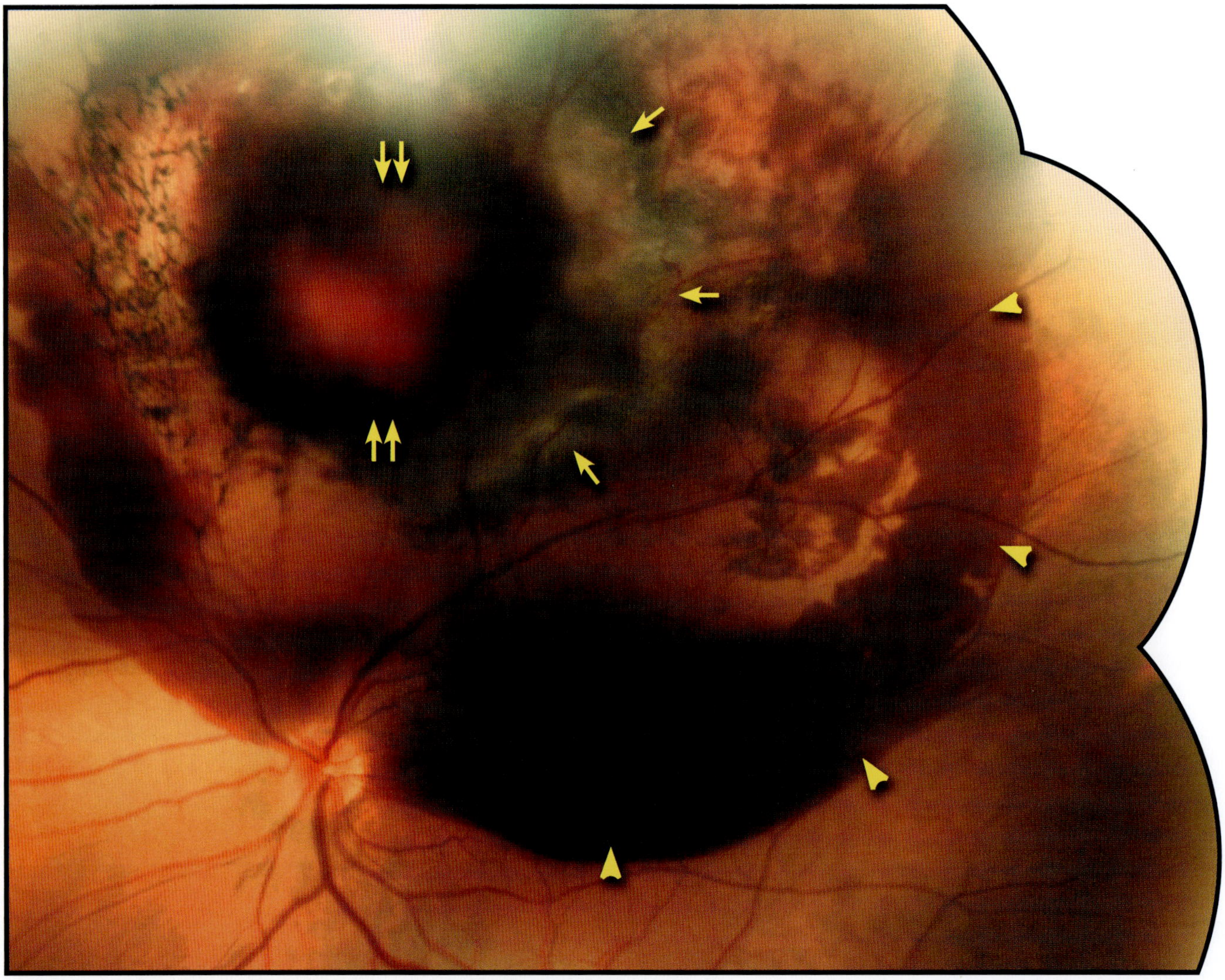

This choroidal melanoma was originally diagnosed as an eccentric peripheral disciform process. The melanoma itself *(arrows)* is obscured by preretinal *(double arrows)* and subretinal hemorrhage *(arrowheads)*. *Courtesy of Dr. Alan Kimura*

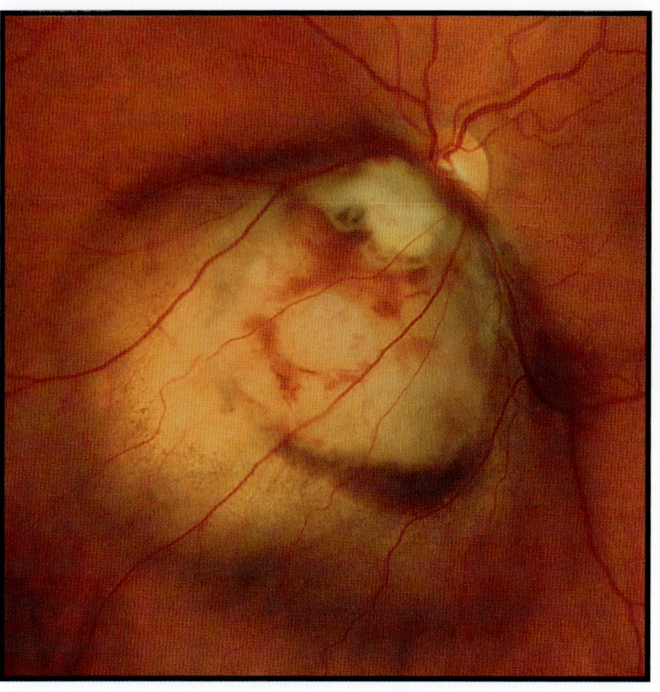

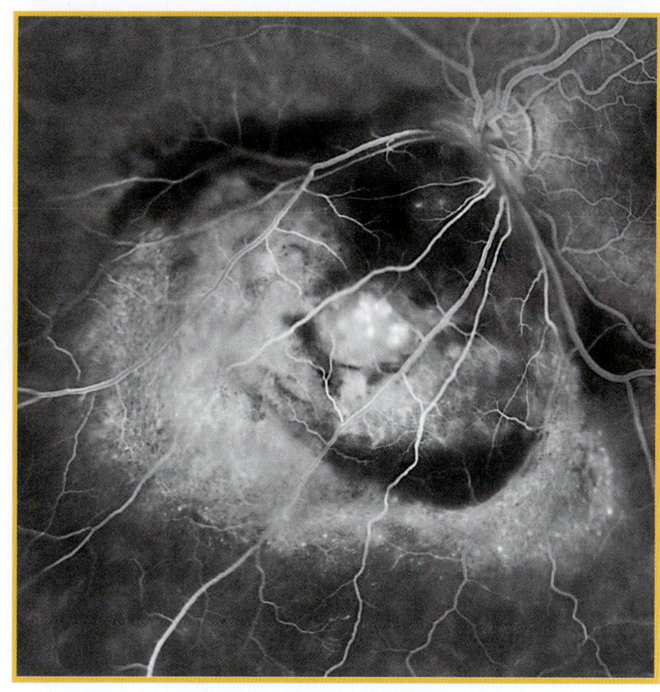

This is a large melanoma that is predominantly amelanotic but fringed with pigmentation at its margins both at the base and the mushroom extension above. The fluorescein angiogram shows that there is vascularity to both sections of the tumor and blockage by blood and pigmentation.
Courtesy of Dr. Mark Johnson

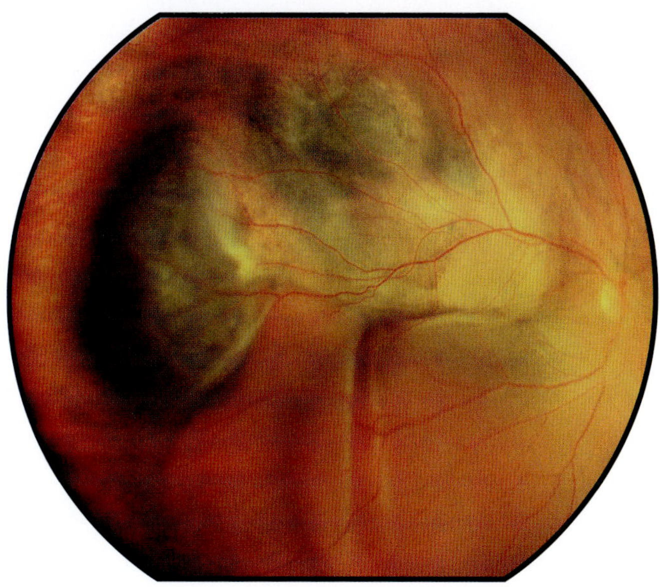

This is a diffuse choroidal melanoma with dependent detachment.

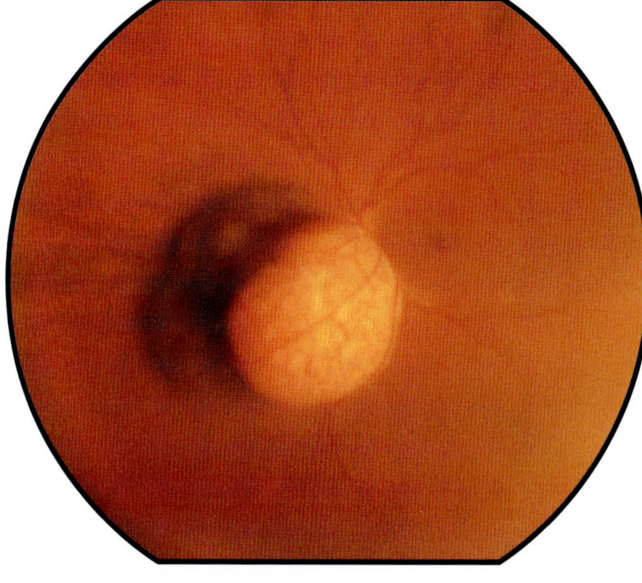

This is a predominantly amelanotic melanoma in a mushroom configuration.

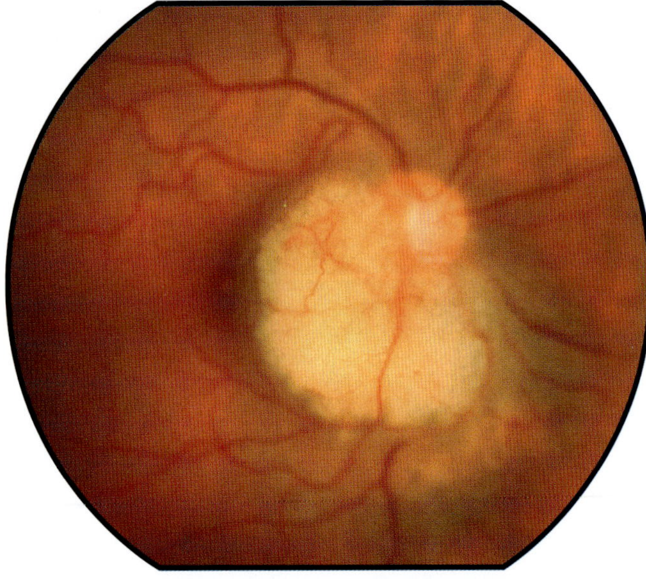

An amelanotic melanoma is contiguous with the optic disk.

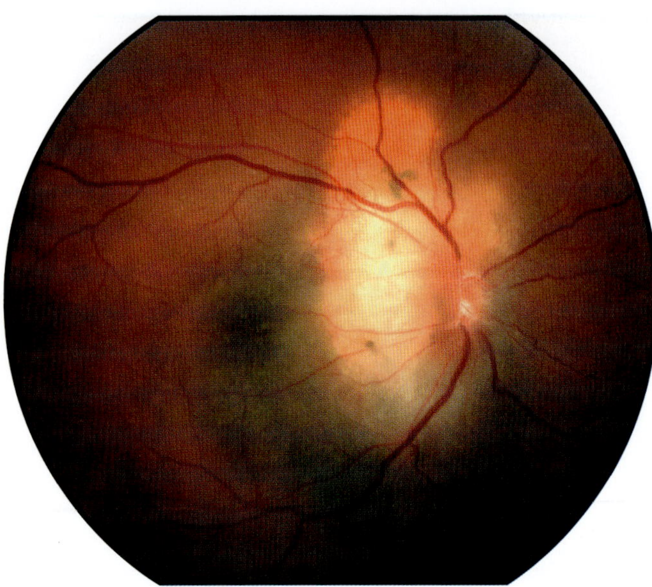

This melanoma presented with amelanotic and melanotic growth encroaching on the optic nerve and with chronic dependent retinal detachment.

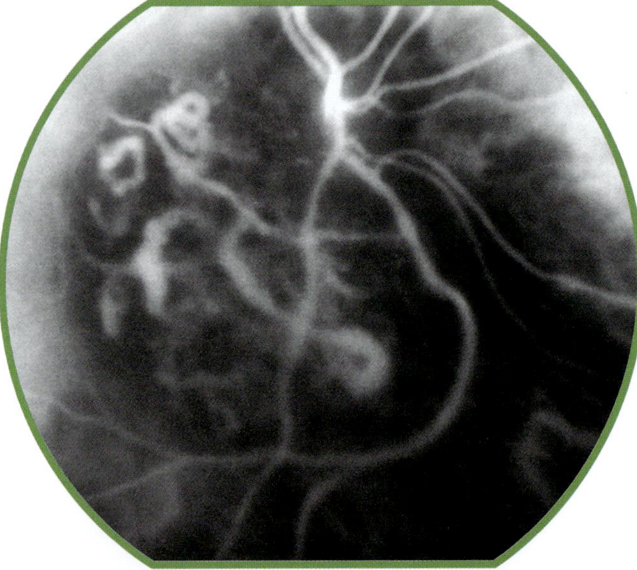

The indocyanine green angiogram of the tumor above shows an internal circulation to the lesion or a so-called double circulation thought to be characteristic of a choroidal melanoma.

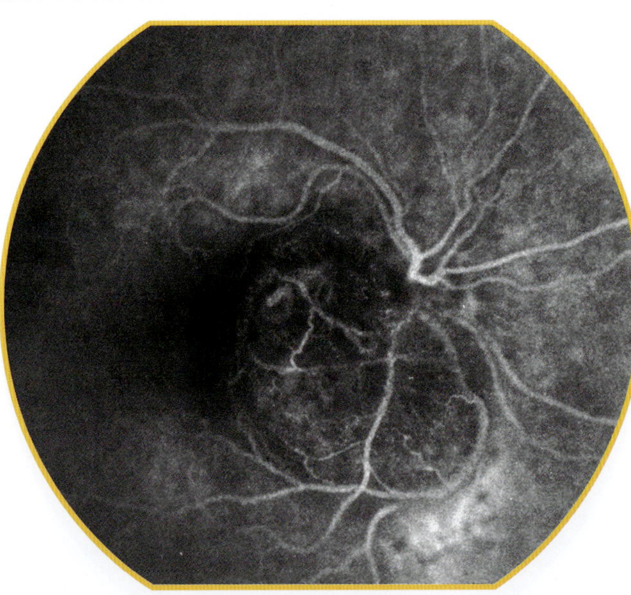

The fluorescein angiogram of the same tumor also shows this double circulation.

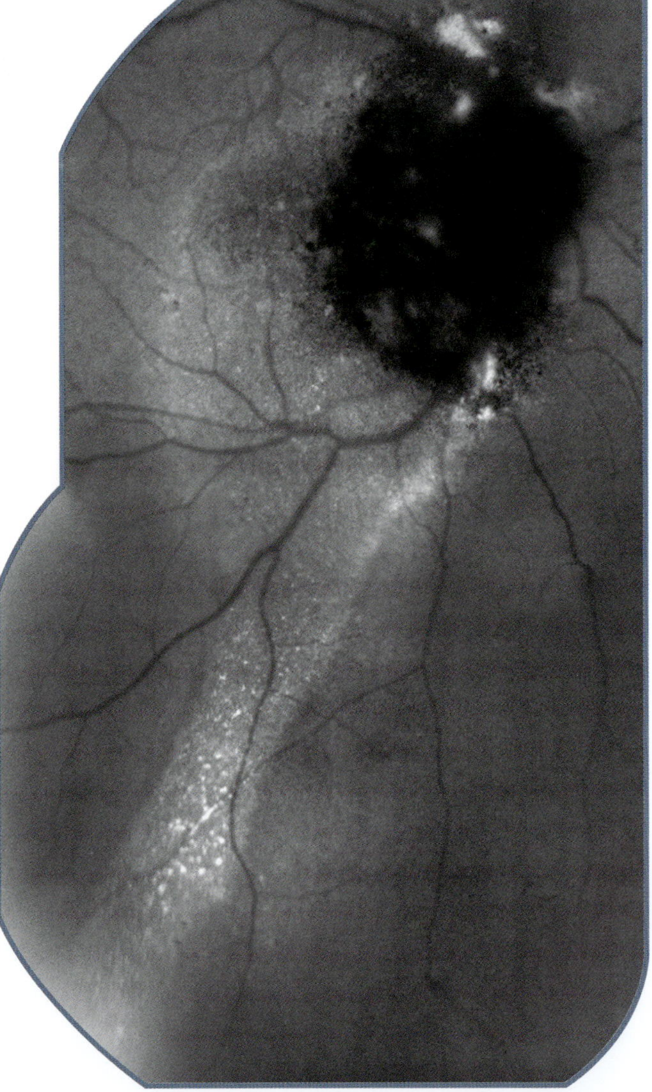

The fundus autofluorescence of the choroidal melanoma above shows a zone of hyperautofluorescence extending inferiorly that corresponds to a dependent neurosensory detachment.

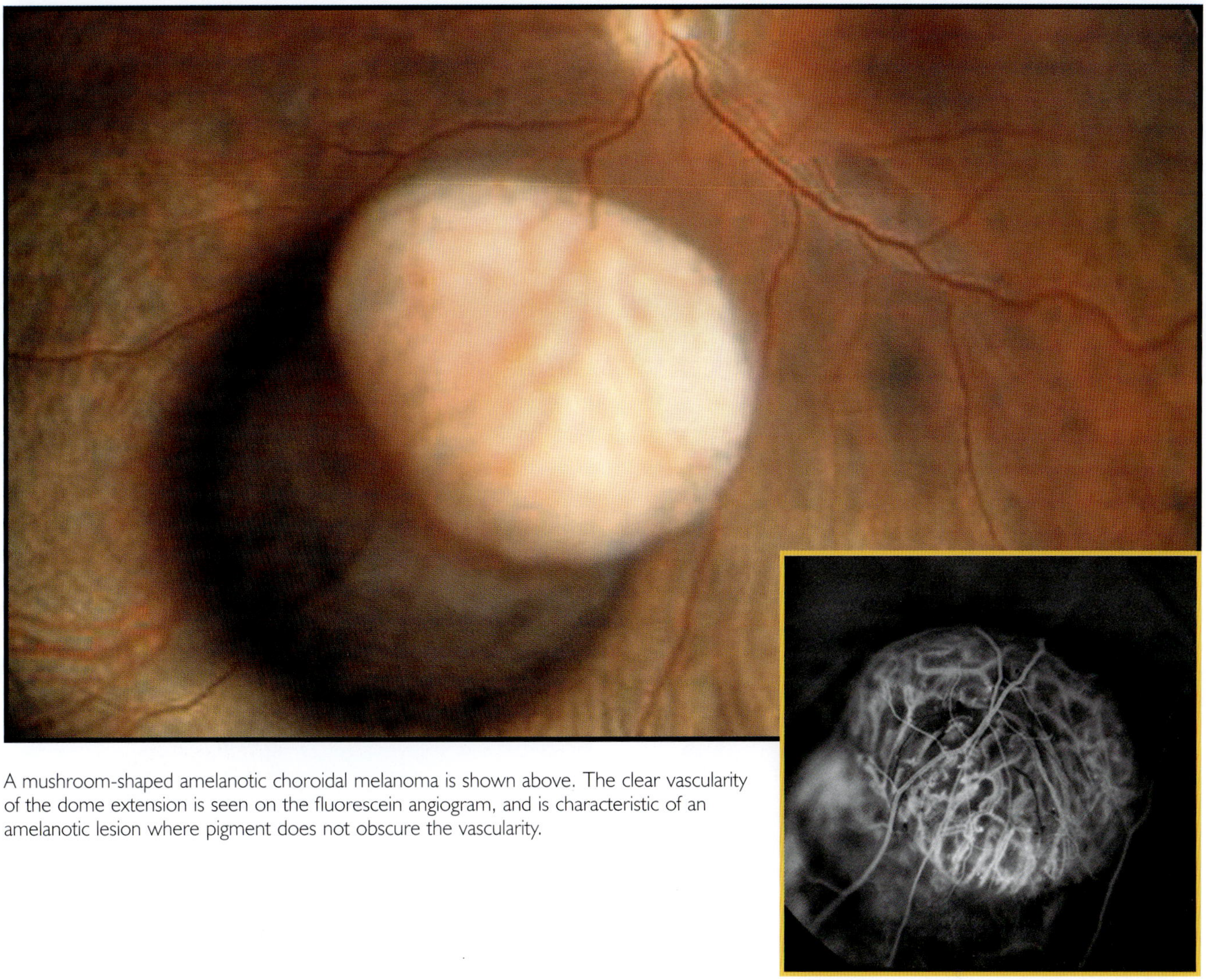

A mushroom-shaped amelanotic choroidal melanoma is shown above. The clear vascularity of the dome extension is seen on the fluorescein angiogram, and is characteristic of an amelanotic lesion where pigment does not obscure the vascularity.

Factors for Early Detection of Choroidal Melanoma

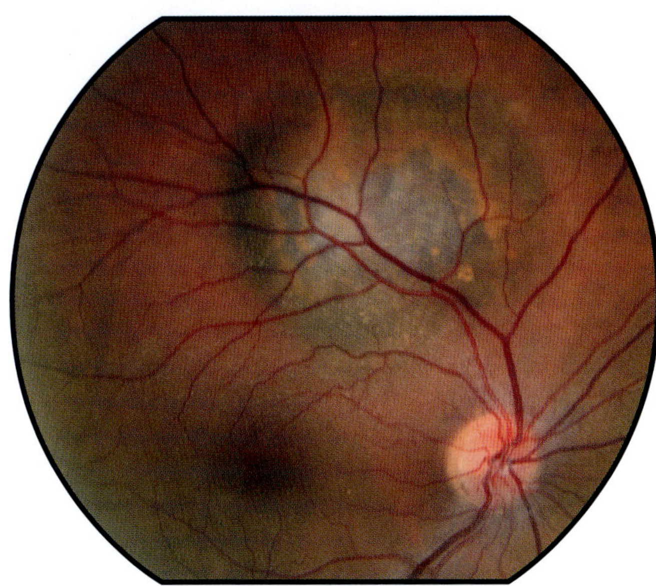

Small choroidal melanoma with overlying orange pigment and shallow subretinal fluid.

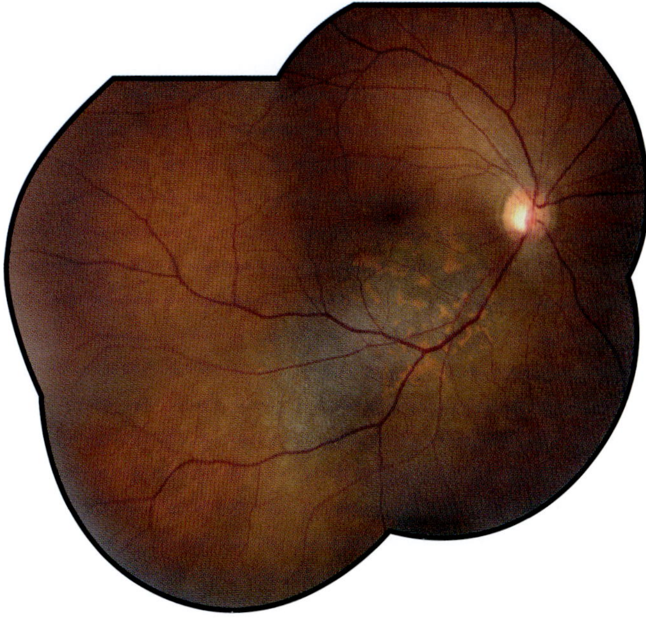

Small choroidal melanoma with overlying orange pigment in an eye with ocular melanocytosis.

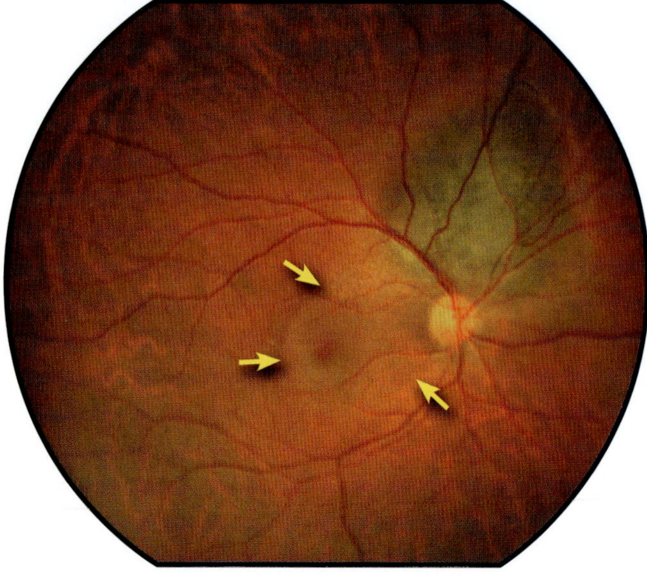

Small choroidal melanoma with subtle overlying orange pigment and subretinal fluid extending under the fovea *(arrows)*.

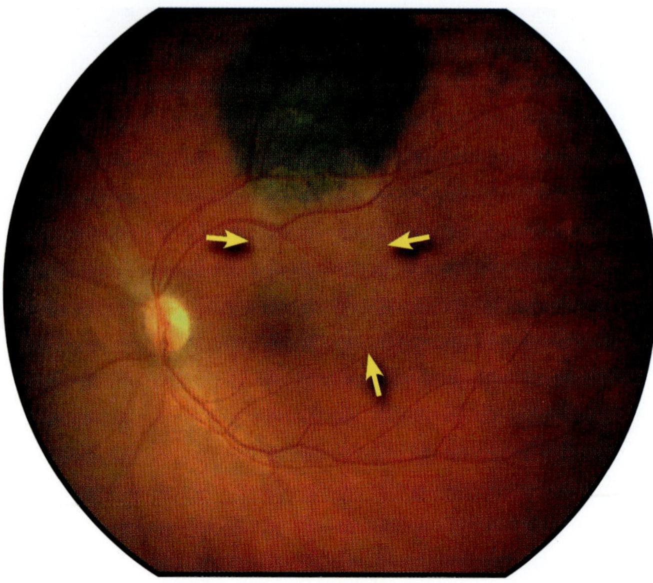

Small choroidal melanoma with subretinal fluid extending under the fovea *(arrows)*.

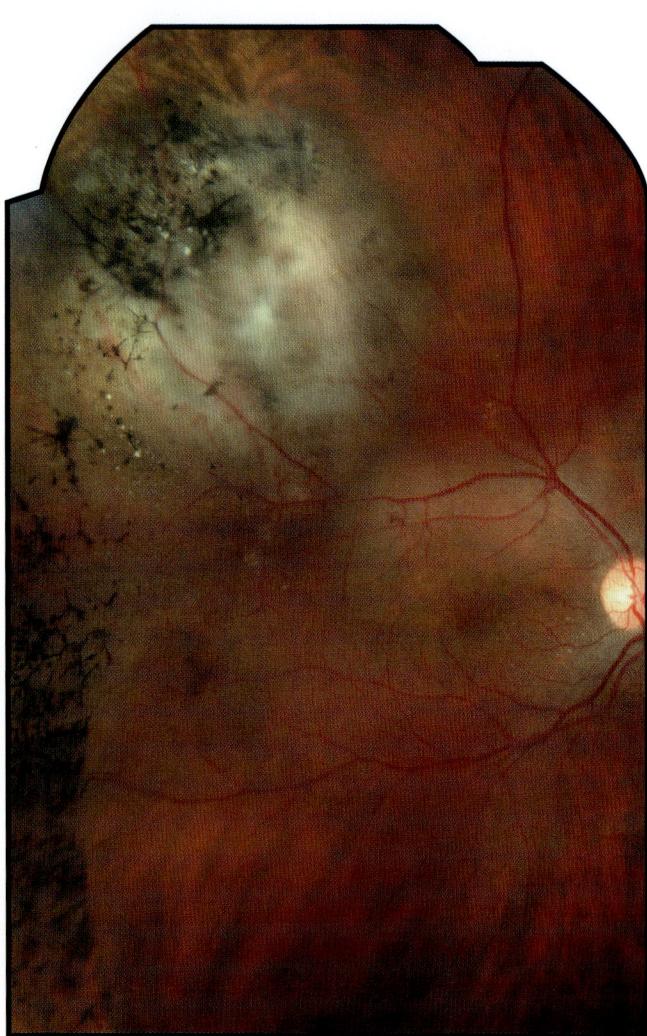

Some suspicious nevi may be associated with chronic leakage, fibrovascular proliferation, and pigment epithelial hyperplastic changes. In this patient, there is a descending retinal pigment epithelial tract, leading from the tumor due to an inferior dependent detachment ("gutter").

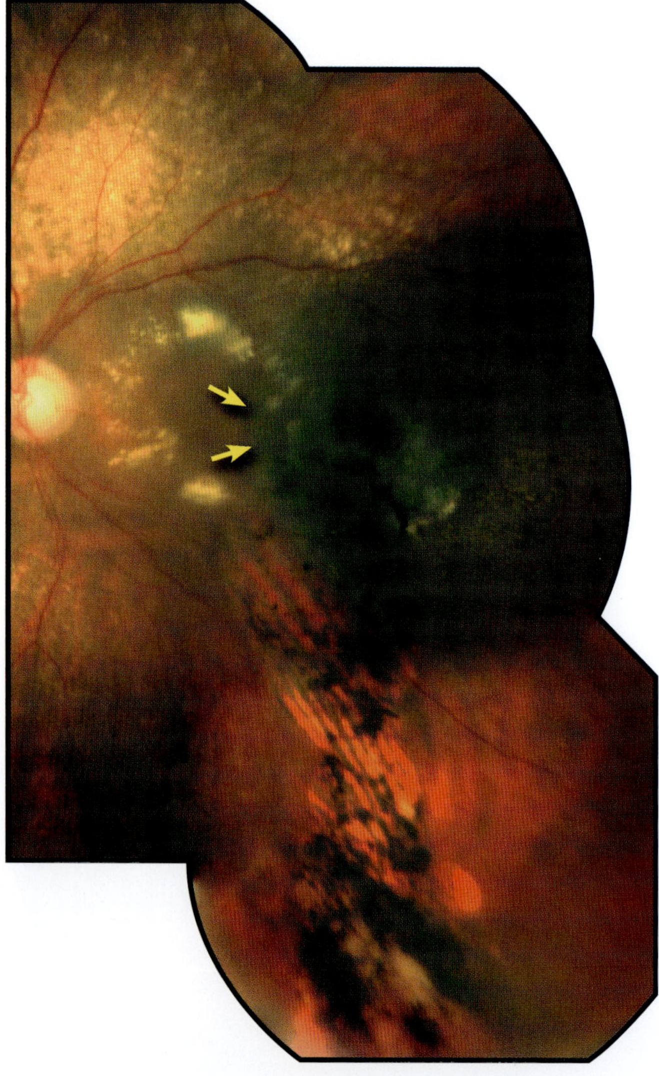

There was choroidal neovascularization *(arrows)* with an inferior exudative detachment extending from the macula to the inferior periphery in this 90-year-old female.

Early Detection of Choroidal Melanoma

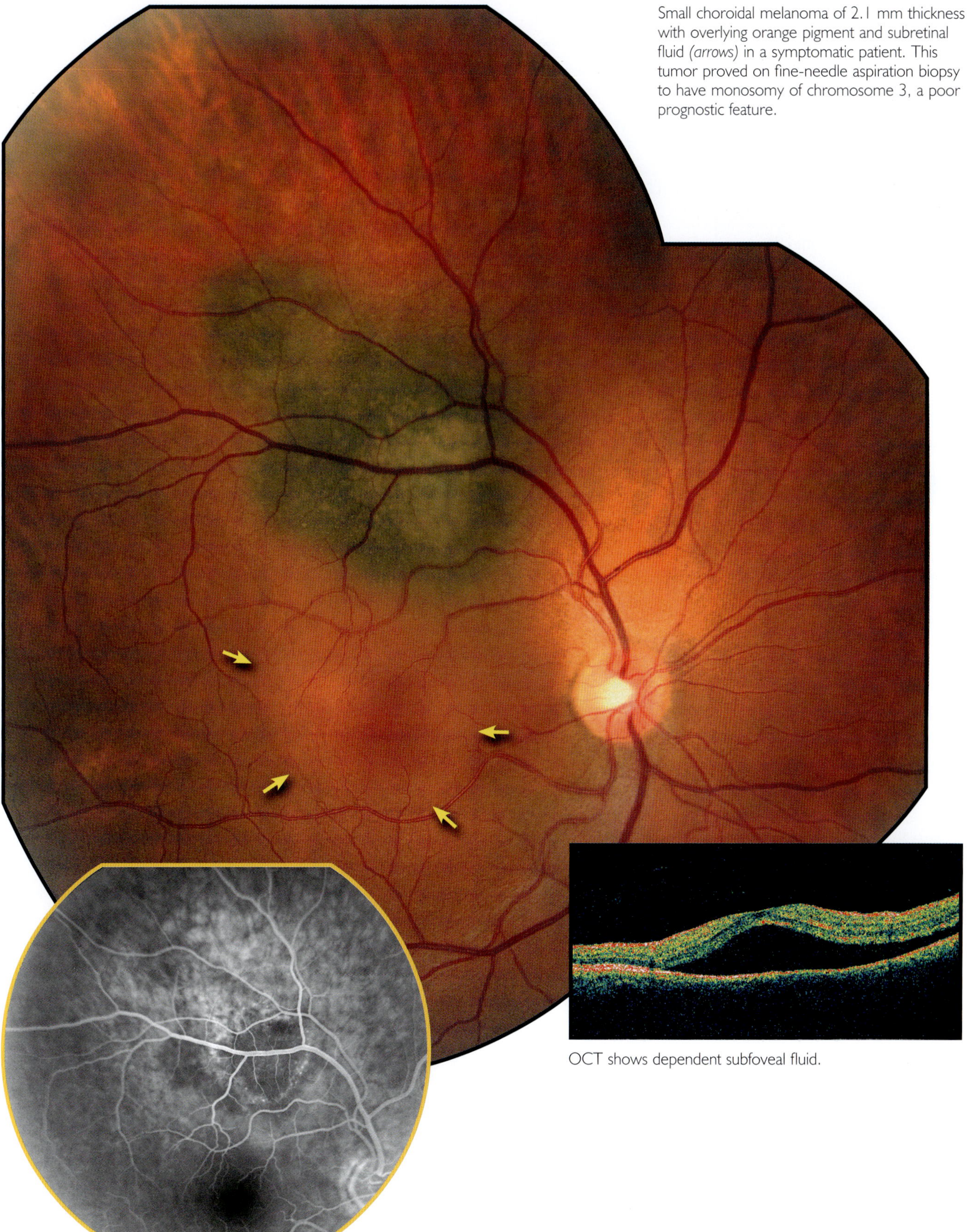

Small choroidal melanoma of 2.1 mm thickness with overlying orange pigment and subretinal fluid *(arrows)* in a symptomatic patient. This tumor proved on fine-needle aspiration biopsy to have monosomy of chromosome 3, a poor prognostic feature.

OCT shows dependent subfoveal fluid.

Fluorescein angiography shows relative hypofluorescence of the choroidal melanoma and overlying multifocal hyperfluorescent spots at the level of the RPE. There is no focal or multifocal RPE leakage. There is a dependent retinal detachment *(arrows in color montage)*.

Early Detection of Small Choroidal Melanoma Using Mnemonic "To Find Small Ocular Melanoma Using Helpful Hints Daily"

Recognizing several important risk factors, as listed in the table below, facilitates early detection of choroidal melanoma. Any lesion manifesting these factors should be evaluated by an ocular oncologist. The mnemonic "To Find Small Ocular Melanoma Using Helpful Hints Daily" helps in early detection of melanoma.

Factors for Detection of Small Choroidal Melanoma at Tumor Thickness ≤ 3 mm Using the Mnemonic "To Find Small Ocular Melanoma Using Helpful Hints Daily"					
Initials	**Mnemonic**	**Features**	**Hazard ratio**	**Nevus growth into melanoma if feature present (%)**	**Nevus growth into melanoma if feature absent (%)**
T	To	Thickness > 2 mm	2	19%	5%
F	Find	Fluid	3	27%	5%
S	Small	Symptoms	2	23%	5%
O	Ocular	Orange pigment	3	30%	5%
M	Melanoma	Margin ≤ 3 mm to disc	2	13%	4%
UH	Using Helpful	Ultrasound hollow	3	25%	4%
H	Hints	Halo absent	6	7%	2%
D	Daily	Drusen absent	na	na	na

na, the risk factor "drusen absent" was identified in other studies to be significant so it was included in this mnemonic for risk factors.

Data adapted from Shields, C.L., Furuta, M., Berman, E.L., et al., 2009. Choroidal nevus transformation into melanoma. Analysis of 2514 consecutive cases. Arch. Ophthalmol. 127 (8), 981–987.

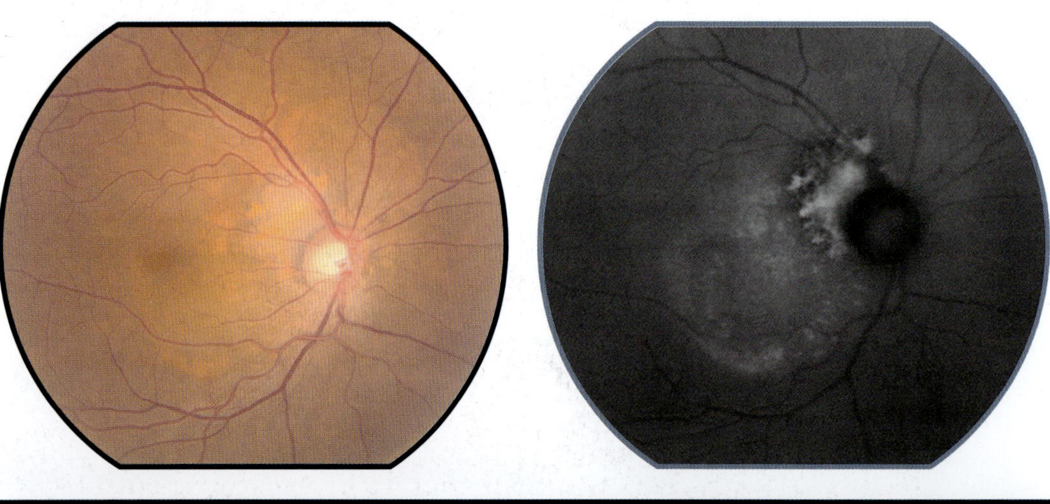

Small juxtapapillary choroidal melanoma with overlying orange pigment, confirmed on fundus autofluorescence and subfoveal fluid, confirmed on OCT. Note the "shaggy" photoreceptors, a sign of fresh subretinal fluid.

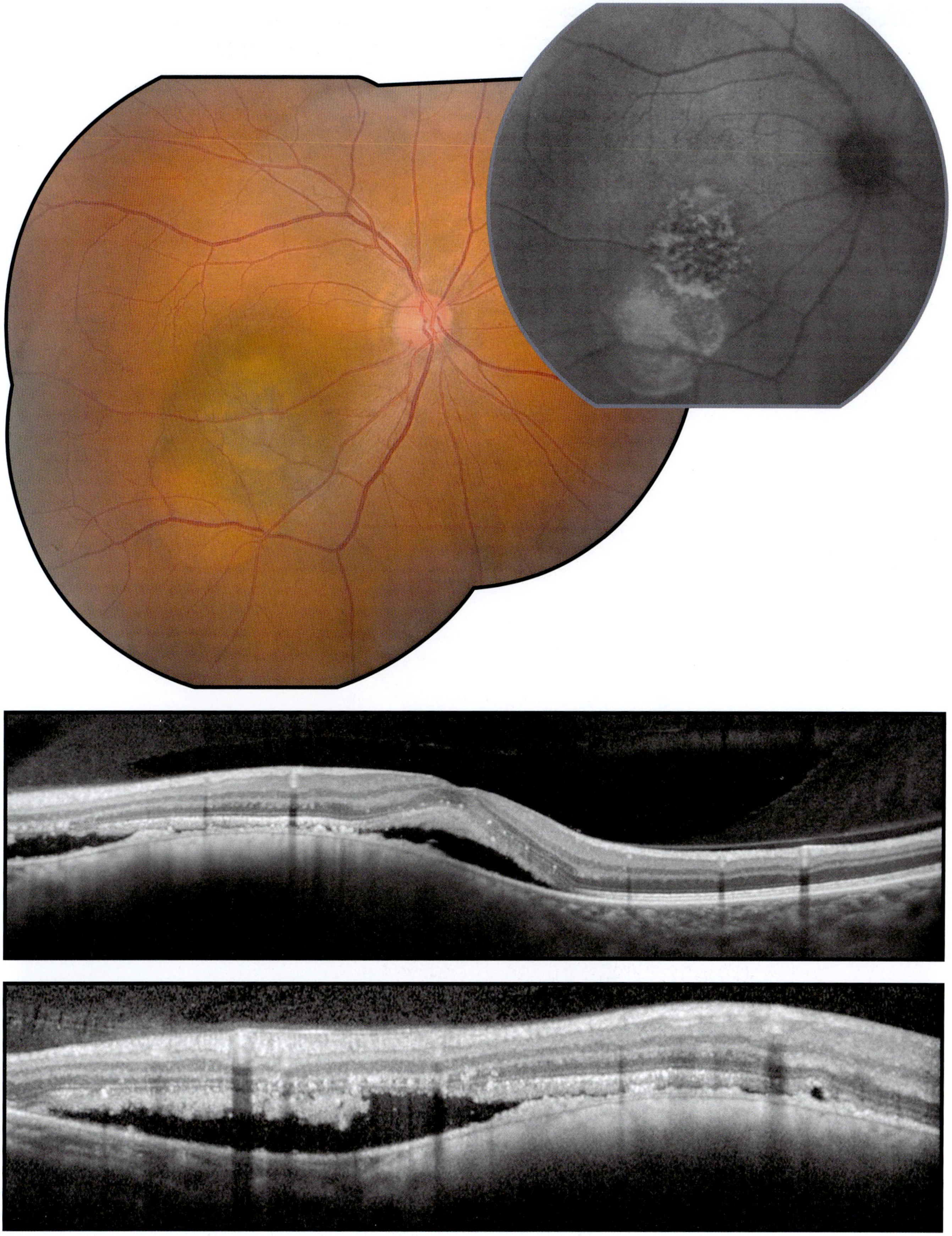

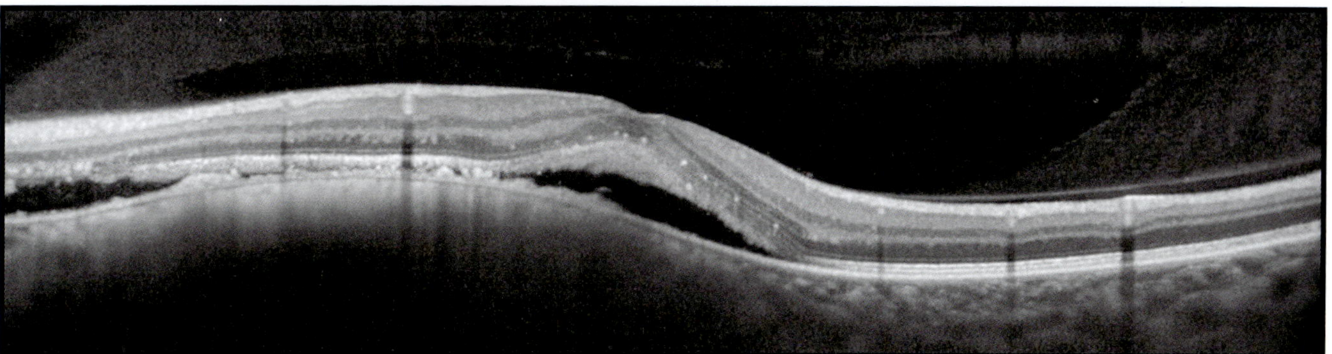

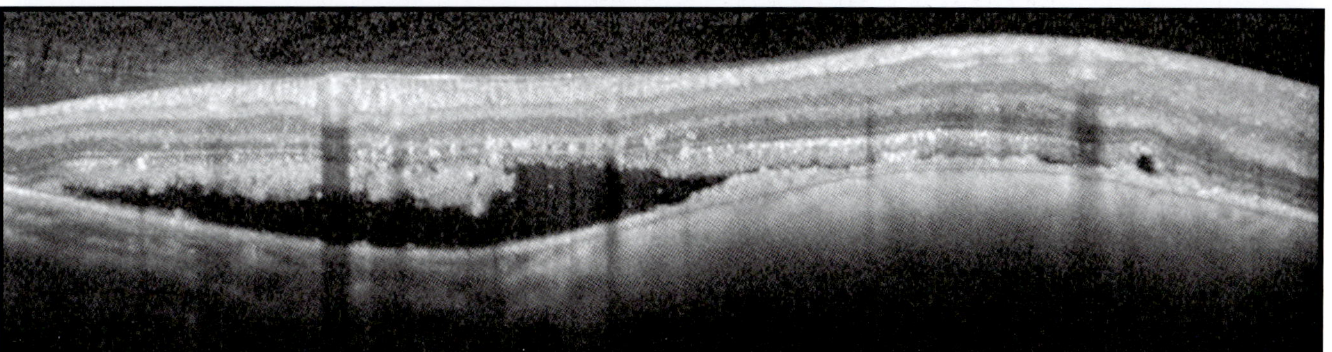

Small submacular choroidal melanoma with overlying prominent orange pigment, confirmed on fundus autofluorescence, and subfoveal fluid, confirmed on OCT. Note again the "shaggy" photoreceptors.

Choroidal Melanoma Before and After Plaque Radiotherapy

The management of posterior uveal melanoma is controversial, with some advocating enucleation and others suggesting more conservative treatment methods designed to save the affected eye. The primary goal of treatment is to eradicate or inactivate the tumor before metastasis occurs. Numerous modalities have been used with this in mind. They include photocoagulation, radiotherapy, local resection, and transpupillary thermal therapy.

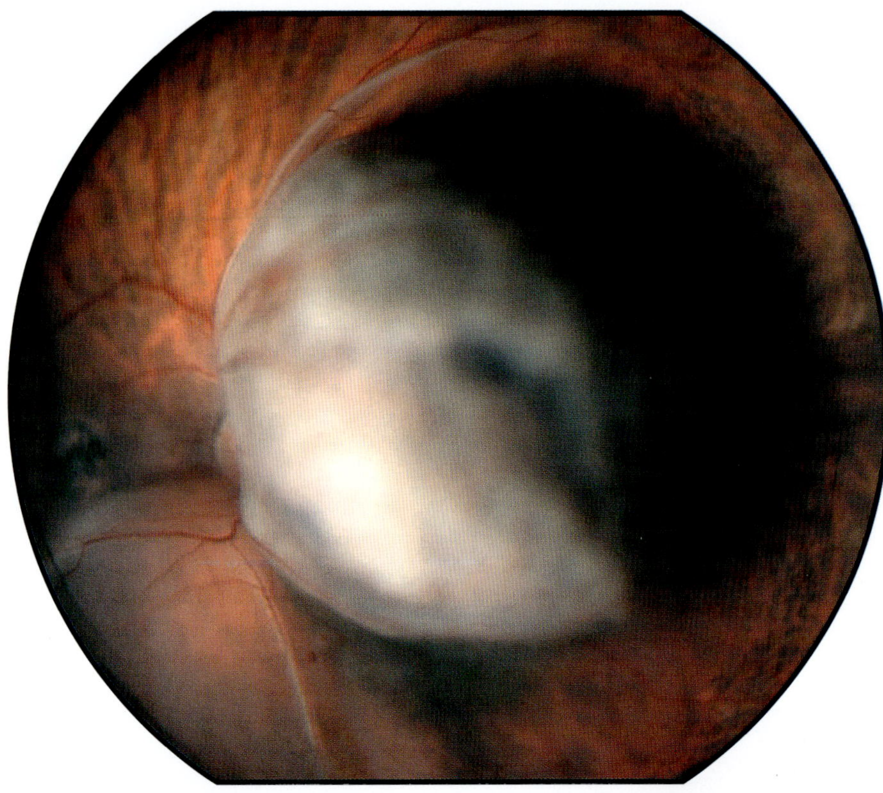

Before treatment, the juxtapapillary choroidal melanoma is noted with extensive subretinal fluid.

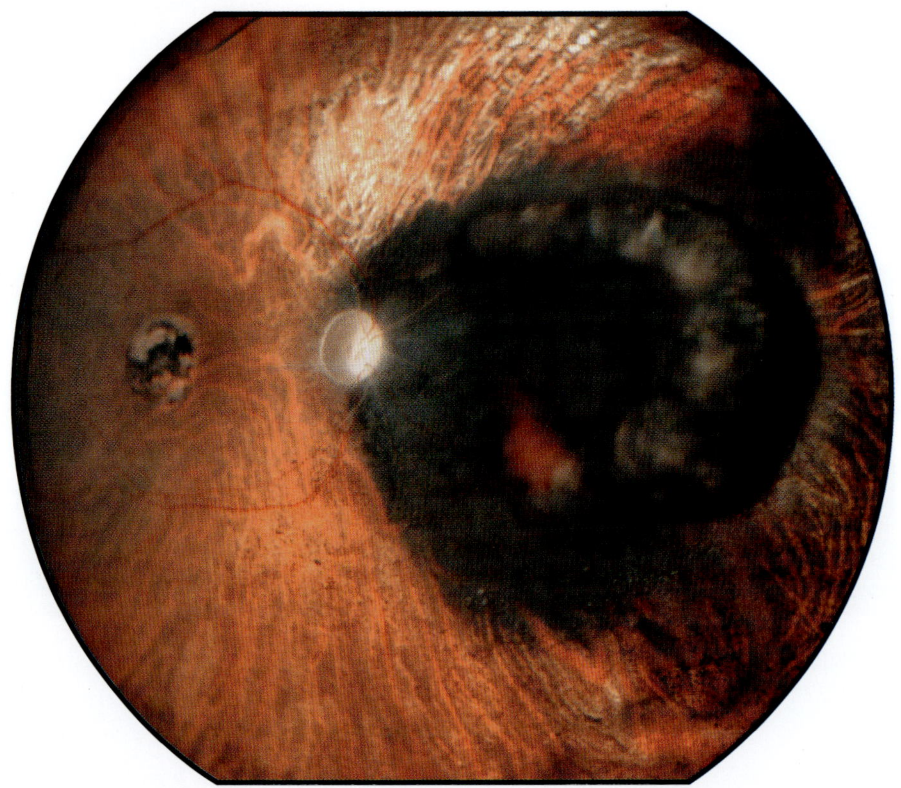

Nine months following treatment, the tumor has regressed to an atrophic scar. There is some optic nerve pallor and radiation-related atrophy. The patient had unrelated ocular histoplasmosis with a foveal scar.

Choroidal Metastasis

Choroidal metastasis appears as a creamy yellow mass, usually in the macula or paramacular region and often with substantial subretinal fluid. Metastatic tumors can be multifocal and bilateral. The most common metastases to the choroid are from the breast and lung. Less often, cancers from the gastrointestinal tract, kidney, and skin (melanoma) spread to the choroid.

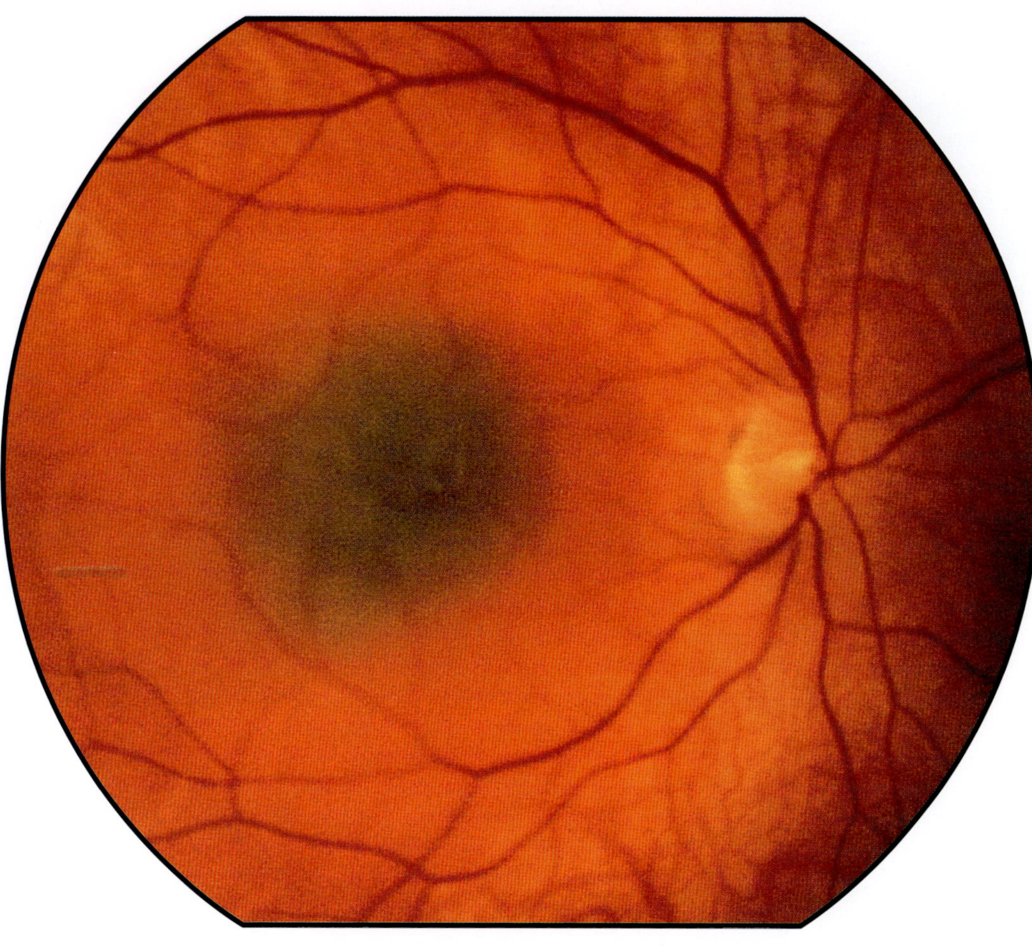

This patient had a metastatic lesion to the choroid from skin melanoma. This choroidal lesion is associated with an overlying and dependent serous detachment and is difficult to distinguish from a choroidal melanoma. A complete medical history and physical examination are essential in patients with choroidal melanoma to ascertain whether the disease is metastatic. *Courtesy of Dr. Evangelos Gragoudas*

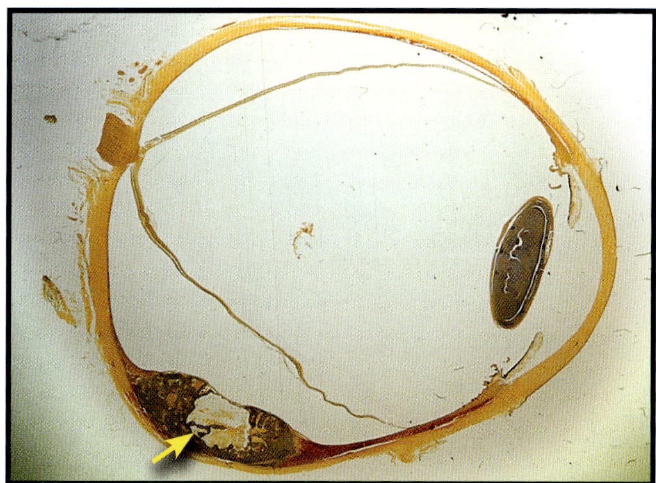

There is a serous detachment of the retina overlying a whitish choroidal mass *(arrow)* with central necrosis that contains neoplastic cells in a patient with breast carcinoma.

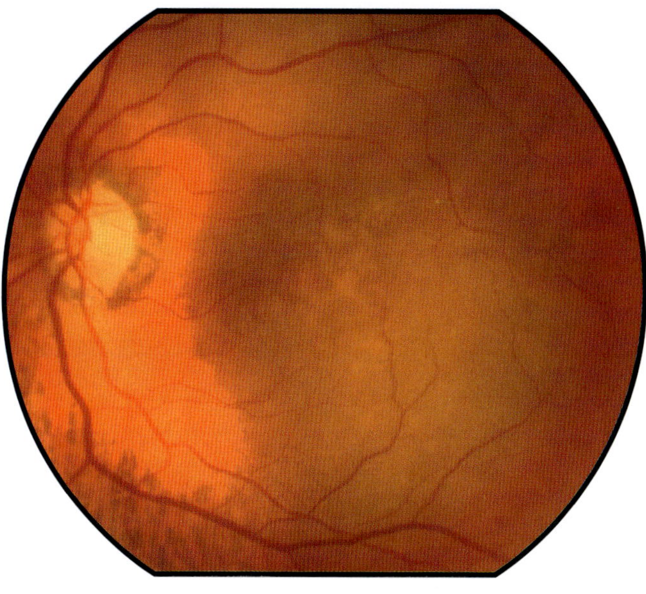

This metastasis was from the breast. *Courtesy of Dr. Martin Pearlman*

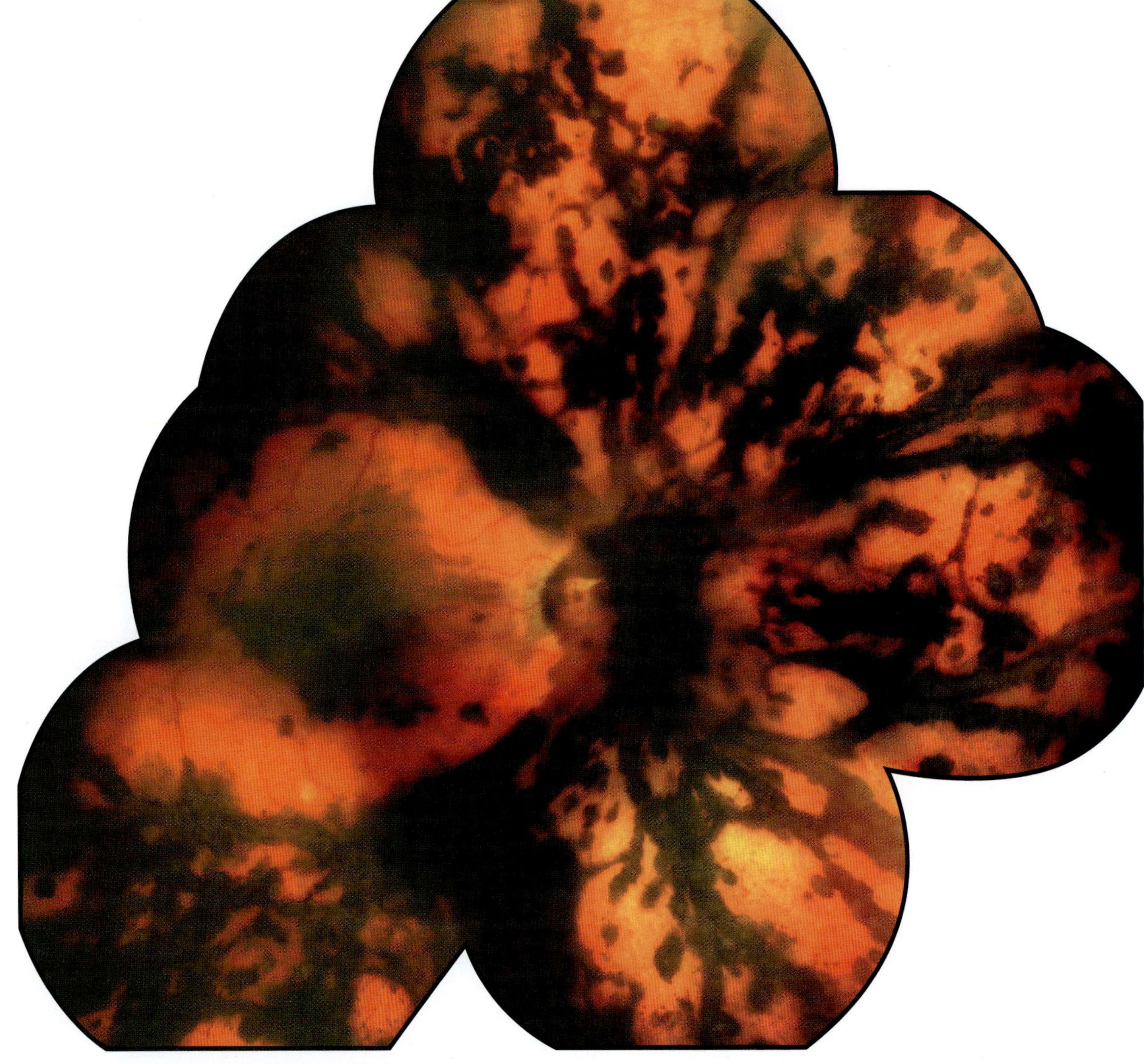

This patient has widespread metastatic choroidal and retinal melanoma from a cutaneous malignant melanoma. *Courtesy of Dr. Naring Rao*

Solitary Choroidal Metastasis in Patients with Carcinoma

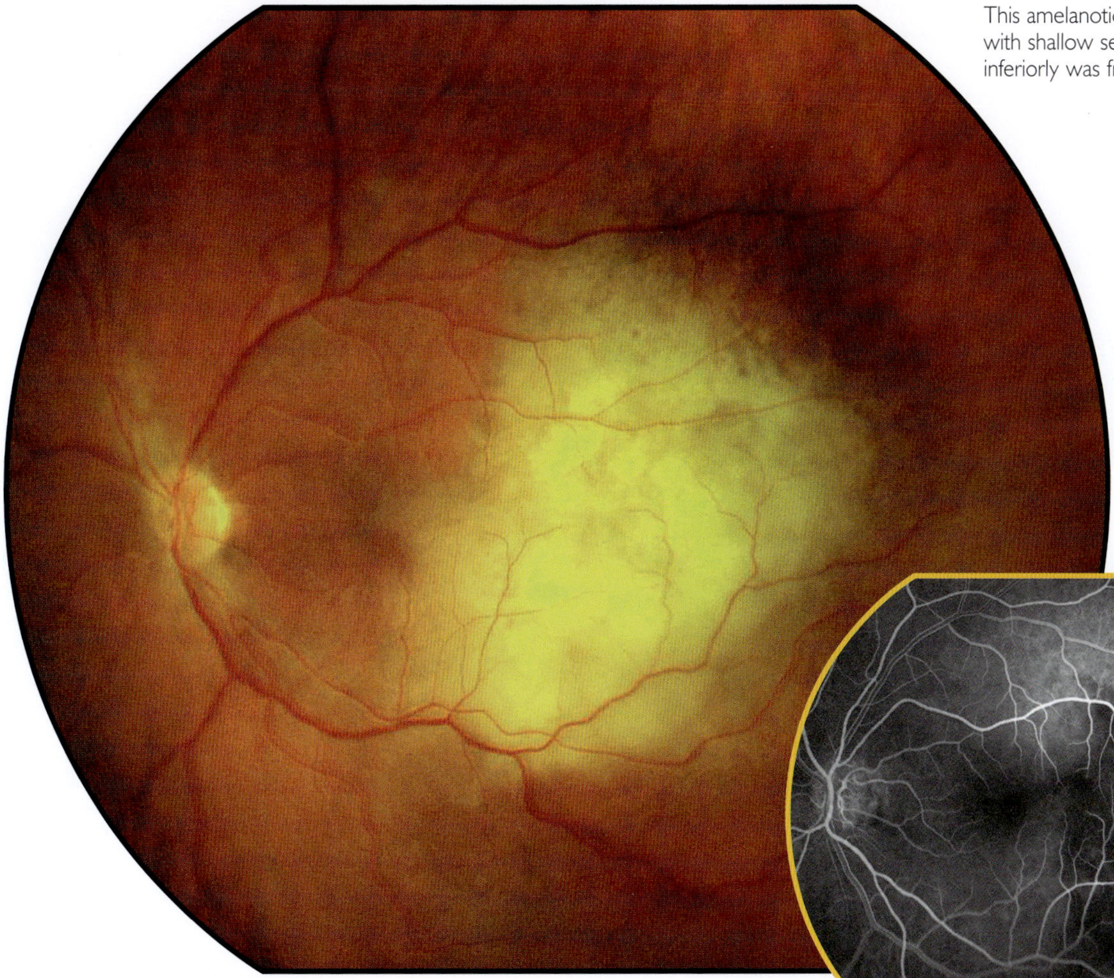

This amelanotic choroidal metastasis with shallow serous retinal detachment inferiorly was from the lung.

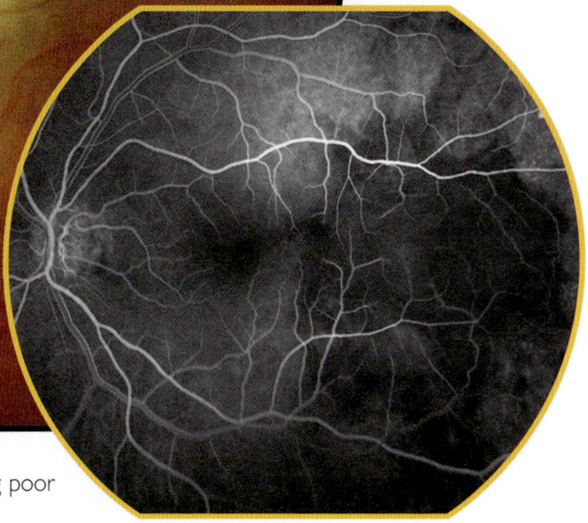

Fluorescein angiography depicts a relative hypofluorescence of the metastasis indicating poor vascularity of the lesion.

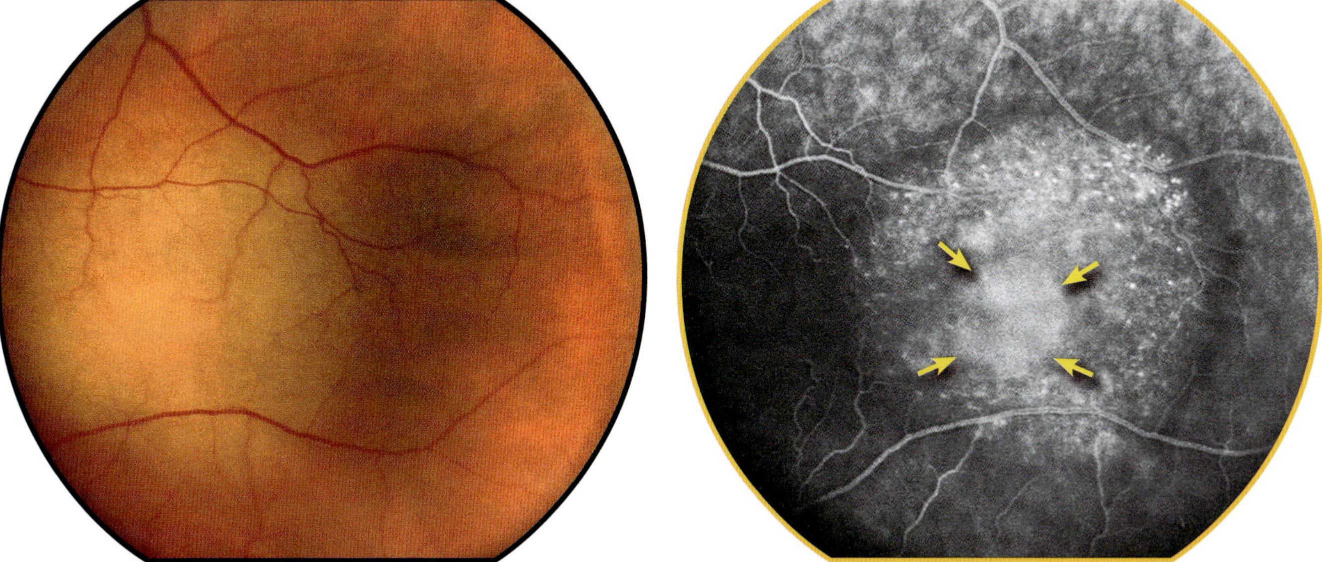

Patients with lung metastasis to the choroid often do not have a documented past history of lung cancer. Note the whitish-yellow elevated mass in this patient. The fluorescein angiogram shows a small serous detachment of the RPE overlying the tumor *(arrows)*. The multiple hyperfluorescent spots are believed to represent infiltration and alteration of the RPE by tumor cells.

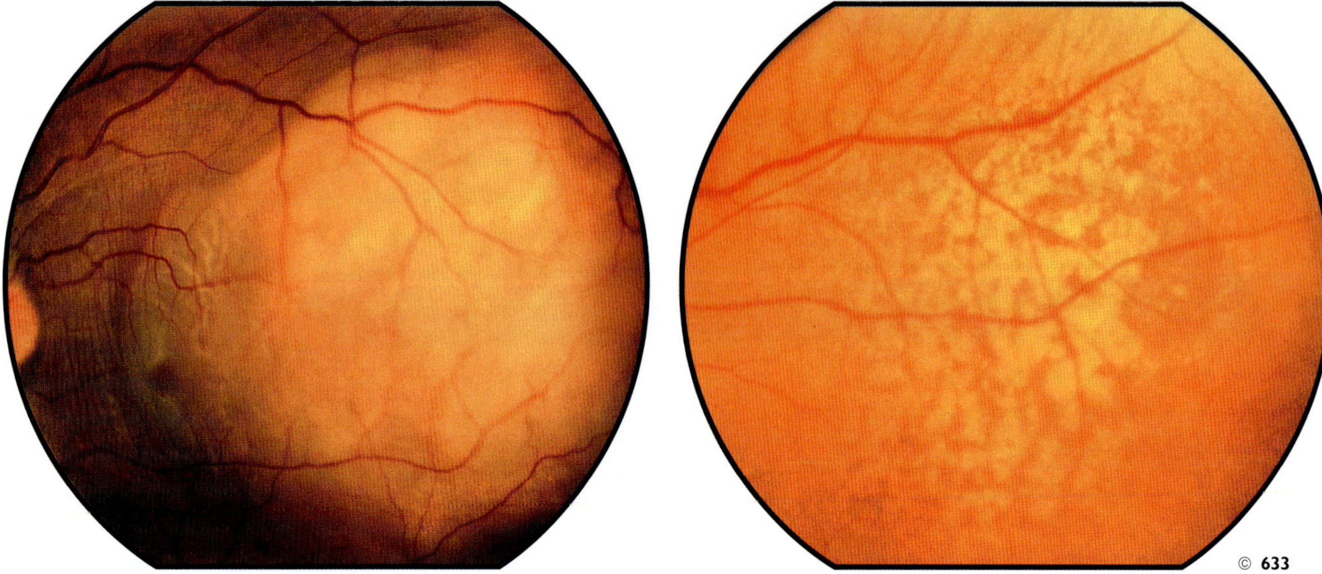

Breast metastasis to the choroid usually occurs in patients with a known history of breast carcinoma. A serous detachment with whitish clumps and retinal folds may be noted in some cases *(left)* and in other cases a leopard-spot configuration may be seen *(right)*. *Left image courtesy of Dr. Evangelos Gragoudas*

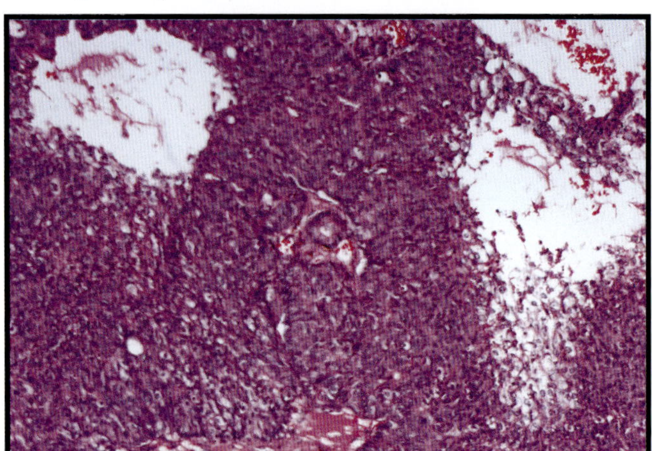

This image shows the histologic appearance of the choroidal metastasis seen in the patient with metastatic breast carcinoma presented in the upper left panel. The neoplastic cells are arranged in an acinar pattern. The white areas represent necrotic tumor cells.

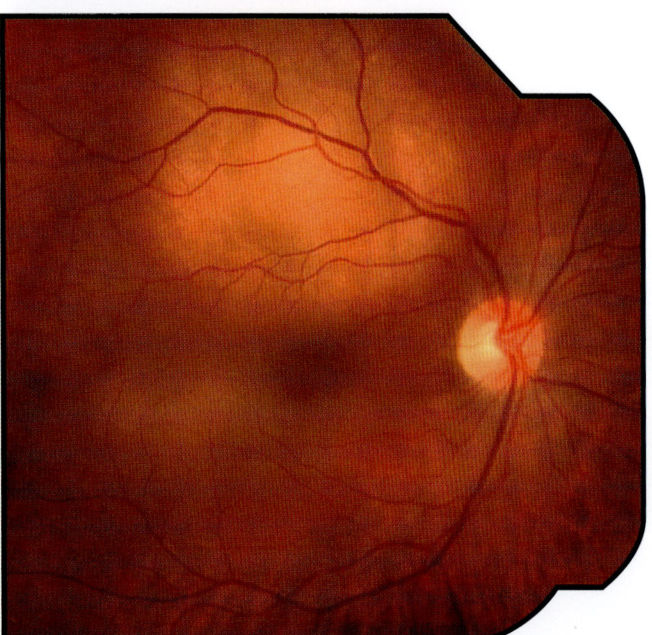

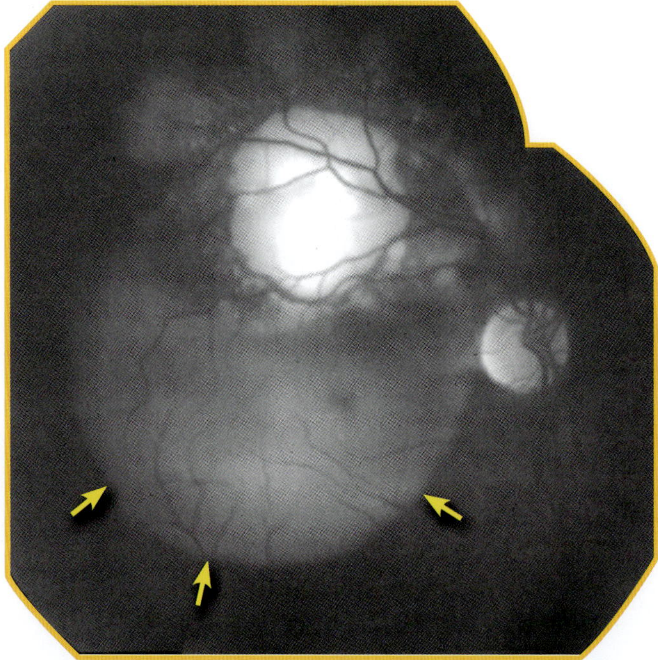

This patient had a creamy-colored mass in the choroid from breast carcinoma. There was an exudative detachment of the retina that is more clearly demonstrated on the late fluorescein angiogram *(arrows)*.

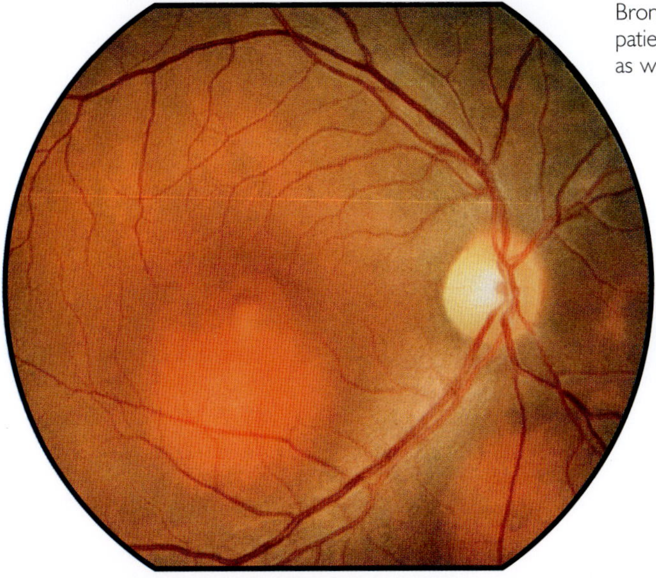

Bronchial carcinoid tumor can rarely metastasize to the choroid, as in this patient. Multifocal, slightly elevated, reddish orange nodules can be seen *(left)*, as well as metastatic lesions to the iris and anterior chamber *(right)*.

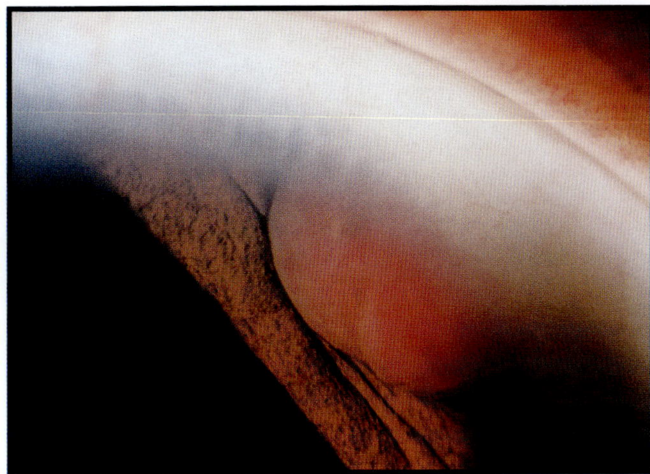

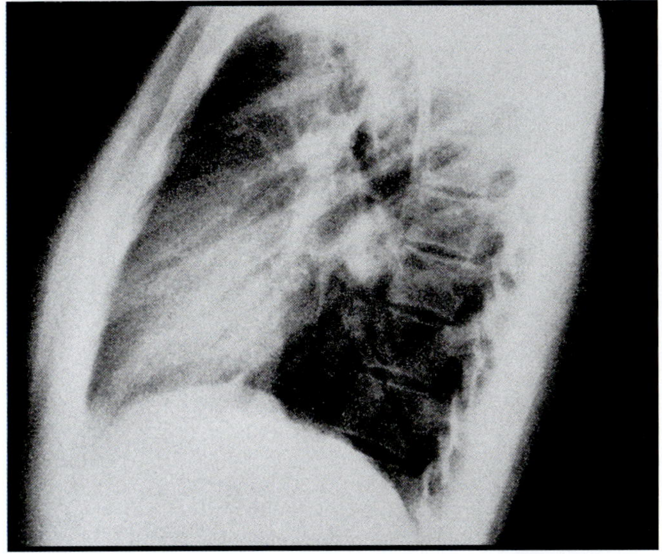

Chest X-ray *(left)* reveals the bronchial lesion. A lung biopsy confirmed bronchial carcinoid *(right)*. *Top two rows courtesy of Dr. Evangelos Gragoudas*

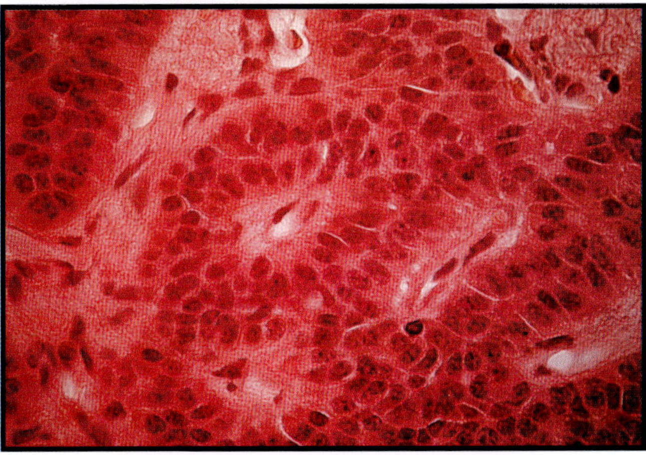

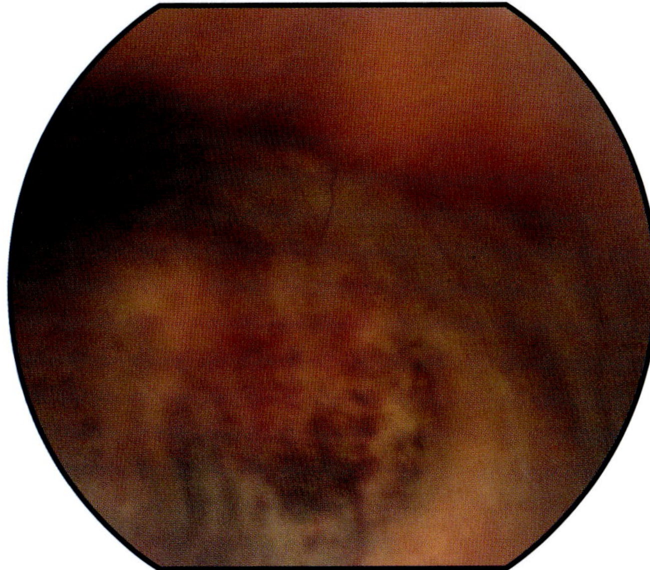

This patient had long-standing renal cell carcinoma with a huge metastatic lesion in the peripheral fundus. There is exudation and bleeding associated with the tumor growth. *Courtesy of Dr. Herbert Cantrill*

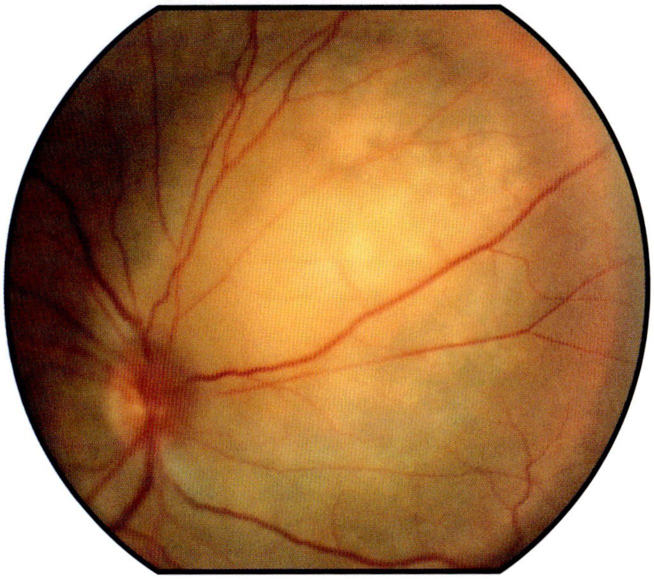

Patients with metastatic lesions from the lung to the choroid frequently do not have a known history of pulmonary cancer.

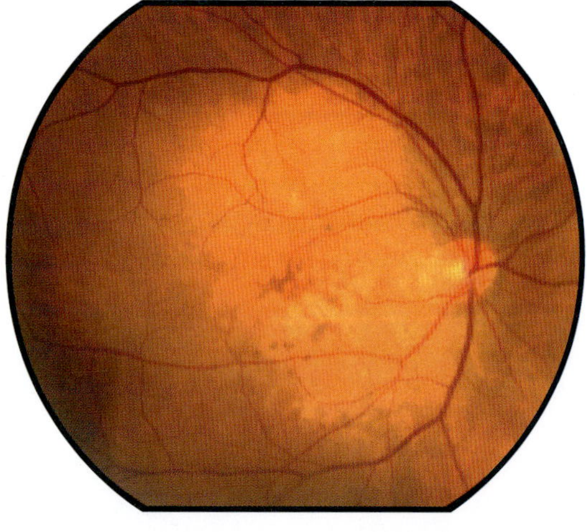

This is a solid, metastatic lesion of the choroid with secondary creamy yellow detachment of the retina.

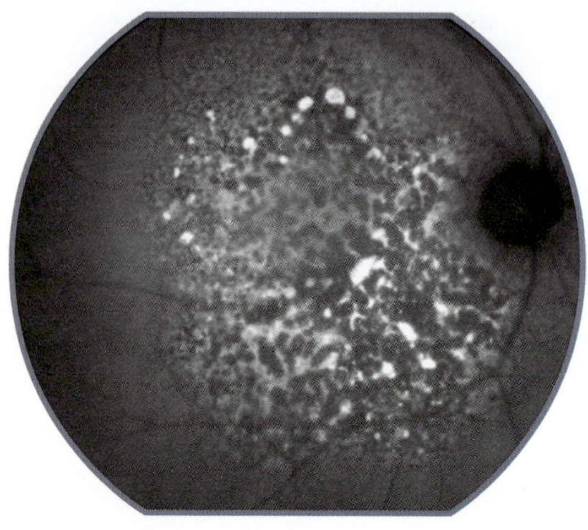

The fundus autofluorescence delineates the mass lesion and its effect on the RPE.

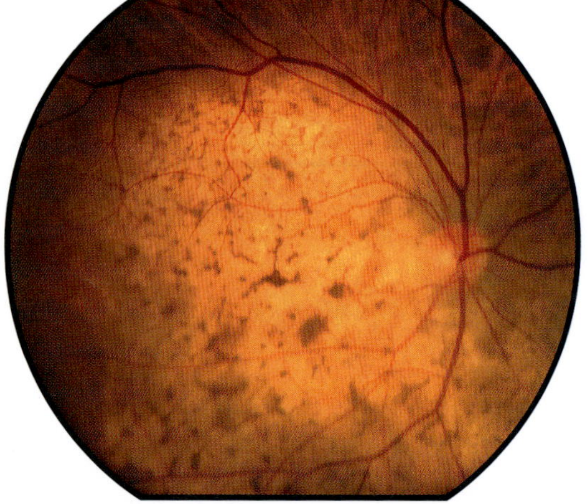

Following radiation treatment, there was flattening of the mass. Residual atrophic and pigmentary changes are present.

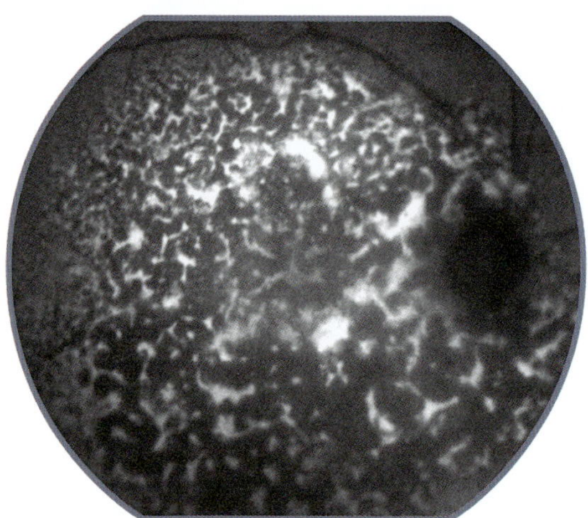

The fundus autofluorescence following regression of the mass shows more extensive retinal pigment epithelial abnormalities. *Top two rows courtesy of Dr. Rama D. Jager*

Bilateral Choroidal Metastasis

Bilateral choroidal metastasis in a female with no known previous cancer. Metastatic lung carcinoma was subsequently confirmed on fine-needle aspiration biopsy.

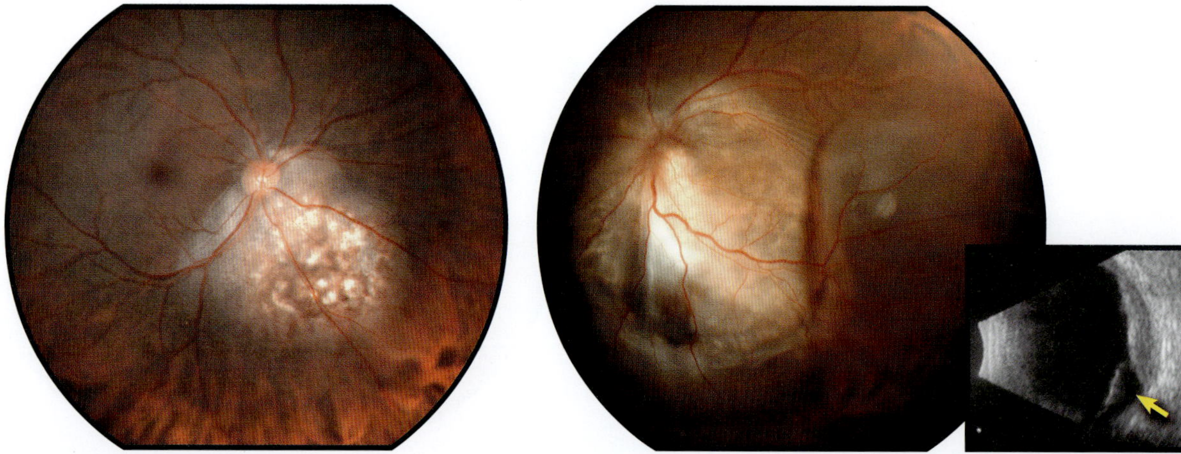

Right eye shows an amelanotic juxtapapillary choroidal mass with shallow retinal detachment. Ocular ultrasonography reveals an acoustically solid choroidal mass with subretinal fluid *(arrow)*. Left eye shows an amelanotic circumpapillary choroidal mass with extensive serous retinal detachment.

Management of Choroidal Metastasis

Choroidal metastasis can be treated with chemotherapy, radiotherapy, hormonal therapy, or photodynamic therapy. Chemotherapy and hormonal therapy are used for those with additional systemic metastasis. Radiotherapy can be in the form of external beam for those with large or multifocal metastasis while plaque radiotherapy is used for those with focal metastasis. Photodynamic therapy is used for patients with small metastasis and this therapy can provide rapid short term recovery of vision as an outpatient treatment.

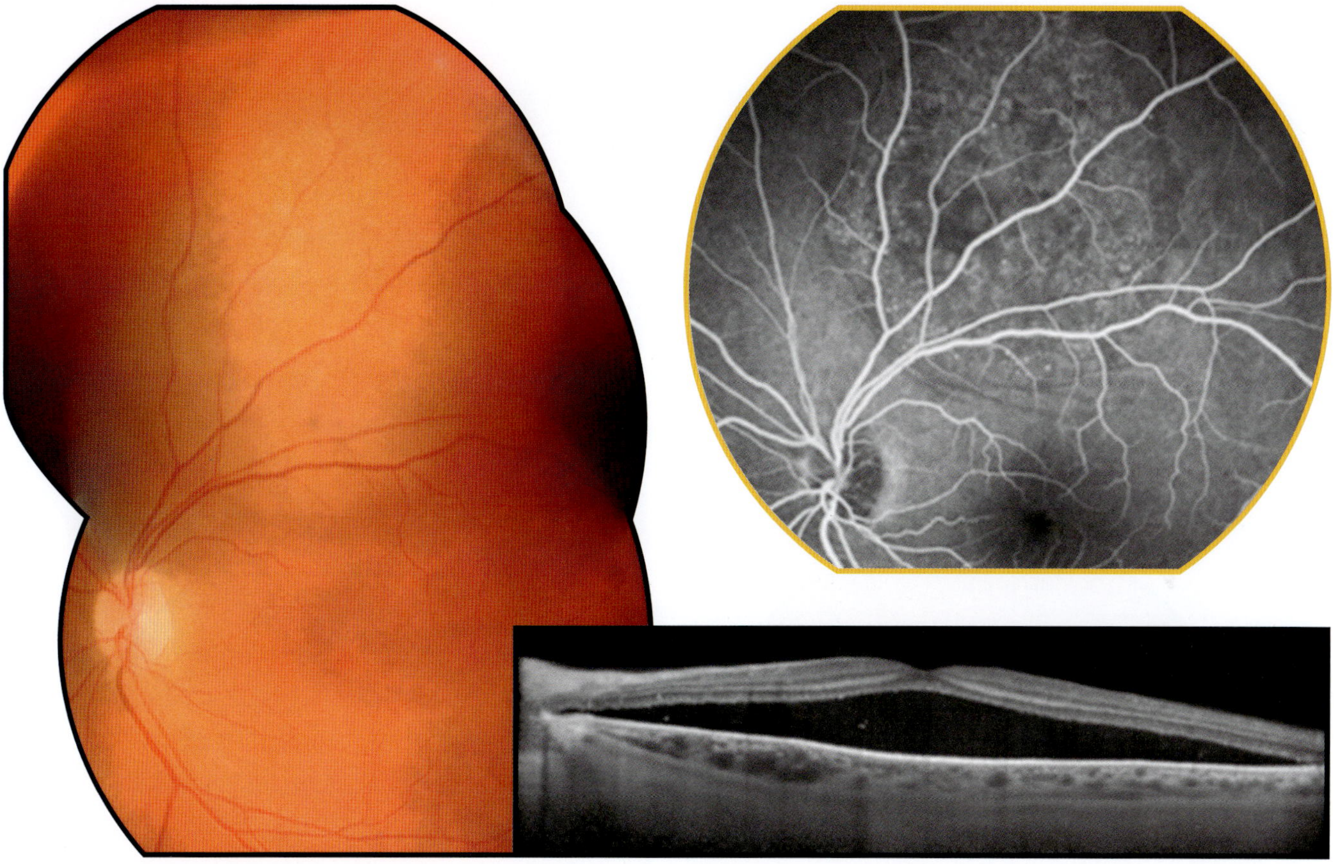

Before photodynamic therapy, the breast metastasis to the choroid appears yellow and is seen to be associated with an inferior tract of subretinal fluid. Neurosensory detachment of the macula is confirmed on OCT. The tumor is hypofluorescent on fluorescein angiography.

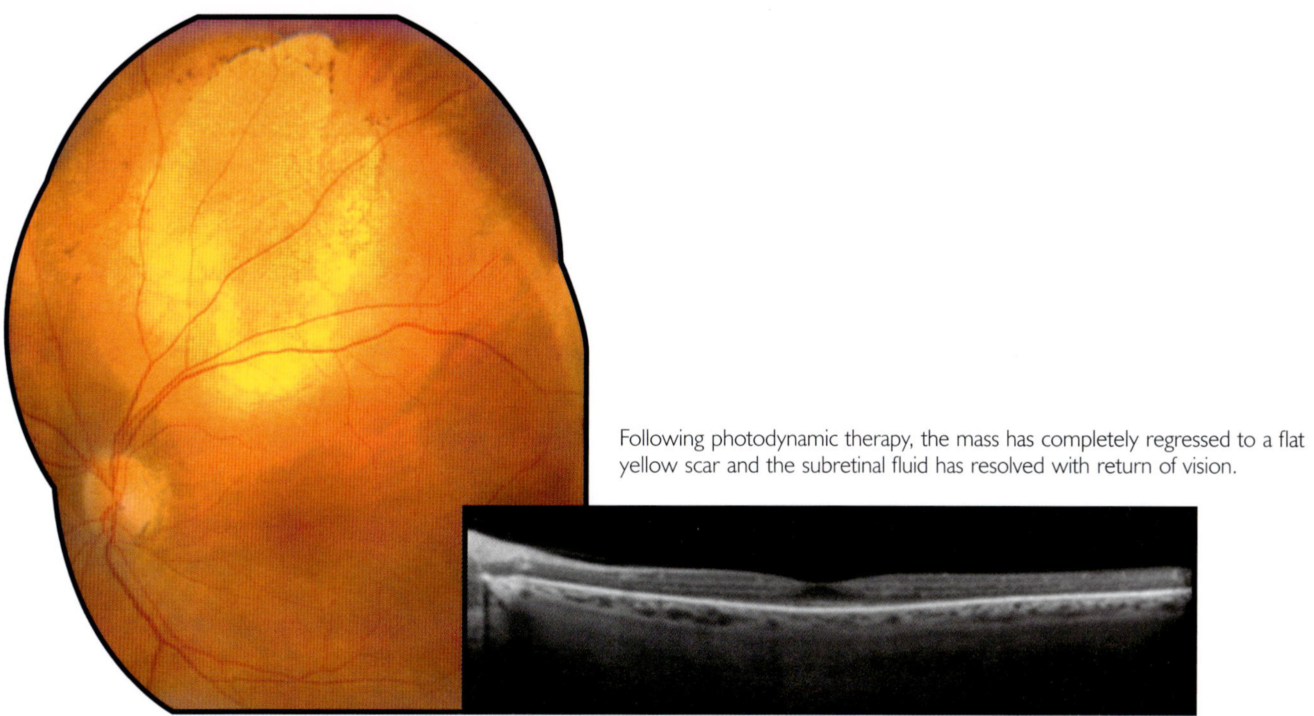

Following photodynamic therapy, the mass has completely regressed to a flat yellow scar and the subretinal fluid has resolved with return of vision.

Bilateral Diffuse Uveal Melanocytic Proliferation

Bilateral diffuse uveal melanocytic proliferation (BDUMP) is a paraneoplastic retinopathy characterized by diffuse uveal thickening due to the occurrence of spindle-shaped melanocytes. Associated systemic neoplasms are noted in these patients, including cancers of the ovary, lung, pancreas, gallbladder, colon, and kidney. Multiple faint orange spots or elevated pigmented choroidal masses are commonly observed in the fundus. BDUMP is sometimes used interchangeably with paraneoplastic melanocytic proliferation.

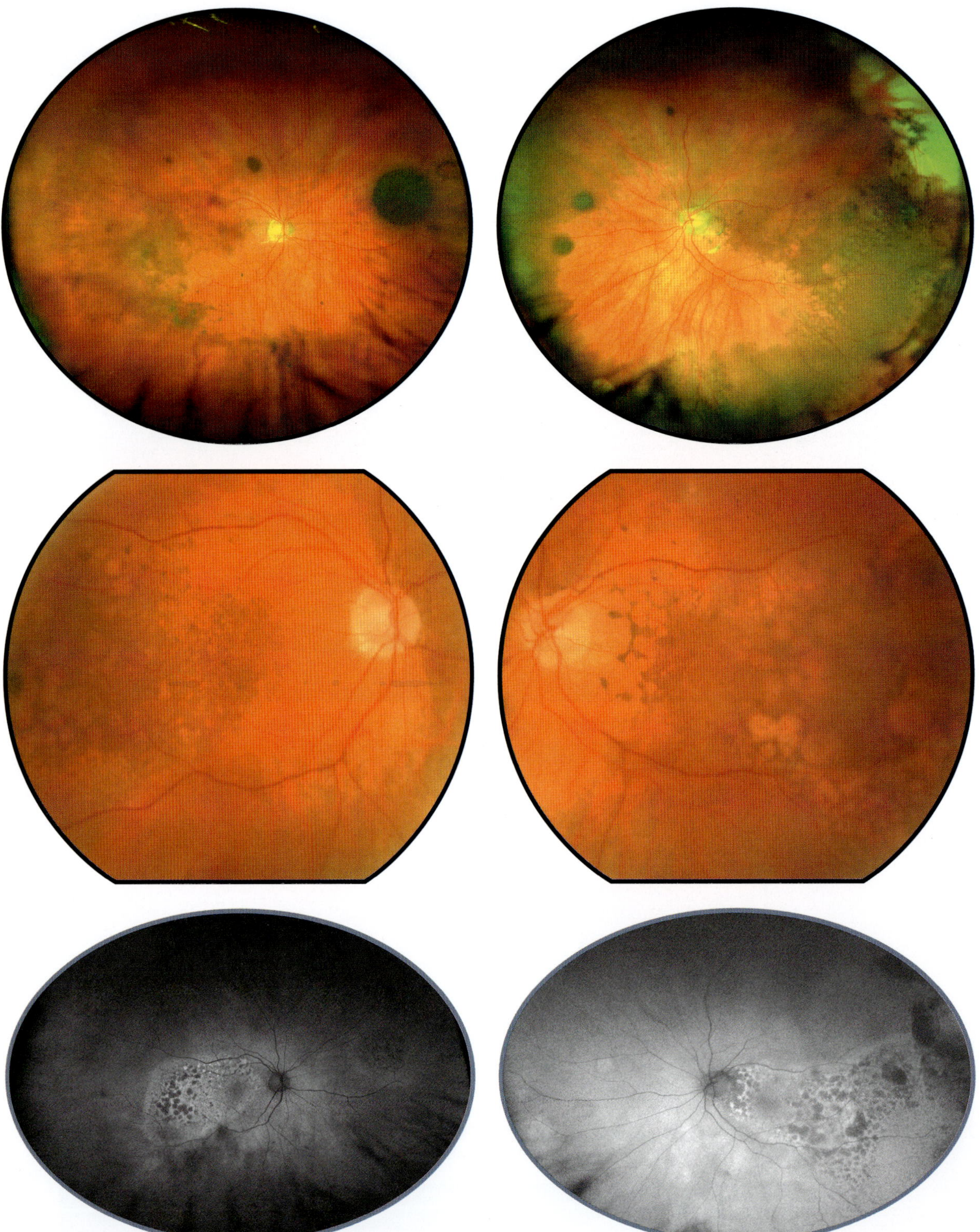

This 73-year-old patient had a history of vaginal adenocarcinoma that was surgically managed. She was also recently diagnosed with metastatic cutaneous melanoma after which she presented with bilateral visual disturbances. In both eyes there were characteristic "giraffe pattern" pigmentary changes that were most marked in the posterior pole and most clearly seen on fundus autofluorescence imaging. Pigmented lesions are seen in the peripheral retina bilaterally. She was subsequently diagnosed with BDUMP. She had scleral buckle surgery and cryopexy in the left eye previously for an unrelated retinal detachment.

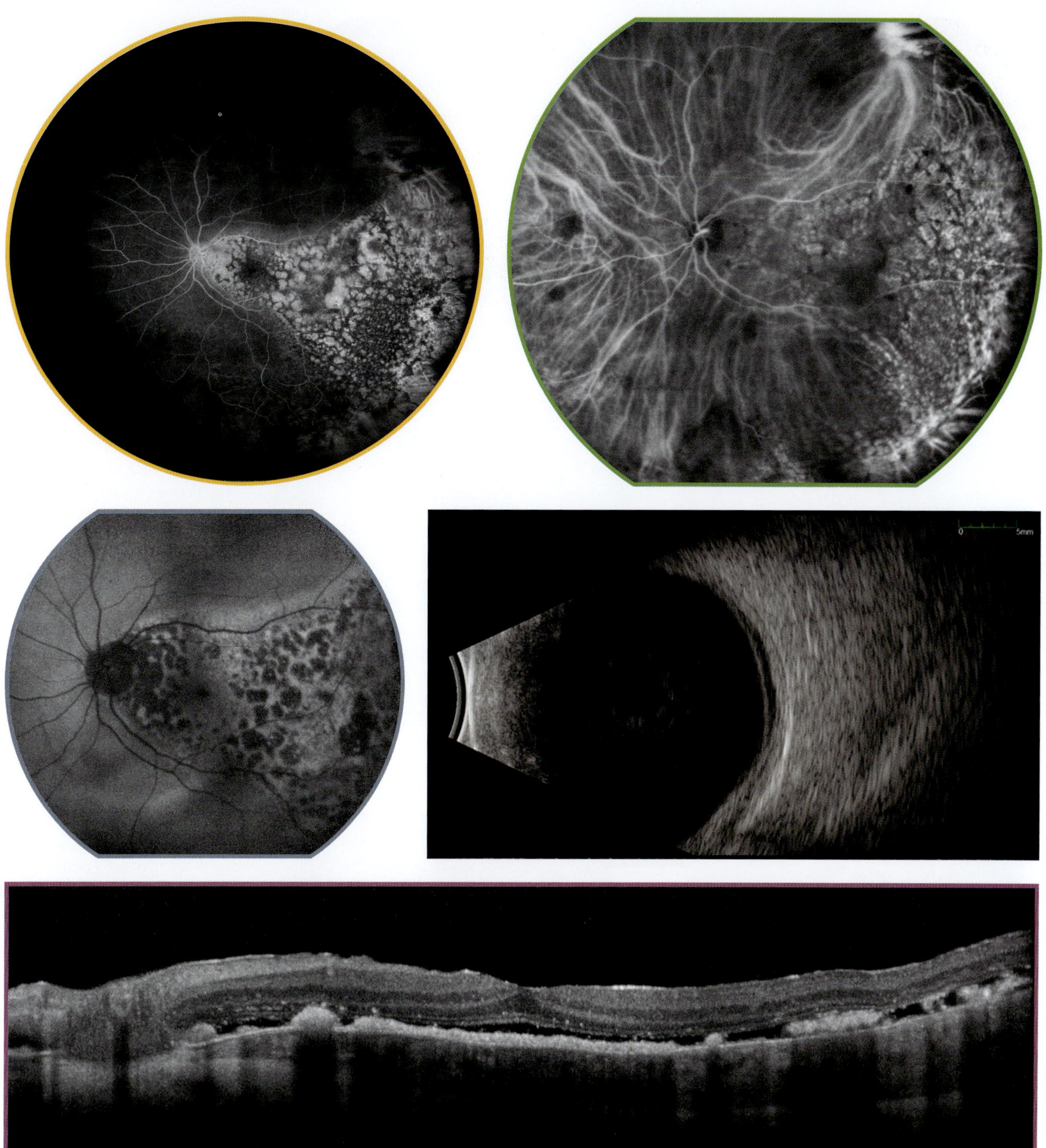

Fluorescein angiography (FA) and indocyanine green angiography of the same patient in the previous page illustrates the "giraffe pattern" of hyperfluorescence that was also seen on fundus autofluorescence (AF) imaging. Note that the giraffe pattern on FA is the inverse of what is seen on AF. Shallow collection of macular subretinal fluid is seen on ultrasonography and OCT. OCT also demonstrates thickened choroid and patches of RPE loss and accumulation. These changes form the basis for the clinical and fluorescence patterns seen on multimodal imaging. *Images courtesy Dr. J. Francis*

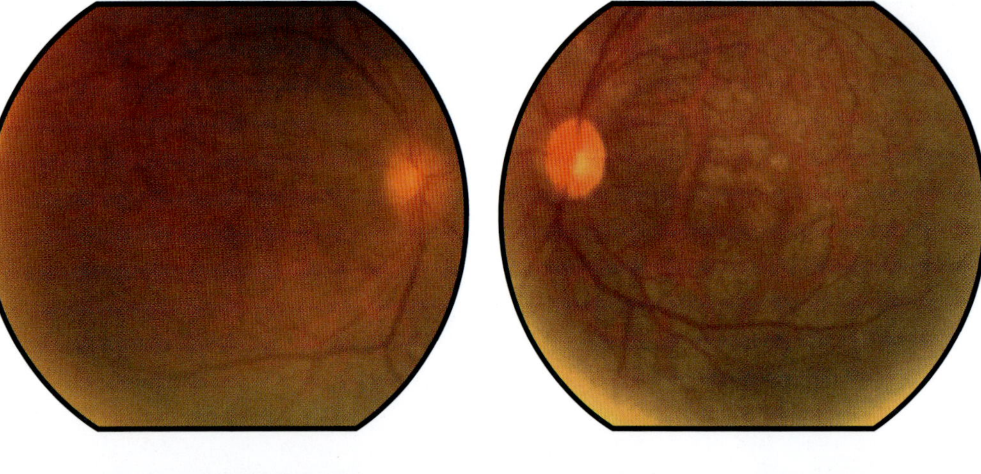

In this patient with BDUMP, there is a rapidly evolving cataract in the right eye more than in the left, obscuring fundus details. Both eyes show the characteristic orange "giraffe pattern" related to the alternating zones of RPE thickening and atrophy.

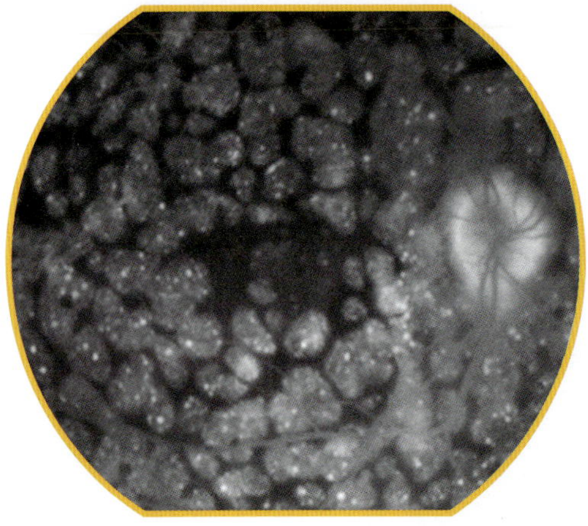

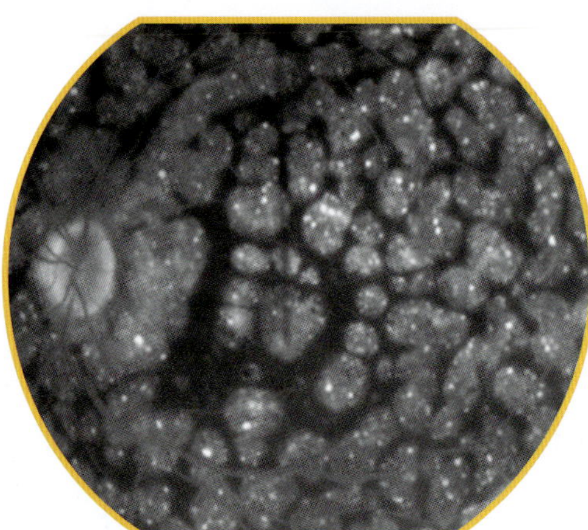

The fluorescein angiogram shows hyperfluorescence in the regions of RPE atrophy indicating an intact underlying choriocapillaris. Dots of more intense hyperfluorescence may correspond to necrosis within the tumor infiltration.

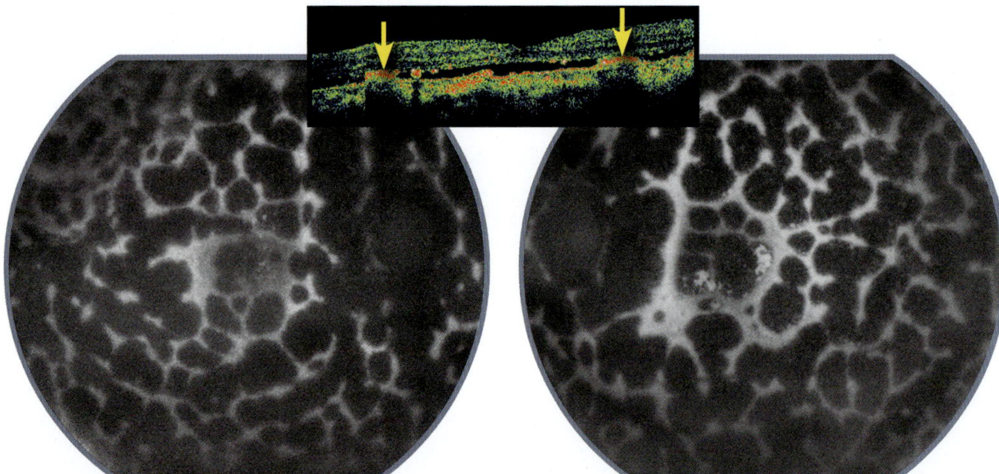

The OCT shows clumps of RPE cells forming an outline around areas of atrophy *(arrows)*. The retinal pigment epithelial atrophic zones are hypoautofluorescent with fundus autofluorescence imaging.

The fundus autofluorescence is an inverse of the fluorescein angiogram: hyperautofluorescence is seen in areas of RPE aggregation due to increased lipofuscin and hypoautofluorescence occurs in areas where there is loss of the RPE. *Above images courtesy of Drs. Jason Slakter and Richard Spaide*

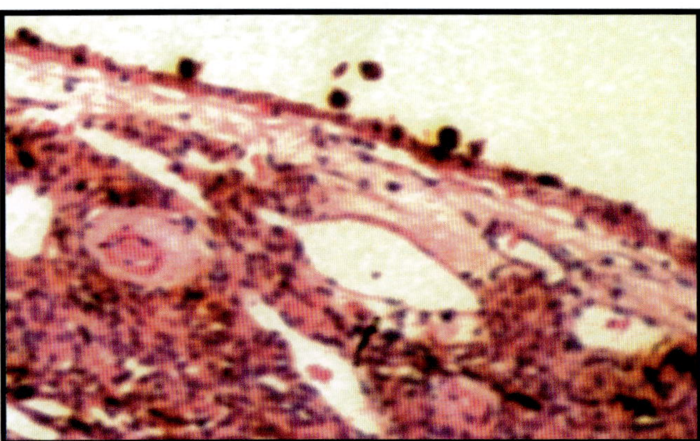

Histopathology of a patient with BDUMP shows RPE hyperpigmentation and atrophy, and an intact choriocapillaris. Infiltration of melanocytic cells occurs posterior to the choriocapillaris. These cells are usually pigmented, but they may be amelanotic as well. A variable degree of pathologic malignancy suggests that the reaction in the fundus may be paraneoplastic rather than a direct infiltrative process. *Courtesy of Dr. Charles Barr*

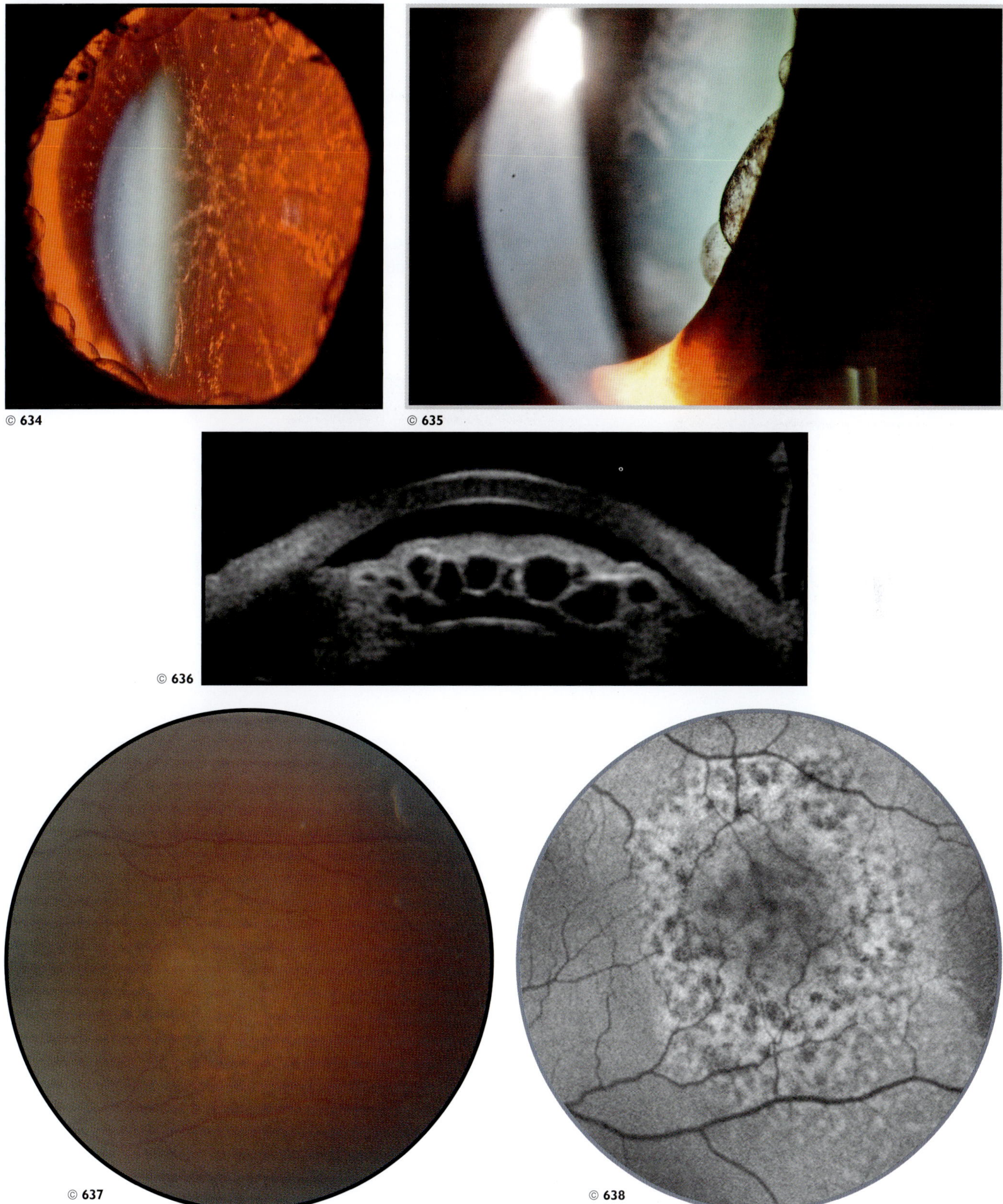

© 634 © 635 © 636 © 637 © 638

Bilateral iris and ciliary body cysts are anterior segment examination findings in some cases of BDUMP *(top panels)*. These findings may be best appreciated on ultrasound biomicroscopy *(middle image)*. The image panel represents the anterior and posterior segment findings of a female with BDUMP that had a prior history of clear cell adenocarcinoma of the endometrium. A "giraffe pattern" of pigmentary changes is seen in the left macula *(bottom panels)*.

Choroidal Hemangioma

Choroidal hemangioma is a benign vascular tumor. It manifests as a circumscribed or diffuse tumor. Circumscribed choroidal hemangioma is generally discovered in mid-life when it produces symptoms of photopsia, floaters, or reduced visual acuity. Decreased visual acuity results from related progressive hyperopia, subretinal fluid, macular edema, or retinal atrophy. Today, photodynamic therapy is used to treat a choroidal hemangioma to resolve secondary detachment and preserve vision. Diffuse choroidal hemangioma manifests as an orange mass involving nearly the entire fundus, typically with extensive thickening of the choroid. Partial or total retinal detachment can occur, usually in the teenage years or soon thereafter. Eventually, neovascular glaucoma can develop. Diffuse choroidal hemangioma is associated with the Sturge–Weber syndrome. External-beam radiotherapy, plaque radiotherapy, multiple spots of photodynamic therapy, or oral propranolol may be used to treat diffuse choroidal hemangiomas associated with retinal detachment.

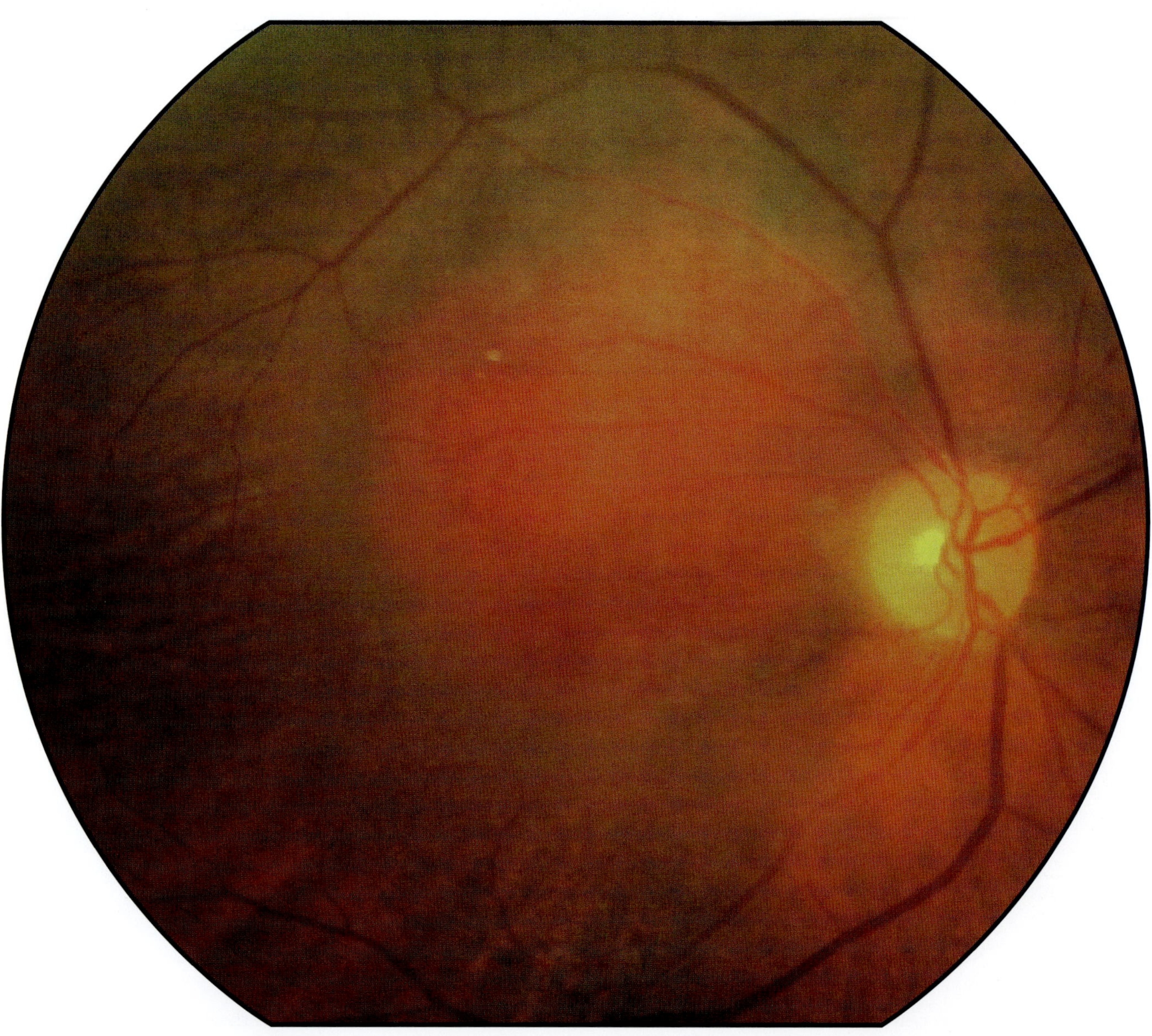

Large choroidal hemangioma of red-orange color.

Choroidal Hemangioma in the Macular Region

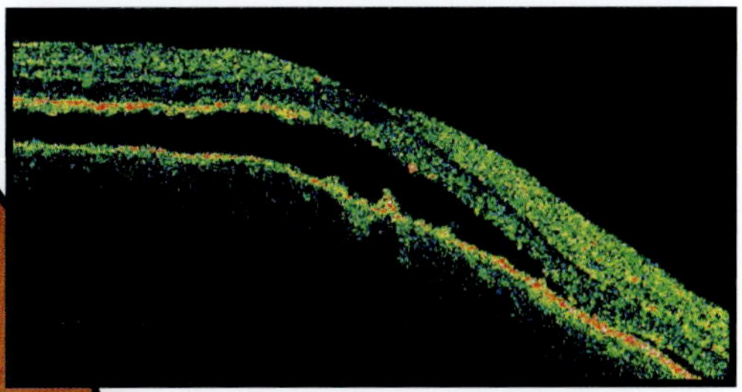

OCT reveals shallow overlying subretinal fluid and hyper-reflective material in the subretinal space.

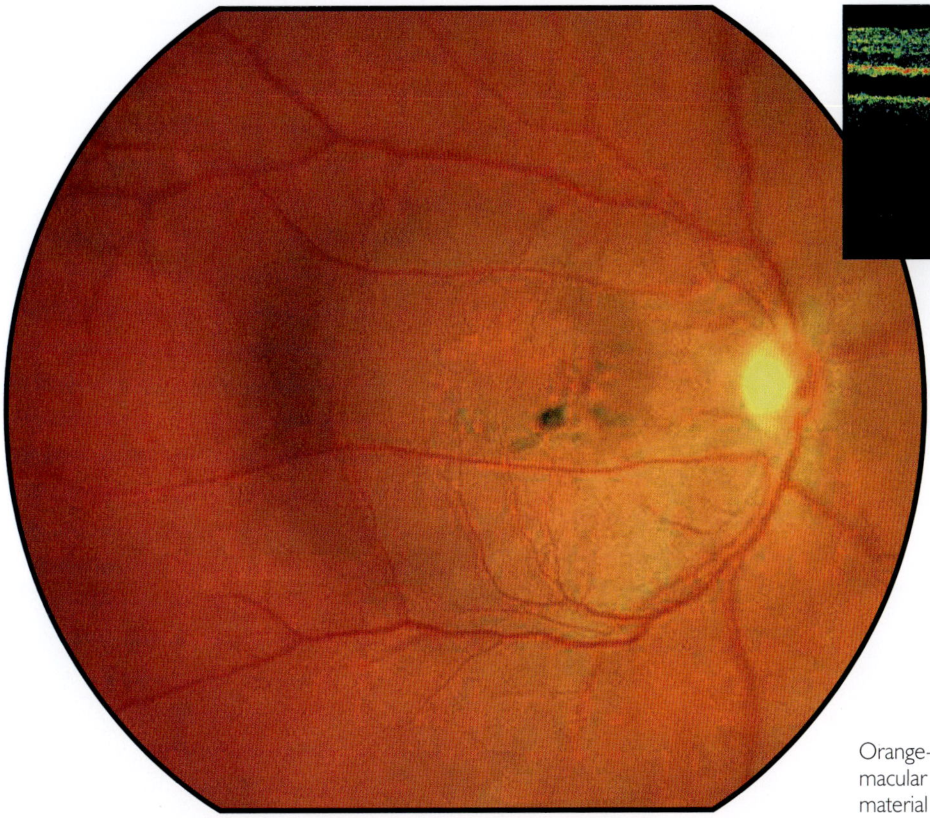

Orange-colored choroidal hemangioma in the macular region with subretinal fluid and pigmented material in the subretinal space.

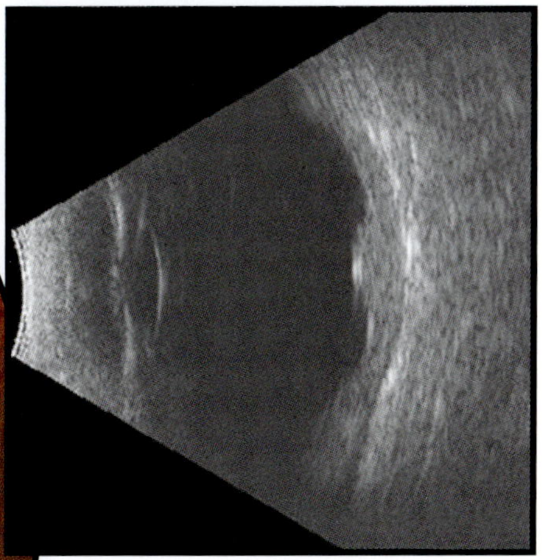

Ocular ultrasonography displays the echogenic choroidal mass and shallow overlying subretinal fluid.

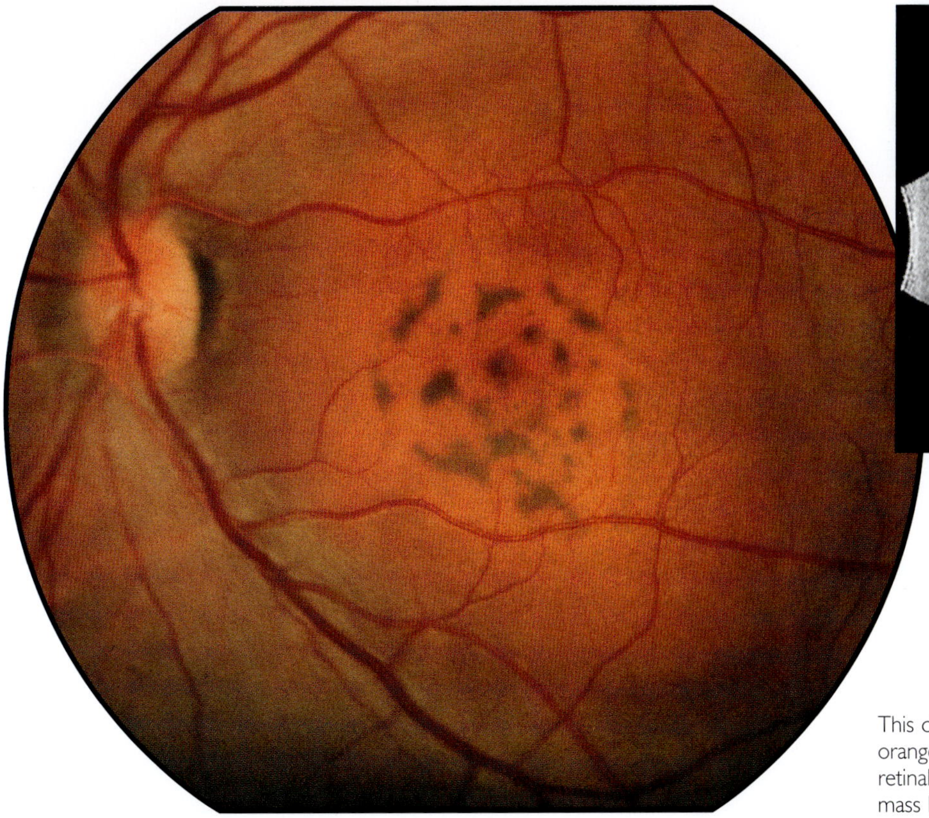

This choroidal hemangioma is a typical reddish-orange color. There is a cluster of focal areas of retinal pigment epithelial hyperplasia overlying the mass lesion.

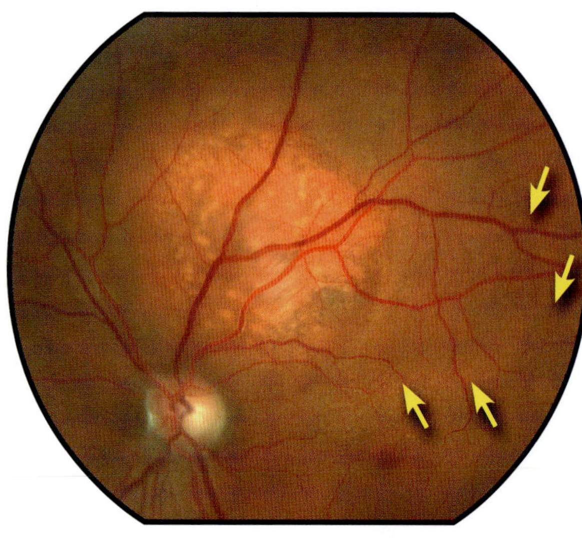

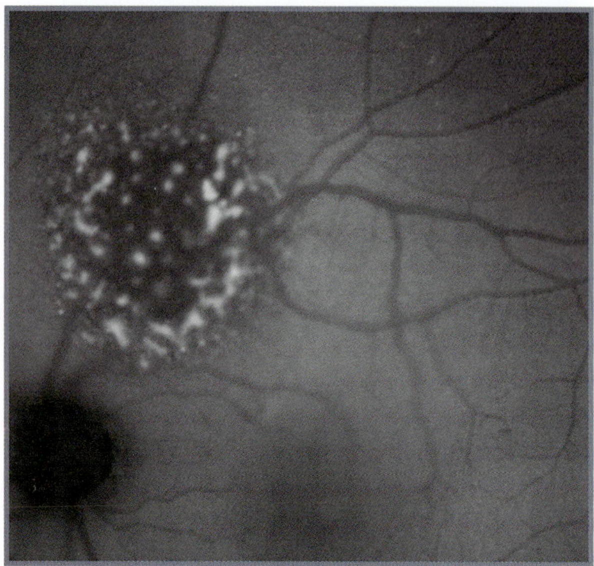

This pale orange choroidal hemangioma is associated with a secondary retinal detachment of the macula *(arrows)*. The fundus autofluorescence shows hyperautofluorescent spots related to overlying RPE changes and clumps of subretinal autofluorescent material.

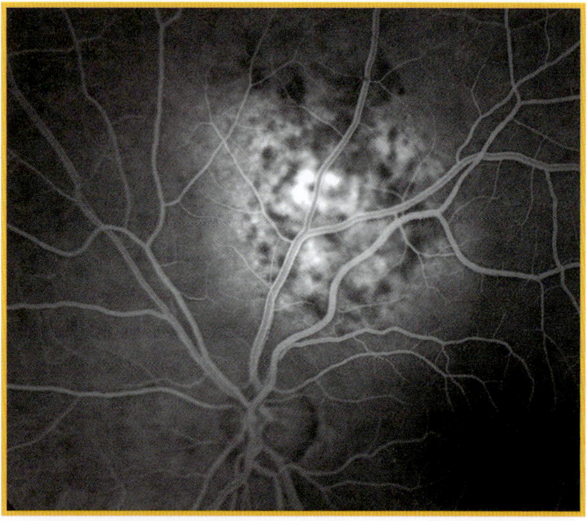

The lesion on fluorescein angiography typically fluoresces early in the prearteriolar filling stage when the prominent vascular elements within the lesion become visible.

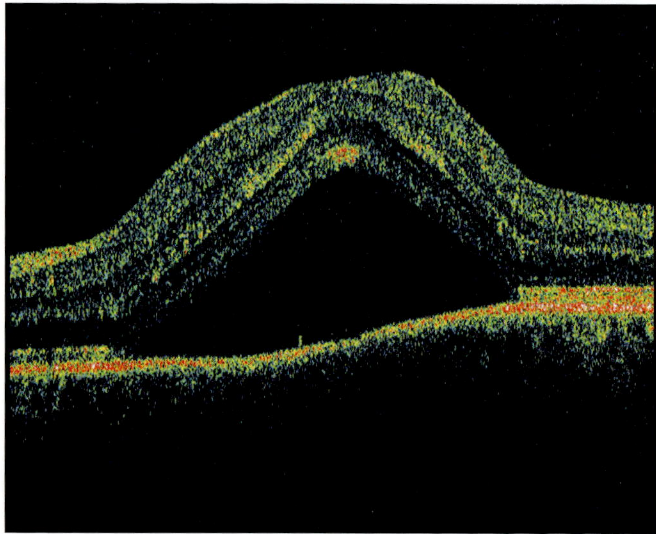

A prominent retinal detachment is seen in association with this lesion.

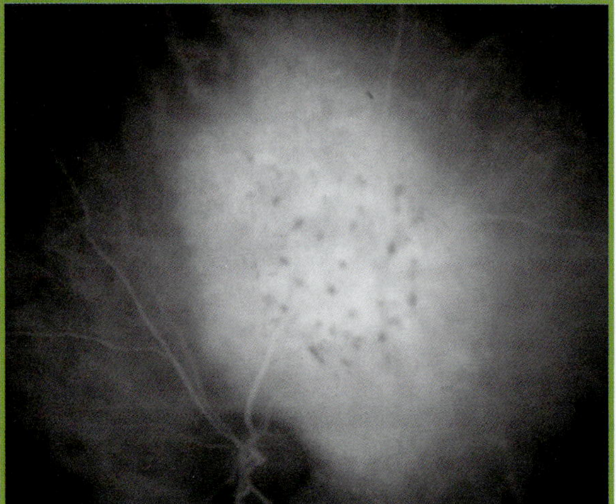

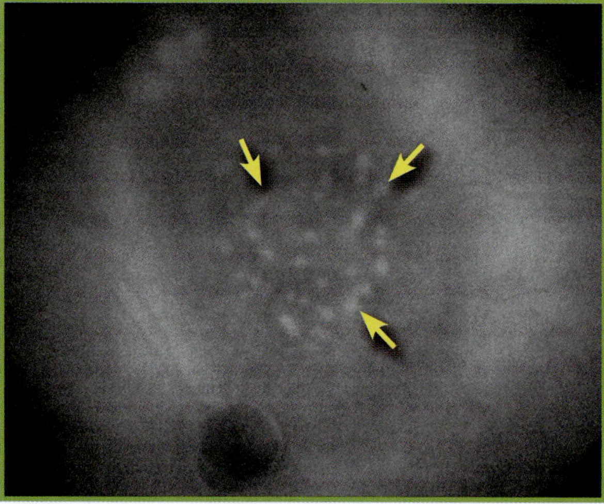

The early ICG angiogram shows diffuse hyperfluorescence of the hemangioma *(left)*. In the late-stage ICG study *(right)*, most of the dye leaves the tumor ("wash-out"), but there is some surrounding hyperfluorescence, like a wreath, and staining of areas within the tumor *(arrows)*.

Choroidal Hemangioma Treated with Photodynamic Therapy

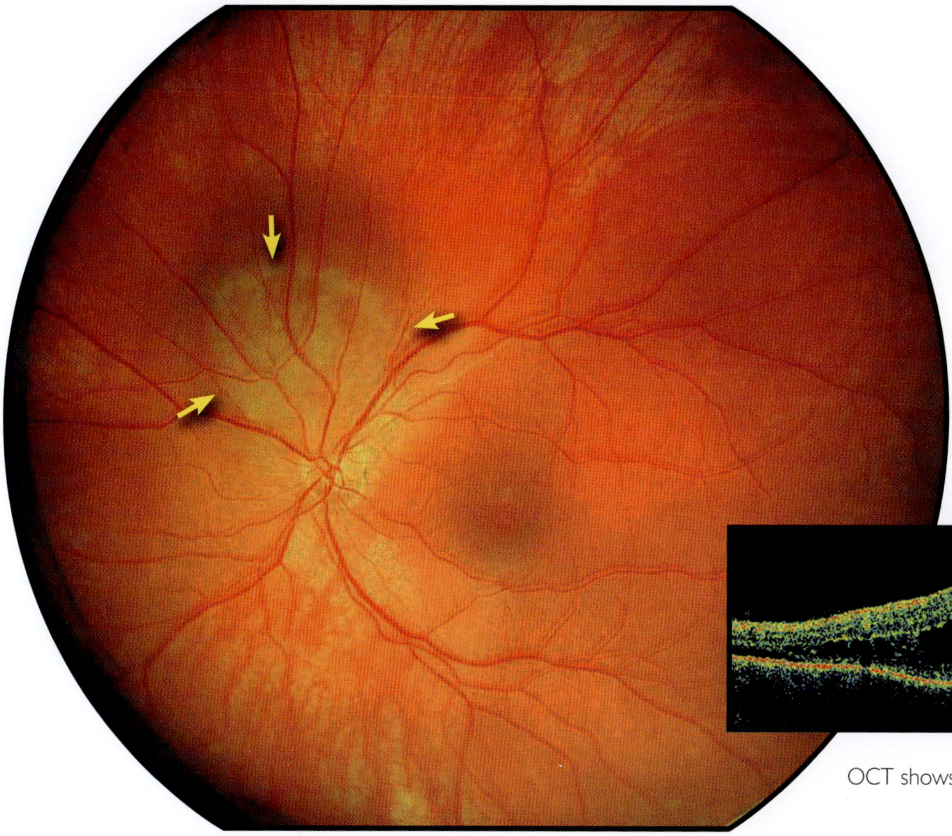

Before photodynamic therapy. An orange-colored choroidal hemangioma is noted superior to the optic disc *(arrows)*.

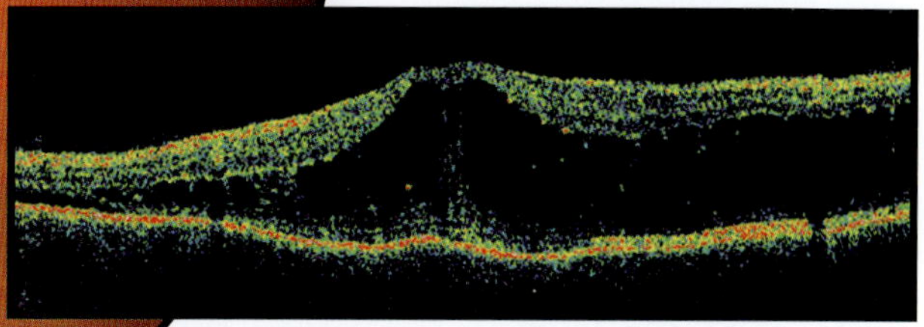

OCT shows related extensive cystoid macular edema.

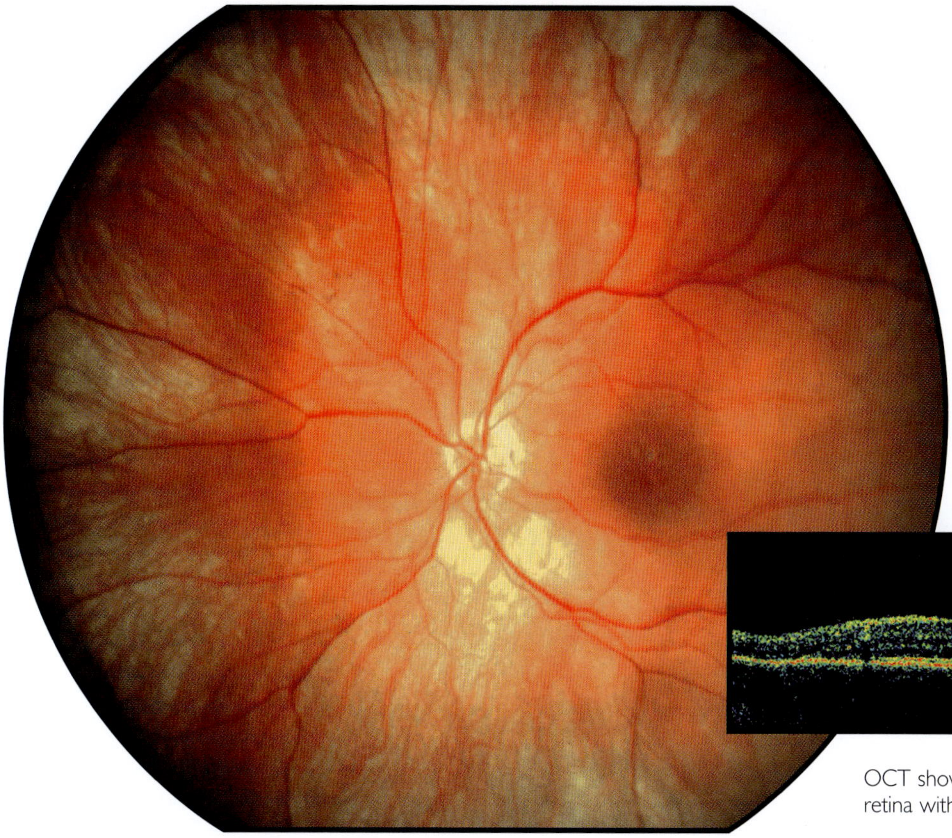

After photodynamic therapy. The hemangioma has flattened.

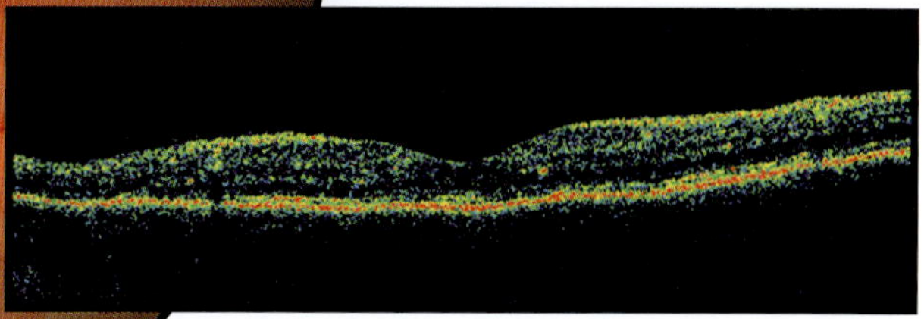

OCT shows resolution of the edema leaving a flat retina with slight photoreceptor atrophy.

Diffuse Choroidal Hemangioma

Diffuse choroidal hemangioma in a 10-year-old boy with Sturge–Weber syndrome that was treated with external-beam radiotherapy.

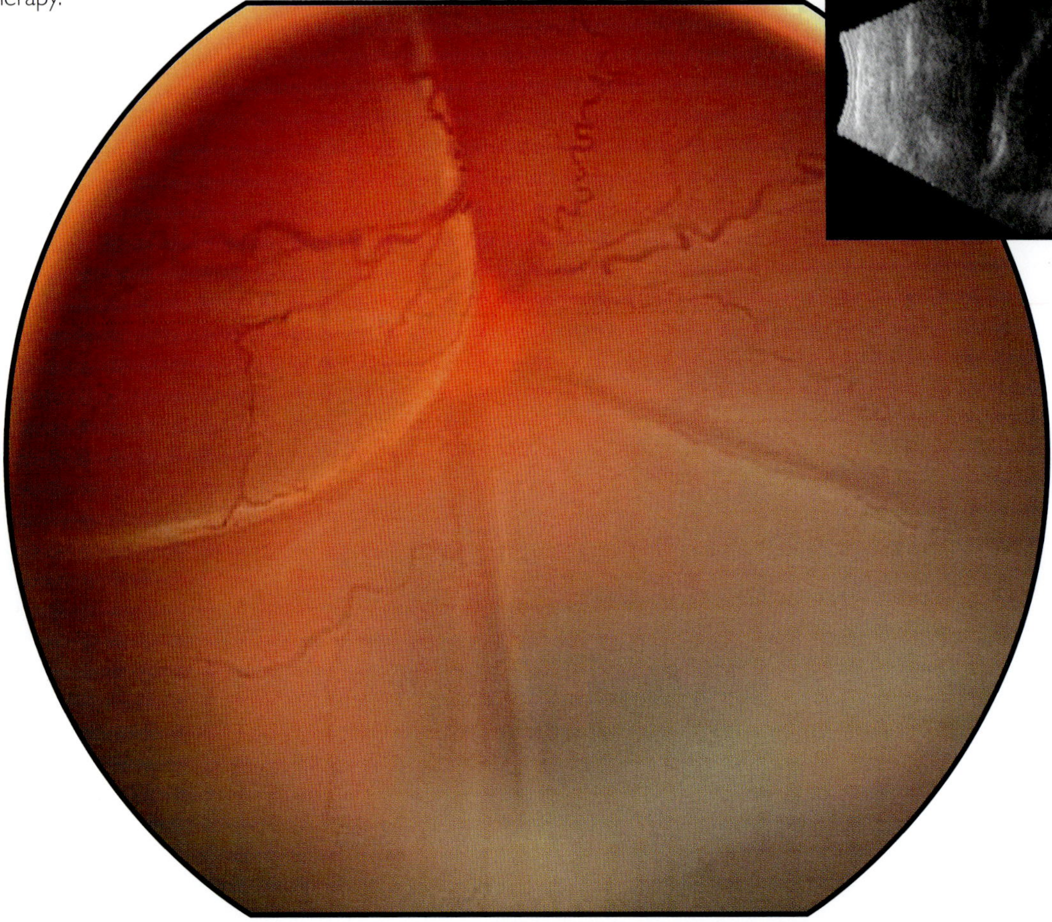

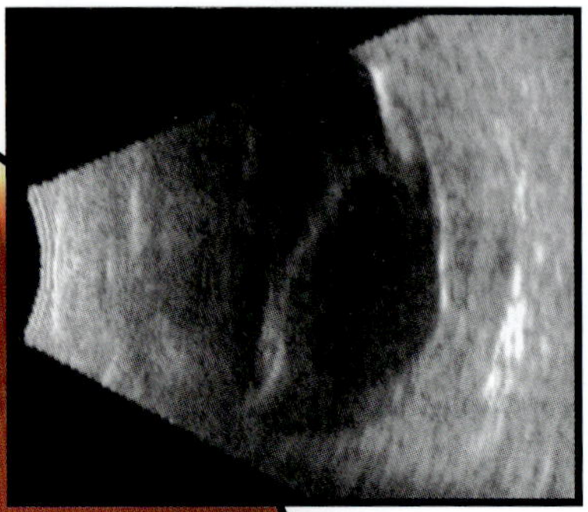

There is a total exudative retinal detachment from the underlying diffuse choroidal hemangioma.
Ocular ultrasonography reveals choroidal thickening related to the hemangioma and overlying extensive retinal detachment.

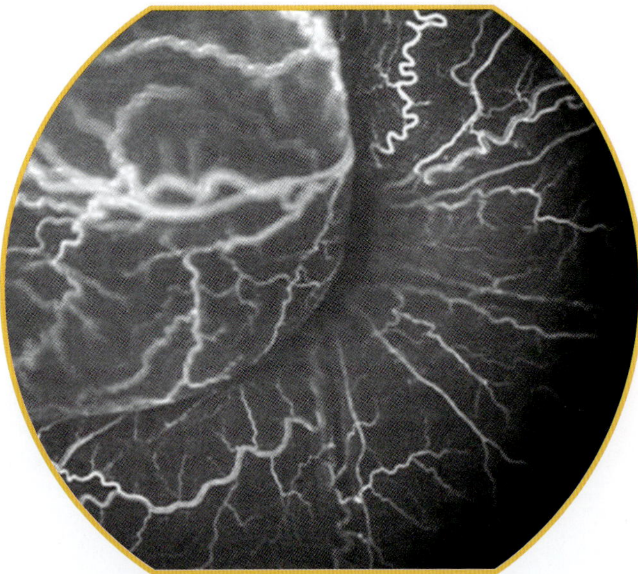

Fluorescein angiography pre-treatment shows the retinal detachment.

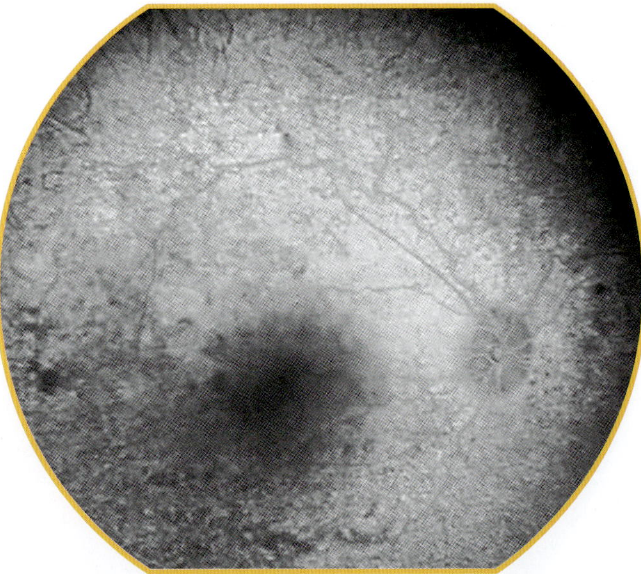

Following external-beam radiotherapy, fluorescein angiography reveals resolution of the retinal detachment and choroidal hemangioma, which leaves scattered areas of retinal pigment epithelial degeneration.

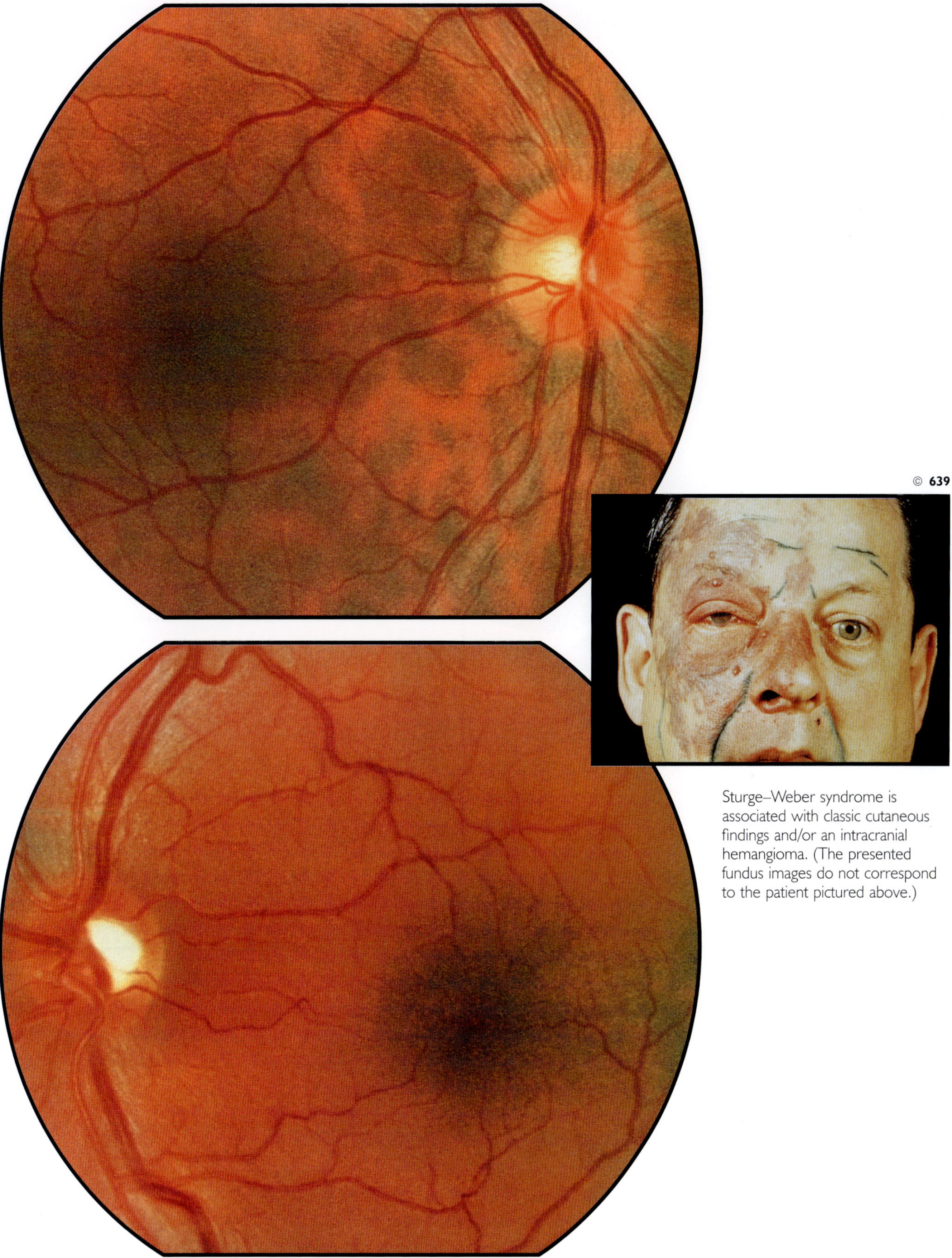

© 639

Sturge–Weber syndrome is associated with classic cutaneous findings and/or an intracranial hemangioma. (The presented fundus images do not correspond to the patient pictured above.)

Diffuse choroidal hemangioma is associated with Sturge–Weber syndrome. The left fundus in this patient is reddish-pink, whereas the right eye has a normal background color. Optic cupping is evident in the left eye from glaucoma, which is a common secondary manifestation in this disease.
Courtesy of Dr. Thomas Burton

Choroidal Osteoma

Choroidal osteoma is a rare tumor comprised of mature bone, classically located in the macular or juxtapapillary region in young women. This tumor can enlarge (osteoblastic change) and produce vision loss from choroidal neovascularization, subretinal fluid, retinal pigment epithelial atrophy, and photoreceptor atrophy. Over time, decalcification of the tumor can ensue (osteoclastic change). Morphologically, pseudopod borders with wedge-shaped edges are often noted with coarse yellowish bony changes.

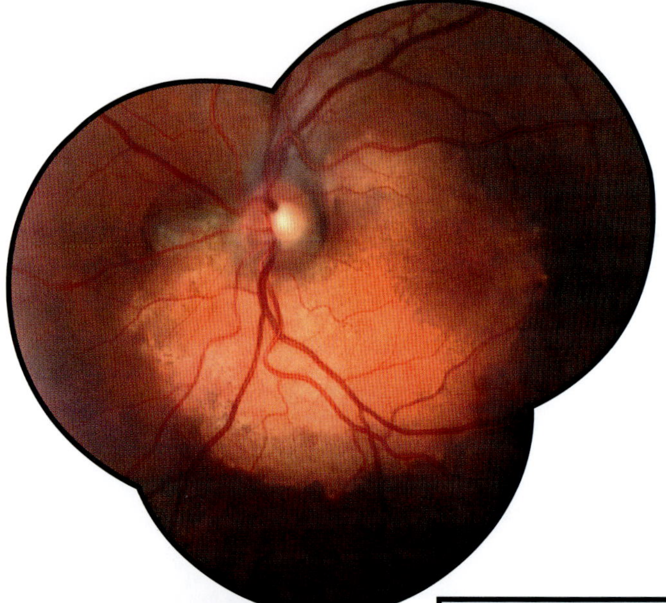

This montage photograph of a choroidal osteoma in a pigmented individual shows the typical orange color The margins have a wedge-shaped appearance, which is very typical of this lesion.

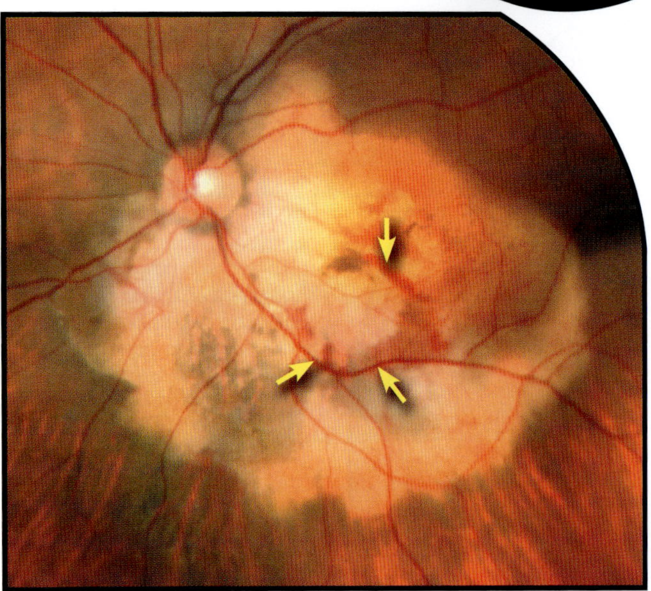

This patient with a choroidal osteoma has a central area of atrophy bordered at its margin by a serosanguineous detachment from choroidal neovascularization *(arrows).*

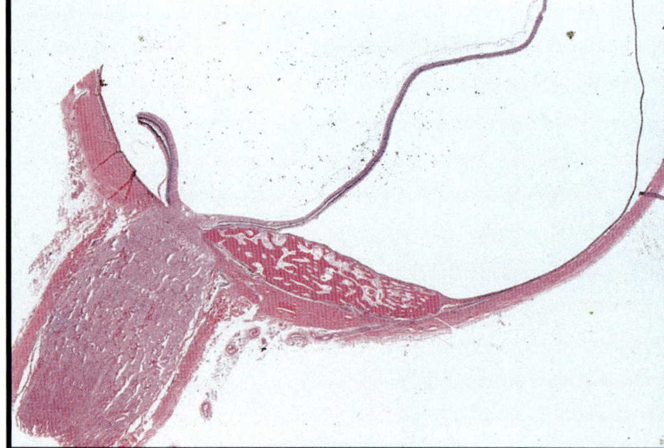

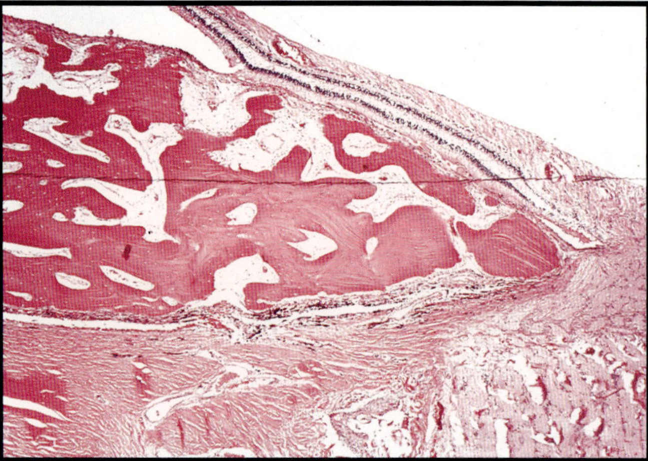

Histopathologic example. A choroidal osteoma is noted near the optic disc. Higher magnification shows that the lesion is composed of compact bone.

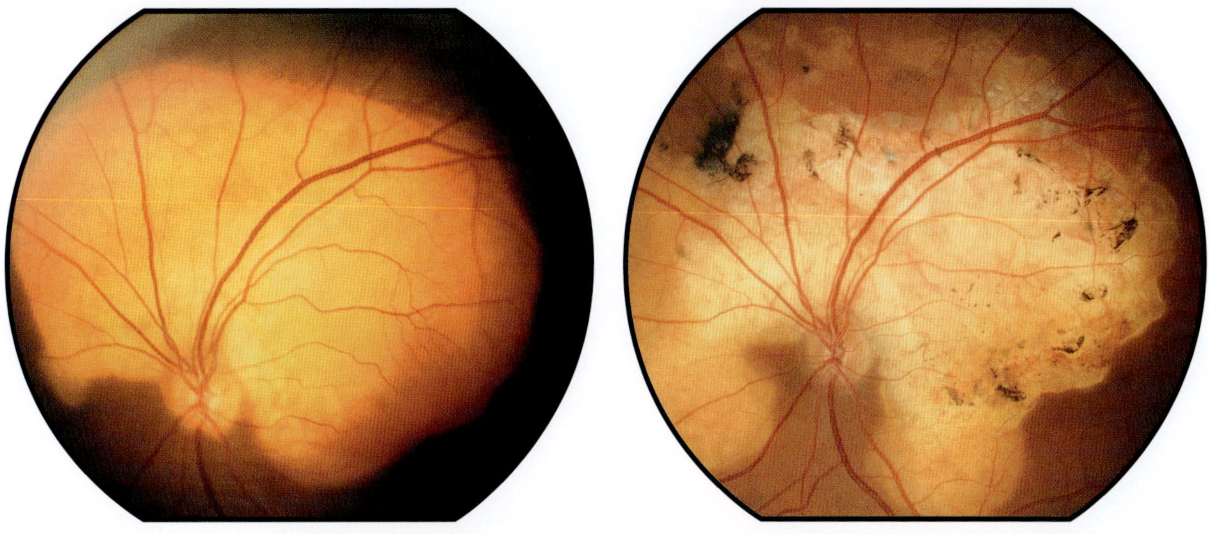

These photographs illustrate progressive change in choroidal osteoma. The patient initially had a lesion demonstrating pure osteoblastic activity *(left)*. Note the sparing of the inferior juxtapapillary area. Seven years later, there is osteoclastic activity with retinal pigment epithelial hyperplasia and scarring in the superior portion of the lesion *(right)*. There has also been some progressive osteoblastic activity along the inferior and superior margins.

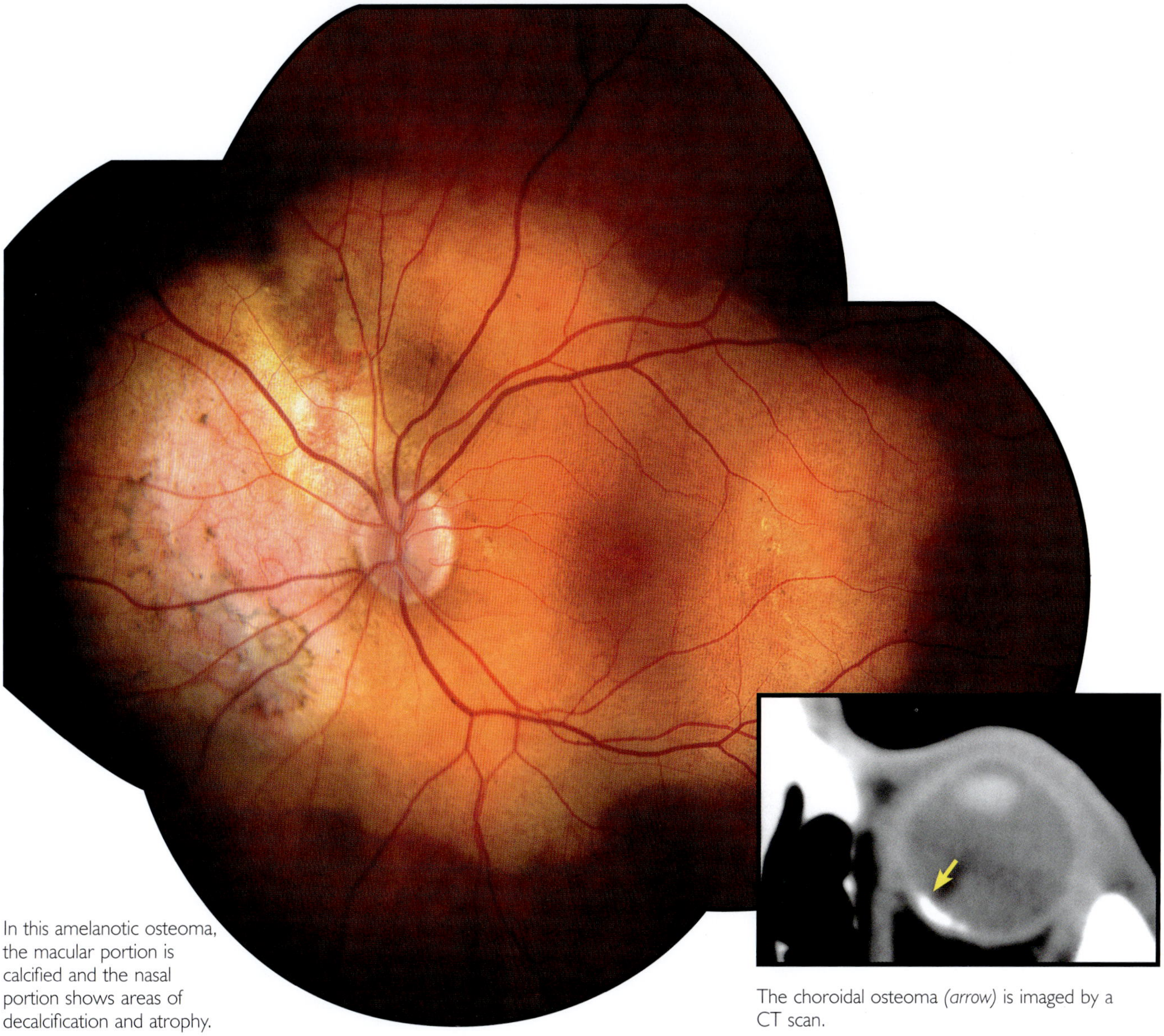

In this amelanotic osteoma, the macular portion is calcified and the nasal portion shows areas of decalcification and atrophy.

The choroidal osteoma *(arrow)* is imaged by a CT scan.

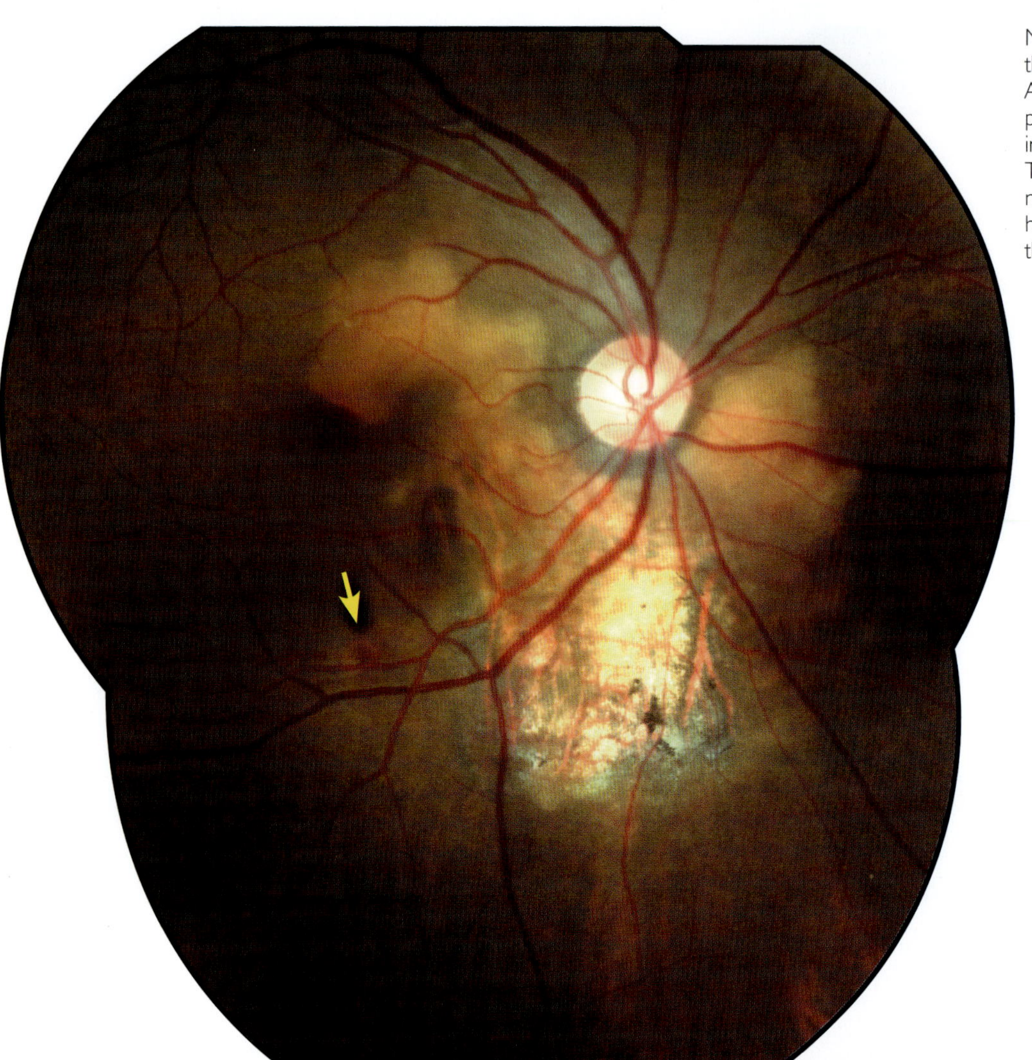

Note the jigsaw morphology of this osteoma in a 50-year-old Asian female. Atrophy and fibrous proliferation are present in the inferior portion of this lesion. There is polypoidal choroidal neovascularization and focal hemorrhage *(arrow)* inferior to the macula.

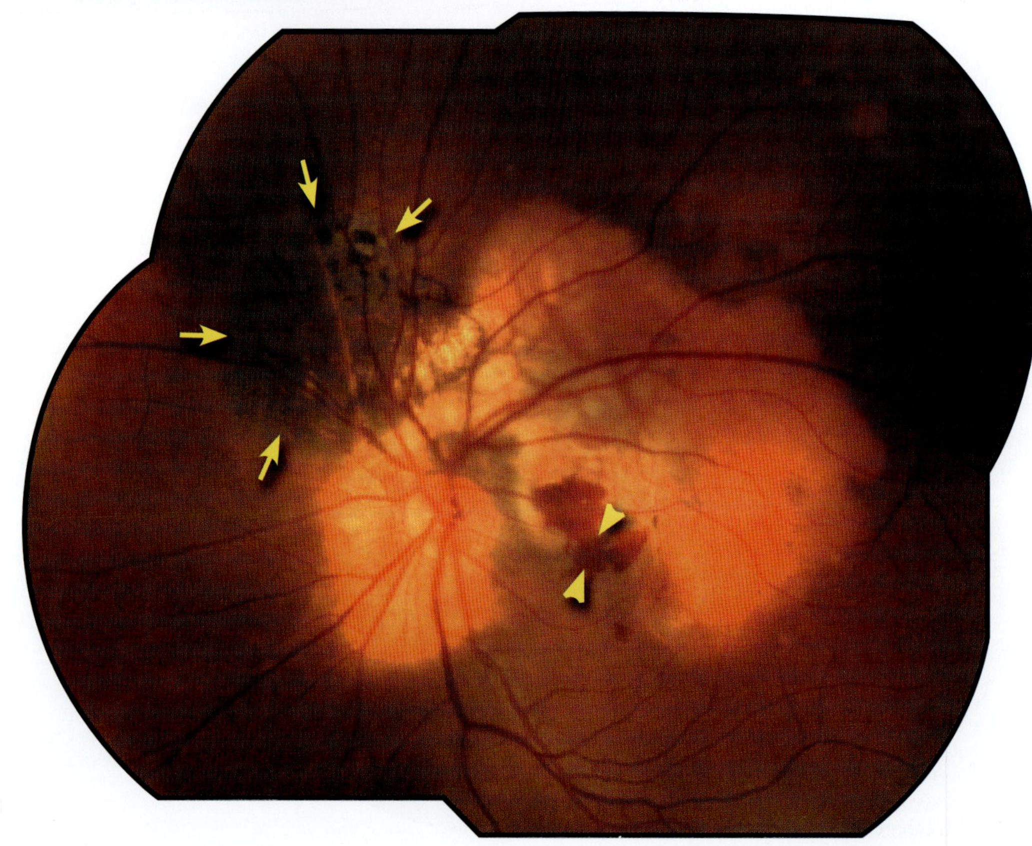

In the left eye, there is a hemorrhagic detachment of the macula from choroidal neovascularization *(arrowheads)*. There is also an ovoid pigmentary area contiguous with the superonasal aspect of the lesion *(arrows)*. These RPE changes are from an antecedent exudative detachment.

Vertical OCT through the calcified and noncalcified macular portion of the tumor reveals fairly intact retina overlying the calcified portion and slightly thickened retina with loss of architecture over the decalcified portion.

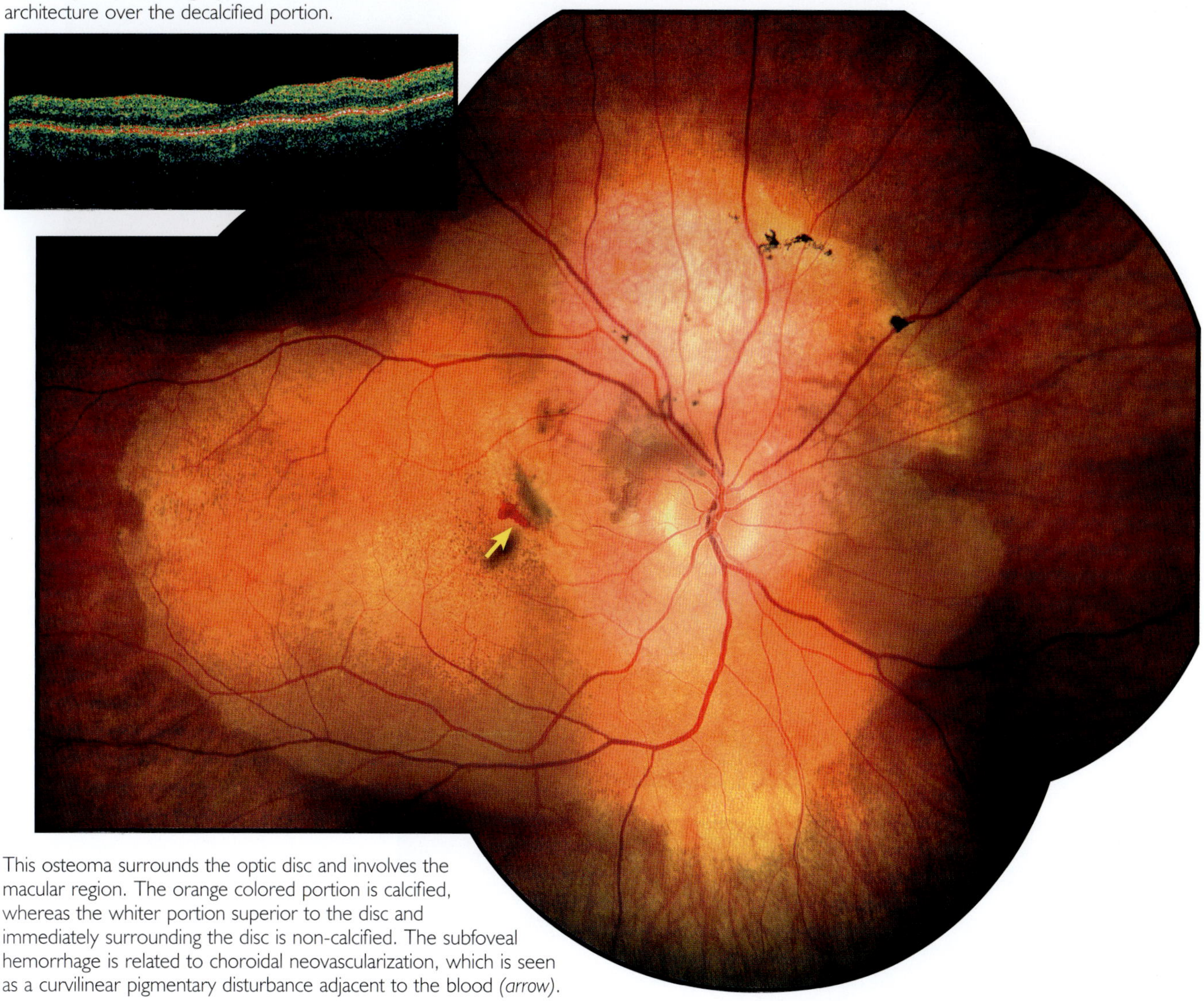

This osteoma surrounds the optic disc and involves the macular region. The orange colored portion is calcified, whereas the whiter portion superior to the disc and immediately surrounding the disc is non-calcified. The subfoveal hemorrhage is related to choroidal neovascularization, which is seen as a curvilinear pigmentary disturbance adjacent to the blood *(arrow)*.

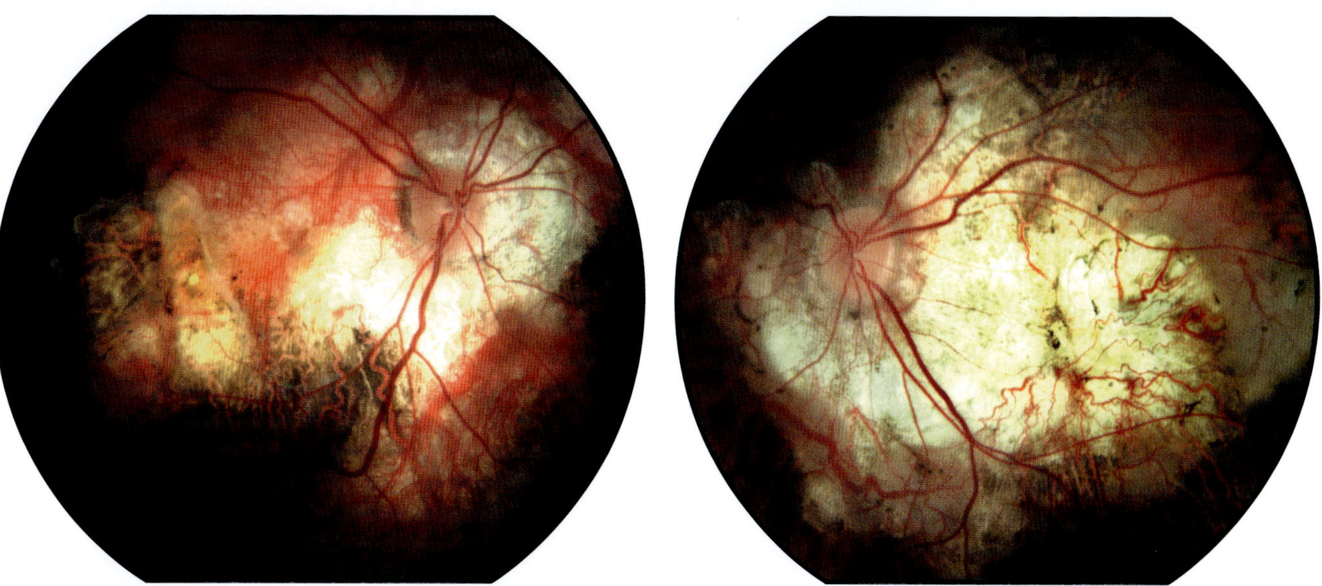

In this patient there is a bilateral severely atrophic and calcified long-standing osteoma.

Optical Coherence Tomography of Choroidal Osteoma

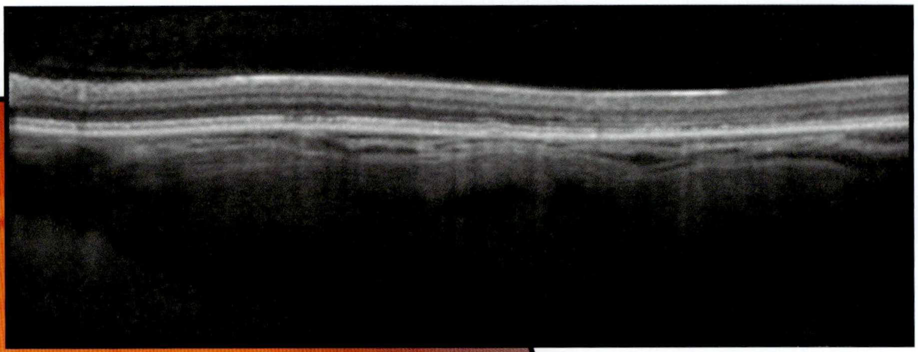

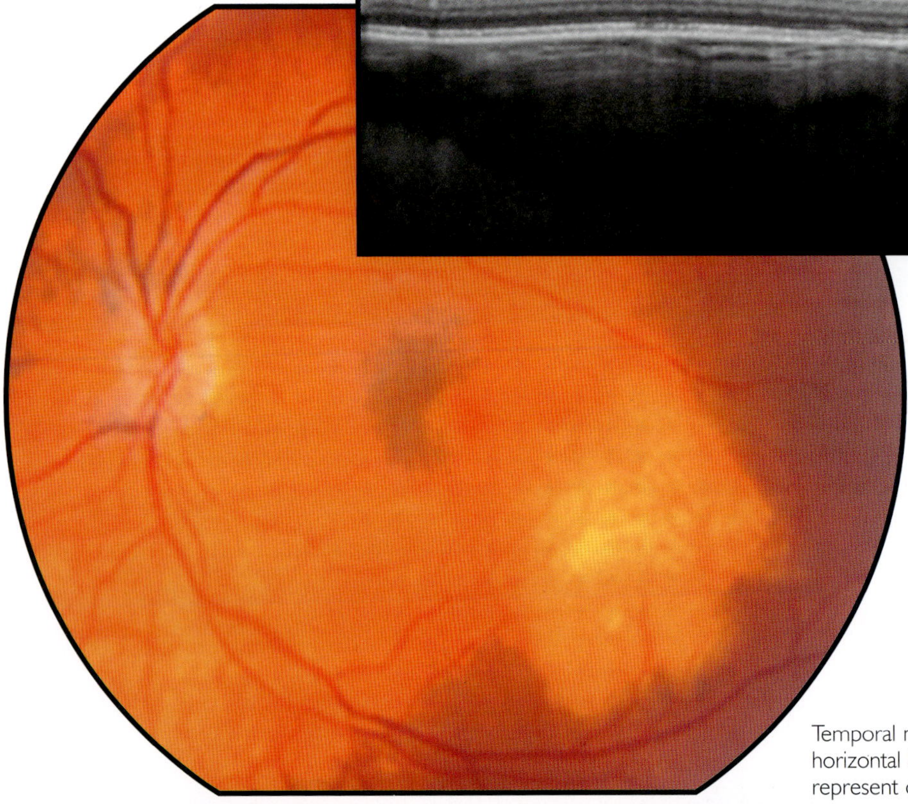

Temporal macular choroidal osteoma with OCT depicting horizontal bone lamella and lucencies that could represent connecting vascular tubules.

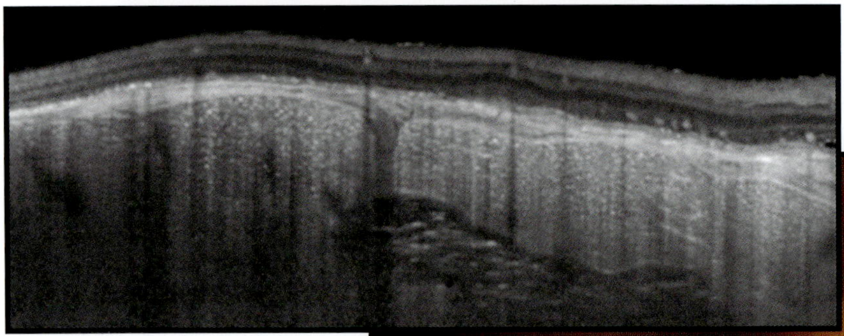

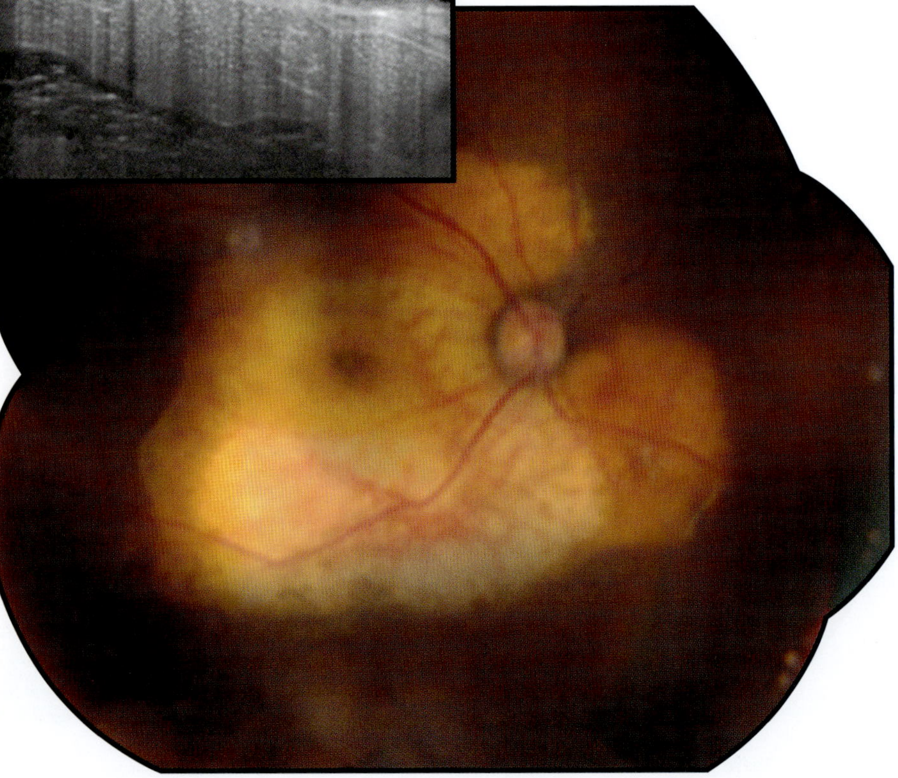

Peripapillary choroidal osteoma with OCT depicting horizontal bone lamella and horizontal and vertical vascular tubules. Spongy bone correlates to the homogenous region.

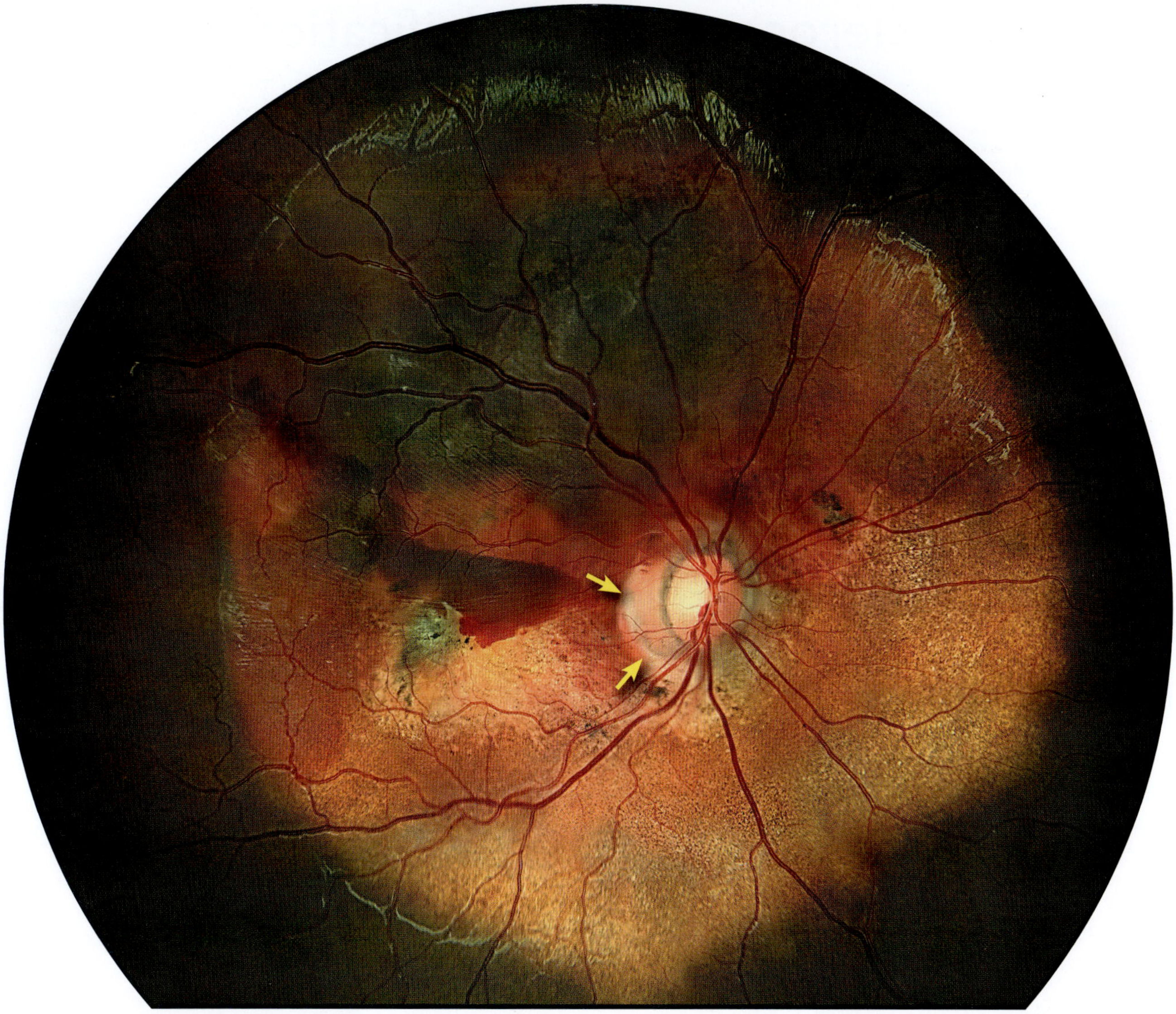

This huge osteoma is associated with several secondary manifestations, including a large area of subretinal hemorrhage, peripapillary fibrosis *(arrows)*, scarring, and atrophy in the macula centrally. More recent osteoblastic activity is present inferiorly.

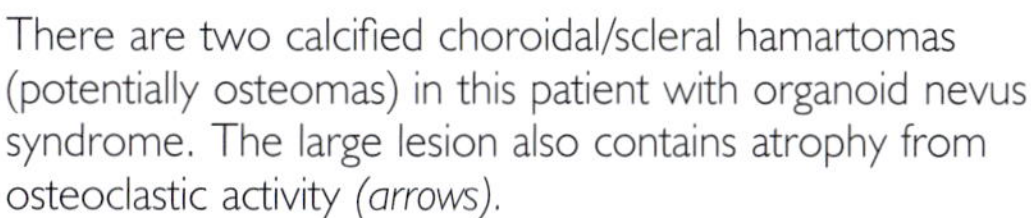
There are two calcified choroidal/scleral hamartomas (potentially osteomas) in this patient with organoid nevus syndrome. The large lesion also contains atrophy from osteoclastic activity *(arrows)*.

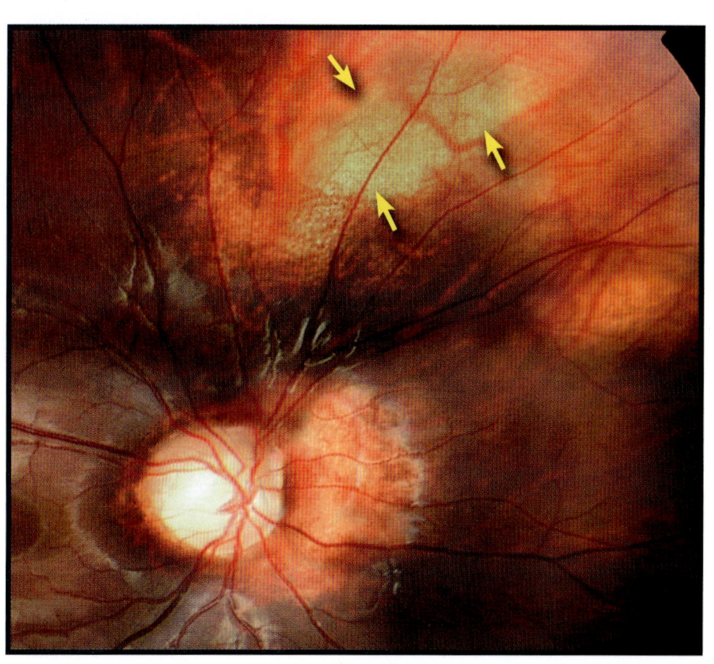

Idiopathic Sclerochoroidal Calcification

Idiopathic sclerochoroidal calcification appears as a collection of calcific scleral nodules with overlying choroidal compression and retinal pigment epithelial alterations. Sometimes there is visible calcification within the lesion. Such calcific changes in patients who do not have clinically detectable clinical manifestations of this disease are fairly common. The overlying retina and vitreous are normal. Abnormalities in calcium metabolism with hyperparathyroidism, parathyroid adenoma, and Gitelman and Bartter syndromes should be investigated.

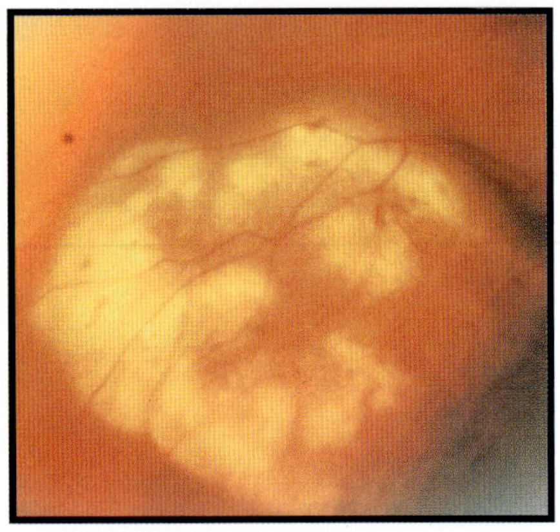
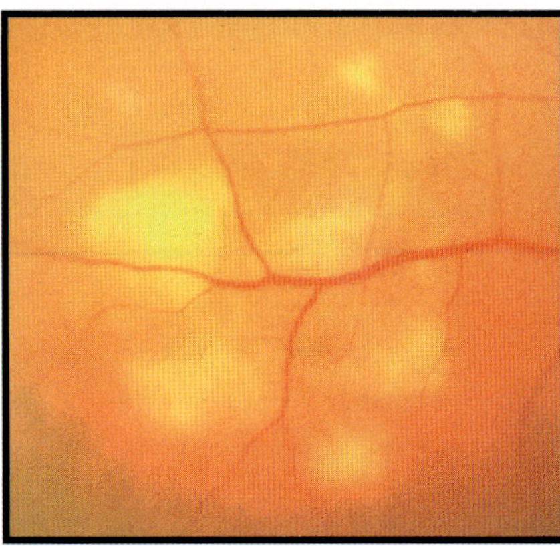
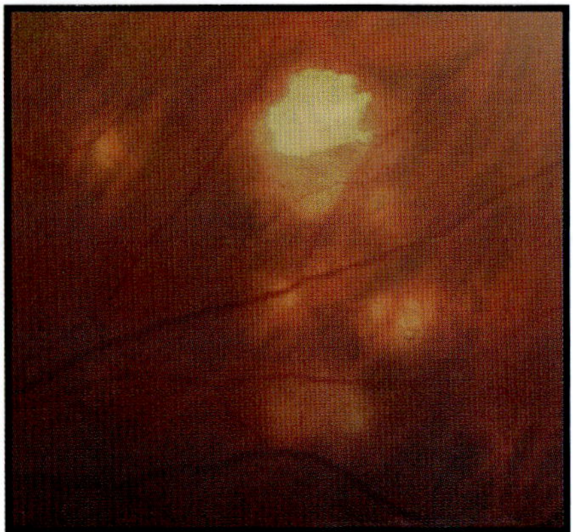

These are examples of idiopathic sclerochoroidal calcification. Yellowish irregular subretinal nodules are noted in these cases. *Left to right: courtesy of Dr. Andrew Schachat, Dr. John Killian, and Dr. James Augsburger*

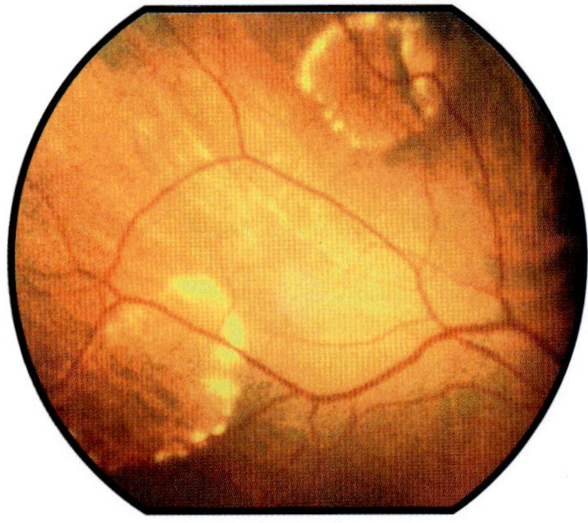
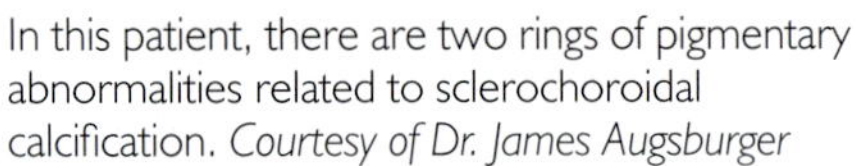

In this patient, there are two rings of pigmentary abnormalities related to sclerochoroidal calcification. *Courtesy of Dr. James Augsburger*

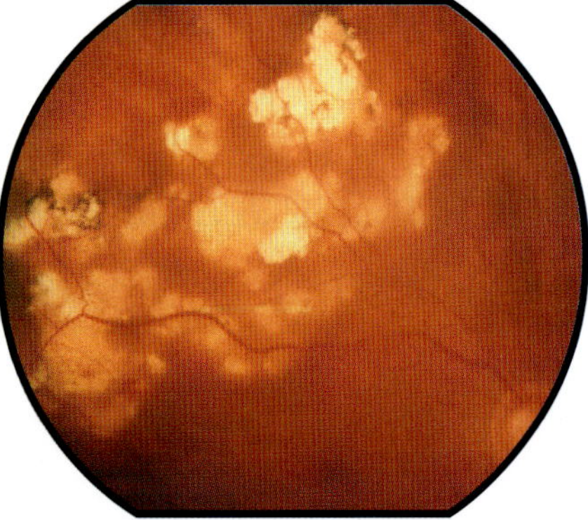

This patient has extensive calcific change with clinically visible mineralization. Sclerochoroidal calcification often shows some degree of bilateral symmetry, as in this patient. *Courtesy of Dr. Martin Perlman*

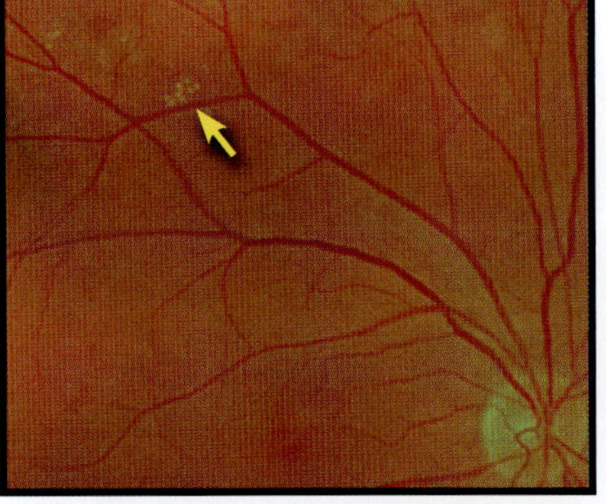
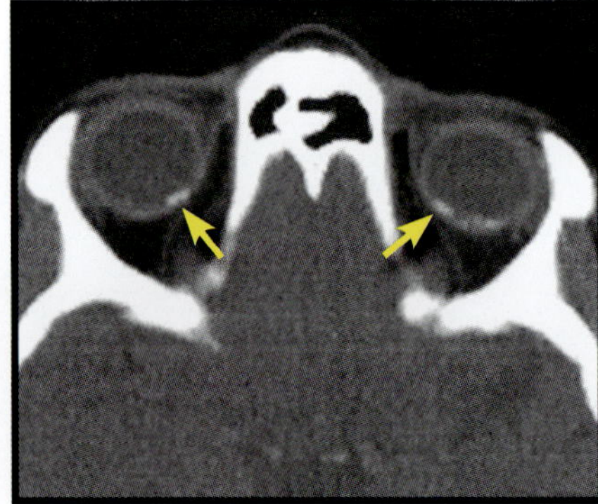
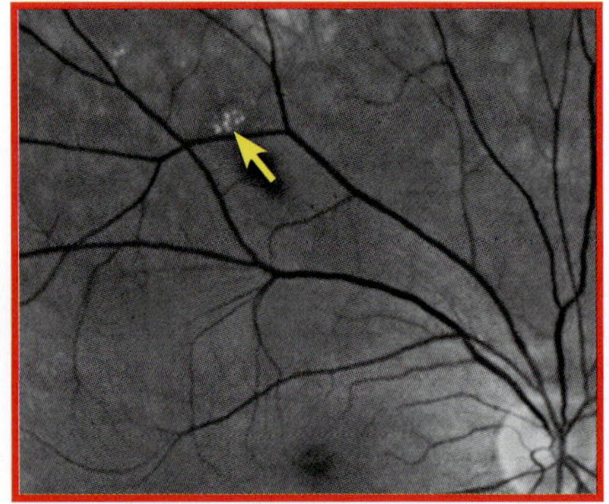

There are virtually no clinical manifestations *(arrows)* in this patient who was noted to have calcific changes within scleral walls on CT scan when scanned for an extraocular problem. The patient was then referred to an ophthalmologist, who detected some subtle pigment epithelial changes in the superotemporal periphery of each eye. Sclerochoroidal calcification may be fairly common. Occult lesions such as those present in this patient are easily overlooked on clinical examination, but are very prominent on CT scan.

Bartter Syndrome and Sclerochoroidal Calcification

Bartter syndrome encapsulates an inherited group of renal diseases that is characterized by hypokalemia and metabolic alkalosis. Bilateral sclerochoroidal calcification is a common manifestation as demonstrated in the 66-year-old patient below.

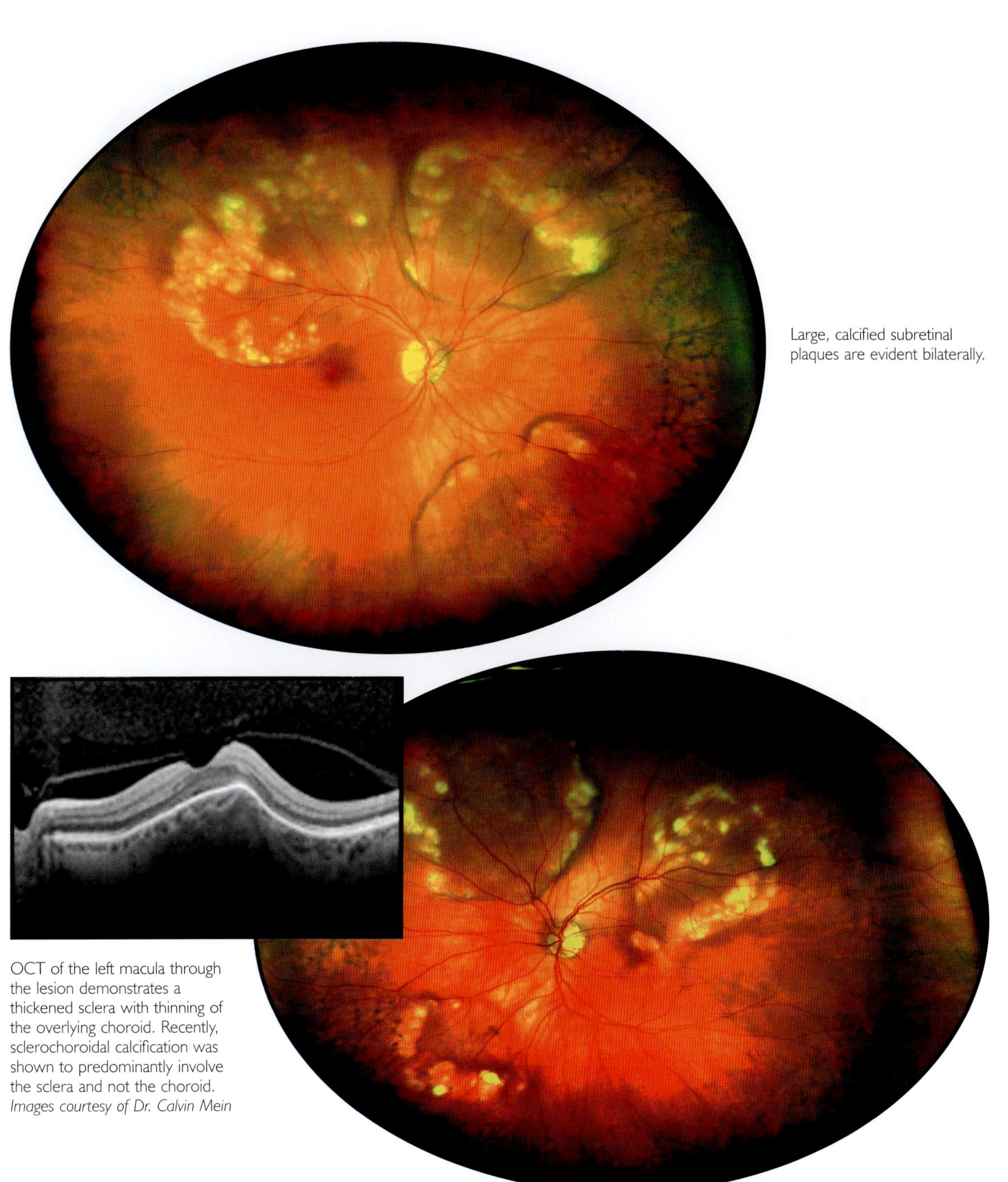

Large, calcified subretinal plaques are evident bilaterally.

OCT of the left macula through the lesion demonstrates a thickened sclera with thinning of the overlying choroid. Recently, sclerochoroidal calcification was shown to predominantly involve the sclera and not the choroid. *Images courtesy of Dr. Calvin Mein*

Choroidal Leiomyoma

Leiomyoma is a tumor of smooth-muscle origin that rarely develops in the uvea. It appears as an amelanotic mass that transmits light on transillumination. It is typically found in the ciliary body region of young women, but can be found rarely in the choroid and in men. It is clinically nonpigmented and frequently involves women with the primary involvement being in the suprauveal space, sparing the uveal stroma itself.

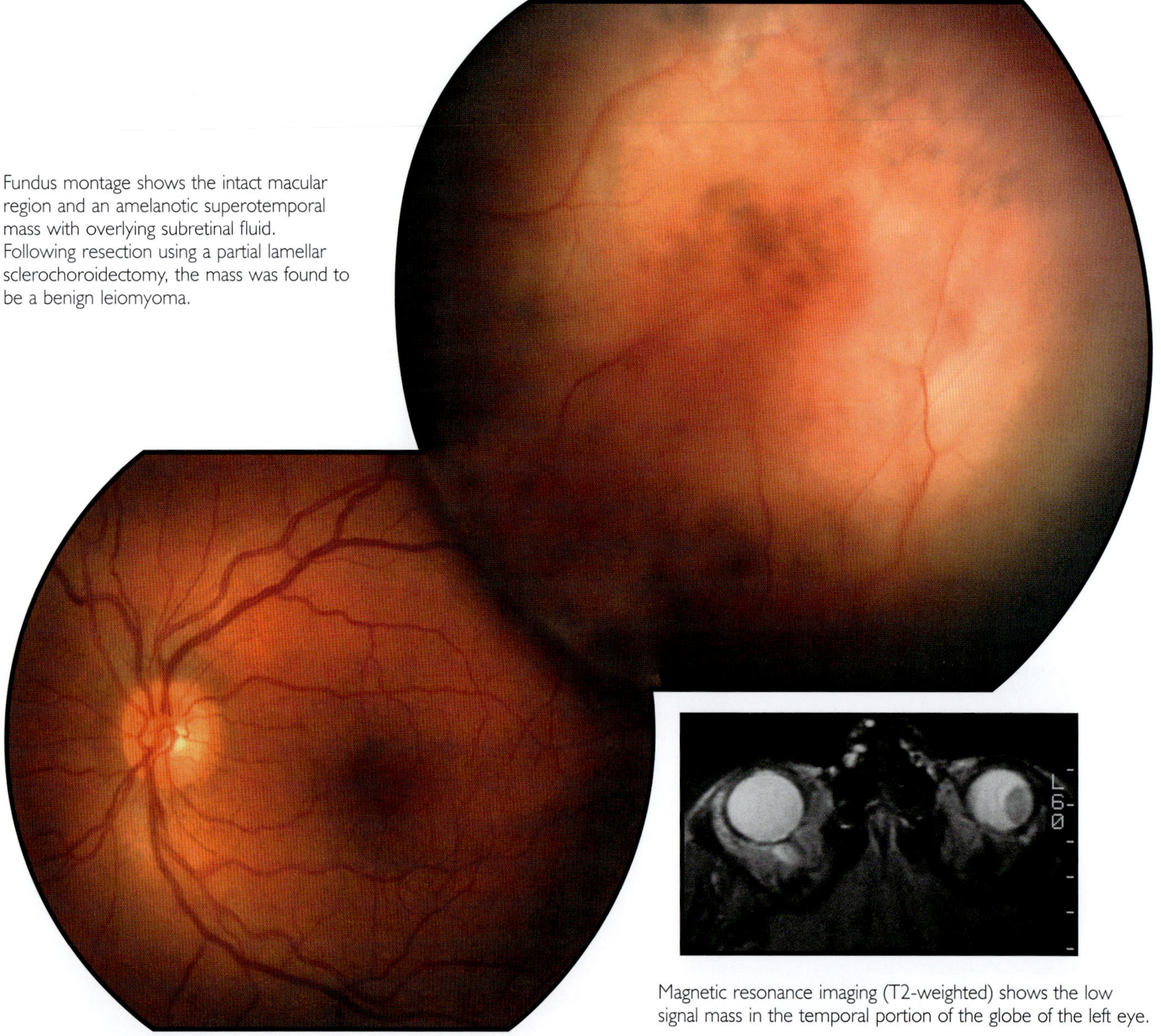

Fundus montage shows the intact macular region and an amelanotic superotemporal mass with overlying subretinal fluid. Following resection using a partial lamellar sclerochoroidectomy, the mass was found to be a benign leiomyoma.

Magnetic resonance imaging (T2-weighted) shows the low signal mass in the temporal portion of the globe of the left eye.

Intraocular Lymphoma

Intraocular lymphoid tumors are rare, compromising less than 1% of ocular oncological tumors. The spectrum of intraocular lymphoid tumors ranges from benign reactive lymphoid hyperplasia to various types of malignant lesions. All of these lymphoid tumors can masquerade as a variety of benign and inflammatory conditions. Very often, they are difficult to diagnose, requiring histological specimens. Intraocular lymphomas are subclassified into primary vitreoretinal lymphoma, primary uveal lymphoma, and secondary intraocular presentation of systemic lymphoma. Primary vitreoretinal lymphomas are typically bilateral and are associated with primary central nervous system lymphoma in a significant number of cases. Primary uveal lymphoma is commonly unilateral and can be further subclassified into choroidal, iridal, and ciliary body lymphomas. Nearly all lymphomas are non-Hodgkin lymphoma of B-cell origin.

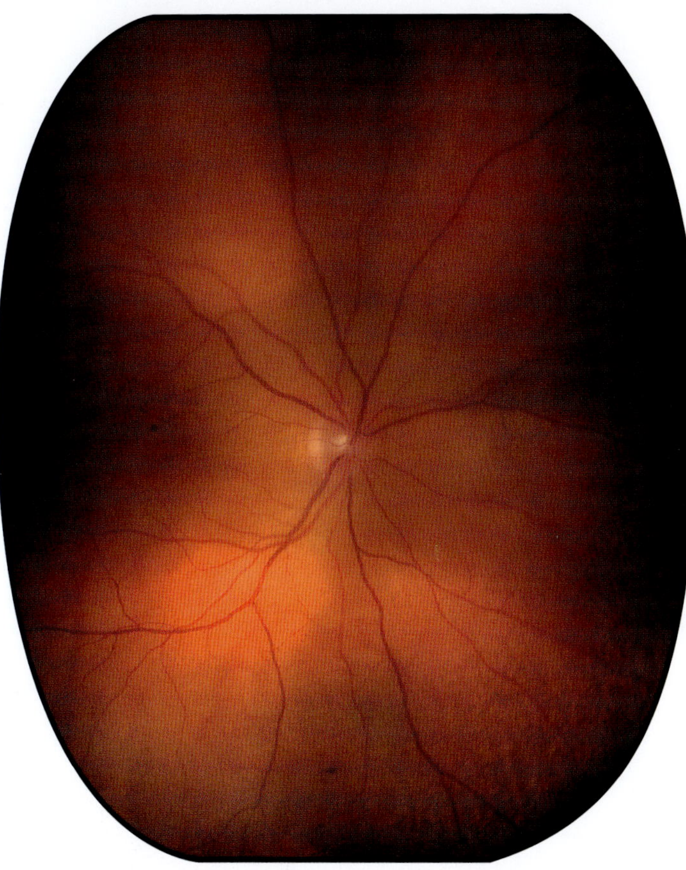

This patient presented with a choroidal lymphoma masquerading as a chronic uveitis. On examination, the right fundus *(left image)* revealed choroidal thickening with loss of choroidal vascular detail. The disc margins appeared blurred nasally.

Externally *(below)*, the right eye showed vascular injection that was present for years and was previously treated with topical steroid eyedrops.

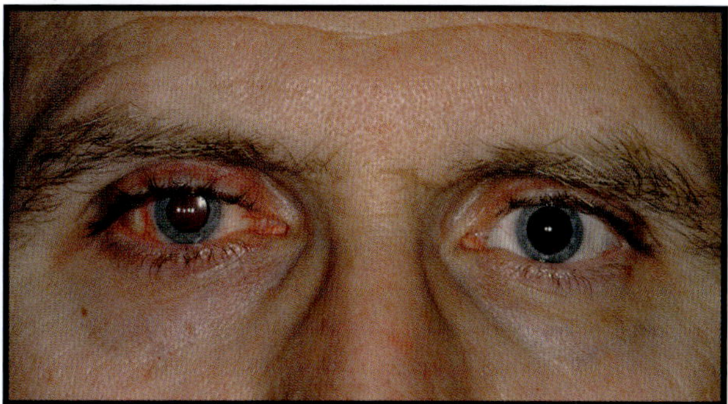

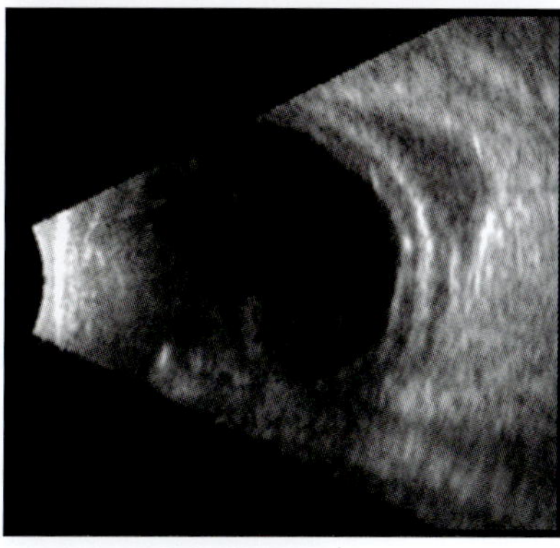

Ocular ultrasonography shows thickening of the choroidal layer and a prominent extra scleral nodule of lymphoma.

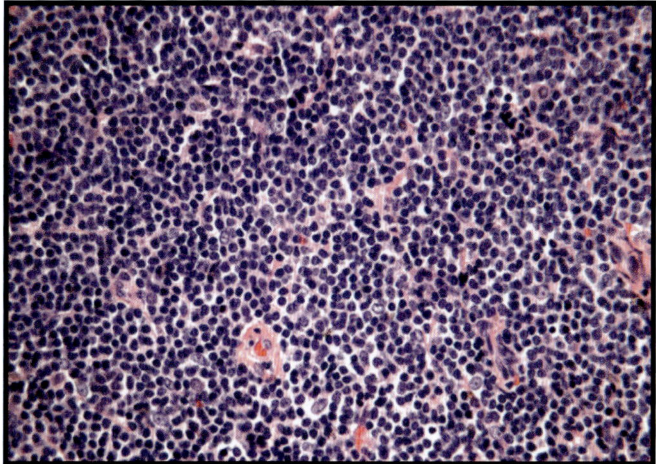

Low-power microscopy of a choroidal biopsy shows monomorphic infiltration by low-grade lymphoma cells.

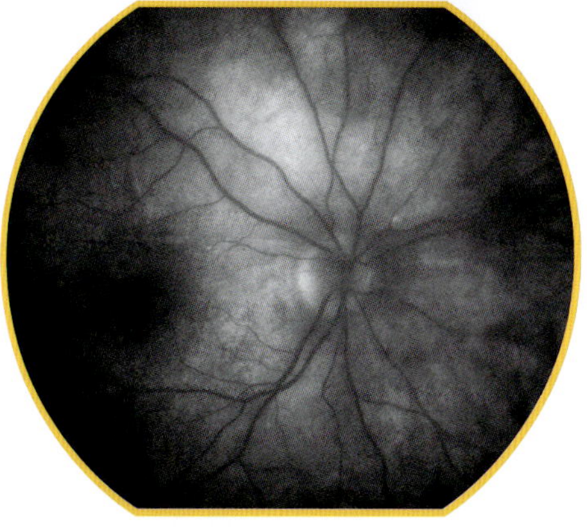

Late phase fluorescein angiogram of the right eye illustrates diffuse choroidal fluorescence.

Vitreoretinal lymphoma associated with central nervous system (CNS) non-Hodgkin lymphomas can present as an isolated intraocular lymphoma, only to develop CNS involvement during long-term follow-up. The usual age of onset is between 55 and 70 years.

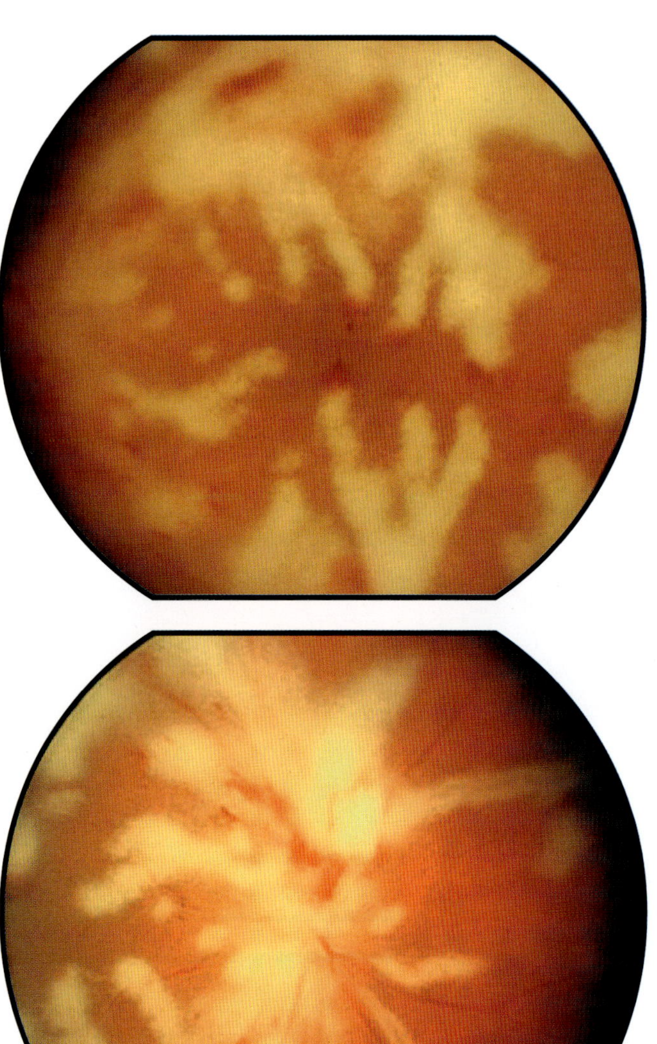

Vitreoretinal lymphoma presenting as frosted angiitis. *Courtesy of Dr. Richard Lewis*

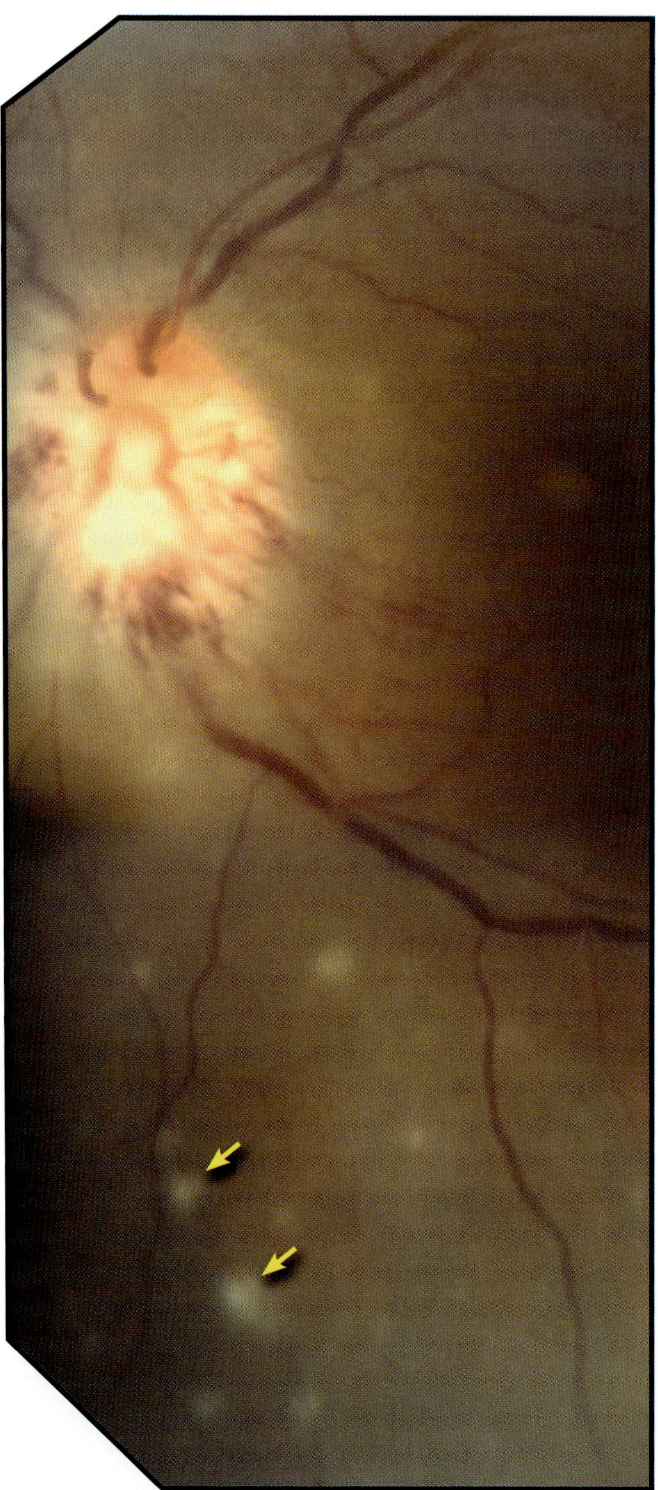

Vitreoretinal lymphoma presenting as optic neuritis and multifocal choroiditis *(arrows)*. *Courtesy of Dr. Darma Ie*

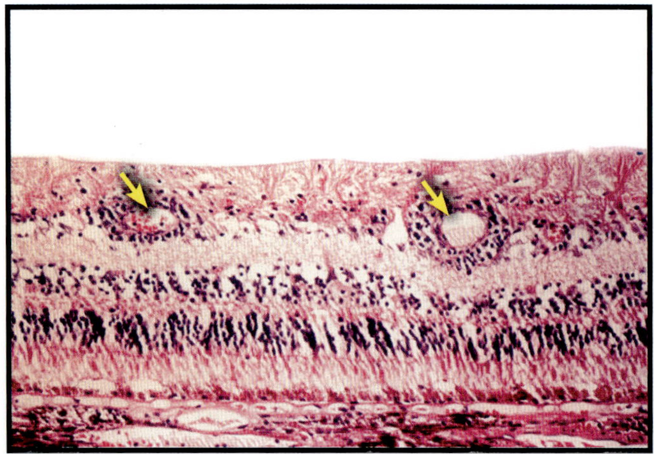

The histopathology in this case of ocular CNS lymphoma shows tumor infiltration in the walls of retinal vessels *(arrows)*.

Paraneoplastic Cloudy Vitelliform Maculopathy

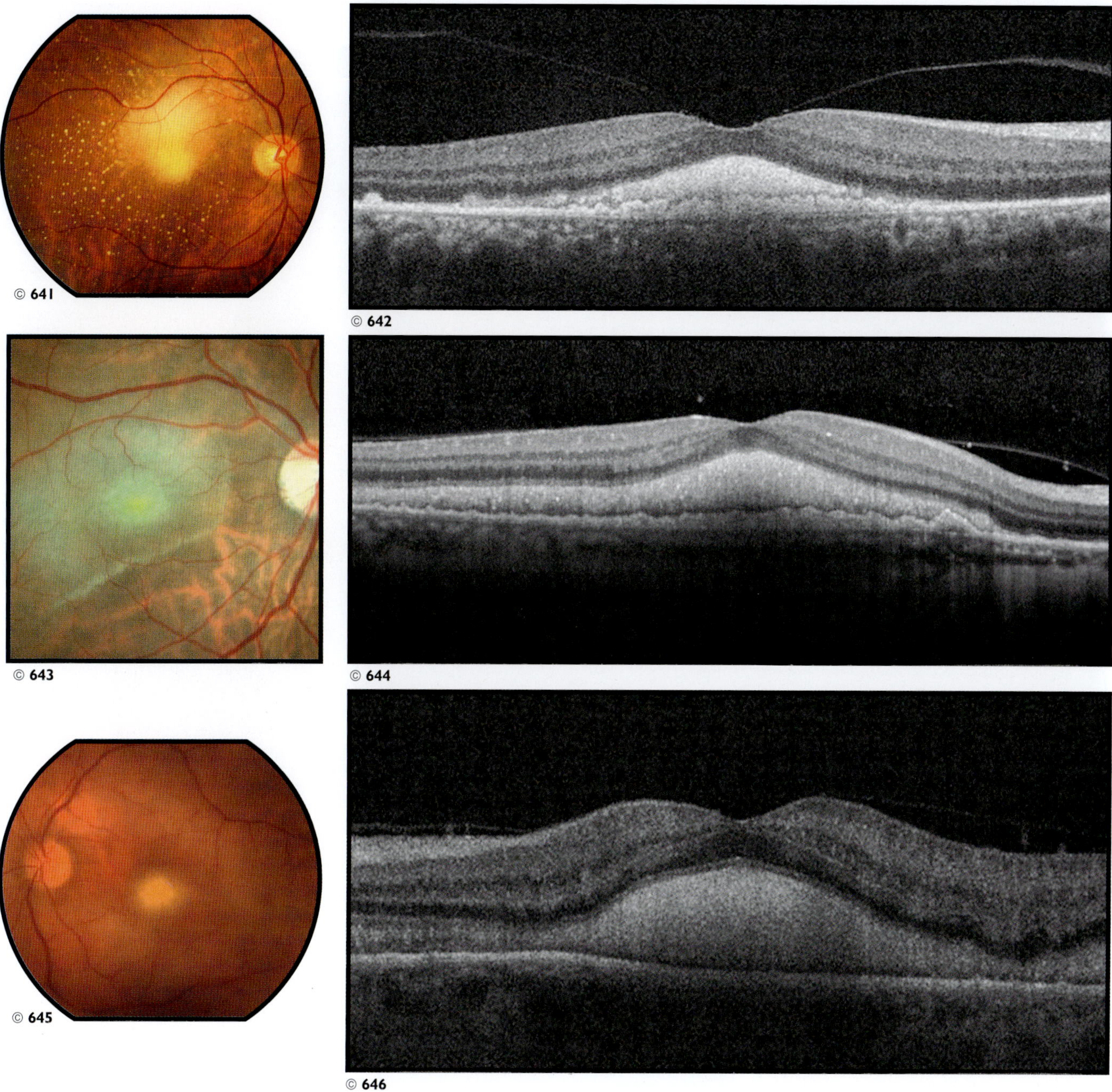

© 641 © 642 © 643 © 644 © 645 © 646

Primary vitreoretinal lymphoma and primary central nervous system lymphoma are uncommonly preceded by a vitelliform retinopathy that can mimic acute exudative polymorphous vitelliform maculopathy. This manifestation, known as paraneoplastic cloudy vitelliform maculopathy, is typically transient and shows spontaneous regression. Vitelliform material is indistinct, located in the subretinal space and associated with a rippled and thickened RPE layer. Three patients that presented with paraneoplastic cloudy vitelliform maculopathy within 6 months of the diagnosis of intraocular lymphoma are presented.

Choroidal Lymphoma Masquerading as Age-Related Macular Degeneration in a 59-year-old Man

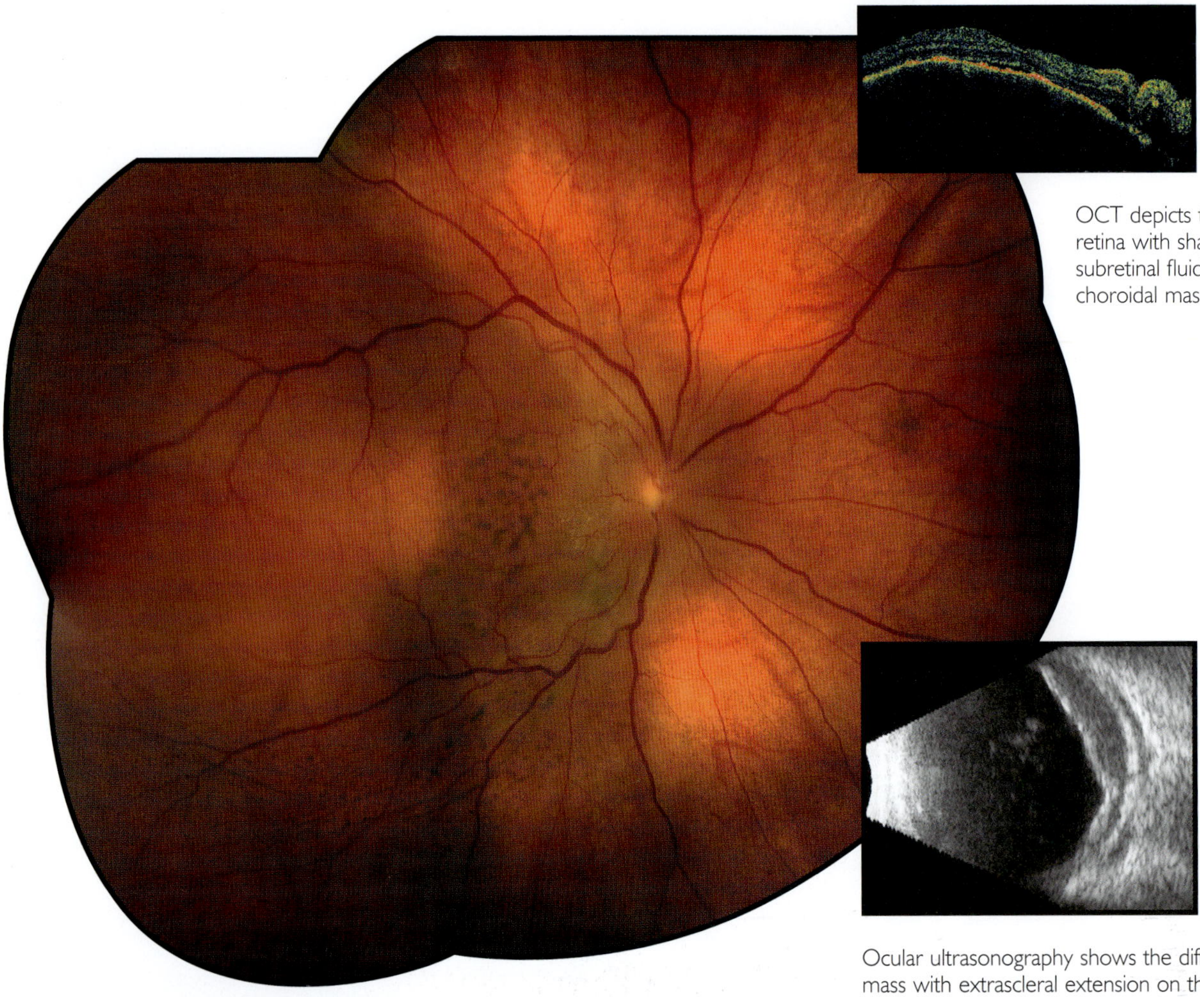

OCT depicts the folded retina with shallow subretinal fluid overlying a choroidal mass.

Ocular ultrasonography shows the diffuse choroidal mass with extrascleral extension on the posterior surface of the globe.

Subtle macular choroidal infiltration by lymphoma with overlying pigment clumps and shallow subretinal fluid are noted. Note the lack of visible choroidal vascular architecture in the macular area.

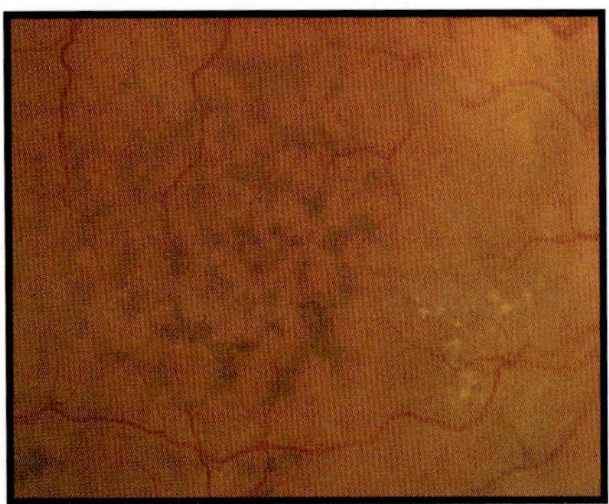

Closer view depicts the pigment clumps and subretinal fluid.

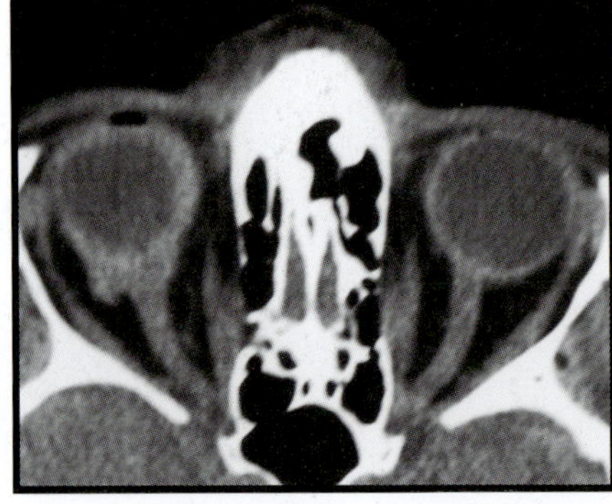

Computed tomography at the level of the optic nerves shows the irregular circumbulbar thickening with perineural mass at the optic disc region of the right eye.

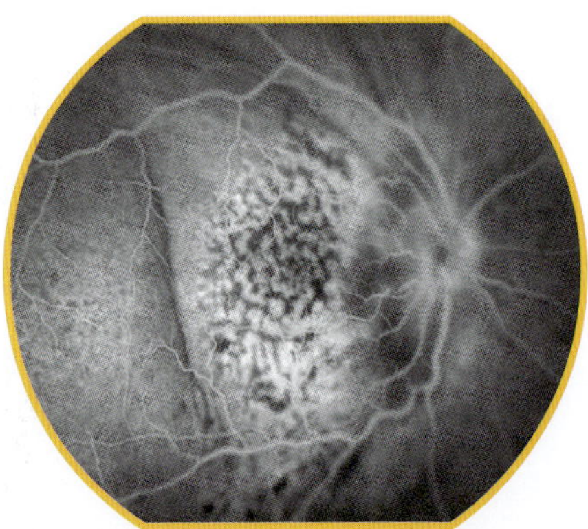

Fluorescein angiography reveals diffuse mottled fluorescence of the choroid, disc staining, and blockage from the overlying pigment clumps. Choroidal folds supertemporally and a large choroidal fold temporally are also seen.

Benign Uveal Lymphoid Hyperplasia

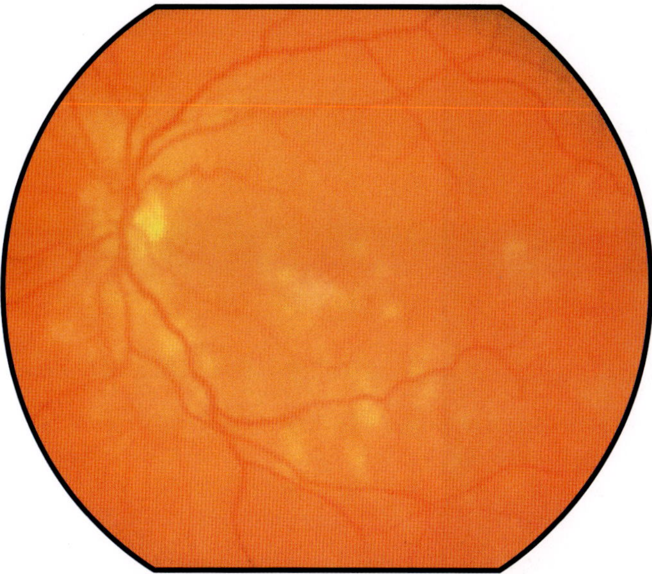

Patients with benign lymphoid hyperplasia may demonstrate focal whitish-yellow choroidal lesions.

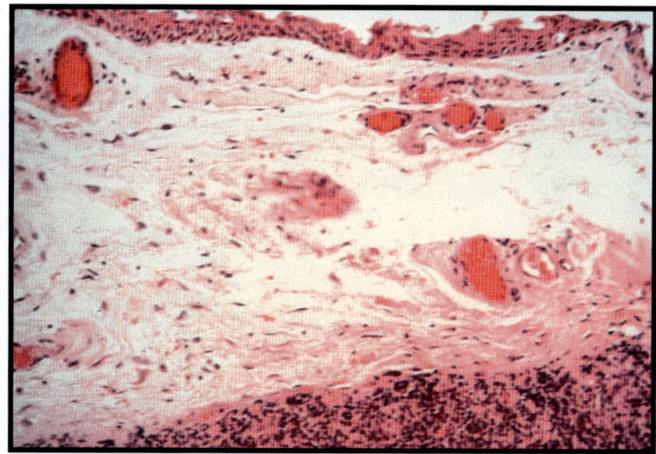

Histopathologic examination of a conjunctival biopsy disclosed a monomorphic infiltrate of well-differentiated lymphocytes. *Top row courtesy of Dr. Evan Sachs*

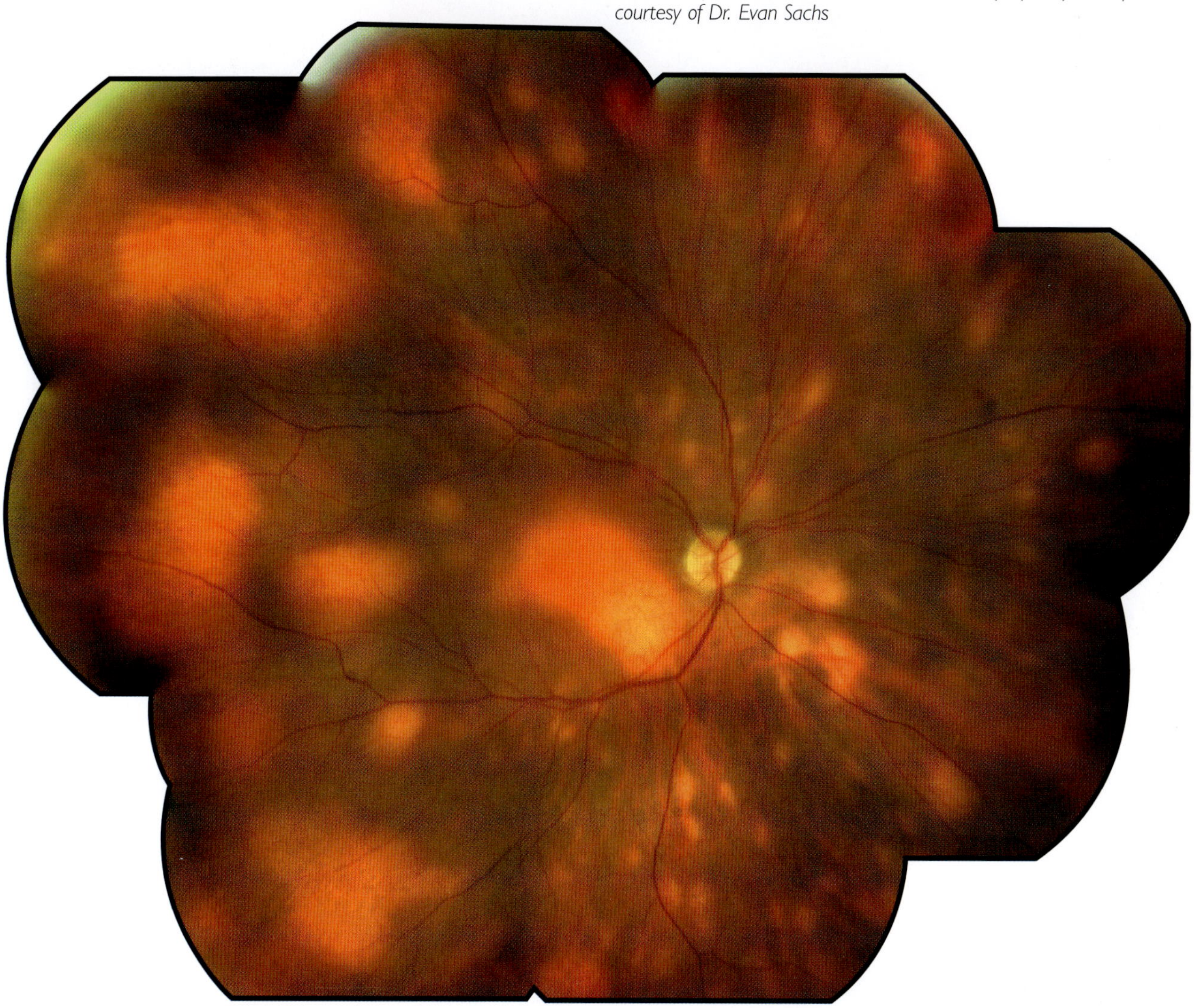

A 77-year-old male with unilateral multifocal reactive lymphoid hyperplasia presenting as orange-colored variably sized mass lesions in the choroid. This patient has been stable for more than 4 years with this presumed low-grade lymphomatous process.

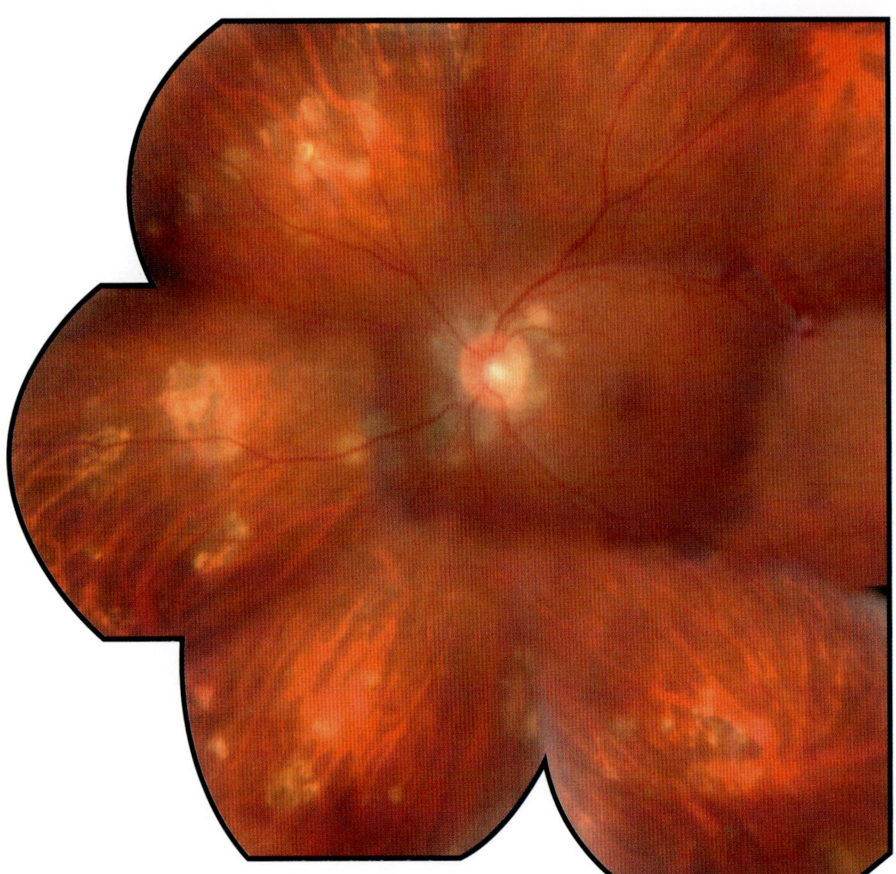

This patient has presumed benign lymphoid hyperplasia with multiple randomly distributed shallowly thickened lesions throughout the fundus. The peripapillary area is involved, but the macula is spared.

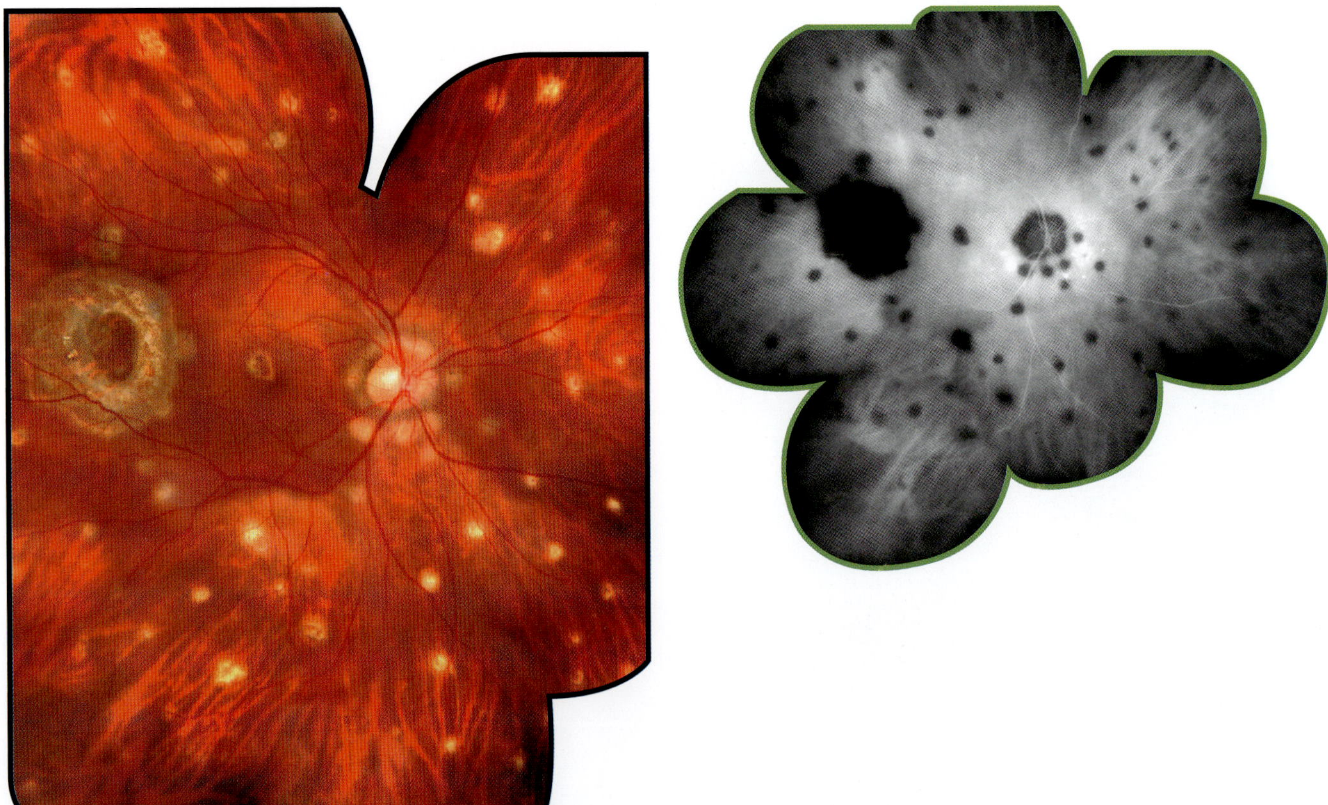

This patient was misdiagnosed as birdshot chorioretinopathy and then as sarcoidosis. Benign lymphoid hyperplasia was proven on biopsy. Indocyanine green angiography shows that these lesions are all hypofluorescent.

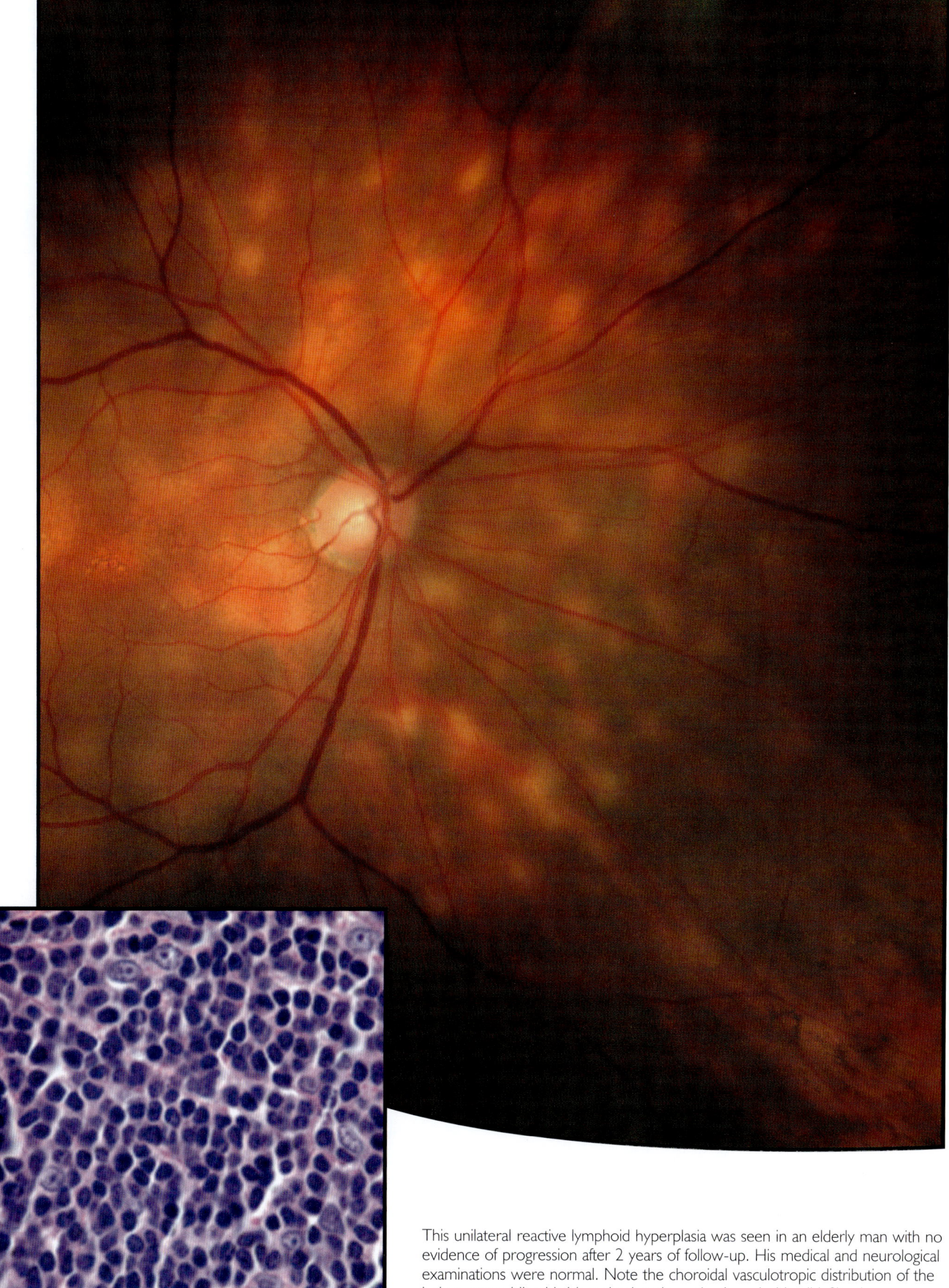

This unilateral reactive lymphoid hyperplasia was seen in an elderly man with no evidence of progression after 2 years of follow-up. His medical and neurological examinations were normal. Note the choroidal vasculotropic distribution of the lesions resembling birdshot chorioretinopathy. Lymphoid cell infiltration was seen on periocular biopsy *(left image)*.

Mucosal-Associated Lymphoid Tumor (MALT Syndrome)

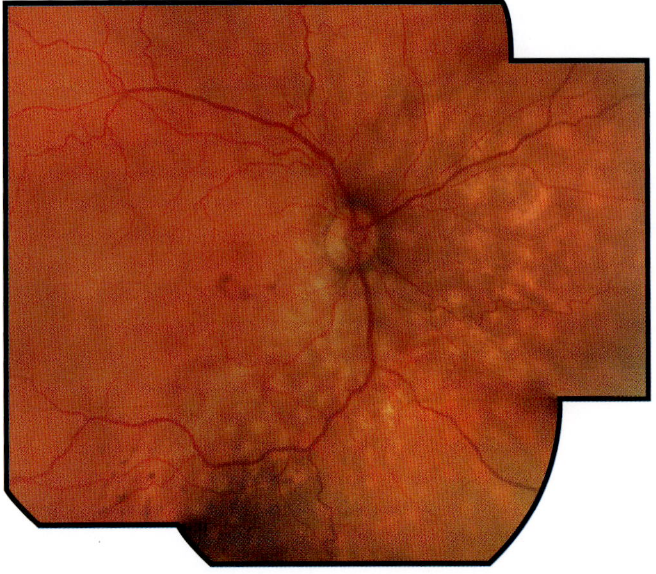

The multifocal progressive lesions in this patient were associated with exudative detachment temporally.

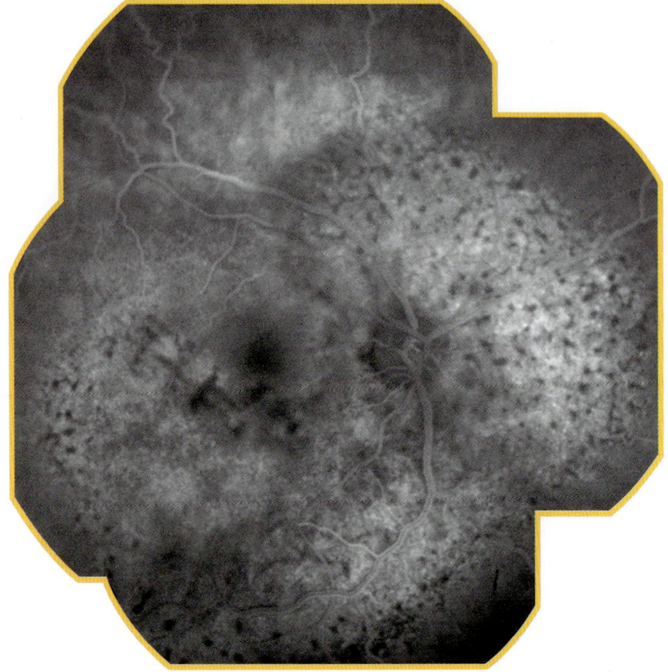

The fluorescein angiogram revealed a mixed hyperfluorescent pattern.

The fundus autofluorescence showed newer hyperfluorescent lesions *(arrows)* and older hypofluorescent lesions in which the RPE became atrophic *(arrowheads)*.

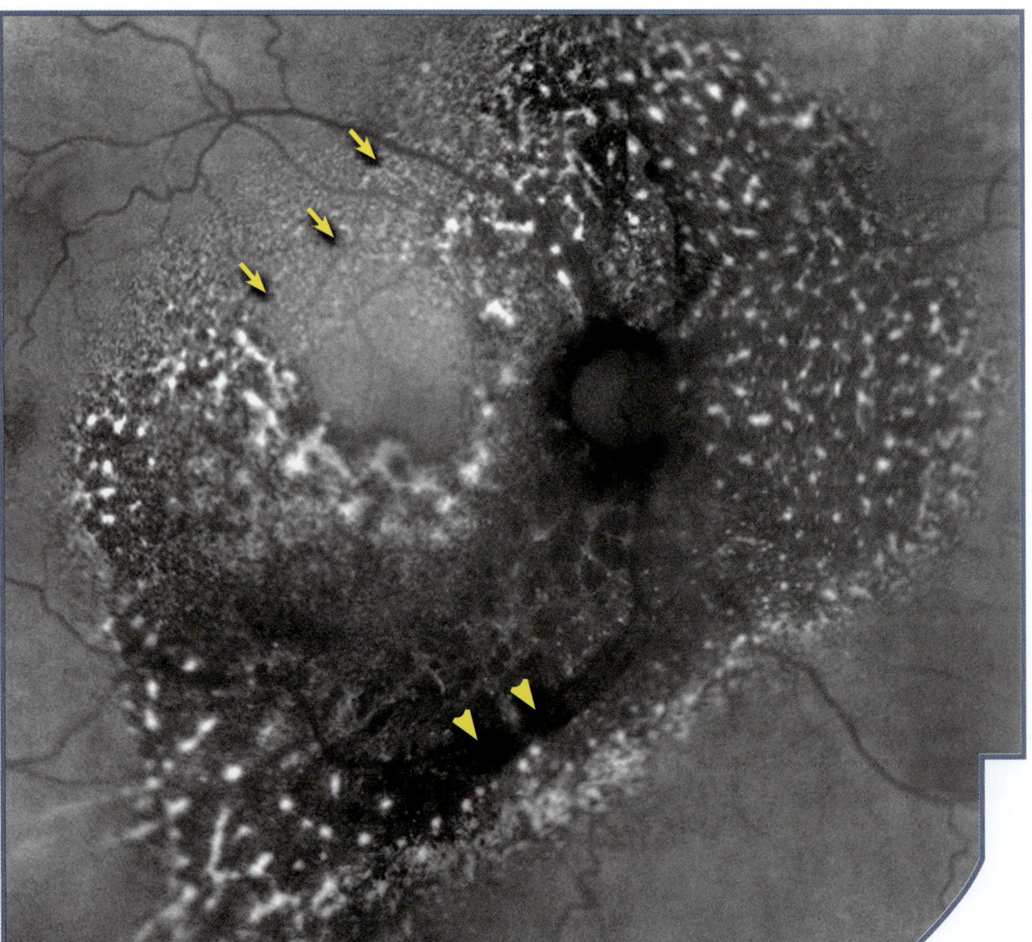

Enhanced Depth Imaging Spectral Domain Optical Coherence Tomography of Choroidal Lymphoma

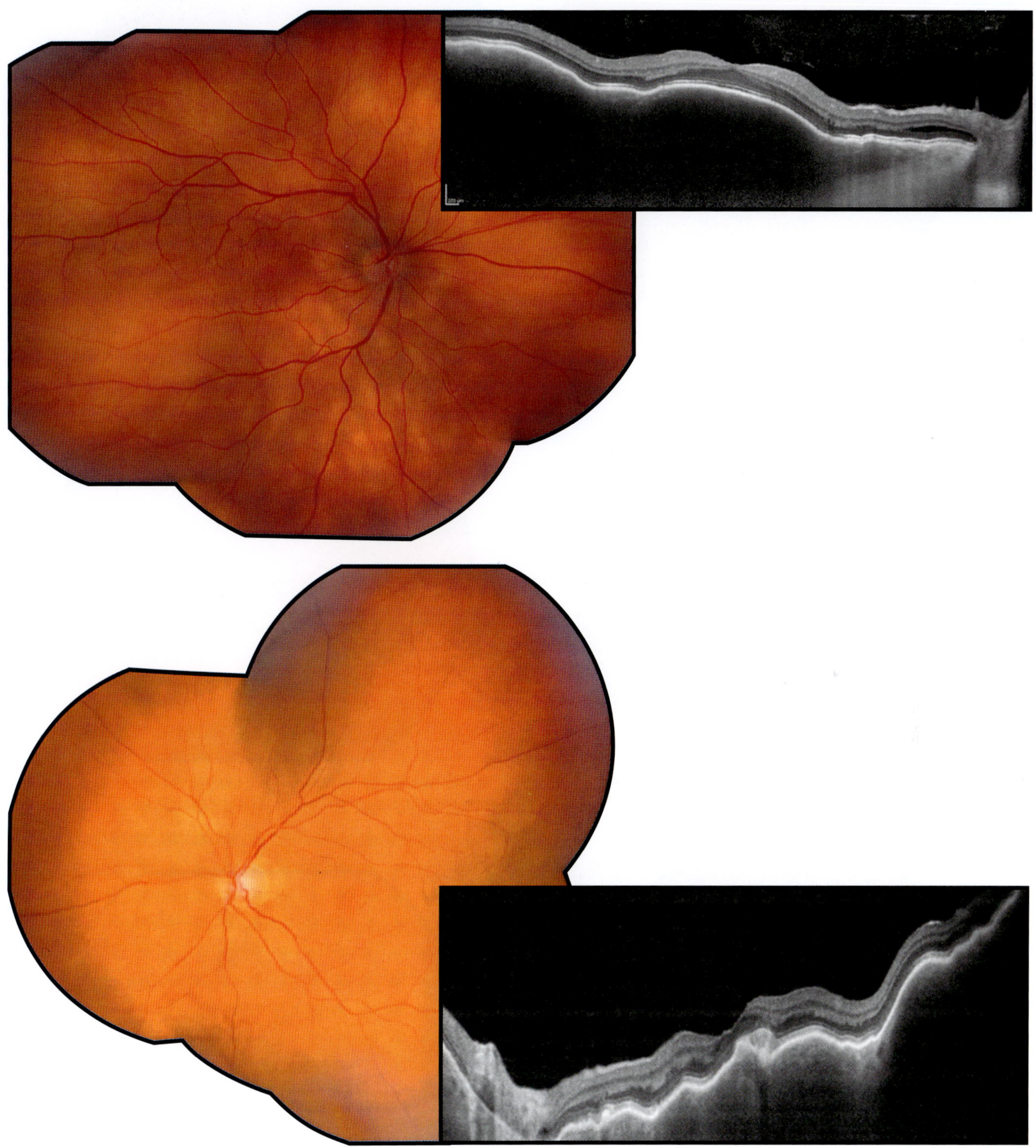

Two different patients with choroidal lymphoma. Both demonstrate the typical, rippled "sea-sick" topography on spectral domain OCT.

Variations in Lymphoma Presentations

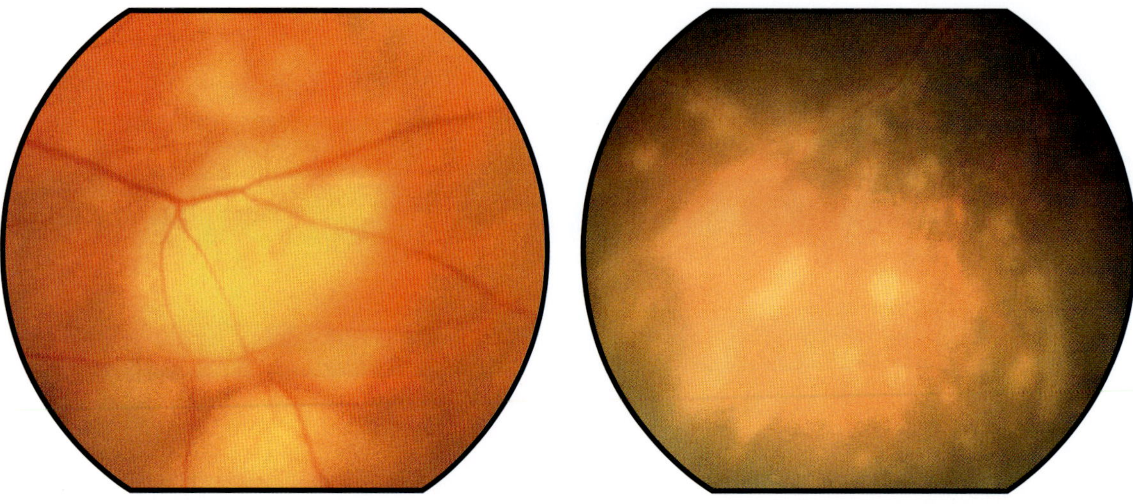

Large-cell vitreoretinal lymphoma can masquerade as primary retinal, vascular, or choroidal disease. Multiple small lesions may masquerade as drusen *(left)*. Larger globular lesions *(right)* may resemble a metastatic mass.

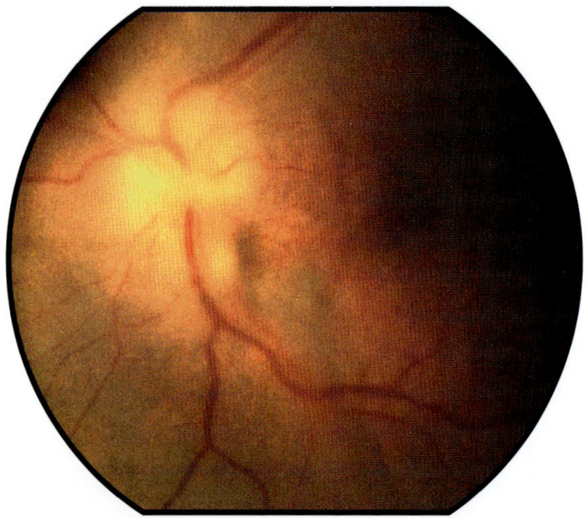

Burkitt lymphoma may also occasionally involve the eye with multifocal chorioretinal spots, vitritis, and optic nerve infiltration.

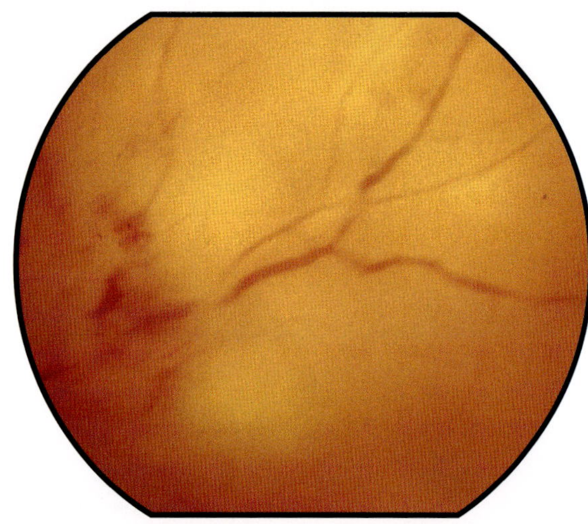

A creamy white deep lesion with secondary hemorrhage is observed in this patient with ocular lymphoma. This patient also has retinal vascular abnormalities.

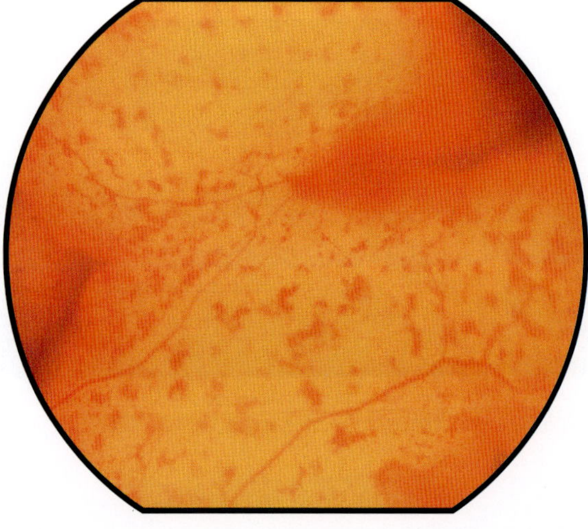

A leopard-type pattern may also be seen as in this patient with large subretinal pigment epithelial infiltrative mass lesion in vitreoretinal lymphoma.

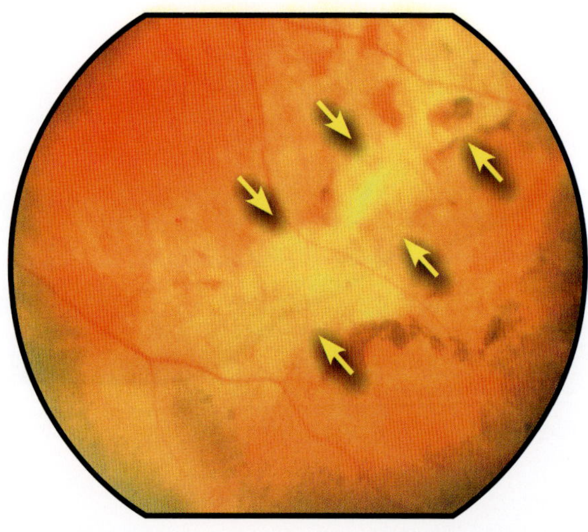

This vitreoretinal case shows scarring *(arrows)* that developed in areas of tumor regression.

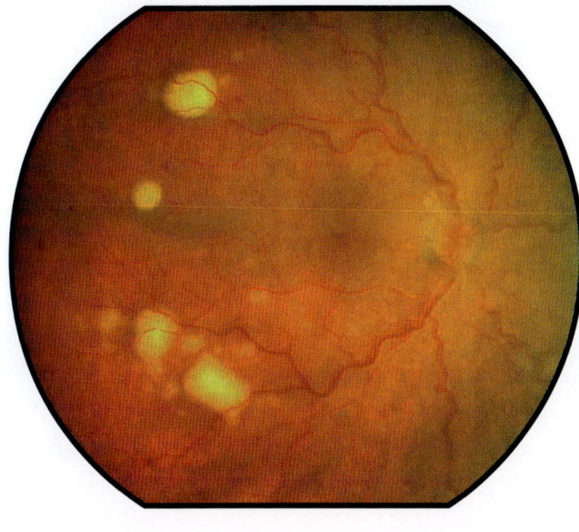

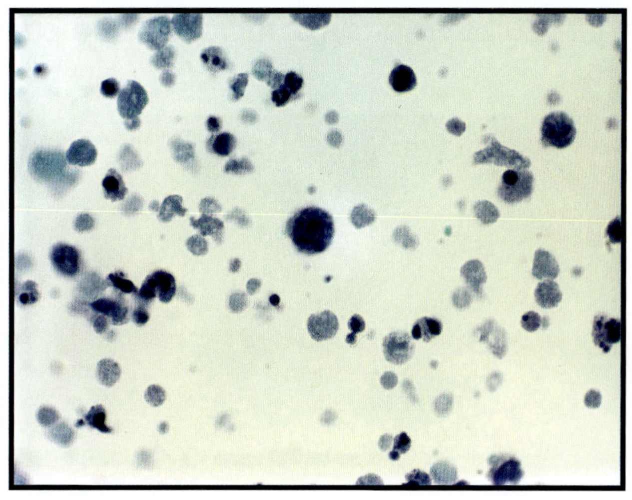

Vitreoretinal large-cell lymphoma infiltration beneath the RPE in an older female. Yellow subpigment epithelial infiltration was scattered throughout the entire fundus *(left)*. Fine-needle aspiration biopsy of the superotemporal lesion showed necrotic and anaplastic lymphoma cells *(right)*.

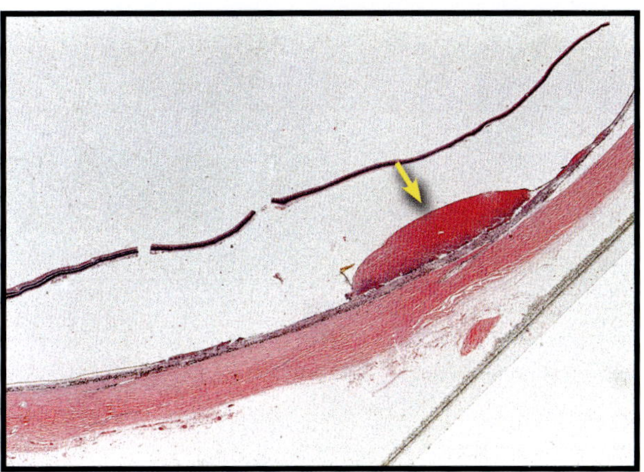

On histopathologic examination, a large area of pigment epithelial detachment secondary to necrotic tumor was noted *(arrow)*.

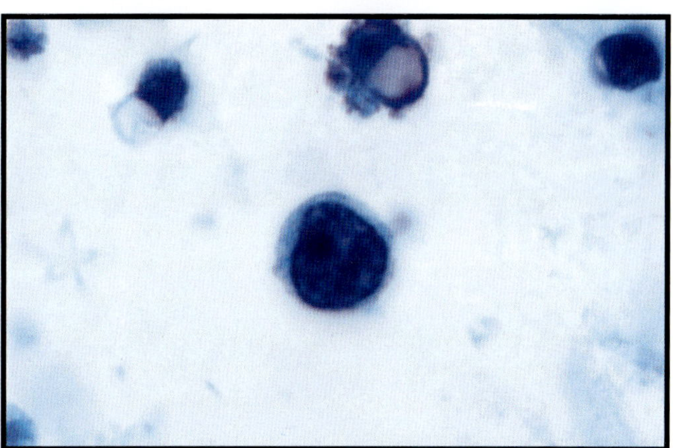

Cytopathologic evaluation of surgically removed vitreous can be useful in the diagnosis of ocular lymphoma. This photograph shows a vitrectomy specimen consisting of characteristic lymphoma cells with scant cytoplasm, nucleolus, and nuclear membrane abnormalities.

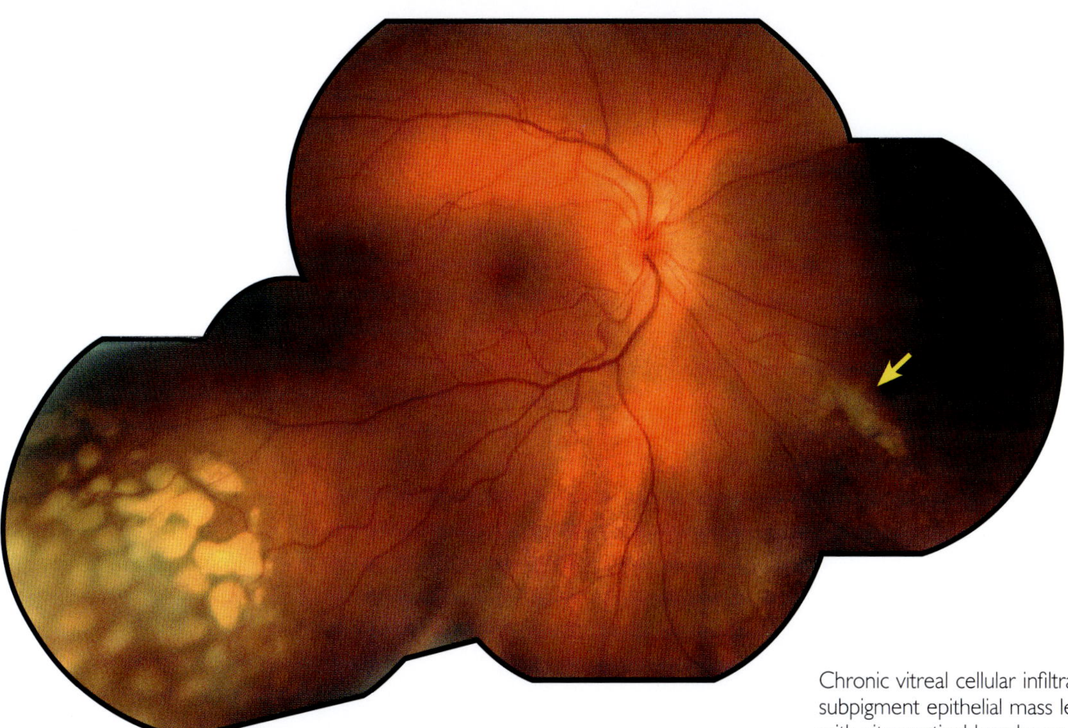

Chronic vitreal cellular infiltration *(arrow)* and multiple subpigment epithelial mass lesions are seen in this patient with vitreoretinal lymphoma. *Courtesy of Dr. James Puklin*

Large-Cell Lymphoma Infiltrating in the Retina and Optic Nerve

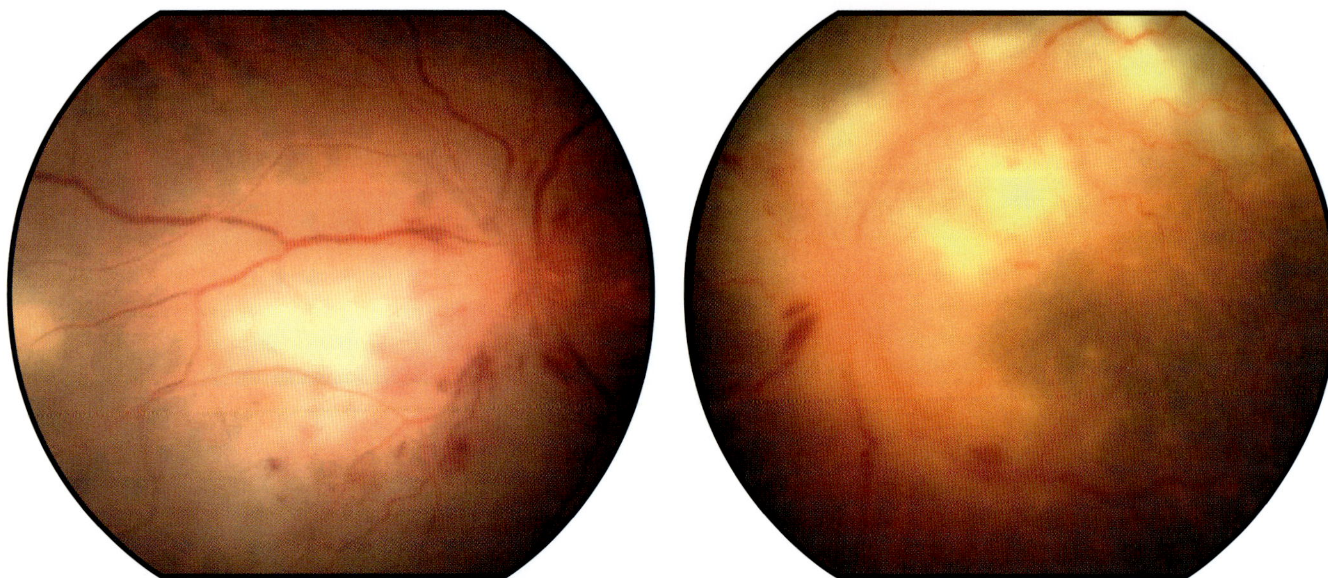

In this patient with lymphoma, white tumor cells are seen to infiltrate the retina. The disc margin is blurred from extension of tumor cells.

Wide-angle photography reveals regression of the infiltrative tumor following ocular radiotherapy.
There is also chorioretinal atrophy in the nasal fundus and optic nerve head atrophy involving the nasal half of the disc.

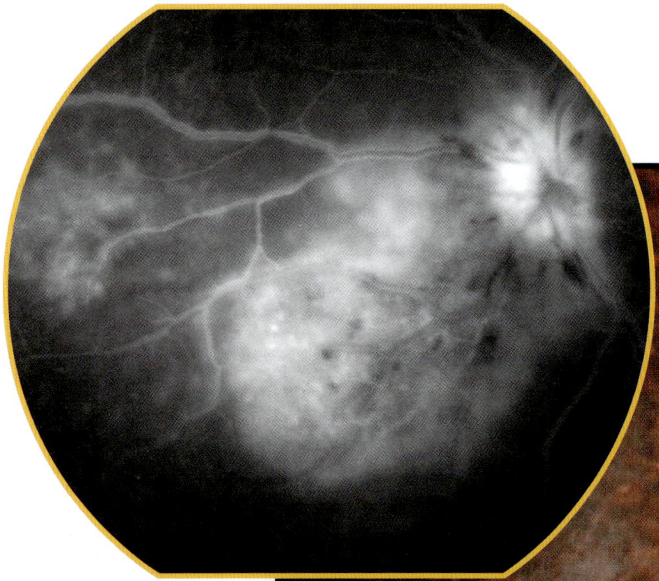

A late fluorescein angiogram shows persistent staining of the retinal vessels, the subretinal mass, and leakage from the disc.

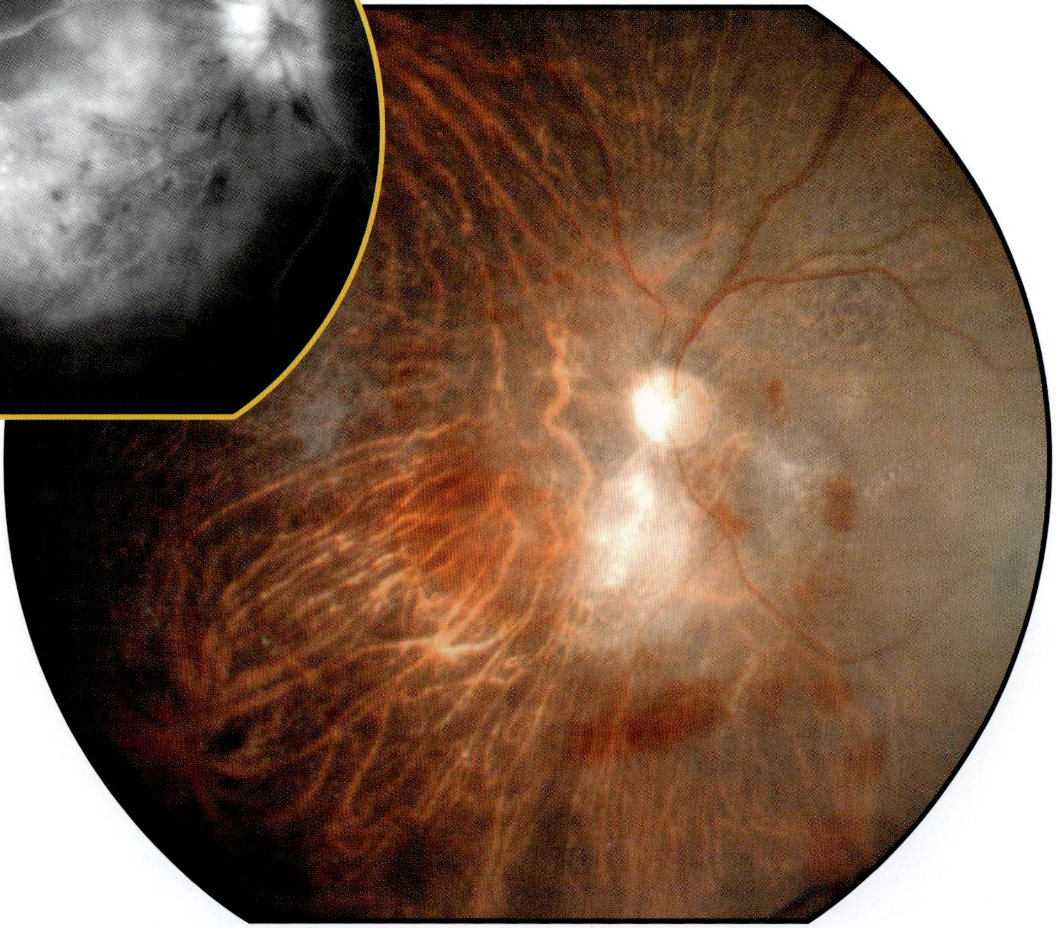

Vitreous, Retinal, Choroidal, and Optic Nerve Involvement in Ocular CNS Lymphoma

There is severe vitreous, retinal, choroidal, and optic nerve tumor infiltration in this patient with ocular CNS lymphoma.

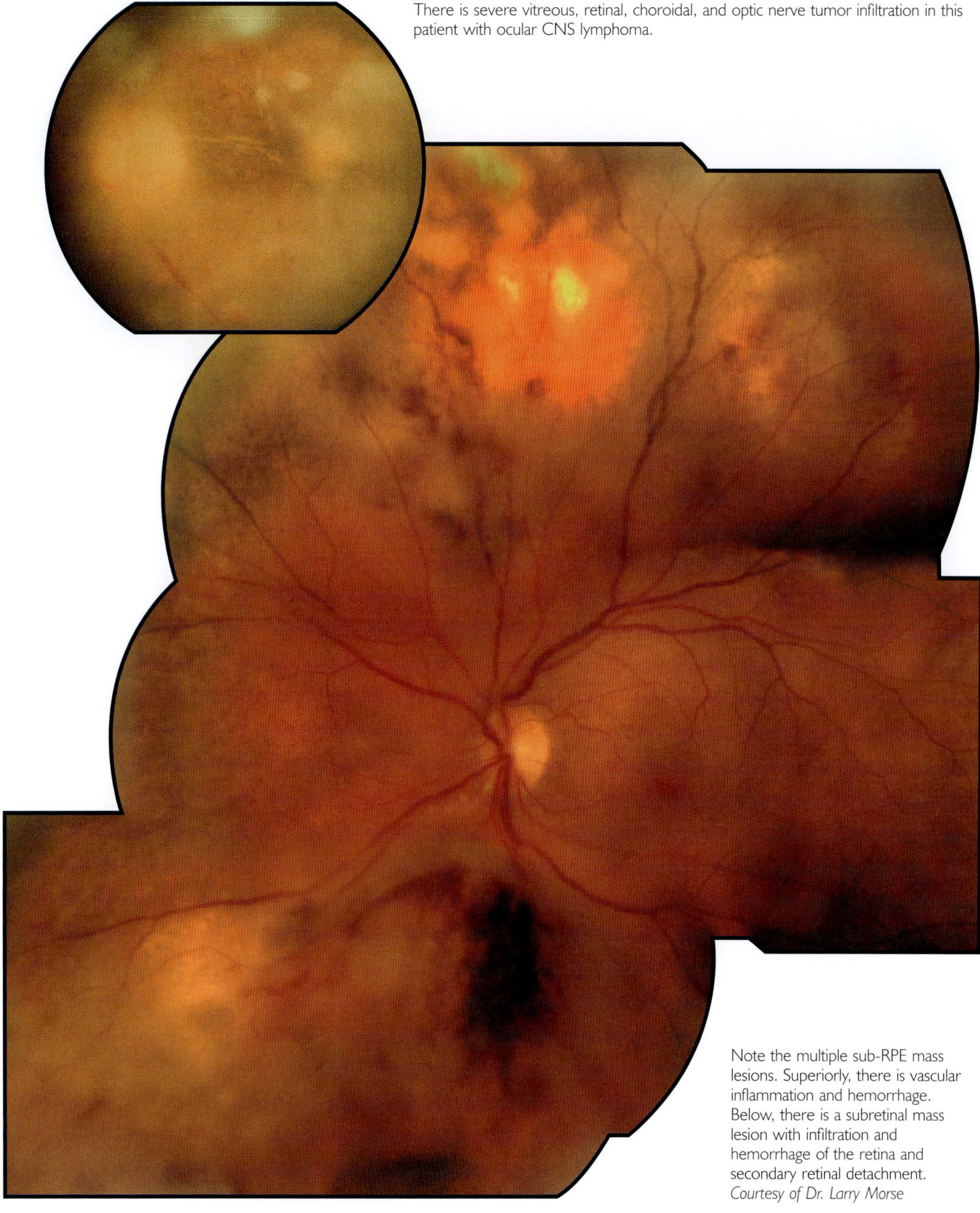

Note the multiple sub-RPE mass lesions. Superiorly, there is vascular inflammation and hemorrhage. Below, there is a subretinal mass lesion with infiltration and hemorrhage of the retina and secondary retinal detachment. *Courtesy of Dr. Larry Morse*

Intraocular Metastatic Testicular Lymphoma

In this patient, testicular lymphoma metastasized to the right eye and eventually to the left eye. The lymphoid proliferation responded to chemotherapy, both intravitreal methotrexate and systemic chemotherapy. In addition to the lymphomatous infiltration, there was an evolving multizonal area of atrophy bordered by heaped-up pigment epithelium resembling a classic BDUMP pattern or "giraffe pattern". Thus, the patient had metastatic intraocular testicular lymphoma, presumably in conjunction with a paraneoplastic process to the choroid.

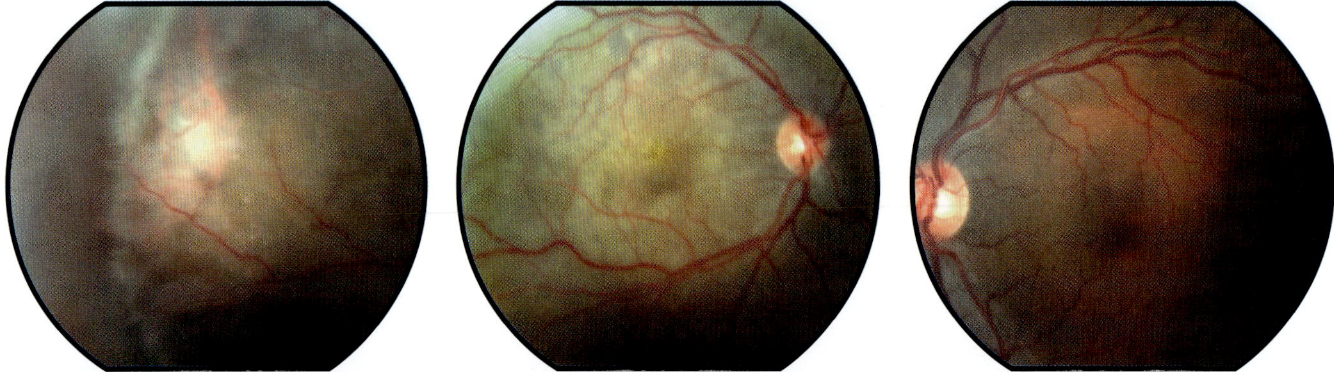

This patient had lymphomatous infiltration of the subretinal space in the peripheral fundus *(left)* and central macular region *(middle)* of the right eye. The left eye showed only very few pigment epithelial abnormalities at that stage *(right)*.

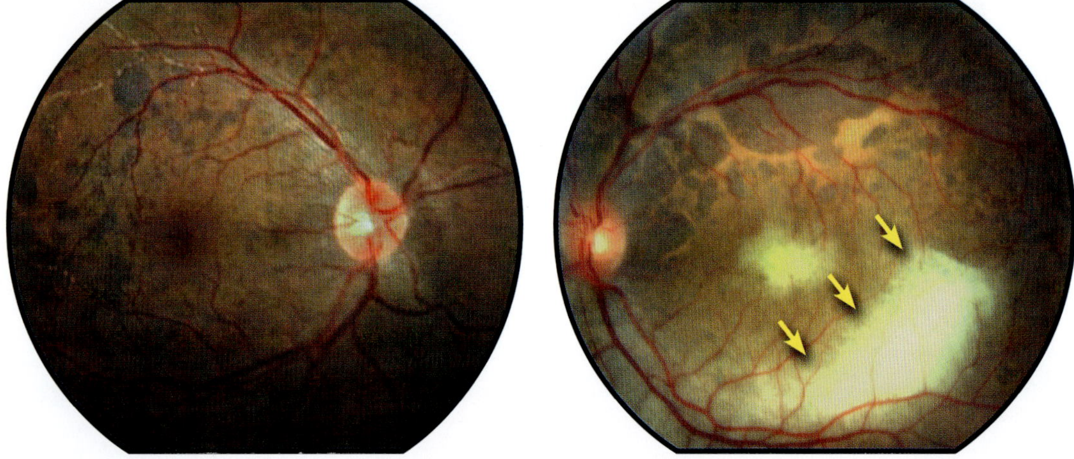

Following a single injection of methotrexate into the right eye, the metastatic lymphoma resolved in 1 week *(left)*. In the same timeframe, there was lymphomatous infiltration in the left eye centrally and along the inferior temporal arcade with extension of an atrophic "giraffe pattern" similar to the right eye.

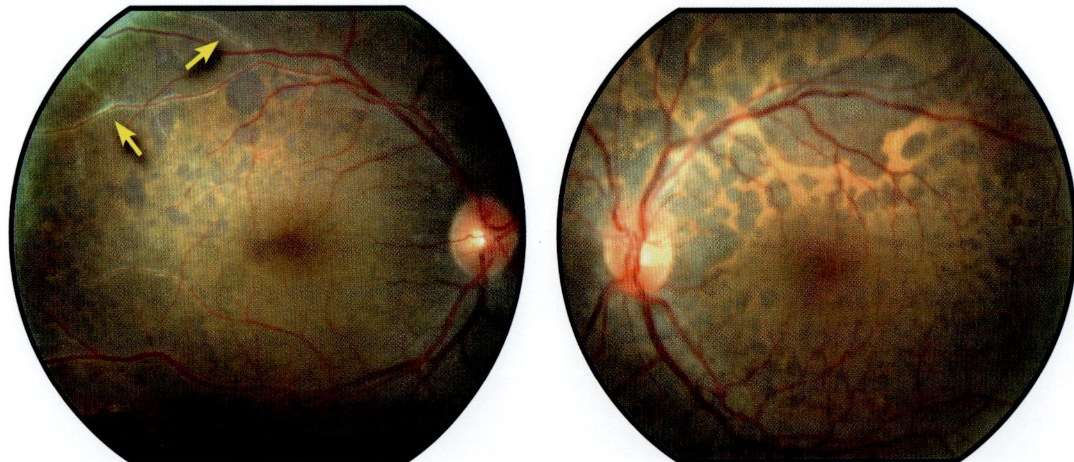

Following additional chemotherapy, there was total remission of the metastatic lymphoma in the right eye, leaving a legacy of retinal vascular ischemic changes and the geographic atrophic "giraffe pattern." The left eye following a single injection of methotrexate also cleared, leaving a more pronounced giraffe pattern characteristic of BDUMP. *All images courtesy of Dr. John Huang*

Treatment of Choroidal Lymphoma with External-Beam Radiotherapy

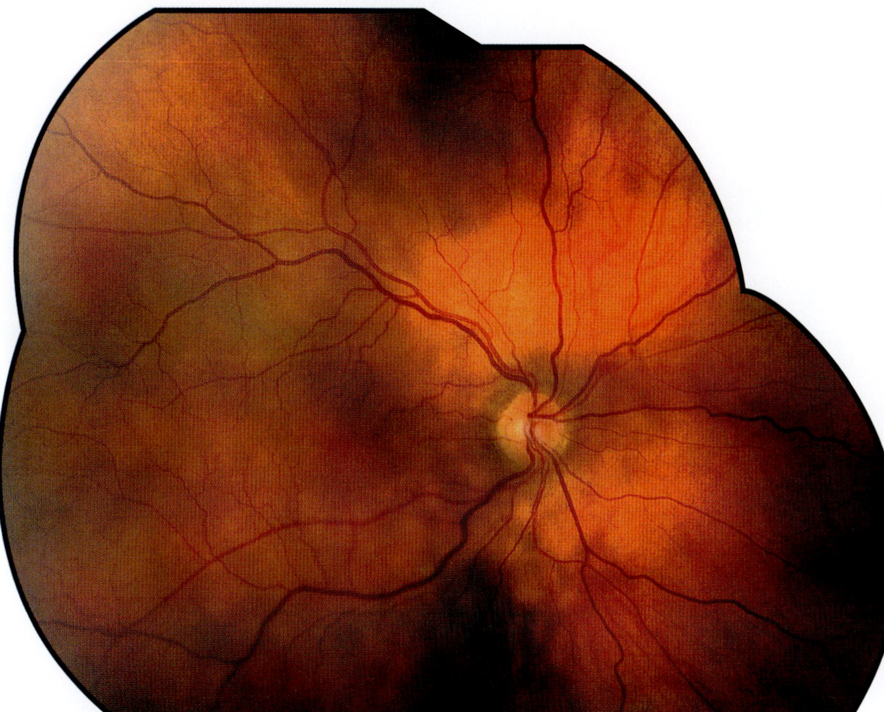

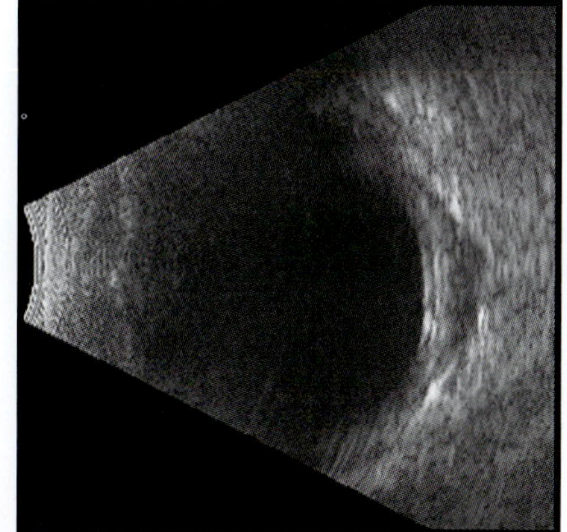

Ocular ultrasonography depicts the extrascleral infiltration.

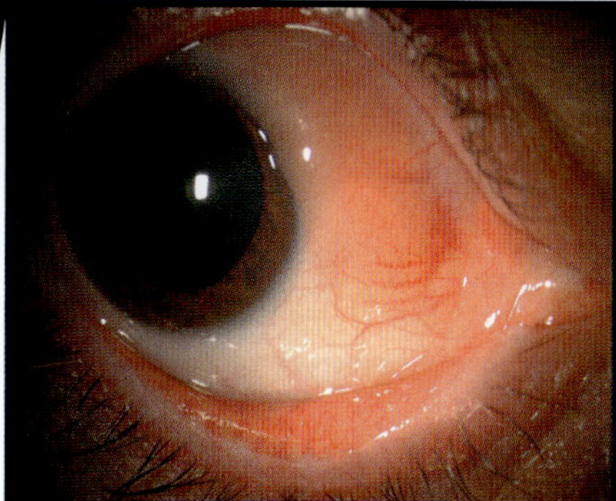

The conjunctiva manifests a "salmon patch" lymphoid infiltrate. Biopsy at this site confirmed mucosal-associated lymphoid tissue (MALT) lymphoma.

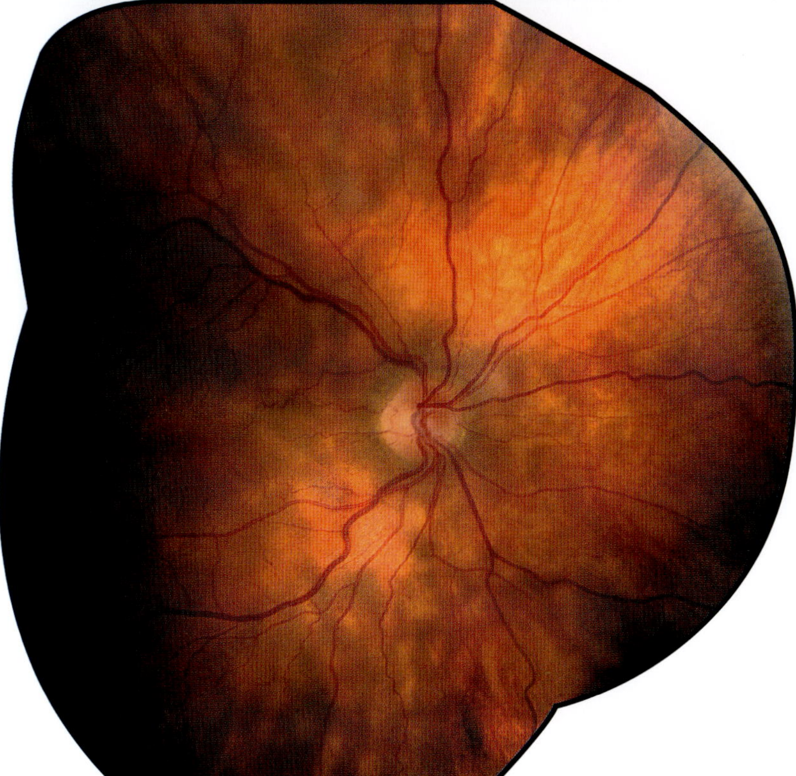

Diffuse choroidal infiltration of the right eye (pre-treament) with classic subtle yellow choroidal infiltrates suggestive of lymphoma.

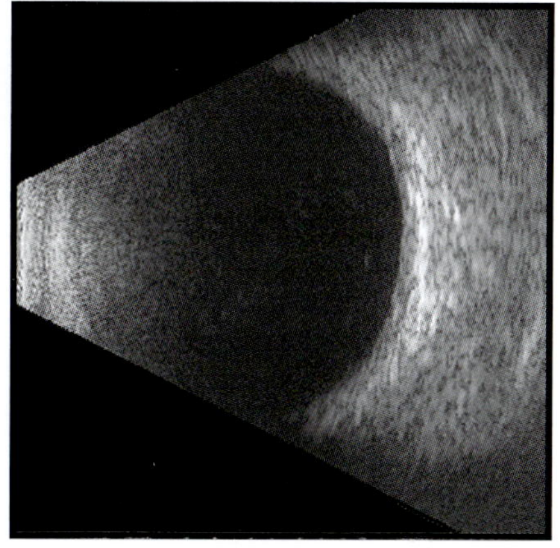

Following radiotherapy, ocular ultrasonography shows marked regression of the mass.

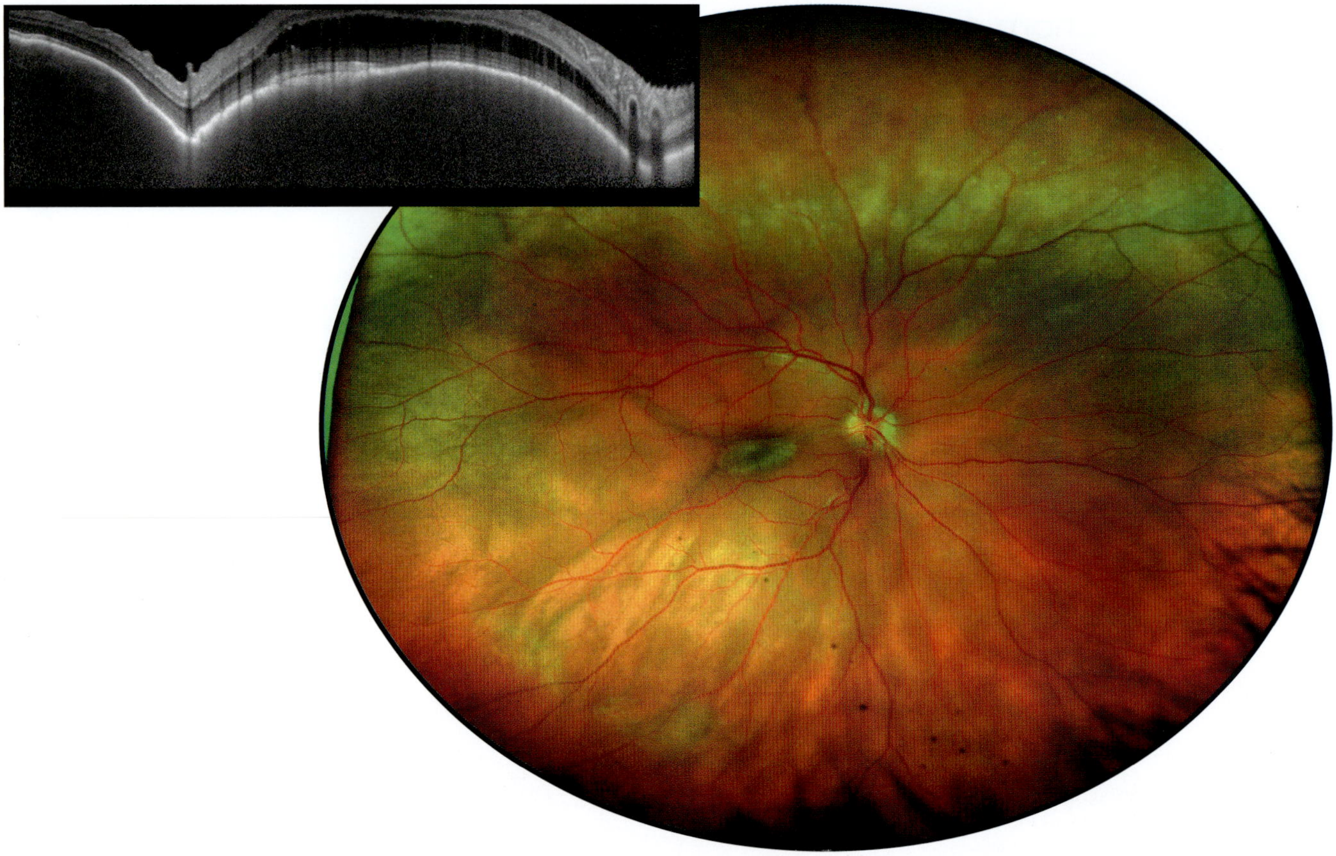

35-year-old male with unilateral vision loss from widespread choroidal lymphoma with direct extraocular extension. Enhanced depth imaging OCT reveals massive choroidal thickening with subretinal and intraretinal fluid.

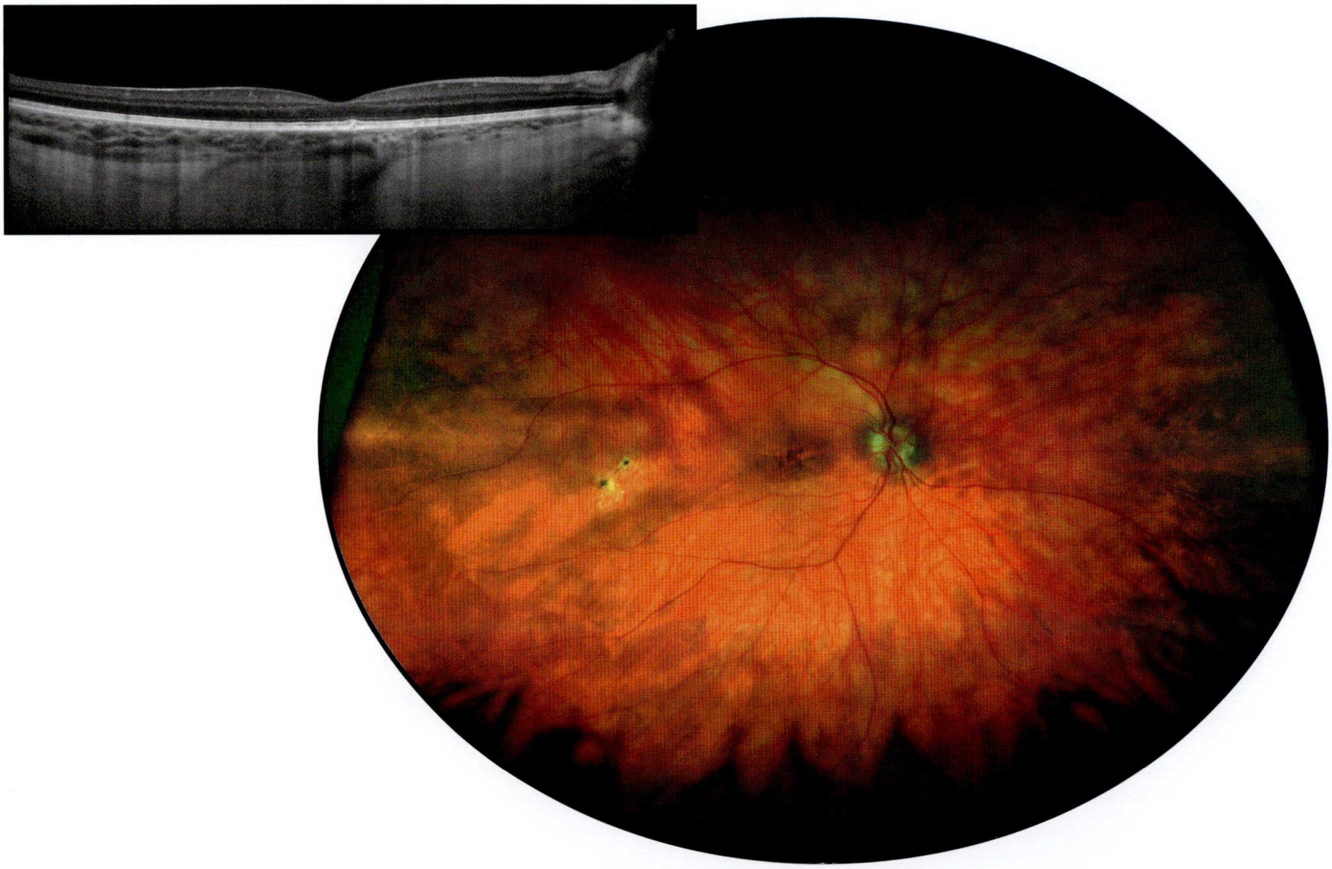

Following multiple sessions of external beam radiotherapy there is total resolution of choroidal infiltration. EDI OCT reveals near-normal choroidal thickness with neurosensory retinal reattachment. Residual pigmentary changes are evident at the macula. *Images courtesy of Dr. John Sorenson*

Tumors of the Optic Disc

Melanocytoma of the Optic Disc

A melanocytoma of the optic nerve appears to be a variant of a choroidal nevus instead located in the optic disc or anywhere else in the uveal tract. It is generally dark brown or black in color and composed histopathologically of deeply pigmented, round to oval cells with small round unifying nuclei. Most melanocytomas do not cause significant visual impairment. As the edge of the melanocytoma is subject to the development of choroidal neovascularization, with resultant serosanguineous detachment, there is a small risk of significant visual compromise. The natural course of the melanocytoma is generally favorable. There is a slight growth potential. Those lesions that experience more dramatic increase in size should be suspected of having malignant transformation and enucleation should be considered.

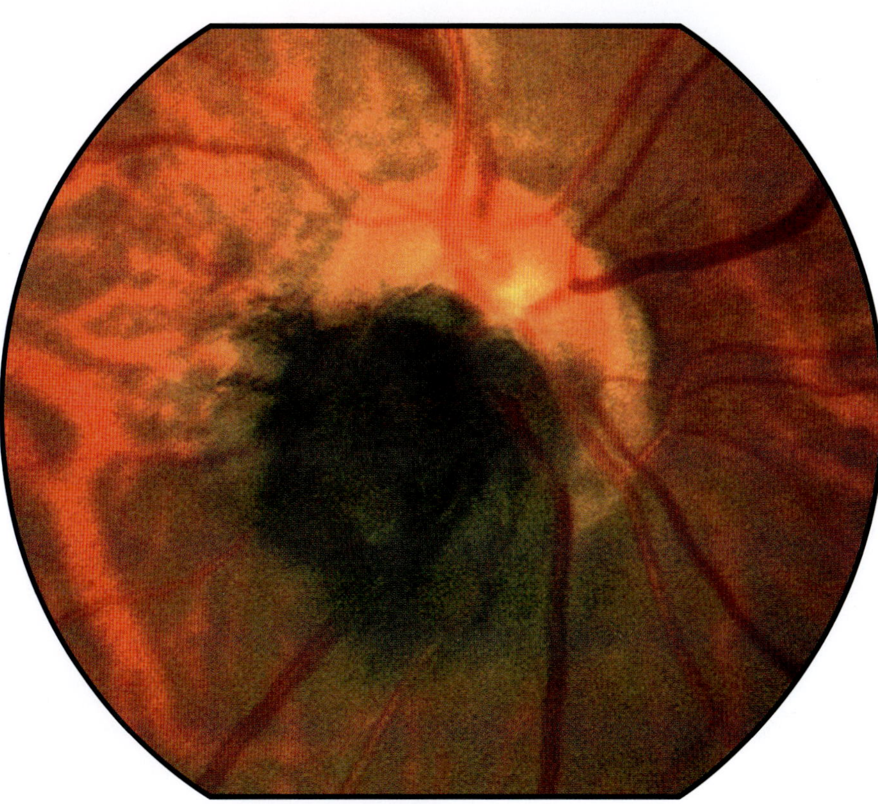

Melanocytomas are benign, densely pigmented tumors that are usually located at the optic nerve head. These lesions vary in size from a small dot of pigment to a large lesion which covers the disc and extends into the vitreous.

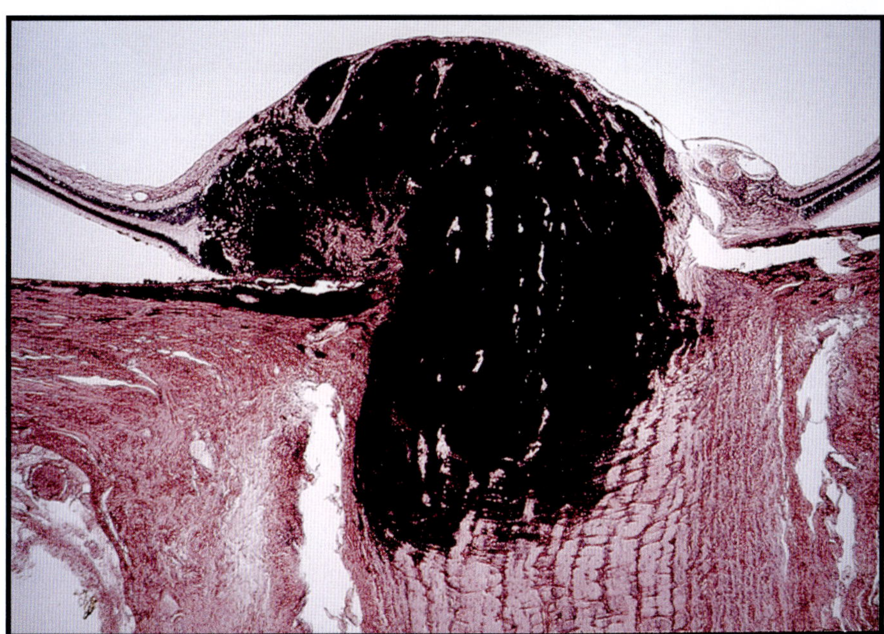

Histopathologic appearance of a melanocytoma involving the optic nerve head, peripapillary retina, and the retrobulbar optic nerve. The eye was enucleated because of a suspected malignant melanoma.

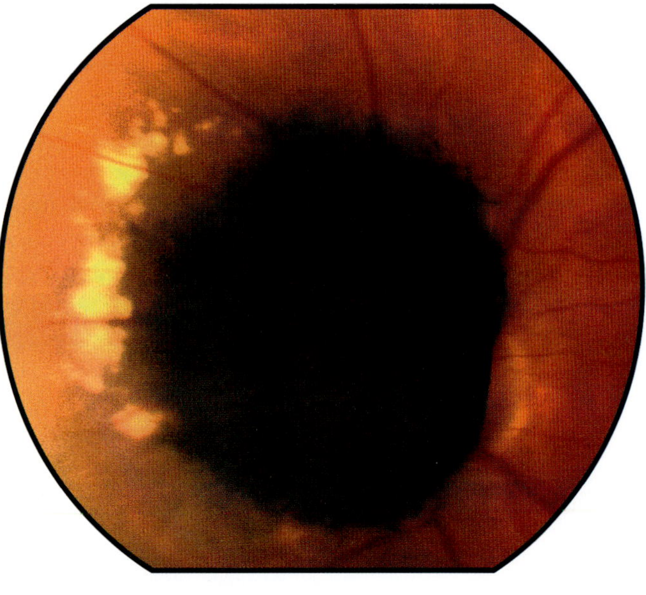

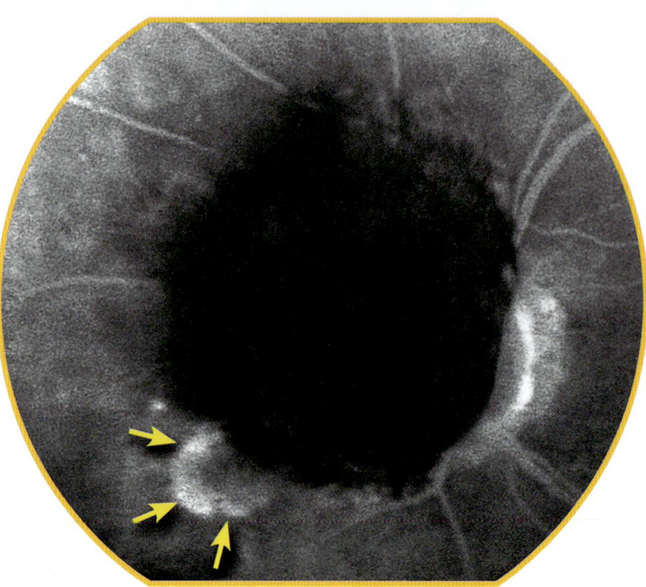

This patient with a melanocytoma was followed for 22 years and developed choroidal neovascularization (CNV) at the inferior margin of the tumor showing hyperfluorescence on the fluorescein study *(arrows)*.

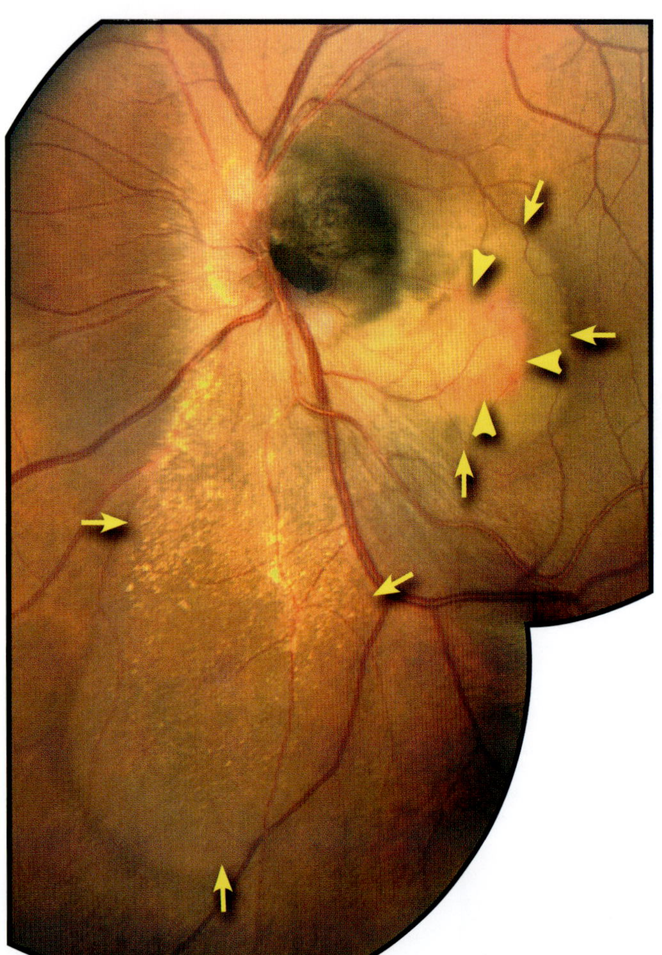

This melanocytoma of the optic nerve is associated with juxtapapillary CNV which is contiguous with the tumor mass *(arrowheads)*. There is a detachment of the retina *(arrowheads)*. There is an associated gravitating neurosensory detachment *(arrows)* extending into the inferior retina due to subretinal fluid arising from the CNV. *Courtesy of Dr. Kourous Rezaei*

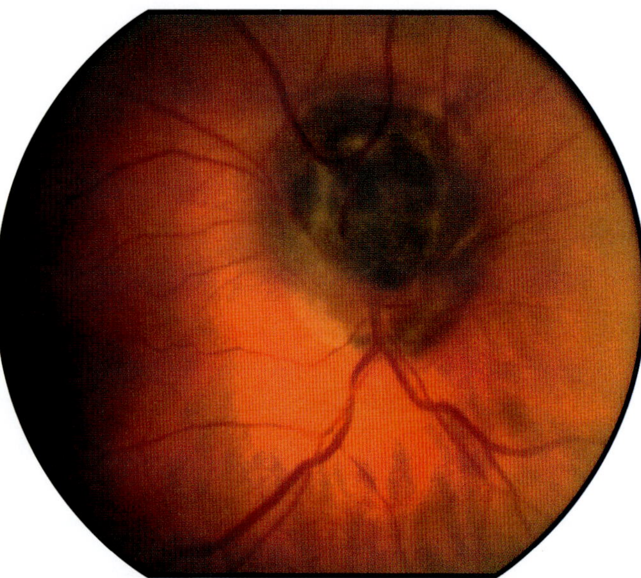

This patient has an RPE adenoma of the optic nerve, which can mimic a melanocytoma. The diagnosis was confirmed by histopathology. It may be very difficult to differentiate an RPE adenoma clinically from a melanocytoma or melanoma. *Courtesy of Dr. Lee Jampol*

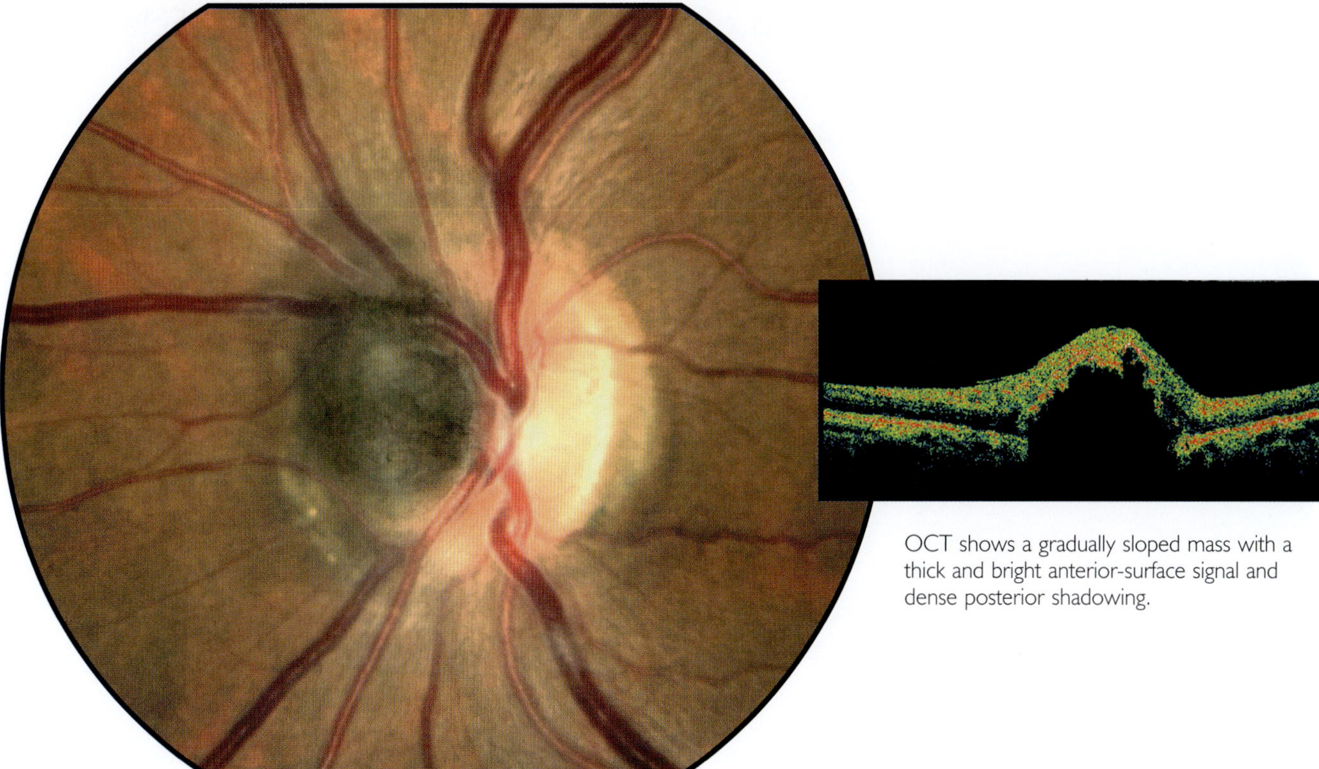

OCT shows a gradually sloped mass with a thick and bright anterior-surface signal and dense posterior shadowing.

Large optic disc melanocytoma with optic nerve infiltration and no light perception vision in a 13-year-old girl.

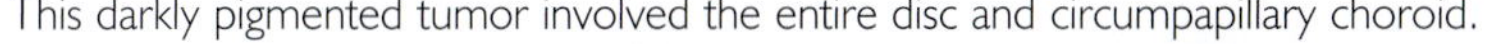

This darkly pigmented tumor involved the entire disc and circumpapillary choroid.

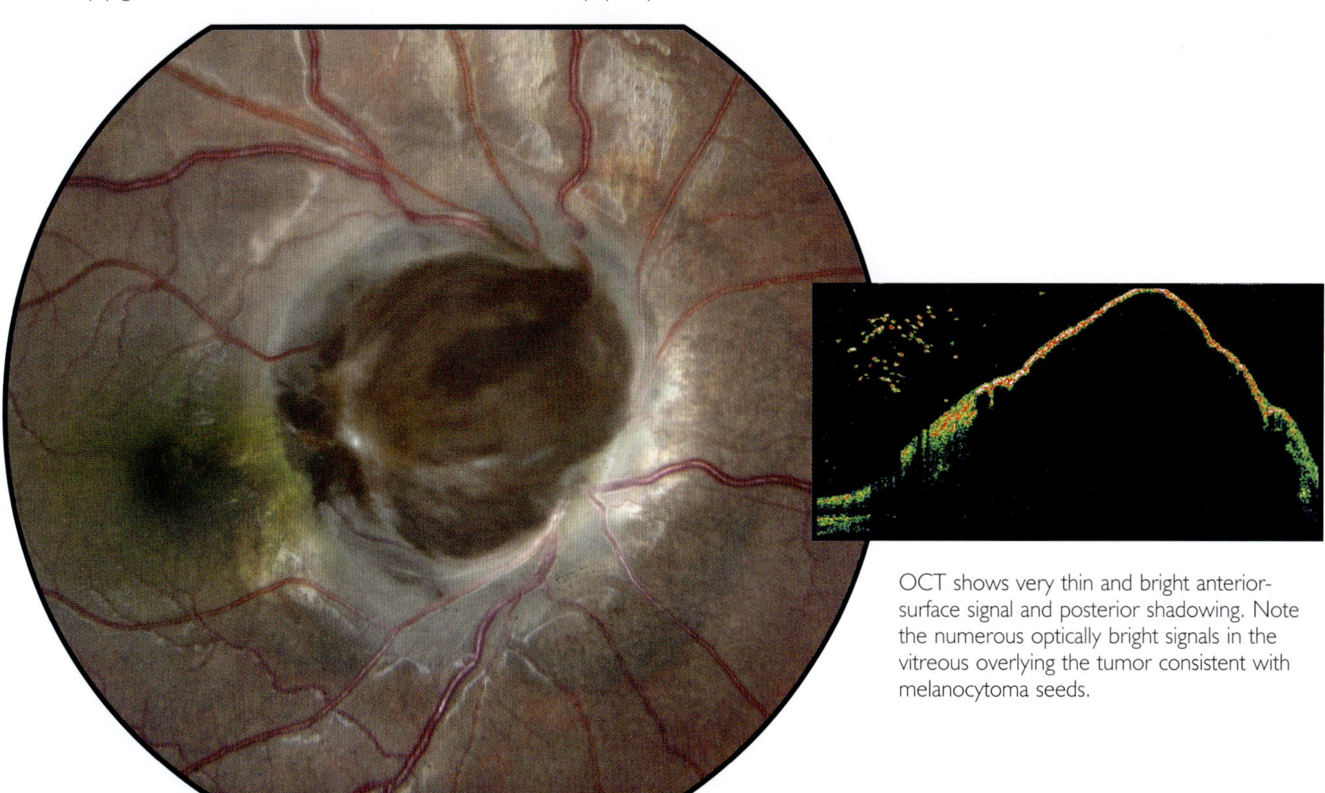

OCT shows very thin and bright anterior-surface signal and posterior shadowing. Note the numerous optically bright signals in the vitreous overlying the tumor consistent with melanocytoma seeds.

Growth of Astrocytic Hamartomas of the Optic Nerve in Tuberous Sclerosis

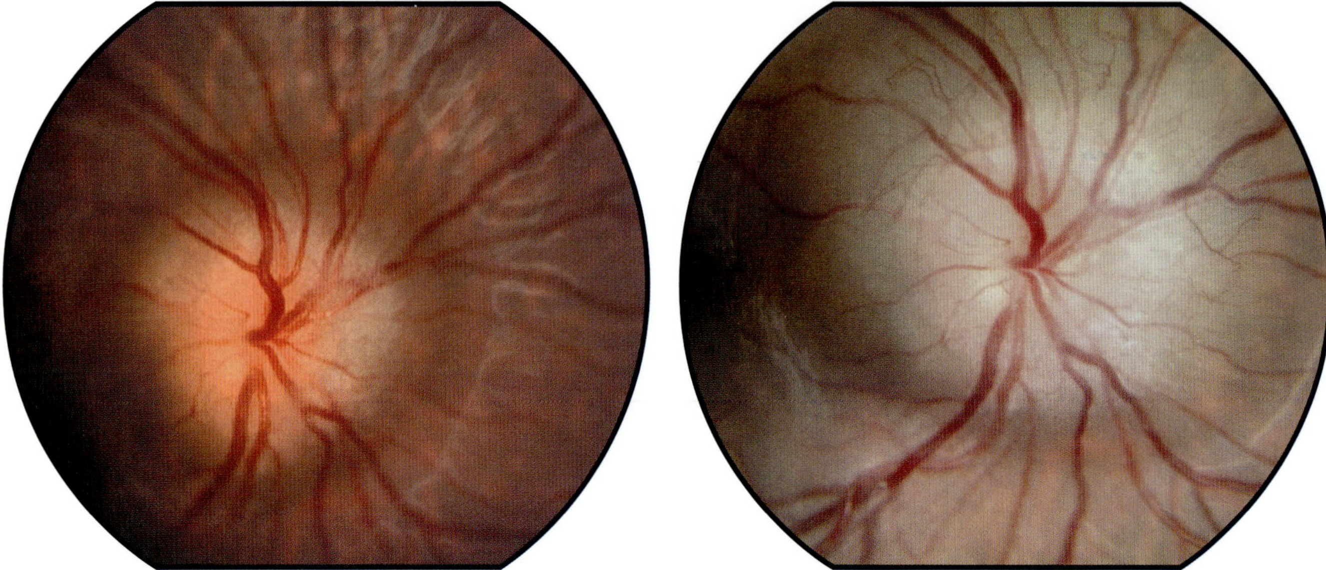

The astrocytic hamartoma involving the disc in this patient with tuberous sclerosis showed progressive enlargement.

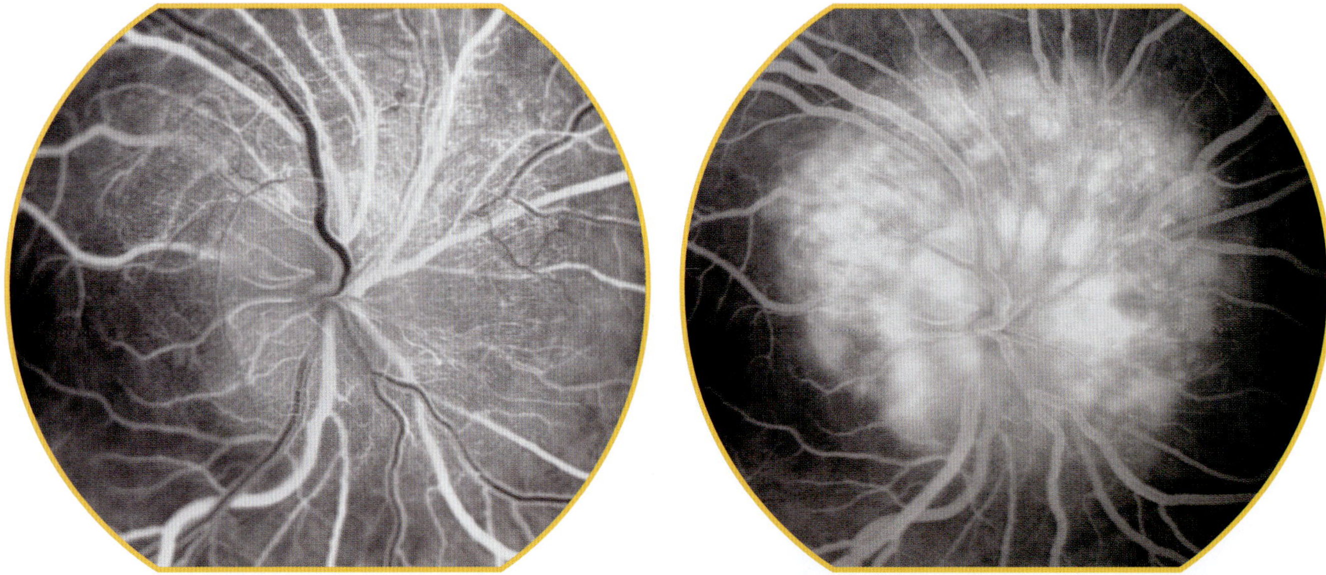

The fluorescein angiogram shows the marked vascular nature of the lesion.

The OCT shows marked shadowing from the calcific components of the lesion as well as retinal thickening from the tumor itself.

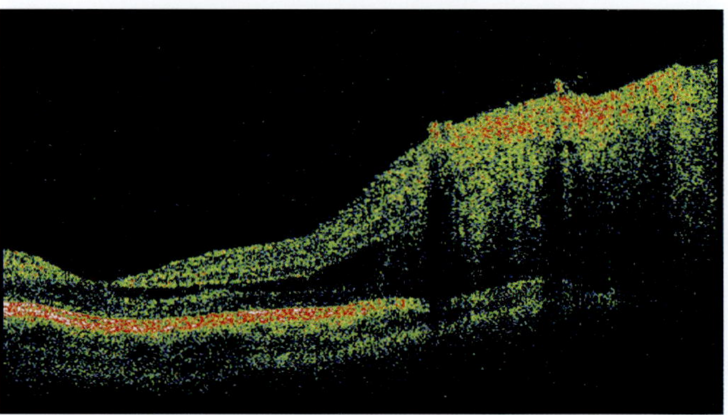

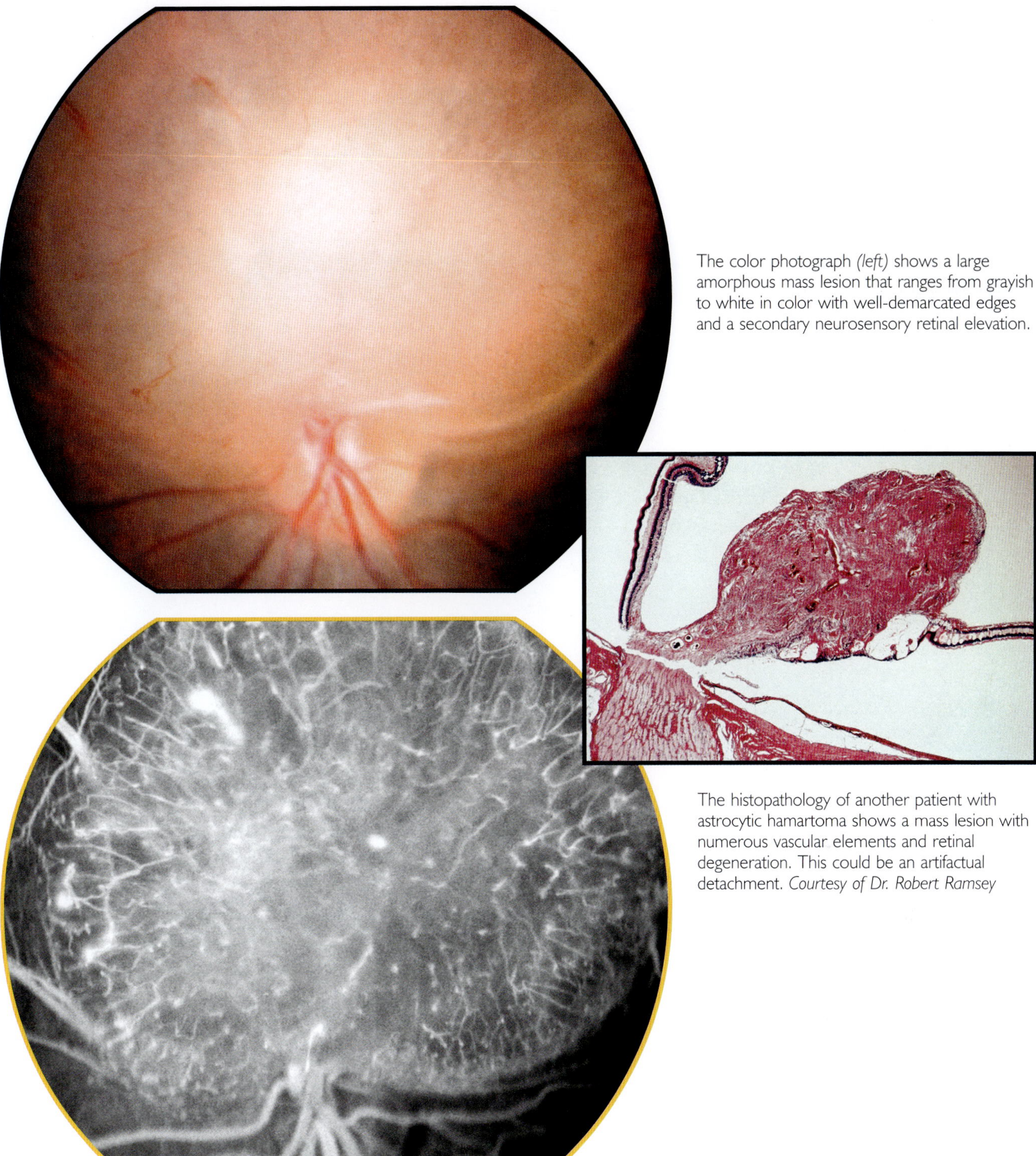

The color photograph *(left)* shows a large amorphous mass lesion that ranges from grayish to white in color with well-demarcated edges and a secondary neurosensory retinal elevation.

The histopathology of another patient with astrocytic hamartoma shows a mass lesion with numerous vascular elements and retinal degeneration. This could be an artifactual detachment. *Courtesy of Dr. Robert Ramsey*

The fluorescein angiogram shows numerous small capillaries throughout the mass lesion. *Fundus images courtesy of Drs. Paul Henkind and Joseph Walsh*

Lymphoma of the Optic Nerve

This 57-year-old white female with non-Hodgkin lymphoma presented with no light perception in both eyes. There was a markedly swollen optic nerve head, cherry-red spot, and vascular non-perfusion of most of the retina. On FA, capillary non-perfusion with attenuated and disrupted blood vessels was noted for 360°.

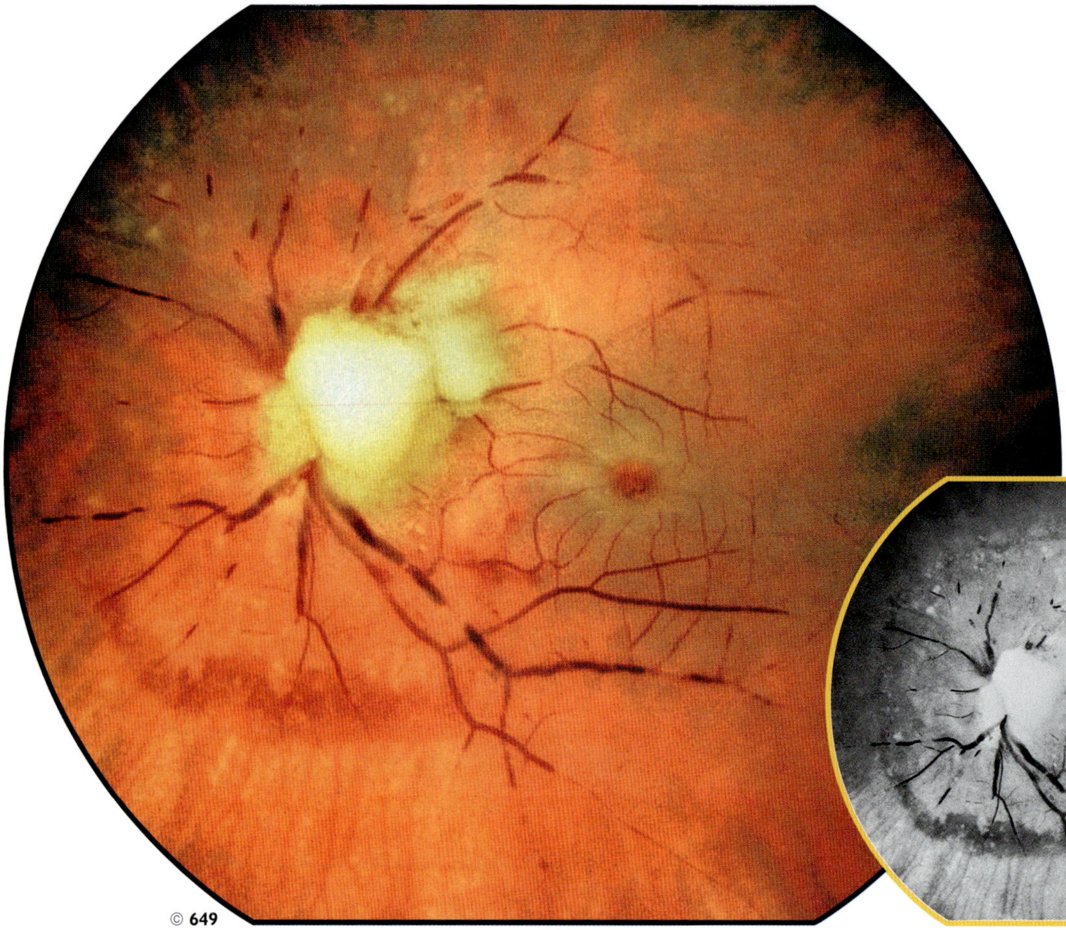

© 649

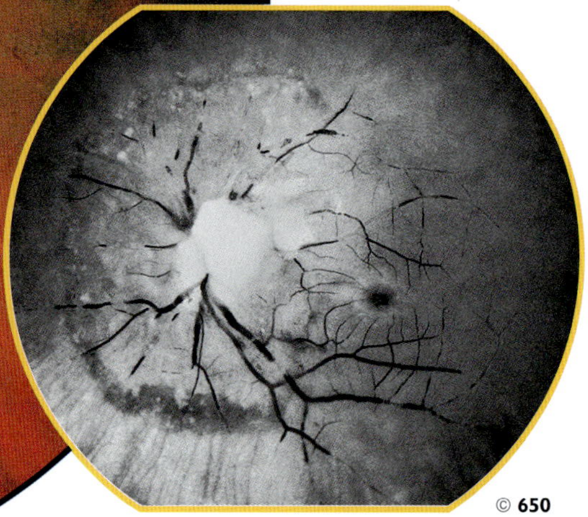

© 650

© 651

© 652

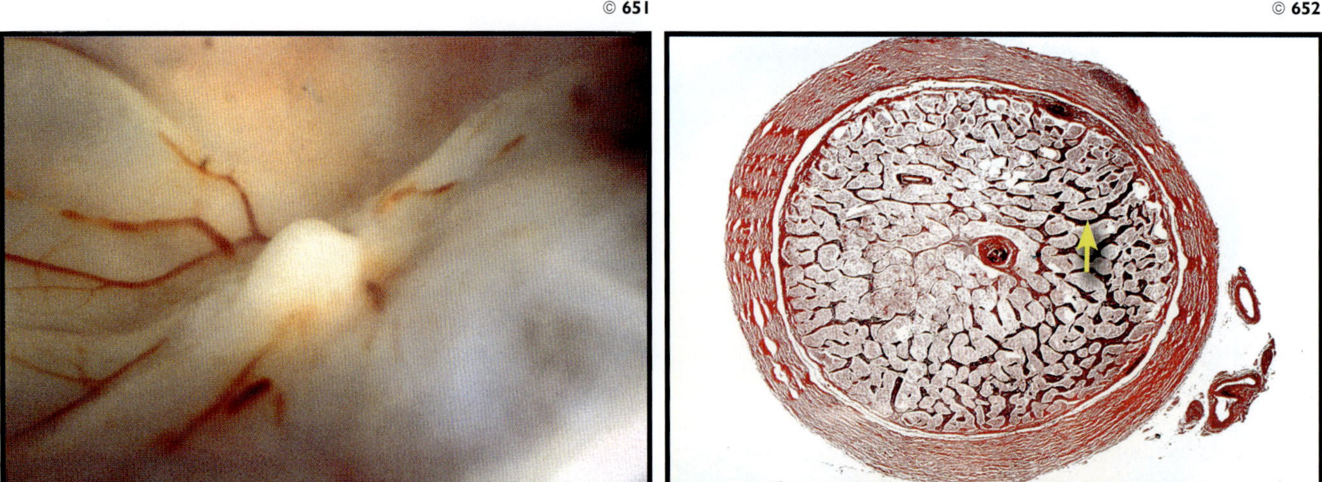

This lymphoma patient expired due to sepsis. Gross examination of the left eye reveals a markedly swollen optic nerve head. Hemorrhage and occluded retinal vessels are noted throughout the fundus on histopathology *(left image)*. Light microscopy reveals tumor invasion of the optic nerve *(right image, arrow)*.

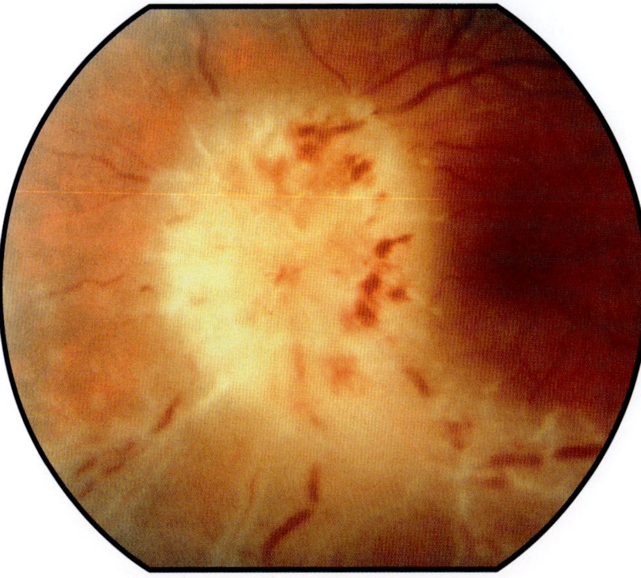

Lymphoma infiltration of the optic nerve is seen here with tumor cells thickening the nerve and obliterating retinal vessels.

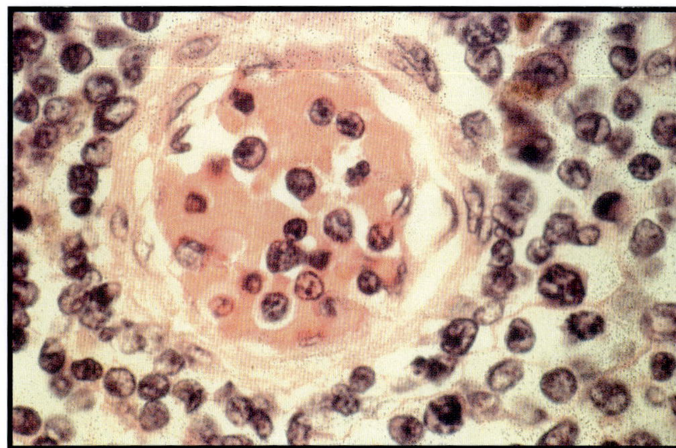

The histopathology shows tumor cells within and surrounding a blood vessel.

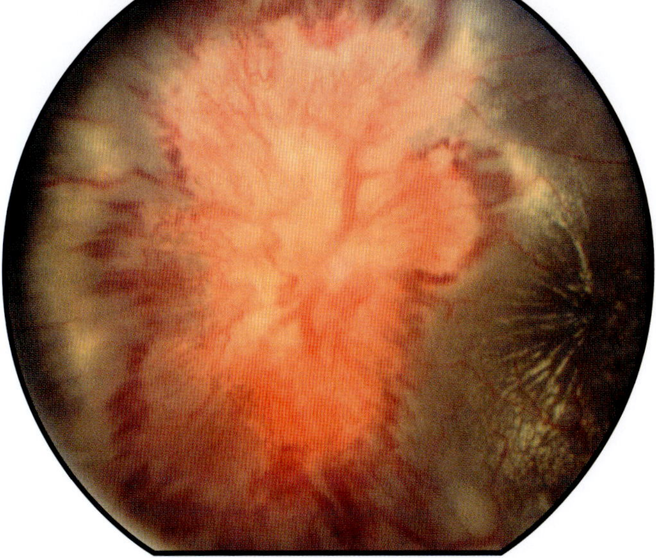

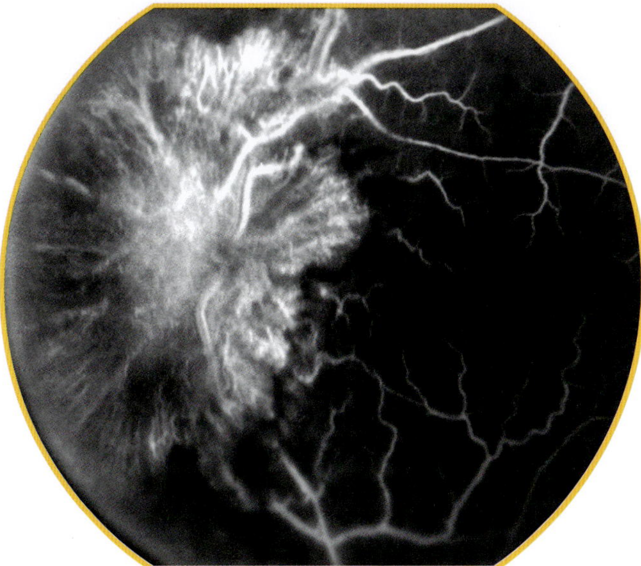

This patient with lymphoma had massive hemorrhagic infiltration of the optic nerve with tumor cells. The fluorescein angiogram shows a prominent vascularity to the infiltration at the nerve head.

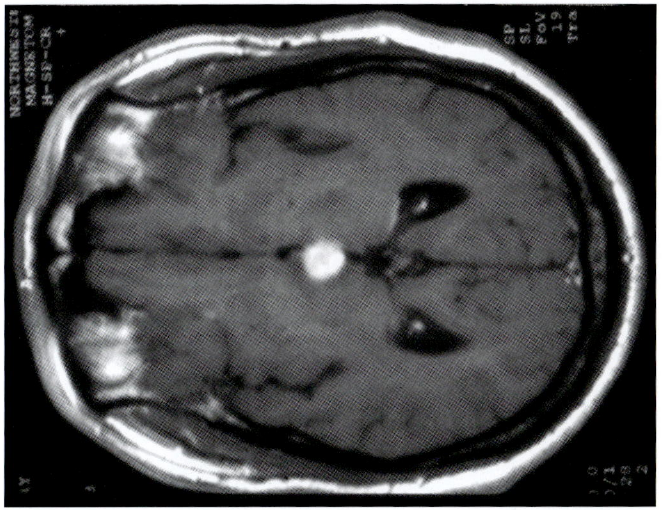

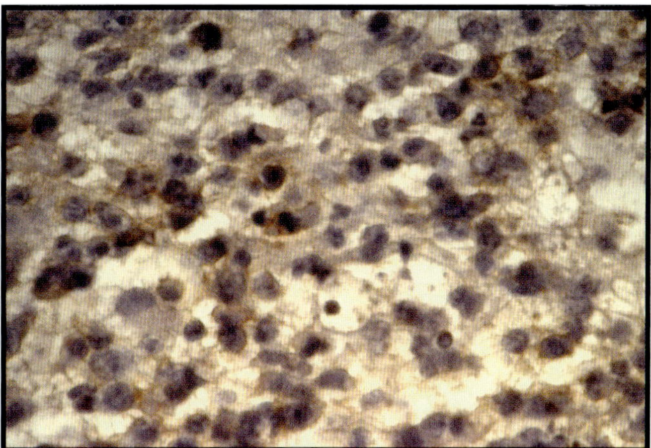

The computed tomography shows a white lesion consistent with lymphoma. The histopathology obtained on brain biopsy shows the typical lymphoma cells with minimal cytoplasm and nucleoli abnormalities. *Courtesy of Dr. Lee Jampol*

Hemangioblastoma (Capillary Hemangioma) of the Optic Disc

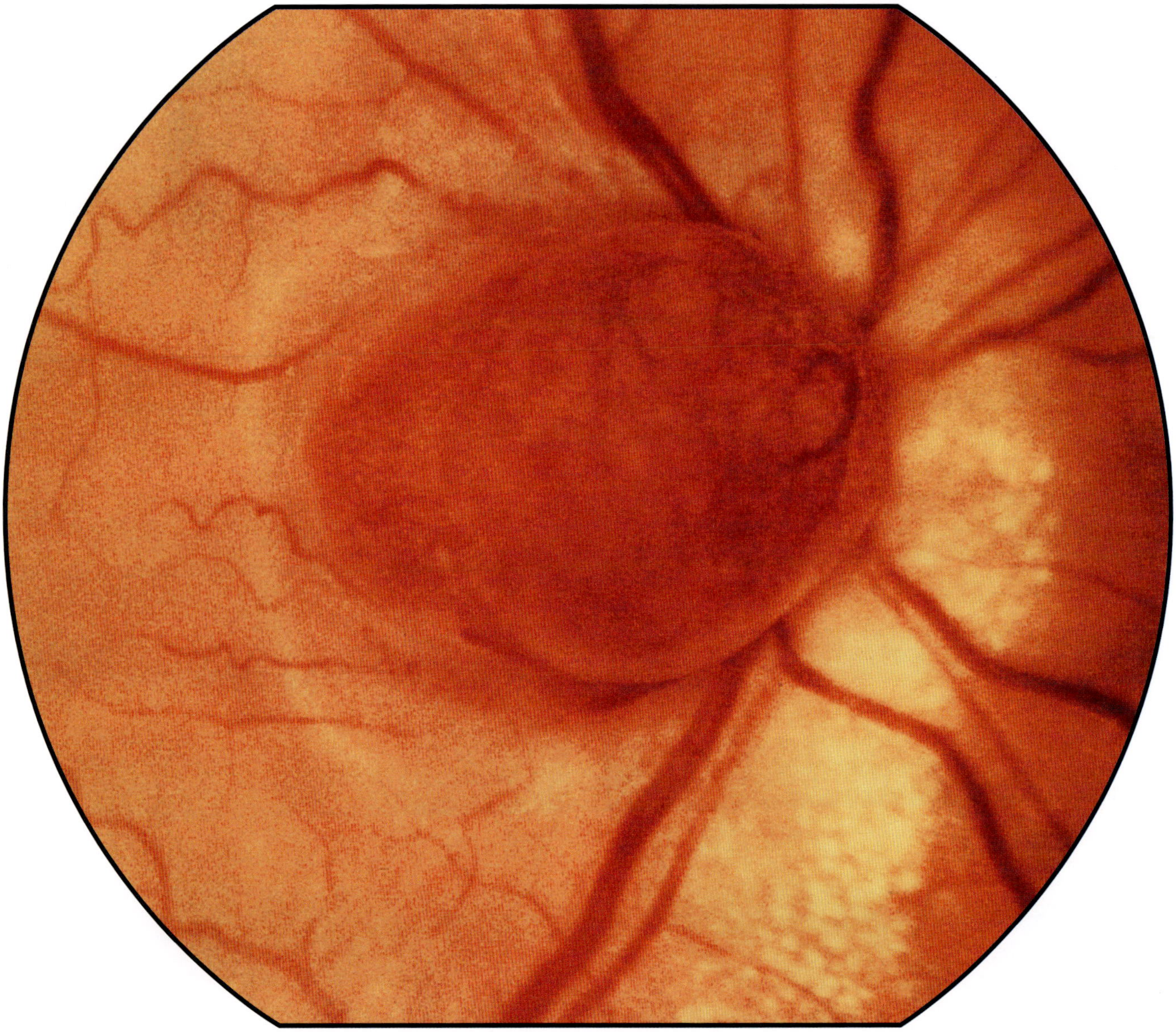

Optic disc hemangioblastomas can be so large that they can obscure the entire optic nerve. *Courtesy of Johnny Justice*

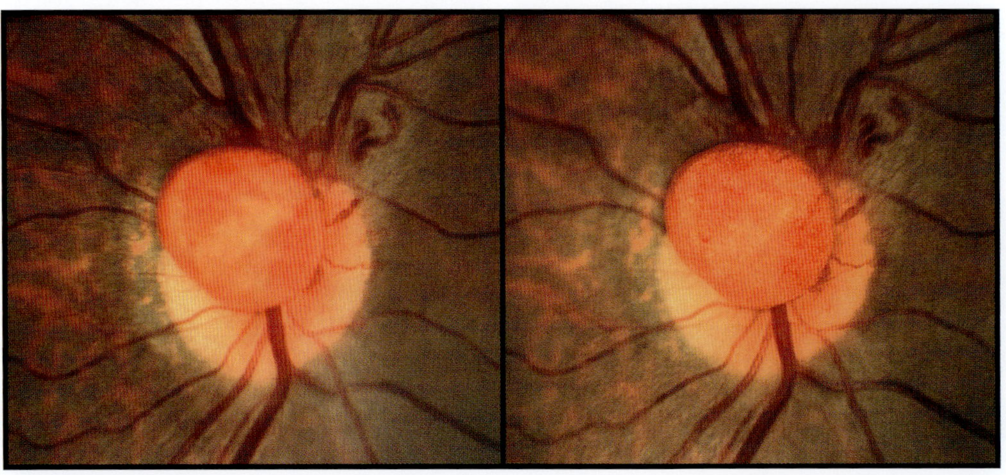

Another patient demonstrates a hemangioblastoma at the optic disc *(stereo pair)*. *Courtesy of Dr. Mark Williams*

Optic Disc Hemangioblastoma with Macular Schisis

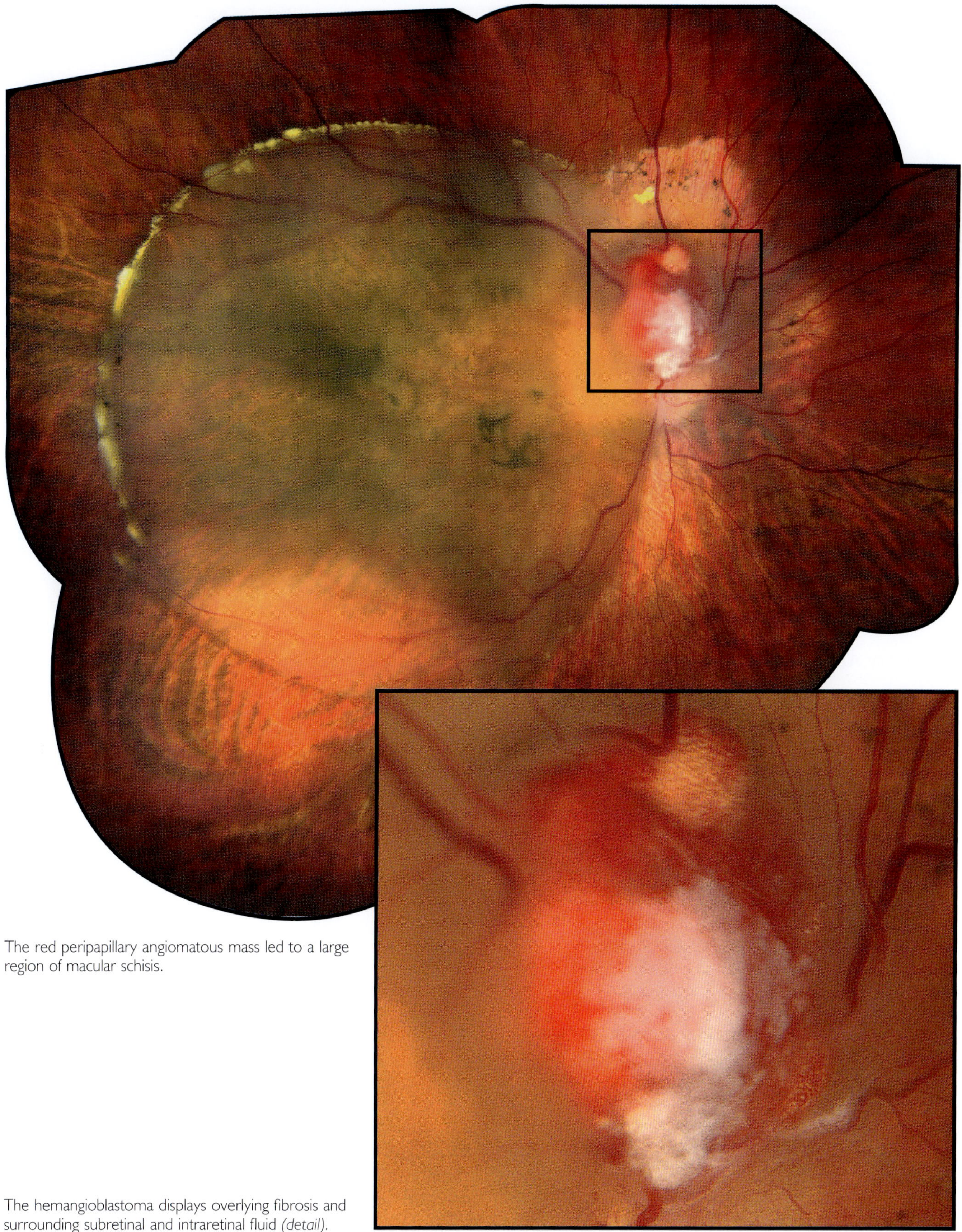

The red peripapillary angiomatous mass led to a large region of macular schisis.

The hemangioblastoma displays overlying fibrosis and surrounding subretinal and intraretinal fluid *(detail)*.

Optic Disc Hemangioblastoma with Macular Hole

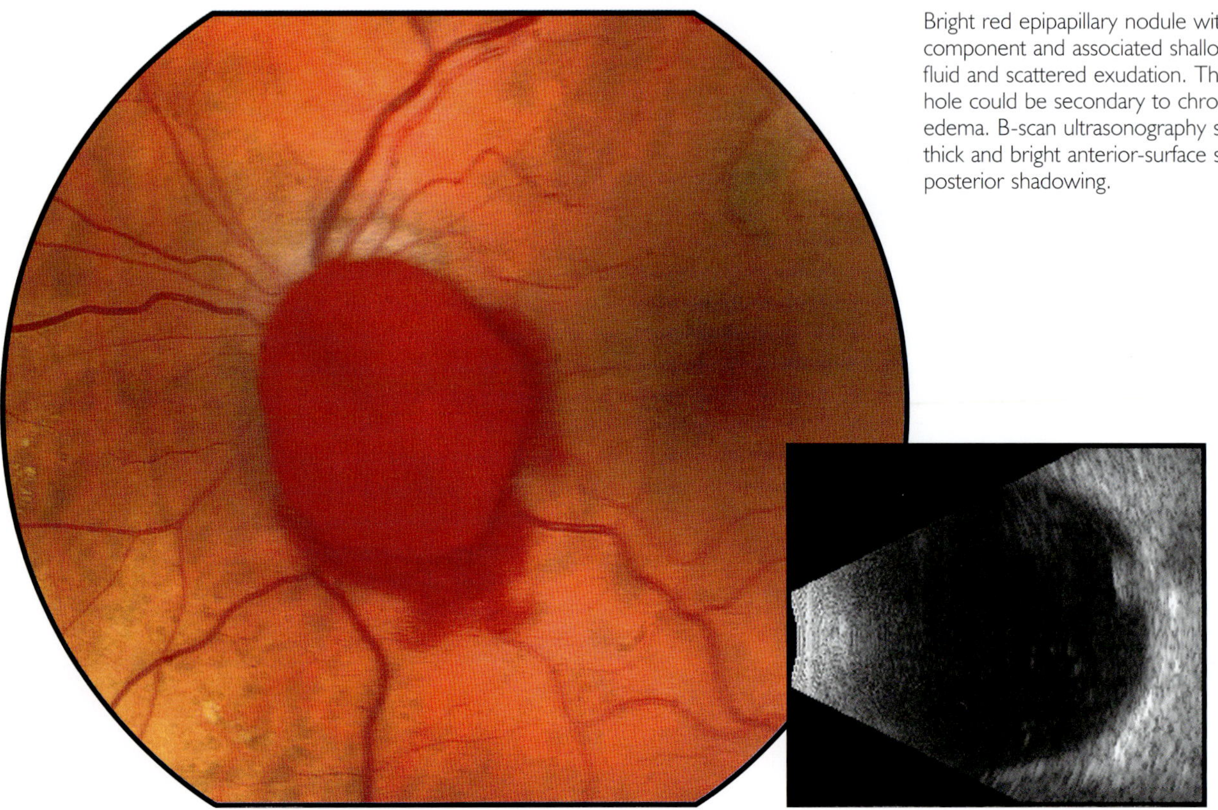

Bright red epipapillary nodule with flat rim component and associated shallow subretinal fluid and scattered exudation. The macular hole could be secondary to chronic cystoid edema. B-scan ultrasonography shows a thick and bright anterior-surface signal and posterior shadowing.

Cavernous Hemangioma

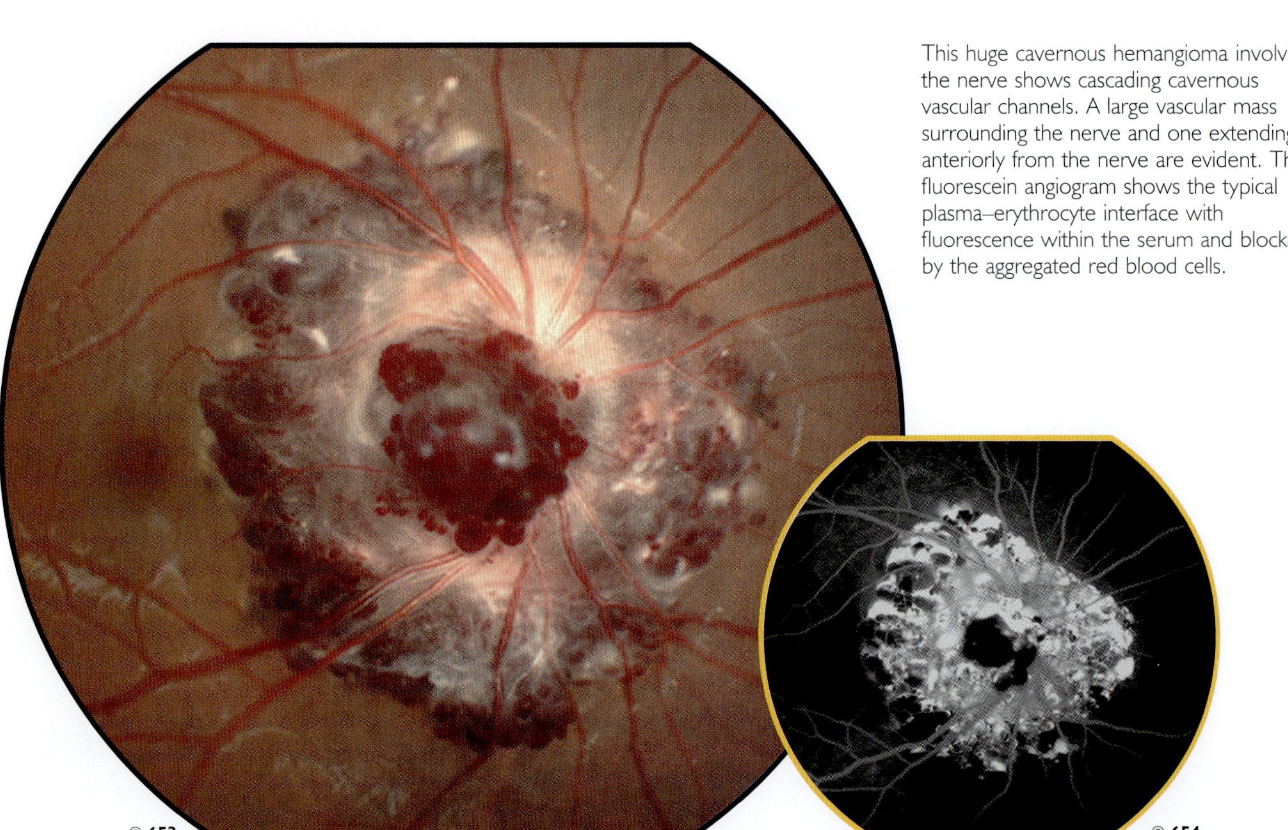

This huge cavernous hemangioma involving the nerve shows cascading cavernous vascular channels. A large vascular mass surrounding the nerve and one extending anteriorly from the nerve are evident. The fluorescein angiogram shows the typical plasma–erythrocyte interface with fluorescence within the serum and blockage by the aggregated red blood cells.

Metastasis to the Optic Disc

Optic Disc Metastasis in Breast Cancer

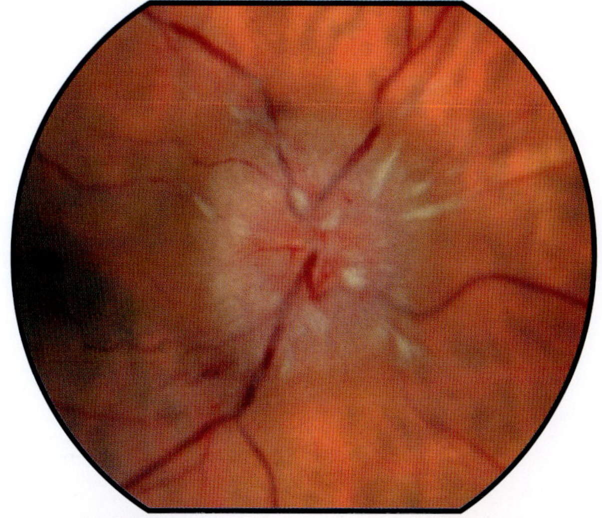

In these three cases, optic nerve metastasis from breast cancer has produced a white swollen nerve head and intraretinal tumor extension with dilated retinal vessels. Breast and lung are the most common sources of optic nerve metastasis. *Courtesy of Dr. Jeffrey Shakin*

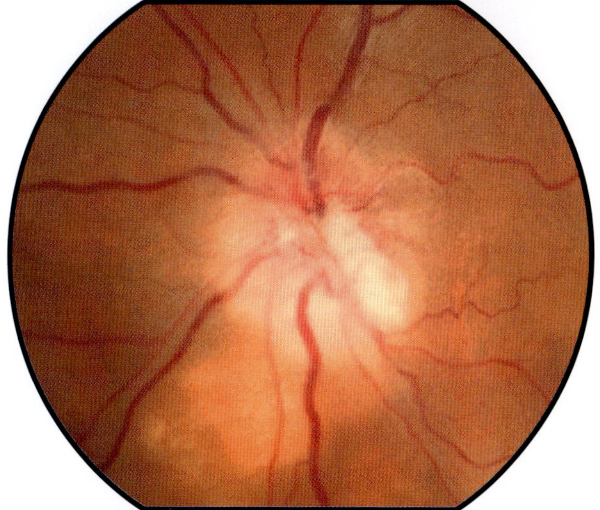

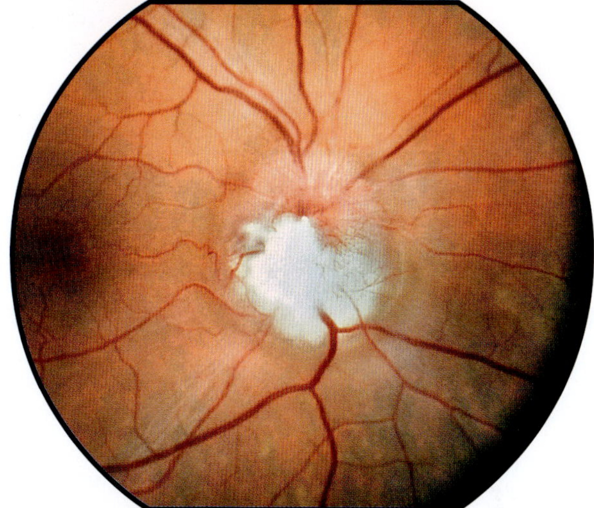

Optic Disc Metastasis in Lung Cancer

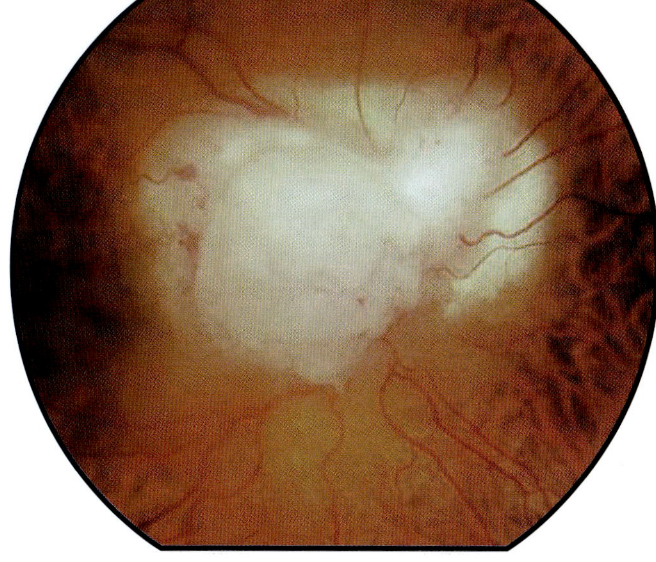

The optic disc is infiltrated with a yellow-white nodular, relatively avascular mass. Circumpapillary choroidal infiltration is noted.

Optic Disc Metastasis from Gastric Carcinoma

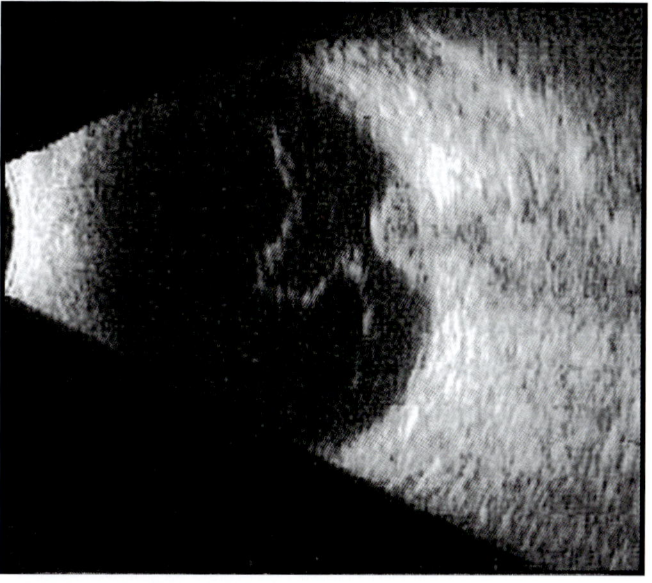

Ultrasonography of a suspected case of optic disc metastasis demonstrated a mass lesion involving the optic nerve which proved to be a gastric carcinoma.

Leukemia

The retinal findings in leukemia typically reflect the overall picture of anemia, leucocytosis and hyperviscosity with intraretinal hemorrhages and nerve fiber layer infarction. In some instances, white leukemic infiltration in the retina, optic disc, or choroid can be found, usually in the circumpapillary region.

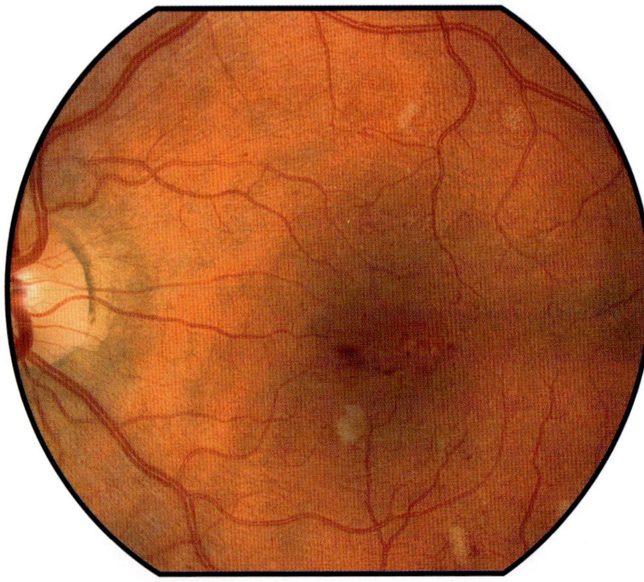

This patient with leukemia shows a microangiopathy in the central macular region with some hemorrhages, exudates, and a few cotton-wool spots.

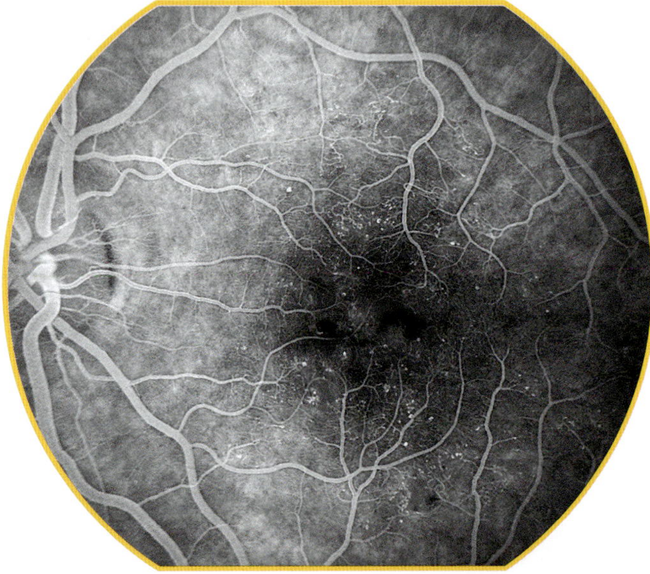

The fluorescein angiogram shows multiple microaneurysms and some areas of non-perfusion. This presentation very much resembles non-proliferative diabetic retinopathy.

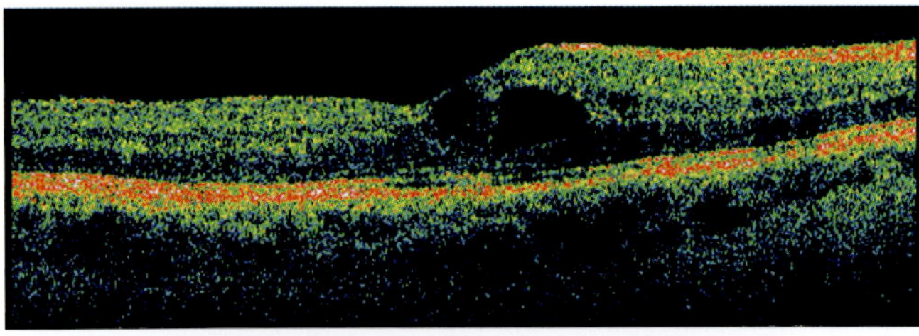

The OCT shows cystic change within the retina as a result of leakage from telangiectatic vessels and aneurysms involving the retinal circulation.

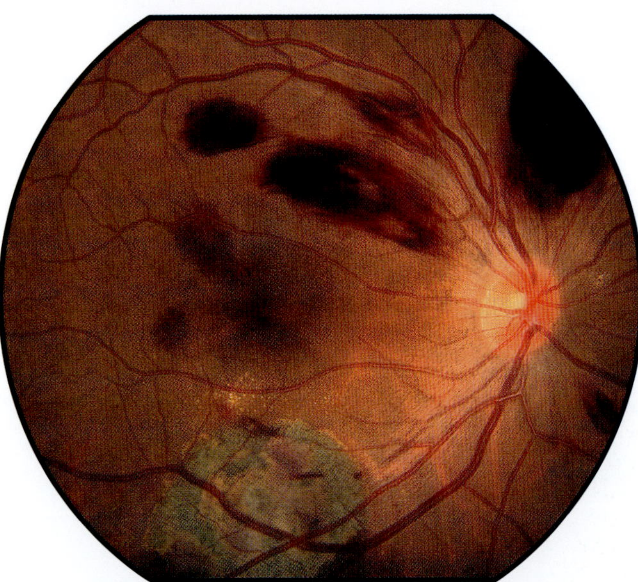

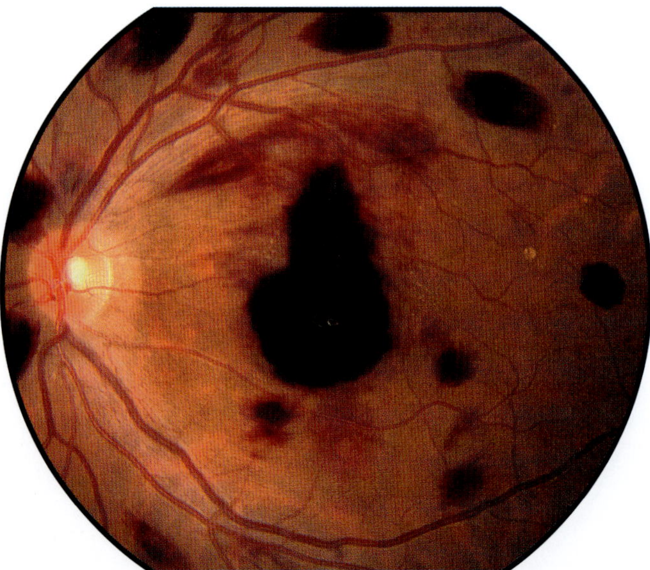

This patient with leukemia presented with a change in vision of the left eye more than the right with widespread hemorrhages, some with white centers. There are no clinically evident aneurysmal, telangiectatic, or ischemic changes. The left eye shows a large preretinal hemorrhage over the fovea. A similar hemorrhage in the right eye occurs superior to the disc. *Courtesy of Ophthalmic Imaging Systems, Inc.*

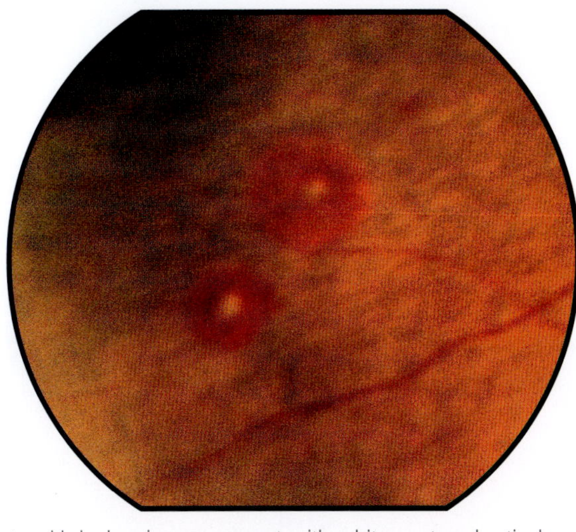

Patients with leukemia may present with white-centered retinal hemorrhages, so-called "Roth spots."

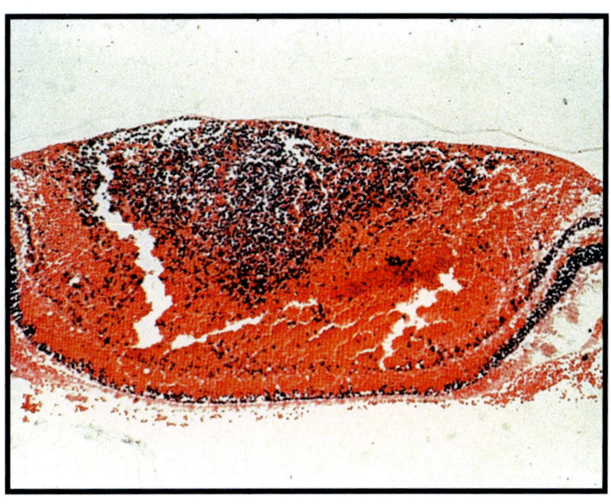

© 655

Histology shows that leukemic cells account for the white center of this hemorrhage.

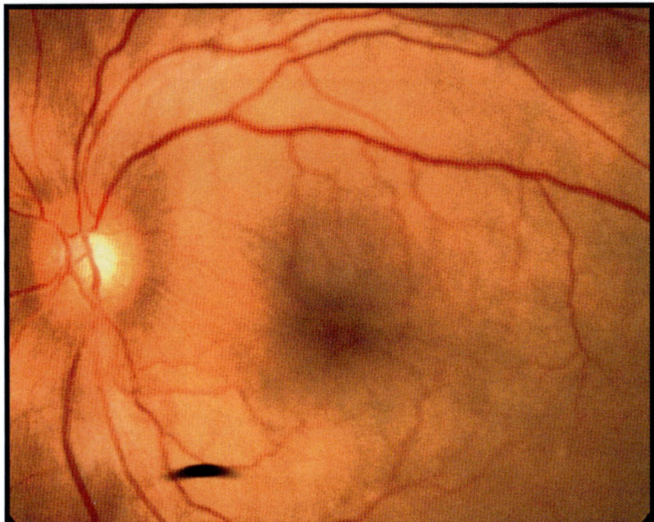

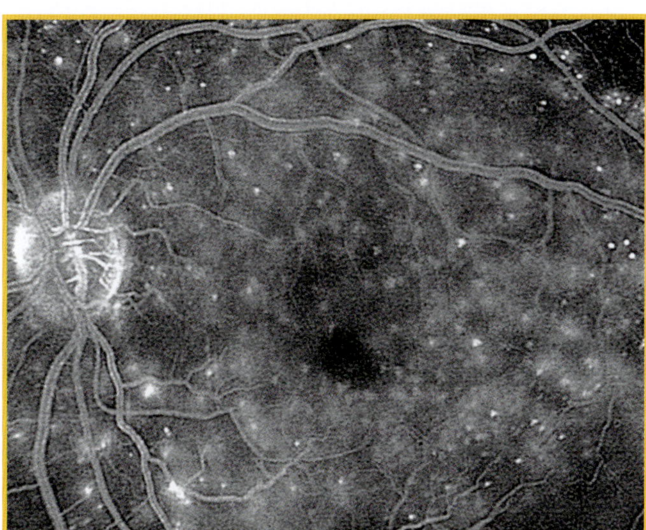

This patient with leukemia has a whitish-yellowish infiltration in the macula with a shallow neurosensory retinal detachment. Multifocal areas of leakage at the level of the RPE present a Harada-like exudative detachment from tumor infiltration of the choroid, inducing decompensation of the posterior blood–retinal barrier. *Courtesy of Dr. Richard Rosen*

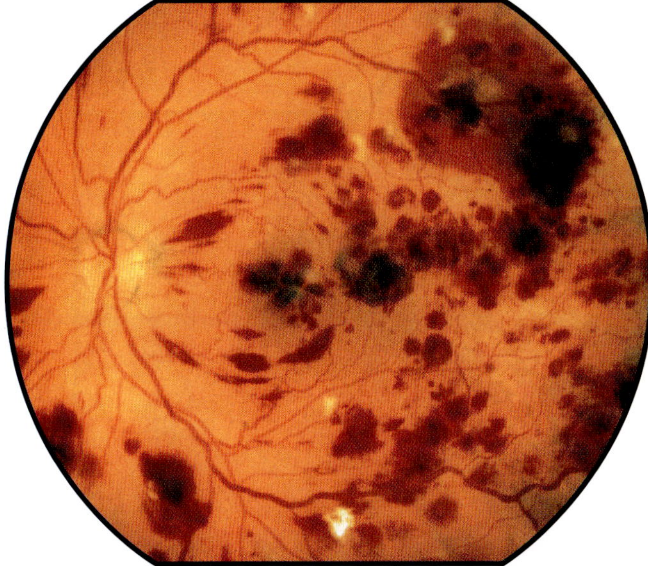

Leukemia in this patient has produced multiple vascular changes in the posterior fundus including various configurations of retinal hemorrhages and scattered cotton-wool spots.

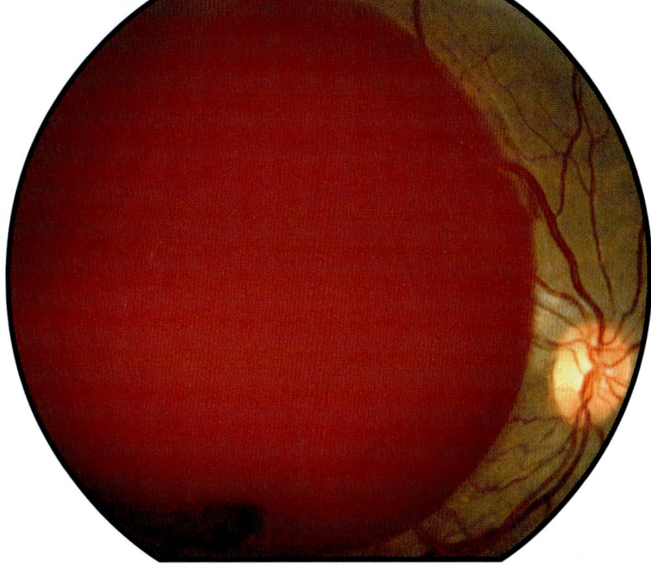

Note the massive pre-retinal hemorrhage in this patient with acute myelogenous leukemia.

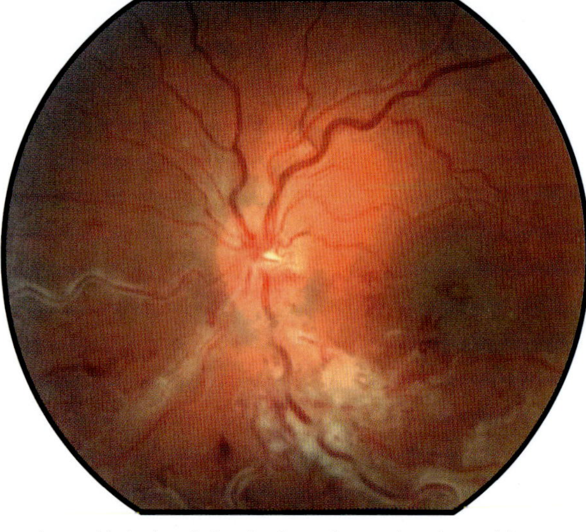

This patient with leukemia has both a microangiopathy and large-vessel involvement producing a frosted angiitis-like picture from tumor infiltration of retinal vessels.

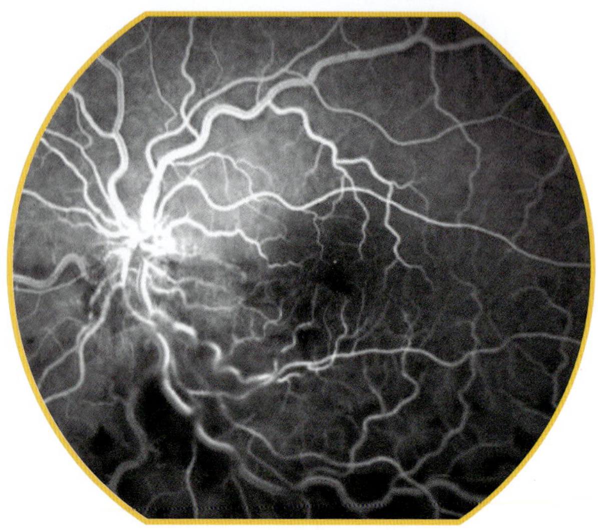

The fluorescein angiogram shows delayed filling of the choroidal circulation due to the tumor cell infiltration and some segmental stain of the veins.

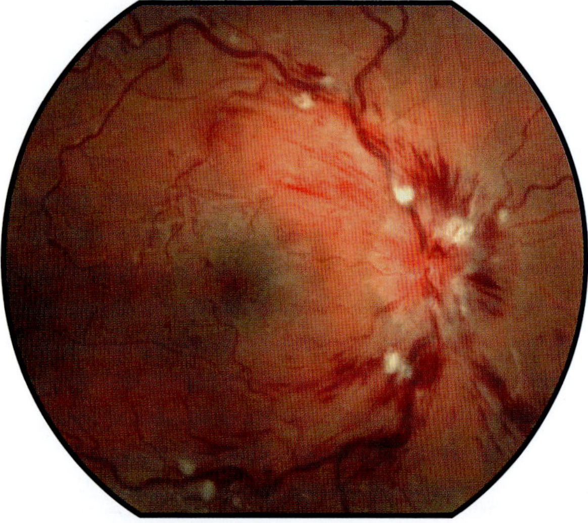

The fellow eye has more advanced changes with hemorrhages along the vascular arcades and optic nerve infiltration by the tumor.

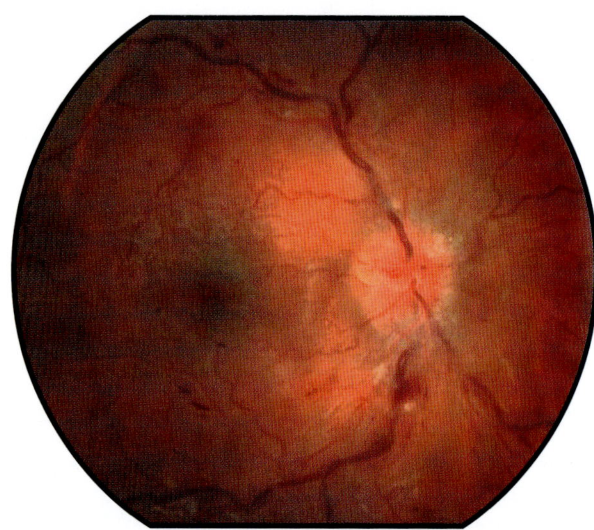

There has been improvement of the retinal vasculature and optic nerve and resolution of the hemorrhages and axoplasmic debris following chemotherapy.

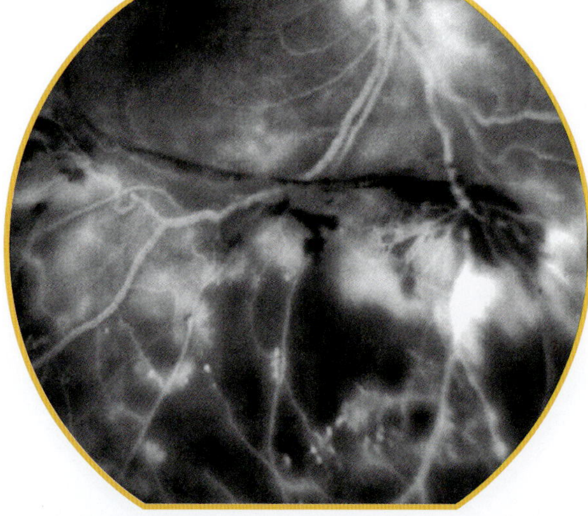

This patient with leukemia has more severe retinal vascular ischemic change with large areas of capillary non-perfusion and an exudative detachment of the inferior retina.

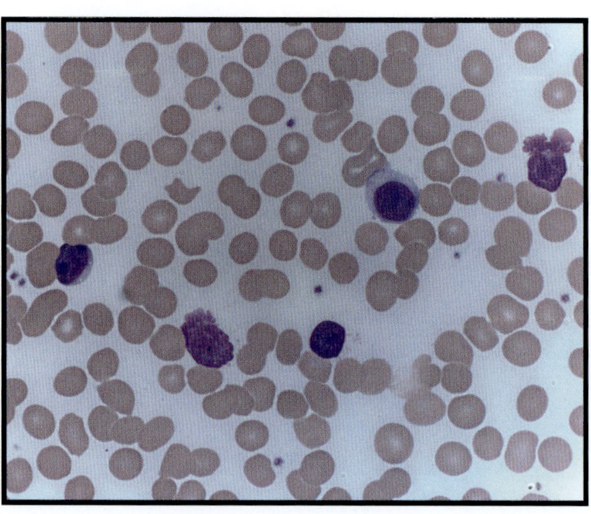

© **656**

The cytology demonstrates chronic lymphocytic leukemic cells.

Spectral Domain Optical Coherence Tomography of Intraocular Leukemia

Using enhanced depth imaging spectral domain OCT, the leukemic infiltration can be visualized in the choroid.

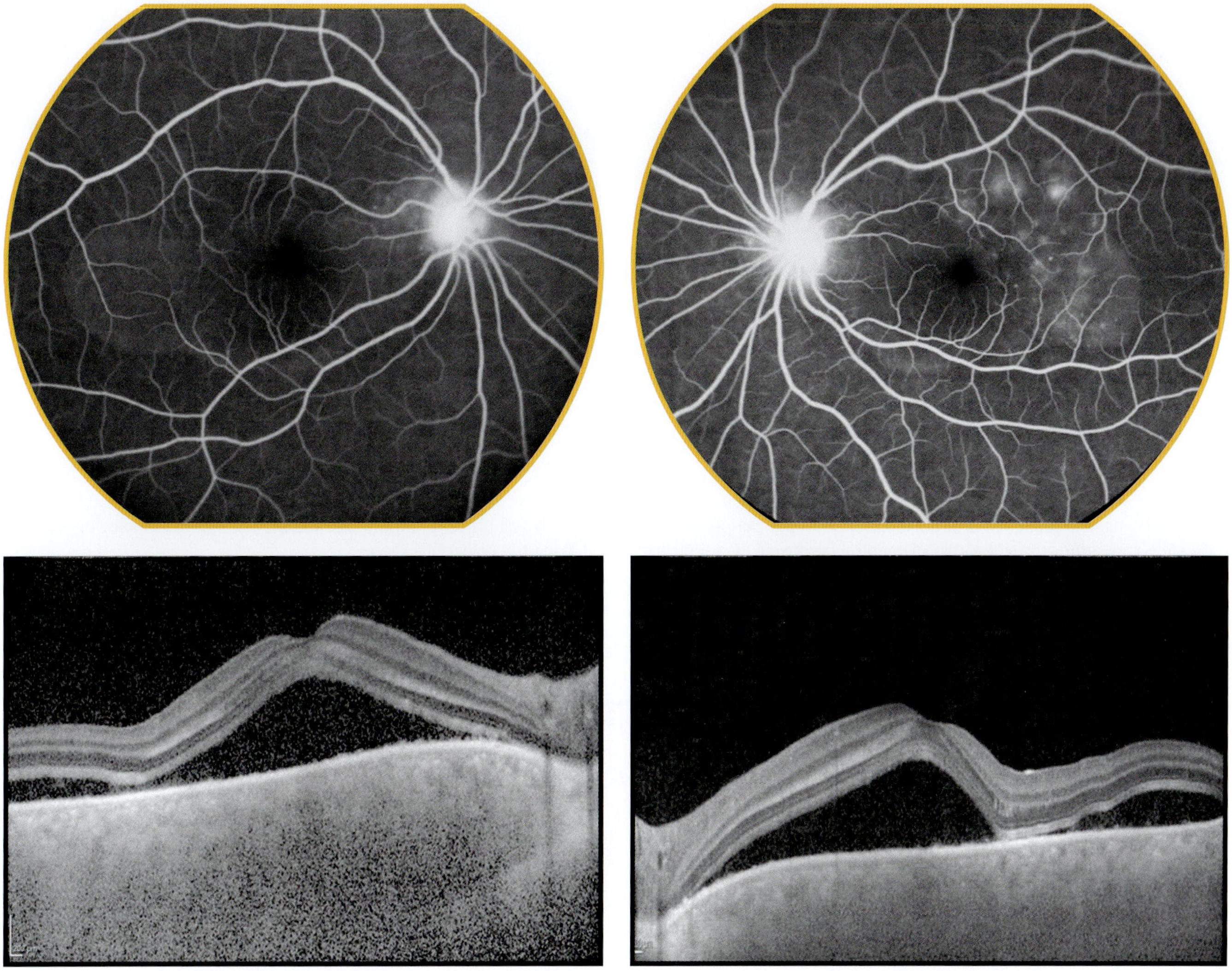

A young man with bilateral visual loss was found to have multifocal leaks on fluorescein angiography. Enhanced depth imaging OCT revealed massive thickening of the choroid with overlying serous retinal detachment. Systemic investigation demonstrated leukemia.

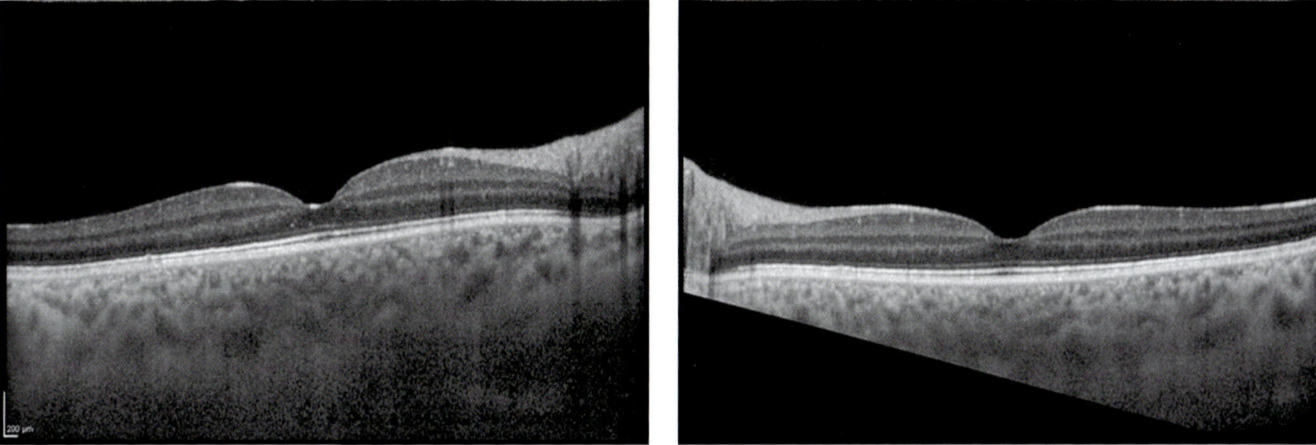

The same patient is shown following treatment with systemic chemotherapy. There is dramatic resolution of the serous detachments.

Perifoveal Ischemia with Leukemia

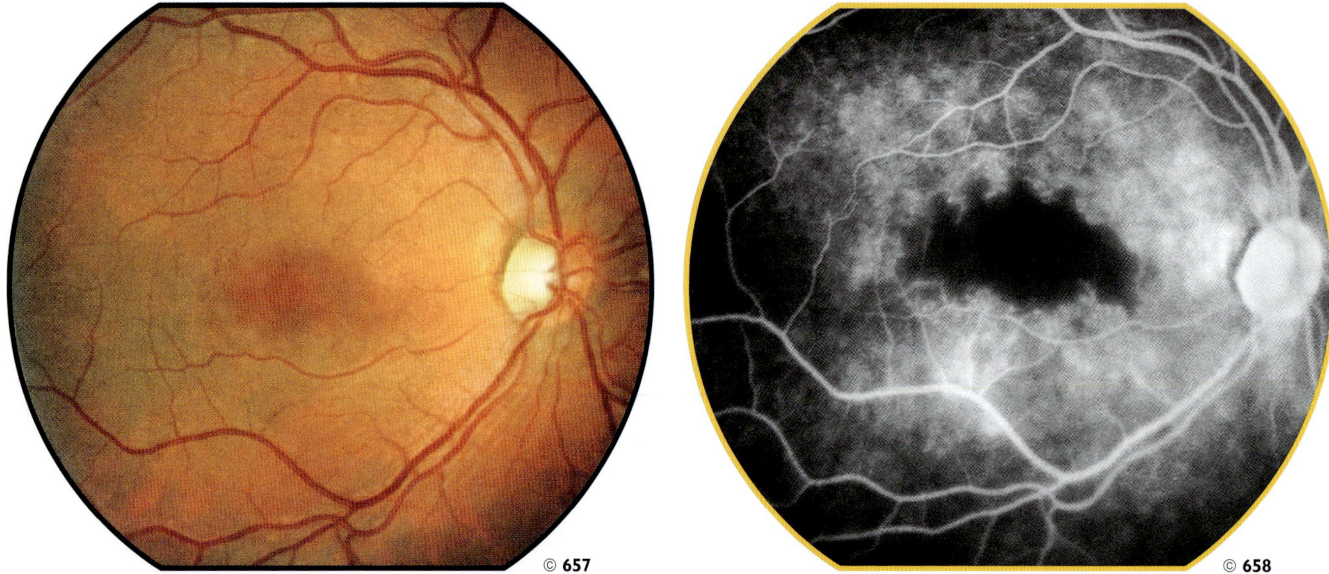

This patient with lymphocytic leukemia presents with permeability abnormalities of the macular circulation and a surrounding a zone of ischemia. Retinal ischemia and leukemia are more common in the peripheral fundus but rarely will present in the macula itself. The fluorescein angiogram shows the capillary non-perfusion in the central perifoveal area with expansion along the horizontal raphe.

Scattered Hemorrhages and Leukemia

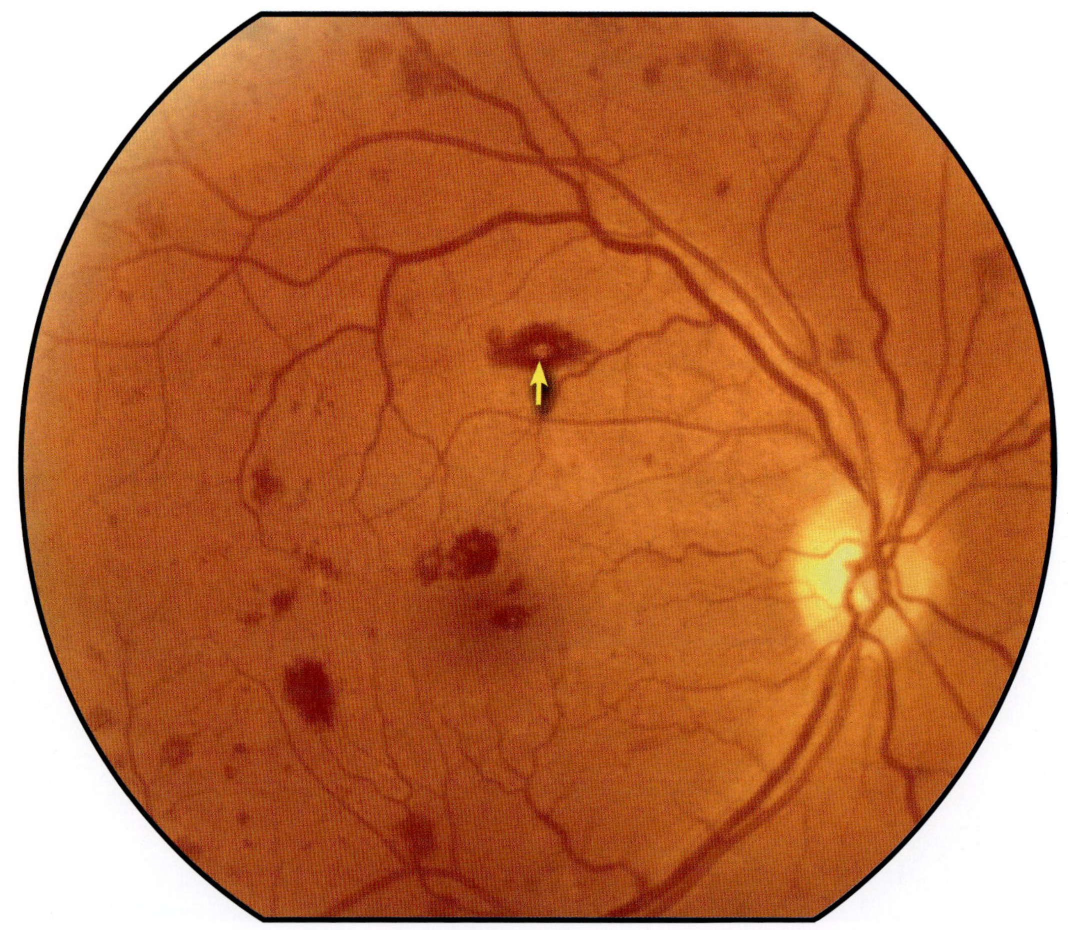

Multiple Roth spots are seen in this patient with leukemia *(arrow)*.

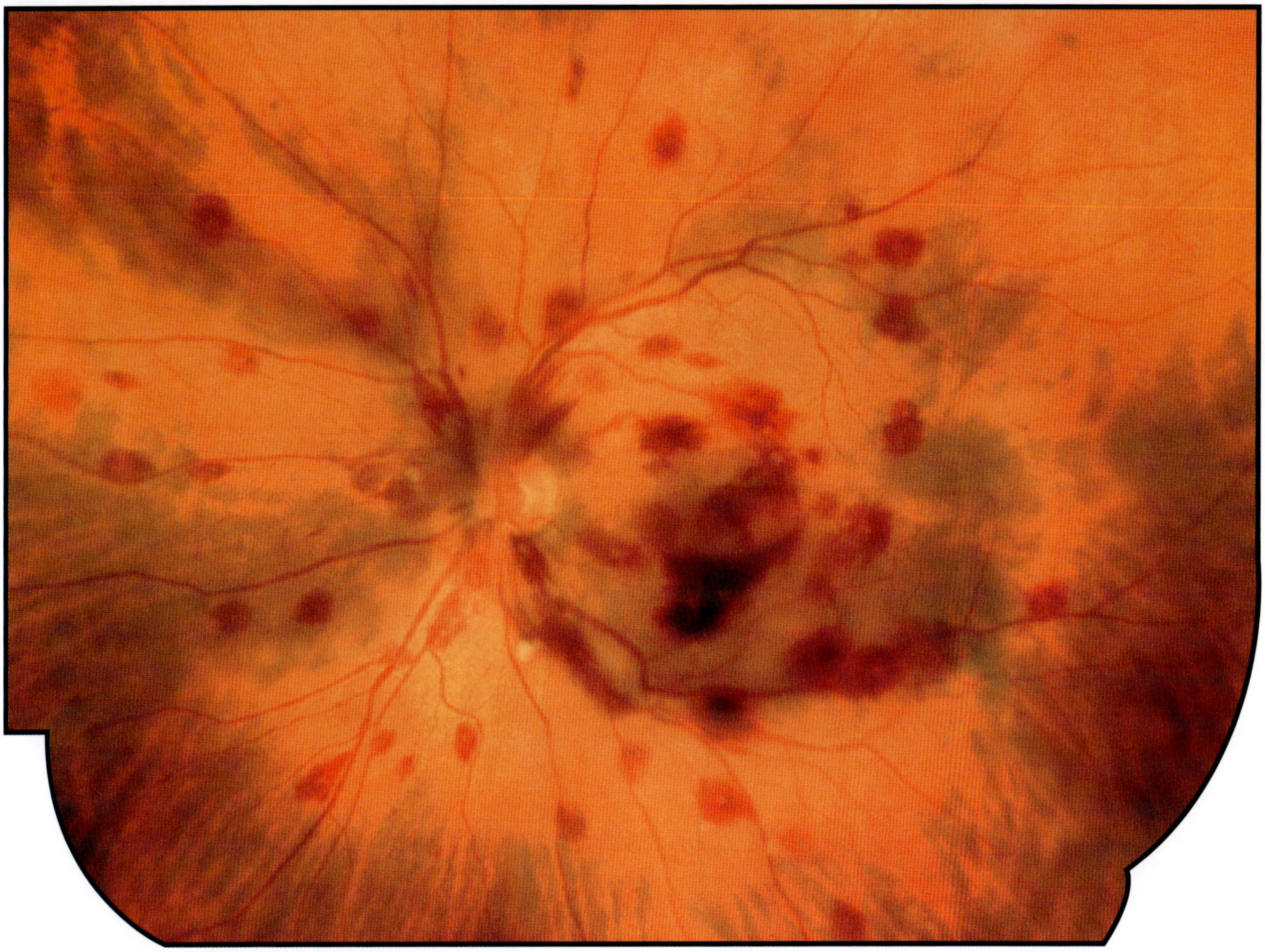

This montage demonstrates widespread retinal vascular hemorrhages in leukemia. The hemorrhages extend out in a multifocal distribution towards the peripheral fundus.

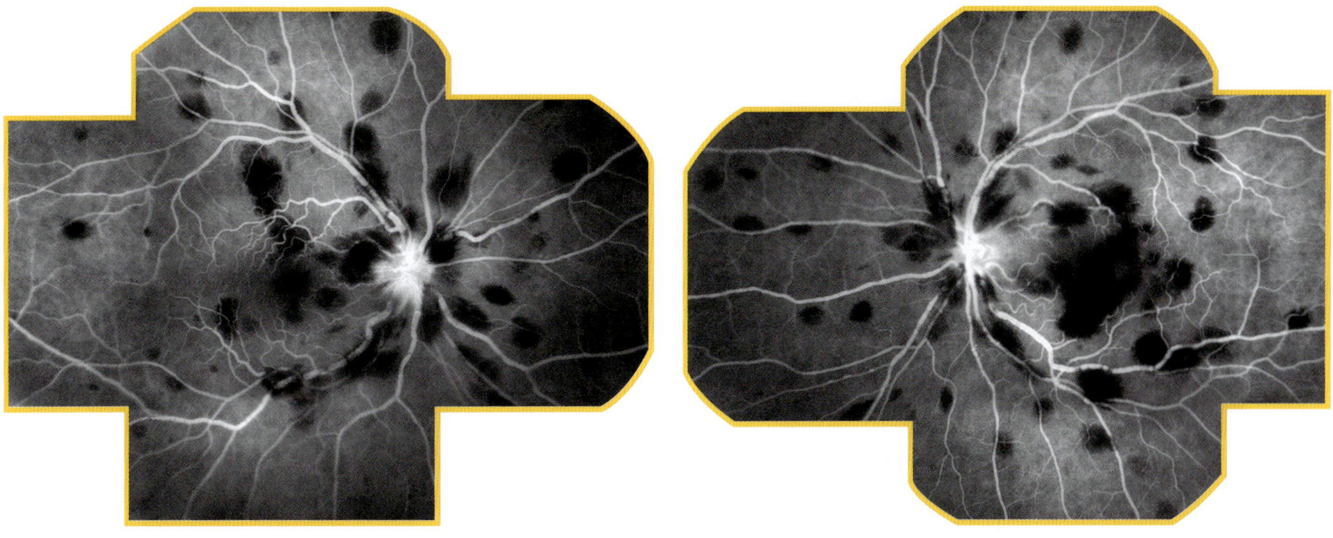

The fluorescein angiogram in this bilateral, symmetrically involved case shows that there are minimal permeability or perfusion abnormalities in association with these widespread, scattered hemorrhages.

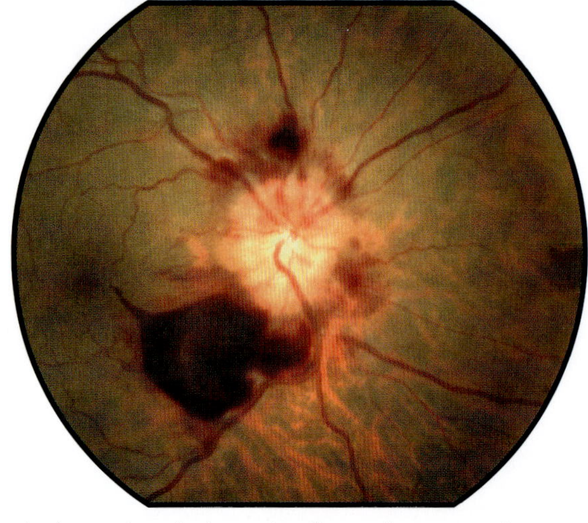

Note the hemorrhage in the peripapillary region surrounding an elevated and infiltrated optic nerve.

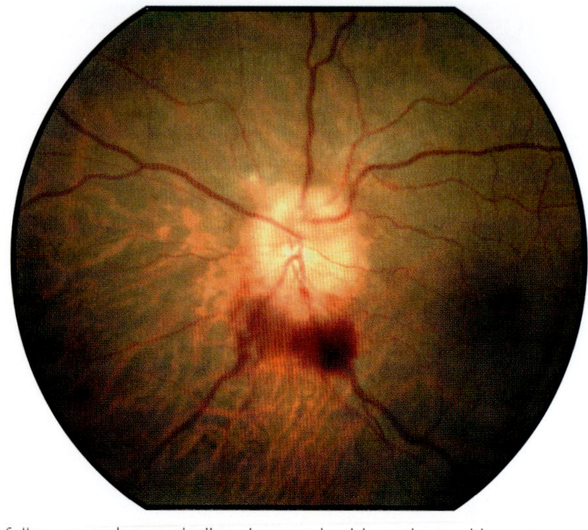

The fellow eye shows similar changes in this patient with acute myelogenous leukemia.

Exudative Detachment in Leukemia

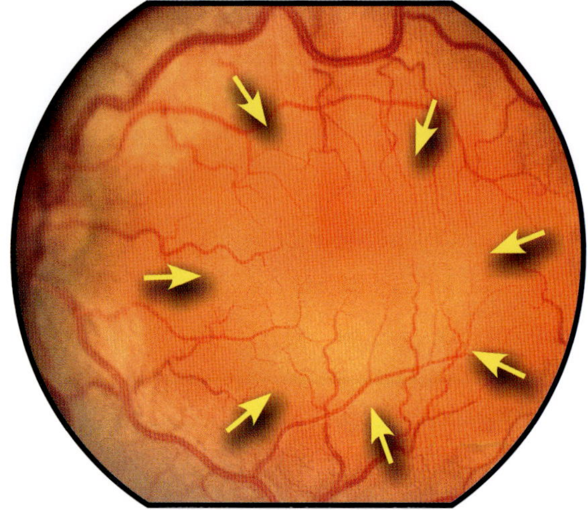

In this leukemic patient, a serous detachment was noted *(arrows)*. Multifocal leakage was seen on fluorescein angiography in this case, which resembled a Harada-like detachment of the macula. *Courtesy of Dr. Stuart L. Fine*

Disc Infiltration and Leukemia

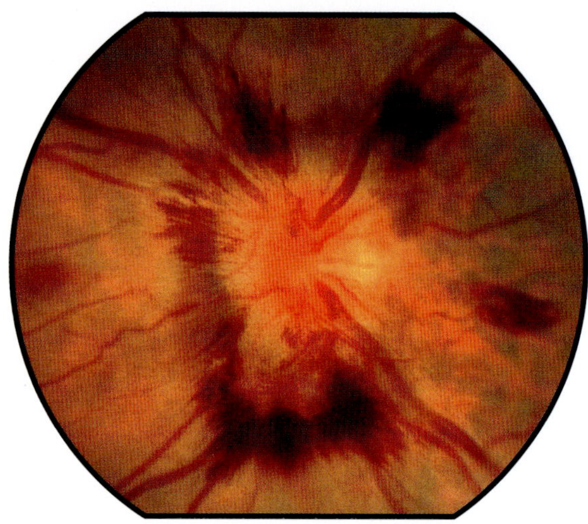

Optic nerve infiltration of tumor cells may occur in leukemia, which produce swelling of the nerve head and retinal vascular occlusive changes with bleeding.

Pre-retinal Infiltration in Leukemia

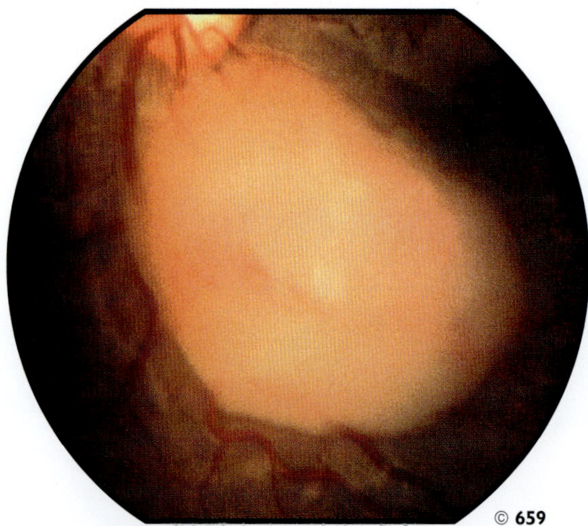

© 659

As seen in this patient, pre-retinal leukemic infiltrations may rarely occur.

Infection and Leukemia

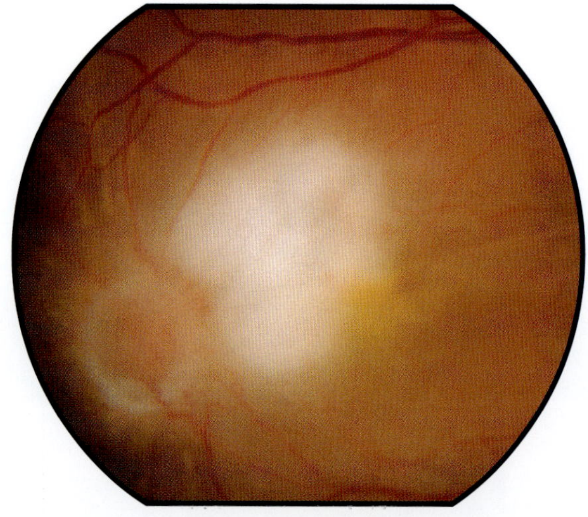

This patient with leukemia developed an opportunistic infection with vitritis and a fluffy white chorioretinal lesion. *Toxoplasma* was identified in this case. *Courtesy of Dr. H. Jay Wisnicki*

Vitreous Hemorrhage and Leukemia

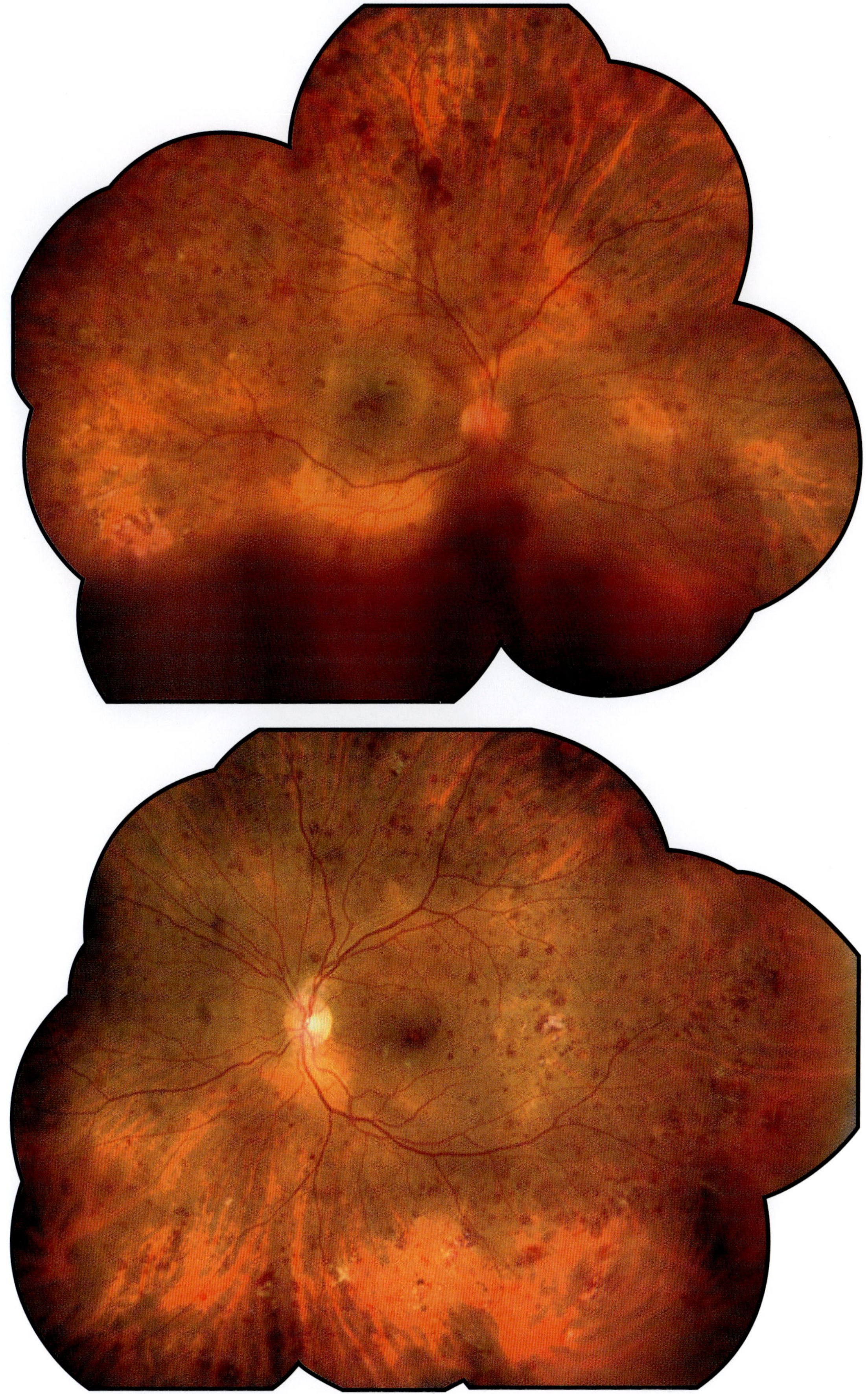

Patients with chronic leukemia are at risk for vitreous hemorrhage, as seen in the right eye of this patient with bilateral scattered retinal hemorrhages. *Courtesy of Dr. Mark Johnson*

Diabetic Retinopathy and Leukemia

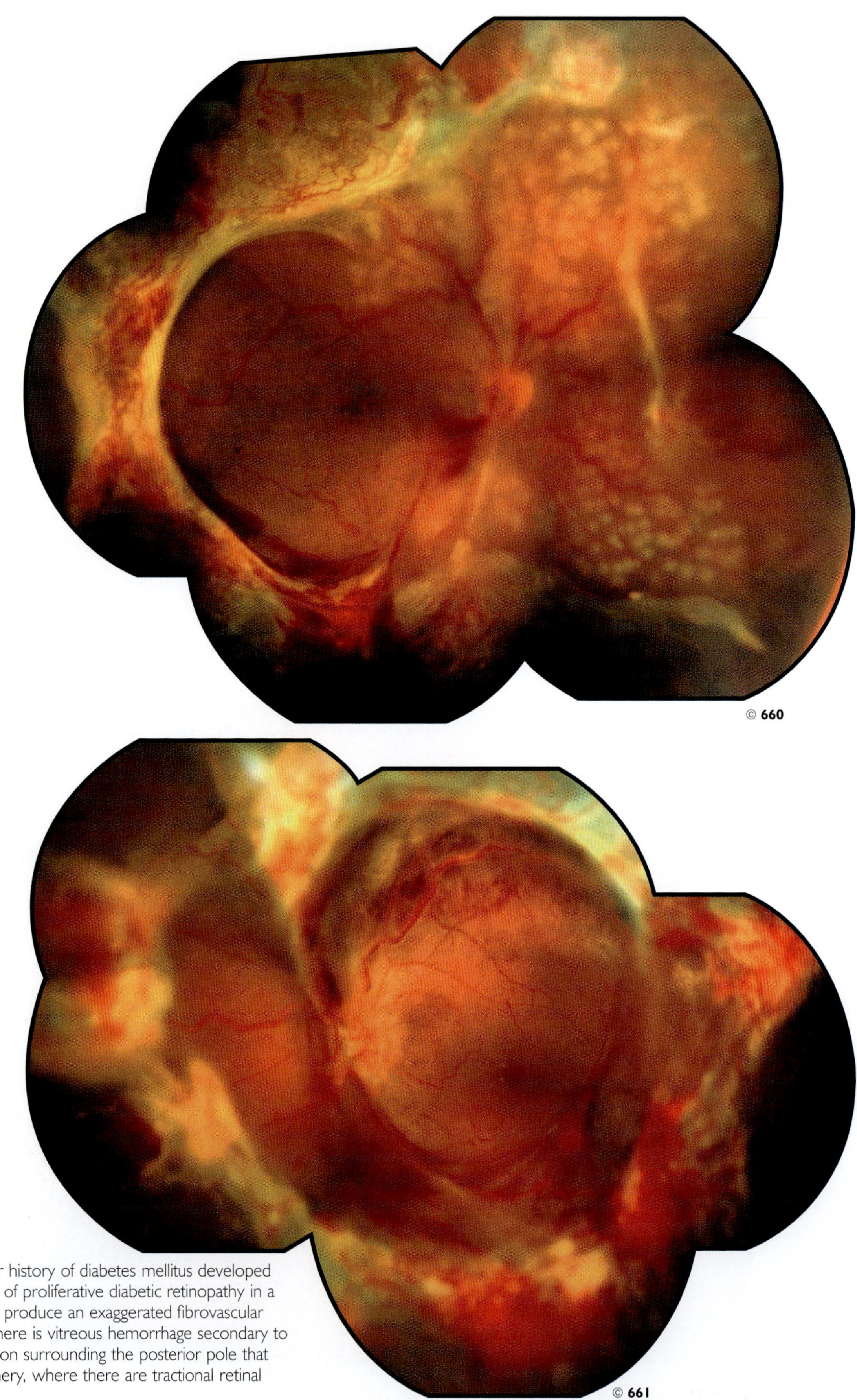

© 660

© 661

This patient with a 14 year history of diabetes mellitus developed leukemia. The occurrence of proliferative diabetic retinopathy in a patient with leukemia may produce an exaggerated fibrovascular response in the fundus. There is vitreous hemorrhage secondary to the fibrovascular proliferation surrounding the posterior pole that extends into the far periphery, where there are tractional retinal detachments.

Suggested Reading

Retinoblastoma

Abramson, D.H., Dunkel, I.J., Brodie, S.E., et al., 2008. A Phase I/II study of direct intraarterial (ophthalmic artery) chemotherapy with melphalan for intraocular retinoblastoma initial results. Ophthalmology 115, 1398–1404.

Abramson, D.H., Marr, B.P., Dunkel, I.J., et al., 2012. Intra-arterial chemotherapy for retinoblastoma in eyes with vitreous and/or subretinal seeding: 2-year results. Br. J. Ophthalmol. 129, 1492–1494.

Francis, J.H., Abramson, D.H., Gaillard, M.C., et al., 2015. The classification of vitreous seeds in retinoblastoma and response to intravitreal melphalan. Ophthalmology 122 (6), 1173–1179.

Ghassemi, F., Shields, C.L., Ghadimi, H., et al., 2014. Combined intravitreal melphalan and topotecan for refractory or recurrent vitreous seeding from retinoblastoma. JAMA Ophthalmol. 132 (8), 936–941.

Kaliki, S., Shields, C.L., Rojanaporn, D., et al., 2013. High-risk retinoblastoma based on international classification of retinoblastoma: analysis of 519 enucleated eyes. Ophthalmology 120 (5), 997–1003.

Kaliki, S., Shields, C.L., Shah, S.U., et al., 2011. Postenucleation adjuvant chemotherapy with vincristine, etoposide and carboplatin for the treatment of high-risk retinoblastoma. Arch. Ophthalmol. 129, 1422–1427.

Munier, F., Gaillard, M.C., Balmer, A., et al., 2012. Intravitreal chemotherapy for vitreous disease in retinoblastoma revisited: from prohibition to conditional indications. Br. J. Ophthalmol. 96, 1078–1083.

Shields, C.L., Au, A.K., Czyz, C., et al., 2006. The International Classification of Retinoblastoma (ICRB) predicts chemoreduction success. Ophthalmology 113, 2276–2280.

Shields, C.L., Bianciotto, C.G., Jabbour, P., et al., 2011. Intra-arterial chemotherapy for retinoblastoma. Report #2: Treatment complications. Arch. Ophthalmol. 129, 1407–1415.

Shields, C.L., Bianciotto, C.G., Ramasubramanian, A., et al., 2011. Intra-arterial chemotherapy for retinoblastoma. Report #1: control of tumor, subretinal seeds, and vitreous seeds. Arch. Ophthalmol. 129, 1399–1406.

Shields, C.L., Fulco, E.M., Arias, J.D., et al., 2013. Retinoblastoma frontiers with intravenous, intra-arterial, periocular and intravitreal chemotherapy. Eye (Lond.) 27, 253–264.

Shields, C.L., Manjandavida, F.P., Arepalli, S., et al., 2014. Intravitreal melphalan for persistent or recurrent retinoblastoma vitreous seeds: preliminary results. JAMA Ophthalmol. 132 (3), 319–325.

Shields, C.L., Manjandavida, F.P., Pieretti, G., et al., 2014. Intra-arterial chemotherapy for retinoblastoma in 70 eyes: outcomes based on the International Classification of Retinoblastoma. Ophthalmology 121 (7), 1453–1460.

Shields, C.L., Schoenfeld, E., Kocher, K., et al., 2013. Lesions simulating retinoblastoma (pseudoretinoblastoma) in 604 cases. Ophthalmology 120, 311–316.

Retinal Astrocytic Hamartoma/ Acquired Retinal Astrocytoma

Aronow, M.E., Nakagawa, J.A., Bupta, A., et al., 2012. Tuberous sclerosis complex: genotype / phenotypecorrelation of retinal findings. Ophthalmology 119, 1917–1923.

Nyboer, J.H., Robertson, D.M., Gomez, M.R., 1976. Retinal lesions in tuberous sclerosis. Arch. Ophthalmol. 94, 1277–1280.

Semenova, E., Veronese, C., Ciardella, A., et al., 2015. Multimodality imaging of retinal astrocytoma. Eur. J. Ophthalmol. 25 (6), 559–564.

Shields, C.L., Benevides, R., Materin, M.A., et al., 2006. Optical coherence tomography of retinal astrocytic hamartoma in 15 cases. Ophthalmology 113, 1553–1557.

Shields, C.L., Reichstein, D.A., Bianciotto, C.G., et al., 2012. Retinal pigment epithelial depigmented lesions associated with tuberous sclerosis complex. Arch. Ophthalmol. 130, 387–390.

Shields, C.L., Shields, J.A., Eagle, R.C. Jr., et al., 2004. Progressive enlargement of acquired retinal astrocytoma in 2 cases. Ophthalmology 111, 363–368.

Zimmer-Galler, I.E., Robertson, D.M., 1995. Long-term observation of retinal lesions in tuberous sclerosis. Am. J. Ophthalmol. 119, 318–324.

Retinal Hemangioblastoma/ Capillary Hemangioma

Ach, T., Thiemeyer, D., Hoeh, A.E., et al., 2010. Intravitreal bevacizumab for retinal capillary hemangioma: long-term results. Acta Ophthalmol. 8, e137–e138.

Chan, C.C., Vortmeyer, A.O., Chew, E.Y., et al., 1999. VHL gene deletion and enhanced VEGF gene expression detected in the stromal cells of retinal angioma. Arch. Ophthalmol. 117, 625–630.

Kreusel, K.M., Bornfeld, N., Lommatzsch, A., et al., 1998. Ruthenium-106 brachytherapy for peripheral retinal capillary hemangioma. Ophthalmology 105, 1386–1392.

Maher, E.R., Neumann, H.P., Richard, S., 2011. von Hippel-Lindau disease: a clinical and scientific review. Eur. J. Hum. Genet. 19, 617–623.

Raja, D., Benz, M.S., Murray, T.G., et al., 2004. Salvage external beam radiotherapy of retinal capillary hemangiomas secondary to von Hippel-Lindau disease: visual and anatomic outcomes. Ophthalmology 111, 150–153.

Singh, A.D., Nouri, M., Shields, C.L., et al., 2002. Treatment of retinal capillary hemangioma. Ophthalmology 109, 1799–1806.

Singh, A.D., Shields, C.L., Shields, J.A., 2001. von Hippel-Lindau disease. Surv. Ophthalmol. 46, 117–142.

Toy, B.C., Agrón, E., Nigam, D., et al., 2012. Longitudinal analysis of retinal hemangioblastomatosis and visual function in ocular von Hippel-Lindau disease. Ophthalmology 119 (12), 2622–2630.

Retinal Cavernous Hemangioma

Couteulx, S.L., Brezin, A.P., Fontaine, B., et al., 2002. A novel KRIT1/CCM1 truncating mutation in a patient with cerebral and retinal cavernous angiomas. Arch. Ophthalmol. 120, 217–218.

Gass, J.D.M., 1971. Cavernous hemangioma of the retina. A neuro-oculocutaneous syndrome. Am. J. Ophthalmol. 71, 799–814.

Goldberg, R.E., Pheasant, T.R., Shields, J.A., 1979. Cavernous hemangioma of the retina. A four-generation pedigree with neuro-oculocutaneous involvement and an example of bilateral retinal involvement. Arch. Ophthalmol. 97, 2321–2324.

Messmer, E., Laqua, H., Wessing, A., et al., 1983. Nine cases of cavernous hemangioma of the retina. Am. J. Ophthalmol. 95, 383–390.

Reddy, S., Gorin, M.B., McCannel, T., et al., 2010. Novel KRIT/CCM1 mutation in a patient with retinal cavernous hemangioma and cerebral cavernous malformation. Graefes Arch. Clin. Exp. Ophthalmol. 248, 1359–1361.

Sarraf, D., Payne, A.M., Kitchen, N.D., et al., 2000. Familial cavernous hemangioma: an expanding ocular spectrum. Arch. Ophthalmol. 118, 969–973.

Retinal Racemose Hemangioma

Archer, D.B., Deutman, A., Ernest, J.T., et al., 1973. Arteriovenous communications of the retina. Am. J. Ophthalmol. 75, 224–241.

Materin, M.A., Shields, C.L., Marr, B.P., et al., 2005. Retinal racemose hemangioma. Retina 25, 936–937.

Papageorgiou, K.I., Ghazi-Nouri, S.M., Andreou, P.S., 2006. Vitreous and subretinal haemorrhage: an unusual complication of retinal racemose haemangioma. Clin. Experiment. Ophthalmol. 34, 176–177.

Qin, X.J., Huang, C., Lai, K., 2014. Retinal vein occlusion in retinal racemose hemangioma: a case report and literature review of ocular complications in this rare retinal vascular disorder. BMC Ophthalmol. 14, 101.

Shah, G.K., Shields, J.A., Lanning, R., 1998. Branch retinal vein obstruction secondary to retinal arteriovenous communication. Am. J. Ophthalmol. 126, 446–448.

Retinal Vasoproliferative Tumor

Anastassiou, G., Bornfeld, N., Schueler, A.O., et al., 2006. Ruthenium-106 plaque brachytherapy for symptomatic vasoproliferative tumours of the retina. Br. J. Ophthalmol. 90, 447–450.

Heimann, H., Bornfeld, N., Vij, O., et al., 2000. Vasoproliferative tumours of the retina. Br. J. Ophthalmol. 84, 1162–1169.

Poole Perry, L.J., Jakobiec, F.A., Zakka, F.R., et al., 2013. reactive retinal astrocytic tumors (so-called vasoproliferative tumors): histopathologic, immunohistochemical, and genetic studies of four cases. Am. J. Ophthalmol. 155, 593–608.

Shields, C.L., Kaliki, S., Al-Daamash, S., et al., 2013. Retinal vasoproliferative tumors. Comparative clinical features of primary versus secondary tumors in 334 cases. JAMA Ophthalmol. 131 (3), 328–334.

Shields, J.A., Decker, W.L., Sanborn, G.E., et al., 1983. Presumed acquired retinal hemangiomas. Ophthalmology 90, 1292–1300.

Shields, J.A., Pellegrini, M., Kaliki, S., et al., 2014. Retinal vasoproliferative tumors in 6 patients with neurofibromatosis type 1. JAMA Ophthalmol. 132 (2), 190–196.

Shields, C.L., Shields, J.A., Barrett, J., et al., 1995. Vasoproliferative tumors of the ocular fundus. Classification and clinical manifestations in 103 patients. Arch. Ophthalmol. 113, 615–623.

Congenital Hypertrophy of the Retinal Pigment Epithelium (CHRPE)

Buettner, H., 1975. Congenital hypertrophy of the retinal pigment epithelium. Am. J. Ophthalmol. 79, 177–189.

Chamot, L., Zografos, L., Klainguti, G., 1993. Fundus changes associated with congenital hypertrophy of the retinal pigment epithelium. Am. J. Ophthalmol. 115, 154–161.

Fung, A.T., Pellegrini, M., Shields, C.L., 2014. Congenital hypertrophy of the retinal pigment epithelium: enhanced depth imaging optical coherence tomography in 18 cases. Ophthalmology 121, 251–256.

Shields, C.L., Mashayekhi, A., Ho, T., et al., 2003. Solitary congenital hypertrophy of the retinal pigment epithelium: clinical features and frequency of enlargement in 330 patients. Ophthalmology 110, 1968–1976.

Shields, C.L., Materin, M.A., Walker, C., et al., 2006. Photoreceptor loss overlying congenital hypertrophy of the retinal pigment epithelium by optical coherence tomography. Ophthalmology 113, 661–665.

Shields, J.A., Shields, C.L., Shah, P., et al., 1992. Lack of association between typical congenital hypertrophy of the retinal pigment epithelium and Gardner's syndrome. Ophthalmology 99, 1705–1713.

Pigmented Ocular Fundus Lesions with Familial Adenomatous Polyposis

Blair, N.P., Trempe, C.L., 1980. Hypertrophy of the retinal pigment epithelium associated with Gardner's syndrome. Am. J. Ophthalmol. 90, 661–667.

Gardner, E.J., Richards, R.C., 1953. Multiple cutaneous and subcutaneous lesions occurring simultaneously with hereditary polyposis and osteomatosis. Am. J. Hum. Genet. 5, 139–148.

Kasner, L., Traboulsi, E.I., De la Cruz, Z., et al., 1992. A histopathologic study of the pigmented fundus lesions in familial adenomatous polyposis. Retina 12, 35–42.

Traboulsi, E.I., Maumenee, I.H., Krush, A.J., et al., 1988. Pigmented ocular fundus lesions in the inherited gastrointestinal polyposis syndromes and in hereditary nonpolyposis colorectal cancer. Ophthalmology 95, 964–969.

Traboulsi, E.I., Maumenee, I.H., Krush, A.J., et al., 1990. Congenital hypertrophy of the retinal pigment epithelium predicts colorectal polyposis in Gardner's syndrome. Arch. Ophthalmol. 108, 525–526.

Congenital Simple Hamartoma of the Retinal Pigment Epithelium

Barnes, A.C., Goldman, D.R., Laver, N.V., et al., 2014. Congenital simple hamartoma of the retinal pigment epithelium: clinical, optical coherence tomography, and histopathological correlation. Eye (Lond.) 28 (6), 765–766.

Laqua, H., 1981. Tumors and tumor-like lesions of the retinal pigment epithelium. Ophthalmologica 183, 34–38.

Shields, C.L., Materin, M.A., Karatza, E., et al., 2004. Optical coherence tomography (OCT) of congenital simple hamartoma of the retinal pigment epithelium. Retina 24, 327–328.

Shields, C.L., Shields, J.A., Marr, B.P., et al., 2003. Congenital simple hamartoma of the retinal pigment epithelium. A study of five cases. Ophthalmology 110, 1005–1011.

Torpedo Maculopathy of the Retinal Pigment Epithelium

Rigotti, M., Babighian, S., Carcereri De Prati, E., et al., 2002. Three cases of a rare congential abnormality of the retinal pigment epithelium: torpedo maculopathy. Ophthalmologica 216, 226–227.

Shields, C.L., Guzman, J., Shapiro, M., et al., 2010. Torpedo maculopathy occurs at the site of the fetal "bulge". Arch. Ophthalmol. 128 (4), 499–501.

Villegas, V.M., Schwartz, S.G., Flynn, H.W. Jr., et al., 2014. Distinguishing torpedo maculopathy from similar lesions of the posterior segment. Ophthalmic Surg. Lasers Imaging Retina 45 (3), 222–226.

Combined Hamartoma of the Retina and Retinal Pigment Epithelium

Arepalli, S., Pellegrini, M., Shields, C.L., et al., 2014. Combined hamartoma of the retina and retinal pigment epithelium. Findings on enhanced depth imaging optical coherence tomography (EDI-OCT) in 8 eyes. Retina 34 (11), 2202–2207.

Destro, M., D'Amico, D.J., Gragoudas, E.S., et al., 1991. Retinal manifestations of neurofibromatosis. Diagnosis and management. Arch. Ophthalmol. 109, 662–666.

Gass, J.D.M., 1973. An unusual hamartoma of the pigment epithelium and retina simulating choroidal melanoma and retinoblastoma. Trans. Am. Ophthalmol. Soc. 71, 171–185.

Kaye, L.D., Rothner, A.D., Beauchamp, G.R., et al., 1992. Ocular findings associated with neurofibromatosis type II. Ophthalmology 99, 1424–1429.

Schachat, A.P., Shields, J.A., Fine, S.L., et al., 1984. Combined hamartoma of the retina and retinal pigment epithelium. Ophthalmology 91, 1609–1615.

Shields, C.L., Mashayekhi, A., Dai, V.V., et al., 2005. Optical coherence tomography findings of combined hamartoma of the retina and retinal pigment epithelium in 11 patients. Arch. Ophthalmol. 123, 1746–17450.

Adenoma/Adenocarcinoma (Epithelioma) of the Retinal Pigment Epithelium

Font, R.L., Zimmerman, L.E., Fine, B.S., 1972. Adenoma of the retinal pigment epithelium. Am. J. Ophthalmol. 73, 544–554.

Shields, J.A., Shields, C.L., Eagle, R.C. Jr., et al., 2001. Adenocarcinoma arising from congenital hypertrophy of the retinal pigment epithelium. Arch. Ophthalmol. 119, 597–602.

Shields, J.A., Shields, C.L., Gunduz, K., et al., 1999. Neoplasms of the retinal pigment epithelium: the 1998 Albert Ruedemann, Sr, memorial lecture, Part 2. Arch. Ophthalmol. 117, 601–608.

Shields, J.A., Shields, C.L., Singh, A.D., 2000. Acquired tumors arising from congenital hypertrophy of the retinal pigment epithelium. Arch. Ophthalmol. 118, 637–641.

Ciliary Body Pigment Epithelium Epithelioma (Adenoma/ Adenocarcinoma)

Bianciotto, C., Shields, C.L., Guzman, J.M., et al., 2011. Assessment of anterior segment tumors with ultrasound biomicroscopy versus anterior segment optical coherence tomography in 200 cases. Ophthalmology 118, 1297–1302.

Chang, M., Shields, J.A., Wachtel, D.I., 1979. Adenoma of the pigmented epithelium of the ciliary body simulating a malignant melanoma. Am. J. Ophthalmol. 88, 40–44.

Dinakaran, S., Rundle, P.A., Parsons, M.A., et al., 2003. Adenoma of ciliary pigment epithelium: a case series. Br. J. Ophthalmol. 87, 504–505.

Lieb, W.E., Shields, J.A., Eagle, R.C., et al., 1990. Cystic adenoma of the pigmented ciliary epithelium: clinical, pathological and immunohistochemical findings. Ophthalmology 97, 1489–1493.

Papale, J.J., Akiwama, K., Hirose, T., et al., 1984. Adenocarcinoma of the ciliary body pigment epithelium in a child. Arch. Ophthalmol. 102, 100–103.

Shields, J.A., Eagle, R.C. Jr., Shields, C.L., et al., 2001. Progressive growth of benign adenoma of the pigment epithelium of the ciliary body. Arch. Ophthalmol. 119, 1859–1861.

Shields, J.A., Shields, C.L., Gunduz, K., et al., 1999. Adenoma of the ciliary body pigment epithelium. The 1998 Albert Ruedemann Sr. Memorial Lecture. Part 1. Arch. Ophthalmol. 117, 592–597.

Medulloepithelioma

Broughton, W.I., Zimmerman, L.E., 1978. A clinicopathologic study of 56 cases of intraocular medulloepitheliomas. Am. J. Ophthalmol. 85, 407–418.

Kaliki, S., Shields, C.L., Eagle, R.C. Jr., et al., 2013. Ciliary body medulloepithelioma: analysis of 41 cases. Ophthalmology 120, 2552–2559.

O'Keefe, M., Fulcher, T., Kelly, P., et al., 1997. Medulloepithelioma of the optic nerve head. Arch. Ophthalmol. 115, 1325–1327.

Shields, J.A., Eagle, R.C. Jr., Shields, C.L., et al., 1996. Congenital neoplasms of the nonpigmented ciliary epithelium (medulloepithelioma). Ophthalmology 103, 1998–2006.

Shields, J.A., Eagle, R.C. Jr., Shields, C.L., et al., 2002. Pigmented medulloepithelioma of the ciliary body. Arch. Ophthalmol. 120, 207–210.

Singh, A., Singh, A.D., Shields, C.L., et al., 2001. Iris neovascularization in children as a manifestation of underlying medulloepithelioma. J. Pediatr. Ophthalmol. Strabismus 38, 224–228.

Choroidal Nevus

Mashayekhi, A., Siu, S., Shields, C.L., et al., 2011. Slow enlargement of choroidal nevi: a long-term follow-up study. Ophthalmology 118, 382–388.

Shah, S.U., Shields, C.L., Kaliki, S., et al., 2012. Enhanced depth imaging optical coherence tomography of choroidal nevus in 104 cases. Ideal case selection, imaging features, and tumor thickness comparison to ultrasonography. Ophthalmology 119, 1066–1072.

Shields, C.L., Cater, J.C., Shields, J.A., et al., 2000. Combination of clinical factors predictive of growth of small choroidal melanocytic tumors. Arch. Ophthalmol. 118, 360–364.

Shields, C.L., Furuta, M., Berman, E.L., et al., 2009. Choroidal nevus transformation into melanoma. Analysis of 2514 consecutive cases. Arch. Ophthalmol. 127 (8), 981–987.

Shields, C.L., Furuta, M., Mashayekhi, A., et al., 2007. Visual acuity in 3422 consecutive eyes with choroidal nevus. Arch. Ophthalmol. 125, 1501–1507.

Shields, C.L., Furuta, M., Mashayekhi, A., et al., 2008. Clinical spectrum of choroidal nevi based on age at presentation in 3422 consecutive eyes. Ophthalmology 115 (3), 546–552.

Shields, C.L., Qureshi, A., Mashayekhi, A., et al., 2011. Sector (partial) oculo(dermal) melanocytosis in 89 eyes. Ophthalmology 118, 2474–2479.

Sumich, P., Mitchell, P., Wang, J.J., 1998. Choroidal nevi in a white population: the Blue Mountains Eye Study. Arch. Ophthalmol. 116, 645–650.

Choroidal Melanoma

Kaliki, S., Shields, C.L., Ganesh, A., et al., 2013. Influence of age on young patients with uveal melanoma: a matched retrospective cohort study. Eur. J. Ophthalmol. 43 (3), 208–216.

Kujala, E., Damato, B., Coupland, S.E., et al., 2013. Staging of ciliary body and choroidal melanomas based on anatomic extent. J. Clin. Oncol. 31, 2825–2831.

Shah, S.U., Shields, C.L., Bianciotto, C.G., et al., 2014. Intravitreal bevacizumab injection at 4-month intervals for prevention of macular edema following plaque radiotherapy of uveal melanoma. Ophthalmology 121, 269–275.

Shields, C.L., Ganguly, A., Bianciotto, C.G., et al., 2011. Prognosis of uveal melanoma in 500 cases using genetic testing of needle aspiration biopsy specimens. Ophthalmology 118, 396–401.

Shields, C.L., Kaliki, S., Furuta, M., et al., 2012. Clinical spectrum and prognosis of uveal melanoma based on age at presentation in 8033 cases. Retina 32, 1363–1372.

Shields, C.L., Kaliki, S., Furuta, M., et al., 2013. American Joint Committee on Cancer classification of uveal melanoma (tumor size category) predicts prognosis in 7731 patients. Ophthalmology 120, 2066–2071.

Shields, C.L., Kaliki, S., Furuta, M., et al., 2013. Diffuse versus non-diffuse small (≤3 millimeters thickness) choroidal melanoma: Comparative analysis in 1751 cases. The 2012 F. Phinizy Calhoun Lecture 2012. Retina 33, 1763–1776.

Shields, C.L., Kaliki, S., Furuta, M., et al., 2015. American Joint Committee on Cancer Classification of Uveal Melanoma (Anatomic Stage) Predicts Prognosis in 7731 Patients: the 2013 Zimmerman Lecture. Ophthalmology 122 (6), 1180–1186.

Shields, C.L., Kaliki, S., Livesey, M., et al., 2013. Association of ocular and oculodermal melanocytosis with rate of uveal melanoma metastasis. Analysis of 7872 consecutive eyes. JAMA Ophthalmol. 131 (8), 993–1003.

Shields, C.L., Kaliki, S., Rojanaporn, D., et al., 2012. Enhanced depth imaging optical coherence tomography of small choroidal melanoma. Comparison with choroidal nevus. Arch. Ophthalmol. 130, 850–856.

Shields, J.A., Shields, C.L., 2015. Management of posterior uveal melanoma: past, present, and future: the 2014 Charles L. Schepens lecture. Ophthalmology 122 (2), 414–428.

Shields, C.L., Shields, J.A., Cater, J., et al., 2000. Plaque radiotherapy for uveal melanoma. Long-term visual outcome in 1106 patients. Arch. Ophthalmol. 118, 1219–1228.

Shields, C.L., Shields, J.A., Kiratli, H., et al., 1995. Risk factors for growth and metastasis of small choroidal melanocytic lesions. Ophthalmology 102, 1351–1361.

The Collaborative Ocular Melanoma Study Group, 1998. The collaborative ocular melanoma study (COMS) randomized trial of pre-enucleation radiation of large choroidal melanoma II: initial mortality findings. COMS report no. 10. Am. J. Ophthalmol. 126, 779–796.

The Collaborative Ocular Melanoma Study Group, 2001. The COMS randomized trial of Iodine 125 brachytherapy for choroidal melanoma, III: initial mortality findings. COMS report no. 18. Arch. Ophthalmol. 119, 969–982.

Choroidal Metastasis

Al Dahmash, S., Shields, C.L., Kaliki, S., et al., 2014. Enhanced depth imaging optical coherence tomography of choroidal metastasis in 14 eyes. Retina 34 (8), 1588–1593.

Arevalo, J.F., Fernandez, C.F., Garcia, R.A., 2005. Optical coherence tomography characteristics of choroidal metastasis. Ophthalmology 112, 1612–1619.

Demirci, H., Shields, C.L., Chao, A.N., et al., 2003. Uveal metastasis from breast cancer in 264 patients. Am. J. Ophthalmol. 136, 264–271.

DePotter, P., Shields, C.L., Shields, J.A., et al., 1993. Uveal metastasis from prostate carcinoma. Cancer 71, 2791–2796.

Ferry, A.P., Font, R.L., 1975. Carcinoma metastatic to the eye and orbit. I. Clinicopathologic study of 227 cases. Arch. Ophthalmol. 92, 276–286.

Kaliki, S., Shields, C.L., Al-Dahmash, S.A., et al., 2011. Photodynamic therapy for choroidal metastasis in 8 cases. Ophthalmology 119, 1218–1222.

Shah, S.U., Mashayekhi, A., Shields, C.L., et al., 2014. Uveal metastasis from lung cancer: clinical features, treatment, and outcome in 194 patients. Ophthalmology 121, 352–357.

Shields, C.L., Shields, J.A., De Potter, P., et al., 1997. Plaque radiotherapy in the management of uveal metastasis. Arch. Ophthalmol. 115, 203–209.

Shields, J.A., Shields, C.L., Ehya, H., et al., 1993. Fine needle aspiration biopsy of suspected intraocular tumors. The 1992 Urwick Lecture. Ophthalmology 100, 1677–1684.

Shields, C.L., Shields, J.A., Gross, N., et al., 1997. Survey of 520 uveal metastases. Ophthalmology 104, 1265–1276.

Stephens, R.F., Shields, J.A., 1979. Diagnosis and management of cancer metastatic to the uvea. A study of 70 cases. Ophthalmology 86, 1336–1349.

Choroidal Hemangioma

Arepalli, S., Shields, C.L., Kaliki, S., et al., 2013. Diffuse choroidal hemangioma management with plaque radiotherapy in 5 cases. Ophthalmology 120, 2358–2359.

Arevalo, J.F., Shields, C.L., Shields, J.A., et al., 2000. Circumscribed choroidal hemangioma: characteristic features with indocyanine green videoangiography. Ophthalmology 107, 344–350.

Blasi, M.A., Tiberti, A.C., Scupola, A., et al., 2010. Photodynamic therapy with verteporfin for symptomatic circumscribed choroidal hemangioma: five-year outcomes. Ophthalmology 117, 1630–1637.

Mashayekhi, A., Shields, C.L., 2003. Circumscribed choroidal hemangioma. Curr. Opin. Ophthalmol. 14, 142–149.

Schmidt-Erfurth, U.M., Michels, S., Kusserow, C., et al., 2002. Photodynamic therapy for symptomatic choroidal hemangioma: visual and anatomic results. Ophthalmology 109, 2284–2294.

Shields, C.L., Honavar, S.G., Shields, J.A., et al., 2001. Circumscribed choroidal hemangioma: clinical manifestations and factors predictive of visual outcome in 200 consecutive cases. Ophthalmology 108, 2237–2248.

Witschel, H., Font, R.L., 1976. Hemangioma of the choroid. A clinicopathologic study of 71 cases and a review of the literature. Surv. Ophthalmol. 20, 415–431.

Choroidal Osteoma

Aylward, G.W., Chang, T.S., Pautler, S.E., et al., 1998. A long-term follow-up of choroidal osteoma. Arch. Ophthalmol. 116, 1337–1341.

Gass, J.D., Guerry, R.K., Jack, R.L., et al., 1978. Choroidal osteoma. Arch. Ophthalmol. 96, 428–435.

Khan, M.A., DeCroos, F.C., Storey, P.P., et al., 2014. Outcomes of anti-vascular endothelial growth factor (VEGF) therapy in the management of choroidal neovascularization associated with choroidal osteoma. Retina 34 (9), 1750–1756.

Shields, C.L., Arepalli, S., Atalay, H.T., et al., 2015. Choroidal osteoma shows bone lamella and vascular channels on enhanced depth imaging optical coherence tomography (EDI-OCT) in 15 eyes. Retina 35 (4), 750–757.

Shields, C.L., Perez, B., Materin, M.A., et al., 2007. Optical coherence tomography of choroidal osteoma in 22 cases. Evidence for photoreceptor atrophy over the decalcified portion of the tumor. Ophthalmology 114, e53–e58.

Shields, C.L., Shields, J.A., Augsburger, J.J., 1988. Choroidal osteoma. Surv. Ophthalmol. 33, 17–27.

Shields, C.L., Sun, H., Demirci, H., et al., 2005. Factors predictive of tumor growth, tumor decalcification, choroidal neovascularization and visual outcome in 74 eyes with choroidal osteoma. Arch. Ophthalmol. 123, 658–666.

Idiopathic Sclerochoroidal Calcification

Fung, A.T., Arias, J.D., Shields, C.L., et al., 2013. Sclerochoroidal calcification is primarily a scleral condition based on enhanced depth imaging optical coherence tomography. JAMA Ophthalmol. 131 (7), 960–963.

Hasanreisoglu, M., Saktanasate, J., Shields, P.W., et al., 2015. Classification of sclerochoroidal calcification based on enhanced depth imaging optical coherence tomography "mountain-like" features. Retina 35 (7), 1407–1414.

Honavar, S.G., Shields, C.L., Demirci, H., et al., 2001. Sclerochoroidal calcification: clinical manifestations and systemic associations. Arch. Ophthalmol. 119, 833–840.

Shields, C.L., Hasanreisoglu, M., Saktanasate, J., et al., 2015. Sclerochoroidal calcification: clinical features, outcomes, and relationship with hypercalcemia and parathyroid adenoma in 179 eyes. Retina 35 (3), 547–554.

Shields, J.A., Shields, C.L., 2002. Sclerochoroidal calcification. Review. The 2001 Harold Gifford Lecture. Retina 22, 251–261.

Sivalingam, A., Shields, C.L., Shields, J.A., et al., 1991. Idiopathic sclerochoroidal calcification. Ophthalmology 98, 720–724.

Choroidal Leiomyoma

Biswas, J., Kumar, S.K., Gopal, L., et al., 2000. Leiomyoma of the ciliary body extending to the anterior chamber: clinicopathologic and ultrasound biomicroscopic correlation. Surv. Ophthalmol. 44 (4), 336–342.

Heegaard, S., Jensen, P.K., Scherfig, E., et al., 1999. Leiomyoma of the ciliary body. Report of 2 cases. Acta Ophthalmol. Scand. 77, 709–712.

Jakobiec, F.A., Font, R.L., Tso, M.O., et al., 1977. Mesectodermal leiomyoma of the ciliary body: a tumor of presumed neural crest origin. Cancer 39, 2102–2113.

Jakobiec, F.A., Witschel, H., Zimmerman, L.E., 1976. Choroidal leiomyoma of vascular origin. Am. J. Ophthalmol. 82, 205–212.

Oh, K.J., Kwon, B.J., Han, M.H., et al., 2005. MR imaging findings of uveal leiomyoma: three cases. Am. J. Neuroradiol. 26, 100–103.

Richter, M.N., Bechrakis, N.E., Stoltenburg-Didinger, G., et al., 2003. Transscleral resection of a ciliary body leiomyoma in a child: case report and review of the literature. Graefes Arch. Clin. Exp. Ophthalmol. 241, 953–957.

Shields, J.A., Shields, C.L., Eagle, R.C. Jr., et al., 1994. Observations on seven cases of intraocular leiomyoma. The 1993 Byron Demorest Lecture. Arch. Ophthalmol. 112, 521–528.

Intraocular Lymphoma

Aronow, M.E., Portell, C.A., Sweetenham, J.W., et al., 2014. Uveal lymphoma: clinical features, diagnostic studies, treatment selection, and outcomes. Ophthalmology 121 (1), 334–341.

Chan, C.C., Buggage, R.R., Nussenblatt, R.B., 2002. Intraocular lymphoma. Curr. Opin. Ophthalmol. 13, 411–418.

Chan, C.C., Sen, H.N., 2013. Current concepts in diagnosing and managing primary vitreoretinal (intraocular) lymphoma. Discov. Med. 15, 93–100.

Cockerham, G.C., Hidayat, A.A., Bijwaard, K.E., et al., 2000. Re-evaluation of "reactive lymphoid hyperplasia of the uvea": an immunohistochemical and molecular analysis of 10 cases. Ophthalmology 107, 151–158.

Coupland, S.E., Foss, H.D., Hidayat, A.A., et al., 2002. Extranodal marginal zone B cell lymphomas of the uvea: an analysis of 13 cases. J. Pathol. 197, 333–340.

Coupland, S.E., Heimann, H., 2004. Primary intraocular lymphoma. Ophthalmologe 101, 87–98.

Grossniklaus, H.E., Martin, D.F., Avery, R., et al., 1998. Uveal lymphoid infiltration. Report of four cases and clinicopathologic review. Ophthalmology 105, 1265–1273.

Mashayekhi, A., Shukla, S.Y., Shields, J.A., et al., 2014. Choroidal lymphoma: clinical features and association with systemic lymphoma. Ophthalmology 121, 342–351.

Nussenblatt, R.B., Chan, C.C., Wilson, W.H., et al., 2006. International Central Nervous System and Ocular Lymphoma Workshop: recommendations for the future. Ocul. Immunol. Inflamm. 14, 139–144.

Pang, C.E., Shields, C.L., Jumper, J.M., et al., 2014. Paraneoplastic cloudy vitelliform submaculopathy in primary vitreoretinal lymphoma. Am. J. Ophthalmol. 158 (6), 1253–1261.

Sagoo, M.S., Mehta, H., Swampillai, A.J., et al., 2014. Primary intraocular lymphoma. Surv. Ophthalmol. 59 (5), 503–516.

Shields, C.L., Arepalli, S., Pellegrini, M., et al., 2014. Choroidal lymphoma appears with calm, rippled, or undulating topography on enhanced depth imaging optical coherence tomography in 14 cases. Retina 34 (7), 1347–1353.

Melanocytoma of the Optic Disc

Reidy, J.J., Apple, D.J., Steinmetz, R.L., et al., 1985. Melanocytoma: nomenclature, pathogenesis, natural history and treatment. Surv. Ophthalmol. 29, 319–327.

Shields, J.A., Demirci, H., Mashayekhi, A., et al., 2004. Melanocytoma of the optic disc in 115 cases. The 2004 Samuel Johnson Memorial Lecture. Ophthalmology 111, 1739–1746.

Shields, C.L., Perez, B., Benavides, R., et al., 2008. Optical coherence tomography of optic disk melanocytoma in 15 cases. Retina 28 (3), 441–446.

Shields, J.A., Shields, C.L., Demirci, H., et al., 2006. Melanocytoma of the optic nerve: review. Surv. Ophthalmol. 51, 93–104.

Shields, J.A., Shields, C.L., Eagle, R.C. Jr., 2007. Melanocytoma (hyperpigmented magnocellular nevus) of the uveal tract. The 34th G. Victor Simpson Lecture. Retina 27, 730–739.

Zimmerman, L.E., 1965. Melanocytes, melanocytic nevi, and melanocytomas: the Jonas S. Friedenwald Memorial Lecture. Invest. Ophthalmol. 4, 11–40.

Hemangioblastoma (Capillary Hemangioma) of the Optic Disc

Garcia-Arumi, J., Sararols, L.H., Cavero, L., et al., 2000. Therapeutic options for capillary papillary hemangiomas. Ophthalmology 107, 48–54.

Golshevsky, J.R., O'Day, J., 2005. Photodynamic therapy in the management of juxtapapilllary capillary hemangiomas. Clin. Experiment. Ophthalmol. 33, 509–512.

McCabe, C.M., Flynn, H.W. Jr., Shields, C.L., et al., 2000. Juxtapapillary capillary hemangiomas. Clinical features and visual acuity outcomes. Ophthalmology 107, 2240–2248.

Schmidt-Erfurth, U.M., Kusserow, C., Barbazetto, I.A., et al., 2002. Benefits and complications of photodynamic therapy of papillary capillary hemangiomas. Ophthalmology 109 (7), 1256–1266.

CHAPTER 9

Vitreomacular Traction, Epiretinal Membranes, and Macular Holes

Epiretinal Membrane

An epiretinal membrane (ERM) is a fibrocellular proliferation occurring on the retinal surface, most commonly in the macular region. ERMs typically occur following a spontaneous partial or complete posterior vitreous detachment, but secondary causes include intraocular surgery, inflammation, ischemic vascular disease, trauma, retinal tear, rhegmatogenous retinal detachment, and intraocular tumors. Cells thought to contribute to ERMs include retinal pigment epithelium (RPE), fibrocytes, myofibrocytes, and intraretinal glial elements.

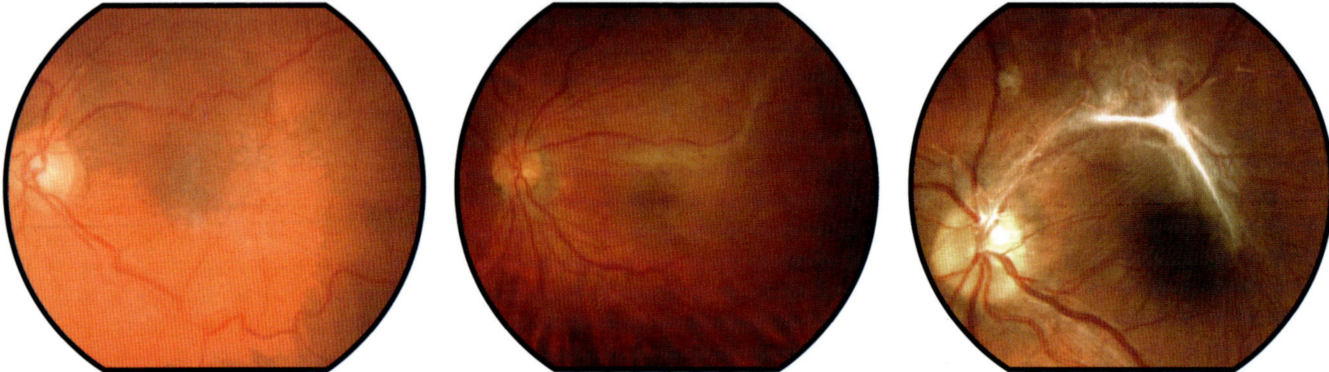

These patients show the variable presentation of ERMs, ranging from semi-translucent gray *(left image)* to opaque white fibrosis *(middle image)*. Some may appear as a fibrotic white band *(right image)*. The appearance during the early stages of an ERM is frequently referred to as "cellophane maculopathy," while prominent surface wrinkling following membrane maturation is referred to as "macular pucker."

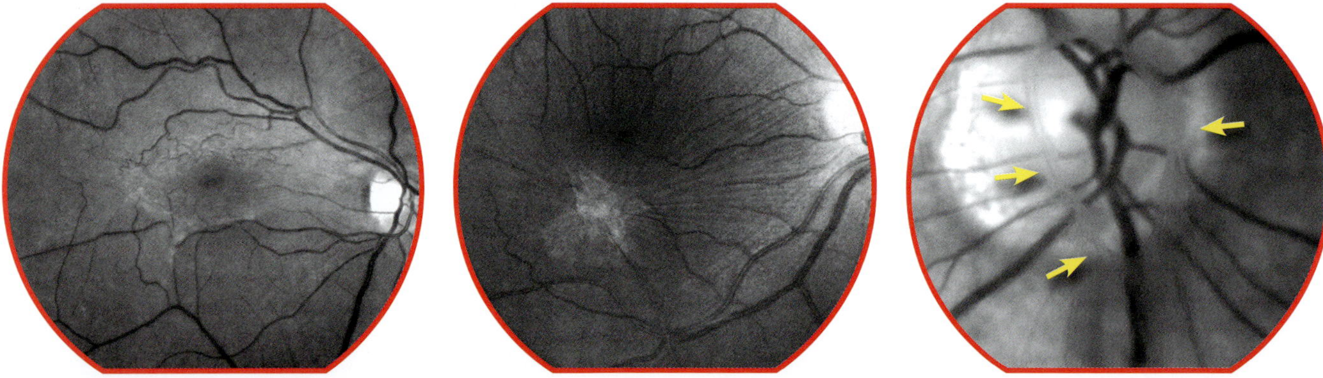

Monochromatic imaging (red-free) can enhance the details of the vitreoretinal interface. Commonly, there is incomplete detachment of the posterior hyaloid with persistent adherence around the disc in the right image *(arrows)*.

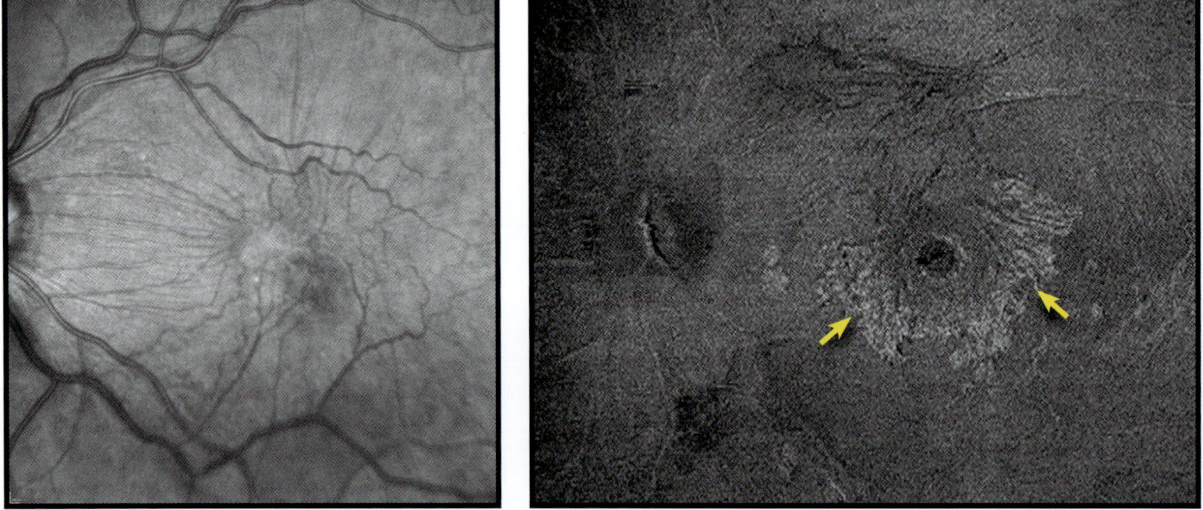

Infrared reflectance imaging *(left)* and *en face* swept source optical coherence tomography (OCT) imaging *(right)* also provide valuable information about the morphologic and topographic features of ERMs. The margins of the ERM are clearly delineated on swept source images *(arrows)*. *Images courtesy of Dr. Michael Engelbert*

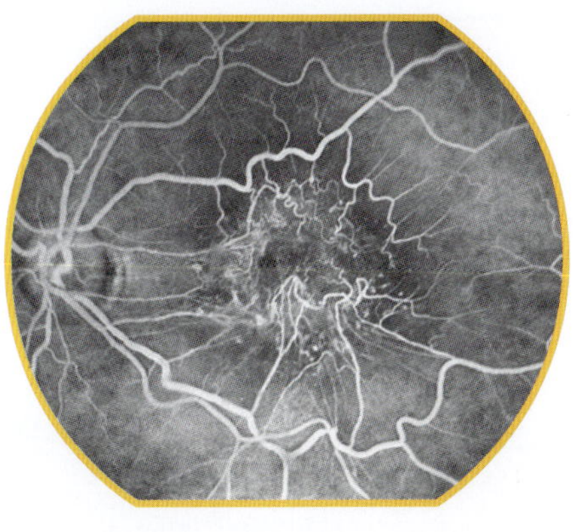
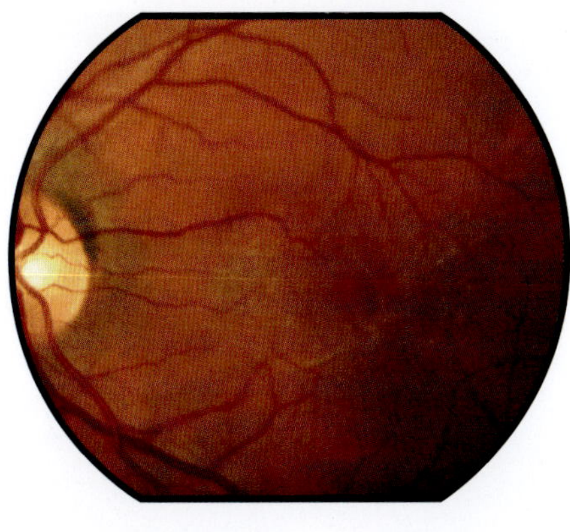
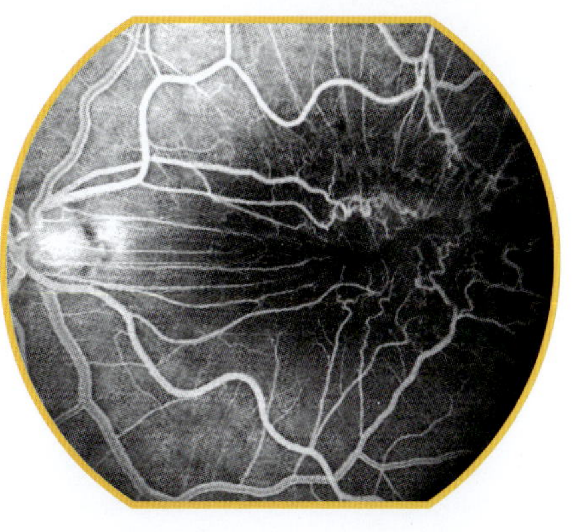

Fluorescein angiography can aid surgical planning and is useful for identifying complex anatomic relationships between retinal vasculature and ERMs. In the above cases, retinal vasculature is observed to be embedded within the ERM tissue complex. Fluorescein angiography is also useful for excluding secondary causes of ERM, such as retinal vein occlusion.

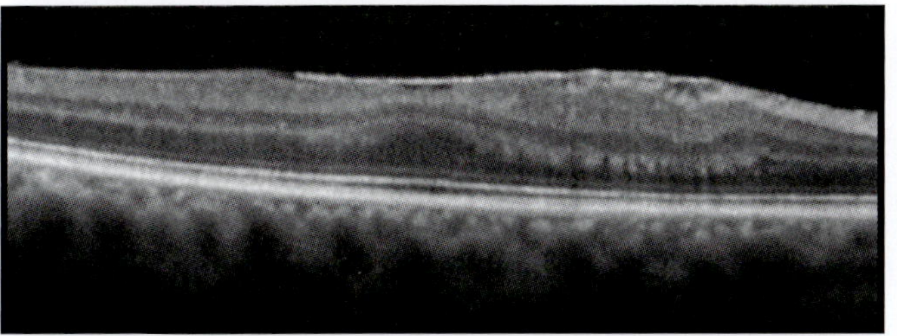
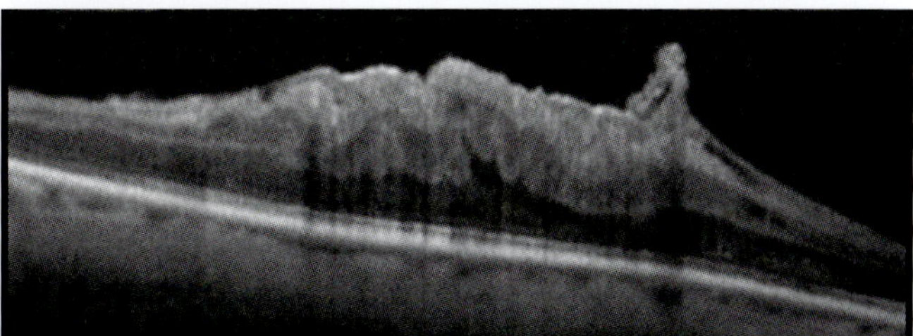
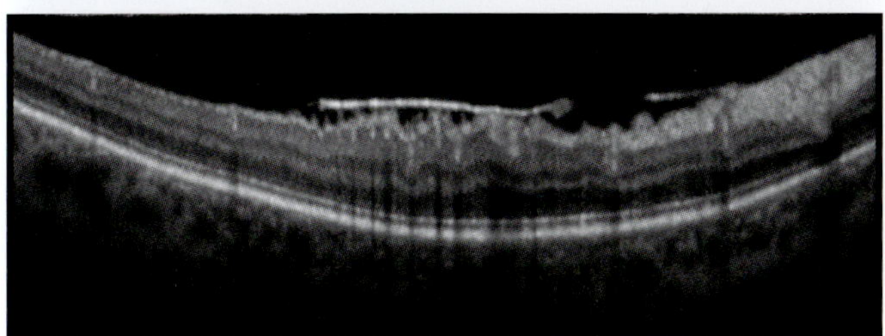
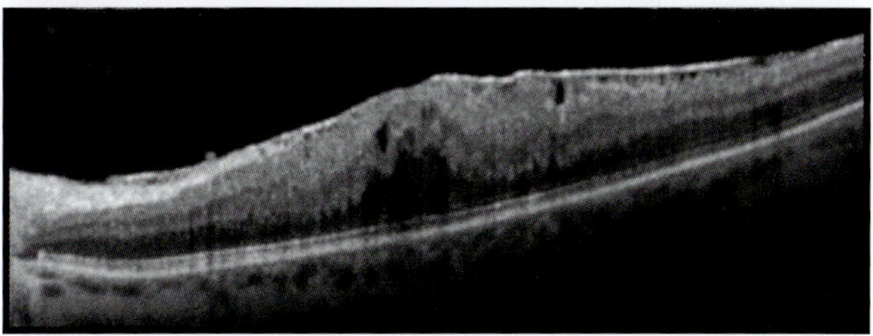

With spectral-domain OCT imaging, an ERM appears as a thin, hyper-reflective line on the inner surface of the retina *(top left image)*. Tractional effects of the membrane include retinal thickening *(top right image)*, wrinkling of the surface of the retina *(bottom left image)*, and intraretinal cystic spaces *(bottom right image)*. These tractional effects are responsible for the patient's symptoms of visual loss and metamorphopsia.

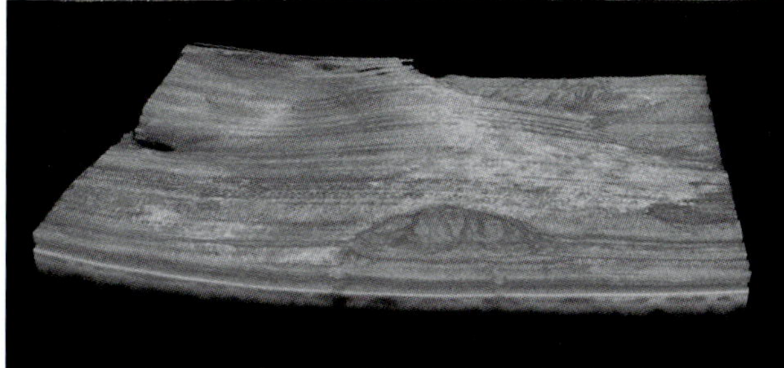

© **662**

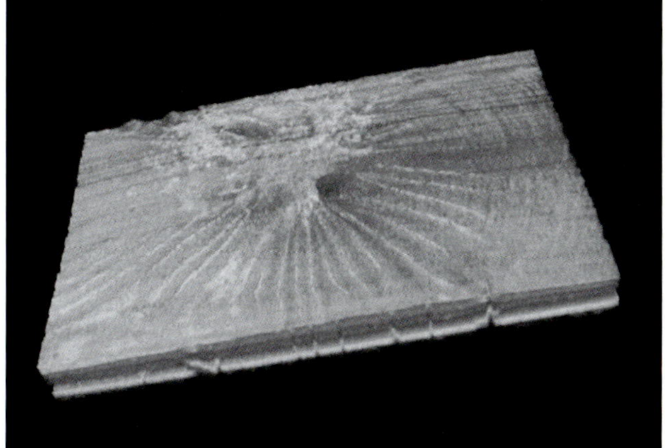

© **663**

Three-dimensional volume rendered OCT images demonstrate wrinkling and traction of the inner surface of the retina due to ERM. *Images courtesy of Dr. Richard Spaide*

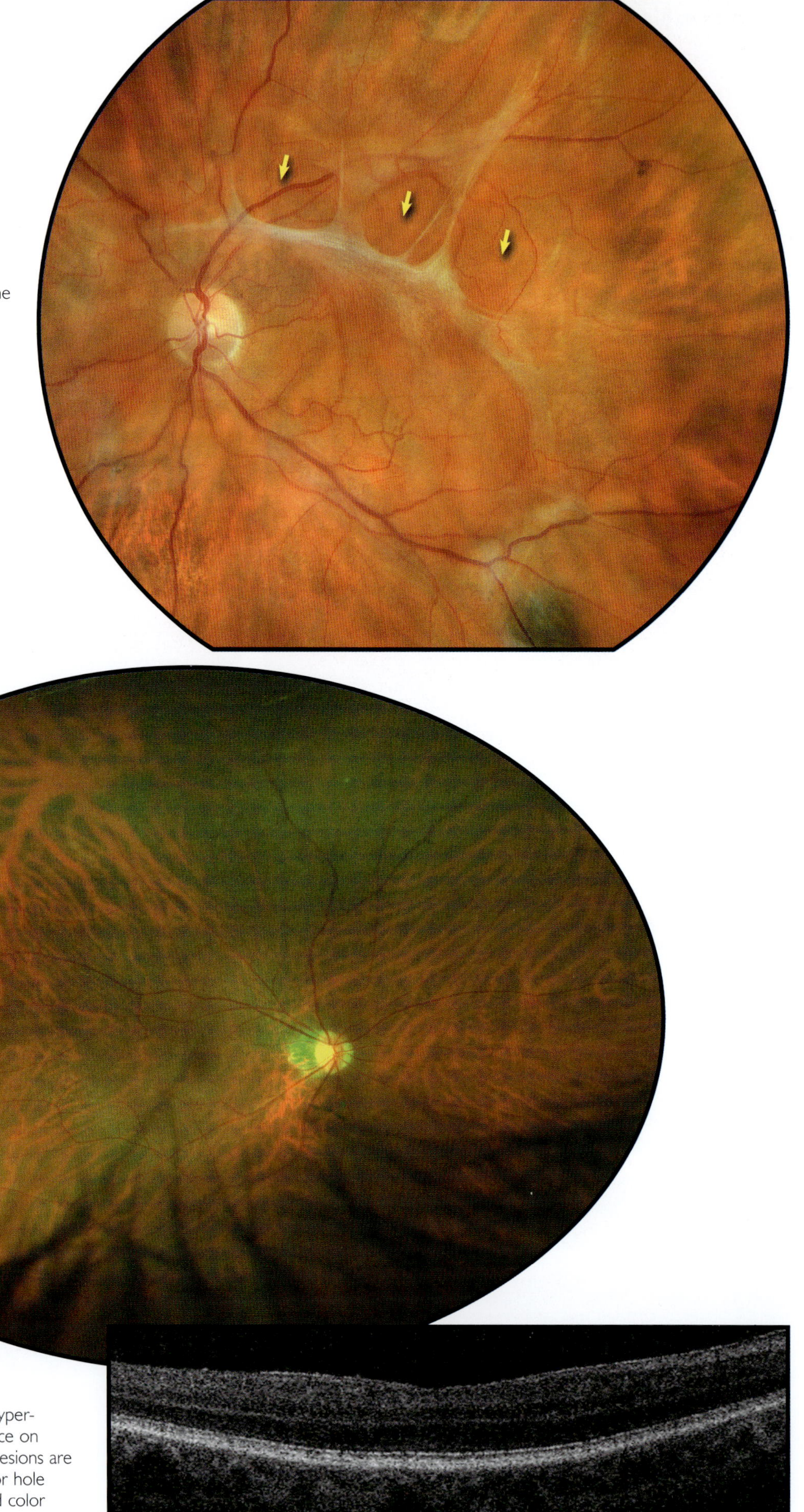

Note the widespread fibrotic membrane in this patient. There are semilunar, ovoid, and circular defects in the epiretinal tissue *(arrows)*.

A subtle ERM may manifest as a thin hyper-reflective line on the inner retinal surface on OCT *(right image)*. Infrequently these lesions are secondary to a peripheral retinal tear or hole *(arrow)* as shown on the ultra-widefield color photograph.

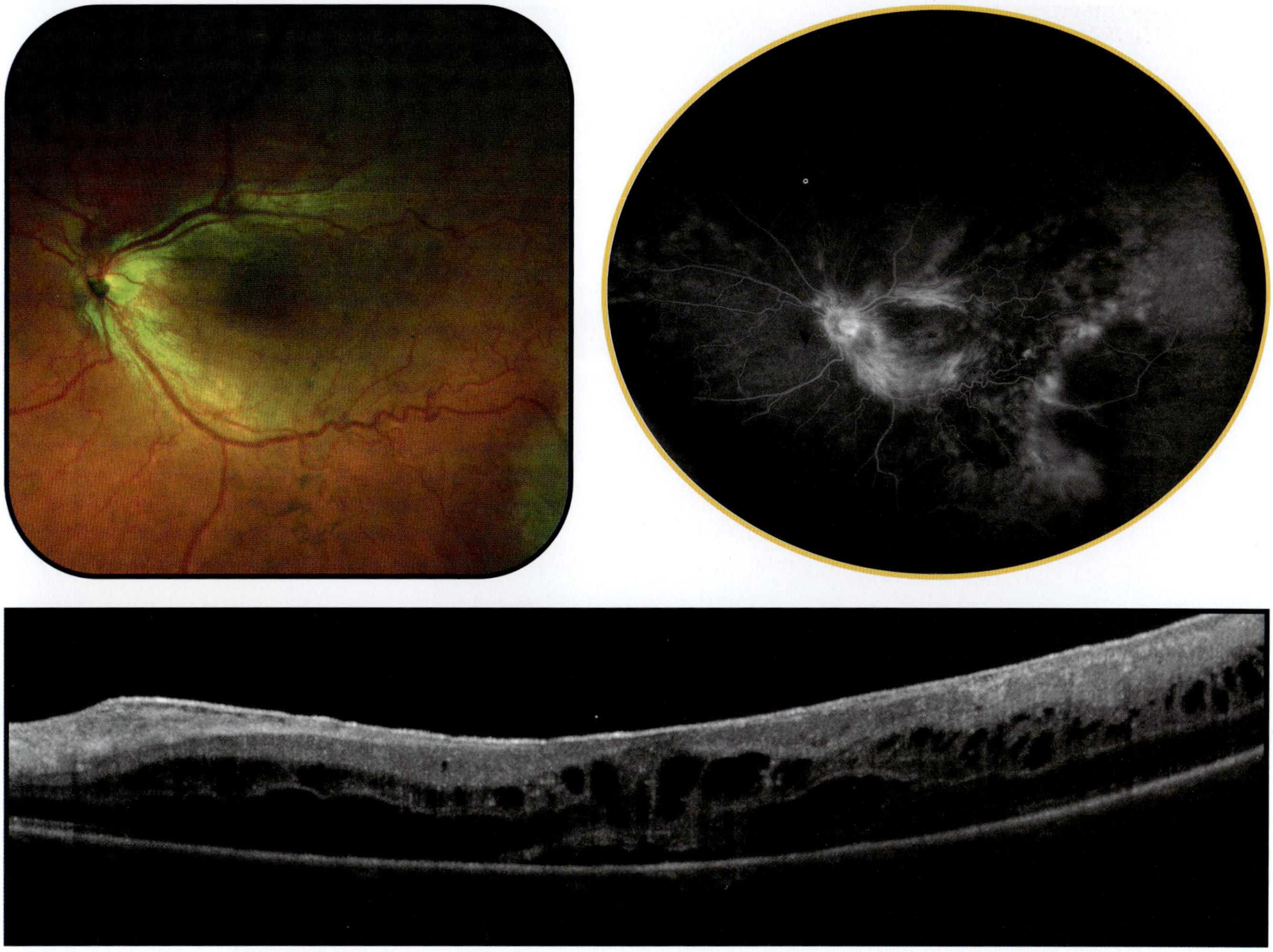

This patient with severe ERM and cystoid macula edema was found to have peripheral occlusive vasculitis in the inferotemporal retina on fluorescein angiography. This case illustrates the importance of a thorough peripheral retina examination to exclude secondary causes of ERM.
Images courtesy of Dr. David Maberley

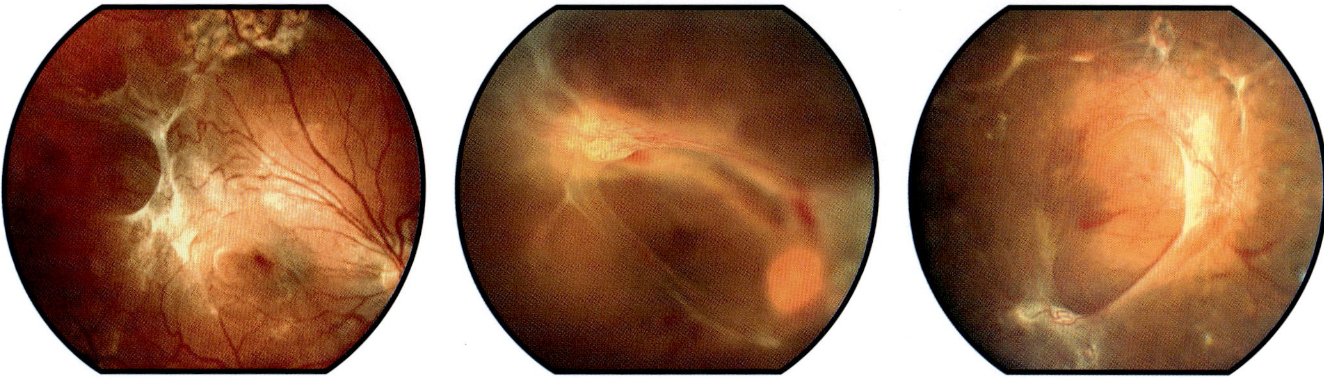

The above patients with proliferative diabetic retinopathy have severe fibrotic proliferation. The fibrovascular tissue usually adopts a curvilinear distribution along the vascular arcades.

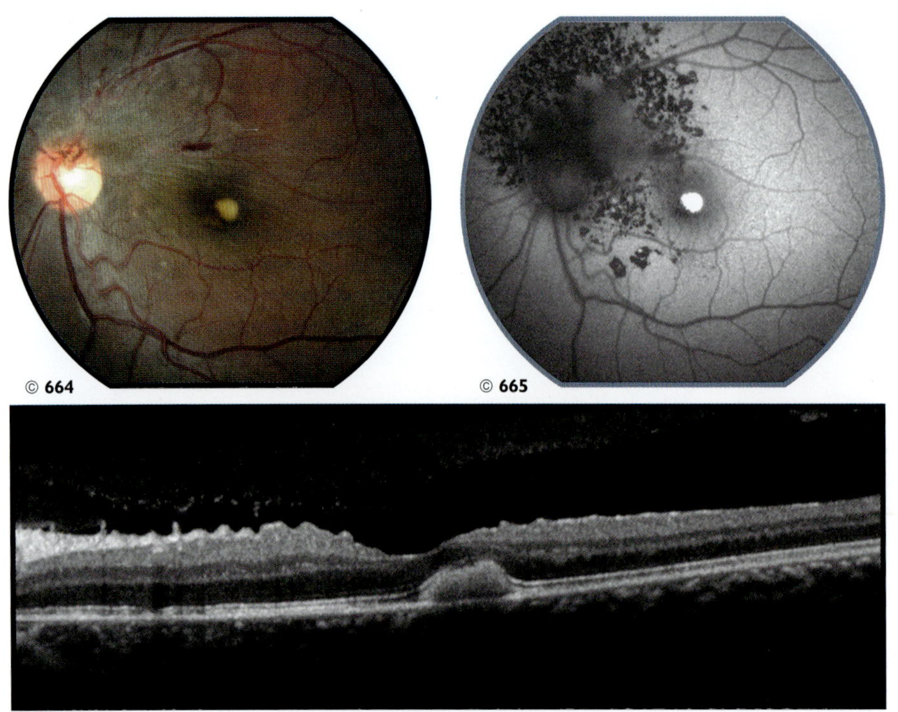

© 664 © 665 © 666

This patient has an ERM surrounding the optic disk secondary to a combined hamartoma of the retina and retinal pigment epithelium. The OCT shows a hyper-reflective vitelliform lesion that exhibits hyperautofluorescence at the fovea with fundus autofluorescence imaging. Folds on the surface of the macula are due to tractional forces around the optic disk.

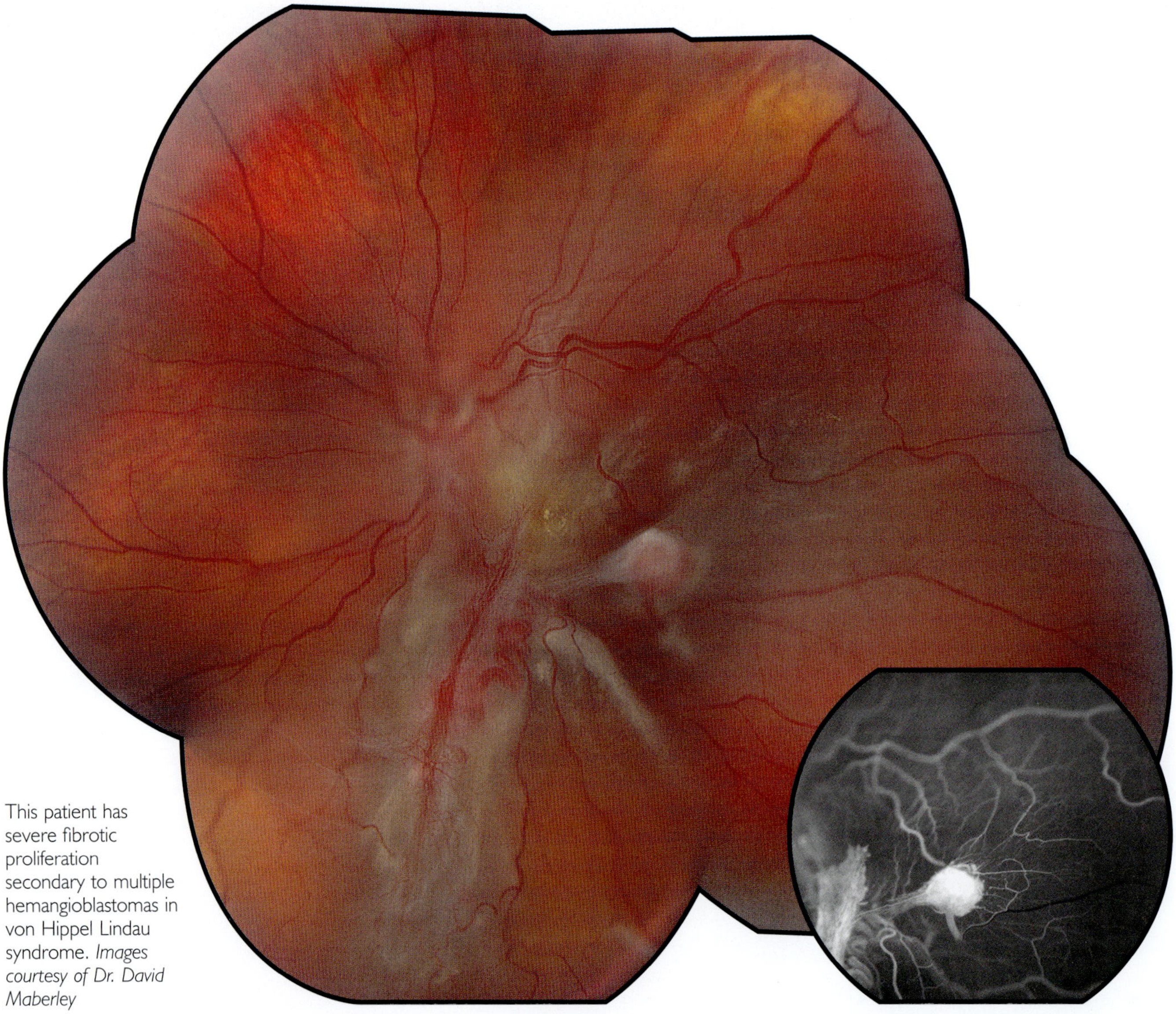

This patient has severe fibrotic proliferation secondary to multiple hemangioblastomas in von Hippel Lindau syndrome. *Images courtesy of Dr. David Maberley*

Spontaneous Release of Epiretinal Membrane

Cases of spontaneous release of ERMs have been reported. Although uncommon, occurring in approximately 1-3% of cases, it is more frequently observed in young, female, myopic patients.

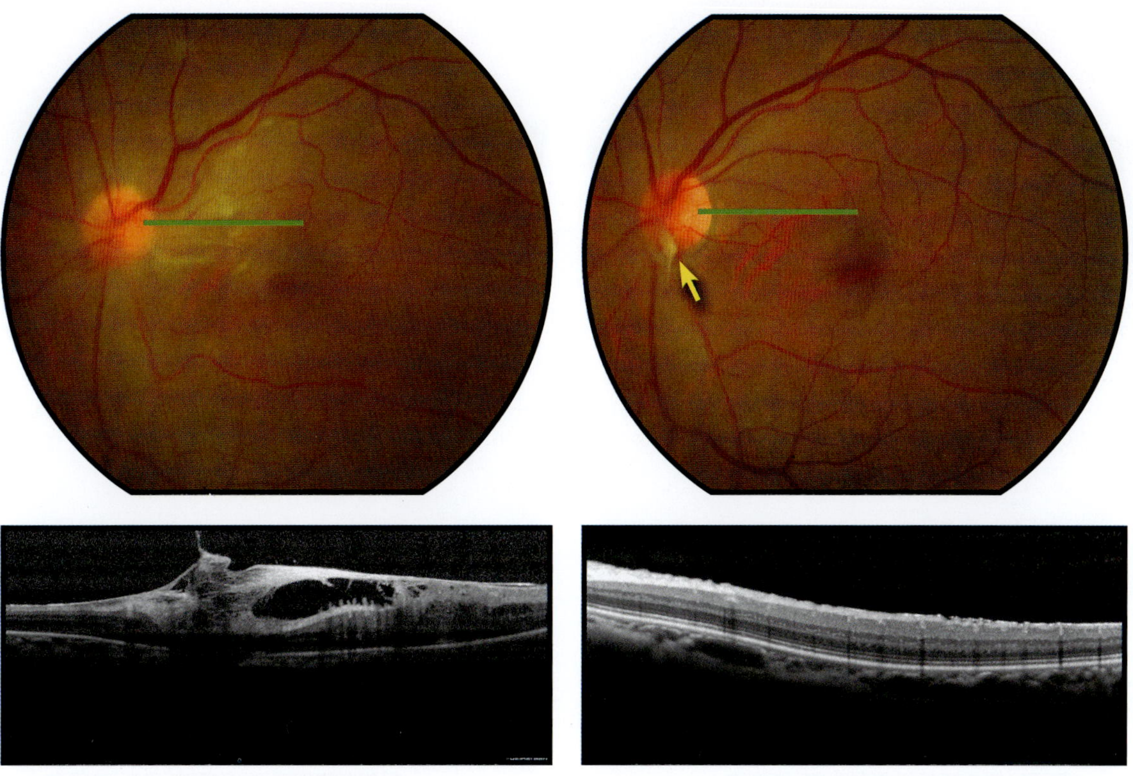

This patient had a thick ERM at the disc and papillomacular bundle *(left)*. The membrane released spontaneously, leaving a legacy of peripapillary fibrous tissue *(arrow)*.

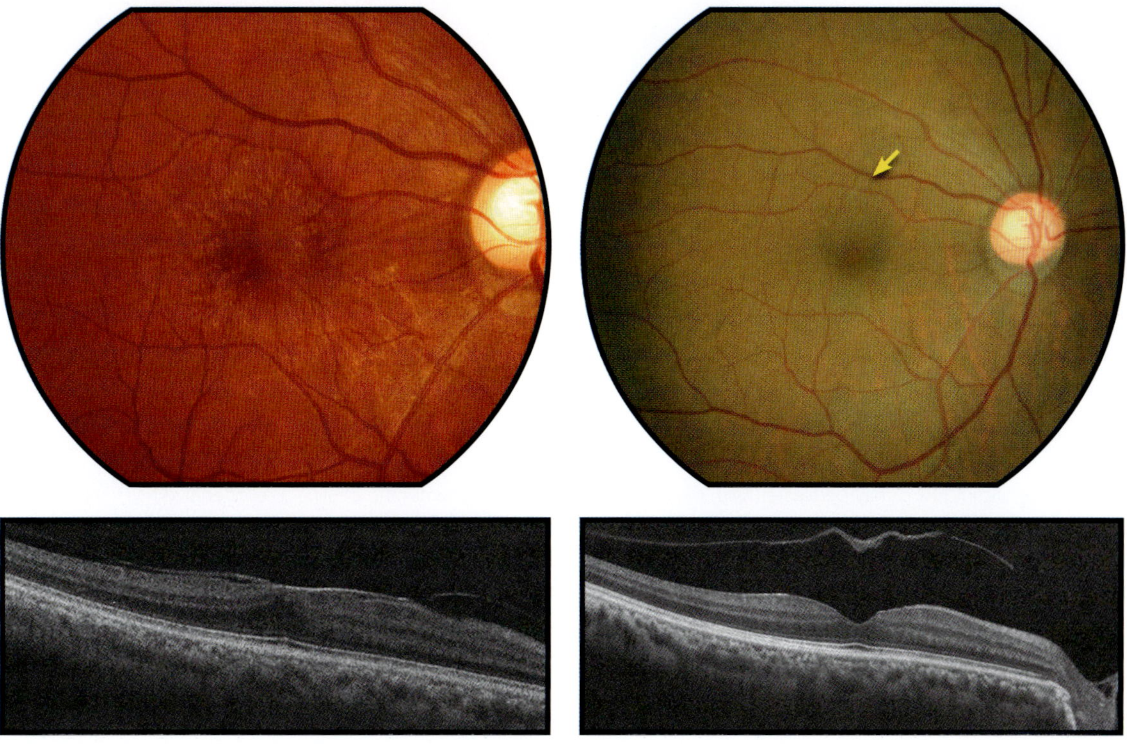

This patient with metamorphopsia due to an ERM experienced spontaneous improvement of symptoms four years later. Color photos and OCT demonstrate spontaneous release of the ERM from the macula. A small remnant of fibrotic tissue is seen along the superior arcade *(arrow)*.

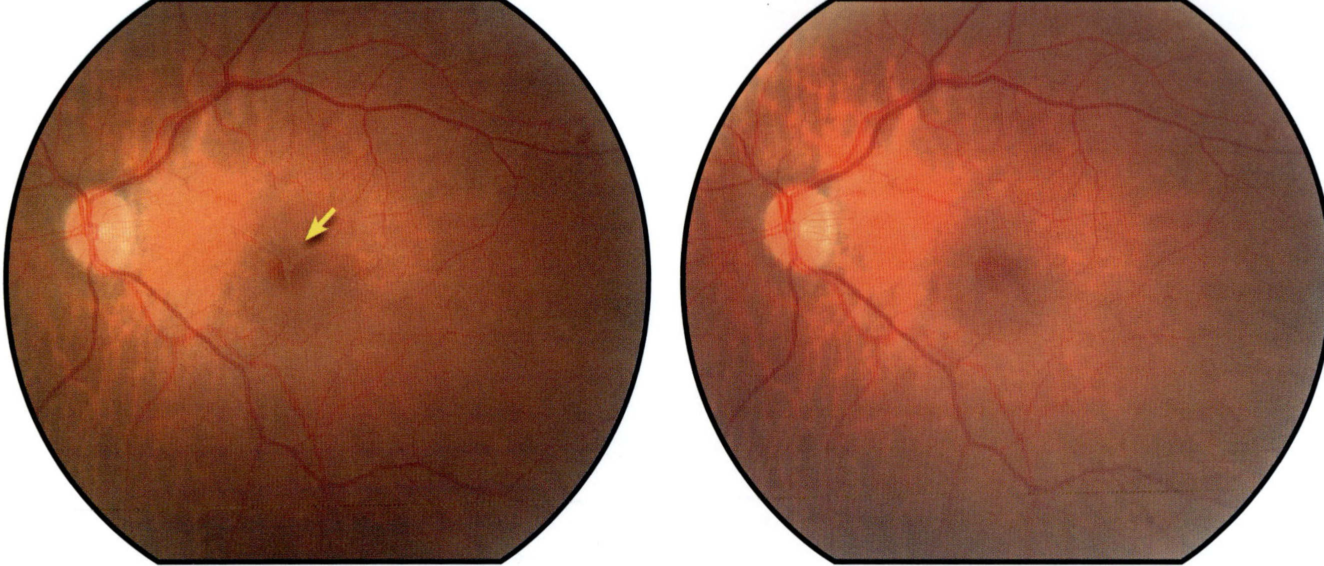

The above patient experienced subjective improvement in metamorphopsia and was noted to have spontaneous release of a macular ERM *(arrow)* that was present on the initial examination. Image on the right was taken 1 month after the baseline examination. *Images courtesy of Dr. Michael Engelbert*

Surgical Treatment

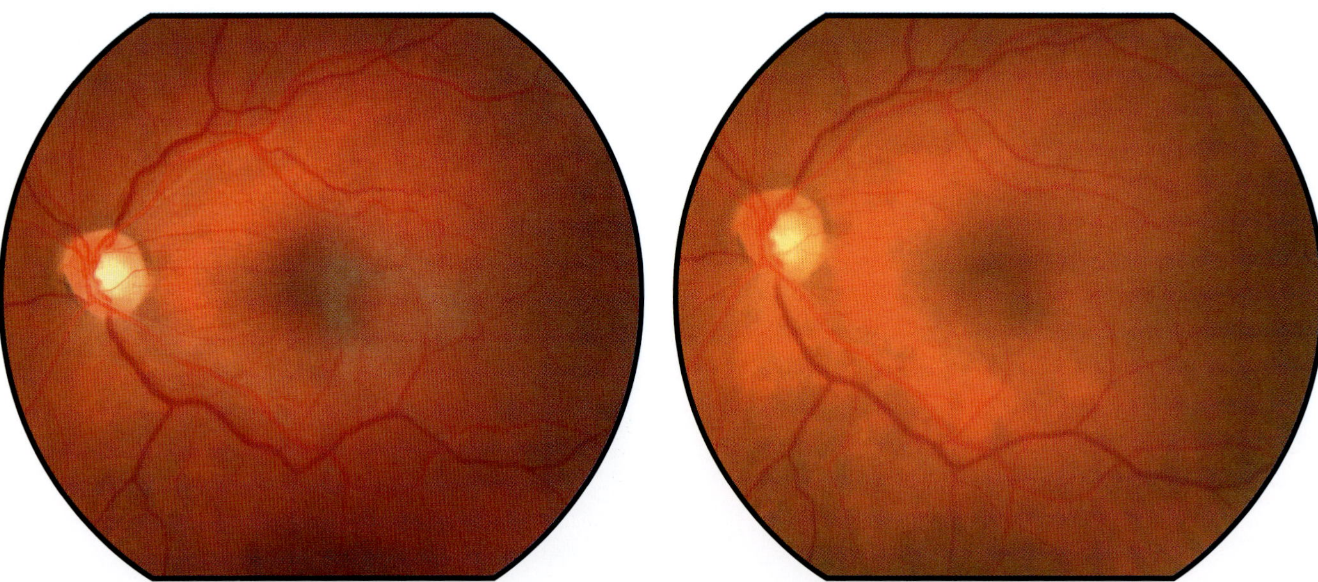

Patients with visually significant ERMs may be treated with pars plana vitrectomy and membrane peeling. Pre-operative *(left)* and post-operative *(right)* images are provided from a patient that presented with a visually significant ERM. Visual acuity was measured as 20/80 pre-operatively and returned to 20/25 following membrane peeling. *Images courtesy of Dr. Michael Engelbert*

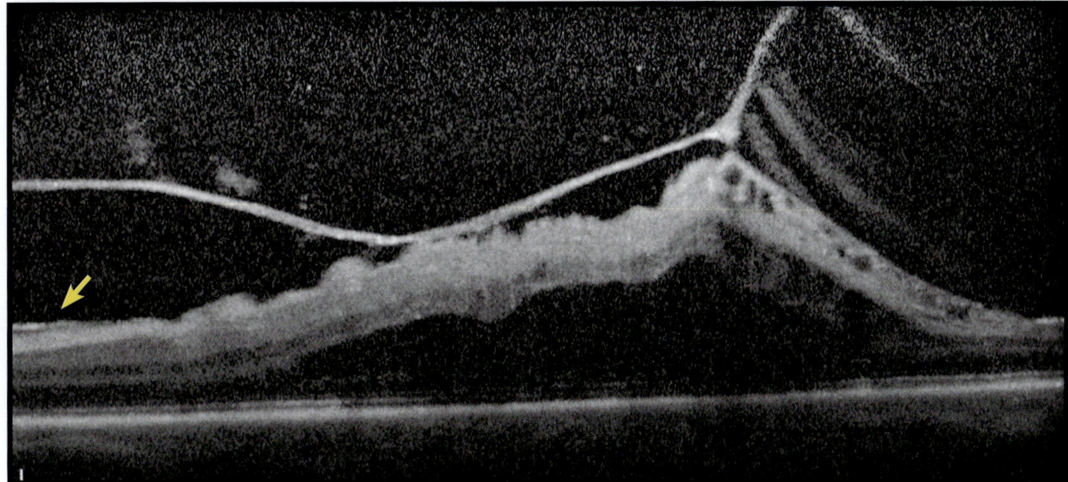

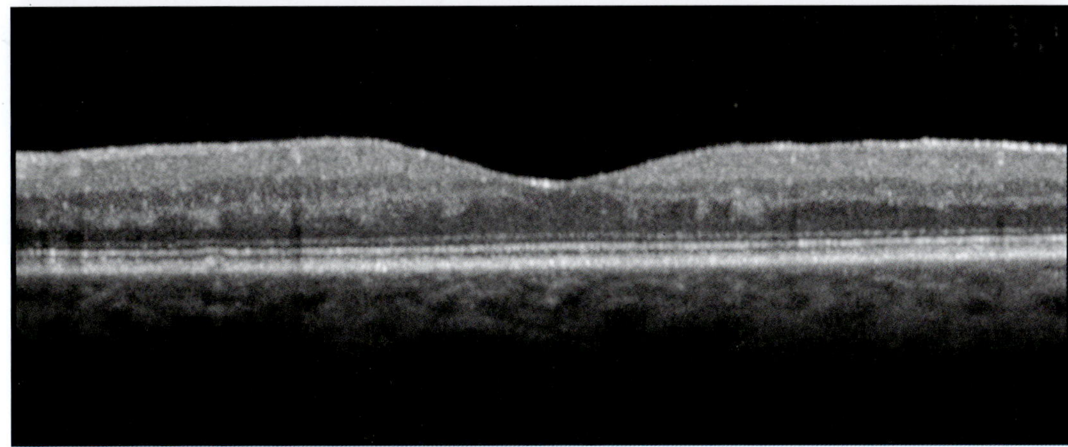

Anatomical outcomes following surgical intervention are best evaluated using OCT. This patient suffered disabling metamorphopsia and visual reduction due to traction from a broad vitreomacular adhesion (VMA). An associated ERM is also seen in the pre-operative OCT *(arrow)* as is frank intraretinal edema. Pre-operative visual acuity was measured as 20/100. Two years following vitrectomy and membrane peeling *(bottom image)*, the normal foveal contour was restored and visual acuity has returned to 20/25. *Images courtesy of Dr. Michael Engelbert*

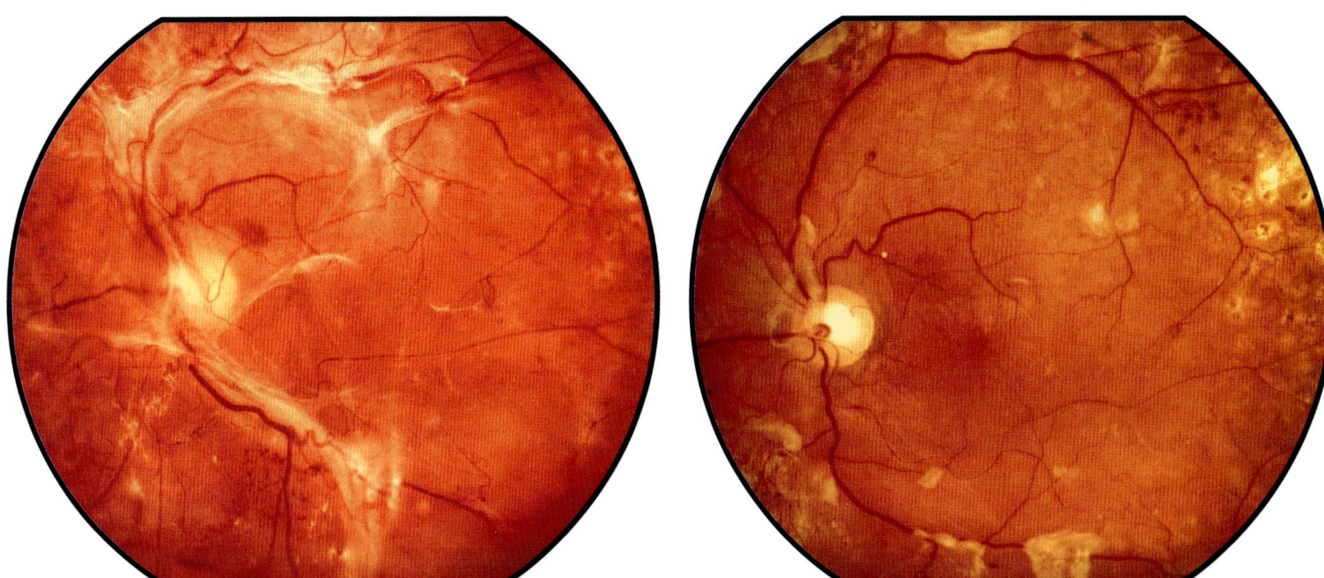

Surgical management of tractional membranes due to systemic vascular diseases such as diabetes mellitus can be more challenging. In the above patient, multiple points of macular traction, secondary to proliferative diabetic retinopathy, are evident. The surgical goal in this instance is to release all points of macular traction as illustrated in the post-surgical image on the right. Remnants of fibrous tissue can be seen on the surface of the retina; however, these structures are typically not visually significant. *Images courtesy of Dr. Yale Fisher*

Vitreomacular Traction (VMT)

Vitreomacular traction (VMT) is defined as persistent vitreous attachment to the central macula due to an incomplete posterior vitreous detachment. Histologically, VMT specimens obtained from surgery show a variety of cell types including fibrous astrocytes, myofibroblasts, and fibrocytes, similar to those found in ERMs. In fact, many eyes with VMT have a concurrent ERM and there is considerable overlap between the two entities. With the advent of spectral-domain OCT and vitreolytic agents, an International Vitreomacular Traction Study Classification System for VMA and VMT has been proposed.

Vitreomacular Adhesion (VMA)

VMA is defined as elevation of the cortical vitreous above the retina surface with the vitreous remaining attached within a 3 mm radius of the fovea. There is no change to the inner retina contour on OCT. VMA can be further subclassified by the size of adhesion into focal or broad.

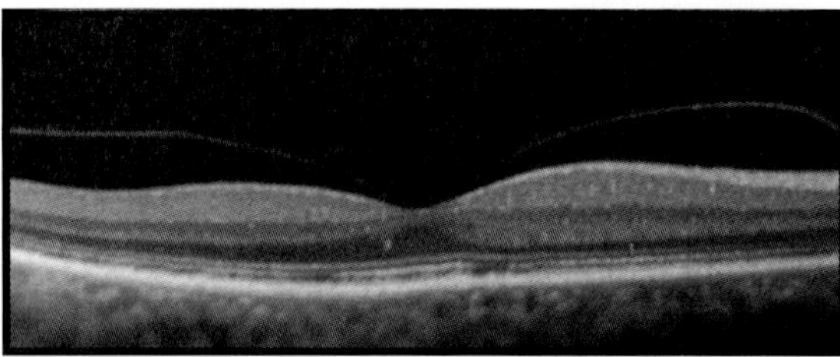

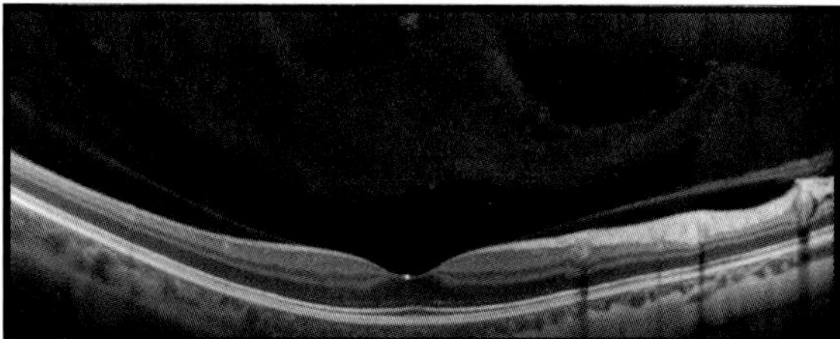

These patients have focal VMA ≤1500 μm *(left image)* and broad VMA > 1500 μm *(right image)*.

Vitreomacular Traction (VMT)

In VMT, all of the following criteria must exist:

(1) Perifoveal vitreous cortex detachment from the retinal surface
(2) Macular attachment of the vitreous cortex within a 3 mm radius of the fovea
(3) Distortion of the foveal surface, intraretinal structural changes, elevation of the fovea above the RPE or a combination thereof, without full-thickness interruption of retinal layers at sites of vitreous adhesion.

Like VMA, VMT can be further subclassified by the size of adhesion into focal or broad.

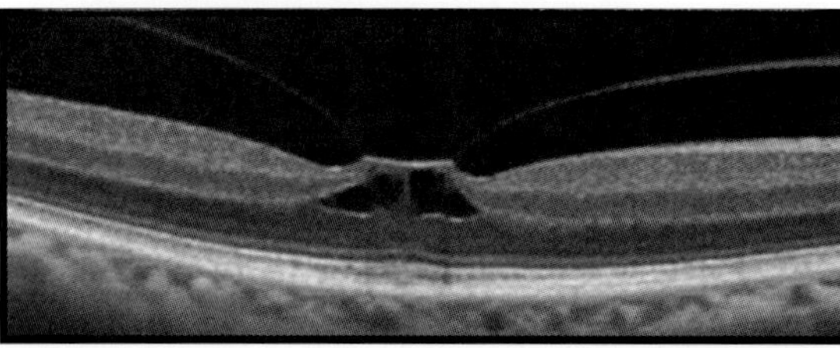

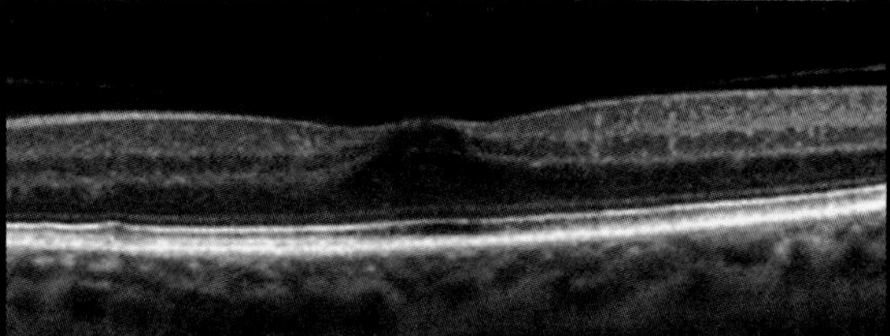

These patients have focal VMT ≤1500 μm *(left image)* and broad VMT > 1500 μm *(right image). Images courtesy of Dr. Jay Duker*

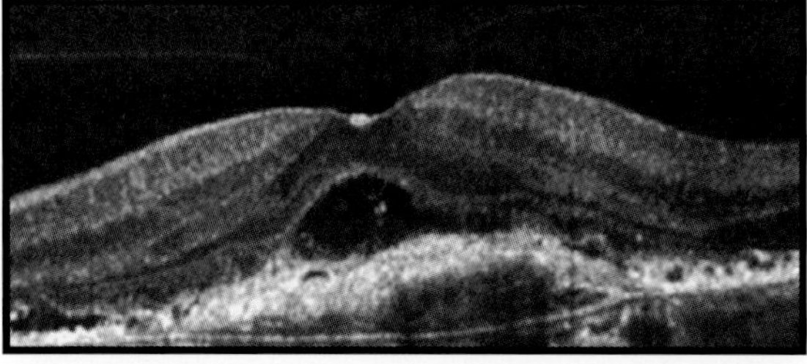

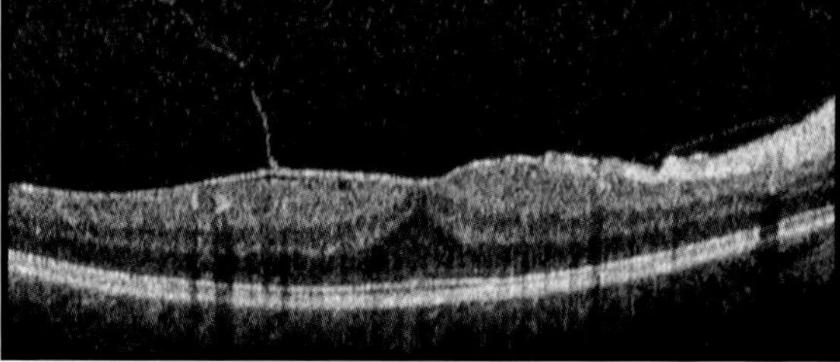

VMA and VMT may occur concurrently with other macular abnormalities including age-related macular degeneration *(left image)*, retinal vein occlusion, or diabetic macular edema. Eyes with VMT frequently have a concurrent ERM *(right image). Images courtesy of Dr. Jay Duker (left) and Dr. Edwin Ryan (right)*

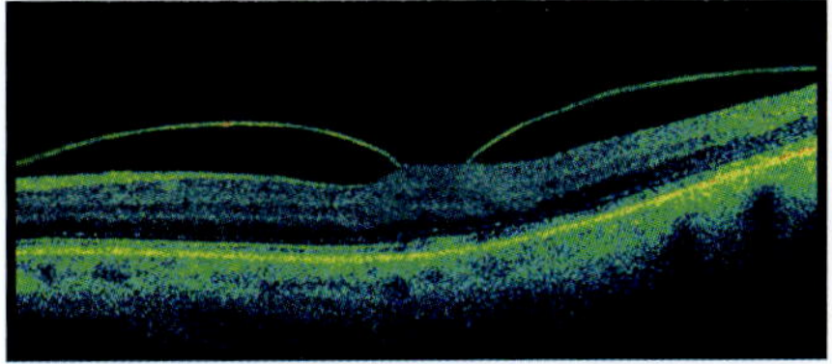
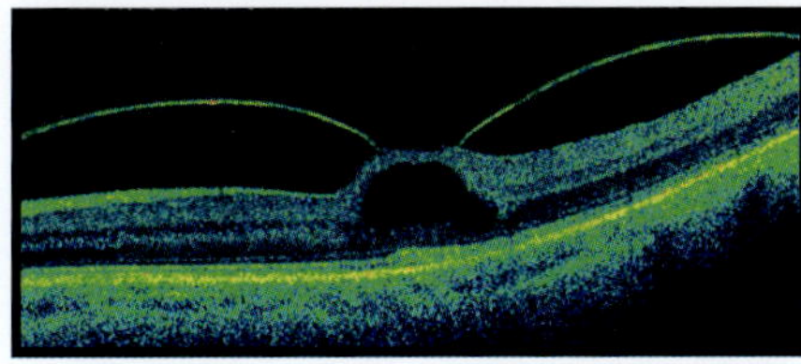
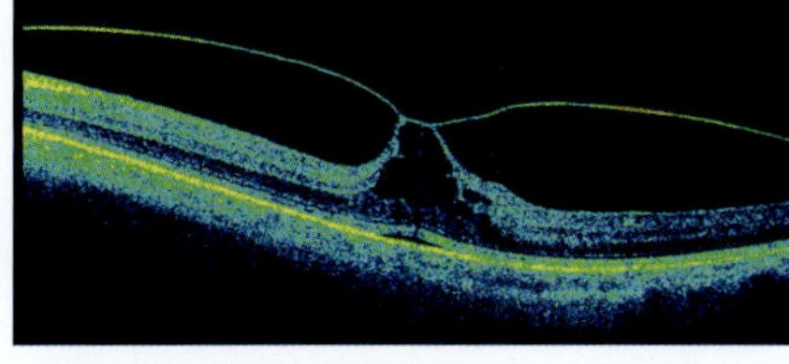

VMT can be graded according to the severity of the tractional effect on the retinal layers. In grade 1, there is elevation of the retina but no split in the retinal layers *(left image)*. In grade 2, there are intraretinal cysts, clefts, or schisis *(middle image)*. In grade 3, there is neurosensory elevation of the retina above the RPE resulting in subretinal fluid *(right image)*. *Images courtesy of Dr. Harry Flynn*

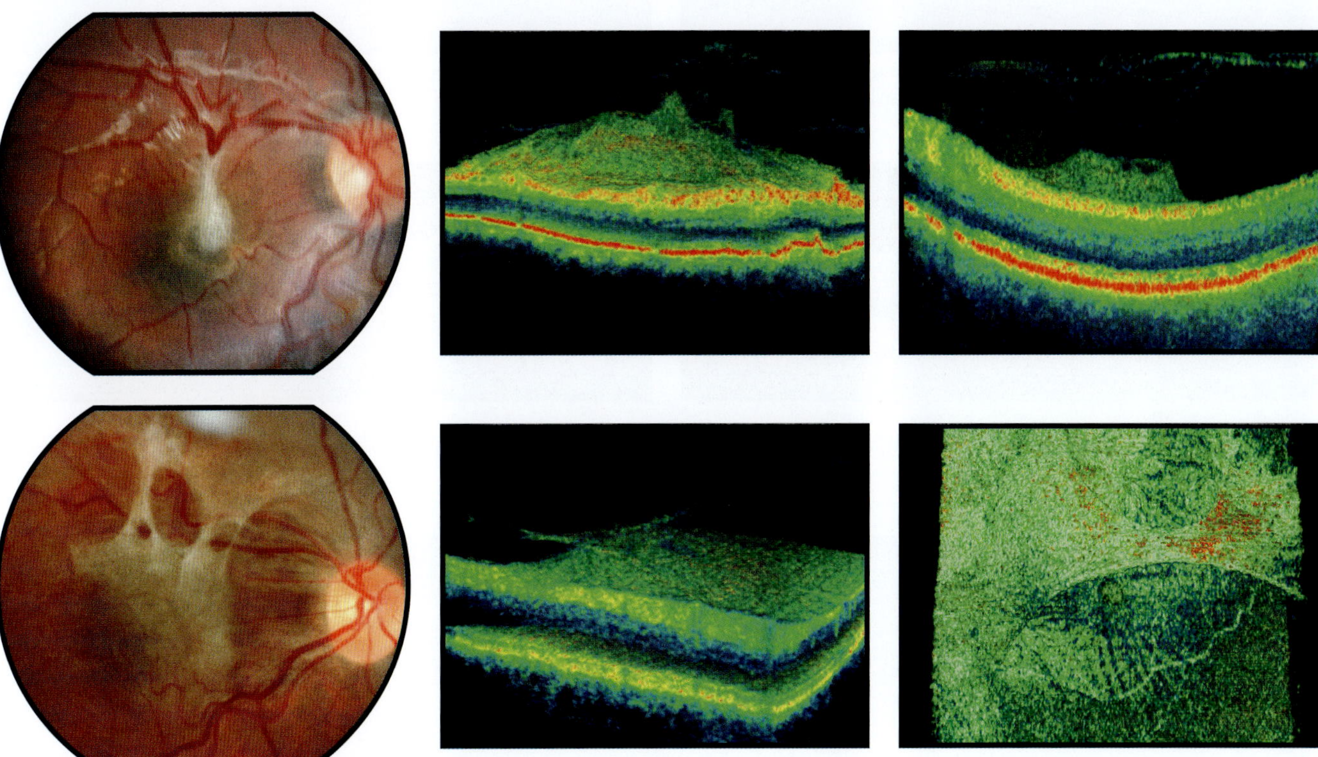

Three-dimensional OCT images show broad-based VMT with retinal thickening. These images may facilitate surgical planning of membrane peeling by the vitreoretinal surgeon. *Images courtesy of Dr. Hideki Koizumi*

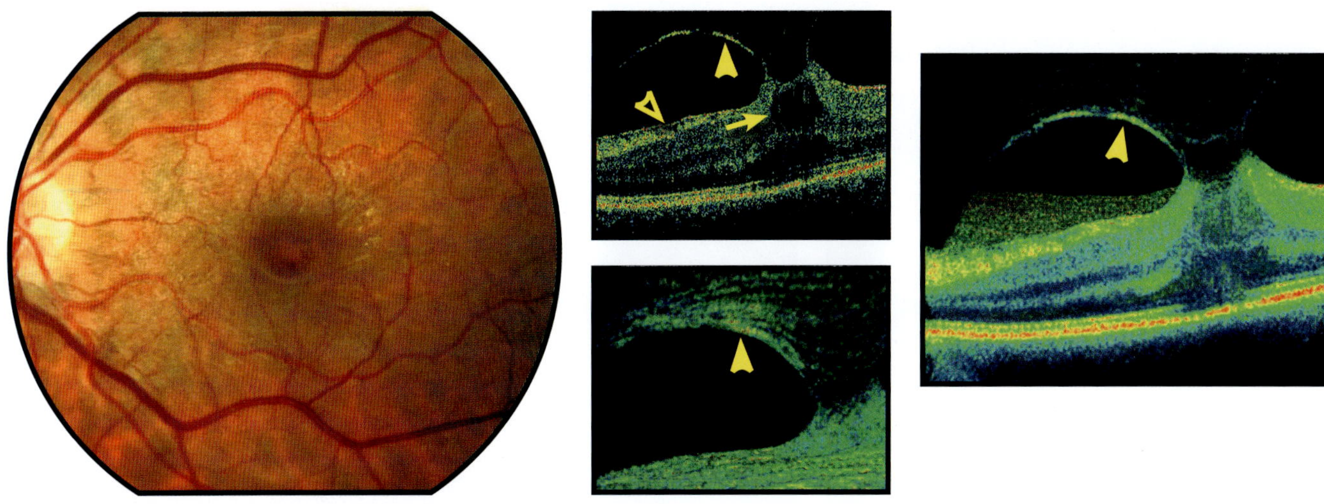

Three-dimensional OCT images show VMT occurring concurrently with an epiretinal membrane. The epiretinal membrane appears as a thin, reflective line above the jagged inner retinal surface *(open arrowhead)*. There is associated retinal thickening, intraretinal cysts *(arrow)*, and subretinal fluid. There are curvilinear bands of fibrous traction or "hourglass" plaques seen with a funnel-like traction on the retina *(arrowheads)*. *Images courtesy of Dr. Hideki Koizumi*

Natural History

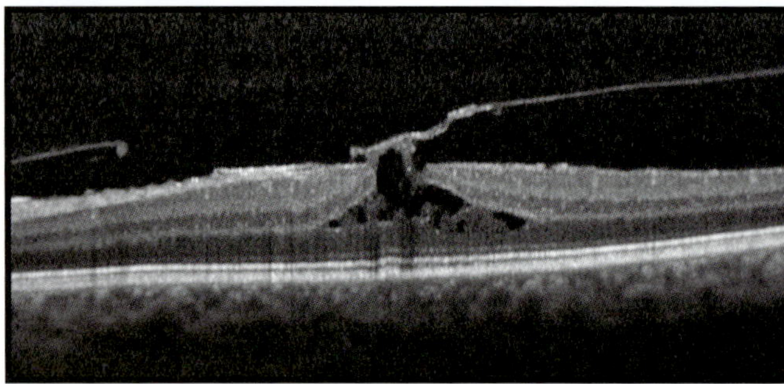
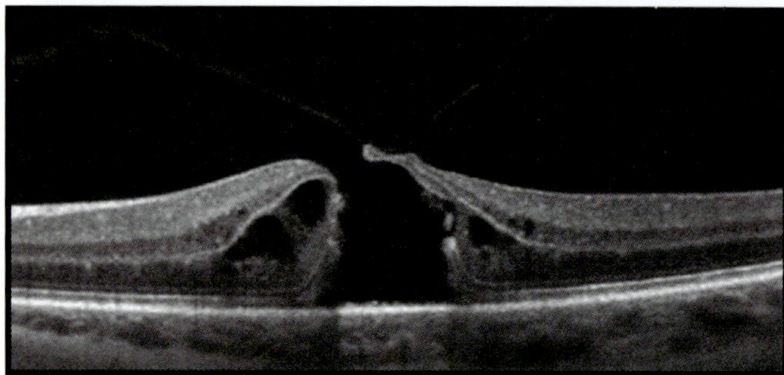

VMT may show progression to a lamellar macular hole *(left image)* or a full-thickness macular hole (FTMH) *(right image)*.

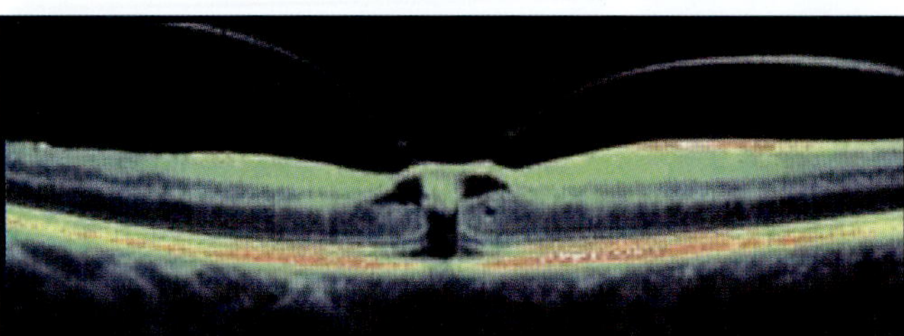
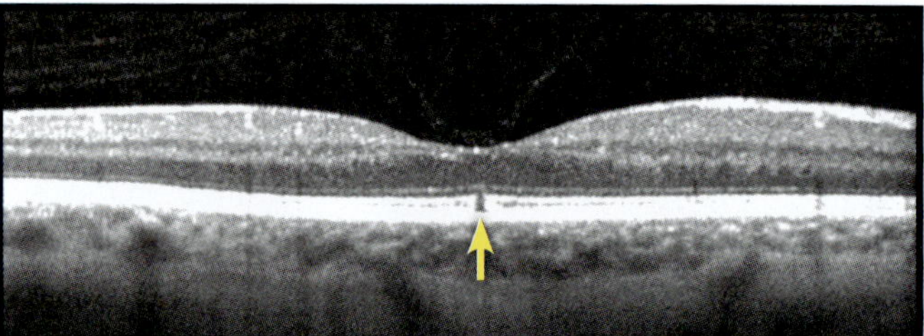

Focal VMT may also result in outer retinal defects, also known as macular microholes, outer lamellar macular holes, or foveal photoreceptor defects *(arrow)*.

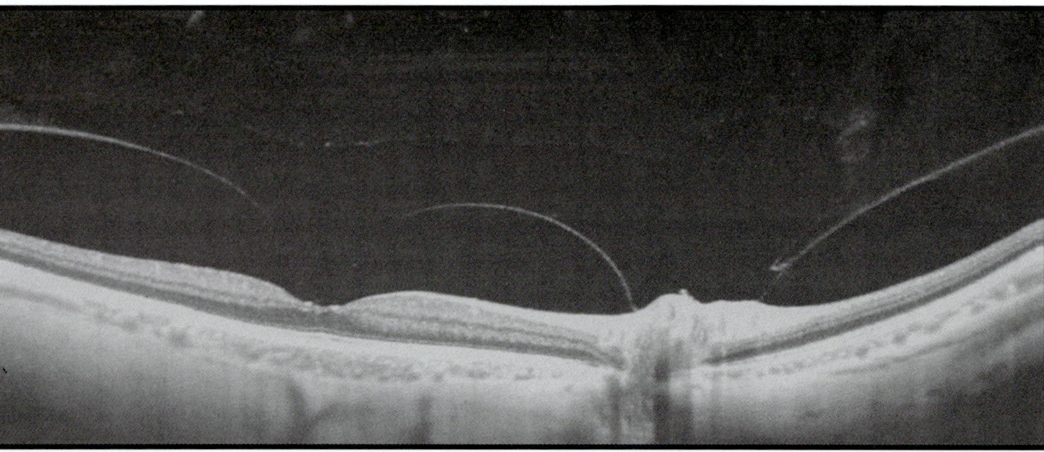
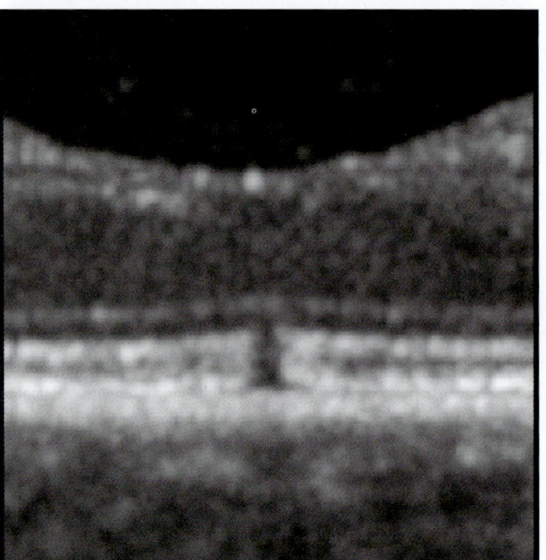

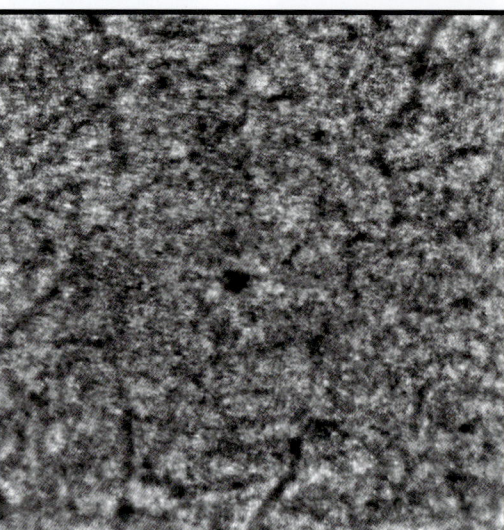

Patients may complain of a microscotoma due to traction-induced foveal lesions. High resolution swept-source OCT imaging *(top image)* clearly demonstrates the VMA in this case but does not identify the foveal abnormality as the density of the volume scan was inadequate. High density OCT imaging *(bottom left image)* at a subsequent visit reveals the foveal defect, which is also seen as a central loss of cones on adaptive optics imaging *(bottom right image)*.

Spontaneous Release of Vitreomacular Traction

Spontaneous release of grade 1 or 2 VMT occurs in approximately 30% of eyes and release of grade 3 VMT occurs in almost 60-70% of cases. The mean time to spontaneous release is approximately 16 months.

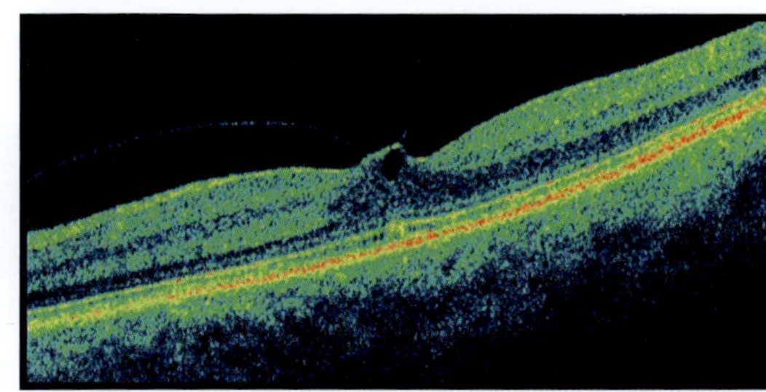
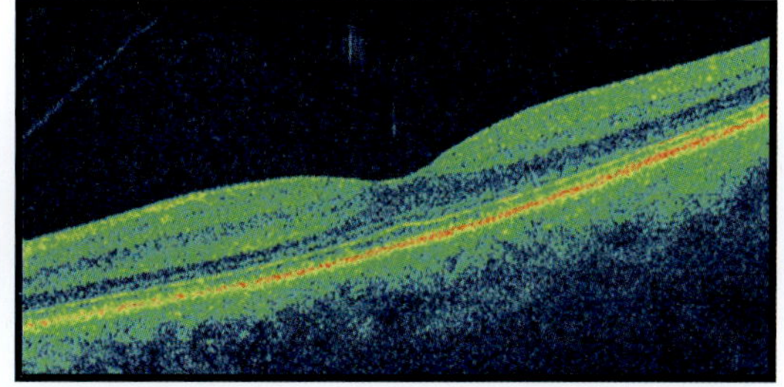

Spontaneous release of VMT may occur with resolution of foveal abnormalities. This patient was found to have spontaneous release of VMT after 4 months. Visual acuity was unchanged and remained at 20/25.

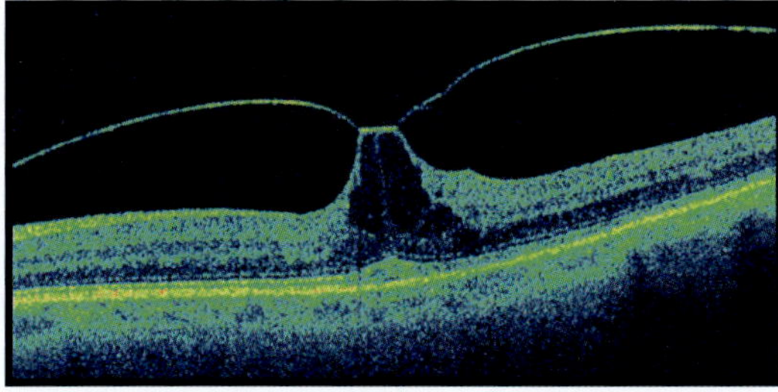
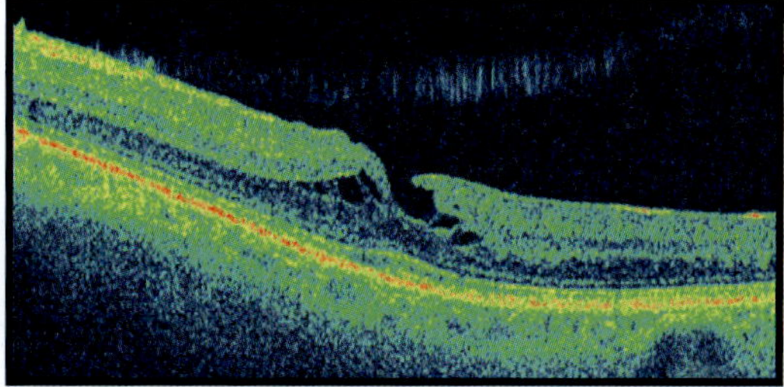

This patient had spontaneous release of VMT 1 year after initial presentation, with resulting intraretinal schisis at the fovea. Visual acuity was unchanged at 20/50.

Vitreomacular Traction and Acquired Vitelliform Lesion

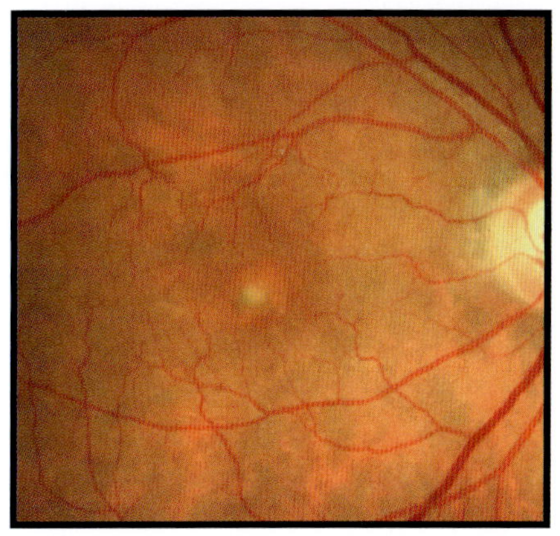
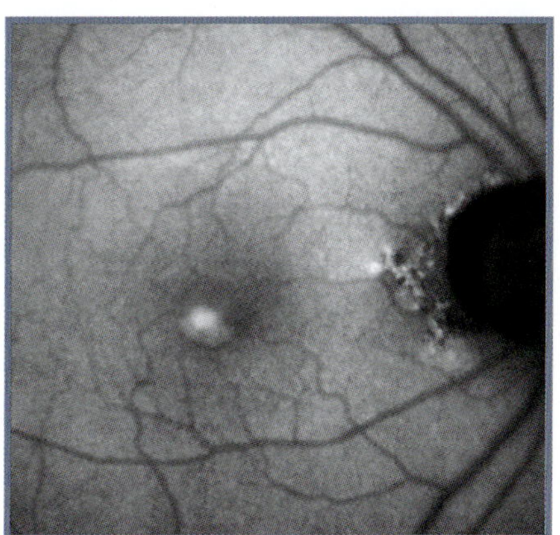
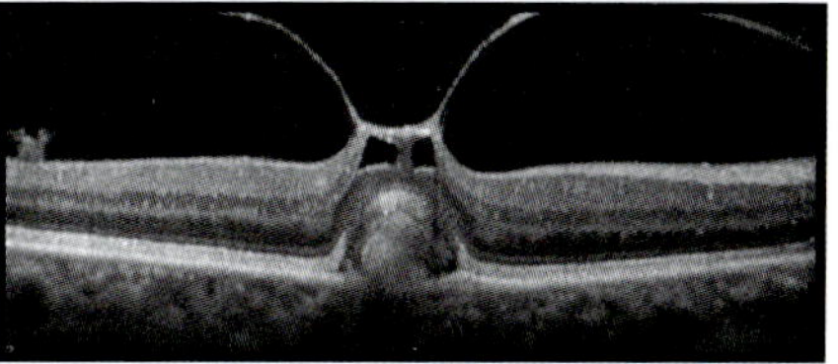

Focal VMT may be associated with an acquired vitelliform lesion. The vitelliform lesion appears yellow on color fundus photographs and is hyperautofluorescent on fundus autofluorescence imaging. The vitelliform lesion appears as hyper-reflective material in the subretinal space with OCT imaging.

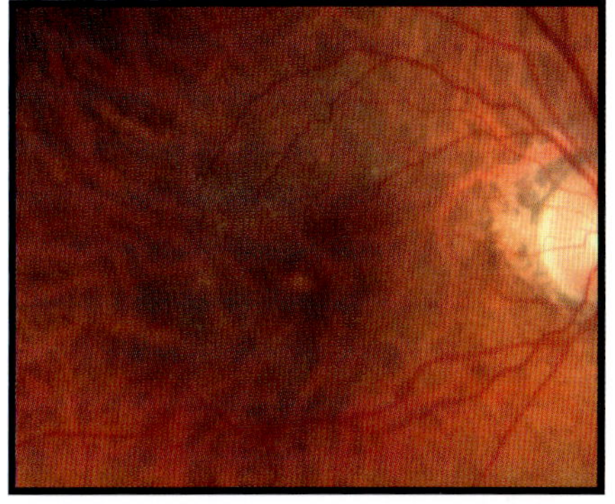
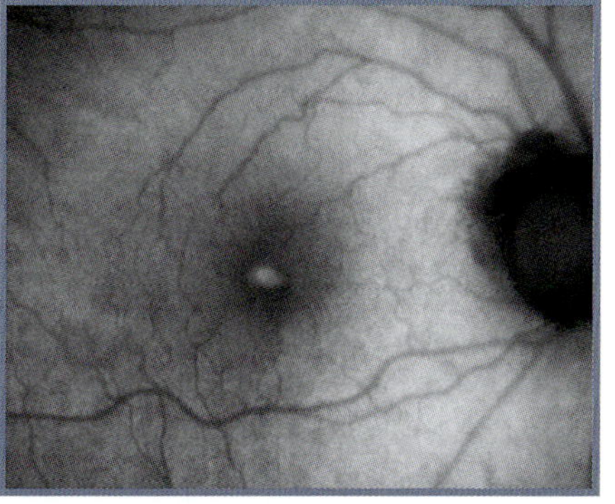
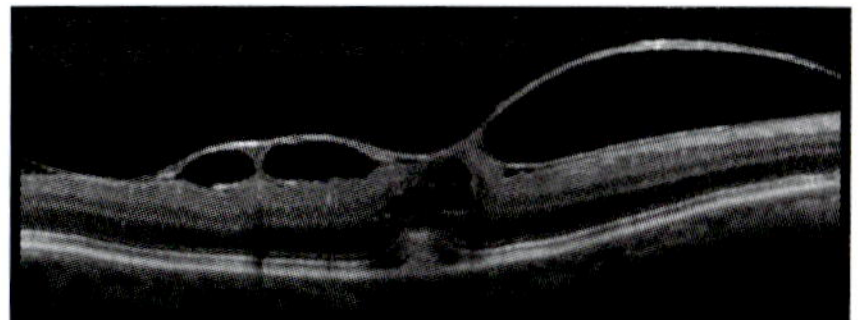

© 667 © 668

A vitelliform lesion was noted in this patient with broad VMT. *Images courtesy of Dr. Richard Spaide*

Vitreolytic Treatment

Recently, ocriplasmin has been employed as an intravitreal vitreolytic agent for focal VMA and focal VMT. Outcomes following treatment with this agent are variable; however, it may be considered as first-line therapy for some symptomatic patients.

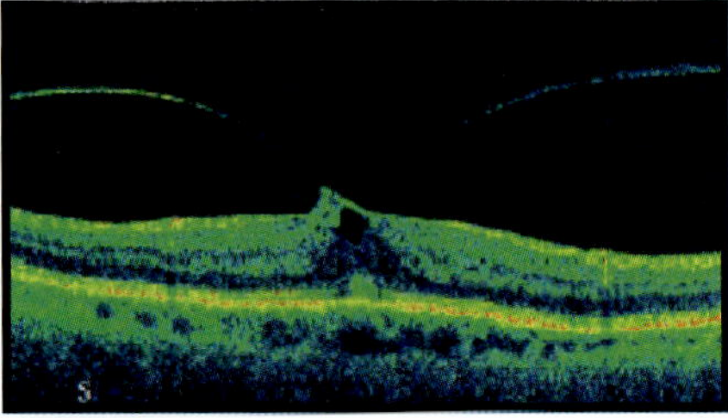
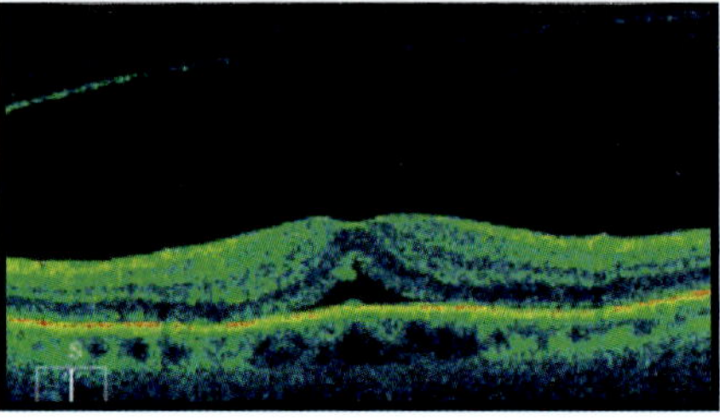
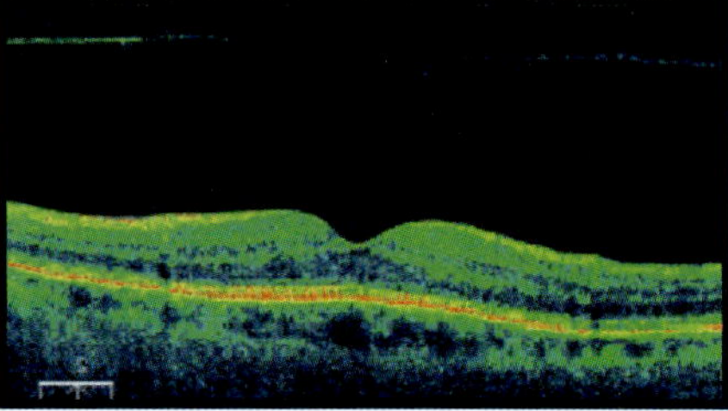

This patient with focal VMT and visual acuity of 20/30 *(left image)* received an intravitreal injection of ocriplasmin, with successful release of the vitreomacular attachment on the first day *(middle image)*. The visual acuity dropped to 20/70 at this time due to subretinal fluid at the fovea. The subretinal fluid resolved by 1 month and the visual acuity improved to 20/20. *Images courtesy of Dr. Rishi Singh*

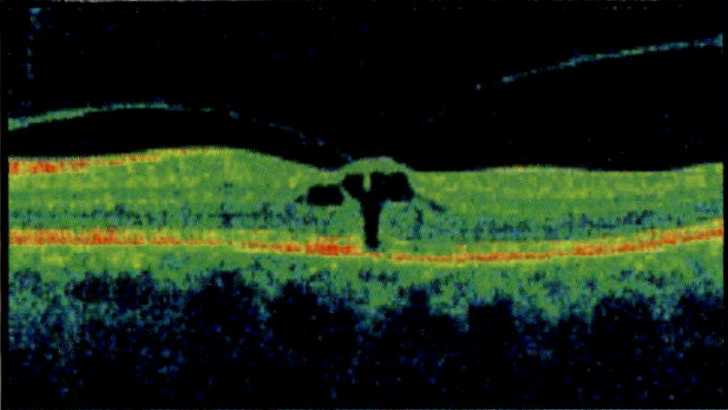
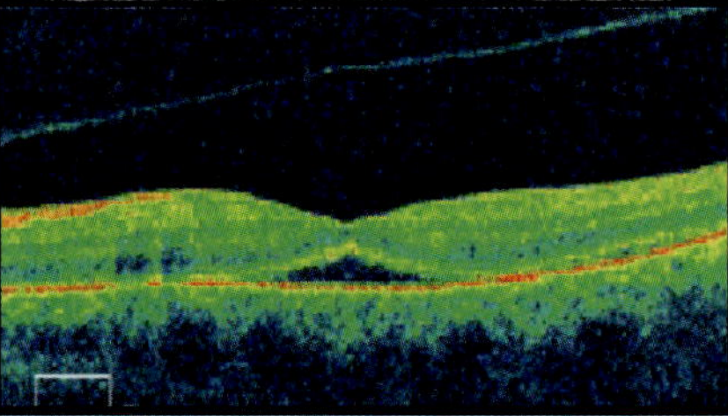
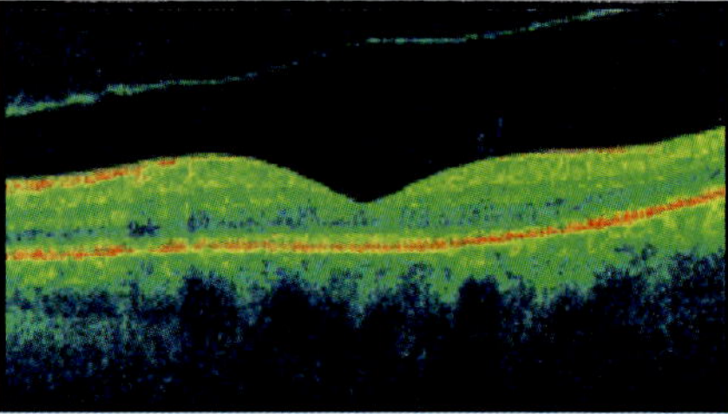

This patient is another example of successful release of focal VMT after intravitreal ocriplasmin injection. The initial visual acuity was 20/50. The release was noted 1 week after the injection *(middle image)*. Again, subretinal fluid at the fovea was noted at this time and visual acuity remained unchanged at 20/40. Subretinal fluid resolved by 3 weeks and visual acuity improved to 20/30 *(right image)*. *Images courtesy of Dr. Rishi Singh*

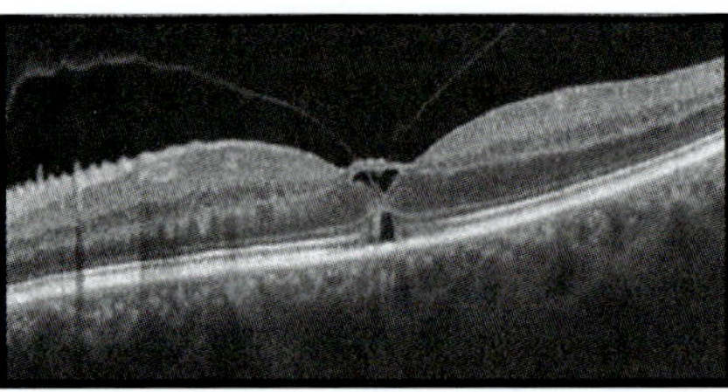
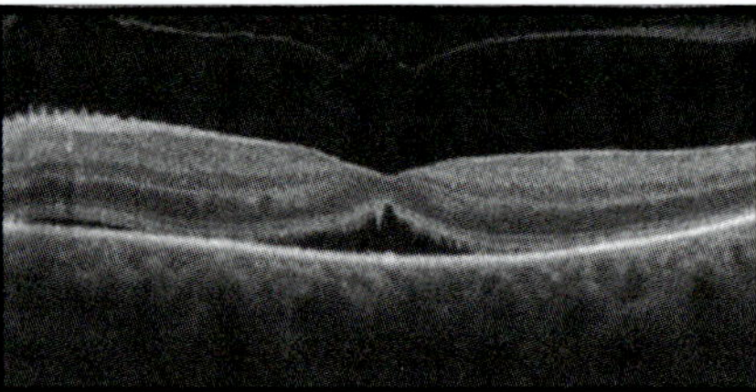
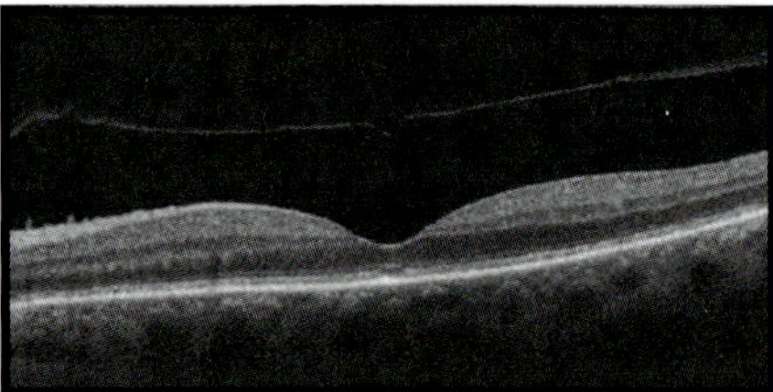

With high resolution OCT, it is possible to appreciate ellipsoid zone disruptions that are a known complication following ocriplasmin injection *(middle image)*. If ellipsoid zone disruption occurs, it usually recovers spontaneously within 1 to 3 months *(right image)*. *Images courtesy of Dr. Rishi Singh*

Full-Thickness Macular Hole

A full-thickness macular hole (FTMH) is a retinal defect that commences at the level of the internal limiting membrane and extends up to, but not including, the RPE. These defects may arise from a number of retinal insults including traction on the inner retina and/or loss of central neurosensory retinal tissue. Primary FTMHs are due to VMT on the fovea from an anomalous posterior vitreous detachment. Secondary FTMHs are due to a range of causes including trauma, lightning strike, myopia, macular telangiectasia type 2, and age-related macular degeneration. VMT may or may not be a pathogenic factor in the formation of secondary macular holes.

Classification

The Gass classification of FTMH comprised 4 stages and was based on clinical examination findings. In contrast, the International Vitreomacular Traction Study Classification of FTMH is based on OCT and describes the size of the hole and the presence or absence of VMT. Correlation between the two schemes is as follows:

Gass Classification	International Vitreomacular Traction Study Classification
Stage 1: Impending hole	VMT
Stage 2: FTMH ≤400 μm, no posterior vitreous detachment (PVD)	Small (≤250 μm) or medium (>250-400 μm) FTMH with VMT
Stage 3: FTMH >400 μm, no PVD	Large (>400 μm) FTMH with VMT
Stage 4: FTMH >400 μm with PVD	Any size FTMH without VMT

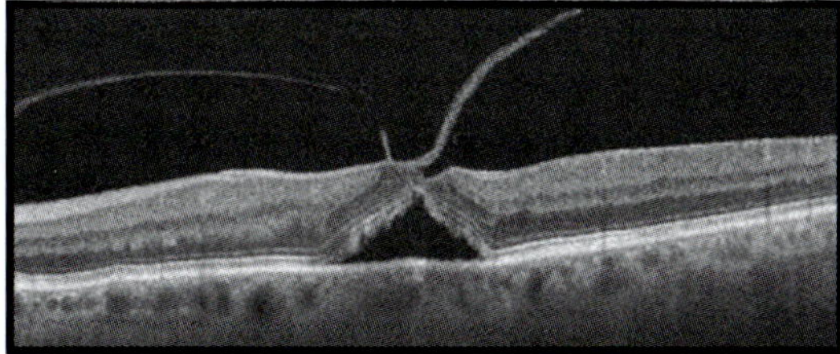

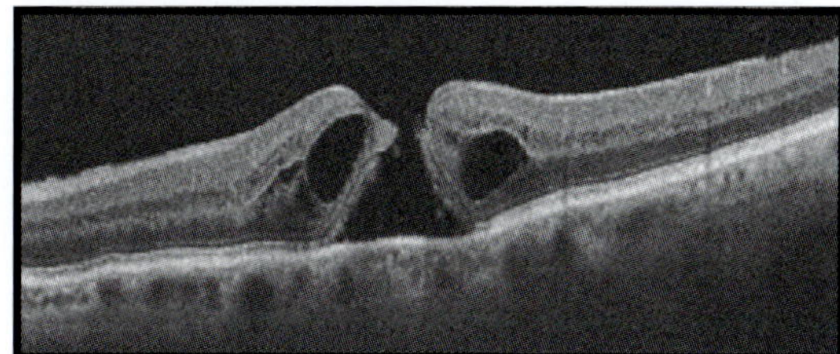

This patient with VMT developed a FTMH 2 years later. The left image illustrates the OCT features of VMT and the right image illustrates the OCT features of FTMH.

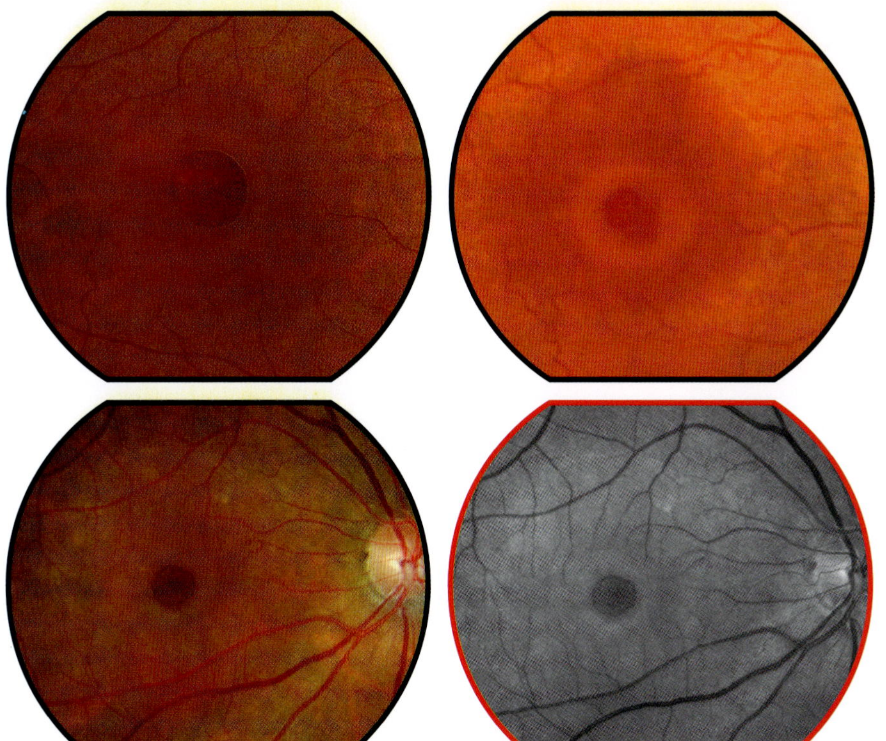

The characteristic clinical findings of FTMHs are illustrated in these cases. A FTMH is typically delineated by a sharp margin and frequently demonstrates a surrounding cuff of cystic change and subretinal fluid.

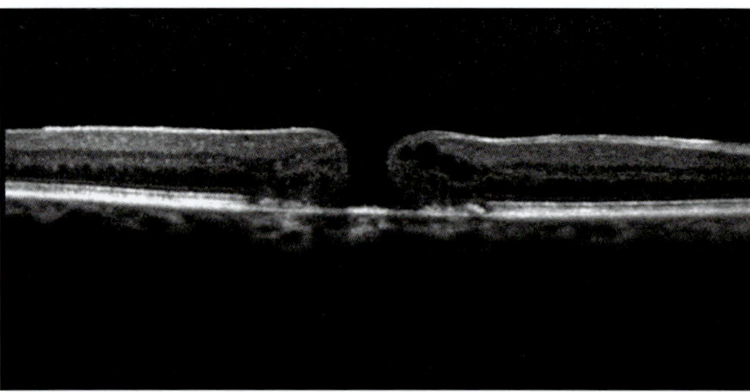

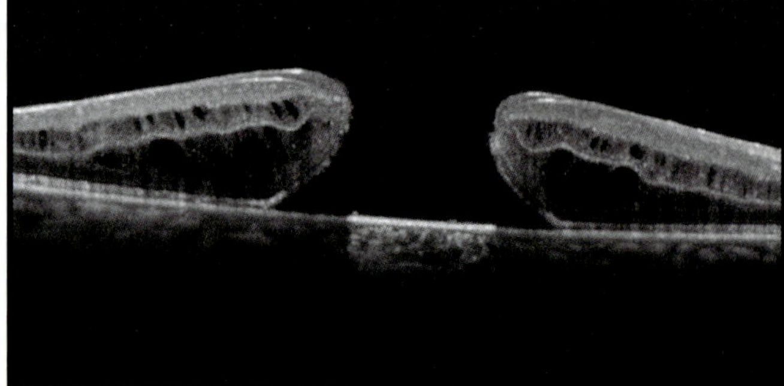

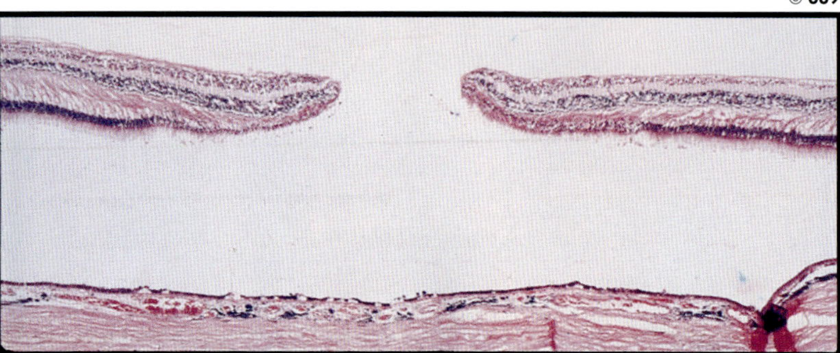

© 669

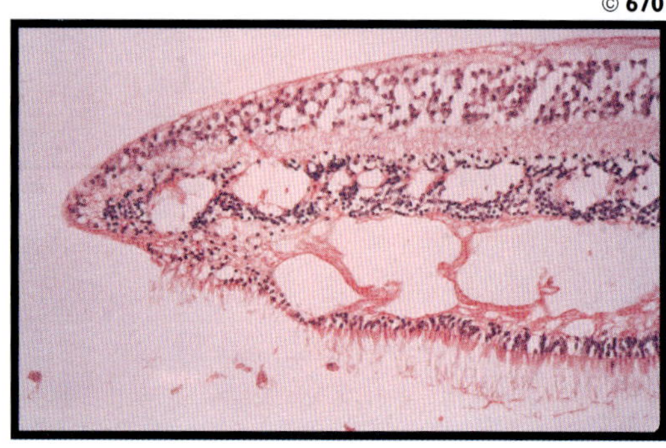

© 670

OCT imaging allows detailed ultrastructural evaluation of macular holes. In the above cases, full-thickness retinal defects are seen as are intraretinal cystic changes at the margins of the hole. Pathology of the margin of the hole shows cystic degeneration of the inner and outer retina and correlates closely to the appearance of macular holes as seen on OCT.

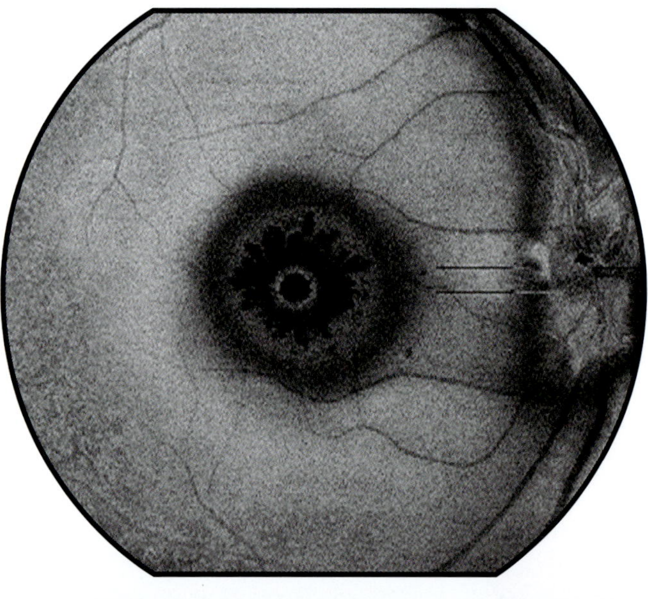

The petalloid morphology of cystic changes surrounding the margins of macular holes are best appreciated with *en face* imaging techniques, as illustrated in this case, which was evaluated with swept source OCT. *Image courtesy of Dr. Michael Engelbert*

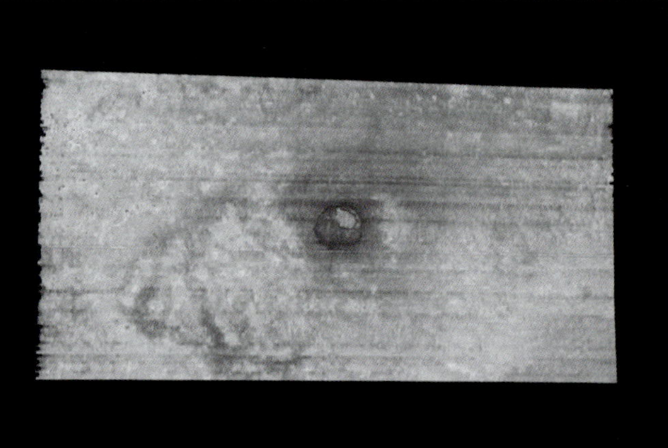

This volume rendered OCT image shows the FTMH in three dimensions. *Image courtesy of Dr. Richard Spaide*

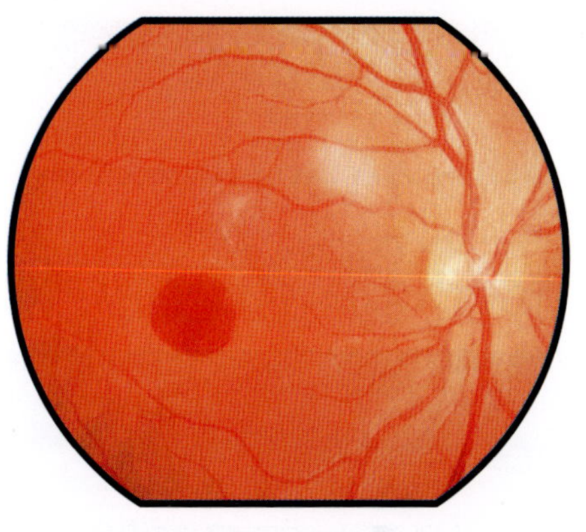
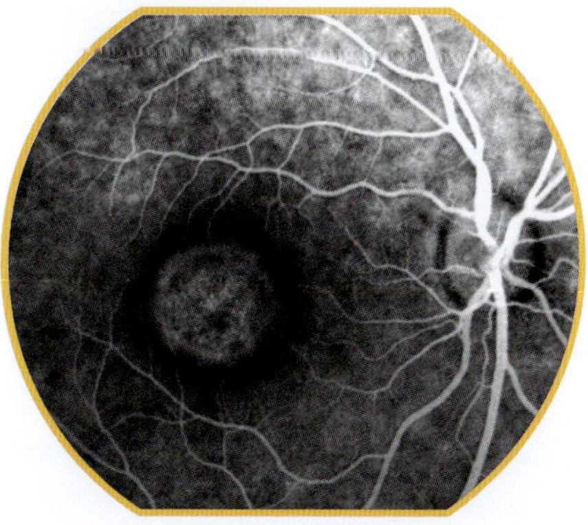
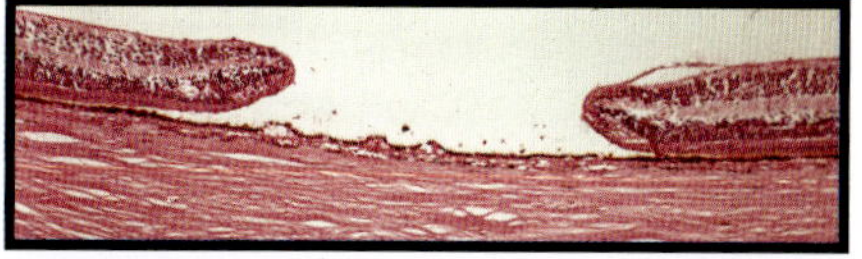

Fluorescein angiography of FTMHs demonstrates hyperfluorescence due to loss of overlying retinal tissue. Attenuation of the RPE at the site of the hole, as seen on the histological specimen *(right image)*, is another reason for this hyperfluorescence.

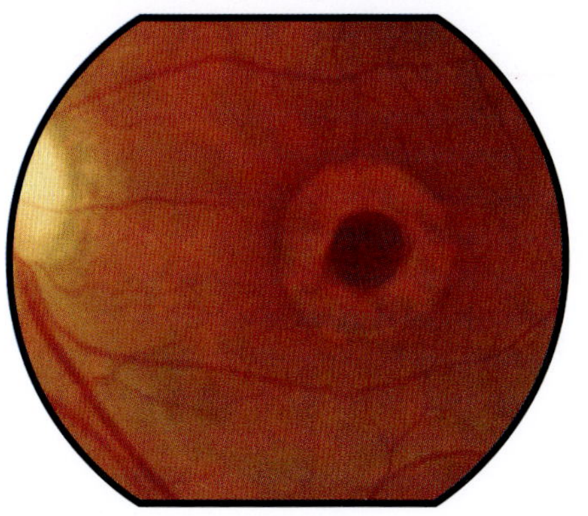
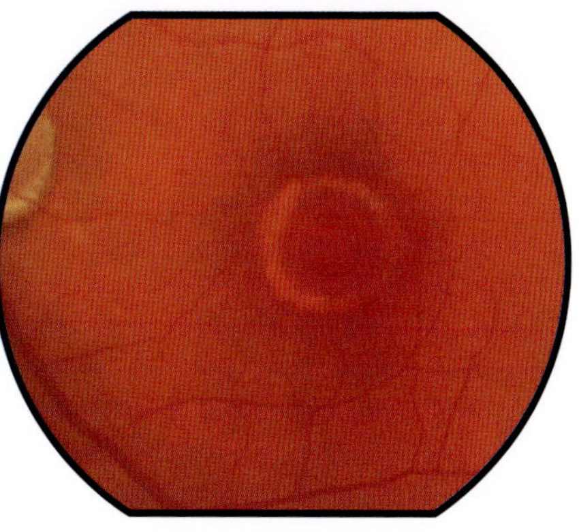
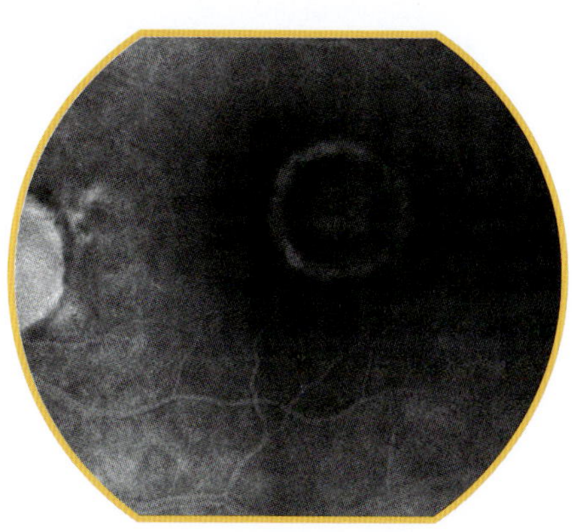

These patients with long-standing macular holes have a demarcation ring that is atrophic in nature. This appears as a hyperfluorescent window defect on fluorescein angiography.

Spontaneous Closure

The rate of spontaneous closure of primary FTMHs has been reported to range from 3% to 6%. The exact mechanism of spontaneous macular hole closure is still unclear, but four different hypotheses have been proposed: (1) complete vitreous detachment over the fovea releasing the tractional forces, (2) formation of an epiretinal membrane resulting in hole shrinkage, (3) glial cell proliferation at the base of the hole, and (4) growth of retinal tissue bridging the hole.

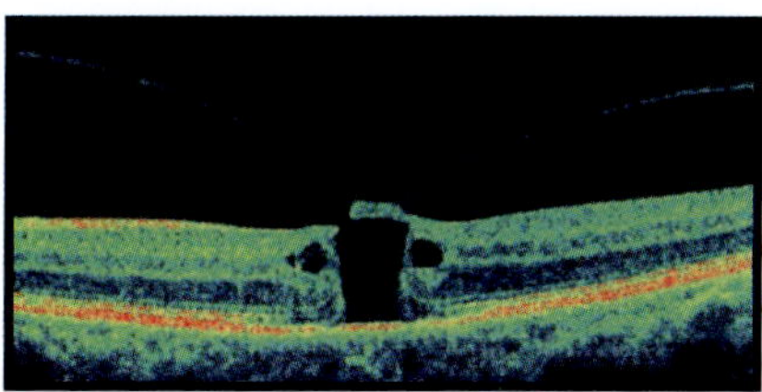
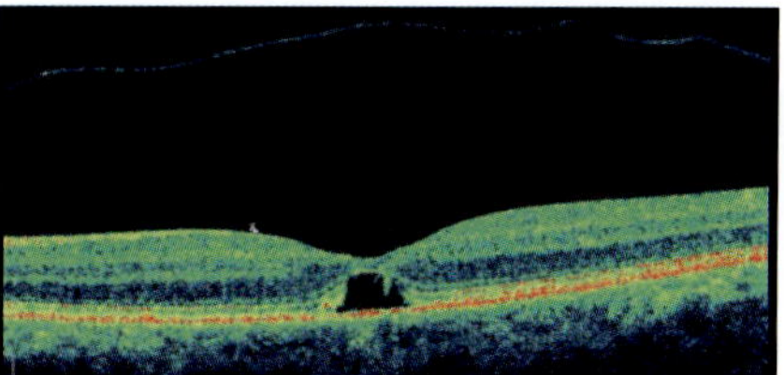
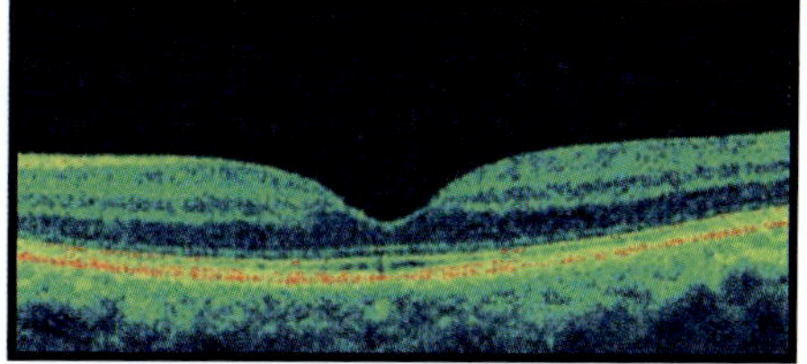

This patient was noted to have VMT with adhesions of the posterior hyaloid to the roof of the macular hole *(left image)*. One week later, there was spontaneous and complete posterior vitreous separation, with bridging of the retinal tissue at the level of the inner retina. Often, there are outer retinal layer defects, which may either persist or recover with time *(middle image)*. After 1 year, foveal architecture appears normal *(right image)*.

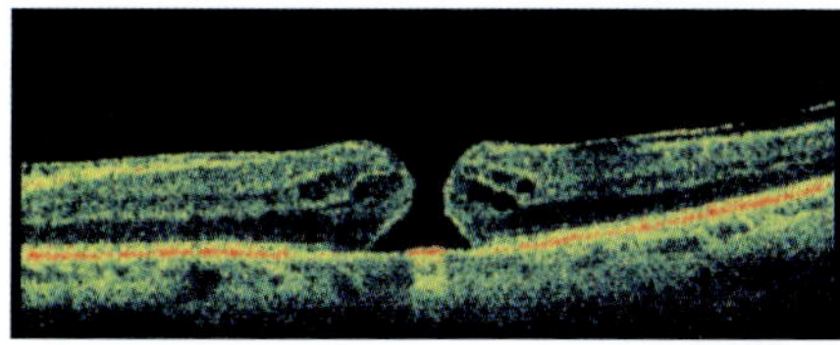
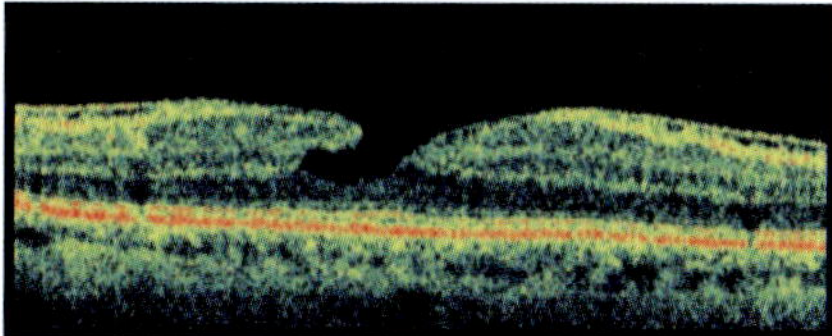
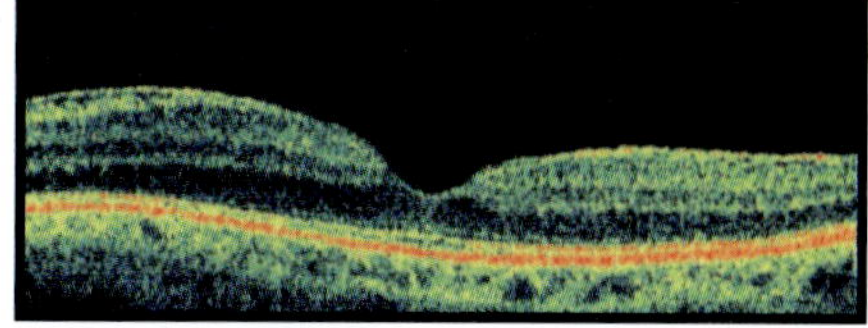

This patient had a FTMH of approximately 200 μm at the narrowest diameter with an epiretinal membrane *(left image)*. Five months later, there was spontaneous apposition of the outer layers of the retina with transformation of the hole into a lamellar configuration *(middle image)*. At 6 months, the foveal architecture appears almost normal *(right image)*. *Images courtesy of Dr. Andrea Scopulo*

Vitreolytic Treatment

Intravitreal ocriplasmin therapy has been shown to have a success rate between 10-40% for small stage 2 FTMHs (≤250 μm). Ocriplasmin therapy is used by some surgeons as first-line therapy for carefully selected cases of FTMH. Eyes that fail vitreolytic therapy are managed surgically.

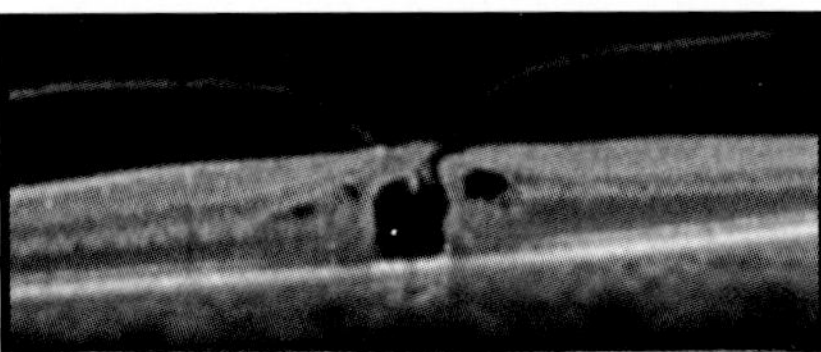
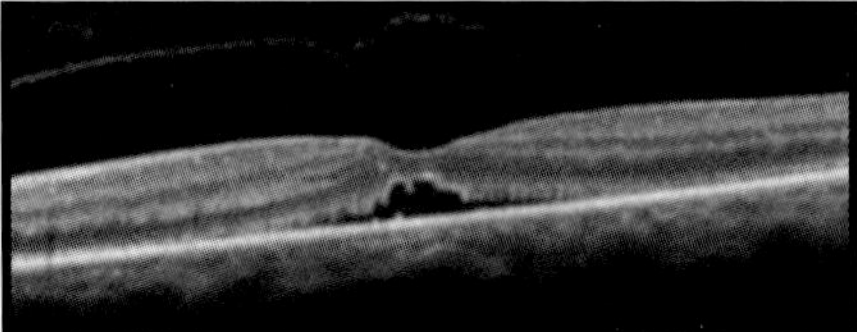
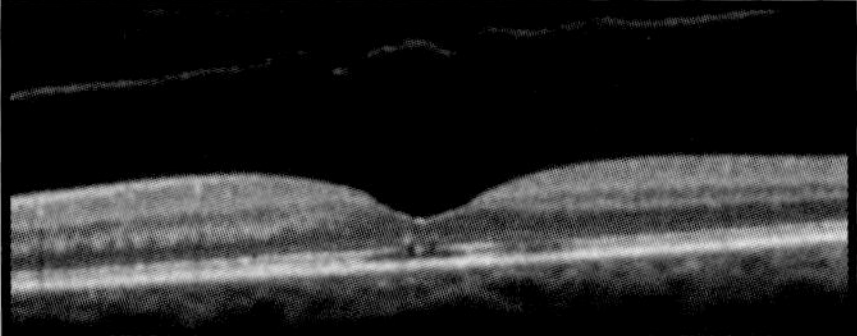

This patient with a stage 2 FTMH was treated with intravitreal ocriplasmin *(left image)*. One week later, there was separation of the posterior hyaloid and closure of the inner retina *(middle image)*. Six months later, there were persistent outer retinal defects and ellipsoid zone disruptions *(right image)*. *Images courtesy of Dr. John Miller*

Surgical Treatment

Patients with FTMHs may be treated with pars plana vitrectomy, internal limiting membrane peeling, and gas tamponade. Post-vitrectomy, inner retinal dimpling is seen on the inner retinal surface in approximately a third of cases and typically appears 3 months after surgery. The exact mechanism is unknown, although it has been proposed that the dimples may represent defects in Müller cell regrowth.

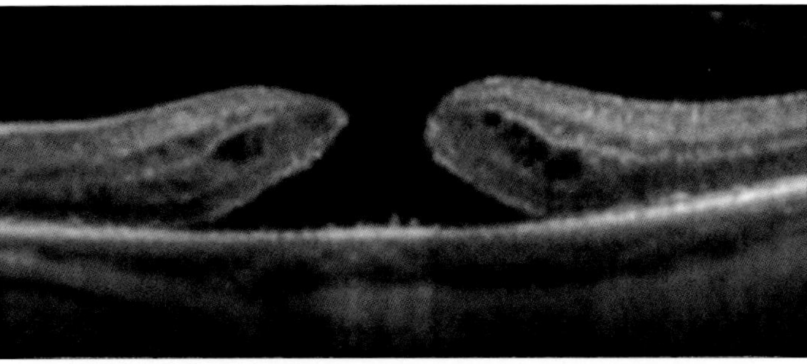
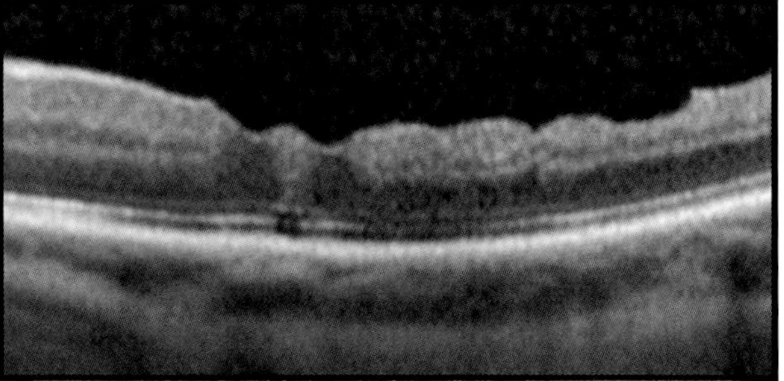

This patient with FTMH underwent pars plana vitrectomy and membrane peeling. Four months after surgery, there is inner retinal dimpling and some disruption at the level of the ellipsoid zone.

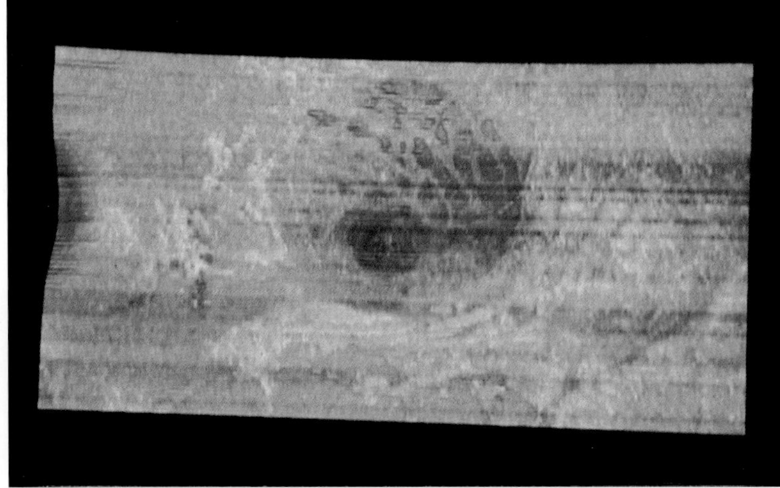

© 671

Three-dimensional volume rendered OCT imaging provides precise spatial visualization of inner retinal dimpling following macular hole surgery. *Image courtesy of Dr. Richard Spaide*

Secondary Macular Holes

The pathogenesis of secondary macular holes is different from primary macular holes. Surgical hole closure rates are lower in eyes with secondary macular holes due to the varied pathophysiology.

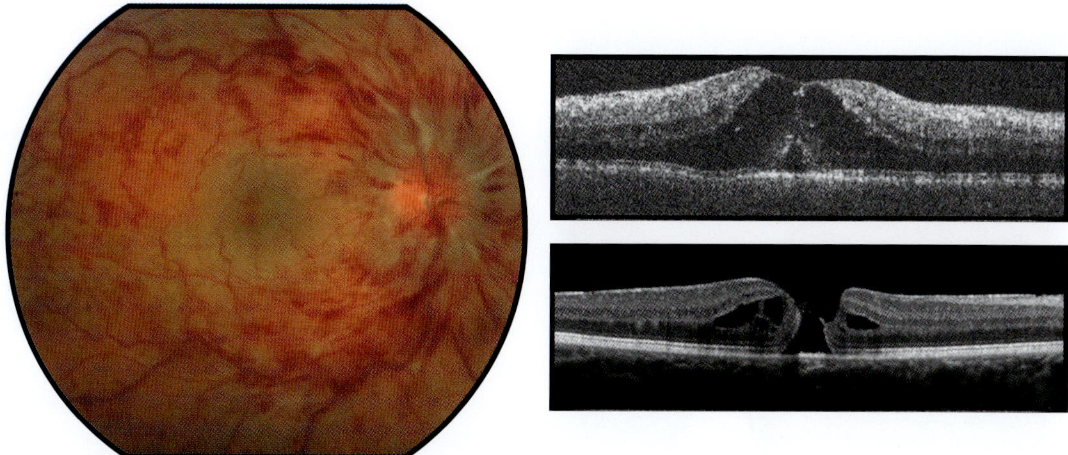

This patient had a central retinal vein occlusion *(left image)* and cystoid macular edema *(top right image)* that was treated with intravitreal steroids and anti-vascular endothelial growth factor therapy. A FTMH appeared after resolution of the central macular edema *(bottom right image). Images courtesy of Dr. Jay Klancnik*

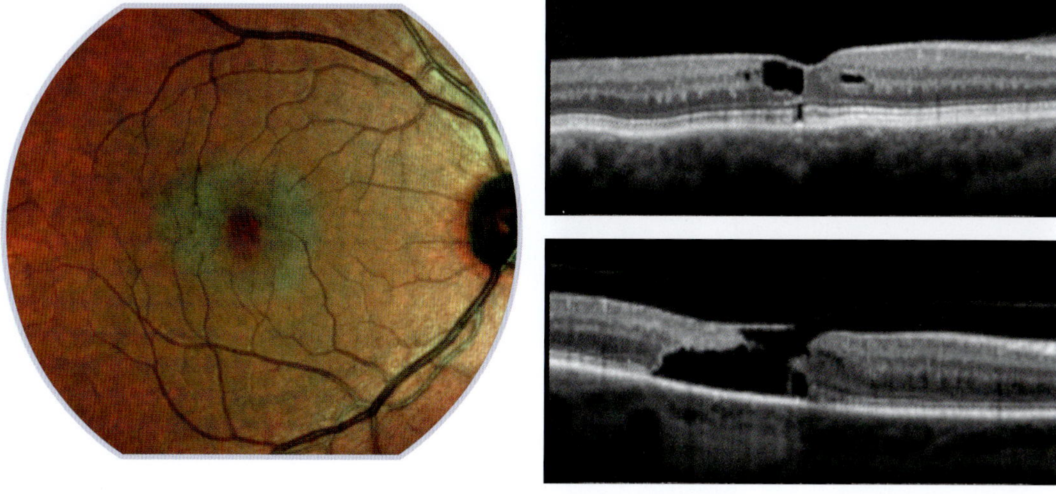

This multicolor image highlights the perifoveal lesion that is characteristic of macular telangiectasia type 2 *(left image).* OCT imaging reveals characteristic atrophic and cavitary retinal defects at the fovea *(top right image).* With time, a FTMH developed as the area of cavitation and atrophy enlarged *(bottom right image).*

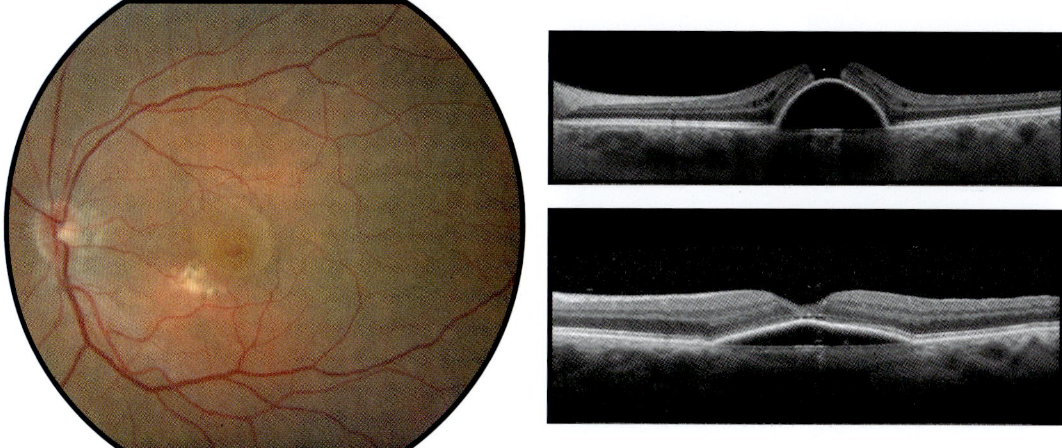

This patient with a macular hole overlying a serous pigment epithelial detachment was treated with multiple intravitreal anti-vascular endothelial growth factor injections and photodynamic therapy over a period of 1 year to induce flattening of the pigment epithelial detachment. A pars plana vitrectomy with peeling of the internal limiting membrane was performed subsequently with successful closure of the macular hole.

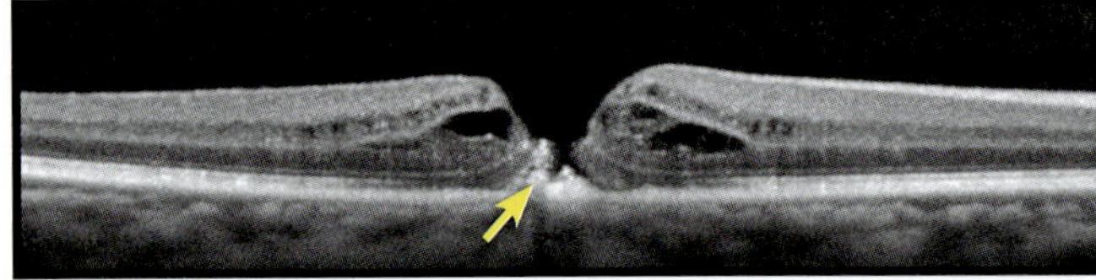

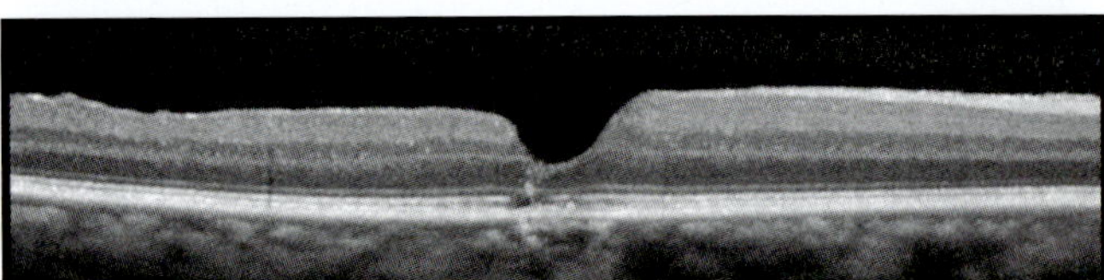

Macular holes may uncommonly develop during the natural course of acquired vitelliform lesions. In this case, a macular hole developed during the process of spontaneous vitelliform reabsorption *(arrow)*. Anatomical closure was achieved following vitrectomy and membrane peeling *(bottom image)*. *Images courtesy of Dr. Michael Engelbert*

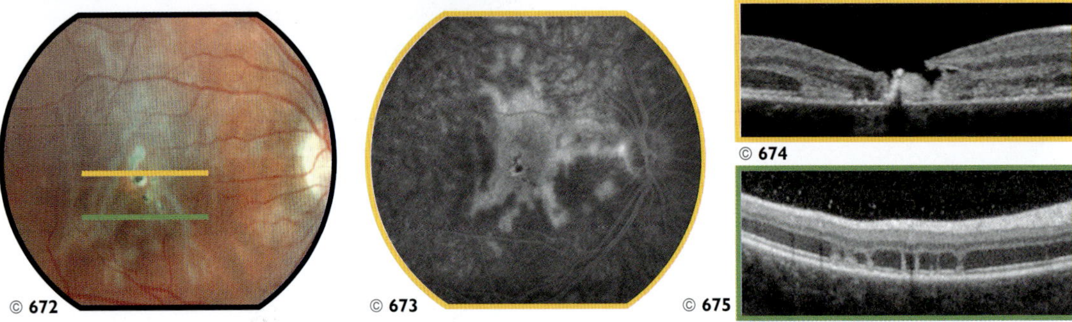

This patient developed a FTMH following self-inflicted injury with a handheld laser pointer. The curvilinear streaks of retinal pigment epithelial damage appear hyperfluorescent on fluorescein angiography. Hyper-reflective vertical steaks in the outer retina, as seen on OCT, characterize the acute stages of laser-induced maculopathy *(bottom right image)*.

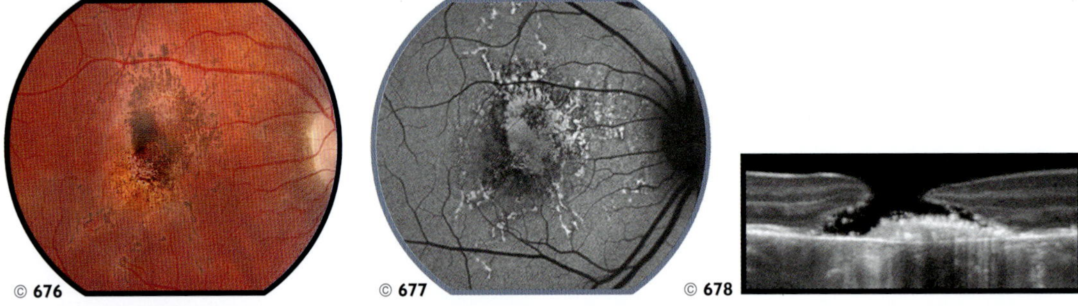

Months later, the patient in the above case developed a pigmented, hyperautofluorescent scar at the site of injury. OCT imaging shows a FTMH at the site of RPE proliferation and scarring.

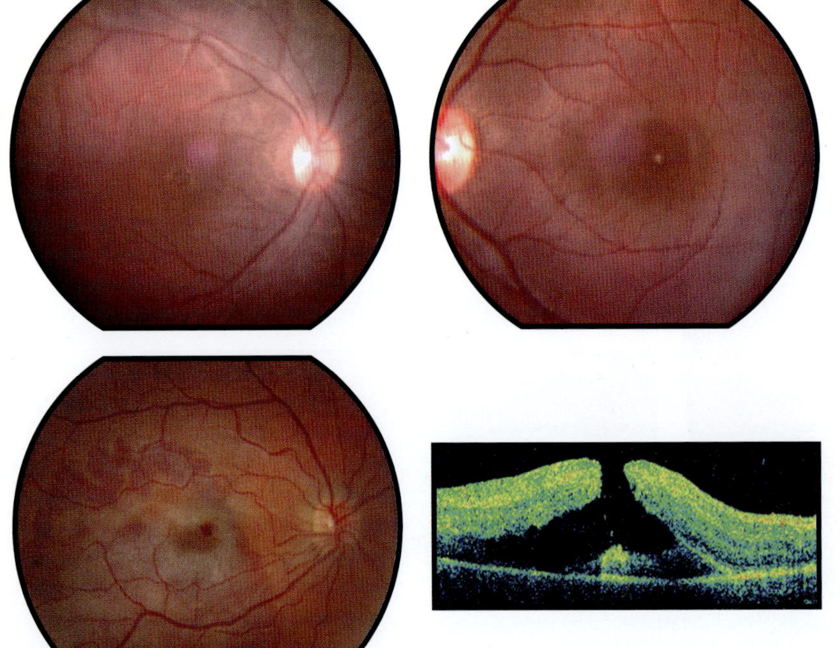

Bilateral macular holes may be induced by lightning strike injury as seen in this case. *Images courtesy of Dr. Vikram Jain*

Blunt trauma may also induce an acute FTMH. Blunt injury in this case resulted in a large, subretinal hemorrhage and a FTMH that was clearly seen on OCT. *Images courtesy of Dr. Carmen Puliafito*

Lamellar Macular Hole

The diagnosis of lamellar macular hole requires the following three criteria to be satisfied: (1) an irregular foveal contour or defect of the inner retina, (2) thinning at the base of the fovea, and (3) absence of a full-thickness defect. Lamellar macular holes may develop following abrupt termination of pathophysiological processes that would otherwise have resulted in a FTMH. Lamellar macular holes may also be due to contraction of an existing perifoveal epiretinal membrane–internal limiting membrane complex. Studies have shown that 80% to 100% of lamellar macular holes are associated with epiretinal membranes. Although lamellar macular holes may progress to FTMHs, approximately 80% were found to be stable, both functionally and morphologically, over time. As such, lamellar macular holes are usually observed and surgical management is considered only if there is visual decline.

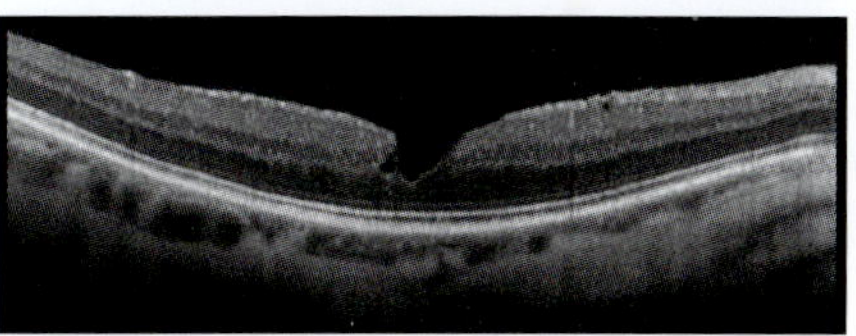

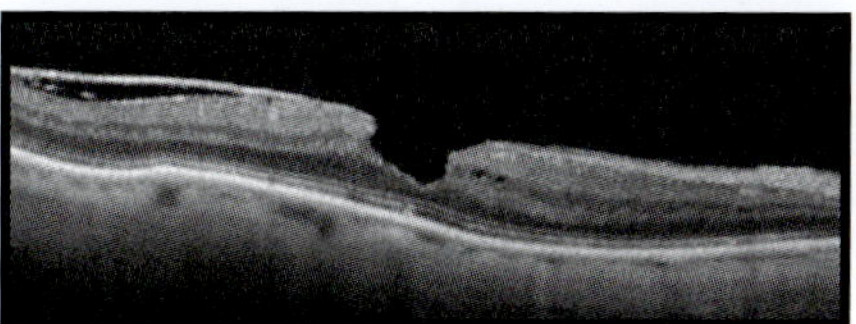

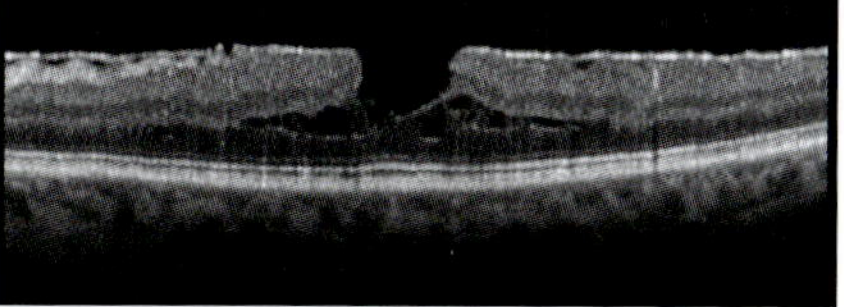

Spectral-domain OCT shows the variable appearance of lamellar macular holes. In these patients, there is an associated epiretinal membrane, an irregularity in the foveal contour, defects in the inner retina, and thinning of the retina at the base of the fovea without a full-thickness defect. There may also be intraretinal schisis due to traction *(right image)*.

Macular Pseudohole

Macular pseudohole is not a true FTMH and is due to contraction of an epiretinal membrane. With spectral-domain OCT, a macular pseudohole has a very similar appearance to a lamellar macular hole, especially when the foveal tissue loss is subtle. Some clinicians believe that lamellar macular hole and macular pseudohole are two distinct entities, best distinguished with fundus autofluorescence by demonstrating foveal tissue loss in true lamellar macular holes. However, other clinicians believe that the two are very similar in that they both possess a perifoveal epiretinal membrane–internal limiting membrane complex, with lamellar macular holes demonstrating centrifugal contraction and macular pseudoholes demonstrating a centripetal contraction. Management of macular pseudoholes is observation unless there is progressive visual decline that warrants surgery.

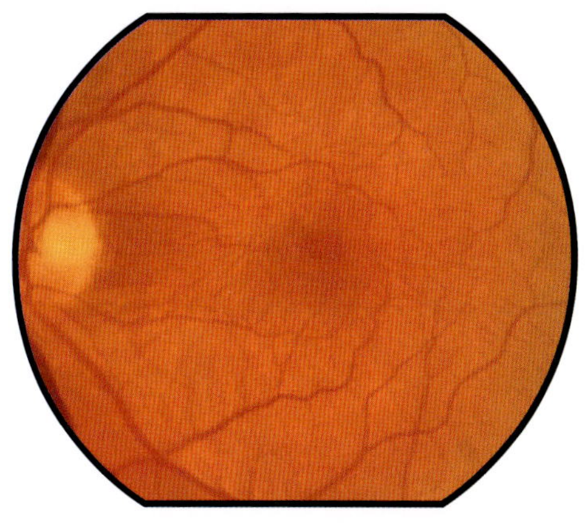

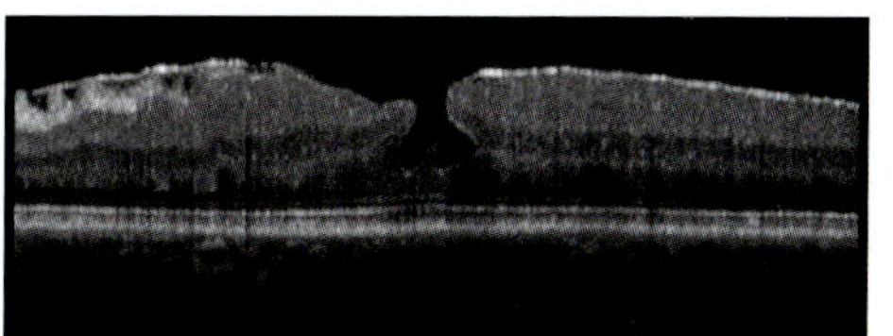

The color fundus photograph shows a macular pseudohole due to an epiretinal membrane *(left image)*. OCT demonstrates an epiretinal membrane with associated tenting of inner retinal tissue due to centripetal contraction *(right image)*.

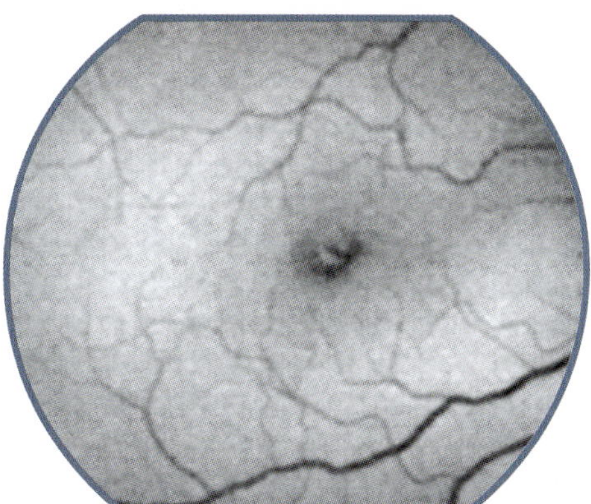

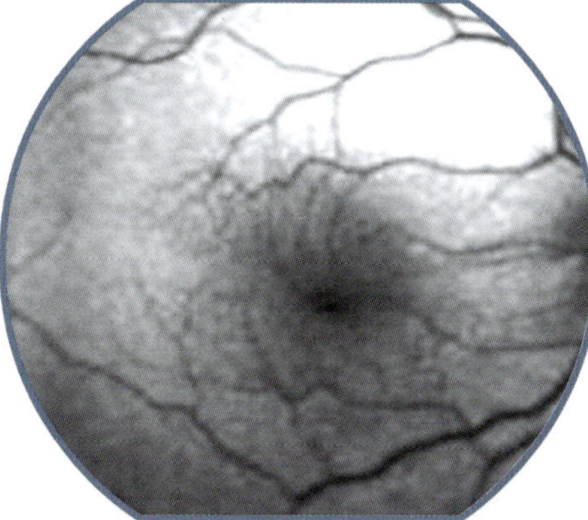

Fundus autofluorescence of a lamellar hole may reveal hyperautofluorescence due to loss of foveal tissue *(left image)* compared to the normal appearance of a macular pseudohole *(right image)*.

Lamellar Hole-Associated Epiretinal Proliferation

Lamellar hole-associated epiretinal proliferation (LHEP) is an OCT finding that is characterized by homogenous material of varying thickness on the retinal surface that is of medium reflectivity. LHEP has been reported in eyes with inner retinal defects and occurs in approximately one-third of lamellar macular holes. With high density and high resolution OCT scans, LHEP is seen to be contiguous with the middle retinal layers and is postulated to be a proliferation of glial cell tissue from the inner retinal defect onto the epiretinal surface. LHEP is differentiated from an epiretinal membrane by its OCT appearance and its non-contractile nature.

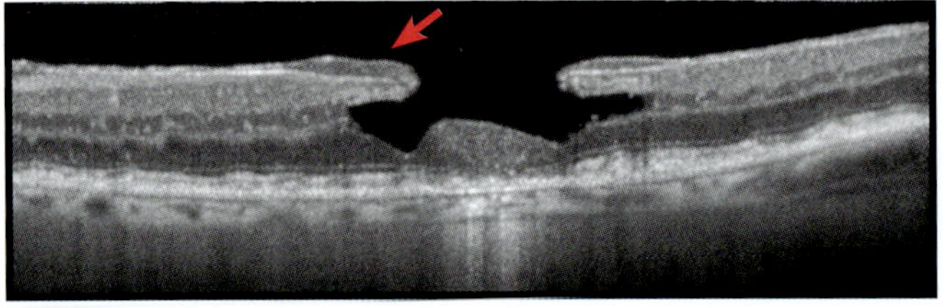

© 679

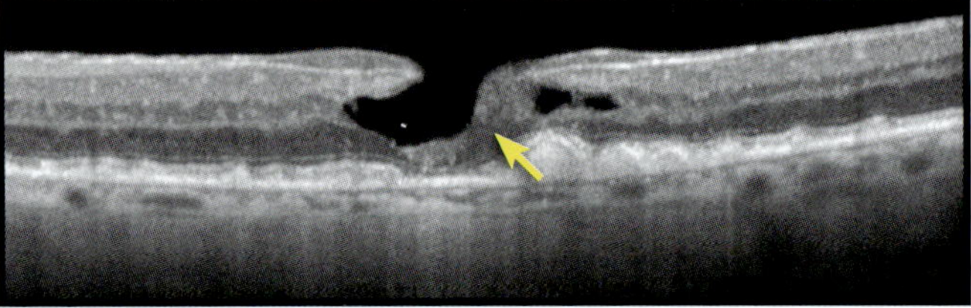

© 680

LHEP typically appears as homogenous, medium-reflective material of varying thickness on SD-OCT *(red arrow)*. The LHEP is present on the epiretinal surface adjacent to the lamellar macular hole and is contiguous with the middle retinal layers *(yellow arrow)*.

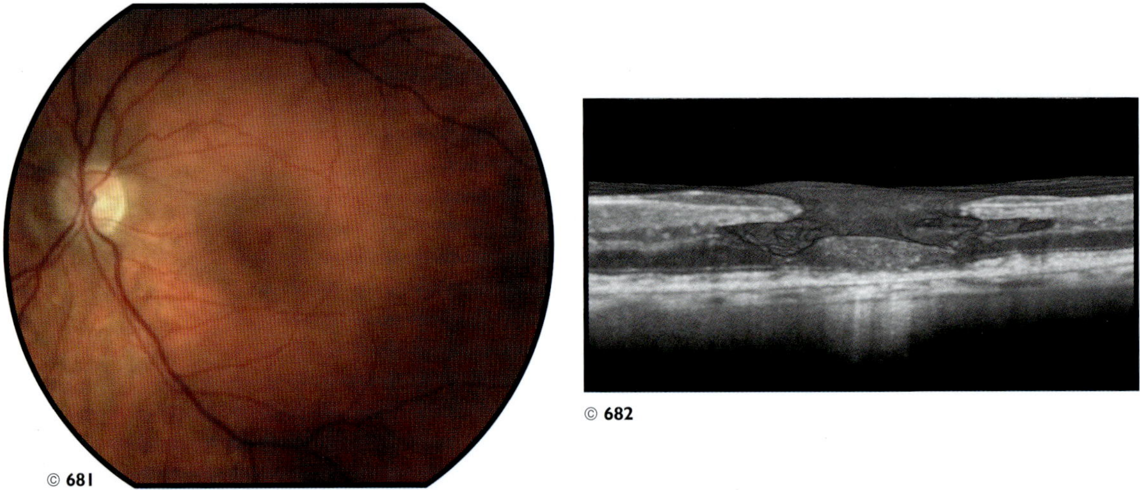

© 681

© 682

LHEP is difficult to distinguish on color photography *(left image)*. Volume rendered OCT imaging *(right image)* demonstrates the relationships between LHEP, the middle retinal layers of the retina, and base of the lamellar macular hole. There is an irregular epiretinal surface contour due to the varying thickness of LHEP but no traction or wrinkling of the retina. *Image courtesy of Dr. Richard Spaide*

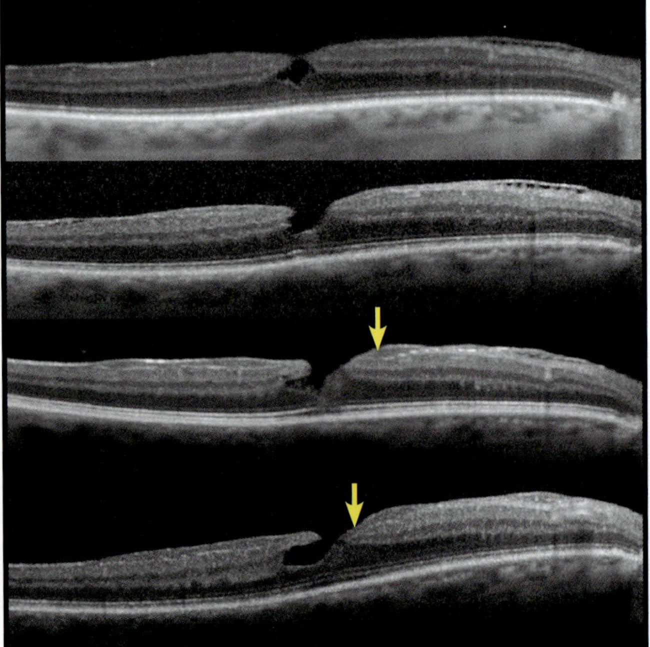

© 683

This serial eye-tracked sequence of OCT scans of the same patient taken over a course of 5 years shows a lamellar macular hole with a thin hyper-reflective epiretinal membrane that develops LHEP over time. There is contiguity between LHEP and the middle retinal layers at the inner retinal defect *(arrow)*.

Suggested Reading

Epiretinal Membrane

Appiah, A.P., 1989. Secondary causes of premacular fibrosis. Ophthalmology 96, 389–392.

Koizumi, H., Spaide, R.F., Fisher, Y.L., et al., 2008. Three-dimensional evaluation of vitreomacular traction and epiretinal membrane using spectral-domain optical coherence tomography. Am. J. Ophthalmol. 145 (3), 509–517.

Pang, C.E., Spaide, R.F., Freund, K.B., 2014. Epiretinal proliferation seen in association with lamellar macular holes: a distinct clinical entity. Retina 34 (8), 1513–1523.

Pang, C.E., Spaide, R.F., Freund, K.B., 2015. Comparing functional and morphologic characteristics of lamellar macular holes with and without lamellar hole-associated epiretinal proliferation. Retina 35 (4), 720–726.

Pesin, S.R., Olk, R.G., Grand, M.G., et al., 1991. Vitrectomy for premacular fibroplasia. Prognostic factors, long-term follow-up, and time course of visual improvement. Ophthalmology 98, 1109–1114.

Scheerlinck, L.M., van der Valk, R., van Leeuwen, R., 2015. Predictive factors for postoperative visual acuity in idiopathic epiretinal membrane: a systematic review. Acta Ophthalmol. 93 (3), 203–212.

Smiddy, W.E., Maguire, A.M., Green, W.R., et al., 1989. Idiopathic epiretinal membranes: ultrastructural characteristics and clinicopathologic correlation. Ophthalmology 96, 811–821.

Tari, S.R., Vidne-Hay, O., Greenstein, V.C., et al., 2007. Functional and structural measurements for the assessment of internal limiting membrane peeling in idiopathic macular pucker. Retina 27, 567–572.

Vitreomacular Traction and Macular Hole

Balaratnasingam, C., Dansingani, K., Dhrami-Gavazi, E., et al., 2015. Documentation of spontaneous macular hole closure in macular telangiectasia type 2 using multimodal imaging. Ophthalmic Surg. Lasers Imaging Retina 46 (8), 883–886.

Bhavsar, K.V., Wilson, D., Margolis, R., et al., 2015. Multimodal imaging in handheld laser-induced maculopathy. Am. J. Ophthalmol. 159 (2), 227–231.

Campo, R.V., Lewis, R.S., 1984. Lightning-induced macular hole. Am. J. Ophthalmol. 97, 792–794.

Chang, L.K., Fine, H.F., Spaide, R.F., et al., 2008. Ultrastructural correlation of spectral-domain optical coherence tomographic findings in vitreomacular traction syndrome. Am. J. Ophthalmol. 146 (1), 121–127.

Chew, E.Y., Sperduto, R.D., Hiller, R., et al., 1999. Clinical course of macular holes: the eye disease case-control study. Arch. Ophthalmol. 117, 248–249.

Duker, J.S., Kaiser, P.K., Binder, S., et al., 2013. The International Vitreomacular Traction Study Group classification of vitreomacular adhesion, traction, and macular hole. Ophthalmology 120 (12), 2611–2619.

Fisher, Y.L., Slakter, J.S., Yannuzzi, L.A., et al., 1994. A prospective natural history study and kinetic ultrasound evaluation of idiopathic macular holes. Ophthalmology 101, 5–11.

Goldberg, N., Freund, K.B., 2012. Progression of an acquired vitelliform lesion to a full-thickness macular hole documented by eye-tracked spectral-domain optical coherence tomography. Arch. Ophthalmol. 130 (9), 1221–1223.

Seider, M.I., Lujan, B.J., Gregori, G., et al., 2009. Ultra-high resolution spectral domain optical coherence tomography of traumatic maculopathy. Ophthalmic Surg. Lasers Imaging 40 (5), 516–521.

Stalmans, P., Benz, M.S., Gandorfer, A., et al., MIVI-TRUST Study Group. 2012. Enzymatic vitreolysis with ocriplasmin for vitreomacular traction and macular holes. N. Engl. J. Med. 367 (7), 606–615.

Steel, D.H., Lotery, A.J., 2013. Idiopathic vitreomacular traction and macular hole: a comprehensive review of pathophysiology, diagnosis, and treatment. Eye (Lond.) 27 (Suppl. 1), S1–S21.

Tzu, J.H., John, V.J., Flynn, H.W. Jr., et al., 2015. Clinical course of vitreomacular traction managed initially by observation. Ophthalmic Surg. Lasers Imaging Retina 46 (5), 571–576.

CHAPTER 10

Central Serous Chorioretinopathy and Other Exudative Detachments

Central Serous Chorioretinopathy

Central serous chorioretinopathy (CSC) is an idiopathic disorder involving a focal or multifocal leak at the level of the retinal pigment epithelium (RPE), usually in conjunction with a serous pigment epithelial detachment (PED). An active leak presents with angiographic pooling of fluorescein dye into the subneurosensory retinal space. The disorder usually occurs unilaterally and asymmetrically in males between the ages of 30 and 50. The natural course of CSC is usually benign with spontaneous resolution of the neurosensory detachment within 3-4 months. However, a small but significant percentage of patients will develop recurrent or persistent detachment with widespread loss of RPE and photoreceptors. These patients are classified as having chronic CSC. Serous detachments in the posterior pole may gravitate inferiorly, resulting in discernible pigment epithelial atrophic tracts and dependent neurosensory detachment.

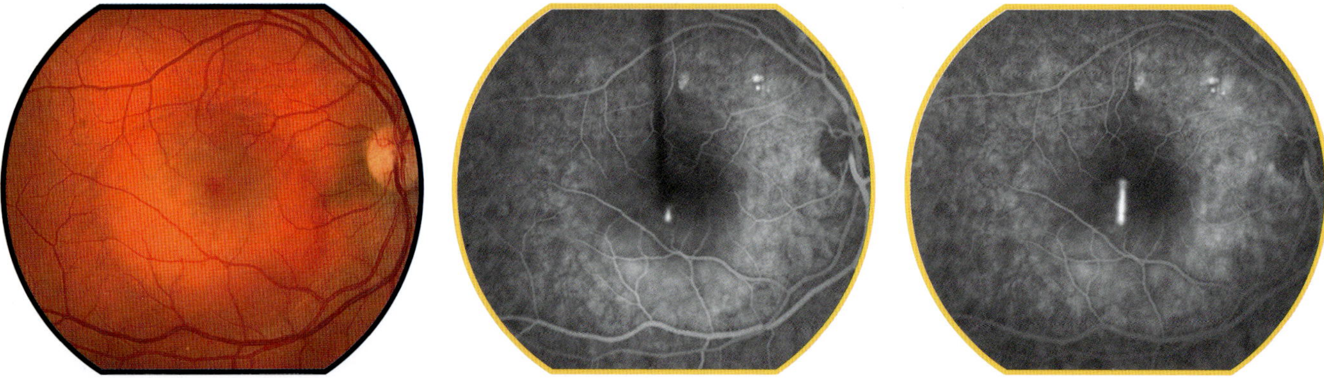

CSC is defined by a focal fluorescein leak at the level of the RPE with pooling of the dye into the subneurosensory retinal space. The characteristics of the focal leak will vary depending on the composition of the subretinal fluid, the morphology of the associated pigment epithelial abnormality, and possibly by convection currents induced by the warmer posterior choroid. A large active leak will rapidly pool into the subneurosensory retinal space. It is sometimes unclear why some fluorescein leaks ascend quickly, as seen in the patient above, while others slowly expand throughout the course of the angiogram.

Fluorescein Angiography in CSC

Smokestack Leak

A "smokestack" leak is associated with a focal pinpoint active RPE leak that ascends vertically in the subretinal space. Once the dye reaches the limiting point of the neurosensory detachment, its hyperfluorescence then expands laterally, constrained by the limits of the fluid compartment.

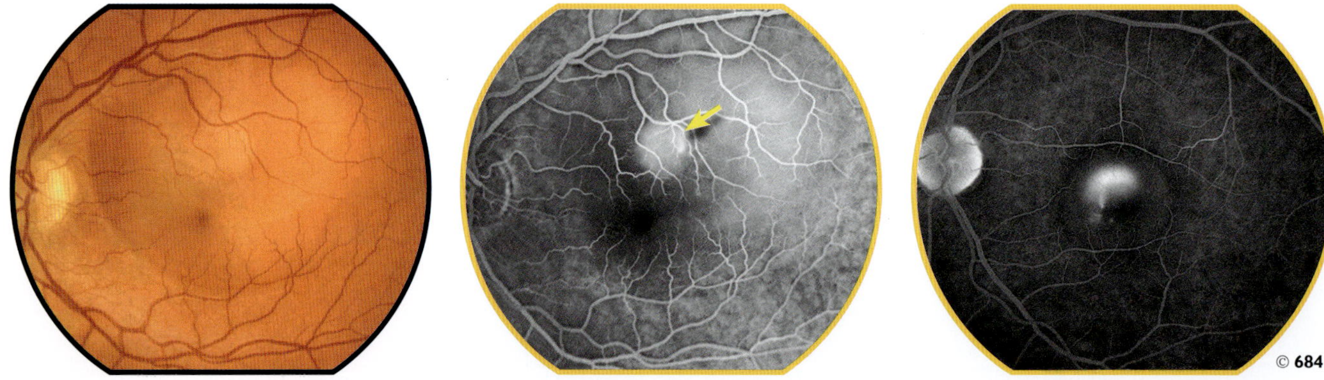

This patient has a focal "smokestack" leak *(arrow)* near the edge of a serous PED beneath a neurosensory retinal detachment. In the late stage of the angiogram there is a pooling of dye superiorly. Hyperfluorescence extends temporally along the same direction as the serous detachment. A "smokestack" pattern of leakage is clearly seen in the angiogram of a different patient *(right image)*.

Mushroom or Umbrella Leak

A "mushroom" or "umbrella" leak will rapidly pool beneath the neurosensory detachment and ascend within the subneurosensory retinal space. Presumably, this angiographic pattern occurs due to molecular weight differences between the dye and the components of the subretinal fluid and due to convection currents within this fluid compartment. The leakage will spread temporally and nasally when it reaches the upper limits of the detachment.

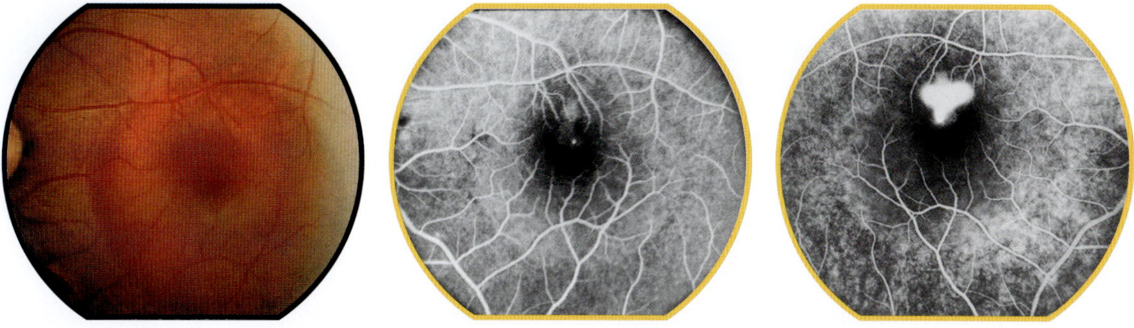

This patient has a focal leak from acute CSC that forms a "mushroom" or "umbrella" appearance in the late angiogram.

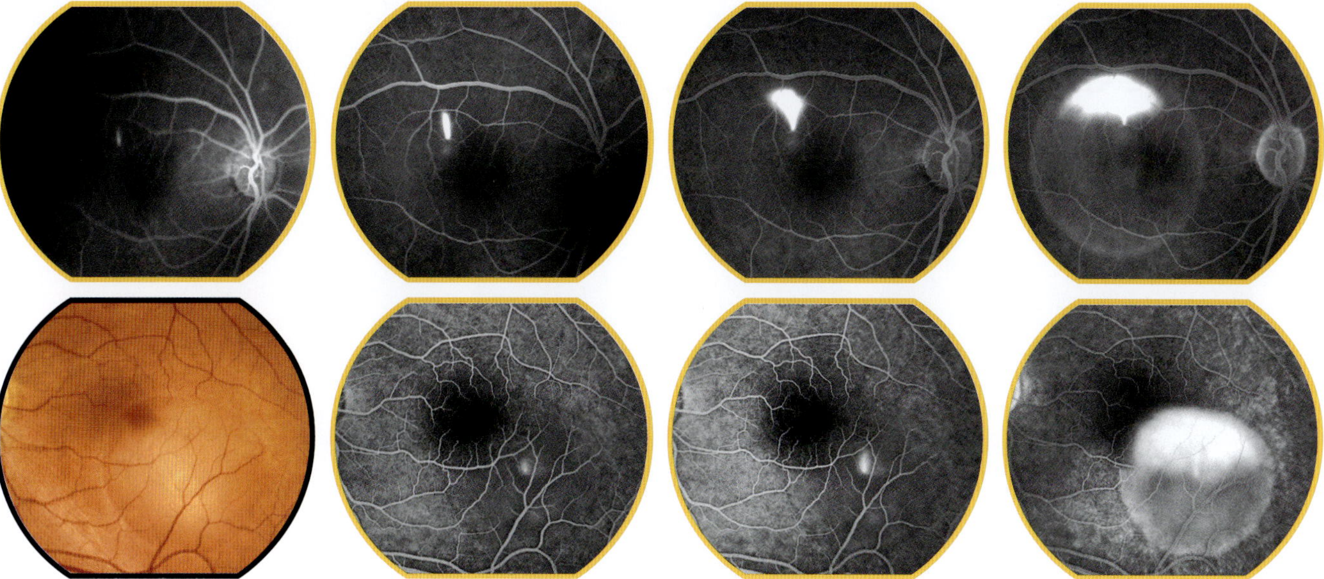

These are two patients who have "mushroom" RPE leaks due to acute CSC. Note that the leaks ascend in the subneurosensory retinal space until they reach the limits of the neurosensory detachments and then extend temporally and nasally to form a "mushroom" or "umbrella" appearance. The leakage of the dye into the subneurosensory retinal space will delineate the neurosensory detachment. The neurosensory detachment in CSC does not fill homogeneously with dye unlike some serous detachments due to other causes. Completely stained subneurosensory retinal spaces may be seen in inflammatory disease and choroidal neovascularization.

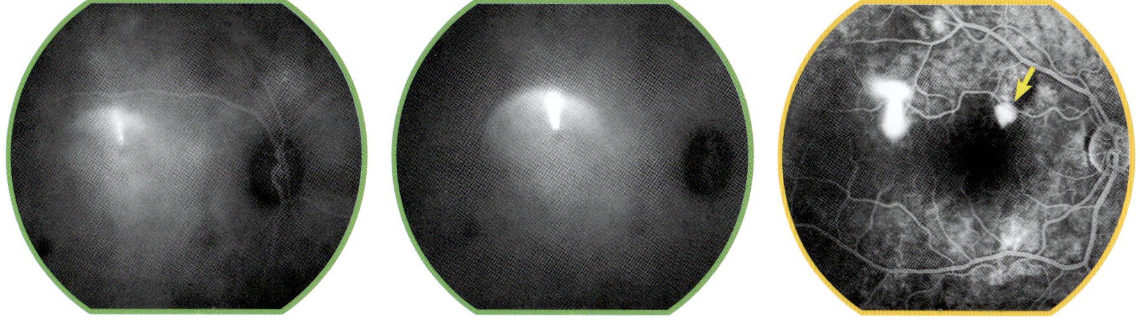

This patient has an "umbrella" leak seen with indocyanine green (ICG) angiography. Note the vertical ascent of the dye in the subneurosensory retinal space. The dye may outline the neurosensory detachment but does not completely fill it *(middle image)*. ICG dye is typically not as useful as fluorescein dye *(right)* in demonstrating leakage in CSC, because fluorescein dye is more permeable and more brilliantly fluorescent (25 times greater than ICG). The right photograph also shows a small serous PED *(arrow)*, which should be differentiated from an active leak.

Inkblot Leak

An "inkblot leak" in CSC is a pinpoint area of hyperfluorescence on the fluorescein angiogram that gradually expands in a localized ovoid fashion. There is no ascent of the fluorescence in the subneurosensory retinal space. This leak usually represents a slow diffusion of the dye through an incomplete or healing defect in the RPE.

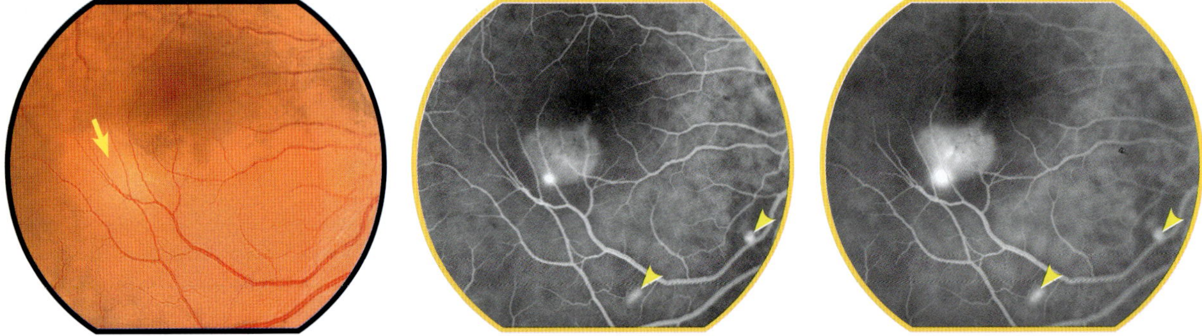

This patient with CSC has a focal "inkblot leak" near the edge of a serous PED. The leak gradually expands in the late stage of the angiogram *(right)*. There is some yellowish discoloration beneath the neurosensory detachment, presumably fibrin *(arrow)*. There are small PEDs that stain without leakage at the bottom right of the fluorescein angiograms *(arrowheads)*.

Indocyanine Green Angiography in CSC

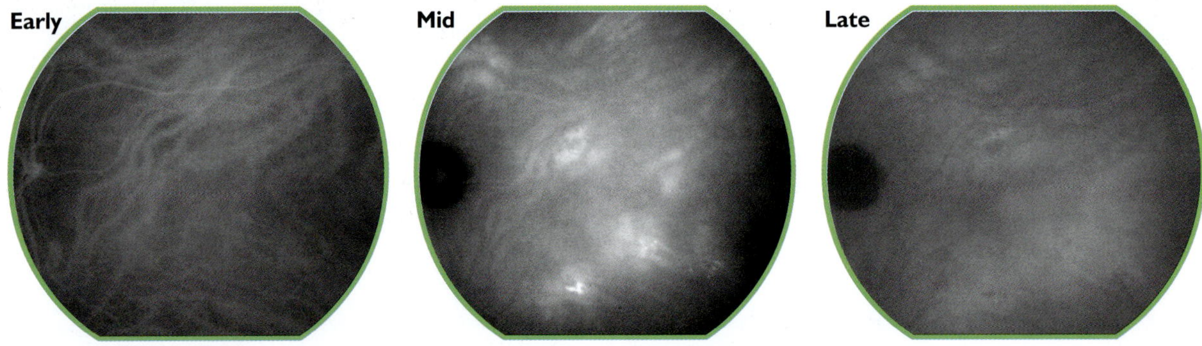

ICG angiography is useful in diagnosing CSC. The characteristic finding is choroidal staining or hyperpermeability, which typically appears in the mid-stage of the angiogram *(middle image)*. It fades in the late study *(right)*, differentiating this leakage from that of choroidal neovascularization.

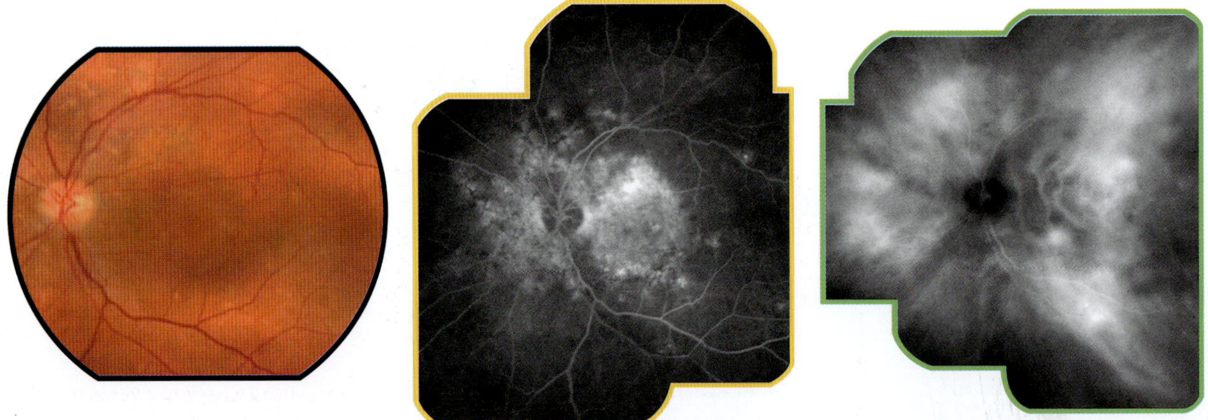

Here there is widespread choroidal leakage seen with ICG angiography *(right)* suggestive of choroidal hyperpermeability, a hallmark of CSC. The ICG angiogram shows choroidal abnormalities that cannot be detected with color photographs or fluorescein angiography *(middle)*. The fluorescein angiogram shows hyperfluorescence due to pigment epithelial atrophy overlying an intact choriocapillaris. The choroidal staining seen with ICG angiography may also be due to the presence of fibrin, which may have an affinity for the ICG molecule. In contrast, fibrin is transparent on fluorescein angiography.

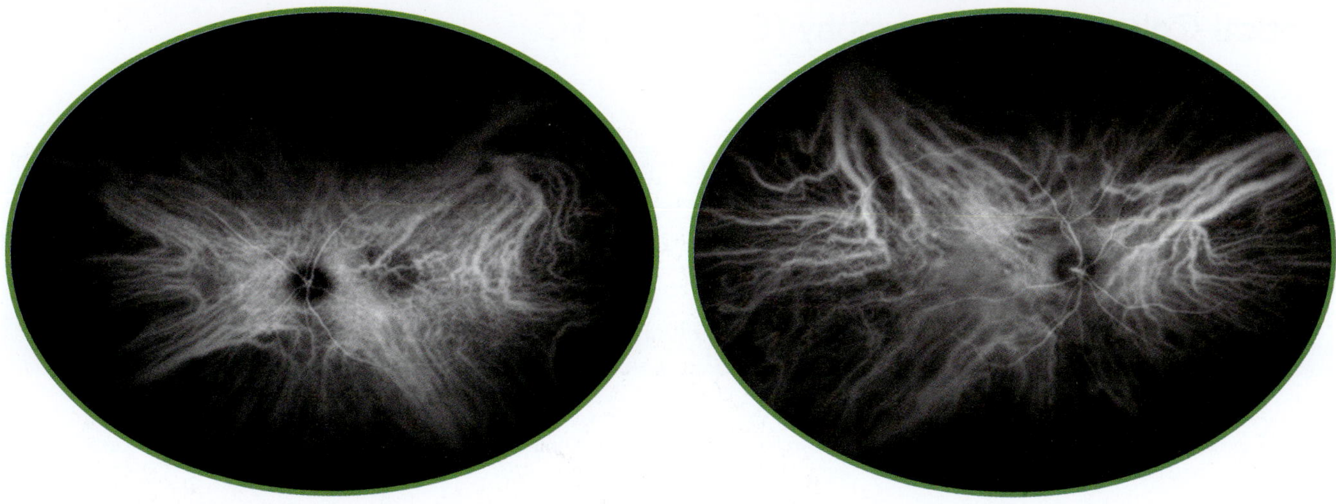

Ultra-widefield ICG angiography in the early- to mid-phase reveals dilation of the choroidal vessels, which may be associated with congestion of all vortex vein ampullas *(left image)* or specific vortex veins, superotemporal and superonasal in this case *(right image)*.

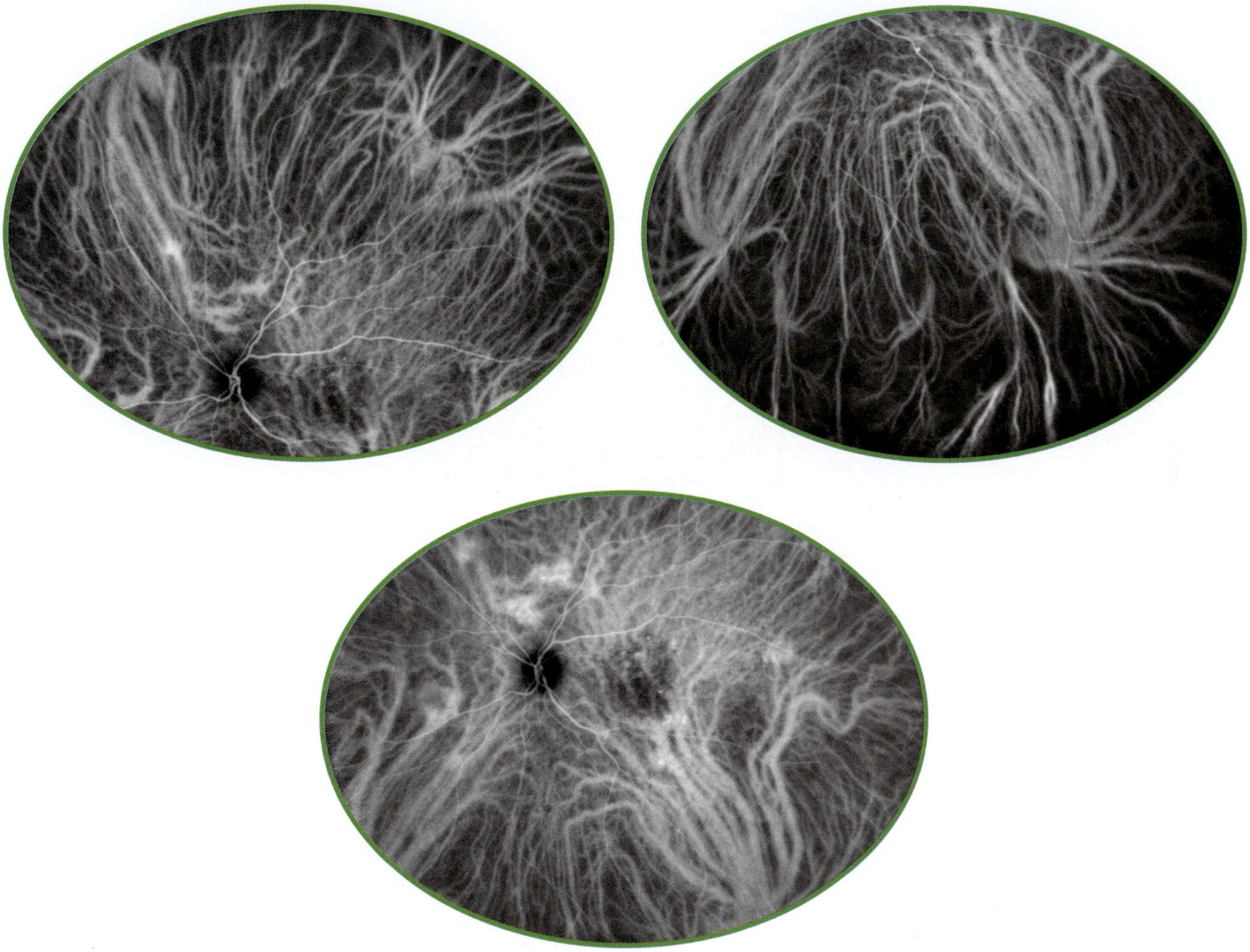

Ultra-widefield ICG angiography in the early- to mid-phase reveals dilation of the choroidal vessels and congestion of the vortex vein ampullas, which may be imaged best in superior gaze *(top left image)* and inferior gaze *(top right image)*.

Optical Coherence Tomography (OCT) in CSC

Serous Retinal Detachment

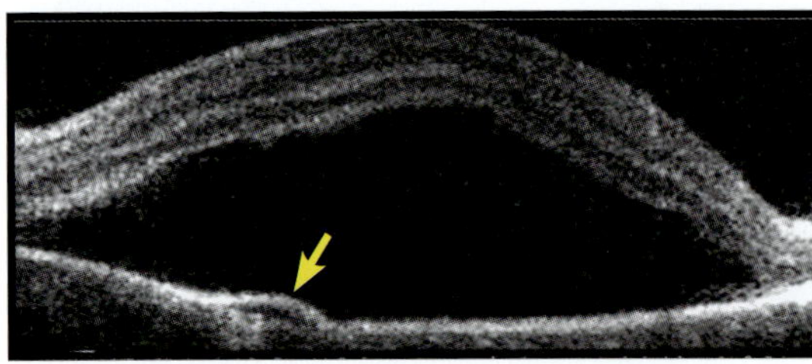

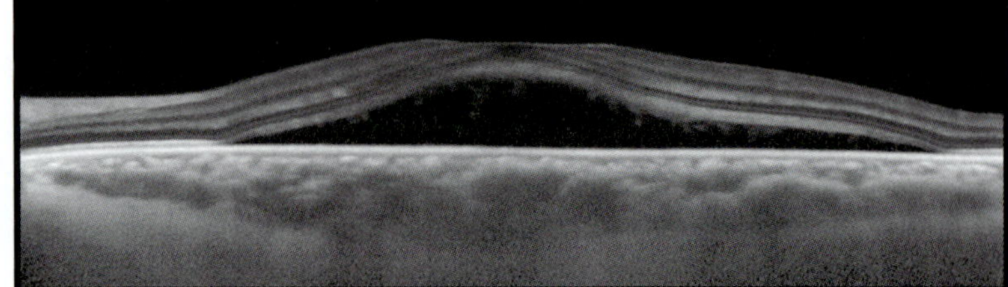

OCT is very helpful in diagnosing and managing CSC. The left image shows a serous detachment overlying a shallow PED *(arrow)*. The right image shows a serous detachment with an accumulation of hyper-reflective material on the undersurface of the retina. This material may represent elongated or shed photoreceptor outer segments or fibrin.

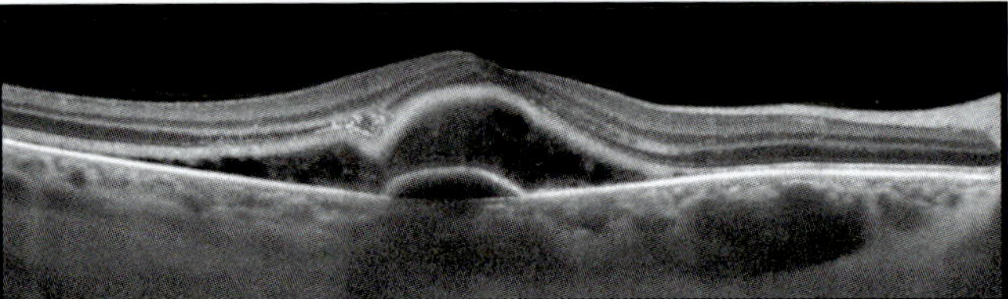

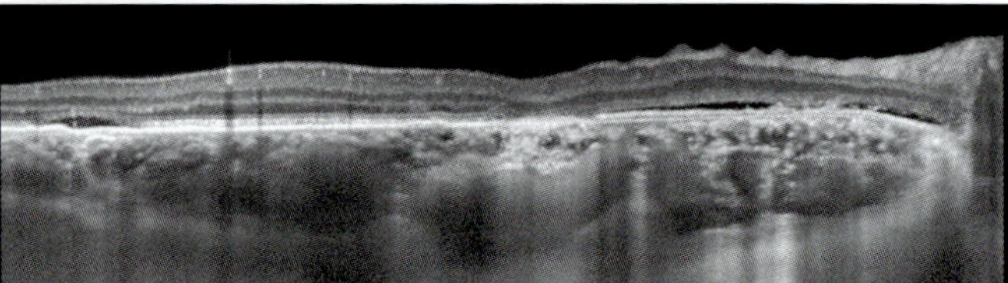

Patients with CSC frequently demonstrate a thickened choroid or "pachychoroid," which is visualized clearly with enhanced depth imaging OCT or swept source OCT as shown in the images above. The left image shows a serous detachment with fibrin overlying a PED. There is thickening of the choroid and large dilated choroidal vessels or "pachyvessels" beneath the area of pathology. The right image shows shallow subretinal fluid in a patient with chronic CSC. Notice the abnormally thickened choroid and grossly dilated pachyvessels.

Pigment Epithelial Detachment (PED)

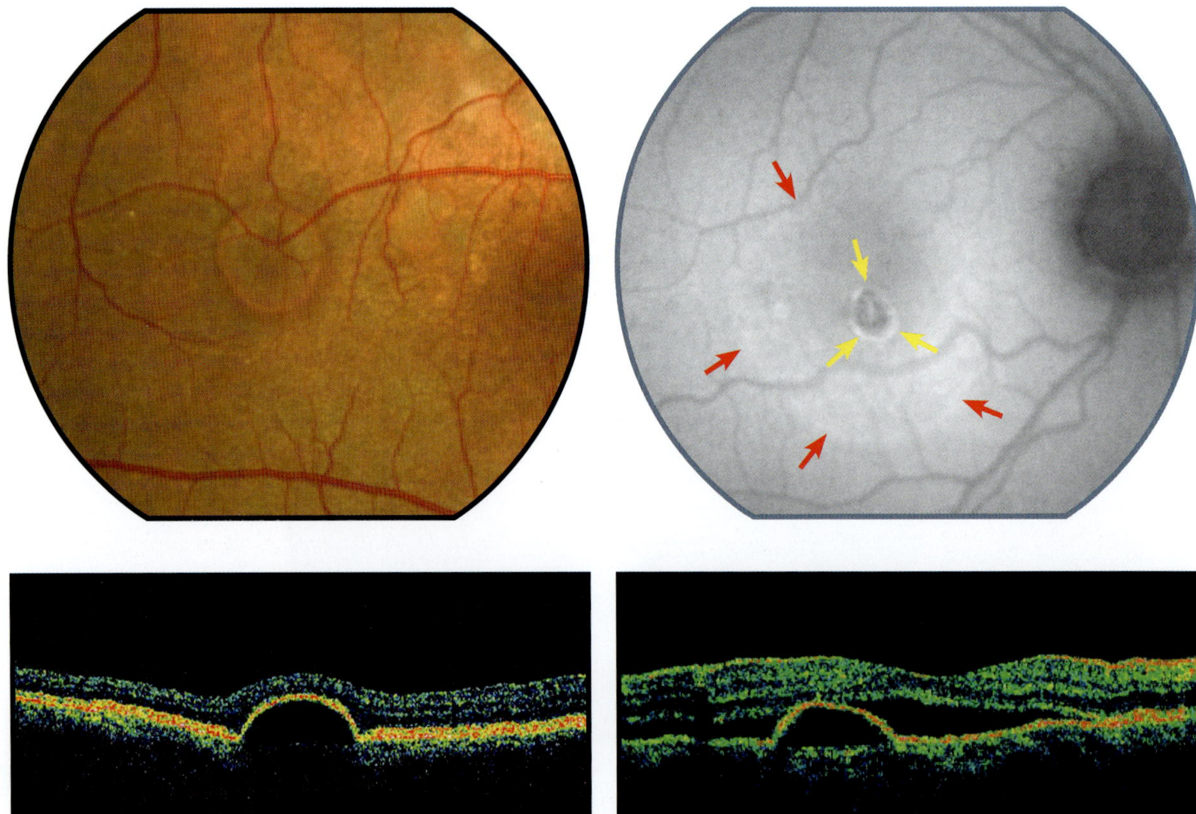

Serous PEDs are a characterisitic feature of CSC. OCT imaging is very useful in detecting serous PEDs. Unlike drusenoid and vascularized PEDs seen in age-related macular degeneration, the sub-RPE space of serous PEDs is uniformly hyporeflective. The color fundus image on the left shows a serous PED with the corresponding OCT below it. The fundus autofluorescence (FAF) image on the right and corresponding OCT below it show a combined PED and serous retinal detachment. A double ring of hyperautofluorescence can be appreciated on the FAF, the larger ring (red arrows) due to the subretinal fluid and the smaller ring (yellow arrows) of the PED.

Cystoid Macular Degeneration

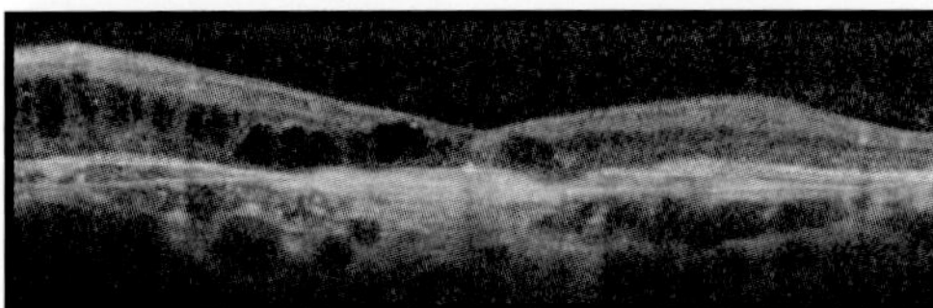

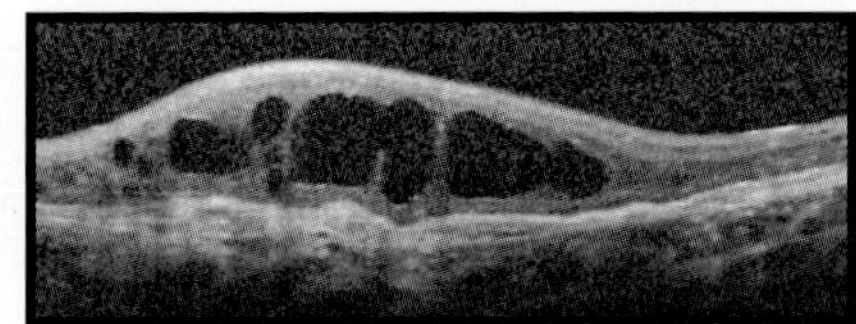

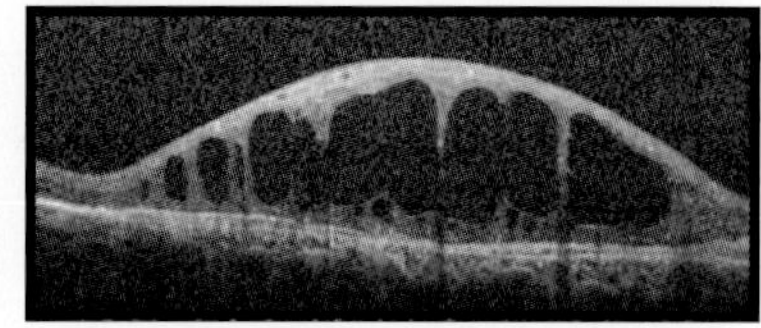

Cystoid macular degeneration is a recognized complication of chronic CSC and occurs in approximately 21% of cases. Cystoid macular degeneration may vary from mild *(left)* to massive in nature *(right)*. Cystoid macular degeneration typically occurs in those eyes that demonstrate irreversible outer retinal damage manifested by disruptions in the external limiting membrane and ellipsoid zone on OCT. Following resolution of cystoid degenerative changes, there is predictable atrophy of the retina.

Fundus Autofluorescence (FAF) in CSC

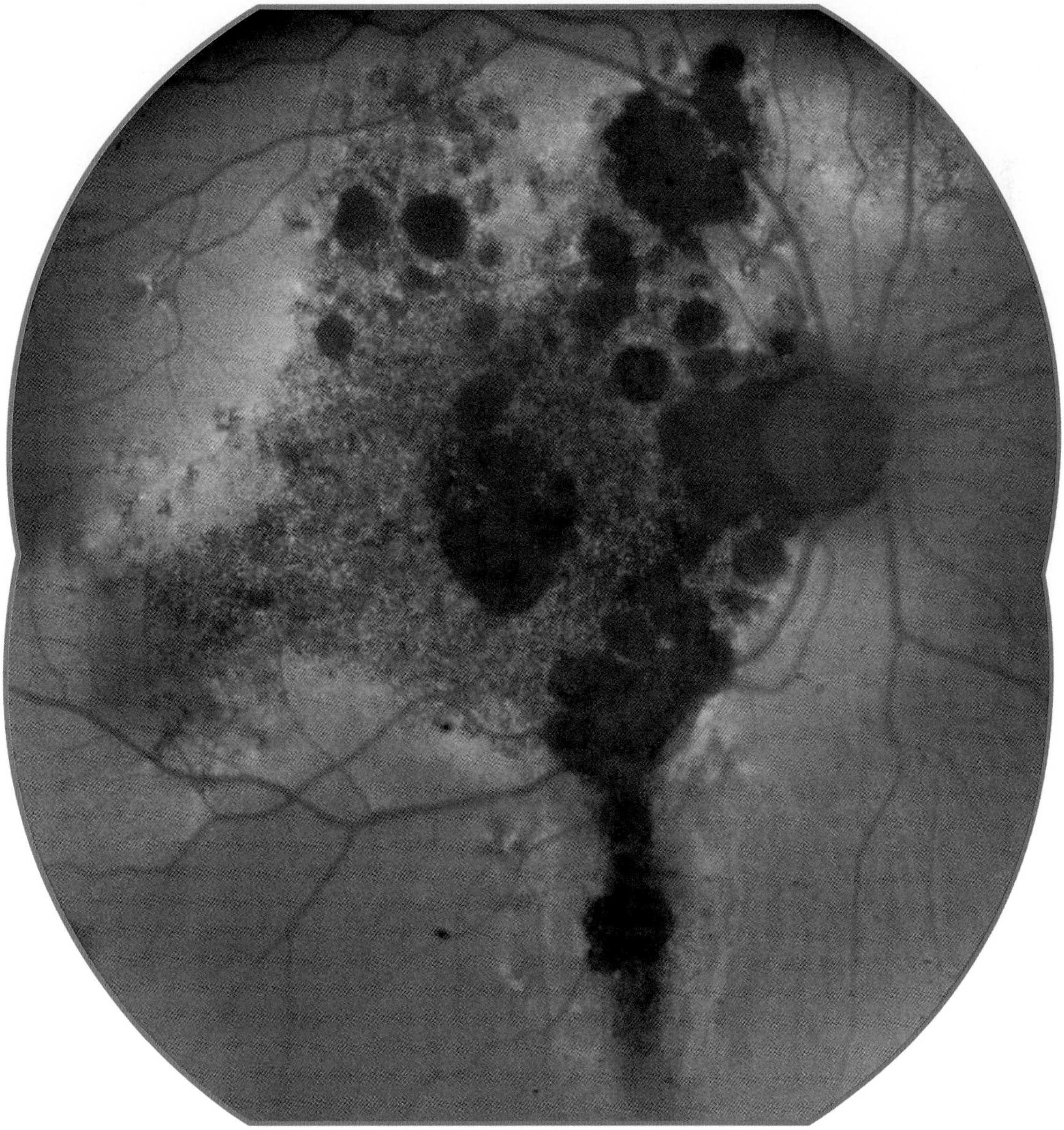

This patient with chronic CSC shows a myriad of FAF abnormalities. The very dark areas correspond to atrophy of the RPE and photoreceptors. The granular autofluorescence represents areas of antecedent detachment, which has resolved with less severe atrophy. Hyperautofluorescent areas on the image represent cells at risk or denote areas of persistent detachment. *Image courtesy of Dr. Richard Spaide*

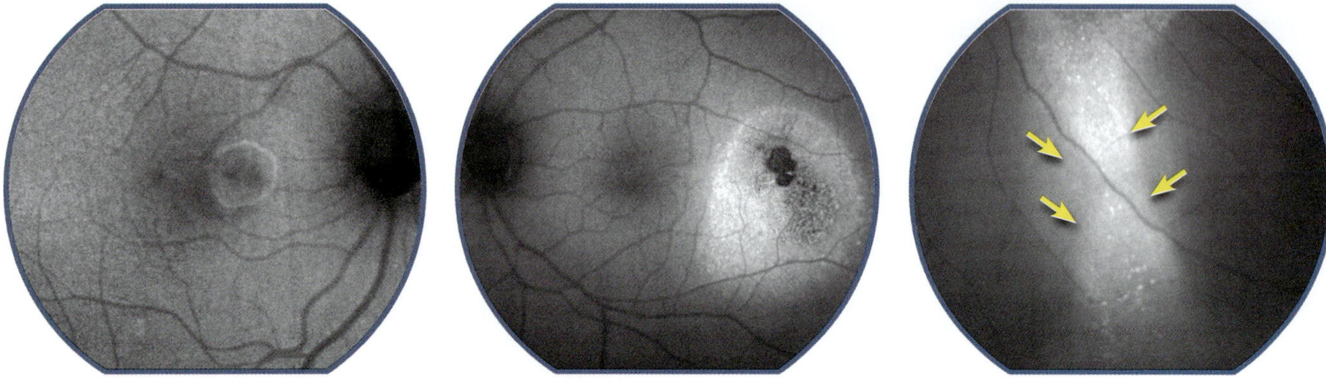

A PED has a ring of hyperautofluorescence *(left image)*. Acute or resolved detachments appear hyperautofluorescent *(middle image)*. The hypoautofluorescent area in this patient corresponds to previous laser photocoagulation treatment. A chronic gravitating neurosensory detachment has an inner column of hyperautofluorescence *(arrows)*.

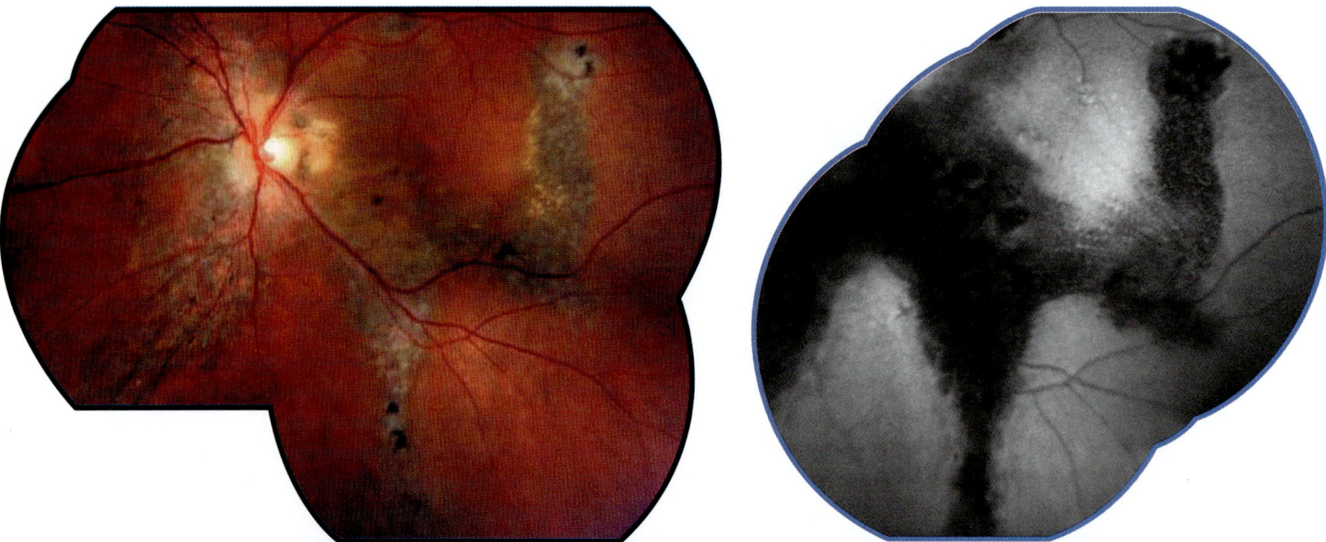

This patient with chronic CSC has gravitating atrophic RPE tracts from chronic detachments. As the neurosensory detachments descend inferiorly, an atrophic and pigmentary degenerative change evolves. These changes are very characteristic of chronic CSC, but they can be produced by other causes of exudation in the central macula, such as leakage from choroidal hemangiomas and disciform disease in age-related macular degeneration.

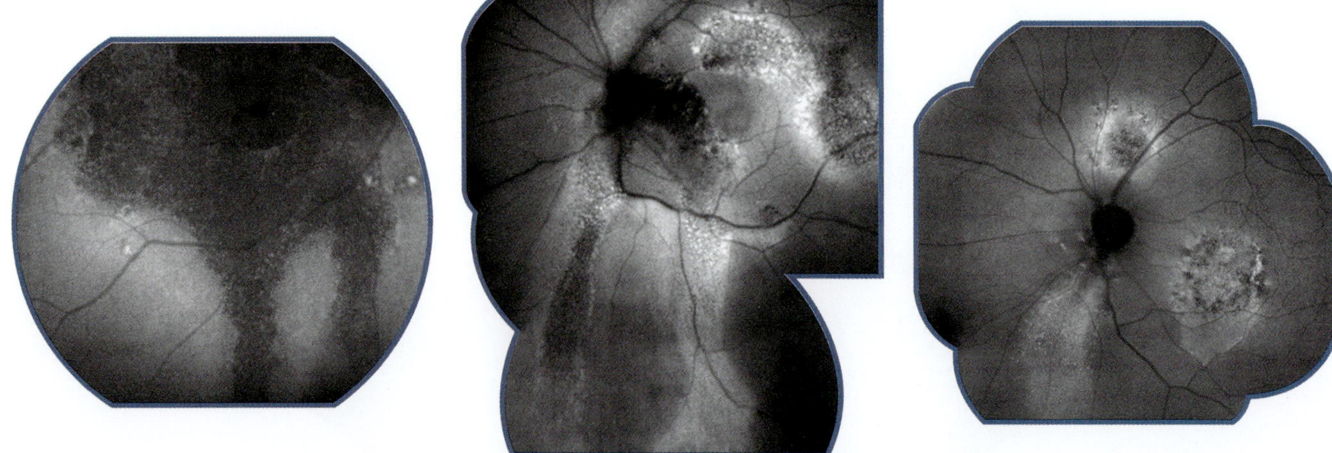

Atrophic RPE appears hypoautofluorescent, whereas areas of with acute or resolved detachments appear hyperautofluorescent, due to the liberation of outer retinal photoreceptors in the subretinal space and unmasking of the normal RPE autofluorescence in areas of outer retinal thinning. *Images courtesy of Dr. Richard Spaide*

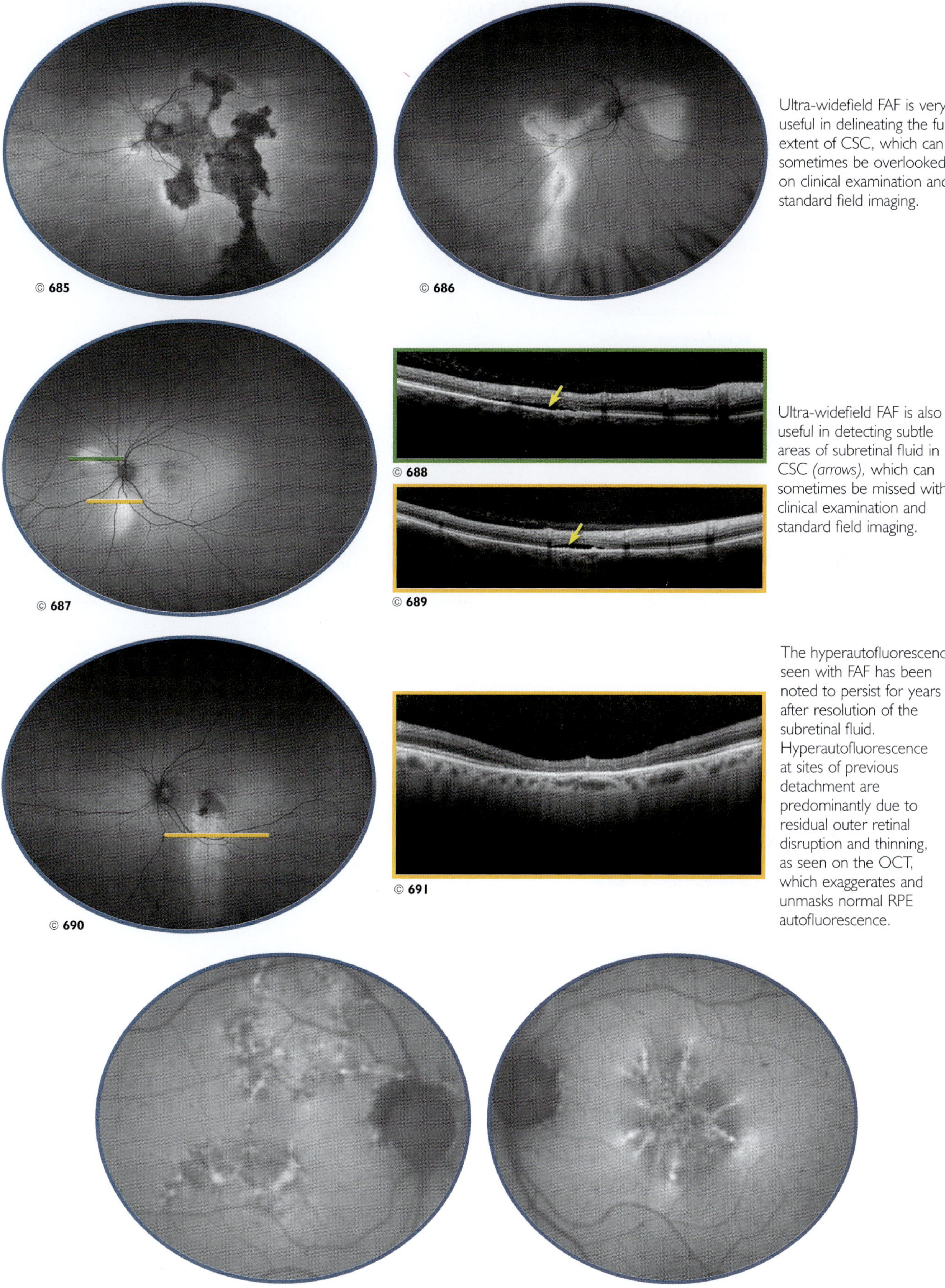

© 685

© 686

Ultra-widefield FAF is very useful in delineating the full extent of CSC, which can sometimes be overlooked on clinical examination and standard field imaging.

© 687

© 688

© 689

Ultra-widefield FAF is also useful in detecting subtle areas of subretinal fluid in CSC *(arrows)*, which can sometimes be missed with clinical examination and standard field imaging.

© 690

© 691

The hyperautofluorescence seen with FAF has been noted to persist for years after resolution of the subretinal fluid. Hyperautofluorescence at sites of previous detachment are predominantly due to residual outer retinal disruption and thinning, as seen on the OCT, which exaggerates and unmasks normal RPE autofluorescence.

Retinal pigment epithelial changes may appear as a reticular pattern, as shown in the above patient, in approximately 25% of CSC patients. Of these, 70% occur bilaterally and are typically asymmetric. The reticular pattern tends to be multifocal, eccentric, and peripapillary. They usually occur over areas of previous or current PEDs. It is important to recognize this reticular pattern of autofluorescence in CSC and distinguish this finding from pattern dystrophy.

CSC Simulating Age-Related Macular Degeneration (AMD)

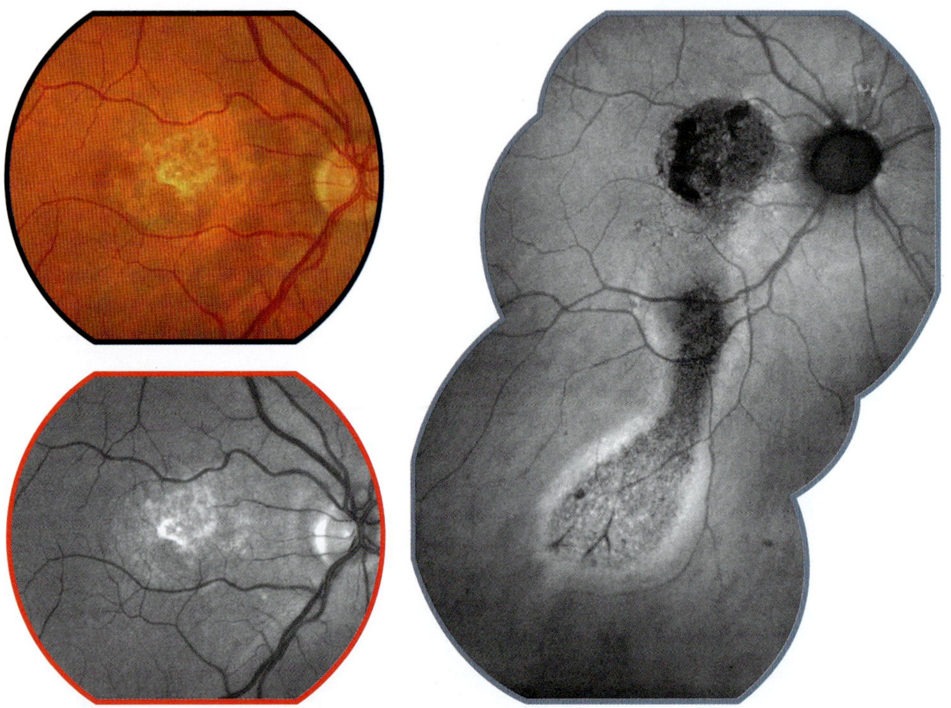

FAF can help distinguish CSC from other entities that may appear similar on clinical examination. This patient has a zone of atrophy with fibrous metaplasia in the central macula and was initially diagnosed as having AMD. However, a gravitating tract of atrophy, coursing into the inferior fundus, is evident on autofluorescence imaging. This autofluorescent pattern is highly characteristic of prior episodes of CSC; a diagnosis that also explains the macular changes.

Asymptomatic Eye

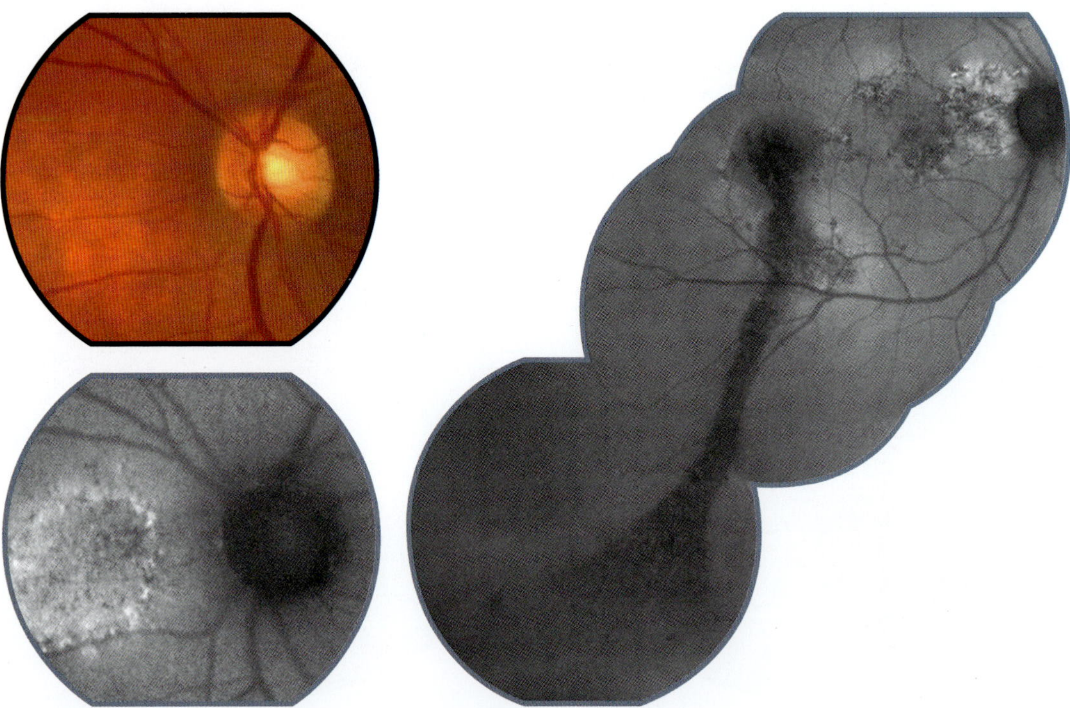

These two patients were asymptomatic. Each had a history of acute CSC in their fellow eye. A zone of autofluorescence abnormalities was noted nasal to the disc *(left images)* in one of the patients. The other patient had widespread autofluorescence changes with an atrophic RPE tract from a previous inferior gravitating detachment. There was relative sparing of the fovea accounting for the asymptomatic state of these patients.

Chronic Central Serous Chorioretinopathy

Chronic CSC is defined as a detachment that persists for more than 6 months or a recurring detachment that produces widespread pigment epithelial alterations including atrophy. Chronic CSC is often associated with an incontinent or a permeable pigment epithelium in widespread areas of the fundus. Focal, recurrent leaks may complicate this form of the disease.

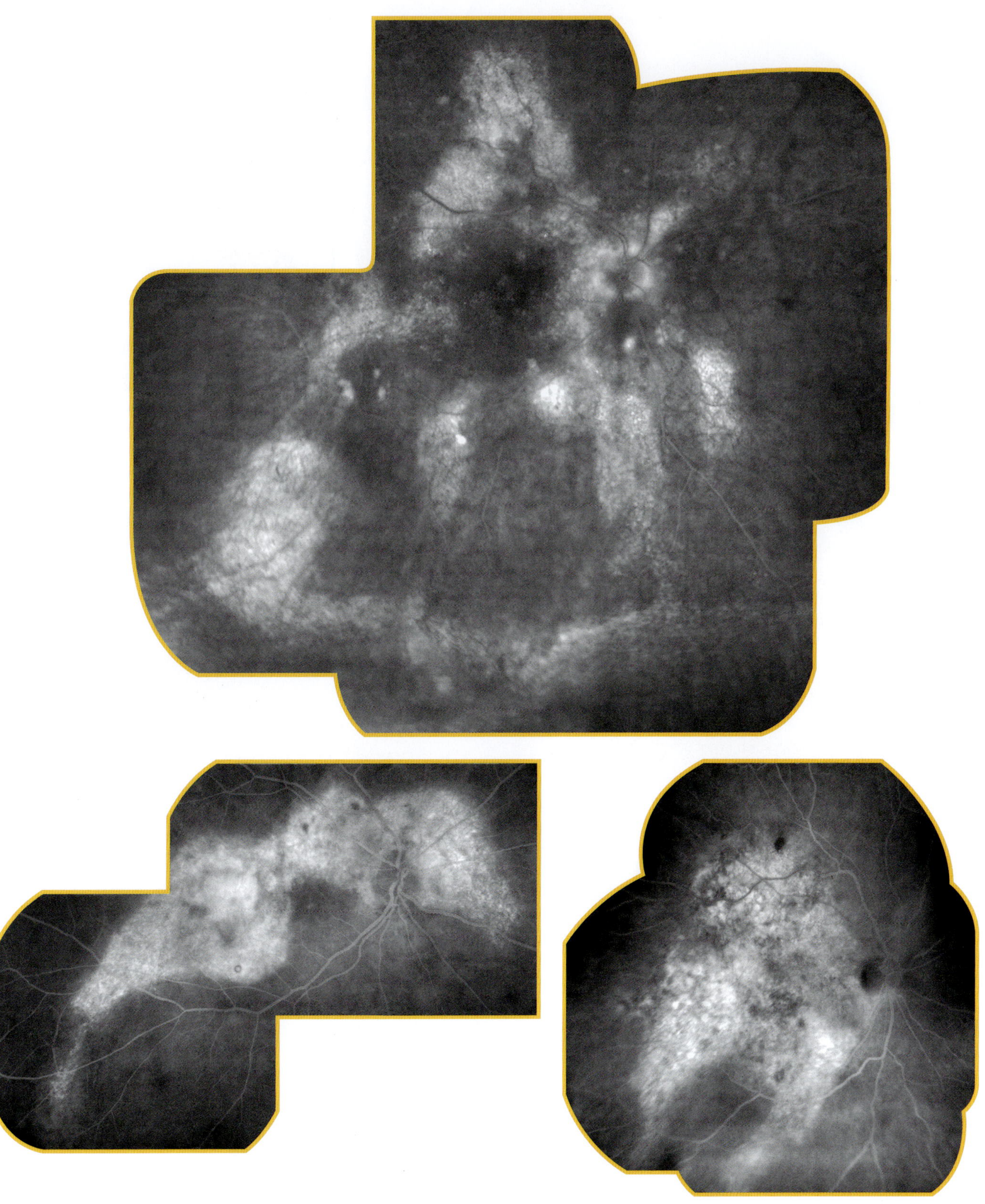

These patients have chronic CSC. There is widespread decompensation of the RPE and descending atrophic retinal pigment epithelial tracts that correspond to active or antecedent gravitating detachments.

Fibrin in CSC

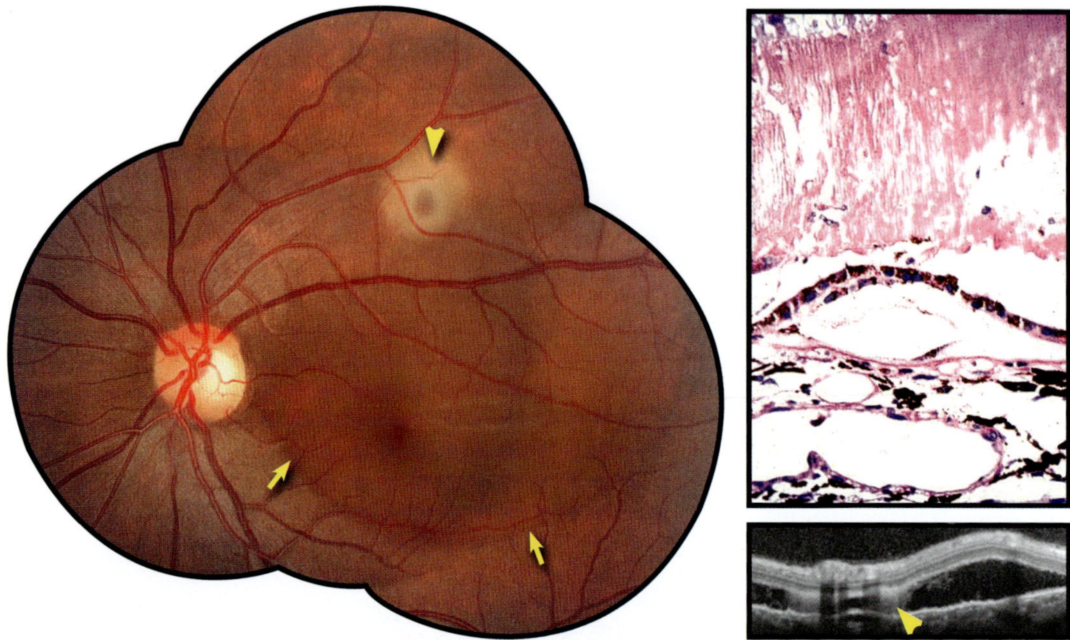

A large serous detachment of the macula is seen in this patient *(arrows)*. The dome of a PED is barely visible within an overlying area of fibrin *(arrowhead)*. The histopathology shows the presence of fibrin beneath the pigment epithelium and neurosensory retina in CSC. The OCT image shows fibrin beneath the detached retina *(arrowhead)*. *Pathology courtesy of Dr. G. de Venecia*

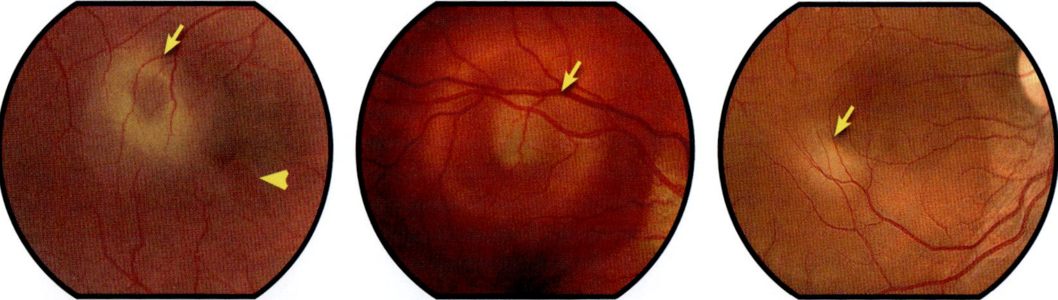

These patients have fibrin in the subneurosensory retinal space *(arrows)*. Fibrin may also occur beneath the RPE. In the left image, there is also a small serous PED *(arrowhead)*, which is not actively leaking.

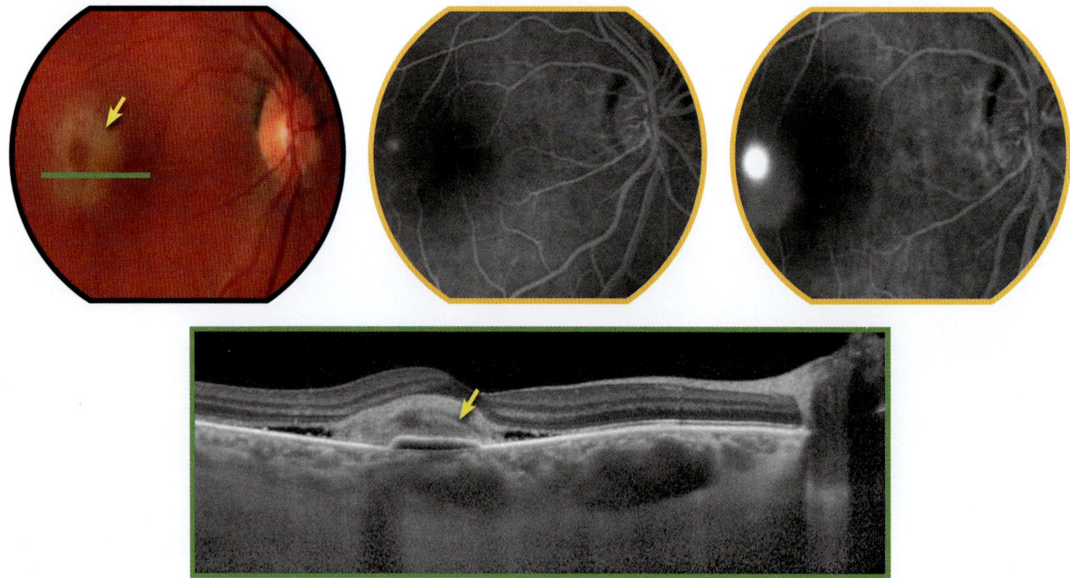

Fibrin is poorly visualized with fluorescein angiography and FAF imaging. However it may stain with ICG angiography and appears as subretinal hyper-reflective material on OCT imaging *(arrow)*.

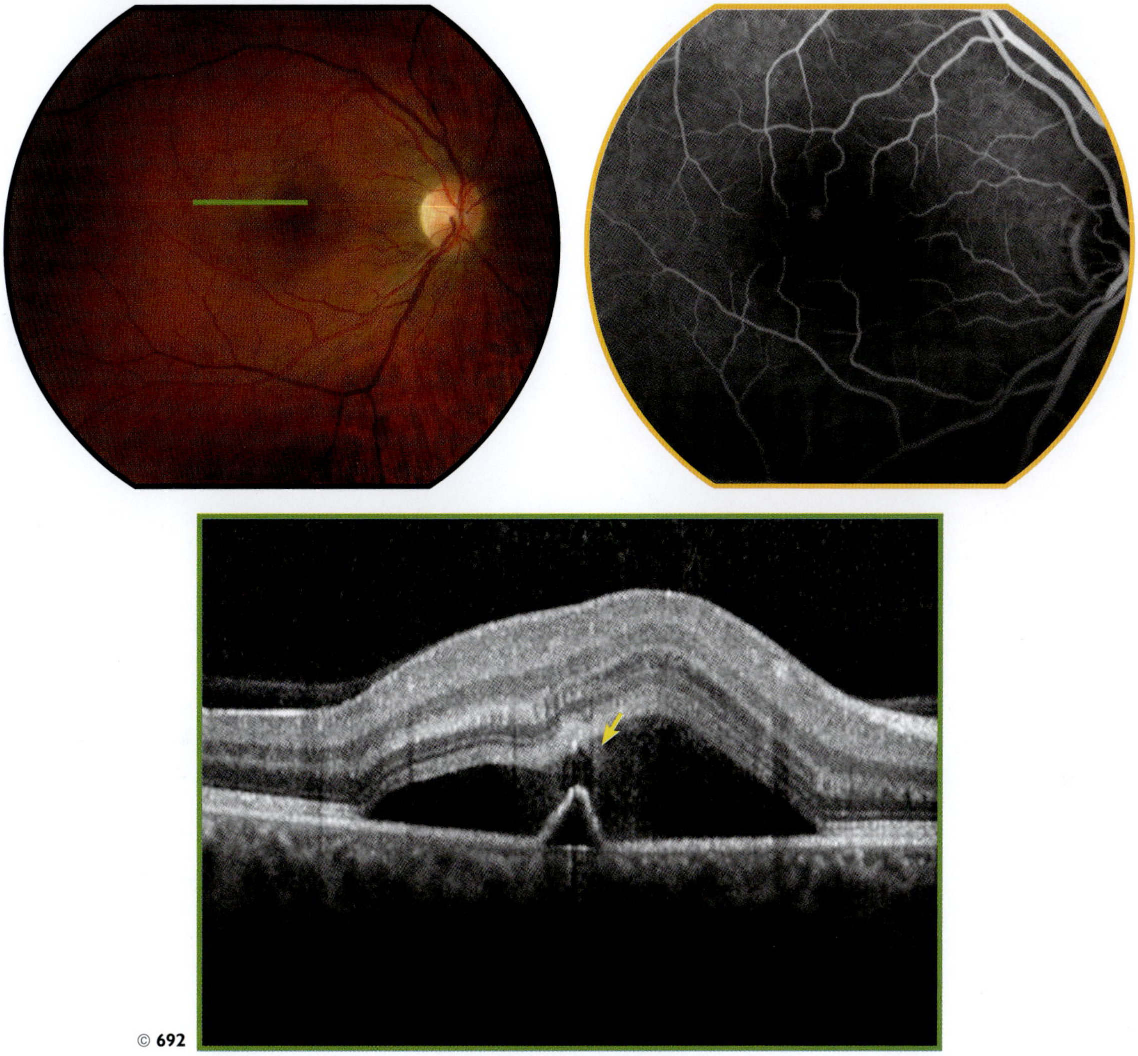

© 692

This patient has subretinal fibrin within an area of neurosensory detachment *(top left image)*. The focal point of leakage appears hyperfluorescent on FA *(top right image)*. Sometimes, on OCT imaging, a round or oval area of lucency *(arrow)* can be seen within the region of subretinal fibrin and this commonly correlates to the defect in the underlying RPE.

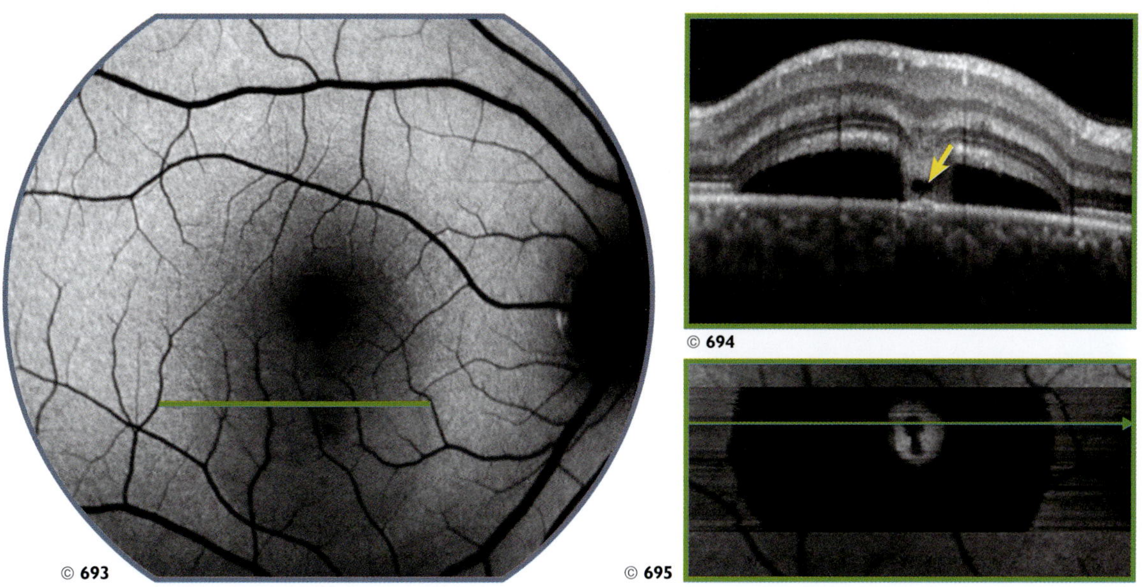

© 693 © 694 © 695

FAF imaging of this patient shows the area of detachment that extends inferior to the fovea. OCT imaging shows the lucency within the fibrin *(arrow)*, which has as a smokestack appearance on *en face* OCT imaging *(bottom right image)*.

PED Microrip (Blow-Out) in CSC

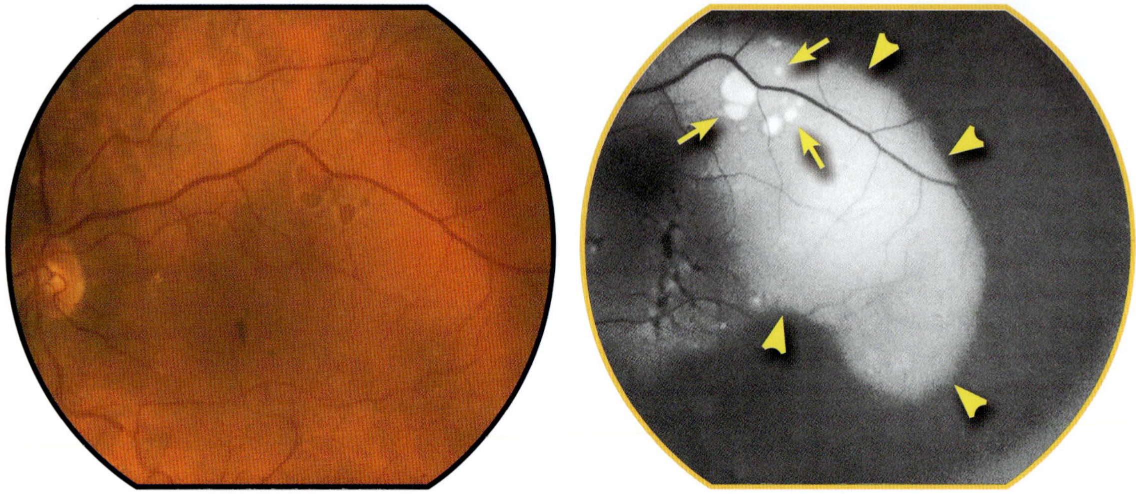

In some cases of CSC, a huge PED will be seen *(arrowheads)*. These PEDs may be associated with one or more microrips or "blow-outs" *(arrows)*. These blow-outs lead to neurosensory detachments but eventually resolve as the pigment epithelium proliferates to close the gap.

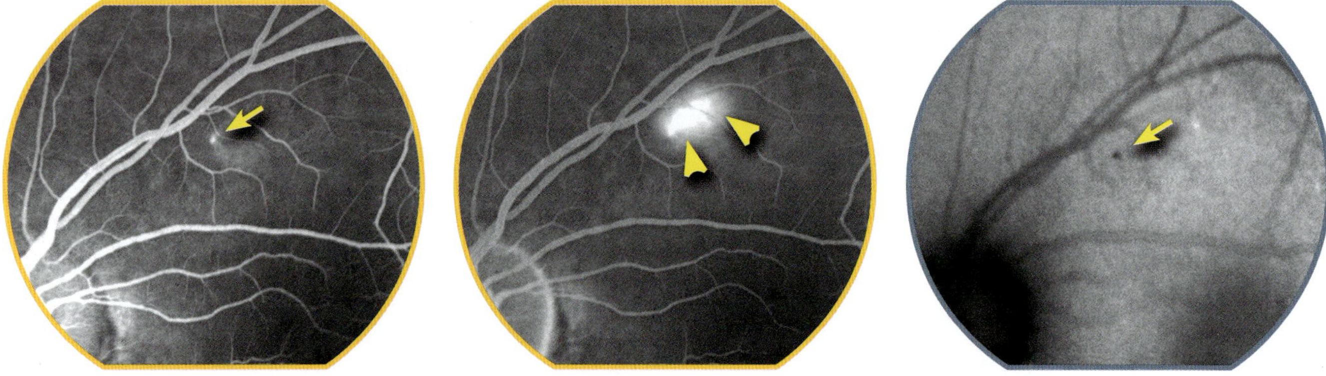

The early-phase FA shows a focal RPE leak *(arrow)* at the edge of a serous PED. The late-phase FA reveals pooling of the dye into the subretinal space *(arrowheads)*. The corresponding FAF image *(right)* shows hypoautofluorescence at the site of the acute RPE leak *(arrow)* from absence of the RPE or a so-called "blow-out" or micro-RPE rip.

RPE Rip in CSC

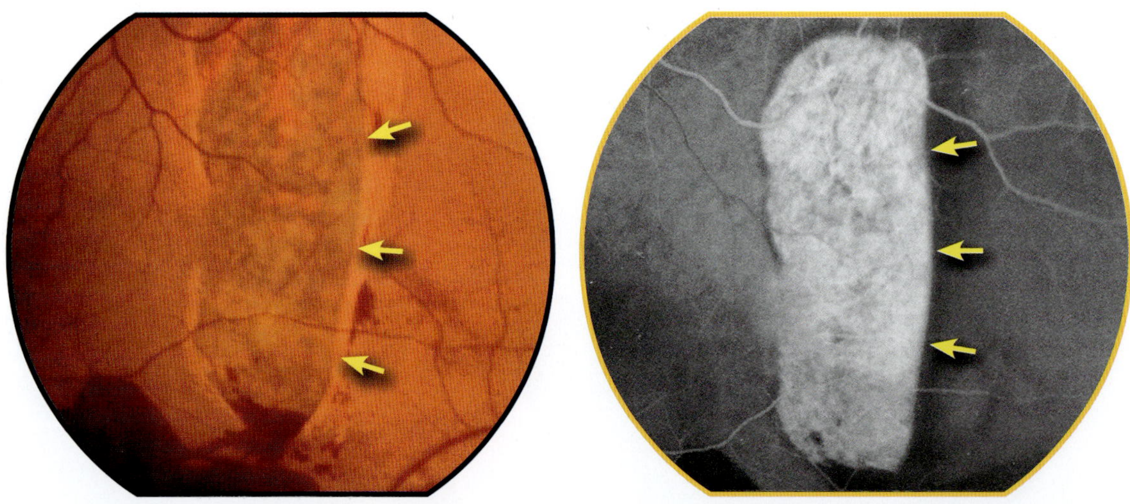

In CSC, large rips *(arrows)* in the RPE may occur with or without subretinal hemorrhage. This patient experienced a huge rip in the RPE with subretinal bleeding. Spontaneous resolution of the serosanguineous changes occurred without evidence of choroidal neovascularization. *Images courtesy of Dr. Stuart Green*

Bullous-Dependent Detachment in CSC

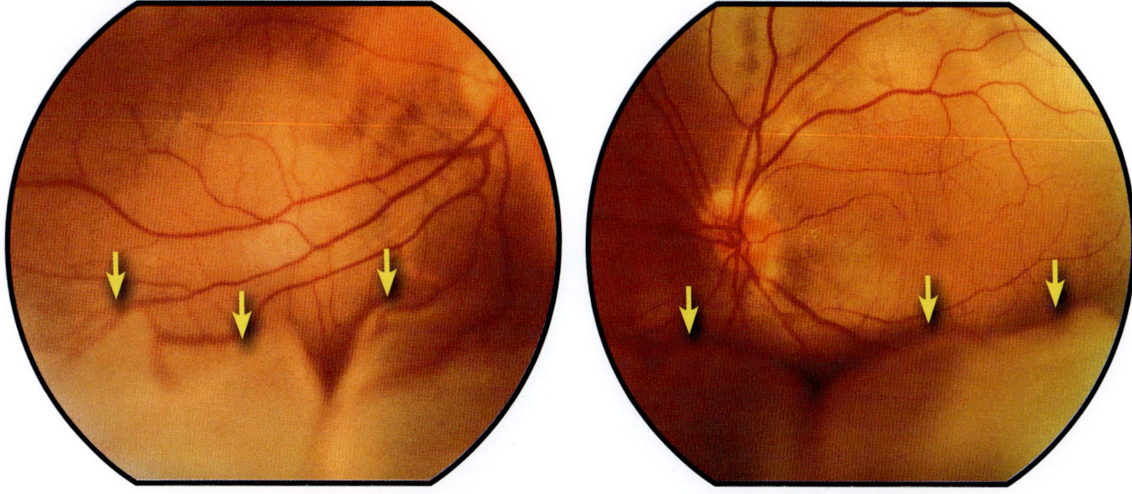

In chronic or severe CSC, a gravitating detachment may be bullous in nature with accumulation of fluid extending into the posterior pole and sometimes reaching the macula *(arrows)*. *Courtesy of Drs Richard Rosen and Joseph Walsh*

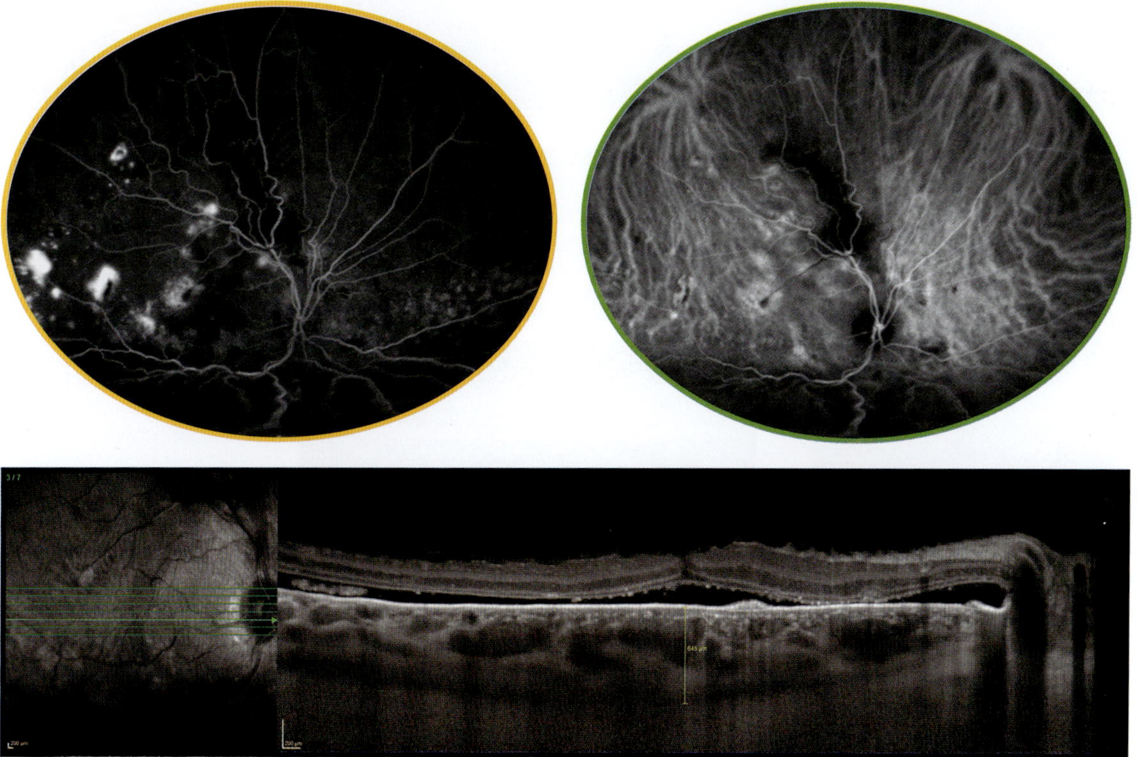

This patient with severe CSC has an inferior bullous retinal detachment. Ultra-widefield fluorescein angiography shows multifocal areas of leakage and ultra-widefield ICG angiography shows hyperpermeability in the choroid with dilated choroidal pachyvessels including the superior vortex vein ampullas. Enhanced depth imaging OCT of the right eye shows subretinal fluid and a thickened choroid with grossly dilated choroidal pachyvessels.

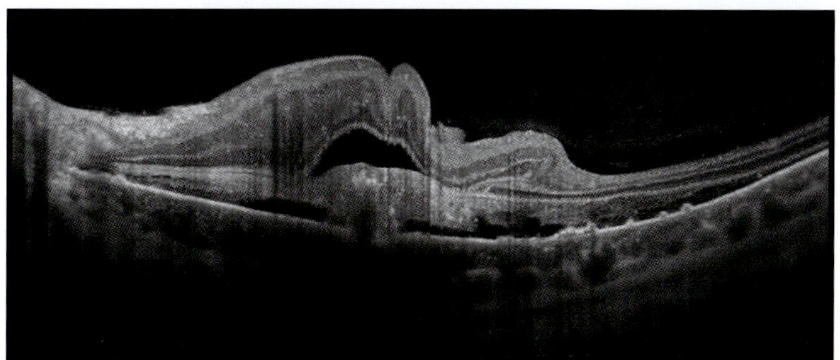

This swept source OCT image of the patient's left eye shows subretinal fluid with retinal folds and subretinal fibrosis. There are dilated choroidal pachyvessels similar to those seen in the fellow eye.

© **696**

Treatment

Laser photocoagulation can be applied to a pigment epithelial leak under the guidance of fluorescein angiography to resolve detachment in CSC. When the leak is close to the center of the macula or if there is diffuse incontinence to the pigment epithelium, photodynamic therapy (PDT) is appropriate in the management of such patients.

Photodynamic Therapy and CSC

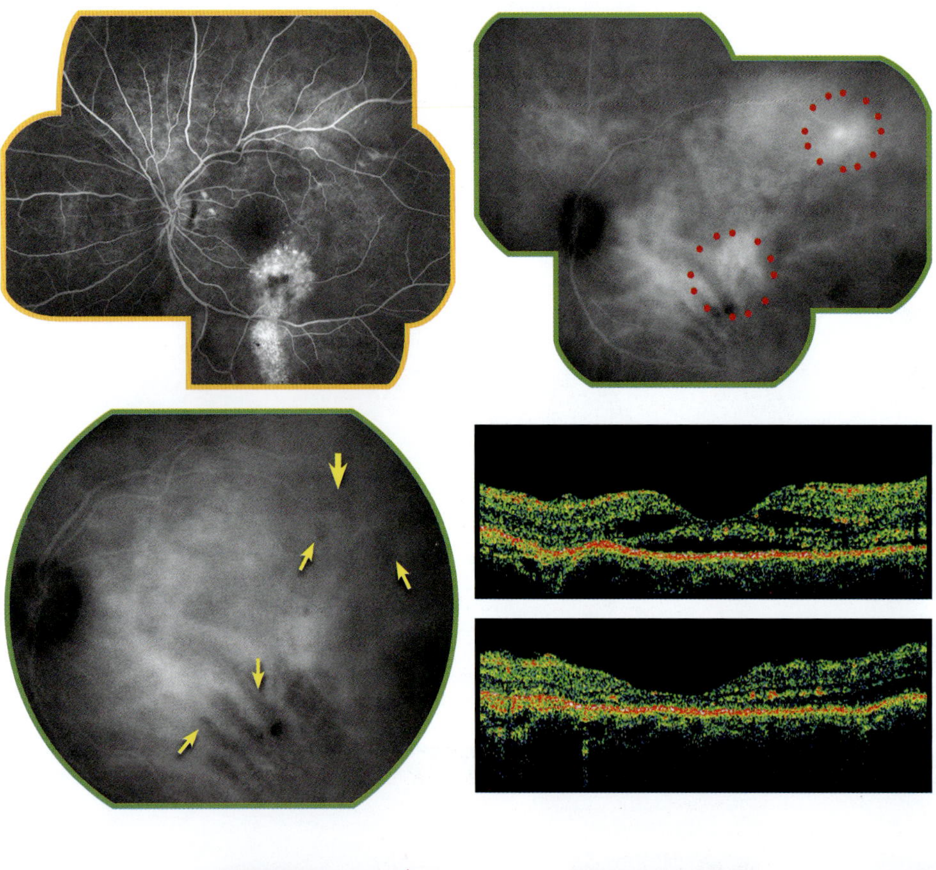

This patient has a gravitating atrophic tract and persistent sensory retinal detachment with cystoid macular degeneration evident with OCT imaging. The ICG angiogram shows multiple areas of choroidal hyperpermeability *(upper right)*. The two areas of leakage were treated with PDT *(red rings)*. There was resolution of the detachment confirmed with OCT imaging. The post-treatment ICG angiogram shows hypofluorescence of the choroid immediately after PDT *(arrows)*. Reperfusion of the choroidal vessels occurs 2-4 weeks after treatment. There was foveal atrophy from the chronic subretinal fluid. Although the detachment often resolves after treatment, recurrent detachment may occur. *Top and bottom left images courtesy of Dr. Lee Jampol*

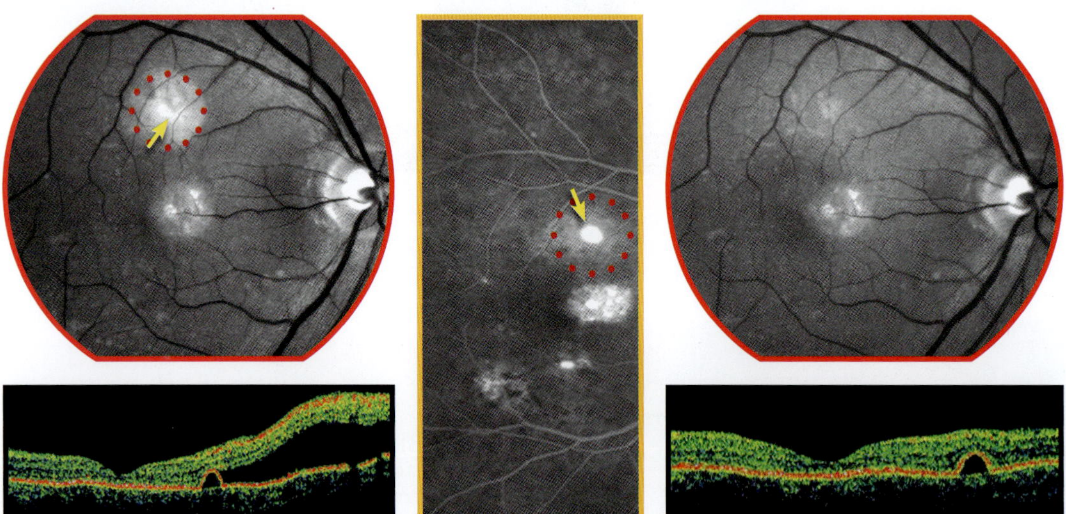

In this patient with chronic CSC there was a focal leak in the superior temporal macula *(arrows)*. The OCT showed a PED and neurosensory retinal detachment. PDT was applied *(red rings)* to the leakage. The detachment resolved, leaving no significant pigment epithelial damage *(upper right)*. The neurosensory retina is flat, but the PED persisted, as seen on the post-treatment OCT *(lower right)*.

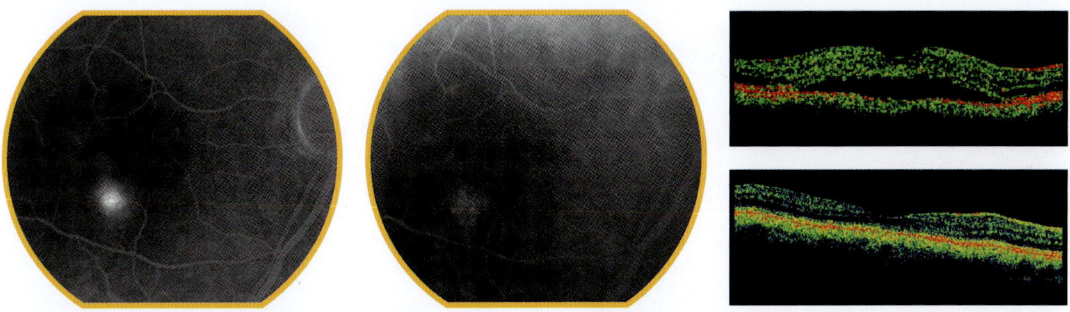

This patient with CSC had a juxtafoveal leak that was treated with half-fluence PDT. There was resolution of the detachment in 2 weeks. Very little clinical change in the pigment epithelium followed the treatment *(right)*. The OCT images show the pretreatment detachment and the post-treatment resolution. Laser photocoagulation of the acute RPE leak is also effective in resolving the associated detachment of the retina. However, thermal laser will leave an atrophic scar that may affect vision when treatment is applied close to fixation.

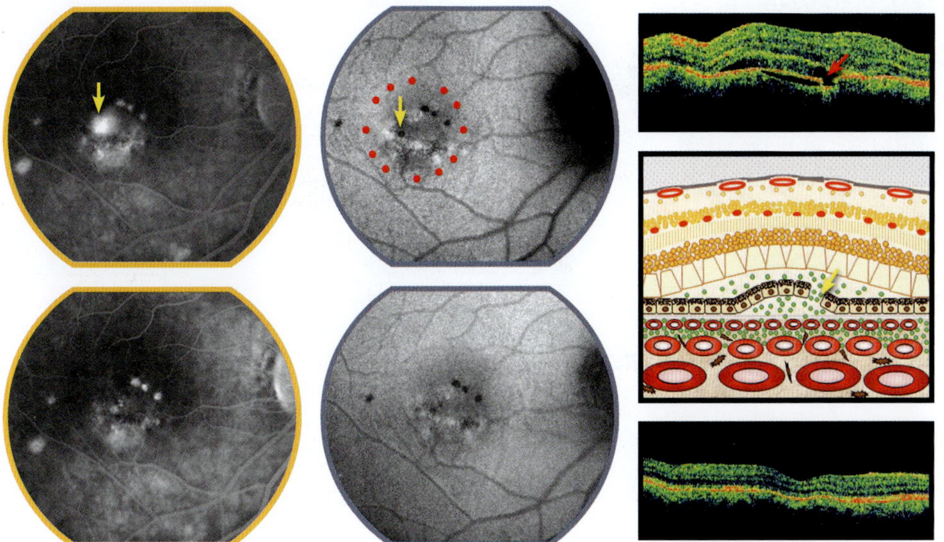

This patient has an active leak near the fovea *(arrow)* with chronic pigment epithelial changes. One focal area of hypoautofluorescence corresponded to the active leak. The OCT shows a "blow-out" in the pigment epithelium *(arrow)*, a shallow pigment epithelial elevation, a neurosensory detachment, and fibrin between the pigment epithelium and the detached retina. Following PDT *(red ring)*, there was closure of the leak, resolution of the detachment, and reconstitution of the RPE. The post-treatment OCT shows resolution of the detachment *(lower right)*. The schematic suggests that there is exudation within the inner choroid *(green dots)* in CSC that causes an elevation of the RPE. There is a "blow-out" or microrip in the pigment epithelium *(arrow)* and leakage of this exudate into the subneurosensory retinal space.

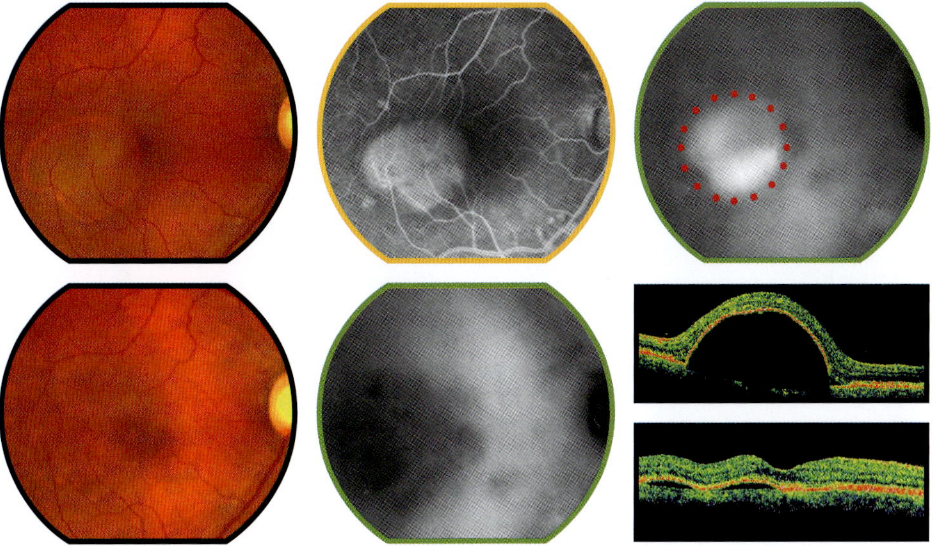

This patient with CSC had a large PED. The fluorescein angiogram showed homogeneous filling. He had severe metamorphopsia compromising his central vision. The ICG angiogram showed leakage under the PED. With ICG guidance, PDT was applied *(red ring)*. The patient had near-complete resolution of the PED in 10 days and the retina has remained flat for 3 years in follow-up. The OCT images demonstrate the pre- and 10-day post-treatment appearances of the PED.

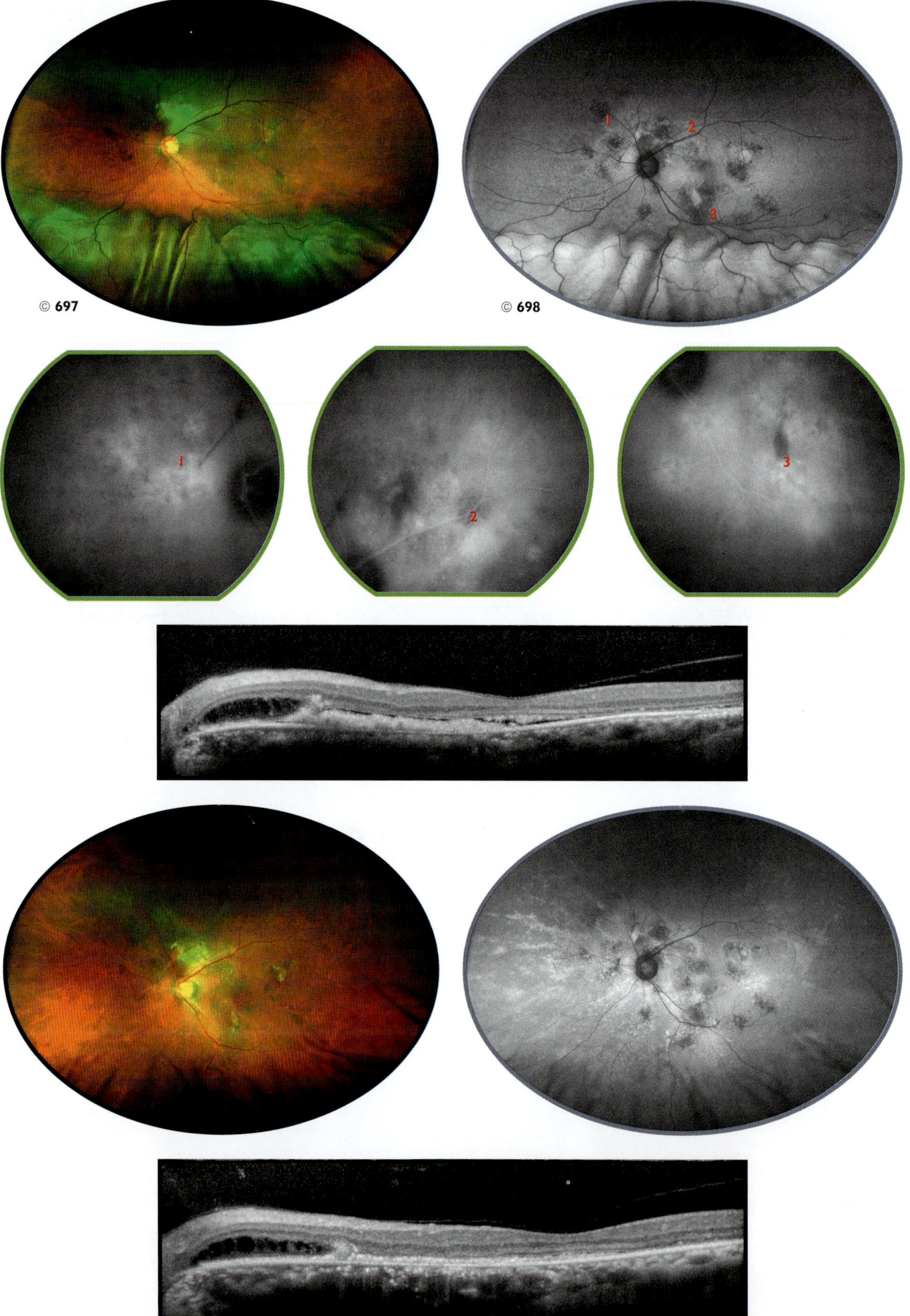

A 50-year-old male presented with an inferior gravitating detachment due to the bullous variant of CSC. Multiple foci of RPE changes are seen on ultra-widefield FAF imaging *(top right)*. ICG angiography *(second row)* reveals three areas of leakage *(1, 2, and 3)*, which are also denoted on FAF imaging. Extensive subretinal fibrin is evident on SD-OCT as is subretinal fluid and intraretinal fluid. Half-fluence PDT was applied to the three sites of leakage and there was complete resolution of subretinal fluid by 4 months *(fourth row)*. Residual hyper- and hypoautofluorescence changes are seen on FAF imaging. SD-OCT demonstrates total resolution of SRF and significant reduction in subretinal fibrin. *Images courtesy of Dr. Irene Barbazetto*

Unusual CSC Cases

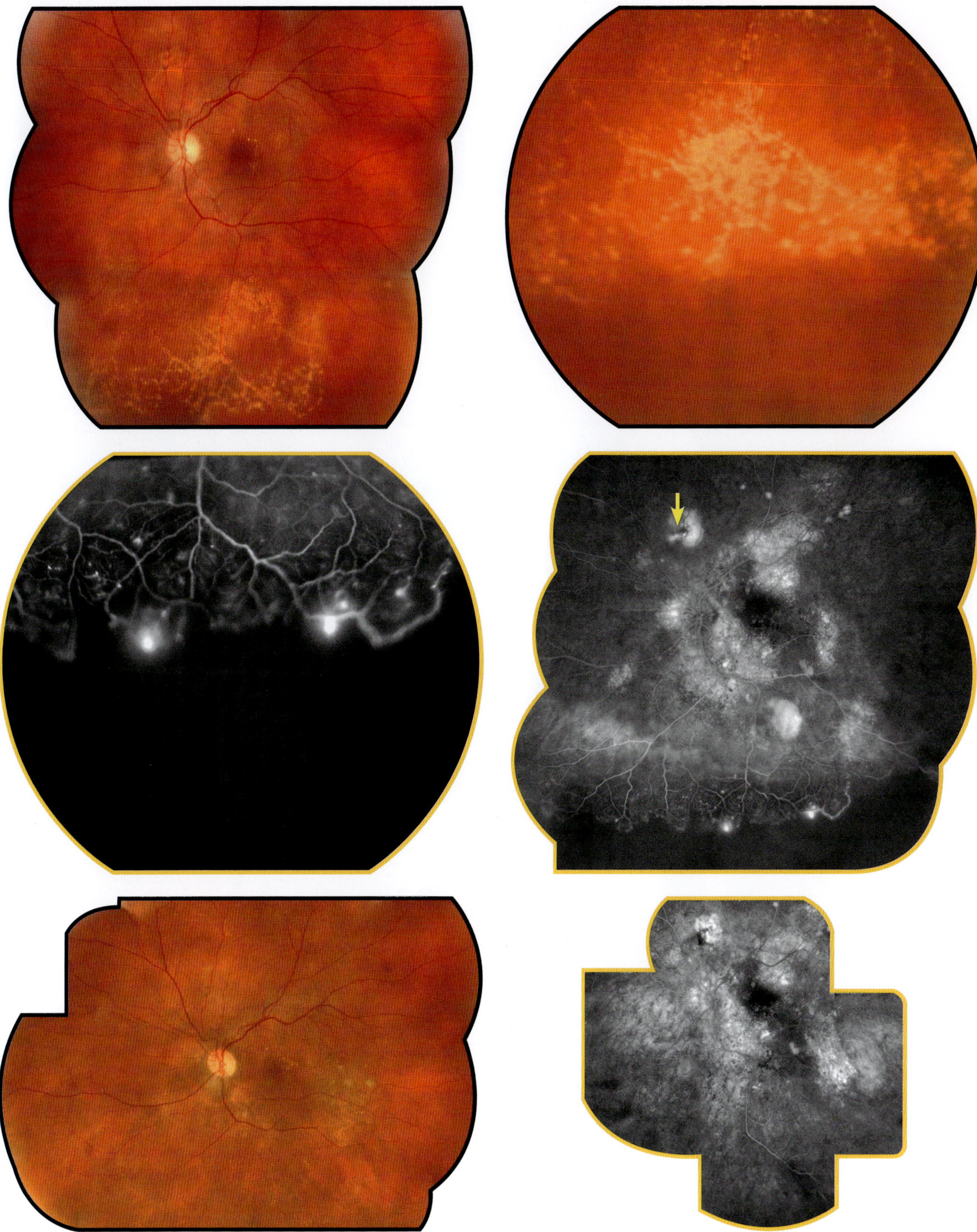

This patient had chronic CSC for a number of years. There is apparent lipid deposition in the peripheral inferior fundus and a persistent dependent detachment. The fluorescein angiogram shows non-perfusion in the peripheral retina and telangiectatic vascular changes at the junction between perfused and non-perfused retina *(middle left)*. Laser treatment was carried out on the PED, where there was a focal leak in the superior juxtapapillary area *(arrow)*. Subsequently, there was complete resolution of the dependent detachment and regression of the telangiectatic changes.

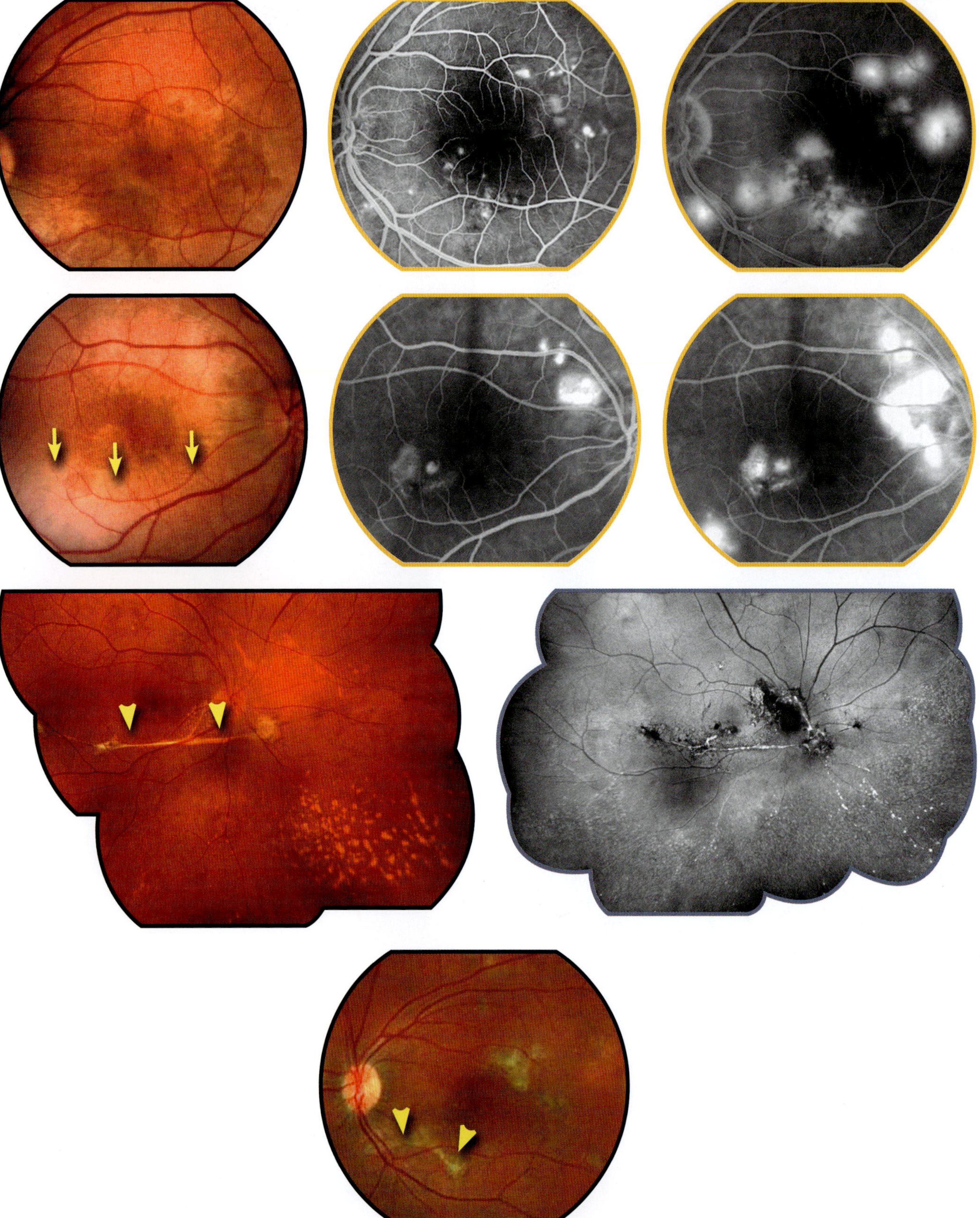

This patient was diagnosed with uveitis. She had idiopathic thrombocytopenic purpura and was administered high doses of steroid, which led to chronic CSC. Multifocal leakage was evident in the posterior segment of each eye on fluorescein angiography *(first and second rows)*. There was a bullous dependent detachment in each eye *(arrows)*. Laser photocoagulation treatment was applied to the active leaks, and there was resolution of the neurosensory detachment but persistence of some of the PEDs. There was a legacy of fibrous proliferation subretinally in each eye *(arrowheads)* and fundus hyperautofluorescence due to residual chromophores in the subretinal space, which gradually cleared.

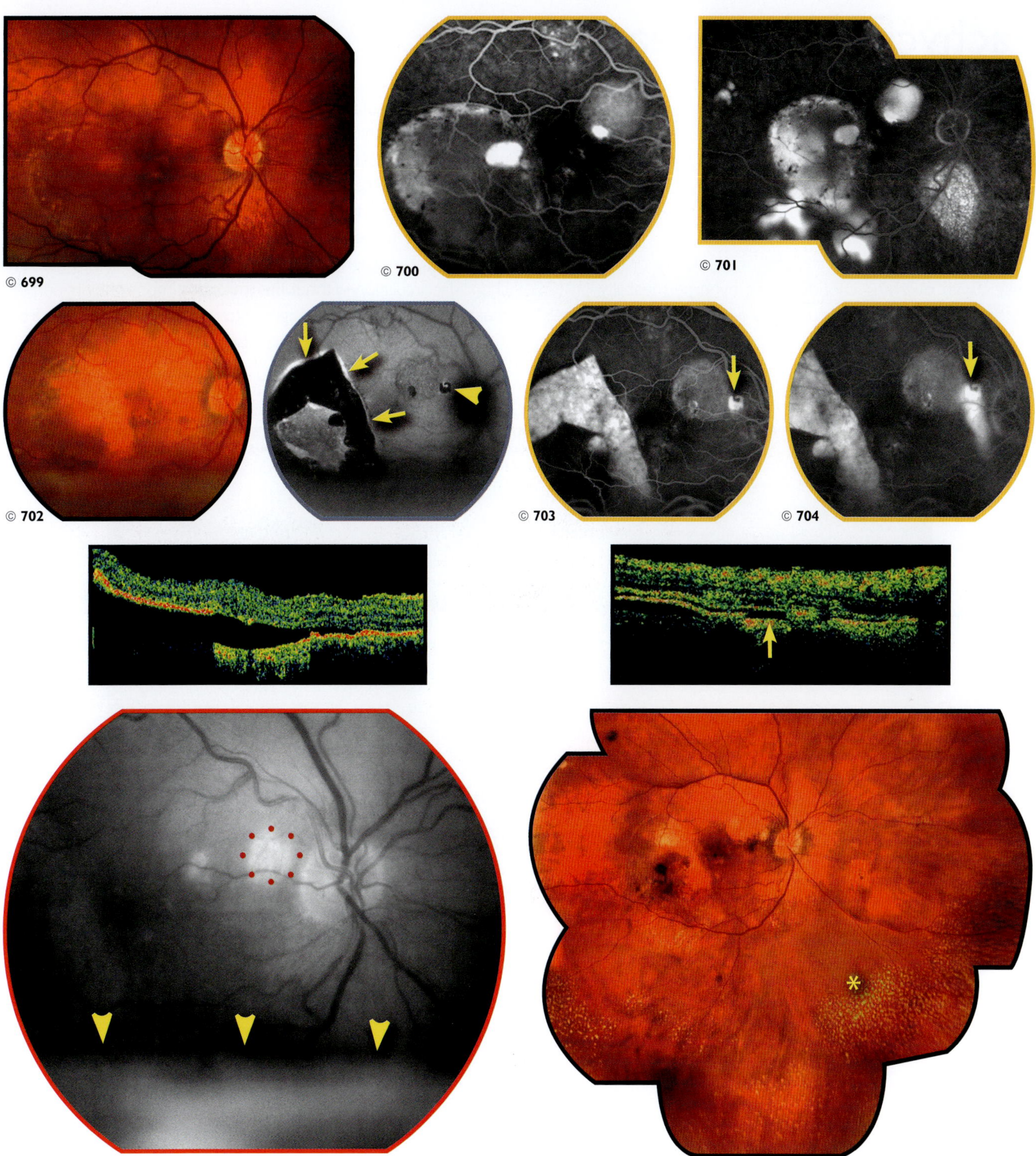

This patient had chronic CSC in both eyes. There were huge PEDs and a bullous neurosensory dependent detachment inferiorly *(arrowheads)*. He experienced a rip to the pigment epithelium *(arrows)*, which was clearly delineated with FA *(second row)*. The edges of the rip were coiled, which produced a margin of hyperautofluorescence. The OCT shows a discontinuity in the RPE corresponding to the rip *(third row, left)*. Eventually, a leak occurred at the edge of the PED near the disc *(second row, arrows)*. Note the fluorescein leakage descending into the bullous inferior detachment ("descending leak"). The OCT showed a pigment epithelial rip in the temporal macula and a "blow-out" at the edge of the pigment epithelium in the nasal macula *(third row, arrow)*, where there was active leakage. Laser treatment was carried out to the "blow-out" leak *(red ring, lower left)*. Eventually, there was total resolution of the bullous detachment with residual exudate in the subretinal space *(asterisk, lower right)*.

Pachychoroid Disease

The term pachychoroid (Greek: παχύ-, pachy-, thick) refers to a choroidal phenotype found in a number of disorders, which unifies them into a spectrum and suggests that they share an underlying mechanism. These disorders include pachychoroid pigment epitheliopathy, CSC, pachychoroid neovasculopathy, and polypoidal choroidal neovasculopathy.

The phenotype is characterized by (1) focally dilated choroid vessels with overlying choriocapillaris hyperpermeability on ICG angiography and (2) dilated outer choroidal vessels ("pachyvessels") on spectral domain OCT with loss of volume in the overlying choriocapillaris and Sattler layers. Fundus tessellation is typically reduced in areas where the choroid is thickened.

Incorporation of novel imaging modalities has refined the definition of the pachychoroid phenotype to emphasize the morphology of pachyvessels over absolute choroidal thickness. Long wavelength swept source OCT rapidly acquires cross-sectional scans of the choroid with a dense raster pattern, which enables the resulting volume scans to be sectioned and segmented in arbitrary image planes. OCT angiography enables depth-resolved imaging of the choroidal circulation without the limitations imposed by hyperpermeability, and offers new insights into understanding pachychoroid neovasculopathy and polypoidal disease.

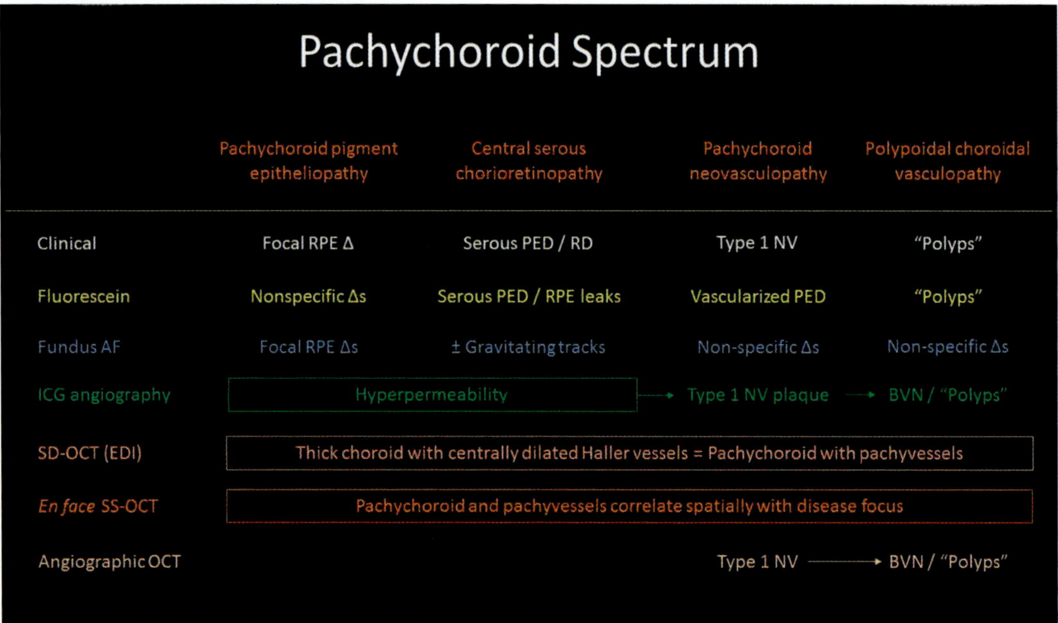

Pachychoroid Spectrum

	Pachychoroid pigment epitheliopathy	Central serous chorioretinopathy	Pachychoroid neovasculopathy	Polypoidal choroidal vasculopathy
Clinical	Focal RPE Δ	Serous PED / RD	Type 1 NV	"Polyps"
Fluorescein	Nonspecific Δs	Serous PED / RPE leaks	Vascularized PED	"Polyps"
Fundus AF	Focal RPE Δs	± Gravitating tracks	Non-specific Δs	Non-specific Δs
ICG angiography	Hyperpermeability		→ Type 1 NV plaque	→ BVN / "Polyps"
SD-OCT (EDI)	Thick choroid with centrally dilated Haller vessels = Pachychoroid with pachyvessels			
En face SS-OCT	Pachychoroid and pachyvessels correlate spatially with disease focus			
Angiographic OCT			Type 1 NV →	BVN / "Polyps"

The table above summarizes the findings on multimodal imaging that unify and distinguish disorders in the pachychoroid spectrum.

Pachychoroid Pigment Epitheliopathy

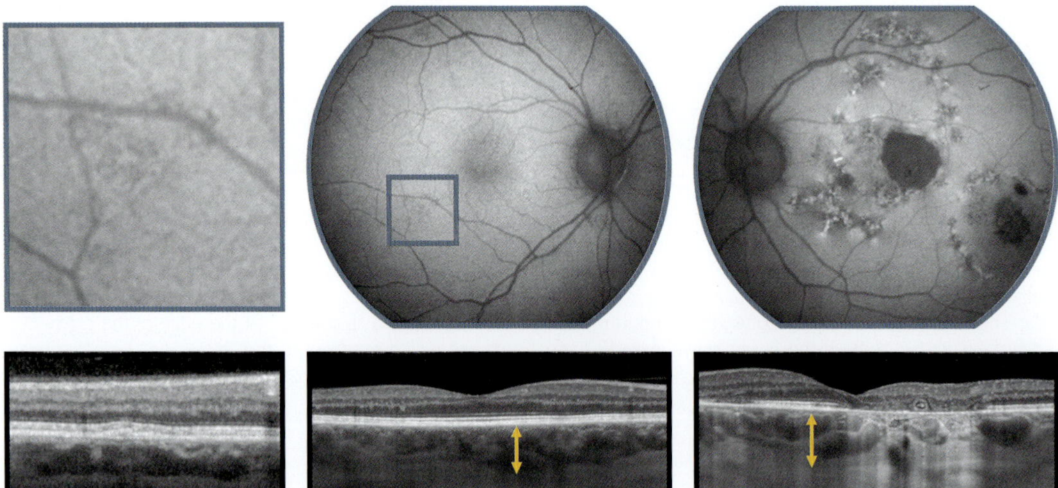

This patient has chronic CSC in the left eye complicated by geographic atrophy and outer retinal tubulations. FAF shows the extent of atrophy at the fovea and extrafoveal reticular RPE changes. The right eye has no history of subretinal fluid but shows extrafoveal RPE changes (magnified). In this area; pachyvessels are seen on cross-sectional OCT with overlying choriocapillaris atrophy. Subfoveal choroidal thickness is 490 μm bilaterally *(double-headed arrows)*. The right eye is therefore classified as having pachychoroid pigment epitheliopathy.

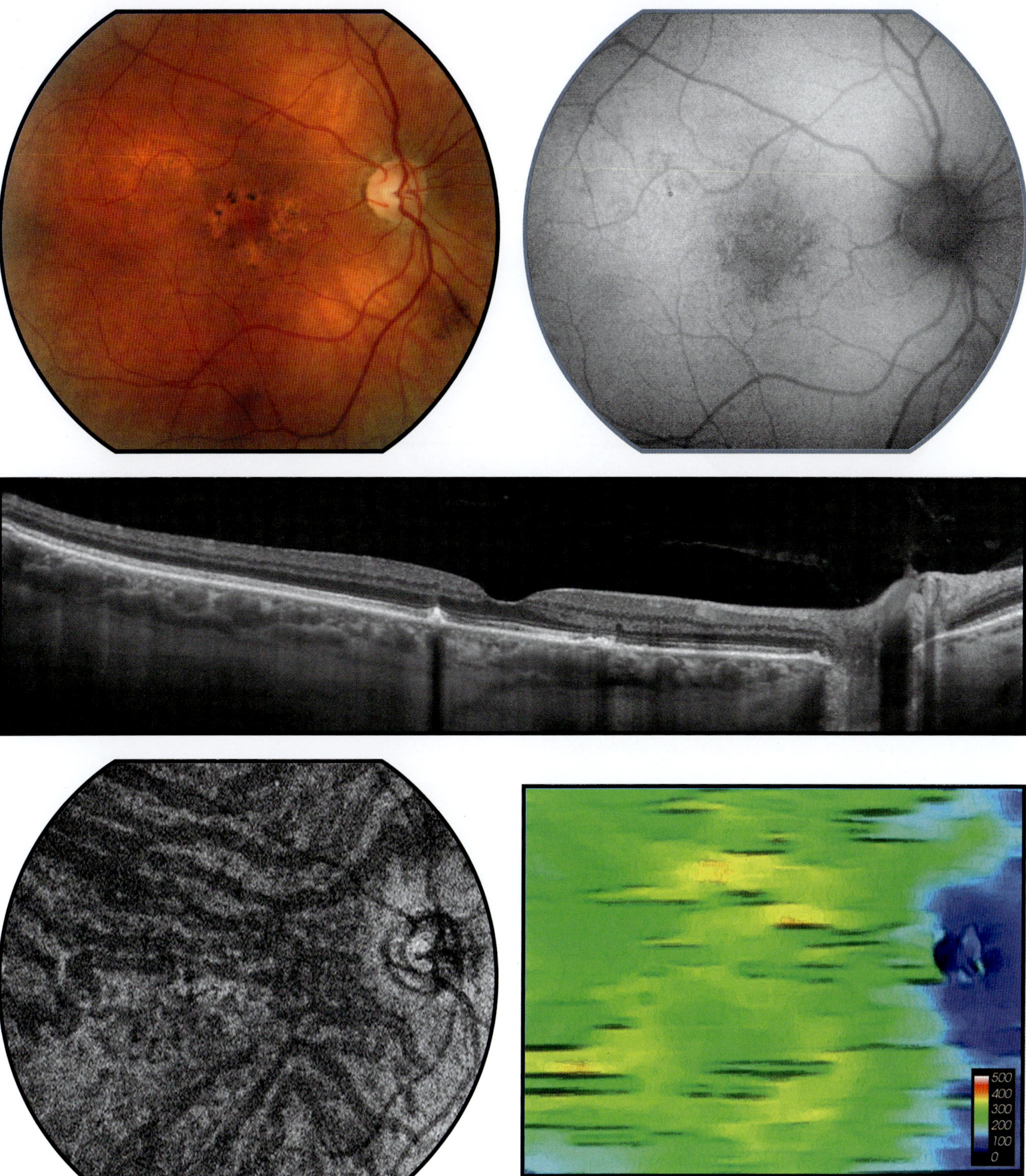

This patient with pachychoroid pigment epitheliopathy has no history of detectable subretinal fluid but has pigment epithelial changes at the fovea in the absence of drusen. Cross sectional swept-source OCT shows subfoveal pachyvessels with choriocapillaris loss in the areas of RPE change. *En face* swept-source OCT (segmented 160 μm below Bruch membrane) shows the distribution and morphology of pachyvessels, which have a large caliber as they traverse the site of pathology. The choroidal thickness map (microns) shows that the choroid is thicker where pachyvessels are most densely present, superior to the fovea.

Pachychoroid Neovasculopathy

Pachychoroid neovasculopathy represents type 1 neovascularization arising in the pachychoroid setting, which may occur even in eyes with no history of frank CSC or neurosensory retinal detachment. Absence or paucity of drusen together with choroidal thickening and pachyvessels distinguish this form of neovascularization from neovascular AMD. The type 1 neovascular tissue itself typically takes the form of a shallow irregular PED. Pachychoroid neovasculopathy may be complicated by polypoidal lesions arising from the type 1 neovascular tissue.

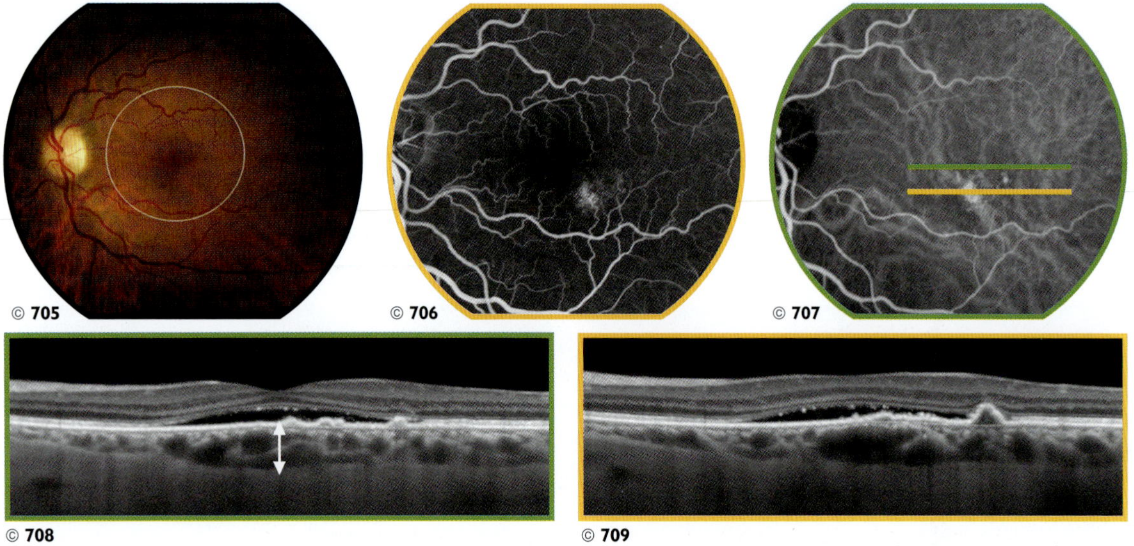

© 705 © 706 © 707 © 708 © 709

This patient has localized choroidal thickening evident clinically by a loss of fundus tessellations within the encircled area of the color image. A focal area of leakage inferior to the fovea, consistent with a type 1 neovascularization, is seen on fluorescein angiography. This area appears hyperfluorescent on ICG angiography. With OCT imaging, the type 1 neovascularization is seen with overlying subretinal fluid. There is localized choroidal thickening and choroidal vessel dilation beneath the type 1 neovascularization.

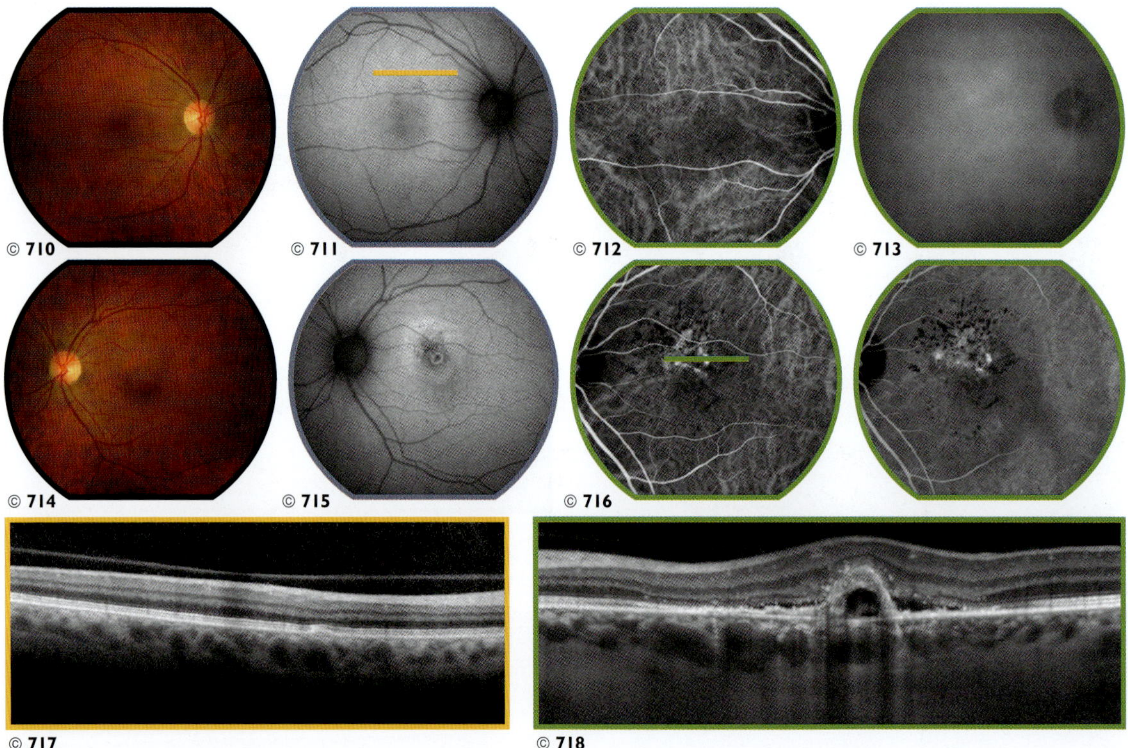

© 710 © 711 © 712 © 713 © 714 © 715 © 716 © 717 © 718

This patient has pachychoroid pigment epitheliopathy in the right eye *(top row images)*, in which pigment epithelial changes are best seen on FAF. The ICG angiogram in the early phase is unremarkable but the late phase shows choroidal hyperpermeability in the area of localized RPE changes. The OCT image *(bottom left image)* also shows focal RPE elevation above an area of dilated choroidal vessels and choroidal thickening. In the left eye *(second row images)*, the patient has pachychoroid neovasculopathy with a hyperfluorescent lesion in the ICG angiogram. The OCT image *(bottom right image)* shows a circular polypoidal lesion arising from the type 1 neovascularization associated with subretinal fluid overlying a pachyvessel cluster.

Optical Coherence Tomography Angiography of Pachychoroid Neovasculopathy

En face OCT angiography of shallow irregular PEDs in pachychoroid neovasculopathy shows the tangled morphology of the type I neovascular tissue.

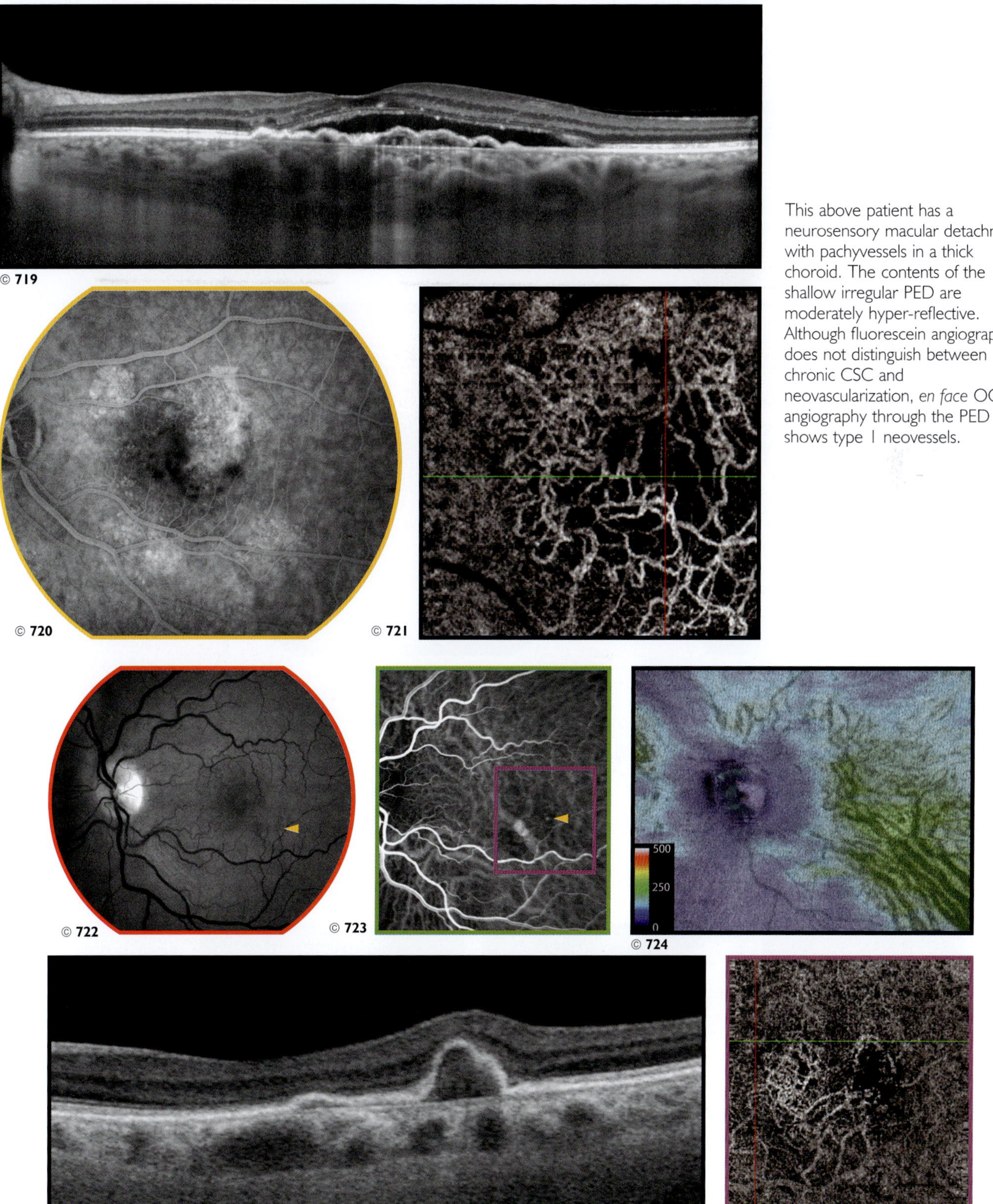

This above patient has a neurosensory macular detachment with pachyvessels in a thick choroid. The contents of the shallow irregular PED are moderately hyper-reflective. Although fluorescein angiography does not distinguish between chronic CSC and neovascularization, *en face* OCT angiography through the PED shows type I neovessels.

This patient has a polypoidal lesion *(arrowhead)* arising from type I neovascularization on a pachychoroid background. The polypoidal lesion is visible on ICG angiography and its type I branching vascular network is seen as an adjacent shallow irregular PED on cross sectional swept source OCT. The *en face* OCT shows the distribution of pachyvessels draining toward the inferotemporal vortex vein, and the overlaid choroidal thickness map shows that choroidal thickness is greatest where pachyvessels occupy its volume. The *en face* OCT angiogram shows the tangled morphology of the type I vascular network, but the polypoidal lesion itself is seen as a flow void.

Acute Exudative Polymorphous Vitelliform Maculopathy

Acute exudative polymorphous vitelliform maculopathy is a disorder associated with multiple serous detachments of the retina in the macular region of both eyes. Multiple pale to yellowish-orange, round or ovoid curvilinear lesions appear in the subretinal space. The fluorescein angiographic features in these patients will vary. Some smaller lesions may stain, while larger accumulations of this substance may block choroidal fluorescence. With fundus autofluorescence, the lesions normally appear hyperautofluorescent. The electrooculogram is normal in these patients and there has been one report of choroidal neovascularization evolving from a disturbance in the pigment epithelium. Slow, but often incomplete resolution of the material in the subretinal space has been known to occur. The pathogenesis of the disorder is unknown, and there is no established treatment.

Although the pathogenesis is unclear, it is important to exclude systemic malignancy, particularly melanoma, because acute polymorphous exudative polymorphous maculopathy has been associated with paraneoplastic retinopathy.

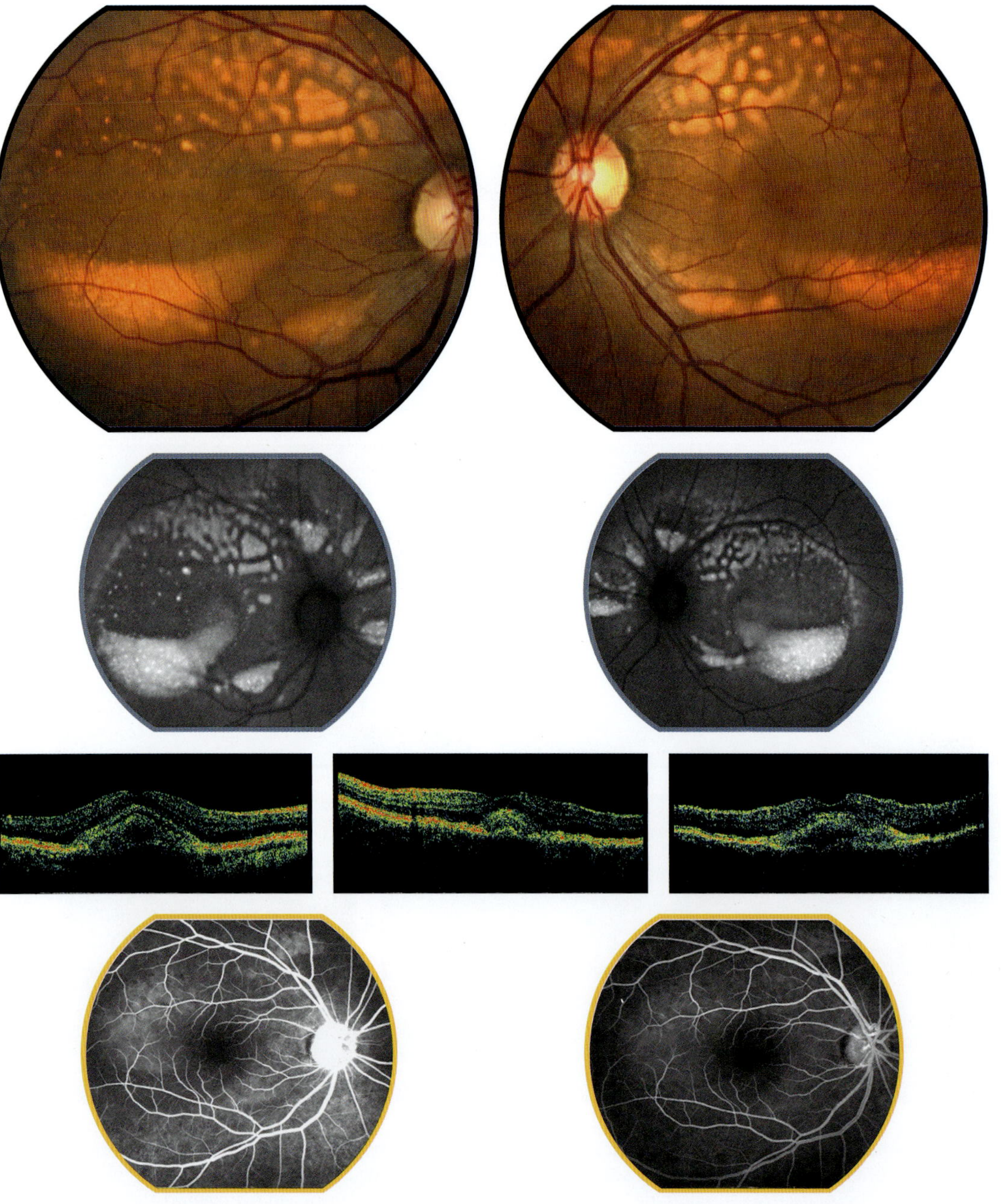

This patient has developed acute exudative polymorphous vitelliform maculopathy. There are multiple yellowish-orange lesions under the retina, within the posterior fundus and slightly beyond the arcades superiorly. These lesions resemble the vitelliform detachments seen in Best disease. The same is true for the FAF photographs, which show hyperautofluorescence *(second row)*. The OCT images show exudative change beneath the neurosensory detachments. The fluorescein angiogram shows a mild degree of fundus hypofluorescence. This is typical of the acute stages of this disease. As the material persists, it will become increasingly yellowish clinically and more hypofluorescent on the angiographic study, similar to Best disease.

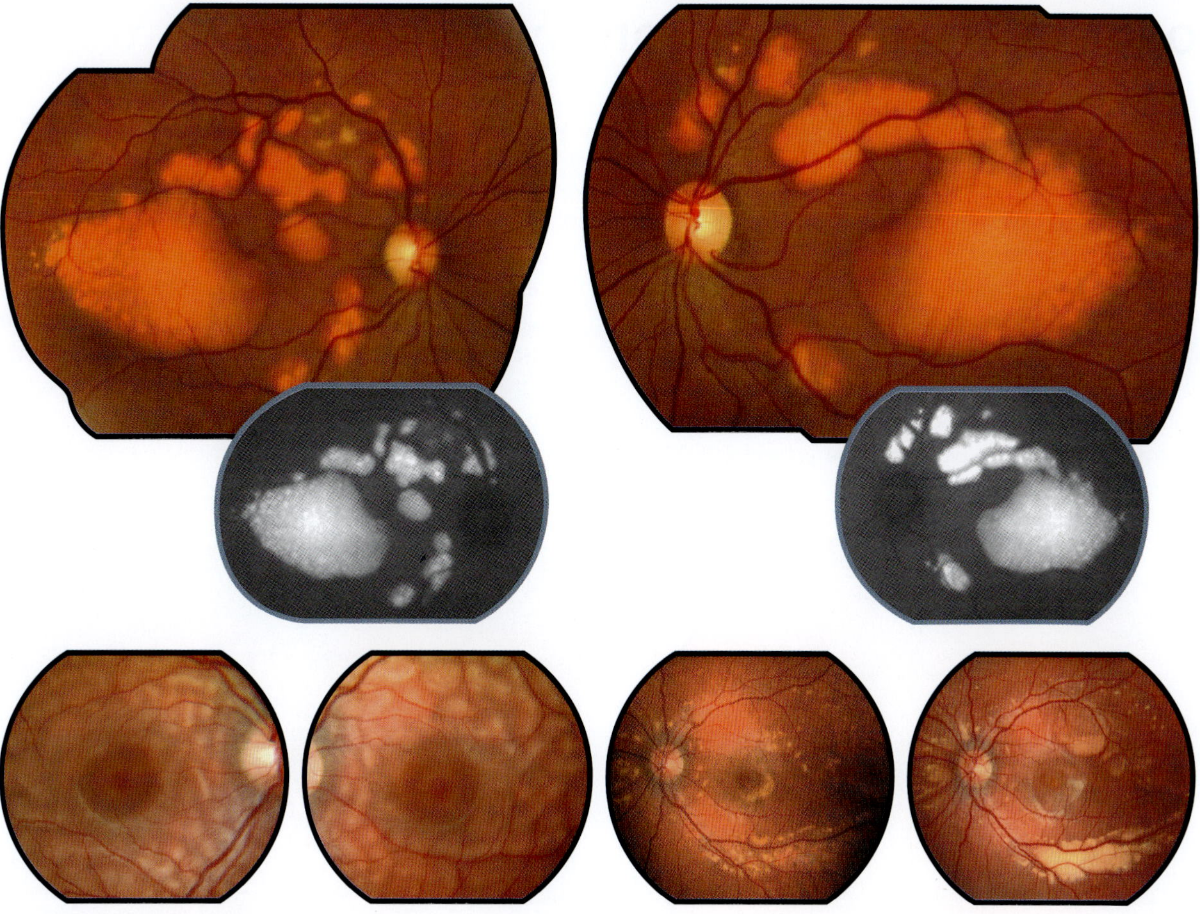

These patients also have acute exudative polymorphous vitelliform maculopathy. Note the variation in the morphology between presentation and later stages of the disease. Subretinal exudation may develop slowly, altering the clinical manifestations originally seen at presentation *(lower row)*.

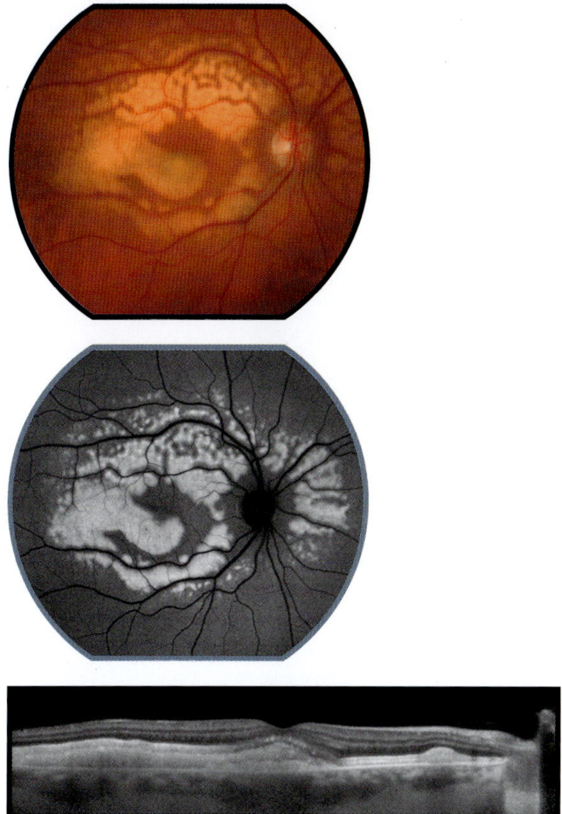

With spectral-domain OCT imaging, the vitelliform material appears as a hyper-reflective material in the subretinal space.

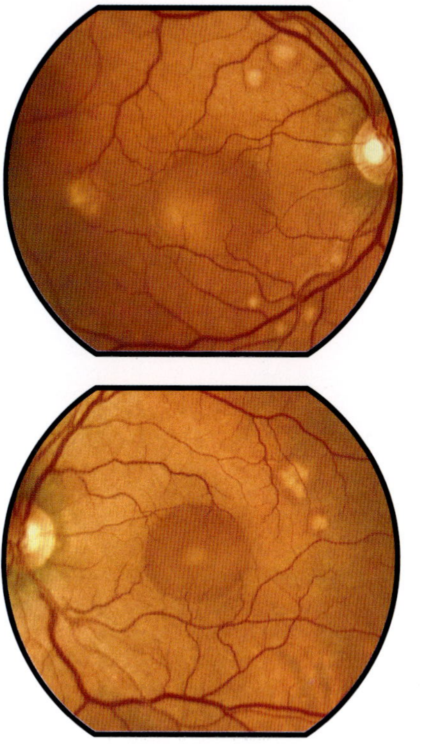

Idiopathic acute exudative polymorphous vitelliform maculopathy may also occur without much evidence of vitelliform-like material under the detachments in a multifocal distribution without fluorescein leakage. These detachments do not block the choroidal fluorescence, as seen with Best disease.

Idiopathic Uveal Effusion Syndrome

Idiopathic uveal effusion syndrome typically presents with loss of vision in one or both eyes, a bullous exudative retinal detachment, and shifting subretinal fluid in healthy middle-aged men with normal-sized eyes. Congenital abnormalities of the sclera and vortex veins may result in intermittent obstruction of the venous outflow, which causes accumulation of extravascular protein in the suprachoroidal space and the high protein content seen in the subretinal fluid and cerebrospinal fluid of these patients. The disease is often characterized by spontaneous remissions and exacerbations in the absence of intraocular inflammation and normal intraocular pressure. Blood may be present in Schlemm canal along with some mild episcleral dilation. The final visual outcome depends on the degree and duration of detachment with spontaneous reattachment requiring weeks to months. Several months after presentation, a "leopard skin" pattern of irregular thinning and RPE clumping may be evident, and is best seen on fluorescein angiography. Full-thickness sclerotomies 1-2 mm in size, left permanently open, may be performed to allow the fluid to absorb over several weeks. In nanophthalmic eyes, the abnormally thick sclera compresses the vortex veins and impedes venous drainage, thus leading to the development of uveal effusions. A sclerotomy procedure can also be utilized for nanophthalmos.

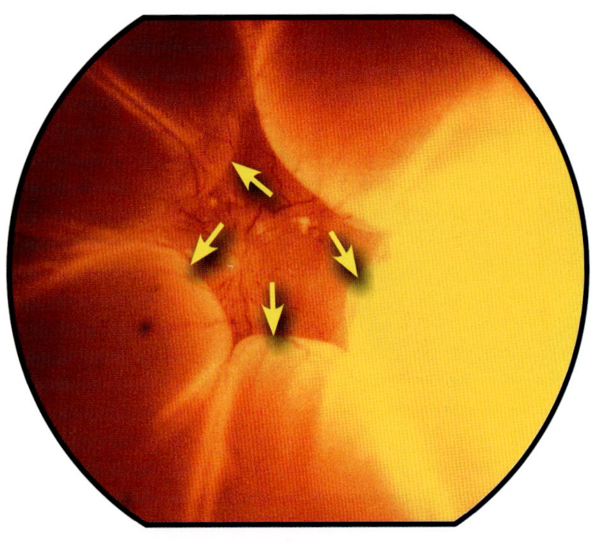

Color image and ultrasound courtesy of Dr. Robert Brockhurst

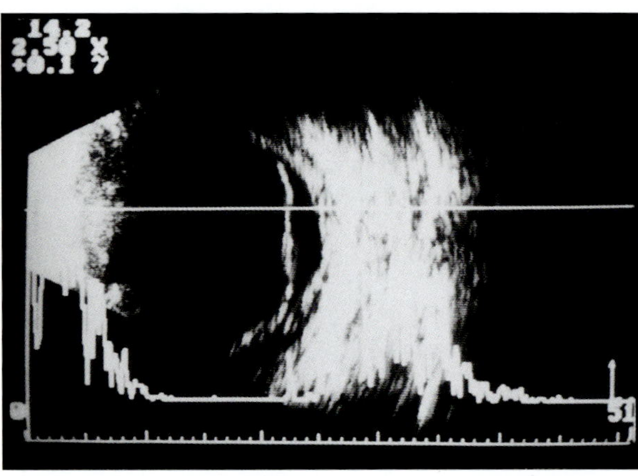

© 727

The ultrasound on this patient with idiopathic uveal effusion syndrome shows a bullous global detachment of the retina and a diffusely thickened choroid. While very small eyes are at risk of this entity, most cases involve normal-sized eyes.

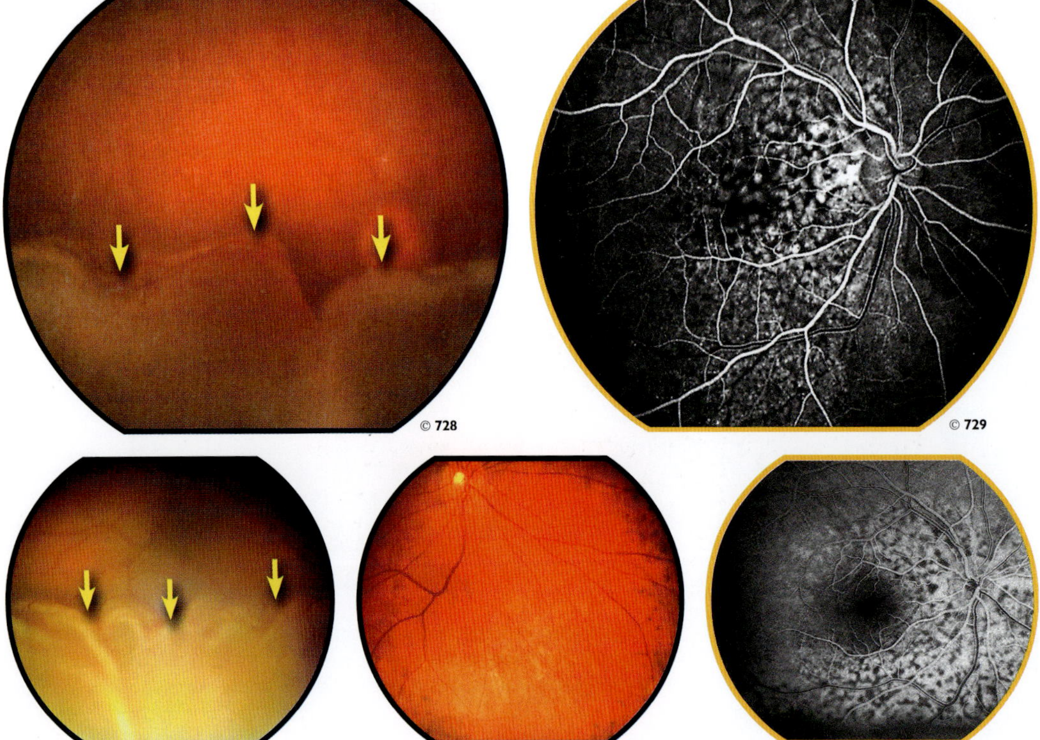

© 728

© 729

These patients with uveal effusion syndrome presented with multiple bullous retinal detachments *(arrows)*. The yellowish area corresponds to the external light source of the camera *(lower left)*. Some bullous detachments contain undulated folds. The pigment epithelium and disc may show some late staining, induced by the surrounding neurosensory detachment. The fluorescein angiogram shows a "leopard skin" appearance of hyper- and hypofluorescence.

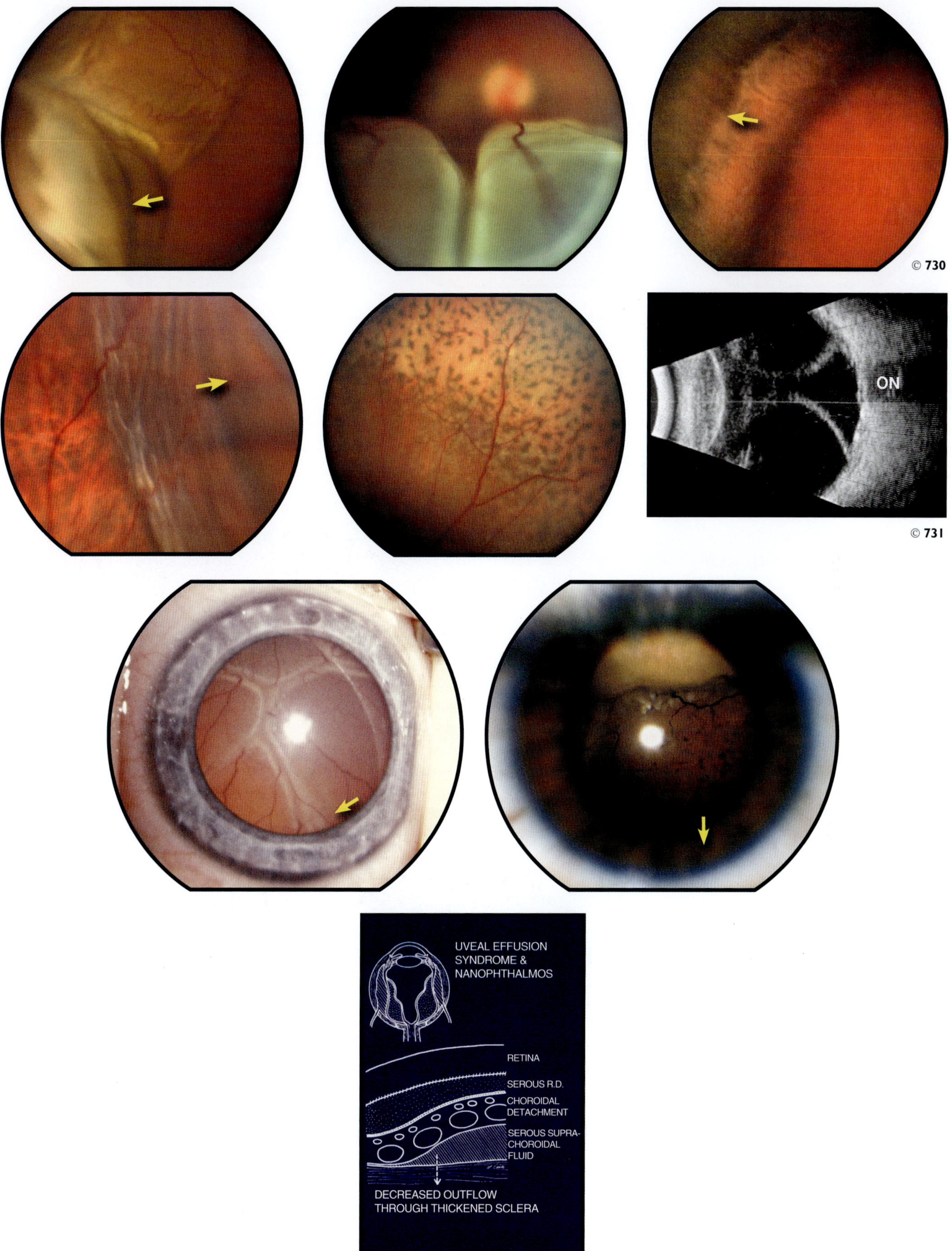

In these cases of idiopathic uveal effusion syndrome, acute choroidal and neurosensory detachments are shown *(first row)*. There are folds in the retina *(second row left)* and a "leopard-like" appearance after resolution *(second row middle)*. The ultrasound shows large serous choroidal detachments without underlying mass lesions *(second row right)*. The bullous retinal detachments can be seen through the dilated pupil *(third row)*. The schematic suggests the mechanism for the effusion in the nanophthalmic eye.

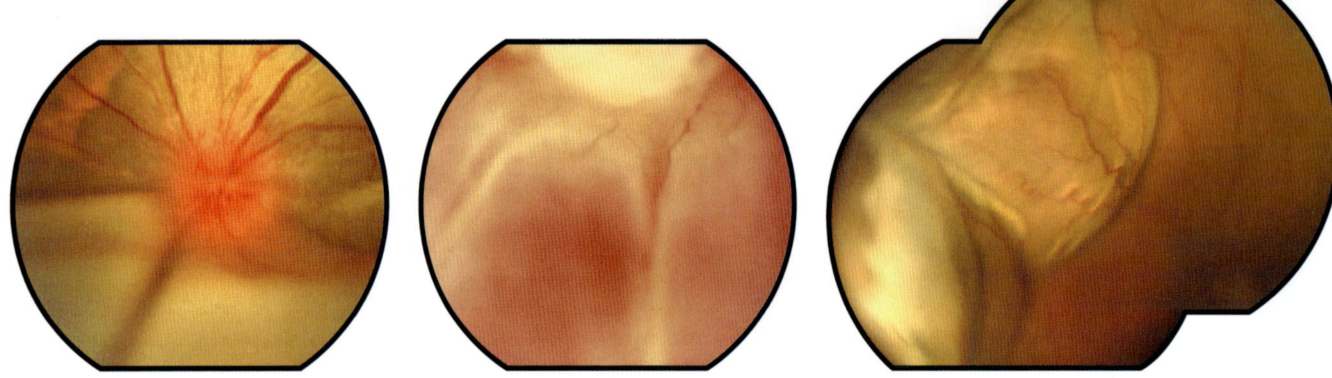

These cases of idiopathic uveal effusion syndrome have occurred in nanophthalmic eyes. Note the extent of the detachment in a bullous configuration in the top row.

Isolated Posterior Uveal Effusion

Isolated posterior uveal effusion is a rare condition that occurs in the absence of peripheral choroidal effusion and is typically associated with hyperopia and focal posterior thickening of the choroid. This may be complicated with serous macular detachment and macular edema, which may be treated successfully with oral or topical carbonic anhydrase inhibitors.

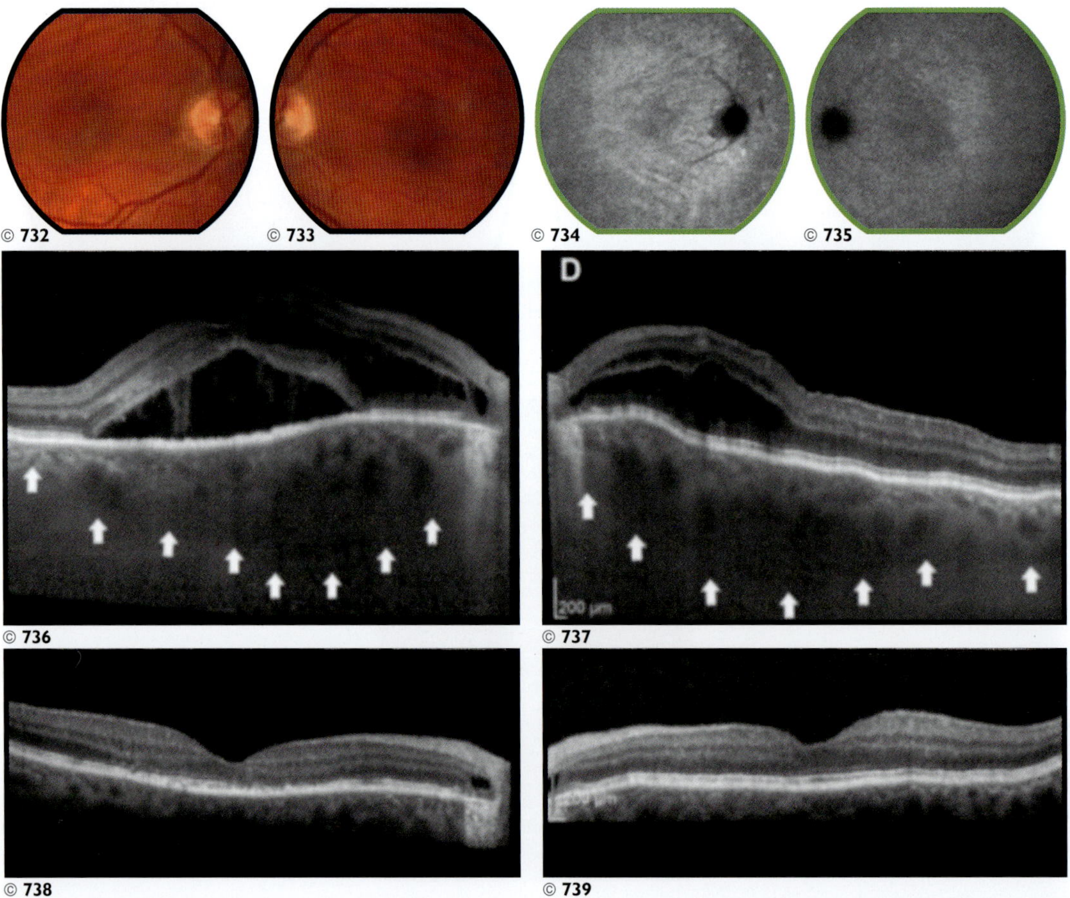

This patient had 7 diopters of hyperopia as a young adult and developed macular edema in late adulthood. Initially diagnosed as having age-related macular degeneration, he was treated with anti-vascular endothelial growth factor and steroid injections without success. ICG angiography shows choroidal hyperpermeability in the posterior pole. Swept source OCT shows macular edema and focal choroidal thickening *(arrows)*. Treatment with oral acetazolamide resulted in resolution of macular edema *(bottom images)*. *Images courtesy of Dr. David Browning*

Idiopathic Organ Transplant Chorioretinopathy

There is a peculiar maculopathy that is associated with organ transplantation of the kidney and heart. These patients develop a chronic detachment of the retina, protein in the subretinal space, and a peculiar "leopard skin" appearance to the pigment epithelium in the posterior pole bilaterally. Such patients are subject to CSC since they are often treated with corticosteroids, but patients with idiopathic organ transplant chorioretinopathy have no serous PED or focal leakage on fluorescein angiography. They also do not have choroidal separations, like patients with the idiopathic uveal effusion syndrome.

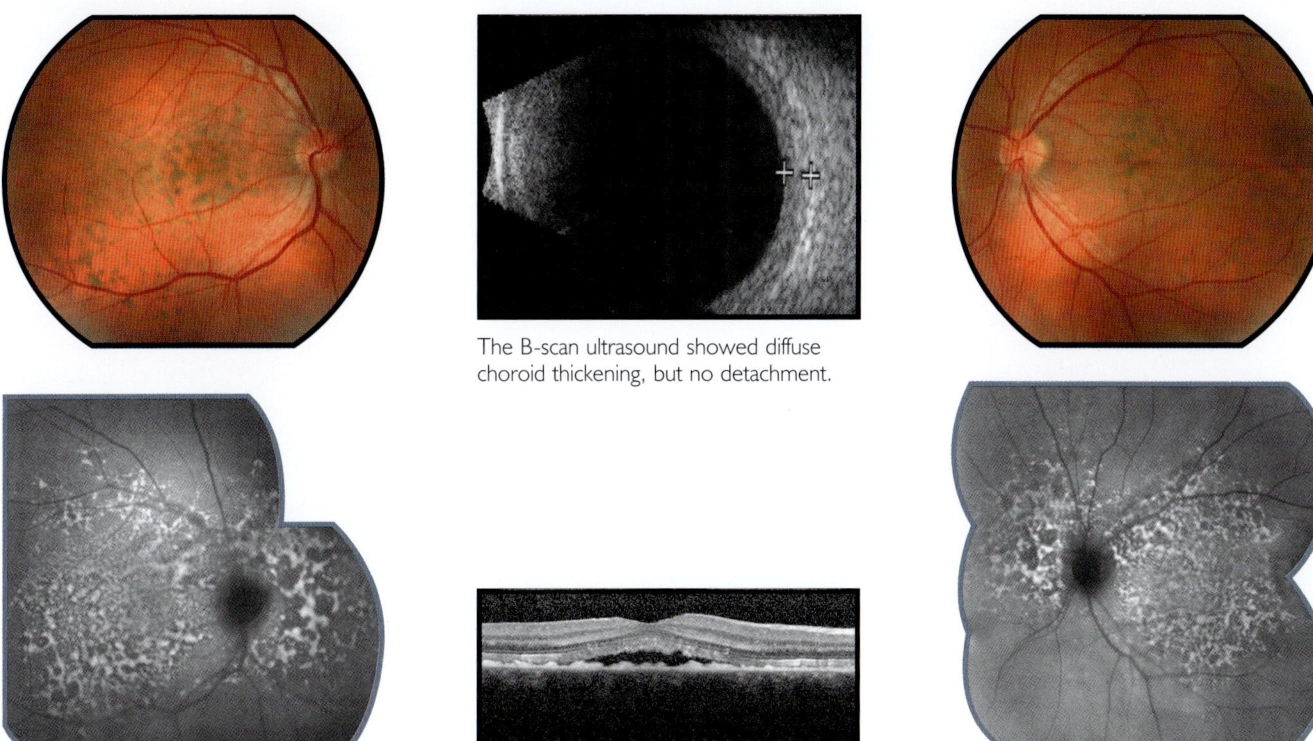

The B-scan ultrasound showed diffuse choroid thickening, but no detachment.

This 38-year-old male had a history of renal disease. He experienced bilateral persistent detachment. Note the leopard skin appearance on FAF in each eye. These changes were more prominent than the manifestations evident on clinical examination where a subtle "leopard skin" appearance was evident bilaterally. High-resolution OCT revealed a protein-enriched exudate without PED underlying a detached central macula, which is characteristic of the disorder.

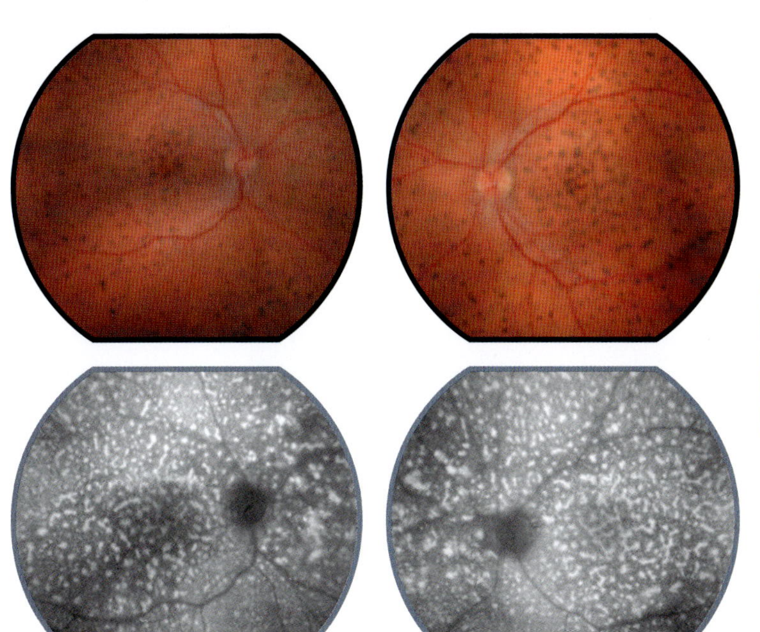

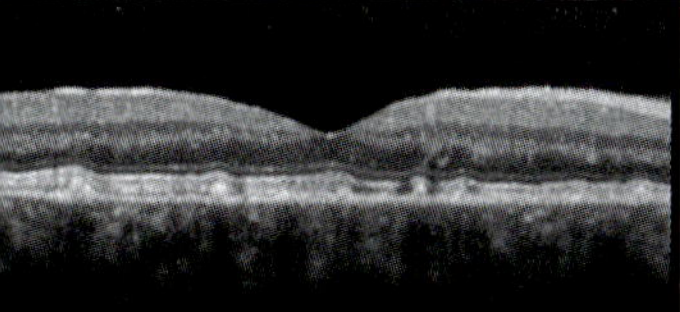

After scleral windows, the same patient as above experienced resolution of the subretinal fluid. However, extensive pigmentary changes of the fundus remained.

Suggested Reading

Carvalho-Recchia, C.A., Yannuzzi, L.A., Negrão, S., et al., 2002. Corticosteroids and central serous chorioretinopathy. Ophthalmology 109, 1834–1837.

Chan, C.K., Gass, J.D., Lin, S.G., 2003. Acute exudative polymorphous vitelliform maculopathy syndrome. Retina 23, 453–462.

Dansingani, K.K., Balaratnasingam, C., Klufas, M.A., et al. 2015. Optical coherence tomography angiography of shallow irregular pigment epithelial detachments in pachychoroid spectrum disease. Am. J. Ophthalmol. 160 (6), 1243–1254.e2.

Dansingani, K., Naysan, J., Balaratnasingam, C., et al., 2016. En face imaging of pachychoroid spectrum disorders with swept-source optical coherence tomography. Retina 36 (3), 499–516.

Elagouz, M., Stanescu-Segall, D., Jackson, T.L., 2010. Uveal effusion syndrome. Surv. Ophthalmol. 55 (2), 134–145.

Fawzi, A.A., Holland, G.N., Kreiger, A.E., et al., 2006. Central serous chorioretinopathy after solid organ transplantation. Ophthalmology 113, 805–813.

Gass, J.D.M., Little, H.L., 1995. Bilateral bullous exudative retinal detachment complicating idiopathic central serous chorioretinopathy during systemic corticosteroid therapy. Ophthalmology 102, 737–747.

Goldstein, B.G., Pavan, P.R., 1987. "Blow outs" in the retinal pigment epithelium. Br. J. Ophthalmol. 71, 676–681.

Guyer, D.R., Yannuzzi, L.A., Slakter, J.S., et al., 1994. Digital indocyanine green videoangiography of central serous chorioretinopathy. Arch. Ophthalmol. 112, 1057–1062.

Iida, T., Yannuzzi, L.A., Spaide, R.F., et al., 2003. Cystoid macular degeneration in chronic central serous chorioretinopathy. Retina 23, 1–7.

Imamura, Y., Fujiwara, T., Spaide, R.F., 2011. Fundus autofluorescence and visual acuity in central serous chorioretinopathy. Ophthalmology 118 (4), 700–705.

Klufas, M.A., Yannuzzi, N.A., Pang, C.E., et al., 2015. Feasibility and clinical utility of ultra-widefield indocyanine green angiography. Retina 35 (3), 508–520.

Lim, J.I., Glassman, A.R., Aiello, L.P., et al., 2014. Collaborative retrospective macula society study of photodynamic therapy for chronic central serous chorioretinopathy. Ophthalmology 121 (5), 1073–1078.

Pang, C.E., Freund, K.B., 2014. Pachychoroid pigment epitheliopathy may masquerade as acute retinal pigment epitheliitis. Invest. Ophthalmol. Vis. Sci. 55 (8), 5252.

Pang, C.E., Freund, K.B., 2015. Pachychoroid neovasculopathy. Retina 35 (1), 1–9.

Pang, C.E., Shah, V.P., Sarraf, D., et al., 2014. Ultra-widefield imaging with autofluorescence and indocyanine green angiography in central serous chorioretinopathy. Am. J. Ophthalmol. 158 (2), 362–371.

Pautler, S.E., Browning, D.J., 2015. Isolated posterior uveal effusion: expanding the spectrum of the uveal effusion syndrome. Clin Ophthalmol 9, 43–49.

Spaide, R.F., Campeas, L., Haas, A., et al., 1996. Central serous chorioretinopathy in younger and older adults. Ophthalmology 103 (12), 2070–2079.

Spaide, R.F., Hall, L., Haas, A., et al., 1996. Indocyanine green videoangiography of older patients with central serous chorioretinopathy. Retina 16, 203–213.

Spaide, R.F., Klancnik, J.M., Jr., 2005. Fundus autofluorescence and central serous chorioretinopathy. Ophthalmology 112, 825–833.

Yannuzzi, L.A., 1987. Type A behavior and central serous chorioretinopathy. Retina 7, 111–131.

Yannuzzi, L.A., Freund, K.B., Goldbaum, M., et al., 2000. Polypoidal choroidal vasculopathy masquerading as central serous chorioretinopathy. Ophthalmology 107, 767–777.

Yannuzzi, L.A., Shakin, J.L., Fisher, Y.L., et al., 1984. Peripheral retinal detachments and retinal pigment epithelial atrophic tracts secondary to central serous pigment epitheliopathy. Ophthalmology 91, 1554–1572.

Yannuzzi, L.A., Slakter, J.S., Gross, N.E., et al., 2003. Indocyanine green angiography-guided photodynamic therapy for treatment of chronic central serous chorioretinopathy. Retina 23, 288–298.

CHAPTER 11

Peripheral Retinal Degenerations and Rhegmatogenous Retinal Detachment

Peripheral Retinal Abnormalities

Each peripheral retinal abnormality poses a different level of risk for retinal detachment. Some of these lesions may be inconsequential manifestations, whereas others represent a high risk for detachment, particularly in patients with high myopia; aphakia or pseudophakia; previous detachment in the fellow eye; or a strong family history of retinal detachment.

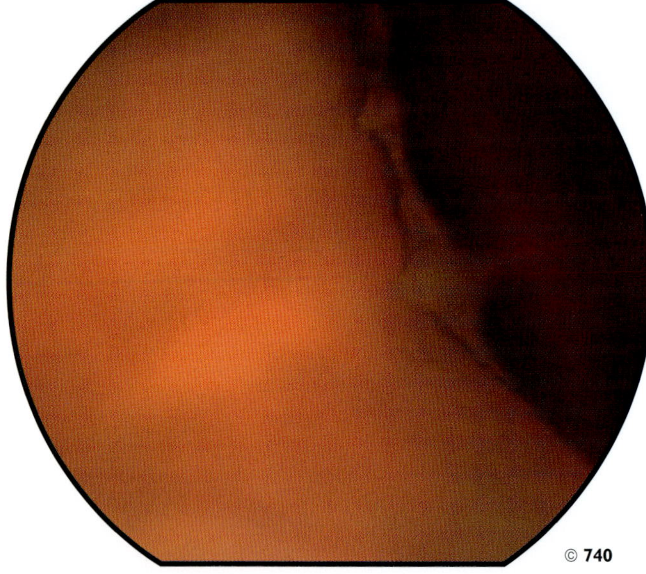

© 740

This patient has a meridional fold in the nasal ora serrata. Meridional folds, which are elevated pleats of peripheral neurosensory retina, occur in 26% of the population and are bilateral in approximately 50% of patients. This feature is generally not of clinical significance.

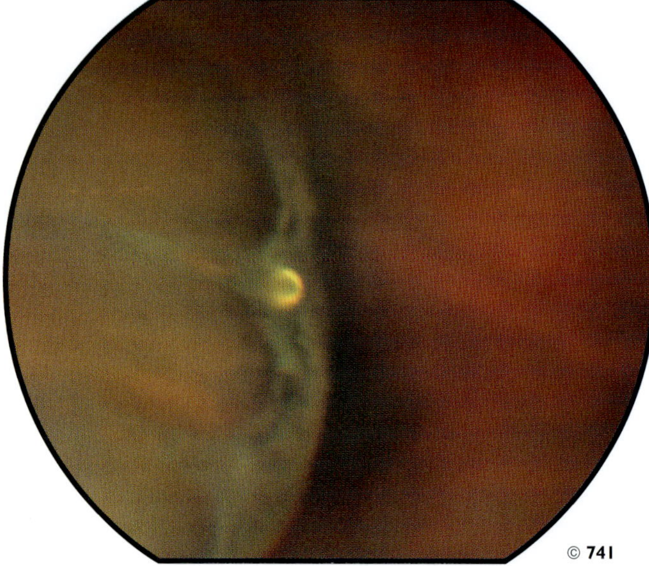

© 741

A whitish-yellow pearl of the ora serrata is demonstrated in this patient. This is not a high-risk factor for detachment. Observation is warranted.

Retinal Holes

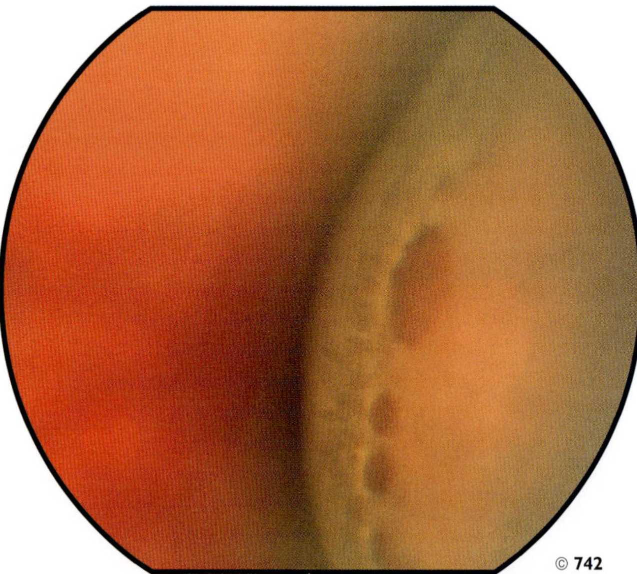

© 742

This patient has four asymptomatic round atrophic holes with a localized subclinical retinal detachment. The holes have been observed for over 20 years, and there has been no appreciable change.

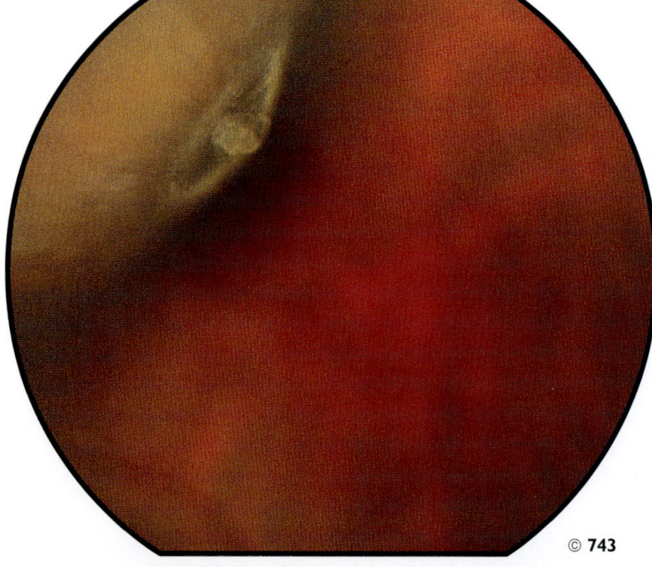

© 743

This 27-year-old white female has a cystic retinal tuft with localized subretinal fluid. Cystic retinal tufts are chalky white, elevated peripheral lesions composed of glial tissue, with associated traction at its apex from condensed vitreous. They are noted in 5% of the population in autopsy studies and are clinically significant in that they are associated with approximately 10% of primary retinal detachments. Approximately 0.28% of patients with these lesions will have retinal detachments secondary to the tuft. Therefore, due to the high prevalence of these tufts in the general population and the low risk of retinal detachment, cystic retinal tufts are not usually required to have prophylactic laser photocoagulation treatment.

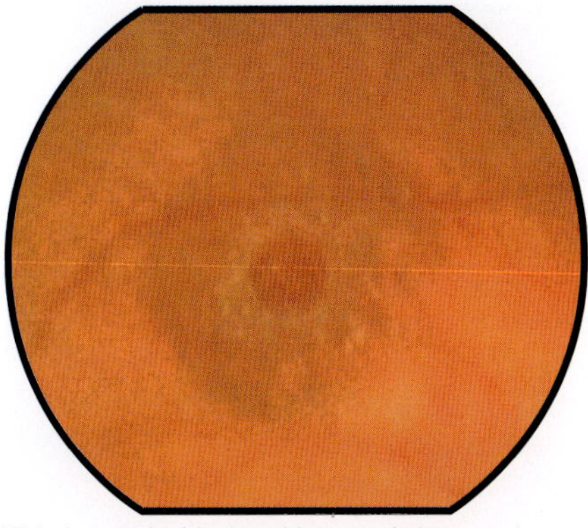
This is a retinal hole without existing traction. There is a surrounding cuff of elevated retina that has lost its transparency.

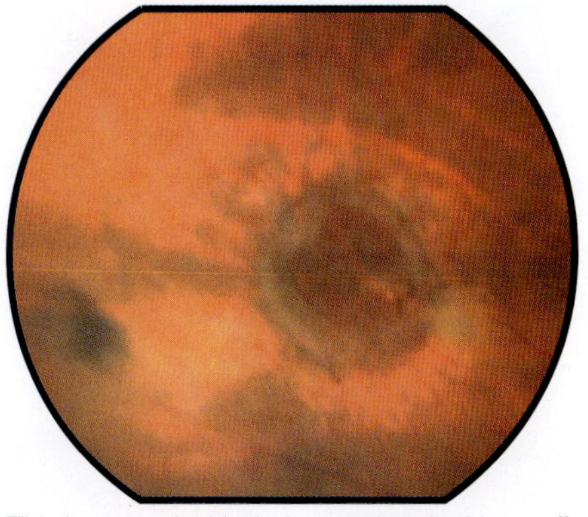
This larger retinal hole is associated with a cuff of subretinal fluid and early pigmentary demarcating boundary.

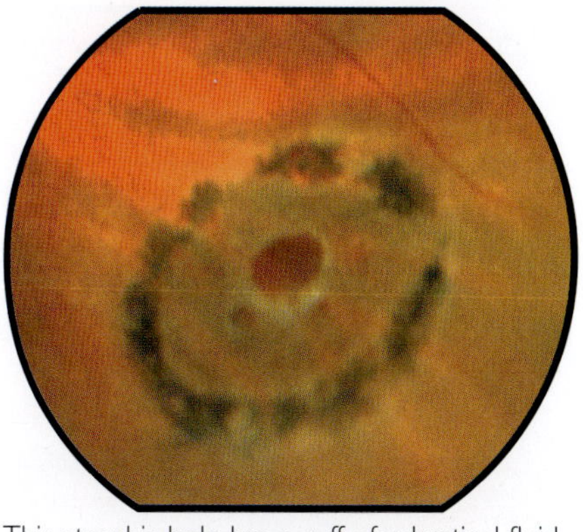
This atrophic hole has a cuff of subretinal fluid that is bordered by a ring of pigment epithelial hyperplasia demarcating the extent of the localized detachment.

Lattice Degeneration

Lattice degeneration is a common peripheral vitreoretinal disorder present in 6-10% of the population. While only 0.5-1% of eyes with lattice degeneration will develop a retinal detachment, approximately 20-30% of patients with rhegmatogenous retinal detachments have lattice degeneration. Lattice degeneration has many morphologies, the most common being circumferentially oriented localized round, linear, or ovoid areas of retinal thinning that are sometimes crossed by whitish lines that represent hyalinized retinal vessels. Other features include superficial whitish yellow flecks; patches of varying degrees of pigmentation; round or linear red craters; round or linear white patches; and small atrophic round holes. On histopathologic examination, lattice degeneration consists of one of three findings: a localized thinning of the inner retinal layers, vitreous liquefaction overlying thinned retina, and vitreous condensation with exaggerated vitreo-retinal attachments at the margins of the lesion. Although lattice degeneration itself is asymptomatic, it can be associated with retinal tears, detachments, or traction, which may cause floaters, photopsias, or other visual disturbances. In some eyes with lattice degeneration, retinal detachment may occur secondary to retinal tears that develop in areas remote from the lattice degeneration. General practice patterns generally recommend observation for asymptomatic lattice degeneration and only consider treatment of the condition in cases where the fellow eye had a previous retinal detachment.

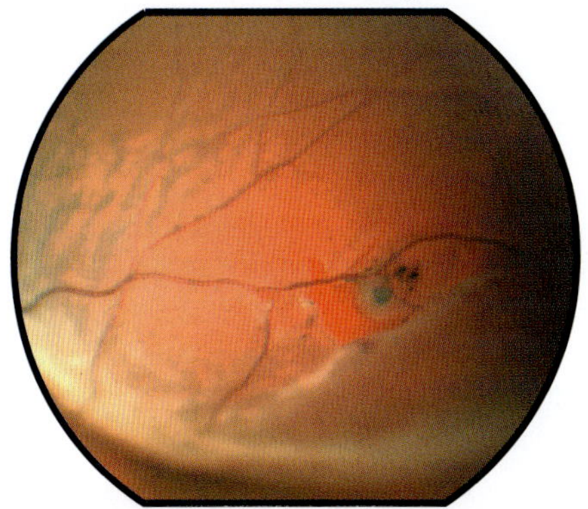
There is a horseshoe retinal break within a patch of lattice degeneration, which resulted in a gravity dependent retinal detachment. Retinal folds with early proliferative vitreoretinopathy (PVR) are seen inferiorly at the border of the detachment.

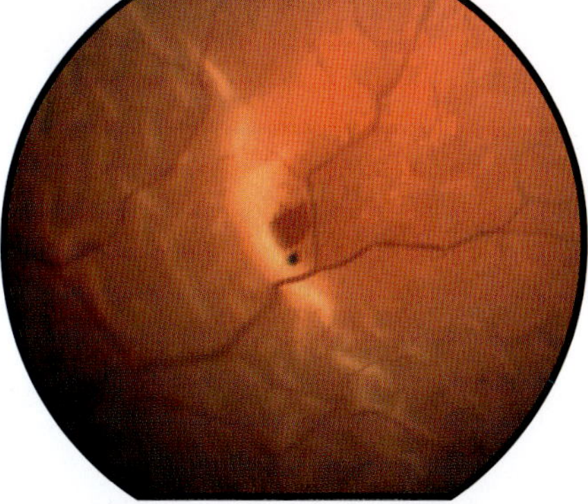
This patient has a break within pigmentary lattice. The hole is round, and the retinal detachment is associated with multiple, irregular folds in the retina. The corresponding OCT image shows the retinal break with traction *(arrow)*, and resulting retinal elevation.

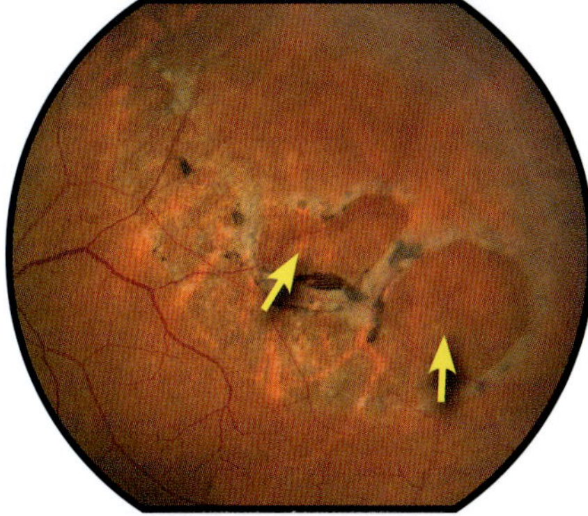
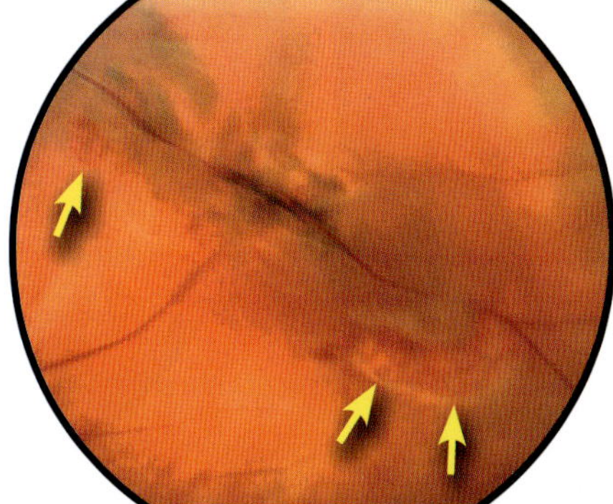
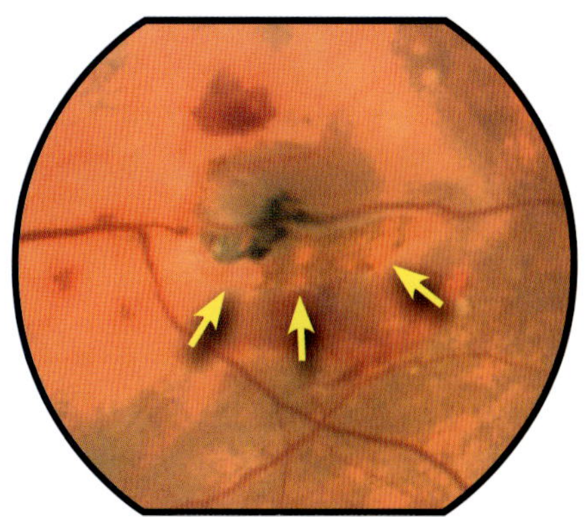
These three cases illustrate different morphologies of lattice degeneration. On the left, there are multiple atrophic holes *(arrows)* bordered by localized fibrosis with a shallow detachment. In the middle, there is radial paravascular pigmentary lattice degeneration with multiple horseshoe breaks *(arrows)*, as well as a localized retinal detachment. In the right image, there is a linear break along the lattice degeneration and localized detachment *(arrows)*. There is also localized hemorrhage within and into the periretinal region.

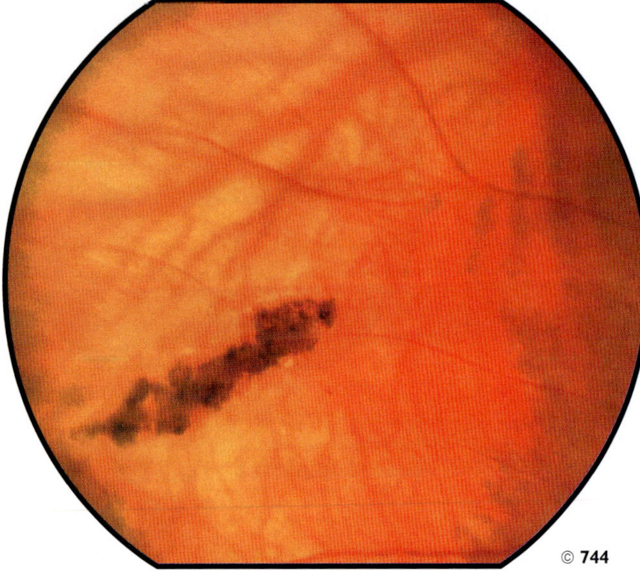
© 744

This patient has pigmentary lattice degeneration without associated pathology.

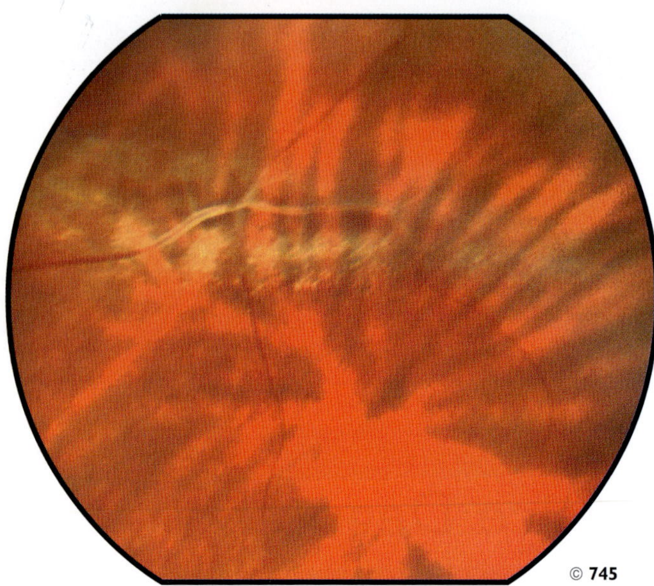
© 745

This patient has lattice degeneration with some atrophic changes, superficial whitish yellow flecks, and sheathing of the retinal vessels.

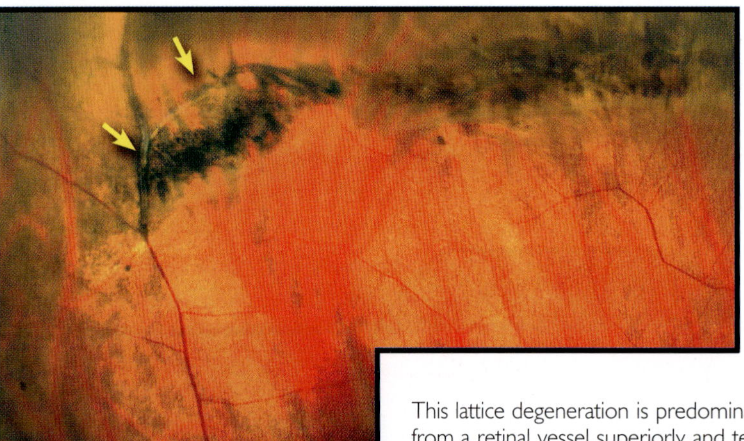

This lattice degeneration is predominantly pigmentary in nature and extends from a retinal vessel superiorly and temporally in an irregular course. The retinal vessels are associated with sclerotic and sheathing abnormalities *(arrows)*.

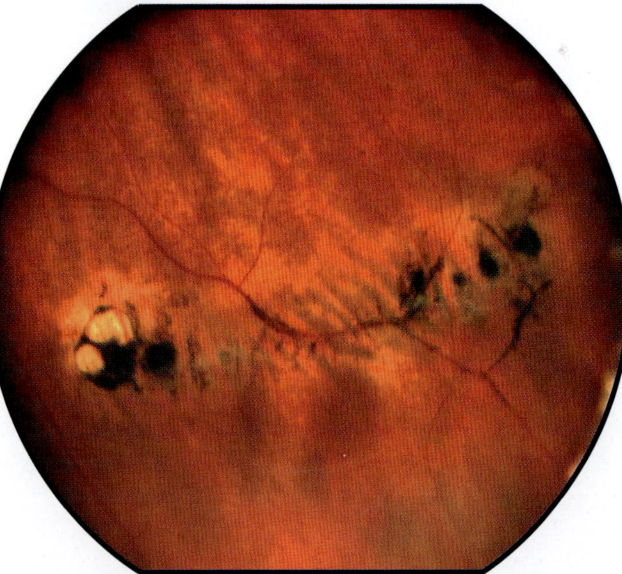

This area of lattice degeneration has intraretinal migration of pigment epithelial cells, areas of pigment epithelial atrophy, and sclerotic vascular changes.

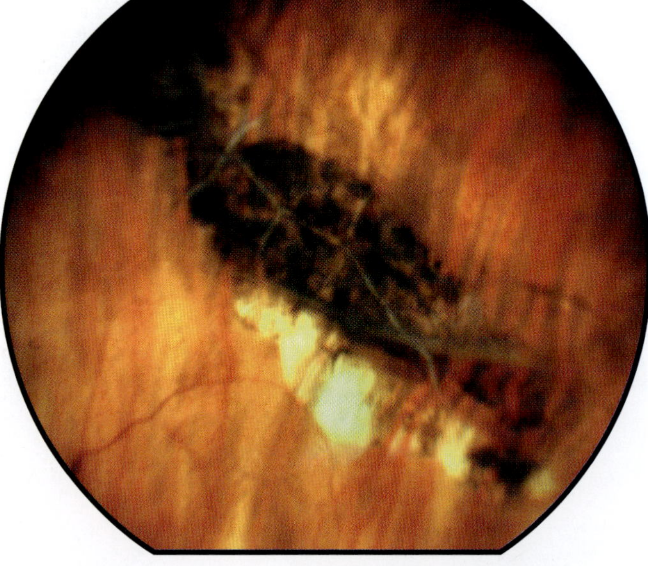

The pigmentation in this area of lattice degeneration is quite intense. A lattice configuration overlying the pigment hyperplasia is evident. There is an adjacent zone of atrophy.

Retinal Tears and Localized Detachments

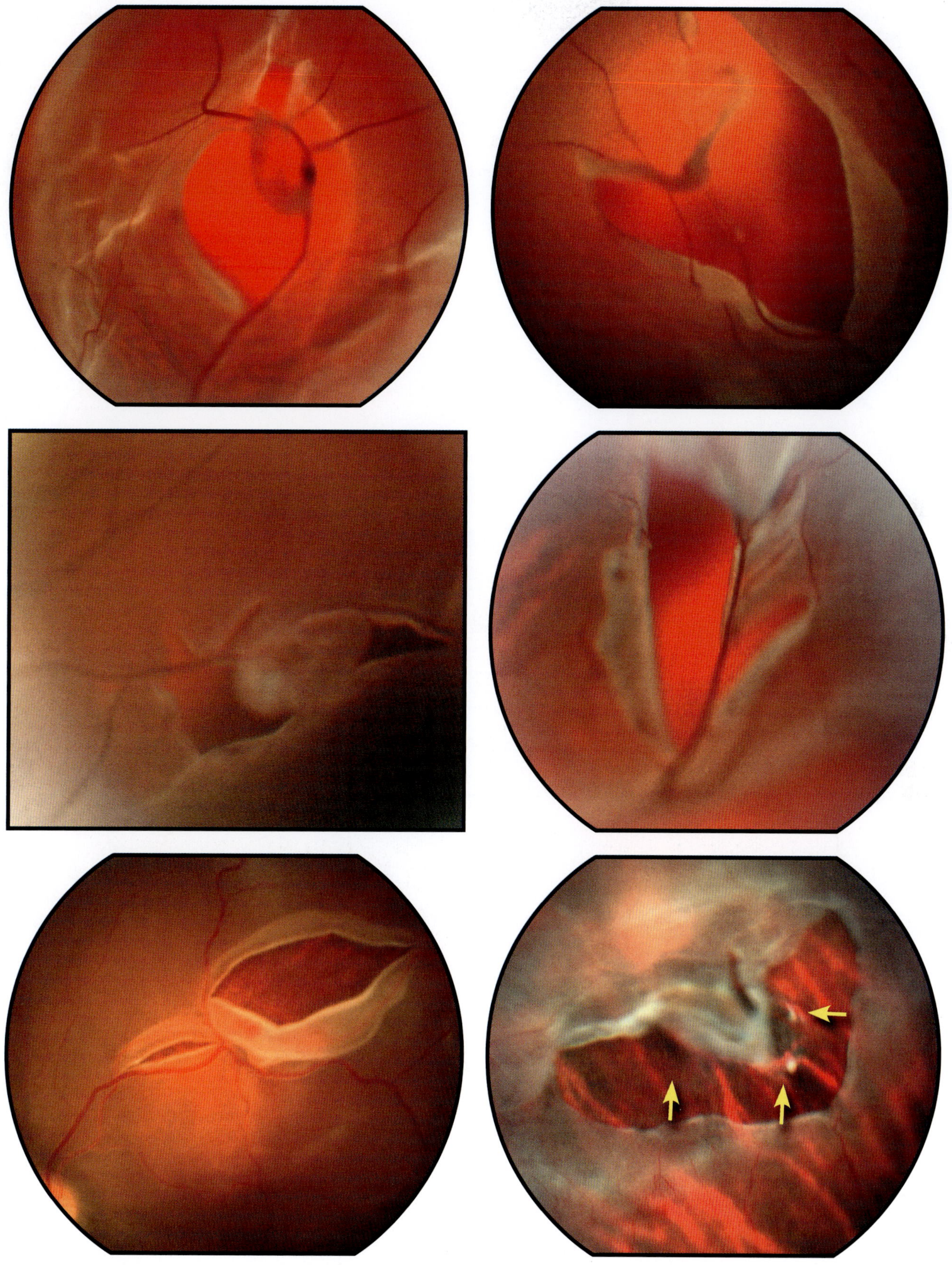

These patients have high-risk retinal breaks with everted edges resulting from vitreous traction and early PVR. Each break has an associated localized detachment, with the detached retina losing its transparency. Bridging retinal vessels are visible traversing the tear in the top four photos, indicative of a high risk for development of vitreous hemorrhage. The choroid can be seen more clearly through the horseshoe breaks, particularly in the lower right photo *(arrows)*.

Retinal Detachments

A rhegmatogenous retinal detachment (RRD) is a sight-threatening condition that occurs in approximately 1 in 10,000 people. Lattice degeneration is the greatest risk factor, but pathologic myopia, previous intraocular surgery, trauma, and family or personal history of retinal detachment are also risk factors. An RRD occurs when fluid accumulates between the sensory retina and retinal pigment epithelium (RPE) through a retinal break caused by vitreous traction. An RRD generally has a classic corrugated appearance and undulates with eye movements. A variety of treatment modalities have evolved to repair RRD, and these include the traditional use of a scleral buckle, pars plana vitrectomy surgery (PPV), or pneumatic retinopexy (PR). Each treatment will influence the appearance of the fundus following treatment, though the general principles for all procedures are essentially the same. The essential steps for repairing RRD are (1) detection of the retinal breaks, (2) closure of the defects, (3) release of vitreous traction, and (4) placement of an adhesive modality (generally photocoagulation and/or cryotherapy). This generally allows for resultant apposition of the retina to the underlying RPE. The most common cause of detachment repair failure, which occurs in 8-10% of patients, is proliferative vitreoretinopathy (PVR), which may require reoperation. There is always the possibility of missing or not fully treating the retinal pathology as well.

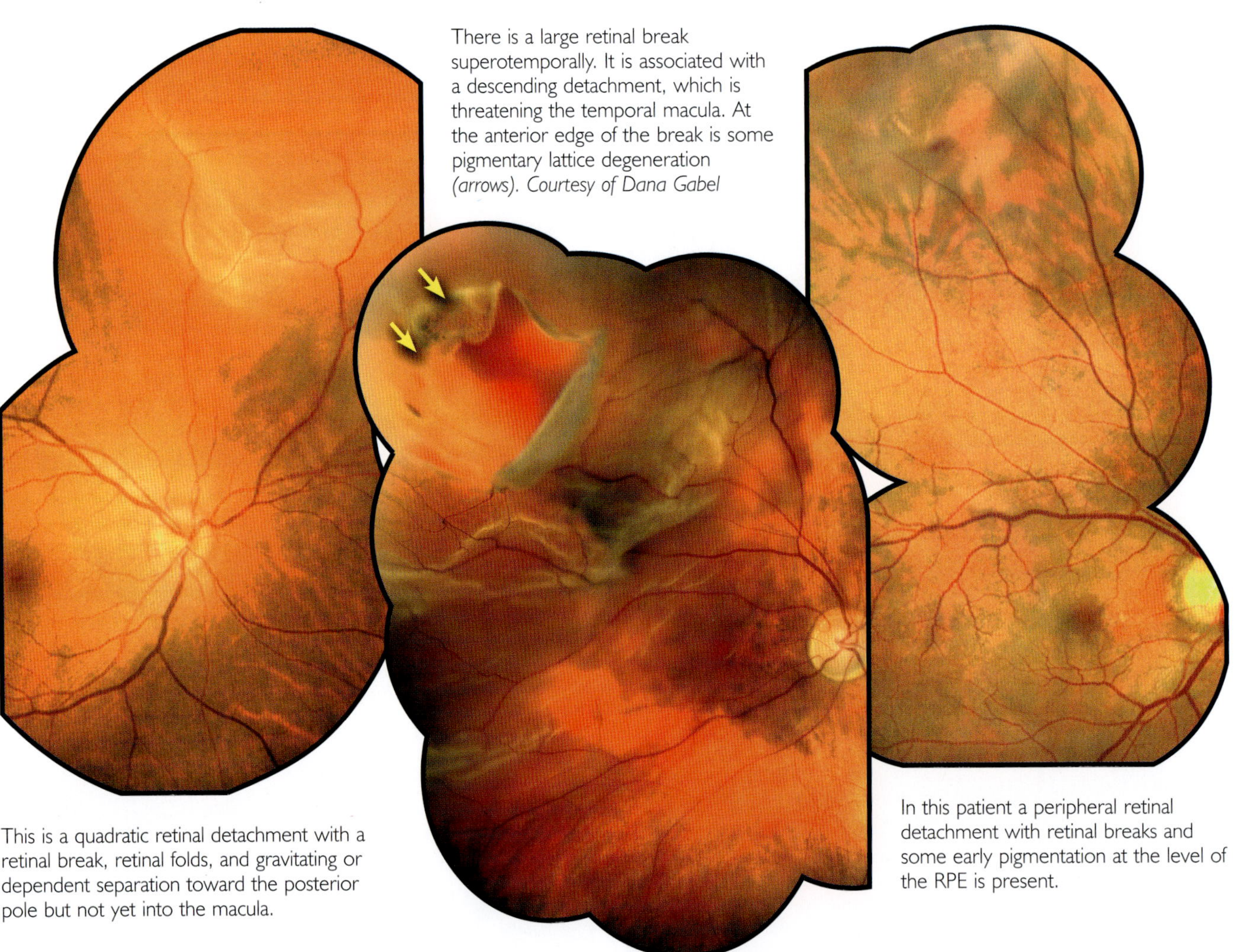

There is a large retinal break superotemporally. It is associated with a descending detachment, which is threatening the temporal macula. At the anterior edge of the break is some pigmentary lattice degeneration *(arrows). Courtesy of Dana Gabel*

This is a quadratic retinal detachment with a retinal break, retinal folds, and gravitating or dependent separation toward the posterior pole but not yet into the macula.

In this patient a peripheral retinal detachment with retinal breaks and some early pigmentation at the level of the RPE is present.

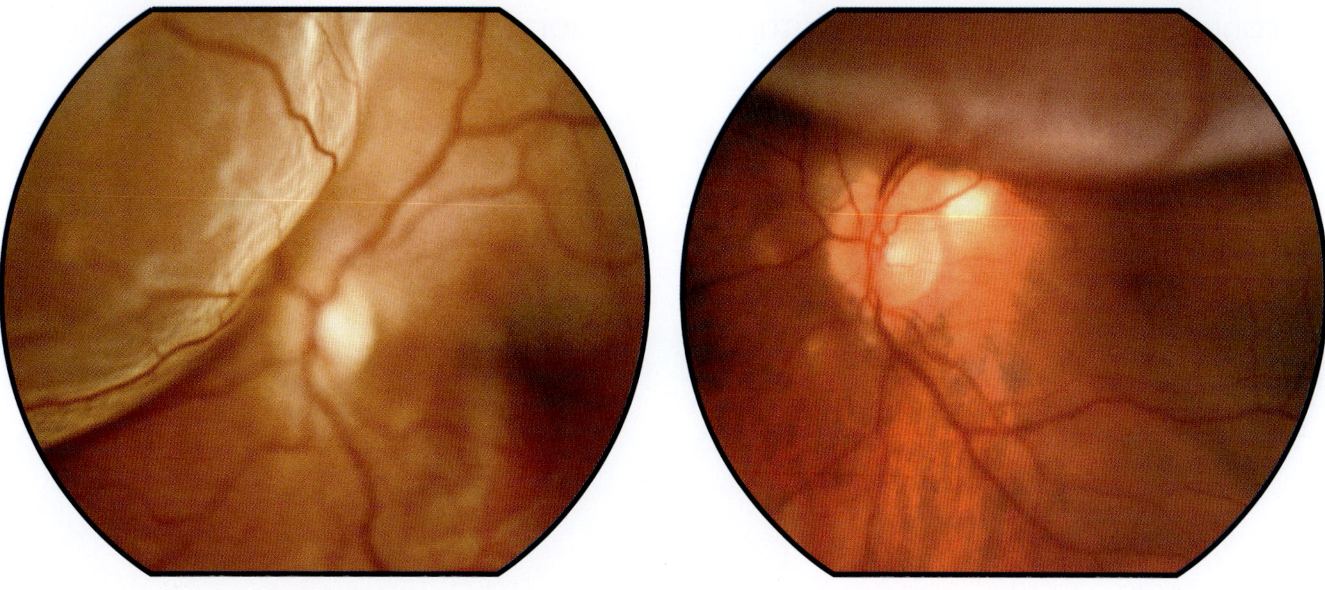

A retinal detachment is encroaching upon the optic nerve in each eye. Note the loss of retinal transparency in the areas of retinal detachment, which obscures visualization of the underlying choroidal vasculature.

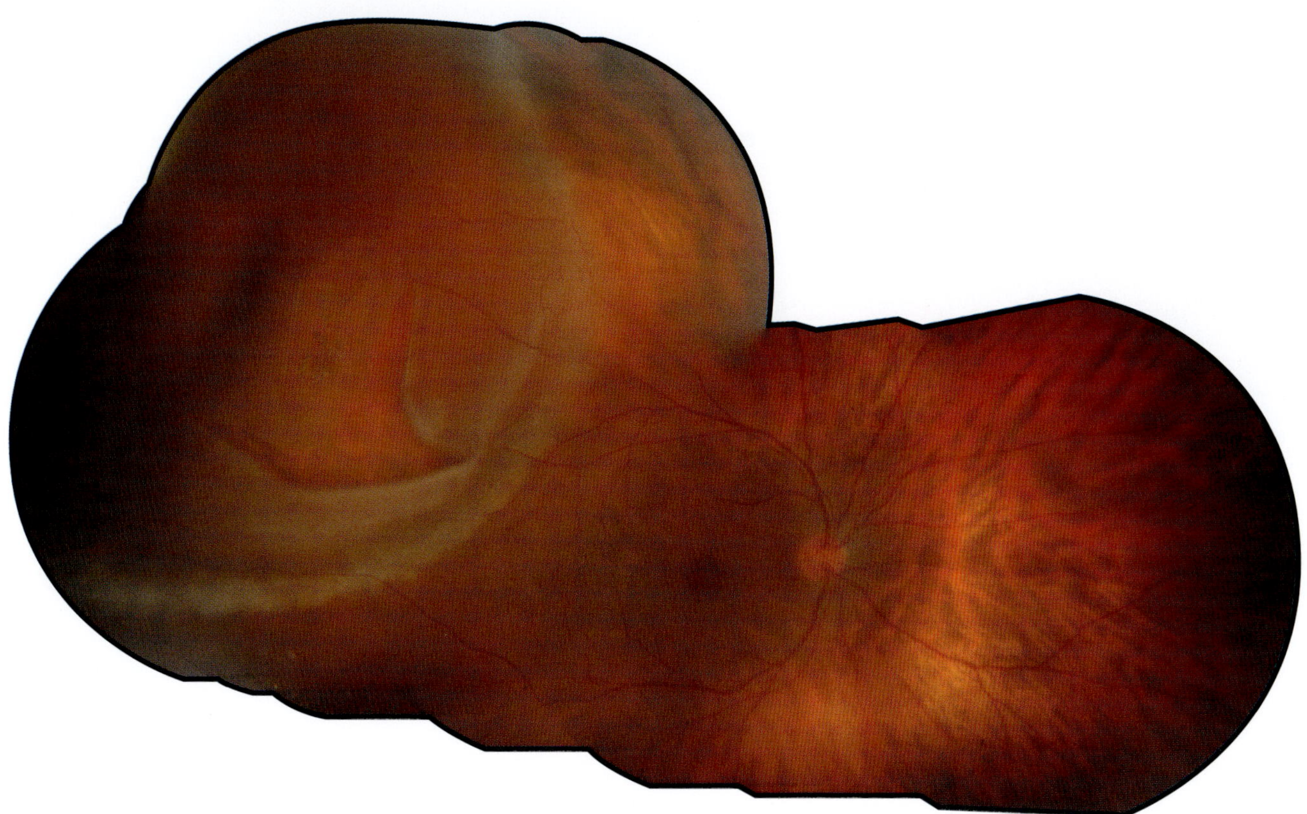

This patient developed a large retinal tear, though with only a limited amount of localized subretinal fluid temporal to the macula. The retina was surgically repaired prior to the detachment extending into the macula.

Chronic Retinal Detachment With Demarcation Lines

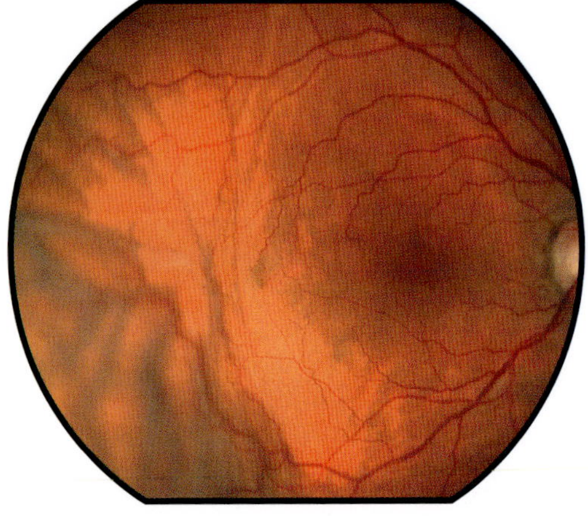

This patient has a chronic detachment that extends to the posterior pole, but not into the central macula. Multiple retinal folds are seen, some concentric with the others and some radiating peripherally in a random fashion.

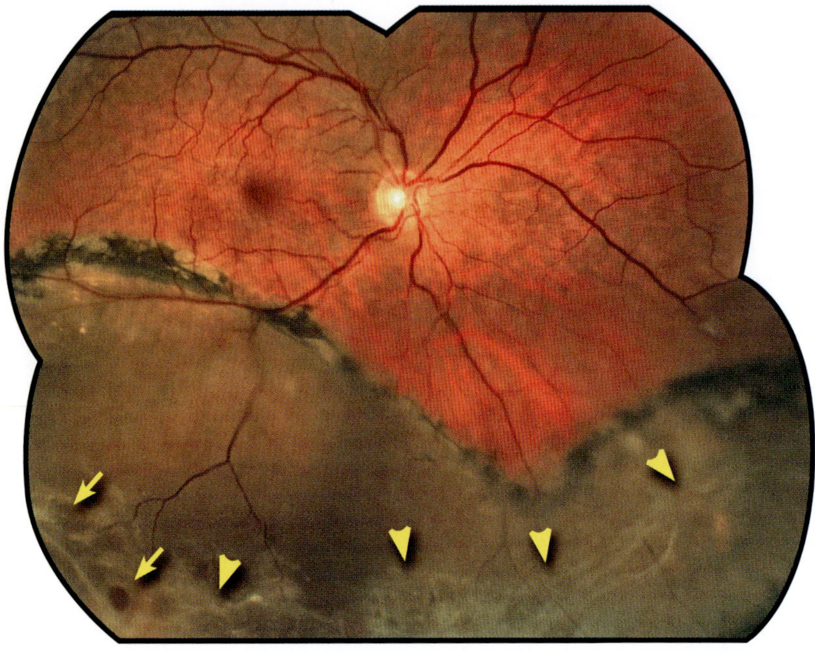

This patient has a dense pigmentary demarcation line bordering a chronic dependent detachment. There are a few retinal breaks *(arrows)* and areas of lattice degeneration *(arrowheads)*.

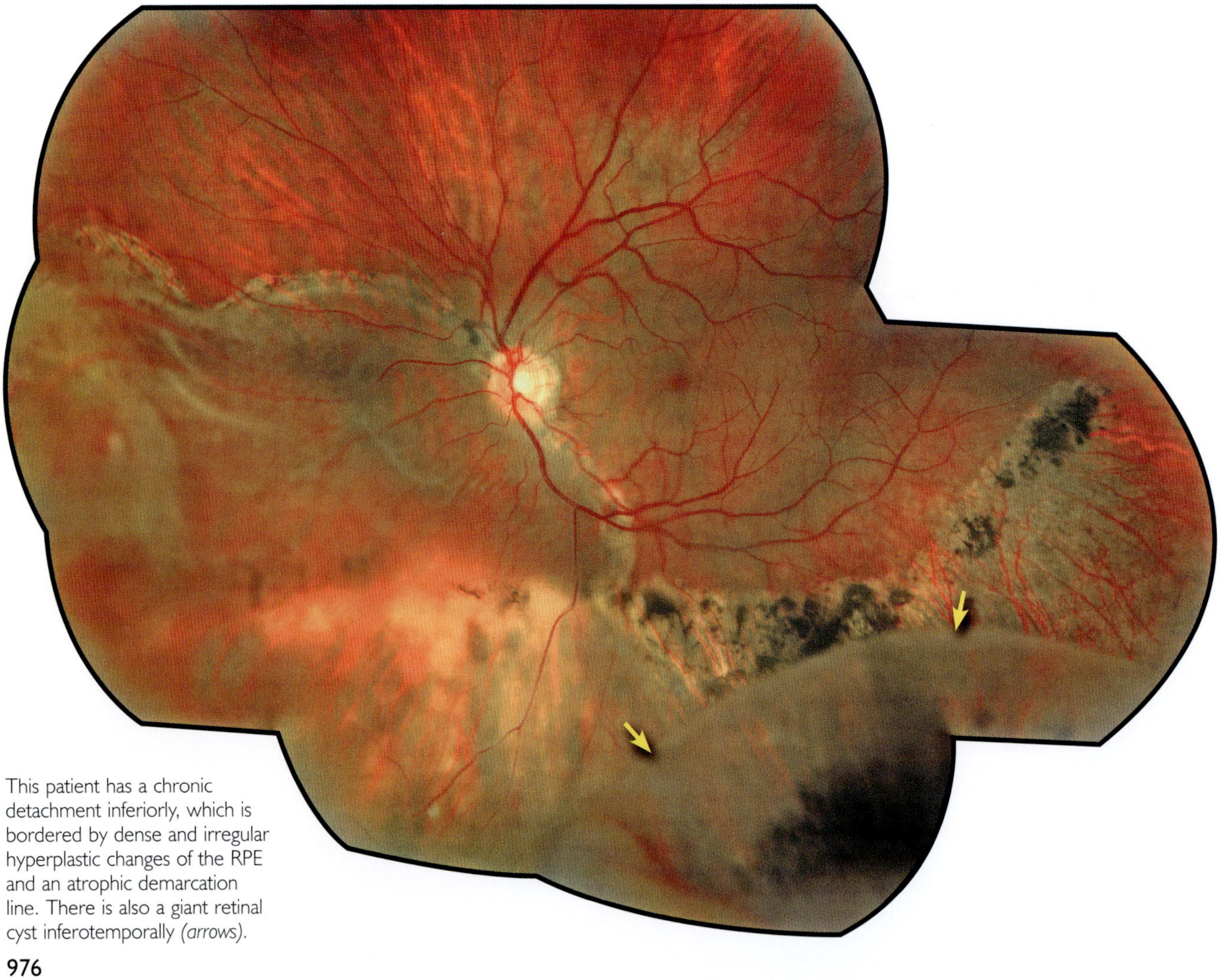

This patient has a chronic detachment inferiorly, which is bordered by dense and irregular hyperplastic changes of the RPE and an atrophic demarcation line. There is also a giant retinal cyst inferotemporally *(arrows)*.

Chronic Retinal Detachment with Retinal Macrocyst

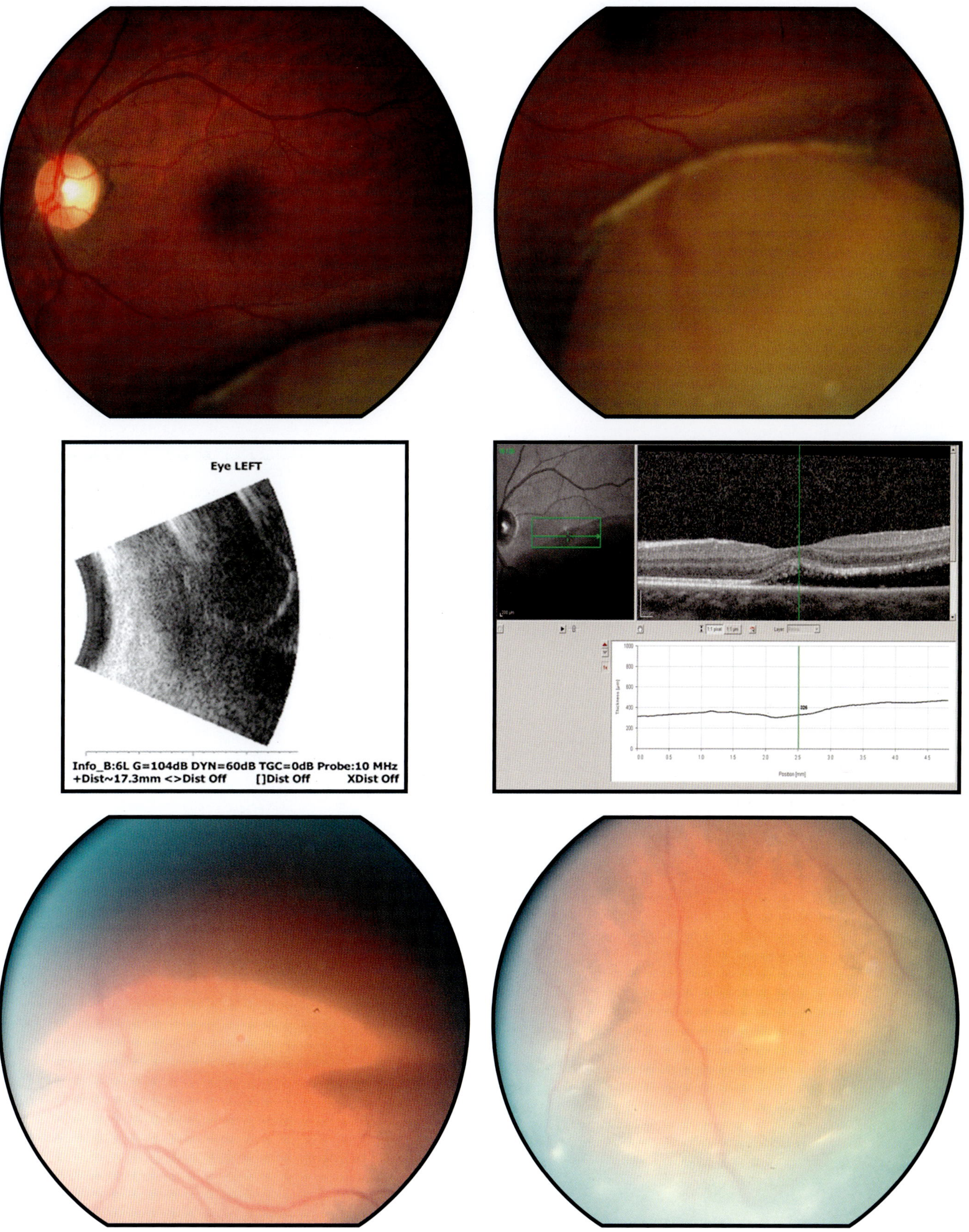

A very prominent macrocyst was noted in conjunction with a low lying retinal detachment (*top row*). Echography *(middle row, left)* confirmed the diagnosis, and SD-OCT showed shallow subretinal fluid encroaching upon the macula. The patient underwent PPV repair of the retinal detachment, with placement of an intraocular air bubble *(bottom row, left)*, though there was no drainage of the cyst. Postoperatively *(bottom row, right)*, the cyst flattened, and vision returned to 20/25.

Retinal Dialysis and Giant Retinal Tear (GRT)

A full-thickness retinal break that involves three or more clock hours is considered a giant retinal tear (GRT). GRTs may be associated with hereditary conditions including Marfan syndrome, Stickler syndrome, and high myopia, though may also occur spontaneously, or result from trauma. Between 80 and 90% of GRTs occur in males.

A retinal dialysis is a tear of the retina that results in disinsertion from the ora serrata. Most retinal dialyses are secondary to trauma and are seen most commonly in the inferotemporal quadrant.

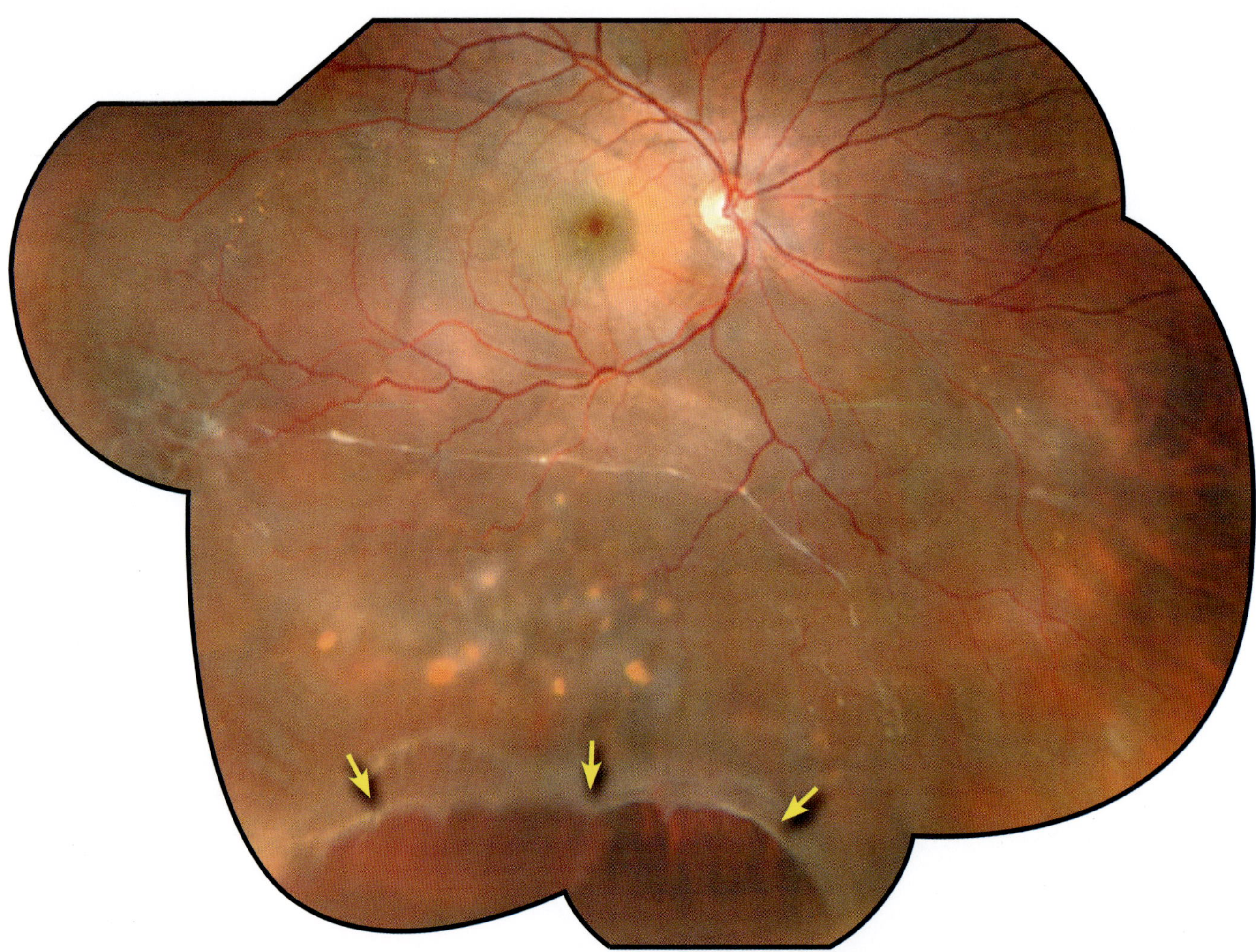

This patient has an inferior retinal detachment caused by a retinal dialysis *(arrows)*. The peripheral retina has separated from the ora serrata and is displaced toward the posterior pole of the fundus. The detached retina has lost some of its transparency due to edema or hydration.

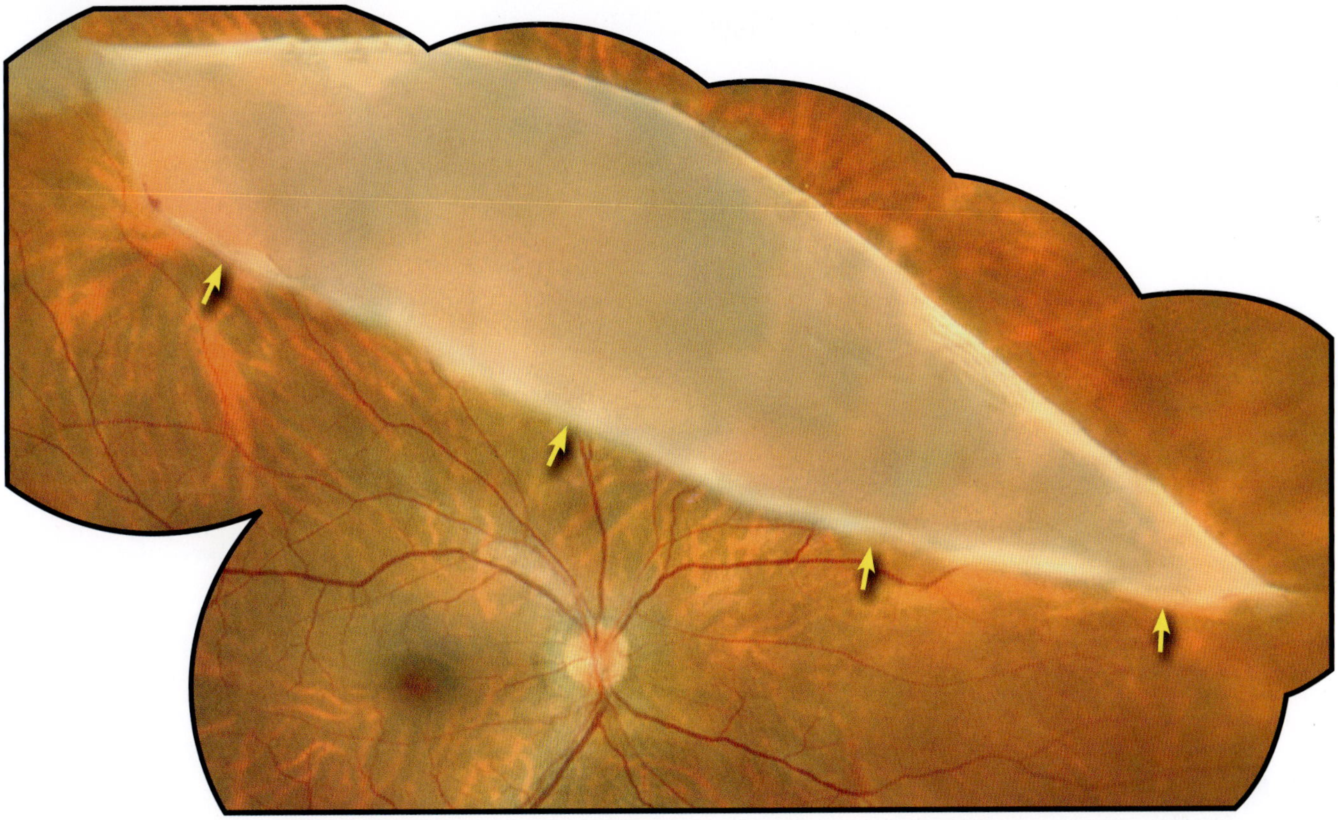

This patient has a retinal detachment from a GRT. The peripheral retina has torn and folded over itself with the anterior edge of the retina now draped over the posterior pole of the fundus *(arrows)*. The detached retina has become hydrated, resulting in loss of retinal transparency.

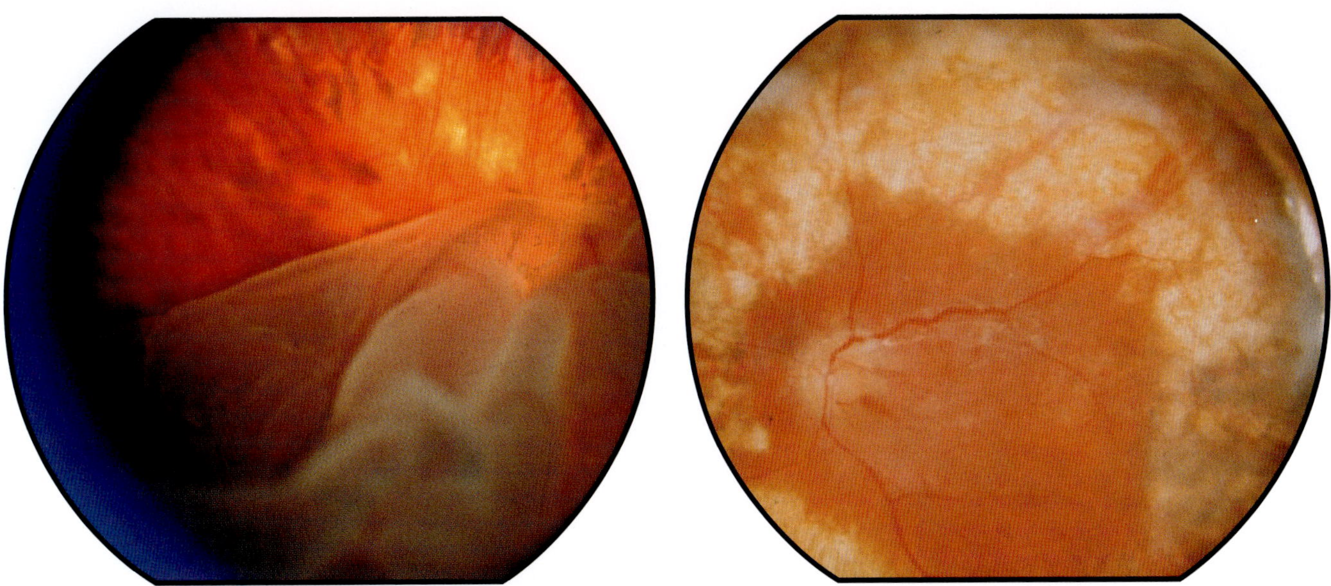

A 180-degree (six clock hours) GRT. The retina is folded upon itself inferiorly, with bare RPE seen superiorly *(left)*. There was minimal PVR. The retina was repaired via a PPV approach, use of intraoperative liquid perfluorocarbon (to unfold the retina), use of extensive peripheral photocoagulation, and placement of an encircling scleral buckle *(right)*. Anatomic success was achieved.

Retinal Detachment and Macular Hole

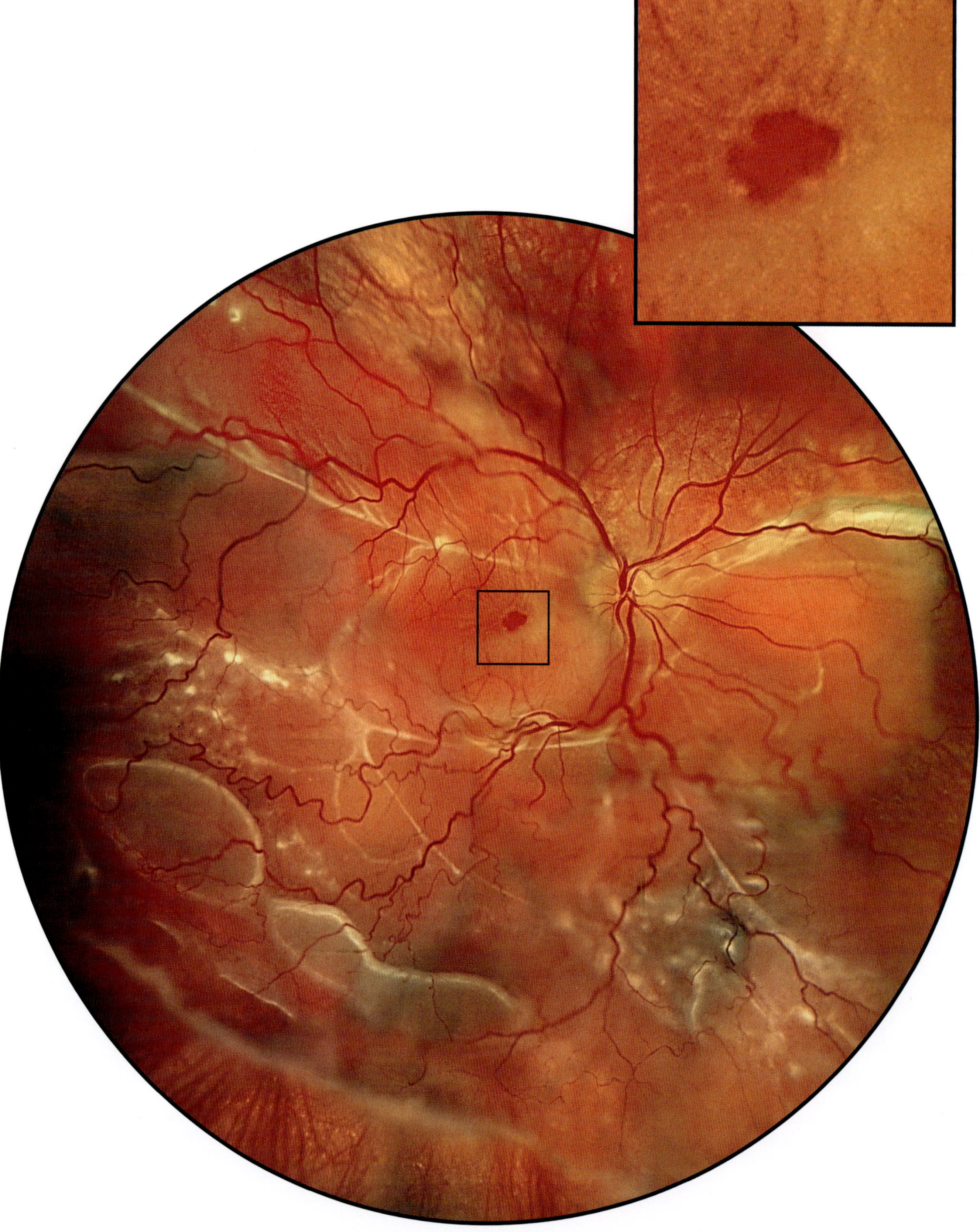

This photo exhibits a bullous retinal detachment with multiple retinal folds in a patient with amyloidosis. A macular hole accounts for the detachment *(inset)*, as no peripheral retinal tears were seen. Most detachments from macular holes occur in pathological myopia or secondary to blunt ocular trauma. This case is an exception.

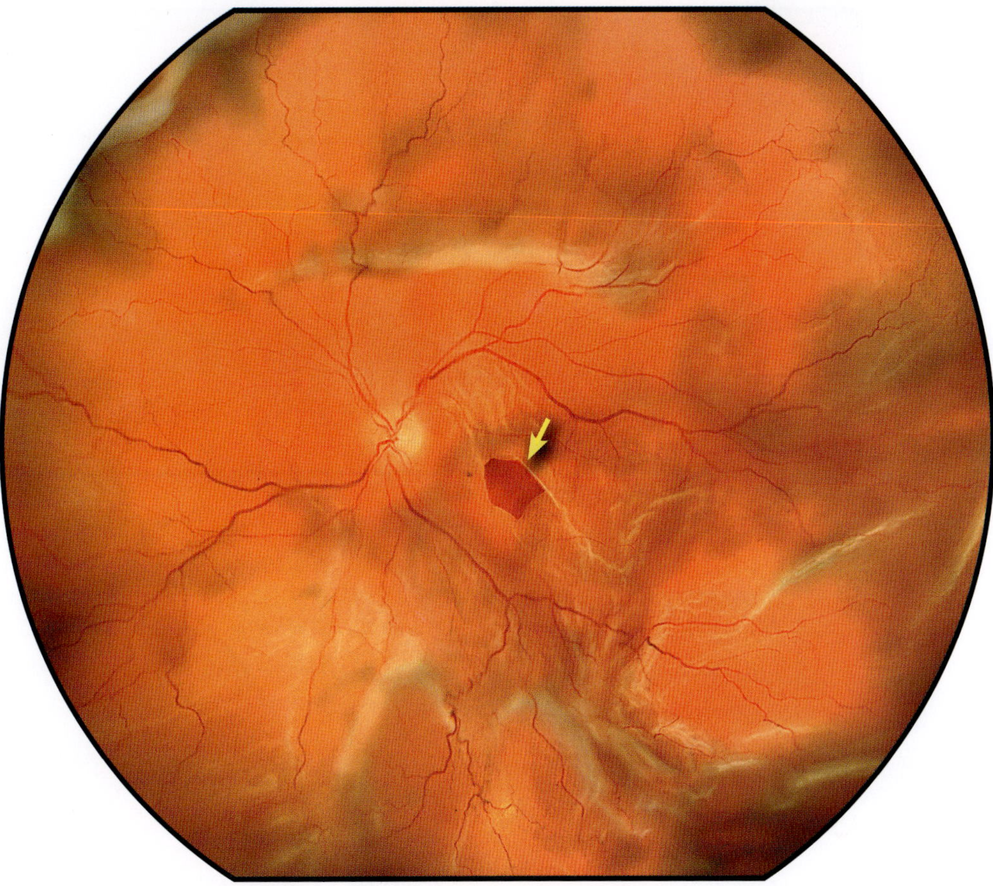

This patient has a macular hole with a bullous retinal detachment. The hole in the macula is clearly evident *(arrow)*. There is early PVR with multiple folds in the retina surrounding the posterior pole.

Proliferative Vitreoretinopathy (PVR)

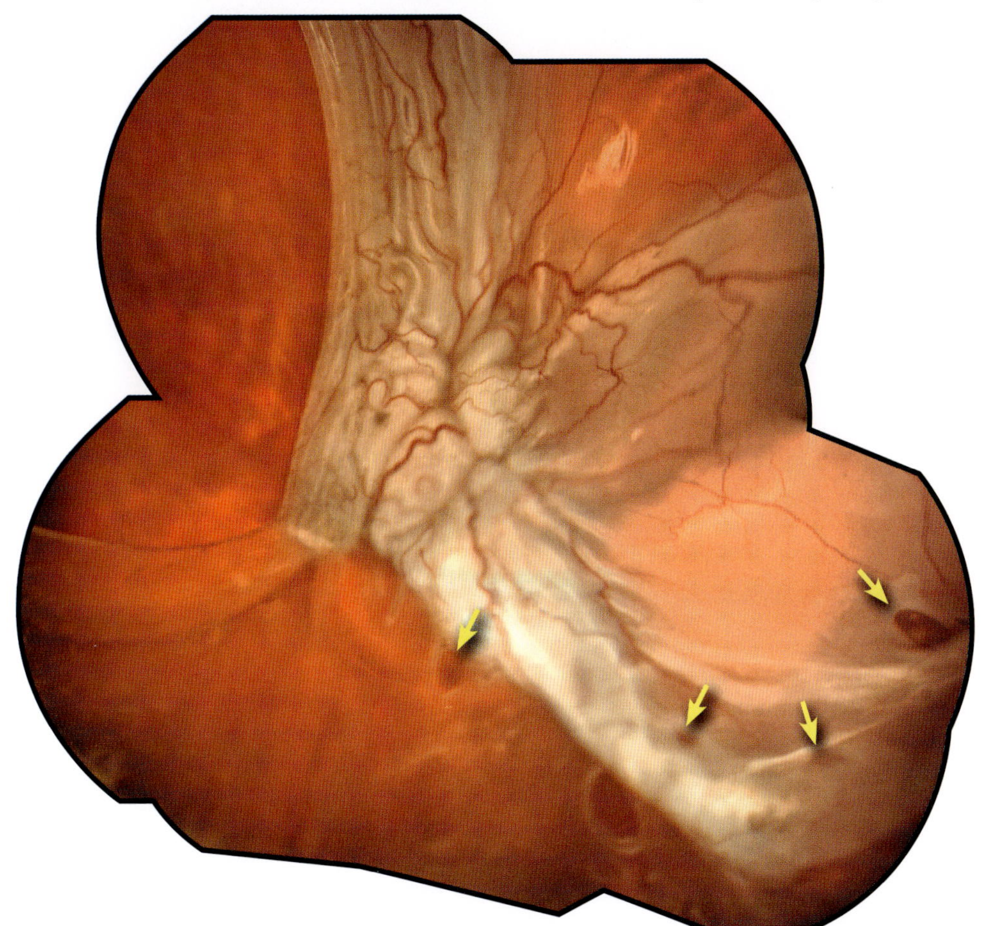

This patient has a bullous retinal detachment with extensive PVR, which is causing contraction of the retina. Multiple retinal breaks are noted throughout the fundus *(arrows)*.

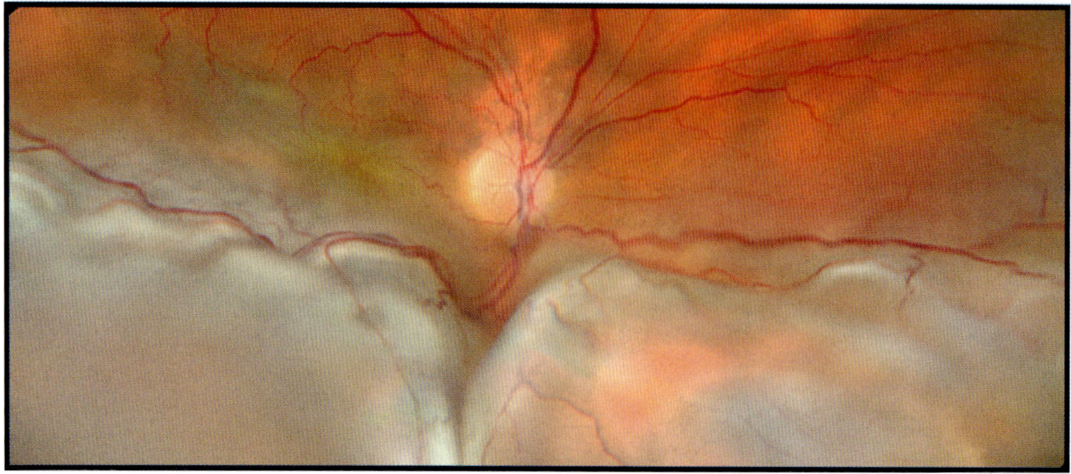

There is a bullous inferior retinal detachment with turbid subretinal fluid in this patient. Note the obscuration of the choroid, the retinal folds, and the biconvex nature of the detached bullous retina.

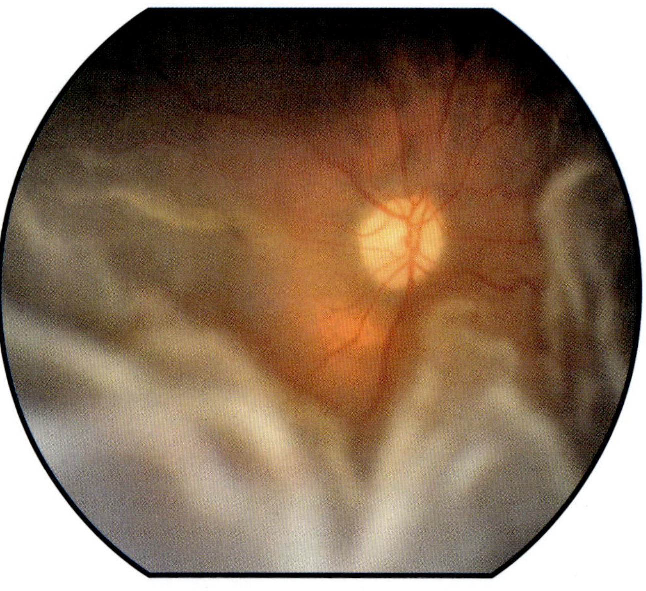

Multiple retinal elevations and folds are seen in this eye with a macular detachment. Retinal folds are very prominent. *Courtesy of Dr. Naresh Mandava*

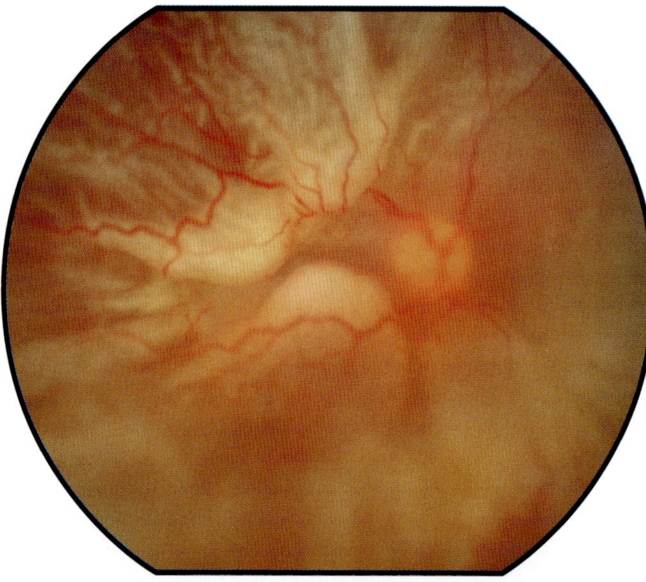

A global detachment is evident in the posterior pole. The dense retinal folds appear to converge on the detached macula.

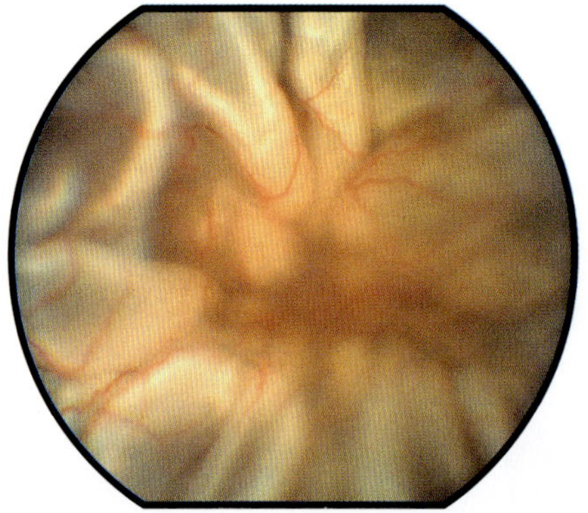

This open funnel-shaped retinal detachment is associated with advanced PVR. Based on the original PVR classification scheme, this is Grade D-1 PVR, as there are retinal folds in all four quadrants, though the funnel is relatively open.

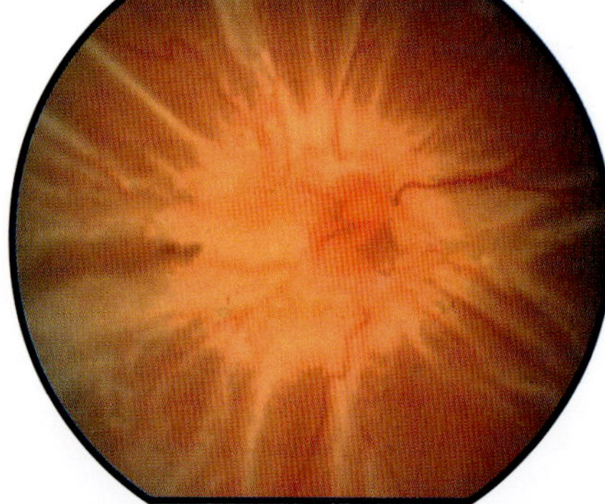

In this eye, PVR is causing a narrow tight funnel configuration with the optic nerve still visible. Based on the original PVR classification scheme, this is Grade D-2 PVR. Fixed retinal folds are present in all four quadrants.

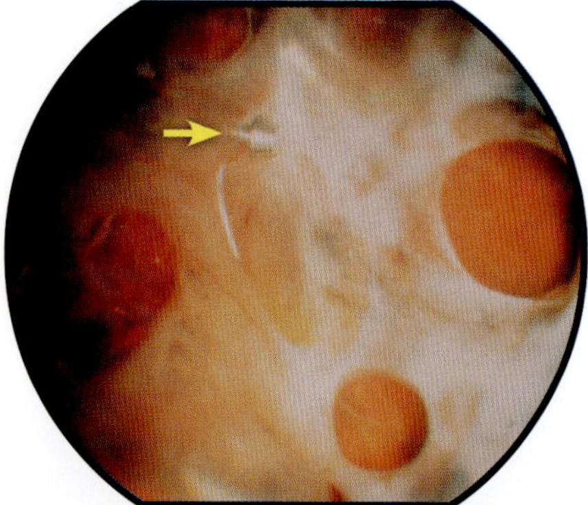

In spite of previous PPV surgery, which included use of silicone oil and even placement of a retinal tack *(arrow)* (which were employed in the 1980s and 1990s), this retina re-detached with massive development of recurrent PVR. In view of the very limited potential for further visual recovery, no additional surgery was recommended.

Retinoschisis

Retinoschisis is an abnormal splitting of the neurosensory layers of the retina, which may resemble the appearance of a retinal detachment. Generally the areas of retinal elevation are smoother and lack the typical corrugated appearance of an RRD. The most common form of retinoschisis is acquired or degenerative retinoschisis, where the retinal split typically occurs in the outer plexiform layer. Acquired retinoschisis occurs in 4-22% of patients over 40 years of age, with both genders being equally impacted. The inferotemporal quadrant is most commonly involved. Most cases of acquired retinoschisis are not visually significant and remain stationary over many years, which therefore require no treatment other than monitoring. Rarely, retinoschisis can progress to RRD. Hereditary retinoschisis, which can be caused by an X-linked genetic defect, is much rarer, predominantly affects young males, and the split typically occurs in the nerve fiber layer. Some individuals with X-linked retinoschisis will develop severely impaired vision.

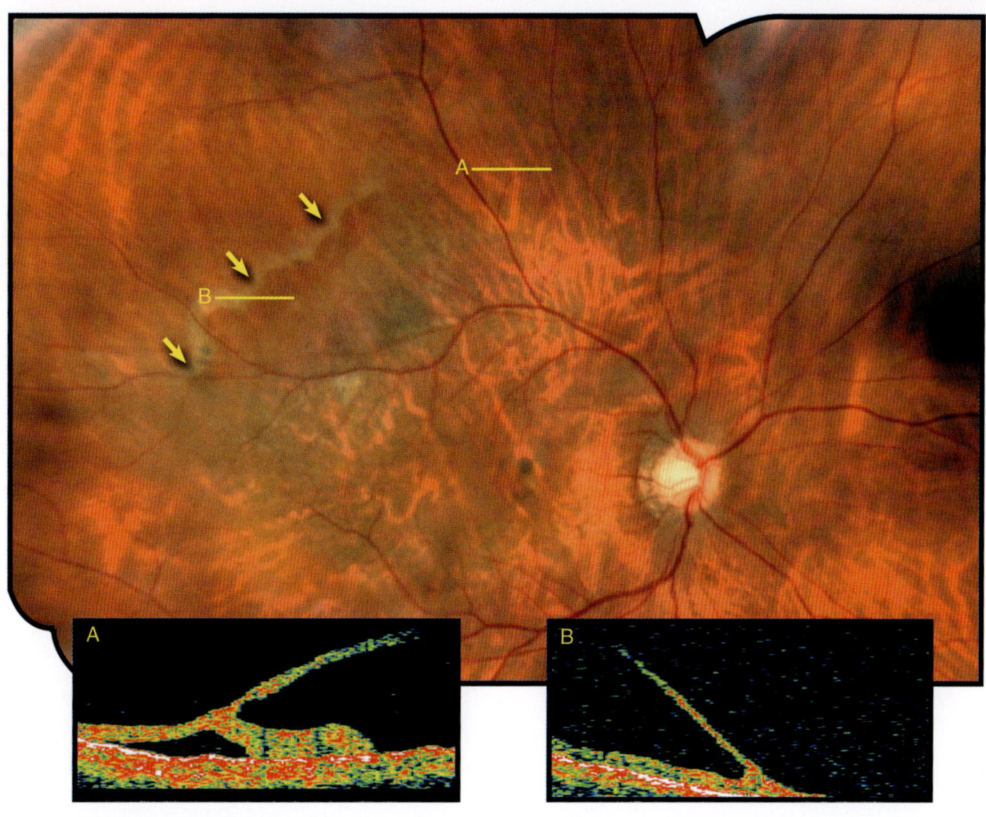

This patient has a retinoschisis and an outer-layer detachment superotemporally. There is an irregular ridge of outer retinal dehiscence *(arrows)*. The OCT A *(inset A)* shows a combined retinal schisis and outer-layer detachment. Straddling the combined schisis detachment is an area of schisis that is represented by OCT B *(inset B)*. In this image, the outer retina is still intact and attached.

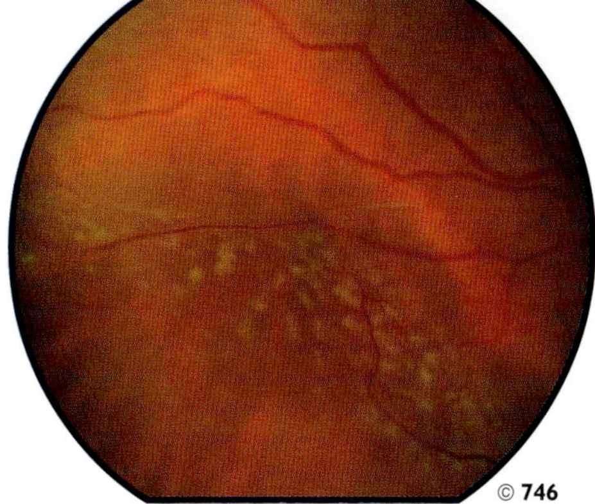

An area of acquired retinoschisis in this patient shows multifocal areas of proteinaceous deposits in the inner retina.

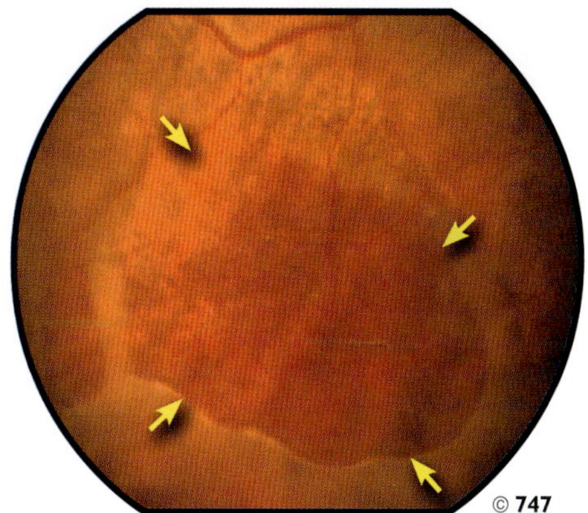

There is a large outer-layer hole *(arrows)* beneath this area of retinoschisis. Outer-layer breaks occur in approximately 6% of patients with acquired retinoschisis. Inner layer breaks are less common. Retinoschisis with isolated outer layer breaks requires no treatment as the subretinal fluid often self-resorbs and rarely progresses posteriorly to involve the macula or transforms into a full thickness break. Rhegmatogenous detachment is estimated to occur in 0.05% of patients with acquired retinoschisis.

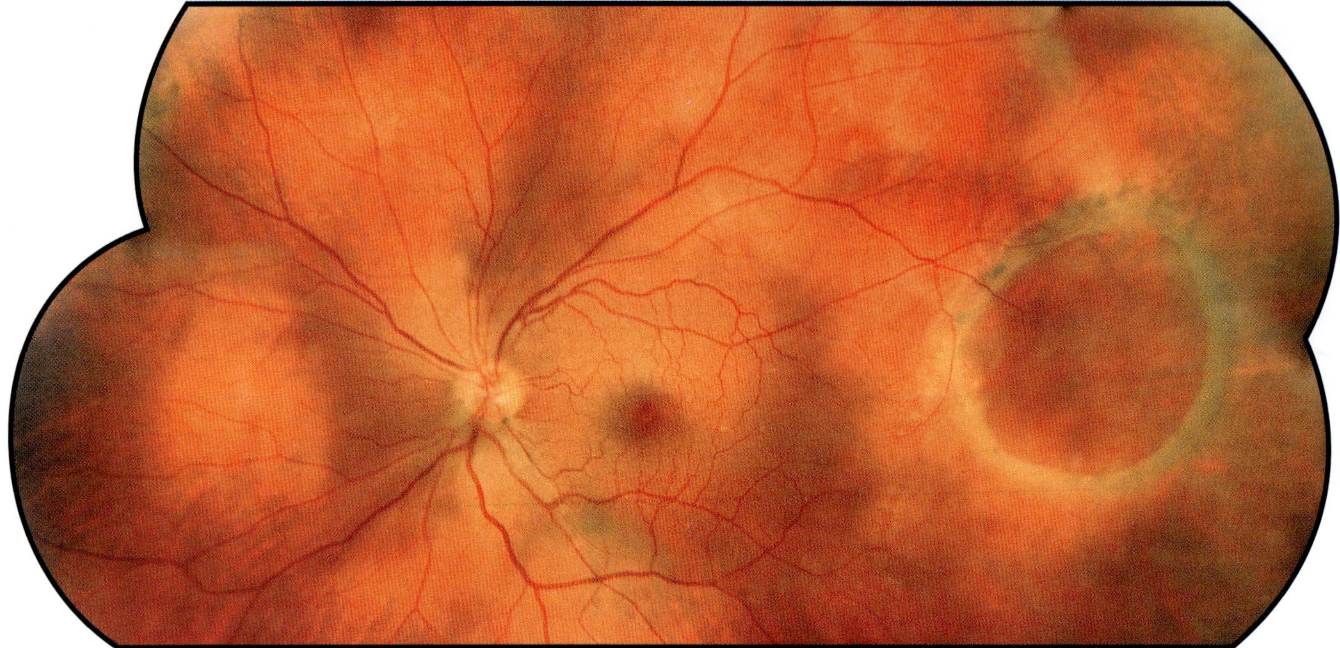

In this patient, there is a large outer-layer break beneath a long-standing area of retinoschisis. A pigmentary demarcation line has formed at the margins of the outer-layer defect.

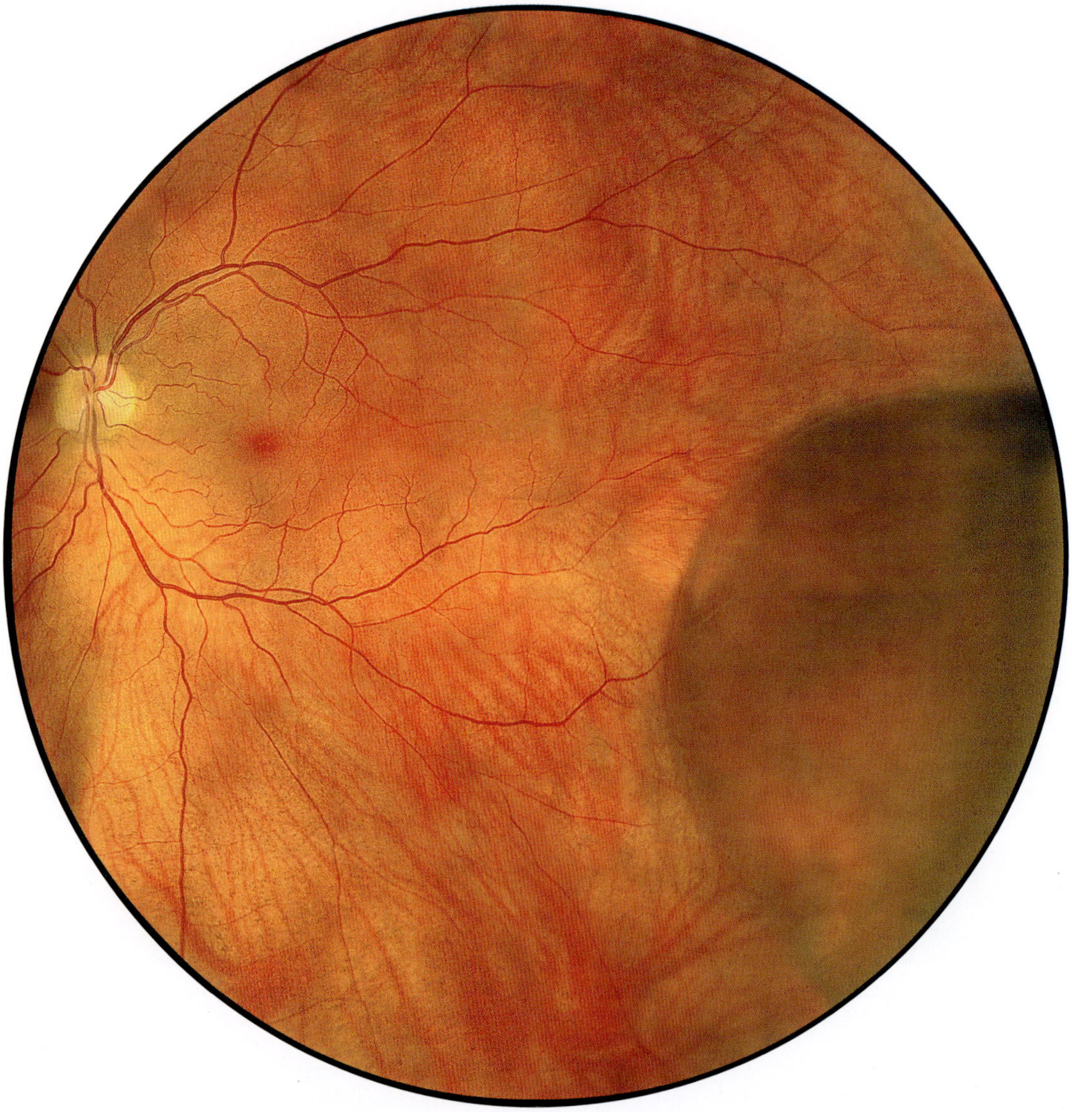

This patient has pigmentary changes within a long-standing, bullous, acquired retinoschisis cavity, presumably from retinal pigment epithelial cells migrating through one or more occult outer-layer retinal breaks.

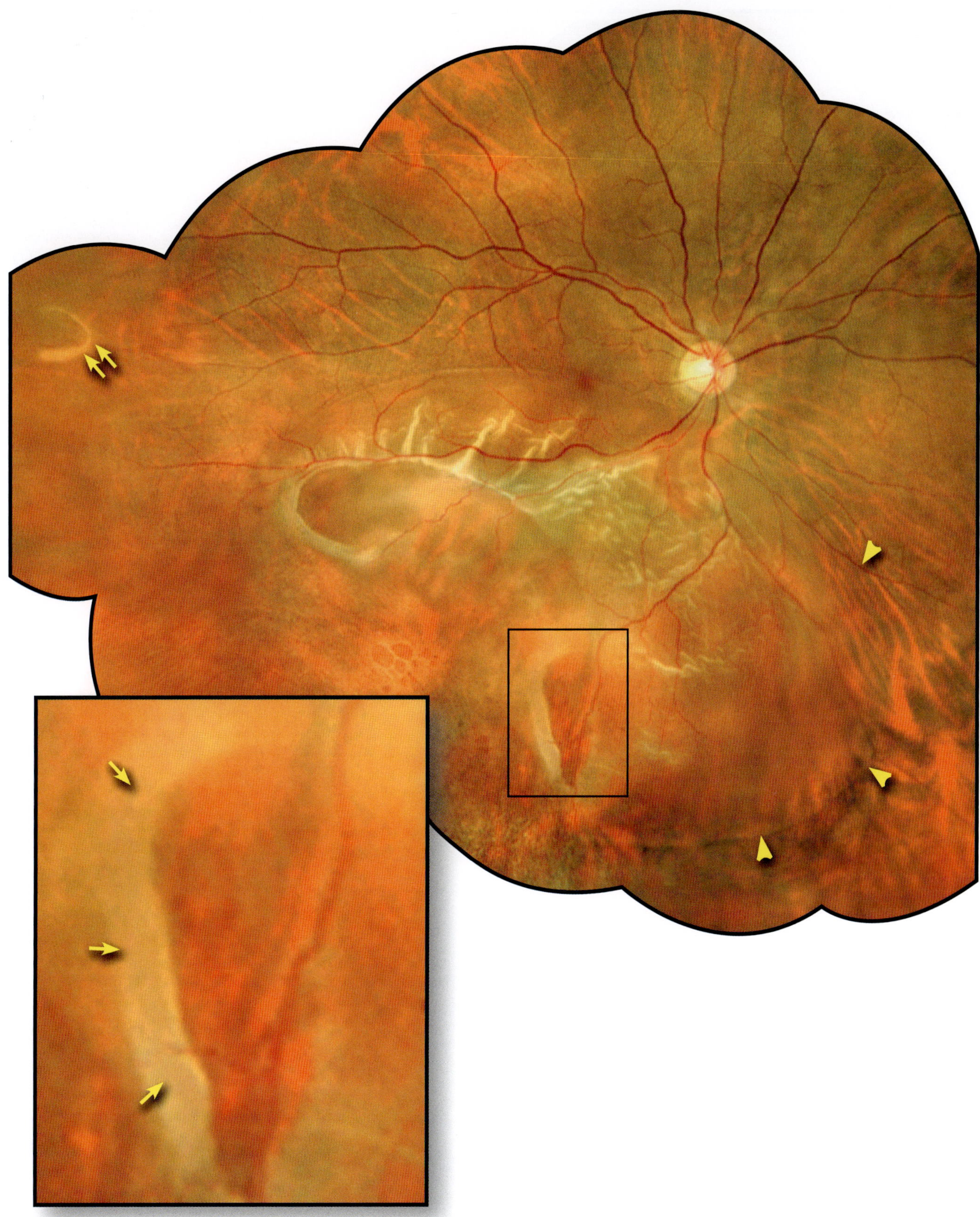

This photo depicts a patient with retinoschisis and an outer-layer detachment in the inferotemporal quadrant. The inset shows a break in the outer retina with hydration and retraction of the torn edge of outer-layer tissue *(arrows)*. When multiple retinal splittings are present, outer-layer breaks usually involve the largest schisis. Inferonasally, there is a faint curvilinear pigmentary line that corresponds to an "early pigmentary demarcation line" at the limits of the outer-layer retinal detachment *(arrowheads)*. A full-thickness horseshoe retinal break is present temporally *(double arrow)*.

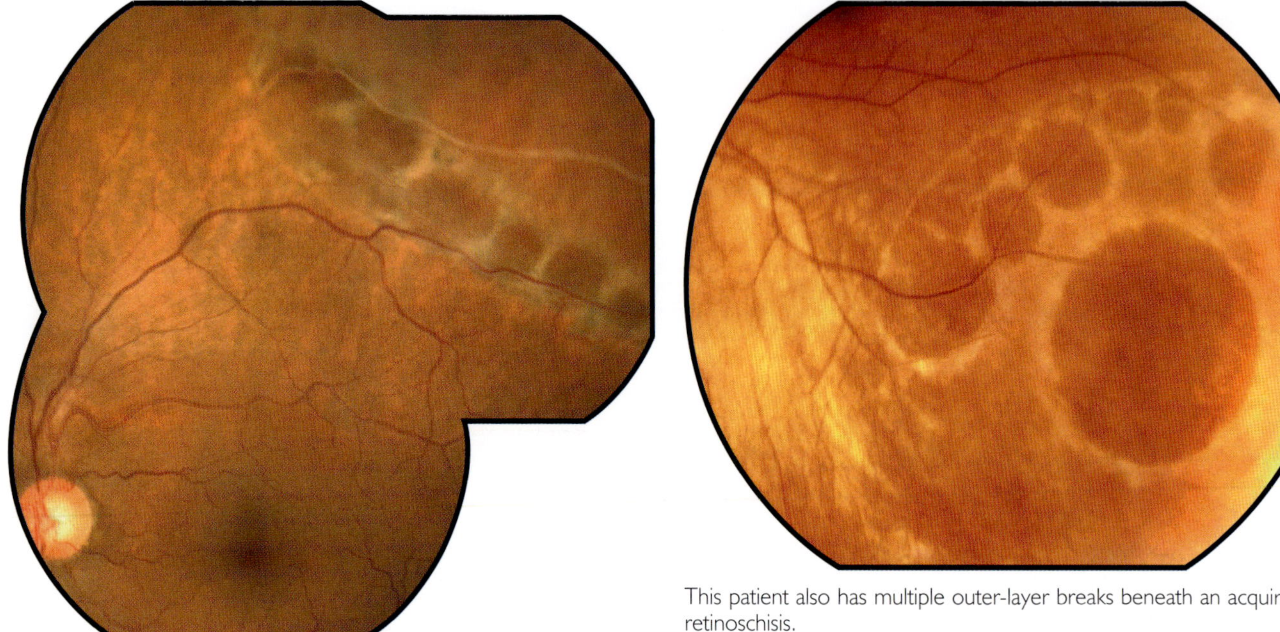

This patient also has multiple outer-layer breaks beneath an acquired retinoschisis.

This patient has superotemporal retinoschisis with multiloculated cavities. There is a traction band anteriorly and a localized peripheral full-thickness retinal detachment. *Courtesy of Dr. Lucian Del Priore*

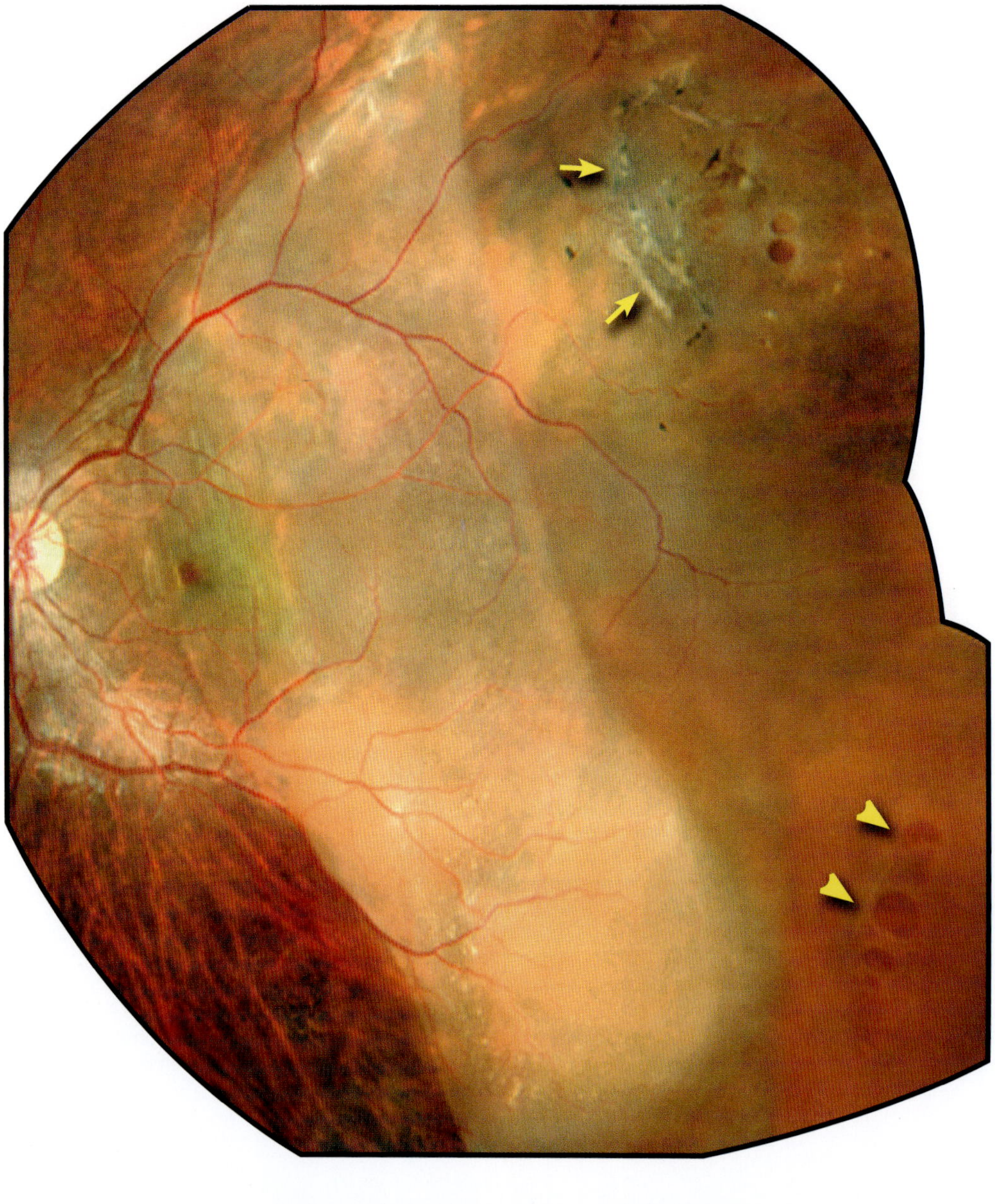

The patient in this photo has a chronic RRD with acquired retinoschisis. There are several outer-layer retinal tears with nasal retraction of the torn outer layers, producing whitening and loss of retinal transparency, as well as detachment and folds in the macula. Superotemporally, there are multiple inner-layer retinal holes associated with an area of lattice degeneration and subretinal pigmentary alterations *(arrows)*. There is a second area of lattice degeneration associated with multiple inner-layer holes inferotemporally *(arrowheads)*.

Juvenile X-Linked Retinoschisis

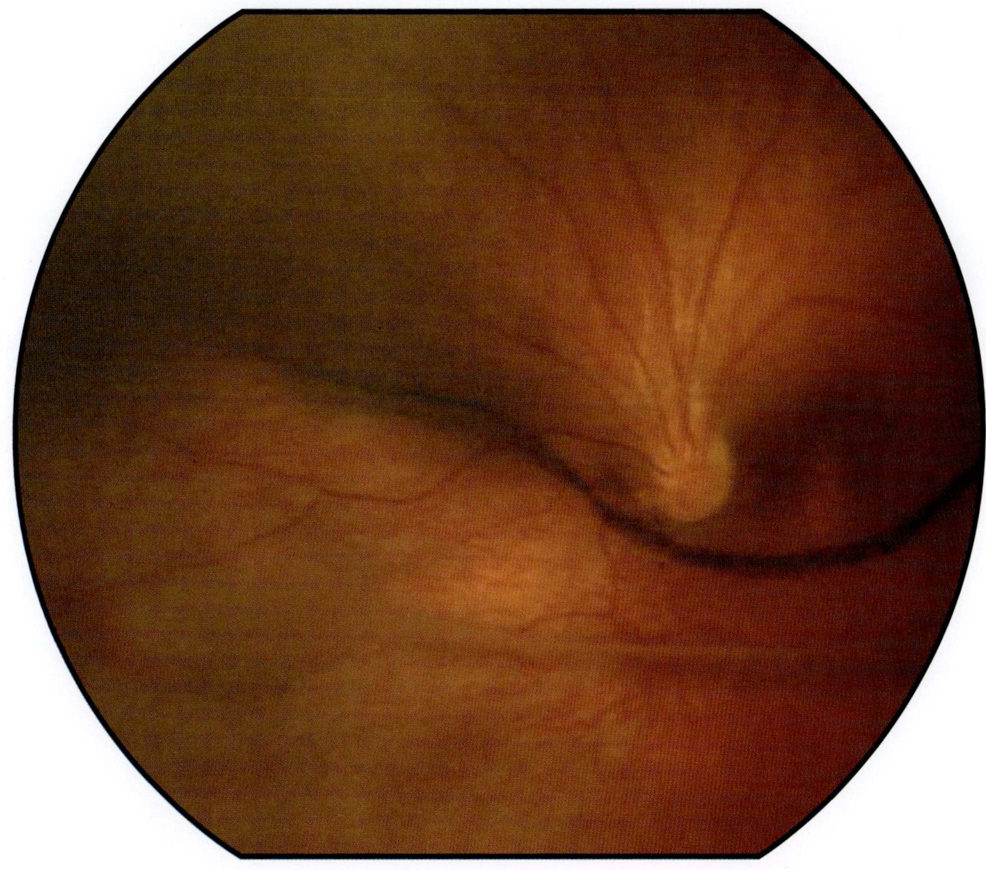

A young male patient with an extensive peripheral schisis cavity encroaching upon the macula. The patient has been monitored for over five years without progression. Visual acuity is 20/70.

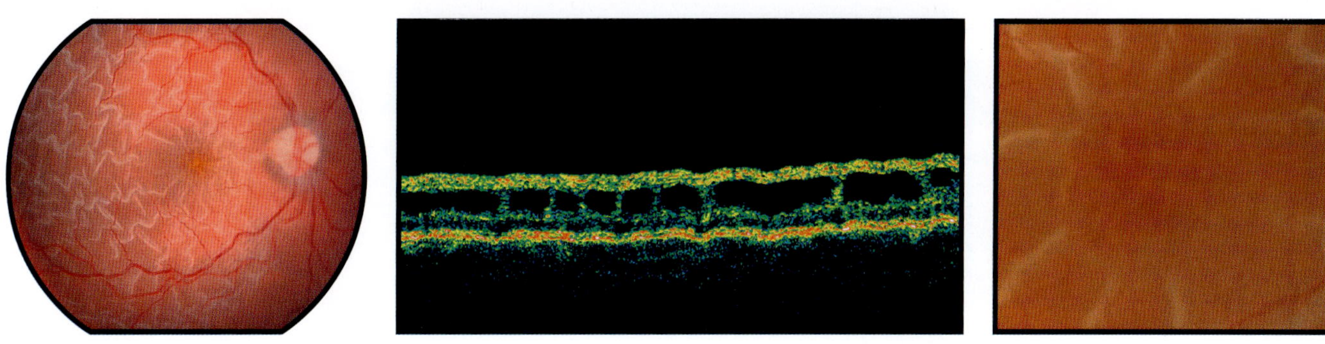

A male patient with juvenile X-linked retinoschisis (JXR). Note the macular schisis and the typical vertically oriented striations on the OCT. *Image courtesy of Henry Lee, MD*

Optic Nerve Pit with Macular Schisis Detachment

An optic nerve pit may lead to a dual detachment in the macula: retinal schisis combined with a full-thickness retinal detachment. It was originally thought that the origin of the fluid was cerebrospinal, gaining access from the subarachnoid space through the optic nerve defect into the subretinal space. However, the more accepted theory is that liquefied vitreous passes through the optic nerve defect and dissects the retinal layers before migrating into the subretinal space to cause a neurosensory detachment. In this setting, an inner lamellar cyst or outer retinal hole may also develop at the fovea.

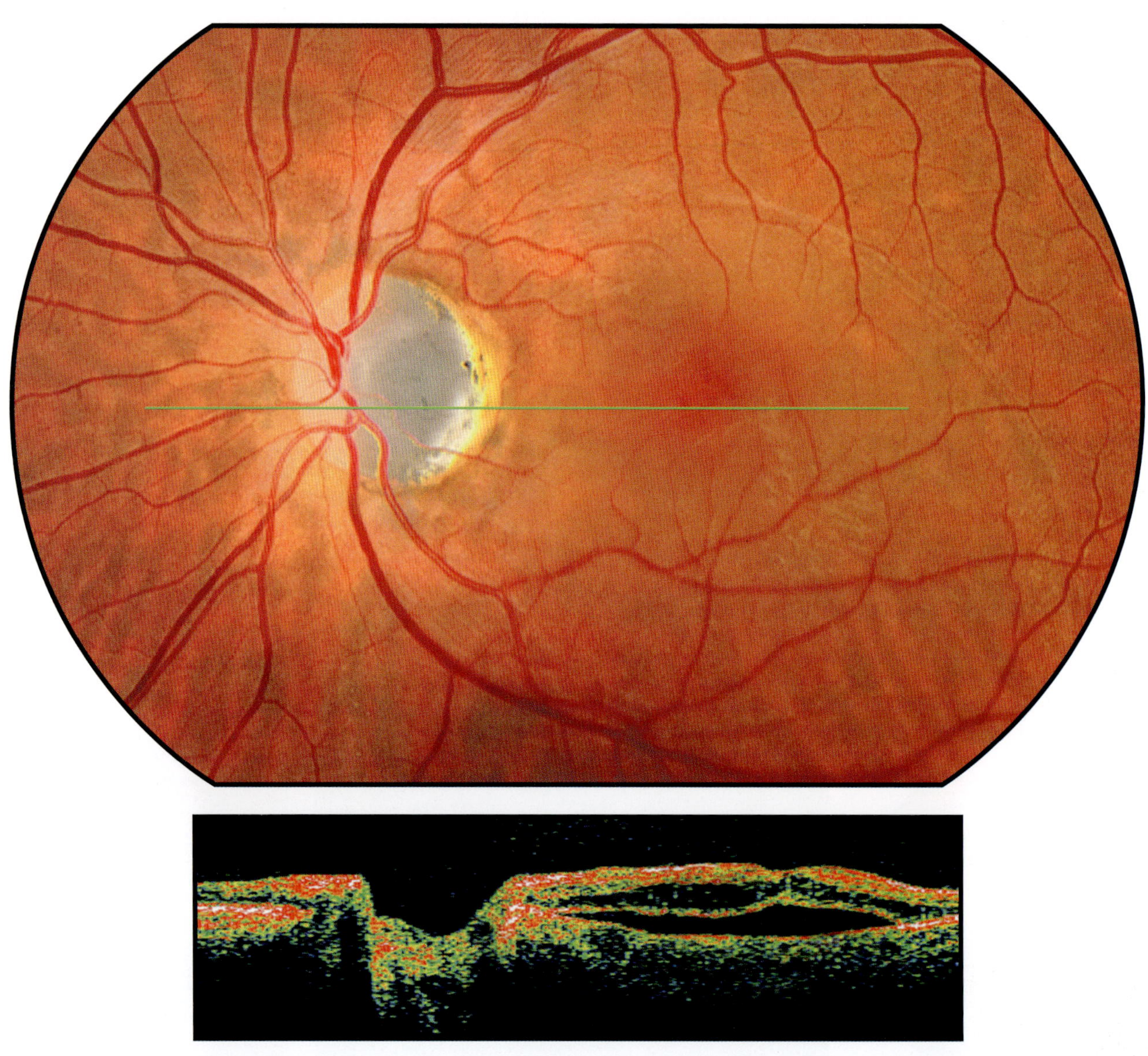

This patient has an optic nerve pit with a combined or dual macular detachment. The OCT shows schisis, as well as an outer-layer neurosensory detachment coursing from the disc through the macula. The overlying schisis generally extends beyond the outer-layer neurosensory detachment, as seen in this patient.

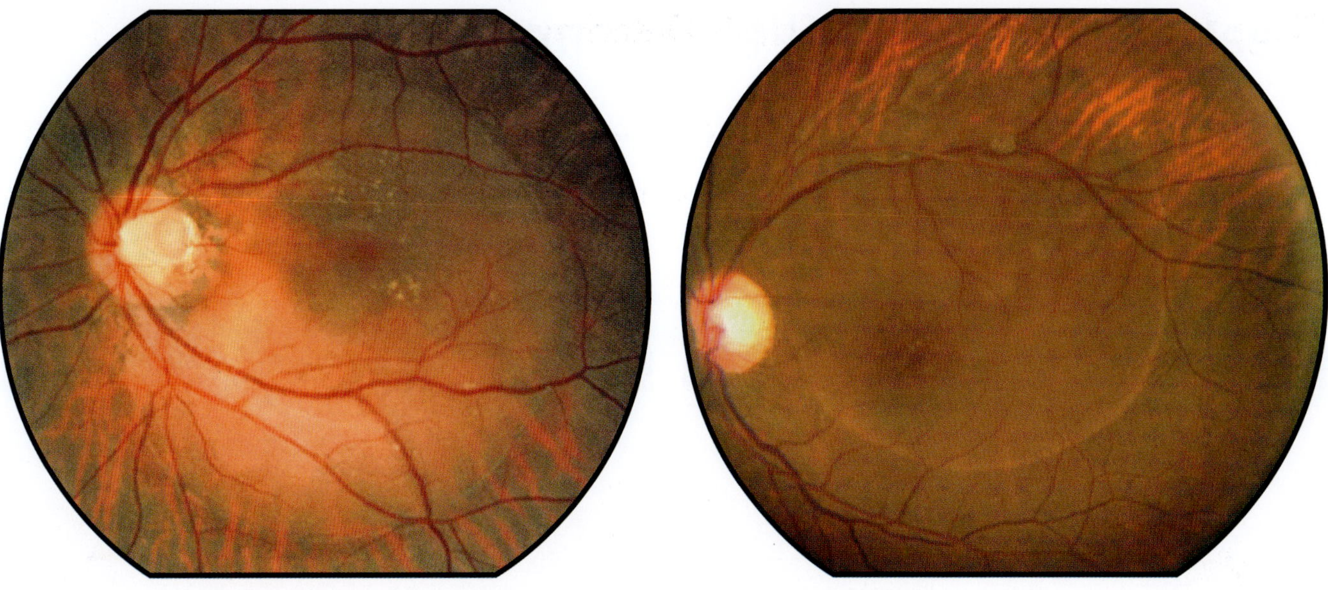

The presence of a proteinaceous demarcation line and the degree of fundus pigmentation will correlate with the duration of the outer-layer detachment.

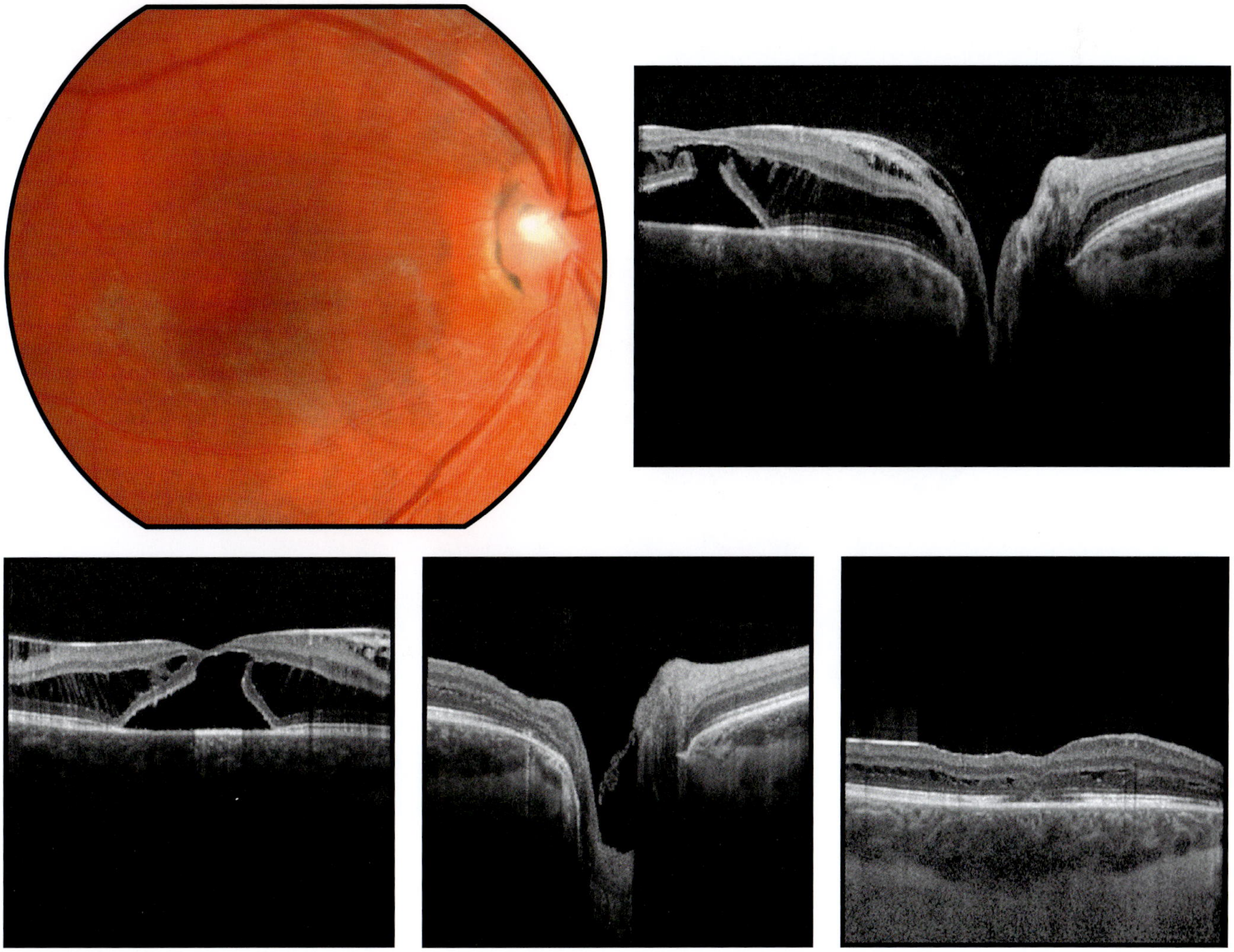

A young female with an optic nerve pit and serous macular detachment. Visual acuity was 20/200. Following a short period of observation during which time there was no change in the ocular examination, vitrectomy surgery was offered, along with peeling of the internal limited membrane, and use of an intraocular air bubble. Following surgery, the serous macular detachment resolved, and vision improved to 20/50 (*bottom right*).

Treatment of Retinal Detachment

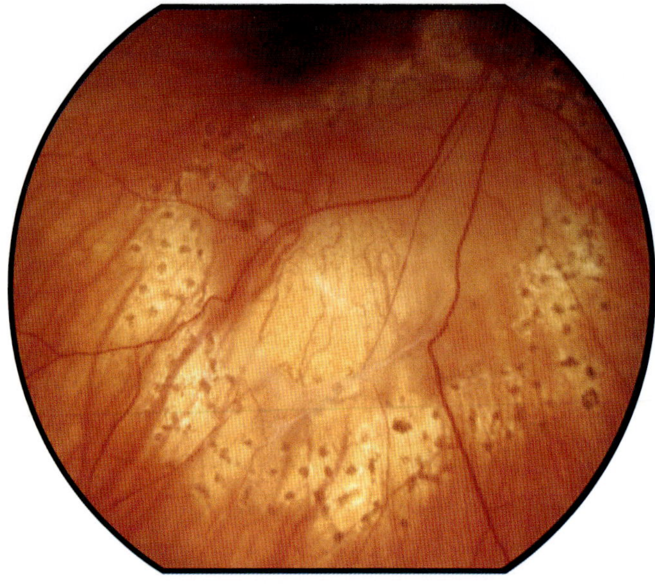

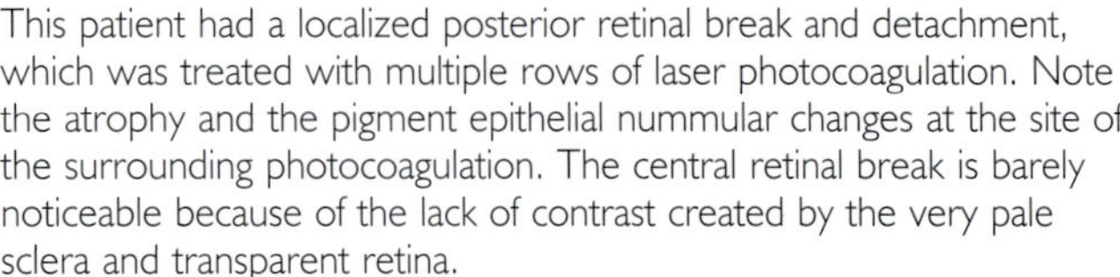

This patient had a localized posterior retinal break and detachment, which was treated with multiple rows of laser photocoagulation. Note the atrophy and the pigment epithelial nummular changes at the site of the surrounding photocoagulation. The central retinal break is barely noticeable because of the lack of contrast created by the very pale sclera and transparent retina.

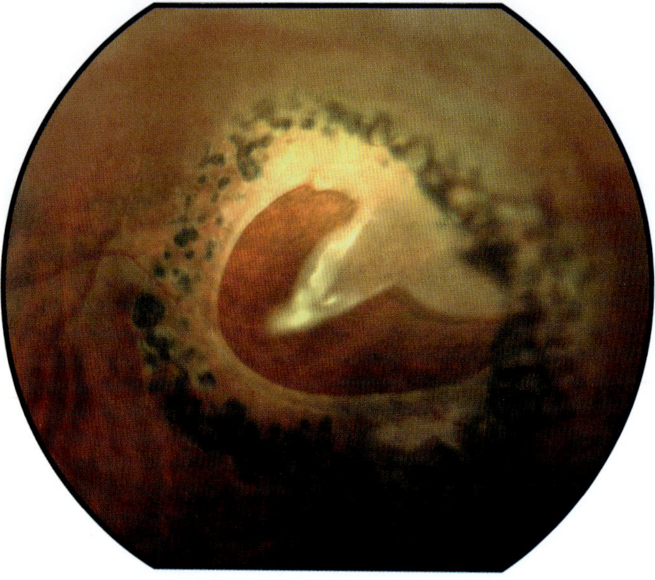

This is a horseshoe retinal tear surrounded with a triple-row of laser photocoagulation therapy. Laser retinopexy decreases the risk of retinal detachment to less than 5%.

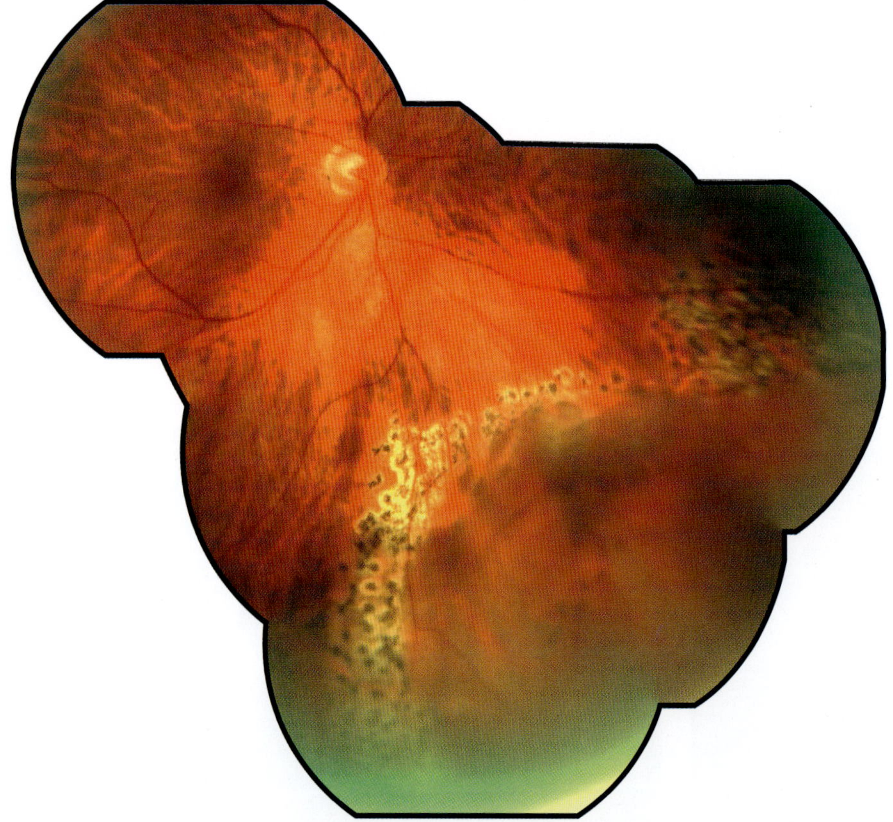

A prominent inferonasal retinal detachment was demarcated with several rows of photocoagulation. The detachment remained stable without extension of the subretinal fluid. *Courtesy of Stephen G. Schwartz, MD*

This is a panoramic image of the fundus following a reattachment surgery with an encircling band. Chorioretinal degenerative changes, likely a result of cryotherapy for retinal breaks, can be seen superiorly, superotemporally, and temporally.

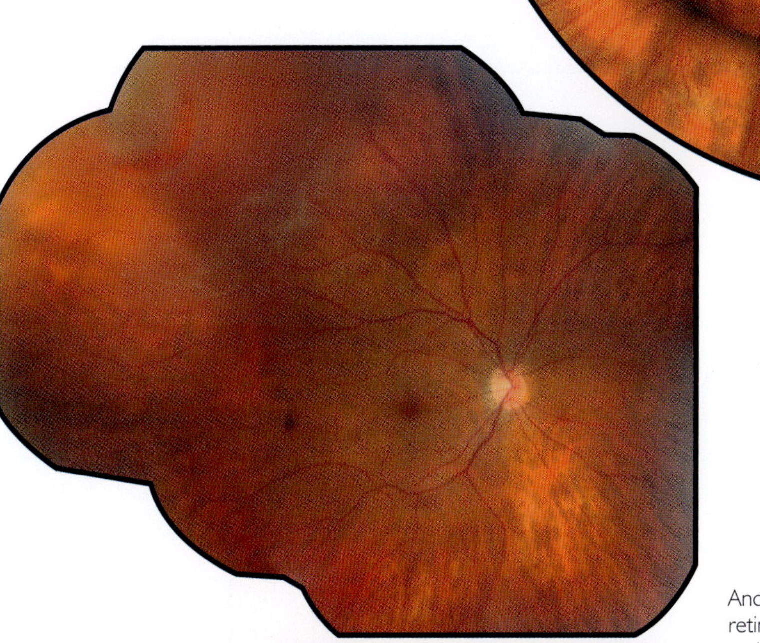

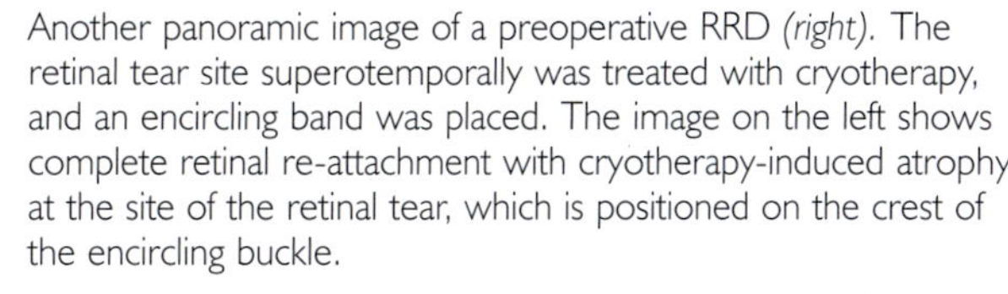

Another panoramic image of a preoperative RRD *(right)*. The retinal tear site superotemporally was treated with cryotherapy, and an encircling band was placed. The image on the left shows complete retinal re-attachment with cryotherapy-induced atrophy at the site of the retinal tear, which is positioned on the crest of the encircling buckle.

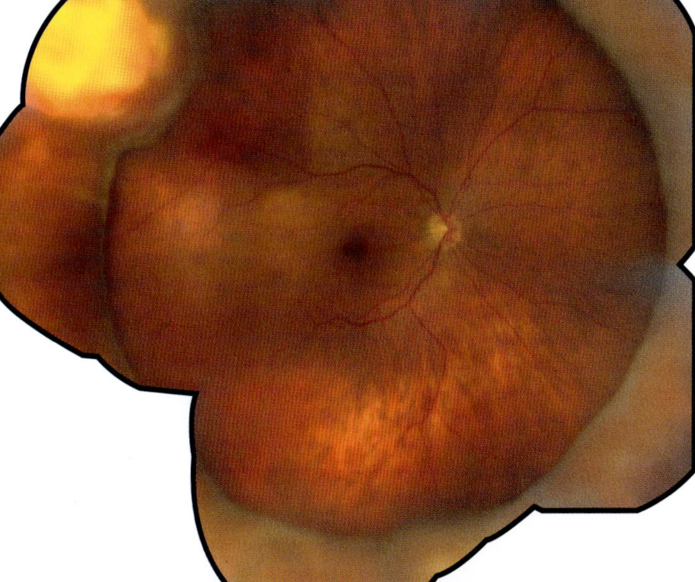

Retinal Detachment: Postsurgery

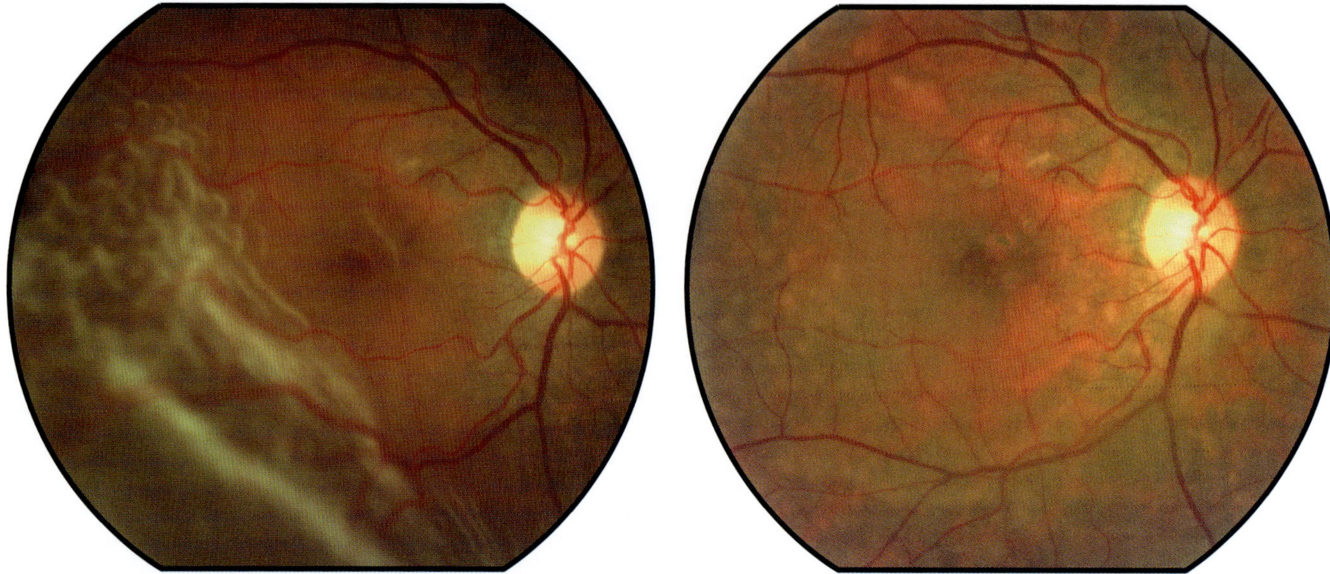

This patient had a large retinal detachment that extended into the macula, which caused multiple white retinal folds inferotemporally and associated serous elevation of the central posterior pole. Following a vitrectomy procedure, the retina is now flat and the retinal folds have resolved *(right)*.

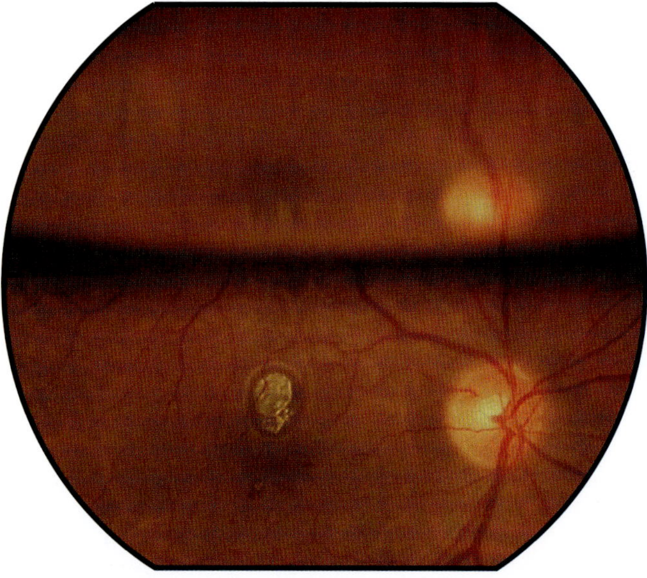

This patient had a pars plana vitrectomy with a long-acting gas tamponade to repair a retinal detachment. Note the reflection created by the gas–fluid interface superiorly. This reflection off the surface of the gas bubble creates a split image, giving the false appearance of a double optic nerve.

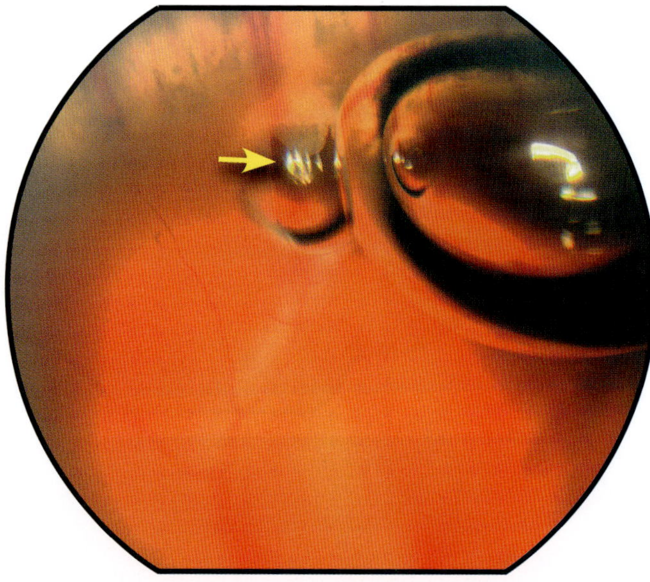

This patient had a PR for a superior horseshoe retinal break and an associated RRD. Note that the smaller gas bubble adjacent to the larger bubble *(arrow)* has migrated through the horseshoe tear into the subretinal space, tenting open the break and temporarily interfering with reattachment of the retina.

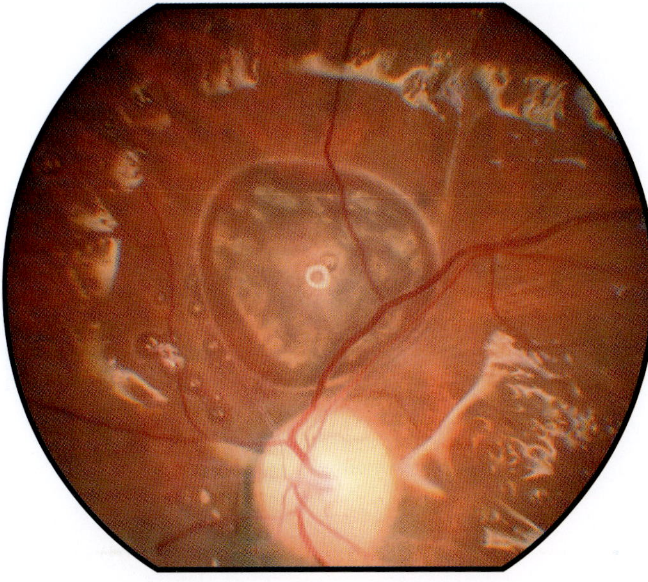

This patient had vitreoretinal surgery with the use of silicone oil as a long-term tamponade. The glistening reflectance off the retinal surface is characteristic of vitrectomized eyes filled with silicone oil. In the center of the photo, just superior to the optic nerve, note the elevated area where silicone oil has migrated into the subretinal space.

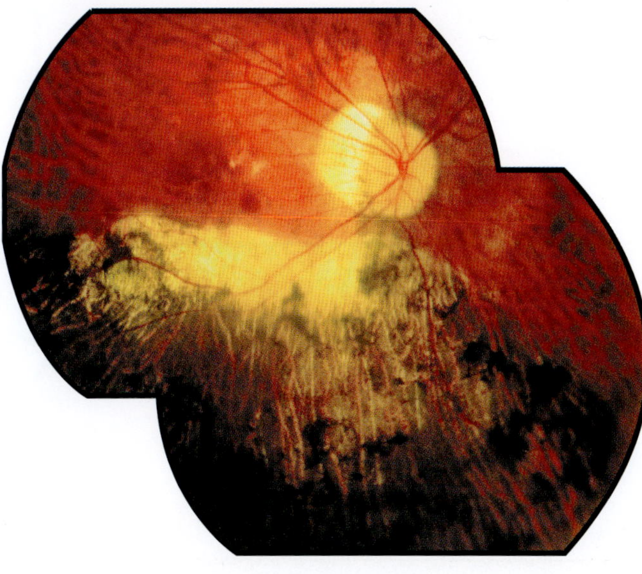

This patient had a chronic inferior retinal detachment, which spontaneously resolved and led to areas of retinal atrophic degeneration (whitening) and significant hyperplastic changes of the RPE inferiorly.

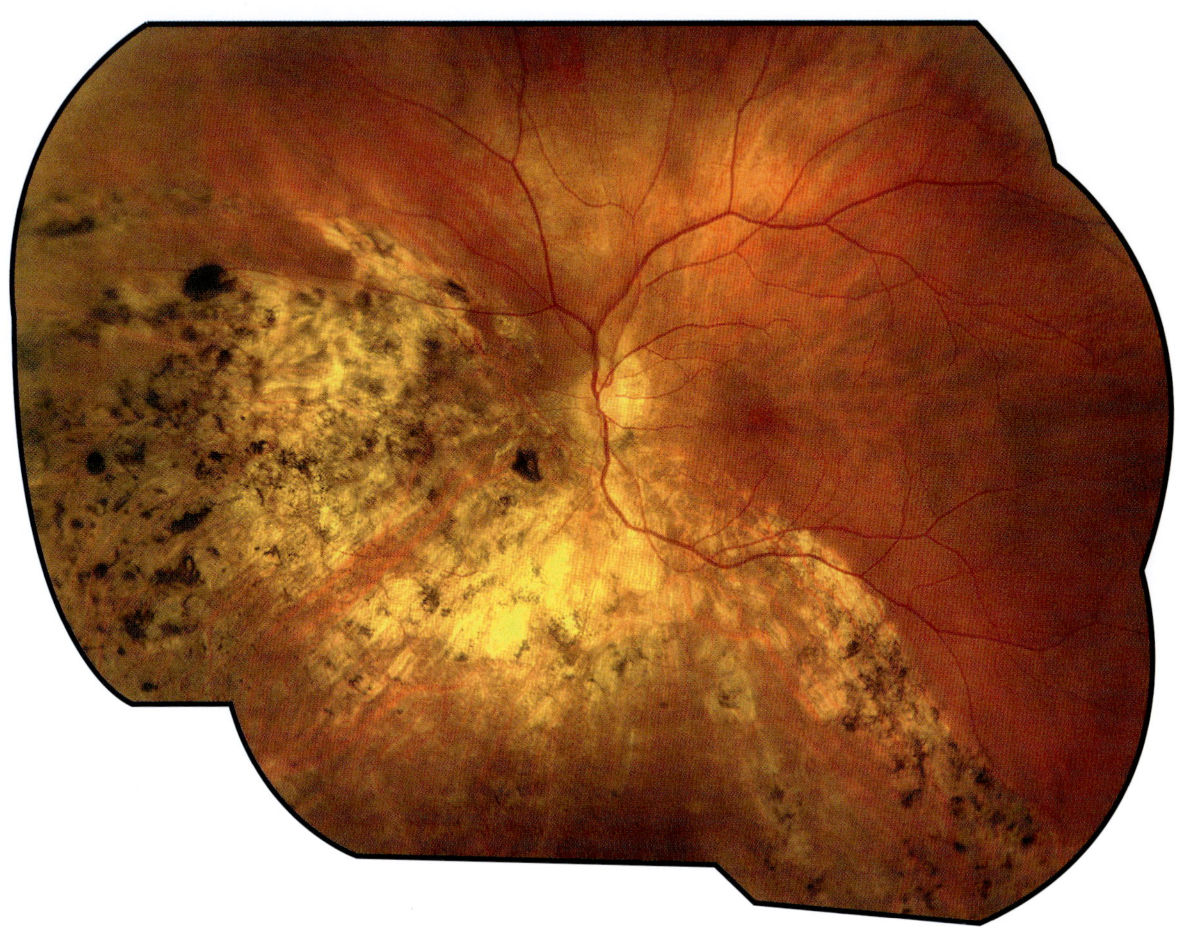

Extension of this chronic detachment centrally led to a transparent, shallow detachment of the macula. The patient became symptomatic because of slowly progressive visual field loss.

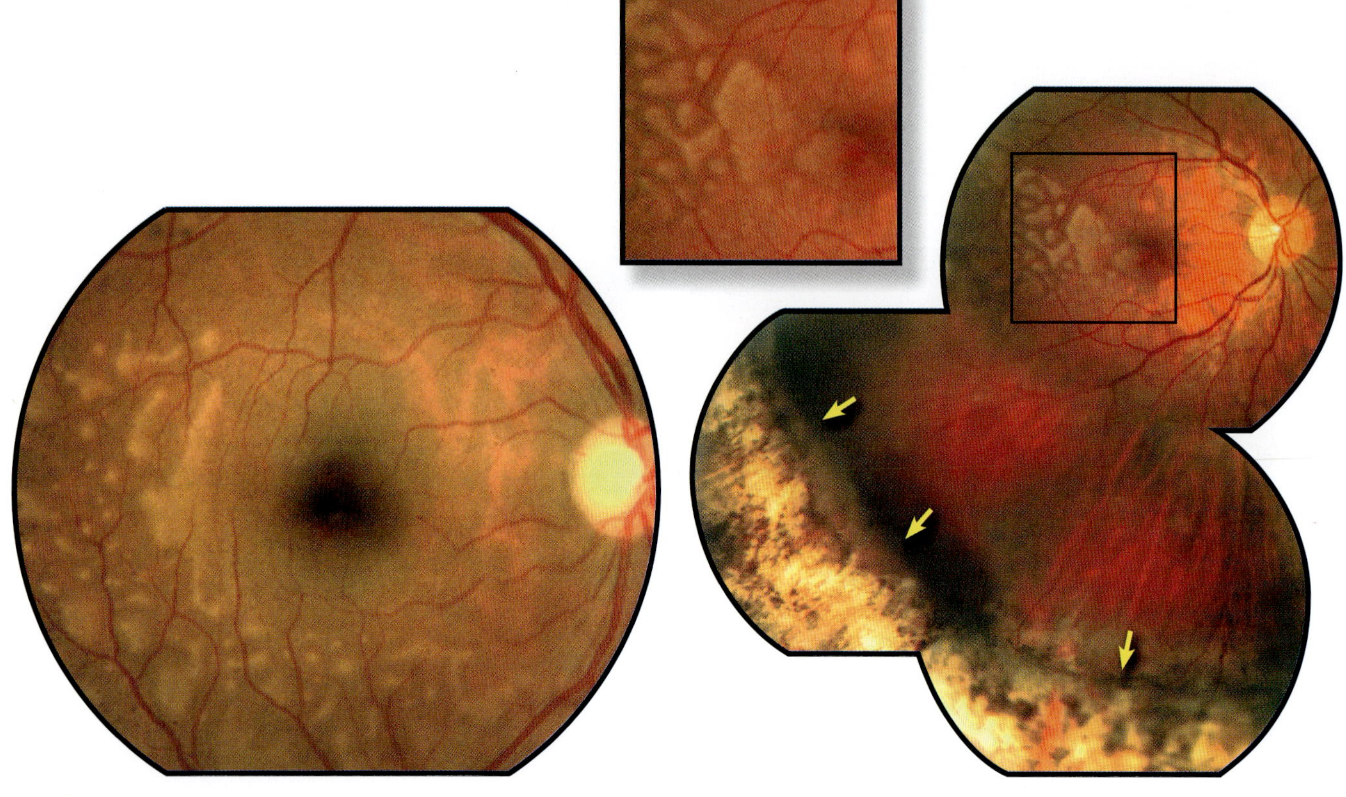

This patient had a bullous retinal detachment that involved the macula. After a re-attachment procedure, there remained multiple small residual pockets of subretinal fluid. These mini-neurosensory retinal detachments eventually resolved spontaneously after many months.

This patient had an inferior scleral buckle *(arrows)* with cryopexy to repair a bullous detachment involving the macula. Following repair, the retina was flat except for multiple small serous elevations involving the fovea and temporal perimacular region *(black box/insert)*. After many months of observation, the fluid resolved spontaneously with eventual recovery of central vision.

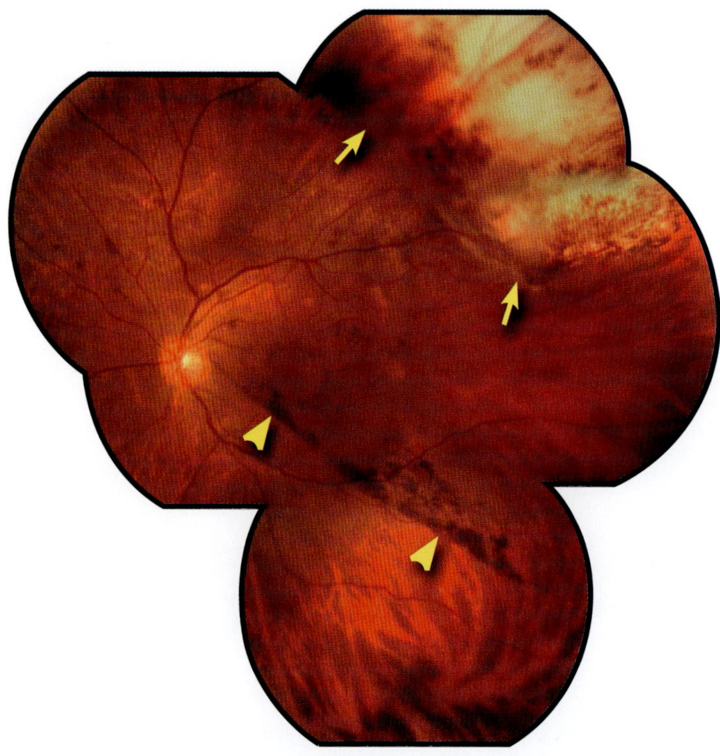

This patient had a scleral buckle placed superotemporally to repair a retinal detachment that had extended into the macula. There are areas of retinal atrophy at the site of the buckle and cryosurgery *(arrows)*. The demarcation line that runs through the macula also has some pigmentary stippling left over from the antecedent detachment *(arrowheads)*.

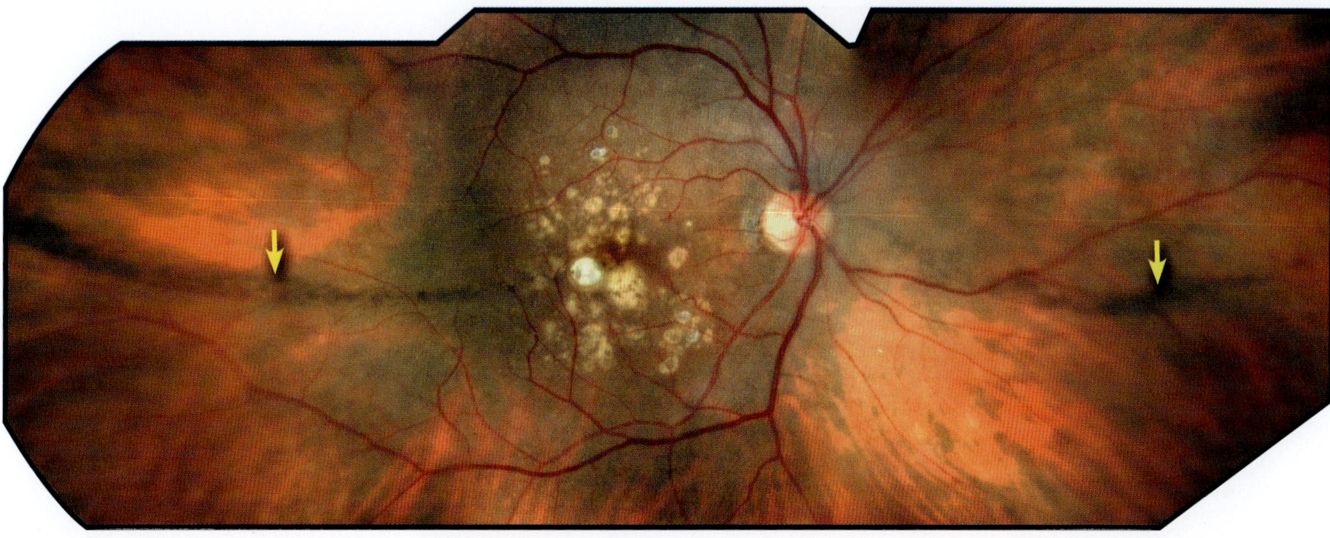

This patient had a large superior bullous retinal detachment that extended into the macula. It left an incomplete pigmentary demarcation line temporally and nasally *(arrows)*. There are also large confluent drusen in the central macula.

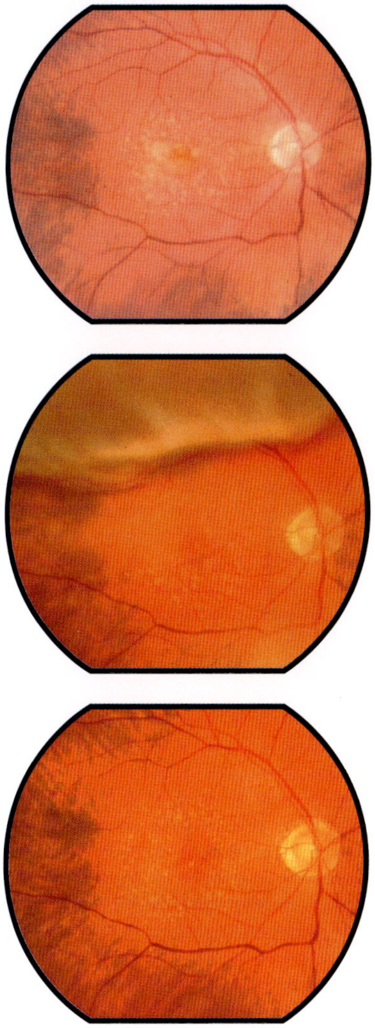

This patient had confluent large drusen in the macula prior to developing a superior bullous RRD with subretinal fluid extending into the macula. One year following repair of the detachment with a PR, most of the larger drusen have disappeared.

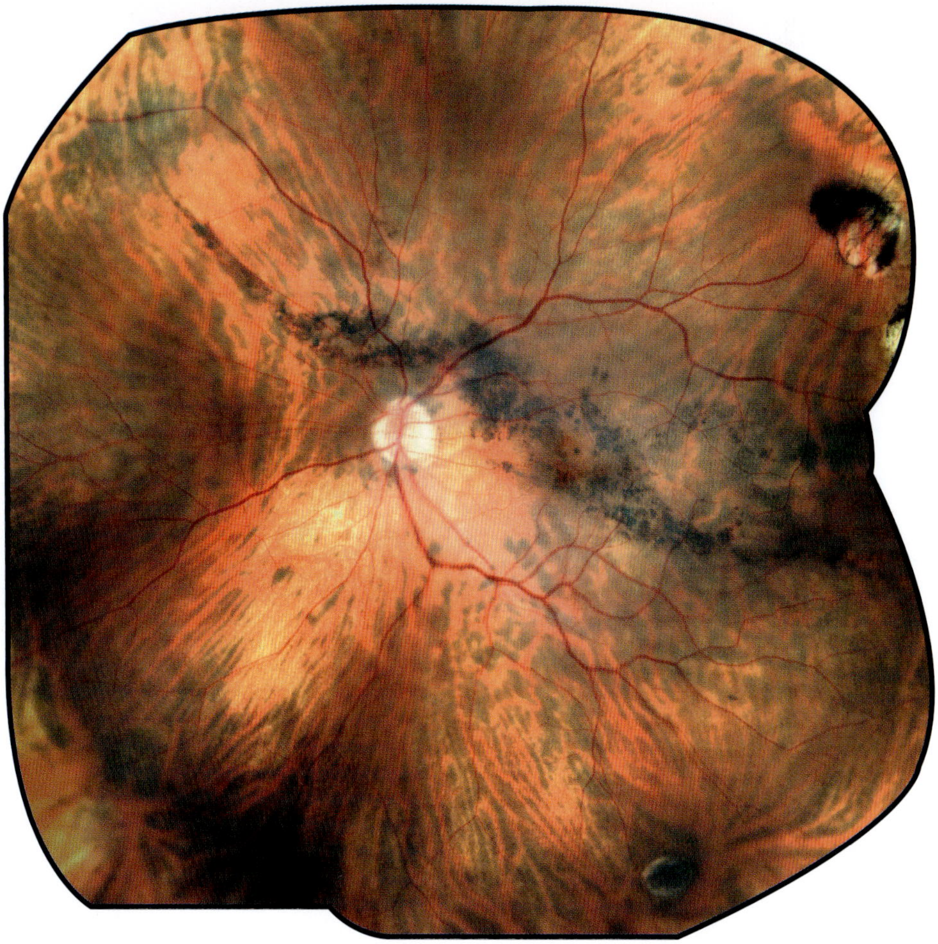

This patient developed a bullous superior retinal detachment from a retinal break superotemporally. Migration of liberated RPE cells subretinally to the posterior margins of the detachment, in conjunction with pigment dispersion as a result of retinal cryopexy, created the curvilinear, pigmented demarcation line through the macula. This has been referred to as a cryodemarcation line in retinal detachment surgery.

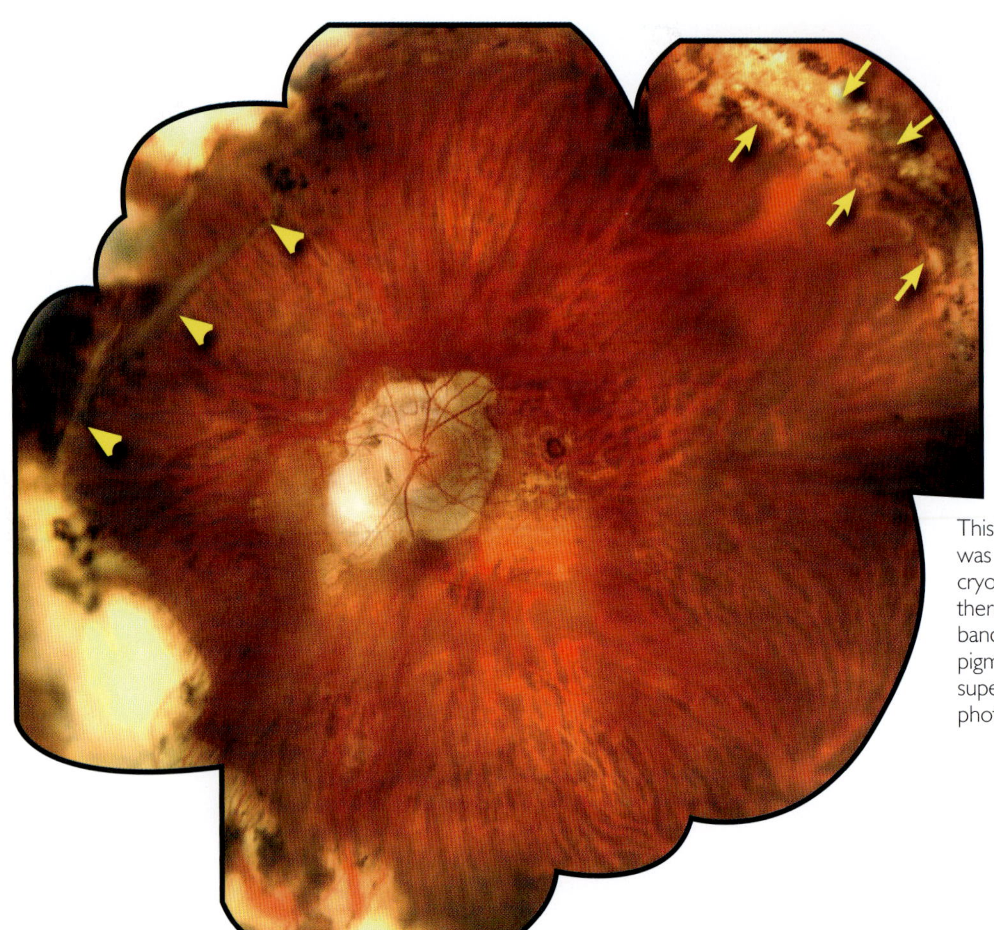

This patient had a global detachment that was repaired by a combination of cryosurgery and vitrectomy. Superonasally, there is still a residual curvilinear traction band *(arrowheads)*. An area of atrophy and pigmentary lattice degeneration superotemporally was treated with laser photocoagulation *(arrows)*.

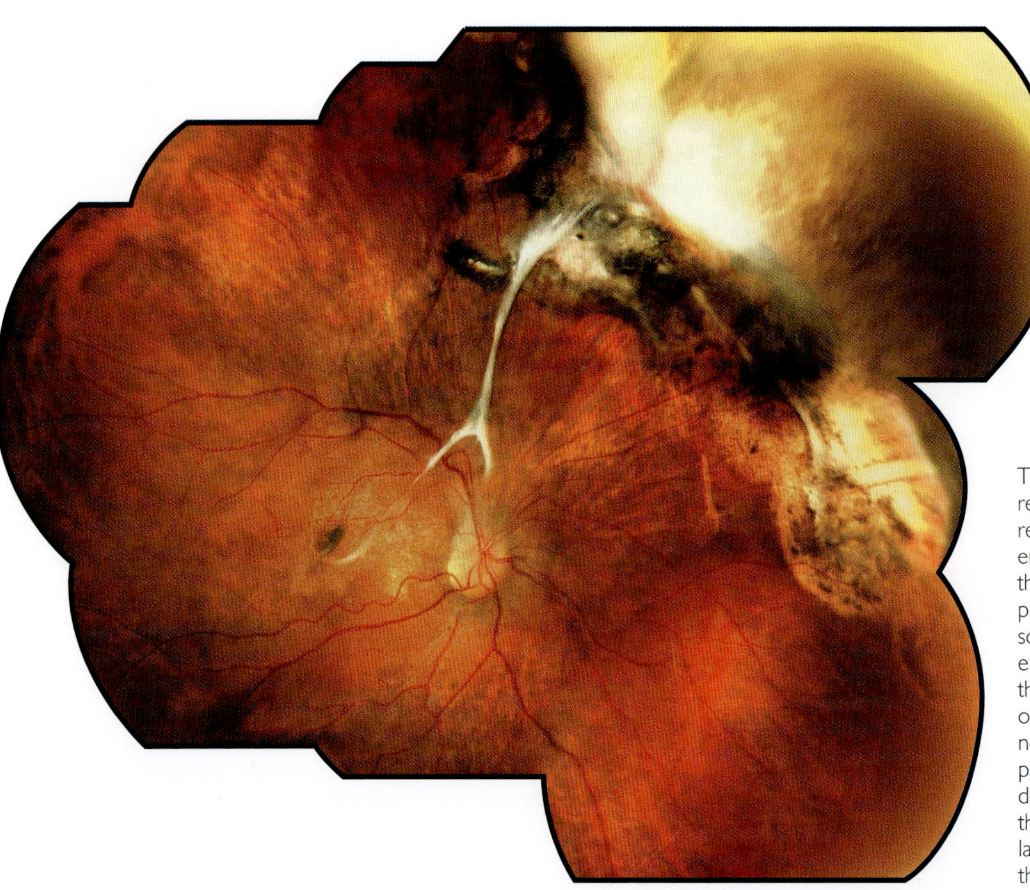

This patient had a traumatic retinal detachment, which was repaired with cryosurgery and an encircling band. Superonasally, there is considerable retinal pigment epithelial hyperplasia and some fibrous proliferation on the encircling element. Also note that there is some residual fluid overlying the encircling band but not posterior to it. Inferiorly, the patient also had a shallow retinal detachment that was treated with the encircling band and scatter laser photocoagulation to close the separate retinal breaks.

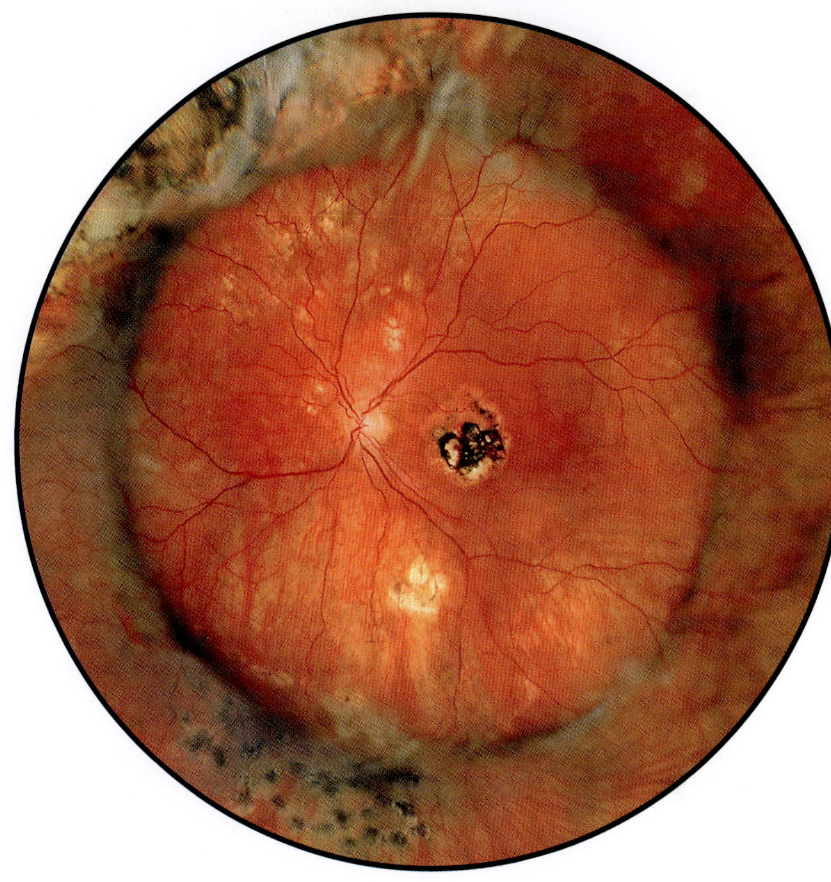

This patient has undergone repair of a retinal detachment with an encircling scleral buckle. There is notable pre-retinal hemorrhage superotemporally, photocoagulation scars overlying the buckle inferiorly, and cryopexy scars superonasally where the thickened margin of the closed retinal break is still visible. There is also a pigmentary scar in the macula.

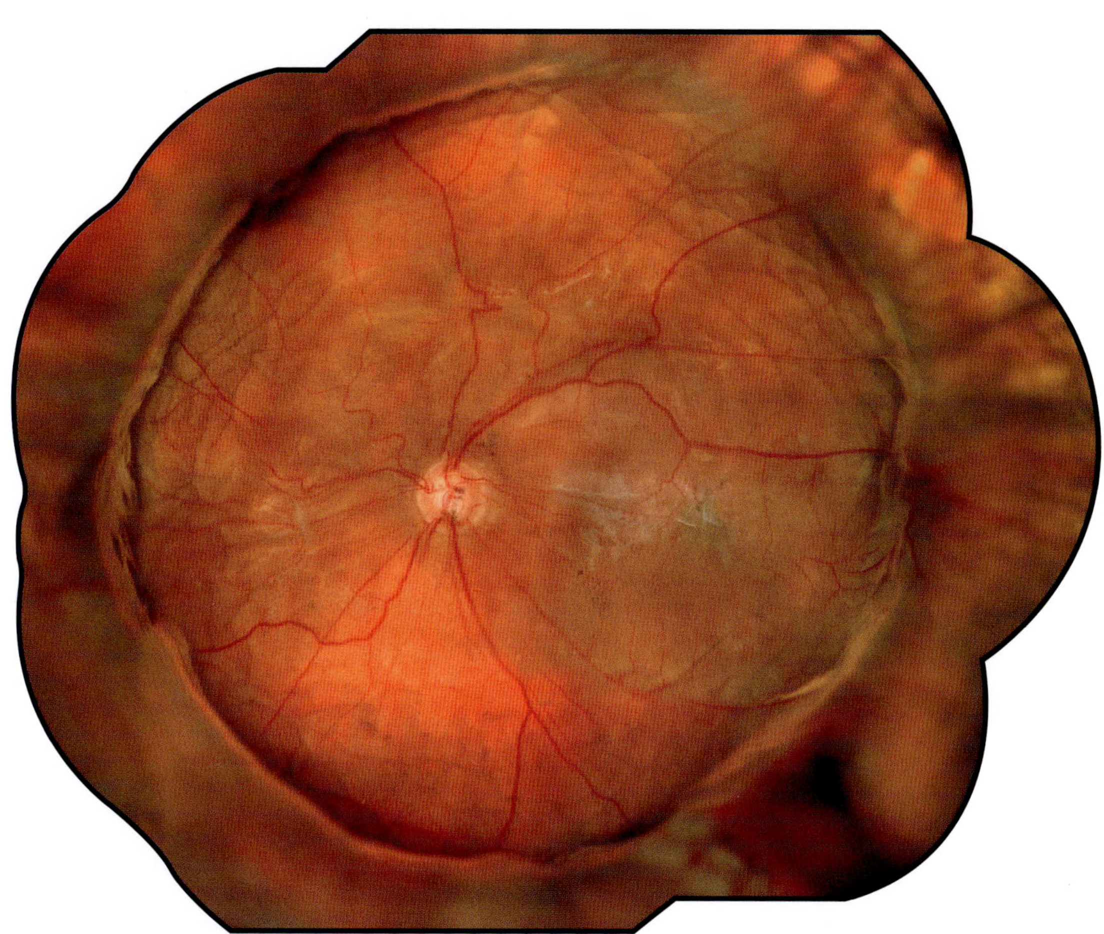

This patient recently had a retinal detachment successfully repaired with an encircling scleral buckle. There are still retinal folds on the posterior slope of the buckle, especially noticeable nasally and superotemporally, related to redundancy of excess tissue induced by a reduced retinal circumference. These folds will often flatten over time without further intervention.

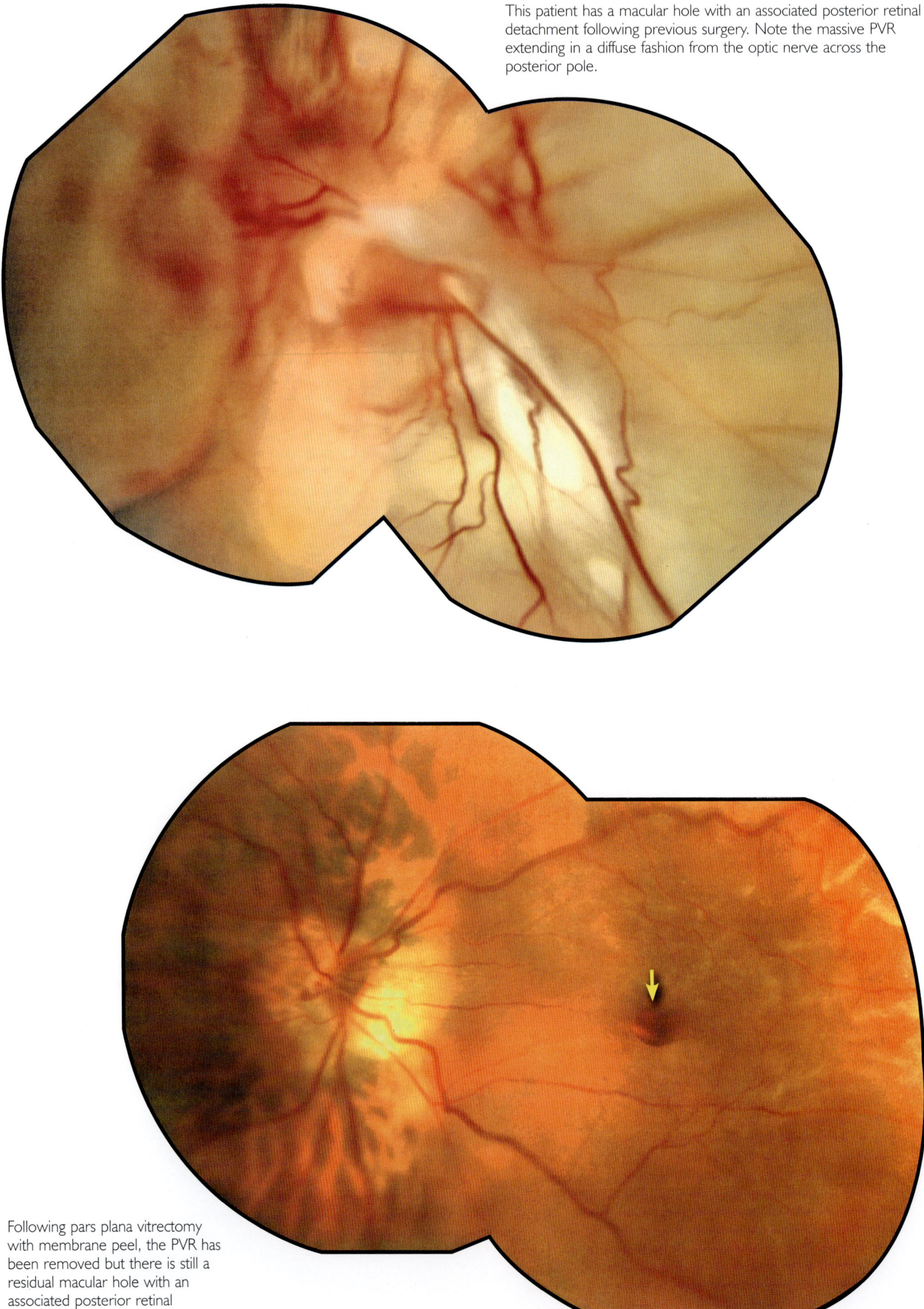

This patient has a macular hole with an associated posterior retinal detachment following previous surgery. Note the massive PVR extending in a diffuse fashion from the optic nerve across the posterior pole.

Following pars plana vitrectomy with membrane peel, the PVR has been removed but there is still a residual macular hole with an associated posterior retinal detachment *(arrow)*.

Macular Translocation Surgery

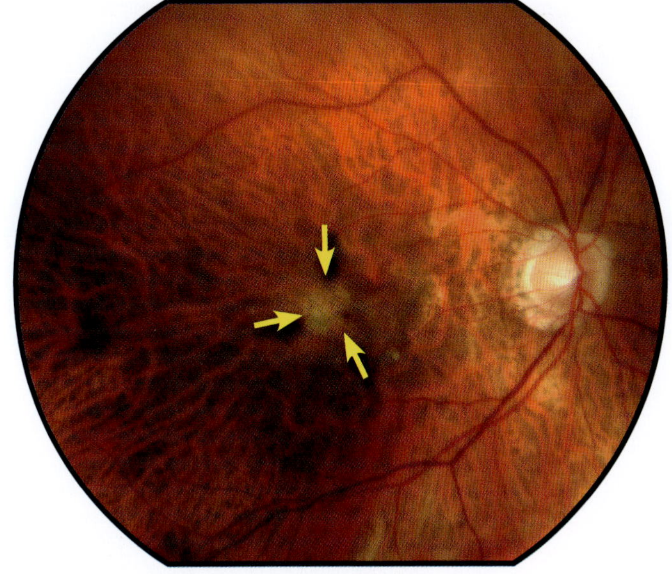

This patient had a subfoveal choroidal neovascularization secondary to age-related macular degeneration *(arrows)*. Vitreoretinal surgery with macular translocation and a 360-degree retinotomy were carried out.

Following macular translocation vitrectomy, with a 360-degree retinotomy and a silicone oil tamponade, the anatomic fovea has been displaced superiorly. The inferotemporal vasculature now rests over what was previously the site of the fovea *(X)*.

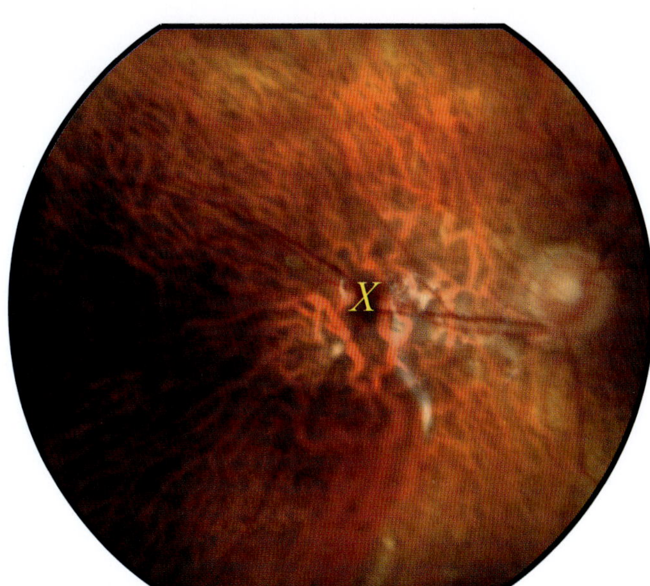

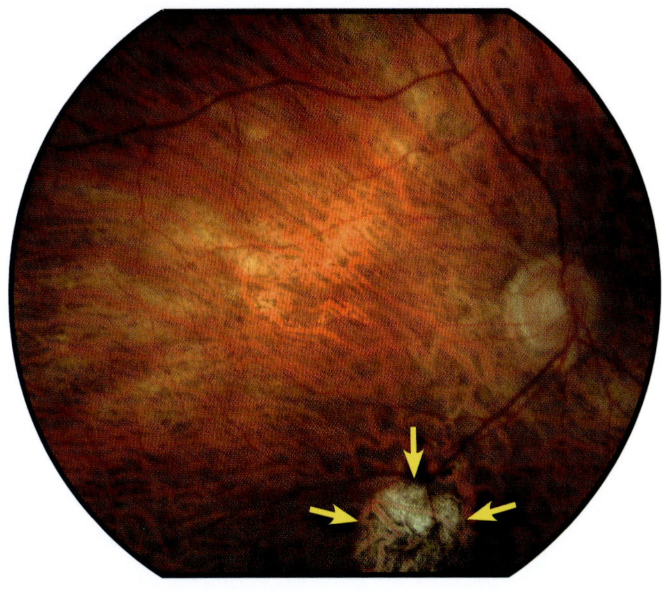

After muscle surgery and removal of the silicone oil, a new foveal region is established at a site of healthy RPE. The choroidal neovascular membrane has been treated with thermal laser, leaving an atrophic scar at the site of the original fovea *(arrows)*. *Courtesy of Dr. James M. Klancnik*

Suggested Reading

Peripheral Retinal Abnormalities

Byer, N.E., 1981. Cystic retinal tufts and their relationship to retinal detachment. Arch. Ophthalmol. 99 (10), 1788–1790.

Choudhry, N., Golding, J., Manry, M.W., et al., 2016. Ultra-widefield steering-based spectral-domain optical coherence tomography imaging of the retinal periphery. Ophthalmology 123, 1368–1374.

Lewis, H., 2003. Peripheral retinal degenerations and the risk of retinal detachment. Am. J. Ophthalmol. 136, 155–160.

Taney, L.S., Baumal, C.R., 2014. Optical coherence tomography of a cystic retinal tuft. JAMA Ophthalmol. 132 (10), 1191.

Lattice Degeneration

Gonzales, C.R., Gupta, A., Schwartz, S.D., et al., 2004. The fellow eye of patients with phakic rhegmatogenous retinal detachment from atrophic holes of lattice degeneration without posterior vitreous detachment. Br. J. Ophthalmol. 88, 1400–1402.

Meguro, A., Ideta, H., Ota, M., et al., 2012. Common variants in the COL4A4 gene confer susceptibility to lattice degeneration of the retina. PLoS ONE 7 (6), e39300.

Straatsma, B.R., Zeegen, P.D., Foos, R.Y., et al., 1974. Lattice degeneration of the retina. Trans. Am. Acad. Ophthalmol. Otolaryngol. 78, 87–113.

Wilkinson, C.P., 2014. Interventions for asymptomatic retinal breaks and lattice degeneration for preventing retinal detachment. Cochrane Database Syst. Rev. (9), CD003170.

Retinal Tears and Localized Detachments

Blindbaek, S., Grauslund, J., 2015. Prophylactic treatment of retinal breaks—a systematic review. Acta Ophthalmol. 93 (1), 3–8.

Byer, N.E., 1981. Cystic retinal tufts and their relationship to retinal detachment. Arch. Ophthalmol. 99 (10), 1788–1790.

Byer, N.E., 1998. What happens to untreated asymptomatic retinal breaks, and are they affected by posterior vitreous detachment? Ophthalmology 105, 1045–1049, discussion 1049-1050.

Coffee, R.E., Westfall, A.C., Davis, G.H., et al., 2007. Symptomatic posterior vitreous detachment and incidence of delayed retinal breaks: case series and meta-analysis. Am. J. Ophthalmol. 144 (3), 409–413.

Davis, M.D., 1974. Natural history of retinal breaks without detachment. Arch. Ophthalmol. 92 (3), 183–194.

El-Sanhouri, A.A., Foster, R.E., Petersen, M.R., et al., 2011. Retinal tears after posterior vitreous detachment and vitreous hemorrhage in patients on systemic anticoagulants. Eye (Lond.) 25 (8), 1016–1019.

Lincoff, H., Gieser, R., 1971. Finding the retinal hole. Arch. Ophthalmol. 85, 565–569.

Richardson, P.S., Benson, M.T., Kirkby, G.R., 1999. The posterior vitreous detachment clinic: do new retinal breaks develop in the six weeks following an isolated symptomatic posterior vitreous detachment? Eye (Lond.) 13, 237–240.

Sharma, M.C., Regillo, C.D., Shuler, M.F., et al., 2004. Determination of the incidence and clinical characteristics of subsequent retinal tears following treatment of the acute posterior vitreous detachment-related initial retinal tears. Am. J. Ophthalmol. 138, 280–284.

Smiddy, W.E., Flynn, H.W., Nicholson, D.H., et al., 1991. Results and complications in treated retinal breaks. Am. J. Ophthalmol. 112, 623–631.

Wilkinson, C.P., 2000. Evidence-based analysis of prophylactic treatment of asymptomatic retinal breaks and lattice degeneration. Ophthalmology 107, 12–15.

Retinal Detachments

Brod, R.D., Flynn, H.W., Lightman, D.A., 1995. Asymptomatic rhegmatogenous retinal detachments. Arch. Ophthalmol. 113, 1030–1032.

Brucker, A.J., Hopkins, T.B., 2006. Retinal detachment surgery: the latest in current management. Retina 26, S28–S33.

Byer, N.E., 1994. Natural history of posterior vitreous detachment with early management as the premier line of defense against retinal detachment. Ophthalmology 101, 1503–1513, discussion 1513-1514.

Byer, N.E., 2001. Subclinical retinal detachment resulting from asymptomatic retinal breaks: prognosis for progression and regression. Ophthalmology 108, 1499–1503, discussion 1503-1504.

Byer, N.E., 1981. Cystic retinal tufts and their relationship to retinal detachment. Arch. Ophthalmol. 99, 1788–1790.

Cohen, S.M., 2005. Natural history of asymptomatic clinical retinal detachments. Am. J. Ophthalmol. 139, 777–779.

Gonzales, C.R., Gupta, A., Schwartz, S.D., et al., 2004. The fellow eye of patients with rhegmatogenous retinal detachment. Ophthalmology 111 (3), 518–521.

Gupta, O.P., Benson, W.E., 2005. The risk of fellow eyes in patients with rhegmatogenous retinal detachment. Curr. Opin. Ophthalmol. 16 (3), 175–178.

Sarrafizadeh, R., Hassan, T.S., Ruby, A.J., et al., 2001. Incidence of retinal detachment and visual outcome in eyes presenting with posterior vitreous separation and dense fundus-obscuring vitreous hemorrhage. Ophthalmology 108 (12), 2273–2278.

Sharma, M.C., Chan, P., Kim, R.U., et al., 2003. Rhegmatogenous retinal detachment in the fellow phakic eyes of patients with pseudophakic rhegmatogenous retinal detachment. Retina 23, 37–40.

Retinal Detachments Following Cataract Surgery

Alldredge, C.D., Elkins, B., Alldredge, O.C., 1998. Retinal detachment following phacoemulsification in highly myopic cataract patients. J. Cataract Refract. Surg. 24, 777–780.

Boberg-Ans, G., Villumsen, J., Henning, V., 2003. Retinal detachment after phacoemulsification cataract extraction. J. Cataract Refract. Surg. 29, 1333–1338.

Dalen, V., Le Pape, A., Heve, D., et al., 2015. Incidence, risk factors, and impact of age on retinal detachment after cataract surgery in France: A national population study. Ophthalmology 122 (11), 2179–2185.

Fan, D.S., Lam, D.S., Li, K.K., 1999. Retinal complications after cataract extraction in patients with high myopia. Ophthalmology 106, 688–691, discussion 691-692.

Nissen, K.R., Fuchs, J., Goldschmidt, E., et al., 1998. Retinal detachment after cataract extraction in myopic eyes. J. Cataract Refract. Surg. 24, 772–776.

Petousis, V., Sallam, A.A., Haynes, R.J., et al., 2016. Risk factors for retinal detachment following cataract surgery: the impact of posterior capsular rupture. Br. J. Ophthalmol. pii: bjophthalmol-2015-307729. doi: 10.1136/bjophthalmol-2015-307729. [Epub ahead of print]

Ranta, P., Tommila, P., Kivela, T., 2004. Retinal breaks and detachment after neodymium: YAG laser posterior capsulotomy: five-year incidence in a prospective cohort. J. Cataract Refract. Surg. 30 (1), 58–66.

Retinal Dialysis and Giant Retinal Tear (GRT)

Ambresin, A., Wolfensberger, T.J., Bovey, E.H., 2003. Management of giant retinal tears with vitrectomy, internal tamponade, and peripheral 360 degrees retinal photocoagulation. Retina 23, 622–628.

Brown, G.C., Benson, W.E., 1989. Use of sodium hyaluronate view drug information for the repair of giant retinal tears. Arch. Ophthalmol. 107, 1246–1249.

Gonzalez, M.A., Flynn, H.W., Jr., Smiddy, W.E., et al., 2013. Giant retinal tears after prior pars plana vitrectomy: management strategies and outcomes. Clin. Ophthalmol. 7, 1687–1691.

Gonzalez, M.A., Flynn, H.W., Jr., Smiddy, W.E., et al., 2013. Surgery for retinal detachment in patients with giant retinal tear etiologies, management strategies, and outcomes. Ophthalmic Surg. Lasers Imaging Retina 44 (3), 232–237.

Jain, N., Kozak, J.A., Niziol, L.M., et al., 2014. Vitrectomy alone in the management of giant retinal tears. Ophthalmic Surg. Lasers Imaging Retina 45 (5), 421–427.

Michels, R.G., Rice, T.A., Blankenship, G., 1983. Surgical techniques for selected giant retinal tears. Retina 3, 139–153.

Randolph, J.C., Diaz, R.I., Sigler, E.J., et al., 2016. 25-gauge pars plana vitrectomy with medium-term postoperative perfluoro-n-octane for the repair of giant retinal tears. Graefes Arch. Clin. Exp. Ophthalmol. 254 (2), 253–257.

Rofail, M., Lee, L.R., 2005. Perfluoro-n-octane as a postoperative vitreoretinal tamponade in the management of giant retinal tears. Retina 25, 897–901.

Scott, I.U., Murray, T.G., Flynn, H.W., Jr., et al., 2002. Outcomes and complications associated with giant retinal tear management using perfluoro-n-octane. Ophthalmology 109 (10), 1828–1833.

Sirimaharaj, M., Balachandran, C., Chan, W.C., et al., 2005. Vitrectomy with short term postoperative tamponade using perfluorocarbon liquid for giant retinal tears. Br. J. Ophthalmol. 89, 1176–1179.

Wolfensberger, T.J., Aylward, G.W., Leaver, P.K., 2003. Prophylactic 360 degrees cryotherapy in fellow eyes of patients with spontaneous giant retinal tears. Ophthalmology 110, 1175–1177.

Retinoschisis

Agarwal, A., Fan, S., Invernizzi, A., et al., 2016. Characterization of retinal structure and diagnosis of peripheral acquired retinoschisis using high-resolution ultrasound B-scan. Graefes Arch. Clin. Exp. Ophthalmol. 254, 69–75.

Byer, N.E., 2002. Perspectives on the management of the complications of senile retinoschisis. Eye (Lond.) 16, 359–364.

Byer, N.E., 2012. Perspectives on the management of the complications of senile retinoschisis. Eye (Lond.) 16, 359–364.

Giansanti, F., Bitossi, A., Giacomelli, G., et al., 2013. Acquired retinoschisis with giant outer layer break and retinal detachment. Eur. J. Ophthalmol. 23 (5), 761–763.

Yeoh, J., Rahman, W., Chen, F.K., et al., 2012. Use of spectral-domain optical coherence tomography to differentiate acquired retinoschisis from retinal detachment in difficult cases. Retina 32 (8), 1574–1580.

Optic Nerve Pit with Macular Schisis Detachment

Gass, J.D.M., 1969. Serous detachment of the macula secondary to congenital pit of the optic nerve head. Am. J. Ophthalmol. 67, 821–841.

Sugar, H.S., 1964. An explanation for the acquired macular pathology associated with congenital pits of the optic disc. Am. J. Ophthalmol. 57, 833–835.

Treatment of Retinal Detachment

Brucker, A.J., Hopkins, T.B., 2006. Retinal detachment surgery: the latest in current management. Retina 26, S28–S33.

Gorovoy, I.R., Porco, T.C., Bhisitkul, R.B., et al., 2014. Same-day versus next-day repair of fovea-threatening primary rhegmatogenous retinal detachments. Semin. Ophthalmol. 21, 1–7.

Kreissig, I., 2000. A Practical Guide to Minimal Surgery for Retinal Detachment, vol. 1: Diagnostics, Segmental Buckling Without Drainage, Case Presentations. Thieme Medical Publishers, New York, pp. 94–122.

Mastropasqua, L., Carpineto, P., Ciancaglini, M., et al., 1999. Treatment of retinal tears and lattice degenerations in fellow eyes in high risk patients suffering retinal detachment: a prospective study. Br. J. Ophthalmol. 83, 1046–1049.

Sudarsky, R.D., Yannuzzi, L.A., 1970. Cryomarcation line and pigment migration after retinal cryosurgery. Arch. Ophthalmol. 83, 395–401.

Vrabec, T.R., Baumal, C.R., 2000. Demarcation laser photocoagulation of selected macula-sparing rhegmatogenous retinal detachments. Ophthalmology 107, 1063–1067.

Wilkinson, C.P., 2000. Evidence-based analysis of prophylactic treatment of asymptomatic retinal breaks and lattice degeneration. Ophthalmology 107 (1), 12–15, discussion 15-8.

CHAPTER 12

Traumatic Chorioretinopathy

Direct Ocular Injury (Nonpenetrating and/or Nonperforating)

Berlin's Edema (Commotio Retinae)

Berlin's edema or so-called commotio retinae is a zonal area of retinal whitening due to outer photoreceptor disruption and retinal pigment epithelial damage from blunt trauma that has led to edema of all retinal layers. There are no intraretinal cystic changes or bleeding in this form of trauma. It is believed that the mechanism is external force transmitted through the vitreous to the chorioretinal area, which induces outer retinal ischemia. These changes gradually resolve spontaneously but can cause late pigment atrophy.

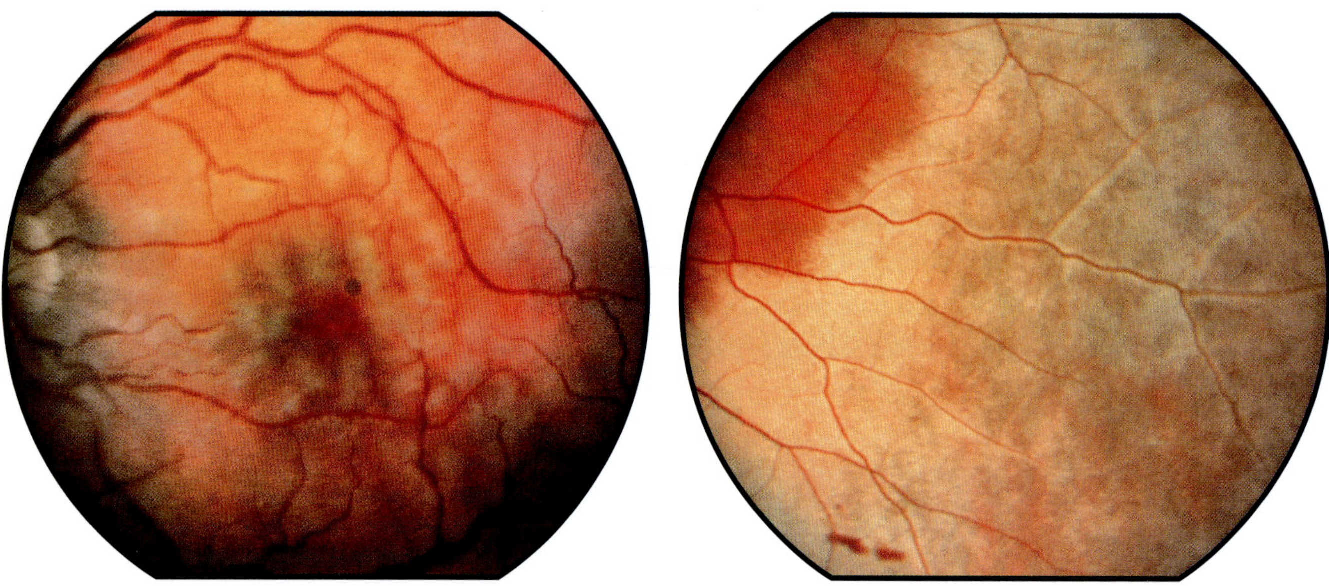

Berlin's edema (commotio retinae) was caused by severe blunt trauma in these patients. The typical outer retinal whitening is shown. It is hypothesized that the blunt trauma has a compressive effect on the inner choroid, which produces outer retinal ischemia or even infarction.

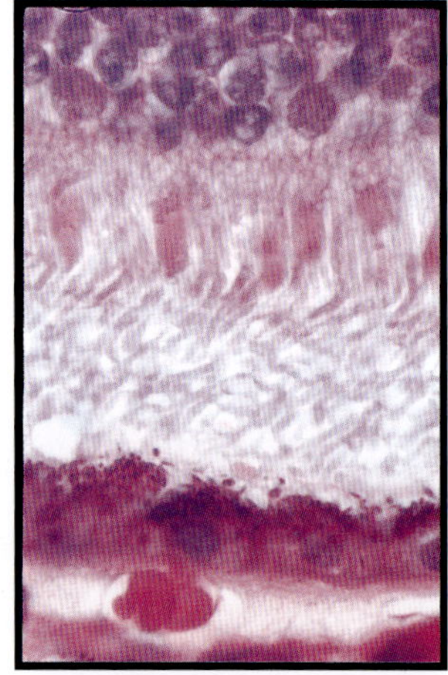

© 748

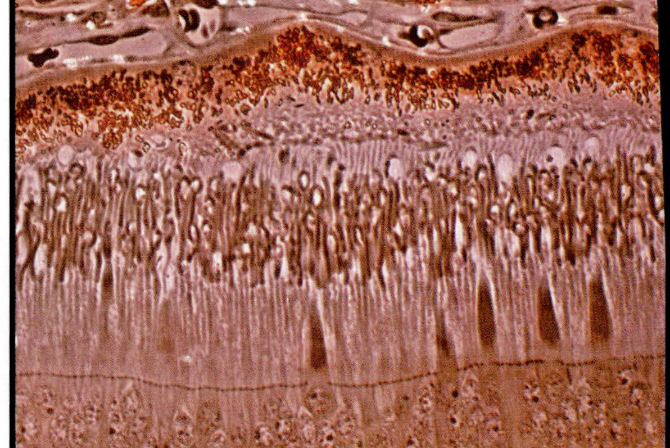

© 749

Microscopically, Berlin's edema (commotio retinae) results in disruption of the outer segments of the photoreceptors. Later, fluid may collect in the outer layers of the retina. When the edema subsides, there may be retinal pigment epithelial degeneration and cystoid retinal degeneration. Coalescence of cystoid areas may produce a large cyst or a macular hole. Visual recovery is uncertain, especially if the macula is involved.

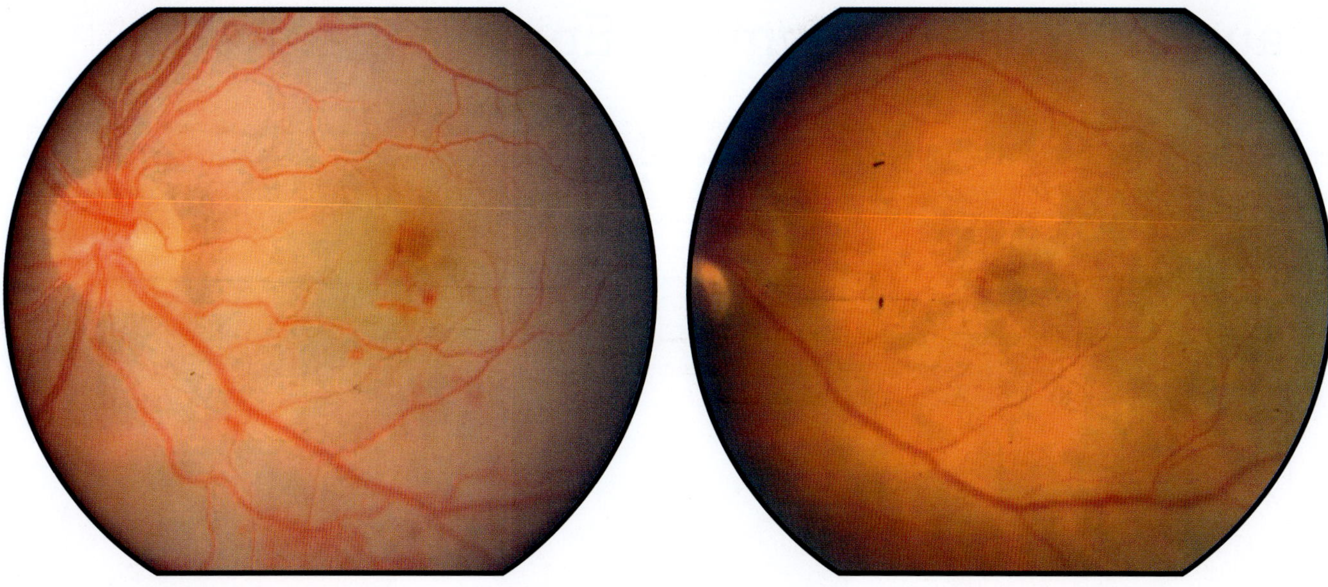

This patient was involved in a motor vehicle accident during which time the air bag deployed. Acute commotio retinae developed along with mild macular hemorrhage OS (*left image*). Over the next two months, there was gradual development of macular pigment mottling (*right image*), though vision recovered to 20/40 OS.

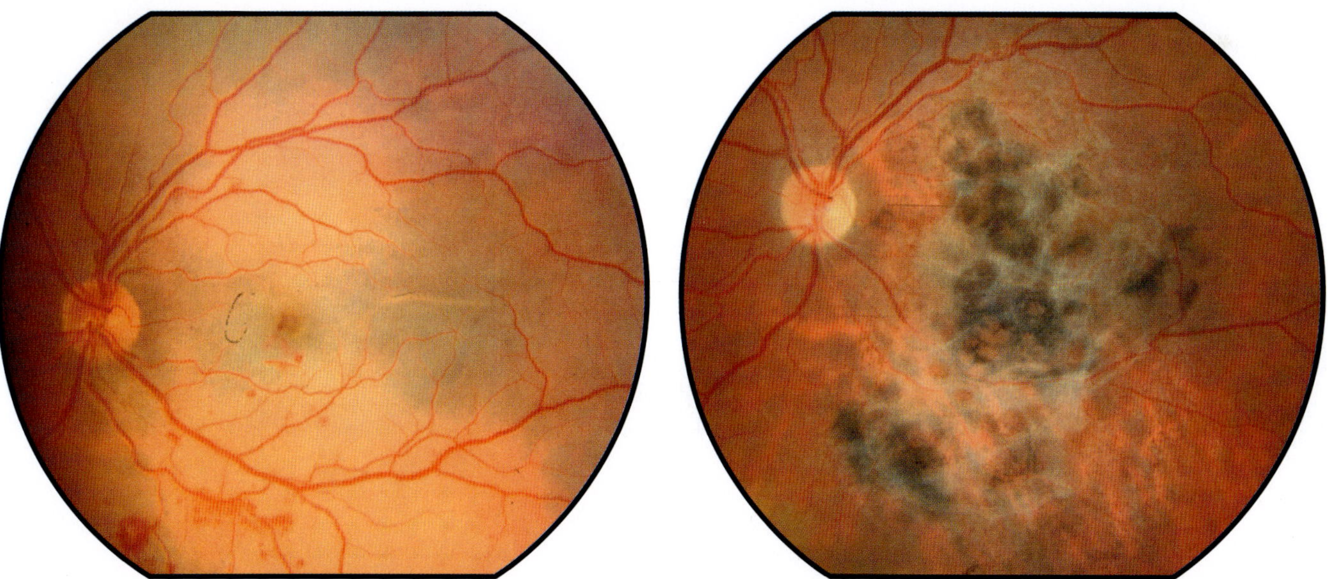

A hockey player sustained a hockey stick injury to his left eye with resultant acute retinal whitening and scattered intraretinal hemorrhages. Two months later, significant reactive hyperplastic pigmentary change developed, which resulted in permanent visual loss.

Traumatic Retinal Pigment Epitheliopathy

Traumatic retinal pigment epitheliopathy may be predominantly atrophic, pigmentary, or fibrotic in nature. Eyes with minimal pigmentation, such as blue eyes, will tend to develop atrophy, while eyes with significant pigmentation in the pigment epithelium and choroid tend to develop hyperpigmentation. Depending on the extent of the trauma, any eye can develop fibrous degeneration.

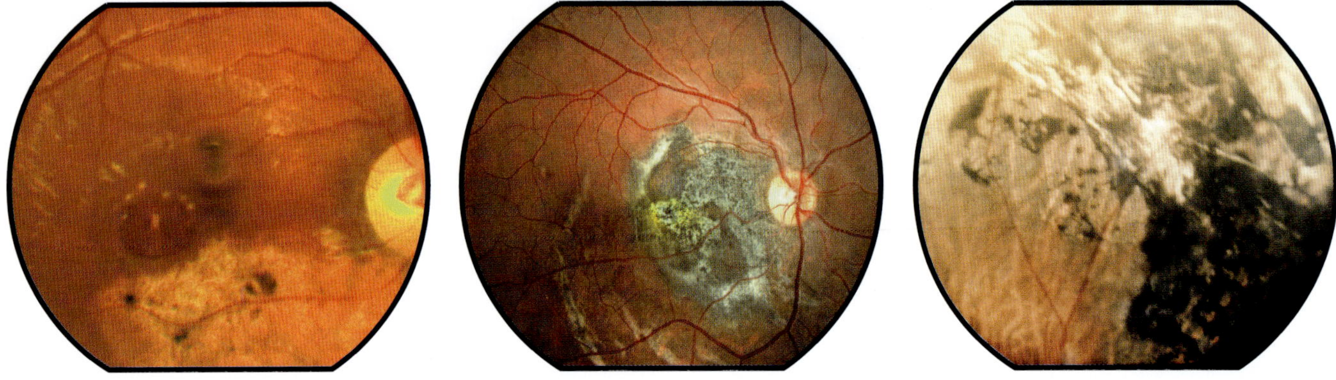

These patients depict the different manifestations of traumatic retinal pigment epitheliopathy. The patient on the left is predominantly atrophic, the one in the middle exhibits pigment epithelial hyperplasia and fibrous metaplasia, and the patient on the right has diffuse severe atrophy, hyperpigmentation, and fibrous scarring. *Right image courtesy of Dr. Howard Schatz*

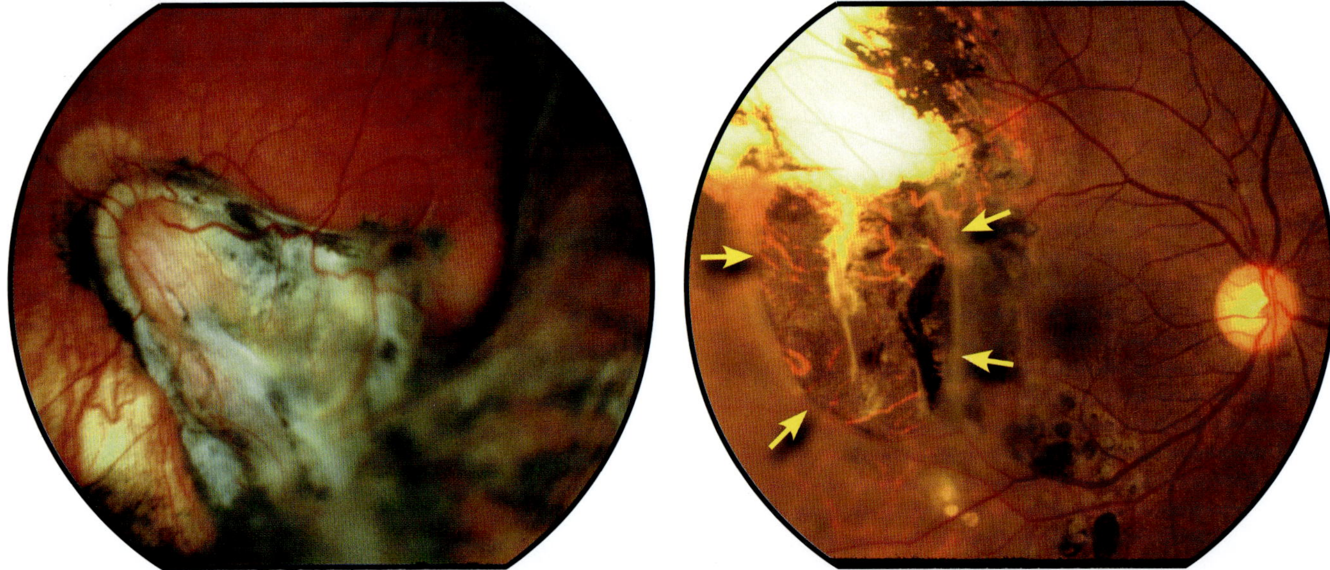

These images are from two professional boxers who sustained ocular injuries from the thumbs of the boxing glove, when they were hit in the eye. The left image shows extensive fibrovascular and pigmentary scarring. In the image on the right, there are areas of atrophy, hyperpigmentation, and fibrosis contiguous with a large retinal break in the temporal macula *(arrows)*. Despite the presence of field loss, the macula was spared and the visual acuity was good, making it possible for the boxer to pass a routine vision test prior to his next bout. The extent of his pathology was detected while he was participating in an ocular boxing complications study. The bout was canceled and the retina was repaired.

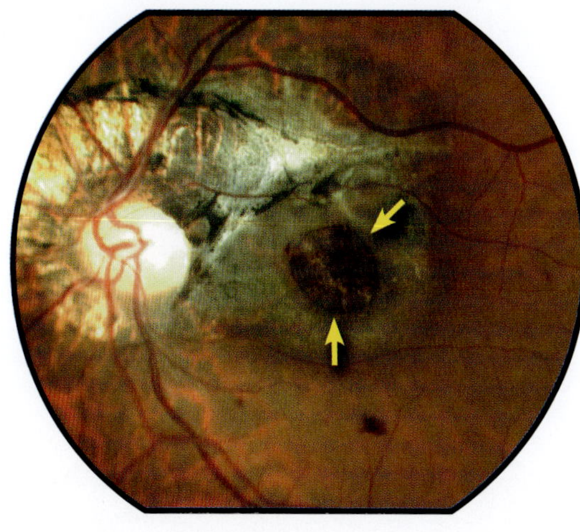

This patient experienced a paintball injury. There is optic nerve atrophy, peripapillary atrophy surrounded by fibro-pigmentary degeneration, and a large macular hole *(arrows)*. This case depicts multiple manifestations of blunt posterior segment trauma.

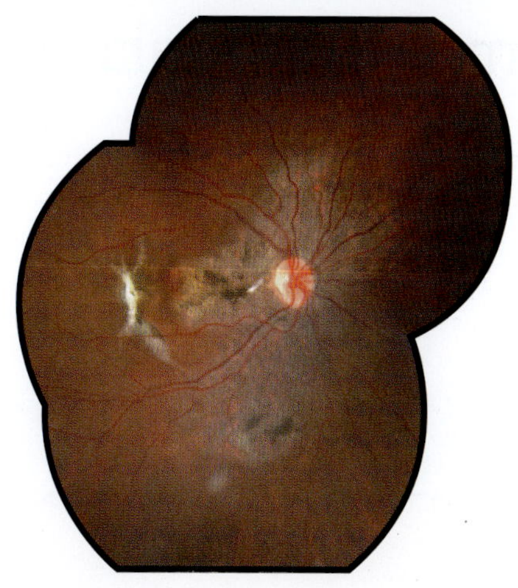

This patient sustained blunt trauma from a bungee cord. He was on anticoagulation medication, which exacerbated the subretinal hemorrhage. Widespread retinal pigment epitheliopathy and a fibrotic choroidal rupture resulted from the injury.

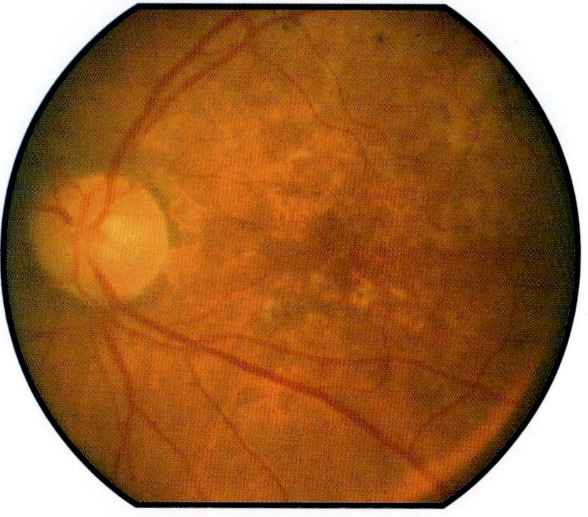

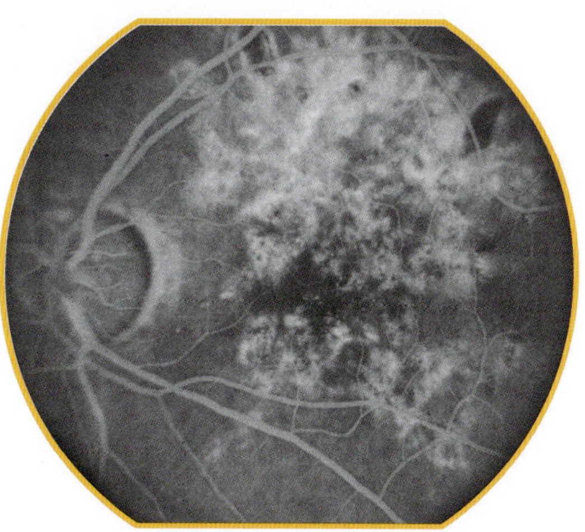

This patient was involved in an altercation, and was struck in the eye with a wooden board. Extensive pigment mottling throughout the posterior pole ensued *(left)*, and the pigmentary changes were highlighted on a fluorescein angiogram *(right)*. Visual acuity was 20/200 in this traumatized eye.

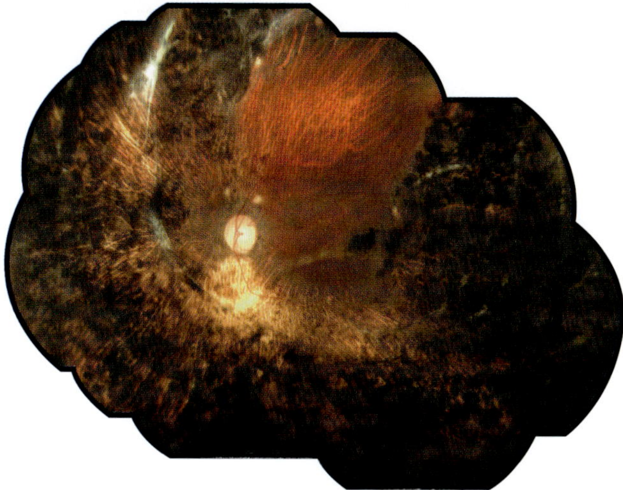

This patient was struck in the eye with a beer bottle. A huge detachment resulted, which left widespread retinal pigmentary epithelial proliferation and atrophy. There was also a band of fibrotic scarring in the supranasal hemisphere and optic atrophy. Only a small area of superior peripheral retina remains relatively intact.

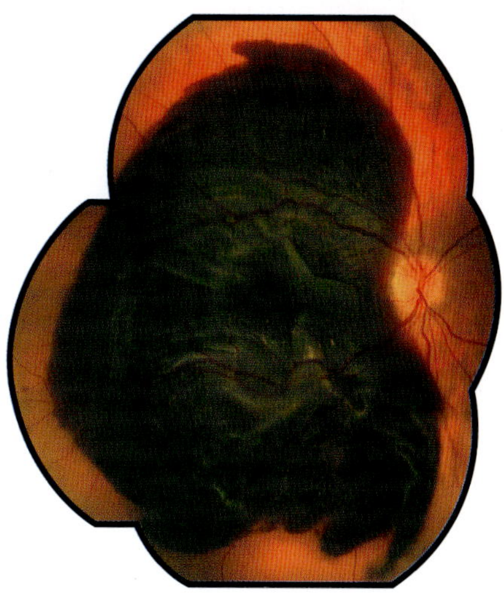

This patient sustained relatively minor blunt trauma in a car accident, but was on anticoagulation medication, which likely contributed to the severe hemorrhage as seen in the photograph. She presented with a huge subretinal hemorrhage and a shallow but discernible retinal detachment with folds.

Traumatic Macular Hole

Ocular trauma quite often results in a macular hole, particularly because the avascularity of the region may predispose a hole to form after a variety of insults. It is often accompanied by other chorioretinal injuries, including commotio retinae, choroidal rupture, and traumatic retinal pigment epitheliopathy. It may occur days to years post-injury. Trauma from a laser or lightning strike has also induced macular holes. While traumatic macular holes may close spontaneously, treatment generally involves the need for vitrectomy surgery with intraocular gas tamponade, and post-operative face-down positioning. The anatomic closure rate is quite comparable to idiopathic age-acquired macular holes, yet visual recovery may be limited due to the holes often being somewhat larger in size.

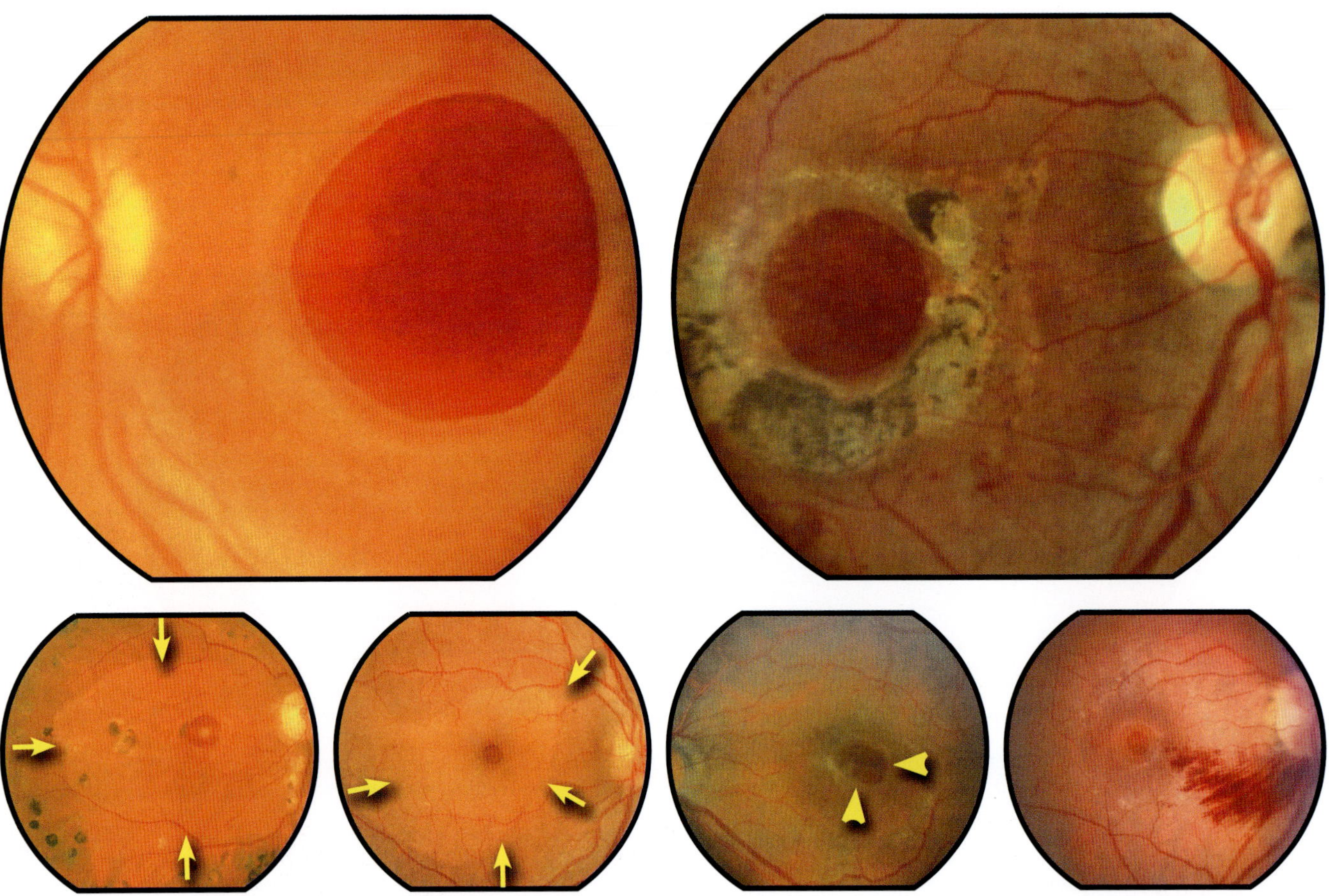

These patients sustained severe trauma and developed macular holes. The hole may be very large, as seen above *(upper left)* and result in a variable reduction in visual acuity, which generally ranges from 20/40 to 20/400. It may be bordered by signs of traumatic pigment epitheliopathy *(upper right)*. Traumatic holes may also result in posterior retinal detachment *(arrows)*, as seen in the two cases on the lower left. Additional traumatic manifestations may be seen with macular holes, as noted by the fibrosis *(arrowheads)* and retinal hemorrhage from a boxing injury *(lower right)*.

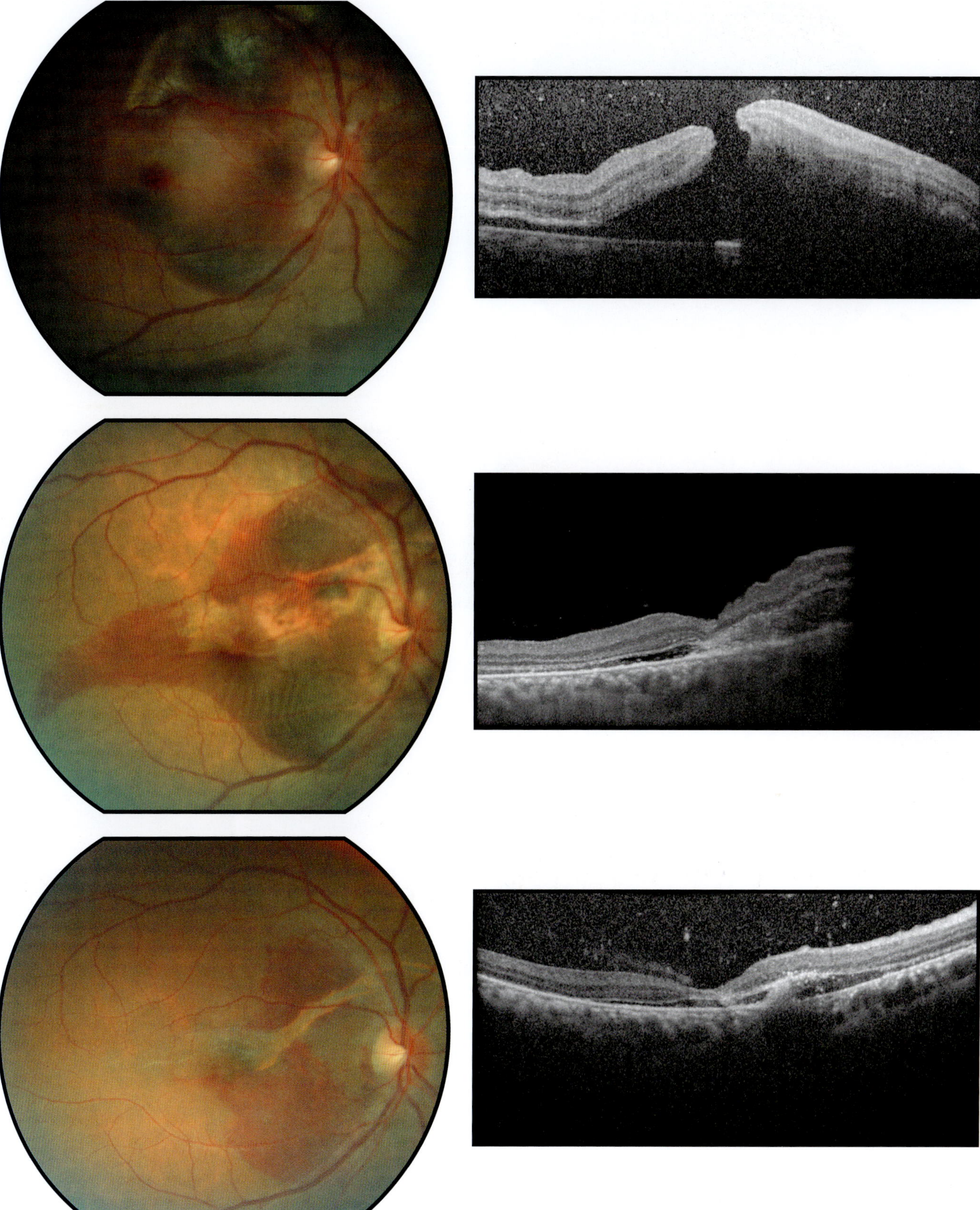

This patient sustained severe blunt trauma to the eye when struck with a piece of metal at work. While there was no open-globe injury, there was extensive submacular hemorrhage (*top left*) and a full-thickness macular hole (*top right*). There was also a peripheral retinal dialysis, which was demarcated by photocoagulation. At one week of follow-up, there was partial resolution of the subretinal hemorrhage (*middle left*), and the macular hole spontaneously closed (*middle right*). By three weeks, more of the hemorrhage cleared, a choroidal rupture became apparent (*bottom left*), and the macular hole remained closed (*bottom right*). Visual acuity improved from hand motions to 20/200 in the traumatized eye.

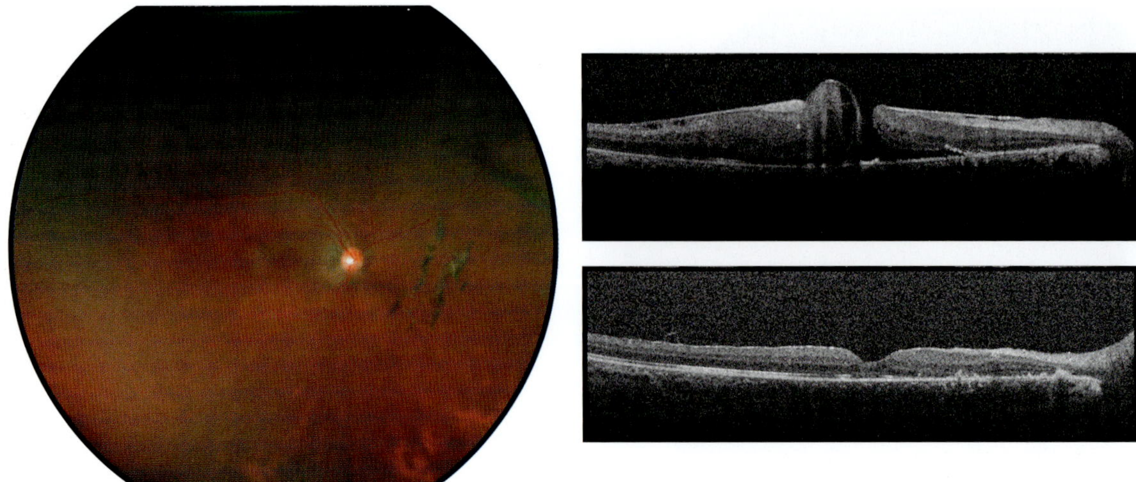

A traumatic injury led to a full-thickness macular hole (*left*) and several nasal concentric choroidal ruptures. A baseline SD-OCT documented the full-thickness macular hole (*upper right*). Following vitrectomy surgery, the hole remained successfully closed (*lower right*).

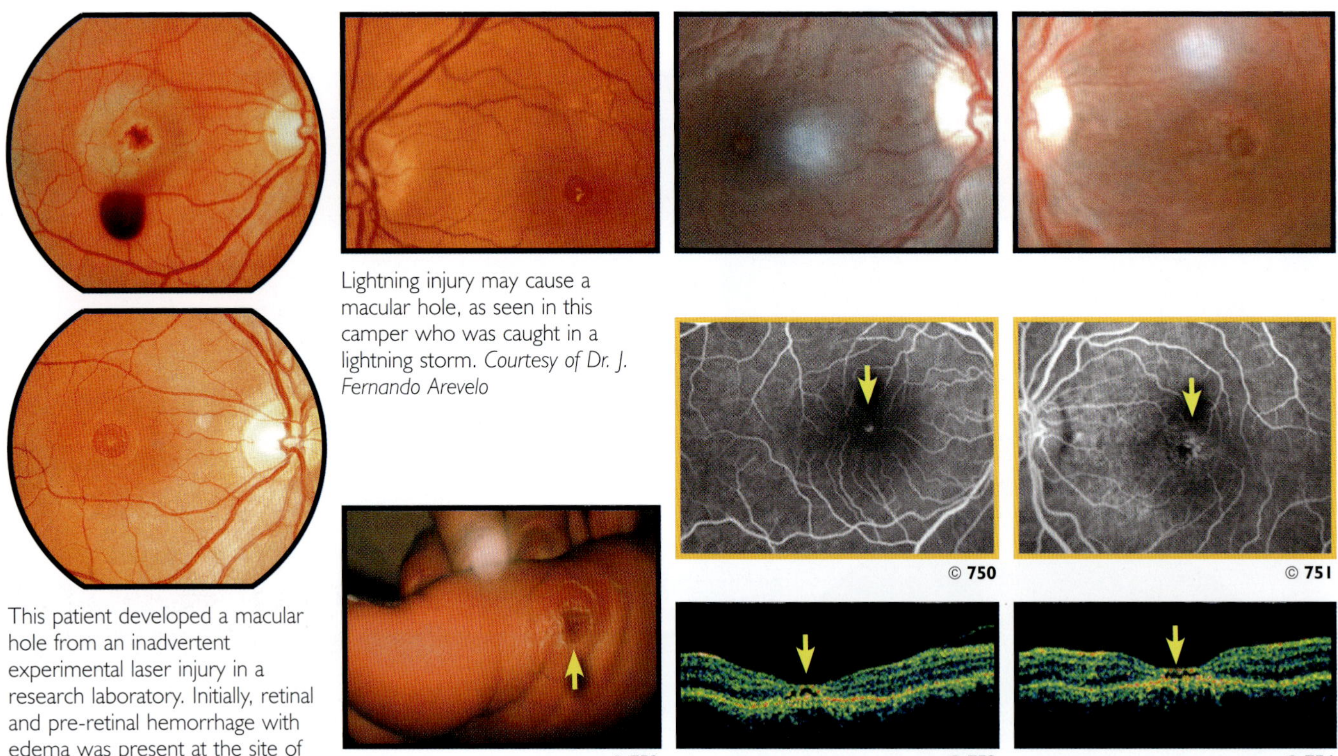

This patient developed a macular hole from an inadvertent experimental laser injury in a research laboratory. Initially, retinal and pre-retinal hemorrhage with edema was present at the site of the injury. Following resolution of the blood and exudate, the patient was noted to have a macular hole *(lower image). Courtesy of Dr. Donald Frambach*

Lightning injury may cause a macular hole, as seen in this camper who was caught in a lightning storm. *Courtesy of Dr. J. Fernando Arevelo*

© 750 © 751 © 752 © 753 © 754

This young child developed lightning-induced macular holes in both eyes after sleeping on the ground in a copper-cement dwelling during a lightning storm. The resolving holes have already evolved into macular cysts bilaterally, as seen on the optical coherence tomography (OCT) images. The entry site on her foot is also evident as an ulcer *(arrow). Courtesy of Dr. J. Fernando Arevelo*

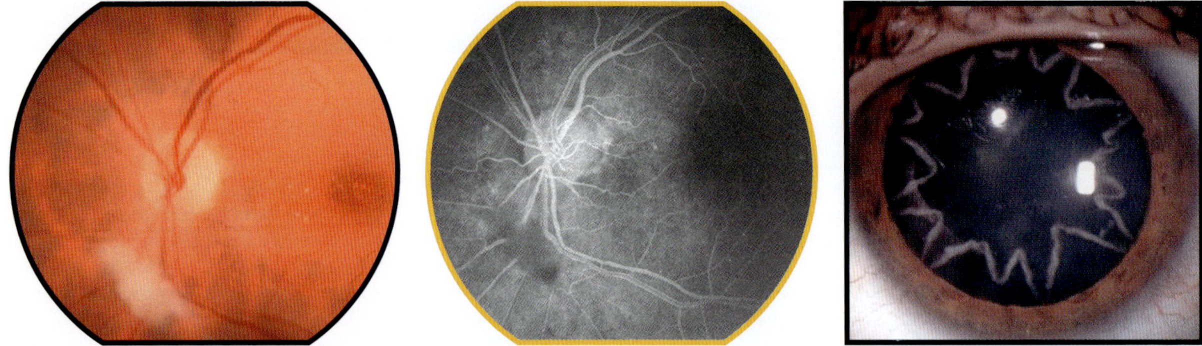

This patient inadvertently sustained a high voltage electrical injury. He developed a full-thickness macular hole *(left and middle)*, along with lenticular peripheral cortical opacities *(right). Courtesy of Michael Goldbaum, MD*

Choroidal Rupture

One or more choroidal ruptures may occur in association with blunt ocular trauma. A choroidal rupture is often associated with uveal and retinal pigment epithelial breaks and most commonly manifests as a white curvilinear streak concentric to the optic nerve temporally, but may have any morphological pattern or location and can even crisscross when multiple breaks occur. The choroid is quite susceptible to energy that gets imparted into the eye and/or orbit in association with an injury. Hemorrhage at the time of injury is common and secondary choroidal neovascularization may develop months to years post-injury, which can result in fibrotic scarring. Other manifestations of trauma are commonly seen in conjunction with a choroidal rupture.

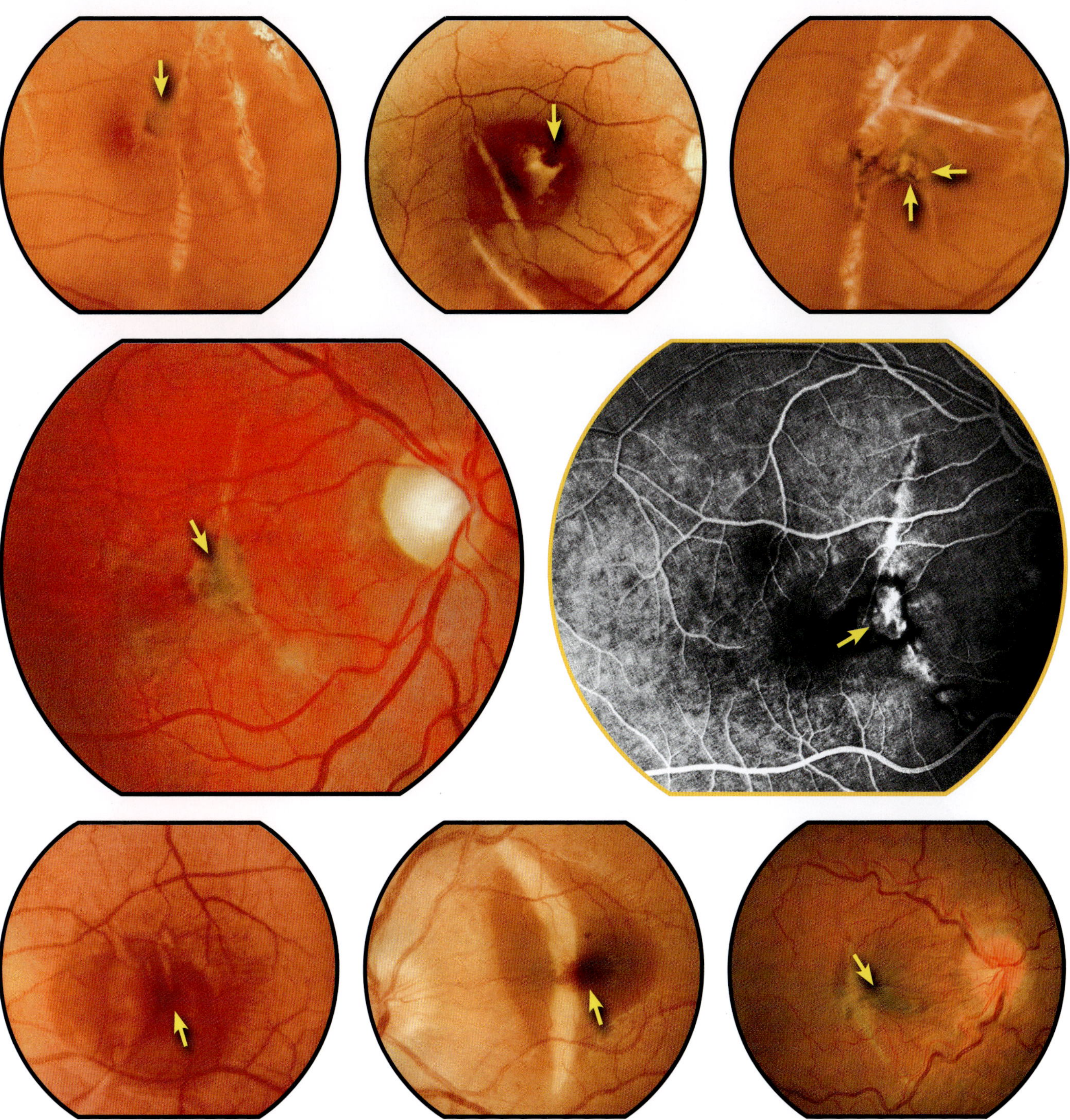

The images shown here are examples of choroidal ruptures following ocular trauma. When there is delayed hemorrhage, there is likely to be choroidal neovascularization *(arrows)*. The fluorescein angiogram *(middle row, right)* reveals actively proliferating blood vessels within a neovascular complex as well as staining of the choroidal rupture where fibrous vascular proliferation has filled the uveal pigmentary defect.

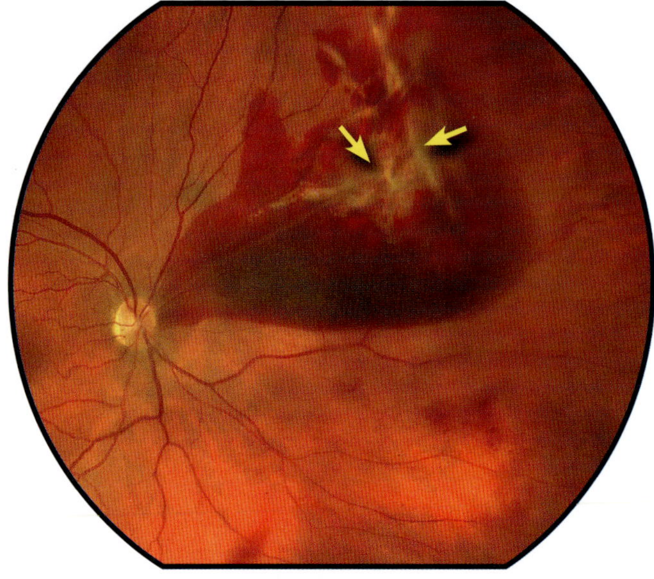

The photograph shows multiple crisscrossing choroidal ruptures *(arrows)* in the supero-temporal paramacular and mid-peripheral region. There is also severe pre-retinal hemorrhage from the trauma.

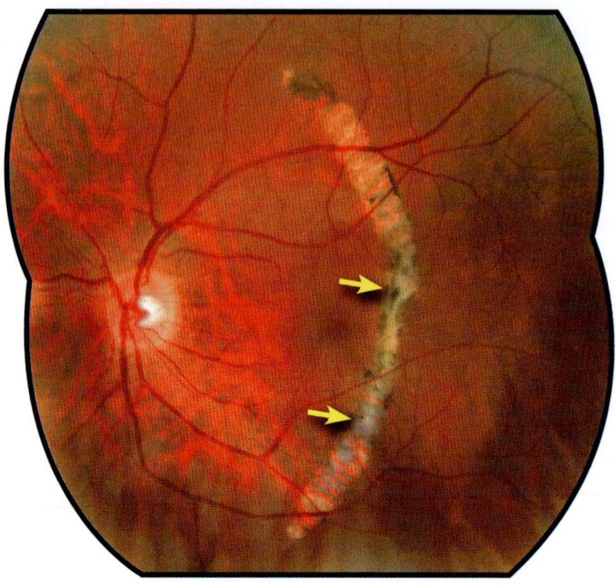

This patient experienced a choroidal rupture curvilinear to the optic nerve, a typical feature of this form of trauma. The superior and inferior sections of the rupture are atrophic in nature with choroidal vessels visible within the lesion. The middle of the rupture contains fibrovascular scarring *(arrows)*, which also occurs in this injury.

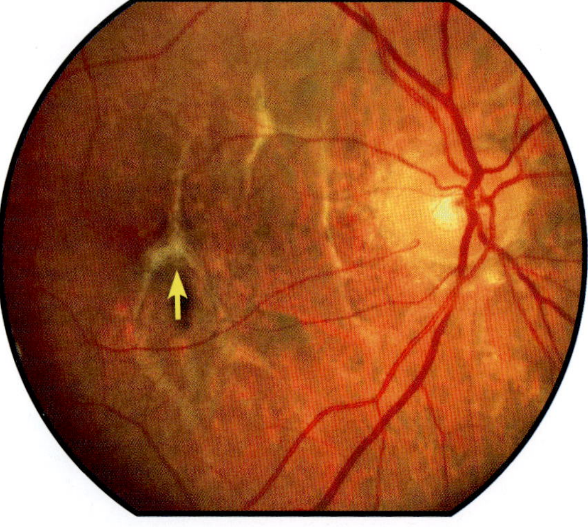

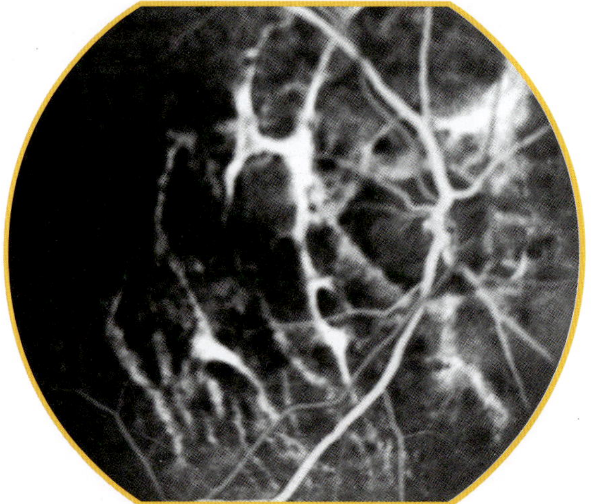

This patient has pseudoxanthoma elasticum (PXE). He experienced blunt trauma and developed multiple choroidal ruptures due to the fragility of the uveal scleral tissue in these patients. The ruptures are especially prominent on fluorescein angiogram *(right)*, with staining of the fibrovascular scar. Secondary choroidal neovascularization *(arrow)* is seen bridging the choroidal ruptures. *Courtesy of Dr. Howard Schatz*

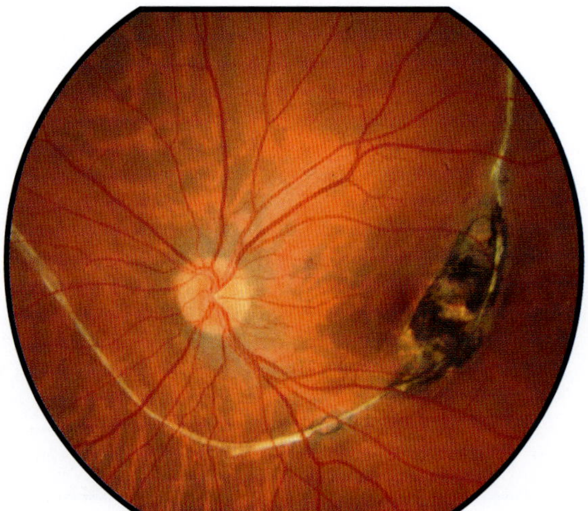

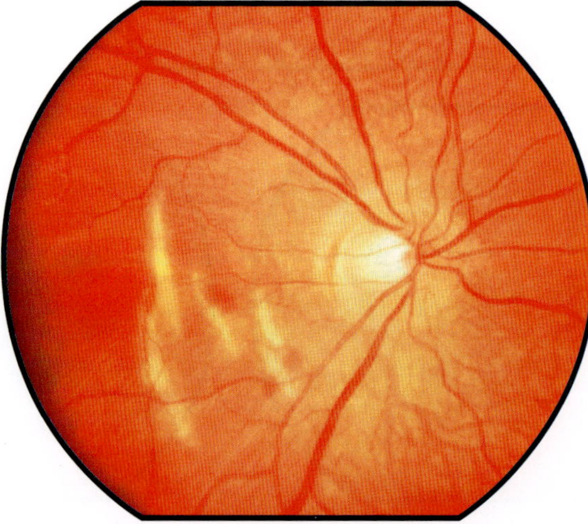

These patients illustrate the phenotypic variability of choroidal ruptures. The first patient sustained a single, large rupture curvilinear to the optic nerve, which is almost completely encircling the nerve *(left)*. The other patient, on the right, has multiple small ruptures curvilinear and concentric to the optic nerve.

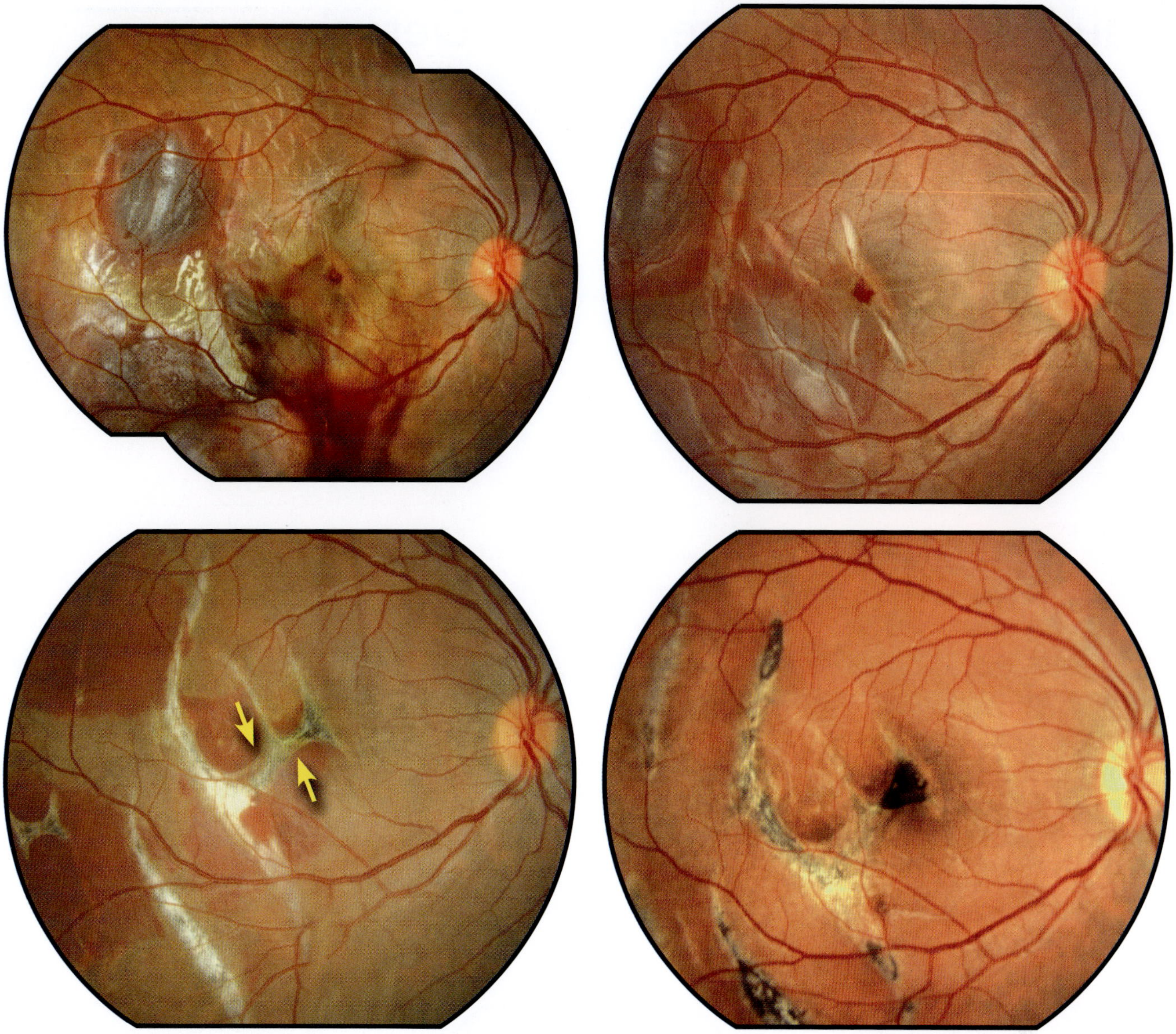

These images are a sequential series of photos taken of one patient who sustained severe trauma that resulted in multiple choroidal ruptures with intraretinal hemorrhage. The acute injury is seen in the upper left image. As the hemorrhage clears, the choroidal ruptures become more visible *(upper right)*. The patient then developed choroidal neovascularization with secondary hemorrhage *(arrows, lower left)*. The proliferating neovascularization is seen bridging adjacent ruptures. As the scars evolve, the ruptures assume a cicatricial or fibrovascular nature with hyperpigmentation *(lower right)*.

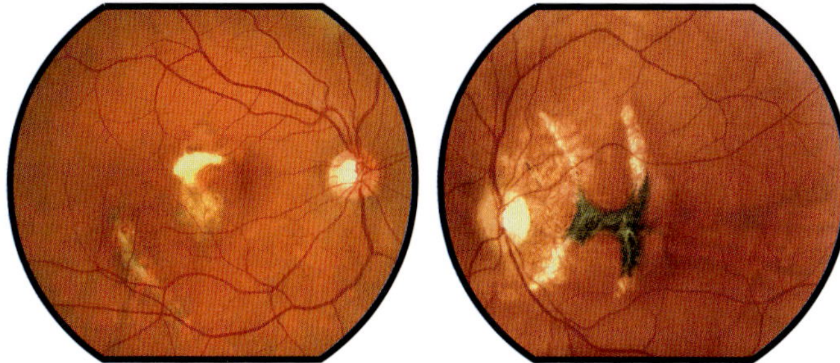

These two patients demonstrate the variability in the healed scar of a choroidal rupture. The patient on the left has a granular ovoid scar in the fovea and a fibrotic choroidal rupture in the inferotemporal paramacular region. There is also deposition of fibrotic tissue in the superior juxtafoveal area. The patient on the right has two curvilinear choroidal ruptures, with one vertically oriented through the fovea. Secondary choroidal neovascularization developed with heavy pigment epithelial hyperplasia enveloping the neovascularization. There is also pigment epithelial atrophy of the juxtapapillary and papillomacular bundles.

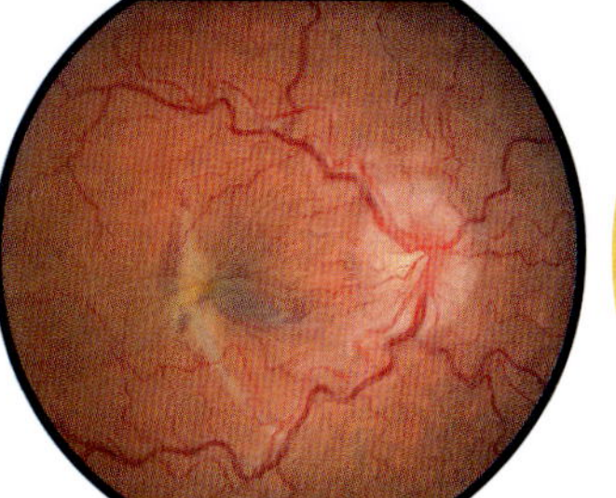

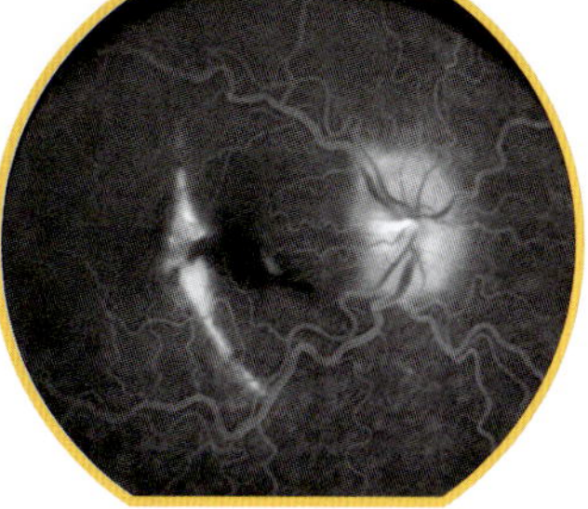

This patient sustained severe trauma and developed a choroidal rupture with hemorrhage. He subsequently developed hypotony from chronically low intraocular pressure, as evidenced by prominent retinal vasculature and staining of the peripapillary area on fluorescein angiography.

Traumatic Retinal Breaks and Detachments

Trauma often leads to retinal breaks and detachment. Trauma generally involves younger, male patients in their second to third decade of life. In the setting of objective findings in association with ocular or periocular trauma (lid ecchymoses, etc.), the risk of retinal detachment is substantially increased. Detachments generally occur within two years of the traumatic event, and in most cases, within three months. Retinal dialysis is most common, and predominantly is located inferotemporally or superotemporally, but giant retinal tears and atypically shaped posterior horseshoe retinal tears are also seen. Very often these rhegmatogenous changes are seen in conjunction with other traumatic manifestations in the fundus. These injuries often lead to the need for scleral buckle and/or pars plana vitrectomy surgery to repair the damage.

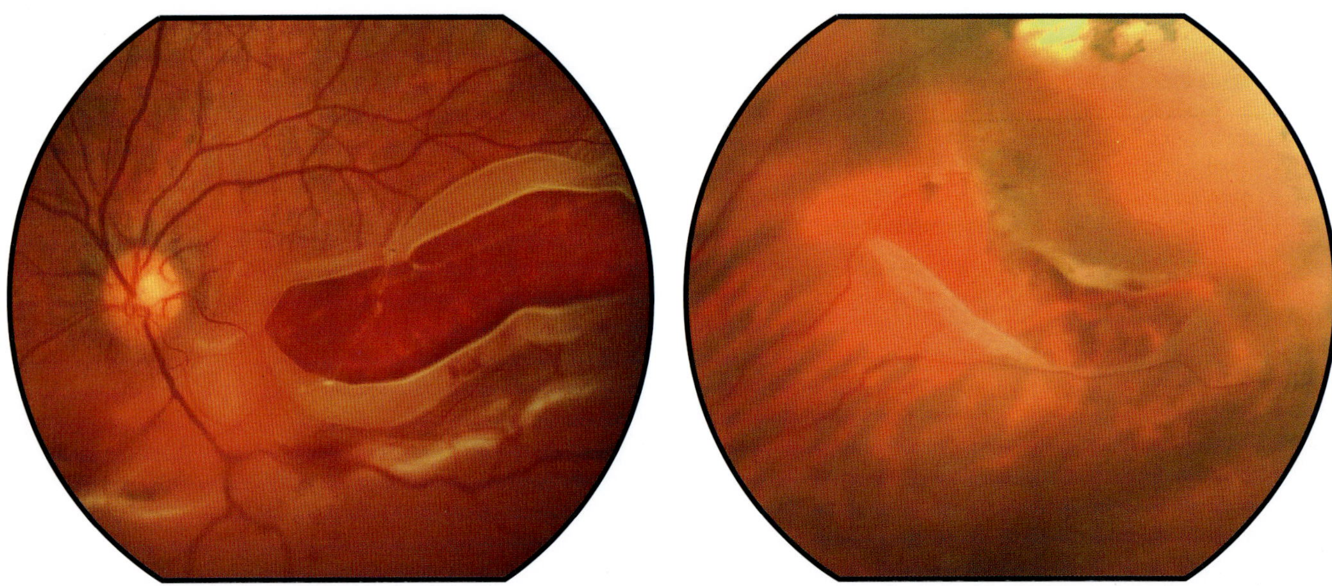

These images are examples of traumatically induced posteriorly located retinal breaks and detachments. As seen here, these tears may be very large with everted or rolled edges and there may be surrounding retinal detachment and associated vitreous hemorrhage. *Left image courtesy of Chris Barry, MD*

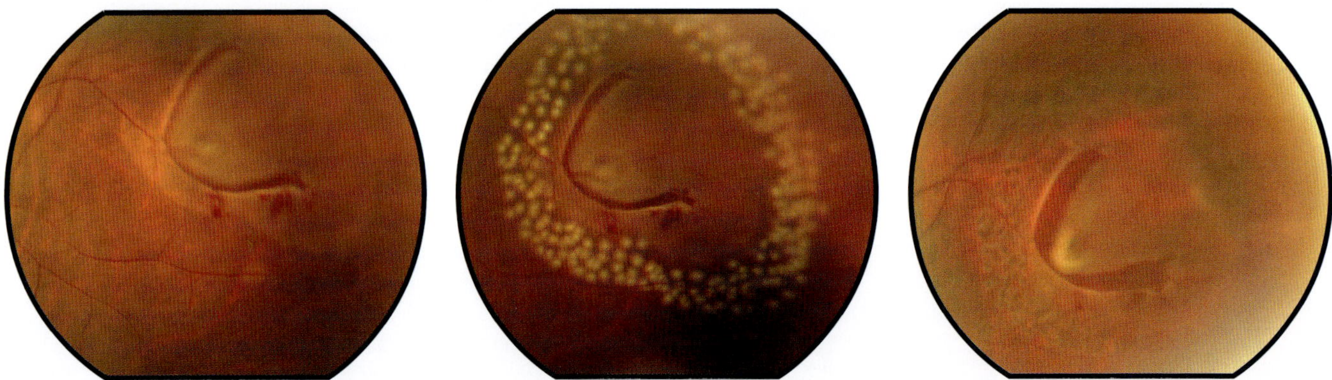

This is a traumatic retinal break *(left)* that was subsequently demarcated with a triple-row of photocoagulation *(middle)*. As the photocoagulation heals, there is a resultant pigmented, atrophic appearance *(right)*.

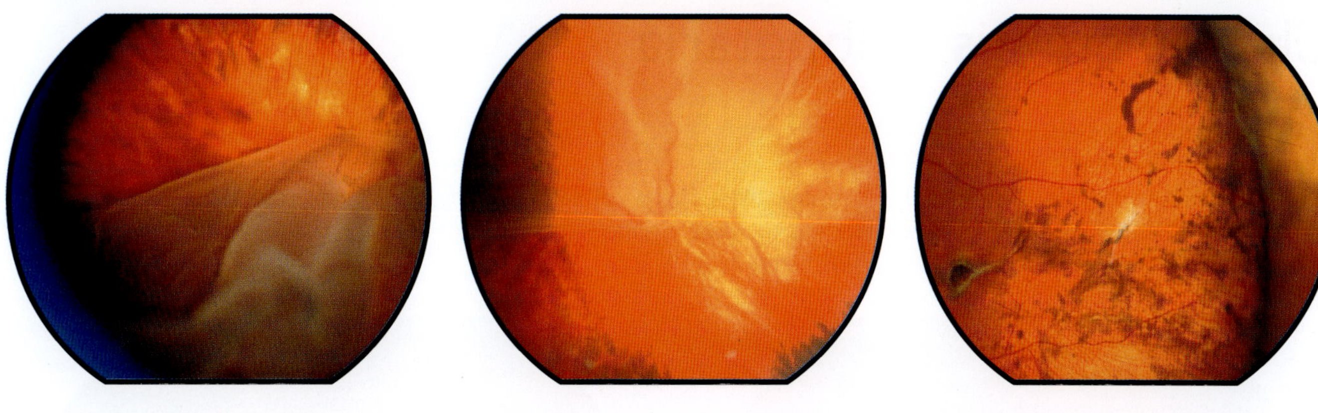

A patient *(left)* sustained a 210 degree giant retinal tear and detachment after being involved in an altercation at a nightclub. Bare retinal pigment epithelium is seen superiorly, with the redundant retina being folded upon itself inferiorly. The retina was repaired via a pars plana vitrectomy approach. A second operation was subsequently required following development of a recurrent retinal detachment with proliferative vitreoretinopathy (PVR). Another patient *(middle)* developed a 270 degree traumatic giant retinal tear and detachment after being involved in a motor vehicle accident and striking his head against the windshield. The detachment was repaired via a scleral buckle and pars plana vitrectomy *(right)*. Anatomically, the patient did well, though vision was limited to 20/100 by a small macular fibrotic scar adjacent to the macula.

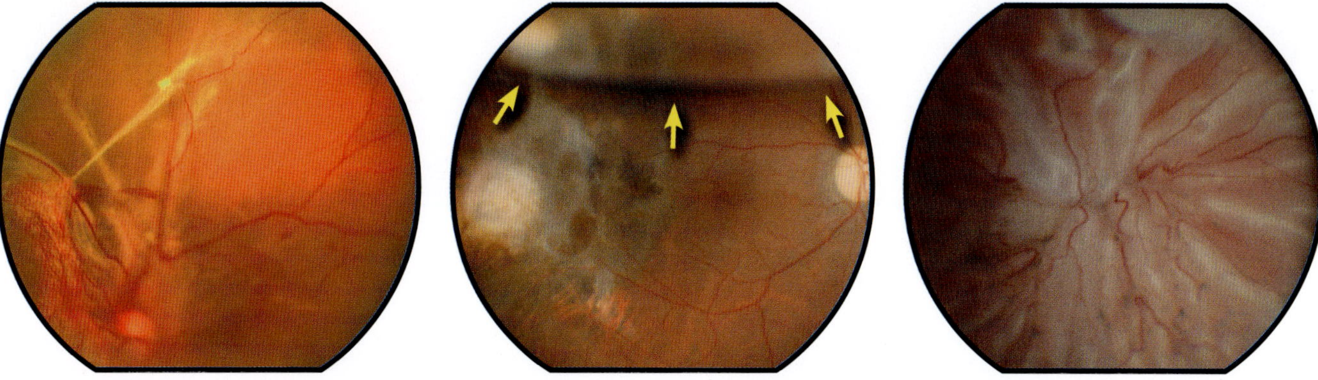

Severe trauma may lead to retinal detachment with pre- and subretinal fibrous proliferation. In the left image, note the band of fibrous tissue inducing traction. The middle image shows an eye that has undergone a retinal re-attachment procedure with injection of air *(arrows)*. Considerable pigmentary and fibrous tissue proliferation from the trauma is noted. In the right image, the patient developed advanced PVR following a traumatic retinal detachment and required further pars plana vitrectomy surgery for stabilization.

Chorioretinitis Sclopetaria

Chorioretinitis sclopetaria is due to the simultaneous rupture of the retina and the choroid from a glancing nonpenetrating high velocity missile to the orbit, such as a bullet or a BB gun. Acutely, there is usually vitreous hemorrhage with extensive retinal and choroidal hemorrhage and widespread retinal necrosis. As the hemorrhage clears, claw-like breaks in Bruch membrane and the choriocapillaris become visible, with late-onset widespread pigmentary disturbances and varying degrees of glial proliferation. By definition, the globe is not ruptured.

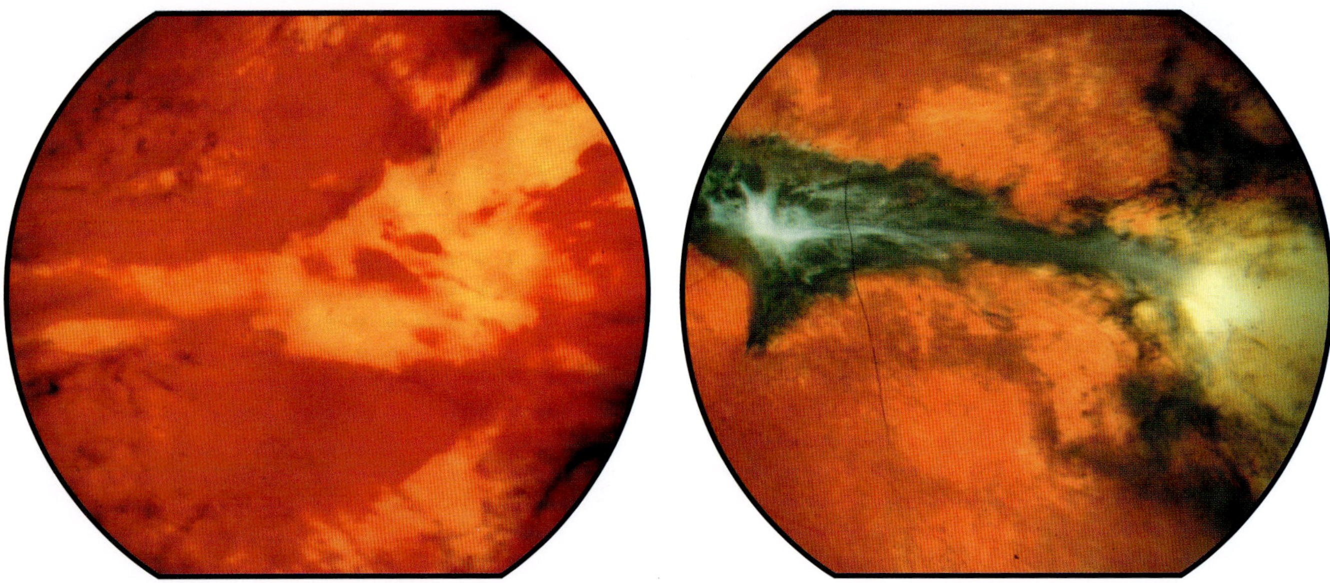

This patient developed chorioretinitis sclopetaria from a bullet injury to the left orbit. Hemorrhage involved all layers of the choroid and retina *(left)*. After three months, the hemorrhages cleared, though the involved areas developed fibrotic scarring and atrophy. While the globe remained intact, the vision only improved to hand motions.

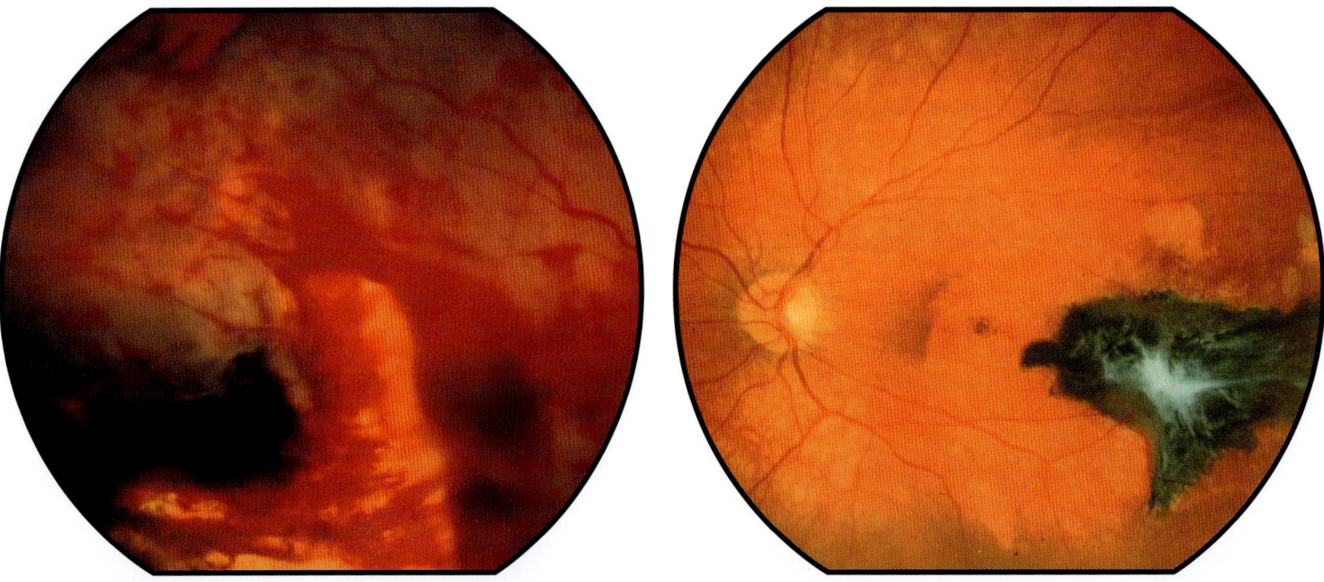

Extensive vitreous and retinal hemorrhage developed in a patient who sustained a gunshot wound to the left orbit *(left)*. Four months later, pigment atrophy was seen in the macular region, along with fibrotic scarring further temporally. Vision was counting fingers.

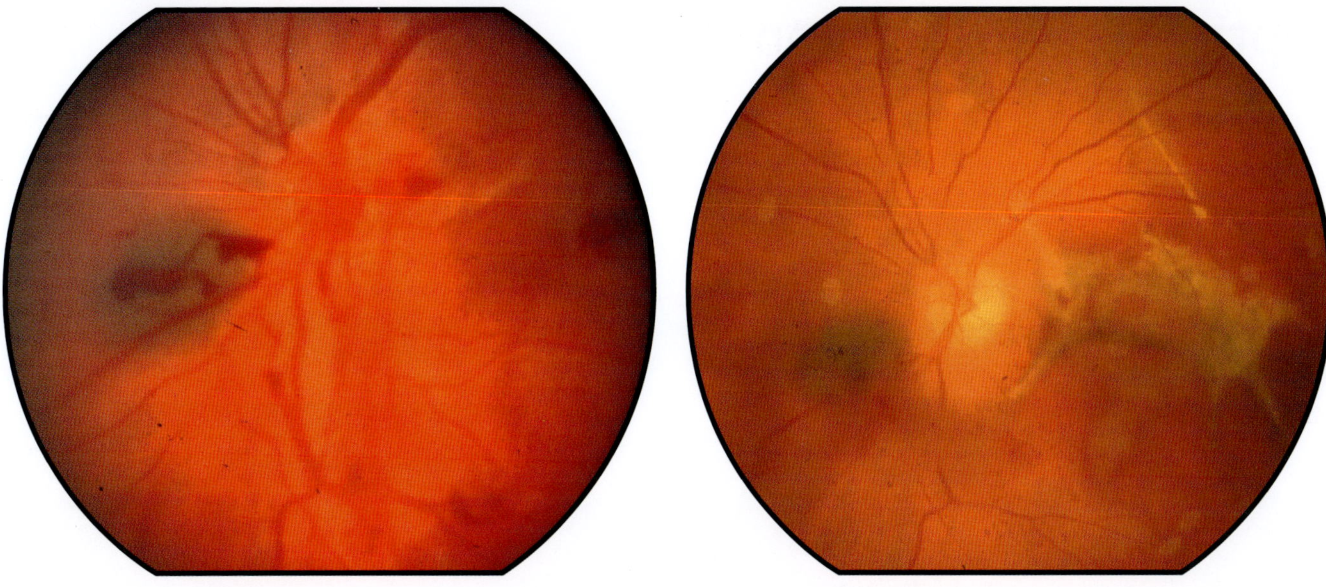

This patient sustained a bullet injury to the left orbit with resultant extensive retinal, subretinal, and vitreous hemorrhage *(left)*. Three months later, the hemorrhages had partially cleared, though vision was limited permanently by development of macular fibrotic scaring *(right)*.

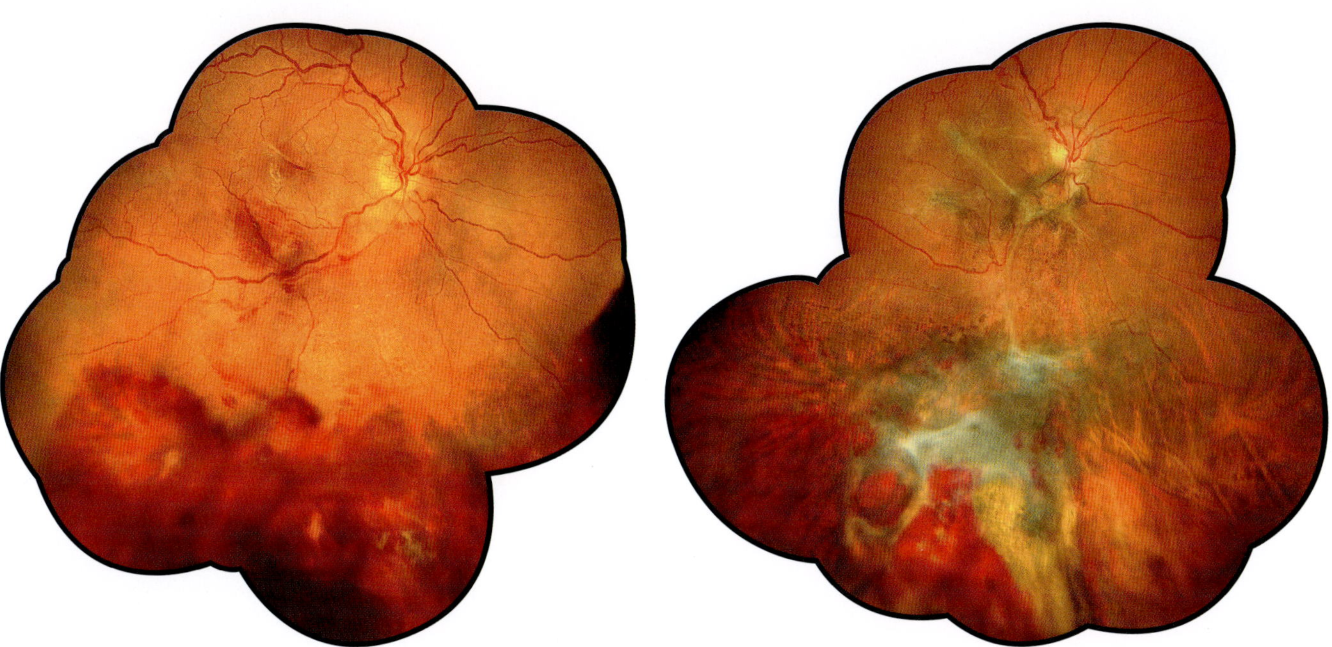

This patient sustained a BB gun injury, which entered the orbit, though did not cause rupture of the globe. The missile produced substantial intraretinal hemorrhage inferiorly, along with disorganization of the retina. Eventually, pigmentary degeneration ensued, along with widespread fibrotic scarring throughout the retina *(right)*.

Optic Nerve Avulsion

Optic nerve avulsion is a coup-contrecoup type injury where the optic nerve is forcibly disinserted from the eye, and the lamina cribrosa is retracted from the scleral rim. It is often accompanied by severe damage to other ocular tissues. However, it may also be the sole manifestation of apparently minor trauma. Patients usually present with symptoms ranging from immediate profound vision loss to no light perception, and fundus examination reveals significant vitreous and retinal hemorrhage overlying the optic disc. Once the media clears, excavation of the optic disc may be seen. Imaging studies, including computed tomography (CT) and magnetic resonance imaging (MRI) generally fail to confirm the diagnosis, though with continued improvements in ocular imaging, the disinsertion may now be seen on MRI.

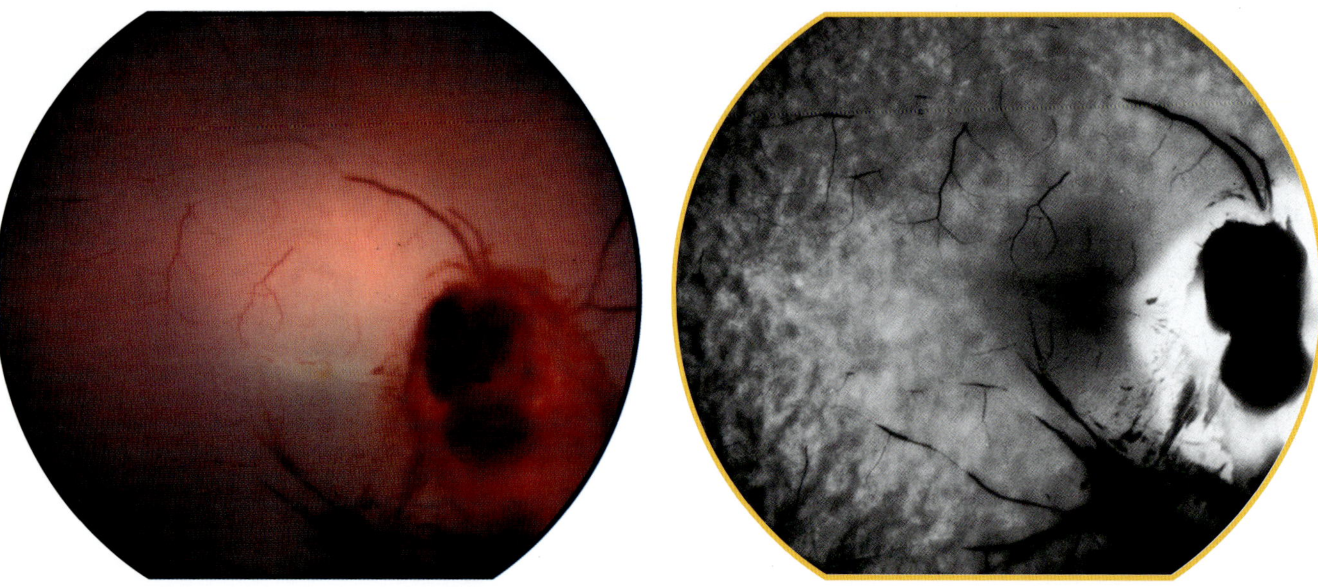

This patient was struck on the right side of his head while playing baseball. He presented with NLP vision, and hemorrhage covering the region of the optic nerve head *(left)*. There was absence of retinal perfusion as seen on fluorescein angiography *(right)*, though there was partial retention of choroidal perfusion. The patient never regained any visual function.

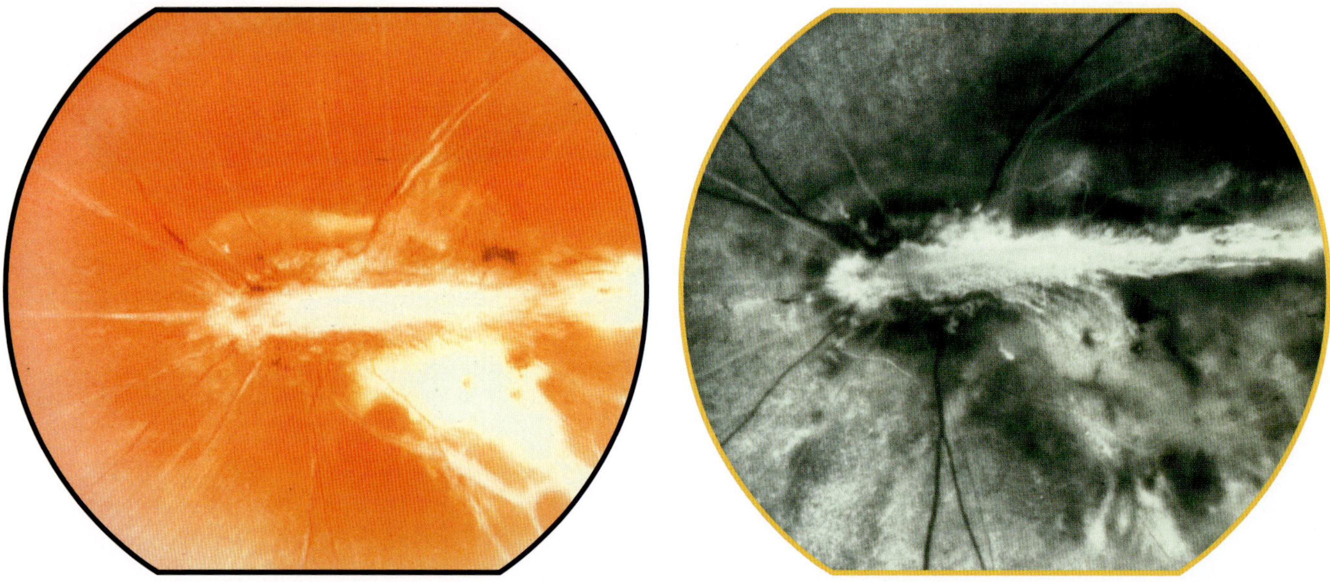

These images are from a patient who sustained an optic nerve avulsion several months earlier. It appears that the disinserted nerve was dragged temporally *(left)*. This region now appears atrophic and slightly fibrotic, and there is total absence of retinal perfusion as seen in the accompanying fluorescein angiogram *(right)*. No specific treatment was possible, and the vision remained NLP. *Images courtesy of J Donald M Gass, MD*

Intraocular Foreign Body (IOFB)

An intraocular foreign body (IOFB) may be found in the vitreous or anywhere in the fundus. Manifestations in the fundus will vary depending on the size of the foreign body and the severity of the impact. Larger and more slowly moving projectiles (such as BB gun injuries) carry a more guarded visual prognosis. Overall, however, eyes with a retained IOFB have an approximate 60% chance of regaining vision of 20/40 or better once the IOFB has been removed and the associated intraocular damage has been repaired. Other than a careful, detailed funduscopic examination, the best way to rule out a metallic IOFB is with a CT scan of the orbits.

These two patients developed metallic IOFBs while hammering metal against metal. The foreign body was found in the vitreous in the first patient *(left)* and embedded in the retina and sclera surrounded by hemorrhage in the second *(right)*. Upon surgical removal of the IOFB, the two patients recovered substantial vision.

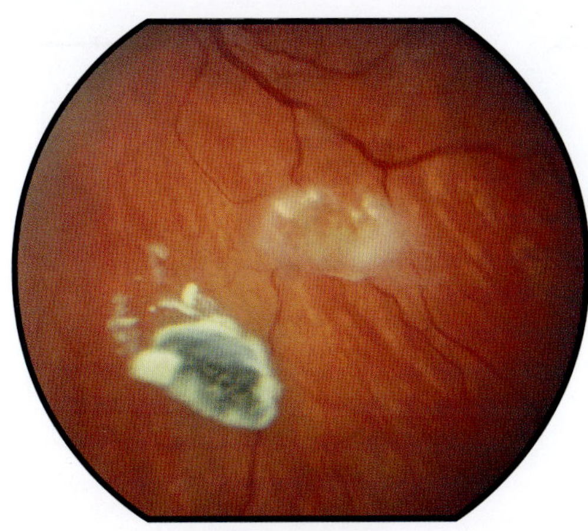

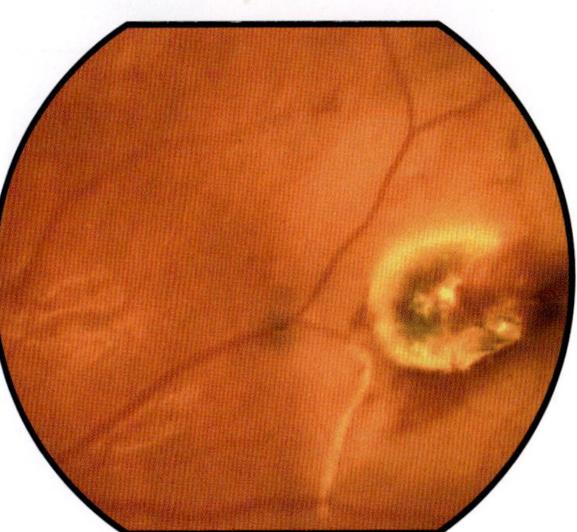

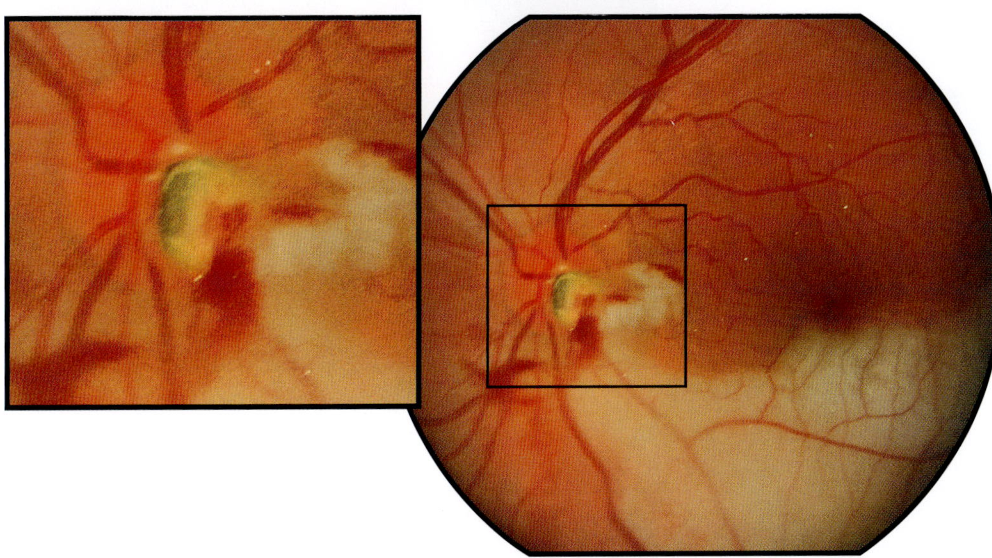

This patient was hammering metal on metal when a foreign body entered the left eye and became embedded in the optic nerve, where it obstructed a retinal arteriole and caused a branch retinal artery occlusion. Whitening of the inner retina from the retinal arteriolar infarction can be seen. *Courtesy of Dr. Keith Zinn*

This patient was changing a glass lighting fixture above her head, when it fell into her face. Glass IOFBs sliced into both eyes, with the IOFB becoming embedded into the retina in her left eye *(left)*. The IOFB was removed surgically via a pars plana vitrectomy approach, and the retinal impact site was treated with demarcating photocoagulation *(right)*. Upon clearing of a small degree of intraoperative hemorrhage, vision returned to 20/20.

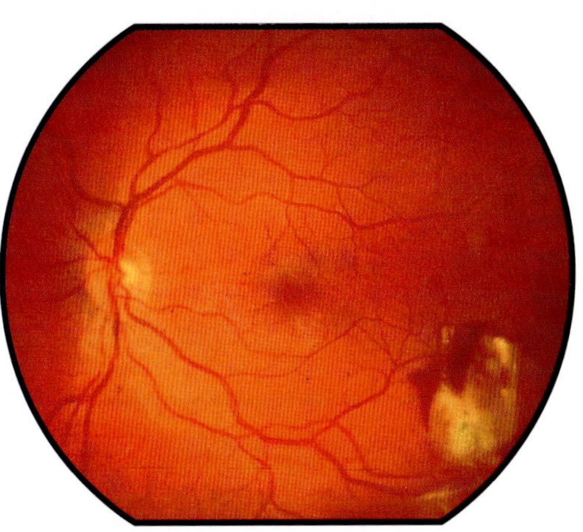

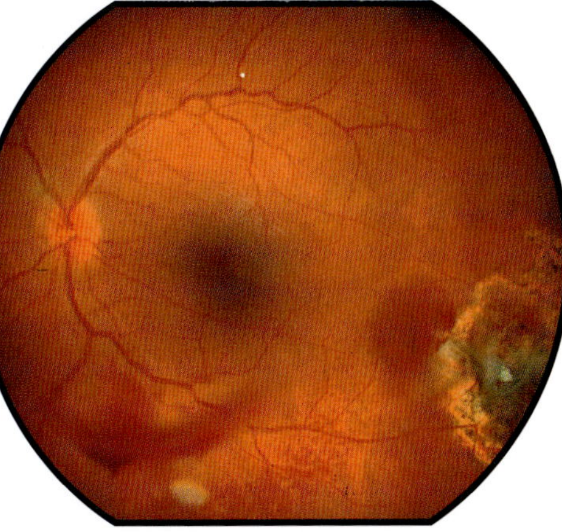

Penetrating and/or Perforating Ocular Injury

Open-globe injuries in the form of penetrating and/or perforating ocular injuries occur in a multitude of settings. The prognosis for visual recovery is extremely variable and dependent upon a multitude of factors. The initial response is to determine the extent of the injury, restore the integrity of the eye, and of course monitor for complications such as endophthalmitis, hypotony, and retinal detachment with PVR.

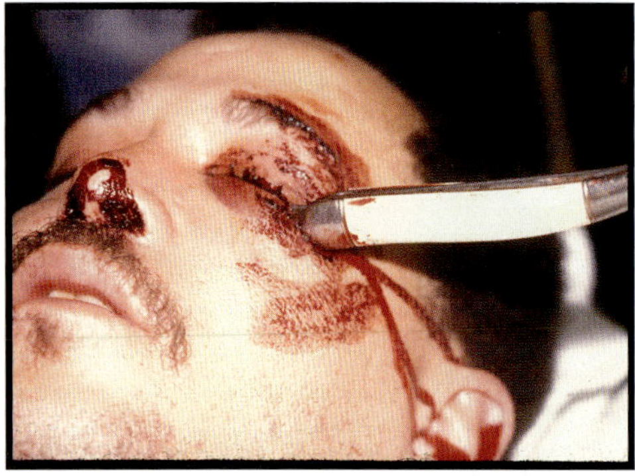

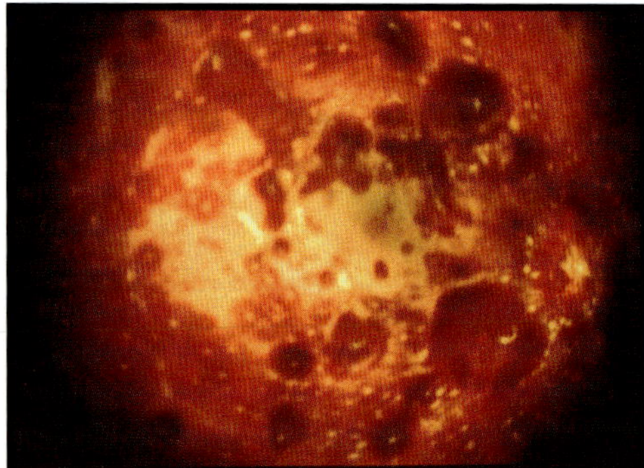

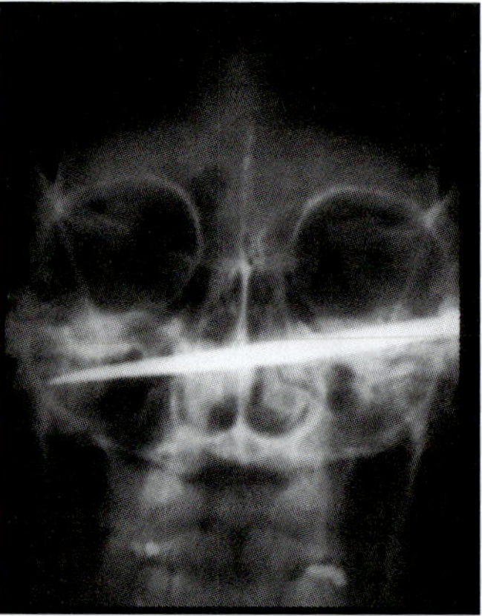

This patient was struck in the eye by a knife *(left)*, visible on external examination and on the X-ray *(right)*. Fundus examination revealed widespread hemorrhage *(middle)*, though the globe was not penetrated.

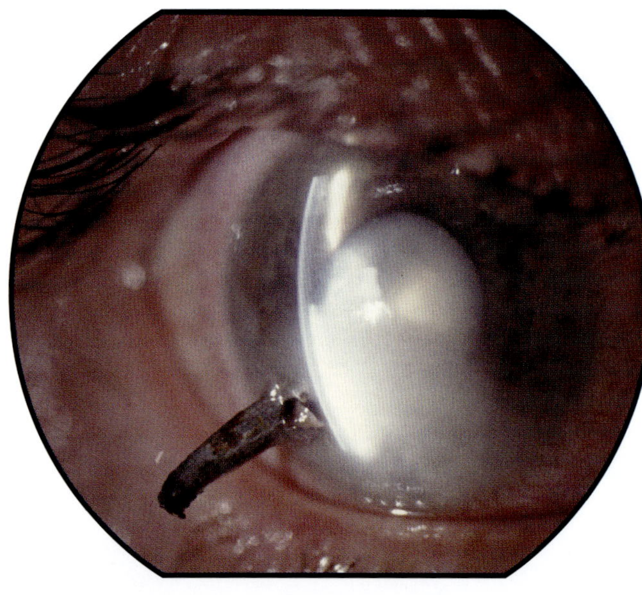

This patient experienced a penetrating injury from a fish hook, which extended into the eye and caused vitreous hemorrhage and retinal detachment.

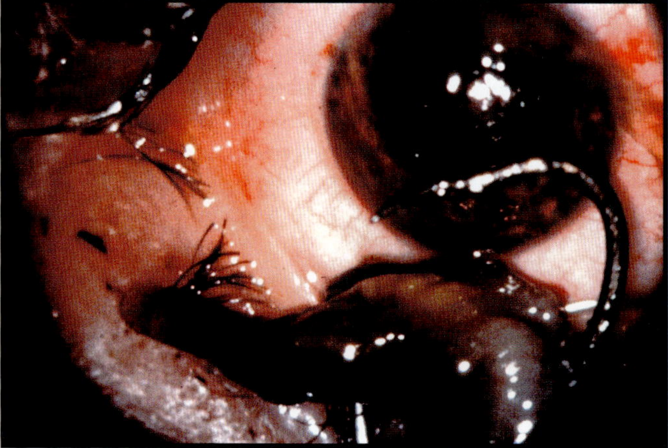

A patient inadvertently embedded a fishing hook into his eye, with an intact worm on the hook.

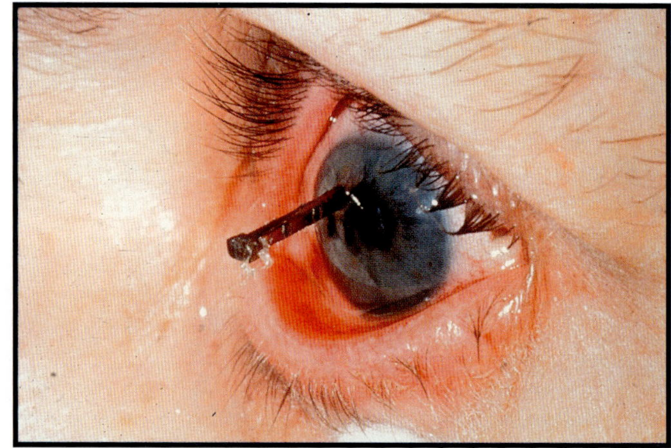

This patient sustained a penetrating corneal injury when a nail from a pneumatic nail gun bounced off a hard surface and entered the superior aspect of his cornea. *Courtesy of Kirk H. Packo, MD*

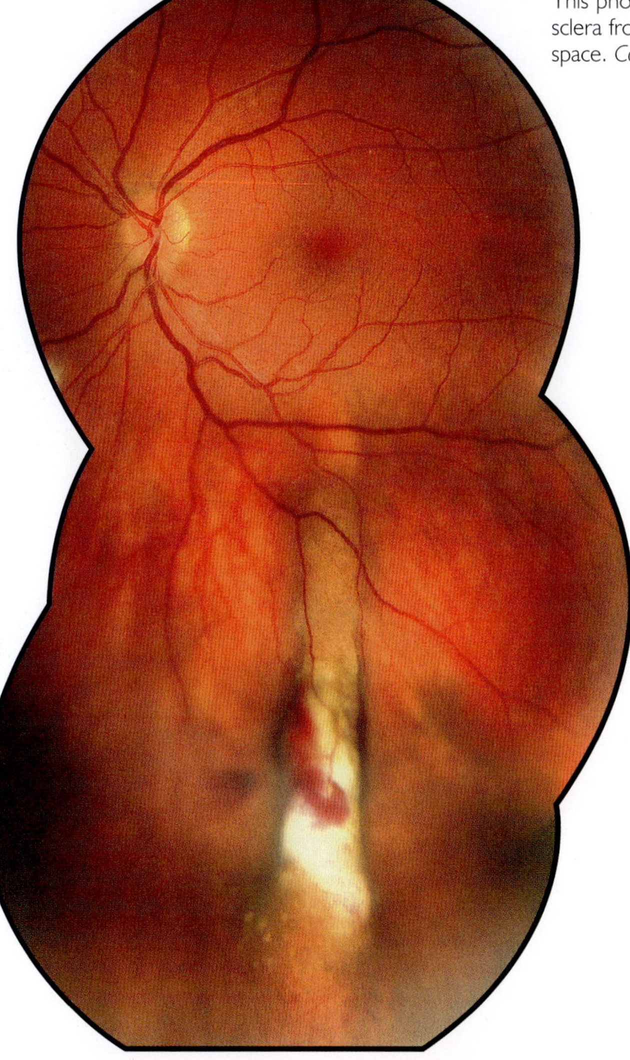

This photograph is of a patient who had a wooden splinter driven into the orbit and sclera from a power saw. The splinter is clearly visible in the inferior subretinal space. *Courtesy of Amanda Moyer, CRA*

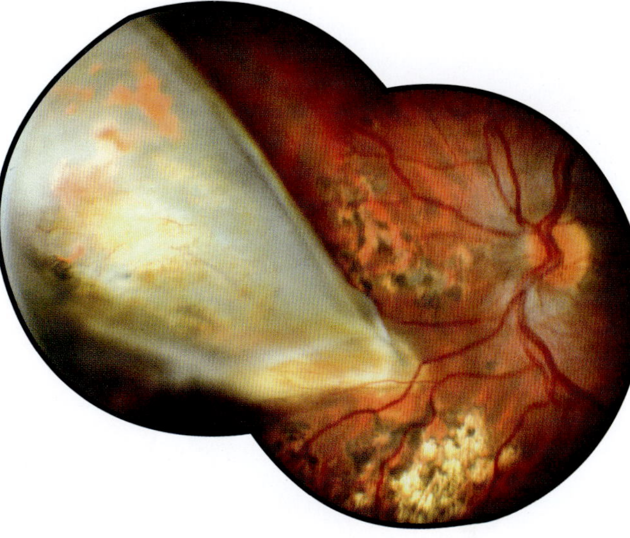

This patient was involved in an automobile accident, after which a huge triangular piece of glass was found in the eye. Laser photocoagulation treatment was applied around it. Despite the presence of the large foreign body, the eye was relatively quiescent. *Courtesy of Dr. Yale Fisher*

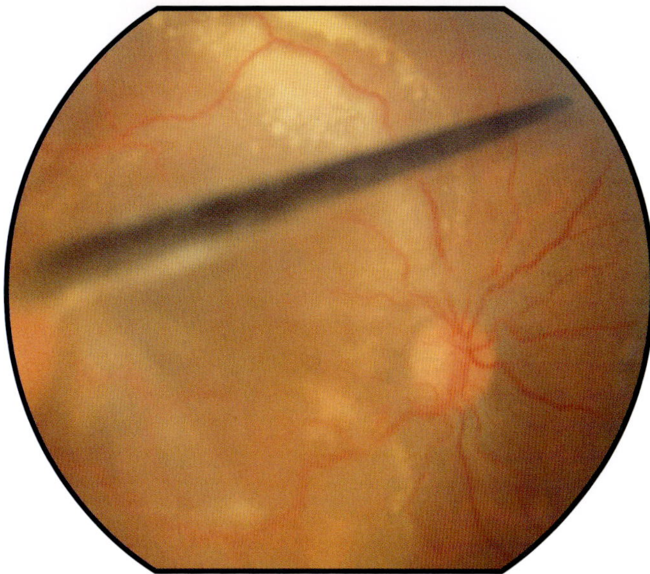

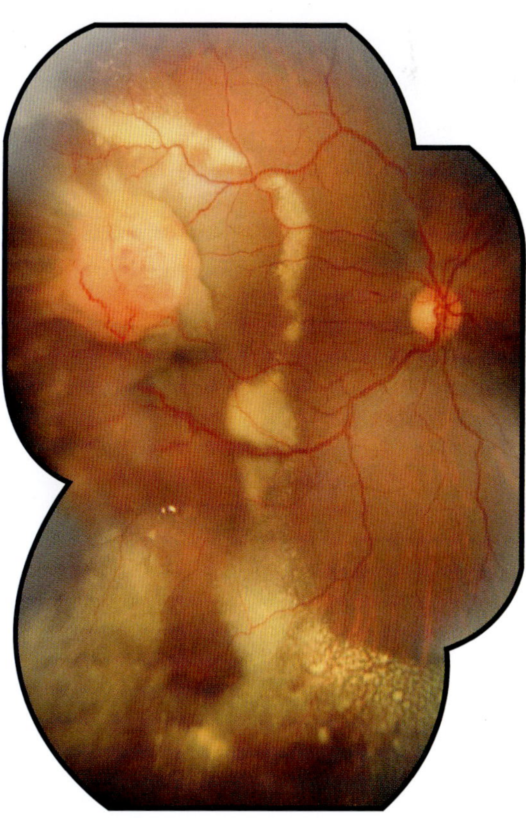

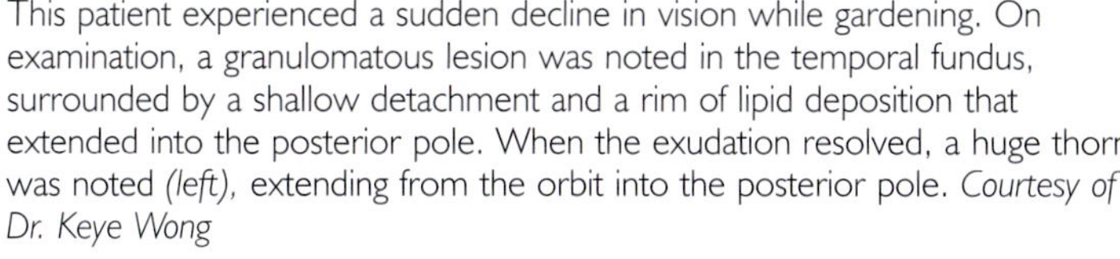

This patient experienced a sudden decline in vision while gardening. On examination, a granulomatous lesion was noted in the temporal fundus, surrounded by a shallow detachment and a rim of lipid deposition that extended into the posterior pole. When the exudation resolved, a huge thorn was noted *(left)*, extending from the orbit into the posterior pole. *Courtesy of Dr. Keye Wong*

Valsalva Retinopathy

Valsalva retinopathy is a particular form of primarily pre-retinal and subhyaloidal hemorrhage, occurring secondary to a sudden increase in intrathoracic and/or intra-abdominal pressure against a closed glottis. The sudden rise in intraocular venous pressure causes retinal capillaries to spontaneously rupture and bleed. Clinically, it presents as a hemorrhagic detachment of the internal limiting membrane (ILM), which may contain a fluid level, intraretinal hemorrhage, and/or vitreous hemorrhage. Multiple etiologies have now been described including pregnancy, general anesthesia, ocular massage, cardiopulmonary cerebral resuscitation (CPR), sexual activity, and heavy exercise. Spontaneous hemorrhage has also been described in patients with familial retinal arteriolar tortuosity. Treatment in most cases involves only observation, though there have been reports of laser treatment release of the hemorrhage.

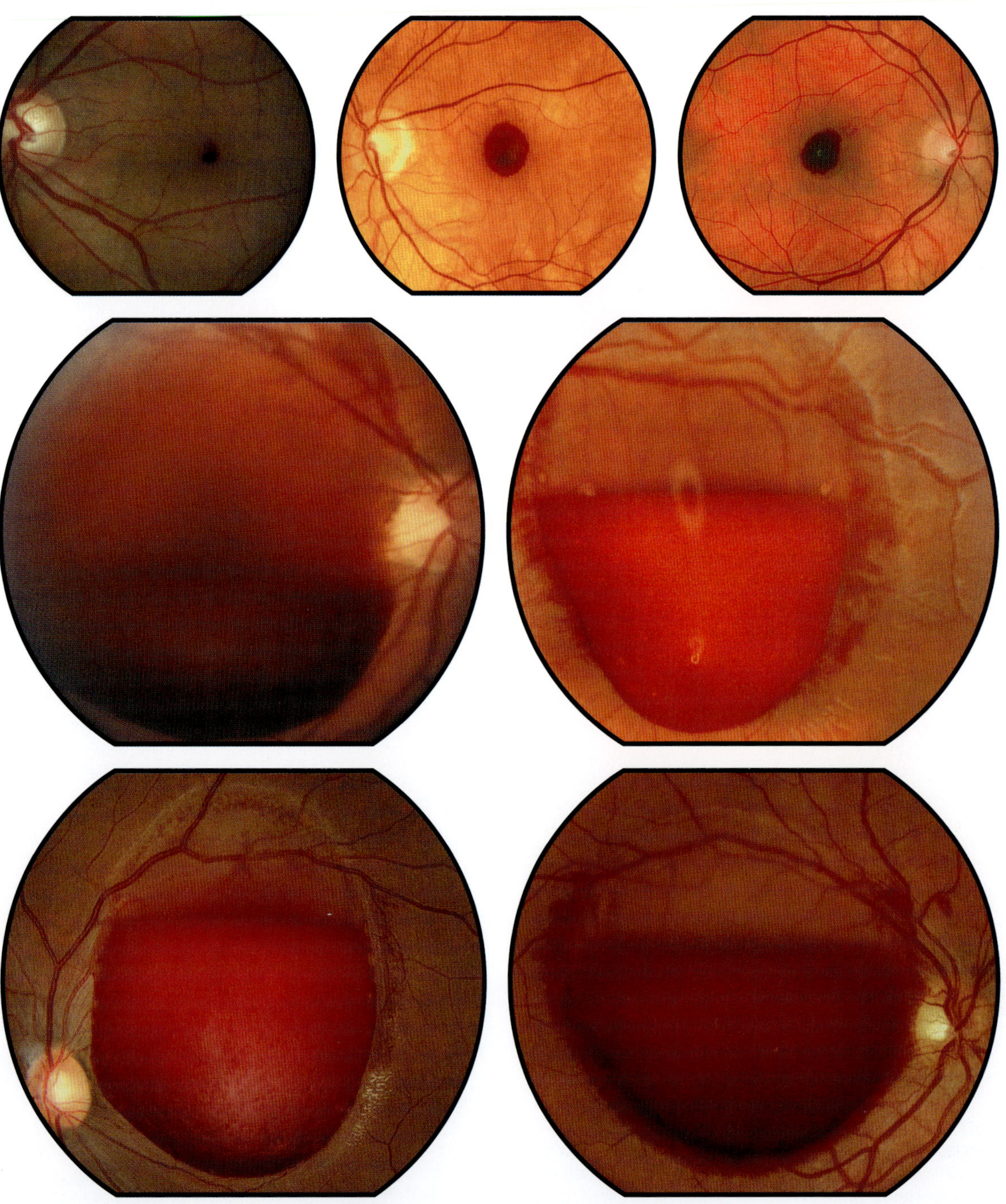

These are patients who experienced Valsalva retinopathy after activities ranging from straining during a bowel movement to an acrobat who was suspended by his legs on a trapeze. The subhyaloidal hemorrhage usually clears spontaneously.

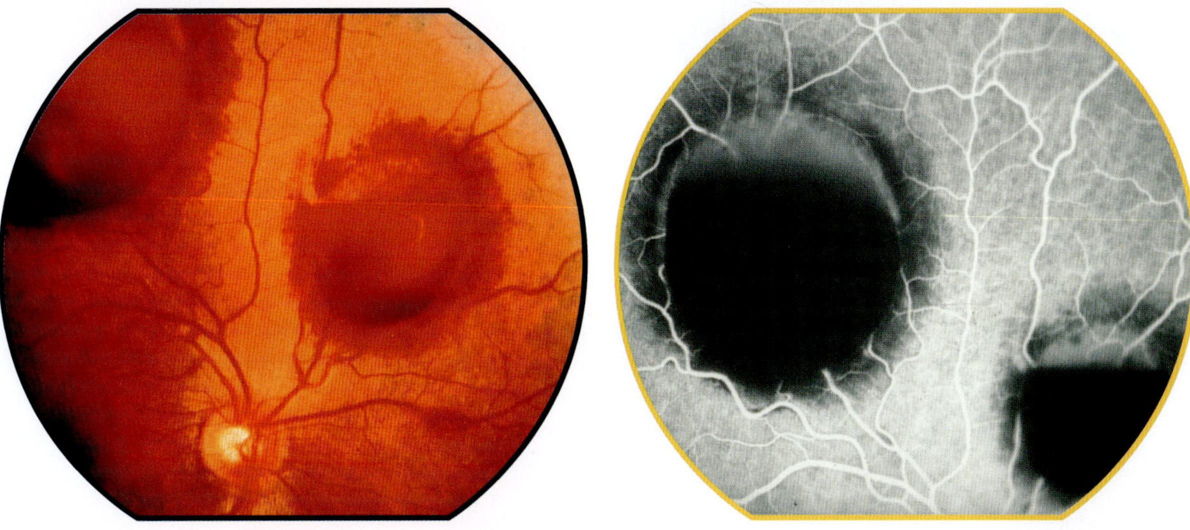

This patient was a prison inmate who was almost choked to death by a fellow inmate. He presented with two scotomas and was noted to have two areas of subhyaloidal hemorrhage with blood-fluid layering. The changes were documented clinically *(left)* and on fluorescein angiography as well *(right)*. While follow-up was requested, the patient was never seen again in the clinic.

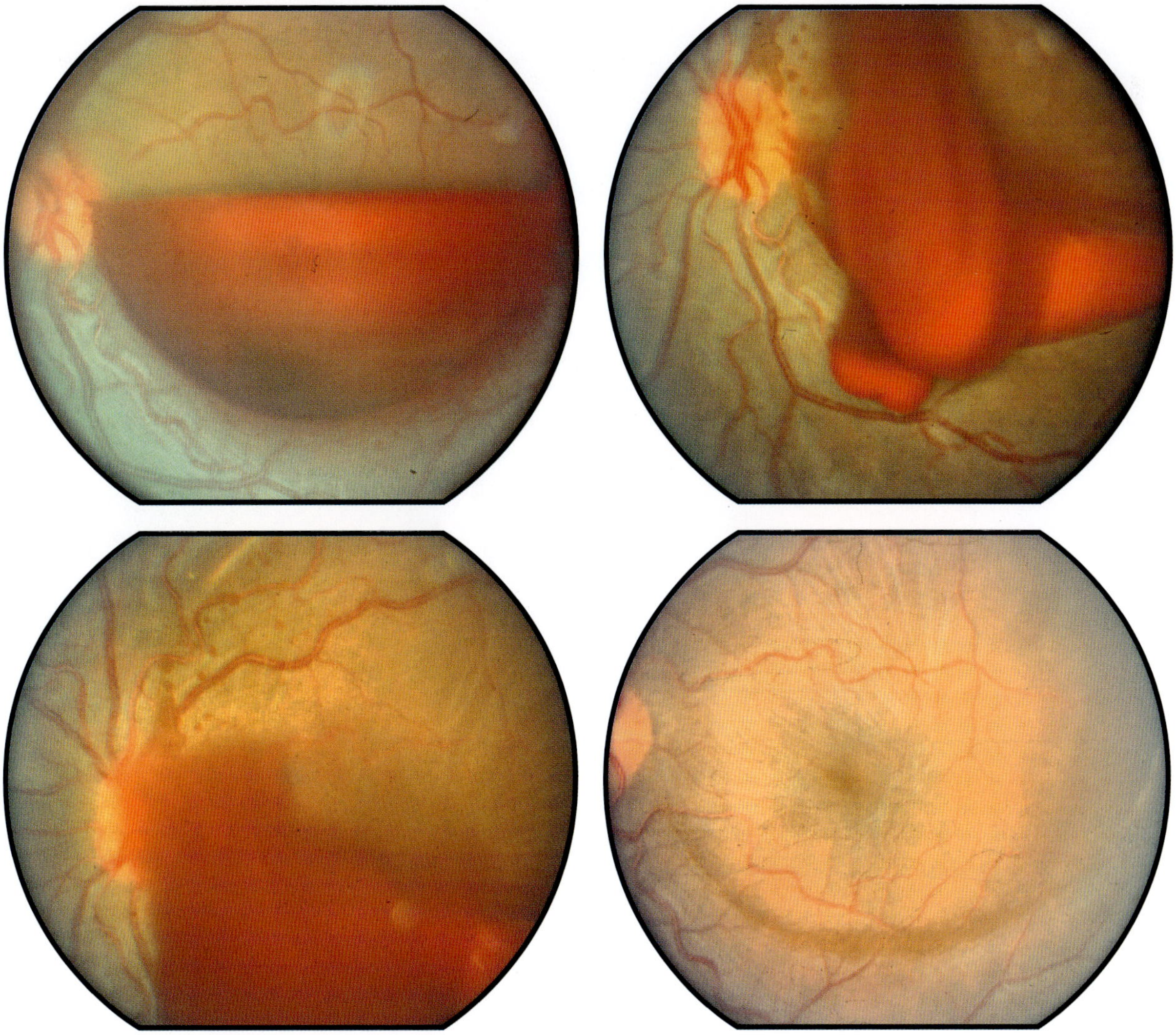

In cases of nonclearing subhyaloidal hemorrhages, accelerated resolution can be carried out with a focal laser to the lower part of the pocket of hemorrhage, which permits it to diffuse or leak into the vitreous cavity *(left)*. Focal laser treatment was performed on this patient, who had a nonresolving hemorrhage that had been monitored for a period of six weeks. Diffusion of the hemorrhage into the vitreous cavity after YAG laser treatment is demonstrated at 5 and 10 minutes *(upper right and lower left)*. Two weeks post-treatment, the hemorrhage has completely resolved *(right)*, though significant retinal striae did remain.

Purtscher Retinopathy

Purtscher retinopathy may occur secondary to numerous systemic conditions. In the realm of trauma, it generally is seen secondary to severe compressive injury to the trunk or head. On clinical examination, there are multiple patches of retinal whitening from axoplasmic debris accumulation (cotton-wool spots), and intraretinal hemorrhage. Patients experience painless loss of central vision in one or both eyes and develop Purtscher flecken (pathognomonic polygonal areas of retinal whitening with a clear demarcating line), and cotton-wool spots around the disc as well as elsewhere in the posterior pole, which represent capillary ischemic changes. Swelling of the macula or optic nerve may sometimes occur. The pathogenesis of the retinal ischemia in Purtscher retinopathy is controversial but the most likely pathogenic processes include complement-mediated granulocyte aggregation or venous reflux and/or arterial spasm from a sudden increase in intrathoracic pressure. The majority of patients do well as the process spontaneously resolves, yet occasionally there can be permanent visual loss.

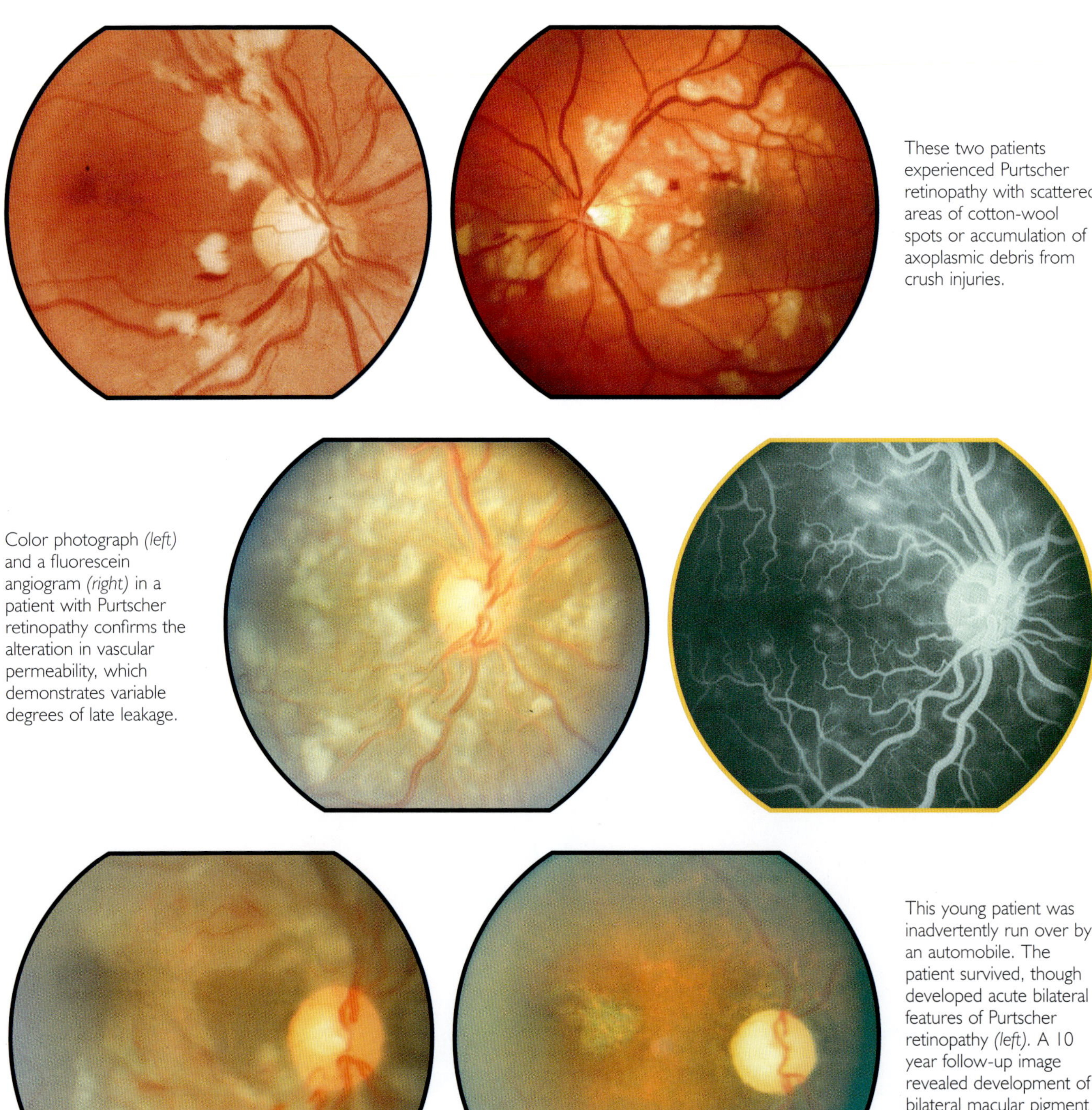

These two patients experienced Purtscher retinopathy with scattered areas of cotton-wool spots or accumulation of axoplasmic debris from crush injuries.

Color photograph *(left)* and a fluorescein angiogram *(right)* in a patient with Purtscher retinopathy confirms the alteration in vascular permeability, which demonstrates variable degrees of late leakage.

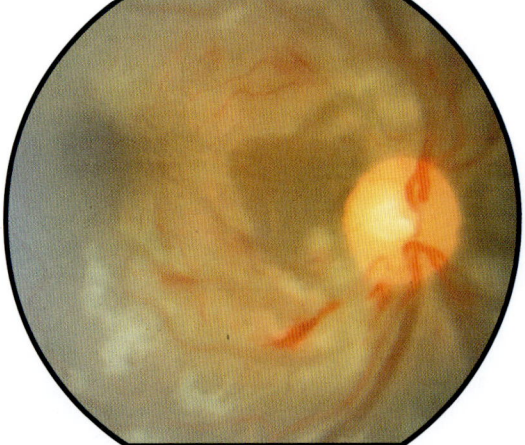

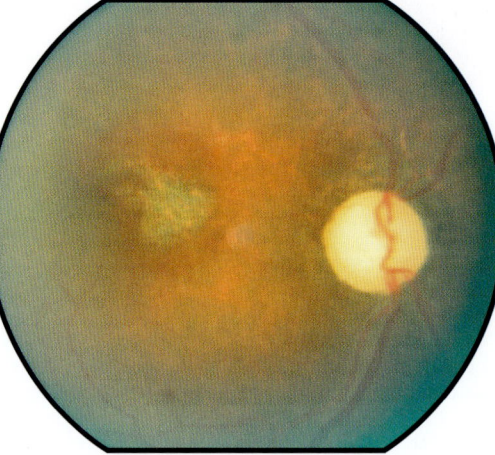

This young patient was inadvertently run over by an automobile. The patient survived, though developed acute bilateral features of Purtscher retinopathy *(left)*. A 10 year follow-up image revealed development of bilateral macular pigment atrophy, presumably from long-standing cystoid macular edema *(right)*.

Terson Syndrome

Terson syndrome is defined as intraocular hemorrhage that is associated with subarachnoid hemorrhage, intracerebral hemorrhage, or traumatic brain injury. The hemorrhage may be located in the vitreous, sub-hyaloid, or sub-ILM spaces. In cases where the hemorrhage spontaneously clears, vision will generally return to normal but vitrectomy may be required in cases of exuberant hemorrhage. The most likely mechanism is the sudden increase in venous pressure from intracranial hypertension, though the true mechanism is still debated.

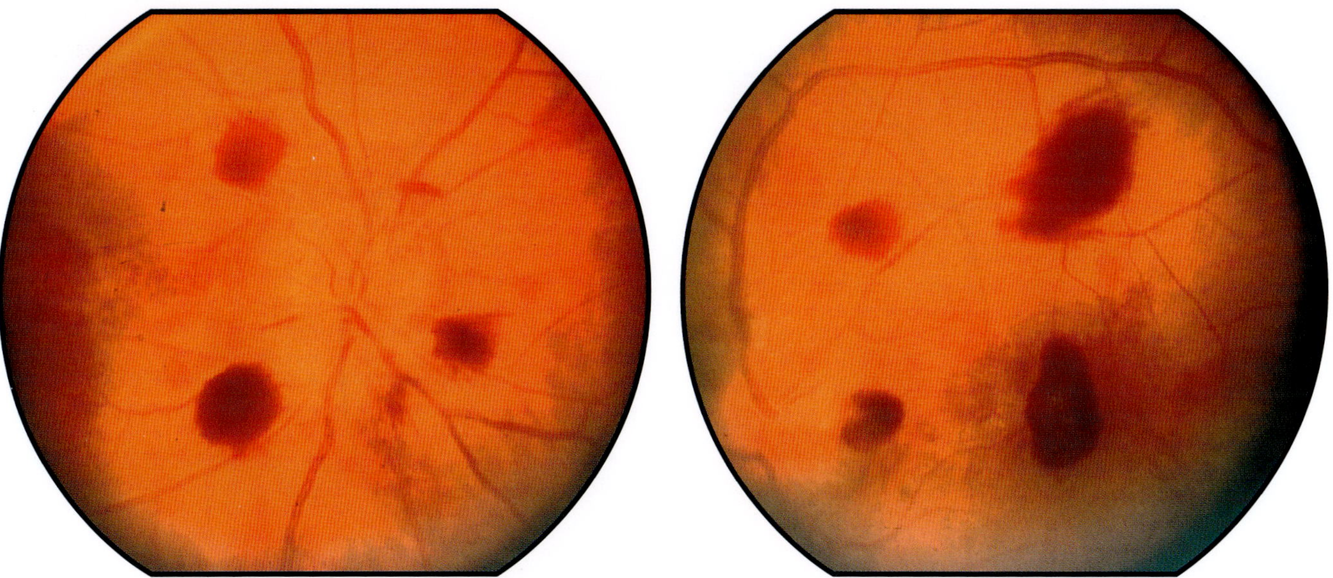

This patient developed Terson syndrome as a result of a traumatic subarachnoid hemorrhage. He developed multiple sub-hyaloid and sub-ILM hemorrhages throughout the macula *(left)* and peripapillary areas *(right)*. Note the presence of optic nerve edema likely indicative of elevated intracranial pressure. Fluorescein angiography generally does not show significant early leakage in these cases. Observation was recommended, and the patient did well with resolution of the hemorrhages and restoration of visual function.

Shaken Baby Syndrome

Infants and children who are subjected to abuse may present with a multitude of ocular findings. Posterior segment abnormalities are generally seen in approximately 30 to 40% of the victims. These findings generally occur after violent shaking, direct ocular or head trauma, chest injuries, and/or choking. The clinical features include diffuse retinal hemorrhages, cotton-wool spots, papilledema, vitreous hemorrhage, and/or perimacular folds. One needs to rule out a ruptured globe. On occasion, pars plana vitrectomy surgery may be required for non-clearing vitreous opacities, or to repair a retinal detachment. If one is suspicious of child abuse, the case needs to be reported to the local authorities.

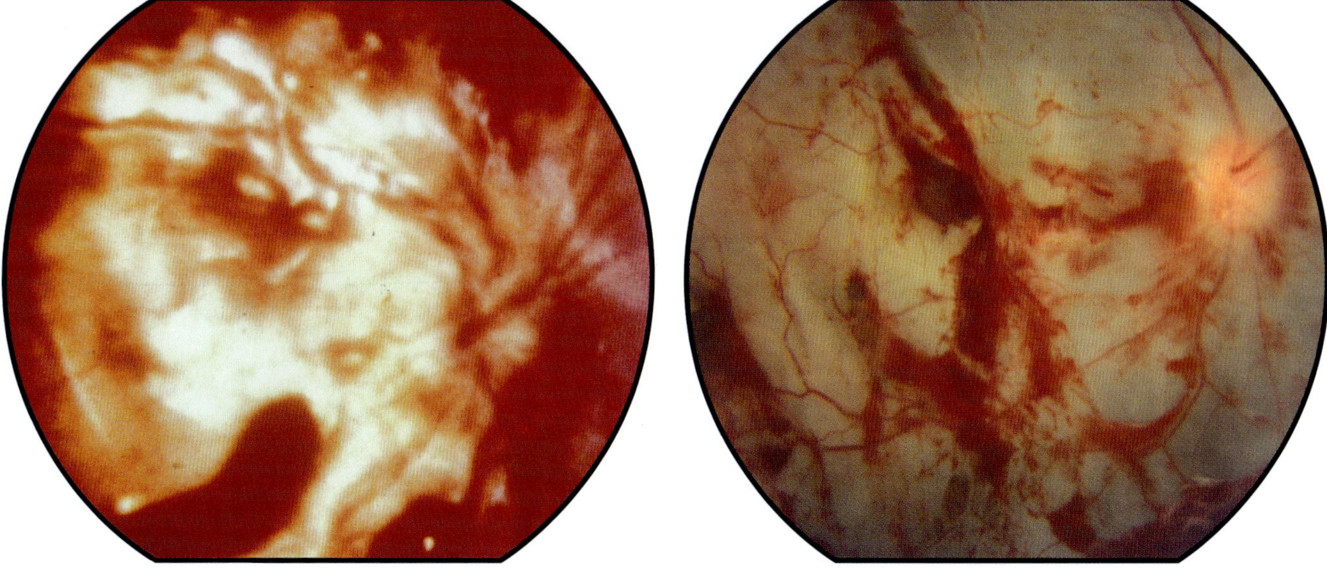

Two infants subjected to child abuse. Hemorrhage at multiple layers was seen *(left)* involving subretinal, preretinal and vitreous hemorrhage. In the second infant *(right)* the degree of retinal and preretinal hemorrhage was less severe. Both infants were observed.

Solar and/or Laser-Induced Retinopathy

Solar retinopathy is a phototoxic reaction in the fundus from light. The reaction is dependent upon duration, intensity, and spectral content. It can be produced by gazing at virtually any source of light but is mainly associated with solar eclipse and religious sun-gazing, or directly viewing a laser pointer. The reaction is photochemical in nature, and generally juxtafoveal, usually bilateral and asymmetric, with more severe disease in the dominant or fixation eye.

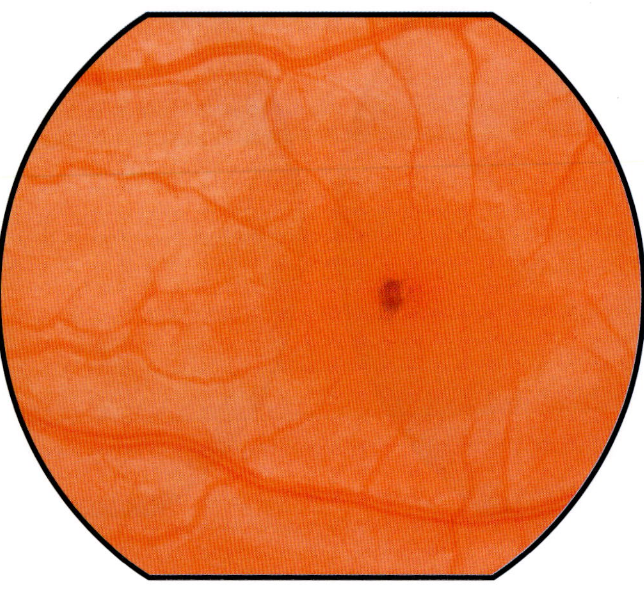

Image of a patient who gazed directly at the sun while on illicit drugs. Note the acute reddish macular lesion. Visual acuity is 20/40. This reddish lesion faded away over a several week time frame and was eventually replaced by a small spot of hypopigmentation.

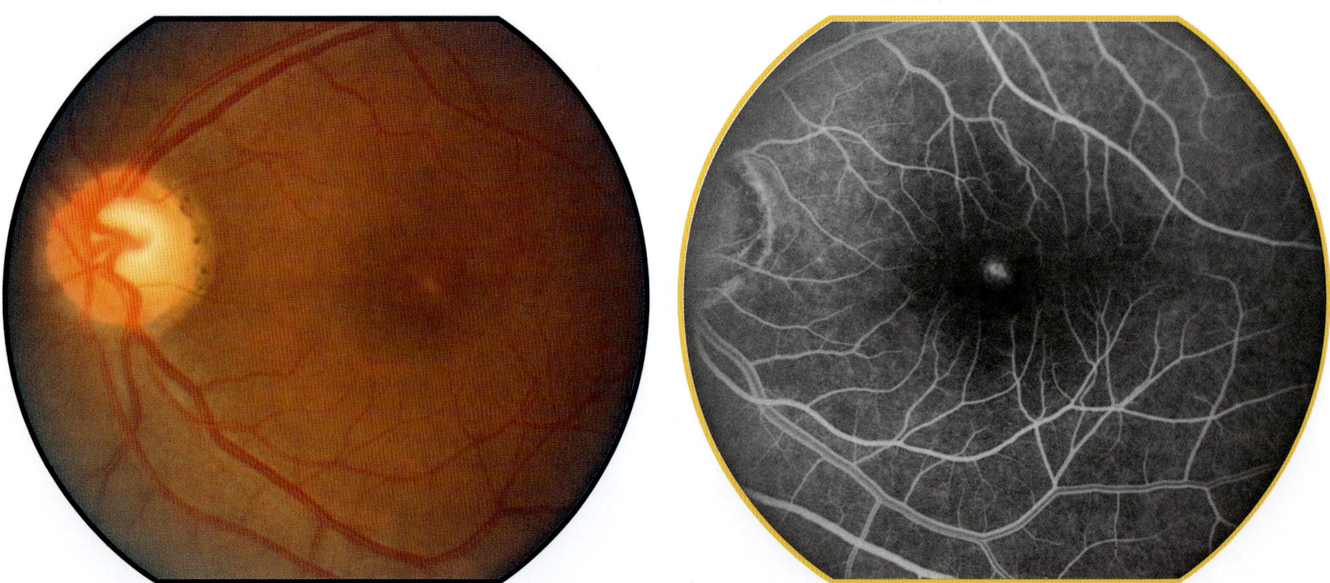

Image of a patient (chronic solar retinopathy) two months after sungazing. The patient has a small area of hypopigmentation just temporal to the fovea *(left)* which appears as a transmission defect on fluorescein angiography *(right)*. Visual acuity is 20/30 OS.

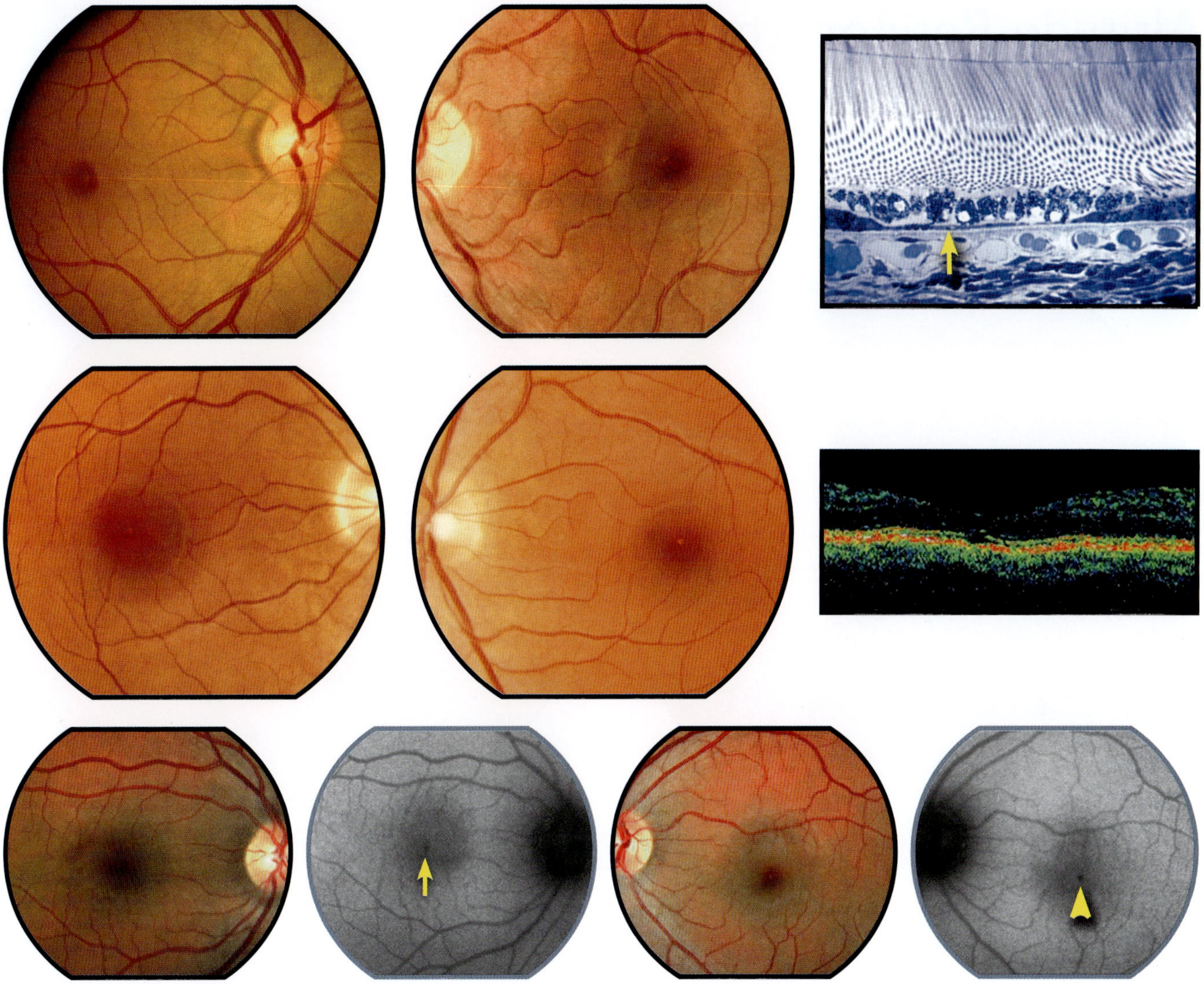

These patients developed solar retinopathy from excessive sun-gazing or eclipse viewing. Note the juxtafoveal yellow lesion that is barely evident on color photographs, accompanied by a small outer retinal disturbance. The OCT shows photoreceptor inner-pigment epithelial focal degeneration corresponding to the clinically evident lesion, which correlates with the focal thinning of the retinal pigment epithelium (RPE) and outer retina seen on histopathology *(arrow)*. Fundus autofluorescence seen in the rightmost image may also demonstrate the juxtafoveal lesion as an area of discrete hypoautofluorescence *(arrowhead)*.

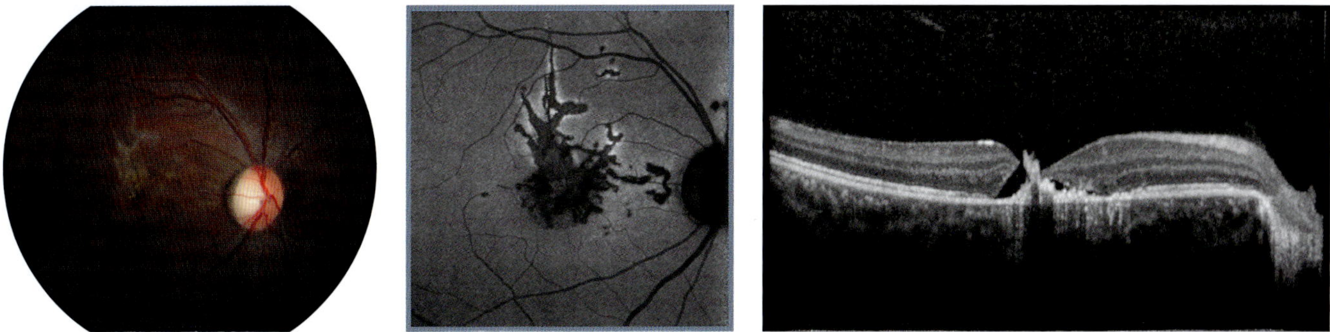

Laser pointer-induced ocular injuries are becoming more common. This patient gazed into a laser pointer bilaterally. The rationale for self-inducement of ocular injury is not clear, though often these patients have underlying psychological issues that need to be explored. Note the multiple streaks of injury to the retina and RPE *(left)* from the repetitive gazing into the laser device. The damage is highlighted on fundus autofluorescence *(middle)*, as well as on SD-OCT imaging *(right)*. *Images courtesy of Amani Fawzi, MD*

Altitude Retinopathy

Altitude retinopathy consists primarily of intraretinal hemorrhages and cotton-wool spots, along with optic nerve edema in patients who exercise vigorously at high altitudes, or are at very high altitude for an extended period of time. Rarely, pre-retinal hemorrhages with extension into the vitreous may also occur. The most likely mechanism involves changes in retinal perfusion due to autoregulation of cerebral blood flow in response to hypoxia at high altitudes.

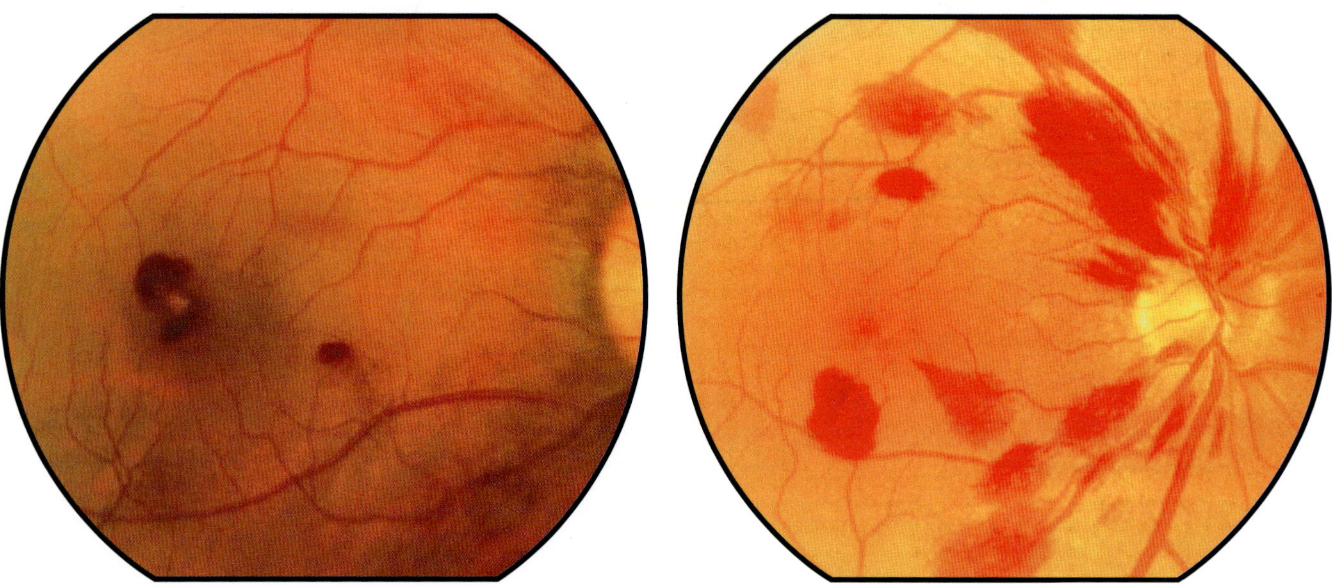

These two patients experienced high-altitude retinopathy, with one patient exhibiting an occasional retinal and pre-retinal hemorrhage *(left)*, while the other patient had more widespread superficial retinal hemorrhages throughout the fundus *(right)*. *Courtesy of Dr. Michael Weiderman*

Suggested Reading

Berlin's Edema (Commotio Retinae)

Ahn, S.J., Woo, S.J., Kim, K.E., et al., 2013. Optical coherence tomography morphologic grading of macular commotion retinae and its association with anatomic and visual outcomes. Am. J. Ophthalmol. 156 (5), 994–1001.

Baath, J., Ells, A.L., Kherani, A., et al., 2007. Severe retinal injuries from paintball projectiles. Can. J. Ophthalmol. 42, 620–623.

Bastek, J.V., Foos, R.Y., Heckenlively, J., 1981. Traumatic pigmentary retinopathy. Am. J. Ophthalmol. 92, 621–624.

Bunt-Milam, A.H., Black, R.A., Bensinger, R.E., 1986. Breakdown of the outer blood–retinal barrier in experimental commotio retinae. Exp. Eye Res. 43, 397–412.

He, D., Blomquist, P.H., Ellis, E. 3rd, 2007. Association between ocular injuries and internal orbital fractures. J. Oral Maxillofac. Surg. 65, 713–720.

Kent, J.S., Eidsness, R.B., Colleaux, K.M., et al., 2007. Indoor soccer-related eye injuries: should eye protection be mandatory? Can. J. Ophthalmol. 42, 605–608.

Kohno, T., Miki, T., Hayashi, K., 1998. Choroidopathy after blunt trauma to the eye: a fluorescein and indocyanine green angiographic study. Am. J. Ophthalmol. 126, 248–260.

Kylstra, J.A., Lamkin, J.C., Runyan, D.K., 1993. Clinical predictors of scleral rupture after blunt ocular trauma. Am. J. Ophthalmol. 115, 530–535.

Lessell, S., 1989. Indirect optic nerve trauma. Arch. Ophthalmol. 107, 382–386.

Mansour, A.M., Green, W.R., Hogge, C., 1992. Histopathology of commotio retinae. Retina 12, 24–28.

Mendes, S., Campos, A., Campos, J., et al., 2015. Cutting edge of traumatic maculopathy with spectral-domain optical coherence tomography—a review. Med. Hypothesis Discov. Innov. Ophthalmol. 4, 56–63.

Pulido, J.S., Blair, N.P., 1987. The blood–retinal barrier in Berlin's edema. Retina 7, 233–236.

Russell, S.R., Olsen, K.R., Folk, J.C., 1988. Predictors of scleral rupture and the role of vitrectomy in severe blunt ocular trauma. Am. J. Ophthalmol. 105, 253–257.

Sipperly, J.O., Quigley, H.A., Gass, J.D.M., 1978. Traumatic retinopathy in primates. The explanation of commotio retinae. Arch. Ophthalmol. 96, 2267–2273.

Sony, P., Venkatesh, P., Gadaginamath, S., et al., 2006. Optical coherence tomography findings in commotio retina. Clin. Experiment. Ophthalmol. 34, 621–623.

Sousa-Santos, F., Lavinsky, D., Moraes, N.S., et al., 2012. Spectral-domain optical coherence tomography in patient with commotio retinae. Retina 32 (4), 711–718.

Steinsapir, K.D., Goldberg, R.A., 1994. Traumatic optic neuropathy. Surv. Ophthalmol. 38, 487–578.

Umeed, S., Shafquat, S., 2004. Commotio-retinae and central retinal artery occlusion after blunt ocular trauma. Eye (Lond.) 18, 333–334.

Williams, D.F., Mieler, W.F., Williams, G.A., 1990. Posterior segment manifestations of ocular trauma. Retina 10 (Suppl. 1), S35–S44.

Traumatic Retinal Pigment Epitheliopathy

Archer, D.B., Canavan, Y.M., 1983. Contusional eye injuries: retinal and choroidal lesions. Aust. J. Ophthalmol. 11, 251–264.

Delori, F., Pomerantzeff, O., Cox, M.S., 1969. Deformation of the globe under high-speed impact: its relation to contusion injuries. Invest. Ophthalmol. 8, 290–301.

Eagling, E.M., 1974. Ocular damage after blunt trauma to the eye: its relationship to the nature of the injury. Br. J. Ophthalmol. 58, 126–140.

Giovinazzo, V.J., Yannuzzi, L.A., Sorenson, J.A., et al., 1987. The ocular complications of boxing. Ophthalmol 94, 587–596.

Traumatic Macular Hole

Armstrong, B., Fecarotta, C., Ho, A.C., et al., 2010. Evolution of severe lightning maculopathy visualized with spectral domain optical coherence tomography. Ophthalmic Surg. Lasers Imaging 41 (Suppl.), S70–S73.

Chow, D.R., Williams, G.A., Trese, M.T., et al., 1999. Successful closure of traumatic macular holes. Retina 19, 405–409.

Frangieh, G.T., Green, W.R., Engel, H.M., 1981. A histopathologic study of macular cysts and holes. Retina 1, 311–336.

Garcia-Arumi, J., Corcostegui, B., Cavero, L., et al., 1997. The role of vitreoretinal surgery in the treatment of posttraumatic macular hole. Retina 17, 372–373.

Ghoraba, H.H., Ellakwa, A.F., Ghali, A.A., 2012. Long term result of silicone oil versus gas tamponade in the treatment of traumatic macular holes. Clin. Ophthalmol. 6, 49–53.

Horn, E.P., McDonald, H.R., Johnson, R.N., et al., 2000. Soccer ball-related retinal injuries: a report of 13 cases. Retina 20, 604–609.

Ismail, R., Tanner, V., Williamson, T.H., 2002. Optical coherence topography imaging of severe commotio retinae and associated macular hole. Br. J. Ophthalmol. 86, 473–474.

Johnson, R.N., McDonald, H.R., Lewis, H., et al., 2001. Traumatic macular hole: observations, pathogenesis, and results of vitrectomy surgery. Ophthalmology 108, 853–857.

Menchini, U., Virgili, G., Giacomelli, G., et al., 2003. Mechanism of spontaneous closure of traumatic macular hole: OCT study of one case. Retina 23, 104–106.

Miller, J.B., Yonekawa, Y., Eliott, D., et al., 2013. A review of traumatic macular hole: diagnosis and treatment. Int. Ophthalmol. Clin. 53, 59–67.

Miller, J.B., Yonekawa, Y., Eliott, D., et al., 2015. Long-term follow-up and outcomes in traumatic macular holes. Am. J. Ophthalmol. 160, 1255–1258.

Moon, S.J., Kim, J.E., Han, D.P., 2005. Lightning-induced maculopathy. Retina 25, 380–382.

Rivas-Aguiño, P.J., Garcia, R.A., Arevalo, J.F., 2006. Bilateral macular cyst after lightning visualized with optical coherence tomography. Clin. Experiment. Ophthalmol. 34, 893–894.

Weichel, E.D., Colyer, M.H., 2009. Traumatic macular holes secondary to combat ocular trauma. Retina 29, 349–354.

Yamashita, T., Uemara, A., Uchino, E., et al., 2002. Spontaneous closure of traumatic macular hole. Am. J. Ophthalmol. 133, 230–235.

Choroidal Rupture

Aguilar, I.P., Green, W.R., 1984. Choroidal rupture: a histopathologic study of 47 cases. Retina 4, 269–275.

Amari, F., Ogino, N., Matsumura, M., et al., 1999. Vitreous surgery for traumatic macular holes. Retina 19, 410–413.

Ament, C.S., Zacks, D.N., Lane, A.M., et al., 2006. Predictors of visual outcome and choroidal neovascular membrane formation after traumatic choroidal rupture. Arch. Ophthalmol. 124, 957–966.

Conrath, J., Forzano, O., Ridings, B., 2004. Photodynamic therapy for subfoveal CNV complicating traumatic choroidal rupture. Eye (Lond.) 18, 946–947.

Francis, J.H., Freund, K.B., 2011. Photoreceptor reconstitution correlates with visual improvement after intravitreal bevacizumab treatment of choroidal neovascularization secondary to traumatic choroidal rupture. Retina 31, 422–424.

Fuller, B., Gitter, K.A., 1973. Traumatic choroidal rupture with late serous detachment of macula: report of successful argon laser treatment. Arch. Ophthalmol. 89, 354–355.

Hart, J.C.D., Natsikos, V.E., Raistrick, E.R., et al., 1980. Indirect choroidal tears at the posterior pole: a fluorescein angiographic and perimetric study. Br. J. Ophthalmol. 64, 59–67.

Kohno, T., Miki, T., Shiraki, K., et al., 2000. Indocyanine green angiographic features of choroidal rupture and choroidal vascular injury after contusion ocular injury. Am. J. Ophthalmol. 129, 38–46.

Levin, D.B., Bell, D.K., 1977. Traumatic retinal hemorrhages with angioid streaks. Arch. Ophthalmol. 95, 1072–1073.

Patel, M.M., Chee, Y.E., Eliott, D., 2013. Choroidal rupture: a review. Int. Ophthalmol. Clin. 53, 69–73.

Smith, R.E., Kelley, J.S., Harbin, T.S., 1974. Late macular complications of choroidal ruptures. Am. J. Ophthalmol. 77, 650–658.

Wyszynski, R.E., Grossniklaus, H.E., Frank, K.E., 1988. Indirect choroidal rupture secondary to blunt ocular trauma: a review of eight eyes. Retina 8, 237–243.

Traumatic Retinal Breaks and Detachments

Yadav, N.K., Bharghav, M., Vasudha, K., et al., 2009. Choroidal neovascular membrane complicating traumatic choroidal rupture managed by intravitreal bevacizumab. Eye (Lond.) 23, 1872–1873.

Archer, D.B., Canavan, Y.M., 1983. Contusional eye injuries: retinal and choroidal lesions. Aust. J. Ophthalmol. 11, 251–264.

Aylward, G.W., Cooling, R.J., Leaver, P.K., 1993. Trauma-induced retinal detachment associated with giant retinal tears. Retina 13, 136–141.

Cox, M.S., Schepens, C.L., Freeman, H.M., 1966. Retinal detachment due to ocular contusion. Arch. Ophthalmol. 76, 678–685.

Cox, M.S., 1980. Retinal breaks caused by blunt non-perforating trauma at the point of impact. Trans. Am. Ophthalmol. Soc. 78, 414–466.

Goffstein, R., Burton, T.C., 1982. Differentiating traumatic from non-traumatic retinal detachment. Ophthalmol 89, 361–368.

Hagler, W.S., 1980. Retinal dialysis: statistical and genetic study to determine pathogenic factors. Trans. Am. Ophthalmol. Soc. 78, 686–733.

Johnston, P.B., 1991. Traumatic retinal detachment. Br. J. Ophthalmol. 75, 18–21.

Nacef, L., Daghfous, F., Chaabini, M., et al., 1997. Ocular contusions and giant retinal tears. J. Fran. d'Ophtalmologie 20, 170–174.

Zion, V.M., Burton, T.C., 1980. Retinal dialysis. Arch. Ophthalmol. 98, 1971–1974.

Chorioretinitis Sclopetaria

Dubovy, S.R., Guyton, D.L., Green, W.R., 1997. Clinocopathologic correlation of chorioretinitis sclopetaria. Retina 17, 510–520.

Goldzieher, W., 1901. Beitrag zur pathologie der orbitalen Schussverletzungen. Z. Augenh. 6, 277–285.

Richard, R.D., West, C.E., Meisels, A.A., 1968. Chorioretinitis sclopetaria. Am. J. Ophthalmol. 66, 852–860.

Hart, J.C., Natsikos, V.E., Raistrick, E.R., et al., 1980. Chorioretinitis sclopetaria. Trans. Ophthalmol. Soc. U. K. 100, 276–281.

Katsumata, S., Takahashi, J., Tamai, M., 1984. Choriortinitis sclopetaria caused by fishing line sinker. Jph. J. Ophthalmol. 28, 69–74.

Perry, H.D., Rahn, E.K., 1977. Chorioretinitis sclopetaria; choroidal and retinal concussion injury from a bullet. Arch. Ophthalmol. 95, 328–329.

Optic Nerve Avulsion

Buchwald, H.J., Otte, P., Lang, G.E., 2003. Evulsion of the optic nerve following blunt bulbar trauma. Klin. Monatsbl. Augenheilkd 220, 303–308.

Chow, A.Y., Goldberg, M.F., Frenkel, M., 1984. Evulsion of the optic nerve in association with basketball injuries. Ann. Ophthalmol. 16, 35–37.

Delaney, W.V. Jr., Geiss, M., 1988. Partial evulsion of the optic nerve. Ann. Ophthalmol. 20, 371–372.

DeVries-Knoppert, W.A., 1989. Evulsion of the optic nerve. Doc. Ophthalmol. 72, 241–245.

Hillman, J.S., Myska, V., Nissim, S., 1975. Complete avulsion of the optic nerve. A clinical, angiographic and electrodiagnostic study. Br. J. Ophthalmol. 59, 503–509.

Kline, L.B., McCluskey, M.M., Skalka, H.W., 1988. Imaging techniques in optic nerve evulsion. J. Clin. Neuroophthalmol 8, 281–282.

Lang, G.K., Bialasiwicz, A.A., Rohr, W.D., 1991. Bilateral traumatic eye avulsion. Klin. Monatsbl. Augenheilkd 198, 112–116.

Morris, W.R., Osborn, F.D., Fleming, J.C., 2002. Traumatic evulsion of the globe. Ophthal. Plast. Reconstr. Surg. 18, 261–267.

Noro, M., Ishikawa, A., Nakanome, Y., et al., 1990. A case of evusion of the optic nerve. Nippon Ganka Gakkai Zasshi 94, 1177–1180.

Park, J.H., Frenkel, M., Dobbie, J.G., et al., 1971. Evulsion of the optic nerve. Am. J. Ophthalmol. 72, 969–971.

Sanborn, G.E., Gonder, J.R., Goldberg, R.E., et al., 1984. Evulsion of the optic nerve: a clinicopathological study. Can. J. Ophthalmol. 19, 10–16.

Temel, A., Sener, A.B., 1988. Complete evulsion of the optic nerve. Acta Ophthalmol. 66, 117–119.

Williams, D.F., Williams, G.A., Abrams, G.W., et al., 1987. Evulsion of the retina associated with optic nerve evulsion. Am. J. Ophthalmol. 104, 5–9.

Intraocular Foreign Body

Agrawal, R., Laude, A., 2012. Predictive factors and outcomes for posterior segment intraocular foreign bodies. Eye (Lond.) 26, 751–752.

Awschalom, L., Meyers, S.M., 1982. Ultrasonography of vitreal foreign bodies in eyes obtained at autopsy. Arch. Ophthalmol. 100, 979–980.

Bai, H.Q., Yao, L., Meng, X.X., et al., 2011. Visual outcome following intraocular foreign bodies: a retrospective review of 5-year clinical experience. Eur. J. Ophthlamol. 21, 98–103.

Bronson, N.R., 1965. Techniques of ultrasonic localization and extraction of intraocular and extraocular foreign bodies. Am. J. Ophthalmol. 60, 596–603.

Colyer, M.H., Weber, E.D., Weichel, E.D., et al., 2007. Delayed intraocular foreign body removal without endophthalmitis during Operations Iraqi Freedom and Enduring Freedom. Ophthalmol 114, 1439–1447.

Ferrari, T.M., Cardascia, N., Di Gesu, I., et al., 2001. Early versus late removal of retained intraocular foreign bodies. Retina 21, 92–93.

Greven, C.M., Engelbrecht, N.E., Slusher, M.M., et al., 2000. Intraocular foreign bodies: management, prognostic factors, and visual outcomes. Ophthalmol 107, 608–612.

Jonas, J.B., Knorr, H.L., Budde, W.M., 2000. Prognostic factors in ocular injuries caused by intraocular or retrobulbar foreign bodies. Ophthalmol 107, 823–828.

Mieler, W.F., Ellis, M.K., Williams, D.F., et al., 1990. Retained intraocular foreign bodies and endophthalmitis. Ophthalmol 97, 1532–1538.

Mittra, R.A., Mieler, W.F., 1999. Controversies in the management of open-globe injuries involving the posterior segement. Surv. Ophthalmol. 44, 215–225.

Shah, C.M., Gentile, R.C., Mehta, M.C., 2016. Perfluorocarbon liquids' ability to protect the macula from intraocular dropping of metallic foreign bodies: a model eye study. Retina 36 (7), 1285–1291.

Thach, A.B., Ward, T.P., Dick, J.S. 2nd, et al., 2005. Intraocular foreign body injuries during Operation Iraqi Freedom. Ophthalmol 112, 1829–1833.

Williams, D.F., Mieler, W.F., Abrams, G.W., 1990. Intraocular foreign bodies in young peiople. Retina 10 (Suppl. 1), S45–S49.

Williams, D.F., Mieler, W.F., Abrams, G.W., et al., 1988. Results and prognostic factors in penetrating ocular injuries with retained intraocular foreign bodies. Ophthalmol 95, 911–916.

Penetrating and/or Perforating Injury

Abrams, G.W., Topping, T.M., Machemer, R., 1979. Vitrectomy for injury: the effect on intraocular proliferation following perforation of the posterior segment of the rabbit eye. Arch. Ophthalmol. 97, 743–748.

Agrawal, R., Shah, M., Mireskandari, K., et al., 2013. Controversies in ocular trauma classification and management: review. Int. Ophthalmol. 33, 435–446.

Alfaro, D.V. III, Jablon, E.P., Fontal, M.R., et al., 2005. Fishing-related ocular trauma. Am. J. Ophthalmol. 139, 488–492.

Campochiaro, P.A., Gaskin, H.C., Vinores, S.A., 1987. Retinal cryopexy stimulates traction retinal detachment formation in the presence of an ocular wound. Arch. Ophthalmol. 105, 1567–1570.

Cardillo, J.A., Stout, J.T., LaBree, L., et al., 1997. Post-traumatic proliferative vitreoretinopathy the epidemiologic profile, onset, risk factors, and visual outcome. Ophthalmol 104, 1166–1173.

Cleary, P.E., Ryan, S.J., 1979. Histology of wound, vitreous and retina in experimental posterior penetrating eye injury in the rhesus monkey. Am. J. Ophthalmol. 88, 221–231.

Cleary, P.E., Ryan, S.J., 1981. Vitrectomy in penetrating eye injury: results of a controlled trial of vitrectomy in an experimental posterior penetrating eye injury in the rhesus monkey. Arch. Ophthalmol. 99, 287–292.

Colyer, M.H., Chun, D.W., Bower, K.S., et al., 2008. Perforating globe injuries during operation Iraqi Freedom. Ophthalmol 115, 2087–2093.

de Bustros, S., Michels, R.G., Glaser, B.M., 1990. Evolving concepts in the management of posterior segment penetrating ocular injuries. Retina 10, 72–75.

De Juan, E., Sternberg, P., Michels, R.G., 1983. Penetrating injuries, types of injuries and visual results. Ophthalmology 90, 1318–1322.

de Juan, E. Jr., Steinberg, P. Jr., Michels, R.G., 1983. Penetrating ocular injuries: types of injuries and visual results. Ophthalmology 90, 1318–1322.

Entezari, M., Rabei, H.M., Badalabadi, M.M., et al., 2006. Visual outcome and ocular survival in open-globe injuries. Injury 37, 633–637.

Esmaeli, B., Elner, S.G., Schork, M.A., et al., 1995. Visual outcome and ocular survival after penetrating trauma: a clinicopathologic study. Ophthalmology 102, 393–400.

Fuller, D.G., Hutton, W.L., 1990. Prediction of postoperative vision in eyes with severe trauma. Retina 10, 20–34.

Gervasio, K.A., Weinstock, B.M., Wu, A.Y., 2015. Prognostic value of ocular trauma scores in patients with combined open globe injuries and facial fractures. Am. J. Ophthalmol. 160, 882–888.

Gregor, Z., Ryan, S.J., 1983. Complete and core vitrectomies in the treatment of epiretinal posterior penetrating eye injury in the rhesus monkey. I. Clinical features. Arch. Ophthalmol. 101, 441–445.

Gregor, Z., Ryan, S.J., 1983. Complete and core vitrectomies in the treatment of experimental posterior penetrating eye injury in the Rhesus monkey. II. Histologic features. Arch. Ophthalmol. 101, 446–450.

Madhusudhana, K.C., Hossain, P., Thiagarajan, M., et al., 2007. Use of anterior segment optical coherence tomography in a penetrating eye injury. Br. J. Ophthalmol. 91, 982–983.

Mieler, W.F., Mittra, R.A., 1997. The role and timing of pars plana vitrectomy in penetrating ocular injuries [editorial]. Arch. Ophthalmol. 113, 1191–1192.

Mittra, R.A., Mieler, W.F., 1999. Controversies in the management of open-globe injuries involving the posterior segement. Surv. Ophthalmol. 44, 215–225.

Moon, C., Lee, J., Sohn, J., et al., 1996. The result of consecutive vitrectomy in penetrating ocular injury. J. Kor. Ophthal. Soc. 37, 1937–1945.

Pieramici, D.J., Sternberg, P., Aaberg, T. Sr., et al., 1997. Perspective: a system for classifying mechanical injuries of the eye (globe). Am. J. Ophthalmol. 123, 820–831.

Pieramici, D.J., Au Eong, K.G., Sternberg, P. Jr., et al., 2003. The prognostic significance of a system for classifying mechanical injuries of the eye (globe) in open-globe injuries. J. Trauma 54, 750–754.

Ryan, S.J., Allen, A.W., 1979. Pars plana vitrectomy in ocular trauma. Am. J. Ophthalmol. 88, 483–491.

Ryan, S.J., 1993. Traction retinal detachment. XLIX Edward Jackson Memorial Lecture. Am. J. Ophthalmol. 115, 1–20.

Sandinha, M.T., Newman, W., Wong, D., et al., 2011. Outcomes of delayed vitrectomy in open-globe injuries in young patients. Retina 31, 1541–1544.

Shock, J.P., Adams, D., 1985. Long-term visual acuity results after penetrating and perforating ocular injuries. Am. J. Ophthalmol. 100, 714–718.

Spalding, S.C., Sternberg, P., 1990. Controversies in the management of posterior segment ocular trauma. Retina 10, 76–82.

Spiegel, D., Nasemann, J., Nawrocki, J., et al., 1997. Severe ocular trauma managed with primary pars plana vitrectomy and silicone oil. Retina 17, 275–285.

Topping, T.M., Abrams, G.W., Machemer, R., 1979. Experimental double perforating injury of the posterior segment in rabbit eyes. The natural history of intraocular proliferation. Arch. Ophthalmol. 97, 735–742.

Ussmann, J.H., Lazarides, E., Ryan, S.J., 1981. Traction retinal detachment: a cell-mediated event. Arch. Ophthalmol. 99, 869–872.

Valsalva Retinopathy

Androudi, S., Ahmed, M., Brazitikos, P., et al., 2005. Valsalva retinopathy: diagnostic challenges in a patient with pars-planitis. Acta Ophthalmol. Scand. 83, 256–257.

De Maeyer, K., Van Ginderdeuren, R., Postelmans, L., et al., 2007. Sub-inner limiting membrane haemorrhage: causes and treatment with vitrectomy. Br. J. Ophthalmol. 91, 869–872.

Durukan, A.H., Kerimoglu, H., Erdurman, C., et al., 2008. Long-term results of Nd:YAG laser treatment for premacular subhyaloid haemorrhage owing to Valsalva retinopathy. Eye (Lond.) 22, 214–218.

Eneh, A., Almeida, D., 2013. Valsalva hemorrhagic retinopathy during labor: a case report and literature review. Can. J. Ophthalmol. 48 (6), e145–e147.

Garcia Fernandez, M., Navarro, J.C., Castano, C.G., 2012. Long-term evolution of Valsalva retinopathy: a case series. J. Med. Case Rep. 6, 346.

Goel, N., Kumar, V., Seth, A., et al., 2011. Spectral-domain optical coherence tomography following Nd:YAG laser membranotomy in valsalva retinopathy. Ophthalmic Surg. Lasers Imaging 42, 222–228.

Hua, R., Liu, L.M., Hu, Y.D., et al., 2013. Combine intravitreal bevacizumab with Nd:YAG laser hyaloidotomy for valsalva pre-macular haemorrhage and observe the internal limiting membrane changes: a spectralis study. Int. J. Ophthalmol. 6, 242–245.

Karagiannis, D., Gregor, Z., 2006. Valsalva retinopathy associated with idiopathic thrombocytopenic purpura and positive antiphospholipid antibodies. Eye (Lond.) 20, 1447–1449.

Ladjimi, A., Zaouali, S., Messaoud, R., et al., 2002. Valsalva retinopathy induced by labour. Eur. J. Ophthalmol. 12, 336–338.

Manche, E.F., Goldberg, R.A., Mondino, B.J., 1997. Air bag-related ocular injuries. Ophthalm. Surg. Lasers 28, 246–250.

Shukla, D., Naresh, K.B., Kim, R., 2005. Optical coherence tomography findings in valsalva retinopathy. Am. J. Ophthalmol. 140, 134–136.

Tatlipinar, S., Shah, S.M., Nguyen, Q.D., 2007. Optical coherence tomography features of sub-internal limiting membrane hemorrhage and preretinal membrane in Valsalva retinopathy. Can. J. Ophthalmol. 42, 129–130.

Purtscher Retinopathy

Agrawal, A., McKibbin, M.A., 2006. Purtscher's and Purtscher-like retinopathies: a review. Surv. Ophthalmol. 51, 129–136.

Agrawal, A., McKibbin, M., 2007. Purtscher's retinopathy: epidemiology, clinical features and outcome. Br. J. Ophthalmol. 91, 1456–1459.

Blodi, B., Johnson, M.W., Gass, J.D.M., et al., 1990. Purtscher's-like retinopathy after childbirth. Ophthalmology 97, 1654–1659.

Burton, T.C., 1980. Unilateral Purtscher's retinopathy. Ophthalmology 87, 1096–1105.

Chan, A., Fredrick, D.R., Leng, T., 2011. Neovascularization in Purtscher's retinopathy. Clin. Ophthalmol. 5, 1585–1587.

Holak, H.M., Holak, S., 2007. Prognostic factors for visual outcome in purtscher retinopathy. Surv. Ophthalmol. 52, 117–118, author reply 118–119.

Kelley, J.S., 1972. Purtscher's retinopathy related to chest compression by safety belts: fluorescein angiographic findings. Am. J. Ophthalmol. 74, 278–283.

Meyer, C.H., Callizo, J., Schmidt, J.C., et al., 2006. Functional and anatomical findings in acute Purtscher's retinopathy. Ophthalmologica 220 (5), 343–346.

Miguel, A.I., Henriques, F., Azevedo, L.F., et al., 2013. Systematic review of Purtscher's and Purtscher-like retinopathies. Eye (Lond.) 27 (1), 1–13.

Nayak, H., Harun, S., Palimar, P., 2005. Purtscher's retinopathy after fracture dislocation of shoulder joint. Emerg. Med. J. 22, 831–832.

Patel, M., Bains, A., O'Hara, J.P., et al., 2001. Purtscher retinopathy as the initial sign of thrombotic thrombocytopenic purpura/hemolytic uremic syndrome. Arch. Ophthalmol. 119, 1388–1390.

Pratt, M.V., De Venecia, G., 1970. Purtscher's retinopathy: a clinicopathological correlation. Surv. Ophthalmol. 14, 417–423.

Shah, G.K., Penne, R., Grand, M.G., 2001. Purtscher's retinopathy secondary to airbag injury. Retina 21, 68–69.

Terson Syndrome

Clarkson, J.G., Flynn, H.W. Jr., Daily, M.J., 1980. Vitrectomy in Terson's syndrome. Am. J. Ophthalmol. 90, 549–552.

Doubler, F.H., Marlow, S.B., 1917. A case of hemorrhage into the optic nerve sheaths as a direct extension from a diffuse intrameningeal hemorrhage caused by rupture of aneurysms of a cerebral artery. Arch. Ophthalmol. 46, 593–596.

Isernhagen, R.D., Smiddy, W.E., Michels, R.G., et al., 1988. Vitrectomy for nondiabetic vitreous hemorrhage: not associated with vascular disease. Retina 8, 81–87.

Keithahn, M.A.Z., Bennett, S.R., Cameron, D., et al., 1993. Retinal folds in Terson's syndrome. Ophthalmology 100, 1187–1190.

Miller, A.J., Cuttino, J.T., 1948. On the mechanism of production of massive preretinal hemorrhage following rupture of a congenital medial defect intracranial aneurysm. Am. J. Ophthalmol. 31, 19–24.

Shaw, H.E. Jr., Landers, M.B. III, Sydnor, C.F., 1977. The significance of intraocular hemorrhages due to subarachnoid hemorrhage. Ann. Ophthalmol. 9, 1403–1405.

Schultz, P.N., Sobol, W.M., Weingeist, T.A., 1991. Long-term visual outcome in Terson syndrome. Ophthalmology 98, 1814–1819.

Terson, A., 1900. De L'hemorrhagie dans le corps vitre au cours de l'hemorrhagie cerebrale. Clin. Ophthalmol. 6, 309.

Tulloh, C.G., 1968. Trauma in retinal detachment. Br. J. Ophthalmol. 52, 317–321.

Weingeist, T.A., Goldman, E.J., Folk, J.C., et al., 1986. Terson's sysdrome: clinicopathologic correlations. Ophthalmology 93, 1435–1442.

Shaken Baby Syndrome

Conway, M.D., Peyman, G.A., Recasens, M., 1999. Intravitreal tPA and SF6 promote clearing of premacular subhyaloid hemorrhages in shaken baby syndrome. Ophthalmic Surg. Lasers 30, 435–441.

Fishman, C.D., Dasher, W.B. 3rd, Lambert, S.R., 1998. Electroretinographic findings in infants with the shaken baby syndrome. J. Pediatr. Ophthalmol. Strabismus 35, 22–26.

Friendly, D.S., 1971. Ocular manifestation of the physical child abuse. Trans. Am. Acad. Ophthalmol. Otolaryngol. 75, 318–332.

Gardner, H.B., 2004. Suspected child abuse victims. Ophthalmol. 111, 1795–1796.

Giangiacomo, J., Khan, J.A., Levine, C., et al., 1988. Sequential cranial computed tomography in infants with retinal hemorrhages. Ophthalmol. 95, 295–299.

Greenwald, M.J., Weiss, A., Oesterle, C.S., 1986. Traumatic retinoschisis in battered babies. Ophthalmol. 93, 618–629.

Harcourt, B., Hopkins, D., 1973. Permanent chorioretinal lesions in childhood of suspected origin. Trans. Ophthalmol. Soc. UK 93, 199–209.

Harley, R.D., 1980. Ocular manifestations of child abuse. J. Pediatr. Ophthalmol. Strabismus 17, 5–13.

Jensen, A.D., 1971. Ocular clues to child abuse. J. Pediatr. Ophthalmol. 8, 270.

Kivlin, J.D., 2001. Manifestations of shaken baby syndrome. Curr. Opin. Ophthalmol. 12, 158–163.

Kivlin, J.D., Simons, K.B., Lazoritz, S., et al., 2000. Shaken baby syndrome. Ophthalmol. 107, 1246–1254.

Massicotte, S.J., Folberg, R., Torczynski, E., et al., 1991. Vitreoretinal traction and perimacular retinal folds in the eyes of deliberately traumatized children. Ophthalmology 98, 1124–1127.

McCabe, C.F., Donahue, S.P., 2000. Prognostic indicators for vision and mortality in shaken baby syndrome. Arch. Ophthalmol. 118, 373–377.

Ober, R.R., 1980. Hemorrhagic retinopathy in infancy: a clinicopathologic report. J. Pediatr. Ophthalmol. Strabismus 17, 17–20.

Paul Chan, R.V., Forbes, B.J., Levin, A.V., 2013. Evaluation and management of nonaccidental head trauma. J. Pediatr. Ophthalmol. Strabismus 50, 262–264.

Spirn, M.J., Lynn, M.J., Hubbard, G.B. 3rd, 2008. Vitreous hemorrhage in children. Ophthalmol. 113, 848–852.

Sturm, V., Landau, K., Menke, M.N., 2008. Optical coherence tomography findings in Shaken Baby Syndrome. Am. J. Ophthalmol. 146, 363–368.

Tongue, A.C., 1991. The ophthalmologist's role in diagnosing child abuse. Ophthalmol. 98, 1009–1010.

Tsao, K., Kazlas, M., Weiter, J.J., 2002. Ocular injuries in shaken baby syndrome. Int. Ophthalmol. Clin. 42, 145–155.

Vincent, A.L., Kelly, P., 2010. Retinal hemorrhages in inflicted traumatic brain injury; the ophthalmologist in court. Clin. Exp. Ophthalmol. 38, 521–532.

Yoshida, M., Yamazaki, J., Mizunuma, H., 2014. A finite element analysis of the retinal hemorrhages accompanied by shaken baby syndrome/abusive head trauma. J. Biomech. 158, 1146–1154.

Solar Retinopathy and/or Laser-Induced Retinopathy

Arda, H., Oner, A., Mutlu, S., et al., 2007. Multifocal electroretinogram for assessing sun damage following the solar eclipse of 29 March 2006: multifocal electroretinography in solar maculopathy. Doc. Ophthalmol. 114, 159–162.

Boldrey, E.E., Little, H.L., Flocks, M., et al., 1981. Retinal injury due to industrial laser burns. Ophthalmology 88, 101–107.

Comander, J., Gardiner, M., Loewenstein, J., 2011. High-resolution optical coherence tomography findings in solar maculopathy and the differential diagnosis of outer retinal holes. Am. J. Ophthalmol. 152 (3), 413–419.

Cordes, F.C., 1944. A type of foveomacular retinitis observed in the US Navy. Am. J. Ophthalmol. 27, 803–816.

Fich, M., Dahl, H., Fledelius, H., et al., 1993. Maculopathy caused by welding arcs. A report of 3 cases. Acta Ophthalmol. (Copenh) 71, 402–404.

Fuller, D., Machemer, R., Knighton, R.W., 1978. Retinal damage produced by intraocular fiber optic light. Am. J. Ophthalmol. 85, 519–537.

Gardner, T.W., Ai, E., Chrobak, M., et al., 1982. Photic maculopathy secondary to short-circuiting of a high-tension electric current. Ophthalmology 89, 865–868.

Glickman, R.D., 2002. Phototoxicity to the retina: mechanisms of damage. Int. J. Toxicol. 21, 473–490.

Gulkilik, G., Taskapili, M., Kocabora, S., et al., 2009. Association between visual acuity loss and optical coherence tomography findings in patients with late solar retinopathy. Retina 29, 257–261.

Ham, W.T. Jr., 1982. Action spectrum for retinal injury from near ultraviolet radiation in the aphakic monkey. Am. J. Ophthalmol. 93, 299–396.

Jain, A., Desai, R.U., Charalel, R.A., et al., 2009. Solar retinopathy: comparison of optical coherence tomography (OCT) and fluorescein angiography (FA). Retina 29 (9), 1340–1345.

Jampol, L.M., Kraff, M.C., Sanders, D.R., et al., 1985. Near-UV radiation from the operating microscope and pseudophakic cystoid macular edema. Arch. Ophthalmol. 103, 28–30.

Mainster, M.A., 1998. Solar eclipse safety. Ophthalmology 105, 9–10.

Mainster, M.A., 2000. Retinal laser accidents: mechanisms, management and rehabilitation. J. Laser Appl. 12, 3–9.

Mainster, M.A., Stuck, B.E., Brown, J. Jr., 2004. Assessment of alleged retinal laser injuries. Arch. Ophthalmol. 122, 1210–1217.

Ong, J.M., Eke, T., 2006. Risk of solar retinopathy: evaluation of newspaper warnings prior to the 2004 Transit of Venus. Eye (Lond.) 20 (3), 397–398.

Stangos, A.N., Petropoulos, I.K., Pournaras, J.A., et al., 2007. Optical coherence tomography and multifocal electroretinogram findings in chronic solar retinopathy. Am. J. Ophthalmol. 144, 131–134.

Symons, R.C., Mainster, M.A., Goldberg, M.F., 2010. Solar maculopathy in a young child. Br. J. Ophthalmol. 94 (9), 1258–1259.

Wu, J., Seregard, S., Algvere, P.V., 2006. Photochemical damage of the retina. Surv. Ophthalmol. 51, 461–481.

Yannuzzi, L.A., Fisher, Y.L., Krueger, A., et al., 1987. Solar retinopathy: a photobiological and geophysical analysis. Trans. Am. Ophthalmol. Soc. 85, 120–158.

Altitude Retinopathy

Ascaso, F.J., Nerin, M.A., Villen, L., et al., 2012. Acute mountain sickness and retinal evaluation by optical coherence tomography. Eur. J. Ophthalmol. 22 (4), 580–589.

Butler, F.K., Harris, D.J. Jr., Reynolds, R.D., 1992. Altitude retinopathy on Mount Everest, 1989. Ophthalmology 99, 739–746.

Chang, B., Nolan, H., Mooney, D., 2004. High altitude flight retinopathy. Eye (Lond.) 18, 653–656.

Frayser, R., Houston, C.S., Bryan, A.C., et al., 1970. Retinal hemorrhage at high altitude. N. Engl. J. Med. 282, 1183–1184.

Ho, T.Y., Kao, W.F., Lee, S.M., et al., 2011. High-altitude retinopathy after climbing Mount Aconcagua in a group of experienced climbers. Retina 31 (8), 1650–1655.

Lubin, J.R., Rennie, D., Hackett, P., et al., 1982. High altitude retinal hemorrhage: a clinical and pathological case report. Ann. Ophthalmol. 14, 1071–1076.

Maclaren, R.E., Ikram, K., Talks, S.J., 2000. Fluorescein angiography in altitude retinopathy. Br. J. Ophthalmol. 84, 339–400.

McFadden, D.M., Houston, C.S., Sutton, J.R., et al., 1981. High-altitude retinopathy. JAMA 245, 581–586.

Shults, W.T., Swan, K.C., 1975. High altitude retinopathy in mountain climbers. Arch. Ophthalmol. 93, 404–408.

Weidman, M., Tabin, G.C., 1999. High-altitude retinopathy and altitude illness. Ophthalmology 106, 1924–1927.

Willmann, G., Fischer, M.D., Schatz, A., et al., 2013. Retinal vessel leakage at high altitude. JAMA 309 (21), 2210–2212.

CHAPTER 13

Complications of Ocular Surgery

Injections
Retrobulbar Anesthetic

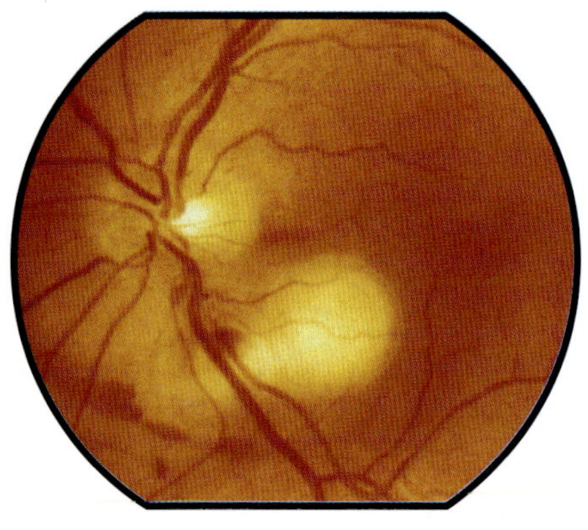
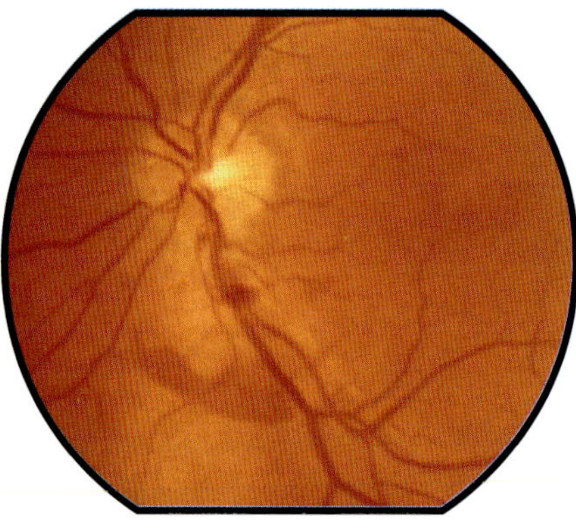

This patient was about to have juxtafoveal laser photocoagulation for a chronic detachment. A retrobulbar anesthetic was used and the needle penetrated the posterior segment. The yellowish material represents the anesthetic agent *(left)*. There is also hemorrhage from the penetration. One day later, the anesthetic resolved and the retina flattened out *(right)*.

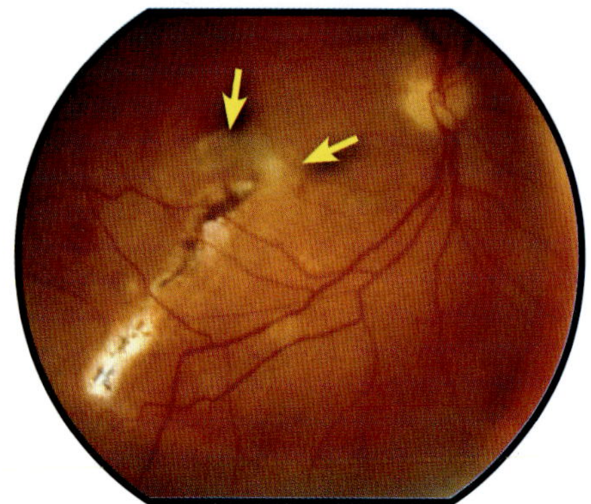

This patient experienced a penetrating injury from a retrobulbar needle. There is exudate at the fovea *(arrows)*, which was the terminal point of the penetration.

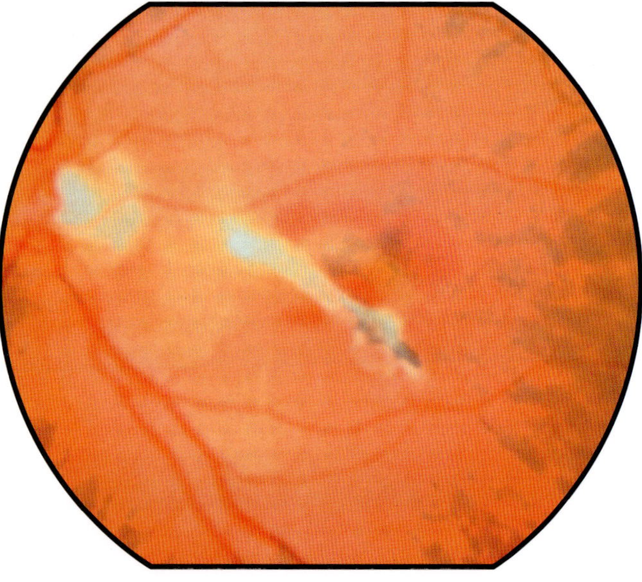
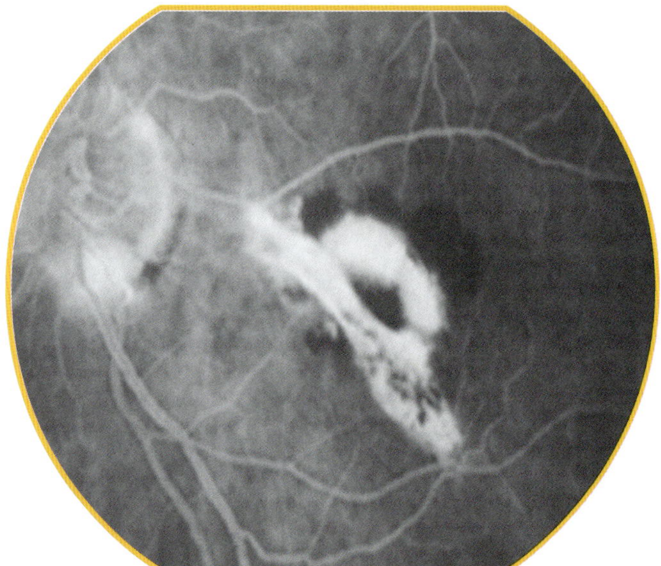

A myopic patient who experienced a needle perforation through the macular region. The track of the needle is clearly visible clinically and angiographically. *Courtesy of David Boyer, MD*

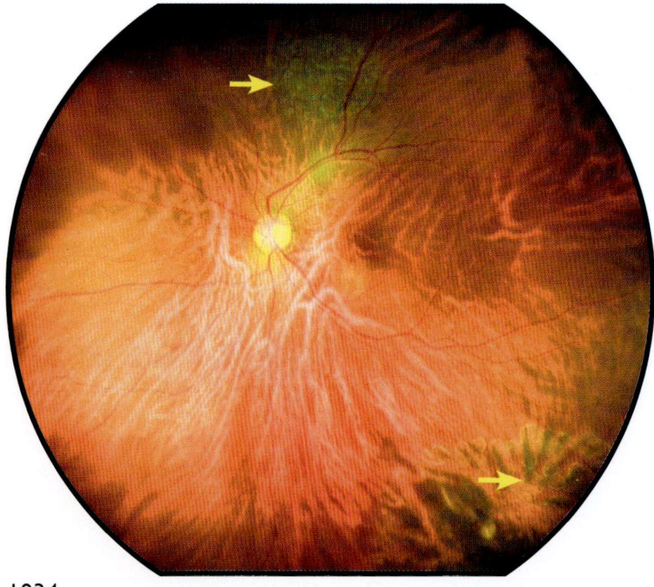

This cataract surgery patient received retrobulbar anesthesia and sustained a double perforating injury. Subsequent vitrectomy surgery for vitreous hemorrhage revealed two perforating sites. There was an entrance site inferotemporally near the equator *(arrow)*, and a second needle exit site superior to the optic disc *(arrow)*. Fortunately, there was no evidence of retinal detachment. Following vitrectomy surgery, the patient recovered vision to 20/30.

Nasopharynx Injection

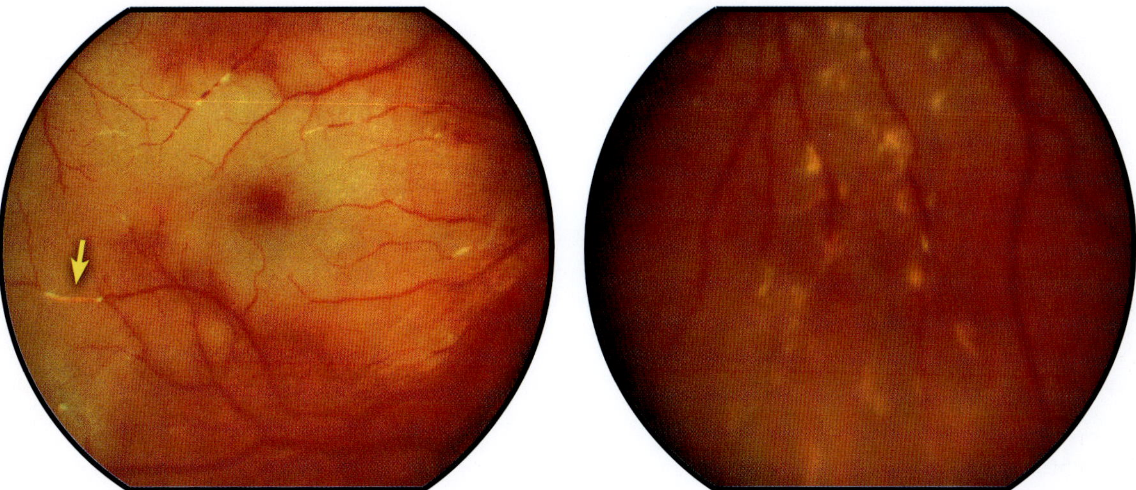

This patient was given a nasopharyngeal injection of a corticosteroid suspension. There was obstruction of retinal arterioles *(left)*, along with whitening of the retina and a plaque of the suspension in a retinal vessel *(arrow)*. The drug can be seen in the choroidal circulation as well *(multiple yellowish particles in the image on the right)*.

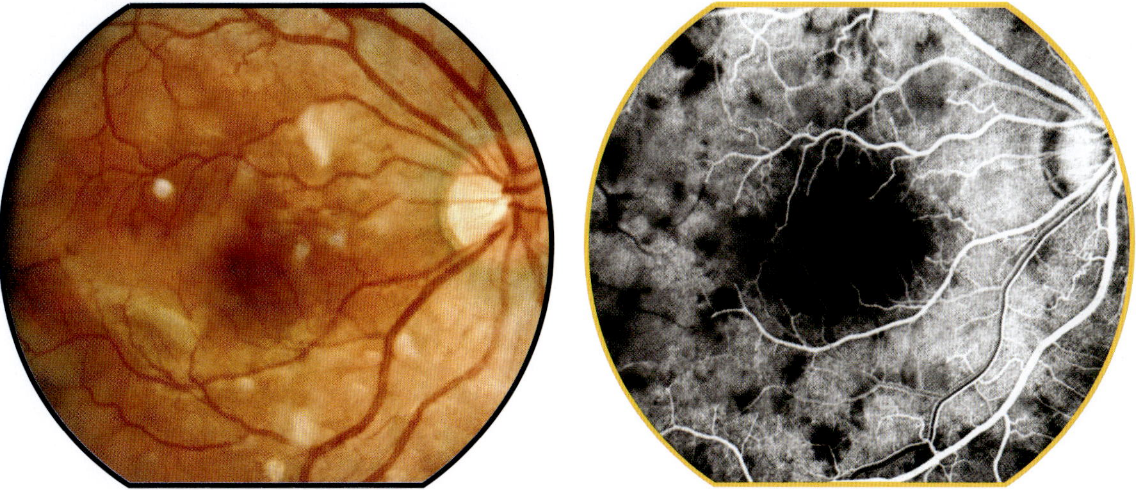

This patient was injected in the nasopharyngeal area for chronic sinusitis. A corticosteroid suspension obstructed arteriolar and choriocapillaris vessels. Note the whitening of the retina on the color photograph and the multifocal areas of absent perfusion on the fluorescein angiogram. *Courtesy of Dr. Kurt Gitter*

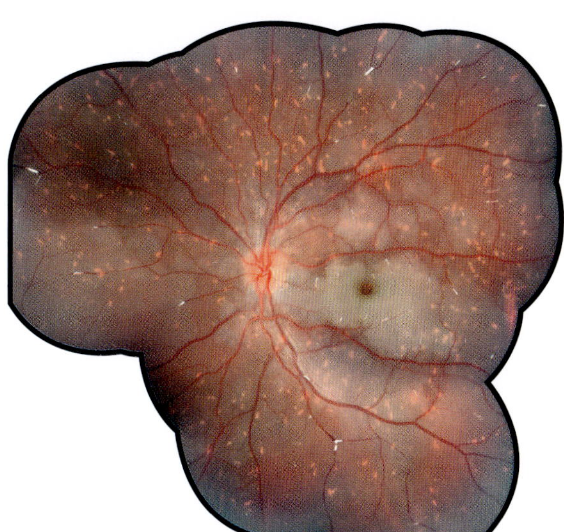

This patient developed epistaxis and received a nasal packing that contained corticosteroids. The patient lost vision and was noted to have corticosteroid particulate matter in the retinal arterioles, along with a central retinal artery occlusion. There was minimal visual recovery. *Courtesy of Scott R. Sneed, MD*

Intravitreal Triamcinolone Injection

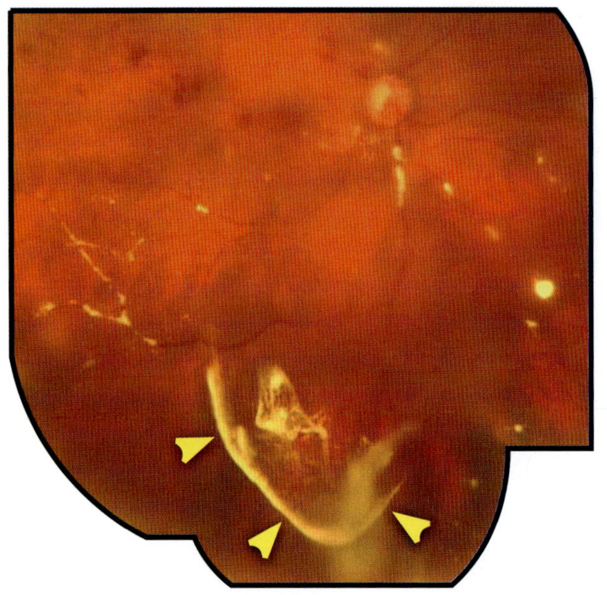

This patient was injected with triamcinolone. This formulation precipitated within the vitreous as irregular lesions *(arrowheads)*. The vitreous is otherwise cloudy from endophthalmitis.

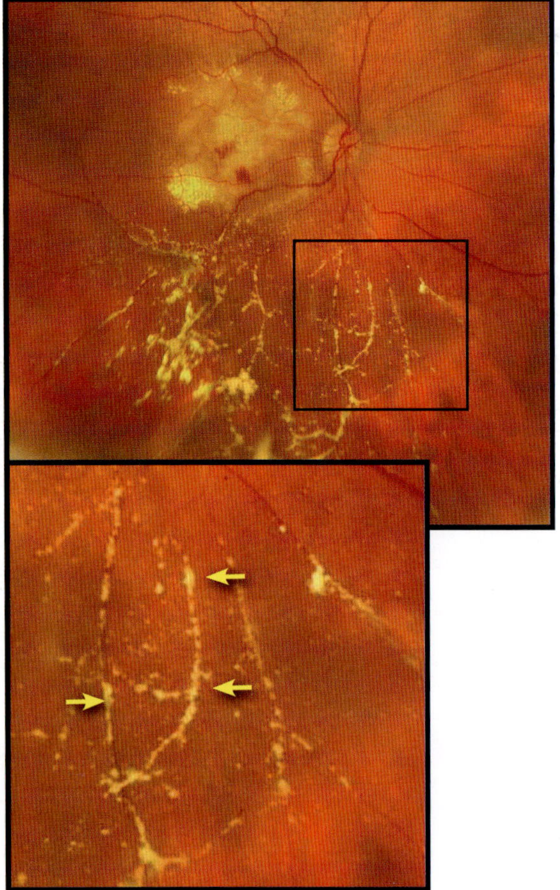

This patient had been administered a triamcinolone suspension for chronic edema and a branch vein occlusion. Note the suspension of the particulate matter in the vitreous. There appears to be a vasotrophic orientation of the drug as it adheres to larger retinal vessels *(arrows)*.

Intravitreal Vancomycin Injection

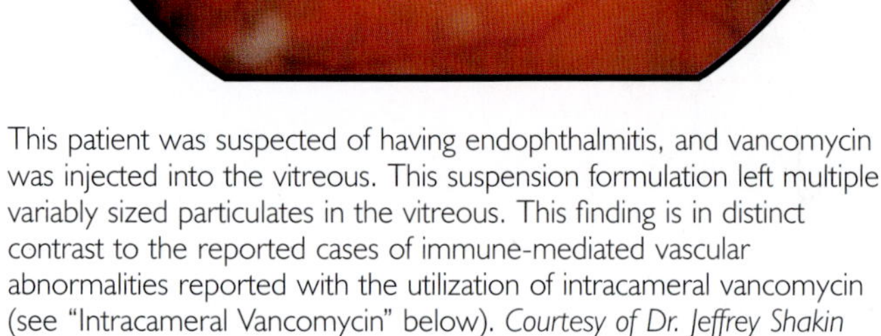

This patient was suspected of having endophthalmitis, and vancomycin was injected into the vitreous. This suspension formulation left multiple variably sized particulates in the vitreous. This finding is in distinct contrast to the reported cases of immune-mediated vascular abnormalities reported with the utilization of intracameral vancomycin (see "Intracameral Vancomycin" below). *Courtesy of Dr. Jeffrey Shakin*

Mechanical Retinal Vascular Obstruction (from Injections)

Mechanical retinal vascular obstruction may occur in the course of ocular surgery from an injection into the optic nerve sheath during anesthesia. Complications range from a retrobulbar hemorrhage with elevation of the intraocular pressure and/or a sudden rise in the intraocular pressure during the course of a closed vitrectomy operation, with resultant central artery occlusion.

Optic Nerve Sheath Injection

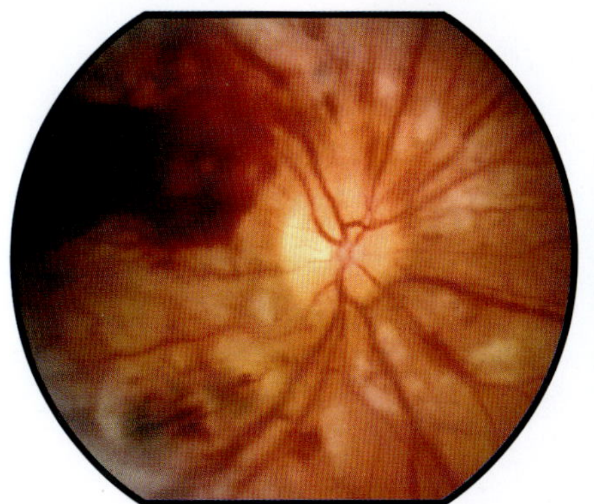

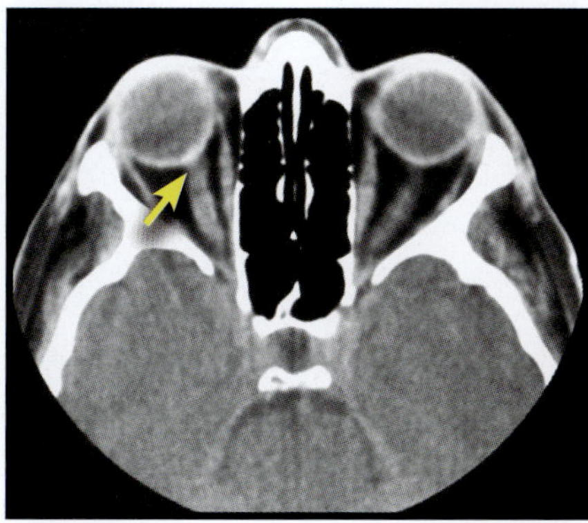

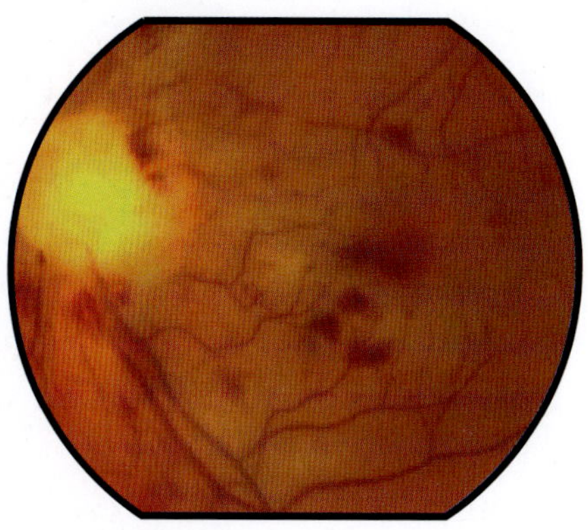

This patient had a combined artery and venous obstruction from an intrasheath injection of the nerve, as captured on a CT scan *(arrow)*. As the pressure in the optic nerve sheath rises, it cuts the venular outflow and eventually the arteriolar inflow will be cut off, resulting in combined whitening of the retina and intraretinal and pre-retinal hemorrhages. In the photo on the right, there is axoplasmic debris within the retina, indicative of retinal ischemia. *Left and middle images courtesy of Dr. Gary Brown*

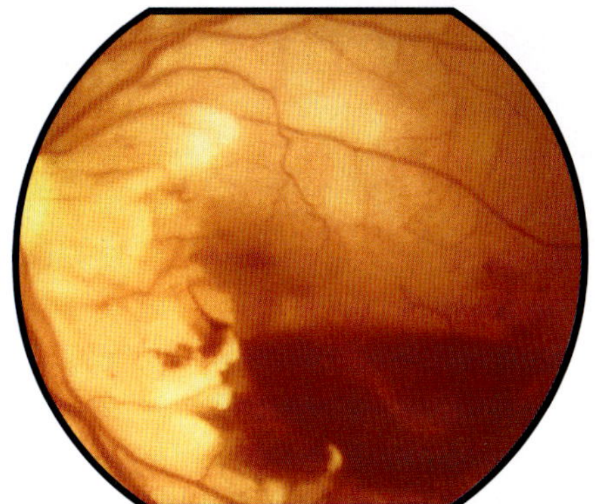

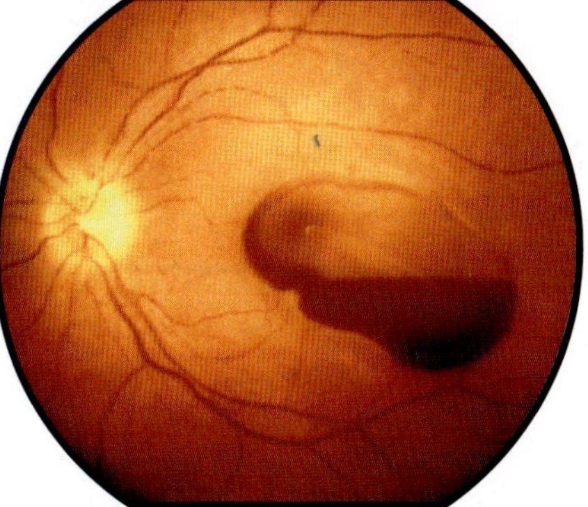

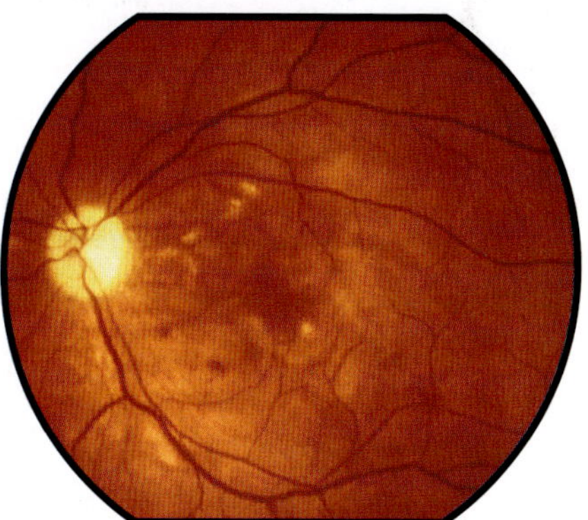

This patient had an inadvertent optic nerve sheath injection that resulted in peripapillary retinal ischemia and pre-retinal hemorrhage or a Terson-like syndrome *(left)*. Eventually the hemorrhage localized in the subhyaloidal area *(middle)*. Three months later, there was complete resolution of the serosanguineous exudative changes, but there was atrophy of the optic nerve *(right)*.

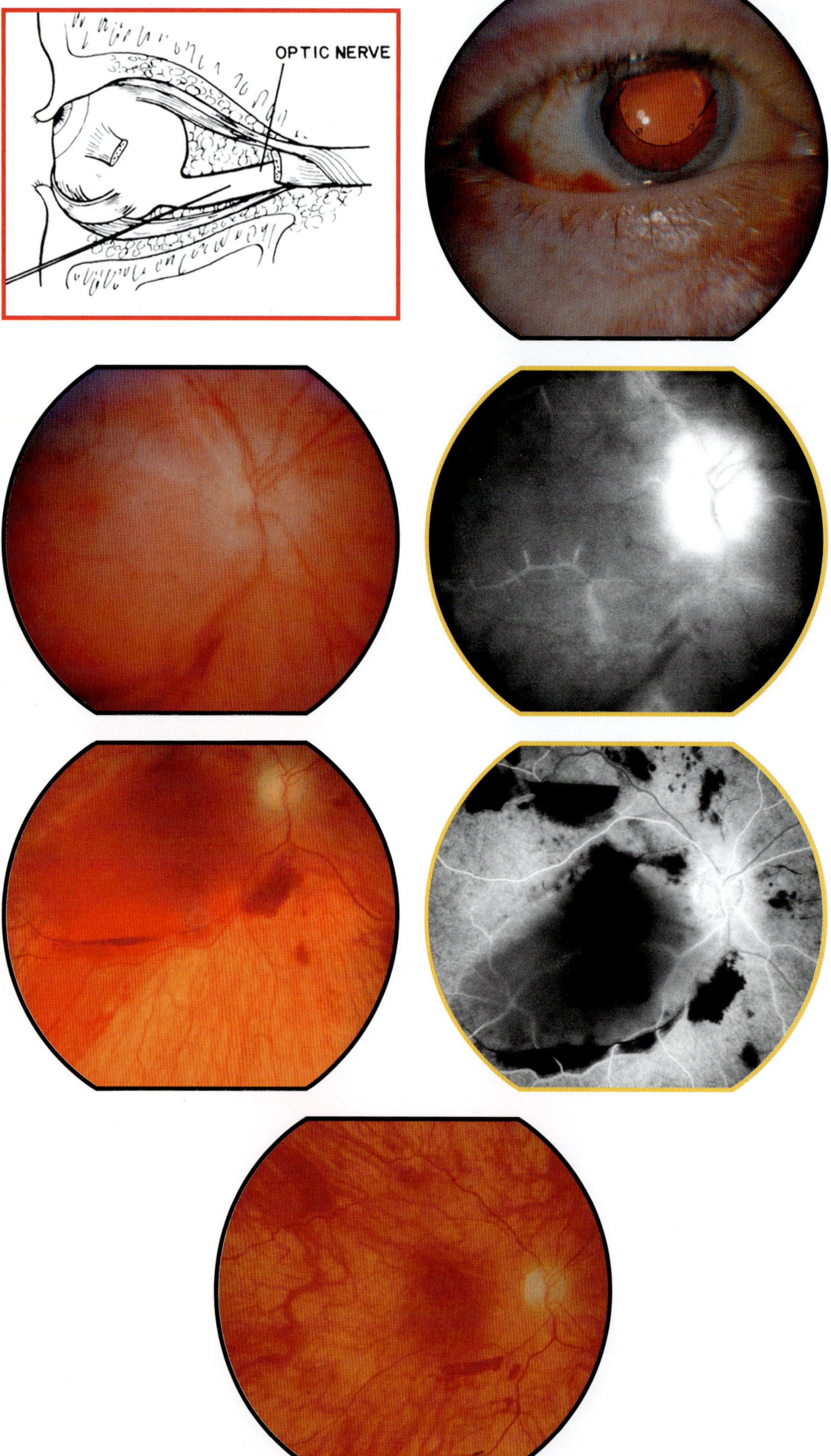

This patient underwent cataract surgery, and no problem was noted until the visit on postoperative day one. The patient sustained a central retinal artery occlusion along with a small amount of intraocular hemorrhage, as is seen in the accompanying color photograph. Visual acuity was bare light perception. MRI of the orbit did not show any definite abnormality (though was obtained two days following the cataract surgery). Vision recovered only to hand motions over the next two months, in spite of eventual reperfusion of the retinal arteries.

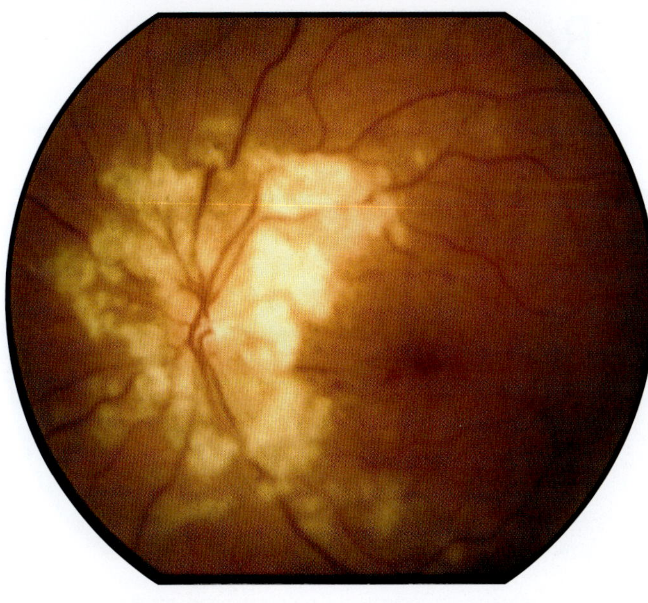

This patient developed a combined retinal artery and vein occlusion presumably from an intrasheath injection prior to cataract surgery. There are elements of Terson syndrome or pre-retinal hemorrhage contiguous with the nerve and extending into the vitreous. A slow rise in intraocular pressure induced the venous obstruction and bleeding, which resulted in arteriolar ischemia.

Retrobulbar Hemorrhage

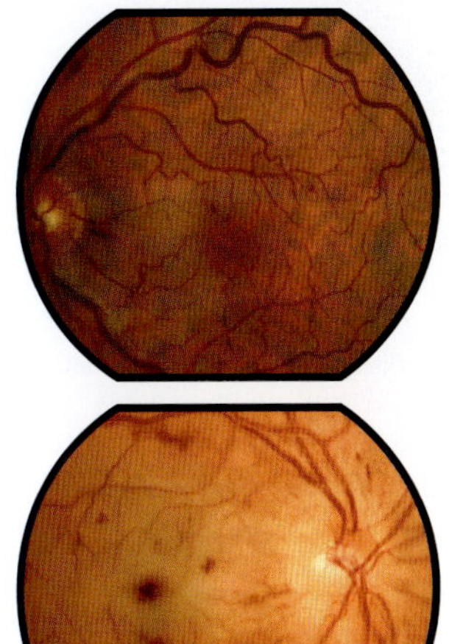

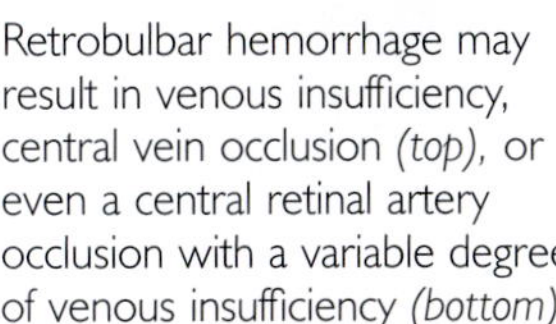

Retrobulbar hemorrhage may result in venous insufficiency, central vein occlusion *(top)*, or even a central retinal artery occlusion with a variable degree of venous insufficiency *(bottom)*.

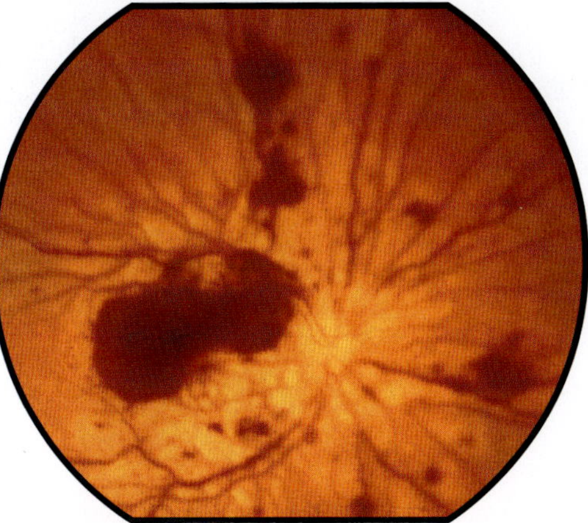

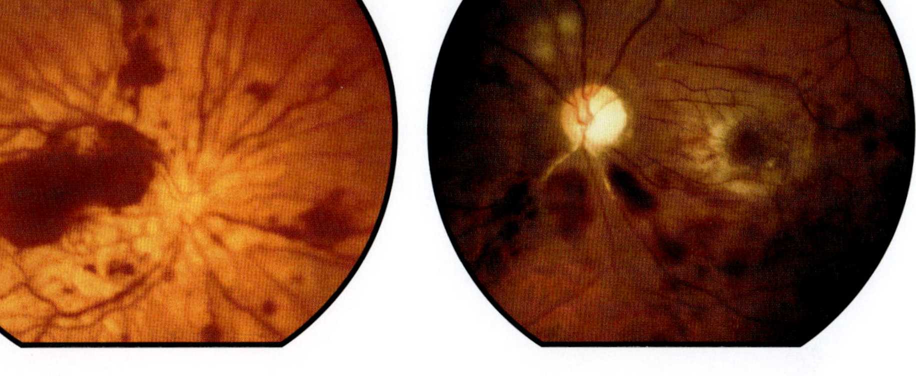

These two patients experienced combined venous and arteriolar occlusion from a retrobulbar hemorrhage. As the intraocular pressure rose there was development of venous occlusion and retinal hemorrhages. Continued elevation of the pressure produced arteriolar obstruction and ischemic whitening of the retina. Each patient ended up with optic atrophy from the antecedent ischemia.

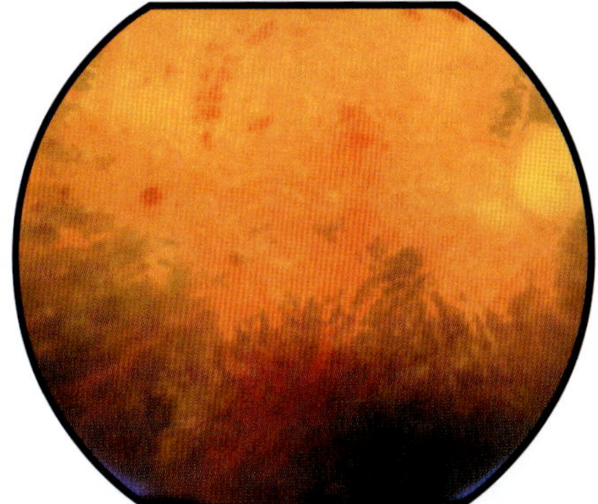

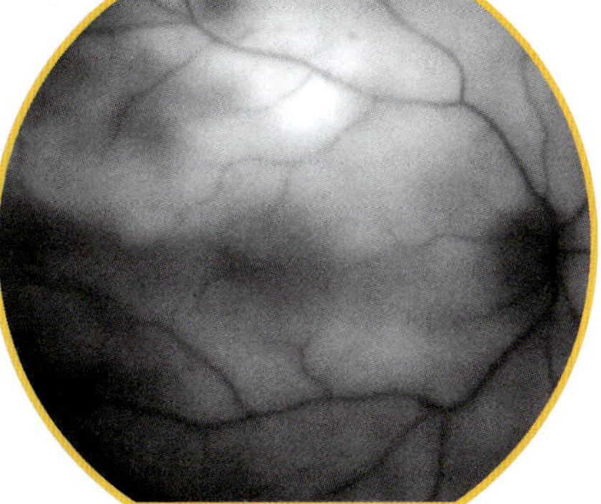

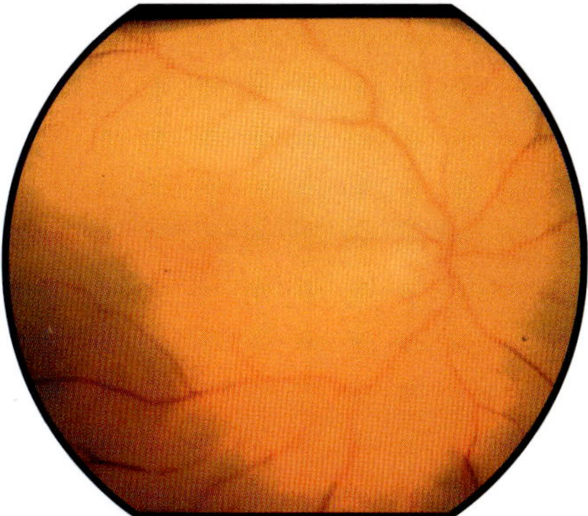

This patient developed an ophthalmic artery occlusion following a retrobulbar injection with localized hemorrhage. Note the complete absence of filling of the choroidal as well as the retinal circulation. There was no visual recovery, and the patient gradually developed optic nerve atrophy, severe vascular attenuation, and diffuse retinal pigment mottling *(right image)*. *Courtesy of David Boyer, MD*

Choroidal Ischemia (Outer Retinal Infarction)

Some intraocular procedures may cause choroidal ischemia, which simulates retinal vascular occlusive disease. While rare, it is particularly known to occur in the course of a closed vitreoretinal procedure.

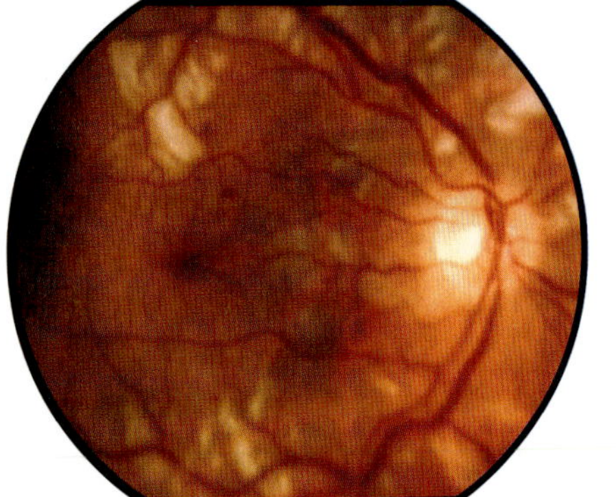

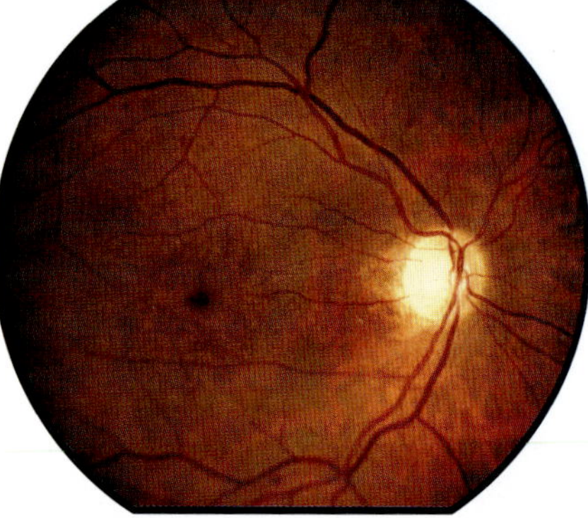

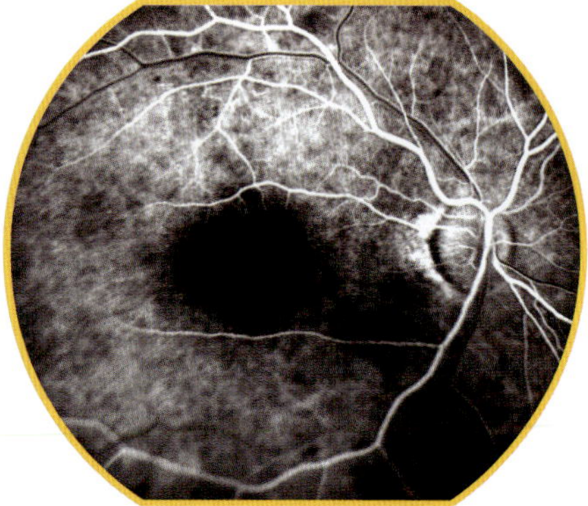

This patient has an accumulation of white subretinal axoplasmic debris from choroidal insufficiency or infarction. The peripapillary insufficiency resulted in a pale nerve *(middle image)*. The fluorescein angiogram shows reperfusion, typical of a compressive event.

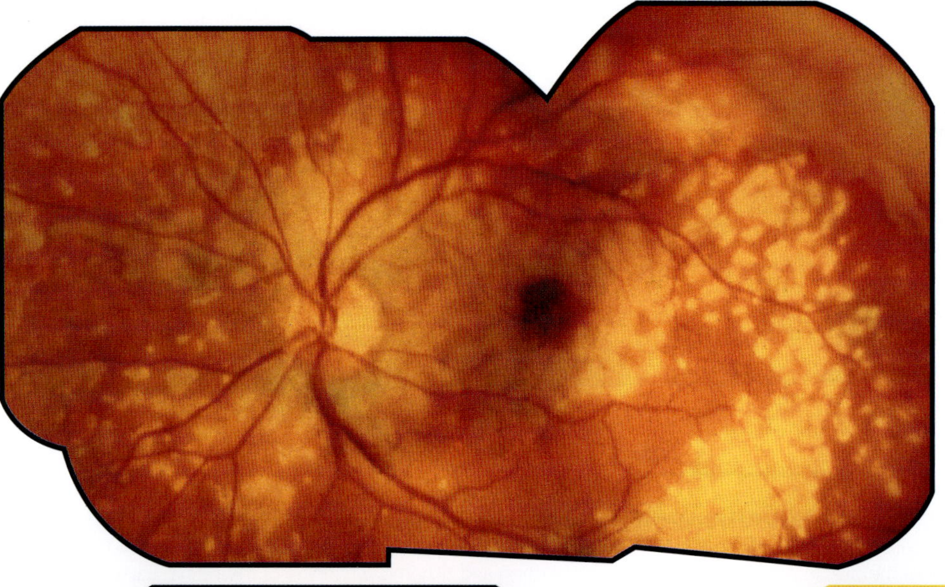

This patient experienced severe inner choroidal vascular insufficiency or outer retinal infarction during phacoemulsification. Notice the relative sparing of the optic nerve and the complete sparing of the perifoveal area, producing a "cherry-red-like" spot.

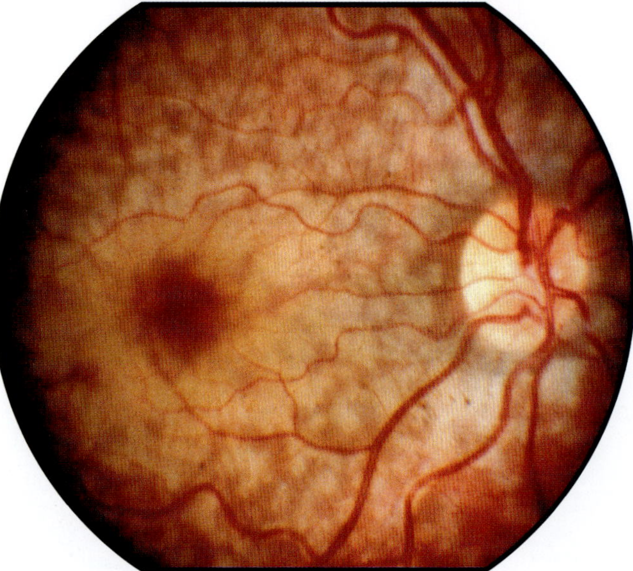

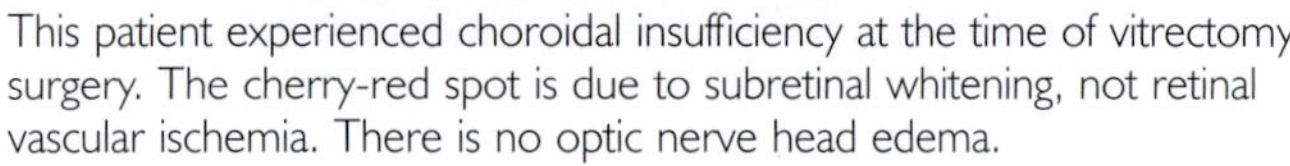

This patient experienced choroidal insufficiency at the time of vitrectomy surgery. The cherry-red spot is due to subretinal whitening, not retinal vascular ischemia. There is no optic nerve head edema.

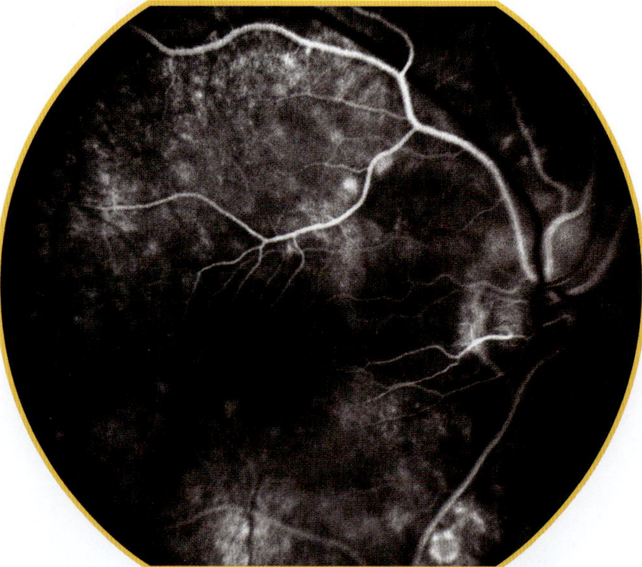

In another patient with choroidal insufficiency, the fluorescein angiogram shows that there is adequate retinal vascular perfusion in this eye.

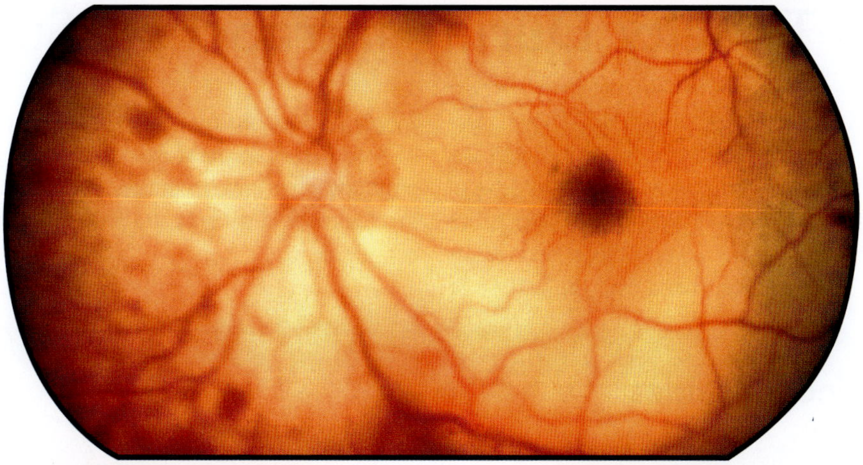

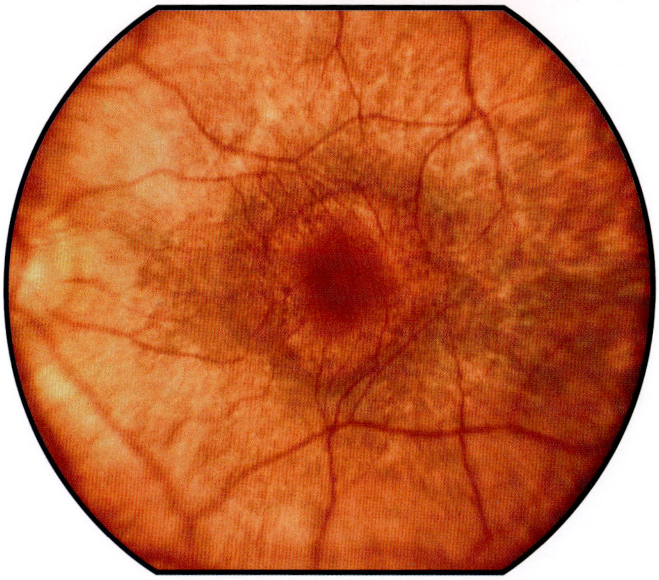

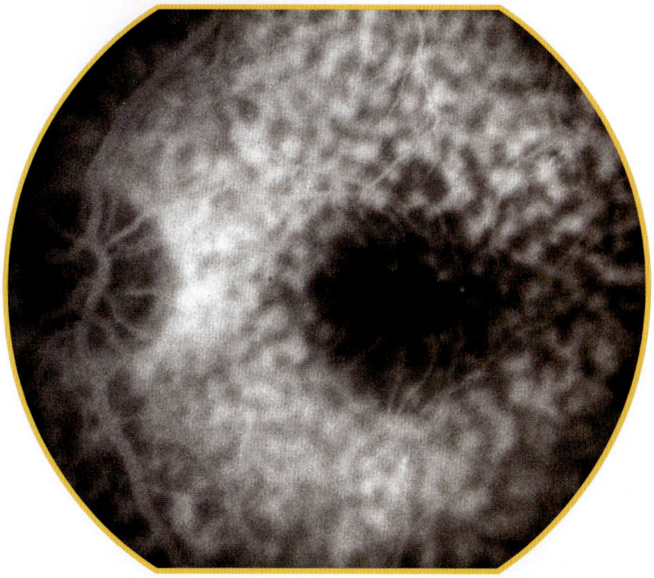

This patient experienced severe choroidal ischemia following a closed vitrectomy. There is outer retinal whitening with hemorrhages, but sparing of the retinal vasculature, optic nerve, and fovea. A "cherry-red-like" spot is seen at the fovea. After reperfusion of the choroid, there are atrophic and pigment epithelial changes, producing a "bull's-eye" pattern. The acuity was not affected, but there was constriction of the peripheral field.

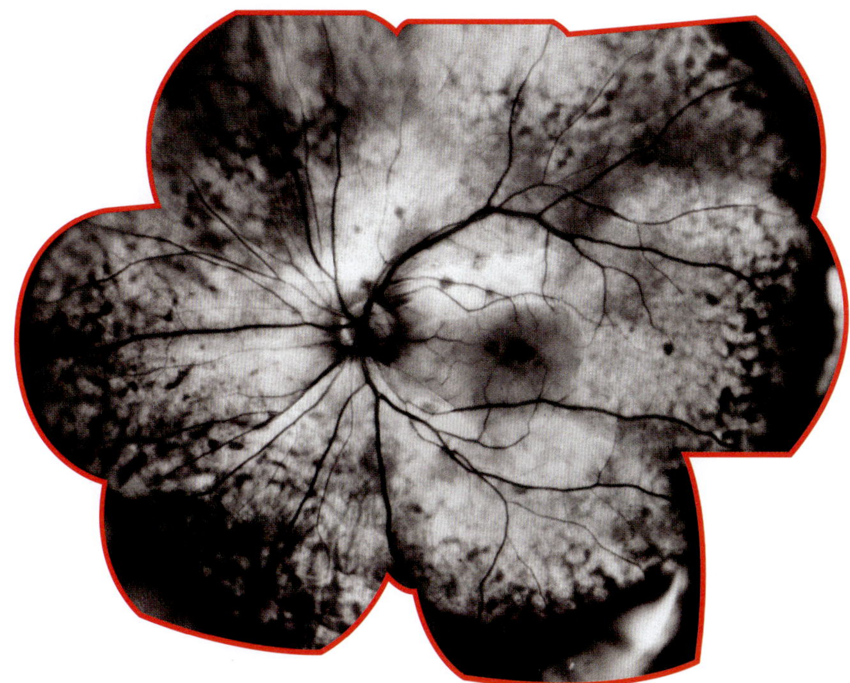

This is a patient who also experienced choroidal insufficiency during a vitrectomy procedure. After resolution of the acute manifestations, there was widespread pigment epithelial atrophy and hyperplasia. The retinal circulation was adequately perfused throughout the course of the complication, and there was sparing of the nerve and disc.
Courtesy of Dr. Sohan Singh Hayreh

Antibiotic Toxicity During Intraocular Surgery

Aminoglycoside toxicity is an uncommon though well-known clinical entity in intraocular surgery. When administered intravitreally, the toxic effect will depend up on the concentration and dose of the drug. Injection into the anterior chamber may also cause prominent uveitis with associated iris complications. Intraocular usage of gentamicin has become quite limited over the past 15 to 20 years. More recently, intracameral vancomycin has been shown to produce an apparent immune-mediated retinal vasculitis, with profound visual impairment. While this has only occurred in a very small number of patients, the precise etiology of this reaction is not entirely clear.

Intraocular Aminoglycosides

When the vitreous is intact, the effect is generally concentrated in a localized area of the posterior pole. The drug can diffusely spread throughout the posterior segment after a vitrectomy procedure. Following resolution of the acute toxic effect of the retina and the associated obliteration of the circulation, there is seldom any reperfusion.

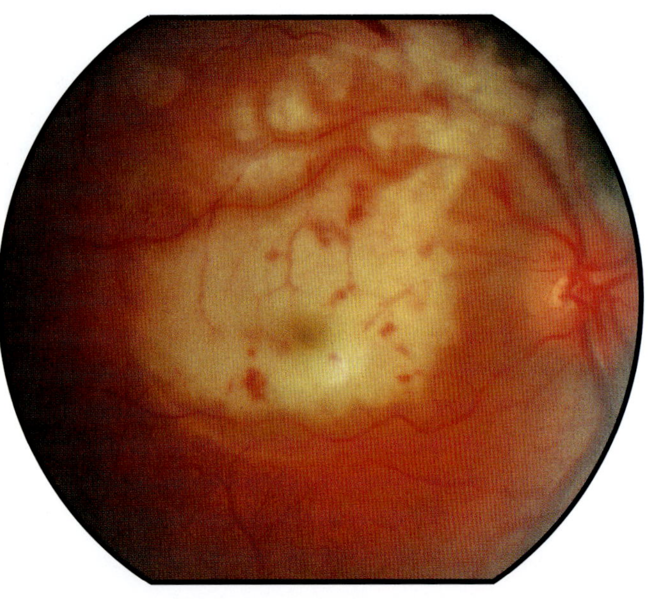

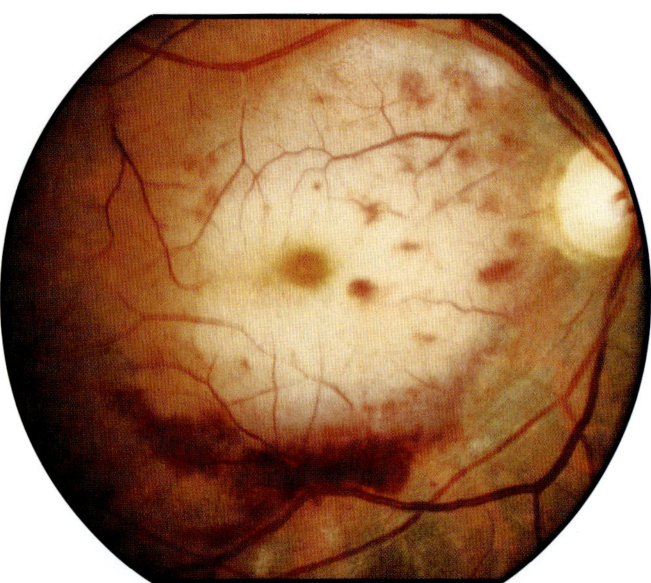

Inadvertent injection of aminoglycosides into the vitreous may gravitate to the posterior pole, producing a necrotizing, obliterative vasculopathy, seen here in these two patients. Often there is a "cookie cutter" distribution of the toxicity producing an ovoid or circular whitening of the retina. There may also be retinal and pre-retinal hemorrhage from necrosis and infarction of retinal vessels. The toxicity specifically does not follow the geographic distribution of the retinal vasculature, though better corresponds to the gravitational effect of the intravitreal injection as the patient is supine during the surgical procedure.

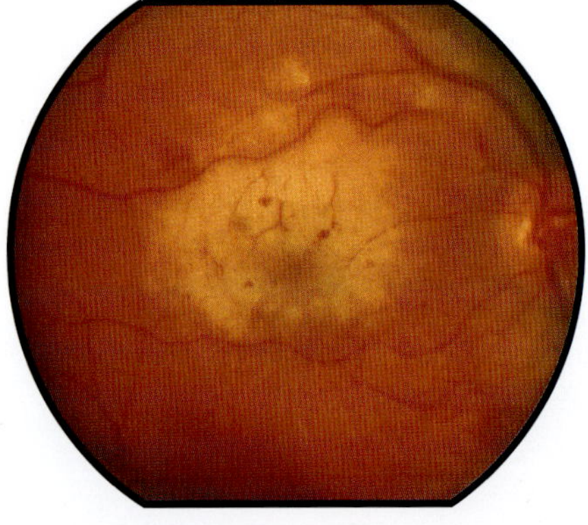

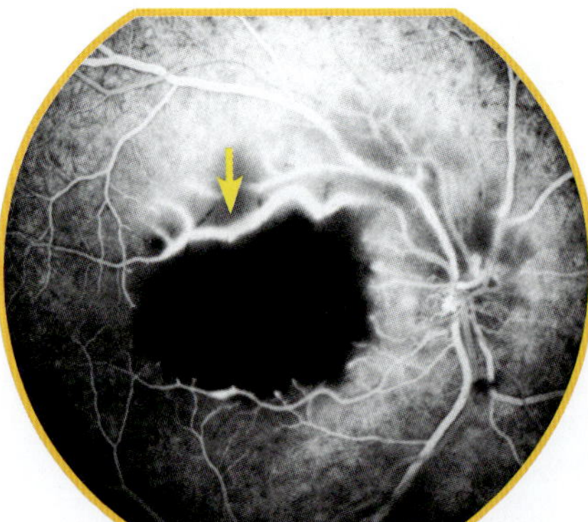

This patient also has a "cookie cutter" necrotizing, ischemic retinopathy centrally. The concentration of the drug may have something to do with the posterior pre-retinal cortical pocket. One of the vessels along the course of the superior temporal vasculature has segmental staining from inflammation, but no obstruction *(arrow)*.

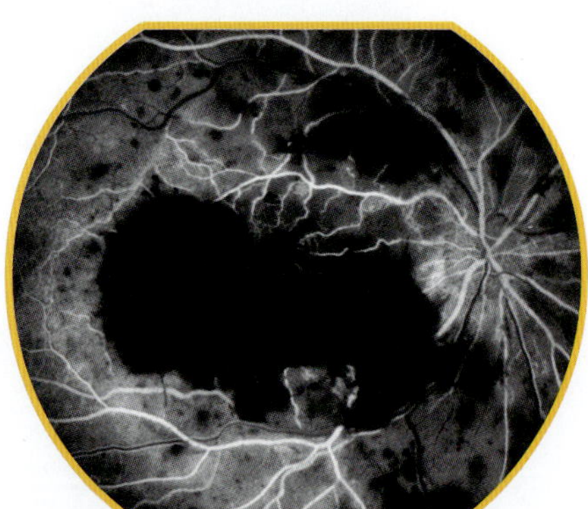

This patient has a necrotizing obliterative vasculopathy centrally, which appears as non-perfusion on the fluorescein angiogram. There are also scattered hemorrhages along the arcades, which produce hypofluorescence.

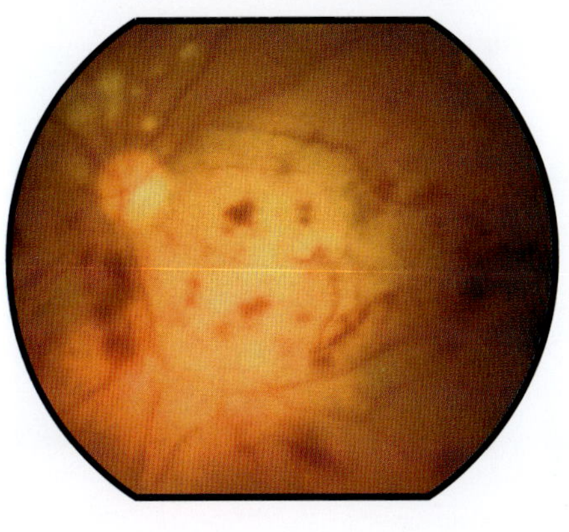
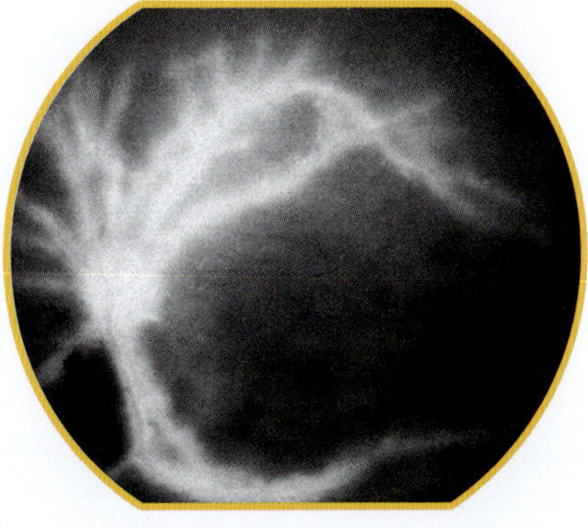
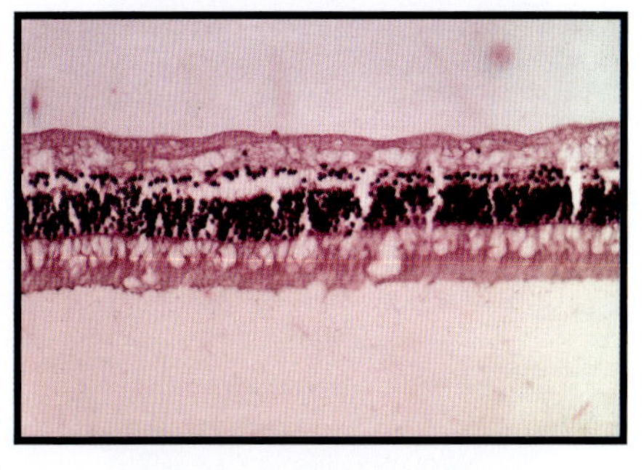

This patient experienced severe aminoglycoside toxicity with diffuse whitening of the retina from infarction *(left)*. Only a few central retinal vessels are perfusing, and they are leaking extensively from inflammation.

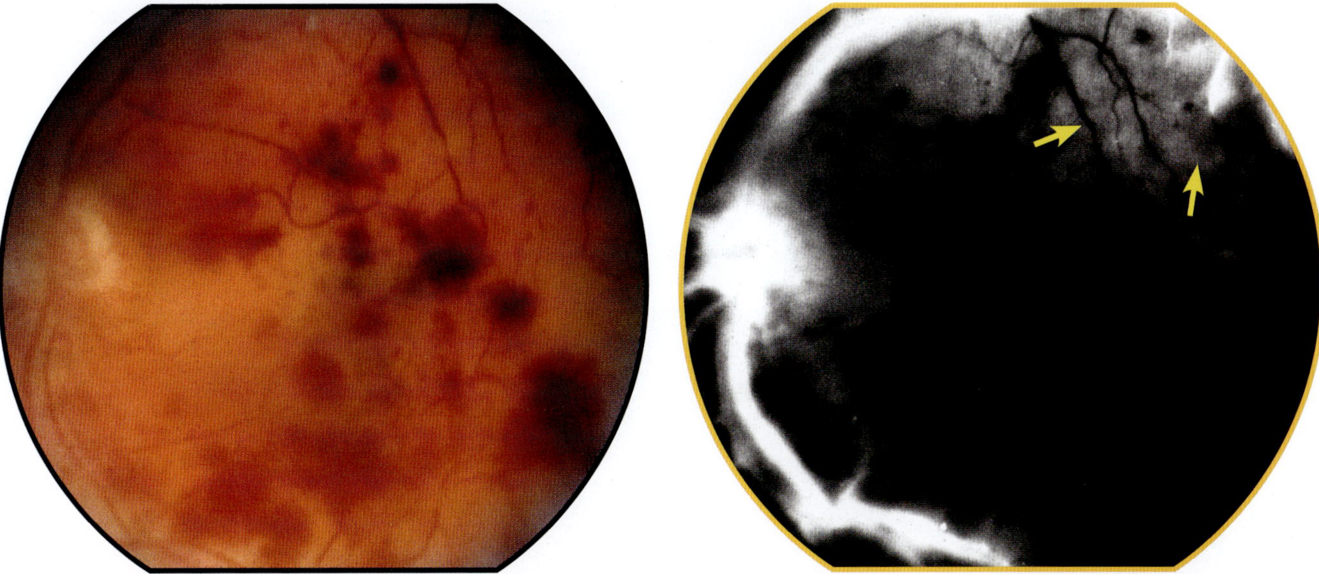

This patient had severe aminoglycoside toxicity (gentamicin) with diffuse whitening of the retina, scattered hemorrhages, and disc edema. There is some sparing of the superior paramacular region *(arrows)*, which received a lower dose of the drug. The fluorescein shows marked hypofluorescence from blockage of the choroid and ischemic necrosis of the retinal vasculature.

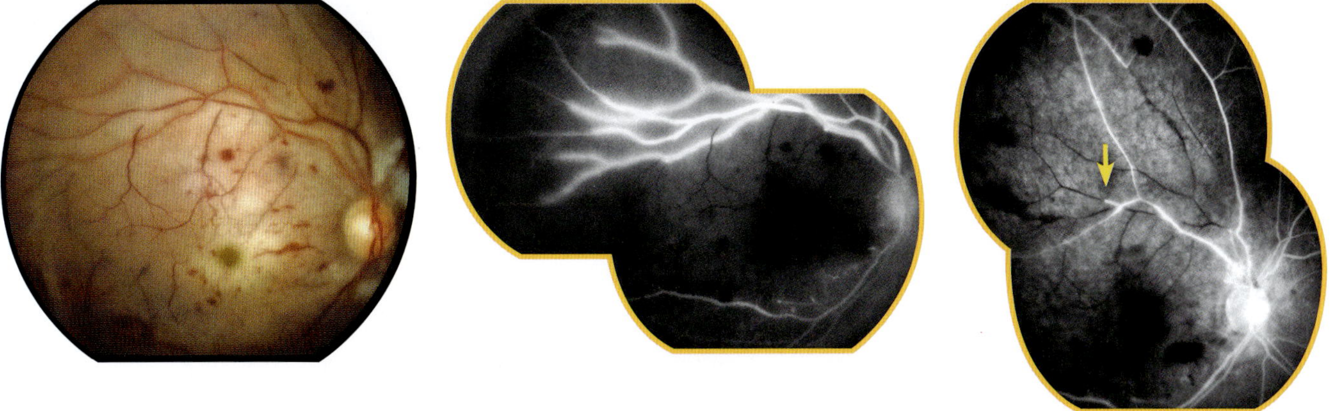

This patient had aminoglycoside toxicity (gentamicin) during a vitrectomy operation. The toxic drug spread toward the peripheral retina due to the removal of the vitreous. There is infarction of the retina and inflammation of the retinal vasculature. There is also pruning of one of the vessels *(arrow)*, presumably from white blood cell aggregation. The fluorescein angiogram *(right)* was carried out after the acute toxic effect resolved. Note that there is limited reperfusion unlike a typical arteriolar infarction.

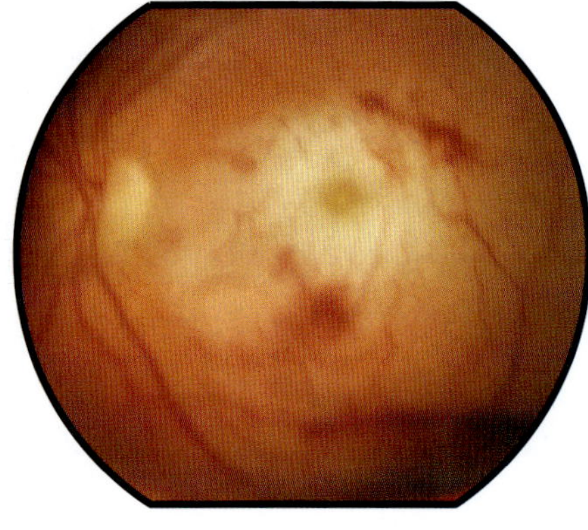

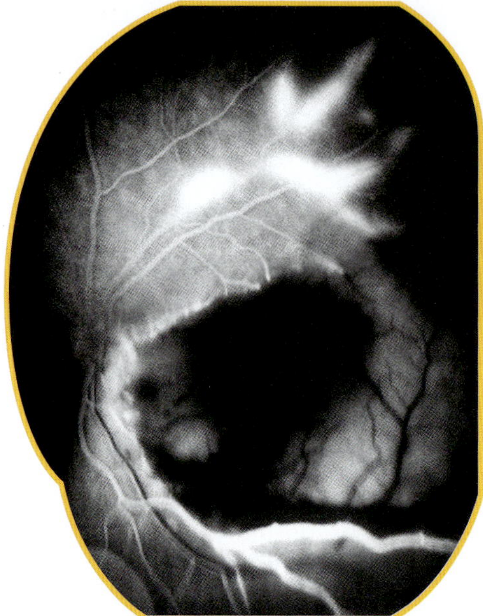

This patient also had aminoglycoside (apramycin) toxicity during cataract surgery. The dark area on the fluorescein angiogram corresponds to necrotizing vascular obliteration and the segmental staining of the arteriolar and venular retinal vessels corresponds to inflammation in the walls of those vessels due to the toxicity.

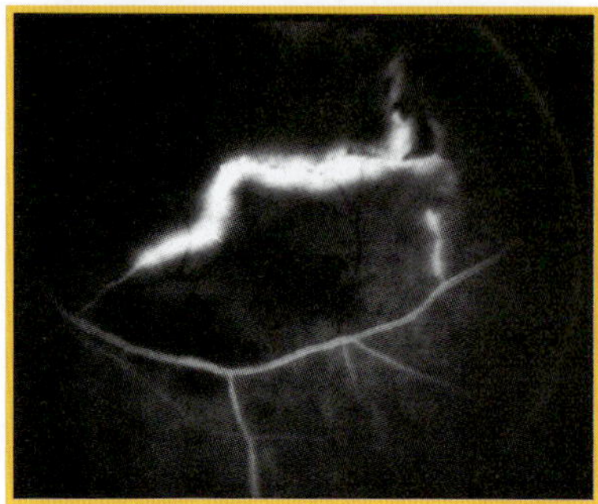

This fluorescein angiogram shows the segmental dilation and staining from aminoglycoside toxicity. It is surrounded by a capillary closure, which appears as hypofluorescence. This vessel was not completely obliterated by the drug, but its wall was compromised to produce a permeability defect or leakage.

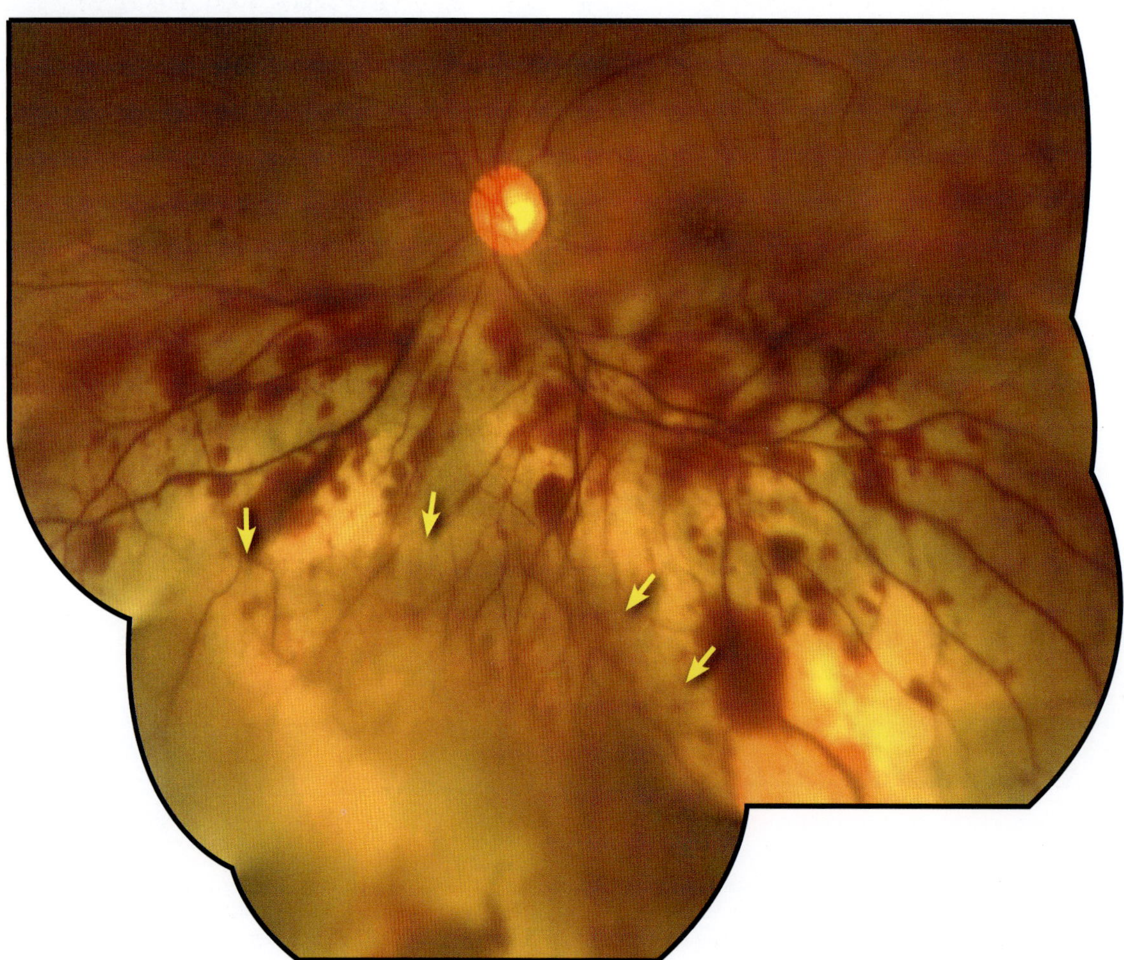

Courtesy of Dr. Antonio Ciardella

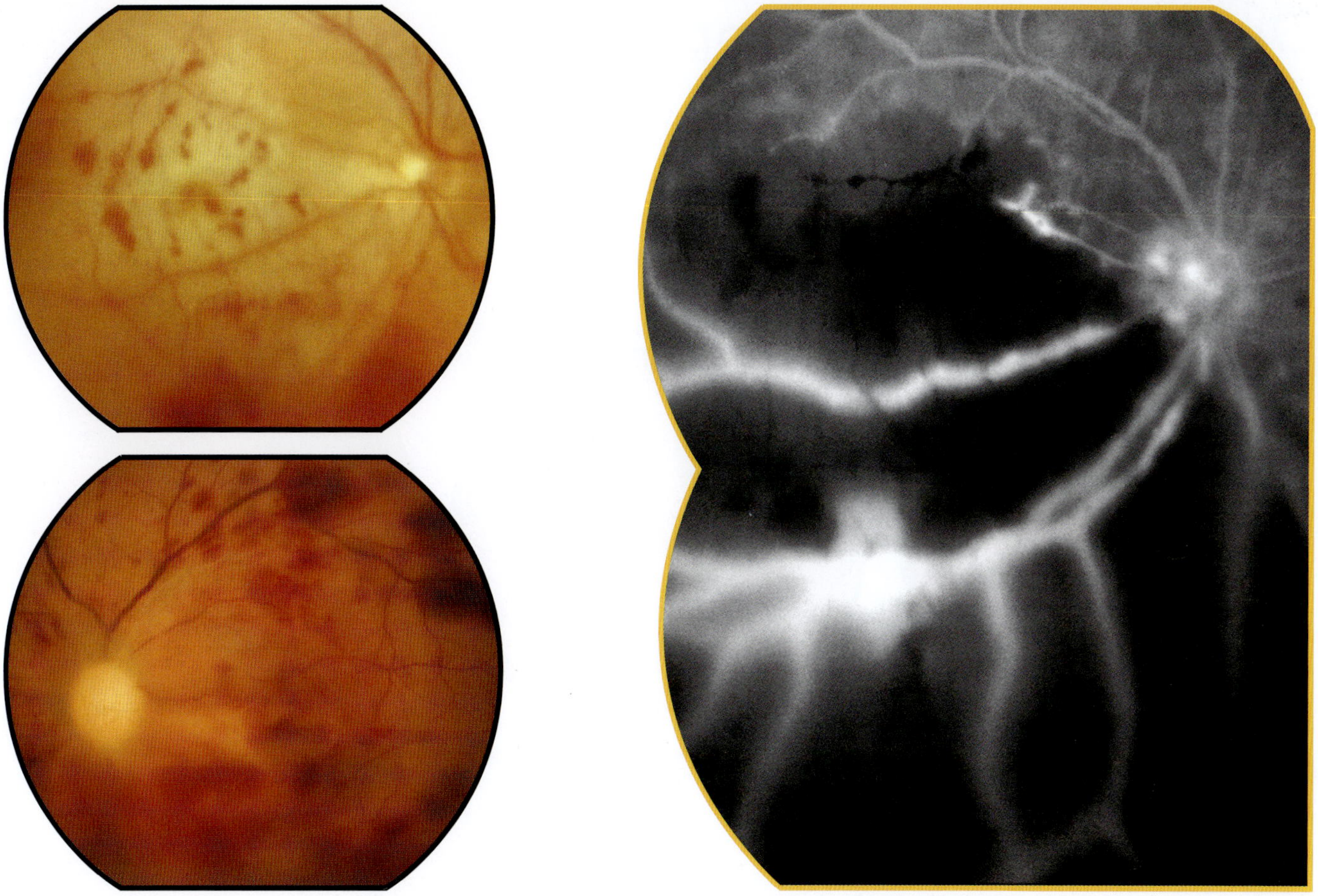

In these three patients with severe aminoglycoside toxicity, the lower half of the retina is more involved. Whitening of the retina and hemorrhage can be seen. There is a detachment *(arrows)* from the necrotizing obliterative retinopathy in the upper image. The fluorescein angiogram shows the absence of perfusion in the necrotic retina and staining vessels.

Intracameral Vancomycin

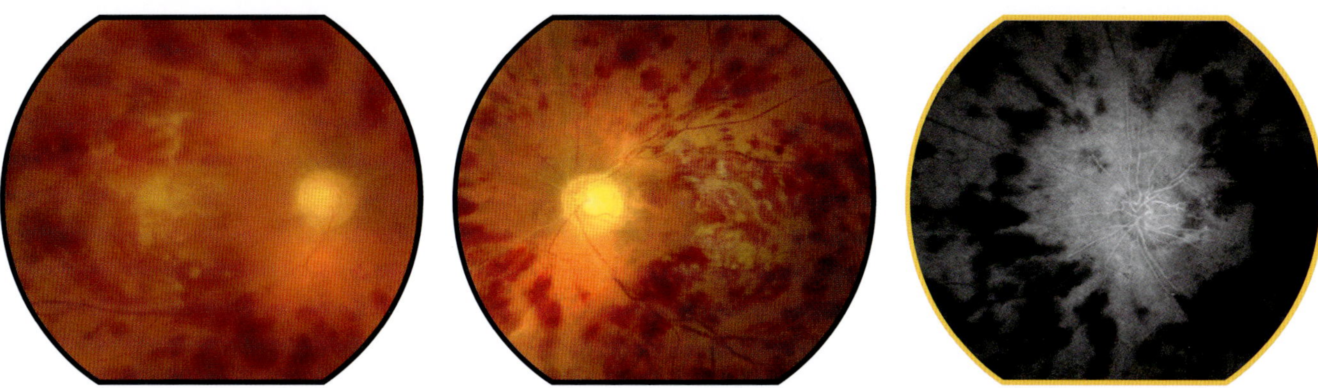

Fundus photograph of both eyes demonstrating a severe bilateral hemorrhagic occlusive retinal vasculitis following cataract surgery with utilization of prophylactic intracameral vancomycin. The cataract surgeries were spaced one week apart. Unfortunately, this immune-mediated event may take a week or so to manifest its features. The fluorescein angiogram exhibits extensive non-perfusion. Visual recovery was very limited. *Courtesy of Stephen Russell, MD*

Decompression Retinopathy

Decompression retinopathy results from a sudden drop in intraocular pressure. It is usually a complication of glaucoma surgery such as trabeculectomy, which is performed under either local or general anesthesia. Hemorrhages, both deep and superficial, may be seen in the posterior segment or diffusely throughout the fundus. There is no venous tortuosity or increased transit time, distinguishing this hemorrhagic event from venous occlusive disease.

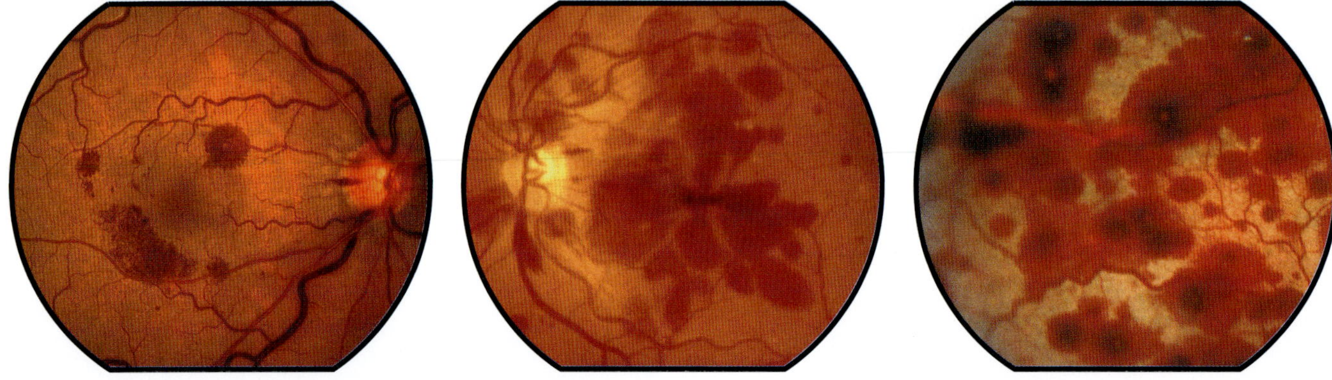

These patients experienced hemorrhage in the posterior segment of the eye and into the vitreous from decompression. The hemorrhages on the venous side of the circulation are presumably caused by a sudden drop in pressure and a compensating surge of blood perfusion into the venous bed. The hemorrhages do not coincide with the geographic distribution of veins.

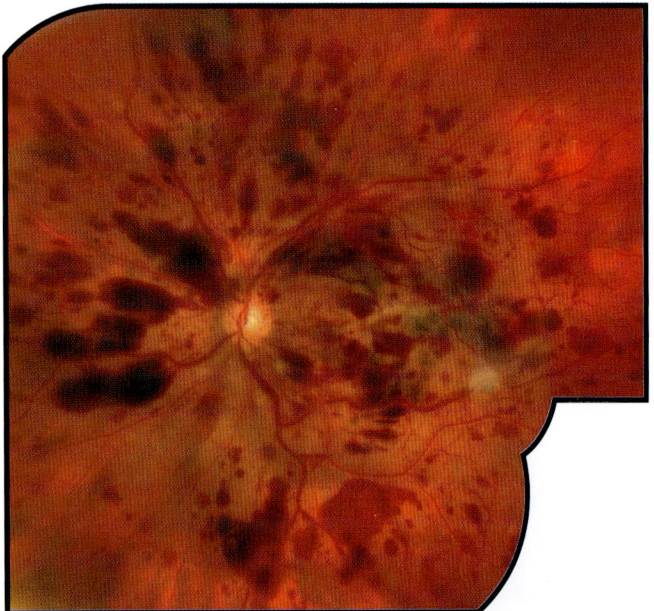

The montage shows decompression retinopathy with widespread hemorrhages involving all four quadrants. The bleeding is pre-retinal and intraretinal, and the hemorrhages vary in size. There is no swelling of the optic nerve, nor is there prominent venous tortuosity, which would be characteristic of venous stasis or a central retinal vein occlusion.

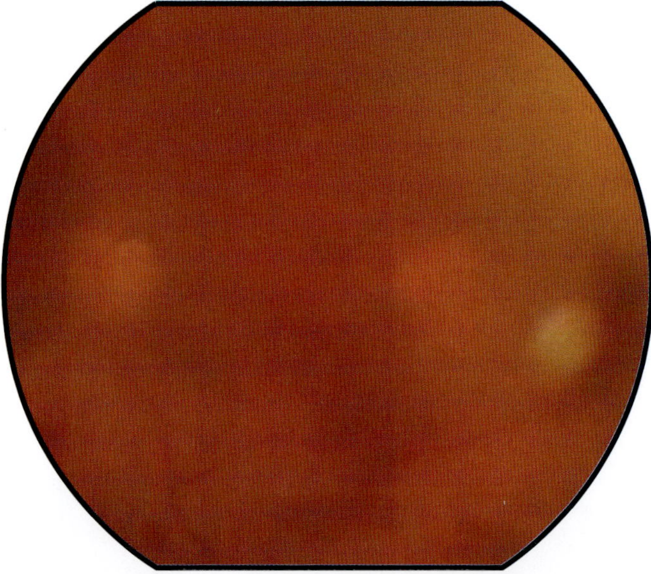

This patient had decompression retinopathy, with hemorrhage breaking through into the vitreous cavity, obscuring fundus details.

Non-Arteritic Anterior Ischemic Optic Neuropathy

Non-arteritic anterior ischemic optic neuropathy is believed by some to be a potential complication of anterior-segment surgery, particularly in patients with small optic cups or so-called "disc at risk." Neuro-ophthalmologists point out that a non-arteritic anterior ischemic optic neuropathy is rarely observed in the fellow eye unless the patient undergoes anterior-segment surgery. This association remains controversial.

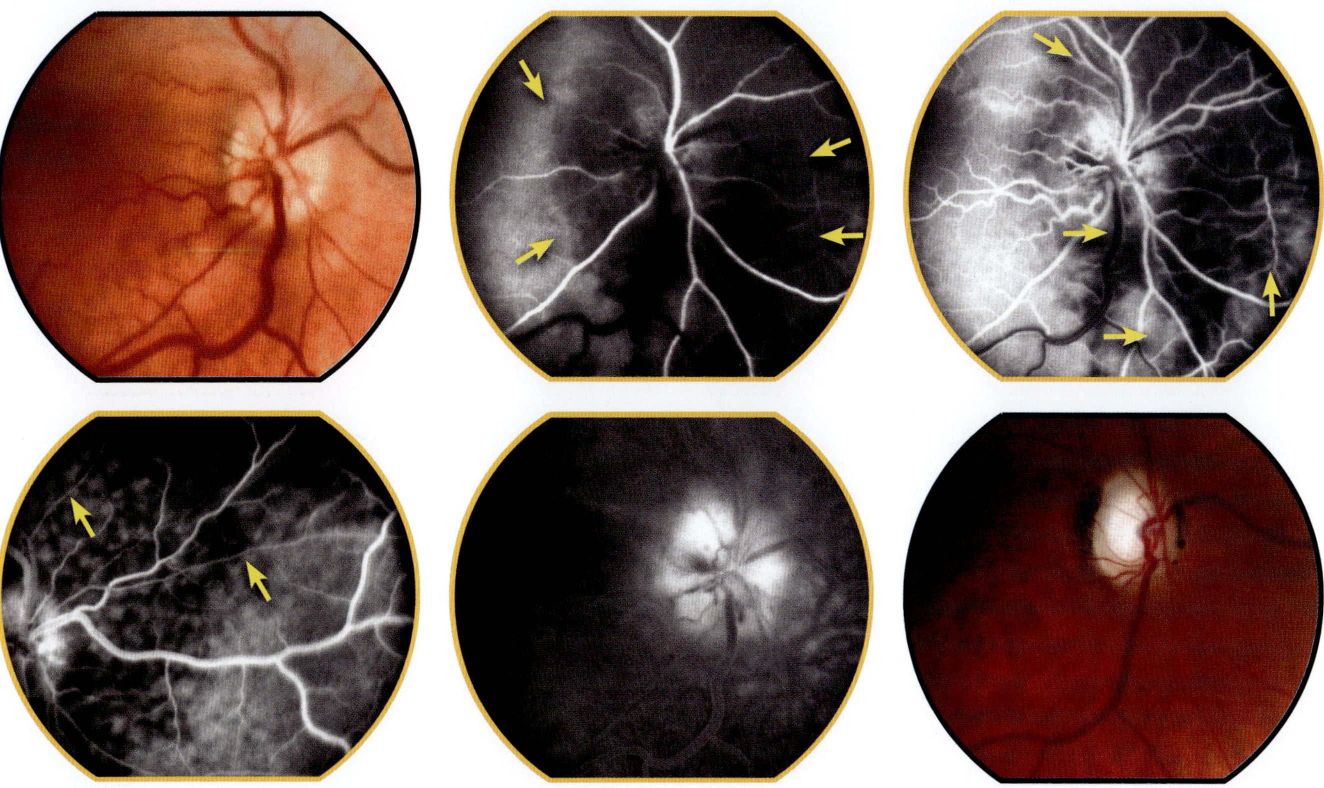

This patient experienced a drop in vision following cataract surgery. There was a swollen disc and prominent dilated retinal vascular changes consistent with venous stasis or obstruction. The fluorescein angiogram reveals a circumpapillary delay in choroidal perfusion, particularly nasal to the disc *(upper row, middle and right)*. In later stages of the angiogram *(lower row, left)*, there are nummular areas of choroidal hyperfluorescence within the hypoperfused choroid that appear to be the cause of the delay in the perfusion of the choriocapillaris *(arrows)*. Late staining of the optic nerve is also evident *(lower row, middle)*. Three months later there was reperfusion of the choroid and resolution of optic nerve swelling and retinal vascular stasis. However, the nerve itself became atrophic and cupped from the antecedent edema and vascular neuropathy *(lower right)*. This patient had a "disc at risk," and a "watershed" choroidal perfusion abnormality located vertically through the disc *(arrows)* – risk factors for the ischemic event.

Phototoxicity

Phototoxicity may be seen following intraocular surgery. It may occur as a result of anterior-segment, as well as posterior, vitreoretinal procedures. The spectral content, duration, and intensity of the illuminating light source or even stimulation from a dye that emits light energy are potential mechanisms for producing these effects. Light produces patterns in the fundus that sometimes correspond to the source of the illumination or vary when there is an internal light source.

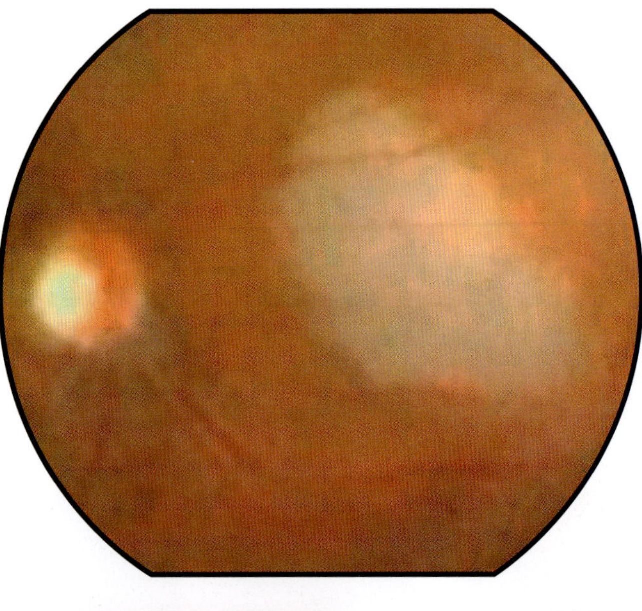

The appearance of a whitish intraretinal lesion eccentric to the macula in the early postoperative time frame was indicative of microscope light-induced phototoxicity. While in this case the lesion is readily apparent clinically, in many cases the area of retinal whitening (damage) is much more subtle and is better seen on a fluorescein angiogram. *Image courtesy of Dr. H. Richard McDonald*

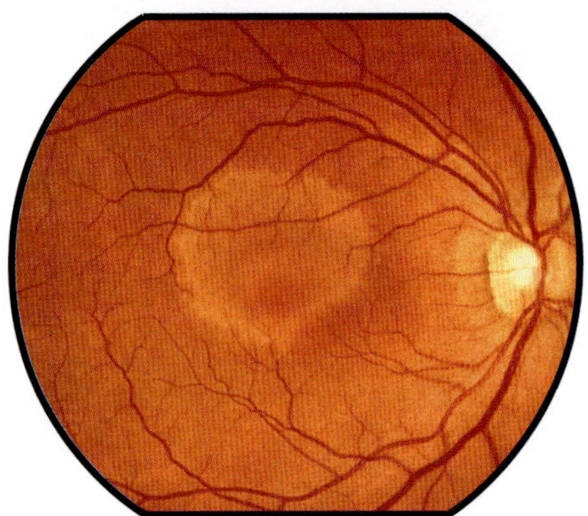

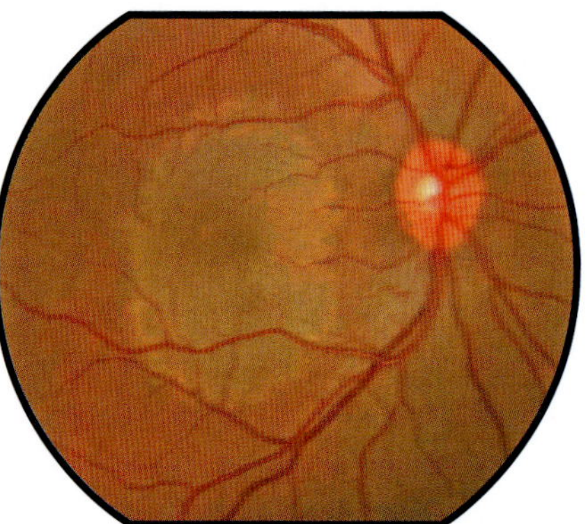

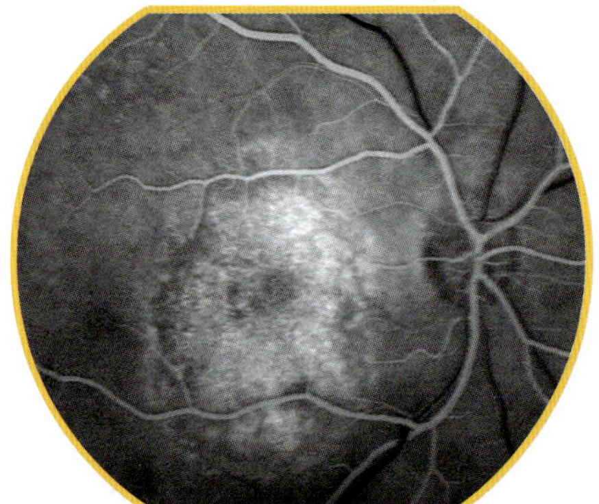

This patient had vitreoretinal surgery. The phototoxic effect is barely visible clinically, but can be seen on fluorescein angiography. An irregular atrophic and pigmentary disturbance was induced as the internal light pipe moved throughout the posterior segment. *Middle and right images courtesy of Dr. Alan Kimura*

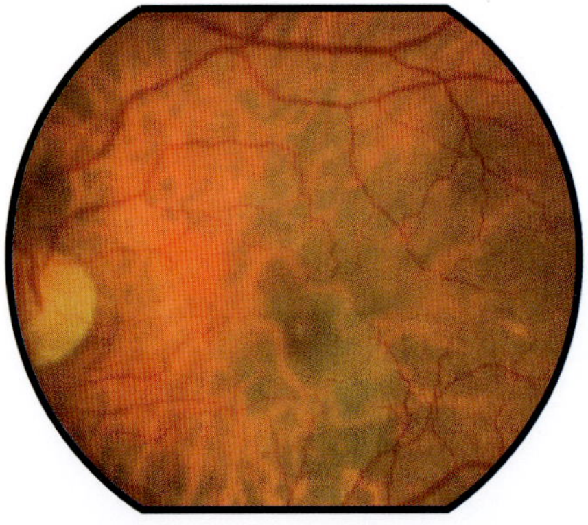

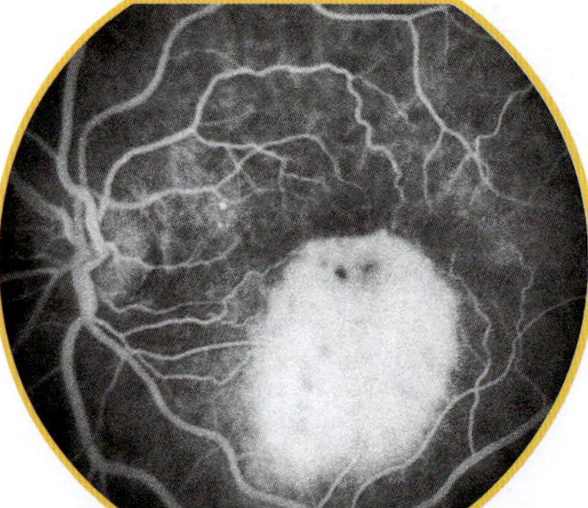

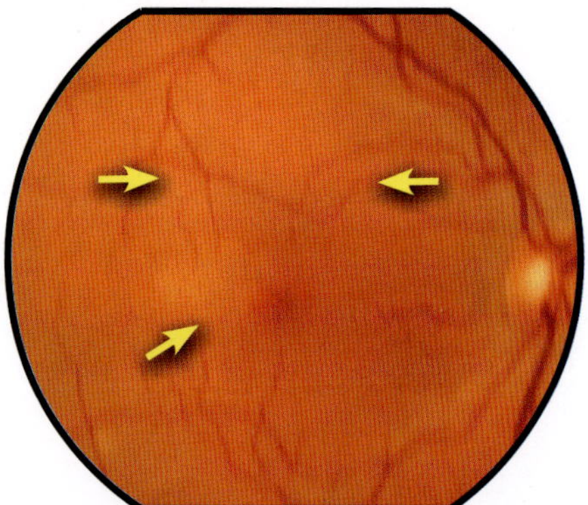

These patients have a zone of acute whitening of the outer retina and pigment epithelium *(arrows)* following cataract surgery. The adverse effect was noted immediately after the procedure. There is a pigment epithelial window defect on the fluorescein angiogram. *Left and middle images courtesy of Dr. H. Richard McDonald*

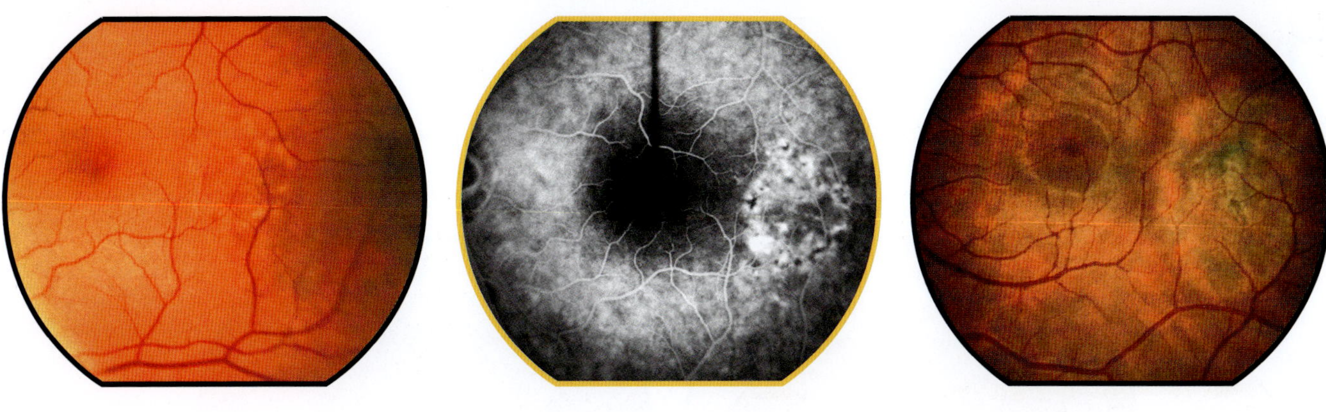

The light toxicity may be seen eccentric to the foveal area and be relatively asymptomatic, such as in these three patients.

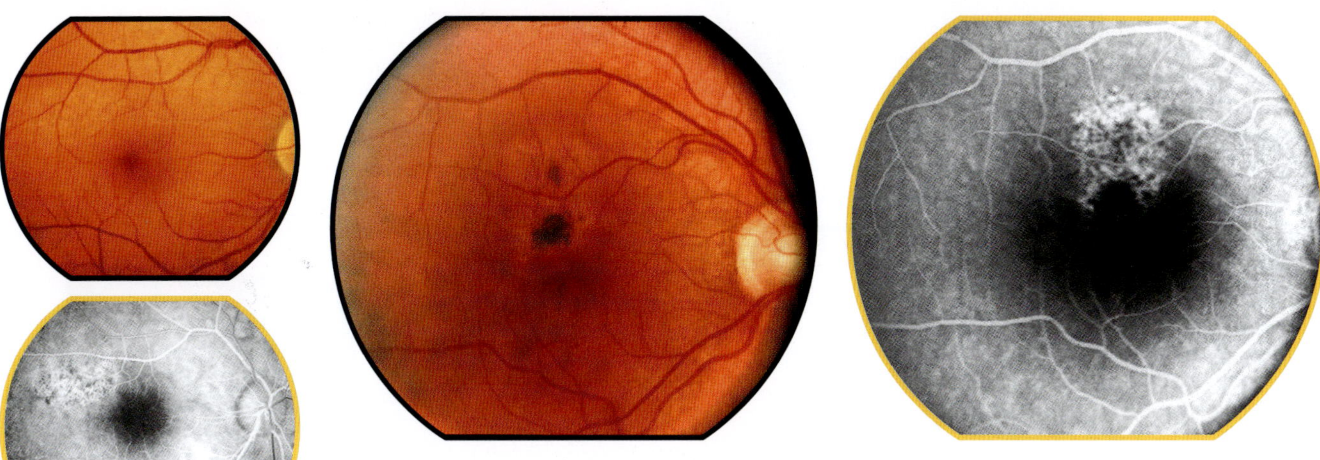

This patient experienced light toxicity during a corneal refractive procedure.

This patient experienced light toxicity during vitreoretinal surgery. The phototoxicity effect is irregular and eccentric to the fovea.

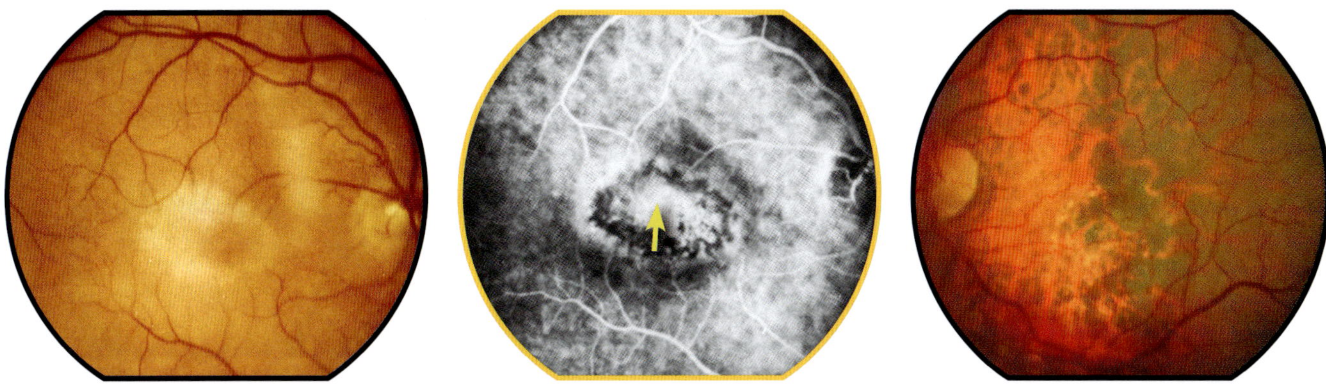

In some cases of severe light toxicity, there is atrophy and pigment epithelial hyperplasia *(left and middle)*. The phototoxic area may become thickened and be associated with fibrous metaplasia *(arrow)*. In an eye with pre-existing atrophy, the phototoxic visual effect may be even more devastating as pigmentary and atrophic degeneration potentiates the pre-existing degenerative changes *(right)*. *Left and middle images courtesy of Dr. E. Bouldrey*

Hypotony

Severe hypotony from a leaking corneal or corneoscleral wound or choroidal separation can result in multiple retinal folds in the posterior fundus, peripapillary detachment, or even disc swelling.

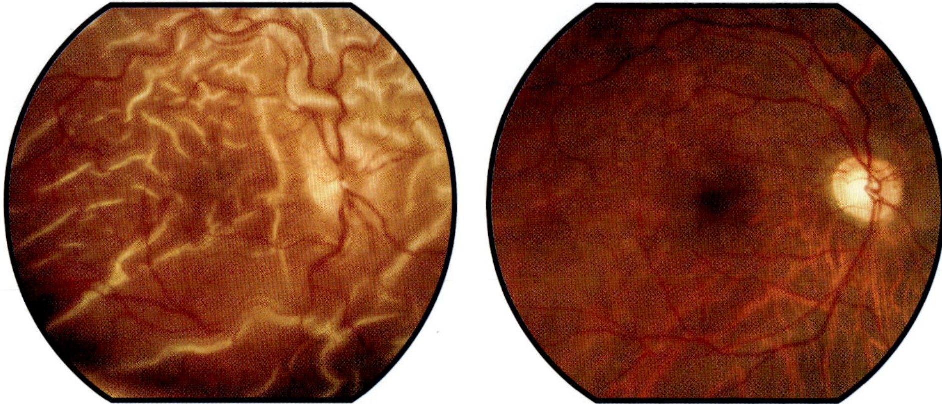

These patients experienced a severe drop in intraocular pressure. Some swelling of the optic nerve and numerous folds of the retina can be seen *(left)*. In time, reconstitution of intraocular pressure will be associated with limited or complete resolution of the detachment and disappearance of the folds *(right)*. Visual recovery generally ensues, though it may not return to normal.

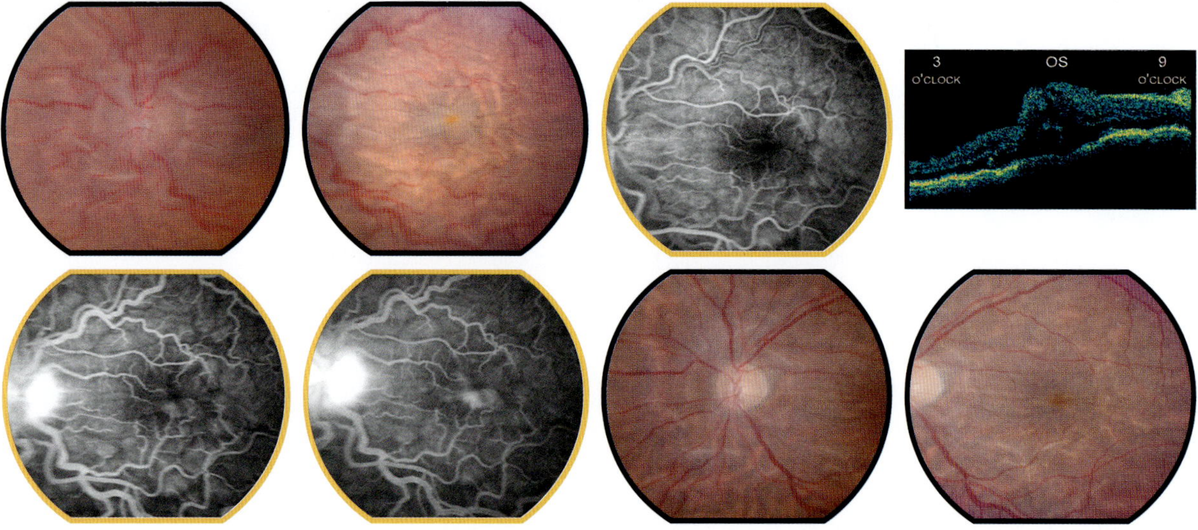

This patient experienced a postoperative cataract wound leak that resulted in hypotony maculopathy/retinopathy. Visual acuity was hand motion. Note the optic disc congestion, retinal and choroidal folds, optic disc edema, cystoid macular edema, and moderate vascular tortuosity. Following closure of the leaking cataract wound, and restoration of normal intraocular pressure, the clinical features normalized after approximately five weeks, and the vision returned to 20/70 *(right two images)*. These features can also be seen following glaucoma filtration surgery (see the images immediately below).

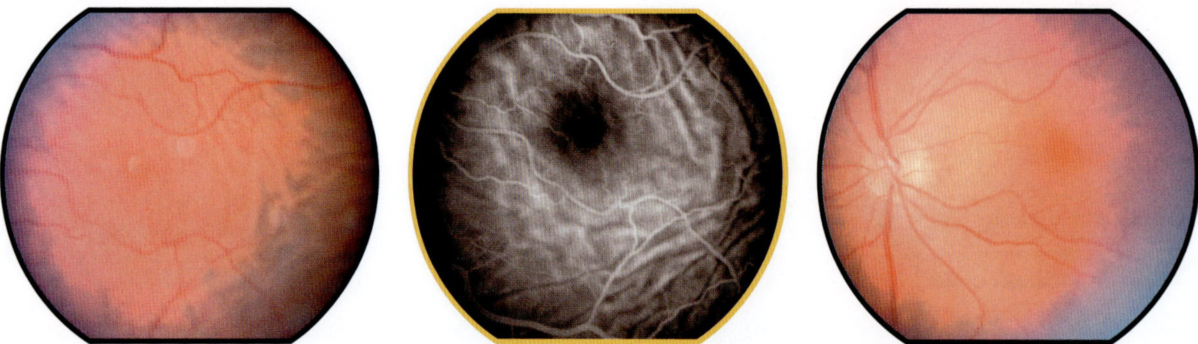

This patient underwent glaucoma filtration surgery. The intraoperative pressure fell to 3 mm Hg. Choroidal folds were noted as part of hypotony maculopathy/retinopathy. The intraocular pressure gradually normalized over several weeks, and the choroidal folds and congestion gradually disappeared *(right image)*.

Choroidal Hemorrhage

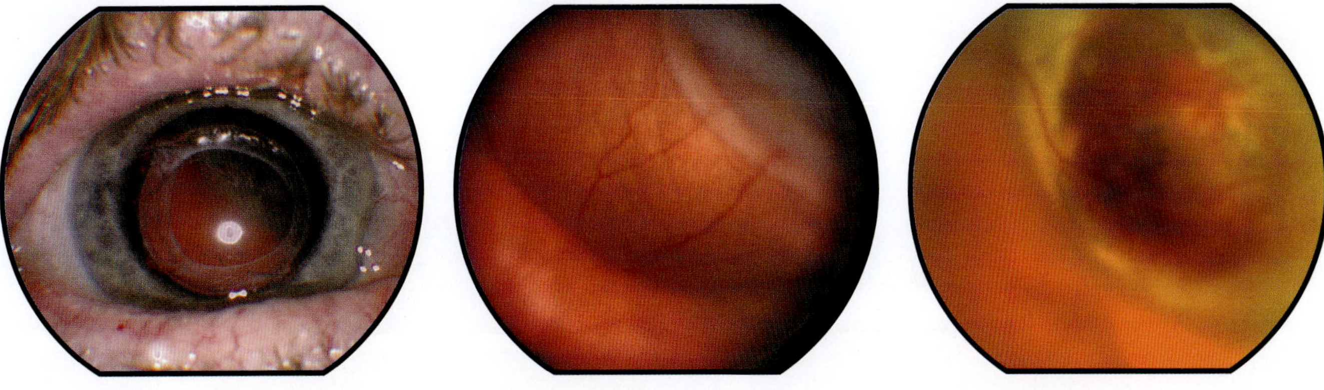

Massive peripheral choroidal hemorrhage may be seen following cataract surgery, as in this patient, through the dilated pupil *(left)* and in the fundus *(middle and right)*.

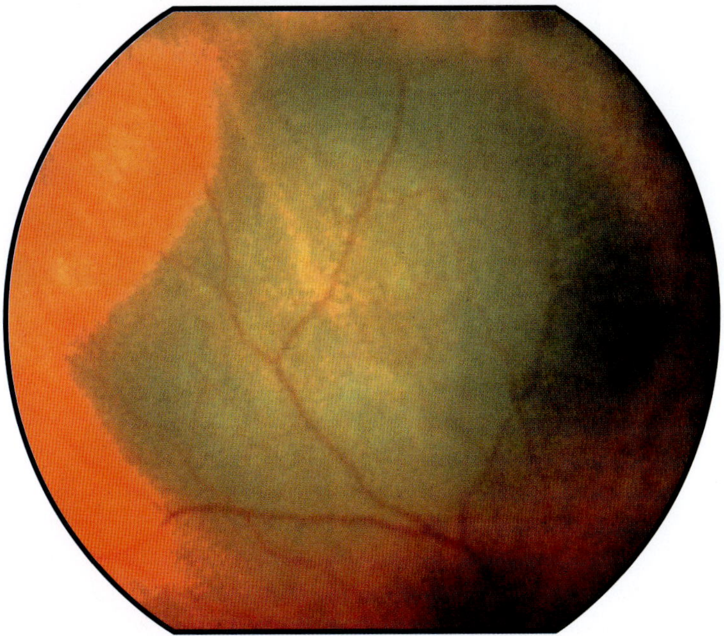

The mass lesion in the periphery, seen post-cataract surgery, was a subretinal choroidal hemorrhage that simulated a choroidal melanoma.

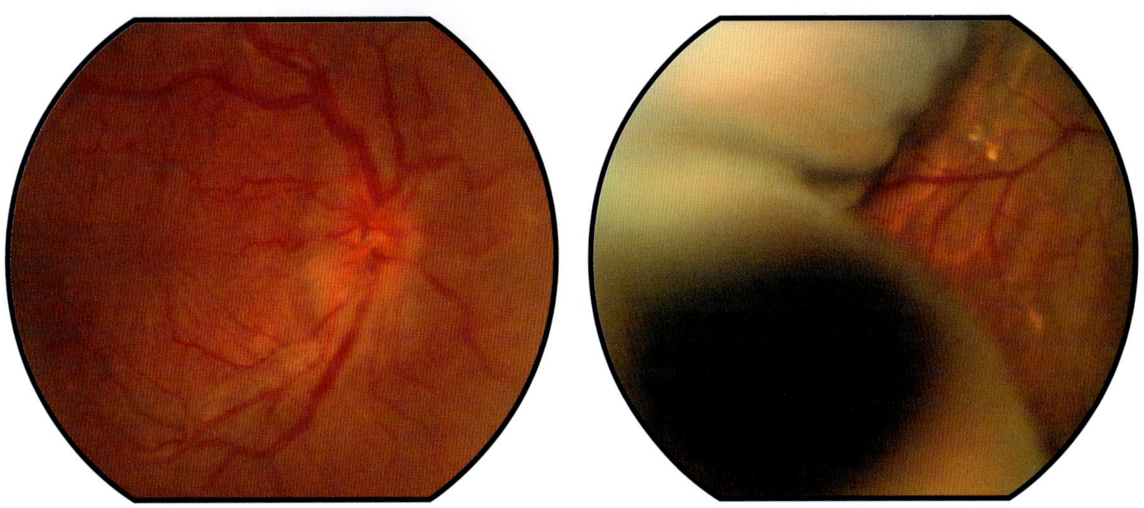

A choroidal detachment may be associated with hypotony and disc edema *(left)*. The peripheral detachment may be in close contact, and on occasion may become appositional ("kissing" choroidals) *(right)*.

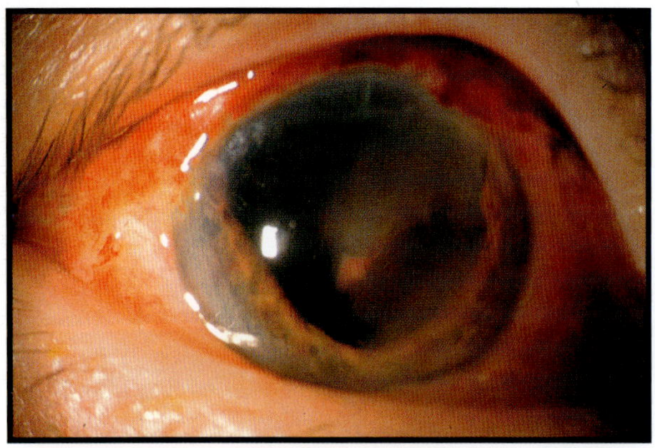
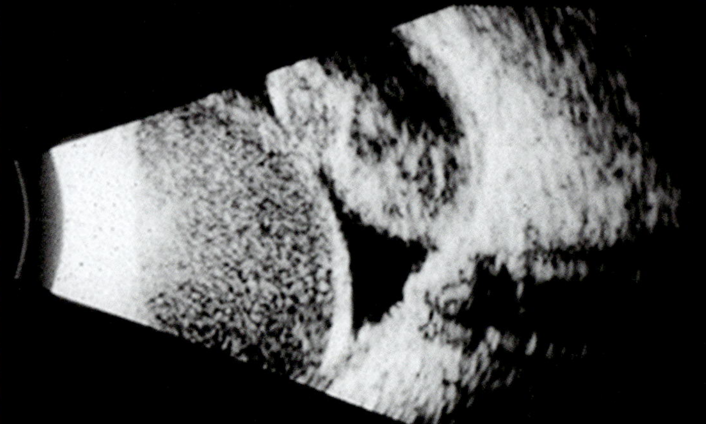
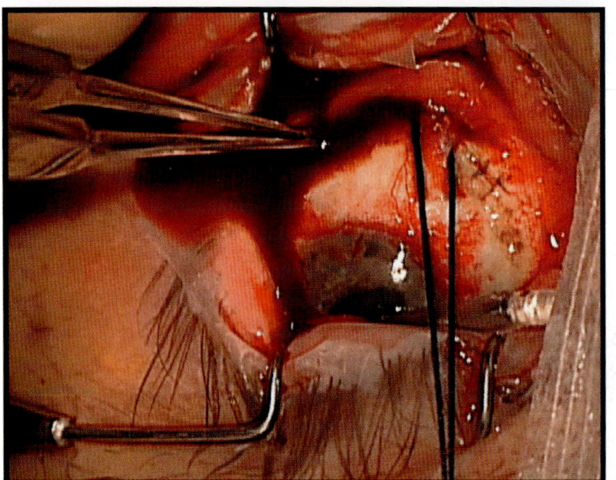
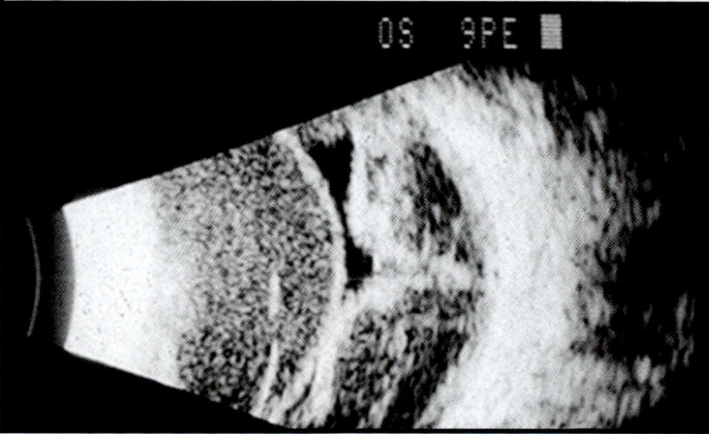

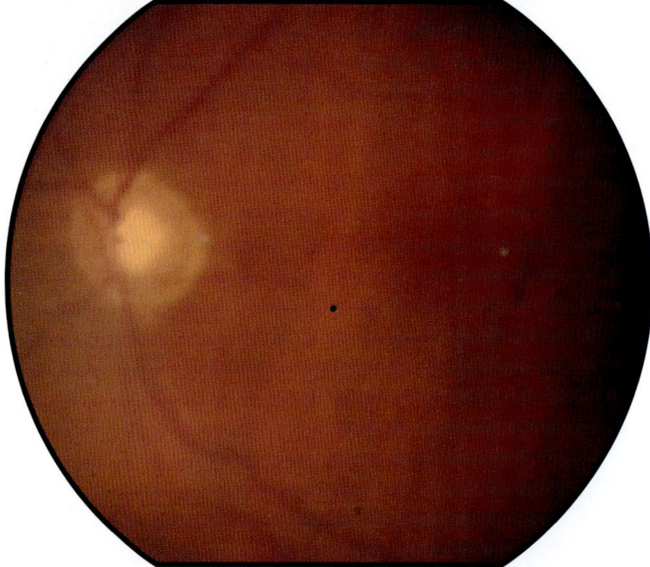

This patient developed a non-expulsive delayed hemorrhagic choroidal detachment seven days following trabeculectomy surgery. The choroidals were appositional as seen echographically *(second image)*. Following liquefaction of the hemorrhagic choroidals over a seven-day time frame, they were drained externally via a sclerotomy approach *(third image)*. The majority of the hemorrhage was alleviated, and the retina remained attached. On post-operative day seven, the visual acuity improved to 20/70, which represented the preoperative level of acuity.

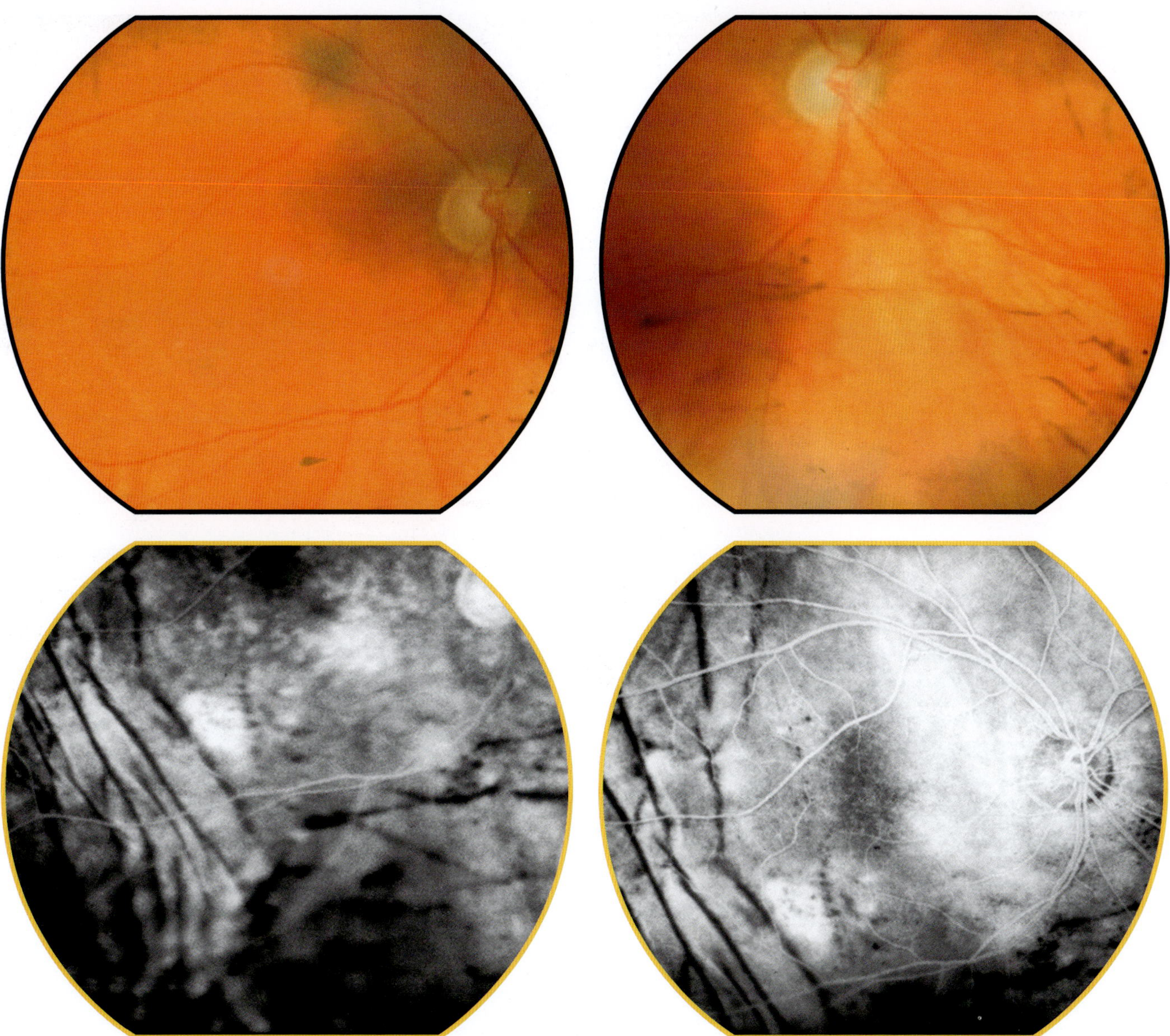

Following drainage of appositional hemorrhagic choroidals, the patient was left with line-like peripheral retinal pigmentary changes, indicative of the extent of the previous retinal elevation by the underlying choroidal hemorrhage

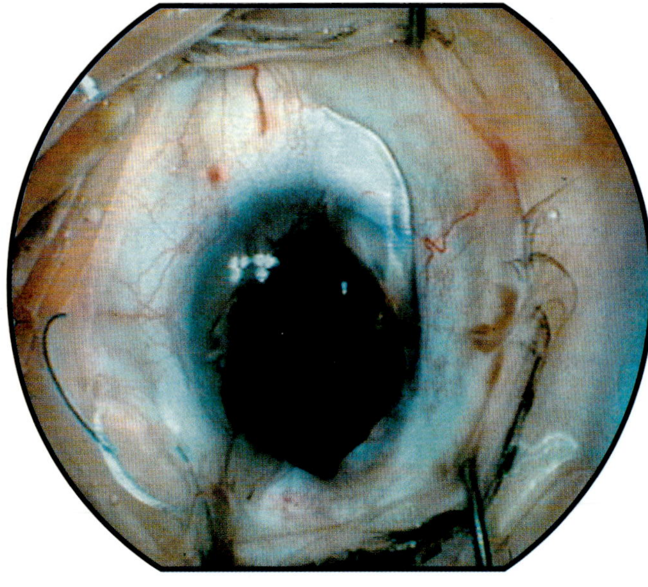

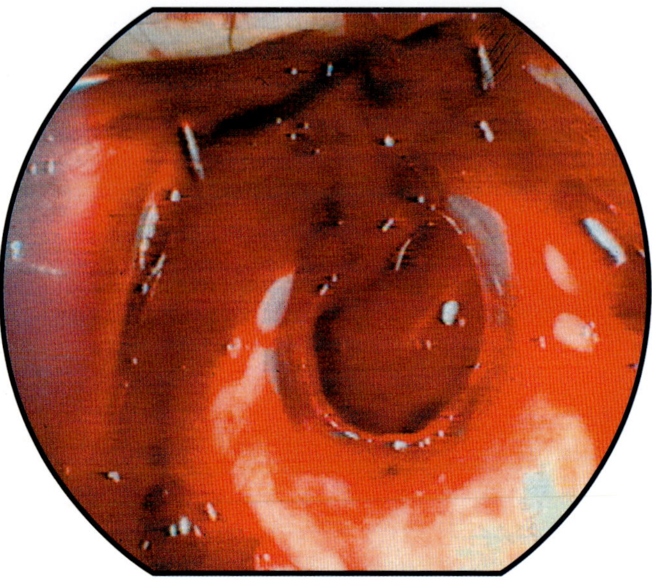

During the course of a penetrating keratoplasty procedure as part of a combined vitrectomy operation, the patient developed rapid expulsion of the vitreous along with the intraocular lens *(left)*, followed immediately by bright red blood. Tamponade was applied digitally, and the corneal graft was sutured in place. The patient did not recover vision.

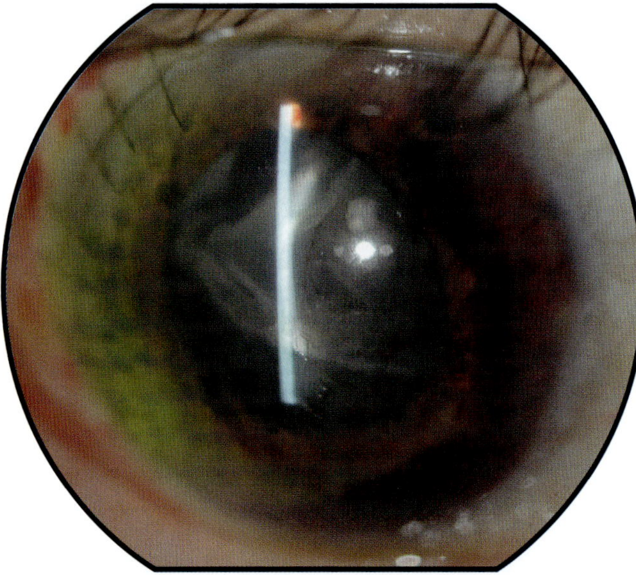

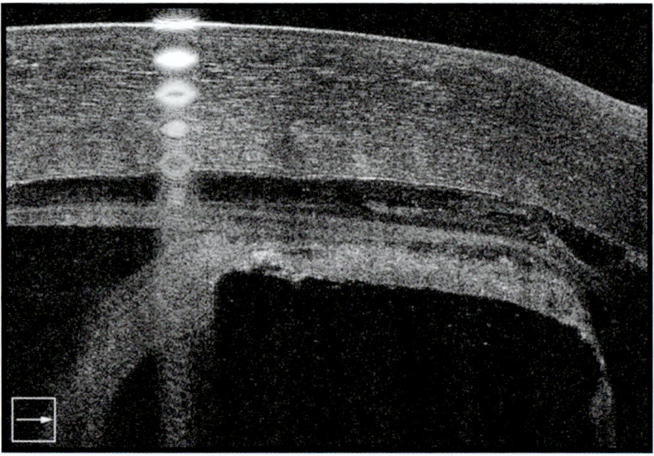

This cataract surgery patient was referred immediately after complicated cataract surgery. Slit lamp examination demonstrated the retina in the anterior chamber, in apposition with the corneal endothelium. Anterior segment OCT emphasized the proximity of the retina to the cornea. The retina was displaced forward by an underlying choroidal detachment.

Spontaneous Choroidal Hemorrhage with Polypoidal Choroidal Vasculopathy (PCV) after Cataract Surgery

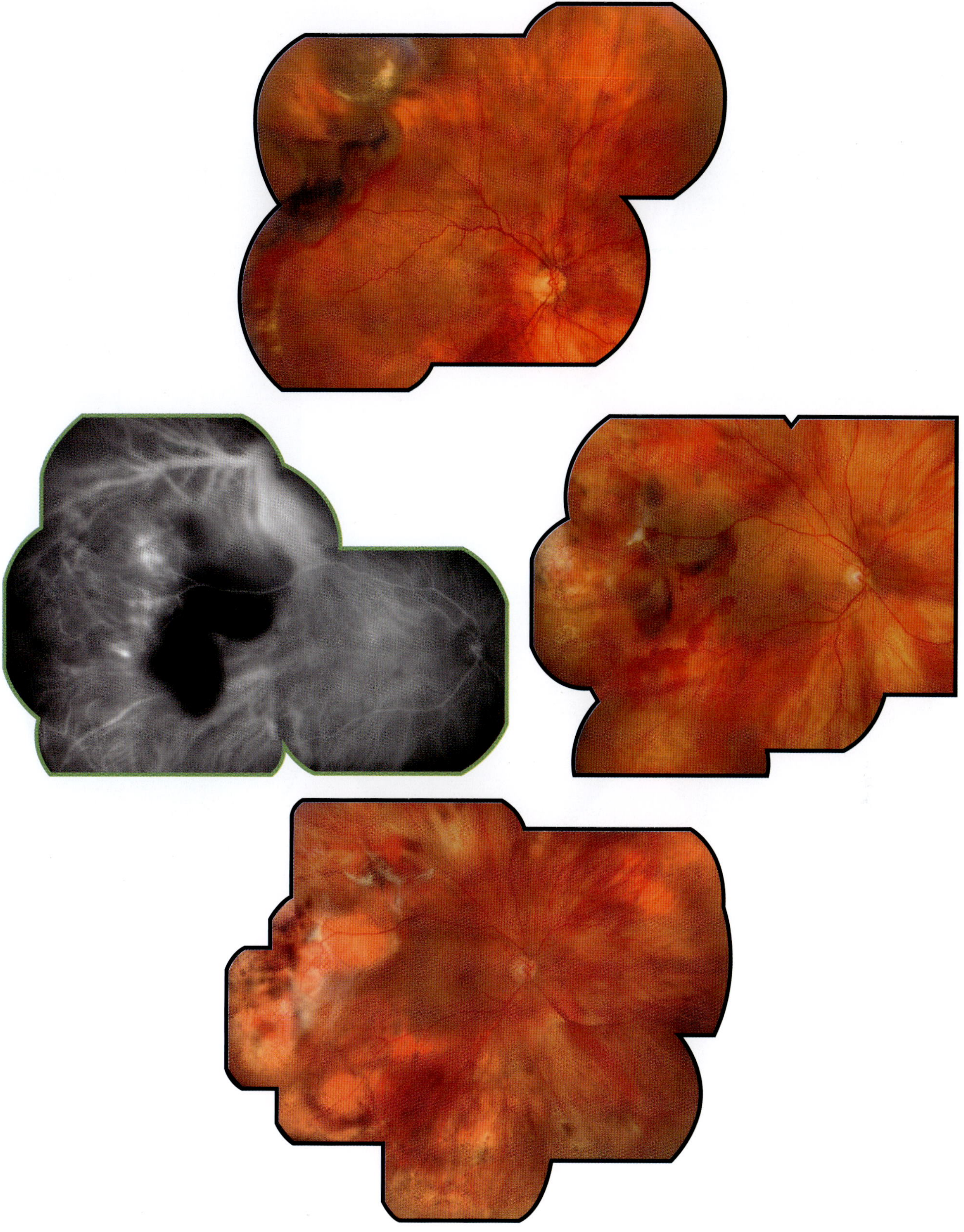

Massive peripheral hemorrhage may be seen following cataract surgery, as in this patient. The indocyanine green (ICG) angiogram shows that the peripheral vessels were polypoidal in nature. This form of choroidal neovascularization is characteristically associated with massive or bullous hemorrhagic detachments of the pigment epithelium and neurosensory retina. In time, there was spontaneous resolution of the blood with a few flecks of residual hemorrhage and scattered fibrosis in the area of hemorrhage. No treatment was administered.

Surgical Materials and Devices

In the course of intraocular surgery, certain devices are implanted and material used to facilitate the operation. These devices and materials may be intentionally or inadvertently left in the eye.

Diamond Particle

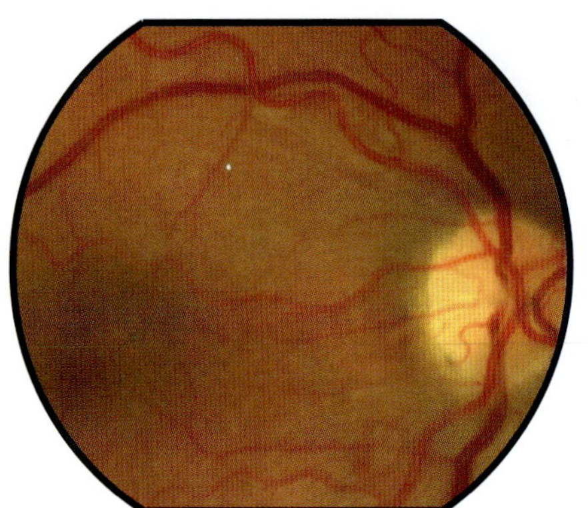

Steel Particles

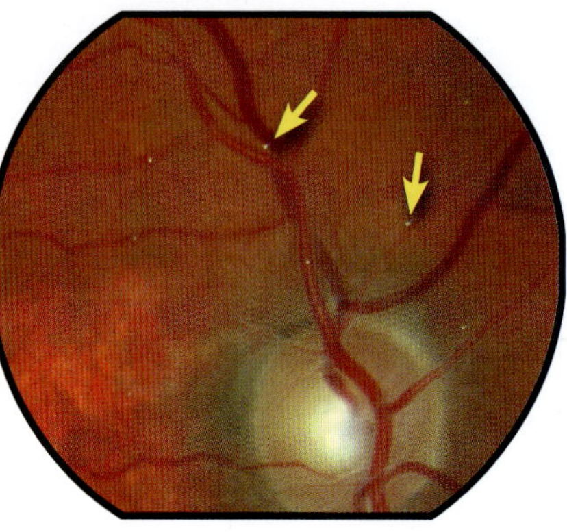

Current instrumentation for vitrectomy procedures contains diamond and steel particles. These are incorporated into solid surgical instruments and brushes. Note the diamond particle *(left)* and the several steel particles seen in the retina *(arrows, right)*. *Left image courtesy of Dr. Belinda Shirkey*

Titanium Tack

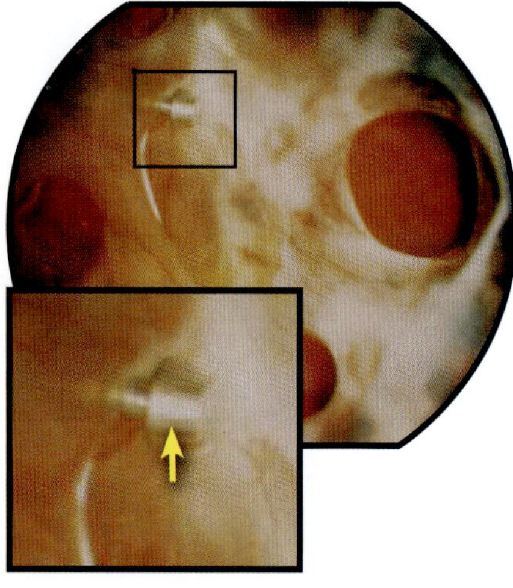

Titanium tacks were used to secure the retina as seen here *(arrow)*.

Silicone Oil

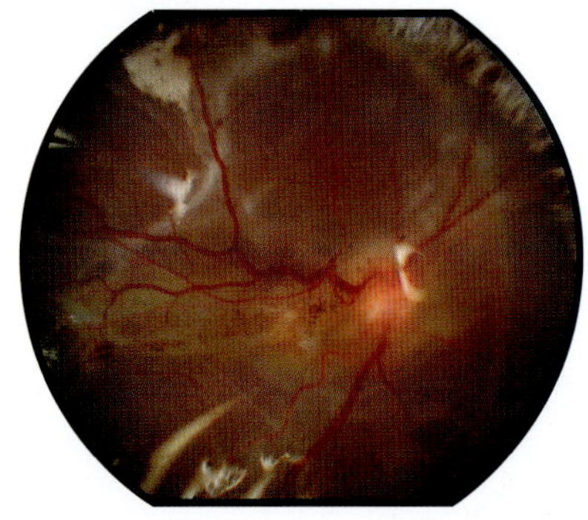

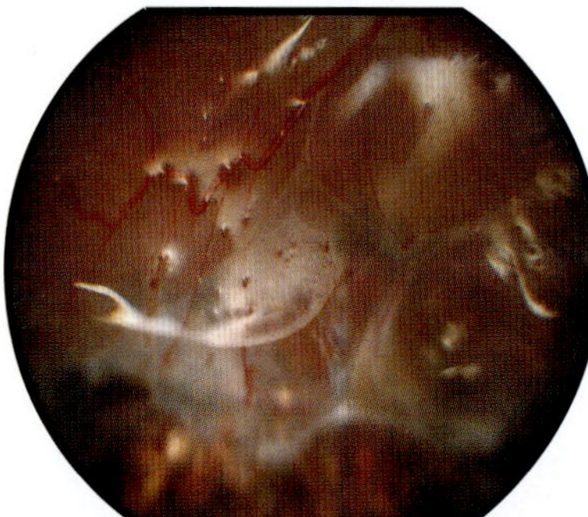

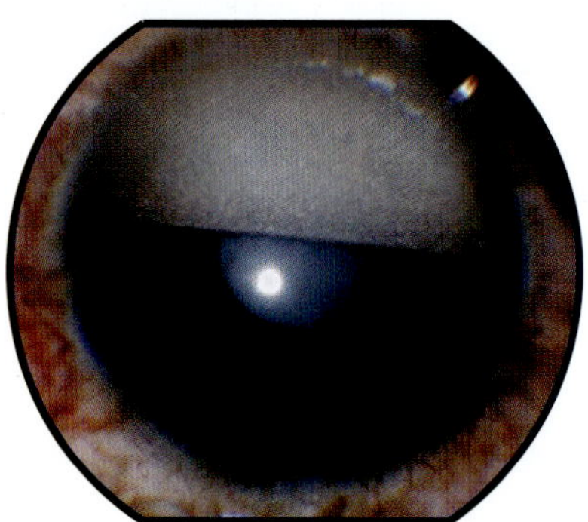

Silicone oil used in vitreoretinal surgery to tamponade the retina can have a variable appearance in the vitreous. Note the cloudiness and opaque polymorphic changes in this patient *(left and middle images)*. Silicone oil has entered the anterior chamber and become emulsified in the patient on the right.

This patient was treated with an intravitreal anti-VEGF agent for neovascular age-related macular degeneration. These two images show a silicone oil droplet from the syringe used to administer the drug *(arrow, left and magnified view, right)*.

Intraocular Gas

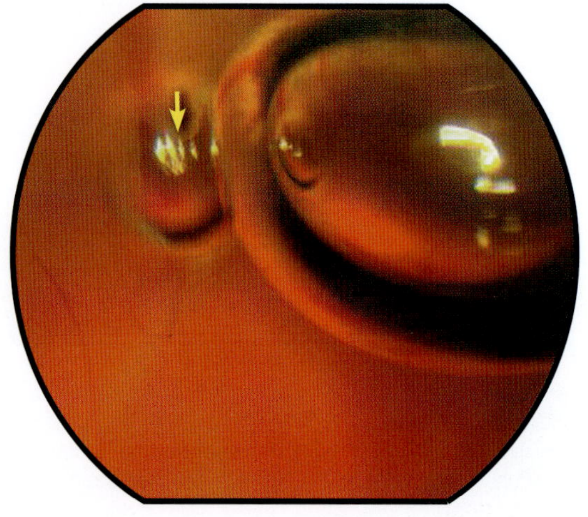

Intraocular gas is used to tamponade the retina in a pneumopexy. A large air bubble can be seen next to a horseshoe tear. A bubble of air has entered through the subretinal space *(arrow)* through the horseshoe tear.

Perfluorocarbon (PFC) Liquid

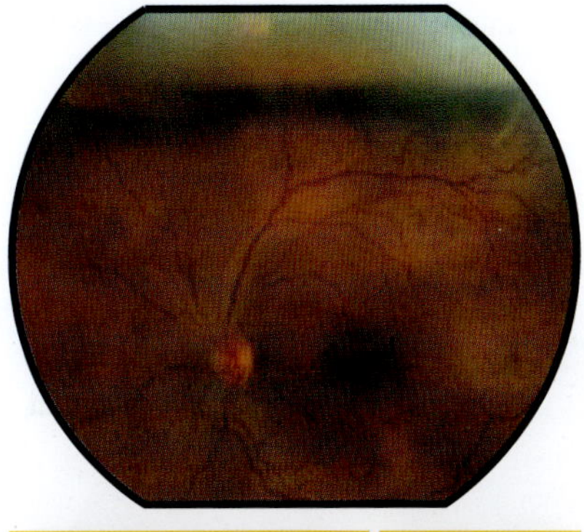

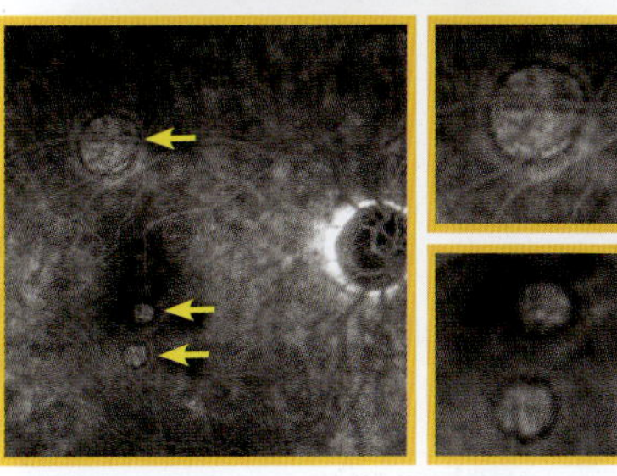

Perfluorocarbon (PFC) liquid is a heavier-than-water agent utilized to help flatten the retina during intraocular surgery. The PFC is removed at the conclusion of the case, though, on occasion, droplets may inadvertently egress under the retina *(arrows)*.

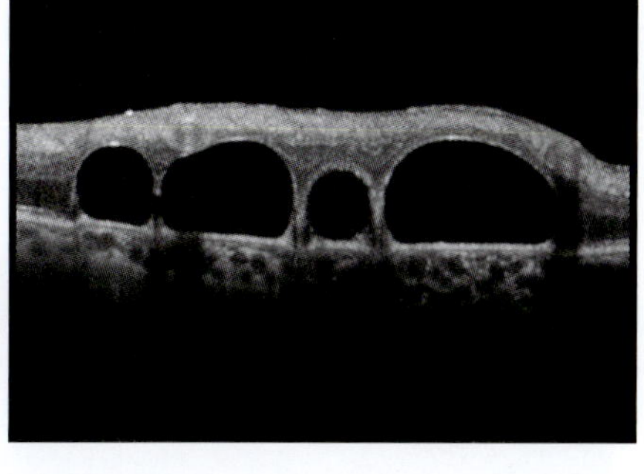

Photograph and an OCT documenting residual subretinal PFC droplets.

Dislocated Implant

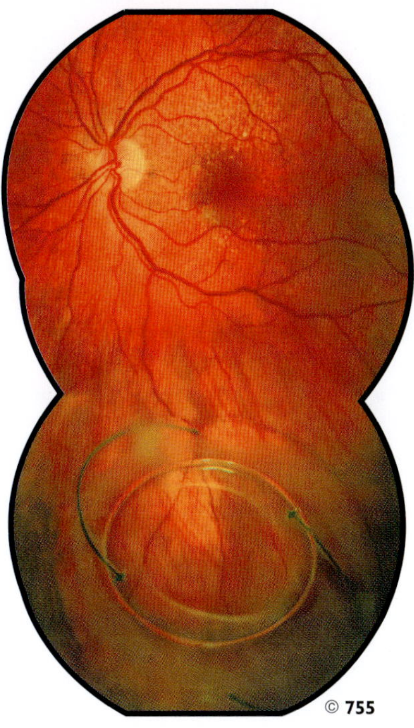

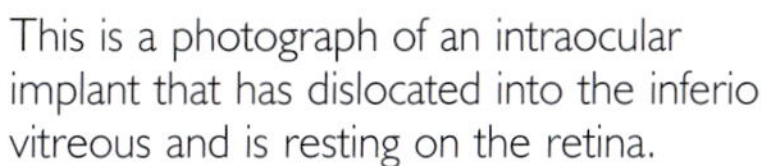

This is a photograph of an intraocular implant that has dislocated into the inferior vitreous and is resting on the retina.

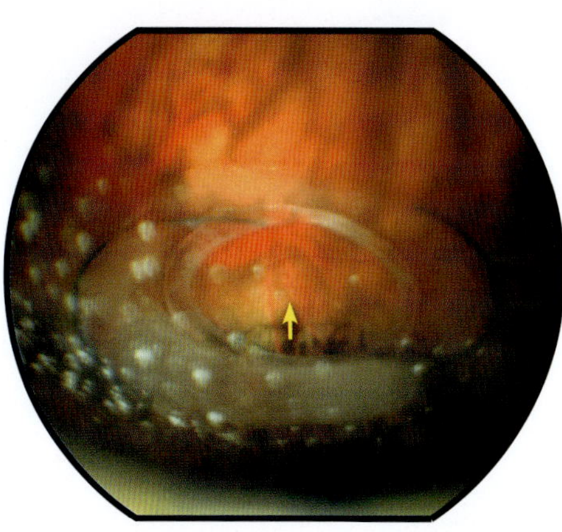

This is an image of an implant that spontaneously dropped into the vitreous months after cataract surgery and lens implantation. A clear area of the fundus can be seen through the optical center of the lens *(arrow)*. The lens was removed via a pars plana vitrectomy approach.

Lens Fragment

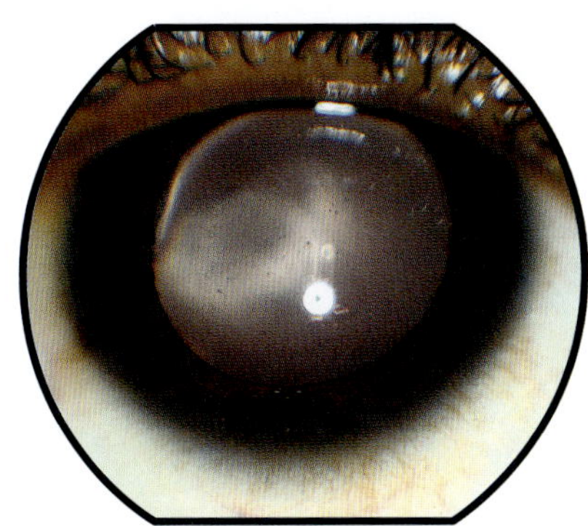

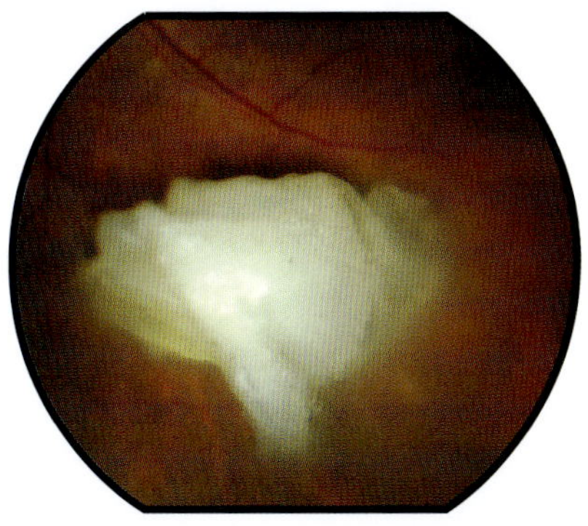

Following cataract surgery, lens fragments can be seen through the pupil *(left)* or in the vitreous *(right)*. *Courtesy of Dr. Kasi Sandhanam*

Retinal Prosthesis

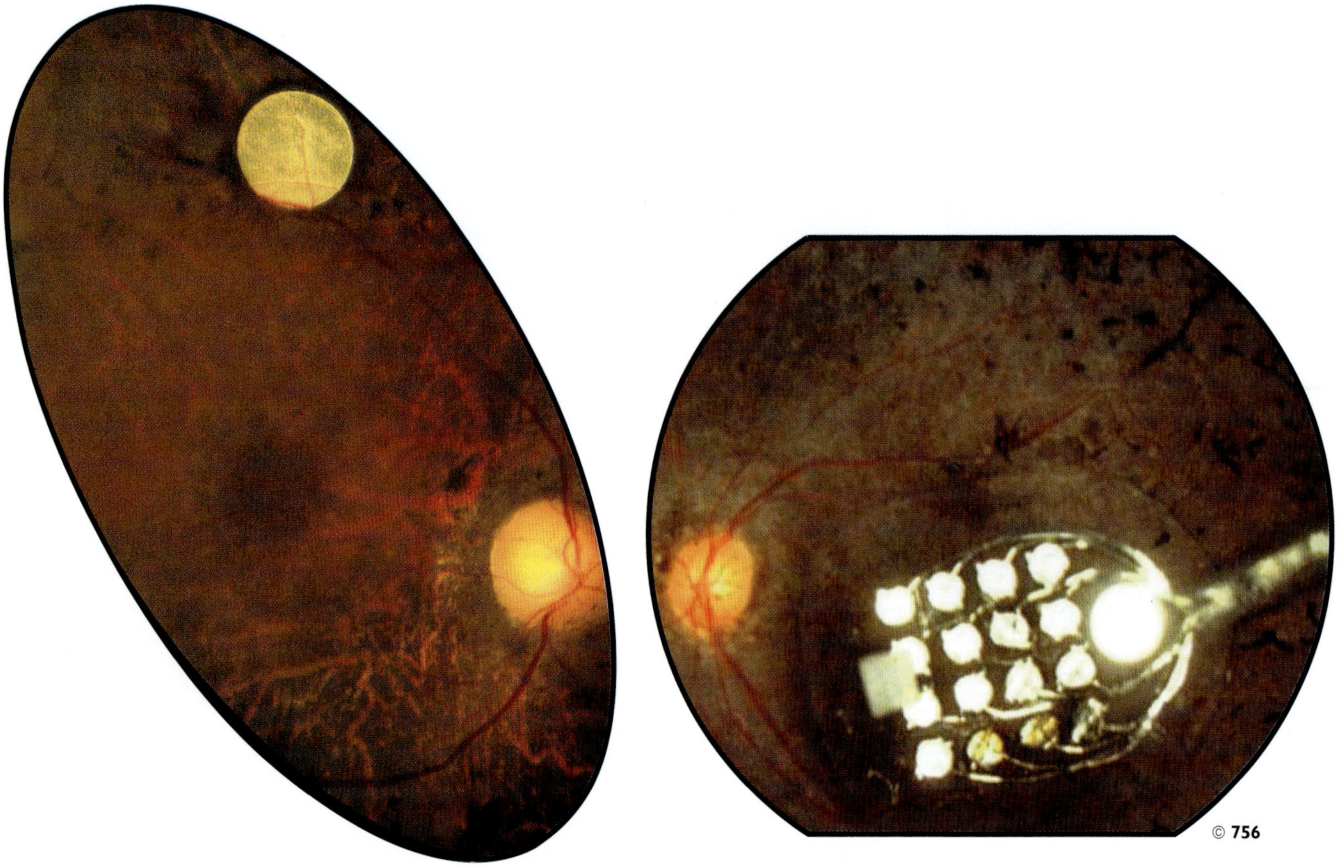

© 756

Retinal prosthetics are under development. They will assume different forms in front of *(right)* and below *(left)* the retina. In these patients with retinitis pigmentosa, these prosthetic implants are designed to deliver drugs, to capture light, and send visual signals to the brain. *Left image courtesy of Robert L. Prusak, CRA*

Transpupillary Thermotherapy (TTT)

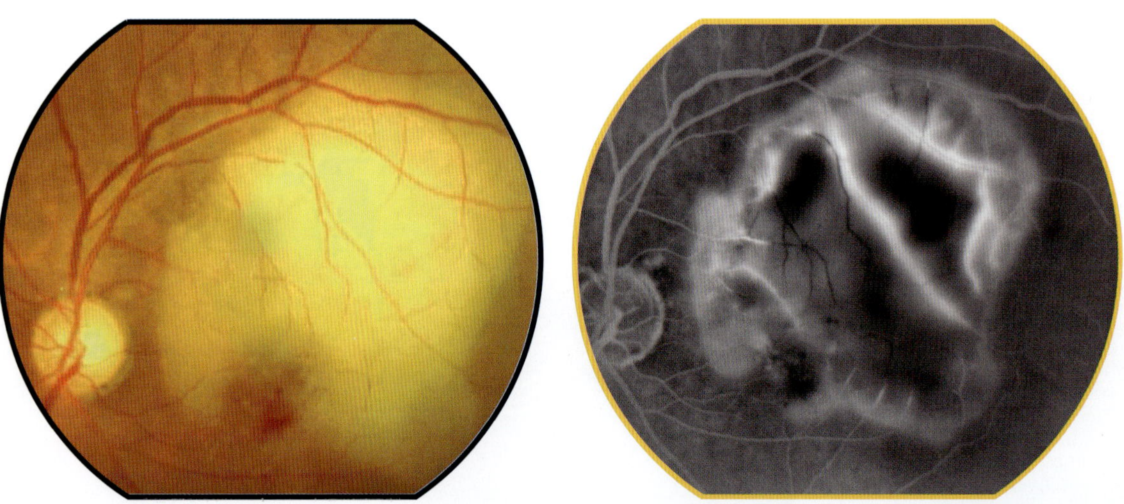

This patient was administered transpupillary thermal therapy to treat a subretinal mass lesion. Note the whitening of the retina and the obliteration of the retinal vasculature on the fluorescein angiogram. Where the vessels are not infarcted, there is some inflammation and segmental permeability in the vasculature. *Courtesy of Dr. Scott Sneed*

Cryodemarcation

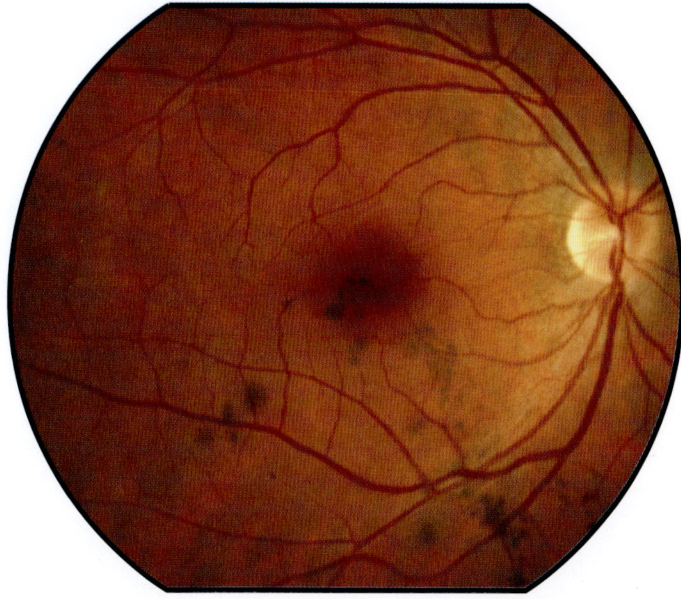

This patient developed a pigmentary line or demarcation following a retinal reattachment operation with a scleral buckle. There was a large peripheral hole. This is a "cryo-demarcation" line, produced by pigmentation that traveled beneath the subretinal space in the detached area toward the fovea. It may also course through the retinal hole into the vitreous to settle in the posterior pole.

Photodynamic Therapy (PDT)

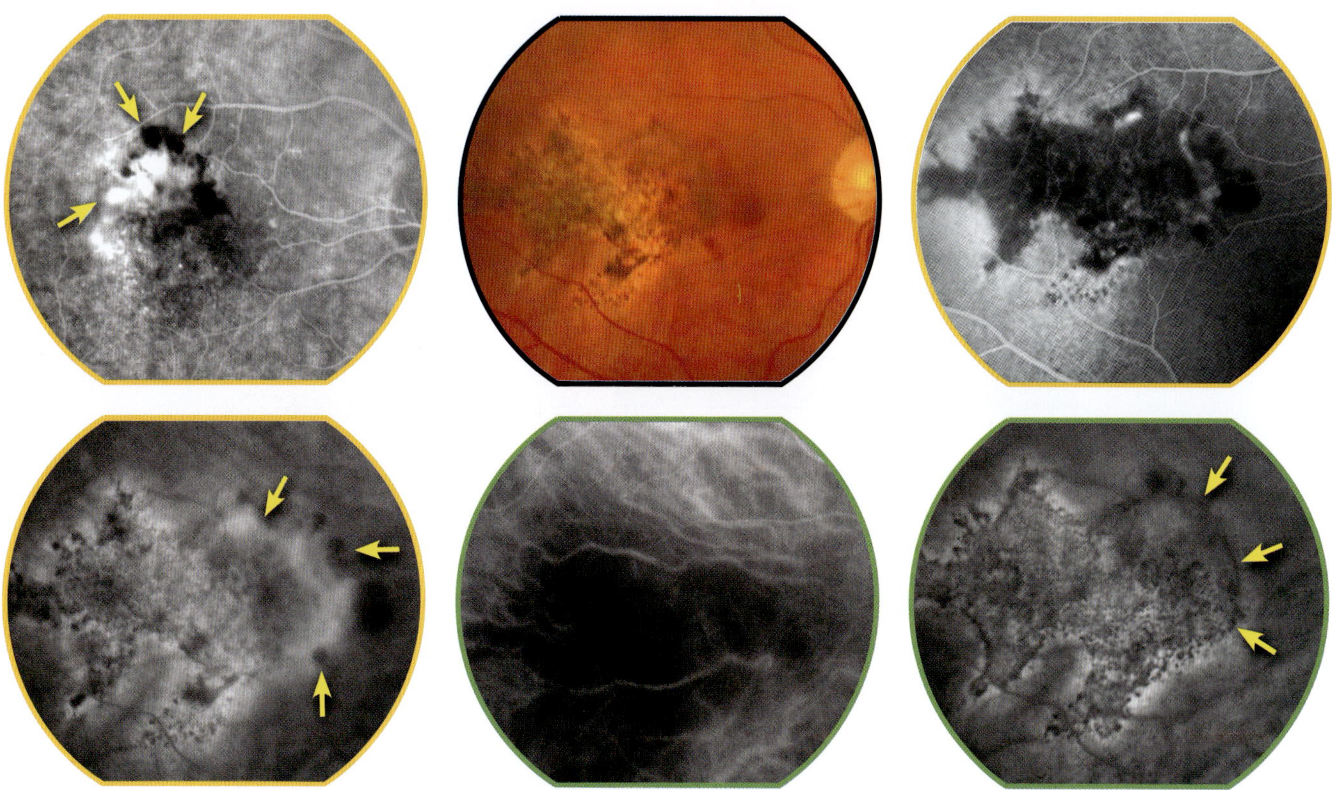

This patient had neovascular age-related macular degeneration and was treated with verteporfin photodynamic therapy *(upper left)*. There is a serosanguineous detachment and choroidal neovascularization on fluorescein angiography *(arrows)*. Following PDT, there is a geographic area of atrophy and pigmentation in the central macula, bordered by a serosanguineous area nasally *(upper right)*. The fluorescein angiogram reveals an infarction of the choroid on the temporal side of the lesion and persistent choroidal neovascularization and leakage on the nasal side *(arrows, lower left image)*. The ICG angiogram shows delayed or absent perfusion of the lesion in the area of infarction *(lower row middle image)* as well as late staining of the pigment epithelium temporally and the neovascularization nasally *(arrows, lower right image)*.

Retinal Cyst on Buckle

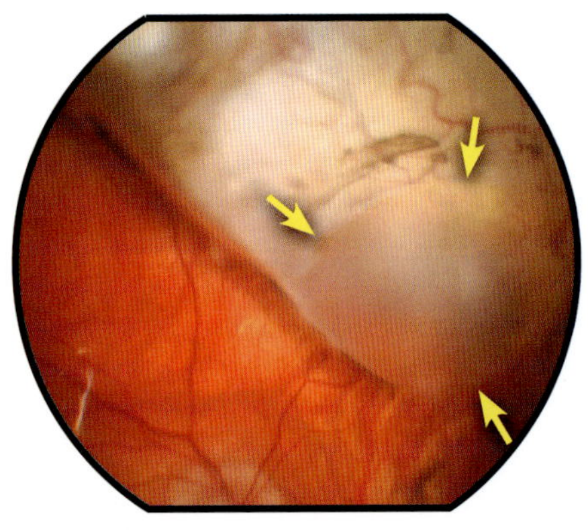

This patient developed a large cyst on a scleral buckle *(arrows)*.

Macular Folds Status Post Scleral Buckling Surgery

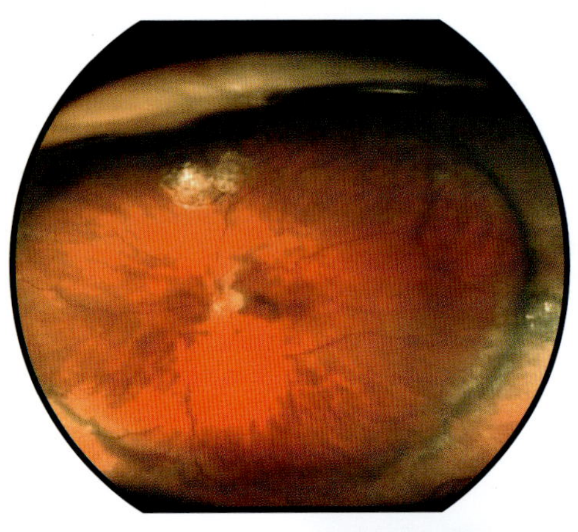

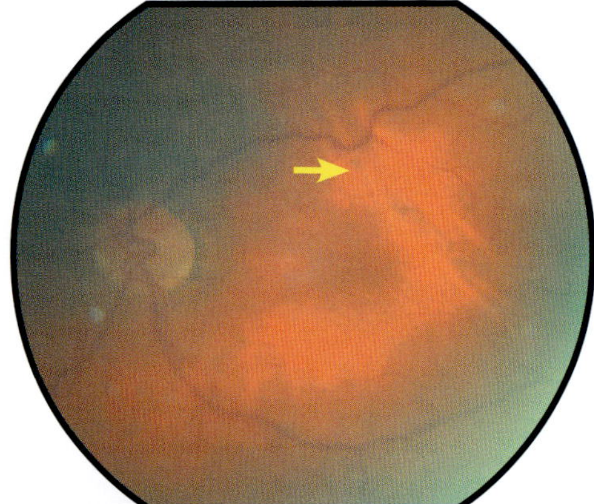

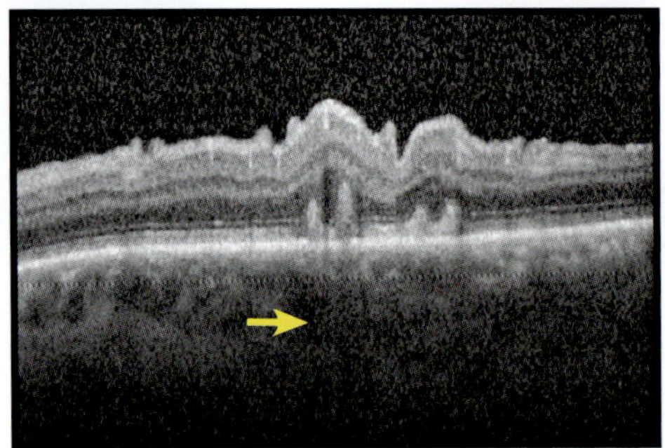

This patient underwent repair of a retinal detachment with placement of a scleral buckle. Postoperatively, the vision was restricted to 20/200 due to development of macular and retinal folds (*arrow* on color photograph and SD-OCT). The folds did not spontaneously resolve, thus vitrectomy surgery was performed with microcatheter-delivered fluid to re-detach the posterior retina, followed by use of an intraoperative air bubble and face-down positioning.

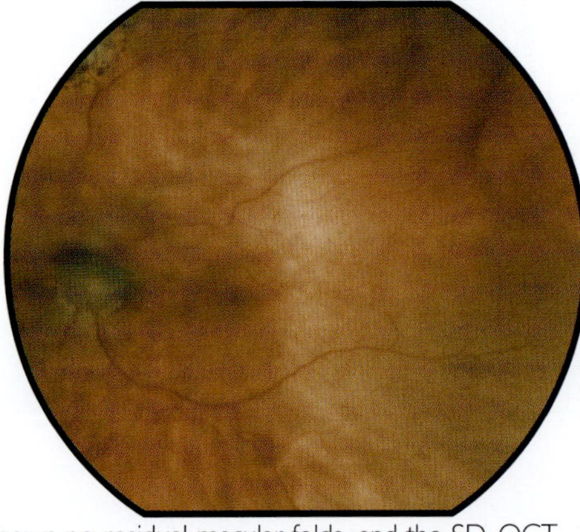

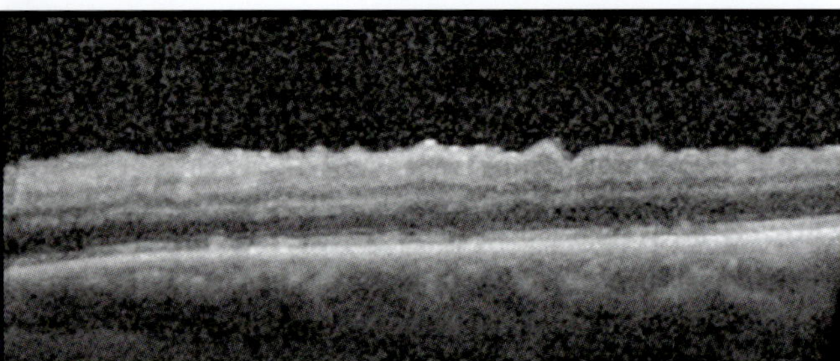

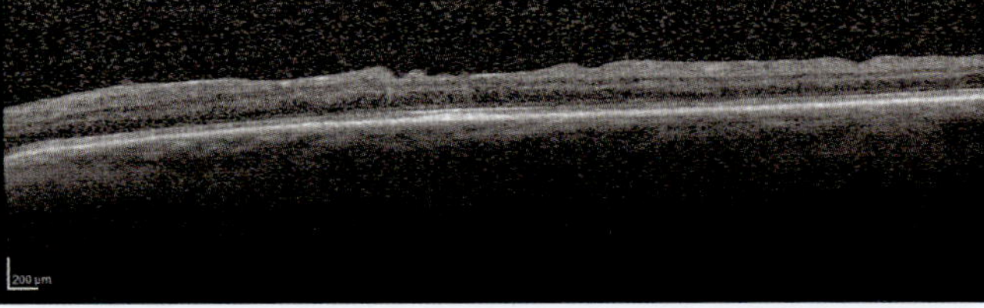

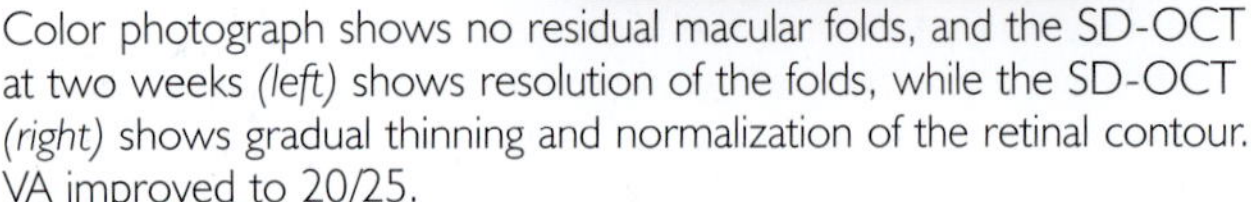

Color photograph shows no residual macular folds, and the SD-OCT at two weeks *(left)* shows resolution of the folds, while the SD-OCT *(right)* shows gradual thinning and normalization of the retinal contour. VA improved to 20/25.

Giant Retinal Pigment Epithelial Tear

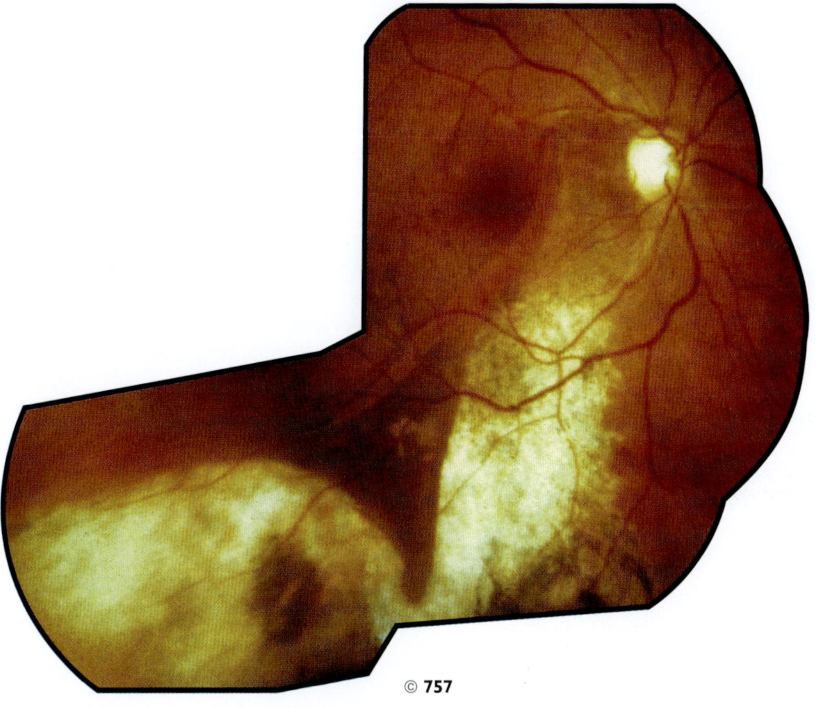

This patient had intraocular surgery and experienced a giant tear of the retinal pigment epithelium.

Extrusion of Buckle

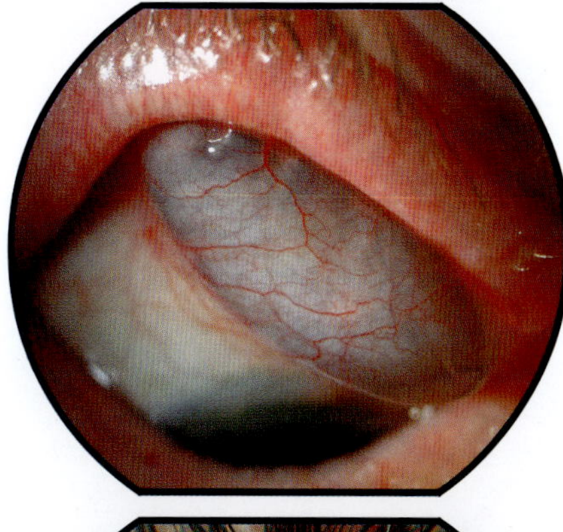

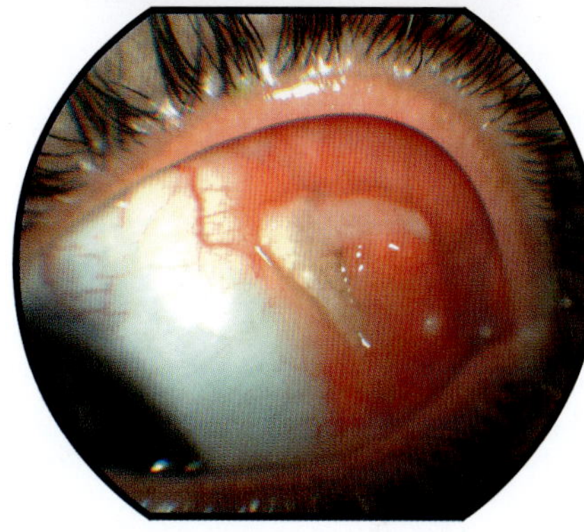

Extrusion of a buckle may also occur, as seen in these two patients after a reattachment procedure.

Laser of Calcific Plaque Arteriole Occlusion

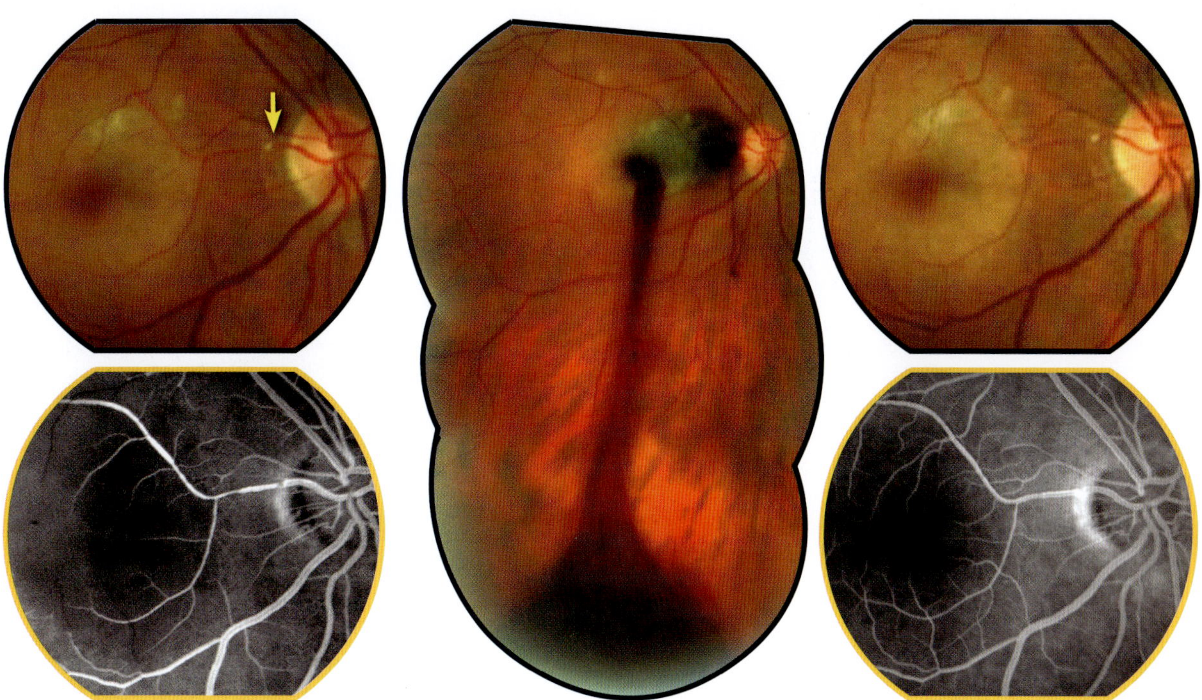

The patient developed a calcific embolus in a temporal arteriole *(arrow left)*. The fluorescein angiogram shows blockage of the affected arteriole. This patient was treated with a Nd:YAG laser for the embolus. Photo microdisruption of the embolus was associated with severe bleeding into the vitreous, including an extension of the hemorrhage and an inverted mushroom configuration from the posterior inferior vitreous *(middle image)*. In time, the hemorrhage cleared, with vision impairment and reperfusion of the obstructed arteriole *(right images). Courtesy of Drs. Michael Cooney and Samira Khan*

Suggested Reading

Injections

Cardascia, N., Boscia, F., Furino, C., et al., 2008. Gentamicin-induced macular infarction in transconjunctival sutureless 25-gauge vitrectomy. Int. Ophthalmol. 28, 383–385.

Duker, J.S., Belmont, J.R., Benson, W.E., et al., 1991. Inadvertent globe perforation during retrobulbar and peribulbar anesthesia. Patient characteristics, surgical management, and visual outcome. Ophthalmology 98, 519–526.

Feibel, R.M., Guyton, D.L., 2003. Transient central retinal artery occlusion after posterior subTenon's anesthesia. J. Cataract Refract. Surg. 29, 1821–1824.

Hay, A., Flynn, H.W., Hoffman, J.I., et al., 1991. Needle penetration of the lobe during retrobulbar and peribulbar injections. Ophthalmology 98, 1017–1024.

Hida, T., Chandler, D., Arena, J.E., et al., 1986. Experimental and clinical observations of the intraocular toxicity of commercial corticosteroid preparations. Am. J. Ophthalmol. 101, 190–195.

Lake, D., Mearza, A., Ionides, A., 2003. Consequence of perforation during peribulbar anesthesia in an only eye. J. Cataract Refract. Surg. 29, 2234–2235.

Lam, D.C., Law, R.W., Leung, A.T., et al., 1999. Intraorbital needle fragment: a rare complication of retrobulbar injection. Arch. Ophthalmol. 117, 1089–1090.

Lau, L.I., Lin, P.K., Hsu, W.M., et al., 2003. Ipsilateral globe penetration and transient contralateral amaurosis following retrobulbar anesthesia. Am. J. Ophthalmol. 135, 251–252.

Mameletzi, E., Pournaras, J.A., Ambresin, A., et al., 2008. Retinal embolisation with localised retinal detachment following retrobulbar anaesthesia. Klin. Monatsbl. Augenheilkd 225, 476–478.

Paulter, S.E., Grizzard, W.S., Thompson, L.N., et al., 1986. Blindness from retrobulbar injection into the optic nerve. Ophthalmic Surg. 17, 334–337.

Pendergast, S.D., Eliott, D., Machemer, R., 1995. Retinal toxic effects following inadvertent intraocular injection of celestone soluspan. Arch. Ophthalmol. 113, 1230–1231.

Ramsey, R.C., Knobloch, W.H., 1978. Ocular perforation following retrobulbar anesthesia for retinal detachment surgery. Am. J. Ophthalmol. 86, 61–64.

Reichstein, D.A., Warren, C.C., Han, D.P., et al., 2016. Local Anesthesia With Blunt SubTenon's Cannula Versus Sharp Retrobulbar Needle for Vitreoretinal Surgery: A Retrospective, Comparative Study. Ophthalmic Surg. Lasers Imaging Retina 47, 55–59.

Roth, S.E., Magargal, L.E., Kimmel, A.S., et al., 1988. Central retinal-artery occlusion in proliferative sickle-cell retinopathy after retrobulbar injection. Ann. Ophthalmol. 20, 221–224.

Schnieder, M.E., Milstein, D.E., Oyakawa, R.T., et al., 1988. Ocular performation from a retrobulbar injection. Am. J. Ophthalmol. 106, 35–40.

Schrader, W.F., Schargus, M., Schneider, E., et al., 2010. Risks and sequelae of scleral perforation during peribulbar or retrobulbar anesthesia. J. Cataract Refract. Surg. 36, 885–889.

Sullivan, K.L., Brown, G.C., Forman, A.R., et al., 1983. Retrobulbar anesthesia and retinal vascular obstruction. Ophthalmology 90, 373–377.

Outer Retinal Infarction

Gass, J.D.M., Parris, R., 1982. Outer retinal ischemic infarction—a newly recognized complication of cataract extraction and closed vitrectomy. Part I. A case report. Ophthalmology 89, 1467.

Cryodemarcation

Hilton, G.F., 1974. Subretinal pigment migration. Effects of cryosurgical retinal reattachment. Arch. Ophthalmol. 91, 445–450.

Sudarsky, R.D., Yannuzzi, L.A., 1974. Cryomarcation line and pigment migration after retinal cryosurgery. Arch. Ophthalmol. 91, 395–401.

Aminoglycoside Toxicity

Brown, G.C., Eagle, R.C., Shakin, E.P., et al., 1990. Retinal toxicity of intravitreal gentamicin. Arch. Ophthalmol. 108, 1740–1744.

Brouzas, D., Moschos, M.M., Koutsandrea, C., et al., 2013. Gentamicin-induced macular toxicity in 25-gauge sutureless vitrectomy. Cutan. Ocul. Toxicol. 32, 258–259.

Hancock, H.A., Guidry, C., Read, R.W., et al., 2005. Acute aminoglycoside retinal toxicity in vivo and in vitro. Invest. Ophthalmol. Vis. Sci. 46, 4804–4808.

Intracameral Vancomycin

Nicholson, L.B., Kim, B.T., Jardon, J., et al., 2014. Severe bilateral ischemic retinal vasculitis following cataract surgery. Ophthalmic Surg. Lasers Imaging Retina 45, 338–342.

Witkin, A.J., Shah, A.R., Engstrom, R.E., et al., 2015. Postoperative hemorrhagic occlusive retinal vasculitis: expanding the clinical spectrum and possible association with vancomycin. Ophthalmology 122, 1438–1451.

Lenci, L.T., Chin, E.K., Carter, C., et al., 2015. Ischemic retinal vasculitis associated with cataract surgery and intracameral vancomycin. Case Rep. Ophthalmol. Med. 2015, 683194.

Dislocated Intraocular Lens/ Retained Lens Fragment

Brod, R.D., Flynn, H.W. Jr., Clarkson, J.G., et al., 1990. Management options for retinal detachment in the presence of a posteriorly dislocated intraocular lens. Retina 10, 50–56.

Chalam, K.V., Murthy, R.K., Priluck, J.C., et al., 2015. Concurrent removal of intravitreal lens fragments after phacoemulsification with pars plana vitrectomy prevents development of retinal detachment. Int. J. Ophthalmol. 8, 89–93.

Ho, L.Y., Doft, B.H., Wang, L., et al., 2009. Clinical predictors and outcomes of pars plana vitrectomy for retained lens material after cataract extraction. Am. J. Ophthalmol. 147, 587–594.

Lai, T.Y., Kwok, A.K., Yeung, Y.S., et al., 2005. Immediate pars plana vitrectomy for dislocated intravitreal lens fragments during cataract surgery. Eye (Lond.) 19, 1157–1162.

Lewis, H., Blumenkranz, M.S., Chang, S., 1992. Treatment of dislocated crystalline lens and retinal detachment with perfluorocarbon liquids. Retina 12, 299–304.

Margherio, R.R., Margherio, A.R., Pendergast, S.D., et al., 1997. Vitrectomy for retained lens fragments after phacoemulsification. Ophthalmology 104, 1426–1432.

Moisseiev, E., Kinori, M., Glovinsky, Y., et al., 2011. Retained lens fragments: nucleus fragments are associated with worse prognosis than cortex or epinucleus fragments. Eur. J. Ophthalmol. 21, 741–747.

Smiddy, W.E., Flynn, H.W. Jr., 1991. Management of dislocated posterior chamber intraocular lenses. Ophthalmology 98, 889–894.

Teo, L., Chee, S.P. 2010. Retained lens fragment in the anterior segment as a cause of recurrent anterioruveitis. Int. Ophthalmol. 30 (1), 89–91.

Extrusion of Scleral Buckle

Brown, D.M., Beardsley, R.M., Fish, R.H., et al., 2006. Long-term stability of circumferential silicone sponge scleral buckling exoplants. Retina 26, 645–649.

Crama, N., Klevering, B.J., 2016. The removal of hydrogel explants: an analysis of 467 consecutive cases. Ophthalmology 123, 32–38.

Hahn, Y.S., Lincoff, A., Lincoff, H., et al., 1979. Infection after sponge implantation for sclera buckling. Am. J. Ophthalmol. 87, 180–185.

Holland, S.P., Pulido, J.S., Miller, D., et al., 1991. Biofilm and scleral buckle-associated infections. A mechanism for persistence. Ophthalmology 98, 933–938.

Decompression Retinopathy

Ben Simon, G.J., Goldberg, R.A., McCann, J.D., 2004. Bilateral decompression retinopathy after orbital decompression surgery. Br. J. Ophthalmol. 88, 1605–1606.

Bui, C.M., Recchia, F.M., Recchia, C.C., et al., 2006. Optical coherence tomography findings in ocular decompression retinopathy. Ophthalmic Surg. Lasers Imaging 37, 333–335.

Danias, J., Rosenbaum, J., Podos, S.M., 2000. Diffuse retinal hemorrhages (ocular decompression syndrome) after trabeculectomy with mitomycin C for neovascular glaucoma. Acta Ophthalmol. Scand. 78, 468–469.

Fechtner, R.D., Minckler, D., Weinreb, R.N., et al., 1992. Complications of glaucoma surgery. Ocular decompression retinopathy. Arch. Ophthalmol. 110, 965–968.

Jung, K.I., Lim, S.A., Lopilly Park, H.Y., et al., 2014. Risk factors for decompression retinopathy after glaucoma surgery. J. Glaucoma 23, 638–643.

Lai, J.S., Lee, V.Y., Leung, D.Y., et al., 2005. Decompression retinopathy following laser peripheral iridoplasty for acute primary angle-closure. Eye (Lond.) 19, 1345–1347.

Rao, S.K., Greenberg, P.B., Macintyre, R.B., et al., 2009. Ocular decompression retinopathy after anterior chamber paracentesis for uveitic glaucoma. Retina 29, 280–281.

Rezende, F.A., Regis, L.G., Kickinger, M., et al., 2007. Decompression retinopathy after 25-gauge transconjunctival sutureless vitrectomy: report of 2 cases. Arch. Ophthalmol. 125, 699–700.

Saricaoglu, M.S., Kalayci, D., Guven, D., et al., 2009. Decompression retinopathy and possible risk factors. Acta Ophthalmol. 87, 94–95.

Wakita, M., Kawaji, T., Ando, E., et al., 2006. Ocular decompression retinopathy following trabeculectomy with mitomycin C associated with familial amyloidotic polyneuropathy. Br. J. Ophthalmol. 90, 515–516.

Non-Arteritic Anterior Ischemic Optic Neuropathy/Ischemia

Elston, J., 2007. Non-arteritic anterior ischaemic optic neuropathy and cataract surgery. Br. J. Ophthalmol. 91, 563.

Hayreh, S.S., 1980. Anterior ischemic optic neuropathy IV. Occurrence after cataract extraction. Arch. Ophthalmol. 98, 1410–1416.

Lam, B.L., Jabaly-Habib, H., Al-Sheikh, N., et al., 2007. Risk of non-arteritic anterior ischaemic optic Neuropathy (NAION) after cataract extraction in the fellow eye of patients with prior unilateral NAION. Br. J. Ophthalmol. 91, 585–587.

McCulley, T.J., Lam, B.L., Feuer, W.J., 2005. A comparison of risk factors for postoperative and spontaneous nonarteritic anterior ischemic optic neuropathy. J. Neuroophthalmol. 25, 22–24.

Rosenblum, P.D., Michels, R.G., Stark, W.J., et al., 1981. Choroidal ischemia after extracapsular cataract extraction by phacoemulsification. Retina 1, 263–270.

Taban, M., Sharma, M.C., Lee, M.S., 2006. Anterior ischemic optic neuropathy after uncomplicated scleral buckling surgery. Graefes Arch. Clin. Exp. Ophthalmol. 244, 1370–1372.

Phototoxicity

Boldrey, E.E., Ho, B.T., Griffith, R.D., 1984. Retinal burns occurring at cataract extraction. Ophthalmology 91, 1297–1302.

Cetinkaya, A., Yilmaz, G., Akova, Y.A., 2006. Photic retinopathy after cataract surgery in diabetic patients. Retina 26, 1021–1028.

Charles, S., 2008. Illumination and phototoxicity issues in vitreoretinal surgery. Retina 28, 1–4.

Kleinmann, G., Hoffman, P., Schechtman, E., et al., 2002. Microscope-induced retinal phototoxicity in cataract surgery of short duration. Ophthalmology 109, 334–338.

Mainster, M.A., 1986. Wavelength selection in macula photocoagulation tissue optics, thermal effects and laser systems. Ophthalmology 93, 952–958.

Mainster, M.A., White, T.J., Tips, J.H., et al., 1970. Retinal temperature increases produced by intense light sources. J. Opt. Soc. Am. A. 60, 264–270.

McDonald, H.R., Harris, M.J., 1988. Operating microscope-induced retinal phototoxicity during pars plana vitrectomy. Am. J. Ophthalmol. 106, 521–523.

Robertson, D.M., Feldman, R.B., 1986. Photic retinopathy from the operating room microscope. Am. J. Ophthalmol. 101, 561–569.

Hypotony

Acar, N., Kapran, Z., Unver, Y.B., et al., 2008. Early postoperative hypotony after 25-gauge sutureless vitrectomy with straight incisions. Retina 28, 545–552.

Hsu, J., Chen, E., Gupta, O., et al., 2008. Hypotony after 25-gauge vitrectomy using oblique versus direct cannula insertions in fluid-filled eyes. Retina 28, 937–940.

Woo, S.J., Park, K.H., Hwang, J.M., et al., 2009. Risk factors associated with sclerotomy leakage and postoperative hypotony after 23-gauge transconjunctival sutureless vitrectomy. Retina 29, 456–463.

Choroidal Hemorrhage

Basti, S., Hu, D.J., Goren, M.B., et al., 2003. Acute suprachoroidal hemorrhage during clear corneal phacoemulsification using topical and intracameral anesthesia. J. Cataract Refract. Surg. 29, 588–591.

Chan, W.C., McGimpsey, S.J., Murphy, M.F., et al., 2005. Suprachoroidal haemorrhage following Nd:YAG laser posterior capsulotomy. Clin. Experiment. Ophthalmol. 33, 334–335.

Chen, C.J., Satofuka, S., Inoue, M., et al., 2008. Suprachoroidal hemorrhage caused by breakage of a 25-gauge cannula. Ophthalmic Surg. Lasers Imaging 39, 323–324.

Ling, R., Cole, M., James, C., et al., 2004. Suprachoroidal haemorrhage complicating cataract surgery in the UK: epidemiology, clinical features, management, and outcomes. Br. J. Ophthalmol. 88, 478–480.

Ling, R., Kamalarajah, S., Cole, M., et al., 2004. Suprachoroidal haemorrhage complicating cataract surgery in the UK: a case control study of risk factors. Br. J. Ophthalmol. 88, 474–477.

Silicone Oil/Perfluorocarbon (PFC) Liquid

Bakri, S.J., Ekdawi, N.S., 2008. Intravitreal silicone oil droplets after intravitreal drug injections. Retina 28, 996–1001.

Chung, J., Spaide, R., 2003. Intraretinal silicone oil vacuoles after macular hole surgery with internal limiting membrane peeling. Am. J. Ophthalmol. 136, 766–767.

Dresp, J.H., Menz, D.H., 2005. Interaction of different ocular endotamponades as a risk factor for silicone oil emulsification. Retina 25, 902–910. Erratum in: Retina; Dec. 25: 1123.

Elsing, S.H., Fekrat, S., Green, W.R., et al., 2001. Clinicopathologic findings in eyes with retained perfluoro-n-octane liquid. Ophthalmology 108, 45–48.

Federman, J.L., Schubert, H.D., 1988. Complications associated with the use of silicone oil in 150 eyes after retina-vitreous surgery. Ophthalmology 95, 870–876.

Figueroa, M.S., Contreras, I., 2012. Characteristics of retained subretinal perfluoro-n-octane on optical coherence tomography. Retina 32, 2177–2178.

Huang, J.Y., Yang, C.M., 2004. Intraocular formation of heavy oil in the subretinal space. Jpn. J. Ophthalmol. 48, 75–77.

Kocabora, M.S., Ozbilen, K.T., Serefoglu, K., 2010. Intravitreal silicone oil droplets following pegaptanib injection. Acta Ophthalmol 88 (2), e44–e45.

Lesnoni, G., Rossi, T., Gelso, A., 2004. Subfoveal liquid perfluorocarbon. Retina 24, 172–176.

Light, D.J., 2006. Silicone oil emulsification in the anterior chamber after vitreoretinal surgery. Optometry 77, 446–449.

Scott, I.U., Murray, T.G., Flynn, H.W. Jr., et al., 2000. Outcomes and complications associated with perfluoro-n-octane and perfluoroperhydrophenanthrene in complex retina detachment repair. Ophthalmology 107, 860–865.

Tien, V.L., Pierre-Kahn, V., Azan, F., et al., 2008. Displacement of retained subfoveal perfluorocarbon liquid after vitreoretinal surgery. Arch. Ophthalmol. 126, 98–101.

Retinal Tacks

de Juan, E. Jr., Hickingbotham, D., Machemer, R., 1985. Retinal tacks. Am. J. Ophthalmol. 99, 272–274.

Javey, G., Schwartz, S.G., Flynn, H.W. Jr., et al., 2009. Lack of toxicity of stainless steel retinal tacks during 21 years of follow-up. Ophthalmic Surg. Lasers Imaging 40, 75–76.

O'Grady, G.E., Parel, J.M., Lee, W., et al., 1988. Hypodermic stainless steel tacks and companion inserter designed for peripheral fixation of retina. Arch. Ophthalmol. 106, 271–275.

Puustjärvi, T.J., Teräsvirta, M.E., 2001. Retinal fixation of traumatic retinal detachment with metallic tacks: a case report with 10 years' follow-up. Retina 21, 54–56.

Diamond/Steel Particles

Dunbar, C.M., Goble, R.R., Gregory, D.W., et al., 1995. Intraocular deposition of metallic fragments during phacoemulsification: possible causes and effect. Eye (Lond.) 9, 434–436.

Harper, T.W., Flynn, H.W. Jr., Berrocal, A., et al., 2008. Lack of toxicity during long-term follow-up of intraocular metallic fragments after pars plana vitrectomy. Ophthalmic Surg. Lasers Imaging 39, 319–322.

Retinal Prosthesis

Chow, A.Y., Chow, V.Y., Packo, K.H., et al., 2004. The artificial silicone retina microchip for the treatment of vision loss from retinitis pigmentosa. Arch. Ophthalmol. 122, 460–469.

Chow, A.Y., Pardue, M.T., Perlman, J.I., et al., 2002. Subretinal implantation of semiconductor-based photodiodes: durability of novel implant designs. J. Rehabil. Res. Dev. 39, 313–321.

Humayun, M.S., de Juan, E. Jr., Weiland, J.D., et al., 1999. Pattern electrical stimulation of the human retina. Vision Res 39, 2569–2576.

Humayun, M.S., Fujii, J., Greenberg, G.Y., et al., 2003. Visual perception in a blind subject with a chronic microelectronic retinal prosthesis. Vision Res. 43, 2573–2581.

Schubert, M., Stelzle, M., Graf, M., et al., 1999. Subretinal Implants for the Recovery of Vision. IEEE International Conf. Systems Man. Cybernetics, Tokyo, Japan, 376–381.

Transpupillary Thermotherapy

Browning, D.J., Antoszyk, A.N., 2003. Retinal tear and detachment after transpupillary thermotherapy for choroidal melanoma. Am. J. Ophthalmol. 135, 729–730.

Currie, Z.I., Rennie, I.G., Talbot, J.F., 2000. Retinal vascular changes associated with transpupillary thermotherapy for choroidal melanomas. Retina 20, 620–626.

Shields, C.L., Shields, J.A., Perez, N., et al., 2002. Primary transpupillary thermotherapy for small choroidal melanoma in 256 consecutive cases:

outcomes and limitations. Ophthalmology 109, 225–234.

Photodynamic Therapy

Arnold, J.J., Blinder, K.J., Bressler, N.M., et al., 2004. Acute severe visual acuity decrease after photodynamic therapy with verteporfin: case reports from randomized clinical trials-TAP and VIP report no. 3. Am. J. Ophthalmol. 137, 683–696.

Blinder, K.J., Bradley, S., Bressler, N.M., et al., 2003. Effect of lesion size, visual acuity, and lesion composition on visual acuity change with and without verteporfin therapy for choroidal neovascularization secondary to age-related macular degeneration: TAP and VIP report no. 1. Am. J. Ophthalmol. 136, 407–418.

Blumenkranz, M.S., Bressler, N.M., Bressler, S.B., et al., 2002. Verteporfin therapy for subfoveal choroidal neovascularization in age-related macular degeneration: three-year results of an open-label extension of 2 randomized clinical trials—TAP report no. 5. Arch. Ophthalmol. 120, 1307–1314.

Bressler, N.M., 2001. Photodynamic therapy of subfoveal choroidal neovascularization in age-related macular degeneration with verteporfin: two-year results of 2 randomized clinical trials-TAP report 2. Arch. Ophthalmol. 119, 198–207.

Klais, C.M., Ober, M.D., Freund, K.B., et al., 2005. Choroidal infarction following photodynamic therapy with verteporfin. Arch. Ophthalmol. 123, 1149–1153.

Miller, J.W., Schmidt-Erfurth, U., Sickenberg, M., et al., 1999. Photodynamic therapy for choroidal neovascularization due to age-related macular degeneration with verteporfin: results of a single treatment in a phase I and II study. Arch. Ophthalmol. 117, 1161–1173.

Schmidt-Erfurth, U.J.M., Bunse, A., Laqua, H., et al., 1998. Photodynamic therapy of subfoveal choroidal neovascularization: clinical and angiographic examples. Graefes Arch. Clin. Exp. Ophthalmol. 236, 365–374.

CHAPTER 14

Chorioretinal Toxicities

Introduction

Numerous exogenous molecules may cause toxic chorioretinitic effects. Some agents cause disruption of the retinal pigment epithelium (RPE), while others produce vascular damage within the retina. Certain agents may also produce edema of the retina, particularly in the macular region, while other agents produce crystalline deposits in the retina from derivatives of their metabolites or even direct deposits as a function of embolic phenomena. An increasing number of drugs are used for the treatment of uveitis or systemic disease and may be associated with toxic effects in the fundus.

Disruption of the Retinal Pigment Epithelium

Chloroquine Derivatives

Chloroquine

Chloroquine is a 4-aminoquinoline derivative used originally as an antimalarial agent, but subsequently for a variety of other diseases, including amebiasis, rheumatoid arthritis, and systemic lupus erythematosus. Its toxicity begins with a very mild, asymptomatic perifoveal granularity at the level of the RPE, followed by progressive loss of pigment epithelium cells and photoreceptors with a peculiar predilection for the inferior perifoveal and paramacular areas, and eventually the entire macula itself. The retinopathy is rarely reported with a total dosage less than 300 g or a daily dosage of less than 250 mg/day. The pigment epithelial degeneration may, in severe cases, extend to involve the near and far peripheral fundus. Following discontinuation of the drug, the retinopathy may still progress as it is slowly metabolized and released by the liver.

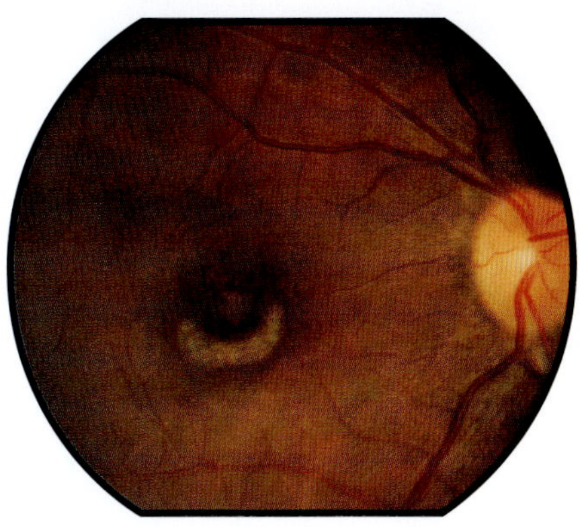

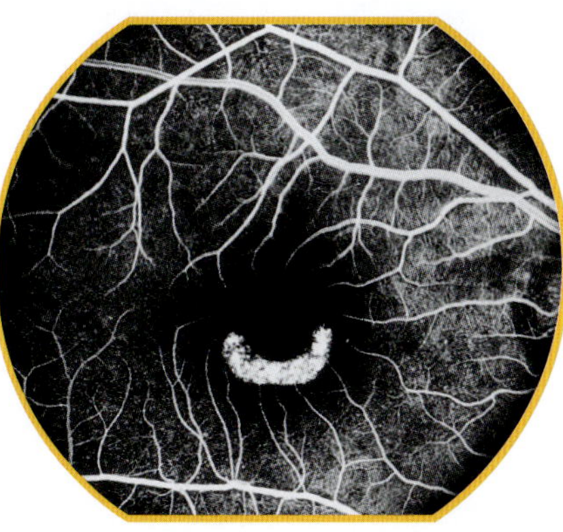

This patient has a typical area of perifoveal atrophy in the inferior portion of the macula from chloroquine toxicity. There is a peculiar predilection for the inferior perifoveal and paramacular region in this disorder.

© 758

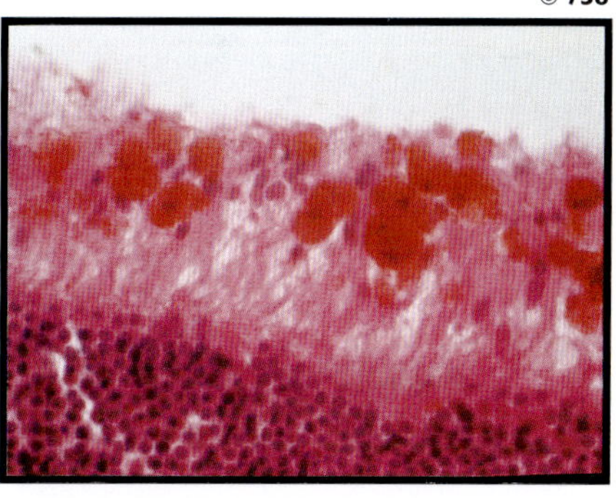

Light microscopy reveals a ring of photoreceptor loss and an aggregation of pigmented cells corresponding to the clinically evident toxicity.

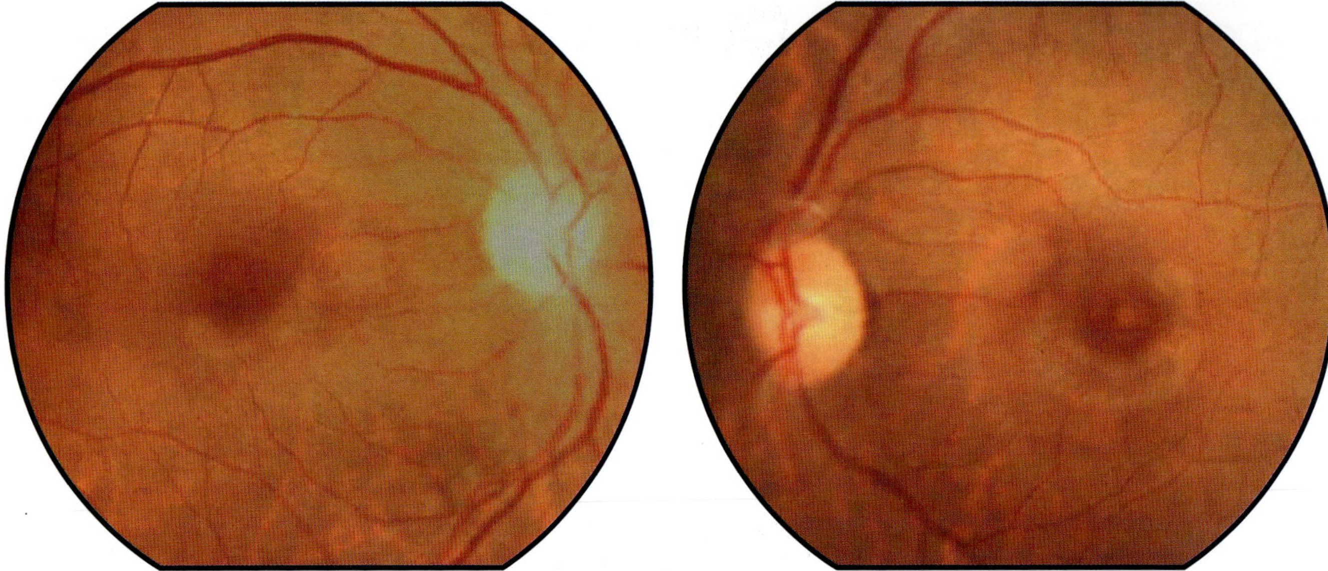

This patient has typical bilateral disease, which is asymmetric with more advanced disease in the left eye and forms a ring or "bull's-eye" appearance. *Courtesy of Dr. Keye Wong*

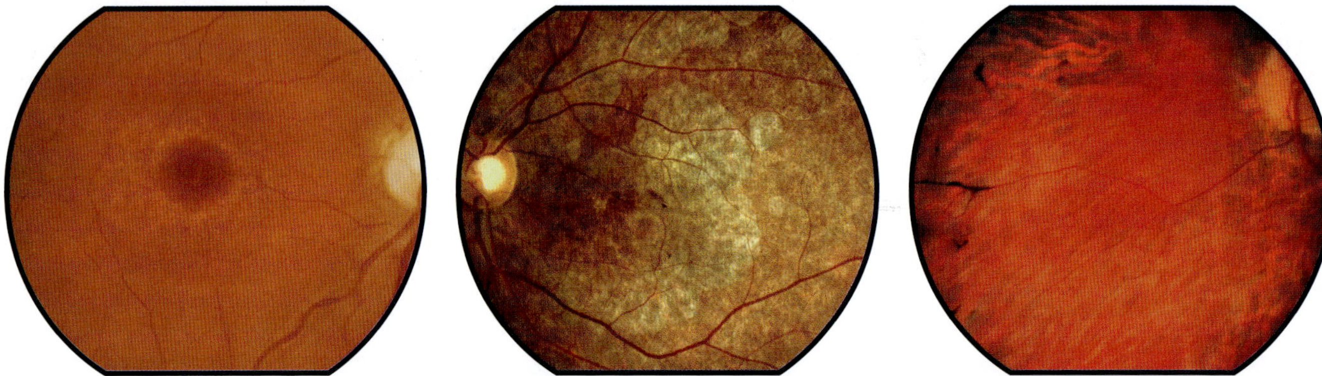

These two patients reveal chloroquine toxicity with a "bull's-eye" atrophy *(left)* and more diffuse pathology through the papillomacular bundle and the paramacular region (*right*).

Chloroquine toxicity can progress to involve the periphery, which shows a retinitis pigmentosa-like fundus. Note the bony spicule appearance with pigment epithelial cell migration into the retina.

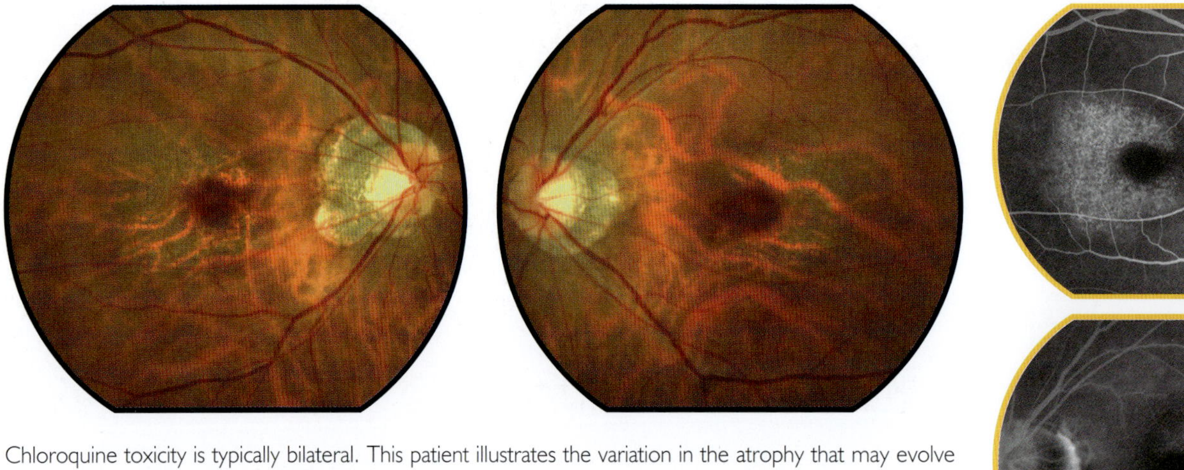

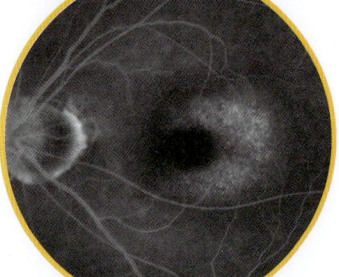

Chloroquine toxicity is typically bilateral. This patient illustrates the variation in the atrophy that may evolve in the course of the toxic response. The fluorescein angiograms show "window defect" or choroidal hyperfluorescence through atrophic defects in the RPE.

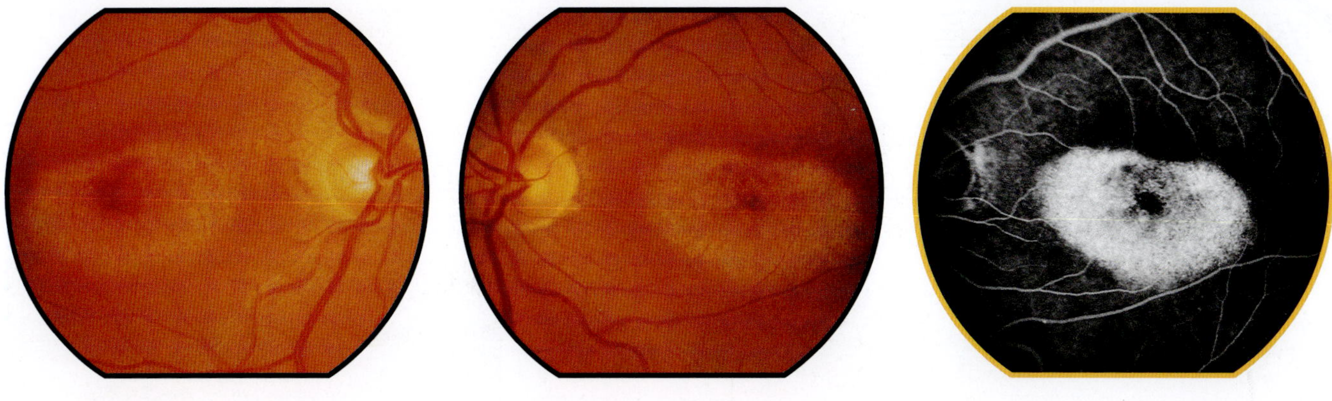

In this patient the area of atrophy forms an ovoid configuration, which is quite typical, again with a more pronounced effect in the inferior juxtafoveal and paramacular areas.

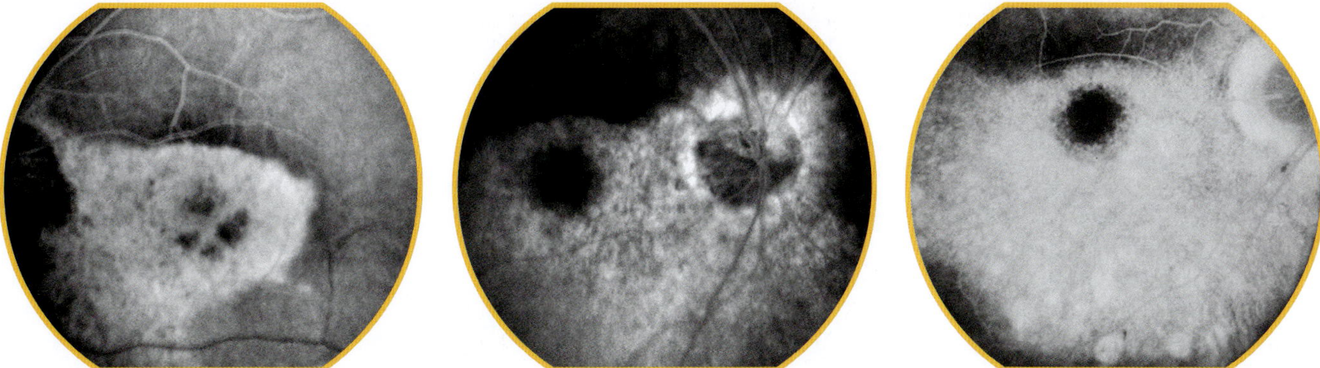

These patients demonstrate the nature of RPE disease in severe chloroquine toxicity. Progressive toxicity extends from the perifoveal area in early cases to more diffuse atrophy in severe toxicity, as above. Again, these patients demonstrate the inferior predilection of the toxic effect. Light exposure may be an explanation for this asymmetric feature.

Hydroxychloroquine

Hydroxychloroquine (Plaquenil) is a derivative of chloroquine and causes similar pathology, but generally less severe than chloroquine. Hydroxychloroquine appears to be significantly safer to use compared to chloroquine, yet it still may be toxic to the retina, producing a similar clinical presentation. Doses up to 5.0 mg/kg/day are typically considered safe. Concurrent tamoxifen therapy or chronic kidney disease may hasten onset of retinopathy. Asian patients may demonstrate a perifoveal pattern of toxicity.

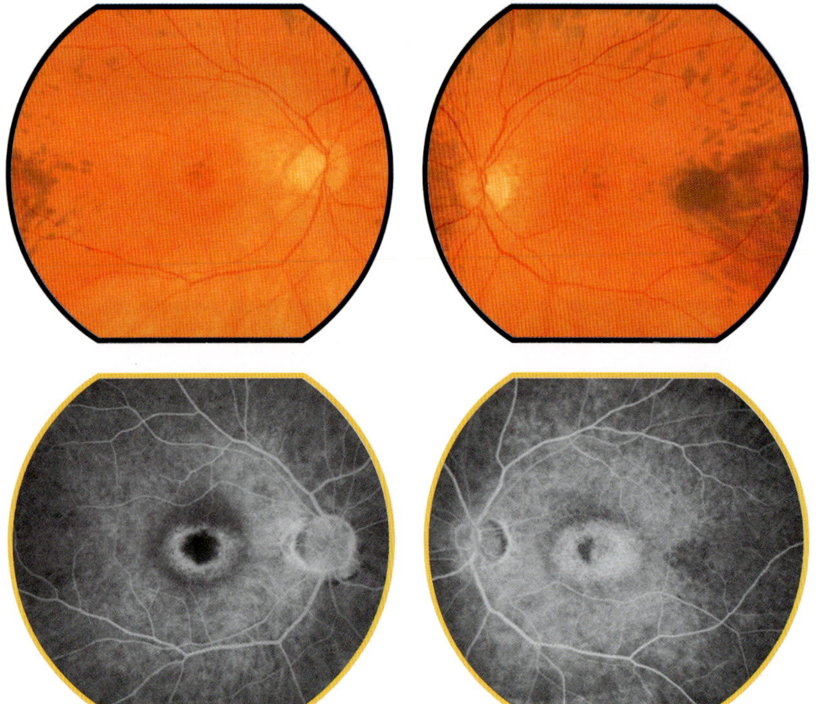

This patient has bilateral hydroxychloroquine toxicity with a "bull's-eye" appearance that is indistinguishable from chloroquine toxicity.

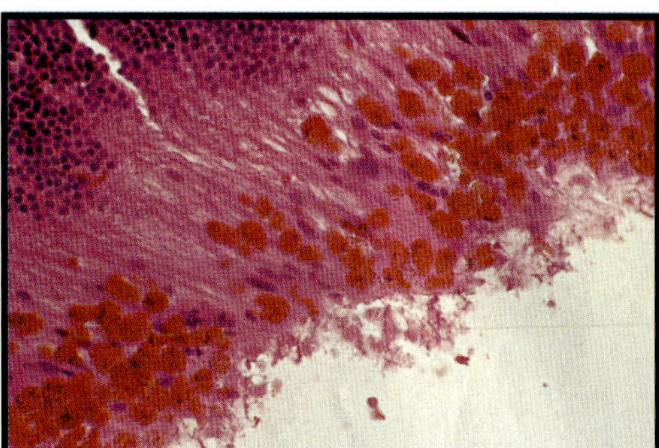

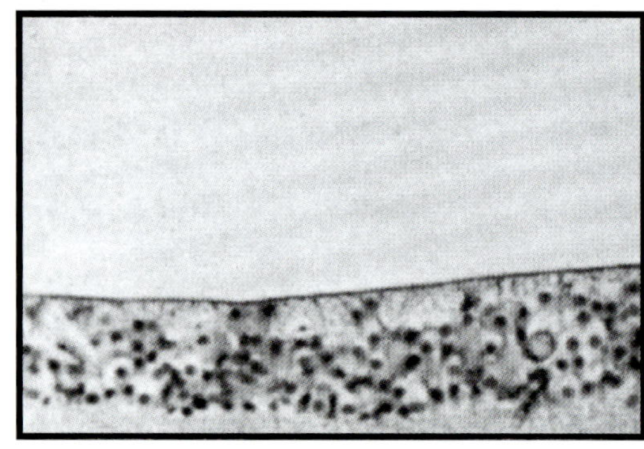

The pathology shows irregular pigment epithelial cell loss and photoreceptor damage.

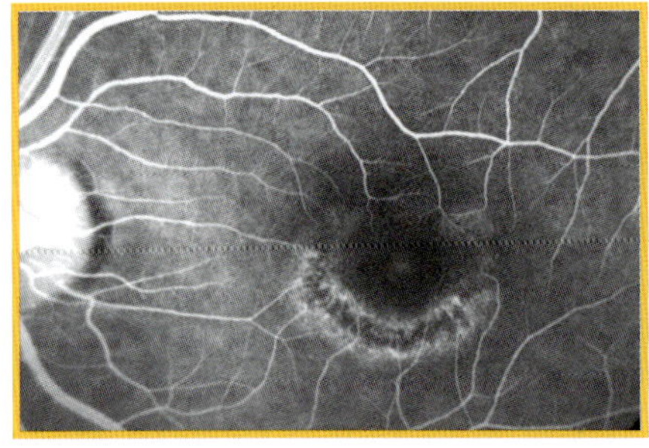

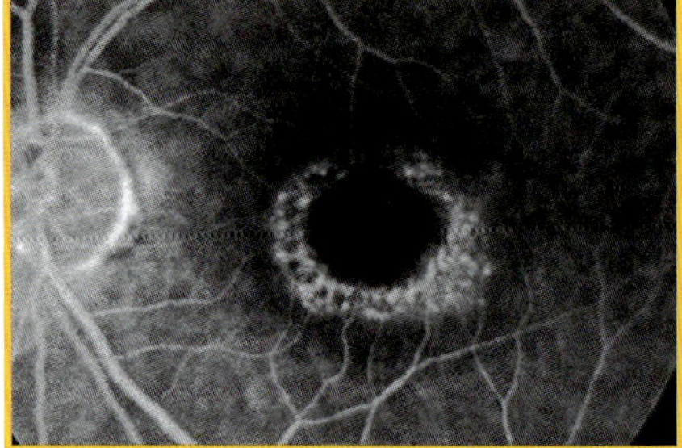

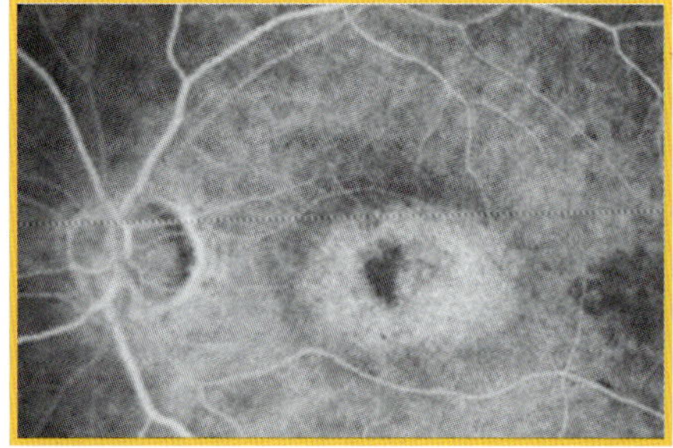

These two patients demonstrate the variation in the atrophic pattern of hydroxychloroquine toxicity with early changes in the inferior juxtafoveal area *(left)* and more prominent disease surrounding the fovea *(middle)*, with advanced toxicity *(right)*.

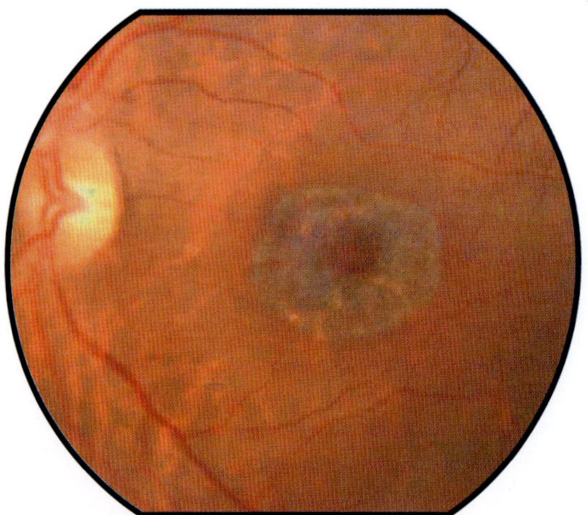

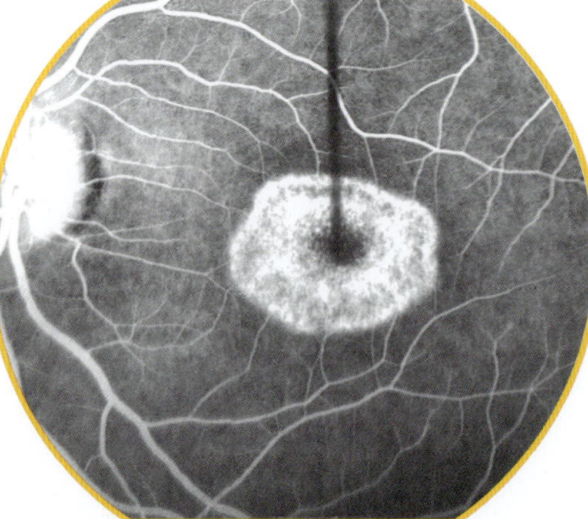

In this more advanced hydroxychloroquine toxicity, there is total involvement of the perifoveal region, forming a "bull's-eye" appearance that is indistinguishable from chloroquine toxicity. *Left image courtesy of Dr. Keye Wong*

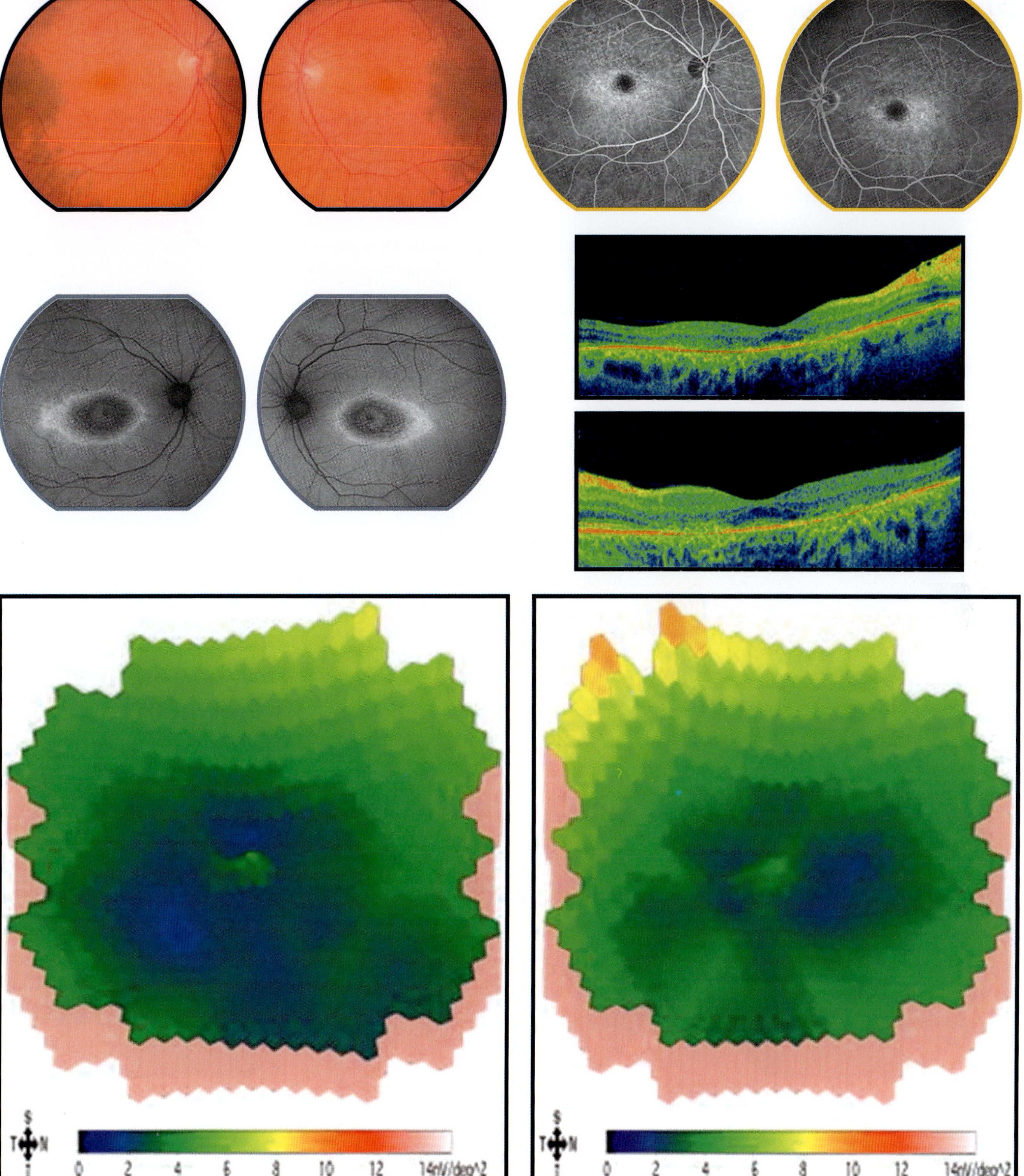

Color photographs *(top left)* showing mild macular pigment mottling in a patient on hydroxychloroquine with corresponding hyperfluorescence on fluorescein angiography *(top right)* in the pattern of a bull's eye. Fundus autofluorescence shows a perifoveal hypoautofluorescence with a border of hyperautofluorescence *(middle left)*. OCT shows atrophy of the outer nuclear layer and disruption of the ellipsoid segment *(middle right)*. Multifocal electroretinogram (mfERG) shows diminished paracentral waveforms *(bottom row)*. *Courtesy of Dr. David Sarraf*

Phenothiazines

Thioridazine

A piperidine initially introduced for treatment of psychoses, thioridazine (Mellaril) is a phenothiazine derivative that may cause damaging effects to the RPE, which can result, in some cases, in a "salt and pepper" appearance of the fundus with zonal atrophy and pigment epithelial clumping. Retinal toxicity is usually seen in doses in excess of 1000 mg/day with a total accumulation of 85-100 g over a 30-50-day period. Severe retinal toxicity may progress even after the drug is discontinued. It is believed that the toxic mechanism is mediated through a piperidyl side chain, which inhibits retinal enzymes and produces subsequent toxicity. Other explanations have been conceptualized, which include a dopamine and oxidative phosphorylation with derangement of rhodopsin. There is no treatment for the disintegration of the outer segments and the accumulation of lipofuscin in the RPE.

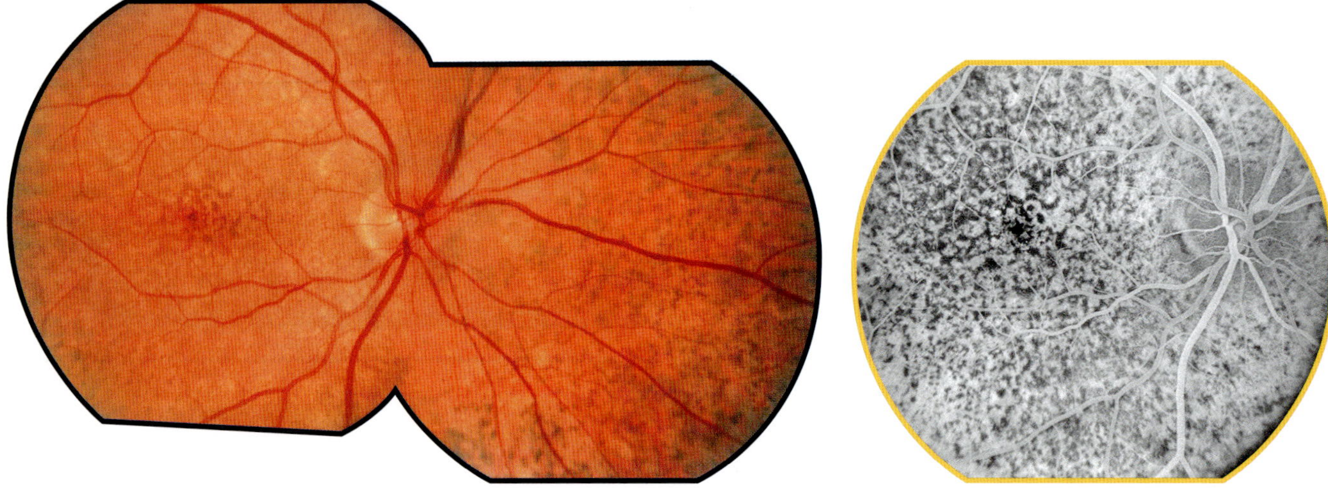

This is a patient with early but diffuse manifestations of thioridazine (Mellaril) toxicity. There is a granular or "salt and pepper"-like appearance to the fundus. The effect on the pigment epithelium is accentuated on the fluorescein angiogram.

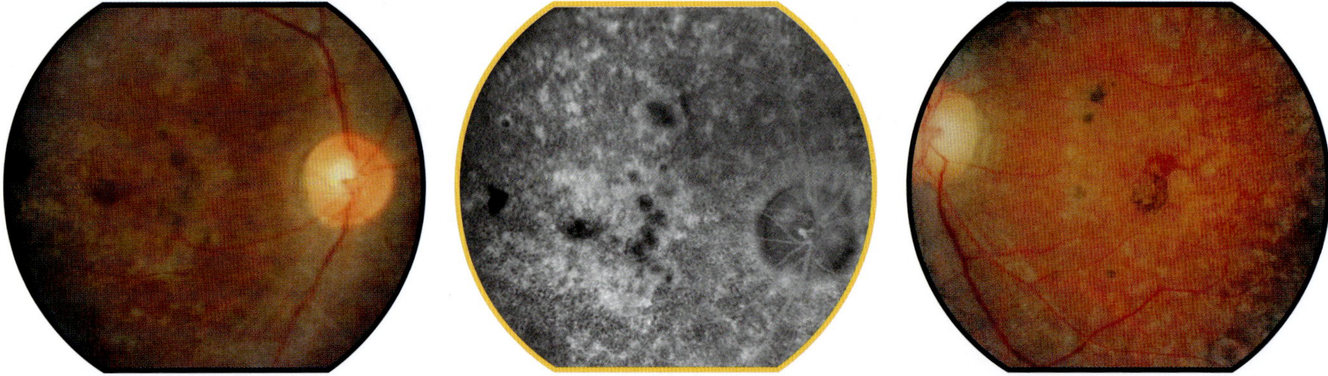

This patient has more advanced thioridazine toxicity with irregular atrophy in the central macula and pigment epithelial hyperplastic clumping.

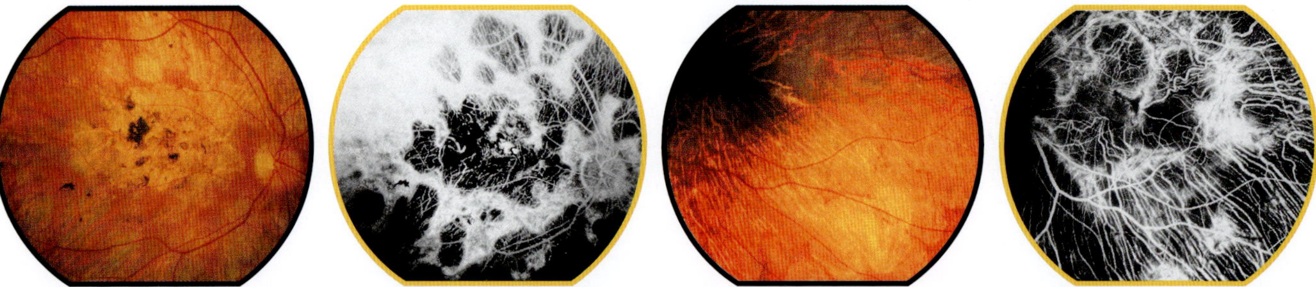

These two patients have progressive atrophy and pigment epithelial hyperplasia. The atrophy is not only in the macula and paramacular area *(left two images)*, but also extends out to the periphery *(right two images)*. The fluorescein angiogram shows pigment epithelial and choriocapillaris atrophy.

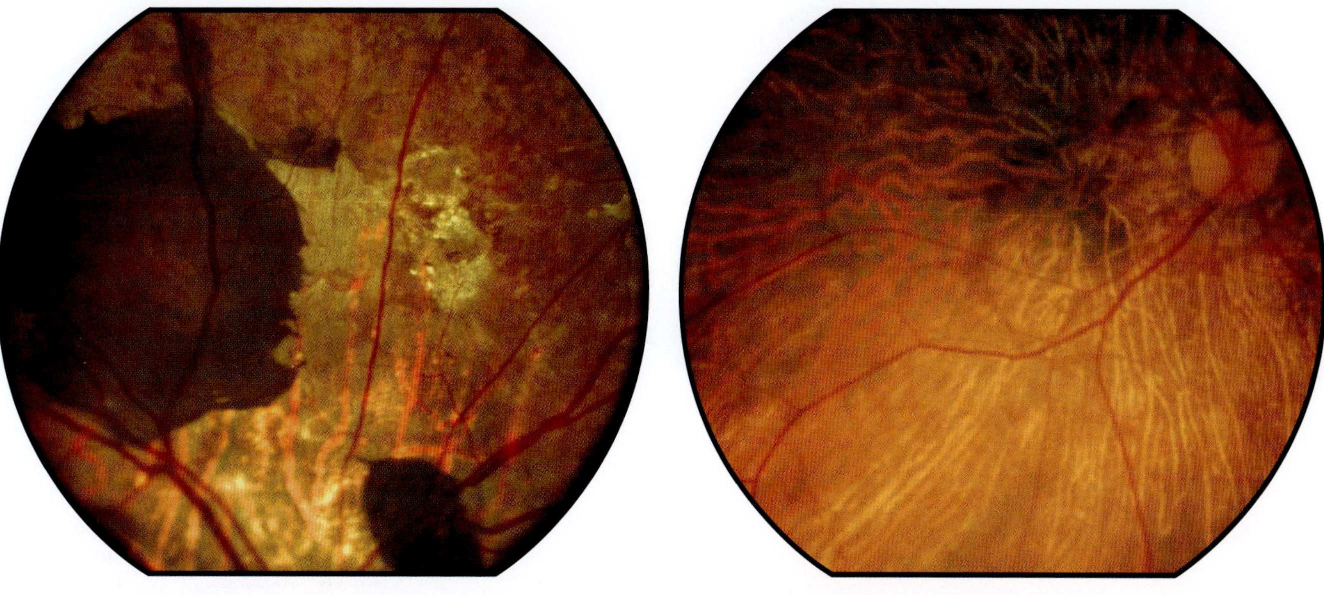

These two patients with thioridazine toxicity have extensive pigment epithelial zonal hyperplasia *(left)* and atrophy *(right)*.

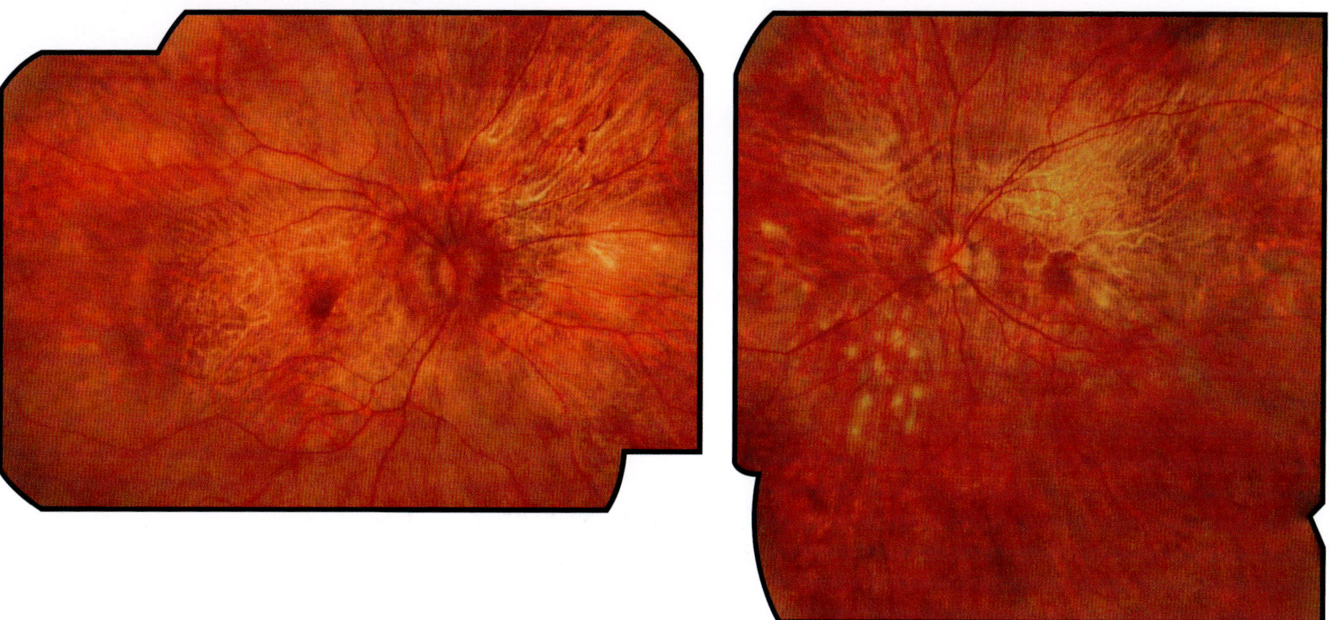

In this case of thioridazine toxicity the montage photos show multizonal areas of atrophy in the mid-peripheral retina with areas of relatively sparse toxicity in the periphery.

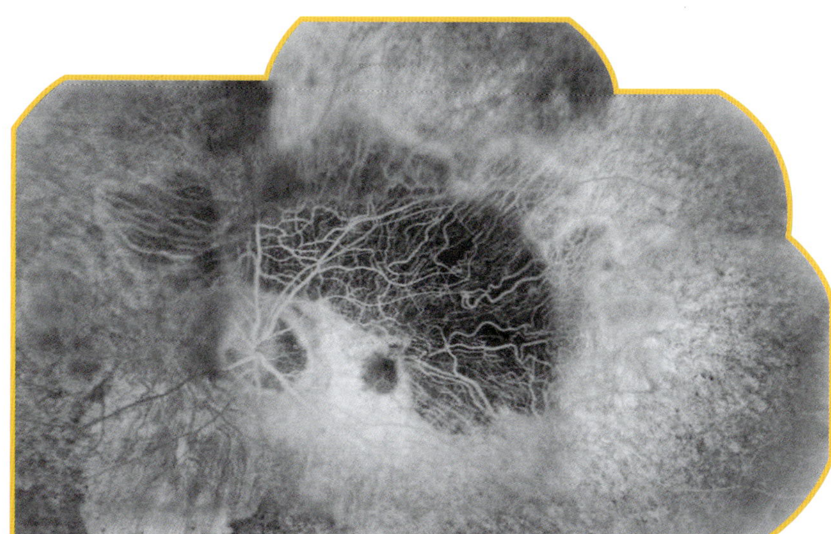

A montage fluorescein angiogram shows a "window defect" through the atrophic pigment epithelium, which is indicative of good perfusion of the choriocapillaris, with the exception of a few zonal areas of pigment aggregation and/or choriocapillaris atrophy that appear hypofluorescent.

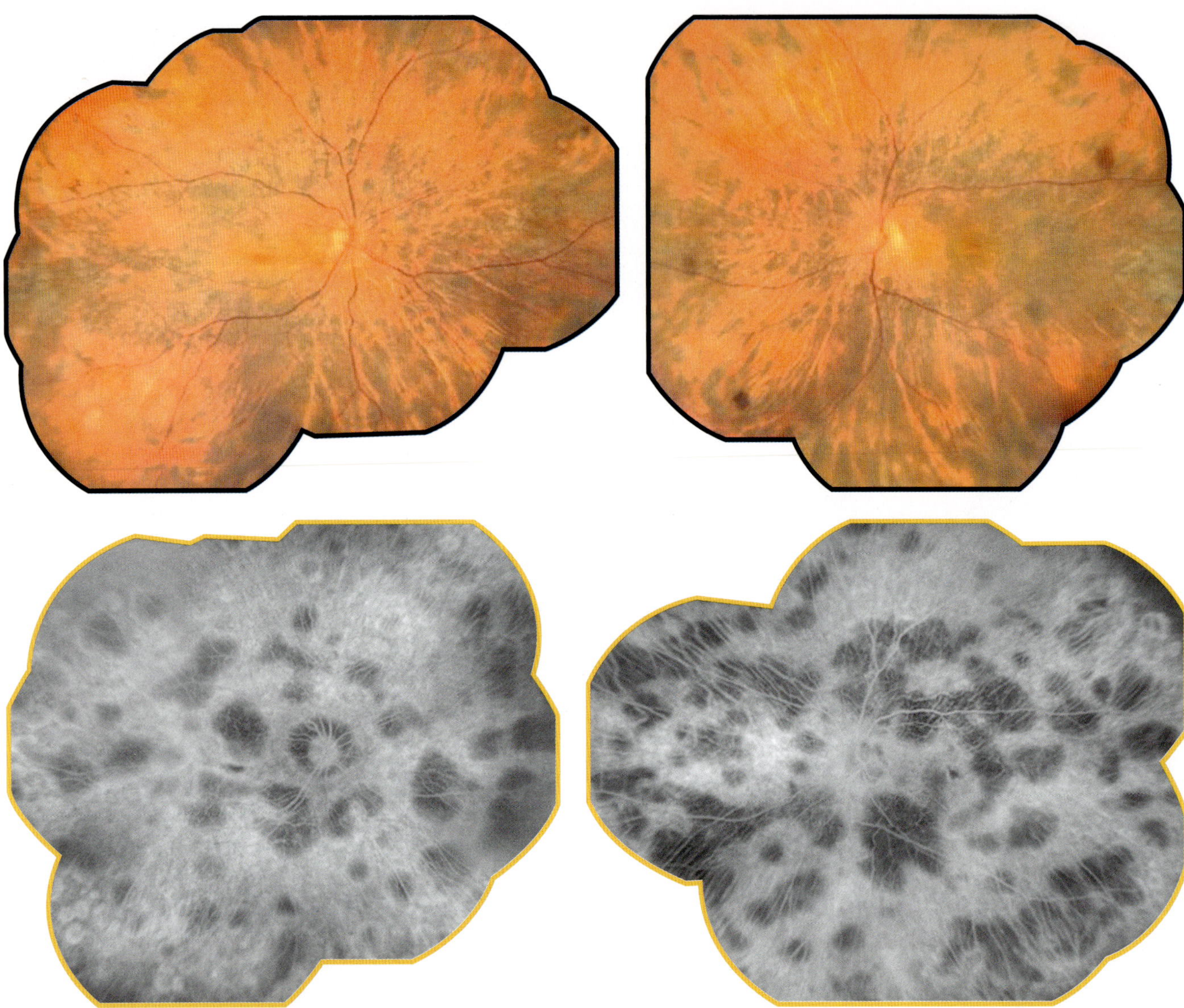

Fundus photographs and fluorescein angiograms show extensive nummular pigmentary changes with atrophy of the choriocapillaris in intermediate thioridazine toxicity. *Courtesy of Dr. David Sarraf*

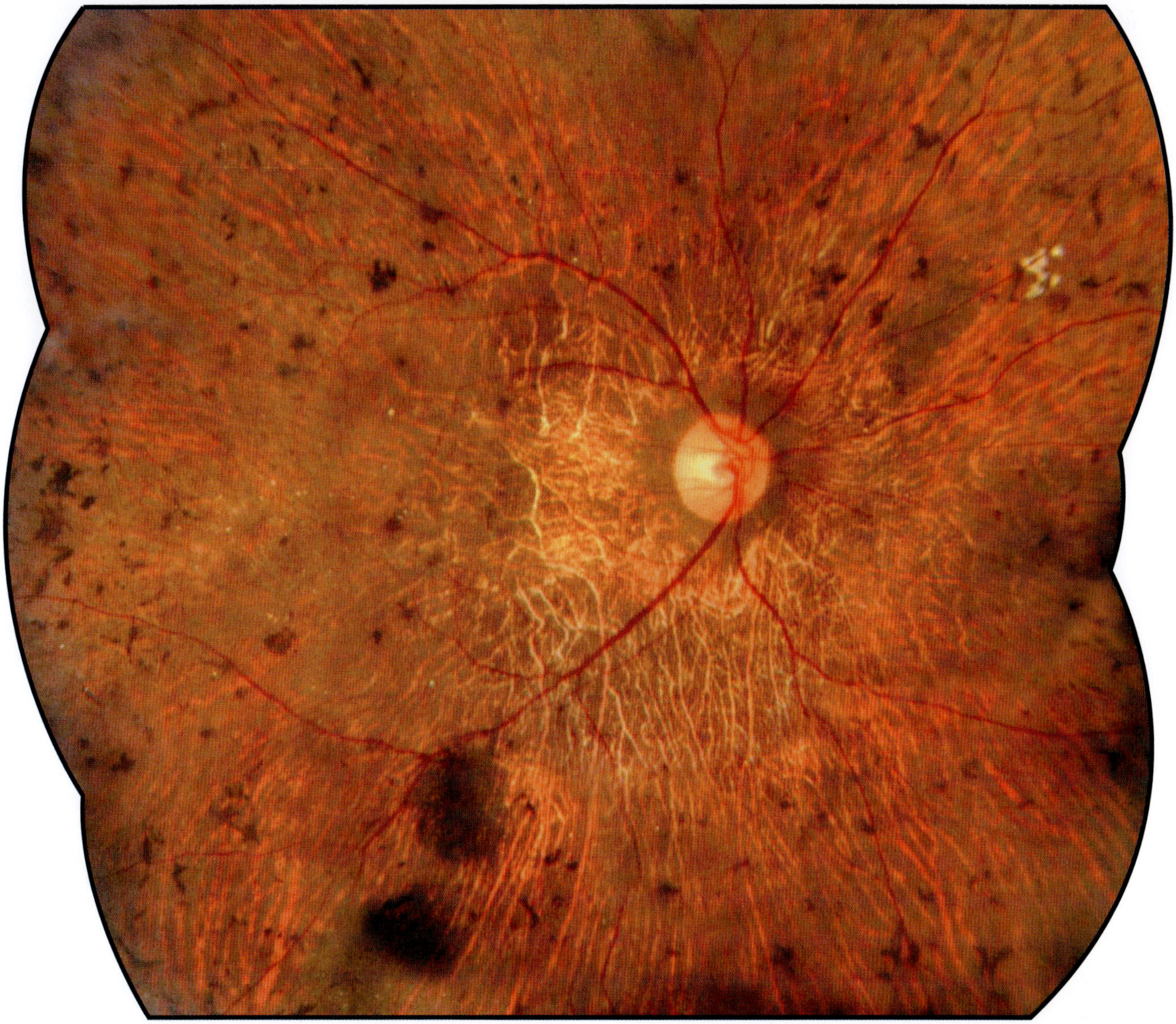

This montage illustrates widespread atrophy and pigment epithelial hyperplastic change in a patient with severe thioridazine toxicity.

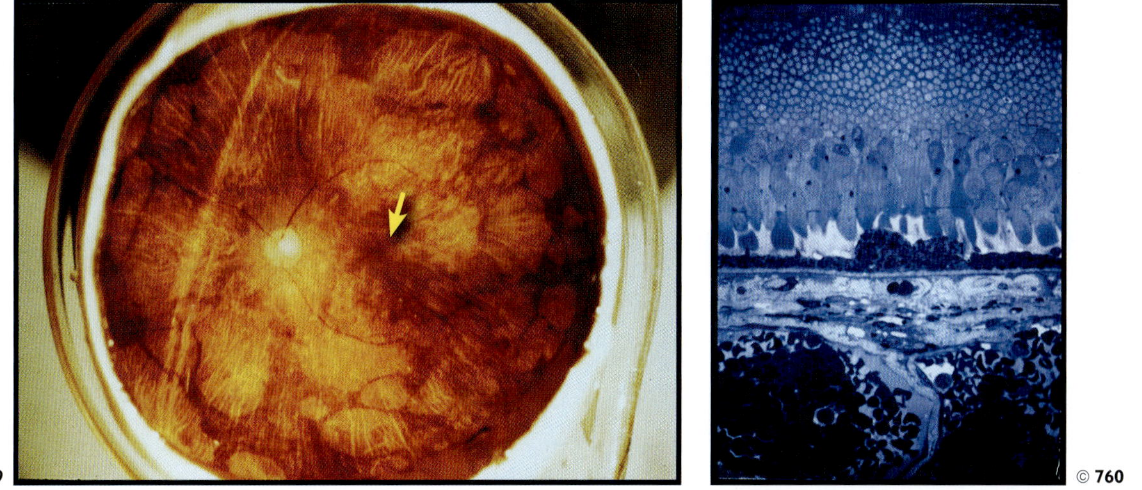

© 759 © 760

The gross appearance of thioridazine retinal toxicity reveals widespread atrophy of the RPE. There is an area of intact RPE near the macula *(arrow)*, as well as only partial atrophy of the photoreceptors. The histology shows photoreceptor and RPE degeneration.

Chlorpromazine

Chlorpromazine is a piperidine similar to thioridazine, but lacks a piperidyl side chain. It is also used in the treatment of psychomotor disorders. The drug itself binds strongly to melanin and very infrequently causes retinal toxicity. The toxic changes include retinal granularity, pigment clumping, and some RPE atrophy. Reversal of the toxic effect may occur with discontinuation of the drug. Crystalline deposits have been described in the lens as cortical opacities.

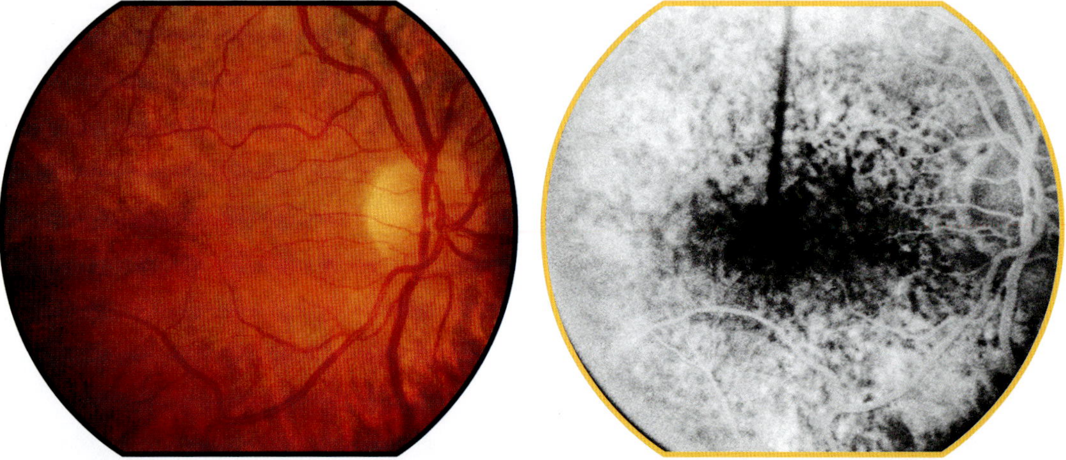

These images show a granular and patchy atrophic effect to the RPE in the central macula and beyond. The fluorescein angiogram reveals pronounced window defect because the choriocapillaris is intact and hyperfluorescent through the atrophic RPE.

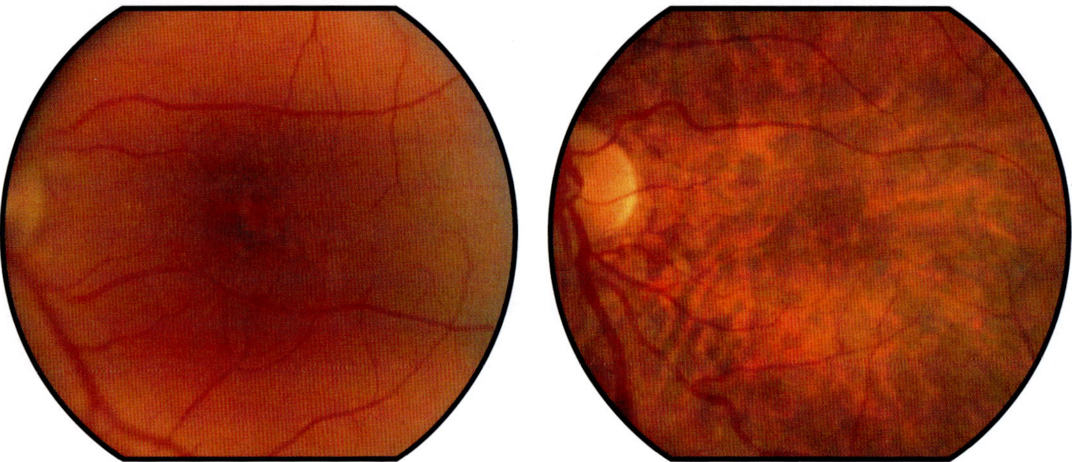

These patients demonstrate early toxicity of the macula *(left)* and more extensive toxicity throughout the posterior pole (*right*) due to chlorpromazine.

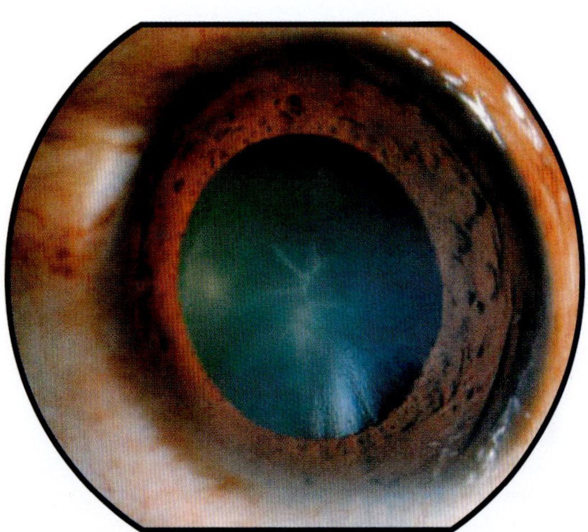

Chlorpromazine toxicity may also produce granular opacities in the lens, as evident in this patient.

Dideoxyinosine (DDI)

A mid-peripheral pigmentary retinopathy has been noted in HIV patients receiving high-dose therapy with the antiviral 2′, 3′-dideoxyinosine. Chorioretinal atrophy is typically noted anterior to the vascular arcades.

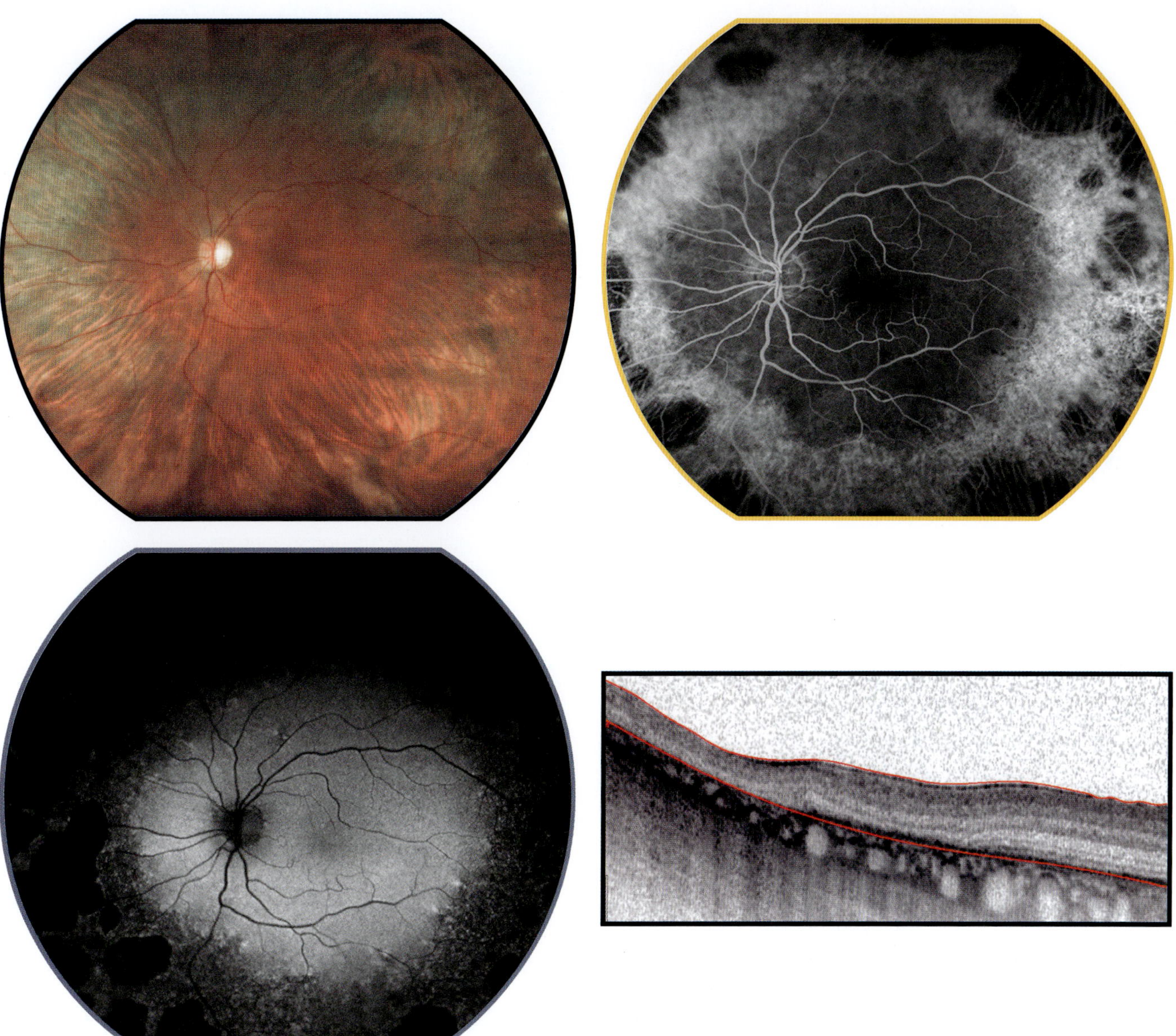

Fundus photograph and fluorescein angiogram exhibiting mid-peripheral retinal pigmentary changes in a patient previously treated with DDI. Fundus autofluorescence demonstrates patches of peripheral hypoautofluorescence. OCT shows outer retinal and RPE atrophy. *Courtesy of Dr. Scott Sneed*

Clofazimine

Clofazimine is a phenazine dye that has been used to treat mycobacteria, psoriasis, pyoderma gangrenosum, and discoid lupus. Toxicity may cause crystal accumulation in the cornea or pigmentary retinopathy.

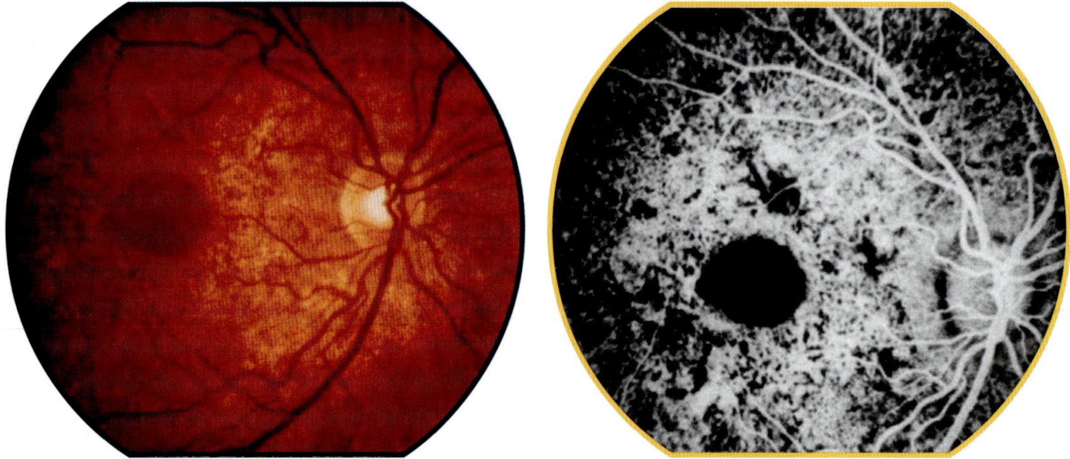

Clofazimine toxicity resembles that of thioridazine toxicity. In this patient, there is peripapillary and posterior polar atrophy with relative sparing of the pigmented perifoveolar zone.

Deferoxamine

Deferoxamine is a drug used for the treatment of excess iron overload generally from chronic transfusions for anemias. Patients may experience reduced vision from RPE atrophy and hyperpigmentation accumulation, a pseudovitelliform detachment, optic neuritis, or cataract.

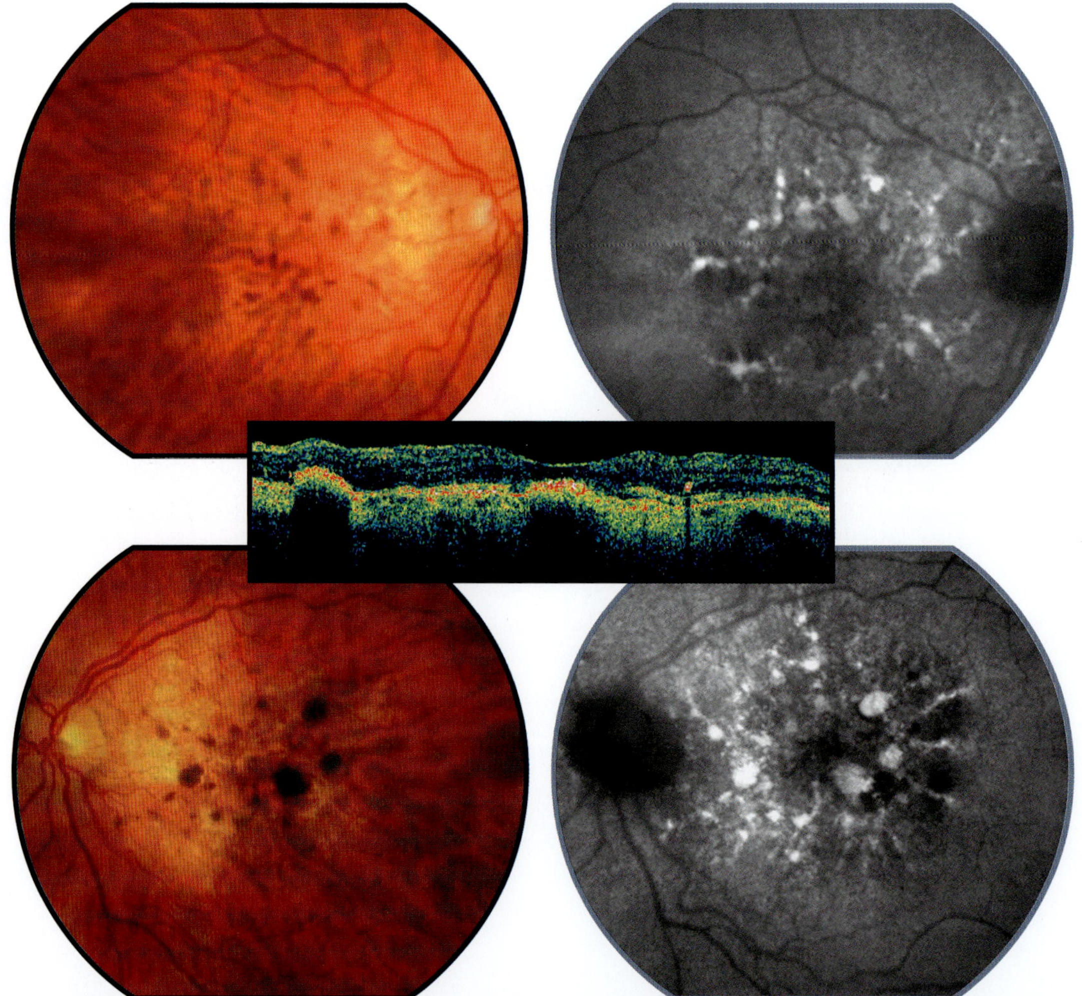

This patient with deferoxamine toxicity has a multifocal pattern dystrophy interspaced with irregular atrophy in the central macula. The fundus autofluorescent photographs shows accumulation of lipofuscin in the darkly pigmented areas, evident clinically. This indicates that the dark, nummular areas actually represent lipofuscin and melanin. The OCT image shows an elevation to the pigment epithelium in the areas where there is excess lipofuscin accumulation and thinning of the pigment epithelium in atrophic zones. There is also photoreceptor loss.

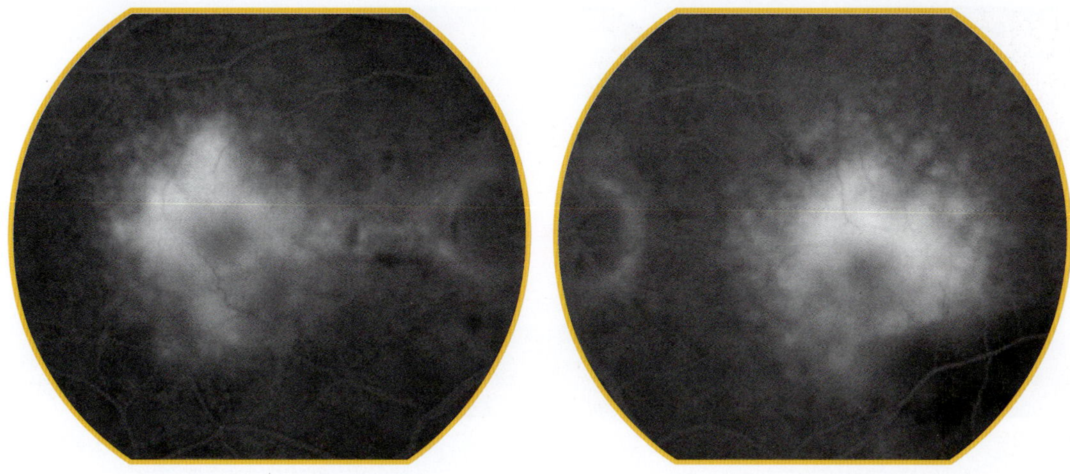

Patients with deferoxamine toxicity may develop a pseudovitelliform detachment like a patient with basal laminar cuticular drusen and/or a pattern dystrophy. The subretinal staining evident on the fluorescein angiogram does not represent underlying choroidal neovascularization. *Courtesy of Dr. Nicole Gross*

Chemotherapeutic Agents

Denileukin Diftitox

This drug is a recombinant protein composed of human interleukin-2 (IL-2) fused to diphtheria toxin. It has a selective cytotoxicity against activated lymphocytes with a high expressivity of the IL-2 receptor. Reports of retinal toxicity have been in patients who were given this drug for steroid-resistant graft-versus-host disease. Vascular leakage producing edema and direct toxicity of selective tissues has been reported with the use of this drug. Extensive RPE mottling and photoreceptor damage may suppress ERG recordings. It may also simulate a cancer-associated retinopathy with diffuse photoreceptor and RPE changes that may not be clearly evident clinically.

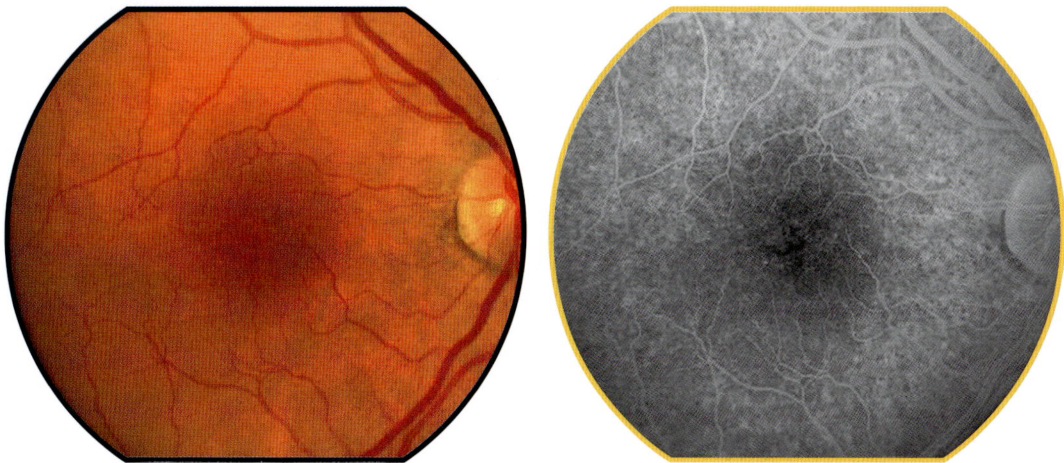

This patient has a generalized, early toxicity to the RPE secondary to denileukin use. Faintly evident atrophy is seen on the fluorescein angiogram as a "window defect" from RPE atrophy.

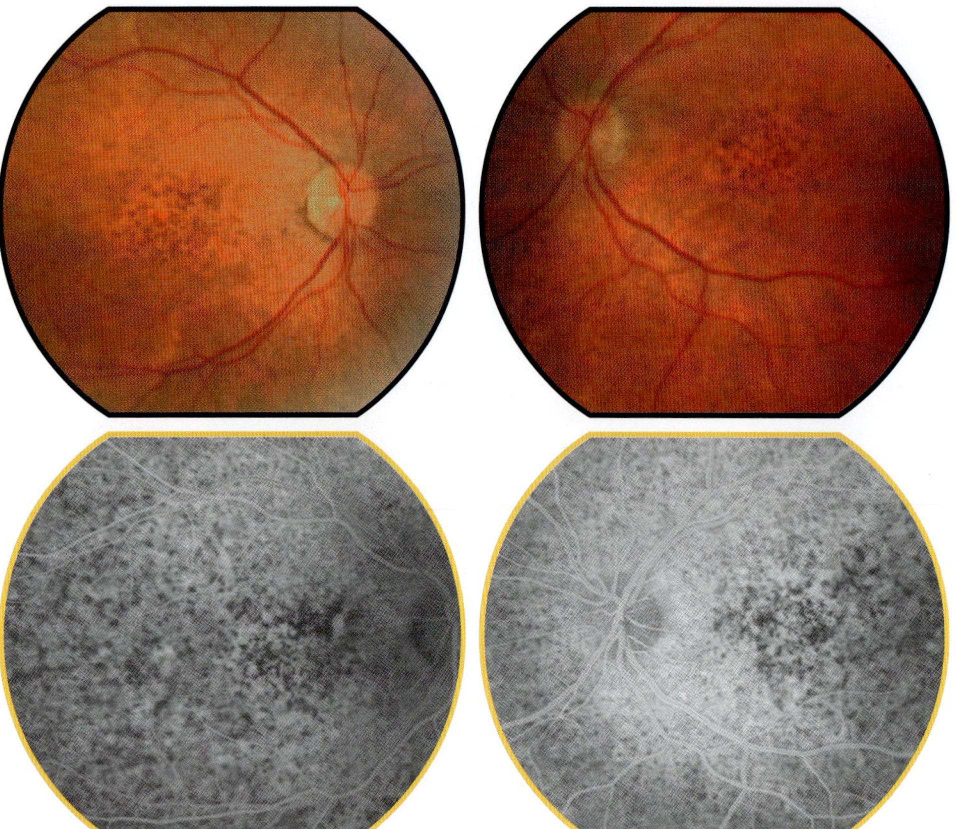

Follow-up of this patient shows more advanced stages of RPE atrophy on fundus photography and fluorescein angiography.

MEK Inhibitors

A new class of chemotherapy agents selectively inhibiting the mitogen-activated protein kinase/extracellular signal-regulated kinase (MAPK/ERK), also referred to as the MEK enzyme, has shown promising results for systemic malignancies including metastatic melanoma. The typical ocular side-effect described is multifocal serous retinal detachment.

However, pigment epithelial detachment, optic neuropathy, retinal vein occlusion, retinal hemorrhage, cystoid macular edema, and anterior chamber inflammation may also be seen.

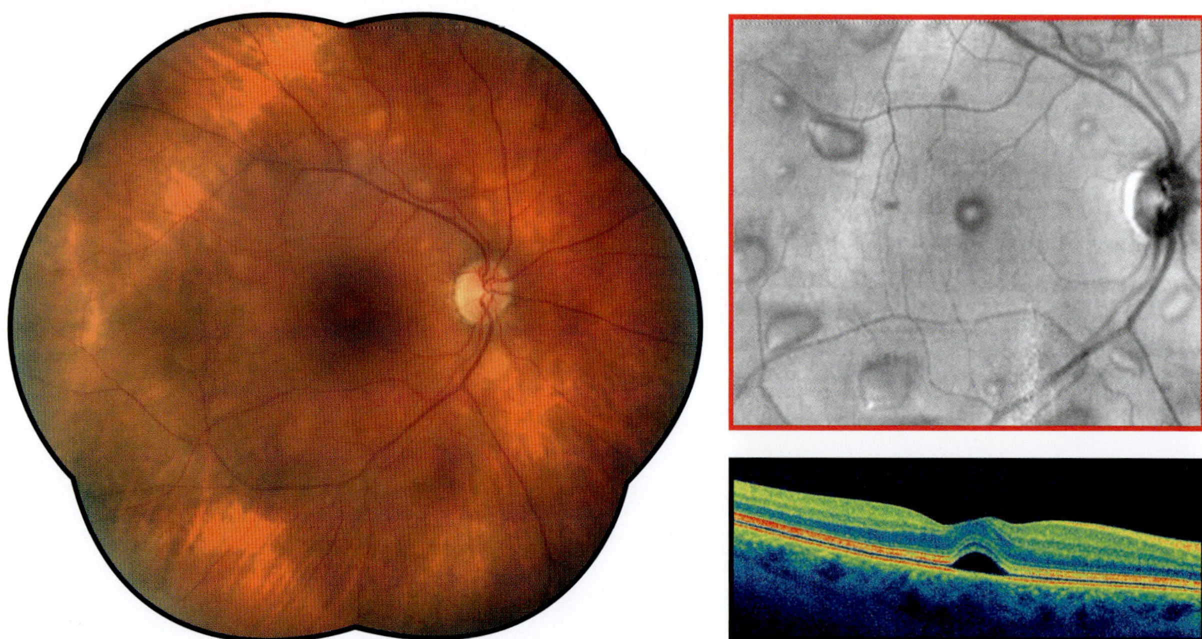

Color photograph, infrared, and OCT demonstrating multiple pigment epithelial detachments while on the MEK inhibitor pimasertib. *Courtesy of Michael Chilov*

Quinine Sulfate

Quinine has been used medically for centuries for a variety of diseases, including the treatment of malaria and muscle spasms. Symptoms of toxicity include blurred vision, visual field loss, nyctalopia, photophobia, and, rarely, transient blindness. Retinal vessel attenuation and disc pallor are early manifestations of toxicity. All layers of the fundus including the pigment epithelium, photoreceptors, and ganglion cell layer, will exhibit secondary adverse effects from damage to the vasculature.

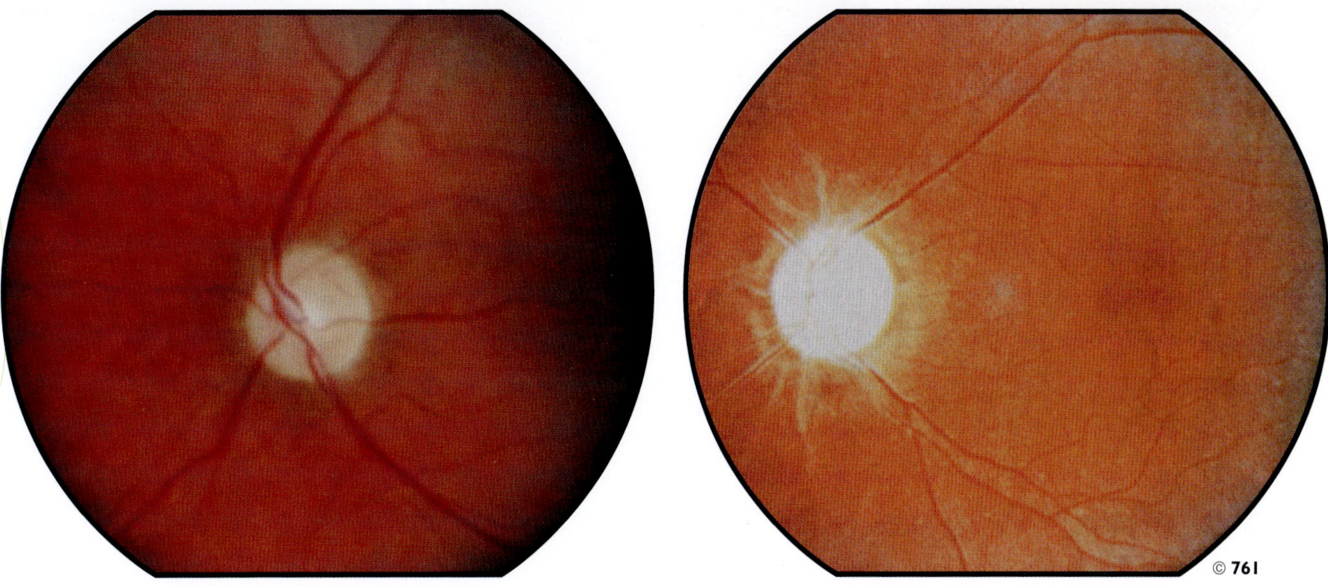

These patients with quinine toxicity developed ischemia of the retina, photoreceptor damage, and optic atrophy. The manifestations are less pronounced in the patient on the left and very severe in the patient on the right.

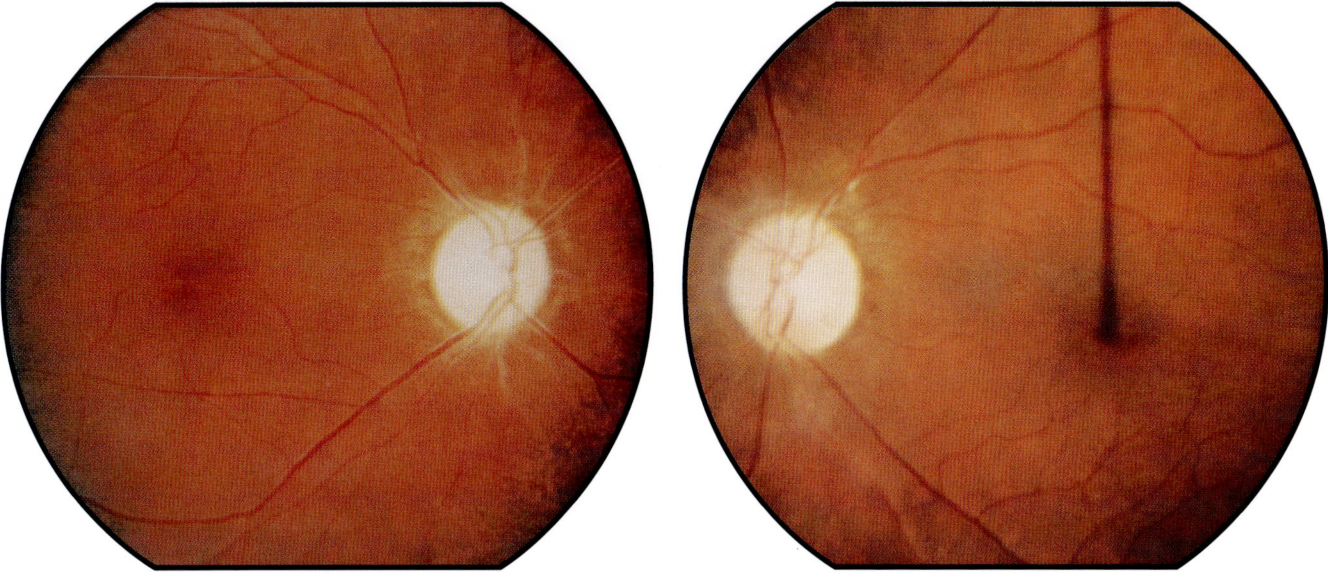

This patient has quinine toxicity with peripapillary retinal vascular ischemia and optic atrophy bilaterally.

Oral Contraceptives

Systemic thromboembolic diseases are known to be associated with the use of oral contraceptives. Retinal adverse effects include arteriolar occlusion, central vein occlusion, retinal hemorrhages, and macular edema. Given this retinal vascular occlusive risk, patients with pre-existing systemic or retinal vascular disease should be extremely cautious about using oral contraceptives.

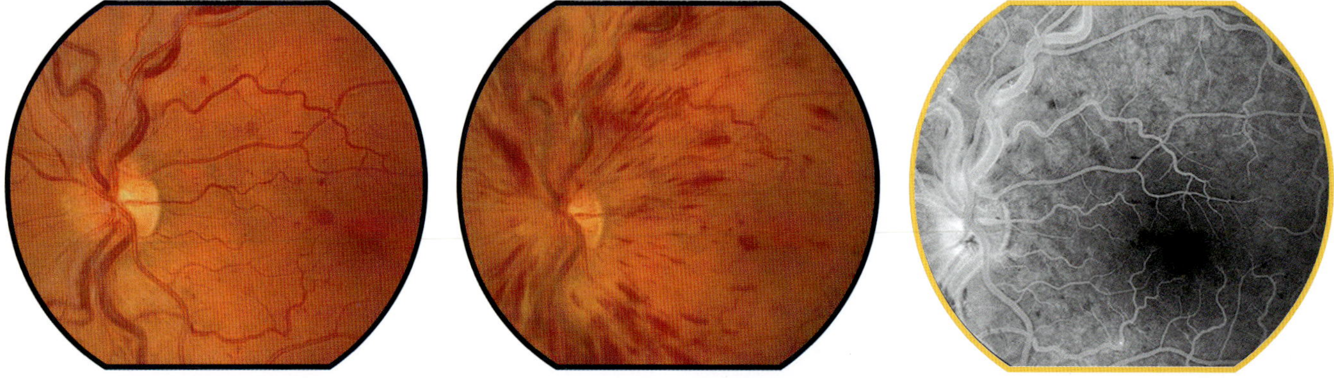

This patient was using oral contraceptives. She experienced a venous stasis retinopathy with marked tortuosity, scattered hemorrhages *(middle)*, segmental venular staining, and macular edema that progressed to a more severe non-ischemic vein occlusion.

Ergot Alkaloids

Ergot alkaloids are adrenergic blockers used to prevent migraine headaches and to control postpartum hemorrhage. Ocular complications have been reported including vasoconstriction of retinal vessels, cystoid macular edema, venous occlusive disease, and optic neuritis.

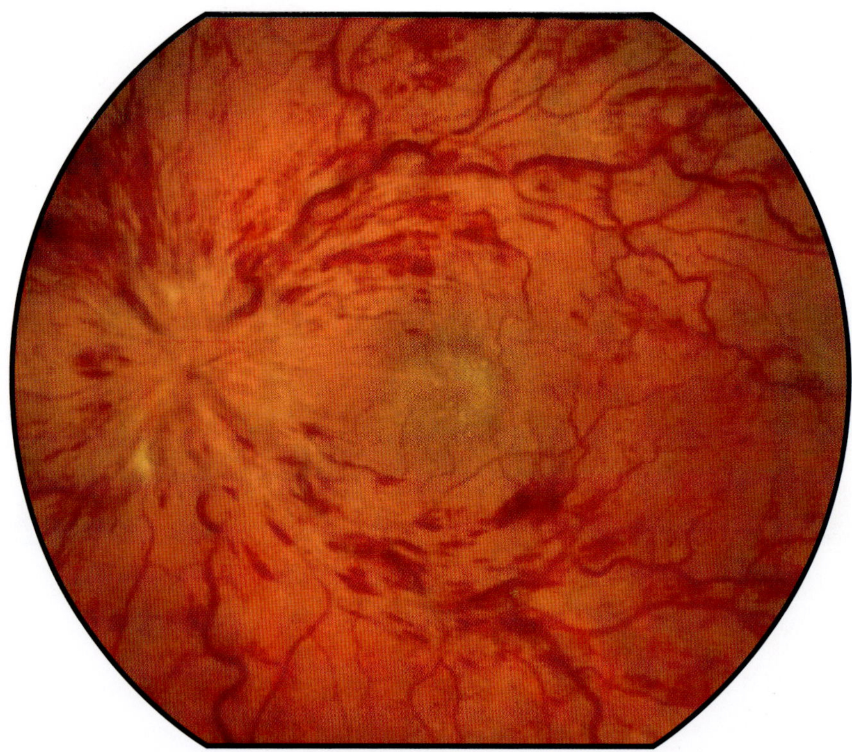

This patient was using ergotamine and experienced a central retinal vein thrombosis and severe macular edema.

Procainamide

Procainamide is an anti-arrhythmic drug used to decrease the incidence of sudden cardiac death. Procainamide depresses the excitability of cardiac muscle to electrical stimulation and slows electrical conduction. It is considered to be a sodium channel blocker. Cases of acute anterior uveitis have been reported, as well as secondary manifestations that may involve the retinal circulation with permeability and ischemic abnormalities. Optic atrophy may also be a rare association.

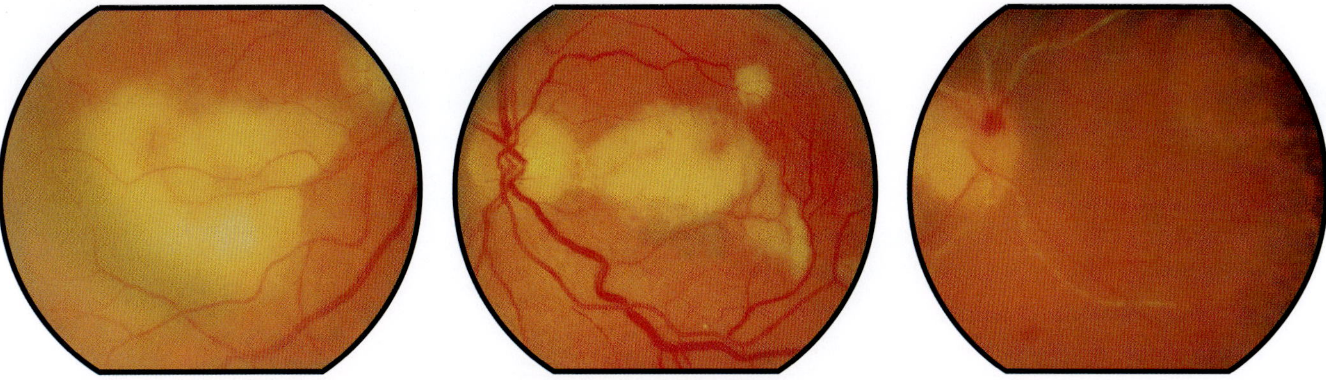

Procainamide toxicity produced zonal areas of retinal whitening secondary to vascular ischemic disease in these two patients. The vascular occlusive disease and optic atrophy can be very severe as in the patient in the image to the right.

Cocaine Abuse

Cocaine is a crystalline tropane alkaloid that is obtained from the leaves of the coca plant. Adverse effects in the eye relate to a carrier substance, which may be used to administer the drug intravenously. The result is a catecholamine systemic hypertensive response that could lead to hypertensive retinal vascular changes and embolic phenomena.

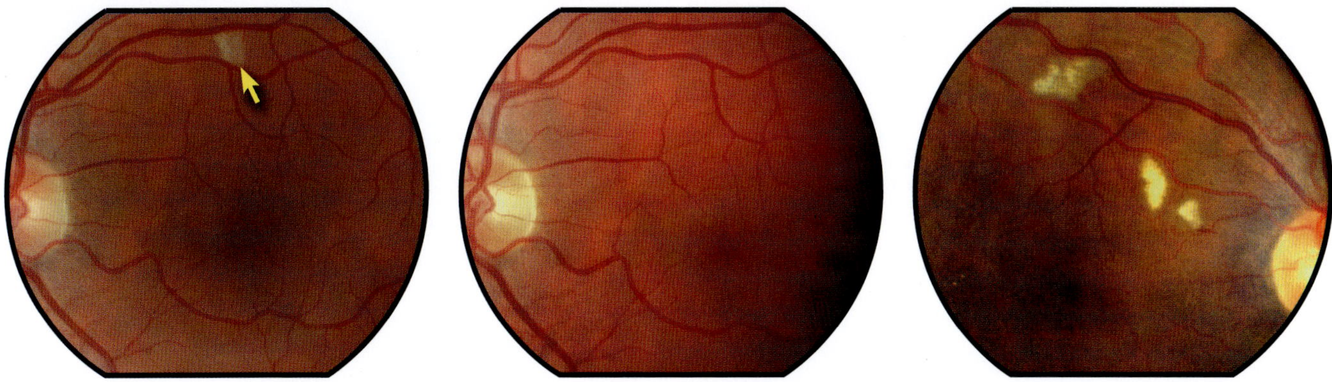

Cocaine use can induce an immediate rise in blood pressure, particularly when inhaled or smoked. This patient noted a sudden change in vision and a focal area of axoplasmic debris *(arrow)* was present. A medical work-up was unrevealing and the cotton-wool spot resolved spontaneously after discontinuation of this illicit drug *(middle)*. More severe ischemia can be seen in some patients using cocaine at higher doses for longer periods, which can result in chorioretinal infarctions. Note the multiple areas of axoplasmic debris *(right)*.

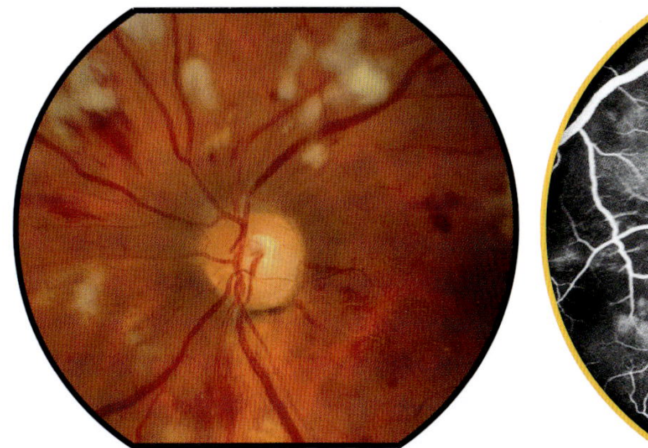

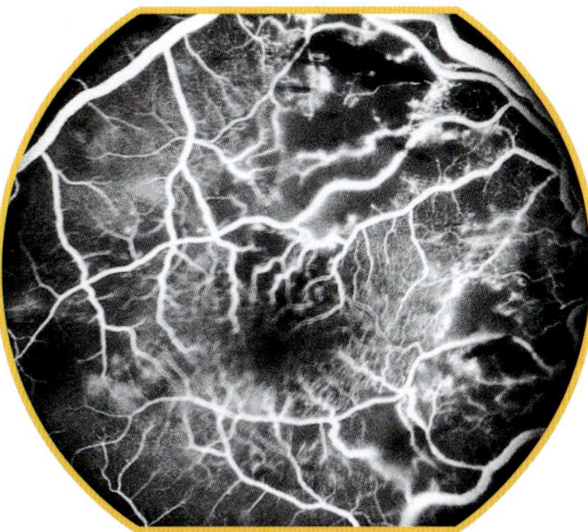

The hemorrhages are intermingled with scattered axoplasmic debris *(left)* and ischemia as seen on fluorescein angiography *(right)*. Some of these changes may be the result of severe, concomitant, systemic hypertension, resulting from drug use. Some of these eyes may also reveal choroidal ischemia. *Left image courtesy of Dr. Matthew Benz*

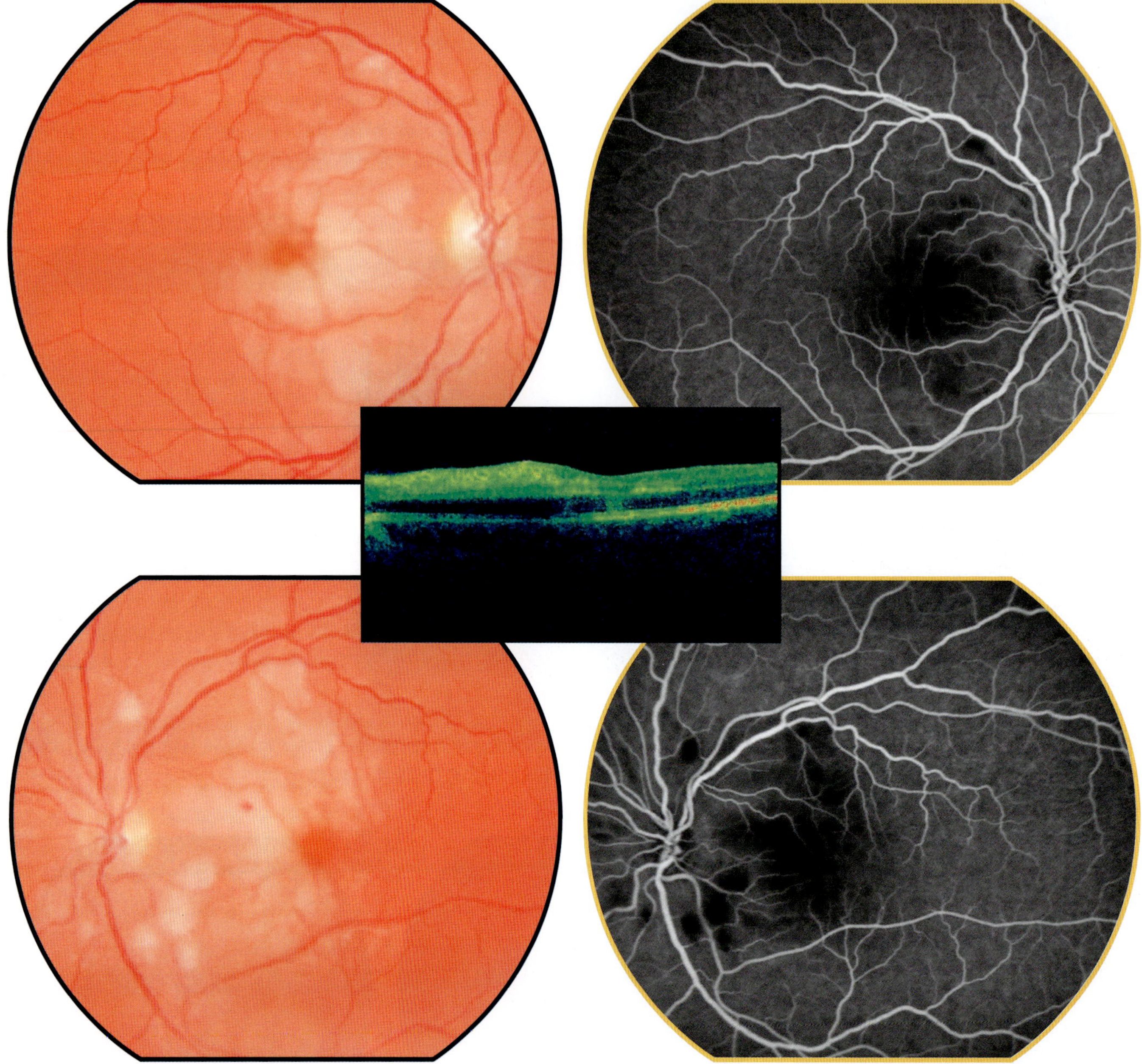

Color fundus photographs and fluorescein angiograms demonstrate areas of choroidal ischemia in a patient abusing cocaine.

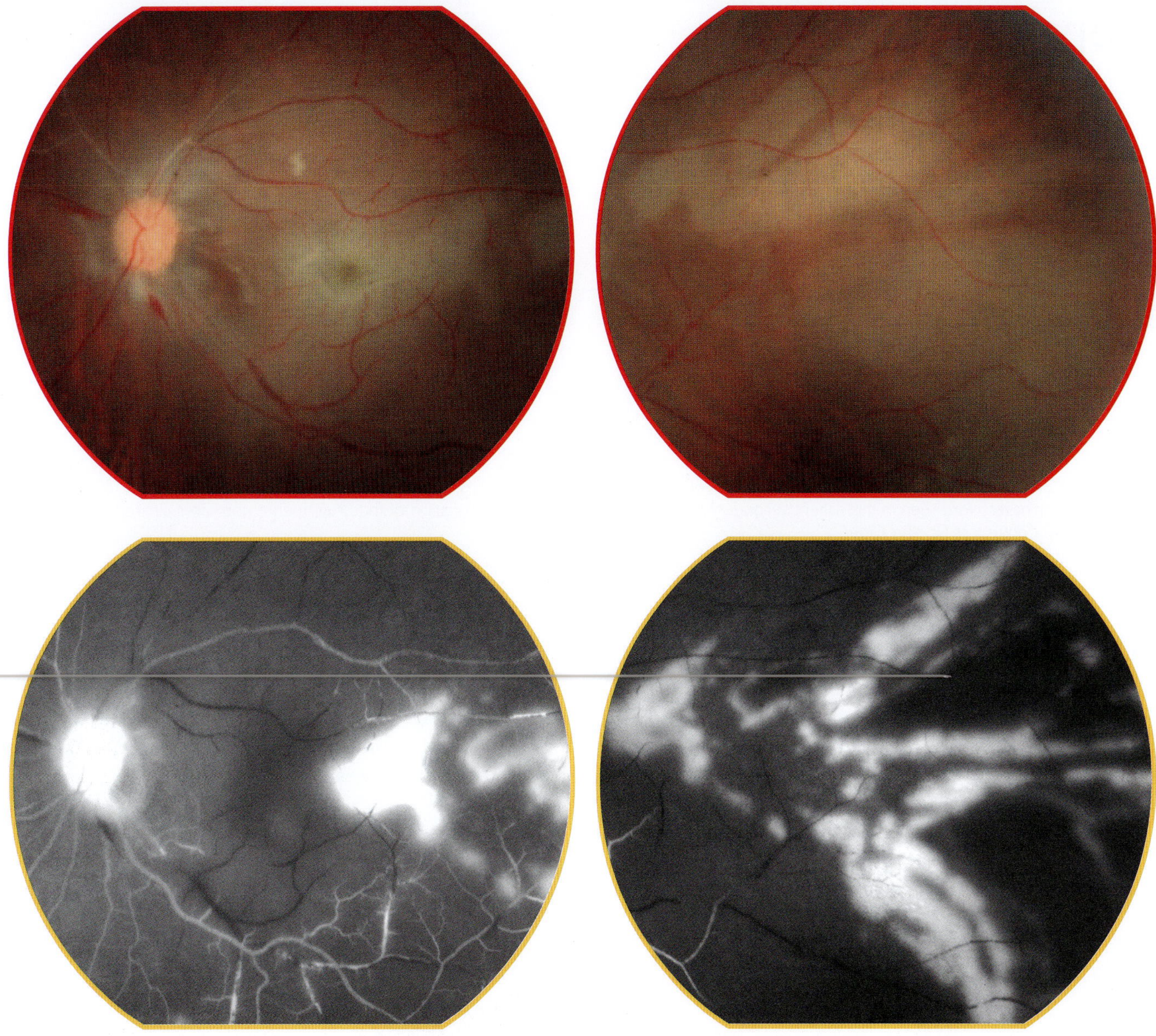

This patient had a history of cocaine abuse and presented with significant choroidal ischemia as seen in the fundus photograph and fluorescein angiogram. The triangular region of infarction is suggestive of the sign of amalric. *Courtesy of Dr. David Sarraf*

Heparin

Heparin is an anticoagulant agent used commonly for a variety of coagulative disorders.

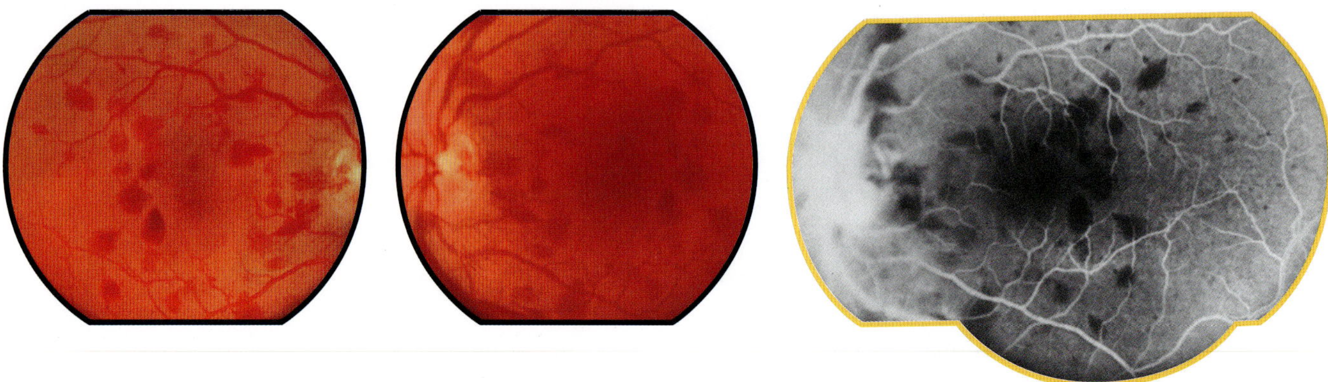

Multiple hemorrhages were seen in this patient secondary to heparin toxicity. On discontinuation of the drug, the hemorrhages cleared spontaneously. *Courtesy of Dr. Kurt Gitter*

Interferon

Alpha-interferon is a natural protein produced by the cells of the immune system of most vertebrates in response to challenges by foreign agents such as viruses, parasites, and tumor cells. Interferon belongs to the large class of glycoproteins known as cytokines. The use of this drug has been associated with retinal vascular ischemic abnormalities such as focal areas of axoplasmic debris or capillary occlusion and hemorrhages.

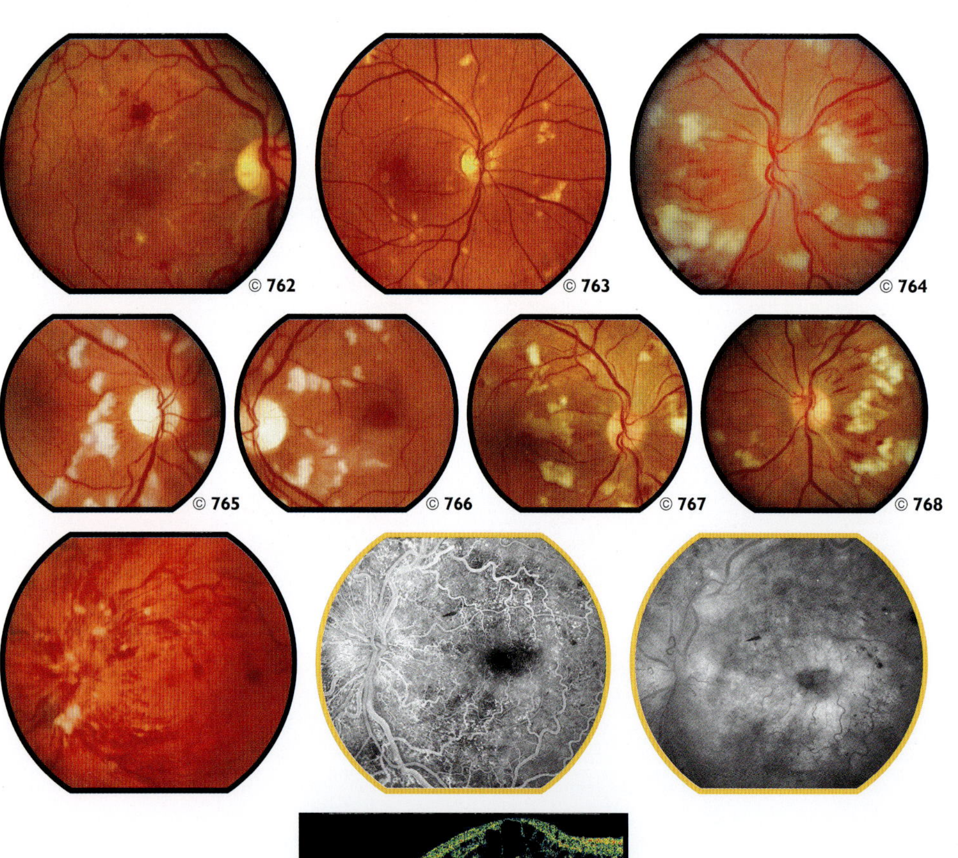

These cases illustrate the variable retinal vascular ischemic effect of interferon. Note the progressive severity in these cases of interferon toxicity, ranging from a few hemorrhages and cotton-wool spots *(top row)* to scattered axoplasmic debris or a Purtscher-like retinopathy *(second row)*, and a central vein occlusion with severe macular edema *(lower rows)*.

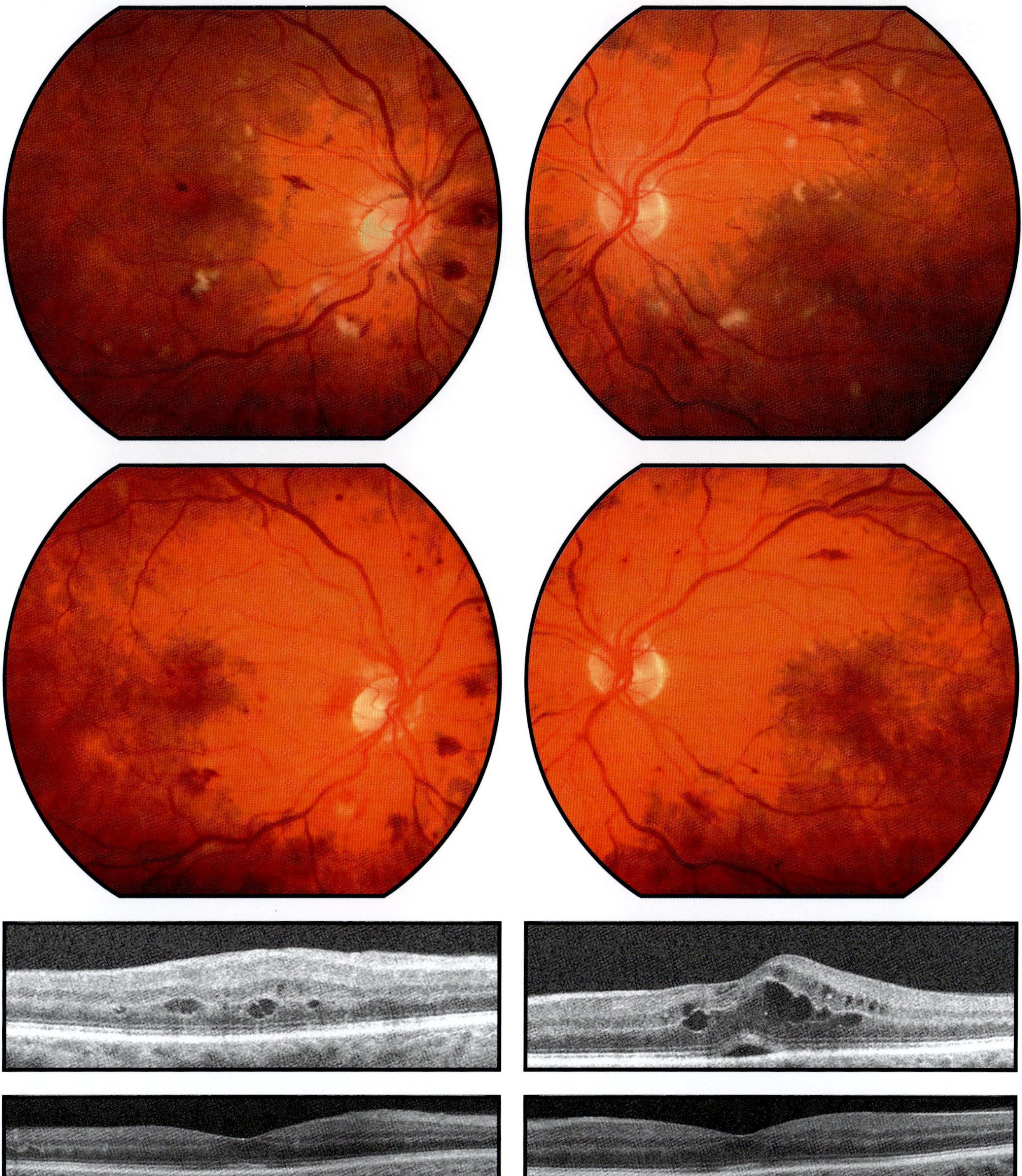

This patient demonstrated moderate intraretinal hemorrhages and cotton wool spots with mild cystoid macular edema on initial examination. The macular edema resolved on OCT after one week after discontinuation of the medication. The fundus showed mild improvement at two months follow-up.

Chemotherapeutic Agents

Gemcitabine

Gemcitabine is a nucleoside analog used in chemotherapy. It is used for various carcinomas such as small-cell lung cancer and pancreatic cancer. Retinal hemorrhages and vascular occlusive manifestations have been observed with the use of this drug systemically. Opportunistic infections and severe neurotoxicity are also included in its toxicity profile.

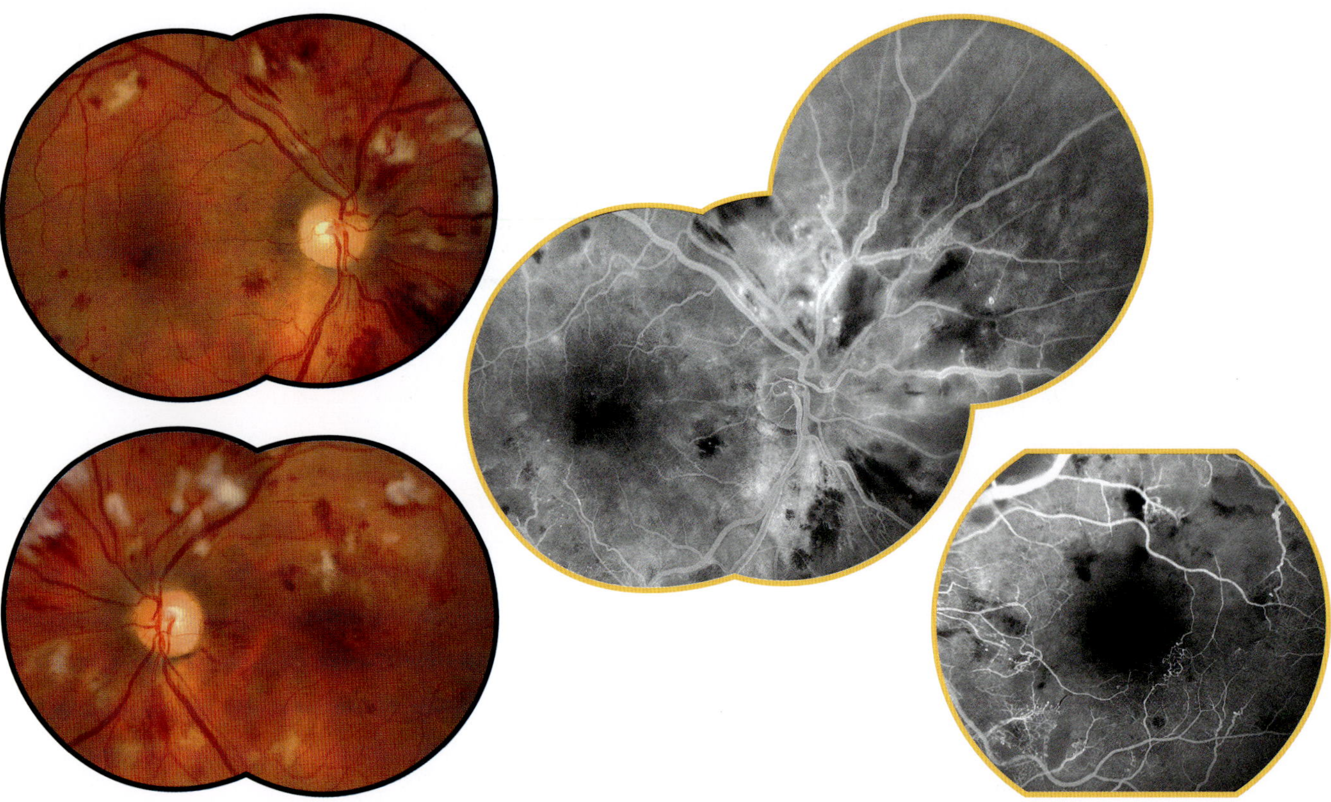

Gemcitabine toxicity was observed in this patient with severe ischemia and is clearly evident on fluorescein angiograms. Widespread cotton-wool spots or axoplasmic debris accumulation and scattered hemorrhages are noted in the posterior segment.

Nicotinic Acid

This agent is used as part of vitamin therapy or at higher doses for the treatment of hypercholesterolemia. Inner or outer retinal cystic change may develop in the retina. With fluorescein angiography, there is no leakage into the cystic cavities, which are clearly apparent with OCT imaging. Toxicity has been seen with dosages greater than 3 g/day. Discontinuation of the drug results in resolution of the cystic changes and improvement of vision.

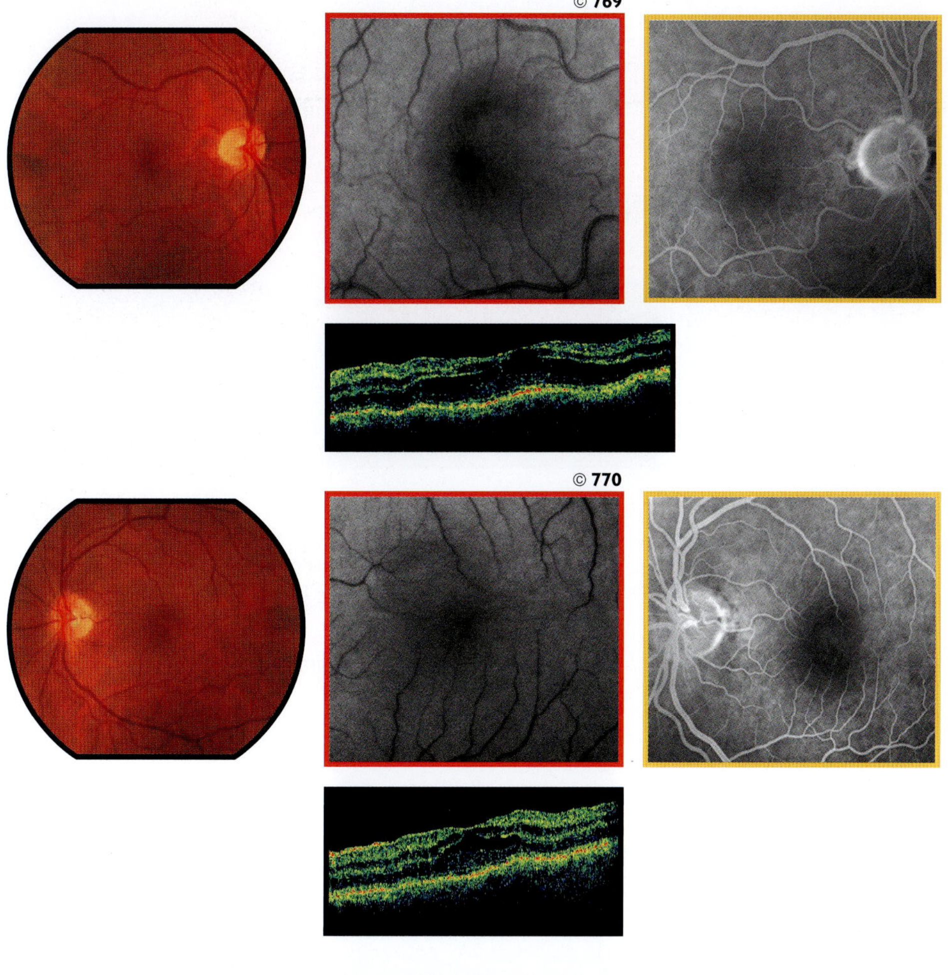

This patient was administered nicotinic acid or niacin as a hypocholesterolemic drug at the level of 3 g/day. The top photographs reveal cystic change in the macula with no fluorescein leakage. The OCT confirmed the presence of inner and outer cystic change in both eyes.

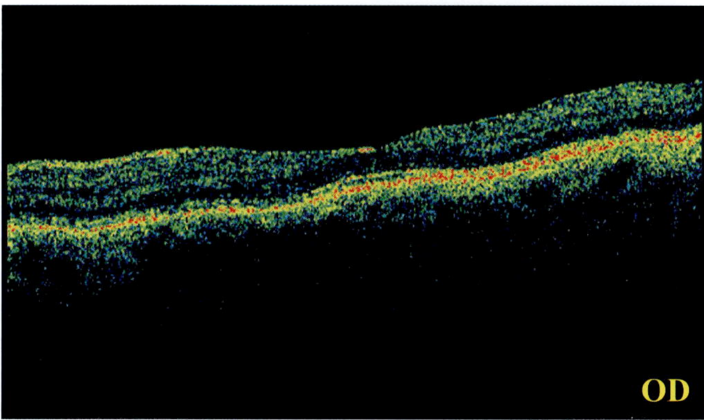

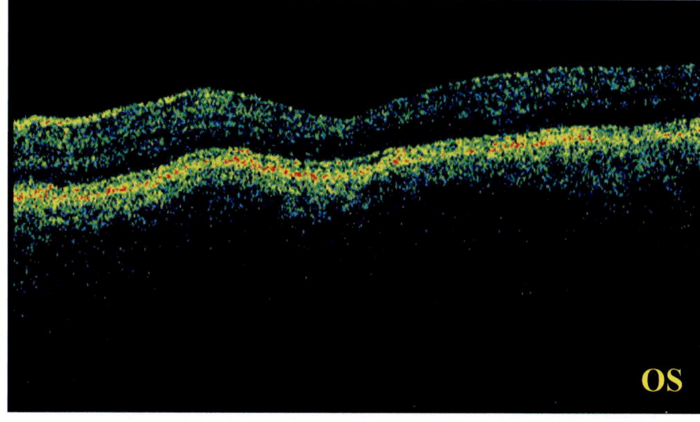

On discontinuation of the medication, there was gradual and complete improvement vision with resolution of the cyst clinically and on OCT imaging.

Drug-Induced Myopia

Various compounds, such as sulfur derivatives, diuretics, and antibiotics, have been associated with transient macular edema with retinal and/or choroidal folds. Chlorthalidone, acetazolamide, hydrochlorothiazide, and other drugs used for menstrual edema have been implicated in such a response. Topiramate, a drug used for refractory epilepsy or migraine headache, has also been shown to induce this phenomenon, which can become associated with anterior displacement of the iris lens diaphragm and may cause alteration in the refractive state. Eicosanoids may also cause the edema. Prostaglandins may actually be responsible for the edema with leukotrienes implicated in the spastic component.

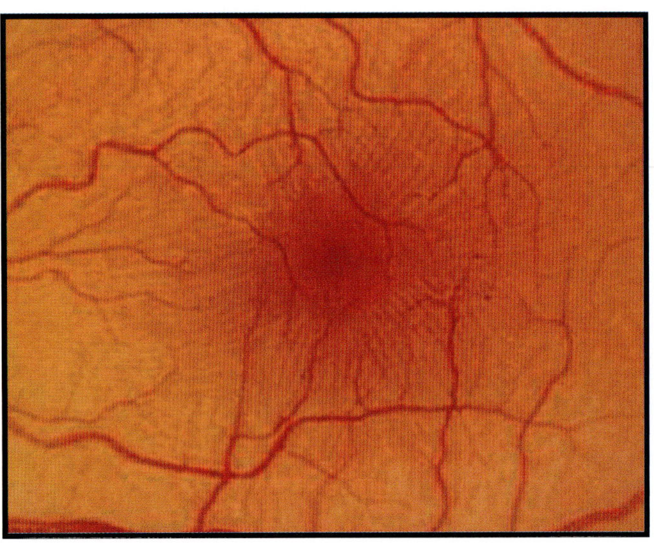

This patient has multiple striating retinal folds, particularly in the superior and inferior paramacular area, and suspected shallow edema. Acetazolamide was considered to be the causative factor for this adverse effect. The folds and the myopia reversed with discontinuation of the drug.

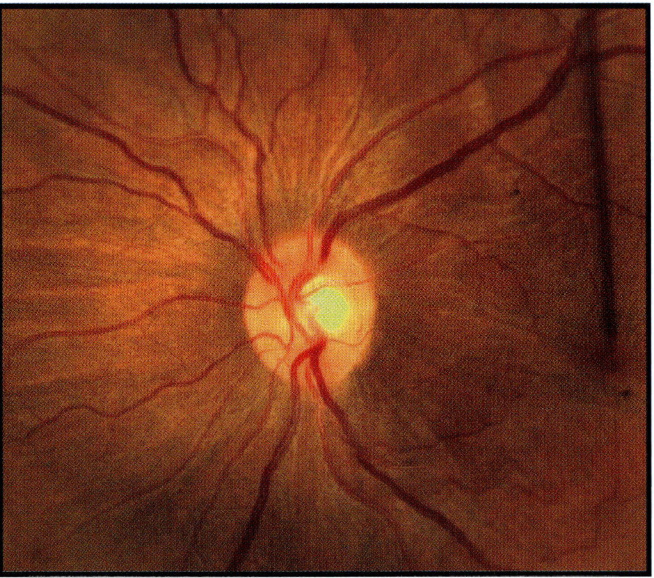

This patient developed radiating folds in the posterior segment nasal to the disc while on hydrochlorothiazide. The drug was suspected of producing this effect when discontinuation resulted in resolution of these changes.

Sulfa Antibiotics, Hydrochlorothiazine, Acetazolamide, Topiramate

Topiramate is an anticonvulsant drug used to treat epilepsy in children and adults. It has also been used for treating obesity and bipolar disorders. Acute myopia and angle closure glaucoma are potential adverse side-effects.

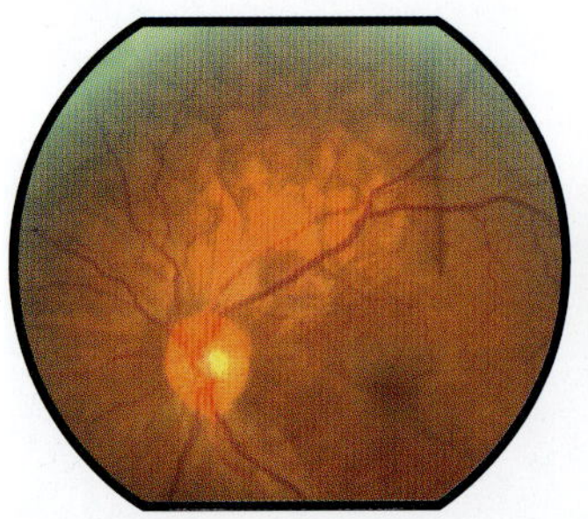

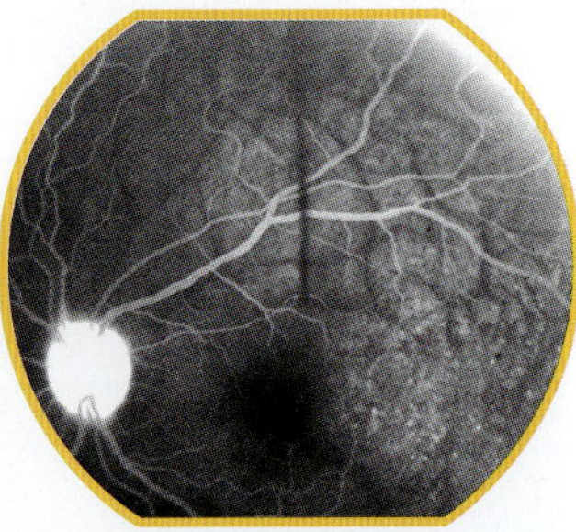

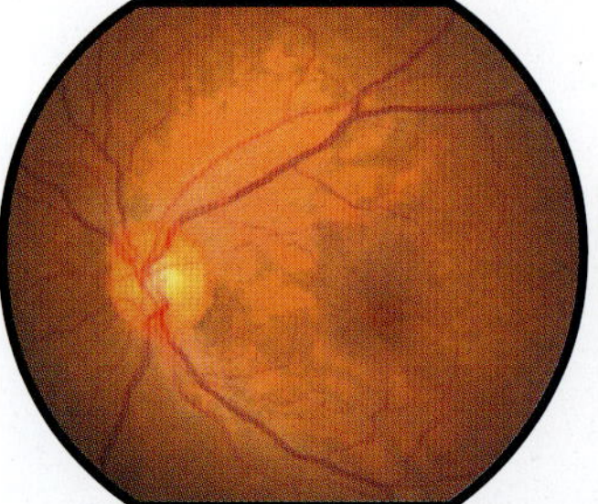

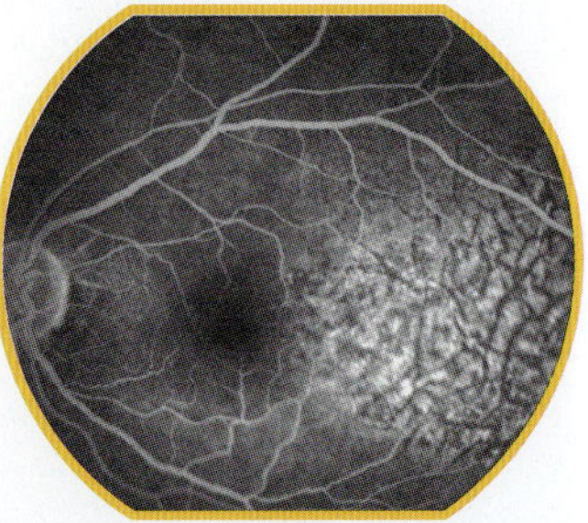

This patient demonstrated retinal striae and choroidal congestion secondary to topiramate treatment, as seen on fundus photography and fluorescein angiography. After discontinuation, the striae and congestion improved. *Courtesy of Dr. Kourous Rezaei*

Imatinib Mesylate

Imatinib is a tyrosine kinase inhibitor that is used as an oral chemotherapeutic agent in the treatment of chronic myelogenous leukemia and gastrointestinal tumors. It can produce generalized fluid retention throughout the body and edema of the macula. It may also cause other retinal vascular abnormalities similar to diabetic retinopathy.

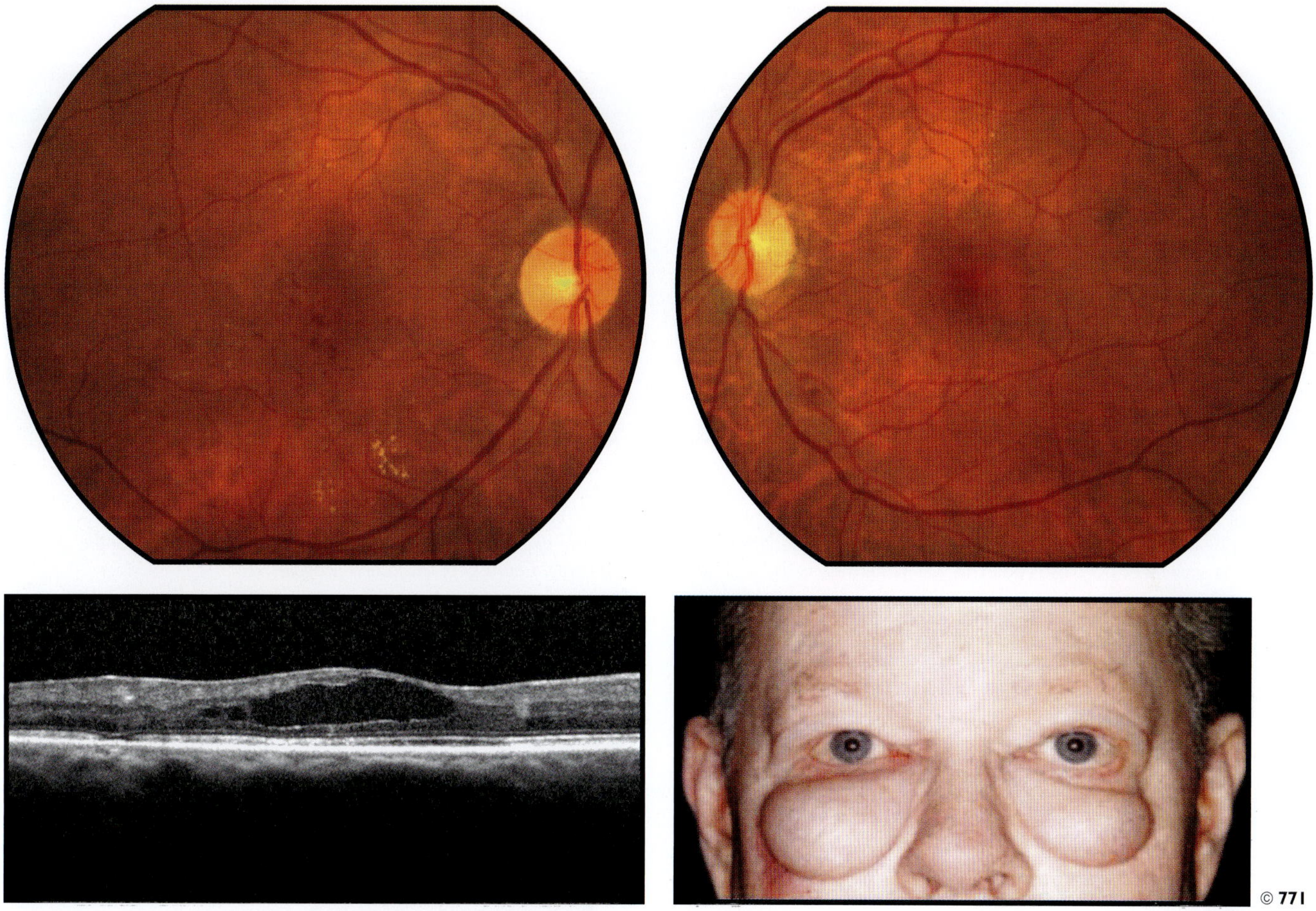

© 771

In this patient, Gleevec toxicity presents as a microangiopathy with manifestations that are indistinguishable from diabetic retinopathy. Note the microaneurysms, the patchy ischemia, and the hemorrhages in the pre-intraretinal and subretinal areas. Severe macular edema is also noted on the OCT. Some of the microangiopathy may be due to the primary disease itself. Gleevec may also cause periocular edema *(bottom right)* which may clear upon discontinuation of the drug.

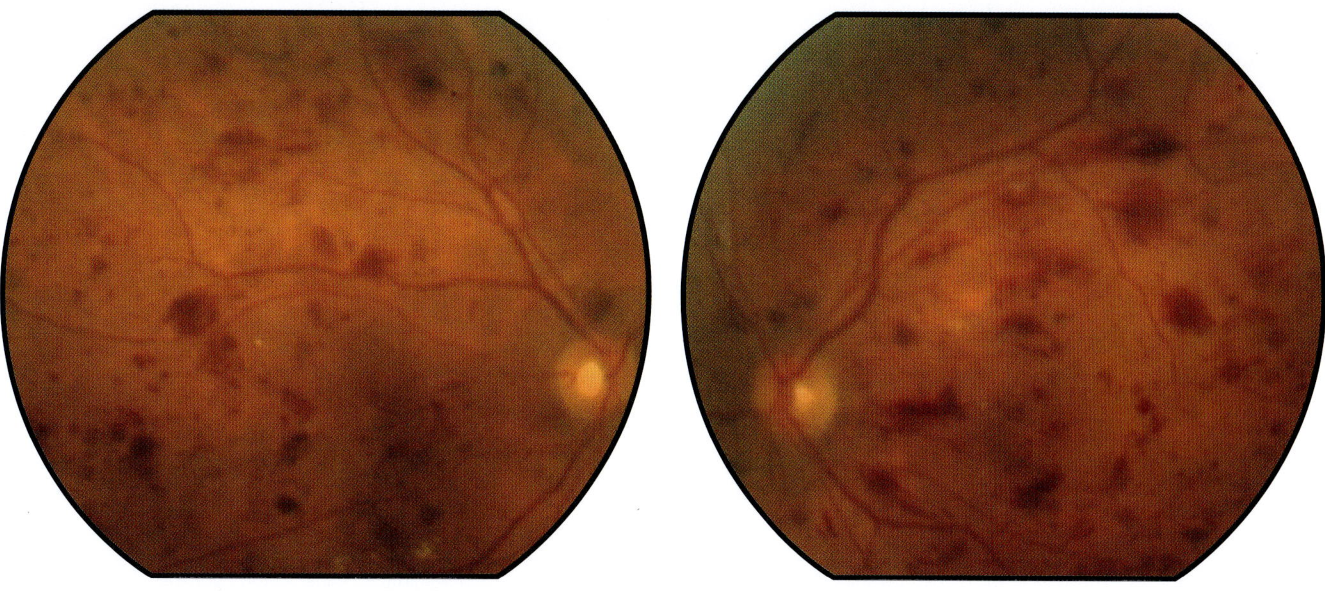

In rare instances, imatinib therapy may result in significant intraretinal hemorrhage, as in this patient.

Glitazones

Pioglitazone

Pioglitazone is an oral hypoglycemic agent in the thiazolidinedione class. It is also an anticancer drug that has a rather well-documented potential for liver toxicity. Thiazolidinediones activate peroxisome proliferator-activated receptors and have been associated with fluid retention, peripheral edema, and macular edema.

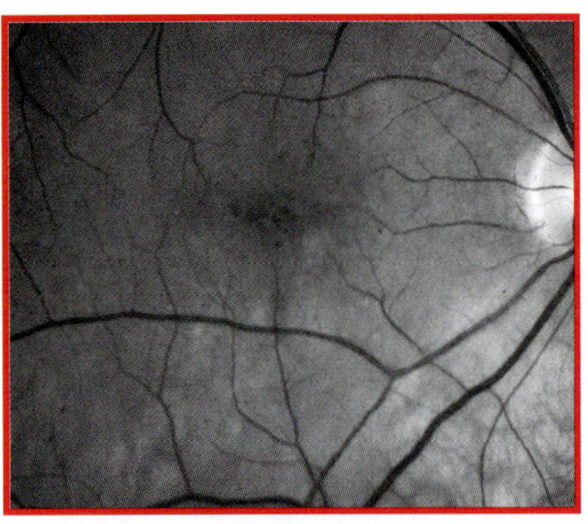

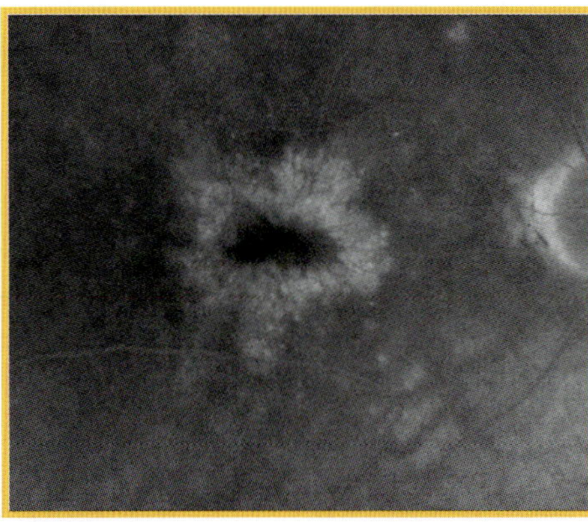

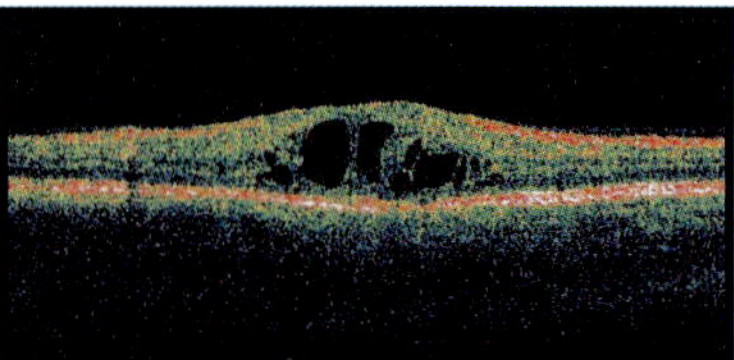

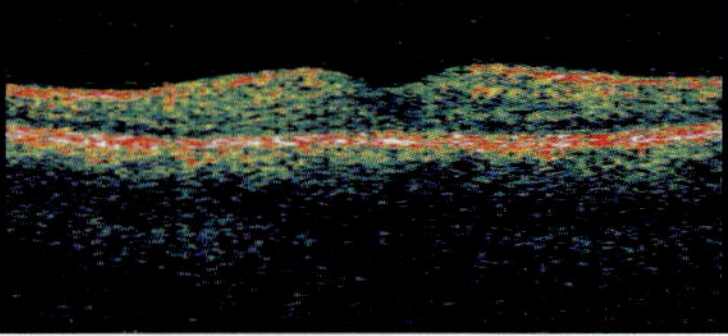

This patient had insulin-dependent diabetes mellitus and was given pioglitazone (Actos). There was a gradual but progressive decline in vision over a period of 2-3 weeks. Macular edema was noted in the clinical photograph *(left)* and confirmed with the OCT *(upper right)* and fluorescein angiography *(middle)*. Associated fluid retention, including peripheral edema, was also experienced by the patient. On discontinuation of the drug, the edema spontaneously resolved. This was confirmed with OCT testing *(lower right)*. *Courtesy of Dr. Joseph Maguire*

Ritonavir

Ritonavir is an anti-HIV protease inhibitor. In the fundus, it is known to cause cystoid macular edema, optic neuritis, and even visual hallucinations.

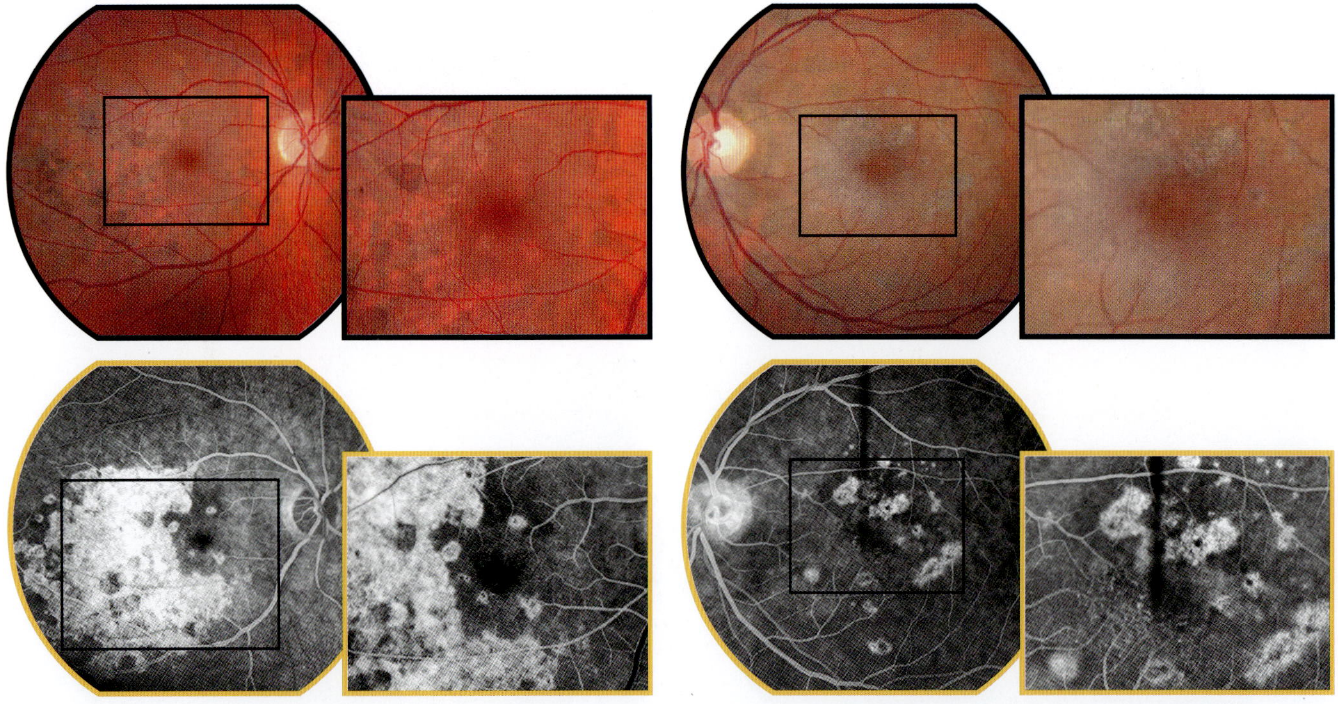

This 45-year-old white male has had HIV for 16 years. He was recently started on multiple drugs, including ritonavir. Thereafter, he developed atrophy of the RPE in the right eye more than the left. There were also crystalline-like dots seen within the retina. In the right eye, there was also nummular pigmentation. *Courtesy of Dr. Richard Roe*

Chemotherapeutic Agents

Paclitaxel, Docetaxel

This drug has been approved in the treatment of metastatic breast and ovarian carcinoma and Kaposi sarcoma. It is a mytotic inhibitor that interferes with microtubule breakdown. Ocular side-effects may include a cystic change in the macula without leakage, manifestations that are similar to those seen with tamoxifen.

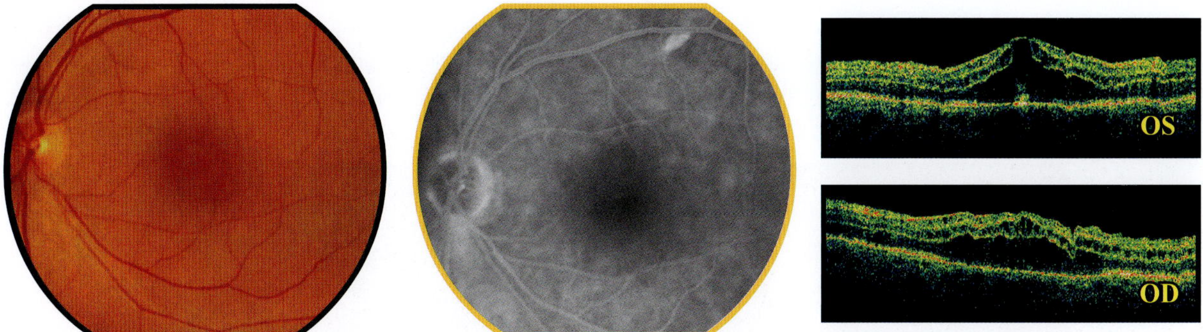

Taxol toxicity also shows a cystic change in the retina, as evident on the OCT study of both eyes. The fluorescein angiogram of the left eye showed no leakage, a characteristic of this toxicity. *Courtesy of Dr. David Weinberg*

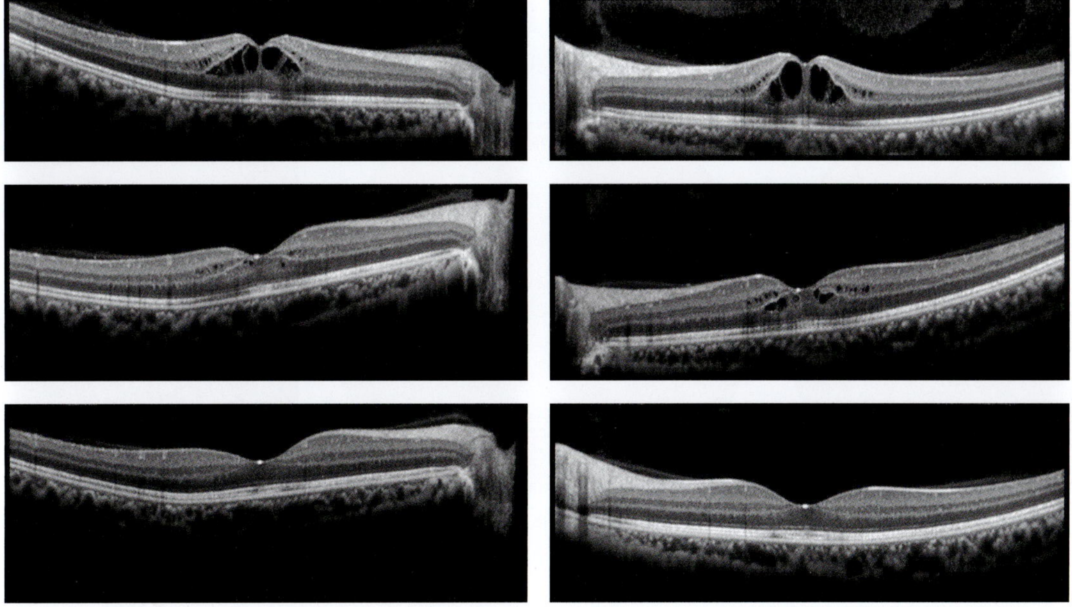

OCT demonstrating moderate cystoid macular edema centered on the fovea on a patient on paclitaxel therapy *(top)*. The macular edema improved 3 weeks *(middle)* after drug discontinuation and completely within 6 weeks *(bottom)*.

Albumin-Bound Paclitaxel

Albumin-bound paclitaxel is a protein-bound, albumin-stabilized nanoparticle formulation of paclitaxel.

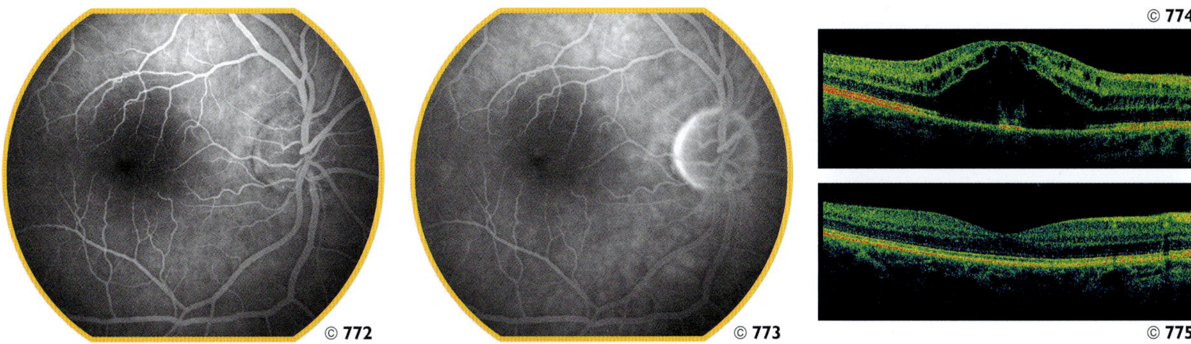

The fluorescein angiogram does not show any leakage in this patient with albumin-bound paclitaxel toxicity. The OCT *(top)* shows intraretinal cystic change, which has pooled beneath the neurosensory retina. Following discontinuation of the drug, there is resolution of the intraretinal cystic degeneration *(bottom)*.

Tamoxifen

Tamoxifen is a non-steroidal anti-estrogen agent used in the treatment of metastatic breast carcinoma. Adverse effects in the retina have been described, including intraretinal refractile opacities at the level of the RPE seen in the perifoveal region, but also in the periphery of the retina. Cystoid macular and retinal edema may also occur. Discontinuation of the medication generally results in improvement of the edema, but the crystalline deposits may remain in perpetuity. The retinal crystals may be seen at lower doses of medication. Histopathology has demonstrated the presence of intracellular spherical lesions in the nerve fiber layer and the inner plexiform layer of the retina.

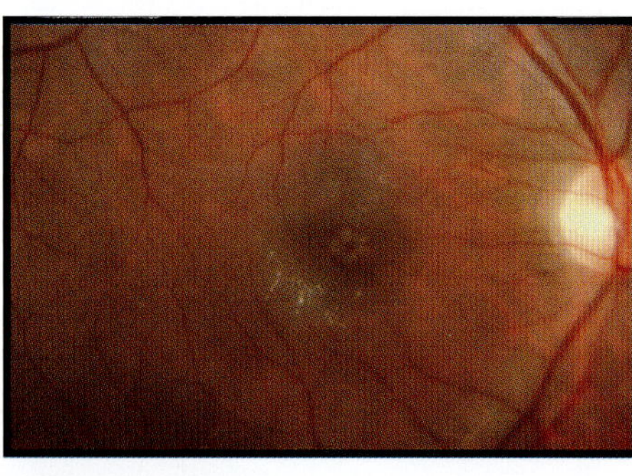

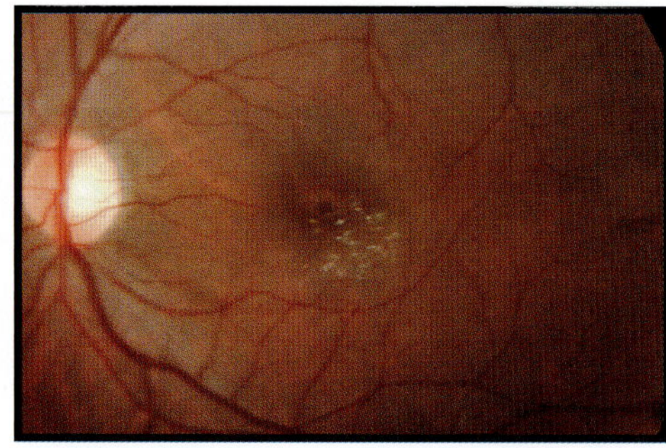

There are very fine crystalline-like deposits near the fovea in the patient on the left who has early tamoxifen toxicity. The patient on the right has slightly more advanced changes with some macular edema.

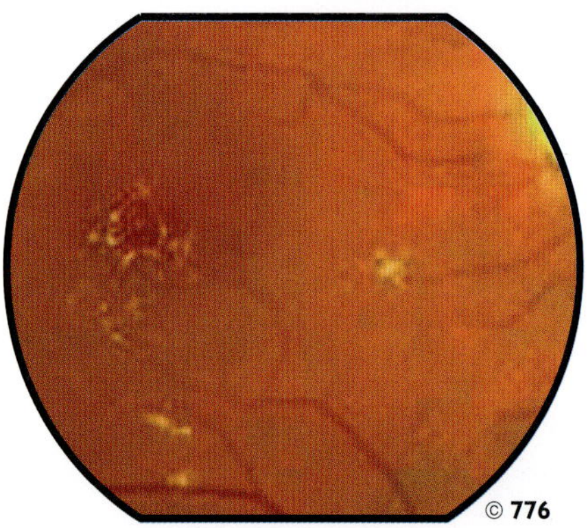

© 776

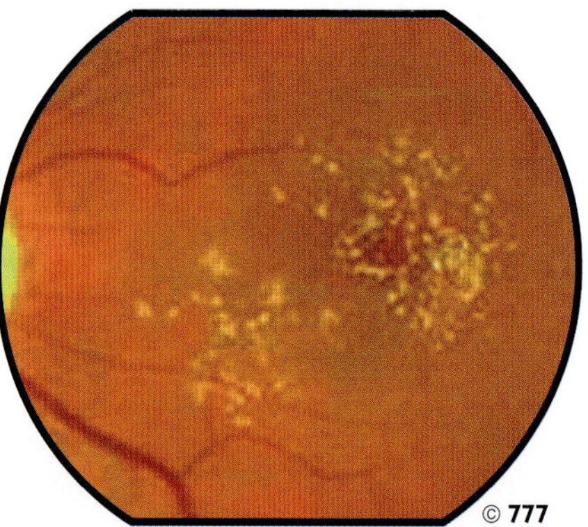

© 777

More advanced tamoxifen toxicity shows crystalline deposits surrounding the paramacular region and in the fovea.

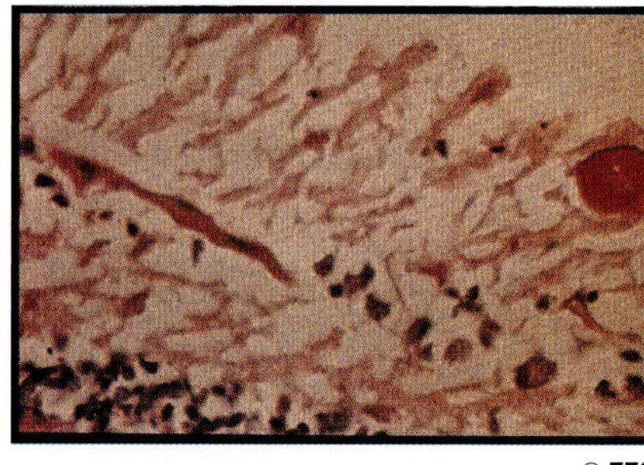

© 778

A large lesion seen as a red globule in the nerve fiber layer temporal to the macular area.

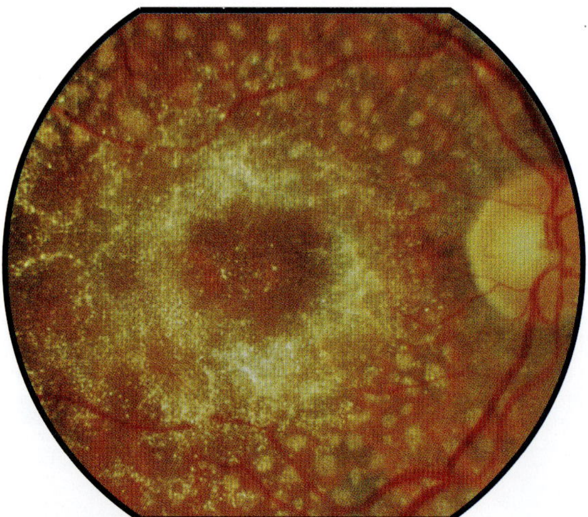

Extremely severe tamoxifen toxicity shows refractive opacities in the entire posterior pole with relative sparing of the fovea, due to its capillary-free nature. Pre-retinal fibrosis has begun to evolve in the paramacular region.

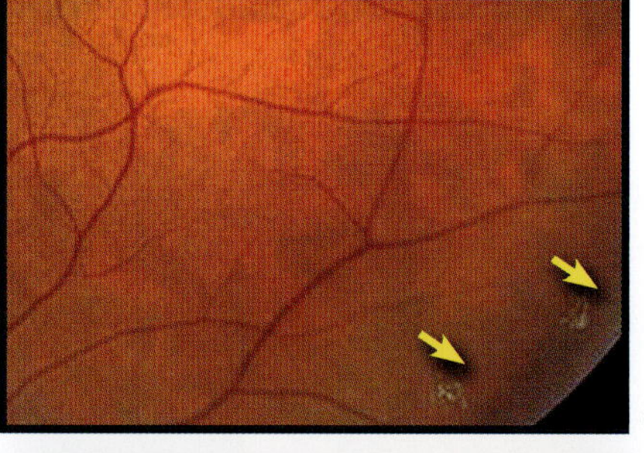

© 779

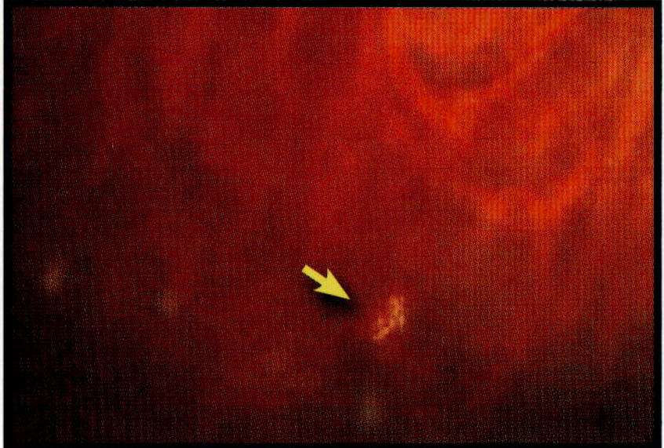

© 780

Tamoxifen crystalline deposits have now been described in the peripheral fundus, as noted here *(arrows)*.

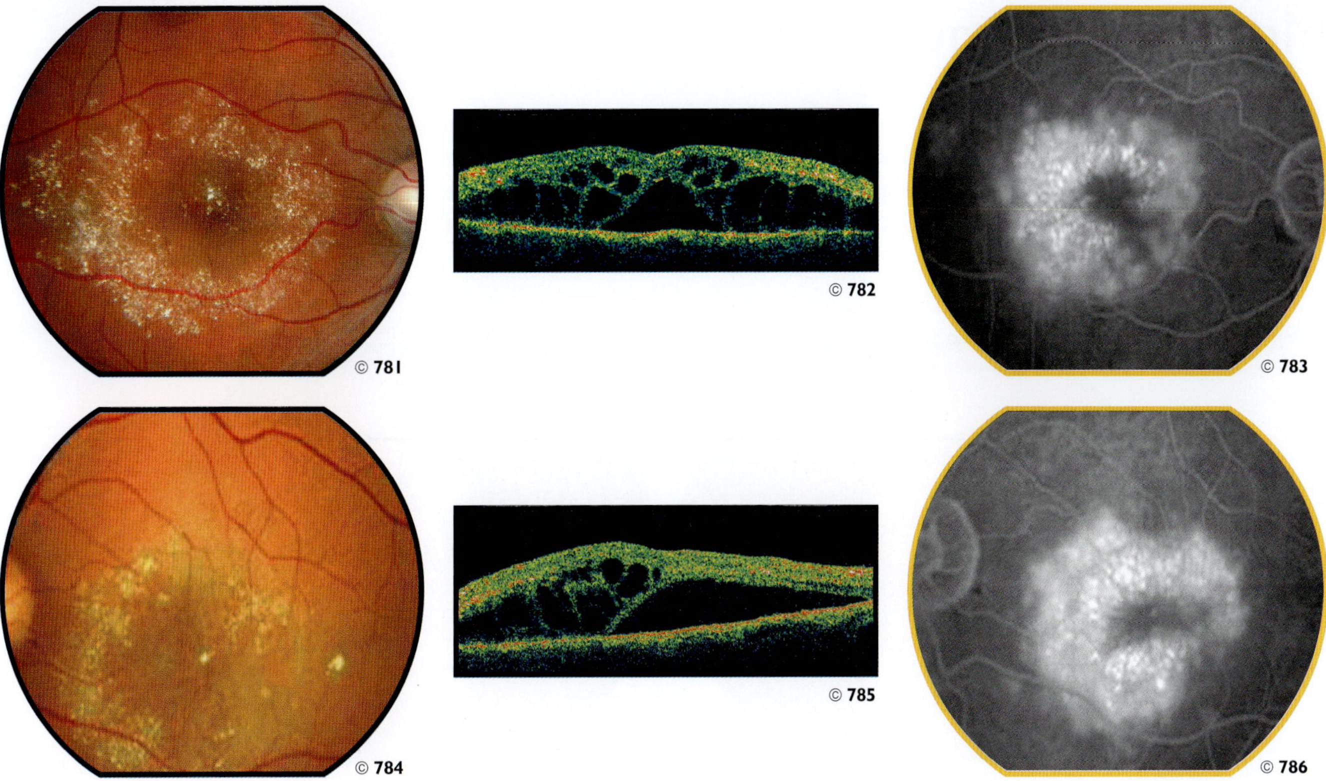

This case of severe tamoxifen toxicity shows a ring of crystalline deposits surrounding the central macula with cystoid retinal and macular edema. Fluorescein angiograms show intense leakage and the OCT images show intraretinal cystic cavities, as well as a neurosensory retinal detachment.

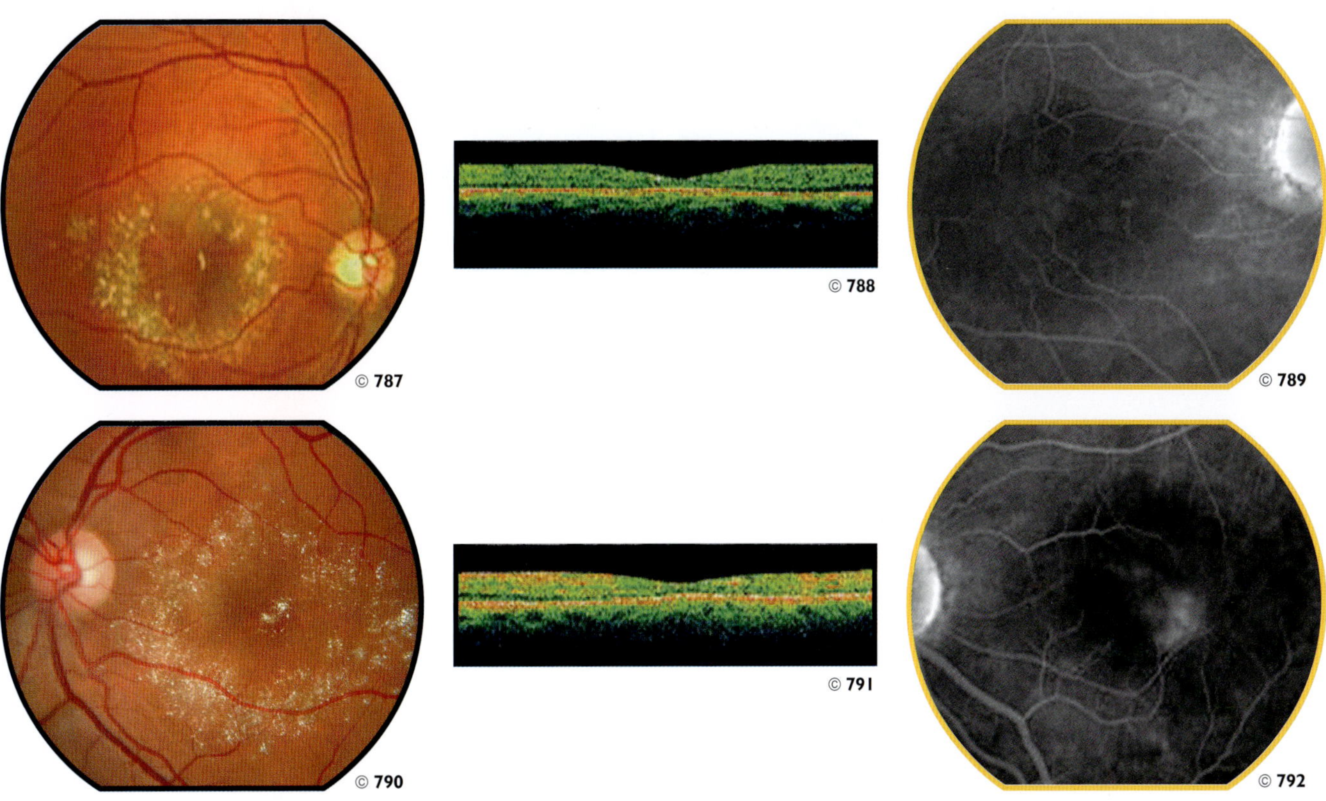

Following discontinuation of the drug, the crystalline deposits have dramatically cleared, although they are still evident in the right eye *(top row)* more than the left *(bottom row)*. Fluorescein leakage has cleared in the right eye, but it is still present in the temporal juxtafoveal region of the left eye. The OCT images show complete resolution of all the intraretinal and subretinal fluid. *Courtesy of Dr. David Sarraf*

Methoxyflurane

Methoxyflurane is an inflammable anesthetic agent with good analgesic properties and a low incidence of cardiac arrhythmias. It may induce a form of secondary hyperoxalosis. Deposition of calcium oxalate crystals at the level of the RPE and inner retina has been noted. These crystals are distributed through chorioretinal tissue via the systemic vasculature. A secondary hyperoxalosis may also occur after a small-bowel resection, renal failure, cirrhosis, or from excessive intake of ethylene glycol, ascorbic acid, and certain amino acids, including tyrosine, phenylalanine, and tryptophan.

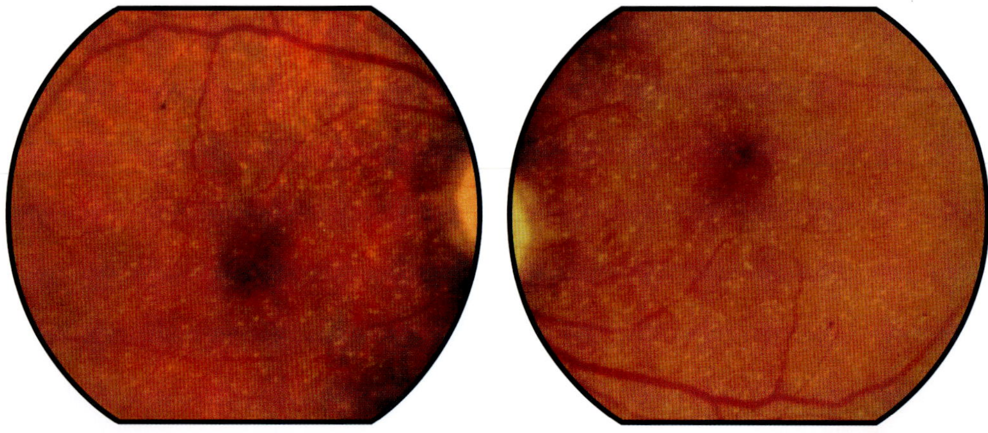

Minimally detectable fine crystals are present in the central macula of this patient with a mild degree of methoxyflurane toxicity.

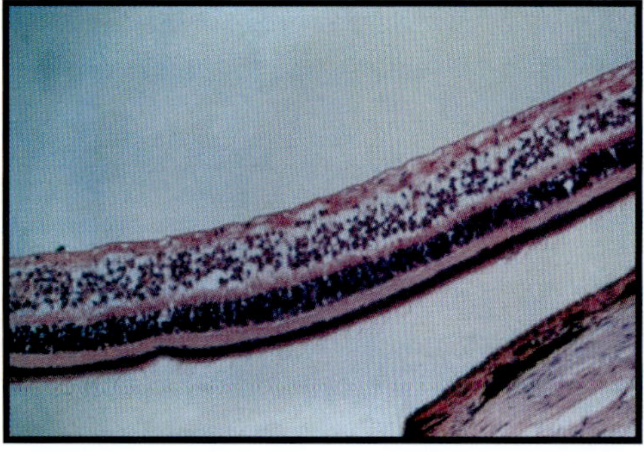

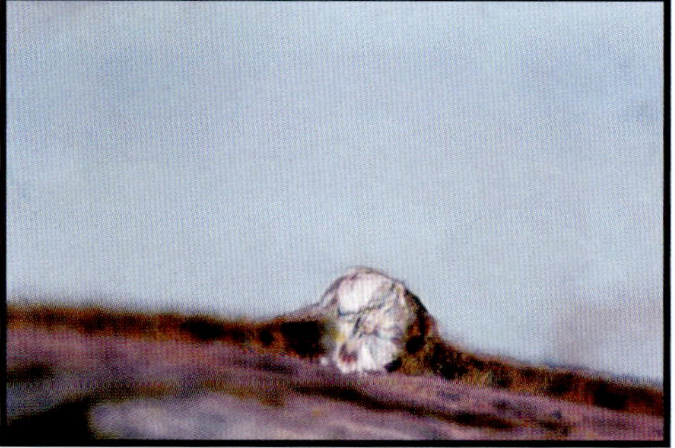

Intraretinal as well as pigment epithelial crystals have been noted histopathologically.

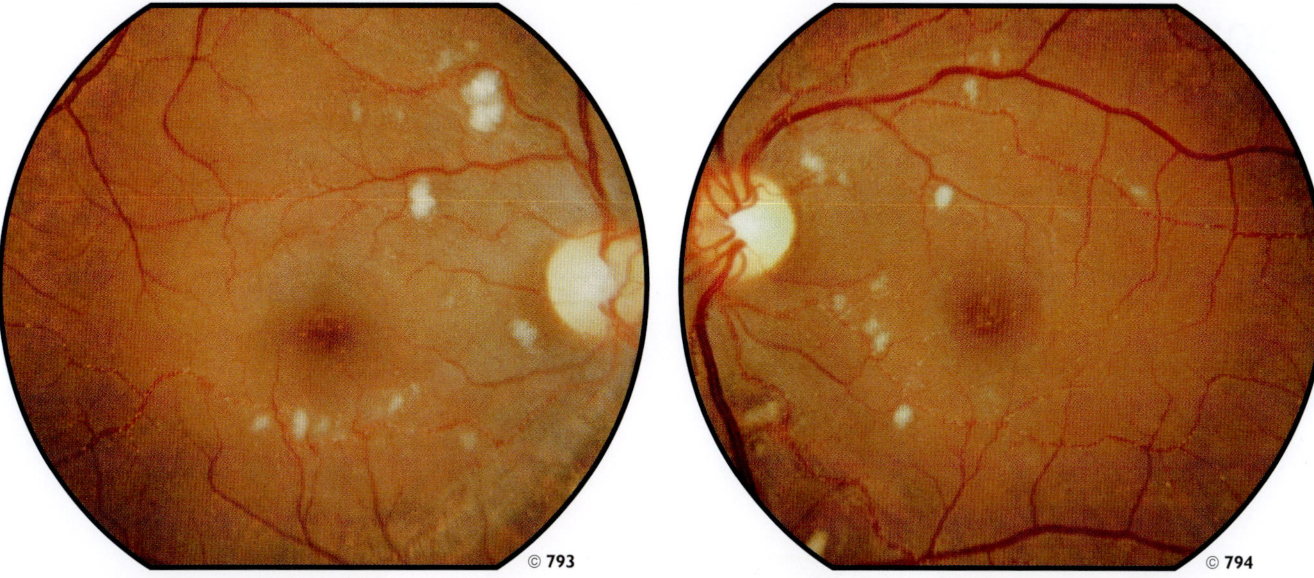

This patient developed crystalline deposition secondary to methoxyflurane ingestion. Initially, cotton-wool spots or axoplasmic debris were noted.

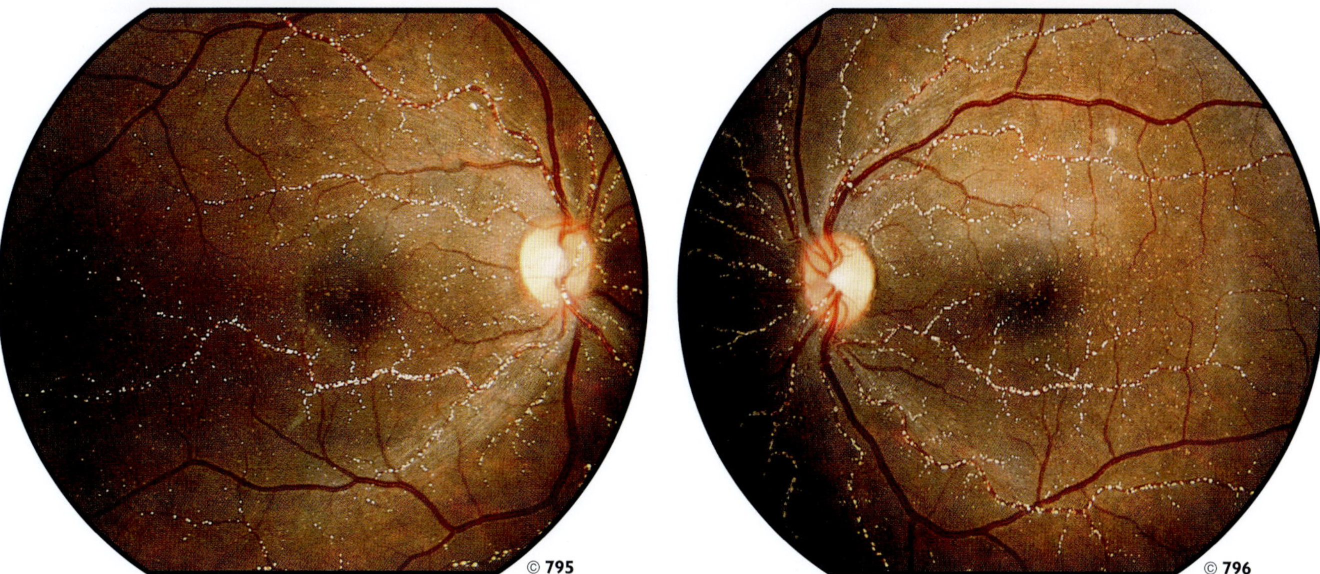

Subsequently, numerous crystalline-like deposits following the retinal vascular distribution, but also in the choriocapillaris, were evident. The deeper regions were modified in their appearance by the RPE.

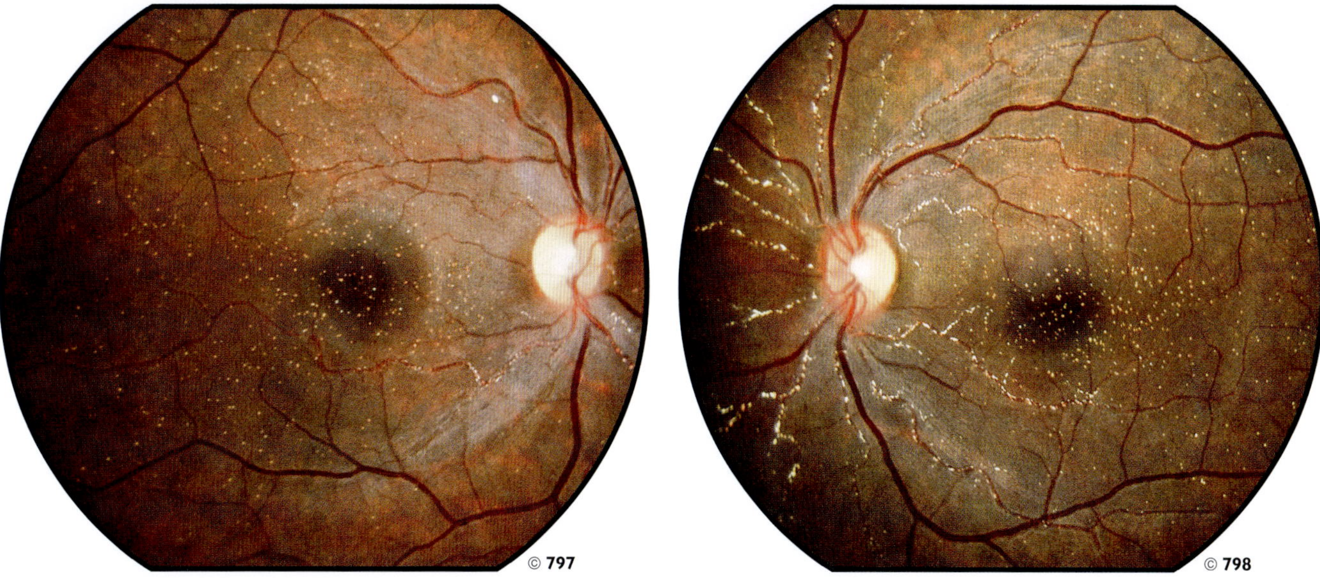

Six months later the crystals have partially resolved. *Courtesy of Dr. Michael Novak*

Canthaxanthin

Canthaxanthin is one of several drugs known to cause a crystalline maculopathy. It is a carotenoid food coloring agent and can be used as a sun-tanning agent although it is not approved for that use by the US Food and Drug Administration. It may be associated with a retinopathy consisting of yellow, glistening dots encircling the macula in an ovoid distribution. Patients are generally asymptomatic.

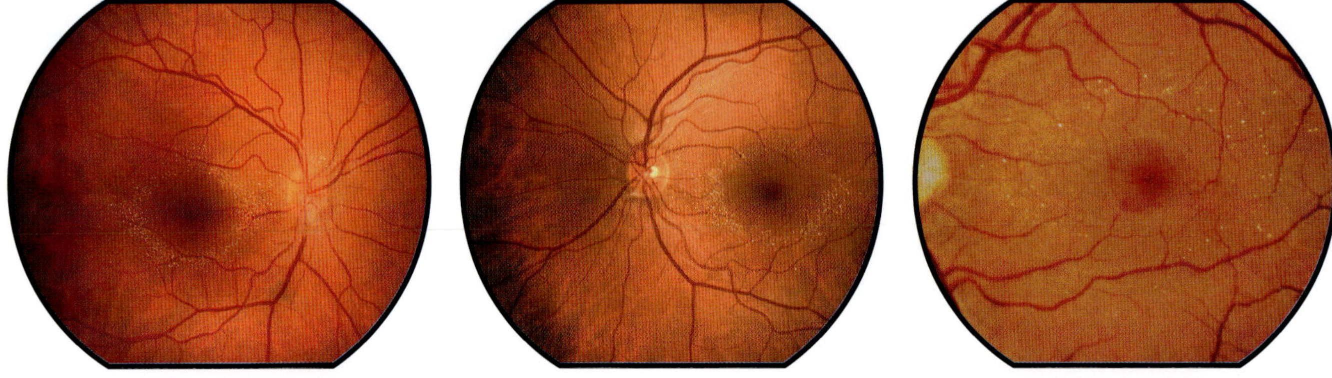

These patients have an early manifestation of canthaxanthine toxicity with scattered crystalline deposits encircling the paramacular region. There is sparing of the fovea and good vision.

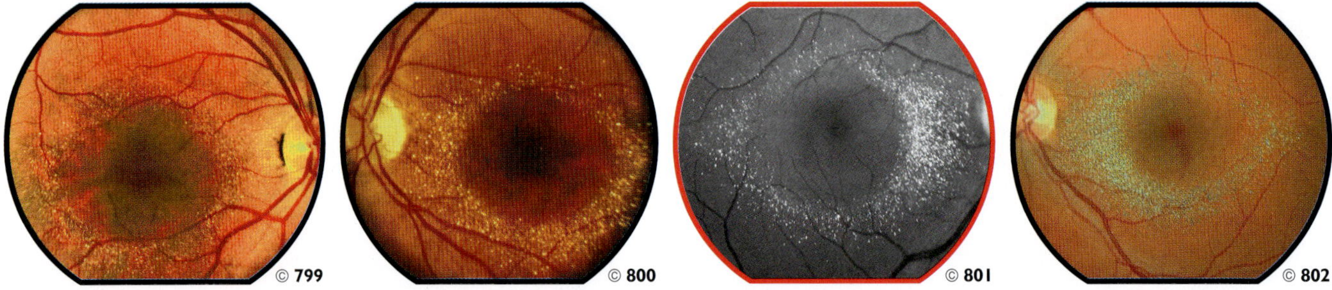

There is often a more prominent crystalline deposit in the inferior macula and also in the papillomacular bundle, as seen in these cases. This distribution of the crystals is not understood. It may be the result of light exposure.

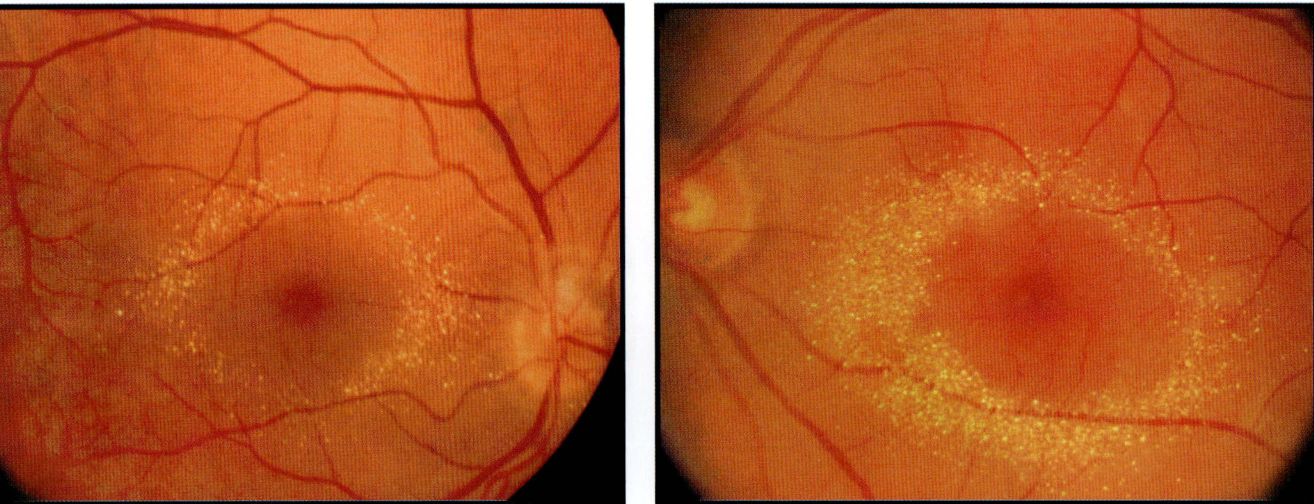

Courtesy of Dr. Dean Eliott

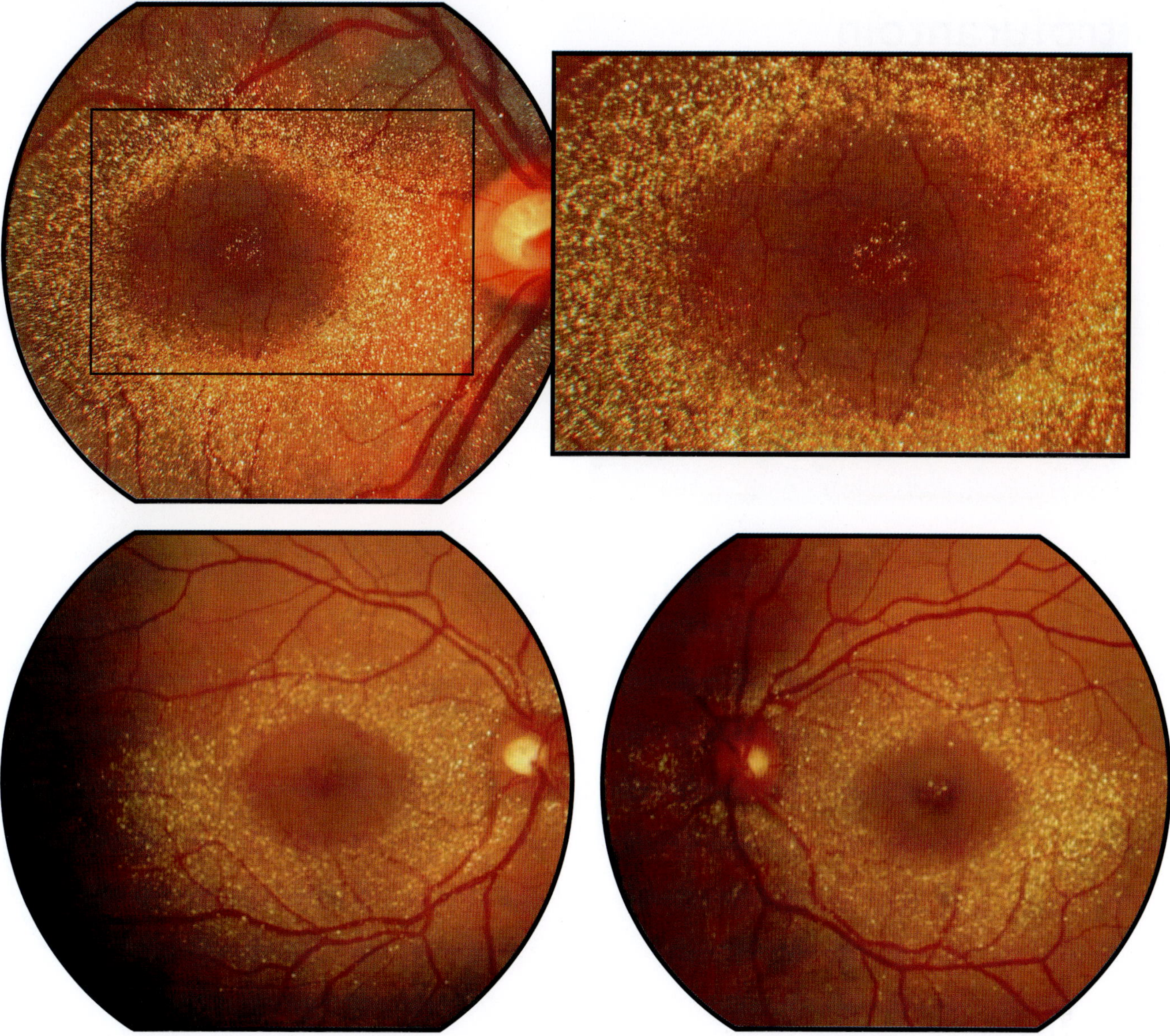

These cases of canthaxanthine toxicity show the variation in the clinical spectrum of this disease, which appears to be related to the dose and the duration of use. *Bottom row courtesy of Dr. Scott Sneed*

Nitrofurantoin

Nitrofurantoin is an antibiotic, generally used for urinary tract infections. Superficial and deep intraretinal crystals have been noted when used for long-term therapy.

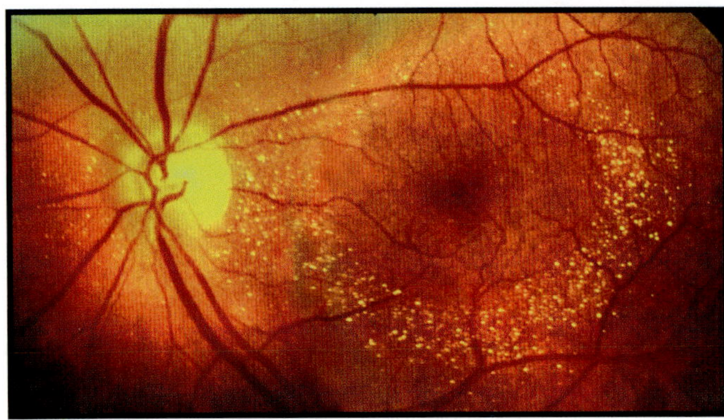

This patient with nitrofurantoin toxicity has crystalline deposits in the fundus, which are virtually indistinguishable from canthaxanthine deposits. This patient had been using nitrofurantoin therapy for 19 years. *Courtesy of Dr. David Williams*

West African Crystalline Maculopathy

West African crystalline maculopathy has been noted in patients in the Ibo tribe of Nigeria and elsewhere in Africa. In this disease, a cluster of highly refractile retinal crystals develops in the central macula. Some of these patients also had diabetic retinopathy. It should be noted that the crystals could be modified by laser treatment of the microangiopathy.

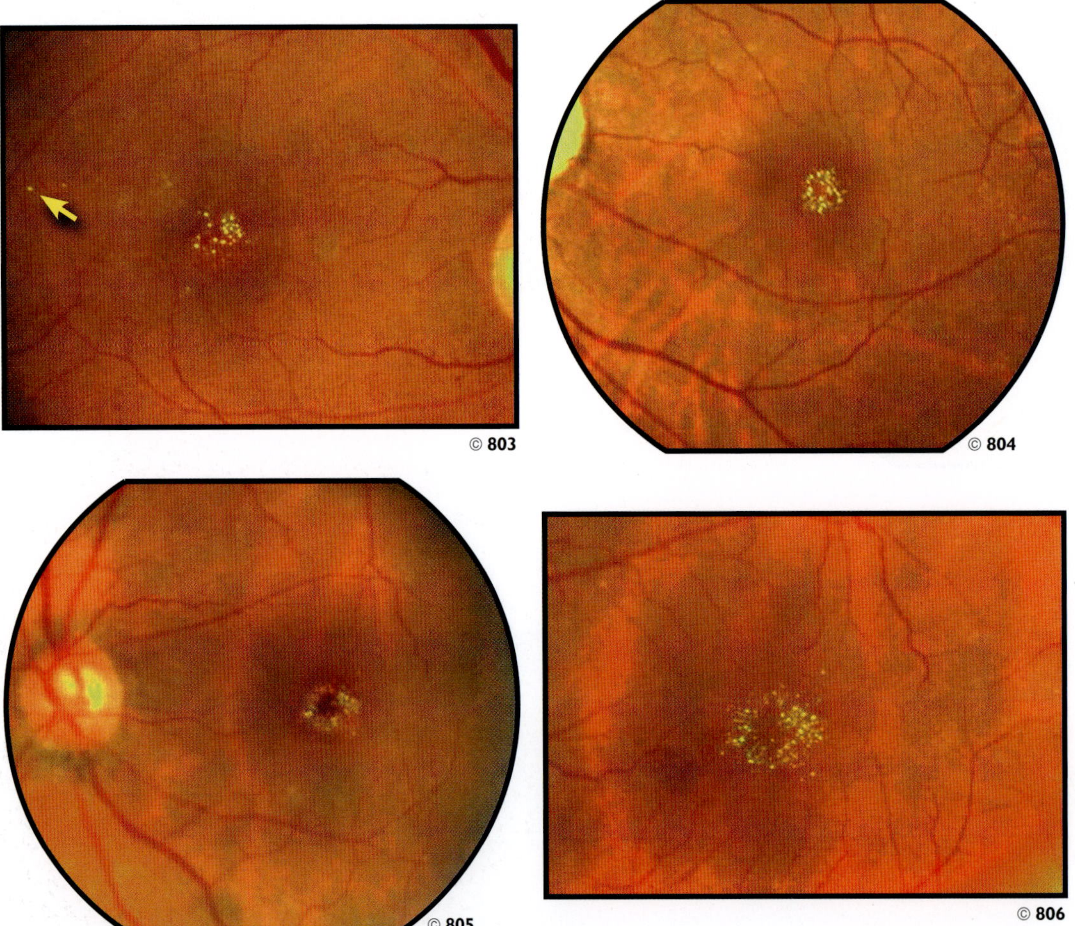

These patients with West African crystalline maculopathy show a clump of crystals randomly around the fovea with a few crystals elsewhere in the paramacular region *(arrow)*. There may be polychromatic reflectance of the crystal. These patients may also have diabetic retinopathy or venous occlusive disease not evident clinically.

Talc Retinopathy

Patients who abuse drugs especially intravenously may experience microembolic phenomena if the agent is combined with talc. Ischemic changes, including the kidney and lung, may be seen systemically but also in the fundus as chorioretinal ischemic abnormalities. Retinal vascular closure in the fundus may also lead to neovascularization and a proliferative retinopathy similar to sickle cell disease or even diabetic retinopathy with hemorrhage into the vitreous and tractional detachments. Cocaine, methamphetamine, and other illicit agents have been implicated in these changes.

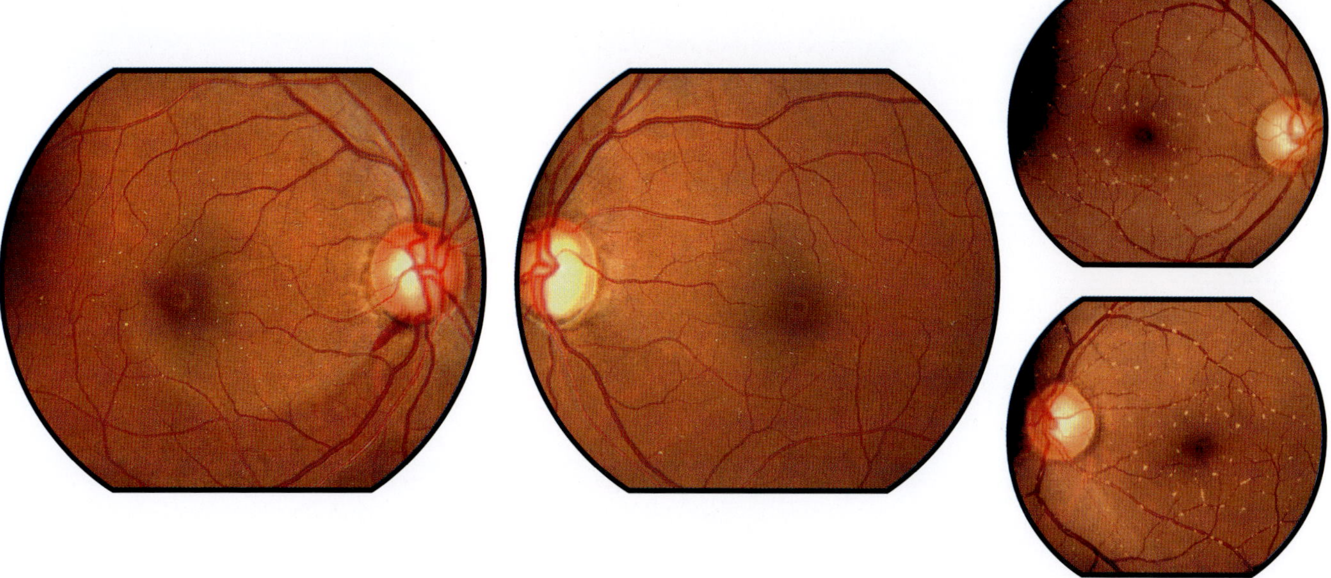

These two patients have very mild to moderate talc deposits in the fundus. A fine granular appearance is evident in the patient shown in the left and middle photographs. The patient on the right has more prominent talc deposits. The size of the deposits is most likely a function of the particles used in the formulation of the drug.

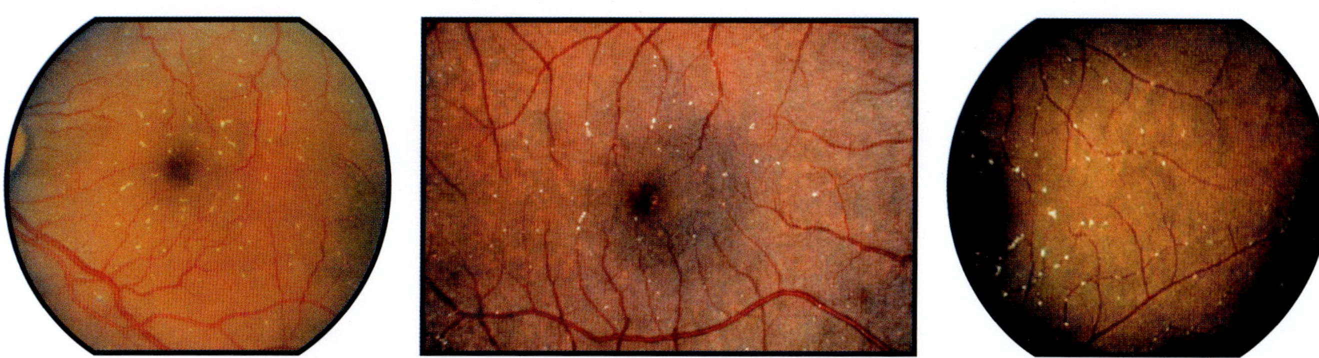

These patients have talc deposits in the posterior pole, which follow a retinal vascular distribution.

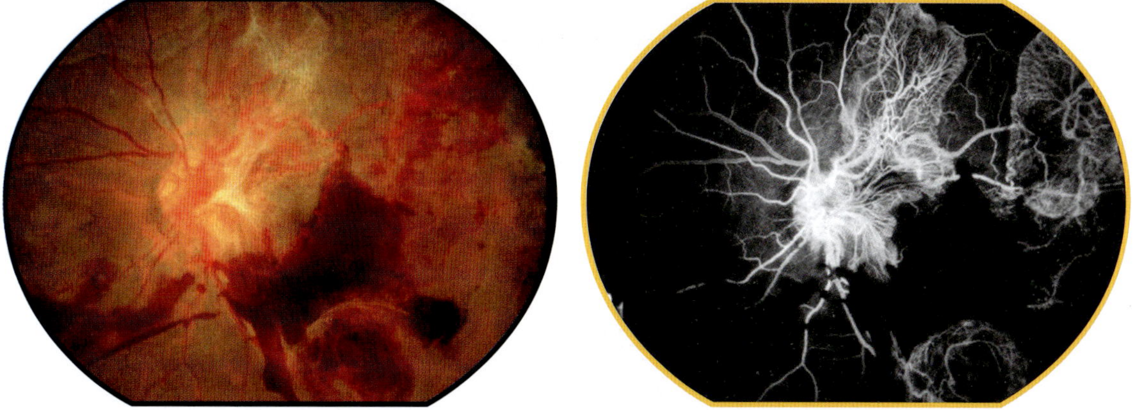

Severe talc toxicity produced ischemia and fibrous proliferation with bleeding into the vitreous in this patient.

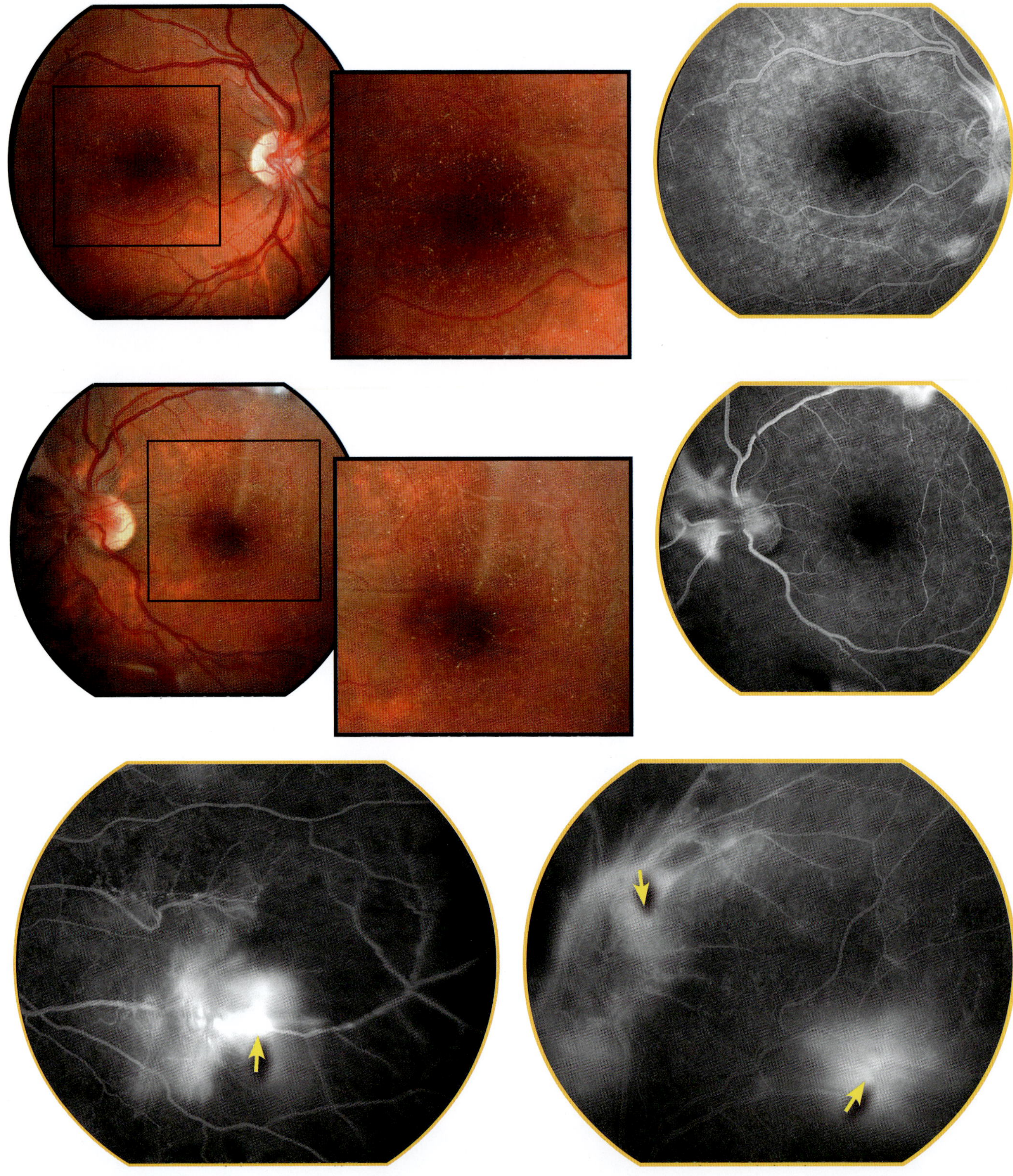

This patient has severe talc toxicity with neovascularization in the posterior pole, as well as in the periphery. There is neovascularization at the disc and peripheral retina *(arrows)*.

Cidofovir

Cidofovir is a nucleotide analog that inhibits viral DNA polymerase and is an effective agent against human cytomegalovirus infection. Profound hypotony and severe uveitis with secondary retinal vascular manifestations are possible adverse effects from the use of this drug.

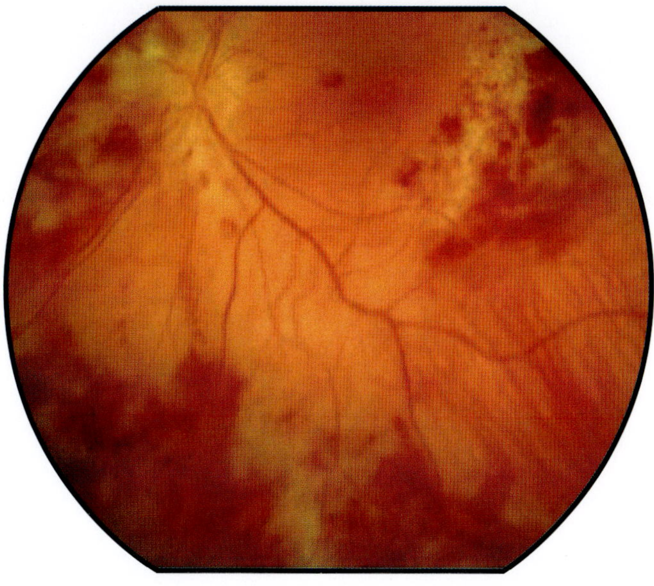

There is widespread retinal hemorrhages and edema of the macula in this patient with cidofovir toxicity.

Rifabutin

Rifabutin is an antimicrobacterial agent utilized for prophylaxis against infections due to *Mycobacterium avium* in patients with AIDS. Uveitis is a rare complication of this drug, and it may be quite extensive, forming a hypopyon. The uveitic response may be seen in the posterior segment as well.

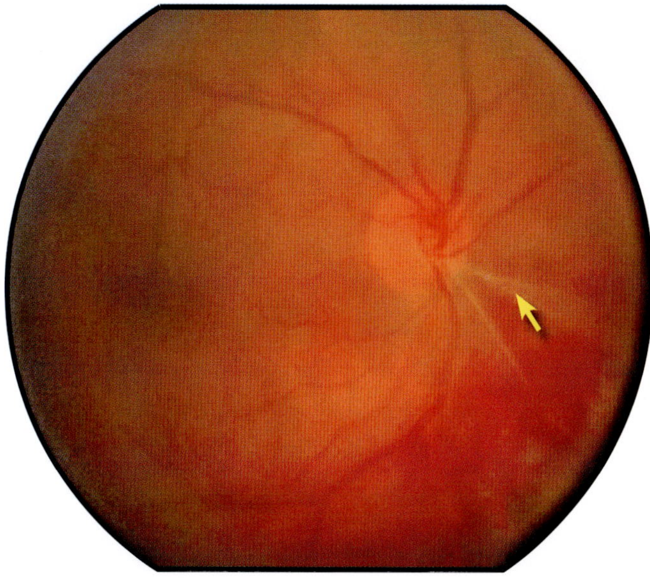

Rifabutin resulted in widespread hemorrhages into the retina as well as the vitreous with elements of retinal vascular ischemia at the inferonasal juxtapapillary area *(arrow)*. There is an intermediate uveitis as well.

Carbon Monoxide

Carbon monoxide poisoning can cause a toxic optic neuropathy that may have a similar etiological mechanism to that of tobacco amblyopia. Other changes in the fundus include engorgement and tortuosity of venules, swelling of the optic nerve, and hemorrhages.

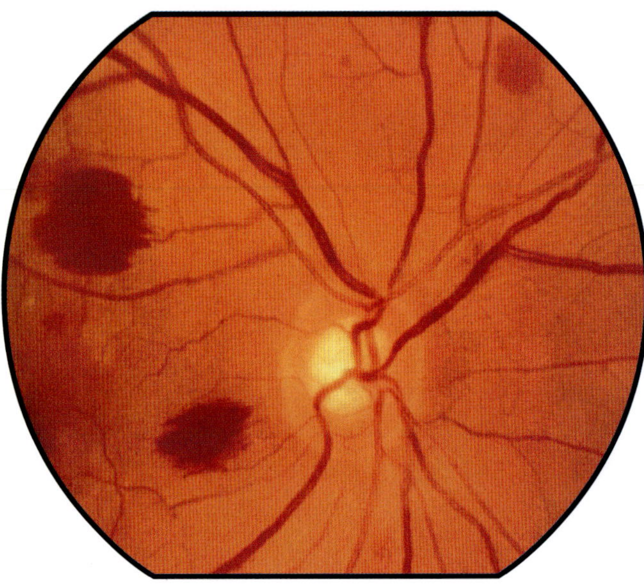

This patient experienced multiple hemorrhages in the fundus and optic atrophy from carbon monoxide toxicity. *Courtesy of Dr. Terry George*

Fludarabine

Fludarabine is a purine analog in an important class of chemotherapeutic agents used to treat a broad spectrum of lymphoid malignancies. Potential toxicity includes myelosuppression, opportunistic infection, immunosuppression, and severe neurotoxicity. The principal ocular toxicity is optic nerve neuropathy and papillitis, although retinal vasculitis and opportunistic infections, including acute retinal necrosis, have been reported.

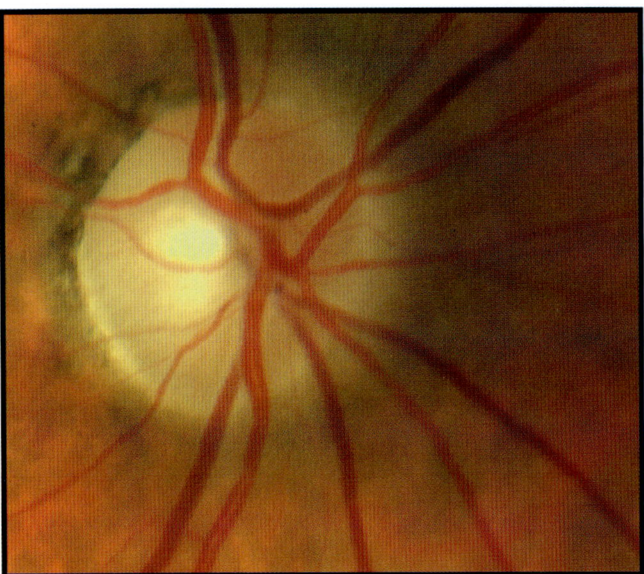

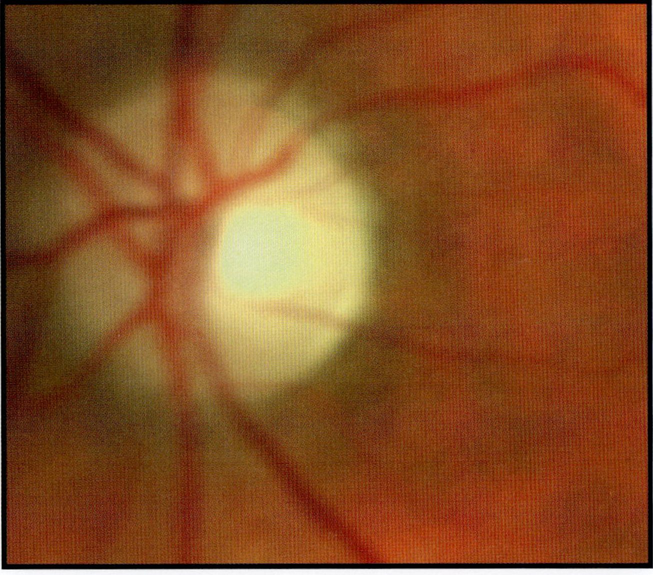

This patient has atrophy of the optic nerve secondary to fludarabine toxicity. There was also some late fluorescein staining of the optic nerve and field loss.

Methanol

Methanol is a highly toxic alcohol commonly found in commercial washing solvents, gasoline and antifreeze. The drug is converted to a highly toxic metabolite that may lead to acidosis and blindness from optic atrophy.

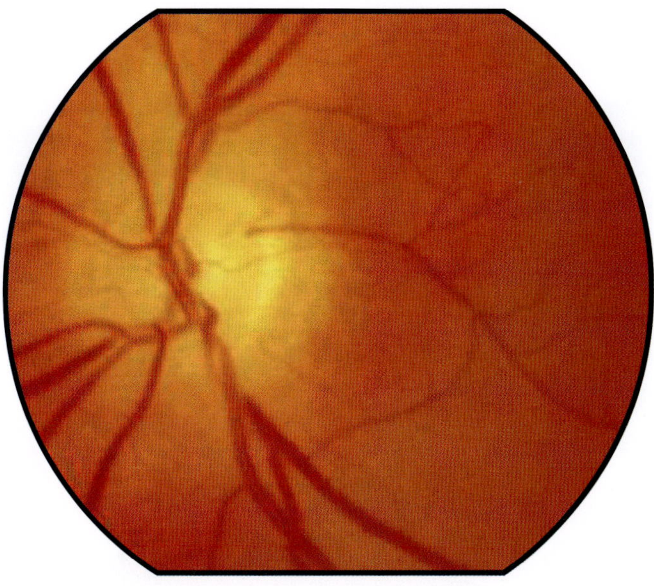

This patient became intoxicated with methanol and developed acute optic atrophy bilaterally.

MISCELLANEOUS

Vitamin A Deficiency

Vitamin A is essential in the metabolism of the retina. Any disease that might inhibit the absorption of vitamin A, such as a malabsorption syndrome from organ transplant surgery, can produce poor absorption, and can lead to a secondary effect on the retina, which includes photoreceptor damage, nyctalopia, and acuity loss. This is essentially a nutritional toxicity.

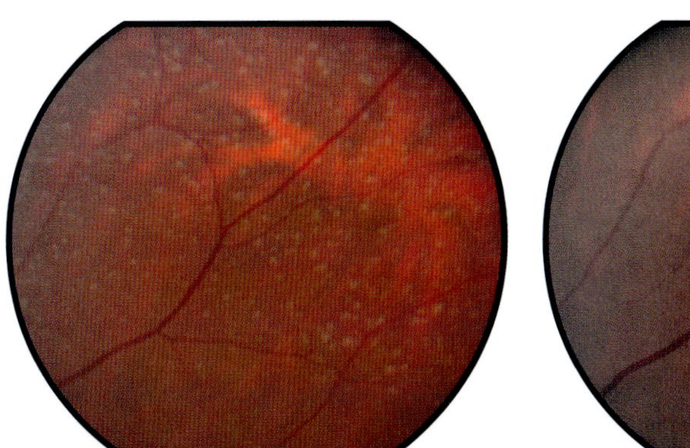

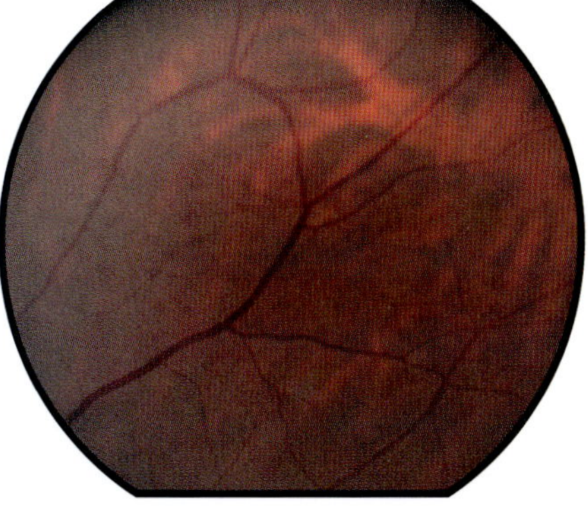

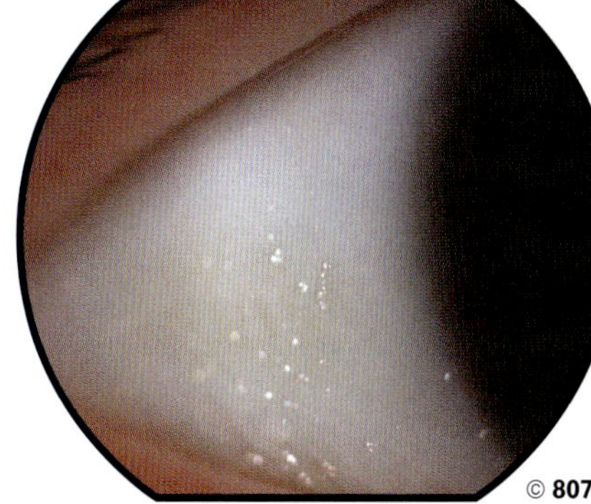

© 807

This patient has vitamin A deficiency from malabsorption. The fundus showed extensive fine dots in the outer retina most pronounced in the periphery, which resolved with treatment as shown in the subsequent image.

The ocular surface may show glistening white spots (Bitot spots) in the conjunctiva.

Celiac Disease

Celiac disease is a gluten-sensitive enteropathy that may lead to inflammatory bowel disease or malabsorption with secondary complications such as vitamin A deficiency, which may affect the eye.

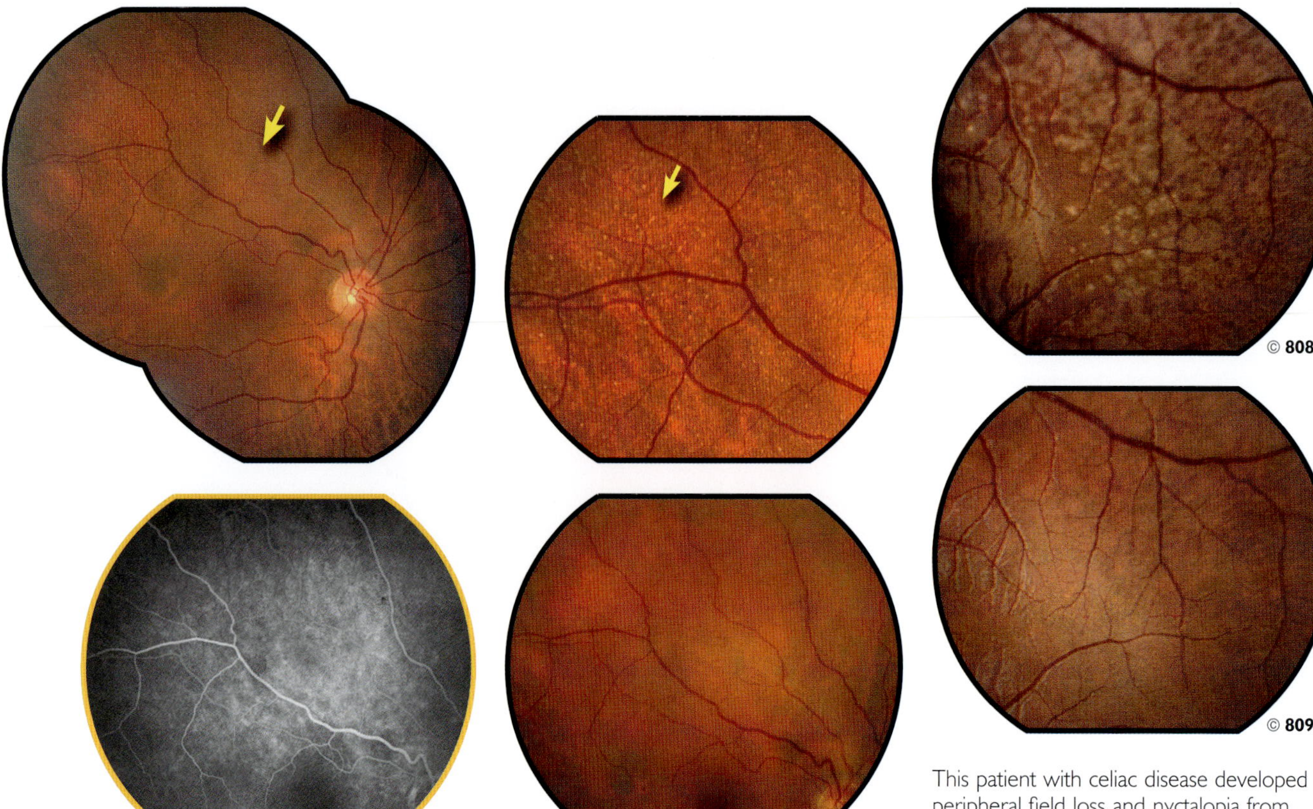

This patient had progressive nyctalopia from malabsorption and vitamin A deficiency. The peripheral spots in the fundus are faintly evident clinically *(arrows)*. The fluorescein angiogram shows no abnormal fluorescence. Crystalline spots were present in the nasal conjunctival area. The bottom photographs show resolution of the fundus spots following administration of parenteral vitamin A.
Courtesy of Dr. Anita Agarwal

This patient with celiac disease developed peripheral field loss and nyctalopia from malabsorption and vitamin A deficiency. Note the spots in the peripheral fundus *(above)*. These cleared on correction of the deficiency *(below)*.

Digoxin

Digoxin is a cardiac glycoside used for chronic heart failure and as an anti-arrhythmic agent. Toxic ocular symptoms include blurred vision or a yellow-tinged alteration in color perception. Minimal posterior-segment abnormalities may occur, and may be the result of a direct toxicity to photoreceptor cells and/or edema.

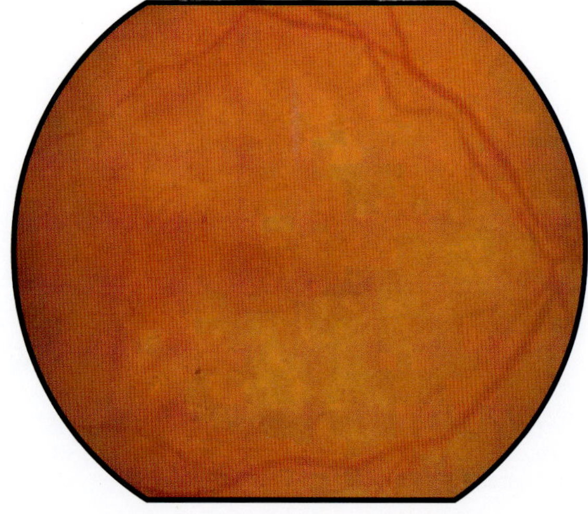

This patient had irregular stippling and atrophy in the macular region. There was also a mild degree of macular edema from digoxin toxicity.

Suggested Reading

Chloroquine

Arden, G.B., Kolb, H.E., 1964. Screening test for chloroquine retinopathy. Lancet 2, 41.

Aylward, J.M., 1993. Hydroxychloroquine and chloroquine: assessing the risk of retinal toxicity. J. Am. Optometric Assoc. 64, 787–797.

Bartel, P.R., Roux, P., Robinson, E., et al., 1994. Visual function and long-term chloroquine treatment. S. Afr. Med. J. 84, 32–34.

Bernstein, H.N., 1967. Chloroquine ocular toxicity. Surv. Ophthalmol. 12, 415.

Bonanomi, M.T., Dantas, N.C., Medeiros, F.A., 2006. Retinal nerve fiber layer thickness measurements in patients using chloroquine. Clin. Experiment. Ophthalmol. 34, 130–136.

Brinkley, J.R., Dubois, E.L., Ryan, S.J., 1979. Long-term course of chloroquine retinopathy after cessation of medication. Am. J. Ophthalmol. 88, 1–11.

Easterbrook, M., 1999. Detection and prevention of maculopathy associated with antimalarial agents. Int. Ophthalmol. Clin. 39, 49–57.

Ehrenfeld, M., Nesher, R., Merin, S., 1986. Delayed onset chloroquine retinopathy. Br. J. Ophthalmol. 70, 281–283.

Finbloom, D.S., Silver, K., Newsome, D.A., et al., 1985. Comparison of hydroxychloroquine and chloroquine use and the development of retinal toxicity. J. Rheumatol. 12, 692–694.

Heckenlively, J.R., Matin, D., Levy, J., 1980. Chloroquine retinopathy. Am. J. Ophthalmol. 89, 150.

Henkind, P., Carr, R., Siegel, I., 1954. Early chloroquine retinopathy: clinical and functional findings. Arch. Ophthalmol. 71, 157.

Kellner, U., Kraus, H., Forester, M.H., 2000. Multifocal ERG in chloroquine retinopathy: regional variance of retinal dysfunction. Graefes Arch. Clin. Exp. Ophthalmol. 238, 94–97.

Lee, D.H., Melles, R.B., Joe, S.G., et al., 2015. Pericentral hydroxychloroquine retinopathy in Korean patients. Ophthalmol. 122, 1252–1256.

Leecharoen, S., Wangkaew, S., Louthrenoo, W., 2007. Ocular side effects of chloroquine in patients with rheumatoid arthritis, systemic lupus erythematosus and scleroderma. J. Med. Assoc. Thai. 90, 52–58.

Mahon, G.J., Anderson, H.R., Gardiner, T.A., et al., 2003. Chloroquine causes lysosomal dysfunction in neural retina and implications for retinopathy. Curr. Eye Res. 28, 277–284.

Neubauer, A.S., Samari-Kermani, K., Schaller, U., et al., 2002. Detecting chloroquine retinopathy: electro-oculogram versus colour vision. Br. J. Ophthalmol. 87, 902–908.

Ochsendorf, F.R., Runne, U., 1996. Chloroquine: consideration of maximum daily dose (3.5 mg/kg ideal weight) prevents retinopathy. Dermatology 192, 382–383.

Tzekov, R., 2005. Ocular toxicity due to chloroquine and hydroxychloroquine. Doc. Ophthalmol. 110, 111–120.

Hydroxychloroquine

Browning, D.J., 2002. Hydroxychloroquine and chloroquine retinopathy: screening for drug toxicity. Am. J. Ophthalmol. 133, 649–656.

Easterbrook, M., 2001. Hydroxychloroquine retinopathy. Ophthalmology 108, 2158–2159.

Elder, M., Rahman, A.M., McLay, J., 2006. Early paracentral visual field loss in patients taking hydroxychloroquine. Arch. Ophthalmol. 124, 1729–1733.

Fiedler, A., Graham, E., Jones, S., et al., 1998. Royal College of Ophthalmologist's guidelines: ocular toxicity and hydroxychloroquine. Eye (Lond.) 12, 907–909.

Grierson, D.J., 1997. Hydroxychloroquine and visual screening in a rheumatology outpatient clinic. Ann. Rheu. Dis 56, 188–190.

Kellner, U., Renner, A.B., Tillack, H., 2006. Fundus autofluorescence and mfERG for the early detection of retinal alterations in patients using chloroquine/hydroxychloroquine. Invest. Ophthalmol. Vis. Sci. 47, 3531–3538.

Lai, T.Y., Chan, W.M., Li, H., et al., 2005. Multifocal electroretinographic changes in patients receiving hydroxychloroquine therapy. Am. J. Ophthalmol. 140, 794–807.

Lai, T.Y., Ngai, J.W., Chan, W.M., et al., 2006. Visual field and multifocal electroretinography and their correlations in patients on hydroxychloroquine therapy. Doc. Ophthalmol. 112, 177–187.

Lyons, J.S., Severns, M.L., 2007. Detection of early hydroxychloroquine retinal toxicity enhanced by ring ratio analysis of multifocal electroretinography. Am J Ophthalmol. 143, 801–809.

Marmor, M.F., 2005. The dilemma of hydroxychloroquine screening: new information from the multifocal ERG. Am. J. Ophthalmol. 140, 894–895.

Marmor, M.F., Kellner, U., Lai, T.Y., et al., 2011. Revised recommendations on screening for chloroquine and hydroxychloroquine retinal toxicity. Ophthalmol. 118, 1242–1252.

Marmor, M.F., Kellner, U., Lai, T.Y., et al., 2016. Recommendations on screening for chloroquine and hydroxychloroquine retinopathy. Ophthalmol. 123, 1386–1394.

Maturi, R.K., Yu, M., Weleber, R.G., 2004. Multifocal electroretinographic evaluation of long-term hydroxychloroquine users. Arch. Ophthalmol. 122, 973–981.

Mavrikakis, I., Sfikakis, P.P., Mavrikakis, E., et al., 2003. The incidence of irreversible retinal toxicity in patients treated with hydroxychloroquine: a reappraisal. Ophthalmol. 110, 1321–1326.

Moschos, M.N., Moschos, M.M., Apostolopoulos, M., et al., 2004. Assessing hydroxychloroquine toxicity by the multifocal ERG. Doc. Ophthalmol. 108, 47–53.

Neubauer, A.S., Stiefelmeyer, S., Berninger, T., et al., 2004. The multifocal pattern electroretinogram in chloroquine retinopathy. Ophthalmic Res. 36, 106–113.

Penrose, P.J., Tzekov, R.T., Sutter, E.E., et al., 2003. Multifocal electroretinography evaluation for early detection of retinal dysfunction in patients taking hydroxychloroquine. Retina 23, 503–512.

Rodriguez-Padrilla, J.A., Hedges, T.R., Monson, B., et al., 2007. High-speed ultra-high-resolution optical coherence tomography findings in hydroxychloroquine retinopathy. Arch. Ophthalmol. 125, 775–780.

Samanta, A., Goh, L., Bawendi, A., 2004. Are evidence-based guidelines being followed for the monitoring of ocular toxicity of hydroxychloroquine? A nationwide survey of practice amongst consultant rheumatologists and implications for clinical governance. Rheumatology 43, 346–348.

Teoh, S.C., Lim, J., Koh, A., et al., 2006. Abnormalities on the multifocal electroretinogram may precede clinical signs of hydroxychloroquine retino-toxicity. Eye (Lond.) 20, 129–132.

Thioridazine

Cerletti, A., Meier-Ruge, W., 1968. Toxicological studies on phenothiazine-induced retinopathy. Excerpt. Med. Internat. Congr. Ser. 145, 170–188.

Chaudhry, T.A., Shamsi, F.A., Weitzman, M.L., 2006. Progressive severe visual loss after long-term withdrawal from thioridazine treatment. Eur. J. Ophthalmol. 16, 651–653.

Cohen, J., Wells, J., Borda, R., 1978. Thioridazine (Mellaril) ocular toxicity. Doc. Ophthalmol. Proc. Ser. 15, 91–94.

Eves, P., Smith-Thomas, L., Hedley, S., et al., 1999. A comparative study of the effect of pigment on drug toxicity in human choroidal melanocytes and retinal pigment epithelial cells. Pigment Cell Res. 12, 22–35.

Fornaro, P., Calabria, G., Corallo, G., et al., 2002. Pathogenesis of degenerative retinopathies induced by thioridazine and other antipsychotics: a dopamine hypothesis. Doc. Ophthalmol. 105, 41–49.

Kozy, D., Doft, B.H., Lipkowitz, J., 1984. Nummular thioridazine retinopathy. Retina 4, 253–256.

Marmor, M.F., 1990. Is thioridazine retinopathy progressive? Relationship of pigmentary changes to visual function. Br. J. Ophthalmol. 74, 739–742.

Oshika, T., 1995. Ocular adverse effects of neuropsychiatric agents. Incidence and management. Drug Saf. 12, 256–263.

Shah, G.K., Auerbach, D.B., Augsburger, J.J., et al., 1998. Acute thioridazine retinopathy. Arch. Ophthalmol. 116, 826–827.

Tekell, J.I., Silva, J.A., Maas, J.A., et al., 1996. Thioridazine-induced retinopathy. Am. J. Psychiat. 153, 1234–1235.

Chlorpromazine

Barrett, S.L., Bell, R., Watson, D., et al., 2004. Effects of amisulpride, risperidone and chloropromazine on auditory and visual latent inhibition, prepulse inhibition, executive function and eye movements in healthy volunteers. J. Psychopharmacol. 18, 156–172.

Gupta, A., Agarwal, A., Ram, J., 2014. Reversal of toxic manifestations of chlorpromazine. JAMA Ophthalmol. 132, 1177.

Mitchell, A.C., Brown, K.W., 1995. Chlorpromazine-induced retinopathy. Br. J. Psychiatry 166, 822–823.

Webber, S.K., Domniz, Y., Sutton, G.L., et al., 2001. Corneal deposition after high-dose chlorpromazine hydrochloride therapy. Cornea 20, 217–219.

Deferoxamine

Bene, C., Manzier, A., Bene, D., et al., 1989. Irreversible ocular toxicity from single "challenge" dose of deferoxamine. Clin. Nephrol. 31, 43–48.

MEK Inhibitors

Duncan, K.E., Chang, L.Y., Patronas, M., 2015. MEK inhibitors: a new class of chemotherapeutic agents with ocular toxicity. Eye (Lond.) 29, 1003–1012.

Infante, J.R., Fecher, L.A., Falchook, G.S., et al., 2012. Safety, pharmacokinetic, pharmacodynamic, and efficacy data for the oral MEK inhibitor trametinib: a phase I dose-escalation trial. Lancet Oncol. 13, 773–781.

McCannel, T.A., Chmielowski, B., Finn, R.S., et al., 2014. Bilateral subfoveal neurosensory retinal detachment associated with MEK inhibitor use for metastatic cancer. JAMA Ophthalmol. 132, 1005–1009.

Niro, A., Strippoli, S., Alessio, G., et al., 2015. Ocular toxicity in metastatic melanoma patients treated with Mitogen activated protein kinase inhibitors: a case series. Am. J. Ophthalmol. 160, 959–967.

Schoenberger, S.D., Kim, S.J., 2013. Bilateral multifocal central serous-like chorioretinopathy due to MEK inhibition for metastatic cutaneous melanoma. Case Rep. Ophthalmol. Med. 2013, 673796.

Urner-Bloch, U., Urner, M., Stieger, P., et al., 2014. Transient MEK inhibitor-associated retinopathy in metastatic melanoma. Ann. Oncol. 25, 1437–1441.

van Dijk, E.H., van Herpen, C.M., Marinkovic, M., et al., 2015. Serous retinopathy associated with mitogen-activated protein kinase kinase inhibition (Binimetinib) for metastatic cutaneous and uveal melanoma. Ophthalmol. 122, 1907–1916.

Quinine Sulfate

Bacon, P., Spacton, D.J., Smith, E., 1988. Blindness from quinine toxicity. Br. J. Ophthalmol. 72, 219–224.

Beare, N.A., Southern, C., Chalira, C., et al., 2004. Prognostic significance and course of retinopathy in children with severe malaria. Arch. Ophthalmol. 122, 1141–1147.

Brinton, G.S., Norton, E.W.D., Zahn, J.R., et al., 1980. Ocular quinine toxicity. Am. J. Ophthalmol. 90, 403–410.

Buchanan, T.A.S., Lyness, R.W., Collins, A.D., et al., 1987. An experimental study of quinine blindness. Eye (Lond.) 1, 522–524.

Canning, C.R., Hague, S., 1988. Ocular quinine toxicity. Br. J. Ophthalmol. 72, 23–26.

Lochhead, J., Movaffaghy, A., Falsini, B., et al., 2003. The effect of quinine on the electroretinogram of children with pediatric cerebral malaria. J. Infect. Dis. 187, 1342–1345.

Mackie, M.A., Davidson, J., Clarke, J., 1997. Quinine-acute self-poisoning and ocular toxicity. Scott. Med. J. 42, 8–9.

Oral Contraceptives

Chizek, D.J., Franceschetti, A.T., 1969. Oral contraceptives: their side effects and ophthalmological manifestations. Surv. Ophthalmol. 14, 90–105.

Fraser-Bell, S., Wu, J., Klein, R., et al., 2006. Smoking, alcohol intake, estrogen use, and age-related macular degeneration in Latinos: the Los Angeles Latino Eye Study. Am. J. Ophthalmol. 141, 79–87.

Garg, S.K., Chase, H.P., Marshall, G., et al., 1994. Oral contraceptives and renal and retinal complications in young women with insulin-dependent diabetes mellitus. JAMA 271, 1099–1102.

Gombos, G.M., Moreno, D.H., Bedrossian, P.B., 1975. Retinal vascular occlusion induced by oral contraceptives. Ann. Ophthalmol. 7, 215–217.

Harris-Yitzhak, M., Harris, A., Ben-Refael, Z., et al., 2000. Estrogen-replacement therapy: effects on retrobulbar hemodynamics. Am. J. Ophthalmol. 129, 623–628.

Petersson, G.J., Fraunfelder, F.T., Meyer, S.M., 1981. Oral contraceptives. Ophthalmology 88, 368–371.

Stowe, G.C., Jakov, A.N., Albert, D.M., 1978. Central retinal vascular occlusion associated with oral contraceptives. Am. J. Ophthalmol. 86, 798–801.

Vessey, M.P., Hannaford, P., Mant, J., et al., 1998. Oral contraception and eye disease: findings in two large cohort studies. Br. J. Ophthalmol. 82, 538–542.

Ergot Alkaloids

Gupta, D.R., Strobos, R.J., 1972. Bilateral papillitis associated with Cafergot therapy. Neurology 22, 793–797.

Mindel, J.S., Rubenstein, A.E., Franklin, B., 1981. Ocular ergotamine tartrate toxicity during treatment of vacor-induced orthostatic hypotension. Am. J. Ophthalmol. 92, 492–496.

Nagaki, Y., Hayasaka, S., Hiraki, S., et al., 1997. Central retinal vein occlusion in a woman receiving bromocriptine. Ophthalmologica 211, 397–398.

Nicotinic Acid

Dajani, H.M., Lauer, A.K., 2006. Optical coherence tomography findings in niacin maculopathy. Can. J. Ophthalmol. 41, 197–200.

Fraunfelder, F.W., Franufelder, F.T., Illingworth, D.R., 1995. Adverse ocular effects associated with niacin therapy. Br. J. Ophthalmol. 79, 54–56.

Gass, J.D.M., 1973. Nicotinic acid maculopathy. Am. J. Ophthalmol. 76, 500–510.

Metelitsina, T.I., Grunwald, J.E., DuPont, J.C., et al., 2004. Effect of niacin on the choroidal circulation of patients with age related macular degeneration. Br. J. Ophthalmol. 88, 1568–1572.

Millay, R.M., Klein, M.L., Illingworth, D.R., 1988. Niacin maculopathy. Ophthalmology 95, 930–936.

Spirn, M.J., Warren, F.A., Guyer, D.R., et al., 2003. Optical coherence tomography findings in nicotinic acid maculopathy. Am. J. Ophthalmol. 135, 913–914.

Drug-Induced Myopia

Bovino, J.A., Marcus, D.F., 1982. The mechanism of transient myopia induced by sulfonamide therapy. Am. J. Ophthalmol. 94, 99–102.

Cereza, G., Pedros, C., Garcia, N., et al., 2005. Topiramate in non-approved indications and acute myopia or angle closure glaucoma. Br. J. Clin. Pharmacol. 60, 578–579.

Craig, J.E., Ong, T.J., Louis, D.L., et al., 2004. Mechanism of topiramate-induced acute-onset myopia and angle closure glaucoma. Am. J. Ophthalmol. 137, 193–195.

Fraunfelder, F.W., Fraunfelder, F.T., Keates, E.U., 2004. Topiramate-associated acute, bilateral, secondary angle-closure glaucoma. Ophthalmol 111, 109–111.

Grinbaum, A., Ashkenazi, I., Avni, I., et al., 1992. Transient myopia following metronidazole treatment for *Trichomonas vaginalis*. JAMA 267, 511–512.

Hook, S.R., Holladay, J.T., Prager, T.C., et al., 1986. Transient myopia induced by sulfonamides. Am. J. Ophthalmol. 101, 495–496.

Medeiros, F.A., Zhang, X.Y., Bernd, A.S., et al., 2003. Angle-closure glaucoma associated with ciliary body detachment in patients using topiramate. Arch. Ophthalmol. 121, 282–285.

Milea, D., Zech, C., Dumontet, C., et al., 1999. Transient acute myopia induced by antilymphocyte globulins. Ophthalmologica 213, 133–134.

Postel, E.A., Assalian, A., Epstein, D.L., 1996. Drug-induced transient myopia and angle closure glaucoma associated with supraciliary choroidal effusion. Am. J. Ophthalmol. 122, 110–112.

Ryan, E.H. Jr., Jampol, L.M., 1986. Drug-induced acute transient myopia with retinal folds. Retina 6, 220–223.

Soylev, M.F., Green, R.L., Feldon, S.E., 1995. Choroidal effusion as a mechanism for transient myopia induced by hydrochlorothiazide and triamterene. Am. J. Ophthalmol. 120, 395–397.

Tamoxifen

Ah-Song, R., Sasco, A.J., 1997. Tamoxifen and ocular toxicity. Cancer Detect. Prev. 21, 522–531.

Ashford, A.R., Donev, I., Tiwari, R.P., et al., 1988. Reversible ocular toxicity related to tamoxifen therapy. Cancer 61, 33–35.

Bourla, D.H., Gonzales, C.R., Mango, C.W., et al., 2007. Intravitreous vascular endothelial growth factor (VEGF) inhibitor therapy for tamoxifen induced macular edema. Semin. Ophthalmol. 22, 87–88.

Bourla, D.H., Sarraf, D., Schwartz, S.D., 2007. Peripheral retinopathy and maculopathy in high-dose tamoxifen therapy. Am. J. Ophthalmol. 144, 126–128.

Flach, A.J., 1994. Clear evidence that long-term, low-dose tamoxifen treatment can induce ocular toxicity: a prospective study of 63 patients. Surv. Ophthalmol. 38, 392–393.

Gorin, M.B., Day, R., Costantino, J.P., et al., 1998. Long-term tamoxifen citrate use and potential ocular toxicity. Am. J. Ophthalmol. 125, 493–501.

Gualino, V., Cohen, S.Y., Delyfer, M.N., et al., 2005. Optical coherence tomography findings in tamoxifen retinopathy. Am. J. Ophthalmol. 140, 757–758.

Kaiser-Kupfer, M.I., Kupfer, C., Rodrigues, M.M., 1981. Tamoxifen retinopathy A clinical pathological report. Ophthalmology 88, 89–91.

Nayfield, S.C., Gorin, M.B., 1996. Tamoxifen-associated eye disease. A review. J. Clin. Oncol. 14, 1018–1026.

Noureddin, B.N., Seoud, M., Bashshur, Z., et al., 1999. Ocular toxicity in low-dose tamoxifen: a prospective study. Eye (Lond.) 13, 729–733.

Yanyali, A.C., Freund, K.B., Sorenson, J.A., et al., 2001. Tamoxifen retinopathy in a male patient. Am. J. Ophthalmol. 131, 386–387.

Zinchuk, O., Watnabe, M., Hayashi, N., et al., 2006. A case of tamoxifen keratopathy. Arch. Ophthalmol. 124, 1046–1048.

Methoxyflurane

Bullock, J.D., Albert, D.M., 1975. Fleck retina: appearance secondary to oxalate crystals from methoxyflurane anesthesia. Arch. Ophthalmol. 93, 26–31.

Fiedler, A.R., Garner, A., Chambers, T.L., 1980. Ophthalmic manifestations of primary oxalosis. Br. J. Ophthalmol. 64, 782–788.

Meredith, T.A., Wright, J.D., Gammon, J.A., et al., 1984. Ocular involvement in primary hyperoxaluria. Arch. Ophthalmol. 102, 584–587.

Novak, M.A., Roth, A.S., Levine, M.R., 1988. Calcium oxalate retinopathy associated with methoxyflurane abuse. Retina 8, 230–236.

Small, K.W., Letson, R., Scheinman, J., 1990. Ocular findings in primary hyperoxaluria. Arch. Ophthalmol. 108, 89–93.

Zak, T.A., Buncic, R., 1983. Primary hereditary oxalosis retinopathy. Arch. Ophthalmol. 101, 78–80.

Canthaxanthine

Boudreault, G., Cortin, P., Corriveau, L.A., et al., 1983. La retinopathies a la canthaxanthine I Etude clinique de 51 consommateurs. Can. J. Ophthalmol. 18, 325–328.

Chang, T.S., Aylward, W., Clarkson, J.G., et al., 1995. Asymmetric canthaxanthine retinopathy. Am. J. Ophthalmol. 119, 801–802.

Espaillat, A., Aiello, L.P., Arrigg, P.G., et al., 1999. Canthaxanthine retinopathy. Arch. Ophthalmol. 117, 412–413.

Fraunfelder, F.W., 2004. Ocular side effects from herbal medicines and nutritional supplements. Am. J. Ophthalmol. 138, 639–647.

Goralczyk, R., Barker, F.M., Buser, S., et al., 2000. Dose dependency of canthaxanthin crystals in monkey retina and spatial distribution of its metabolites. Invest. Ophthalmol. Vis. Sci. 41, 1513–1522.

Harnois, C., Samson, J., Malenfant, M., et al., 1989. Canthaxanthine retinopathy: anatomic and functional reversibility. Arch. Ophthalmol. 107, 538–540.

Hueber, A., Rosentreter, A., Severin, M., 2011. Canthaxanthine retinopathy: long-term observations. Ophthalmic Res. 46, 103–106.

Nitrofurantoin

Ibanez, H.E., Williams, D.F., Boniuk, I., 1994. Crystalline retinopathy associated with long-term macrodantin therapy A case report. Arch. Ophthalmol. 112, 304–305.

Wasserman, B.N., Chronister, T.E., Stark, B.I., et al., 2000. Ocular myasthenia and nitrofurantoin. Am. J. Ophthalmol. 130, 531–533.

Talc Retinopathy

Atlee, W.E., 1972. Talc and cornstarch emboli in eyes of drug users. JAMA 219, 49–51.

Bluth, L.L., Hanscom, T.A., 1981. Retinal detachment and vitreous hemorrhage due to talc emboli. JAMA 246, 980–981.

Cidofovir

Banker, A.S., Arevalo, J.F., Munguia, D., et al., 1997. Intraocular pressure and aqueous humor dynamics in patients with AIDS treated with intravitreal cidofovir (HPMPC) for cytomegalovirus retinitis. Am. J. Ophthalmol. 124, 168–180.

Davis, J.L., Taskintuna, I., Freeman, W.R., et al., 1997. Iritis and hypotony after treatment with intravenous cidofovir for cytomegalovirus retinitis. Arch. Ophthalmol. 115, 785–786.

Jabs, D.A., 1997. Cidofovir. Arch. Ophthalmol. 115, 785–786.

Kirsch, L.S., Arevalo, J.F., Chavez de la Paz, E., et al., 1995. Intravitreal cidofovir (HPMPC) treatment of cytomegalovirus retinitis in patients with acquired immune deficiency syndrome. Ophthalmol. 102, 533–542.

Lin, A.P., Holland, G.N., Engstrom, R.E. Jr., 1999. Vitrectomy and silicone tamponade for cidofovir-associated hypotony with ciliary body detachment. Retina 19, 75–76.

Song, M.K., Azen, S.P., Buley, A., et al., 2003. Effect of anti-cytomegalovirus therapy on the incidence of immune recovery uveitis in AIDS patients with healed cytomegalovirus retinitis. Am. J. Ophthalmol. 136, 696–702.

Taskintuna, I., Rahhal, F.M., Arevalo, J.F., et al., 1997. Low-dose intravitreal cidofovir (HPMPC) therapy of cytomegalovirus retinitis in patients with acquired immune deficiency syndrome. Ophthalmol. 104, 1049–1057.

Rifabutin

Arevalo, J.F., Freeman, W.R., 1999. Corneal endothelial deposits in children positive for human immunodeficiency virus receiving rifabutin prophylaxis for *Mycobacterium avium* complex bacteremia. Am. J. Ophthalmol. 127, 164–169.

Becker, K., Schimkat, M., Jablonowski, H., et al., 1996. Anterior uveitis associated with rifabutin medication in AIDS patients. Infection 24, 36–38.

Bhagat, N., Read, R.W., Rao, N.A., et al., 2001. Rifabutin-associated hypopyon uveitis in human immunodeficiency virus-negative immunocompetent individuals. Ophthalmol. 108, 750–752.

Chaknis, M.J., Brooks, S.E., Mitchell, K.T., et al., 1996. Inflammatory opacities of the vitreous in rifabutin-associated uveitis. Am. J. Ophthalmol. 122, 580–582.

Fraunfelder, F.W., 2007. Drug-induced ocular inflammatory diseases. Drugs Today 43, 117–123.

Golchin, B., McClellan, K., 2003. Corneal endothelial deposits secondary to rifabutin prophylaxis for *Mycobacterium avium* complex bacteraemia. Br. J. Ophthalmol. 87, 798–799.

Jewelewicz, D.A., Schiff, W.M., Brown, S., et al., 1998. Rifabutin-associated uveitis in an immuno suppressed pediatric patient without acquired immunodeficiency syndrome. Am. J. Ophthalmol. 125, 872–873.

Saha, N., Bansal, S., Bishop, F., et al., 2009. Bilateral hypopyon and vitritis associated with rifabutin therapy in an immunocompetent patient taking itraconazole. Eye (Lond.) 23, 1481.

Saran, B.R., 1997. Rifabutin-associated uveitis. Ann. Pharmacother. 31, 1405.

Smith, J.A., Mueller, B.U., Nussenblatt, R.B., et al., 1999. Corneal endothelial deposits in children positive for human immunodeficiency virus receiving rifabutin prophylaxis for *Mycobacterium avium* complex bacteremia. Am. J. Ophthalmol. 127, 164–169.

Cardiac Glycosides

Blair, J.R., Mieler, W.F., 1995. Retinal toxicity associated with commonly encountered systemic agents. Int. Ophthalmol. Clin. 35, 137–156.

Robertson, D.M., Hollenhorst, T.W., Callahan, J.A., 1966. Ocular manifestations of digitalis toxicity. Discussion and report of three cases of central scotoma. Arch. Ophthalmol. 76, 640–645.

Weleber, R.G., Shults, W.T., 1981. Digoxin retinal toxicity: clinical and electrophysiologic evaluation of a cone dysfunction syndrome. Arch. Ophthalmol. 99, 1568–1572.

Methanol

Baumbach, G.L., Cancilla, P.A., Martin-Amat, G., et al., 1977. Methyl alcohol poisoning, IV: alterations of the morphological findings of the retina and optic nerve. Arch. Ophthalmol. 95, 1859–1865.

Eells, J.T., 1991. Methanol-induced visual toxicity in the rat. J. Pharmacol. Exp. Ther. 257, 56–63.

Frisen, L., Malmgren, K., 2003. Characterization of vigabatrin-associated optic atrophy. Acta Ophthalmol. Scand. 81, 466–473.

Fujihara, M., Kikuchi, M., Kurimoto, Y., 2006. Methanol-induced retinal toxicity patient examined by optical coherence tomography. Jpn. J. Ophthalmol. 50, 239–241.

Hayreh, M.S., Hayreh, S.S., Baumbach, G.L., et al., 1977. Methyl alcohol poisoning, III: Ocular toxicity. Arch. Ophthalmol. 95, 1851–1858.

Treichel, J.L., Murray, T.G., Lewandowski, M.F., et al., 2004. Retinal toxicity in methanol poisoning. Retina 24, 309–312.

CHAPTER 15

Congenital and Developmental Anomalies of the Optic Nerve

Optic Nerve Hypoplasia

Optic nerve hypoplasia appears to be the result of excessive pruning of the optic nerve bundles during its development. The disc is pale and may be surrounded by a variably pigmented yellow–white ring. This appearance has been referred to as the "double ring" sign. While the nerve head is small, the retinal vessels are usually of normal caliber. It may occur in one or both eyes and be associated with mild to severe visual impairment, including limited visual acuity and visual field deficits.

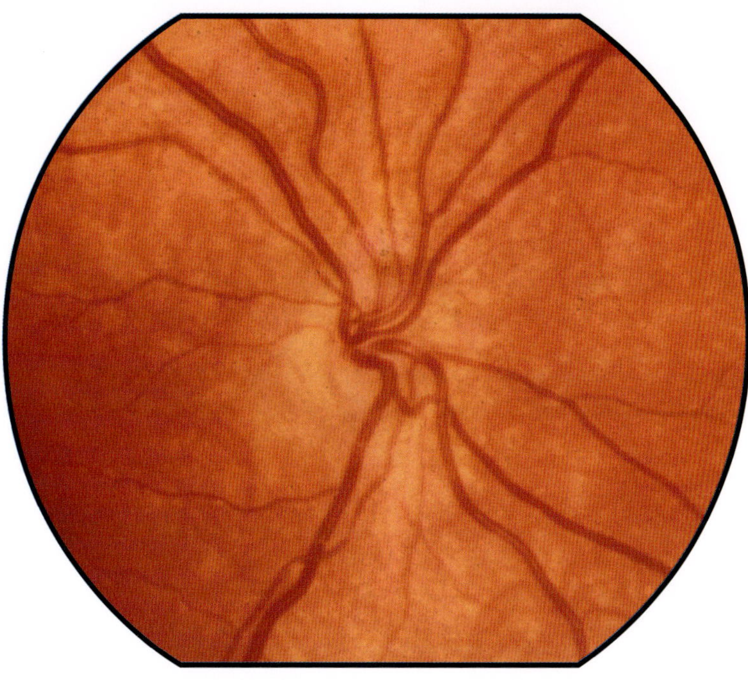

This patient has a hypoplastic right optic disc. An incomplete "double ring" is present on the temporal aspect of the nerve. The retinal arteries and veins appear of normal caliber and exit and enter centrally. The crowded central cup places these nerves at risk for vascular occlusive disease, including large retinal venous and arterial occlusions, as well as ischemic papillopathy.

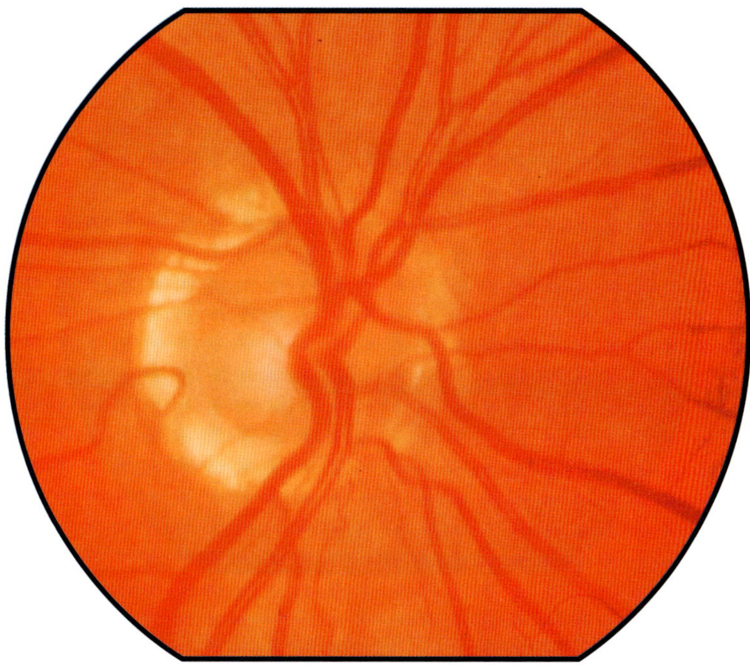

This patient exhibits the classic complete "double ring" sign of optic nerve hypoplasia.

Megalopapilla

Megalopapilla classically presents as an enlarged, but otherwise normal appearing optic disc. Patients often present with good visual acuity, but mild to moderate visual deficits may be seen.

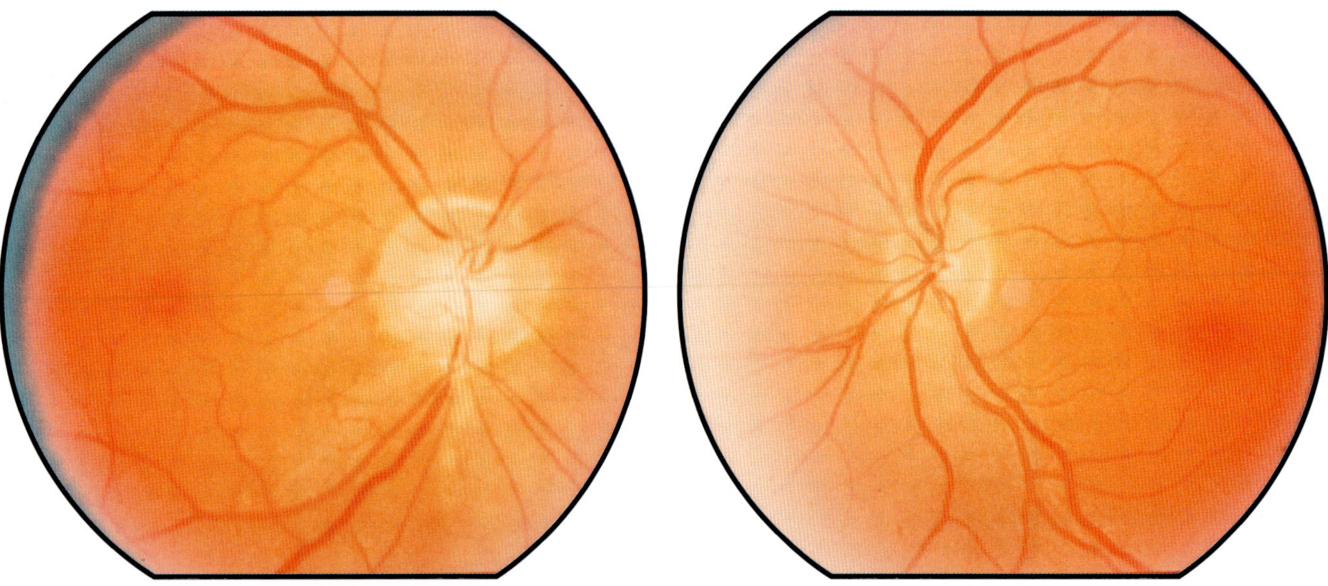

This patient exhibits distinct asymmetry between the sizes of the optic discs compatible with megalopapilla. Visual function was normal.

Optic Nerve Aplasia

Optic nerve aplasia denotes total absence of the optic nerve, retinal blood vessels, and retinal ganglion cells. It is a rare condition, most commonly unilateral, and associated with microphthalmos, retinochoroidal colobomas, and cataracts. No light perception visual acuity and an afferent pupillary defect are common findings.

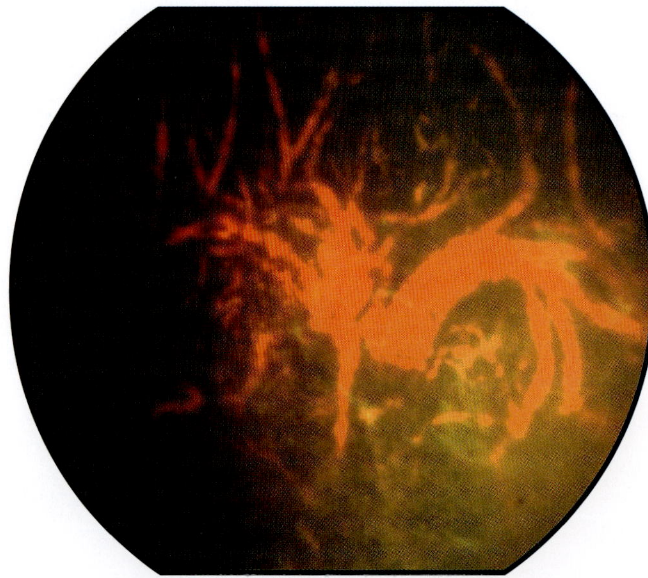

This patient has unilateral optic nerve aplasia. This photograph was taken in the region where the optic nerve should have been located. Note the complete absence of the optic nerve and associated blood vessels, and the extensive thinning of the retinal pigment epithelium (RPE).

Congenital Prepapillary Vascular Loops

Congenital vascular anomalies, or congenital prepapillary vascular loops, usually appear as tortuous loops of an arteriole or venule that extend above the plane of the optic nerve and into the vitreous cavity. It may have a corkscrew or spiral shape and is often encased in a white fibroglial sheath as it enters the vitreous cavity. They are usually found in eyes with good visual acuity, though may be associated with retinal arterial obstruction in the distribution of the retina supplied by the loop. Amaurosis fugax and vitreous hemorrhage have also rarely been reported.

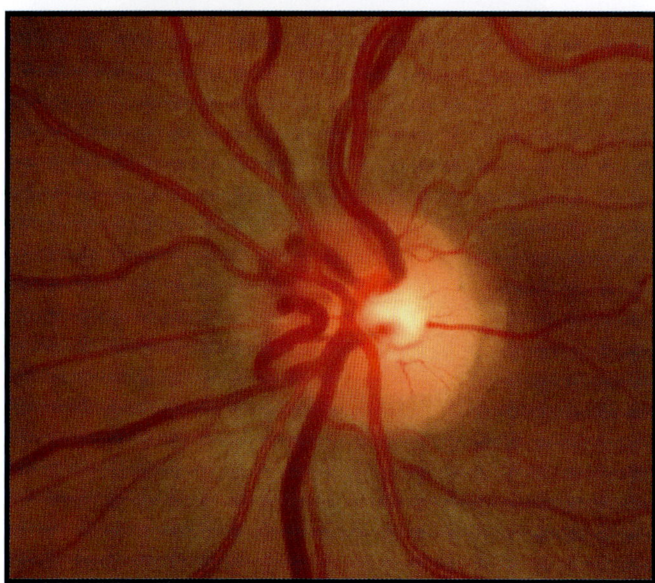

A congenital vascular loop with a "hairpin" configuration is seen on the nasal aspect of the optic nerve extending into the vitreous cavity. The vast majority of congenital vascular loops are arteriolar malformations. Visual function was normal in this patient.

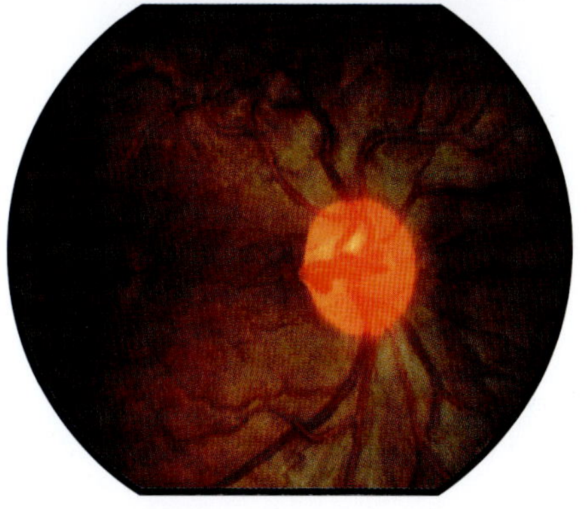

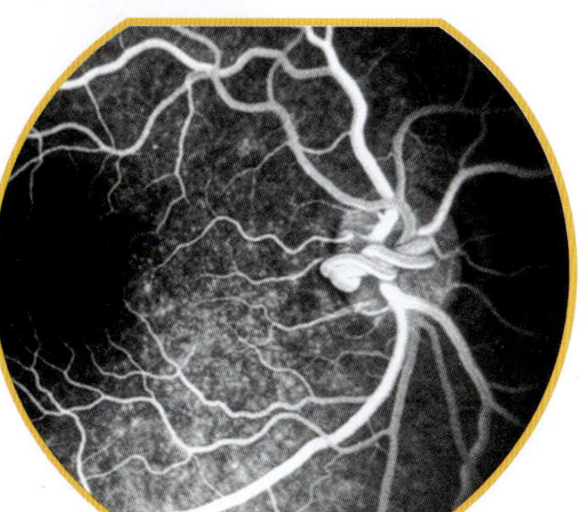

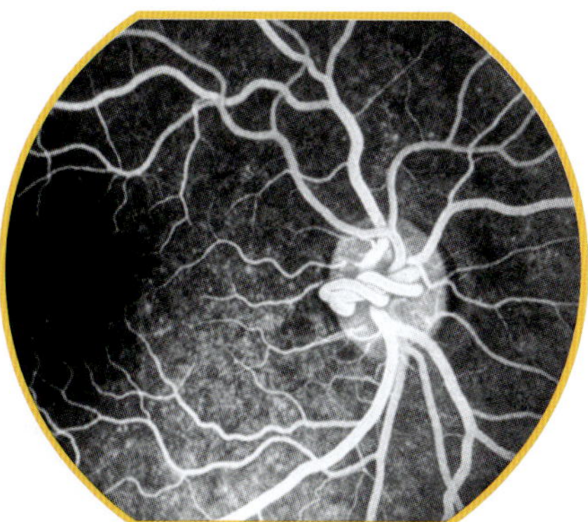

A corkscrew-shaped retinal arterial loop is seen overlying the center of the optic nerve in this asymptomatic patient.

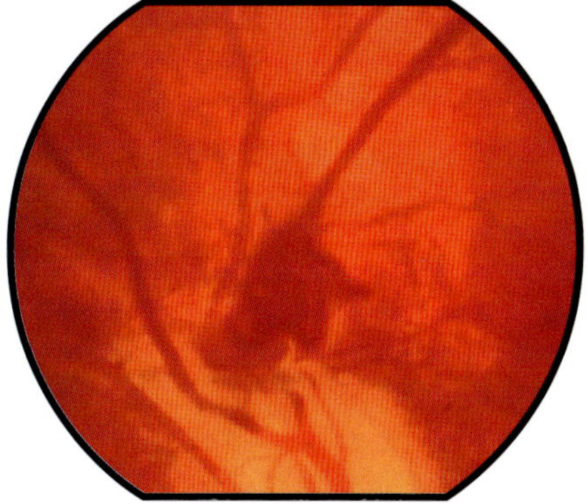

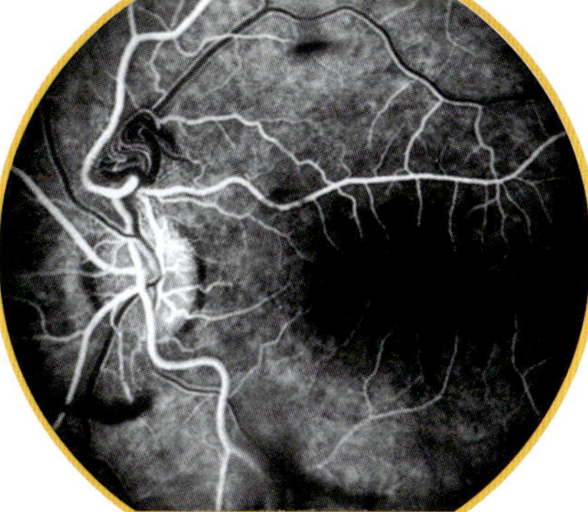

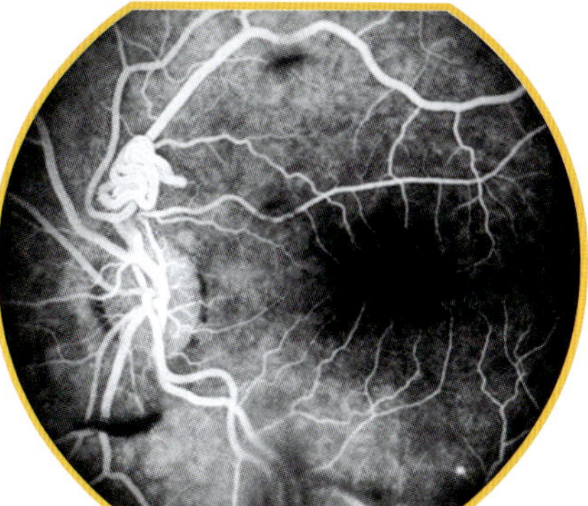

A patient with a congenital prepapillary venous loop located along the superior border of the optic disc. Note the slow venous filling. There is no leakage or evidence of vascular compromise within the vascular arcades.

Persistent Fetal Vasculature (PFV)

Regression of the hyaloid artery usually begins in the third month of gestation and is complete by the eighth month of gestation. Failure of regression may result in variable findings, from only threadlike remnants protruding from the optic nerve to a grossly visible vessel attached to the posterior capsule of the lens, usually in an inferonasal location. If the hyaloid artery is encased by a glial sheath of neuroectodermal cells it is known as Bergmeister papilla.

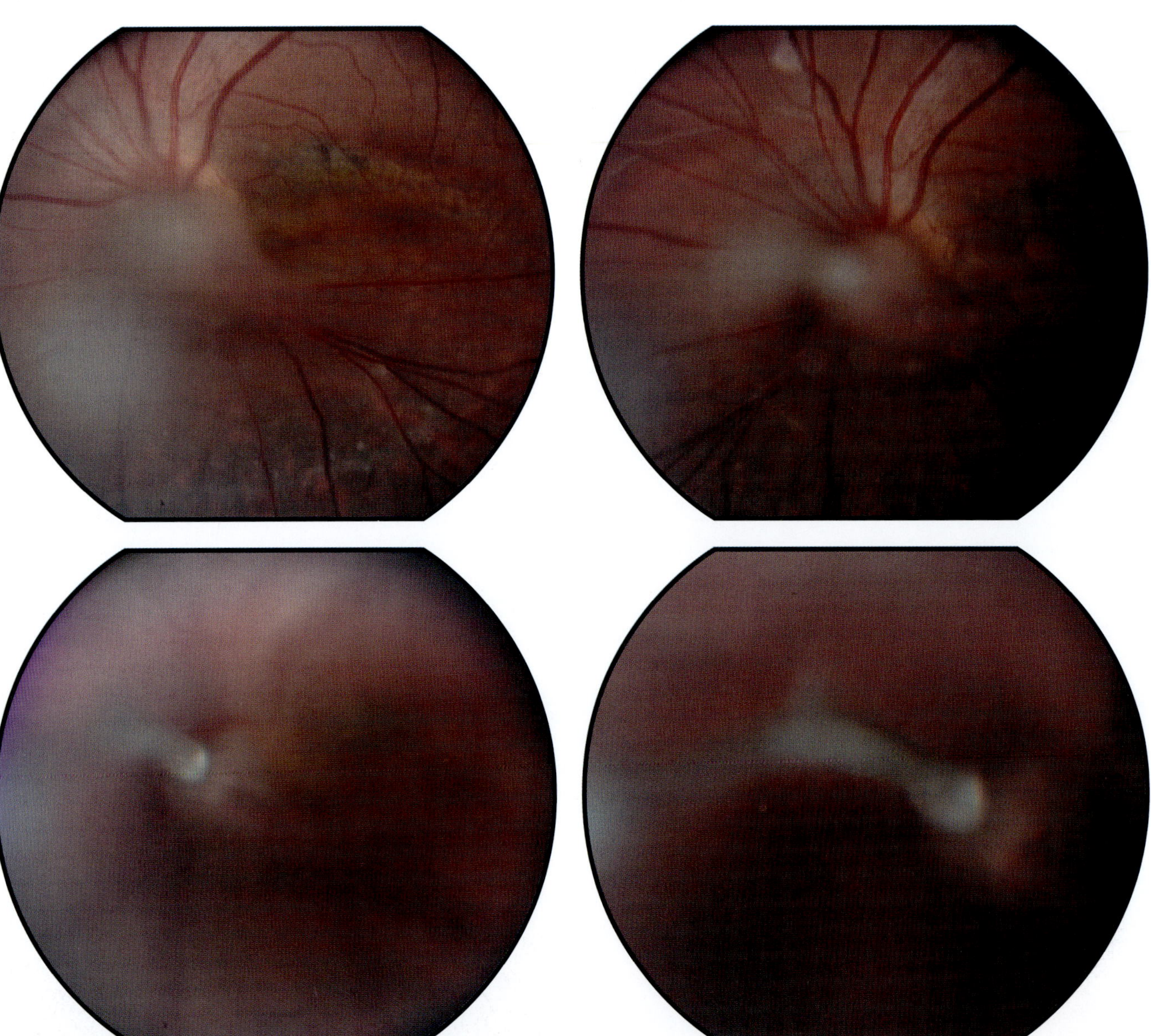

Incomplete regression of the hyaloid artery, with an attachment to the posterior surface of the lens. This patient also had a localized posterior retinal detachment. This 5-month-old patient underwent lensectomy/vitrectomy surgery, with stabilization of the anatomic abnormalities. Dense amblyopia limited visual recovery in spite of ocular patching and utilization of a corrective contact lens.

Bergmeister Papilla

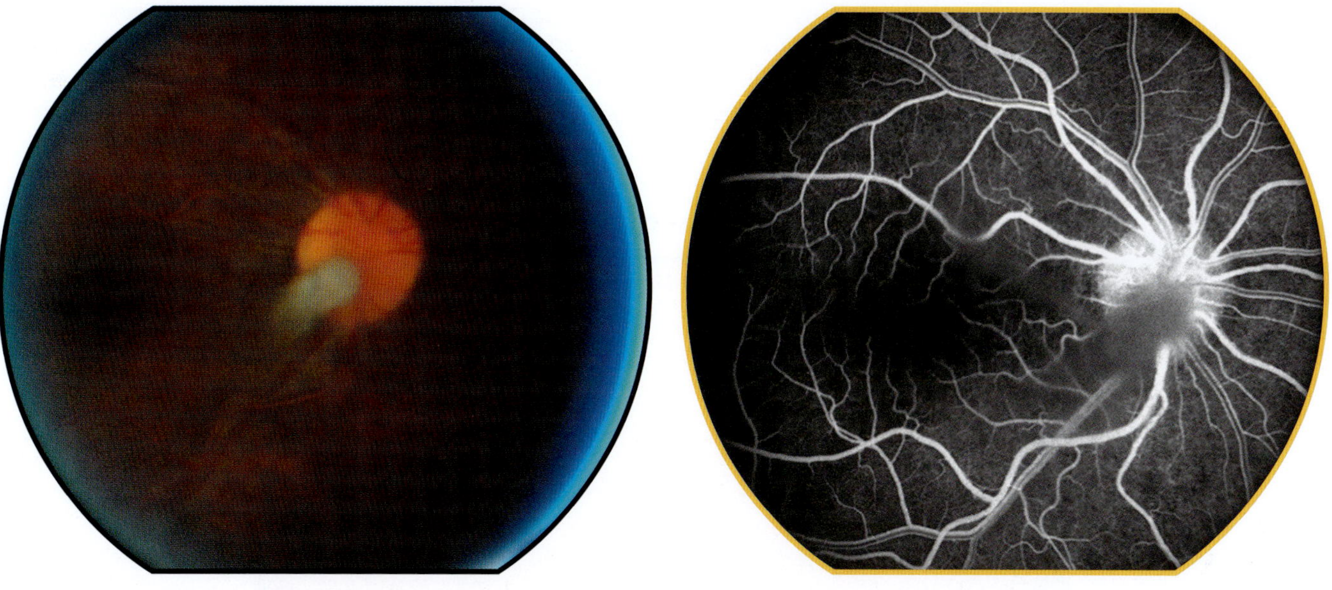

A fibrous encased vascular stalk coursing above the plane of the optic disc, though not reaching the posterior surface of the lens. This finding was of no visual consequence.

Congenital Retinal Macrovessel

A congenital retinal macrovessel is a rare vascular anomaly that appears as an enlarged vessel exiting the optic nerve and traversing the macula with several first-order tributaries extending superior and inferior to its horizontal course. The optic nerve itself is generally normal. Venous macrovessels are more common than arterial and are most commonly located in an inferotemporal location. Visual acuity is usually preserved despite the vessel crossing over or through the foveal avascular zone.

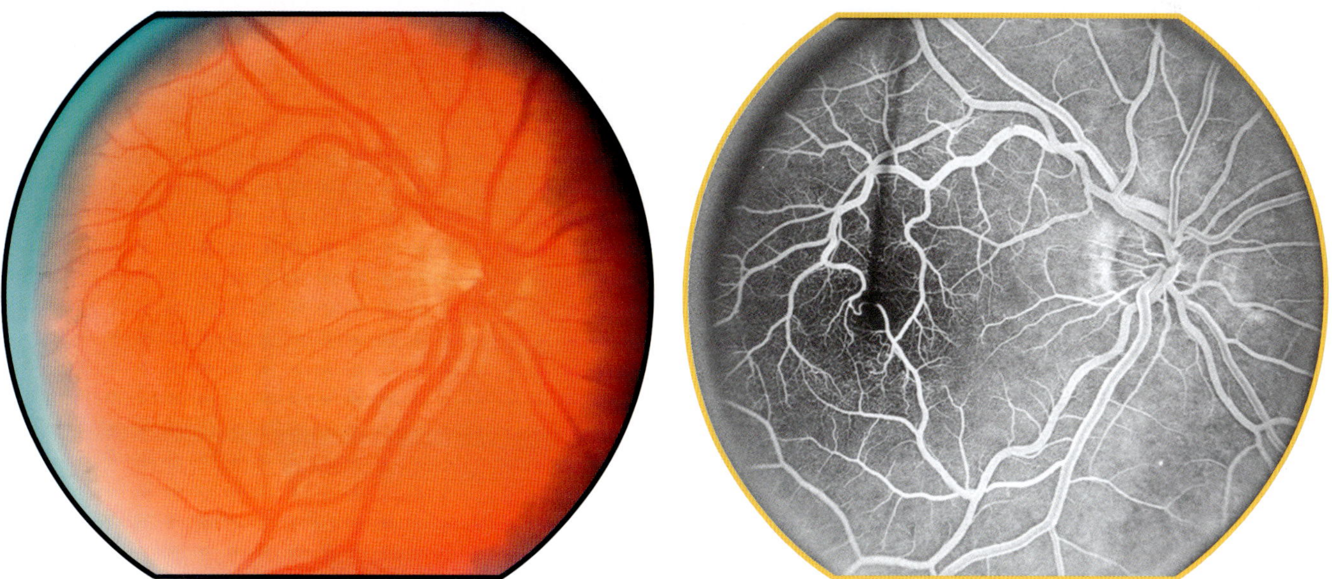

A congenital retinal macrovessel emanates from the superior aspect of the optic nerve and courses along the superior vascular arcade. The vessels then cross the macular region and extend inferiorly. While visual function was normal, there appears to be slight enlargement of the macular capillary free zone. The optic nerve was normal.

Cilioretinal Artery Occlusion

A cilioretinal artery is seen in approximately 5 to 10% of patients and is generally temporal in location. It emerges from the optic nerve separately from the vessels derived from the central retinal artery. It often has a hook-like appearance and exits from the nerve substance and/or the edge of the nerve with approximate equal frequency. A cilioretinal artery becomes significant when an occlusion occurs. This may occur by itself or in conjunction with a central retinal vein occlusion. If the artery supplies blood to the papillomacular bundle and the macular region, significant visual loss may occur. The converse scenario may also be seen, in that in the setting of a central retinal artery occlusion, a cilioretinal artery may be protective in the preservation of central visual function.

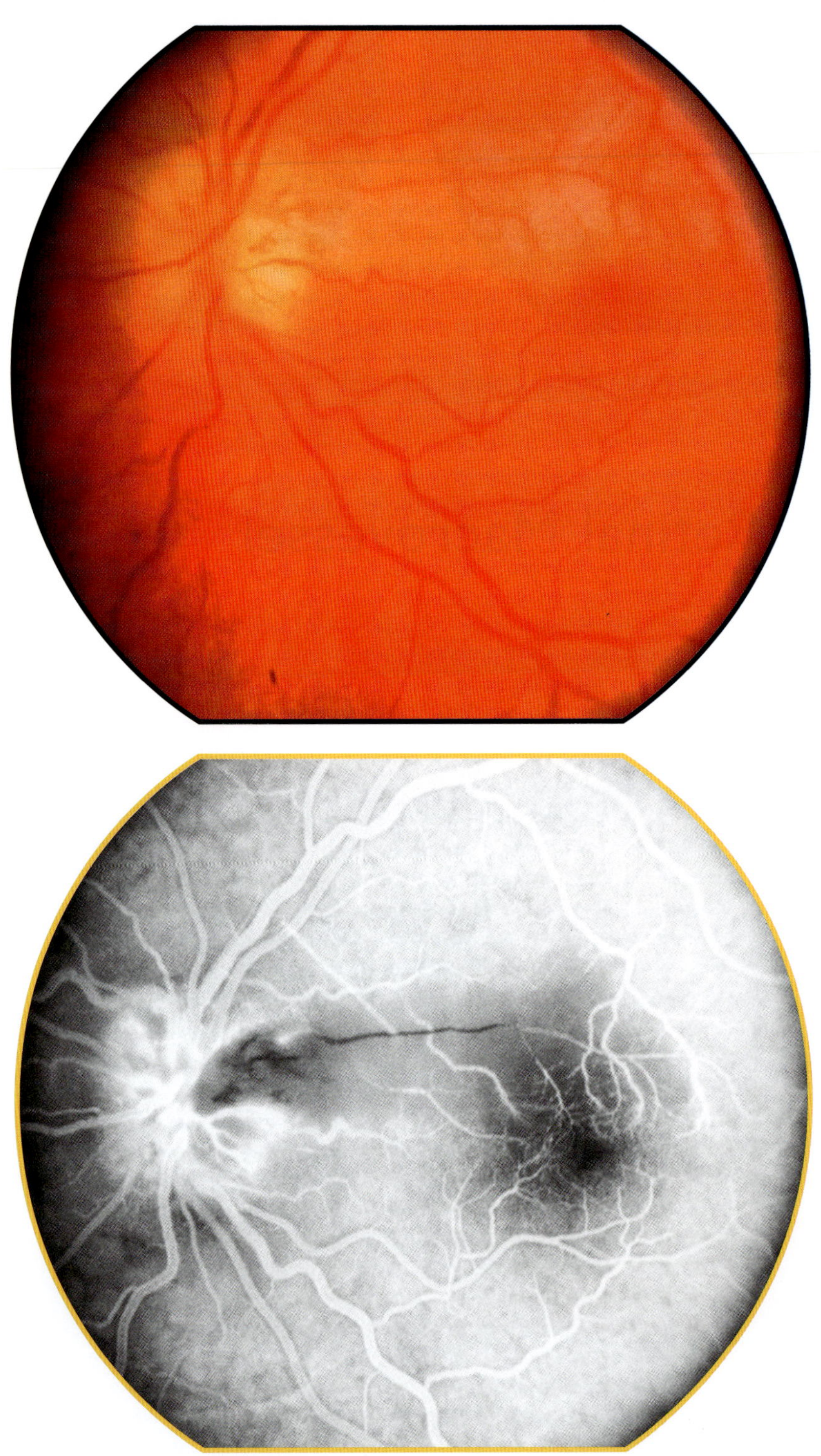

A cilioretinal artery occlusion is seen in this patient, with ischemia along the superior portion of the papillomacular bundle. While the patient was aware of a pericentral visual field deficit, the central vision remained 20/25.

Optic Nerve, Retinochoroidal, and Iris Colobomas

Congenital coloboma of the optic nerve is characterized by absent tissue and may show enlargement of the papillary area, partial or total excavation with a white surface, and retinal vessels that enter and exit from the borders of the defect. The affected nerve is commonly larger than normal in diameter. The coloboma may be unilateral or bilateral, and it is thought to be secondary to a failure of fusion of the posterior part of the embryonic fissure. Coloboma of the optic nerve may be caused by a mutation in the PAX6 gene.

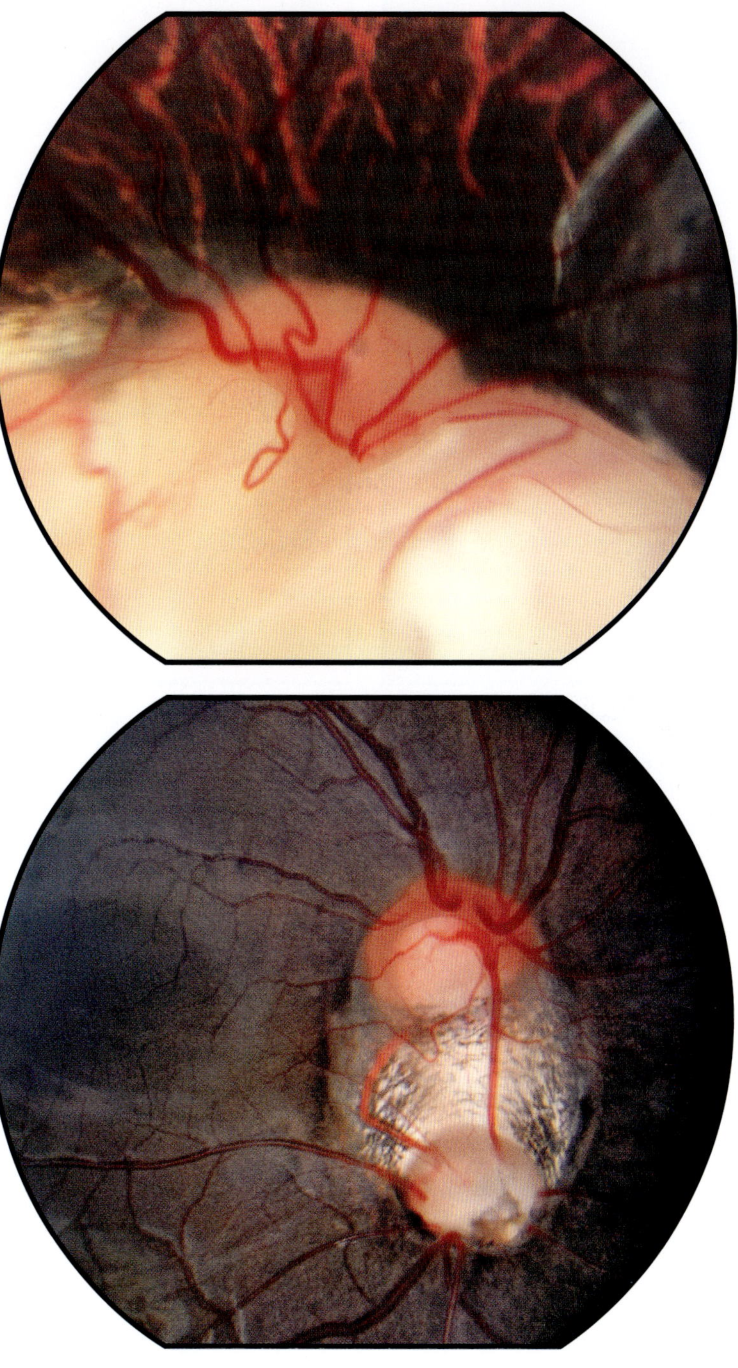

These two patients have a coloboma of the optic nerve in conjunction with a contiguous coloboma of the choroid. In the lower photo, there is a fistulous tract that extends posteriorly, simulating a second optic nerve in appearance.

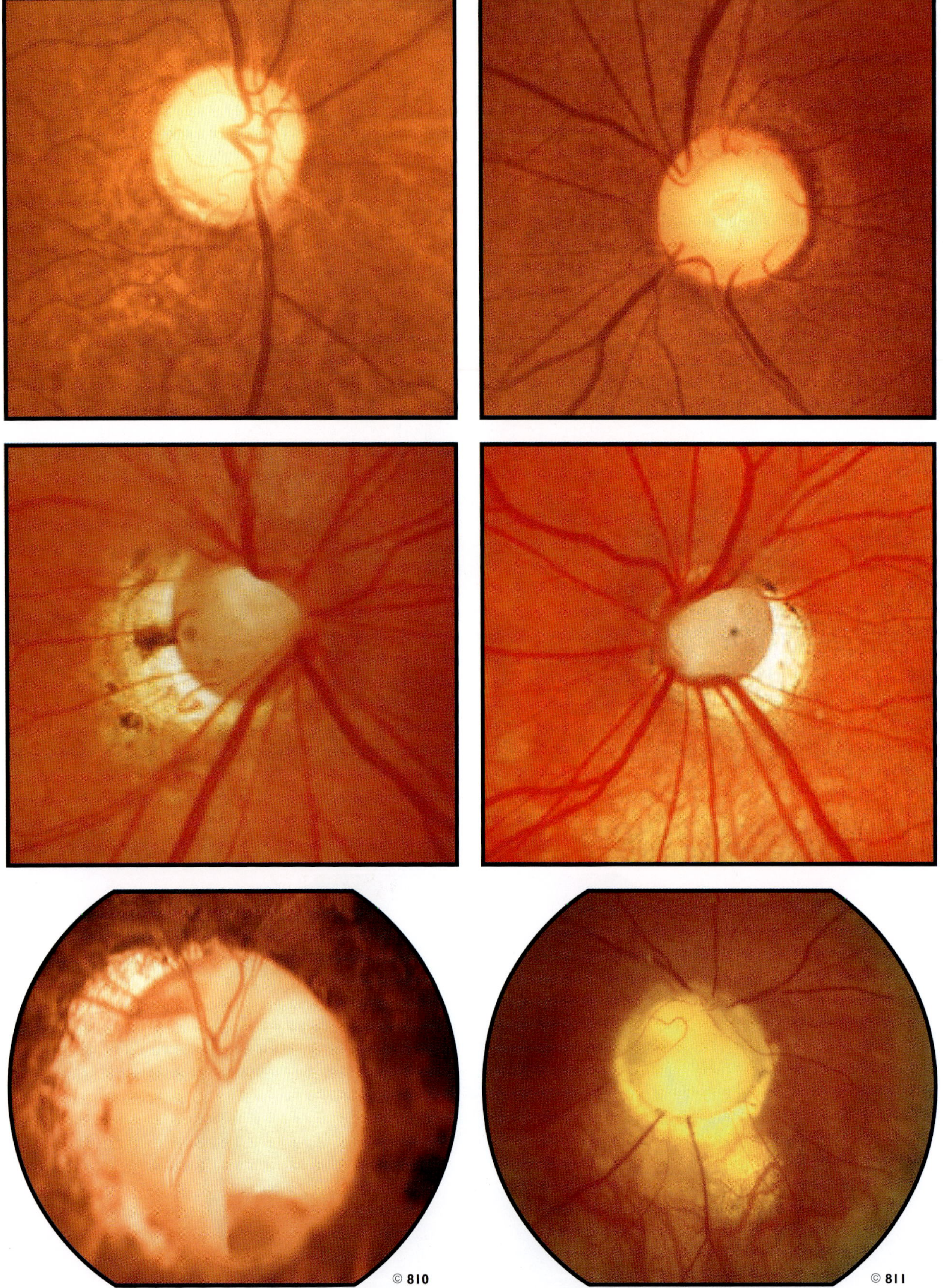

Excavation of the optic nerve, essentially a coloboma of the optic nerve secondary to cupping from glaucoma *(top and middle rows)*. In some patients, the colobomatous nature with fibrous proliferation and additional retinal vascular anomalous changes serve to differentiate this group of patients from other congenital anomalies and acquired disorders, such as glaucoma, trauma, or acquired ischemia.

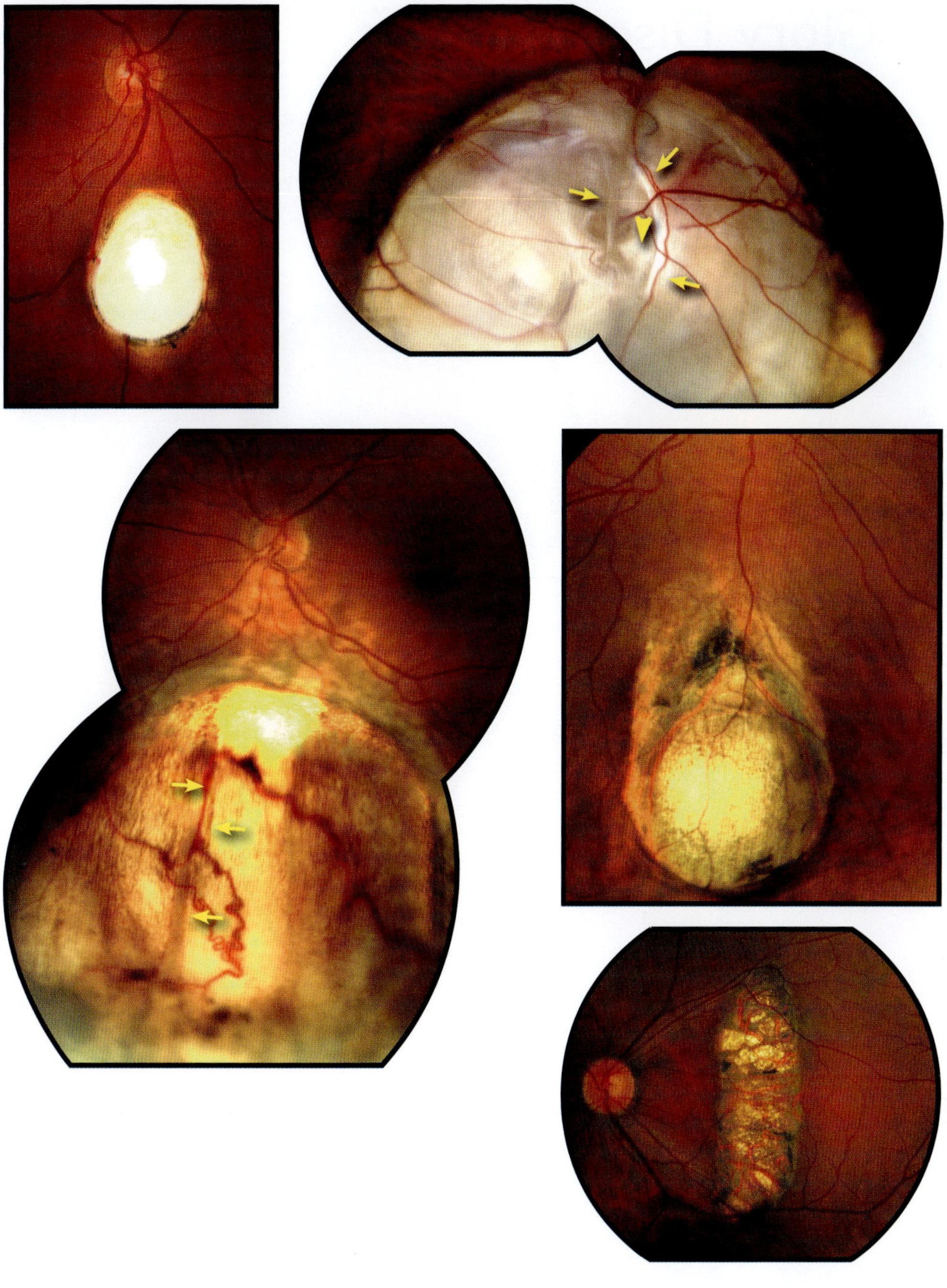

A coloboma may involve the retinochoroid with or without concurrent optic nerve involvement. In this patient, there is a ridge of fibrous tissue bordering the superior aspect of the coloboma *(middle left, arrows)*. There is pre- and subretinal fibrosis *(upper right, arrows)* and a fissure through the sclera *(arrowhead)*. Colobomas may be associated with non-rhegmatogenous serous retinal detachments of the macula. Pigment epithelial hyperplasia is often seen at the margins of such a coloboma, sometimes in conjunction with a zonal area of atrophy from a resolved antecedent detachment.

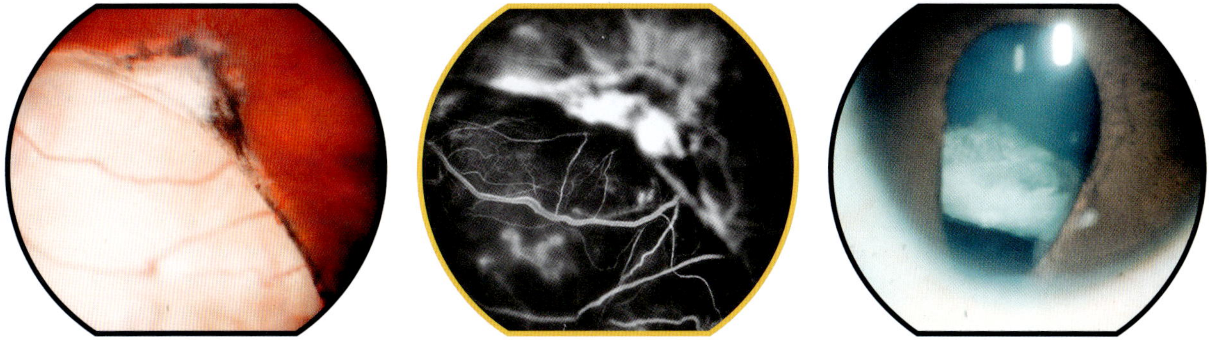

A patient with a very large inferonasal retinochoroidal coloboma and an associated iris coloboma. The fluorescein angiogram documents almost complete hypofluorescence due to lack of RPE and choriocapillaris within the confines of the coloboma.

Morning Glory Disc Anomaly

The morning glory disc anomaly is a variant of an optic nerve coloboma. It is classically an enlarged, unilateral, funnel-shaped excavation of the optic nerve head with a central core of pale glial tissue. The margins are raised and chorioretinal pigmentary changes are commonly present at its border. Retinal vessels course near the margins, but are obscured centrally by glial tissue. It is more common in females and affects right eyes to a slightly greater degree than left eyes. There may be persistent hyaloidal remnants in the base of the excavation.

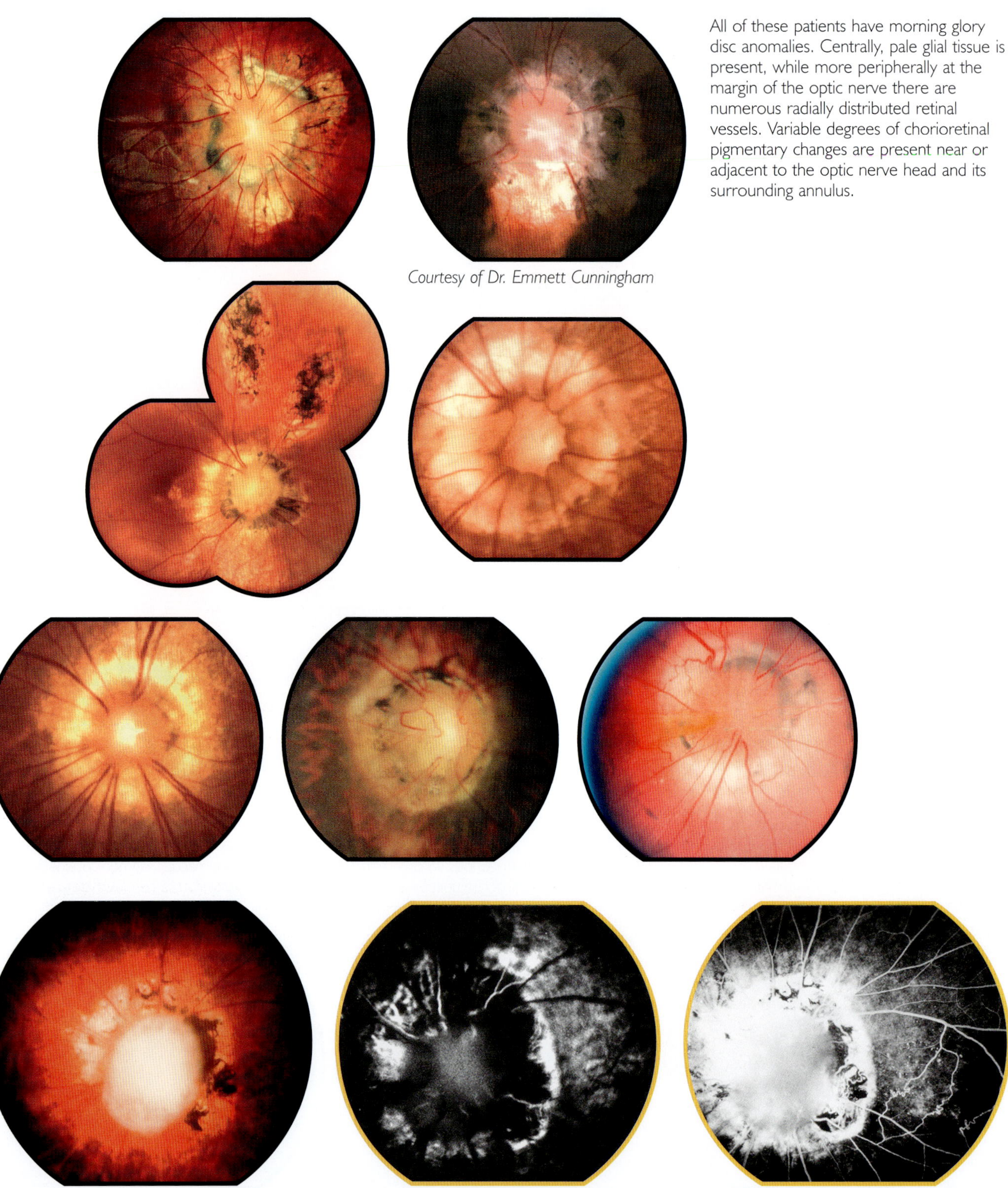

All of these patients have morning glory disc anomalies. Centrally, pale glial tissue is present, while more peripherally at the margin of the optic nerve there are numerous radially distributed retinal vessels. Variable degrees of chorioretinal pigmentary changes are present near or adjacent to the optic nerve head and its surrounding annulus.

Courtesy of Dr. Emmett Cunningham

A patient with a morning glory disc anomaly showing a glial cap over the optic nerve. The retinal vessels appear to exit the nerve in a more peripheral location, and this is seen quite readily on the accompanying fluorescein angiograms.

Optic Nerve Pit

(Also see Chapter 11, Peripheral Retinal Degenerations and Rhegmatogenous Retinal Detachment)

An optic nerve head pit is an uncommon congenital anomaly that may result from imperfect closure of the superior edge of the embryonic fissure. It appears as a grey-white round or oval-shaped depression on the inferotemporal aspect of the optic nerve, often with adjacent peripapillary chorioretinal atrophy or retinal pigment epithelial pigment changes. Associated non-rhegmatogenous serous retinal detachments of the macula and schisis cavities are common. The origin of the subretinal fluid is controversial, but may arise from the vitreous cavity, leakage from retinal vessels within the pit or adjacent choroid, or may be cerebrospinal fluid leaking into the subretinal space via the subarachnoid space. In the presence of a long-standing serous macular detachment, pars plana vitrectomy surgery is often offered as treatment.

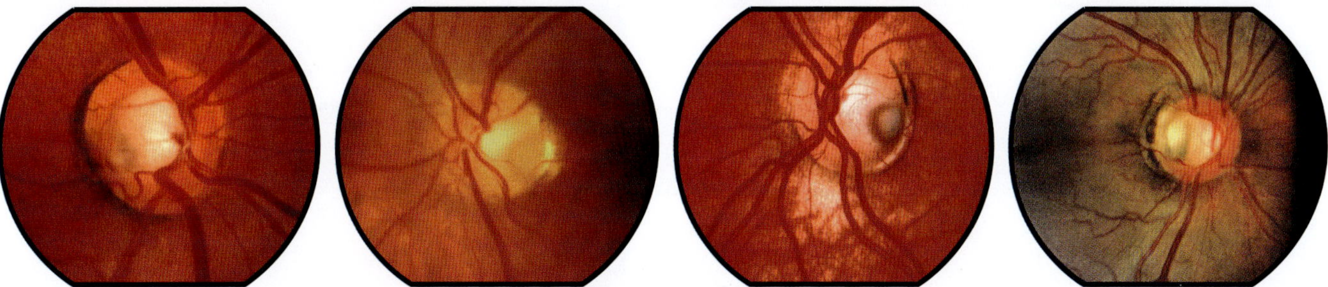

Several patients with optic nerve pits are shown. The pits are round, pale depressions most commonly found in a temporal location with adjacent chorioretinal pigmentary changes. Visual acuity is typically excellent except in cases of non-rhegmatogenous serous detachments. There is an association between optic nerve pits and glaucoma. *Third image courtesy of Dr. Eric Shrier*

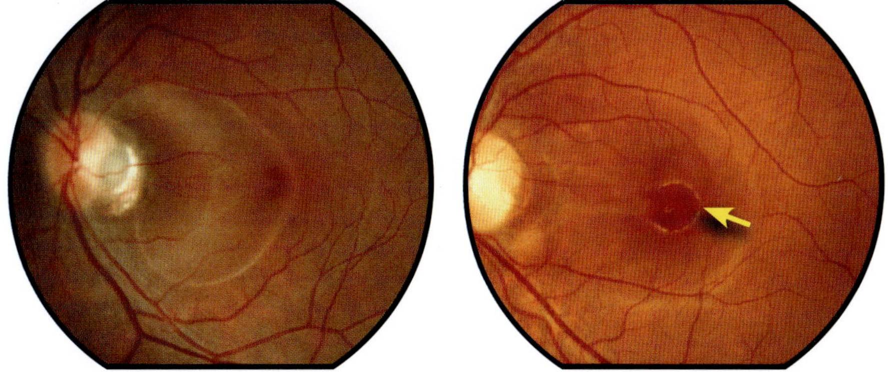

Two patients have an optic nerve head pit with a macular detachment, consisting of schisis and neurosensory elevation. Thinning of the inner limiting membrane is present in the fovea in the patient on the right, which gives the appearance of a macular hole *(arrow)*. Chronic serous detachments may result in localized formation of subretinal precipitates and mimic the appearance of central serous chorioretinopathy.

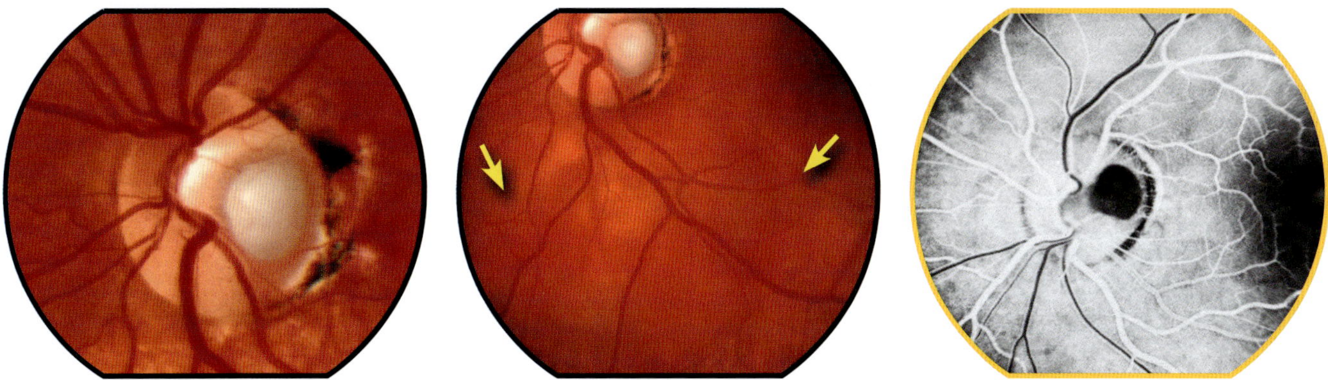

This patient has an optic nerve head pit in association with a dual macular detachment composed of intraretinal schisis and a neurosensory elevation. The middle image shows a serous detachment inferior to the nerve *(arrows)*. The detachment resolved following photocoagulation to the temporal edge of the disc. The fluorescein angiogram shows no leakage from the pit.

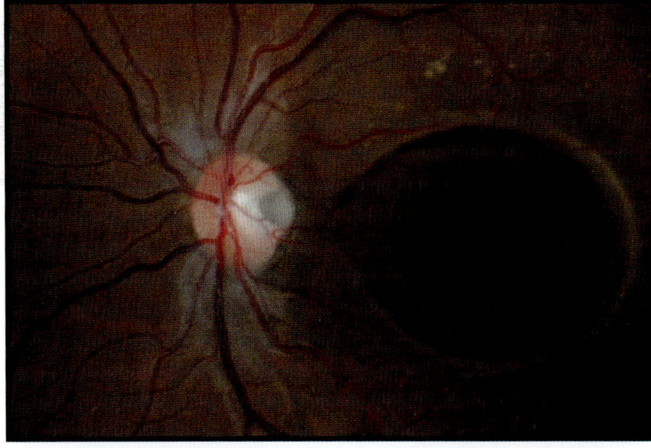

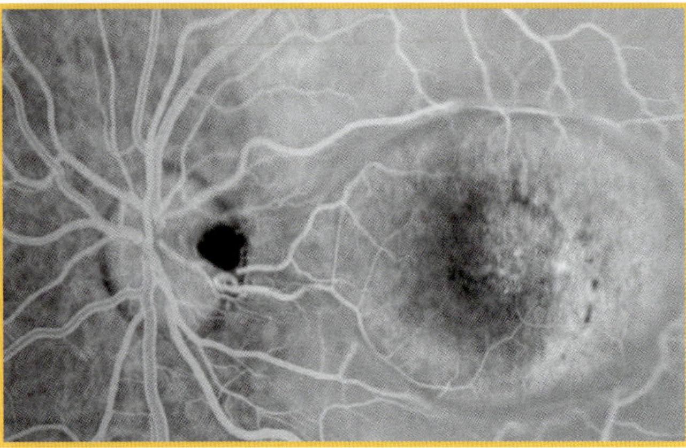

A color fundus photo and associated fluorescein angiogram in a patient with an optic nerve pit and serous macular detachment demonstrates no leakage near the pit or beneath the detachment. The optic pit is hypofluorescent on fluorescein angiography. *Courtesy of Dr. Jonathan G. Williams*

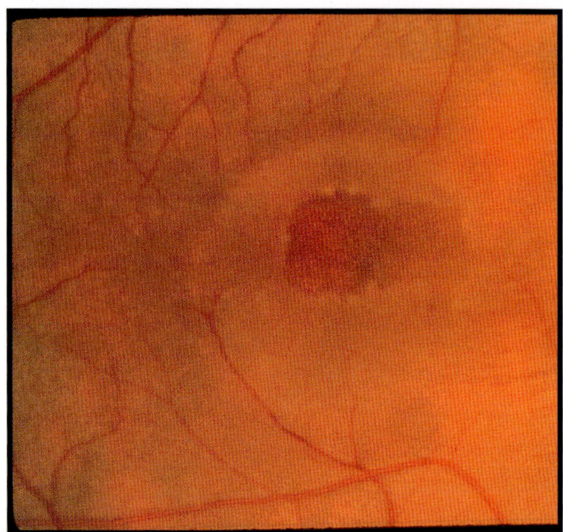

© **812**

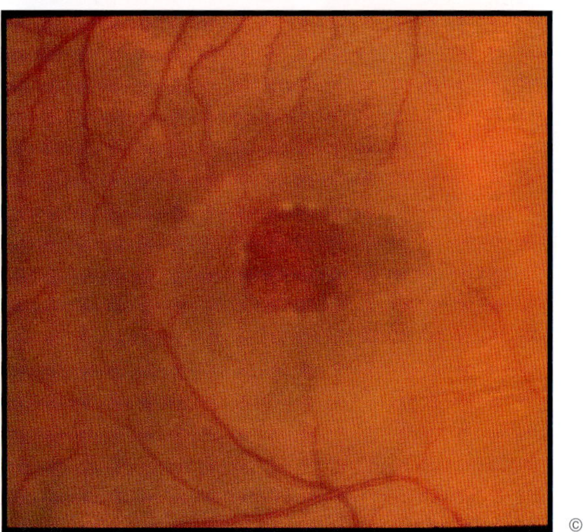

© **813**

A patient with an optic pit developed a serous neurosensory detachment and a lamellar hole. An external lamellar or full-thickness macular hole may develop within the detached retina of patients with optic pits.

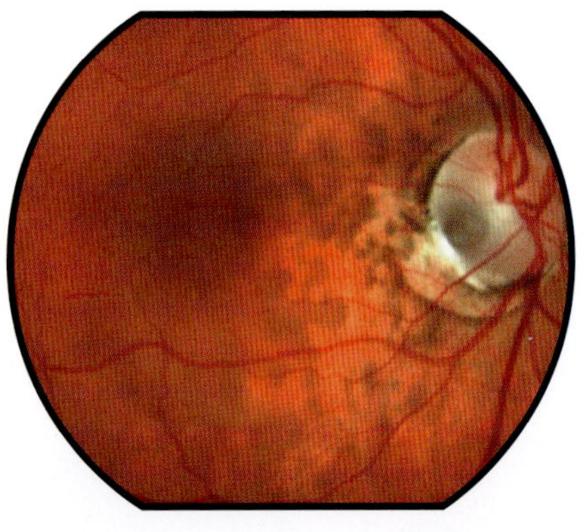

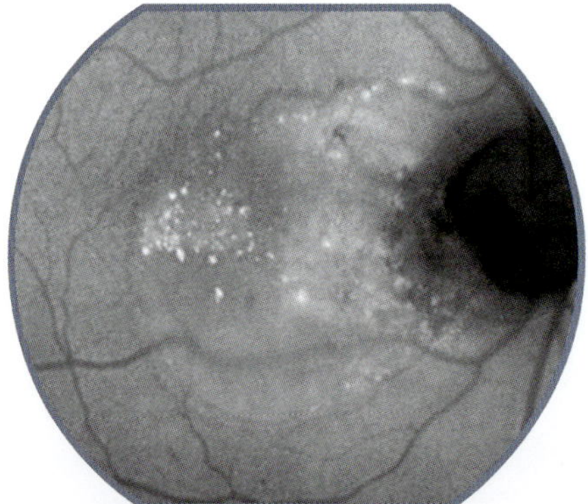

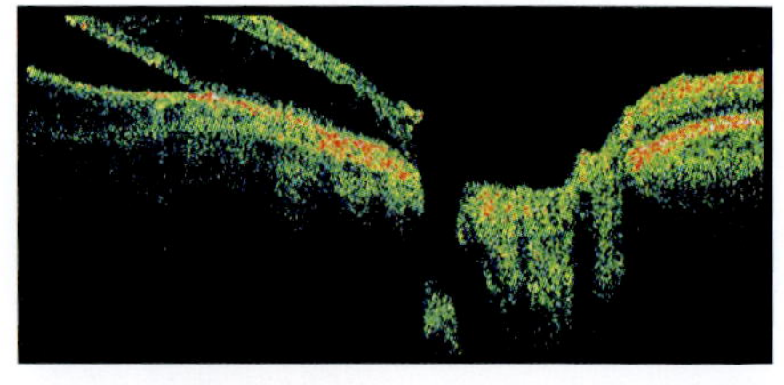

Chronic serous detachments may result in localized formation of subretinal precipitates and chorioretinal pigmentary changes. The optic pit leaves degenerated photoreceptors in the subretinal space that contain chromophores detectable with fundus autofluorescence (FAF) *(middle)*. The optical coherence tomography (OCT) shows the pit of the retina combined with a schisis cavity.

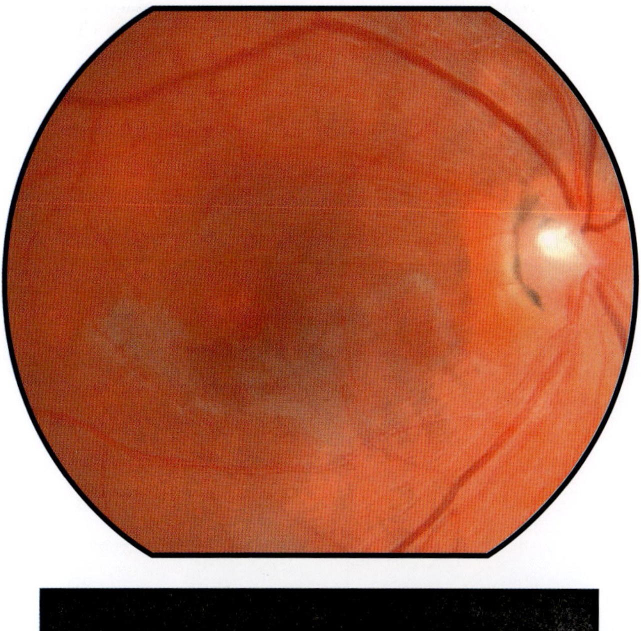

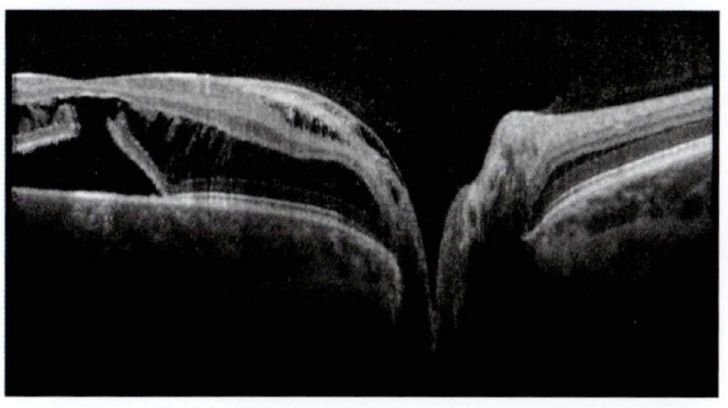

A patient with an optic nerve pit and an associated serous schisis macular detachment. The detachment did not improve spontaneously, so therefore the patient underwent eventual pars plana vitrectomy surgery, which led to successful resolution of the serous macular detachment and improvement in visual function.

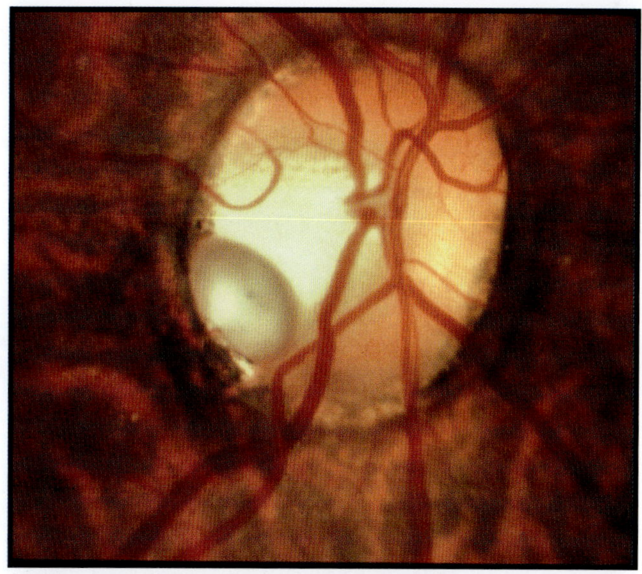

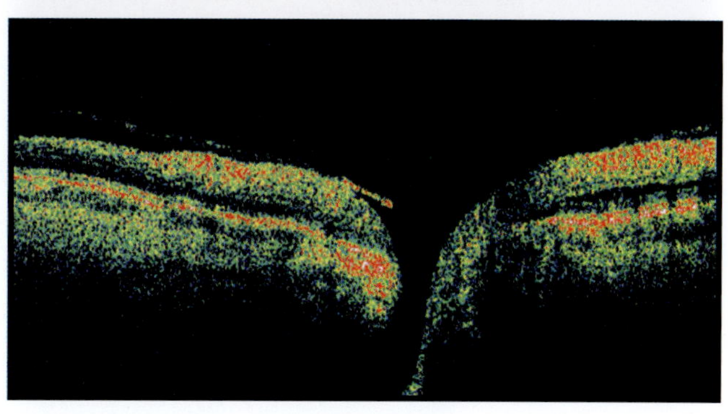

A patient with an optic disc pit in the inferotemporal location. The OCT shows a deep excavation of the optic nerve pit in this patient.

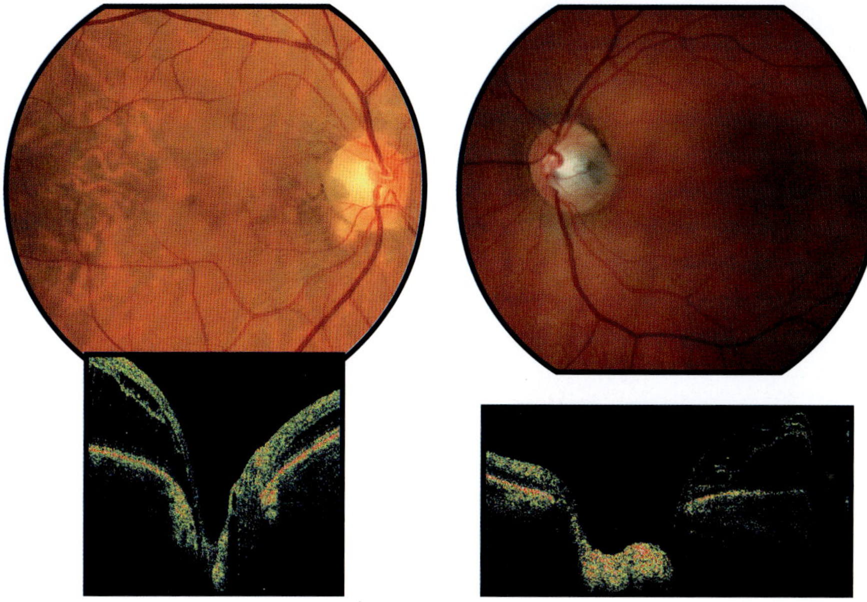

This patient presented with bilateral optic nerve pits and combined detachments. A schisis cavity and full-thickness retinal separation in contiguity with an excavation on the nerve head is readily apparent on the OCT image. *Bottom left image courtesy of Dr. Hideki Koizumi*

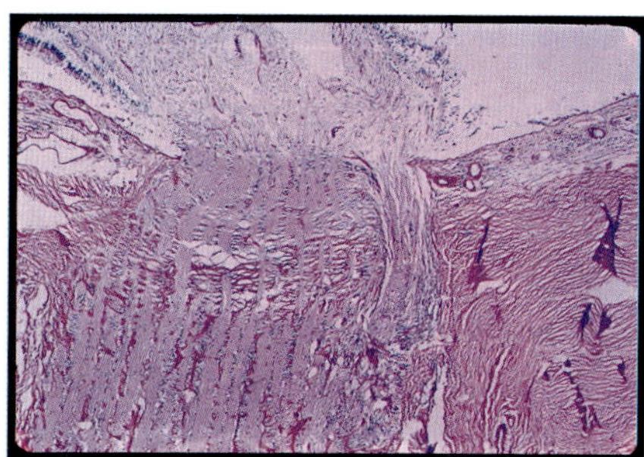

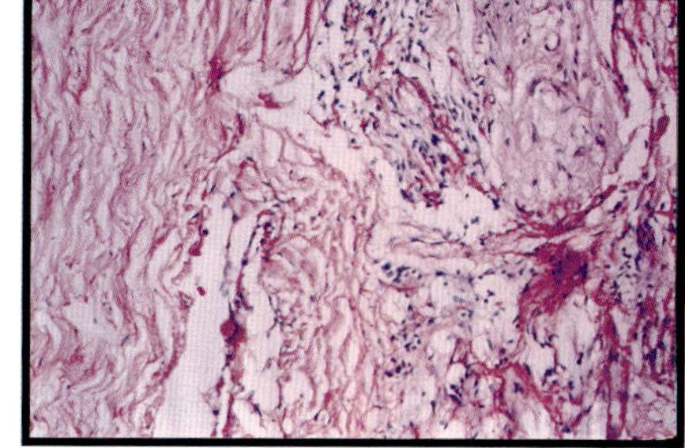

Histopathologic light microscopy of an optic nerve head pit in the temporal aspect of the optic nerve head. Neuronal tissue can be seen entering the pit from the adjacent retina and extends far below the lamina cribrosa. Only a thin diaphanous tissue separates the optic pit from the subarachnoid space.

Situs Inversus

The retinal vessels exiting from the optic nerve generally progress directly temporally. However, on occasion they take a nasal bend, prior to heading temporally. The temporal half of the nerve generally appears full, and the optic cup is generally absent. Optic nerve hypoplasia may also be seen. This finding is also referred to as tilted disc syndrome (see below), nasal fundus ectasia, and Fuchs coloboma. Patients are generally asymptomatic.

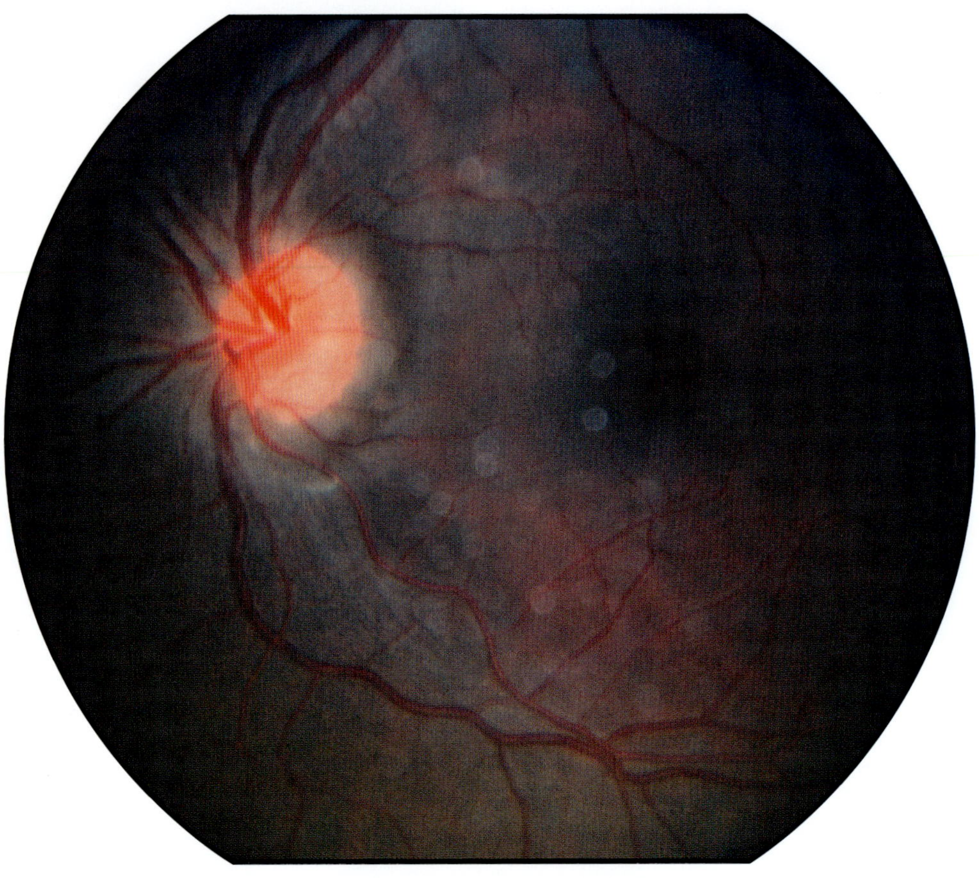

The retinal vessels in this patient exit this optic nerve in a nasal direction prior to turning temporally. The patient was visually asymptomatic. Note the absence of a central optic nerve cup.

Tilted Disc Syndrome

Features of tilted disc syndrome include inferonasal tilting, an inferior or inferonasal crescent, situs inversus of the retinal vessels, fundus ectasia, myopia, and astigmatism. About 75% of cases are bilateral. Choroidal neovascularization may occur due to weakness in Bruch membrane, usually near the crescent of a staphyloma in myopic eyes.

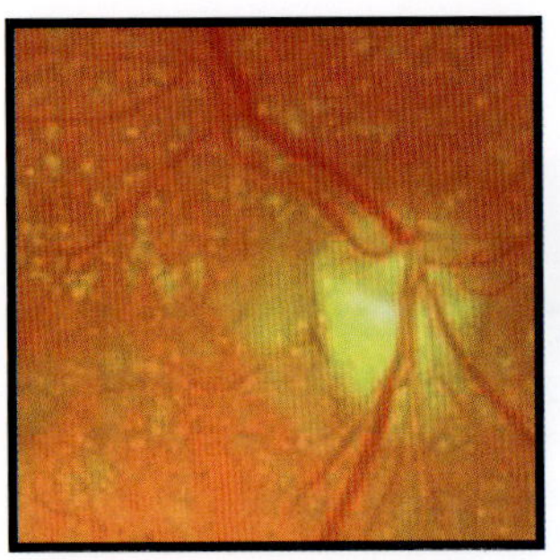

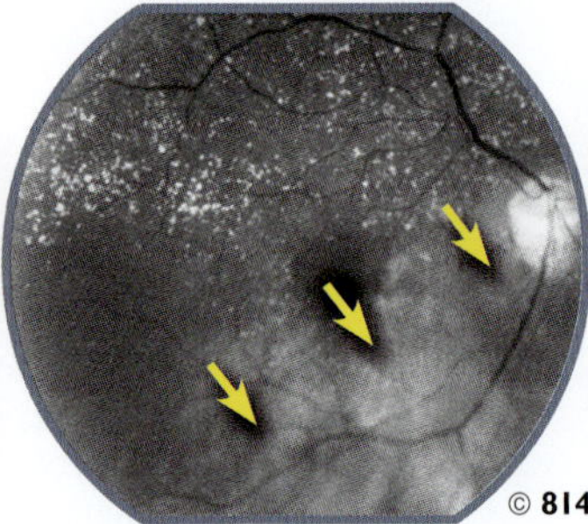

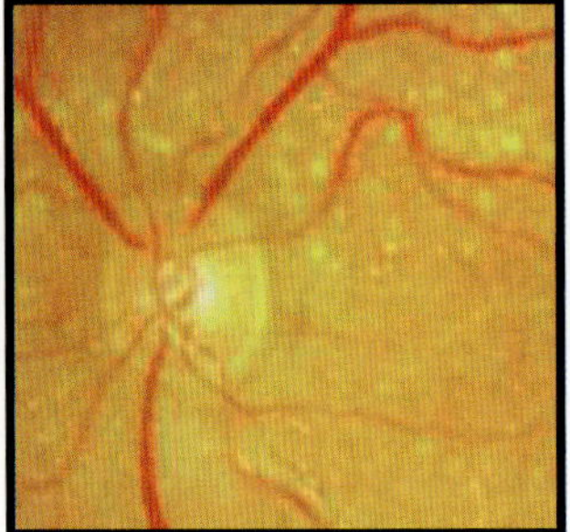

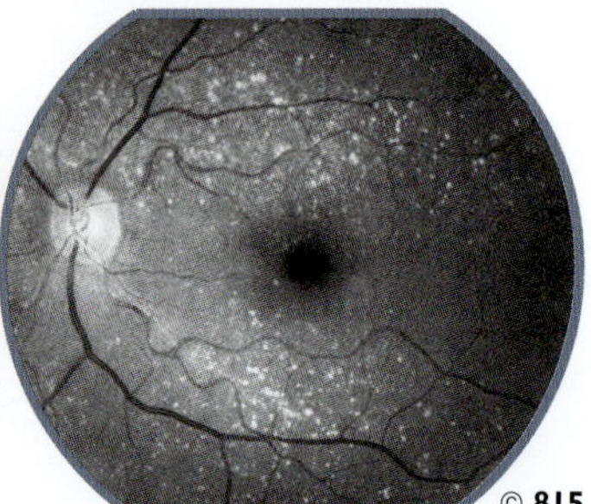

In this patient with tilted disc syndrome, there is an absence of drusenoid change within a staphylomatous area *(arrows)* of the right eye. The nerve in the fellow eye *(left)* is only mildly tilted. *Left and second from right image, courtesy of Dr. Salomen Cohen*

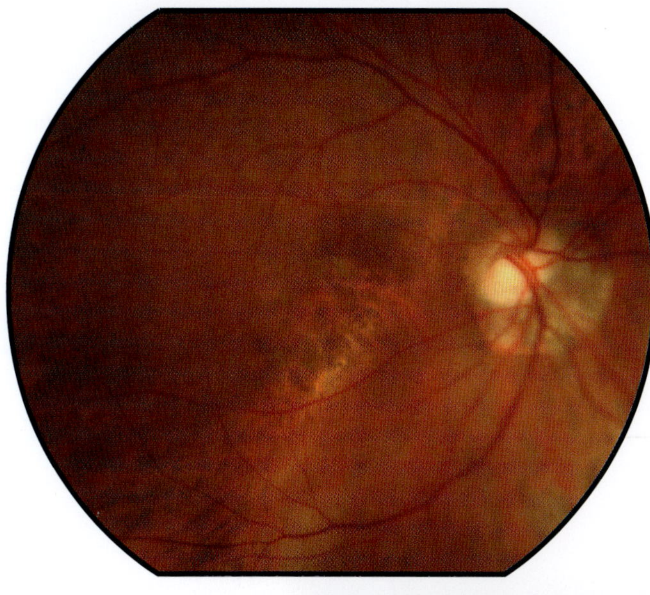
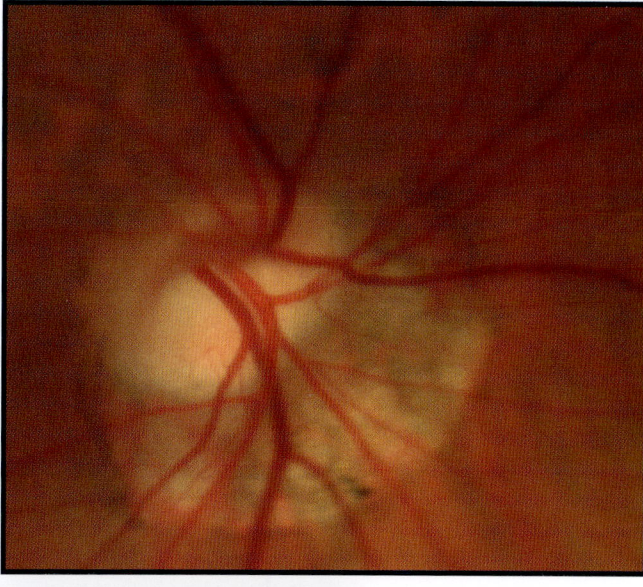
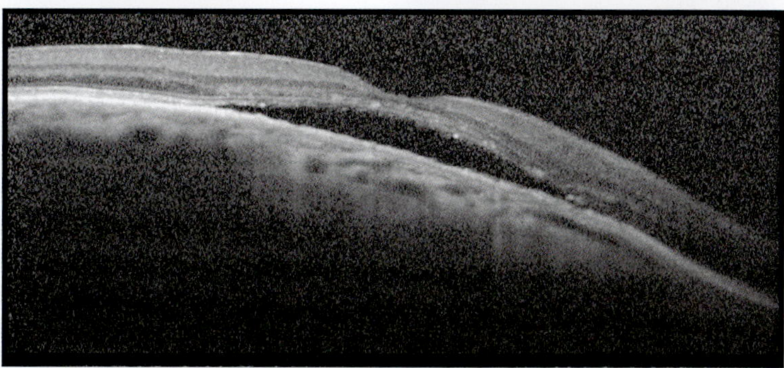

This patient has an inferonasal tilted disc with a crescent bordering on a staphyloma. There is a myopic conus on the inferior nasal margin of the disc. These patients are susceptible to exudative retinal detachments simulating central serous chorioretinopathy without serous pigment epithelial detachment. They may also experience choroidal neovascularization, usually at or near the crest of the staphyloma. The OCT shows a serous elevation of the retina in this patient.

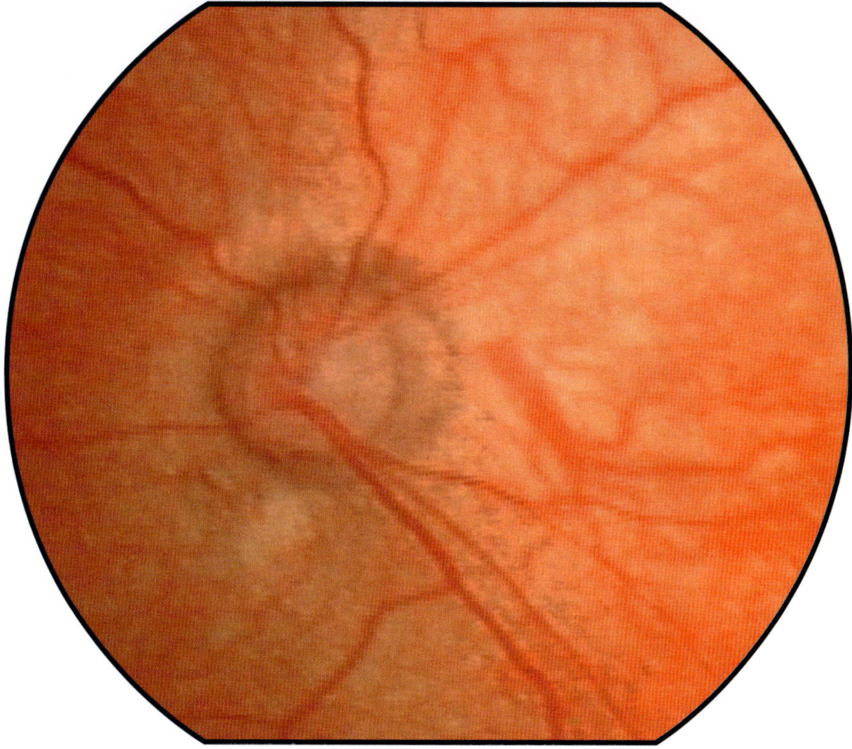

A patient with a tilted disc and a classic myopic conus temporally.

Peripapillary Staphyloma

Peripapillary staphylomas are rare congenital anomalies characterized by a normal appearing optic nerve surrounded by a zone of staphylomatous excavation. Chorioretinal degeneration is a universal finding within the walls of the staphyloma. It is differentiated from myopic conus and staphyloma by a relatively normal refraction, normal appearing optic disc, absence of a progressive chorioretinal degeneration, and lack of a temporal predilection of the peripapillary pigmentary alterations.

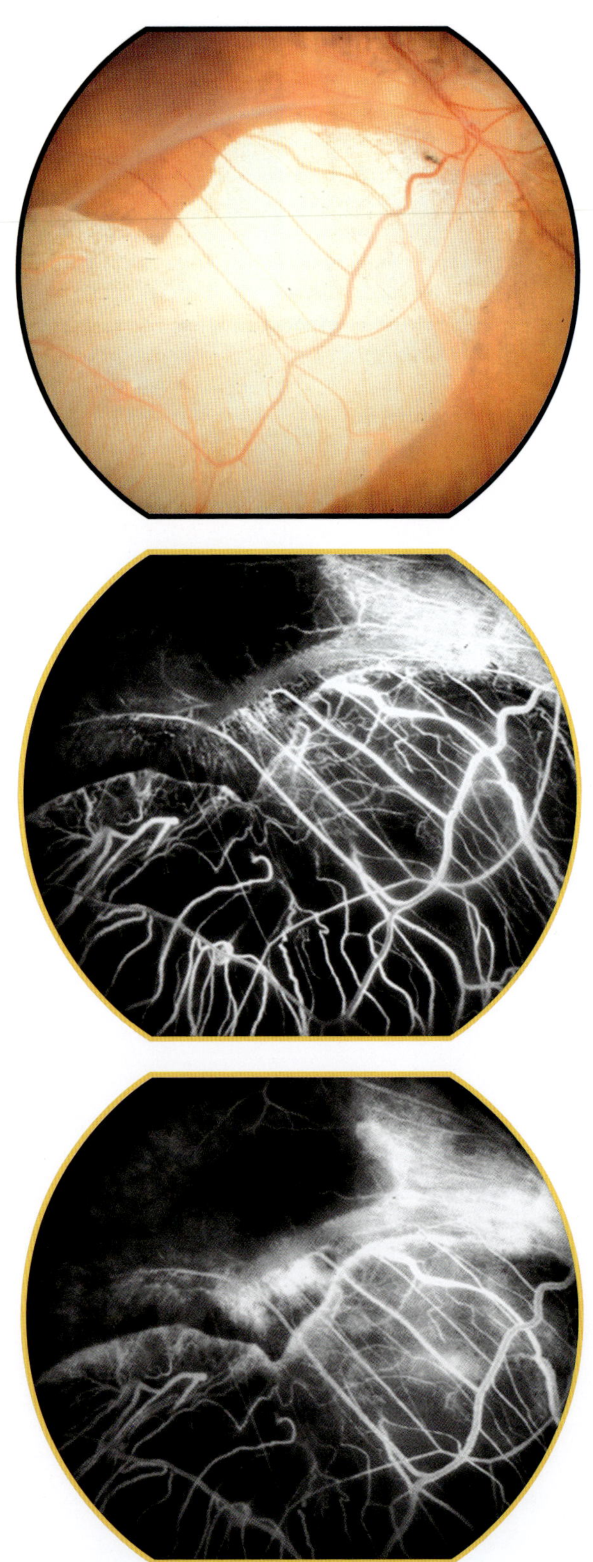

A typical posterior staphyloma in a highly myopic patient (–20 diopter myope).

Optic Nerve Head Drusen

Optic nerve head drusen are congenital intrapapillary refractile bodies unrelated to choroidal drusen. They occur in approximately 1% of the general population, are more common in Caucasian races, and are frequently bilateral. They may mimic papilledema of the optic nerve and are associated with spontaneous disc hemorrhages and arcuate visual field deficits. The drusen become increasingly visible with age and are rare before the teenage years. Buried drusen are readily detectable with B-scan ultrasonography and on spectral domain optical coherence tomography (SD-OCT) scans as well.

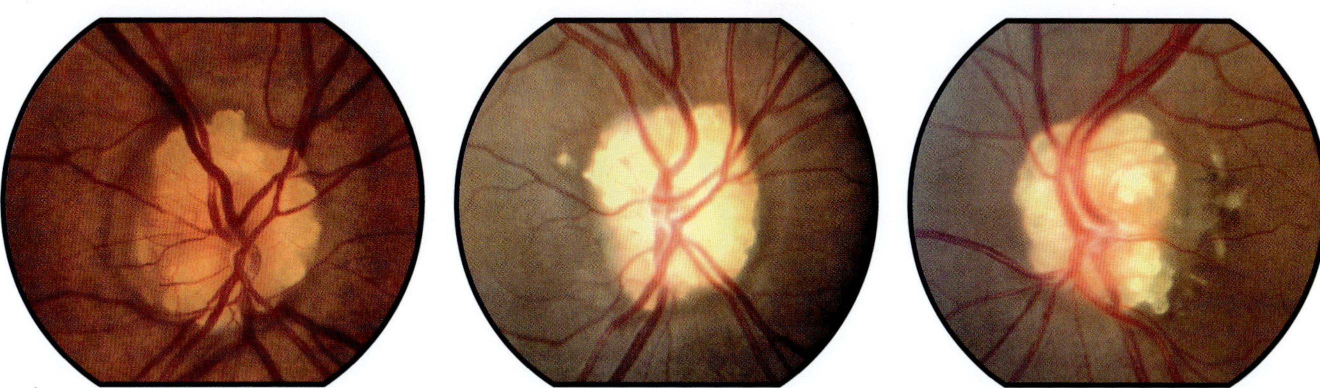

Optic nerve head drusen in several eyes are shown. Note that they extend beyond the margin of the normal nerve, as well as in a cascade fashion anteriorly. They may mimic papilledema of the optic nerve and may be associated with spontaneous disc hemorrhages and arcuate visual field deficits. *Left image courtesy of Mark Croswell*

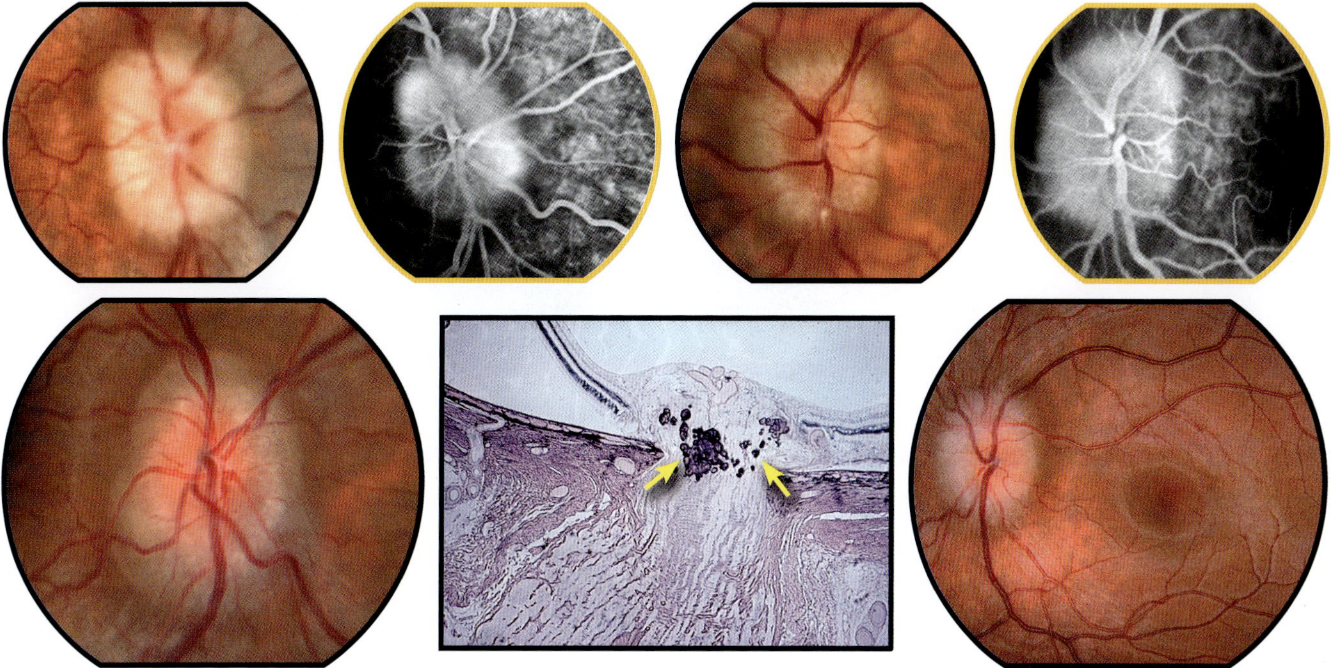

Subpapillary optic nerve head drusen may create irregular peripapillary margins that may masquerade as papilledema (pseudopapilledema). Differentiating true papilledema from buried optic nerve head drusen is critical because true papilledema requires an extensive neurological assessment. The fluorescein angiogram stains those lesions, simulating edema. The histopathology shows the calcific deposits within the nerve head *(arrows)*. B-scan echography, SD-OCT, and/or FAF are useful imaging modalities to detect the presence of optic nerve head drusen not readily visualized on funduscopic examination.

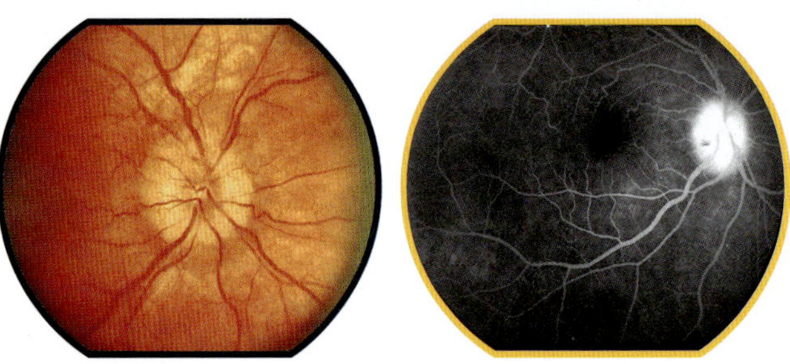

This patient with subpapillary drusen mimicking pseudo-papilledema shows no prominence to the vasculature emerging to and from the optic nerve head.

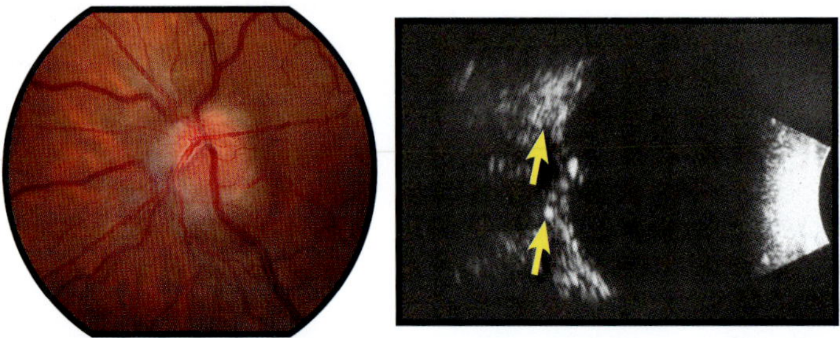

Subpapillary drusen may be visible echographically with a B-scan ultrasound device. In this image, persistent acoustical reflectance with low-sensitivity B-scan echography delineates the location of buried optic nerve head drusen *(arrows)*. Acoustic shadows from the calcified drusen are also visible.

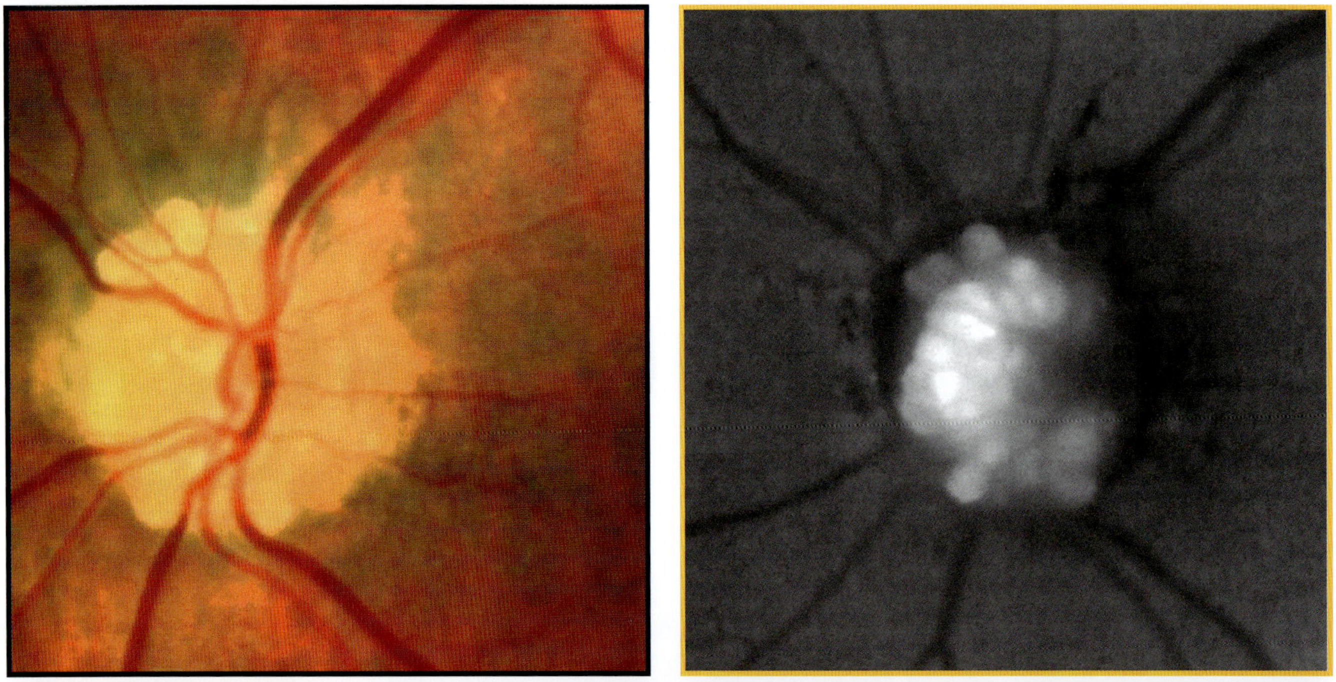

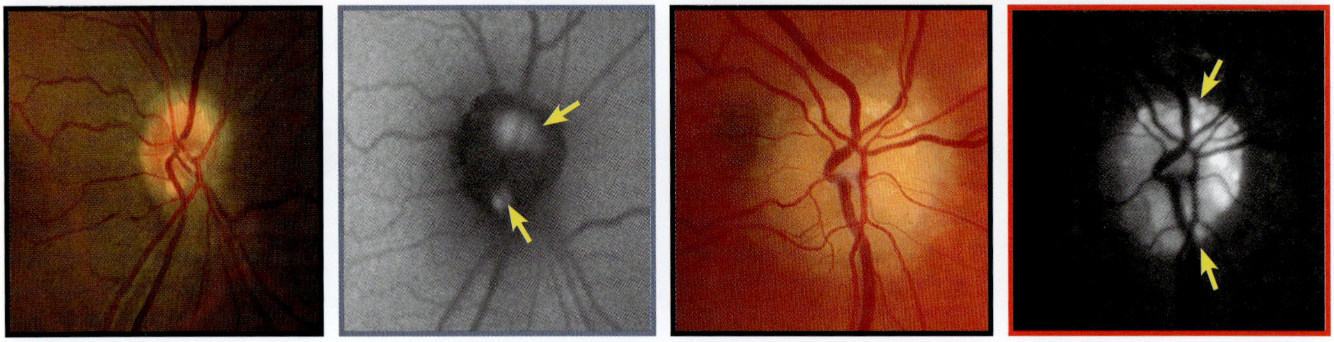

FAF is a non-invasive imaging modality that records the natural fluorescent properties of intraocular structures, most readily the RPE. Subpapillary optic nerve head drusen not easily detectable clinically are readily visualized with FAF *(arrows)*.

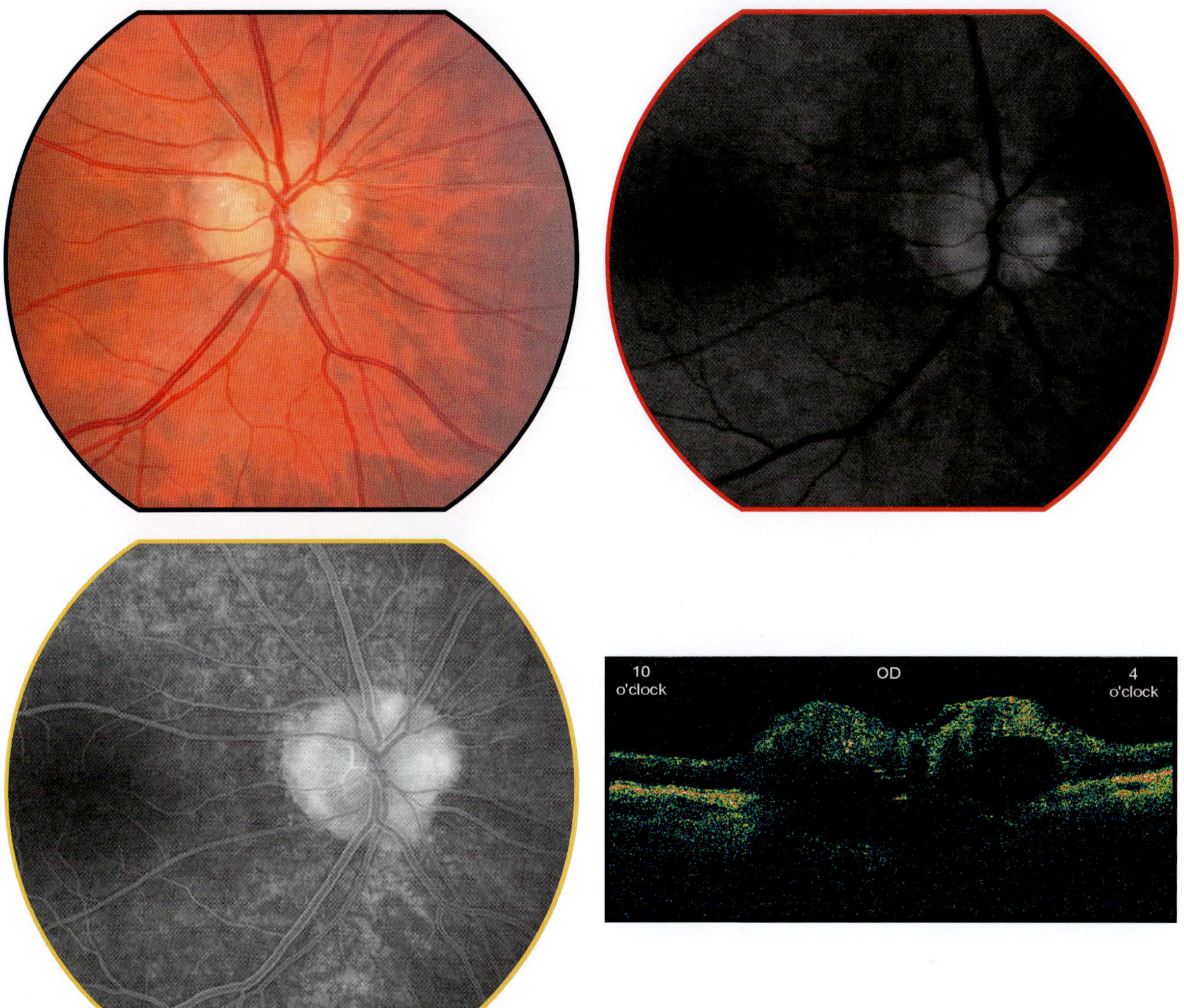

Optic nerve head drusen can be imaged with OCT as prominent tissue masses extending above the plane of the retina and optic nerve.

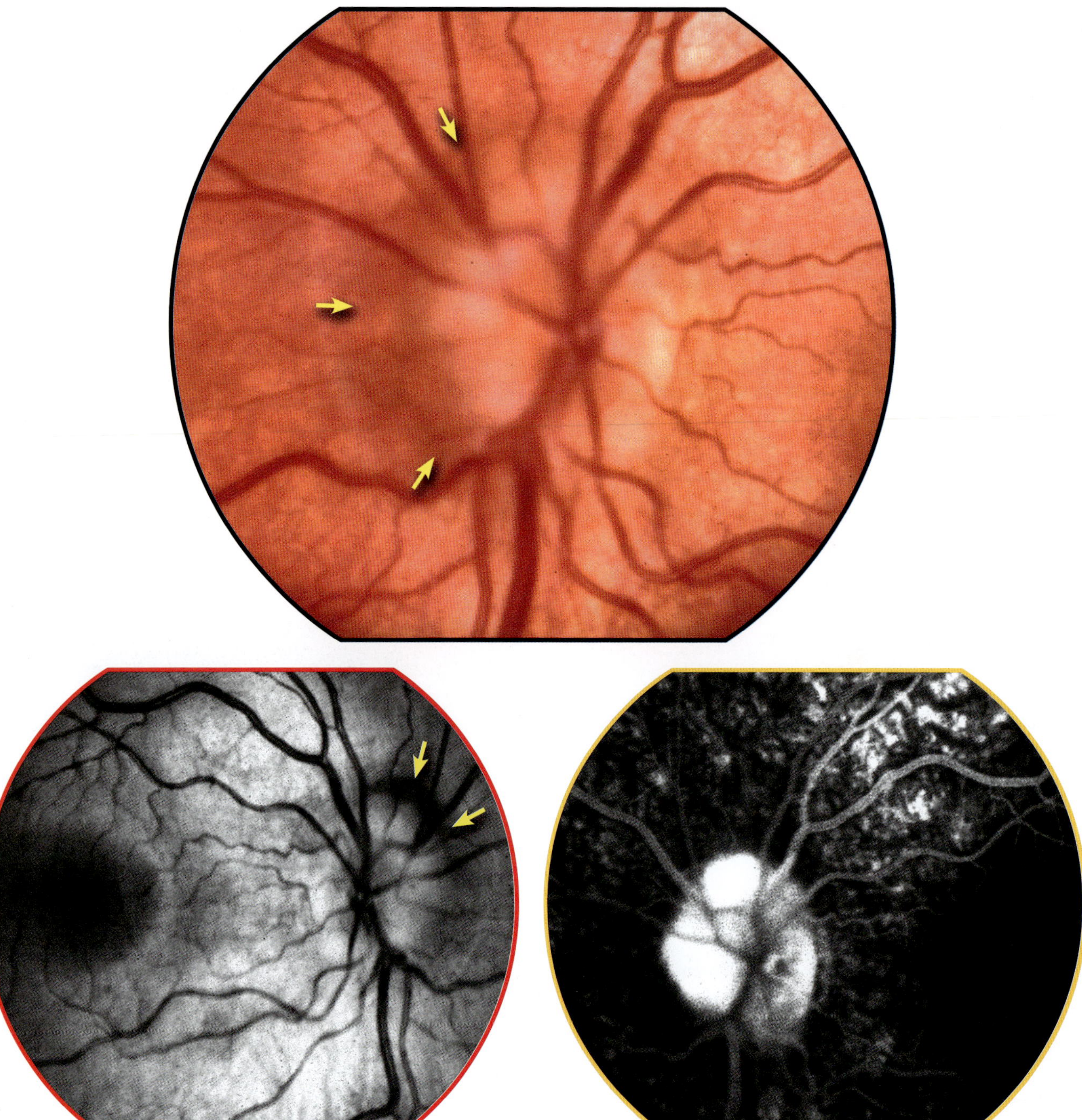

Patients with optic nerve head drusen are at risk for developing crescent shaped peripapillary hemorrhages and subretinal neovascular membrane formation. Note the hemorrhage surrounding the temporal border of the right optic nerve *(arrows)* and the superior nasal edge of the disc in the left eye *(left)*. Fluorescein angiography shows hyperfluorescence of the nasal margin of the disc with blockage by the hemorrhage *(right)*.

Optic Nerve Head Drusen with Juxtapapillary Choroidal Neovascularization (CNV)

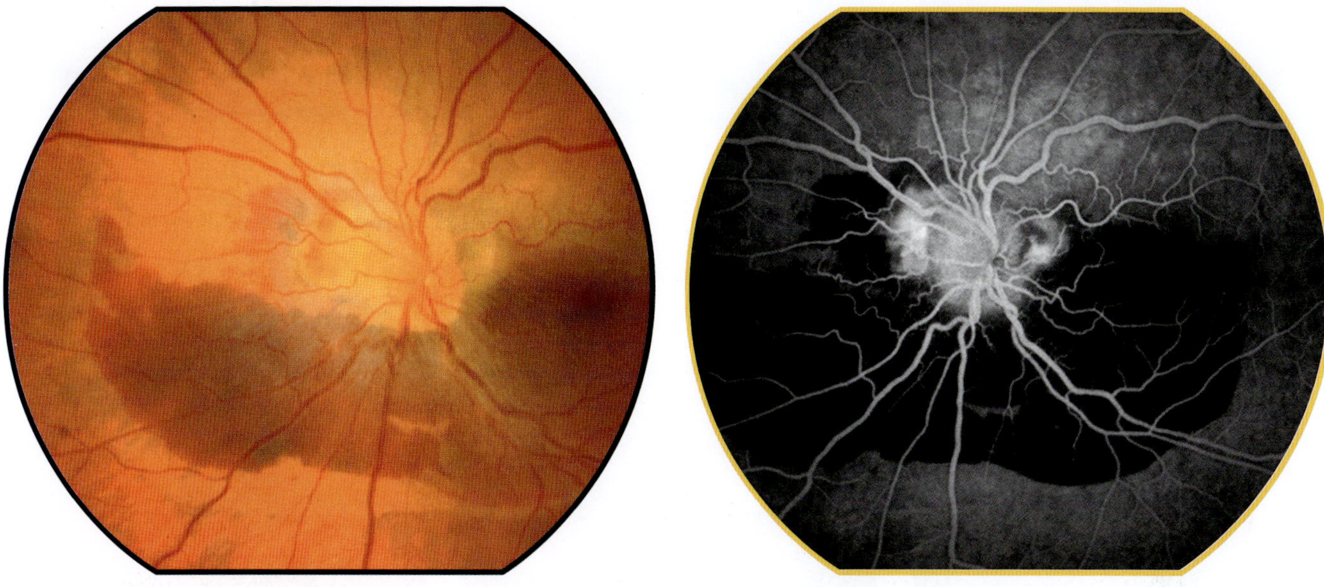

A young patient with optic nerve head drusen developed juxtapapillary subretinal hemorrhage, secondary to CNV. The optic nerve head drusen were confirmed echographically. The subretinal hemorrhage spontaneously cleared and visual function improved.

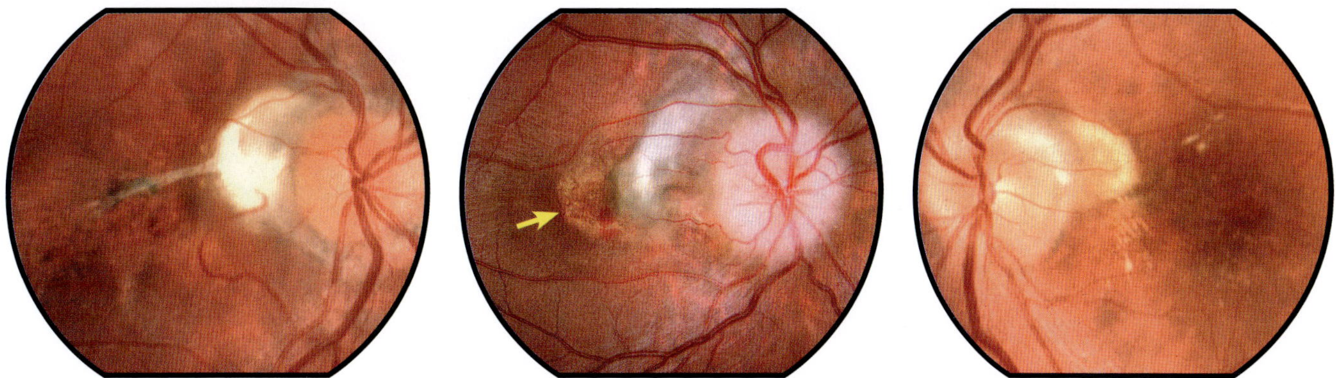

Optic nerve head drusen may provide a route for capillary proliferation and choroidal neovascularization to penetrate the subretinal space. This may result in type 2 CNV with associated serosanguineous fluid accumulation. Eventually, fibrous infiltration and disciform scar formation evolved in the macular region *(arrow)*.

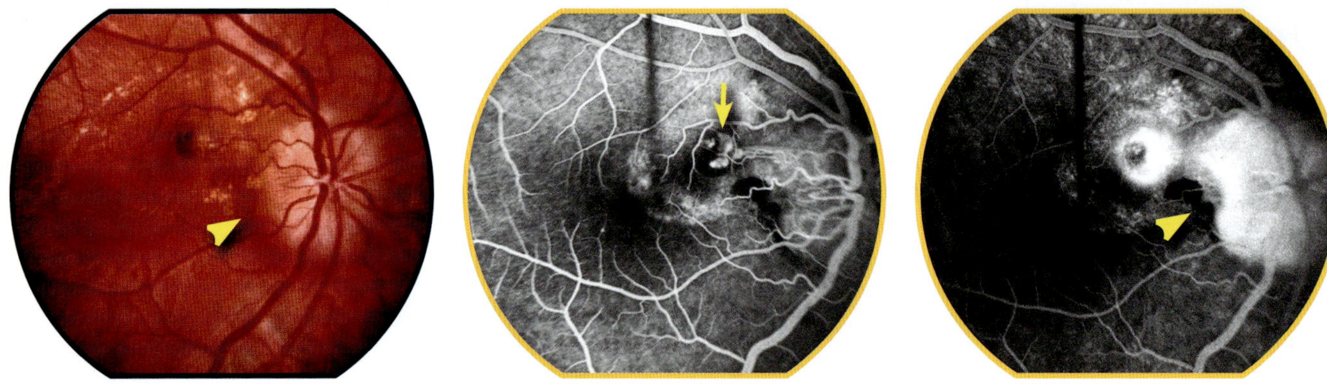

This patient with optic nerve head drusen has a pigmentary scar in the macula *(arrowhead, left)* that is the result of abnormal choroidal neovascularization extending from the edge of the disc, around Bruch membrane, and into the subretinal space *(arrow, middle)*. There is late staining on fluorescein angiography from pooling into the subneurosensory detachment. Peripapillary hemorrhage is also present *(arrowhead, right)*.

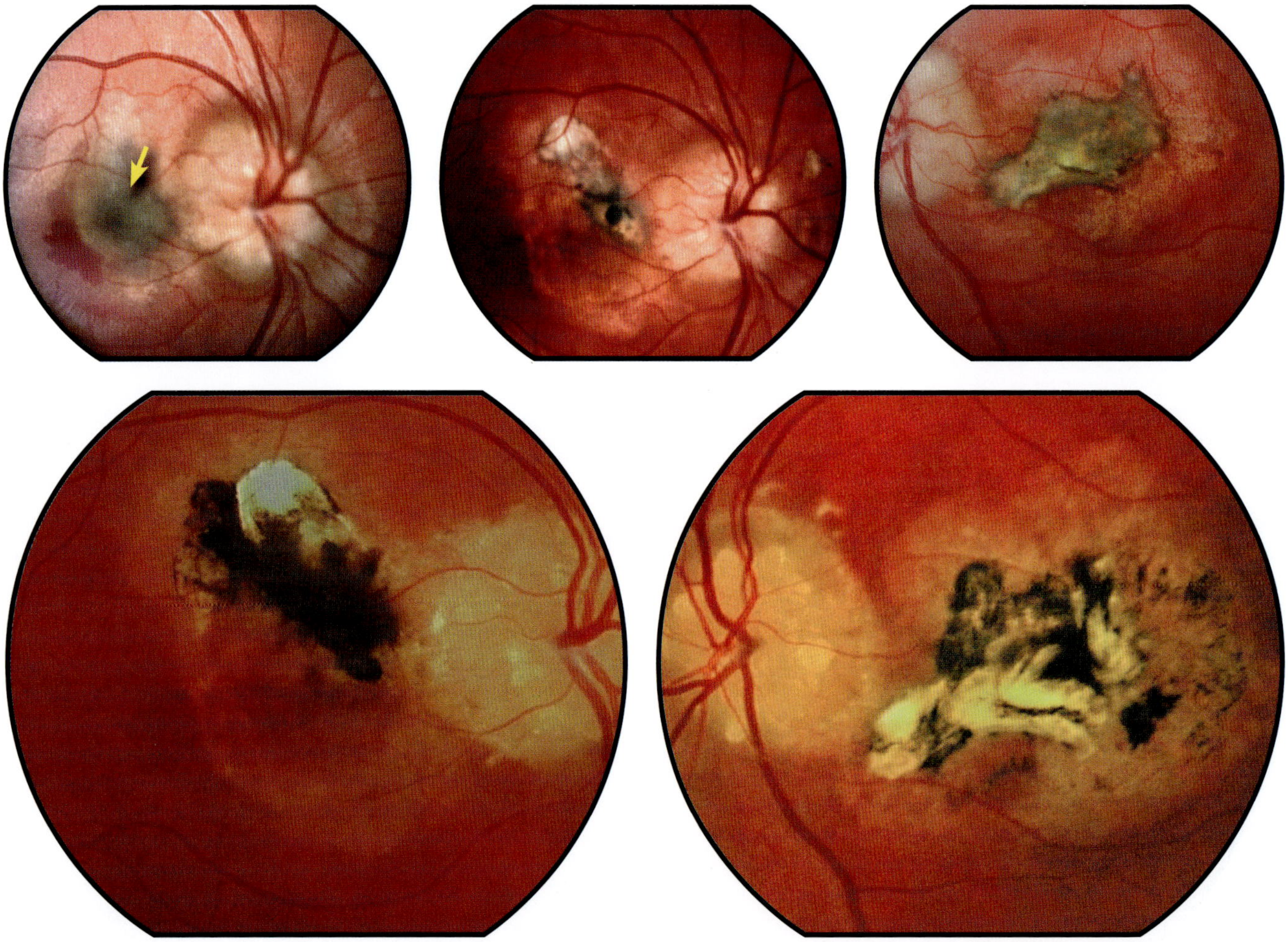

This patient experienced an acute serosanguineous detachment of the macula in the right eye *(upper left)* from CNV associated with hemorrhage surrounding the optic nerve head drusen and in the subretinal space *(arrow)*. Regression of the neovascularization left a fibrous, atrophic hyperpigmented disciform scar (as seen in the middle upper photograph). The left eye also experienced choroidal neovascularization resulting in a fibrotic scar involving the fovea *(upper right)*. Follow-up on this patient 26 years later showed stabilization of the scar and visual function, though with an increase in the fibrous and pigmentary degenerative lesions in each eye.

Optic Nerve Trauma

Also see Chapter 12 Traumatic Chorioretinopathy

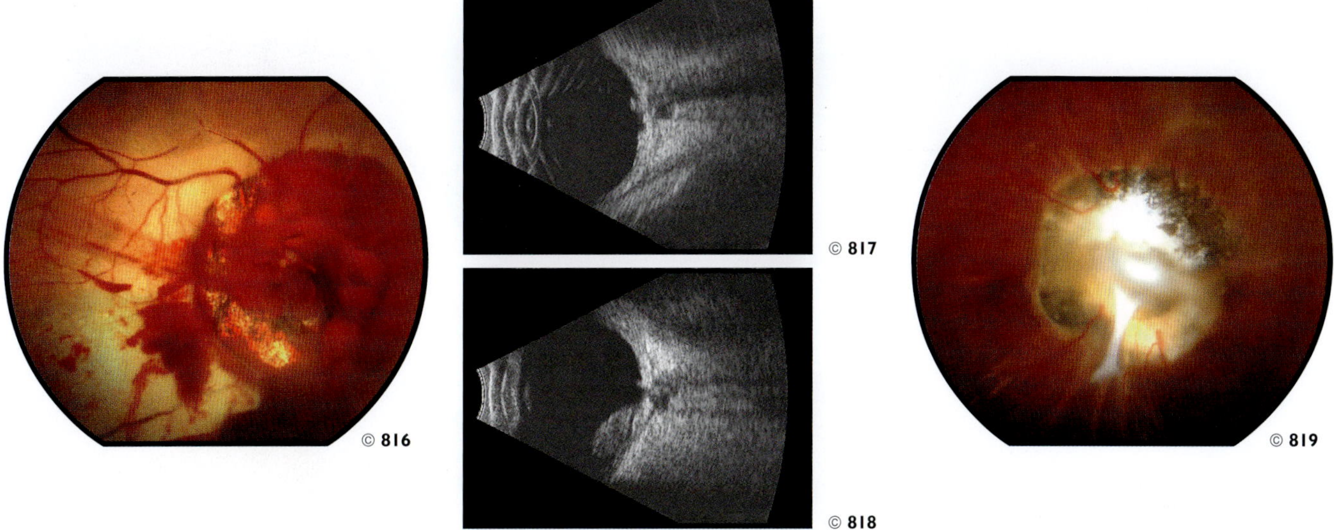

This patient experienced an avulsion of the optic nerve from severe blunt trauma. Note the hemorrhage surrounding the optic nerve head. There is also whitening of the retina from cleavage of perfusing arterioles. B-scan echography is often helpful in demonstrating the avulsed nerve head. In time, the hemorrhage resolves, though ischemia prevails. There may also be fibrous and pigmentary proliferation as a scar fills the avulsed defect.

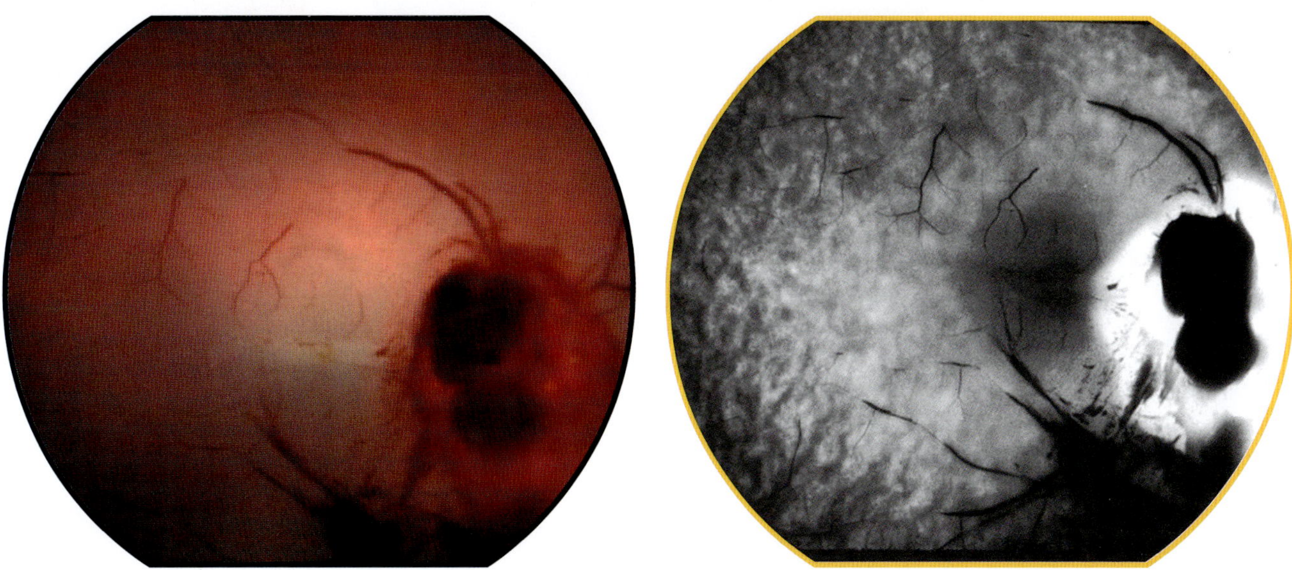

In this patient with avulsion of the optic nerve there is severance of the retinal vasculature following blunt trauma. This is confirmed on the fluorescein angiogram, where there is complete lack of filling of the retinal vasculature, with the only observed fluorescence being from the choroid. The patient had no light perception (NLP) vision.

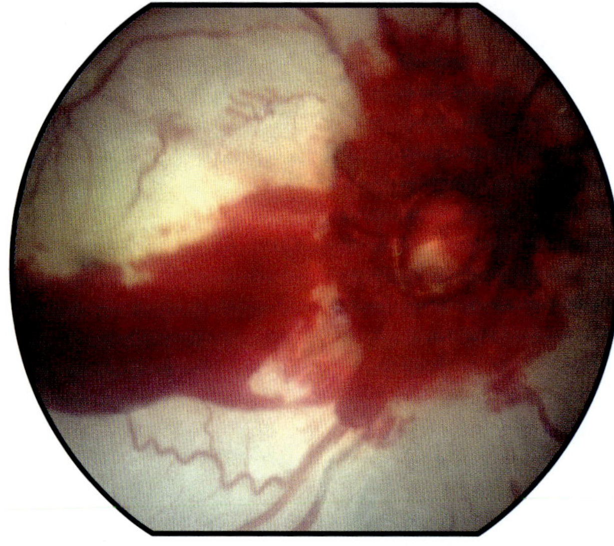

This patient suffered an avulsion of the optic nerve. Note the circumferential ring of hemorrhage surrounding the optic nerve and the adjacent pale, ischemic retina.

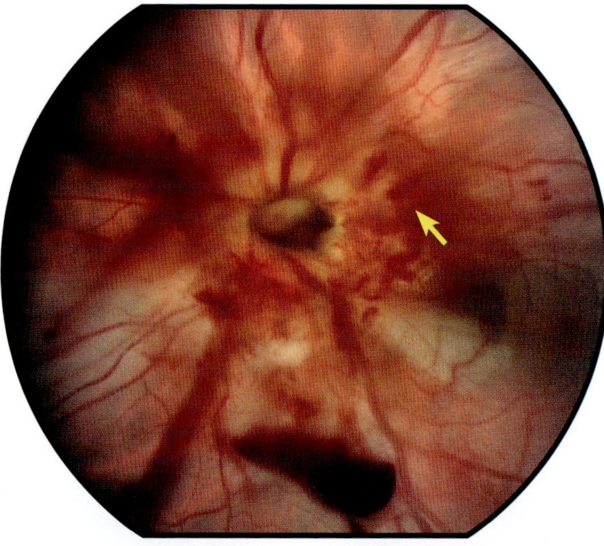

In this patient with avulsion of the optic nerve, a gap corresponding to the avulsed area is clinically apparent *(arrow)*. Fibrous scarring eventually will seal the gap at the nerve head and in the peripapillary area as well.

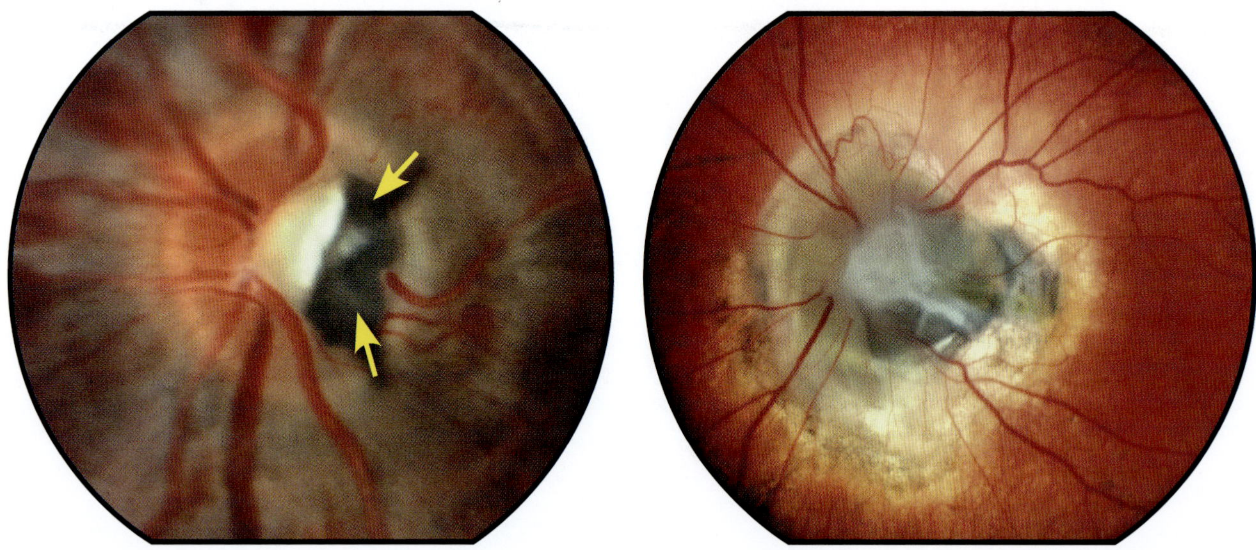

In this patient with avulsion of the optic nerve, the gap created is in the center of the disc *(arrows)* with ischemia of the adjacent retina and widespread hemorrhages throughout the fundus. The fundus is characterized predominantly by hemorrhage.

Select Optic Nerve Ischemic, Inflammatory, and Infectious Processes

Non-Arteritic Anterior Ischemic Optic Neuropathy (NAION)

Non-arteritic anterior ischemic optic neuropathy (NAION) is a common optic neuropathy affecting primarily adults over the age of 50 years. Classically, the condition affects hyperopic, small discs, with a crowded central cup ("disc-at-risk"). It may result in altitudinal or arcuate visual field defects, disc hemorrhage, or edema of the optic nerve. These eyes must be differentiated from a vasculitis or temporal arteritis, which has a more threatening prognosis and generally necessitates intervention with systemic corticosteroid and/or other immunosuppressive agents.

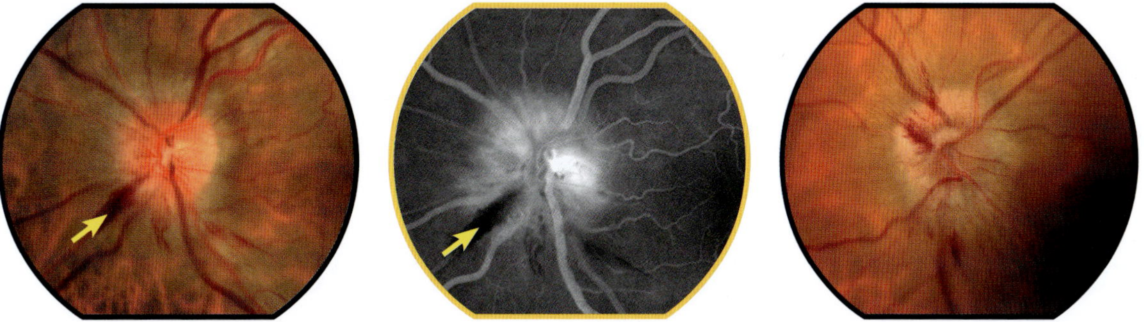

This patient has a small, crowded optic nerve, which placed the patient at risk for development of NAION. At presentation, the nerve is hyperemic with a prominent microvascular papillopathy and flame-shaped hemorrhages *(arrows)*. The image on the right shows optic nerve edema in an eye with a similar process.

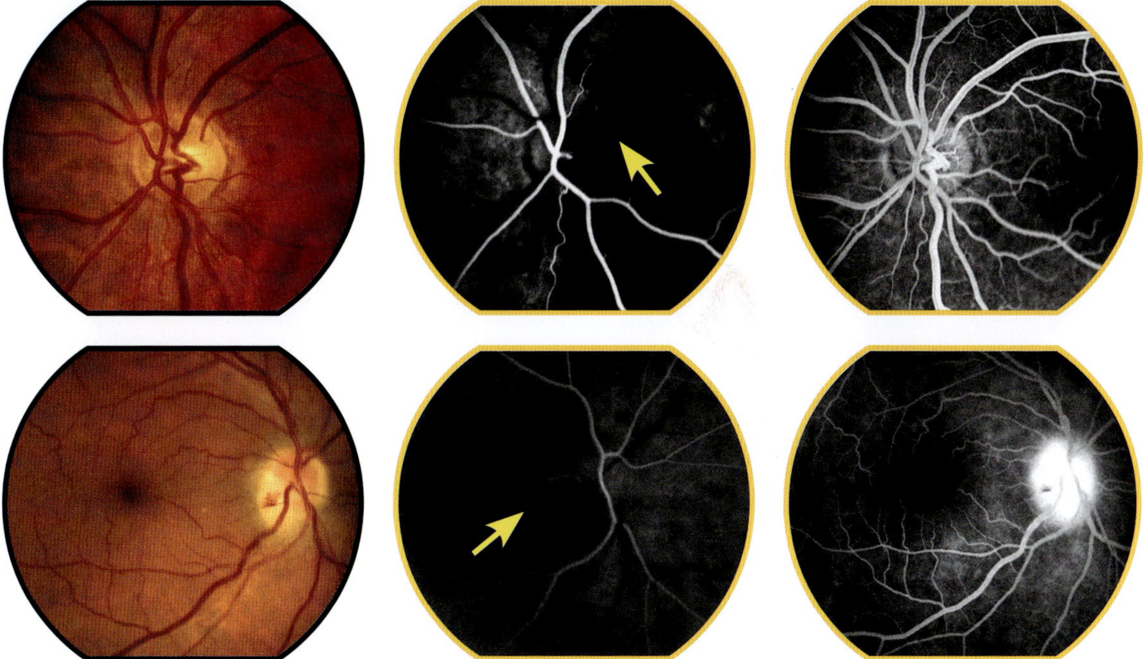

These two patients have non-arteritic anterior ischemic optic neuropathy. Fluorescein angiography in anterior ischemic optic neuropathy may demonstrate a "watershed abnormality," or a zone of delayed vertical hypoperfusion of the choriocapillaris *(arrow)*. These capillaries eventually perfuse and are homogeneously fluorescent compared to the other surrounding small vessels of the choroid *(right)*. In the acute stages, the optic nerve head will have late leakage *(lower right image)*.

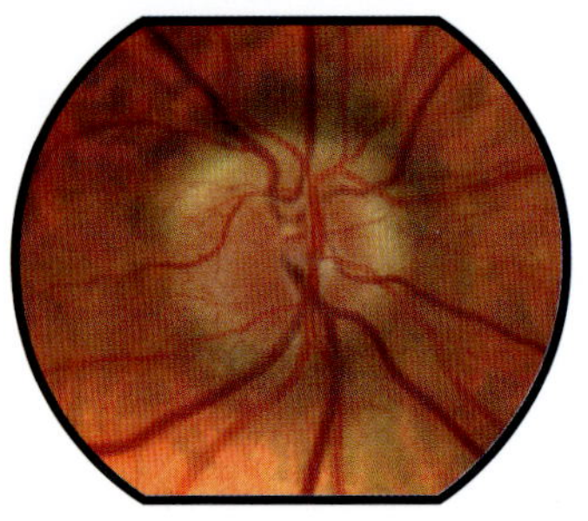
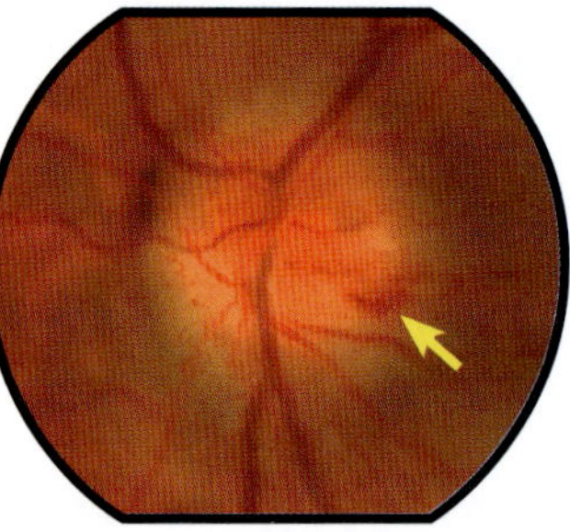

This patient had a history of non-arteritic anterior ischemic optic neuropathy in the right eye followed by acute manifestations in the left eye. The right eye shows a pale, ischemic nerve with central crowding of the small cup from retinal blood vessels. The left eye demonstrates an acute presentation, with swelling of the optic nerve, blurring of the disc margins, and juxtapapillary hemorrhage *(arrow)*.

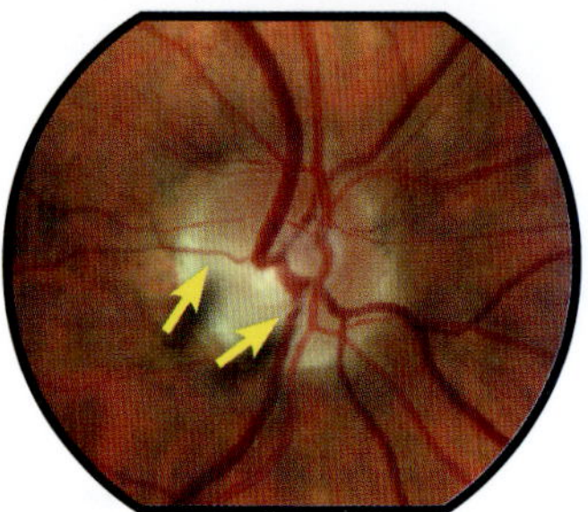
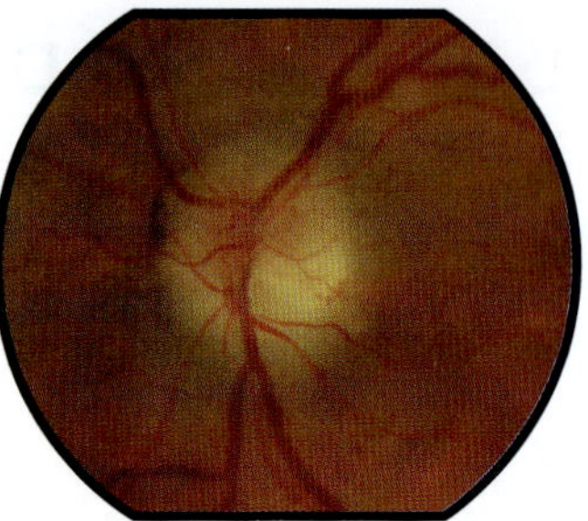

Bilateral non-arteritic anterior ischemic optic neuropathy may occur. This patient has a history of segmental atrophy from an antecedent acute episode of non-arteritic anterior ischemic optic neuropathy *(arrows)*. The left eye *(right)* now has acute manifestations of the disease with edema of the lower half of the nerve and a corresponding superior altitudinal field defect.

Optic Nerve Papillitis

Papillitis describes swelling of the optic disc caused by local inflammation of the optic nerve head. It is most commonly secondary to demyelinating disease in younger patients and ischemic optic neuropathy in patients older than 50 years of age. Infectious, inflammatory, autoimmune, and neoplastic entities must also be considered.

Acute Neuroretinitis *(Bartonella henselae)*

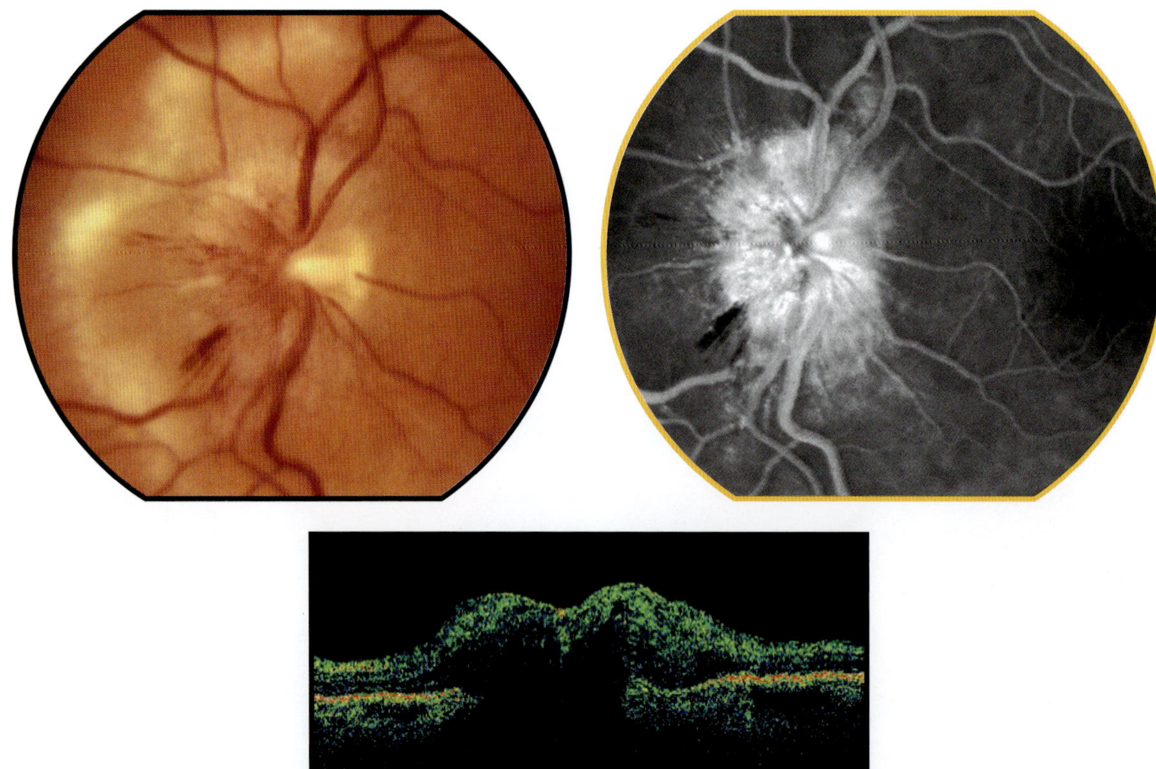

Bartonella henselae is a gram negative rod and a common cause of acute neuroretinitis characterized by inflammation of the optic disc vasculature with exudation of fluid into the peripapillary retina. In this patient, optic nerve edema is present with flame hemorrhages and deposition of exudate. OCT confirms the acute swelling.

Leber Idiopathic Stellate Neuroretinitis

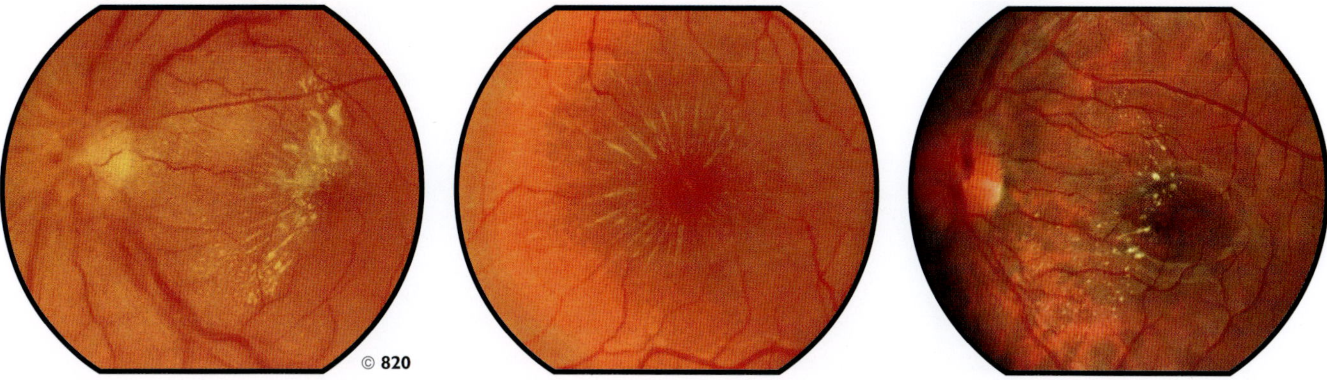

Leber idiopathic stellate neuroretinitis is characterized by a papillitis, prominent optic nerve vessels and a maculopathy with macular star formation from deposition of intraretinal lipid exudates. Serous retinal detachment may occur in some cases. The majority of patients previously classified with acute macular neuroretinitis most likely had a *Bartonella henselae* infection.

Chronic Papillitis

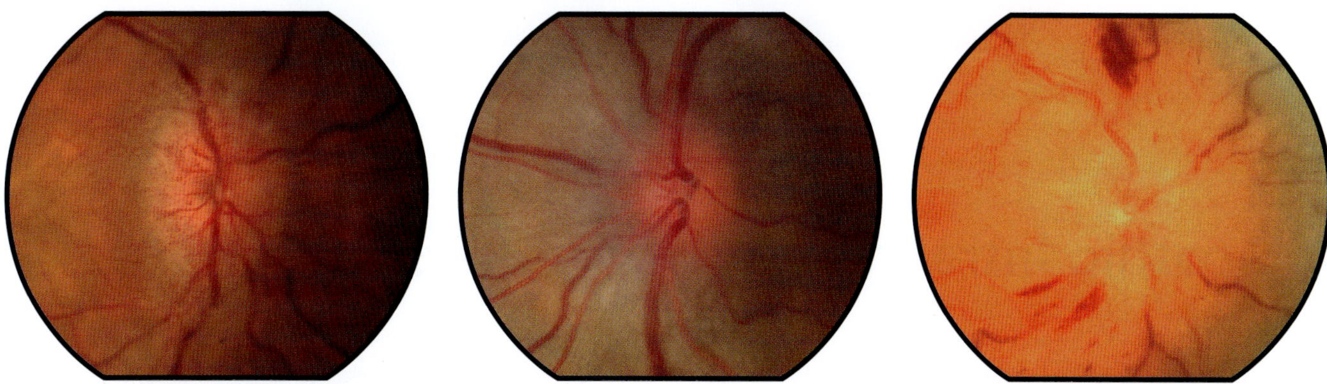

These patients have chronic papillitis with different associated manifestations. There is pure edema and erythematous prominence to the papillary circulation *(left)*, peripapillary neurosensory detachment *(middle)*, as well as scattered hemorrhages and prominent retinal vessels from obstructive venous disease *(right)*.

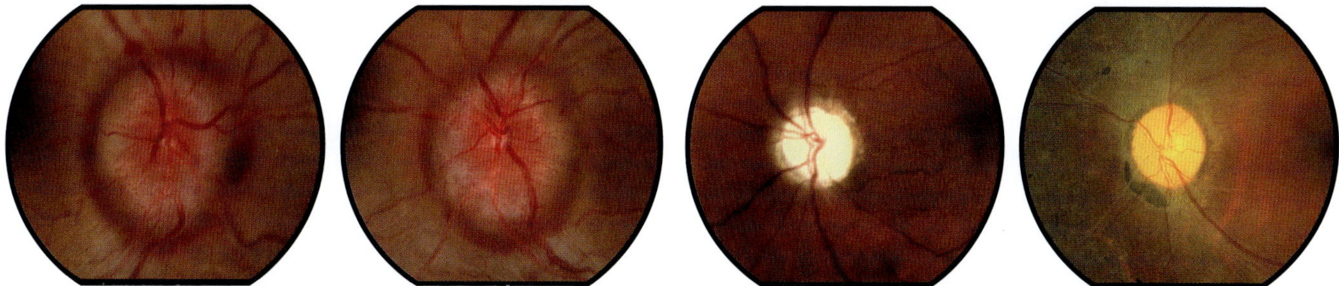

Chronic papillitis may be severe and result in a persistently swollen disc with blurred margins, peripapillary hemorrhage, occlusive vasculopathy, and obliteration of the normal physiologic cup, as seen in the accompanying image.

Chronic papillitis can result in optic atrophy with residual swelling and pallor of the optic nerve. Residual arterial attenuation may be present. The pallor is not usually associated with significant cupping, though it can be confused in certain cases with a glaucomatous optic neuropathy. The visual fields will be irreversibly constricted with poor visual acuity.

Ocular Syphilis

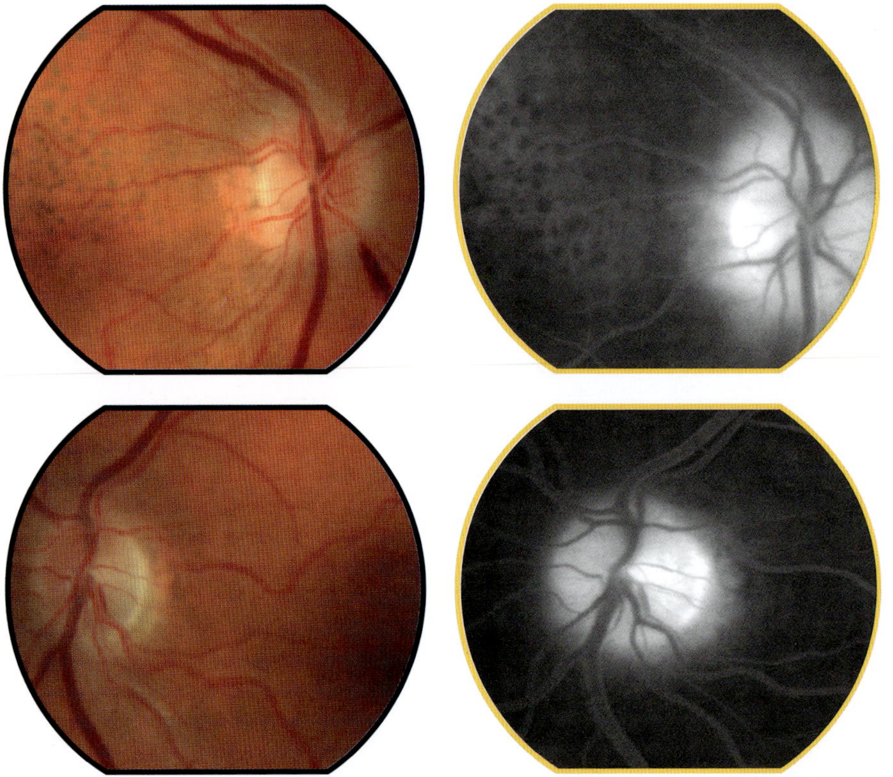

Syphilis is a sexually transmitted infection caused by the spirochete bacterium *Treponema pallidum* that may involve almost any intraocular structure. It may present as an acute papillitis with associated serous retinal detachment. Syphilitic papillitis may resolve to leave optic disc pallor and adjacent retinal pigment epithelial atrophy.

Idiopathic Intracranial Hypertension (IIH)

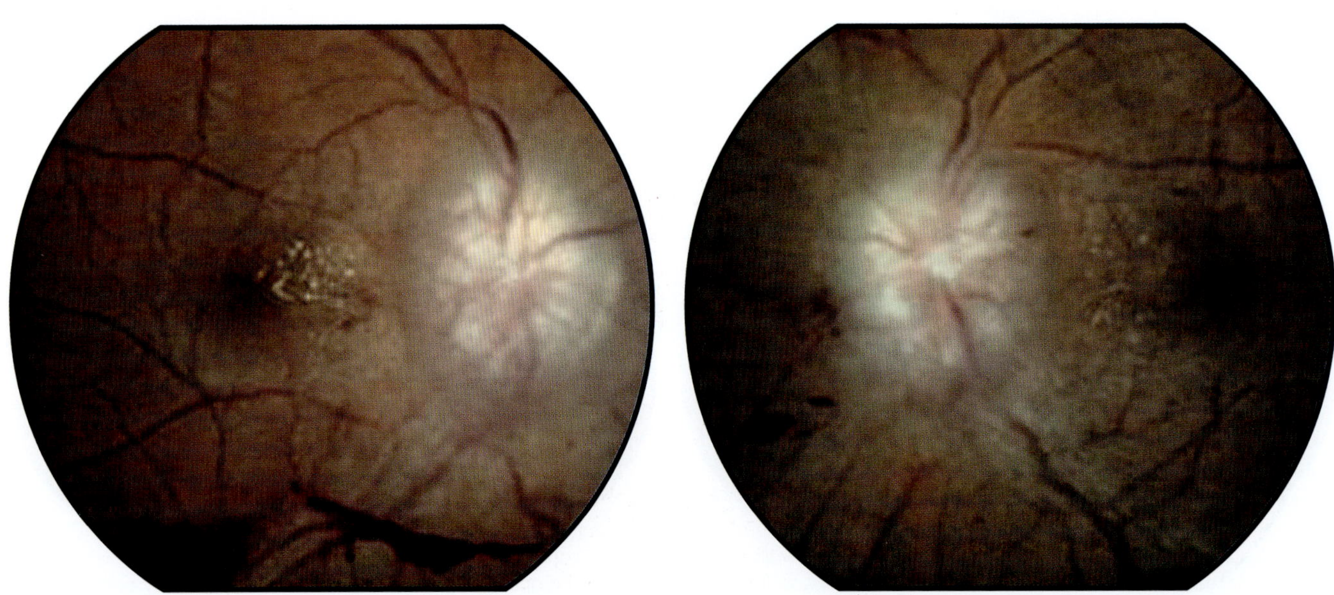

Papilledema, or idiopathic intracranial hypertension (IIH), implies optic disc swelling due to raised intracranial pressure. This patient has papilledema, which has led to swelling of the optic nerve, peripapillary detachment, lipid deposition extending toward the fovea, and pre-retinal hemorrhage bilaterally. *Courtesy of Dr. Blake Cooper*

Also see Chapter 8 Oncology

Optic Nerve Glioma

Optic nerve gliomas are most commonly seen in children or young adults and present with unilateral proptosis and decreased visual acuity. They are strongly associated with neurofibromatosis.

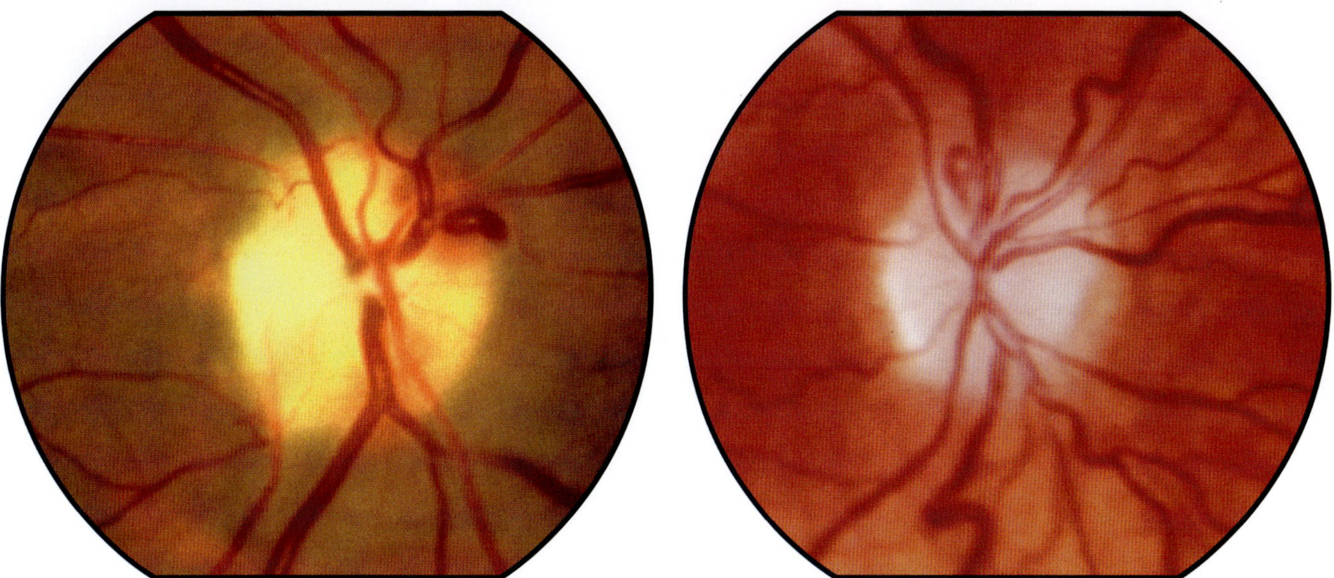

These two patients have an optic nerve glioma, which has led to atrophy of the nerve head and dilated venous–venous collateralization to compensate for posterior retrobulbar venous obstructive disease. The pale disc with collateralization can be compared to ciliary retinal collaterals following central retinal vein thrombosis where the nerve head is pink from prominence of the lamellar circulation of the nerve head. *Right image courtesy of Dr. James Bollings*

Meningioma of the Optic Nerve

Primary optic nerve meningiomas are rare tumors that arise from the arachnoid within the dura and infiltrate the subarachnoid and subdural space to compress the nerve. There often is prominent glial extension in the preliminary area, bordered by atrophy and hyperpigmentation.

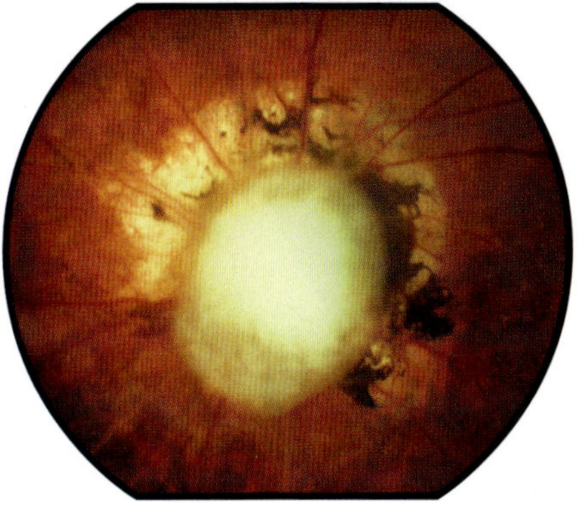

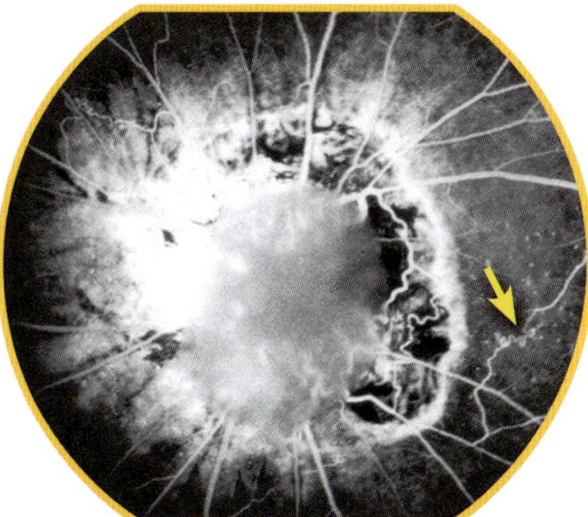

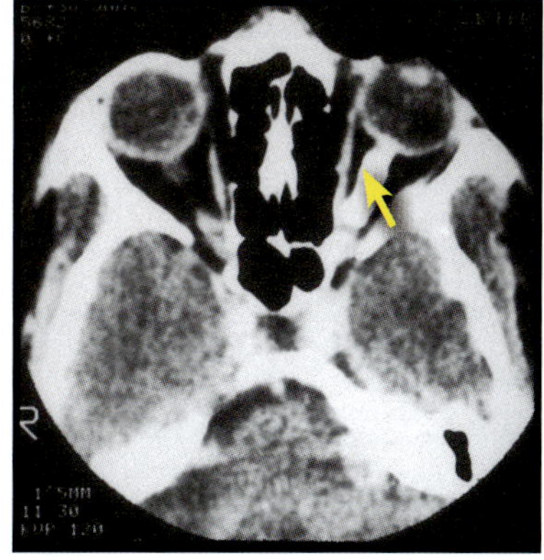

This young patient has an optic nerve meningioma. There are venous–venous collaterals in the fundus *(arrow, middle image)* compensating for the retrobulbar obstructive mass. The corresponding MRI shows the classic "tram-track" sign referring to the parallel thickening and enhancement around the optic nerve *(arrow, right)*.

Metastatic Tumors of the Optic Nerve

While the majority of metastatic disease in the eye occurs in the choroid or iris, occasionally systemic cancers may metastasize to the optic nerve.

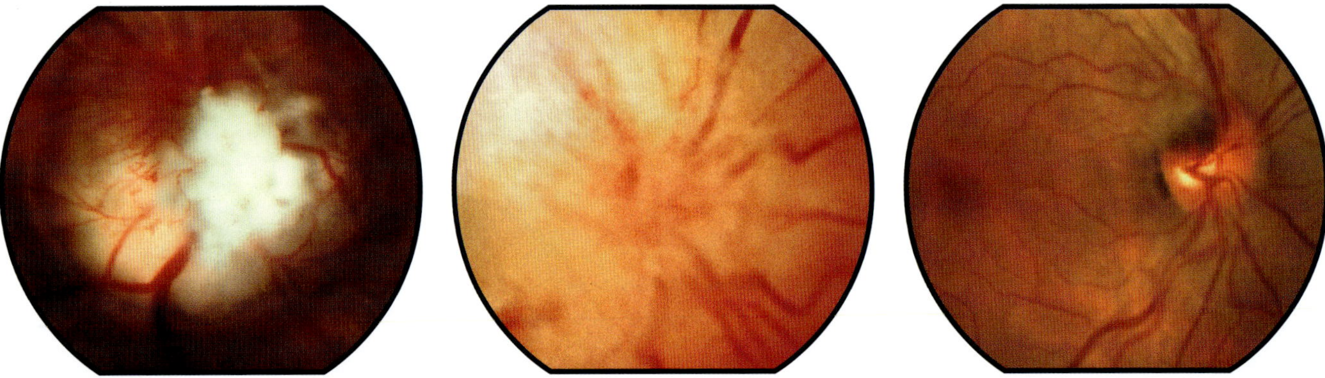

The left and center images demonstrate optic nerve metastatic disease from lung cancer, while the right image reveals metastatic disease from breast cancer. The underlying systemic cancers were known prior to the time of ocular involvement. *Left image courtesy of Dr. Jeffrey Shakin*

Optic Nerve Melanocytoma

Melanocytomas are benign, jet-black lesions of variable size and shape located on the optic disc, oftent eccentric in location. They are typically unilateral and may be confused with malignant melanomas. Patients are generally asymptomatic, though visual field testing may reveal an enlarged blind spot.

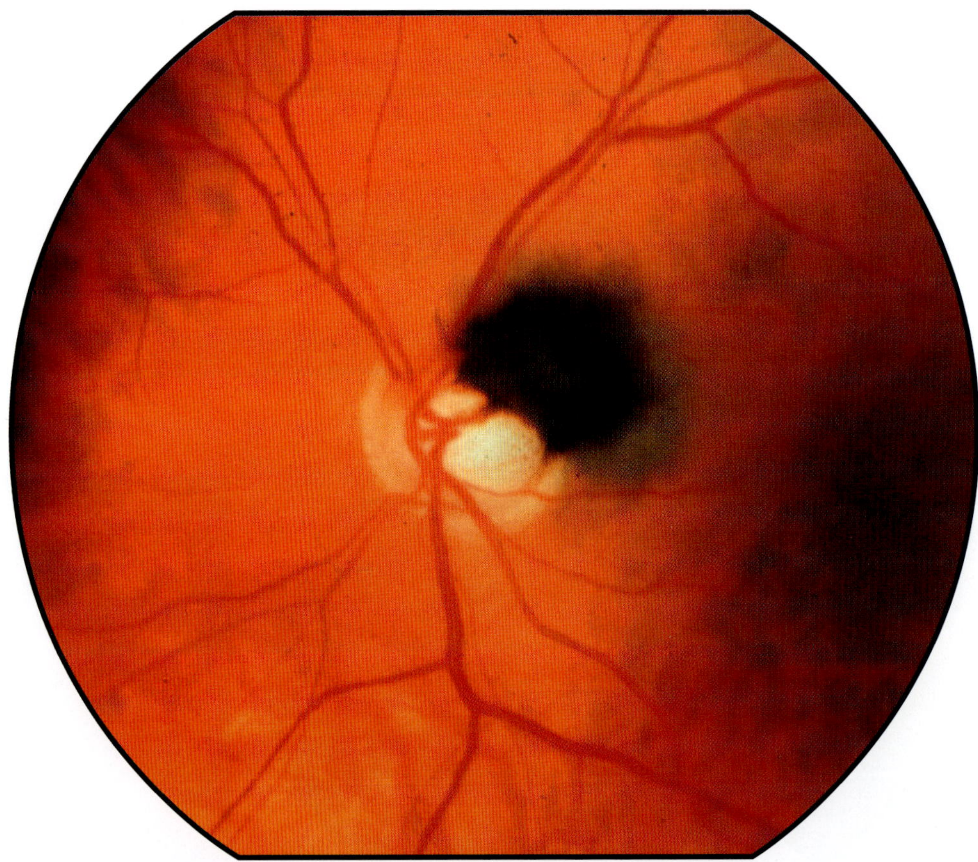

This patient exhibited an eccentrically located jet black lesion on the superotemporal border of the optic nerve. The lesion has fibrillated borders, and there is a small contiguous juxtapapillary choroidal nevus as well. The patient was visually asymptomatic, and the lesion has remained unchanged for 10 years.

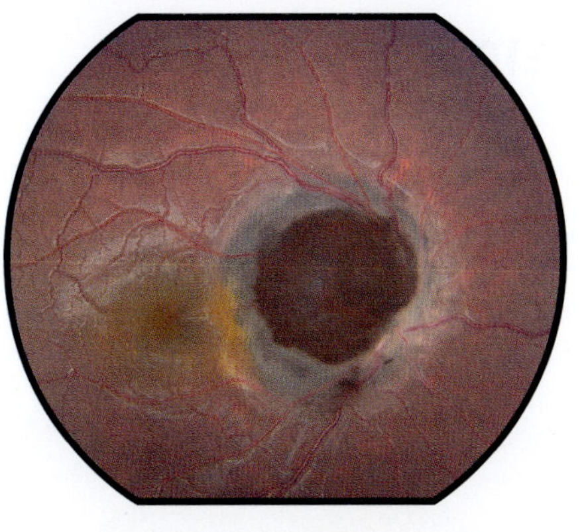

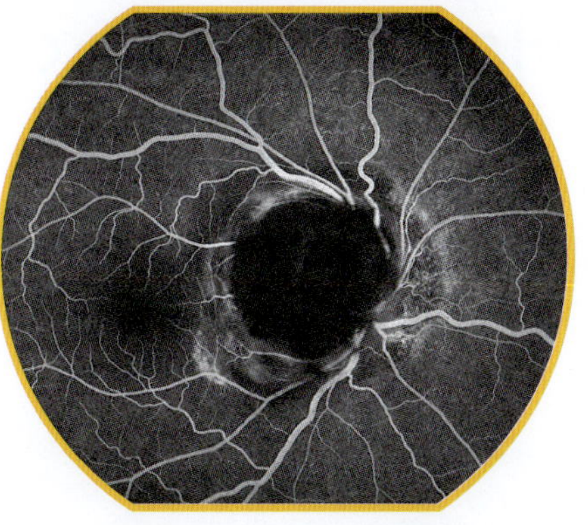

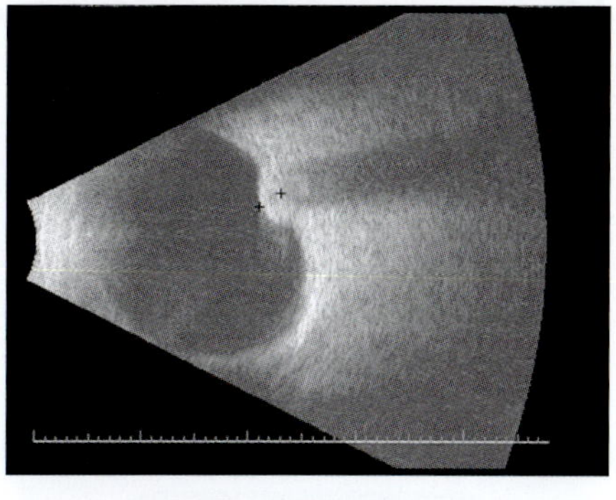

A more prominent jet black lesion overlying the majority of the optic nerve. The fibrillated borders are not as readily seen. On the fluorescein angiogram, there is complete blockage of fluorescence, and the accompanying echogram shows thickness of approximately 1.5 mm. These lesions generally have medium to high internal reflectivity. *Images courtesy of Jerry A Shields, MD*

Retinal Capillary Hemangioma

Retinal capillary hemangiomas are classified as benign hamartomas. They may occur in an isolated fashion, or more commonly in association with the oculoneurocutaneous syndrome (phakomatosis) of von Hippel–Lindau. They commonly appear as a large, orange-to-red dilated retinal vessel emerging from the optic nerve. Lipid exudates and subretinal fluid surrounding the tumor are common and can affect visual function if the macula is involved.

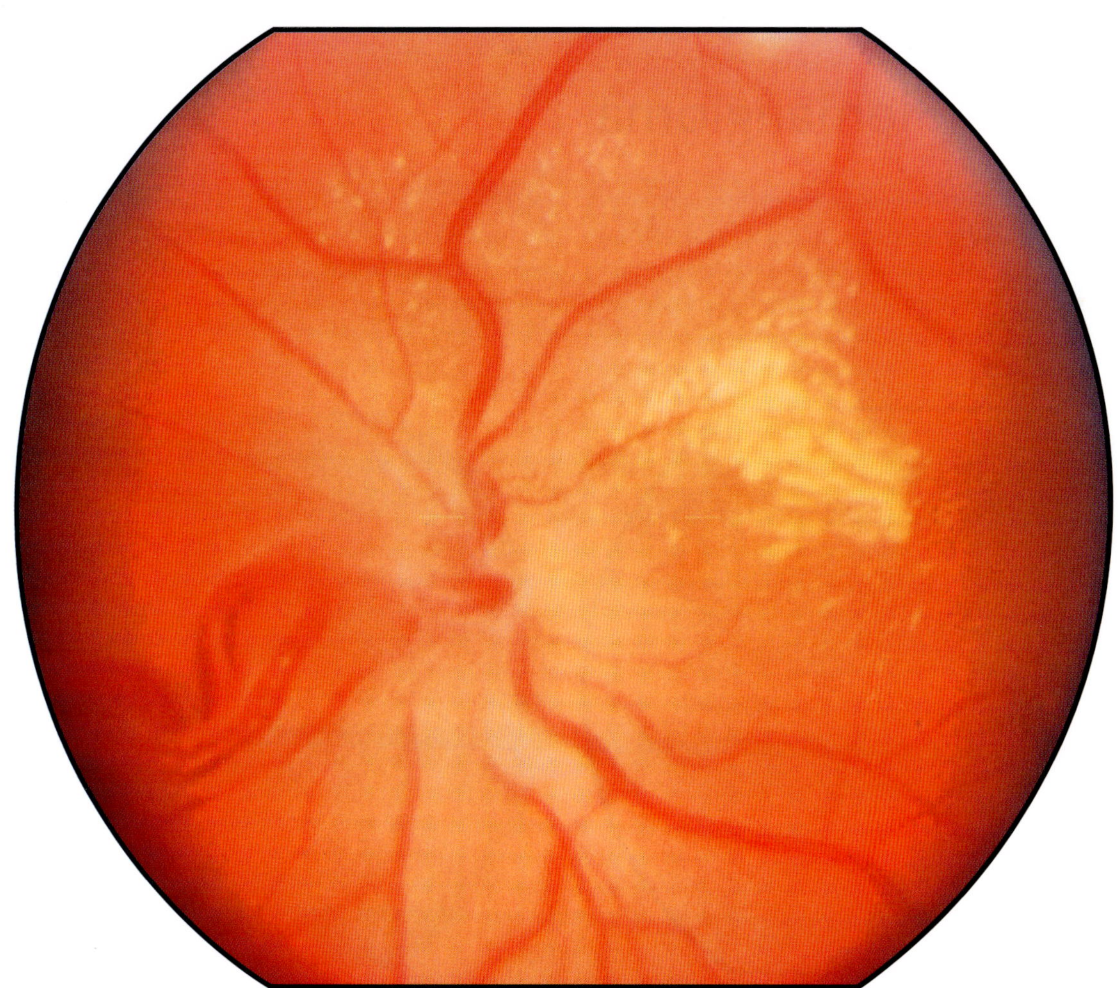

A prominent dilated feeder vessel is seen exiting the optic nerve head toward the inferonasal periphery, where a retinal capillary hemangioma was located. There is moderate exudation in the macular region with decreased visual acuity.

Retinal Capillary Hemangioma of the Optic Nerve Head

Retinal capillary hemangiomas may be seen on the optic nerve head. They may be encapsulated or occur in a more diffuse form. The hemangioma may be isolated or occur in conjunction with the von Hippel–Lindau syndrome. When there is leakage into the macular region, treatment is challenging as one needs to be careful not to impair the function of the optic nerve.

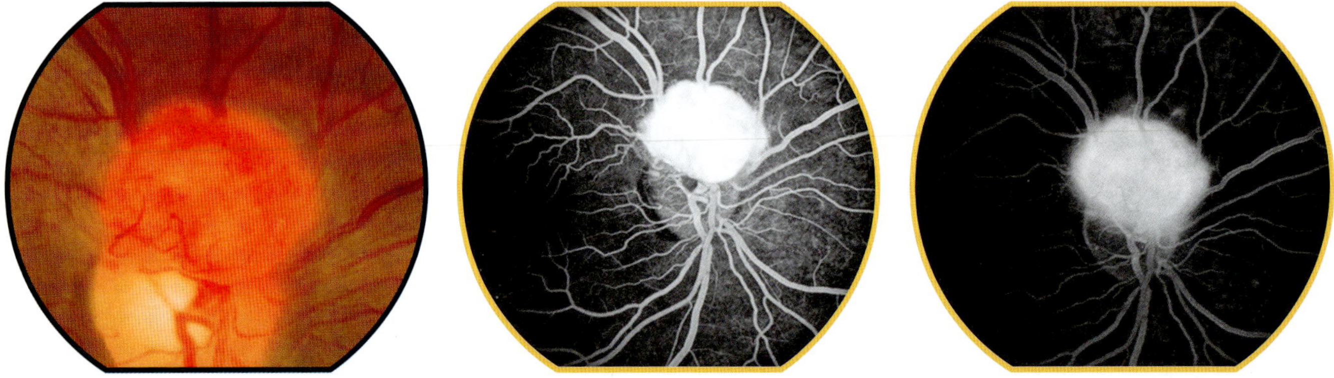

A well-delineated hemangioma is seen along the superior border of the optic nerve. There was no appreciable leakage from the lesion clinically or angiographically. Observation was recommended and there was no change in the appearance of the lesion over a 5 year time frame.

Racemose Hemangioma

A racemose hemangioma is a retinal vascular malformation with a dilated vessel (or vessels) that leaves the optic disc, travels through the retina, and returns to the disc without an intervening capillary plexus. One or all four quadrants of the retina may be involved. Larger lesions may be part of the Wyburn–Mason syndrome and involve the central nervous system, facial, and/or orbital regions as well. This condition at times has been classified as a systemic phakomatosis.

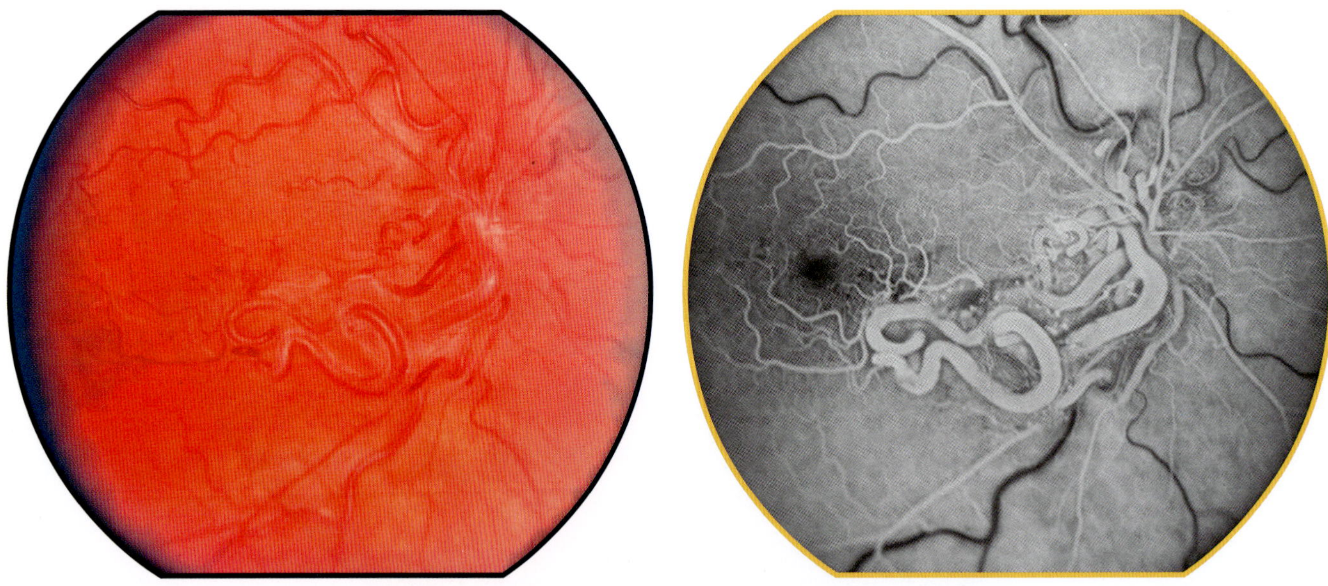

A single dilated, markedly tortuous vessel coursing over the inferior portion of the papillomacular bundle, stopping just short of the macula, and then returning to the optic nerve. No vascular compromise was noted, and the patient was visually asymptomatic.

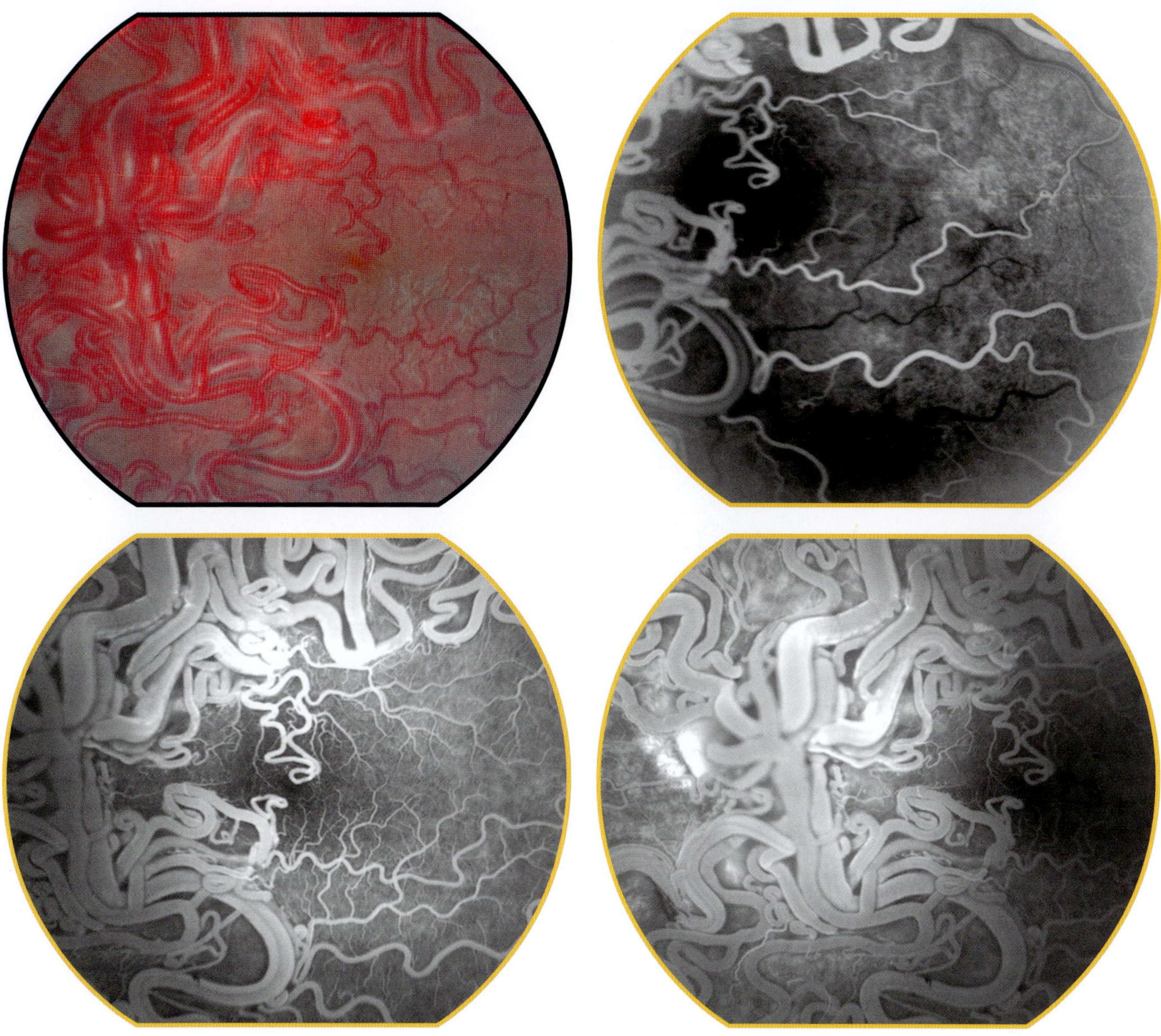

A more extensive racemose hemangioma involving portions of all four retinal quadrants. Note the extreme vascular tortuosity and dilation of the retinal vessels.

Astrocytic Hamartoma

Astrocytic hamartomas are benign, mulberry-type lesions associated with tuberous sclerosis (and occasionally neurofibromatosis) that most commonly appear in a juxtapapillary location or directly on the surface of the optic nerve. They appear as round or oval-shaped masses with a yellow–white color that project into the vitreous cavity. They may contain calcium and these are echographically dense on B-scan echography.

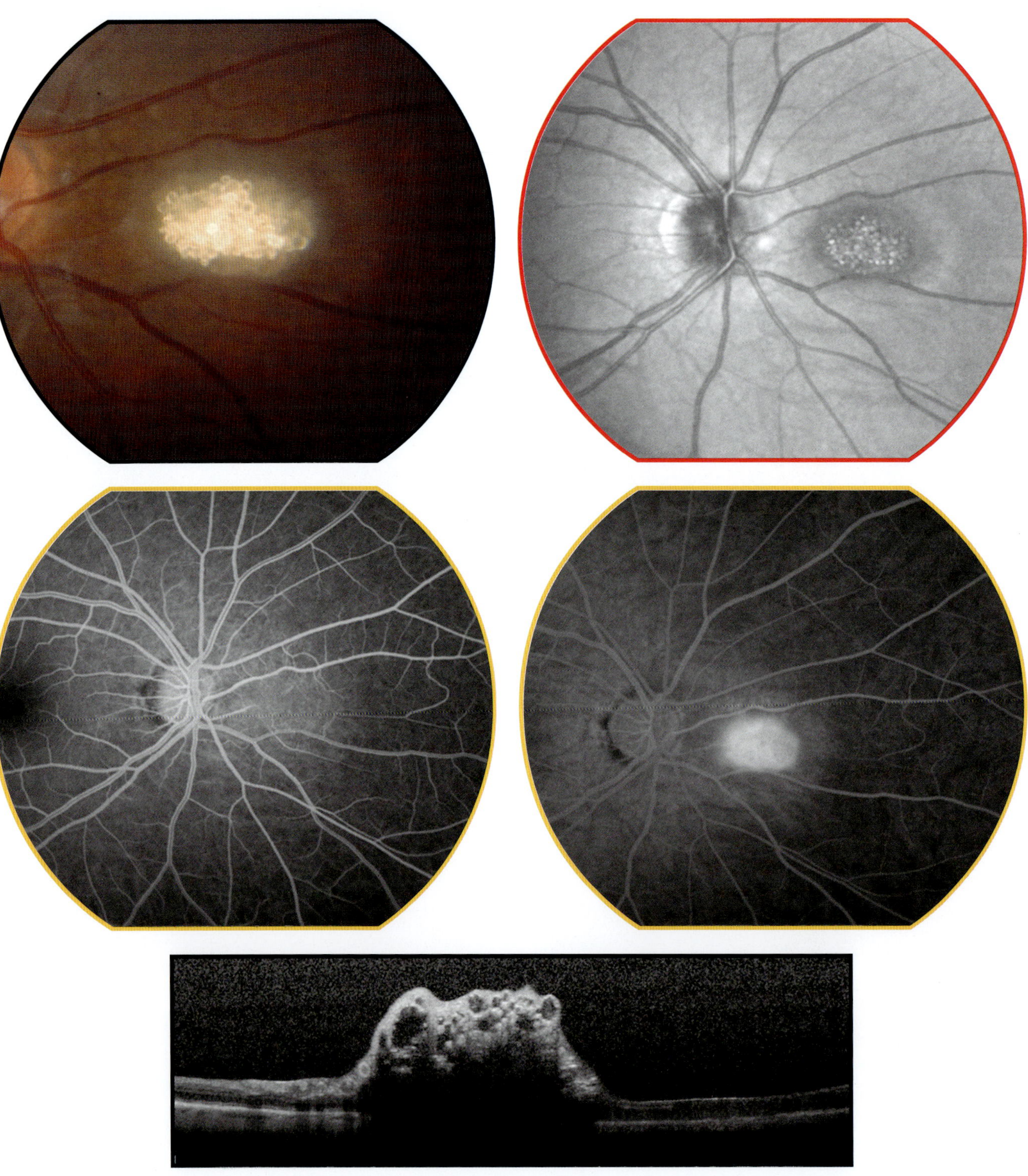

A nasal juxtapapillary retinal lesion containing multiple foci of calcium, seen clinically and echographically, fully compatible with an astrocytic hamartoma. The lesion mildly stains on fluorescein angiography, though there are no enlarged retinal feeder vessels. This patient had a systemic diagnosis of tuberous sclerosis. Observation was recommended.

Combined Hamartoma of Retina and Retinal Pigment Epithelium (RPE)

A combined hamartoma is a congenital lesion of the retina and RPE characterized by the presence of retinal vascular tortuosity, epiretinal membrane formation, hyperpigmentation, and slight elevation. The average age at presentation is 15 years of age. These lesions are most commonly found in a juxtapapillary location, though also are seen in the far anterior periphery of the retina. There frequently are signs of retinal traction and fluorescein angiography demonstrates numerous dilated capillaries within the hamartoma that leak to varying degrees.

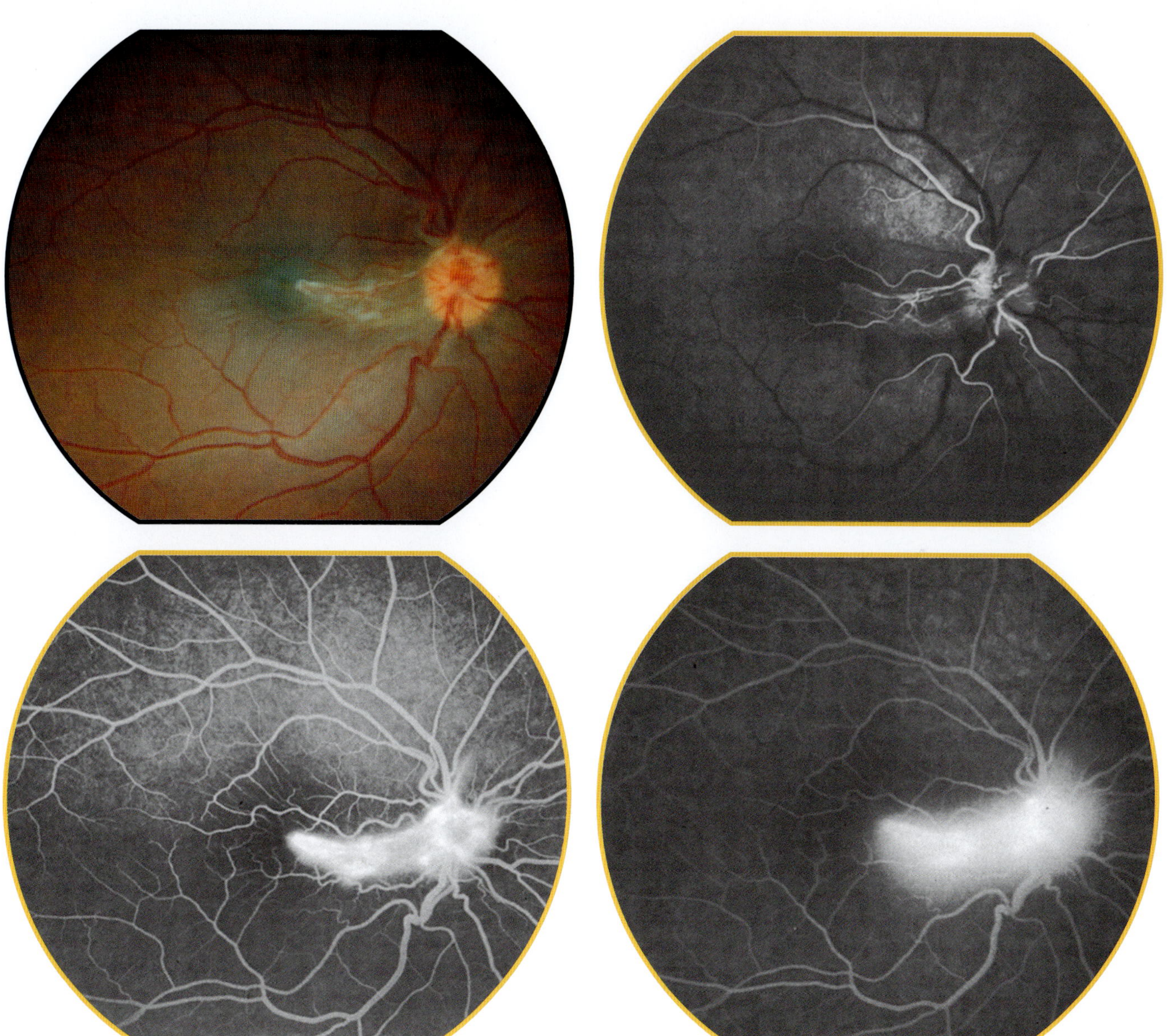

A localized combined hamartoma overlying the papillomacular bundle. Note the prominent vascularity, epiretinal membrane formation, mild hyperpigmentation, and angiographic leakage.

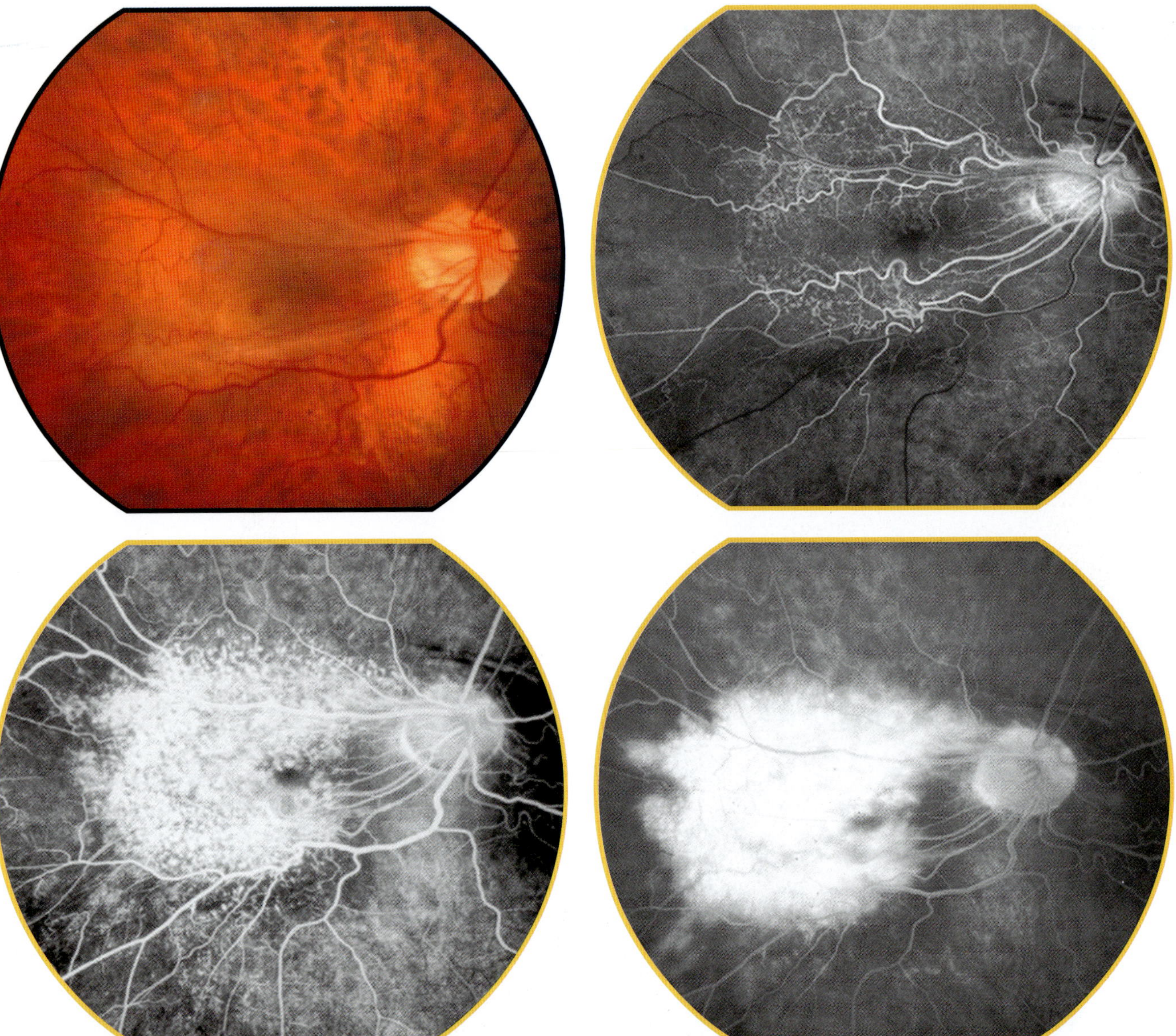

A more prominent combined hamartoma of the retina and RPE occupying the entire posterior pole of the retina including the macular region. There was very prominent vascularity and fluorescein angiographic leakage.

Retinoblastoma

Retinoblastoma is the most common primary malignancy of childhood. Retina tumors may be found through the entire retina and may involve the optic nerve as well.

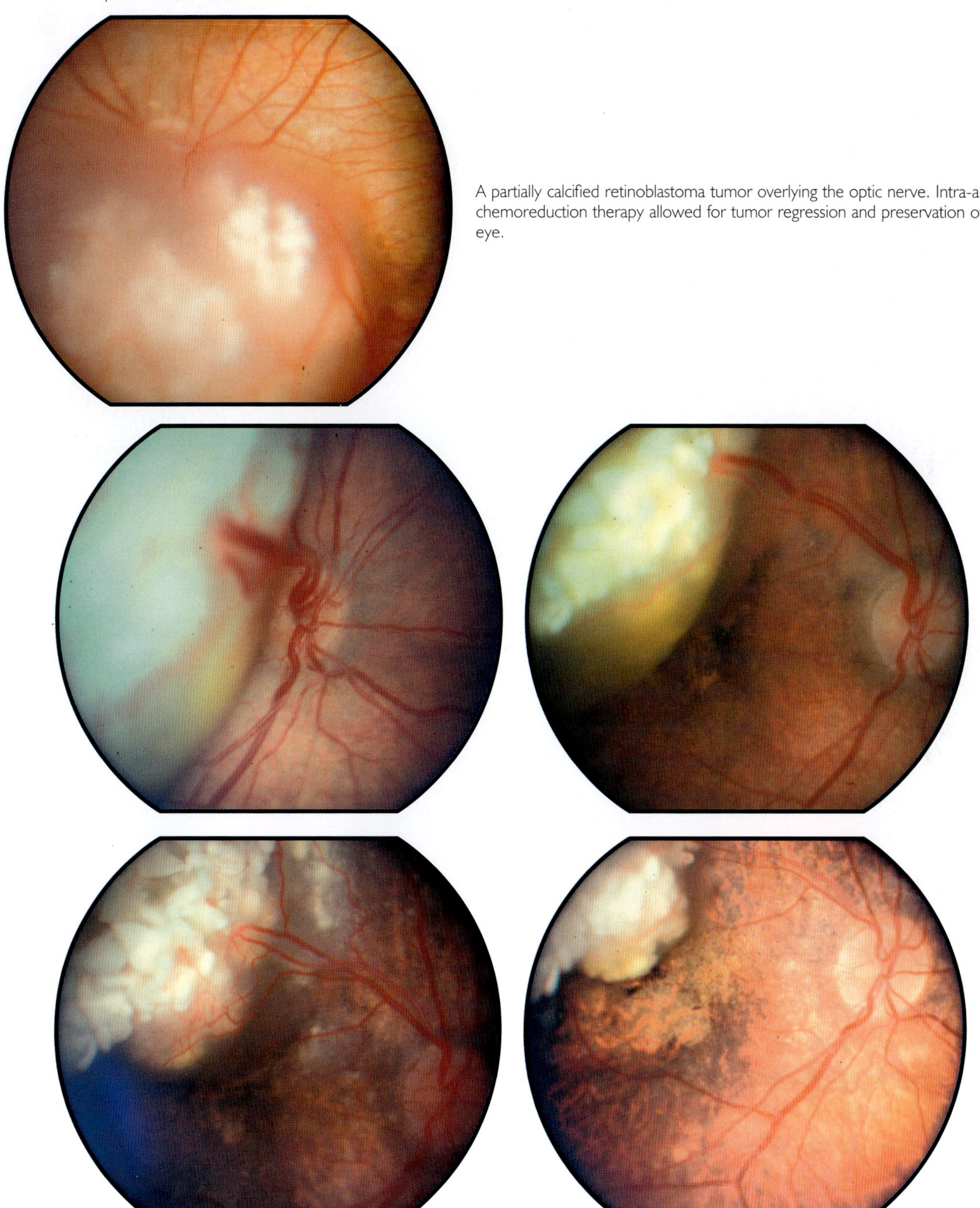

A partially calcified retinoblastoma tumor overlying the optic nerve. Intra-arterial chemoreduction therapy allowed for tumor regression and preservation of the eye.

A very prominent retinoblastoma in the right eye adjacent to the optic nerve *(upper left)*. The left eye was enucleated due to massive tumor involvement. This right eye was salvaged with external beam radiation therapy (prior to the advent of intra-arterial chemoreduction therapy). While the eye was preserved, and the child has remained healthy systemically, visual function was eventually compromised by optic nerve pallor and macular pigmentary atrophy *(bottom right)*.

Paraneoplastic Disorders

Paraneoplastic disorders may impact the choroid and less commonly the optic nerve. They are triggered by systemic malignancies and give the choroid a thickened, reddish or brownish discoloration, along with possible multiple serous detachments. The optic nerve is variably involved.

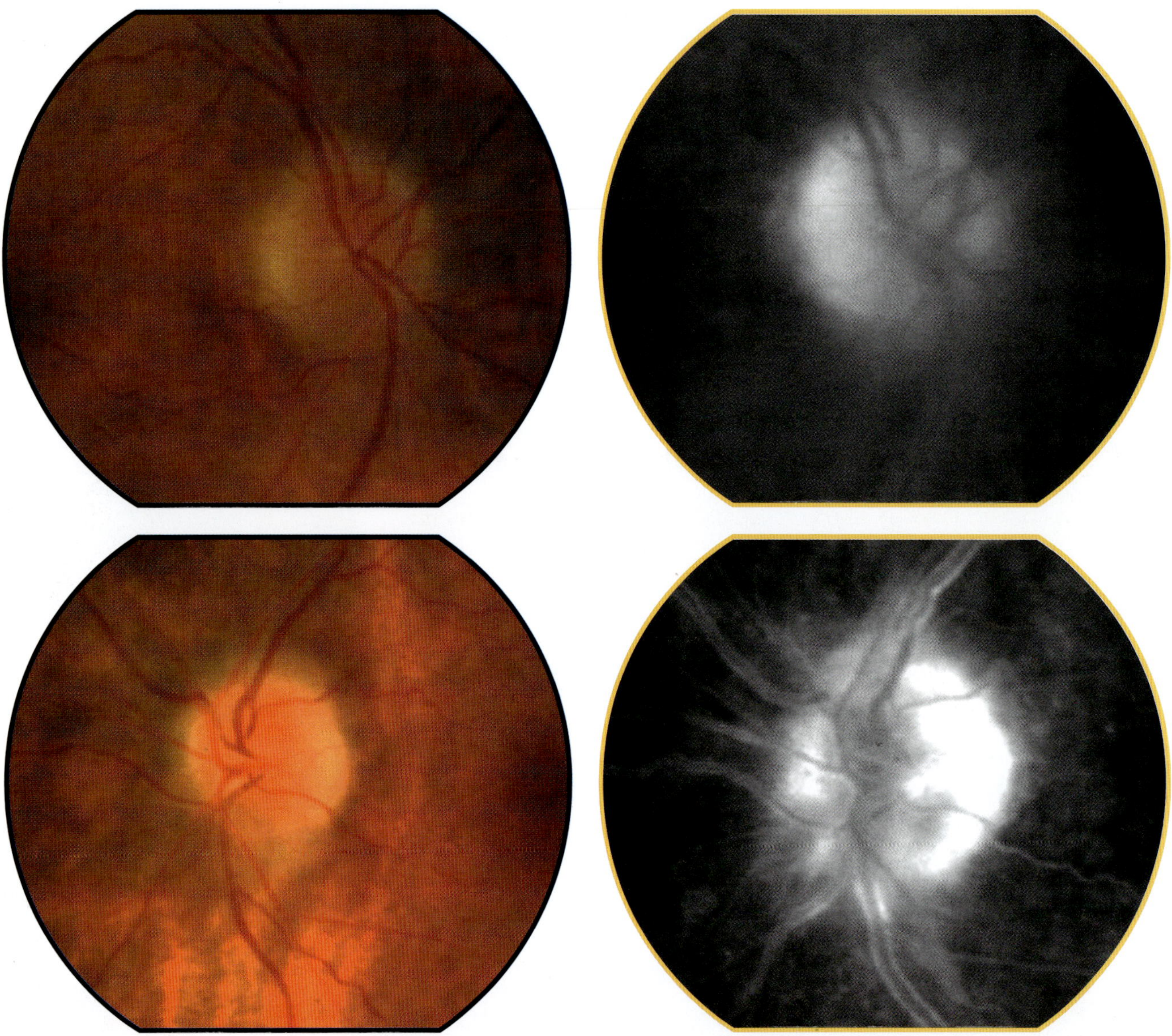

This patient has optic nerve inflammation (papillitis) as part of a paraneoplastic disorder from lung cancer. There are optic nerve and retinal vascularities. The visual acuity is 20/25 in each eye, as the macula does not have significant cystoid macular edema.

Myelinated Nerve Fibers (MNF)

Myelinated retinal nerve fibers (MNFs) are relatively common and occur in about 1% of the population. They most commonly appear contiguous with the optic nerve as white or gray–white patches with feathered or fibrillated borders distributed in an arcuate configuration coincident with the distribution of the retinal nerve fiber layer. MNFs may also be seen along the vascular arcades, separated from the optic nerve. Myelination may be associated with a relative or absolute visual field defect. Generally, eyes with MNFs are otherwise normal in structure and function.

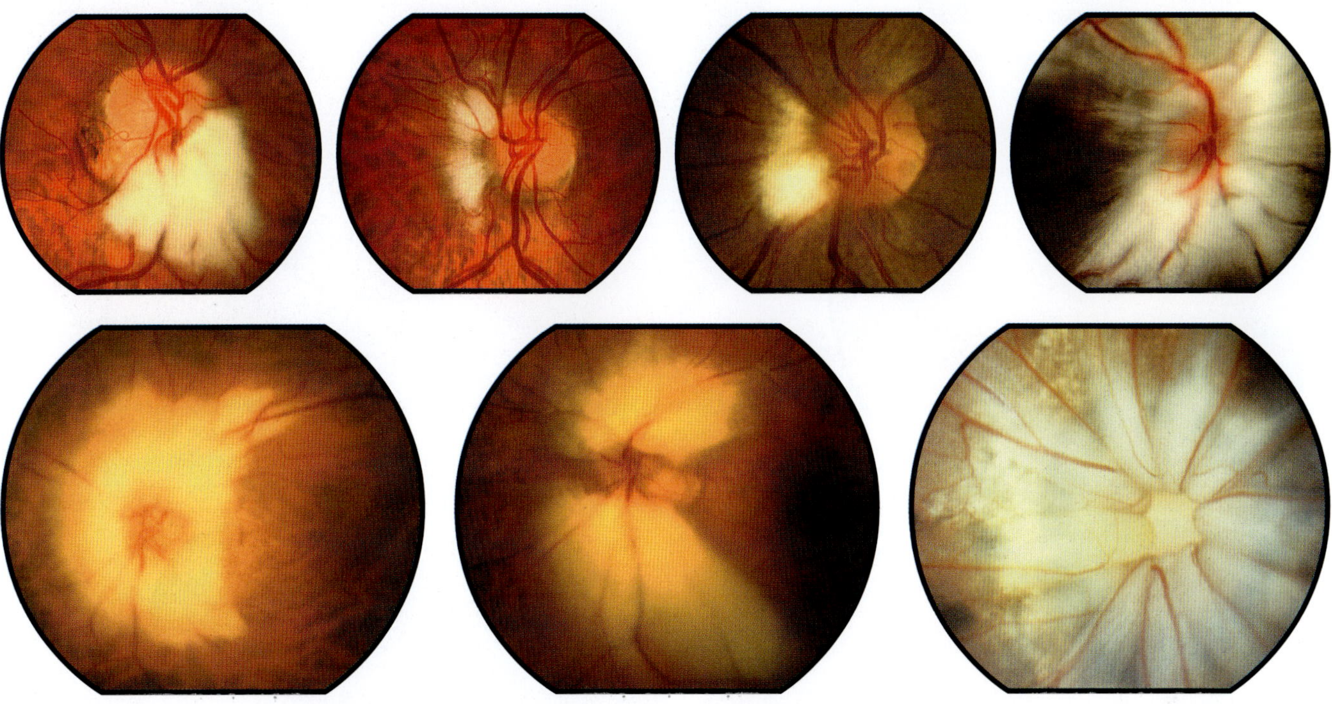

MNFs may range from small, asymptomatic feathery lesions to large, encompassing abnormalities that obscure the entire optic nerve. Relative or absolute visual field defects may be associated with MNFs.

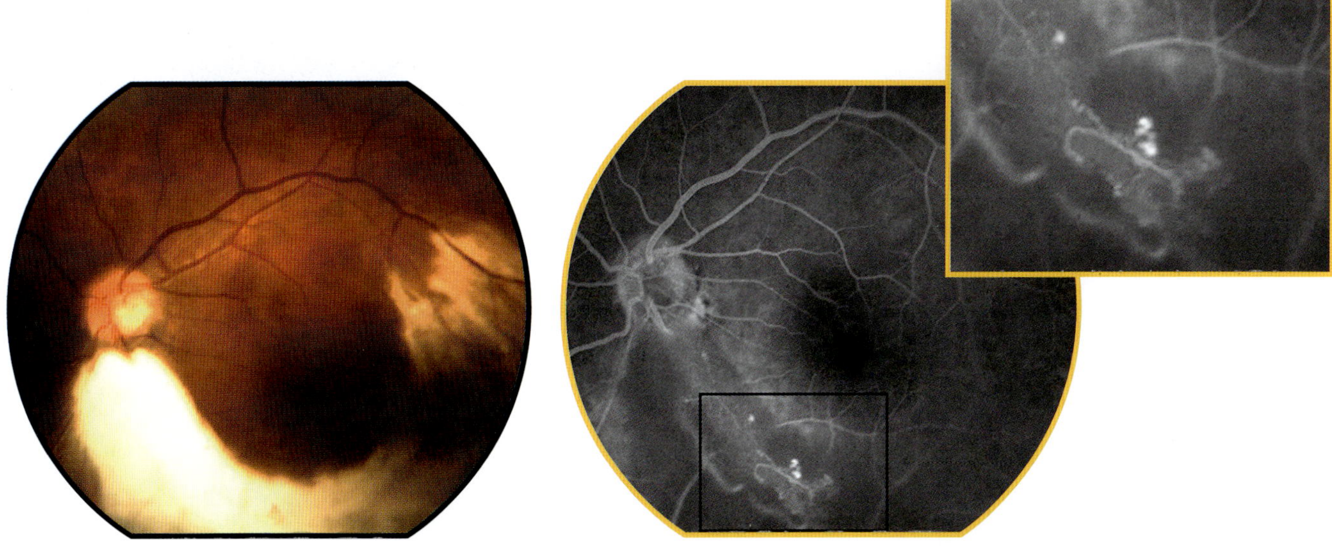

This patient has a large area of MNFs extending from the peripapillary region inferiorly in an arcuate configuration around the macula. Fluorescein angiography demonstrates retinal vascular microangiopathy including dilated, telangiectatic vessels, aneurysms, and ischemia. *Courtesy of Dr. Alfonso Ponce*

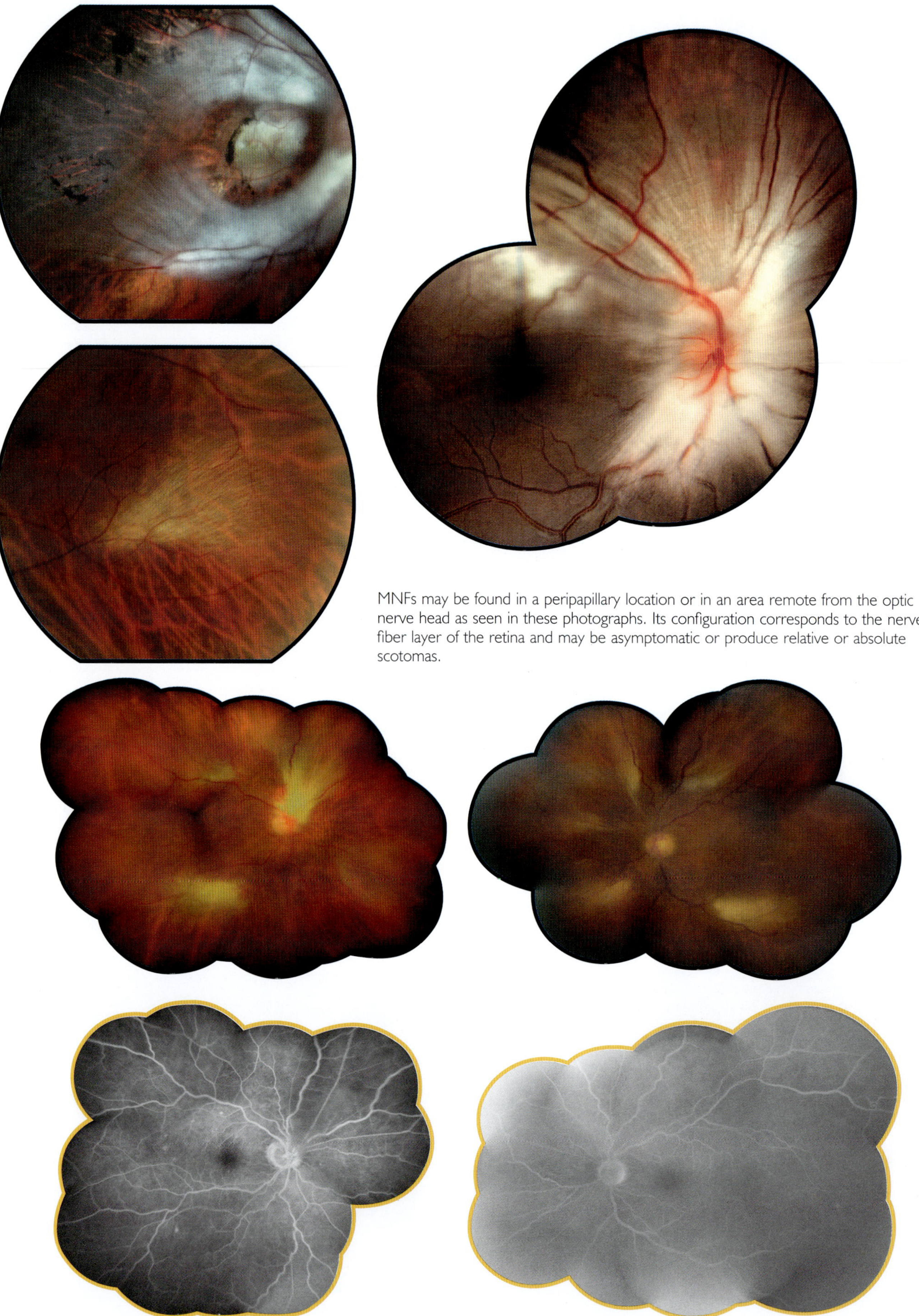

MNFs may be found in a peripapillary location or in an area remote from the optic nerve head as seen in these photographs. Its configuration corresponds to the nerve fiber layer of the retina and may be asymptomatic or produce relative or absolute scotomas.

Multiple patches of MNFs in a patient referred for assessment of possible endogenous fungal endophthalmitis. The appearance is classic for MNFs, and there was no infection. The fluorescein angiogram reveals several punctate dots of hyperfluorescence within the areas of the MNFs.

Suggested Reading

General References

Brown, G.C., Shields, J.A., 1985. Tumors of the optic nerve head. Surv. Ophthalmol. 29, 239–264.

Brown, G.C., Tasman, W.S., 1983. Congenital Anomalies of the Optic Disc. Grune & Stratton, New York.

Byrne, S.F., 1986. Evaluation of the Optic Nerve with Standardized Echography. In: Smith, J.L. (Ed.), Neuro-Ophthalmology Now! Field, Rich & Associates, New York.

Jensen, P.E., Kalina, R.E., 1976. Congenital anomalies of the optic disc. Am. J. Ophthalmol. 82, 27–31.

Optic Nerve Hypoplasia

Acers, T.E., 1981. Optic nerve hypoplasia: septo-optic-pituitary dysplasia syndrome. Trans. Am. Ophthalmol. Soc. 79, 425–457.

Ahmad, T., Borchert, M., Geffner, M., 2008. Optic nerve hypoplasia and hypopituitarism. Pediatr. Endocrinol. Rev. 5, 772–777.

Ahuja, Y., Traboulsi, E.I., 2010. Unilateral megalopapilla and contralateral optic nerve hypoplasia: a case report and review of the literature. J. AAPOS 14, 83–84.

Borchert, M., 2012. Reappraisal of the optic nerve hypoplasia syndrome. J. Neuroophthalmol. 32, 58–67.

Borchert, M., Garcia-Filion, P., 2008. The syndrome of optic nerve hypoplasia. Curr. Neurol. Neurosci. Rep. 8, 395–403.

Borchert, M., Garcia-Filion, P., 2008. The syndrome of optic nerve hypoplasia. Curr. Neurol. Neurosci. Rep. 8, 395–403.

Brodsky, M.C., Phillips, P.H., 2000. Optic nerve hypoplasia and congenital hypopituitarism. J. Pediatr. 136, 850.

Dutton, G.N., 2004. Congenital disorders of the optic nerve: excavations and hypoplasia. Eye (Lond.) 18, 1038–1048.

Edwards, W.C., Layden, W.E., 1970. Optic nerve hypoplasia. Am. J. Ophthalmol. 70, 950–959.

Fard, M.A., Wu-Chen, W.Y., Man, B.L., et al., 2010. Septo-optic dysplasia. Pediatr. Endocrinol. Rev. 8, 18–24.

Gaur, A., Squirell, D., Burke, J.P., et al., 2006. Optic nerve diastasis in a patient with congenital optic nerve hypoplasia. J. AAPOS 10, 482–483.

Hoyt, C.S., Good, W.V., 1992. Do we really understand the difference between optic nerve hypoplasia and atrophy? Eye (Lond.) 6 (Pt 2), 201–204.

Kaur, S., Jain, S., Sodhi, H.B., et al., 2013. Optic nerve hypoplasia. Oman J Ophthalmol. 6, 77–82.

Lambert, S.R., Hoyt, C.S., Narahara, M.H., 1987. Optic nerve hypoplasia. Surv. Ophthalmol. 32, 1–9.

Lempert, P., 2000. Optic nerve hypoplasia and small eyes in presumed amblyopia. J. AAPOS 4, 258–266.

Ouvrier, R., Billson, F., 1986. Optic nerve hypoplasia: a review. J. Child Neurol. 1, 181–188.

Ragge, N.K., Hoyt, W.F., Lambert, S.R., 1991. Big discs with optic nerve hypoplasia. J. Clin. Neuroophthalmol 11, 137.

Skarf, B., Hoyt, C.S., 1984. Optic nerve hypoplasia in children. Arch. Ophthalmol. 102, 62–67.

Sowka, J., Vollmer, L., Reynolds, S., 2008. Superior segmental optic nerve hypoplasia: the topless disc syndrome. Optometry 79, 576–580.

Zeki, S.M., Dutton, G.N., 1990. Optic nerve hypoplasia in children. Br. J. Ophthalmol. 74, 300–304.

Zion, V., 1976. Optic Nerve Hypoplasia. Ophthalmic Semin. 1, 171–196.

Megalopapilla

Ahuja, Y., Traboulsi, E.I., 2010. Unilateral megalopapilla and contralateral optic nerve hypoplasia: a case report and review of the literature. J. AAPOS 14, 83–84.

Franceschetti, A., Bock, R.H., 1950. Megalopapilla: a new congenital anomaly. Am. J. Ophthalmol. 33, 227–235.

Goldhammer, Y., Smith, J.L., 1975. Optic nerve anomalies in basal encephalocele. Arch. Ophthalmol. 93, 115–118.

Lee, H.S., Park, S.W., Heo, H., 2015. Megalopapilla in children: a spectral domain optical coherence tomography analysis. Acta Ophthalmol. 93, e301–e305.

Randhawa, S., Shah, V.A., Kardon, R.H., 2007. Megalopapilla, not glaucoma. Arch. Ophthalmol. 125, 1134–1135.

Sampaolesi, R., Sampaolesi, J.R., 2001. Large optic nerve heads: megalopapilla or megalodiscs. Int. Ophthalmol. 23, 251–257.

Strieff, B., 1961. Uber Megalopapille. Klin. Monatsbl. Augenheilkd 139, 824–827.

Swann, P.G., Coetzee, J., 1999. Megalopapilla. Clin. Exp. Optom. 82, 200–202.

Optic Nerve Aplasia

Brodsky, M.C., Atreides, S.P., Fowlkes, J.L., et al., 2004. Optic nerve aplasia in an infant with congenital hypopituitarism and posterior pituitary ectopia. Arch. Ophthalmol. 122 (1), 125–126.

Caputo, R., Sodi, A., Menchini, U., 2009. Unilateral optic nerve aplasia associated with rudimental retinal vasculature. Int. Ophthalmol. 29 (6), 517–519.

Floyd, M.S., Kwon, Y.H., Shah, S., et al., 2011. Unilateral congenital glaucoma in a child with optic nerve aplasia. J. AAPOS 15 (2), 200–202.

Ghassemi, F., Bazvand, F., Hosseini, S.S., et al., 2015. Optic nerve aplasia: case report and literature review. J. Ophthalmic Vis. Res. 10 (2), 187–192.

Ginsberg, J., Bove, K.E., Cuesta, M.G., 1980. Aplasia of the optic nerve with aniridia. Ann. Ophthalmol. 12 (4), 433–439.

Hotchkiss, M.L., Green, W.R., 1970. Optic nerve aplasia and hypoplasia. J. Pediatr. Ophthalmol. 84, 572–578.

Lee, B.L., Bateman, J.B., Schwartz, S.D., 1996. Posterior segment neovascularization associated with optic nerve aplasia. Am. J. Ophthalmol. 122 (1), 131–133.

Little, L.E., Whitmore, P.V., Wells, T.W., 1950. Aplasia of the optic nerve. J. Pediatr. Ophthalmol. 33, 227–235.

Mannan, R., Chandra, P., 2015. Rare case of unilateral optic nerve aplasia. BMJ Case Rep. 23, 2015.

Margo, C.E., Hamed, L.M., Fang, E., 1992. Optic nerve aplasia. Arch. Ophthalmol. 110 (11), 1610–1613.

Scott, I.U., Warman, R., Altman, N., 1997. Bilateral aplasia of the optic nerves, chiasm, and tracts in an otherwise healthy infant. Am. J. Ophthalmol. 124 (3), 409–410.

Silver, J., Puck, S.M., Albert, D.M., 1984. Development and aging of the eye in mice with inherited optic nerve aplasia: histopathological studies. Exp. Eye Res. 38 (3), 257–266.

Storm, R.L., PeBenito, R., 1984. Bilateral optic nerve aplasia associated with hydranencephaly. Ann. Ophthalmol. 16 (10), 988–992.

Tang, D.C., Man, E.M., Cheng, S.C., 2015. Aplasia of the optic nerve. Hong Kong Med. J. 21 (4), 366–368.

Weiter, J.J., McLean, I.W., Zimmerman, L.E., 1977. Aplasia of the optic nerve and disk. Am. J. Ophthalmol. 83, 569–576.

Congenital Prepapillary Vascular Loops

Degenhart, W., Brown, G.C., Augsburger, J.J., et al., 1981. Prepapillary vascular loops. Ophthalmology 88, 1126–1131.

Fujiwara, T., Machida, S., Herai, T., et al., 2004. Case of subretinal hemorrhage that developed from a prepapillary vascular loop. Jpn J. Ophthalmol. 48, 175–177.

Grossniklaus, H., Thall, E., Annable, W., 1986. Familial prepapillary vascular loops. Arch. Ophthalmol. 104, 1755–1756.

Misra, A., Flanagan, D.W., Martin, K.R., 2008. Recurrent transient visual loss due to intermittent occlusion of a prepapillary vascular loop. Br. J. Ophthalmol. 92, 431–432.

Romano, P.E., 2001. Prepapillary vascular loops. Clin. Experiment. Ophthalmol. 29, 90–91.

Shakin, E.P., Shields, J.A., Augsburger, J.J., et al., 1988. Clinicopathologic correlation of a prepapillary vascular loop. Retina 8, 55–58.

Sipperley, J.O., 1987. Familial association of prepapillary vascular loops. Arch. Ophthalmol. 105, 614.

Strassman, I.B., Desai, U.R., 1997. Prepapillary vascular loop and a recurrent vitreous hemorrhage. Retina 17, 166–167.

Wygnanski-Jaffe, T., Desatnik, H., Treister, G., et al., 1997. Acquired prepapillary vascular loops. Arch. Ophthalmol. 115, 1329–1330.

Persistent Fetal Vasculature

Acers, T.E., Coston, T.O., 1967. Persistent hyperplastic primary vitreous. Early surgical management. Am. J. Ophthalmol. 64, 734–735.

Dass, A.B., Trese, M.T., 1999. Surgical results of persistent hyperplastic primary vitreous. Ophthalmol 106, 280–284.

Edward, D.P., Mafee, M.F., Garcia-Valenzuela, E., et al., 1998. Coats' disease and persistent hyperplastic primary vitreous. Role of MR imaging and CT. Radiol. Clin. North Am. 36 (6), 1119–1131.

Federman, J.L., Shields, J.A., Altman, B., et al., 1982. The surgical and nonsurgical management of persistent hyperplastic primary vitreous. Ophthalmology 89 (1), 20–24.

Font, R.L., Yanoff, M., Zimmerman, L.E., 1969. Intraocular adipose tissue and persistent hyperplastic primary vitreous. Arch. Ophthalmol. 82 (1), 43–50.

Gass, J.D., 1970. Surgical excision of persistent hyperplastic primary vitreous. Arch. Ophthalmol. 83 (2), 163–168.

Gieser, D.K., Goldberg, M.F., Apple, D.J., et al., 1978. Persistent hyperplastic primary vitreous in an adult: case report with fluorescein angiographic findings. J. Pediatr. Ophthalmol. Strabismus 15 (4), 213–218.

Goldberg, M.F., 1997. Persistent fetal vasculature (PFV): an integrated interpretation of signs and symptoms associated with persistent hyperplastic primary vitreous (PHPV). LIV Edward Jackson Memorial Lecture. Am. J. Ophthalmol. 124 (5), 587–626.

Haddad, R., Font, R.L., Reeser, F., 1978. Persistent hyperplastic primary vitreous. A clinicopathologic study of 62 cases and review of the literature. Surv. Ophthalmol. 23 (2), 123–134.

Jampol, L.M., 2007. Persistent fetal vasculature. Arch. Ophthalmol. 125 (3), 432.

Jensen, O.A., 1968. Persistent hyperplastic primary vitreous. Cases in Denmark 1942-1966. A mainly histopathological study. Acta Ophthalmol. (Copenh) 46 (3), 418–429.

Joseph, N., Ivry, M., Oliver, M., 1972. Persistent hyperplastic primary vitreous at the optic nerve head. Am. J. Ophthalmol. 73 (4), 580–583.

Kumar, A., Jethani, J., Shetty, S., et al., 2010. Bilateral persistent fetal vasculature: a study of 11 cases. J. AAPOS 14 (4), 345–348.

Laatikainen, L., Tarkkanen, A., 1982. Microsurgery of persistent hyperplastic primary vitreous. Ophthalmologica 185 (4), 193–198.

Lloyd, R.I., 1940. Variations in the development and regression of Bergmeister's papilla and the hyaloid artery. Trans. Am. Ophtalmol. Soc. 38, 326–332.

Mann, I.C., 1957. Developmental Abnormalities of the Eye, second ed. JB Lippincott, Philadepphia, pp. 116–121.

Mann, I.C., 1969. Development of the Human Eye, third ed. Grune & Stratton, New York, pp. 27–28, 228–231.

Manschot, W.A., 1958. Persistent hyperplastic primary vitreous; special reference to preretinal glial tissue as a pathological characteristic and to the development of the primary vitreous. AMA Arch. Ophthalmol. 59 (2), 188–203.

Meisels, H.I., Goldberg, M.F., 1979. Vascular anastomoses between the iris and persistent hyperplastic primary vitreous. Am. J. Ophthalmol. 88 (2), 179–185.

Muen, W.J., Roberts, C., Sagoo, M.S., et al., 2012. Persistent fetal vasculature. Ophthalmology 119 (9), 1944–1945.e1-2.

Nankin, S.J., Scott, W.E., 1977. Persistent hyperplastic primary vitreous: roto-extraction and other surgical experience. Arch. Ophthalmol. 95 (2), 240–243.

Peyman, G.A., Sanders, D.R., Nagpal, K.C., 1976. Management of persistent hyperplastic primary vitreous by pars plana vitrectomy. Br. J. Ophthalmol. 60 (11), 756–758.

Pollard, Z.F., 1997. Persistent hyperplastic primary vitreous: diagnosis, treatment and results. Trans. Am. Ophthalmol. Soc. 95, 487–549.

Raskind, R.H., 1966. Persistent hyperplastic primary vitreous. Necessity of early recognition and treatment. Am. J. Ophthalmol. 62 (6), 1072–1076.

Reese, A.B., 1955a. Persistent hyperplastic primary vitreous. Trans. Am. Acad. Ophthalmol. Otolaryngol. 59 (3), 271–295.

Reese, A.B., 1955b. Persistent hyperplastic primary vitreous. Am. J. Ophthalmol. 40 (3), 317–331.

Rosen, D.A., Yamashita, T., 1964. Persistent hyperplastic primary vitreous. Am. J. Ophthalmol. 57, 1002–1007.

Spaulding, A.G., 1967. Persistent hyperplastic primary vitreous humor; a finding in a 71-year-old man. Surv. Ophthalmol. 12 (5), 448–452.

Spaulding, A.G., Naumann, G., 1967. Persistent hyperplastic primary vitreous in an adult. A brief review of the literature and a histopathologic study. Arch. Ophthalmol. 77 (5), 666–671.

Stark, W.J., 1981. Surgical management of persistent hyperplastic primary vitreous. Dev. Ophthalmol. 5, 115–121.

Stark, W.J., Fagadau, W., Lindsey, P.S., et al., 1983. Management of persistent hyperplastic primary vitreous. Aust. J. Ophthalmol. 11 (3), 195–200.

Stark, W.J., Lindsey, P.S., Fagadau, W.R., et al., 1983. Persistent hyperplastic primary vitreous. Surgical treatment. Ophthalmology 90 (5), 452–457.

Traboulsi, E.I., Maumenee, I.H., 1992. Peters' anomaly and associated congenital malformations. Arch. Ophthalmol. 110 (12), 1739–1742.

Wang, M.K., Phillips, C.I., 1973. Persistent hyperplastic primary vitreous in non-identical twins. Acta Ophthalmol. (Copenh) 51 (4), 434–437.

Wegener, J.K., Sogaard, H., 1968. Persistent hyperplastic primary vitreous with resorption of the lens. Acta Ophthalmol. (Copenh) 46 (2), 171–175.

Zhao, Y.E., Chen, D., Li, J.H., 2010. Bilateral persistent fetal vasculature in an adult: clinical manifestations and surgical outcomes. J. Cataract Refract. Surg. 36 (8), 1421–1426.

Bergmeister Papilla

Giuffrè, G., 1987. Remnants of Bergmeister's papilla and retinochoroidal colobomas. Ann. Ophthalmol. 19 (8), 316–318.

Lloyd, R.I., 1940. Variations in the Development and Regression of Bergmeister's Papilla and the Hyaloid Artery. Trans. Am. Ophthalmol. Soc. 38, 326–332.

Petersen, H.P., 1968. Persistence of the Bergmeister papilla with glial overgrowth. Various diagnostic problems. Acta Ophthalmol. (Copenh) 46 (3), 430–440.

Santos-Bueso, E., Asorey-García, A., Vinuesa-Silva, J.M., et al., 2015. Bergmeister's papilla. Arch. Soc. Esp. Oftalmol. 90 (8), 395–396.

Congenital Retinal Macrovessel

Brown, G.C., 1977. Congenital fundus abnormalities. In: Duane, T.D. (Ed.), Clinical Ophthalmology. Harper & Row, Hagerstown.

Brown, G.C., Donoso, L.A., Magargal, L.E., et al., 1982. Congenital retinal macrovessels. Arch. Ophthalmol. 100 (9), 1430–1436.

Bruè, C., Vance, S.K., Yannuzzi, L.A., et al., 2011. Cavernous hemangioma associated with retinal macrovessels. Retin Cases Brief Rep. 5 (4), 323–325.

Ceylan, O.M., Gullulu, G., Akin, T., et al., 2011. Congenital retinal macrovessel: atypical presentation using optical coherence tomography. Int. Ophthalmol. 31 (1), 55–58.

Choudhry, N., Rao, R.C., 2016. Enhanced depth imaging features of a choroidal macrovessel. Retin Cases Brief Rep. 10 (1), 18–21.

de Crecchio, G., Alfieri, M.C., Cennamo, G., et al., 2006. Congenital macular macrovessels. Graefes Arch. Clin. Exp. Ophthalmol. 244 (9), 1183–1187.

de Crecchio, G., Mastursi, B., Alfieri, M.C., et al., 1986. Congenital retinal macrovessel. Ophthalmologica 193 (3), 143–145.

de Crecchio, G., Pacente, L., Alfieri, M.C., et al., 1999. Congenital retinal macrovessels: a "low visual acuity" case report with a 14-year follow-up. Acta Ophthalmol. Scand. 77 (4), 474–475.

de Crecchio, G., Pacente, L., Alfieri, M.C., et al., 2000. Valsalva retinopathy associated with a congenital retinal macrovessel. Arch. Ophthalmol. 118 (1), 146–147.

Jager, R.D., Timothy, N.H., Coney, J.M., et al., 2005. Congenital retinal macrovessel. Retina 25 (4), 538–540.

Kovach, J.L., 2016. Unilateral Choroidal Macrovessel. JAMA Ophthalmol 134 (3), e153678.

Lima, L.H., Laud, K., Chang, L.K., et al., 2011. Choroidal macrovessel. Br. J. Ophthalmol. 95 (9), 1333–1334.

Petropoulos, I.K., Petkou, D., Theoulakis, P.E., et al., 2008. Congenital retinal macrovessels: description of three cases and review of the literature. Klin Monbl Augenheilkd. 225 (5), 469–472.

Pichi, F., Nucci, P., Srivastava, S.K., 2016. Choroidal macrovessel. Ophthalmology 123 (3), 531.

Polk, T.D., Park, D., Sindt, C.W., et al., 1997. Congenital retinal macrovessel. Arch. Ophthalmol. 115 (2), 290–291.

Sanfilippo, C.J., Sarraf, D., 2015. Congenital macrovessel associated with cystoid macular edema and an ipsilateral intracranial venous malformation. Retin Cases Brief Rep. 9 (4), 357–359.

Soltau, J.B., Olk, R.J., Gordon, J.M., 1996. Prepapillary arterial loop associated with vitreous hemorrhage and venous retinal macrovessel. Retina 16 (1), 74–75.

Souissi, K., El Afrit, M.A., Kraiem, A., 2006. Congenital retinal arterial macrovessel and congenital hamartoma of the retinal pigment epithelium. J. Pediatr. Ophthalmol. Strabismus 43 (3), 181–182.

Volk, P., 1956. Visual function studies in a case of large aberrant vessels in the macula. Arch. Ophthalmol. 55, 119–122.

Cilioretinal Artery Occlusion

Ahmadieh, H., Javadi, M.A., 2005. Cilioretinal artery occlusion following laser in situ keratomileusis. Retina 25 (4), 533–537.

Brosnan, D.W., 1962. Occlusion of a cilioretinal artery with permanent central scotoma. Am. J. Ophthalmol. 53, 687–688.

Brown, G.C., Moffat, K., Cruess, A., et al., 1983. Cilioretinal artery obstruction. Retina 3 (3), 182–187.

Dori, D., Gelfand, Y.A., Brenner, B., et al., 1997. Cilioretinal artery occlusion: an ocular complication of primary antiphospholipid syndrome. Retina 17 (6), 555–557.

Friedman, M.W., 1959. Occlusion of the cilioretinal artery. Am. J. Ophthalmol. 47 (5 Pt 1), 684–686.

Galasso, J.M., Jay, W.M., 2004. An occult case of giant cell arteritis presenting with combined anterior ischemic optic neuropathy and cilioretinal artery occlusion. Semin. Ophthalmol. 19 (3–4), 75–77.

Gangwar, D.N., Grewal, S.P., Jain, I.S., et al., 1984. Cilioretinal artery occlusion: a case report. Ann. Ophthalmol. 16 (11), 1022–1024.

Greven, C.M., Slusher, M.M., Weaver, R.G., 1995. Retinal arterial occlusions in young adults. Am. J. Ophthalmol. 120 (6), 776–783.

Hayreh, S.S., Fraterrigo, L., Jonas, J., 2008. Central retinal vein occlusion associated with cilioretinal artery occlusion. Retina 28 (4), 581–594.

Hayreh, S.S., Podhajsky, P.A., Zimmerman, B., 1998. Ocular manifestations of giant cell arteritis. Am. J. Ophthalmol. 125 (4), 509–520.

Hayreh, S.S., Zimmerman, M.B., 2005. Central retinal artery occlusion: visual outcome. Am. J. Ophthalmol. 140 (3), 376–391.

Hwang, J.F., Chen, S.N., Chiu, S.L., et al., 2004. Embolic cilioretinal artery occlusion due to carotid artery dissection. Am. J. Ophthalmol. 138 (3), 496–498.

Keyser, B.J., Duker, J.S., Brown, G.C., et al., 1994. Combined central retinal vein occlusion and cilioretinal artery occlusion associated with prolonged retinal arterial filling. Am. J. Ophthalmol. 117 (3), 308–313.

Kunikata, H., Tamai, M., 2006. Cilioretinal artery occlusions following embolization of an artery to an intracranial meningioma. Graefes Arch. Clin. Exp. Ophthalmol. 244 (3), 401–403.

Levitt, J.M., 1948. Occlusion of the cilioretinal artery. Arch Ophthal. 40 (2), 152–156.

Mehre, K.S., 1965. Incidence of cilio-retinal artery in Indians. Br. J. Ophthalmol. 49, 52–53.

Nicholson, L., Bizrah, M., Hussain, B., et al., 2016. Video Angiography of Cilioretinal Artery Infarction in Central Retinal Vein Occlusion. Retina 36 (5), e33–e35.

Noble, K.G., 1994. Central retinal vein occlusion and cilioretinal artery infarction. Am. J. Ophthalmol. 118 (6), 811–813.

Perry, H.D., Mallen, F.J., 1977. Cilioretinal artery occlusion associated with oral contraceptives. Am. J. Ophthalmol. 84 (1), 56–58.

Rubenzik, R., Selezinka, W., Wolter, J.R., 1975. Embolism of a cilioretinal artery following cardiac surgery. Ann. Ophthalmol. 7 (2), 209–211.

Sahu, D.K., Rawoof, A.B., 2000. Cilioretinal artery occlusion in posterior scleritis. Retina 20 (3), 303–305.

Schatz, H., Fong, A.C., McDonald, H.R., et al., 1991. Cilioretinal artery occlusion in young adults with central retinal vein occlusion. Ophthalmology 98 (5), 594–601.

Stoffelns, B.M., Laspas, P., 2015. Cilioretinal artery occlusion. Klin Monbl Augenheilkd. 232 (4), 519–524.

Zylbermann, R., Rozenman, Y., Ronen, S., 1981. Functional occlusion of a cilioretinal artery. Ann. Ophthalmol. 13 (11), 1269–1272.

Optic Nerve, Retinochoroidal, and Iris Colobomas

Ahmad, N., Sheard, R.M., 2010. Management of macular hole with choroidal coloboma. Retin Cases Brief Rep. 4 (1), 78–80.

Brodsky, M.C., Ford, R.E., Bradford, J.D., 1991. Subretinal neovascular membrane in an infant with a retinochoroidal coloboma. Arch. Ophthalmol. 109 (12), 1650–1651.

Cionni, R.J., Karatza, E.C., Osher, R.H., et al., 2006. Surgical technique for congenital iris coloboma repair. J. Cataract Refract. Surg. 32 (11), 1913–1916.

Cogan, D.G., 1978. Coloboma of the optic nerve with overlay of the peripapillary retina. Br. J. Ophthalmol. 62, 347–350.

Dailey, J.R., Cantore, W.A., Gardner, T.W., 1993. Peripapillary choroidal neovascular membrane associated with an optic nerve coloboma. Arch. Ophthalmol. 111 (4), 441–442.

Fine, H.F., Sorenson, J.J., Spaide, R.F., et al., 2008. Spontaneous scleral rupture adjacent to retinochoroidal coloboma. Retin Cases Brief Rep. 2 (4), 296–298.

Gupta, A., Narang, S., Gupta, V., et al., 2001. Successful closure of spontaneous scleral fistula in retinochoroidal coloboma. Arch. Ophthalmol. 119 (8), 1220–1221.

Hall, B.D., 1989. Iris coloboma, ptosis, hypertelorism, and mental retardation. J. Med. Genet. 26 (1), 69.

Leff, S.R., Britton, W.A. Jr., Brown, G.C., et al., 1985. Retinochoroidal coloboma associated with subretinal neovascularization. Retina 5 (3), 154–156.

Morrison, D.A., FitzPatrick, D.R., Fleck, B.W., 2000. Iris coloboma with iris heterochromia: a common association. Arch. Ophthalmol. 118 (11), 1590–1591.

Murphy, B.L., Griffin, J.F., 1994. Optic nerve coloboma (morning glory syndrome): CT findings. Radiology 191 (1), 59–61.

Pagon, R.A., 1981. Ocular coloboma. Surv. Ophthalmol. 25 (4), 223–236.

Perkins, S.L., Han, D.P., Gonder, J.R., et al., 2005. Dynamic atypical optic nerve coloboma associated with transient macular detachment. Arch. Ophthalmol. 123 (12), 1750–1754.

Pyhtinen, J., Lindholm, E.L., 1996. Imaging in optic nerve coloboma. Neuroradiology 38 (2), 171–174.

Rahimy, E., Rahimy, E., 2016. Bilateral optic nerve coloboma and macular schisis in papillorenal syndrome. Ophthalmology 123 (5), 990.

Rouland, J.F., Constantinides, G., 1991. Retinochoroidal coloboma and subretinal neovascularization. Ann. Ophthalmol. 23 (2), 61–62.

Shami, M., McCartney, D., Benedict, W., et al., 1992. Spontaneous retinal reattachment in a patient with persistent hyperplastic primary vitreous and an optic nerve coloboma. Am. J. Ophthalmol. 114 (6), 769–771.

Slusher, M.M., Weaver, R.G., Greven, C.M., et al., 1989. The spectrum of cavitary optic disc anomalies in a family. Ophthalmol 96, 342–347.

Soong, H.K., Raizman, M.B., 1986. Corneal changes in familial iris coloboma. Ophthalmology 93 (3), 335–339.

Spitzer, M., Grisanti, S., Bartz-Schmidt, K.U., et al., 2006. Choroidal neovascularization in retinochoroidal coloboma: thermal laser treatment achieves long-term stabilization of visual acuity. Eye (Lond.) 20 (8), 969–972.

Steahly, L.P., 1986. Laser treatment of a subretinal neovascular membrane associated with retinochoroidal coloboma. Retina 6 (3), 154–156.

Steahly, L.P., 1990. Retinochoroidal coloboma: varieties of clinical presentations. Ann. Ophthalmol. 22 (1), 9–14.

Theodossiadis, P., Moschos, M., Theodossiadis, G., 2000. Optic nerve coloboma with retinal degeneration associated with cystic microphthalmia of the other eye. Acta Ophthalmol. Scand. 78 (2), 235–236.

Tormene, A.P., Riva, C., 1998-1999. Electroretinogram and visual-evoked potentials in children with optic nerve coloboma. Doc. Ophthalmol. 96 (4), 347–354.

Traboulsi, E.I., 1986. Corneal changes in familial iris coloboma. Ophthalmology 93 (10), 1369–1370.

van Dalen, J.T., Delleman, J.W., Yogiantoro, M., 1983. A discussion of 61 cases of optic nerve coloboma. Doc. Ophthalmol. 56 (1–2), 177–181.

Wiggins, R.E., von Noorden, G.K., Boniuk, M., 1991. Optic nerve coloboma with cyst: a case report and review. J. Pediatr. Ophthalmol. Strabismus 28 (5), 274–277.

Yamashita, T., Kawano, K., Ohba, N., 1988. Autosomal dominantly inherited optic nerve coloboma. Ophthalmic Paediatr. Genet. 9 (1), 17–24.

Ying, M.S., Fuller, J., Young, J., et al., 2004. Spontaneous resolution of optic nerve coloboma-associated retinal detachment. J. Pediatr. Ophthalmol. Strabismus 41 (6), 358–360.

Morning Glory Disc Anomaly

Adam, P., Bec, P., Mathis, A., et al., 1984. Morning glory syndrome: CT findings. J. Comput. Assist. Tomogr. 8 (1), 134–136.

Akamine, T., Doi, M., Takahashi, H., et al., 1997. Morning glory syndrome with peripheral exudative retinal detachment. Retina 17, 73–74.

Akiyama, K., Azuma, N., Hida, T., et al., 1984. Retinal detachment in morning glory syndrome. Ophthalmic Surg. 15 (10), 841–843.

Beyer, W.B., Quencer, R.M., Osher, R.H., 1982. Morning glory syndrome. A functional analysis including fluorescein angiography, ultrasonography and computerized tomography. Ophthalmology 89, 1362–1367.

Caprioli, J., Lesser, R.L., 1983. Basal encephalocele and morning glory syndrome. Br. J. Ophthalmol. 67 (6), 349–351.

Cennamo, G., de Crecchio, G., Iaccarino, G., et al., 2010. Evaluation of morning glory syndrome with spectral optical coherence tomography and echography. Ophthalmology 117 (6), 1269–1273.

Cennamo, G., Sammartino, A., Fioretti, F., 1983. Morning glory syndrome with contractile peripapillary staphyloma. Br. J. Ophthalmol. 67 (6), 346–348.

Chang, S., Gregory-Roberts, E., Chen, R., 2012. Retinal detachment associated with optic disc colobomas and morning glory syndrome. Eye (Lond.) 26 (4), 494–500.

Chaudhuri, Z., Grover, A.K., Bageja, S., et al., 2007. Morning glory anomaly with bilateral choroidal colobomas in a patient with Goldenhar's syndrome. J. Pediatr. Ophthalmol. Strabismus 44, 187–189.

Coll, G.E., Chang, S., Flynn, T.E., et al., 1995. Communication between the subretinal space and the vitreous cavity in the morning glory syndrome. Graefes Arch. Clin. Exp. Ophthalmol. 233, 441–443.

Eustis, H.S., Sanders, M.R., Zimmerman, T., 1994. Morning glory syndrome in children. Association with endocrine and central nervous system anomalies. Arch. Ophthalmol. 112 (2), 204–207.

Fei, P., Zhang, Q., Li, J., et al., 2013. Clinical characteristics and treatment of 22 eyes of morning glory syndrome associated with persistent hyperplastic primary vitreous. Br. J. Ophthalmol. 97 (10), 1262–1267.

Giuffrè, G., 1986. Morning glory syndrome: clinical and electrofunctional study of three cases. Br. J. Ophthalmol. 70 (3), 229–236.

Harasymowycz, P., Chevrette, L., Décarie, J.C., et al., 2005. Morning glory syndrome: clinical, computerized tomographic, and ultrasonographic findings. J. Pediatr. Ophthalmol. Strabismus 42, 290–295.

Ho, T.C., Tsai, P.C., Chen, M.S., et al., 2006. Optical coherence tomography in the detection of retinal break and management of retinal detachment in morning glory syndrome. Acta Ophthalmol. Scand. 84 (2), 225–227.

Irvine, A.R., Crawford, J.B., Sullivan, J.H., 1986. The pathogenesis of retinal detachment with morning glory disk and optic pit. Retina 6, 146–150.

Jackson, W.E., Freed, S., 1985. Ocular and systemic abnormalities associated with morning glory syndrome. Ophthalmic Paediatr. Genet. 5 (1–2), 111–115.

Kindler, P., 1970. Morning glory syndrome: unusual congenital optic disc anomaly. Am. J. Ophthalmol. 69, 376.

Koenig, S.B., Naidich, T.P., Lissner, G., 1982. The morning glory syndrome associated with sphenoidal encephalocele. Ophthalmology 89 (12), 1368–1373.

Krause, U., 1972. Three cases of the morning glory syndrome. Acta Ophthalmol. (Copenh) 50 (2), 188–198.

Lee, B.J., Traboulsi, E.I., 2008. Update on the morning glory disc anomaly. Ophthalmic Genet. 29, 47–52.

Lenhart, P.D., Lambert, S.R., Newman, N.J., et al., 2006. Intracranial vascular anomalies in patients with morning glory disk anomaly. Am. J. Ophthalmol. 142, 644–650.

Manschot, W.A., 1990. Morning glory syndrome: a histopathological study. Br J Ophthalmol 74 (1), 56–58.

Matsumoto, H., Enaida, H., Hisatomi, T., et al., 2003. Retinal detachment in morning glory syndrome treated by triamcinolone acetonide-assisted pars plana vitrectomy. Retina 23 (4), 569–572.

Murphy, B.L., Griffin, J.F., 1994. Optic nerve coloboma (morning glory syndrome): CT findings. Radiology 191 (1), 59–61.

Nagasawa, T., Mitamura, Y., Katome, T., et al., 2014. Swept-source optical coherence tomographic findings in morning glory syndrome. Retina 34 (1), 206–208.

Rosenberg, A.M., Gole, G.A., 1981. Morning glory syndrome: a report of two cases. Aust. J. Ophthalmol. 9 (4), 263–265.

Rubinstein, K., 1983. Acute morning glory syndrome: report of a case. Br. J. Ophthalmol. 67 (6), 343–345.

Srinivasan, G., Venkatesh, P., Garg, S., 2007. Optical coherence tomographic characteristics in morning glory disc anomaly. Can. J. Ophthalmol. 42, 307–309.

Steinkuller, P.G., 1980. The morning glory disk anomaly: case report and literature review. J. Pediatr. Ophthalmol. Strabismus 17 (2), 81–87.

Taşkintuna, I., Oz, O., Teke, M.Y., et al., 2003. Morning glory syndrome: association with moyamoya disease, midline cranial defects, central nervous system anomalies, and persistent hyaloid artery remnant. Retina 23 (3), 400–402.

von Fricken, M.A., Dhungel, R., 1984. Retinal detachment in the Morning Glory syndrome. Pathogenesis and management. Retina 4 (2), 97–99.

Wu, Y.K., Wu, T.E., Peng, P.H., et al., 2008. Quantitative optical coherence tomography findings in a 4-year-old boy with typical morning glory disk anomaly. J. AAPOS 12, 621–622.

Yamana, T., Nishimura, M., Ueda, K., et al., 1983. Macular involvement in morning glory syndrome. Jpn J. Ophthalmol. 27 (1), 201–209.

Optic Nerve Pit

Annesley, W., Brown, G.C., Bolling, J., et al., 1987. Treatment of retinal detachment with congenital optic pit with krypton laser photocoagulation. Graefes Arch. Clin. Exp. Ophthalmol. 225, 3–4.

Cox, M.S., Witherspoon, C.D., Morris, R.E., et al., 1988. Evolving techniques in the treatment of macular detachment caused by optic nerve pits. Ophthalmology 95, 889–896.

Doyle, E., Trivedi, D., Good, P., et al., 2009. High-resolution optical coherence tomography demonstration of membranes spanning optic disc pits and colobomas. Br. J. Ophthalmol. 93, 360–365.

Ferry, A.P., 1963. Macular detachment associated with congenital pit of the optic nerve head: pathologic findings in two cases simulating malignant melanoma of the choroid. Arch. Ophthalmol. 70, 346–357.

Krivoy, D., Gentile, R., Liebmann, J.M., et al., 1996. Imaging congenital optic disc pits and associated maculopathy using optic coherence tomography. Arch. Ophthalmol. 114, 165–170.

Kunjam, V., Sekhar, G.C., 2004. Optic disc imaging by Heidelberg retinal tomogram in congenital optic disc anomaly. Indian J. Ophthalmol. 52, 149–151.

Lincoff, H., Lopez, R., Kreissig, I., et al., 1988. Retinoschisis associated with optic nerve pits. Arch. Ophthalmol. 106, 61–67.

Lincoff, H., Yannuzzi, L., Singerman, L., et al., 1993. Improvement in visual function after displacement of the retinal elevations emanating from optic pits. Arch. Ophthalmol. 111, 1071–1079.

Meyer, C.H., Rodrigues, E.B., Schmidt, J.C., 2003. Congenital optic nerve head pit associated with reduced retinal nerve fibre thickness at the papillomacular bundle. Br. J. Ophthalmol. 87, 1300–1301.

Singerman, L.J., Mittra, R.A., 2001. Hereditary optic pit and iris coloboma in three generations of a single family. Retina 21, 273–275.

Sobol, W.M., Boldi, C.F., Folk, J.C., et al., 1990. Long-term visual outcome in patients with optic nerve pit and serous retinal detachment of the macula. Ophthalmology 97, 1539–1542.

Tilted Disc Syndrome

Alexander, L.J., 1978. The tilted disc syndrome. J. Am. Optom. Assoc. 49 (9), 1060–1062.

Apple, D.J., Rabb, M.F., Walsh, P.M., 1982. Congenital anomalies of the optic disc. Surv. Ophthalmol. 27 (1), 3–41.

Brazitikos, P.D., Safran, A.B., Simona, F., et al., 1990. Threshold perimetry in tilted disc syndrome. Arch. Ophthalmol. 108 (12), 1698–1700.

Cohen, S.Y., Quentel, G., 2006. Chorioretinal folds as a consequence of inferior staphyloma associated with tilted disc syndrome. Graefes Arch. Clin. Exp. Ophthalmol. 244, 1536–1538.

Cohen, S.Y., Quentel, G., 2008. Uneven distribution of drusen in tilted disc syndrome. Retina 28, 1361–1362.

Giuffrè, G., 1991. Chorioretinal degenerative changes in the tilted disc syndrome. Int. Ophthalmol. 15 (1), 1–7. Erratum in: Int Ophthalmol 1991; 145(4):285.

Giuffrè, G., Anastasi, M., 1986. Electrofunctional features of the tilted disc syndrome. Doc. Ophthalmol. 62 (3), 223–230.

Hamada, T., Tsukada, T., Hirose, T., 1987. Clinical and electrophysiological features of tilted disc syndrome. Jpn J. Ophthalmol. 31 (2), 265–273.

Moschos, M.M., Triglianos, A., Rotsos, T., et al., 2009. Tilted disc syndrome: an OCT and mfERG study. Doc. Ophthalmol. 119 (1), 23–28.

Nakanishi, H., Tsujikawa, A., Gotoh, N., et al., 2008. Macular complications on the border of an inferior staphyloma associated with tilted disc syndrome. Retina 28, 1493–1501.

Prost, M., De Laey, J.J., 1988. Choroidal neovascularization in tilted disc syndrome. Int. Ophthalmol. 12 (2), 131–135.

Semes, L., 2000. The tilted disc syndrome. Optom. Vis. Sci. 77 (2), 67.

Sowka, J., Aoun, P., 1999. Tilted disc syndrome. Optom. Vis. Sci. 76 (9), 618–623.

Tosti, G., 1999. Serous macular detachment and tilted disc syndrome. Ophthalmology 106 (8), 1453–1455.

Vuori, M.L., Mäntyjärvi, M., 2007. Tilted disc syndrome and colour vision. Acta Ophthalmol. Scand. 85 (6), 648–652.

Vuori, M.L., Mäntyjärvi, M., 2008. Tilted disc syndrome may mimic false visual field deterioration. Acta Ophthalmol. 86 (6), 622–625.

Wijngaarde, R., van Lith, G.H., 1981. Electrodiagnostics of the tilted disc syndrome. Doc. Ophthalmol. 50 (2), 365–369.

Peripapillary Staphyloma

Blair, M.P., Blair, N.P., Rheinstrom, S.D., et al., 2000. A case of peripapillary staphyloma. Arch. Ophthalmol. 118 (8), 1138–1139.

Burvenich, H., 1981. Peripapillary staphyloma and optical pit with serous detachment of the macula. Bull. Soc. Belge Ophtalmol. 193, 143–146.

Caldwell, J.B., Sears, M.L., Gilman, M., 1971. Bilateral peripapillary staphyloma with normal vision. Am. J. Ophthalmol. 71 (1 Pt 2), 423–425.

Cennamo, G., Sammartino, A., Fioretti, F., 1983. Morning glory syndrome with contractile peripapillary staphyloma. Br. J. Ophthalmol. 67 (6), 346–348.

Donaldson, D.D., Bennett, N., Anderson, D.R., et al., 1969. Peripapillary staphyloma. Arch. Ophthalmol. 82 (5), 704–705.

Gottlieb, J.L., Prieto, D.M., Vander, J.F., et al., 1997. Peripapillary staphyloma. Am. J. Ophthalmol. 124 (2), 249–251.

Kim, S.H., Choi, M.Y., Yu, Y.S., et al., 2005. Peripapillary staphyloma: clinical features and visual outcome in 19 cases. Arch. Ophthalmol. 123 (10), 1371–1376. Erratum in: Arch Ophthalmol. 2005; 123 (12):1740.

Kim, B.M., Shapiro, M.J., Miller, M.T., et al., 2011. Peripapillary staphyloma with associated retinopathy of prematurity. Retin Cases Brief Rep. 5 (2), 146–148.

Konstas, P., Katikos, G., Vatakas, L.C., 1976. Contractile peripapillary staphyloma. Ophthalmologica 172 (5), 379–381.

Kral, K., Svarc, D., 1971. Contractile peripapillary staphyloma. Am. J. Ophthalmol. 71 (5), 1090–1092.

Sanjari, M.S., Falavarjani, K.G., Kashkouli, M.B., 2006. Bilateral peripapillary staphyloma, a clinicoradiological report. Br. J. Ophthalmol. 90 (10), 1326–1327.

Seybold, M.E., Rosen, P.N., 1977. Peripapillary staphyloma and amaurosis fugax. Ann. Ophthalmol. 9 (9), 1139–1141.

Singh, D., Verma, A., 1978. Bilateral peripapillary staphyloma (ectasia). Indian J. Ophthalmol. 25 (4), 50–51.

Wang, J.K., Huang, T.L., 2015. Spectral-domain optical coherence tomography findings of peripapillary staphyloma. BMJ Case Rep. 22, 2015.

Wise, J.B., MacLean, A.L., Gass, J.D., 1966. Contractile peripapillary staphyloma. Arch. Ophthalmol. 75 (5), 626–630.

Woo, S.J., Hwang, J.M., 2009. Spectral-domain optical coherence tomography of peripapillary staphyloma. Graefes Arch. Clin. Exp. Ophthalmol. 247 (11), 1573–1574.

Optic Nerve Head Drusen

Beck, R.W., Corbett, T.I., Thompson, H.S., et al., 1985. Decreased visual acuity from disc drusen. Arch. Ophthalmol. 103, 1155–1159.

Boldt, H.C., Byrne, S.F., DiBernardo, C., 1991. Echographic evaluation of optic disc drusen. J. Clin. Neuroophthalmol. 11, 85–91.

Chern, S., Magargal, L.E., Atmesley, W.H., 1991. Central retinal vein occlusion associated with drusen of the optic disc. Ann. Ophthalmol. 23, 66–69.

Choi, S.S., Zawadzki, R.J., Greiner, M.A., et al., 2008. Fourier-domain optical coherence tomography and adaptive optics reveal nerve fiber layer loss and photoreceptor changes in a patient with optic nerve drusen. J. Neuroophthalmol. 28, 120–125.

Cohen, D.N., 1971. Drusen of the optic disc and the development of field defects. Arch. Ophthalmol. 85, 224–226.

Coleman, K., Ross, M.H., McCabe, M., et al., 1991. Disk drusen and angioid streaks in pseudoxanthoma elasticum. Ophthalmology 112, 166–170.

Dinakaran, S., Talbot, J.F., 2005. Optic disc drusen associated with neovascularization of optic disc. Eye (Lond.) 19, 816–818.

Erkkila, H., 1976. The central vascular pattern of the eye ground in children with drusen of the optic disc. Albrecht. Von. Graefes. Arch. Klin. Exp. Ophthalmol. 199, 1–10.

Floyd, M.S., Katz, B.J., Digre, K.B., 2005. Measurement of the scleral canal using optical coherence tomography in patients with optic nerve drusen. Am. J. Ophthalmol. 139, 664–669.

Friedman, A.H., Beckerman, B., Gold, D.H., et al., 1977. Drusen of the optic disc. Surv. Ophthalmol. 21, 375–390.

Frisén, L., 2008. Evolution of drusen of the optic nerve head over 23 years. Acta Ophthalmol. 86, 111–112.

Frisen, L., Scholdstrom, G., Svendsen, P., 1978. Drusen in the optic nerve head. Verification by computerized tomography. Arch. Ophthalmol. 96, 1611–1614.

Gartner, S., 1987. Drusen of the optic disc in retinitis pigmentosa. Am. J. Ophthalmol. 103 (6), 845.

Gaynes, P.M., Towle, P.S., 1967. Hemorrhage in hyaline bodies (drusen) of the optic disc in an attack of migraine. Am. J. Ophthalmol. 63, 1693–1696.

Grippo, T.M., Shihadeh, W.A., Schargus, M., et al., 2008. Optic nerve head drusen and visual field loss in normotensive and hypertensive eyes. J. Glaucoma 17, 100–104.

Hu, K., Davis, A., O'Sullivan, E., 2008. Distinguishing optic disc drusen from papilloedema. BMJ 337, a2360.

Johnson, L.N., Diehl, M.L., Hamm, C.W., et al., 2009. Differentiating optic disc edema from optic nerve head drusen on optical coherence tomography. Arch. Ophthalmol. 127, 45–49.

Kapur, R., Pulido, J.S., Abraham, J.L., et al., 2008. Histologic findings after surgical excision of optic nerve head drusen. Retina 28, 143–146.

Katz, B.J., Pomeranz, H.D., 2006. Visual field defects and retinal nerve fiber layer defects in eyes with buried optic nerve drusen. Am. J. Ophthalmol. 141, 248–253.

Kelley, J.S., Hoover, R.E., Robin, A., et al., 1979. Laser scotometry in drusen and pits of the optic nerve head. Ophthalmology 86, 442–447.

Lee, A.G., Zimmerman, M.B., 2005. The rate of visual field loss in optic nerve head drusen. Am. J. Ophthalmol. 139, 1062–1066.

Michaelson, C., Behrens, M., Odel, J., 1989. Bilateral anterior ischaemic optic neuropathy associated with optic disc drusen and systemic hypotension. Br. J. Ophthalmol. 73, 762–764.

Novack, R.L., Foos, R.Y., 1987. Drusen of the optic disc in retinitis pigmentosa. Am. J. Ophthalmol. 103, 44–47.

Pierro, L., Brancato, R., Minicucci, M., et al., 1994. Echographic diagnosis of drusen of the optic nerve head in patients with angioid streaks. Ophthalmologica 208, 239–242.

Reese, A.B., 1940. Relation of drusen of the optic nerve to tuberous sclerosis. Arch. Ophthalmol. 24, 369–371.

Shiono, T., Noro, M., Iamai, M., 1991. Presumed drusen of optic nerve head in siblings with Usher syndrome. Jpn J. Ophthalmol. 35, 300–305.

Tso, M.O.M., 1981. Pathology and pathogenesis of drusen of the optic nervehead. Ophthalmology 88, 1066–1080.

Optic Nerve Trauma

Berestka, J.S., Rizzo, J.F. 3rd., 1994. Controversy in the management of traumatic optic neuropathy. Int. Ophthalmol. Clin. 34 (3), 87–96.

Bilyk, J.R., Joseph, M.P., 1994. Traumatic optic neuropathy. Semin. Ophthalmol. 9 (3), 200–211.

Cook, M.W., Levin, L.A., Joseph, M.P., et al., 1996. Traumatic optic neuropathy. A meta-analysis. Arch. Otolaryngol. Head Neck Surg. 122 (4), 389–392.

de Vries-Knoppert, W.A., 1989. Evulsion of the optic nerve. Doc. Ophthalmol. 72, 241–245.

Foster, B.S., March, G.A., Lucarelli, M.J., et al., 1997. Optic nerve avulsion. Arch. Ophthalmol. 115, 623–630.

Goldenberg-Cohen, N., Miller, N.R., Repka, M.X., 2004. Traumatic optic neuropathy in children and adolescents. J. AAPOS 8 (1), 20–27.

Hart, J.C.D., Pilley, S.F.J., 1970. Partial evulsion of optic nerve: a fluorescein angiographic study. Br. J. Ophthalmol. 54, 781–785.

Leino, M., 1986. Optic nerve injury after sudden traumatic rotation of the eye. Acta Ophthalmol. (Copenh) 64, 364–365.

Levin, L.A., Baker, R.S., 2003. Management of traumatic optic neuropathy. J. Neuroophthalmol. 23 (1), 72–75.

Levin, L.A., Beck, R.W., Joseph, M.P., et al., 1999. The treatment of traumatic optic neuropathy: the International Optic Nerve Trauma Study. Ophthalmology 106 (7), 1268–1277.

Mauriello, J.A., DeLuca, J., Krieger, A., et al., 1992. Management of traumatic optic neuropathy—a study of 23 patients. Br. J. Ophthalmol. 76 (6), 349–352.

Oliver, S.C.N., Mandava, N., 2007. Ultrasonographic signs in complete optic nerve avulsion. Arch. Ophthalmol. 125, 716–717.

Pomeranz, H.D., Rizzo, J.F., Lessell, S., 1999. Treatment of traumatic optic neuropathy. Int. Ophthalmol. Clin. 39 (1), 185–194.

Sanborn, G.E., Gonder, J.R., Goldberg, R.E., et al., 1984. Evulsion of the optic nerve: a clinicopathological study. Can. J. Ophthalmol. 19, 10–16.

Seiff, S.R., 1991. Therapy for traumatic optic neuropathy. Arch. Ophthalmol. 109 (5), 610.

Steinsapir, K.D., 1999. Traumatic optic neuropathy. Curr. Opin. Ophthalmol. 10 (5), 340–342.

Steinsapir, K.D., Goldberg, R.A., 1994. Traumatic optic neuropathy. Surv. Ophthalmol. 38 (6), 487–518.

Tandon, R., Vanathi, M., Verma, L., et al., 2003. Traumatic optic nerve avulsion: role of ultrasonography. Eye (Lond.) 17, 667–670.

Temel, A., Sener, A.B., 1988. Complete evulsion of the optic nerve. Acta. Ophthalmol. (Copenh) 66, 117–119.

Williams, D.F., Williams, G.A., Abrams, G.W., et al., 1987. Evulsion of the retina associated with optic nerve evulsion. Am. J. Ophthalmol. 104, 5–9.

Non-Arteritic Anterior Ischemic Optic Neuropathy (NAION)

Arnold, A.C., 2003. Pathogenesis of nonarteritic anterior ischemic optic neuropathy. J. Neuroophthalmol. 23 (2), 157–163.

Arnold, A.C., Helper, R.S., 1994. Fluorescein angiography in acute nonarteritic anterior ischemic optic neuropathy. Am. J. Ophthalmol. 117, 220–230.

Arnold, A.C., Levin, L.A., 2002. Treatment of ischemic optic neuropathy. Semin. Ophthalmol. 17 (1), 39–46.

Atkins, E.J., Bruce, B.B., Newman, N.J., et al., 2010. Treatment of nonarteritic anterior ischemic optic neuropathy. Surv. Ophthalmol. 55 (1), 47–63.

Bernstein, S.L., Johnson, M.A., Miller, N.R., 2011. Nonarteritic anterior ischemic optic neuropathy (NAION) and its experimental models. Prog. Retin. Eye Res. 30 (3), 167–187.

Borchert, M., Lessell, S., 1988. Progressive and recurrent nonarteritic anterior ischemic optic neuropathy. Am. J. Ophthalmol. 106, 443–449.

Buono, L.M., Foroozan, R., Sergott, R.C., et al., 2002. Nonarteritic anterior ischemic optic neuropathy. Curr. Opin. Ophthalmol. 13 (6), 357–361.

Burde, R.M., 1993. Optic disk risk factors for nonarteritic anterior ischemic optic neuropathy. Am. J. Ophthalmol. 116, 759–764.

Dickersin, K., Li, T., 2015. Surgery for nonarteritic anterior ischemic optic neuropathy. Cochrane Database Syst. Rev. (3), CD001538.

Dickersin, K., Manheimer, E., 2000. Surgery for nonarteritic anterior ischemic optic neuropathy. Cochrane Database Syst. Rev. (2), CD001538.

Dickersin, K., Manheimer, E., Li, T., 2006. Surgery for nonarteritic anterior ischemic optic neuropathy. Cochrane Database Syst. Rev. (1), CD001538.

Dickersin, K., Manheimer, E., Li, T., 2012. Surgery for nonarteritic anterior ischemic optic neuropathy. Cochrane Database Syst. Rev. (1), CD001538.

Giusti, C., 2010. Bilateral non-arteritic anterior ischemic optic neuropathy (NA-AION): case report and review of the literature. Eur. Rev. Med. Pharmacol. Sci. 14 (2), 141–144.

Guyer, D.R., Miller, N.R., Auer, C.L., et al., 1985. The risk of cerebrovascular and cardiovascular disease in patients with anterior ischemic optic neuropathy. Arch. Ophthalmol. 103, 1136–1142.

Hayreh, S.S., Zimmerman, M.B., 2008. Nonarteritic anterior ischemic optic neuropathy: natural history of visual outcome. Ophthalmology 115, 298–305. e2.

Johnson, L.N., Kuo, H.C., Arnold, A.C., 1993. HLA-A29 as a potential risk factor for nonarteritic anterior ischemic optic neuropathy. Am. J. Ophthalmol. 115, 540–542.

Kaderli, B., Avci, R., Yucel, A., et al., 2007. Intravitreal triamcinolone improves recovery of visual acuity in nonarteritic anterior ischemic optic neuropathy. J. Neuroophthalmol. 27, 164–168.

Kalenak, J.W., Kosmorsky, G.S., Rockwood, E.J., 1991. Nonartertic anterior ischemic optic neuropathy and intraocular pressure. Arch. Ophthalmol. 109, 660–661.

Katz, B., Spencer, W.B., 1993. Hyperopia as a risk factor for nonarteritic anterior ischemic optic neuropathy. Am. J. Ophthalmol. 166, 754–758.

Katz, D.M., Trobe, J.D., 2015. Is there treatment for nonarteritic anterior ischemic optic neuropathy. Curr. Opin. Ophthalmol. 26 (6), 458–463.

Kellett, S.C., Madonna, R.J., 1997. Current perspectives on nonarteritic anterior ischemic optic neuropathy. J. Am. Optom. Assoc. 68 (7), 413–424.

Kerr, N.M., Chew, S.S., Danesh-Meyer, H.V., 2009. Non-arteritic anterior ischaemic optic neuropathy: a review and update. J. Clin. Neurosci. 16 (8), 994–1000.

Lessell, S., 1999. Nonarteritic anterior ischemic optic neuropathy: enigma variations. Arch. Ophthalmol. 117 (3), 386–388.

Mathews, M.K., 2005. Nonarteritic anterior ischemic optic neuropathy. Curr. Opin. Ophthalmol. 16 (6), 341–345.

Repka, M.X., Savino, P.J., Schatz, N.J., et al., 1983. Clinical profile and long-term implications of anterior ischemic optic neuropathy. Am. J. Ophthalmol. 96, 478–483.

Worrall, B.B., Moazami, G., Odel, J.G., et al., 1997. Anterior ischemic optic neuropathy and activated protein C resistance. A case report and review of the literature. J. Neuroophthalmol. 17 (3), 162–165.

Optic Nerve Papillitis

Browning, D.J., Fraser, C.M., 2005. Ocular conditions associated with peripapillary subretinal neovascularization, their relative frequencies, and associated outcomes. Ophthalmology 112, 1054–1061.

Cohen, B.M., Davis, J.L., Gass, J.D.M., 1995. Branch retinal arterial occlusions in multifocal retinitis with optic nerve edema. Arch. Ophthalmol. 113, 1271–1276.

Collett-Solberg, P.F., Liu, G.T., Satin-Smith, M., et al., 1998. Pseudopapilledema and congenital disc anomalies in growth hormone deficiency. J. Pediatr. Endocrinol. Metab. 11, 261–265.

Hollander, D.A., Hoyt, W.F., Howes, E.L., et al., 2004. The pseudopapilledema of neonatal-onset multisystem inflammatory disease. Am. J. Ophthalmol. 138, 894–895.

Hoyt, W.F., Pont, M.E., 1962. Pseudopapilledema: anomalous elevation of optic disk. Pitfalls in diagnosis and management. JAMA 181, 191–196.

Maitland, C.G., Miller, N.R., 1984. Neuroretinitis. Arch. Ophthalmol. 102, 1146–1150.

Rosenberg, M.A., Savino, P.J., Glaser, J.S., 1979. A clinical analysis of pseudopapilledema: I. Population, laterality-acuity, refractive error, ophthalmoscopic characteristics, and coincident disease. Arch. Ophthalmol. 97, 65–70.

Shams, P.N., Davies, N.P., 2010. Pseudopapilloedema and optic disc haemorrhages in a child misdiagnosed as optic disc swelling. Br. J. Ophthalmol. 94 (10), 1398–1399.

Trick, G.L., Bhatt, S.S., Dahl, D., et al., 2001. Optic disc topography in pseudopapilledema: a comparison to pseudotumor cerebri. J. Neuroophthalmol. 21, 240–244.

Acute Neuroretinitis *(Bartonella henselae)*

Ando, R., Shinmei, Y., Nitta, T., et al., 2005. Central serous retinal detachment detected by optical coherence tomography in Leber's idiopathic stellate neuroretinitis. Jpn J. Ophthalmol. 49, 547–548.

Brazis, P.W., Lee, A.G., 1996. Optic disk edema with a macular star. Mayo Clin. Proc. 71 (12), 1162–1166.

Carroll, D.M., Franklin, R.M., 1982. Leber's idiopathic stellate retinopathy. Am. J. Ophthalmol. 93, 96–101.

Casson, R.J., O'Day, J., Crompton, J.L., 1999. Leber's idiopathic stellate neuroretinitis: differential diagnosis and approach to management. Aust. N. Z. J. Ophthalmol. 27 (1), 65–69.

Conrad, D.A., 2001. Treatment of cat-scratch disease. Curr. Opin. Pediatr. 13 (1), 56–59.

Cunningham, E.T., Koehler, J.E., 2000. Ocular bartonellosis. Am. J. Ophthalmol. 130 (3), 340–349.

De Schryver, I., Stevens, A.M., Vereecke, G., et al., 2002. Cat scratch disease (CSD) in patients with stellate neuroretinitis: 3 cases. Bull. Soc. Belge Ophtalmol. 286, 41–46.

Dreyer, R.F., Hopen, G., Gass, J.D., et al., 1984. Leber's idiopathic stellate neuroretinitis. Arch. Ophthalmol. 102, 1140–1145.

Ormerod, L.D., Dailey, J.P., 1999. Ocular manifestations of cat-scratch disease. Curr. Opin. Ophthalmol. 10 (3), 209–216.

Ormerod, L.D., Skolnick, K.A., Menosky, M.M., et al., 1998. Retinal and choroidal manifestations of cat-scratch disease. Ophthalmology 105 (6), 1024–1031.

Papastratigakis, B., Stavrakas, E., Phanouriakis, C., et al., 1981. Leber's idiopathic stellate maculopathy. Ophthalmologica 183, 68–71.

Purvin, V.A., 2000. Optic neuropathies for the neurologist. Semin. Neurol. 20 (1), 97–110.

Purvin, V., Sundaram, S., Kawasaki, A., 2011. Neuroretinitis: review of the literature and new observations. J. Neuroophthalmol. 31 (1), 58–68.

Ray, S., Gragoudas, E., 2001. Neuroretinitis. Int. Ophthalmol. Clin. 41 (1), 83–102.

Sadun, A.A., Currie, J.N., Lessell, S., 1984. Transient visual obscurations with elevated optic discs. Ann. Neurol. 16, 489–494.

Smith, J.R., Cunningham, E.T. Jr., 2002. Atypical presentations of ocular toxoplasmosis. Curr. Opin. Ophthalmol. 13 (6), 387–392.

Idiopathic Intracranial Hypertension (IIH)

Arnold, A.C., 2003. Pathogenesis of nonarteritic anterior ischemic optic neuropathy. J. Neuroophthalmol. 23 (2), 157–163.

Arnold, A.C., Levin, L.A., 2002. Treatment of ischemic optic neuropathy. Semin. Ophthalmol. 17 (1), 39–46.

Atkins, E.J., Bruce, B.B., Newman, N.J., et al., 2010. Treatment of nonarteritic anterior ischemic optic neuropathy. Surv. Ophthalmol. 55 (1), 47–63.

Baker, R.S., Baumann, R.J., Buncic, J.R., 1989. Idiopathic intracranial hypertension (pseudotumor cerebri) in pediatric patients. Pediatr. Neurol. 5 (1), 5–11.

Ball A.K., Clarke, C.E., 2006. Idiopathic intracranial hypertension. Lancet Neurol. 5 (5), 433–442.

Bernstein, S.L., Johnson, M.A., Miller, N.R., 2011. Nonarteritic anterior ischemic optic neuropathy (NAION) and its experimental models. Prog. Retin. Eye Res. 30 (3), 167–187.

Binder, D.K., Horton, J.C., Lawton, M.T., et al., 2004. Idiopathic intracranial hypertension. Neurosurgery 54 (3), 538–551, discussion 551–552.

Brodsky, M.C., Vaphiades, M., 1998. Magnetic resonance imaging in pseudotumor cerebri. Ophthalmology 105, 1686–1693.

Buono, L.M., Foroozan, R., Sergott, R.C., et al., 2002. Nonarteritic anterior ischemic optic neuropathy. Curr. Opin. Ophthalmol. 13 (6), 357–361.

Burde, R.M., 1993. Optic disk risk factors for nonarteritic anterior ischemic optic neuropathy. Am. J. Ophthalmol. 116 (6), 759–764.

Carter, S.R., Seiff, S.R., 1995. Macular changes in pseudotumor cerebri before and after optic nerve sheath fenestration. Ophthalmology 102, 937–941.

Corbett, J.J., Thompson, H.S., 1989. The rational management of idiopathic intracranial hypertension. Arch. Neurol. 46 (10), 1049–1051.

Dickersin, K., Li, T., 2015. Surgery for nonarteritic anterior ischemic optic neuropathy. Cochrane Database Syst. Rev. (3), CD001538.

Dickersin, K., Manheimer, E., 2000. Surgery for nonarteritic anterior ischemic optic neuropathy. Cochrane Database Syst. Rev. (2), CD001538.

Dickersin, K., Manheimer, E., Li, T., 2006. Surgery for nonarteritic anterior ischemic optic neuropathy. Cochrane Database Syst. Rev. (1), CD001538.

Dickersin, K., Manheimer, E., Li, T., 2012. Surgery for nonarteritic anterior ischemic optic neuropathy. Cochrane Database Syst. Rev. (1), CD001538.

Friedman, D.I., Jacobson, D.M., 2002. Diagnostic criteria for idiopathic intracranial hypertension. Neurology 59 (10), 1492–1495.

Friedman, D.I., Jacobson, D.M., 2004. Idiopathic intracranial hypertension. J. Neuroophthalmol. 24, 138–145.

Giusti, C., 2010. Bilateral non-arteritic anterior ischemic optic neuropathy (NA-AION): case report and review of the literature. Eur. Rev. Med. Pharmacol. Sci. 14 (2), 141–144.

Katz, D.M., Trobe, J.D., 2015. Is there treatment for nonarteritic anterior ischemic optic neuropathy. Curr. Opin. Ophthalmol. 26 (6), 458–463.

Kellett, S.C., Madonna, R.J., 1997. Current perspectives on nonarteritic anterior ischemic optic neuropathy. J. Am. Optom. Assoc. 68 (7), 413–424.

Kerr, N.M., Chew, S.S., Danesh-Meyer, H.V., 2009. Non-arteritic anterior ischaemic optic neuropathy: a review and update. J. Clin. Neurosci. 16 (8), 994–1000.

Lessell, S., 1992. Pediatric pseudotumor cerebri (idiopathic intracranial hypertension). Surv. Ophthalmol. 37 (3), 155–166.

Lessell, S., 1999. Nonarteritic anterior ischemic optic neuropathy: enigma variations. Arch. Ophthalmol. 117 (3), 386–388.

Lueck, C., McIlwaine, G., 2002. Interventions for idiopathic intracranial hypertension. Cochrane Database Syst. Rev. (3), CD003434.

Mathews, M.K., 2005. Nonarteritic anterior ischemic optic neuropathy. Curr. Opin. Ophthalmol. 16 (6), 341–345.

Morse, P.H., Leveille, A.S., Antel, J.P., et al., 1981. Bilateral juxtapapillary subretinal neovascularization associated with pseudotumor cerebri. Am. J. Ophthalmol. 91, 312.

Randhawa, S., Van Stavern, G.P., 2008. Idiopathic intracranial hypertension (pseudotumor cerebri). Curr. Opin. Ophthalmol. 19 (6), 445–453.

Randhawa, S., Yonker, J.M., Van Stavern, G.P., 2007. Idiopathic intracranial hypertension. Ophthalmology 114, 827–828.

Rangwala, L.M., Liu, G.T., 2007. Pediatric idiopathic intracranial hypertension. Surv. Ophthalmol. 52, 597–617.

Shah, V.A., Fung, S., Shahbaz, R., et al., 2007. Idiopathic intracranial hypertension. Ophthalmology 114, 617.

Spoor, T.C., McHenry, J.G., 1993. Long-term effectiveness of optic nerve sheath decompression for pseudotumor cerebri. Arch. Ophthalmol. 111, 632–635.

Taktakishvili, O., Shah, V.A., Shahbaz, R., et al., 2008. Recurrent idiopathic intracranial hypertension. Ophthalmology 115, 221.

Uretsky, S., 2009. Surgical interventions for idiopathic intracranial hypertension. Curr. Opin. Ophthalmol. 20 (6), 451–455.

Wall, M., 1991. Idiopathic intracranial hypertension. Neurol. Clin. 9 (1), 73–95.

Wall, M., 1995. Idiopathic intracranial hypertension. Semin. Ophthalmol. 10 (3), 251–259.

Wall, M., 2000. Idiopathic intracranial hypertension: mechanisms of visual loss and disease management. Semin. Neurol. 20 (1), 89–95.

Worrall, B.B., Moazami, G., Odel, J.G., et al., 1997. Anterior ischemic optic neuropathy and activated protein C resistance. A case report and review of the literature. J. Neuroophthalmol. 17 (3), 162–165.

Ocular Syphilis

Aldave, A.J., King, J.A., Cunningham, E.T. Jr., 2001. Ocular syphilis. Curr. Opin. Ophthalmol. 12 (6), 433–441.

Butler, N.J., Thorne, J.E., 2012. Current status of HIV infection and ocular disease. Curr. Opin. Ophthalmol. 23 (6), 517–522.

Chao, J.R., Khurana, R.N., Fawzi, A.A., et al., 2006. Syphilis: reemergence of an old adversary. Ophthalmology 113 (11), 2074–2079.

Davis, J.L., 2014. Ocular syphilis. Curr. Opin. Ophthalmol. 25 (6), 513–518.

Eandi, C.M., Neri, P., Adelman, R.A., et al., 2012. Acute syphilitic posterior placoid chorioretinitis: report of a case series and comprehensive review of the literature. Retina 32 (9), 1915–1941.

Gaudio, P.A., 2006. Update on ocular syphilis. Curr. Opin. Ophthalmol. 17 (6), 562–566.

Kiss, S., Damico, F.M., Young, L.H., 2005. Ocular manifestations and treatment of syphilis. Semin. Ophthalmol. 20 (3), 161–167.

Levy, J.H., Liss, R.A., Maguire, A.M., 1989. Neurosyphilis and ocular syphilis in patients with concurrent human immunodeficiency virus infection. Retina 9 (3), 175–180.

Margo, C.E., Hamed, L.M., 1992. Ocular syphilis. Surv. Ophthalmol. 37 (3), 203–220.

Tucker, J.D., Li, J.Z., Robbins, G.K., et al., 2011. Ocular syphilis among HIV-infected patients: a systematic analysis of the literature. Sex. Transm. Infect. 87 (1), 4–8.

Optic Nerve Glioma

Bianchi-Marzoli, S., Brancato, R., 1994. Tumors of the optic nerve and chiasm. Curr. Opin. Ophthalmol. 5 (6), 11–17.

Dario, A., Iadini, A., Cerati, M., et al., 1999. Malignant optic glioma of adulthood. Case report and review of the literature. Acta Neurol. Scand. 100 (5), 350–353.

Dutton, J.J., 1994. Gliomas of the anterior visual pathway. Surv. Ophthalmol. 38 (5), 427–452.

Fried, I., Tabori, U., Tihan, T., et al., 2013. Optic pathway gliomas: a review. CNS Oncol. 2 (2), 143–159.

Hayasaka, S., Miyagawa, M., Ugomori, S., et al., 1992. Optic nerve glioma in Japanese patients with neurofibromatosis 1. Case reports and literature review. Jpn J. Ophthalmol. 36 (3), 315–322.

Hwang, J.M., Cheon, J.E., Wang, K.C., 2008. Visual prognosis of optic glioma. Childs Nerv. Syst. 24 (6), 693–698.

Jahraus, C.D., Tarbell, N.J., 2006. Optic pathway gliomas. Pediatr. Blood Cancer 46 (5), 586–596.

Lynch, T.M., Gutmann, D.H., 2002. Neurofibromatosis 1. Neurol. Clin. 20 (3), 841–865.

Miller, N.R., 2004. Primary tumours of the optic nerve and its sheath. Eye (Lond.) 18 (11), 1026–1037.

Nair, A.G., Pathak, R.S., Iyer, V.R., et al., 2014. Optic nerve glioma: an update. Int. Ophthalmol. 34 (4), 999–1005.

Okuno, T., Prensky, A.L., Gado, M., 1985. The moyamoya syndrome associated with irradiation of an optic glioma in children: report of two cases and review of the literature. Pediatr. Neurol. 1 (5), 311–316.

Sadun, F., Hinton, D.R., Sadun, A.A., 1996. Rapid growth of an optic nerve ganglioglioma in a patient with neurofibromatosis 1. Ophthalmology 103 (5), 794–799.

Schnur, R.E., 2012. Type I neurofibromatosis: a geno-oculo-dermatologic update. Curr. Opin. Ophthalmol. 23 (5), 364–372.

Shapey, J., Danesh-Meyer, H.V., Kaye, A.H., 2011. Diagnosis and management of optic nerve glioma. J. Clin. Neurosci. 18 (12), 1585–1591.

Shofty, B., Ben-Sira, L., Kesler, A., et al., 2015. Optic pathway gliomas. Adv. Tech. Stand. Neurosurg. 42, 123–146.

Stieber, V.W., 2008. Radiation therapy for visual pathway tumors. J. Neuroophthalmol. 28 (3), 222–230.

Sylvester, C.L., Drohan, L.A., Sergott, R.C., 2006. Optic-nerve gliomas, chiasmal gliomas and neurofibromatosis type 1. Curr. Opin. Ophthalmol. 17 (1), 7–11.

Taphoorn, M.J., de Vries-Knoppert, W.A., Ponssen, H., et al., 1989. Malignant optic glioma in adults. Case report. J Neurosurg. 70 (2), 277–279.

Tekkök, I.H., Tahta, K., Saglam, S., 1994. Optic nerve glioma presenting as a huge intrasellar mass. Case report. J. Neurosurg. Sci. 38 (2), 137–140.

Traber, G.L., Pangalu, A., Neumann, M., et al., 2015. Malignant optic glioma—the spectrum of disease in a case series. Graefes Arch. Clin. Exp. Ophthalmol. 253 (7), 1187–1194.

Walker, D., 2003. Recent advances in optic nerve glioma with a focus on the young patient. Curr. Opin. Neurol. 16 (6), 657–664.

Wilhelm, H., 2009. Primary optic nerve tumours. Curr. Opin. Neurol. 22 (1), 11–18.

Meningioma of the Optic Nerve

Alper, M.G., 1981. Management of primary optic nerve meningiomas; current status–therapy in controversy. J. Clin. Neuroophthalmol. 1, 101–117.

Brodsky, M.C., Safar, A.N., 2007. Optic disc tuber. Arch. Ophthalmol. 125, 710–712.

Eddleman, C.S., Liu, J.K., 2007. Optic nerve sheath meningioma: current diagnosis and treatment. Neurosurg. Focus 23, E4.

Garcia, J.P., Finger, P.T., Kurli, M., et al., 2005. 3D ultrasound coronal C-scan imaging for optic nerve sheath meningioma. Br. J. Ophthalmol. 89, 244–245.

Harold Lee, H.B., Garrity, J.A., Cameron, J.D., et al., 2008. Primary optic nerve sheath meningioma in children. Surv. Ophthalmol. 53, 543–558.

Hart, W.M., Burde, R.M., Klingele, T.G., et al., 1980. Bilateral optic nerve sheath meningiomas. Arch. Ophthalmol. 98, 149–151.

Imes, R.K., Schatz, H., Hoyt, W.F., et al., 1985. Evolution of optociliary veins in optic nerve sheath meningioma; evolution. Arch. Ophthalmol. 103, 59–60.

Islam, N., Best, J., Mehta, J.S., et al., 2005. Optic disc duplication or coloboma? Br. J. Ophthalmol. 89, 26–29.

Kim, J.W., Rizzo, J.F., Lessell, S., 2005. Controversies in the management of optic nerve sheath meningiomas. Int. Ophthalmol. Clin. 45, 15–23.

Lin, C.C.L., Tso, M.O.M., Vygantas, C.M., 1984. Coloboma of the optic nerve associated with serous maculopathy: a clinicopathologic correlative study. Arch. Ophthalmol. 102, 1651–1654.

Melian, E., Jay, W.M., 2004. Primary radiotherapy for optic nerve sheath meningioma. Semin. Ophthalmol. 19, 130–140.

Miller, N.R., 2006. New concepts in the diagnosis and management of optic nerve sheath meningioma. J. Neuroophthalmol. 26, 200–208.

Moschos, M., Ladas, I.D., Zafirakis, P.K., et al., 2001. Recurrent vitreous hemorrhages due to combined pigment epithelial and retinal hamartoma: natural course and indocyanine green angiographic findings. Ophthalmologica 215, 66–69.

Moster, M.L., 2005. Detection and treatment of optic nerve sheath meningioma. Curr. Neurol. Neurosci. Rep. 5, 367–375.

Perkins, S.L., Han, D.P., Gonder, J.R., et al., 2005. Dynamic atypical optic nerve coloboma associated with transient macular detachment. Arch. Ophthalmol. 123, 1750–1754.

Rosca, T.I., Carstocea, B.D., Vlădescu, T.G., et al., 2006. Cystic optic nerve sheath meningioma. J. Neuroophthalmol. 26, 121–122.

Sawaya, R.A., Sidani, C., Farah, N., et al., 2008. Presumed bilateral optic nerve sheath meningiomas presenting as optic neuritis. J. Neuroophthalmol. 28, 55–57.

Smee, R.I., Schneider, M., Williams, J.R., 2009. Optic nerve sheath meningiomas–non-surgical treatment. Clin. Oncol. (R. Coll. Radiol.) 21, 8–13.

Sughrue, M.E., McDermott, M.W., Parsa, A.T., 2009. Vision salvage after resection of a giant meningioma in a patient with a loss in light perception. J. Neurosurg. 110, 109–111.

Theodossiadis, P.G., Panagiotidis, D.N., Baltatzis, S.G., et al., 2001. Combined hamartoma of the sensory retina and retinal pigment epithelium involving the optic disk associated with choroidal neovascularization. Retina 21, 267–270.

Vagefi, M.R., Larson, D.A., Horton, J.C., 2006. Optic nerve sheath meningioma: visual improvement during radiation treatment. Am. J. Ophthalmol. 142, 343–344.

Wilhelm, H., 2009. Primary optic nerve tumours. Curr. Opin. Neurol. 22, 11–18.

Wright, J.E., McNab, A.A., McDonald, W.I., 1989. Optic nerve glioma and the management of optic nerve tumors in the young. Br. J. Ophthalmol. 73, 967–974.

Retinal Capillary Hemangioma and Hemangioma of the Optic Nerve Head

Atebara, N.H., 2002. Retinal capillary hemangioma treated with verteporfin photodynamic therapy. Am. J. Ophthalmol. 134 (5), 788–790.

Atebara, N.H., Shields, J.A., 1993. Capillary hemangioma of the optic disc associated with a total retinal detachment. Ophthalmic Surg. 24 (10), 686–688.

Brown, G.C., Shields, J.A., 1985. Tumors of the optic nerve head. Surv. Ophthalmol. 29 (4), 239–264.

Costa, R.A., Meirelles, R.L., Cardillo, J.A., et al., 2003. Retinal capillary hemangioma treatment by indocyanine green-mediated photothrombosis. Am. J. Ophthalmol. 135 (3), 395–398.

Gass, J.D., Braunstein, R., 1980. Sessile and exophytic capillary angiomas of the juxtapapillary retina and optic nerve head. Arch. Ophthalmol. 98 (10), 1790–1797.

Johnston, P.B., Lotery, A.J., Logan, W.C., 1995. Treatment and long-term follow up of a capillary angioma of the optic disc. Int. Ophthalmol. 19 (2), 129–132.

Malecha, M.A., Haik, B.G., Morris, W.R., 2000. Capillary hemangioma of the optic nerve head and juxtapapillary retina. Arch. Ophthalmol. 118 (2), 289–291.

Milewski, S.A., 2002. Spontaneous regression of a capillary hemangioma of the optic disc. Arch. Ophthalmol. 120 (8), 1100–1101.

Miller, N.R., 2004. Primary tumours of the optic nerve and its sheath. Eye (Lond.) 18 (11), 1026–1037.

Mochizuki, Y., Noda, Y., Enaida, H., et al., 2004. Retinal capillary hemangioma managed by transpupillary thermotherapy. Retina 24 (6), 981–984.

Nielsen, P.G., 1979. Capillary haemangioma of the optic disc. A case report. Acta Ophthalmol. (Copenh) 57 (1), 63–68.

Papastefanou, V.P., Pilli, S., Stinghe, A., et al., 2013. Photodynamic therapy for retinal capillary hemangioma. Eye (Lond.) 27 (3), 438–442.

Parmar, D.N., Mireskandari, K., McHugh, D., 2000. Transpupillary thermotherapy for retinal capillary hemangioma in von Hippel-Lindau disease. Ophthalmic Surg. Lasers 31 (4), 334–336.

Pierro, L., Guarisco, L., Zaganelli, E., et al., 1992. Capillary and cavernous hemangioma of the optic disc. Echographic and histological findings. Acta Ophthalmol. Suppl. 204, 102–106.

Rubio, A., Meyers, S.P., Powers, J.M., et al., 1994. Hemangioblastoma of the optic nerve. Hum. Pathol. 25 (11), 1249–1251.

Schindler, R.F., Sarin, L.K., McDonald, P.R., 1975. Hemangiomas of the optic disc. Can. J. Ophthalmol. 10, 305–318.

Shields, J.A., 1993. Response of retinal capillary hemangioma to cryotherapy. Arch. Ophthalmol. 111 (4), 551.

Singh, A.D., Nouri, M., Shields, C.L., et al., 2001. Retinal capillary hemangioma: a comparison of sporadic cases and cases associated with von Hippel-Lindau disease. Ophthalmology 108 (10), 1907–1911.

Singh, A.D., Nouri, M., Shields, C.L., et al., 2002. Treatment of retinal capillary hemangioma. Ophthalmology 109 (10), 1799–1806.

Singh, A., Shields, J., Shields, C., 2001. Solitary retinal capillary hemangioma: hereditary (von Hippel-Lindau disease) or nonhereditary? Arch. Ophthalmol. 119 (2), 232–234.

Sykora, K.W., Weiss, R.A., Ellsworth, R.M., et al., 1990. Ophthalmic neoplasms in infancy and childhood. Pediatrician 17 (3), 163–172.

Takahashi, T., Wada, H., Tani, E., et al., 1984. Capillary hemangioma of the optic disc. J. Clin. Neuroophthalmol. 4 (3), 159–162.

Racemose Hemangioma

Barreira, A.K. Jr., Nakashima, A.F., Takahashi, V.K., et al., 2016. Retinal racemose hemangioma with focal macular involvement. Retin Cases Brief Rep. 10 (1), 52–54.

Elizalde, J., Vasquez, L., 2011. Spontaneous regression in a case of racemose haemangioma archer's type 2. Retin Cases Brief Rep. 5 (4), 294–296.

Eskandari, M.R., Rahimi-Ardabili, B., Javadzade, A., 2013. Racemose hemangioma type 2: the first case report from the Middle East. Int. Ophthalmol. 33 (1), 95–97.

Kaliki, S., Tyagi, M., Kumar, H.P., 2016. Bilateral peripapillary racemose hemangioma: an unusual presentation. Ophthalmology 123 (2), 323.

Materin, M.A., Shields, C.L., Marr, B.P., et al., 2005. Retinal racemose hemangioma. Retina 25 (7), 936–937.

Nadal, J., Delás, B., 2010. Temporal branch retinal vein occlusion secondary to a racemose hemangioma. Retin Cases Brief Rep. 4 (4), 323–325.

Panagiotidis, D., Karagiannis, D., Tsoumpris, I., 2011. Spontaneous development of macular ischemia in a case of racemose hemangioma. Clin Ophthalmol. 5, 931–932.

Qin, X.J., Huang, C., Lai, K., 2014. Retinal vein occlusion in retinal racemose hemangioma: a case report and literature review of ocular complications in this rare retinal vascular disorder. BMC Ophthalmol. 14, 101.

Shields, J.A., Bianciotto, C., Kligman, B.E., et al., 2010. Vascular tumors of the iris in 45 patients: the 2009 Helen Keller Lecture. Arch. Ophthalmol. 128 (9), 1107–1113.

Optic Nerve Melanocytoma

Apple, D.J., Craythorn, J.M., Reidy, J.J., et al., 1984. Malignant transformation of an optic nerve melanocytoma. Can. J. Ophthalmol. 19 (7), 320–325.

Balestrazzi, E., 1973. Melanocytoma of the optic disk. Ophthalmologica 166 (4), 289–292.

Brown, G.C., 1983. Congenital Anomalies of the Optic Disc. Grune & Stratton, New York, pp. 217–222.

Chaudhary, R., Arora, R., Mehta, D.K., et al., 2006. Optical coherence tomography study of optic disc melanocytoma. Ophthalmic Surg. Lasers Imaging 37 (1), 58–61.

De Potter, P., Shields, C.L., Eagle, R.C. Jr., et al., 1996. Malignant melanoma of the optic nerve. Arch. Ophthalmol. 114 (5), 608–612.

Eldaly, H., Eldaly, Z., 2015. Melanocytoma of the optic nerve head, thirty-month follow-up. Semin. Ophthalmol. 30 (5–6), 464–469.

François, J., de Laey, J.J., Kluyskens, J., et al., 1980. Melanocytoma of the optic disc. Ophthalmologica 180 (6), 314–327.

Gupta, V., Gupta, A., Dogra, M.R., et al., 1995. Progressive growth in melanocytoma of the optic nerve head. Indian J. Ophthalmol. 43 (4), 198–200.

Joffe, L., Shields, J.A., Osher, R.H., et al., 1979. Clinical and follow-up studies of melanocytomas of the optic disc. Ophthalmology 86 (6), 1067–1083.

Juarez, C.P., Tso, M.O., 1980. An ultrastructural study of melanocytomas (magnocellular nevi) of the optic disk and uvea. Am. J. Ophthalmol. 90 (1), 48–62.

Kadayifcilar, S., Akman, A., Aydin, P., 1999. Indocyanine green angiography of optic nerve head melanocytoma. Eur. J. Ophthalmol. 9 (1), 68–70.

Mansour, A.M., Zimmerman, L., La Piana, F.G., et al., 1989. Clinicopathological findings in a growing optic nerve melanocytoma. Br. J. Ophthalmol. 73 (6), 410–415.

Meyer, D., Ge, J., Blinder, K.J., et al., 1999. Malignant transformation of an optic disk melanocytoma. Am. J. Ophthalmol. 127 (6), 710–714.

Osher, R.H., Shields, J.A., Layman, P.R., 1979. Pupillary and visual field evaluation in patients with melanocytoma of the optic disc. Arch. Ophthalmol. 97 (6), 1096–1099.

Rai, S., Medeiros, F.A., Levi, L., et al., 2007. Optic disc melanocytoma and glaucoma. Semin. Ophthalmol. 22 (3), 147–150.

Reidy, J.J., Apple, D.J., Steinmetz, R.L., et al., 1985. Melanocytoma: nomenclature, pathogenesis, natural history and treatment. Surv. Ophthalmol. 29 (5), 319–327.

Salvanos, P., Utheim, T.P., Moe, M.C., et al., 2015. Autofluorescence imaging in the differential diagnosis of optic disc melanocytoma. Acta Ophthalmol. 93 (5), 476–480.

Servodidio, C.A., Abramson, D.H., Romanella, A., 1990. Melanocytoma. J. Ophthalmic Nurs. Technol. 9 (6), 255–263.

Shanmugam, M.P., Khetan, V., Sinha, P., 2004. Optic disk melanocytoma with neuroretinitis. Retina 24 (2), 317–318.

Shields, C.L., Perez, B., Benavides, R., et al., 2008. Optical coherence tomography of optic disk melanocytoma in 15 cases. Retina 28 (3), 441–446.

Shields, J.A., 1978. Melanocytoma of the optic nerve head: a review. Int. Ophthalmol. 1 (1), 31–37.

Shields, J.A., Demirci, H., Mashayekhi, A., et al., 2004. Melanocytoma of optic disc in 115 cases: the 2004 Samuel Johnson Memorial Lecture, part 1. Ophthalmology 111 (9), 1739–1746.

Shields, J.A., Demirci, H., Mashayekhi, A., et al., 2006. Melanocytoma of the optic disk: a review. Surv. Ophthalmol. 51 (2), 93–104.

Shields, J.A., Shields, C.L., Piccone, M., et al., 2002. Spontaneous appearance of an optic disk melanocytoma in an adult. Am. J. Ophthalmol. 134 (4), 614–615.

Shuey, T.F., Blacharski, P.A., 1988. Pigmented tumor and acute visual loss. Surv. Ophthalmol. 33 (2), 121–126.

Takahashi, T., Isayama, Y., Okuzawa, I., 1984. Unusual case of melanocytoma in optic disk. Jpn J. Ophthalmol. 28 (2), 171–175.

Thomas, C.I., Purnell, E.W., 1969. Ocular melanocytoma. Am. J. Ophthalmol. 67 (1), 79–86.

Usui, T., Shirakashi, M., Kurosawa, A., et al., 1990. Visual disturbance in patients with melanocytoma of the optic disk. Ophthalmologica 201 (2), 92–98.

Walsh, T.J., Packer, S., 1971. Bilateral melanocytoma of the optic nerve associated with intracranial meningioma. Ann. Ophthalmol. 3 (8), 885–888.

Wiznia, R.A., Price, J., 1974. Recovery of vision in association with a melanocytoma of the optic disk. Am. J. Ophthalmol. 78 (2), 236–238.

Zimmerman, L.E., 1965. Melanocytes, melanocytic nevi, and melanocytomas. Invest. Ophthalmol. 4, 11–40.

Zimmerman, L.E., Garron, L.K., 1962. Melanocytoma of the optic disc. Int. Ophthalmol. Clin. 2, 431–440.

Astrocytic Hamartoma

Destro, M., D'Amico, D.J., Gragoudas, E.S., et al., 1991. Retinal manifestations of neurofibromatosis. Diagnosis and management. Arch. Ophthalmol. 109 (5), 662–666.

Drewe, R.H., Hiscott, P., Lee, W.R., 1985. Solitary astrocytic hamartoma simulating retinoblastoma. Ophthalmologica 190 (3), 158–167.

Giles, J., Singh, A.D., Rundle, P.A., et al., 2005. Retinal astrocytic hamartoma with exudation. Eye (Lond.) 19 (6), 724–725.

Iaccheri, B., Fiore, T., Cagini, C., et al., 2007. Retinal astrocytic hamartoma with associated macular edema: report of spontaneous resolution of macular edema as a result of increasing hamartoma calcification. Semin. Ophthalmol. 22 (3), 171–173.

Kimoto, K., Kishi, D., Kono, H., et al., 2008. Diagnosis of an isolated retinal astrocytic hamartoma aided by optical coherence tomography. Acta Ophthalmol. 86 (8), 921–922.

Kiratli, H., Bilgiç, S., 2002. Spontaneous regression of retinal astrocytic hamartoma in a patient with tuberous sclerosis. Am. J. Ophthalmol. 133 (5), 715–716.

Leroy, B.P., Carton, D., De Laey, J.J., 1996. Ophthalmological signs of tuberous sclerosis. Bull. Soc. Belge Ophtalmol. 262, 115–121.

Mennel, S., Meyer, C.H., Eggarter, F., et al., 2005. Autofluorescence and angiographic findings of retinal astrocytic hamartomas in tuberous sclerosis. Ophthalmologica 219 (6), 350–356.

Moschos, M.M., Chamot, L., Schalenbourg, A., et al., 2005. Spontaneous regression of an isolated retinal astrocytic hamartoma. Retina 25 (1), 81–82.

Nyboer, J.H., Robertson, D.M., Gomez, M.R., 1976. retinal lesions in tuberous sclerosis. Arch. Ophthalmol. 94, 1277–1280.

Pichi, F., Massaro, D., Serafino, M., et al., 2016. Retinal astrocytic hamartoma: optical coherence tomography classification and correlation with tuberous sclerosis complex. Retina 36 (6), 1199–1208.

Reeser, F.H., Aaberg, T.M., Van Horn, D.L., 1978. Astrocytic hamartoma of the retina not associated with tuberous sclerosis. Am. J. Ophthalmol. 86 (5), 688–698.

Schwartz, P.L., Beards, J.A., Maris, P.J., 1980. Tuberous sclerosis associated with a retinal angioma. Am. J. Ophthalmol. 90 (4), 485–488.

Shields, C.L., Benevides, R., Materin, M.A., et al., 2006. Optical coherence tomography of retinal astrocytic hamartoma in 15 cases. Ophthalmology 113 (9), 1553–1557.

Shields, C.L., Materin, M.A., Shields, J.A., 2005. Review of optical coherence tomography for intraocular tumors. Curr. Opin. Ophthalmol. 16 (3), 141–154.

Soliman, W., Larsen, M., Sander, B., et al., 2007. Optical coherence tomography of astrocytic hamartomas in tuberous sclerosis. Acta Ophthalmol. Scand. 85 (4), 454–455.

Trincão, R., Cunha-Vaz, J.G., Pires, J.M., 1973. Astrocytic hamartoma of the optic disc in localized ocular neurofibromatosis (von Recklinghausen's disease). Ophthalmologica 167 (5), 465–469.

Trojman, C., Zografos, L., Dirani, A., et al., 2016. Multimodal imaging of retinal astrocytic hamartoma associated with congenital hypertrophy of retinal pigment epithelium. Klin. Monbl. Augenheilkd. 233 (4), 530–533.

Veronese, C., Pichi, F., Guidi, S.G., et al., 2011. Cystoid changes within astrocytic hamartomas of the retina in tuberous sclerosis. Retin Cases Brief Rep. 5 (2), 113–116.

Yung, M., Iafe, N., Sarraf, D., 2016. Optical coherence tomography angiography of a retinal astrocytic hamartoma. Can. J. Ophthalmol. 51 (2), e62–e64.

Combined Hamartoma of Retina and RPE

Avitabile, T., Franco, L., Reibaldi, M., et al., 2007. Combined pigment epithelial and retinal hamartoma: long-term follow-up of three cases. Can. J. Ophthalmol. 42 (2), 318–320.

Brown, G.C., 1983. Congenital Anomalies of the Optic Disc. Grune & Stratton, New York, pp. 206–207.

Cilliers, H., Harper, C.A., 2006. Photodynamic therapy with Verteporfin for vascular leakage from a combined hamartoma of the retina and retinal pigment epithelium. Clin. Experiment. Ophthalmol. 34 (2), 186–188.

Font, R.L., Moura, R.A., Shetlar, D.J., et al., 1989. Combined hamartoma of sensory retina and retinal pigment epithelium. Retina 9 (4), 302–311.

Gass, J.D.M., 1973. An unusual hamartoma of the pigment epithelium and retina simulating choroidal melanoma and retinoblastoma. Trans. Am. Ophthalmol. Soc. 71, 171.

Harper, C.A., Gole, G.A., 1986. Combined hamartoma of the retina and RPE: an unusual cause of the dragged disc appearance. Aust. N. Z. J. Ophthalmol. 14 (3), 235–238.

Palmer, M.L., Carney, M.D., Combs, J.L., 1990. Combined hamartomas of the retinal pigment epithelium and retina. Retina 10 (1), 33–36.

Sandhu, H.S., Kim, B.J., 2016. Combined hamartoma of the retina and RPE: A spectrum of presentation with epiretinal membrane masquerade. Can. J. Ophthalmol. 51 (1), e10–e13.

Shields, C.L., Shields, J.A., Marr, B.P., et al., 2003. Congenital simple hamartoma of the retinal pigment epithelium: a study of five cases. Ophthalmol 110, 1005–1011.

Shields, C.L., Thangappan, A., Hartzell, K., et al., 2008. Combined hamartoma of the retina and retinal pigment epithelium in 77 consecutive patients visual outcome based on macular versus extramacular tumor location. Ophthalmology 115 (12), 2246–2252.

Theodossiadis, P.G., Panagiotidis, D.N., Baltatzis, S.G., et al., 2001. Combined hamartoma of the sensory retina and retinal pigment epithelium involving the optic disk associated with choroidal neovascularization. Retina 21, 267–270.

Vogel, M.H., Zimmerman, L.E., Gass, J.D.M., 1969. Proliferation of the juxtapapillary retinal pigment epithelium simulating malignant melanoma. Doc. Ophthalmol. 26, 461.

Xue, K., Mellington, F., Gout, I., et al., 2012. Combined hamartoma of the retina and retinal pigment epithelium. BMJ Case Rep. 15, 2012.

Retinoblastoma

Brown, G.C., Shields, J.A., 1985. Tumors of the optic nerve head. Surv. Ophthalmol. 29 (4), 239–264.

Chantada, G., Schaiquevich, P., 2015. Management of retinoblastoma in children: current status. Paediatr. Drugs 17 (3), 185–198.

de Jong, M.C., de Graaf, P., Noij, D.P., et al., 2014. Diagnostic performance of magnetic resonance imaging and computed tomography for advanced retinoblastoma: a systematic review and meta-analysis. Ophthalmology 121 (5), 1109–1118.

De Potter, P., 2002. Current treatment of retinoblastoma. Curr. Opin. Ophthalmol. 13 (5), 331–336.

Finger, P.T., Harbour, J.W., Karcioglu, Z.A., 2002. Risk factors for metastasis in retinoblastoma. Surv. Ophthalmol. 47 (1), 1–16.

Jaradat, I., Mubiden, R., Salem, A., et al., 2012. High-dose chemotherapy followed by stem cell transplantation in the management of retinoblastoma: a systematic review. Hematol. Oncol. Stem. Cell. Ther. 5 (2), 107–117.

Makimoto, A., 2004. Results of treatment of retinoblastoma that has infiltrated the optic nerve, is recurrent, or has metastasized outside the eyeball. Int. J. Clin. Oncol. 9 (1), 7–12.

Sastre, X., Chantada, G.L., Doz, F., et al., 2009. Proceedings of the consensus meetings from the International Retinoblastoma Staging Working Group on the pathology guidelines for the examination of enucleated eyes and evaluation of prognostic risk factors in retinoblastoma. Arch. Pathol. Lab. Med. 133, 1199–1202.

Shields, C.L., Meadows, A.T., Leahey, A.M., et al., 2004. Continuing challenges in the management of retinoblastoma with chemotherapy. Retina 24, 849–862.

Shields, C.L., Shields, J.A., 1999. Recent developments in the management of retinoblastoma. J. Pediatr. Ophthalmol. Strabismus 36 (1), 8–18, quiz 35–36.

Shields, C.L., Shields, J.A., De Potter, P., 1996. New treatment modalities for retinoblastoma. Curr. Opin. Ophthalmol. 7 (3), 20–26.

Shields, J.A., Shields, C.L., Donoso, L.A., et al., 1989. Current treatment of retinoblastoma. Trans. Pa Acad. Ophthalmol. Otolaryngol. 41, 818–822.

Smith, M.M., Strottmann, J.M., 2001. Imaging of the optic nerve and visual pathways. Semin. Ultrasound CT MR 22 (6), 473–487.

Paraneoplastic Disorders

Alabduljalil, T., Behbehani, R., 2007. Paraneoplastic syndromes in neuro-ophthalmology. Curr. Opin. Ophthalmol. 18 (6), 463–469.

Arruga, J., 2000. Metastatic and paraneoplastic lesions of the optic nerve. Rev. Neurol. 31 (12), 1256–1258.

Bataller, L., Dalmau, J., 2004. Neuro-ophthalmology and paraneoplastic syndromes. Curr. Opin. Neurol. 17 (1), 3–8.

Chan, J.W., 2003. Paraneoplastic retinopathies and optic neuropathies. Surv. Ophthalmol. 48 (1), 12–38.

Jacobson, D.M., 1996. Paraneoplastic disorders of neuro-ophthalmologic interest. Curr. Opin. Ophthalmol. 7 (6), 30–38.

Ko, M.W., Dalmau, J., Galetta, S.L., 2008. Neuro-ophthalmologic manifestations of paraneoplastic syndromes. J. Neuroophthalmol. 28 (1), 58–68.

Thambisetty, M.R., Scherzer, C.R., Yu, Z., et al., 2001. Paraneoplastic optic neuropathy and cerebellar ataxia with small cell carcinoma of the lung. J. Neuroophthalmol. 21 (3), 164–167.

Volpe, N.J., Rizzo, J.F. 3rd., 1995. Retinal disease in neuro-ophthalmology: paraneoplastic retinopathy and the big blind spot syndrome. Semin. Ophthalmol. 10 (3), 234–241.

Myelinated Nerve Fibers (MNF)

Ellis, G.S., Frey, T., Gouterman, R.Z., 1987. Myelinated nerve fibers, axial myopia and refractory amblyopia: an organic disease. J. Pediatr. Ophthalmol. Strabismus 24, 111–119.

Funnell, C.L., George, N.D., Pai, V., 2003. Familial myelinated retinal nerve fibres. Eye (Lond.) 17 (1), 96–97.

Gharai, S., Prakash, G., Ashok Kumar, D., et al., 2010. Spectral domain optical coherence tomographic characteristics of unilateral peripapillary myelinated retinal nerve fibers involving the macula. J. AAPOS 14 (5), 432–434.

Hittner, H.M., Antoszyk, J.K., 1987. Unilateral peripapillary myelinated nerve fibers with myopia and/or amblyopia. Arch. Ophthalmol. 105, 943–948.

Käsmann-Kellner, B., Ruprecht, K.W., 1998. Unilateral peripapillary myelinated retinal nerve fibers associated with strabismus, amblyopia, and myopia. Am. J. Ophthalmol. 126 (6), 853.

Kodama, T., Hayasaka, S., Setogawa, T., 1990. Myelinated retinal nerve fibers: prevalence, location and effect on visual acuity. Ophthalmologica 200 (2), 77–83.

Lee, J.C., Salchow, D.J., 2008. Myelinated retinal nerve fibers associated with hyperopia and amblyopia. J. AAPOS 12 (4), 418–419.

Lee, M.S., Gonzalez, C., 1998. Unilateral peripapillary myelinated retinal nerve fibers associated with strabismus, amblyopia, and myopia. Am. J. Ophthalmol. 125 (4), 554–556.

Leys, A.M., Leys, M.J., Mooymans, J.M., et al., 1996. Myelinated nerve fibers and retinal vascular abnormalities. Retina 16, 89–96.

Rosen, B., Barry, C., Constable, I.J., 1999. Progression of myelinated retinal nerve fibers. Am. J. Ophthalmol. 127 (4), 471–473.

Shelton, J.B., Digre, K.B., Gilman, J., et al., 2013. Characteristics of myelinated retinal nerve fiber layer in ophthalmic imaging: findings on autofluorescence, fluorescein angiographic, infrared, optical coherence tomographic, and red-free images. JAMA Ophthalmol 131 (1), 107–109.

Straatsma, B.R., Foos, R.Y., Heckenlively, J.R., et al., 1981. Myelinated retinal nerve fibers. Am. J. Ophthalmol. 91 (1), 25–38.

Straatsma, B.R., Heckenlively, J.R., Foos, R.Y., et al., 1979. Myelinated retinal nerve fibers associated with ipsilateral myopia, amblyopia, and strabismus. Am. J. Ophthalmol. 88 (3 Pt 1), 506–510.

Tarabishy, A.B., Alexandrou, T.J., Traboulsi, E.I., 2007. Syndrome of myelinated retinal nerve fibers, myopia, and amblyopia: a review. Surv. Ophthalmol. 52 (6), 588–596.

Index

Page numbers followed by "*f*" indicate figures, and "*t*" indicate tables.

C

D

E

F

G

K

L

M

N

O

Q

R

S

T

U

V

W

X

Z